FIFTH EDITION

Yaffe and Aranda's Neonatal and Pediatric Pharmacology

Therapeutic Principles in Practice

FIFTH EDITION

Yaffe and Aranda's Neonatal and Pediatric Pharmacology

Therapeutic Principles in Practice

JACOB (JACK) V. ARANDA, MD, PHD, FRCPC, FAAP
Professor of Pediatrics and Ophthalmology
Director of Neonatology and the New York Pediatric Developmental Pharmacology Research Center
Program Director, Neonatal Perinatal Medicine Fellowship
State University of New York Downstate Health Sciences University
Brooklyn, New York

JOHANNES (JOHN) N. VAN DEN ANKER, MD, PHD, FCP, FAAP
Evan and Cindy Jones Endowed Chair in Pediatric Clinical Pharmacology
Vice Chair of Pediatrics for Experimental Therapeutics
Chief Division of Clinical Pharmacology
Children's National Hospital and Professor of Pediatrics
Pharmacology & Physiology, Genomics & Precision Medicine
The George Washington University School of Medicine and Health Sciences
Washington, District of Columbia
Eckenstein-Geigy Distinguished Professor of Pediatric Pharmacology and Pharmacometrics
University Children's Hospital Basel
University of Basel
Basel, Switzerland
Intensive Care and Department of Pediatric Surgery
Erasmus Medical Center-Sophia Children's Hospital
Rotterdam, the Netherlands

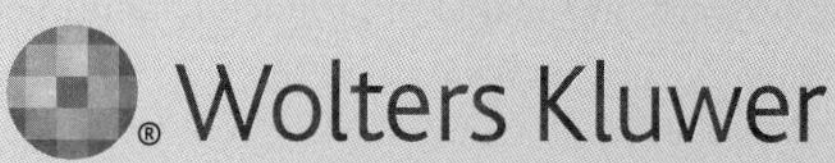

Philadelphia • Baltimore • New York • London
Buenos Aires • Hong Kong • Sydney • Tokyo

Acquisitions Editor: Colleen Dietzler/Nicole Dernoski
Development Editor: Robyn Alvarez/Thomas Celona
Editorial Coordinator: Julie Kostelnik
Marketing Manager: Kirsten Watrud
Production Project Manager: Kirstin Johnson
Design Coordinator: Holly McLaughlin
Manufacturing Coordinator: Beth Welsh
Prepress Vendor: S4Carlisle Publishing Services

Fifth edition

9 8 7 6 5 4 3 2 1

Printed in China

Library of Congress Cataloging-in-Publication Data

Names: Aranda, Jacob V., author. | Van den Anker, Johannes, author.
Title: Yaffe and Aranda's neonatal and pediatric pharmacology : therapeutic principles in practice / Jacob Aranda, MD, PhD, FRCPC, FAAP, Professor of Pediatrics and Ophthalmology, Director of Neonatology, Director: New York Pediatric Developmental Pharmacology Research Consortium, Program Director: Neonatal -Perinatal Medicine Fellowship, State Univ of New York Downstate Health Sciences University, Johannes van den Anker, MD, PhD, FCP, FAAP, Evan and Cindy Jones Endowed Chair in Pediatric Clinical Pharmacology, Vice Chair of Pediatrics for Experimental Therapeutics, Chief Division of Clinical Pharmacology, Children's National Hospital and Professor of Pediatrics, Pharmacology & Physiology, Genomics & Precision Medicine, The George Washington University School of Medicine and Health Sciences, Washington, DC, USA, Eckenstein-Geigy Distinguished Professor of Pediatric Pharmacology and Pharmacometrics, University Children's Hospital Basel, University of Basel, Basel, Switzerland, Intensive Care and Department of Pediatric Surgery, Erasmus Medical Center-Sophia Children's Hospital, Rotterdam, the Netherlands.
Description: Fifth edition. | Philadelphia : Lippincott Williams & Wilkins, [2021] | Revision of: Neonatal and pediatric pharmacology / [edited by] Sumner J. Yaffe, Jacob V. Aranda. c2010. 4th ed. | Includes bibliographical references and index. | Summary: "textbook in pediatric pharmacology and provides evidence-based guidelines for safe, effective, and rational drug therapy in newborns, children, and adolescents"— Provided by publisher.
Identifiers: LCCN 2020028621 | ISBN 9781975112486 (hardcover)
Subjects: LCSH: Pediatric pharmacology. | Children—Diseases—Chemotherapy.
Classification: LCC RJ560 .P4 2021 | DDC 615.1083—dc23
LC record available at https://lccn.loc.gov/2020028621

shop.lww.com

CCS1020

To our loved ones
Kenneth Frederic and Christopher James Aranda

and

John Nicolaas Yuri van den Anker and Natella Yurievna Rakhmanina

and the Editorial and Production Team:

Julie Kostelnik, Robyn Alvarez, Collen Dietzler, Nicole Dernoski, Thomas Celona, and Kirstin Johnson

For their dedication, enthusiasm, guidance, and invaluable assistance in the preparation of the fifth edition

Tribute to Sumner J. Yaffe, MD

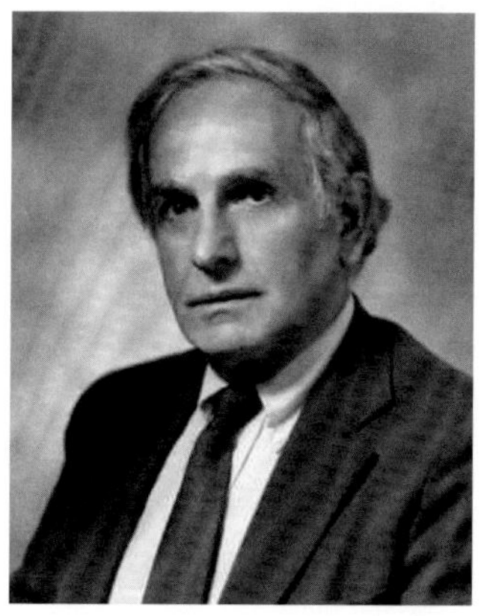

The fifth edition of this textbook, *Yaffe and Aranda's Neonatal and Pediatric Pharmacology: Therapeutic Principles in Practice*, pays tribute to its founding editor, Dr. Sumner J. Yaffe. He is acknowledged as the Father of Pediatric Clinical Pharmacology and on his passing in 2011, the international community of neonatal and pediatric clinical pharmacologists lost a true pioneer, a long-standing leader, a preeminent scholar, and an unwavering advocate for pediatric therapeutics. Those of us who were privileged to have known, worked, and/or interacted with him, many of whom are authors of the chapters in this edition, were all impacted by Sumner in so many ways. His academic history, professional life, and immense impact on pediatric pharmacotherapeutics have been comprehensively reviewed (Giacoia G, Reed MD. Sumner J. Yaffe: The father of pediatric clinical pharmacology. *J Pediatr Pharmacol Ther* 2011;16:162–166) and what follows is our personal reflections on our colleague, mentor, and dear friend, Sumner J. Yaffe, MD.

Accolades are often used to describe individuals from all walks of life describing courageous actions, game-changing accomplishments, out-of-the-box innovations but at times many can ring hollow. In the case of Dr. Yaffe, these accolades describing his illustrious career are well earned, unembellished, and enduring. A sampling of our list includes the following:

Pioneer and Trailblazer. Sumner was an early leader in the scientific and clinical research of the ontogeny of drug metabolism and action in the maturing infant and child with a special interest in the prematurely born infant. Early in his academic career, he studied the age-dependent differences in cardiac responses to digitalis, recognizing that understanding the mechanism(s) of drug action provided the path to optimal therapeutics and evolving innovations. His pioneering efforts in scientifically sound clinical pharmacology and toxicology research techniques in infants and children across the age continuum were foundational, as were his insightful, visionary approaches to education, teaching, and clinical research. His career included many important firsts and landmarks in the field of pediatric pharmacotherapeutics, with components and variants emulated throughout the world today. Sumner was the first director of the then-newly established Clinical Research Center for Premature Infants at Stanford University and the first division director of the then-newly established Division of Pediatric Clinical Pharmacology at the Children's Hospital of Philadelphia. He joined the National Institute of Child Health and Human Development (NICHD) of the National Institutes of Health (NIH) as its director of the Center for Research for Mothers and Children in 1980 and became a tireless advocate in the field.

Advocate. As the NIH/NICHD director of the Center for Research for Mothers and Children, he recognized very early on the power and synergy of clinical research networks and was instrumental in leading the establishment of the neonatal and fetal/maternal medicine network and then to his personal crowning achievement, the establishment of the Pediatric Pharmacology Research Units (PPRUs) network. He ensured that drugs in newborns and children were addressed in national and international forums and congresses. The international communities of educators, students, practitioners, organizational leaders, and government agencies embracing multiple disciplines focused on improving the health of children of all ages continue to flourish, innovate, and direct forward actions and road maps.

Visionary. From his early laboratory-based work in identifying the mechanism of drug action to his clinical pharmacology and toxicology research and bedside application of evolving age-dependent, age-directed therapeutics and to then operationalize these life-altering activities through continuously successful enduring, ever-expanding clinical research collaboratives is a testament to the person he was. These accomplishments reflected not only his visionary abilities but also his unbiased and boundless inquisitiveness, intelligence, and unwavering commitment to do what he knew was right, combined with his ability to accept each setback as a new challenge to overcome—all peppered with a healthy dose of common sense! He always looked forward to the day when newborns, children, and adolescents will be therapeutic orphans no more.

Mentor. Sumner embodied the true meaning of a mentor. Although extremely busy and consumed by a multitude of complex, dynamic issues, he would always make time to speak directly with you, uninterrupted, with his focus on you. He offered thoughtful, insightful, practical advice, always following up to determine outcome, next steps, and lessons learned. Above all, he expected nothing in return other than your success. His success was your success.

The fifth edition of this book is not only a tribute but also a testament of the foundation that Sumner prepared for our specialty so many years ago to ensure safe and effective drug therapies for newborns and children. He prepared our community to meet the challenges and to expand the dynamic evolution of neonatal and pediatric clinical pharmacology research and practice now and in the future. He helped shorten the timeline until newborns, children, and adolescents will be therapeutic orphans no more. With such a legacy, it is easy to understand, appreciate, and acknowledge Dr. Yaffe as the Father of Pediatric Clinical Pharmacology.

Michael D. Reed
George Giacoia
Johannes N. van den Anker
Jacob V. Aranda

Reprinted with permission from Giacoia G, Reed MD. Sumner J. Yaffe: The father of pediatric clinical pharmacology. *J Pediatr Pharmacol Ther* 2011;16(3):162–166.

Foreword

It has been almost 10 years since the publication of the fourth edition of *Neonatal and Pediatric Pharmacology: Therapeutic Principles in Practice*, and we continue to make great strides in the evaluation of pediatric therapeutics. Since the last edition, advancements have been made in cell and gene therapy and treatments available for rare diseases, with data available for a range of pediatric patients that could potentially benefit from therapy. New drug and biologic products have been evaluated in pediatric patients for most of the therapeutic areas, including infectious diseases, cancer, and chronic diseases.

Dr. Sumner J. Yaffe was a visionary in his appreciation of the importance of clinical pharmacology in the study of products to treat children when he established a network of Pediatric Pharmacology Research Units in 1994, funded by the National Institute of Child Health and Development (NICHD). These efforts have been supported by the legislative mandates, the Best Pharmaceuticals for Children Act (BPCA), and the Pediatric Research Equity Act (PREA). The BPCA and PREA, initiated in 2002 and 2003, respectively, were made permanent by the Food and Drug Administration Safety and Innovation Act (FDASIA) in 2012. The BPCA encourages the developers of drug and biologic products to undertake studies in the pediatric population in exchange for an exclusivity incentive. There is also a part of the BPCA to support the study of off-patent drugs through NICHD. The Pediatric Trials Network, coordinated by the Duke Clinical Research Institute as part of the NICHD/BPCA program, has enrolled more than 7,000 children in studies of more than 70 drugs. The PREA requires a pediatric assessment for certain drug and biologic products unless a waiver or deferral has been obtained. Between 1998 and 2019, there have been more than 800 pediatric labeling changes, with approximately two-thirds having studies done under the PREA.

Significant work in the basic sciences continues to support the development of pediatric therapeutics. New information on the ontogeny of systems involved in the absorption, distribution, metabolism, and excretion (ADME) of drugs and biologics has been especially important in efforts to identify optimal dosing for neonates and infants and has been critical in the establishment of physiologically based pharmacokinetic models. Innovative approaches to study pediatric therapeutics, such as novel trial designs, modeling, and simulation of doses, and the development of age-appropriate formulations and therapeutic drug monitoring assays that require small blood volumes, have encouraged the ability to obtain information in neonatal and pediatric patients. As with all the previous editions of this book, key subject matter experts have contributed to this edition, detailing information on therapeutic approaches to neonatal brain injury, seizures, hyperbilirubinemia, apnea, cancer, and pain and withdrawal syndromes, as well as approaches to treatment and prevention of diseases in the areas of ophthalmology, infectious diseases, gastroenterology, endocrinology, neurology, psychology, and pulmonology. Although it is an exciting time in the development of therapeutics for pediatric patients, potential safety issues must be evaluated. Unique considerations include length of therapy, exposure during vulnerable periods of growth and development, and the ontogeny of ADME characteristics that might influence the approach to dosing. To efficiently study new pediatric therapeutics, collaborative global resources, including sites with experience in collecting regulatory-ready data, are being established.

This book, with its unique and comprehensive approach to neonatal and pediatric pharmacology, will help guide treatment of newborns and children with information on optimal dosing approaches and benefit–risk considerations associated with therapeutic use in pediatric patients.

Dr. Susan McCune, MD

Preface to the Fourth Edition

Neonatal and pediatric pharmacology and drug therapy may be viewed as corrective and manipulative physiology and biochemistry for the fetus, newborn infant, and growing child using drugs, biologic and molecular entities. Drugs are used to correct physiologic, molecular, and biochemical as well as disease-related abnormalities that occur during pre- and postnatal periods, extrauterine adaptation, and growth and development to adulthood.

As advances in the knowledge of diseases and their diagnoses are made, the complexities of treatment, particularly by drugs, increase in tandem. Therapeutic drug exposure and administration in the newborn and children has increased over the years. Moreover, the number of drugs available to physicians and health care givers continues to increase. There is an increasing variety of antimicrobials, cardiovascular drugs, diuretics, immunosuppressants and immunomodulators, antivirals, biologic, and other drugs for the management of sick newborn and children. Safe and effective use of these agents in infants and children requires adequate knowledge of their pharmacologic properties, including drug action, metabolism, and disposition.

The fourth edition of *Neonatal and Pediatric Pharmacology: Therapeutic Principles in Practice* has been substantially revised to meet the current needs of clinicians, pharmacologists, pharmacists, and other health care givers. The book has expanded to 66 chapters in this edition, plus drug formularies for newborns and children. This edition is designed to provide relevant information on drugs and their uses in newborn infants, older infants, children, and adolescents. It was proposed as a quick reference for busy clinicians, house staff, students, nurses, pharmacists, and health care providers. It may also serve as a general and basic reference for teaching neonatal and pediatric pharmacology. It is also hoped that researchers will find it useful to understand the unique characteristics and dynamic changes in drug requirements and action during a period of intense growth and development. The mechanisms of drug actions, the evidence of drug efficacy in certain disease states, dose, therapeutic guidelines, and drug toxicities are emphasized. The book was organized to parallel the distinct periods of early human development. Special sections useful in drug therapy such as therapeutic drug monitoring, adverse drug reactions, and epidemiologic considerations are also included. The unraveling of some of the secrets of the human genome has resulted in major progress and challenges in the understanding of drug disposition and pharmacologic effects in humans and personalized drug therapies. A chapter is devoted to this issue in this book. The importance of pharmacogenetics and pharmacogenomics in clinical therapeutics in children and in pediatric drug trials and drug development can no longer be ignored. Developmental changes in receptors, drug-metabolizing enzymes, transporters, and ion channels may have impact on the efficacy and safety of drugs in children. The determinants of drug action, metabolism, and disposition are multifaceted, and the impact of the variations in the human genome, the environment demographics, and other factors will remain a major challenge in the immediate future.

Drugs are double-edged swords; although they can cure illnesses and restore health and well-being, they can also produce unwanted and, at times, unanticipated toxicities. The rational, intelligent, and safe use of drugs springs mainly from understanding their actions, uses, problems, and limitations. This understanding, in turn, will permit selection of the appropriate drug and prescription of the optimal dosage. It is our utmost desire that this textbook can help those providers of care to newborns and children to maximize the benefits of pharmacologic agents while averting their adverse effects. Identified areas of ignorance or concern should stimulate further research to minimize the unknowns in neonatal and pediatric drug therapy. Thus, this book will advance and promote the health and wellness in newborns and children.

Sumner J. Yaffe
Jacob V. Aranda

Preface to the Fifth Edition

Developmental pharmacotherapeutics may be simplistically viewed as the use of drugs, biologics, and molecular entities to correct, restore, and manipulate aberrant molecular biology, physiology, and biochemistry in the fetus, newborn infant, growing child, and adolescent. Drugs preserve wellness as they rectify and amend physiologic, molecular, and biochemical lesions as well as disease-related abnormalities that may occur during pre- and postnatal periods, extrauterine adaptation, growth, and development to adulthood. The knowledge on diseases and their diagnoses and therapies inexorably advances. Drug exposures in newborns and children have also increased over the years. There is an increasing variety and number of antimicrobials, cardiovascular drugs, diuretics, immunosuppressants and immunomodulators, antivirals, biologics, and other drugs for the management of sick newborns, children, and adolescents. Safe and effective use of these agents in these populations requires adequate knowledge of their pharmacologic properties, including drug action, metabolism, disposition, and safe and efficacious drug dosing regimens that are appropriate for age and maturity.

The fifth edition of *Yaffe and Aranda's Neonatal and Pediatric Pharmacology: Therapeutic Principles in Practice* has been substantially revised to meet the current needs of clinicians, nurses, pharmacologists, pharmacists, researchers, and other health care providers. A completely new section on biologic pharmacology reflects the knowledge explosion and development of biologic entities, including monoclonal antibodies, vaccines, stem cells, erythropoietin, and pulmonary surfactant in neonatal and pediatric therapies. As novel diseases like the Coronavirus (COVID-19) or SARS-CoV-2 global pandemic emerge, new and old drugs must be developed, tested, and "repurposed" to prevent viral entry and replication as well as to avert or modulate severe pathophysiologic states such as the cytokine storm. New chapters in the fifth edition such as antimalarial drugs, cardiovascular pharmacology, antiarrhythmic drugs, and others provide new information that may improve therapeutic outcomes.

This edition is designed to provide relevant information on drugs and their uses in newborns, children, and adolescents. It may serve as a quick reference for busy clinicians, house staff, students, nurses, pharmacists, and all health care providers. It may be used as a general and basic reference for teaching neonatal and pediatric pharmacology. It is also hoped that researchers will find it useful to understand the unique characteristics and dynamic changes in drug requirements and action during a period of intense growth and development. The mechanisms of drug actions, the evidence of drug efficacy in certain disease states, dose, therapeutic guidelines, and drug toxicities are emphasized. The book was organized to parallel the distinct periods of early human development. Special sections useful in drug therapy such as therapeutic drug monitoring, adverse drug reactions, epidemiologic considerations, clinical trials, and pediatric drug development are also included. The unraveling of the many secrets of the human genome has resulted in major progress and challenges in the understanding of drug disposition and pharmacologic effects in humans and personalized drug therapies. A chapter is again devoted to this issue in this book. The importance of pharmacogenetics and pharmacogenomics in clinical therapeutics in children, in pediatric drug trials, and in drug development can no longer be ignored. Developmental changes in receptors, drug-metabolizing enzymes, transporters, and ion channels may affect the efficacy and safety of drugs in children. The determinants of drug action, metabolism, and disposition are multifaceted, and the impact of the variations in the human genome, the environment demographics, and other factors remain as major challenges in pharmacotherapeutics.

Drugs can heal or kill; drugs can cure or harm. Indeed, they are double-edged swords. They can not only restore health and well-being but also produce unwanted and unanticipated toxicities. The effective and safe use of drugs arises from fully understanding their actions, uses, problems, limitations, and selection of the appropriate drug, using the correct dosing regimen. This textbook may help care providers to maximize the benefits of pharmacologic agents while averting their adverse effects. Identified gaps in knowledge and areas of concern should stimulate further research to bridge these gaps and to minimize the unknowns in neonatal and pediatric drug therapy. As in the past four decades, we hope that this book will continue to help advance and promote the health and wellness in newborns, children, and adolescents through the safe and wise use of pharmacologic agents.

Jacob V. Aranda
Johannes N. van den Anker

Contributors

Nahed Abdel-Haq, MD
Professor of Pediatrics
Wayne State University/Children's Hospital of Michigan
Detroit, Michigan

Susan M. Abdel-Rahman, PharmD
Marion Merrell Dow/Missouri Chair in Pediatric Clinical Pharmacology
Chief, Section of Therapeutic Innovation, Children's Mercy Kansas City
Director, Health Care Innovation, Children's Mercy Research Institute
Professor of Pediatrics, University of Missouri Kansas City School of Medicine
Kansas City, Missouri

Elissa M. Abrams, MD
Assistant Professor
University of Manitoba
Winnipeg, Manitoba, Canada

Homa K. Ahmadzia, MD/MPH
Assistant Professor
Division of Maternal-Fetal Medicine
Department of Obstetrics & Gynecology
The George Washington University
Washington, District of Columbia

Tageldin M. Ahmed, MBBS, MRCP, MRCPCH
Assistant Professor of Pediatrics
Wayne State University School of Medicine
Division of Pediatric Critical Care
Children's Hospital of Michigan,
Detroit, Michigan

Zahraa H. Al-Lawati, MD
Physician
Pulmonary Critical Care
Children's Hospital of Michigan
Detroit, Michigan

Mohammad H. Al-Shaer, PharmD, PhD
Research Assistant Professor
University of Florida
Gainesville, Florida

Wael A. Alghamdi, PharmD, PhD
Assistant Professor
Department of Clinical Pharmacy
College of Pharmacy
King Khalid University
Abha, Saudi Arabia

Karel Allegaert, MD, PhD
Professor
Department of Development and Regeneration
Department of Pharmaceutical and Pharmacological Sciences
Leuven, Belgium
Senior Consultant
Clinical Pharmacy
Erasmus Medical Center
Rotterdam, the Netherlands

Sasha A. Alvarado, DO
Allergy and Immunology Section
Louisiana State University Health Sciences Center
Shreveport, Louisiana

Johannes (John) N. van den Anker, MD, PHD, FCP, FAAP
Evan and Cindy Jones Endowed Chair in Pediatric Clinical Pharmacology
Vice Chair of Pediatrics for Experimental Therapeutics
Chief Division of Clinical Pharmacology
Children's National Hospital and Professor of Pediatrics
Pharmacology & Physiology, Genomics & Precision Medicine
The George Washington University School of Medicine and Health Sciences
Washington, District of Columbia
Eckenstein-Geigy Distinguished Professor of Pediatric Pharmacology and Pharmacometrics
University Children's Hospital Basel
University of Basel
Basel, Switzerland
Intensive Care and Department of Pediatric Surgery
Erasmus Medical Center-Sophia Children's Hospital
Rotterdam, the Netherlands

Jacob (Jack) V. Aranda, MD, PhD, FRCPC, FAAP
Professor of Pediatrics and Ophthalmology
Director of Neonatology and the New York Pediatric Developmental Pharmacology Research Center
Program Director, Neonatal Perinatal Medicine Fellowship
State University of New York Downstate Health Sciences University
Brooklyn, New York

Elizabeth A. Ashley, MBBS, PhD
Director
Lao-Oxford-Mahosot Hospital-Wellcome Trust Research Unit,
Microbiology Laboratory Mahosot Hospital
Vientiane, Lao PDR
Centre for Tropical Medicine and Global Health, Nuffield
Department of Medicine, University of Oxford
Oxford, United Kingdom

Basim I. Asmar, MD
Professor of Pediatrics
Director, Division of Infectious Diseases
Wayne State University, School of Medicine
Children's Hospital of Michigan
Detroit, Michigan

Gerri R. Baer, MD
Medical Officer
U.S. Food and Drug Administration/Office of Pediatric Therapeutics
Silver Spring, Maryland

Sami L. Bahna, MD, DrPH
Professor of Pediatrics & Medicine
Chief of Allergy & Immunology Section
Louisiana State University Health Sciences Center
Shreveport, Louisiana

Suruchi Batra, MD
Fellow
Division of Gastroenterology
Hepatology and Nutrition
Children's National Hospital
Washington, District of Columbia

Frank van Bel, MD, PhD
EM Professor of Neonatology
Former Director of the Perinatal Center
University Medical Center Utrecht
Utrecht, the Netherlands

Manon J.N.L. Benders, MD, PhD
Professor/Head of Department Neonatology
University Utrecht/University Medical Center Utrecht
Utrecht, the Netherlands

Daniel K. Benjamin, Jr., MD, PhD
Distinguished Professor of Pediatrics
Deputy Director of Duke Clinical Research Institute
Duke University Medical Center
Durham, North Carolina

Stacey L. Berg, MD
Professor of Pediatrics and Medical Ethics
Director, Developmental Therapeutics Program
Texas Children's Cancer Center
Associate Dean for Research Assurances
Baylor College of Medicine
Houston, Texas

Brookie M. Best, PharmD, MAS
Associate Dean for Pharmacy Education
Professor of Clinical Pharmacy and Pediatrics
UC San Diego
San Diego, California

Adrianne Rahde Bischoff, MD
Clinical Assistant Professor of Pediatrics
University of Iowa Stead Family Children's Hospital
Iowa City, Iowa

Lisa R. Bomgaars, MSc, MD
Professor
Texas Children's Hospital/Baylor College of Medicine
Houston, Texas

Jan Bonhoeffer, MD, PhD
Vice-Chair, Paediatric Infectious Diseases & Vaccines
University of Basel Children's Hospital
Basel, Switzerland

Gerbrich E. van den Bosch, MD, PhD
Pediatrician, fellow-Neonatology
Erasmus Medical Center-Sophia Children's Hospital
Rotterdam, the Netherlands

Stephanie M. Boyd, MBBS (Hons), BSc (Med), MPHTM, FRACP
Neonatologist
Grace Centre for Newborn Intensive Care
Children's Hospital at Westmead
Sydney, New South Wales, Australia

John S. Bradley, MD
Distinguished Professor, Infectious Diseases/Pediatrics
University of California, San Diego School of Medicine
San Diego, California

Jörg Breitkreutz, MD
APV President
Director Institute of Pharmaceutics and Biopharmaceutics
Heinrich-Heine-University Duesseldorf
Duesseldorf, Germany

David M. Burger, PharmD, PhD
Head Research Department of Pharmacy
Radboud University Medical Center
Nijmegen, the Netherlands

Edmund V. Capparelli, PharmD
Professor of Clinical Pediatrics and Pharmacy
Host-Microbe Systems and Therapeutics
UC San Diego
La Jolla, California

Gabrielle Sky Cardwell, BA
Clinical Research Assistant
Children's National Health System
Washington, District of Columbia

Bruce Carleton, BSc, PharmD
Professor and Division Chief
Translational Therapeutics
Department of Pediatrics, Faculty of Medicine
University of British Columbia
Director
Pharmaceutical Outcomes Programme, BC Children's Hospital
Senior Clinician Scientist
BC Children's Hospital Research Institute
Vancouver, British Columbia, Canada

Eda Cengiz, MD, MHS, FAAP
Associate Professor
Yale School of Medicine
New Haven, CT
Visiting Professor
Bahcesehir University
Istanbul, Turkey

James M. Chamberlain, MD
Director, Data Analytics and Informatics
Division of Emergency Medicine
Children's National Hospital
Washington, District of Columbia

Alenka Chapron, MPharm, PhD
Postdoctoral Research Scholar
Children's Mercy Hospital
Kansas City, Missouri

Brian D. Chapron, PharmD, PhD
Pediatric Fellow
Children's Mercy Kansas City
Kansas City, Missouri

Sylvain Chemtob, MD, PhD
Professor of Pediatrics, Ophthalmology and Pharmacology
University of Montreal
Centre Hospitalier Universitaire Ste Justine
Montreal, Quebec, Canada

Vivian L. Chin, MD
Assistant Professor of Pediatrics
Associate Program Director, Pediatric Residency Program
Division of Pediatric Endocrinology, Department of Pediatrics,
SUNY Downstate Medical Center
Brooklyn, New York

George P. Chrousos
Division of Endocrinology, Metabolism and Diabetes
First Department of Pediatrics
National and Kapodistrian University of Athens Medical School
'Aghia Sophia' Children's Hospital
Division of Endocrinology and Metabolism Center of Clinical Experimental Surgery and Translational Research
Biomedical Research Foundation of the Academy of Athens
University Research Institute of Maternal and Child Health and Precision Medicine
UNESCO Chair of Adolescent Health Care, National and Kapodistrian University of Athens
Athens, Greece

Michael Cohen-Wolkowiez, MD, PhD
Kiser-Arena Distinguished Professor of Pediatrics
Duke University
Durham, North Carolina

Laurie S. Conklin, MD
Associate Professor of Pediatrics
Children's National Hospital
Washington, District of Columbia

André Dallmann, PhD
Scientist Systems Pharmacology
Clinical Pharmacometrics
Bayer AG
Leverkusen, Germany

Jonathan M. Davis, MD
Vice-Chair of Pediatrics
Chief of Newborn Medicine
The Floating Hospital for Children at Tufts Medical Center
Professor of Pediatrics
Tufts University School of Medicine
Associate Director Tufts CTSI and Director of the Tufts CTSA Trial Innovation Network Center
Chair, Neonatal Advisory Committee, Office of the Commissioner, FDA
Director, International Neonatal Consortium (INC), FDA/European Medicines Agency/Critical Path Institute
Boston, Massachusetts

David J. Diemert, MD, FRCP(C)
Professor
Department of Medicine
George Washington University School of Medicine and Health Sciences
Washington, District of Columbia

Bram A. Dolcourt, MD
Assistant Professor, Emergency Medicine/Medical Toxicology
Wayne State University
Detroit, Michigan

Nikola Dragisic, MD
Associate
University of Iowa Stead Family Children's Hospital
Iowa City, Iowa

Thomas J. Duggan, MD, FAAP
Assistant Professor of Pediatrics
Division of Neonatology
SUNY Downstate Health Sciences University
Brooklyn, New York

Abdelbaset A. Elzagallaai, BSc, Pharm, MSc, PhD
Adjunct Professor
Department of Physiology and Pharmacology
Western University
London, Ontario, Canada

Robert L. Findling, MD, MBA
Chair
Department of Psychiatry
Virginia Commonwealth University
Richmond, Virginia

Delbert A. Fisher, M.D.
Professor Emeritus, Pediatrics and Medicine
UCLA David Geffen School of Medicine
Los Angeles, California
Academic Associate
Quest Diagnostics Nichols Institute
San Juan Capistrano, California

Jennifer H. Foster, MD MPH
Assistant Professor
Texas Children's Hospital, Baylor College of Medicine
Houston, Texas

Densley Francois, PharmD, BCPS, BCPPS
Clinical Pharmacist – Neonatal Intensive Care Unit
New York Presbyterian Hospital/Morgan Stanley Children's Hospital
New York, New York

Kendell R. German, MD
Assistant Professor
Department of Pediatrics
Division of Neonatology
University of Washington/Seattle Children's Hospital
Seattle, Washington

Regan E. Giesinger, MD, FRCPC
Clinical Associate Professor
University of Iowa
Iowa City, Iowa

Bradley R. Grant, DO
Assistant Professor
Johns Hopkins University School of Medicine
Baltimore, Maryland

Floris Groenendaal
Neonatoloog/Associate Professor
Division Woman and Baby, MS Neonatologie
Wilhelmina Children's Hospital
Utrecht, the Netherlands

Jean-Pierre Guignard, MD
Honorary Professor of Pediatrics
Lausanne University Medical School
Lausanne, Switzerland

Margaret R. Hammerschlag, MD
Professor of Pediatrics and Medicine
Director, Pediatric Infectious Diseases Fellowship Program
SUNY Downstate Medical Center
New York, New York

L. M. Hanff, PharmD, PhD
Hospital Pharmacist, Clinical Pharmacologist
Director of Pharmacy
Princess Maxima Center for Pediatric Oncology
Utrecht, the Netherlands

Ulrich Heininger, MD
Head of Division of Pediatric Infectious Diseases and Vaccinology
University of Basel Children's Hospital
Basel, Switzerland

Steven Hirschfeld, MD, PhD
Professor of Pediatrics
F. Edward Hebert School of Medicine
Uniformed Services University of the Health Sciences
Bethesda, Maryland

Britta Höcker, MD
Associate Professor
University Children's Hospital of Heidelberg
Heidelberg, Germany

Silvia Iacobelli, MD, PhD
Full Professor of Pediatrics
Réanimation Néonatale et Pédiatrique, Néonatologie
CHU La Réunion - Site Sud (Saint Pierre)
Centre d'Études Périnatales de l'Océan Indien (CEPOI)
Université de la Réunion
Saint Pierre Cedex, France

Shinya Ito, MD, FRCPC
Professor
Departments of Paediatrics and Pharmacology & Toxicology
University of Toronto
Head
Division of Clinical Pharmacology and Toxicology
Department of Paediatrics
The Hospital for Sick Children
Toronto, Canada

Sota Iwatani, MD, PhD
Post-Doctoral Fellow
Pediatrics
Stanford University
Stanford, California

Kim Jackson, MD
Allergist/Immunologist
Little Rock Asthma and Allergy Clinic (LRAAC)
Little Rock, Arkansas

Nynke G. L. Jager, PharmD, PhD
Hospital Pharmacist and Clinical Pharmacologist
Department of Clinical Pharmacy
Radboud University Medical Center and Radboud Institute for Health Sciences
Nijmegen, the Netherlands

Alan H. Jobe, MD, PhD
Professor of Pediatrics
Cincinnati Children's Hospital
University of Cincinnati
Cincinnati, Ohio

Bridgette L. Jones, MD, MS
Associate Professor of Pediatrics
Division of Pediatric Clinical Pharmacology and Therapeutic Innovation and Section of Allergy/Asthma/Immunology
University of Missouri-Kansas City School of Medicine
Kansas City, Missouri

Sandra E. Juul, MD, PhD
Professor of Pediatrics
University of Washington and Seattle Children's Hospital
Seattle, Washington

Jamil M. Kazma, MD
Project Lead
Division of Maternal-Fetal-Medicine
Department of Obstetrics and Gynecology
The George Washington University
Washington, District of Columbia

H. William Kelly, PharmD
Professor Emeritus of Pediatrics
University of New Mexico Health Sciences Center
Albuquerque, New Mexico

Aditi Khokhar, MBBS
Assistant Professor
Rutgers New Jersey Medical School
Newark, New Jersey

David W. Kimberlin, MD
Professor of Pediatrics
University of Alabama at Birmingham
Birmingham, Alabama

Tomoshige Kino
Department of Human Genetics
Division of Translational Medicine
Sidra Medicine
Education City North Campus
Doha, Qatar

Stephan A. Kohlhoff, MD
Director, Pediatric Infectious Diseases
Associate Professor, Pediatrics and Medicine
SUNY Downstate Medical Center
Brooklyn, New York

Sarah Kolnik, MD, FAAP
Neonatal-Perinatal Fellow
University of Washington, Seattle Children's Hospital
Division of Neonatology
Department of Pediatrics
Seattle, Washington

Walter K. Kraft, MD
Professor of Pharmacology
Surgery and Medicine
Thomas Jefferson University
Philadelphia, Pennsylvania

John D. Lantos, MD
Professor of Pediatrics
Director, Children's Mercy Hospital Bioethics Center
University of Missouri-Kansas City and Children's Mercy Kansas City
Kansas City, Missouri

Anie Lapointe, MD
Associate Professor (Clinical) of Pediatrics
University of Montreal
Centre Hospitalier Universitaire Ste Justine
Montreal, Quebec, Canada

Ian H. Law, MD
Professor
University of Iowa Stead Family Children's Hospital
Iowa City, Iowa

Jennifer Le, PharmD, MAS, FIDSA, FCCP, FCSHP, BCPS-ID
Professor of Clinical Pharmacy
University of California San Diego
Skaggs School of Pharmacy and Pharmaceutical Sciences
La Jolla, California

J. Steven Leeder, PharmD, PhD
Deputy Director, Children's Mercy Research Institute
Children's Mercy Hospital
Kansas City, Missouri

Victoria Tutag Lehr, BSPharm, PharmD
Professor
Department of Pharmacy Practice
Eugene Applebaum College of Pharmacy and Health Sciences
Wayne State University
Detroit, Michigan

Mary W. Lieh-Lai, MD, FAAP, FCCP
Professor of Pediatrics (Vol)
Wayne State University School of Medicine
Chicago, Illinois

Jose Maria de Andrade Lopes, MD, PhD
Post Graduate Program
Instituto Fernandes Figueira - Oswaldo Cruz Foundation
Clinical Director
Perinatal Maternity Group
Rio de Janeiro, Brazil

Mirjana Lulic-Botica, PharmD, BCPS
Adjunct Assistant Professor
Wayne State University
Neonatal Clinical Pharmacy Specialist
Hutzel Women's Hospital- Detroit Medical Center
Detroit, Michigan

Shannon F. Manzi, PharmD, BCPPS, FPPA
Director, Safety & Quality, Department of Pharmacy
Assistant Professor, Pediatrics
Boston Children's Hospital
Harvard Medical School
Boston, Massachusetts

Maryann E. Mazer-Amirshahi, PharmD, MD, MPH, PhD, BCPS, FACEP, FACMT, FASAM, FCP
Associate Professor of Emergency Medicine
Georgetown University School of Medicine
Department of Emergency Medicine
MedStar Washington Hospital Center
Washington, District of Columbia

Susan McCune, MD
Director, Office of Pediatric Therapeutics
Office of Clinical Policy and Programs
Office of the Commissioner
U.S. Food and Drug Administration

Patrick J. McNamara, MB, BCh, BAO, MSc, MRCPCH, DCH
Professor
University of Iowa Stead Family Children's Hospital
Iowa City, Iowa

Bernd Meibohm, PhD, FCP, FAAPS
Associate Dean for Research & Graduate Programs
Professor of Pharmaceutical Sciences
The University of Tennessee Health Science Center
College of Pharmacy
Memphis, Tennessee

Jorge Mejia-Corletto, MD
Clinical Assistant Professor of Pediatrics
NYU Langone Health
Mineola, New York

Mark Mirochnick, MD
Professor of Pediatrics
Boston University/Boston Medical Center
Boston, Massachusetts

Tomoyuki Mizuno, PhD
Assistant Professor of Pediatrics
Division of Clinical Pharmacology
Cincinnati Children's Hospital Medical Center
Department of Pediatrics
University of Cincinnati College of Medicine
Cincinnati, Ohio

Hussain Mulla, MD
Senior Clinical Pharmacist
Researcher in Clinical Pharmacy/Pharmacology
Department of Pharmacy, University Hospitals of Leicester
Glenfield Hospital
Honorary Senior Lecturer
College of Life Sciences
University of Leicester
Leicester, United Kingdom

Diana Muñoz-Mendoza, MD
Allergist-Immunologist
Assistant Professor of Pediatrics
University of Arkansas for Medical Sciences (UAMS)
Arkansas Children's Hospital
Clinical Investigator
Arkansas Children's Research Institute
Little Rock, Arkansas

Mathieu Nadeau-Vallée, MD, PhD
Resident
University of Montreal
Montreal, Quebec, Canada

Girija Natarajan, MD
Professor, Central Michigan University
Co-Chief, Division of Neonatology
Children's Hospital of Michigan and Hutzel Women's Hospital
Detroit, Michigan

Josef Neu, MD
Professor of Pediatrics
University of Florida
Miami, Florida

Nicolas C. Nicolaides
Division of Endocrinology, Metabolism and Diabetes
First Department of Pediatrics
National and Kapodistrian University of Athens Medical School
'Aghia Sophia' Children's Hospital
Division of Endocrinology and Metabolism
Center of Clinical
Experimental Surgery and Translational Research
Biomedical Research Foundation of the Academy of Athens
University Research Institute of Maternal and Child Health and Precision Medicine
Athens, Greece

Luis A. Ochoa, MD
Assistant Professor
University of Iowa Stead Family Children's Hospital
Iowa City, Iowa

Charles A. Peloquin, PharmD, FCCP
Professor
Director
Infectious Disease Pharmacokinetics Lab
College of Pharmacy
Emerging Pathogens Institute
University of Florida
Gainesville, Florida

Sheila Perez-Colon, MD
Assistant Professor
Pediatrics, Division of Pediatric Endocrinology
SUNY Downstate Medical Center
Brooklyn, New York

Mary Frances Picciano, PhD (Deceased)

Claudette L. Poole, MD
Assistant Professor of Pediatrics, Division of Pediatric Infectious Diseases
University of Alabama at Birmingham
Birmingham, Alabama

Geoffrey A. Potts, MD
Assistant Professor of Dermatology
Wayne State University
Dearborn, Michigan

Hengameh H. Raissy, PharmD
Research Professor and Vice Chair of Research
Interim Division Chief Pediatric Pulmonary
Department of Pediatrics
University of New Mexico, School of Medicine
Albuquerque, New Mexico

Natella Rakhmanina, MD, PhD, FAAP, FCP, AAHIVS
Professor of Pediatrics
The George Washington University School of Medicine and Health Sciences
Director of HIV Services & Special Immunology
Children's National Hospital
Washington, District of Columbia
Senior Technical Advisor
Elizabeth Glaser Pediatric AIDS Foundation
Washington, District of Columbia

John Jeffrey Reese, MD
Professor of Pediatrics and Cell and Developmental Biology
Vanderbilt University
Children's Hospital at Vanderbilt
Nashville, Tennessee

Michael Rieder, MD, PhD, FRCPC, FAAP, FRCP(Edinburgh)
CIHR-GSK Chair in Paediatric Clinical Pharmacology
University of Western Ontario
London, Ontario, Canada

Desirée Rivera-Nieves, MD
Pediatric Gastroenterology, Hepatology, and Nutrition
John Hopkins All Children's Hospital
St. Petersburg, Florida

John D. Roarty, MD, MPH
Assistant Professor
Children's Hospital of Michigan
Detroit, Michigan

Adelaide S. Robb, MD
Distinguished Endowed Professor and Chair, Division of Psychiatry and Behavioral Sciences
The George Washington University School of Medicine, Children's National Hospital
Washington, District of Columbia

Paul H. Saenger, MD, MACE
Professor of Pediatrics Emeritus
NYU Langone Health
Mineola, New York

Ayman Saleh, MD
Child and Adolescent Psychiatrist
Assistant Professor
Medical Director of Children's National Takoma Theatre Clinic
Medical Director of Ambulatory Psychiatry Clinic
George Washington University
Children's National Hospital
Washington, District of Columbia

Ashok P. Sarnaik, MD
Professor of Pediatrics
Wayne State University School of Medicine
Former Chief, Critical Care Medicine
Children's Hospital of Michigan
Detroit, Michigan

Rachel K. Scott, MD, MPH, FACOG
Associate Chair for Research
Scientific Director of Women's Health Research
Georgetown University/MedStar Health Research Institute
Washington, District of Columbia

Roopali Sharma, BS, PharmD, AAHIVP, BCPS (AQ-ID)
Associate Professor, Pharmacy Practice
2090 Adam Clayton Powell Jr Blvd, Room 514
New York, New York

Kelly P. Shaw, RPh, PharmD
Pharmacist
University Health Network
Toronto General Hospital
Toronto, Ontario, Canada

Sinno H. P. Simons, MD, PhD
Pediatrician—Neonatologist—Clinical Pharmacologist
Pediatrics, Neonatology
University Medical Center Rotterdam
Erasmus Medical Center
Rotterdam, the Netherlands

Michael J. Smith, MD, MSCE
Associate Professor of Pediatrics
Pediatric Infectious Diseases
Medical Director Pediatric Antimicrobial Stewardship
Duke University Medical Center
Durham, North Carolina

Anne Smits, MD, PhD
Assistant Professor
Department of Development and Regeneration
KU Leuven
Neonatologist
University Hospitals Leuven
Leuven, Belgium

Susan C. Smolinske, PharmD, DABAT
Professor
College of Pharmacy
University of New Mexico
Albuquerque, New Mexico

Wayne R. Snodgrass, MD, PhD
Professor
Pediatrics, Pharmacology-Toxicology, & Obstetrics (Research)
Head
Clinical Pharmacology-Toxicology Unit
Medical Director
Texas Poison Center-Houston/Galveston
University of Texas Medical Branch
Galveston, Texas

Donna L. Snyder, MD, MBE
Senior Pediatric Ethicist
US Food and Drug Administration
Silver Spring, Maryland

Stephani L. Stancil, PhD, APRN
Postdoctoral Research Fellow and Nurse Practitioner
Divisions of Adolescent Medicine and Clinical Pharmacology
Children's Mercy Kansas City
Kansas City, Missouri

Amy H. Stanford, MD
Neonatal Hemodynamics Fellow
University of Iowa
Iowa City, Iowa

William J. Steinbach, MD
Samuel L. Katz Professor of Pediatrics
Professor in Molecular Genetics and Microbiology
Chief, Pediatric Infectious Diseases
Director, International Pediatric Fungal Network
Duke University
Durham, North Carolina

Ekaterina Stepanova, MD, PhD
Assistant Professor, Medical Director of the Children's Mental Health Center
Johns Hopkins University
Baltimore, Maryland

David K. Stevenson, MD
Harold K. Faber Professor of Pediatrics
Senior Associate Dean for Maternal and Child Health
Co-Director, Maternal and Child Health Research Institute
Stanford University School of Medicine
Stanford, California

Satyendra Suryawanshi, MPharm, PhD
Director
Bristol-Myers Squibb
Princeton, New Jersey

Stanley J. Szefler, MD
Professor of Pediatrics
Research Medical Director and Director of the Pediatric Asthma Research Program,
The Breathing Institute, Interim Medical Director of the Research Institute
University of Colorado School of Medicine, Children's Hospital Colorado, Anschutz Medical Campus
Aurora, Colorado

William V. Tamborlane, MD
Professor and Chief of Pediatric Endocrinology
Yale University School of Medicine
New Haven, Connecticut

Zaid H. Temrikar, MS
PhD Student
The University of Tennessee Health Science Center
Memphis, Tennessee

Dick Tibboel, MD, PhD
Professor Emeritus Research Intensive Care in Childhood
Erasmus Medical Center-Sophia Children's Hospital
Rotterdam, the Netherlands

Joseph D. Tobias, MD
Chief, Department of Anesthesiology & Pain Medicine
Nationwide Children's Hospital
Professor of Anesthesiology & Pediatrics
The Ohio State University
Columbus, Ohio

Burkhard Tönshoff, MD, PhD
Vice Chairman
Department of Pediatrics
University Children's Hospital Heidelberg
Heidelberg, Germany

Vatcharapan Umpaichitra, MD
Assistant Professor of Pediatrics
SUNY Downstate Health Sciences University
Brooklyn, New York

Ruud Verstegen, MD, PhD
Clinical Fellow
Division of Clinical Pharmacology and Toxicology
Department of Paediatrics
The Hospital for Sick Children
Toronto, Canada

Alexander A. Vinks, PharmD, PhD, FCP
Professor of Pediatrics and Pharmacology
Endowed Chair
Division of Clinical Pharmacology
Cincinnati Children's Hospital Medical Center
Department of Pediatrics
University of Cincinnati College of Medicine
Cincinnati, Ohio

Linda S. de Vries, MD, PhD
Emeritus Professor Neonatology
University Medical Center Utrecht
Utrecht, the Netherlands

Philip D. Walson, MD
Visiting Professor
Department of Clinical Pharmacology
University Medical Center Goettingen
Goettingen, Germany

Thomas G. Wells, MD, MBA
Professor
Department of Pediatrics
University of Arkansas for Medical Sciences/Arkansas Children's Hospital
Little Rock, Arkansas

Sir Nicholas J. White, FRS
Chairman, Wellcome Trust South East Asian Research Units
Faculty of Tropical Medicine, Mahidol University
Bangkok, Thailand
Centre for Tropical Medicine and Global Health, Nuffield
Department of Medicine
University of Oxford
Oxford, United Kingdom

Richard J. Whitley, MD
Distinguished Professor
Professor of Pediatrics, Microbiology, Medicine and Neurosurgery
The University of Alabama at Birmingham
Birmingham, Alabama

Mitchel T. Williams, MD
Assistant Professor
Children's Hospital of Michigan
Detroit, Michigan

Ronald J. Wong, MD
Senior Research Scientist
Stanford University School of Medicine
Stanford, California

Lynne Yao, MD
Director
Division of Pediatric and Maternal Health
Center for Drug Evaluation and Research
US Food and Drug Administration
Silver Spring, Maryland

Elizabeth Yen, MD, MA
Assistant Professor of Pediatrics/Neonatologist
Tufts University School of Medicine
Floating Hospital for Children at Tufts Medical Center
Boston, Massachusetts

Karen C. Young, MD, MS, FAHA
Associate Director Neonatology Fellowship Program
Associate Professor of Pediatrics
University of Miami Miller School of Medicine
Miami, Florida

Anne Zajicek, MD, PharmD
Deputy Director, Office of Clinical Research
National Institutes of Health
Bethesda, Maryland

Contents

SECTION III: Pharmacology in Special Settings and Population

SECTION IV: Antimicrobial Pharmacology

SECTION VI: Immunopharmacology, Allergy, and Inflammation

SECTION VII: Pharmacology of Biologic Drugs

SECTION VIII: Cardiorenal Drugs

SECTION IX: Gastrointestinal Pharmacology

SECTION X: Endocrine and Hematologic Pharmacology

SECTION XI: Nutritional Pharmacology, Pharmacotoxidromes, Adverse Drug Reactions, and Interactions

Introduction to the Fifth Edition and Historical Highlights

In 1968, Dr. Harry Shirkey wrote the following: "By an odd and unfortunate twist of fate, infants and children are becoming therapeutic or pharmaceutical orphans." His observation was based on the very low number of drugs that were appropriately labeled for use in children caused by laws regulating drug manufacturing, testing, and distribution, which were, paradoxically, often introduced as a response to therapeutic misadventures in children. These early regulatory laws advocated for the practice of restriction as the primary means to maximize drug safety in pediatric patients, resulting in the exclusion of pediatric patients from the study of therapeutic drugs, many of which were intended for pediatric use. Consequently, these laws resulted in drug labeling practices that included warnings for most new drugs stating that because of inadequate (or nonexistent) data in children, the majority of drugs were not recommended for use in children. This led Dr. Shirkey in 1968 to issue a call to academia, industry, and government to actively take the responsibility for including children in the development programs of drugs intended for pediatric use. Despite a profound unmet need, little progress was made in almost two decades after this call to action was issued.

All of the regulatory preparation for pediatric drug development was accomplished in the 1970s by the Food and Drug Administration (FDA), the American Academy of Pediatrics, and the National Institutes of Health (NIH). In 1974, Congress passed the National Research Act and established the National Commission for the Protection of Human Subjects of Medical and Behavioral Research. The same year the American Academy of Pediatrics issued a report commissioned by the FDA called "General Guidelines for the Evaluation of Drugs to be Approved for Use during Pregnancy and for Treatment of Infants and Children." In 1977, the FDA issued a Pediatric Guidance called "General Considerations for the Clinical Evaluation of Drugs in Infants and Children." In the same year, the American Academy of Pediatrics, reacting to the paucity of information for children on drug labels, asserted that it was unethical to adhere to a system that forced physicians to use drugs in what was basically an uncontrolled experiment whenever they wrote prescriptions for children. The Academy stated that it was imperative for new drugs that were to be used in children to be studied in children under controlled circumstances so that the benefits of therapeutic advances would become available to all who would need them. This was a powerful, yet simple statement: Children deserve the same standard as adults. If adequate and well-controlled studies were required to determine the efficacy of the products used in adults, then the same should be true for products used to treat children. It was now considered unethical *not* to study children. Following this unprecedented statement, in 1979, the FDA confirmed the need to have information on how best to use a product in the pediatric population and issued a Regulation on the *Pediatric Use* Subsection of Product Package Insert *Precautions* Section (21 CFR 201.57 (f)).

Thereafter, a number of milestones in Pediatric Drug Development in the United States and in Europe occurred (see Table FM 1.1). The FDA issued a regulation in 1994 that required that statements on pediatric use of a drug for an indication approved for adults must be based on substantial evidence derived from adequate and well-controlled studies conducted in children, unless the requirement was waived.

The intent of the initial regulation (1994 rule) was to encourage manufacturers to conduct the necessary trials so that adequate prescribing information would be available to physicians. Unfortunately, it did not generate the response intended. Few clinical trials were initiated in the pediatric population. Manufacturers cited financial, medicolegal, and methodologic disincentives, especially for products already approved for adults. These products were available to physicians for prescription use outside of labeled indications through the practice of medicine. The FDA could encourage but not require that a sponsor conduct the appropriate trials to support pediatric labeling.

At the time this rule was issued, approximately 80% of drugs listed in the *Physicians' Desk Reference* did not have directions for use in the pediatric population based on clinical trials. This disturbing situation was heightened by the AIDS epidemic, which served to contrast the disparity between the pace of drug development between adults and children. In 1994, the FDA issued a final, slightly modified rule requiring drug manufacturers to survey the existing data and determine whether those data were sufficient to support additional pediatric use information in a drug's labeling. In addition, the rule explicitly stated that controlled clinical studies need not be carried out in pediatric patients when the course of the disease and the response to treatment were similar in adults and children. Extrapolation from adult efficacy data to pediatric patients was permitted. Therefore, controlled clinical studies in adults, together with other information, such as pharmacokinetic and adverse reaction data in pediatric patients, could be found to be sufficient to establish pediatric safety and efficacy. Under the 1994 rule, the manufacturer could determine that existing data permitted modification of the label's pediatric use. The manufacturer, however, had to submit a supplemental new drug application to the FDA, seeking approval of the labeling change.

It is important to recognize that the 1994 rule did not require that manufacturers conduct pediatric studies if existing information was not adequate to support a labeling change. Instead, where there was insufficient information to support a pediatric indication or pediatric use statement, the 1994 rule allowed the manufacturer to include in the drug's labeling the statement, "safety and effectiveness in pediatric patients have not been established."

The FDA was hopeful and enthusiastic about this regulation. Unfortunately, well over half of the responses to the rule concluded that there were insufficient data, and the resulting labeling change consisted of inclusion of the statement just given. Only 23% of the responses resulted in improved labeling for pediatrics.

Clearly, if the goal of ensuring the safe and effective use of therapeutic agents in children was to be met, additional steps had to be taken. Two pieces of legislation underscored the commitment of the FDA to the safe and effective use of therapeutic agents in children. The first of these was Section 111 of the FDA Modernization Act (FDAMA). Congress passed this act in November 1997 (see Table FM 1.1). Section 111 of this act created a financial incentive (called "pediatric exclusivity") consisting of an additional 6 months of marketing exclusivity for conducting pediatric studies on new drugs and drugs already on the market and under patent. The second advance was the 1998 Final Pediatric Rule, which was to become effective in 1999. This regulation required that pediatric studies be conducted for certain new as well as marketed drugs and biologic products. Requiring studies in the pediatric population represented a significant departure from the previous regulations, which were voluntary. Both the final rule and the pediatric exclusivity provision were critical to ensuring that necessary and timely pediatric drug development occurred and that improved pediatric labeling would be the result. The financial incentive of an additional 6 months of marketing exclusivity could apply to both new drugs and marketed drugs as defined by the FDAMA. If the 6 months of additional marketing exclusivity was granted, all the sponsor's products that contain the drug ("active moiety" formulations of the drug) might receive this extension. Because of this wide application, this was seen as a significant "carrot" in getting manufacturers to conduct pediatric studies. To qualify for pediatric exclusivity, the drug manufacturer had to receive a written request for pediatric studies from the FDA. This written request outlines the studies that the drug manufacturer must conduct and complete, and which complete study reports must be submitted by an agreed-on date. New and approved drugs that this law applied to were those that had been determined as likely to produce health benefits in the pediatric population. For any given drug, the FDA evaluated every indication under development or that had been previously approved and requested that the appropriate studies were performed. Conducting pediatric studies in response to a written request was voluntary. To obtain pediatric exclusivity, final reports of the submitted studies had to meet the terms of the written request and the drug needed to have existing patent protection or exclusivity.

Because voluntary efforts such as the 1994 Pediatric Rule did not substantially increase the number of products entering the market with adequate pediatric labeling, the FDA concluded that additional steps were necessary to ensure the safety and effectiveness of drugs and biologic products for pediatric patients. In addition, even though the pediatric exclusivity offered by the FDAMA was expected to provide a substantial incentive for sponsors to conduct pediatric studies, that provision did not apply to drugs that no longer had existing patent protection or exclusivity or to biologics or "old" antibiotics. It was a voluntary program, making it likely that manufacturers might elect not to conduct studies in products with smaller markets, even though there might be a great medical need for the product in pediatric patients. Therefore, it was felt that there were still many situations where there was a need to require the collection of data in children.

The 1998 Pediatric Rule required the manufacturers of new and marketed drugs and biologic products to evaluate the safety and effectiveness of their products in pediatric patients. It was designed to ensure that new drugs and biologic products contained adequate pediatric labeling for the claimed indication at the time of, or soon after, approval. This rule established a presumption that all new drugs and biologics would be studied in pediatric patients, but allowed manufacturers to obtain a waiver of the requirement in some circumstances (e.g., if the indication was not applicable to the pediatric population). This rule applied to new chemical entities, new indications, new dosage forms, new dosing regimens, and new routes of administration.

This rule also authorized the FDA to require pediatric studies of marketed drugs and biologic products where there was a compelling need for studies (defined as situations in which the product is used in a substantial number of pediatric patients) and the absence of adequate labeling could pose significant risks for pediatric patients, or the product would provide a meaningful therapeutic benefit over existing treatments. Thus, this rule was mandatory and gave the FDA additional power to require studies in children. Although this rule was being implemented, the rule was considered by the Federal courts to be illegal and not within the FDA's authority.

FDAMA was authorized for 5 years. At its termination in 2002, because of its unprecedented success, it was reauthorized for 5 to 7 additional years. In doing so, Congress incorporated the pediatric exclusivity provisions of FDAMA into the Best Pharmaceuticals for Children Act (BPCA). This legislation had important provisions for infants and children. The BPCA identified the NIH as a major player together with the FDA in supporting drug studies in infants and children. The act made provisions to address new (on-patent) drugs, but also asked the NIH and FDA to identify off-patent drugs that need to be evaluated in the pediatric population.

In 2003, the Pediatric Research Equity Act (PREA) was passed into US law as an enactment of the Pediatric Rule of 1998. The provisions of PREA mandated the conduct of pediatric clinical trials for drugs under development that had the indications which also occurred in pediatric patients. Under the 2007 Food and Drug Administration Amendments Act (FDAAA), provisions in BPCA and PREA were renewed in addition to a section pertaining to the study of pediatric devices, a requirement for FDA to actively monitor safety for all drugs studied under the provisions of this legislation, and the formation of an FDA Pediatric Review Committee to standardize pediatric drug development programs. After another 5 years, BPCA and PREA were finally made permanent under the 2012 FDA Safety and Innovation Act (FDASIA). FDASIA also focused on one of the neglected pediatric groups in drug development, the neonates.

In 2017, the FDA Reauthorization Act (FDARA) focused on another neglected pediatric patient group in drug development, namely pediatric oncology patients. Because cancer indications in adults frequently do not pertain to pediatric patients, studies cannot be required under PREA, which is indication based. Therefore, the Research to Accelerate Cures and Equity (RACE) for Children Act was passed as part of FDARA and changed the basis for PREA inclusion to be molecular targets for pediatric oncology instead of indication. The RACE Act for Children also removes the PREA exemption for orphan drug products, which is critical in small oncology patient groups.

TABLE FM 1.1 Milestones in Pediatric Drug Development
1977—AAP Statement concerning the need to conduct clinical trials in children
1979—The US Food and Drug Administration (FDA) establishes a section for drug labels and requires trials in children parallel to adult process
1994—FDA requirement for sponsors or drug manufacturers to update drug labels, to evaluate existing data, and to determine whether these data are sufficient to support information for pediatric drug labeling. The FDA also implements a voluntary collection of data on pediatric use before and after a drug is approved. FDA introduces the "extrapolation concept"
1997—US Congress passes FDAMA (FDA Modernization Act) and prolongs patent exclusivity for 6 months to pharmaceuticals that voluntarily perform studies on the drug in children
1998—The FDA publishes the Pediatric Rule, which requires manufacturers to assess the safety and efficacy of drugs and biologic products in children in specified circumstances
2002—The Best Pharmaceuticals for Children Act (BPCA) was signed into law by President G. W. Bush. BPCA renewed exclusivity or patent protection for an additional 6 months. Provides additional mechanisms, such as studies funded by the National Institutes of Health to obtain drug data from "off-patent" or patented drugs (which manufacturers decline to study in children). BPCA provides process for "off-patent" drug development, public posting of results, and reporting of all AEs for 1 year after exclusivity is granted
2003—Pediatric Research Equity Act (PREA) is passed, which requires the study of drugs and biologics for pediatric population except in defined situations and also creates a Pediatric Advisory Committee
2006—European Parliament passes the Best Medicines for Children Act on December 12, 2006, which became law in January 2007. The law requires studies of drug in newborns and children and a pediatric investigation plan (PIP) for all drugs being developed. It creates a pediatric committee to decide priority drugs to study and to review protocol proposals and study plans for drug development in children. It also provides procedures to study drugs for newborns and children and funding mechanisms. EMEA (European Medication Evaluation Agency) reviews data for approval and marketing licensure
2007—US Congress reauthorized BPCA. Thereafter, the number of clinical pharmacology studies in newborns and children increased followed by several labeling changes
2012—US Congress made BPCA and PREA permanent under the 2012 FDA Safety and Innovation Act (FDASIA). FDASIA also focused on one of the neglected pediatric groups in drug development, the neonates
2017—US Congress approved the FDA Reauthorization Act (FDARA) and the Research to Accelerate Cures and Equity (RACE) for Children Act. FDARA also focused on another neglected pediatric patient group in drug development, namely, pediatric oncology patients

AAP, American Academy of Pediatrics; AEs, adverse events.

This change to PREA-based pediatric drug development study requirements will take place in August 2020.

In Europe, parallel regulatory developments were also occurring. On December 12, 2006, the European Parliament passed the Best Medicines for Children Act, which became law in January 2007. The law requires studies of drug in newborns and children and a pediatric investigation plan (PIP) for all drugs being developed. It provides for the creation of a pediatric committee to decide priority drugs to study. The pediatric committee also reviews protocol proposals and study plans for drug development in children. It also provides procedures and funding mechanisms to foster studies of drugs for newborns and children. Thus, there is an increasingly concerted effort in Europe and North America to ensure that requisite data for the safe and effective drug use in children are obtained.

All of this work can only be done through collaborative efforts. One model for this is the development of public–private partnerships or consortia that bring together stakeholders from academia, industry, patient/parent advocacy groups, regulators, and other government entities. In October 2014, a workshop sponsored by the Critical Path Institute, Burroughs-Wellcome Fund, and the FDA was held at the FDA to discuss the logistics to support a neonatal consortium. Based on this initial meeting, the International Neonatal Consortium (INC) was launched in May 2015 at a workshop in London. In its first year, the INC focused on four key areas: clinical pharmacology, seizures, bronchopulmonary dysplasia, and databases.

Another consortium working on neonatal issues is the International Life Sciences Institute (ILSI)—Health and Environmental Sciences Institute (HESI) Developmental and Reproductive Toxicology (DART) Committee. ILSI-HESI DART is a multisector collaborative research effort to identify and explore nonclinical models to inform the efficacy and long-term safety of drugs as they apply to neonatal disease. The working groups are surveying established nonclinical neonatal disease models, identifying nonclinical models to inform efficacy and safety of neonatal drug therapy in neonatal-specific conditions and physiology as it pertains to neonatal absorption, distribution, metabolism, and excretion (ADME), and reviewing case studies to highlight the uses of nonclinical data to inform the selection of safe starting doses for neonatal studies.

These consortia provide opportunities for the scientific community to work together to develop innovative trial designs, new biomarkers, new outcome assessment tools, and clinically meaningful short- and long-term endpoints.

Collaborative efforts are needed to support the infrastructure for the actual trials in neonates. A successful example of these collaborative efforts is the Pediatric Trials Network (PTN), an alliance of clinical research sites sponsored by the NICHD and managed through the Duke Clinical Research Institute that has focused on conducting clinical trials to support studies of off-patent drugs prioritized by the NICHD under BPCA, leading to several labeling changes of drugs used in newborns and children.

Since the publication of the previous editions of this book, neonatal and pediatric pharmacology has grown and flourished. Indeed, the future appears bright, and we welcome the day when therapeutic orphans will no longer be applicable to drug use in infants and children.

Johannes N. van den Anker
Jacob V. Aranda

SECTION

I General Principles

Steven Hirschfeld
Susan McCune
Lynne Yao
Donna L. Snyder
Gerri R. Baer
Bridgette L. Jones
Anne Zajicek

CHAPTER

1 Clinical Trials Involving Children: History, Rationale, Regulatory Framework, and Technical Considerations

INTRODUCTION

The premise for this chapter is that clinical trials are a justifiable activity to guide decision-making. Clinical trials are formal mechanisms to evaluate interventions by capturing observations and measurements about exposure to the intervention in a structured manner from individuals with a particular phenotype that are selected to represent the larger population of all people, current and future, with the phenotype of interest. A phenotype may be characterized as individuals with or at risk for a particular condition, whether it is chronic or temporary, whether it is life threatening or a mild annoyance. The data that represent the signals from the individual observations and measurements are subsequently pooled and analyzed to infer a generalization about the effects of the intervention under evaluation.

The decision types that are supported by the analysis of clinical trials include whether a patient might receive benefit with acceptable risk if exposed to an intervention or whether a body of data about an intervention support marketing authorization or whether cumulative data warrant further development of an intervention. In all cases, the amount, type, and quality of collected data generated from a clinical trial will be important components of the credibility, validity, and confidence in any analysis and the inferences and decisions that are influenced by that analysis.

The general paradigm is illustrated in Figure 1.1.

The concept of exposure includes the concepts of amplitude or intensity, duration, and frequency. All are variables and must be described. The concept of structured measurements includes the concepts of methodology, precision, sensitivity, specificity, receiver-operator characteristics, and other factors to be discussed in further detail subsequently. These must also be described to properly interpret the signals and perform informative analyses.

A historical asymmetry characterizes the role of children in exposure to interventions that are either untried or have a history but no formal body of evidence establishing the benefit and potential risks to children. Just as the perception of children evolved from one of being the property of adults to individuals worthy of special protections, the role children played in the history of research is complex and, prior to the mid-20th century, often unfavorable to the individual.

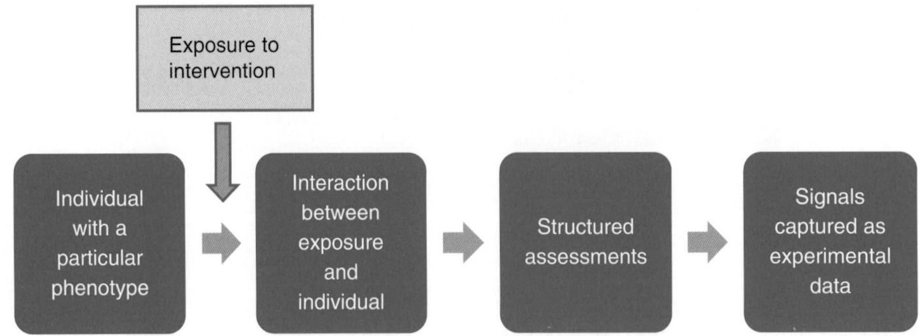

Figure 1.1 General paradigm for individual data capture in a clinical trial showing a person with a defined phenotype with or without a defined genotype exposed to an intervention followed by a structured measurement. The signal from the structured measurement is captured and the collection of the data from all individuals is pooled and analyzed.

BRIEF HISTORY OF RESEARCH INVOLVING CHILDREN

Children have been utilized to test new therapies for thousands of years, but the first documented prospective structured clinical investigations to test scientific hypotheses were a development of the 18th century during the period known in Europe as the Age of Enlightenment. While living in Constantinople in 1718, Lady Mary Montague, daughter of the Duke of Kinston, observed the Turkish procedure of inoculation against smallpox and had her 6-year-old son inoculated. Upon her return to London, she requested a surgeon to inoculate her 5-year-old daughter. The surgeon used a thread soaked in pustular secretions bound to the skin. This technique was replaced by scarring with a lance tip dipped in pus. The resulting plaque was then covered until it healed, and experimental research in pediatric preventive medicine began in Europe.[1]

The American clergyman Cotton Mather also became interested in the procedure after hearing from the slave Onesimus about the practice of using fluid from a patient with mild smallpox to inoculate uninfected people in Africa. Subsequently, he read about the European experience in his correspondence with members of the Royal Society of London. An outbreak of smallpox in Boston in 1721, despite efforts at quarantining the index case, provided an opportunity to experiment. Mather persuaded Boston physician Zabdiel Boylston to proceed with what may have been the first clinical trial in North America. Boylston inoculated his 6-year-old son by lancing the skin and applying to it 9- to 14-day-old pustular material from a smallpox patient, then wrapped the skin in a cabbage leaf. Subsequently, he inoculated 280 people, including 65 children. Unfortunately, six of the adults, although none of the children, subsequently died, with a case fatality rate of approximately 2%. Despite the fact that the smallpox fatality rate for the general population in Boston was 14%, a great controversy about the value of inoculation followed, including the hurling of a bomb into Rev. Mather's home. Fortunately, the explosive did not detonate, but the practice of inoculation did not become public policy.[2]

Experimental immunotherapy evolved further with the work of Edward Jenner in England. In 1796 Jenner injected James Phipps, an 8-year-old boy, with extract from pustules from the hand of Sarah Nelmes, a milkmaid. Jenner had been told by milkmaids that cowpox protected them against smallpox. The word "vaccination" is derived from the Latin word for cow—*vacca*. Jenner examined his patient every day and then 2 weeks after the cowpox injection; Jenner applied a challenge of smallpox extract and found that the boy was protected. He expanded his study from the initial child to "a number" of others ranging in age from 11 months to 8 years. None of the children became ill. Over the course of the next 50 years, vaccination became compulsory in some areas of England.[3]

During the 19th century children's hospitals were established in Europe and the United States in cities including Paris, Vienna, London, Philadelphia, Boston, and New York. Concurrently, pediatrics became an academic specialty, and textbooks were published. Ludwig Friedrich Meissner of Leipzig, Germany, published a survey of texts and monographs pertaining to pediatric medicine in 1826 noting that prior to 1775 there were 200 publications, and subsequently there were at least almost 7,000.[1]

In 1828 Charles-Michel Billard of the Hospice des Infants-Trouvés in Paris published a revolutionary treatise classifying pediatric diseases on the basis of tissue pathology rather than patient symptoms. In addition, he included a catalogue of height, weight, and vital signs.[4] This was followed by surveys by Quetelet in Belgium and Chadwick in England on growth rates of children showing that lower socioeconomic class was associated with less growth, most probably due to nutritional deficiencies.[5,6] Comparative pharmacology began in about the middle of the 19th century.

In 1834 the first periodical devoted entirely to the care of children, *Aizalekteiz über Kinderkrankheiten* (*Annals of Diseases of Children*), was published in Stuttgart; it ceased publication in 1837 after publishing 12 volumes. Over the course of the following decades, many journals appeared in several countries as academic societies and publishing houses developed interest in the field of pediatric research.

In 1847 John Snow began to administer anesthesia with ether to children aged 4 through 16 years. He also experimented with chloroform and, by 1857, had successfully anesthetized hundreds of children, including 186 infants under the age of 1 year. He first described differences in metabolism between adults and children, noting that the effects of chloroform were more quickly produced and also subsided more quickly in children, explaining the observation in terms of the quicker breathing and circulation in pediatric patients.[1]

Frederik Theodor Berg was appointed the first European professor of pediatrics at the Karolinska Institute in Stockholm, Sweden, in 1845. In 1858, he resigned the post to become director of the Central Bureau of Statistics. In that capacity, he expanded the bureau's data banks to include not only population, but also welfare, agricultural, and industrial data. He founded a statistical journal in 1869, and in the same year, utilizing parish records, he published a paper analyzing infant mortality rates in Sweden.[7]

The first course in the United States at an academic institution devoted to pediatrics was offered at the Yale College of Medicine in 1813 by Eli Ives.[8] In 1860, Abraham Jacobi, an émigré from Germany, was appointed as professor of infantile pathology and therapeutics at the New York Medical College, which may have been the first full academic pediatric appointment in America. A pediatric clinic with the first use of bedside teaching was founded in 1862.[9,10]

The first institution for sick children in the United States was founded in 1855 in Philadelphia. Boston and New York followed in 1869 and the District of Columbia in 1871. By 1880, Jacobi had been instrumental in the establishment of several hospitals for children in the United States—Chicago, San Francisco, St. Louis, and Cincinnati—so that by 1895 there were 26 children's hospitals in this country. In 1868, Jacobi wrote an article on croup in the first issue of the *American Journal of Obstetrics and Diseases of Women and Children*, published by the American Medical Association (AMA). The first American journal dedicated totally to pediatric research, *Archives of Pediatrics*, began publication in 1884.

In 1880, Jacobi organized the pediatric section of the AMA and in 1885 he became president of the New York Academy of Medicine. In 1888, he became a founding member of the American Pediatric Society, which limited membership to 110. The society published its *Transactions*, which, for the first third of the 20th century, was the major American journal devoted to pediatric research. Jacobi was among the first to recognize the potential of using government resources to advance clinical science. He is credited with persuading the U.S. Congress to appropriate funds for the first printing of *Index Medicus*, compiled by his friend John Shaw Billings.

TRANSITION INTO THE 20TH CENTURY AND THE BEGINNING OF RESEARCH REGULATION

Claude Bernard wrote in 1865, "It is our duty and our right to perform experiments on man whenever it can save his life, cure him or give him some personal benefit".[11] This statement has been subsequently interpreted that on an ethical basis only studies that provide direct benefit to the participants should be undertaken, but the principle had no legal authority. The question of prior permission to participate was not addressed.

The last decades of the 19th century saw further experimentation in immunotherapy for the treatment of infectious diseases, with many of the major advances resulting from studies on children. In 1885, Pasteur injected 9-year-old Joseph Meister of Alsace, who had been bitten by a rabid dog, with extract of rabbit spinal cord from a rabbit that had died of rabies 2 weeks before. Thirteen inoculations were given daily, with the last an extract from a rabid dog. The boy recovered, and a second shepherd boy was similarly cured.[12]

In 1892, an immunologic approach to reduce transmission of venereal disease was attempted in a study by Albert Neisser, Professor of Dermatology and Syphilis in Breslau and discoverer of the organism responsible for gonorrhea. He subcutaneously and intravenously injected eight women and girls, the youngest being 10 years old, with cell-free extract of syphilis in an attempt to stimulate an immune response. Subsequently, four of the women became infected, leading to the speculation that the cause of their illness could have been Neisser and his experiment, and a subsequent public scandal followed.[13]

The debate continued primarily in the press for several years until December 19, 1900, when the Prussian Ministry of Education and Medicine issued a policy statement about human experimentation. The proclamation stated that research may not be performed without the permission of the patient and that research on children was forbidden. It further stated that research should have as its goal the diagnosis, treatment, or prevention of disease.

This was probably the first government edict about human research, and although a potent statement had been made, enforcement powers did not follow.[14,15] The rise of the chemical industry, particularly in Germany, fed the hope of targeting diseases through the administration of manufactured compounds. As an example, the recognition of genital infections as a source of infant morbidity led Karl Sigmund Franz Crede in 1884 to use silver nitrate solution to prevent gonorrhea infections of the eyes of the newborn.[16,17]

There was a rush to examine the medical (and potential commercial) activity of many newly synthesized products, spurred by Paul Ehrlich's vision of a "magic bullet" and a permissive social climate. In 1902 the psychiatrist Albert Moll published a monograph, *Aertzliche Ethik*,[18,19] in which he catalogued some 600 publications of medical experiments where, he argued, there was no possible benefit to the subject. Moll criticized not only the dangers of the experiments, but also the lack of advantage to the research participant. Despite the Prussian edict and Moll's book, however, there would be no translation of research participant protection into public policy for another third of a century.

EVOLUTION OF ETHICAL PRINCIPLES AND THEIR APPLICATION TO RESEARCH

Health crises involving children have played a major role in the evolution of food and drug law in the United States. The first major domestic controls occurred early in the 20th century, following more than 100 attempts in the 19th century to pass federal legislation regulating the manufacture and sale of foods and drugs. In the autumn of 1901 in St. Louis, more than a dozen children died of tetanus after receiving diphtheria antitoxin that had been recovered from a tetanus-infected horse. Subsequently, another 100 cases of tetanus were reported, including the deaths of 9 more children. This led to the passage of the Biologics Control Act of 1902, which called for the licensing, labeling, and supervision of biologic products intended for humans.[20]

In the autumn of 1905, Collier's Weekly published an expose of fraud in the manufacture and sale of patent medicines, citing cases of infants who died following administration of syrup that contained morphine that was intended to treat colic. Although concern was widespread, public documentation of specific cases of death or morbidity due to commercial drugs was lacking due to contract clauses on publications by drug manufacturers threatening to cancel advertisements if legislation regulating drug marketing was passed. Nevertheless, through the efforts of a coalition of chemists, women's clubs, state officials, civic organizations, and writers, in June 1906, President Theodore Roosevelt signed the first Pure Food and Drug Act into law. The Act established the need for product labels, prohibited interstate commerce in adulterated or misbranded drugs, and established the need to maintain standards.[20,21] There was, however, a provision in the Act that permitted deviation from the standards if they were stated on the label. Enforcement was to be by the courts.

This led to the case of *US v Johnson* in 1911, in which a majority of the Supreme Court ruled in favor of the defendant, the manufacturer of Dr. Johnson's Mild Combination Treatment for Cancer, that claimed as its ingredients a mixture of substances with names like Cancerine tablets, Antiseptic tablets, Blood purifier, Special No. 4, Cancerine No. 17, and Cancerine No. 1. The Court stated that prosecution was to be limited to false and misleading statements about the ingredients or the identity of a product and was not intended to extend to false therapeutic claims.[22] In an effort to address the gap, the 1912 Sherley Amendment to the Pure Food and Drug Act stated that false therapeutic claims could be prosecuted, but only if intent to defraud could be proven in court.[23] The rising political prominence of pediatrics led to the first White House Conference on the Care of Dependent Children in 1909. Based on a recommendation from the Conference, the United States Children's Bureau was established by Congress in 1912 to coordinate health care policy.[24]

World War I had multiple aftereffects, including recognition of the poor physical condition of many of the young men recruited to serve in the armed forces. A political response was the Sheppard-Towner Bill in 1921 to provide funding for the health care of poor mothers and infants and extend health supervision from infancy to preschool children (Reference Sheppard Towner Bill, Public Law 67–97: Statutes at Large: 42 Stat. 224, Chap 135: November 23, 1921). The question of the role of government and how much support it should provide for health care and children's issues was debated for much of the 20th century, primarily on philosophical and political grounds.

The next major change in regulations occurred in 1927 when the Federal Caustic Poisons Act was passed in an effort to protect children from lye and other dangerous chemicals by requiring labeling with warnings and antidotes (Reference United States Code: Federal Caustic Poison Act, 15 U.S.C. §§ 401-411 [Suppl. 1 1925]).

The AMA was not sheltered from the discussion of pediatric safety, and at the 1928 meeting there was plan for a society that would be open to any physician trained in pediatrics. Two years later, a schism occurred within the AMA on the issue of government support for clinics to treat infants and children with the goal of reducing mortality. A group of pediatricians withdrew and formed a new organization, the American Academy of Pediatrics (AAP).[25]

In 1930, the U.S. Congress established the National Institutes of Health (NIH) by renaming the U.S. Hygiene Laboratory in Washington, DC.[26] In addition, the Food, Drug and Insecticide Administration was established as an enforcement agency.[20] The name was shortened in 1930 to the Food and Drug Administration (FDA). Legislation to revise the 1906 Food and Drug Act was proposed in 1933 but became mired in Congress.[20]

In 1931 the German Ministry of the Interior issued the first guidelines published for the conduct of research on children. These were part of general guidelines for the conduct of clinical research that were issued in response to allegations by the press and members of the national legislature of questionable and even unethical conduct by physicians. The guidelines were the initial governmental statement of requirements for the ethical conduct of clinical research, which are found in subsequent statements such as the Helsinki Declaration.

The general principles were the primary obligation and duty of the experimenter to protect the subject, the need for informed consent in all circumstances, the principle of preclinical testing in animals prior to human use, and the principle of accurate publication of findings. An experimental compound was defined as any intervention that did not contribute directly to the treatment of an individual patient. No mention is made of peer review in either the experimental or the publication process, although the Berlin Medical Board, which earlier in the century had issued its own recommendations on protection of research subjects, had proposed a regulatory oversight body. This proposal was not incorporated into the final guidelines.

The German guidelines contained two sentences specifically about children: "Application of the new treatment must be considered particularly carefully if it involves infants or adolescents of less than 18 years" and "Experimentation on infants or persons of less than 18 years is forbidden even if it will only expose them to a very slight danger".[27]

In September 1937, the Samuel E. Massengill Pharmaceutical Company in St. Louis marketed the newly discovered antibiotic sulfanilamide as a 10% solution, substituting 72% diethylene glycol for the usual solute of ethanol and sweetening it with sugar and raspberry syrup. The resulting elixir killed more than 100 people including many children, due to glycol-induced renal failure, and resulted in the suicide of the chemist who made it. The product was only labeled as an elixir, which implied ethyl alcohol and did not state the full list of ingredients, and thus the company was charged with misbranding. The absence of an applicable law meant that there was no culpability for the deaths.

This tragedy led to the passage of the Food, Drug and Cosmetic Act, which was signed into law by President Franklin Roosevelt in June 1938. The Act gave authority to the FDA to require that safety is established prior to marketing, required disclosure of all active ingredients, required directions for use and warnings about misuse unless the product was sold by prescription, allowed federal inspections of manufacturing facilities, established procedures for the formal review of applications for marketing, explicitly prohibited false claims, and extended the scope of the regulation to cosmetics and devices. There were no provisions for premarketing review, and only those products that were to be sold for interstate commerce were covered. All applications were automatically approved if the FDA did not act within 60 days. The regulation of advertising of therapeutics was assigned to the Federal Trade Commission.[28]

International recognition of the need to protect participants in clinical experiments surfaced during the Nuremberg Military Tribunals in 1946. Evidence was given that up to 200 German doctors had performed experiments with prisoners of war and civilians that had no protections for the participants and caused harm without any prospect of benefit. The subsequent court proceedings led to the development of the Nuremberg Code, which established international standards for the treatment of one human by another. The guiding principle was that "The voluntary consent of the human subject is absolutely essential." This statement has been widely interpreted as precluding research on children, although the Nuremberg Code is silent on the specific subject of pediatric research.[29]

In 1962, the tragedy of the births of malformed children, primarily in Europe and Canada due to thalidomide taken as a sedative by their mothers while pregnant, resulted in part in Congress passing the Kefauver–Harris amendment to the Food, Drug and Cosmetic Act.[30]

This amendment added an important new facet—the requirement that a product demonstrate efficacy prior to approval of a marketing claim. Additional provisions in the amendment were the need to establish good manufacturing practice (GMP) and maintain production records, the requirement to file an application with the FDA prior to clinical testing (Investigational New Drug application, or IND), an increase in the time for FDA marketing authorization review from 60 to 180 days, the transferal of regulatory authority for drug advertising to the FDA, and withdrawal of approval if new evidence indicated lack of safety or effectiveness.[31] The addition of an efficacy requirement prompted a retrospective study by the National Academy of Sciences of FDA approvals between 1938 and 1962 that showed that 40% of the approved products lacked evidence that they were effective.[32] The new aspect in analysis of product use by adding an efficacy requirement was that benefit and risk could be assessed and acceptable ratios of risk to benefit determined for the intended use at the prescribed dose.

To summarize, the three principles of drug regulation—labeling, safety, and efficacy—were formalized during the first two-thirds of the 20th century. Formal guidelines for the protection of participants in research, and children in particular, are a product of the last third of the 20th century.

As a point of reference, protection for animals goes back to the 19th century. For example, in the United Kingdom, the Cruelty to Animals Act became law in 1876.[31] In 1960, Louis G. Welt, of the Department of Medicine at Yale University, sent a questionnaire regarding practices for clinical research to university departments of medicine. Sixty-six replied, of which 24 (36%) either already had or were in favor of establishing a committee to review studies involving human experimentation.[32] In 1962, the Medical Research Council of the United Kingdom made a statement in its annual report that drew a distinction between research interventions intended to be of direct benefit to the subject of the research and those that are not so intended. These two categories of research were referred to as "therapeutic" and "nontherapeutic", respectively. The report went on to state that "In the strict view of the law, parents and guardians of minors cannot give consent on their behalf to any procedures which are of no particular benefit to them and which may carry some risk of harm." This statement has regularly been interpreted as placing a complete embargo on nontherapeutic research on children. A follow-up report in 1963 addressed some of the perceived legal and ethical problems in clinical research.[33]

The World Medical Association adopted in 1964 the Declaration of Helsinki: Recommendations Guiding Medical Doctors in Biomedical Research Involving Human Subjects. The document made a distinction between therapeutic and nontherapeutic research and stated that protocols, independent review of the proposed research, and informed consent should be part of the protection of participants in research. Third-party consent for a participant unable to give consent was described, thus offering an approach to pediatric research.[34]

Henry Beecher, Professor of Anesthesia at Harvard Medical School, published an article entitled "Ethics and clinical research" in the *New England Journal of Medicine* in 1966.[35] He drew attention to 22 reports that contained clinical research with a variety of ethical problems, most of which put patients at considerable risk. One of these was the Willowbrook study in New York, which exposed institutionalized children to serum infected with hepatitis. The study was performed with institutional approval, and parents gave permission. The rationale was that hepatitis was so prevalent that the children were likely to become infected and that it was scientifically important to study the early phases of the infectious process.

The Willowbrook approach of using institutionalized children as experimental subjects was not unprecedented. Other studies with institutionalized children in Massachusetts during the 1950s exposed children to radioactive compounds, in one case to study mineral absorption and in another case to study the protective effect of nonradioactive iodine in blocking radioactive iodine in the event of a nuclear explosion. Both studies had federal funding, and the former study had additional funding from the Quaker Oats Company because one of the study questions was to examine the effect of cereal composition on mineral absorption.[36]

In 1966 the Surgeon General of the United States, Dr. William H. Stewart, issued a memo based on recommendations by his predecessor, Dr. Luther Terry, and the NIH director, Dr. James Shannon, requiring institutions accepting federal funds to certify to establish independent review of research projects before they were started. In addition, institutions had to provide the relevant federal funding agency assurance that procedures were in place for consent and review.

In December 1966, the policy was expanded to include behavioral as well as medical research.[37] In 1967, the Public Health Service required that intramural research, including that conducted at NIH, abide by similar requirements.[38] Even institutions with existing review committees had to improve their procedures to comply with the new regulations.

Also in 1967, the U.K. Royal College of Physicians Committee on the Supervision of the Ethics of Clinical Investigation in Institutions published a first report recommending that every hospital or institution in which clinical research was undertaken have a research committee that should satisfy itself of the ethics of all proposed investigations. The proposed research committees, with at least one lay member, should be established in every region to review the ethics of proposed investigation, and by law they should be responsible to the General Medical Council.[39] In the same year, M. H. Pappworth published Human Guinea Pigs, which detailed several hundred reports of questionable ethics in human experimentation.[40,41]

In 1973 in Great Britain, the chief medical officer of the Department of Health and Social Security requested the Royal College of Physicians Committee to again make a recommendation. The subsequent committee report reflected a shift in attitude. It stated, "If advances in medical treatment are to continue, so must clinical research investigation. It is in this light, therefore that it is recommended that clinical research investigations of children or mentally handicapped adults which is not of direct benefit to the patients should be conducted, only when the procedures entail negligible risk or discomfort and subject to the provisions of any common and statute law prevailing at the time. The parent or guardian should be consulted and his agreement recorded." This revision appears to suggest that it is permissible to conduct nontherapeutic research on children provided this is perceived to be of negligible risk.[42] In 1974, the U.S. Department of Health, Education, and Welfare issued regulations requiring institutions that receive federal funds for research to establish institutional review boards (IRBs) and described procedures and criteria for informed consent.[43]

Also in 1974, Congress passed the National Research Act. All federally funded clinical research proposals as well as the adequacy of informed consent had to be reviewed by an IRB with oversight and enforcement dependent on the particular federal funding agency, meaning there was no global oversight of federally funded research.[44]

The National Research Act also established a National Commission for the Protection of Human Subjects of Medical and Behavioral Research. The National Commission had a mandate to develop ethical guidelines for the conduct of research on human subjects, in particular children, and to make recommendations to the secretary of Health, Education, and Welfare.

When the U.K. Department of Health and Social Security issued a circular entitled "Supervision of the Ethics of Clinical Research Investigations and Fetal Research" in 1975, it drew attention to this point, stating, "(one) ought not to infer from this recommendation that the fact that consent has been given by the parent or guardian and that the risk involved is considered negligible will be sufficient to bring such clinical research investigation within the law as it stands".[45] The British chief medical officer wrote in another publication that it was not legitimate to perform an experiment on a child that was not in the child's interests.

The 1975 revision of the Declaration of Helsinki addresses this point by stating, "the potential benefits, hazards and discomfort of a new method should be weighed against the advantage of the best current diagnostic and therapeutic methods." It provides no clear guidance on the subject of nontherapeutic research on children or any other potential subject deemed legally incompetent. The final statement of the Declaration concerning nontherapeutic research states, "In research on man, the interest of science and society should never take precedence over considerations related to the well-being of the subject."[46]

The U.S. National Commission for the Protection of Human Subjects of Biomedical and Behavioral Research established by the National Research Act in 1974 and in 1977 published its report on research involving children. To prepare the report, the National Commission, over the next several years, held public hearings, commissioned papers and other reports, commissioned a survey of the practice of more than 400 investigators engaged in pediatric research, and convened a national conference to ensure that the views of various constituencies were heard. The report contains an analysis of law as it applies to research of children and considerable discussion of the ethical bases of various viewpoints.[47]

The conclusions were that research involving children was important for the health of all children and that such research could be conducted ethically within the general conditions outlined in documents such as the Helsinki Declaration. The rationale for pediatric research was based on two factors: (a) children are different than adults and animals in general and some diseases only occur in children, and (b) the risk of harm from treatments and practices is increased without research. Part of the mission was to develop guidelines. These included a determination by an institutional ethical review board that the proposed study is scientifically sound and significant; that appropriate studies must be conducted first on animals, subsequently in adult humans, and then on older children prior to involving infants; and that the risks must be minimized by using the safest method consistent with sound research design and by using procedures performed for diagnostic or treatment purposes whenever feasible.

Parents must provide permission for children to participate in research and the child, when feasible, should provide assent. Assent was considered feasible for a normal child at 7 years of age. The Commission report, in an innovative approach, categorized risk and made the following recommendations:

1. Research not involving greater than minimal risk might be conducted on children subject to permission obtained from parents.
2. Research greater than minimal risk might be conducted if it held out the prospect of direct benefit to the subject.
3. Research not holding the prospect of benefit to the subject might be conducted so long as the risk involved was no more than a minor increase over minimal.
4. An additional category for research that was not included in the previous categories is research that carries no prospect of direct benefit to the subject but carries a risk greater than a small increase over minimal. Such research could be carried out provided it was approved by a national ethics advisory board and was open to public review and comment.

The Commission also recommended that adolescents could have the requirement for parental permission waived in specific circumstances. The Commission published a report in 1978 on IRBs, and in 1979 the Belmont Report (named after the donor of the conference room where the Commission met) reviewed the Commission's findings and outlined the ethical basis for clinical research.[48,49] The Commission's recommendations can be summarized in three principles:

1. Respect for the personal dignity and autonomy of individuals, with special protection for those with diminished autonomy
2. Beneficence to maximize benefit and minimize harm
3. Justice to distribute fairly and equitably the benefits and burdens of research

The recommendations of the Commission were adopted in June 1983 as federal regulations that apply to all federally funded research (45 CFR 46), with only some minimal changes, for example, excluding the waivers for parental permission for adolescents. Subpart A applies to all research participants, Subpart B applies to research enrolling fetuses and pregnant women, Subpart C applies to research with prisoners, and Subpart D applies to research with children. Sections within Subpart D describe the risk categories and are shown in Figure 1.2.[50]

Tyson and colleagues published a study in 1983 that evaluated the quality of perinatal research. The object of the investigation was to determine the quality of the studies because the treatment methods recommended were widely and rapidly incorporated into clinical practice after publication in a respected obstetric and pediatrics journal. They found that many of the studies failed to meet the criteria for quality perinatal therapeutic research, as shown in Table 1.1.[51]

HISTORIC LACK OF BENEFITS TO CHILDREN OF PHARMACEUTICAL RESEARCH

The U.S. federal government has been systematically supporting clinical trials with children since the 1950s. Early studies on childhood leukemia were sponsored by the National Cancer Institute; on rheumatic heart disease by the National Heart, Blood

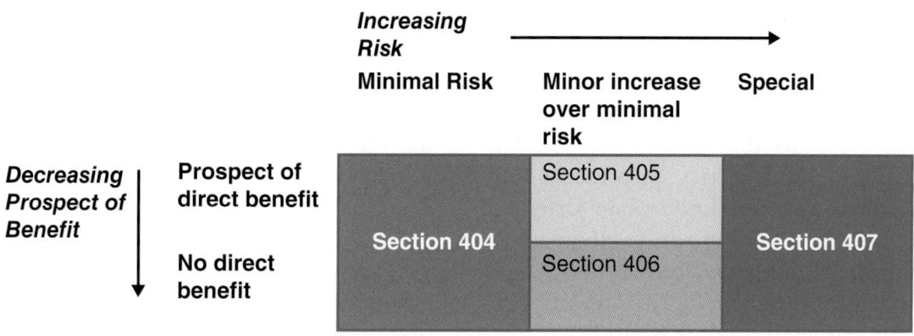

Figure 1.2 Risk categories and applicable sections of Subpart D Title 45 CFR Part 46, the subpart of the Common Rule of the Federal Regulations Governing Federally Funded Research that applies to children.

and Lung Institute; on retrolental fibroplasia by the National Institute of Neurological Diseases and Blindness; on diabetic retinopathy by the National Eye Institute; on diabetes by the National Institute of Arthritis and Metabolic Diseases; on extracranial to intracranial arterial anastomosis (a clinical trial) by the National Institute of Neurological and Communicative Disorders and Stroke; and on hereditary angioedema (a clinical trial) by the National Institute of Allergy and Infectious Diseases.[52] An NIH institute dedicated to pediatric investigation was founded in 1960, the National Institute of Child Health and Human Development (NICHD). The first director was Dr. Robert Aldrich.[53]

As noted earlier, in 1962, the Food, Drug and Cosmetic Act was amended to include efficacy data in the FDA approval process and in the approved product package insert. Despite the growing interest in pediatric research, the majority of medications used in children were not studied in children. In 1968 Dr. Harry Shirkey coined the term "therapeutic orphan" to refer to the situation in which sick children were deprived of access to medications because the drugs had not been adequately tested in children.[54]

TABLE 1.1 Summary of Review of 88 Therapeutic Trials in Perinatal Research

% of Studies Fulfilling Criteria	*Yes*	*Unclear*	*No*
Statement of purpose	94	6	0
Clearly defined outcome variables	74	1	25
Planned prospective data collection	48	30	22
Predetermined sample size (or a sequential trial)	3	16	71
Sample size specified	93	6	1
Disease/health status of subjects specified ($n = 85$)	51	20	29
Exclusion criteria specified ($n = 81$)	46	9	45
Randomization (if feasible) appropriately performed and documented ($n = 69$)	9	12	79
Blinding used, or lack or blinding unlikely to have biased results ($n = 83$)	49	47	4
Adequate sample size	15	44	41
Statistical methods identified, appropriately used, and interpreted	26	0	74
Recommendations/conclusions justified	10	71	19

Tyson JE, Furzan JA, Reisch JS, et al. An evaluation of the quality of therapeutic studies in perinatal medicine. *J Pediatr* 1983;102(1):10–13.

In 1972, at the annual meeting of the AAP Dr. Charles Edwards, former commissioner of the FDA, stated that a large percentage of the drugs used in sick infants and children are prescribed on empirical grounds.[55] In 1973, a report from the National Academy of Sciences emphasized the different nature of the response of an immature organ to pharmacologic agents and suggested that innovative investigative programs were needed to supply information on the use of pharmacologic agents in the pediatric population. Among the reasons cited was that children are different from adults in the process of drug disposition and receptor sensitivity. As an example: the plasma concentrations of the drug theophylline change with the age of the patient.

In 1974, the AAP issued a report commissioned by the FDA: General Guidelines for the Evaluation of Drugs to Be Approved for Use during Pregnancy and, for the Treatment of Infants and Children.[56] In the following year, Dr. John Wilson found that 78% of prescription drugs had a statement in the package insert that its use in infants and children had not been adequately studied or there was no statement and the label was silent on the issue.[57]

The FDA adapted the AAP report and in 1977 published it as a guidance document entitled "General Considerations for the Clinical Evaluation of Drugs in Infants and Children." The major points were an emphasis on anticipating and describing unexpected toxicities in the pediatric population, an expectation that reasonable evidence for efficacy should exist prior to study in infants and children, that only sick children should be enrolled in studies, a preference for active or historical controls over placebo controls, and a recommendation for studying patients in decreasing age order so that experience is gained with older children first.[58] Concurrently, the AAP issued "Guidelines for the Ethical Conduct of Studies to Evaluate Drugs in Pediatric Populations".[59]

In 1979, the FDA issued a regulation adding a Pediatric Use Subsection to the Product Package Insert Precautions Section.[60] The intent was to highlight differences in adverse event profiles and to note whether any pediatric use information existed.

Although not directed exclusively at pediatric patients, an important regulatory change occurred in 1983 with the passage of the Orphan Drug Act.[61] The Act outlined criteria whereby rare diseases, many of them pediatric and defined as having a prevalence of less than 200,000 in the United States, could benefit from incentives to develop new therapeutics. The program is administered by the FDA and provides both a longer period of marketing exclusivity (7 years for an "orphan" indication compared to 5 years for the first approved indication of a new molecular entity) and subsidies in the way of grants and technical advice for clinical development. An orphan designation is given to the combination of a rare disease and a product. This allows the same disease to have multiple products qualify for orphan designation and does not restrict a product to only being used to treat an orphan disease. The Orphan Drug Act established the principle of government incentives to promote product development in areas of public health need.

Despite the initiative to encourage pediatric data, in 1988 Dr. Franz Rosa, an FDA epidemiologist, surveyed product labels for drugs that are used in infants and found that only 50% had been formally evaluated. Of these, half had been considered safe and effective and the other half had a caution or risk statement in the product label. Of the 50% that had not been evaluated, 60% had a disclaimer about not being indicated for use in children and 40% had no information.[62] An independent survey in 1991 found that, just as in 1975, about 80% of product labels had either limited pediatric dosing information or had a disclaimer for use in children.[63]

FEDERAL PEDIATRIC INITIATIVES

To further encourage pediatric therapeutic development and the inclusion of pediatric information in product package inserts (product labels), in 1994, the FDA revised the Pediatric Use section of the regulations, adding a Subsection (iv) permitting extrapolation of efficacy data if the disease course in adult and pediatric patients was similar.[64]

An FDA guidance document issued in 1996 on the Content and Format of Pediatric Use Section noted that extrapolation should be considered, that the effects of the drugs, both beneficial and adverse, in adult and pediatric patients should be described, and that critical literature references should be included. Compliance was voluntary and did not result in an increase in the proportion of products with pediatric labeling.[65]

Also in 1995, the AAP Committee on Drugs issued a revision of its Guidelines for the Ethical Conduct of Studies to Evaluate Drugs in Pediatric Populations with detailed discussion of IRBs, informed consent, risk and benefit determination, investigator competence, scientific validity and special cases of the dying patient, the newly dead patient, and patients with chronic progressive and potentially fatal diseases.[66]

The NICHD established the Pediatric Pharmacology Research Unit Network in 1994 as the first national network for pediatric research, with seven institutions. The network was expanded to 13 institutions in 2001 and ran until 2010, when it was replaced by the Pediatric Trials Network. A guiding principle was that children are not small adults.[67,68]

As part of the 1997 Food and Drug Administration Modernization Act (FDAMA), an incentive, similar in spirit to the Orphan Drug Act, was added as an option for certain types of products for which pediatric data were submitted to the FDA in response to a written request from the agency.

The incentive was a 6-month extension to existing marketing or patent exclusivity for any product that had the active moiety that was studied in the written request. To qualify for the incentive, a study report must be submitted to the FDA that fairly responds to the terms of the written request. Written requests can be initiated by a sponsor through submission of a proposal for pediatric studies to the FDA or internally by the FDA when a perceived public health need exists. Not all sponsors that received an FDA written request accepted the opportunity. Some of the reasons sponsors declined were because the product was a generic drug that lacks exclusivity, the requested indication was for a hard to study small population for a rare condition, reluctance to conduct studies in populations such as neonates or premature infants, or a business decision that the exclusivity extension was not useful.

The results of the submitted studies must be interpretable and informative, but do not need to demonstrate a positive outcome. A negative study can be part of the submission and still contribute to the granting of pediatric exclusivity because the intent is to provide appropriate pediatric information. At the time, existing and newly approved products could qualify with the exception of biologics, certain antibiotics, and devices.[69]

In 1998, the FDA issued a Pediatric Rule that mandated pediatric studies based on the proposed labeling claim. If the adult indication occurred in children, the Pediatric Rule would apply. If the adult disease or condition did not apply to children, a waiver from compliance could be granted. If the adult indication did not apply to a pediatric subpopulation, for example, children younger than 5 years, a partial waiver could be granted. In contrast, the pediatric incentive program in the FDAMA could apply to any pediatric disease independent of the adult indication.

One of two additional conditions had to be met before the Pediatric Rule would apply. Either the product had to be a therapeutic advance or it likely had to have widespread use defined as 50,000 or more children with the relevant disease or condition. The Pediatric Rule did apply to biologics, but products with Orphan Drug designation were exempted.[70]

In October 2002, the Rule was invalidated in a court decision that ruled that the FDA did not have authority to mandate studies in a population to which a drug sponsor did not intend to market.[71] In November 2003, the FDA gained the statutory authority to mandate pediatric studies with the signing of Public Law 108-155, the Pediatric Research Equity Act, into law. The Pediatric Research Equity Act was an updated version of the Pediatric Rule that continued as a principle that the linkage between an adult and pediatric indication is flexible and may evolve over time as biologic, genetic, and physiologic knowledge advances.[72]

The death of a patient with an inherited metabolic deficiency, Jesse Gelsinger, in a gene therapy experiment in Philadelphia in September 1999[73] was a catalyst for the formation of a new agency within the Department of Health and Human Services, the Office for Human Research Protection, in June 2000.[74]

The responsibilities for supervising federally funded research were previously in the Office of Protection from Research Risks in the NIH. The Office of Human Research Protection has both enforcement and educational roles. The FDA published an adaptation of Subpart D of 45 CFR 46 in the Federal Register in 2001 that would extend the principles and risk categories of the original regulations with some modification to all FDA-regulated research and not just federally funded research.[75]

The Best Pharmaceuticals for Children Act (BPCA), signed into law in January 2002, renewed the incentive program contained in the FDAMA and extended the time for the FDA to issue written requests until October 2007. Study reports were due whenever the written request stated and were independent of the last date for issuing written requests. Additionally, the BPCA in 2002 endorsed the principle of public disclosure of information regarding the effects of medications in children and provided mechanisms such as Federal Register notices, posting of FDA review summaries on the Internet, product labeling, and advisory committee discussion to promote this goal. A further provision in the BPCA provides mechanisms for the study of off-patent drugs in pediatric populations and a plan for adverse event tracking and reporting.[76]

The federal pediatric initiatives were renewed, revised, and extended in September 2007 with enactment of Public Law 110-85, The Food and Drug and Administration Amendment Act of 2007 (FDAAA). Within FDAAA, Title IV, The Pediatric Medical Device Safety and Improvement Act; Title V, The Pediatric Research Equity Act; and Title VI, The BPCA are all directed at pediatric populations, while Title VIII, Clinical Trial Databases, has implications for pediatric research through the mandatory listing and posting of summary results of clinical studies using FDA-regulated products. FDAAA also established an FDA Pediatric Review Committee.[77]

The Pediatric Medical Device Safety and Improvement Act extended the general principles of pediatric initiatives to medical devices. The definition of child in that Act for research purposes is up to and including 21 years of age. The interpretation of the definition is that if other pediatric populations are enrolled, the upper limit should include patients through 21 years. The law does not state or imply that a study that enrolls patients between 18 and 21 years is a pediatric study nor that such a study would be responsive to any of the federal pediatric initiatives. The law recognizes that some studies of childhood diseases and conditions that enroll patients through 21 years acknowledge late physiologic and developmental changes at the end of adolescence and that inclusion of such patients can be scientifically and medically informative. The primary features of the Pediatric Medical Device Safety and Improvement Act are:

1. Requirement to perform pediatric studies in relevant populations
2. Applicability of the law to "patients" who "suffer from" a disease or condition
3. Specific monitoring requirements
4. Funding of demonstration projects
5. Development of a federal pediatric medical device plan
6. Designation of a pediatric medical device point of contact at the NIH

In July 2012, Public Law 112-144, the Food and Drug Administration Safety and Innovation Act (FDASIA), made the BPCA and the Pediatric Research Equity Act (PREA) permanent and therefore no longer subject to a term limited expiration. In Section 508 the law required that every 5 years the secretary of Health and Human Services report to Congress on various activities related to Sections 505A and 505B of the Food, Drug, and Cosmetic Act. Additional provisions include:

- Establishment of a permanent position of a neonatologist in the Office of Pediatric Therapeutics and as a member of the Pediatric Review Committee
- For products granted pediatric exclusivity under the BPCA, in addition to the medical and clinical pharmacology reviews, a statistical review be posted

On August 18, 2017, Public Law 115-52, the FDA Reauthorization Act (FDARA), was signed into law. This included the Research to Accelerate Cures and Equity (RACE) for Children Act, which requires evaluation of new molecularly targeted drugs and biologics "intended for the treatment of adult cancers and directed at a molecular target substantially relevant to the growth or progression of a pediatric cancer." It also eliminated the orphan exemption from pediatric studies for cancer drugs directed at relevant molecular targets. FDARA permanently authorized the requirement for neonatology expertise in the Office of Pediatric Therapeutics at the FDA and required the development of draft guidance on clinical pharmacology considerations for neonatal studies for drugs and biologics.[78]

As of mid-2019, the FDA recorded about 785 labeling changes, of which 715 were based on new pediatric studies. Attributions for which pediatric initiative supported the label change are PREA alone 430, PREA + BPCA 119, and BPCA alone 187. Another 49 are attributed to the Pediatric Rule. An inference from these results is that the mandate accounted in whole or in part for almost 600 label changes. The incentive program accounted in whole or in part for approximately 300 label changes. The combined programs triggered new pediatric studies to support 91% of the label changes.

The package insert or label changes include information on pediatric doses, safety information, and in some cases extended or established indications for pediatric use.[79]

GENERAL SCIENTIFIC AND ETHICAL RATIONALE FOR CLINICAL STUDIES

For thousands of years medicine relied on tradition and eminence-based practices, that is, practice based on authority that was not questioned. Interventions that were thought to be highly active were readily adopted, but other treatments were promulgated without formal establishment of their effectiveness. As a result, the history of medicine is populated with practices that harmed patients and diverted resources. General acceptance that a demonstration of effectiveness based on scientific principles is a necessity for marketing authorization and acceptance into clinical practice came in the mid-20th century.

The current status of knowledge of biology and pharmacology is insufficient to allow deduction of therapeutic effects, risk, and clinical outcome. Empirical observations are necessary to predict potential risks and benefits, and observations are often limited for technical and psychological reasons including false expectations, inability to observe events, and bias. The goals of clinical research are to maximize the validity of the observations so that they can be generalized to other relevant populations and minimize the major confounding influences of bias and uncertainty.

Bias is the tendency, intentionally or unintentionally, to influence the outcome by factors such as the study design or implementation. Uncertainty is a measure of the confidence in a result. It is defined as the amount that the apparent result differs from what would be a "true" result. The larger the uncertainty, the less confidence there is in the apparent result. Even if the "true" result is not known, there are various analytic methods to determine the level or degree of uncertainty.

Among the ethical reasons for striving for unbiased research are minimizing exposure of patients to unjustified risk and avoiding the consequences of disseminating misleading results, which include not only unjustified risk, but the potential delay of the development or implementation of superior alternatives.

For many years, multiple definitions of the terms "clinical research" and "clinical trial" were published by different organizations, but the NIH attempted to consolidate the definition of "clinical trial" in 2014. The current definition is "A research study in which one or more human participants are prospectively assigned to one or more interventions (which may include placebo or other control) to evaluate the effects of those interventions on health-related biomedical or behavioral outcomes".[80] For this discussion, a clinical trial will be a bit more broadly defined as a systematic investigation for the evaluation of an intervention regarding potential risks and benefits for a defined target population or phenotype. The broader definition is more aligned with international usage of the concept. The linkage to biomedical outcomes noted in the NIH definition will apply when referencing U.S. government scientific funding programs to maintain consistency, but for other discussions, the emphasis will be on the evaluation of the intervention without specific linkage to meeting a specific definition for the type of outcome.

CONCEPTUAL PARADIGM FOR CLINICAL TRIALS

A clinical trial in an abstract form is an activity designed to capture data to support solving a problem for a target population. Operationally, a clinical trial is a series of coordinated encounters where a person, an intervention, a context, and relevant measurement methods coincide in time and space (Fig. 1.3). The major conceptual differences between a clinical trial encounter and health care delivery encounter are that in a clinical trial:

- The intervention is provided in the context of a protocol.
- The intervention is under evaluation.
- Participation is voluntary with documented permission.
- The data will be pooled and analyzed systematically.
- The results will be disseminated.
- The clinical trial process has greater stringency and oversight than standard health care delivery.

MINIMIZING BIAS AND UNCERTAINTY

Clinical trials should be undertaken with the concept of equipoise, that is, the expectation that the results are unknown prior to the clinical trial and can only be known after a clinical trial is properly conducted and analyzed. The concept of equipoise has multiple interpretations and may vary with perspective but is generally taken to reflect that the information needed to make a critical decision is not available and the planned study is intended to contribute to that information.[81]

Among the methods to reduce bias and uncertainty are:

- the integration of controls or comparators in the design and analysis to properly interpret the signals generated by data capture. The most precise controls or comparators have their data generated concurrent with the study data, usually by exposing one group of participants to the intervention under evaluation and exposing another group of participants to the control or comparator. The control or comparator is typically a placebo, an alternative intervention, or nothing at all.
- selection of measurement techniques and outcomes that are objective, quantitative, validated for the specific population of interest, and have characteristics that are well defined and precise over a known range
- utilization of qualified and trained personnel with specific training on the study protocol, techniques, and quality management
- a risk-adjusted quality management plan and infrastructure for study implementation
- a data security plan with audit tracking
- use of an ontology and terminology that provides the detail and precision needed to objectively describe the phenotypes and events that will be captured[82–84]
- a prospective data analytic plan with potential adjustments in the study protocol prespecified
- a data sharing plan to allow independent access to the data for confirmation and validation of study-specified analyses

CONSIDERATIONS REGARDING CONTROLS

A controlled clinical trial will have a comparator integrated into the design. The most precise controls are concurrent with the time frame and context of the study because data generated at other times or in other contexts, even other clinical trials, can be skewed or biased due to differences in definitions, measurement techniques, and general secular trends that affect people in general and health care delivery and technology. As an example, imaging techniques continue to evolve and improve so measurements of masses such as tumors or cysts will vary in precision based on the type of apparatus, the calibration technique, the version of the analytic software, and the date and location it was measured. Microbiologic diagnosis will vary based on when, from where, and what type of processing a sample may have had; the identification methodology such as morphologic, immunologic, genetic, or other criteria; and the characteristics and calibration of the equipment.

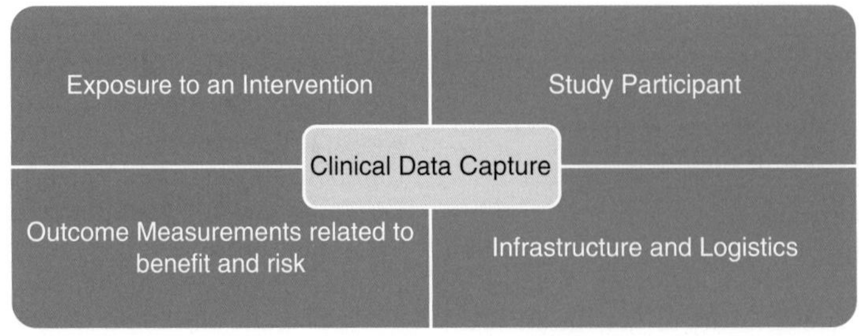

Figure 1.3 Conceptual framework for clinical trial data capture with the intersection of the study participant, the intervention, measurements, and infrastructure and logistics in time and space.

An important goal of any scientific study is to reduce the number of variables that can affect the outcome to a minimum. Using concurrent controls that employ the same methodology with personnel trained in the same way and risk-adjusted quality management are among the most effective and pragmatic approaches to minimize variability in data capture.

RANDOMIZED CONTROLLED TRIALS

Randomized controlled clinical trials, where individual participants were assigned to receive either an intervention to be evaluated or a comparator, were developed in the United States and the United Kingdom during the 1920s and 1930s, but Dr. Austin Bradford Hill initiated the practice of using random numbers to assign patients to treatment arms to study infectious disease therapy, which grew out of a need to treat malaria during World War II.[85]

In 1948 the Medical Research Council of Britain reported on the use of streptomycin to treat pulmonary tuberculosis in a randomized controlled trial.[86] Following World War II, randomized controlled studies began in the United States in academia with a study at Johns Hopkins University comparing tetracycline to penicillin for the treatment of pneumococcal pneumonia and in government with the Veterans Administration study of tuberculosis.[87,88]

The first randomized controlled pediatric study, as noted previously, was organized by the U.S. NIH as a multicenter trial for rheumatic heart disease in 1951.[89]

In 1954, Congress established the Cancer Chemotherapy National Service Center (CCNSC). Subsequently a clinical trial network was initiated with one section devoted to pediatrics. In the establishment of the clinical program, the CCNSC agreed upon the importance of the following principles:

1. Combination of data from all institutions to rapidly accumulate the necessary number of patients
2. Standard criteria of diagnosis, treatment, and measurement of effect
3. Statistical design of the study with randomly assigned patients to different treatment groups
4. Statistical analysis and collaborative reporting of results

The rationale for these principles was that randomized studies generally provide more persuasive evidence of benefit than alternative study designs such as single-arm studies. Improvements in outcomes ascribed to treatment may be due to other factors such as patient selection (selection bias), other medications or therapies, diet, genetics, and other environmental factors. In addition, historical control populations may differ from current study populations regarding demographics, precision of diagnosis, and changes in the general practice of medicine.[90,91]

The design and analysis of clinical trials continue to evolve, but the value of careful observation and recording of results is timeless. Independent of trial design, clinical studies must address ethical requirements. The varied published international documents have overlapping characteristics and elements, and these have been analyzed by Emanuel, Wendler, and Grady of the NIH, leading to a recommendation of seven requirements for ethically conducting a clinical study. They are value, scientific validity, fair subject selection, favorable risk–benefit ratio, independent review, informed consent, and respect.[92] Regarding children, the issue of informed consent, as previously discussed, is redirected to parental or guardian permission and assent.

SPECIFIC RATIONALE FOR CLINICAL STUDIES IN CHILDREN

One of the prevalent justifications for studying interventions in children is that children are not small adults. Indeed, results of studies in one adult population may not be translatable to another adult population. The differences between children and adults are many and vary according to age and developmental stage. Examples are listed in Table 1.2.

The continuing metabolic changes and alterations in surface-to-volume ratio, lymphatic structure and function, and other anatomic and physiologic factors limit the use of fixed doses in children and are the basis for the need to study dosing in people of different sizes and developmental stages. Among the reasons are the increased risk of adverse reactions or decreased effectiveness due to inappropriate dose and the potential reluctance of practitioners to prescribe potentially useful products without adequate information.

Additional general factors to address in pediatric studies are the sampling challenges of obtaining meaningful clinical material such as blood, serum, tissue, and images in patients of various sizes; degrees of maturation; and developmental stages.[93]

The AAP issued updated Guidelines for the Ethical Conduct of Studies to Evaluate Drugs in the Pediatric Population in 1995, which can be summarized as follows[66]:

The premise of studying drugs in children is that it is ethically imperative so that children can have equal access to therapeutic agents. In most cases, therapeutic agents should be studied in adults prior to children except for agents that are specific for pediatric diseases. Proposed pediatric research must by design protect children and encompass six conditions:

- The proposed research must be of value to children in general and, in most instances, to the individual child subject. The value may be a potential benefit in the treatment of the subject's disease or may be improved understanding of basic biology of the disease state or of children in general.
- The research design must be appropriate for the stated purposes. Poorly designed research may not provide scientifically valid or useful data and may place the subjects at risk with no potential benefits.
- The research design must take into consideration the unique physiology, psychology, and pharmacology of children and their special needs and requirements as research subjects.
- The design should minimize risk while maximizing potential benefit.

TABLE 1.2 Factors That Vary With Age and Developmental Age
Continuing changes in physiologic development and metabolic function such as renal and hepatic function
Evolving surface-to-volume ratio
Changes in integrity of the skin and other anatomic barriers
Alterations in penetrability of the central nervous system barriers
Maturation of the neurohumoral-immune axis
Alterations in protein binding and displacement
Continuing anatomic changes such as skull shape, size, and proportion of passages such as eustachian tubes, mineralization of cartilage, structure and location of lymphatic organs including the thymus

- The study design must take into account the racial, ethnic, gender, and socioeconomic characteristics of the children and their parents and, when appropriate, should include input from the community or appropriate advocacy representatives.
- The study must be designed to conform to the local, state, and federal laws of the jurisdiction of the study's location and the investigators' home jurisdiction, and to their local and national ethical guidelines.

The document further states that research studies may be considered ethically permissible when they can be shown to have a potential benefit to the individual child or provide generalizable knowledge, and when potential benefits outweigh potential risks. Benefits should be construed broadly. The investigator's competence and ethical conduct are the most important safeguards for the protection of the child. The primary responsibility of the IRB is to protect the rights of the research participant.

Additional subsections address specific populations that may be at increased risk for abuse and exploitation, including the child with handicaps, institutionalized children, patients requiring emergency care, the dying patient, patients with chronically progressive or potentially fatal disease, and the brain dead patient. The following paragraphs have brief comments for each population.

The child with handicaps (mentally, physically, or emotionally) must be stringently protected from disproportionate representation in research studies through either exclusion or inclusion. Institutionalized children should rarely be considered for participation in research studies because of the possibility of not having sufficient safeguards.

The International Conference on Harmonization (ICH) document on pediatric studies, discussed later, is consistent with the AAP guidelines, noting that information that can be obtained in a less vulnerable, consenting population should not be obtained in a more vulnerable population or one in which the patients are unable to provide individual consent. Studies in populations with handicaps or institutionalized pediatric populations should be limited to diseases or conditions found principally or exclusively in these populations, or to situations in which the disease or condition in these pediatric patients would be expected to alter the disposition or pharmacodynamic effects of a medicinal product.

Patients requiring emergency care may participate in research and have the usual procedures for informed consent or permission or assent altered or waived if

- the clinical condition is potentially life threatening or permanently disabling
  AND
- permission cannot be obtained in a timely way
  AND
- the only available therapy is investigational or not validated
  AND
- no accepted therapy is known to be superior to the proposed experimental therapy

The Code of Federal Regulations in Title 21 Part 50.24 provides the authority to proceed, and compliance with Subpart D of the Common Rule Title 45 Part 46 is still required.

In addition, the relevant IRB should receive assurance that the risk is not more than a minimal added risk, equipoise exists among therapeutic alternatives, participants and parents or guardians will be provided with pertinent information regarding the study as soon as feasible, and the waiver will not affect the rights and welfare of participants.

The dying patient may be enrolled in a study if the question being addressed is extremely important, the therapy being proposed is well founded in animal and clinical research, or there is good expectation that the therapy may be beneficial and the potential benefits exceed the potential risks. In addition, physicians not involved in the research must document that death appears inevitable and that standard therapy has not improved the patient's prognosis.

Patients with chronically progressive or potentially fatal disease and their parents or guardians are potentially prone to feel an obligation to participate in research proposed by physicians that care for these patients due to the dependent relationship that can develop. Investigators who are not involved in the care of the patient should obtain approval for participation.

The brain dead patient is legally dead in most jurisdictions. The circumstance of considering research would involve some measurements on remaining body functions. The AAP document stipulates that research may proceed if the death certificate has been signed by a physician independent of the planned research, the medical question addressed by the research is of utmost importance, permission is received from the parents, the research procedure is brief, the drugs are intended for human use, and the research will not compromise either organ donation or an autopsy, if either is planned.

DESIGNING CLINICAL TRIALS: GENERAL CONSIDERATIONS

To be ethical, a clinical trial must be informative. To be informative, a trial must measure an outcome in an unbiased, valid, and interpretable manner. The sequence of steps can vary, but an effective approach to designing a clinical trial is to

- first decide what the potential benefit may be as it relates to mitigating or solving a problem for a population with a phenotype (condition or disease) of interest
- select an intervention to evaluate
- determine whether there is an outcome measure or small collection of measures that could inform the nature, magnitude, and duration of the benefit
- assess the reproducibility and applicability of the outcome measure to the phenotype (disease or condition) of interest
- decide what type of study design would be most resource effective, minimize bias, and maximize certainty
- select the appropriate elements to write a study protocol

ADDITIONAL PEDIATRIC-SPECIFIC CONSIDERATIONS FOR TRIAL DESIGN

Studies in pediatric populations require additional considerations on ethical, technical, and scientific grounds. For these reasons, pediatric research should be led by investigators trained and experienced in studying children and performed at facilities that have the staffing and infrastructure to support and comfort children. In such a facility, children can feel positive about participation in clinical research.[94]

The ideal circumstance in clinical research is that consent, risk, and benefit are vested in the same individual. This is the case with adult volunteers. In pediatric research, formal consent does not apply, but permission is provided by a third party—usually parents or legal guardians, the risk is always borne by the child, and the benefit may or may not accrue to the child. The consequence of permission process is always imperfect, especially in multiarm studies, because if neither the subject nor the researcher knows which therapy is being consented to or what the possible risks may be, the process of being "informed" cannot be considered complete. A need to educate parents and patients about clinical trials should be a component of the process.[95,96]

The institutional approval of pediatric studies is also a challenge and would require pediatric expertise on IRBs and ethics committees. The question of whether children who are not affected by a disease or condition under study should be enrolled was formally addressed by an FDA Advisory Subcommittee on November 15, 1999.

The Pediatric Subcommittee of the Anti-Infectives Drugs Advisory Committee, supplemented by ethicists, was charged with providing guidance on the ethical consideration for the conduct of pediatric clinical trials, namely the role of pediatric volunteers who do not have the disease under study.[97] The consensus areas of the discussion were as follows:

1. In general, pediatric studies should be conducted in subjects who may benefit from participation in the trial. Usually this implies the participant has or is susceptible to the disease under study. The Pediatric Subcommittee utilized a broad definition of potential benefit. For example, almost any child has the potential to benefit from a treatment for otitis media due to the likely risk of developing the condition.
2. In general, children who can give assent should be enrolled in a study in preference to, or prior to, children who cannot give assent. Careful consideration must be given to the importance of the potential benefit of the study. In certain circumstances, the potential benefit that may be derived from studying children who cannot give assent may override the preference for first enrolling assenting children.

As a result of the subcommittee discussions, it is considered appropriate and preferable to refer to children enrolled in clinical research as patients rather than subjects or participants to emphasize the expectation of potential benefit. The subcommittee also recommended that the federal regulations that apply to protecting children enrolled in research studies that receive federal funding, 45CFR46, be adapted and extended to studies that receive other sources of funding.

In April 2001, the FDA published in the Federal Register an adaptation of 45CFR46 Subpart D that applies to all children enrolled in studies that are FDA regulated.[98] The regulation was finalized in 2013.[99]

Placebo-controlled studies have been formally addressed by the AAP 1995 guidelines, which state that placebo or untreated observational control groups can be used in pediatric studies if their use does not place children at increased risk.

The International Conference on Harmonisation Efficacy Document 11 (E-11), which the FDA contributed to and accepts as guidance, also comments on placebo-controlled studies. Acceptable conditions include when there is no commonly accepted therapy for the condition, or when the commonly used therapy is of questionable efficacy, or when the commonly used therapy has a high frequency of undesirable side effects and the risk may be greater than the benefits. A placebo is also considered acceptable in a comparative add-on study design where a new treatment or placebo is added to an established regimen.[100]

As a consequence of the prior discussions and recommendations, current thinking is that comparison with a placebo may be acceptable if there are no approved or adequately studied therapies for children with the condition under study. For serious or life-threatening illness, a data monitoring committee with planned interim analysis and study-topping rules should be used.

In all studies, each patient should have escape criteria to minimize exposure to ineffective treatment. For serious and life-threatening illnesses or when other risks to study conduct or completion exist, such as a major efficacy study that is intended to define policy or be submitted for FDA labeling or enrolls a population that requires additional protections or addresses a condition about which controversy or social sensitivity may be present or a multinational study, a data monitoring committee may be advisable. For minor illness or discomfort symptoms, a randomized withdrawal study may minimize exposure to placebo. Individual patient escape rules should be defined. A data monitoring committee would generally not be needed unless there was a specific safety concern.

Criteria for enrolling children in Phase 1 or initial exposure studies were commented upon by the Pediatric Subcommittee of the FDA Oncologic Drugs Advisory Committee in 2002 as it pertains to children with cancer who have relapsed or who are refractory to available anticancer therapy and would be candidates for investigational drugs. The consensus was that the evidence for initiating clinical studies in children with cancer should include biologic plausibility of the product having activity against a pediatric tumor (which could be obtained from preclinical data), some expectation of potential benefit, a reasonable expectation of safety, and sufficient information to choose an appropriate starting dose.

If a scientific rationale and a population of pediatric cancer patients with no available anticancer therapy exists, then pediatric oncology clinical studies should be initiated, in most cases, immediately following adult Phase 1 studies.[101] Although the committee only commented on children with cancer, the same principles may be applicable to children with diseases other than cancer that may also be life threatening and have limited therapeutic options.

The ICH began work on a guideline for pediatric research in 1998. These guidelines were adopted as a recommendation by all participating regions in the year 2000 and subsequently updated in 2017.[100] The document is identified as E11, which is the eleventh document in a series of recommendations related to the conduct of clinical studies. The letter E stands for efficacy. Major provisions of the document, due to its global importance, are summarized in the following paragraphs.

The general principles are that pediatric patients should be given medicines that have been properly evaluated for their use in the intended population. The product development programs should include pediatric studies when pediatric use is anticipated, that pediatric development should not delay adult studies or adult availability, and that pediatric therapeutic development is a shared responsibility among companies, regulatory authorities, health professionals, and society as a whole.

The default state is that data on the appropriate use of medicinal products in the pediatric population should be generated unless the use of a specific medicinal product in pediatric patients is clearly inappropriate. Factors to consider when deciding to begin a pediatric development program are the prevalence and seriousness of the condition to be treated in the pediatric population, whether there are unique pediatric indications, age ranges of probable patients, availability and suitability of alternatives (including adverse events and pediatric-specific safety concerns), pediatric knowledge about the class of compounds, potential need for a pediatric formulation, and the need to develop pediatric-specific endpoints for study.

The timing of initiation of pediatric studies will depend on the prevalence, seriousness, availability, and suitability of alternatives. E11 states that the most important factor is the presence of a serious or life-threatening disease for which the medicinal product represents a potentially important advance in therapy and should initiate an urgent and early introduction of pediatric studies in the development program. For products that are predominantly or exclusively intended for pediatric use, all phases of development may occur in children.

Products intended for serious or life-threatening conditions occurring in adults and children for which there are no or limited therapies should begin pediatric studies following initial adult safety and preliminary evidence of potential benefit (early Phase 2). This recommendation differs from the FDA Advisory Committee recommendation of October 2002 that those pediatric studies begin immediately after adult Phase 1.

For all other conditions, pediatric studies should begin when safety and efficacy have sufficient data to justify exposing children to a product. Exposure of children to a product that will be of no benefit should be avoided. In all studies, accurate dosing and patient compliance must be assured: thus, a pediatric formulation may be required. In developing a formulation, the variability of susceptibility of patients of different ages and developmental stages to the toxicity of excipients must be addressed.

Four types of studies are discussed: pharmacokinetics, pharmacokinetics/pharmacodynamics, efficacy, and safety. A pharmacokinetic study in pediatric patients with additional safety data may be adequate to establish pediatric use when the disease process is similar in adults and children and the outcome of therapy is likely to be comparable. In such a case, extrapolation from adult efficacy data may be appropriate. An approach based only on pharmacokinetics is likely to be insufficient when product blood levels are known or expected not to correspond with efficacy or when there is concern those concentration–response relationships vary with age.

If the comparability of the disease and outcome of therapy are similar, a combined pharmacokinetic/pharmacodynamic approach may be possible. Although relative bioavailability comparisons of formulations should be done in adults, definitive pharmacokinetic studies for dose selection for pediatric patients should be done in the intended population.

In general, dosing should be based on a per-kilogram basis (body weight) because errors in measuring height or length are common and lead to errors in the calculation of body surface area. However, some medications with a narrow therapeutic index may require dosing based on body surface area. In all studies, principles of good clinical practice, design and statistical considerations, and principles of safety monitoring and adverse event reporting in ICH apply.

Clinical endpoints must be age and developmentally appropriate and validated. Endpoints that rely on patient self-assessment may be unreliable. Age-appropriate laboratory and clinical values should be used. Some efficacy studies may be simplified by extrapolation of efficacy findings from older to younger patients. The pediatric adverse event profile of a product may differ from the adult profile in types of events and magnitude of severity or duration due to different surface-to-volume ratio in children of varying ages and different levels of maturation of organ function and metabolism.

Unintended exposure such as accidental ingestion may provide additional opportunity for dose and safety information. Long-term or surveillance studies should be considered, particularly for chronic therapies, to observe effects on growth and development. Dimensions to consider are skeletal growth, cognitive function, and maturation. Postmarketing surveillance and/or long-term follow-up studies may provide safety and/or efficacy information for subgroups within the pediatric population or additional information for the entire pediatric population.

ICH E11 discusses age classification and the ICH E11 addendum (R1) pays particular attention to the neonate.

- Neonatal period for term newborn infants—0 to 27 days of age
- Neonatal period for preterm newborn infants—day of birth through expected date of delivery plus 27 days
- Infants and toddlers—28 days to 23 months
- Children—2 to 11 years
- Adolescents—12 years to 16 or 18 years, depending on region

Any age classification is arbitrary, and therefore decisions on how to stratify studies and data by age should take into consideration developmental biology and pharmacology. The category of preterm newborn infants is not a homogeneous group of patients, and protocol development should incorporate expert input from neonatologists and neonatal pharmacologists. A child of 25 weeks gestational age and weighing 500 g is very different in terms of metabolism and response to therapy than a newborn of 30 weeks gestational age weighing 1,500 g.

A distinction should also be made for low-birth-weight newborns (<2,500 g) as to whether they are immature or were growth restricted in utero. Extrapolation of study findings from other populations is generally not feasible. This is due to the immaturity of renal and hepatic clearance mechanisms, protein binding and displacement issues (particularly bilirubin), the integrity of the blood–brain barrier, subsequent penetration of medicinal products into the central nervous system, transdermal absorption, and rapid and variable maturation of all physiologic and pharmacologic processes leading to different dosing regimens with chronic exposure. Neonatal disease states and morbidities such as respiratory distress syndrome of the newborn, patent ductus arteriosus, primary pulmonary hypertension, necrotizing enterocolitis, intraventricular hemorrhage, and retinopathy of prematurity add further complexity. Adolescence has a variable upper age limit that depends on the context.

CONSIDERATIONS RELATED TO AGE

The ICH Guidance E-11 notes that pediatrics extends up to age 16 to 18 years depending upon the region. The World Health Organization notes that the age may be up to 20 years.[102]

The Food and Drug Administration Amendments Act of 2007 in Section 303 includes people till 21 years as a target population for pediatric device product development. The intent is

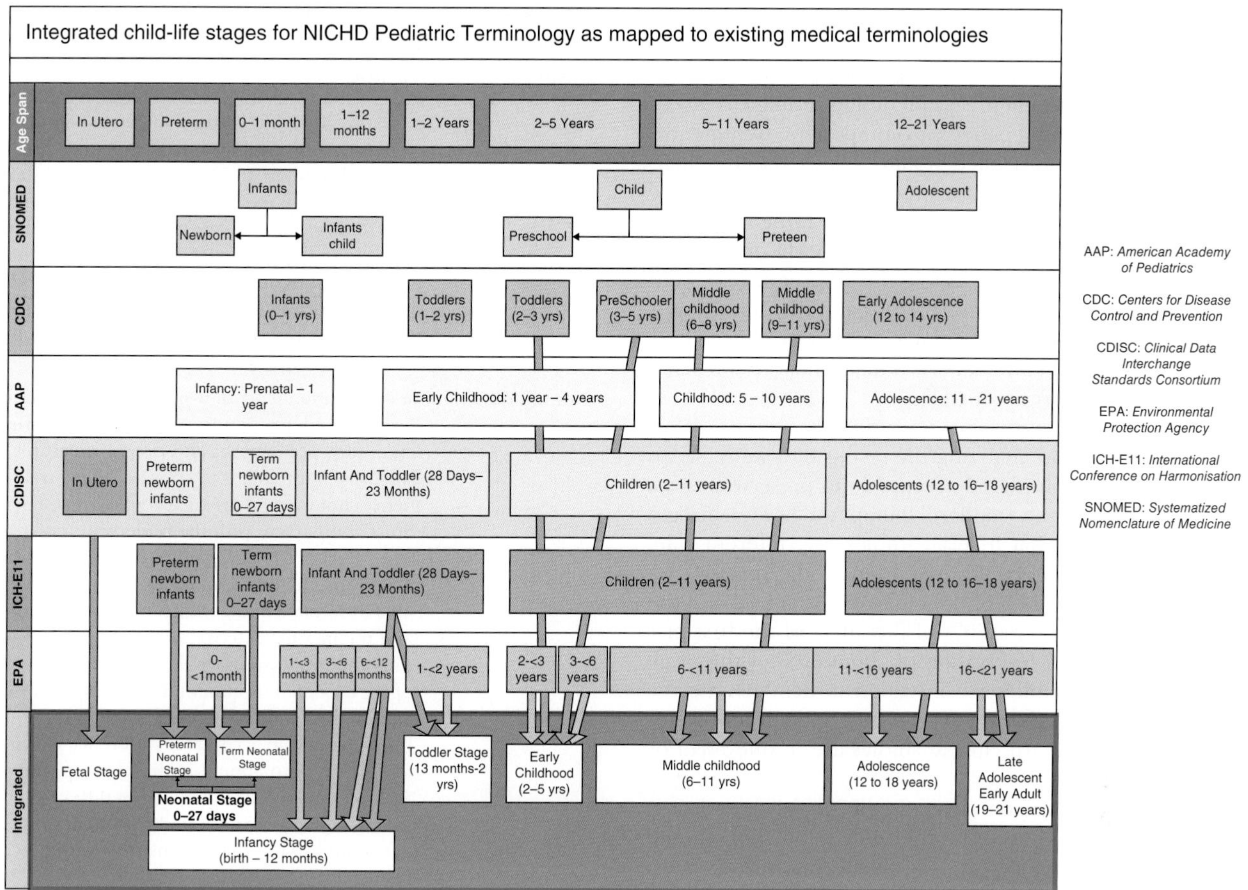

Figure 1.4 Variability of boundaries of ages and stages schema for human development during childhood. Ages and stages are generally guided by cognitive and behavioral criteria. (From Hirschfeld S, Zajicek A. What could the future of safety monitoring look like? *Ther Innov Regul Sci* 2019;53(5):590–600.)

not to recast the 16- or 18-year-old to 21-year-old population as a pediatric population that would be responsive to regulatory expectations, but rather allow extension of the upper age limit in pediatric studies, particularly for chronic diseases or those with growth delay, to gain additional follow-up information.

Figure 1.4 shows a comparison of different classification systems for pediatric age groups.

For all age groups, risk, discomfort, and distress can be minimized if studies are designed and conducted by investigators trained and experienced in the treatment of pediatric patients. Specific suggestions on minimizing distress include the use of trained personnel, the use of topical anesthetics, minimization of sample collection volume and frequency, comforting physical settings, and the availability and cooperation of parents.

Age has limitations in that children of the same chronologic age can be at different physiologic and developmental stages. In many cases, using a size parameter such as weight or surface area with or without a developmental stage indicator may be more precise and preferable than simply an age range.

CHARACTERIZATION OF STUDY GOALS

Study goals will depend upon the question being asked, the expectations for the size of the effect, the available resources, and the feasibility of implementation of the study design. Studies are often categorized by type based on the goals.

Pharmacokinetic studies have a series of predefined parameters that describe the fate of a drug and its metabolites at different doses in different patient populations. Exposure response studies examine the relationship between exposures to a product and physiologic or clinical events (both beneficial and adverse) associated with its use. If pharmacodynamics are also measured, then the study may be considered a pharmacokinetic/pharmacodynamic study. Pharmacokinetic studies and exposure response studies are generally considered exploratory. A case where they may not be considered exploratory is when extrapolation of efficacy is feasible between two populations and pharmacokinetic and exposure response studies are used to extend the use of the product to the new population.

Efficacy studies are by design adequate with regard to power and planned analysis to demonstrate patient benefit and to assess risks. The results of efficacy studies are usually expressed as a calculated number, often called the point estimate, with associated confidence intervals. Confidence intervals are by convention based on the 95% probability that the true result is within a range between an upper and a lower limit.

Efficacy studies may be designed to demonstrate superiority to available therapies or no inferiority. To demonstrate superiority, the 95% confidence intervals of a therapy should not overlap with a comparator; that is, the lower limit of one result must be greater than the upper limit of the comparator. All studies have by implication a historical comparator, although historical comparators can be difficult to determine and not appropriate for direct comparison due to differences in study populations and standards of medical care. The most persuasive and credible comparator is one that is measured concurrently with the study regimen. Several design strategies exist to minimize bias in assigning patients to comparative treatments.

To demonstrate equivalence would usually require large numbers of patients and precise measurements. To conserve resources and maintain a level of confidence in being able to substitute one product for another, a noninferiority approach is employed. Noninferiority implies that the difference in benefit and outcome between a standard therapy and the new therapy is within a predefined and acceptable margin of effect. It requires that the standard have an effect that is measurable, clinically meaningful, and reproducible.

There are several approaches to setting the margin of acceptable difference and analyzing the results of a study. As an example, it may be considered acceptable to preserve at least 80% of the effect of the standard therapy or have a margin of 20%. A caution is that if serial studies use different standards, the efficacy effect could drift down. To be specific, if a new product preserves 80% of the effect of a standard and the next new product preserves 80% of the effect of the first new product, the result is a reservation of about 60% of the original standard. Safety studies are intended to demonstrate the relationship between exposure to a product and adverse events associated with its use. All clinical studies are in one form or another safety studies.

Vaccine studies enlarged in scope in the late 1990s and early 2000s due to the realization that the study population should have sufficient exposures to the candidate vaccine to detect rare but medically significant events.

In general, the sensitivity of signal detection is based on and expressed in logarithmic or semi-logarithmic scales. For example, if the typical range is based on logarithmic 10, then semi-logarithmic factors would be based on the square root of 10. To an approximation, that number is 3, so a semi-logarithmic scale would have sample sizes that correspond to 1, 3, 10, 30, 100, 300, 1,000, 3,000,10,000, 30,000, 100,000, etc.

To provide the public assurance that a vaccine is safe, with the assumption that millions of people will be administered the product, the initial studies are sized to detect rare but medically significant events. Thus, a vaccine safety study may be on the order of magnitude of 30,000 to 60,000+ participants in order to detect such events with a frequency of <0.1%.

Vaccine efficacy can be based on three general types of outcomes. They are:

- use of a biomarker or surrogate such as immune response like generation of specific antibodies above a specific level
- use of randomized controlled trials with a precise case definition of the condition of interest and comparison of the rates that meet the definition
- use of animals to demonstrate efficacy for a rare or life-threatening condition and then applying extrapolation of a relevant biomarker to the human population

Since the 1950s clinical studies have been classified into phases based on this study. Initial drug dose finding and safety studies have been termed Phase 1. Exploratory studies to determine biologic or clinical activity of a drug have been termed Phase 2. Confirmatory studies to compare an investigational regimen with an established regimen that are powered to establish efficacy have been termed Phase 3. Studies that have been requested by the FDA to comply with postmarketing commitments following approval of a claim for marketing exclusivity have been termed Phase 4.

Alternative nomenclature such as learning phase and confirming study[94,103] or initial exposure phase, development phase, and validation phase may also be acceptable as shown in Table 1.3.

TABLE 1.3 Types of Clinical Trial Goals

Type	*Comment*
Superiority	The test treatment is better than a comparator. The confidence intervals around the measurement for the test treatment and for the comparator should not overlap. For example, if the standard treatment shows that median survival for a population is 22 mo and the confidence intervals are ±3 mo, then the test treatment must have a lower confidence interval that is greater than 25 mo (22 + 3) to be considered superior. Results of 29 ± 3 mo or 28 ± 2 mo would qualify.
Noninferiority	The test treatment is not worse than a comparator. Exact equivalence is difficult to prove requiring large study populations and precise measures. The usual approach is to consider that a treatment is not worse than an accepted treatment by direct comparison with the understanding that: 1. The effect of the accepted treatment is measurable, reproducible, and meaningful. An acceptable difference between the accepted treatment and the new treatment is defined prior to beginning the study and is smaller than the total effect of the accepted treatment. For example, if the accepted treatment increases median survival by 6 mo and the acceptable difference is 1 mo, then the new treatment in direct comparison to the accepted treatment must not differ by more than 1 mo and the accepted treatment must have a median survival that is consistent with previous results.
Exploratory	A study to examine biologic or clinical activity but not designed to establish efficacy.

STUDY POPULATION SELECTION

As noted previously, the FDA held public hearings and issued guidance in the early 2000s to clarify that children that are considered healthy should not be enrolled in clinical trials that exceed minimal risk; however, children that have a disease or condition that compromises their health or are at risk for the development of such a disease or condition may be enrolled in clinical trials that offer no direct benefit and are a minor increase over minimal risk. The perspective both clarifies what populations are appropriate for interventional studies and provides an ethical and regulatory framework for preventive or prophylactic studies such as vaccine inoculation.

Study population selection is based on the Belmont Report principles of beneficence, justice, and respect for persons. All three principles apply, and implementation decisions are rarely limited to a single criterion. For example, integration of the principles in a balanced manner supports enrollment of children on the basis of justice and respect for persons, yet limits enrollment to children with or at high risk of a disease or condition on the basis of beneficence and respect for persons.

While the specific target population may not be the only population enrolled, both justification for including others and the formal mechanism to apply the clinical trial results to the relevant populations are part of the planning and implementation process.

The principle of justice is nuanced using the examples of enrollment and subsequent analysis. For enrollment, the demographics of the enrolled population should reflect the demographics of the future population to which the analytic inferences will apply. For enrollment purposes, not only should a broad and diverse population that meet the health-related phenotypic characteristics of the target populations be included, but it may be necessary to actively initiate measures to remove barriers to enrollment. Selection based on race typically utilizes the U.S. Census Bureau classification as declared by the study participant or, most often in the case of children, declaration of the mother of the child. However, analyses based on race can introduce complexities related to the variability of biologic and demographic factors within the standard classifications of race, which show as much or greater differences within a race as between races. Thus, analyses should reflect the biologic and demographic characteristics of the individual. If the selection process for a study included a broad and diverse population, then the high-level aggregate inferences from the study results should also apply to a broad and diverse population.

Age and, perhaps more critically, developmental stage are additional factors to include in eligibility criteria if an intervention is likely to be widely used in a defined population, such as neonates or premature infants. Although efforts to include children in studies of regulated products have resulted in enhanced activity and label changes, the youngest and least mature children have received disproportionately fewer benefits. Consequently, recent legislation, regulatory initiatives, and international cooperation generated additional focus and resources to include neonates and premature infants.

OUTCOME MEASURES—GENERAL CONSIDERATIONS

Outcome assessments, sometimes called endpoints, are the measures taken to determine benefit or risk in a clinical trial. If the goal of a clinical trial is to evaluate an intervention, then the evaluation is expected to be based on reproducible objective results. It is the reproducibility and objectivity that make the results of a clinical trial generalizable. Therefore, the selection of outcome assessments should be based on the characteristics of objectivity, reproducibility, and, whenever feasible, a quantity. In some cases, the quantity can be continuous over a known range while in other cases the quantity may place the outcome into a category such as mild, moderate, or substantial.

The general concept of benefit is that people with a particular phenotype, more commonly referred to as a condition or a status, are through an intervention able to alter the natural history of the condition of interest and either live longer or live better. Sometimes living better is further subdivided into functioning better or feeling better, but for the topic of outcome assessments, the principles and practice are the same.

Living longer is objective and quantifiable, but unless the condition under study is rapidly progressive and fatal, survival often is not practical to measure in the time frame and context of most clinical trials.

The objective, quantifiable assessment of living better can be challenging and is often performed using indirect measures such as structured questionnaires, functional tests, images, or other modalities. Thus, benefit, in general, is inferred from indirect measures and both the objective and subjective perception of living better can be relatively imprecise, but still acceptable. For example, hearing function is often assessed through an audiogram using pure tones, but the results of the audiogram may not be informative regarding the ability to understand table conversation in a crowded restaurant or enjoy a piece of music.

All outcome assessments have characteristics or properties that provide some information about the precision of the measure. Laboratory or functional assessments usually have a range over which the measurements are considered accurate and predictable. In other words, changes in values over the informative range will reflect improvement or deterioration for some physiologic function or anatomic structure. The properties usually linked to an assessment are the sensitivity, meaning the ability to detect true positives, the specificity, meaning the ability to reject false positives, and the receiver operating characteristics, meaning how much input produces how much signal across the range. The properties for survey questions and other testing relying on communication skills regarding feelings or perceptions have other measures such as interclass correlation, reliability, and validity for the specific populations that were tested. Generally, survey instruments are validated as a whole, and taking sections out of the whole or changing the sequence will require new validation studies in the population of interest.

The characteristics of individual assessments can be a guide to the type and size of clinical trial. An outcome assessment with high precision that has been validated specifically in the population of interest will provide the best results for constructing analytic datasets and interpreting the overall trial outcome. In general, the larger the effect size coupled with high reproducibility, the smaller the clinical trial needs to be to provide the requisite data. The smaller the effect size and the lower the reproducibility or consistency, the larger the clinical trial needs to be to have confidence in the results.

If a clinical trial is at a preliminary phase of the evaluation of the intervention, that is, there is little prior knowledge and the intervention is new or innovative, then it is necessary to establish the preliminary effect size. The effect size can have at least two components—one for benefit and one for safety or tolerability. Additional measures can be taken to evaluate various types of benefit measures and various types of safety or tolerability measures. An early phase study will typically vary the exposure of an individual to the intervention to determine if there are changes in the benefit or safety with different exposures and identify, if possible, an optimal exposure that provides the greatest benefit with acceptable risk. To achieve that goal may require more than one study.

If a clinical trial is at a more advanced phase of the evaluation of an intervention, that is, there is prior experience using the intervention of interest in the population with the phenotype of interest, then the goals will shift from preliminary characterization of the effects of the intervention to capturing enough data to reliably predict the benefit and risks using some of the same outcome assessments as used previously. In addition, the introduction of new supplemental outcome assessments may be of value for purposes of either

- Initial characterization of the supplemental outcome assessment in the population of interest exposed to the intervention of interest or
- Establishing consistency in the benefit and safety measures using different outcome assessments to broaden understanding of the overall effects and to different dimensions of those effects

Later phase clinical trials that are intended to formally and quantitatively establish benefit and risk, sometimes known as efficacy studies, must be designed to provide greater precision and reliability on the initial estimated effect size of the outcome assessment of primary interest. Introducing a new outcome assessment that has not been at least initially validated in the population of interest with the intervention of interest will complicate the design and interpretation because there are no prior data to guide either the design or the analysis.

Evaluating an intervention is a systematic objective process where all the clinical trials exploring the use of the intervention will contribute to a general body of knowledge about both the intervention and the population of interest. Thus, components of prior studies must be included in any new study to properly calibrate and interpret the results.

A trial may have more than one outcome measure, but as the number of outcome measures increases, the complexity of the study and the analysis increases. Clinical outcomes that directly demonstrate patient benefit such as improvement in survival, improvement of functioning, improvement of symptoms, or delay of disease progression are generally preferable because interpretation is simplest.

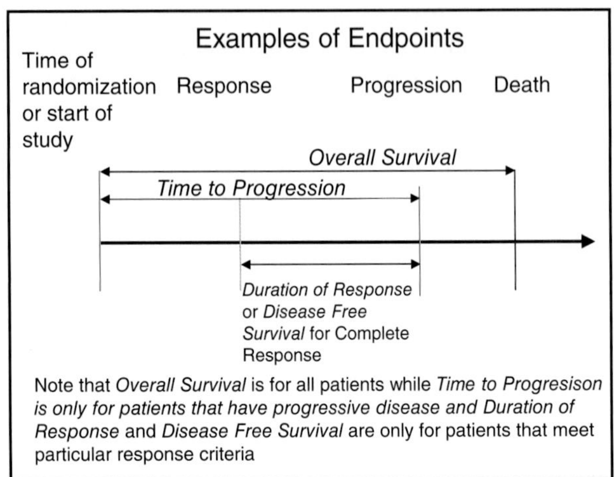

Figure 1.5 Typical definitions of some time-dependent endpoints.

Tables 1.4 and 1.5 list endpoints based on their relationship to time. If time is variable (Table 1.4), then the outcome that is being measured is usually expressed in units of time and duration. In general, the longer the therapeutic effect or benefit, the more favorable is the outcome. Another way to express the concept is time to event, where the event is either the duration of benefit or the appearance of an unfavorable outcome.

Examples include overall survival, time to disease progression, and duration of favorable response (Figs. 1.5 and 1.6).

If time is fixed (Table 1.5), then the outcome that is being measured is a rate of events, where, in general, the more events that occur in a population during the study period or some other predefined time interval, the more favorable is the

TABLE 1.4 Types of Time-Dependent Endpoints

Time-Dependent or Variable Time Expressed as Units of Time (Usually the Median Time to an Event for a Population)	*Population*	*Comment*
Pharmacokinetics	All patients	A series of parameters that describe the absorption, distribution, metabolism, and elimination of a drug as a function of time and exposure.
Overall survival	All patients	Typically time between study entry and death. Measurement is usually unambiguous. Cause of death may be difficult to determine. Effective therapies can result in long follow-up times for completing studies.
Progression-free survival/time to progression	All patients that progress	Typically, time between study entry and first date of disease progression with death being considered as progression. The parameters for progression must be reliably defined and the assay validated—may be symptom based, imaging study, biomarker, or patient-reported outcome.
Disease-free survival	Only complete responders	Parameter for progression must be reliably defined and assay validated—may be symptom based, imaging study, biomarker, or patient-reported outcome.
Time to treatment failure	All patients that change treatment	Treatment failure must be reliably defined and may include disease progression or unacceptable toxicity. Unacceptable toxicity can be a highly individual assessment and treatment failure can be due to multiple factors, not all of which are objective. Time to treatment failure is particularly difficult to interpret.
Duration of response	Only responders	Typically, time between first date of response and first date of disease progression. Response is usually defined as having a minimum duration (typically 4 wk) to be considered a response.
Time to response	Only responders	Typically, time between date of study entry and first date of response. Response is usually defined as having a minimum duration (typically 4 wk) to be considered a response.

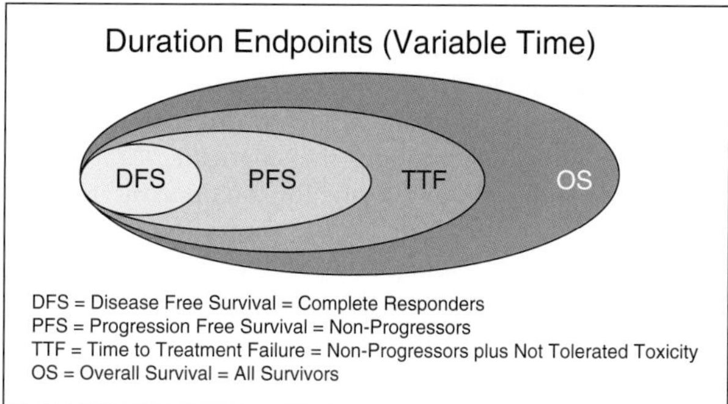

Figure 1.6 Relative proportions of population size of some time-dependent endpoints.

outcome. Examples include percentage of responders, survival at 5 years, and percentage of patients not progressing at 2 years (Fig. 1.7).

BIOMARKERS AND SURROGATE ENDPOINTS

The NIH Definition Working Group defined the terms *clinical endpoint, biomarker,* and *surrogate endpoint* in 2001 as:

1. A clinical endpoint is a characteristic or variable that reflects how a patient feels, functions, or survives.
2. A biomarker is a characteristic that is objectively measured and evaluated as an indicator of normal biologic processes, pathogenic processes, or pharmacologic responses to a therapeutic intervention.
3. A surrogate endpoint is a biomarker intended to substitute for a clinical endpoint that should predict clinical benefit or harm or lack of both.[104]

The Biomarkers Consortium, a public–private partnership dedicated to developing biomarkers for general use, defines biomarkers as "characteristics that are objectively measured and evaluated as indicators of normal biological processes, pathogenic processes, or pharmacologic responses to therapeutic intervention."[105–107]

Biomarkers may be submitted for formal FDA qualification, which helps ensure that the assessment results are reproducible and consistent and independent of who is performing the assessment or where the assessment is done. Qualification usually involves the establishment of standard operating procedures, calibration of the outcome measures, a training procedure, and, if applicable, specifications for reagents and equipment. The Food and Drug Administration Center for Drug Evaluation and Research Biomarker Qualification Program (https://www.fda.gov/drugs/drug-development-tool-qualification-programs/cder-biomarker-qualification-program) will provide guidance on the qualification of candidate biomarkers. The process of establishing the properties, utility, and validity of a biomarker is a structured orderly one.[106]

(A)

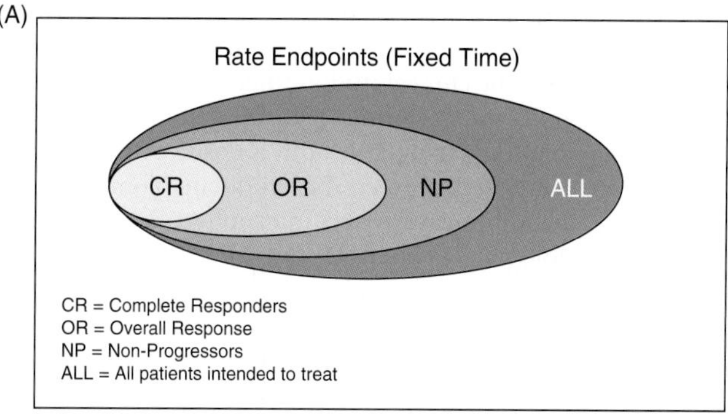

(B)

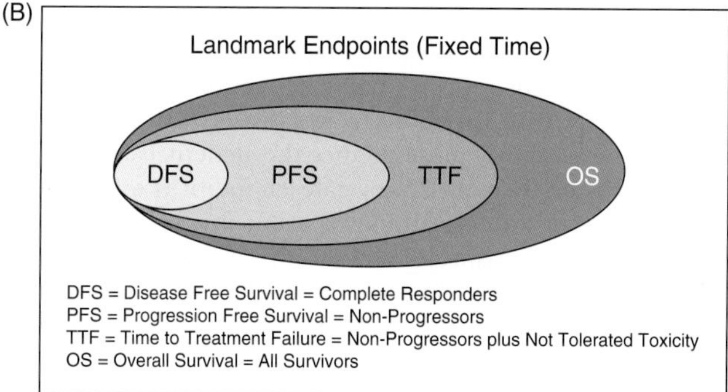

Figure 1.7 Relative proportions of population size of some time-independent endpoints: **(A)** rate endpoints and **(B)** landmark endpoints.

TABLE 1.5 Types of Time-Independent Endpoints

Time-Independent or Time Is Fixed Expressed as a Rate of Events Per Unit Time (Usually Length of the Study) Such As Percent of the Population with An Event During the Fixed Time Period	*Population*	*Comment*
Pharmacokinetic/pharmacodynamic relationships	All patients where measurements are taken	Description of relationship between drug exposure and a clinical or biochemical effect
Response	% of all patients or a continuous variable such as a drug level	Criteria are extremely variable; may be drug levels, symptom based, imaging study, biomarker, or patient-reported outcome. Response is often subdivided into categories that may be ordered (e.g., complete response, partial response, stable disease, progression). Ordered categories require additional analyses and in some cases are combined
Adverse events	Usually % of all patients	Standard reporting criteria are available from several sources
Landmark	% of all patients	Highly variable—paradigm—an example would be % of patients alive at 2 y for a life-threatening illness, but must be meaningful with regard to disease and patient population

Once a biomarker is qualified, it may be a candidate for a surrogate clinical trial endpoint. Validation of a surrogate endpoint requires specific clinical studies where the direct measure of the clinical outcome is statistically compared to values of the candidate biomarker. Changes in both a positive and negative direction are correlated between the candidate biomarker and the clinical outcome measure and interpreted in the context of plausible biologic mechanisms and what is known about the causal pathway of the intended clinical outcome. The validation process may not apply to all populations, so should be accepted only for the population in which the surrogate was studied and validated. This caveat is particularly relevant for pediatric populations.

Operationally, a surrogate endpoint substitutes for another outcome variable. The ideal surrogate endpoint is a disease marker that directly reflects what is happening, both positively and negatively, with the underlying disease. A surrogate endpoint, to be credible, must predict the benefit based on scientific evidence. Usually a surrogate endpoint is a laboratory measurement or an observation or event that serves as a substitute for direct measure of a clinically meaningful endpoint. Some examples of surrogates are blood glucose or hemoglobin A_{1c} for diabetes, intraocular pressure for glaucoma, and blood pressure for hypertension.

Surrogates are often employed as substitutes for efficacy variables but may also serve as substitutes for safety variables. Among the reasons to use surrogate endpoints in a study are that a clinical event may be difficult to measure, a clinical event may have a low event rate, and it may be faster or cheaper to measure a surrogate. The use of surrogates in an overall development plan can accelerate the determination of benefit and provide patients earlier access to therapy than waiting for a direct demonstration of clinical benefit.

Presumptive surrogate markers can be misleading. Patients who have a positive outcome based on the surrogate may not have true clinical benefit. This can arise in several circumstances when the association of a surrogate endpoint with clinical outcome may not be causal but is based on a statistical correlation. Possibilities include alternate mechanisms or multiple pathways for the pathophysiology and alternate or multiple pathways for the action of a drug. A misleading surrogate assumes patient benefit yet exposes patients to risk.[108]

In addition, the safety of long-term exposure may not be adequately assessed. Unexpected results relying on surrogates can occur in almost any clinical setting, such as cardiology (flosequinan for the treatment of heart failure [PROFILE study]; encainide, flecainide, and moricizine for the treatment of arrhythmias in patients after a myocardial infarction [CAST study]; milrinone for the treatment of heart failure [PROMISE Study]); infectious diseases (interferon gamma for chronic granulomatous disease), and metabolism (sodium fluoride for osteoporosis).[108]

In the heart failure study, the surrogate endpoints were cardiac output and ejection fraction; whereas the clinical endpoint was survival. The lack of correlation between changes in the surrogates and survival could be due to actions of the drug that are independent of the disease process, such as postulated for flosequinan on survival in chronic heart failure.[109–112]

A similar scenario may exist for arrhythmia studies, where the surrogate endpoints were electrocardiographic readings, whereas the clinical endpoint was survival.[113–117] For chronic granulomatous disease, the endpoint was superoxide production and in vitro bacterial killing, whereas the clinical endpoint was incidence of serious infection. The lack of correlation may be due to the disease process having an effect on clinical outcome that is independent of the pathway that the drug acts on and which contains the surrogate.[118–120] The metabolism study with sodium fluoride for osteoporosis used bone mineral density as a surrogate for the clinical outcome of fractures. The lack of correlation could be due to the surrogate not being in the causal pathway of the disease process.[121,122]

The importance of having consistency and alignment is illustrated by several studies supported by the U.S. NIH to evaluate the impact of inhaled nitric oxide (iNO) on survival and pulmonary morbidities associated with preterm birth. There was no effect of iNO on the composite primary endpoint, death or chronic lung disease (CLD) of prematurity, in two of the large trials, and a marginal improvement was seen in one trial.[123,124]

Each trial had different enrollment criteria, including gestational age at birth and postnatal age at randomization, dose, and duration of treatment. International multicenter trials were also underway at the time of the NIH-supported studies, adding to the body of available data on this therapy. Subsequent meta-analyses have examined the impact of iNO on death or CLD, and the heterogeneity in trial designs is apparent.[125,126] An NIH consensus panel considered all the available evidence and determined that the data did not support routine use of iNO in premature infants to prevent or treat pulmonary morbidities, although additional studies to define subgroups that appeared to benefit were supported.[127]

The experience of these trials and analyses emphasizes the need for well-characterized, precise, and accepted standards to minimize heterogeneity, potential bias, and uncertainty. Without agreement on key protocol and data elements, the return on the substantial investment of time, resources, and risk is unlikely to enhance our knowledge or advance the field.[83]

To summarize, understanding the characteristics of the outcome assessments with regard to sensitivity, specificity, receiver-operator characteristics, interclass correlation, validity, reproducibility, or any additional relevant parameters is necessary to describe in detail the study protocol and the study statistical analytic plan. These characteristics in turn will inform the design, including the target enrollment, of the clinical trial.

Clinical trial protocols and statistical analytic plans should acknowledge the phase of therapeutic development, whether it is early with a goal to better understand the characteristics and effects of an intervention or whether it is a later phase with a goal to refine the precision of prior knowledge to formally establish benefit and risk in a consistent and generalizable manner for a population of interest.

There are multiple statistical approaches to clinical trial analysis, with the distinctions dependent on whether a normal, or parametric, distribution of results is expected and whether prior information is incorporated.

All measurements have associated confidence intervals, which are calculated from statistical tables. The smaller or narrower the confidence intervals, the greater is the certainty of the result. This can be achieved through either a large study population size or a large therapeutic effect. The most difficult results to interpret are from a small population size with a small effect. It is unlikely that the most informative high-quality design will be the least resource intensive. A truism in clinical research, as it is for software development, is "good, fast, cheap-pick any two."[128]

ADDITIONAL CONSIDERATIONS FOR PEDIATRIC STUDY OUTCOMES

Pediatric clinical trials are easiest to implement and interpret when the outcome measures are objective and do not require active patient participation. Outcome measures that are physical signs may be sufficiently precise and reproducible to substitute for symptom evaluation in some cases (e.g., respiratory rate and presence, and extent of retractions for shortness of breath). However, when objective outcomes are not available, trials with subjective outcome measures or outcome measures that require active patient participation may be the most feasible option.

Patient-reported outcomes can be direct or indirect, particularly in younger children. Indirect or proxy reporting can be complex to design, analyze, and interpret. Rigorous statistical analyses apply, although the methods to analyze pediatric patient-reported outcomes may differ from the analyses for other types of clinical trial endpoints.

Several variables can affect patient-reported outcome. Using pain as a paradigm can be instructive. Pain is a combination of perception plus sensation. Therapy can usually be effective, and there are multiple scales available for assessment by the patient or an observer. A literature review shows that age,[129–136] gender,[137–140] and type of instrument[130,131,141] are variables that affect outcome in published studies. These reports collectively demonstrate that particular variables can affect patient-reported outcome and must be accounted for in the design and analysis of studies. Validation is context and treatment specific.

EXTRAPOLATION OF EFFICACY

The goal in pediatric clinical studies is to follow Einstein's dictum of making things as simple as possible, but not simpler. In 1994 the FDA published a Pediatric Rule that allowed extrapolation of adult efficacy to a pediatric population if the course of the disease and the beneficial and adverse effects of the drug are "sufficiently similar" in the pediatric and adult populations.[64] The goal was to reduce the barrier to pediatric labeling of products by encouraging the use of borrowed data under appropriate circumstances to eliminate the need for separate adequate and well-controlled studies in children.

A 1996 FDA guidance document on the subject notes that the determination of "sufficiently similar" will depend on numerous factors including pathophysiology, natural history, drug action, and metabolism and would be easier to conclude for brief or acute disorders than for chronic disorders or those with a lengthy and variable history.[65] More recent explorations into factors that may provide a basis for extrapolation have identified four domains that could provide supporting evidence:

- nonclinical evidence
- pathophysiology
- natural history
- response to therapy

Establishing a consistent framework for extrapolation is an ongoing area of development and, if done effectively, could contribute to the sharing of data among study populations that would diminish the resource burden for conducting clinical trials.[142–148] Extrapolation is a subset of the more general case of borrowing data from one or more sources and applying those data to a new context or target population. The selection of the source data must align with biologic plausibility and the quality and stringency of the collected data.

Some important principles related to extrapolation are:

- the datasets for both the source population and the target population must be of high quality and stringency
- the outcome measures need to be validated in the populations of interest as extrapolating data brings additional risks of imprecision and error
- extrapolation of efficacy or benefit data is the usual paradigm as safety data are likely to vary based on physiologic function and developmental stage

The Center for Drug Evaluation and Research of the FDA published a flowchart for pediatric extrapolation to guide the types of studies that could be acceptable for drugs and the Center for Devices and Radiological Health published a separate flowchart for devices.[142,144] The European Medicines Agency published a reflection on extrapolation with its own flowchart.[146]

The flowcharts all acknowledge adherence to the principle of linking the biologic basis for extrapolation along with the age-appropriate outcome measures to use. What is not included in any of the documents are technical criteria to assess the data quality, limitations, and robustness of the source dataset and the target dataset in a manner that is used in other contexts such as meta-analyses or Cochrane evaluations.[149]

PATIENT-REPORTED OUTCOMES

Patient-reported outcomes are descriptions of what happens to the patient based on his or her own direct assessment, usually through answering a list of standard questions or indicating a perception on some type of a scale. Patient-reported outcomes can also be captured indirectly through a trained observer completing the questions or scale on behalf of a study participant that lacks capacity to do so directly. Examples include young children or people with impairment of communication or understanding. Patient-reported outcomes generally address the goals of how an individual feels or improvement in function or improvement in symptoms.

From a scientific perspective, desirable properties of patient-reported outcomes are that they be disease related, specifically validated for the disease and population including improvement and worsening of clinically meaningful changes, have real-time assessments (not based on recall), can have confirmation by other assessments, and can be measured in controlled studies.

Some examples are changes in pain or changes in symptoms that are disease related and limit activity or function. Valid reproducible measurements are still required to interpret the results. General advice about the systematic collection of patient-reported outcomes is available from the FDA in the form of a guidance document (https://www.regulations.gov/docket?D=FDA-2006-D-0362).

The general principles are that a series of questions are structured during an interview or administration of a questionnaire and organized according to topic. Pediatric-specific aspects of patient-reported outcomes are discussed later.

PROTOCOL CONSTRUCTION

The mechanics of implementing a study begins with writing a study protocol consistent with the International Conference of Harmonization guidelines and relevant regulations. A summary of applicable FDA regulations may be found at https://www.fda.gov/science-research/clinical-trials-and-human-subject-protection/preambles-gcp-regulations.

The general features of a study protocol are that it poses a question, identifies a study population for which the question is relevant, proposes an intervention, has safety monitoring and escape rules for individual patients, assesses outcome based on meaningful and validated endpoints, utilizes systematic and validated measurement techniques to assess the endpoints, and contains an analytic plan that minimizes bias and uncertainty. Some elements to address in trial design and protocol writing are listed in Table 1.6.

A protocol must be approved by an IRB and, if an investigational agent is used or if an FDA-approved product is used under some conditions, then an IND application must be filed and the protocol reviewed by the FDA. Detailed information can be found at: http://www.fda.gov/BiologicsBloodVaccines/DevelopmentApprovalProcess/InvestigationalNewDrugINDorDeviceExemptionIDEProcess/default.htm.

There are many possible and plausible design variations that include having multiple stages where continuation of the trial from an early to a later stage is dependent on interim results.

Such an approach is termed an adaptive design. Among the more common is a two-stage design for clinical activity where an initial cohort of patients is assessed with prespecified rules for a minimum level of activity to justify an expansion of the study to enroll more patients. Another variation on an adaptive design would assign subsequent interventions or observations

TABLE 1.6 Trial Design Elements

Element	*Comment*
TIME FRAME	
Prospective	A protocol is written and the study is performed following the approval of the protocol. Opportunity to collect all data that are required to test the hypothesis.
Retrospective	A protocol is written to systematically analyze historical data. Often unable to locate all the data required to test the hypothesis.
CONTROLS	
Historical	Comparison is made with either a specific study that is considered to be an appropriate match for the current therapy or with a valid meta-analysis of a series of previous studies. Major problems are: 1. Changes in medical practice (secular effect) that affect results over time 2. Differences in eligibility criteria in different protocols 3. Differences in assessment in different studies 4. Differences in analysis in different studies
PLACEBO	
Supportive care	If no active therapy exists for the patient population then it may be ethical to provide supportive care plus a placebo vs. supportive care plus the test therapy. Examples may include testing a symptom benefit therapy.
Add-on	All arms receive the same standard therapy with the control arm receiving in addition a placebo and the experimental arm receiving in addition the test therapy.
ACTIVE	
Standard therapy	Direct comparison between a standard therapy and the test therapy.
Add-on	All arms receive the same standard therapy with the experimental arm receiving in addition the test therapy.
Withdrawal	All arms receive the same therapy until a predetermined time when one arm has the test therapy withdrawn. The endpoint of interest is usually the appearance of an event that would be prevented if the test therapy were still present. This type of design is often used in measuring the effect of lowering blood pressure.
Dose comparison	Different doses of the same drug are compared. Generally a trend in benefit or response that follows the exposure to the drug is considered evidence of activity—the greater the exposure the greater the response.
ARMS	
Single	A single series of patients
Multiple	Treatment arms are compared concurrently to one another.
Crossover	Patients can change from one treatment arm to another based on predetermined criteria. If the critical evaluation occurs after the crossover it may be difficult to interpret due to factors such as the sequence of therapy having an effect or one therapy having a delayed effect.
ANALYSES	
Single	Study analysis occurs when either a particular time or predefined landmark is reached.
Multiple	Study analysis will incorporate one or more interim analyses triggered by events, landmarks, or time schedule.
Adaptive	The study design may alter in a prospectively defined manner based on the outcome of an interim analysis; e.g., a study arm may be closed to accrual, the overall sample size may be increased, or a new study arm may open. All adaptive designs are based on rules described in detail in the original protocol and are not based on protocol amendments developed subsequent to any data analysis.

to patients depending on the results of the initial intervention or other events.

Some study designs are not intended to assess a specific intervention but are intended to systematically collect data in a prospective manner to describe natural history or make long-term observations. Such a study design may be applicable as a follow-up study to a study that assessed an intervention.

A study design that emerged during the last decade called the "wedge-step" is a variation on a randomized controlled study where multiple arms are constructed, with each arm having a run-in period of different lengths prior to exposure to the experimental intervention. The rationale of such a design is to collectively generate enough time in enough people without the intervention exposure to serve as a control dataset yet ensure that everyone in the study is exposed to the intervention.[150–152]

CLINICAL TRIAL MONITORING

The risks of investigational therapy can be unknown. Extrapolation from preclinical models for safety are about 65% predictive.[153] The predictive value of preclinical models for children is a field under development. Although preclinical models for teratogenicity exist, several acceptable preclinical models for pediatric-specific toxicities such as the impact on growth and organ maturation are still being developed.

In addition, children, particularly the youngest, may not be able to communicate adverse effects. As a consequence, the monitoring of clinical studies in children merits greater vigilance than monitoring in adult populations.[70,84,153–158]

The rationale for monitoring is based on two general research principles:

- Ensuring and enhancing the safety of the study, that is, to protect the study participant from unacceptable risk; and
- Assuring the scientific validity of the study, that is, to protect the data and preserve its integrity.

The most critical component is investigator integrity, which can be actualized by a proactive, comprehensive, and integrated monitoring plan.

To uphold and implement these principles, a monitoring plan must:

- Be proactive and anticipate a range of outcomes and responses; and
- Include a communication plan to support dynamic interaction between relevant parties, including monitors, investigators, sponsors, regulatory authorities, and others.

Monitoring is assuming responsibility for reviewing events and outcomes during the implementation of a study in two domains: (1) safety of participants and (2) integrity and quality of data including study accrual. Study monitoring encompasses comparing events and outcomes to predefined criteria. If the study events and outcomes indicate deviance from those criteria, study monitoring would mandate making a recommendation to alter the study implementation.

Routine monitoring is when the study team has primary responsibility for monitoring the study typically based on a monitoring plan incorporated in the study protocol or study plan; IRB oversight; institutional oversight in compliance with applicable institutional, state, and federal guidelines, policies, regulations, and laws.

Each study should develop a monitoring plan that is included in the overall study plan or protocol that defines:

- How the study will comply with regulatory requirements
- The specific events and activities that will be monitored
- The roles and responsibilities for everyone on the team who is involved in monitoring
- Who has responsibility for reporting (and who they report to)
- A schedule for monitoring
- Any escape and stopping rules

Escape rules are criteria for an individual patient to leave the study based on disease progression, toxicity, or lack of efficacy. Escape rules may define alternative regimens. Stopping rules are criteria for either halting accrual or closing a study for toxicity, lack of efficacy, or sufficient efficacy that further enrollment is not required to determine a conclusion. If applicable, the type and number of events that would halt accrual and would generate a review of eligibility, monitoring, assessments, intervention, and how the resumption of accrual would occur in each study plan or protocol will include a list of expected adverse events regardless of whether these adverse events are referenced or explained in other types of study documentation.

A list or description of *expected events* should be in the following forms:

- A description of the scope of expected adverse events of the underlying condition based on either a recent literature review or textbook. If none are expected during the study time frame, simply state that no adverse events are expected;
- If interventional products are administered, a description of the safety profile for *each* product administered in the study (investigational and marketed) including, if known, the frequency, severity, and duration of adverse events;
- If assessments (e.g., a blood test, imaging study, survey instrument) that are not part of the routine care of the disease or underlying condition are scheduled in the study, then the known risks and complications from those assessments should be listed in the study protocol.

The best quality information to include in the study protocol regarding research-specific assessments would be individual institutional experience using the assessment at the study site, which includes the total number of people that received the assessment plus the complication rates. If institutional experience is not available, published data from similar studies and published data on the general use of the assessment tool or technique may be substituted.

An integrated listing of adverse events containing those anticipated from the natural history plus those anticipated from any and all interventions and assessments that may occur on study should conclude the anticipated risks section of the study plan or protocol. The potential advantages of an integrated list of expected events are that IRBs could readily assess the overall risks from a study, the informed consent process and documents could be prepared to better inform prospective study participants of potential risks, and adverse event reporting could be simplified by comparison of an event with a single source document.

Risk-adjusted supplemental monitoring can be implemented in addition to routine monitoring, and depending on the nature of the research, monitoring can be effectively augmented through mechanisms and independent external entities such as a single-person Medical Monitor, a small Study Monitoring Committee, a multidisciplinary committee, or a chartered multidisciplinary team such as an Independent Data Monitoring Committee (IDMC). Alternative terms include Data and Safety Monitoring Board, Data Monitoring Board, or Data Monitoring Committee.

Study characteristics that have risks that can trigger supplemental monitoring include, but are not limited to:

- Late phase clinical trials statistically powered to establish efficacy. Late phase clinical trials are generally large studies, but not necessarily so, and are designed to affect current medical practice, product labeling if applicable, or public health policy.
- Multisite/multicenter clinical trials. Multisite/multicenter clinical trials involve separate institutions using the same study protocol. Several sites that are within the same legally established institution are not generally considered to be a multisite study.
- Clinical trials involving randomized treatments. Multiarm clinical trials that use randomization are designed to minimize potential bias in the interpretation of the results. Randomization implies scrupulous attention to the details of study implementation to avoid any compromise in data integrity.
- Clinical trials involving vulnerable populations, such as those who are children, elderly and ill, terminally ill, or of diminished mental capacity, or any population otherwise unable or unlikely to provide informed consent that are at greater than minimal risk. If the clinical trial involves only minimal risk to participants, as defined by 45 CFR Subpart A, Sec. 46.102 and minimal risk to data integrity and quality (e.g., small number of sites, small sample size, few data elements, short duration), monitoring can be accomplished through alternative mechanisms, such as the use of a detailed monitoring plan in the protocol.
- Clinical trials in which the treatment is particularly invasive or has other serious safety concerns that may result in serious toxicity.
- Clinical research studies in which an assessment that is used solely for research purposes is considered greater than minimal risk.
- Clinical research studies, including observational studies in which participants are already at elevated risk of: (1) death; (2) life-threatening conditions (i.e., immediate risk of death); (3) in-patient hospitalization or prolongation of existing hospitalization; (4) persistent or significant disability/incapacity; or (5) congenital anomaly or birth defect. These events are considered serious adverse events by regulatory authorities.
- A clinical research project that is of sufficiently long duration that protocol changes may need to be considered based on changing medical practice or interim analyses.
- Any clinical trial in which members of the study team have a stated or perceived conflict of interest.

An IDMC is a structured multidisciplinary mechanism for supplemental monitoring that may be dedicated to a single study or may serve multiple studies. The role of the Board or Committee is established before a clinical trial begins. Its functions typically include review of the protocol before it is implemented, review of study implementation and progress, and ongoing review of the accumulating data to detect evidence of early, significant benefit or harm for participants while the trial is in progress. This latter review serves as an additional protection for participants, beyond that provided by the IRB, but does not take the place of regulatory requirements for investigators to report serious and unanticipated adverse events to the FDA. Examples of IDMC responsibilities are:

- Review the research protocol, review model informed consent documents, and plans for data and safety monitoring, including all proposed revisions.
- Review methodology used to help maintain the confidentiality of the study data and the results of monitoring by reviewing procedures put in place by investigators to ensure confidentiality.
- Monitor study design, procedures, and events that will maximize the safety of the study participants and minimize the risks.
- Evaluate the progress of the study, including periodic assessments of data quality and timeliness, participant recruitment, accrual and retention, participant risk versus benefit, performance of the study site(s), and other factors that may affect the study outcome.
- Consider factors external to the study when relevant information becomes available, such as scientific or therapeutic developments that may have an impact on the safety of the participants or the ethics of the studies.
- Review serious adverse event documentation and safety reports and make recommendations regarding protection of the safety of the study participants.
- Report on the safety and progress of the study.
- Evaluate and report on any perceived problems with study conduct, enrollment, sample size, and/or data collection.
- Provide a recommendation regarding continuation, termination, or other modifications of the study based on the cumulative experience including the observed beneficial or adverse effects.

An IDMC operates under a charter outlining the roles, responsibilities, and standard operating procedures for the group. The charter will:

- Define the roles, responsibilities, and relationships for each of the members, such as who are voting members or advisory members, who may attend open and closed sessions, the line of authority for reviews and decision making, who is granted access to certain data (e.g., blinded and unblinded), the compensation for IDMC members, and any potential conflicts of interest.
- Outline the responsibilities of the group including: familiarizing group members with the study protocol and monitoring of adverse events, data quality, participant recruitment and enrollment, the risks and benefits, reporting, etc.
- May also include an organizational chart depicting the relationships between all of the major stakeholders of the study team, the study sponsor, the funding organization, and the IDMC.
- Identify the standard procedures for each items such as meeting frequency and format, including logistics and required attendees/quorum, procedures for unscheduled evaluations, including types of events that would trigger an unscheduled evaluation, expected information, involvement of the study chair, required number of members, and communication of recommendations.

- Identify statistical procedures that may be utilized by the IDMC, including any stopping rules based on benefit or harm, futility analysis, or decision points in adaptive designs.
- Monitor recruitment goals.
- Identify methods for making recommendations to the study sponsor and investigators, funding organization, and other relevant parties.

INTERNATIONAL STUDIES

Performing a study in several countries could have multiple advantages including faster accrual, potentially greater confidence in the results due to replicability, and sharing of resources. Engagement in international studies could also provide opportunities for professional development and cooperation as well as

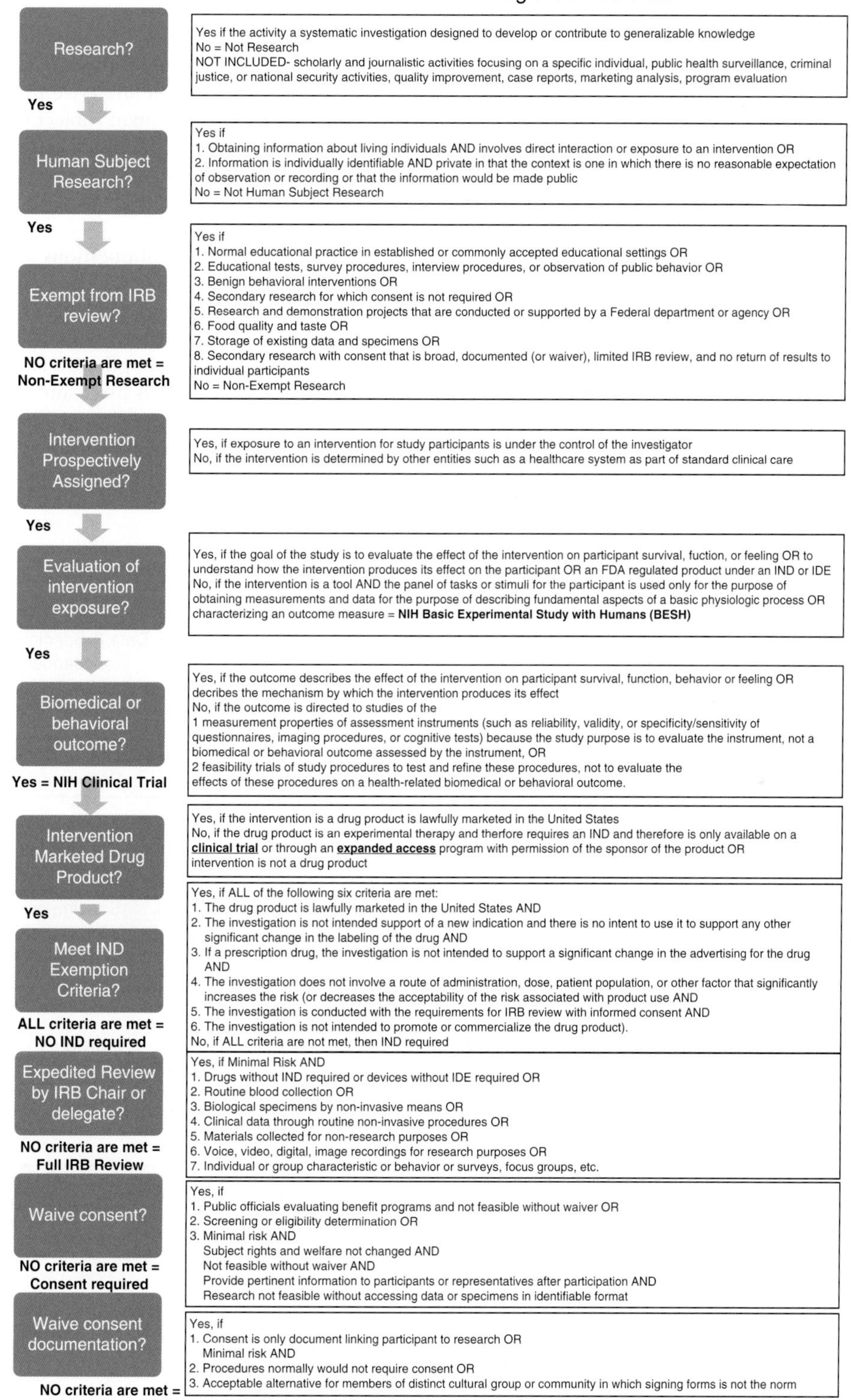

Figure 1.8 Integrated clinical research flowchart.

support better acceptance of study findings. In addition, best practices could be disseminated based on the clinical trial experience, which would quickly and directly benefit pediatric patients. The implementation of international studies, to be informative for all participants, should meet several criteria. The study question should be of value to all communities that participate. All assessment techniques should be available and validated at all sites. Eligibility criteria should be standardized. The data repository and analysis should be centralized.

Among the considerations in the design and implementation of an international study are the types of diseases relevant to each region, priority of any new proposed agents, types of studies, and incorporation of study endpoints that are demonstrative or predictive of clinical benefit. There are also several barriers that include, but are not limited to, regional differences in health care systems and practice, lack of common informatics standards, different languages and different medical terms, logistics and speed of protocol development, regulatory requirements and inconsistencies, compliance with good clinical practice and assurances, logistical challenges to sample processing, access to new agents, data sharing and credit, and funding.[158]

Cooperative and collaborative studies in the 21st century will be feasible on the basis of development and acceptance of international standards for data acquisition, data transmission, and adherence to infrastructure and systems that are interoperable as a result of standards.[145,159–161]

COMPLEXITIES OF CLINICAL TRIAL IMPLEMENTATION

Clinical trials have a life cycle with a repetitive series of activities that can be summarized as

- Submission of a structured document for peer review evaluation
- Evaluation of the document based on established criteria
- Response to evaluation

If the evaluation is favorable, the clinical trial process proceeds to the next step, often with some modification.

Examples of steps in the life cycle process include funding review, scientific review, human subject protection review, FDA review, data monitoring committee review, funding agency review, and publication review.

The process has multiple steps and each review focuses on different criteria.

Examples of the types of questions and subsequent actions to be taken include a formal determination of whether the activity is research, if it is human subject research, if IRB review is required, what type of IRB review may be required, classification if the activity is funded by the US NIH, IND requirement if an FDA-regulated product is used, and expectations regarding the informed consent process.

Figure 1.8 outlines in schematic form one feasible sequence of decisions to approach the multiple decisions.

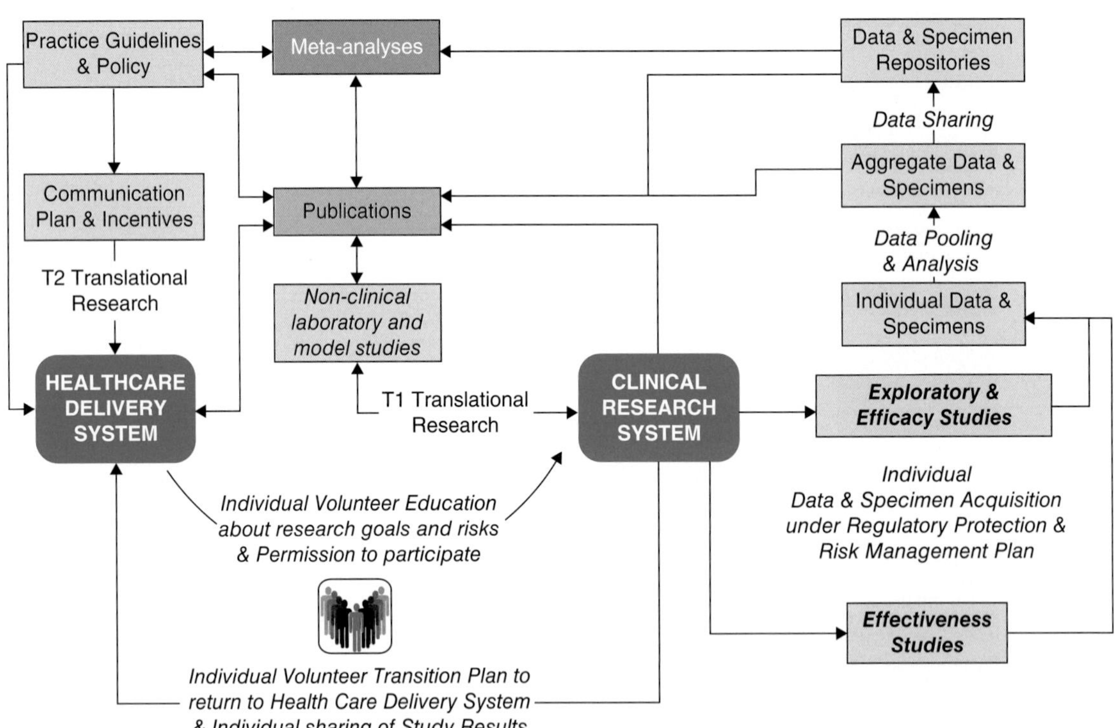

Figure 1.9 Linkages between health care delivery and research. The flow of information is in black. The transition of individuals is in blue. Permission is a generic term to indicate either consent from individuals legally capable of providing consent or the permission process by a parent or legal guardian or authorized representative to provide permission for an individual to participate in research. The permission process may or may not include an assent component.

COMMON WEAKNESSES OR ERRORS IN TRIAL DESIGN OR ANALYSIS

It is rare for a pediatric study to enroll large numbers of patients outside vaccine trials, so designs and analytic plans must anticipate a limited patient population size. Techniques are available to address the problems associated with limited population size.[162]

Hayden and colleagues noted a trend over the prior 30 years of pediatric research to increasingly use a variety of statistical techniques and offered a critique of published studies.[163] Pocock later published a survey of statistical problems in clinical trials that noted that studies tended to have excessive hypothesis testing, which increased the number of false-positive findings.[164]

An FDA survey in 1999 noted several consistent weaknesses in submissions of clinical trial data for review. These included invalid assumptions, analytic methods, incomplete data, no dictionary for data fields, absence of a protocol with the submission, no statistical plan stated in the protocol, incomplete submissions of data, inconsistent field names across studies, multiple terms for the same type of adverse event, unexplained dropouts, lack of follow-up, treating categorical data as continuous data, mixing dose exposure and dose response, inventing new response variables, unspecified subgroup analysis, analyzing only "evaluable" patients displaying only adjusted analyses, stating results as percentage change or percentage change in hazard ratio, site bias, expressing efficacy per patient and adverse events per dose, and pooling analyses of distinct patient populations.[165] Given the preciousness of the resource of pediatric patients, it is imperative that studies be informative and include an analytic plan that minimizes assumptions, is consistent with the endpoints, adheres to accepted statistical principles, and is prospective.

CONCLUSION

On an abstract level, health care delivery is based on the principle of an information flow that integrates general and specific information to support a decision intended to benefit a patient. While some of the information comes from direct observation including a history and physical findings, and some comes from real- or near-time assessments such as images or laboratory studies, guidance is provided by upstream sources such as cumulative experience and research data.

A system schema of the information flow is outlined in Figure 1.9 illustrating the linkages between the health care delivery system and the clinical research system.

Within the research process, a similar abstraction of a study, whether it involves primary data collection or not, is the need to produce a quality analytic dataset.

From both an abstract and a practical perspective, the goal of any research activity is to produce inferences that support decision making. The general method is to assemble either previously collected or capture de novo primary data to construct analytic datasets. Primary means line level or patient level or participant level, as in this context these terms indicate the same concept. The quality and stringency of the primary data determine the quality, stringency, and robustness of the analytic dataset. High-quality, high-stringency primary data can be used multiple times and contribute to multiple analyses to address questions of interest and relevance. Once an analytic dataset is properly constructed, that dataset can be used to produce inferences with estimates of confidence around the inferences. The inferences in turn are used to support decision making, whether it is a sponsor deciding on the next step in a development program or describing a use claim for a regulatory submission, a regulator making a determination if a use claim is adequately supported with regard to benefit and acceptable risk, or a practitioner selecting an intervention for a patient. There are many other examples, but the general paradigm holds (Fig. 1.10).

For historical and practical reasons, the need for high-quality, high-stringency data to support the use of medicinal products in children is an imbalance between need and supply.

A key distinction between research decisions and health care decisions is that research addresses populations, while health care delivery addresses individuals. An analogy may be between classical quantum mechanics as described by Schrödinger, which is directed at system states, and quantum trajectory theory, which is directed at individual particle states. To invoke quantum trajectory theory, near complete system information is required, which is now feasible with sufficient precision to permit the relevant calculations. Classical quantum mechanics is not intended or capable of predicting individual particle states and trajectories.

In the case of human physiology and the contextual influences on the most probable responses for an individual, we do not have the knowledge or the assessment tools to predict the probable response with a high level of precision. Thus, research results can support decision making but are not expected to inform the trajectory of the status of an individual.

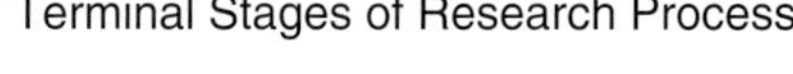

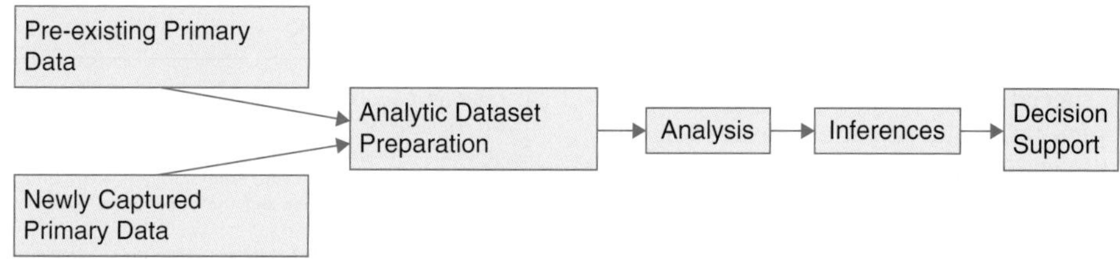

Figure 1.10 Terminal stages of research process showing the flow from data collection to decision support.

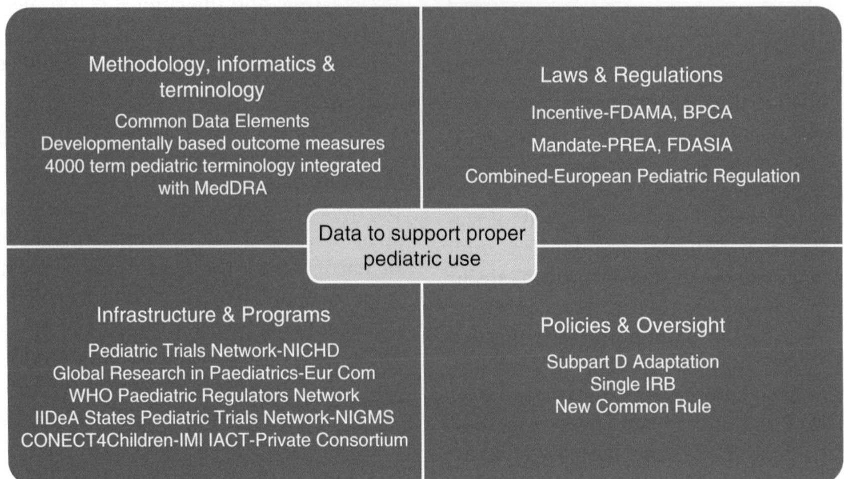

Figure 1.11 Integrated activities to support pediatric research showing how resources, policies, culture, and training intersect to produce quality data.

What research results can support are population results regarding health care and specific results within the research system for the trajectory of a research project. Examples include Go–No Go decisions. Contexts for Go–No Go decisions include:

- Issuing licenses where passing a test results in receiving the license, whereas not passing the test results in no license.
- FDA approval for a product use claim where establishing efficacy that can be reasonably mapped to clinical benefit and providing sufficient evidence to infer an acceptable safety profile can result in marketing authorization. Failing to establish efficacy results in no approval. Establishing efficacy without an acceptable safety profile also results in no approval.
- A Master Protocol will continue to enroll study participants on each arm until an arm meets criteria for discontinuation.
- Multiple applications within a cohort are submitted for a funding review with only a subset selected for funding.
- Multiple product candidates under development are evaluated for continuation to the next stage of development.

The common factor is that criteria are established to guide the decision making and research data provide the enabling information to make the assessment.

Scientific and ethical rationales support the use of clinical investigations to minimize risk and maximize benefit for the use of therapeutic products or interventions. Children of various ages have sufficient differences in metabolism, organ maturation and function, emotional and psychological function that studies are necessary to extend the benefits of therapeutics while minimizing the potential for harm.

Clinical studies in pediatric patients should be designed to minimize risk, distress, and discomfort. This is best done by trained and experienced pediatric investigators at facilities that can support the special needs of pediatric patients and by adherence to accepted principles of patient protection and respect for persons. Enrolling children in studies is a combination of educating and gaining the permission of parents or legal guardians and educating the child while obtaining assent if appropriate.

There are conditions when the permission/assent process can be postponed or waived due to emergent circumstances. Approaches to minimize nontherapeutic interventions such as sparse population sampling for pharmacokinetics and special imaging studies in lieu of tissue sampling are preferred. Study design should incorporate escape rules for individual patients, stopping rules for the entire population, and an IDMC, if appropriate, particularly for life-threatening diseases. Assessments, both clinical and laboratory, need to be age and developmental stage appropriate. Multiple factors may affect study results. Patient-reported outcomes are generally not sufficiently reliable to serve as the only endpoint and should be confirmed by other objective findings. Strategies to minimize exposure and risk include studying older populations before younger ones and using extrapolation of efficacy when scientific evidence warrants.

Diseases or conditions that are specific to a particular age group require studies in that population. Study designs and analytic approaches need to address the limitations of small numbers of patients and variability among patient populations. International cooperation can share resources but has many challenges to address before multinational pediatric studies become routine (Fig. 1.11).

Clinical studies in pediatric patients are a necessary component of therapeutic development unless the product is unsafe or addresses only a condition that does not exist in children. The responsibility for clinical studies in pediatrics is shared with pharmaceutical firms, regulatory authorities, health professionals, and society as a whole. The most vulnerable populations merit the most protection and deserve the benefits available to others, which is achieved through careful and persistent pursuit of further knowledge.

REFERENCES

1. Colon AR, Cowan CP. Nurturing children: a history of pediatrics. In: Cowan CP, Colon AR, eds. *Nurturing children: a history of pediatrics.* Westport, CT: Greenwood, 1999:189, 201, 210.
2. Aronson S, Newman L. Smallpox in the Americas 1492 to 1815 contagion and controversy. 2002. https://www.brown.edu/Administration/News_Bureau/2002-03/02-017t.html.
3. Roddis L. Edward Jenner and the discovery of smallpox vaccination. *Ann Intern Med* 1930;4(5):512.
4. Beckwith JB. Charles-Michel Billard (1800-1832): pioneer of infant pathology. *Pediatr Dev Pathol* 2002;5(3):248–256.
5. Quetelet A. Sur l'homme et le développement de ses facultés: ou, Essai de physique sociale. Paris, France: Bachelier, imprimeur-libraire, quai des Augustins, no 55, 1835.
6. Bogin B. *Patterns of human growth.* Cambridge, England: Cambridge University Press, 1999:455.

7. Rydelius P-A. Child and adolescent psychiatry in Sweden—from yesterday until today. *Nord J Psychiatry* 2009;47(6):395–404.
8. Pearson HA. Lectures on the diseases of children by Eli Ives, MD, of Yale and New Haven: America's first academic pediatrician. *Pediatrics* 1986;77(5):680–686.
9. Burke EC. Abraham Jacobi, MD: the man and his legacy. *Pediatrics* 1998;101(2):309–312.
10. Haggerty RJ. Abraham Jacobi, MD, respectable rebel. *Pediatrics* 1997;99(3):462–466.
11. Bernard C. *An introduction to the study of experimental medicine.* New York, NY: Dover Publications, 1865:226.
12. Geison GL. Chapter seven. From boyhood encounter to "private patients" pasteur and rabies before the vaccine. In: *The private science of Louis Pasteur.* Princeton, NJ: Princeton University Press, 1996:177–205.
13. Silver JR. The decline of German medicine, 1933-45. *J R Coll Phys Edinb* 2003;33(1):54–66.
14. Vollmann J, Winau R. The Prussian regulation of 1900: early ethical standards for human experimentation in Germany. *IRB* 1996;18(4):9–11.
15. Vollmann J, Winau R. Informed consent in human experimentation before the Nuremberg code. *BMJ* 1996;313(7070):1445–1449.
16. Credé. Die Verhütung der Augenentzündung der Neugeborenen. *Archiv für Gynaekologie* 1881;17(1):50–53.
17. Schaller UC, Klauss V. Is Crede's prophylaxis for ophthalmia neonatorum still valid? *Bull World Health Organ* 2001;79(3):262–263.
18. Moll A. Ärztliche Ethik; die Pflichten des Arztes in allen Beziehungen seiner Thätigkeit. Suttgart, Germany: Enke, 1902:650.
19. Maehle AH. 'God's ethicist': Albert Moll and his medical ethics in theory and practice. *Med Hist* 2012;56(2):217–236.
20. FDA Consumer. 100 Years of biologics regulation. In: *FDA consumer magazine.* Rockville, MD: FDA, 2002.
21. Janssen WF. The story of the laws behind he labels. In: *FDA consumer magazine.* Rockville, MD: FDA, 1981.
22. United States v Johnson, in Oliver Wendall Holmes. 1910, US. Supreme Court. p. 488.
23. A brief history of the Center for Drug Evaluation and Research. 2019. https://www.fda.gov/about-fda/virtual-exhibits-fda-history/brief-history-center-drug-evaluation-and-research.
24. US Department of Health, Education, and Welfare. The story of the White House conferences on children and youth. In: *White House Conferences on children and youth.* Washington, DC: The White House, 1967.
25. Gartner L, Gartner C. Founding of the American Academy of Pediatrics. https://www.aap.org/en-us/about-the-aap/Gartner-Pediatric-History-Center/Pages/AAP-Founding.aspx.
26. Swain DC. The rise of a research empire: NIH, 1930 to 1950. *Science* 1962;138(3546):1233–1235.
27. Sass HM. Reichsrundschreiben 1931: pre-Nuremberg German regulations concerning new therapy and human experimentation. *J Med Philos* 1983;8(2):99–111.
28. Ballentine C. Taste of raspberries, taste of death: the 1937 elixir sulfanilamide incident. In: FDA *consumer magazine.* Rockville, MD: Food and Drug Administration, 1981:5.
29. Kopelman LM. Children as research subjects: a dilemma. *J Med Philos* 2000;25(6):745–764.
30. Trent Stephens RB. *Dark remedy: the impact of thalidomide and its revival as a vital medicine.* New York, NY: Basic Books, 2009:240.
31. Nicholson R. Children as research subjects: science, ethics and law. *J Med Ethics* 1996;22(2):124–125.
32. Welt LG. Reflections on the problems of human experimentation. *Conn Med* 1961;25:75–78.
33. Rickham PP. Responsibility in investigations on human subjects. Statements by Medical Research Council. *Br Med J* 1964;2(5402):178–179.
34. World Medical Association. Delcaration of Helsinki. 1964. https://www.fda.gov/science-research/clinical-trials-and-human-subject-protection/preambles-gcp-regulations.
35. Beecher HK. Ethics and clinical research. *N Engl J Med* 1966;274(24):1354–1360.
36. *Advisory Committee on human radiation experiments. Supplemental Volume 2a, Sources and documentation appendices. Final report.* 1995. Office of Scientific and Technical Information (OSTI).
37. Surgeon General, H.a.H. Services, ed. Public Health Service to the heads of the institutions contracting research with Public Health Service grants. Washington, DC: Bureau of Medical Services Curriculum, 1966.
38. Department of Health Education, and Welfare, ed. PHS policy for intramural programs and for contracts when investigations involving human subjects are included. Washington, DC: Department of Health, Education, and Welfare, 1966.
39. Royal College of Physicians. Supervision of clinical investigations. *The Lancet* 1967;290(7511):357–358.
40. Kelsey FO. Human guinea pigs experimentation on man. By M. H. Pappworth. Beacon Press, Boston. 228 pp. 1967. *Teratology* 1971;4(2):215–216.
41. Pappworth MH. "Human guinea pigs"—a history. *BMJ* 1990;301(6766):1456–1460.
42. Royal College of Physicians. *Supervision of the ethics of clinical research investigation in institutions.* London, England: Royal College of Physicians, 1973.
43. Department of Health Education, and Welfare, ed. Protection of human subjects. Washington, DC: Federal Register, 1974:18914–18920.
44. Culliton BJ. National research act: restores training, bans fetal research. *Science* 1974;185(4149):426–427.
45. Department of Health and Social Security, ed. Supervision of the ethics of clinical research investigations and fetal research. London, England: National Health Service (United Kingdom), 1975.
46. World Medical Association. Declaration of Helsinki revised. 1975. https://www.wma.net/what-we-do/medical-ethics/declaration-of-helsinki/doh-oct1975/.
47. National Commission for the Protection of Human Subjects of Biomedical and Behavioral Research. Research involving children: report and recommendations. Washington, DC: Department of Health Education, and Welfare, 1977.
48. National Commission for the Protection of Human Subjects of Biomedical and Behavioral Research. *Institutional review boards: report and recommendations.* Washington, DC, 1978.
49. National Commission for the Protection of Human Subjects of Biomedical and Behavioral Research. *Belmont report: principles and guidelines for the protection of human subjects of research.* Washington, DC: E.a.W. Health, 1979.
50. US Department of Health and Human Services. Code of federal regulations title 45 part 46 common rule. 1983. http://www.hhs.gov/ohrp/humansubjects/guidance/45cfr46.html.
51. Tyson JE, Furzan JA, Reisch JS, et al. An evaluation of the quality of therapeutic studies in perinatal medicine. *J Pediatr* 1983;102(1):10–13.
52. Greenhouse SW. Some historical and methodological developments in early clinical trials at the National Institutes of Health. *Stat Med* 1990;9(8):893–901; discussion 903–906.
53. Bock R. NICHD Renamed for Eunice Kennedy Shriver, advocate for institute's founding. In: *NIH record.* Bethesda, MD: NIH, 2008.
54. Shirkey H. Editorial comment: therapeutic orphans. *J Pediatr* 1968;72(1):119–120.
55. Marks I. Drugs (e.g., hexachlorophene), the FDA, and the AAP. *Pediatrics* 1972;50(2):338.
56. American Academy of Pediatrics Committee on Drugs. *General guidelines for the evaluation of drugs to be approved for use during pregnancy and for the treatment of infants and children.* Chicago, IL: American Academy of Pediatrics, 1974.
57. Wilson JT. Pragmatic assessment of medicines available for young children and pregnant or breast-feeding women. In: Garattini S, Morselli PL, Sereni F, eds. *Basic and therapeutic aspects of perinatal pharmacology.* New York, NY: Raven, 1975:411–421.
58. Food and Drug Administration. General considerations for the clinical evaluation of drugs in infants and children. Washington, DC: Department of Health, Education, and Welfare, 1977.
59. American Academy of Pediatrics, Committee on Drugs. Guidelines for the ethical conduct of studies to evaluate drugs in pediatric populations. *Pediatrics* 1977;60:91–101.
60. Food and Drug Administration. Labeling and prescription drug advertising: content and format for labeling for human prescription drugs. Washington, DC: Federal Register, 1979:37434–37462.
61. US Congress. *Orphan drug act public law* 97-414. Washington, DC: US Government, 1983.
62. House Committee on Energy and Commerce. Health care reform, hearing before the Committee on Energy and Commerce, House of Representatives, One Hundred Third Congress, first session, on President Clinton's Proposal to Reform the Nation's Health Care System—United States. Congress. House. Committee on Energy and Commerce. Washington, DC: Government Printing Office, 1994:622–623.
63. Gilman JT, Gal P. Pharmacokinetic and pharmacodynamic data collection in children and neonates. A quiet frontier. *Clin Pharmacokinet* 1992;23(1):1–9.
64. Food and Drug Administration. Specific requirements on content and format of labeling for human prescription drugs; revision of "pediatric use" subsection in the labeling. Washington, DC: Federal Register, 1994:64240–64250.
65. Food and Drug Administration. The *content and format for pediatric use supplements.* Washington, DC: Food and Drug Adminsitration, 1996.
66. American Academy of Pediatrics, Committee on Drugs. Guidelines for the ethical conduct of studies to evaluate drugs in the pediatric population. *Pediatrics* 1995;95(2):288–294.
67. NICHD. Pediatric Pharmacology Research Units (PPRU) Network. 2017. https://www.nichd.nih.gov/research/supported/ppru.
68. NICHD. Making medicines safer for children: NICHD-supported research in pediatric pharmacology. 2013. https://www.nichd.nih.gov/newsroom/resources/spotlight/120313-pediatric-pharmacology.
69. US Congress. *Public Law 105-115 Food and Drug Administration Modernization Act.* Washington, DC: Government Printing Office, 1997:86.
70. Food and Drug Administration. Regulations requiring manufacturers to assess the safety and effectiveness of new drugs and biological products in pediatric patients. Washington, DC: Federal Register, 1998:66631.
71. US District Count for the District of Columbia. Civil Action130-02898 October 17. 2002. Washington, DC: US District Court, 2002.
72. US Congress. *Public Law 108-155 Pediatric Research Equity Act.* Washignton, DC: Government Printing Office, 2003.
73. Stolbeg SG. The biotech death of Jesse Gelsinger. *New York Times.* New York, NY: New York Times, 1999:149–150.
74. Office of Public Health and Science and National Institutes of Health-Office of the Director. Statement of organization, functions, and delegations of authority. Washington, DC: Federal Register, 2000:37136.
75. Food and Drug Administration. Additional safeguards for children in clinical investigations of FDA regulated products. Washington, DC: Federal Register, 2001:20589.
76. US Congress. *Best Pharmaceuticals for Children Act. Public Law No. 107-109.* 2002.
77. US Congress. *Public Law 110-85, The Food and Drug and Administration Amendment Act of 2007 (FDAAA).* Washington, DC: US Federal Government, 2007.
78. US Congress. FDA Reauthorization Act (FDARA). Washington, DC: US Federal Government, 2017.
79. Food and Drug Administration. FDA pediatric exclusivity statistics. 2019. http://www.fda.gov/Drugs/DevelopmentApprovalProcess/DevelopmentResources/ucm049867.htm.
80. National Institutes of Health. Clinical trial definition. https://grants.nih.gov/policy/clinical-trials/CT-Definition-Case-Studies_1.7.19.pdf.
81. Ashcroft R. Equipoise, knowledge and ethics in clinical research and practice. *Bioethics* 1999;13(3–4):314–326.
82. Sioutos N, de Coronado S, Haber MW, et al. NCI Thesaurus: a semantic model integrating cancer-related clinical and molecular information. *J Biomed Inform* 2007;40(1):30–43.
83. Kahn MG, Bailey LC, Forrest CB, et al. Building a common pediatric research terminology for accelerating child health research. *Pediatrics* 2014;133(3):516–525.
84. Gipson DS, Kirkendall ES, Gumbs-Petty B, et al. Development of a pediatric adverse events terminology. *Pediatrics* 2017;139(1):e20160985.
85. Hill AB. *Conrolled clinical trials.* Oxford, England: Blackwell, 1960.
86. Council MR. Streptomycin treatment of pulmonary tuberculosis: a medical research council investigation. *BMJ* 1948;2(4582):769–782.
87. Austrian R, Mirick GS, Rogers DE, et al. The efficacy of modified oral penicillin therapy of pneumococcal lobar pneumonia. *Bull Johns Hopkins Hosp* 1951;88(3):264–269.
88. Tucker WB. *Experiences with controls in the study of the chemotherapy of tuberculosis.* in *Transactions of the 13th Veterans Administration Conference on chemotherapy of tuberculosis.* 1954.
89. Rheumatic Fever Working Party of the Medical Research Council of Great Britain and the Subcommittee of Principal Investigators of the American Council on Rheumatic Fever and Congenital Heart Disease. The evolution of rheumatic heart disease in children. *Circulation* 1960;22(4):503–515.

90. Stanley A. The cancer chemotherapy national service center antitumor testing program for antibiotics. In: *Developments in industrial microbiology*. Springer Science + Business Media, 1960:86–90.
91. Gehan EA, Schneiderman MA. Historical and methodological developments in clinical trials at the National Cancer Institute. *Stat Med* 1990;9(8):871–880; discussion 903–906.
92. Emanuel EJ, Wendler D, Grady C. What makes clinical research ethical? *JAMA* 2000;283(20):2701–2711.
93. Sutcliffe AG. Testing new pharmaceutical products in children. *BMJ* 2003;326(7380):64–65.
94. Sheiner LB. Learning versus confirming in clinical drug development. *Clin Pharmacol Ther* 1997;61(3):275–291.
95. Kauffman RE. Clinical research involving children. *Bioethics Forum* 2000;16(4):45–46.
96. Hirschfeld S. Comment—disclosing a diagnosis of HIV in pediatrics: providing the best possible care. *J Clin Ethics* 2001;12(2):158–160.
97. Henney J. Remarks to Pediatric Academic Socieites and American Academy of Pediatrics. 1999. https://wayback.archive-it.org/7993/20170406163039/https://www.fda.gov/NewsEvents/Speeches/ucm054212.htm.
98. Food and Drug Administration. Additional safeguards for children in clinical investigations of FDA regulated products. Washington, DC: Federal Register, 2001:20589–20600.
99. Food and Drug Administration. Additional safeguards for children in clinical investigations of food and drug administration-regulated products. Washington, DC: Federal Register, 2013:12937–12951.
100. International Conference on Harmonisation of Technical Requiremeents for Registration of Pharmaceuticals for Human Use. E11 Clinical investigation of medicinal products in the pediatric population. 2017. https://database.ich.org/sites/default/files/E11_R1_Addendum.pdf.
101. Food and Drug Administration. *Pediatric oncology subcommittee meeting notice*. Washington, DC: Federal Register, 2002:61344.
102. Harvey A, Towner E, Peden M, et al. Injury prevention and the attainment of child and adolescent health. *Bull World Health Organ* 2009;87(5):390–394.
103. Sheiner LB, Steimer JL. Pharmacokinetic/pharmacodynamic modeling in drug development. *Annu Rev Pharmacol Toxicol* 2000;40(1):67–95.
104. Biomarkers Definitions Working Group. Biomarkers and surrogate endpoints: preferred definitions and conceptual framework. *Clin Pharmacol Ther* 2001;69(3):89–95.
105. Menetski JP, Austin CP, Brady LS, et al. The FNIH Biomarkers Consortium embraces the BEST. *Nat Rev Drug Discov* 2019;18(8):567–568.
106. Leptak C, Menetski JP, Wagner JA, et al. What evidence do we need for biomarker qualification? *Sci Transl Med* 2017;9(417):eaal4559.
107. Menetski JP, Hoffmann SC, Cush SS, et al. The foundation for the National Institutes of Health Biomarkers consortium: past accomplishments and new strategic direction. *Clin Pharmacol Ther* 2019;105(4):829–843.
108. Fleming TR, DeMets DL. Surrogate end points in clinical trials: are we being misled? *Ann Intern Med* 1996;125(7):605–613.
109. Massie BM, Berk MR, Brozena SC, et al. Can further benefit be achieved by adding flosequinan to patients with congestive heart failure who remain symptomatic on diuretic, digoxin, and an angiotensin converting enzyme inhibitor? Results of the flosequinan-ACE inhibitor trial (FACET). *Circulation* 1993;88(2):492–501.
110. Packer M, Narahara KA, Elkayam U, et al. Double-blind, placebo-controlled study of the efficacy of flosequinan in patients with chronic heart failure. Principal Investigators of the REFLECT Study. *J Am Coll Cardiol* 1993;22(1):65–72.
111. Massie BM, Shah NB, Pitt B, et al. Importance of assessing changes in ventricular response to atrial fibrillation during evaluation of new heart failure therapies: experience from trials of flosequinan. *Am Heart J* 1996;132(1 Pt 1):130–136.
112. Packer M, Pitt B, Rouleau JL, et al. Long-term effects of flosequinan on the morbidity and mortality of patients with severe chronic heart failure: primary results of the PROFILE trial after 24 years. *JACC Heart Fail* 2017;5(6):399–407.
113. Cardiac Arrhythmia Suppression Trial Investigators. Preliminary report: effect of encainide and flecainide on mortality in a randomized trial of arrhythmia suppression after myocardial infarction. *N Engl J Med* 1989;321(6):406–412.
114. Flecainide and CAST. *Lancet* 1989;2(8661):481–482.
115. Bigger JT Jr. The events surrounding the removal of encainide and flecainide from the Cardiac Arrhythmia Suppression Trial (CAST) and why CAST is continuing with moricizine. *J Am Coll Cardiol* 1990;15(1):243–245.
116. Echt DS, Liebson PR, Mitchell LB, et al. Mortality and morbidity in patients receiving encainide, flecainide, or placebo. The Cardiac Arrhythmia Suppression Trial. *N Engl J Med* 1991;324(12):781–788.
117. Akiyama T, Pawitan Y, Greenberg H, et al. Increased risk of death and cardiac arrest from encainide and flecainide in patients after non-Q-wave acute myocardial infarction in the Cardiac Arrhythmia Suppression Trial. CAST Investigators. *Am J Cardiol* 1991;68(17):1551–1555.
118. The International Chronic Granulomatous Disease Cooperative Study Group. A controlled trial of interferon gamma to prevent infection in chronic granulomatous disease. The International Chronic Granulomatous Disease Cooperative Study Group. *N Engl J Med* 1991;324(8):509–516.
119. Mouy R, Seger R, Bourquin JP, et al. Interferon gamma for chronic granulomatous disease. *N Engl J Med* 1991;325(21):1516–1517.
120. Gallin JI. Interferon-gamma in the treatment of the chronic granulomatous diseases of childhood. *Clin Immunol Immunopathol* 1991;61(2 Pt 2):S100–S105.
121. Riggs BL, Seeman E, Hodgson SF, et al. Effect of the fluoride/calcium regimen on vertebral fracture occurrence in postmenopausal osteoporosis. Comparison with conventional therapy. *N Engl J Med* 1982;306(8):446–450.
122. Riggs BL, Hodgson SF, O'Fallon WM, et al. Effect of fluoride treatment on the fracture rate in postmenopausal women with osteoporosis. *N Engl J Med* 1990;322(12):802–809.
123. Kinsella JP, Cutter GR, Walsh WF, et al. Early inhaled nitric oxide therapy in premature newborns with respiratory failure. *N Engl J Med* 2006;355(4):354–364.
124. Ballard RA, Truog WE, Cnaan A, et al. Inhaled nitric oxide in preterm infants undergoing mechanical ventilation. *N Engl J Med* 2006;355(4):343–353.
125. Barrington KJ, Finer N, Pennaforte T, et al. Nitric oxide for respiratory failure in infants born at or near term. *Cochrane Database Syst Rev* 2017;1:CD000399.
126. Barrington KJ, Finer N, Pennaforte T. Inhaled nitric oxide for respiratory failure in preterm infants. *Cochrane Database Syst Rev* 2017;1:CD000509.
127. Cole FS, Alleyne C, Barks JD, et al. NIH Consensus Development Conference statement: inhaled nitric-oxide therapy for premature infants. *Pediatrics* 2011;127(2):363–369.
128. Noel CJ. Pick any two-fast, good, cheap. http://mercury.lcs.mit.edu/~jnc/.
129. Arts SE, Abu-Saad HH, Champion GD, et al. Age-related to lidocaine-prilocaine (EMLA) emulsion and effect of music distraction on the pain of intravenous cannulation. *Pediatrics* 1994;93(5):797–8010.
130. Chambers CT, Craig KD. An intrusive impact of anchors in children's faces pain scales. *Pain* 1998;78(1):27–37.
131. Johnston CC, Stevens B, Arbess G. The effect of the sight of blood and use of decorative adhesive bandages on pain intensity ratings by preschool children. *J Pediatr Nurs* 1993;8(3):147–151.
132. Kotiniemi LH, Ryhanen PT, Moilanen IK. Behavioural changes in children following day-case surgery: a 4-week follow-up of 551 children. *Anaesthesia* 1997;52(10):970–976.
133. Lander J, Fowler-Kerry S. TENS for children's procedural pain. *Pain* 1993;52(2):209–216.
134. Ljungman G, Kreuger A, Andréasson S, et al. Midazolam nasal spray reduces procedural anxiety in children. *Pediatrics* 2000;105(1 Pt 1):73–78.
135. Santavirta N, Björvell H, Solovieva S, et al. Coping strategies, pain, and disability in patients with hemophilia and related disorders. *Arthritis Rheum* 2001;45(1):48–55.
136. Goodenough B, Thomas W, Champion GD, et al. Unravelling age effects and sex differences in needle pain: ratings of sensory intensity and unpleasantness of venipuncture pain by children and their parents. *Pain* 1999;80(1):179–190.
137. Aho AC, Erickson MT. Effects of grade, gender, and hospitalization on children's medical fears. *J Dev Behav Pediatr* 1985;6(3):146–153.
138. Bruusgaard D, Smedbråten BK, Natvig B. Bodily pain, sleep problems and mental distress in schoolchildren. *Acta Paediatr* 2007;89(5):598–600.
139. Hirschfeld S. Pain as a complication of HIV disease. *AIDS Patient Care STDS* 1998;12(2):91–108.
140. Guite JW, Walker LS, Smith CA, et al. Children's perceptions of peers with somatic symptoms: the impact of gender, stress, and illness. *J Pediatr Psychol* 2000;25(3):125–135.
141. Chambers CT, Craig KD, Bennett SM. The impact of maternal behavior on children's pain experiences: an experimental analysis. *J Pediatr Psychol* 2002;27(3):293–301.
142. Food and Drug Administration. *General clinical pharmacology considerations for pediatric studies for drugs and biological products*. Silver Spring, MD: Food and Drug Administration, 2014.
143. Turner MA, Catapano M, Hirschfeld S, et al. Paediatric drug development: the impact of evolving regulations. *Adv Drug Deliv Rev* 2014;73:2–13.
144. Food and Drug Administration. *Leveraging existing clinical data for extrapolation to pediatric uses of medical devices*. Silver Spring, MD: Food and Drug Admininistration, 2016.
145. Turner MA, Hirschfeld S. Frameworks for evaluating medicines in children. *Clin Ther* 2017;39(10):1949–1958.
146. European Medicines Agency. Reflection paper on the use of extrapolation in the development of medicines for paediatrics. London, England: European Medicines Agency, 2018:20.
147. Dunne J, Rodriguez WJ, Murphy MD, et al. Extrapolation of adult data and other data in pediatric drug-development programs. *Pediatrics* 2011;128(5):e1242–e1249.
148. Ollivier C, Thomson A, Manolis E, et al. Commentary on the EMA Reflection Paper on the use of extrapolation in the development of medicines for paediatrics. *Br J Clin Pharmacol* 2019;85(4):659–668.
149. Higgins JPT, Chandler J, Cumpston M, et al. *Cochrane handbook for systematic reviews of interventions*, 2nd ed. Chichester, England: John Wiley & Sons, 2019:720.
150. Brown CA, Lilford RJ. The stepped wedge trial design: a systematic review. *BMC Med Res Methodol* 2006;6:54.
151. Mdege ND, Man MS, Taylor Nee Brown CA, et al. Systematic review of stepped wedge cluster randomized trials shows that design is particularly used to evaluate interventions during routine implementation. *J Clin Epidemiol* 2011;64(9):936–948.
152. Hargreaves JR, Copas AJ, Beard E, et al. Five questions to consider before conducting a stepped wedge trial. *Trials* 2015;16(1):350.
153. Johnson DE, Wolfgang GH. Predicting human safety: screening and computational approaches. *Drug Discov Today* 2000;5(10):445–454.
154. Hirschfeld S, Zajicek A. What could the future of safety monitoring look like? *Ther Innov Regul Sci* 2019;53(5):590–600.
155. Hirschfeld S. Pediatric patients and drug safety. *J Pediatr Hematol Oncol* 2005;27(3):122–124.
156. Bonhoeffer J, Kochhar S, Hirschfeld S, et al. Global alignment of immunization safety assessment in pregnancy—The GAIA project. *Vaccine* 2016;34(49):5993–5997.
157. Jones CE, Munoz FM, Spiegel HM, et al. Guideline for collection, analysis and presentation of safety data in clinical trials of vaccines in pregnant women. *Vaccine* 2016;34(49):5998–6006.
158. Kochhar S, Bonhoeffer J, Jones CE, et al. Immunization in pregnancy clinical research in low-and middle-income countries—study design, regulatory and safety considerations. *Vaccine* 2017;35(48 Pt A):6575–6581.
159. Connor EM, Smoyer WE, Davis JM, et al. Meeting the demand for pediatric clinical trials. *Sci Transl Med* 2014;6(227):227fs11.
160. Sheehan J, Hirschfeld S, Foster E, et al. Improving the value of clinical research through the use of Common Data Elements. *Clin Trials* 2016;13(6):671–676.
161. Hirschfeld S, Saint-Raymond A. Pediatric regulatory initiatives. *Handb Exp Pharmacol* 2011;205:245–268.
162. White IR. Book review: Nonparametric statistics for health care research. Statistics for small samples and unusual distributions. Marjorie A. Pett, Page Publications. Thousand Oaks, 1997. No. of pages: 305. Price: £22. ISBN 0-8039-7039-0. *Stat Med* 1998;17(19):2287–2288.
163. Hayden GF. Biostatistical trends in pediatrics: implications for the future. *Pediatrics* 1983;72(1):84–87.
164. Pocock SJ, Hughes MD, Lee RJ. Statistical problems in the reporting of clinical trials. A survey of three medical journals. *N Engl J Med* 1987;317(7):426–432.
165. Hirschfeld S. *Common errors associated with FDA submissions*. In: *DIA Conference on Electronic Submissions*, Washington DC, 1999.

CHAPTER

2

Edmund V. Capparelli

Clinical Pharmacokinetics in Infants and Children

INTRODUCTION

Considerable growth has occurred in a number of new chemical and biologic pediatric treatments during the last 30 years. Appropriate use of these agents in pediatric patients requires determining the safe and effective dosage for infants and children. A rational approach to determining appropriate dosage requires understanding the pharmacokinetic (PK) and pharmacodynamic (PD) properties of a drug in the population in which it is being used. Optimal therapy uses knowledge of a drug's PK to determine the dosage with a given formulation that will achieve desired drug concentrations and effects for a particular infant or child. In this setting, PK represents the mathematical description of drug metabolism and movement through a pediatric patient. PD describes the relationship of drug concentrations at the site of action and the magnitude of responses, both therapeutic and toxic. In simplified terms, PK describes what the body does to the drug, and PD describes what the drug does to the body (Fig. 2.1).

Knowing the right dosage for an individual is as important as selection of the correct drug. Determining the dosage for an individual patient that maximizes clinical benefit yet minimizes toxicity requires knowledge of the general PK and PD properties of the drug in the population, the variability of these properties, and the important physiologic determinants of this variability. Some of the PK and PD variability may be explained by formulation-, genetic-, age-, size-, and disease-related effects. Even when the sources of PK and PD variability cannot be identified or linked to clinical characteristics, understanding the range of concentrations and responses to a dosing regimen is necessary in the development of rational treatment strategies.

The PK of most drugs can be well described by a few key parameters. The two most important are volume of distribution, V_d, and clearance, CL. The elimination half-life, $t_{1/2}$, and associated elimination rate constant, K, are also widely determined and useful to determine dosing frequency. Following nonparenteral administration (such as oral, intramuscular, subcutaneous, or inhaled), bioavailability and absorption rate parameters are also necessary to describe a drug's PK behavior. Through these PK parameters, a dosing regimen can be derived to achieve target drug concentrations or range of concentrations where the desirable effect is likely and toxicity is minimal. Clinical PD endpoint measurements and related biomarkers are often highly variable and can require study of many individuals in multiple studies to understand the exposure–effect relationship. To develop appropriate target concentrations, PD models that describe the maximal effect, E_{max}, and concentration that achieves half of the maximal effect, EC_{50}, as either inhibitory or stimulatory influences on disease processes can be used. Methods for calculating these parameters and clinical (physiologic and pathologic) factors that affect them are presented in this chapter.

VOLUME OF DISTRIBUTION

After a drug is administered, it does not stay confined in the circulating blood pool. The drug diffuses into tissues, organs, and other fluid spaces, where it exerts its actions. However, when measuring drug concentrations, we are usually limited to collecting serum or plasma samples from the circulating blood pool and determining drug concentrations in these matrices. This serves as a surrogate for the drug concentration at the site of action. Therefore, it is useful to relate drug concentration measured in plasma to the total amount of drug in the body. The volume of distribution, V_d, is a proportionality constant that relates the drug concentration to the total amount of drug in the body and can be represented as

$$V_d = \frac{A}{C_p}$$

where A is the total amount of drug in the body and C_p is the drug concentration in plasma. The direct clinical application of this PK parameter is that it can determine a loading dose:

$$\text{Loading dose} = C_{\text{p-desired}} \cdot V_d$$

It can be defined in relation to blood concentrations, plasma or serum concentrations, or unbound concentrations (V_{db}, V_{dp}, or V_{du}, respectively). For a given drug, each of these drug concentration measurements may have different values; thus, V_d is relative to the matrix from which concentrations were measured. If, after bolus administration, a drug were to equilibrate incautiously between plasma and tissues, V_{dp} can easily be estimated as

$$V_{dp} = \frac{\text{Dose}}{C_{p0}}$$

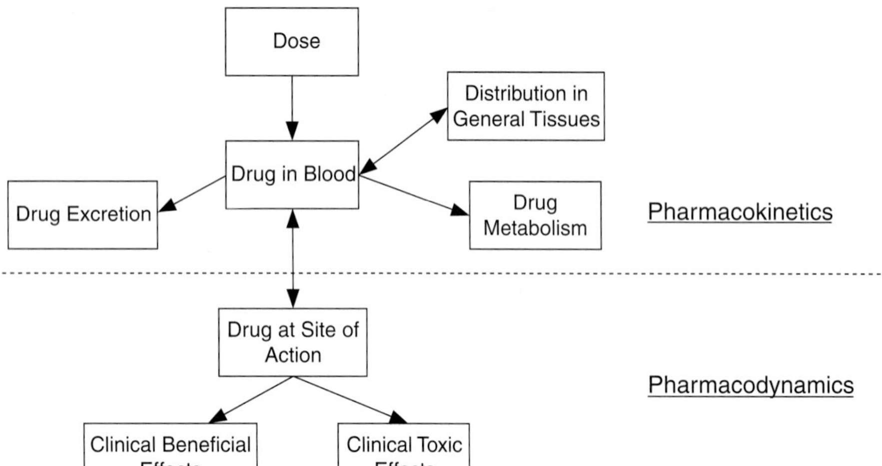

Figure 2.1 Schematic representation of the components that make up the pharmacokinetic–pharmacodynamic interface.

where C_{p0} is the drug concentration in plasma at time zero or immediately after drug administration (Fig. 2.2). This represents a *one-compartment* model with a single fixed V_{dp} value. Distribution of drug out of blood and into other fluids and tissues takes time; so "true" one-compartment drug behavior is almost never encountered. However, if distribution is very rapid relative to elimination or absorption (following oral administration), a one-compartment model can adequately describe the drug concentration-versus-time profile. More commonly, after intravenous administration, a rapid fall in drug concentrations is followed by a slower disappearance of drug. This multiphasic pattern of drug concentrations requires more complicated models characterized by multiple compartments with differential equations describing the movement of the drug between compartments and overall drug elimination. The most common model in this situation is the *two-compartment model* (Fig. 2.3). In this setting, drug concentrations initially fall rapidly because of distribution of the drug out of blood into tissues followed by a slower decline because of elimination. The initial distribution phase is also known as the alpha (α) phase and the elimination period as the beta (β) phase. For a few drugs, the redistribution out of tissues is a slower process than elimination through metabolism or excretion. In these settings, the terminal β phase may represent redistribution rather than elimination. It is important to recognize that these V_ds do not represent true physical tissue or fluid spaces per se but are greatly influenced by body composition, physiologic processes, and the chemical and physical properties of the drug. Therefore, a drug that has a much higher affinity for extravascular tissue than for plasma may have a V_d that is in excess of true body size (greater than 1 L per kg). However, it is possible to set a minimum value for V_d at the blood or plasma volume. Thus, no drug can have a V_d less than total intravascular plasma volume, or about 50 mL per kg. In multicompartment models, various methods can be used to calculate V_d. A common approach is to estimate V_d from the terminal β phase as follows:

$$V_{d\beta} = \frac{\text{Dose}}{(\text{AUC} \cdot \beta)}$$

where *AUC* is the area under the concentration–time curve after a single dose. An alternative method used to calculate V_d is the noncompartmental approach. With this method, V_d is defined as V_d at a steady state, V_{dss}; this is calculated using the following equation:

$$V_{dss} = \frac{\text{Dose} \cdot \text{AUMC}}{\text{AUC}^2}$$

where *AUMC* is the area under the first moment curve (concentration × time vs. time). The related fraction *AUMC/AUC* equals the mean time that drug molecules remain in the body and is referred to as the mean residence time (*MRT*). From a theoretical basis, $V_{dss} = V_{dc} + V_{dp}$, where c and p are the central and peripheral compartments, respectively. Although this method has the advantage of being relatively independent of terminal slope determination, it requires a much longer sample collection duration to characterize the *AUMC* from the first moment curve (because this curve is less "steep" than the concentration vs. time curve, Fig. 2.4). It also requires estimating an absorption input parameter (mean absorption time, *MAT*) as a correction factor when estimating V_d for drugs that are not administered as an intravenous bolus.

Although the volume of distribution does not represent a true physical space, changes in body composition seen throughout infancy and childhood can have a predictable impact on the volume of distribution based on a drug's chemical and physical properties. Newborn infants have a higher proportion of

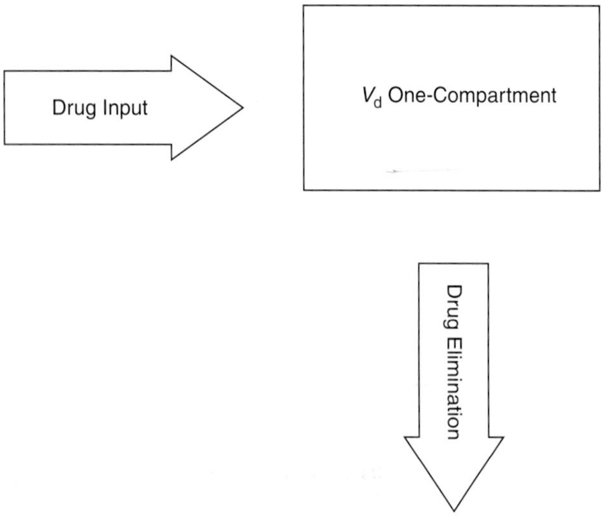

Figure 2.2 Basic one-compartment model.

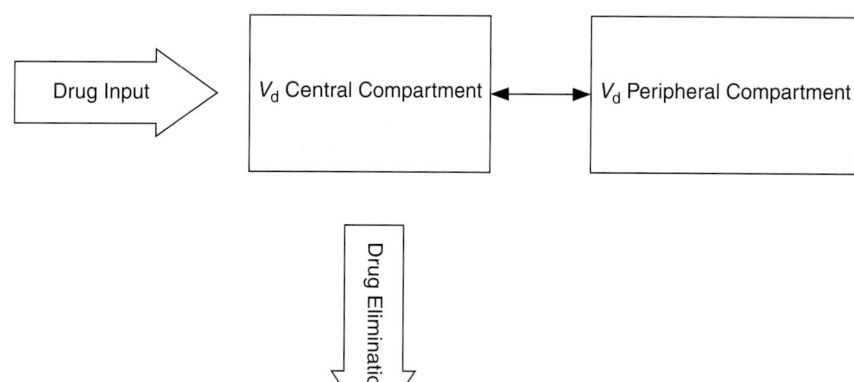

Figure 2.3 Basic two-compartment model. Drug distributes between central and peripheral compartments and is eliminated from the central compartment.

extracellular and total body water than older populations, and thus drugs that are distributed freely in water have larger volumes of distribution in newborns. Accordingly, aminoglycoside antibiotics, which are highly polar and hydrophilic and are distributed primarily into extracellular fluid, have approximately double the volume of distribution in newborns as in adults. Preterm newborns have a reduced percentage of total body fat. Thus, for lipophilic drugs, the volume of distribution may be reduced compared to that in adults.

Differences in drug binding across age groups can affect its V_d. Whereas drugs can bind to tissue components and plasma proteins, only the free (unbound) drug equilibrates. Thus, with newborns and certain diseases in which albumin and α-1-acid glycoprotein levels are low, highly bound drugs will have a greater free fraction (unbound/total drug concentration) in plasma, and more drug will distribute out of the plasma compartment into tissues. This will have the net effect of a higher V_d for total drug, although the V_{du} may be similar. While unbound drug concentrations may be more representative of the "effective" concentration seen at the site of action, they are not routinely measured because their measurements require more sensitive, time-consuming, and expensive assays. In most clinical situations, alterations in protein binding will not have a significant impact on therapy but can greatly impact the interpretation of measured (total) drug concentrations.

DISTRIBUTION INTO SPECIFIC TISSUES

When acute drug effects are of critical importance, such as in induction of anesthesia or in treatment of shock, the distribution characteristics of a drug are integral to its therapeutic utility. In general, distribution characteristics for drugs used in the treatment of chronic diseases are of lesser clinical importance. One important exception relates to target sites that a drug may not access easily. Whereas most distribution is based on concentration gradients and passive diffusion, in some tissues drug access is limited by tight junctions in the endothelium and active drug transport. For many drugs, free concentrations do not come into true equilibrium within the central nervous system due to these processes. P-glycoprotein and other active transporters pump various drugs out of the central nervous system and greatly reduce the overall effective penetration into this site.

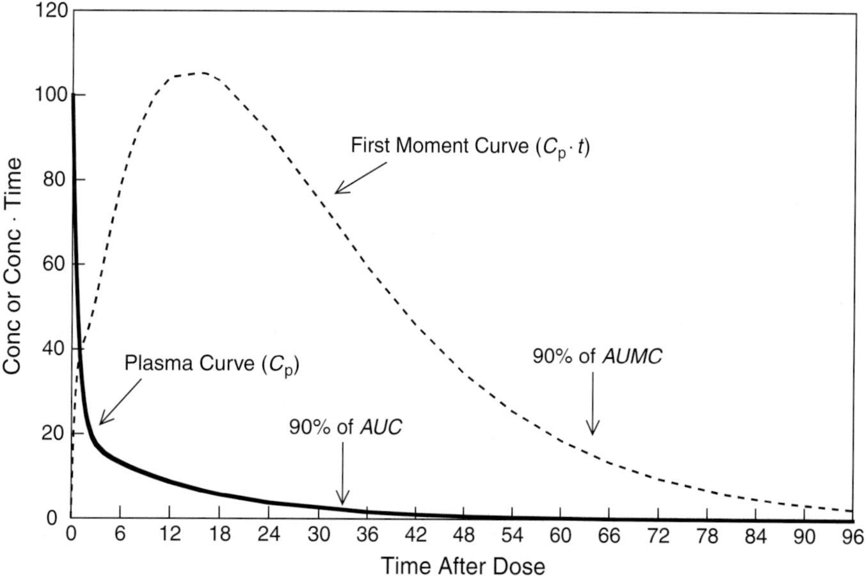

Figure 2.4 Concentration-versus-time and first moment curve (concentration × time vs. time) for a drug exhibiting pronounced multicompartment pharmacokinetics. Ninety percent of the area under the concentration-versus-time curve (*AUC*) can be captured with sampling out to 36 hours. To characterize the same portion of the first moment curve (*AUMC*) requires collecting samples nearly twice as long.

CLEARANCE

Drug clearance (CL) is a measure of drug elimination. It represents the volume of blood or plasma from which the drug is completely removed per unit of time. It is analogous to creatinine clearance as an assessment of renal function. It is the ratio of the rate of elimination or extraction divided by the drug concentration and can be mathematically defined as

$$CL = \frac{\text{Rate of elimination}}{C_p}$$

At steady state, whereby definition drug input equals drug elimination, this equation can be rearranged to

$$\text{Dose (rate in)} = CL \cdot C_{pave}$$

Thus, CL dictates the average steady-state concentration, C_{pave}, that will be achieved from a given dosing regimen. It can also be expressed in terms of mass balance for the organ of elimination. The rate of drug clearance from an eliminating organ is the product of the blood flow, Q, and the extraction ratio (ER) from arterial blood of that organ. An organ's ER is determined from arterial concentration, C_{pA}, reaching the organ and venous concentration, C_{pV}, leaving the organ of elimination and can be expressed as

$$ER = \frac{(C_{pA} - C_{pV})}{C_{pA}}$$

It can range from 0 (no extraction) to 1 (complete extraction). An important mathematical property regarding CL is that it can be separated into its individual components. The two most common organs of drug elimination are the liver and the kidney. The liver metabolizes drugs and can also excrete drugs and drug metabolites in bile. The kidney filters and excretes drugs and drug metabolites. Occasionally, other tissues contribute significantly to a drug's clearance. Therefore, overall CL can be expressed as

$$CL_{total} = CL_{hepatic} + CL_{renal} + CL_{other}$$

For most drugs, CL is constant over the range of concentration encountered clinically. When a drug's CL is independent of concentration, the elimination is referred to as first order. In this setting, there is a linear relationship between the logarithm of drug concentration and time during drug elimination. With first-order elimination, changes in dosing lead to proportional changes in drug concentrations. Clearance can be estimated by model-based methods through fitting the observed concentration-versus-time profile to an appropriate PK model. Following intravenous administration, CL (and V_d) can be determined using a *one-compartment* model through iterative fitting of drug concentrations to the following equation:

$$C_{p(t)} = \frac{\text{Dose}}{V_d} e^{-t \cdot CL/V_d}$$

Alternatively, CL can be estimated using noncompartmental methods from AUC. The AUC can be approximated following intensive sampling using the trapezoidal method. This is the summation of the area of trapezoids estimated from sequential, intensively collected plasma concentrations with the area of each individual trapezoid equal to $[(C_{pi} + C_{pi+1})/2] \cdot (t_{i+1} - t_i)$, and the final area after the last trapezoid can be estimated as $C_{p\text{-}last}/\lambda_z$, where λ_z is the terminal slope of the log plasma concentration-versus-time curve. From the AUC, the CL following a single intravenous dose can be calculated as

$$CL = \frac{\text{Dose}}{\text{AUC}_{0-\infty}}$$

Clearance may also be defined with respect to unbound drug concentrations. For drugs with protein binding, unbound drug concentrations are always less than the total drug concentrations, and thus AUC for unbound drug concentration is always lower than AUC for total drug concentration. Because clearance is inversely related to AUC, the calculated clearance for unbound drug is greater than that for total drug.

RENAL CLEARANCE

Many drugs undergo elimination into the urine by the kidneys. This occurs via filtration through the glomerulus and active secretion of acids and bases, which occurs primarily in the proximal tubule. Typically, only free or unbound drugs are filtered by the glomerulus into the urine; thus, renal elimination via filtration equals glomerular filtration rate (GFR) $\cdot$ f_u, where f_u is the unbound fraction of the drug in serum. Separate active transport systems exist for acid (anion) and base (cation) secretion by the kidneys. Drug elimination by filtration and active secretion can be mitigated by reabsorption of the drug along the proximal and distal tubules as well as the collecting duct. Reabsorption is primarily a passive process; however, its impact can be pronounced. Because the great majority of water that is filtered by the glomerulus is reabsorbed, drugs with favorable physical–chemical properties (small, nonpolar) will follow the water and be reabsorbed as well. The reabsorption of drugs with pK_a values in the range of urinary pH can be markedly influenced by acidification or alkalinization of urine. Mathematically, renal clearance equals renal excretion rate divided by average plasma concentration and can be determined from serial blood and urine collections using the equation:

$$CL_{renal} = \frac{A_{e0-t}}{\text{AUC}_{0-t}}$$

where A_e is the cumulative drug excreted unchanged in the urine and AUC is derived from the plasma concentration-versus-time profile.

GFR can be estimated from serum creatinine or cystatin C in adults and is used to individualize dosing of drugs eliminated by renal mechanisms. Although GFR can also be estimated from serum creatinine in children, the relationship between measured serum creatinine and GFR is different between pediatric and adult populations. Age-specific equations have been developed for estimating GFR in pediatric populations; however, lower serum creatinine concentrations in children reduce the precision of these equations. In newborn infants, estimating the GFR from serum creatinine is confounded by the transplacental creatinine that infants receive from their mothers in utero. This additional maternally derived creatinine may bias estimates of GFR in newborns during the first few days of life.

HEPATIC CLEARANCE

The liver is the primary site of drug metabolism. Drug biotransformation is influenced by a drug's chemical and structural properties, which determine its affinity to various drug-metabolizing enzymes in the liver. Drug metabolism may also be influenced by hepatic blood flow and protein binding. Drugs with a great affinity for metabolizing enzymes are highly extracted and their metabolism is limited primarily by hepatic perfusion. Their hepatic clearance approaches and parallels hepatic blood flow. Changes in hepatic blood flow have much less impact on the clearance of those drugs with lower affinity for metabolizing enzymes or low hepatic extraction. However, for low-hepatic-extraction drugs, their total hepatic clearance is sensitive to changes in protein binding. Hepatic clearance of unbound drug can be used as a measure of the liver's overall ability to metabolize that drug. Hepatic clearance of unbound drug is also frequently referred to as intrinsic clearance, CL_{hu}. It is mathematically related to total hepatic clearance, CL_h, by multiplying with the fraction unbound:

$$CL_h = CL_{hu} \cdot f_u$$

Understanding the hepatic extraction of a compound aids in determining the impact that patient-specific factors, including age, genotype, drug–drug interactions, liver disease, and cardiac status, may have on hepatic clearance. Although it is easiest to think of hepatic extraction as fixed in an individual, drugs may impact their own metabolism either by autoinduction or by autoinhibition. In these settings, the hepatic extraction and CL_h will increase or decrease with exposure to the drug of interest; thus, single-dose PK studies will not accurately predict steady-state concentrations.

SATURABLE ELIMINATION

In some instances, CL is not independent of drug concentration, as the metabolizing enzyme or secretory pump gets overwhelmed by excessive drug. This is often referred to as nonlinear or Michaelis–Menten elimination. It is mathematically expressed as

$$\text{Rate of elimination} = \frac{V_{max} \cdot C_p}{(K_m + C_p)} \quad \text{or} \quad CL = \frac{V_{max}}{(K_m + C_p)}$$

where V_{max} is the maximum capacity of drug metabolism and K_m is the concentration at which metabolism is half of maximal. This equation is analogous to equations describing enzyme kinetic behavior. An important characteristic of this equation is that as drug input approaches V_{max}, small increases in dose can lead to very large increases in steady-state drug concentrations. Another category of nonlinear PK is zero-order elimination, where metabolism is constant regardless of drug concentration. This represents an extreme version of Michaelis–Menten kinetics where the drug concentration greatly exceeds K_m such that elimination is essentially equal to V_{max} at all experienced concentrations. This PK behavior is seen with ethanol.

PHARMACOKINETICS OF BIOLOGICS

The development of biologics as drugs has gained increased interest in the past 10 years. Most notably monoclonal antibodies (mAbs) are becoming important therapies for use in adults with oncology, inflammatory bowel disease, and other disorders. These agents are typically administered intravenously because of the volume. However, the injection volume of infant doses is much smaller and can be administered subcutaneously. Adults may also be able to receive larger doses subcutaneously in conjunction with hyaluronidase. mAb metabolism follow the metabolic fate of endogenous immunoglobulin s (IgGs) and are governed by different processes than typical standard small molecule drugs and are relatively slow. IgGs are not metabolized by typical drug-metabolizing enzymes (cytochrome P450 [CYP]s or uridine diphospho-glucuronosyltransferases [UGTs]) in the liver, nor are they eliminated renally or exhibit blood flow dependent PK. Instead their elimination is through the reticuloendothelial system (RES) where they are taken up via endocytosis. Within the endosome, they develop into lysosome where they undergo proteolysis. Of interest during this process is the fact that mAbs can bind to FcRn intracellularly, which protects them from metabolism, and a portion of these protected mAbs are returned intact to the circulation. Another unique characteristic of mAb PK is that they can be affected by the relative concentration of their antigen (Ag) target with a saturable elimination pathway because of mAb–Ag interactions. So, at mAb concentrations that greatly exceed the target Ag concentrations (high mAb/Ag ratio), the elimination of mAb is primarily dictated by the linear, nonspecific RES uptake and metabolism. However, at low mAb or high Ag concentrations, the mAb–Ag-mediated elimination may play a more prominent role and the PK will appear very nonlinear. This phenomenon is referred to as *target-mediated drug disposition* (TMDD).

DRUG ABSORPTION

Whereas drugs that are administered intravenously are completely available to the systemic circulation, drugs administered by other routes may not enter into the systemic circulation intact. The proportion of a dose that enters into the systemic circulation intact is defined as the drug's bioavailability. By definition, the bioavailability following intravenous administration equals 1. *Absolute bioavailability* F is calculated as the ratio of exposures from an extravenous dose to an intravenous dose, or

$$F = \frac{AUC_{extravenous}}{AUC_{iv}}$$

If extravenous and intravenous doses are of different sizes, then

$$F = \frac{(AUC_{extravenous} \cdot Dose_{iv})}{(AUC_{iv} \cdot Dose_{extravenous})}$$

When PK data following intravenous administration are not available, the *relative bioavailability* between various formulations and routes of administration can be compared. PK parameters estimated exclusively from oral data are confounded by not knowing the dose of drug absorbed intact. Thus, the relative contribution of bioavailability in estimating CL and V_d cannot be determined. PK parameters from oral data are typically presented as apparent or oral parameters, specifically CL/F and V_d/F. Bioavailability less than 100% following oral administration can occur for a number of physiologic and drug formulation–related issues, including problems with drug dissolution or solubility and instability in gastric acid. In addition, gastrointestinal transit time, gastric acid secretion, and biliary and pancreatic exocrine function all can affect drug absorption. These are dynamic processes during the first years of life and can result in age-dependent bioavailability differences. Oral drugs may also undergo metabolism in the gut and liver before reaching the systemic circulation. Blood from the intestinal tract that contains the absorbed drug is carried to the liver by the portal vein, where it can be metabolized before reaching the general systemic circulation. The combined drug metabolism in the gut and in the liver via portal circulation before the drug has reached the systemic circulation is termed first-pass metabolism. Therefore, drugs exhibiting first-pass metabolism, such as morphine, may have excellent absorption but low bioavailability. Whereas most drug absorption from the gut is passive, active transport of drugs in enterocytes back into the lumen of the gut may also limit bioavailability. Other routes of drug administration, including intramuscular, subcutaneous, rectal, and inhaled, may have bioavailability less than 1.

Bioavailability characterizes the extent of absorption but drug entry into the body can also be characterized by the rate of drug absorption. Absorption rate is sometimes confused with bioavailability, as it can be influenced by some of the same formulation and physiologic processes that affect bioavailability. Intuitively, the rate of absorption dictates the onset of effect for rapidly acting drugs, but it can also determine the duration of effect for drugs that are also rapidly eliminated (Fig. 2.5). Absorption rate is most commonly characterized by peak time, t_{max}. Although this is relatively easy to obtain graphically, it reflects both absorption and elimination processes and is different following single-dose and multiple-dose administration. The most common mathematical model used to characterize oral drug absorption is the first-order absorption. This model is characterized by an absorption rate constant K_A, with the amount of drug absorbed per unit of time equal to K_A times the amount of drug remaining in the gut. Because very little drug absorption occurs in the stomach, a delay in the detection of drug in the systemic circulation is often observed during the first few minutes after oral drug administration. In this setting, a lag time can be utilized in conjunction with a first-order absorption model to describe this absorption pattern. Alternative absorption models with multiple first-order absorption compartments in serial (transit compartments), constant drug absorption (zero order), and convoluted functions with multiple rate constants affecting various fractions of the dose can also be used to describe drug input.

The rate and extent of oral drug absorption are dependent on a drug's chemical properties and formulation as well as physiologic characteristics of the patient and administration circumstances. Oral drug administration to infants and young children requires either liquid or chewable product formulations. These pediatric formulations may have significantly different absorption properties than solid oral dosage forms used in older populations. Extemporaneous compounding liquid pediatric formulations from adult dosage forms may also alter drug stability and thus limit the intended dose administered. The bioavailability of a drug may also be altered by the presence and composition of coadministered food. A true fasting state is difficult to achieve for drug administration in infants and the limited variety in their dietary intake can limit bioavailability of compounds that require high-fat meals for optimal absorption. Based on these factors, large, unanticipated differences between oral absorption in young pediatric and adult populations can be encountered.

HALF-LIFE

The elimination half-life, $t_{1/2}$, is defined as the time necessary for the drug concentration to decrease by 50%. After one half-life, 50% of the initial concentration remains; after two half-lives, 25% of the initial concentration remains; and so on. A related parameter is the elimination rate constant, K, that is related to $t_{1/2}$ by $K = 0.693/t_{1/2}$. During the elimination phase, K can be used to predict concentrations at any time t from the following equation (Fig. 2.6):

$$C_{pi\delta t} = C_{pi} \cdot e^{-K \cdot \Delta t}$$

where Δt is the time between the two concentrations C_{pi} and C_{pi+1} measured during the elimination phase. Half-life can also be used to describe drug accumulation. After one half-life, the drug concentration will be 50% of the ultimate steady-state value; after two half-lives, 75% of the steady-state value; and so on (Fig. 2.7 and Table 2.1). Drug accumulation approaches steady state asymptotically; after 3.3 to 5 half-lives on a constant-dosage regimen, drug concentrations are 90% to 97% of final steady-state values and can be effectively considered steady state. The exact proportion of steady-state concentration at any time t can be determined from

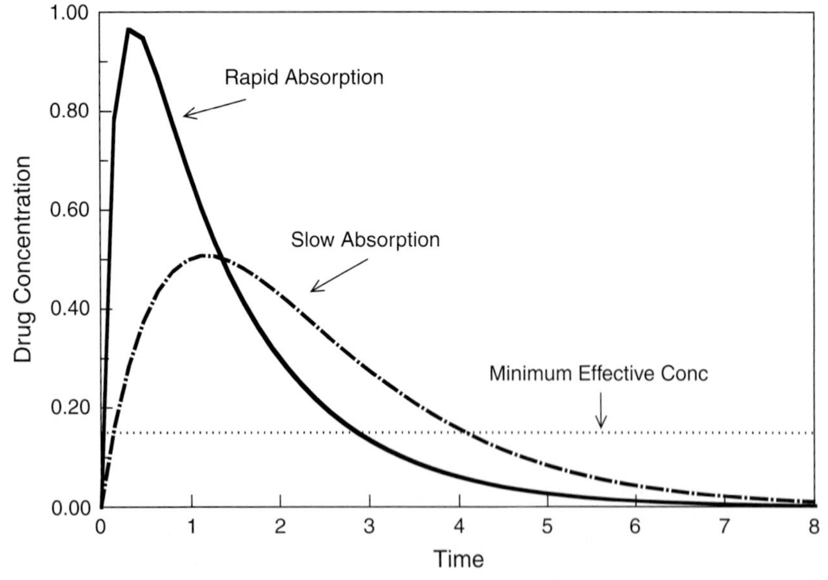

Figure 2.5 The impact of absorption rate on duration of action for drugs with rapid elimination. The slower absorption (K_A = 0.9 hour^{-1}) results in later and much lower peak than the rapidly absorbed formulation (K_A = 6.5 hour^{-1}). However, the more slowly absorbed formulation maintains higher concentrations later in the dose interval (the area under the curve [AUC]s are identical). This results in a longer total time above the minimum effective concentration.

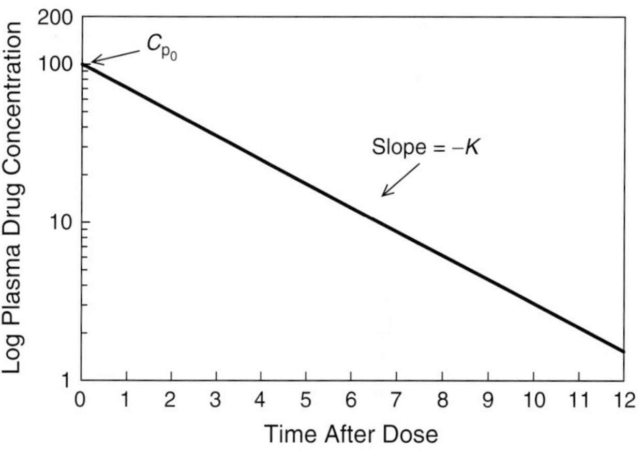

Figure 2.6 Concentration-versus-time profile for one-compartment drug, plotted as log concentration versus time, with the slope representing the elimination rate constant ($-K$).

$$\text{Proportion of steady state} = 1 - e^{-K \cdot t}$$

For drugs exhibiting first-order elimination (which includes most drugs), $t_{1/2}$ is independent of dose. It is mechanistically dependent on CL and V_d and can be described as

$$T_{1/2} = \frac{0.693 \cdot V_d}{CL}$$

For drugs with saturable or Michaelis–Menten elimination, $t_{1/2}$ has limited utility as a PK parameter because it is dynamic, increasing at higher drug concentrations. Whereas the general concept of half-life is easily grasped, it is often assumed that any change in half-life reflects a change in drug elimination. This is not necessarily true, as half-life alterations may be entirely due to changes in drug distribution. It is clear from the above equation that clinical situations that reduce a drug's CL or increase its V_d will be associated with an increase in that drug's $t_{1/2}$. Whereas $t_{1/2}$ does not indicate what drug concentrations will result from a given dosage, it is used to determine dosing intervals. Half-life dictates the peak/trough ratio and needs to be considered when constructing an appropriate dosing regimen for a drug.

TABLE 2.1 Relationship Between Half-Life and Portion of Drug Remaining and Accumulation

Half-Lives	*Percentage Remaining*	*Percentage Accumulation*
0.5	71	29
1	50	50
2	25	75
3.3	10	90
4	6	94
5	3	97
6.6	1	99

The elimination $t_{1/2}$ is most commonly determined from the terminal slope or "washout" portion of the concentration–time profile. For drugs that exhibit multicompartment PK, $t_{1/2}$ and the apparent elimination rate constant (λ_z or β for a two-compartment model) can also be determined in this manner (Fig. 2.8). However, care must be taken in estimating β to ensure that a sufficiently long portion of the log-linear concentration-versus-time profile is captured and that concentrations influenced by ongoing absorption or distribution are not included. The elimination rate constant and half-life can also be estimated from drug accumulation or urinary excretion profiles as well as derived from the area under the first moment curve ($K = 1/MRT$ and $t_{1/2} = 0.693 \cdot MRT$).

APPLICATION OF PHARMACOKINETIC PRINCIPLES TO MULTIPLE-DOSE REGIMENS

In most clinical situations, drugs are administered repeatedly at fixed intervals rather than as single doses. The goal is to maintain drug concentrations above a minimum effective target concentration associated with clinical benefit and below concentrations that are likely to result in toxicity, keeping drug concentrations

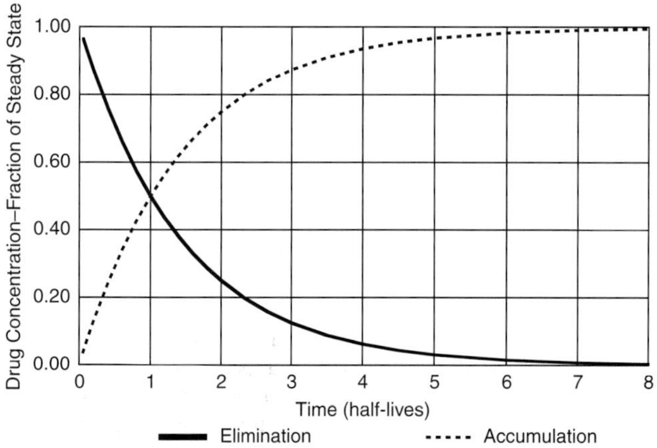

Figure 2.7 Symmetry and relationship between half-life and portion of drug remaining and accumulation with continuous infusion to steady state. After one half-life, the drug concentration is 50% of its initial value and the drug has accumulated to 50% of the steady-state level.

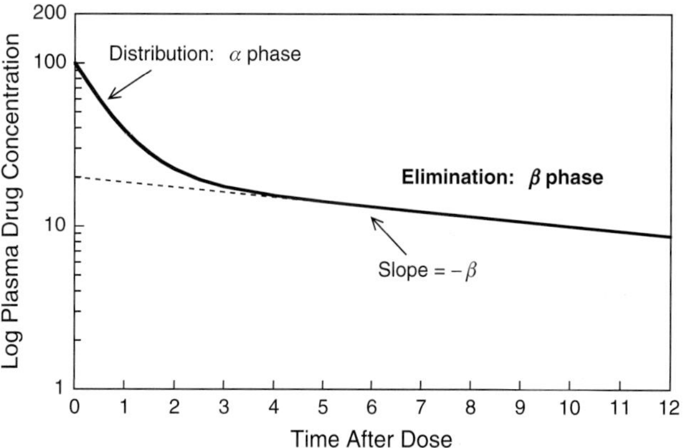

Figure 2.8 Concentration-versus-time profile for a two-compartment drug, plotted as log concentration versus time. The initial slope represents the distribution phase and rate constant, α, and the terminal, linear portion of the curve represents the elimination phase and rate constant β.

in this "therapeutic range" throughout the dosage interval. For drugs that exhibit linear or dose-independent PK, the PK parameters from a single dose can be used to predict drug concentrations that will result from various multiple-dose regimens. The contribution of each individual dose can be calculated and summed to determine the total concentration following multiple doses. This method of superposition can be used to determine non–steady-state and steady-state concentrations but becomes cumbersome if the number of doses included for steady-state determination is large. However, because the *AUC* during a dosing interval at steady state equals the sum of *AUCs* contributed from single doses at dosing intervals of τ ($AUC_{0-\tau}$ + $AUC_{\tau-2\tau}$ + $AUC_{2\tau-3\tau}$ + ⋯), the total $AUC_{0-\tau}$ (at steady state) is equal to AUC_{0-inf} for a single dose. Thus, steady-state clearance can be calculated from the following equation:

$$CL = \frac{\text{Dose}}{\text{AUC}_{0-\tau}}$$

Once steady state is achieved, an accumulation factor can determine concentrations at various times in the dosing interval. The rate of accumulation is independent of the dosing interval, but the magnitude of the peak/trough ratio increases with increasing dosing intervals (Fig. 2.9). Peak, trough, and average steady-state concentrations following repeated intravenous boluses can be easily determined using a one-compartment model from the following equations:

$$C_{\text{peak,ss}} = \frac{\text{Dose}}{V_d \cdot (1 - e^{-K \cdot \tau})}$$

$$C_{\text{trough,ss}} = C_{\text{peak,ss}} \cdot e^{-K \cdot \tau}$$

$$C_{\text{ave,ss}} = \frac{\text{Dose}}{CL \cdot \tau}$$

For example, for a drug with V_d = 2.0 L per kg and CL = 0.10 L per hour per kg (K = 0.05 hour^{-1}), a bolus dose of 100 mg per kg every 8 hours yields the following steady-state peak and trough concentrations:

$$C_{\text{peak,ss}} = \frac{100 \text{ mg/kg}}{[(2.0 \text{ L/kg}) \cdot (1 - e^{-0.05 \cdot 8})]} = 152 \text{ mg/L}$$

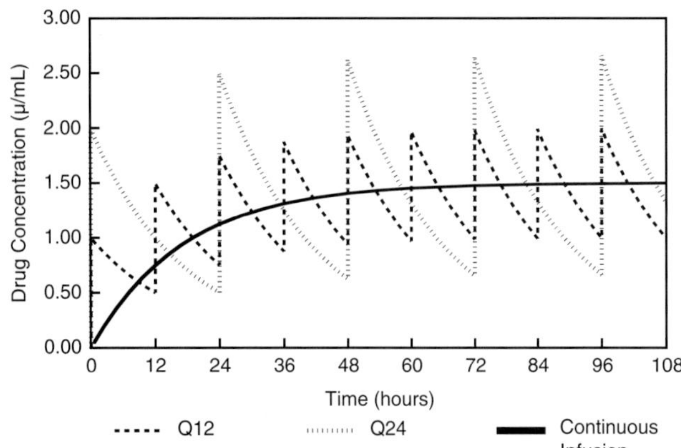

Figure 2.9 Impact of various dosing intervals on concentration-versus-time profile following multiple doses and same total daily dose. Average concentrations for all three regimens are identical, with peak/trough differences increasing with larger dose intervals.

$$C_{\text{trough,ss}} = 152 \cdot e^{-0.05 \cdot 8} = 102 \text{ mg/L}$$

$$C_{\text{ave,ss}} = \frac{100 \text{ mg/kg}}{(0.10 \text{ L/h/kg} \cdot 8 \text{ hr})} = 125 \text{ mg/L}$$

Whereas these equations predict drug concentrations after intravenous bolus administration, they can also approximate drug concentrations following oral administration if bioavailability, *F*, is added to the numerator and drug absorption is much more rapid than drug elimination (K_A much greater than K). If the absorption rate does not greatly exceed the elimination rate, use of these equations will result in overestimating the true peak and underestimating the true trough concentrations. To characterize drug concentrations following a single-dose oral administration using a one-compartment model with first-order absorption, the following equation can be used:

$$C_p(t) = \frac{F \cdot K_A \cdot \text{Dose} \cdot (e^{-K \cdot t} - e^{-K_A \cdot t})}{[V_d \cdot (K_A - K)]}$$

SIZE AND AGE EFFECTS ON PHARMACOKINETICS

Size is a critical element in understanding, analyzing, and applying principles of PK in pediatrics. Weight (*WT*) can range more than 100-fold between premature infants and adolescents and correlates strongly with age and other clinical characteristics that may also impact a drug's disposition. Pediatric PK parameters are most often scaled by body weight. This scaling approach has the advantage of being easy to calculate and apply to dosing resulting in milligram per kilogram dosing. However, many physiologic functions that affect drug clearance (renal function, cardiac output, and hepatic blood flow) do not scale directly to weight in a linear manner. Estimated body surface area (*BSA*) is an alternative scalar for many physiologic processes that affect drug disposition. Using *BSA* rather than weight to scale for size in children has been found empirically to provide a more linear relationship with clearance for many drugs. However, scaling volume of distribution with *BSA* may not be as linear as it is with weight. The use of *BSA* requires height measurements to estimate, is prone to calculation errors, and is primarily reserved for antineoplastic and other agents with very narrow therapeutic indices. A third approach to scaling clearance is the allometric method. Allometric scaling is used extensively in evaluating physiologic and preclinical PK data across animal species. Since the 1940s, it has been applied to adjusting drug doses in humans and is based on relating physiologic functions and morphology to body size. This approach suggests that $WT^{0.75}$ be used to scale clearance, and this scalar correlates closely with percentage of liver weight relative to body weight during the first 18 years of life (Fig. 2.10). It also suggests V_d be scaled by $WT^{1.0}$, which results in shorter half-lives in smaller, younger individuals, which is consistent with what is generally observed. The allometric approach produces similar clearance results to scaling by *BSA* without requiring a height measurement. However, like *BSA*, this method is prone to calculation errors and has limited clinical application for estimating dosage in individual children. It is important to recognize that these sizing approaches do not account for additional maturational effects on processes that impact PK during human development. Thus, in addition to

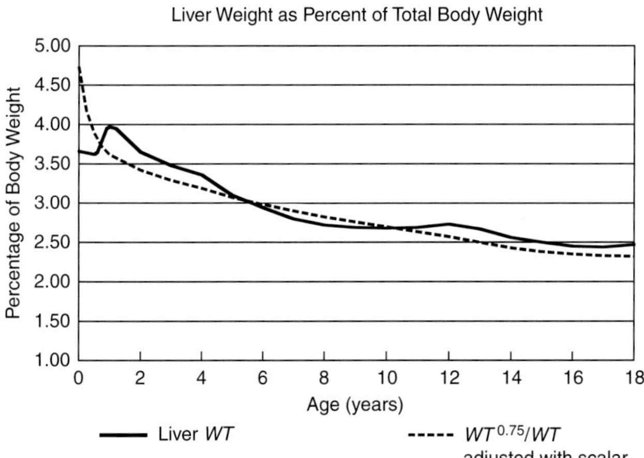

Figure 2.10 Liver size as function of age. The relative liver weight (WT) as percentage of total body weight shows decrease during infancy and childhood. This relationship closely mirrors the shape of the allometric scaling factor $WT^{0.75}/WT$ (adjusted by a scalar to superimpose the two curves).

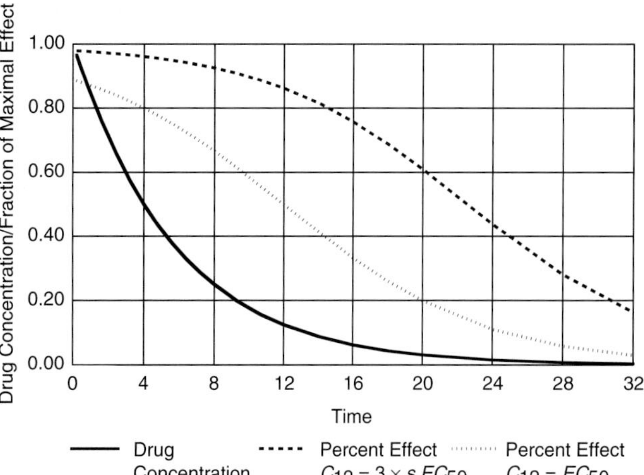

Figure 2.11 The pharmacokinetic–pharmacodynamic relationship of a sigmoid E_{max} model. Although the drug concentrations fall rapidly ($t_{1/2}$ = 4 hours), the pharmacodynamic effect persists and drops more slowly when the concentrations are well above the EC_{50}. At 12 hours postdose, the concentration is only 12.5% of the peak value, yet only 50% of the effect has been lost if the 12-hour concentration equals EC_{50}. If the 12-hour concentration is higher (three times the EC_{50}), less than 15% of the effect is lost in this interval. This persistence of effect allows dosing less frequently than half-life.

these size effects, additional components that account for developmental PK differences are necessary, especially in younger populations. Linked allometric scaling with maturation models for development of elimination pathways may be helpful to describe pediatric PK.

A more mechanistic approach can be used to describe pediatric PK based on changes in body composition through physiologic-based PK (PBPK). This approach incorporates organ sizes and tissue-specific drug partitioning along with organ blood flows to describe drug disposition in the human body as a system of blood flows and tissue partitioning. These models require a large number of differential equations to characterize the drug concentration-versus-time profile and thus cannot be used to estimate PK parameters based on individual patient's PK data. However, the PBPK approach is very useful for predicting the impact of physiologic and maturational changes on drug exposure in plasma and tissues. PBPK modeling is widely used in environmental toxicology to predict the disposition of chemicals in pediatric populations.

PHARMACODYNAMICS

A number of different PD models are used to describe drug action, and most include a monotonic component linking drug exposure and action. The most common are the E_{max} and related sigmoid E_{max} models, which are represented mathematically as

$$\text{Effect} = \frac{E_{max} \cdot C_p^{\gamma}}{(EC_{50}^{\gamma} + C_p^{\gamma})}$$

where E_{max} is the maximum effect, EC_{50} is the concentration that produces half-maximal effect, and γ is a shape constant. When γ equals 1, the sigmoid E_{max} simplifies to the E_{max} model. This model has its origins in receptor–ligand binding relationships and predicts that effects increase nearly in proportion to drug concentrations at low concentrations (well below EC_{50}), and effects increase in proportion to the logarithm of drug concentrations around EC_{50}. In situations in which drug concentrations greatly exceed EC_{50}, drug effects can be maintained despite relatively dramatic changes in drug concentrations (Fig. 2.11).

In some situations, E_{max} and related models can be directly linked to serum concentrations to describe rapidly occurring drug effects. However, a lag or hysteresis between serum drug concentrations and effects often exists. This can be due to two separate phenomena. The first type of lag can be due to distribution. This can be encountered with central nervous system–active drugs, which require distribution into the brain to produce their effects. The second delay occurs when the effects of drugs are mediated through synthesis or metabolism of endogenous moieties. In the latter situation, drug effects can occur through a cascade of processes, and overall homeostasis is altered only after the drug has caused endogenous intermediaries of effects to be synthesized or depleted. A group of indirect response PD models with E_{max} equation components can be used to describe these processes. Examples of drugs that have delayed effects through this mechanism include anti-inflammatory effects of glucocorticoids and anticoagulant effects of warfarin. PD effects may also be related to total drug exposure. In these situations, either very slow accumulation or irreversible changes accrue with continued exposure. This PD relationship commonly describes toxic effects, including those from heavy metals and antineoplastic agents that irreversibly bind to DNA.

Determining the PD parameters for a drug requires selection of appropriate effect measurements and mechanistically plausible models. PD parameter estimates are most robust when the effects are relatively direct and reproducible. The range of drug concentrations used to determine the PD parameters is also important. The use of a narrow range of concentrations may limit the ability to fully characterize the concentration–response relationship. A single paired drug concentration and associated response can be described by a variety of E_{max}–EC_{50} value combinations, so broad concentration–response measurements are desired. Although this broad dose range approach is used in the early phases of drug development for adults, PD studies in pediatrics typically have limited concentration–effect ranges. In addition, the use of indirect markers of drug effects, such as surrogate or biomarkers, can result in different PD parameter values based on the specific biomarker measured. Whereas methods to determine drug concentration are typically consistent across the age continuum studied, biomarkers appropriate in one age group may not be appropriate in another or may change with human development. These potential confounders should be addressed when calculating pediatric PD parameters. Lastly, even with high-quality surrogate markers, disease presentation and progression differences in pediatric subpopulations can lead to PD changes, particularly when the organ system affected undergoes significant development during infancy and childhood.

POPULATION PHARMACOKINETICS/ PHARMACODYNAMICS

Whereas detailed description of PK in individual subjects is determined for regulatory and research purposes, in most clinical circumstances precise determination of an individual's PK to optimize therapy is impractical. Summary data generated from intensive phase 1 PK studies are used to infer individual patient's PK characteristics and drug exposure from a specific dosing regimen. However, most of these studies are performed in relatively healthy and homogeneous populations with limited age ranges and are conducted under tightly controlled environments. Although this approach results in rapid generation of PK data, the patients studied may not reflect subpopulations that will frequently receive the drug clinically. Concomitant drugs, diseases, and patient characteristics encountered clinically with drug use, but avoided in intensive studies, may alter a drug's PK and PD. Thus, the dosing derived from tightly controlled phase 1 and phase 2a clinical trials may provide biased estimates of the larger population of subjects that will ultimately receive therapy. In addition, these studies provide little insight into the extreme PK/PD responses likely to be encountered on a given dose to the larger population. Accordingly, most phase 1 PK studies focus on average or median CL and V_d values with little attention directed to variability and sources of variability.

The use of sparse PK sampling in larger pediatric populations has been emphasized to better describe PK and PD using population analysis approaches. In this approach, the precision in the PK parameter estimates for individual participants is reduced by taking fewer evaluations per subject. However, less intensive sampling allows inclusion of a wider spectrum of participants likely to receive the drug clinically. Although reduction in frequency and number of samples has obvious appeal in pediatric populations, the ability of population methods to analyze unbalanced data collected at various times is also attractive in these populations. This method allows pooling of data across studies to provide a uniform, robust, single PK analysis rather than attempting to compare results of separate, smaller studies that are complicated by significant analysis methodology differences. The population PK method also regards variability differently than does the traditional intensive approach. Instead of avoiding variability by design, one goal of the population approach is to quantify both within- and between-participant variability and examine clinical characteristics that can explain between-participant variability to indicate alternative dosing requirements for specific subpopulations. It is a robust method and can be used to characterize the impact of age and development on drug PK (Fig. 2.12).

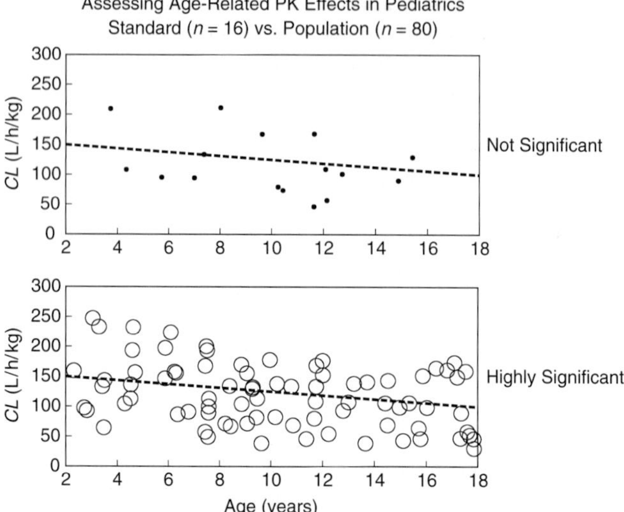

Figure 2.12 A comparison of intensive two-stage and population pharmacokinetic (PK) methods for detecting sources of PK variability such as age. This represents a typical simulation using 240 concentrations. In the intensive evaluation, 15 samples were used to precisely calculate the clearance in each of 16 subjects. In the population analysis, three samples collected in 80 subjects were used to describe the population PK. Individual clearance estimates were generated for graphical comparison by a Bayesian method. The size of the symbols is proportional to the relative error of the parameter estimate in each subject. Having fewer samples reduced individual subject parameter precision in the population analysis, but the population analysis was robust in detecting the age effect on clearance.

The population PK approach in pediatrics has been most widely applied in the newborn population, although there has been growing use in older pediatric populations. The ability to accommodate unbalanced designs allows one to incorporate both longitudinal and cross-sectional elements to assess maturation within a study. Whereas traditional PK studies have uniformly been unable to distinguish differences between in utero and postnatal maturation, appropriately designed population studies are able to tease out these different influences. The population method is also particularly useful for drugs with long half-lives or for drugs whose steady-state PK may be difficult to predict from a single-dose PK evaluation (autoinduction or inhibition of metabolism or excretion). In these instances, the logistics and ethical constraints of waiting for the drug to "wash out" to capture $AUC_{0\text{-inf}}$ following a single dose for a traditional PK analysis may preclude its study. Although clearance can be estimated from classically intensive steady-state data collected over a dosage interval, the resulting analyses assume dosing and collection times that are performed exactly on schedule. Even in experienced pediatric study environments, these assumptions can be violated. Although the classical intensive analysis has difficultly accounting for these variations, even when they are known, the population approach does not need to make the assumption of steady state if an exact dosing history is collected. The study of drug interactions is another area where population PK methods have significant value in pediatrics. The logistics of conducting traditional PK drug interaction studies is extremely difficult in pediatric populations, and these studies can often be more easily done using population approaches. However, potential drug interactions identified by population methods must be interpreted cautiously. Unless randomized, the relationship between concomitant therapies and altered PK is not causal and may serve only as a marker for other patient characteristics that may be responsible for the PK differences.

Whereas the primary goal of most population PK analyses is to describe the overall PK of the study group, estimates of individual subjects' PK parameters can be obtained through Bayesian post hoc analyses. This allows population PK studies to be nested into traditional phase 3 efficacy studies and provide estimates of individual drug exposure that can be used for exploratory analysis of potential PD relationships. This paradigm is being extensively used for regulatory purposes to look at drug exposure in subjects who experience toxicity or lack clinical benefit. Another outcome from population PK studies is the ability to get more accurate estimates of PK variability. Accurate estimates of the variance and covariance of PK parameters are essential for realistic simulations to evaluate the impact of various dosing strategies on drug exposure and ultimately clinical outcome.

Like other analysis methods, the population PK approach has limitations. It requires a high degree of expertise to perform these analyses, and the analysis process can be time-consuming. The underlying mathematical principles are complex, and if the data are not appropriate for the complexity of the drug, adequate characterization may not be possible. Thus, PK samples that are informative of all of the PK parameters to be estimated must be collected. Random samples or only trough samples may not be sufficient. Frequently, these samples are taken in outpatient settings, so there are additional assumptions of adherence to therapy that are not encountered in single-dose intensive studies. Assessing adherence in younger pediatric populations, where multiple caregivers may be involved, is challenging. Although population analyses allow collection of fewer samples per individual, this reduction of information per subject is compensated by collecting information from a larger number of subjects. As pediatric studies try to maximize the information generated, there is temptation to perform population PK studies from sparse samples in a small number of subjects. The results from these small studies must be viewed critically because they can generate unreliable parameter estimates.

The population method attempts to determine the sources of between-participant variability. As age, size, and many laboratory measures are highly correlated, it is important that pediatric population–based models have a mechanistic basis. Maturational changes may impact multiple PK parameters simultaneously and can be nonlinear. Thus, standard correlation screens of potential covariates and PK parameters may underappreciate important factors that drive pediatric PK variability. Even after accounting for age, gender, size, renal function, and pharmacogenomic differences, unexplained pediatric between-participant variability may still be largely due to unidentifiable causes.

SUMMARY

Understanding the PK and PD behavior of a drug for its use in the intended patient population is needed for rational and optimal drug therapy. Application of general PK principles, equations, and models is essential to determining appropriate pediatric dosages. Because the ontogeny of various elimination pathways can differ, detailed knowledge of a drug's PK behavior is important in determining when to expect significant age-specific PK. Significant variability in PK parameters exists and can result in variable drug exposure with similar doses. Defining the determinants of between-participant variability by developmental, genetic, and other clinical characteristics allows optimization of treatment for individual patients. Linking dosing information to population PK/PD (pop PK/PD) and disease models can facilitate informed and improved therapeutic decision making.

SUGGESTED READINGS

Anderson BJ, Meakin GH. Scaling for size: some implications for paediatric anaesthesia dosing. *Paediatr Anaesth* 2002;12:205–219.

Barrett JS, Della Casa Alberighi O, Läer S, et al. Physiologically based pharmacokinetic (PBPK) modeling in children. *Clin Pharmacol Ther* 2012;92(1):40–49.

Benet L, Galeazzi R. Noncompartmental determination of the steady-state volume of distribution. *J Pharm Sci* 1979;68:1071–1074.

Benet LZ, Hoener BA. Changes in plasma protein binding have little clinical relevance. *Clin Pharmacol Ther* 2002;71:115–121.

Capparelli EV, Lane JR, Romanowski GL, et al. The influences of renal function and maturation on vancomycin elimination in newborns and infants. *J Clin Pharmacol* 2001;41(9):927–934.

Capparelli EV, Mirochnick M, Dankner WM, et al. Pharmacokinetics and tolerance of zidovudine in preterm infants. *J Pediatr* 2003;142(1):47–52.

Chiba K, Ishizaki T, Miura H, et al. Michaelis–Menten pharmacokinetics of diphenylhydantoin and application in the pediatric age patient. *J Pediatr* 1980;96:479–484.

Edginton AN, Schmitt W, Voith B, et al. A mechanistic approach for the scaling of clearance in children. *Clin Pharmacokinet* 2006;45:683–704.

Gadkar K, Kirouac D, Parrott N, et al. Quantitative systems pharmacology: a promising approach for translational pharmacology. *Drug Discov Today Technol* 2016;21–22:57–65.

Gibaldi M, Boyes R, Feldman S. Influence of first-pass on the availability of drugs on oral administration. *J Pharm Sci* 1971;60:1338–1340.

Gibaldi M, Perrier D. *Pharmacokinetics*, 2nd ed. New York, NY: Marcel Dekker, 1982.

Gibiansky L, Gibiansky E. Target-mediated drug disposition model: approximations, identifiability of model parameters and applications to the population pharmacokinetic-pharmacodynamic modeling of biologics. *Expert Opin Drug Metab Toxicol* 2009;5(7):803–812.

Haddad S, Restieri C, Krishnan K. Characterization of age-related changes in body weight and organ weights from birth to adolescence in humans. *J Toxicol Environ Health* 2001;64:453–464.

Hoskin PJ, Hanks GW, Aherne GW, et al. The bioavailability and pharmacokinetics of morphine after intravenous, oral and buccal administration in healthy volunteers. *Br J Clin Pharmacol* 1989;27:499–505.

Johnson TN, Tucker GT, Tanner MS, et al. Changes in liver volume from birth to adulthood: a meta-analysis. *Liver Transpl* 2005;11(12):1481–1493.

Kearns GL, Reed MD. Clinical pharmacokinetics in infants and children. A reappraisal. *Clin Pharmacokinet* 1989;17(suppl 1):29–67.

Kim RB. Transporters and xenobiotic disposition. *Toxicology* 2002;181–182:291–297.

Lundeberg S, Beck O, Olsson GL, et al. Rectal administration of morphine in children. Pharmacokinetic evaluation after a single-dose. *Acta Anaesthesiol Scand* 1996;40:445–451.

Mahmood I. Pharmacokinetic considerations in designing pediatric studies of proteins, antibodies, and plasma-derived products. *Am J Ther* 2016;23(4):e1043–e1056.

Malik P, Edginton A. Pediatric physiology in relation to the pharmacokinetics of monoclonal antibodies. *Expert Opin Drug Metab Toxicol* 2018;14(6):585–599.

Murray DJ, Crom WR, Reddick WE, et al. Liver volume as a determinant of drug clearance in children and adolescents. *Drug Metab Dispos* 1995;23:1110–1116.

Nicolas JM, Bouzom F, Hugues C, et al. Oral drug absorption in pediatrics: the intestinal wall, its developmental changes and current tools for predictions. *Biopharm Drug Dispos* 2017;38(3):209–230.

Norberg A, Jones WA, Hahn RG, et al. Role of variability in explaining ethanol pharmacokinetics: research and forensic applications. *Clin Pharmacokinet* 2003;42:1–31.

Oie S. Drug distribution and binding. *J Clin Pharmacol* 1986;26:583–586.

Pelekis M, Gephart L, Lerman S. Physiologic-model-based derivation of the adult and child pharmacokinetic intraspecies uncertainty factors for volatile organic compounds. *Regul Toxicol Pharmacol* 2001;33:12–20.

Schwartz GJ, Brion LP, Spitzer A. The use of plasma creatinine concentration for estimating glomerular filtration rate in infants, children, and adolescents. *Pediatr Clin North Am* 1987;34(3):571–590.

Sheiner LB, Ludden TM. Population pharmacokinetics/dynamics. *Annu Rev Pharmacol Toxicol* 1992;32:185–209.

Sheiner LB, Rosenberg B, Marathe V. Estimation of population characteristics of pharmacokinetic parameters from routine clinical data. *J Pharmacokinet Biopharm* 1977;5:445–479.

Takasawa K, Terasaki T, Suzuki H, et al. Distributed model analysis of 3⊠-azido-3⊠-deoxythymidine and 2⊠,3⊠-dideoxyinosine distribution in brain tissue and cerebrospinal fluid. *J Pharmacol Exp Ther* 1997;282:1509–1517.

Tozer TN, Rowland M. *Introduction to pharmacokinetics and pharmacodynamics. The quantitative basis of drug therapy*. Philadelphia, PA: Lippincott Williams & Wilkins, 2006.

Wu CY, Benet LZ, Hebert MF, et al. Differentiation of absorption and first-pass gut and hepatic metabolism in humans: studies with cyclosporine. *Clin Pharmacol Ther* 1995;58(5):492–497.

Yun YE, Edginton AN. Model qualification of the PK-Sim® pediatric module for pediatric exposure assessment of CYP450 metabolized compounds. *J Toxicol Environ Health A* 2019;12:1–26.

CHAPTER

3

Hussain Mulla

Developmental Pharmacodynamics, Receptor Function, and Drug Action in Newborns and Children

ONTOGENY OF DRUG ACTION (PHARMACODYNAMICS)

A rational use of drugs is based on knowledge of their pharmacokinetic (PK) and pharmacodynamic (PD) properties.[1] Key to understanding drug response and, therefore, optimizing drug therapy both in populations and individuals is defining the relationship between PK and PD. This relationship is affected by many factors, including age, genotype, comorbidities, and comedications. It is only from a thorough understanding of the age-dependent PK–PD relationship that optimal doses for the pediatric population can be defined.

Although most basic cellular and physiologic processes and receptors are common to all mammals, irrespective of age or stage of development,[2] structural and functional characteristics of biologic systems constantly evolve from birth to adulthood. Alongside developmental changes in drug metabolism and other physiologic processes affecting PK, developmental changes also affect the therapeutic targets and receptors that mediate drug action and response.

Developmental PD is the study of age-related maturation of the structure and function of biologic systems and how this affects response to drug therapy. Age-dependent changes in potency and efficacy may be a consequence of maturational changes in receptor affinity, density, or signal transduction, and so even if the nature of the pharmacologic response is predicted to be the same in children, the magnitude of the response may not be (Fig. 3.1). In some cases, receptors or mediators may be absent altogether so that no response is observed. In others, altered response is a consequence of changes further downstream in the biochemical pathway.

STUDIES OF DEVELOPMENTAL PHARMACODYNAMICS

Unfortunately, to date, there is a dearth of studies reported in the literature on developmental PD. Whereas developmental PK has been and continues to be studied extensively, preclinical and clinical studies of developmental PD are relatively rare.

ANIMAL MODELS

Juvenile animal models can potentially help in the understanding of the maturation of human biologic systems and how this maturation affects both the disease process and drug response in neonates through to adolescence and adulthood. A limited number of juvenile animal studies (mostly in rodents) have been conducted, but these are quite rare, largely because of a lack of suitable models.[3,4] But even with juvenile animal models, extrapolating findings to children is hampered because correlating the postnatal age of the experimental animals with the corresponding stages of human development is not straightforward. The maturational rate of each developmental process varies across species; hence, cross-species extrapolation may not be very accurate. For example, it is assumed that the 7th to 13th postnatal days in rodents approximately correlate with the human full-term newborn, based on gross measures of brain growth, whereas the birth of the macaque coincides approximately with the 172nd to 217th postconceptual days of human development, depending on the brain region.[3]

STUDIES IN CHILDREN

There is a large evidence gap in the pediatric population, a consequence of a general insufficiency of studies in children but also lower quality clinical research relative to adults.[5] Special ethical considerations in children, for example, relating to consent and number of biologic samples, increase the complexity and reduce the feasibility of research studies. Direct comparison between control groups and severely diseased children is also limited because of ethical constraints regarding the inclusion of healthy children in clinical trials. In addition, the lack of age-appropriate, disease-specific, and validated PD endpoints makes assessing efficacy and safety in infants and young children particularly challenging (Table 3.1).

To increase the efficiency of clinical studies and limit unnecessary evaluations in children, regulatory authorities have issued guidelines to aid the pharmaceutical industry on the nature of clinical data required from pediatric drug development programs for marketing authorization.[6]

TABLE 3.1 Examples of Age-Dependent Pharmacodynamic Responses by Therapeutic Class

			Ontogeny Data from	
Therapeutic Class	*Effect in Children*	*Developmental Difference*	*Animals (Reference)*	*Humans (Reference)*
DRUGS ACTING ON THE CENTRAL NERVOUS SYSTEM				
Antidepressants	Lack of efficacy of tricyclics	Neurodevelopmental delay in norepinephrine system	9, 10	
Anticonvulsants	Paradoxical seizures in neonates	Excitatory GABA-A receptor and increased receptor density	3, 4	20[a]
Opioid analgesics	Increased sensitivity in neonates	Changes in opioid receptor expression	16, 17	
DRUGS ACTING ON THE CARDIOVASCULAR SYSTEM				
ACE inhibitors	Unknown	Angiotensin I, angiotensin II elevated at birth, decreasing into adolescence		21
Angiotensin receptor antagonists	Unknown	AT2 receptor highly and transiently expressed in fetal tissues	27, 28	
Drugs prolonging QT interval	Increased propensity for QT prolongation	Maturation of myocardial potassium channels, autonomic nervous system	38, 39	
Dopaminergic system	Renal vasoconstriction and no natriuretic effect in neonates	Difference in receptor density, affinity, and coupling to secondary messengers	43	Clinical data suggest urine output increases in human neonates 44
Oral anticoagulants	Increased sensitivity to warfarin	Decreased plasma concentration of vitamin K–dependent factors		46, 47
Heparin	Reduced sensitivity to UFH and LMWH	Low antithrombin 3 levels, high α-2-macroglobulin		45
Antiplatelet	Increased sensitivity to clopidogrel			45
DRUGS ACTING ON/WITH THE IMMUNE SYSTEM				
Immunosuppressants	Increased sensitivity	Qualitative and quantitative differences in immune system		51, 53–58
Antibiotics	Reduced efficacy	Immature immune system less effective at clearing infection		

[a]Data on receptor density.
ACE, angiotensin-converting enzyme; AT2, angiotensin receptor type 2; GABA-A, γ-aminobutyric acid receptor A; LMWH, low-molecular weight heparin; UFH, unfractionated heparin.

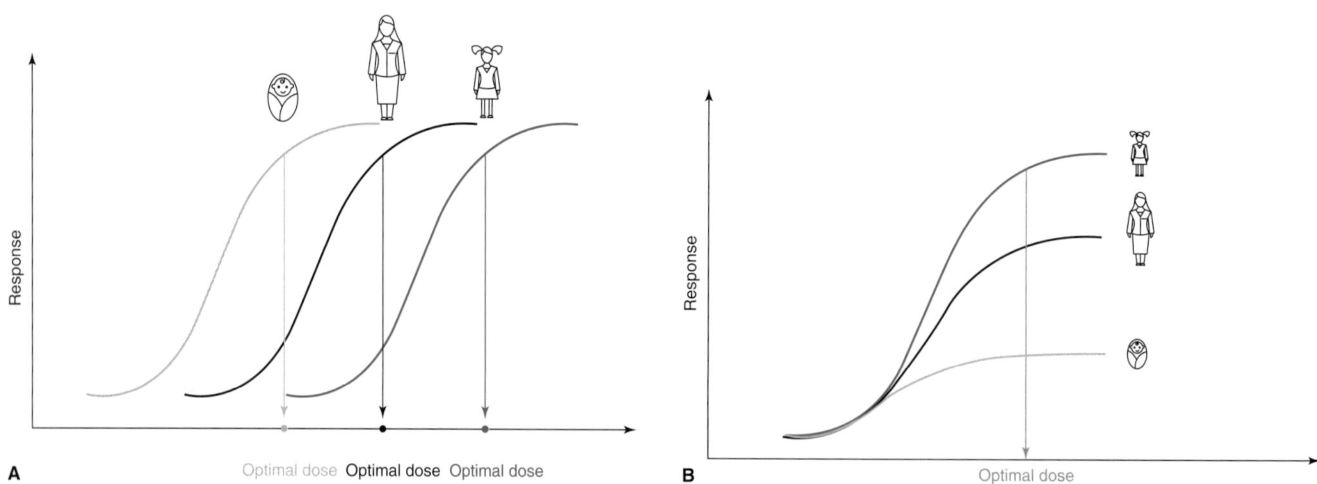

Figure 3.1 Hypothetical age-dependent changes in **(A)** drug potency and **(B)** efficacy.

These guidelines address the circumstances under which data from adult studies can be extrapolated to children, given a similar disease process and PK–PD response to intervention. But few example drugs exist where pediatric use could be completely extrapolated from adult data, because in the vast majority of cases, there is a lack of a validated, pediatric-specific biomarker. The paucity of validated biomarkers in neonates and children for use as endpoints in clinical trial settings and clinical practice has made it difficult to establish the PK–PD response in children and contributed to the knowledge gap.

The ideal PD endpoint should be "relevant, responsive, reproducible, and reliable."[7] The PD endpoint must be able to consistently quantify the clinical response to a specific intervention, at a given stage of development. The PD endpoint must also be acceptable and not burdensome to children and caregivers and ideally combined with routine tests. The development of dedicated age-specific PD measures is challenging, however, with the absence of established normal ranges/values in healthy children and the target population. Diligently compiled PD data from literature could be used as supportive reference for pediatric clinical trials.

The following sections provide strong evidence for changes in drug response during development with examples from animal reports on receptor ontogeny and clinical studies of age-related changes in PD (Table 3.1).

DRUGS ACTING ON THE CENTRAL NERVOUS SYSTEM

PSYCHOTROPIC DRUGS

Although psychological treatments are considered the first-line treatment of a major depressive episode in children, and despite the U.S. Food and Development Administration (FDA) cautions of increased suicide risk in children and adolescents, antidepressants are widely used in the treatment of childhood depression, and the rate of prescription has increased over time. However, according to current evidence comparing antidepressants (tricyclics, selective serotonin reuptake inhibitors [SSRIs], serotonin and norepinephrine reuptake inhibitors [SNRIs], atypical agents) with placebo or another active antidepressant as oral monotherapy in the acute treatment of major depressive disorder in children and adolescents (mean age 9 to 18 years), only fluoxetine is significantly more efficacious than placebo and some other active drugs at reducing depressive symptoms or the number of discontinuations owing to adverse events over 8 weeks.[8]

A common view is that delayed maturation of the norepinephrine neurotransmitter system relative to serotonin is one factor as to why tricyclics and SNRIs are not effective in children and adolescents.[9] Several indicators of maturation including the extent of innervation, the levels of serotonin and norepinephrine and their biosynthetic enzymes, receptor density, and the levels of reuptake transporters suggest that serotonergic system reaches adult stages of development more rapidly than the norepinephrine system. For example, in the rat, the serotonin system reaches maturity at about 3 weeks of age, whereas the norepinephrine system is not fully developed until sexual maturity is reached, at about 5 weeks of age. Although studies in humans are relatively scant, those that exist, together with studies in nonhuman primates, suggest that the serotonin system matures faster than the noradrenergic system.[10]

Even so, it is clear that the antidepressant response of children and adolescents is less than that of adults.[11] The complexity of the neural systems means that the reasons for the age dependency of antidepressant response remain poorly understood, and therefore, safety and efficacy of psychopharmacologic medicines cannot be readily extrapolated from adults. The developing brain is a highly malleable structure that is susceptible to environmental influences.[12] The adolescent brain development is characterized by synaptic regression and pruning, increases in myelination, strengthening of connections between limbic and cortical regions, and maturation of monoaminergic systems. Given the malleability of the adolescent brain to environmental stimuli, exposure to psychotropic drugs during the adolescent period can have lasting consequences on brain development, as well as having unexpected behavioral and neural outcomes in the short term. Antidepressant administration during adolescence may also modify normal developmental neurotrophic processes, thus having lasting effects on the maturation of the brain regions involved in emotional regulation. In the absence of more certain conclusions on the short term and enduring behavioral and neural consequences of antidepressant exposure during adolescence, the treatment of young persons with these agents should be approached with caution.

Dopamine is an important catecholamine with wide-ranging effects peripherally as well as in the central nervous system (CNS). It acts through a family of receptors that includes at least five subtypes: D_1, D_2, D_3, D_4, and D_5. Studies of D_1 and D_2 ontogeny in the CNS are inconclusive. Most studies have been done in rats, with some studies of D_1 receptors showing an increasing number of receptors during maturation and others showing an increase to 35 to 40 days of age followed by a decline. Studies of D_2 receptors in the CNS are also inconsistent, but more recent studies have shown peak expression in the rat at 28 days with subsequent decline to adult levels.[12] In correspondence with a higher density of dopamine receptors in childhood, clinical observations of increased extrapyramidal effects from antipsychotic medication in children and adolescents can be traced back to an imbalance of dopaminergic and cholinergic innervation of the basal ganglia regions. Extrapyramidal effects are believed to be related to postsynaptic D_2 receptor antagonism in the nigrostriatal pathway. Thus, a heightened D_2 receptor density may lead to a greater vulnerability in children.[12]

OPIOID ANALGESICS

For a long time, pain management in neonates and infants was suboptimal, often justified by the belief that infants do not feel pain because of immaturity of the CNS and because there were no long-term outcomes to infant suffering.[13] Perhaps, previous underappreciation of the impact of noxious stimulation and neonatal pain was because, in part, of the variable and sometimes conflicting data reported, not least, the inadequacy and limited sensitivity of pain assessment tools. In fact, preterm infants demonstrate an exaggerated acute response to pain and worse behavioral and sensory long-term outcomes when compared to term neonates.[14]

It is now known that the neurotransmitters and structures required for pain sensation as well as structures needed for long-term memory are developed adequately in the neonate. Though the absence of inhibitory descending spinothalamic fibers and an underdeveloped cortical pain memory system point to differences in pain thresholds and perception in the newborn infant, there is consensus that pain assessment and treatment should be part of current standard medical care.[13,15] There is growing evidence to show that controlling pain in the newborn period is beneficial, improving physiologic, behavioral, and hormonal outcomes.

Pain conduction and modulation at the synapse are mediated through opioid receptors located in both the CNS (reticular formation, hypothalamus, thalamus, globus pallidus, and cortex) and the peripheral nervous system.[16] Studies in animals show that opioid receptor expression and binding undergoes considerable postnatal reorganization. The three main opioid receptors are *mu* (MOR), κ, and δ. All three receptors exhibit rapid developmental changes over the first 3 postnatal weeks. In general, MOR is the predominant opioid receptor during development as in adulthood, but it is exuberantly expressed at birth decreasing to adult levels by postnatal day 21. Both the MOR and κ receptor present similar patterns of ontogeny, whereas the δ receptor is first observed on day 7 postnatally. Moreover, the ontogeny of opioid receptors and their ligands is not uniform. The endogenous opioid ligands (endorphins, enkephalins, and dynorphins) appear before receptors are present.[17]

The developmental changes in opioid receptor pharmacology studied in rats provide a possible explanation for the age-related differences in opioid sensitivity and selectivity. Spinal MOR activation produces profound analgesia in neonatal rats, and analgesic efficacy decreases as the animals age.[18] Morphine induced a 75% depression of respiration in immature rats with no analgesia, whereas adult rats given the same weight-adjusted dose exhibited complete analgesia with only a 33% decrease in respiratory rate. In contrast, supraspinal MOR activation results in pronociceptive effects in younger rats; a switch in function occurs at around postnatal day 21, and in matured rats, only inhibitory effects can be observed.[18]

The increased expression of functional MOR is also likely to be a significant factor in the increased responsiveness of human neonates to opioids, although receptor expression may not necessarily correlate with receptor activation.[17,19] Receptor density varies by brain region, with earlier development of caudal and later development in rostral parts of the CNS. Earlier development of opioid receptors in the medulla and pons, where respiratory and cardiovascular centers are located, is consistent, with clinically observed higher incidence of opioid-related respiratory depression and bradycardia in the neonate who receives opioids.

These observations have important implications for response to opioid analgesics in the infant and the young child, independent of age-dependent PK. But they also suggest that changes in the normal pattern of maturation could result in long-term alterations in nociceptive processing that may be irreversible. The quality of pain treatment and management in the neonatal units can be improved by clinicians being aware of the changes that occur during this sensitive period and not disrupt the normal endogenous activity where possible.[18]

ANTICONVULSANTS

γ-Aminobutyric acid (GABA) is the most prevalent inhibitory neurotransmitter in the mature brain interacting with postsynaptic GABA receptors. However, it has a different role during early development, acting as a trophic factor influencing proliferation, migration, differentiation, synapse maturation, and cell death.[20]

There are two types of GABA receptors: GABA-A and GABA-B. The GABA-A receptor incorporates binding sites not only for GABA but also for benzodiazepines, barbiturates, steroid anesthetics, volatile general anesthetics, and possibly alcohols. These agents are allosteric modulators at the receptors, resulting in increased GABA affinity and increased frequency of chloride channel opening.[3,4]

Studies in nonhuman primates and, more recently, in children with seizure disorders have shown that major changes in GABA-A receptor binding and subunit expression occur during postnatal development. During early development, the chloride concentration in nerve cells is high. Opening of the chloride channels by GABA results in a depolarization (i.e., excitation). During maturation, possibly because of changes in the GABA-A receptor subunit composition, the intracellular chloride concentration decreases, so that the effect of GABA to open up the chloride channels causes the cell to become hyperpolarized, thus interrupting impulse conduction (i.e., inhibition). In this way, GABA switches from excitatory to an inhibitory neurotransmitter. This switch occurs around 1 to 2 weeks postnatally in the rat, but it is not known when it occurs in humans.[3,4]

A change in the density and distribution of GABA-A receptor with age has been shown in humans.[21] By applying positron emission tomography using the tracer [^{11}C] flumazenil, a ligand that binds to a subunit of the GABA-A receptor complex, all brain regions showed the highest distribution of the tracer at 2 years of age (which was the youngest age measured) and the values subsequently decreased with age. The greatest differences between children and adults occur in the temporal lobe, visual cortex, and thalamus. The developmental changes in GABA-A receptor subunit composition, distribution, or abundance, therefore, could have a significant impact on the efficacy of anticonvulsant drugs in the pediatric population. Increased apoptotic death and reduced neurogenesis are observed in 1-week-old rats exposed to benzodiazepines or phenobarbital. Similar findings were observed with other anticonvulsant drugs, suggesting that the immature brain may be more dependent upon a higher level of neuronal activity for survival than the adult brain is. Midazolam is reported to decrease the mechanical reflex threshold and increase the magnitude of mechanical and thermal reflexes in neonatal rats, but had no effect in juvenile rats. In the same study, midazolam had sedative effects in postnatal age day 10 and 21 rats, but not in postnatal age day 3 rats.[4]

Excitatory mode of GABA-A receptors may help to explain seizures experienced by preterm infants and newborns after exposure to benzodiazepines. The hypothesis could also be extended to febrile convulsions in young children. Although differences in anticonvulsant doses between adults and children are largely because of PK, the requirement for larger doses in children may also be partly attributed to changes in receptor density and subunit composition (which affect binding affinity) during maturation.

Since GABA has a trophic role during early brain development, it is important that future studies in preterm and young infants evaluate how interference with the function of GABAergic transmission during this period affects the development of neuronal wiring, plasticity of neuronal network, and neuronal organization, all of which could have long-term behavioral effects.[20]

DRUGS ACTING ON THE CARDIOVASCULAR SYSTEM

RENIN–ANGIOTENSIN–ALDOSTERONE SYSTEM

The renin–angiotensin–aldosterone system (RAAS) plays a major role in pathophysiology of cardiovascular disease and organ damage across the cardiovascular continuum. It controls cardiovascular, renal, and adrenal function by regulating body fluids, electrolyte balance, and arterial pressure. It is a commonly used target for pharmacotherapy of cardiovascular diseases in adults. However, the efficacy of this pharmacotherapy can only be inferred in children in a limited way. The vast collection of information on physiologic and therapeutic effects of drugs acting on the RAAS derived from adult populations may not be entirely applicable to children.[22]

Comprehensive knowledge of the peptides acting in the pediatric RAAS (e.g., angiotensin I, angiotensin II, angiotensin 1 to 7, angiotensin III, and angiotensin IV) might facilitate a more effective and rational pharmacotherapy in children. Age has a major impact on circulating angiotensin I and angiotensin II, with both being significantly elevated at birth and decreasing into adolescence, from a median of 302 to 98 pg per mL.[22] The sex hormones that are believed to play a regulatory role in the adult RAAS do not appear to be influential in children, suggesting that the gender-specific differences in the RAAS develop after childhood. The effect of addition of antihypertensive medication appears to increase angiotensin I and decrease angiotensin II, whereas cardiac and renal surgery seems to decrease both angiotensin I and angiotensin II.[22] Elevated levels of aldosterone and 18-hydroxycorticosterone have also been reported in children.[23,24]

Angiotensin-converting enzyme (ACE) inhibitors are known to play a role in cardiovascular remodeling and, in adults, have shown to regress left ventricular hypertrophy and improve systolic function. Such effects are beneficial in patients with ventricular hypertrophy who have achieved most of their somatic growth potential. But there is concern that similar effects may be detrimental in young children.[25] A study of the newborn pig heart shows that rapid growth of the left ventricle can be diminished by ACE inhibitors.[26] Thus, in the actively growing child with other etiologies of congestive heart failure, inhibiting hypertrophy, the mechanism by which the heart grows in humans beyond the age of 6 months, could limit cardiac growth potential. The findings of a large randomized controlled trial (RCT) in children with single ventricle physiology did not support the routine use of enalapril.[27]

There also appears to be an age influence on the expression of two main angiotensin receptor subtypes: AT1 and AT2. AT1 is believed to mediate the classic actions of angiotensin II, such as vasoconstriction, sodium and water retention, and cardiovascular remodeling. AT2 is highly and transiently expressed in fetal tissues, with receptor density falling significantly in all tissues soon after birth and AT1 becoming dominant by 3 months of age. This has led to the speculation that the AT2 receptor has an important role in cell growth, differentiation, and adhesion. The neonatal decrease and simultaneously higher AT2 receptor density is a point of concern with regard to the use of angiotensin receptor blockers in the developing child.[28,29]

CARDIAC ELECTROPHYSIOLOGY

The developing heart demonstrates significant differences in calcium regulation mechanisms and in responses to physiologic and pharmacologic interventions.[30]

Digoxin

Children appear to require and tolerate higher doses of digoxin to achieve therapeutic endpoints comparable with adults.[31–33] The developmental PD effects of digoxin have been demonstrated in the myocardium of various species.[34–36] One possible explanation for the relative resistance of children to digoxin may lie in the developmental changes in Na K-ATPase isoform expression (the binding site of digoxin), which have been shown to alter electrophysiologic properties and cardiac glycoside sensitivity.[37]

QT Interval Prolongation

The QT interval reflects ventricular repolarization on an electrocardiogram, and prolongation is associated with ventricular arrhythmias. During infancy, it has been shown that the QT interval is related to postmenstrual age and progressively increases after birth, reaching a maximum value in the second month of life, and thereafter progressively decreases until 6 months of age to reach values similar to those of adults.[38] The changes in QT interval according to postmenstrual age may be due to developmental changes in repolarizing potassium currents.[39] Another possible mechanism of QT developmental changes is the maturation of the autonomic nervous system.[40] These data suggest that electrocardiogram monitoring should be implemented in premature newborns who have reached 30 to 32 weeks' postmenstrual age and are exposed potentially to QT lengthening.[38]

There is actual evidence that infants are more sensitive to drugs with proarrhythmic tendencies. Cisapride, a prokinetic agent widely used in the 1980s and early 1990s for gastrointestinal disorders, especially esophageal reflux, was withdrawn from the market after publication of multiple reports of QT prolongation in children and adults.[41] A PK–PD study of sotalol in the treatment of children with supraventricular tachycardia (SVT) showed that neonates exhibited a higher sensitivity toward QTc interval prolongation compared with older children.[42] In a study of oral domperidone in neonates, advanced gestational age and serum potassium at the upper limit of normal were two risk factors associated with QT prolongation.[43]

DOPAMINERGIC SYSTEM

Studies in several animal species have demonstrated an important difference in cardiovascular response to dopamine between newborn and mature animals.[44] Dopamine does not elicit D_1-mediated renal vasodilatation in the newborn as it does in the adult animal. In fact, low doses of dopamine that produce renal vasodilatation in the adult actually may induce vasoconstriction in the newborn from stimulation of α-adrenergic receptors, which are well developed at term. Likewise, the natriuretic response to D_1 agonists is blunted in the newborn. It is unclear whether the decreased response to dopamine in immature animals is due to differences in receptor density, affinity for the agonist, coupling to second messengers, or distal intracellular mechanisms. In addition, the ontogenic profile of the different dopamine receptor subgroups in various organs and tissues beyond the newborn period is not known. However, differences in response to dopamine between the newborn and the adult animal do not appear to translate to humans. A number of studies in premature neonates show that a dose-dependent increase in urine output *is* observed with dopamine infusions.[45]

HEMOSTATIC SYSTEM

The hemostatic system is a dynamic, evolving, age-dependent system.[46] Synthesis of clotting factors by the fetus starts during the fifth week of gestation for fibrinogen, and blood is capable of clotting after 11 weeks. At birth, the plasma levels of most coagulation proteins are around half that measured in adults, preterm neonates having lower levels than term neonates. Although there is continuous maturation of the hemostatic system postnatally, it is still significantly different from adults at 6 months of age. For example, plasma concentrations of vitamin K–dependent coagulation factors (FII, FVII, FIX, FX) are approximately 20% lower than the corresponding values in adults until the late teenage years. Plasma prothrombin concentrations during childhood are 10% to 20% lower than adults. In addition, plasma concentrations of the thrombin inhibitor, α-2-macroglobulin was twice the adult value in early childhood and remained elevated throughout childhood. In contrast, mean plasma concentrations of protein C and heparin cofactor II were significantly lower than for adults until early teenage years.

Primary hemostasis is far less studied, but the platelet count is usually normal or elevated at birth, reaching adult values within 1 year.[46] Platelets are hyporeactive in neonates, but despite this, the bleeding time and the platelet closure time (platelet function assay) were found to be shorter in newborns and normalized before the end of the first month of life. Levels of von Willebrand factor appear to be associated with the physiologic development of the ABO(H) and I blood group system and are reported to be significantly higher in newborns and decreasing to adult values after 1 year of life.[46]

The effect of these developmental differences on the relationship between anticoagulants and the hemostatic system has been explored in a limited number of studies.

Warfarin

An ex vivo study revealed that the capacity of plasma to generate thrombin was decreased and delayed in children receiving warfarin therapy compared to adults with similar international normalized ratio (INR) values. Increased inhibition of thrombin was attributed to elevated α-2-macroglobulin levels in children. The in vivo relevance of these observations was highlighted with decreased plasma concentrations of prothrombin fragment 1 + 2 in children compared to adults at equivalent doses of warfarin.[47] The increased sensitivity of children to warfarin has also been reported in an in vivo PK–PD study. Children and adults (age range 1 to 76 years) on a constant maintenance dose of warfarin for at least 1 month were investigated for plasma concentrations of unbound warfarin, CYP2C9 genotype, vitamin K, and various coagulation parameters. Accounting for the developmental changes in PK and genotype, comparable unbound concentrations of (S)-warfarin, showed significantly lower plasma concentrations for protein C and prothrombin fragments 1 + 2 and greater INR in children.[48]

Heparin

Unfractionated heparin (UFH), an antithrombin activator, remains one of the most commonly used drugs in pediatric secondary care. Neonates have low antithrombin levels, high levels of α-2-macroglobulin, and an increased volume of distribution because of increased binding of UFH to heparin-binding proteins. The overall effect, at least at lower doses, appears to be heparin resistance, with UFH dosage usually higher in neonates and younger children than in older children or adults. Because activated partial thromboplastin time (aPTT) ratio is physiologically prolonged in the younger patients, treatment with UFH should preferably be monitored using anti-FXa activity.[46]

Age dependency of the dose of low-molecular weight heparin (LMWH) has also been observed. Younger patients required higher doses of enoxaparin to achieve target anti-FXa level on a per-kg basis: 1.5 to 2.0 mg per kg in infants versus 1.0 mg per kg in older children and adults. Similarly, pediatric doses for tinzaparin administered once daily decrease with age: 280 IU per kg between 0 and 2 months, 245 IU per kg between 2 and 12 months, 240 IU per kg between 1 and 5 years, 200 IU per kg between 5 and 10 years, and 175 IU per kg (adult dosage) between 10 and 16 years.[46]

Antiplatelets

There are limited literature data on the use of antiplatelet agents in children.[46] Aspirin antiplatelet doses (1 to 5 mg per kg per d) appear to have been extrapolated linearly from adults, although there are no supporting data. In contrast, the antiplatelet effects of clopidogrel have been evaluated in a study of children aged 0 to 24 months and appeared to exhibit age-dependent PD with a lower dose of 0.2 mg per kg per d, achieving a platelet inhibition level similar to that in adults taking 75 mg per d.[49] This dose was subsequently evaluated in a randomized, double-blind, placebo-controlled trial in neonates and infants with cyanotic congenital heart disease. The study concluded that clopidogrel treatment of young infants with cyanotic congenital heart disease does not reduce all-cause mortality or shunt-related morbidity. Consequently, there have been some question marks around whether the 0.2 mg per kg per d dose was actually too low dose.[50,51]

DRUGS ACTING ON/WITH THE IMMUNE SYSTEM

The normal neonatal immune response is relatively hypoinflammatory, characterized by the production of anti-inflammatory cytokines, negative regulators of Toll-like receptor signaling, and decreased innate-adaptive immune system communication.[52] This functional immaturity of the immune system in neonates, especially preterm neonates, makes them susceptible to bacterial and viral infections often presenting as sepsis.

In the early postnatal immune system, neonates have lower numbers and/or decreased functional capacity of leukocytes (T and B lymphocytes, natural killer cells, and myeloid-lineage cells). There is a predisposition in the perinatal period to Th-2 skewed immunity and suboptimal Th1 responses so that early-life adaptive T-cell immunity is characterized by tolerogenic reactivity, reduced alloantigen recognition, and poor responses to foreign antigens. Suboptimal B-cell response contributes to blunted humoral immune responses with incomplete immunoglobulin class switching. The ability of B cells to produce various immunoglobulins matures at different rates. Serum immunoglobulin M (IgM) concentrations are only approximately 10% of adult levels at birth and do not reach adult levels until 1 to 2 years of age. Similarly, concentrations of IgG in serum do not reach adult levels for 4 to 6 years after birth.[53]

Compared to adult innate cells, neonatal cells are much less polyfunctional, and each individual cell produces fewer cytokines. Neonatal cells produce high levels of superoxide and display an increased production of chemotactic interleukin-8 (IL8). In contrast, a low production of classic pro-inflammatory cytokines is detected. Monocytes from children have the capacity to produce tumor necrosis factor (TNF) and IL6 to the same levels as adult monocytes around the age of 3 years, but a number of other cytokines such as interferon-γ (IFNγ) and IL12 remain low until the teenage years.[54] Low cytokine production in response to infectious stimulus continues for years and increases children's susceptibility to microbial infections.

Newborn serum concentrations of almost all circulating components of the complement system are 10% to 80% lower than in adults, with diminished biologic activity. Complement levels increase after birth, with some serum factors reaching adult concentration within a month (e.g., factor B), but others evolve more slowly.[55]

IMMUNOSUPPRESSANTS

There is some evidence that lymphocyte ontogeny corresponds to a variable and age-related response to immune-modulating agents. In humans, it has been shown that there is a difference in sensitivity of adult and infant T cells to inhibition of their proliferative response by dexamethasone. T cells from cord blood of preterm and term neonates are more sensitive to inhibition by dexamethasone than were adult peripheral blood cells. The heightened sensitivity to dexamethasone gradually decreases throughout infancy, and the adult response pattern is reached at 1 year of age.[56] Similarly, an ex vivo study investigating the effect of age on the immunosuppressive effects of cyclosporine revealed markedly enhanced sensitivity in infants compared with older children and adults. The concentration at which 50% inhibition occurs (IC_{50}) for peripheral blood monocyte proliferation was less than half that in older children and adults. In addition, inhibition of IL2 expression by peripheral blood monocytes was significantly greater in infants than that in adults. This is likely related to immaturity of the T-lymphocyte response in the infant and has important therapeutic implications for dosing cyclosporine in infants independent of PK differences.[57]

Perturbation of the developmental sequence of events can lead to immune dysfunctions that may be life-threatening. Studies in mice suggest that administration of certain drugs during early postnatal life can also result in altered immune function later in life. For example, 1-day-old mice exposed to cortisol or hydrocortisone displayed thymic atrophy and reduced antibody responses to sheep red blood cells.[58]

ANTIMICROBIALS AND VACCINES

Despite the general recognition of the important role of the host's defense in contributing to clearance of microorganisms, most clinical studies focus almost exclusively on the PK/PD of the antimicrobial drug and microorganism and neglect the contribution of the immune system.[59] Therefore, the exposure that yields the desired microbiologic and clinical cure in adults is assumed to be similar in all pediatric age categories, and adjusting doses in children to achieve equivalent exposure to that observed in adult studies is the main objective.[60]

This, however, ignores the possibility that, particularly in neonates due to their immature immune function, to achieve microbiologic and clinical cure, age-specific exposure in children may differ from the exposure needed in adults. Currently, no prospective data exist in children to validate the exposures required for microbiologic and clinical cure.

The immaturity of the neonatal immune system is also relevant to vaccination development programs because infants are the target age group for many of the vaccines in development, including tuberculosis (TB), malaria, and HIV vaccines. A better understanding of the intrinsic factors influencing maturation and development of the neonatal immune system can inform the development of effective and safe vaccines, which can elicit protective responses against these organisms.

GROWTH, DEVELOPMENT, AND DRUG TOXICITY

Age-dependent PD, of course, does apply not only to the desired pharmacologic response but also to adverse effects. The complex processes involved in growth and development frequently make the child uniquely vulnerable to mechanisms of toxicity that are not present in mature individuals. There are periods of vulnerability in the developing infant, when they are much more sensitive to toxic effects of drugs than later in life. This phenomenon is particularly relevant to the nervous, endocrine, reproductive, immune, and visual systems.[61] This may have the consequence of narrowing or widening the therapeutic window so that for a given exposure, an adverse effect is more or less likely to occur in children compared to adults (Table 3.2 and Fig. 3.2).

EXAMPLES OF INCREASED TOXICITY

In the growing child, chronic treatment with corticosteroids impedes linear growth, and similar concerns have been expressed about stimulants such as amphetamine and methylphenidate used for attention deficit/hyperactivity disorder (ADHD).[62,63] Tetracycline antibiotics are not recommended for children younger than 8 years of age because they cause enamel dysplasia in developing teeth.[64] The use of the fluoroquinolone antibiotics in children is limited because of potential toxicity to growing cartilage.[65]

The incidence of metoclopramide-induced dystonias and bradykinetic reactions diminishes strikingly with maturation from ages 10 years to adulthood, whereas neuroleptic-induced akathisia is less common in children.[66] Neuroleptic-withdrawal dyskinesias are also more common in children.[9] This may be related to greater concentration of dopamine-2 receptors in the brain of young patients.[12] Alternatively, the intensity of adverse effect maybe increased because of enhanced tissue sensitivity.

There are also examples of paradoxical responses reflecting the different roles that neurotransmitters, receptors, and hormones play in infancy and in the developed adult. Children younger than 1 year of age are more susceptible to respiratory

TABLE 3.2 Examples of Age-Dependent Toxicity

Drug	*Toxicity*	*Mechanism for Age-Dependent Effect*	*Reference*
INCREASED SUSCEPTIBILITY			
Corticosteroids	Growth suppression	Suppressive effect on osteoblastogenesis in the bone marrow, apoptosis of osteoblasts and osteocytes	62
Amphetamine/ methylphenidate	Growth suppression	Effect on appetite?	63
Tetracycline	Teeth staining in children <8 y	Binding to calcium ions during tooth mineralization	64
Fluoroquinolones	Arthotoxicity	Effect on growing cartilage	65
Metoclopramide	Acute dystonia	Increased D_2 receptor density	9, 12, 66
Opioids	Respiratory depression in neonates, mortality in children <12 y	Opioid receptor distribution and sensitivity	67
Verapamil	Severe bradycardia, hypotension, and cardiovascular collapse in neonates and infants <1 y of age	Deficiency of calcium channels	68
Valproic acid	Acute hyperammonemia, encephalopathy	Effect on urea cycle, neurotransmitters and neuronal toxicity	69, 70
REDUCED SUSCEPTIBILITY			
Aminoglycosides	Reduced ototoxicity and nephrotoxicity	Reduced accumulation in tubular epithelial cells	71, 72
Halothane	Reduced rate of hepatotoxicity	No information available	73
Isoniazid	Reduced hepatitis	No information available	74, 75

depression from weight-adjusted doses of opioid drugs, which are generally safe in older children and adults. Codeine is now contraindicated in children under the age of 12 years, following the identification of cases of respiratory depression, including deaths when codeine was used as an analgesic for postoperative pain, general pain, and cough and cold.[67]

Verapamil is used for the treatment of supraventricular arrhythmias in older children and adult patients. However, infants with supraventricular tachyarrhythmias appear to be at increased risk of sudden cardiac arrest. The neonatal myocardium appears to be especially sensitive to calcium-channel blockade with a relative deficiency of calcium channels compared with adult myocytes, predisposing to conduction block complications. In addition, the dynamics of calcium in excitation–contraction coupling are different in the immature fetal and neonatal heart to those in the older child and adult. Hence, blocking of calcium channels may have a pronounced negative effect on the intracellular calcium concentration responsible for contraction. Verapamil is not recommended for the treatment of acute arrhythmias in infants younger than 1 year of age.[68]

Valproic acid is one of the anticonvulsants most commonly used in children. In rare cases, it can cause acute hyperammonemia associated with encephalopathy. Children younger than 5 years of age are at highest risk for developing this life-threatening adverse reaction, particularly if they are receiving concurrent therapy with other anticonvulsant drugs.[69,70]

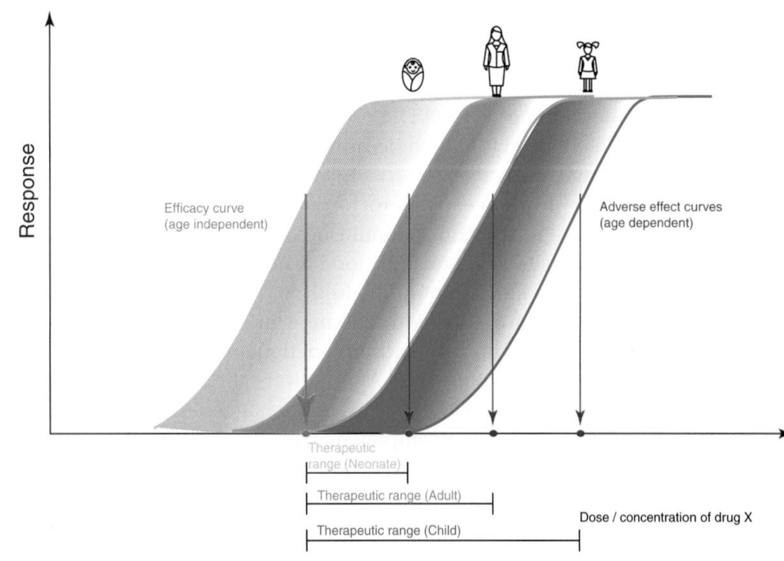

Figure 3.2 Hypothetical age-dependent changes in the therapeutic margin.

EXAMPLES OF DECREASED TOXICITY

Immaturity does not invariably predispose to increased risk of toxicity. Although infants and children may be more susceptible than adults to certain types of drug toxicity, there are important examples in which differences in drug disposition appear to result in decreased risk of toxicity in immature individuals.

Infants and young children appear to be less susceptible to ototoxicity and renal toxicity from aminoglycoside antibiotics compared with older patients.[71] This may be due, in part, to reduced intracellular accumulation of the aminoglycoside in renal tubular epithelial cells.[72]

Hepatotoxicity from halothane is relatively rare in children, even following multiple exposures, whereas it is not uncommon in adults.[73] The risk of isoniazid-induced hepatitis is age related.[74] An incidence of 0 per 1,000 patients younger than 20 years of age was reported by the FDA, whereas the incidence was 23 per 1,000 in patients 50 to 65 years of age.[75] It is usually unnecessary to routinely check liver function tests in children receiving isoniazid.

SUMMARY

The prepubescent child is clearly different from the newborn infant and the adolescent. From a pharmacotherapy perspective, the dynamic processes of growth and development create a moving target for the prescriber. The developmental changes in infants and children affect organ responses to both diseases and drugs. To employ, drug therapy across the population requires a thorough understanding of the PK–PD relationship. Hence, the key to successful drug therapy in children is to understand the age dependency of this relationship. This, in turn, requires that drugs are appropriately evaluated in the pediatric population and that appropriate dosage regimens are designed to compensate for developmental changes.

Whereas the age dependency of PK processes such as absorption, distribution, metabolism, and excretion are extensively studied and delineated for many commonly prescribed drugs, thus far, much less effort has been afforded to investigating the age dependency of PD responses. Similar efforts to increase and establish data on developmental PD are urgently required to achieve optimal drug therapy in children and to ensure long-term success of pediatric drug development. Key to such efforts is the availability of clinically relevant and validated, age-specific PD endpoints.

Sparsely reported experimental data from animal models provide some insight into developmental changes affecting the structure and function of receptors, cells, tissues, and organs and, therefore, some explanation for age-related differences in PD response. Though clinical study data are extremely limited, together with empirical data, there is convincing evidence from a number of therapy areas of altered efficacy in children. Also, children may be uniquely susceptible to some types of drug toxicity while being protected from other toxic mechanisms by their immaturity. Finally, it is also important to remember that structure and function of organ systems, particularly the developing brain, may be permanently affected by interaction of pharmacologic agents with receptors during early crucial phases of development. Therefore, the decision to use pharmacologic agents in young children must follow careful consideration of potential long-term impact.

REFERENCES

1. Holford NHG, Sheiner LB. Understanding the dose-effect relationship: clinical application of pharmacokinetic-pharmacodynamic models. *Clin Pharmacokinet* 1981;6:429–453.
2. Stephenson T. How children's responses to drugs differ from adults. *Br J Clin Pharmacol* 2005;59(6):670–673.
3. Kilb W. Development of the GABAergic system from birth to adolescence. *Neuroscientist* 2012;18(6):613–630
4. McGoldrick MK, Galanopoulou AS. Developmental pharmacology of benzodiazepines under normal and pathological conditions. *Epileptic Disord* 2014;16 (Suppl 1):S59–S68.
5. Sampson MR, Benjami DK, Cohen-Wolkowiez M. Evidence-based guidelines for pediatric clinical trials: focus on StaR Child Health. *Expert Rev Clin Pharmacol* 2012;5(5):525–531.
6. U.S. Department of Health and Human Services Food and Drug Administration, Center for Drug Evaluation and Research (CDER). *Draft guidance: general clinical pharmacology considerations for pediatric studies for drugs and biological products guidance for industry.* Silver Spring, MD: Author, 2014.
7. Kelly LE, Sinha Y, Barker CIS, et al. Useful pharmacodynamic endpoints in children: selection, measurement, and next steps. *Pediatr Res* 2018;83(6):1095–1103.
8. Cipriani A, Xinyu Z, Del Giovane C, et al. Comparative efficacy and tolerability of antidepressants for major depressive disorder in children and adolescents: a network meta-analysis. *Lancet* 2016;388:881–890.
9. Bylund DB, Reed AL. Childhood and adolescent depression: why do children and adults respond differently to antidepressant drugs? *Neurochem Int* 2001;51:246–253.
10. Murrin LC, Sanders JD, Bylund DB. Comparison of the maturation of the adrenergic and serotonergic neurotransmitter systems in the brain: implication for differential drug effects on juveniles and adults. *Biochem Pharmacol* 2007;73:1225–1236.
11. Bowman MA, Daws LC. Targeting serotonin transporters in the treatment of juvenile and adolescent depression. *Front Neurosci* 2019;13:1–14.
12. Pitzer M. The development of monoaminergic neurotransmitter systems in childhood and adolescence *Int J Dev Neurosci* 2019;74:49–55.
13. McClain BC, Kain ZN. Procedural pain in neonates: the new millennium. *Pediatrics.* 2005;115:1073–1075.
14. Simons SHP, Tibboel D. Pain perception development and maturation. *Semin Fetal Neonatal Med* 2006;11:227–231.
15. Witt N, Coynor S, Edwards C et al. A guide to pain assessment and management in the neonate. *Curr Emerg Hosp Med Rep* 2016;4:1–10.
16. Kretz FJ, Reimann B. Ontogeny of receptors relevant to anaesthesiology. *Curr Opin Anaesthesiol* 2003;16:281–284.
17. Nandi R, Fitzgerald M. Opioid analgesia in the newborn. *Eur J Pain* 2005;9(2):105–108.
18. Kwok CHT, Devonshire IM, Bennett AJ, et al. Postnatal maturation of endogenous opioid systems within the periaqueductal grey and spinal dorsal horn of the rat. *Pain.* 2014;155(1):168–178.
19. Bouwmeester NJ, Hop WC, van Dijk M, et al. Postoperative pain in the neonate: age-related differences in morphine requirements and metabolism. *Intensive Care Med* 2003;29(11):2009–2015.
20. Herlenius E, Lagercrantz H. Development of neurotransmitter systems during critical periods. *Exp Neurol* 2004;190:S8–S21.
21. Chugani DC, Muzik O, Juhasz C, et al. Postnatal maturation of human GABAA receptors measured with positron emission tomography. *Ann Neurol* 2001;49:618–626.
22. Suessenbach FK, Burckhardt BB. Levels of angiotensin peptides in healthy and cardiovascular/renal-diseased paediatric population—an investigative review. *Heart Fail Rev.* 2019;24(5):709–723.
23. Hattangady NG, Olala LO, Bollag WB, et al. Acute and chronic regulation of aldosterone production. *Mol Cell Endocrinol* 2012;350:151–162.
24. Häkkinen MR, Heinosalo T, Saarinen N, et al. Analysis by LC-MS/MS of endogenous steroids from human serum, plasma, endometrium and endometriotic tissue. *J Pharm Biomed Anal* 2018;152:165–172.
25. Grenier MA, Fioravanti J, Truesdell SC, et al. Angiotensin-converting enzyme inhibitor therapy for ventricular dysfunction in infants, children and adolescents: a review. *Prog Pediatr Cardiol* 2000;12(1):91–111
26. Beinleich CJ, Rissinger CJ, Vitkauskis KJ, et al. Role of bradykinin in the antihypertrophic effects of enalapril in the newborn pig heart. *Mol Cell Biochem* 1996;63/164:77–83.
27. Hsu DT, Zak V, Mahony L, et al. Enalapril in infants with single ventricle: results of a multicenter randomized trial. *Circulation* 2010;122(4):333–340.
28. Cox BE, Rosenfeld CR. Ontogeny of vascular angiotensin 2 receptor subtype expression in ovine development. *Pediatr Res* 1999;45(3):414–424.
29. Samyn ME, Petershack JA, Kurt AB, et al. Ontogeny and regulation of cardiac angiotensin types 1 and 2 receptors during fetal life in sheep. *Pediatr Res* 1998;44(3):323–329.
30. Auslender M. New drugs in the treatment of heart failure. *Prog Pediatr Cardiol* 2000;12:119–124.
31. McCulloch H, Rupe WA. The tolerance of children for digitalis. *S Med J* 1922;15:381–385.
32. Mathes S, Greiner T, Messeloff C, et al. Comparison of the sensitivity of children and adults to digoxin. *Fed Proc* 1951;10:323.
33. Kearin M, Kelly J, O'Malley K. Digoxin 'receptors' in neonates: an explanation of less sensitivity to digoxin than in adults. *Clin Pharmacol Ther* 1980;28:346–349.
34. Kelliher G, Roberts J. Effect of age on the cardiotoxic action of digitalis. *J Pharmacol Exp Ther* 1976;197:10–18.
35. Haag HB, Corbell RL Jr. The effect of age of cats on susceptibility to digitalis. *J Pharmacol Exp Ther* 1940;68:45–49.
36. Weinhouse E, Kaplanski J, Warszawski D, et al. Cardiac toxicity of digoxin in newborn and adult rats. *Pediatr Pharmacol* 1980;1:97–103.
37. Lucchesi PA, Sweadner KJ. Postnatal changes in NaK-ATPase isoform expression in rat cardiac ventricle: conservation of biphasic ouabain affinity. *J Biol Chem* 1991;266:9327–9331.
38. Seguela PE, Roze J, Gournay V. Evolution of the QT interval in premature infants: a preliminary study. *Cardiol Young* 2012;22:430–435.

39. Tanaka H, Namekata I, Nouchi H, et al. New aspects for the treatment of cardiac diseases based on the diversity of functional controls on cardiac muscles: diversity in the excitation–contraction mechanisms of the heart. *J Pharmacol Sci* 2009;109:327–333.
40. De Rogalski Landrot I, Roche F, Pichot V, et al. Autonomic nervous system activity in premature and full-term infants from theoretical term to 7 years. *Auton Neurosci* 2007;136:105–109.
41. Dubin A, Kikkert M, Mirmiran M, et al. Cisapride associated with QTc prolongation in very low birth weight preterm infants. *Pediatrics* 2001;107:1313–1316.
42. Läer S, Elshoff JP, Meibohm B, et al. Development of a safe and effective pediatric dosing regimen for sotalol based on population pharmacokinetics and pharmacodynamics in children with supraventricular tachycardia. *J Am Coll Cardiol* 2005;46(7):1322–1330.
43. Djeddi D, Kongolo G, Lefaix C, et al. Effect of domperidone on QT interval in neonates. *J Pediatr* 2008;153(5):663–666.
44. Cheung PY, Barrington KJ. Renal dopamine receptors: mechanisms of action and developmental aspects. *Cardiovasc Res* 1996;31:2–6.
45. Crouchley JL, Smith PB, Cotton CM et al. Effects of low-dose dopamine on urine output in normotensive very low birth weight neonates. *J Perinatol* 2013;33(8):619–621.
46. Toulon P. Developmental hemostasis: laboratory and clinical implications. *Int J Lab Hematol* 2016;38(Suppl 1):66–77.
47. Massicotte P, Leaker M, Marzinotto V, et al. Enhanced thrombin regulation during warfarin therapy in children compared to adults. *Thromb Haemost* 1998;80:570–574.
48. Takahashi H, Ishikawa S, Nomoto S, et al. Developmental changes in pharmacokinetics and pharmacodynamics of warfarin enantiomers in Japanese children. *Clin Pharmacol Ther* 2000;68:541–555.
49. Jennings LK, Michelson AD, Jacoski MV et al. Pharmacodynamic effects of clopidogrel in pediatric cardiac patients: a comparative study of platelet aggregation response. *Platelets* 2012;23(6):430–438.
50. Caruthers RL, Dorsch MP. Letter by Caruthers and Dorsch regarding article, "Dosing of clopidogrel for platelet inhibition in infants and young children: primary results of the platelet inhibition in children on cLOpidogrel (PICOLO) trial". *Circulation* 2008;118(7):e120.
51. Michelson AD. Antiplatelet drugs in the management of thrombotic/ischemic events in children. In: Michelson AD, ed. *Platelets,* 4th ed. San Diego, CA: Academic Press, 2019:1079–1083.
52. Adkins B, Leclerc C, Marshall-Clarke S. Neonatal adaptive immunity comes of age. *Nat Rev Immunol* 2004;4(7):553–556.
53. Basha S, Surendran N, Pichichero M. Immune responses in neonates. *Expert Rev Clin Immunol* 2014;10(9):1171–1184.
54. Ygberg S, Nilsson A. The developing immune system – from foetus to toddler. *Acta Paediatr* 2012;101(2):120–127.
55. Simon AK, Hollander GA, McMichael A. Evolution of the immune system in humans from infancy to old age. *Proc Biol Sci* 2015;282(1821):20143085.
56. Kavelaars A, Cats B, Visser GHA, et al. Ontogeny of the response of human peripheral blood t cells to glucocorticoids. *Brain Behav Immun* 1996;10:288–297.
57. Marshall JD, Kearns GL. Developmental pharmacodynamics of cyclosporine. *Clin Pharmacol Ther* 1999;66(1):66–75.
58. Holladay SD, Smialowicz RJ. Development of the murine and human immune system: differential effects of immunotoxicants depend on time of exposure. *Environ Health Perspect* 2000;108 (Suppl 3):463–473.
59. Handel A, Margolis E, Levin BR. Exploring the role of the immune response in preventing antibiotic resistance. *J Theor Biol* 2009;256(4):655–662.
60. Le J, Bradley JS. Optimizing antibiotic drug therapy in pediatrics: current state and future needs. *J Clin Pharmacol* 2018;58(S10):S108–S122.
61. Koch, SC, Fitzgerald M, Hathway GJ. Midazolam potentiates nociceptive behavior, sensitizes cutaneous reflexes, and is devoid of sedative action in neonatal rats. *Anesthesiology* 2008;108:122–129.
62. Mushtaq T, Ahmed S. The impact of corticosteroids on growth and bone health. *Arch Dis Child* 2002;87(2):93–96.
63. Faraone SV, Biederman J, Morley CP, et al. Effect of stimulants on height and weight: a review of the literature. *J Am Acad Child Adolesc Psychiatry* 2008;47(9):994–1009.
64. Stewart DJ. Prevalence of tetracyclines in children's teeth. II. Resurvey after five years. *Br Med J* 1973;3:320–322.
65. Bradley JS, Jackson MA; Committee on Infectious Diseases, American Academy of Pediatrics. The use of systemic and topical fluoroquinolones. *Pediatrics* 2011;128:e1034–e1045.
66. Campbell M, Adams P, Perry R, et al. Tardive and withdrawal dyskinesia in autistic children: a prospective study. *Psychopharmacol Bull* 1988;24:251–255.
67. https://www.fda.gov/drugs/drug-safety-and-availability/fda-drug-safety-communication-fda-restricts-use-prescription-codeine-pain-and-cough-medicines-and
68. Kugler JD, Danford DA. Management of infants, children, and adolescents with paroxysmal supraventricular tachycardia. *J Pediatr* 1996;129:324–338.
69. Yamamoto Y, Takahashi Y, Imai K et al. Risk factors for hyperammonemia in pediatric patients with epilepsy. *Epilepsia* 2013;54(6):983–989.
70. Ghodke-Puranik Y, Thorn CF, Lamba JK, et al. Valproic acid pathway: pharmacokinetics and pharmacodynamics. *Pharmacogenet Genomics* 2013;23(4):236–241.
71. Kent A, Turner MA, Sharland M, et al. Aminoglycoside toxicity in neonates: something to worry about? *Expert Rev Anti Infect Ther* 2014;12(3):319–331
72. Hermann G. Renal toxicity of aminoglycosides in the neonatal period. *Pediatr Pharmacol* 1983;3:251–254.
73. Warner LO, Beach TP, Garvin JP. Halothane and children: the first quarter century. *Anesth Analg* 1984;63:838–842.
74. Chang SH, Hanid P, Eitzman SR. Hepatotoxicity in children receiving isoniazid therapy for latent tuberculosis infection. *J Pediatr Infect Dis Soc* 2014;3(3):221–227.
75. Food and Drug Administration. Hepatitis associated with isoniazid-warning. *FDA Drug Bull* 1978;8:11.

CHAPTER

4

Stephani L. Stancil
Alenka Chapron
Susan M. Abdel-Rahman

Drug Absorption, Distribution, Metabolism, Excretion, and Transporters in Newborns and Children

INTRODUCTION

Between the time that a drug is prescribed and the time it elicits an effect in the human body, it will have encountered numerous physiologic processes that determine the extent to which it gets in, where it goes once it enters, and how it will be removed. Success in choosing the right drug at the right dose for the pediatric patient is best achieved by understanding how these processes influence the relationship between dose and exposure and, by extension, between exposure and response. For the vast majority of therapeutic agents administered to children, treatment focuses solely on the dose necessary to achieve a desired response (e.g., cure from infection). Yet, any provider will tell you that children administered the same weight-adjusted dose of a drug do not always respond in the same way. In many cases, this can be attributed to variations in systemic exposure that arise because of the unique constitution of each patient and their current stage of growth and development. In this chapter, we explore the physiologic drivers that influence absorption, distribution, metabolism, excretion, and transport (ADMET) and describe the current state of knowledge as to how these processes change across the continuum of age. Prior to exploring these data, however, it is important to comment on their strengths and limitations so as to ensure their interpretation in the most judicious manner possible.

The source of truth with respect to pharmacokinetic (PK) phenotype in children derives from carefully conducted pediatric clinical studies. Powered adequately, these studies can also confer insights into the role that demographic, pathologic, and environmental factors play in the disposition of the drug under investigation. Unfortunately, the relatively limited number of pediatric PK trials that are undertaken often requires us to predict pediatric exposures from preexisting adult PK data combined with nonclinical data generated in animal- or cell-based systems. Juvenile animal studies provide an avenue for predicting drug disposition in children, but caution is advised when extrapolating data from animals to humans. First, the overall physiology between animal models and humans can differ as can the developmental trajectory of key disposition processes[1] (for a meaningful interpretation of animal studies, the developmental stages of selected animals relative to human are presented in Table 4.1). Second, interspecies differences occur for protein isoforms of various drug-metabolizing enzymes (DMEs) and transporters.[2] Despite these discrepancies, some animal models can provide important insights into age-dependent changes in plasma and tissue concentrations following drug administration.

Research conducted in vitro in human tissues can also contribute to our understanding of pediatric drug disposition. Though largely devoid of ancillary physiologic influences, these models allow us to characterize developmental variations in the expression levels and activity of DMEs and transporters and to define the mechanistic basis behind intrinsic and extrinsic modulators of activity that may be present at discrete ages. Quantitation of gene and protein expression is accomplished by measuring messenger RNA (mRNA) and protein content, respectively, whereas protein activity is determined via direct measurement of drug biotransformation or transport. Notably, correlations between transcript copy number, protein levels, and functional protein activity range from poor to strong. Thus, mRNA and protein levels are inconsistent surrogates for protein function. Nevertheless, their expression profiles can still offer insight into age-dependent changes that may influence the disposition of drugs that serve as substrates for these proteins. As exemplified in the sections below, human, animal, and in vitro studies are often used in a complementary manner to paint a comprehensive picture of the impact of ontogeny on drug disposition.

TABLE 4.1 Analogous Developmental Stages Between Humans and Selected Animal Species

Developmental Stage	*Human*	*Rat*	*Dog*	*Pig*
Neonate	Birth to 1 mo	Birth to 1 wk	Birth to 3 wk	Birth to 2 wk
Infant	1 mo to 2 y	1–3 wk	3–6 wk	2–4 wk
Child	2–12 y	3–6 wk	6 wk to 6 mo	4 wk to 4 mo
Adolescent	12–18 y	6–9 wk	6 mo–18 mo	4–7 mo
Adult	>18 y	>9 wk	>18 mo	>7 mo

ABSORPTION

Generally speaking, absorption is defined as the process by which drugs pass into the intravascular space (systemic circulation) from the site of application or administration. Bioavailability, more specifically, describes the extent to which unchanged drug enters the systemic circulation. For drugs administered by routes other than parenteral, both the rate and the extent of absorption are influenced by physicochemical and mechanical processes that are susceptible to age-dependent influences.

ORAL ADMINISTRATION

A sample of processes that impact oral absorption is detailed in Figure 4.1. However, all of these presuppose that the drug has passed through the oral cavity, not a guarantee in children. It is not uncommon for children to reject medications based on taste, smell, or texture, each of which demonstrates a unique developmental trajectory. The capacity to discriminate sour, salty, and bitter appears to mature around the age of 2 years preceded by texture, temperature, and piquancy at 1 to 2 years and sweet and umami which actually appear to be present in utero. Olfactory development, by contrast, does not fully mature until a child reaches 5 to 7 years of age.[3–5] These teleologic drivers influence a child's willingness to accept newly introduced foods and, by extension, medicines. Consequently, thoughtful consideration of a child's age or age group is necessary when making therapeutic decisions, or designing masking strategies, for drugs with aversive palatability characteristics for no drug that fails to make it past the oropharynx will be effective.

Immediately past the oral cavity, the drug encounters the stomach which, for many drugs, serves as the site of disintegration and dissolution. Whereas the gastric milieu is highly acidic in the adult (pH ≤3), a combination of factors contributes to higher gastric pH in neonates and young infants. These include reduced hydrochloric acid production (despite a state of relative hypergastrinemia) and increased feeding frequencies where food contents effectively buffer the gastric fluid. As the stomach is not the primary site of absorption for orally administered drugs, the impact of altered pH on the ionization state of drugs holds limited relevance.[6–8] More important is the impact of gastric pH on the stability of drug. With an elevated pH, acid-labile drugs (e.g., β-lactam antibiotics) are afforded an element of protection, making more of the drug available for absorption. Figure 4.2 illustrates this phenomenon, showing that comparable weight-based doses of penicillin demonstrate five to six times higher concentrations in newborns compared with older infants and children.[9] These findings can be extrapolated to other acid-labile drugs not otherwise formulated in a manner which protects the active compound from gastric acid. These pH differences can also impact formulations designed to liberate their contents under selected physiologic pH. Those designed to release drug in an acidic environment may exhibit incomplete or delayed release profiles in younger children,[10] whereas those designed to release their contents at the more basic intestinal pH may experience faster release characteristics in this population.[11]

From the stomach, drugs migrate into the intestines where the time required for emptying of the gastric contents and motility along the intestinal lumen can influence the rate of drug absorption. Owing to irregular peristaltic activity at the time

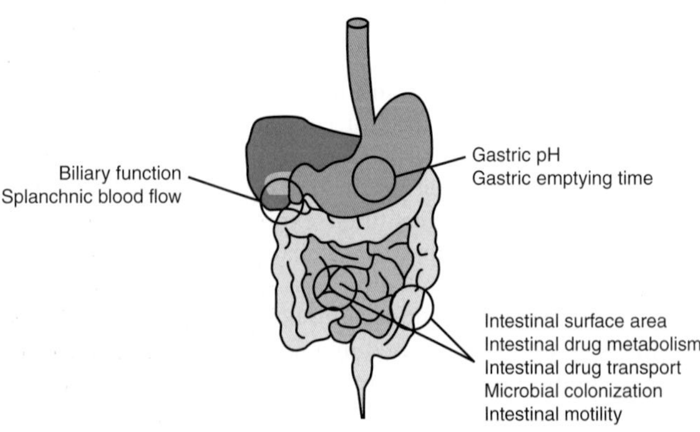

Figure 4.1 Physicochemical and mechanical factors influencing oral drug absorption.

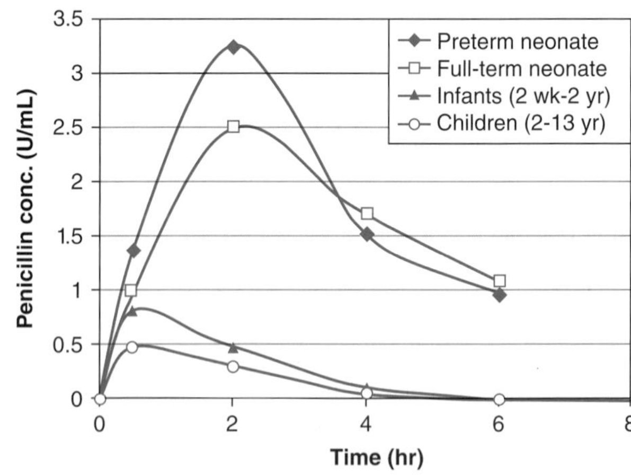

Figure 4.2 Impact of age on weight-based dosing of penicillin. (Reprinted with permission from Brown JT, Abdel-Rahman SM. *Pediatric pharmacokinetics. Pediatric pharmacotherapy.* Lenexa, KS: American College of Clinical Pharmacy, 2013:19.)

of birth, the rate of gastric emptying and intestinal transit is prolonged in the first few days of life, but quickly approaches adult values within weeks to months.[7,12,13] Consequently, it is not unusual to see slower absorption rates and delayed T_{max} for selected drugs during this time frame.[7,14] Since these physiologic changes normalize relatively quickly after birth, the physicochemical properties of a drug (i.e., solubility and permeability) should more heavily influence absorption profiles after the first month of life. Other contributors to altered rates of drug absorption in children that persist beyond the first month of life include underlying disease (e.g., prematurity, respiratory, gastroesophageal, congenital heart disease) and diet.[15]

In contrast to intestinal transit, age-dependent differences in the maturation of intestinal structures are not expected to negatively influence drug absorption rates in children. Finger-like projections of villi populating the intestinal wall immensely expand intestinal surface area, making it the primary absorptive site for orally administered drugs. Importantly, these villi and their corresponding microvilli are essentially fully mature by 20 weeks of gestational age.[16,17] In addition, intestinal length relative to body length is greater in neonates and children as compared with adults (Fig. 4.3). Consequently, the available absorptive surface area for drugs in the intestine of children is comparable to or greater than that of adults when adjusted for size.

Despite the rapid maturation of intestinal motility and expanded intestinal surface area early in life, absorption rates for some passively absorbed compounds still demonstrate delays through the first 3 to 6 months of life.[7] The iatrogenic administration of prokinetic agents can enhance absorption rates in young infants, but not to the extent experienced by older infants, suggesting that additional factors contribute to slower rates of absorption in young infants[7] (Fig. 4.4). Though not well characterized, other explanations may include alterations in splanchnic blood flow. In both preterm and full-term neonates, preprandial mesenteric blood flow volume increases markedly over the first few weeks of life.[18–20] Whether this can be offset by the changes in splanchnic blood flow that accompany the increased feeding frequency at this age is unclear.[21,22]

The extent of oral absorption can also be influenced by maturational changes occurring in tissues and organs

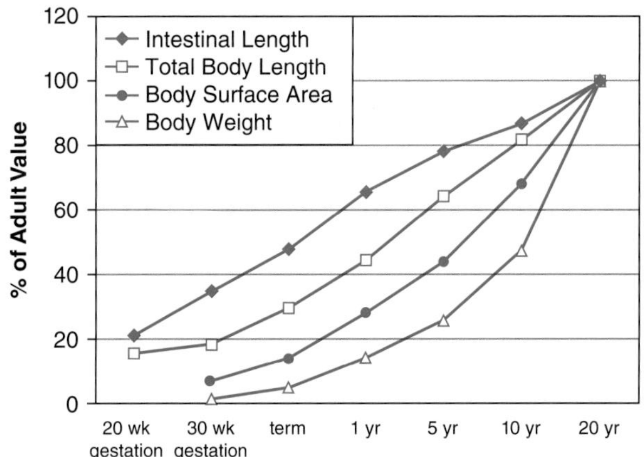

Figure 4.3 Anthropometric data relative to adult values as a function of age. (Reprinted with permission from Brown JT, Abdel-Rahman SM. *Pediatric pharmacokinetics. Pediatric pharmacotherapy.* Lenexa, KS: American College of Clinical Pharmacy, 2013:20.)

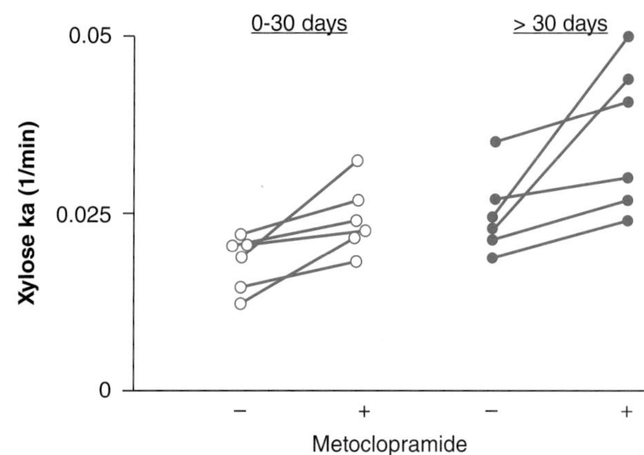

Figure 4.4 The impact of metoclopramide, a prokinetic agent, on the rate of absorption in neonates versus older infants. (Adapted from Heimann G. Enteral absorption and bioavailability in children in relation to age. *Eur J Clin Pharmacol* 1980;18:43–50.)

affiliated with the intestine. Through the first 6 months of life, postprandial sampling of two major bile salts demonstrates high circulating plasma concentrations, yet lower concentrations in the intestinal lumen as compared with older children and adults. This is likely the consequence of an immature bile salt transport mechanism.[23–27] The pharmacologic relevance is a reduced capacity for the absorption of drugs that require solubilization by bile acids prior to absorption. The impact can be seen in the example of pleconaril, a highly lipophilic antiviral, where dose escalation in adults is accompanied by a dose-proportional increase in total body exposure, yet dose escalation in neonates fails to show increase exposure.[28,29] The lipid-based chloramphenicol palmitate serves as another example[30] as do the dietary fatty acids, palmitate and stearate, for which absorption increases steadily through the first 3 to 4 months of life.[31]

Role of the Microbiome on Oral Absorption

Although the biology and function of the microbiome, particularly in neonates and children, has yet to be fully described, its impact on drug absorption cannot be discounted. An infant's mode of delivery (e.g., vaginal vs. Cesarean) and diet are two factors that contribute to the composition of the gut microbiome fostering the diversity that appears to increase with age.[32,33] These organisms can play a role in drug biotransformation, including conversion of orally administered drugs into metabolites with different activity profiles and deconjugation of enterohepatically recycled compounds liberating an active moiety for reabsorption. Digoxin offers one example of the impact that age-dependent changes in the microflora have on drug disposition. Anaerobic bacteria, which predominate in adult intestines, mediate the inactivation of digoxin into digoxin reduction products (DRPs). The recovery of DRPs in the urine of patients receiving digoxin increases steadily from birth to adulthood, with the biggest increase seen near the time of weaning. This occurs in concert with an increase in the presence of DRP forming bacteria in stool.[34] Because of the complexity of factors influencing the composition of the intestinal microbiome, the full impact of developmental trajectories of the microbiome on drug absorption has yet to be elucidated.

Role of Transporters in Oral Absorption

Drug transporters that reside in the membrane of intestinal epithelial cells localized either apically (i.e., facing the gut lumen) or basolaterally (i.e., facing the gut vasculature) can also contribute to age-dependent changes in drug disposition. The primary role of intestinal transporters, as it relates to drug disposition, is to modulate the transcellular passage of drugs from the gut lumen to the presystemic circulation by either facilitating or preventing the process. This is particularly important in the disposition of drugs that demonstrate poor passive diffusion characteristics (i.e., those that are large, hydrophilic, and charged at intestinal pH). The two major superfamilies present in the intestines include the ATP (adenosine triphosphate)-binding cassette (ABC) family or the solute carrier (SLC) family (Table 4.2).

The ontogeny of transporters is typically assessed via measurement of mRNA or protein expression in human pediatric biopsy tissues, postmortem human tissues, or animal models. A fairly robust example of intestinal transporter ontogeny is available with permeability glycoprotein (P-gp). The absence of detectable mRNA levels during the first 12 weeks of gestation are followed by measurable and stable mRNA expression after the completion of the first trimester (i.e., >12 weeks' gestation). Limited data suggest that adult levels of expression are reached at, or shortly after, birth. Not unexpectedly, these investigations also document marked interindividual variation in P-gp expression.[35] Multidrug resistance protein 2 (MRP2) is similarly detected in neonatal tissue, appearing constant through adulthood and characterized by marked interindividual variation.[35] Expression and cellular localization of the transporter, breast cancer resistance protein (BCRP), was detected as early as 5.5 weeks of gestation and remains unchanged up to 28 weeks. P-gp, MRP2, and BCRP are located on the apical membrane and function as efflux transporters restricting the passage of a drug into an intestinal epithelial cell. The organic anion transporting polypeptide 2 (OATP2B1) is also located apically, but functions as an uptake transporter by facilitating drug or solute entry into the intestinal epithelial cell. Significantly higher levels of OATP2B1 mRNA are detected in neonates than in adults, suggesting that levels decrease as the child develops.[35]

Although less frequently available, the strongest evidence for developmental patterns of intestinal transporter activity is provided by studies that utilize probe transporter substrates. For example, a study examining age-dependent changes in the PK of the H2-receptor antagonist, nizatidine, reveals a clear age-dependent reduction in apparent oral clearance unaccompanied by a change in the elimination rate constant. The authors hypothesize that this finding may be accounted for by age-dependent expression of the transporter(s) that mediate translocation of the drug into the presystemic blood circulation.[36] Other studies allude to age-dependent differences in intestinal transporter expression by examining nutrient uptake. Iron absorption, for example, mediated by the divalent metal transporter 1 (DMT1), increases linearly with age, attaining adult levels in early childhood[37,38] (Fig. 4.5).

TABLE 4.2 Clinically Relevant Drug Transporters

Common	*Gene*	*Substrates*	*Inhibitors*
OATP1A2	*SLCO1A2*	Imatinib, fexofenadine, ouabain, rocuronium	Dexamethasone, erythromycin, lovastatin, naloxone, naltrindole, quinidine, verapamil
OATP1B1	*SLCO1B1*	Atorvastatin, pravastatin, rosuvastatin, valsartan	Amikacin, cyclosporine, lopinavir, nicardipine, rifampin
OATP1B3	*SLCO1B3*	Atorvastatin, pitavastatin, pravastatin, rosuvastatin	Amoxicillin, cyclosporine, etoposide, rifampin, ritonavir
OATP2B1	*SLCO2B1*	Benzylpenicillin, methotrexate, pemetrexed	Amoxicillin, rifampin, streptomycin, linezolid
OCT1	*SLC22A1*	Metformin, acyclovir, ganciclovir, morphine	Acebutolol, amantadine, cimetidine, clonidine, disopyramide, midazolam, procainamide, prazosin, quinine, quinidine, vecuronium, verapamil
OCT2	*SLC22A2*	Metformin, amantadine, memantine	Desipramine, cimetidine, cisplatin, procainamide, quinine
OCT3	*SLC22A3*	Metformin, disopyramide	Clonidine, desipramine, imipramine, prazosin, procainamide
OCTN1	*SLC22A4*	Gabapentin, entecavir	Verapamil
OCTN2	*SLC22A5*	Oxaliplatin, tiotropium	Amiodarone, cephalosporins, cimetidine, desipramine, quinidine, quinine
OAT1	*SLC22A6*	Methotrexate, acyclovir, tenofovir	β-Lactam antibiotics, NSAIDs, diuretics
OAT2	*SLC22A7*	Zidovudine, penciclovir	β-Lactam antibiotics, NSAIDs, diuretics
OAT3	*SLC22A8*	Zidovudine, cimetidine, methotrexate, salicylate, oseltamivir carboxylate	β-Lactam antibiotics, diuretics, NSAIDs, quinidine
OAT4	*SLC22A11*	Methotrexate, olmesartan	β-Lactam antibiotics, diuretics, NSAIDs
P-gp	*ABCB1*	Atorvastatin, cyclosporine, digoxin, tacrolimus	Cyclosporine, miconazole, rifampin
MRP1	*ABCC1*	Methotrexate	Indomethacin, sulfinpyrazone
MRP2	*ABCC2*	Furosemide, methotrexate, vinblastine	Cyclosporine, indomethacin, probenecid
MRP3	*ABCC3*	Methotrexate, rosuvastatin	Rifampin, verapamil
MRP4	*ABCC4*	Adefovir, methotrexate, oseltamivir carboxylate	Flurbiprofen, sildenafil, probenecid
BCRP	*ABCG2*	Rosuvastatin, topotecan, imatinib, methotrexate	Cyclosporine, ketoconazole

ABC, ATP (adenosine triphosphate)-binding cassette; MRP, multidrug resistance protein; NSAIDs, nonsteroidal anti-inflammatory drugs; OAT, organic anion transporter; OCT, organic cation transporter; SLC, solute carrier.

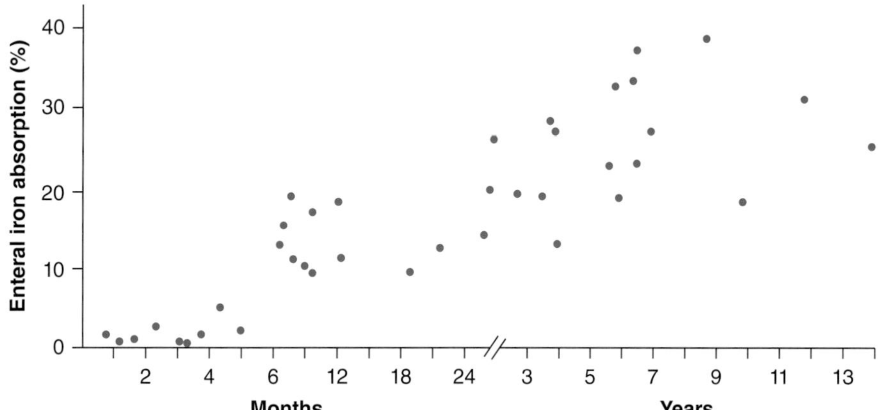

Figure 4.5 Enteral iron absorption as a percentage of the dose administered. (Adapted with permission from Gladtke E, Rind H. Iron therapy during childhood. *Ger Med Mon* 1966;11:438–442.)

It is important to recognize that current data suggest no single, unified developmental pattern of intestinal transporter expression in children. It is also important to point out that age-dependent changes in feeding frequency and composition can alter the expected activity of intestinal transporters. For example, the consumption of milk-based feeds delivered every few hours in the young infant may interfere with the uptake of substrates for intestinal peptide transporters (e.g., PEPT1),[39] and the exceedingly large quantities of apple juice consumed by young children can influence the uptake of substrates for organic anion-transporting polypeptides. The extent to which these interactions are relevant in children will largely depend on the level of expression for these and other transport proteins.

EXTRAORAL ADMINISTRATION

The rate and extent of extraoral drug absorption is similarly affected by physicochemical and mechanical factors that are susceptible to age-dependent changes (Fig. 4.6). Rectal administration is favored for the delivery of drugs to children when oral or intravenous routes are unavailable or contraindicated.[40–42] Unless delivered as a rectal solution, the absorption of rectally administered drugs depends on the characteristics of the formulation and the age of the child. Slow-melt suppositories, for example, will likely be expelled before releasing the entirety of their drug contents in young infants who experience far more high-amplitude pulsatile contractions of the lower gastrointestinal (GI) tract than do older children or adults.[40–44]

Transdermal drug delivery is employed for protracted delivery of chronic medications (e.g., clonidine, methylphenidate, hormonal contraception). The systemic exposure of medications applied to the skin is often increased in infants and young children due to a more expansive body surface area (BSA) that exhibits a higher degree of hydration and an increased extent of perfusion.[45–47] Skin thickness has been implicated as a reason for enhanced percutaneous absorption; however, only the preterm neonate demonstrates a thinner stratum corneum. Neonates born at term demonstrate stratum corneum thickness comparable to older children as do preterm newborns by 2 weeks of age.[48] While the dermis and epidermis may be thinner during the neonatal period, the primary barrier to drug absorption (i.e., the stratum corneum) is intact and fully developed. This potential for enhanced bioavailability needs to be considered not only for drugs intended for systemic delivery but even for drugs delivered with topical intent. There are countless cases of significant and life-threatening toxicities in infants and children after exposure to topical formulations (e.g., testosterone, other steroids, sulfadiazine, laundry detergent, talcum powder).[49–51]

Subcutaneous drug delivery has historically been used with insulin to treat diabetes and, more recently, to delivery abortive therapy for migraines. However, newer, protein-based biologics may also be expected to utilize this mode of delivery. Entry into

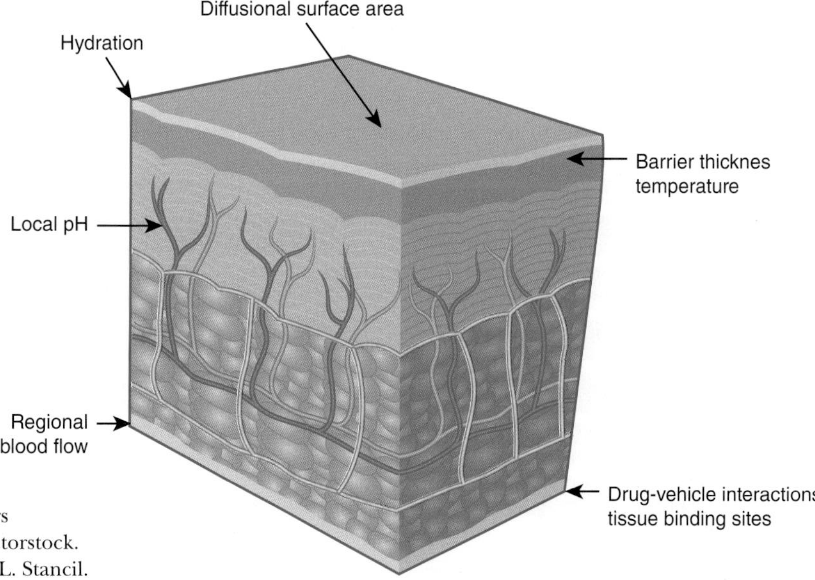

Figure 4.6 Physicochemical and mechanical factors influencing extraoral drug absorption. Image from vectorstock.com/1858074. Adapted by Sue Rahman and Stephani L. Stancil.

systemic circulation after subcutaneous administration is granted through absorption into blood vessels (drug molecules <10 nM) or lymphatic capillaries (drug molecules ~10 to 100 nM).[52] Studies of insulin describe significant inter- and intraindividual variability in subcutaneous absorption.[53,54] Though the factors influencing this variability are not well defined, developmental changes in capillary organization and composition of the hypodermis may play a role.[53,55–57]

Finally, the intramuscular (IM) route of delivery is chosen for vaccines and depot formulations of medications (e.g., medroxyprogesterone, ceftriaxone). Drug is typically absorbed through the capillaries that are perfusing the muscle. Though IM absorption is often touted as erratic in young children, infants exhibit greater muscle capillary density compared with older children (+25%) and adults (+56%), making this an effective means of drug delivery in young children.[58–60] Other issues influencing the efficiency of this route include muscle contractility, drug pK_a, and solubility.

DISTRIBUTION

Once absorbed into the systemic circulation, a drug is available for distribution throughout the body. The rate and extent of distribution is equally dependent on the physiologic factors of the host (e.g., fraction of weight constituted by water, circulating protein composition, expression of tissue transporters, pH of body fluids) and the physicochemical characteristics of the drug (e.g., molecular weight, lipophilicity, protein-binding affinity, acid–base properties) (Fig. 4.7).

Developmental changes in body water stores reflect the most well-characterized age-dependent factor influencing drug distribution. The fraction of total body weight accounted for by water is highest in preterm and full-term neonates, approaching adult values by 1 year of age (Fig. 4.8). The implication of these changes is most evident for hydrophilic drugs (i.e., those with a V_d <0.7 to 1 L per kg) where higher weight-based doses are required in infants and young children to achieve systemic exposures comparable to those seen in adults. For example, infants experience peak concentrations of gentamicin that are 33% to 50% lower than children and adults after comparable weight-based doses.[61] With their corresponding reduction in renal clearance, infants in whom doses have not been adjusted to compensate for the expanded volumes would

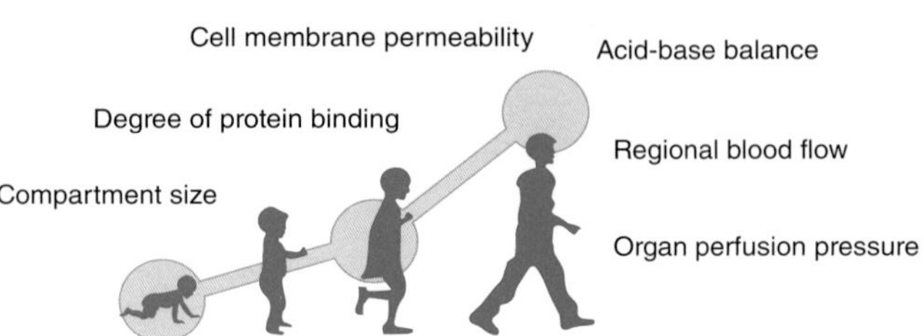

Figure 4.7 Factors influencing the rate and extent of drug distribution volume (Vd).

eventually achieve gentamicin concentrations equivalent to, or in excess of, adults once steady state is achieved. However, this delay could have significant clinical consequences, given the concentration-dependent nature of this drug.[62,63] Another example can be seen with linezolid where distribution volume is expanded but clearance is increased. This antibiotic demonstrates 15% to 25% higher V_d values in neonates corresponding with 25% to 37% lower C_{max}. In concert with a more rapid rate of clearance, the drug if administered at the same weight-based dose and dosing interval would spend only 20% to 35% of the time above the minimum inhibitory concentration (*MIC*) in infants compared with 35% to 70% in children and 70% to 100% in adults.[64] The impact of these findings on the recommended dosing regimens for both of these drugs is reflected in their labeling.

Though neonates and infants have decreased body fat stores relative to adults (normalizing by 2 to 3 years of age, Fig. 4.8), there is little evidence to suggest a meaningful contribution to differences in the V_d for highly lipophilic drugs. Such drugs are impacted, to a greater extent, by developmental changes that influence protein binding. For highly protein-bound drugs, changes in V_d can be clinically meaningful when the absolute amounts of plasma protein (e.g., albumin, globulin, α-1 acid glycoprotein, lipoprotein) are reduced, when conformational changes in the protein reduce the affinity for the drug, and when endogenous substrates capable of displacing drugs from their binding sites are present in the circulation.

Albumin is the most abundant protein circulating in the plasma. Acidic drugs (those negatively charged at physiologic pH 7.4) bind almost exclusively to albumin, while basic drugs (those positively charged at physiologic pH 7.4) can bind to

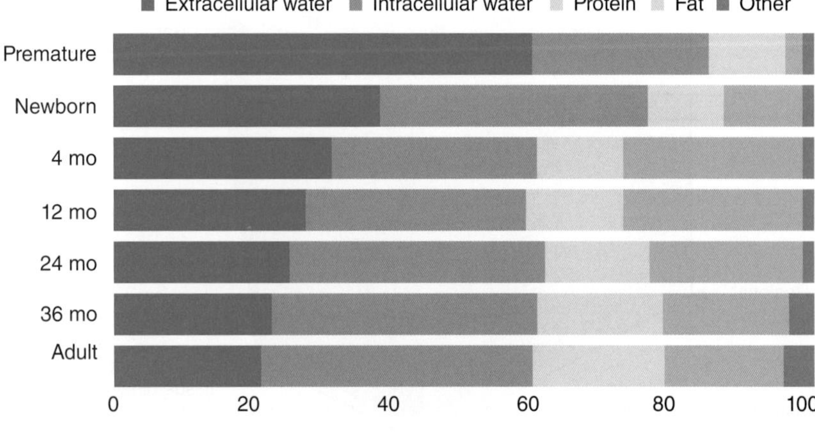

Figure 4.8 Total body weight accounted for by various compartments as a function of age. (Reprinted with permission from Brown JT, Abdel-Rahman SM. *Pediatric pharmacokinetics. Pediatric pharmacotherapy*. Lenexa, KS: American College of Clinical Pharmacy, 2013:23.)

albumin as well as to other plasma proteins (e.g., α-1 acid glycoprotein, lipoproteins). Neonates have reduced albumin levels relative to adults, as well as isoforms of albumin with lower drug-binding affinity (e.g., fetal albumin). Neonates and young infants also demonstrate reduced concentrations of α-1 acid glycoprotein and other lipoproteins. Circulating levels of bilirubin and free fatty acids, which functionally reduce protein binding via displacement of drugs from their binding site, are also increased in neonates. Collectively, these developmental alterations lead to reduced overall drug protein binding in the newborn and young infant. The implications of these alterations are an increase in fraction unbound for many drugs shortly after birth (e.g., propranolol, verapamil, ampicillin, phenytoin, phenobarbital, thiopental, sufentanil).[65–68] Notably, these effects can be bidirectional, where high-affinity drugs displace bilirubin from its binding site, increasing the risk of kernicterus in the neonate.

As it is the free drug that is responsible for eliciting pharmacologic effects, the impact of changes in protein binding is greatest for highly protein-bound drugs and, more specifically, those with a narrow therapeutic index. One of the best examples of this principle is illustrated by phenytoin, a drug that is 99% bound in adults. A small shift in protein binding from 99% to 98% effectively doubles the free phenytoin from 1% to 2%. Thus, very small changes in protein binding can significantly increase the risk of toxicity. By contrast, a minimally protein-bound drug such as ampicillin shows small increases in free drug available (~15%) and negligible change in risk profile when percentage of protein bound decreases from 22% in neonates to 10% in adults.

To our knowledge, no investigations to date have assessed alterations in drug tissue protein binding during pediatric growth and development. However, there have been attempts to explore differences in tissue distribution that are driven by transporters. For many drugs, protein transporters may represent a rate-limiting step in the overall distribution across body tissues, regulating access to the therapeutic site of action. Due to the limitations of experimental clinical approaches currently available to explore tissue distribution, our understanding relies on the findings from animal studies or human tissues collected postmortem. A study investigating developmental expression of P-gp, MRP1, and BCRP in postmortem brain tissues of neonates born at 22 to 42 weeks' gestation revealed that, by late gestation, the localization pattern is similar to that of adults; however, the adult tissues exhibit greater quantitative expression of these transport proteins.[69] Additional investigations into P-gp ontogeny in the brain reveal that infants between the ages of 3 and 6 months exhibit comparable levels of this protein to adults.[70] For the neonate and young infant, it is possible that reduced expression of P-gp contributes to increased central exposure to the P-gp substrate morphine and the enhanced opioid effects observed in neonates compared to older infants and adults.[71–73] However, this is also likely influenced by other ontogenic changes relevant to morphine disposition [i.e., reduced UGT2B7-mediated metabolism, reduced hepatic uptake mediated by organic cation transporter (OCT1)].

Other examples of transporter ontogeny that merit consideration when discussing V_d are hepatic OCT1 and OATP1B1/3, located on the sinusoidal membrane of the hepatocyte, that mediate the entry of drugs into the hepatocyte. Studies of OCT1 and OATP1B3 protein expression report that neonates and infants demonstrate significantly lower levels of these transport proteins compared with older children, who exhibit protein levels comparable to adults.[74,75] For OCT1, the ontogenic pattern of protein expression is supported by lower transporter activity in pediatric versus adult hepatocytes.[35] These data may explain the age-dependent changes in the volume of distribution for drugs that are primarily transported by hepatic OCT1 (e.g., metformin) and may lay the foundation for further investigations into relationships between hepatic transporter ontogeny and response for drugs that exert therapeutic actions within the liver. However, these age-dependent changes may be obscured by the contribution of genetic variations that account for more of the interindividual variability observed with these proteins.[74,76,77]

Lastly, the distribution of drugs can also be impacted by factors specifically associated with critically ill neonates and children. Pathophysiologic changes such as systemic inflammation or end-organ dysfunction may lead to a higher volume of distribution. For a child requiring extracorporeal oxygenation (ECMO) or hemodialysis, drug *ad*sorption to the circuit's tubing or membrane may lead to an observed increase in V_d depending on the age of the ECMO circuit.[78] Further studies are needed to expand our understanding of the impact these processes have on drug disposition.

METABOLISM

The purpose of metabolism, as it relates to drug therapy, is to biotransform an exogenously administered substrate into a more readily excretable form. The resulting metabolites may be wholly inactive, retain some activity, or become pharmacologically activated. Phase I reactions are typically responsible for oxidation, reduction, and hydrolysis of relevant substrates, while phase II processes links the substrate with a functional group intended to increase its water solubility. Drug metabolizing enzymes (DME) mediating biotransformation are implicated in drug–drug, drug–nutrient, and drug–gene interactions. Accordingly, understanding the impact of development on DME expression and activity is important not only to anticipate changes in drug clearance but to accurately interpret the clinical significance of potential interactions.

The majority of drug metabolism occurs in the liver, though age-dependent changes in liver mass, alone, do not account for ontogenic profile of most DMEs.[79] Each DME has its own developmental profile that contributes to clearance of medications as is discussed in the following sections.

PHASE I METABOLISM

The most prominent DMEs involved in phase I metabolism are the cytochrome P450 enzymes (CYPs). These enzymes are highly expressed in the liver, but also expressed at lower levels in a variety of human tissue, including the lung, oropharynx, intestine, kidney, and reproductive organs. The most clinically relevant of these CYPs is CYP3A4, responsible for metabolism of 30% of drugs on the market, followed by CYP2D6 and CYP2C8/9/19[80] (Fig. 4.9). Shortly after birth, a shift occurs, triggering a steady increase in CYP3A4 expression and a decline in the fetal isoform CYP3A7, through the first year of life. CYP3A4 activity increases to 30% to 60% of adult levels within the first week of life, with full adult values reached by 1 year of age. Clinically relevant examples of the impact of CYP3A ontogeny on drug metabolism

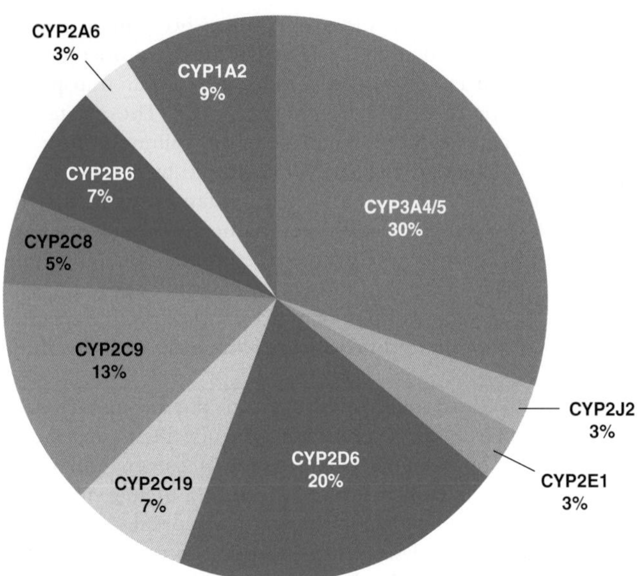

Figure 4.9 Contribution of individual CYP450 enzymes to the metabolism of clinically used drugs. (Adapted from Zanger UM, Schwab M. Cytochrome P450 enzymes in drug metabolism: regulation of gene expression, enzyme activities, and impact of genetic variation. *Pharmacol Ther* 2013;138(1):103–141).

exist with numerous medications (e.g., sildenafil, cisapride) that demonstrate marked reductions in half-life as children mature.[14,81,82]

CYP2D6 displays a different developmental trajectory, plateauing to adult levels by 2 weeks of life.[83] Though age may be relevant shortly after birth, genetic polymorphisms rapidly assume the role as predominant contributors to variability after 2 weeks. CYP2C9 displays expression and activity profiles in microsomal samples that are similar between young infant (0 to 5 months) and older child (5 months to 18 years); however, PK data paint a slightly different story. The terminal half-life of phenytoin, a CYP2C9 substrate, decreases from 20 hours at birth to 8 hours at 2 weeks of life.[84,85] Microsomal data suggest that CYP2C19 expression and activity in vitro gradually increases over the first 6 months of life.[86] Yet, intravenously administered omeprazole, a CYP2C19 substrate, has been found to have high clearance in the young infant that normalizes in the first 5 years of life.[87,88] These examples of the discrepancy between in vitro and in vivo data regarding the impact of age on activity in the pediatric population underscore the complexity of metabolism in the developing child and the need for substrate-specific investigations.

CYPs that are qualitatively and quantitatively less relevant include CYP2E1, CYP1A2, and CYP2A6. CYP2E1 is involved in the metabolism of a variety of anesthetic agents and has shown negligible activity in the prenatal period, increasing to 80% of adult expression and activity by the first year of life.[89] Following a similar developmental profile, CYP1A2 (contributing to caffeine and theophylline metabolism) has minimal activity in the prenatal and neonatal period (<4% to 5% of adult values), with gradual increase to 10% to 15%, 20% to 25%, and 50% to 55% of adult values by 1 to 3 months, 3 to 12 months, and 1 to 9 years respectively.[90] The activity of CYP2A6, responsible for the metabolism of nicotine, cotinine, and metronidazole, appears to reach adult levels by 2 to 3 months of age; however, ontogeny in the neonate and young infant (up to 1 to 2 months of age) is not yet well described. Examining metronidazole as a surrogate for CYP2A6, the hydroxyl metabolite is only present in neonates greater than 35 weeks' gestational age and metronidazole half-life is two to four times longer in neonates compared with adults,[91,92] suggesting negligible activity in preterm infants and reduced CYP2A6 activity in the first 1 to 2 months after birth.

The intestinal brush border is rich with digestive enzymes and DMEs. Individual digestive enzymes demonstrate unique developmental trajectories, and the same is expected for DMEs.[93] Pediatric intestinal biopsies demonstrate an age-dependent increase in CYP3A4 protein expression and activity (via 6-OH-testosterone formation) from neonate to older children.[94] In addition, CYP1A1 activity in intestinal biopsies also shows an age-dependent effect.[95] Importantly, breast-fed infants whose mothers take herbal supplements known to alter DME activity (e.g., St. John's wort, ginkgo biloba) may experience sufficient exposures to alter DME activity.[96]

PHASE II METABOLISM

Phase II metabolism is typically carried out by uridine 5-diphospho-glucuronosyltransferases (UGTs), glutathione *S*-transferases (GSTs), *N*-acetyltransferases (NATs), and sulfotransferases (SULTs), each of which has multiple isoforms with varying developmental trajectories.

UGT1A4, UGT1A6, UGT1A9, and UGT2B7 display activity in vitro that is 10-fold lower in neonatal tissue compared with adult. Neonates dosed with medications primarily metabolized by these enzymes may have reduced intrinsic clearance.[97] UGT1A1 (involved in the metabolism of acetaminophen, ibuprofen, and warfarin as well as bilirubin) is absent in fetal liver, then quickly ramps up expression to adult values by 3 to 6 months of life.[98] Transcript levels of UGT1A9 (involved in the metabolism of ethinyl estradiol, ibuprofen, and acetaminophen) ramp up a bit more slowly, demonstrating 44% and 64% of adult values by 6 months and 2 years of life, respectively.[99] UGT2B7 (responsible for 3- and 6-glucuronidation of morphine and glucuronidation of naloxone) demonstrates differential expression and activity with age. For example, naloxone glucuronidation was two- to 2.5-fold lower in adolescents than adults, highlighting the continuation of an ontogenic effect through development.[97] Although typically associated with the liver, there is considerable extrahepatic expression of UGTs with tissue-specific levels of activity. For example, estrone conjugation by UGT is an order of magnitude higher in the small intestine compared with the liver, while *p*-nitrophenol conjugation is fivefold higher in the liver compared with the small intestine.[100]

Given their role in the metabolism of endogenous compounds such as steroid hormones, catecholamines, and thyroid hormone, the SULTs represent another important phase II pathway. For SULT1A1, expression profiles do not appear to differ significantly between infancy and adulthood. SULT2A1, by contrast, demonstrates a significant increase in activity from birth to 3 months, when values equal those seen in adults.[101] Interestingly, protein expression of SULT1E1, an enzyme responsible for estrogen inactivation, declines from fetal life to adulthood.

GSTs are responsible for glutathione conjugation of cisplatin, busulfan, and endogenous compounds, such as leukotrienes and prostaglandins.[102] GST1 reaches adult expression levels by 1 to 2 years of age.[103] However, GSTA1 and GSTA2 are present in fetal liver and increase 1.5- to twofold at the time of birth without evidence of significant further increase through adulthood. Yet, busulfan conjugation by GSTA1-1 from intestinal biopsies appears to be increased at 1 year of age and then slowly declines until adulthood. In parallel, busulfan apparent oral clearance in vivo also shows an age-dependent decrease.[104]

The phase II DME also provides an illustrative example of compensatory metabolism that occurs when primary drug metabolism pathways have yet to fully develop. UGT1A6 and SULT1A1 are both responsible for primary metabolism of acetaminophen. In the adult, the glucuronide metabolite is recovered in majority with a glucuronide-to-sulfate ratio of 1.80 ± 0.32. In contrast, the sulfate conjugate is recovered in majority in the newborn with glucuronide-to-sulfate ratio of 0.34 ± 0.08, suggesting lack of full activity of UGT1A6.[105] However, because SULT1A1 is a less efficient clearance pathway, young infants have a longer acetaminophen half-live than do older children and adults.[106]

NON–PHASE I/PHASE II METABOLISM

Large molecules (e.g., biologics) are often metabolized by non–phase I and non–phase II DMEs. Limited data are available on the role of ontogeny in the clearance of large molecules; however, some assumptions can be made from the examples that do exist. Factor VIII, a clotting cascade protein, is associated with shorter half-lives in children 1 to 6 years of age (9.2 hours) compared with older individuals 10 to 65 years (12.2 hours).[107] PK studies of insulin, growth hormone, and erythropoietin demonstrate age-dependent changes in clearance as well. Growth hormone has lower metabolic clearance rates in prepubertal children compared with adult men and women.[108,109] Erythropoietin clearance is elevated in premature infants compared with adults.[110] Insulin demonstrates higher systemic exposures in diabetic adolescents compared with diabetic children with PK profiles that are specific to the insulin isoform.[111–113] With a trend toward increased approval and use of large molecule agents, an understanding of their distinct disposition pathways and the impact of development is critical.

EXCRETION

Though excretion can occur through a variety of organ systems, the kidneys are responsible for the majority of xenobiotic elimination. Passive filtration occurs in the glomerulus, while secretion and reabsorption (both passive and active) occur at the level of the proximal and distal tubule, respectively.[114] Developmentally, nephrogenesis is complete by 36 weeks of gestation; however, maturation of the kidney continues well into childhood. The newborn kidney contains the same number of nephrons as in adults (~1,000,000 per kidney), yet is anatomically, morphologically, and functionally distinguishable from the mature adult organ.[115] From birth to 12 years of age, the kidney undergoes nearly a doubling in length and corresponding increase in weight, growth that is noticeable in the microstructures as well. The average diameter of a glomerulus in a newborn is approximately one-third of the adult. During the first 3 months of life, the radius of small pores in the glomerulus increases from 19.6 to 25 Å (~25% increase). During this period, the proportion of large pores relative to small pores increases as well. Remarkable development of proximal tubules is also observed. The average length of proximal tubules at birth is only one-tenth of the adult (2 mm vs. 20 mm), and the variability in their length is much more pronounced, with 11-fold difference between the shortest and the longest measured proximal tubule in tissue samples versus twofold difference in adult. Finally, increased vascular resistance and reduced renal blood flow occur in the newborn with a subsequent increase in fractional cardiac output to the kidney of nearly fourfold during the first year of life.[114,116]

These age-dependent anatomic differences are, as expected, accompanied by functional differences (Fig. 4.10). Glomerular filtration rate (GFR) increases strikingly after birth and continues to increase until the completion of growth in the child. However, when normalized to BSA, filtration appears similar to that observed in adults within first 1 to 2 years.[117] Interestingly, premature newborns have a significantly reduced GFR, which exhibits its own developmental trajectory[118] (Fig. 4.11). With respect to tubular reabsorption, urine concentrating ability is significantly lower at birth (600 mOsm per kg water), and it increases slowly to 900 mOsm per kg water during the first month of life, ultimately reaching 1,200 mOsm per kg in adolescence.[118]

The implication of these functional differences manifests as a significant reduction in renal clearance, often resulting in a longer elimination half-lives, for many renally cleared drugs. In premature infants, for example, the half-life of fluconazole is 88 hours. In contrast, fluconazole half-life in term newborns is reported in the range of 19.5 to 25 hours.[119] Vancomycin and amikacin clearances are also reduced in premature infants and, irrespective of gestational age, increase with postnatal age.[120,121] Typically, dosing is less frequent (i.e., dosing interval is extended) for these medications in newborns and infants in order to accommodate for the immature renal glomerular filtration and maintain appropriate systemic exposures.

Age-dependent changes in clearance of *p*-aminohippurate (PAH), a substrate for renal transport and marker of renal plasma flow, are also well described. At birth, clearance of PAH is low and gradually increases until age 2 when the adult values are reached.[122] Whether this is the result of increasing renal plasma flow or developmental changes in the expression

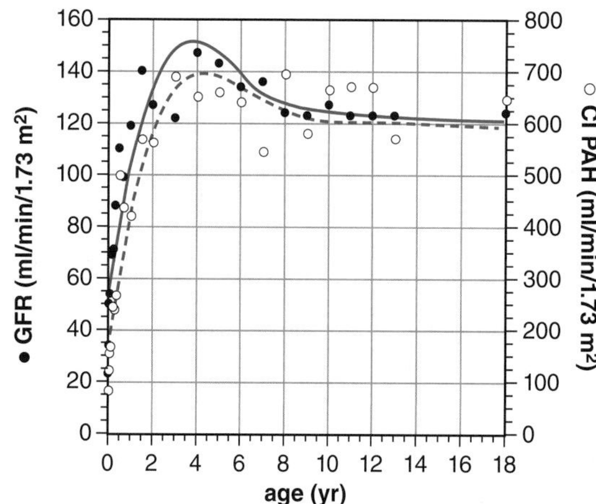

Figure 4.10 Changes in glomerular filtration (solid circles, solid line) rate and *p*-aminohippurate clearance (open circles, dashed line) as a function of age. (Reprinted with permission from Brown JT, Abdel-Rahman SM. *Pediatric pharmacokinetics. Pediatric pharmacotherapy.* Lenexa, KS: American College of Clinical Pharmacy, 2013:26.)

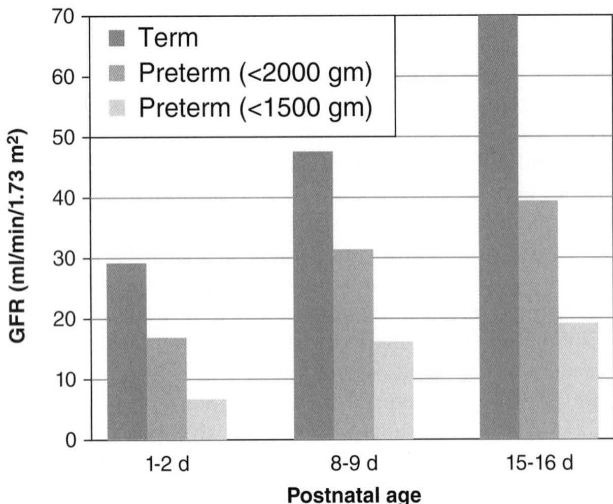

Figure 4.11 Postnatal acquisition of functional renal filtration capacity as a function of gestational age. (Reprinted with permission from Brown JT, Abdel-Rahman SM. *Pediatric pharmacokinetics. Pediatric pharmacotherapy.* Lenexa, KS: American College of Clinical Pharmacy, 2013:26.)

of relevant transporters (e.g., basolateral uptake OAT1/3 and apical efflux MRP2/4, Table 4.2) is unclear. This finding signals that the complementary transport of drugs may also change as a function of age. Recently, extensive information on the ontogeny of human renal drug transporters residing in basolateral and apical membranes of proximal tubule cells became available via quantitation of these proteins in pediatric kidney tissues.[123] The expression of basolateral uptake OAT1, OAT3, OCT2, and apical efflux P-gp transport proteins were significantly reduced in term newborn and infants compared to children, adolescents, and adults. On the other hand, expression of other apical efflux transporters (e.g., MATE1, MATE2-K, BCRP, MRP2, MRP4) demonstrated little age dependency. A summary of drugs that are representative substrates of renal transporters is presented in Table 4.2.[124–127] Based on these findings, it is reasonable to conclude which substrates may be susceptible to age-dependent changes. However, it is important to note that a fraction of this increase in renal clearance may also be due to concomitant maturation of glomerular filtration function (as discussed above). Dedicated prospective PK studies in children will help determine the extent of age-dependent PK and appropriate dosing modifications for renal transport substrates that are primarily excreted via the kidney. Given the important role of the kidneys in maintaining electrolyte homeostasis, it is not unexpected to observe age-dependent changes in expression and function of transporters mediating passage of the electrolytes across the proximal tubule. The apically located Na^+/H^+ and Cl^-/OH^- transporters and basolaterally located Na^+/K^+ ATPase, as well as several different chloride transporters, show very reduced activity in fetal and young animal models. The reduction in activity associated with age appears to be due to the lower protein abundance along the entire length of the nephron tubule in the young animals. To date, evidence implicating the presence of unique transporter isoforms or different affinities for these transporters during growth and development is lacking.[124,128–131]

Hepatobiliary clearance serves as another route of excretion. As discussed in the distribution section, a clear ontogenic profile has been demonstrated for sinusoidally located hepatic OCT1 and OATP1B3 transporters. Importantly, immature functioning of transporters located on the canalicular membrane of the hepatocyte is evident during the first few weeks of life.[132] Investigations of age-dependent expression for canalicular transporters of bile salts have, thus far, been most extensive for P-gp and MRP2.[35] Transcript and protein expression for both transporters have been detected in 14-week-old fetuses. Compared with the adult, P-gp transcript expression is approximately 20- to 30-fold lower in the fetus; however, a rapid increase occurs in the first 12 months of life, bringing expression values to within fivefold of the adult by 1 year of age. Importantly, mRNA and protein expression for P-gp may not be concordant, since protein expression levels of P-gp are reported to be constant between the ages of 1 month and 12 years,[35,133] or even through adulthood.[134] This finding was corroborated by a separate study demonstrating relatively stable expression of P-gp protein in livers from donors between 7 and 70 years old,[35] although it is important to note that the absence of age-dependent changes in P-gp expression has not been uniformly reproduced.[74] With regard to MRP2, relatively low mRNA expression has been found in fetal tissue, followed by an increase in expression seen after birth. The relative difference between fetal MRP2 mRNA and adult MRP2 mRNA is quite dramatic—approximately 200-fold. In contrast, protein expression of MRP2 was either shown not to be affected by age[74,134] or showed a reduced expression in infants less than 8 months of age compared to children older than 12 years.[35] Data on protein expression for other efflux transporter proteins residing on the canalicular membrane are similarly somewhat nonconsistent between studies; BCRP, BSEP, and MATE1 expression was shown not to be age dependent.[74] A second study showed distinct increased (BSEP) or decreased (BCRP) protein expression pattern though smaller in sample size with reduced statistical power.[134]

In following with developmental expression profiles, reduced biliary excretion may be expected for drugs that are known substrates of hepatic transporters, suggesting the need to consider dose adjustments in infants and young children.[35] Interestingly, renal clearance can compensate for this reduction in biliary clearance for some drugs that are otherwise excreted into the bile. For example, approximately 70% of the ceftriaxone dose is recovered in the urine of neonates compared to older children and adults (40% to 60%).[135] Analogous to ceftriaxone, the renal excretion of cefoperazone in premature infants is more extensive than in full-term neonates (55% vs. 18%).[136]

CONCLUSIONS

Once a drug enters the body of a child, its disposition is governed by developmental physiology and pathophysiology. Successful and rational drug dosing requires a comprehensive understanding of (a) the developmental trajectories of enzyme and transporter function, (b) the physiology of a growing and maturing body, and (c) the pathology of the underlying disease, its presentation, and progression. Due to the existing gaps in knowledge (and with limited data in the drug product label), clinicians are often presented with a challenging task, to provide the best dosing recommendation for an individual child. It is, therefore, imperative that the knowledge of underlying mechanisms that govern drug disposition continues to expand, paving the way for individualized pharmacotherapy in the neonate, child, and adolescent.

REFERENCES

1. Gad SC. Regulatory requirements for INDs/FIH (first in human) studies. In: Gad SC, ed. *Preclinical development handbook: ADME and biopharmaceutical properties.* Hoboken, NJ: John Wiley & Sons, 2008:1267–1303.
2. Giacomini KM, Huang SM, Tweedie DJ, et al. Membrane transporters in drug development. *Nat Rev Drug Discov* 2010;9(3):215–236.
3. Ventura AK, Worobey J. Early influences on the development of food preferences. *Curr Biol* 2013;23(9):R401–R408.
4. Abdel-Rahman SM, Reed MD, Wells TG, et al. Considerations in the rational design and conduct of phase I/II pediatric clinical trials: avoiding the problems and pitfalls. *Clin Pharmacol Ther* 2007;81(4):483–494.
5. Lawless H. Sensory development in children: research in taste and olfaction. *J Am Diet Assoc* 1985;85(5):577–582, 585.
6. Hogben CA, Schanker LS, Tocco DJ, et al. Absorption of drugs from the stomach. II. The human. *J Pharmacol Exp Ther* 1957;120(4):540–545.
7. Heimann G. Enteral absorption and bioavailability in children in relation to age. *Eur J Clin Pharmacol* 1980;18(1):43–50.
8. Milsap RL, Jusko WJ. Pharmacokinetics in the infant. *Environ Health Perspect* 1994;102(Suppl 11):107–110.
9. Huang NN, High RH. Comparison of serum levels following the administration of oral and parenteral preparations of penicillin to infants and children of various age groups. *J Pediatr* 1953;42(6):657–658.
10. Chen R, Takahashi H, Okamoto H, et al. Particle design of three-component system for sustained release using a 4-fluid nozzle spray-drying technique. *Chem Pharm Bull* 2006;54(11):1486–1490.
11. Patra S, Samantaray R, Pattnaik S, et al. Taste masking of Etoricoxib by using ion-exchange resin. *Pharm Dev Technol* 2010;15(5):511–517.
12. Gupta M, Brans YW. Gastric retention in neonates. *Pediatrics* 1978;62(1):26–29.
13. Berseth CL. Gestational evolution of small intestine motility in preterm and term infants. *J Pediatr* 1989;115(4):646–651.
14. Kearns GL, Robinson PK, Wilson JT, et al. Cisapride disposition in neonates and infants: in vivo reflection of cytochrome P450 3A4 ontogeny. *Clin Pharmacol Ther* 2003;74(4):312–325.
15. Bonner JJ, Vajjah P, Abduljalil K, et al. Does age affect gastric emptying time? a model-based meta-analysis of data from premature neonates through to adults. *Biopharm Drug Dispos* 2015;36(4):245–257.
16. Grand RJ, Watkins JB, Torti FM. Development of the human gastrointestinal tract. A review. *Gastroenterology* 1976;70(5 Pt1):790–810.
17. Weaver LT, Austin S, Cole TJ. Small intestinal length: a factor essential for gut adaptation. *Gut* 1991;32(11):1321–1323.
18. Yanowitz TD, Yao AC, Pettigrew KD, et al. Postnatal hemodynamic changes in very low-birth weight infants. *J Appl Physiol* 1999;87(1):370–380.
19. Martinussen M, Brubakk AM, Linker DT, et al. Mesenteric blood flow velocity and its relation to circulatory adaptation during the first week of life in healthy term infants. *Pediatr Res* 1994;36(3):334–339.
20. Martinussen M, Brubakk AM, Vik T, et al. Mesenteric blood flow velocity and its relation to transitional circulatory adaptation in appropriate for gestational age preterm infants. *Pediatr Res* 1996;39(2):275–280.
21. Brundin T. Whole body and splanchnic metabolic, circulatory, and thermal effects of oral vs. intravenous fat administration. *Am J Physiol* 1998;274(4):E684–E691.
22. Lane AJ, Coombs RC, Evans DH, et al. Effect of feed interval and feed type on splanchnic haemodynamics. *Arch Dis Child Fetal Neonatal Ed* 1998;79(1):F49–F53.
23. Poley JR, Dower JC, Owen CA Jr, et al. Bile acids in infants and children. *J Lab Clin Med* 1964;63:838–846.
24. Suchy FJ, Balistreri WF, Heubi JE, et al. Physiologic cholestasis: elevation of the primary serum bile acid concentrations in normal infants. *Gastroenterology* 1981;80(5 Pt 1):1037–1041.
25. Filer LJ Jr, Mattson FH, Fomon SJ. Triglyceride configuration and fat absorption by the human infant. *J Nutr* 1969;99(3):293–298.
26. Lee PC, Borysewicz R, Struve M, et al. Development of lipolytic activity in gastric aspirates from premature infants. *J Pediatr Gastroenterol Nutr* 1993;17(3):291–297.
27. Hamosh M, Bitman J, Liao TH, et al. Gastric lipolysis and fat absorption in preterm infants: effect of medium-chain triglyceride or long-chain triglyceride-containing formulas. *Pediatrics* 1989;83(1):86–92.
28. Abdel-Rahman SM, Kearns GL. Single oral dose escalation pharmacokinetics of pleconaril (VP 63843) capsules in adults. *J Clin Pharm* 1999;39(6):613–618.
29. Kearns GL, Bradley JS, Jacobs RF, et al. Single dose pharmacokinetics of pleconaril in neonates. Pediatric Pharmacology Research Unit Network. *Pediatr Infect Dis J* 2000;19(9):833–839.
30. Shankaran S, Kauffman RE. Use of chloramphenicol palmitate in neonates. *J Pediatr* 1984;105(1):113–116.
31. Rings EH, Minich DM, Vonk RJ, et al. Functional development of fat absorption in term and preterm neonates strongly correlates with ability to absorb long-chain fatty acids from intestinal lumen. *Pediatr Res* 2002;51(1):57–63.
32. Orrhage K, Nord CE. Factors controlling the bacterial colonization of the intestine in breastfed infants. *Acta Paediatr* 1999;88(430):47–57.
33. Kundu P, Blacher E, Elinav E, et al. Our gut microbiome: the evolving inner self. *Cell* 2017;171(7):1481–1493.
34. Linday L, Dobkin JF, Wang TC, et al. Digoxin inactivation by the gut flora in infancy and childhood. *Pediatrics* 1987;79(4):544–548.
35. Brouwer KL, Aleksunes LM, Brandys B, et al. Human ontogeny of drug transporters: review and recommendations of the Pediatric Transporter Working Group. *Clin Pharmacol Ther* 2015;98(3):266–287.
36. Abdel-Rahman SM, Johnson FK, Connor JD, et al. Developmental pharmacokinetics and pharmacodynamics of nizatidine. *J Pediatr Gastroenterol Nutr* 2004;38(4):442–451.
37. Garrick MD. Human iron transporters. *Genes Nutr* 2011;6(1):45–54.
38. Gladtke E, Rind H. Iron therapy during childhood. *Ger Med Mon* 1966;11(11):438–442.
39. Ogihara T, Kano T, Wagatsuma T, et al. Oseltamivir (tamiflu) is a substrate of peptide transporter 1. *Drug Metab Dispos* 2009;37(8):1676–1681.
40. Beck DH, Schenk MR, Hagemann K, et al. The pharmacokinetics and analgesic efficacy of larger dose rectal acetaminophen (40 mg/kg) in adults: a double-blinded, randomized study. *Anesth Analg* 2000;90(2):431–436.
41. Coulthard KP, Nielson HW, Schroder M, et al. Relative bioavailability and plasma paracetamol profiles of Panadol suppositories in children. *J Paediatr Child Health* 1998;34(5):425–431.
42. van Lingen RA, Deinum JT, Quak JM, et al. Pharmacokinetics and metabolism of rectally administered paracetamol in preterm neonates. *Arch Dis Child Fetal Neonatal Ed* 1999;80(1):F59–F63.
43. Di Lorenzo C, Flores AF, Hyman PE. Age-related changes in colon motility. *J Pediatr* 1995;127(4):593–596.
44. Stratchunsky LS, Nazarov AD, Firsov AA, et al. Age dependence of erythromycin rectal bioavailability in children. *Eur J Drug Metab Pharmacokinet* 1991;Spec No 3:321–323.
45. Fluhr JW, Pfisterer S, Gloor M. Direct comparison of skin physiology in children and adults with bioengineering methods. *Pediatr Dermatol* 2000;17(6):436–439.
46. Okah FA, Wickett RR, Pickens WL, et al. Surface electrical capacitance as a noninvasive bedside measure of epidermal barrier maturation in the newborn infant. *Pediatrics* 1995;96(4 Pt 1):688–692.
47. Amato M, Huppi P, Isenschmid M, et al. Developmental aspects of percutaneous caffeine absorption in premature infants. *Am J Perinatol* 1992;9(5–6):431–434.
48. Rutter N. Percutaneous drug absorption in the newborn: hazards and uses. *Clin Perinatol* 1987;14(4):911–930.
49. West DP, Worobec S, Solomon LM. Pharmacology and toxicology of infant skin. *J Invest Dermatol* 1981;76(3):147–150.
50. Nelson D, Ho J, Pacaud D, et al. Virilization in two pre-pubertal children exposed to topical androgen. *J Pediatr Endocrinol Metab* 2013;26(9–10):981–985.
51. Parekh D, Miller MA, Borys D, et al. Transdermal patch medication delivery systems and pediatric poisonings, 2002–2006. *Clin Pediatr* 2008;47(7):659–663.
52. Swartz MA. The physiology of the lymphatic system. *Adv Drug Deliv Rev* 2001;50(1–2):3–20.
53. Richter WF, Bhansali SG, Morris ME. Mechanistic determinants of biotherapeutics absorption following SC administration. *AAPS J* 2012;14(3):559–570.
54. Kim H, Park H, Lee SJ. Effective method for drug injection into subcutaneous tissue. *Sci Rep* 2017;7(1):9613.
55. Heinemann L. Variability of insulin absorption and insulin action. *Diabetes Technol Ther* 2002;4(5):673–682.
56. King A, Balaji S, Keswani SG. Biology and function of fetal and pediatric skin. *Facial Plast Surg Clin North Am* 2013;21(1):1–6.
57. Ruan Y, Elleri D, Allen JM, et al. Pharmacokinetics of diluted (U20) insulin aspart compared with standard (U100) in children aged 3–6 years with type 1 diabetes during closed-loop insulin delivery: a randomised clinical trial. *Diabetologia* 2015;58(4):687–690.
58. Carry MR, Ringel SP, Starcevich JM. Distribution of capillaries in normal and diseased human skeletal muscle. *Muscle Nerve* 1986;9(5):445–454.
59. Sheng KT, Huang NN, Promadhattavedi V. Serum concentrations of cephalothin in infants and children and placental transmission of the antibiotic. *Antimicrob Agents Chemother (Bethesda)* 1964;10:200–206.
60. Kafetzis DA, Sinaniotis CA, Papadatos CJ, et al. Pharmacokinetics of amikacin in infants and pre-school children. *Acta Paediatr Scand* 1979;68(3):419–422.
61. Siber GR, Echeverria P, Smith AL, et al. Pharmacokinetics of gentamicin in children and adults. *J Infect Dis* 1975;132(6):637–651.
62. Gerber AU, Craig WA. Aminoglycoside-selected subpopulations of *Pseudomonas aeruginosa*: characterization and virulence in normal and leukopenic mice. *J Lab Clin Med* 1982;100(5):671–681.
63. Blaser J, Stone BB, Groner MC, et al. Comparative study with enoxacin and netilmicin in a pharmacodynamic model to determine importance of ratio of antibiotic peak concentration to MIC for bactericidal activity and emergence of resistance. *Antimicrob Agents Chemother* 1987;31(7):1054–1060.
64. Kearns GL, Abdel-Rahman SM, Blumer JL, et al. Single dose pharmacokinetics of linezolid in infants and children. *Pediatric Infect Dis J* 2000;19(12):1178–1184.
65. Holt DW, Hayler AM, Healey GF. Effect of age and plasma concentrations of albumin and alpha 1-acid glycoprotein on protein binding of disopyramide. *Br J Clin Pharm* 1983;16(3):344–345.
66. Kingston HG, Kendrick A, Sommer KM, et al. Binding of thiopental in neonatal serum. *Anesthesiology* 1990;72(3):428–431.
67. Meistelman C, Benhamou D, Barre J, et al. Effects of age on plasma protein binding of sufentanil. *Anesthesiology* 1990;72(3):470–473.
68. Fredholm BB, Rane A, Persson B. Diphenylhydantoin binding to proteins in plasma and its dependence on free fatty acid and bilirubin concentration in dogs and newborn infants. *Pediatr Res* 1975;9(1):26–30.
69. Daood M, Tsai C, Ahdab-Barmada M, et al. ABC transporter (P-gp/ABCB1, MRP1/ABCC1, BCRP/ABCG2) expression in the developing human CNS. *Neuropediatrics* 2008;39(4):211–218.
70. Lam J, Baello S, Iqbal M, et al. The ontogeny of P-glycoprotein in the developing human blood-brain barrier: implication for opioid toxicity in neonates. *Pediatr Res* 2015;78(4):417–421.
71. Koren G, Butt W, Chinyanga H, et al. Postoperative morphine infusion in newborn infants: assessment of disposition characteristics and safety. *J Pediatr* 1985;107(6):963–967.
72. Way WL, Costley EC, Leongway E. Respiratory sensitivity of the newborn infant to meperidine and morphine. *Clin Pharmacol Ther* 1965;6:454–461.
73. Bouwmeester NJ, van den Anker JN, Hop WC, et al. Age-and therapy-related effects on morphine requirements and plasma concentrations of morphine and its metabolites in postoperative infants. *Br J Anaesth* 2003;90(5):642–652.

74. Prasad B, Gaedigk A, Vrana M, et al. Ontogeny of hepatic drug transporters as quantified by LC-MS/MS proteomics. *Clin Pharmacol Ther* 2016;100(4):362–370.
75. Hahn D, Emoto C, Vinks AA, et al. Developmental changes in hepatic organic cation transporter OCT1 protein expression from neonates to children. *Drug Metab Dispos* 2017;45(1):23–26.
76. Wagner JB, Abdel-Rahman S, Van Haandel L, et al. Impact of SLCO1B1 genotype on pediatric simvastatin acid pharmacokinetics. *J Clin Pharm* 2018;58(6):823–833.
77. Fukuda T, Chidambaran V, Mizuno T, et al. OCT1 genetic variants influence the pharmacokinetics of morphine in children. *Pharmacogenomics* 2013;14(10):1141–1151.
78. Zuppa AF, Zane NR, Moorthy G, et al. A population pharmacokinetic analysis to study the effect of extracorporeal membrane oxygenation on cefepime disposition in children. *Pediatr Crit Care Med* 2019;20(1):62–70.
79. Pineiro-Carrero VM, Pineiro EO. Liver. *Pediatrics* 2004;113(Suppl 4):1097–1106.
80. Zanger UM, Schwab M. Cytochrome P450 enzymes in drug metabolism: regulation of gene expression, enzyme activities, and impact of genetic variation. *Pharmacol Ther* 2013;138(1):103–141.
81. Maya MT, Domingos CR, Guerreiro MT, et al. Comparative bioavailability of two immediate release tablets of cisapride in healthy volunteers. *Eur J Drug Metab Pharmacokinet* 1998;23(3):377–381.
82. Mukherjee A, Dombi T, Wittke B, et al. Population pharmacokinetics of sildenafil in term neonates: evidence of rapid maturation of metabolic clearance in the early postnatal period. *Clin Pharmacol Ther* 2009;85(1):56–63.
83. Blake MJ, Gaedigk A, Pearce RE, et al. Ontogeny of dextromethorphan O- and N-demethylation in the first year of life. *Clin Pharmacol Ther* 2007;81(4):510–516.
84. Bourgeois BF, Dodson WE. Phenytoin elimination in newborns. *Neurology* 1983;33(2):173–178.
85. Whelan HT, Hendeles L, Haberkern CM, et al. High intravenous phenytoin dosage requirement in a newborn infant. *Neurology* 1983;33(1):106–108.
86. Koukouritaki SB, Manro JR, Marsh SA, et al. Developmental expression of human hepatic CYP2C9 and CYP2C19. *J Pharmacol Exp Ther* 2004;308(3):965–974.
87. Faure C, Michaud L, Shaghaghi EK, et al. Intravenous omeprazole in children: pharmacokinetics and effect on 24-hour intragastric pH. *J Pediatr Gastroenterol Nutr* 2001;33(2):144–148.
88. Jacqz-Aigrain E, Bellaich M, Faure C, et al. Pharmacokinetics of intravenous omeprazole in children. *Eur J Clin Pharmacol* 1994;47(2):181–185.
89. Vieira I, Sonnier M, Cresteil T. Developmental expression of CYP2E1 in the human liver. Hypermethylation control of gene expression during the neonatal period. *Eur J Biochem* 1996;238(2):476–483.
90. Sonnier M, Cresteil T. Delayed ontogenesis of CYP1A2 in the human liver. *Eur J Biochem* 1998;251(3):893–898.
91. Suyagh M, Collier PS, Millership JS, et al. Metronidazole population pharmacokinetics in preterm neonates using dried blood-spot sampling. *Pediatrics* 2011;127(2):e367–e374.
92. Upadhyaya P, Bhatnagar V, Basu N. Pharmacokinetics of intravenous metronidazole in neonates. *J Pediatr Surg* 1988;23(3):263–265.
93. Lacroix B, Kedinger M, Simon-Assmann P, et al. Early organogenesis of human small intestine: scanning electron microscopy and brush border enzymology. *Gut* 1984;25(9):925–930.
94. Johnson TN, Tanner MS, Taylor CJ, et al. Enterocytic CYP3A4 in a paediatric population: developmental changes and the effect of coeliac disease and cystic fibrosis. *Br J Clin Pharmacol* 2001;51(5):451–460.
95. Stahlberg MR, Hietanen E, Maki M. Mucosal biotransformation rates in the small intestine of children. *Gut* 1988;29(8):1058–1063.
96. Cho HJ, Yoon IS. Pharmacokinetic interactions of herbs with cytochrome p450 and p-glycoprotein. *Evid Based Complement Alter Med* 2015;2015:736431.
97. Bhatt DK, Mehrotra A, Gaedigk A, et al. Age-and genotype-dependent variability in the protein abundance and activity of six major uridine diphosphate-glucuronosyltransferases in human liver. *Clin Pharmacol Ther* 2019;105(1):131–141.
98. de Wildt SN, Kearns GL, Leeder JS, et al. Glucuronidation in humans. Pharmacogenetic and developmental aspects. *Clin Pharmacokinet* 1999;36(6):439–452.
99. Strassburg CP, Vogel A, Kneip S, et al. Polymorphisms of the human UDP-glucuronosyltransferase (UGT) 1A7 gene in colorectal cancer. *Gut* 2002;50(6):851–856.
100. Tukey RH, Strassburg CP. Genetic multiplicity of the human UDP-glucuronosyltransferases and regulation in the gastrointestinal tract. *Mol Pharmacol* 2001;59(3):405–414.
101. Duanmu Z, Weckle A, Koukouritaki SB, et al. Developmental expression of aryl, estrogen, and hydroxysteroid sulfotransferases in pre- and postnatal human liver. *J Pharmacol Exp Ther* 2006;316(3):1310–1317.
102. Allocati N, Masulli M, Di Ilio C, et al. Glutathione transferases: substrates, inhibitors and pro-drugs in cancer and neurodegenerative diseases. *Oncogenesis* 2018;7(1):8.
103. Strange RC, Davis BA, Faulder CG, et al. The human glutathione S-transferases: developmental aspects of the GST1, GST2, and GST3 loci. *Biochem Genet* 1985;23(11–12):1011–1028.
104. Gibbs JP, Liacouras CA, Baldassano RN, et al. Up-regulation of glutathione S-transferase activity in enterocytes of young children. *Drug Metab Dispos* 1999;27(12):1466–1469.
105. Miller RP, Roberts RJ, Fischer LJ. Acetaminophen elimination kinetics in neonates, children, and adults. *Clin Pharmacol Ther* 1976;19(3):284–294.
106. Allegaert K, Van der Marel CD, Debeer A, et al. Pharmacokinetics of single dose intravenous propacetamol in neonates: effect of gestational age. *Arch Dis Child Fetal Neonatal Ed* 2004;89(1):F25–F28.
107. Bjorkman S, Oh M, Spotts G, et al. Population pharmacokinetics of recombinant factor VIII: the relationships of pharmacokinetics to age and body weight. *Blood* 2012;119(2):612–618.
108. Rosenbaum M, Gertner JM. Metabolic clearance rates of synthetic human growth hormone in children, adult women, and adult men. *J Clin Endocrinol Metab* 1989;69(4):820–824.
109. Kearns GL, Kemp SF, Frindik JP. Single and multiple dose pharmacokinetics of methionyl growth hormone in children with idiopathic growth hormone deficiency. *J Clin Endocrinol Metab* 1991;72(5):1148–1156.
110. Brown MS, Jones MA, Ohls RK, et al. Single-dose pharmacokinetics of recombinant human erythropoietin in preterm infants after intravenous and subcutaneous administration. *J Pediatr* 1993;122(4):655–657.
111. Mortensen HB, Lindholm A, Olsen BS, et al. Rapid appearance and onset of action of insulin aspart in paediatric subjects with type 1 diabetes. *Eur J Pediatr* 2000;159(7):483–488.
112. Danne T, Becker RH, Heise T, et al. Pharmacokinetics, prandial glucose control, and safety of insulin glulisine in children and adolescents with type 1 diabetes. *Diabetes Care* 2005;28(9):2100–2105.
113. Danne T, Lupke K, Walte K, et al. Insulin detemir is characterized by a consistent pharmacokinetic profile across age-groups in children, adolescents, and adults with type 1 diabetes. *Diabetes Care* 2003;26(11):3087–3092.
114. Spitzer A. Renal physiology and functional development. In: Edelman CM, ed. *Pediatric kidney disease*. Boston, MA: Little, Brown and Company, 1978:25–128.
115. Chen N, Aleksa K, Woodland C, et al. Ontogeny of drug elimination by the human kidney. *Pediatr Nephrol (Berlin, Germany)* 2006;21(2):160–168.
116. McCrory WM. Embryonic development and prenatal maturation of the kidney. In: Edelman CM, ed. *Pediatric kidney disease*. Boston, MA: Little, Brown and Company, 1978:3–25.
117. Schwartz GJ, Feld LG, Langford DJ. A simple estimate of glomerular filtration rate in full-term infants during the first year of life. *J Pediatr* 1984;104(6):849–854.
118. John TR, Moore WM, Jeffries JE, eds. *Children are different: developmental physiology*, 2nd ed. Columbus, OH: Ross Laboratories, 1978.
119. Saxen H, Hoppu K, Pohjavuori M. Pharmacokinetics of fluconazole in very low birth weight infants during the first two weeks of life. *Clin Pharmacol Therapeut* 1993;54(3):269–277.
120. Capparelli EV, Lane JR, Romanowski GL, et al. The influences of renal function and maturation on vancomycin elimination in newborns and infants. *J Clin Pharmacol* 2001;41(9):927–934.
121. Kenyon CF, Knoppert DC, Lee SK, et al. Amikacin pharmacokinetics and suggested dosage modifications for the preterm infant. *Antimicrob Agents Chemother* 1990;34(2):265–268.
122. Kearns GL, Abdel-Rahman SM, Alander SW, et al. Developmental pharmacology–drug disposition, action, and therapy in infants and children. *N Engl J Med* 2003;349(12):1157–1167.
123. Cheung KWK, van Groen BD, Spaans E, et al. A comprehensive analysis of ontogeny of renal drug transporters: mRNA analyses, quantitative proteomics and localization. *Clin Pharmacol Ther* 2019;106(5):1083–1092.
124. Lee W, Kim RB. Transporters and renal drug elimination. *Ann Rev Pharmacol Toxicol* 2004;44:137–166.
125. Tsuji A. Transporter-mediated drug interactions. *Drug Metab Pharmacokinet* 2002;17(4):253–274.
126. Wright SH, Dantzler WH. Molecular and cellular physiology of renal organic cation and anion transport. *Physiol Rev* 2004;84(3):987–1049.
127. University of Washington Drug Interaction Database. www.druginteractioninfo.org. Accessed May, 2019.
128. Shah M, Quigley R, Baum M. Maturation of proximal straight tubule NaCl transport: role of thyroid hormone. *Am J Physiol Renal Physiol* 2000;278(4):F596–F602.
129. Guillery EN, Karniski LP, Mathews MS, et al. Maturation of proximal tubule Na+/H+ antiporter activity in sheep during transition from fetus to newborn. *Am J Physiol* 1994;267(4 Pt 2):F537–F545.
130. Petershack JA, Nagaraja SC, Guillery EN. Role of glucocorticoids in the maturation of renal cortical Na+-K+-ATPase during fetal life in sheep. *Am J Physiol* 1999;276(6):R1825–R1832.
131. Shah M, Quigley R, Baum M. Neonatal rabbit proximal tubule basolateral membrane Na+/H+ antiporter and Cl-/base exchange. *Am J Physiol* 1999;276(6):R1792–R1797.
132. Rollins DE, Klaassen CD. Biliary excretion of drugs in man. *Clin Pharmacokinet* 1979;4(5):368–379.
133. Schuetz EG, Furuya KN, Schuetz JD. Interindividual variation in expression of P-glycoprotein in normal human liver and secondary hepatic neoplasms. *J Pharmacol Exp Ther* 1995;275(2):1011–1018.
134. Mooij MG, van de Steeg E, van Rosmalen J, et al. Proteomic analysis of the developmental trajectory of human hepatic membrane transporter proteins in the first three months of life. *Drug Metab Dispos* 2016;44(7):1005–1013.
135. Hayton WL, Stoeckel K. Age-associated changes in ceftriaxone pharmacokinetics. *Clin Pharmacokinet* 1986;11(1):76–86.
136. Rosenfeld WN, Evans HE, Batheja R, et al. Pharmacokinetics of cefoperazone in full-term and premature neonates. *Antimicrob Agents Chemother* 1983;23(6):866–869.

CHAPTER

5

Brian D. Chapron
J. Steven Leeder

Pharmacogenetics, Pharmacogenomics, and Pharmacoproteomics in Newborns and Children

INTRODUCTION

It is readily accepted that genetic factors play an important role in influencing a child's potential physical characteristics, such as height, weight, or hair color. Genetic factors are also important (although not sole) determinants of interindividual and intraindividual variability in susceptibility to pediatric diseases as well as in the disposition of and response to medications used to treat those diseases. Pharmacotherapy in adults has benefited from knowledge of pharmacogenetic principles acquired over the past 60 to 70 years, but application to pediatric therapeutics is still in its infancy. In 2003, the International Human Genome Sequencing Consortium announced the successful completion of the Human Genome Project initiated in 1990, 2 years after being presented in draft form.[1] Since then, whole genomic sequencing has become dramatically more accessible and affordable. Numerous companies now offer full genomic sequencing services both to clinicians and directly to consumers, often at a cost of under a thousand dollars (compared to the $2.7B cost of the first genome by the Human Genome Project Consortium). More targeted approaches, focusing on predetermined subsets of genes with potential implications for human health, can be purchased for even less. Following the vanguard of genomics has been a host of other "-omics" sciences. In 2002, the Human Plasma Proteome Project was initiated. As of the time of the writing this chapter, over 3,500 proteins have been conclusively identified as part of the Human Plasma Proteome Project, and there is inconclusive evidence for at least 1,000 additional proteins.[2] Comparable advances in characterizing the human lipidome and metabolome have also been made. A truly enormous and progressively expanding amount patient-specific data is now at our fingertips, but precisely how to interpret and clinically apply these data has proved a persistent challenge. Nevertheless, there is continued hope that investments in these "-omics" fields will decrease morbidity and mortality through the development of more effective strategies to diagnose, treat, and prevent human disease. Society has every right to expect that children and adults will benefit equally from this investment of public funds. However, children present unique challenges in this context because developmental changes in drug disposition and response are superimposed upon a basal level of pharmacogenetic variability. The purpose of this chapter is to introduce the concepts of pharmacogenetics and pharmacogenomics and to describe how pharmacoproteomics (and other "-omic" fields of endeavor spawned in the genome era) can be employed to navigate the complex relationship between genotype and phenotype at a given stage of childhood development.

HISTORICAL CONSIDERATIONS

In 1841, Alexander Ure reported that hippuric acid was formed from benzoic acid in the body, leading physiologic chemists to discover that many foreign substances excreted by humans were chemically altered relative to the forms that had been administered—the process we now refer to as drug biotransformation (or less properly, drug metabolism). At the beginning of the 20th century, Archibald Garrod proposed that enzymes were implicated in the detoxification of foreign substances. A key element of his later work was the concept that disproportionate responses to foreign substances could result from deficiency of the required detoxifying enzyme. A variation in the theme of altered responses to foreign substances (*xenobiotics*) became apparent with the synthesis of phenylthiocarbamide in 1931 when, in the process searching out artificial sweeteners, A. L. Fox discovered that some people found the chemical intensely bitter while others found it tasteless.[3] It was not until the 1950s, however, that certain adverse drug reactions, such as unusually prolonged respiratory muscle paralysis due to succinylcholine, hemolysis associated with antimalarial therapy, and isoniazid-induced neurotoxicity, were recognized to be a consequence of inherited variation in enzyme activities, as reviewed by Arno Motulsky in 1957.[4]

In 1959, Fridriech Vogel coined the term *pharmacogenetics* to describe the study of genetically determined variations in drug response, and the first book on the subject was published in 1962 by Werner Kalow.[5] Through a series of twin studies conducted during the late 1960s and early 1970s, Elliott Vesell illustrated the importance of genetic variation in drug disposition by observing that the half-lives of several drugs were more similar in monozygotic twins than those in dizygotic twins.[6] With the discovery of the debrisoquine/sparteine hydroxylase polymorphism,[7,8] due to inherited defects in the cytochrome P450 2D6 gene (*CYP2D6*) and mephenytoin hydroxylase deficiency (*CYP2C19*)[9] in the late 1970s and early 1980s, the importance of genetic polymorphisms in drug-metabolizing enzymes has become increasingly apparent. This is particularly true in recent years due to an enhanced awareness of the number of clinically useful drugs that are metabolized by polymorphically expressed enzymes and the proportion of treated patients who are affected.

In the 1970s, an increasing appreciation of genetic influences on variability in drug disposition and response was accompanied by heightened awareness that environmental factors (e.g., diet, smoking status, concomitant drug or toxicant exposure), physiologic variables (e.g., age, gender, disease, pregnancy), and patient compliance also played important roles. Advances in analytic tools to accurately measure drugs and drug metabolites in biologic fluids and the development of mathematical models to characterize and predict changes in drug concentration over time (*pharmacokinetics*) led to the application of pharmacokinetic principles to optimize drug therapy in individual patients. Introduction of *therapeutic drug monitoring* (TDM) programs was the first application of personalized medicine—recognition that all patients were unique and that serum concentration–time data for an individual patient theoretically could be used to optimize pharmacotherapy was a significant advance over the concept of "one-dose-fits-all." However, routine TDM does not necessarily translate to improved patient outcome in all situations.[10]

At a molecular level, the pharmacokinetic properties of a drug are determined by the genes that control its disposition in the body (e.g., absorption, distribution, metabolism, excretion), with drug-metabolizing enzymes and drug transporters assuming particularly important roles. Over the past 25 years, the functional consequences of genetic variation in several drug-metabolizing enzymes have been described in individuals representative of different ethnic groups.[11] Whereas the most common clinical manifestation of pharmacogenetic variability in drug biotransformation is an increased risk of concentration-dependent toxicity due to reduced clearance and drug accumulation, it has become more apparent in recent years that the concentration–effect relationship (*pharmacodynamics*) is perhaps more relevant for optimizing drug efficacy. Therefore, the pharmacogenetics of drug receptors and other target proteins involved in signal transduction or disease pathogenesis can also be expected to contribute significantly to interindividual variability in drug response.[12,13] However, the most important concept is that the pharmacogenetic determinants of drug response involve multiple genes, and therefore, for a particular individual, polymorphisms in a single gene are unlikely to be predictive of response.

In 1987, the term *genomics* was introduced to describe the study of the structure and function of the entire complement of genetic material—the genome—including chromosomes, genes, and DNA.[14] In 1990, the Human Genome Project was initiated as a nearly three billion dollar public investment with the goal of sequencing the entire complement of human genes by the year 2005 but, more importantly, with the expectation that decreased morbidity and mortality through the development of more effective strategies to diagnose, treat, and prevent human disease would be the return on that investment (Fig. 5.1). The publicly funded initiative was forced to accelerate its efforts when J. Craig Venter announced that his company, Celera Genomics, would sequence the human genome first. The two efforts resulted in simultaneous publication of initial draft sequences in 2001,[1,15] and the International Human Genome Sequencing Consortium announced completion of the task on April 15, 2003, with an estimated accuracy of one error in 100,000 bases.[16] The human genome consists of three gigabases (three billion bases) of DNA sequence that code for approximately 30,000 genes, far fewer than was originally expected. However, it appears that this number of genes encodes 100,000 proteins through the process of *alternative splicing* whereby a gene's *exons* or coding regions are spliced together in different ways to produce variant messenger RNA (mRNA) molecules that are translated into different proteins or isoforms of the same protein. Thus, the vast amounts of genomic data generated by the Human Genome Project have laid the foundation for an "-omic" revolution that includes, but is not limited to, the *transcriptome*, the set of expressed genes from a genome[17,18]; the *proteome*, the set of proteins encoded by the genome[19]; and the *physiome*, in which biochemical, biophysical, and anatomic information from cells, tissues, and organs will be integrated using computational methods to provide a model of the human body.[20] Metabolomics and metabonomics are related terms that are sometimes used interchangeably in the literature. *Metabolomics* refers to the complete set of low-molecular weight molecules (metabolites) present in a living system (cell, tissue, organ, or organism) at a particular developmental or pathologic state. *Metabonomics* has been defined as the study of how the metabolic profile of biologic systems change in response to perturbations due to pathophysiologic stimuli, toxic exposures, and dietary changes, among others.[21,22] *Pharmacometabonomics* has been defined as "the prediction of the outcome, efficacy, or toxicity of a drug or xenobiotic intervention in an individual based on a mathematical model of preintervention metabolite signatures."[23] *Chemogenomics* is the application of combinatorial chemistry to generate libraries of small molecular weight compounds that can serve both as probes to investigate biologic mechanisms and as lead compounds for drug development.[24] *Lipidomics* has been defined as the study of "cellular lipids on a large scale based on analytical chemistry principles."[25] Several resources that define pharmacogenetics, pharmcogenomics, and to some extent related "-omics" fields and their potential application to human health and disease are available on the Internet (Table 5.1).

BASIC CONCEPTS AND DEFINITIONS

Genetic variability results from gene mutation and the exchange of genetic information between chromosomes that occurs during meiosis. With the exception of sex-linked genes (genes occurring on the X or Y chromosomes), every individual carries two copies of each gene they possess. All copies of a specific gene present within a population may not have identical nucleotide sequences, and these genetic *polymorphisms* contribute to the variability observed in that population. The presence of different nucleotides at a given position within a gene is called a *single-nucleotide polymorphism* (SNP), and SNPs are rapidly becoming an important component of the genomics lexicon. More recently, focus has shifted to characterizing *haplotypes*, collections of SNPs and other allelic variations that are located close to each

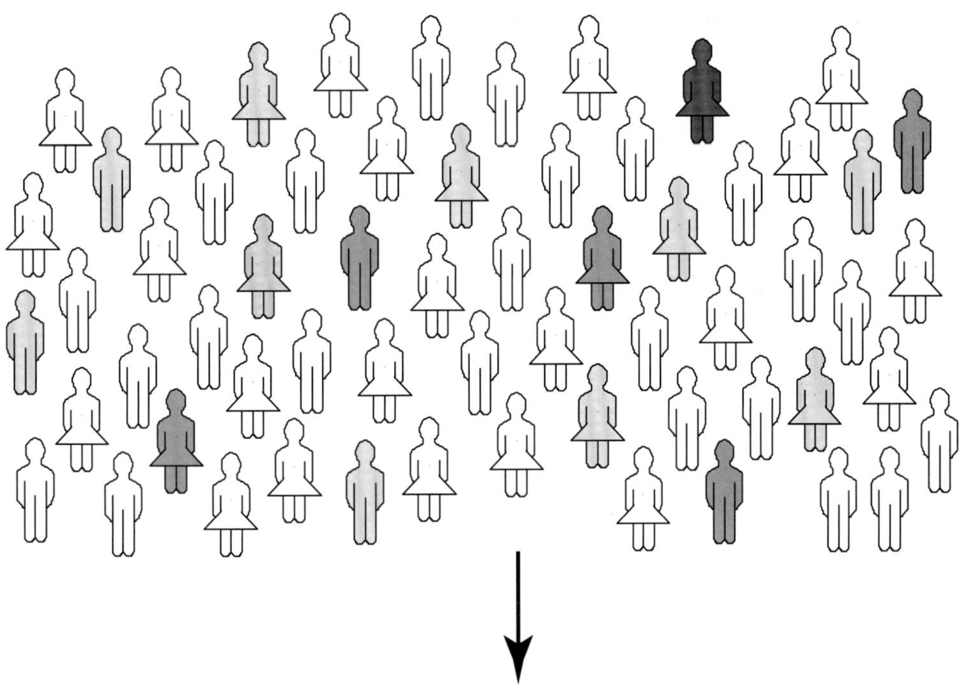

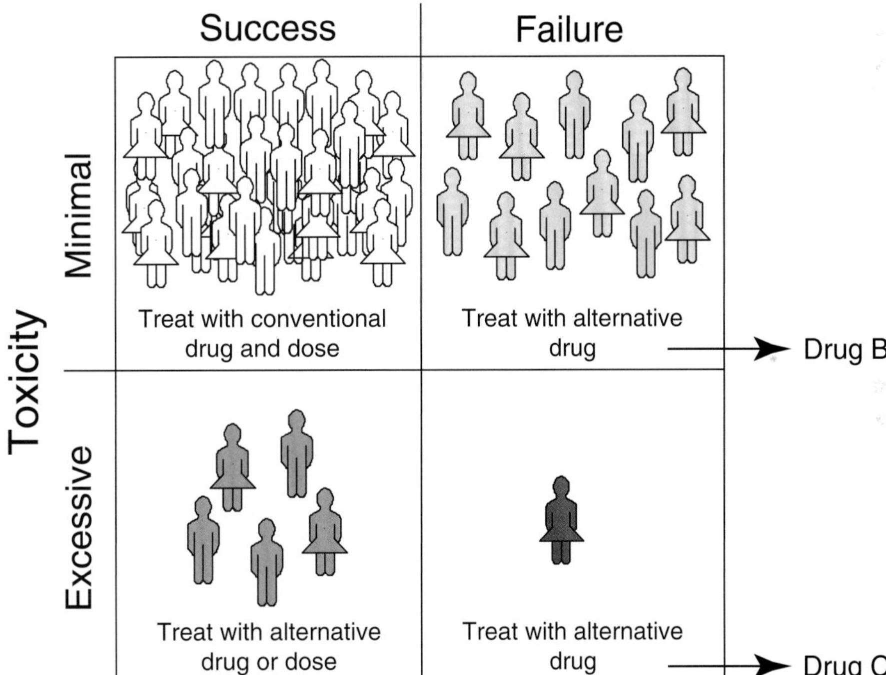

Figure 5.1 The promise of genomic medicine to human health and disease. The goal of personalized medicine will be achieved by identifying subgroups of patients who will respond favorably to a given drug with a minimum of side effects, as well as those who will not respond or who will show excessive toxicity with standard doses. A further benefit of pharmacogenomics will be the ability to select the most appropriate alternative drug for those patients who fail treatment with conventional drugs and doses.

other and inherited together; creating a catalog of haplotypes is also a goal of the Human Genome Project, referred to as the HapMap Project.[26] In genes where polymorphisms have been detected, alternative forms of the gene are called *alleles*. Individual alleles are designated by the italicized gene name (e.g., *CYP2D6*) followed by an asterisk and an Arabic number, with **1* typically designating, by convention, the fully functional wild-type allele. When the alleles at a particular gene locus are identical, a *homozygous* state exists, whereas the term *heterozygous* refers to the situation in which different alleles are present at the same gene locus. The term *genotype* refers to an individual's genetic constitution, while the observable characteristics or physical manifestations constitute the *phenotype*, which is the net consequence of genetic and environmental effects.

Human genetic variation can take many forms, but is broadly divided into two general classes of variation: single-nucleotide variations and *structural variations.* SNPs are the most prevalent class of genetic variation, and it has been estimated that there are approximately 11 million SNPs in the human genome. Structural variations encompass all differences in DNA sequence that involve more than one nucleotide. Insertions–deletions variants (*indels*) occur when a contiguous set of one or more nucleotides is absent in some individuals and present in others. *Block substitutions* involve variation of a string of contiguous nucleotides (or "block") that differs between two genomes. Sequence *inversions* occur when the order of an entire block of nucleotides is reversed in a specific region of the genome. Finally, *copy number variations* (CNVs) refer to the deletion or duplication of identical or near-identical DNA sequences that may be thousands to millions of bases in size. Although they occur less frequently than SNPs, structural variations may constitute 0.5% to 1% of an individual's genome and thus are the subject of intensive investigation for their contribution to phenotypic variation.[27,28]

Pharmacogenetics, the study of the role of genetic factors in drug disposition, response, and toxicity, essentially relates allelic variation in human genes to variability in drug responses at the level of the individual patient. In other words, the promise of pharmacogenetics is to identify the right drug at the right dose for the right patient. The field of pharmacogenetics classically has focused on the phenotypic consequences of allelic variation in single genes, but often in the past, there was confusion between genotypic and phenotypic definitions of "polymorphism" and thus a need to clarify the relationship between genetic concepts and the clinical relevance of a given phenotype. In 1991, Meyer proposed that *pharmacogenetic polymorphism* be defined as a monogenic trait caused by the presence in the same population of more than one allele at the same locus and more than one phenotype with regard to drug interaction with the organism. The frequency of the least common allele should be at least 1%.[29] According to this definition, the key elements of pharmacogenetic polymorphisms are heritability, the involvement of a single-gene locus, and the fact that distinct phenotypes are observed within the population *only after drug challenge.*

The vast majority of our current understanding of pharmacogenetic polymorphisms involves enzymes responsible for drug biotransformation. Clinically, individuals are classified as being "fast," "rapid," or "extensive" metabolizers, at one end of the spectrum, and "slow" or "poor" metabolizers, at the other end of a continuum, that may, depending on the specific enzyme, also include an intermediate-metabolizer group. *Pediatric pharmacogenetics* involves an added measure of complexity since fetuses and newborns may be phenotypically "slow" or "poor" metabolizers for certain drug-metabolizing pathways, acquiring a phenotype traditionally consistent with their genotype at some point later in the developmental process as those pathways mature (e.g., glucuronidation, some cytochrome P450 activities).[30–32]

Although some authors use the terms *pharmacogenetics* and *pharmacogenomics* interchangeably, the latter term represents the marriage of pharmacology with genomics and is, therefore, considerably broader in scope. *Pharmacogenomics* can be defined as the study of the genome-wide response to small molecular weight compounds administered with therapeutic intent—finding the right drug for the right disease. *Proteomics* represents the systematic investigation of qualitative and quantitative changes in protein expression in a cell or tissue in response to disease or disease treatment. In this context, *pharmacoproteomics* involves characterizing the response of the proteome to therapeutic agents. Similarly, *toxicogenomics* and *toxicoproteomics* investigate the analogous response to environmental contaminants and other toxicants.[33,34] In contrast to the focus of "pharmacogenetics" on single-gene events, "pharmacogenomics" involves understanding how interacting systems or networks of genes influence drug responses.[35] This definition is particularly appealing to pediatric health and disease since the concept of many genes acting in concert captures the essence of the developmental processes that characterize maturation from the time of birth through adulthood while retaining a focus on the individual.

It is safe to say that application of pharmacogenomic principles to pediatric medicine has received far less attention than its application to diseases affecting adults, and the scope of the field remains to be completely defined. However, *developmental* and *pediatric pharmacogenomics* necessarily must take into consideration the dynamic changes in gene expression that accompany maturation from embryonic life through fetal development, the neonatal period, infancy, childhood, and adolescence (e.g., during organogenesis, as receptor systems and neural networks become established, and functional drug biotransformation capacity is acquired, among others). In other words, patterns of gene expression and the nature of the gene interactions that contribute to the pathogenesis of pediatric diseases (and thereby serve as potential targets for pharmacologic intervention) may only be discernable or relevant at specific critical points in the developmental continuum. Furthermore, variability in drug disposition (i.e., pharmacokinetics) and action (i.e., pharmacodynamics) that ultimately impact drug response in pediatric patients can also be expected to change as children grow and develop. Finally, developmental and pediatric pharmacogenomic investigations can be distinguished from similar studies conducted in adults by the fact that drug or toxicant exposure at critical points in development may disrupt or alter the normal patterns of development—a genome-wide response to drug/toxicant exposure. This may have immediate, observable consequences, for example, fetal demise or major structural abnormalities such as those associated with retinoids[36] or other human teratogens. Of equal concern, however, is the possibility that drug exposure, or lack of effective drug treatment,[37] may have unintended consequences on cognitive or behavior development that do not manifest until much later in maturation. The remainder of this chapter highlights examples of how pharmacogenomic approaches are currently improving pediatric pharmacotherapy and presents several opportunities for future application.

PHARMACOGENETIC, PHARMACOGENOMIC, PHARMACOPROTEOMIC, AND METABOLOMIC TOOLS

Completion of the Human Genome Project was facilitated by several technological advances, and the demands of pharmacoproteomic, metabolomic, pharmacogenetic, and pharmacogenomic analyses have driven the development of an industry dedicated to the discovery and refinement of technologies capable of generating large data sets of information derived from DNA, RNA, proteins, and small molecules that are present in the body from endogenous sources. These tools are used widely to investigate disease pathogenesis but are equally applicable to investigations of variability in drug disposition and response.

PHENOTYPING TOOLS

Historically, pharmacogenetic analyses have been dependent upon phenotyping studies to estimate enzyme activity in vivo at a specific time point as well as genotyping strategies to identify and characterize SNPs and other forms of genetic variation. Phenotyping studies are best conducted with a probe compound carefully selected to ensure that its biotransformation is primarily dependent upon a single target enzyme and varies quantitatively with the level of protein expression.[38] An ideal probe should involve noninvasive sampling strategies, such as collection of urine or expired air rather than blood samples, especially when phenotyping studies are to be conducted in children. Finally, candidate phenotyping probes should be widely available (nonprescription status, preferably) and have a wide margin of safety. For pediatric studies, the phenotyping probe should be selected from compounds that are likely to be administered to children and perceived as safe by parents, caregivers, and ethics committees (e.g., dextromethorphan as opposed to debrisoquine or sparteine for CYP2D6).

The advantages and disadvantages of phenotyping probes commonly used in adult studies have been comprehensively and critically evaluated by Streetman et al.[39] Dextromethorphan and caffeine are commonly used in pediatric phenotyping studies with nontherapeutic intent.[40–43] However, other accepted phenotyping probes, such as midazolam for CYP3A4 and omeprazole for CYP2C19, may be utilized in selected patient populations where their use is required for therapeutic purposes. Because of the rigorous demands for enzymatic specificity, safety, and clinical feasibility, very few drugs have been identified that meet the criteria of a useful probe compound, particularly for non-P450 drug-metabolizing enzymes. Fortunately, recent advances in technologies for metabolomic analysis have shifted focus toward the measurement of endogenous biomarkers for phenotyping studies. Including endogenous biomarkers among the phenotyping tools at our disposal may greatly expand the breadth of drug disposition pathways we can evaluate; some drug-metabolizing enzymes or transporters exist for which no currently marketed drug is a sufficiently specific probe. Furthermore, endogenous biomarkers offer a number of advantages to exogenously administered probe substrates. They do not require a potentially invasive administration and do not subject a patient to any compounds that are not already present in circulation at the time of phenotyping. Their minimal invasiveness makes them better suited for phenotyping studies in children.

GENOTYPING TOOLS

The genotyping component of pharmacogenetic studies has undergone tremendous change over the past 30 years. Historically, studies were conducted at the level of individual genes using rather insensitive DNA hybridization techniques[44] to detect differences in the patterns of DNA fragments generated following digestion of genomic DNA with restriction endonucleases (enzymes that cleave DNA molecules at specific nucleotide sequences). The restriction fragment length polymorphism (RFLP) technique was later coupled with polymerase chain reaction (PCR) (PCR-RFLP) to allow a specific region surrounding the SNP of interest to be amplified from small amounts of genomic DNA followed by endonuclease digestion to identify the allelic variant(s) present.[45] PCR-RFLP techniques have been widely used to study cytochrome P450 polymorphisms,[46] among others, but they are too labor-intensive for routine use in genomic applications, such as fine-mapping of disease loci or candidate gene association studies, which involve the analysis of multiple SNPs in thousands of genes. Instead, *microarray* or *gene-chip technology* was developed for the purpose. These whole-genome genotyping technologies now make it possible to interrogate genetic variation at more than a million sites throughout an individual genome for SNP and CNV analyses using a single "chip." Most genome-wide association studies (GWASs) have been conducted with "SNP chips" utilizing one of two commercial platforms, and the approach has been applied to several pediatric diseases. A study of Kawasaki disease identified a set of functionally related genes potentially related to inflammation, apoptosis, and cardiovascular pathology.[47] The results of the study provide novel insights into the pathogenesis of the disorder and lead to the possibility of identifying new targets for therapeutic intervention. Similarly, GWASs in patients with early-onset asthma[48] and pediatric inflammatory bowel disease[49] have been implemented as a new strategy to identify novel genes in disease pathogenesis. GWASs are also being applied to identify genetic associations with drug dosing, response, and efficacy, as reported for warfarin[50] and clopidogrel[51] and risk for drug-induced toxicity, as has been described for statin-induced myopathy.[52] A defining feature of GWAS is the use of Manhattan plots, and an example is presented in Figure 5.2. Chips targeting the pharmacogenome are now in use by several institutions, with a focus on genes broadly involved in drug disposition and response (various cytochromes P450, transporters, and targets of drug action, such as neurotransmitter receptors or reuptake pumps).

The most recent addition to the genomic toolbox is next-generation sequencing technology.[53] The major difference between next-generation sequencing methods and the older, more established Sanger capillary sequencing method is the vast amount of sequencing data that can be generated by the next-generation technologies, which utilize massively parallel and short-read strategies to sequence DNA and RNA templates. Whereas it has been estimated that 500 days of runtime were required to generate one gigabase (one billion nucleotides) of data, the newer next-generation sequencers can produce these same amount of data in half a day at one-hundredth the cost. However, the short 50 to 75 bp read lengths provide computational challenges related to assembly of the short sequence reads to produce an accurate contiguous genomic sequence. Despite the computational challenges, genotyping strategies utilizing next-generation sequencing show considerable promise for routine application, even for complex genes like *CYP2D6*.[54]

Recommendations and requirements for pharmacogenetics testing are now a regular part of the Food and Drug Administration (FDA) drug approval process, and international groups

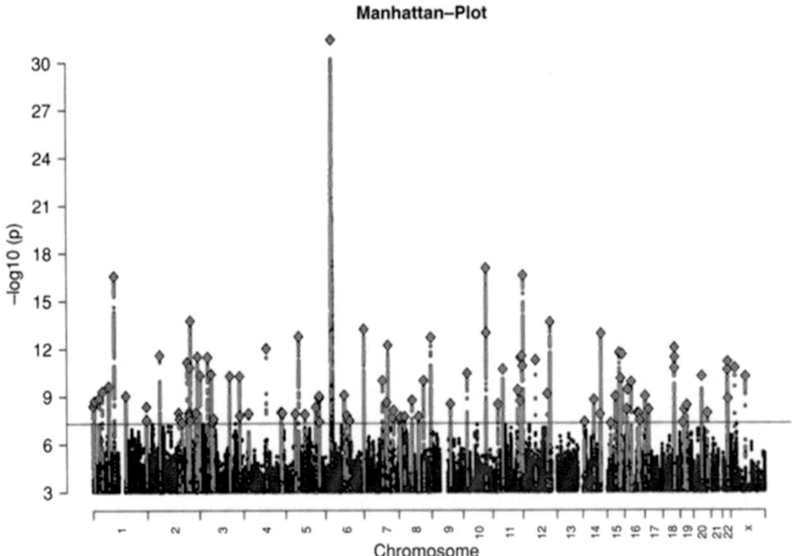

Figure 5.2 Example of a Manhattan Plot from a genome-wide association study. This type of plot gains its name from the similarity of such a plot to the Manhattan skyline and presents the genome-wide significance of several hundred thousand single-nucleotide polymorphisms (SNPs) distributed throughout the genome with the trait or phenotype of interest. Along the *x*-axis, each SNP is plotted according to its chromosomal coordinate, with each shade representing an individual chromosome from chromosome 1 to the X chromosome. The *y*-axis represents the inverse $\log_{10}$ of the *p* value for the association. SNPs exceeding a particular threshold are subject to further verification and validation. (From Schizophrenia Working Group of the Psychiatric Genomics Consortium. Biological insights from 108 schizophrenia-associated genetic loci. *Nature* 2014;511(7510):421–427.

of experts like the Clinical Pharmacogenetics Implementation Consortium (CPIC) have been established to help identify further "actionable" polymorphic genes. Health care providers, who serve as gatekeepers, use this pharmacogenetics information to lead discussions with patients and guide evidence-based drug and dosage selection with the patient. However, continuing innovations that expand the accessibility of at home genetic testing and the gradual loosening of regulations related to what information can be provided directly to patients may upend this long-standing model. In 2018, a major change occurred within the regulatory landscape of pharmacogenetic testing. For the first time, the FDA approved direct-to-consumer at home pharmacogenetic testing for drug biotransformation pathways.[55] It is critical now more than ever before that health care practitioners be informed about the utility and limitations of pharmacogenetics testing as patients become increasingly more likely to approach practitioners with personal pharmacogenetic testing results already in hand. Important ethical questions regarding who owns patient data, what level of data interpretation and reporting by vendors could be described as practicing medicine, what legal protections should be afforded patients from discrimination by medical insurance or health care providers, and what respective roles should children and parents have in providing consent to testing in the absence of trained intermediary health care providers must also be addressed.

PROTEOMIC TOOLS

Genetic mutations in genes are like atypical features in a relatively static blueprint, and the *penetrance* is the proportion of individuals with a given genetic mutation who exhibit a phenotypic change. While some mutations, such as those contributing to complete loss of CYP2D6 activity, have high penetrance, functional differences for many mutations may never come to bear or they may manifest differentially over the course of years, weeks, or even across the span of a single day. Furthermore, polymorphic genes interact with environmental conditions or other genes, often in complex and unanticipated ways. It is with this understanding that considerable research has been undertaken in the related fields of transcriptomics, proteomics, and metabolomics. Each of these fields represents a successive step toward a more accurate "snapshot" of true functional differences in a given individual at a given time, and each offer unique opportunities and limitations in the realm of personalized medicine. Following in the wake of advancements in technologies for studying genomics, great investments have been made to improve other "-omics" technologies. The field of pharmacoproteomics has benefited considerably with improvements across the entire workflow from sample preparation to analysis, but perhaps the most enabling advancements have been the development of more sensitive and accurate mass spectrometers.[56] This is because, unlike with sequences of nucleotides, no amplification method analogous to PCR exists to increase the quantity of protein from small amounts of starting material. Regardless of specific requirements for sample processing, whether whole proteins (i.e., *top-down proteomics*) or proteolytically digested protein fragments (i.e., *bottom-up proteomics*) are being assessed, highly sensitive mass spectrometers are crucial for the identification and quantification of proteins in human tissues. While it is important to note that traditional antibody-based methods such as Western blots and enzyme-linked immunosorbent assays (ELISA) do still offer liquid chromatography–mass spectrometry (LC/MS)–independent means to detect and quantify amounts of proteins in human tissues, these techniques are increasingly falling out of favor due to their generally reduced throughput, specificity, sensitivity, and severely limited capacity for simultaneous measurement of multiple proteins (i.e., multiplexing) when compared to techniques using mass spectrometers.[57,58] Furthermore, neither ELISA nor Western blots are capable of identifying or detecting proteins beyond those for which the assays have been designed to measure. As such, they cannot be used to truly characterize novel proteins or to agnostically evaluate the contribution of proteins that are not designated a priori to any sort of outcome, such as drug responsiveness. Conversely, mass spectrometer–based proteomics can be used to detect a set of proteins that are defined a priori (i.e., *targeted proteomics*) and those that are not (i.e., *global proteomics*). The incorporation of calibration curves consisting of labeled proteins or peptides, in conjunction with targeted proteomic analysis, further permits relative or absolute quantification of proteins in human tissues.

The use of quantitatively targeted proteomics has proved to be of considerable value to the field pediatric clinical pharmacology, in that it has provided important information regarding the ontogeny of proteins important in drug disposition. Most recently, quantitative proteomic data are making significant contributions in the area of modeling and simulation as protein abundance of drug-metabolizing enzymes and transporters is crucial information for the construction of physiologically based pharmacokinetic (PBPK) models that can estimate an exposure range for a given drug as function of age and other patient-specific variables. The coupling of accurate proteomic data to PBPK models has been used to estimate doses for first-in-children studies of drugs seeking pediatric dosing indications and even to simulate the results of clinical pharmacokinetic studies where difficulties in enrollment prohibit conducting properly powered pediatric clinical studies. Notably, the FDA approval of both valganciclovir dosing for infants under 4 months and nilotinib dosing in children over 2 years of age was based, in part, on results from PBPK simulations incorporating targeted proteomic data relating to the ontogeny of protein expression of drug-metabolizing enzymes and transporters.[59,60] However, much of the current data for the maturation of drug-metabolizing enzymes and transporters span a very wide age range and are not sufficiently descriptive of the early years where the most dramatic changes in the expression of these proteins often occur. More detailed, pediatric-focused, targeted proteomic studies into the ontogeny of proteins important in drug disposition and response are warranted to adequately refine these pediatric PBPK models.

There is also considerable interest in using pediatric PBPK models as the basis for clinical decision support tools for the precision dosing of medications in children.[61] The measurement of protein abundance in organs of interest often requires obtaining biopsies, which are typically acquired from large tissue repositories available to scientific researchers. However, it is neither ethical nor feasible to obtain tissue biopsies in the clinic for the sole purposes of generating a tailored PBPK model. Even biopsies acquired as a part of routine care would not be of great utility for this purpose as enzyme and transporters expression change with age and environmental exposures. One approach is to rely on more readily accessible tissues, such as the blood, and use global proteomics approaches to characterize signature protein abundance patterns reflective the protein expression of various drug-metabolizing enzymes and transporters in other tissues like the liver. The application of other targeted quantitative approaches to blood samples is also being explored, such as the quantification of *exosomes*, secreted circulating vesicles that are derived from the cellular endosomal compartment, that contain drug-metabolizing enzyme and transporters. Exosomes of hepatic origin may offer a snapshot of expression of these drug-metabolizing enzymes in the liver and potentially serve as a measure of individual drug biotransformation capacity in vivo.[62]

Finally, it is important to remember there are key limitations to proteomic analyses, even when tissue samples are available. Protein quantitation is not a perfect surrogate for function. Concomitant medications and post-translational conformational modifications that may go unnoticed in a quantitative proteomic analysis have the potential to impact enzyme activity. Furthermore, trafficking of proteins to sites of action may not be completely efficient or may exist in the form of a dynamic equilibrium. This is particularly relevant for drug transporters, many of which have endogenous ligands and participate in homeostatic processes regulating their localization on cellular membranes. To quantify the amount of drug transporters on cellular surfaces (i.e., those that may be capable of regulating intracellular drug concentration), additional approaches are currently being developed to supplement targeted proteomic analysis. Application of purification procedures allows transporters to be selectively measured in the purified plasma membrane fraction, thereby excluding any transporters present in internalized membrane vesicles from the analysis. Use of reference proteins, such as aquaporin, can further confirm transporter regional localization in tissues like the kidney, leading to higher confidence in the robustness of the data.[63] The potential importance of quantitative proteomics to link in vitro studies with in vivo outcomes in translational pharmacology research and the subsequent clinical applications has been recognized, and efforts have been initiated to establish best practices for this important new tool.[58]

METABOLOMIC TOOLS

Several analytical approaches can be utilized for metabolomic and metabonomic investigations, depending on the analytes of interest, but the most used platforms are nuclear magnetic resonance (NMR) spectroscopy and LC or gas chromatography coupled with mass spectral detection.[64] Analogous to proteomics, one popular strategy for conducting these metabolomic studies is to use a global profiling approach (i.e., *global metabolomics*) to measure the concentrations of all detectable small molecules in a biologic sample. Evaluated holistically, the relative levels of these compounds from one individual to the next constitute what is often referred to as an individual unique “metabolomic fingerprint.” Using a statistical approach known as principle component analysis (PCA), the differentness of groups of individual metabolomic fingerprints can be evaluated and related to drug responsiveness or the functional activity of the biologic pathways relevant to drug disposition. If associations are discovered, a patient’s unique metabolomic fingerprint could then be compared for similarities to these predetermined patterns to identify the optimal drug to use and to guide dose selection. Global metabolomics, when coupled with small molecule libraries, can also be used to identify a promising subset of small molecules within the biologic matrix that may reflect an outcome of interest. *Targeted metabolomics*, the assessment of these discrete small molecule groups, can be subsequently applied and may even result in the discovery of singular endogenous biomarkers that reflect the activity of drug-metabolizing enzymes and transporters. The identification of endogenous biomarkers to replace exogenously administered probes for phenotyping drug disposition pathways would be of great utility for pediatric medicine where nontherapeutic pharmacologic effects of probes drugs should be minimized. A metabolomic approach was applied to identify an endogenous compound with a molecular mass of 444.3 Da as a potential biomarker of CYP2D6 activity from pediatric urine samples.[65]

Combining metabolomic and genome-wide genotyping data has revealed common genetic variations that are associated with variability in metabolic phenotypes involving the corresponding biochemical pathways.[66] Metabolomics in conjunction with simultaneous gene expression analysis of the transcriptome provides additional mechanistic insights, leading to a more "systems-based" understanding of cellular processes, especially in the context of drug-related perturbations.[67] A particularly exciting application of pharmacometabolomics is the identification of metabolic signatures and corresponding cellular pathways to predict drug response[68,69]; the approach has not been applied to drug response in pediatrics to any appreciable extent so far.

APPLICATIONS OF PEDIATRIC PHARMACOGENETICS AND PHARMACOGENOMICS

DRUG BIOTRANSFORMATION AND CONCENTRATION-DEPENDENT TOXICITY

Clinical observation of patients with high drug concentrations/excessive or prolonged drug responses together with the realization that the biochemical traits (subsequently identified as proteins involved in drug biotransformation) were inherited provided the origins of the concept of pharmacogenetics. Indeed, with few exceptions, the major consequence of pharmacogenetic polymorphisms in drug-metabolizing enzymes is concentration-dependent toxicity due to impaired drug clearance and, to a lesser extent, reduced conversion of prodrugs to therapeutically active compounds. For most cytochromes P450, genotype–phenotype relationships are influenced by development in that fetal expression is limited (with the exception of CYP3A7) and functional activity is acquired postnatally in isoform-specific patterns. Furthermore, clearance of some compounds appears to be greater in children relative to adults, obscuring the correlation between genotype and phenotype in neonatal life through adolescence.[30] The ontogeny of several phase I and phase II drug biotransformation pathways has been exhaustively reviewed.[70] Comprehensive reviews of cytochromes P450 pharmacogenetics in general,[71] and for individual drug biotransformation enzymes, such as CYP2B6,[72] CYP2C9,[73] CYP2C19,[74] CYP2D6,[75–77] the CYP3A subfamily,[78] glucuronosyl transferases (UGT),[79,80] sulfotransferases (SULTs),[81] *N*-acetyltransferases (NATs),[82] and thiopurine *S*-methyltransferase (TPMT)[83] are also available. Salient features of the more common polymorphisms of clinically relevant drug-metabolizing enzymes are discussed briefly below.

CYP2C9

Although several clinically useful compounds are substrates for CYP2C9, the effects of allelic variation are most profound for drugs with narrow therapeutic indices, such as phenytoin,[84,85] warfarin,[86] and tolbutamide.[87,88] Several allelic variants of CYP2C9 have been observed in population studies, and an up-to-date listing is maintained by the Pharmacogene Variation (PharmVar) Consortium (https://www.pharmvar.org/gene/CYP2C9). Individual alleles are designated by the gene name (*CYP2C9*) followed by an asterisk and an Arabic number; *CYP2C9*1* designates, by convention, the fully functional wild-type allele. The *CYP2C9*2* allele results in an amino acid substitution at position 144 of the CYP2C9 protein and is associated with an approximately 5.5-fold decreased intrinsic clearance for (*S*)-warfarin relative to the wild-type enzyme.[89] The conservative isoleucine to leucine change at position 359 characteristic of the CYP2C9*3 allele occurs within a region of the protein that affects substrate orientation in the active site and, as a result, produces a considerable (27-fold) decrease in intrinsic (*S*)-warfarin clearance.[90] The risk of bleeding complications in patients treated with warfarin and concentration-dependent phenytoin toxicity is most pronounced for individuals with a *CYP2C9*3/*3* genotype. A decrease in activity has been observed for the relatively rarer *CYP2C9*5* allele due to an aspartate to glutamate change at position 360, also within the active site of the enzyme.[91] Interestingly, the *CYP2C9*8* allele, resulting in a substitution of arginine with histidine at position 150, demonstrated increased activity for metabolizing tolbutamide in vitro.[92] However, the allele was associated with reduced in vivo phenytoin and warfarin clearance in subsequent clinical studies. Additional uncommon CYP2C9 alleles with evidence suggesting reduced activity in vivo are *CYP2C9*6*, *CYP2C9*11*, and *CYP2C9*12*.[73]

Approximately one-third of the Caucasian population carries a variant *CYP2C9* allele (**2* and **3* alleles, most commonly), whereas the **2* and **3* alleles are less common in African Americans, Chinese, Japanese, or Korean populations. In contrast, the **5* and **6* alleles have been detected in African Americans but are each found in less than 0.01% of Caucasians. The **8* and **11* alleles are also more common in individuals of African ancestry, but the differences in allele frequency compared to other populations are less pronounced than for the **5* and **6* alleles.[73]

A pediatric case illustrating the clinical relevance of CYP2C9 pharmacogenetics involved the administration of phenytoin to a 2-year-old child who was homozygous for the *CYP2C9*2* allele.[93] During standard-of-care administration of phenytoin to treat status epilepticus, the patient developed acute toxicity. Measurement of phenytoin plasma levels revealed phenytoin concentrations in excess of threefold the upper therapeutic limit. Symptoms of phenytoin intoxication took over 5 days to abate, and monitoring of drug levels in the patient revealed that it took almost a week for phenytoin concentrations to fall within the normal range, thus illustrating the fact that in addition to the potential for genetic polymorphisms to result in dramatic elevations in drug concentrations, they can also extend the duration of time a patient is exposed to potentially toxic drug concentrations relative to patients with an extensive metabolizer phenotype who may for other reasons (e.g., greater dose) achieve the same elevated concentrations. Another important contributor to the marked increases in phenytoin levels experienced by this patient was the presence of a nonfunctional allele for *CYP2C19*. Whereas CYP2C19 only accounts for about 10% of phenytoin clearance in CYP2C9 extensive metabolizers,[94] it can play a much more dominant role in CYP2C9 poor metabolizers. Cases like this highlight the importance of considering polymorphisms in secondary pathways of drug metabolism, especially when a patient is genetically deficient in or taking an inhibitor of the major pathways of drug metabolism.

CYP2C19

Originally reported as "mephenytoin hydroxylase" deficiency, the CYP2C19 poor-metabolizer phenotype is present in 3% to

5% of the Caucasian population and 20% to 25% of Asians. Although several defective alleles have been identified, the two most common variant alleles, *CYP2C19*2* and *CYP2C19*3*, result from single-base substitutions that introduce premature stop codons and, consequently, truncated polypeptide chains that possess no functional activity.[95] In Japanese adults treated with lansoprazole, amoxicillin, and clarithromycin for *Helicobacter pylori* infection, the eradication rate for CYP2C19 poor metabolizers (97.8%) and heterozygous extensive metabolizers (one functional *CYP2C19* allele; 92.1%) was significantly greater than that observed in homozygous extensive metabolizers (72.7%; $p < 0.001$). Of the 35 patients in whom initial treatment failed to eradicate *H. pylori*, 34 had at least one functional *CYP2C19* allele, and eradication could be achieved with higher lansoprazole doses in almost all cases.[96] Given that the frequency of the functional *CYP2C19*1* allele is considerably greater in Caucasians (~84%) compared to Japanese (~55%),[95] eradication failure can be expected to occur more frequently in Caucasians.

The *CYP2C19*17* allele, characterized by two variants in the 5′-upstream region of the *CYP2C19* gene, occurs at a frequency of 18% in Swedish and Ethiopian populations and approximately 4% in a Chinese population.[97] *CYP2C19*17* is associated with "ultrarapid" activity as measured by omeprazole metabolite ratio[97] and decreased serum concentrations of substrates, such as escitalopram.[98] Both *CYP2C19*2* and *CYP2C19*4*, an uncommon allele resulting in loss of function via impaired gene transcription, have been observed to be in linkage disequilibrium with *CYP2C19*17* in some populations. The **17* allele is believed to be unable to impact phenotype when present on the same chromosome as the **2* or **4* allele. Additional uncommon alleles resulting in loss of function in CYP2C19 are **5*, **6*, **7*, and **8*. A detailed summary of *CYP2C19* allelic variants reported to date can be found at https://www.pharmvar.org/gene/CYP2C19.

CYP2C19 substrates, such as proton pump inhibitors, voriconazole, and escitalopram, are used clinically in pediatric patient populations, and therefore, it is reasonable to expect that pharmacogenetic considerations should guide dosing strategies in children as well as in adults. The 2018 CPIC recommends that voriconazole not be administered to children who are either CYP2C19 poor or ultrarapid metabolizers whenever an appropriate alternative drug (e.g., amphotericin B) is available.[99] Among children receiving escitalopram or citalopram, CYP2C19 poor-metabolizer status has been associated with greater incidence of adverse drug reactions and drug discontinuation. Conversely, faster metabolizer status was associated with more rapid treatment response.[100] Simulations leveraging *CYP2C19* pharmacogenetics and clinical pharmacokinetic data suggest poor metabolizers require, on average, only 50% of the dose administered to extensive metabolizers to achieve comparable systemic exposure, and ultrarapid metabolizers were estimated to require an approximately 50% greater dose.[101] Although CPIC has provided dosing recommendations for CYP2C19 antidepressant substrates, actual experience to support recommendations in children is limited.[102]

CYP2D6

The *CYP2D6* gene locus is highly polymorphic with more than 130 allelic variants identified to date (https://www.pharmvar.org/gene/CYP2D6; Table 5.1).[77] For CYP2D6, allelic variants are the consequence of point mutations, single-base pair deletions or additions, and gene rearrangements or deletion of the entire gene that result in a reduction or complete loss of activity. Inheritance of two recessive loss-of-function alleles results in the "poor-metabolizer phenotype," which is found in about 5% to 10% of Caucasians and about 1% to 2% of Asian subjects. In Caucasians, the **3*, **4*, **5*, and **6* alleles are the most common loss of functional alleles and account for approximately 98% of poor-metabolizer phenotypes.[103] CYP2D6 activity is lower, on a population basis, in Asian and African American populations due to a lower frequency of nonfunctional alleles (**3*, **4*, **5*, and **6*) and a relatively high frequency of alleles that are associated with decreased activity relative to the wild-type *CYP2D6*1* allele. In Asians, *CYP2D6*10* has an allele frequency of approximately 50%, whereas *CYP2D6*17* and *CYP2D6*29* occur at relatively high frequencies in subjects of black African origin.[104] A schematic representation of some of the more common allelic variants is presented in Figure 5.3. At the other end of the spectrum, the presence of *CYP2D6* gene duplication/multiplication events, which occur at a frequency of 1% to 2% in Caucasians,[75–77] most often is associated with enhanced clearance

TABLE 5.1 Internet Resources for Pharmacogenetics and Pharmacogenomics

	Topic	*URL*
General pharmacogenetic sites	Pharmacogenetics Knowledge Base	https://www.pharmgkb.org/
	Pharmacogene Variation Consortium	https://www.pharmvar.org/
Pharmacogenetics: allelic variants of drug-metabolizing enzymes	CYP2C9	https://www.pharmvar.org/gene/CYP2C9
	CYP2C19	https://www.pharmvar.org/gene/CYP2C19
	CYP2D6	https://www.pharmvar.org/gene/CYP2D6
	CYP3A4	https://www.pharmvar.org/gene/CYP3A4
	CYP3A5	https://www.pharmvar.org/gene/CYP3A5
	CYP3A7	https://www.pharmvar.org/gene/CYP3A7
	UGTs	https://www.pharmacogenomics.pha.ulaval.ca/ugt-alleles-nomenclature/
	NAT1	http://nat.mbg.duth.gr/Human%20NAT1%20alleles_2013.htm
	NAT2	http://nat.mbg.duth.gr/Human%20NAT2%20alleles_2013.htm
	NUDT15	https://www.pharmvar.org/gene/NUDT15

All sites were accessible on September 5, 2019.

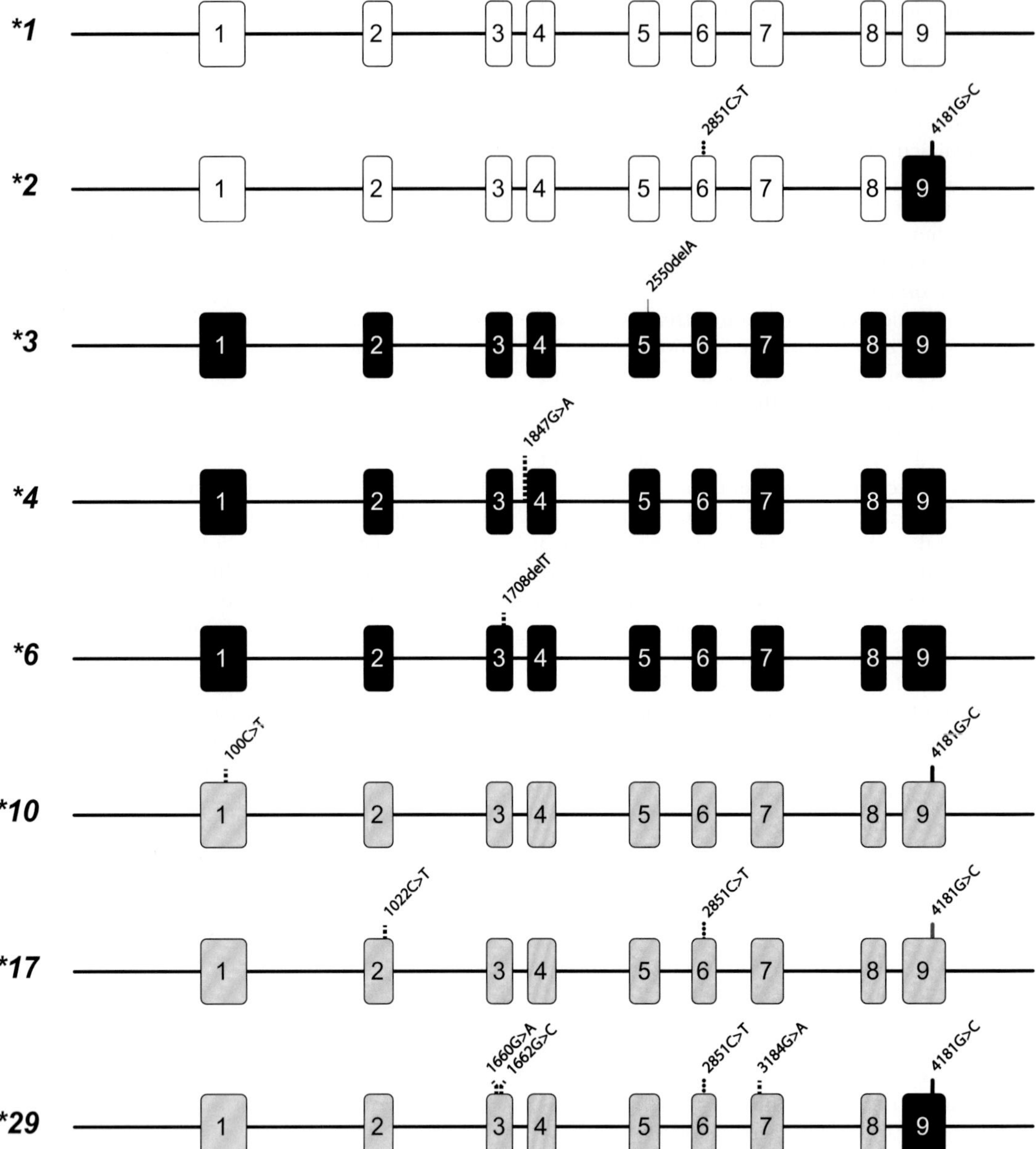

Figure 5.3 Common *CYP2D6* allelic variants. The *CYP2D6* gene consists of nine exons, and individual alleles are defined by the presence of key single-nucleotide variants, such as single-nucleotide polymorphisms, insertions, and deletions, throughout the gene relative to the reference *CYP2D6*1* allele (top of figure). The different types of dashed lines refers to the functional consequence of allelic variants of the activity of the protein, with solid line representing fully functional activity (*CYP2D6*1, CYP2D6*2*), dashed line representing complete loss of activity (*CYP2D6*3, CYP2D6*4, CYP2D6*6*), and dotted line representing partial activity (*CYP2D6*10, CYP2D6*17, CYP2D6*29*).

of CYP2D6 substrates, although cases of increased toxicity due to increased formation of pharmacologically active metabolites have also been reported.[105] In addition to gene duplication/multiplication events, the *CYP2D6* gene locus is also subject to gene rearrangements, hybrid structures, and tandem arrangements involving two or more nonidentical gene copies.[77] Examples of relatively frequent structural variants are presented in Figure 5.4.

CYP2D6 is involved in the biotransformation of more than 40 therapeutic entities, including several β-receptor antagonists, antiarrhythmics, antidepressants, antipsychotics and morphine derivatives. Of these, atomoxetine, codeine, dextromethorphan, diphenhydramine, fluoxetine, imipramine, risperidone, and tramadol are commonly encountered in pediatrics. In vitro studies indicate that fetal liver microsomes have very limited CYP2D6 activity (~1% of adult values), but CYP2D6 protein is detectable in all samples from newborns.[106] A second study utilizing a relatively large number of pediatric liver samples revealed that CYP2D6 protein and activity were similar between fetal liver samples obtained during the third trimester of pregnancy and liver samples obtained from infants in the first week of life, and both protein and activity remained relatively constant after 1 week of age up to 18 years. The data further imply that genetic variability, rather than ontogeny, is primarily responsible for the observed variability in catalytic activity.[107] Similar results have been observed in an in vivo longitudinal phenotyping study involving more than 100 infants over the first year of life. This study utilized dextromethorphan as a

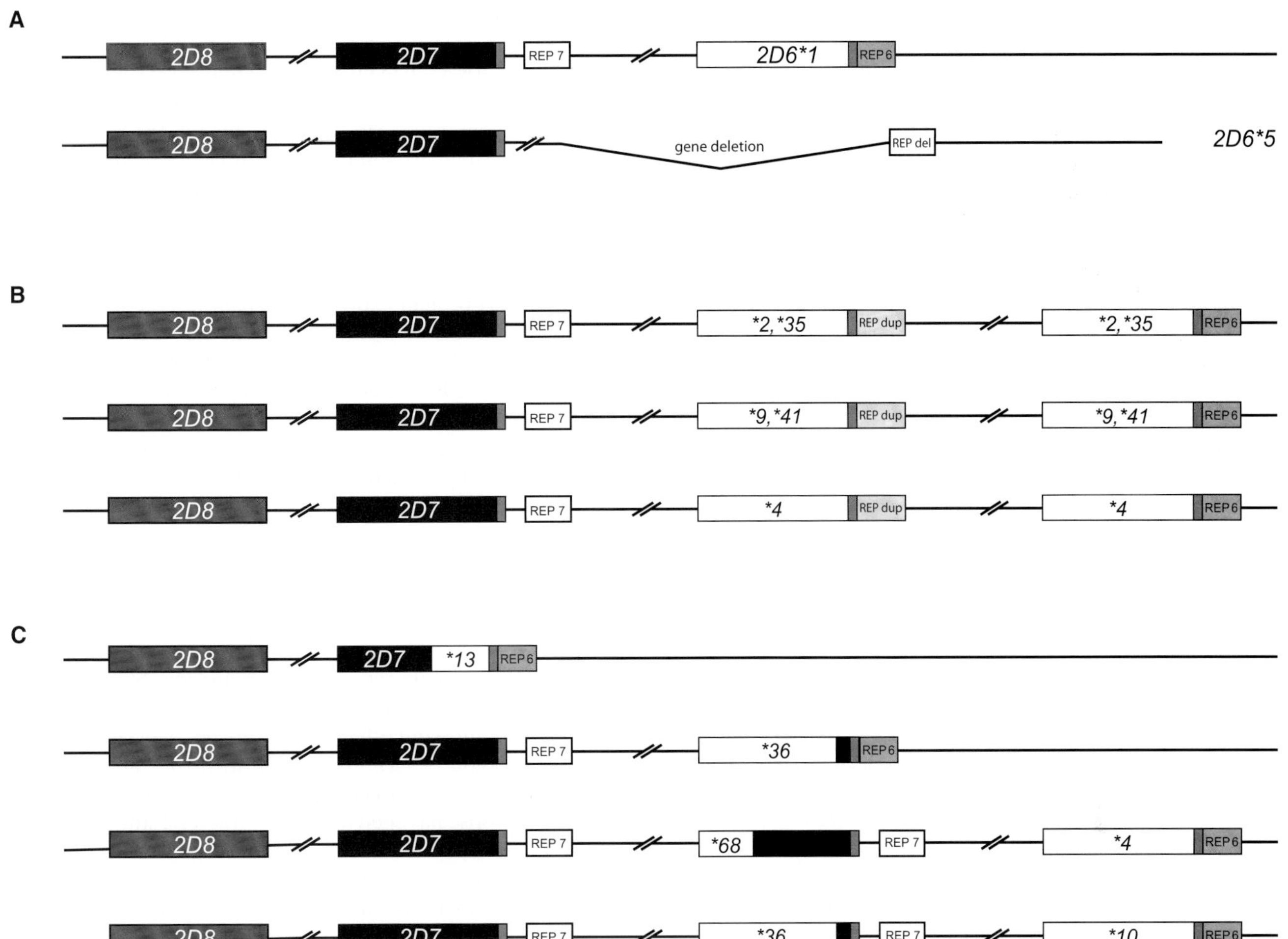

Figure 5.4 Structural variation in the *CYP2D6* locus. **A:** The reference gene locus containing a single copy of the *CYP2D6* gene downstream of the *CYP2D8* and *CYP2D7* pseudogenes. A gene deletion event results in the complete loss of *CYP2D6*, resulting in the *CYP2D6*5* allele. **B:** Gene duplication and multiplication events. Two or more (multiple) copies of a *CYP2D6* allelic variant may be present in tandem on a single chromosome. Duplication/multiplication events may involve fully functional alleles (*CYP2D6*2xN, CYP2D6*35xN*, where *N* represents the number copies present, e.g., *CYP2D6*2x2* for a duplication), decreased function (*CYP2D6*9xN, CYP2D6*41xN*), or nonfunctional (*CYP2D6*4xN*) gene copies. **C:** Hybrid and tandem events. Rearrangements involving two or more nonidentical gene copies can also occur within the *CYP2D* locus. The top two lines represent examples of hybrid genes. *CYP2D6*13* is considered a *CYP2D7–CYP2D6* hybrid as it is composed of DNA sequence from the *CYP2D7* pseudogene and DNA derived from the downstream *CYP2D6* genes (top line). The *CYP2D6*36* allele is an example of a *CYP2D6–CYP2D7* hybrid and consists primarily of *CYP2D6* sequence with a 3′-region derived from *CYP2D7* (second line). These hybrid structures generally do not code for functional protein. The bottom two lines represent examples of two commonly observed tandem events: *CYP2D6*68+*4* (inactive) and *CYP2D6*36+*10*, a partial function allele with an activity score of 0.25 due to the presence of the partial function **10* allele. REP6, REP7, REPdup, and REPdel refer to repeat elements within the locus. (Adapted from Nofziger C, Turner AJ, Sangkuhl K, et al. PharmVar GeneReview: CYP2D6. *Clin Pharmacol Ther* 2020; 107:154-170.)

probe compound and the urinary ratio of dextromethorphan to dextrorphan as a measure of CYP2D6 activity. Although considerable interindividual variability in CYP2D6 activity was observed, no relationship between CYP2D6 activity and postnatal age was apparent between the ages of 2 weeks and 12 months.[108] Similarly, a cross-sectional study involving 586 children (480 Caucasians and 106 African Americans) indicated that the distribution of CYP2D6 phenotypes in children was comparable to that observed in adults by at least 10 years of age, and probably much earlier.[40] Cumulatively, these in vitro and in vivo indicate that developmental factors are less important than genetic variation as determinants of CYP2D6 variability in children.

Drug accumulation with an increased risk of concentration-dependent toxicity is of particular concern in CYP2D6 poor metabolizers. Indeed, a fluoxetine-related death has been reported in a 9-year-old child with multiple neuropsychiatric disorders who was subsequently determined to be a CYP2D6 poor metabolizer by genotype analysis. Measurements of blood and liver concentrations of fluoxetine at autopsy were several-fold higher than expected, consistent with *CYP2D6* genotype.[109] On the other hand, poor metabolizers may experience decreased efficacy or therapeutic failure when prescribed drugs are dependent upon functional CYP2D6 activity for conversion to the pharmacologically active species, such as codeine and tramadol.[110,111] Infants and children appear capable of converting codeine to morphine,[112] achieving morphine-to-codeine ratios comparable to those of adults.[113] However, in one study, morphine and its metabolites were not detected in 36% of children receiving codeine, and codeine analgesia was found to be unreliable in the studied pediatric population and not related to

CYP2D6 phenotype.[114] At the other end of the phenotypic spectrum, an ultrarapid metabolizer genotype and phenotype has been associated with much greater morphine formation from codeine than anticipated, with potentially fatal consequences. The index case for this phenomenon was a child exposed to excessively high morphine concentrations through breast milk from his codeine-treated mother with three functional CYP2D6 alleles.[105] Since the initial case report, several additional case reports and case series or morphine toxicity from codeine prescribed to children have been reported. Due to the potential for both lack of efficacy and serious adverse events, the U.S. FDA limits the use of codeine and tramadol to patients older than 18 years (https://www.fda.gov/drugs/drug-safety-and-availability/fda-drug-safety-communication-fda-requires-labeling-changes-prescription-opioid-cough-and-cold). CPIC guidelines for codeine and tramadol have been published and updated,[115] but do not reflect the most recent (2018) FDA recommendations.

In addition to the codeine example described above, *CYP2D6* pharmacogenomics has been incorporated into dosing algorithms for additional medications, including atomoxetine and pimozide. One of the more relevant examples for pediatrics is atomoxetine, a nonstimulant drug used in the treatment of attention-deficit/hyperactivity disorder (ADHD). Atomoxetine pharmacokinetics is associated with *CYP2D6* genotype, and increased incidence of a number of adverse drug reactions have been observed in children taking atomoxetine who are CYP2D6 poor metabolizers, but concern has also been raised that extensive and ultrarapid CYP2D6 metabolizers may be at risk for poor response and require doses greater than approved doses.[116] As such, CPIC has published genotype-stratified guidelines for initial atomoxetine doses in children, and time until dosage escalation can proceed.[117] The genotype-stratified dosing recommendations for all CYP2D6-based CPIC guidelines are based on the concept of *activity score*, an ordinal system that converts CYP2D6 genotype calls into a predicted phenotype based on the relative activity the CYP2D6 protein encoded by the allelic variant, with values of “0” assigned to nonfunctional alleles, such as **3, *4, *5,* and **6*; a value of “0.5” assigned to partial function alleles **9, *17, *29,* and **41*; and a score of “1” assigned to fully functional **1, *2,* and **35* alleles.[118,119] Each allele in the diplotype is assigned a value, such that poor-metabolizer individuals with two nonfunctional alleles (e.g., *CYP2D6* diplotypes such as *CYP2D6*3/*4, CYP2D6*4/*6*, or *CYP2D6*5/*5*) are assigned an activity score of 0, whereas individuals with diplotypes consisting of fully functional **1, *2,* or *35 alleles (e.g., *CYP2D6*1/*2, CYP2D6*2/*35*) are assigned an activity score of 2. For gene duplication/multiplication events, the allele value is multiplied by the number of copies present: *CYP2D6*1/*2x2* would be assigned an activity score of *1 = 1 plus *2×2 = 1×2 for a total activity score of 1+2 = 3. Similarly, a CYP2D6 diplotype of *CYP2D6 *4x2/*17* would have a score of 0×2 = 0 plus 0.5 for a total score of 0.5. In 2019, the score assigned to *10 was downgraded from a partial function allele with a value of 0.5 to a new value of 0.25,[77] and a recent study confirms that inclusion of structural variants in the calculation of the activity score provides an improved estimate of activity from genotype data.[120]

CYP3A4, CYP3A5, and CYP3A7

The CYP3A subfamily consists of four members in humans (CYP3A4, CYP3A5, CYP3A7, and CYP3A43) and is quantitatively the most important group of CYPs in terms of human hepatic drug biotransformation. These isoforms catalyze the oxidation of many different therapeutic entities, several of which are of potential importance to pediatric practice. CYP3A7 is the predominant CYP isoform in fetal liver and can be detected in embryonic liver as early as 50 to 60 days' gestation.[121,122] CYP3A7 activity is maximal in the early neonatal period with a progressive decline thereafter. In contrast, CYP3A4 activity, the major CYP3A isoform in adults, is essentially absent in fetal liver but increases during the first week of postnatal life.[123,124] CYP3A4 is also abundantly expressed in the intestine where it contributes significantly to the first-pass metabolism of orally administered substrates, such as midazolam and tacrolimus.[125–127] Similar to the liver, the ontogeny of CYP3A4 protein expression in the intestine has also been described as progressively increasing in the first few years of life before plateauing to levels comparable to those seen in adults.[128]

Several methods have been proposed for CYP3A phenotyping, and the advantages and limitations of each have been reviewed in detail.[38,39] Using these various phenotyping probes, CYP3A4 activity has been reported to vary widely (up to 50-fold) among individuals, but the population distributions of activity are essentially unimodal and evidence for polymorphic activity has been elusive. Several allelic variants have been identified (https://www.pharmvar.org/gene/CYP3A4; see Table 5.1), but they occur relatively infrequently, and data are conflicting regarding clinical significance. One variant that has received attention is *CYP3A4*22*, originally reported as an intronic SNP associated with improved clinical response to simvastatin, a CYP3A4 substrate,[129] and subsequently reported to be associated with reduced expression of CYP3A4 protein in vitro[130] and activity in vivo.[131] The potential effect of *CYP3A4*22* on tacrolimus exposure and response has been described in several studies since the original report,[132] but currently, the CPIC guideline for tacrolimus dosing does not include any recommendations CYP3A4*22 genotype.[133] Prospective studies will need to be conducted to validate whether inclusion of *CYP3A4*22* allele truly has a clinically meaningful role in achieving appropriate systemic tacrolimus exposure. In the interim, the Immunosuppressive Drugs Scientific Committee of the International Association of Therapeutic Drug Monitoring and Clinical Toxicity (IATDMCT) has recognized the potential importance of the **22* allele and recommend its inclusion as a covariate of interest in future pharmacokinetic studies to determine the drivers of interindividual variability in tacrolimus disposition and guide dose selection.[134]

Of interest to pediatrics is the *CYP3A4*1B* allele present in the CYP3A4 promoter region.[135,136] The clinical significance of this allelic variant appears limited with respect to drug biotransformation activity,[137–139] despite being associated with two-fold increased activity over the wild-type *CYP3A4*1* allele in reporter gene assays in vitro.[140] Although there does not appear to be an association between the *CYP3A4*1B* allele and age of menarche as recalled in adulthood in one study,[141] a significant relationship does exist between the number of **1B* alleles and onset of puberty as defined by Tanner breast score (odds ratio = 3.21; 95% confidence interval 1.62–6.89).[142] In this study, 90% of 9-year-old girls with a *CYP3A4*1B/*1B* genotype had a Tanner breast score ≥2 compared to 56% of *CYP3A4*1A/*1B* heterozygotes and 40% of girls homozygous for the *CYP3A4*1A* allele. Since CYP3A4 plays an important role in testosterone catabolism, the authors of the latter study proposed that the estradiol-to-testosterone ratio may be shifted toward higher values in the presence of the *CYP3A4*1B* allele and trigger the hormonal cascade that accompanies puberty.

CYP3A5 is polymorphically expressed, being present in approximately 25% of adult liver samples studied in vitro.[143,144]

Expression of CYP3A5 is greatest in individuals of African ancestry, and loss of function in Caucasian livers is largely due to an SNP in intron 3 that creates a cryptic splice site and gives rise to splice variants that carry premature stop codons.[144] Even more so than with CYP3A4, genetic polymorphisms in CYP3A5 have shown to be associated with tacrolimus pharmacokinetics, but as with CYP3A4, IATDMCT guidelines do not currently include CYP3A5 genotype in the dosage selection process.[134] Conversely, the guidelines issued by CPIC call for increasing the starting dosage of tacrolimus, in conjunction with TDM, in adult CYP3A5 intermediate and normal metabolizers relative to CYP3A5 nonexpressers.[133] While CPIC has not released official *CYP3A5* genotype–guided recommendations for tacrolimus dosing in the pediatric population, they conclude that based on the available data, extrapolation of the adult recommendations to children "seems appropriate."[133]

CYP3A7 is unusual in that it is expressed at high levels in human fetal liver[124] and plays a critical role during pregnancy through the formation of the 16α-hydroxy metabolite of dehydroepiandrosterone sulfate (DHEA-S), the process by which a third hydroxyl group is added to DHEA-S prior to final formation of estriol by placental syncytiotrophoblasts. Other substrates of CYP3A7 include retinoic acid and a wide range of foreign compounds that gain access to the fetus from the maternal circulation. Many drugs prescribed during pregnancy, such as glyburide for gestational diabetes, have been shown to cross the placenta, and residual drug in the child following delivery may be dependent on CYP3A7 for metabolic clearance.[145] Therefore, variability in CYP3A7 activity following delivery may be a determinant of postnatal hypoglycemia in neonates exposed to glyburide in utero. Genetic polymorphisms have been identified in *CYP3A7* that have yielded conflicting results regarding their contribution to enzymatic function. A notable example is the *CYP3A7*2* allele that occurs at a relatively low frequency in Caucasians (8%) and Asians (28%) compared with Africans (68%). Although the CYP3A7.2 protein product has been associated with 20% to 25% higher activity than the CYP3A7.1 enzyme in vitro,[146] no significant differences in DHEA 16α-hydroxylation activity were observed in livers genotyped for *CYP3A7*1* and *CYP3A7*2*.[147] Given the recent observation of sex-dependent effects of genetic variants in *CYP3A4* and *CYP3A7*,[148] the functional consequences of genetic variation in fetal liver *CYP3A7* warrant further investigation. Persistence of fetal CYP3A7 mRNA in adult liver has been partially attributed to the *CYP3A7*1C* allele in which a set of seven tightly linked variants essentially replace 60 bp of the *CYP3A7* promoter with the identical sequence from *CYP3A4*.[144]

Glucuronosyl Transferases

The UGT gene superfamily catalyzes the conjugation of substrates with glucuronic acid. The ontogeny of protein abundance for several UGTs in the human liver has been characterized, with expression of UGT1A1, UGT1A4, UGT1A6, UGT1A9, UGT2B7, and UGT2B15 all reported to increase with age.[149] Both drugs and endogenous compounds[150] have been identified as substrates for UGTs, and the implications of genetic variation in UGTs on drug dosing have been extensively reviewed.[151] UGT1A1 is the major *UGT* gene product responsible for bilirubin glucuronidation, and more than 60 genetic alterations have been reported, most of which are rare and are more properly considered mutations rather than gene polymorphisms. Inheritance of two defective alleles is associated with reduced bilirubin-conjugating activity and gives rise to clinical conditions such as Crigler-Najjar syndrome and Gilbert syndrome. More frequently occurring polymorphisms involve a dinucleotide (TA) repeat in the atypical TATA box of the *UGT1A1* promoter. The wild-type *UGT1A1*1* allele has six repeats (TA_6), and the TA_5 (*UGT1A1*33*), TA_7 (*UGT1A1*28*), and TA_8 (*UGT1A1*34*) variants are all associated with reduced activity. *UGT1A1*28* is the most frequent variant and is a contributory factor to prolonged neonatal jaundice[152,153] and toxicity of the irinotecan-active metabolite, SN-38.[154,155] Currently, the FDA recommends reductions in irinotecan dose in patients who are homozygous for the **28* allele.[156] The antiretroviral, atazanavir, is known to inhibit UGT1A1 and lead to hyperbilirubinemia. This adverse event is more common in poor metabolizers, presumably due to reduced basal UGT1A1-mediated clearance of bilirubin.[157] As such, CPIC has issued a recommendation that atazanavir not be used in adults who possess two reduced function alleles.[158] While specific pediatric recommendations are not included, they state that the adult guidelines may be directly adapted to children.[158]

Polymorphisms in UGT1A4 have also been identified, with the *UGT1A4*2* allele resulting in the substitution of a proline to a threonine residue upstream of the normal cleavage site for the formation of the mature protein. Diminished catalytic activity has been observed for the mature *UGT1A4*2* protein product.[159] Conversely, another variant allele, *UGT1A4*3*, may have enhanced activity of its mature protein product. The *UGT1A4*3* allele has been associated with increased glucuronidation of olanzapine and 25-hydroxyvitamin D_3.[160,161] However, one study evaluating the effects of the *UGT1A4*3* allele on dose-normalized concentrations of lamotrigine in children yielded conflicting results, complicating the interpretation of the genotype–phenotype relationship.[162] Several allelic variants of other important UGTs involved in drug biotransformation (UGT1A6 and UGT2B7) have also been reported,[151] but the lack of isoform-specific probe compounds analogous to dextromethorphan for CYP2D6 has precluded a clear understanding of the clinical impact of polymorphisms in these genes, with some exceptions[80]; issues related to developmental trajectory adding further complexity to genotype–phenotype associations. Nevertheless, from a pediatric perspective, genetic variation in the promoter region of *UGT1A9* has been reported to influence glucuronidation of acetaminophen in newborns administered intravenous acetaminophen. Specifically, insertion of an extra thymidine in a run of nine sequential thymidine residues (T_9) to form a T_{10} motif was associated in a 42% reduction in the formation of acetaminophen glucuronide.[163] Expression of UGT2B17 protein is perhaps the most variable of the UGTs in children and adolescents, being influenced by sex (~2.6-fold higher in males and females), age (minimally expressed in children less than 9 years of age and increases during puberty), and genetic variation (SNPs and CNV).[164] Its primary function is sex hormone homeostasis, especially androgens such as testosterone and dihydrotestosterone. Although a limited number of drugs are also UGT2B17 substrates, the consequences of variable activity on clearances of these agents have not been investigated in pediatric patients.

Arylamine N-Acetyltransferases

One the earliest discovered and most widely recognized genetic polymorphisms is the arylamine *N*-acetyltransferase-2 (NAT2) polymorphism. Approximately 50% of Caucasians and African Americans residing on the North American continent are phenotypically slow metabolizers placing a substantial number of individuals at increased risk for the development of adverse drug effects, such as sulfasalazine-induced hemolysis, hydrazine- or arylamine-induced peripheral neuropathy, procainamide- or isoniazid-induced lupus erythematosus, and Stevens-Johnson syndrome (SJS) or toxic epidermal necrolysis (TEN) associated with sulfonamide administration.[165] NAT2 function is inherited in an autosomal dominant manner with the inheritance of two "slow" alleles required for expression of the slow-metabolizer phenotype. The relative proportion of rapid and slow metabolizers varies considerably with ethnic or geographic origin. For example, the percentage of slow acetylators among Canadian Eskimos is 5% but approaches 90% in some Mediterranean populations.[166] According to the standardized NAT2 nomenclature, the wild-type and three additional "fast" alleles give rise to the rapid acetylator phenotype, while nine "slow" alleles have been described.[82]

In vivo, using caffeine as a phenotyping probe, all infants between the ages of 0 and 55 days appear to be phenotypically slow acetylators, while 50% and 62% of infants between the ages of 122 to 224 and 225 to 342 days, respectively, can be characterized as fast acetylators.[41] Several independent studies indicate that maturation of the NAT2 phenotype occurs during the first 4 years of life.[40,167,168] Thus, phenotype–genotype discordance is likely to be most apparent in the first 2 to 4 months of life, and drugs highly dependent on NAT2 function for their elimination should be used with caution.

Thiopurine S-methyltransferase

TPMT is a cytosolic enzyme that catalyzes the S-methylation of aromatic and heterocyclic sulfur-containing compounds, such as 6-mercaptopurine, azathioprine, and 6-thioguanine, that are used in the treatment of several pediatric diseases and disorders including acute lymphoblastic anemia (ALL), inflammatory bowel disease, and juvenile arthritis and to prevent renal allograft rejection. To exert its cytotoxic effects, 6-mercaptopurine requires metabolism to thioguanine nucleotides (TGNs) by a multistep process that is initiated by hypoxanthine guanine phosphoribosyl transferase. TPMT prevents TGN production by methylating 6-mercaptopurine (Fig. 5.5A). TPMT activity is usually measured in blood with activity in erythrocytes reflecting that found in other tissues, including liver and leukemic blasts. While approximately 89% of Caucasians and African Americans have high TPMT activity and 11% have intermediate activity, 1 in 300 individuals inherit TPMT deficiency as an autosomal recessive trait (Fig. 5.5B).[83] In patients with intermediate or low activity, more drug is shunted toward production of cytotoxic TGNs. TPMT can also methylate 6-thioinosine 5′-monophosphate (TIMP) to generate a methylated metabolite that is capable of inhibiting de novo purine synthesis (Fig. 5.5C).

Conflicting relationships between age and TPMT activity have been reported in children. In one study, peripheral blood TPMT activity in newborns was reported to be 50% greater than in race-matched adults and demonstrated a distribution of activity consistent with the polymorphism characterized in adults.[169] In contrast, TPMT activities were comparable to previously reported adult values in a population of Korean school children (n = 309) aged 7 to 9 years[170] and in French Caucasian children (n = 165) hospitalized for day surgery.[171] Considerable interindividual variability in TPMT activity exists for both pediatric and adult populations consistently, with genetic variation being the primary driver of the observed variability.

Several genetic variants contribute to the TPMT poor-metabolizer phenotype. The **2, *3A, *3B, *3C,* and **4* alleles are all considered nonfunctional and clinically actionable under CPIC thiopurine dosing guidelines.[172] Although the **3A* allele has only a frequency of 0.03% in the general population, it is the most common variant and represents 55% of all mutant alleles. *TMPT*3A* is characterized by two nucleotide transition mutations, G460A and A719G, that lead to two amino acid substitutions Ala154Thr and Tyr240Cys (Fig. 5.5D). Either variant alone results in loss of functional activity through the production of unstable proteins that are subject to accelerated proteolytic degradation.[173,174] Less frequent allelic variants involve SNPs that produce amino acid substitutions in the coding region and defective intron–exon splicing.

A polymorphic locus has been identified in the promoter region of the *TPMT* gene involving a variable number of tandem repeats (VNTR) in which three to nine repeats of a specific nucleotide sequence occur in tandem.[175,176] The VNTR polymorphism modulates TPMT activity when expressed in vitro,[177] apparently by a mechanism involving gene transcription.[178] In vivo, the VNTR occurs most commonly as four (*V4) or five (*V5) repeats, and the *V4/*V5 diplotype has been associated with higher erythrocyte TPMT activity compared to *V4/*V4 or *V5/*V5 diplotypes in one study,[176] and *V6 was associated with decreased levels of TPMT in another study.[179] In childhood ALL patients, TPMT expression has been observed to increase 1.5- to 7.9-fold during the maintenance phase relative to the beginning of treatment, with VNTR*5a/*5a carriers having the highest levels of TPMT expression during maintenance treatment, even though they exhibited low expression prior to treatment. In contrast, carriers of the VNTR*7a allele had the lowest level of enzyme expression prior to treatment and the lowest increase in activity during the maintenance phase.[180] Thus, the VNTR polymorphism in the regulatory region of the *TPMT* gene affects the level of gene expression, whereas allelic variation in the coding region of the *TPMT* gene primarily affects the catalytic activity of the expressed enzyme.

The small percentage of patients with low to absent TPMT activity is at increased risk for developing severe myelosuppression if treated with routine doses of thiopurines, and the most recent CPIC guideline recommends a 10-fold reduction of dose and reduced frequency from daily to three times per week to minimize the risk of toxicity; CPIC also recommends decreases in dosing and adjustment based on the degree of myelosuppression for TPMT intermediate metabolizers as well.[172] Furthermore, poor metabolizers may be at increased risk of relapse consequent to inadequate or absent treatment with the thiopurines. In the context of the expanding use of 6-mercaptopurine and azathioprine in pediatrics to treat inflammatory bowel disease and juvenile arthritis and to prevent renal allograft rejection, TPMT deficiency is not a trivial matter, and risk-to-benefit considerations will differ compared to ALL.

The 2019 thiopurine pharmacogenomics-based dosing guidelines have also incorporated *NUDT15* polymorphisms alongside *TPMT*.[172] Nudix hydrolase 15, the protein product of *NUDT15*, acts as a nucleoside diphosphatase capable of transforming genotoxic thioguanine triphosphate compounds into less toxic monophosphates. Among the identified genetic variants, the *NUDT15*2* and *NUDT15*3* alleles are currently the

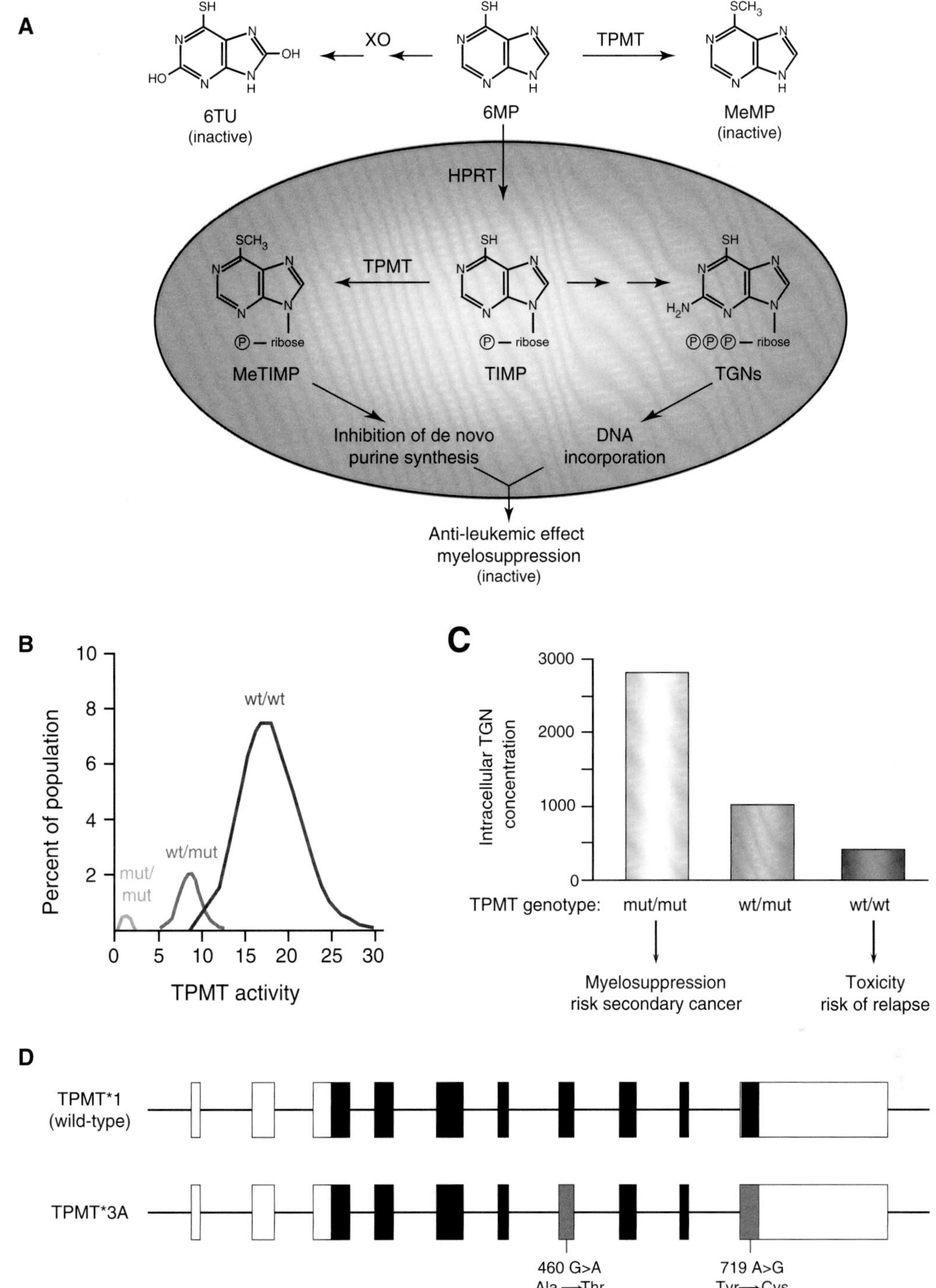

Figure 5.5 The 6-thioinosine 5′-monophosphate (TPMT) polymorphism. **A:** 6-Mercaptopurine (6MP) undergoes metabolism to thioguanine nucleotides (TGNs) to exert its cytotoxic effects. TPMT and xanthine oxidase reduce the amount of 6MP available for the bioactivation pathway to TGNs. TPMT can also methylate TIMP to generate a methylated compound capable of inhibiting de novo purine synthesis. **B:** Distribution of TPMT activity in humans. In all, 89% of the population has high activity, while 11% have intermediate activity. Approximately 1 in 300 individuals. A is homozygous for two loss of functional alleles and thus has very low activity. **C:** Correlation between TPMT genotype and intracellular TGN concentrations. In TPMT poor metabolizers, more 6MP is available to go down the bioactivation pathway to form TGNs and is associated with an increased risk of myelosuppression. **D:** The most common variant TPMT allele is the result of two mutations that give rise to an unstable protein product that undergoes proteolytic degradation. (Modified with permission from *Nature Reviews Cancer* 1:99–108 copyright 2001, Macmillan Magazines Ltd; Kim SH, Kim M, Lee KW, et al. HLA-B*5901 is strongly associated with methazolamide-induced Stevens-Johnson syndrome/toxic epidermal necrolysis. *Pharmacogenomics* 2010;11:879–884.)

most understood with regard to functional impact. Patients who possess two copies of these alleles or one of each are considered poor metabolizers, while those with one copy of **2* or **3* and a function allele (e.g., **1*) are classified as intermediate metabolizers. Deficiencies in both pathways should be considered for thiopurine dosing. For instance, the likelihood of requiring a dosing adjustment would be expected to be greater in a TPMT intermediate metabolizer who is also a nudix hydrolase 15 intermediate metabolizer when compared to an individual with solely a TPMT intermediate-metabolizer status.[172]

An association between TPMT deficiencies and cisplatin-mediated toxicity in cancer patients has been reported, with children apparently at a disproportionate risk of developing hearing loss after taking cisplatin.[181] This finding has been replicated by some investigators,[182] but not others,[183] and remains controversial.[184,185]

Carboxylesterases

The observation that heritable butyrylcholinesterase deficiency resulted in prolonged paralysis following succinylcholine administration was one of the foundational discoveries in the field of pharmacogenetics. Since then, our understanding of the role of esterases in metabolism and bioactivation of drugs and prodrugs has greatly expanded. While multiple esterases are now recognized to affect the disposition of drugs, attention has been directed toward carboxylesterases 1 (CES1) and 2 (CES2) in particular. CES1 and CES2 are part of a broader family of esterases and are responsible for the cleavage of carboxylic esters into an alcohol and a carboxylate moiety. While there exists extensive substrate overlap between the two isoforms, CES1 preferentially hydrolyzes esters with relatively small alcohol substituents and larger acyl substituent, while CES2 generally favors the reverse.[186] In humans, CES2 is extensively present in both the liver and the intestine, while CES1 is preferentially expressed in the liver.[186] Expression of both CES1 and CES2 increases fivefold and threefold, respectively, in the liver from birth to adulthood.[187,188]

While genetic polymorphisms have been identified for both carboxylesterases, there is currently more evidence supporting the clinical importance of *CES1* genetics. It has been observed that children with a reduced function polymorphism resulting in an amino acid substitution from glycine to glutamic acid at position 143 in the CES1 protein require a higher dose of methylphenidate than those with the wild-type allele.[189] Increased exposure to the active metabolite of clopidogrel, which is cleared by CES1, and subsequent clinical responsiveness, has also been observed in adults with this variant.[190] The underlying mechanism of these associations was elucidated by independent observations of substantially reduced catalytic activity in the CES1 protein product of this genetic polymorphism.[191] It is worth noting that genetic polymorphisms in *CES1* have also been associated with alterations in the biotransformation of oseltamivir, a drug frequently reserved for use in infants and other populations at high risk for influenza-related complications.[192,193]

DRUG TRANSPORTERS AND LOCAL DRUG CONCENTRATIONS

While somewhat overshadowed by the abundance of information on the pharmacogenomics of drug-metabolizing enzymes, there exists a number of convincing examples of the importance of transporter pharmacogenomics in drug action and disposition. Some transporters represent direct targets for therapeutic agents. Examples include the sodium glucose transporter 2 inhibitors used in the treatment of diabetes and ivacaftor for cystic fibrosis. When a transporter is a direct target of pharmacologic action, polymorphisms in the genes encoding for the transporter can play a role in determining the presence or magnitude of drug response. A particularly relevant example for pediatrics involves the treatment of cystic fibrosis with ivacaftor. Ivacaftor is a potentiator of cystic fibrosis transmembrane conductance regulator (CFTR), an ATP-binding cassette (ABC) transporter, and chloride channel that is defective in individuals with cystic fibrosis. Only certain mutations that impair CFTR function will respond to potentiation via ivacaftor. As such, the CPIC guidelines for ivacaftor state that a patient should be genotyped as positive for the G551D mutation in CFTR in order to receive the drug.[194] While examples of genotype-dependent requirements for pharmacologic action are especially compelling in making a case for the utility of transporter pharmacogenetics, most of the known instances where transporter pharmacogenetics influences drug therapy relate to their role in modulating systemic pharmacokinetics. Over the past two decades, research in the field of drug transporters has expanded to also include an equally important emphasis on their role in modulating local drug concentrations at intracellular sites of metabolic clearance, toxicity, and therapeutic action. This effect is most pronounced in the case of active transporters (i.e., those directly or indirectly dependent upon cellular energy sources to function), which can operate against drug concentration gradients and are, therefore, capable of maintaining intracellular drug concentrations that are many-fold greater or less than those of the surrounding extracellular environment. In their role in modulating local concentrations, a useful functional classification for discussing drug transporters is to divide them into uptake transporters, those that bring drug molecules into cells, and efflux transporters, those that remove drug molecules from cells. Uptake transporters are typically members of the solute carrier (SLC) superfamily, but members of ABC transporter family also mediate the active cellular uptake of drugs.

Organic Anion Transporter Polypeptides

Organic anion–transporting polypeptides (OATPs) are a subfamily of SLC uptake transporters, and four OATP transporters, OATP1A2, OATP1B1, OATP1B3, and OATP2B1, are widely recognized for their importance in drug disposition. Targeted proteomics and more traditional immunoblot-based methods have revealed that OATPs are expressed in a diversity of tissues, with OATP1A2 and OATP2B1 being almost ubiquitously expressed.[195] By comparison, OATP1B1 and OATP1B3 protein expression is largely restricted to the liver.[196–198] According to recent studies utilizing targeted proteomics, hepatic OATP1B3 expression is present at birth and increases as a child approaches adulthood, whereas OATP1B1 and OATP2B1 expression remains relatively unchanged.[199] It is worth noting that prior studies relying upon Western Blot, real-time PCR (for mRNA), and transporter activity assays in primary hepatocytes suggest differing maturation profile, and further confirmatory studies are warranted.

OATP1B1 has a particularly well-defined role in modulating the pharmacokinetics of statins and other substrates. A considerable amount of attention has been paid to assessing the impact of genetic polymorphisms in *SLCO1B1*, the gene encoding OATP1B1, on statin pharmacotherapy. In particular, the 521T>C SNP resulting in a change from valine to an alanine at residue 174 has repeatedly been associated with greater plasma concentrations and increased risk of myopathies in individuals taking statins.[200–204] Based on this and other *SLCO1B1* polymorphisms, over 30 haplotypes have been assigned. Alterations in in vivo drug disposition or response have been observed for several haplotypes, including **1B, *5, *14, *15, *17,* and **27*.[205,206] Interestingly, while most of the variant *SLCO1B1* haplotypes are associated with reductions in OATP1B1-mediated transport, the **14* haplotype was found to be associated with increased OATP1B1 protein expression in the liver.[207] Not all statins are affected to the same extent by *SLCO1B1* haplotypes, and of the currently marketed statins, simvastatin acid is most affected.[208–211] Current CPIC guidelines recommend the carriers of the **5, *15,* or **17* haplotype receive a reduced dose of simvastatin acid or an alternate HMG-CoA reductase inhibitor.[212] Generally speaking, genotype–phenotype associations for *SLCO1B1*5* and systemic exposure of simvastatin acid and pravastatin are similar between children/adolescents and adults,[204,213] but interindividual variability *within* a genotype group is greater than the difference *between* genotype groups, indicating that additional nongenetic factors are also important.

Organic Cation Transporters

Organic cation transporters (OCTs) are a group of uptake transporters within subfamily 22 of the SLC family (i.e., SLC22A). OCTs have been implicated in the modulation of the pharmacokinetics and pharmacodynamics of cationic drugs, such as cisplatin, citalopram, lamivudine, metformin, morphine, ondansetron, and sumatriptan. Some drugs are transported preferentially by certain OCTs, but there exists considerable substrate overlap among isoforms. Whereas OCT1 and OCT2 are enriched in the liver and kidney proximal tubule, respectively, OCT3 is expressed more ubiquitously across tissues.[195] Genetic polymorphisms have been identified in *SLC22A1, SLC22A2,* and *SLC22A3,* the genes encoding for OCT1, OCT2, and OCT3, respectively.

Six haplotypes (**1* through **6*) have been described for *SLC22A1* based on the five reduced function polymorphisms (262T>C, 286C>T, 1306G>A, 1365GAT>del, and 1498G>C), and their impact on pharmacokinetics has been evaluated. Reduced clearance of morphine was observed in children who carry two reduced function variants (**2, *3, *4,* or **5*); the **6* haplotype was not evaluated.[214] A subsequent study in neonates demonstrated similar findings relating to the **2* through **5* haplotypes and additionally observed reduced morphine clearance with the **6* variant.[215] The **3* through **6* variants, but not **2*, have also been associated with decreased clearance of fenoterol and sumatriptan in adults.[216,217] For *SLC22A1* polymorphisms, associations between the decreased function haplotypes and alterations in pharmacokinetics have been attributed to impaired OCT1-mediated uptake into the liver, the principle organ of elimination for most of the implicated drugs. However, in addition to the liver, OCT1 is also present in the intestinal epithelia, and the potential for OCT1 polymorphisms to alter oral bioavailability and absorption rate should also be considered.[196]

Because the intestine and liver are the sites of pharmacologic effects for many drugs, impairments in OCT1 function have the potential to alter the apparent pharmacodynamics of substrates. Associations have been observed between *SLC22A1* polymorphisms and reduced tolerability to metformin, an OCT1 substrate with adherence issues related to gastrointestinal irritation.[218] Considering the liver is a major site where metformin exerts its therapeutic effects, it has also been suggested that reduced hepatic uptake, secondary to *SLC22A1* polymorphisms, may result in relatively reduced glycemic control. However, experimental results investigating this hypothesis have been inconsistent.[219] Variants of the gene encoding OCT2 (i.e., *SLC22A2*) that may be relevant in metformin therapy have also been identified. In particular, the nonsynonymous 808G>T polymorphism results in a reduced function allele and has been associated with impaired renal tubular secretion of metformin.[220,221] Reduced incidence of nephrotoxicity to cisplatin, another substrate of renal OCT2, has also been in observed in carriers of the 808G>T SNP.[222] While variants of *SLC22A3* (i.e., OCT3) have been identified, their capacity to impact drug disposition and response remains relatively unclear.

Breast Cancer Resistance Protein

Breast cancer resistance protein (BCRP) is a member of the ABC family of active transporters. It is encoded by the *ABCG2* gene and is expressed in many epithelial and endothelial cells in humans. Oriented outwardly, BCRP transports substrates out of cells and contributes to the critical restrictive functions of the testis, placenta, and the blood–brain barrier (BBB). In the liver, BCRP is expressed on the canalicular membrane of hepatocytes and contributes to the biliary secretion of drugs, such as nitrofurantoin and rosuvastatin.[223] Targeted proteomic studies have revealed that BCRP expression in the liver is relatively stable from birth to adulthood and that age may not be a substantial independent source of interindividual variability.[199]

Most of the genetic polymorphisms in *ABCG2* for which a functional impact has been established are rare, with the notable exception of 421G>T, a particularly common SNP among individuals of Han Chinese ancestry.[224] The 421G>T SNP results in a reduced function allele and has been associated with increased exposure to rosuvastatin and greater reductions in low-density lipoprotein (LDL) cholesterol.[202,225–227] This association presumably is a consequence of impaired secretion of rosuvastatin into the bile via hepatic BCRP. Conversely, it has been observed that patients with the relatively reduced function GT or TT genotypes appear to have reduced effectiveness of allopurinol in gout.[228,229] However, a mechanism has yet to be established, and the association may be the result of the 421G>T SNP being in linkage disequilibrium with another genetic polymorphism.

Whereas rosuvastatin and allopurinol provide the most convincing examples of a role for the clinical utility of BCRP pharmacogenetics, they are not frequently used drugs in the pediatric population, and studies specifically investigating the impact of BCRP genetic polymorphisms on drug exposure and response in children have been limited. Clearance and incidence of adverse events in children receiving tacrolimus for hematopoietic stem cell transplants have been observed to be unaffected by the 421G>T variant.[230] In a study of methotrexate pharmacokinetics in a pediatric population, another relatively more common BCRP SNP, -24C>T, was not found to have a detectable effect.[231] Other pediatric-relevant drugs, such as lamotrigine and sulfasalazine, have been identified as BCRP substrates, and although clinical studies in adults suggest a potential effect of the 421G>T SNP on their pharmacokinetics, no pediatric data are currently available.[232–234]

Multidrug Resistance–Associated Proteins

The multidrug resistance–associated protein (MRP) transporters are a subfamily of ABC efflux transporters with an affinity for organic anionic compounds. A variety of drugs and endogenous substrates, such as bile acids, are transported by MRPs. Broadly speaking, MRPs have an affinity for conjugated compounds, including phase II drug metabolites (e.g., glucuronide, glutathione, and sulfate conjugates). In humans, MRPs are expressed in all tissues traditionally considered important in governing pharmacokinetics. In the small intestine, MRP2, and, possibly, MRP4 are localized to the apical membrane of the enterocytes, whereas MRP1, MRP3, and MRP5 are expressed on the basolateral membranes.[235] In the liver, MRP2 is present in the bile canalicular membrane, and MRP1, MRP3, MRP4, and MRP5 are expressed in the sinusoidal membranes of the hepatocytes.[235] In the kidney, MRP2 and MRP4 are found on the apical membranes of the proximal tubule epithelial cells, whereas MRP1 and MRP3 are expressed in the basolateral membranes.[235] In the BBB, MRP1, MRP4, and MRP5 are expressed along the luminal membranes of the capillary endothelial cells, thereby restricting access of substrates to the cerebrospinal fluid.[235] Broadly speaking, MRPs are oriented outwardly, and their action results in reduced intracellular concentrations of their respective substrates.

MRP1 is encoded by the *ABCC1* gene and is perhaps the most studied MRP transporter regarding protein structure–function relationships. It has an affinity for transporting phase II drug metabolites (e.g., glucuronide and glutathione conjugates), anthracyclines, and vincristine. Much of the focus of *ABCC1* pharmacogenetic studies in children has related to the effect of allelic variation on adverse drug reactions to anticancer agents. For the most part, no associations of clinical consequence have been found in pediatric trials. Notably, the intronic 825T>C SNP, present in approximately 10% of the African populations, was associated with incidence of anthracycline-induced cardiotoxicity in children.[236] However, a follow-up study could not confirm the association.[237]

MRP2 shares a high degree of substrate overlap with MRP1. In humans, MRP2 is extensively expressed in the apical brush border of the kidney proximal tubule. In conjunction with other transporters, including MRP4, it plays an important role in secreting substrates from inside proximal tubule epithelial cells out into the glomerular ultrafiltrate. A reduced function variant resulting from the -24C>T SNP in *ABCC2*, the gene encoding for MRP2, has been associated with tenofovir-induced nephrotoxicity in adults.[238,239] However, the mechanism underlying a role of MRP2 genetics is less clear, given that tenofovir has not been consistently shown to be a substrate of MRP2. In the pediatric population, the -24C>T SNP has also been associated with elevated trough concentrations of voriconazole and increased incidence of toxicities to methotrexate.[231,240]

MRP3 has an affinity for phase II drug metabolites, particularly glucuronide conjugates. In perfused livers isolated from *ABCC3* (i.e., MRP3) knockout mice, secretion of acetaminophen glucuronide into the blood was decreased, and secretion into the bile was increased.[241] Similar findings have reported for morphine. In *ABCC3* knockout mice, morphine-3-glucuronide concentrations are increased in the bile, while plasma concentrations are dramatically reduced (~50-fold).[242] In humans, reduced expression of *ABCC3* mRNA has been observed in individuals who are homozygous for the -211C>T SNP,[243] and the presence of the T allele also has been associated with reduced systemic exposure to morphine-glucuronide metabolites in children.[244]

MRP4 is predominantly responsible for transporting nucleoside drugs, such as tenofovir and ganciclovir. Like many other MRPs, it is also capable of transporting methotrexate and phase II drug metabolites. One of the clearer examples of an impact of MRP genetics on drug disposition is the 3463T>C polymorphism in *ABCC4*, the gene encoding MRP4. The variant is quite common, occurring in 10% to 20% of individuals, and is associated with increased plasma and cellular tenofovir exposure and decreased tenofovir renal clearance in adults.[245,246] Other studies have also connected the relatively common 4131A>C and 4976A>G SNPs in *ABCC4* with increased tenofovir clearance and incidence of tenofovir-induced nephrotoxicity, respectively.[247,248] MRP5 has a substrate profile that is similar to MRP4, consisting of nucleosides, nucleotides, and methotrexate. However, relatively less is known about the pharmacogenetics of *ABCC5* (i.e., MRP5), particularly in pediatrics. There is some evidence suggesting MRP5 may play a role mitigating the severity of 5-fluorouracil (5-FU) and irinotecan-induced gastrointestinal toxicity.[249]

P-Glycoprotein

P-glycoprotein (P-gp) is an ABC efflux transporter encoded by the *ABCB1*, also known as the *MDR1*, gene. Generally, it transports lipophilic and cationic compounds and has a high substrate overlap with the drug-metabolizing enzyme CYP3A. In humans, P-gp is expressed extensively in the intestines, kidneys, BBB, placenta, and liver.[250] In the small intestine and liver, where CYP3A and P-gp are co-expressed, evidence suggests the two proteins operate synergistically.[251] As such, reductions in P-gp function due to factors including genetic polymorphisms may also reduce the apparent activity of CYP3A. Much like CYP3A4, hepatic protein expression of P-gp has been shown to increase from birth to adulthood and that age may be a determinant in the functional consequences of interplay between the two proteins. Polymorphic expression of CYP3A5 adds an additional layer of complexity, and CYP3A5 polymorphisms may represent effect modifiers on associations between *ABCB1* polymorphisms and drug exposure. Enzyme-transporter interplay may even explain the results of one study where the CC genotype (1236C>T SNP) for *ABCB1* was associated with decreased tacrolimus blood concentrations *only* in children who also possessed at least one copy of the active *CYP3A5*1* allele.[252]

P-gp also plays a critical role in restricting drug transit across the BBB. Functional impairment of P-gp at the BBB could result in increased efficacy and toxicity of drugs that exert pharmacologic actions in the central nervous system (CNS), presumably through reduced efflux from the CNS. With this in mind, it is interesting to note that 1236C>T has been associated with increased response to risperidone and combined anesthetic regimens (e.g., remifentanil–sevoflurane and remifentanil–propofol).[253–255] Both 1236C>T and 3435C>T in *ABCB1* have been found to be associated with increased incidence of methotrexate-induced toxicities in children,[256] and 3435C>T has also been associated with increased neuropsychiatric adverse events in children taking oseltamivir.[257] Generally speaking, efforts to demonstrate a clear relationship between discrete genetic polymorphisms and transporter function have been complicated by the tremendous degree of variation in the *ABCB1* gene. While some utility has been found in aggregating multiple polymorphisms into haplotypes, much more work is needed to clarify P-gp pharmacogenetics.

HYPERSENSITIVITY REACTIONS

Many drugs and their metabolites can bind to proteins in the body and elicit hypersensitivity reactions. The potential for hypersensitivity reactions is especially great when drug or drug-modified peptides bind to the major histocompatibility complex (MHC) proteins that are important in T-cell recognition of antigens. Genetic variation in the *HLA* genes that encode MHC proteins has been shown to be reliable predictors of risk for hypersensitivity reactions to certain drugs. Hypersensitivity reactions to abacavir commonly result from the presence of the *HLA-B*57:01* allele, which occurs in approximately 5% of individuals of European ancestry.[258] Prospective screening for the *HLA-B*57:01* allele has dramatically reduced incidence of abacavir-induced hypersensitivity reactions.[259] The presence of *HLA-B*15:02*, an allele that is much more commonly encountered in individuals of Asian ancestry, has been associated with the incidence of SJS/TEN in children treated with carbamazepine and oxcarbazepine.[260] The FDA-approved product label recommends testing for *HLA-B*15:02* be conducted for patients with ancestry in populations with increased frequency of the allele prior to treatment with carbamazepine and oxcarbazepine.[261,262] While the *HLA-B*15:02* allele has also been associated with severe cutaneous adverse reactions to phenytoin, pharmacogenetics testing is currently not indicated prior to imitating therapy. However, alternative medications (other than fosphenytoin, carbamazepine, or oxcarbazepine) should be considered if a patient is known to carry the *HLA-B*15:02* allele and is phenytoin naïve.[263] The *HLA-A*31:01* allele is found in most populations worldwide and may also be a risk factor for SJS/TEN, although it seems to be more strongly associated with other carbamazepine-induced reactions, such as DRESS and maculopapular eruptions. As such, CPIC guidelines recommend carbamazepine not be used in carbamazepine-naïve patients who are positive for *HLA-B*15:02* or any *HLA-A*31:01* genotype.[264] Alternative antiseizure medications other than oxcarbazepine or phenytoin (or its prodrug fosphenytoin) should be used for any *HLA-B*15:02* carrier.[264] The presence of the *HLA-B*58:01* allele is associated with allopurinol-induced severe cutaneous adverse reactions, and CPIC guidelines recommend carriers of the allele not receive the drug.[265] Additional *HLA-B* variants have been implicated in cutaneous adverse reactions to nevirapine (*HLA-B*35:05*),[266,267] dapsone (*HLA-B*13:01*),[268,269] and methazolamide (*HLA-B*59:01*)[270,271]; the FDA has not issued guidelines for pharmacogenetic screening for these drugs at this time. Although most data for HLA associations with idiosyncratic drug reactions have been based on data from adults, the guidelines should be considered applicable to pediatric patients as well.

IMPROVING UPON ROUTINE THERAPEUTIC MONITORING WITH "-OMICS" DATA

The introduction of routine TDM has improved patient safety and efficacy for a number of drugs, and application of "-omics" data, such as pharmacogenomics, has the potential to lead to more precise therapy. For example, the relative activities of multiple contributing metabolic pathways, through measurement of metabolites in addition to the parent drug, are not typically captured in routine TDM. When one or more of these pathways is polymorphic, or the competing pathways have differing developmental trajectories, an understanding of the relationship between pharmacogenomics and metabolite-to-parent ratios can help in the translation of measurements taken during routine TDM into relatively more clinically meaningful numbers. Furthermore, understanding the relationship between pharmacogenomics and the contribution of individual pathways can provide insight into individual's unique sensitivity for drug–drug interactions (DDIs). PBPK models, leveraging data on the relationship between genotype and phenotype and known trends in the ontogeny of drug-metabolizing enzymes and transporters, provides a potential means to estimate full concentration–time course of drugs in the pediatric population. Similarly, metabolomics offers the prospect of identifying metabolomic signatures or discrete urinary biomarkers that could aid in the prediction of patient-specific pharmacokinetics and adverse event profile of a drug in a given patient.

INDIVIDUALIZED DRUG–DRUG INTERACTION RISK

Drugs are typically cleared from the body via multiple metabolic and excretory pathways that may or may not be dependent upon the effects of genetic polymorphisms. There is often a generally recognized major clearance pathway, but the specific contribution of each pathway will vary from individual to individual based on their relative expression levels for the participating enzymes. The risks of inappropriate drug exposure presented by this underlying interindividual variability can be somewhat mitigated by the practice of adjusting the dose to achieve a particular effect, such as is done with warfarin, or with the implementation of routine TDM. Nevertheless, the magnitude of change in drug exposure upon coadministration of an interacting medication will vary greatly from patient to patient, even among patients who have previously been dosed to the same systemic exposure or pharmacologic effect. When a clear genotype–phenotype relationship exists, pharmacogenomics can offer insight into an individual's unique propensity to experience a particular DDI. Furthermore, enzyme expression within a given genotype may vary considerably as a function of age and environmental factors. Here, identification of endogenous biomarkers of activity through metabolomic screening offers an attractive avenue for determining the compliment of drug-metabolizing enzymes in a given person at a given point in time, and to predict an individualized fold-change in drug as exposure with the addition of a concomitant medication. While the use multiple concomitant medications has traditionally been associated with the adult population, the rate of polypharmacy in pediatric population has been progressively expanding. In recent years, our understanding of the interplay between pharmacogenetics and DDIs has been leveraged to quantitatively predict changes in relative drug exposure. However, refinement and clinical implementation of these predictive models, in the form of decision support tools for dose adjustment, is still outstanding. Furthermore, the incorporation of parameters reflecting the ontogeny of drug-metabolizing enzymes and transporters will be required to produce accurate estimates in the pediatric population.

PEDIATRIC PHARMACOGENETICS: CHALLENGES FOR THE FUTURE

Challenges for pediatric pharmacogenetics in the future and considerations for the design of studies to improve the quality of pharmacogenomic data in children are well exemplified by the progress in warfarin pharmacogenetics over the past 10 years.

Warfarin is a 4-hydroxycoumarin anticoagulant that exerts its pharmacologic actions via the antagonism of vitamin K epoxide reductase (VKOR), the enzyme responsible for the bioactivation of vitamin K and downstream synthesis of vitamin K–dependent clotting factors II, VII, IX, and X. Warfarin is well known to be a CYP2C9 substrate, and historically, prepubertal children have been reported to require larger weight-based doses of warfarin to achieve the same target international normalized ratio (INR),[137] as older children and adults.[272] This observation is now attributed to age-dependent changes in the ratio of liver mass to total body mass,[273] but hints that the pharmacodynamic response to warfarin may differ between younger children and adults were also present. Studies of warfarin pharmacogenetics in children have lagged behind those of adults, but the results of at least seven studies consistently have found that genetic variation in CYP2C9 *and* the target of warfarin action, vitamin K oxidoreductase complex 1 (VKORC1), are the most important determinants of warfarin dose in studied populations. Although these studies consistently reveal that children with *VKORC1* -1639AA genotypes require significantly lower doses of warfarin to achieve the same target INR as children with -1639GG genotypes, a major inconsistency among the various studies is the relative importance of genetic (primarily *VKORC1* and *CYP2C9* genotype) and "nongenetic/developmental" factors as determinants of variability in the warfarin dose required to achieve a stable INR target therapeutic goal. For example, age was reported to account for 28.3% of dose variability, and genetic factors contributed approximately 4% (3.7% for *VKORC1* and 0.4% for *CYP2C9*) in one study, whereas in six subsequent studies, the genetic contribution (predominantly *VKORC1* genotype) was larger (11.9% to 52% of dose variability), but in four of these studies, the "developmental" component still exceeded the genetic contribution (reviewed in reference [274]). It has been proposed that the composition of individual study cohorts may contribute to the discrepancy between relative contributions of genetic and nongenetic factors.[274] For example, in a subgroup analysis, patients receiving warfarin after a Fontan surgery, genetic factors accounted for approximately 50% of variability in dose and developmental factors were <10%, whereas for patients receiving warfarin for a thromboembolic disorder, developmental factors were most important, accounting for approximately 60% of variability, and genetic factors were negligible.[274]

This case of pediatric warfarin pharmacogenetics provides important insights that should be considered in the design of future pharmacogenetic studies in children. First, treatment with warfarin was the primary inclusion criterion for the pediatric warfarin studies to ensure adequate cohorts for analysis. In fact, the practice of enrolling all pediatric patients based primarily on use of a specific medication, without consideration of underlying disease process is a fairly common practice in pediatrics where the numbers of affected patients generally are much smaller than adult populations. Including patients who are receiving a drug for different indications—for primary prevention of a thromboembolic event or for prophylaxis to prevent recurrent thromboembolic events, both of which may be cardiac or noncardiac in origin, and post-Fontan procedure—risks confounding the analysis when different disease mechanisms may be operative. Second, the warfarin case illustrates the importance of improved mechanistic insights into the effects of increasing age—specifically, potential differences in the influence of the processes involved in growth (e.g., changes in height, weight, and body composition) and development, such as progression through the various Tanner stages to achieve full sexual maturity—on drug disposition and response.[274]

SUMMARY AND CONCLUSIONS

The postgenomic era represents an unprecedented opportunity to translate the increasing volume of untapped genomic, transcriptomic, proteomic, and metabonomic data into discoveries that favorably impact the care and treatment of children. Many diseases have their onset during childhood, and effective early intervention may have unforeseen benefits later in life. On the other hand, pharmacologic management of disease or unintended exposure to environmental toxins at critical stages of development may have consequences that are not immediately apparent due to the profound changes that occur as a fetus develops, and as newborn infants mature through childhood to adolescence and, ultimately, adulthood. Given the complexity of human development, a focus on the influence of a single gene or gene product is likely to be of limited value in terms of understanding the consequences of small molecule interactions with a dynamic developmental environment. Rather, the developmental process should be perceived, at a minimum, as networks of interacting genes and different networks being operative at different developmental stages. Furthermore, the repertoire of genes operative within a given network may vary at different developmental stages, and the phenotypic manifestations of gene variants may not manifest until much later in the process of maturation. In the context of identifying new target genes or gene networks for therapeutic intervention, the most compelling challenge to pediatric pharmacogenomic research will be to identify the essential network or pathway (knowing where to look) at the appropriate developmental stage (knowing when to look). There is reason to be optimistic that new strategies and technologies will help unravel the complexities of pediatric disorders since this new knowledge is essential for children to benefit as much as adults from new treatment modalities.

REFERENCES

1. Lander ES, Linton LM, Birren B, et al. Initial sequencing and analysis of the human genome. *Nature* 2001;409:860–921.
2. Schwenk JM, Omenn GS. The human plasma proteome draft of 2017: building on the human plasma peptide atlas from mass spectrometry and complementary assays. *J Proteome Res* 2017;16:4299–4310.
3. Guo SW, Reed DR. The genetics of phenylthiocarbamide perception. *Ann Hum Biol* 2001;28:111–142.
4. Motulsky AG. Drug reactions, enzymes, and biochemical genetics. *J Am Med Assoc* 1957;165:835–837.
5. Kalow W. *Pharmacogenetics: heredity and the response to drugs.* Philadelphia, PA: W.B. Saunders, 1962.
6. Vesell ES. Twin studies in pharmacogenetics. *Hum Genet* 1978;1:19–30.
7. Mahgoub A, Idle JR, Dring LG, et al. Polymorphic hydroxylation of debrisoquine in man. *Lancet* 1977;2:584–586.
8. Eichelbaum M, Spannbrucker N, Steincke B, et al. Defective N-oxidation of sparteine in man: a new pharmacogenetic defect. *Eur J Clin Pharmacol* 1979;16:183–187.
9. Küpfer A, Preisig R. Pharmacogenetics of mephenytoin: a new drug hydroxylation polymorphism in man. *Eur J Clin Pharmacol* 1984;26:753–759.
10. Ensom MH, Davis GA, Cropp CD, et al. Clinical pharmacokinetics in the 21st century. Does the evidence support definitive outcomes. *Clin Pharmacokinet* 1998;34:265–279.
11. Weinshilboum R. Inheritance and drug response. *N Engl J Med* 2003;348:529–537.
12. Johnson JA. Drug target pharmacogenomics: an overview. *Am J Pharmacogenomics* 2001;1:271–281.
13. Evans WE, McLeod HL. Pharmacogenomics—drug disposition, drug targets, and side effects. *N Engl J Med* 2003;348:538–549.
14. McKusick VA, Ruddle FH. A new discipline, a new name, a new journal. *Genomics* 1987;1:1–2.
15. Venter JC, Adams MD, Myers EW, et al. The sequence of the human genome. *Science* 2001;291:1304–1351.

16. Pennisi E. Reaching their goal early, sequencing labs celebrate. *Science* 2003;300:409.
17. Velculescu VE, Zhang L, Zhou W, et al. Characterization of the yeast transcriptome. *Cell* 1997;88:243–251.
18. Velculescu VE, Madden SL, Zhang L, et al. Analysis of human transcriptomes. *Nat Genet* 1999;23:387–388.
19. Kahn P. From genome to proteome: looking at a cell's proteins. *Science* 1995;270:369–370.
20. Hunter PJ, Borg TK. Integration from proteins to organs: the physiome project. *Nat Rev Mol Cell Biol* 2003;4:237–243.
21. Tweedale H, Notley-McRobb L, Ferenci T. Effect of slow growth on metabolism of *Escherichia coli*, as revealed by global metabolite pool ('metabolome') analysis. *J Bacteriol* 1988;180:5109–5116.
22. Nicholson JK, Lindon JC, Holmes E. 'Metabonomics': understanding the metabolic responses of living systems to pathophysiologic stimuli via multivariate analysis of biological NMR data. *Xenobiotica* 1999;29:1181–1189.
23. Clayton TA, Lindon JC, Clorec O, et al. Pharmaco-metabonomic phenotyping and personalized drug treatment. *Nature* 2006;440:1073–1077.
24. Agrafiotis DK, Lobanov VS, Salemme FR. Combinatorial informatics in the post-genomics era. *Nat Rev Drug Discov* 2002;1:337–346.
25. Yang K, Han X. Lipidomics: techniques, applications, and outcomes related to biomedical sciences. *Trends Biochem Sci* 2016;41:954–969.
26. Daly MJ, Rioux JD, Schaffner SF, et al. High-resolution haplotype structure in the human genome. *Nat Genet* 2001;2:229–232.
27. Beckmann JS, Estivill X, Antonarakis SE. Copy number variants and genetic traits: closer to the resolution of phenotypic to genotypic variability. *Nat Rev Genet* 2007;8:639–646.
28. Frazer KA, Murray SS, Schork NJ, et al. Human genetic variation and its contribution to complex traits. *Nat Rev Genet* 2009;10:241–251.
29. Meyer UA. Genotype or phenotype: the definition of a pharmacogenetic polymorphism. *Pharmacogenetics* 1991;1:66–67.
30. Leeder JS. Pharmacogenetics and pharmacogenomics. *Pediatr Clin North Am* 2001;48:756–781.
31. Hines RN, McCarver DG. The ontogeny of human drug-metabolizing enzymes: phase I oxidative enzymes. *J Pharmacol Exp Ther* 2002;300:355–360.
32. McCarver DG, Hines RN. The ontogeny of human drug metabolizing enzymes: phase II conjugation enzymes and regulatory mechanisms. *J Pharmacol Exp Ther* 2002;300:361–366.
33. Nuwaysir EF, Bittner M, Trent J, et al. Microarrays and toxicology: the advent of toxicogenomics. *Mol Carcinog* 1999;24:153–159.
34. Kennedy S. The role of proteomics in toxicology: identification of biomarkers of toxicity by protein expression analysis. *Biomarkers* 2002;7:269–290.
35. Klein TE, Chang JT, Cho MK, et al. Integrating genotype and phenotype information: an overview of the PharmGKB project. *Pharmacogenomics J.* 2001;1:167–170.
36. Collins MD, Mao GE. Teratology of retinoids. *Annu Rev Pharmacol Toxicol.* 1999;39:399–430.
37. Nulman I, Rovet J, Stewart DE, et al. Child development following exposure to tricyclic depressants or fluoxetine throughout fetal life: a prospective, controlled study. *Am J Psychiatry* 2002;159:1889–1895.
38. Watkins PB. Role of cytochromes P450 in drug metabolism and hepatotoxicity. *Semin Liver Dis* 1990;10:235–250.
39. Streetman DS, Bertino JS, Nafziger AN. Phenotyping of drug-metabolizing enzymes in adults: a review of in-vivo cytochrome P450 phenotyping probes. *Pharmacogenetics* 2000;10:187–216.
40. Evans WE, Relling MV, Petros WP, et al. Dextromethorphan and caffeine as probes for simultaneous determination of debrisoquin-oxidation and N-acetylation phenotypes in children. *Clin Pharmacol Ther* 1989;45:568–573.
41. Pariente-Khayat A, Pons G, Rey E, et al. Caffeine acetylator phenotyping during maturation in infants. *Pediatr Res* 1991;29:492–495.
42. Relling MV, Cherrie J, Schell MJ, et al. Lower prevalence of the debrisoquin oxidative poor metabolizer phenotype in American black versus white subjects. *Clin Pharmacol Ther* 1991;50:308–313.
43. Bosso JA, Liu Q, Evans WE, et al. CYP2D6, N-acetylation, and xanthine oxidase activity in cystic fibrosis. *Pharmacotherapy* 1996;16:749–753.
44. Skoda RC, Gonzalez FJ, Demierre A, et al. Two mutant alleles of the human cytochrome P450dbl gene associated with genetically deficient metabolism of debrisoquine and other drugs. *Proc Natl Acad Sci U S A.* 1988;85:5240–5243.
45. Heim MH, Meyer UA. Genetic polymorphism of debrisoquine oxidation: restriction fragment analysis and allele-specific amplification of mutant alleles of CYP2D6. *Methods Enzymol* 1991;206:173–183.
46. Gaedigk A, Bradford LD, Marcucci KA, et al. Unique CYP2D6 activity distribution and genotype-phenotype discordance in black Americans. *Clin Pharmacol Ther* 2002;72:76–89.
47. Burgner D, Davila S, Breunis WB, et al. A genome-wide association study identifies novel and functionally related susceptibility loci for Kawasaki disease. *PLoS Genet* 2009;5:e1000319.
48. Moffatt MF, Kabesch M, Liang L, et al. Genetic variants regulating ORMDL3 expression contribute to the risk of childhood asthma. *Nature* 2007;448:470–473.
49. Kugathasan S, Baldassano RN, Bradfield JP, et al. Loci on 20q13 and 21q22 are associated with pediatric-onset inflammatory bowel disease. *Nat Genet* 2008;40:1211–1215.
50. Takeuchi F, McGinnis R, Bourgeois S, et al. A genome-wide association study confirms VKORC1, CYP2C9, and CYP4F2 as principal genetic determinants of warfarin dose. *PLoS Genet* 2009;5(3):e1000433.
51. Shuldiner AR, O'Connell JR, Bliden KP, et al. Association of cytochrome P450 2C19 genotype with the antiplatelet effect and clinical efficacy of clopidogrel therapy. *JAMA* 2009;302:849–857.
52. Search Collaborative Group. SLCO1B1 variants and statin-induced myopathy—a genomewide study. *N Engl J Med* 2008;359:789–799.
53. Marguerat S, Wilhelm BT, Bähler J. Next-generation sequencing: applications beyond genomes. *Biochem Soc Trans* 2008;36:1091–1096.
54. Twist GP, Gaedigk A, Miller NA, et al. Constellation: a tool for rapid, automated phenotype assignment of a highly polymorphic pharmacogene, CYP2D6, from whole genome sequences. *NPJ Genom Med* 2016;1:15007.
55. U.S. Food and Drug Administration, ed. *FDA authorizes first direct-to-consumer test for detecting genetic variants that may be associated with medication metabolism.* https://www.fda.gov/news-events/press-announcements/fda-authorizes-first-direct-consumer-test-detecting-genetic-variants-may-be-associated-medication
56. Iwamoto N, Shimada T. Recent advances in mass spectrometry-based approaches for proteomics and biologics: great contribution for developing therapeutic antibodies. *Pharmacol Therapeut* 2018;185:147–154.
57. Aebersold R, Burlingame AL, Bradshaw RA. Western blots versus selected reaction monitoring assays: time to turn the tables? *Mol Cell Proteomics* 2013;12:2381–2382.
58. Prasad B, Achour B, Artursson P, et al. Toward a consensus on applying quantitative liquid chromatography-tandem mass spectrometry proteomics in translational pharmacology research: a white paper. *Clin Pharmacol Ther* 2019;106:525–543.
59. Heimbach T, Lin W, Hourcade-Potelleret F, et al. Physiologically based pharmacokinetic modeling to supplement nilotinib pharmacokinetics and confirm dose selection in pediatric patients. *J Pharm Sci* 2019;108:2191–2198.
60. Jorga K, Chavanne C, Frey N, et al. Bottom-up meets top-down: complementary physiologically based pharmacokinetic and population pharmacokinetic modeling for regulatory approval of a dosing algorithm of Valganciclovir in very young children. *Clin Pharmacol Ther* 2016;100:761–769.
61. Johnson TN, Rostami-Hodjegan A. Resurgence in the use of physiologically based pharmacokinetic models in pediatric clinical pharmacology: parallel shift in incorporating the knowledge of biological elements and increased applicability to drug development and practice. *Pediatr Anesth* 2011;21:291–301.
62. Rowland A, Ruanglertboon W, van Dyk M, et al. Plasma extracellular nanovesicle (exosome)-derived biomarkers for drug metabolism pathways: a novel approach to characterize variability in drug exposure. *Br J Clin Pharmacol* 2019;85:216–226.
63. Li CY, Hosey-Cojocari C, Basit A, et al. Optimized renal transporter quantification by using aquaporin 1 and aquaporin 2 as anatomical markers: application in characterizing the ontogeny of renal transporters and its correlation with hepatic transporters in paired human samples. *AAPS J* 2019;21:88.
64. Kaddurah-Douk R, Kristal BS, Weinshilboum RM. Metabolomics: a global biochemical approach to drug response and disease. *Annu Rev Pharmacol Toxicol* 2008;48:653–683.
65. Tay-Sontheimer JC, Shireman L, Beyer RP, et al. Discovery of an endogenous urinary biomarker of CYP2D6 activity. *Pharmacogenomics* 2014;15:1947–1962.
66. Geiger C, Geistlinger L, Altmaier E, et al. Genetics meets metabolomics: a genome-wide association study of metabolite profiles in human serum. *PLoS Genet* 2008;4(11):E1000282.
67. Xu EY, Perlina A, Vu H, et al. Integrated pathway analysis of rat urine metabolic profiles and kidney transcriptomic profiles to elucidate the systems toxicology of model nephrotoxicants. *Chem Res Toxicol* 2008;21:1548–1561.
68. Bhattacharyya S, Ahmed AT, Arnold M, et al. Metabolomic signature of exposure and response to citalopram/escitalopram in depressed outpatients. *Transl Psychiatry* 2019;9:173.
69. Kaddurah-Daouk R, Boyle SH, Matson W, et al. Pretreatment metabotype as a predictor of response to sertraline or placebo in depressed outpatients: a proof of concept. *Transl Pscychiatry* 2011;1:e26.
70. Hines RN. The ontogeny of drug metabolism enzymes and implications for adverse drug events. *Pharmacol Ther* 2008;118:250–267.
71. Zanger UM, Turpeinen M, Klein K, et al. Functional pharmacogenetics/genomics of human cytochromes P450 involved in drug biotransformation. *Anal Bioanal Chem* 2008;392:1093–1108.
72. Zanger UM, Klein K, Saussele T, et al. Polymorphic CYP2B6: molecular mechanisms and emerging clinical significance. *Pharmacogenomics* 2007;8:743–759.
73. Daly AK, Rettie AE, Fowler DM, et al. Pharmacogenomics of CYP2C9: Functional and clinical considerations. *J Pers Med* 2017;8:1.
74. Furuta T, Sugimoto M, Shirai N, et al. CYP2C19 pharmacogenomics associated with therapy of *Helicobacter pylori* infection and gastro-esophageal reflux diseases with a proton pump inhibitor. *Pharmacogenomics* 2007;8:1199–1210.
75. Zanger UM, Raimundo S, Eichelbaum M. Cytochrome P450 2D6: overview and update on pharmacology, genetics and biochemistry. *Naunyn-Schmiedebergs Arch Pharmacol* 2004;369:23–37.
76. Sistonen J, Sajantila A, Lao O, et al. CYP2D6 worldwide genetic variation shows high frequency of altered activity variants and no continental structure. *Pharmacogenet Genomics* 2007;17:93–101.
77. Nofziger C, Turner AJ, Sangkuhl K, et al. PharmVar genereview: CYP2D6. *Clin Pharmacol Ther* 2019. doi:10.1002/cpt.1643.
78. Lee S-J, Goldstein JA. Functionally defective or altered CYP3A4 and CYP3A5 single nucleotide polymorphisms and their detection with genotyping tests. *Pharmacogenomics* 2005;6:357–371.
79. Guillemette C. Pharmacogenomics of human UDP-glucuronosyltransferase enzymes. *Pharmacogenomics J* 2003;3:136–158.
80. Nagar S, Blanchard RL. Pharmacogenetics of uridine diphosphoglucuronsyltransferase (UGT) 1A family members and its role in patient response to irinotecan. *Drug Metab Rev* 2006;38:393–409.
81. Hildebrandt MA, Carrington DP, Thomae BA, et al. Genetic diversity and function in the human cytosolic sulfotransferases. *Pharmacogenomics J* 2007;7:133–143.
82. Sim E, Lack N, Wang CJ, et al. Arylamine N-acetyltransferases: structural and functional implications of polymorphisms. *Toxicology* 2008;254:170–183.
83. Wang L, Weinshilboum R. Thiopurine S-methyltransferase pharmacogenetics: insights, challenges and future directions. *Oncogene* 2006;25:1629–1638.
84. Kutt H, Wolk M, Scherman R, et al. Insufficient parahydroxylation as a cause of diphenylhydantoin toxicity. *Neurology (NY)* 1964;14:542–548.
85. Kidd RS, Curry TB, Gallagher S, et al. Identification of a null allele of CYP2C9 in an African-American exhibiting toxicity to phenytoin. *Pharmacogenetics* 2001;11:803–808.
86. Steward DJ, Haining RL, Henne KR, et al. Genetic association between sensitivity to warfarin and expression of CYP2C9*3. *Pharmacogenetics* 1997;7:361–367.

87. Sullivan-Klose TH, Ghanayem BI, Bell DA, et al. The role of the CYP2C9-Leu[359] allelic variant in the tolbutamide polymorphism. *Pharmacogenetics* 1996;6:341–349.
88. Bhasker CR, Miners JO, Coulter S, et al. Allelic and functional variability of cytochrome P4502C9. *Pharmacogenetics* 1997;7:51–58.
89. Rettie AE, Wienkers LC, Gonzalez FJ, et al. Impaired (S)-warfarin metabolism catalysed by the R144C allelic variant of CYP2C9. *Pharmacogenetics* 1994;4:39–42.
90. Haining RL, Hunter AP, Veronese ME, et al. Allelic variants of human cytochrome P4502C9: baculovirus-mediated expression, purification, structural characterization, substrate stereospecificity and prochiral selectivity of the wild-type and I359L mutant forms. *Arch Biochem Biophys* 1996;333:447–458.
91. Dickman LJ, Rettie AE, Kneller MB, et al. Identification and functional characterization of a new CYP2C9 variant (CYP2C9*5) expressed among African Americans. *Mol Pharmacol* 2001;60:382–387.
92. Blaisdell J, Jorge-Nebert LF, Coulter S, et al. Discovery of new potentially defective alleles of human CYP2C9. *Pharmacogenetics* 2004;14:527–537.
93. Dorado P, Lopez-Torres E, Penas-Lledo EM, et al. Neurological toxicity after phenytoin infusion in a pediatric patient with epilepsy: influence of CYP2C9, CYP2C19 and ABCB1 genetic polymorphisms. *Pharmacogenomics J* 2013;13:359–361.
94. Silvado CE, Terra VC, Twardowschy CA. CYP2C9 polymorphisms in epilepsy: influence on phenytoin treatment. *Pharmacogenomics Pers Med* 2018;11:51–58.
95. Goldstein JA. Clinical relevance of genetic polymorphisms in the human CYP2C subfamily. *Br J Clin Pharmacol* 2001;52:349–355.
96. Furuta T, Shirai N, Takashima M, et al. Effect of genotypic differences in CYP2C19 on cure rates for *Helicobacter pylori* infection by triple therapy with a proton pump inhibitor, amoxicillin, and clarithromycin. *Clin Pharmacol Ther* 2001;69:158–168.
97. Sim SC, Risinger C, Dahl ML, et al. A common novel CYP2C19 gene variant causes ultrarapid drug metabolism relevant for the drug response to proton pump inhibitors and antidepressants. *Clin Pharmacol Ther* 2006;79:103–113.
98. Rudberg I, Mohebi B, Hermann M, et al. Impact of the ultrarapid CYP2C19*17 allele on serum concentration of escitalopram in psychiatric patients. *Clin Pharmacol Ther* 2008;83(2):322–327.
99. Moriyama B, Obeng AO, Barbarino J, et al. Clinical pharmacogenetics implementation consortium (CPIC) guidelines for CYP2C19 and voriconazole therapy. *Clin Pharmacol Ther* 2017;102:45–51.
100. Aldrich SL, Poweleit EA, Prows CA, et al. Influence of CYP2C19 metabolizer status on escitalopram/citalopram tolerability and response in youth with anxiety and depressive disorders. *Front Pharmacol* 2019;10:99.
101. Strawn JR, Poweleit EA, Ramsey LB. CYP2C19-guided escitalopram and sertraline dosing in pediatric patients: a pharmacokinetic modeling study. *J Child Adolesc Psychopharmacol* 2019;29:340–347.
102. Hicks JK, Bishop JR, Sangkuhl K, et al. Clinical pharmacogenetics implementation consortium (CPIC) guideline for CYP2D6 and CYP2C19 genotypes and dosing of selective serotonin reuptake inhibitors. *Clin Pharmacol Ther* 2015;98:127–134.
103. Gaedigk A, Gotschall RR, Forbes NS, et al. Optimization of cytochrome P450 2D6 (CYP2D6) phenotype assignment using a genotyping algorithm based on allele frequency data. *Pharmacogenetics* 1999;9:669–682.
104. Gaedigk A, Sangkuhl K, Whirl-Carrillo M, et al. Prediction of CYP2D6 phenotype from genotype across world populations. *Genet Med* 2017;19:69–76.
105. Koren G, Cairns J, Chitayat D, et al. Pharmacogenetics of morphine poisoning in a breastfed neonate of a codeine-prescribed mother. *Lancet* 2007;368:704–705.
106. Treluyer J-M, Jacqz-Aigrain E, Alvarez F, et al. Expression of CYP2D6 in developing human liver. *Eur J Biochem* 1991;202:583–588.
107. Stevens JC, Marsh SA, Zaya MJ, et al. Developmental changes in human liver CYP2D6 expression. *Drug Metab Disp* 2008;36:1587–1593.
108. Blake MJ, Gaedigk A, Pearce RE, et al. Ontogeny of dextromethorphan O and N-demethylation in the first year of life. *Clin Pharmacol Ther* 2007;81:510–516.
109. Sallee FR, DeVane CL, Ferrell RE. Fluoxetine-related death in a child with cytochrome P-450 2D6 genetic deficiency. *J Child Adol Psychopharmacol* 2000;10:27–34.
110. Sindrup SH, Brøsen K. The pharmacogenetics of codeine hypoalgesia. *Pharmacogenetics* 1995;5:335–346.
111. Poulsen L, Arendt-Nielsen L, Brøsen K, et al. The hypoalagesic effect of tramadol in relation to CYP2D6. *Clin Pharmacol Ther* 1996;60:636–644.
112. Quiding H, Olsson GL, Boreus LO, et al. Infants and young children metabolise codeine to morphine. A study after single and repeated rectal administration. *Br J Clin Pharmacol* 1992;33:45–49.
113. Quiding H, Anderson P, Bondesson U, et al. Plasma concentrations of codeine and its metabolite, morphine, after single and repeated oral administration. *Eur J Clin Pharmacol* 1986;30:673–677.
114. Williams DG, Patel A, Howard RF. Pharmacogenetics of codeine metabolism in an urban population of children and its implications for analgesic reliability. *Br J Anaesth* 2002;89:839–845.
115. Crews KR, Gaedigk A, Dunnenberger HM, et al.; Clinical Pharmacogenetics Implementation Consortium. Clinical pharmacogenetics implementation consortium guidelines for cytochrome P450 2D6 genotype and codeine therapy: 2014 update. *Clin Pharmacol Ther* 2014;95:376–382.
116. de Leon J. Translating pharmacogenetics to clinical practice: do cytochrome P450 2D6 ultrarapid metabolizers need higher atomoxetine doses? *J Am Acad Child Adolesc Psychiatry* 2015;54:532–534.
117. Brown JT, Bishop JR, Sangkuhl K, et al. Clinical pharmacogenetics implementation consortium (CPIC) guideline for CYP2D6 genotype and atomoxetine therapy. *Clin Pharmacol Ther* 2019;106:94–102.
118. Gaedigk A, Dinh JC, Jeong H-Y, et al. Ten years' experience with the CYP2D6 activity score: a perspective on future investigations to improve clinical predictions for precision therapeutics. *J Pers Med* 2018;8:15.
119. Gaedigk A, Simon SD, Pearce RE, et al. The CYP2D6 activity score: translating genotype information into a qualitative measure of phenotype. *Clin Pharmacol Ther* 2008;83:234–242.
120. Dalton R, Lee SB, Claw KG, et al. Interrogation of CYP2D6 structural variant alleles improves the correlation between CYP2D6 genotype and CYP2D6-mediated metabolic activity. *Clin Transl Sci* 2019.doi:10.1111/cts.12695.
121. Wrighton SA, VandenBranden M. Isolation and characterization of human fetal liver cytochrome P450HLp2: a third member of the P450III gene family. *Arch Biochem Biophys* 1989;268:144–151.
122. Yang H-Y, Lee QP, Rettie AR, et al. Functional cytochrome P4503A isoforms in human embryonic tissues: expression during organogenesis. *Mol Pharmacol* 1994;46:922–928.
123. Lacroix D, Sonnier M, Moncion A, et al. Expression of CYP3A in the human liver. Evidence that the shift between CYP3A7 and CYP3A4 occurs immediately after birth. *Eur J Biochem* 1997;247:625–634.
124. Stevens JC, Hines RN, Gu C, et al. Developmental expression of the major human hepatic CYP3A enzymes. *J Pharmacol Exp Ther* 2003;307:573–582.
125. Thummel KE, O'Shea D, Paine MF, et al. Oral first-pass elimination of midazolam involves both gastrointestinal and hepatic CYP3A-mediated metabolism. *Clin Pharmacol Ther* 1996;59:491–502.
126. Paine MF, Shen DD, Kunze KL, et al. First-pass metabolism of midazolam by the human intestine. *Clin Pharmacol Ther* 1996;60:14–24.
127. Gertz M, Harrison A, Houston JB, et al. Prediction of human intestinal first-pass metabolism of 25 CYP3A substrates from in vitro clearance and permeability data. *Drug Metab Dispos* 2010;38:1147–1158.
128. Johnson TN, Tanner MS, Taylor CJ, et al. Enterocytic CYP3A4 in a paediatric population: developmental changes and the effect of coeliac disease and cystic fibrosis. *Br J Clin Pharmacol* 2001;51:451–460.
129. Wang D, Guo Y, Wrighton SA, et al. Intronic polymorphism in CYP3A4 affects hepatic expression and response to statin drugs. *Pharmacogenomics J* 2011;11:274–286.
130. Okubo M, Murayama N, Shimizu M, et al. CYP3A4 intron 6 C>T polymorphism (CYP3A4*22) is associated with reduced CYP3A4 protein level and function in human liver microsomes. *J Toxicol Sci* 2013;38:349–354.
131. Elens L, Nieuweboer A, Clarke SJ, et al. CYP3A4 intron 6 C>T SNP (CYP3A4*22) encodes lower CYP3A4 activity in cancer patients, as measured with probes midazolam and erythromycin. *Pharmacogenomics* 2013;14:137–149.
132. Elens L, Bouamar R, Hesselink DA, et al. A new functional CYP3A4 intron 6 polymorphism significantly affects tacrolimus pharmacokinetics in kidney transplant recipients. *Clin Chem* 2011;57:1574–1583.
133. Birdwell KA, Decker B, Barbarino JM, et al. Clinical pharmacogenetics implementation consortium (CPIC) guidelines for CYP3A5 genotype and tacrolimus dosing. *Clin Pharmacol Ther* 2015;98:19–24.
134. Brunet M, van Gelder T, Asberg A, et al. Therapeutic drug monitoring of tacrolimus-personalized therapy: second consensus report. *Ther Drug Monit* 2019;41:261–307.
135. Rebbeck TR, Jaffe JM, Walker AH, et al. Modification of clinical presentation of prostate tumors by a novel genetic variant in CYP3A4. *J Natl Cancer Inst* 1998;90:1225–1229.
136. Felix CA, Walker AH, Lange BJ, et al. Association of CYP3A4 genotype with treatment-related leukemia. *Proc Natl Acad Sci U S A* 1998;95:13176–13181.
137. Ball SE, Scatina J, Kao J, et al. Population distribution and effects on drug metabolism of a genetic variant in the 5′ promoter region of CYP3A4. *Clin Pharmacol Ther* 1999;66:288–294.
138. Westlind A, Löfberg L, Tindberg N, et al. Interindividual differences in hepatic expression of CYP3A4: relationship to genetic polymorphism in the 5′-upstream regulatory region. *Biochem Biophys Res Commun* 1999;259:201–205.
139. Wandel C, Witte JS, Hall JM, et al. CYP3A activity in African American and European American men: population differences and functional effect of the CYP3A4*1B 5′-promoter region polymorphism. *Clin Pharmacol Ther* 2000;68:82–91.
140. Amirimani B, Weber BL, Rebbeck TR. Regulation of reporter gene expression by a CYP3A4 promoter variant in primary human hepatocytes. *Proc Am Assoc Cancer Res* 2000;60:114.
141. Lai J, Vesprini D, Chu W, et al. CYP gene polymorphisms and early menarche. *Mol Genet Metab* 2001;74:449–457.
142. Kadlubar FF, Berkowitz GS, Delongchamp RR, et al. The CYP3A4*1B variant is related to the onset of puberty, a known risk factor for the development of breast cancer. *Cancer Epidemiol Biomarkers Prev* 2003;12:327–331.
143. Wrighton SA, Ring BJ, Watkins PB, et al. Identification of a polymorphically expressed member of the human cytochrome P-450III family. *Mol Pharmacol* 1989;36:97–105.
144. Kuehl P, Zhang J, Lin Y, et al. Sequence diversity in CYP3A promoters and characterization of the genetic basis of polymorphic CYP3A5 expression. *Nat Genet* 2001;27:383–391.
145. Shuster DL, Risler LJ, Prasad B, et al. Identification of CYP3A7 for glyburide metabolism in human fetal livers. *Biochem Pharmacol* 2014;92:690–700.
146. Rodríguez-Antona C, Jande M, et al. Identification and phenotype characterization of two CYP3A haplotypes causing different enzymatic capacity in fetal livers. *Clin Pharmacol Ther* 2005;77:259–270.
147. Leeder JS, Gaedigk R, Marcucci KA, et al. Variability of CYP3A7 in human fetal liver. *J Pharmacol Exp Ther* 2005;314:626–635.
148. Schirmer M, Rosenberger A, Klein K, et al. Sex-dependent genetic markers of CYP3A4 expression and activity in human liver microsomes. *Pharmacogenomics* 2007;8:443–453.
149. Bhatt DK, Mehrotra A, Gaedigk A, et al. Age and genotype-dependent variability in the protein abundance and activity of six major uridine diphosphate-glucuronosyltransferases in human liver. *Clin Pharmacol Ther* 2019;105:131–141.
150. Bock KW. Roles of human UDP-gluronosyltransferases in clearance and homeostasis of endogenous substrates, and functional implications. *Biochem Pharmacol* 2015;96:77–82.
151. Stingl JC, Bartels H, Viviani R, et al. Relevance of UDP-glucuronosyltransferase polymorphisms for drug dosing: a quantitative systematic review. *Pharmacol Ther* 2014;141:92–116.
152. Monaghan G, McLellan A, McGeehan A, et al. Gilbert's syndrome is a contributory factor in prolonged unconjugated hyperbilirubinemia of the newborn. *J Pediatr* 1999;134:441–446.
153. Kadakol A, Sappal BS, Ghosh SS, et al. Interaction of coding region mutations and the Gilbert-type promoter abnormality of the UGT1A1 gene causes moderate degrees of unconjugated hyperbilirubinaemia and may lead to neonatal kernicterus. *J Med Genet* 2001;38:244–249.

154. Gagne JF, Montminy V, Belanger P, et al. Common human UGT1A polymorphisms and the altered metabolism of irinotecan active metabolite 7-ethyl-10-hydroxycamptothecin (SN-38). *Mol Pharmacol* 2002;62:608–617.
155. Iyer L, Das S, Janisch L, et al. UGT1A1*28 polymorphism as a determinant of irinotecan disposition and toxicity. *Pharmacogenomics J* 2002;2:43–47.
156. Dean L. Irinotecan therapy and UGT1A1 genotype. In: Pratt V, McLeod H, Rubinstein W, et al., eds. *Medical genetics summaries*. Bethesda, MD: National Center for Biotechnology Information (US), 2012.
157. Culley CL, Kiang TK, Gilchrist SE, et al. Effect of the UGT1A1*28 allele on unconjugated hyperbilirubinemia in HIV-positive patients receiving Atazanavir: a systematic review. *Ann Pharmacother* 2013;47:561–572.
158. Gammal RS, Court MH, Haidar CE, et al. Clinical pharmacogenetics implementation consortium (CPIC) guideline for UGT1A1 and atazanavir prescribing. *Clin Pharmacol Ther* 2016;99:363–369.
159. Troberg J, Finel M. The polymorphic variant P24T of UDP-glucuronosyltransferase 1A4 and its unusual consequences. *Drug Metab Dispos* 2015;43:1769–1772.
160. Haslemo T, Loryan I, Ueda N, et al. UGT1A4*3 encodes significantly increased glucuronidation of olanzapine in patients on maintenance treatment and in recombinant systems. *Clin Pharmacol Ther* 2012;92:221–227.
161. Wang Z, Wong T, Hashizume T, et al. Human UGT1A4 and UGT1A3 conjugate 25-hydroxyvitamin D3: metabolite structure, kinetics, inducibility, and interindividual variability. *Endocrinology* 2014;155:2052–2063.
162. Liu L, Zhao L, Wang Q, et al. Influence of valproic acid concentration and polymorphism of UGT1A4*3, UGT2B7-161C> T and UGT2B7*2 on serum concentration of lamotrigine in Chinese epileptic children. *Eur J Clin Pharmacol* 2015;71:1341–1347.
163. Linakis MW, Cook SF, Kumar SS, et al. Polymorphic expression of UGT1A9 is associated with variable acetaminophen glucuronidation in neonates: a population pharmacokinetic and pharmacogenetic study. *Clin Pharmacokinet* 2018;57:1325–1336.
164. Bhatt DK, Basit A, Zhang H, et al. Hepatic abundance and activity of androgen-and drug-metabolizing enzyme UGT2B17 are associated with genotype, age, and sex. *Drug Metab Dispos* 2018;46:888–896.
165. May G. Genetic differences in drug disposition. *J Clin Pharmacol* 1994;34:881–897.
166. Meyer UA. Genetic polymorphisms of drug metabolism. *Fund Clin Pharmacol* 1990;4:595–615.
167. Hadasova E, Brysova V, Kadlcakova E. N-Acetylation in healthy and diseased children. *Eur J Clin Pharmacol* 1990;39:43–47.
168. Pariente-Khayat A, Rey E, Gendrel D, et al. Isoniazid acetylation metabolic ratio during maturation in children. *Clin Pharmacol Ther* 1997;62:377–383.
169. McLeod HL, Krynetski EY, Wilimas JA, et al. Higher activity of polymorphic thiopurine S-methyltransferase in erythrocytes from neonates compared to adults. *Pharmacogenetics* 1995;5:281–286.
170. Park-Hah JO, Klemetsdal B, Lysaa R, et al. Thiopurine methyltransferase activity in a Korean population sample of children. *Clin Pharmacol Ther* 1996;60:68–74.
171. Ganiere-Monteil C, Medard Y, Lejus C, et al. Phenotype and genotype for thiopurine methyltransferase activity in the French Caucasian population: impact of age. *Eur J Clin Pharmacol* 2004;60:89–96.
172. Relling MV, Schwab M, Whirl-Carrillo M, et al. Clinical pharmacogenetics implementation consortium guideline for thiopurine dosing based on TPMT and NUDT15 genotypes: 2018 update. *Clin Pharmacol Ther* 2019;105:1095–1105.
173. Tai HL, Krynetski EY, Schuetz EG, et al. Enhanced proteolysis of thiopurine S-methyltransferase (TPMT) encoded by mutant alleles in humans (TPMT*3A, TPMT*2): mechanisms for the genetic polymorphism of TPMT activity. *Proc Natl Acad Sci U S A* 1997;94:6444–6449.
174. Tai HL, Fessing MY, Bonten EJ, et al. Enhanced proteasomal degradation of mutant human thiopurine S-methyltransferase (TPMT) in mammalian cells: mechanism for TPMT protein deficiency inherited by TPMT*2, TPMT*3A, TPMT*3B or TPMT*3C. *Pharmacogenetics* 1999;9:641–650.
175. Spire-Vayron de la Moureyre C, Debuysère H, Sabbagh N, et al. Detection of known and new mutations in the thiopurine S-methyltransferase gene by single-strand conformation polymorphism analysis. *Hum Mutat.* 1998;12:177–185.
176. Yan L, Zhang S, Eiff B, et al. Thiopurine methyltransferase polymorphic tandem repeat: genotype-phenotype correlation analysis. *Clin Pharmacol Ther* 2000;68:210–219.
177. Spire-Vayron de la Moureyre C, Debuysère H, Fazio F, et al. Characterization of a variable number tandem repeat region in the thiopurine S-methyltransferase gene promoter. *Pharmacogenetics* 1999;9:189–198.
178. Zukic B, Radmilovic M, Stojiljkovic M, et al. Functional analysis of the role of the TPMT gene promoter VNTR polymorphism in TPMT gene transcription. *Pharmacogenomics* 2010;11:547–557.
179. Alves S, Amorim A, Ferreira F, et al. Influence of the variable number of tandem repeats located in the promoter region of the thiopurine methyltransferase gene on enzymatic activity. *Clin Pharmacol Ther* 2001;70:165–174.
180. Kotur N, Dokmanovic L, Janic D, et al. TPMT gene expression is increased during maintenance therapy in childhood acute lymphoblastic leukemia patients in a TPMT gene promoter variable number of tandem repeat-dependent manner. *Pharmacogenomics* 2015;16:1701–1712.
181. Ross CJ, Katzov-Eckert H, Dube MP, et al. Genetic variants in TPMT and COMT are associated with hearing loss in children receiving cisplatin chemotherapy. *Nat Genet* 2009;41:1345–1349.
182. Pussegoda K, Ross CJ, Visscher H, et al. Replication of TPMT and ABCC3 genetic variants highly associated with cisplatin-induced hearing loss in children. *Clin Pharmacol Ther* 2013;94:243–251.
183. Thiesen S, Yin P, Jorgensen AL, et al. TPMT, COMT and ACYP2 genetic variants in paediatric cancer patients with cisplatin-induced ototoxicity. *Pharmacogenet Genomics* 2017;27:213–222.
184. Ratain MJ, Cox NJ, Henderson TO. Challenges in interpreting the evidence for genetic predictors of ototoxicity. *Clin Pharmacol Ther* 2013;94:631–635.
185. Carleton BC, Ross CJ, Pussegoda K, et al. Genetic markers of cisplatin-induced hearing loss in children. *Clin Pharmacol Ther* 2014;96:296–298.
186. Wang D, Zou L, Jin Q, et al. Human carboxylesterases: a comprehensive review. *Acta Pharm Sin B* 2018;8:699–712.
187. Boberg M, Vrana M, Mehrotra A, et al. Age-dependent absolute abundance of hepatic carboxylesterases (CES1 and CES2) by LC-MS/MS proteomics: application to PBPK modeling of oseltamivir in vivo pharmacokinetics in infants. *Drug Metab Dispos* 2017;45:216–223.
188. Hines RN, Simpson PM. Age-dependent human hepatic carboxylesterase 1 (CES1) and carboxylesterase 2 (CES2) postnatal ontogeny. *Drug Metab Dispos* 2016;44:959–966.
189. Nemoda Z, Angyal N, Tarnok Z, et al. Carboxylesterase 1 gene polymorphism and methylphenidate response in ADHD. *Neuropharmacology* 2009;57:731–733.
190. Lewis JP, Horenstein RB, Ryan K, et al. The functional G143E variant of carboxylesterase 1 is associated with increased clopidogrel active metabolite levels and greater clopidogrel response. *Pharmacogenet Genomics* 2013;23:1–8.
191. Zhu HJ, Patrick KS, Yuan HJ, et al. Two CES1 gene mutations lead to dysfunctional carboxylesterase 1 activity in man: clinical significance and molecular basis. *Am J Hum Genet* 2008;82:1241–1248.
192. Oh J, Lee S, Lee H, et al. The novel carboxylesterase 1 variant c.662A>G may decrease the bioactivation of oseltamivir in humans. *PLoS One* 2017;12:e0176320.
193. Shi J, Wang X, Eyler RF, et al. Association of oseltamivir activation with gender and carboxylesterase 1 genetic polymorphisms. *Basic Clin Pharmacol Toxicol* 2016;119:555–561.
194. Clancy JP, Johnson SG, Yee SW, et al. Clinical pharmacogenetics implementation consortium (CPIC) guidelines for ivacaftor therapy in the context of CFTR genotype. *Clin Pharmacol Ther* 2014;95:592–597.
195. Roth M, Obaidat A, Hagenbuch B. OATPs, OATs and OCTs: the organic anion and cation transporters of the SLCO and SLC22A gene superfamilies. *Br J Pharmacol* 2012;165:1260–1287.
196. Drozdzik M, Busch D, Lapczuk J, et al. Protein abundance of clinically relevant drug transporters in the human liver and intestine: a comparative analysis in paired tissue specimens. *Clin Pharmacol Ther* 2019;105:1204–1212.
197. Hagenbuch B, Gui C. Xenobiotic transporters of the human organic anion transporting polypeptides (OATP) family. *Xenobiotica* 2008;38:778–801.
198. Obaidat A, Roth M, Hagenbuch B. The expression and function of organic anion transporting polypeptides in normal tissues and in cancer. *Annu Rev Pharmacol Toxicol* 2012;52:135–151.
199. Prasad B, Gaedigk A, Vrana M, et al. Ontogeny of hepatic transporters as quantified by LC-MS/MS proteomics. *Clin Pharmacol Ther* 2016;100:362–370.
200. de Keyser CE, Peters BJ, Becker ML, et al. The SLCO1B1 c.521T>C polymorphism is associated with dose decrease or switching during statin therapy in the Rotterdam Study. *Pharmacogenet Genomics* 2014;24:43–51.
201. DeGorter MK, Tirona RG, Schwarz UI, et al. Clinical and pharmacogenetic predictors of circulating atorvastatin and rosuvastatin concentrations in routine clinical care. *Circ Cardiovasc Genet* 2013;6:400–408.
202. Lee HK, Hu M, Lui S, et al. Effects of polymorphisms in ABCG2, SLCO1B1, SLC10A1 and CYP2C9/19 on plasma concentrations of rosuvastatin and lipid response in Chinese patients. *Pharmacogenomics* 2013;14:1283–1294.
203. Marciante KD, Durda JP, Heckbert SR, et al. Cerivastatin, genetic variants, and the risk of rhabdomyolysis. *Pharmacogenet Genomics* 2011;21:280–288.
204. Wagner JB, Abdel-Rahman S, van Haandel L, et al. Impact of SLCO1B1 genotype on pediatric simvastatin acid pharmacokinetics. *J Clin Pharmacol* 2018;58:823–833.
205. Gong IY, Kim RB. Impact of genetic variation in OATP transporters to drug disposition and response. *Drug Metabol Pharmacokinet* 2013;28:4–18.
206. Zhang B, Lauschke VM. Genetic variability and population diversity of the human SLCO (OATP) transporter family. *Pharmacol Res* 2019;139:550–559.
207. Nies AT, Niemi M, Burk O, et al. Genetics is a major determinant of expression of the human hepatic uptake transporter OATP1B1, but not of OATP1B3 and OATP2B1. *Genome Med* 2013;5:1.
208. Neuvonen PJ, Backman JT, Niemi M. Pharmacokinetic comparison of the potential over-the-counter statins simvastatin, lovastatin, fluvastatin and pravastatin. *Clin Pharmacokinet* 2008;47:463–474.
209. Niemi M, Pasanen MK, Neuvonen PJ. SLCO1B1 polymorphism and sex affect the pharmacokinetics of pravastatin but not fluvastatin. *Clin Pharmacol Ther* 2006;80:356–366.
210. Pasanen MK, Fredrikson H, Neuvonen PJ, et al. Different effects of SLCO1B1 polymorphism on the pharmacokinetics of atorvastatin and rosuvastatin. *Clin Pharmacol Ther* 2007;82:726–733.
211. Pasanen MK, Neuvonen M, Neuvonen PJ, et al. SLCO1B1 polymorphism markedly affects the pharmacokinetics of simvastatin acid. *Pharmacogenet Genomics* 2006;16:873–879.
212. Ramsey LB, Johnson SG, Caudle KE, et al. The clinical pharmacogenetics implementation consortium guideline for SLCO1B1 and simvastatin-induced myopathy: 2014 update. *Clin Pharmacol Ther* 2014;96:423–428.
213. Wagner J, Abdel-Rahman SM, Gaedigk R, et al. Impact of genetic variation on pravastatin systemic exposure in pediatric hypercholesterolemia. *Clin Pharmacol Ther* 2019;105:1501–1512.
214. Fukuda T, Chidambaran V, Mizuno T, et al. OCT1 genetic variants influence the pharmacokinetics of morphine in children. *Pharmacogenomics* 2013;14:1141–1151.
215. Hahn D, Emoto C. Influence of OCT1 ontogeny and genetic variation on morphine disposition in critically ill neonates: lessons from PBPK modeling and clinical study. *Clin Pharmacol Ther* 2019;105:761–768.
216. Matthaei J, Kuron D, Faltraco F, et al. OCT1 mediates hepatic uptake of sumatriptan and loss-of-function OCT1 polymorphisms affect sumatriptan pharmacokinetics. *Clin Pharmacol Ther* 2016;99:633–641.
217. Tzvetkov MV, Matthaei J, Pojar S, et al. Increased systemic exposure and stronger cardiovascular and metabolic adverse reactions to fenoterol in individuals with heritable OCT1 deficiency. *Clin Pharmacol Ther* 2018;103:868–878.

218. Dawed AY. Variation in the plasma membrane monoamine transporter (PMAT) (encoded by SLC29A4) and organic cation transporter 1 (OCT1) (encoded by SLC22A1) and gastrointestinal intolerance to metformin in type 2 diabetes: an IMI DIRECT study. *Diabetes Care* 2019;42:1027–1033.
219. Chan P, Shao L, Tomlinson B. Metformin transporter pharmacogenomics: insights into drug disposition—where are we now? *Expert Opin Drug Metab Toxicol* 2018;14:1149–1159.
220. Chen Y, Li S, Brown C, et al. Effect of genetic variation in the organic cation transporter 2 on the renal elimination of metformin. *Pharmacogenet Genomics* 2009;19:497–504.
221. Wang ZJ, Yin OQ, Tomlinson B, et al. OCT2 polymorphisms and in-vivo renal functional consequence: studies with metformin and cimetidine. *Pharmacogenet Genomics* 2008;18:637–645.
222. Filipski KK, Mathijssen RH, Mikkelsen TS, et al. Contribution of organic cation transporter 2 (OCT2) to cisplatin-induced nephrotoxicity. *Clin Pharmacol Ther* 2009;86:396–402.
223. Mao Q, Unadkat JD. Role of the breast cancer resistance protein (BCRP/ABCG2) in drug transport—an update. *AAPS J* 2015;17:65–82.
224. de Jong FA, Marsh S, Mathijssen RH, et al. ABCG2 pharmacogenetics: ethnic differences in allele frequency and assessment of influence on irinotecan disposition. *Clin Cancer Res* 2004;10:5889–5894.
225. Keskitalo JE, Zolk O, Fromm MF, et al. ABCG2 polymorphism markedly affects the pharmacokinetics of atorvastatin and rosuvastatin. *Clin Pharmacol Ther* 2009;86:197–203.
226. Wan Z, Wang G, Li T, et al. Marked alteration of rosuvastatin pharmacokinetics in healthy Chinese with ABCG2 34G>A and 421C>A homozygote or compound heterozygote. *J Pharmacol Exp Ther* 2015;354:310–315.
227. Zhang W, Yu BN, He YJ, et al. Role of BCRP 421C>A polymorphism on rosuvastatin pharmacokinetics in healthy Chinese males. *Clin Chim Acta* 2006;373:99–103.
228. Roberts RL, Wallace MC, Phipps-Green AJ, et al. ABCG2 loss-of-function polymorphism predicts poor response to allopurinol in patients with gout. *Pharmacogenomics J* 2017;17:201–203.
229. Wen CC, Yee SW, Liang X, et al. Genome-wide association study identifies ABCG2 (BCRP) as an allopurinol transporter and a determinant of drug response. *Clin Pharmacol Ther* 2015;97:518–525.
230. Yanagisawa R, Katsuyama Y, Shigemura T, et al. Engraftment syndrome, but not acute GVHD, younger age, CYP3A5 or MDR1 polymorphisms, increases tacrolimus clearance in pediatric hematopoietic SCT. *Bone Marrow Transplant* 2011;46:90–97.
231. Liu Y, Yin Y, Sheng Q, et al. Association of ABCC2-24C>T polymorphism with high-dose methotrexate plasma concentrations and toxicities in childhood acute lymphoblastic leukemia. *PLoS One* 2014;9:e82681.
232. Klarica Domjanovic I, Lovric M, Trkulja V, et al. Interaction between ABCG2 421C>A polymorphism and valproate in their effects on steady-state disposition of lamotrigine in adults with epilepsy. *Br J Clin Pharmacol* 2018;84:2106–2119.
233. Shen CH, Zhang YX, Lu RY, et al. Specific OCT1 and ABCG2 polymorphisms are associated with Lamotrigine concentrations in Chinese patients with epilepsy. *Epilepsy Res* 2016;127:186–190.
234. Zhou Y, Wang X, Li H, et al. Polymorphisms of ABCG2, ABCB1 and HNF4alpha are associated with Lamotrigine trough concentrations in epilepsy patients. *Drug Metab Pharmacokinet* 2015;30:282–287.
235. Giacomini KM, Huang SM, Tweedie DJ, et al. Membrane transporters in drug development. *Nat Rev Drug Discov* 2010;9:215–236.
236. Visscher H, Ross CJ, Rassekh SR, et al. Pharmacogenomic prediction of anthracycline-induced cardiotoxicity in children. *J Clin Oncol* 2012;30:1422–1428.
237. Visscher H, Ross CJ, Rassekh SR, et al. Validation of variants in SLC28A3 and UGT1A6 as genetic markers predictive of anthracycline-induced cardiotoxicity in children. *Pediatr Blood Cancer* 2013;60:1375–1381.
238. Nishijima T, Komatsu H, Higasa K, et al. Single nucleotide polymorphisms in ABCC2 associate with tenofovir-induced kidney tubular dysfunction in Japanese patients with HIV-1 infection: a pharmacogenetic study. *Clin Infect Dis* 2012;55:1558–1567.
239. Rodriguez-Novoa S, Labarga P, Soriano V, et al. Predictors of kidney tubular dysfunction in HIV-infected patients treated with tenofovir: a pharmacogenetic study. *Clin Infect Dis* 2009;48:e108–e116.
240. Allegra S, Fatiguso G, Francia S, et al. Pharmacogenetic of voriconazole antifungal agent in pediatric patients. *Pharmacogenomics* 2018;19:913–925.
241. Manautou JE, de Waart DR, Kunne C, et al. Altered disposition of acetaminophen in mice with a disruption of the Mrp3 gene. *Hepatology* 2005;42:1091–1098.
242. Zelcer N, van de Wetering K, Hillebrand M, et al. Mice lacking multidrug resistance protein 3 show altered morphine pharmacokinetics and morphine-6-glucuronide antinociception. *Proc Natl Acad Sci U S A* 2005;102:7274–7279.
243. Lang T, Hitzl M, Burk O, et al. Genetic polymorphisms in the multidrug resistance-associated protein 3 (ABCC3, MRP3) gene and relationship to its mRNA and protein expression in human liver. *Pharmacogenetics* 2004;14:155–164.
244. Venkatasubramanian R, Fukuda T, Niu J, et al. ABCC3 and OCT1 genotypes influence pharmacokinetics of morphine in children. *Pharmacogenomics* 2014;15:1297–1309.
245. Kiser JJ, Aquilante CL, Anderson PL, et al. Clinical and genetic determinants of intracellular tenofovir diphosphate concentrations in HIV-infected patients. *J Acquir Immune Defic Syndr* 2008;47:298–303.
246. Kiser JJ, Carten ML, Aquilante CL, et al. The effect of lopinavir/ritonavir on the renal clearance of tenofovir in HIV-infected patients. *Clin Pharmacol Ther* 2008;83:265–272.
247. Likanonsakul S, Suntisuklappon B, Nitiyanontakij R, et al. A single-nucleotide polymorphism in ABCC4 is associated with tenofovir-related beta2-microglobulinuria in Thai patients with HIV-1 infection. *PLoS One* 2016;11:e0147724.
248. Rungtivasuwan K, Avihingsanon A, Thammajaruk N, et al. Influence of ABCC2 and ABCC4 polymorphisms on tenofovir plasma concentrations in Thai HIV-infected patients. *Antimicrob Agents Chemother* 2015;59:3240–3245.
249. Chen S, Villeneuve L, Jonker D, et al. ABCC5 and ABCG1 polymorphisms predict irinotecan-induced severe toxicity in metastatic colorectal cancer patients. *Pharmacogenet Genomics* 2015;25:573–583.
250. Hodges LM, Markova SM, Chinn LW, et al. Very important pharmacogene summary: ABCB1 (MDR1, P-glycoprotein). *Pharmacogenet Genomics* 2011;21:152–161.
251. van Waterschoot RA, ter Heine R, Wagenaar E, et al. Effects of cytochrome P450 3A (CYP3A) and the drug transporters P-glycoprotein (MDR1/ABCB1) and MRP2 (ABCC2) on the pharmacokinetics of lopinavir. *Br J Pharmacol* 2010;160:1224–1233.
252. Yang TH, Chen YK, Xue F, et al. Influence of CYP3A5 genotypes on tacrolimus dose requirement: age and its pharmacological interaction with ABCB1 genetics in the Chinese paediatric liver transplantation. *Int J Clin Pract Suppl* 2015:53–62.
253. Correia CT, Almeida JP, Santos PE, et al. Pharmacogenetics of risperidone therapy in autism: association analysis of eight candidate genes with drug efficacy and adverse drug reactions. *Pharmacogenomics J* 2010;10:418–430.
254. Shi NJ, Zhang WX, Zhang N, et al. Correlation of MDR1 gene polymorphisms with anesthetic effect of sevoflurane-remifentanil following pediatric tonsillectomy. *Medicine* 2017;96:e7002.
255. Zhang Y, Li Y, Wang H, et al. Correlation of MDR1 gene polymorphism with propofol combined with remifentanil anesthesia in pediatric tonsillectomy. *Oncotarget* 2018;9:20294–20303.
256. Zgheib NK, Akra-Ismail M, Aridi C, et al. Genetic polymorphisms in candidate genes predict increased toxicity with methotrexate therapy in Lebanese children with acute lymphoblastic leukemia. *Pharmacogenet Genomics* 2014;24:387–396.
257. L'Huillier AG, Ing Lorenzini K, Crisinel PA, et al. ABCB1 polymorphisms and neuropsychiatric adverse events in oseltamivir-treated children during influenza H1N1/09 pandemia. *Pharmacogenomics* 2011;12:1493–1501.
258. Small CB, Margolis DA, Shaefer MS, et al. HLA-B*57:01 allele prevalence in HIV-infected North American subjects and the impact of allele testing on the incidence of abacavir-associated hypersensitivity reaction in HLA-B*57:01-negative subjects. *BMC Infect Dis* 2017;17:256.
259. Mallal S, Phillips E, Carosi G, et al. HLA-B*5701 screening for hypersensitivity to abacavir. *N Engl J Med* 2008;358:568–579.
260. Sun D, Yu CH, Liu ZS, et al. Association of HLA-B*1502 and *1511 allele with antiepileptic drug-induced Stevens-Johnson syndrome in central China. *J Huazhong Univ Sci Technolog Med Sci* 2014;34:146-50.
261. Tegretol package insert. U.S. Food and Drug Administration, 2014. https://www.accessdata.fda.gov/drugsatfda_docs/label/2014/016608s103,018281s051,018927s044,020234s035lbl.pdf
262. Trileptal package insert. U.S. Food and Drug Administration, 2017. https://www.accessdata.fda.gov/drugsatfda_docs/label/2017/021014s036lbl.pdf
263. Caudle KE, Rettie AE, Whirl-Carrillo M, et al. Clinical pharmacogenetics implementation consortium guidelines for CYP2C9 and HLA-B genotypes and phenytoin dosing. *Clin Pharmacol Ther* 2014;96:542–548.
264. Phillips EJ, Sukasem C, Whirl-Carrillo M, et al. Clinical pharmacogenetics implementation consortium guideline for HLA genotype and use of carbamazepine and oxcarbazepine: 2017 update. *Clin Pharmacol Ther* 2018;103:574–581.
265. Hershfield MS, Callaghan JT, Tassaneeyakul W, et al. Clinical pharmacogenetics implementation consortium guidelines for human leukocyte antigen-B genotype and allopurinol dosing. *Clin Pharmacol Ther* 2013;93:153–158.
266. Chantarangsu S, Mushiroda T, Mahasirimongkol S, et al. HLA-B*3505 allele is a strong predictor for nevirapine-induced skin adverse drug reactions in HIV-infected Thai patients. *Pharmacogenet Genomics* 2009;19:139–146.
267. Tsuchiya N, Pathipvanich P, Wichukchinda N, et al. Incidence and predictors of regimen-modification from first-line antiretroviral therapy in Thailand: a cohort study. *BMC Infect Dis* 2014;14:565.
268. Chen WT, Wang CW, Lu CW, et al. The function of HLA-B*13:01 involved in the pathomechanism of dapsone-induced severe cutaneous adverse reactions. *J Invest Dermatol* 2018;138:1546–1554.
269. Tempark T, Satapornpong P, Rerknimitr P, et al. Dapsone-induced severe cutaneous adverse drug reactions are strongly linked with HLA-B*13: 01 allele in the Thai population. *Pharmacogenet Genomics* 2017;27:429–437.
270. Kim SH, Kim M, Lee KW, et al. HLA-B*5901 is strongly associated with methazolamide-induced Stevens-Johnson syndrome/toxic epidermal necrolysis. *Pharmacogenomics* 2010;11:879–884.
271. Yang F, Xuan J, Chen J, et al. HLA-B*59:01: a marker for Stevens-Johnson syndrome/toxic epidermal necrolysis caused by methazolamide in Han Chinese. *Pharmacogenomics J* 2016;16:83–87.
272. Streif W, Andrew M, Marzinatto V, et al. Analysis of warfarin therapy in pediatric patients: a retrospective cohort study of 319 patients. *Blood* 1999;94:3007–3014.
273. Takahashi H, Ishikawa S, Nomoto S, et al. Developmental changes in pharmacokinetics and pharmacodynamics of warfarin enantiomers in Japanese children. *Clin Pharmacol Ther* 2000;68:541–555.
274. McLaughlin MJ, Wagner JB, Carleton B, et al. Considerations for implementing precision therapeutics in children. *Clin Transl Sci* 2019;12:140–15

CHAPTER

6

John D. Lantos

Ethics of Drug Research in Newborns and Children

In the prior edition of this textbook, Russell and colleagues noted the ongoing concern and debate about the moral, ethical, and legal issues that surround drug research and evaluation in infants and children. They noted tension that can exist between our ongoing quest for new knowledge, on the one hand, and, our obligation to adhere to the highest ethical standards in protecting research participants, on the other. Those tensions have gotten more complex.

Children are a uniquely vulnerable population for medical research because they can be easily exploited. This became apparent when ethicists scrutinized research done by Saul Krugman and colleagues in the 1950s and the Willowbrook State School in New York. Willowbrook was a residential facility for children with a variety of neurocognitive problems. In order to better understand the natural history and etiology of hepatitis, Krugman studied hepatitis transmission in these children. Some of his study designs involved deliberate infection of children with bodily fluids from other children who had active hepatitis. Although these studies were done with parental permission, Beecher argued that they were unacceptable because the risks to the children were too high and the informed consent process lacked details about those risks.[1]

The controversies over Willowbrook continued for decades and would eventually lead to regulations that mandated special protections for children. In 1970, theologian Paul Ramsey wrote of the Willowbrook studies, "Such use of captive populations of children for purely experimental purposes ought to be made legally impossible... stopped by legal acknowledgement of the moral invalidity of parental or legal proxy consent for the child to procedures having no relation to a child's own diagnosis or treatment."[1] Ramsey's important qualification—that special attention should be paid to studies "having no relation to the child's diagnosis or treatment"—would later become one pillar of federal regulation of pediatric research. Goldby supported Ramsey's concerns and also argued that "it was indefensible to give potentially dangerous infected material to children." Goldby highlighted that extra protection was especially important for children with cognitive defects and in studies that were not designed to provide direct benefit to the child.[2]

Krugman defended the studies on the grounds that the children involved did, in fact, benefit, because, instead of being admitted to the overcrowded wards at the underfunded facility, children in the studies were admitted to a clinical research unit where they would be isolated from exposure to pathogens. He wrote, "Their exposure in the hepatitis unit would be associated with less risk than the type of institutional exposure where multiple infections could occur."[3]

In 1982, medical historian David Rothman wrote of Willowbrook that the parental consent was meaningless because "[t]he consent form that parents signed to allow their children to be infected with the virus read as though their children were to receive a vaccine against the virus."[4] Furthermore, he argued, parents often consented to the studies in order to get their children out of the overcrowded wards at Willowbrook and into the far superior accommodations of the research wing. This, he argued, was coercive and possibly discriminatory because it would more likely attract poor children than rich children whose parents could afford places other than Willowbrook.

The debate over Willowbrook illustrates the central tension in pediatric research. The tension is between two noble goals. Everyone fervently hopes to discover new effective treatments childhood illnesses, and they also want to protect children from the harms of research. The tension between these two goals—protection and progress—is inevitable. Reasonable people can disagree about the proper balance in any particular intervention.

Current federal guidelines are a nuanced attempt to find the right balance. Because they are nuanced, however, they can also be difficult to interpret. Reasonable people can look at a study, look at the regulations, and draw different conclusions.

THE REGULATORY OVERSIGHT OF PEDIATRIC RESEARCH

Most research regulations include special requirements for studies involving children. In the United States, the Common Rule governing research defines four levels of riskiness in pediatric research studies, each of which is subject to a different level of regulation and oversight. The lowest level of risk is "minimal risk," which is defined as "the probability and magnitude of physical or psychological harm that is normally encountered in the daily lives, or in the routine medical or psychological examination of health children."[5] Studies that entail only minimal risk can be carried out, even if they do not offer any prospect of direct benefit to the research subjects.

Unfortunately, the category of "minimal risk" is problematic because the definition of minimal risk is somewhat vague. It does not specify, for example, whether the risks of everyday life should be those encountered by normal, healthy children growing up in safe homes and safe neighborhoods or, instead, should be those of sick children or children living in less optimal environments. The "normal daily lives" of sick children often include invasive procedures and dangerous drugs. Furthermore, the daily life of a child can be quite risky. Children are at risk of injury when they ride a bike, play competitive sports, take ballet lessons, or climb trees, but these risks seem different from those to which a child is exposed in a research study. This vagueness creates variable interpretations by investigators and institutional review boards (IRBs).[6] Shah and colleagues showed that IRB chairs vary in their assessment of whether a procedure is minimal risk. For example, allergy skin testing was found by 23% of those surveyed to be minimal risk, whereas 70% thought it was greater than minimal risk.[7]

The second level of risk in the U.S. federal regulations is an even vaguer category, "a minor increase over minimal risk." Research with this level of risk—and with no prospect of direct benefit to the research subjects—may be approved only if the research is likely to yield knowledge that is of vital importance to understand or ameliorate the child's disorder or condition. These greater-than-minimal risks should be commensurate with those in the child's actual or expected medical, dental, psychological, social, or educational situations.

Russell and colleagues noted that, although there is some disagreement about the exact boundaries of "minimal risk" or "minor increase over minimal risk," the disagreements focus on a narrow range of studies and tend to be resolved in a conservative manner. They note, "It is never morally acceptable to enroll a child in a study that involves significant pain *when there is no prospect of direct benefit to that child*, even when that child is already subjected to painful treatments/procedures as a part of a therapeutic regimen."

A third risk category is for studies that include the prospect of direct benefit to the child. Such studies may entail higher risks if the potential benefit is judged to balance out the risks. Because many studies involve new drugs or innovative procedures, we often do not know the risks or the benefits. The reason we are doing the study is to quantify the risks and benefits.[8] Thus, judgments about the relative risks and benefits are always tentative and require constant monitoring as the study is proceeding.

The fourth risk category is the most complex. It is for studies that involve more than a minor increase over minimal risk and no prospect of direct benefit for the child, but that are judged to be so important, in terms of the knowledge that they might yield that they ought, perhaps, to be conducted anyway. IRBs cannot approve these studies, but if they decide that the studies should be approved, they can ask the federal government to convene an expert panel to review them. The expert panel can decide that such studies should be permitted. They may also modify the protocol or the consent process.

THE COMPLICATED CONCEPT OF "ASSENT"

Children who are old enough (and neurocognitively capable) must give their assent before they can be enrolled in research studies. Assent is a complicated topic because assent is different from consent. William Bartholome, a pediatrician who was a strong advocate for children's right to refuse to participate in research, broke assent down into four elements. First, he said, the child must have "a developmentally appropriate understanding" of the nature of the condition. Second, investigators must disclose the nature of the proposed study, including what interventions it will involve. Third, those seeking assent must assess the child's understanding of the information provided and the influences on the child's evaluation of the situation. Finally, investigators must solicit the child's expression of willingness to participate.[9] These elements require subjective assessments of each child's capacities. Roth-Cline and colleagues point out that controversies arise about two different aspects of assent. First, researchers have to judge how much information to give. Too little will lead to decisions that are not well informed. Too much can be cognitively and emotionally overwhelming. Then, researchers must decide whether patients and parents understand the information. For this, they must develop "methods for assessing both children's understanding of disclosed information and of the assent process itself and what constitutes an effective, practical, and realistically applicable decision-making model."[10]

We often fall short of the ideal of child assent. Unguru and colleagues showed that many children who assent and are then enrolled in cancer clinical trials do not understand basic aspects of the research (e.g., that there might be added risk compared to standard treatments) and do not actually feel that they were able to play a significant role in decision-making.[11] The process of obtaining assent before enrolling children in research studies is difficult and often flawed.

A deeper problem with assent arises when parents and their children disagree about whether the child should be enrolled in a research study. For studies in which the anticipated benefit is thought to outweigh the risk—such as clinical trials of cancer chemotherapy—the parents may claim the right to override the child's dissent. In such situations, two fundamental moral principles clash: the research paradigm that protects children's autonomy-based right to refuse and the clinical paradigm in which the principle of beneficence generally guides doctors' and parents' choices.

Not surprisingly, IRB chairs are as variable in their interpretations of assent as they are in their interpretations of minimal risk. Whittle et al. found that half of IRB chairs rely on the investigators' judgments about when assent must be sought; the other half had a required method for investigators to determine whether obtaining assent was appropriate, most commonly based on age, but the age cutoff for requiring investigators to obtain assent from the child ranged from ages 5 years or younger to 10 years or older.[12]

CONTROVERSIAL RESEARCH IN CHILDREN

There are many examples of the difficulties in following the current regulations for pediatric research. This chapter briefly discusses four areas of controversy: studies involving genetic testing, the enrollment of healthy children in studies of sibling bone marrow donation, studies of the use of hypothermia for neonates with asphyxia, and comparative effectiveness research (CER).

GENETIC TESTING RESEARCH IN CHILDREN

Studies of genetic testing in children have been ethically controversial. Controversies arose in different domains. Some focused on population-based newborn screening programs and questions of whether the information that is gained from testing is of direct benefit to the child. For example, screening newborns for sickle cell disease was controversial when there was no beneficial treatment that could be offered to newborns with the disease. Once it became clear that prophylactic penicillin saved lives, the ethical controversy receded and screening became widely accepted. This has happened with many other newborn tests. However, controversy continues to grow around many newborn screening tests that diagnose genetic diseases for which there is no widely accepted beneficial treatment.

Some of the earliest debates arose with the advent of population-based newborn screening for autosomal recessive conditions, such as sickle cell disease or cystic fibrosis. Newborn screening is an unusual form of clinical testing. In most states, it is mandated and done without parental consent. Some states allow parents to opt-out, but most do not explicitly inform parents of this right.[13] Testing without consent is only possible when the benefits of testing are so clear and the harms so egregious that it would not be harmful to the child not to be tested and treated. When newborn screening was first developed, tests targeted severe disorders that were relatively prevalent and treatable.

The advent of new technology that made screening easier and less expensive led to the expansion of screening panels that can include diseases that are untreatable.[14] Tests for such diseases were initiated before there was any empirical assessment of long-term outcomes, harms, and benefits. But it is difficult to study the harms and benefits of a screening program because, in many cases, there is no treatment or the treatment itself is experimental.

In addition to population screening, genetic testing has also been used to test for carriers of genetic disease in carefully selected high-risk populations. Usually, people are selected for testing based on their race, ethnicity, and family history. For example, screening for Tay-Sachs was originally carried out in Ashkenazi Jewish communities and screening for sickle cell in people of African descent. People responded to the results with differing emotions. Studies of screening for Tay-Sachs,[15] muscular dystrophy,[16] cystic fibrosis,[17] and many other conditions reveal that such testing is predictably associated with anxiety and guilt in some people, euphoria or relief in others.

The latest form of genetic testing is whole-genome sequencing (WGS) or whole-exome sequencing. This type of testing raises a host of new issues. These arise, in part, because it can be used for a variety of purposes and for a variety of contexts. It can be used to diagnose symptomatic children whose conditions have eluded diagnosis with standard testing. It can be used to predict later-onset disease in healthy children. It can be used in population screening to diagnose disease or detect carrier status. In each of these cases, controversies arise because genome sequencing results are difficult to interpret. Interpretation will get better only with further study, but studying genome sequencing also requires some decisions about which results to disclose and how to interpret those results.

A recent summary of the ethical issues in genome sequencing by Johnston et al. made specific recommendations regarding such testing in different contexts.[18] In the clinical context, they recommended, whole-exome sequencing or WGS may be used to assist in diagnosis of symptomatic newborns. This should be done in a research context and only with parental consent and with access to genetic counseling.

The benefits of sequencing in a clinical context are deemed to outweigh the risks. For affected children and families who participate in these types of genetic testing research, the benefits of this kind of research outweigh the risks. It may yield an etiologic diagnosis that may inform future treatments and reproductive decisions. However, there are concerns about the psychological harms caused by the identification of a genetic condition.[19,20]

Attitudes within the professional community are quite divided as to whether or not genome sequencing, even for diagnosis, is valuable. On one hand, WGS is a potentially powerful tool that could transform the way that we diagnose disease and estimate prognosis. WGS may allow difficult diagnoses to be made in a timely way that would be impossible to make using any other diagnostic tools. Bieseker and colleagues, proponents of such testing, note, "...some of these variants can be not only highly predictive of disease but their return can enable life-saving treatment."[21] Green imagines "the routine use of genomics for disease prevention."[22]

On the other hand, many are skeptical about WGS's clinical benefit, in part, because they fear that it generates too much information, making its interpretation difficult, especially because it creates a very low signal-to-noise ratio.[23] Bieseker and colleagues recognized the problems of information overload, "A whole-genome or -exome result is overwhelming for both the clinician and the patient...(because).... variants from genome or exome range from those that are extremely likely to cause disease to those that are nearly certain to be benign, and every gradation between these two extremes."[23]

Barrington is among the skeptics who worry that this vast amount of information is not only of no clinical benefit, but actually harmful. He worries that such testing might lead to ambiguous results that cause anxiety but have no clinical benefit for the child. He concludes, "I certainly wouldn't have whole genome sequencing, nor accept it for my children."[22]

Careful studies of the ways in which doctors and parents use and react to DNA-based sequencing and analysis might help resolve the debate about whether such testing is perceived overall as helpful, harmful, or simply expensive and irrelevant. However, the studies themselves raise many of the same ethical questions as do the tests.

Any potential benefits from genetic testing research in childhood are significantly tempered when the child will not develop disease until adulthood. A commonly cited case is identification of children with a genetic predisposition to breast cancer. Many professional societies recommend deferring such testing and allowing the child to grow up and then make the decision about testing for himself or herself.[24,25]

Johnston et al. warned, however, that, given the state of knowledge in 2018, gene sequencing should not be used as a sole screen in state-sponsored newborn screening programs. The reason was because, in that context, there were too many false-positive and false-negative tests, and even more ambiguous findings as a result of genomic variants of unknown significance. Instead, the group recommended targeted testing for specific diseases, as is done today with population-based newborn screening. In some cases, genome sequencing can be used in conjunction with newborn screening to confirm specific genomic variants as a cause of disease. Research in this area will likely continue to be controversial for decades to come.

RESEARCH ON HEALTHY CHILDREN WHO DONATE STEM CELLS TO SIBLINGS

Hematopoietic stem cell transplantation has become standard treatment for a number of oncologic and hematologic illnesses. The human leukocyte antigen (HLA)–matched children may be identified as potential stem cell donors for these pediatric patients.[26] It is difficult to evaluate the risks and benefits to a child of donating bone marrow to a sibling because the benefits are psychological and the risks are physical. Research regulations stipulate that children can participate in research if the benefits of participating balance the risks. A recent protocol made the questions even more complex. Investigators proposed to give the donors granulocyte-macrophage colony-stimulating factor (GM-CSF), a treatment generally thought to be safe but one with potential long-term risks, in order to improve the likelihood of success for the recipient.[27] In 2008, the U.S. Food and Drug Administration (FDA) Pediatric Advisory Committee's Pediatric Ethics Subcommittee reviewed this protocol and considered whether a third party should advocate for the donor, whether parental discretion can credibly be based on assessment of risk and benefit to the donor, and what implications the committee findings would have on future research on healthy sibling stem cell donation. They concluded that

1. The potential research represented more than minor increase over minimal risk.
2. There were potential benefits, but these were indirect. They should not be considered a benefit of research.
3. The protocol offered an opportunity to address a serious problem affecting the health of children. Thus, potential donors would be allowed to participate provided that they had no identifiable risk factors for complications from GM-CSF administration, that an independent third party was available as an advocate for the potential donor, that the life-threatening nature of some of the potential risks (acute respiratory distress syndrome and leukemia) were disclosed in the informed consent document, and that "all things being equal, preference should go to an older sibling donor."[28]

RESEARCH ON THERAPEUTIC HYPOTHERMIA FOR PERINATAL HYPOXIC–ISCHEMIC ENCEPHALOPATHY

Research on therapeutic hypothermia for newborns with perinatal asphyxia illustrates a variety of ethical issues. The earliest clinical trials of hypothermia for babies with neonatal hypoxic–ischemic encephalopathy (HIE) were conducted in the late 1990s. Gunn and colleagues in New Zealand showed that hypothermia could be administered safely.[29] A few years later, Shankaran and colleagues drew on Gunn's research and on animal studies to suggest that a prospective randomized trial offered a prospect of direct benefit to research participants.[30] Over the next few years, many such randomized trials were conducted. A 2007 meta-analysis of eight randomized controlled trials involving 638 term infants concluded that therapeutic hypothermia improved both survival and neurodevelopmental outcomes.[31] Some adverse effects of hypothermia included an increase in the need for inotrope support of borderline significance and a significant increase in thrombocytopenia.

At that point, the debate shifted. Initially, it had been about whether or not a randomized trial would be ethically permissible because some thought the risks were too high and the prospect of direct benefit too low. After studies showed that hypothermia had benefits, some investigators wanted to refine the treatment by continuing to test different protocols for hypothermia against placebo. Others argued that hypothermia should be considered the standard of care and that, in future studies, it would be unethical not to offer it to patients in the control arm. The debate polarized the neonatal research community. In 2005, the American Academy of Pediatrics Committee on the Fetus and Newborn noted, "Therapeutic hypothermia is a promising therapy that should be considered investigational until the short-term safety and efficacy have been confirmed in the additional human trials underway. Long-term safety and efficacy remain to be defined."[32] Kirpalani and colleagues similarly called for more studies before accepting therapeutic hypothermia as an efficacious therapeutic modality.[33]

Others, however, took a different view. Wilkinson and associates, writing in 2007, noted, "We believe that the strength of the existing evidence warrants careful consideration of whether the risks to participants involved in continuing trials are justified."[34] The next year, Gunn and colleagues noted that the evidence of benefit was strong enough so that practicing physicians, in consultation with patients and families, should routinely use hypothermia as a treatment for neonatal encephalopathy.[35]

The debate about hypothermia illustrates the difficulty in reaching an answer to two different questions. One is deciding when a clinical trial of an innovative therapy is justifiable. For this, we have to extrapolate from animal data or small pilot studies. The second question arises as evidence from such trials accumulates. Then, we have to decide when further studies are no longer necessary. For both questions, reasonable people—and reasonable IRBs—can disagree.[36] Such debates frequently arise around intensive care interventions.[37]

For all such studies, we need a careful assessment of risk and benefit and then a laborious and often impossibly complex process of informed consent. The problems in assessing risks and benefits and then conveying them in a consent form led to a controversy about a comparative effectiveness study in neonates.

STUDYING OUTCOMES AFTER USING DIFFERENT TARGETS FOR OXYGEN SATURATION IN PREMATURE BABIES

CER is done to ascertain which of two treatments that are in widespread use is safer and more effective. It usually involves a prospective randomized trial. In the early 2000s, there was genuine uncertainty among experts in neonatology about the optimum level of oxygen saturation to target in adjusting ventilators and oxygen concentrations for critically ill premature babies.

Some prominent voices see CER as a disingenuous effort "to blur or eliminate the distinctions between research and therapy, scientist and physician, and subject and patient."[38] Proponents disagree and instead believe that CER can be conceptually distinguished from what we might call "innovative therapy research" (where a new treatment is compared against a placebo or a standard-of-care practice).[39] Debates about the ethical appropriateness of CER, generally, and about the study of oxygen saturation targets, in particular, highlight long-standing and fundamental tensions in the conduct of human subject research.

Supplemental oxygen is uniquely toxic to premature babies, and yet it is essential for their survival. Thus, they must be given some oxygen or they die. But if they are given too much oxygen for too long, then they can end up with brain damage, blindness, visual impairment, or chronic lung disease. Thus, it has been crucial for neonatologists to discover just how much oxygen to give to these fragile babies. But the research studies that would allow them to test different approaches to oxygen therapy in different subpopulations of babies are methodologically challenging and ethically controversial.

In order for any prospective study to be ethically appropriate, there must be uncertainty about the relative risks and benefits of the different treatments being studied. If clinicians and investigators knew that one treatment was better, there would be no scientific reason to do the study and it would be unethical at the outset. The requirement for genuine uncertainty dictates, to a certain extent, what must be included in the informed consent form and discussion.

Parents need information about the potential harms and benefits of enrolling their child in a study. Informed consent for CER is different from informed consent for studies of previously untested therapies in at least three important ways. First, in studies of new therapies, the potential harms are, generally, not completely known. For a CER study, by contrast, all the treatments are in widespread use. We know a lot about the risks and benefits. We just do not know the relative risks and benefits. Thus, as part of the consent process, we must explain what is known, what is not known, and what we hope to learn by doing the study.

Second, in studies of new therapies, the treatment that patients will get if they do not enroll in the study is clear. They will get the same treatment as patients in the control arm, that is, the existing standard of care. In CER, by contrast, there is no obvious "default" position. Prospective study subjects must be told that if they do not enroll in the study, they might get the exact same treatment that they would have gotten if they had enrolled in the trial. They should also be told whether and how treatment will be different if they enroll in the study.

Finally, in any clinical situation, prospective study subjects must be told about the potential harms that they (or their child) face from their underlying disease, regardless of whether or not they enroll in the trial. For premature babies, all parents should be told of the long-term complications of prematurity. They need to understand that premature babies can die or can survive with eye disease, blindness, chronic lung disease, and neurodevelopmental impairment. This is not an easy conversation to have. There has been much discussion and debate among expert clinicians about how to explain these potential harms.[40,41]

The process of informed consent for any prospective randomized trial is difficult. We know from studies of consent in other situations that parents often have trouble understanding randomization. For example, Kodish and colleagues have shown that half of parents who consented for their children to be in a study of cancer chemotherapy did not understand randomization.[42,43]

Part of the problem may be that consent forms themselves, while designed to inform and empower parents, are often long and confusing. They could be simplified. Lantos and Feudtner suggest that it would have been sufficient, and perhaps more informative, to replace the traditional consent form with one that simply said the following:

> *Your baby was born extremely prematurely. Many babies who are born this early die. Many of those who survive have long-term complications, including eye disease, chronic lung disease, cerebral palsy, and brain damage. Most survivors, however, do not have any of these problems. We are doing a study to try to learn the best ways to prevent these things from happening. The study involves giving babies two different levels of oxygen: higher and lower. Some babies in the study may do better—and some babies worse—than other babies in the study. But we don't know which group will have better outcomes. (If we knew, we wouldn't be doing the study.) Right now, babies in NICUs across the United States receive both levels of oxygen and many levels in between. We also don't know whether babies in the study will have better or worse outcomes than babies who are not in the study. For babies in the study, we will decide what oxygen level to provide by a random choice (similar to flipping a coin.) Every baby will have a 50-50 chance of getting either low or high oxygen levels. Babies who are not in the study are treated according to our NICU protocol. You can decide whether to be in the study or not. If you decide to be in the study, this decision will only determine the level of oxygen that we use and will not affect the care that your baby gets in any other way.*[44]

CONCLUSION

Our regulations governing research in children offer general guidelines that are designed to protect children from harm or exploitation. These important protections can sometimes lead to disagreements about whether particular studies are ethically permissible. Controversies arise in studies that involve genomics, healthy children, and sick babies. They focus on psychological harms and benefits as well as physical ones. In some cases, they turn on subtle issues of epistemology—that is, when do we know enough and when are we uncertain enough that randomization is justifiable.

In each controversial area, the challenge for researchers and policy makers is to use the framework of minimal risk or acceptable risk–benefit ratio in order to determine whether the study is permissible. We then need to pay meticulous attention to informing parents and older children. The application of the basic principles of research ethics to the practicalities of the specific research projects requires careful attention to the details of the study, flexibility in the application of the principles, and open deliberation about the complex judgments that must be made.

REFERENCES

1. Beecher HK. Ethics and clinical research. *N Engl J Med* 1966;274(24):1354–1360.
2. Ramsey, P. *The patient as person: explorations in medical ethics.* New Haven, CT: Yale University Press, 1970.
3. Goldby S. Experiments at the Willowbrook State School. *Lancet.* 1971;1(7702):749.
4. Krugman S. Experiments at the Willowbrook State School. *Lancet.* 1971;1(7706):966–967.
5. Rothman DJ. Were Tuskegee & Willowbrook 'studies in nature'? *Hastings Cent Rep* 1982;12(2):5–7.
6. National Commission for the Protection of Human Subjects of Biomedical and Behavioral Research. *Report and recommendations on research involving children.* Washington, DC: U.S. Department of Health Education and Welfare, 1977.

7. Westra AE, Wit JM, Sukhai RN, et al. How best to define the concept of minimal risk. *J Pediatr.* 2011;159(3):496–500.
8. Shah S, Whittle A, Wilfond B, et al. How do institutional review boards apply the federal risk and benefit standards for pediatric research? *JAMA* 2004;291(4):476–482.
9. Jonsen AR. Research involving children: recommendations of the National Commission for the Protection of Human Subjects of Biomedical and Behavioral Research. *Pediatrics* 1978;62(2):131–136.
10. Bartholme W. Ethical issues in pediatric research. In: Vanderpooo H, ed *The ethics of research involving human subjects.* Frederick, MD: University Publishing Group, 1996.
11. Roth-Cline MDGJ, Bright P, Lee CS, et al. Ethical considerations in conducting pediatric research. In: Seyberth HW, Rane A, Schwab M, eds. *Pediatric clinical pharmacology.* Heidelberg, Germany: Springer, 2011.
12. Unguru Y, Sill AM, Kamani N. The experiences of children enrolled in pediatric oncology research: implications for assent. *Pediatrics* 2010;125(4):e876–e883.
13. Whittle A, Shah S, Wilfond B, et al. Institutional review board practices regarding assent in pediatric research. *Pediatrics* 2004;113:1747–1752.
14. Dhanda RK, Reilly PR. Legal and ethical issues of newborn screening. *Pediatr Ann* 2003;32:540–546.
15. Plass AM, van El CG, Pieters T, et al. Neonatal screening for treatable and untreatable disorders: prospective parents' opinions. *Pediatrics* 2010;125:e99–106.
16. Marteau TM, van Duijn M, Ellis I. Effects of genetic screening on perceptions of health: a pilot study. *J Med Genet* 1992;29(1):24–26.
17. James CA, Hadley DW, Holtzman NA, et al. How does the mode of inheritance of a genetic condition influence families? A study of guilt, blame, stigma, and understanding of inheritance and reproductive risks in families with X-linked and autosomal recessive diseases. *Genet Med* 2006;8(4):234–242.
18. Lakeman P, Plass AM, Henneman L, et al. Three-month follow-up of Western and non-Western participants in a study on preconceptional ancestry-based carrier couple screening for cystic fibrosis and hemoglobinopathies in the Netherlands. *Genet Med* 2008:10(11):820–830.
19. Johnston J, Lantos JD, Goldenberg A, et al. Sequencing newborns: a call for nuanced use of genomic technologies. *Hastings Cent Rep* 2018;48(4): S2:1–20 doi:10.1002/hast.874.
20. Lehmann A, Speight BS, Kerzin-Storrar L. Extended family impact of genetic testing: the experiences of X-linked carrier grandmothers. *J Genet Couns* 2011;20(4):365–373.
21. Tabor HK, Cho MK. Ethical implications of array comparative genomic hybridization in complex phenotypes: points to consider in research. *Genet Med* 2007;9(9):626–631.
22. Biesecker L. Opportunities and challenges for the integration of massively parallel genomic sequencing into clinical practice: lessons from the ClinSeq project. *Genet Med* 2012;14:393–398.
23. Green ED, Guyer MS, National Human Genome Research Institute. Charting a course for genomic medicine from base pairs to bedside. *Nature* 2011;470:204–213.
24. Barrington KJ. Who benefits from whole genome sequencing in the NICU? Who suffers? http://neonatalresearch.org/2012/10/07/who-benefits-from-whole-genome-sequencing-in-the-nicu-who-suffers/. Accessed November 3, 2012.
25. Davis DS. Genetic dilemmas and the child's right to an open future. *Rutgers Law J* 1997;28:549–592.
26. Wilfond B, Ross LF. From genetics to genomics: ethics, policy, and parental decision-making. *J Pediatr Psychol* 2009;34(6):639–647.
27. American Academy of Pediatrics, Bioethics Committee. Children as hematopoietic stem cell donors. *Pediatrics* 2010;125(2):392–404.
28. Pulsipher MA, Nagler A, Iannone R, et al. Weighing the risks of G-CSF administration, leukopheresis, and standard marrow harvest: ethical and safety considerations for normal pediatric hematopoietic cell donors. *Pediatr Blood Cancer* 2006;46(4):422–433.
29. https://wayback.archive-it.org/7993/20170405042537/https://www.fda.gov/ohrms/dockets/ac/08/briefing/2008-4406b1-14%20(ASCT0631%20Initial%20Review%20APM%20Letter).pdf. Accessed May 3, 2018.
30. Gunn AJ, Gluckman PD, Gunn TR. Selective head cooling in newborn infants after perinatal asphyxia: a safety study. *Pediatrics* 1998;102:885–892.
31. Shankaran S, Laptook A, Wright L, et al. Whole-body hypothermia for neonatal encephalopathy: animal observations as a basis for a randomized, controlled pilot study in term infants. *Pediatrics* 2002;110(2):377–385.
32. Jacobs S, Hunt R, Tarnow-Mordi W, et al. Cooling for newborns with hypoxic ischaemic encephalopathy. *Cochrane Database Syst Rev* 2007;(4):CD003311.
33. Blackmon LR, Stark AR, American Academy of Pediatrics Committee on Fetus and Newborn. Hypothermia: a neuroprotective therapy for neonatal hypoxic-ischemic encephalopathy. *Pediatrics* 2006;117(3):942–948.
34. Kirpalani H, Barks J, Thorlund K, et al. Cooling for neonatal hypoxic ischemic encephalopathy: do we have the answer? *Pediatrics* 2007;120(5):1126–1130.
35. Wilkinson D, Casalaz D, Watkins A, et al. Hypothermia: a neuroprotective therapy for neonatal hypoxic-ischemic encephalopathy. *Pediatrics* 2007;119(2):422–423.
36. Gunn A, Hoehn T, Hansmann G, et al. Hypothermia: an evolving treatment for neonatal hypoxic ischemic encephalopathy. *Pediatrics* 2008;121:648–649.
37. Laventhal N, Tarini B, Lantos J. Ethical issues in neonatal and pediatric clinical trials. *Pediatr Clin North Am* 2012;59(5):1205–1220. doi:10.1016/j.pcl.2012.07.007.
38. Lantos JD, Frader J. Extracorporeal membrane oxygenation and the ethics of clinical research in pediatrics. *N Engl J Med* 1990;323:409–413.
39. Annas GJ, Questing for grails: duplicity, betrayal and self-deception in postmodern medical research. *J Contemp Health Law Policy* 1996;12:297.
40. Faden R, Kass N, Whicher D, et al. Ethics and informed consent for comparative effectiveness research with prospective electronic clinical data. *Med Care* 2013;51(8 Suppl 3):S53–S57.
41. Janvier A, Lorenz JM, Lantos JD. Antenatal counselling for parents facing an extremely preterm birth: limitations of the medical evidence. *Acta Paediatr* 2012;101:800–804.
42. Haward MF, Murphy RO, Lorenz JM. Default options and neonatal resuscitation decisions. *J Med Ethics* 2012;38:713–718.
43. Kodish E, Eder M, Noll RB, et al. Communication of randomization in childhood leukemia trials. *JAMA* 2004;291:470–475.
44. Greenley RN, Drotar D, Zyzanski SJ, et al. Stability of parental understanding of random assignment in childhood leukemia trials: an empirical examination of informed consent. *J Clin Oncol* 2006;24:891–897.
45. Lantos JD, Feudtner C. SUPPORT and the ethics of study implementation: lessons for comparative effectiveness research from the trial of oxygen therapy for premature babies. *Hastings Cent Rep* 2015;45(1):1–11. doi:10.1002/hast. 407.

CHAPTER 7

Tomoyuki Mizuno
Philip D. Walson
Alexander A. Vinks

Precision Medicine and Therapeutic Drug Monitoring

INTRODUCTION

Most medical treatments currently on the market come with recommendations for the average patient. However, there is often substantial between- and within-patient variability in drug exposure and response to many medications when administered at the labeled dose. In addition, children (especially infants) undergo rapid dynamic changes in their body size and physiology, which have an impact on the variability in drug exposure and response. Therefore, when using a "one-size-fits-all" approach, treatments can be successful for some patients, but not for others. Precision medicine is an innovative approach to this problem which tailors drug treatments to individual needs based on patient-specific factors, including genotype, demographic, and clinical characteristics; environment; and lifestyle. The simplest way to identify and adjust for interindividual variability in drug response is to objectively measure the degree of effect and then adjust the dosing regimen accordingly. However, such a straightforward approach is seldom feasible, as simple and reliable therapeutic effect measures are not always available in routine clinical situations. In addition, many serious conditions require rapid attainment of adequate clinical effect while avoiding excessive dosing in clinical conditions where drug effects are especially difficult to measure. This is particularly true in newborns and other nonverbal or noncommunicative patients. Rational pharmacotherapy requires a basic understanding of the way patients handle drugs (pharmacokinetics, PK) and their response (effect) to specific drug concentrations (pharmacodynamics, PD).[1] PK may be simply defined as what the body does to the drug, as opposed to PD, which may be defined as what the drug does to the body.[2] During the past decades, significant advances have been made in the field of pediatric and neonatal PK and PD, including a better understanding of the effects of growth (size) and development (or maturation) on organ function and drug dose–exposure–effect relationships.[3] The ultimate goal of the study of dose–exposure–effect relationships is to allow clinicians to derive optimal, individualized dosing regimens, which produce maximal therapeutic and minimal side effects with the simplest dosing regimen possible. This can best be achieved by linking PK and PD information to better understand or predict the exposure–effect relationship in a time-dependent (dynamic) manner. The proper measurement and interpretation of drug concentrations [therapeutic drug monitoring (TDM) or the more proactive term "management"[4]] in a specific patient can help us better understand how a particular drug is behaving and is required for further individualization of the dosing regimen in that patient as well as how to best select an initial dosing regimen in future patients.[5]

PRECISION MEDICINE

Doctors have always recognized that every patient is unique, and doctors have always tried to tailor their treatments as best they can to individuals. You can match a blood transfusion to a blood type—that was an important discovery. What if matching a cancer cure to our genetic code was just as easy, just as standard? What if figuring out the right dose of medicine was as simple as taking our temperature?

—President Barack Obama, State of the Union Address, January 20, 2015

The statement in the 2015 State of the Union that most medical treatments are designed for the average patient initiated the rollout of the Precision Medicine Initiative, a broad research effort to revolutionize how health care and treatment of disease can be more precise, personalized, and improved.[6] Precision medicine is an innovative approach that considers individual differences in patient's genes, environments, and lifestyles for better clinical decision-making in treatment of disease and in health care. Progress in precision medicine has already led to powerful new discoveries and several new treatments that are tailored to specific characteristics, such as a patient's genotype or the genetic profile of an individual's tumor.

Therapeutic optimization can be viewed as the continuum of improving practice-changing paradigms across the spectrum of disease-specific pharmacologic interventions and, as such, forms an important keystone of precision medicine.[7] In the pediatric and neonatal populations, therapeutic optimization is more challenging than in the adult population as evidence for dosing, efficacy, and safety of many medications is sparser. Therefore, the dosage regimen is frequently determined by extrapolation from adult clinical data and by a "trial-and-error" paradigm. This can be successful for some patients and some medications but may lead to unsafe or ineffective dosing for others, especially in very young children. The biggest challenge for implementation of precision medicine in the pediatric populations is to identify age-appropriate and evidence-based safe and effective dose ranges across the age spectrum from newborns to adolescents. A better understanding of the age-related dynamic changes in PK/PD characteristics is important to establish dosing strategy and implement therapeutic optimization in the pediatric populations.

THE TARGET CONCENTRATION STRATEGY

Drug actions (effects) are directly related to the drug concentration at the site(s) of action. Although imperfect, there is almost always a better relationship between the effect of a given drug and its concentration in the blood than between the dose of the drug given and the effect. PK is the science that can explain and predict the relationship between a dosing regimen and the concentration of a drug in various body compartments over time. A basic understanding of PK principles and how these principles are altered in the developing child is required to better understand and predict drug actions. The interrelationship between drug input (dose), PK, PD, and clinical effects is schematically conceptualized in Figure 7.1.[8]

There are many practical, physiologic, and pathophysiologic factors that determine how much drug effect will be associated with a drug prescription. Clinicians make a diagnosis and then prescribe a dosing regimen: drug, dose, formulation, route, frequency, and duration. Once a drug is prescribed, there are many factors that determine how much effect, either therapeutic or toxic, is seen in the individual patient. Prescriptions must be filled correctly, the prescription filled must contain the correct drug and amount, the dosage regimen must be taken/given (adherence), and the drug must get into the patient and reach the site(s) of action. There are many reasons why concentrations and drug exposure (and therefore the effects) that result from prescriptions differ among patients. Even if taken or given exactly as desired, effects produced will depend on many factors, including the patient's physiology, prior history, and other drugs present. Patients/parents may never fill the prescription. Up to 25% of patients do not fill prescriptions, and even more do not take medication as indicated. Children and adolescents with chronic illness have great difficulty completing prescribed treatment regimens, which can be complex and burdensome. High rates of nonadherence to treatment (up to 50% or more) have been reported for various pediatric chronic conditions, such as asthma, epilepsy, transplantation, juvenile rheumatoid arthritis (JRA), and diabetes.[9–11] Different formulations of the same drug may have different absorption characteristics. Manufacturing problems can and do occur. Pharmacy or pharmaceutical errors can alter the amount of drug delivered or in fact which drug is given, and parents or patients may or may not comply with instructions. All of these factors can alter the amount of drug that reaches the site of action. Several studies have documented unpredictable drug delivery in neonates. This is especially relevant for antibiotics such as aminoglycosides that are used frequently to treat bacterial infections in this population. A lack of appreciation of drug delivery issues such as the small volumes and low infusion rates used in these patients can result in a much lower-than-expected blood concentrations and much lower than what is required for optimal antimicrobial therapy.[12] Drug concentration measurements can provide an objective way to identify, explain, or eliminate uncertainty caused by a number of these factors, especially in patients who have unusual or unexpected drug responses. However, even patients who actually take or are given the same amount of a drug may also have very different amounts of drug in their body or blood at different times after dosing. The ability to predict and explain the inter- and intraindividual differences in drug concentrations over time requires knowledge of basic PK principles.

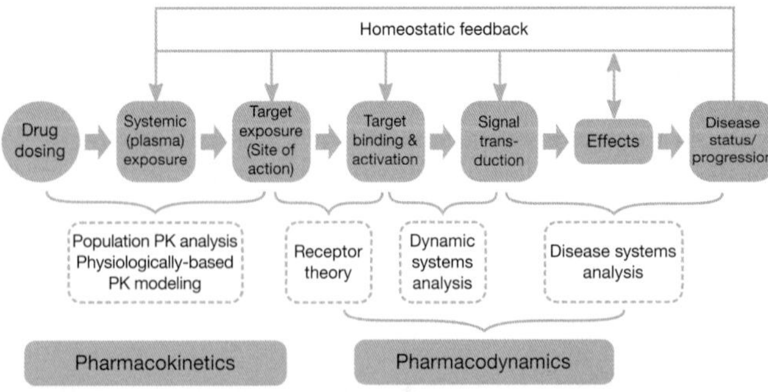

Figure 7.1 Schematic representation of the interrelationships between drug input (dose), pharmacokinetics (concentration), pharmacodynamics, and clinical effects. (Adapted from Danhof M. Kinetics of drug action in disease states: towards physiology-based pharmacodynamic (PBPD) models. *J Pharmacokinet Pharmacodyn* 2015;42:447–462.)

THE CONCEPT OF THERAPEUTIC DRUG MONITORING

TDM is a multidisciplinary clinical specialty aimed at improving treatment of disease and patient health care by individually tailoring a dosage regimen of drugs based on the measurement made in the laboratory with appropriate interpretation.[13] The measurement can be a genotype, demographic and clinical data, drug concentration in a biologic matrix (e.g., blood), and/or biomarkers to represent drug response. *A priori TDM* is defined by the International Association of Therapeutic Drug Monitoring and Clinical Toxicology (IATDMCT; www.iatdmct.org) as the determination of a medication's initial dosing regimen based on patient-specific baseline information, such as body size, laboratory data, and genetic makeup. In recent years, significant progress has been made in quantitative pharmacology using PK/PD modeling and simulation (M&S). This has facilitated the establishment of population-specific starting dosing regimens based on specific factors that are predictive of exposure and response. PK/PD models serve as *a priori* knowledge that link the drug dose to exposure and subsequent effects. Especially in pediatrics, where growth and maturation are correlated, age-related variation in PK/PD can be taken into account quantitatively with the M&S approach[3,14] (see "Model-Informed Precision Dosing" section). *A posteriori TDM* as defined by IATDMCT includes dose adjustment after the start of therapy based on treatment-related feedback data collected from a particular patient, such as blood concentration measurements and/or clinical biomarkers indicating drug response. Proper *a posteriori* TDM requires interpretation of drug concentration measurements and/or biomarker data with consideration of preanalytical conditions, clinical information, and the clinical efficiency of the current dosage

TABLE 7.1	Indications for Therapeutic Drug Monitoring
Drugs with a narrow therapeutic index (NTI)	
Inadequate response	
Higher than standard dose required	
Serious, unexpected, or persistent side effects	
Suspected toxicity	
Suspected nonadherence	
Suspected drug–drug or drug–diet interactions	
New preparation, changing brands	
Other illnesses, for example, hepatic/renal problems, inflammatory diseases	

regimen. Although frequently dose adjustments are made based on a simple comparison of the observed concentration versus therapeutic target range, using a population PK/PD model in combination with individualized forecasting techniques such as Bayesian estimation can facilitate more precise and rapid target attainment (see later examples).

The rationale for using TDM to optimize dosing of a given drug is contingent on three important requirements: (a) there is a better association between the concentration and the therapeutic effect than between the dose and the effect, (b) TDM and dose individualization will reduce variability and will better predict the patient's concentration–time profile, and (c) maintenance of drug concentrations within desired target ranges (see later discussion) improves clinical outcome by either increasing efficacy or reducing toxicity or both.[15] Proper TDM requires that dosing regimens are then further individualized based on individual measured concentrations and responses. The criteria for monitoring (managing) drugs in children are similar to those in adults. Generally accepted indications for concentration measurements are summarized in Table 7.1.

The cost-effectiveness of TDM has also been demonstrated as a result of dose reduction and the reduced duration of hospitalization for many treatments.[16] In addition, it is suggested that the use of TDM potentially reduces relapse rates as it is helpful to detect nonadherence to medication before rehospitalization.

In pediatrics, the use of TDM has been common in (a) the treatment of epilepsy,[17–19] (b) transplantation,[20] and (c) drug therapy in neonates.[21] In recent years, TDM has also been increasingly implemented in other important therapeutic areas in pediatrics, such as psychiatry,[22] HIV,[23] and inflammatory diseases,[24,25] including therapies involving monoclonal antibodies. Oncology is another emerging therapeutic area where TDM is increasingly being used for dose optimization. However, TDM implementation in children is still not as common as in adult populations.[26]

THE THERAPEUTIC RANGE CONCEPT

Despite decades of TDM, recommended target concentrations (therapeutic ranges) are largely empirical, population rather than individually based, independent of assay method used, seldom consider time after dosing, and seldom are the result of evidence-based studies. The therapeutic range is also commonly misunderstood even for commonly monitored drugs such as digoxin, aminoglycosides, phenobarbital, phenytoin, and theophylline. Interpretation of TDM results is still almost exclusively focused on altering dosing to get measured concentrations within a published "therapeutic range".[27] The "therapeutic range" is defined as the range of drug concentrations associated with a *high* degree of efficacy and a *low* risk of dose-related toxicity in the *majority* of patients. This is not the same as the optimal concentration for each individual patient. Furthermore, the emphasis in measuring drug concentrations has been mostly toxicity oriented and for drugs with a narrow therapeutic index (NTI). NTI drugs are defined as those drugs where small differences in dose or blood concentration may lead to dose and blood concentration dependent, serious therapeutic failures, or adverse drug reactions.

The "therapeutic range" concept is hampered by some important problems.[28] First, defining a single, time-independent concentration range leaves the physician with the uncertainty of how to choose the optimal dose when in fact a range of dosing regimens would produce a "therapeutic concentration" at some time in the regimen. Second, the definition of a therapeutic range does not differentiate among concentrations but assumes that all concentrations within the range may be equally desirable. Third, the ranges depend on a number of other things, including time after a dose, time on a particular regimen, the condition being treated, the assay used, and the possibility of active metabolites. Problems created by assays with different specificity for active and inactive metabolites or interfering substances are more commonly a problem in pediatric than in adult patients. Poor understanding of the therapeutic range has led to a rather naive and even potentially dangerous "numbers-only," three-step, all-or-nothing interpretation of the concentration–effect relationship. This simplistic approach assumes that any concentration below the lower end of the range will be of no benefit to the patient, that anywhere within the range the patient will be okay, and that above the upper end of the range the patient will experience unacceptable adverse reactions. None of these may be true in any given patient.

DISTRIBUTION PHASE

Immediately after administration, drugs must distribute into the blood and then to tissues in the body. This results in initial concentrations that are much higher than, and which do not show a log-linear correlation with, postdistributional concentrations. This is true for most, if not all, drugs given intravenously, and for several drugs (e.g., digoxin and clonazepam), this phenomenon also occurs after oral administration. There are large differences between trough and distribution concentrations even for drugs with a very long half-life. Digoxin, for example, can have postdose peak concentrations of 3 to 5 ng per mL in patients with trough concentrations of less than 1 ng per mL. There are also greatly different concentration–effect relationships between distribution and postdistributional concentrations at the site of action.[29] If not appreciated, this can lead to inappropriate decreases in digoxin doses or even use of Digibind, digoxin antigen-binding fragments (personal experience). Unfortunately, many physicians believe, and teach, that sampling time is not important for drugs with long half-lives because concentrations are not expected to change much when dosing intervals are much shorter than the drug's half-life. Although true well after completion of the distribution phase, this is not true when comparing trough values with concentrations obtained during distribution. Randomly collected clonazepam concentrations have been used to claim that there is a poor relationship between concentrations and effect. However, it is highly likely that this conclusion is based on the fact that clonazepam, despite having relatively slow clearance, also has very high distribution concentrations relative to predose (trough) concentrations even after oral administration.[30] Concentrations drawn during the distribution phase (4 to 6 hours after dosing) will not correlate with effects because they do not reflect the effect site concentration. PK modeling of digoxin or clonazepam with respect to concentrations at their sites of action (heart muscle and brain, respectively) is needed to attempt to correlate concentrations and effect. Bayesian modeling, but not linear correlation methods, can deal with sampling during the distribution phase, but sampling and accurate information on administration time become even more critical.[29,31] Unfortunately, in pediatrics, the time of drug administration is not as easy to determine as it is in adults. Decades ago, Leff and Roberts showed that it can take hours for drugs put into an intravenous setup to actually reach the patient.[32] This is still true to date, as the delivery of drugs administered by intravenous infusion in extremely low-birth-weight neonates can be substantially extended due to the small volumes and low infusion rates used in these patients.[12] Appreciation of both distribution phase sampling as well as the practical problems of ascertaining actual drug administration time for different intravenous setups, fluids and administration rates, and sites is required to properly interpret some drug concentrations.

THE STEADY-STATE CONCEPT

Steady state is another commonly misunderstood PK principle. Drug concentrations fluctuate over a defined range once a patient reaches steady state. If the clearance of a drug which follows first-order PK stays the same, then the patient receiving the drug will reach one half (50%) of eventual concentrations after one half-life, 3/4 (75%) after two half-lives, 7/8 (87.5%) after three half-lives, 15/16 (94%) after four half-lives, and so on. This is commonly misinterpreted to mean that drug concentrations should be measured after three to four doses have been given. However, drugs are seldom given every half-life. Drugs with much shorter half-lives than the dosing interval reach steady state long before three to four doses, and drugs with very long half-lives may not reach steady state until after many dozens of doses unless a loading dose is given. A patient with a gentamicin half-life of 1 to 2 hours who is given a dose every 8 hours is very close to steady state after a single dose, whereas a patient receiving a drug with a half-life of 36 hours every 8 hours without a loading dose does not reach steady state for almost a week. Routine orders to measure a drug concentration after three or four doses demonstrate a lack of understanding of basic PK principles let alone any appreciation for the effects of individual differences in drug clearance. In addition, attainment of steady state described above assumes that the patient's clearance is not changing over time; something which is almost never true in a critically ill patient or even in a healthy newborn or young child.

DEVELOPMENTAL ASPECTS OF DRUG DISPOSITION AND RESPONS

Proper PK/PD guidance is especially important in patients with rapidly changing PK (clearance) and responses (PD). Although this applies to most critically ill, hospitalized patients, it applies especially to neonates and children because of large, often rapid developmental changes in both PK and PD.[33,34] It has been well documented that development of physiology and organ function (e.g., liver and kidney) mostly occurs in the early phases of life up to approximately 2 years of age.[33] In children aged 2 years and older, maturation is mostly completed, and the changes in PK parameters such as clearance and volume of distribution can be well described using an appropriate body size scaling factor, such as allometric scaling.[35–37] The developmental changes in PK of medications that occur between birth and infancy create challenges for physicians who desire to prescribe medications on a rational, age-appropriate, individual basis. Routine TDM of prescribed drugs and their active metabolites can be of great help to individualize dose requirements during long-term treatment.[15] In addition, the ratio of metabolite(s) to parent drug can also give important information on (non)adherence and can reveal unusual metabolic patterns.

Increasingly, proper interpretation of measured drug concentrations is being used to provide important insights into the different PK behavior in neonates, children, and adolescents.[38] Of all routinely monitored drugs, the aminoglycosides have been studied most extensively. PK data for gentamicin, tobramycin, netilmicin, and amikacin are available across (arbitrary) pediatric age categories: preterm newborns, term newborn infants (0 to 27 days), infants and toddlers (28 days to 23 months), children (2 to 11 years), and adolescents (12 to 16 or 18 years).[39,40] These studies have demonstrated that in the premature neonate, drug clearance is reduced and volume of distribution increased as compared with older children and adults, and glomerular filtration (the predominant route of elimination) by the immature kidney is reduced.[41,42] Volumes of distribution are larger than those in older pediatric patients because of larger body water fat content and higher body surface-to-weight ratios. Such increased volume of distribution in newborns has also been observed for other drugs.[43] An overview of age-related PK changes and PK parameter estimates for gentamicin and vancomycin[44,45] as index drugs is summarized in Table 7.2. Drug clearance rapidly increases with age as the kidney develops and the total body water decreases. Although the limitations of serum creatinine or creatinine clearance as a diagnostic biomarker of kidney function has been recognized,[46] the creatinine concentration in plasma or calculated creatinine clearance remains a good *a priori* indicator of individual renal drug elimination.[47,48] Individual differences in renal drug clearance can, therefore, be predicted before or during dosing and used to individualize dosing (both dose and dosing frequency). In addition, however, clearance of renally cleared drugs such as gentamicin can be used to predict renal function more accurately than creatinine clearance calculations used in adults.[49] This is especially useful in the newborn, where maternal creatinine contributes to neonatal creatinine concentration in the first days after birth (see case presentation in later discussion). Besides renally cleared drugs, recent studies have provided evidence on the developmental changes in clearance of drugs that are predominantly metabolized. Anderson and Holford in a series of articles quantitatively describe the relationship between young age and the developmental trajectory of clearance as a percentage of adult clearance.[35–37,50]

Drugs that are metabolized often show large, unpredictable interindividual and sometimes intraindividual differences in PK

TABLE 7.2 Age-Related Differences in Pharmacokinetic Parameters for Aminoglycosides and Vancomycin

	CL	V_d	$t_{1/2}$	*Targets*
Aminoglycosides				
Neonates	↓	↑↑	↑	↓
Children	↑	↑	↓/~	↓/~
Cystic fibrosis patients	↑↑	↑	↓/~	↑↑
Vancomycin				
Neonates	↓	↑	↑	↓/~
Children	↑	↑/~	↓	~

CL, clearance; $t_{1/2}$, half-life; V_d, volume of distribution.

behavior. This interpatient as well as intrapatient variability may be further increased if the drug is taken orally, because of differences in absorption, transport, as well as intestinal metabolism. TDM can detect such interindividual as well as intraindividual variations. However, a single measurement will only describe the net results of all the different underlying processes (e.g., bioavailability, absorption, distribution, metabolism, excretion) involved. For instance, a concentration that is lower-than-expected based on data for that patient population can be the result of poor adherence, absorption problems, increased metabolism and excretion, or any combination of these.

DOSE ADJUSTMENTS BASED ON THERAPEUTIC DRUG MONITORING DATA

The decision to alter a generally accepted dosing regimen either before or during ongoing therapy is frequently based on an empirical trial-and-error decision-making process where different pieces of clinical information are considered. Patients in whom a rapid onset of effect is required or patients who exhibit lower or higher effects than expected after initiation or alteration of therapy can clearly benefit from proper TDM. In the nonresponding patient, concentration measurements will help the clinician decide whether nonadherence is present, whether a medication error is possible, whether a drug–drug or drug–diet interaction has occurred, or whether individual differences in PK or PD require a different dose or frequency of dosing or whether alternate therapy is indicated. This is true even for drugs for which a well-described "therapeutic range" is unknown.

Appropriate timing of sample collection is crucial for the appropriate interpretation of drug concentrations. Within a dosing interval, the predose or trough concentration is usually the sampling time after steady state is achieved, but efficacy is questioned. In the case of adverse events or (suspected) toxicity, sampling is preferably done at the time maximal side effects are experienced. Other sampling strategies may be required for drugs that exhibit a complex PK profile and poor correlation between the trough concentration and the area under the concentration–time curve (*AUC*). An example of this is mycophenolic acid (MPA), a drug with complex absorption characteristics and which exhibits enterohepatic recycling.[51,52] Lack of all necessary information, such as the actual time of drug intake, how long after dosing was started, whether a loading dose was used, timing of concomitant medications, and time of sampling, makes it more difficult, or sometimes impossible, to interpret results. TDM laboratories and services can play an important role in improving patient outcomes and the efficient use of TDM by providing up-to-date guidelines and educating physicians and other health care providers about what information is necessary to properly interpret any result. This information must either be accurately provided with laboratory requests or obtained by TDM service personnel. Unless the ordering professional is thoroughly familiar with PK and analytical principles, all drug concentrations should include an individualized PK interpretation.[53–57] For several drug classes, the use of population models and the application of Bayesian optimization algorithms have been shown to be a clinically useful and cost-effective way to provide such interpretations.[29,58] These algorithms are quite different from dosing nomograms, which are used to predict "average" or initial doses in various populations.

REACTIONARY THERAPEUTIC DRUG MONITORING

Many clinical laboratories offer some form of TDM menu. However, test results are commonly reported as "numbers only" (i.e., without PK-appropriate interpretation), in a similar manner as general chemistry test results are reported (result with a reference range). This type of reporting is misleading and does not optimally use what is known about the drug's PK characteristics. As opposed to most endogenous compounds, drug concentrations are not stable over time and are governed by known and predictable PK principles. In addition, more in-depth interpretations (i.e., PK consultation), with the possible exception of aminoglycosides and vancomycin, are seldom offered. As a result, dose adjustments frequently are made on an ad hoc basis relying on one or more "numbers" (i.e., concentration measurements) that are within or outside a "therapeutic range." This can best be described as "reactionary TDM," where a standard dose is administered, and a concentration is checked to verify whether it is "therapeutic." The process is often toxicity driven; if the concentration is "toxic" (i.e., above the "therapeutic range"), the dose will be empirically lowered, and the concentration will be checked again. If "subtherapeutic," the dose may be empirically increased, with measurements being repeated until "therapeutic." If the first measurement is within the therapeutic range, things are considered "okay," and no further action is taken. It is obvious that such reactionary TDM does not take into consideration PK principles or the full concentration–time profile, individual PK/PD differences, time to attain steady state, or patient-specific PD targets. It does not lead to efficient use of resources and has not been shown to produce optimal outcomes. However, many studies have documented that proper PK/PD guidance, but not "reactionary TDM," is effective.[58] Such guidance can improve overall use of resources and produce better and more cost-efficient outcomes, fewer inappropriately drawn samples, more concentrations within the desired range, fewer dose adjustments, and reduction in the incidence of adverse events.[58–60]

MODEL-INFORMED PRECISION DOSING

To overcome the shortcomings of reactionary TDM, the implementation of population PK/PD model–based prediction and the application of Bayesian adaptive control have been advocated as clinically useful strategies and cost-effective ways to improve precision dosing and rapid target attainment. It is of interest to note that the model-based approaches using Bayesian estimation were pioneered in the late seventies but never found the broad clinical acceptance they deserved.[61,62] In recent years, with the advent of more powerful and easier-to-use software tools, renewed interest has been sparked for the implementation of model-based therapeutic optimization and clinical pharmacometrics.[4] Such strategy and approach to therapeutic optimization is now being coined as "model-informed precision dosing" (MIPD) and is part of a wider context of precision medicine.[63] MIPD is designed to identify optimal dosage regimens in a particular patient(s) using statistical and/or mathematical models representing drug responses, including individual PK/PD. MIPD provides a quantitative framework to use prior experience accumulated from previous patients and/or subjects who participated in clinical trials for dose optimization in a current and future patient. As part of the TDM process, MIPD is particularly useful for both *a priori* TDM (initial dosage regimen optimization based on identifiable patient characteristics) and *a posteriori* TDM (real-time dose individualization based on measurements, such as drug concentrations and response biomarkers) (see later discussion and examples). MIPD can provide an important extension of TDM. Application of PK/PD models that relate drug exposure to changes in biomarkers (whether microbiologic, immunologic, neoplastic, neurologic, or other) and ultimately to clinical outcomes will provide a better rationale for proper individualized dose selection and other therapeutic interventions in multiple patient populations.

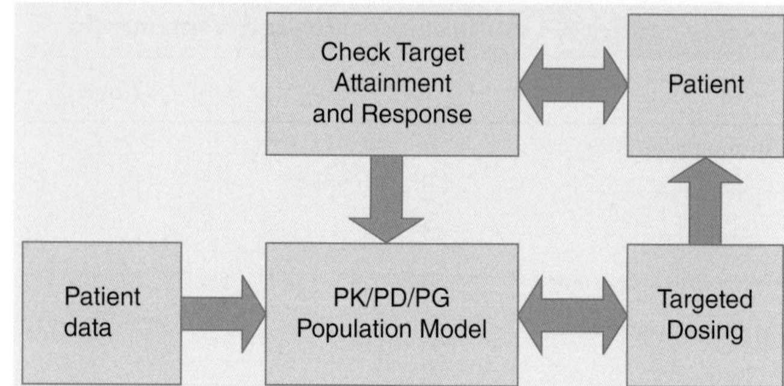

Figure 7.2 Flow diagram of the goal-oriented, model-informed strategy. A computer program is used with a patient-specific population model describing absorption, distribution, and elimination of the drug in relation to patient-specific parameters. Patient data and desired target concentrations are entered into the system. Next, a model-based loading dose and maintenance dosing regimen required to optimally achieve the target concentrations is selected. This regimen is administered to the patient, and subsequent concentration measurements and clinical effect observations are used as feedback to update the initial model and design a new dosing regimen if necessary. PD, pharmacodynamic; PG, pharmacogenetic; PK, pharmacokinetic.

BAYESIAN FORECASTING

Bayesian forecasting is derived from Bayes' theorem and is based on the concept that prior PK knowledge of a drug, in the form of a population model, can be combined with individual patient data, such as drug concentrations (Bayesian feedback)[4,31,64,65] (Table 7.3). The idea is to make an individualized model of the behavior of the drug in a particular patient to see how the drug will be or has been handled and to obtain the necessary information to make rational dose adjustments so as to best achieve the selected target goal(s).

Figure 7.2 shows a diagram of the goal-oriented, model-informed optimization process. Drug dosage optimization requires (a) population PK parameters (PK model), defined as mean values, standard deviations, covariates, and information on the statistical distribution necessary to select the initial dosing regimen for that particular patient based on chosen goals; (b) measurement of a performance index related to the therapeutic goal, generally one or more plasma concentrations or effects as feedback information to update the system; and (c) availability of reliable software for an adaptive control strategy [maximum a posteriori probability (*MAP*) Bayesian fitting] and calculation of the subsequent optimal dosage regimen.

Figure 7.3 illustrates an example of the use of a population MIPD with Bayesian feedback. This process was successfully implemented in a concentration-controlled clinical study of sirolimus in pediatric patients with acute lymphoblastic leukemia.[66] First, a population model–based predicted concentration profile is generated based on patient-specific dosing data and body weight as a covariate of clearance and volume of distribution (Fig. 7.3A). Next, individual PK parameter estimates are generated using Bayesian estimation based on the measured concentrations (Fig. 7.3B). Lastly, the dosing regimen(s) to best attain the concentration target is identified based on simulation using the individual PK parameters (Fig. 7.3C). In this trial, the initial

TABLE 7.3 Flow Scheme for Bayesian Goal-Oriented, Model-Informed Dosing

Bayes Theorem	Prior probability	→ New information	→ Consider prior and new information	→ Posterior probability	→ Therapeutic goals	→ Control
PK/PD Model–Informed Guidance	Population model	→ Drug concentration, biomarker data	→ Objective function	→ Individual model	→ Look at patient. Set your goals and targets	→ Calculate new dosing regimen

PD, pharmacodynamic; PK, pharmacokinetic.
Data from Jelliffe RW, Schumitzky A, Bayard D, et al. Model-based, goal-oriented, individualised drug therapy. Linkage of population modelling, new 'multiple model' dosage design, Bayesian feedback and individualised target goals. *Clin Pharmacokinet* 1998;34:57–77.

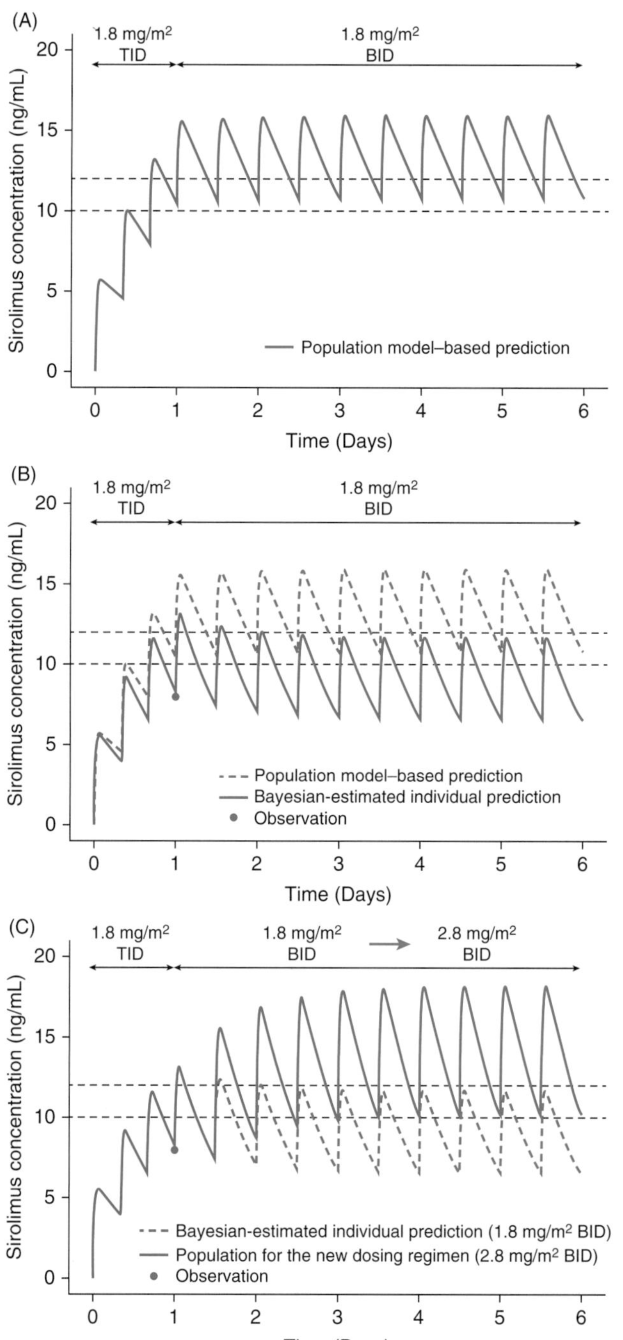

Figure 7.3 The process of Bayesian adaptive precision dosing. **A:** The concentration–time profile represents population model–based prediction for an average patient treated with the initial loading (1.8 mg per m^2 per dose three times daily) and maintenance doses (1.8 mg per m^2 per dose twice daily). Dashed lines indicate the target trough concentration range of 10 to 12 ng per mL. **B:** The concentration–time profile (solid line) represents the individual pharmacokinetic (PK) profile estimates generated using Bayesian estimation based on the measured concentration(s) (closed circle). The predicted trough concentrations are below the target of 10 ng per mL, suggesting that the patient needs a higher dose to attain the target concentration. **C:** The concentration–time profile (solid line) represents the individual's predicted PK profile with the new dosing regimen (2.8 mg per m^2 per dose twice daily) identified based on simulations using the individual PK parameters. (Reused from Mizuno T, O'Brien MM, Vinks AA. Significant effect of infection and food intake on sirolimus pharmacokinetics and exposure in pediatric patients with acute lymphoblastic leukemia. *Eur J Pharm Sci* 2019;128:209–214 with permission from Elsevier.)

loading and maintenance doses were identified based on the population PK model–based simulation using the pediatric sirolimus PK model.

Bayesian methods can be more cost-effective than other techniques because they require fewer drug measurements for individual PK parameter estimation. They can also handle sparse, random and distribution phase samples.[67] TDM, when applied appropriately, can also be used to detect and quantify clinically relevant drug–drug or drug–diet interactions[68,69] as well as medication errors.

However, regardless of which PK dose individualization technique is being used, all are superior to a simple reactionary comparison of a reported result to a "therapeutic range." Simply reporting results as "numbers" that are below, within, or above a published range is usually uninformative, not cost saving, and can lead to inappropriate or even dangerous actions.

REAL-TIME DOSE INDIVIDUALIZATION WITH BAYESIAN ADAPTIVE CONTROL

Real-time MIPD can refer to the direct prospective implementation of M&S in a patient care setting based on real-time feedback about the patient, such as drug concentrations or biomarker effect data.[63] The approach can be particularly useful for treatments requiring continuous monitoring of efficacy/toxicity to control for variability in drug response. Large interindividual PK variability (variability between patients) has been documented for many drugs. This variability is incorporated in many useful population PK models. Intraindividual variability (the variability in the same patient), however, is equally important, especially when interpreting TDM data during lifelong treatments, such as for epilepsy, transplantation, and HIV/AIDS patients. Causes of intraindividual PK variability have not all been systematically studied but can be attributed to temporary changes in physiology, drug absorption, enterohepatic recycling, or, sometimes, as part of the clinical noise in the system. Population model–based methods, with the additional use of a graphical presentation of the concentration–time profile, can be of great help in the clinical management of patients. It can also identify outliers, patients with unusual PK and other candidates who would benefit from more intensive monitoring.

Figure 7.4 shows an example of MIPD process that was implemented in the concentration-controlled phase 2 sirolimus study in pediatric patients with complicated vascular anomalies.[70,71] The process includes data on patient visits and PK sample collection, sample shipment, and the specific assay used to measure blood concentrations. It generates interpretative reports for assay results and a final model-based dosing recommendation. In this study, sirolimus was initiated at a dose of 0.8 mg per m^2 twice a day (BID). Subsequent dosing was individually adjusted using the drug concentration measurements in combination with population model–based Bayesian forecasting to target a sirolimus trough concentration of 10 to 15 ng per mL. The first sirolimus blood concentration was measured at 8 to 14 days after start of treatment. This was followed by weekly measurements throughout the rest of the 28-day treatment course. During subsequent courses, sirolimus concentrations were measured weekly until stable, which was defined as two subsequent concentration results within the target range. After any dose modification, subsequent sirolimus concentrations were measured every 7 to 14 days until stable. During the study, patients kept a dosing diary, recording exact dosing times and

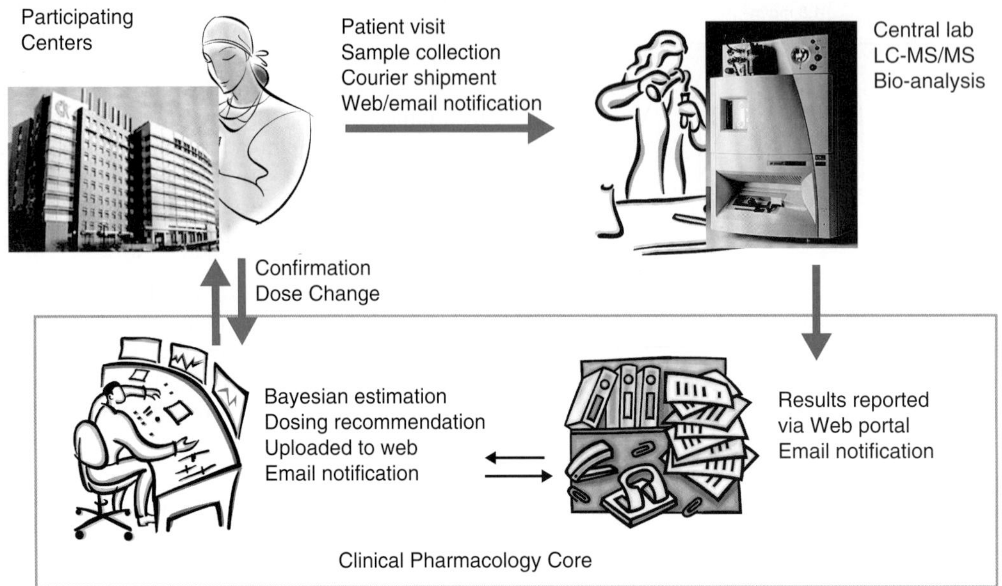

Figure 7.4 Outline of the different steps in the sirolimus precision dosing process from patient visit and sampling, sample shipment, analysis, reporting of assay results, and the final communication of the model-based dosing recommendations. (Reused from Mizuno T, Emoto C, Fukuda T, et al. Model-based precision dosing of sirolimus in pediatric patients with vascular anomalies. *Eur J Pharm Sci* 2017;109S:S124–S131 with permission from Elsevier.)

any missed doses for 5 days before each visit. This diary was reviewed before the drawing of blood for sirolimus concentration measurements to document adherence and provided the actual dosing time information for the PK assessments.

Figure 7.5 shows representative examples of the model-based predictions and dosing recommendations reported for patients in the concentration-controlled phase 2 sirolimus study.[70,71] The profile depicted in Figure 7.5A represents the concentration–time data for a 3-year-old male patient (11.9 kg, 90.5 cm, 0.54 m^2) with a kaposiform hemangioendothelioma who was started on 0.8 mg per m^2 BID. The first sirolimus concentration was 4.9 ng per mL after which the dose was increased to 0.9 mg BID (1.67 mg per m^2) and eventually to 1.3 mg BID (2.4 mg per m^2). Figure 7.5B shows the sirolimus concentration–time course for a 2-month-old patient born with a congenital lymphaticovenous malformation who received sirolimus in the neonatal intensive care unit (NICU). This 2-month-old (4.7 kg, 52 cm, 0.24 m^2) was started on 0.2 mg BID (also 0.8 mg per m^2). The first sirolimus concentration came back as 22 ng per mL after which the dose was empirically reduced by 50% (2 days later) and another sirolimus measurement was ordered. The second sirolimus concentration result was 27 ng per mL after which subsequent doses were held. A PK consult was performed, and a new maintenance dose regimen of 0.06 mg (0.25 mg per m^2) was suggested. A loading dose (0.2 mg) was also suggested based on the model-based simulation to reachieve the rapid target attainment. After this loading dose, the new regimen provided sirolimus concentrations that remained on target. This baby had a clearance of 3.4 L per h per 70 kg; approximately 35% lower than the median predicted clearance for a newborn of this age. Based on a maturation model, sirolimus clearance was predicted to increase by 50% over the next month, requiring a dose increase to 0.09 mg BID.

TABLE 7.4 Practical Problems in Neonatal and Pediatric Therapeutic Drug Monitoring
Sample collection—access, volume, skin contamination, line or catheter draws
Interference—maternal (Cr, DLIS, maternal Rx)
Altered metabolic patterns as well as rates
Dietary differences, fasting, stomach emptying, gastrointestinal transit-prolonged release, inappropriate dosage alteration
Position or infusion apparatus changes
Administration uncertainty—cooperation, spillage, measurement, extemporaneous formulation, inappropriate concentrations, measurement errors
Analytical differences (e.g., phenobarbital glucuronide interference missed in adult samples)
Day-to-day variation—weight, pharmacokinetics
Intravenous administration problems, no dose or sample before dose

Cr, serum creatinine; DLIS, digoxin-like immunoreactive substances; maternal Rx, maternal drug therapy.

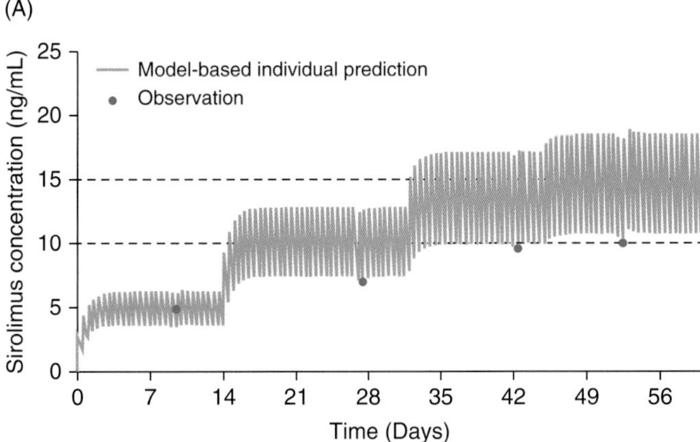

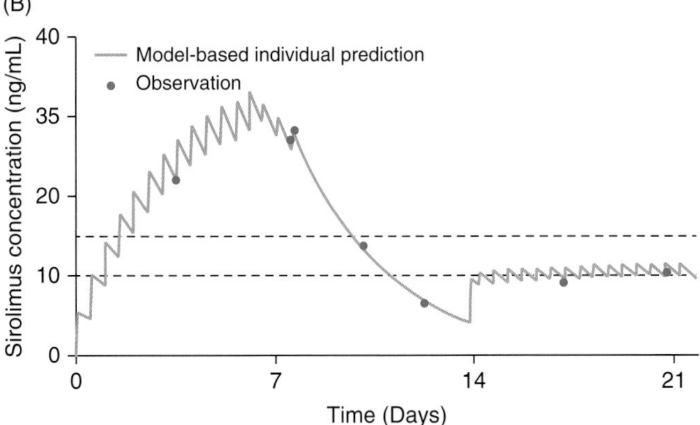

Figure 7.5 Reporting of model-based pharmacokinetic (PK) profiles during the clinical trial and as part of off-label treatment with subsequent dosing recommendations. This 3-year-old male patient was enrolled, and sirolimus dosing was initiated at a dose of 0.8 mg per m^2 twice a day. **A:** The model predicted concentration–time profile resulting from the subsequent recommended dose increases (0.9, 1.2, and 1.3 mg twice daily) based on the measured sirolimus concentrations (closed circles) are shown. **B:** The sirolimus concentration–time profile of a 2-month-old baby who was started on 0.8 mg per m^2 twice a day. The dose was reduced by 50% after the first sirolimus result came back (22 ng per mL), and another concentration was checked. As the second blood concentration was higher than the first (27 ng per mL), subsequent doses were held, and another PK evaluation was performed based on the measured sirolimus concentrations (closed circles). After a loading dose, subsequent sirolimus concentrations were on target. (Reused from Mizuno T, Emoto C, Fukuda T, et al. Model-based precision dosing of sirolimus in pediatric patients with vascular anomalies. *Eur J Pharm Sci* 2017;109S:S124–S131 with permission from Elsevier.)

OVERCOMING PRACTICAL PROBLEMS IN NEONATAL AND PEDIATRIC THERAPEUTIC DRUG MONITORING

INCOMPLETE INFORMATION FOR INTERPRETATION OF THE DOSE–CONCENTRATION–EFFECT RELATIONSHIP

Unfortunately, incorrect sample collection, handling, or analysis as well as improper interpretation of results can diminish the clinical value of TDM results and have negative clinical and economic implications. This can, and has, lead to incorrect attitudes about the usefulness of TDM. There are multiple studies showing that, when properly ordered, assayed, and interpreted, TDM can often be useful in all patients and is always useful in specific clinical situations.[17] Although there are few studies of the cost-effectiveness of TDM, those that have been done have shown very positive results.[58,59,72–76] When poorly done, TDM can be useless or even harmful.

Despite the fact that TDM concepts are relatively simple, most laboratories are not set up to perform the necessary data collection that would allow unambiguous clinical interpretation of drug concentration measurements.[77] For instance, simple information such as the time of sampling in relation to the time of last dose needs to be known to properly interpret the result. In addition, demographic data (date of birth, weight, height), route of administration, and dosing regimen (time and dates of recent intake, duration of use, whether loading doses were given, concomitant medications taken) should also be available. Additional factors that may influence proper TDM interpretation are summarized in Table 7.4. Over the years, institutions have struggled with ways of collecting and reporting this type of information. In the outpatient setting, a useful method to collect these data is the use of a questionnaire administered by laboratory staff or filled out by the patients, parents, or guardians while waiting for phlebotomy. Figure 7.6 shows an example of a questionnaire that has been successfully used in a PK consult service at the author's institutions.[78] The TDM system should be set up in such a way that information from the questionnaire is processed with the test request and ultimately reported in a user-friendly format. An important item on this questionnaire is space for patient, parent, or guardian feedback on any issues related to medication effects. This is a valuable tool for adverse event monitoring as well as documenting therapeutic response.

ADHERENCE AND VARIATIONS IN PHARMACOKINETICS ARE DIFFICULT TO CONTROL

In an outpatient setting, nonadherence can represent a major problem in patient management.[79] TDM can contribute to detecting nonadherence, although this will be dependent on the clearance of the drug. For instance, skipping doses and only taking medication shortly before a visit may not be obvious for highly cleared drugs but will result in much lower-than-expected concentrations for more slowly eliminated drugs. Metabolite profiles, when measured, will almost always change and be indicative for poor or nonadherence. For inpatients, poor adherence should not be an issue, but can occur, and inaccurate recording of the timing of the dose in relation to the blood draw may result in confusion and mistakes. For instance, samples drawn supposedly as "peaks" but actually taken before the actual dose was given will give lower-than-expected results and may sometimes have people question adherence, whereas a PK consult would clearly predict the measured concentration when assuming a "missed" dose. Over adherence, such as in drug overdose, can also be identified.

DETERMINATION OF UNBOUND CONCENTRATIONS OF DRUGS

Typically, in routine TDM, total drug concentrations (protein bound and unbound or "free") are measured. Because only the unbound concentration can diffuse to the extracellular and

TABLE 7.5 Menu for Pediatric Therapeutic Drug Management[a]

Drug	*Target Range*	*Comments*
Antiepileptic drugs[5,18,19]		
Carbamazepine	4–9 mg/L	More favorable adverse events profile; has active CBZ-10,11-epoxide metabolite; autoinduction and in combination with other AEDs
Ethosuximide	40–100 mg/L	Treatment of absence (petit mal) seizures; poorly established concentration–effect relationship
Phenobarbital	20–40 mg/L	Negative effects on cognitive and psychomotor function; relatively slow clearance; half-life 4–5 d in neonate and $\sim$2 d in children; inactive glucuronide metabolite may accumulate in newborn. Ranges differ for seizure prophylaxis, for treatment of hyperbilirubinemia (undetectable), and sedation. Long-term treatment leads to tolerance causing the concentration–effect relationship to change over time.
Phenytoin	5–20 mg/L	Concentration-dependent elimination; slower elimination at high concentrations; highly protein bound; free level monitoring useful in specific cases
Primidone	5–12 mg/L	Metabolized to phenobarbital
Valproic acid	50–100 mg/L	Complex concentration–effect relation; several drug–drug interactions with other AEDs
Antibiotics[5,92]		
Gentamicin	MDD: >5–10 mg/L peak <1–2 mg/L trough >20 mg/L peak ODD: <0.1–0.5 mg/L	Use short courses; preferably maximal duration of therapy 5–7 d; toxicity may occur despite therapeutic drug management
Tobramycin	MMD: >5–10 mg/L peak <1–2 mg/L trough ODD: >20 mg/L peak <0.1–0.5 mg/L	Better intrinsic activity against *Pseudomonas aeruginosa* use short courses; preferably maximal duration of therapy 5–7 d; toxicity may occur despite therapeutic drug management
Vancomycin	<10–15 mg/L trough 20–40 mg/L peak	Rapid infusion may give "red man" syndrome; increased toxicity when combined with aminoglycoside
Immunosuppressants		Ranges depend on time post-transplant as well as transplant organ (kidney, liver, heart, or bone marrow)
Cyclosporine	100–200 µg/L (trough)	Target *AUC*[174]: <D30: 6.0 ± 2.2; D30–M3: 5.5 ± 1.7; M3–1 y: 4.7 ± 1.2; >1 y: 3.8 ± 1.0 mg/h/L In pediatric patients, ranges have been reported as: <M30: 7.4 ± 2.4; D30–1 y: 5.2 ± 1.4; >1 y: 3.9 ± 1.2 mg/h/L
Sirolimus	4–12 µg/L (with CsA) 10–20 µg/L (without CsA)	No *AUC* target consensus range has been established yet.[123,175]
Tacrolimus	5–20 µg/L	Target *AUC*[125,176]: First week post-transplantation: 0.15–0.21 mg/h/L Long term: 0.12–0.15 mg/h/L
Mycophenolic acid	1–3.5 mg/L	Target *AUC*[52,177]: 30–60 mg/h/L
Mycophenolic acid glucuronide	35–100 mg/L	
Miscellaneous[5]		
Caffeine	5–15 mg/L	Prevention of apneas in premature neonates
Digoxin	0.8–2.0 µg/L	Concentration–effect relationship with peripheral compartment; detection of accumulation in renal compromised patient; endogenous digoxin-like immunoreactive substances are present in neonates and may interfere with assay
Methotrexate	Depends on therapeutic regimen	Light sensitive; protect sample from daylight
Theophylline	5–20 mg/L	Saturation kinetics; *Note 1*: methylation to caffeine in neonate will lead to two active drugs—theophylline and caffeine. Depending on the assay method, only one will be detected and reported[122] *Note 2*: Target range depends on condition (asthma requires much lower concentrations than apnea)[123,124]

[a]This table is included as an example of what a basic TDM service could provide in terms of routine assays. For more comprehensive service overview, the reader is referred to the following websites: http://www.clinchem.med.uni-goettingen.de/downloads/Referenzwerte-2008_06_25.pdf; http://www.umcg.nl/Professionals/dienstverlening/85932/157322/Pages/Default.aspx

AED, antiepileptic drug; *AUC*, area under the curve; CBZ, carbamazepine; CsA, cyclosporin A (cyclosporine); D30, first 30 d post-transplantation; D30–M3, 30 d to 3 mo post-transplant; MDD, multiple-daily dosing (dosing interval, 8 or 12 h); ODD, once-daily dosing.

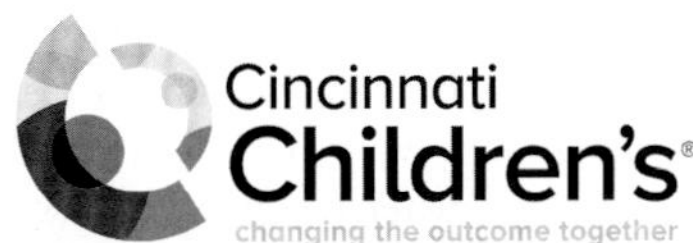

Division of Clinical Pharmacology
Sirolimus PK consult from

PATIENT INFORMATION	Visit 1	Visit 2	Visit 3
Patient Name (or subject ID)			
Gender			
Date of Birth (or age)			
Race			
Weight (most recent) kg			
Height (most recent) cm			
DOSING DATA			
Start of Therapy (or date of last dose adjustment)			
Dosing Regimen (mg)			
Number of doses per day			
Date of last sirolimus dose			
Time of last sirolimus dose			
Regular time of sirolimus doses			
In the past 2 days has the dosing varied by greater than 1 hour from typical timing:			
Any missed doses in past 5 days			
BLOOD LEVEL INFORMATION			
Date Sample obtained			
Time pre-dose sample obtained			
Time 1HR-post sample obtained			
Time 3HR-post sample obtained			
Pre-dose test result (ng/mL)			
1HR-post test result (ng/mL)			
3HR-post test result (ng/mL)			
Current target trough concentration (ng/mL)			
CONCOMITANT DRUGS			
1			
2			
3			
4			
5			
OTHER CONDITIONS			
Any suspected infection?			
Any toxicity/drug related adverse events?			
Hematocrit (%)			

Figure 7.6 Questionnaire that has been successfully used in an antiepileptic therapeutic drug management service at Cincinnati Children's Hospital Medical Center

intracellular space to exert its pharmacologic action, measurement of unbound concentrations may be of value for highly protein-bound drugs, for example, phenytoin (~90%), valproic acid (~90%), and, possibly, carbamazepine (~75%). Changes in unbound concentration may be the result of hypoalbuminemia, displacement due to endogenous compounds (such as bilirubin), or a drug–drug interaction (e.g., phenytoin–valproic acid). Several methods are available to measure unbound concentrations even in microsamples. Some of the reasons to measure unbound concentrations as well as some problems with interpretation are given in a later discussion of phenytoin. A TDM service should be helpful in deciding which patients would benefit from unbound measurements, but clinicians should consider such monitoring for drugs with high binding, especially if there is clinical suspicion of abnormal binding protein concentrations, including albumin and α acid glycoprotein.

SUGGESTIONS FOR MODEL-INFORMED THERAPEUTIC DRUG MANAGEMENT: A TEAM APPROACH

Proper TDM requires cooperation among informed patients or parents/caregivers and skilled nursing, pharmacy, medical, and laboratory staff. It is best done by a team approach with everyone involved helping to provide accurate information; proper sample collection, handling, and analysis; proper interpretation; as well as correct clinical response and follow-up.[80] The best computed PK/PD modeling and interpretation cannot overcome inaccurate information or incorrect laboratory analysis. The most accurate laboratory analysis is not useful without all the necessary information, proper interpretation, and appropriate clinical response and follow-up. The most cost-efficient, clinically effective TDM will result when all members of the health care team (and this should include patients and their parents/guardians as well) are familiar with, and provide, what is necessary to properly collect, analyze, interpret, and follow up drug concentration measurements.

There are a number of components of an effective pediatric PK consultation or therapeutic drug management service. Table 7.5 presents the drugs that should be routinely monitored. Most of these drugs have reasonably well-established concentration–effect and adverse events relationships. The suggested target concentration ranges are not to be viewed as "fixed," but rather as a useful starting point in a new patient. Several drugs and important drug classes have not been included because their assay is not readily available or because there is no consensus on the clinical utility of routine TDM. For instance, we have not included HIV drugs such as the protease inhibitors, as additional pediatric data are needed to establish child-specific reference values and to assess the optimal method of TDM.[23,81] Yet, TDM is considered a useful tool in the treatment of HIV-infected children. TDM has clearly been useful in individual patients, including those with poor adherence or who experience unexpected toxic side effects.[82] Also not included are antifungal[83] and drugs routinely used in pediatric oncology.[84] These drugs are, however, rapidly becoming part of TDM menus and should be more commonly monitored/managed in the near future.

GENTAMICIN AND OTHER ANTIBIOTICS

For decades, TDM of the aminoglycosides (gentamicin, tobramycin, amikacin, and netilmicin) has been primarily focused on avoiding potential nephrotoxicity and ototoxicity.[5] With intermittent dosing (e.g., every 8 hours or every 12 hours), a trough concentration of 2 mg per L is broadly used as the cutoff point above which toxicity is likely to occur, although good clinical evidence-based studies are lacking.[85] In addition, it must be realized that aminoglycoside-related toxicity typically develops slowly and that reducing the duration of exposure to a maximum of 7 to 10 days will reduce the incidence of adverse events.[86,87] Few early studies documented clinically effective concentrations, which resulted in the commonly used 5 to 10 mg per L postdose target concentrations.[88,89] However, later better understanding of the PD of aminoglycosides has shifted focus to optimizing efficacy as well.[90,91] The new paradigm for this class of "concentration-dependent" drugs is to achieve rapid bacterial killing with as high as possible initial concentrations. The new target concentrations include high peak concentrations (i.e., ten times the *MIC*) and virtually nondetectable trough concentrations. These targets can be achieved with once-daily dosing regimens, where the traditional total daily dose is given in one dose instead of as multiple doses. Other even more extended intervals have also been used. The transition to higher doses given less frequently is ongoing and has generated ongoing discussion about whether to keep using the well-established peak-and-trough monitoring concept, which is still being used in many institutions, or to go back to less informative midpoint nomogram methods or trough-only strategies for the sake of simplicity.[92] The traditional dosing interval in newborns and children is every 8 to 12 hours, but once-daily dosing is also now being used in the pediatric population.[93,94] Much of the increased efficacy of once-daily dosing arises because it results in less underdosing of seriously ill patients. It was not generally appreciated that such children were underdosed because of the much higher (0.5 to 1.0 L per kg) volumes of distribution (V_d) aminoglycosides have in septic adults and children. Giving a single 5 mg per kg dose is the only way to achieve 10 mg per L concentrations in someone with a V_d = 0.5 L per kg. Renal patients were also often underdosed when given usual doses. This underdosing was the result of not understanding the difference between low clearance and high V_d in renal patients. Clearance determines the interval needed between doses. Whereas the V_d determines how much should be given to achieve a given concentration. We have seen renal patients given only 1 mg per kg gentamicin "because they have slow clearance." This is not a problem if the patient is not septic, but a fatal mistake if the patient is really infected, especially with more resistant bacteria as demonstrated by Moore et al. many years ago.[89] Although a number of studies in adults have reported equivalent efficacy and equal or less toxicity with once-daily dosing, this approach has not yet become standard of practice in all hospitals treating pediatric patients. Limited clinical and efficacy data in children and the difference in PK (e.g., higher clearance) are among the reasons for lack of general acceptance.[95] As a result of several recent studies, the extended interval-dosing concept has received much broader acceptance in specific pediatric populations, such as neonates and patients with cystic fibrosis.[96–101] In our view, aminoglycosides are particularly suited for PK model–based monitoring using aminoglycoside concentration-predicted clearance, serum creatinine, or creatinine clearance PK methods.[102] This will also require (as mentioned previously) that "therapeutic ranges" be adjusted so that they are specific for the dosing regimen used. If the goal is to truly individualize therapy, then a TDM strategy should be adopted that will enable this to occur. This is not the case when nomograms are implemented. Recently, efficacy of MIPD has been established for aminoglycosides in very young pediatric populations[103–105] and obese patients.[106,107] For instance, a model-based dosing regimen was developed using an amikacin PK model in preterm and term neonates.[105] The developed dosing regimen has been prospectively evaluated.[104] Similar strategies have been implemented for vancomycin[45] and other antibiotics[108] in infants and children.

Bacterial *MIC*s have been used for years to individualize drug concentration targets, such as peaks, troughs, and *AUC*s. A similar method is being used for other infectious agents, such as viruses and fungi. Pharmacogenetics offers the promise of individualizing patient-specific targets as well. For example, genetic predisposition to aminoglycoside ototoxicity has been well described.[109] Studies are beginning to demonstrate that determination of individual susceptibility can be used to predict and eventually prevent both drug- and patient-specific toxicity. For aminoglycoside ototoxicity, susceptibility is transmitted by maternal mitochondrial DNA. It should, therefore, be possible to predict or prevent such toxicity by maternal testing and altering maternal or newborn dosing or exposure.

ANTIEPILEPTIC DRUGS

Antiepileptic drugs (AEDs) have been monitored since the 1950s and are some of the medications for which TDM is most commonly used.[18,19] The marketing of 18 new AEDs to the epilepsy treatment armamentarium since 1989 has led to increasingly widespread implementation of TDM in AED therapy.[19] Indeed, a recent review article indicated that TDM is now performed for the 27 AEDs approved for the treatment of epilepsy, which are also used for a number of other medical conditions such as bipolar disorder and pain.[19] TDM is well established and important in the clinical management of epilepsy because (a) plasma AED concentrations are correlated better than dose with efficacy, (b) assessment of therapeutic response is difficult in most cases as AED treatment is prophylactic and there are no laboratory markers for clinical efficacy of AEDs, (c) AEDs exhibit substantial PK variability that results in the highly variable dosages among patients, and (d) the ranges of therapeutic plasma concentrations have been defined for most AEDs based on population data, summarizing the exposure–response relationships observed in clinical studies.[19] These AED reference ranges are generally useful for the majority patients; however, the optimal therapeutic target may be different in some patients due to variability in disease severity, seizure type, the use of multiple AEDs, and individual sensitivity to the drug(s). In most cases, the total concentration (both protein bound and unbound) is being analyzed for TDM; however, it is suggested that the free concentration is more suitable for some patients, especially for those who exhibit an irregular protein-binding profile (e.g., pregnant patients and patients after surgery) and who are taking highly protein-bound AEDs (e.g., phenytoin carbamazepine and valproic acid).[19] When an AED is displaced from its binding sites, the amount of unbound and pharmacologic active drug increases, whereas the total concentration may stay the same or go down as a result of increased metabolism and elimination. Thus, published therapeutic ranges cannot necessarily be applied in case of patients with a protein binding different from that of the population used to generate these ranges. Alternative sample matrices and assay methodologies including dried blood sport (DBS) and saliva have been increasingly studied for managing AEDs. Population PK/PD model–based approaches have been evaluated for many AEDs to control for the large interindividual variability in drug disposition and response.[110] In a publication, van Dijkman et al.[111] proposed dosing regimens developed with model-based simulations for 11 commonly used AEDs in both adults and children. The authors indicated that the AED target concentrations are unlikely to be attained without the use of dosing algorithms and individualized dosing recommendations, given the large PK variability. The model-based dosing algorithms in conjunction with TDM have the advantage of being able to personalize and optimize treatments.[111] It has also been shown that the toxicity of some AEDs is associated with specific, identifiable genetic characteristics. This provides a way to avoid some concentration-dependent as well as concentration-independent AED toxicities. Pharmacogenetic differences in both causes of epilepsy as well as AED targets (e.g., transporters or receptors) are playing an increasing role in the design of more personalized AED therapy, but this topic is beyond the scope of this chapter.

IMMUNOSUPPRESSANTS

One of the most rapidly advancing areas in TDM in recent years has been the measurement of immunosuppressive drugs used to avert rejection of transplanted organs.[112–115] Cyclosporine has been available and routinely measured for over 20 years. Despite the fact that its concentration–effect relationship is not well established, clear associations have been made between predose or trough cyclosporine concentration (C_0) monitoring and clinical end points. In recent years, there have been major changes in cyclosporine TDM with the advent of *AUC* and especially C_2 monitoring strategies.[116–118] Bayesian methods have shown great potential and allow more flexible sampling.[74,119,120] Trough (C_0) monitoring of tacrolimus has also been well established. However, there appears to be an emerging consensus that tacrolimus, too, may benefit from alternatives to C_0 monitoring. MPA was originally marketed as "not requiring monitoring." However, the evidence supports the benefits of MPA TDM as well,[20,121] as illustrated by a consensus document on the routine monitoring of MPA published by The Transplantation Society (TTS) Consensus Group on TDM of MPA in 2010.[52] Sirolimus monitoring has fewer sampling time issues because there is a reasonable relationship between C_0 and *AUC*. The most optimal way to establish immunosuppressant dose–exposure relationships is by using Bayesian estimation with a limited sampling strategy.[122] The limitations for routine TDM of immunosuppressants are the current lack of a reliable immunoassays, metabolite activity, and interferences.[123] This is especially relevant in children, as developmental changes may result in different age-dependent metabolite patterns. For instance, the metabolism of sirolimus in children is very different from that reported in adults. This should be considered when monitoring sirolimus exposure using immunoassays, as metabolite cross-reactivity issues may interfere with assay accuracy and influence interpretation of results.[124] Tacrolimus drug monitoring has been used in solid-organ transplantation for many years. The latest consensus document on tacrolimus TDM was published by the Immunosuppressive Drugs Scientific Committee of the IATDMCT in 2019.[125] The relationship between tacrolimus exposure and the risk of acute rejection and drug-related adverse events has been well documented. Although *AUC* is considered the PK exposure parameter best associated with clinical effects, no prospective studies of clinical outcomes have been conducted in adult or pediatric transplant recipients to properly investigate the potential benefits of *AUC* monitoring compared with C_0-guided therapy.[125] Therefore, predose trough concentration is still being monitored in most transplant centers for routine tacrolimus TDM.

HIV THERAPY

HIV therapy has much to gain from properly applied TDM.[126–128] Protease inhibitor monitoring can be an especially valuable tool as part of therapeutic optimization as demonstrated by several groups, largely because even brief exposure of the virus to low protease concentrations is associated with rapid development of tolerance and poor therapeutic outcome. Additionally, exposure to excessive protease concentrations is associated with increased risk of toxicity. Measuring multiple protease concentrations can help clinicians identify causes of low (including "none detected") or excessive concentrations, leading to more effective and less toxic individualized dosing regimens, less resistance, better outcomes, fewer adverse effects, and some cost savings. In adult patients, suggested target concentration ranges have also been established for other antiretroviral drugs, such as non-nucleoside reverse transcriptase inhibitors (NNRTIs) and integrase strand transfer inhibitors (InSTIs).[129] More recently introduced antiretroviral drugs have broader therapeutic windows with improved benefit–risk ratios and reduced intersubject variability; thus, the need for TDM of these drugs is currently limited to specific clinical scenarios.[129] The dosing recommendations for HIV-infected children are not always uniform among regulatory agencies or HIV management guidelines as the current pediatric doses are often based on small sample size studies.[129]

NEUROPSYCHIATRIC DRUGS

The use of TDM in support of neuropsychopharmacology treatments has been increasing over the past few decades. The first TDM consensus guidelines in psychiatry were issued by the TDM task force of the working group on neuropsychopharmacology (Arbeitsgemeinschaft für Neuropsychopharmakologie und Pharmakopsychiatrie, AGNP) in 2004.[130] The guidelines were updated in 2011[131] and 2017.[22] For TDM in psychiatry, the regular monitoring of blood drug concentrations is recommended during maintenance therapy and at least every 3 to 6 months to prevent relapses and rehospitalizations, The frequency of TDM measurements may be increased in patients suspected of being nonadherent, when there are changes in comedications or when smoking is likely to affect the PK of the drugs prescribed. Reference therapeutic concentration ranges have been published for many psychopharmacological drugs (over 150 medications). The ranges for older drugs are based on clinical studies which documented the relationships between drug concentration and clinical improvement (e.g., lithium and tricyclic antidepressants).[22] These reference ranges were derived based on average population data and may not necessarily be applicable to all patients. Any individual patient may benefit from using a different therapeutic target, and treatment can best be further guided by identifying the exposure or concentration to which the patient best responds while adverse event free. It has also been suggested that the arithmetic mean and standard deviation of blood concentration in responders could be used as an initial therapeutic reference range or drugs for which further studies are needed to establish a range.

BIOLOGICS

In recent years, therapies with biologics, including monoclonal antibodies and therapeutic proteins, have had major impact on disease management and prevention, improving overall clinical outcomes in a large number of disease areas, especially in cancer, infectious diseases, and autoimmune-mediated inflammatory diseases. TDM has emerged as a potential useful tool to optimize the use of many biologic therapies. The benefits of TDM have been especially well demonstrated in inflammatory bowel diseases (IBD), including Crohn disease and ulcerative colitis.[24,25,132] Infliximab is a chimeric monoclonal antibody against tumor necrosis factor α (TNF-α) that was approved in 1998 by the U.S. Food and Drug Administration (FDA) for treatment of adult IBD and subsequently approved in 2006 for pediatric IBD patients. The labeled dose of infliximab is 5 mg per kg given at 0, 2, and 6 weeks followed by a maintenance dose of 5 mg per kg every 8 weeks. Primary response to infliximab induction therapy was reportedly achieved in 75% to 90% of pediatric patients with IBD.[133,134] However, over 30% of patients require dose intensifications because of the loss of initial response (LOR).[135] Multiple studies have documented the association of LOR with low infliximab trough concentrations during maintenance therapy in both adults[136–139] and in children.[140–142] A meta-analysis demonstrated that lower infliximab trough concentrations were found in nonremitters than in patients in clinical remission (0.9 mg per L vs. 3.1 mg per L).[143] IBD practice guidelines suggest a trough concentration of 3 to 10 mg per L as the target range for maintenance therapy.[144] In patients with infliximab concentrations below this target, dose escalation has been shown to result in a better clinical response rather than is changing to another anti-TNF therapy.[145] Recent studies have indicated that low drug exposure is also a risk factor for the development of antidrug antibodies (ADAs). ADAs are associated with an increased risk of infusion reactions and a reduced response to treatment.[146] In addition, there is substantial evidence that disease progression and worsening of inflammation increase infliximab clearance, which result in lower drug exposure.[147–153] Therefore, concentration monitoring and dose individualization of infliximab have been recommended to prevent subtherapeutic exposure and help with the achievement of a sustained and durable remission. Mould and colleagues developed a promising model-informed dosing strategy using Bayesian estimation for infliximab dose optimization.[154] Their Bayesian decision support tool is designed to integrate a population PK model with clinical TDM data to predict the individual patient's PK profile and the dose required to achieve the desired target concentration.

DRUG DETERMINATION IN ALTERNATIVE FLUIDS

Blood, either serum or plasma, has been the preferred biologic matrix for TDM.[155] However, a number of other fluids can and have been used, including tears, saliva, and urine.[156] In addition, transcutaneous and continuous microdialysis sampling techniques hold promise for the future, especially for small children, where sampling can be problematic.

FUTURE DEVELOPMENTS

A number of recent developments promise to improve the use and broader implementation of TDM. These include the development of therapeutic drug management teams, decision support tools that are integrated with the electronic medical record (EMR), cost-effectiveness studies, and emerging data on new drug classes, such as biologics, antifungal, antiviral, and anticancer drugs. TDM is also likely to become more effective and broadly applied with the implementation of advanced analytical techniques, such as less invasive microsampling devices, DBS technology, rapid drug quantification assays with paper spray ionization technology, and more sensitive liquid chromatography/tandem mass spectrometry, which can rapidly and reliably quantify a large number of drugs and metabolites simultaneously (e.g., metabolomics). The impact of these technologies will increase as the cost and complexity of the instrumentation decreases and their reliability increases. The high sensitivity of such methods promises to allow noninvasive (e.g., sweat, transcutaneous, or respiratory) real-time monitoring of multiple drug and metabolite concentrations simultaneously. When combined with stable isotope techniques, these techniques make it possible to also simultaneously measure absorption from multiple sites and quantify bioavailability in individual patients. Linkage of such advanced analytical techniques with powerful computer modeling, innovative wearable electronic devices, and drug sensors, along with patient management software including smartphone applications promises to revolutionize MIPD. Eventual linkage with individual pharmacogenetic and pharmacogenomic information, physiology- and mechanism-based PK/PD, and quantitative systems pharmacology platforms could revolutionize how individual patients are dosed, both initially and repetitively, prophylactically or therapeutically.[157,158]

As indicated, MIPD approaches have already been successfully used to personalize the drug treatment at the point of care in individual patients. However, those efforts are mostly confined to relatively few academic institutions and have not found broad application throughout the health care systems.[63] One of the biggest unmet needs which would facilitate the implementation of MIPD at the bedside is the development and verification of more user-friendly tools to integrate a patient's clinical information (e.g., dosing history, laboratory results, PK measurements) with PK/PD estimations to identify the optimal dosing regimen. Model-informed dose optimization uses patient-specific data that are predictive of the target drug's PK/PD in an individual. Standalone clinical TDM software application requires collection and manual entry of the clinical information into the program. This is often time-consuming, prone to errors, and not always feasible in clinical settings with limited resources. Given that clinical data as well as dosing histories are now documented in the EMR in many hospitals, leveraging the EMR as part of decision support systems should reduce the workload and time required to generate model-based precision dosing guidance. This would facilitate the availability of MIPD capabilities to all clinical care providers and increase the number of patients who would benefit from more precise, personalized drug treatment.

One of the first-generation integrated decision support tools for TDM was a "Dashboard" system developed by Barrett et al.[159] at the Children's Hospital of Philadelphia (CHOP) in the 2000s for the management of leucovorin rescue utilized for high-dose methotrexate (MTX) therapy in pediatric oncology patients. This MTX dashboard system was designed to integrate individual patient data from the medical record with a population PK model and then graphically display the most relevant clinical data needed for the management of methotrexate therapy. MTX plasma concentrations are used as feedback to generate the individual MTX PK profile which is depicted together with the leucovorin rescue nomogram to guide leucovorin dose intensity based on MTX concentration cutoffs. The dashboard forecasting algorithm was retrospectively evaluated and shown to be reasonably accurate in predicting MTX concentrations while facilitating leucovorin rescue dose management.[160] Another compelling example of a "dashboard" for children is the busulfan PK decision support tool recently developed by Abdel-Rahman et al.[161] at the Children's Mercy Hospital, Kansas City. Busulfan exhibits an NTI for which clinicians routinely employ TDM. Abdel-Rahman et al.[161] developed and tested a clinical decision support tool embedded in their EMR designed to streamline the TDM process. Patient and busulfan concentration results automatically populate the tool. Data are then visualized, fitted, and inspected utilizing color-coded indicators signaling goodness of fit. The tool provides clinicians the ability to seamlessly transition from patient assessment, to PK M&S, and subsequent prescription order entry. The usability of the tool was tested by 28 content experts as end users and produced a high level of satisfaction.[161] Another Bayesian dashboard system for biologics therapy was the previously mentioned first infliximab dashboard described by Mould et al.[154] for use in patients with IBD. A small cohort study demonstrated that patients dosed according to the Bayesian dashboard recommendations had longer disease remissions than did those dosed according to standard of care (51.5 months vs. 4.6 months).[162] Model-informed decision support tools have been utilized not only for PK but also for PK/PD-guided dose individualization. Hamberg et al.[163] developed a Bayesian decision support tool using a published warfarin PK/PD model in adult and pediatric patients. The tool is designed to estimate an initial dosage regimen based on patient's body weight, age, baseline, and target INR and optionally also including the presence of specific genetic variants of cytochrome P450 (CYP) 2C9 and vitamin K epoxide reductase (VKORC1). After institution of the model predicted optimal, individual starting dose, subsequent dosing regimens can be optimized using Bayesian, forecasting with INR results as feedback.

Another EMR-linked decision support platform for morphine precision dosing in neonates treated in an NICU was developed and implemented at Cincinnati Children's Hospital Medical Center.[164] This platform is set up as a dashboard and translates morphine dose into a predicted PK profile, which allows the clinical team to follow morphine exposure together with pain scores, heart rate, and breathing frequency in real time.[165] Figure 7.7 shows an example of a morphine PK prediction using the platform based on the infant's weight, gestational and postnatal age, and dosing regimen administered (continuous infusion plus bolus doses as needed, based on the pain scores). In this case, two measured morphine concentrations (open circles) revealed the concentration to be less than the population model–based (mean) predictions (dotted curved line). Based on these measured morphine concentrations, a new individual PK profile was predicted (blue line) using Bayesian estimation. The lower observed concentrations compared with the population model–based predictions suggest that this infant's morphine clearance was higher than clearance in the average neonate. The horizontal dotted lines represent the tentative target range of 10 to 30 ng per mL (mean 20 ng per mL in red) as suggested by Anderson and van den Anker.[166]

TDM teams and model TDM services have been in existence for decades, but in only a few institutions. However, as modern quality control methods are applied (belatedly) to medicine and more data become available on the cost-effectiveness of TDM in terms of outcomes rather than laboratory revenue, there is hope that such services will become more common. An interesting recent development in terms of data management, reporting of TDM results, and interpretation has been the use of information technology and the design of web-based tools that allow health care providers to access real-time data for their patients 24/7 from any place in the world. An example of such a web-based approach is the ImmunoSuppressants Bayesian dose Adjustment (ISBA) support platform offered through the Department of Pharmacology and Toxicology at the University Hospital of Limoges, France.[167] Through this resource, population model–based data interpretation is being provided using Bayesian estimators, which includes a numerical report and graphical representation of the predicted exposure–time relationship. This program provides support for several different immunosuppressive drugs and transplant indications and uses drug- and transplant-specific validated sparse sampling strategies to estimate dose–exposure relationships. Other Bayesian estimators have been developed and validated for MPA therapeutic drug management in the treatment of multiple diseases.[168–173]

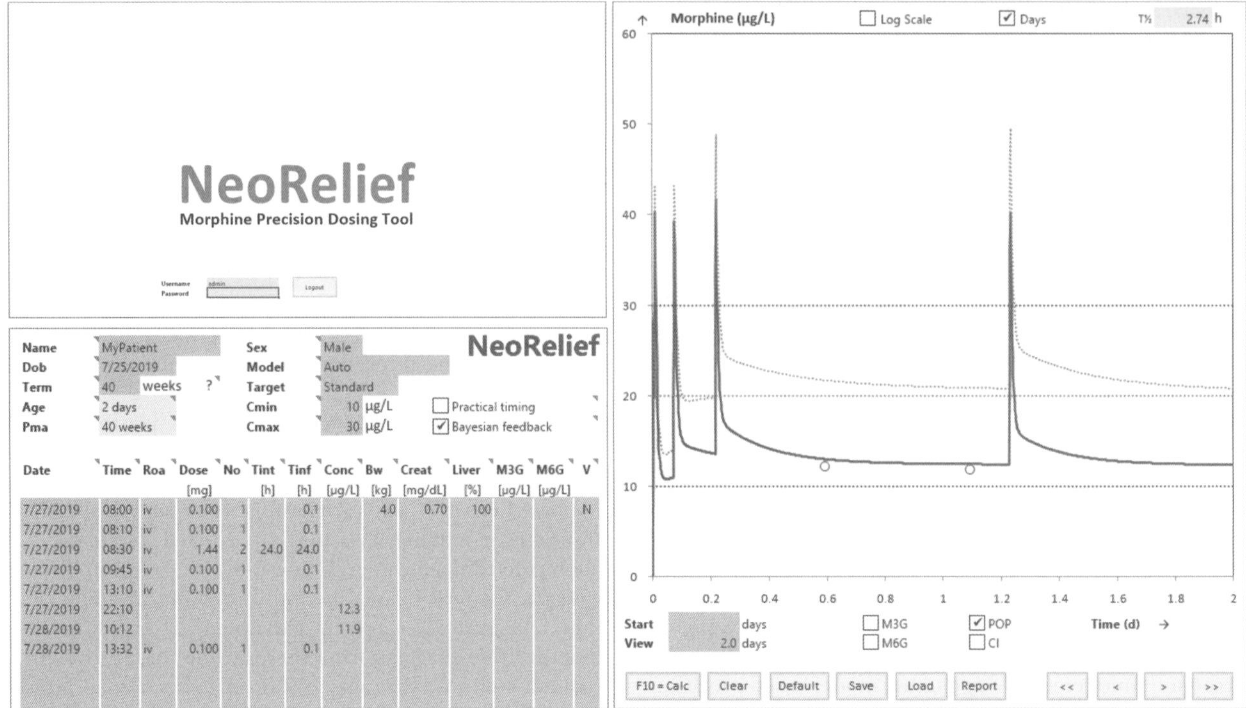

Figure 7.7 Decision support tool using Bayesian estimation integrated within the electronic health record (EHR) for morphine precision dosing in neonates.[164] The dotted curved line represents the population model–based (average) predicted morphine concentration profile. The open circles indicate measured morphine concentrations. The solid line represents the Bayesian estimated individual predicted profile. The horizontal dotted lines represent the tentative target concentration range of 10 to 30 ng per mL (mean 20 ng per mL) as suggested by Anderson and van den Anker.[166]

CONCLUSION

Properly done, TDM has been and will continue to be useful, especially in pediatric populations. However, there are many knowledge and performance deficits that must be corrected for TDM to reach its full potential. Simple-minded, reactionary TDM is often not useful and can even be dangerous. However, modern modeling, prediction, and control when combined with modern medical information and laboratory analytical technologies can clearly provide better, more cost-effective precision medicine for pediatric patients. In addition, in the future, the combination of analytical, PK/PD and systems pharmacology modeling, pharmacogenetics, and information technology techniques offers tremendous promise for truly individualized optimization of therapy, beginning with the initial dose of a medication and the continuation of tailored precision dosing thereafter.

REFERENCES

1. Ritschel WA, Kearns GL, American Pharmacists Association. *Handbook of basic pharmacokinetics—including clinical applications*, 7th ed. Washington, DC: American Pharmacists Association, 2009.
2. Benet LZ. Pharmacokinetics: basic principles and its use as a tool in drug metabolism. In: Mitchell JR, Horning MG, eds. *Drug metabolism and drug toxicity*. New York, NY: Raven Press, 1984:199.
3. Vinks AA, Emoto C, Fukuda T. Modeling and simulation in pediatric drug therapy: application of pharmacometrics to define the right dose for children. *Clin Pharmacol Ther* 2015;98:298–308.
4. Neely M, Jelliffe R. Practical, individualized dosing: 21st century therapeutics and the clinical pharmacometrician. *J Clin Pharmacol* 2010;50:842–847.
5. Burton ME. *Applied pharmacokinetics & pharmacodynamics: principles of therapeutic drug monitoring*, 4th ed. Baltimore, MD: Lippincott Williams & Wilkins, 2006.
6. The Precision Medicine Initiative. https://obamawhitehouse.archives.gov/precision-medicine. Accessed April 23, 2019.
7. Vinks AA. Therapeutic optimization as part of the precision medicine paradigm. *Clin Pharmacol Ther* 2016;99:340–342.
8. Danhof M. Kinetics of drug action in disease states: towards physiology-based pharmacodynamic (PBPD) models. *J Pharmacokinet Pharmacodyn* 2015;42:447–462.
9. Kahana S, Drotar D, Frazier T. Meta-analysis of psychological interventions to promote adherence to treatment in pediatric chronic health conditions. *J Pediatr Psychol* 2008;33:590–611.
10. Modi AC, Morita DA, Glauser TA. One-month adherence in children with new-onset epilepsy: white-coat compliance does not occur. *Pediatrics* 2008;121:e961–e966.
11. Quittner AL, Modi AC, Lemanek KL, et al. Evidence-based assessment of adherence to medical treatments in pediatric psychology. *J Pediatr Psychol* 2008;33:916–936; discussion 937–938.
12. Sherwin CM, McCaffrey F, Broadbent RS, et al. Discrepancies between predicted and observed rates of intravenous gentamicin delivery for neonates. *J Pharm Pharmacol* 2009;61:465–471.
13. International Association of Therapeutic Drug Monitoring and Clinical Toxicology. Definitions of TDM and CT. 2011. https://www.iatdmct.org/about-us/about-association/about-definitions-tdm-ct.html. Accessed April 23, 2019.
14. Neely M, Bayard D, Desai A, et al. Pharmacometric modeling and simulation is essential to pediatric clinical pharmacology. *J Clin Pharmacol* 2018;58(Suppl 10):S73–S85.
15. Soldin OP, Soldin SJ. Review: therapeutic drug monitoring in pediatrics. *Ther Drug Monit* 2002;24:1–8.
16. Touw DJ, Neef C, Thomson AH, et al. Cost-effectiveness of therapeutic drug monitoring: a systematic review. *Ther Drug Monit* 2005;27:10–17.
17. Walson PD. Role of therapeutic drug monitoring (TDM) in pediatric anti-convulsant drug dosing. *Brain Dev* 1994;16:23–26.
18. Patsalos PN, Berry DJ, Bourgeois BF, et al. Antiepileptic drugs—best practice guidelines for therapeutic drug monitoring: a position paper by the subcommission on therapeutic drug monitoring, ILAE Commission on Therapeutic Strategies. *Epilepsia* 2008;49:1239–1276.
19. Patsalos PN, Spencer EP, Berry DJ. Therapeutic drug monitoring of antiepileptic drugs in epilepsy: a 2018 update. *Ther Drug Monit* 2018;40:526–548.
20. Filler G. Value of therapeutic drug monitoring of MMF therapy in pediatric transplantation. *Pediatr Transplant* 2006;10:707–711.
21. Pauwels S, Allegaert K. Therapeutic drug monitoring in neonates. *Arch Dis Child* 2016;101:377–381.
22. Hiemke C, Bergemann N, Clement HW, et al. Consensus guidelines for therapeutic drug monitoring in neuropsychopharmacology: update 2017. *Pharmacopsychiatry* 2018;51:e1.
23. Waalewijn H, Turkova A, Rakhmanina N, et al. Optimizing pediatric dosing recommendations and treatment management of antiretroviral drugs utilizing therapeutic drug monitoring data in children living with HIV. *Ther Drug Monit* 2019;41(4):431–443.

24. Carman N, Mack DR, Benchimol EI. Therapeutic drug monitoring in pediatric inflammatory bowel disease. *Curr Gastroenterol Rep* 2018;20:18.
25. Singh N, Dubinsky MC. Therapeutic drug monitoring in children and young adults with inflammatory bowel disease: a practical approach. *Gastroenterol Hepatol (NY)* 2015;11:48–55.
26. Paci A, Veal G, Bardin C, et al. Review of therapeutic drug monitoring of anticancer drugs part 1—cytotoxics. *Eur J Cancer* 2014;50:2010–2019.
27. Shenfield GM. Therapeutic drug monitoring beyond 2000. *Br J Clin Pharmacol* 2001;52(Suppl 1):3S–4S.
28. Holford NH. Target concentration intervention: beyond Y2K. *Br J Clin Pharmacol* 1999;48:9–13.
29. Jelliffe RW, Schumitzky A, Van Guilder M, et al. Individualizing drug dosage regimens: roles of population pharmacokinetic and dynamic models, Bayesian fitting, and adaptive control. *Ther Drug Monit* 1993;15:380–393.
30. Walson PD, Edge JH. Clonazepam disposition in pediatric patients. *Ther Drug Monit* 1996;18:1–5.
31. Jelliffe RW, Schumitzky A, Bayard D, et al. Model-based, goal-oriented, individualised drug therapy. Linkage of population modelling, new 'multiple model' dosage design, Bayesian feedback and individualised target goals. *Clin Pharmacokinet* 1998;34:57–77.
32. Leff RD, Roberts RJ. Methods of intravenous drug administration in the pediatric patient. *J Pediatr* 1981;98:631–635.
33. Kearns GL, Abdel-Rahman SM, Alander SW, et al. Developmental pharmacology—drug disposition, action, and therapy in infants and children. *N Engl J Med* 2003;349:1157–1167.
34. Kearns GL, Reed MD. Clinical pharmacokinetics in infants and children. A reappraisal. *Clin Pharmacokinet* 1989;17(Suppl 1):29–67.
35. Anderson BJ, Holford NH. Mechanism-based concepts of size and maturity in pharmacokinetics. *Annu Rev Pharmacol Toxicol* 2008;48:303–332.
36. Anderson BJ, Holford NH. Mechanistic basis of using body size and maturation to predict clearance in humans. *Drug Metab Pharmacokinet* 2009;24:25–36.
37. Anderson BJ, Holford NH. Understanding dosing: children are small adults, neonates are immature children. *Arch Dis Child* 2013;98:737–744.
38. Loebstein R, Koren G. Clinical pharmacology and therapeutic drug monitoring in neonates and children. *Pediatr Rev* 1998;19:423–428.
39. Guidance for Industry. E11 clinical investigation of medical products in the pediatric population. U.S. Department of Health and Human Services, Food and Drug Administration, Center for Drug Evaluation and Research (CDER), Center for Biologics Evaluation and Research (CBER), 2000.
40. De Cock RF, Allegaert K, Brussee JM, et al. Simultaneous pharmacokinetic modeling of gentamicin, tobramycin and vancomycin clearance from neonates to adults: towards a semi-physiological function for maturation in glomerular filtration. *Pharm Res* 2014;31:2643–2654.
41. Paap CM, Nahata MC. Clinical pharmacokinetics of antibacterial drugs in neonates. *Clin Pharmacokinet* 1990;19:280–318.
42. Butler DR, Kuhn RJ, Chandler MH. Pharmacokinetics of anti-infective agents in paediatric patients. *Clin Pharmacokinet* 1994;26:374–395.
43. McLay JS, Engelhardt T, Mohammed BS, et al. The pharmacokinetics of intravenous ketorolac in children aged 2 months to 16 years: a population analysis. *Paediatr Anaesth* 2018;28:80–86.
44. Balch AH, Constance JE, Thorell EA, et al. Pediatric vancomycin dosing: trends over time and the impact of therapeutic drug monitoring. *J Clin Pharmacol* 2015;55:212–220.
45. Janssen EJ, Valitalo PA, Allegaert K, et al. Towards rational dosing algorithms for vancomycin in neonates and infants based on population pharmacokinetic modeling. *Antimicrob Agents Chemother* 2016;60:1013–1021.
46. Slocum JL, Heung M, Pennathur S. Marking renal injury: can we move beyond serum creatinine? *Transl Res* 2012;159:277–289.
47. Rhodin MM, Anderson BJ, Peters AM, et al. Human renal function maturation: a quantitative description using weight and postmenstrual age. *Pediatr Nephrol* 2009;24:67–76.
48. Bhongsatiern J, Stockmann C, Yu T, et al. Renal function descriptors in neonates: which creatinine-based formula best describes vancomycin clearance? *J Clin Pharmacol* 2016;56:528–540.
49. Koren G, James A, Perlman MA. Simple method for the estimation of glomerular filtration rate by gentamicin pharmacokinetics during routine drug monitoring in the newborn. *Clin Pharmacol Ther* 1985;38:680–685.
50. Anderson BJ, Holford NH. Tips and traps analyzing pediatric PK data. *Paediatr Anaesth* 2011;21:222–237.
51. Sherwin CM, Fukuda T, Brunner HI, et al. The evolution of population pharmacokinetic models to describe the enterohepatic recycling of mycophenolic acid in solid organ transplantation and autoimmune disease. *Clin Pharmacokinet* 2011;50:1–24.
52. Kuypers DR, Le Meur Y, Cantarovich M, et al. Consensus report on therapeutic drug monitoring of mycophenolic acid in solid organ transplantation. *Clin J Am Soc Nephrol* 2010;5:341–358.
53. Burton ME, Vasko MR, Brater DC. Comparison of drug dosing methods. *Clin Pharmacokinet* 1985;10:1–37.
54. Erdman SM, Rodvold KA, Pryka RD. An updated comparison of drug dosing methods. Part III: Aminoglycoside antibiotics. *Clin Pharmacokinet* 1991;20:374–388.
55. Erdman SM, Rodvold KA, Pryka RD. An updated comparison of drug dosing methods. Part II: Theophylline. *Clin Pharmacokinet* 1991;20:280–292.
56. Pryka RD, Rodvold KA, Erdman SM. An updated comparison of drug dosing methods. Part IV: Vancomycin. *Clin Pharmacokinet* 1991;20:463–476.
57. Pryka RD, Rodvold KA, Erdman SM. An updated comparison of drug dosing methods. Part I: Phenytoin. *Clin Pharmacokinet* 1991;20:209–217.
58. van Lent-Evers NA, Mathot RA, Geus WP, et al. Impact of goal-oriented and model-based clinical pharmacokinetic dosing of aminoglycosides on clinical outcome: a cost-effectiveness analysis. *Ther Drug Monitoring* 1999;21:63–73.
59. Ensom MH, Davis GA, Cropp CD, et al. Clinical pharmacokinetics in the 21st century. Does the evidence support definitive outcomes? *Clin Pharmacokinet* 1998;34:265–279.
60. Sjoqvist F, Eliasson E. The convergence of conventional therapeutic drug monitoring and pharmacogenetic testing in personalized medicine: focus on antidepressants. *Clin Pharmacol Ther* 2007;81:899–902.
61. Jelliffe RW. Computer-controlled administration of cardiovascular drugs. *Prog Cardiovasc Dis* 1983;26:1–14.
62. Sheiner LB, Beal S, Rosenberg B, et al. Forecasting individual pharmacokinetics. *Clin Pharmacol Ther* 1979;26:294–305.
63. Darwich AS, Ogungbenro K, Vinks AA, et al. Why has model-informed precision dosing not yet become common clinical reality? lessons from the past and a roadmap for the future. *Clin Pharmacol Ther* 2017;101:646–656.
64. Jelliffe R, Bayard D, Milman M, et al. Achieving target goals most precisely using nonparametric compartmental models and "multiple model" design of dosage regimens. *Ther Drug Monit* 2000;22:346–353.
65. Jelliffe R. Goal-oriented, model-based drug regimens: setting individualized goals for each patient. *Ther Drug Monit* 2000;22:325–329.
66. Mizuno T, O'Brien MM, Vinks AA. Significant effect of infection and food intake on sirolimus pharmacokinetics and exposure in pediatric patients with acute lymphoblastic leukemia. *Eur J Pharm Sci* 2019;128:209–214.
67. Merle Y, Mentre F. Optimal sampling times for Bayesian estimation of the pharmacokinetic parameters of nortriptyline during therapeutic drug monitoring. *J Pharmacokinet Biopharm* 1999;27:85–101.
68. Gex-Fabry M, Balant-Gorgia AE, Balant LP. Therapeutic drug monitoring databases for postmarketing surveillance of drug-drug interactions: evaluation of a paired approach for psychotropic medication. *Ther Drug Monit* 1997;19:1–10.
69. Jerling M, Bertilsson L, Sjoqvist F. The use of therapeutic drug monitoring data to document kinetic drug interactions: an example with amitriptyline and nortriptyline. *Ther Drug Monit* 1994;16:1–12.
70. Adams DM, Trenor CC 3rd, Hammill AM, et al. Efficacy and safety of sirolimus in the treatment of complicated vascular anomalies. *Pediatrics* 2016;137:e20153257.
71. Mizuno T, Emoto C, Fukuda T, et al. Model-based precision dosing of sirolimus in pediatric patients with vascular anomalies. *Eur J Pharm Sci* 2017;109S:S124–S131.
72. Destache CJ, Meyer SK, Bittner MJ, et al. Impact of a clinical pharmacokinetic service on patients treated with aminoglycosides: a cost-benefit analysis. *Ther Drug Monit* 1990;12:419–426.
73. Destache CJ, Meyer SK, Rowley KM. Does accepting pharmacokinetic recommendations impact hospitalization? a cost-benefit analysis. *Ther Drug Monit* 1990;12:427–433.
74. Le Meur Y, Buchler M, Thierry A, et al. Individualized mycophenolate mofetil dosing based on drug exposure significantly improves patient outcomes after renal transplantation. *Am J Transplant* 2007;7:2496–2503.
75. Destache CJ. Economic aspects of pharmacokinetic services. *Pharmacoeconomics* 1993;3:433–436.
76. Bertino JS Jr, Rodvold KA, Destache CJ. Cost considerations in therapeutic drug monitoring of aminoglycosides. *Clin Pharmacokinet* 1994;26:71–81.
77. Bates DW, Soldin SJ, Rainey PM, et al. Strategies for physician education in therapeutic drug monitoring. *Clin Chem* 1998;44:401–407.
78. Cox S, Team T. *Gathering outpatient data for therapeutic drug monitoring.* Third International Congress of Therapeutic Drug Monitoring and Clinical Toxicology, Philadelphia, PA, 1993.
79. Blaschke TF, Osterberg L, Vrijens B, et al. Adherence to medications: insights arising from studies on the unreliable link between prescribed and actual drug dosing histories. *Annu Rev Pharmacol Toxicol* 2012;52:275–301.
80. Vinks AA. From molecule to patient and ways to get the dose precisely right. *Clin Pharmacol Ther* 2019;105:534–537.
81. Fraaij PL, Rakhmanina N, Burger DM, et al. Therapeutic drug monitoring in children with HIV/AIDS. *Ther Drug Monit* 2004;26:122–126.
82. Walson PD, Cox S, Utkin I, et al. Clinical use of a simultaneous HPLC assay for indinavir, saquinavir, ritonavir and nelfinavir in children and adults. *Ther Drug Monit* 2003;25:650–656.
83. Smith J, Andes D. Therapeutic drug monitoring of antifungals: pharmacokinetic and pharmacodynamic considerations. *Ther Drug Monit* 2008;30:167–172.
84. Rousseau A, Marquet P, Debord J, et al. Adaptive control methods for the dose individualisation of anticancer agents. *Clin Pharmacokinet* 2000;38:315–353.
85. McCormack JP, Jewesson PJ. A critical reevaluation of the "therapeutic range" of aminoglycosides. *Clin Infect Dis* 1992;14:320–339.
86. De Broe ME, Giuliano RA, Verpooten GA. Choice of drug and dosage regimen. Two important risk factors for aminoglycoside nephrotoxicity. *Am J Med* 1986;80:115–118.
87. Rougier F, Claude D, Maurin M, et al. Aminoglycoside nephrotoxicity: modeling, simulation, and control. *Antimicrob Agents Chemother* 2003;47:1010–1016.
88. Moore RD, Smith CR, Lietman PS. Association of aminoglycoside plasma levels with therapeutic outcome in gram-negative pneumonia. *Am J Med* 1984;77:657–662.
89. Moore RD, Smith CR, Lietman PS. The association of aminoglycoside plasma levels with mortality in patients with gram-negative bacteremia. *J Infect Dis* 1984;149:443–448.
90. Nicolau DP, Freeman CD, Belliveau PP, et al. Experience with a once-daily aminoglycoside program administered to 2,184 adult patients. *Antimicrob Agents Chemother* 1995;39:650–655.
91. Craig W. Pharmacodynamics of antimicrobial agents as a basis for determining dosage regimens. *Eur J Clin Microbiol Infect Dis* 1993;12(Suppl 1):S6–S8.
92. Maglio D, Nightingale CH, Nicolau DP. Extended interval aminoglycoside dosing: from concept to clinic. *Int J Antimicrob Agents* 2002;19:341–348.
93. Hansen A, Forbes P, Arnold A, et al. Once-daily gentamicin dosing for the preterm and term newborn: proposal for a simple regimen that achieves target levels. *J Perinatol* 2003;23:635–639.
94. Contopoulos-Ioannidis DG, Giotis ND, Baliatsa DV, et al. Extended-interval aminoglycoside administration for children: a meta-analysis. *Pediatrics* 2004;114:e111–e118.
95. Knoderer CA, Everett JA, Buss WF. Clinical issues surrounding once-daily aminoglycoside dosing in children. *Pharmacotherapy* 2003;23:44–56.
96. de Hoog M, Mouton JW, Schoemaker RC, et al. Extended-interval dosing of tobramycin in neonates: implications for therapeutic drug monitoring. *Clin Pharmacol Ther* 2002;71:349–358.

97. Touw DJ, Vinks AA, Mouton JW, et al. Pharmacokinetic optimisation of antibacterial treatment in patients with cystic fibrosis. Current practice and suggestions for future directions. *Clin Pharmacokinet* 1998;35:437–459.
98. Hennig S, Norris R, Kirkpatrick CM. Target concentration intervention is needed for tobramycin dosing in paediatric patients with cystic fibrosis—a population pharmacokinetic study. *Br J Clin Pharmacol* 2008;65:502–510.
99. Lam W, Tjon J, Seto W, et al. Pharmacokinetic modelling of a once-daily dosing regimen for intravenous tobramycin in paediatric cystic fibrosis patients. *J Antimicrob Chemother* 2007;59:1135–1140.
100. Touw DJ, Knox AJ, Smyth A. Population pharmacokinetics of tobramycin administered thrice daily and once daily in children and adults with cystic fibrosis. *J Cyst Fibros* 2007;6:327–333.
101. Burkhardt O, Lehmann C, Madabushi R, et al. Once-daily tobramycin in cystic fibrosis: better for clinical outcome than thrice-daily tobramycin but more resistance development?. *J Antimicrob Chemother* 2006;58:822–829.
102. Vinks AA. The application of population pharmacokinetic modeling to individualized antibiotic therapy. *Int J Antimicrob Agents* 2002;19:313–322.
103. Valitalo PA, van den Anker JN, Allegaert K, et al. Novel model-based dosing guidelines for gentamicin and tobramycin in preterm and term neonates. *J Antimicrob Chemother* 2015;70:2074–2077.
104. Smits A, De Cock RF, Allegaert K, et al. Prospective evaluation of a model-based dosing regimen for amikacin in preterm and term neonates in clinical practice. *Antimicrob Agents Chemother* 2015;59:6344–6351.
105. De Cock RF, Allegaert K, Schreuder MF, et al. Maturation of the glomerular filtration rate in neonates, as reflected by amikacin clearance. *Clin Pharmacokinet* 2012;51:105–117.
106. Smit C, Wasmann RE, Wiezer MJ, et al. Tobramycin clearance is best described by renal function estimates in obese and non-obese individuals: results of a prospective rich sampling pharmacokinetic study. *Pharm Res* 2019;36:112.
107. Smit C, Wasmann RE, Goulooze SC, et al. A prospective clinical study characterizing the influence of morbid obesity on the pharmacokinetics of gentamicin: towards individualized dosing in obese patients. *Clin Pharmacokinet*; 58: 1333–1343.
108. Downes KJ, Hahn A, Wiles J, et al. Dose optimisation of antibiotics in children: application of pharmacokinetics/pharmacodynamics in paediatrics. *Int J Antimicrob Agents* 2014;43:223–230.
109. Guan MX, Fischel-Ghodsian N, Attardi G. A biochemical basis for the inherited susceptibility to aminoglycoside ototoxicity. *Hum Mol Genet* 2000;9:1787–1793.
110. van Dijkman SC, Rauwe WM, Danhof M, et al. Pharmacokinetic interactions and dosing rationale for antiepileptic drugs in adults and children. *Br J Clin Pharmacol* 2018;84:97–111.
111. van Dijkman SC, Wicha SG, Danhof M, et al. Individualized dosing algorithms and therapeutic monitoring for antiepileptic drugs. *Clin Pharmacol Ther* 2018;103:663–673.
112. Filler G. Optimization of immunosuppressive drug monitoring in children. *Transplant Proc* 2007;39:1241–1243.
113. Kahan BD, Keown P, Levy GA, et al. Therapeutic drug monitoring of immunosuppressant drugs in clinical practice. *Clin Ther* 2002;24:330–350; discussion 329.
114. Oellerich M, Armstrong VW, Schutz E, et al. Therapeutic drug monitoring of cyclosporine and tacrolimus. Update on Lake Louise Consensus Conference on cyclosporin and tacrolimus. *Clin Biochem* 1998;31:309–316.
115. del Mar Fernandez De Gatta M, Santos-Buelga D, Dominguez-Gil A, et al. Immunosuppressive therapy for paediatric transplant patients: pharmacokinetic considerations. *Clin Pharmacokinet* 2002;41:115–135.
116. David O, Johnston A. Limited sampling strategies. *Clin Pharmacokinet* 2000;39:311–313.
117. Johnston A, Chusney G, Schutz E, et al. Monitoring cyclosporin in blood: between-assay differences at trough and 2 hours post-dose (C2). *Ther Drug Monit* 2003;25:167–173.
118. Morris RG, Ilett KF, Tett SE, et al. Cyclosporin monitoring in Australasia: 2002 update of consensus guidelines. *Ther Drug Monit* 2002;24:677–688.
119. Monchaud C, Rousseau A, Leger F, et al. Limited sampling strategies using Bayesian estimation or multilinear regression for cyclosporin AUC(0-12) monitoring in cardiac transplant recipients over the first year post-transplantation. *Eur J Clin Pharmacol* 2003;58:813–820.
120. Rousseau A, Monchaud C, Debord J, et al. Bayesian forecasting of oral cyclosporin pharmacokinetics in stable lung transplant recipients with and without cystic fibrosis. *Ther Drug Monit* 2003;25:28–35.
121. Oellerich M, Shipkova M, Schutz E, et al. Pharmacokinetic and metabolic investigations of mycophenolic acid in pediatric patients after renal transplantation: implications for therapeutic drug monitoring. German Study Group on Mycophenolate Mofetil Therapy in Pediatric Renal Transplant Recipients. *Ther Drug Monit* 2000;22:20–26.
122. Djebli N, Rousseau A, Hoizey G, et al. Sirolimus population pharmacokinetic/pharmacogenetic analysis and Bayesian modelling in kidney transplant recipients. *Clin Pharmacokinet* 2006;45:1135–1148.
123. Shaw LM, Kaplan B, Brayman KL. Advances in therapeutic drug monitoring for immunosuppressants: a review of sirolimus. Introduction and overview. *Clin Ther* 2000;22(Suppl B):B1–B13.
124. Filler G, Bendrick-Peart J, Strom T, et al. Characterization of sirolimus metabolites in pediatric solid organ transplant recipients. *Pediatr Transplant* 2009;13:44–53.
125. Brunet M, van Gelder T, Asberg A, et al. Therapeutic drug monitoring of tacrolimus-personalized therapy: second consensus report. *Ther Drug Monit* 2019;41:261–307.
126. Rakhmanina NY, van den Anker JN, Soldin SJ. Therapeutic drug monitoring of antiretroviral therapy. *AIDS Patient Care STDS* 2004;18:7–14.
127. Aarnoutse RE, Schapiro JM, Boucher CA, et al. Therapeutic drug monitoring: an aid to optimising response to antiretroviral drugs? *Drugs* 2003;63:741–753.
128. van Rossum AM, Bergshoeff AS, Fraaij PL, et al. Therapeutic drug monitoring of indinavir and nelfinavir to assess adherence to therapy in human immunodeficiency virus-infected children. *Pediatr Infect Dis J* 2002;21:743–747.
129. Ford D, Turner R, Turkova A, et al. optimizing clinical trial design to maximize evidence generation in pediatric HIV. *J Acquir Immune Defic Syndr* 2018;78(Suppl 1):S40–S48.
130. Baumann P, Hiemke C, Ulrich S, et al. The AGNP-TDM expert group consensus guidelines: therapeutic drug monitoring in psychiatry. *Pharmacopsychiatry* 2004;37:243–265.
131. Hiemke C, Baumann P, Bergemann N, et al. AGNP consensus guidelines for therapeutic drug monitoring in psychiatry: update 2011. *Pharmacopsychiatry* 2011;44:195–235.
132. Lega S, Bramuzzo M, Dubinsky MC. Therapeutic drug monitoring in pediatric IBD: current application and future perspectives. *Curr Med Chem* 2018;25:2840–2854.
133. Hyams J, Crandall W, Kugathasan S, et al. Induction and maintenance infliximab therapy for the treatment of moderate-to-severe Crohn's disease in children. *Gastroenterology* 2007;132:863–873, quiz 1165–1166.
134. Hyams J, Damaraju L, Blank M, et al. Induction and maintenance therapy with infliximab for children with moderate to severe ulcerative colitis. *Clin Gastroenterol Hepatol* 2012;10:391–399, e391.
135. Qiu Y, Chen BL, Mao R, et al. Systematic review with meta-analysis: loss of response and requirement of anti-TNFalpha dose intensification in Crohn's disease. *J Gastroenterol* 2017;52:535–554.
136. Maser EA, Villela R, Silverberg MS, et al. Association of trough serum infliximab to clinical outcome after scheduled maintenance treatment for Crohn's disease. *Clin Gastroenterol Hepatol* 2006;4:1248–1254.
137. Bortlik M, Duricova D, Malickova K, et al. Infliximab trough levels may predict sustained response to infliximab in patients with Crohn's disease. *J Crohns Colitis* 2013;7:736–743.
138. Vande Casteele N, Ferrante M, Van Assche G, et al. Trough concentrations of infliximab guide dosing for patients with inflammatory bowel disease. *Gastroenterology* 2015;148:1320–1329.e3.
139. Vande Casteele N, Khanna R, Levesque BG, et al. The relationship between infliximab concentrations, antibodies to infliximab and disease activity in Crohn's disease. *Gut* 2015;64:1539–1545.
140. Choi SY, Kang B, Lee JH, et al. Clinical use of measuring trough levels and antibodies against infliximab in patients with pediatric inflammatory bowel disease. *Gut Liver* 2017;11:55–61.
141. Merras-Salmio L, Kolho KL. Clinical use of infliximab trough levels and antibodies to infliximab in pediatric patients with inflammatory bowel disease. *J Pediatr Gastroenterol Nutr* 2017;64:272–278.
142. Rolandsdotter H, Marits P, Sundin U, et al. Serum-infliximab trough levels in 45 children with inflammatory bowel disease on maintenance treatment. *Int J Mol Sci* 2017;18:575.
143. Moore C, Corbett G, Moss AC. Systematic review and meta-analysis: serum infliximab levels during maintenance therapy and outcomes in inflammatory bowel disease. *J Crohns Colitis* 2016;10:619–625.
144. Zandvliet ML, van Bezooijen JS, Bos MA, et al. Monitoring antigen-specific biologics: current knowledge and future prospects. *Ther Drug Monit* 2013;35:588–594.
145. Afif W, Loftus EV Jr, Faubion WA, et al. Clinical utility of measuring infliximab and human anti-chimeric antibody concentrations in patients with inflammatory bowel disease. *Am J Gastroenterol* 2010;105:1133–1139.
146. Baert F, Noman M, Vermeire S, et al. Influence of immunogenicity on the long-term efficacy of infliximab in Crohn's disease. *N Engl J Med* 2003;348:601–608.
147. Kevans D, Murthy S, Mould DR, et al. Accelerated clearance of infliximab is associated with treatment failure in patients with corticosteroid-refractory acute ulcerative colitis. *J Crohns Colitis* 2018;12:662–669.
148. Brandse JF, Mould D, Smeekes O, et al. A real-life population pharmacokinetic study reveals factors associated with clearance and immunogenicity of infliximab in inflammatory bowel disease. *Inflamm Bowel Dis* 2017;23:650–660.
149. Dotan I, Ron Y, Yanai H, et al. Patient factors that increase infliximab clearance and shorten half-life in inflammatory bowel disease: a population pharmacokinetic study. *Inflamm Bowel Dis* 2014;20:2247–2259.
150. Ordas I, Mould DR, Feagan BG, et al. Anti-TNF monoclonal antibodies in inflammatory bowel disease: pharmacokinetics-based dosing paradigms. *Clin Pharmacol Ther* 2012;91:635–646.
151. Fasanmade AA, Adedokun OJ, Blank M, et al. Pharmacokinetic properties of infliximab in children and adults with Crohn's disease: a retrospective analysis of data from 2 phase III clinical trials. *Clin Ther* 2011;33:946–964.
152. Fasanmade AA, Adedokun OJ, Olson A, et al. Serum albumin concentration: a predictive factor of infliximab pharmacokinetics and clinical response in patients with ulcerative colitis. *Int J Clin Pharmacol Ther* 2010;48:297–308.
153. Fasanmade AA, Adedokun OJ, Ford J, et al. Population pharmacokinetic analysis of infliximab in patients with ulcerative colitis. *Eur J Clin Pharmacol* 2009;65:1211–1228.
154. Mould DR, D'Haens G, Upton RN. Clinical decision support tools: the evolution of a revolution *Clin Pharmacol Ther* 2016;99:405–418.
155. Gorodischer R, Koren G. Salivary excretion of drugs in children: theoretical and practical issues in therapeutic drug monitoring. *Dev Pharmacol Ther* 1992;19:161–177.
156. Langman LJ. The use of oral fluid for therapeutic drug management: clinical and forensic toxicology. *Ann NY Acad Sci* 2007;1098:145–166.
157. Danhof M. Systems pharmacology-Towards the modeling of network interactions. *Eur J Pharm Sci* 2016;94:4–14.
158. Lesko LJ, Schmidt S. Individualization of drug therapy: history, present state, and opportunities for the future. *Clin Pharmacol Ther* 2012;92:458–466.
159. Barrett JS, Mondick JT, Narayan M, et al. Integration of modeling and simulation into hospital-based decision support systems guiding pediatric pharmacotherapy. *BMC Med Inform Decis Mak* 2008;8:6.
160. Dombrowsky E, Jayaraman B, Narayan M, et al. Evaluating performance of a decision support system to improve methotrexate pharmacotherapy in children and young adults with cancer. *Ther Drug Monit* 2011;33:99–107.
161. Abdel-Rahman SM, Breitkreutz ML, Bi C, et al. Design and testing of an EHR-integrated, busulfan pharmacokinetic decision support tool for the point-of-care. *Clin Front Pharmacol* 2016;7:65.
162. Eser A, Primas C, Reinisch S, et al. Prediction of individual serum infliximab concentrations in inflammatory bowel disease by a Bayesian dashboard system. *J Clin Pharmacol* 2018;58:790–802.

163. Hamberg AK, Hellman J, Dahlberg J, et al. Bayesian decision support tool for efficient dose individualization of warfarin in adults and children. *BMC Med Inform Decis Mak* 2015;15:7.
164. Vinks AA, Punt NC, Menke F, Kirkendall, E, Butler, D, Duggan, T. J., Cortezzo, D. E., Kiger, S., Dietrich, T., Spencer, P., Keefer, R., Setchell, K. D. R., Zhao, J., Euteneuer, J. C., Mizuno, T., Dufendach, K. R. Electronic Health Record-Embedded Decision Support Platform for Morphine Precision Dosing in Neonates. *Clin Pharmacol Ther* 2020;107:186–94.
165. Euteneuer JC, Kamatkar S, Fukuda T, et al. Suggestions for model-informed precision dosing to optimize neonatal drug therapy. *J Clin Pharmacol* 2019;59:168–176.
166. Anderson BJ, van den Anker J. Why is there no morphine concentration-response curve for acute pain? *Paediatr Anaesth* 2014;24:233–238.
167. Department of Pharmacology and Toxicology at the University Hospital of Limoges F. ISBA: Access portal to the websites of routine and clinical trials of the Limoges University Hospital laboratory of Pharmacology. https://pharmaco.chu-limoges.fr/. Accessed July 24, 2019.
168. Tellier S, Dallocchio A, Guigonis V, et al. Mycophenolic acid pharmacokinetics and relapse in children with steroid-dependent idiopathic nephrotic syndrome. *Clin J Am Soc Nephrol* 2016;11:1777–1782.
169. Woillard JB, Bader-Meunier B, Salomon R, et al. Pharmacokinetics of mycophenolate mofetil in children with lupus and clinical findings in favour of therapeutic drug monitoring. *Br J Clin Pharmacol* 2014;78:867–876.
170. de Winter BC, Monchaud C, Premaud A, et al. Bayesian estimation of mycophenolate mofetil in lung transplantation, using a population pharmacokinetic model developed in kidney and lung transplant recipients. *Clin Pharmacokinet* 2012;51:29–39.
171. Saint-Marcoux F, Vandierdonck S, Premaud A, et al. Large scale analysis of routine dose adjustments of mycophenolate mofetil based on global exposure in renal transplant patients. *Ther Drug Monit* 2011;33:285–294.
172. Saint-Marcoux F, Guigonis V, Decramer S, et al. Development of a Bayesian estimator for the therapeutic drug monitoring of mycophenolate mofetil in children with idiopathic nephrotic syndrome. *Pharmacol Res* 2011;63:423–431.
173. Le Guellec C, Bourgoin H, Buchler M, et al. Population pharmacokinetics and Bayesian estimation of mycophenolic acid concentrations in stable renal transplant patients. *Clin Pharmacokinet* 2004;43:253–266.
174. Oellerich M, Armstrong VW, Kahan B, et al. Lake Louise Consensus Conference on cyclosporin monitoring in organ transplantation: report of the consensus panel. *Ther Drug Monit* 1995;17:642–654.
175. Schubert M, Venkataramanan R, Holt DW, et al. Pharmacokinetics of sirolimus and tacrolimus in pediatric transplant patients. *Am J Transplant* 2004;4:767–773.
176. Wallemacq P, Armstrong VW, Brunet M, et al. Opportunities to optimize tacrolimus therapy in solid organ transplantation: report of the European consensus conference. *Ther Drug Monit* 2009;31:139–152.
177. van Gelder T, Le Meur Y, Shaw LM, et al. Therapeutic drug monitoring of mycophenolate mofetil in transplantation. *Ther Drug Monit* 2006;28:145–154.

CHAPTER

8

Jörg Breitkreutz

Drug Formulations for Children

Prior to prescribing a drug product for a child, the pediatrician has to consider whether the clinically required drug substance can be administered completely, conveniently, and safely to the child. A critical review of available drugs has shown, however, that this is hardly the case for many authorized medicinal products.[1] The route of drug administration, the dosage form, the composition of the drug formulation, the condition, and child-appropriate mode of drug administration have to be carefully evaluated. Within this process, it has to be realized that the pediatric population is heterogeneous by nature and undergoes continuing growth and maturation.

There are various reasons why pharmaceutical industry has been reluctant in developing pediatric drug products. Enormous costs of drug development, a relatively small market, plenty of specific requirements for children, quite comprehensive clinical studies on efficacy and safety, related ethical concerns, and—for many years—unknown regulatory requirements have been impediments to developing and marketing new pediatric drug products. Raised awareness of these problems has led to various regulatory incentives for pediatric drug development in the European Union (EU) and the United States.[2] Whereas for new chemical compounds, it is generally mandatory to develop and test pediatric drug formulations in clinical practice, it remains a voluntary task for the off-patent drug substances, which are the majority of used active pharmaceutical ingredients (APIs) in pediatric clinical practice today.

As a consequence of the still existing lack of child-appropriate medicines, the pediatrician might consider alternatives to the authorized medicines for the pediatric population. This should be carefully performed, reflecting the different levels of drug quality, scientific knowledge, and experience.

APPROPRIATENESS OF DRUG DOSAGE FORMS

The pediatric population has been divided by age into five to six categories. In the International Conference of Harmonization (ICH) E 11 guideline,[3] the age groups of preterm neonates, neonates, infants and toddlers, children, and adolescents have been defined based on physiologic and pharmacokinetic differences, for example, metabolic capacity, organ maturation, and drug clearance.[4] These variations affect not only the API but also the entire drug product. The pharmaceutical excipients, which are required to generate a child-appropriate drug dosage form out of the pure API, may be absorbed into the body, distribute into different body tissues, may interfere with the API or its metabolites, and are eliminated by different pathways.[4] Some of these may be safe for adults, but clearly show some adverse effects or at least safety signals for the use in children, including organic diluents, preservatives, antioxidants, and plasticizers.[5] Term, and in particular preterm, neonates are at highest risk for toxic reactions to pharmaceutical excipients, which are often underestimated.[6]

The European Medicines Agency (EMA) has further divided the group of "children" into two subgroups, "preschool children" between the ages of 2 and 6 years and "school children" from 6 to 12 years old, in order to reflect the capability of children to swallow or at least to accept solid oral drug dosage forms, such as tablets or capsules.[7] Recent clinical studies on the acceptability of small-sized tablets, the so-called mini-tablets, in pediatric patients,[8] have raised some doubts, however, on the widely accepted age-dependent ratings that have been followed for years by academia and pharmaceutical industry. By these groundbreaking studies, it was shown that even neonates may take a mini-tablet orally,[9] and older children may take a couple of mini-tablets as a resulting single dose[10] without significant problems. In all cases, the mini-tablets were at least equally suitable, but often superior to the liquid control, a sweet syrup. As a consequence, EMA now encourages pharmaceutical companies within its most recent "Guideline on pharmaceutical development of medicines for pediatric use" to develop small-sized solid drug carriers such as mini-tablets or pellets for the use in children, including the very young children.[11] Earlier, the World Health Organization (WHO) had recommended the development of "multiparticulates" for the pediatric population.[12] Acceptability of these multiparticulates, including pellets or mini-tablets, has been demonstrated for both children and adults.[13] Besides the superior acceptability, the higher stability and more precise dosing are advantageous for the multiparticulate formulations. Some experts have, therefore, claimed a shift of paradigm using small-sized solid preparations instead of liquid drug formulations.[14] Other alternatives to liquid drug formulations are dispersible drug dosage forms. In the best case, these solid dosage forms dissolve in the oral cavity immediately after administration and are, therefore, called "orodispersible formulations."[15] These new formulation concepts comprise orodispersible tablets,[16] oral lyophilisates,[17] and orodispersible films.[18]

NEW MEDICINAL PRODUCTS FOR ORAL USE WITH ADVANCED DOSAGE FORMS

The change of mindset toward solid dosage forms can be observed best in the most recent drug authorizations in Europe concerning Pediatric Use Marketing Authorizations (PUMAs) for off-patent drug substances (Table 8.1).

The first PUMA product, Buccolam, initially appeared on the market in 2011 as a drug formulation of midazolam hydrochloride preserved by methyl paraben and propyl paraben. Due to concerns about the safety of propyl paraben use in young children, the pharmaceutical sponsor changed the composition and manufacturing procedure. Now it comes as a sterilized oral liquid without preservation system, which is prefilled into an oral syringe for single use and tightly sealed (see Table 8.1). The next two PUMA products were oral liquid formulations: propranolol hydrochloride oral solution without preservation system (Hemangiol), but high propylene glycol content (2.60 mg per mL), and glycopyrronium bromide oral solution with sodium benzoate as preservative (Sialanar). Sodium benzoate is considered a relatively safe preservation agent at low doses. Propylene glycol has been associated with serum hyperosmolality and also seizures[6,19,20] as it may pass the blood–brain barrier in neonates and young infants, but not in adolescents and adults.

The next PUMA products contain solid drug formulations. Dispersible vigabatrin tablets (Kigabeq 100 and 500 mg) are dissolved in water on a spoon in order to facilitate the drug administration. Alkindi contains small-sized pellets with hydrocortisone which are taste-masked by an ethyl cellulose/hypromellose coating. By accumulating different counts of taste-masked pellets in hypromellose capsules, different dose strengths (0.5, 1.0, 2.0, and 5.0 mg) are obtained. The capsule is to be opened before use, and the pellets can be sprinkled onto semisolid or liquid food. The newest PUMA product, Slenyto, is a melatonin formulation with prolonged-release coated mini-tablets which are filled into hard capsules at different quantities (1 and 5 mg dose strengths). Orodispersible mini-tablet formulations with 0.25 and 1.00 mg enalapril maleate are close to a PUMA filing.[21] Orodispersible mini-tablets offer various beneficial features: precise dosing, high content uniformity, good drug stability during storage as a solid dosage form, and safe administration, resulting in a liquid dispersion in the saliva with ease of swallowing.[22]

Although the PUMA approach is not applicable in the United States, many products with off-patent drug substances, but innovative drug dosage forms,[23] have been introduced to the market (Table 8.2). Many of these are available in other countries outside the United States or EU, too.[24]

Chewable tablets (e.g., Isentress) have been designed for school-aged children and adolescents. Dispersible tablets for preparation of a solution or suspension prior to administration are a good compromise between the benefits of solid dosage forms in the package and liquid dosage forms at the time point of administration. Advanced tablet geometries enable more flexible dosing by splitting the dispersible tablets (e.g., Coartem, Tracleer, Carbaglu, Siklos) before the liquid preparation. The remaining parts of the tablets should not be reused as they lack primary packaging after breaking, which may impact drug stability. Orodispersible films, for example, with desloratadine or ondansetron, are sealed water-soluble polymeric films in aluminum sachets for single use. These small thin strips immediately dissolve on the tongue within a few seconds. Further, dose flexibility could be increased by precise cutting or ad hoc preparation in hospital pharmacies in general. However, these types of dose adjustments for pediatric use have not been authorized yet.[25] Spheronized granules ("pellets") mini-tablets offer multiple opportunities of modified drug release and sprinkling onto food materials to facilitate swallowing.[26] Mini-tablets are superior to pellets in the precision of dosing, even at very small diameter like 1 or 2 mm, and, therefore, qualify as a very flexible dosing system for pediatric use.[27–29] Some pharmaceutical companies call mini-tablets in a primary package "granules," for example, for the product Kalydeco, because they are not monographed in the pharmacopoeias and quality test specifications have not been authorized so far. If flexible dosing is required because of a required dose titration step or a narrow therapeutic window, a specific counting device may be required to enable correct dosing.

MANIPULATING OR COMPOUNDING OF DRUG PRODUCTS

The majority of commercially available drug products in the United States and EU are not labeled for use in all subgroups of children.

TABLE 8.1 PUMA Products Authorized in the EU[a]

Product	*Drug Substance*	*Drug Dosage Form*	*Indication*
Buccolam	Midazolam hydrochloride, 2.5/5/7.5/10 mg midazolam	Oral liquid in prefilled syringe, preservative free	Epilepsy
Hemangiol	Propranolol hydrochloride, 3.75 mg/mL propranolol	Oral liquid, preservative free (2.60 mg/mL propylene glycol)	Hemangioma
Sialanar	Glycopyrronium bromide, 320 µg/mL glycopyrronium	Oral liquid, preserved with sodium benzoate	Sialorrhea
Alkindi	Hydrocortisone, 0.5/1/2/5 mg	Hard capsules (to be opened) containing taste-masked pellets	Adrenal insufficiency
Kigabeq	Vigabatrin, 100/500 mg	Dispersible tablets	Infantile spasms
Slenyto	Melatonin, 1/5 mg	Hard capsules (to be opened) containing prolonged-release mini-tablets	Insomnia

[a]Presented in the order of authorization.
EU, European Union; PUMA, Pediatric Use Marketing Authorizations.

TABLE 8.2 Recently Introduced Medicinal Products with Innovative Drug Dosage Forms[a]

Product	*Drug Substance*	*Drug Dosage Form*	*Indication*
Isentress	Raltegravir 25/100 mg	Chewable tablets	HIV infection
Afinitor Disperz/Votubia	Everolimus 2/3/5 mg	Dispersible tablets	Epilepsy
Coartem/Riamet	Artemether/Lumefantrine 20/120 mg	Dispersible, single-scored tablets	Malaria
Tracleer	Bosentan 32 mg	Dispersible, cross-scored tablets (revealing quarters at 8 mg)	Pulmonary arterial hypertension
Carbaglu	Carglumic acid 200 mg	Dispersible, triple-scored tablets (revealing quarters at 50 mg)	*N*-Acetyl-glutamate synthase deficiency
Siklos	Hydroxyurea 1,000 mg	Dispersible, triple-scored tablets (revealing quarters at 250 mg)	Sickle cell anemia
Zofran	Ondansetron hydrochloride 4/8 mg ondansetron	Oral lyophilizates (Zydis technology)	Vomiting, cytostatics induced
Zuplenz, Setofilm	Ondansetron hydrochloride 4/8 mg ondansetron	Orodispersible films	Vomiting, cytostatics induced
Zmax/Sumamed	Azithromycin 27 mg/mL	Prolonged-release granules (pellets) for preparing a suspension	Bacterial infections
Kalydeco	Ivacaftor 50/75 mg	Sachets with "granules" (actually mini-tablets)	Cystic fibrosis
Orfiril long	Valproic acid 150/300 mg capsules 500/1,000 mg sachets	Capsules/sachets with prolonged-release mini-tablets	Epilepsy
Levetiracetam Desitin	Levetiracetam 250/500/1,000 mg	Sachets with taste-masked mini-tablets	Epilepsy

[a]Includes examples, sorted by dosage forms as they appear in the text.

When an appropriate drug product for the child is not available, the options of the pediatrician include the following:

- to refuse or delay the intended drug therapy
- to change to another product/another drug substance even if the efficacy and safety might be potentially inferior or unknown
- to call the pharmaceutical manufacturer for scientific evidence on manipulation or compounding of the authorized drug to make it more child appropriate
- to request the compounding of an extemporaneous drug formulation based on different scientific evidence and quality levels.

Manipulation has been defined to happen close to the bedside, for example, splitting or crushing a tablet before mixing with food. Compounding means the preparation of a new drug formulation in advance, for example, in a compounding center, a hospital, or a community pharmacy.[30] It has to be distinguished between authorized and nonauthorized manipulations or compounding steps.

Authorized medicinal products have been approved by the competent authorities after evaluation of all submitted data on quality, efficacy, and safety. The Summary of Product Characteristics (SmPC) of the authorized product reflects the approved practices for medical use. Further, the product is subjected to a mandatory pharmacovigilance procedure after approval. Authorized manipulations or compounding of the medicine include reconstitution of a "dry syrup" (powder or granule) into a liquid formulation or dissolution of a tablet for preparing a liquid for drug administration if these procedures are described in the SmPC of the authorized medicinal product. As the compounding is always performed by health care professionals in the pharmacies, it can be assumed that the risk of failures is lower than the manipulation procedures performed by naïve caregivers, such as parents or grandparents (see Fig. 8.1).

If the SmPC comprises the required information, it can be assumed that the quality of the resulting preparation has been tested and approved by the competent authority. Splitting of tablets into pieces can only be accepted if the breaking notches (scores) have been designed for dividing the tablet and if there is evidence that this procedure reveals the intended doses. Splitting

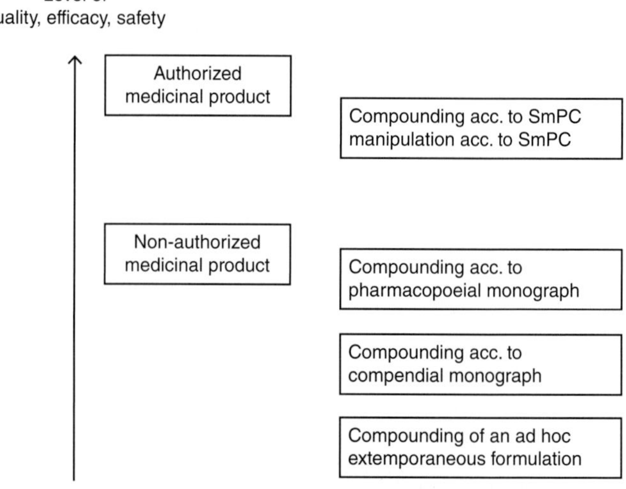

Figure 8.1 Levels of evidence and quality of drug preparations for children. SmPC, Summary of Product Characteristics.

devices as marketed in many variations usually do not improve the uniformity of the resulting pieces.[31] Crushing of tablets is unacceptable if a functional coating (enteric or prolonged-release coating) is applied to the tablet core or if there is a sophisticated technology for improving drug solubility or dissolution in place, for example, by an amorphous solid dispersion. Crushing would accelerate the forming of water-insoluble crystals by increased surface and reduce the bioavailability by far as it has been demonstrated for lopinavir and ritonavir with an exposure of less than 50% after crushing.[32] Sprinkling drug carriers onto food can be an issue if the food material interacts with the drug product and impacts the stability or dosing accuracy. Instructions provided in the SmPC should be strictly followed therefore. It has to be noted that the pharmacovigilance program in place only covers authorized use of the medicinal product.

If the SmPC does not include the required information (and this happens in the majority of cases), the manipulation or compounding is called "nonauthorized" use of approved medicines. Often, this has been called "unlicensed use"; however, most national drug laws allow this pharmaceutical practice in order to prepare child-appropriate drug formulations and to bridge the gaps in pediatric health care. The quality of the preparations obtained by nonauthorized manipulation or compounding is generally inferior to the authorized variations as it always lacks official approval and, in most cases, scientific evidence. Bioavailability is mostly unknown when administering extemporaneous preparations.

If the composition and preparation procedure are monographed by a pharmacopoeia, the higher quality can be assumed. The European Directorate for the Quality of Medicines and Healthcare (EDQM) has launched a public Pediatric Formulary in December 2019, which will be continuously enlarged (paedform.edqm.eu). So far, it contains—beside some general provision and texts—monographs on "hydrochlorothiazide 0.5 mg per mL oral solution" and "sotalol 20 mg per mL oral solution." Sources of these monographs are compendial recipes. The composition of the drug formulation, according to recent EMA guidelines, including the safety of excipients, the quality of the drug substance, and the manufacturing procedure, has been evaluated by the scientific committee, and the quality testing of the compounded preparations has been performed by laboratory testing of competent authorities. The new pediatric formulary will only contain monographs on drug substances for which no authorized pediatric medicine is available within the member states of the Council of Europe.

A major concern in compounding medicines is the quality of starting materials. In the best case, pharmaceutical grades of the drug substance are used, ideally indicated by a certificate of compliance from the authority. However, costs are high for these qualities, and package sizes are often not appropriate for a preparation in a hospital or community pharmacy. Therefore, substances of questionable quality are often used, for example, by purchasing from a catalog of chemicals. It should be noted that these qualities may not be necessarily produced for pharmaceutical purposes, are not monitored by pharmaceutical companies or authorities, and are often quality controlled in a different way. In these cases and if the drug substance is not available at all, the use of an authorized medicine, for example, a tablet or capsule, may be superior. However, it should be noted that the actual drug content of the products varies around the labeled claim and may be reduced already over storage in an unknown magnitude. Impurities may be increased already, and the compatibility of the excipients with the intended diluent is unproven (as long as this is not described in the SmPC).

In order to facilitate the compounding, there are different commercial diluents or dispersing agents available, for example, Ora Plus, Ora Sweet, and SyrSpend. Stability studies for a number of drug preparations using these standard materials are available in textbooks and scientific literature.[33,34] However, in some countries, the legal status of the suspending agents is unclear, and their use is, therefore, not recommended or even illegal in those countries. Further, some of them contain excipients, such as propyl paraben, which are not recommended for young children. Included sweeteners like sucrose and fructose increase blood sugar concentration and may cause cariogenic effects. Sorbitol and xylitol may cause osmotic diarrhea. In total, only a very limited number of these products matches the recommendations for safe excipients of the EMA. The U.S. Pharmacopoeia has monographed a number of these bases which can be prepared from pharmaceutical excipients, mainly hypromellose and methylcellulose, but, in most cases significant, time is just spent for the manufacturing of the diluents. Various recipes for different pH values and preservative-free bases are available.

Intravenous medicinal products for adult patients are often too concentrated for accurate dosing young children, in particular newborns. Measurement of small volumes can be associated with inaccurate administration of these drugs. In fact, intoxication has been reported in infants with the use of concentrated digoxin and morphine.[35,36] When diluting commercial intravenous products at the pharmacies, additional quality testing, for example, on sterility and pyrogens, applies.

The need for extemporaneous formulations will continue despite recent efforts to stimulate drug development and research for pediatric medicines. There will be never a complete coverage of all the needs of pediatric patients from different age groups. Compatibility and stability studies are still required to improve the quality of extemporaneously prepared medicines. Studies on the bioavailability, efficacy, and safety would be desirable, but are scarce due to limited financial resources. The available information should be made public as it has been started for the European Pediatric Formulary to improve scientific evidence and knowledge on extemporaneous drug formulations.

PALATABILITY OF MEDICINES

The child's acceptance of a drug formulation is dependent on its palatability.[37–39] Palatability includes the sensation of taste, flavor, and texture (mouthfeel). Better tasting usually improves the ease of administration and the loss of drug substance by spitting out. Liquid formulations often require the addition of sweeteners and flavors in order to improve the taste or flavor of the medicines. The risk–benefit balance between the toxicity of the added pharmaceutical excipients and the improved taste perception has to be carefully considered. In principle, different approaches for taste-masking are feasible[40]:

- Modify the pH of a liquid formulation
- Add sweeteners and/or flavors in order to mimic another liquid
- Increase the viscosity of the formulation to reduce drug diffusion to the taste receptors
- Add complexation agents (e.g., cyclodextrins or ion-exchange resins)
- Add a pharmacologic taste blocker (e.g., adenosine monophosphate)
- Introduce a barrier (e.g., using a polymer, wax, or fat coating)
- Mix with food or beverage

Natural sweeteners may cause diarrhea and cariogenic effects. Chemical sweeteners may show toxicity in children. Artificial or natural flavors sometimes contain allergenic components that are often not fully disclosed by the flavor manufacturer. Most cyclodextrins and ion-exchange resins display low amounts for acceptable intake. A pharmacologically active taste blocker has not been licensed for a pediatric product so far. Hence, in most cases, the introduction of a diffusion barrier for the poorly tasting API is the last chance, which automatically leads to a solid drug dosage form. Mixing or sprinkling solid multiparticulates onto food usually results in short contact time and poor diffusion of the unpleasant tasting API. If the stability or the bioavailability is not impacted by using food as a vehicle, it can be an excellent choice for improving the palatability and adherence. Just the texture of a multiparticulate can be an issue as the child may perceive a "sandy" mouthfeel.[41] Therefore, palatability is another driving force for the shift of paradigm toward solid drug formulations for children as these preparations offer more potential for the pharmaceutical technologist to improve the palatability.

In pharmaceutical development of new medicines for children, a major issue is how to predict the child's aversion to an API or a drug formulation. Taste panel results from adults usually cannot be extrapolated to children, because children prefer more sweet and less bitter sensations of taste. Pediatric taste data are only available in the clinical studies, usually obtained in a hedonic scale approach,[40] but then reformulation is hardly possible as it would cause a loop in the drug development and some loss of time until the authorization of the product. Predictive tools such as the Brief-Access Taste Aversion (BATA) model[42] and chemical taste sensing system (the so-called "electronic tongues")[43] are very popular. They cannot replace taste results from real pediatric patients, but enable better decision-making in the drug development process.

SUMMARY

Availability of a child-appropriate formulation is a limiting step for the clinical use of medicines in newborn, infants, and children. New products with advanced dosage forms, especially multiparticulate formulations as pellets and mini-tablets, have appeared on the market. These new solid dosage forms offer more opportunities in regard to taste-masking, safety of used excipients, stability, dose uniformity, and flexibility than the previously preferred liquid formulations. However, various gaps in pediatric medicines are still existing. Therefore, manipulating authorized products or compounding extemporaneous formulations is still common practice. In order to further improve the quality, efficacy, and safety of compounded products, more research is needed, and the results should be collected and published in the public domain. Spontaneous "ad hoc" preparations without scientific evidence should be abandoned unless there is not a single alternative for the use in children.

REFERENCES

1. Breitkreutz J, Boos J. Paediatric and geriatric drug delivery. *Expert Opin Drug Deliv* 2007;4:37–45.
2. Breitkreutz J. European perspectives on pediatric formulations. *Clin Ther* 2008;30:2146–2154.
3. International Council for Harmonisation of Technical Requirements for Pharmaceutical for Human Use. Addendum to ICH E11 (R1) clinical investigations of medicinal products in the paediatric population (EMA/CPMP/ICH/2711/1999). 2017. database.ich.org/sites/default/files/E11_R1_Addendum.pdf
4. Kearns GL, Abdel-Rahman SM, Alander SW, et al. Developmental pharmacology-drug disposition, action, and therapy in infants and children. *N Engl J Med* 2003;349:1157–1167.
5. Salunke S, Brandys B, Giacoia G, et al. The STEP (Safety and Toxicity of Excipients for Paediatrics) database: Part 2—The pilot version. *Int J Pharm* 2013;457:310–322.
6. Valeur KS, Holst H, Allegaert K. Excipients in neonatal medicinal products: never prescribed, commonly administered. *Pharm Med* 2018;32:251–258.
7. European Medicines Agency. Reflection paper: formulations of choice for the paediatric population (EMEA/CHMP/PEG/194810/2005). 2006. www.ema.europa.eu/en/documents/scientific-guideline/reflection-paper-formulations-choice-paediatric-population_en.pdf
8. Klingmann V, Spomer N, Lerch C, et al. Favourable acceptance of mini-tablets compared with syrup: a randomised controlled trial in infants and preschool children. *J Pediatr* 2013;163:1728–1732.
9. Klingmann V, Seitz A, Meissner T, et al. Acceptability of uncoated mini-tablets in neonates—a randomized controlled trial. *J Pediatr* 2015;167:893–896.
10. Klingmann V, Linderskamp H, Meissner T, et al. Acceptability of multiple uncoated minitablets in infants and toddlers: a randomized controlled trial. *J Pediatr* 2018;201:202–207.
11. European Medicines Agency. Guideline on pharmaceutical development of medicines for paediatric use (EMA/CHMP/QWP/805880/2012 Rev. 2). 2013. www.ema.europa.eu/en/documents/scientific-guideline/guideline-pharmaceutical-development-medicines-paediatric-use_en.pdf
12. World Health Organization. Report of the informal expert meeting on dosage forms of medicines for children. 2008. www.who.int/childmedicines/progress/Dosage_form_reportDEC2008.pdf.
13. Lopez FL, Mistry P, Batchelor HK, et al. Acceptability of placebo multiparticulate formulations in children and adults. *Sci Rep* 2018;8:9210.
14. Hoppu K. Time to change the paradigm of children's medicines from liquid formulations to flexible solid oral dosage forms. *Ceylon Med J* 2016;61:93–95.
15. Slavkova M, Breitkreutz J. Orodispersible drug formulations for children and elderly. *Eur J Pharm Sci* 2015;75:2–9.
16. Brniak W, Jachowicz R, Krupa A, et al. Evaluation of co-processed excipients used for direct compression of orally disintegrating tablets (ODT) using novel disintegration apparatus. *Pharm Dev Technol* 2013;18:464–474.
17. Seeger H. Drug-delivery products and the Zydis fast-dissolving dosage form. *J Pharm Pharmacol* 1998;50:375–382.
18. Hoffmann EM, Breitenbach A, Breitkreutz J. Advances in orodispersible films for drug delivery. *Exp Opin Drug Deliv* 2011;8:299–316.
19. Macdonald MG, Getson PR, Glasgow AM, et al. Propylene glycol: increased incidence of seizures in low birth weight infants. *Pediatrics* 1987;79:622–625.
20. Glasgow AM, Boeckx RL, Miller MK, et al. Hyperosmolarity in small infants due to propylene glycol. *Pediatrics* 1983;72:353–355.
21. Thabet Y, Slavkova M, Breitkreutz J. 10 years EU regulation of pediatric medicines—impact on cardiovascular drug formulations. *Exp Opin Drug Deliv* 2018;15:261–270.
22. Stoltenberg I, Breitkreutz J. Orally disintegrating mini-tablets (ODMTs)—a novel solid dosage form for paediatric use. *Eur J Pharm Biopharm* 2011;78:462–469.
23. Zajicek A, Fossler M, Barret JS, et al. A report from the pediatric formulations task force: perspectives on the state of child-friendly oral dosage forms. *AAPS J* 2013;15:1072–1081.
24. Strickley RG. Pediatric oral formulations: an updated review of commercially available pediatric oral formulations since 2007. *J Pharm Sci* 2019;108:1335–1365.
25. Visser JC, Woerdenbag HJ, Hanff LM, et al. Personalized medicine in pediatrics: the clinical potential of orodispersible films. *AAPS PharmSciTech* 2017;18:267–272.
26. Gaber DM, Nafee N, Abdallah OY. Mini-tablets versus pellets as promising multiparticulate modified release delivery systems for highly soluble drugs. *Int J Pharm* 2015;488:86–94.
27. Tissen C, Woertz C, Breitkreutz J, et al. Development of mini-tablets with 1 mm and 2 mm diameter. *Int J Pharm* 2011;416:164–170.
28. Hagen E, Loding FS, Mattsson S, et al. Use of interactive mixtures to obtain mini-tablets with high dose homogeneity for paediatric drug delivery. *J Drug Deliv Sci Technol* 2016;34:51–59.
29. Mitra B, Chang J, Wu SJ, et al. Feasibility of mini-tablets as a flexible drug delivery tool. *Int J Pharm* 2017;525:149–159.
30. Ernest TB, Craig J, Nunn A, et al. Preparation of medicines for children—a hierarchy of classification. *Int J Pharm* 2012;435:124–130.
31. Jacques ER, Alexandridis P. Tablet scoring: current practice, fundamentals, and knowledge gaps. *Appl Sci* 2019;9:3390.
32. Best BM, Capparelli EV, Diep H, et al. Pharmacokinetics of lopinavir/ritonavir crushed versus whole tablets in children. *J Acquir Immune Defic Syndr* 2011;58:385–391.
33. Nahata MC, Pai VB. *Pediatric drug formulations*, 7th ed. Cincinnati, OH: Harvey Whitney Books, 2018.
34. Trissel LA, Ashworth LD, Ashworth J. *Trissel's stability of compounded formulations*, 6th ed. Washington, DC: American Pharmacists Association, 2018.
35. Berman W Jr, Whitman V, Marks KH, et al. Inadvertent over administration of digoxin to low birth weight infants. *J Pediatr* 1978;92:1024–1025.
36. Zenk KE, Anderson S. Improving the accuracy of mini-volume injections. *Infusion* 1982;6:7–11.
37. Kozarewicz P. Regulatory perspectives on acceptability testing of dosage forms in children. *Int J Pharm* 2014;469:245–248.
38. Mistry P, Batchelor H. Evidence of acceptability of oral paediatric medicines: a review. *J Pharm Pharmacol* 2016;69:361–376.
39. Van Riet-Nales DA, de Neef BJ, Schobben AF, et al. Acceptability of different oral formulations in infants and preschool children. *Arch Dis Child* 2013;98:725–731.
40. Walsh J, Cram A, Woertz K, et al. Playing hide and seek with poorly tasting paediatric medicines: do not forget the excipients. *Adv Drug Deliv Rev* 2014;73:14–33.
41. Ranmal S, Cram A, Tuleu C. Age-appropriate and acceptable paediatric dosing forms: insights into end-user perceptions, preferences and practices from the Children's acceptability of oral formulations (CALF) study. *Int J Pharm* 2016;514:296–307.
42. Soto J, Winzenburg G, Turner R, et al. Assessing the bitter taste of medicines: a comparison between rat taste panels (via the brief-access taste aversion (BATA) model) and human taste panels. *Int J Pharm* 2016;511:1127–1128.
43. Woertz K, Tissen C, Kleinebudde P, et al. Taste sensing systems (electronic tongues) for pharmaceutical applications. *Int J Pharm* 2011;417:256–271.

SECTION

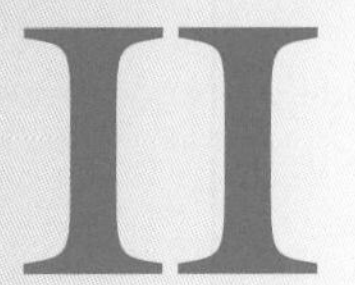

Pharmacology in Special Settings and Population: The Newborn

Jamil M. Kazma
Johannes N. van den Anker
Karel Allegaert
André Dallmann
Homa K. Ahmadzia

CHAPTER

9

Role of Placenta in Drug Metabolism and Drug Transfer

INTRODUCTION

The placenta is an ephemeral organ that is pivotal for the development of the fetus.

In some cultures, it is believed that burying the placenta after birth reinforces the baby's belonging to earth. Since the 16th century, in its powdered form "Placenta Hominis," the placenta has been used in traditional Chinese medicine to treat a myriad of symptoms.[1] The ground-breaking work of Mossman, published in 1937, on the developmental comparison of the placenta across species,[2] paved the way for more sophisticated delineations of its anatomic and physiologic architecture. He simplified the definition of the placenta as "fusion of the fetal membrane to the uterine mucosa for physiologic exchange."

The placenta's growth from a few cells into a multifunctional organ is unmatched by any other organ. It serves as an interface connecting the mother and fetus. However, the wording "placental barrier" holds a false notion since the placenta is the entry through which the fetus is exposed to compounds as well as the exit to eliminate compounds. In addition, it plays an important role in the synthesis of hormones (progesterone, estrogen) and peptides (human chorionic gonadotropin, placental growth hormone, insulin growth factor) that are vital for a successful pregnancy, while its dysfunction has been associated with preeclampsia.[3–7] Furthermore, the placenta has metabolic functions, including metabolic processes related to medicines, like for some steroids. The "barrier" or "filter" function of the placenta includes passive diffusion, facilitated diffusion, active transport, and pinocytosis/endocytosis.[7]

Historically, it took several articles[8–10] to discredit the notion that the placenta is an impermeable barrier against xenobiotics. Some reasons that corroborated the original belief of impermeability were the perceived idealization of the womb and a general disinterest in stillborn outcomes.[11] It was not until the thalidomide disaster in 1961 that the scientific community embraced the fact that the placenta is a permeable barrier to molecules and drugs, some of which can result in fetal teratogenicity.[12,13] Since then, it has been the target of research despite the countless challenges accompanying it. Understanding the underlying mechanism of the transport of drugs and molecules across the placenta and its physiology is essential in paving the way for experiments conducted by researchers and pharmaceutical companies to unravel the real mystery of this interface and improve our understanding of pharmacotherapy in pregnancy.

This chapter reviews the function of the placenta in drug transfer, focusing on the mechanisms and factors that mediate it. In addition, the chapter expands on the biotransformation and metabolism of compounds that cross the placenta, highlighting the enzymes and chemical reactions involved.

ANATOMY OF THE HUMAN PLACENTA

There is extensive variability in the placenta among different species. This variability is based on the four categories: shape, placental interdigitation, maternal–fetal interface, and the arrangement of the maternal and fetal circulation.[14] The human placenta is of discoid shape, which provides the lowest surface area.[15] As for the placental interdigitation in humans, it is best described as villous, which may offer a metabolic advantage in requiring less energy and thus the ability to sustain a longer gestation.[16] The human placenta is of the hemochorial type where

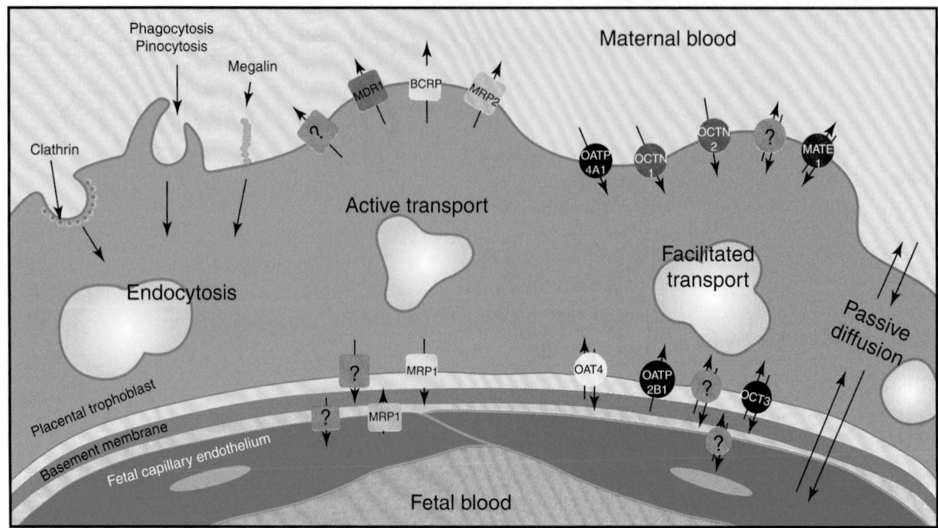

Figure 9.1 Normal anatomy of the maternal–fetal placental interface and overview of important transport mechanisms across the placenta. BRCP, breast cancer resistance protein; MATE1, multidrug and toxin extruding protein 1; MDR1, multidrug-resistant protein 1; MRP1, multidrug resistance-associated protein 1; MRP2, multidrug resistance-associated protein 2; OAT4, organic anion transporter 4; OATP4A1, organic anion transporting polypeptide 4A1; OATP2B1, organic anion transporting polypeptide 2B1; OCT1, organic cation transporter 1; OCT3, organic cation transporter 3; OCTN1, organic cation/carnitine transporter 1; OCTN2, organic cation/carnitine transporter 2; Question marks indicate transport process required characterization. (Reprinted with permission from Al-Enazy S, Ali S, Albekairi N, et al. Placental control of drug delivery. *Adv Drug Deliv Rev* 2017;116:63–72.)

one syncytiotrophoblast layer is in direct contact with the maternal blood and is the most intimate form.[17] The predicament of this type of interface is that it is dependent on the development of tolerance in the maternal immune system to the paternal antigens present on the placenta.[18] The difference in the anatomic structure of the placenta among animal species complicates the design of animal experiments to study human diseases.[14]

The placenta, on average, measures approximately 22 cm in diameter and weighs about 470 g at delivery[19]; however, the weight may vary at term, with a median of 475 g at 37 weeks to 515 g at 40 weeks, and by disease status, such as in the case of pregnancy in women with diabetes.[20] Also, it is polarized with two plates, the basal plate, which is in contact with the uterine endometrium and maternal circulation, and the chorionic plate to which the umbilical cord attaches.[19]

At implantation (day 6), the trophoblast cells, surrounding the inner cell mass at the embryonic pole of the blastocyst, interact with the epithelial cells of the endometrium. This interaction triggers the remodeling of the extracellular matrix of the endometrium and the interweaving of the syncytiotrophoblast (multinucleated cells of the trophoblast) between endometrial cells. As a result, the arterioles and capillaries are eroded, allowing maternal blood to perfuse to what is referred to as the intervillous space,[21,22] eventually surrounding the conceptus where the blastocyst is covered with maternal blood, forming the trophoblastic lacunae.[23,24] This intervillous circulation is not evident until 9 weeks and becomes continuous across the placenta by 12 weeks of gestation.[25] The placenta thus develops in a low O_2 milieu, which minimizes the production of reactive oxygen species that has been linked to causing damage to the syncytiotrophoblast.[26]

The cytotrophoblasts (unicellular cells of the trophoblast) covered with syncytiotrophoblast cells penetrate the lacunae to form the primary villi and subsequently differentiate to the anchoring villi as they reach the uterine decidua.[27] These differentiated villi are made up of two cell lineages: cytotrophoblast and syncytiotrophoblast. The basic structure of the placenta is complete by 4 weeks of gestation. The syncytiotrophoblast layer is also polarized with a maternal-facing brush border membrane (apical) and fetal-facing (basal) membrane that share different molecular compositions. In addition, the syncytiotrophoblast layer is continuous, whereas the underlying cytotrophoblast is discontinuous.[28,29] It is important to note that normally maternal and fetal blood do not mix directly, but exchange of nutrients and drugs occurs across these various cellular layers (Fig. 9.1).

MATERNAL PHYSIOLOGIC CHANGES IN PREGNANCY

Pregnancy results in notable physiologic changes to the maternal body and placenta to accommodate the metabolic demands of the mother and the growing fetus. Several of these changes may affect variables governing pharmacokinetics of drugs, including absorption, distribution, metabolism, and excretion.[30] Among the most critical changes is an increase in plasma volume, which is first evident around 6 to 8 weeks, and continues to increase with a peak around the 32nd week of gestation.[31–33] This expansion leads to an increased volume of distribution of hydrophilic drugs, similar to the increase in fat mass in pregnancy and its effect on lipophilic drugs. In addition, the blood flow to the uteroplacental circulation reaches its peak in the third trimester, ranging from 50 to 60 mL per minute at first trimester to the peak of 185 mL per minute before hitting another peak at term reaching between 450 and 750 mL per minute.[34–36] The proportion of the cardiac output flowing into the uteroplacental circulation at early pregnancy also increases from 3% to 6% to about 12% at term.[35,36]

Furthermore, the concentration of albumin, an important protein carrier of many drugs, decreases by 25% as pregnancy progresses, causing drugs that are highly protein bound to have a higher concentration of the unbound form.[37–40] Another binding protein for many basic drugs, α-1 acid glycoprotein, also decreases by 15% by the third trimester.[40,41]

Changes in the gastrointestinal tract, including decreased gastric pH, increased volume of gastric secretions, and a

TABLE 9.1 Major Pharmacokinetic Changes during Pregnancy

Change in Pregnancy	*Pharmacokinetic Effect*	*Potential Clinical Effect*
Increased body weight	Lower serum concentrations	Smaller effects if dose not increased
Lower serum albumin levels	Higher free (unbound) fraction leads to greater transport, clearance	No change in the steady-state concentration of the free drug (e.g., phenytoin)
Increased hepatic metabolic rate	Faster clearance rate of some drugs metabolized by the liver	Smaller effects if the dose is not increased; for example, dexamethasone is not metabolized in the liver and hence is more likely to cross the placenta at higher concentrations
Decreased hepatic metabolic rate	Slower clearance rate	For example, theophylline metabolized more slowly
Higher liver blood flow	Faster clearance rate of high-extraction ratio drugs	Smaller effects if dose is not increased
Higher glomerular filtration rate	Faster clearance rate of renally excreted drugs or their active metabolites	Smaller effects if dose is not increased (e.g., lithium, digoxin)
Lower compliance (because of fears of teratogenicity)	Lower drug concentrations	More therapeutic failures

Data from Koren G, Klinger G, Ohlsson A. Fetal pharmacotherapy. *Drugs* 2002;62(5):757–773 and Loebstein R, Lalkin A, Koren G. Pharmacokinetic changes during pregnancy and their clinical relevance. *Clin Pharmacokinet* 1997;33(5):328–343.

relaxed esophageal sphincter tone, not only contribute to increased nausea and vomiting but may also affect the absorption and bioavailability of oral drugs.[42,43] Despite controversy as to whether there is a decrease in gastric motility during pregnancy across different studies,[44,45] theoretically, these hormonally induced changes would decrease the peak concentration of oral drugs in the maternal circulation.[46] Moreover, the liver enzymes responsible for phase I and phase II metabolism are altered in pregnancy.[47,48] These enzymatic alterations may affect drug clearance and excretion, which in response may require dose adjustments for certain drugs. Renally cleared drugs can be particularly affected as pregnancy causes an increase in renal plasma flow and glomerular filtration rate.[49,50] Table 9.1 summarizes the key physiologic changes during pregnancy.

The placenta itself undergoes physical changes during pregnancy. The placental barrier thickness decreases by up to 95% from late first trimester to term, the surface area increases by 140% from the late second trimester to term, and the cytotrophoblast layer becomes more discontinuous as the pregnancy progresses.[51–53] Moreover, placental transport and exchange is altered as pregnancy progresses, shifting from histotrophic nutrition under anaerobic conditions during first trimester to supplementation by maternal arterial circulation that perfuses the intervillous space for the remainder of the pregnancy.[54–56] Gestational-specific uterine perfusion to the placental compartment increases by about 12-fold at term.[43] However, there is limited information on whether there is a change in placental drug transport with gestation.[57] The complexity of placental and physiologic changes during pregnancy makes it challenging to conduct clinical drug trials to identify optimal dosing regimens. In addition, concerns about fetal safety hinder further advancements in this field.

MECHANISMS OF PLACENTAL TRANSFER OF DRUGS

Transplacental therapy has been a low-profile research field for some time. Decades ago, Ampola and colleagues were the first to treat methylmalonic acidemia of a fetus by administering large doses of vitamin B_{12} to the mother.[58] More recently, transplacental therapy has been used to treat several fetal disorders, including fetal arrhythmias, human immunodeficiency virus (HIV) mother-to-child transmission, fetal lung maturity, and passive fetal immunity.[59] Also, fetomaternal alloimmune thrombocytopenia can be managed by giving intravenous immunoglobulins (IVIgs) to the mother, saturating the receptors on the placenta, and preventing further transfer of the antibodies targeting platelets across the syncytiotrophoblast membrane and into the fetal circulation.[60] In addition, drug therapy can target placental dysfunction such as the case of sildenafil used in the management of early-onset fetal growth restriction and preeclampsia; a promising but experimental therapy so far.[61]

Endogenous and exogenous compounds may cross the placenta to various degrees and are best characterized as an unequal bidirectional transfer. The crossing is governed by several factors intrinsically related to the nature of the compound and the need for transport shuttle and energy expenditure across the syncytiotrophoblast, the basement membrane, and the endothelium of fetal capillaries.[51] Maternal diseases such as preeclampsia may also affect placental drug transfer in ex vivo models.[61] An increase in oxidative stress seen in conditions such as fetal growth restriction, diabetes, and preeclampsia may also affect the transport of nutrients and the permeability of the membrane.[62] With the advancements in transplacental pharmacokinetics and the need to have accurate and safe pharmacotherapy during gestation, it became important to understand the function and expression of transport proteins and drug interaction at this interface.

CHEMICAL AND PHYSICAL FACTORS AFFECTING PLACENTAL TRANSFER

Size

Any molecule with a molecular weight (MW) of more than 1,000 Da rarely crosses the placenta, those with MW of less than 500 Da generally cross readily, and the remaining cross at a slower rate.[63] This property does not limit transport, however, as most drugs are less than 500 Da, except e.g. for the various forms of heparin, which are known not to cross the placenta.[64] Insulin (5,734 Da) is another example where the placenta is an effective barrier against its transport.[65]

Blood Flow

For lipophilic drugs, the blood flow is critical in determining the rate of exchange across the placenta. It limits the availability of the drug at the interface, making them flow limited, as opposed to the hydrophilic drugs, which are permeability limited.[66] Any change from the maternal blood flow (uterine) and fetal blood flow (umbilical), such as hypertensive disorders in the mother or severe cardiac insufficiency in the fetus (like fetal end-diastolic reversed blood flow), may result in an altered drug exposure and thus affect the diffusion rate.[67,68] During labor and delivery, the decrease in blood flow to the placenta due to regular uterine contractions may contribute to a delay in the clearance of drugs already in the fetal circulation and affect the delivery of the drug from maternal circulation.[66]

Protein Binding

Protein-bound drugs cannot readily cross the placenta. Two essential plasma proteins are responsible for the majority of protein binding of drugs, albumin and α-1 acid glycoprotein, which, generally speaking, bind acidic and basic drugs, respectively.[69,70] Valproic acid, for example, binds to albumin,[71] whereas drugs such as cocaine and sufentanil, both weak bases, bind predominantly to α-1 acid glycoprotein. Diazepam, a weak base, does not comply with the general rule as it is shown to bind albumin.[72] Bupivacaine, a common anesthetic used in spinal anesthesia for cesarean delivery, is highly protein bound to albumin.[73] Both α-1 acid glycoprotein and albumin concentration decrease in pregnancy, yet albumin does so at a far greater degree.[39] In the fetus, the concentration of both albumin and α-1 acid glycoprotein increases from the first trimester until term, but α-1 acid glycoprotein concentration in the fetus reaches only 50% of that found in maternal blood.[66,74] This differential translates into having more unbound drugs readily available to cross the placenta across the gradient. Propofol is a highly protein-bound drug to albumin and red blood cells, and its placental transfer is affected by both increased maternal blood flow and decreased albumin concentration, such that there is an increased uptake by the placenta and transfer to the fetus.[75] The use of propofol has been associated with lower Apgar scores at 1 and 5 minutes compared to thiopental, when used for induction of anesthesia in cesarean delivery.[76] However, in other studies, this has not shown to be true.[77,78] This phenomenon of protein binding is subject to competition by endogenous molecules like free fatty acids, which are three times higher in the mother compared to fetal concentration at term. However, the saturation of proteins like albumin by free fatty acids is negligible when compared to the protein concentration effect on the placental transfer of drugs.[79–81]

pH and Ion Trapping

A drug cannot pass the placental barrier in its ionized or charged form. Most drugs are either weak acids or weak bases, which cause them to be charged at physiologic pH. The maternal pH (pH = 7.4) is higher than fetal pH (pH = 7.3) by 0.1 log units, allowing the fetal concentration of basic drugs to exceed the maternal concentration at equilibrium.[82] Clinically, this is important to consider during fetal acidemia, as fetal pH decreases further, allowing for more basic drug accumulation such as lidocaine, bupivacaine, and other amide anesthetics during delivery, possibly leading to neonatal side effects.[83–8]

Neerheles, studieshve shown that the phenomenon of ion trapping merely contributes as a sole factor for controlling placental transfer. Weak acid drugs such as salicylates and valproate, which are ionized at physiologic pH, appear to transfer across the placenta readily.[87,88] Similarly, antibiotics such as ampicillin and methicillin seem to follow the same flow.[89] However, neuromuscular blockade drugs, which are large quaternary ammonium compounds that are highly ionized at physiologic pH, cannot cross the placenta.[90]

Placental Binding

In vitro studies illustrate how the placenta can serve as a depot for some drugs, particularly with very lipophilic drugs which can readily cross the lipid bilayer of the syncytiotrophoblast cell.[91] The change in serum protein concentration has an implication on the drug transfer by affecting its binding to tissue protein. If the drug binds tissue proteins with a higher affinity than serum proteins, this allows the drug to be removed from the protein binding in plasma and cross more readily to the placenta.[92] One study was able to show that the increasing fetal circulation of albumin enhances the uptake of steroids and freeing them from entrapment by tissue proteins in the placenta.[93] The immunosuppressive drug tacrolimus is used during pregnancy for renal transplant patients, and it has been shown that it can be entrapped in the placenta. Clinically, placental insufficiency has been associated with the use of calcineurin inhibitors of which tacrolimus is an example, and this entrapment maybe one of the causes.[94,95] Sildenafil, a phosphodiesterase-5 inhibitor given to treat pulmonary hypertension during pregnancy, has also been shown to accumulate in the placenta.[96] Interestingly, the accumulation of drugs in the placenta can be advantageous, such as the case of treating placental toxoplasmosis infection with spiramycin, a drug that concentrates in the placenta to help reduce maternal-to-fetal transmission.[97] The importance of placental perfusion studies that specifically investigate the effect of maternal and fetal protein concentrations is imperative in understanding yet another layer of complexity in the transfer of drugs across the placental barrier.

MECHANISM OF TRANSPORT

Simple Diffusion

Most drugs cross the placenta by simple diffusion, which is a passive process that is dependent on the concentration gradient of the drug. Antipyrine is a classic example of this type of transplacental diffusion and is the most important molecule used in ex vivo perfusion studies because it serves as an indicator of experimental validity.[98] Passive diffusion over a biologic membrane is typically described by Fick's first law of diffusion. Assuming a time-independent linear concentration profile, the diffusion rate of a drug across the placental membrane can be expressed as follows[99]:

$$dC_m/dt = D \times \alpha \times SA/(\Delta x \times V_m) \times (C_m - C_f) = P \times SA/V_m \times (C_m - C_f)$$

where C_m and C_f is the concentration of unbound, uncharged drug on the maternal and fetal side, respectively; D is the drug's diffusion coefficient; α is the partition coefficient of the drug into the membrane; SA the surface area of the cell membrane of exchange; Δx is the width of the cell membrane; V_m is the volume of the fluid in which the drug is dissolved on the maternal side (i.e., the volume of the maternal blood plasma filling the intervillous space); and P is the drug's permeability coefficient. Likewise, the equation for the fetal concentration is as follows:

$$dC_f/dt = -P \times SA/V_f \times (C_m - C_f)$$

The rate of diffusion of a drug is directly proportional to the surface area of exchange (SA) and the concentration gradient across the membrane $(C_m - C_f)$ and inversely proportional to the thickness of the membrane (Δx). The thickness and surface area of exchange undergo gestation-specific changes during pregnancy. Several studies showed that the thickness decreases, while the surface area increases as pregnancy progress, resulting in an increased placental transfer during gestation.[100,101] Extrapolating this into in vivo studies is challenging as the anatomic changes are more complex. Thornburg and Faber[102] were able to show the importance of the fetal endothelium layer, which is not much altered during pregnancy, in limited drug diffusion, and is responsible for the resistance to compounds with large MWs.[100,101]

The syncytiotrophoblast barrier is a lipid bilayer that favors molecules that are of low MW, unionized, and relatively hydrophobic (lipophilic).[82] However, extremely lipophilic drugs can get stuck and become constituents of the cell membrane (e.g., thyroid hormones) requiring other forms of transfer across the membrane, such as active transport.[103,104] Measuring lipophilicity by means of the compound's partition ratio between octanol and water (log *P* value) or aqueous buffer with a pH of 7.4 (log *D* value) can be used as a first screening tool to assess whether a given compound is likely to cross the placenta readily.[105] Also, toxic waste products from the fetus are transferred across the placenta by simple diffusion, including urea, bilirubin, and carbon dioxide.[91]

Facilitated Transport

This transport mechanism is similar to simple diffusion. It does not require energy expenditure, and the direction of flow is dependent on the concentration gradient but differs in that it requires a carrier or transporter.[106] The goal of the transporters is to facilitate the transfer of nonlipid-soluble compounds down their concentration gradient. Although Fick's law does not apply here, this mechanism is under the influence of competitive and noncompetitive inhibition, stereoselectivity, and saturation kinetics.[107] Maternal disease states such as preeclampsia or elevated steroid levels may affect transporter function.[108] The most commonly studied transporters of the placenta belong to the solute carrier family (SLC), which constitutes several subgroups including organic anion transporters (OATs), organic anion transporting polypeptides (OATPs), organic cation transporters (OCTs), organic cation/carnitine transporters (OCTNs), multidrug and toxin extruding protein 1 (MATE1), and nucleoside transporters (NTs).[106] Ganciclovir is an antiviral drug that utilizes this mechanism by entering the basolateral side (maternal) into the syncytiotrophoblast but follows a passive diffusion after that to reach the fetal circulation.[109] Studies showed the presence of carrier proteins for cephalexin and glucocorticoids. Other compounds that resemble endogenous substances are assumed to be transported by this mechanism as well.[110,111]

Organic Anion Transporters

The OAT family includes seven members (OAT1 to OAT7), of which OAT4 is specific to humans. OAT4 is localized at the basolateral membrane of the syncytiotrophoblast, in addition to its presence in the kidneys and the liver.[112] Small, amphiphilic organic anions, including antibiotics, angiotensin-converting enzyme inhibitors, diuretics, and nonsteroidal anti-inflammatory drugs, are known substrates.[113] This transporter also plays an important role in the placental synthesis of estrogen by transporting C-19 precursor compounds necessary for the pathway and protect the fetus from toxicity of steroid sulfates.[114] A study showed that olmesartan undergoes bidirectional transport at the basolateral membrane.[115] Newly developed anti-HIV and anti-HCV drugs are anionic compounds and may play part in drug–drug interaction at the level of this transport.[116]

Organic Anion Transporting Polypeptides

The OATP family includes two important membranes in placental transport, the basolateral OATP2B1 (OATP-B) and the apical OATP4A1 (OATP-E).[114,117] The former is involved with OAT4 in the estrogen synthesis in the placenta in addition to transporting drugs such as pravastatin, fexofenadine glyburide, methotrexate, imatinib, and repaglinide.[118–122] On the other hand, OATP-E plays an important physiologic role in transplacental transport of endogenous substances, particularly thyroid hormones.[117]

Organic Cation Transporters

The OCT is a uniporter in which its substrates are hydrophilic, organic cations and that its transport is electrogenic and dependent on the electrochemical gradient of the transported substrate.[123] Among the three OCTs (OCT1 to OCT3), OCT3 is most abundant in the placenta and is located on the basolateral membrane.[112] The physiologic role of OCT3 is limited to transfer of catecholamines from the fetal circulation and the release of acetylcholine from the placenta along with OCT1.[124,125] Metformin is one of the substrates of OCT3.[126]

Organic Cation/Carnitine Transporters

The OCTNs are also members of the same family of OCTs, which is SLC22A, and have three different transporters OCTN1, OCTN2, and OCTN3. It is responsible for the influx of carnitine in addition to the cationic molecules and is localized at the apical membrane.[127] Carnitine is important in oxidation of fatty acids in the mitochondria of the fetus.[128] OCTN2 is expressed early in pregnancy and continues to be expressed unchanged till term; however, carnitine transport can be affected by preeclampsia.[129] Substrates for OCTN1 include quinine, quinidine, and verapamil, whereas OCTN2 involves the transport of spironolactone, cephaloridine, and valproic acid.[130] OCTN3 is not well known to be involved in xenobiotic transport and is suggested that its function is limited to carnitine transport.[112]

Multidrug and Toxin Extrusion Proteins

The MATEs are antiporters that utilize the H^+ concentration gradient to transfer molecules across the cell membrane.[131] Characteristically, this class of transporters is located on the apical side and collaborates with OCTs to make an efficient transport mechanism that limits fetal exposure to drugs. In one study, Ahmadimoghaddam et al. have shown that OCT3 transports cationic compounds from the fetal circulation into the placenta, and the MATE transporters pump those back to the maternal circulation.[132] There is a wide variety of substrates that are shared, including many endogenous molecules (estrogen, progesterone, corticosteroids) and exogenous drugs (acyclovir, metformin, procainamide, imipramine).[133]

Nucleoside Transporters

NTs are bidirectional transporters that are divided into two categories, equilibrative NTs (ENTs) and concentrative NTs (CNTs), and their function is uptake of natural nucleoside needed for physiologic processes.[112] Isoforms of the ENTs, ENT1 and ENT2, are expressed on the apical and basolateral sides of the syncytiotrophoblast membrane, respectively.[134] They play a role in the effect of the pharmacokinetics of nucleoside reverse transcriptase inhibitors (didanosine and zalcitabine), antihepatitis therapy (ribavirin and entecavir), and antineoplastic drugs (gemcitabine and cladribine).[135–137]

Pinocytosis and Endocytosis

This is an endocytosis-driven process, facilitating transfer of large molecules like (endogenous) immunoglobulins or exogenous monoclonal antibodies. PEGylation of monoclonal antibodies, such as certolizumab, reduces its placental transfer.[138] Megalin, a known endocytic receptor, is responsible for the transfer of aminoglycosides such as gentamicin, which is used for the treatment of intra-amniotic infections. From a clinical perspective, fetal exposure to gentamicin is known to result in nephrotoxicity, which is believed to be mediated by megalin-mediated endocytosis and accumulation of the drug in fetal renal epithelium.[139,140]

Active Transport

Primary active transport is an adenosine triphosphate (ATP)-dependent process that can primarily work against a concentration gradient, while a secondary active transport utilizes the energy stored in the electrochemical gradient of a cotransported ion like Na^+, Cl^-, and H^+.[141] These transporters play an essential physiologic role in the exchange of nutrients from the mother to the fetus and waste products from the fetus to the mother. It is believed to be the mechanism which many amino acids, vitamins, and glucose utilize. It is also incorporated in the protective role of the placenta by facilitating the efflux of xenobiotics that might be harmful to the fetus.[66,142–144]

Most of the transports belong to the ATP-binding cassette (ABC) protein family, which contains several subfamilies that have been shown to exist on both basolateral and apical membranes of the syncytiotrophoblast.[145] Of those, the most studied in the placenta are P-glycoprotein, multidrug resistance-associated proteins (MRPs), and breast cancer resistance proteins (BRCPs).[146,147] Initially, these transporters were identified in cancer patients resistant to chemotherapy; more studies have been shown that these transporters are found in the placenta and that drug interaction with these transporters is implicated in controlling several factors of pharmacokinetics, including absorption, distribution, and elimination.[146] Some other transporters have also been described and are present in the placenta, including OCTs, serotonin transporter, norepinephrine transporter, sodium/multivitamin transporters, and monocarboxylate and dicarboxylate transporters. Knowledge of their role in modulating drug transport across the placenta and fetal pharmacology is limited. Figure 9.1 illustrates the distribution of the transporters across the basolateral and apical sides of the placental interface.

P-glycoprotein (MDR1)

The P-glycoprotein, or "permeability" protein, was first discovered in 1976 in an ovarian cell.[148] It is encoded by the *ABCB1* (MDR1) gene in humans and serves to protect cells and tissues from harmful xenobiotics.[149] P-glycoproteins are mainly found on the apical side facing the maternal circulation in the placental syncytiotrophoblast, and its physiologic function is the transfer of hydrophobic cationic compounds from the fetus to the maternal circulation.[150] Their expression is higher during the first trimester and decreases at term,[151,152] and in the placenta than in the liver.[153]

The implications of P-glycoprotein in the placenta are evident from the transfer of vincristine, vinblastine, and digoxin into the trophoblast cells showing preferential uptake in the fetal-to-maternal direction[154] and from an in vitro study showing trophoblasts pumping cyclosporin out of the cells.[155] Substrates for this enzyme are not structurally related; they include a wide array of drugs, such as cardiovascular (digoxin, statins), HIV protease inhibitors (tenofovir disoproxil fumarate, saquinavir), anticancer drugs (paclitaxel), cyclosporin, and others.[57,147,156] Also, some drugs may serve as inhibitors, including cyclosporin and verapamil. As such, their intake might affect the exposure of the fetus to toxic compounds.[157] One example of this inhibition can be illustrated in the antenatal therapy of fetal supraventricular tachycardia using digoxin for the mother. When treatment with digoxin as monotherapy fails, verapamil is usually added. Since digoxin is a good substrate to P-glycoprotein, the addition of verapamil is thought to increase fetal exposure to digoxin by inhibiting the P-glycoprotein.[66,154]

Clinically, the understanding of how P-glycoprotein works at the level of syncytiotrophoblast membrane can lead to potential advances in pharmacotherapy during pregnancy. In case of HIV transmission, the current regimen involves zidovudine, which has been shown to cross the placenta and accumulate in the fetal circulation to ensure the protection of the fetus. However, protease inhibitors, which have been an essential component of highly active antiretroviral therapy (HAART) for HIV patients, cannot cross the placenta readily because of several factors, including the effect of the efflux transporter P-glycoprotein, and thus limiting its clinical effectiveness. In the future, it may prove beneficial to administer an inhibitor of the transporter in conjunction with a protease inhibitor to achieve adequate levels of the latter in the fetal circulation.[158]

The efficacy of glucocorticoids in lung maturation has been proven to be a critical measure in reducing respiratory distress syndrome in preterm babies, among other important reductions in neonatal morbidity.[159] Antenatal glucocorticoid, being a substrate of P-glycoprotein, can cross the placenta rapidly via passive diffusion to reach fetal circulation aided by the concentration gradient. P-glycoprotein may play a role in the development of this gradient by pumping glucocorticoid from the fetus into the maternal circulation.[160]

Furthermore, several antidepressants have been substrates for P-glycoprotein, and studies showed umbilical cord concentration is lower than the maternal concentration, thus highlighting yet another benefit of P-glycoprotein in reducing exposure of antidepressants to the fetus.[147,161] Thus, drug–drug interaction and drug–transporter interaction are both crucial parameters to be explored in order to improve drug choice in pregnancy.

Methadone is also another known drug to be transported by the P-glycoprotein across the placenta in which the activity and expression affect the fetal concentration.[162] Genetic variation in transport gene expression results in variability of fetal drug exposure.[163] The clinical picture of neonatal abstinence syndrome depends on the understanding of how the placenta regulates the pharmacokinetics and pharmacodynamics of opiates crossing and that is one contributor to its complexity, as several other variables such as polypharmacy, dosage, or use of alcohol and smoking also contribute.[163]

Multidrug Resistance Proteins

The MRP family belongs to the ABC protein family of transporters that plays an essential role in regulating the active transport of substrates in the placenta, specifically the unconjugated, amphiphilic anions and conjugated lipophilic compounds (glutathione, glucuronate, and sulfate).[164] There are several members of this family, of which MRP3 is the most expressed in the placenta and plays an essential role in the transport of drugs from the fetal to the maternal side. Other MRPs can be found on the apical membrane, basolateral membrane, and/or on fetal endothelial cells.[165] Apical and basolateral localization of MRPs may indicate their role in placental transport from fetuses to the mother and from mother to fetus, respectively.[166] The physiologic role of the MRPs is limited to the removal of waste products and bilirubin from the fetus to the mother.[124,157] Several drugs serve as substrates for this active transporter, including anticancer agents (methotrexate, etoposide, vinca alkaloids, platinum-based compounds), HIV protease inhibitors, acetaminophen, and antibacterial agents (grepafloxacin and ampicillin).[66,167]

Breast Cancer Resistance Proteins

This ATP-dependent transport is present on the apical side of the syncytiotrophoblast and the fetal endothelial cells since the first trimester; thus, it has a role in the efflux of many endogenous and exogenous compounds.[165] Among all tissues, the expression of BRCP is highest in the placenta, making it an exciting target for research to elucidate its function in the maternal–fetal interface.[150] Although its physiologic function remains ambiguous, it plays a vital role in the efflux transport of anticancer drugs (methotrexate, doxorubicin, daunorubicin, mitoxantrone, topotecan, irinotecan), antiretroviral (zidovudine, lamivudine), glyburide, nitrofurantoin, cimetidine, and several others.[17,112,165,168] Interestingly, glyburide, a prominent oral antidiabetic medication that has been suggested for the treatment of gestational diabetes in the mother, was less popular among physicians due to the side effects in the neonate, including hypoglycemia. However, studies have shown that there is little transfer of glyburide across the placenta and that the fetal concentration in treated women is minimal, suggesting a more complex interplay between different efflux transporters and their expression in the membrane of the syncytiotrophoblast.[169]

PLACENTAL METABOLISM

One of the placenta's critical roles, which may be of concern in pharmacotherapy, is the ability to process endogenous and exogenous compounds into their metabolites through phase I and phase II biotransformation. This function of the placenta has not been well studied, and its importance is yet limited. The enzymes responsible are mainly localized in the endoplasmic reticulum and mitochondrial membrane of the syncytiotrophoblast, and their expression varies by gestational age, where the maximal expression is often believed to be in the first trimester.[170–172]

PHASE I BIOTRANSFORMATION

The placenta utilizes a myriad of enzymes from the cytochrome P450 (CYP) system that has been extensively studied in the liver. The most commonly expressed enzyme is CYP19, which is responsible for metabolizing many of the xenobiotics that cross the placenta, in addition to its physiologic role.[173] Other enzymes commonly expressed include members of CYP1, CYP2, and CYP3 enzymes. CYP2 and CYP3 enzymes have not been well studied as their expression in the placenta is relatively unnoticeable.

Cytochrome P450 CYP19 Family

CYP19 enzymes, also known as the aromatase enzymes, play an important role in steroid synthesis, particularly of estrogen necessary for the maintenance of pregnancy.[174–176] It is responsible for the metabolism of buprenorphine into norbuprenorphine, an alternative drug to methadone in treating opiate abuse patients. Of clinical relevance, both drugs have been prescribed during pregnancy and have been linked to neonatal abstinence syndrome, even though risk was minimal in the buprenorphine therapy.[177–180] It has been shown that both methadone and buprenorphine may affect the physiologic function of CYP19 in estrogen biosynthesis.[181] CYP19 has been shown to metabolize glyburide.[182] The metabolite generated can cross into the fetal tissue in in vitro studies. It is yet unclear whether this metabolism holds true in vivo and the extent of its effect on the imbalance of the fetal euglycemia state.[183]

Cytochrome P450 CYP1 Family

CYP1 enzymes, including CYP1A1, CYP1B1, and CYP1A2, are expressed in the placenta of women who have been smoking during pregnancy, particularly the form CYP1A1. On the other hand, CYP1A2 is mainly expressed in the liver.[184,185] Physiologically, these are involved in the biosynthesis of steroids such as estradiol. CYP1B1 plays a role in the metabolism of testosterone and progesterone and also in retinoic acid, an essential compound in the formation of the eye.[186–189] Clinically, CYP1B1 mutation has been linked to primary congenital glaucoma as the enzyme is known to metabolize retinoic acid.[190] However, the involvement of CYP1B1 in the biotransformation of drugs is relatively minimal.[171] Smoking has been shown to play a role in regulating metabolic genes, particularly that of *CYP1A1* and *GSTT1*, which, in turn, are associated with the pathogenesis of low birth weight in mothers who smoke.[191,192] CYP1A1 is induced by polycyclic aromatic hydrocarbons and other environmental pollutants present, leading to the creation of DNA adducts in the placenta.[193] Of particular interest in this enzyme is the fact that it is inducible under the aryl hydrocarbon receptor (Ah receptor) activity, which is abundantly present in the placenta.[194,195] This enzyme has a low level of activity at baseline but is inducible in smoking mothers. Its activity is highest at the end of pregnancy.[185,196] The role of this enzyme in mediating fetal toxicity from smoking, such as intrauterine growth restriction, has not been explored yet.[197,198] However, mothers who smoked cigarettes and delivered low birth weight babies had a higher activity of placental aryl hydrocarbon hydroxylase (an indicator of high activity of CYP1A1) and thus are at increased risk of having DNA adducts.[199–201] Interestingly, patients who delivered infants with anencephaly had a lower activity of CYP1A1 and the activity of this enzyme was lower in older mothers, suggesting that the activity of this enzyme may explain the association of fetal abnormalities with advanced maternal age.[172,202]

Cytochrome P450 CYP3A Family

This particular group of metabolic enzymes is the most commonly expressed drug metabolizing enzyme in the liver.[203] Its expression in the placenta has been studied; however, its contribution to metabolism of drugs is limited.[66] CYP3A in the placenta may play a role in the teratogenicity of thalidomide.[204] Glyburide is another substrate that is metabolized by CYP3A7 in the fetal liver. However, metabolism of drugs by placental CYP3A7 is poorly understood.[205,206]

PHASE II BIOTRANSFORMATION

Uridine 5′-diphosphate Glucuronosyltransferase

The fetoprotective role of the uridine 5′-diphosphate glucuronosyltransferase (UGT) enzymes is to conjugate glucuronic acid to the drug, increasing its polarity and thus enhancing its excretion.[207] There are more than 15 isoforms that are present ubiquitously throughout the pregnancy with high interindividual variability.[208] Olanzapine is an example for a UGT1A4 substrate, whereby the drug is partially converted into its glucuronide conjugate, which has a lower rate of transfer across the placenta compared to its parent compound due to placental UGT1A4 metabolism.[209] Lamotrigine is metabolized by UGT1A4, which may explain why its level may fall in pregnant women and dose adjustments are necessary to achieve optimal therapeutic effect.[210]

Glutathione-S-Transferases

The glutathione-*S*-transferase (GST) is responsible for the conjugation of a glutathione group to compounds, diminishing their toxicity. The only isoform in the placenta is the GST-π, and this is present throughout the pregnancy.[211] Its role in the detoxification of drugs in the placenta is not clear. However, it is implicated in hormone metabolism and may play a role in protecting the fetus from oxidative stress.[66] Fluoxetine, an antidepressant, and its metabolite can inhibit the GST-π in the placenta, exposing the fetus to unknown electrophiles and toxins.[212] In addition, mutations in other forms have been associated with an increased risk of unexpected recurrent pregnancy loss, suggesting an important role of detoxification for this enzyme early in pregnancy.[213]

Others

The role of sulfotransferases in drug metabolism is not well known. However, it is a crucial enzyme in the process of estrogen production, removing the sulfate group from estrone sulfate and from 3β-hydroxysteroids.[214,215] The epoxide hydrolase enzyme is responsible for transforming epoxides into trans-glycols or trans-dihydrodiols.[216] Epoxide metabolites of anticonvulsant drugs (e.g., phenytoin) are known to be associated with the pathway of teratogenicity and fetal hydantoin syndrome. However, little is known about the role of the placental epoxide hydroxylase in the detoxification process.[214,215]

TERATOGENICITY OF DRUGS

The critical period of pregnancy for teratogenic effects is organogenesis between the third and eighth week of gestation; however, other developmental toxicity may occur after the first trimester. Major malformations, particularly anatomic, can arise in that period due to drug exposures or other exogenous compounds. Exposure to drugs later on in pregnancy may induce malformation that affects neurobiologic development.[217] Fetal exposure to drugs is dependent on the fetal concentration, which is, in turn, a factor determined by maternal concentration. However, the toxicity due to a drug may be from the direct exposure of the drug or perhaps other secondary consequences due to the drug exposure. For example, one theory highlights misoprostol-associated Moebius syndrome secondary to uterine contractions, instead of direct effects on the fetus.[218] Another theory linked misoprostol-associated congenital abnormalities in early pregnancy to its vasoconstrictive effects.[219] The importance of identifying teratogenicity comes into play during physician counseling and selection of pharmacotherapy. Especially in the era of advertising new pharmacotherapy, this is a developing field and postmarket surveillance of adverse effects aids in available data. However, limited case reports or series in humans, if any data in humans at all, are often referenced by online platforms, such as Reprotox.org. Table 9.2 provides a list of common drugs and their teratogenic effect on fetal development.

STUDYING DRUG TRANSFER ACROSS THE PLACENTA

With the advancement of technology and the expanding research in the field of pharmacotherapy in pregnancy, researchers are facing the predicament of extrapolating data from animal studies to the human species in addition to the limited inclusion of pregnant women as human subjects in pharmacology clinical trials. In the past 60 years, more attention has been placed on the placenta and its ability to serve as a conduit for drugs from the mother to the fetus and vice versa. The ability of the placenta to metabolize many endogenous and exogenous substances adds a level of complexity to the understanding of the mechanism behind drug transfer and, ultimately, the impact on the developing fetus. There are several important experimental techniques utilized by researchers in an effort to decrease the knowledge gaps using in vitro experiments performed on the human placenta. These techniques aim to overcome the ethical and logistic challenges when dealing with human clinical trials.

IN VITRO STUDIES

Cell and Tissue Culture

With the use of this technique, researchers attempt to delineate the details of the placenta to better understand the interaction of cells and their phenotypes. Primary undifferentiated cytotrophoblast cells can be isolated from the term placenta,[220] then supported to differentiate into a syncytiotrophoblast. The cells will form a monolayer on semipermeable support and thus can be beneficial to study the transfer of molecules across its membrane and cellular metabolism.[221] A disadvantage of this model is the loss of tight junctions when growing on semipermeable support. Alternatively, another method of cell culture, as described by Hemmings et al.,[222] solves this problem by forming confluent monolayers, including the human BeWo, JEG-3, and Jar cell lines.[165,223,224]

TABLE 9.2 Drugs with Proven Teratogenic or Other Adverse Effects in Humans

Drug	*Teratogenic Effect*
Aminopterin, methotrexate	Skull and limb malformations
Angiotensin-converting enzyme inhibitors	Prolonged renal failure in neonates, skull dysgenesis, Potter sequence
Carbamazepine	Neural tube defects
Danazol and other androgenic drugs	Masculinization of the female fetus
Diethylstilbestrol	Vaginal carcinoma and other genitourinary defects in female and male offspring
Hypoglycemic drugs	Neonatal hypoglycemia
Lithium	Heart defects
Mycophenolate mofetil	Microtia, cleft lip/palate, hypoplastic fingers and toenails, heart defects, micrognathia
Misoprostol	Moebius sequence
Nonsteroidal anti-inflammatory drugs	Constriction of the ductus arteriosus, necrotizing enterocolitis, oligohydramnios
Paramethadione	Facial and CNS defects
Phenytoin	Growth restriction, CNS and heart defects
Psychoactive drugs (e.g., barbiturates, opioids, benzodiazepines)	Neonatal withdrawal syndrome when a drug is taken in late pregnancy
Systemic retinoids (isotretinoin, etretinate)	Craniofacial, cardiovascular, and other defects related to neural crest migration failure
Tetracycline	Discolored teeth, hypoplastic fibula
Thalidomide	Phocomelia (limb-shortening defects), internal organ defects, autism
Trimethadione	Facial and CNS defects
Valproic acid	Lumbar meningomyelocele, limb defects, cognitive impairment, autism
Warfarin	Cartilage hypoplasia, porencephaly

CNS, central nervous system.
Data from Briggs GG, Freeman RK, Towers CV, et al. *Drugs in pregnancy and lactation: a reference guide to fetal and neonatal risk*, 8th ed. Philadelphia, PA: Lippincott Williams & Wilkins, 2017 and Koren G, Pastuszak A, Ito S. Drugs in pregnancy. *N Engl J Med* 1998;338(16):1128–1137.

Ex vivo Placental Perfusion

This method was first described by Panigel in 1967, then later adapted and improved.[98,225,226] The advantage of this method is that it provides the closest model to an in vivo study, making it an ideal model to study drug transfer across the placenta. Several other functions can be elucidated from this experiment, including the production of endogenous substances and the effect of drugs on vascular resistance.[66] The placental circulation is reestablished by running a physiologic perfusate through the maternal and fetal blood vessels in the placenta in a closed (recirculating) or open (single-pass or nonrecirculating) circuit (Fig. 9.2). The advantage of the former is that it allows studying the transfer of drugs and the production of metabolites, whereas the latter is useful for studying fetal–maternal clearance.[165] One limitation of this study is the need to use a placenta after a cesarean or vaginal delivery at term gestation, thus limiting generalizability to earlier in the pregnancy.[165] However, its importance remains unchallenged, as a recent review showed that 26 drugs had comparable results in the placenta perfusion studies and in vivo studies.[227] Figure 9.2 provides an illustration of the setup of the ex vivo perfusion experiment.

Placenta-on-a-chip Model

Recently, researchers were able to create a device that recapitulates the placental barrier in an attempt to further our understanding on transport mechanism.[228] This innovative work entails growing a trophoblast and endothelial cell population and depicting the specific architecture of the membrane with careful evaluation of cell–cell junctions and expression of various active transports, including the BRCP.[228,229] The drug glyburide was tested in one model which showed an active transport from fetal to mother circulation, recapitulating that the placenta transport mechanism limits fetal exposure to glyburide taken by the mother for gestational diabetes.[229] This promising technology can serve as a reproductive model that will highlight the

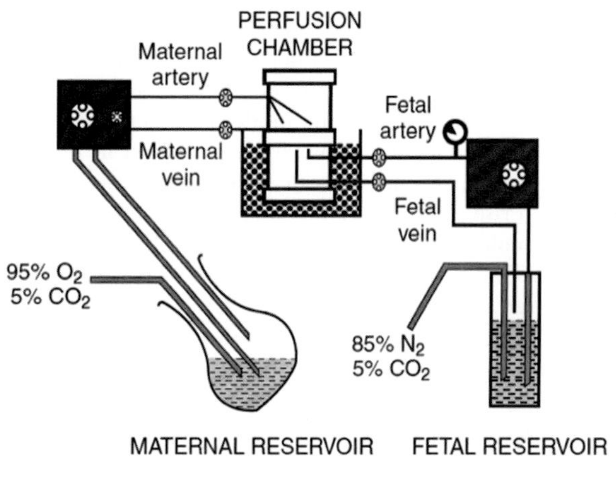

Figure 9.2 Experimental setup for perfusing a human placental lobule ex vitro.

transport mechanism and may explain several key links between a drug and its toxicity in fetal exposure.

IN VIVO STUDIES

The difficulty of incorporating pregnant women in pharmacology clinical trials is often related to primarily logistical challenges and at times ethical concerns when dealing with unknown exposures to the fetus that are difficult to study in utero.[230] The only available study methodology of placental transfer measures drug levels in the mother and cord blood of the fetus after drug administration to the mother. This provides very little information on kinetics and the mechanism behind the transfer. However, the importance of this method is by obtaining the fetal-to-maternal concentration ratio, which can be utilized to guide therapy. Ceftriaxone has a high fetal-to-maternal concentration ratio, making it an ideal drug for the treatment of chorioamnionitis where you need the antibiotic to accumulate in both the mother and the fetus who are at risk of complications.[231] However, if therapy is needed for the mother, it is better only to use a drug with a low fetal-to-maternal ratio such as cyclosporine in patients with a liver transplant.[232] Concerns of confounding the maternal concentration of drugs due to surgery, anesthesia, or the physiologic changes in pregnancy should be taken into consideration. Researches have also been looking for other tools such as biomarkers found in hair and meconium to assess long-term exposure of drugs in the fetus, particularly intrauterine exposure to drug of abuse.[233] Table 9.3 presents some important drugs that can cross the placenta with their fetal-to-maternal ratio obtained from in vivo studies.

PHYSIOLOGICALLY BASED PHARMACOKINETIC MODELS

While the ex vivo placental perfusion experiment provides insight into maternal–fetal transfer in a cotyledon, this information can be leveraged within a physiologically based pharmacokinetic (PBPK) modeling framework to simulate and predict pharmacokinetics in the fetus.

PBPK models are compartmental models consisting of a plethora of differential equations describing the processes of absorption, distribution, metabolism, and excretion (ADME) of a xenobiotic in the body. Importantly, these models are mechanistic, that is, the ADME processes are mathematically described based on the understanding of underlying physical, chemical, and biologic principles. Put differently, the relationship between the observed data and the model parameters (and the interplay between model parameters) is specified in terms of the physical, chemical, and biologic processes that are thought to have given rise to the observed data. The model parameters thus have a biologic meaning; model parameterization, that is, the process of assigning a numerical value to a parameter, can be done based on experimentally measuring or studying relevant model parameters. In a PBPK model, tissues and organs are hence compartmentalized with knowledge of their size and composition and structurally arranged in a parallel circuit to reflect the circulatory system; drug exchange between these organ compartments is described through the blood flow.[280] Of note, PBPK models are rarely purely mechanistic, but may contain empirical components; yet, major parts of the model follow mechanistic principles. Mechanistic models are especially powerful in that they are more likely to work correctly under perturbation of the underlying system, meaning that they can be used to predict the expected outcome in a new scenario.[281] More specifically, PBPK models have been successfully used to predict drug pharmacokinetics in special populations, such as preterm neonates,[282] children,[283] and pregnant women.[284]

As previously demonstrated by various groups,[285,286] the experimental results obtained from the ex vivo placental perfusion experiment can be harnessed in PBPK models. Specifically, these groups used a compartmental model to first describe the drug transfer in the ex vivo experiment by fitting unknown parameters (e.g., the transfer clearance, partition coefficient, potentially elimination rate constants) to the observed data. Thereafter, the transfer clearance for the single cotyledon is scaled to the whole placenta and then integrated in a PBPK model. Using this approach, pharmacokinetics in the umbilical vein observed at delivery in the third trimester could be adequately predicted for several drugs, including acyclovir, emtricitabine, tenofovir, and nevirapine.[286–288]

Other approaches for informing placental drug transfer in a PBPK model that circumvent the use of the ex vivo placental perfusion experiment have also been proposed in the literature. For example, Zhang and Unadkat have suggested an approach for drugs crossing the placenta exclusively via passive diffusion that relies on the drug's apparent membrane permeability measured, for example, in Caco-2 cells.[289] Specifically, the authors developed an empirical equation for scaling the transplacental passive diffusion clearance of midazolam to other drugs by means of their apparent membrane permeability that was reported in the literature. Integration of the scaled diffusion clearances in a PBPK model showed that the pharmacokinetics of theophylline and zidovudine could be adequately predicted in the umbilical vein at term delivery. Recently, Codaccioni et al. elegantly reviewed various placental transfer submodels and approaches to inform the relevant transfer parameters in PBPK models that have been applied to both animals and humans.[290]

SUMMARY

Although tremendous advancements have been made in elucidating the anatomic and physiologic changes in the placenta, there remains a gap in identifying all transporters and their interaction with different exogenous and endogenous compounds at the interface between the mother and the fetus. Understanding the mechanism behind placental transport and metabolism is paramount as more pregnant women are receiving medical therapy throughout their pregnancy. This empowers clinicians to better tailor drug therapy used for treating maternal medical conditions and minimize fetal exposure. In addition, dosing adjustments to some medications are made with the intention to treat fetal conditions and minimize maternal toxicity. Adding to this complexity is the fact that maternal diseases can also contribute to changes in transporter expression and may alter physiologic pathways occurring at the cellular level.

The use of in vitro and in vivo studies to explore the pharmacokinetics and pharmacodynamics of drugs and enumerate the fetal-to-maternal ratio has been a cornerstone in pharmacometric studies. Newer techniques such as the placenta-on-a-chip uses a microengineered interface made to mimic the syncytiotrophoblast membrane, with expression and production of transports and molecule bathed in an environment similar

TABLE 9.3 Examples of In Vitro and In Vivo Transplacental Transfer of Drugs of Therapeutic Interest

Group	Drug	Transfer	Fetal-to-Maternal Ratio[a] In Vitro	In Vivo	References
Cardiac glycoside	Digoxin		0.36–1.00	1.00, 0.35	234, 235
Antiarrhythmic	Amiodarone		0.30	0.03	236, 237
	Verapamil		<0.25	0.35	238
	Flecainide		0.6–0.8		239, 240
	Propranolol		0.1–0.3		241, 242
	Atenolol	$T = 3.1\%–3.4\%$			242
	Timolol	$T = 17\%–21\%$			242
Analgesic	Aspirin	$T = 15\%$			243, 244
	Indomethacin	$T = 36\%$			243
	Naproxen			0.002	245
Antibiotic	Penicillins	$CL_A = 0.13–0.22$			246
	Cephalosporins	$CL_A = 0.04–0.03$			247, 248
	Sulfonamide	$CL_A = 0.06$			249
	Trimethoprim	$T_f = 0.08\%$			249
β-Agonist	Salbutamol	$T = 2.8\%$			250
	Ritodrine	$T = 2.4\%$		0.69	251, 252
	Fenoterol	$T = 2.3\%$			250
Corticosteroid	Dexamethasone	$CL_A = 0.37$			253
	Prednisolone	$CL_A = 0.38$			254
	Cortisol	$CL_A = 0.48$			255
	Betamethasone	$CL_A = 0.41$			255
Respiratory	Theophylline	$T = 22\%$	0.45		256
Gastrointestinal	Cimetidine	$CL_A = 0.23–0.4$	0.46		257
Minor tranquilizer	Diazepam	$T_f = 0.85\%$		1.0	258–260
	Clorazepate	$T_f = 0.84\%$			260
	Midazolam			0.6–0.7	261
Selective serotonin uptake inhibitor	Fluoxetine	$T(SS) = 5.6\%$			262
	Citalopram	$T(SS) = 9.1\%$			262
Anticonvulsant	Phenytoin	$CL_A = 1.08, 1.6$	0.94	0.91	263–265
	Carbamazepine	$CL_A = 0.24$		0.73	265, 266
	Valproic acid	$CL_A = 0.95$		1.59	265–268
	Phenobarbital	$CL_A = 0.12–52$	1	~1, 0.86	265
Antiviral	Acyclovir	$CL_A = 0.18$		0.3	269
	Ganciclovir	$CL_A = 0.18$			109, 270
	AZT + 3TC + NFV			0–0.3	158
	Nelfinavir			0.0.2	158
	Ritonavir	$CL_G = 0.08$			158, 271
	Saquinavir			0.0.1	271
Systemic pain medication	Fentanyl			0.57	272
	Morphine	$CL_A = 0.89$		0.92	273, 274
	Bupivacaine			0.3	275, 276
Miscellaneous	Heparin	$CL_A = 0.02$	0.12		277
	Propofol			0.65–0.85	278
	Cyclosporine	$T < 5\%$			279

[a]In vitro study: the fetal-to-maternal ratio is the mean fetal-to-maternal concentration ratio of the drug of interest in the fetal and maternal reservoir in the placental perfusion model. In vivo study (cord blood sampling): the fetal-to-maternal ratio is the mean fetal-to-maternal concentration ratio of the drug of interest in cord blood and maternal venous sample.

AZT + 3TC + NFV, zidovudine plus lamivudine plus nelfinavir; *CL*, clearance index; CL_A, *CL* compound/antipyrine; CL_G, *CL* compound/L-glucose; *T*, percentage transfer from maternal to fetal direction; T_f, percentage transfer from fetal to maternal direction; *T*(SS), percentage mean steady-state transfer from maternal to fetal direction.

to the physiologic matrix in the human placenta. This would help identify drugs that can cross the placental barrier and the mechanism governing the process in hopes that this information can be taken into consideration when prescribing medical therapy for pregnant patients and ensuring patient safety and reducing fetotoxicity.

ACKNOWLEDGMENTS

This work was supported by the National Heart, Lung and Blood Institute grant to HKA (K23HL141640).

The authors express the gratitude to Dr. Anthony Scialli for his assistance in reviewing the manuscript. The authors deeply acknowledge the insightful contributions of Nada Djokanociv, Rada Boskovic, Gideon Koren, Olga Zharikova, Tatiana Nanovskaya, and Mahmoud S. Ahmed in preparing the previous versions of this chapter.

REFERENCES

1. Lo YT, Yik MH, Shaw PC. Effective authentication of Placenta Hominis. *Chin Med* 2018;13:32.
2. Mossman HW. Classics revisited: comparative morphogenesis of the fetal membranes and accessory uterine structures. *Placenta* 1991;12(1):1–5.
3. Burton GJ, Fowden AL. Review: the placenta and developmental programming: balancing fetal nutrient demands with maternal resource allocation. *Placenta* 2012;33(Suppl):S23–S27.
4. Burton GJ, Jauniaux E. What is the placenta? *Am J Obstet Gynecol* 2015;213(4 Suppl):S6.e1, S6–8.
5. Clabault H, Laurent L, Sanderson JT, et al. Isolation and purification of villous cytotrophoblast cells from term human placenta. In: Murthi P, Vaillancourt C, eds. *Preeclampsia: methods and protocols.* New York, NY: Springer, 2018:219–231.
6. Costa MA. The endocrine function of human placenta: an overview. *Reprod Biomed Online* 2016;32(1):14–43.
7. Wu JL, Jia J, He MZ, et al. Placental origins of preeclampsia: potential therapeutic targets. *Curr Med Sci* 2019;39(2):190–195.
8. Baker JB. The effects of drugs on the foetus. *Pharmacol Rev* 1960;12:37–90.
9. Jones KL, Smith DW. The fetal alcohol syndrome. *Teratology* 1975;12(1):1–10.
10. McAlister Gregg N. Congenital cataract following German measles in the mother. 1942. [classical article]. *Rev Med Virol* 2001;11(5):277–283; discussion 284–275.
11. Dally A. Thalidomide: was the tragedy preventable? *Lancet* 1998;351(9110):1197–1199.
12. Grafmuller S, Manser P, Krug HF, et al. Determination of the transport rate of xenobiotics and nanomaterials across the placenta using the ex vivo human placental perfusion model. *J Vis Exp* 2013;(76) doi:10.3791/50401.
13. Koren G, Ornoy A. The role of the placenta in drug transport and fetal drug exposure. *Expert Rev Clin Pharmacol* 2018;11(4):373–385.
14. Gundling WE, Jr, Wildman DE. A review of inter-and intraspecific variation in the eutherian placenta. *Philos Trans R Soc Lond B Biol Sci* 2015;370(1663):20140072.
15. Wooding P, Burton G. *Comparative placentation: structures, functions and evolution.* Berlin, Germany: Springer, 2008.
16. Wildman DE, Chen C, Erez O, et al. Evolution of the mammalian placenta revealed by phylogenetic analysis. *Proc Natl Acad Sci U S A* 2006;103(9):3203–3208.
17. Han LW, Gao C, Mao Q. An update on expression and function of P-gp/ABCB1 and BCRP/ABCG2 in the placenta and fetus. *Expert Opin Drug Metab Toxicol* 2018;14(8):817–829.
18. Moffett A, Loke C. Immunology of placentation in eutherian mammals. *Nat Rev Immunol* 2006;6(8):584–594.
19. Huppertz B. The anatomy of the normal placenta. *J Clin Pathol* 2008;61(12):1296–1302.
20. O'Brien O, Higgins MF, Mooney EE. Placental weights from normal deliveries in Ireland. *Ir J Med Sci* 2020; 189(2): 581–583.
21. Meekins JW, Luckas MJ, Pijnenborg R, et al. Histological study of decidual spiral arteries and the presence of maternal erythrocytes in the intervillous space during the first trimester of normal human pregnancy. *Placenta* 1997;18(5–6):459–464.
22. Burrows TD, King A, Loke YW. Trophoblast migration during human placental implantation. *Hum Reprod Update* 1996;2(4):307–321.
23. Herzog M. A contribution to our knowledge of the earliest known stages of placentation and embryonic development in man. *Am J Anat* 1909;9(1):361–400.
24. Enders AC. Trophoblast differentiation during the transition from trophoblastic plate to lacunar stage of implantation in the rhesus monkey and human. *Am J Anat* 1989;186(1):85–98.
25. Jauniaux E, Gulbis B, Burton GJ. The human first trimester gestational sac limits rather than facilitates oxygen transfer to the foetus: a review. *Placenta* 2003;24(Suppl A):S86–S93.
26. Jauniaux E, Watson AL, Hempstock J, et al. Onset of maternal arterial blood flow and placental oxidative stress. A possible factor in human early pregnancy failure. *Am J Pathol* 2000;157(6):2111–2122.
27. Sadler TW. *Langman's medical embryology,* 13th ed. Philadelphia, PA: Wolters Kluwer, 2015.
28. Sideri M, de Virgiliis G, Rainoldi R, et al. The ultrastructural basis of the nutritional transfer: evidence of different patterns in the plasma membranes of the multilayered placental barrier. In: Miller RK, Thiede HA, eds. *Fetal nutrition, metabolism, and immunology.* Boston, MA: Springer, 1984:15–25.
29. Smith CH, Moe AJ, Ganapathy V. Nutrient transport pathways across the epithelium of the placenta. *Annu Rev Nutr* 1992;12:183–206.
30. Zhao Y, Hebert MF, Venkataramanan R. Basic obstetric pharmacology. *Semin Perinatol* 2014;38(8):475–486.
31. Hytten FE, Paintin DB. Increase in plasma volume during normal pregnancy. *J Obstet Gynaecol Br Emp* 1963;70:402–407.
32. Pritchard JA. Changes in the blood volume during pregnancy and delivery. *Anesthesiology* 1965;26:393–399.
33. Chesley LC. Plasma and red cell volumes during pregnancy. *Am J Obstet Gynecol* 1972;112(3):440–450.
34. Assali NS, Rauramo L, Peltonen T. Measurement of uterine blood flow and uterine metabolism. VIII. Uterine and fetal blood flow and oxygen consumption in early human pregnancy. *Am J Obstet Gynecol* 1960;79:86–98.
35. Flo K, Wilsgaard T, Vartun A, et al. A longitudinal study of the relationship between maternal cardiac output measured by impedance cardiography and uterine artery blood flow in the second half of pregnancy. *BJOG* 2010;117(7):837–844.
36. Thaler I, Manor D, Itskovitz J, et al. Changes in uterine blood flow during human pregnancy. *Am J Obstet Gynecol* 1990;162(1):121–125.
37. Pacheco LD, Costantine MM, Hankins GDV. Physiologic changes during pregnancy. In: Mattison DR, ed. *Clinical pharmacology during pregnancy.* New York, NY: Academic Press, 2013:5–16.
38. Frederiksen MC. Physiologic changes in pregnancy and their effect on drug disposition. *Semin Perinatol* 2001;25(3):120–123.
39. Murphy MM, Scott JM, McPartlin JM, et al. The pregnancy-related decrease in fasting plasma homocysteine is not explained by folic acid supplementation, hemodilution, or a decrease in albumin in a longitudinal study. *Am J Clin Nutr* 2002;76(3):614–619.
40. Dallmann A, Ince I, Meyer M, et al. Gestation-specific changes in the anatomy and physiology of healthy pregnant women: an extended repository of model parameters for physiologically based pharmacokinetic modeling in pregnancy. *Clin Pharmacokinet* 2017;56(11):1303–1330.
41. Hayashi M, Ueda Y, Hoshimoto K, et al. Changes in urinary excretion of six biochemical parameters in normotensive pregnancy and preeclampsia. *Am J Kidney Dis* 2002;39(2):392–400.
42. Richter JE. Review article: the management of heartburn in pregnancy. *Aliment Pharmacol Ther* 2005;22(9):749–757.
43. Feghali M, Venkataramanan R, Caritis S. Pharmacokinetics of drugs in pregnancy. *Semin Perinatol* 2015;39(7):512–519.
44. Sandhar BK, Elliott RH, Windram I, et al. Peripartum changes in gastric emptying. *Anaesthesia* 1992;47(3):196–198.
45. Levy DM, Williams OA, Magides AD, et al. Gastric emptying is delayed at 8-12 weeks' gestation. *Br J Anaesth* 1994;73(2):237–238.
46. Parry E, Shields R, Turnbull AC. Transit time in the small intestine in pregnancy. *J Obstet Gynaecol Br Commonw* 1970;77(10):900–901.
47. Hodge LS, Tracy TS. Alterations in drug disposition during pregnancy: implications for drug therapy. *Expert Opin Drug Metab Toxicol* 2007;3(4):557–571.
48. Tukey RH, Strassburg CP. Human UDP-glucuronosyltransferases: metabolism, expression, and disease. *Annu Rev Pharmacol Toxicol* 2000;40:581–616.
49. Danielson LA, Conrad KP. Acute blockade of nitric oxide synthase inhibits renal vasodilation and hyperfiltration during pregnancy in chronically instrumented conscious rats. *J Clin Invest* 1995;96(1):482–490.
50. Conrad KP, Davison JM. The renal circulation in normal pregnancy and preeclampsia: is there a place for relaxin? *Am J Physiol Renal Physiol* 2014;306(10):F1121–F1135.
51. Al-Enazy S, Ali S, Albekairi N, et al. Placental control of drug delivery. *Adv Drug Deliv Rev* 2017;116:63–72.
52. Audus KL. Controlling drug delivery across the placenta. *Eur J Pharm Sci* 1999;8(3):161–165.
53. Mori M, Ishikawa G, Luo SS, et al. The cytotrophoblast layer of human chorionic villi becomes thinner but maintains its structural integrity during gestation. *Biol Reprod* 2007;76(1):164–172.
54. Gude NM, Roberts CT, Kalionis B, et al. Growth and function of the normal human placenta. *Thromb Res* 2004;114(5–6):397–407.
55. Glazier JD, Jansson T. Placental transport in early pregnancy: a workshop report. *Placenta* 2004;25(Suppl A):S57–S59.
56. Burton GJ, Watson AL, Hempstock J, et al. Uterine glands provide histiotrophic nutrition for the human fetus during the first trimester of pregnancy. *J Clin Endocrinol Metab* 2002;87(6):2954–2959.
57. Schinkel AH, Jonker JW. Mammalian drug efflux transporters of the ATP binding cassette (ABC) family: an overview. *Adv Drug Deliv Rev* 2003;55(1):3–29.
58. Ampola MG, Mahoney MJ, Nakamura E, et al. Prenatal therapy of a patient with vitamin-B12-responsive methylmalonic acidemia. *N Engl J Med* 1975;293(7):313–317.
59. Hui L, Bianchi DW. Prenatal pharmacotherapy for fetal anomalies: a 2011 update. *Prenat Diagn* 2011;31(7):735–743.
60. Espinoza JP, Caradeux J, Norwitz ER, Illanes SE. Fetal and neonatal alloimmune thrombocytopenia. *Rev Obstet Gynecol* 2013;6(1):e15–e21.
61. Hitzerd E, Broekhuizen M, Mirabito Colafella KM, et al. Placental effects and transfer of sildenafil in healthy and preeclamptic conditions. *EBioMedicine* 2019;45:447–455.
62. Araujo JR, Pereira AC, Correia-Branco A, et al. Oxidative stress induced by tert-butylhydroperoxide interferes with the placental transport of glucose: in vitro studies with BeWo cells. *Eur J Pharmacol* 2013;720(1–3):218–226.
63. Ward RM. Drug therapy of the fetus. *J Clin Pharmacol* 1993;33(9):780–789.

64. Forestier F, Daffos F, Capella-Pavlovsky M. Low molecular weight heparin (PK 10169) does not cross the placenta during the second trimester of pregnancy study by direct fetal blood sampling under ultrasound. *Thromb Res* 1984;34(6):557–560.
65. Buse MG, Roberts WJ, Buse J. The role of the human placenta in the transfer and metabolism of insulin. *J Clin Invest* 1962;41:29–41.
66. Syme MR, Paxton JW, Keelan JA. Drug transfer and metabolism by the human placenta. *Clin Pharmacokinet* 2004;43(8):487–514.
67. Gembruch U, Hansmann M, Bald R. Direct intrauterine fetal treatment of fetal tachyarrhythmia with severe hydrops fetalis by antiarrhythmic drugs. *Fetal Ther* 1988;3(4):210–215.
68. Bourget P, Roulot C, Fernandez H. Models for placental transfer studies of drugs. *Clin Pharmacokinet* 1995;28(2):161–180.
69. Kragh-Hansen U. Molecular aspects of ligand binding to serum albumin. *Pharmacol Rev* 1981;33(1):17–53.
70. Paxton JW, Briant RH. Alpha 1-acid glycoprotein concentrations and propranolol binding in elderly patients with acute illness. *Br J Clin Pharmacol* 1984;18(5):806–810.
71. Nau H, Krauer B. Serum protein binding of valproic acid in fetus-mother pairs throughout pregnancy: correlation with oxytocin administration and albumin and free fatty acid concentrations. *J Clin Pharmacol* 1986;26(3):215–221.
72. Zakowski MI, Geller A. The placenta: anatomy, physiology, and transfer of drugs. In: Chestnut DH, ed. *Chestnut's obstetric anesthesia*. Philadelphia, PA: Saunders, 2020:56–76.
73. Souza MCO, Marques MP, Duarte G, et al. Analysis of bupivacaine enantiomers in plasma as total and unbound concentrations using LC-MS/MS: application in a pharmacokinetic study of a parturient with placental transfer. *J Pharm Biomed Anal* 2019;164:268–275.
74. Yang YQ, Lee MP, Schenken RS, et al. Effects of binding on human transplacental transfer of cocaine. *Am J Obstet Gynecol* 1995;172(2 Pt 1):720–722.
75. Gin T, Yau G, Chan K, et al. Disposition of propofol infusions for caesarean section. *Can J Anaesth* 1991;38(1):31–36.
76. Celleno D, Capogna G, Tomassetti M, et al. Neurobehavioural effects of propofol on the neonate following elective caesarean section. *Br J Anaesth* 1989;62(6):649–654.
77. Montandrau O, Espitalier F, Bouyou J, et al. Thiopental versus propofol on the outcome of the newborn after caesarean section: an impact study. *Anaesth Crit Care Pain Med* 2019;38(6):631–635.
78. Tumukunde J, Lomangisi DD, Davidson O, et al. Effects of propofol versus thiopental on Apgar scores in newborns and peri-operative outcomes of women undergoing emergency cesarean section: a randomized clinical trial. *BMC Anesthesiol* 2015;15:63.
79. Hill MD, Abramson FP. The significance of plasma protein binding on the fetal/maternal distribution of drugs at steady-state. *Clin Pharmacokinet* 1988;14(3):156–170.
80. Nau H, Luck W, Kuhnz W. Decreased serum protein binding of diazepam and its major metabolite in the neonate during the first postnatal week relate to increased free fatty acid levels. *Br J Clin Pharmacol* 1984;17(1):92–98.
81. Ridd MJ, Brown KF, Nation RL, et al. Differential transplacental binding of diazepam: causes and implications. *Eur J Clin Pharmacol* 1983;24(5):595–601.
82. Allegaert K, Van den Anker JN. Physicochemical and structural properties regulating placental drug transfer. In: Polin RA, Abman SH, Rowitch DH, et al., eds. *Fetal and neonatal physiology*. Philadelphia, PA: Elsevier, 2017:208–221.e204.
83. Garland M. Pharmacology of drug transfer across the placenta. *Obstet Gynecol Clin North Am* 1998;25(1):21–42.
84. Biehl D, Shnider SM, Levinson G, et al. Placental transfer of lidocaine: effects of fetal acidosis. *Anesthesiology* 1978;48(6):409–412.
85. Carson RJ, Reynolds F. Elimination of bupivacaine and pethidine from the rabbit feto-placental unit. *Br J Anaesth* 1992;69(2):150–153.
86. Nau H. Clinical pharmacokinetics in pregnancy and perinatology. II. Penicillins. *Dev Pharmacol Ther* 1987;10(3):174–198.
87. Nau H, Rating D, Koch S, et al. Valproic acid and its metabolites: placental transfer, neonatal pharmacokinetics, transfer via mother's milk and clinical status in neonates of epileptic mothers. *J Pharmacol Exp Ther* 1981;219(3):768–777.
88. Tagashira E, Nakao K, Urano T, et al. Correlation of teratogenicity of aspirin to the stage specific distribution of salicylic acid in rats. *Jpn J Pharmacol* 1981;31(4):563–571.
89. Pacifici GM, Nottoli R. Placental transfer of drugs administered to the mother. *Clin Pharmacokinet* 1995;28(3):235–269.
90. Reynolds F. Drug transfer across the term placenta. *Placenta* 1998;19:239–255.
91. Sastry BV. Techniques to study human placental transport. *Adv Drug Deliv Rev* 1999;38(1):17–39.
92. Barre J, Urien S, Albengres E, et al. Plasma and tissue binding as determinants of drug body distribution. Possible applications to toxicological studies. *Xenobiotica* 1988;18(Suppl 1):15–20.
93. Dancis J, Jansen V, Levitz M. Placental transfer of steroids: effect of binding to serum albumin and to placenta. *Am J Physiol* 1980;238(3):E208–E213.
94. Morgan TK. Role of the placenta in preterm birth: a review. *Am J Perinatol* 2016;33(3):258–266.
95. Freriksen JJM, Feyaerts D, van den Broek PHH, et al. Placental disposition of the immunosuppressive drug tacrolimus in renal transplant recipients and in ex vivo perfused placental tissue. *Eur J Pharm Sci* 2018;119:244–248.
96. Russo FM, Conings S, Allegaert K, et al. Sildenafil crosses the placenta at therapeutic levels in a dually perfused human cotyledon model. *Am J Obstet Gynecol* 2018;219(6):619.e1–619.e10.
97. Stray-Pedersen B. Treatment of toxoplasmosis in the pregnant mother and newborn child. *Scand J Infect Dis Suppl* 1992;84:23–31.
98. Schneider H, Panigel M, Dancis J. Transfer across the perfused human placenta of antipyrine, sodium and leucine. *Am J Obstet Gynecol* 1972;114(6):822–828.
99. Brodin B, Steffansen B, Nielsen CU. Passive diffusion of drug substances: the concepts of flux and permeability. In: Brodin B, Steffansen B, Nielsen CU, eds. *Molecular biopharmaceutics*. London, England: Pharmaceutical Press, 2010:135–152.
100. Mirkin BL, Singh S. Placental transfer of pharmacologically active molecules In: Mirkin BL, ed. *Perinatal pharmacology and therapeutics*. New York, NY: Academic Press, 1976:1–69.
101. Green TP, O'Dea RF, Mirkin BL. Determinants of drug disposition and effect in the fetus. *Annu Rev Pharmacol Toxicol* 1979;19:285–322.
102. Thornburg KL, Faber JJ. The steady state concentration gradients of an electron-dense marker (ferritin) in the three-layered hemochorial placenta of the rabbit. *J Clin Invest* 1976;58(4):912–925.
103. Hillier AP. The binding of thyroid hormones to phospholipid membranes. *J Physiol* 1970;211(3):585–597.
104. Lai CS, Korytowski W, Niu CH, et al. Transverse motion of spin-labeled 3,3',5-triiodo-L-thyronine in phospholipid bilayers. *Biochem Biophys Res Commun* 1985;131(1):408–412.
105. Dickinson RG, Fowler DW, Kluck RM. Maternofetal transfer of phenytoin, p-hydroxy-phenytoin and p-hydroxy-phenytoin-glucuronide in the perfused human placenta. *Clin Exp Pharmacol Physiol* 1989;16(10):789–797.
106. Roth M, Obaidat A, Hagenbuch B. OATPs, OATs and OCTs: the organic anion and cation transporters of the SLCO and SLC22A gene superfamilies. *Br J Pharmacol* 2012;165(5):1260–1287.
107. Hall JE. *Guyton and hall textbook of medical physiology*, 13th ed. Philadelphia, PA: Elsevier, 2015.
108. Ghosh C, Marchi N. Drug permeation across the fetal maternal barrier. In: Janigro D, ed. *Mammalian brain development*. New York, NY: Humana Press, 2009:153–170.
109. Henderson GI, Hu ZQ, Yang Y, et al. Ganciclovir transfer by human placenta and its effects on rat fetal cells. *Am J Med Sci* 1993;306(3):151–156.
110. Kudo Y, Urabe T, Fujiwara A, et al. Carrier-mediated transport system for cephalexin in human placental brush-border membrane vesicles. *Biochim Biophys Acta* 1989;978(2):313–318.
111. Fant ME, Yeakley J, Harrison RW. Evidence for carrier-mediated transport of glucocorticoids by human placental membrane vesicles. *Biochim Biophys Acta* 1983;731(3):415–420.
112. Staud F, Cerveny L, Ceckova M. Pharmacotherapy in pregnancy; effect of ABC and SLC transporters on drug transport across the placenta and fetal drug exposure. *J Drug Target* 2012;20(9):736–763.
113. Burckhardt BC, Burckhardt G. Transport of organic anions across the basolateral membrane of proximal tubule cells. *Rev Physiol Biochem Pharmacol* 2003;146:95–158.
114. Ugele B, Bahn A, Rex-Haffner M. Functional differences in steroid sulfate uptake of organic anion transporter 4 (OAT4) and organic anion transporting polypeptide 2B1 (OATP2B1) in human placenta. *J Steroid Biochem Mol Biol* 2008;111(1–2):1–6.
115. Noguchi S, Nishimura T, Fujibayashi A, et al. Organic anion transporter 4-mediated transport of olmesartan at basal plasma membrane of human placental barrier. *J Pharm Sci* 2015;104(9):3128–3135.
116. Nabekura T, Kawasaki T, Kamiya Y, et al. Effects of antiviral drugs on organic anion transport in human placental BeWo cells. *Antimicrob Agents Chemother* 2015;59(12):7666–7670.
117. Sato K, Sugawara J, Sato T, et al. Expression of organic anion transporting polypeptide E (OATP-E) in human placenta. *Placenta* 2003;24(2–3):144–148.
118. Tertti K, Petsalo A, Niemi M, et al. Transfer of repaglinide in the dually perfused human placenta and the role of organic anion transporting polypeptides (OATPs). *Eur J Pharm Sci* 2011;44(3):181–186.
119. Nozawa T, Imai K, Nezu J, et al. Functional characterization of pH-sensitive organic anion transporting polypeptide OATP-B in human. *J Pharmacol Exp Ther* 2004;308(2):438–445.
120. Satoh H, Yamashita F, Tsujimoto M, et al. Citrus juices inhibit the function of human organic anion-transporting polypeptide OATP-B. *Drug Metab Dispos* 2005;33(4):518–523.
121. Obaidat A, Roth M, Hagenbuch B. The expression and function of organic anion transporting polypeptides in normal tissues and in cancer. *Annu Rev Pharmacol Toxicol* 2012;52:135–151.
122. Tetro N, Moushaev S, Rubinchik-Stern M, et al. The placental barrier: the gate and the fate in drug distribution. *Pharm Res* 2018;35(4):71.
123. Koepsell H, Endou H. The SLC22 drug transporter family. *Pflugers Arch* 2004;447(5):666–676.
124. Ganapathy V, Prasad PD. Role of transporters in placental transfer of drugs. *Toxicol Appl Pharmacol* 2005;207(2 Suppl):381–387.
125. Wessler I, Roth E, Deutsch C, et al. Release of non-neuronal acetylcholine from the isolated human placenta is mediated by organic cation transporters. *Br J Pharmacol* 2001;134(5):951–956.
126. Gong L, Goswami S, Giacomini KM, et al. Metformin pathways: pharmacokinetics and pharmacodynamics. *Pharmacogenet Genomics* 2012;22(11):820–827.
127. Koepsell H, Lips K, Volk C. Polyspecific organic cation transporters: structure, function, physiological roles, and biopharmaceutical implications. *Pharm Res* 2007;24(7):1227–1251.
128. Rytting E, Audus KL. Novel organic cation transporter 2-mediated carnitine uptake in placental choriocarcinoma (BeWo) cells. *J Pharmacol Exp Ther* 2005;312(1):192–198.
129. Chang TT, Shyu MK, Huang MC, et al. Hypoxia-mediated down-regulation of OCTN2 and PPARalpha expression in human placentas and in BeWo cells. *Mol Pharm* 2011;8(1):117–125.
130. Klaassen CD, Aleksunes LM. Xenobiotic, bile acid, and cholesterol transporters: function and regulation. *Pharmacol Rev* 2010;62(1):1–96.
131. Tsuda M, Terada T, Asaka J, et al. Oppositely directed H+ gradient functions as a driving force of rat H+/organic cation antiporter MATE1. *Am J Physiol Renal Physiol* 2007;292(2):F593–F598.
132. Ahmadimoghaddam D, Hofman J, Zemankova L, et al. Synchronized activity of organic cation transporter 3 (Oct3/Slc22a3) and multidrug and toxin extrusion 1 (Mate1/Slc47a1) transporter in transplacental passage of MPP+ in rat. *Toxicol Sci* 2012;128(2):471–481.
133. Nies AT, Koepsell H, Damme K, et al. Organic cation transporters (OCTs, MATEs), in vitro and in vivo evidence for the importance in drug therapy. *Handb Exp Pharmacol* 2011(201):105–167.
134. Errasti-Murugarren E, Diaz P, Godoy V, et al. Expression and distribution of nucleoside transporter proteins in the human syncytiotrophoblast. *Mol Pharmacol* 2011;80(5):809–817.
135. Yamamoto T, Kuniki K, Takekuma Y, et al. Ribavirin uptake by cultured human choriocarcinoma (BeWo) cells and *Xenopus laevis* oocytes expressing recombinant plasma membrane human nucleoside transporters. *Eur J Pharmacol* 2007;557(1):1–8.

136. Molina-Arcas M, Casado FJ, Pastor-Anglada M. Nucleoside transporter proteins. *Curr Vasc Pharmacol* 2009;7(4):426–434.
137. Ma Z, Yang X, Jiang T, et al. Multiple SLC and ABC transporters contribute to the placental transfer of entecavir. *Drug Metab Dispos* 2017;45(3):269–278.
138. Tun GS, Lobo AJ. Evaluation of pharmacokinetics and pharmacodynamics and clinical efficacy of certolizumab pegol for Crohn's disease. *Expert Opin Drug Metab Toxicol* 2015;11(2):317–327.
139. Nagai J, Takano M. Entry of aminoglycosides into renal tubular epithelial cells via endocytosis-dependent and endocytosis-independent pathways. *Biochem Pharmacol* 2014;90(4):331–337.
140. Akour AA, Kennedy MJ, Gerk PM. The role of megalin in the transport of gentamicin across BeWo cells, an in vitro model of the human placenta. *AAPS J* 2015;17(5): 1193–1199.
141. Forrest LR, Kramer R, Ziegler C. The structural basis of secondary active transport mechanisms. *Biochim Biophys Acta* 2011;1807(2):167–188.
142. Hahn T, Desoye G. Ontogeny of glucose transport systems in the placenta and its progenitor tissues. *Early Pregnancy* 1996;2(3):168–182.
143. Moe AJ. Placental amino acid transport. *Am J Physiol* 1995;268(6 Pt 1):C1321–C1331.
144. Bissonnette JM. Placental transport of carbohydrates. *Mead Johnson Symp Perinat Dev Med* 1981(18):21–23.
145. Vahakangas K, Myllynen P. Drug transporters in the human blood-placental barrier. *Br J Pharmacol* 2009;158(3):665–678.
146. Leslie EM, Deeley RG, Cole SP. Multidrug resistance proteins: role of P-glycoprotein, MRP1, MRP2, and BCRP (ABCG2) in tissue defense. *Toxicol Appl Pharmacol* 2005;204(3):216–237.
147. Wang JS, Newport DJ, Stowe ZN, et al. The emerging importance of transporter proteins in the psychopharmacological treatment of the pregnant patient. *Drug Metab Rev* 2007;39(4):723–746.
148. Juliano RL, Ling V. A surface glycoprotein modulating drug permeability in Chinese hamster ovary cell mutants. *Biochim Biophys Acta* 1976;455(1):152–162.
149. Schinkel AH. The physiological function of drug-transporting P-glycoproteins. *Semin Cancer Biol* 1997;8(3):161–170.
150. Ceckova-Novotna M, Pavek P, Staud F. P-glycoprotein in the placenta: expression, localization, regulation and function. *Reprod Toxicol* 2006;22(3):400–410.
151. Mylona P, Hoyland JA, Sibley CP. Sites of mRNA expression of the cystic fibrosis (CF) and multidrug resistance (MDR1) genes in the human placenta of early pregnancy: No evidence for complementary expression. *Placenta* 1999;20(5–6):493–496.
152. Sun M, Kingdom J, Baczyk D, et al. Expression of the multidrug resistance P-glycoprotein, (ABCB1 glycoprotein) in the human placenta decreases with advancing gestation. *Placenta* 2006;27(6–7):602–609.
153. Leazer TM, Klaassen CD. The presence of xenobiotic transporters in rat placenta. *Drug Metab Dispos* 2003;31(2):153–167.
154. Ushigome F, Takanaga H, Matsuo H, et al. Human placental transport of vinblastine, vincristine, digoxin and progesterone: contribution of P-glycoprotein. *Eur J Pharmacol* 2000;408(1):1–10.
155. Pavek P, Fendrich Z, Staud F, et al. Influence of P-glycoprotein on the transplacental passage of cyclosporine. *J Pharm Sci* 2001;90(10):1583–1592.
156. Holtzman CW, Wiggins BS, Spinler SA. Role of P-glycoprotein in statin drug interactions. *Pharmacotherapy* 2006;26(11):1601–1607.
157. St-Pierre MV, Serrano MA, Macias RI, et al. Expression of members of the multidrug resistance protein family in human term placenta. *Am J Physiol Regul Integr Comp Physiol* 2000;279(4):R1495–R1503.
158. Marzolini C, Rudin C, Decosterd LA, et al. Transplacental passage of protease inhibitors at delivery. *AIDS* 2002;16(6):889–893.
159. Ward RM. Pharmacologic enhancement of fetal lung maturation. *Clin Perinatol* 1994;21(3):523–542.
160. Varma DR. Investigation of the maternal to foetal serum concentration gradient of dexamethasone in the rat. *Br J Pharmacol* 1986;88(4):815–820.
161. Hendrick V, Stowe ZN, Altshuler LL, et al. Placental passage of antidepressant medications. *Am J Psychiatry* 2003;160(5):993–996.
162. Nanovskaya T, Nekhayeva I, Karunaratne N, et al. Role of P-glycoprotein in transplacental transfer of methadone. *Biochem Pharmacol* 2005;69(12):1869–1878.
163. Lewis T, Dinh J, Leeder JS. Genetic determinants of fetal opiate exposure and risk of neonatal abstinence syndrome: knowledge deficits and prospects for future research. *Clin Pharmacol Ther* 2015;98(3):309–320.
164. Borst P, Evers R, Kool M, et al. A family of drug transporters: the multidrug resistance-associated proteins. *J Natl Cancer Inst* 2000;92(16):1295–1302.
165. Dallmann A, Liu XI, Burckart GJ, et al. Drug transporters expressed in the human placenta and models for studying maternal-fetal drug transfer. *J Clin Pharmacol* 2019;59(Suppl 1): S70–S81.
166. Evseenko D, Paxton JW, Keelan JA. Active transport across the human placenta: impact on drug efficacy and toxicity. *Expert Opin Drug Metab Toxicol* 2006;2(1):51–69.
167. Gerk PM, Vore M. Regulation of expression of the multidrug resistance-associated protein 2 (MRP2) and its role in drug disposition. *J Pharmacol Exp Ther* 2002;302(2):407–415.
168. Francois LN, Gorczyca L, Du J, et al. Down-regulation of the placental BCRP/ABCG2 transporter in response to hypoxia signaling. *Placenta* 2017;51:57–63.
169. Schwartz RA, Rosenn B, Aleksa K, et al. Glyburide transport across the human placenta. *Obstet Gynecol* 2015;125(3):583–588.
170. Pavek P, Smutny T. Nuclear receptors in regulation of biotransformation enzymes and drug transporters in the placental barrier. *Drug Metab Rev* 2014;46(1):19–32.
171. Hakkola J, Pasanen M, Pelkonen O, et al. Expression of CYP1B1 in human adult and fetal tissues and differential inducibility of CYP1B1 and CYP1A1 by Ah receptor ligands in human placenta and cultured cells. *Carcinogenesis* 1997;18(2):391–397.
172. Collier AC, Tingle MD, Paxton JW, et al. Metabolizing enzyme localization and activities in the first trimester human placenta: the effect of maternal and gestational age, smoking and alcohol consumption. *Hum Reprod* 2002;17(10):2564–2572.
173. Fournet-Dulguerov N, MacLusky NJ, Leranth CZ, et al. Immunohistochemical localization of aromatase cytochrome P-450 and estradiol dehydrogenase in the syncytiotrophoblast of the human placenta. *J Clin Endocrinol Metab* 1987;65(4):757–764.
174. Thompson EA Jr, Siiteri PK. The involvement of human placental microsomal cytochrome P-450 in aromatization. *J Biol Chem* 1974;249(17):5373–5378.
175. Simpson ER, Mahendroo MS, Means GD, et al. Aromatase cytochrome P450, the enzyme responsible for estrogen biosynthesis. *Endocr Rev* 1994;15(3):342–355.
176. Kragie L. Aromatase in primate pregnancy: a review. *Endocr Res* 2002;28(3):121–128.
177. Nanovskaya TN, Deshmukh SV, Nekhayeva IA, et al. Methadone metabolism by human placenta. *Biochem Pharmacol* 2004;68(3):583–591.
178. Marquet P, Chevrel J, Lavignasse P, et al. Buprenorphine withdrawal syndrome in a newborn. *Clin Pharmacol Ther* 1997;62(5):569–571.
179. Fischer G, Johnson RE, Eder H, et al. Treatment of opioid-dependent pregnant women with buprenorphine. *Addiction* 2000;95(2):239–244.
180. Deshmukh SV, Nanovskaya TN, Ahmed MS. Aromatase is the major enzyme metabolizing buprenorphine in human placenta. *J Pharmacol Exp Ther* 2003;306(3):1099–1105.
181. Zharikova OL, Deshmukh SV, Nanovskaya TN, et al. The effect of methadone and buprenorphine on human placental aromatase. *Biochem Pharmacol* 2006;71(8):1255–1264.
182. Zharikova OL, Ravindran S, Nanovskaya TN, et al. Kinetics of glyburide metabolism by hepatic and placental microsomes of human and baboon. *Biochem Pharmacol* 2007;73(12):2012–2019.
183. Zharikova OL, Fokina VM, Nanovskaya TN, et al. Identification of the major human hepatic and placental enzymes responsible for the biotransformation of glyburide. *Biochem Pharmacol* 2009;78(12):1483–1490.
184. Shimada T, Yamazaki H, Mimura M, et al. Interindividual variations in human liver cytochrome P-450 enzymes involved in the oxidation of drugs, carcinogens and toxic chemicals: studies with liver microsomes of 30 Japanese and 30 Caucasians. *J Pharmacol Exp Ther* 1994;270(1):414–423.
185. Pasanen M, Pelkonen O. The expression and environmental regulation of P450 enzymes in human placenta. *Crit Rev Toxicol* 1994;24(3):211–229.
186. Jonsson A, Hallengren B, Rydberg T, et al. Effects and serum levels of glibenclamide and its active metabolites in patients with type 2 diabetes. *Diabetes Obes Metab* 2001;3(6):403–409.
187. Spink BC, Fasco MJ, Gierthy JF, et al. 12-O-tetradecanoylphorbol-13-acetate upregulates the Ah receptor and differentially alters CYP1B1 and CYP1A1 expression in MCF-7 breast cancer cells. *J Cell Biochem* 1998;70(3):289–296.
188. Spink DC, Eugster HP, Lincoln DW II, et al. 17 beta-estradiol hydroxylation catalyzed by human cytochrome P450 1A1: a comparison of the activities induced by 2,3,7,8-tetrachlorodibenzo-p-dioxin in MCF-7 cells with those from heterologous expression of the cDNA. *Arch Biochem Biophys* 1992;293(2):342–348.
189. Spink DC, Spink BC, Cao JQ, et al. Differential expression of CYP1A1 and CYP1B1 in human breast epithelial cells and breast tumor cells. *Carcinogenesis* 1998;19(2):291–298.
190. Choudhary D, Jansson I, Sarfarazi M, et al. Characterization of the biochemical and structural phenotypes of four CYP1B1 mutations observed in individuals with primary congenital glaucoma. *Pharmacogenet Genomics* 2008;18(8):665–676.
191. Wang X, Zuckerman B, Pearson C, et al. Maternal cigarette smoking, metabolic gene polymorphism, and infant birth weight. *JAMA* 2002;287(2):195–202.
192. Suter M, Abramovici A, Showalter L, et al. In utero tobacco exposure epigenetically modifies placental CYP1A1 expression. *Metabolism* 2010;59(10):1481–1490.
193. Manchester DK, Bowman ED, Parker NB, et al. Determinants of polycyclic aromatic hydrocarbon-DNA adducts in human placenta. *Cancer Res* 1992;52(6):1499–1503.
194. Dolwick KM, Schmidt JV, Carver LA, et al. Cloning and expression of a human Ah receptor cDNA. *Mol Pharmacol* 1993;44(5):911–917.
195. Manchester DK, Gordon SK, Golas CL, et al. Ah receptor in human placenta: stabilization by molybdate and characterization of binding of 2,3,7,8-tetrachlorodibenzo-p-dioxin, 3-methylcholanthrene, and benzo(a)pyrene. *Cancer Res* 1987;47(18):4861–4868.
196. Juchau MR. Human placental hydroxylation of 3,4-benzpyrene during early gestation and at term. *Toxicol Appl Pharmacol* 1971;18(3):665–675.
197. Beresford AP. CYP1A1: friend or foe? *Drug Metab Rev* 1993;25(4):503–517.
198. Hakkola J, Pasanen M, Hukkanen J, et al. Expression of xenobiotic-metabolizing cytochrome P450 forms in human full-term placenta. *Biochem Pharmacol* 1996;51(4):403–411.
199. Everson RB, Randerath E, Santella RM, et al. Quantitative associations between DNA damage in human placenta and maternal smoking and birth weight. *J Natl Cancer Inst* 1988;80(8):567–576.
200. Naeye RL. The duration of maternal cigarette smoking, fetal and placental disorders. *Early Hum Dev* 1979;3(3):229–237.
201. Pelkonen O, Maenpaa J, Taavitsainen P, et al. Inhibition and induction of human cytochrome P450 (CYP) enzymes. *Xenobiotica* 1998;28(12):1203–1253.
202. Manchester D, Jacoby E. Decreased placental monooxygenase activities associated with birth defects. *Teratology* 1984;30(1):31–37.
203. Murray M. P450 enzymes. Inhibition mechanisms, genetic regulation and effects of liver disease. *Clin Pharmacokinet* 1992;23(2):132–146.
204. Kazuki Y, Akita M, Kobayashi K, et al. Thalidomide-induced limb abnormalities in a humanized CYP3A mouse model. *Sci Rep* 2016;6:21419.
205. Maezawa K, Matsunaga T, Takezawa T, et al. Cytochrome P450 3As gene expression and testosterone 6 beta-hydroxylase activity in human fetal membranes and placenta at full term. *Biol Pharm Bull* 2010;33(2):249–254.
206. Shuster DL, Risler LJ, Prasad B, et al. Identification of CYP3A7 for glyburide metabolism in human fetal livers. *Biochem Pharmacol* 2014;92(4):690–700.
207. Mackenzie PI, Owens IS, Burchell B, et al. The UDP glycosyltransferase gene superfamily: recommended nomenclature update based on evolutionary divergence. *Pharmacogenetics* 1997;7(4):255–269.
208. Collier AC, Ganley NA, Tingle MD, et al. UDP-glucuronosyltransferase activity, expression and cellular localization in human placenta at term. *Biochem Pharmacol* 2002;63(3):409–419.
209. Schenker S, Yang Y, Mattiuz E, et al. Olanzapine transfer by human placenta. *Clin Exp Pharmacol Physiol* 1999;26(9):691–697.

210. Reimers A, Ostby L, Stuen I, et al. Expression of UDP-glucuronosyltransferase 1A4 in human placenta at term. *Eur J Drug Metab Pharmacokinet* 2011;35(3–4):79–82.
211. Pasanen M, Pelkonen O. Xenobiotic and steroid-metabolizing monooxygenases catalysed by cytochrome P450 and glutathione S-transferase conjugations in the human placenta and their relationships to maternal cigarette smoking. *Placenta* 1990;11(1):75–85.
212. Dalmizrak O, Kulaksiz-Erkmen G, Ozer N. Fluoxetine-induced toxicity results in human placental glutathione S-transferase-pi (GST-pi) dysfunction. *Drug Chem Toxicol* 2016;39(4):439–444.
213. Polimanti R, Piacentini S, Lazzarin N, et al. Glutathione S-transferase genes and the risk of recurrent miscarriage in Italian women. *Fertil Steril* 2012;98(2):396–400.
214. Finnell RH, Buehler BA, Kerr BM, et al. Clinical and experimental studies linking oxidative metabolism to phenytoin-induced teratogenesis. *Neurology* 1992;42(4 Suppl 5):25–31.
215. Buehler BA, Bick D, Delimont D. Prenatal prediction of risk of the fetal hydantoin syndrome. *N Engl J Med* 1993;329(22):1660–1661.
216. Pacifici GM, Rane A. Epoxide hydrolase in human placenta at different stages of pregnancy. *Dev Pharmacol Ther* 1983;6(2):83–93.
217. Holmes LB. Human teratogens: update 2010. *Birth Defects Res A Clin Mol Teratol* 2011;91(1):1–7.
218. Shepard TH. Mobius syndrome after misoprostol: a possible teratogenic mechanism. *Lancet* 1995;346(8977):780.
219. Yip SK, Tse AO, Haines CJ, et al. Misoprostol's effect on uterine arterial blood flow and fetal heart rate in early pregnancy. *Obstet Gynecol* 2000;95(2):232–235.
220. Kliman HJ, Nestler JE, Sermasi E, et al. Purification, characterization, and in vitro differentiation of cytotrophoblasts from human term placentae. *Endocrinology* 1986;118(4):1567–1582.
221. Bode CJ, Jin H, Rytting E, et al. In vitro models for studying trophoblast transcellular transport. *Methods Mol Med* 2006;122:225–239.
222. Hemmings DG, Lowen B, Sherburne R, et al. Villous trophoblasts cultured on semi-permeable membranes form an effective barrier to the passage of high and low molecular weight particles. *Placenta* 2001;22(1):70–79.
223. Liu F, Soares MJ, Audus KL. Permeability properties of monolayers of the human trophoblast cell line BeWo. *Am J Physiol* 1997;273(5):C1596–C1604.
224. Pattillo RA, Gey GO. The establishment of a cell line of human hormone-synthesizing trophoblastic cells in vitro. *Cancer Res* 1968;28(7):1231–1236.
225. Miller RK, Wier PJ, Shah Y, et al. Criteria for in vitro dual perfusions in the human placental lobule: perfusions in excess of 12 hours. In: Genbačev O, Klopper A, Beaconsfield R, eds. *Placenta as a model and a source.* Boston, MA: Springer, 1989:27–38.
226. Panigel M. Placental perfusion experiments. *Am J Obstet Gynecol* 1962;84(11):1664–1683.
227. Hutson JR, Garcia-Bournissen F, Davis A, et al. The human placental perfusion model: a systematic review and development of a model to predict in vivo transfer of therapeutic drugs. *Clin Pharmacol Ther* 2011;90(1):67–76.
228. Blundell C, Tess ER, Schanzer AS, et al. A microphysiological model of the human placental barrier. *Lab Chip* 2016;16(16):3065–3073.
229. Blundell C, Yi YS, Ma L, et al. Placental drug transport-on-a-chip: a microengineered in vitro model of transporter-mediated drug efflux in the human placental barrier. *Adv Healthc Mater* 2018;7(2) doi:10.1002/adhm.201700786.
230. Dallmann A, Mian P, Van den Anker J, et al. Clinical pharmacokinetic studies in pregnant women and the relevance of pharmacometric tools. *Curr Pharm Des* 2019;25(5):483–495.
231. Bourget P, Quinquis-Desmaris V, Fernandez H. Ceftriaxone distribution and protein binding between maternal blood and milk postpartum. *Ann Pharmacother* 1993;27(3):294–297.
232. Bourget P, Fernandez H, Bismuth H, et al. Transplacental passage of cyclosporine after liver transplantation. *Transplantation* 1990;49(3):663.
233. Delano K, Koren G. Emerging biomarkers of intrauterine neonatal and pediatric exposures to xenobiotics. *Pediatr Clin North Am* 2012;59(5):1059–1070.
234. Kanhai HH, van Kamp IL, Moolenaar AJ, et al. Transplacental passage of digoxin in severe Rhesus immunization. *J Perinat Med* 1990;18(5):339–343.
235. Derewlany LO, Leeder JS, Kumar R, et al. The transport of digoxin across the perfused human placental lobule. *J Pharmacol Exp Ther* 1991;256(3):1107–1111.
236. Schmolling J, Renke K, Richter O, et al. Digoxin, flecainide, and amiodarone transfer across the placenta and the effects of an elevated umbilical venous pressure on the transfer rate. *Ther Drug Monit* 2000;22(5):582–588.
237. Azancot-Benisty A, Jacqz-Aigrain E, Guirgis NM, et al. Clinical and pharmacologic study of fetal supraventricular tachyarrhythmias. *J Pediatr* 1992;121(4):608–613.
238. Wolff F, Breuker KH, Schlensker KH, et al. Prenatal diagnosis and therapy of fetal heart rate anomalies: with a contribution on the placental transfer of Verapamil. *J Perinat Med* 1980;8(4):203–208.
239. Wren C, Hunter S. Maternal administration of flecainide to terminate and suppress fetal tachycardia. *Br Med J (Clin Res Ed)* 1988;296(6617):249.
240. Allan LD, Chita SK, Sharland GK, et al. Flecainide in the treatment of fetal tachycardias. *Br Heart J* 1991;65(1):46–48.
241. Erkkola R, Lammintausta R, Liukko P, et al. Transfer of propranolol and sotalol across the human placenta. Their effect on maternal and fetal plasma renin activity. *Acta Obstet Gynecol Scand* 1982;61(1):31–34.
242. Schneider H, Proegler M. Placental transfer of beta-adrenergic antagonists studied in an in vitro perfusion system of human placental tissue. *Am J Obstet Gynecol* 1988;159(1):42–47.
243. Akbaraly R, Leng JJ, Brachet-Liermain A, et al. [Trans-placental transfer of four anti-inflammatory agents. A study carried out by in vitro perfusion (author's transl)]. *J Gynecol Obstet Biol Reprod (Paris)* 1981;10(1):7–11.
244. Jacobson RL, Brewer A, Eis A, et al. Transfer of aspirin across the perfused human placental cotyledon. *Am J Obstet Gynecol* 1991;165(4 Pt 1):939–944.
245. Siu SS, Yeung JH, Lau TK. An in-vivo study on placental transfer of naproxen in early human pregnancy. *Hum Reprod* 2002;17(4):1056–1059.
246. Akbaraly JP, Guibert S, Leng JJ, et al. [Transplacental transfer of 5 antibiotics by in vitro human placental perfusion]. *J Pathol Biol (Paris)* 1985;33(5):368–372.
247. Fortunato SJ, Bawdon RE, Maberry MC, et al. Transfer of ceftizoxime surpasses that of cefoperazone by the isolated human placenta perfused in vitro. *Obstet Gynecol* 1990;75(5):830–833.
248. Fortunato SJ, Bawdon RE, Baum M. Placental transfer of cefoperazone and sulbactam in the isolated in vitro perfused human placenta. *Am J Obstet Gynecol* 1988;159(4):1002–1006.
249. Bawdon RE, Maberry MC, Fortunato SJ, et al. Trimethoprim and sulfamethoxazole transfer in the in vitro perfused human cotyledon. *Gynecol Obstet Invest* 1991;31(4):240–242.
250. Sodha RJ, Schneider H. Transplacental transfer of beta-adrenergic drugs studied by an in vitro perfusion method of an isolated human placental lobule. *Am J Obstet Gynecol* 1983;147(3):303–310.
251. Fujimoto S, Tanaka T, Akahane M. Levels of ritodrine hydrochloride in fetal blood and amniotic fluid following long-term continuous administration in late pregnancy. *Eur J Obstet Gynecol Reprod Biol* 1991;38(1):15–18.
252. Urbach J, Mor L, Fuchs S, et al. Transplacental transfer of ritodrine and its effect on placental glucose and oxygen consumption in an in vitro human placental cotyledon perfusion. *Gynecol Obstet Invest* 1991;32(1):10–14.
253. Smith MA, Thomford PJ, Mattison DR, et al. Transport and metabolism of dexamethasone in the dually perfused human placenta. *Reprod Toxicol* 1988;2(1):37–43.
254. Addison RS, Maguire DJ, Mortimer RH, et al. Metabolism of prednisolone by the isolated perfused human placental lobule. *J Steroid Biochem Mol Biol* 1991;39(1):83–90.
255. Levitz M, Jansen V, Dancis J. The transfer and metabolism of corticosteroids in the perfused human placenta. *Am J Obstet Gynecol* 1978;132(4):363–366.
256. Omarini D, Barzago MM, Bortolotti A, et al. Placental transfer of theophylline in an in vitro closed perfusion system of human placenta isolated lobule. *Eur J Drug Metab Pharmacokinet* 1993;18(4):369–374.
257. Schenker S, Dicke J, Johnson RF, et al. Human placental transport of cimetidine. *J Clin Invest* 1987;80(5):1428–1434.
258. Jauniaux E, Jurkovic D, Lees C, et al. In-vivo study of diazepam transfer across the first trimester human placenta. *Hum Reprod* 1996;11(4):889–892.
259. Crawford JS. Premedication for elective caesarean section. *Anaesthesia* 1979;34(9):892–897.
260. Guerre-Millo M, Challier JC, Rey E, et al. Maternofetal transfer of two benzodiazepines. Effect of plasma protein binding and placental uptake. *Dev Pharmacol Ther* 1982;4(3–4):158–172.
261. Wilson CM, Dundee JW, Moore J, et al. A comparison of the early pharmacokinetics of midazolam in pregnant and nonpregnant women. *Anaesthesia* 1987;42(10):1057–1062.
262. Heikkine T, Ekblad U, Laine K. Transplacental transfer of citalopram, fluoxetine and their primary demethylated metabolites in isolated perfused human placenta. *Bjog* 2002;109(9):1003–1008.
263. Shah YG, Miller RK. The pharmacokinetics of phenytoin in perfused human placenta. *Pediatr Pharmacol (New York)* 1985;5(3):165–179.
264. Kluck RM, Cannell GR, Hooper WD, et al. Disposition of phenytoin and phenobarbitone in the isolated perfused human placenta. *Clin Exp Pharmacol Physiol* 1988;15(11):827–836.
265. Takeda A, Okada H, Tanaka H, et al. Protein binding of four antiepileptic drugs in maternal and umbilical cord serum. *Epilepsy Res* 1992;13(2):147–151.
266. Pienimaki P, Hartikainen AL, Arvela P, et al. Carbamazepine and its metabolites in human perfused placenta and in maternal and cord blood. *Epilepsia* 1995;36(3):241–248.
267. Fowler DW, Eadie MJ, Dickinson RG. Transplacental transfer and biotransformation studies of valproic acid and its glucuronide(s) in the perfused human placenta. *J Pharmacol Exp Ther* 1989;249(1):318–323.
268. Barzago MM, Bortolotti A, Stellari FF, et al. Placental transfer of valproic acid after liposome encapsulation during in vitro human placenta perfusion. *J Pharmacol Exp Ther* 1996;277(1):79–86.
269. Henderson GI, Hu ZQ, Johnson RF, et al. Acyclovir transport by the human placenta. *J Lab Clin Med* 1992;120(6):885–892.
270. Gilstrap LC, Bawdon RE, Roberts SW, et al. The transfer of the nucleoside analog ganciclovir across the perfused human placenta. *Am J Obstet Gynecol* 1994;170(4):967–972;discussion 972–973.
271. Casey BM, Bawdon RE. Placental transfer of ritonavir with zidovudine in the ex vivo placental perfusion model. *Am J Obstet Gynecol* 1998;179(3 Pt 1):758–761.
272. Loftus JR, Hill H, Cohen SE. Placental transfer and neonatal effects of epidural sufentanil and fentanyl administered with bupivacaine during labor. *Anesthesiology* 1995;83(2):300–308.
273. Gerdin E, Rane A, Lindberg B. Transplacental transfer of morphine in man. *J Perinat Med* 1990;18(4):305–312.
274. Kopecky EA, Simone C, Knie B, et al. Transfer of morphine across the human placenta and its interaction with naloxone. *Life Sci* 1999;65(22):2359–2371.
275. Johnson RF, Cahana A, Olenick M, et al. A comparison of the placental transfer of ropivacaine versus bupivacaine. *Anesth Analg* 1999;89(3):703–708.
276. Datta S, Camann W, Bader A, et al. Clinical effects and maternal and fetal plasma concentrations of epidural ropivacaine versus bupivacaine for cesarean section. *Anesthesiology* 1995;82(6):1346–1352.
277. Bajoria R, Contractor SF. Transfer of heparin across the human perfused placental lobule. *J Pharm Pharmacol* 1992;44(12):952–959.
278. Gin T, Gregory MA, Chan K, et al. Maternal and fetal levels of propofol at caesarean section. *Anaesth Intensive Care* 1990;18(2):180–184.
279. Nandakumaran M, Eldeen AS. Transfer of cyclosporine in the perfused human placenta. *Dev Pharmacol Ther* 1990;15(2):101–105.
280. Nestorov I. Whole body pharmacokinetic models. *Clin Pharmacokinet* 2003;42(10):883–908.
281. Thakur AK. Model: mechanistic vs empirical. In: Rescigno A, Thakur AK, eds. *New trends in pharmacokinetics.* Boston, MA: Springer, 1991:41–51.
282. Claassen K, Thelen K, Coboeken K, et al. Development of a physiologically-based pharmacokinetic model for preterm neonates: evaluation with in vivo data. *Curr Pharm Des* 2015;21(39):5688–5698.
283. Edginton AN, Schmitt W, Willmann S. Development and evaluation of a generic physiologically based pharmacokinetic model for children. *Clin Pharmacokinet* 2006;45(10):1013–1034.
284. Dallmann A, Pfister M, van den Anker J, et al. Physiologically based pharmacokinetic modeling in pregnancy: a systematic review of published models. *Clin Pharmacol Ther* 2018;104(6):1110–1124.

285. Schalkwijk S, Buaben AO, Freriksen JJM, et al. Prediction of fetal darunavir exposure by integrating human ex-vivo placental transfer and physiologically based pharmacokinetic modeling. *Clin Pharmacokinet* 2018;57(6):705–716.
286. Liu XI, Momper JD, Rakhmanina N, et al. Physiologically based pharmacokinetic models to predict maternal pharmacokinetics and fetal exposure to emtricitabine and acyclovir. *J Clin Pharmacol* 2019;60(5):240–255.
287. De Sousa Mendes M, Lui G, Zheng Y, et al. A physiologically-based pharmacokinetic model to predict human fetal exposure for a drug metabolized by several CYP450 pathways. *Clin Pharmacokinet* 2017;56(5):537–550.
288. De Sousa Mendes M, Hirt D, Vinot C, et al. Prediction of human fetal pharmacokinetics using ex vivo human placenta perfusion studies and physiologically based models. *Br J Clin Pharmacol* 2016;81(4):646–657.
289. Zhang Z, Unadkat JD. Development of a novel maternal-fetal physiologically based pharmacokinetic model ii: verification of the model for passive placental permeability drugs. *Drug Metab Dispos* 2017;45(8):939–946.
290. Codaccioni M, Bois F, Brochot C. Placental transfer of xenobiotics in pregnancy physiologically-based pharmacokinetic models: structure and data. *Comput Toxicol* 2019;12:100111.

CHAPTER

10

Shinya Ito
Ruud Verstegen

Maternal Medications During Pregnancy and Lactation

PHARMACOKINETIC CHARACTERISTICS IN PREGNANCY: ITS IMPLICATIONS IN FETAL DRUG EXPOSURE

Medication use in pregnancy poses two main pharmacologic challenges: pharmacokinetics (PK) changes during pregnancy and fetal drug safety. In this chapter, we provide an overview on these two aspects.

MATERNAL PHYSIOLOGIC CHANGES OF PREGNANCY

Pregnancy is associated with drastic changes in hemodynamics, including fluid volume expansion, vasodilation, and hyperperfusion (i.e., increased blood flow to most organs, except for the brain). The percentage increase in water compartment sizes during pregnancy is in the range of 30% to 40% from the prepregnancy levels.[1–4] Increase in blood/plasma volume, heart rate, and stroke volume contributes to nearly 40% rise of cardiac output[5] and resultant increase in blood/plasma flow to drug-eliminating organs (Table 10.1). In addition, glomerular filtration rate (*GFR*) increases,[6–8] and intrinsic activity of some drug-metabolizing enzymes in the liver changes during pregnancy.[9,10] Along with decreased plasma protein binding, these changes cause alterations in the PK parameters of many drugs.

Gastrointestinal motility also changes during pregnancy. Gastric emptying time remains relatively unchanged during pregnancy, but total gastrointestinal transit time (mouth-to-cecum) is longer in pregnancy than in nonpregnant state, suggesting that intestinal transit time is prolonged significantly.[11–13] This may increase oral bioavailability of some drugs, which do not undergo intestinal metabolism, although its clinical significance may not be obvious.

During pregnancy, total plasma protein concentrations decrease,[14] and colloid osmotic pressure is reduced.[15] Although concentrations of some proteins such as globulins are increased,[14] concentrations of major drug-binding proteins (i.e., albumin and α-1-acid glycoprotein) are decreased in pregnancy, leading to an increased fraction of unbound drug (f_u).[14–17] The impact of an increased f_u on total and free (unbound) drug concentrations varies among drugs, depending on the magnitude of the increase and the elimination characteristics of the drug.

PHARMACOKINETIC PARAMETER CHANGES

Pharmacokinetic Determinants of Plasma Drug Concentration at Steady State

In order to predict the impact of pregnancy-associated physiologic changes on drug concentration–time profiles, it is important to understand PK determinants of drug concentrations in plasma at steady state. A simplified picture of their relation is described below on the assumption of a one-compartment model with instant distribution. Note that precise interpretation of PK theories is outside the scope of this chapter.

First, at a given dose (*D*) and a dosing interval (τ), plasma clearance (*CL*) and oral bioavailability (*F*) define an average concentration of drug at steady state ($[C]_{mean}$), but volume of distribution (V_d) does not influence $[C]_{mean}$; the higher the *CL*, the lower the $[C]_{mean}$.

$$[C]_{mean} = \frac{F \times (D/\tau)}{CL}$$

Note that drug concentrations and PK parameters here are based on total drug concentrations in plasma (i.e., bound plus unbound), unless stated otherwise. The ratio of *CL* to V_d also defines an elimination rate constant (*k*), and an elimination half-life ($t_{1/2}$) is a function of *k*: the higher the *CL*, the shorter the $t_{1/2}$; the larger the V_d, the longer the $t_{1/2}$.

$$\frac{CL}{V_d} = k = \frac{\ln 2}{t_{1/2}}$$

The two primary parameters (i.e., *CL* and V_d) and their ratio (k or $\ln 2 / t_{1/2}$) are mathematically interdependent, and if any two of the three parameters are known, then one can calculate the remaining one. However, *CL* and V_d are physiologically determined independent parameters, while *k* and $t_{1/2}$ depend on these two parameters because it is a ratio of the two. Therefore, *k* and $t_{1/2}$ may be viewed as secondary parameters. These secondary parameters cannot be primarily altered without changing one of the two primary parameters: *CL* and V_d. Also, the mathematical relationship ($CL = V_d \times k$) is correct but only

TABLE 10.1 Main Hemodynamic and Physiologic Changes in Pregnancy

Parameter	*Change (Prepregnancy → Peak Level in Pregnancy)*	*References*
Body weight	+15% (60 kg → 70 kg)	
Cardiac output	+40% (5 L/min → 7 L/min)	Robson et al.[5]
Organ blood/plasma flow		Moran et al.,[6] Nakai et al.[21]
Total liver blood flow (portal vein plus hepatic artery)	+50% (2 L/min → 3 L/min)	
Renal plasma flow	+50% (0.6 L/min → 0.9 L/min)	
Drug elimination systems		Odutayo and Hladunewich,[7] Cheung and Lafayette,[8] Pariente et al.[30]
Liver:		
Intrinsic hepatic metabolism	Variable (enzyme specific)	
Biliary excretion	Not well characterized	
Kidney:		
Glomerular filtration rate	+50% (120 mL/min → 180 mL/min)	
Net tubular secretion	Not well characterized (transporters)	
Volume compartment		Lukaski et al.,[1] Van Loan et al.,[2] Silver et al.,[3] Wadsworth[4]
Total blood volume	+40% (4L → 5.7 L)	
Plasma volume	+40% (2.8L → 4 L)	
Total body water	+30% (32L → 40 L)	
Extracellular fluid	+30% (15L → 20 L)	
Plasma protein		Notarianni[14], Chen et al.[17]
Albumin	−20% (47 g/L → 38 g/L)	
α-1-Acid glycoprotein	−30% (0.7 g/L → 0.5 g/L)	
Gastrointestinal function		Wald et al.,[11] Lawson et al.,[12] Chiloiro et al.[13]
Gastric emptying time	Unchanged	
Gastrointestinal transit time	Prolonged	

on a mathematical term. Physiologically, *CL* is not dependent upon V_d and vice versa.

Second, at steady state during repeated dosing (e.g., every 12-hour oral dose), V_d determines an amplitude of a rise from a trough ($[C]_{min}$) to a peak concentration ($[C]_{max}$); the larger the V_d, the smaller is the difference between $[C]_{max}$ and $[C]_{min}$. As described before, changes in V_d per se do not affect $[C]_{mean}$, but *CL* changes do.

Third, *CL* through a main drug-eliminating organ can be expressed as a function of plasma protein binding [i.e., unbound fraction (f_u), blood flow rate (Q), and intrinsic clearance (CL_{int})], according to the well-stirred model. In this chapter, we approximate *CL* as plasma clearance and *Q* as organ plasma flow. Note that this scheme does not fully address the bioavailability and intestinal metabolism in oral drug administration and the potential impact of additional factors including the fetoplacental unit on plasma clearance of drugs. Although further refinement of such a theoretical model is necessary, the simple scheme facilitates our conceptual understanding of the pregnancy-associated changes in drug concentration profiles.

Efficiency of drug elimination is expressed as extraction ratio (*ER*), ranging from 0 to 1.

$$\mathrm{ER} = \frac{f_u \times CL_{int}}{Q + (f_u \times CL_{int})}$$

$$CL = Q \times ER$$

If ($f_u \times CL_{int}$) is sufficiently higher than *Q*, *ER* approaches the maximum value of 1, which is the characteristic of high *ER* drugs (i.e., $ER > 0.7$). In this case, *CL* almost equals and becomes highly dependent on *Q*, as long as high *ER* status is maintained. For high *ER* drugs, if *Q* increases by a factor of 0.5 (i.e., 50% increase), such as in pregnancy (and if [$f_u \times CL_{int}$] is not significantly decreased), then *CL* will increase by nearly 40% to 50%. Because physiologic increase in *Q* of the liver and kidney in pregnancy is within a range of about 1.5-fold, it will not alter the high *ER* status of the drug. This *CL* increase occurs irrespective of their elimination routes, unless responsible transporters and/or drug-metabolizing enzymes are significantly downregulated.

On the other hand, if ($f_u \times CL_{int}$) is sufficiently smaller than *Q*, then *ER* becomes far lower than 1 (i.e., $ER = [f_u \times CL_{int}]/Q$), which defines low *ER* drugs (i.e., $ER < 0.3$). For these low *ER* drugs, *CL* equals ($f_u \times CL_{int}$), and increases of *Q* have no impact on *CL*, but changes of ($f_u \times CL_{int}$) do. As discussed later, drugs that are mainly eliminated via *GFR* from the kidney are low *ER* drugs (because *GFR* represents CL_{int} that is much smaller than renal plasma flow), and therefore, their *CL* is elevated in pregnancy due to pregnancy-associated *GFR* increase (by 50%) and f_u elevation (the magnitude depends on drugs). For low *ER* drugs mainly metabolized by the liver, CL_{int} represents each of the enzymatic processes unique to the respective drugs, and therefore, their *CL* changes during pregnancy become drug specific. In addition, overall reduction of plasma protein binding leads to an increase in f_u, which becomes a factor to increase *CL* of low *ER* drugs. These two examples above are extreme ends of the spectrum, and there are drugs in the intermediate *ER* category (e.g., *ER*: 0.3 to 0.7), which show mixed patterns.

On the whole, pregnancy-associated PK changes stem from (a) increased organ blood/plasma flow to the liver and kidney, the main drug-eliminating organs; (b) increased f_u due to lower plasma protein concentrations; (c) increased *GFR*; and (d) increased sizes of water compartments. Intrinsic activity changes of hepatic drug-metabolizing enzymes (i.e., CL_{int} of the enzyme) are variable and enzyme specific. Also, pregnancy-associated changes of transporter expression in renal tubular cells are not well understood. With some exceptions, the above changes tend to result in decreased $[C]_{mean}$ due to increased *CL*, and a smaller amplitude between $[C]_{max}$ and $[C]_{min}$ due to increased V_d. As described before, changes in *k* and $t_{1/2}$ are dependent on *CL* and V_d. The clinical implications of these PK changes will be illustrated by examples later.

The simple conceptual understanding described above is not sufficient for accurate description of the observations in vivo. For this purpose, physiologically based PK modeling is necessary, which is outside the scope of this chapter.

Drugs Metabolized by the Liver

Hepatic Blood/Plasma Flow

The liver receives blood supply from two systems: the hepatic artery and the portal vein. Although food intake alters their relative contribution to total liver blood flow,[18,19] about one-third of total liver blood flow is from hepatic artery, and the remaining two-thirds are from portal vein.[20–22] Total hepatic blood flow measured by Doppler ultrasonography reaches approximately 3 L per minute in the third trimester (>50% increase from the prepregnancy level, Table 10.1), mainly due to significant increase in portal venous blood flow.[21] While this is consistent with the overall increase in cardiac output during pregnancy, liver blood flow estimated from clearance of indocyanine green (ICG)[23] or bromsulphalein (bromsulphthalein, BSP)[24] does not show significant pregnancy-associated increase.

Both ICG and BSP are substrates for hepatic uptake transporters[25,26] and have a high *ER*.[27] Their clearance depends mainly on hepatic blood flow, at least in nonpregnant women and male subjects. Reduced function of uptake transporters for ICG/BSP during pregnancy is likely to result in lower *ER*, which has been shown in animal experiments.[28] In addition, the presence of endogenous substances during pregnancy, such as progesterone metabolites, interferes with the transporters.[29] ICG and BSP may not represent flow-dependent high *ER* compounds during pregnancy. Therefore, it is fair to assume that total liver blood/plasma flow is significantly increased during pregnancy as the imaging studies using Doppler ultrasonography demonstrated.[21,22]

Table 10.2 presents *CL* changes of drugs during pregnancy,[30] according to the three categories of *ER*. Assuming that total liver blood/plasma flow is increased during pregnancy by 50% to 60%, one may expect similar increases in *CL* of drugs metabolized by the liver with high *ER*, unless responsible uptake systems and/or metabolizing enzymes are significantly downregulated, such as the case of ICG and BSP described above. Although *CL* increase often gives an impression of increased "intrinsic activity" of respective drug-metabolizing enzymes, increase in liver blood/plasma flow during pregnancy is likely to be the main mechanism for those high *ER* drugs. It is also important to note that this flow-dependent *CL* increase occurs in any enzymatic system as long as the *ER* is high. Examples include metoprolol (CYP2D6 substrate) and indinavir (CYP3A4 substrate), which show 50% to 100% increase in *CL* and resultant decrease in steady-state serum concentrations during pregnancy.[31–34] Although the pregnancy-associated increase in their *CL* and resultant reduction in serum concentrations can be explained mainly by increased liver blood flow, minor changes in the intrinsic enzyme activity may exist. In contrast, some high *ER* drugs, such as propranolol (CYP1A2 and CYP2D6 substrate),[35,36] do not show clear increase in *CL* during pregnancy.[30] This is likely a result of reduced intrinsic activity of the enzyme (e.g., CYP1A2 for propranolol) or transporters during pregnancy as discussed below.

Intrinsic Activity of Drug-Metabolizing Enzymes and Plasma Protein Binding

CL of a low *ER* drug depends on the product of intrinsic activity of responsible enzymes (CL_{int}) and f_u, and therefore, changes in $[CL_{int} \times f_u]$ are reflected on *CL* changes. Lamotrigine is a low *ER* drug, and its plasma protein binding is also not high. Therefore, the reported *CL* increase during pregnancy[30] is likely a result of significant increase in CL_{int} (i.e., increased expression of UGT1A4), which is consistent with the findings from experiments of humanized UGT1 mice.[37] Phenytoin is a CYP2C9 substrate with low *ER* but has relatively high plasma protein binding. Phenytoin *CL* during pregnancy is increased by an average of 40% as well as f_u by about 20%.[30] Because its oral bioavailability remains unchanged in pregnancy,[38] *CL* increase in phenytoin may indicate an increase in both unbound fraction and intrinsic activity of hepatic CYP2C9. Carbamazepine, a CYP3A4 substrate, is another low *ER* drug with an f_u of 0.2 (i.e., 80% bound). During pregnancy, its f_u may increase by about 50% to 0.3,[39] which is likely to account for the relative increase of its *CL* of 10% to 30%.[30] However, a small increase in intrinsic activity of CYP3A4 may coexist.

Pregnancy-associated increases in *CL* are also reported in other CYP3A4 substrates, such as midazolam.[40,41] They are characterized by intermediate *ER* (midazolam 0.43) and relatively high plasma protein binding (>95%).[42] This suggests that *CL* of midazolam is dependent on all three factors (i.e., organ blood flow, protein binding, and intrinsic activity of CYP3A4). For example, pregnancy-associated relative increase in midazolam *CL* is about 1.8- to twofold from the nonpregnant level for both intravenous and oral administration.[40,41] Because the 50% increase in liver plasma flow in pregnancy cannot account for the entire twofold increase in midazolam *CL*, it is likely that $[CL_{int} \times f_u]$ is also increased substantially, but evidence is scarce to define the relative contribution of f_u and CL_{int} increase (i.e., CYP3A4 activity).

By contrast, *CL* of caffeine, a CYP1A2 substrate, is decreased in pregnancy.[10] Because it has a low-intermediate *ER* with low plasma protein binding, its *CL* decrease is likely a result of decreased CYP1A2 activity. Whether this is due to decreased expression or other factors has yet to be determined, but it provides a clue to the fact that propranolol, which is a high *ER* drug in nonpregnant state and a partial CYP1A2 substrate, does not show elevated *CL* in pregnancy.[30]

TABLE 10.2 Clearance Changes during Pregnancy

Drug	*Peak CL[a] Change in Pregnancy*	*Main Eliminating Organ*	*Elimination System*	*Plasma Protein Binding [f_u]*	*Presumed Primary Mechanisms of CL Changes during Pregnancy*
High *ER* drug (*ER*[b]: >0.7): *CL* change is dependent mainly on changes in organ blood flow.					
Indinavir	215%	Liver	CYP3A4	60% [0.4]	Increased liver blood flow
Labetalol	160%[90]	Liver	UGT1A1, UGT2B7	50% [0.5]	Increased liver blood flow
Metformin	131%	Kidney	*GFR*, net tubular secretion	0% [1.0]	Increase in renal blood flow and CL_{int} (*GFR*)
Metoprolol	180%[91]	Liver	CYP2D6	10% [0.9]	Increased liver blood flow
Proguanil	116%	Liver	CYP2C19	75% [0.25]	CYP2C19 activity may be reduced, offsetting effects of increase in liver blood flow.
Propranolol	106%	Liver	CYP1A2, CYP2D6	90% [0.1]	Pregnancy-associated reduction of CYP1A2 activity offsets effects of increase in liver blood flow.
Intermediate *ER* drug (*ER*: 0.3–0.7): *CL* change depends on both organ blood flow and $f_u \times CL_{int}$					
Acetaminophen	142%	Liver	UGT1A6, UGT1A9	20% [0.8]	Increase in liver blood flow and CL_{int} (UGT1A6/9 activity)
Amoxicillin	140%	Kidney	*GFR*, net tubular secretion	20% [0.8]	Increase in renal blood flow and CL_{int} (*GFR*)
Digoxin	157%	Kidney	*GFR*, net tubular secretion	25% [0.75]	Increase in renal blood flow and CL_{int} (*GFR*)
Darunavir	150%	Liver	CYP3A4	95% [0.05]	Increase in liver blood flow and $f_u \times CL_{int}$ (CYP3A4 activity)
Efavirenz	123%	Liver	CYP2B6	99% [0.01]	Increase in liver blood flow and $f_u \times CL_{int}$ (CYP2B6 activity)
Midazolam	184%	Liver	CYP3A4	97% [0.03]	Increase in liver blood flow and $f_u \times CL_{int}$ (CYP3A4 activity)
Low *ER* drug (*ER*: <0.3): *CL* change is dependent mainly on changes in $f_u \times CL_{int}$					
Caffeine	35%[10]	Liver	CYP1A2	30% [0.7]	CYP1A2 activity reduction
Carbamazepine	127%	Liver	CYP3A4	80% [0.2]	f_u increase (CYP3A4 activity may be also increased).
Ketorolac	150%	Kidney	*GFR*	99% [0.01]	*GFR* (CL_{int}) increase and f_u increase
Lamotrigine	212%	Liver	UGT1A4	50% [0.5]	UGT1A4 activity increase
Phenytoin	145%	Liver	CYP2C9	90% [0.1]	Increase in CYP2C9 activity and f_u
Sotalol	160%	Kidney	*GFR*	0% [1.0]	*GFR* (CL_{int}) increase

[a]Total plasma clearance expressed as mean percentages of the nonpregnant state (Shuster DL, Bammler TK, Beyer RP, et al. Gestational age-dependent changes in gene expression of metabolic enzymes and transporters in pregnant mice. Drug Metab Dispos 2013;41:332–342, unless otherwise stated).
[b]Extraction ratio in nonpregnant state.
CL, clearance; *ER*, extraction ratio; *GFR*, glomerular filtration rate; Fu, unbound fraction; CLint, intrinsic clearance.

Drugs Eliminated from the Kidney

Renal Plasma Flow

Hemodynamics of normal pregnancy is characterized by volume expansion, vasodilation, and increase in organ blood flow. Renal blood/plasma flow reaches a peak of about 140% compared to the prepregnancy level in the first and second trimesters, before gradually returning to the prepregnancy level in the early postpartum period.[7] For drugs mainly eliminated through kidney, the processes of glomerular filtration and net secretion (i.e., secretion minus reabsorption) are equivalent to CL_{int} according to the well-stirred model. Because normal *GFR* (100 to 120 mL per minute) in the nonpregnant state is much lower than renal plasma flow (500 to 700 mL per minute), *GFR*-dependent drugs without net secretion are low *ER* drugs. Conversely, drugs with high *ER* through renal elimination must have significant tubular secretion, which overwhelms reabsorption processes, causing substantial net secretion. Pregnancy-associated increase in renal plasma flow raises the *CL* of drugs with relatively high *ER*, such as metformin. Metformin is eliminated through kidney via filtration and net tubular secretion[43,44] and shows no appreciable plasma protein binding. Renal *CL* of metformin is as high as renal plasma flow, indicating its high *ER*. Renal *CL* of metformin rises by nearly 50% in mid-pregnancy and by 30% in late pregnancy,[45,46] which is consistent with the time profile of renal plasma flow change in pregnancy.[7]

Filtration and Net Secretion

In contrast to high *ER* drugs such as metformin, *GFR*-dependent drugs with no or minor net secretion are low *ER* drugs because *GFR* (i.e., CL_{int}) is much smaller than renal plasma flow (Q); therefore, its *CL* is insensitive to plasma flow increase but depends on changes in f_u and CL_{int}.

Increase in *GFR* during pregnancy is observed as early as in the first trimester. In the second and third trimesters, it reaches 150% of the prepregnancy level (e.g., 120 mL per minute in prepregnancy and 180 mL per minute in the second and third trimesters; Table Table 10.1). Note that this time profile is different from that of renal plasma flow, which shows a peak increase in mid-pregnancy.[7] As a result, *CL* of drugs, which are eliminated mainly through kidney by filtration such as amoxicillin (low-intermediate *ER*), becomes significantly higher in the second and third trimesters (>50% increase), which is consistent with the profile of *GFR* change. Digoxin is another example, showing similar changes.

Drug Concentrations in Plasma and Clinical Impact

The PK changes in pregnancy described above often lead to decreased drug concentrations in plasma, with some exceptions. Given that the f_u is usually increased in pregnancy, reduced total drug concentrations (bound plus unbound drug) somewhat offset an increased f_u, thereby unbound drug concentrations (not the fraction) may remain relatively unchanged compared to nonpregnant state. Although this suggests that plasma concentrations of pharmacologically active drug molecules (i.e., unbound) remain unchanged, there are clinical examples of reduced therapeutic effects.

Because pregnancy is not only characterized by PK changes but also alterations in disease courses and drug responses, clinical consequences of the PK changes are difficult to predict. Data are slowly accumulating, nonetheless. For example, pregnancy-associated PK changes of lamotrigine (increased *CL* and decreased $[C]_{mean}$) were reportedly associated with unfavorable clinical outcomes.[47,48] For antimicrobial drugs including anti-HIV drugs such as indinavir, failure to achieve target plasma concentrations is a major concern in the treatment of pregnant patients.[32] Another example are atazanavir-, elvitegravir-, or darunavir-cobicistat combinations for anti-HIV treatment. These anti-HIV protease inhibitors are CYP3A4 substrates. In order to acquire adequate plasma concentration profiles, cobicistat is coadministered as a PK enhancer by blocking CYP3A4. Although cobicistat is not extensively metabolized and its PK is complex, plasma concentrations of cobicistat become low in pregnant patients.[49] The failure of CYP3A4 inhibition results in substantial increase in *CL* and decreased $[C]_{mean}$ of these anti-HIV protease inhibitors. Because of this, instead of teratogenic effects on the fetus, the combination is considered a contraindication during pregnancy.

DRUG SAFETY IN PREGNANCY

THE THALIDOMIDE DISASTER

In November 22, 1961, at the meeting of West German Pediatricians, Widukind Lenz, a pediatrician in former West Germany, reported the outbreak of phocomelia (i.e., reduction defects of the limbs) in infants exposed in utero to thalidomide that was used as a sedative to relieve symptoms of morning sickness during pregnancy. Followed by the letter to the editor in the *Lancet* by an Australian obstetrician, William McBride, published on December 16, 1961, the "thalidomide" disaster became widely recognized, leaving more than 10,000 infants worldwide to face the consequences of the rare birth defects. The hardship of the survivors of this tragedy marks one of the darkest moments in the history of pharmacotherapy. Thalidomide was then withdrawn from the market, but later reintroduced and presently used for other indications, including multiple myeloma, as an immune modulator. In the past, thalidomide was also used to control a leprosy complication known as erythema nodosum leprosum. Although this is no longer a recommended practice, inadvertent exposure during pregnancy continues to occur, posing significant challenges to drug regulation.

TERATOGENICITY OF DRUG

A human teratogen is broadly defined as a medical condition, infection, or substance that causes harm to an embryo (10 weeks' gestational age or 8 weeks' postconceptional age) and/or fetus (Table 10.3). Data obtained in developed countries indicate that the prevalence of congenital anomalies of all causes is about 2% to 4% of live births.[50–53] Because of the background occurrence of fetal abnormality in the absence of intrauterine exposures to drugs, signal detection of drug-induced fetal toxicity is challenging. Teratogenicity of thalidomide and some others such as isotretinoin for intractable acne can be recognized relatively easily because their signals of fetal adverse effects are very high compared to the background occurrence. This is due to their characteristic fetal toxicity (i.e., phocomelia for thalidomide and ear plus other facial deformity for isotretinoin), which is considered highly specific to the intrauterine exposures to these drugs in the first trimester. As a result of their extremely low background occurrence, the toxicity signals of these exposures become distinct and pathognomonic. In contrast, if a resultant abnormality is not specific (e.g., ventricular septal defect, which is a relatively common congenital heart defect), it is more challenging to confirm exposure–defect causality in individual cases.

SHEPARD CRITERIA

The teratogenicity criteria proposed in 1994 by Thomas Shepard set a foundation for assessment of fetal drug toxicity (Table 10.4).[54] The seven-item criteria for proof of human teratogenicity are an amalgamation of several other criteria and deeply embedded in the framework of Hill criteria for causation. The first criterion stipulates a presence of proven exposure within the critical period of organ development in question because vulnerable periods of fetal development differ among different organs, although the first trimester is often the most vulnerable period for malformations. The second criterion describes required consistency/reproducibility of the findings, which should have a sufficiently high effect size of the signal of abnormality. Although the original Shepard criteria proposed a relative risk of 6 (compared to the nonexposure) as a necessary signal for a teratogen, smaller risks of 1.5 to 3 in well-executed studies may be considered sufficient as a clinically meaningful attribute of a teratogen. The third criterion calls for clear definition of resultant phenotypes. The fourth criterion is an extreme case of the spectrum, exemplifying a rare abnormality with a large effect size (i.e., relative risk) and, therefore, considered as a special case of the second criterion. A teratogen is expected to

TABLE 10.3 Major Human Teratogens

	Phenotypes	*Critical Period*	*Estimated Incidence*	*Reference*
Isotretinoin[a]	Spontaneous abortions, stillbirth, microtia/anotia, micrognathia, cleft palate, heart defects, thymic defects, retinal or optic-nerve abnormalities, and central nervous system malformations	First trimester	30%	Lammer et al.[92]
Thalidomide	Limb reduction defects, facial hemangiomata, esophageal and duodenal atresia, tetralogy of Fallot, renal agenesis, and anomalies of the ear	20–36 d after fertilization/34–50 d after LMP	20%–50%	Vargesson[93]
Phenytoin	Major congenital malformations	First trimester	6%	Weston et al.[94]
	Vitamin K deficiency–related abnormalities of hemostasis	Third trimester	50%	Cornelissen et al.[95]
Carbamazepine	Major congenital malformations	First trimester	3%–9%	Weston et al.[94]
	Vitamin K deficiency–related abnormalities of hemostasis	Third trimester	50%	Cornelissen et al.[95]
Valproic acid	Major congenital malformations (mainly neural tube defects, atrial septum defect, cleft palate, hypospadias, polydactyly, craniosynostosis)	Week 4–7 after LMP	7.5%	Jentink et al.,[96] Deshmukh et al.,[97] Tanoshima et al.[98]
	Neurodevelopmental delay	NA	15%–40%	Meador et al.[99]
	Autism	NA	5%	Christensen et al.[100]
Lithium	Major congenital malformations	First trimester	7%	Munk-Olsen et al.[101]
	Cardiac malformations	First trimester	2%	Munk-Olsen et al.[101]
Angiotensin-converting enzyme (ACE) inhibitors/angiotensin receptor blockers (ARB)	Major congenital malformations	First trimester	5%	Walfisch et al.[102]
	Impaired renal function, oligohydramnios, fetal death	Second/third trimester	50%–90%	Bullo et al.[103]
Ethanol[a] (heavy drinker)	Fetal alcohol syndrome [growth deficiency, CNS dysfunction including mental retardation and behavioral abnormalities, a distinctive pattern of facial features (short palpebral fissures, hypoplastic philtrum, flattened maxilla), and major organ system malformations]	First trimester	4%	Abel[104]
Warfarin[a]	Major congenital malformations	Until wk 8 after LMP	5%	Schaefer et al.[105]
Indomethacin[a]	Premature constriction of ductus arteriosus (potentially irreversible)	Third trimester	>50%	Moise et al.[106]
Organic mercury	Cerebral palsy characterized by ataxia, athetosis, and dysarthria (Minamata disease)	NA	Unknown	
Lead[a]	Neurodevelopmental delay	NA	Unknown	
Methotrexate[a]	Major congenital malformations	6–8 wk	7%	Weber-Schoendorfer et al.[107]

[a]These teratogens have been associated with increased rates of spontaneous abortions.
LMP, last menstrual period; NA, Not available.

TABLE 10.4 Shepard Criteria for Teratogenicity

1. Proven exposure to agent at critical time(s) in prenatal development (prescriptions, physicians' records, dates).
2. Consistent findings by two or more epidemiologic studies of high quality
   a. Control of confounding factors
   b. Sufficient numbers
   c. Exclusion of positive and negative bias factors
   d. Prospective studies, if possible
   e. Relative risk of six or more (?).
3. Careful delineation of the clinical cases. A specific defect or syndrome, if present, is very helpful.
4. Rare environmental exposure associated with rare defect. Probably three or more cases (e.g., oral anticoagulants and nasal hypoplasia, methimazole and scalp defects (?), and heart block and maternal rheumatism).
5. Teratogenicity in experimental animals important, but not essential.
6. The association should make biologic sense.
7. Proof in an experimental system that the agent acts in an unaltered state. Important information for prevention.

A teratogen is expected to satisfy the criteria 1, 2, and 3 or criteria 1, 3, and 4. The remaining three criteria are nonessential.

Reprinted with permission from Shepard TH. "Proof" of human teratogenicity. *Teratology* 1994;50:97–8.

satisfy the criteria 1, 2, and 3 or criteria 1, 3, and 4. The remaining three criteria are nonessential but important nonetheless, which include biologic plausibility and findings in animal experiments. In addition to drug-associated fetal toxicity, the Shepard criteria have been applied to positively identify Zika virus as a human teratogen.[55]

IMPACT OF MATERNAL DISEASE: CONFOUNDING BY INDICATION

While some infectious agents are teratogenic, *noninfectious* maternal disease conditions may have an impact on fetal development and/or normal functioning, modifying an association between a drug exposure and an outcome (e.g., diabetes mellitus). This factor, known as *confounding by indication*, is another reason why teratogenicity of drug is difficult to assess, although there are ways to minimize this bias, including a control group with the same indication but without drug exposure, or with a different indication.

DRUGS IN LACTATION

Breastfeeding is a standard method for feeding for most infants, but infant safety of maternal medication use and exposures to nonmedicinal compounds including environmental toxins is an important clinical issue. Here, we describe key pharmacologic elements essential for safety assessment of those maternal exposures during breastfeeding.

EPIDEMIOLOGY OF MATERNAL MEDICATION USE DURING BREASTFEEDING

Although the majority of women initiate breastfeeding,[56] in developed countries, more than half of them require medication.[57,58] Safety-risk balance in these circumstances is difficult to evaluate because basic information on PK in milk is often lacking. This is in part due to noninclusion of pregnant as well as breastfeeding patients in the drug development processes. The lack of PK data in milk continues after marketing. As a result, poor adherence occurs,[59] and unnecessary discontinuation or noninitiation of breastfeeding is observed.[60,61] Given the tangible benefits of human milk,[62–72] consequences of the information gap appear substantial, although they may not be readily recognized. On the other hand, reports of serious infant toxicity through breastfeeding by women on drugs or other substances continue to emerge.[73,74]

BENEFITS OF BREASTFEEDING

When drug safety during lactation is assessed, benefits of human milk for both mother and infant must be made explicit.[62] The evidence of the benefits is generated mostly from cohort studies and epidemiologic analyses, as randomized trials are not possible under most circumstances. However, biologic plausibility and frequently observed associations between breastfeeding and various health benefits support the presence of causal relationship. Table 10.5 lists those benefits, including infection resistance and better cognitive development in the infant.[62,64–68,71,72] Also, maternal benefits have been observed, including reduced rates of malignancies affecting the reproductive organs.[75,76]

CELLULAR MECHANISM OF DRUG EXCRETION INTO MILK

The mammary gland epithelia are comprised of the ducts and the secreting alveoli, surrounded by contractile myoepithelial cells.[77,78] These secretory systems and blood vessels are contained in the interstitium of the breast tissue, forming a drug excretion unit.

Lactation is regulated by the hypothalamo–pituitary–mammary axis. Prolactin stimulates milk synthesis by alveolar cells, whereas milk ejection by myoepithelial cells is stimulated by oxytocin. Within this pathway, dopamine is an important inhibitory factor of the release of prolactin.

Multiple mechanisms exist for drug excretion into milk, including passive and facilitated diffusion and active transport.[79] Also, during exocytosis, vesicles are formed that contain newly synthesized proteins and lactose, as well as water and electrolytes, including small molecule drugs in the cytoplasm. Once excreted into a milk compartment, slightly acidic pH in milk compared to maternal plasma makes cationic compounds to be more ionized in milk than plasma, preventing them from freely diffusing back to plasma through lipid bilayers. This phenomenon of ion trapping of cationic compounds in the milk compartment explains relatively high milk-to-(maternal) plasma concentration ratio (*MP* ratio) of basic drugs. Other factors that may increase *MP* ratio include low plasma protein binding and high lipophilicity of drug. As described later, however, *MP* ratio by itself does not fully define the level of infant drug exposure through milk. Therefore, selecting medications for breastfeeding women, based only on relatively low values of *MP* ratio alone, has little clinical significance.

A complete picture of mammary drug excretion remains to be fully elucidated, particularly regarding carriers involved in transport. However, a combined model of diffusion and breast cancer resistance protein (BCRP)—mediated efflux into milk explains milk disposition profiles of BCRP substrate drugs, including cimetidine and nitrofurantoin.[80–84] This model of combined diffusion and active transport indicates importance of both diffusion-related factors (e.g., ionization characteristics, plasma protein binding, and lipophilicity, as described above) and substrate specificity to the transporter such as BCRP in defining drug excretion into milk.

BCRP is highly induced in the lactating mammary gland epithelia, as an efflux transporter reducing exposures to drugs and toxins.[82] High-level expression and function are also observed in tissues of barrier function, including vascular endothelial cells in the brain (i.e., blood–brain barrier), placental syncytiotrophoblast, and intestinal epithelia. Importantly, the lactation-associated induction of mammary gland BCRP is specific to the mammary gland responding to a lactation-related prolactin surge in plasma and resultant activation of the JAK2/STAT5 pathway.[85] While BCRP is known for toxin excretion function in general, its role in the mammary gland appears to be the transporter for vitamin B2 (riboflavin),[84] which is enriched in milk. In contrast to BCRP, other ATP-binding cassette transporter P-glycoprotein (ABCB1) and MRP1 (ABCC1) are downregulated during lactation.[83]

PHASES OF MILK EXPRESSION

Milk composition varies depending on temporal profiles within the feeding (i.e., foremilk vs. hindmilk) and across the entire

TABLE 10.5 Benefits of Human Milk

Outcome	*Parameters Associated with Breastfeeding Compared to Formula Feeding/Nonbreastfeeding*
Rates of infection in the infant	
Acute otitis media	50% lower
Lower respiratory infection	70% lower
NEC	80% lower
Gastroenteritis	60% lower
Inflammatory bowel disease	30% lower
Obesity	20% lower
SIDS	40% lower
Cognitive function of the infant	
IQ	8 points higher
Rates of malignancies in the mother	
Breast cancer	60% lower
Ovarian cancer	30% lower

NEC, necrotizing enterocolitis; SIDS, sudden infant death syndrome. Data from Johnston M, Landers S, Noble L, et al. Breastfeeding and the use of human milk. *Pediatrics* 2012;129:e827–e841 and Stuebe A. The risks of not breastfeeding for mothers and infants. *Rev Obstet Gynecol* 2009;2:222–231 and Collaborative Group on Hormonal Factors in Breast Cancer. Breast cancer and breastfeeding: collaborative reanalysis of individual data from 47 epidemiological studies in 30 countries, including 50302 women with breast cancer and 96973 women without the disease. *Lancet* 2002;360:187–195.

breastfeeding period (i.e., colostrum, transition milk, and mature milk). Foremilk is defined as milk expressed at the beginning of a feeding. Milk toward the end of a feeding is called hindmilk. From a pharmacologic point of view, the foremilk–hindmilk distinction is important with regard to the relative composition of the milk. Namely, foremilk is rich in lactose, and hindmilk is rich in lipid fractions. Lipophilic drugs may achieve higher concentrations in hindmilk than in foremilk, assuming that other properties of milk remain the same, such as pH. Because it is difficult to mimic actual feeding in experimental settings of milk PK studies, description of how milk was collected is considered practical and sufficient. Colostrum is milk during the first few days of the postpartum period, which is rich in immune cells and factors. For ethical reasons, milk PK studies are rarely performed using colostrum, and because milk intake is not so high during the first couple of days, drug exposure through milk is relatively small during the colostrum period. In general, mature milk is used for milk PK research.

RELATIVE INFANT DOSE AND MILK-TO-PLASMA CONCENTRATION RATIO

There are two PK indices that are useful in characterizing drug disposition in milk: relative infant dose (*RID* or %*RID*) and milk-to-(maternal) plasma drug concentration ratio (*MP* ratio).

The *MP* ratio indicates a drug concentration in milk relative to that in maternal plasma and is expressed as a ratio of *AUC* (area under the curve) between milk and maternal plasma.[79] As a simplified surrogate, a single time point is often used to derive *MP* ratio. However, concentration–time profiles may be different between milk and maternal plasma, rendering this approach grossly inaccurate. This parameter represents a relative concentration of the drug in milk in relation to maternal plasma/serum, providing information on drug disposition across the mammary gland epithelia. As described below, interpretation of *MP* ratio requires caution because it is a ratio and not an absolute concentration of drug in milk.

MP ratio is sometimes misinterpreted as a single determinant of the infant drug exposure level.[73] For example, *MP* ratio of greater than 1 indicates accumulation of the drug in milk relative to maternal plasma concentration and often interpreted as an indicator of toxic exposure. However, this interpretation is not necessarily correct because infant exposure levels to drug in milk are determined by not only *MP* ratio but also drug clearance.[73]

While *MP* ratio relates drug concentrations in the two distinct compartments (i.e., milk and maternal plasma), *RID* (or %*RID*) relates infant dose of the drug via milk-to-maternal therapeutic doses on a weight basis. It is a weight-adjusted, time-averaged (e.g., daily) dose of drug in milk the infant would take, expressed as a fraction or a percentage of the time-averaged therapeutic dose on a body weight basis. *RID* (or %*RID*) of 100% is the same as receiving a full therapeutic dose per weight; *RID* 10% means that infant receives the drug in milk at 10% of the therapeutic dose per body weight.

RID (also known as %*RID*) of 10% is often viewed as a safety threshold for dose-dependent effects in risk assessment,[79] but some consider 5% as a threshold of compatibility for psychoactive drugs.[86] Distribution of *RID* among the current therapeutic drugs indicates that *RID* is 10% or lower for most drugs. The exceptions are those with relatively low CL (<1 mL per kg per minute, such as phenobarbital, ethosuximide, and lithium), which result in relatively high *RID* (20% to 50% of the levels of exposure at therapeutic doses),[73] but this does not mean that they are contraindicated in breastfeeding because risk–benefit analyses are specific to circumstances of individual patients.

These cutoff values (i.e., *RID* of 5% to 10%) are not thresholds of toxicity but rather theoretical reference points for risk assessment. Although infant drug exposure through milk should be compared to a neonatal therapeutic dose as a reference point, rather than a maternal dose, information on neonatal therapeutic doses is often unknown.

PHARMACOKINETICS OF DRUG IN MILK

RID is a function of *MP* ratio and *CL* as described below.[73] Table 10.6 summarizes definitions of some parameters necessary to derive key PK equations of drug disposition in milk.

By definition described above, infant dose (*ID*) of the drug through milk is:

$$ID = \left[C\right]_{\text{milk}} \times MV$$

Because $[C]_{\text{milk}}$ can be also expressed as a product of *MP* ratio and $[C]_{\text{plasma}}$,

$$ID = MP \text{ ratio} \times \left[C\right]_{\text{plasma}} \times MV \qquad (1)$$

By the definition,

$$RID = \frac{ID}{MoD}$$

TABLE 10.6 Pharmacokinetic Parameters of Drug Excretion in Milk

Parameter (Symbol)	*Definition*
Infant dose (*ID*)	Amount of drug the infant ingests via milk/body weight/day
Mother's dose (*MoD*)	Mother's dose of drug/body weight/day
Milk volume (*MV*)	Milk volume for an infant/body weight/day
Drug concentration in milk ($[C]_{milk}$) and in maternal plasma ($[C]_{plasma}$)	Average drug concentration at steady state over a 24-h period.
Relative infant dose (*RID* or %*RID*)	*ID* divided by *MoD*, expressed as percentage
Milk-to-plasma concentration ratio (*MP* ratio)	*AUC* (area under the curve) ratio between milk and maternal plasma

Replacing *ID* in the above formula with Equation (1),

$$RID = \frac{MP \text{ ratio} \times [C]_{plasma} \times MV}{MoD} \quad (2)$$

At steady state, $[C]_{plasma}$ can be expressed as:

$$[C]_{plasma} = \frac{F \times MoD}{CL}$$

where *F* is bioavailability and *CL* is total body clearance of the drug in the mother. Therefore, Equation (2) can be rewritten as:

$$RID = \frac{MP \text{ ratio} \times \left(\frac{F \times MoD}{CL}\right) \times MV}{MoD}$$

$$= MP \text{ ratio} \times \left(\frac{F}{CL}\right) \times MV$$

Assuming that $F = 1$, *RID* can be rewritten as a percentage parameter:

$$RID(\%) = \left(\frac{MP \text{ ratio}}{CL}\right) \times MV \times 100$$

MV of an infant is usually assumed to be 150 mL per kg per day (about 0.1 mL per kg per minute).[79,87] Therefore,

$$RID(\%) = \frac{MP \text{ ratio} \times 10}{CL} \quad (3)$$

where the unit of *CL* is mL per kg per minute.

Figure 10.1 shows Equation (3) as the logarithmic relationship between *CL* and *RID* (*RID* can be depicted as "exposure index",[73] because they are equivalent by definition) in three *MP* ratio categories. Because observed *MP* ratios and *CL* show limited ranges of values, drugs are distributed into a relatively confined space. For example, reported *MP* ratios of most drugs are around 1 or lower, and most drugs have a clearance of greater than 1 mL per kg per minute,[88] indicating that most drugs are in the shaded area of Figure 10.1. In addition, it is noted that *RID* dependence on *MP* ratio is pronounced for drugs with relatively low *CL*; drugs with low *CL* (e.g., <1 mL per kg per minute) have relatively high *RID*, which is further accentuated if their *MP* ratios become high due to intra- or interindividual variations. Therefore, clinical significance of *MP* ratio to define *RID* depends on maternal *CL* of the drug. In other words, most drugs are *unlikely* to achieve *RID* of greater than 10%, but those with low *CL* (e.g., <1 mL per kg per minute) may achieve higher *RID*, especially if *MP* ratio is high.

Figure 10.2 contrasts a high *CL* drug with a low *CL* drug, illustrating a higher degree of *MP* ratio dependence of *RID* in low *CL* drug than in high *CL* drugs. In clinical settings, this indicates that inter- or intraindividual variations of *MP* ratio have a bigger impact on *RID* of low *CL* drugs, compared to high *CL* drugs.

These concepts, including Equation (3), are based on *CL* in the mother, and *RID* estimation in a clinical setting often uses mother's dose (*MoD*) in the absence of neonatal therapeutic dosing recommendations. If infant drug clearance per body weight is markedly lower than that of an adult (e.g., liver dysfunction or renal failure), then this must be further taken into account, when *RID* is interpreted as a risk assessment tool for dose-dependent effects.

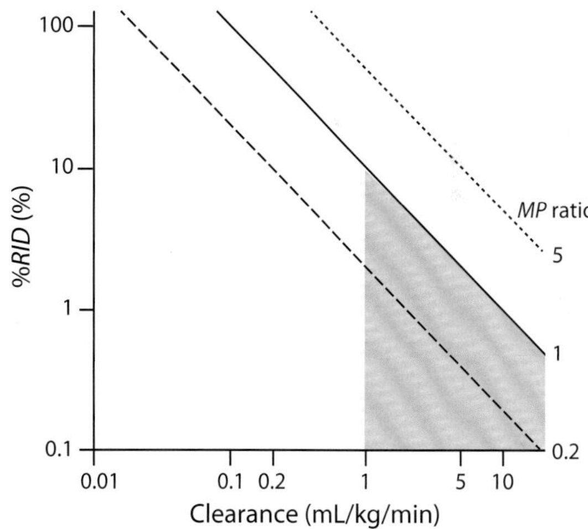

Figure 10.1 Percent relative infant dose (%*RID*) as a logarithmic function of clearance and milk-to-plasma concentration (*MP*) ratio. %*RID* is infant dose of drug through milk (mg per kg per day) expressed as a percentage of a weight-adjusted therapeutic dose of drug in the mother. With three different *MP* ratio scenarios (0.2, 1, and 5), the graph shows Equation (3) (see text) in a logarithmic scale, which defines %*RID* as a function of *MP* ratio and maternal drug clearance. The shaded area indicates a space where most drugs belong. Note that drugs with relatively low clearance (e.g., <1 mL per kg per minute) tend to achieve high %*RID* compared to high clearance drugs. Also, variations in *MP* ratio have more significant impact on %*RID* in low clearance drugs.

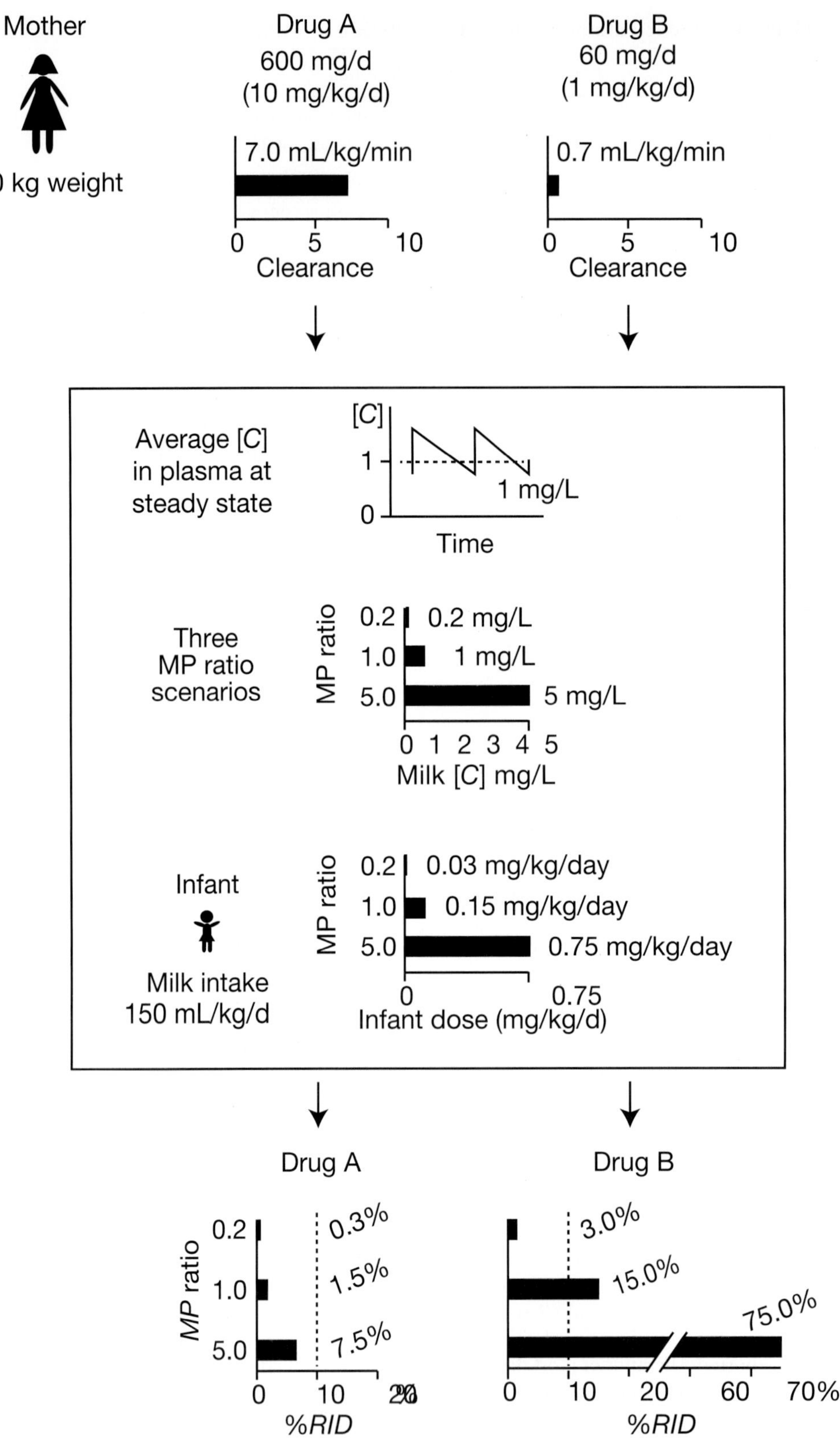

Figure 10.2 Examples of high and low clearance drugs and their percent relative infant dose (%*RID*). Drug A (clearance of 7 mL per kg per minute) and Drug B (clearance of 0.7 mL per kg per minute) are assumed to have the same therapeutic plasma concentration (1 mg per L). Therapeutic doses to achieve the target concentration at steady state are 600 mg per day for Drug A and 60 mg per day for Drug B. Because maternal plasma concentrations are the same (1 mg per L) for both drugs, their milk concentrations become equal under a given *MP* ratio. There are three different scenarios of *MP* ratio (i.e., 0.2, 1, and 5), and each of these scenarios lead to three scenarios of infant dose for both Drug A and Drug B. Derived %*RID* are shown at the bottom of the figure, demonstrating that %*RID* of Drug A (high clearance drug) does not exceed a threshold of 10% even at an *MP* ratio of as high as 5. This is in sharp contrast with Drug B (low clearance drug). (Adapted from Ito S. Emerging research paradigm for infant drug exposure through breast milk. *Curr Pharm Des* 2019;25:528–533.)

TABLE 10.7 Main Factors That Require Cautious Risk–Benefit Assessment during Breastfeeding

Maternal medications

- **Radioactive compounds.** Duration of breastfeeding interruption depends on dose and elimination half-life of the compounds. Because of thyroid accumulation, radioactive iodine needs particular caution.
- **Cancer chemotherapy.** Amount excreted into milk may be small, and/or gastrointestinal absorption may be marginal, but human data are often lacking. Each drug needs careful risk analysis in the context of individual circumstances.
- **Opioids.** Although a short-term use for 2–3 days is usually acceptable, its serious toxicity profiles including respiratory depression justify close monitoring of infant conditions. In an unsupervised outpatient setting, maternal regular use of opioids for more than 2–3 days is not recommended. The U.S. Food and Drug Administration (FDA) advises against the use of codeine and tramadol for breastfeeding women, partly because their metabolism depends on highly polymorphic CYP2D6 causing wide individual variations in plasma (and milk) concentration profiles.[74]

Infant factor

- **Dysfunction of drug-eliminating organs of infant.** Reduced function of liver and kidney, two major drug-eliminating organs, may decrease clearance of drug, posing a risk of drug accumulation over time.
- **Neonates.** More than half of reported toxicity involves neonates with neurologic or gastrointestinal symptoms.[108]

EFFECTS OF DRUG ON LACTATION

Some drugs may affect lactation by changing prolactin secretion. As previously described, dopamine is an important inhibitory factor of the release of prolactin. As a result, dopamine agonists such as bromocriptine and ergotamine diminish breast milk production, while dopamine antagonists, including domperidone and some antipsychotics, stimulate prolactin production and thus increase milk volume. Indeed, domperidone is sometimes used as a galactogogue.

ADVERSE EFFECTS OF DRUG IN MILK

Infants may experience adverse effects from maternal medication used in breastfeeding. Such cases are rare but reported, although causality assessment is difficult. Because *RID* is relatively low for most drugs, acute toxicity is unlikely for otherwise healthy infants. However, if infant drug clearance is low and its age-dependent development is compromised, even small doses through milk may cause accumulation over time. Table 10.7 presents drug groups and infant factors, which necessitate an even more cautious approach in the risk assessment, compared to other medications and healthy infants. Particularly important is maternal use of opioids because their profiles of adverse effects include serious events such as respiratory depression.[74]

RESOURCES

There are a variety of resources available that provide information on the use of drugs in lactation. In general, product monographs contain limited information, because pregnant and lactating women are usually excluded from clinical trials. Fortunately, regulatory bodies increasingly acknowledge the importance of this information. As a result, the U.S. Food and Drug Administration (FDA) introduced the Pregnancy and Lactation Labeling Rule (PLLR) in 2014, which outlines how available information should be presented and updated in product monographs.[89] Several databases are available in printed and digital formats to guide clinicians in determining drug safety during lactation. LactMed is the largest online database that contains lactation safety data on approximately 1,500 drugs and substances. The database, which is supported by the National Institute of Health (NIH), is constantly updated and can be accessed online free of charge (https://www.ncbi.nlm.nih.gov/books/NBK501922/).

REFERENCES

1. Lukaski HC, Siders WA, Nielsen EJ, et al. Total body water in pregnancy: assessment by using bioelectrical impedance. *Am J Clin Nutr* 1994;59:578–585.
2. Van Loan MD, Kopp LE, King JC, et al. Fluid changes during pregnancy: use of bioimpedance spectroscopy. *J Appl Physiol (1985)* 1995;78:1037–1042.
3. Silver HM, Seebeck M, Carlson R. Comparison of total blood volume in normal, preeclamptic, and nonproteinuric gestational hypertensive pregnancy by simultaneous measurement of red blood cell and plasma volumes. *Am J Obstet Gynecol* 1998;179:87–93.
4. Wadsworth GR. The blood volume of normal women. *Blood* 1954;9:1205–1207.
5. Robson SC, Hunter S, Boys RJ, et al. Serial study of factors influencing changes in cardiac output during human pregnancy. *Am J Physiol* 1989;256:H1060–H1065.
6. Moran P, Baylis PH, Lindheimer MD, et al. Glomerular ultrafiltration in normal and preeclamptic pregnancy. *J Am Soc Nephrol* 2003;14:648–652.
7. Odutayo A, Hladunewich M. Obstetric nephrology: renal hemodynamic and metabolic physiology in normal pregnancy. *Clin J Am Soc Nephrol* 2012;7:2073–2080.
8. Cheung KL, Lafayette RA. Renal physiology of pregnancy. *Adv Chronic Kidney Dis* 2013;20:209–214.
9. Tran TA, Leppik IE, Blesi K, et al. Lamotrigine clearance during pregnancy. *Neurology* 2002;59:251–255.
10. Tracy TS, Venkataramanan R, Glover DD, et al. Temporal changes in drug metabolism (CYP1A2, CYP2D6 and CYP3A activity) during pregnancy. *Am J Obstet Gynecol* 2005;192:633–639.
11. Wald A, Van Thiel DH, Hoechstetter L, et al. Effect of pregnancy on gastrointestinal transit. *Dig Dis Sci* 1982;27:1015–1018.
12. Lawson M, Kern F Jr, Everson GT. Gastrointestinal transit time in human pregnancy: prolongation in the second and third trimesters followed by postpartum normalization. *Gastroenterology* 1985;89:996–999.
13. Chiloiro M, Darconza G, Piccioli E, et al. Gastric emptying and orocecal transit time in pregnancy. *J Gastroenterol* 2001;36:538–543.
14. Notarianni LJ. Plasma protein binding of drugs in pregnancy and in neonates. *Clin Pharmacokinet* 1990;18:20–36.
15. Wu PY, Udani V, Chan L, et al. Colloid osmotic pressure: variations in normal pregnancy. *J Perinat Med* 1983;11:193–199.
16. Krauer B, Dayer P, Anner R. Changes in serum albumin and alpha 1-acid glycoprotein concentrations during pregnancy: an analysis of fetal-maternal pairs. *Br J Obstet Gynaecol* 1984;91:875–881.
17. Chen SS, Perucca E, Lee JN, et al. Serum protein binding and free concentration of phenytoin and phenobarbitone in pregnancy. *Br J Clin Pharmacol* 1982;13:547–552.
18. Lycklama à Nijeholt GJ, Burggraaf K, Wasser MN, et al. Variability of splanchnic blood flow measurements using MR velocity mapping under fasting and post-prandial conditions—comparison with echo-Doppler. *J Hepatol* 1997;26:298–304.
19. Burggraaf J, Schoemaker HC, Cohen AF. Assessment of changes in liver blood flow after food intake—comparison of ICG clearance and echo-Doppler. *Br J Clin Pharmacol* 1996;42:499–502.
20. Williams LR, Leggett RW. Reference values for resting blood flow to organs of man. *Clin Phys Physiol Meas* 1989;10:187–217.
21. Nakai A, Sekiya I, Oya A, et al. Assessment of the hepatic arterial and portal venous blood flows during pregnancy with Doppler ultrasonography. *Arch Gynecol Obstet* 2002;266:25–29.
22. Clapp JF 3rd, Stepanchak W, Tomaselli J, et al. Portal vein blood flow-effects of pregnancy, gravity, and exercise. *Am J Obstet Gynecol* 2000;183:167–172.
23. Robson SC, Mutch E, Boys RJ, et al. Apparent liver blood flow during pregnancy: a serial study using indocyanine green clearance. *Br J Obstet Gynaecol* 1990;97:720–724.
24. Munnell EW, Taylor HC. Liver blood flow in pregnancy-hepatic vein catheterization. *J Clin Invest* 1947;26:952–956.
25. Hata S, Wang P, Eftychiou N, et al. Substrate specificities of rat oatp1 and ntcp: implications for hepatic organic anion uptake. *Am J Physiol Gastrointest Liver Physiol* 2003;285:G829–G839.
26. de Graaf W, Hausler S, Heger M, et al. Transporters involved in the hepatic uptake of (99m)Tc-mebrofenin and indocyanine green. *J Hepatol* 2011;54:738–745.

27. De Gasperi A, Mazza E, Prosperi M. Indocyanine green kinetics to assess liver function: Ready for a clinical dynamic assessment in major liver surgery? *World J Hepatol* 2016;8:355–367.
28. Shuster DL, Bammler TK, Beyer RP, et al. Gestational age-dependent changes in gene expression of metabolic enzymes and transporters in pregnant mice. *Drug Metab Dispos* 2013;41:332–342.
29. Dixon PH, Williamson C. The pathophysiology of intrahepatic cholestasis of pregnancy. *Clin Res Hepatol Gastroenterol* 2016;40:141–153.
30. Pariente G, Leibson T, Carls A, et al. Pregnancy-associated changes in pharmacokinetics: a systematic review. *PLoS Med* 2016;13:e1002160.
31. Hogstedt S, Rane A. Plasma concentration-effect relationship of metoprolol during and after pregnancy. *Eur J Clin Pharmacol* 1993;44:243–246.
32. Cressey TR, Best BM, Achalapong J, et al. Reduced indinavir exposure during pregnancy. *Br J Clin Pharmacol* 2013;76:475–483.
33. Kosel BW, Beckerman KP, Hayashi S, et al. Pharmacokinetics of nelfinavir and indinavir in HIV-1-infected pregnant women. *AIDS* 2003;17:1195–1199.
34. Unadkat JD, Wara DW, Hughes MD, et al. Pharmacokinetics and safety of indinavir in human immunodeficiency virus-infected pregnant women. *Antimicrob Agents Chemother* 2007;51:783–786.
35. Yoshimoto K, Echizen H, Chiba K, et al. Identification of human CYP isoforms involved in the metabolism of propranolol enantiomers—N-desisopropylation is mediated mainly by CYP1A2. *Br J Clin Pharmacol* 1995;39:421–431.
36. Johnson JA, Herring VL, Wolfe MS, et al. CYP1A2 and CYP2D6 4-hydroxylate propranolol and both reactions exhibit racial differences. *J Pharmacol Exp Ther* 2000;294:1099–1105.
37. Chen S, Yueh MF, Evans RM, et al. Pregnane-x-receptor controls hepatic glucuronidation during pregnancy and neonatal development in humanized UGT1 mice. *Hepatology* 2012;56:658–667.
38. Lander CM, Smith MT, Chalk JB, et al. Bioavailability and pharmacokinetics of phenytoin during pregnancy. *Eur J Clin Pharmacol* 1984;27:105–110.
39. Johnson EL, Stowe ZN, Ritchie JC, et al. Carbamazepine clearance and seizure stability during pregnancy. *Epilepsy Behav* 2014;33:49–53.
40. Hebert MF, Easterling TR, Kirby B, et al. Effects of pregnancy on CYP3A and P-glycoprotein activities as measured by disposition of midazolam and digoxin: a University of Washington specialized center of research study. *Clin Pharmacol Ther* 2008;84:248–253.
41. Wilson CM, Dundee JW, Moore J, et al. A comparison of the early pharmacokinetics of midazolam in pregnant and nonpregnant women. *Anaesthesia* 1987;42:1057–1062.
42. Thummel KE, O'Shea D, Paine MF, et al. Oral first-pass elimination of midazolam involves both gastrointestinal and hepatic CYP3A-mediated metabolism. *Clin Pharmacol Ther* 1996;59:491–502.
43. Tucker GT, Casey C, Phillips PJ, et al. Metformin kinetics in healthy subjects and in patients with diabetes mellitus. *Br J Clin Pharmacol* 1981;12:235–246.
44. Graham GG, Punt J, Arora M, et al. Clinical pharmacokinetics of metformin. *Clin Pharmacokinet* 2011;50:81–98.
45. Eyal S, Easterling TR, Carr D, et al. Pharmacokinetics of metformin during pregnancy. *Drug Metab Dispos* 2010;38:833–840.
46. Hughes RC, Gardiner SJ, Begg EJ, et al. Effect of pregnancy on the pharmacokinetics of metformin. *Diabet Med* 2006;23:323–326.
47. de Haan GJ, Edelbroek P, Segers J, et al. Gestation-induced changes in lamotrigine pharmacokinetics: a monotherapy study. *Neurology* 2004;63:571–573.
48. Pennell PB, Peng L, Newport DJ, et al. Lamotrigine in pregnancy: clearance, therapeutic drug monitoring, and seizure frequency. *Neurology* 2008;70:2130–2136.
49. Boyd SD, Sampson MR, Viswanathan P, et al. Cobicistat-containing antiretroviral regimens are not recommended during pregnancy: viewpoint. *AIDS* 2019;33:1089–1093.
50. Dastgiri S, Stone DH, Le-Ha C, et al. Prevalence and secular trend of congenital anomalies in Glasgow, UK. *Arch Dis Child* 2002;86:257–263.
51. Moorthie S, Blencowe H, Darlison MW, et al. Estimating the birth prevalence and pregnancy outcomes of congenital malformations worldwide. *J Community Genet* 2018;9:387–396.
52. Parker SE, Mai CT, Canfield MA, et al. Updated National Birth Prevalence estimates for selected birth defects in the United States, 2004–2006. *Birth Defects Res A Clin Mol Teratol* 2010;88:1008–1016.
53. Canadian Perinatal Surveillance System (CPSS). Perinatal Health Indicators for Canada 2017. Ottawa, Canada, 2017.
54. Shepard TH. "Proof" of human teratogenicity. *Teratology* 1994;50:97–98.
55. Rasmussen SA, Jamieson DJ, Honein MA, et al. Zika virus and birth defects—reviewing the evidence for causality. *N Engl J Med* 2016;374:1981–1987.
56. OECD. Doing Better for Children. 2009.
57. Schirm E, Schwagermann MP, Tobi H, et al. Drug use during breastfeeding. A survey from the Netherlands. *Eur J Clin Nutr* 2004;58:386–390.
58. Stultz EE, Stokes JL, Shaffer ML, et al. Extent of medication use in breastfeeding women. *Breastfeed Med* 2007;2:145–151.
59. Ito S, Koren G, Einarson TR. Maternal noncompliance with antibiotics during breastfeeding. *Ann Pharmacother* 1993;27:40–42.
60. Ito S, Moretti M, Liau M, et al. Initiation and duration of breast-feeding in women receiving antiepileptics. *Am J Obstet Gynecol* 1995;172:881–886.
61. Lee A, Moretti ME, Collantes A, et al. Choice of breastfeeding and physicians' advice: a cohort study of women receiving propylthiouracil. *Pediatrics* 2000;106:27–30.
62. Johnston M, Landers S, Noble L, et al. Breastfeeding and the use of human milk. *Pediatrics* 2012;129:e827–e841.
63. Ip S, Chung M, Raman G, et al. A summary of the Agency for Healthcare Research and Quality's evidence report on breastfeeding in developed countries. *Breastfeed Med* 2009;4(Suppl 1):S17–S30.
64. Chantry CJ, Howard CR, Auinger P. Full breastfeeding duration and associated decrease in respiratory tract infection in US children. *Pediatrics* 2006;117:425–432.
65. Nishimura T, Suzue J, Kaji H. Breastfeeding reduces the severity of respiratory syncytial virus infection among young infants: a multi-center prospective study. *Pediatr Int* 2009;51:812–816.
66. Duijts L, Jaddoe VW, Hofman A, et al. Prolonged and exclusive breastfeeding reduces the risk of infectious diseases in infancy. *Pediatrics* 2010;126:e18–e25.
67. Quigley MA, Kelly YJ, Sacker A. Breastfeeding and hospitalization for diarrheal and respiratory infection in the United Kingdom Millennium Cohort Study. *Pediatrics* 2007;119:e837–e842.
68. Sullivan S, Schanler RJ, Kim JH, et al. An exclusively human milk-based diet is associated with a lower rate of necrotizing enterocolitis than a diet of human milk and bovine milk-based products. *J Pediatr* 2010;156:562.e1–567.e1.
69. Hauck FR, Thompson JM, Tanabe KO, et al. Breastfeeding and reduced risk of sudden infant death syndrome: a meta-analysis. *Pediatrics* 2011;128:103–110.
70. Greer FR, Sicherer SH, Burks AW. The effects of early nutritional interventions on the development of atopic disease in infants and children: the role of maternal dietary restriction, breastfeeding, hydrolyzed formulas, and timing of introduction of allergenic complementary foods. *Pediatrics* 2019;143.
71. Kramer MS, Aboud F, Mironova E, et al. Breastfeeding and child cognitive development: new evidence from a large randomized trial. *Arch Gen Psychiatry* 2008;65:578–584.
72. Belfort MB, Anderson PJ, Nowak VA, et al. Breast milk feeding, brain development, and neurocognitive outcomes: a 7-year longitudinal study in infants born at less than 30 weeks' gestation. *J Pediatr* 2016;177:133.e1–139.e1.
73. Ito S. Drug therapy for breast-feeding women. *N Engl J Med* 2000;343:118–126.
74. Ito S. Opioids in breast milk: pharmacokinetic principles and clinical implications. *J Clin Pharmacol* 2018;58(Suppl 10):S151–S163.
75. Stuebe A. The risks of not breastfeeding for mothers and infants. *Rev Obstet Gynecol* 2009;2:222–231.
76. Collaborative Group on Hormonal Factors in Breast Cancer. Breast cancer and breastfeeding: collaborative reanalysis of individual data from 47 epidemiological studies in 30 countries, including 50302 women with breast cancer and 96973 women without the disease. *Lancet* 2002;360:187–195.
77. Hennighausen L, Robinson GW. Information networks in the mammary gland. *Nat Rev Mol Cell Biol* 2005;6:715–725.
78. Inman JL, Robertson C, Mott JD, et al. Mammary gland development: cell fate specification, stem cells and the microenvironment. *Development* 2015;142:1028–1042.
79. Anderson PO, Sauberan JB. Modeling drug passage into human milk. *Clin Pharmacol Ther* 2016;100:42–52.
80. Koshimichi H, Ito K, Hisaka A, et al. Analysis and prediction of drug transfer into human milk taking into consideration secretion and reuptake clearances across the mammary epithelia. *Drug Metab Dispos* 2011;39:2370–2380.
81. Ito N, Ito K, Ikebuchi Y, et al. Prediction of drug transfer into milk considering Breast Cancer Resistance Protein (BCRP)-mediated transport. *Pharm Res* 2015;32:2527–2537.
82. Leslie EM, Deeley RG, Cole SP. Multidrug resistance proteins: role of P-glycoprotein, MRP1, MRP2, and BCRP (ABCG2) in tissue defense. *Toxicol Appl Pharmacol* 2005;204:216–237.
83. Jonker JW, Merino G, Musters S, et al. The breast cancer resistance protein BCRP (ABCG2) concentrates drugs and carcinogenic xenotoxins into milk. *Nat Med* 2005;11:127–129.
84. van Herwaarden AE, Wagenaar E, Merino G, et al. Multidrug transporter ABCG2/breast cancer resistance protein secretes riboflavin (vitamin B2) into milk. *Mol Cell Biol* 2007;27:1247–1253.
85. Wu AM, Yang M, Dalvi P, et al. Role of STAT5 and epigenetics in lactation-associated upregulation of multidrug transporter ABCG2 in the mammary gland. *Am J Physiol Endocrinol Metab* 2014;307:E596–E610.
86. Larsen ER, Damkier P, Pedersen LH, et al. Use of psychotropic drugs during pregnancy and breast-feeding. *Acta Psychiatr Scand Suppl* 2015:1–28.
87. Anderson PO, Valdes V. Variation of milk intake over time: clinical and pharmacokinetic implications. *Breastfeed Med* 2015;10:142–144.
88. Ito S, Koren G. A novel index for expressing exposure of the infant to drugs in breast milk. *Br J Clin Pharmacol* 1994;38:99–102.
89. United States Food and Drug Administration: Pregnancy and Lactation Labeling Rule (PLLR). https://www.federalregister.gov/d/2014-28241.
90. Fischer JH, Sarto GE, Hardman J, et al. Influence of gestational age and body weight on the pharmacokinetics of labetalol in pregnancy. *Clin Pharmacokinet* 2014;53:373–383.
91. Hogstedt S, Lindberg B, Peng DR, et al. Pregnancy-induced increase in metoprolol metabolism. *Clin Pharmacol Ther* 1985;37:688–692.
92. Lammer EJ, Chen DT, Hoar RM, et al. Retinoic acid embryopathy. *N Engl J Med* 1985;313:837–841.
93. Vargesson N. Thalidomide-induced teratogenesis: history and mechanisms. *Birth Defects Res C Embryo Today* 2015;105:140–156.
94. Weston J, Bromley R, Jackson CF, et al. Monotherapy treatment of epilepsy in pregnancy: congenital malformation outcomes in the child. *Cochrane Database Syst Rev* 2016;11:CD010224.
95. Cornelissen M, Steegers-Theunissen R, Kollee L, et al. Increased incidence of neonatal vitamin K deficiency resulting from maternal anticonvulsant therapy. *Am J Obstet Gynecol* 1993;168:923–928.
96. Jentink J, Loane MA, Dolk H, et al. Valproic acid monotherapy in pregnancy and major congenital malformations. *N Engl J Med* 2010;362:2185–2193.
97. Deshmukh U, Adams J, Macklin EA, et al. Behavioral outcomes in children exposed prenatally to lamotrigine, valproate, or carbamazepine. *Neurotoxicol Teratol* 2016;54:5–14.
98. Tanoshima M, Kobayashi T, Tanoshima R, et al. Risks of congenital malformations in offspring exposed to valproic acid in utero: a systematic review and cumulative meta-analysis. *Clin Pharmacol Ther* 2015;98:417–441.
99. Meador KJ, Baker GA, Browning N, et al. Cognitive function at 3 years of age after fetal exposure to antiepileptic drugs. *N Engl J Med* 2009;360:1597–1605.

100. Christensen J, Gronborg TK, Sorensen MJ, et al. Prenatal valproate exposure and risk of autism spectrum disorders and childhood autism. *JAMA* 2013;309:1696–1703.
101. Munk-Olsen T, Liu X, Viktorin A, et al. Maternal and infant outcomes associated with lithium use in pregnancy: an international collaborative meta-analysis of six cohort studies. *Lancet Psychiatry* 2018;5:644–652.
102. Walfisch A, Al-maawali A, Moretti ME, et al. Teratogenicity of angiotensin converting enzyme inhibitors or receptor blockers. *J Obstet Gynaecol* 2011;31:465–472.
103. Bullo M, Tschumi S, Bucher BS, et al. Pregnancy outcome following exposure to angiotensin-converting enzyme inhibitors or angiotensin receptor antagonists: a systematic review. *Hypertension* 2012;60:444–450.
104. Abel EL. An update on incidence of FAS: FAS is not an equal opportunity birth defect. *Neurotoxicol Teratol* 1995;17:437–443.
105. Schaefer C, Hannemann D, Meister R, et al. Vitamin K antagonists and pregnancy outcome. A multi-centre prospective study. *Thromb Haemost* 2006;95:949–957.
106. Moise KJ Jr, Huhta JC, Sharif DS, et al. Indomethacin in the treatment of premature labor. Effects on the fetal ductus arteriosus. *N Engl J Med* 1988;319:327–331.
107. Weber-Schoendorfer C, Chambers C, Wacker E, et al. Pregnancy outcome after methotrexate treatment for rheumatic disease prior to or during early pregnancy: a prospective multicenter cohort study. *Arthritis Rheumatol* 2014;66:1101–1110.
108. Anderson PO, Manoguerra AS, Valdes V. A review of adverse reactions in infants from medications in breastmilk. *Clin Pediatr (Phila)* 2016;55:236–244.
109. Ito S. Emerging research paradigm for infant drug exposure through breast milk. *Curr Pharm Des* 2019;25:528–533.

CHAPTER

11

Karel Allegaert
Johannes N. van den Anker

Principles of Neonatal Pharmacology

INTRODUCTION

Pharmacotherapy is a very powerful intervention to improve outcomes in neonates.[1] Prescription of a given drug should result in a safe and effective intervention to treat or prevent a specific disease or risk in an individual patient or population, while avoiding disproportional side effects. Clinical pharmacology supports these aims in predicting drug-related effects and side effects, driven by pharmacokinetics (PK) and pharmacodynamics (PD). The dynamic changes related to maturation and growth in newborns result in a unique setting with extensive variability.[2] Nonmaturational changes (e.g., disease characteristics, drug–drug interactions, pharmacogenetics) further add to this variability.[1,2] Consequently, neonates are a particularly vulnerable subgroup, covering the time interval from birth up to 28 days of postnatal life, although this definition has been adapted to the maturational age of 44 weeks' postmenstrual age (term-equivalent age + 4 weeks) to cover the subpopulation of preterm neonates.[3]

Unfortunately, the potential impact of drugs to improve outcome in neonates is still underexplored. A recent meta-analysis (2015) confirmed that off-label drug prescription remains common practice (90%) in neonates,[4,5] despite legal initiatives to stimulate pediatric studies, and additional initiatives like the Food and Drug Administration Safety and Innovation Act (FDASIA) to stimulate drug research in neonates.[3] Compared to adults, available information to make informed decisions on pharmacotherapy (choice, dose, indication) in neonates is much more limited.[6]

Throughout the years, it has been repeatedly shown that newborns are more prone to adverse drug reactions (Table 11.1), while some of these events could have been anticipated based on the available knowledge on neonatal pharmacology. A knowledge-driven approach requires understanding of human developmental biology and insights in the ontogeny of drug absorption, distribution, metabolism, and excretion (PK). In addition, there must be a rigorous appreciation of the developmental aspects of drug–receptor (number, affinity, modulation, and regulation) interactions (PD). The purpose of this chapter is to provide information on the foundations for neonatal drug therapy, based on their physiologic characteristics. This chapter focuses on absorption and distribution as PK determinants in neonates, since the impact of hepatic and renal function (metabolism and elimination) is discussed in Chapters 4 and 12. This is followed by a reflection on the need to also assess maturational PD.

ABSORPTION

Absorption describes the movement of a drug into the systemic circulation. Drugs administered by nonintravenous (e.g., sublingual, oral, rectal, buccal) routes may not enter the systemic circulation completely and intact. Although the primary focus of interest is on absorption, these barriers can have effects on distribution, metabolism, and excretion. This is because barriers (like intestinal mucosa and skin) can avoid, delay, or limit, but also drugs during passage by first-pass metabolism, and are not just filters.

Absorption describes the concentration–time profile following nonintravenous administration, captured by the rate of absorption and bioavailability (translocation). The absorption rate is most commonly reflected by the time to reach the peak concentration (t_{max}).[2] To assess bioavailability, the area under the drug concentration–time curve (*AUC*) is a measure of the total amount of drug that reaches the systemic circulation, as absolute bioavailability (compared to intravenous administration) or—when compared to a nonintravenous route—relative bioavailability. Absorption depends on physicochemical (drug specific) factors and host factors (patient specific) (Table 11.2).

ONTOGENY OF GASTRIC ACID PRODUCTION

The gastric and duodenal pH affect drug solubility and ionization, as well as gastrointestinal motility, and this will also affect absorption and bioavailability.[7–9] An acid pH favors absorption of acid drugs (low pK_a) because the drug will largely be unionized and more lipid soluble. In contrast, a relatively high pH (as in achlorhydria) enhances translocation of basic drugs and restricts acidic drug absorption. The relevance of maturational changes in gastric acid production has been illustrated by Huang and High, documenting that oral penicillin G absorption is much more pronounced in the newborn when compared to infants or children because less penicillin G is destroyed by the lower amount of gastric acid in the neonate.[10]

At birth, gastric pH is neutral,[6–8] but falls rapidly to 1.5 to 3 within hours.[11] This gastric pH fall is quite variable, but appears to be independent of birth weight or age. Data on gastric fluid composition (reflecting *gastric acid production* and *feeding pattern*) throughout childhood were recently reported, and these authors confirmed that differences were most prominent in preterm and term neonates when compared to other pediatric subpopulations or adults.[6,12] In this context, the fact that

TABLE 11.1 Illustrations of Adverse Drug Reactions in Neonates with the Mechanisms Involved and the Clinical Relevance

Compound	*Clinical Syndrome*	*Mechanism Involved*	*Clinical Relevance*
Sulfisoxazole	Kernicterus	Antibiotic highly bound to albumin, competitive with endogenous compounds like bilirubin. This results in higher free bilirubin and a higher risk for kernicterus.	Similar effects can be anticipated for other high protein-bound drugs (e.g., ceftriaxone, phenytoin, ibuprofen).
Chloramphenicol	Gray baby syndrome	Impaired glucuronidation capacity resulted in chloramphenicol accumulation and subsequent mitochondrial dysfunction, circulatory collapse, and death.	Glucuronidation capacity in early neonatal life is limited and can be relevant for drug PK and elimination (e.g., propofol, paracetamol, morphine).
Lopinavir/ ritonavir	Alcohol intoxication	Kaletra syrup contains ethanol and propylene glycol. Impaired metabolic clearance results in accumulation, and subsequent hyperosmolality, lactic acidosis, renal toxicity, central nervous system impairment, cardiac arrhythmia, hemolysis, and collapse.	This event is explained by ethanol/propylene glycol, competition for hepatic metabolic elimination. The extent of excipient exposure is difficult to assess in neonates, and cumulative exposure can be relevant.
Codeine (by breastfeeding)	Sudden infant death syndrome	Exposure to morphine after conversion from codeine, related to an ultrafast metabolizer maternal genotype. The newborn has a poor glucuronidation and renal elimination capacity, resulting in accumulation, sedation, and death.	Similar effects can be anticipated by other opioid analgesics. This reillustrates that exposure by human milk occurs and has effects, either positive (e.g., to treat neonatal abstinence syndrome) or negative.
Ceftriaxone/ calcium	Collapse	Simultaneous administration of calcium infusions and ceftriaxone resulted in intravascular precipitation.	May be similar for other "mixtures" with calcium-containing formulations (low-flow rate, low volumes).
Topical iodide	Hypothyroidism	More pronounced skin permeability and higher body surface area results in more effective absorption of iodine with subsequent suppression of thyroid function.	Similar events can occur for other topical compounds such as steroids and hexachlorophene.
Dexamethasone	Cerebral palsy	High-dose dexamethasone exposure in neonatal life results in an increased risk to subsequently develop cerebral palsy during infancy, likely due to increased neuroapoptosis.	Developmental vulnerability results in a population-specific risk (e.g., bumetanide and subsequent hearing impairment or exposure to narcotics and neurodevelopmental risk).

PK, pharmacokinetics.

neonates are rarely fasted because of frequent feedings affects the gastric fluid composition. When we focus on the ontogeny of gastric acid production, Kelly et al. described the presence of gastric acid secretion in preterm infants from 24 to 29 weeks of gestational age.[13] All 22 preterm infants studied on multiple occasions (71 recordings) from 1 to 17 days' postnatal life were able to produce and maintain an intragastric median pH less than 4, with an inverse relationship between age and initial acid production.[13] Grahnquist et al. documented gastric H,K-adenosine triphosphatase activity in stomach biopsies from infants of 25 to 42 weeks' gestation, with increasing activity with age.[14] The initiation of gastric acid production likely relates to extrauterine factors (such as nutrition) and correlates with postnatal age.[7–9]

TABLE 11.2 Factors Affecting Gastrointestinal Drug Absorption

Physicochemical factors = issues likely not specific to neonates
Formulation characteristics
- Disintegration of tablets or solid phase
- Dissolution of drug in gastric or intestinal fluid
- Release from sustained-release preparations

Molecular weight
pK_a and number of ionizable groups
Degree of lipid solubility
Patient factors = *issues more specific to neonates*
Gastric content and gastric emptying time: *frequent feeding, delayed gastric emptying*
Gastric and duodenal pH: *frequent feeding, delayed gastric emptying*
Intestinal surface area: *intestinal growth and maturation (like enzymes, transporters)*
Tube feeding: *potential adherence to the plastic tubing used*
Size of bile salt pool: *maturational changes*
Bacterial colonization of the lower intestines: *microbiome patterns depend on nutrition (formula vs. human milk), perinatal antibiotic exposure, and type of delivery*
Underlying disease states: *necrotizing enterocolitis, short-bowel syndrome, intestinal motility including drug-related changes (opioids, erythromycin)*

Its subsequent pattern is still somewhat controversial. Initial descriptions suggested that the acid secretion capacity displays a biphasic pattern with an initial low gastric pH in the first 8 to 10 days, followed by relatively higher pH values between the first and fourth week of postnatal life. Using betazole stimulation, Agunod et al. confirmed these patterns since the gastric fluid volume and its acidity are related to postnatal age to reach the lower limit of adult values by 3 months of age. Secretion of pepsin and intrinsic factor was also found to parallel that of gastric acid.[15] In contrast, the longitudinal data of Kelly et al. suggest a more constant intragastric pH (0.6 to 3.9) over the first 2 weeks of life in very premature infants.[13] As mentioned earlier, this is likely because gastric fluid composition reflects both gastric acid production and the feeding pattern.[6,16]

GASTRIC EMPTYING

The stomach serves as a reservoir, with subsequent titrated emptying to the duodenum and small intestines. Because most orally administered drugs are absorbed in the small intestines, the rate of gastric emptying is an important determinant of the rate and extent of absorption. Assuming intestinal motility and absorption capacity remain stable, slower gastric emptying will result in delayed and lower peak serum drug concentrations. In contrast, nasoduodenal tube feeding bypasses the stomach and may result in earlier and higher peak serum drug concentrations shortly after administration.[2,6] Observations on maturational changes should be interpreted cautiously because maturational changes display collinearity with the type of feeding (milk for neonates; different types of foods for infants, and beyond), so observations on maturation of peristalsis do not always reflect the phenotypic gastric emptying patterns. An overview on the covariates of faster or slower gastric emptying is provided in Table 11.3.

When based on peristaltic activity, the gastric emptying rate in neonates is variable and characterized by irregular and unpredictable peristaltic activity.[8,16–19] It is prolonged relative to adults and appears to be affected by gestational and postnatal age, as well as by type of feeding to attain adult values at 6 to 8 months.[16,17,19–21] An inverse relationship between gestational age and the amount of gastric retention 30 minutes after a 5% glucose feeding has been demonstrated. Similar, slower gastric emptying times have been reported with increasing caloric density in premature infants (age 25 to 35 weeks). Significant differences were noted between formulas containing 0, 6.5, 13, or 20 calories per 100 g. These differences were significant at all times (20, 40, 60, 80, and 100 minutes) after feeding. Interestingly, although reduction in emptying rate is observed with higher caloric density substrates, the quantity of calories delivered to the duodenum from the stomach increased with increasing formula concentration.[8,9] Long-chain compared to medium-chain fatty acids result in slower gastric emptying, whereas osmolality is not relevant.[8,17] In contrast, when based on breath tests, gastric emptying in neonates is mainly driven by the type of food (regular formula < partially hydrolyzed < extensively hydrolyzed < human milk), with the fastest gastric emptying for human milk.[19] Consequently, when using mean gastric residence time (MGRT) of age-adjusted liquid and solid food, Bonner et al. concluded that the meal type and not the maturational changes determines gastric emptying.[6,20]

EXOCRINE PANCREATIC FUNCTIONS, SECRETION OF BILE ACIDS, AND INTESTINAL MOTILITY

The ontogeny of other intestinal physiologic processes can further influence the gastrointestinal absorption of drugs and other compounds.[7,8,21,22]

TABLE 11.3 Factors Affecting Gastric Emptying Rate in Neonates

Faster	*Slower*	*No Effect*
Human milk > formula Hypocaloric feedings *Drugs*: erythromycin	Prematurity Gastroesophageal reflux Respiratory distress syndrome Congenital heart disease Long-chain fatty acids Congenital malformations: esophageal atresia, congenital diaphragmatic hernia *Drugs*: opioids, feed thickeners	Osmolality Posture

At birth, pancreatic enzyme activity is low and is even lower in premature neonates. Interestingly, at 1 week of postnatal age, pancreatic fluid output and enzyme activity are higher in preterm than those in full-term neonates. Lipase activity is present by 34 to 36 weeks of gestation. This increases fivefold during the first week and 20-fold during the first 9 months.[7,8,16,21,22] Importantly, human milk also has lipase activity (bile salt–stimulated lipase, or BSSL) that disappears when pasteurized. However, substitution by recombinant BSSL formulation had no effect on lipid absorption, growth, or weight gain.[23] Human milk and colostrum also contain bile salts, predominately cholate and chenodeoxycholate.[24] In contrast, amylase activity has been detected as early as 23 weeks of gestation but remains very low even after birth (10% of adult values). Decreased duodenal amylase activity in fasting and fed infants has been observed in the first year of life. This is only in part compensated by salivary amylase. It has been documented that salivary amylase produces significant glucose polymer digestion in the stomach and small intestine (acid resistant), but falls substantially short of that accomplished by pancreatic amylase.[25] Trypsin secretion in response to pancreozymin and secretin administration is blunted in term infants to develop throughout infancy.[7,8,16,21,22]

The pool size, the rate of synthesis, and the intestinal reabsorption of bile acids are lower in neonates than in adults.[22,26,27] These factors result in overall lower duodenal bile acid concentrations and can affect the dissolution and solubility of lipophilic drugs.[28,29] Duodenal contractions in term neonates appear to occur at rates similar to those observed in fasting adults, although the number of contractions per burst may be less, while fasting or interdigestive motor activity also appears to be shorter.[9,27]

MATURATION OF INTESTINAL BARRIERS, INTESTINAL DRUG-METABOLIZING ENZYMES, AND TRANSPORTERS

The intestinal barrier is not a passive filter, but an active organ that displays maturation for permeability, enzymes, and transporter activities.

Permeability

The potential age-related changes in the intestinal paracellular and transcellular permeability of drugs did not receive the necessary attention they deserved for a long time.[28] Using lactulose/rhamnose as a biomarker of intestinal permeability in preterm neonates, the intestinal barrier maturation related to gestational and postnatal age was investigated. This permeability was influenced by feeding and showed an age-driven maturational effect, with additional effects related to exposure to human milk or antibiotics, two of the covariates that affect the microbiome.[30] The same lactulose/rhamnose biomarker has also been used to assess intestinal permeability after necrotizing enterocolitis.[31]

Drug-Metabolizing Enzymes

There are preliminary data on age-related patterns for several drug-metabolizing enzymes and transporter proteins in the intestines, but the exact ontogeny still remains to be elucidated. Although the liver is commonly considered to be the main organ for drug metabolism, first-pass effects are not limited to the liver but also involve the gut. Even more relevant for neonates, the ontogenic profile of drug-metabolizing enzymes varies across organs.[32] Cytochrome P-450 enzymes (CYPs) are also expressed in the intestinal wall, and this can alter the oral bioavailability of drugs such as midazolam.[33] CYP3A4/5 accounts for 80% of the total immuno-quantifiable intestinal CYPs, with its expression decreasing from duodenum to ileum.[33] The clinical relevance of these ontogenic processes has been illustrated by the ontogeny of oral midazolam bioavailability: this is substantially higher in preterm infants when compared to adults, because of the more limited intestinal drug metabolism.[34]

Transporters

The ontogeny of P-glycoprotein (P-gp) and other transporters like breast cancer resistance protein (BCRP), multidrug resistance proteins 1 to 3 (MRP1, MRP2, MRP3), organic anion transporting polypeptide (OATP)2B1-1A2, organic cation transporter (OCT)1, or peptide transporter (PEPT1) has recently been summarized.[35] Multidrug resistance (MDR) 1 P-gp (P-gp *ABCB1*) is the intestinal transport protein for which most data are available.[35] Initially considered to be responsible for primary drug resistance in tumors (cellular resistance to "cancer" chemotherapeutics), studies subsequently confirmed that P-gp is expressed in the cellular membranes of the intestinal tract (duodenum, ileum, jejunum, and colon), apical hepatic membranes, renal proximal tubular cells, and on the luminal side of the capillary endothelial cells of the blood–brain barrier. The overall developmental pattern of intestinal P-gp expression revealed a change from undetectable expression in the first trimester of fetal life to being present from approximately 12 weeks of gestation onward. Very limited data suggest that P-gp expression subsequently increases slowly to reach adult levels at or very shortly after birth.[35] In contrast, Lam et al. documented that P-gp expression on the meningeal endothelial cells (blood–brain barrier) is limited at birth and reaches an adult level of expression at 3 to 6 months.[36]

BEYOND MATURATIONAL CHANGES IN INTESTINAL ABSORPTION

Absorption-related changes are not only affected by age (i.e., maturation) but are also driven by nonmaturational covariates such as disease, microbiologic flora, or the type and extent of enteral nutrition. These nonmaturational covariates interrelate as nutrition or exposure to antibiotics will both affect the intestinal flora.

Disease States

Table 11.4 provides an illustrative list of disease states affecting gastrointestinal drug absorption. The diseases that likely have the greatest impact on oral drug absorption are those affecting the total intestinal surface area, such as short-bowel syndrome.[37] This syndrome results from massive bowel resection complicating necrotizing enterocolitis, from volvulus, or from congenital anomalies like gastroschisis or multiple intestinal atresia. Multiple systemic diseases may also affect gastrointestinal drug absorption. Congestive heart failure may cause mucosal edema or—by means of various hemodynamic compensations—affect drug absorption by delaying gastric emptying or by shunting blood flow away from visceral organs. Hypothyroidism or hyperthyroidism also influences drug absorption by its effects on the intestinal transit.

TABLE 11.4 Selected Disease States Affecting Gastrointestinal Absorption of Drugs

Affected Factor	*Disease State*
Decreased surface area	Short-bowel syndrome Protein-calorie malnutrition
Delayed gastric emptying	Pyloric stenosis Congestive heart failure Protein-calorie malnutrition
Bile salt excretion	Cholestatic liver disease Extrahepatic biliary obstruction
Intestinal transit time	Protein-calorie malnutrition Thyroid disease Diarrheal disease
Gastric acid secretion	Proximal small-bowel resection

Microbiologic Flora

The microbiologic flora affects bile salt metabolism, intestinal motility, intestinal barriers, intestinal drug-metabolizing enzymes and transporter proteins.[30,38] To further illustrate this, the production of secondary bile acids requires enzymatic modification by colonic bacteria. This is, therefore, affected by the development of the microbiologic flora.[38] Besides age-driven maturation, there is an increasing interest in the metabolic activity of the intestinal tract through intestinal drug-metabolizing enzymes, the gut microflora, and the interaction between both of these.[39] These interactions are not limited to drug metabolism but may also affect drug transporter activity, as well as bioactivation, biotransformation, or biodegradation.

Type and Extent of Enteral Nutrition

A gastrointestinal growth spurt occurs in early neonatal life, mainly driven by the trophic effects of enteral nutrition. Early feeding with a non-nutritive (like water alone) delays the enteric motor activity, impairs gastrointestinal growth, and slows clinical progress.[38]. This has also resulted in the practice of minimal enteral feeding to enhance enteral feeding tolerance in preterm neonates.[40] It has been reported that the type of feeding, either human milk or formula, affects both the intestinal bacterial flora and drug metabolism.[2,6] Using in vivo probe drugs, the type of feeding (human milk vs. formula) also affected CYP3A4 (dextromethorphan) and CYP1A2 (caffeine) metabolism.[2,6] Formula feeding appears hereby to accelerate maturation.[2,6,38] Similarly, enteral nutrition affects the duration and extent of hyperbilirubinemia, whereas parenteral nutrition is associated with an increased likelihood to develop cholestasis, including an elevated conjugated bilirubin.

ABSORPTION FOLLOWING NONORAL ROUTES OF ADMINISTRATION

When oral therapy is precluded because of maturational- or disease-related causes, or when the bioavailability of an oral formulation is too poor, parenteral or nonoral routes are used. Parenteral (i.e., intravenous) route is the most commonly used in neonates and is preferred over intramuscular injection. Other routes are percutaneous or rectal. Irrespective of the extravascular route used, the physiochemical and physiologic constraints mentioned in Table 11.2 will affect the rate and/or extent of drug bioavailability and absorption. This also includes unintentional and inadvertent absorption.

Absorption of Intramuscular Drugs

The serum concentration–time profile following intramuscular drug administration depends on factors related to the drug, the site of administration, the presence of concomitant pathophysiology, and the developmental status of the neonate (Table 11.5). These differences may result in differences in bioavailability and PK and, therefore, should be considered when this route is used in neonates. Lipophilicity of a drug favors rapid diffusion into the capillaries. However, the drug must retain some water solubility at physiologic pH to prevent precipitation at the injection site. The impact of these characteristics on absorption is used in clinical care like for intramuscular vitamin K injection to prevent neonatal bleeding (delayed, to attain sufficient exposure over 2 to 3 months),[41] or for respiratory syncytial virus (RSV) or human immunodeficiency virus (HIV) infection prophylaxis (palivizumab and nevirapine, respectively).[2,42] In contrast, intramuscular aminoglycoside administration is effective in the AFRINEST studies in neonates with suspected infection in limited-resource settings.[43]

A relevant physiologic factor that influences drug absorption from an intramuscular injection site is the blood flow to and from the injection site and the muscle mass. As a consequence, the muscle activity and its microcirculation matters.[2] This may be compromised in newborns with poor peripheral perfusion with low cardiac output states or respiratory distress. The absorption rate and extent from an intramuscular injection site is also influenced by the total surface area of muscle coming into contact with the injected solution, similar to the dependence of oral absorption on the absorptive intestinal area. The ratio of skeletal muscle mass to body mass is lower in neonates.[2] The muscle activity may also display both maturational (age) and nonmaturational (critical illness, neuromuscular diseases, muscle relaxants) covariates. This may affect the absorption rate and, therefore, the peak concentration.

TABLE 11.5 Considerations for Extravascular Routes, Nongastrointestinal Routes of Drug Administration that May Affect Drug Absorption

Physicochemical factors = ***issues likely not specific to neonates***
Molecular weight
pK_a and degree of ionization
Lipid-water partition coefficient
pH and viscosity at the site(s) membrane translocation
Particle size
Physiologic factors = ***issues likely more specific to neonates***
Membrane permeability, "leakiness"
Thickness and surface area of membranes at the site(s) of translocation
Relative differences in solute concentration around membranes
Presence or absence of facilitated or active transport mechanisms
Relative surface area at the site(s) of membrane translocation
Volume of fluid at administration site
Presence or absence of metabolic pathways and/or enzymes necessary for biotransformation
Determination of residence time at absorptive sites (like gastrointestinal motility, bulk flow of cerebrospinal fluid)
Blood supply to the site(s) of membrane translocation
Affinity of drug for binding to plasma and/or tissue constituents
Concomitant pathophysiology, like cutaneous lacerations, inflammation at the site of administration (conjunctiva, nasal, buccal, or retinal), muscular activity (in the setting of muscular administration), or bronchial tree and alveolar surface (inhalation)

Percutaneous Absorption

Postnatal life accelerates the skin barrier functions (e.g., stratum corneum thickness and hydration, pH, sebum) so that even preterm neonates have barrier functions similar to term neonates from 2 to 3 weeks of postnatal age onward, although there are differences between anatomic regions.[44] Nachman and Esterly studied the blanching response to topical 10% phenylephrine in (pre)term neonates. At 28 to 34 weeks of gestational age, there was a rapid (30 minutes) and lasting (6 to 8 hours) response, no longer observed at 21 days of postnatal age. In near-term newborns at birth, there was a blunted response with a longer latency period, and term infants failed to demonstrate any blanching response.[45] This suggests that neonatal skin adjusts to extrauterine life, irrespective of the age at birth.[45,46] Antenatal glucocorticoid exposure is another covariate of neonatal skin maturation.[47] Obviously, if the skin integrity is compromised, percutaneous translocation will be enhanced, as illustrated for topical timolol to treat infantile hemangiomas.[48]

Besides skin maturation, the larger body surface area to weight (BSA per kg) ratio in (pre)term neonates is also relevant. Using the Mosteller formula, the BSA per kg ratio in neonates of 26, 30, 34, and 38 weeks is 0.090, 0.087, 0.075, and 0.064, respectively, as compared to infants (0.046) or adults (0.025).[2] Based on this BSA per kg ratio, the systemic availability per kilogram of body weight is 3.6 to 2.5 (0.09 to 0.064/0.025) times greater in the newborn, if both receive the same percutaneous dose per kg.

Because of this permeability and the BSA/kg ratio, the skin represents an often overlooked but important organ for drug absorption in neonates.[49] There are numerous reports on neonatal toxicity related to cutaneous drug exposure. These reports include cases on hexachlorophene, pentachlorophenol-containing laundry detergents, excipients, hydrocortisone, lidocaine-prilocaine, and iodine- or aniline-containing disinfectant solutions–related toxicity.[2,49] Extreme caution should be exercised in using topical therapy in newborns.

Rectal Absorption

Rectal absorption is erratic with unpredictable absorption that depends on the formulation (liquid or solid suppository) and retention time within the rectal vault. The predominant mechanism for rectal absorption is passive diffusion, with faster absorption from aqueous or alcoholic solutions than from suppositories.[50,51] Acetaminophen observations illustrated that the rectal route results in more limited bioavailability and more extensive variability.[52] Compared to oral, the relative bioavailability was 0.67 (30%) and 0.61 (21%) for triglyceride base elixir and capsule suppositories, respectively.[52] This necessitates higher doses to attain a similar median plasma concentration, be it with still poor predictability, making the rectal route less suitable for repeated administration.

The inferior and middle rectal veins drain the anus and lower rectum, connected to the systemic circulation by the inferior vena cava. In contrast, the superior rectal vein drains the upper part of the rectum to empty into the portal vein by the inferior mesenteric vein. Therefore, drugs administered into the upper rectal part will undergo hepatic first-pass, whereas drugs administered in the lower rectal part will initially bypass the liver.[51] Because of these anatomic findings, rectal administration is associated with higher and earlier peak concentrations of lipophilic compounds (pK_a values 7 to 8) like thiopentone, methohexitone, or benzodiazepines.[2,51] The rapid attainment of effective systemic drug concentrations after rectal administration has been applied to treat seizures, although this recently has shifted to the buccal or nasal route.[53]

Observations on Other Routes Involved in Absorption

Alternative routes reported in neonates cover—among others—the endotracheal, epidural, intrathecal, intraperitoneal, buccal, nasal, or intravitreal route. Overall, there is still limited knowledge on drug absorption via these routes, although some drug-specific observations have been reported.[2,51,54]

Inhalational absorption is of relevance for inhalational anesthetic agents. Their absorption relates to the functional residual capacity and alveolar surface area. This results in faster absorption in neonates.[54] Conjunctival absorption is commonly nonintentional, but mydriatics (for retinopathy of prematurity screening) have been associated with cardiorespiratory events, feeding intolerance, and paralytic ileus in preterm neonates.[55] Absorption after intravitreal injection of anti–vascular epithelial growth factor (VEGF) results in systemic appearance. This may be relevant because preterm infants treated with bevacizumab had higher odds of severe neurodevelopmental disability.[56] *The buccal route f*or midazolam (buccolam) has been mentioned earlier,[53] although there is increasing interest in the nasal route.[57]

Finally, locoregional anesthesia techniques (epidural, intrathecal) result in lower but quantifiable systemic exposure to analgesics or adjuvants, such as clonidine.[54]

For any extravascular route, the physiochemical and physiologic constraints will affect the absorption rate and extent.[51] In neonates, this is even the case for the intravenous route.[58] To attain a target exposure, any method should enable the drug to reach its site of action at the desired time and concentration. Appreciation of the substantial delay and variability in the rate of drug delivery from the intravenous line is often lacking. Other challenges relate to slow intravenous flow rates, small drug volumes, dead space volumes, and limitations of the flush volume in neonates.[58] The lack of awareness to critical aspects of drug administration techniques can lead to therapeutic misadventures (Table 11.6).

DISTRIBUTION

Distribution describes the passage of compounds in the systemic circulation and to other compartments. Distribution depends on maturational (e.g., body composition), drug (e.g., molecular size, ionization, lipophilicity, protein binding), or disease factors (e.g., regional perfusion, membrane permeability).[6,59] Mathematically, the distribution volume (V_d) describes the relationship between the amount of drug in the body and its plasma concentration. Although affected by physiologic covariates, V_d does not necessary reflect a physiologic compartment, since V_d is the volume needed to contain the total body store of drug if the concentration in the whole body were the same as in plasma. This is described by the following equation:

$$V_d = \frac{DF}{C_0}$$

TABLE 11.6 Potential Errors in Drug Administration Techniques

Factors Involved	*Potential Errors*
Drug (dose) preparation	Inappropriate dilutions Similarity in appearance of dose units Loss of potentially large amounts of drug dose in the dead space of a syringe or infusion Y site Unsuitable drug formulations for administration Unlabeled or undesirable ingredients in dose forms Undesirable drug concentrations and/or osmolality Errors in interpreting drug orders and/or dose calculations
Intravenous drug administration	Loss of drug consequent to routine changing of intravenous sets Reduction in serum concentration for drugs with rapid plasma clearance that are infused slowly Extreme increase in plasma drug concentrations consequent to rapid infusion with small central compartment volume of distribution Delayed infusion of total dose when intravenous line is not flushed Inadvertent admixture of drugs by the manual intravenous retrograde method Large distance between the site of drug infusion into an intravenous line and the insertion of the line in the patient Potential loss of large volume doses in the overflow syringe with the intravenous retrograde technique Possible loss of drug because of binding to tubing Use of large intraluminal diameter tubing for small patients Infiltrations not detected by pump alarms Infusion of multiple medications/fluids at different rates by a single access Oscillations in fluid/dose rate of potent medication infused with piston-type pumps
Other routes of drug administration	Loss in delivery (nasogastric tube dead space) or from oral cavity Leakage of drug from intramuscular or subcutaneous injection site Expulsion of drug from the rectum Misapplication to external sites (i.e., ophthalmic ointment in young infants)

where D = dose administered, F = bioavailability, and C_0 is derived by extrapolating the slope of the curve of plasma concentration versus time to time 0. Several factors, including plasma protein concentration and tissue binding, affect V_d. This is described by the following equation:

$$V_d = \frac{V_b + V_t f_B}{f_t}$$

where V_b= blood volume, V_t = tissue volume, f_B = unbound blood drug fraction, and f_t = unbound tissue drug fraction. Therefore, any factor that *increases* the blood volume or the unbound blood drug fraction, or *reduces* the unbound tissue drug fraction will increase V_d. Differences in drug-specific distribution are mainly driven by differences in protein binding or body composition.

DEVELOPMENTAL ASPECTS OF PROTEIN BINDING IN NEONATES

Drug binding of plasma proteins depends on the protein concentrations, the affinity constant of the relevant protein(s), the number of available binding sites, and the presence of pathophysiologic conditions or endogenous compounds that may alter the drug–protein-binding interaction.[60] Table 11.7 provides an overview on to what extent these variables are different in neonates. Total plasma protein increases in early infancy to reach adult levels at 10 to 12 months.[61] Albumin may reach adult levels earlier, while the albumin concentration is proportional to gestational age. Within the neonatal age range, albumin significantly increases with postmenstrual age, but this only explained 20% of the variability, illustrating that there are also nonmaturational covariates.[59,62] Albumin is not the only plasma protein that binds drugs. Basic drugs are bound by plasma proteins like α_1-acid glycoprotein, and a sigmoidal maturational pattern for this glycoprotein has recently been described.[63] The significant lower concentrations result in lower binding capacity and higher free concentrations for drugs like lidocaine or propranolol.

TABLE 11.7 Physiologic Variables Influencing Drug–Protein Binding in Neonates, Compared to Infants or Children, Relative to Adult Values

	Value Relative to Adult Values		
Parameter	Neonates	Infants	Children
Total plasma protein	Decreased	Decreased	Equivalent
Plasma albumin	Decreased	Equivalent	Equivalent
Fetal albumin	Present	Absent	Absent
Plasma globulin	Decreased	Decreased	Equivalent
Plasma IgA	Decreased	Decreased	Equivalent
Unconjugated bilirubin	Increased	Equivalent	Equivalent
Free fatty acids	Increased	Equivalent	Equivalent
Blood pH	Decreased	Equivalent	Equivalent
α_1-Acid glycoprotein[a]	Decreased[a]	Equivalent[a]	Equivalent[a]

[a]Besides maturational changes, α_1-acid glycoprotein is significantly increased during inflammation or after surgery (nonmaturational covariates).

From Maharaj AR, Gonzalez D, Cohen-Wolkowiez M, et al. Improving pediatric protein binding estimates: an evaluation of α1-acid glycoprotein maturation in healthy and infected subjects. *Clin Pharmacokinet* 2018;57:577–589.

IgA, immunoglobulin A.

TABLE 11.8 Comparative Protein Binding of Some Representative Drugs

	Percentage Bound	
Drug	Newborn	Adult
Ampicillin	10	18
Cefazolin	60	80
Diazepam	84	99
Lidocaine	20	70
Phenytoin	80	90
Propranolol	60	93
Theophylline	36	56
Vancomycin	10	40

Table 11.8 provides data on comparative protein binding (newborns to adults) for eight specific drugs. Differences are not only driven by the protein concentration (Table 11.7) but are also explained by other mechanisms like (a) displacement of drugs from binding sites by bilirubin, (b) different binding properties of albumin, (c) different binding properties of globulins, and (d) decreased binding properties of albumin because of interaction with globulins in newborns.

INFLUENCE OF ENDOGENOUS SUBSTANCES ON PROTEIN BINDING

There are different endogenous compounds that also bind to plasma proteins and may displace (*competitive binding*) drugs from these binding sites, or alter the protein structure, and its binding places and affinity (*allosteric effects*). If the drug is displaced, this results in an increase in distribution volume. More relevant, the increased free drug concentration may result in a transient intensified pharmacologic response at the same serum total drug concentration and may also affect clearance.[60,63] The clinical significance of protein displacement-related drug–compound interactions is usually very limited owing to the increased V_d and concurrent change in body clearance.[64] However, in neonates, this interaction may be of greater importance because of their immature clearance.[60,63,64]

Clinically significant protein-binding displacement reactions occur when (a) a drug is more than 80% to 90% protein (un)bound, (b) the clearance is capacity limited, (c) the clearance is binding sensitive, and (d) the V_d is small, usually less than 0.15 L per kg. Above this value, only a small percentage of total drug in the body is present in plasma. Under these conditions, the following sequence of events may occur: displacement increases the free drug concentration, which may result in a heightened pharmacologic response if the drug's concentration–effect curve is reasonably steep. Such intensified pharmacologic effect is often transient because the displacement increases the amount of free drug available for clearance. Once a steady state is achieved, the result is a decreased total and an unchanged free drug concentration.[61]

FREE FATTY ACIDS AND UNCONJUGATED BILIRUBIN

Free fatty acids (FFAs) and unconjugated bilirubin are both illustrations of endogenous compounds that can display competitive binding and drug displacement at the albumin sites. This can affect the variability in binding capacity, especially in neonates.[65,66]

Nonesterified fatty acids are reversibly bound to albumin and may have allosteric effects.[67] FFA is present at relatively high concentrations in neonatal plasma. Significant reductions in albumin binding of phenylbutazone, dicoumarol (bishydroxycoumarin), and phenytoin have been demonstrated at high serum levels of FFAs and at a FFA-to-albumin molar ratio of greater than 3.5. Although these values are rarely attained, they have been observed under certain pathophysiologic conditions, such as Gram-negative septicemia. Bilirubin is also noncovalently bound to albumin and can display competitive binding. The bilirubin-binding affinity of albumin at birth is independent of gestational age and is lower in the newborn than in the adult to reach adult capacity by approximately 5 months of age.[68,69] The lower bilirubin-binding affinity of albumin in neonates is believed to be a contributing factor in their susceptibility to kernicterus.[68,69] However, other covariates like hypothermia, acidosis, hypoglycemia, hypoxemia, sepsis, birth asphyxia, and hypercapnia, and their effect on bilirubin–albumin binding and on the blood–brain barrier permeability must be considered.[70] The apparent importance of P-gp maturation on the blood–brain barrier to bilirubin transport has recently been described.[36] A number of drugs are thought to be able to compete with and displace bilirubin from the albumin-binding sites, increasing the risk to develop kernicterus. This includes not only sulfonamides, ceftriaxone, ibuprofen, or indomethacin but also some X-ray contrast agents.[68,70,71]

DEVELOPMENTAL ASPECTS OF BODY COMPARTMENTS

Alterations in body water compartments affect the distribution volume, especially when drugs are water soluble. Age-dependent changes in the various body water compartments are summarized in Table 11.9.[72,73] This reflects the very high body water content in fetal and neonatal life (75% to 90%), with a subsequent decrease to reach adult values (50% to 60%) after the first year of life. This decrease is almost completely explained by a simultaneous decrease in extracellular water, partially mirrored by a proportional increase in body fat.[72,73]

The clinical relevance of this gradual reduction in the size of body water compartments and a gradual increase in body fat with age cannot be overemphasized. To achieve comparable plasma and tissue concentrations of drugs distributed into the extracellular fluid, higher doses per kilogram of body weight must be given to neonates, as compared to children or adults for water-soluble drugs, such as acetaminophen or aminoglycosides, whereas the reverse occurs for highly lipophilic drugs, such as propofol (Table 11.10).[74–77] This is reflected in the higher dose (mg per kg) for aminoglycosides to attain a similar peak concentration, with a subsequent further extended time interval between doses to enable sufficient time for clearance.[75,76] Besides maturational changes, fluid retention related to diseases (such as sepsis and respiratory distress) or treatment modalities (such as extracorporeal membrane oxygenation) further contributes to the inter- and intrapatient variability in drug distribution.[73,78]

TABLE 11.9 Body Water Compartment Sizes (Percentage of Body Weight, Median Estimates) as a Function of Age[a]

Age	*Total Body Water*	*Extracellular Water*	*Intracellular Water*
Fetus, first trimester	92	65	25
Preterm, 2 kg	82	44	34
Term, at birth	78	40	32
1–30 d	74	32	43
1–3 mo	73	30	42
3–6 mo	70	30	42
6–12 mo	60	27	35
1–2 y	58	26	34
2–3 y	63	27	38
3–5 y	62	21	46
5–10 y	61	22	43
10–15 y	57	18	42
Adulthood	59	19	40

[a]Because of the sometimes limited number of observations, the sum of the median values of extracellular and intracellular water does not always equal the median total body water.

From Friis-Hansen B. Body water compartments in children: changes during growth and related changes in body composition. *Pediatrics* 1961;28:169–181; and Shaffer SG, Bradt SK, Hall RT. Postnatal changes in total body water and extracellular volume in the preterm infant with respiratory distress syndrome. *J Pediatr* 1986;109:509–514.

TABLE 11.10 Impact of Maturational Changes in Body Composition on Distribution Volume (L/kg) of Frequently Used Drugs

Age	*Acetaminophen*	*Amikacin*	*Propofol*
Preterm (1–1.5 kg)	0.62	0.66	5.5
Term (3–3.5 kg)	0.55	0.52	5.5
1–3 y (10–15 kg)	0.45	0.25–0.35	8.2
8–10 y (25–35 kg)	0.43	0.25–0.35	8.1

From Anderson BJ, Pons G, Autret-Leca E, et al. Pediatric intravenous paracetamol (propacetamol) pharmacokinetics: a population analysis. *Paediatr Anaesth* 2005;15:282–292; Langhendries JP, Battisti O, Bertrand JM, et al. Adaptation in neonatology of the once-daily concept of aminoglycoside administration: evaluation of a dosing chart for amikacin in an intensive care unit. *Biol Neonate* 1998;74:351–362; Illamola SM, Sherwin CM, van Hasselt JGC. Clinical pharmacokinetics of amikacin in pediatric patients: a comprehensive review of population pharmacokinetic analyses. *Clin Pharmacokinet* 2018;57:1217–1228; and Allegaert K, Peeters MY, Verbesselt R, et al. Inter-individual variability in propofol pharmacokinetics in preterm and term neonates. *Br J Anaesth* 2007;99:864–870.

METABOLISM

Drug removal from the body occurs by metabolism or primary (renal) elimination. The primary organ for drug metabolism is the liver, but kidneys, intestine, lungs, or skin may contribute.[59,79] Although metabolism generally results in pharmacologically weaker, inactive, and water-soluble compounds, parent compounds may be transformed into active metabolites (like theophylline to caffeine, codeine to morphine) or prodrugs may be converted to their active moiety (like chloramphenicol-succinate or chloramphenicol-palmitate to chloramphenicol base).

Hepatic metabolism commonly determines the PK and PD properties of a drug. The PK parameter of estimated clearance describes the overall rate of drug removal and can be described as plasma clearance, organ clearance, or total body clearance. Plasma clearance is the volume of plasma from which a drug is completely removed per unit of time. Drugs can be cleared by several mechanisms, with hepatic biotransformation, renal excretion, and exhalation representing the primary routes. Drug clearance (*CL*) by an individual organ depends on the organ-specific blood flow (Q). The organ's extraction ratio (E) can be described as follows:

$$CL = Q \times E$$

where E is the ratio of the arteriovenous concentration difference, divided by the arterial concentration, expressed by:

$$E = \frac{C_a - C_v}{C_a}$$

where C_a and C_v are the arterial and venous concentration, respectively. Hepatic clearance depends on hepatic blood, plasma free drug concentration, cellular uptake, hepatic metabolism, and biliary excretion. The hepatic drug clearance can be expressed by the following equation:

$$\mathrm{CL_H} = Q\frac{f_B \times \mathrm{CL_{int}}}{Q + (f_B \times \mathrm{CL_{int}})}$$

where CL_H = hepatic clearance, Q = hepatic blood flow, f_B = fraction of free drug, and CL_{int} = intrinsic clearance, as measure of hepatocellular metabolism. Drugs that are primarily cleared by the liver can be classified as *flow limited* or *capacity limited*. If a drug displays a high CL_{int} and E, then doubling the CL_{int} will have little effect on CL_H, whereas a change in blood flow will produce a proportional CL_H change. In other words, for drugs that are highly extracted (>80%) and undergo hepatic metabolism, CL_H reflects the amount and rate of drug delivered to the liver. High extraction ratios drugs will be subjected to the *first-pass effect* when administered orally. This signifies that a drug is rapidly metabolized or altered when passing through the intestinal mucosa or liver after absorption. Therefore, the parent compound is found in lower concentrations in the systemic circulation compared to intravenous administration, whereas metabolites are the predominant form of the drug retrieved in the circulation. Examples of drugs that exhibit high extraction are lidocaine, propranolol, acetylsalicylic acid, and isoproterenol.

In contrast, capacity-limited drugs display low extraction ratios (<20%) and low intrinsic metabolic clearance. Hepatic clearance depends on the degree of hepatic uptake and metabolism, independent of hepatic blood flow. Capacity-limited drugs can be further subdivided into binding-sensitive and binding-insensitive drugs. For *binding-sensitive drugs* (such as clindamycin), extraction ratios approach the free drug concentration ($E = f_B$). Therefore, factors that increase f_B, such as decreased protein binding, will increase hepatic clearance. In contrast, other drugs may display extraction ratios that are much less than that of the free drug, and therefore, the hepatic clearance is only a function of the intrinsic clearance, independent of protein binding. These drugs are referred to as *binding insensitive* (such as chloramphenicol).

Ontogenetic and pathophysiologic changes in hepatic blood flow, portal oxygen tension, developmental alterations in protein binding, and metabolizing enzyme activities all affect processes associated with hepatic clearance. Significant developmental changes in the physiologic and biochemical processes that govern drug disposition occur during infancy. The description of the ontogeny of hepatic drug–related functions, including cytochrome P-450 hepatic enzymes (phase I) and conjugation (phase II), is addressed in Chapter 4.

ELIMINATION CLEARANCE

Most drugs and their metabolites are eliminated by the kidneys or, more rarely, by exhalation or biliary excretion. Renal excretion depends not only on glomerular filtration but also on tubular reabsorption and tubular secretion. The amount of drug that is cleared is influenced by the extent of protein binding and the renal plasma flow. If the latter is constant, then greater protein binding will result in a smaller fraction that is filtered. The influence of renal function maturation and its covariates on drug clearance is addressed in Chapter 12.

DEVELOPMENTAL PHARMACODYNAMICS

We do not give drugs to neonates to reach a given concentration–time profile, but with the intention to treat or prevent a specific disease or risk, while avoiding disproportional side effects. Consequently, the concentration–effect profile is the real target.[80,81] Assumptions are hereby commonly made that a systemic drug exposure similar to that associated with desired drug action in adults will produce the same response in neonates. A review of the literature suggests that this assumption may—frequently—be wrong.[82] As discussed earlier in this chapter, most of the variability observed relates to differences in PK. In addition to these PK differences, differences in neonatal physiology may also result in population-specific PD. There is little information on how human development and growth, and its intersection with disease, have its impact on PD. This may result in differences in efficacy, potency, or toxicity, because age-related developmental changes in the functionality and expression of receptors and differences in disease status may alter the response to a given drug concentration.[6,80–82] Perhaps, the greatest obstacle and challenge in characterizing developmental PD aspects is to measure drug effects, using valid outcome measurements or biomarkers.

SUMMARY

There are relevant differences in drug disposition in newborns compared to adults with respect to all PK processes. Besides age, (patho)physiologic covariates also contribute to the variability in drug disposition. In this chapter, we mainly have focused on absorption and distribution to illustrate its relevance for neonatal pharmacotherapy.

REFERENCES

1. Allegaert K, van den Anker J. Neonatal drug therapy: the first frontier of therapeutics for children. *Clin Pharmacol Ther* 2015;98:288–297.
2. Allegaert K, Mian P, van den Anker JN. Developmental pharmacokinetics in neonates: maturational changes and beyond. *Curr Pharm Des* 2017;23:5769–5778.
3. Ward RM, Benjamin D, Barrett JS, et al. Safety, dosing, and pharmaceutical quality for studies that evaluate medicinal products (including biological products) in neonates. *Pediatr Res* 2017;81:692–711.
4. Magalhaes J, Rodrigues AT, Roque F, et al. Use of off-label and unlicenced drugs in hospitalised paediatric patients: a systematic review. *Eur J Clin Pharmacol* 2015;71:1–13.
5. Hsieh EM, Hornik CP, Clark RH, et al. Medication use in the neonatal intensive care unit. *Am J Perinatol* 2014;31:811–821.
6. van den Anker J, Reed MD, Allegaert K, et al. Developmental changes in pharmacokinetics and pharmacodynamics. *J Clin Pharmacol* 2018;58:S10–S25.
7. Lin L, Wong H. Predicting oral absorption: minireview on physiologically-based pharmacokinetic models. *Pharmaceutics* 2017;9:E41.
8. Yu G, Zheng QS, Li GF. Similarities and differences in gastrointestinal physiology between neonates and adults: a physiologically based pharmacokinetic modeling perspective. *AAPS J* 2014;16:1162–1166.
9. Somani AA, Thelen K, Zheng S, et al. Evaluation of changes in oral drug absorption in preterm and term neonates for Biopharmaceutics Classification System (BCS) class I and II compounds. *Br J Clin Pharmacol* 2016;81:137–147.
10. Huang NN, High RH. Comparison of serum levels following the administration of oral and parenteral preparations of penicillin to infants and children of various age groups. *J Pediatr* 1953;42:657–658.
11. Hess AF. The gastric secretion of infants at birth. *Am J Dis Child* 1913;6:264–284.
12. Van Den Abeele J, Rayyan M, Hoffman I, et al. Gastric fluid composition in a paediatric population: age-dependent changes relevant for gastrointestinal drug disposition. *Eur J Pharm Sci* 2018;123:301–311. doi: 10.1016/j.ejps.2018.07.022.
13. Kelly EJ, Newell SJ, Brownlee KG, et al. Gastric acid secretion in preterm infants. *Early Hum Dev* 1993;35:215–220.
14. Grahnquist L, Ruuska T, Finkel Y. Early development of human gastric H,K-adenosine triphosphatase. *J Pediatr Gastroenterol Nutr* 2000;30:533–537.
15. Agunod M, Yamaguchi N, Lopez R, et al. Correlative study of hydrochloric acid, pepsin and intrinsic factor secretion in newborns and infants. *Am J Dig Dis* 1969;14:400–414.
16. Cavell B. Gastric emptying in infants fed human milk or infant formula. *Acta Paediatr Scand* 1981;70:639–641.
17. Dumont RC, Rudolph CD. Development of gastrointestinal motility in the infant and child. *Gastroenterol Clin North Am* 1994;23:655–671.
18. Carlos MA, Babyn PS, Marcon MA, et al. Changes in gastric emptying in early postnatal life. *J Pediatr* 1997;130:931–937.
19. Staelens S, Van den Driessche M, Barclay D, et al. Gastric emptying in healthy newborns fed an intact protein formula, a partially and an extensively hydrolysed formula. *Clin Nutr* 2008;27:264–268.
20. Bonner JJ, Vajjah P, Abduljalil K, et al. Does age affect gastric emptying time? A model-based meta-analysis of data from premature neonates through to adults. *Biopharm Drug Dispos* 2015;36:245–257.
21. Johnson TN, Bonner JJ, Tucker GT, et al. Development and applications of a physiologically-based model of paediatric oral drug absorption. *Eur J Pharm Sci* 2018;115:57–67.
22. Fernandez E, Perez R, Hernandez A, et al. Factors and mechanisms for pharmacokinetic differences between pediatric population and adults. *Pharmaceutics* 2011;3:53–72.
23. Casper C, Hascoet JM, Ertl T, et al. Recombinant bile salt-stimulated lipase in preterm infant feeding: a randomized phase 3 study. *PLoS One* 2016;11:e0156071.
24. Forsyth JS, Donnet L, Ross PE. A study of the relationship between bile salts, bile salt-stimulated lipase, and free fatty acids in breast milk: normal infants and those with breast milk jaundice. *J Pediatr Gastroenterol Nutr* 1990;11:205–210.
25. Murray RD, Kerzner B, Sloan HR, et al. The contribution of salivary amylase to glucose polymer hydrolysis in premature infants. *Pediatr Res* 1986;20:186–191.
26. Heubi JE, Balistreri WF, Suchy FJ. Bile salt metabolism in the first year of life. *J Lab Clin Med* 1982;100:127–136.
27. Milla PJ, Fenton TR. Small intestinal motility patterns in the perinatal period. *J Pediatr Gastroenterol Nutr* 1983;2(Suppl 1):S141–S144.
28. Nicolas JM, Bouzom F, Hugues C, et al. Oral drug absorption in pediatrics: the intestinal wall, its developmental changes and current tools for predictions. *Biopharm Drug Dispos* 2017;38:209–230.
29. Watkins JB, Ingall D, Szczepanik P, et al. Bile-salt metabolism in the newborn. Measurement of pool size and synthesis by stable isotope technic. *N Engl J Med* 1973;288:431–434.
30. Saleem B, Okogbule-Wonodi AC, Fasano A, et al. Intestinal barrier maturation in very low birthweight infants: relationship to feeding and antibiotic exposure. *J Pediatr* 2017;183:31–36.e1.
31. Piena-Spoel M, Albers MJ, ten Kate J, et al. Intestinal permeability in newborns with necrotizing enterocolitis and controls: does the sugar absorption test provide guidelines for the time to (re-)introduce enteral nutrition? *J Pediatr Surg* 2001;36:587–592.
32. Brussee JM, Yu H, Krekels EHJ, et al. First-pass CYP3A-mediated metabolism of midazolam in the gut wall and liver in preterm neonates. *CPT Pharmacometrics Syst Pharmacol* 2018;7:374–383.
33. Johnson TN, Thomson M. Intestinal metabolism and transport of drugs in children: the effects of age and disease. *J Pediatr Gastroenterol Nutr* 2008;47:3–10.
34. de Wildt SN, Kearns GL, Hop WC, et al. Pharmacokinetics and metabolism of oral midazolam in preterm infants. *Br J Clin Pharmacol* 2002;53:390–392.
35. Brouwer KL, Aleksunes LM, Brandys B, et al. Human ontogeny of drug transporters: review and recommendations of the pediatric transporter working group. *Clin Pharmacol Ther* 2015;98:266–287.
36. Lam J, Baello S, Iqbal M, et al. The ontogeny of P-glycoprotein in the developing human blood-brain barrier: implication for opioid toxicity in neonates. *Pediatr Res* 2015;78:417–421.
37. Cohran VC, Prozialeck JD, Cole CR. Redefining short bowel in the 21st century. *Pediatr Res* 2017;81:540–549.
38. Neal-Kluever A, Fisher J, Grylack L, et al. Physiology of the neonatal gastrointestinal system relevant to the disposition of orally administered medications. *Drug Metab Dispos* 2018;47(3):296–313 doi: 10.1124/dmd.118.084418.
39. Stojančević M, Bojić G, Salami HA, et al. The influence of intestinal tract and probiotics on the fate of orally administered drugs. *Curr Issues Mol Biol* 2014;16:55–68.
40. Lenfestey MW, Neu J. Gastrointestinal development: implications for managements of preterm and term infants. *Gastroenterol Clin North Am* 2018;47:773–791.
41. Mihatsch WA, Braegger C, Bronsky J, et al. Prevention of vitamin K deficiency bleeding in newborn infants: a position paper by the ESPGHAN committee on nutrition. *J Pediatr Gastroenterol Nutr* 2016;63:123–129.
42. Cortez JM Jr, Quintero R, Moss JA, et al. Pharmacokinetics of injectable, long-acting nevirapine for HIV prophylaxis in breastfeeding infants. *Antimicrob Agents Chemother* 2015;59:59–66.
43. Dewez JE, Chellani HK, Halim A, et al. Simplified antibiotic regimens for neonatal sepsis—AFRINEST. *Lancet* 2015;386:1337–1338.
44. Kanti V, Bonzel A, Stroux A, et al. Postnatal maturation of skin barrier function in premature infants. *Skin Pharmacol Physiol* 2014;27:234–241.
45. Nachman RL, Estlerly NB. Increased skin permeability in preterm infants. *J Pediatr* 1971;79:628–632.
46. Chiou YB, Blume-Peytavi U. Stratum corneum maturation. A review of neonatal skin function. *Skin Pharmacol Physiol* 2004;17:57–66.
47. August D, Kandasamy Y. The effects of antenatal glucocorticoid exposure on fetal and neonatal skin maturation. *J Perinat Med* 2017;45:969–975.
48. Weibel L, Barysch MJ, Scheer HS, et al. Topical timolol for infantile hemangiomas: evidence for efficacy and degree of systemic absorption. *Pediatr Dermatol* 2016;33:184–190.
49. Choonara I. Percutaneous drug absorption and administration. *Arch Dis Child* 1994;71:F73–F74.
50. Choonara IA. Giving drugs per rectum for systemic effect. *Arch Dis Child* 1987;62:771–772.
51. Linakis MW, Roberts JK, Lala AC et al. Challenges associated with route of administration in neonatal drug delivery. *Clin Pharmacokinet* 2016;55:185–196.
52. Anderson BJ, van Lingen RA, Hansen TG, et al. Acetaminophen developmental pharmacokinetics in premature neonates and infants: a pooled population analysis. *Anesthesiology* 2002;96:1336–1345.
53. Maglalang PD, Rautiola D, Siegel RA et al. Rescue therapies for seizure emergencies: new modes of administration. *Epilepsia* 2018;59(Suppl 2):207–215.
54. Anderson BJ, Allegaert K. The pharmacology of anaesthetics in the neonate. *Best Pract Res Clin Anaesthesiol* 2010;24:419–431.
55. Lux AL, Mouriaux F, Guillois B, et al. Serious adverse side effects after pupillary dilation in preterm infants. *J Fr Ophtalmol* 2015;38:193–198.
56. Morin J, Luu TM, Superstein R, et al. Neurodevelopmental outcomes following bevacizumab injections for retinopathy of prematurity. *Pediatrics* 2016;137:e20153218.
57. Milési C, Baleine J, Mura T, et al. Nasal midazolam vs ketamine for neonatal intubation in the delivery room: a randomised trial. *Arch Dis Child Fetal Neonatal Ed* 2018;103:F221–F226.
58. Sherwin M, Medlicott NJ, Reith DM, et al. Intravenous drug delivery in neonates: lessons learnt. *Arch Dis Child* 2014;99:590–594.
59. Smits A, de Cock P, Vermeulen A, et al. Physiologically based pharmacokinetic (PBPK) modeling and simulation in neonatal drug development: how clinicians can contribute. *Expert Opin Drug Metab Toxicol* 2019;15(1):25–34. doi: 10.1080/17425255.2019.1558205.
60. Dalhoff A. Seventy-five years of research on protein binding. *Antimicrob Agents Chemother* 2018;62:e01663–17.
61. Grandison MK, Boudinot FD. Age-related changes in protein binding of drugs: implications for therapy. *Clin Pharmacokinet* 2000;38:271–290.
62. Sethi PK, White CA, Cummings BS, et al. Ontogeny of plasma proteins, albumin and binding of diazepam, cyclosporine, and deltamethrin. *Pediatr Res* 2016;79:409–415.
63. Maharaj AR, Gonzalez D, Cohen-Wolkowiez M, et al. Improving pediatric protein binding estimates: an evaluation of α1-acid glycoprotein maturation in healthy and infected subjects. *Clin Pharmacokinet* 2018;57:577–589.
64. T'jollyn H, Vermeulen A, Van Bocxlaer J, et al. A physiologically based pharmacokinetic perspective on the clinical utility of albumin-based dose adjustments in critically ill patients. *Clin Pharmacokinet* 2018;57:59–69.
65. Nau H, Luck W, Kuhnz W. Decreased serum protein binding of diazepam and its major metabolite in the neonate during the first postnatal week relate to increased free fatty acid levels. *Br J Clin Pharmacol* 1984;17:92–98.

66. Notarianni LJ. Plasma protein binding of drugs in pregnancy and in neonates. *Clin Pharmacokinet* 1990;18:20–36.
67. Thiessen H, Jacobsen J, Brodersen R. Displacement of albumin-bound bilirubin by fatty acids. *Acta Paediatr Scand* 1972;61:285–288.
68. Ahlfors CE, Bhutani VK, Wong RJ, et al. Bilirubin binding in jaundiced newborns: from bench to bedside? *Pediatr Res* 2018;84:494–498.
69. Kapitulnik J, Horner-Mibashan R, Blondheim SH, et al. Increase in bilirubin-binding affinity of serum with age of infant. *J Pediatr* 1975;86:442–445.
70. Watchko JF, Spitzer AR, Clark RH. Prevalence of hypoalbuminemia and elevated bilirubin/albumin ratios in a large cohort of infants in the neonatal intensive care unit. *J Pediatr* 2017;188:280–286;e4.
71. Amin SB. Bilirubin binding capacity in the preterm neonate. *Clin Perinatol* 2016;43:241–257.
72. Friis-Hansen B. Body water compartments in children: changes during growth and related changes in body composition. *Pediatrics* 1961;28:169–181.
73. Shaffer SG, Bradt SK, Hall RT. Postnatal changes in total body water and extracellular volume in the preterm infant with respiratory distress syndrome. *J Pediatr* 1986;109:509–514.
74. Anderson BJ, Pons G, Autret-Leca E, et al. Pediatric intravenous paracetamol (propacetamol) pharmacokinetics: a population analysis. *Paediatr Anaesth* 2005;15:282–292.
75. Langhendries JP, Battisti O, Bertrand JM, et al. Adaptation in neonatology of the once-daily concept of aminoglycoside administration: evaluation of a dosing chart for amikacin in an intensive care unit. *Biol Neonate* 1998;74:351–362.
76. Illamola SM, Sherwin CM, van Hasselt JGC. Clinical pharmacokinetics of amikacin in pediatric patients: a comprehensive review of population pharmacokinetic analyses. *Clin Pharmacokinet* 2018;57:1217–1228.
77. Allegaert K, Peeters MY, Verbesselt R, et al. Inter-individual variability in propofol pharmacokinetics in preterm and term neonates. *Br J Anaesth* 2007;99:864–870.
78. Lingvall M, Reith D, Broadbent R. The effect of sepsis upon gentamicin pharmacokinetics in neonates. *Br J Clin Pharmacol* 2005;59:54–61.
79. Kearns GL, Abdel-Rahman SM, Alander SW, et al. Developmental pharmacology—drug disposition, action, and therapy in infants and children. *N Engl J Med* 2003;349:1157–1167.
80. Stephenson T. How children's responses to drugs differ from adults. *Br J Clin Pharmacol* 2005;59:670–673.
81. Mulla H. Understanding developmental pharmacodynamics: importance for drug development and clinical practice. *Paediatr Drugs* 2010;12:223–233.
82. Kearns GL, Artman M. Functional biomarkers: an approach to bridge pharmacokinetics and pharmacodynamics in pediatric clinical trials. *Curr Pharm Design* 2015;21:5636–5642.

CHAPTER

12

Johannes N. van den Anker
Karel Allegaert

Renal Function and Excretion of Drugs in the Newborn

INTRODUCTION

The final destiny of the majority of drugs and their metabolites is elimination by the renal route. Consequently, a thorough understanding of the developmental changes in neonatal renal function is needed to estimate the renal clearing capacity for these drugs and their metabolites in neonates. At birth, anatomic and functional immaturity limits glomerular and tubular functional renal capacity, which results in lower drug elimination and a prolonged elimination half-life.[1,2]

In early neonatal life, rapid increases in glomerular and tubular functions occur, greatly enhancing renal drug elimination. The main factors involved in the development of renal function are gestational age (GA) and the dramatic sequential hemodynamic changes after birth following a fetal setting dominated by high vascular resistance and lower renal blood flow. This increase is due to increased cardiac output and reduced renal vascular resistance, resulting in increased renal blood flow, changes in intrarenal blood flow distribution, and higher permeability of the glomerular membrane.[1–4] The kidney of a term neonate already possesses a full set of nephrons, approximately 850,000 to 1,200,000 per kidney, further reflecting the relevance of these perfusion-related aspects on renal maturation.

In addition to these rapid developmental glomerular filtration rate (*GFR*) changes, new information concerning mechanisms of tubular drug transport has become available.[5] Transporter protein science is a rapidly evolving field of pharmacology. However, the ontogeny and clinical implications of many of these findings for neonatal renal drug handling are not yet fully established.[5–7]

RENAL CLEARANCE

Renal clearance contributes to the elimination of a significant number of water-soluble drugs and their metabolites. The *renal clearance* rate (CL_R) is expressed as the sum of the *rate of GFR* and the rate of *tubular secretion* (CL_S) minus the rate of *tubular reabsorption* (CL_{RA}). This relationship between CL_R and these processes can be expressed as

$$CL_R = f_u \times GFR + CL_S - CL_{RA}$$

where f_u is the unbound fraction of the drug in plasma. All these mechanisms exhibit independent rates and patterns of development. Glomerular filtration involves the unidirectional diffusion of unbound drug from the glomerular blood supply into the glomerular filtrate and is dependent on renal blood flow, the extent of plasma protein binding of drugs, and the net ultrafiltration pressure across the glomerulus. Tubular reabsorption and secretion are bidirectional processes involving active transport mechanisms and—in the case of tubular reabsorption—passive transport processes. Arterial blood passes through the glomerulus, the part of the nephron that filters plasma. The pores within the capillary endothelium and the glomerular ultrafiltration membrane allow only small molecules (<400 to 600 Å in diameter, about <5 kDa in molecular weight) to be filtered into the glomerular filtrate. Therefore, large macromolecules, such as most proteins and hence drugs bound to them, cannot pass through this filter.

Although the *GFR* is about 120 mL per min in adults, reabsorption along the proximal, distal, and collecting tubules leads to only 1 to 2 mL per min of filtered water being eliminated as urine.[7] The tubular epithelium is the site of reabsorption of many substances, with the net effect that these molecules pass through the renal interstitial fluid back to the plasma. Lipid-soluble or nonionized substances are able to diffuse across cell membranes, whereas charged molecules (including most drugs) are usually not and are subsequently excreted in the urine. The tubular fluid pH is an important factor influencing drug reabsorption, because this may affect the nonionized/ionized drug ratio. For example, urine alkalinization may be used to promote drug excretion in cases of acidic drug overdose, such as with salicylates. Renal secretion is mostly an active process because the transport of drugs is against a concentration gradient.[8] Therefore, transporter proteins must be located within the tubules and so must the sources of energy, cotransporters, and countertransport molecules. Furthermore, saturation and competition of these transport mechanisms may affect the renal drug elimination rate and result in drug interactions and toxicity.[7,8]

GLOMERULAR FILTRATION RATE

The newborn kidney's main physiologic limitation is its very low *GFR*, maintained by a delicate balance between vasodilatory (afferent) and vasoconstrictor (efferent) renal forces (Fig. 12.1). This setting results in a maximal attainable glomerular filtration pressure despite an overall low mean arterial blood pressure. This *GFR* is sufficient for growth and development under normal conditions, but limits the postnatal renal functional adaptation to endogenous and exogenous stressors.[1,3,4] Such stressors may be renal hypoperfusion caused by asphyxia, sepsis, or exposure to nephrotoxic medications. Nonspecific cyclooxygenase (COX) inhibitors such as aspirin, indomethacin, or ibuprofen, but also new selective COX-2 inhibitors such as rofecoxib can induce renal hypoperfusion due to the reduction in dilation of the afferent arteriole.[9,10] When prostaglandin (PG) synthesis is inhibited, the vasoconstrictor state of the newborn kidney (efferent) is unopposed. This phenomenon appears to be specific for the newborn and young infant, but is most prominent in the preterm newborn.[9,10] These observations are of clinical relevance, because COX inhibitors are prescribed during pregnancy to manage preeclampsia, polyhydramnios, or preterm labor. These drugs easily pass the placenta, so the fetus is readily exposed. Consequently, COX inhibition in utero may lead to renal morphologic changes and even end-stage renal disease at birth.[11] Postnatally, COX inhibitors are administered to induce closure of a hemodynamically significant patent ductus arteriosus (PDA). Indomethacin has traditionally been the drug of choice. More recently, ibuprofen is more commonly used because of its decreased renal toxicity.[10,12] However, any (non) specific COX inhibitor exposure will result in some degree of transient renal impairment, so caution is advised when administering any of these drugs to the newborn.

The most important factors that influence the *GFR* in neonates are *maturation until birth* (GA, birth weight), *postnatal maturation* (postnatal age), *prenatal events* like drug exposure (e.g., betamethasone, angiotensin I (AT1)-converting enzyme (ACE) inhibitors, angiotensin II (ANG II) receptor inhibitors, COX inhibitors) or congenital malformations, and *postnatal events* (PDA, asphyxia, sepsis) or *pharmacologic interventions* (COX inhibitors, dopamine, furosemide, ACE inhibitors). More recently, *genetic polymorphisms* of proteins related to neonatal renal physiology have been linked to *GFR* function and its variability.[5,13,14]

THE EFFECT OF GESTATIONAL AGE ON THE GLOMERULAR FILTRATION RATE

Developmental *GFR* changes have been the subject of many studies.[7,9,15] Almost all reports showed a pattern of a GA-dependent (or birth weight) increase in the *GFR* at birth,[7,9,16,17] with a trend line similar but not equal to the increase in fetal GFR during gestation.[17] To further illustrate the postnatal differences, the effects of GA and body weight on the *GFR* on day 3 of life were studied.[18] *GFR* measurements were performed in 147 preterm (GA 23.4 to 37 weeks) infants by means of a continuous inulin infusion technique. Mean *GFR* values increased significantly with GA and body weight. Multivariate analysis indicated that GA was the major determinant for this *GFR* increase.[18]

The clinical implications of this GA-dependent maturation become apparent when one considers drugs primarily eliminated by *GFR*.[7,9,19] Recent studies showed that ceftazidime, amoxicillin, aminoglycoside, or vancomycin clearance increase significantly with GA or birth weight, necessitating GA-based dosage adjustments to attain similar exposure and avoid toxicity related to overexposure.[9,19–23]

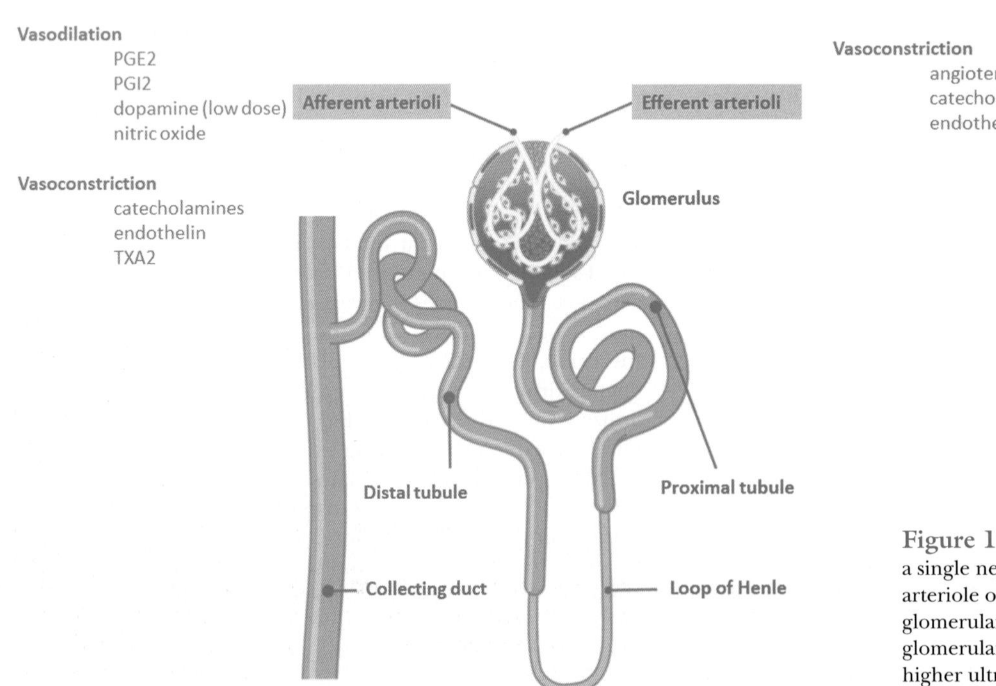

Figure 12.1 Anatomic representation of a single nephron. Vasodilation at the afferent arteriole or vasoconstriction at the efferent glomerular arteriole will result in higher glomerular capillary hydraulic pressure and higher ultrafiltration if the postglomerular tubular pressure remains similar.

THE EFFECT OF POSTNATAL AGE ON THE GLOMERULAR FILTRATION RATE

The recommendation used to be not to adjust dosage regimens for drugs throughout the first 4 weeks of life. This recommendation was based on the assumption that no significant postnatal *GFR* increment occurred in preterm infants. Previous studies on the postnatal *GFR* development in preterm infants indeed showed conflicting data.

GFR values in infants increase with a mean of 0.19 mL per min during the 7-day period between day 3 and day 10 after birth.[18] During fetal life, the increase is 0.035 mL per min per week.[17] This indicates that the postnatal increase of the *GFR* between days 3 and 10 after birth is 5.4 times higher compared to the intrauterine changes. Median *GFR* reference values in infants aged 27 to 31 weeks GA ranged from 7.9 to 30.3 on postnatal day 7, 10.7 to 33.1 on postnatal day 14, 12.5 to 34.9 on postnatal day 21, to raise to 15.5 to 37.9 mL per min per 1.73 m^2 on postnatal day 28.[3] Therefore, postnatal age is associated with an acceleration of the *GFR* maturation and results in about a fivefold (7.9 to 37.9 mL per min per 1.73 m^2) difference in *GFR* in this cohort.

This postnatal *GFR* increase is also relevant to estimate clearance for drugs that are mainly eliminated by glomerular filtration, integrated in semiphysiologic models.[7,9,19,20,23] Data on maternal, fetal, and neonatal renal clearance can even be integrated in physiology-based pharmacokinetic models (PB-PK), as illustrated for maternal, fetal, and neonatal ceftazidime PK.[21,22]

THE EFFECT OF PRENATAL BETAMETHASONE EXPOSURE ON THE GLOMERULAR FILTRATION RATE

Betamethasone is a synthetic glucocorticoid with a potency equivalent to dexamethasone. The drug is prescribed to pregnant women with an increased risk of preterm delivery before week 34 of gestation to prevent hyaline membrane disease.[24] Much of the data regarding the renal responses to antenatal glucocorticoid treatment are derived from animal studies in lambs and rats.[25,26] Prolonged fetal betamethasone infusions have been shown to increase *GFR* and urine flow in both near-term fetal and newborn lambs.[25,26] Although fetal cortisol infusion may increase fetal renal blood flow, betamethasone-induced increases in *GFR* result primarily from an increase in filtration fraction.[26] Thus, although glucocorticoids increase blood pressure and thus will indirectly alter renal perfusion pressure, glucocorticoid-induced *GFR* increases primarily relate to changes in renal vasculature resistance. This is of interest because an increase in filtration fraction, rather than total renal blood flow, appears to be the primary mechanism for the marked perinatal increase in *GFR* observed in term newborn lambs.[27] Antenatal betamethasone treatment significantly increases *GFR* in preterm newborn lambs supported by mechanical ventilation.[28]

The effects of prenatal betamethasone exposure on the *GFR* of preterm infants have been studied.[18,29–31] The majority of these studies did not show an increase of *GFR* during the first week of life after prenatal exposure to glucocorticoids. However, in three of these studies, creatinine clearance was used as a less reliable marker for the *GFR* in preterm infants, and a small number of children were studied.[29–31] This might have prevented the authors from demonstrating an increase in the *GFR* in the first week of life. The only study that showed an increase in *GFR* was hampered by the fact that the majority of pregnant women (21/27) who were treated with betamethasone were also treated with indomethacin.[18] However, betamethasone reversed the indomethacin-induced *GFR* decrease.[18] It was hypothesized that an increase in renal plasma flow due to betamethasone may overcome the intrarenal vasoconstriction secondary to the decreased synthesis of intrarenal PGs by indomethacin. Allegaert and Anderson reported no impact of prenatal exposure to betamethasone on postnatal amikacin clearance in preterm neonates, indicating the need for prospective studies on the impact of prenatal betamethasone exposure on short-term neonatal PKs,[32] as well as on the long-term renal and cardiovascular outcome.[33]

THE EFFECT OF ANGIOTENSIN I-CONVERTING ENZYME INHIBITORS OR ANGIOTENSIN II-RECEPTOR INHIBITORS EXPOSURE ON THE GLOMERULAR FILTRATION RATE

All components of the renin–angiotensin system (RAS) exist within the fetal kidney during the early stages of development and participate as promoting factors for the growth of this organ, more specifically its angiogenesis, and have an important role in controlling intrarenal hemodynamics.[34,35] In the early fetal stage, renin-containing cells are present in the developing intrarenal branches of the renal artery. Renin is also distributed in other vascular parts including the arcuate, interlobar, and afferent arterioles. Renin mRNA gene expression markedly increases throughout fetal life to peak in the perinatal period.[36,37] In early life, renin is almost exclusively detected in the juxtaglomerular apparatus. Renin acts on plasma angiotensinogen to form AT1.[36,37] Similarly, (pro)renin receptors are highly expressed in the developing kidney, even more pronounced in the preterm when compared to the term newborn.

ACE is a dipeptidyl carboxypeptidase that releases the pressor peptide ANG II from AT1 and inactivates bradykinin as well.[34] ACE is present in both vascular and extravascular tissues (brush border) of the kidney. Although the extravascular localization of ACE is not fully known, this enzyme is found on glomerular endothelial cells where the capillary invades the inferior cleft of the S-shaped body. ACE may participate in the tubular handling process of ANG II, as it has been found on the apical and basolateral membranes already in the early nephron stage. This glomerular distribution in the fetal kidney looks different as compared with the more mature kidney, where ACE is essentially found in the peritubular endothelial cells.[34,38–40] The switch of ACE from glomerular to peritubular vessels with maturation has been well documented and occurs progressively during infancy. In addition to renal hemodynamic regulation, the ANG II locally generated in the glomerulus also stimulates angiogenesis through the stimulation of its receptors. ANG II acts as a growth factor for renal cells and therefore plays a crucial role in the development of the kidney through its two receptors: AT1-R and ANG II receptor 2 (AT2-R).[38–40]

Both receptors are indeed independently present in mammalian fetal kidney tissues, and AT2-R seems to predominate.[38–40] AT2-R mRNA has been observed in almost all fetal tissues, including the metanephros and undifferentiated mesenchymal and connective tissues. AT1-R has been found more specifically in the adrenal glands, liver, and kidney. Within the kidney, both AT1-R and AT2-R mRNAs are expressed in the metanephros at 14 days of gestation, when branching of the ureter bud already started. AT1-R expression in the immature glomeruli coincides with mesangial cell differentiation from the pericyte and continues throughout adulthood in the glomeruli and the tubular interstitium, whereas AT2-R expression decreases after birth except in large cortical blood vessels. AT1-R mRNA is expressed in mature glomeruli, in maturing S-shaped bodies, and in the proximal and distal tubule as well. Early in the embryologic period, AT2-R mRNA is first expressed in mesenchymal cells adjacent to the ureter epithelial stalk. The expression is then extended in the mesenchyme cells of the nephrogenic area and in the collecting ducts. AT2-R is also invariantly expressed in the epithelial cells of the macula densa.

Studies to determine the localization of AT1-R and AT2-R will help identify the roles of ANG II for kidney development.[38–40] Via AT1-R, ANG II stimulates proliferation, regulates nitric oxide synthase expression, has growth-promoting effects, and acts on glomerular mesangial and tubular cell differentiation during nephrogenesis.[34] It further mediates biologic actions such as maintenance of circulatory homeostasis and cell proliferation.[34] Furthermore, ANG II participates in downregulation of AT2-R and renin gene expression. In the growth-retarded fetus, AT2-R expression has been downregulated, and it has been postulated that this is associated with a higher risk of hypertension in adulthood. Given the fundamental role of the RAS for renal morphogenesis, administration of drugs with ACE inhibitory effects or acting as AT1-R or AT2-R inhibitors during pregnancy is contraindicated.[41,42] Impaired fetal renal growth and glomerulogenesis are associated with cardiovascular and renal morbidity in later life.[33]

THE EFFECT OF PRENATAL NONSTEROIDAL ANTI-INFLAMMATORY DRUG EXPOSURE ON THE GLOMERULAR FILTRATION RATE

Three COX isoforms are known: COX-1 is expressed constitutively in almost all organs, COX-2 can be induced by various stimuli, and COX-3 is still considered not to be relevant in humans. These enzymes have a key role in the biosynthesis of prostanoids.[11,43] Renal PG synthesis counterbalances at the afferent arteriole by vasodilation for the vasoconstrictive agents (like ANG II) (see Fig. 12.1). Renal vasodilatory prostanoids (like PGE_2 or PGI_2) are primarily derived from COX-2.[10,11] In the fetus, PGs are crucial in glomerulogenesis and subsequent differentiation of these nephrons. For example, metabolites of arachidonic acid modulate the Na^+/K^+/ATPase activity along the nephron, and this action is age dependent.[44] Vasodilatory prostanoids counteract the high vascular resistance in utero and during the first days of life. PGE_2 and PGI_2 could also act as potent and rapid stimulators of renin secretion through PG receptors located on renal juxtamedullary cells, as demonstrated in more mature animals.[37,45] Experimental studies show that constitutive cortical as well as medullary COX-2 are overexpressed in fetal life and during the first days of life, and this accounts for the high excretion of vasodilatory PGs.[46,47]

Numerous PG receptors have been identified, and their role in renal development has become increasingly clearer.[48,49] Four PGE_2 receptor subtypes have been identified in the kidney as well: EP1, EP2, EP3, and EP4. They are localized on glomerular vessels (EP1, EP2, and EP4) and on different parts of the tubule (EP1, EP3, and EP4). Overexpression of some PG receptors (EP2 and EP4) has been demonstrated in the glomerular afferent vessels of the developmental kidney, allowing for increased activity of vasodilator prostanoids. The vasodilation of the afferent vessels via these receptors is the way by which PGs counteract the high vascular resistance generated by ANG II–mediated vasoconstriction of efferent vessels (see Fig. 12.1). It is the main mechanism to maintain glomerular filtration in fetal and early postnatal life.

Tubular EP3 receptor overexpression (located in the distal tubule and collecting duct) is needed for amniotic fluid formation and to excrete water (higher free water clearance) during the first days of life.[50–52] In addition, the downregulation of the apical collecting duct water channel aquaporin-2 (AQP2) also results in the excretion of hypotonic urine in utero and during the first days of life.[53] Embryonic calcium-sensing receptor expression is another mechanism involved in arginine vasopressin action blockade, resulting in hypotonic fetal urine.[54]

THE EFFECT OF A PATENT DUCTUS ARTERIOSUS AND POSTNATAL ADMINISTRATION OF COX INHIBITORS ON THE GLOMERULAR FILTRATION RATE

PDA is a common clinical problem among preterm infants.[12,55] The ductus arteriosus is a normal fetal vascular connection between the left pulmonary artery and the descending aorta. In utero, the ductus serves to allow the majority of blood flow leaving the right ventricle to circumvent the high-resistance pulmonary circulation and flow directly into the descending aorta. This directs oxygen-deprived blood to flow toward the placenta, the fetal source for reoxygenation. After birth, the elimination of the low-resistance placenta results in an increase in systemic vascular resistance, and the exchange of air for fluid in the lungs results in decreased pulmonary resistance. Constriction of the ductus arteriosus and functional closure generally are spontaneous after birth, redirecting blood flow toward the lungs, which then assumes oxygenation. Factors crucial to the closure of this vessel appear to be oxygen tension, concentrations of circulating PGs, and available muscle mass in the ductus. In preterm infants, higher circulating concentrations of PGs, an immature ductus, and/or an immature respiratory system contribute to continued patency of the ductus.[12,55] After birth, the increased systemic vascular resistance combined with the fall in pulmonary vascular resistance result in a shift of blood flow across the ductus from what previously was a right-to-left shunt (before birth) to a left-to-right shunt (after birth) if the ductus remains patent. This hemodynamic change can lead to a left ventricular overload, increased left ventricular end-diastolic pressure and volume, increased left atrial pressure, and congestive heart failure.[12,55] The physiologic consequences of PDA relate primarily to hypoxia, hypoperfusion, fluid overload, and acidosis.[12,55]

Although PK studies directly examining the differences between newborns with and without PDAs are sparse, potential PK changes (distribution volume, clearance) can be easily predicted, as observed for vancomycin or aminoglycosides.[56,57] However, it is difficult to disentangle the diagnosis and its hemodynamic consequence from pharmacologic interventions, most commonly nonselective COX inhibitors, or more recently, acetaminophen.[12] Our data showed that a PDA and postnatal exposure to indomethacin altered the aforementioned rapid postnatal increase in *GFR*.[18] This phenomenon will probably delay the need for dosage adjustment during the first 2 postnatal weeks in these preterm infants.

The volume of drug distribution may be altered in neonates with a PDA.[56,57] Drugs that distribute primarily into body water may demonstrate an increased volume of distribution, as fluid overload is common in newborns with a PDA. Other mechanisms may relate to the presence of acidosis with an effect on drug protein binding. Concurrent acidosis may alter the ionization of agents with a pK_a close to 7.4 (like phenobarbital), resulting in increased concentrations of unionized molecules. Unionized molecules cross biologic membranes more freely and potentially distribute more extensively into tissues.

Even in healthy term newborns, elimination of most drugs is usually diminished because of immature excretory functions.[1] In the presence of a hemodynamically significant PDA, decreased renal and hepatic blood flow can be anticipated, potentially leading to further reductions in drug elimination capacity.[22] The interpretation of (renal) drug clearance data in neonates with PDA often is confounded by the effects of mechanical ventilation, indomethacin or ibuprofen therapy, or surgical ligation, which may also influence regional renal or hepatic blood flow.[9,55,58,59] The pharmacologic treatment of PDA with indomethacin further confounds PK interpretations because drug disposition changes related to drug interactions may be difficult to separate from those altered by the underlying disease state.[22] The same holds true for ibuprofen, but is likely less relevant for acetaminophen.[9,10,55]

The reduced clearance of drugs like gentamicin, amikacin, and vancomycin with concurrent use of indomethacin appears to be the consequence of a dual effect of decreasing renal elimination secondary to indomethacin and a decreased volume of distribution once the PDA closes. As either or both interactions may play a role, drug concentrations should be monitored closely (therapeutic drug monitoring) when indomethacin therapy is started and after it is discontinued.

A relevant number of studies with ibuprofen for the treatment of PDA in preterm infants have meanwhile been performed. However, it was concluded from studies in neonates that ibuprofen as compared with indomethacin is effective at closing the duct and is associated with fewer cerebral and renal adverse effects.[10,12]

Both ibuprofen and indomethacin have a quantifiable impact on renal function. However, compared to ibuprofen, the negative impact of indomethacin is more pronounced. Based on the available study cohorts, the number-needed-to-harm (NNH, avoidance of oliguria) has been calculated to be 8 in favor of ibuprofen.[10] In the most recent meta-analysis on observations in 386 preterm neonates, serum creatinine on day 3 after administration was significantly lower (−8.2 mmol per L, or −0.1 mg per dL) in the ibuprofen when compared to the indomethacin-exposed neonates.[60] Finally, indomethacin and ibuprofen reduced vancomycin renal clearance by 46% and 28%, respectively.[61]

THE EFFECT OF DOPAMINE OR METHYLXANTHINES ON THE GLOMERULAR FILTRATION RATE

Although based on limited evidence, dopamine is widely used to treat hypotension or oliguria in critically ill neonates.[62] Through stimulation of adrenergic and dopaminergic receptors, dopamine exerts dose-dependent cardiovascular, renal, and endocrine effects that combat the clinical manifestations of shock. This discussion will only focus on its renal aspects. As long as renal perfusion pressure is within the autoregulatory range, the direct tubular rather than the renal hemodynamic action of dopamine is mostly responsible for its diuretic and natriuretic effects.[63]

The renal hemodynamic effects are brought about by activation of the renal tubular dopamine receptors. Data indicate the presence and functional integrity of these receptors and postreceptor mechanisms in the human kidney from 24 weeks GA onward.[63,64,65] In a controlled animal experimental setting, selective activation of the renal DA_1 and DA_2 receptors with low doses of dopamine induces 20% to 40% increase in renal blood flow and a concomitant rise of 5% to 20% in *GFR*, without significantly influencing systemic blood pressure.[61] Micropuncture studies indicated that this dopamine-induced *GFR* increase was due to enhancement of glomerular ultrafiltration pressure, caused by a more pronounced vasodilation of the afferent than the efferent arteriole (see Fig. 12.1).[66] Despite these pharmacologic findings that suggest a relevant effect on *GFR*, the currently available evidence on the clinical value of low-dose dopamine strategies is—at best—very limited.

Theoretically, a strategy to protect *GFR* function in settings like asphyxia, or administration of aminoglycosides, contrast agents, or COX inhibitors may be useful. However, the currently available meta-analytic evidence in adults, but also in children and neonates, has resulted in moving away from using this low-dose dopamine concept.[67,68] To further illustrate this, a Cochrane analysis concluded that there is no evidence to support the use of dopamine to prevent renal dysfunction (primarily *GFR*) in indomethacin-treated preterm infants. Similar, dopamine administration had no effect on amikacin clearance.[69]

Along the same line, the use of theophylline or caffeine to prevent renal dysfunction has been explored in the setting of perinatal asphyxia and in preterm newborn, respectively. The available data consistently showed that a single dose of theophylline shortly (<1 hour) after birth was effective to reduce the severity of renal impairment (lower creatinine, higher creatinine clearance) in early neonatal life (from day 2 onward).[70] However, the relevance of this biomarker to the overall outcome is questionable. In preterm neonates, the diuretic effect of caffeine and the potential link with the incidence of bronchopulmonary dysplasia (BPD) has been described, but also in this indication, the renal outcome effect is more of a safety marker than the primary indication.[71,72]

THE EFFECT OF THE ADMINISTRATION OF FUROSEMIDE ON THE GLOMERULAR FILTRATION RATE

Furosemide is the most commonly administered loop diuretic to augment urine output, decrease pulmonary edema, or, rarely, to treat hypercalcemia, but not the GFR itself. It inhibits chloride reabsorption, thereby inhibiting passive reabsorption of sodium and, related to this, also calcium. Because loop diuretics also result in increased calciuria, exposure to furosemide is a strong risk factor for nephrocalcinosis in preterm infants.[73] Along the same line, metabolic bone disease is associated with exposure to loop diuretics. Because furosemide exerts this diuretic effect on the luminal side of the renal tubule at the thick ascending limb of the loop of Henle, loop diuretics have to be filtered by the glomerulus into the tubular fluid to be effective.[74–76] In addition to the distal tubular action, free water clearance is increased by inhibition of carbonic anhydrase activity in the proximal tubule.[76]

A number of hemodynamic responses contribute to the diuretic action of furosemide.[77] Total renal vascular blood flow is increased, renal cortical blood flow is redistributed, and renin secretion is stimulated from the juxtaglomerular cells to the kidney. The mechanisms controlling each of these responses to furosemide are, at least in part, mediated by PGs, as furosemide administration also in critically ill pediatric patients resulted in a prompt increase in PGs and renin production.[78,79] The furosemide-induced increase in PGs likely is a intermediator of the hemodynamic, diuretic, and neurohormonal changes.

Diuresis may occur in response to increased renal blood flow induced by an increase in renal PG production. Furosemide causes a rapid diuresis in newborns of all GAs after parenteral administration. In premature infants, the onset of action is evident within 1 hour, but peak diuresis does not occur until 1 to 3 hours after dosing, with a duration of diuresis of approximately 6 hours.[76,80] The mediating effect of PG on the furosemide-related pharmacologic effects also explains the association with the occurrence of PDA in preterm infants.[81] Furosemide coadministration with indomethacin resulted in a more pronounced increase in creatinine and a higher incidence of hyponatremia, without an increase in urine output.[82] In addition, it was recently shown in a study of critically ill pediatric infants that administration of furosemide can induce a decrease in cardiac output and an increase in systemic vascular resistance, potentially increasing the risk for paradoxical pulmonary edema.[79] The clinician needs to consider such hemodynamic alterations when administering furosemide in critically ill preterm infants. Continuous furosemide infusion may perhaps lead to more controlled diuresis with fewer hemodynamic alterations, as has been investigated in near-term neonates on extracorporeal membrane oxygenation.[83] Loop diuretics have been associated with an increased risk of hearing impairment, but this seems to be a multifactorial risk, more prominent when compared to furosemide.[76,84] Using a propensity scoring in 1,020 preterm (23 to 29 weeks GA) infants with prolonged (28 days) furosemide exposure matched to controls who were never exposed, no statistically significant difference in abnormal hearing screening was observed.[85]

ASSESSMENT OF GLOMERULAR FILTRATION RATE

Besides assessment of *GFR* based on exogenous compounds like ^{51}Cr-EDTA (ethylenediaminetetraaceticacid), ^{99m}Tc-DTPA (diethylenetriaminepentaaceticacid), iohexol, and inulin, creatinine clearance (CL_{crea}) or estimated creatinine clearance (*eGFR*) can be used to quantify *GFR*.[7,86,87] Alternatively, patterns of clearance of renally excreted drugs and its covariates can be used to estimate *GFR* and its covariates.[9,19–21,23]

CL_{crea} is calculated based on paired serum and urine creatinine observations [CL_{crea} = $Crea_{ur}$ (mg per dL) × urine volume (mL per minute) per S_{cr}], preferably based on 24-hour urine collections.[7,86,87] Creatinine clearance remains a widely used clinical tool for evaluating renal glomerular function. Creatinine was chosen as biomarker to estimate *GFR* because serum creatinine can be easily measured, and creatinine is totally filtered at the glomerulus, not reabsorbed by the renal tubule, and only slightly secreted by the tubular cells. CL_{crea} is an excellent endogenous estimate of *GFR*. However, measures of renal clearance using CL_{crea} do not account for tubular secretion or reabsorption of drugs. Moreover, quantitative measures of the contributions of tubular and glomerular function are not available for most drugs, and CL_{crea} remains the only guiding factor for drug dosing in renal failure. Finally, CL_{crea} is cumbersome and unreliable in neonates and young children, unless a bladder catheterization is used to ensure urine collection. This invasive procedure is not indicated for routine use. Therefore, it became standard of care to follow renal function in neonates using repeated serum creatinine concentrations. Indirect calculations (*eGFR*) based on single S_{cr} values are much more convenient to monitor renal function. The National Kidney Foundation even strongly recommends automatic calculation when S_{cr} measurements are performed and has defined kidney damage stages (stage 1 to 5). Obviously, population-specific reference values are needed because these adult values do not yet apply to neonates, and there are some other analytical and maturational aspects that result in extensive variability within the neonatal population.

This likely also explains the absence of an universally adopted definition of acute kidney injury (AKI) in infants. Different threshold S_{cr} values (1.13 to 2 mg per dL) are suggested, whereas the modified pediatric RIFLE (pRIFLE = pediatric Risk, Injury, Failure, Loss, End-stage) recommends diagnostic criteria based on the S_{cr} increase (stage 1 = +0.3 mg per dL or 150% to 200% increase from trough S_{cr} value; stage 2 = increase of 200% to 300% from trough S_{cr} value; stage 3 = increase in S_{cr} >300%, or 2.5 mg per dL or dialysis) and the urine output.[88] Other definitions have been suggested by the Acute Kidney Injury Network (AKIN), or the Neonatal Modified Kidney Disease Improving Global Outcomes (KDIGO) project. In essence, it remains difficult to disentangle physiology from pathophysiology. The use of these definitions classifies 56% to 60% of ELBW (extremely low birth weight, <1 kg) neonates as AKI cases. Although this serves as a risk factor for mortality and morbidity, these definitions do not provide sufficient granularity to describe a specific risk population.[89,90] It seems much more reasonable to use age-dependent assay-specific reference intervals or centiles as threshold values.

AKI affects approximately 10% of severely ill neonates.[91] The majority of AKI cases are prerenal, also called vasomotor nephropathy. Hypovolemia, hypotension, and hypoxemia are some of the main causes of prerenal AKI.[91] In addition to these well-known risk factors (like PDA, intracerebral hemorrhage, respiratory distress syndrome, necrotizing enterocolitis, pharmacotherapy), there is also a growing body of evidence that genetic polymorphisms may contribute to the risk for AKI in neonates.[14,92,93] Intriguingly, the major pathways implicated in the pathogenesis of AKI in the neonate are vasoactive agents such as ANG II, adenosine or renal PGs, and factors participating in the regulation of inflammatory pathways, called cytokines, earlier described in the chapter. In this way, research on polymorphisms in early life may also inform us on the phenotypic activity and the relevance of a given pathway.[93]

Some reference values for serum creatinine values are provided in Table 12.1.[87,93–98] At birth, S_{cr} reflects maternal concentrations.[99] In term neonates, serum creatinine decreases rapidly to reach stable neonatal levels close to 0.4 mg per dL by 1 to 2 weeks of age. In very premature infants, there is a transient increase in S_{cr} followed by a progressive decline toward normal neonatal values by 3 to 4 weeks of life. This decline is probably

TABLE 12.1 Reference Values of Plasma Creatinine Concentrations in the Newborn

References	*Gestational Age (wk)*	*Postnatal Age*	*n*	*Creatinine Concentration (μmol/L)*
96	28–32	4–5 d	7	60 (54–85)[a]
		8–10 d	5	73 (65–86)[a]
	33–37	4–5 d	13	63 (60–70)[a]
		8–10 d	6	53 (50–60)[a]
97	25–28	1 wk	10	123 ± 70[b]
		2–8 wk	26	79 ± 44[b]
		>8 wk	9	35 ± 18[b]
	29–34	1 wk	27	79 ± 26[b]
		2–8 wk	27	62 ± 26[b]
		>8 wk	1	31
98	30–40	6–30 d	34	35 (12–62)[a]
99	26–34	1 wk	34	97 (69–141)[c]
		2 wk	34	70 (45–99)[c]
		3–4 wk	34	57 (39–71)[c]
		5–6 wk	34	51 (42–62)[c]
		7–9 wk	34	44 (39–48)[c]
95	28–31	1–2 d	11	95 ± 5[d]
		8–9 d	10	64 ± 5[d]
		15–16 d	8	49 ± 4[d]
		22–23 d	8	35 ± 3[d]
87	32–34	1–2 d	15	90 ± 5[d]
		8–9 d	11	58 ± 7[d]
		15–16 d	11	50 ± 8[d]
		22–23 d	9	30 ± 2[d]
	<28	3 d	26	92 ± 24[b]
	28–32	3 d	76	77 ± 21[b]
	28–32	3 d	42	64 ± 19[b]

[a]Median and range.
[b]Mean and standard deviation.
[c]Mean and 10th–90th percentile.
[d]Mean and the standard error of the mean.

caused by the passive back-diffusion of creatinine across leaky tubules.[100] Finally, it is important to use an appropriate assay for creatinine assessment to prevent interferences with cephalosporins, bilirubin, and keto-acids.[101] The practical conclusion, therefore, is that repeated determinations of serum creatinine is the only clinically applicable, but a less than ideal, approach to assess *GFR* trends.

To illustrate the impact of maturational (weight at birth and postnatal age) and assay-related (an uncompensated creatinine Jaffe assay versus an enzymatic creatinine assay) aspects of serum creatinine observations, a retrospective study on such observations with the Jaffe assay collected as part of their routine care in 1,140 neonates admitted between 2001 and 2006 was analyzed, compared to values obtained by using the enzymatic method in 1,023 neonates admitted between 2007 and 2011 in the same neonatal intensive care unit.[102] The pooled results on postnatal trends (days 1 to 28) for median creatinine values in neonates of different birth weight (<1 kg, 1 to 2 kg, 2 to 3 kg, or >3 kg) with the Jaffe (Fig. 12.2A) or enzymatic assay (Fig. 12.2B) are provided. In essence, creatinine values and its trends depend on the weight at birth, the postnatal age, and the assay.

Recently, cystatin C, a 13-kDa protein produced at a constant rate by all nucleated cells, has been suggested to be a more reliable *GFR* marker. However, insufficient data are available to recommend the routine use of cystatin C in neonates, and issues similar to creatinine (weight at birth, postnatal age, but also assay) also apply to cystatin C.[103]

Patterns of clearance of renally excreted drugs and its covariates can also be used to estimate *GFR* and its covariates, or to develop models to predict disposition of drugs exclusively or mainly eliminated by renal route.[9,19,20,23]

Following evaluation of predictive performance of population models to predict renal clearance in neonates and young infants for eight different drugs, Wang et al. concluded that a postmenstrual age (PMA)-based sigmoidal Emax model, in combination with body weight–based scaling and kidney function assessment, can be used in population PK modeling for drugs that are primarily eliminated via the renal pathway to inform initial dose selection for newborns and infants *with normal renal function.*[19] Similarly, a covariate model characterizing

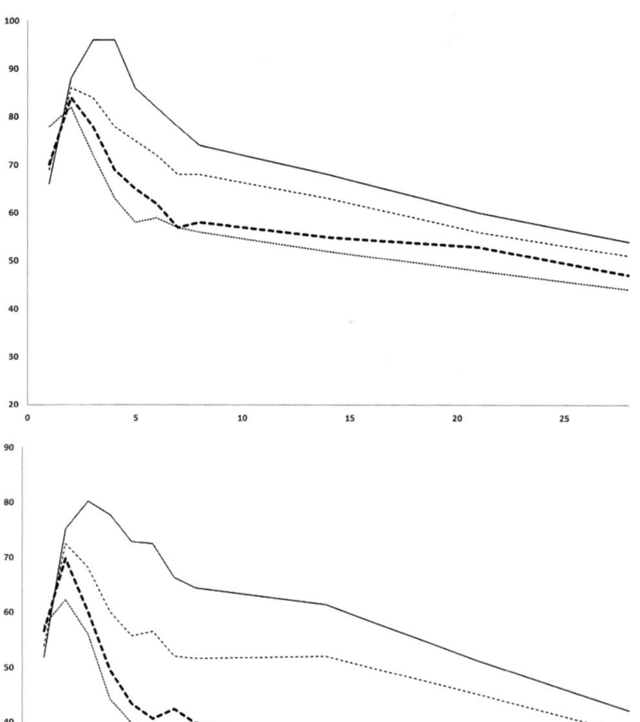

Figure 12.2 The postnatal trends (days 1 to 28) for median creatinine values in neonates of different birth weight (<1 kg, 1 to 2 kg, 2 to 3 kg, or >3 kg) with the **(A)** Jaffe or **(B)** enzymatic assay. (Data from Allegaert K, Kuppens M, Mekahli D, et al. Creatinine reference values in ELBW infants: impact of quantification by Jaffe or enzymatic method. *J Matern Fetal Neonatal Med* 2012;25:1678–1681.)

amikacin clearance predicted reasonably well clearance of other renally excreted drugs (netilmicin, vancomycin, tobramycin, gentamicin) in neonates.[23]

DRUG TRANSPORTERS AND RENAL TUBULAR HANDLING OF DRUGS

The term "drug transporter" refers to any protein that affects how drugs get in or out or—when combined—across cells. Secretion or reabsorption of compounds may be against a concentration gradient and needs energy, so adenosine triphosphate (ATP) must be consumed by ATPases to enable the uphill concentration flow. The movement of molecules that requires ATP consumption is referred to as active transport, whereas passive transport is not energy dependent. Sometimes exchanger molecules are required that replace one ion or atom with another to provide enough substrate to drive cotransport or to maintain isoelectricity or pH. Cotransporters move two molecules in the same direction across cell membranes, whereas countertransporters move two molecules in opposite directions. The sodium/hydrogen (Na^+/H^+) transporter is an example of such a countertransporter that exchanges sodium for hydrogen ions.

A variety of human transport proteins have meanwhile been described, including proteins for the transport of organic cations [human organic cation transporter (OCT) 1, human OCT2, human OCT3][104,105]; proton–organic cation exchangers [organic cation transporter novel type (OCTN) 1, OCTN2][104,106]; a protein for transport of neutral and cationic hydrophobic compounds, the ATP-dependent drug efflux protein [multidrug resistance (MDR) 1-type P-glycoprotein][107]; proteins for the transport of organic anions, including a sodium-independent organic anion transport protein (OATP)[108]; nucleoside transporters (sodium-dependent purine nucleoside transporter); concentrative nucleoside transporter (CNT) 1 and CNT2[109,110]; a PG transporter[111]; and proteins for the transport of anionic conjugates, such as the ATP-dependent drug efflux transporters [MRP1, MRP2, canalicular multispecific organic anion transporter (cMOAT), MRP3/cMOAT3, MRP6].[112,113]

All these transporters display maturational changes and can affect drug disposition or toxicity in a population-specific manner.[8,71,93,114,115] In general, the knowledge on transporter ontogeny is lagging behind and—based on a recent systematic review—information on the ontogeny of human drug transporters is even limited as it relates to the kidney. Major knowledge gaps still exist regarding gene expression, protein abundance, and actual transporter ontogeny.[93] At least, based on the clinical experience on endogenous compounds, tubular functions are not functioning in a mature way either shortly after birth. This may lead to increased urinary loss of water, sodium, bicarbonate, or glucose necessitating additional temporary supplementation in preterm neonates.[71] The immaturity of the renal tubular activities may also result in additional renal loss of drugs. As an example, intravenous administration of epoetin-β leads to a loss of approximately 5% via the urine in preterm infants.[116] Based on the currently available animal experimental and some evidence in the human setting, it seems that organic anion transporters mature faster than organic cation transporters, whereas P-glycoprotein expression is already mature between 2 and 3 weeks of postnatal age, reaching adult levels.[5]

It must be remembered that for renal tubular secretion to occur, a molecule must first pass from the extracellular fluid (ECF) (blood) into the renal tubular cell and then from the renal tubular cell into the tubular lumen to be excreted in the urine, or the other way around. Thus, two distinct transporters are required, one at the basolateral membrane of the tubular cell to accept molecules from the blood and one at the apical (brush border) membrane to mediate the exit of the molecule into the tubular lumen (urine).

TRANSPORTERS AT THE BASOLATERAL MEMBRANE

A proton concentration gradient exists among the three compartments involved in renal drug secretion. The concentration of protons is greater in the urine and lowest in the ECF. Furthermore, an electrical gradient is maintained between the renal tubular lumen (0 mV), renal tubular cell (−70 mV), and blood (−3 mV). The basolateral membrane is in contact with the ECF. Electrogenic pH-independent transport systems located here are able to transport organic cations from ECF into the renal tubular cells.[117,118] The transporters are believed to be the proteins coded by the *OCT1*, *OCT2*, and *OCT3* genes. These OCTs are supposed to mediate the first step in organic cation secretion from the blood into the renal tubule and translocate a variety of organic cations such as endogenous cationic metabolites, creatinine, monoamine transmitters, cationic drugs, and xenobiotics. Recently, polymorphisms in OCT2 have been linked to adversely affect transporter function, indicating that future studies in humans with OCT2 variants will elucidate the relationship between genetic variation in OCT2 and renal drug elimination and toxicities.[119]

At the brush border membrane is an electroneutral pH-dependent hydrogen/organic cation antiporter system energized by the transmembrane hydrogen gradient that is sustained by a Na^+/H^+ exchanger and/or hydrogen ATPase. Thus, organic cation transport is mediated by a variety of transmembrane proteins that either sustain or depend on both pH and an electrical gradient.

Organic anions are able to enter renal tubular cells from the ECF via the dicarboxylate–organic anion exchanger.[120] This entry of anions is coupled with a sodium–dicarboxylate (α-ketoglutarate) exchanger, which moves dicarboxylates outward. This exchange process constitutes the first step in the proximal tubular excretion of a large number of organic anions, including widely used drugs such as ACE inhibitors (captopril, enalapril), angiotensin receptor blockers (losartan and related compounds), β-lactam antibiotics (penicillins, cephalosporins), antiviral drugs (like acyclovir, amantadine, azidothymidine), diuretics (bumetanide, furosemide, thiazides), sedatives (barbiturates), nonsteroidal anti-inflammatory drugs (NSAIDs; like acetylsalicylate, diclofenac, ibuprofen), and a number of test agents such as *p*-aminohippurate, phenol red, and some X-ray contrast agents.[108,121,122] These examples underline the physiologic and pharmacologic importance of proximal tubules in the handling of organic anions of diverse chemical structures. The process is driven by an inward sodium gradient established by a sodium–potassium ATPase.

TRANSPORTER AT THE APICAL (BRUSH BORDER) MEMBRANE

The apical membrane is on the luminal side of the tubular cell in contact with urine. At the luminal membrane, organic cations are exchanged with protons from the urine by transporters such as OCTN1 and OCTN2. Although OCTN2 is coupled with sodium-independent OAT, there also appears to be a sodium-dependent, high-affinity carnitine transport function. Protons for these exchangers are supplied by a Na^+/H^+ antiporter and hydrogen-ATPases. Organic anions that have been exchanged with dicarboxylic acid at the basal membranes are believed to be excreted into urine by two postulated mechanisms, either a potentially sensitive facilitated diffusion system or a hydroxyl ion exchanger. Such a hydroxyl exchange pump is believed to be coded by the OATP gene.[108] OATs have been described to function at a reduced level after birth but increase functionally over the first weeks of life and reach adult levels around 7 to 8 months of life.[71,114,123]

Peptide transporters (PEPTs) involved in the absorption of oligopeptides are also expressed in the apical membrane. These PEPTs are involved in the electrogenic hydrogen-coupled cotransport of dipeptides and tripeptides. The drive for this comes from an inward hydrogen gradient and a negative transmembrane potential difference. Two homologous PEPTs have been described, PEPT1 and PEPT2, with the latter showing higher affinity for a variety of substrates. PEPTs mediate transport of peptide-like drugs, including β-lactam antibiotics, ACE inhibitors, and the dipeptide chemotherapeutic drug bestatin.[104]

Amphipathic anionic conjugates such as glucuronide, sulfate, and glutathione S-conjugates are believed to be moved by ATP-dependent pumps called glutathione S-conjugate export (GS-X) pumps, which belong to the ABC (ATP-binding cassette) family of transporters. The ABC family of transport proteins includes MRP, the cystic fibrosis transmembrane regulator, and P-glycoprotein. GS-X pumps are forms of MRP, and two isoforms have been identified, MRP1 at the basolateral membrane and MRP2 and cMOAT at the apical membrane. These ATP-dependent pumps are able to move conjugated drugs within renal tubular cells either into the urine or back to the ECF. There is also evidence to suggest that cisplatin and daunorubicin may be handled by GS-X transporters.[124]

Also known as MDR, P-glycoprotein is an ATP-dependent, 170-kDa membrane glycoprotein that belongs to the ABC family of transport proteins. Two human isoforms of P-glycoprotein have been identified: MDR1 can be found on the apical membrane of renal tubular cells and MDR3 is found mostly in liver cells.[124] Although the exact mechanism of drug translocation by P-glycoprotein MDR1 is speculative, it is known that drug transport is unidirectional into the urine. In a landmark study by Schinkel et al.,[125] genetically altered knockout mice without the *MDR1α* gene (the murine equivalent to human MDR1) had plasma concentrations of a variety of drugs that were two to three times higher than those measured in the wild-type mice.[125]

THE CLINICAL SIGNIFICANCE OF RENAL TUBULAR SECRETORY MECHANISMS

Drugs can affect the renal excretion of other drugs leading to PK drug interactions.[71,126] If two drugs are eliminated through the same tubular secretion protein, then one or both drugs may have reduced excretion, increased serum concentrations, and thus a greater chance for causing side effects. Examples of such interactions in the newborn are outlined in Table 12.2. There is also the possibility that a drug may induce or inhibit the expression or function of a particular transport protein. A drug that can cause an altered action or elimination of another drug is often called the precipitant drug in a drug–drug interaction. Table 12.3 lists some examples of common precipitant drugs implicated in drug interactions due to altered active tubular secretion used in the neonatal period.

Tables 12.4 and 12.5 provide a summary of the major cloned human renal tubular transport systems, grouped as having either anionic or cationic substrates, that are relevant to the neonate. Knowing the basic properties of these transport systems may be useful in predicting potential drug interactions. Methotrexate and NSAIDs are organic anions believed to be transported by

TABLE 12.2 Renal Tubular Pharmacokinetic Interactions in the Newborn

Transporter	*Sample Drug*	*Precipitant*[a]	*Effect of Interaction*
Organic anion	Benzyl penicillin	Probenecid	Increased penicillin levels
Organic cation	Triamterene	Histamine-2 blockers	Decreased triamterene secretion
P-glycoprotein	Digoxin	Quinidine	Increased digoxin levels

[a]Refers to a drug that causes an alteration of the action or pharmacokinetics of another drug.

TABLE 12.3 Precipitant Drugs in Tubular Secretion–Related Pharmacokinetic Drug Interactions in the Newborn

Amphotericin B
Cephalosporins
Cimetidine
Nonsteroidal anti-inflammatory drugs
Penicillins
Probenecid
Salicylates
Thiazides

TABLE 12.4 Human Organic Anion Transport Proteins Relevant to the Newborn

Transporter	*Substrates*
OAT1	NSAIDs, uric acid, β-lactam antibiotics, and prostaglandin E_2
OAT2	Salicylates and prostaglandin E_2
OAT3	Cimetidine
PEPT1	β-Lactam antibiotics, ACE inhibitors, and valacyclovir
PEPT2	β-Lactam antibiotics and ACE inhibitors
PGT	Prostanoids

ACE, angiotensin-converting enzyme; NSAIDs, nonsteroidal anti-inflammatory drugs; OAT, organic anion transporter; PEPT, peptide transporter; PGT, prostaglandin transporter.

TABLE 12.5 Human Renal Organic Cation Transport Proteins Relevant to the Newborn

Transporter	*Substrates*
OCT1	Dopamine
OCT2	Dopamine, epinephrine, norepinephrine
OCTN1	L-Carnitine, quinidine, verapamil
OCTN2	L-Carnitine

OCT, organic cationic transporter; OCTN, organic cationic transporter novel type.

OAT1. Animal models suggest that OATs are involved in the methotrexate–NSAID interaction.[127] Trimethoprim, procainamide, triamterene, and histamine-2 receptor antagonists appear to interact via OCTs. Cimetidine and trimethoprim can inhibit renal secretion of procainamide, whereas ranitidine and famotidine can inhibit renal secretion of triamterene.[108]

THE IMPORTANCE OF RENAL P-GLYCOPROTEIN

Immunohistochemistry studies reveal that P-glycoprotein is localized at the apical brush border membrane of the proximal renal tubule, the major site of renal secretion. The finding of the localization of renal P-glycoprotein has led to recognition of the importance of this transporter in tubular secretion of drugs. P-glycoprotein has been shown to transport a variety of drugs including vinca alkaloids, cyclosporine, colchicine, tacrolimus, anthracyclines, etoposide, verapamil, diltiazem, nifedipine, propafenone, digoxin, chloroquine, and protease inhibitors, including saquinavir, ritonavir, and nelfinavir.[128–131] P-glycoprotein-mediated drug interactions may be anticipated when P-glycoprotein substrates and P-glycoprotein inhibitors (or inducers) are coadministered. Inhibition and induction of P-glycoprotein have been reported.[71,126] The best known and most relevant observation on drug–drug interaction in neonates with P-glycoprotein as target relates to digoxin.[71,126] Because P-glycoprotein transport changes significantly during maturation and matures quickly, these interactions are also already of relevance in neonates.[5] Tables 12.6, 12.7 and 12.8 list drugs used in the neonatal period that are P-glycoprotein substrates, inducers, and inhibitors, respectively.

TABLE 12.6 P-Glycoprotein Substrates in the Newborn

Cimetidine
Dexamethasone
Digoxin
Morphine
Nifedipine
Erythromycin
Hydrocortisone
Lidocaine
Propanolol

TABLE 12.7 P-Glycoprotein Inducers in the Newborn

Dexamethasone
Rifampin

TABLE 12.8 P-Glycoprotein Inhibitors

Nifedipine
Erythromycin
Hydrocortisone
Lidocaine
Propranolol
Clarithromycin
Ketoconazole
Local anesthetics

SUMMARY

Renal clearance of drugs in the newborn is a complex dynamic process involving glomerular filtration, but also tubular secretion and reabsorption. The variability (both inter- and intrapatient) in *GFR* is extensive and is driven by maturational (like weight, age) and nonmaturational covariates (like nonselective COX, asphyxia). Unfortunately, the most commonly used biomarkers to assess renal function (like creatinine, cystatin C) have their limitations in neonates. Patterns of clearance of renally excreted drugs and its covariates in neonates can also be used to estimate *GFR* or to develop models to predict disposition of drugs exclusively or mainly eliminated by the renal route.

Besides *GFR*, there is a growing field of knowledge on renal tubular maturation. Its relevance in neonates is reflected in the clinical observations on renal losses of endogenous compounds like water, sodium, or bicarbonate in preterm neonates, as well as in observations of drug-specific (like digoxin) maturational pattern. Improved insights in these combined maturational changes (*GFR*, renal tubular) should ultimately lead to individualized pharmacotherapy for the neonate and result in optimal treatment and improved short- and long-term clinical outcome.

REFERENCES

1. van den Anker J, Reed MD, Allegaert K, et al. Developmental changes in pharmacokinetics and pharmacodynamics. *J Clin Pharmacol* 2018;58:S10–S25.
2. Ward RM, Benjamin D, Barrett JS, et al. Safety, dosing, and pharmaceutical quality for studies that evaluate medicinal products (including biological products) in neonates. *Pediatr Res* 2017;81:692–711.
3. Vieux R, Hascoet JM, Merdariu D, et al. Glomerular filtration rate reference values in very preterm infants. *Pediatrics* 2010;125:e1186–e1192.
4. Allegaert K, Mian P, van den Anker JN. Developmental pharmacokinetics in neonates: maturational changes and beyond. *Curr Pharm Des* 2017;23:5769–5778.
5. De Gregori S, De Gregori M, Ranzani GN, et al. Drug transporters and renal drug disposition in the newborn. *J Matern Fetal Neonatal Med* 2009;22:31–37.
6. Morrissey KM, Stocker SL, Wittwer MB, et al. Renal transporters in drug development. *Annu Rev Pharmacol Toxicol* 2013;53:503–529.
7. Rhodin MM, Anderson BJ, Peters AM. Human renal function maturation: a quantitative description using weight and postmenstrual age. *Pediatr Nephrol* 2009;24:67–76.
8. Ivanyuk A, Livio F, Biollaz J, et al. Renal drug transporters and drug interactions. *Clin Pharmacokinet* 2017;56:825–892.

9. Rodieux F, Wilbaux M, van den Anker JN, et al. Effect of kidney function on drug kinetics and dosing in neonates, infants, and children. *Clin Pharmacokinet* 2015;54:1183–1204.
10. Allegaert K, De Hoon J, Debeer A, et al. Renal side effects of non-steroidal anti-inflammatory drugs in neonates. *Pharmaceuticals* 2010;3:393–405.
11. Antonucci R, Zaffanello M, Puxeddu E, et al. Use of non-steroidal anti-inflammatory drugs in pregnancy: impact on the fetus and newborn. *Curr Drug Metab* 2012;13:474–490.
12. Mitra S, Florez ID, Tamayo ME, et al. Association of placebo, indomethacin, ibuprofen, and acetaminophen with closure of hemodynamically significant patent ductus arteriosus in preterm infants: a systematic review and meta-analysis. *JAMA* 2018;319:1221–1238.
13. Girardi A, Raschi E, Galletti S, et al. Drug-induced renal damage in preterm neonates: state of the art and methods for early detection. *Drug Saf* 2015;38:535–551.
14. Kapur G, Mattoo T, Aranda JV. Pharmacogenomics and renal drug disposition in the newborn. *Semin Perinatol* 2004;28:132–140.
15. Guignard JP. Postnatal development of glomerular filtration rate in neonates. In: Polin RA, Abman SH, et al., eds. *Fetal and neonatal physiology*. 5th ed. Philadelphia, PA: Elsevier, 2017:993–1002.
16. van der Heijden AJ, Grose WF, Ambagstheer JJ, et al. Glomerular filtration rate in the preterm infant: the relation to gestational and postnatal age. *Eur J Pediatr* 1988;148:24–28.
17. Haycock GB. Development of glomerular filtration and tubular sodium reabsorption in the human fetus and newborn. *Br J Urol* 1998;81(Suppl 2):33–38.
18. van den Anker JN, Hop WC, de Groot R, et al. Effects of prenatal exposure to betamethasone and indomethacin on the glomerular filtration rate in the preterm infant. *Pediatr Res* 1994;36:578–581.
19. Wang J, Kumar SS, Sherwin CM, et al. Renal clearance in newborns and infants: predictive performance of population based modeling for drug development. *Clin Pharmacol Ther* 2018;105:1462–1470. doi: 10.1002/cpt.1332.
20. Wilbaux M, Fuchs A, Samardzic J, et al. Pharmacometric approaches to personalize use of primarily renally eliminated antibiotics in preterm and term neonates. *J Clin Pharmacol* 2016;56:909–935.
21. Dallmann A, van den Anker J, Pfister M, et al. Characterization of maternal and neonatal pharmacokinetic behavior of ceftazidime. *J Clin Pharmacol* 2019;59:74–82.
22. van den Anker JN, Hop WC, Schoemaker RC, et al. Ceftazidime pharmacokinetics in preterm infants: effect of postnatal age and postnatal exposure to indomethacin. *Br J Clin Pharmacol* 1995;40:439–443.
23. de Cock RF, Allegaert K, Sherwin CM, et al. A neonatal amikacin covariate model can be used to predict ontogeny of other drugs eliminated through glomerular filtration in neonates. *Pharm Res* 2014;31:754–767.
24. Roberts D, Brown J, Medley N, et al. Antenatal corticosteroids for accelerating fetal lung maturation for women at risk of preterm birth. *Cochrane Database Syst Rev* 2017;3:CD004454.
25. Stonestreet BS, Hansen NB, Laptook AR, et al. Glucocorticoid accelerates renal functional maturation in fetal lambs. *Early Hum Dev* 1983;8:331–341.
26. Ortiz LA, Quan A, Weinberg A, et al. Effect of prenatal dexamethasone on rat renal development. *Kidney Int* 2001;59:1663–1669.
27. Nakamura KT, Matherne GP, McWeeny OJ, et al. Renal hemodynamics and functional changes during the transition from fetal to newborn life in sheep. *Pediatr Res* 1987;21:229–234.
28. Berry LM, Ikegami M, Woods E, et al. Postnatal renal adaptation in preterm and term lambs. *Reprod Fertil Dev* 1995;7:491–498.
29. MacKintosh D, Baird-Lambert J, Drage D, et al. Effects of prenatal glucocorticoids on renal maturation in newborn infants. *Dev Pharmacol Ther* 1985;8:107–114.
30. Al-Dahhan J, Stimmler L, Chantler C, et al. The effect of antenatal dexamethasone administration on glomerular filtration rate and renal sodium excretion in premature infants. *Pediatr Nephrol* 1987;1:131–135.
31. Zanardo V, Giacobbo F, Zambon P, et al. Antenatal aminophylline and steroid exposure: effects of glomerular filtration rate and renal sodium excretion in preterm newborns. *J Perinat Med* 1990;18:283–288.
32. Allegaert K, Anderson B. Antenatal steroids and neonatal renal function. *Arch Dis Child* 2006;91:451.
33. Luyckx VA, Perico N, Somaschini M, et al. A developmental approach to the prevention of hypertension and kidney disease: a report from the low birth weight and nephron number working group. *Lancet* 2017;390:424–428.
34. Smith FG. Development of the renin-angiotensin system. In: Polin RA, Abman SH, Rowitch DH, et al., eds. *Fetal and neonatal physiology*. 5th ed. Philadelphia, PA: Elsevier, 2017:983–992.
35. Tufro-McReddie A, Gomez RA. Ontogeny of the renin–angiotensin system. *Semin Nephrol* 1993;13:519–530.
36. Wang J, Rose JC. Developmental changes in renal renin mRNA half-life and responses to stimulation in fetal lambs. *Am J Physiol* 1999;277:R1130–R1135.
37. Schnermann J, Briggs JP. Tubular control of renin synthesis and secretion. *Pflugers Arch* 2013;465:39–51.
38. Vinturache AE, Smith FG. Angiotensin type 1 and type 2 receptors during ontogeny: cardiovascular and renal effects. *Vascul Pharmacol* 2014;63:145–154.
39. Robillard JE, Page WV, Mathews MS, et al. Differential gene expression and regulation of renal angiotensin II receptor subtypes (AT1 and AT2) during fetal life in sheep. *Pediatr Res* 1995;38:896–904.
40. Butkus A, Albiston A, Alcorn D, et al. Ontogeny of angiotensin II receptors, types 1 and 2, in ovine mesonephros and metanephros. *Kidney Int* 1997;52:628–636.
41. Pandey R, Koshy RG, Dako J. Angiotensin converting enzyme inhibitors induced acute kidney injury in the newborn. *J Matern Fetal Neonatal Med* 2017;30:748–750.
42. Bullo M, Tschumi S, Bucher BS, et al. Pregnancy outcome following exposure to angiotensin-converting enzyme inhibitors or angiotensin receptor antagonists: a systematic review. *Hypertension* 2012;60:444–450.
43. Smyth EM, Grosser T, Wang M, et al. Prostanoids in health and disease. *J Lipid Res* 2009;50 (Suppl):S423–S428.
44. Li D, Belusa R, Nowicki S, et al. Arachidonic acid metabolic pathways regulating activity of renal Na(+)-K(+)-ATPase are age dependent. *Am J Physiol Renal Physiol* 2000;278:F823–F829.
45. Jensen BL, Schmid C, Kurtz A. Prostaglandins stimulate renin secretion and renin mRNA in mouse renal juxtaglomerular cells. *Am J Physiol* 1996;271:F659–F669.
46. Khan KN, Stanfield KM, Dannenberg A, et al. Cyclooxygenase-2 expression in the developing human kidney. *Pediatr Dev Pathol* 2001;4:461–466.
47. Smith FG, Wade AW, Lewis ML, et al. Cyclooxygenase (COX) inhibitors and the newborn kidney. *Pharmaceuticals* 2012;5:1160–1176.
48. Hao CM, Breyer MD. Physiological regulation of prostaglandins in the kidney. *Annu Rev Physiol* 2008;70:357–377.
49. Breyer MD, Breyer RM. Prostaglandin E receptors and the kidney. *Am J Physiol Renal Physiol* 2000;279:F12–F23.
50. Bonilla-Felix M, Jiang W. Expression and localization of prostaglandin EP3 receptor mRNA in the immature rabbit kidney. *Am J Physiol* 1996;271:F30–F36.
51. Joppich R, Häberle DA, Weber PC. Studies of the immaturity of the ADH-dependent cAMP system in conscious newborn piglets–possible impairing effects of renal prostaglandins. *Pediatr Res* 1981;15:278–281.
52. Bonilla-Felix M, John-Phillip C. Prostaglandins mediate the defect in AVP-stimulated cAMP generation in immature collecting duct. *Am J Physiol* 1994;267:F44–F48.
53. Feng J, Chen Y, Yan S, et al. The relationship between aquaporin-2 protein levels in amniotic fluid and the fetal kidney in humans. *Biochem Biophys Res Commun* 2018;506:585–589.
54. Chattopadhyay N, Baum M, Bai M, et al. Ontogeny of the extracellular calcium-sensing receptor in rat kidney. *Am J Physiol* 1996;271:F736–F743.
55. Deshpande P, Baczynski M, McNamara PJ, et al. Patent ductus arteriosus: the physiology of transition. *Semin Fetal Neonatal Med* 2018;23:225–231.
56. de Hoog M, Mouton JW, van den Anker JN. Vancomycin: pharmacokinetics and administration regimens in neonates. *Clin Pharmacokinet* 2004;43:417–440.
57. Touw DJ, Proost JH, Stevens R, et al. Gentamicin pharmacokinetics in preterm infants with a patent and a closed ductus arteriosus. *Pharm World Sci* 2001;23:200–204.
58. Collins C, Koren G, Crean P, et al. Fentanyl pharmacokinetics and hemodynamic effects in preterm infants during ligation of patent ductus arteriosus. *Anesth Analg* 1985;64:1078–1080.
59. Jones LJ, Craven PD, Attia J, et al. Network meta-analysis of indomethacin versus ibuprofen versus placebo for PDA in preterm infants. *Arch Dis Child Fetal Neonatal Ed* 2011;96:F45–F52.
60. Fanos V, Benini D, Verlato G, et al. Efficacy and renal tolerability of ibuprofen vs indomethacin in preterm infants with patent ductus arteriosus. *Fundam Clin Pharmacol* 2005;19:187–193.
61. Allegaert K. The impact of ibuprofen or indomethacin on renal drug clearance in neonates. *J Matern Fetal Neonatal Med* 2009;22(Suppl 3):88–91.
62. Ergenekon E, Rojas-Anaya H, Bravo MC, et al. Cardiovascular drug therapy for human newborn: review of pharmacodynamic data. *Curr Pharm Des* 2017;23:5850–5860.
63. Seri I, Rudas G, Bors Z, et al. Effects of low-dose dopamine infusion on cardiovascular and renal functions, cerebral blood flow, and plasma catecholamine levels in sick preterm neonates. *Pediatr Res* 1993;34:742–749.
64. Seri I. Cardiovascular, renal, and endocrine actions of dopamine in neonates and children. *J Pediatr* 1995;126:333–344.
65. Felder RA, Felder CC, Eisner GM, et al. The dopamine receptor in adult and maturing kidney. *Am J Physiol* 1989;257:F315–F327.
66. Seri I, Aperia A. Contribution of dopamine 2 receptors to dopamine-induced increase in glomerular filtration rate. *Am J Physiol* 1988;254:F196–F201.
67. Joannidis M, Druml W, Forni LG, et al. Prevention of acute kidney injury and protection of renal function in the intensive care unit: update 2017: expert opinion of the working group on prevention, AKI section, European Society of Intensive Care Medicine. *Intensive Care Med* 2017;43:730–749.
68. Barrington K, Brion LP. Dopamine versus no treatment to prevent renal dysfunction in indomethacin-treated preterm newborn infants. *Cochrane Database Syst Rev* 2002;(3):CD003213.
69. Allegaert K, Debeer A, Cossey V, et al. Dopamine is not an independent risk factor for reduced amikacin clearance in extremely low-birth-weight infants. *Pediatr Crit Care Med* 2006;7(2):143–146.
70. Askenazi D. Should neonates with perinatal asphyxia receive a single dose of IV theophylline to prevent acute kidney injury? *Acta Paediatr* 2016;105:1125–1126.
71. Schreuder MF, Bueters RR, Allegaert K. The interplay between drugs and the kidney in premature neonates. *Pediatr Nephrol* 2014;29:2083–2091.
72. Osswald H, Schnermann J. Methylxanthines and the kidney. *Handb Exp Pharmacol* 2011;200:391–412.
73. Gimpel C, Krause A, Franck P, et al. Exposure to furosemide as the strongest risk factor for nephrocalcinosis in preterm infants. *Pediatr Int* 2010;52:51–56.
74. Burg M, Stoner L, Cardinal J, et al. Furosemide effect on isolated perfused tubules. *Am J Physiol* 1973;225:119–124.
75. Brenner BM, Keimowitz RI, Wright FS, et al. An inhibitory effect of furosemide on sodium reabsorption by the proximal tubule of the rat nephron. *J Clin Invest* 1969;48:290–300.
76. Pacifici GM. Clinical pharmacology of the loop diuretics furosemide and bumetanide in neonates and infants. *Paediatr Drugs* 2012;14:233–246.
77. Dormans TP, Pickkers P, Russel FG, et al. Vascular effects of loop diuretics. *Cardiovasc Res* 1996;32:988–997.
78. Weber PC, Scherer B, Larsson C. Increase of free arachidonic acid by furosemide in man as the cause of prostaglandin and renin release. *Eur J Pharmacol* 1977;41:329–332.
79. Yetman AT, Singh NC, Parbtani A, et al. Acute hemodynamic and neurohormonal effects of furosemide in critically ill pediatric patients. *Crit Care Med* 1996;24:398–402.
80. Ross BS, Pollak A, Oh W. The pharmacologic effects of furosemide therapy in the low-birth-weight infant. *J Pediatr* 1978;92:149–152.
81. Green TP, Thompson TR, Johnson DE, et al. Furosemide promotes patent ductus arteriosus in premature infants with the respiratory-distress syndrome. *N Engl J Med* 1983;308:743–748.

82. Andriessen P, Struis NC, Niemarkt H, et al. Furosemide in preterm infants treated with indomethacin for patent ductus arteriosus. *Acta Paediatr* 2009;98:797–803.
83. van der Vorst MM, den Hartigh J, Wildschut E, et al. An exploratory study with an adaptive continuous intravenous furosemide regimen in neonates treated with extracorporeal membrane oxygenation. *Crit Care* 2007;11(5):R111.
84. Allegaert K, Lahav A, van den Anker JN. A mechanism to explain ototoxicity in neonates exposed to bumetanide: lessons to help improve future product development in neonates. *Paediatr Drugs* 2016;18:331–333.
85. Wang LA, Smith PB, Laughon M, et al. Prolonged furosemide exposure and risk of abnormal newborn hearing screen in premature infants. *Early Hum Dev* 2018;125:26–30.
86. Levey AS, Inker LA, Coresh J. GFR estimation: from physiology to public health. *Am J Kidney Dis* 2014;63:820–834.
87. Van den Anker JN, de Groot R, Broerse HM, et al. Assessment of glomerular filtration rate in preterm infants by serum creatinine: comparison with inulin clearance. *Pediatrics* 1995;96:1156–1158.
88. Akcan-Arikan A, Zappitelli M, Loftis LL, et al. Modified RIFLE criteria in critically ill children with acute kidney injury. *Kidney Int* 2007;71:1028–1035.
89. Chowdhary V, Vajpeyajula R, Jain M, et al. Comparison of different definitions of acute kidney injury in extremely low birth weight infants. *Clin Exp Nephrol* 2018;22:117–125.
90. Raaijmakers A, Ortibus E, van Tienoven TP, et al. Neonatal creatinemia trends as biomarker of subsequent cognitive outcome in extremely low birth weight neonates. *Early Hum Dev* 2015;91:367–372.
91. Perico N, Askenazi D, Cortinovis M, et al. Maternal and environmental risk factors for neonatal AKI and its long-term consequences. *Nat Rev Nephrol* 2018;14:688–703.
92. Zaza G, Granata S, Sallustio F, et al. Pharmacogenomics: a new paradigm to personalize treatments in nephrology patients. *Clin Exp Immunol* 2010;159:268–280.
93. Brouwer KL, Aleksunes LM, Brandys B, et al. Human ontogeny of drug transporters: review and recommendations of the pediatric transporter working group. *Clin Pharmacol Ther* 2015;98:266–287.
94. Bueva A, Guignard JP. Renal function in preterm neonates. *Pediatr Res* 1994;36:572–577.
95. Gordjani N, Burghard R, Leititis JU, et al. Serum creatinine and creatinine clearance in healthy neonates and prematures during the first 10 days of life. *Eur J Pediatr* 1988;148:143–145.
96. Brion LP, Fleischman AR, McCarton C, et al. A simple estimate of glomerular filtration rate in low birth weight infants during the first year of life: noninvasive assessment of body composition and growth. *J Pediatr* 1986;109:698–707.
97. Feldman H, Guignard JP. Plasma creatinine in the first month of life. *Arch Dis Child* 1982;57:123–126.
98. Sonntag J, Prankel B, Waltz S. Serum creatinine concentration, urinary creatinine excretion and creatinine clearance during the first 9 weeks in preterm infants with a birth weight below 1500 g. *Eur J Pediatr* 1996;155:815–819.
99. Kuppens M, George I, Lewi L, et al. Creatinaemia at birth is equal to maternal creatininaemia at delivery: does this paradigm still hold? *J Matern Fetal Neonatal Med* 2012;25:978–980.
100. Guignard JP, Drukker A. Why do newborn infants have a high plasma creatinine? *Pediatrics* 1999;103:e49.
101. Ceriotti F. Establishing pediatric reference intervals: a challenging task. *Clin Chem* 2012;58:808–810.
102. Allegaert K, Kuppens M, Mekahli D, et al. Creatinine reference values in ELBW infants: impact of quantification by Jaffe or enzymatic method. *J Matern Fetal Neonatal Med* 2012;25:1678–1681.
103. Allegaert K, Mekahli D, van den Anker J. Cystatin C in newborns: a promising renal biomarker in search for standardization and validation. *J Matern Fetal Neonatal Med* 2015;28:1833–1838.
104. Inui K, Masuda S, Saito H. Cellular and molecular aspects of drug transport in the kidney. *Kidney Int* 2000;58:944–958.
105. Gorboulev V, Ulzheimer JC, Akhoundova A, et al. Cloning and characterization of two human polyspecific organic cation transporters. *DNA Cell Biol* 1997;16:871–881.
106. Tamai I, Yabuuchi H, Nezu J, et al. Cloning and characterization of a novel human pH-dependent organic cation transporter, OCTN1. *FEBS Lett* 1997;419:107–111.
107. Gros P, Ben Neriah YP, Croop JM, et al. Isolation and expression of a complimentary DNA that confers multidrug resistance. *Nature* 1986;323:728–731.
108. Kullak-Ublick GA, Hagenbuch B, Stieger B, et al. Molecular and functional characterization of an organic anion transporting polypeptide cloned from human liver. *Gastroenterology* 1995;109:1274–1282.
109. Wang J, Su SF, Dresser MJ, et al. Na(+)-dependent purine nucleoside transporter from human kidney: cloning and functional characterization. *Am J Physiol* 1997;273:F1058–F1065.
110. Van Aubel RA, Masereeuw R, Russel FG. Molecular pharmacology of renal organic anion transporters. *Am J Physiol Renal Physiol* 2000;279:F216–F232.
111. Lu R, Kanai N, Bao Y, et al. Cloning, *in vitro* expression, and tissue distribution of a human prostaglandin transporter cDNA (hPGT). *J Clin Invest* 1996;98:1142–1149.
112. Cole SP, Bhardwaj G, Gerlach JH, et al. Overexpression of a transporter gene in a multidrug-resistant human lung cancer cell line. *Science* 1992;258:1650–1654.
113. Evers R, Kool M, van Deemter L, et al. Drug export activity of the human canalicular multispecific organic anion transporter in polarized kidney MDCK cells expressing cMOAT (MRP2) cDNA. *J Clin Invest* 1998;101:1310–1319.
114. Sweeney DE, Vallon V, Rieg T, et al. Functional maturation of drug transporters in the developing, neonatal, and postnatal kidney. *Mol Pharmacol* 2011;80:147–154.
115. . Momper JD, Nigam SK. Developmental regulation of kidney and liver solute carrier and ATP-binding cassette drug transporters and drug metabolizing enzymes: the role of remote organ communication. *Expert Opin Drug Metab Toxicol* 2018;14:561–570.
116. Langer J, Obladen M, Dame C. Urinary loss of erythropoietin after intravenous versus subcutaneous epoetin-beta in preterm infants. *J Pediatr* 2008:152:728–730.
117. Schlatter E, Mönnich V, Cetinkaya I, et al. The organic cation transporters rOCT1 and hOCT2 are inhibited by cGMP. *J Membr Biol* 2002;189:237–244.
118. Goralski KB, Lou G, Prowse MT, et al. The cation transporters rOCT1 and rOCT2 interact with bicarbonate but play only a minor role for amantadine uptake into rat renal proximal tubules. *J Pharmacol Exp Ther* 2002;303:959–968.
119. Leabman MK, Huang CC, Kawamoto M, et al. Polymorphisms in a human kidney xenobiotic transporter, OCT2, exhibit altered function. *Pharmacogenetics* 2002;12:395–405.
120. Burckhardt BC, Drinkuth B, Menzel C, et al. The renal Na(+)-dependent dicarboxylate transporter, NaDC-3, translocates dimethyl-and disulfhydryl-compounds and contributes to renal heavy metal detoxification. *J Am Soc Nephrol* 2002;13:2628–2638.
121. Sekine T, Watanabe N, Hosoyamada, et al. Expression, cloning and characterization of a novel multispecific organic anion transporter. *J Biol Chem* 1997;272:18526–18529.
122. Dresser MJ, Leabman MK, Giacomini KM. Transporters involved in the elimination of drugs in the kidney: organic anion transporters and organic cation transporters. *J Pharm Sci* 2001;90:397–421.
123. Sweet DH, Bush KT, Nigam SK. The organic anion transporter family: from physiology to ontogeny and the clinic. *Am J Physiol Renal Physiol* 2001;281:F197–F205.
124. Ito S. Drug secretion systems in renal tubular cells: functional models and molecular identity. *Pediatr Nephrol* 1999;13:980–988.
125. Schinkel AH, Wagenaar E, van Deemter L, et al. Absence of the mdr1a P-glycoprotein in mice affects tissue distribution and pharmacokinetics of dexamethasone, digoxin, and cyclosporin A. *J Clin Invest* 1995;96:1698–1705.
126. Masuda S, Saito H, Inui KI. Interactions of nonsteroidal anti-inflammatory drugs with rat renal organic anion transporter, OAT-K1. *J Pharmacol Exp Ther* 1997;283:1039–1042.
127. Shapiro AB, Ling V. The mechanism of ATP-dependent multidrug transport by P-glycoprotein. *Acta Physiol Scand* 1998;643:227–234.
128. Vezmar M, Georges E. Direct binding of chloroquine to the multidrug resistance protein (MRP); possible role for MRP in chloroquine drug transport and resistance in tumor cells. *Biochem Pharmacol* 1998;56:733–742.
129. Washington CB, Duran GE, Man MC, et al. Interaction of anti-HIV protease inhibitors with the multidrug transporter P-glycoprotein (P-gp) in human cultured cells. *J Acquir Immune Defic Syndr Hum Retrovirol* 1998;19:203–209.
130. Rebbeor JF, Senior AE. Effects of cardiovascular drugs on ATPase activity of P-glycoprotein in plasma membranes and in purified reconstituted form. *Biochim Biophys Acta* 1998;1369:85–93.

Floris Groenendaal
Manon J.N.L. Benders
Linda S. de Vries
Frank van Bel

CHAPTER 13

Neuroprotective Drugs and Perinatal Brain Injury

OUTLINE

In this chapter, we summarize pharmacologic neuroprotective interventions that are already established or have potential value to reduce or prevent perinatal and neonatal brain damage due to perinatal and postnatal ischemia–hypoxia and/or premature birth. We subsequently discuss pharmacologic add-on therapy for moderate hypothermia in moderately and severely asphyxiated term neonates, emerging pharmacologic therapies to reduce or even prevent the consequences of periventricular–intraventricular hemorrhages and (diffuse) white matter injury in the preterm neonate and pharmacologic interventions in case of perinatal ischemic arterial stroke. We end this chapter with the potential role autologous and allogeneic stem cell therapy can have for the repair of perinatal and postnatal brain injury.

INTRODUCTION

An adverse outcome is still encountered in 40% to 45% of full-term neonates with perinatal hypoxia–ischemia[1,2] and up to 60% of very and extremely preterm infants.[3] About 75% of infants with perinatal arterial ischemic stroke (PAIS) develop sequelae.[4,5] At present, pharmacologic therapies are being developed to be added to hypothermia after moderate-to-severe encephalopathy due to perinatal hypoxia–ischemia,[6] to reduce or prevent brain injury related to preterm birth,[7] and to reduce PAIS-related brain damage.[8] In the present chapter, promising neuroprotective pharmacologic interventions to help reduce or prevent brain injury to the developing brain are summarized, and, where possible, a dosing advice is provided. Important to state here is to realize that, to date, clinical research related to pharmacologic reduction of neonatal brain injury is still in its preliminary phase.

PERINATAL HYPOXIA–ISCHEMIA IN THE TERM NEONATE

Hypoxic–ischemic encephalopathy (HIE) due to birth asphyxia in the (near) term neonate is still one of the most prominent causes for neonatal mortality and morbidity. Depending on the site and setting of birth, HIE has an incidence ranging from 1 to 20 children in every 1,000 live-born neonates and is responsible for about 25% of the neonatal mortality worldwide.[1,2,9] Long-term consequences might be cerebral palsy, cognitive impairment, seizure disorders, hearing deficits, and cerebral visual impairment.[10]

The etiology of HIE includes those circumstances that can affect cerebral blood flow in the fetus and newborn, compromising oxygen supply to the brain. The neonatal brain is increasingly dependent on optimal perfusion as pregnancy progresses because of its increasing metabolic demands.[11] Moreover, the immature brain is more prone to damage, given its high amount of fatty acids and unbound ions like iron (Fe^{2+}), which makes it more vulnerable to free radical stress and lipid peroxidation.[11,12] About 60% of perinatal asphyxia is due to an acute HI insult, affecting especially the basal ganglia, thalamus, and brain stem, whereas a subacute or chronic HI insult, occurring in about 15% of perinatal asphyxia, is associated with damage of gray and white matter in the watershed areas of the territories of the anterior, middle, and posterior cerebral arteries.[13,14] A minority of perinatal HI insults is extremely severe and results in a global pattern of brain damage.[14]

HI may develop antepartum (20%), intrapartum (30%), antepartum and intrapartum (35%), or postpartum (10%).[15] The specific mechanism of pathologic processes preceding the onset of cerebral dysfunction is complex and determined by subsequent occurring destructive molecular pathways.[6,12] There is ample evidence now that not only the actual episode of (fetal) hypoxia and consequent ischemia damage the vulnerable developing brain, but that recovery of perfusion and oxygenation upon and after birth with an initial recovery from the oxidative metabolism of the brain can lead to "secondary" energy failure and delayed brain damage.[11,12] This derailment of the oxidative metabolism leading to secondary energy failure starts between 6 and 12 hours and lasts up to 72 hours after birth with consequent (delayed) necrotic and apoptotic neuronal cell death which can last for days or even weeks.[16,17] This postnatal process of cell death adds substantially to the total amount of brain damage due to perinatal asphyxia.[17]

This biphasic response "creates" a therapeutic window up to about 6 hours after the insult during which it may be possible to reduce or even prevent the abovementioned reperfusion/

reoxygenation injury to the developing brain with neuroprotective drugs or other strategies.[6,18] At present, moderate hypothermia during the first 72 hours after birth and starting before 6 hours after the HI insult is the only established neuroprotective therapy which reduced death and/or adverse outcome from about 60% to 45%.[18] However, early pharmacologic interference in the destructive molecular pathways that lead to secondary energy failure and delayed brain damage is now a hot topic[6,19] and may reduce the complication rate of birth asphyxia-induced encephalopathy further.

This chapter does not discuss therapeutic hypothermia and the effects thereof on pharmacokinetics,[20] but is a critical appraisal of promising drugs and compounds which potentially can be used as an add-on intervention for further reduction in composite adverse outcome due to (severe) birth asphyxia.

A detailed knowledge of the basic cellular mechanisms about the destructive molecular pathways set in motion by fetal hypoxia–ischemia and, later on, by reperfusion and oxygenation and their subsequent patterns in relation to postnatal time is very important in relation with pharmacologic add-on therapy.

During the actual (fetal) hypoxia–ischemia, oxidative metabolism will be curtailed, and hypoxanthine will accumulate. Furthermore, hypoxia-driven excessive production of excitatory neurotransmitters, such as glutamate, will activate the *N*-methyl-D-aspartate (NMDA) and voltage-regulated receptors, resulting in an influx of extracellular calcium into the neuronal cell, leading to a huge increase in intracellular and intranuclear Ca^{2+}.[21,22] The result of all this is direct damage to the cell membranes and eventually (necrotic) death of neurons, oligodendrocytes, and astrocytes and a direct drop in interstitial and intracellular pH with liberation of ions from their binding proteins, such as iron (Fe^{2+}), which becomes a free proradical.[21–23]

After resuscitation, when perfusion and oxygenation gradually recover, there is an early surge of free radical formation overwhelming the antioxidant defenses. The metabolization of hypoxanthine, which accumulated during fetal hypoxia, to uric acid catalyzed by the xanthine oxidase enzyme generates an excessive amount of the superoxide free radical ($O_2\cdot$) early after recovery of perfusion and oxygenation.[22,24] Reoxygenation also gives rise to a huge production of the neuronal nitric oxide (NO·) free radical. $O_2\cdot$ formation, which is already maximal in the first 30 minutes after reoxygenation, plays a central role in the total free radical formation and production of toxic compounds in this early stage: it reacts with proradicals like free or non–protein-bound iron generating the very aggressive hydroxyl free radical (OH·) and with (neuronal) NO· to form the very toxic peroxynitrite (ONOO–).[25–27]

The free radicals and toxic compounds are damaging in itself for the developing brain, but contribute also to an inflammatory response by activation of the transcription factors of nuclear factor κB (NF-κB), leading to a huge production of pro- and anti-inflammatory cytokines starting mostly 6 to 12 hours after the actual HI insult and often lasting for days, even weeks.[25–27] This inflammatory response is also responsible for the formation of inducible nitric oxide synthase (iNOS), leading to more free radical production.[27]

A late effect of the birth asphyxia-induced free radical formation and activation of the inflammatory response is the precarious inhibition of neurogenesis and repair by downregulation of maturational, neurotrophic, and growth factors, giving rise to a delayed loss of neurons, oligodendrocytes, and astrocytes.[28,29] Figure 13.1 provides a graphical and schematic pattern of the above-described molecular pathways as a function of (post-)ictal time.

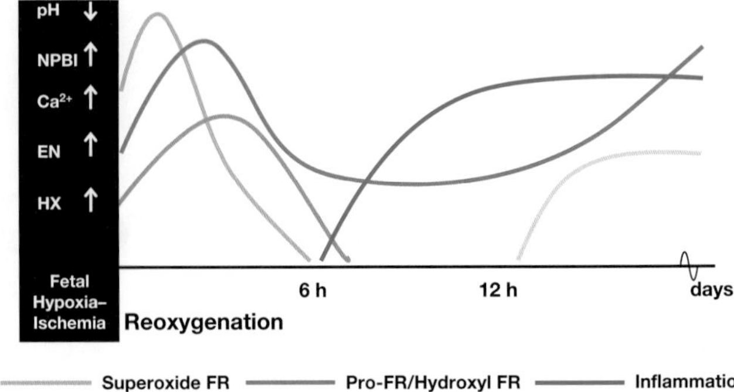

Figure 13.1 Formation of (potentially) harmful events/compounds during fetal hypoxia and the time profiles of the potentially destructive molecular pathways induced by reoxygenation and reperfusion. During fetal hypoxia–ischemia, hypoxanthine (HX) and excitatory neurotransmitters (ENs) increase, causing activation of *N*-methyl-D-aspartate receptors, leading to calcium influx into neuronal cells and formation of proradicals (non–protein-bound iron, NPBI) due to lowering of the interstitial pH. Upon reoxygenation and reperfusion during the early postictal phase, formation of superoxide, hydroxyl free radicals (FR), and nitric oxide synthase–induced peroxynitrite occurs. These events activate also the inflammatory pathway with increased production of cytokines from about 6 to 8 hours after reperfusion, inducing an inappropriate apoptotic activity; eventually, neurotrophic factors needed for the repair of perinatal and postnatal brain injury are downregulated. (Reprinted from van Bel F, Groenendaal F. Drugs for neuroprotection after birth asphyxia: pharmacologic adjuncts to hypothermia. *Semin Perinatol* 2016;40:152–159 with permission from Elsevier.)

This chapter primarily focuses on the latest information of neuroprotective agents that have been suggested to be effective in human clinical studies on top of moderate hypothermia. Dosages used in clinical studies reported in this chapter are merely systematically summarized in Table 13.1, but not extensively mentioned in the text.

NEUROPROTECTIVE PHARMACOLOGIC THERAPY DURING FETAL HYPOXIA

In the brain, excessive formation of excitatory neurotransmitters and free radicals and liberation of metal ions from their binding proteins (such as iron) because of a low interstitial and intracellular pH start already during the actual fetal hypoxia and accelerate upon reperfusion and reoxygenation. This leads to early damage of neuronal cells, oligodendrocytes, and astrocytes in the fetal brain. Antenatal therapy via the mother can then be considered as a "first line of defense" after recognition of fetal hypoxia.

Allopurinol (and its active metabolite oxypurinol), a xanthine oxidase inhibitor, was investigated in a blinded randomized clinical trial in term pregnant women diagnosed with fetal hypoxia just before delivery.[30] Allopurinol and oxypurinol readily pass the placenta, and therapeutic concentrations in umbilical blood are detectable as early as 20 minutes after oral or

TABLE 13.1 Neuroprotective Agents Effective in Human Clinical Studies

Treatment and Study	*Dose*
Perinatal Hypoxic–Ischemic Encephalopathy	
MATERNAL/FETAL THERAPY	
Maternal allopurinol	
Torrance et al.[39]	500 mg iv; IT 10 min
Kaandorp et al.[34]	500 mg iv; IT 10 min
EARLY NEONATAL THERAPY	
Allopurinol	
van Bel et al.[54]	20 mg/kg iv <4 h (IT 10 min); second dose of 20 mg/kg iv after 12 h
Benders et al.[202]	20 mg/kg iv <4 h (IT 10 min); second dose of 20 mg/kg iv after 12 h
Gunes et al.[55]	20 mg/kg iv <6 h (IT 10 min); repeat every 12 h (total 120 mg/kg)
ALBINO Trial (NT & HT) (CT: NCT03162653)	20 mg/kg iv <4 h (IT 10 min); second dose of 10 mg/kg iv after 12 h (if on HT)
Xenon ventilation	
TOBYXe study (HT)[64] (CT: NCT00934700)	30% xenon gas for 24 h (start <6 h)
CoolXeno 3 study (HT) (CT: NCT02071394)	50% xenon gas for 18 h (start <5 h)
2-Iminobiotin	
2-STEP study www.trialregister.nl (NTR5221)	0.08 mg/kg iv started <6 h; in total, 8 doses every 6 h
Melatonin	
Fulia et al.[80]	10 mg/kg orally <6 h, 8 doses separated by 2-h intervals
Aly et al.[81] (HT)	10 mg/kg, daily for 5 d
$MgSO_4$	
Levene et al.[86]	250 mg/kg iv <6 h (IT 10 min) or 400 mg/kg iv (IT 20 min)
Ichiba et al.[90]	250 mg/kg iv <6 h (IT 60 min); repeat on days 2 and 3
Groenendaal et al.[87]	250 mg/kg iv <6 h (IT 30 min); repeat on days 2 and 3
Bhat et al.[88]	250 mg/kg iv <6 h (IT 60 min); repeat on days 2 and 3
Hemen study (HT) (CT: NCT02499393)	250 mg/kg iv <6 h (IT 60 min); repeat on days 2 and 3
MagCool (HT) (CT: NCT01646619)	250 mg/kg iv <6 h; repeat on days 2 and 3
Topiramate	
NeoNATI study[83] (HT)	10 mg/kg orally at admission; repeat on days 2 and 3
RhEPO	
Elmahdy et al.[113]	2,500 U/kg sc <6 h; repeated daily for 5 d
ANTI-INFLAMMATORY/TROPHIC THERAPY	
rhEPO/Darbepoetin	
Zhu et al.[114] (NT)	300 U/kg or 500 U/kg sc <48 h; every other day for 2 wk
Wu et al.[115,117] (HT)	250, 500, 1,000 or 2,500 U/kg iv <24 h; up to 6 doses every 48 h
Avasiloaiei et al.[120] (HT)	1,000 U/kg sc days 1, 2, and 3
El Shimi et al.[121] (HT)	1,500 U/kg sc; single dose on day 1
Wu et al.[117] (HT)	1,000 U/kg iv; days 1, 2, 3, 5, and 7 (cumulative 5,000 U/kg)
Malla et al.[119] (HT)	500 U/kg iv; every other day for 10 d (cumulative 2,500 U/kg)
Baserga et al.[118] (HT)	2 or 10 μg/kg iv <12 h; second dose at day 7 (Darbepoetin)

(*continued*)

TABLE 13.1 Neuroprotective Agents Effective in Human Clinical Studies (*continued*)

Treatment and Study	*Dose*
Brain Injury in the Preterm Neonate	
Maternal $MgSO_4$	
Crowther et al.[85]	Initial dose: 4–6 g iv (10–30 min); maintenance: no, up to 3 g/h iv 12–24 h
Indomethacin	
Fowlie et al.[149]	From once 0.2 mg/kg iv, up to 0.1 mg/kg iv daily for first 6 d after birth (first dose recommended before 6 h after birth)
Caffeine	
Schmidt et al.[176]	Initial dose: 20 mg/kg iv caffeine citrate; maintenance: 5 mg/kg daily
rhIGF-1/rhIGF1BP-3	
Prevention of ROP (23–27 wk, CT: NCT01096784)	250 µg/kg in 24 h (continuous); day 0 up to 30.0 wk PMA
RhEPO	
Ohls et al.[166] (≤32 wk)	400 U/kg iv or sc 3 times weekly, up to 35.0 wk PMA
Ohls et al.[167] (any GA)	400 U/kg iv or sc 3 times weekly, up to 35.0 wk PMA
Natalucci et al.[169] (26–32 wk)	3,000 U/kg iv at birth, at 12–18 h, and at 36–42 h
Song et al.[168] (≤32 wk)	500 U/kg iv; every other day for 2 wk
PENUT study (≤32 wk) (NCT01378273)	1,000 U/kg/dose iv; 6 doses at 48-h intervals; Thereafter 400 U/kg/dose sc 3 times a week until 32-6/7 wk PMA
Perinatal Arterial Ischemic Stroke	
rhEPO/Darbepoetin	
Benders et al.[8]	1,000 U/kg iv at 0, 24, and 48 h after confirmation of stroke
DINOSAUR study (NCT03171818)	10 µg/kg iv at 0 and 7 d after confirmation of stroke (Darbepoetin), first dose starting within 7 d after birth

HT, moderate hypothermia; IT; infusion time; iv, intravenous; NT, normothermia; PMA, postmenstrual age; sc, subcutaneous.

intravenous (IV) administration of the drug to the mother.[31] In high dosages, allopurinol is thought to be a free or non-protein-bound iron chelator and free radical (hydroxyl) scavenger.[32,33] Based on chemical biomarkers, allopurinol appeared to be potentially effective. There was a gender-specific effect: only females showed potential benefit from fetal therapy with allopurinol.[34] Sex differences with respect to neuroprotective therapy after HI were already suggested in earlier reports.[35–37] The long-term results of this investigated cohort, where the vast majority of included fetuses experienced probably mild hypoxic stress, found no proof that allopurinol administered to laboring women with suspected fetal hypoxia improved long-term and behavioral outcome.[38] An earlier pilot study preceding the randomized trial by the same investigators in fetuses with more severe hypoxia showed the potency of allopurinol as a neuroprotective agent.[39]

Maternal treatment with ascorbic acid (vitamin C[40,41]), tetrahydrobiopterin (BH4[42]), phenobarbital,[43] *N*-acetylcysteine,[44] and melatonin[45] was investigated for their potential fetal neuroprotection, but inconclusive disappointing clinical results or lack of clinical studies prevent clinical use of these compounds up to now.

Magnesium reduces excitotoxicity following hypoxia–ischemia by inhibition of the NMDA-receptor/ion channel complex.[46] However, the mode of action of magnesium in fetal hypoxia remains unknown, since the in vivo reached fetal concentrations are much lower than those needed for inhibition of the NMDA receptor.[47] In term pregnant women, no definite beneficial effects of maternal magnesium have been demonstrated.[48]

Xenon, a noble gas and antagonist of the NMDA receptor, has also strong antiapoptotic properties.[49–51] The use of this noble gas may, therefore, be a potential neuroprotective agent. Since xenon is considered to be a safe anesthetic rapidly crossing the placenta,[52] this makes it very attractive for its use in mothers undergoing an emergency cesarean section because of severe fetal hypoxia.[53] To date, no studies were performed to confirm its neuroprotective action, unlike the situation in the (early) postnatal period (see below).

NEUROPROTECTIVE PHARMACOLOGIC THERAPY DURING THE EARLY POST-HYPOXIC–ISCHEMIC PERIOD

The early post-HI reoxygenation–reperfusion phase intensifies the activation of formation of free radicals (O_2; OH·), NMDA-receptor–induced calcium influx in neurons, and nNOS-related $ONOO^-$ production.

Therefore, inhibition of free radical formation and xanthine oxidase, inhibition of NMDA/ion channel antagonists, prevention of nNOS (and subsequently also of iNOS) formation, and chelation of proradicals may be critical to reduce reperfusion–reoxygenation damage to the brain in this early post-HI phase.[6,12]

Especially allopurinol, an inhibitor of xanthine oxidase and by that of O_2 formation, may exert its optimal impact in the very early post-HI period because O_2 formation is assumed to reach its top within the first 30 minutes after reoxygenation–reperfusion. Although several clinical studies using IV allopurinol in the postnatal period suggested a beneficial effect on short-term cerebral biomarkers and even on long-term developmental outcome, especially in moderately asphyxiated infants without serious adverse effects,[54–56] a Cochrane review in 2008 could not confirm that allopurinol was an effective neuroprotective therapy in the post-HI neonatal brain since the clinical trials reported up to now were underpowered.[57] The mostly relatively late treatment regimen in these clinical studies, up to 4 hours after the actual HI insult, may be an important cause for these ambiguous results. A large European double-blind randomized trial in 13 countries (ALBINO trial), treating birth asphyxiated babies (>36 weeks' gestation) with IV allopurinol or placebo on the resuscitation table within 45 minutes after birth, is currently including patients (ClinicalTrials.gov NCT03162653).

Xenon, see also above, has been tested in several experiments as an add-on therapy for asphyxiated neonatal species.[58–60] It shows a rapid passage of the blood–brain barrier and has no reported negative cardiovascular side effects. Xenon, as such, did not appear to be effective as a single therapy, but, in combination with moderate hypothermia neuroprotection, has been demonstrated in several species.[61] In a feasibility study, neonates with perinatal asphyxia and therapeutic hypothermia received 30% to 50% xenon for 18 hours without side effects.[62] The drawbacks of xenon use in neonates are its costs and the need for a closed-loop system, necessitating adjustments in neonatal ventilators and the use of cuffed tracheal tubes to prevent loss of xenon.[63] The only published clinical study with xenon as add-on therapy in asphyxiated neonates requiring moderate hypothermia showed no side effects but also no additional neuroprotective effect of xenon ventilation, although the allowed therapeutic window of 12 hours in this study might have been too long.[64] A possible alternative here is the use of argon, another noble gas which showed neuroprotective properties in experimental studies in the neonatal animal.[65–67] It is much cheaper and easier to use since it does not need a closed-loop system. Up to now, no adverse effects were detected.[68]

(Selective) NOS inhibition in case of birth asphyxia was considered since it was demonstrated in the early 90s of the past century that upregulation of neuronal NOS (nNOS) and iNOS could contribute to brain cell injury following perinatal asphyxia and reperfusion. All isoforms are upregulated after asphyxia; nNOS and endothelial NOS (eNOS) immediately after reperfusion and iNOS from several hours onward.[69] NOS is an enzyme catalyzing the production of nitric oxide (NO) from L-arginine.

eNOS is important in maintaining pulmonary blood flow, preventing pulmonary hypertension, and maintaining adequate oxygenation. In contrast, activation of nNOS and iNOS is associated with deleterious effects on the brain.[70] In eNOS knockout mice, infarct size after middle cerebral artery occlusion is larger compared to wild-type animals, due to a reduction in regional cerebral blood flow.[71]

After perinatal asphyxia, NO can react with the superoxide free radical to form toxic peroxynitrite, setting a preapoptotic pathway in motion, resulting in neuronal loss.[72] Nitrotyrosine, an end product of this process, has been demonstrated postmortem in neonatal brain and spinal cord tissue in infants who died due to severe HIE.[73,74] Protection against HI brain injury is seen in nNOS knockout mice,[75] and iNOS upregulation augments brain injury.[76] Therefore, selective inhibition of these isoforms of NOS could be a potential target for neuroprotection. This was confirmed in a recent review of experimental studies on NOS inhibition.[70] Combined inhibition of nNOS and iNOS started as soon as possible after birth and in a repeated dosing regimen seems to have the best potential based on the combined outcome parameters. 2-Iminobiotin is a selective nNOS and iNOS inhibitor, studied in several species during the past two decades.[77] Recently, pharmacokinetics of 2-iminobiotin was studied in human infants with perinatal asphyxia and therapeutic hypothermia (submitted).

Melatonin is a neuroendocrine hormone, which easily crosses membranes due to lipophilic and hydrophilic properties. Melatonin is involved in the circadian rhythm. In addition, it has neuroprotective effects in the developing brain as a result of reduction of oxidative stress, anti-inflammatory, and antiapoptotic activity.[78]

Maternal melatonin crosses the placenta and the (fetal) blood–brain barrier. In animal models, melatonin levels are increased following hypoxia–ischemia.[79] In a small study, melatonin was given by gastric tube within 6 hours after birth to infants following perinatal asphyxia (eight doses of 10 mg each separated by 2-hour intervals). This resulted in reductions in malondialdehyde and nitrite/nitrate levels at both 12 and 24 hours.[80] In another study, 15 infants received the combination of hypothermia and melatonin for 5 consecutive days, resulting in neurologic improvement compared to hypothermia.[81] Although the first results were positive, these studies were underpowered, preventing confirmation of the neuroprotective effects of melatonin after birth asphyxia.

Topiramate is an anticonvulsant exerting it effects through inhibition of glutamate receptors. Animal studies have demonstrated neuroprotective effects likely due to a combination of glutamate receptor (AMPA, kainate) inhibition, blockade of Na^+ channels, high-voltage activated calcium currents, carbonic anhydrase, and mitochondrial permeability transition pore.[82]

Recently, potential neuroprotective effects of topiramate have been explored in human infants.[83] Oral topiramate in a dose of 10 mg per kg by nasogastric tube once daily during 3 days after the start of hypothermia was well tolerated. The relatively small study did not reveal any difference in outcome.

At present, no IV form of topiramate is commercially available. Resorption of topiramate following perinatal asphyxia during therapeutic hypothermia may be unpredictable depending on the severity of gastrointestinal involvement of the infant and the administration of opioids during therapeutic hypothermia.

As a result of perinatal asphyxia, concentrations of glutamate are elevated in the synaptic cleft, resulting in an increased activity of the NMDA-receptor/ion channel complex and calcium influx into neurons. Thereby, multiple intracellular pathways will be activated, resulting in the production of reactive oxygen species.[84] Magnesium has been shown to alleviate this so-called excitotoxic activity in vitro by binding to the magnesium site on the NMDA glutamate channel. This may stabilize cell membranes, inhibit free radical production, and improve cardiovascular stability with a subsequent reduction of secondary inflammation and associated injury. Randomized controlled trials have shown that antenatal administration of magnesium sulfate ($MgSO_4$) is associated with a reduction in the risk of cerebral palsy in early childhood after preterm birth.[48] Meta-analyses confirmed the effectivity of magnesium to reduce the composite outcome of death and cerebral palsy.[85] The mechanisms through which magnesium exerts its neuroprotective effect in the preterm fetus and infant have not been elucidated in much detail (see also below).

Magnesium in term infants has been tested in several trials.[86–91] The results were summarized in a meta-analysis demonstrating a reduction in the unfavorable short-term composite outcome, but no difference in mortality or seizures.[92] In the Mag Cool trial, (near-)term infants (≥35 weeks) with HIE qualifying for therapeutic hypothermia were randomized to either $MgSO_4$ or placebo. In this trial of 60 infants, no differences in short-term outcome could be demonstrated.[93] At present, there is no conclusive evidence that $MgSO_4$ in combination with hypothermia provides neuroprotection in (near-)term infants with HIE, which is in line with animal models.[94]

N-Acetylcysteine (NAC), a precursor of glutathione, has the properties of an antioxidant and exerts also a direct free radical scavenging activity.[95] Neuroprotective properties of NAC have been reported in rodent pups and piglets with and without additional hypothermia.[96,97] However, the neuroprotective actions are controversial, and there are reports of (hemodynamic) adverse reactions.[61] NAC has been clinically used in preterm babies to prevent or reduce bronchopulmonary dysplasia. One feasibility study in preterm fetuses and neonates was performed for neuroprotection after chorioamnionitis, showing its safety and potential benefits.[98] Clinical studies in asphyxiated newborns are scarce and nonconclusive.[98] NAC is used in older children to treat intoxications of paracetamol in a loading dose of 150 mg per kg IV over 60 minutes.[99]

Tetrahydrobiopterin has known neuroprotective actions, but its research and use in the field of perinatal asphyxia are actually nonexistent, although its safety profile is very attractive for further study in relation with perinatal hypoxia–ischemia.[61]

Cannabinoids ameliorate the neurotoxic[100] and inflammatory responses.[101] Gray and white matter protection after neonatal hypoxia–ischemia are reported in the experimental setting.[102–104] Cannabinoids seem to achieve neuroprotection in part through hypothermia.[105] Up to now, no clinical studies are reported in neonates.

ANTI-INFLAMMATORY THERAPY AND SUPPLETION OF NEUROTROPHIC FACTORS

Inflammation and apoptotic activity are driven by the transcription factor NF-κB, which regulates expression of genes involved in inflammation and apoptosis. Activation of NF-κB starts abundant formation of pro- and anti-inflammatory cytokines, starts production of iNOS, and induces inappropriate apoptosis.[106]

Melatonin is also supposed to have anti-inflammatory properties by preventing activation and translocation of NF-κB to the nucleus, in addition to its antioxidative and free radical scavenging actions.[78] However, no clinical studies have been performed with respect to its anti-inflammatory actions (see also above).

Erythropoietin (EPO) and its derivatives, such as asialo-EPO and darbepoetin, are potentially important neuroprotective agents with anti-inflammatory, antiapoptotic, and neurotrophic properties and are candidates for clinical application in the near future.[105,107] EPO exerts its neuroprotective action after hypoxia–ischemia by its formation in neurons and other brain cells such as oligodendrocytes and astrocytes by hypoxia-mediated activation of the transcription factor hypoxia-inducible factor-1α (HIF-1α).[108] This HIF-1α–related production of EPO triggers induction of antiapoptotic genes by binding to the EPO receptors (EPORs) on the cell membranes of neurons, oligodendrocytes, and astrocytes.[107–109] EPO also has anti-inflammatory properties[110] and is thought to have definite neurotrophic properties.[111] Recombinant human EPO (rhEPO) has a safe pharmacologic profile and is already used in preterm infants below 32 gestational weeks and in term neonates with PAIS[8,112] (see also below).

Extensive experimental studies in different neonatal species confirmed its neuroprotective actions, especially in case of HI-induced brain damage.[107] Clinically, a pilot study of 45 patients showed that treatment of asphyxiated newborns with rhEPO appeared safe and feasible.[113] Before the era of moderate hypothermia after birth asphyxia in China, a phase III trial (double-blinded and randomized) in moderately and severely asphyxiated term newborns showed that repeated (low) dosages of IV administered rhEPO decreased the incidence of disabilities at 18 months of age, although there was a suggestion that females, but not necessarily males, benefited from this therapy.[114] A pharmacokinetic study in 24 severely asphyxiated newborns who underwent hypothermia, treated with additional rhEPO, reported that repeated high dosages up to 1,000 U per kg were well tolerated. Plasma concentrations were similar as reported in earlier neuroprotective studies in newborn animals.[115,116] A randomized phase II trial with moderate hypothermia and add-on therapy with high-dose rhEPO was safe and feasible and suggested to reduce magnetic resonance imaging (MRI)–derived brain injury and improve 1-year motor function.[117] A recent systemic review and meta-analysis of six randomized controlled trials[114,117–121] concluded that administration of EPO or EPO derivatives as add-on therapy by moderate hypothermia in case of perinatal hypoxia–ischemia reduces the risk of brain damage, cerebral palsy, and cognitive outcome, although they advocate larger powered trials to confirm these conclusions.[122] To summarize the results of clinical studies up to now, it can be concluded that at present, no serious adverse effects are published during the clinical use of rhEPO in asphyxiated term newborns. However, especially when higher dosages are used and/or administered for longer periods of time (e.g., ≥1,000 IU per kg), the safety of EPO therapy needs more confirmation, and more research is warranted here. Therefore, as already stated by others, appropriately powered studies in newborns undergoing hypothermia are necessary to confirm neuroprotective properties of rhEPO add-on therapy and to determine optimal timing, dosing, and duration of rhEPO treatment. A phase III double-blind randomized study (HEAL trial), treating birth asphyxiated babies with IV rhEPO, is currently including patients (ClinicalTrials.gov NCT02511263).

EPO derivatives which may have less unwanted effects such as asialo-EPO[123] or longer half-life such as darbepoetin[118] are less well investigated but may be clinically interesting because of their specific properties.

Azithromycin, an antibiotic, is a macrolide derivative of erythromycin and is frequently used in children.[124] Preliminary studies in preterm neonates, investigating its positive effects on bronchopulmonary dysplasia, showed it to be safe and free of major side effects.[124] In a HI neonatal rodent model, azithromycin improved functional and neuropathology outcomes, probably based on its anti-inflammatory properties.[125] More experimental and clinical research is needed to study its efficacy in neuroprotection after neonatal HI brain injury.

The development of specific inhibitors of pro-inflammatory cytokines[126] or antiapoptotic strategies (NF-κB inhibition)[127] are extremely interesting and potentially very forceful but beyond the focus of this review.

Neurotrophic, maturational, and growth factors are important for normal development of the immature brain by stimulation of the endogenous neurogenesis.[128] Downregulation of these factors occurs after severe perinatal HI may be deleterious for recovery and proper development of the postasphyxiated newborn brain. Besides the antioxidative and anti-inflammatory actions of EPO, as described above, it has been supposed that

EPO has also important neurotrophic properties.[129–131] As already mentioned above, it has been suggested that EPO has a sustained effect on neurogenesis and angiogenesis, improving developmental outcome, especially when higher doses (up to 5,000 U per kg) for prolonged periods are used. This may raise safety issues.[82,132] In this respect, the role of HIF-1α, activated during and upon hypoxia–ischemia and giving rise to formation of transcriptional targets, enhanced the production of EPO, endothelial growth factor, and, consequently, brain repair, is of utmost interest.[108]

Neurotrophic factors such as insulin-like growth factor 1 (IGF-1), basic fibroblast growth factor (BFGF), and brain-derived neurotrophic factor (BDNF) investigated in experimental studies in neonatal species are said to reduce (post) HI injury of the neonatal brain,[133,134] but their use in the clinical setting is still far away.

OPTIMAL RESULTS BY COMBINING THERAPIES AT THE RIGHT POINT OF TIME

The ultimate answer toward a further reduction of brain damage after perinatal asphyxia by pharmacologic neuroprotection is not yet available. However, if calcium influx can be reduced, free (pro-) radical production and toxic compounds in the fetal and early postictal phase can be reduced or even prevented, and, subsequently, the inflammatory activation and loss of trophic factors can be restrained, which requires multiple drugs and interventions, a substantial improvement of developmental outcome after moderate and severe HIE may be possible. This requires appropriate dosing, optimal timing, and optimal duration of treatment for each drug depending on its specific action on the destructive molecular pathways. This is the next challenge in this field of research. Questions such as a possible gender specificity of the drugs used also need ongoing research. However, when we can solve abovementioned questions, a major achievement can be added to the treatment of hypoxia–ischemia-induced neonatal encephalopathy.

BRAIN INJURY IN THE PRETERM NEONATE

Periventricular–intraventricular hemorrhages (PIVHs) and diffuse white matter injury (dWMI) dominate nowadays the incidence of acquired brain lesions and adverse outcome of the preterm neonate.[135,136]

The occurrence of PIVH is linked to immaturity of the cerebral vascular bed, especially of the germinal matrix vasculature, and immature lungs manifesting itself as the idiopathic respiratory distress syndrome (IRDS).[137,138] The fragility and functional immaturity of cerebral vessels with IRDS-related abnormal blood gasses leads to lack of autoregulation of the cerebral vascular bed with consequent fluctuation and hyperperfusion of the immature brain, which are thought to be important mechanisms for the occurrence and extension of PIVH.[137–139]

On the other hand, extremely and very preterm neonates have a substantial risk to develop white matter damage.[140,141] Although, in the earlier days, WMI was related to the so-called cystic periventricular leukomalacia, dWMI and "punctate white matter lesions" are the norm nowadays.[142] It has been suggested that arrest in maturation of oligodendrocyte precursors is responsible for hypomyelination as seen in dWMI.[143] Several causes of dWMI have been suggested, from which perinatal and early postnatal hypoxia with or without inflammation are dominating.[144,145]

PHARMACOLOGIC THERAPY FOR PREVENTION AND REDUCTION OF PERIVENTRICULAR–INTRAVENTRICULAR HEMORRHAGE

In the past, maternal corticosteroid treatment during imminent preterm birth and postnatal application of surfactant, aimed to accelerate neonatal lung maturation, contributed, indirectly, to a decrease in the incidence of PIVH.[146,147] Although numerous interventions, including pharmacologic ones, are suggested to be related to a lower incidence and less severe grades of PIVH,[7] causative pharmacologic PIVH-reducing therapies are scarce and mostly not yet proven. Only prophylactic treatment with the nonselective cyclooxygenase inhibitor indomethacin during the first days of life starting within 6 hours after preterm birth reduced the incidence of especially severe PIVH.[148,149] Indomethacin promotes maturation of the cerebral vascular bed[137,150] and has a stabilizing effect on the cerebral vascular bed.[151] Indomethacin prophylaxis is indeed used in a vast minority of neonatal intensive care units in the United States.[152]

Postnatal neuroprotective therapy with trophic factors such as EPO and IGF-1 and its binding protein 3 (IGF-1-BP3) is suggested to have neuroprotective and, possibly, PIVH-preventing properties.[153,154]

EPO supports cell survival, and its receptors (EPORs) are detected on endothelial, glia, neuronal cells, and oligodendrocytes.[107,155–157] EPO has also antioxidative properties and anti-inflammatory effects, preventing apoptotic death of the endothelial cells.[158–160] This suggests a positive impact on the PIVH incidence in premature neonates. A recent meta-analysis including 3,643 extremely and very preterm infants receiving early EPO therapy reported a reducing effect on PIVH incidence.[161,162]

IGF-1 has been suggested to exert a positive effect on proper vascularization and brain development and is, therefore, considered important for a normal neurodevelopment.[154] IGF-1 levels in extremely preterm neonates are much lower than in utero serum concentrations at corresponding gestational ages, indicating that the immature fetus is dependent on maternal IGF-1 levels. Intranasal IGF-1 suppletion reduced indeed germinal matrix hemorrhages in a preterm rat pup model.[163] This motivated investigators to administer exogenous IGF-1 and its IGF-1–binding protein BP3 to extremely prematurely born neonates to induce maturational effects on vascularization and the immature brain.[164] A clinical study of Hellström et al.[154] aim at a reduction of retinopathy of prematurity and may reduce the incidence of PIVH and bronchopulmonary dysplasia simultaneously (ClinicalTrials.gov: NCT01096784).

PHARMACOLOGIC THERAPY FOR PREVENTION AND REDUCTION OF DIFFUSE WHITE MATTER INJURY

Magnesium sulfate given antenatally to women with imminent preterm birth reduced the incidence of cerebral palsy of the infant.[85] Although the mechanism of this neuroprotective action is unknown, stabilization of uterine perfusion (vasodilation) and reduction of PIVH have been the proposed mechanisms. Blockade of NMDA receptors or other excitotoxic pathways, which is an important neuroprotective action of magnesium however, seems less probable, given that the concentrations achieved in mothers and fetuses are much lower than those measured in studies in neonatal animals.[85]

Postnatal pharmacologic actions to reduce the incidence of dWMI are scarce. As already suggested earlier, EPO and IGF-1 and its IGF-1–binding protein BP3 are supposed to reduce or even prevent WMI, given their anti-inflammatory and trophic properties. EPO inhibits glutamate release, reduces accumulation of intracellular calcium, is antiapoptotic, and reduces inflammation and NO-mediated injury and, finally, has regenerative properties.[107,156,157] In the EpoKids study in very preterm infants, MRI at term equivalent age showed less WMI in the EPO group compared to the placebo group.[165] As already stated above, a meta-analysis including four studies showed improved cognitive development of very preterm infants treated with rhEPO without affecting other neurodevelopmental outcomes.[161,166–169] IGF-1 stimulates oligodendrocyte maturation and, by that, myelination.[170–174] Studies in IGF-1 knockout mice[174] reported lower total brain volumes and hypomyelination. Human studies relating serum IGF-1 levels to brain development show a positive association between postnatal serum IGF-1 concentrations and head circumference, brain volume measures, and developmental scores at 2 years of age.[173] Further studies are needed to confirm the suggested neuroprotective effects of IGF-1.

Early postnatal dexamethasone therapy is associated with a decrease in cerebral palsy, but further studies are necessary to confirm its benefits.[175] Postnatal use of caffeine to prevent apnea resulted in improved motor outcome at 11 years of age.[176] It further has been suggested that nutrition may contribute to a proper development of the immature brain. The microbiome–gut–brain axis may be the mechanism of interaction, with a positive effect on neuronal, endocrine, and immunologic pathways.[177] Especially fatty acids, proteins, and probiotics may support the development of the preterm brain.[178,179] Finally, avoiding pain and stress with the use of opioids may reduce WMI. Alternative strategies for stress and pain reduction, such as sucrose or nonsedative analgesics, need, therefore, to be explored further.

PERINATAL ARTERIAL ISCHEMIC STROKE

PAIS occurs in 1/2,300 to 1/5,000 live-born term newborns.[180] It is associated with a variety of adverse outcomes, with unilateral spastic cerebral palsy in around 30% of all affected infants. More accurate prediction of motor outcome is possible using neonatal MRI and taking site and size of the lesion into account. Involvement of the corticospinal tracts (posterior limb of the internal capsule and cerebral peduncle) and the basal ganglia can be best recognized using diffusion-weighted imaging, and when restricted diffusion is present, this is now referred to as "pre–Wallerian degeneration."[4,181] Impaired cognitive outcome, postneonatal epilepsy, language, visual, and behavioral problems may also be diagnosed in 50% to 75% of the children during infancy and childhood.[4,5,180] Many studies have looked at risk factors, and a comparison was also made between newborns with PAIS and HIE.[182] Similar rates of intrapartum complications were found, but with different patterns. Maternal fever, PROM, prolonged second stage, tight nuchal cord, and failed ventouse delivery were more common in PAIS, and thick meconium, sentinel events, and shoulder dystocia were more often seen in HIE.[182] Perinatal inflammation is also considered to play an important role in the development of PAIS.[183] In contrast to HIE where the delivery is complicated and resuscitation is usually required and the criteria are met to start neuroprotective therapy within the therapeutic window, PAIS does not become symptomatic during the first 12 hours, even though the insult is also considered to have its onset at or around delivery. When the children do present at 12 to 48 hours after birth, mostly with focal seizures, it is too late to start therapeutic hypothermia. Management is, therefore, at present still supportive, with control of hypoglycemia, anticonvulsant therapy, and respiratory and circulatory support.

EPO and its derivatives such as darbepoetin, as mentioned in the HIE section, are potentially important neuroprotective agents with acutely, anti-inflammatory, antiapoptotic and neurotrophic, and antioxidant effects.[153] Infants with PAIS may also benefit from possible long-term effects of EPO, promoting brain development and brain recovery, including angiogenesis, neurogenesis, and oligodendrogenesis. Several in vitro studies have been performed, showing neuroprotection by reducing free radical formation, inflammation, and apoptosis in neuronal cultures.[184] In a review from our group, the neuroregenerative effects of EPO in neonatal experimental in vivo studies, including MCAO models, were summarized.[107] EPO administration after MCAO in postnatal day (P) 7 to 10 rat pups was noted to improve neurogenesis, as measured by increased brain volume up to 70%.[107] Using EPO, several rodent studies have shown not only a substantial reduction in infarct volume in neonatal stroke models but also an improvement in motor and cognitive function.[185–188] In a subsequent study, the same group demonstrated that EPO treatment after neonatal stroke in rats stimulated neural progenitor cells' proliferation in the subventricular zone and migration of these progenitors to the site of the injury, again emphasizing the neuroregenerative effects of EPO.[189] Recently, they were able to show that delayed EPO treatment, up to 1 week after the onset of neonatal stroke, improved histologic as well as functional outcome, which further supports the involvement of EPO as a trophic factor stimulating neurogenesis.[189]

In view of these experimental data, EPO was considered a promising neuroprotective agent for the newborn infant with PAIS. This resulted in a phase 1 trial in infants with PAIS.[8] In this study, 21 full-term infants were treated with rhEPO immediately after diagnosis and 24 and 48 hours after the first dose. An MRI was performed in the acute phase to confirm the diagnosis and repeated at 3 months of age to assess the area of cavitation. No adverse effects were noted on red blood cells, white blood cells, platelets count, or coagulation. No beneficial effect of rhEPO was shown for stroke volume when compared to historic non–rhEPO-treated neonates with PAIS, which was most likely due to the small sample size.

Darbepoetin alfa is more potent, exhibits a lower clearance and longer terminal half-life in serum than rhEPO, and is more universally available.[190–192] Safety and pharmacokinetic data have been published in full-term infants with HIE.[118] Darbepoetin was chosen for a placebo-controlled phase 2 trial (NCT03171818), which is now enrolling infants in the Netherlands and Canada.

In this phase 2 trial of (near-)term newborns ≥36 weeks' gestation with MRI-confirmed PAIS in the middle cerebral artery territory, two doses of darbepoetin alfa or placebo are administered IV: the first dose within the first week after birth, the second 1 week later. Primary outcome measure is change in lesion size between the time of onset of the insult and 6 to 8 weeks of age, estimated using advanced volumetric MRI techniques. Secondary outcome measures are reorganization of the corticospinal connectivity detected using MRI and neurodevelopmental outcome measures of cognition and motor development at 18 months of age using the BSID-III.

NEONATAL BRAIN INJURY AND CELL THERAPY

Increasing experimental evidence shows that regeneration of the injured neonatal brain with stem cell therapy may serve as an effective "repair" strategy. Stem cells have a potential for self-renewal and are able to differentiate into different cellular phenotypes.[193] The omnipotent embryonic stem cells seem to be the obvious choice for repair of neonatal brain injury, but a reliable ethical concern is that this cell type can induce formation of teratomas after cell transplantation.[194,195] The fate of embryonic stem cells is to become a hematopoietic, neural, or mesenchymal stem cell (MSC). A major advantage of multipotent neural stem cells is of course their ability to derive all neural lineages, but their accessibility in humans is limited, and, even more important, they also carry a significant risk of tumor formation.[196] As a detailed discussion of the potential benefits and hazards of several types of stem cells is beyond the scope of this review, we refer to recent review papers published for an overview of the safety aspects and therapeutic values of major stem cell types.[197]

Among all progenitor cells, the MSC seems to be most promising for near-future use in human neonates, given its excellent neuroregenerative and favorable immunomodulating properties and its excellent safety profile.[198] Although it is obvious that MSCs can differentiate into mesodermal tissue cells (e.g., bone, cartilage, fat), recent studies showed that MSCs are also capable to induce profound proliferation of endogenous neural stem cells.[199,200] In vivo administration of MSCs is associated with increasing numbers of neurons, astrocytes, and oligodendrocytes, and it is hypothesized that MSCs stimulate this formation of new brain cells by paracrine effects rather than by transformation into various cell types themselves.[193,200,201] A detailed description of the repairing abilities of MSCs after neonatal brain injury is beyond the aims of this chapter, but is extensively discussed in a recent review paper of our group by Wagenaar et al.[193]

CONCLUDING REMARKS

Ongoing research in pharmacologic neuroprotection of the perinatal brain brought us potentially strong drugs and compounds to further reduce and even prevent neonatal brain injury, after perinatal hypoxia–ischemia, in very and extremely preterm born infants and after PAIS. Appropriate dosing of drugs, the optimal time and duration of treatment, and a possible gender specificity of these drugs needs ongoing research. Subsequent repair by cell therapy of the developing brain is a rather new but exciting field of research.

ACKNOWLEDGMENTS

The authors have based the text of this chapter on the excellent version in previous editions by Maria Delivoria-Papadopoulos, Agustín Legido, Ignacio Valencia, and Om Prakash Mishra.

DISCLOSURE STATEMENT

Herewith, the authors of this manuscript, Floris Groenendaal, MD; Manon Benders, MD; Linda de Vries, MD; and Frank van Bel, MD, declare that Frank van Bel and Floris Groenendaal are, together with Cacha Peeters-Scholte, inventors of 2-iminobiotin as a neuroprotective agent for neonates with cerebral hypoxia–ischemia. They have no financial or personal relationships with other people or organizations that could potentially and inappropriately influence their work and conclusions. They further declare to have no proprietary or commercial interest in any product mentioned or concept discussed in this article.

REFERENCES

1. Kurinczuk JJ, White-Koning M, Badawi N. Epidemiology of neonatal encephalopathy and hypoxic-ischaemic encephalopathy. *Early Hum Dev* 2010;86:329–338.
2. Aminu M, Unkels R, Mdegela M, et al. Causes of and factors associated with stillbirth in low- and middle-income countries: a systematic literature review. *BJOG* 2014;121(Suppl 4):141–153.
3. Norman M, Hallberg B, Abrahamsson T, et al. Association between year of birth and 1-year survival among extremely preterm infants in Sweden during 2004–2007 and 2014–2016. *JAMA* 2019;321:1188–1199.
4. Wagenaar N, Martinez-Biarge M, van der Aa NE, et al. Neurodevelopment after perinatal arterial ischemic stroke. *Pediatrics* 2018;142:e20174164.
5. Chabrier S, Peyric E, Drutel L, et al. Multimodal outcome at 7 years of age after neonatal arterial ischemic stroke. *J Pediatr* 2016;172:156.e3–161.e3.
6. van Bel F, Groenendaal F. Drugs for neuroprotection after birth asphyxia: pharmacologic adjuncts to hypothermia. *Semin Perinatol* 2016;40:152–159.
7. van Bel F, Vaes J, Groenendaal F. Prevention, reduction and repair of brain injury of the preterm infant. *Front Physiol* 2019;10:181.
8. Benders MJ, van der Aa NE, Roks M, et al. Feasibility and safety of erythropoietin for neuroprotection after perinatal arterial ischemic stroke. *J Pediatr* 2014;164:481.e1–e2–486.e1–e2.
9. Liu L, Oza S, Hogan D, et al. Global, regional, and national causes of child mortality in 2000–13, with projections to inform post-2015 priorities: an updated systematic analysis. *Lancet* 2015;385:430–440.
10. Badawi N, Felix JF, Kurinczuk JJ, et al. Cerebral palsy following term newborn encephalopathy: a population-based study. *Dev Med Child Neurol* 2005;47:293–298.
11. Saugstad OD, Oei JL, Lakshminrusimha S, et al. Oxygen therapy of the newborn from molecular understanding to clinical practice. *Pediatr Res* 2019;85:20–29.
12. Qin X, Cheng J, Zhong Y, et al. Mechanism and treatment related to oxidative stress in neonatal hypoxic-ischemic encephalopathy. *Front Mol Neurosci* 2019;12:88.
13. Miller SP, Ramaswamy V, Michelson D, et al. Patterns of brain injury in term neonatal encephalopathy. *J Pediatr* 2005;146:453–460.
14. de Vries LS, Groenendaal F. Patterns of neonatal hypoxic-ischaemic brain injury. *Neuroradiology* 2010;52:555–566.
15. Glass HC, Ferriero DM. Treatment of hypoxic-ischemic encephalopathy in newborns. *Curr Treat Options Neurol* 2007;9:414–423.
16. Hope PL, Costello AM, Cady EB, et al. Cerebral energy metabolism studied with phosphorous NMR spectroscopy in normal and birth asphyxiated infants. *Lancet* 1984;8399:366–370.
17. Fleiss B, Gressens P. Tertiary mechanisms of brain damage: a new hope for treatment of cerebral palsy? *Lancet Neurol* 2012;11:556–566.
18. Jacobs SE, Berg M, Hunt R, et al. Cooling for newborns with hypoxic ischaemic encephalopathy. *Cochrane Database Syst Rev* 2013;1:CD003311.
19. Parikh P, Juul SE. Neuroprotective strategies in neonatal brain injury. *J Pediatr* 2018;192:22–32.
20. van den Broek MP, Groenendaal F, Egberts AC, et al. Effects of hypothermia on pharmacokinetics and pharmacodynamics: a systematic review of preclinical and clinical studies. *Clin Pharmacokinet* 2010;49:277–294.
21. Ferriero DM. Neonatal brain injury. *N Engl J Med* 2004;351:1985–1995.
22. Saugstad OD. Role of xanthine oxidase and its inhibitor in hypoxia: reoxygenation injury. *Pediatrics* 1996;98:103–107.
23. Hilton GD, Nunez JL, Bambrick L, et al. Glutamate-mediated excitotoxicity in neonatal hippocampal neurons is mediated by mGluR-induced release of Ca^{++} from intracellular stores and is prevented by estradiol. *Eur J Neurosci* 2006;24:3008–3016.
24. Mink R, Johnston J. The effect of infusing hypoxanthine or xanthine on hypoxic-ischemic brain injury in rabbits. *Brain Res* 2007;1147:256–264.
25. Shouman BO, Mesbah A, Aly H. Iron metabolism and lipid peroxidation products in infants with hypoxic ischemic encephalopathy. *J Perinatol* 2008;28:487–491.

26. van den Tweel ERW, Nijboer C, Kavelaars A, et al. Expression of nitric oxide synthase isoforms and nitrotyrosine formation after hypoxia-ischemia in the neonatal rat brain. *J Neuroimmunol* 2005;167:64–71.
27. Suzuki M, Tabuchi M, Ikeda M, et al. Concurrent formation of peroxynitrite with the expression of inducible nitric oxide synthase in the brain during middle cerebral artery occlusion and reperfusion in rats. *Brain Res* 2002;951:113–120.
28. Scheepens A, Wassink G, Blanco CE. The effect of a global birth asphyxia on the ontogeny of BDNF and NGF protein expression in the juvenile brain. *Brain Res Dev Brain Res* 2003;140:215–221.
29. Skoff RP, Bessert D, Barks JD, et al. Plasticity of neurons and glia following neonatal hypoxic-ischemic brain injury in rats. *Neurochem Res* 2007;32:331–342.
30. Boda D. Results of and further prevention of hypoxic fetal brain damage by inhibition of xanthine oxidase enzyme with allopurinol. *J Perinat Med* 2011;39:441–444.
31. Boda D, Nemeth I, Kiss P, et al. Treatment of mothers with allopurinol to produce therapeutic blood levels in newborns. *Prenatal Neonatal Med* 1999;4:130–134.
32. Ko KM, Godin DV. Inhibition of transition metal ion-catalysed ascorbate oxidation and lipid peroxidation by allopurinol and oxypurinol. *Biochem Pharmacol* 1990;40:803–809.
33. Moorhouse PC, Grootveld M, Halliwell B, et al. Allopurinol and oxypurinol are hydroxyl radical scavengers. *FEBS Lett* 1987;213:23–28.
34. Kaandorp JJ, Benders MJ, Schuit E, et al. Maternal allopurinol administration during suspected fetal hypoxia: a novel neuroprotective intervention? A multicentre randomised placebo controlled trial. *Arch Dis Child Fetal Neonatal Ed* 2015;100:F216–F223.
35. Nijboer CH, Kavelaars A, Van Bel F, et al. Gender-dependent pathways of hypoxia-ischemia-induced cell death and neuroprotection in the immature P3 rat. *Dev Neurosci* 2007;29:385–392.
36. Weis SN, Pettenuzzo LF, Krolow R, et al. Neonatal hypoxia-ischemia induces sex-related changes in rat brain mitochondria. *Mitochondrion* 2012;12:271–279.
37. Hill CA, Fitch RH. Sex differences in mechanisms and outcome of neonatal hypoxia-ischemia in rodent models: implications for sex-specific neuroprotection in clinical neonatal practice. *Neurol Res Int* 2012;2012:867531.
38. Klumper J, Kaandorp JJ, Schuit E, et al. Behavioral and neurodevelopmental outcome of children after maternal allopurinol administration during suspected fetal hypoxia: 5-year follow up of the ALLO-trial. *PLoS One* 2018;13:e0201063.
39. Torrance HL, Benders MJ, Derks JB, et al. Maternal allopurinol treatment during fetal hypoxia lowers cord blood levels of the brain injury marker protein S-100B. *Pediatrics* 2009;124:350–357.
40. Jackson TS, Xu A, Vita JA, et al. Ascorbate prevents the interaction of superoxide and nitric oxide only at very high physiological concentrations. *Circ Res* 1998;83:916–922.
41. Poston L, Briley AL, Seed PT, et al. Vitamin C and Vitamin E in pregnant women at risk for pre-eclampsia (VIP trial): randomised placebo-controlled trial. *Lancet* 2006;367: 1145–1154.
42. Vasquez-Vivar J, Whitsett J, Derrick M, et al. Tetrahydrobiopterin in the prevention of hypertonia in hypoxic fetal brain. *Ann Neurol* 2009;66:323–331.
43. Reinisch JM, Sanders SA, Mortensen EL, et al. In utero exposure to phenobarbital and intelligence deficits in adult men. *JAMA* 1995;274:1518–1525.
44. Xu DX, Chen YH, Wang H, et al. Effect of N-acetylcysteine on lipopolysaccharide-induced intra-uterine fetal death and intra-uterine growth retardation in mice. *Toxicol Sci* 2005;88:525–533.
45. Jahnke G, Marr M, Myers C, et al. Maternal and developmental toxicity evaluation of melatonin administered orally to pregnant Sprague-Dawley rats. *Toxicol Sci* 1999;50:271–279.
46. Lipton SA, Rosenberg PA. Excitatory amino acids as a final common pathway for neurologic disorders. *N Engl J Med* 1994;330:613–622.
47. Crowther CA, Brown J, McKinlay CJ, et al. Magnesium sulphate for preventing preterm birth in threatened preterm labour. *Cochrane Database Syst Rev* 2014;(8):CD001060.
48. Nguyen TM, Crowther CA, Wilkinson D, et al. Magnesium sulphate for women at term for neuroprotection of the fetus. *Cochrane Database Syst Rev* 2013;(2):CD009395.
49. Franks NP, Dickinson R, de Sousa SL, et al. How does xenon produce anaesthesia? *Nature* 1998;396:324.
50. Ma D, Williamson P, Januszewski A, et al. Xenon mitigates isoflurane-induced neuronal apoptosis in the developing rodent brain. *Anesthesiology* 2007;106:746–753.
51. Ma D, Lim T, Xu J, et al. Xenon preconditioning protects against renal ischemic-reperfusion injury via HIF-1alpha activation. *J Am Soc Nephrol* 2009;20:713–720.
52. Goto T, Saito H, Shinkai M, et al. Xenon provides faster emergence from anesthesia than does nitrous oxide-sevoflurane or nitrous oxide-isoflurane. *Anesthesiology* 1997;86:1273–1278.
53. Lane GA, Nahrwold ML, Tait AR, et al. Anesthetics as teratogens: nitrous oxide is fetotoxic, xenon is not. *Science* 1980;210:899–901.
54. Van Bel F, Shadid M, Moison RM, et al. Effect of allopurinol on postasphyxial free radical formation, cerebral hemodynamics, and electrical brain activity. *Pediatrics* 1998;101:185–193.
55. Gunes T, Ozturk MA, Koklu E, et al. Effect of allopurinol supplementation on nitric oxide levels in asphyxiated newborns. *Pediatr Neurol* 2007;36:17–24.
56. Kaandorp JJ, van Bel F, Veen S, et al. Long-term neuroprotective effects of allopurinol after moderate perinatal asphyxia: follow-up of two randomised controlled trials. *Arch Dis Child Fetal Neonatal Ed* 2012;97(3):F162–F166.
57. Chaudhari T, McGuire W. Allopurinol for preventing mortality and morbidity in newborn infants with suspected hypoxic-ischaemic encephalopathy. *Cochrane Database Syst Rev* 2008;(2):CD006817.
58. Thoresen M, Hobbs CE, Wood T, et al. Cooling combined with immediate or delayed xenon inhalation provides equivalent long-term neuroprotection after neonatal hypoxia-ischemia. *J Cereb Blood Flow Metab* 2009;29:707–714.
59. Faulkner S, Bainbridge A, Kato T, et al. Xenon augmented hypothermia reduces early lactate/N-acetylaspartate and cell death in perinatal asphyxia. *Ann Neurol* 2011;70:133–150.
60. Liu X, Dingley J, Scull-Brown E, et al. Adding 5 h delayed xenon to delayed hypothermia treatment improves long-term function in neonatal rats surviving to adulthood. *Pediatr Res* 2015;77:779–783.
61. Robertson NJ, Tan S, Groenendaal F, et al. Which neuroprotective agents are ready for bench to bedside translation in the newborn infant? *J Pediatr* 2012;160:544–552.
62. Dingley J, Tooley J, Liu X, et al. Xenon ventilation during therapeutic hypothermia in neonatal encephalopathy: a feasibility study. *Pediatrics* 2014;2014:809–818.
63. Chakkarapani E, Thoresen M, Hobbs CE, et al. A closed-circuit neonatal xenon delivery system: a technical and practical neuroprotection feasibility study in newborn pigs. *Anesth Analg* 2009;109:451–460.
64. Azzopardi D, Robertson NJ, Bainbridge A, et al. Moderate hypothermia within 6 h of birth plus inhaled xenon versus moderate hypothermia alone after birth asphyxia (TOBY-Xe): a proof-of-concept, open-label, randomised controlled trial. *Lancet Neurol* 2016;15:145–153.
65. Zhuang L, Yang T, Zhao H, et al. The protective profile of argon, helium, and xenon in a model of neonatal asphyxia in rats. *Crit Care Med* 2012;40:1724–1730.
66. Ryang YM, Fahlenkamp AV, Rossaint R, et al. Neuroprotective effects of argon in an in vivo model of transient middle cerebral artery occlusion in rats. *Crit Care Med* 2011;39:1448–1453.
67. Broad KD, Fierens I, Fleiss B, et al. Inhaled 45–50% argon augments hypothermic brain protection in a piglet model of perinatal asphyxia. *Neurobiol Dis* 2016;87:29–38.
68. Alderliesten T, Favie LM, Neijzen RW, et al. Neuroprotection by argon ventilation after perinatal asphyxia: a safety study in newborn piglets. *PLoS One* 2014;9:e113575.
69. Liu H, Li J, Zhao F, et al. Nitric oxide synthase in hypoxic or ischemic brain injury. *Rev Neurosci* 2015;26:105–117.
70. Favie LMA, Cox AR, van den Hoogen A, et al. Nitric oxide synthase inhibition as a neuroprotective strategy following hypoxic-ischemic encephalopathy: evidence from animal studies. *Front Neurol* 2018;9:258.
71. Huang Z, Huang PL, Ma J, et al. Enlarged infarcts in endothelial nitric oxide synthase knockout mice are attenuated by nitro-L-arginine. *J Cereb Blood Flow Metab* 1996;16:981–987.
72. Beckman JS, Viera L, Estevez AG, et al. Nitric oxide and peroxynitrite in the perinatal period. *Semin Perinatol* 2000;24:37–41.
73. Groenendaal F, Lammers H, Smit D, et al. Nitrotyrosine in brain tissue of neonates after perinatal asphyxia. *Arch Dis Child Fetal Neonatal Ed* 2006;91:F429–F433.
74. Groenendaal F, Vles J, Lammers H, et al. Nitrotyrosine in human neonatal spinal cord after perinatal asphyxia. *Neonatology* 2008;93:1–6.
75. Ferriero DM, Holtzman DM, Black SM, et al. Neonatal mice lacking neuronal nitric oxide synthase are less vulnerable to hypoxic-ischemic injury. *Neurobiol Dis* 1996;3:64–71.
76. Brown GC, Vilalta A. How microglia kill neurons. *Brain Res* 2015;1628:288–297.
77. Zitta K, Peeters-Scholte C, Sommer L, et al. 2-Iminobiotin superimposed on hypothermia protects human neuronal cells from hypoxia-induced cell damage: an in vitro study. *Front Pharmacol* 2017;8:971.
78. Colella M, Biran V, Baud O. Melatonin and the newborn brain. *Early Hum Dev* 2016;102:1–3.
79. Robertson NJ, Faulkner S, Fleiss B, et al. Melatonin augments hypothermic neuroprotection in a perinatal asphyxia model. *Brain* 2013;136:90–105.
80. Fulia F, Gitto E, Cuzzocrea S, et al. Increased levels of malondialdehyde and nitrite/nitrate in the blood of asphyxiated newborns: reduction by melatonin. *J Pineal Res* 2001;31:343–349.
81. Aly H, Elmahdy H, El-Dib M, et al. Melatonin use for neuroprotection in perinatal asphyxia: a randomized controlled pilot study. *J Perinatol* 2015;35:186–191.
82. Cilio MR, Ferriero DM. Synergistic neuroprotective therapies with hypothermia. *Semin Fetal Neonatal Med* 2010;15:293–298.
83. Filippi L, Fiorini P, Catarzi S, et al. Safety and efficacy of topiramate in neonates with hypoxic ischemic encephalopathy treated with hypothermia (NeoNATI): a feasibility study. *J Matern Fetal Neonatal Med* 2018;31:973–980.
84. Hagberg H, Edwards AD, Groenendaal F. Perinatal brain damage: the term infant. *Neurobiol Dis* 2016;92:102–112.
85. Crowther CA, Middleton PF, Voysey M, et al. Assessing the neuroprotective benefits for babies of antenatal magnesium sulphate: an individual participant data meta-analysis. *PLoS Med* 2017;14:e1002398.
86. Levene M, Blennow M, Whitelaw A, et al. Acute effects of two different doses of magnesium sulphate in infants with birth asphyxia. *Arch Dis Child Fetal Neonatal Ed* 1995;73:F174–F177.
87. Groenendaal F, Rademaker CMA, Toet MC, et al. Effects of magnesium sulfate on amplitude-integrated continuous EEG in asphyxiated term neonates. *Acta Paediatr* 2002;91:1073–1077.
88. Bhat MA, Charoo BA, Bhat JI, et al. Magnesium sulfate in severe perinatal asphyxia: a randomized, placebo-controlled trial. *Pediatrics* 2009;123:e764–e769.
89. Khashaba MT, Shouman BO, Shaltout AA, et al. Excitatory amino acids and magnesium sulfate in neonatal asphyxia. *Brain Dev* 2006;28:375–379.
90. Ichiba H, Tamai H, Negishi H, et al. Randomized controlled trial of magnesium sulfate infusion for severe birth asphyxia. *Pediatr Int* 2002;44:505–509.
91. Ichiba H, Yokoi T, Tamai H, et al. Neurodevelopmental outcome of infants with birth asphyxia treated with magnesium sulfate. *Pediatr Int* 2006;48:70–75.
92. Tagin M, Shah PS, Lee KS. Magnesium for newborns with hypoxic-ischemic encephalopathy: a systematic review and meta-analysis. *J Perinatol* 2013;33:663–669.
93. Rahman SU, Canpolat FE, Oncel MY, et al. Multicenter randomized controlled trial of therapeutic hypothermia plus magnesium sulfate versus therapeutic hypothermia plus placebo in the management of term and near—term infants with hypoxic ischemic encephalopathy (The Mag Cool Study): a pilot study. *J Clin Neonatol* 2015;4:158–163.
94. Galinsky R, Bennet L, Groenendaal F, et al. Magnesium is not consistently neuroprotective for perinatal hypoxia-ischemia in term-equivalent models in preclinical studies: a systematic review. *Dev Neurosci* 2014;36:73–82.
95. Aruoma OI, Halliwell B, Hoey BM, et al. The antioxidant action of N-acetylcysteine: its reaction with hydrogen peroxide, hydroxyl radical, superoxide, and hypochlorous acid. *Free Radic Biol Med* 1989;6:593–597.
96. Plaisant F, Clippe A, Vander Stricht D, et al. Recombinant peroxiredoxin 5 protects against excitotoxic brain lesions in newborn mice. *Free Radic Biol Med* 2003;34:862–872.
97. Jatana M, Singh I, Singh AK, et al. Combination of systemic hypothermia and N-acetylcysteine attenuates hypoxic-ischemic brain injury in neonatal rats. *Pediatr Res* 2006;59:684–689.

98. Jenkins DD, Wiest DB, Mulvihill DM, et al. Fetal and neonatal effects of N-acetylcysteine when used for neuroprotection in maternal chorioamnionitis. *J Pediatr* 2016;168:67.e6–76.e6.
99. White ML, Liebelt EL. Update on antidotes for pediatric poisoning. *Pediatr Emerg Care* 2006;22:740–746.
100. Freund TF, Katona I, Piomelli D. Role of endogenous cannabinoids in synaptic signaling. *Physiol Rev* 2003;83:1017–1066.
101. Klein TW. Cannabinoid-based drugs as anti-inflammatory therapeutics. *Nat Rev Immunol* 2005;5:400–411.
102. Alonso-Alconada D, Alvarez A, Alvarez FJ, et al. The cannabinoid WIN 55212-2 mitigates apoptosis and mitochondrial dysfunction after hypoxia ischemia. *Neurochem Res* 2012;37:161–170.
103. Lafuente H, Alvarez FJ, Pazos MR, et al. Cannabidiol reduces brain damage and improves functional recovery after acute hypoxia-ischemia in newborn pigs. *Pediatr Res* 2011;70:272–277.
104. Pazos MR, Mohammed N, Lafuente H, et al. Mechanisms of cannabidiol neuroprotection in hypoxic-ischemic newborn pigs: role of 5HT(1A) and CB2 receptors. *Neuropharmacology* 2013;71:282–291.
105. Hassell KJ, Ezzati M, Alonso-Alconada D, et al. New horizons for newborn brain protection: enhancing endogenous neuroprotection. *Arch Dis Child Fetal Neonatal Ed* 2015;100:F541–F552.
106. Nijboer CH, Heijnen CJ, Groenendaal F, et al. A dual role of the NF-{kappa}B pathway in neonatal hypoxic-ischemic brain damage. *Stroke* 2008;39:2578–2586.
107. van der Kooij MA, Groenendaal F, Kavelaars A, et al. Neuroprotective properties and mechanisms of erythropoietin in in vitro and in vivo experimental models for hypoxia/ischemia. *Brain Res Rev* 2008;59:22–33.
108. Fan X, Heijnen CJ, van der Kooij MA, et al. The role and regulation of hypoxia-inducible factor-1alpha expression in brain development and neonatal hypoxic-ischemic brain injury. *Brain Res Rev* 2009;62:99–108.
109. Digicaylioglu M, Lipton SA. Erythropoietin-mediated neuroprotection involves cross-talk between Jak2 and NF-kappaB signalling cascades. *Nature* 2001;412:641–647.
110. Sun Y, Calvert JW, Zhang JH. Neonatal hypoxia/ischemia is associated with decreased inflammatory mediators after erythropoietin administration. *Stroke* 2005;36:1672–1678.
111. Dame C, Juul SE, Christensen RD. The biology of erythropoietin in the central nervous system and its neurotrophic and neuroprotective potential. *Biol Neonate* 2001;79:228–235.
112. Fauchere JC, Koller BM, Tschopp A, et al. Safety of early high-dose recombinant erythropoietin for neuroprotection in very preterm infants. *J Pediatr* 2015;167:52.e1–e3–57.e1–e3.
113. Elmahdy H, El-Mashad AR, El-Bahrawy H, et al. Human recombinant erythropoietin in asphyxia neonatorum: pilot trial. *Pediatrics* 2010;125:e1135–e1142.
114. Zhu C, Kang W, Xu F, et al. Erythropoietin improved neurologic outcomes in newborns with hypoxic-ischemic encephalopathy. *Pediatrics* 2009;124:e218–e226.
115. Wu YW, Bauer LA, Ballard RA, et al. Erythropoietin for neuroprotection in neonatal encephalopathy: safety and pharmacokinetics. *Pediatrics* 2012;130:683–691.
116. Frymoyer A, Juul SE, Massaro AN, et al. High-dose erythropoietin population pharmacokinetics in neonates with hypoxic-ischemic encephalopathy receiving hypothermia. *Pediatr Res* 2017;81:865–872.
117. Wu YW, Mathur AM, Chang T, et al. High-dose erythropoietin and hypothermia for hypoxic-ischemic encephalopathy: a phase II trial. *Pediatrics* 2016;137(6):e20160191.
118. Baserga MC, Beachy JC, Roberts JK, et al. Darbepoetin administration to neonates undergoing cooling for encephalopathy: a safety and pharmacokinetic trial. *Pediatr Res* 2015;78:315–322.
119. Malla RR, Asimi R, Teli MA, et al. Erythropoietin monotherapy in perinatal asphyxia with moderate to severe encephalopathy: a randomized placebo-controlled trial. *J Perinatol* 2017;37:596–601.
120. Avasiloaiei A, Dimitriu C, Moscalu M, et al. High-dose phenobarbital or erythropoietin for the treatment of perinatal asphyxia in term newborns. *Pediatr Int* 2013;55:589–593.
121. El Shimi MS, Awad HA, Hassanein SM, et al. Single dose recombinant erythropoietin versus moderate hypothermia for neonatal hypoxic ischemic encephalopathy in low resource settings. *J Matern Fetal Neonatal Med* 2014;27:1295–1300.
122. Razak A, Hussain A. Erythropoietin in perinatal hypoxic-ischemic encephalopathy: a systematic review and meta-analysis. *J Perinat Med* 2019;47:478–489.
123. Siren AL, Fasshauer T, Bartels C, et al. Therapeutic potential of erythropoietin and its structural or functional variants in the nervous system. *Neurotherapeutics* 2009;6:108–127.
124. Smith C, Egunsola O, Choonara I, et al. Use and safety of azithromycin in neonates: a systematic review. *BMJ Open* 2015;5:e008194.
125. Barks JDE, Liu Y, Wang L, et al. Repurposing azithromycin for neonatal neuroprotection. *Pediatr Res* 2019;86(4):444–451.
126. Nijboer CH, Heijnen CJ, Groenendaal F, et al. Alternate pathways preserve tumor necrosis factor-{alpha} production after nuclear factor-{kappa}B inhibition in neonatal cerebral hypoxia-ischemia. *Stroke* 2009;40(10):3362–3368.
127. Nijboer CH, Heijnen CJ, Groenendaal F, et al. Strong neuroprotection by inhibition of NF-{kappa}B after neonatal hypoxia-ischemia involves apoptotic mechanisms but is independent of cytokines. *Stroke* 2008;39:2129–2137.
128. Alagappan D, Lazzarino DA, Felling RJ, et al. Brain injury expands the numbers of neural stem cells and progenitors in the SVZ by enhancing their responsiveness to EGF. *ASN Neuro* 2009;1(2):e00009.
129. Campana WM, Misasi R, O'Brien JS. Identification of a neurotrophic sequence in erythropoietin. *Int J Mol Med* 1998;1:235–241.
130. Iwai M, Stetler RA, Xing J, et al. Enhanced oligodendrogenesis and recovery of neurological function by erythropoietin after neonatal hypoxic/ischemic brain injury. *Stroke* 2010;41:1032–1037.
131. Reitmeir R, Kilic E, Kilic U, et al. Post-acute delivery of erythropoietin induces stroke recovery by promoting perilesional tissue remodelling and contralesional pyramidal tract plasticity. *Brain* 2011;134:84–99.
132. Ehrenreich H, Weissenborn K, Prange H, et al. Recombinant human erythropoietin in the treatment of acute ischemic stroke. *Stroke* 2009;40:e647–e656.
133. Lin S, Fan LW, Rhodes PG, et al. Intranasal administration of IGF-1 attenuates hypoxic-ischemic brain injury in neonatal rats. *Exp Neurol* 2009;217:361–370.
134. Galvin KA, Oorschot DE. Continuous low-dose treatment with brain-derived neurotrophic factor or neurotrophin-3 protects striatal medium spiny neurons from mild neonatal hypoxia/ischemia: a stereological study. *Neuroscience* 2003;118:1023–1032.
135. Hamilton BE, Hoyert DL, Martin JA, et al. Annual summary of vital statistics: 2010–2011. *Pediatrics* 2013;131:548–558.
136. Pierrat V, Marchand-Martin L, Arnaud C, et al. Neurodevelopmental outcome at 2 years for preterm children born at 22 to 34 weeks' gestation in France in 2011: EPIPAGE-2 cohort study. *BMJ* 2017;358:j3448.
137. Ballabh P. Pathogenesis and prevention of intraventricular hemorrhage. *Clin Perinatol* 2014;41:47–67.
138. Krediet TG, Kavelaars A, Vreman HJ, et al. Respiratory distress syndrome-associated inflammation is related to early but not late peri/intraventricular hemorrhage in preterm infants. *J Pediatr* 2006;148:740–746.
139. Perlman JM, Goodman S, Kreusser KL, et al. Reduction in intraventricular hemorrhage by elimination of fluctuating cerebral blood-flow velocity in preterm infants with respiratory distress syndrome. *N Engl J Med* 1985;312:1353–1357.
140. Volpe JJ. Brain injury in premature infants: a complex amalgam of destructive and developmental disturbances. *Lancet Neurol* 2009;8:110–124.
141. Chau V, Synnes A, Grunau RE, et al. Abnormal brain maturation in preterm neonates associated with adverse developmental outcomes. *Neurology* 2013;81:2082–2089.
142. Kersbergen KJ, Benders MJ, Groenendaal F, et al. Different patterns of punctate white matter lesions in serially scanned preterm infants. *PLoS One* 2014;9:e108904.
143. van Tilborg E, de Theije CGM, van Hal M, et al. Origin and dynamics of oligodendrocytes in the developing brain: implications for perinatal white matter injury. *Glia* 2018;66:221–238.
144. Groenendaal F, de Vries LS. Hypocarbia and white matter echolucencies in newborns <28 weeks gestation. *Pediatr Res* 2001;50:772–773.
145. Hagberg H, Mallard C, Ferriero DM, et al. The role of inflammation in perinatal brain injury. *Nat Rev Neurol* 2015;11:192–208.
146. Norman M, Piedvache A, Borch K, et al. Association of short antenatal corticosteroid administration-to-birth intervals with survival and morbidity among very preterm infants: results from the EPICE cohort. *JAMA Pediatr* 2017;171:678–686.
147. Ng E, Taddio A, Ohlsson A. Intravenous midazolam infusion for sedation of infants in the neonatal intensive care unit. *Cochrane Database Syst Rev* 2017;1:CD002052.
148. Nelin TD, Pena E, Giacomazzi T, et al. Outcomes following indomethacin prophylaxis in extremely preterm infants in an all-referral NICU. *J Perinatol* 2017;37:932–937.
149. Fowlie PW, Davis PG, McGuire W. Prophylactic intravenous indomethacin for preventing mortality and morbidity in preterm infants. *Cochrane Database Syst Rev* 2010;(7):CD000174.
150. Ment LR, Stewart WB, Ardito TA, et al. Indomethacin promotes germinal matrix microvessel maturation in the newborn beagle pup. *Stroke* 1992;23:1132–1137.
151. Van Bel F, Bartelds B, Teitel DF, et al. Effect of indomethacin on cerebral blood flow and oxygenation in the normal and ventilated fetal lamb. *Pediatr Res* 1995;38:243–250.
152. Jensen EA, Foglia EE, Schmidt B. Association between prophylactic indomethacin and death or bronchopulmonary dysplasia: a systematic review and meta-analysis of observational studies. *Semin Perinatol* 2018;42:228–234.
153. Juul SE, Pet GC. Erythropoietin and neonatal neuroprotection. *Clin Perinatol* 2015;42:469–481.
154. Hellström A, Ley D, Hansen-Pupp I, et al. Role of insulin-like growth factor 1 in fetal development and in the early postnatal life of premature infants. *Am J Perinatol* 2016;33:1067–1071.
155. Koulnis M, Porpiglia E, Hidalgo D, et al. Erythropoiesis: from molecular pathways to system properties. *Adv Exp Med Biol* 2014;844:37–58.
156. Chateauvieux S, Grigorakaki C, Morceau F, et al. Erythropoietin, erythropoiesis and beyond. *Biochem Pharmacol* 2011;82:1291–1303.
157. Rangarajan V, Juul SE. Erythropoietin: emerging role of erythropoietin in neonatal neuroprotection. *Pediatr Neurol* 2014;51:481–488.
158. Yamaji R, Okada T, Moriya M, et al. Brain capillary endothelial cells express two forms of erythropoietin receptor mRNA. *Eur J Biochem* 1996;239:494–500.
159. Bernaudin M, Marti HH, Roussel S, et al. A potential role for erythropoietin in focal permanent cerebral ischemia in mice. *J Cereb Blood Flow Metab* 1999;19:643–651.
160. Kawakami M, Sekiguchi M, Sato K, et al. Erythropoietin receptor-mediated inhibition of exocytotic glutamate release confers neuroprotection during chemical ischemia. *J Biol Chem* 2001;276:39469–39475.
161. Fischer HS, Reibel NJ, Buhrer C, et al. Prophylactic early erythropoietin for neuroprotection in preterm infants: a meta-analysis. *Pediatrics* 2017;139(5):e20164317.
162. Ohlsson A, Aher SM. Early erythropoiesis-stimulating agents in preterm or low birth weight infants. *Cochrane Database Syst Rev* 2017;11:CD004863.
163. Lekic T, Flores J, Klebe D, et al. Intranasal IGF-1 reduced rat pup germinal matrix hemorrhage. *Acta Neurochir Suppl* 2016;121:209–212.
164. Ley D, Hansen-Pupp I, Niklasson A, et al. Longitudinal infusion of a complex of insulin-like growth factor-I and IGF-binding protein-3 in five preterm infants: pharmacokinetics and short-term safety. *Pediatr Res* 2013;73:68–74.
165. Leuchter RH, Gui L, Poncet A, et al. Association between early administration of high-dose erythropoietin in preterm infants and brain MRI abnormality at term-equivalent age. *JAMA* 2014;312:817–824.
166. Ohls RK, Ehrenkranz RA, Das A, et al. Neurodevelopmental outcome and growth at 18 to 22 months' corrected age in extremely low birth weight infants treated with early erythropoietin and iron. *Pediatrics* 2004;114:1287–1291.
167. Ohls RK, Kamath-Rayne BD, Christensen RD, et al. Cognitive outcomes of preterm infants randomized to darbepoetin, erythropoietin, or placebo. *Pediatrics* 2014;133:1023–1030.
168. Song J, Sun H, Xu F, et al. Recombinant human erythropoietin improves neurological outcomes in very preterm infants. *Ann Neurol* 2016;80:24–34.

169. Natalucci G, Latal B, Koller B, et al. Effect of early prophylactic high-dose recombinant human erythropoietin in very preterm infants on neurodevelopmental outcome at 2 years: a randomized clinical trial. *JAMA* 2016;315:2079–2085.
170. Cao Y, Gunn AJ, Bennet L, et al. Insulin-like growth factor (IGF)-1 suppresses oligodendrocyte caspase-3 activation and increases glial proliferation after ischemia in near-term fetal sheep. *J Cereb Blood Flow Metab* 2003;23:739–747.
171. Pang Y, Zheng B, Campbell LR, et al. IGF-1 can either protect against or increase LPS-induced damage in the developing rat brain. *Pediatr Res* 2010;67:579–584.
172. Cai Z, Fan LW, Lin S, et al. Intranasal administration of insulin-like growth factor-1 protects against lipopolysaccharide-induced injury in the developing rat brain. *Neuroscience* 2011;194:195–207.
173. Hansen-Pupp I, Hovel H, Hellström A, et al. Postnatal decrease in circulating insulin-like growth factor-I and low brain volumes in very preterm infants. *J Clin Endocrinol Metab* 2011;96:1129–1135.
174. O'Kusky J, Ye P. Neurodevelopmental effects of insulin-like growth factor signaling. *Front Neuroendocrinol* 2012;33:230–251.
175. Doyle LW, Cheong JL, Ehrenkranz RA, et al. Early (<8 days) systemic postnatal corticosteroids for prevention of bronchopulmonary dysplasia in preterm infants. *Cochrane Database Syst Rev* 2017;10:CD001146.
176. Schmidt B, Roberts RS, Davis P, et al. Long-term effects of caffeine therapy for apnea of prematurity. *N Engl J Med* 2007;357:1893–1902.
177. Cryan JF, Dinan TG. Mind-altering microorganisms: the impact of the gut microbiota on brain and behaviour. *Nat Rev Neurosci* 2012;13:701–712.
178. Uauy R, Mena P. Long-chain polyunsaturated fatty acids supplementation in preterm infants. *Curr Opin Pediatr* 2015;27:165–171.
179. Coviello C, Keunen K, Kersbergen KJ, et al. Effects of early nutrition and growth on brain volumes, white matter microstructure, and neurodevelopmental outcome in preterm newborns. *Pediatr Res* 2018;83:102–110.
180. Dunbar M, Kirton A. Perinatal stroke: mechanisms, management, and outcomes of early cerebrovascular brain injury. *Lancet Child Adolesc Health* 2018;2:666–676.
181. Kirton A, Shroff M, Visvanathan T, et al. Quantified corticospinal tract diffusion restriction predicts neonatal stroke outcome. *Stroke* 2007;38:974–980.
182. Martinez-Biarge M, Cheong JL, Diez-Sebastian J, et al. Risk factors for neonatal arterial ischemic stroke: the importance of the intrapartum period. *J Pediatr* 2016;173:62.e1–68.e1.
183. Giraud A, Guiraut C, Chevin M, et al. Role of perinatal inflammation in neonatal arterial ischemic stroke. *Front Neurol* 2017;8:612.
184. Chong ZZ, Kang JQ, Maiese K. Erythropoietin fosters both intrinsic and extrinsic neuronal protection through modulation of microglia, Akt1, Bad, and caspase-mediated pathways. *Br J Pharmacol* 2003;138:1107–1118.
185. Sola A, Wen TC, Hamrick SE, et al. Potential for protection and repair following injury to the developing brain: a role for erythropoietin? *Pediatr Res* 2005;57:110r–117r.
186. Chang YS, Mu D, Wendland M, et al. Erythropoietin improves functional and histological outcome in neonatal stroke. *Pediatr Res* 2005;58:106–111.
187. Gonzalez FF, McQuillen P, Mu D, et al. Erythropoietin enhances long-term neuroprotection and neurogenesis in neonatal stroke. *Dev Neurosci* 2007;29:321–330.
188. Gonzalez FF, Abel R, Almli CR, et al. Erythropoietin sustains cognitive function and brain volume after neonatal stroke. *Dev Neurosci* 2009;31:403–411.
189. Gonzalez FF, Larpthaveesarp A, McQuillen P, et al. Erythropoietin increases neurogenesis and oligodendrogliosis of subventricular zone precursor cells after neonatal stroke. *Stroke* 2013;44:753–758.
190. Egrie JC, Dwyer E, Browne JK, et al. Darbepoetin alfa has a longer circulating half-life and greater in vivo potency than recombinant human erythropoietin. *Exp Hematol* 2003;31:290–299.
191. Padhi D, Ni L, Cooke B, et al. An extended terminal half-life for darbepoetin alfa: results from a single-dose pharmacokinetic study in patients with chronic kidney disease not receiving dialysis. *Clin Pharmacokinet* 2006;45:503–510.
192. Patel S, Ohls RK. Darbepoetin administration in term and preterm neonates. *Clin Perinatol* 2015;42:557–566.
193. Wagenaar N, Nijboer CH, van Bel F. Repair of neonatal brain injury: bringing stem cell-based therapy into clinical practice. *Dev Med Child Neurol* 2017;59:997–1003.
194. Itskovitz-Eldor J, Schuldiner M, Karsenti D, et al. Differentiation of human embryonic stem cells into embryoid bodies compromising the three embryonic germ layers. *Mol Med* 2000;6:88–95.
195. Bjorklund LM, Sanchez-Pernaute R, Chung S, et al. Embryonic stem cells develop into functional dopaminergic neurons after transplantation in a Parkinson rat model. *Proc Natl Acad Sci U S A* 2002;99:2344–2349.
196. Comi AM, Cho E, Mulholland JD, et al. Neural stem cells reduce brain injury after unilateral carotid ligation. *Pediatr Neurol* 2008;38:86–92.
197. Fleiss B, Guillot PV, Titomanlio L, et al. Stem cell therapy for neonatal brain injury. *Clin Perinatol* 2014;41:133–148.
198. Uccelli A, Moretta L, Pistoia V. Mesenchymal stem cells in health and disease. *Nat Rev Immunol* 2008;8:726–736.
199. Dezawa M, Kanno H, Hoshino M, et al. Specific induction of neuronal cells from bone marrow stromal cells and application for autologous transplantation. *J Clin Invest* 2004;113:1701–1710.
200. van Velthoven CT, Kavelaars A, van Bel F, et al. Mesenchymal stem cell treatment after neonatal hypoxic-ischemic brain injury improves behavioral outcome and induces neuronal and oligodendrocyte regeneration. *Brain Behav Immun* 2010;24:387–393.
201. van Velthoven CT, Kavelaars A, van Bel F, et al. Mesenchymal stem cell transplantation changes the gene expression profile of the neonatal ischemic brain. *Brain Behav Immun* 2011;25:1342–1348.
202. Benders MJ, Bos AF, Rademaker CM, et al. Early postnatal allopurinol does not improve short-term outcome after severe birth asphyxia. *Arch Dis Child Fetal Neonatal Ed* 2006;91:F163–F165.

CHAPTER

14

David K. Stevenson
Ronald J. Wong
Sota Iwatani

Pharmacologic Agents for Neonatal Hyperbilirubinemia

INTRODUCTION

Hyperbilirubinemia is a natural and essentially ubiquitous transitional phenomenon among human newborns. Approximately 60% to 70% of all term infants, and nearly all premature infants, become visibly jaundiced during the first week of life after birth. For term infants, the serum or plasma total bilirubin (TB) concentration typically peaks 3 to 4 days after birth in the range of 5 to 6 mg per dL (86 to 103 μmol per L). For premature infants, TB levels peak later and higher after the first several days of life. Although much uncertainty and debate remain concerning the range of TB considered as benign physiologic jaundice, the consensus places the maximal "safe" peak TB threshold at approximately 17 mg per dL (291 μmol per L) for otherwise healthy term and late preterm infants. Because hyperbilirubinemia above this threshold is considered to be pathologic, the etiology of the hyperbilirubinemia should be investigated and appropriate therapy considered or initiated depending on the clinical circumstances.[1] In immature infants, treatment to decrease TB levels is often initiated at lower TB levels because of lower albumin (Alb) levels and diminished affinity of Alb for bilirubin in these infants. Moreover, binding to Alb is least avid in the early transitional period after birth and is influenced adversely by any confounding conditions, such as infection or acidosis, that increase free or unbound bilirubin (UB) in circulation and the likelihood of movement into tissues.

Historically, the main therapies for neonatal hyperbilirubinemia have been phototherapy and exchange transfusion. Light should be considered a drug for hyperbilirubinemia, but most physicians pay little attention to the radiometric qualities (effective spectral width and peak emission) and quantities [irradiance (μW per cm^2 per nm)] involved or the factors that affect the dose of phototherapy (duration, body surface area exposure).[2,3] Finally, issues that are involved in producing phototherapy-related side effects (riboflavin destruction, erythema, and photosensitizing drugs) also deserve attention. A discussion of these topics should include reference to the qualities of light-emitting diodes (LEDs) because of their high intensity and narrow-band light in the spectrum of choice with minimal heat generation,[3–6] but these issues are beyond the scope of this chapter. In spite of the proven benefits of phototherapy and maximal spatial limitations, the understanding of the biology of newborn hyperbilirubinemia and the existence and further development of alternative pharmacologic therapies are an integral part of its management and consequences.

NEONATAL JAUNDICE

Neonatal jaundice is the result of an imbalance between the production of bilirubin and its elimination.[7–9] Bilirubin production on a body weight basis is increased in the newborn by approximately two to three times that of an adult.[10,11] This relative increase in bilirubin production in the newborn is the result of an increased circulating red blood cell (RBC) mass and a shortened RBC life span. Consequently, all newborn infants have increased bilirubin production as a contributing cause of their transitional or pathologic jaundice. The pattern of hyperbilirubinemia (its peak and duration) is influenced further by the efficiency with which the pigment is eliminated. The major factor contributing to impaired elimination in the transitional period after birth is decreased hepatic conjugation of bilirubin. The gradual induction of uridine diphosphoglucuronate glucuronosyltransferase (UGT) contributes most importantly to the pattern of hyperbilirubinemia after birth because changes in bilirubin production are slower and more gradual within the time frame of the rapid elevation in TB levels after birth and the decline in the latter part of the first week and into the second week of life. Thus, because all newborn babies have temporarily impaired conjugation, any pathologic state associated with increased bilirubin production, such as hemolysis, represents a serious risk to the newborn infant, especially in the first several days of life. Even without pathologic elevations in bilirubin production, greater impairments in conjugation associated with conditions such as Gilbert syndrome[12–14] and the Asian G71R mutation in the *UGT1A1* gene[14–16] can place infants at risk for kernicterus because of unexpected alterations in the pattern of hyperbilirubinemia, including its peak and duration. In particular, the coexpression of gene polymorphisms involved in bilirubin production, such as $(GT)_n$, repeats in the HO-1 promoter region and glucose-6-phosphate dehydrogenase (G6PD) mutations, and metabolisms, such as OATP1A1 and *UGT1A1* and the TATAA box variants, may provide genetic markers for clinical risk assessments, as well as potential therapeutic targets.[17,18]

The imbalances in the production of the pigment and its elimination have been well studied, and various methods have been proposed to identify infants at risk for severe hyperbilirubinemia. Because the predominant source of carbon monoxide (CO) in the body is the degradation of heme, which ultimately leads to the production of equimolar amounts of bilirubin, increased bilirubin production can be estimated by measuring the end-tidal CO in breath, or carboxyhemoglobin in circulation, after these measurements are corrected for ambient CO (ETCOc or COHbc, respectively).[19,20] The normalization of COHbc to hemoglobin concentration (COHbc/Hb) can serve as an even more sensitive index of excessive RBC destruction.[21] For example, the infant with hemolytic anemia would have a higher COHbc/Hb ratio than the infant with anemia caused by blood loss. By measuring the conjugated fraction of bilirubin, another index can be applied, which assesses the relative balance between bilirubin production and conjugation [COHbc/TCB (%)], where TCB is the total conjugated bilirubin.[9] Finally, a nomogram plotting hour-specific TB levels is also informed by the balance of bilirubin production and elimination over time.[22] Because all infants have impaired conjugation during the transitional period, deviations from the percentile tracks in the first several days of life are most often related to a relative increase in bilirubin production, whereas deviations after the first week of life are more likely the result of persistent impairment in bilirubin conjugation and therefore elimination.

The logic of removing bilirubin from circulation after it has been produced is clear, but it is also only reactionary and may not avoid potential neurologic injury in every circumstance. Another more rational treatment strategy would be to directly inhibit bilirubin production, thus ameliorating the primary contributing factor in neonatal hyperbilirubinemia and the risk for kernicterus. If a safe drug for inhibiting bilirubin production could be identified, its use could be universalized. However, another alternative preventive strategy could involve the early rapid and accurate identification of infants at risk for increased bilirubin production or at least with an imbalance between the production and the elimination of bilirubin. One approach would be to measure ETCOc or COHbc as an index of bilirubin formation and, thus, identify high producers of the pigment for targeted therapy. Another approach would be to plot hour-specific TB levels and be cognizant of early deviations from the nomogram suggestive of increased bilirubin production or the combination of relatively insufficient conjugation for a given bilirubin load.[23] Whether the approach is targeted would depend, at least in part, on the safety, efficacy, and cost of the chemotherapeutic agent.

HEME DEGRADATION PATHWAY

Heme is degraded in a two-step enzymatic pathway, which requires molecular oxygen and nicotinamide adenine dinucleotide phosphate (NADPH; see Fig. 14.1). The first step is rate limiting and catalyzed by heme oxygenase (HO), a membrane-bound enzyme.[24] In this first step, the porphyrin macrocycle is broken at the 9-α-meso carbon bridge after a series of oxidations and reductions and liberates CO, iron, and biliverdin in equimolar amounts. In the second enzymatic step, biliverdin is immediately reduced in the cytosol by biliverdin reductase in an NADPH-dependent reaction to generate bilirubin. Because HO is the rate-limiting enzyme in the pathway, its inhibition results in decreased production of CO, iron, and biliverdin, thus leading to decreased bilirubin production.[25,26]

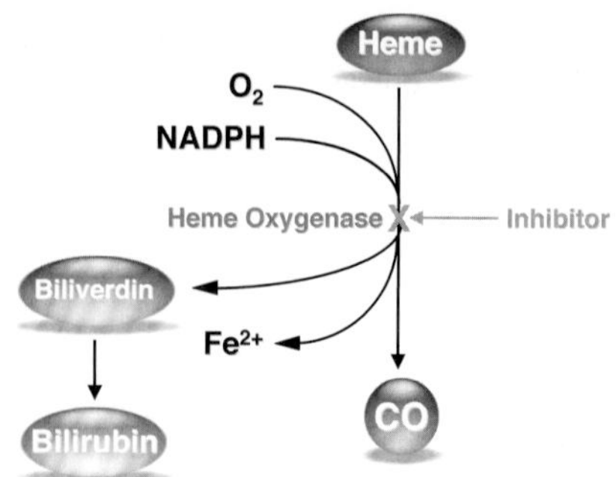

Figure 14.1 Heme catabolic pathway.

HEME OXYGENASE INHIBITORS

METALLOPORPHYRINS

Many synthetic structural analogues or metalloporphyrins of heme (ferroprotoporphyrin) are effective in vitro and in vivo competitive inhibitors of HO (Fig. 14.2 and Table 14.1). The original idea for using heme analogues [i.e., zinc protoporphyrin (ZnPP)] as drugs for modulating bilirubin production was pioneered in 1981 by Maines[27] and has driven over three decades of intensive investigation of a variety of potential chemopreventive agents in this class of compounds. They have variable efficacies with respect to the two primary and well-described isoforms of HO, the inducible form (HO-1) and the constitutive form (HO-2), which occur in different relative proportions in tissues.[28] Moreover, some of these compounds have been found to also inhibit other enzymes, such as nitric oxide synthase (NOS) and soluble guanylyl cyclase (sGC), as well as processes such as lipid peroxidation.[29,30] In fact, the products of heme degradation, CO, iron, biliverdin, and bilirubin, have all been shown to play important biologic roles as antioxidants and anti-inflammatory agents.[20,31–33] Thus, the deliberate attenuation of heme degradation for the purpose of controlling the production of bilirubin must be considered in the context of the potential side effects on other important biologic processes in the transitional period and their effects beyond.[34]

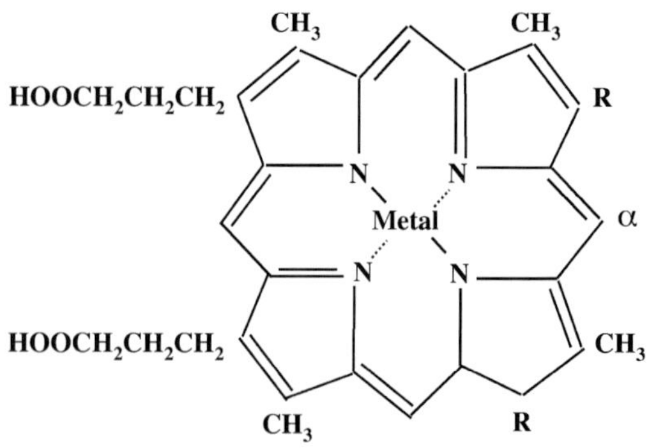

Figure 14.2 Metalloporphyrin structure. (From Vreman HJ, Wong RJ, Stevenson DK. Alternative metalloporphyrins for the treatment of neonatal jaundice. *J Perinatol* 2001;21(Suppl 1):S108–S113, with permission.)

TABLE 14.1 Porphyrin Type Based on Chelated Metal and Ring Substituent

Metal	*Deuteroporphyrin (DP)* *(R = –H)*	*Mesoporphyrin (MP)* *(R = $-CH_2-CH_3$)*	*Protoporphyrin (PP)* *(R = $-CH=CH_2$)*	*Bis Glycol Porphyrin (BG)* *(R = $-CHOH-CH_2OH$)*
Metal free	MfDP	MfMP	MfPP	MfBG
Iron (Fe^{2+})	FeDP	FeMP	FePP (hemin)	FeBG
Zinc (Zn^{2+})	ZnDP	ZnMP	ZnPP	ZnBG
Tin (Sn^{4+})	SnDP	SnMP	SnPP	SnBG
Chromium (Cr^{2+})	CrDP	CrMP	CrPP	CrBG
Manganese (Mn^{2+})	MnDP	MnMP	MnPP	MnBG
Copper (Cu^{2+})	CuDP	CuMP	CuPP	CuBG
Nickel (Ni^{2+})	NiDP	NiMP	NiPP	NiBG

Tin protoporphyrin (SnPP) was the first synthetic heme analogue used for the purpose of inhibiting HO in human neonates after intensive investigation in rodents and nonhuman primates.[35–37] Although highly efficacious, the photoreactivity of this metalloporphyrin made it a less desirable drug.[38–40] Tin mesoporphyrin (SnMP), which is also photoreactive and more potent, however, has been used in several randomized controlled trials in human neonates at considerably lower doses than was possible with SnPP.[41,42] In fact, a single intramuscular dose of 6- and 4.5-µM SnMP per kg body weight has been shown to eliminate the need for phototherapy[41] or for exchange transfusion,[43] respectively, during the postnatal period. The efficacy of the compound has been well established, but it still may not represent the ideal therapeutic agent because it is photoreactive and contains a foreign (non-essential) metal, induces the HO-1 gene, and can inhibit other enzyme systems such as NOS and sGC. ZnPP has been proposed as an alternative drug, but its inhibitory potency is much lower and its formulation for administration has been more difficult.[26] Nonetheless, it is a naturally occurring metalloporphyrin and has both in vitro and in vivo inhibitory properties for both HO-1 and HO-2 and has been shown to suppress hyperbilirubinemia in neonatal rodents and nonhuman primates.[39] Moreover, this naturally occurring heme analogue has no apparent photoreactivity in vivo. Recently, we have designed a formulation of ZnPP (10%) incorporated in lipid microspheres [45% 1,2-dipalmitoyl-sn-glycero-3-phosphocholine (DPPC) and 45% 1,2-distearoyl-sn-glycero-3-phosphocholine (DSPC)] to enhance its oral absorptivity and found that it has sufficient potency in inhibiting liver and spleen HO activity in vitro[44] and in vivo.[44,45] In addition, incorporation of ZnPP into the microspheres did not affect its selectivity for the HO-1 isozyme, but increased its in vitro potency up to 10-fold.[46] With respect to photoreactivity, many of the heme analogues have already been characterized along with their inhibitory potency.[26,39,40,47] Importantly, no photo- or chemical toxicity was observed in newborn pups treated with the ZnPP microspheres.[44] Thus, the use of ZnPP microspheres has potential for oral use in the treatment of neonatal hyperbilirubinemia.

In addition to screening for potential phototoxicity, the impact of these metalloporphyrins on the induction of HO-1 is also important to consider.[26,48–50] In fact, the various compounds also differ in their ability to upregulate the HO-1 gene. For example, ZnPP and zinc bis glycol porphyrin (ZnBG) appear to cause minimal induction. The latter compound is a very potent inhibitor, which is orally absorbable.[48,49,51–53] Although ZnBG is photoreactive, its substantial potency would allow for its use with minimal clinical risk similar to what has been observed for SnMP. The other characteristics of the unique metabolite ZnPP have been reviewed in detail elsewhere.[54] Besides its therapeutic potential, it also has clinical applications for assessing nutritional iron status in pediatric patients, pregnant women, and blood donors and for diagnosing other disorders in iron metabolism including lead toxicity.[54] With respect to the potential for inducing HO-1, preliminary data on cadmium-induced HO-1 transcription suggest a possible programming effect, with a second exposure to the drug resulting in less of an induction. However, ZnPP has shown minimal effects of HO-1 transcriptional activity in adult HO-1-*luc* transgenic mice, whose transgene consists of the HO-1 promoter driving expression of the reporter gene *luciferase* (*luc*) using in vivo bioluminescence imaging.[53,55] Additionally, ZnPP microspheres did not significantly increase liver and brain HO-1 mRNA and protein in 3-day-old mouse pups given a heme load to mimic an acute hemolytic condition.[45] Whether such an effect is observable and consequential with the other structural analogues of heme, some of which are also strong inducers of HO-1, would be important to understand in the context of selecting a safe drug with a short duration of action, no lingering side effects on other biologic processes, and no long-term alterations in HO-1 gene expression secondary to drug exposure in a critical period.

Besides a wide spectrum of HO inhibitory potential among the different metalloporphyrins, for the two isozymes, the route of administration can also influence the bioavailability and efficacy of the drugs. For example, oral administration may be possible with ZnBG and with chromium mesoporphyrin (CrMP),[51,53,56,57] but with the current formulations, it is unlikely to be possible for SnMP or ZnPP. The packaging of metalloporphyrins for targeting particular tissues, such as the spleen, is also possible. Liposomes have been reported as useful for this purpose.[58] As described above, incorporation of metalloporphyrins, such as ZnPP, into lipid microspheres can enhance oral bioavailability, gastric passage, and intestinal absorption of these compounds.[45] There are probably other targeting approaches that could alter distribution by the various routes of administration.

Another factor to consider when choosing a drug for hyperbilirubinemia is the fact that inhibition of HO in the liver and spleen leads to the proportional excretion of undegraded heme in bile.[59] Thus, it is important to inhibit HO activity in the intestine so that heme reaching the intestine is not catabolized to bilirubin, which can be recirculated via the enterohepatic circulation of bilirubin. Little is known about the effect that most of these drugs have on intestinal HO; however, it is likely that inhibition occurs sufficiently to ensure the overall attenuation of bilirubin production in the clinical setting.

The ideal chemotherapeutic agent should have a relatively short duration of action and have a limited residence time. Unfortunately, little is known about the distribution and duration of action and metabolism of most of the metalloporphyrins.[53,60,61] Of the synthetic analogues, only cobalt protoporphyrin, besides heme, appears to be a substrate for HO and is therefore metabolized like heme. It is also likely that developmental changes may affect the pharmacokinetics of the various heme analogues, and more information is needed, in particular, about the retention of SnMP after administration.

In summary, the ideal compound should have a low I_{50} (dose for 50% inhibition of HO activity); should not be a photosensitizer; should be orally absorbable; should not cross the blood–brain barrier; should be short acting and easily excretable; should not be degraded with subsequent release of the sequestered metal iron; should not substantially upregulate HO-1, mRNA, protein, or activity; and should not affect other enzyme systems.[26,40,53] To date, no compound seems to meet all the ideal characteristics, and compounds vary in their fulfillment of these criteria. Nonetheless, SnMP is the only compound approved as an investigational drug. It has a low I_{50}, it does not appear to cross the blood–brain barrier, but it possesses photoreactive properties and upregulates HO-1.[26,49,53] ZnPP is naturally occurring but has only moderate inhibitory potency. Nevertheless, it is the least likely to be toxic and is not a photosensitizer in vivo. However, it is also unstable under acid (gastric) conditions, cannot be absorbed orally, and upregulates HO-1, but only very briefly. However, its incorporation into lipid microspheres makes it possible for oral use. ZnBG has very high potency, is orally absorbable, but it is a photosensitizer[52] and increases HO-1 transcription minimally.[50] Thus, this compound has a promising potential, as it also contains a biocompatible, essential metal. CrMP is also an interesting compound, which may have promise. It has high inhibitory potency, is orally absorbable, does not cross the blood–brain barrier, and is photochemically inactive. It also does not upregulate HO-1.[56,57] At low doses, it affects only HO-1 and does not affect the activity of NOS or sGC, like the zinc and tin analogues and their derivatives.[53]

D-PENICILLAMINE

D-penicillamine is a chelating agent in use since the 1950s in the treatment of Wilson disease and heavy metal intoxication. It has also been used to treat cystinuria and rheumatoid arthritis. In the early 1970s, D-penicillamine was described as a therapy for neonatal hyperbilirubinemia in Europe.[62] Further studies provided a likely mechanism of action for its use in the treatment of hyperbilirubinemia, indicating that a 3-day course of the drug significantly reduced HO activity levels in neonatal, but not adult rats.[63] A study of D-penicillamine to reduce severe hyperbilirubinemia was conducted in 120 full-term infants with ABO hemolytic disease over a 5-year period, using 60 untreated infants from the first part of the study period as historical controls.[62] If initiated within the first 24 hours of life, treatment with D-penicillamine was associated with significantly reduced TB levels and a decreased need for exchange transfusion in this population. Although the proposed mechanism of its action in decreasing TB levels may be through inhibition of HO activity, this finding has not been confirmed through direct measurement. Its administration (300 to 400 mg per kg per day) has been associated with amelioration of neonatal hyperbilirubinemia; however, its efficacy has not been well proven, especially in light of the considerable risks associated with its use in neonates.

Numerous cutaneous lesions, including urticaria, macular or papular reactions, pemphigoid lesions, and dermatomyositis, have been reported with long-term use of D-penicillamine.[64] Furthermore, significant renal, hepatic, and hematologic complications, including nephrotic syndrome, Goodpasture syndrome, elevation of liver enzymes, aplastic anemia, and thrombocytopenia, have been associated with prolonged therapy for rheumatoid arthritis. The effect of short-term therapy on liver function has been reported in 20 term or near-term infants and on renal function in 30 term or near-term infants.[65] Liver function tests were found to be unchanged after 4.3 ± 1.7 days of treatment with D-penicillamine at a dose of 300 mg per kg per day. Cholesterol, blood urea nitrogen, and creatinine levels were also unaffected after 2.8 ± 1.1 days of D-penicillamine treatment at the same dose. The in vitro effect of the drug on human peripheral granulocytes was also investigated. Superoxide anion generation and β-glucuronidase release were both found to be significantly increased at all concentrations of D-penicillamine; however, phagocytic or killing activity of the granulocytes appeared to be unaffected by the drug.

A decreased incidence of retinopathy of prematurity (ROP) was unexpectedly noted among very low-birth-weight (VLBW) infants treated with D-penicillamine in later studies.[66,67] Recently, a meta-analysis of the effect of prophylactic D-penicillamine on the incidence of ROP in infants of less than 2,000 g BW was undertaken.[68] This review concluded that treatment was unlikely to affect survival and may reduce the incidence of ROP among survivors. It is important to note, however, that these conclusions were based on the findings of only two randomized trials, and that no conclusion could be reached regarding the effect of D-penicillamine on severity of ROP. Further studies are required to fully evaluate the possible efficacy and potential side effects of D-penicillamine in the neonatal population before including this drug in the therapeutic armamentarium.

OTHER NONMETALLOPORPHYRIN INHIBITORS

Peptide inhibitors, originally developed for use in transplantation survival studies from the immunomodulatory peptide 2702.75–84, have been shown to be immunosuppressive in vitro and in vivo.[69] Some of these compounds, such as D2702.75–84, can bind heat shock protein 70 and have also been found to inhibit HO activity in vitro in a dose-dependent manner. However, similar to what has been found with some metalloporphyrins, administration of peptides in mice results in an upregulation of HO-1 mRNA and protein, as well as HO activity in liver, spleen, and kidney. Consequently, human studies using these peptides for the treatment of hyperbilirubinemia have not been performed.

Originally designed to inhibit cholesterol production,[70–72] imidazole dioxolanes, which are structurally different from metalloporphyrins, have also been found to inhibit in vitro[73–76] and in vivo[77] HO activity. These compounds have been observed to have a high selectivity for inhibiting the inducible HO-1.[78] Some of these compounds have been found to affect other important enzymes, such as NOS and sGC, in rat tissues,[74] whereas others, such as Azalanstat, inhibit in vivo HO activity, but only at high doses and also can induce HO-1 gene transcription.[56] However, Hum et al. have shown that the effects of these compounds on HO activity are different between mice and rats and were not due to differences in HO expression.[79] The effects of these compounds have not been evaluated in humans to date.

Inhibition of the downstream step in the generation of bilirubin, the conversion of biliverdin to bilirubin, can be a potential option to reduce bilirubin production without affecting heme catabolism. A recent paper has identified compounds (e.g., disulfiram and montelukast) that can inhibit biliverdin reductase activity in vitro. However, these compounds have been shown to not lower TB levels in the *Ugt1a1*-deficient (Gunn) rat, a model for chronic hyperbilirubinemia.[80]

DRUGS INCREASING CONJUGATION OF BILIRUBIN

Several pharmacologic compounds have been found to induce UGT activity in hepatocytes and thereby increase the conjugation and excretion of bilirubin. Phenobarbital and nicotinamide were the first of such agents used for the prevention and treatment of hyperbilirubinemia. Phenobarbital continues to be used in the treatment of Gilbert syndrome and Crigler–Najjar syndrome type II (Arias) disease. Crigler–Najjar syndrome type I disease does not respond well to this therapy.[81]

PHENOBARBITAL

A state of limited bilirubin clearance exists in the immediate neonatal period. The associated causes for this phenomenon include a relatively immature neonatal hepatic enzyme system in general, including UGT, as demonstrated by studies in both humans and animal models.[82–86] In addition, it has been suggested that the lack of bilirubin in the in utero environment, owing to mature maternal bilirubin conjugation and elimination systems in the normal state, results in the absence of a potent natural inducer of UGT.[87,88]

Phenobarbital has been shown to induce a number of hepatic enzymes, including UGT.[89–91] The phenobarbital response enhancer sequence of the *UGT1A1* gene has recently been delineated.[92] Further research demonstrated a successful reduction of TB levels with phenobarbital therapy in patients with mild or moderate Crigler–Najjar syndrome.[93–96] These studies, and a retrospective analysis demonstrating a decreased incidence of neonatal jaundice in infants of mothers treated with phenobarbital for seizure disorders,[97] led to additional clinical investigations of the efficacy of antenatal and postnatal phenobarbital for neonatal hyperbilirubinemia.

Antenatal Phenobarbital

The available studies of antenatal phenobarbital for the prevention of neonatal hyperbilirubinemia differ broadly in terms of dose, length of treatment, target patient population, and sample size.[98–103] Comparison of studies is therefore less than optimal. In general, the studies indicate that antenatal phenobarbital treatment was associated with a lower incidence of neonatal jaundice. A daily dose of 30 mg[98,103] was less effective than a daily dose of 60 to 100 mg in both reducing neonatal TB levels at 48 hours to 4 days of age and decreasing incidence of significant hyperbilirubinemia or need for phototherapy. In the randomized trial by Rayburn et al.,[101] which focused on VLBW infants, a daily dose of 90 mg of phenobarbital was given to women with arrested premature labor at 26 to 33 weeks of gestation. Conjugated bilirubin levels were found to be significantly higher among infants of the phenobarbital-treated group, and need for phototherapy significantly decreased. Initiation of phototherapy was also delayed among infants of treated mothers. In the very large randomized controlled trial of antenatal phenobarbital therapy in Greece by Valaes et al.,[104] a highly significant decrease in neonatal TB levels was demonstrated among infants of treated mothers; however, this effect was dependent on the mothers' receipt of at least 10 daily doses of 100 mg of phenobarbital prior to delivery. Among infants exposed to this phenobarbital regimen in utero, the need for exchange transfusion was all but eliminated (1.4% vs. 0.23%, $p < 0.001$). The three infants who required exchange transfusion in the treatment group were all noted to have hemolytic diseases.

The true need for and actual applicability of such a prophylactic therapy for neonatal hyperbilirubinemia is questionable. For populations at very high risk for severe neonatal hyperbilirubinemia, this approach appears attractive, although alternative therapies have been more recently proposed. Metalloporphyrin treatment for infants would have the advantage of a much shorter course of therapy and would eliminate the need for early prenatal identification of high-risk mothers. It is unclear whether the cost of a single postnatal metalloporphyrin injection would outweigh that of a full course of antenatal phenobarbital. Similarly, the safety of each therapy remains to be established definitively; however, data regarding the neurodevelopmental outcome of infants exposed to antenatal phenobarbital suggest that risks in this regard are limited. In the Greek antenatal phenobarbital study by Valaes et al.,[104] no difference in neurodevelopmental outcome was seen between treated and untreated infants among a small subgroup of infants who were examined at 61 to 82 months of age. Long-term follow-up studies have also been published of premature infants enrolled in a National Institute of Child Health and Human Development (NICHD) Neonatal Research Network–sponsored randomized controlled trial of antenatal phenobarbital for reducing the incidence of intraventricular hemorrhage (IVH).[105–107] There were no significant differences in Bayley Scales of Infant Development scores or incidence of cerebral palsy between treatment and control groups at 18 to 22 months corrected age.[108] Furthermore, there were no significant differences in McCarthy Scales of Children's Abilities scores or the incidence of neurologic deficits noted on examination at 36 months.[107] It is crucial to note, however, that although 93% of women enrolled received the entire first infusion dose of 10 mg per kg body weight, only 33% received one or more oral maintenance doses of 100 mg per day.[105] Therefore, the cumulative phenobarbital exposure in this study is unlikely to approach what would be required for significant reduction in neonatal TB levels.

Other potential risks of treatment are of more concern. Antenatal phenobarbital is known to significantly decrease vitamin K–dependent clotting factors in the newborn, as demonstrated by reports of hemorrhagic complications of infants born to epileptic women[108–110] and in the Greek antenatal phenobarbital trial.[111] Vitamin K injection at birth was shown to correct these clotting abnormalities at 48 to 72 hours, but there were significant hemorrhagic findings in two of the phenobarbital-exposed infants, including one with subgaleal hemorrhage. None of the control infants had hemorrhagic complications. Increased somnolence was reported among phenobarbital-treated mothers compared with controls in the trial of antenatal phenobarbital for IVH reduction[107]; however, no significant sedation effects have been observed among infants born to mothers treated with phenobarbital to prevent neonatal jaundice.

Postnatal Phenobarbital

The mechanistic basis for postnatal phenobarbital is the same as that for antenatal treatment: UGT activity is induced, enhancing bilirubin conjugation and subsequent elimination. In addition, an increase in bile flow with phenobarbital treatment has been reported, putatively mediated by the induction of multidrug resistance protein-2 (MRP-2).[112] Unfortunately, it is clear that there is a delay from initiation of phenobarbital treatment to clinical effectiveness. From a practical standpoint, the usefulness of phenobarbital for the treatment of neonatal hyperbilirubinemia is therefore limited in the era of phototherapy.

Comparison of studies of postnatal phenobarbital therapy are limited by many of the same shortcomings that were described in relation to antenatal treatment studies: sample size in most studies is very small, patient population and treatment regimen differ from study to study, and timing of study enrollment or endpoints and main outcomes, such as neonatal TB levels or the need for particular therapy, are not consistent among reports. Studies from the late 1960s and early 1970s[100,102,113–119] reported decreased TB levels at 3 to 7 days of age, although statistically significant differences between treatment and control groups were not observed in all studies. In general, a decrease in the need for exchange transfusion was also observed in phenobarbital-treated infants compared with control, especially among the low-birth-weight (LBW) population. Phenobarbital doses used in these studies ranged from 2 to 10 mg per kg per day, and drug was administered intramuscularly or orally. Because of the numerous differences in study designs, it is difficult to ascertain which would be the most efficacious phenobarbital dosage regimen. A randomized controlled study of the effect of different single phenobarbital doses (0 to 12 mg per kg) in preventing neonatal hyperbilirubinemia[120] indicated that patients only in the 12 mg per kg group had a significantly improved TB disappearance rate, which was not evident until day 7 of life. However, sample size was extremely small (approximately 10 patients in each of the four groups), and dosing regimen was arguably limited in terms of consistency with clinical practice.

Although postnatal phenobarbital alone is inappropriate for the treatment of neonatal hyperbilirubinemia in the current era, the therapeutic combination of phototherapy and phenobarbital has been suggested. Blackburn et al.[121] reported no advantage to phenobarbital with phototherapy compared with phototherapy alone in the premature population. However, in scenarios of ongoing hemolysis, such as clinically significant ABO incompatibility or Rh sensitization, the addition of phenobarbital to the treatment regimen may be of potential benefit.

MINOCYCLINE

Minocycline, a semisynthetic second-generation tetracycline, has been shown to exert beneficial anti-inflammatory effects that are independent of its antimicrobial actions.[122] It has also been shown to inhibit matrix metalloproteinases, superoxide production, and iNOS expression.[123] In a recent study by Lin et al.,[124] minocycline was shown to afford neuroprotection against cerebellar damage due to hyperbilirubinemia in the Gunn rat. In 2007, also using the Gunn rat model, Shapiro and colleagues[125] reported that minocycline protects the central auditory system from acute bilirubin neurotoxicity. However, the exact mechanism by which minocycline might be protective is largely speculative.[124,126]

CLOFIBRATE

Clofibrate, the ethyl ester of 2-chlorophenoxy-2-methylpropionic acid, has been primarily used as an antilipemic agent in adult patients with hyperlipoproteinemia.[127,128] The drug is an activator of peroxisome proliferator–activated receptors[129] and has also been shown to enhance UGT activity in rats,[130] significantly increasing hepatic clearance of bilirubin within hours. Subsequently, clofibrate was shown to decrease unconjugated TB levels in adult patients with Gilbert syndrome.[127] Two randomized controlled trials of clofibrate for the treatment or prophylaxis of neonatal jaundice have been performed in Europe. In the first of these studies,[131] 93 term infants with hyperbilirubinemia before day 5 of life were randomized to receive either a single 50 mg per kg oral dose of clofibrate or an equal volume of placebo. The treatment group had significantly lower TB levels than controls from 16 hours after drug or placebo administration. In a later study,[132] 89 infants of 31 to 36 weeks estimated gestational age were randomized to receive either a single 100 mg per kg dose of clofibrate or placebo during day 2 of life. Significantly reduced TB levels were reported in the treatment group compared with controls from 48 hours after drug or placebo dosing.

Concerns regarding the safety of clofibrate in the neonatal population have been raised.[133] Studies in rats have demonstrated carcinogenic properties primarily affecting the liver and pancreas by an unknown mechanism. However, these properties are likely to be observed only after prolonged therapy and furthermore, two multicenter studies of clofibrate in adults demonstrated no significant increase in cancer-related mortality in treated compared with untreated patients after analyses of long-term follow-up data.[134,135] No long-term follow-up studies were undertaken in the two neonatal studies noted previously.[131,132] An acute muscular syndrome has also been described but reportedly only in the presence of high serum levels of clofibric acid. Finally, concerns regarding displacement of bilirubin from Alb by clofibric acid have been raised, which have been refuted by Gabilan et al.[136] Many more neonatal-specific pharmacokinetic, safety, and efficacy studies would likely be required before clofibrate treatment for neonatal jaundice could be routinely considered. Given the relatively ready accessibility to phototherapy in the United States, this would seem to be a highly unlikely prospect.

CHINESE HERBAL REMEDIES

A number of traditional Chinese herbal medicines have properties of inducing UGT activity similar to that of phenobarbital.[137] It has been common practice among Chinese women to take herbal remedies during pregnancy. These herbs have been shown to accelerate plasma clearance and conjugation of bilirubin but have different effects on other liver enzymes, most likely due to different mechanisms of action. Exposure to herbs either before or after birth has been suspected to be a cause of hemolysis and jaundice in newborns, such that a number of herbs have been implicated in causing hemolysis in infants with G6PD deficiency. It can be concluded that although herbal treatment has been practiced for a long time in China, its effectiveness remains doubtful with no convincing evidence without properly controlled randomized clinical studies.

Herbs and Chinese herbal combinations have for centuries been used for the treatment of neonatal jaundice. Only relatively recently, however, have these traditional remedies been critically studied by Western medical researchers. In a review of the Chinese literature,[138] *Artemisia* (*Yin-chin*, or Oriental wormwood) was the most commonly used herb for neonatal jaundice. Other commonly used herbs included *Glycyrrhiza* (*Gan-coa*, or licorice), *Scutellaria baicalensis* (*Huang-qin*, or skullcap root), *Rheum officinale* (*Da-huang*, or rhubarb), and *Coptis chinensis* (*Huang-lian*, or goldthread rhizome). In the 1980s, treatment with the herbal combination known as *Yin zhi huang* (YZH), consisting of *Artemisia*, *Gardenia*, *Rheum*, and *Scutellaria*, as well as another traditional herbal combination, was shown to decrease neonatal TB levels after 3 to 4 days.[139,140] Subsequent studies revealed increased conjugation and clearance of bilirubin in animal models after YZH similar to that seen after phenobarbital,[141,142] although the pattern of hepatic enzyme induction was different.[137] Further delineation of the individual components of YZH revealed that *Artemisia* and *Rheum*, but not *Gardenia* or *Scutellaria*, were potent inducers of UGT.[143] Cytochrome P450 levels of animals treated with individual component herbs of YZH were shown to be similar to control and lower among those animals treated with *Gardenia*. This is in sharp contrast to the significant elevation of cytochrome P450 levels seen among animals treated with phenobarbital.

The safety of these traditional remedies has not been adequately studied. However, some of these herbs have been shown to possess potentially extremely dangerous properties in the setting of neonatal hyperbilirubinemia. *Artemisia*, for example, can displace bilirubin from Alb, which could lead to enhanced neurotoxicity.[144,145] The alkaloid berberine, which is contained in *Huang-lian*, can cause severe acute hemolysis in patients with G6PD deficiency.[138] Contamination of herbal medicines with heavy metals has also been reported.[146] In light of the unregulated atmosphere in which these herbal remedies are currently produced, inconsistencies in preparation, and inability to reliably assess concentrations of individual herbal components or presence of contaminants, the use of these therapies cannot be recommended.

ACTIGALL

Actigall, or ursodeoxycholic acid (UDCA), is primarily used for the treatment of cholestatic liver diseases but has been suggested to be useful for the treatment of hyperbilirubinemia in patients with Crigler–Najjar syndrome.[147] Experimental evidence suggests that its mechanisms of action may be mediated through the stimulation of hepatobiliary secretion, via Ca^{2+}- and protein kinase C-α-dependent mechanisms and/or activation of p38 (mitogen-activated protein kinase) and extracellular signal-regulated kinases, resulting in insertion of transporter molecules [e.g., bile salt export pump and conjugate export pump (MRP-2)]. Future studies need to be performed to investigate dosage regimens as well as to elucidate the mechanisms of action of UDCA at the molecular level[148] and potential toxicities in the newborn.

George et al.[149] conducted a retrospective study reviewing the efficacy of Actigall in the treatment of hyperbilirubinemia in a pediatric intensive care unit population. Actigall administered at a dose of 20 mg per kg per day to five pediatric intensive care unit patients resulted in a decrease in TB levels with no adverse effects in four patients. These preliminary findings suggest that Actigall is effective in the treatment of hyperbilirubinemia. However, a prospective, randomized trial is warranted to further assess the efficacy of this therapy before use in the neonatal population.

REDUCTION OF ENTEROHEPATIC CIRCULATION OF BILIRUBIN

Neonatal hyperbilirubinemia is exacerbated and may be caused by enhanced reabsorption of bilirubin in the enterohepatic circulation. The absence of intestinal flora in neonates prevents the degradation of bilirubin in meconium and stool to products such as urobilinogen, which can be excreted. Bilirubin glucuronides entering the intestines are readily deconjugated to bilirubin and subsequently reabsorbed. To circumvent this process, various strategies have been developed to bind the bilirubin in the intestinal lumen to substances that resist absorption.

BILIRUBIN OXIDASE

Bilirubin oxidase (BOX), derived from the fungus *Myrothecium verrucaria*, has been found to interrupt bilirubin reabsorption by oxidizing bilirubin to biliverdin and other less toxic and more water-soluble products in order to be excreted.[150,151] A study by Soltys et al.[151] showed that the in vivo administration of 0.1 to 2.0 mg per day of BOX to chronically jaundiced Gunn rats over a 4-day period effectively decreased TB levels from 11.3 to 6.3 mg per dL (193 to 108 μmol per L) (−40%, $n = 5$; $p < 0.05$). However, the decrease was observed only when the molar ratio of TB to rat serum Alb was greater than 0.35. When BOX was administered to rats with a ratio less than 0.35 ($n = 10$), there was no statistically significant change in TB levels. Because large-scale human studies are lacking, the potential for use of BOX for the treatment of neonatal hyperbilirubinemia is still under investigation.[152]

ORAL FEEDING

Initiation of oral feedings can ameliorate the accumulation of bilirubin in the intestines and its enterohepatic recirculation. Formula feeding is most influential in this regard, but successful breastfeeding has a similar effect.

CHARCOAL

Activated charcoal administered by gavage feeding can reduce TB levels by binding bilirubin in the intestinal lumen and reducing the enterohepatic circulation of unconjugated bilirubin. The effectiveness of activated charcoal as an adjunct to phototherapy in reducing TB levels has been studied in the jaundiced rat.[153,154] The administration of charcoal by feeding or gavage was shown to be effective in reducing TB levels in both the adult and the suckling jaundiced rat. Charcoal feeding and phototherapy administered jointly in the adult rat was shown to be additive in significantly lowering TB levels when compared with reductions in TB levels of those given charcoal alone. In the suckling rat, TB levels were also significantly reduced after the administration of either charcoal alone or charcoal in combination with phototherapy; however, the combination of treatments did not appear to be additive. These findings suggest that charcoal can be used as an adjunct to phototherapy and that charcoal used in combination with phototherapy may also reduce the intensity of phototherapy needed to effectively lower TB levels.

Amitai et al.[155] prospectively studied the efficacy of multiple-dose oral activated charcoal (OAC) therapy for neonatal hyperbilirubinemia in 30 jaundiced newborns receiving phototherapy. For newborns under phototherapy who received OAC before meals with a total amount of 8.5 ± 0.85 g (mean ± SE, $n = 14$) and for infants receiving phototherapy only (controls, $n = 16$), TB levels on initiation of phototherapy were 265 ± 8 and 253 ± 4 μmol per L (15.5 ± 0.5 and 14.7 ± 0.2 mg per dL), respectively. After 24 hours, there was no significant decrease in TB levels in the control group [240 ± 8 μmol per L (14.0 ± 0.5 mg per dL)], but TB levels of the study group decreased [235 ± 7 μmol per L (13.7 ± 1.0 mg per dL); $p < 0.02$]. For both groups, TB levels were significantly lower than baseline values 48 hours after initiation of phototherapy. However, the decline in TB levels in the study group [56 ± 10 μmol per L (3.3 ± 0.6 mg per dL)] was greater than that of the controls [21 ± 10 μmol per L (1.2 ± 0.6 mg per dL); $p < 0.02$]. It was concluded that OAC seems to be an effective adjunct to phototherapy in the treatment of neonatal hyperbilirubinemia.

AGAR

Plain dried agar, an extract of seaweed, has been shown to effectively decrease TB levels by binding to bilirubin in the gut and increasing stool frequency. Consequently, the enterohepatic circulation of bilirubin is decreased, which in turn leads to an enhanced clearance of intraluminal bilirubin and decreased TB levels.

An early study[156] investigating the efficacy of oral agar supplementation (600 mg per kg) in LBW infants (1,500 to 2,500 g) at 12 hours of age for 7 days found that TB levels were not significantly lower in the agar-fed infants. It was concluded that agar-supplemented oral feeding is not indicated in the management of hyperbilirubinemia in LBW infants. In 1977, Ebbesen and Moller[157] evaluated the ingestion of agar used as an adjunct to phototherapy and found that TB levels were decreased regardless of agar ingestion and concluded that oral agar does not supplement the effect of phototherapy alone.

In another study that investigated the effect of oral agar in term and preterm newborns,[158] it was observed that agar ingestion decreased TB levels and increased fecal elimination of the pigment ($p < 0.001$) only in term newborns and not in preterm newborns.

Odell et al.[159] tested the hypothesis that sequestration of luminal unconjugated bilirubin by enteral agar administration would enhance the efficacy of phototherapy in jaundiced infants. They found that the rate of decline of TB concentrations after 24 hours of phototherapy was greater and significantly more uniform in the agar-supplemented infants [−1.59 ± 2.3 vs. −2.51 ± 1.44 mg per dL (−27 ± 39 vs. −429 ± 25 μmol per L)]. Stool frequencies were greater in control infants (5.5 vs. 4.3 mg per kg per 24 hours), whereas fecal bilirubin excretions were greater in agar-supplemented infants during the second day of phototherapy (1.32 vs. 3.29 mg per kg per 24 hours). In addition, agar supplementation reduced the duration of phototherapy by 23% (37.6 ± 3.2 vs. 48.1 ± 5.0 hours).

The value of oral agar in the treatment of neonatal hyperbilirubinemia was determined and compared with phototherapy alone and phototherapy plus oral agar.[160] Oral agar was found to be as effective as phototherapy, with the most significant decrease in TB levels in infants treated with both phototherapy and oral agar. It was concluded that the efficacy of phototherapy in decreasing the TB levels could be enhanced with the use of oral agar. In addition, oral agar can also be used alone for the treatment of neonatal hyperbilirubinemia because it is as effective as phototherapy.

A meta-analysis of nine prospective clinical trials evaluating agar therapy found these studies at risk for biased treatment allocation.[161] Although the pooled data analysis suggests that prophylactic agar treatment is associated with reduced peak TB levels, this observation must be interpreted cautiously in light of heterogeneous patient populations and the methodologic problems. Based on this meta-analysis, agar therapy for neonatal jaundice can neither be recommended nor rejected.

BILIRUBIN BINDING

Bilirubin in circulation is predominantly bound to Alb. Although the binding ratio is potentially 1:1 and avid, Alb levels are lower in premature and sick infants, and binding affinity is often diminished.[162] Furthermore, some drugs (e.g., sulfisoxazole, benzoate) can compete with bilirubin for binding to Alb, causing displacement of bilirubin.[163,164] Therefore, prior to exchange transfusion, Alb can be administered (1 g per kg) to improve the efficacy of the exchange.

A method has been described by Ahlfors[165–167] for measuring the unconjugated fraction of the UB concentration in plasma by combining the peroxidase method for determining UB with a diazo method for measuring conjugated and unconjugated bilirubin. The accuracy of the UB determination is improved by decreasing sample dilution, eliminating interference by conjugated bilirubin, monitoring changes in bilirubin concentration, and correcting for rate-limiting dissociation of bilirubin from Alb. It was found that the unbound unconjugated bilirubin concentration by this method in plasma from 20 jaundiced newborns was significantly greater than and poorly correlated ($r = 0.7$) with the UB determined by the existing peroxidase method.[168] This may be possibly due to differences in sample dilution between the two methods. The unbound unconjugated bilirubin was an unpredictable fraction of the UB in plasma samples from patients with similar TB concentrations but varying levels of conjugated bilirubin. A bilirubin-binding competitor was readily detected at a sample dilution typically used for the combined test but not at the dilution used for the existing peroxidase method. The combined method is ideally suited to measuring unbound unconjugated bilirubin in jaundiced human newborns or animal models of kernicterus.[169]

SUMMARY

Besides phototherapy, the HO inhibitors are the most promising therapeutic agents for the prevention and treatment of neonatal jaundice. Whether any of these compounds would be suitable for universal prophylaxis for the essentially ubiquitous phenomenon of transitional hyperbilirubinemia of the neonate would depend upon the relative frequency of pathologic jaundice [>17 mg per dL (291 µmol per L)] in the population and the relative safety and efficacy of the compounds. A targeted approach for infants at higher risk for pathologic jaundice is a more likely scenario. Nonetheless, chemotherapeutic approaches for the management of hyperbilirubinemia may become more important if phototherapy applied to small, very immature, and relatively translucent neonates (<1,500 g) were found to pose previously unrecognized risks.[170] Most likely, phototherapy will remain the mainstay of therapy for most jaundiced neonates, but understanding the biology of newborn jaundice and further development of alternative pharmacologic therapies for neonatal hyperbilirubinemia will broaden the options for the management of neonatal jaundice and its consequences.

ACKNOWLEDGMENTS

This work was supported by the National Institutes of Health, grants HL68703 and HD/HL58013, the Christopher Hess Research Fund, the L. H. M. Lui Research Fund, and the Mary L. Johnson Research Fund.

REFERENCES

1. American Academy of Pediatrics. Management of hyperbilirubinemia in the newborn infant 35 or more weeks of gestation. *Pediatrics* 2004;114(1):297–316.
2. Maisels MJ. Phototherapy – traditional and nontraditional. *J Perinatol* 2001;21(Suppl 1):S93—S97; discussion S104—S107.
3. Vreman HJ, Wong RJ, Stevenson DK. Phototherapy: current methods and future directions. *Semin Perinatol* 2004;28(5):326–333.
4. Seidman DS, Moise J, Ergaz Z, et al. A new blue light-emitting phototherapy device: a prospective randomized controlled study. *J Pediatr* 2000;136(6):771–774.
5. Vreman HJ, Wong RJ, Stevenson DK. Light emitting diodes for phototherapy for the control of jaundice. In: Holick MF, ed. *Biology of light*. Boston, MA: Kluwer Academic Publishers, 2001:355–367.
6. Wong RJ, Stevenson DK, Ahlfors CE, et al. Neonatal jaundice: bilirubin physiology and clinical chemistry. *NeoReviews* 2007;8:e58–67.
7. Yao TC, Stevenson DK. Advances in the diagnosis and treatment of neonatal hyperbilirubinemia. *Clin Perinatol* 1995;22(3):741–758.
8. Dennery PA, Seidman DS, Stevenson DK. Neonatal hyperbilirubinemia. *N Engl J Med* 2001;344(8):581–590.
9. Kaplan M, Muraca M, Hammerman C, et al. Imbalance between production and conjugation of bilirubin: a fundamental concept in the mechanism of neonatal jaundice. *Pediatrics* 2002;110(4):e47
10. Stevenson DK, Vreman HJ, Oh W, et al. Bilirubin production in healthy term infants as measured by carbon monoxide in breath. *Clin Chem* 1994;40(10):1934–1939.
11. Vreman HJ, Rodgers PA, Gale R, et al. Carbon monoxide excretion as an index of bilirubin production in rhesus monkeys. *J Med Primatol* 1989;18(6):449–460.
12. Kaplan M, Renbaum P, Levy-Lahad E, et al. Gilbert syndrome and glucose-6-phosphate dehydrogenase deficiency: a dose-dependent genetic interaction crucial to neonatal hyperbilirubinemia. *Proc Natl Acad Sci U S A* 1997;94(22):12128–12132.
13. Koiwai O, Nishizawa M, Hasada K, et al. Gilbert's syndrome is caused by a heterozygous missense mutation in the gene for bilirubin UDP-glucuronosyltransferase. *Hum Mol Genet* 1995;4(7):1183–1186.
14. Kaplan M, Hammerman C, Maisels MJ. Bilirubin genetics for the nongeneticist: hereditary defects of neonatal bilirubin conjugation. *Pediatrics* 2003;111(4 Pt 1):886–893.
15. Akaba K, Kimura T, Sasaki A, et al. Neonatal hyperbilirubinemia and mutation of the bilirubin uridine diphosphate-glucuronosyltransferase gene: a common missense mutation among Japanese, Koreans and Chinese. *Biochem Mol Biol Int* 1998;46(1):21–26.
16. Beutler E, Gelbart T, Demina A. Racial variability in the UDP-glucuronosyltransferase 1 (UGT1A1) promoter: a balanced polymorphism for regulation of bilirubin metabolism? *Proc Natl Acad Sci U S A* 1998;95(14):8170–8174.
17. Lin Z, Fontaine J, Watchko JF. Coexpression of gene polymorphisms involved in bilirubin production and metabolism. *Pediatrics* 2008;122(1):e156–162.
18. Huang CS, Chang PF, Huang MJ, et al. Glucose-6-phosphate dehydrogenase deficiency, the UDP-glucuronosyl transferase 1A1 gene, and neonatal hyperbilirubinemia. *Gastroenterology* 2002;123(1):127–133.
19. Vreman HJ, Mahoney JJ, Stevenson DK. Carbon monoxide and carboxyhemoglobin. *Adv Pediatr* 1995;42:303–325.
20. Vreman HJ, Wong RJ, Stevenson DK. Carbon monoxide in breath, blood, and other tissues. In: Penney DG, ed. *Carbon monoxide toxicity*. Boca Raton, FL: CRC Press, 2000:19–60.
21. Widness JA, Lowe LS, Stevenson DK, et al. Direct relationship of fetal carboxyhemoglobin with hemolysis in alloimmunized pregnancies. *Pediatr Res* 1994;35(6):713–719.
22. Bhutani VK, Johnson L, Sivieri EM. Predictive ability of a predischarge hour-specific serum bilirubin for subsequent significant hyperbilirubinemia in healthy term and near-term newborns. *Pediatrics* 1999;103(1):6–14.
23. Stevenson DK, Fanaroff AA, Maisels MJ, et al. Prediction of hyperbilirubinemia in near-term and term infants. *Pediatrics* 2001;108(1):31–39.
24. Tenhunen R, Marver HS, Schmid R. The enzymatic conversion of heme to bilirubin by microsomal heme oxygenase. *Proc Natl Acad Sci U S A* 1968;61(2):748–755.
25. Stevenson DK, Rodgers PA, Vreman HJ. The use of metalloporphyrins for the chemoprevention of neonatal jaundice. *Am J Dis Child* 1989;143(3):353–356.
26. Wong RJ, Bhutani VK, Vreman HJ, et al. Tin mesoporphyrin for the prevention of severe neonatal hyperbilirubinemia. *NeoReviews* 2007;8:e77—e84.
27. Maines MD. Zinc•protoporphyrin is a selective inhibitor of heme oxygenase activity in the neonatal rat. *Biochim Biophys Acta* 1981;673(3):339–350.
28. Wong RJ, Vreman HJ, Schulz S, et al. *In vitro* inhibition of heme oxygenase isoenzymes by metalloporphyrins. *J Perinatol* 2011;31(Suppl 1):S35—S41.
29. Appleton SD, Chretien ML, McLaughlin BE, et al. Selective inhibition of heme oxygenase, without inhibition of nitric oxide synthase or soluble guanylyl cyclase, by metalloporphyrins at low concentrations. *Drug Metab Dispos* 1999;27(10):1214–1219.
30. Wong RJ, Vreman HJ, Stevenson DK. (Metallo)porphyrin inhibitors of heme oxygenase also inhibit lipid peroxidation (LP). *Pediatr Res* 2000;47:465–465.
31. Dore S, Snyder SH. Neuroprotective action of bilirubin against oxidative stress in primary hippocampal cultures. *Ann NY Acad Sci* 1999;890:167–172.
32. Stocker R, McDonagh AF, Glazer AN, et al. Antioxidant activities of bile pigments: Biliverdin and bilirubin. *Methods Enzymol* 1990;186:301–309.
33. Stocker R, Yamamoto Y, McDonagh AF, et al. Bilirubin is an antioxidant of possible physiological importance. *Science* 1987;235(4792):1043–1046.
34. Stevenson DK, Vreman HJ, Wong RJ, et al. Carbon monoxide detection and biological investigations. *Trans Am Clin Climatol Assoc* 2000;111:61–75.
35. Drummond GS, Galbraith RA, Sardana MK, et al. Reduction of the C2 and C4 vinyl groups of Sn-protoporphyrin to form Sn-mesoporphyrin markedly enhances the ability of the metalloporphyrin to inhibit *in vivo* heme catabolism. *Arch Biochem Biophys* 1987;255(1):64–74.
36. Drummond GS, Kappas A. Prevention of neonatal hyperbilirubinemia by tin protoporphyrin IX, a potent competitive inhibitor of heme oxidation. *Proc Natl Acad Sci U S A* 1981;78(10):6466–6470.
37. Drummond GS, Kappas A. Sn-protoporphyrin inhibition of fetal and neonatal brain heme oxygenase. Transplacental passage of the metalloporphyrin and prenatal suppression of hyperbilirubinemia in the newborn animal. *J Clin Invest* 1986;77(3):971–976.
38. Vreman HJ, Cipkala DA, Stevenson DK. Characterization of porphyrin heme oxygenase inhibitors. *Can J Physiol Pharmacol* 1996;74(3):278–285.
39. Vreman HJ, Ekstrand BC, Stevenson DK. Selection of metalloporphyrin heme oxygenase inhibitors based on potency and photoreactivity. *Pediatr Res* 1993;33(2):195–200.
40. Vreman HJ, Wong RJ, Stevenson DK. Alternative metalloporphyrins for the treatment of neonatal jaundice. *J Perinatol* 2001;21(Suppl 1):S108–113.
41. Martinez JC, Garcia HO, Otheguy LE, et al. Control of severe hyperbilirubinemia in full-term newborns with the inhibitor of bilirubin production Sn-mesoporphyrin. *Pediatrics* 1999;103(1):1–5.
42. Valaes T, Petmezaki S, Henschke C, et al. Control of jaundice in preterm newborns by an inhibitor of bilirubin production: studies with tin-mesoporphyrin. *Pediatrics* 1994;93(1):1–11.
43. Reddy P, Najundaswamy S, Mehta R, et al. Tin-mesoporphyrin in the treatment of severe hyperbilirubinemia in a very-low-birth-weight infant. *J Perinatol* 2003;23(6):507–508.
44. Wong RJ, Schulz S, Espadas C, et al. Effects of light on metalloporphyrin-treated newborn mice. *Acta Paediatr* 2014;103(5):474–479.
45. Fujioka K, Kalish F, Wong RJ, et al. Inhibition of heme oxygenase activity using a microparticle formulation of zinc protoporphyrin in an acute hemolytic newborn mouse model. *Pediatr Res* 2016;79(2):251–257.
46. Jacobsen D, Iwatani S, Onderdonk Z, et al. *In vitro* inhibitory potency of zinc protoporphyrin microspheres on heme oxygenase isozyme activity. *J Invest Med* 2019;67:63–288.
47. Vreman HJ, Gillman MJ, Stevenson DK. *In vitro* inhibition of adult rat intestinal heme oxygenase by metalloporphyrins. *Pediatr Res* 1989;26(4):362–365.
48. Morioka I, Wong RJ, Abate A, et al. Systemic effects of orally-administered zinc and tin (IV) metalloporphyrins on heme oxygenase expression in mice. *Pediatr Res* 2006;59(5):667–672.
49. Wong RJ, Abate A, Dennery PA, et al. Direct intestinal administration of metalloporphyrins and heme oxygenase expression. *J Invest Med* 2003;51:S140.
50. Zhang W, Contag PR, Hardy J, et al. Selection of potential therapeutics based on *in vivo* spatiotemporal transcription patterns of heme oxygenase-1. *J Mol Med* 2002;80(10):655–664.
51. Vallier HA, Rodgers PA, Stevenson DK. Oral administration of zinc deuteroporphyrin IX 2,4 bis glycol inhibits heme oxygenase in neonatal rats. *Dev Pharmacol Ther* 1991;17(3–4):220–222.
52. Vreman HJ, Lee OK, Stevenson DK. *In vitro* and *in vivo* characteristics of a heme oxygenase inhibitor: ZnBG. *Am J Med Sci* 1991;302(6):335–341.
53. Schulz S, Wong RJ, Vreman HJ, et al. Metalloporphyrins – an update. *Front Pharmacol* 2012;3:68.
54. Labbé RF, Vreman HJ, Stevenson DK. Zinc protoporphyrin: a metabolite with a mission. *Clin Chem* 1999;45(12):2060–2072.
55. Hajdena-Dawson M, Zhang W, Contag PR, et al. Effects of metalloporphyrins on heme oxygenase-1 transcription: correlative cell culture assays guide *in vivo* imaging. *Mol Imaging* 2003;2(3):138–149.
56. Morisawa T, Wong RJ, Xiao H, et al. Inhibition of heme oxygenase activity by chromium mesoporphyrin in the heme-loaded newborn mouse. *E-PAS2008*;2008:6130.6139.
57. Xiao H, Morisawa T, Wong RJ, et al. Short-and long-term effects of heme oxygenase activity by chromium mesoporphyrin in newborn mice. *EPAS2008*;2008:6130.6138.

58. Hamori CJ, Lasic DD, Vreman HJ, et al. Targeting zinc protoporphyrin liposomes to the spleen using reticuloendothelial blockade with blank liposomes. *Pediatr Res* 1993;34(1):1–5.
59. Hintz SR, Kwong LK, Vreman HJ, et al. Recovery of exogenous heme as carbon monoxide and biliary heme in adult rats after tin protoporphyrin treatment. *J Pediatr Gastroenterol Nutr* 1987;6(2):302–306.
60. Anderson KE, Simionatto CS, Drummond GS, et al. Tissue distribution and disposition of tin-protoporphyrin, a potent competitive inhibitor of heme oxygenase. *J Pharmacol Exp Ther* 1984;228(2):327–333.
61. Anderson KE, Simionatto CS, Drummond GS, et al. Disposition of tin-protoporphyrin and suppression of hyperbilirubinemia in humans. *Clin Pharmacol Ther* 1986;39(5):510–520.
62. Lakatos L, Kover B, Peter F. D-penicillamine therapy of neonatal hyperbilirubinaemia. *Acta Paediatr Acad Sci Hung* 1974;15(1):77–85.
63. Oroszlan G, Lakatos L, Szabo L, et al. Heme oxygenase activity is decreased by D-penicillamine in neonates. *Experientia* 1983;39(8):888–889.
64. Levy RS, Fisher M, Alter JN. Penicillamine: review and cutaneous manifestations. *J Am Acad Dermatol* 1983;8(4):548–558.
65. Lakatos L, Szabo I, Csathy L. The effects of D-penicillamine on the renal and liver functions in neonates and the *in vitro* influence on granulocytes. *Acta Paediatr Scand Suppl* 1989;360:135–139.
66. Lakatos L. D-penicillamine and retinopathy of prematurity. *Pediatrics* 1988;82(6):951–953.
67. Lakatos L, Hatvani I, Oroszlan G, et al. D-penicillamine in the prevention of retrolental fibroplasia. *Acta Paediatr Acad Sci Hung* 1982;23(3):327–335.
68. Phelps DL, Lakatos L, Watts JL. D-Penicillamine for preventing retinopathy of prematurity in preterm infants. *Cochrane Database Syst Rev* 2001;(1):CD001073.
69. Iyer S, Woo J, Cornejo MC, et al. Characterization and biological significance of immunosuppressive peptide D2702.75-84(E-> V) binding protein. Isolation of heme oxygenase-1. *J Biol Chem* 1998;273(5):2692–2697.
70. Burton PM, Swinney DC, Heller R, et al. Azalanstat (RS-21607), a lanosterol 14 alpha-demethylase inhibitor with cholesterol-lowering activity. *Biochem Pharmacol* 1995;50(4):529–544.
71. Swinney DC, So OY, Watson DM, et al. Selective inhibition of mammalian lanosterol 14 alpha-demethylase by RS-21607 *in vitro* and *in vivo*. *Biochemistry* 1994;33(15):4702–4713.
72. Walker KA, Kertesz DJ, Rotstein DM, et al. Selective inhibition of mammalian lanosterol 14 alpha-demethylase: a possible strategy for cholesterol lowering. *J Med Chem* 1993;36(15):2235–2237.
73. DeNagel DC, Verity AN, Madden FE, et al. Identification of non-porphyrin inhibitors of heme oxygenase-1. *Neuroscience* 1998;24:2058.
74. Kinobe RT, Vlahakis JZ, Vreman HJ, et al. Selectivity of imidazole-dioxolane compounds for *in vitro* inhibition of microsomal haem oxygenase isoforms. *Br J Pharmacol* 2006;147(3):307–315.
75. Vlahakis JZ, Kinobe RT, Bowers RJ, et al. Imidazole-dioxolane compounds as isozyme-selective heme oxygenase inhibitors. *J Med Chem* 2006;49(14):4437–4441.
76. Vreman HJ, Wong RJ, Stevenson DK, et al. Azalanstat (RS-1607): Evidence for a novel class of potential heme oxygenase inhibitors. *Pediatr Res* 2002;51:341A.
77. Morisawa T, Wong RJ, Bhutani VK, et al. Inhibition of heme oxygenase activity in newborn mice by Azalanstat. *Can J Physiol Pharmacol* 2008;86:651–659.
78. Csongradi E, Vera T, Rimoldi JM, et al. In vivo inhibition of renal heme oxygenase with an imidazole-dioxolane inhibitor. *Pharmacol Res* 2010;61(6):525–530.
79. Hum M, McLaughlin BE, Kong X, et al. Differential inhibition of rat and mouse microsome heme oxygenase by derivatives of imidazole and benzimidazole. *Can J Physiol Pharmacol* 2017;95(12):1454–1461.
80. van Dijk R, Aronson SJ, de Waart DR, et al. Biliverdin reductase inhibitors did not improve severe unconjugated hyperbilirubinemia *in vivo*. *Sci Rep* 2017;7(1):1646.
81. Rubaltelli FF, Griffith PF. Management of neonatal hyperbilirubinaemia and prevention of kernicterus. *Drugs* 1992;43(6):864–872.
82. Gartner LM, Lee KS, Vaisman S, et al. Development of bilirubin transport and metabolism in the newborn rhesus monkey. *J Pediatr* 1977;90(4):513–531.
83. Gow PJ, Ghabrial H, Smallwood RA, et al. Neonatal hepatic drug elimination. *Pharmacol Toxicol* 2001;88(1):3–15.
84. Pacifici GM, Rane A. Intestinal and hepatic morphine glucuronidation in immature and pregnant rats. *Dev Pharmacol Ther* 1981;3(3):160–167.
85. Pasleau F, Kolodzici C, Kremers P, et al. Ontogenic development of steroid 16 alpha-hydroxylase as a tool for the study of the multiplicity of cytochrome P-450. *Eur J Biochem* 1981;120(2):213–220.
86. Yaffe SJ. Antimicrobial therapy and the neonate. *Obstet Gynecol* 1981;58(5 Suppl):85S–94S.
87. Thaler MM. Substrate-induced conjugation of bilirubin in genetically deficient newborn rats. *Science* 1970;170(957):555–556.
88. Valaes T. Bilirubin metabolism. Review and discussion of inborn errors. *Clin Perinatol* 1976;3(1):177–209.
89. Conney AH, Davison C, Gastell R, et al. Adaptive increases in drug-metabolizing enzymes induced by phenobarbital and other drugs. *J Pharmacol Exp Ther* 1960;130:1–8.
90. Hollman S, Touster O. Alterations in tissue levels of uridine diphosphate glucose dehydrogenase, uridine diphosphate glucuronic acid pyrophosphatase and glucuronyl transferase induced by substances influencing the production of ascorbic acid. *Biochim Biophys Acta* 1962;26:338.
91. Inscoe JK, Axelrod J. Some factors affecting glucuronide formation *in vitro*. *J Pharmacol Exp Ther* 1960;129:128–131.
92. Sugatani J, Kojima H, Ueda A, et al. The phenobarbital response enhancer module in the human bilirubin UDP-glucuronosyltransferase UGT1A1 gene and regulation by the nuclear receptor CAR. *Hepatology* 2001;33(5):1232–1238.
93. Berthelot P, Erlinger S, Dhumeaux D, et al. Mechanism of phenobarbital-induced hypercholeresis in the rat. *Am J Physiol* 1970;219(3):809–813.
94. Crigler JF Jr., Gold NI. Effect of sodium phenobarbital on bilirubin metabolism in an infant with congenital, nonhemolytic, unconjugated hyperbilirubinemia, and kernicterus. *J Clin Invest* 1969;48(1):42–55.
95. Kreek MJ, Sleiseng MH. Reduction of serum-unconjugated-bilirubin with phenobarbitone in adult congenital non-haemolytic unconjugated hyperbilirubinaemia. *Lancet* 1968;2:73.
96. Yaffe SJ, Levy G, Matsuzawa T, et al. Enhancement of glucuronide-conjugating capacity in a hyperbilirubinemic infant due to apparent enzyme induction by phenobarbital. *N Engl J Med* 1966;275(26):1461–1466.
97. Trolle D. Phenobarbitone and neonatal icterus. *Lancet* 1968;1:251.
98. Halpin TF, Jones AR, Bishop HL, et al. Prophylaxis of neonatal hyperbilirubinemia with phenobarbital. *Obstet Gynecol* 1972;40(1):85–90.
99. Maurer HM, Wolff JA, Finster M, et al. Reduction in concentration of total serum-bilirubin in offspring of women treated with phenobarbitone during pregnancy. *Lancet* 1968;2(7560):122–124.
100. Ramboer C, Thompson RP, Williams R. Controlled trials of phenobarbitone therapy of neonatal jaundice. *Lancet* 1969;1(7602):966–968.
101. Rayburn W, Donn S, Piehl E, et al. Antenatal phenobarbital and bilirubin metabolism in the very low birth weight infant. *Am J Obstet Gynecol* 1988;159(6):1491–1493.
102. Valaes T, Petmezaki S, Doxiadis SA. Effect on neonatal hyperbilirubinemia of phenobarbital during pregnancy or after birth: practical value of the treatment in a population with high risk of unexplained severe neonatal jaundice. *Birth Defects Orig Artic Ser* 1970;6(2):46–54.
103. Yeung CY, Tam LS, Chan A, et al. Phenobarbitone prophylaxis for neonatal hyperbilirubinemia. *Pediatrics* 1971;48(3):372–376.
104. Valaes T, Karaklis A, Stravrakakis D, et al. Incidence and mechanism of neonatal jaundice related to glucose-6-phosphate dehydrogenase deficiency. *Pediatr Res* 1969;3(5):448–458.
105. Shankaran S, Papile LA, Wright LL, et al. The effect of antenatal phenobarbital therapy on neonatal intracranial hemorrhage in preterm infants. *N Engl J Med* 1997;337(7):466–471.
106. Shankaran S, Papile LA, Wright LL, et al. Neurodevelopmental outcome of premature infants after antenatal phenobarbital exposure. *Am J Obstet Gynecol* 2002;187(1):171–177.
107. Shankaran S, Woldt E, Nelson J, et al. Antenatal phenobarbital therapy and neonatal outcome. II: neurodevelopmental outcome at 36 months. *Pediatrics* 1996;97(5):649–652.
108. Mountain KR, Hirsh J, Gallus AS. Neonatal coagulation defect due to anticonvulsant drug treatment in pregnancy. *Lancet* 1970;1(7641):265–268.
109. Bleyer WA, Skinner AL. Fatal hemorrhage after maternal anticonvulsant therapy. *JAMA* 1976;235:626.
110. Srinivasan G, Seeler RA, Tiruvury A, et al. Maternal anticonvulsant therapy and hemorrhagic disease of the newborn. *Obstet Gynecol* 1982;59(2):250–252.
111. Valaes T, Kipouros K, Petmezaki S, et al. Effectiveness and safety of prenatal phenobarbital for the prevention of neonatal jaundice. *Pediatr Res* 1980;14(8):947–952.
112. Johnson DR, Habeebu SS, Klaassen CD. Increase in bile flow and biliary excretion of glutathione-derived sulfhydryls in rats by drug-metabolizing enzyme inducers is mediated by multidrug resistance protein 2. *Toxicol Sci* 2002;66(1):16–26.
113. Cao A, Falorni A, Fracassini F, et al. Phenobarbital effect on serum bilirubin levels in underweight infants. *Helv Paediatr Acta* 1973;28(3):231–238.
114. Carswell F, Kerr MM, Dunsmore IR. Sequential trial of effect of phenobarbitone on serum bilirubin of preterm infants. *Arch Dis Child* 1972;47(254):621–625.
115. Dortmann A, Haupt H, Kuster F. Barbiturate treatment of neonatal icterus. *Z Kinderheilkd* 1972;112(2):163–170.
116. Stern L, Khanna NN, Levy G, et al. Effect of phenobarbital on hyperbilirubinemia and glucuronide formation in newborns. *Am J Dis Child* 1970;120(1):26–31.
117. Valdes OS, Maurer HM, Shumway CN. Controlled clinical trial of phenobarbital and/or light in reducing neonatal hyperbilirubinemia in a predominantly Negro population. *J Pediatr* 1971;79:1015.
118. Vest M, Signer E, Weisser K, et al. A double blind study of the effect of phenobarbitone on neonatal hyperbilirubinaemia and frequency of exchange transfusion. *Acta Paediatr Scand* 1970;59(6):681–684.
119. Zwacka G, Frenzel J. The influence of short time phenobarbital treatment on neonatal jaundice. *Padiatr Padol* 1971;6(1):102–107.
120. Wallin A, Boreus LO. Phenobarbital prophylaxis for hyperbilirubinemia in preterm infants. A controlled study of bilirubin disappearance and infant behavior. *Acta Paediatr Scand* 1984;73(4):488–497.
121. Blackburn MG, Orzalesi MM, Pigram P. The combined effect of phototherapy and phenobarbital on serum bilirubin levels of premature infants. *Pediatrics* 1972;49(1):110–112.
122. Ryan ME, Ashley RA. How do tetracyclines work? *Adv Dent Res* 1998;12(2):149–151.
123. Gabler WL, Smith J, Tsukuda N. Comparison of doxycycline and a chemically modified tetracycline inhibition of leukocyte functions. *Res Commun Chem Pathol Pharmacol* 1992;78(2):151–160.
124. Lin S, Wei X, Bales KR, et al. Minocycline blocks bilirubin neurotoxicity and prevents hyperbilirubinemia-induced cerebellar hypoplasia in the Gunn rat. *Eur J Neurosci* 2005;22(1):21–27.
125. Geiger AS, Rice AC, Shapiro SM. Minocycline blocks acute bilirubin-induced neurological dysfunction in jaundiced Gunn rats. *Neonatology* 2007;92(4):219–226.
126. Arvin KL, Han BH, Du Y, et al. Minocycline markedly protects the neonatal brain against hypoxic-ischemic injury. *Ann Neurol* 2002;52(1):54–61.
127. Kutz K, Kandler H, Gugler R, et al. Effect of clofibrate on the metabolism of bilirubin, bromosulphophthalein and indocyanine green and on the biliary lipid composition in Gilbert's syndrome. *Clin Sci (Lond)* 1984;66(4):389–397.
128. Thorp JM, Waring WS. Modifcation of metabolism and distribution of lipids by ethyl chlorophenoxyisobutyrate. *Nature (Lond)* 1962;194:948–949.
129. Brun S, Carmona MC, Mampel T, et al. Activators of peroxisome proliferator-activated receptor-alpha induce the expression of the uncoupling protein-3 gene in skeletal muscle: a potential mechanism for the lipid intake-dependent activation of uncoupling protein-3 gene expression at birth. *Diabetes* 1999;48(6):1217–1222.
130. Foliot A, Drocourt JL, Etienne JP, et al. Increase in the hepatic glucuronidation and clearance of bilirubin in clofibrate-treated rats. *Biochem Pharmacol* 1977;26(6):547–549.
131. Lindenbaum A, Hernandorena X, Vial M, et al. Clofibrate for the treatment of hyperbilirubinemia in neonates born at term: a double blind controlled study (author's transl). *Arch Fr Pediatr 1981*;38(Suppl):867–873.

132. Lindenbaum A, Delaporte B, Benattar C, et al. Preventive treatment of jaundice in premature newborn infants with clofibrate. Double-blind controlled therapeutic trial. *Arch Fr Pediatr* 1985;42(9):759–763.
133. Erkul I, Yavuz H, Ozel A. Clofibrate treatment of neonatal jaundice. *Pediatrics* 1991;88(6):1292–1294.
134. Coronary Drug Project Research Group. Clofibrate and niacin in coronary heart disease. *JAMA* 1975;231(4):360–381.
135. World Health Organization. WHO cooperative trial on primary prevention of ischaemic heart disease with clofibrate to lower serum cholesterol: final mortality follow-up. Report of the Committee of Principal Investigators. *Lancet* 1984;2(8403):600–604.
136. Gabilan JC, Benattar C, Lindenbaum A. Clofibrate treatment of neonatal jaundice. *Pediatrics* 1990;86(4):647–648.
137. Yin J, Miller M, Wennberg RP. Induction of hepatic bilirubin-metabolizing enzymes by the traditional Chinese medicine *yin zhi huang*. *Dev Pharmacol Ther* 1991;16(3):176–184.
138. Ho NK. Traditional Chinese medicine and treatment of neonatal jaundice. *Singapore Med J* 1996;37(6):645–651.
139. Chen ZL, Guan WH. Approach to the effect and indication of *Yin Zhi Huang* to treat neonatal jaundice (Chinese). *J Clin Pediatr* 1985;3:302–303.
140. Yang SH, Lu CF. Effects of *Artemisia, Rheum, Gardenia, Coptidis*, and *Rhizoma* on neonatal jaundice in Chinese newborn infants. *J Chin Child Med* 1984;25:144–148.
141. Roberts RJ, Plaa GL. Effect of phenobarbital on the excretion of an exogenous bilirubin load. *Biochem Pharmacol* 1967;16(5):827–835.
142. Yin J, Wennberg RP, Xia YC, et al. Effect of a traditional Chinese medicine, *yin zhi huang*, on bilirubin clearance and conjugation. *Dev Pharmacol Ther* 1991;16(1):59–64.
143. Yin J, Wennberg RP, Miller M. Induction of hepatic bilirubin and drug metabolizing enzymes by individual herbs present in the traditional Chinese medicine, *yin zhi huang*. *Dev Pharmacol Ther* 1993;20(3–4):186–194.
144. Dennery PA. Pharmacological interventions for the treatment of neonatal jaundice. *Semin Neonatol* 2002;7(2):111–119.
145. Yeung CY, Leung CS, Chen YZ. An old traditional herbal remedy for neonatal jaundice with a newly identified risk. *J Paediatr Child Health* 1993;29(4):292–294.
146. Chan TY. The prevalence use and harmful potential of some Chinese herbal medicines in babies and children. *Vet Hum Toxicol* 1994;36(3):238–240.
147. Strauss KA, Robinson DL, Vreman HJ, et al. Management of hyperbilirubinemia and prevention of kernicterus in 20 patients with Crigler-Najjar disease. *Eur J Pediatr* 2006;165(5):306–319.
148. Paumgartner G, Beuers U. Ursodeoxycholic acid in cholestatic liver disease: mechanisms of action and therapeutic use revisited. *Hepatology* 2002;36(3):525–531.
149. George R, Stevens A, Berkenbosch JW, et al. Ursodeoxycholic acid in the treatment of cholestasis and hyperbilirubinemia in pediatric intensive care unit patients. *South Med J* 2002;95(11):1276–1279.
150. Murao S, Tanaka N. A new enzyme "bilirubin oxidase" produced by *Myrothecium verrucarea* MT-1. *Agric Biol* 1981;45:2383–2385.
151. Soltys PJ, Mullon C, Langer R. Oral treatment for jaundice using immobilized bilirubin oxidase. *Artif Organs* 1992;16(4):331–335.
152. Johnson LH, Dworanczyk R, Abbasi M, et al. Bilirubin oxidase (BOX) feedings significantly decrease serum bilirubin (B) in jaundiced infant Gunn rats. *Pediatr Res* 1988;22:412A.
153. Davis DR, Yeary RA. Activated charcoal as an adjunct to phototherapy for neonatal jaundice. *Dev Pharmacol Ther* 1987;10(1):12–20.
154. Davis DR, Yeary RA, Lee K. Activated charcoal decreases plasma bilirubin levels in the hyperbilirubinemic rat. *Pediatr Res* 1983;17(3):208–209.
155. Amitai Y, Regev M, Arad I, et al. Treatment of neonatal hyperbilirubinemia with repetitive oral activated charcoal as an adjunct to phototherapy. *J Perinat Med* 1993;21(3):189–194.
156. Romagnoli C, Polidori G, Foschini M, et al. Agar in the management of hyperbilirubinaemia in the premature baby. *Arch Dis Child* 1975;50(3):202–204.
157. Ebbesen F, Moller J. Agar ingestion combined with phototherapy in jaundiced newborn infants. *Biol Neonate* 1977;31(1–2):7–9.
158. Bueno A, Perez-Gonzalez J, Bueno M. Effect on agar on neonatal bilirubin seric levels (author's transl). *An Esp Pediatr* 1977;10(10):721–730.
159. Odell GB, Gutcher GR, Whitington PF, et al. Enteral administration of agar as an effective adjunct to phototherapy of neonatal hyperbilirubinemia. *Pediatr Res* 1983;17(10):810–814.
160. Caglayan S, Candemir H, Aksit S, et al. Superiority of oral agar and phototherapy combination in the treatment of neonatal hyperbilirubinemia. *Pediatrics* 1993;92(1):86–89.
161. Kemper K, Horwitz RI, McCarthy P. Decreased neonatal serum bilirubin with plain agar: a meta-analysis. *Pediatrics* 1988;82(4):631–638.
162. Brodersen R, Stern L. Deposition of bilirubin acid in the central nervous system – a hypothesis for the development of kernicterus. *Acta Paediatr Scand* 1990;79(1):12–19.
163. Ahlfors CE. Benzyl alcohol, kernicterus, and unbound bilirubin. *J Pediatr* 2001;139(2):317–319.
164. Ahlfors CE. Bilirubin-albumin binding and free bilirubin. *J Perinatol* 2001;21(Suppl 1):S40–S42; discussion S59–S62.
165. Ahlfors CE. Measurement of plasma unbound unconjugated bilirubin. *Anal Biochem* 2000;279(2):130–135.
166. Ahlfors CE, Marshall GD, Wolcott DK, et al. Measurement of unbound bilirubin by the peroxidase test using Zone Fluidics. *Clin Chim Acta* 2006;365(1–2):78–85.
167. Ahlfors CE, Vreman HJ, Wong RJ, et al. Effects of sample dilution, peroxidase concentration, and chloride ion on the measurement of unbound bilirubin in premature newborns. *Clin Biochem* 2007;40(3–4):261–267.
168. Nakamura H, Yonetani M, Uetani Y, et al. Determination of serum unbound bilirubin for prediction of kernicterus in low birthweight infants. *Acta Paediatr Jpn* 1992;34(6):642–647.
169. McDonagh AF, Vreman HJ, Wong RJ, et al. Photoisomers — obfuscating factors in clinical peroxidase measurements of unbound bilirubin? *Pediatrics* 2009;123(1):67–76.
170. Morris BH, Oh W, Tyson JE, et al. A Multi-center randomized trial of aggressive versus conservative phototherapy for extremely low birth weight infants. *N Engl J Med* 2008;359(18):1885–1896.

CHAPTER

15

Girija Natarajan
Jose Maria de Andrade Lopes
Jacob V. Aranda

Pharmacologic Treatment of Neonatal Apnea

METHYLXANTHINES

Neonatal apnea or cessation of breathing occurs in almost all extremely low gestational age newborns. It is often clinically referred to as arterial desaturations or more recently intermittent hypoxia. As in the initial reports of a decrease in the frequency of apneic episodes in 10 preterm neonates given theophylline rectally in 1973[1] and in 18 preterm neonates given caffeine citrate by Aranda et al.,[4] numerous studies have demonstrated the usefulness of the methylated xanthines in the treatment of neonatal apnea. Thus, caffeine and theophylline have gained universal acceptance in the last few decades as the first-line therapy of neonatal apnea. Moreover, the substantial beneficial impact of caffeine on many neonatal morbidities appropriately made caffeine as the silver bullet in neonatology.

MECHANISM OF ACTION

Several mechanisms appear to be involved in the decrease in apnea frequency found after methylxanthine administration. These include the following:

1. Respiratory center stimulation.
2. Improvement in respiratory muscle contraction.
3. Others: altered sleep states, metabolic rate, cardiac output, metabolic homeostasis, and potentiation of catecholamine effect.

Respiratory Center Stimulation

Both caffeine and theophylline produce an increase in minute ventilation, a decrease in the partial pressure of arterial carbon dioxide (P_aCO_2), and an increase in most indices of neural respiratory drive. Davi et al. investigated the effect of theophylline on the control of breathing in newborn infants and found a decreased CO_2 threshold and increased CO_2 sensitivity.[2] Gerhardt et al. observed a parallel shift in the slope of the CO_2 response curve after aminophylline administration.[3] In both newborn infants and cats, caffeine has a potent effect on central neural drive.[4,5] Caffeine increases mean inspiratory flow (tidal volume/inspiratory time) (V_t/T_i), the pressure generated after airway occlusion ($p < 0.01$), and minute ventilation. In the cat, when isocapnic conditions were maintained, ventilation was threefold greater, suggesting an interaction between caffeine and CO_2. In the newborn baby, doses as low as 2.5 mg per kg of caffeine increase tidal volume. However, the optimal ventilatory response is observed only with doses of 10 mg per kg.[6] The central respirogenic effect of the xanthines is further supported by the observation that they antagonize the depressant effects of narcotics such as codeine, morphine, and meperidine.[7–9]

Improved Respiratory Muscle Function

The effect of caffeine and theophylline on muscle contraction has been known for many years.[10] However, it was only in the last decade that the effects of these drugs were investigated in relation to respiratory muscle function. Several reports in the literature have described the effects of caffeine and theophylline on diaphragmatic contraction both in vivo and in vitro.[11–13] Theophylline improves diaphragmatic efficiency and increases force production with electric stimulation. The drug not only affects muscle contraction but also decreases the recovery time of fatigued muscles.[14] In the newborn, fatigue of the respiratory muscles has been associated with apnea, which is effectively treated by xanthine administration.[15–17] Therefore, it is possible that part of the anti-apneic effect of these drugs is owing to improvement in respiratory muscle function.[15–17]

Other Mechanisms

In addition to the increase in respiratory drive, increased CO_2 sensitivity, and improvement in respiratory muscle contraction, other factors that may facilitate the action of the xanthines include increased neuromuscular transmission, catecholamine release, improved metabolic homeostasis, and changes in sleep states.[18–22] The increase in metabolic rate and catecholamine levels after xanthine administration may lead to improved oxygenation and increased cardiac output. Improvement in metabolic homeostasis, such as increased blood glucose, may also lessen the frequency of apneic spells. A decrease in apnea frequency has been described at low doses of theophylline that do not alter ventilation or the CO_2 response curve but may impact the sleep–wake pattern. Increased neuromuscular transmission may lead to improved muscle tone, a well-known in vitro effect of the xanthines. Improved respiratory muscle tone has been related to increased functional residual capacity and better oxygenation in the newborn.[23]

Adenosine Receptor Blockade

The methylxanthines exert their effects by (a) blocking adenosine receptors A1 and A2a, (b) the inhibition of phosphodiesterase with increased 3′,5′-cyclic adenosine monophosphate (AMP), and (c) the translocation of intracellular calcium and interaction with gamma-aminobutyric acid receptors. Prostaglandin antagonism and upregulation of γ-aminobutyric acid receptor A subunit expression (opposing the effect of hypoxia) have also been described.[24,25] Both caffeine and theophylline are able to bind to adenosine receptors; adenosine is a neurotransmitter or neuromodulator with a role in the control of breathing.[21,22,26] Adenosine and its analogues have potent inhibitory effects on respiration. The administration of L-phenylisopropyl adenosine, a stable adenosine analogue, causes respiratory depression in laboratory animals in a dose-dependent manner.[27] This effect has been described in several species, including rat, rabbit, cat, and newborn piglet, and in both the anesthetized state (cat, rabbit, and piglet models) and the awake state (rat model).[28–30] The inhibition of respiration can be partially or completely reversed by the administration of theophylline and caffeine, both of which antagonize adenosine at the receptor level.

The role of intracerebral adenosine levels in the control of ventilatory response to hypoxia was explored in 15 spontaneously breathing piglets, 1 to 5 days old, sedated with chloral hydrate. Animals exposed to 12% oxygen showed a typical biphasic ventilatory response with an initial increase in ventilation followed by a late decrease. Both intravenous caffeine citrate (20 mg per kg) and inhaled CO_2 separately and independently abolished or attenuated the late respiratory depression associated with hypoxia. In the same experiment, the administration of dipyridamole, a competitive inhibitor of adenosine receptors, potentiated the ventilatory depression.[30] These observations suggest that part of the efficacy of the xanthines in reducing apnea frequency in the neonate may be owing to adenosine blockade with consequent central nervous system (CNS) stimulation.

PHARMACOKINETICS AND THERAPEUTIC DRUG MONITORING

Several studies have shown that the plasma clearance and elimination of theophylline and caffeine are both prolonged in newborn babies compared with adults.[31–33] The representative kinetic profiles of these two drugs are shown in Table 15.1. The obvious difference between the two drugs is the remarkably slow elimination of caffeine relative to theophylline. The plasma half-life is about 100 hours for caffeine and about 30 hours for theophylline. This difference in drug elimination indicates that caffeine can be given more sparingly (i.e., once daily) and that drug monitoring is probably not as crucial with caffeine as with theophylline. Caffeine half-life may be further prolonged in infants with cholestatic jaundice and in breastfed infants.[34] The recommended therapeutic plasma concentrations for theophylline and caffeine are about 5 to 15 and 5 to 20 mg per L, respectively. To achieve and maintain these plasma concentrations, a loading dose of 4 to 8 mg per kg of theophylline (active base) followed by a maintenance dose of 2 to 4 mg per kg per day in two to four divided doses may be required. There exists substantial interindividual variability in the pharmacokinetic properties of theophylline; thus, it is necessary to monitor plasma concentrations and adjust the dose accordingly (saliva has been proposed as an alternative site for therapeutic drug monitoring in the preterm, with good correlation with blood levels).[35,36] Similarly, caffeine is recommended as a loading dose of 10 to 20 mg per kg of active base or 20 to 40 mg per kg of caffeine citrate salt, intravenously or orally. A maintenance dose of 2.5 to 4 mg per kg per day (or 5 to 8 mg per kg per day of caffeine citrate) is usually needed to maintain plasma concentrations of 5 to 20 mg per L of caffeine (Table 15.2). About 25% of theophylline is methylated to caffeine,[37,38] with plasma theophylline-to-caffeine ratios sometimes reaching 0.30 to 0.40 at a steady state. A small (3% to 8%) proportion of caffeine is converted to theophylline via CYP1A2. Thus, the overall methylxanthine effect has to account for the sum of the two drugs because both agents are pharmacologically active.

The methylxanthines are powerful CNS stimulants and may interact with anticonvulsants such as phenobarbital at a kinetic or a pharmacodynamic level. Babies given theophylline and phenobarbital have been shown to require higher doses of theophylline to control apnea and higher doses of phenobarbital to control seizures.[39] The methylxanthines also have the potential to interact with drugs that are substrates for CYP1A2, such as cimetidine and ketoconazole.

TABLE 15.1 Pharmacokinetics of Theophylline and Caffeine Used in the Neonatal Period

	Theophylline	*Caffeine*
Plasma half-life (h)	30	100
Range	12–64	40–230
Mean adult value	6.7	6
Apparent volume of distribution (L/kg)	0.69	0.9
Range	0.2–2.8	0.4–1.3
Mean adult value	0.5	0.6
Clearance (mL/kg/h)	22	8.9
Range	4.3–68	2.5–17
Adult value	66	94
Dose (mg/kg)		
Loading	5–6	10[a]
	2.5[b]	
Maintenance	1 q8 h	2.5 q24 h
	0.66 q8 h+	
Route of administration	IV, PO	IV, PO
Desired plasma level (mg/L)	5–15	5–20
	3–4[c]	

Note: q8 h, every 8 h; q24 h, every 24 h; IV, intravenous; PO, oral.
[a]Active base.
[b]Low-dose regimen.
[c]Adjusted according to plasma level.

TABLE 15.2 Suggested Guidelines for Respiratory Stimulants in Neonatal Apnea

	Theophylline	*Caffeine*	*Doxapram*
Plasma half-life (h)	30	100	7
Loading dose (mg/kg)	5–6	10	2.5[a]
Maintenance dose (mg/kg/d)[b]	2–4	2.5	1.0[c]
Therapeutic blood level (mg/L)	5–15	5–20	1.5–3
TDM	EMIT/HPLC	EMIT/HPLC	HPLC

[a]Intravenous infusion only for 15 min. All doses are in active base.
[b]All doses are in active base.
[c]As intravenous infusion per hour.
EMIT, enzyme-multiplied immunoassay technique; HPLC, high-performance liquid chromatography; TDM (Therapeutic Drug Monitoring).

CHOICE OF METHYLXANTHINES

Caffeine and theophylline exert similar pharmacodynamic effects but may vary in their potency concerning a specific organ receptor. Moreover, the differences in their kinetic properties alter the dosing schedules and the need for therapeutic drug monitoring. Table 15.3 lists some of the differences between the two drugs. Controlled comparative trials between theophylline and caffeine indicate that although both drugs are effective in the management of apnea, more adverse effects such as tachycardia are observed with theophylline.[40–48] Henderson-Smart and Steer reviewed five trials comparing theophylline and caffeine in reducing recurrent apnea and the need for mechanical ventilation.[44] There was no difference in the failure rate (<50% reduction in apnea/bradycardia) of treatment with caffeine or theophylline at 1 to 3 days (two studies) or at 5 to 7 days (one study). There was no difference in the mean rate of apnea after 1 to 3 days (five studies) or at 5 to 7 days (four studies). Side effects, as indicated by tachycardia or feed intolerance leading to dose change, were lower with caffeine, relative risk (*RR*) = 0.17 (0.04 to 0.72). Because caffeine has a more prolonged plasma half-life, the dosing schedule is less frequent and the need for therapeutic monitoring is less crucial. Although frequent monitoring is advisable for theophylline, routine serum caffeine measurement is not warranted.[49–52] Therapeutic drug monitoring may be needed during the neonatal period only if there is a lack of clinical response or unexplained tachycardia.[49–52] In cases of overdosing with caffeine, the prolonged drug elimination may result in sustained high plasma concentrations of caffeine for a prolonged period. However, observations suggest that caffeine plasma concentrations of up to 50 mg per L may occur with no adverse effects, whereas plasma concentrations of theophylline greater than 15 mg per L may be associated with tachycardia. Some investigators even suggest much higher doses of caffeine to achieve a therapeutic effect. This suggests that caffeine might have a wider therapeutic index relative to theophylline. In practice, caffeine has emerged as the preferred alternative in infants with apnea of prematurity.

TABLE 15.3 Theophylline and Caffeine in Neonatal Apnea

Variable	*Theophylline*	*Caffeine*
Efficacy	+++	+++
Peripheral side effects	+++	+/−
Drug clearance	Slow ($t_{1/2}$ = 30 h)	Very slow ($t_{1/2}$ = 100 h)
Plasma level at steady state	Fluctuating	Stable
Need for drug monitoring	+++	−
Dosing interval	1–3×/d	Once/day

+ or − indicates the relative potency of the pharmacologic effect or need for therapeutic drug monitoring.

CLINICAL EFFECTS

EFFICACY OF METHYLXANTHINES IN NEONATAL APNEA AND WEANING FROM MECHANICAL VENTILATION

The capability of caffeine to stimulate respiration has been known for a century, and the ability of aminophylline to regulate breathing in adult patients with Cheyne–Stokes respiration was noted in 1927. Kuzemko and Paala first described the use of aminophylline in 10 neonates.[53] Since then, several clinical trials have confirmed the efficacy of xanthines in decreasing the number of apneas, cyanotic spells, and episodes of bradycardia[4,54–61] (Table 15.4). Shannon et al. described a reduced incidence of severe apnea, lasting more than 30 seconds, and bradycardia associated with theophylline serum concentrations between 6 and 11 µg per mL.[54] Peabody et al. observed less apnea and bradycardia associated with regulating the breathing pattern and less fluctuation in transcutaneous partial pressure of oxygen (PO_2) in infants treated with aminophylline.[56] Roberts et al. described a significant reduction in all types of apnea, suggesting that theophylline may act to improve the coordination between upper airway and respiratory muscles.[58] This has also been observed in premature infants where diaphragmatic electromyelography (EMG) and laryngeal muscle EMG were recorded simultaneously.[62] Similarly, caffeine, which has potent CNS stimulant properties with fewer peripheral effects than theophylline, has also been shown to be effective in neonatal apnea. Caffeine stimulates respiration and decreases episodes of apnea, produces regular breathing patterns, and increases alveolar ventilation. Henderson-Smart and De Paoli reviewed randomized controlled trials to evaluate the efficacy of methylxanthines for the treatment of apnea.[63] In six studies (three with theophylline and three with caffeine) including a total of 192 infants, they found that, compared with control (placebo or no drug), methylxanthine administration to preterm infants with recurrent apnea was associated with a reduction in apnea and the use of mechanical ventilation in the first 2 to 7 days. The post hoc analysis of the large multicenter Caffeine for Apnea of Prematurity (CAP) trial showed that positive airway pressure was discontinued one week earlier in the caffeine-treated infants (median postmenstrual age, 31.0 weeks; interquartile

TABLE 15.4 Clinical Studies and Drug Regimens of Methylxanthines in Neonatal Apnea

			Frequency of Apnea		
Reference (year)	Drug Preparation	Dose and Route	Before	After	Success Rate
53 (1973)	Aminophylline suppositories	5 mg q6 h × 3 doses, then q6 h PRN	63	6	24/24
54 (1975)	Theophylline alcohol elixir (10%)	4 mg/kg q6 h orally	5.9/13 h	0/13 h	17/17
55 (1975)	Theophylline alcohol solution (20%)	4 mg/kg q6 h orally	10.6/d	0.9/d	15/15
145 (1976)	Aminophylline suppositories	5 mg q6 h (1.7–4 mg/kg/d) rectally	1.7/h	0.39/h	10/13
4 (1977)	Caffeine citrate	I.D.: 20 mg/kg IV or orally M.D.: 5–140 mg/kg every day or twice daily	13.6/d	2.1/d	17/18
56 (1978)	Aminophylline	I.D.: 8 mg/kg q12 h; M.D.: 4 mg/kg q12 h rectally	115/12 h	26/12 h	4/4
2 (1978)	Theophylline	3 mg/kg q6 h IV or orally	55/h+	11/h+	8/10
16 (1980)	Theophylline	2 mg/kg/d by nasogastric tube	16.1/h	5.2/h	6/7
57 (1981)	Caffeine citrate	20 mg/kg loading IM, then 5 mg/kg q24 h PO	1.17/h day 1	0.11/h day 5	9/9
58 (1982)	Theophylline	6 mg/kg/d orally	80	46	5/20
59 (1985)	Theophylline	6.8 mg/kg IV loading, then 1.4 mg/kg q8 h	11/24 h	1/24 h day 5	19/22
60 (1990)	Theophylline	8.0 mg/kg IV continuous infusion of 0.5 mg/kg/h	0.72/h	0.34/h	8/10
61 (2000)	Caffeine citrate	10 mg/kg loading, 2.5 mg/kg q24 h			

I.D., initial dose; IM, intramuscular; IV, intravenous; M.D., maintenance dose; PO, oral; PRN, as the situation demands; q6 h, every 6 h; q8 h, every 8 h; q12 h, every 12 h; q24 h, every 24 h.

range, 29.4 to 33.0), compared with the placebo group (median postmenstrual age, 32.0 weeks; interquartile range, 30.3 to 34.0; $p < 0.001$).[64]

Despite optimal plasma concentrations of theophylline, however, significant apnea reduction has been reported in only about 75% of neonates.[65] When used as prophylaxis to prevent apnea in preterm infants, two placebo-controlled studies involving 104 infants found no differences between the groups in the proportion of infants with apnea, bradycardia, hypoxemic episodes, or the use of positive pressure ventilation (PPV) or adverse effects.[66,67] The sample sizes in the studies were small, however, and caffeine was used for a total duration of 96 hours in one. A subgroup of infants treated with prophylactic caffeine in the CAP trial did not demonstrate any significant differences in clinical outcomes except for a decrease in the risk of patent ductus arteriosus (PDA) ligation.[68]

Caffeine and theophylline are also effective respiratory stimulants during weaning from mechanical ventilation. Several clinical trials have suggested that the success rate of extubation is improved if theophylline/caffeine is administered prior to extubation.[69–72] The effect is presumed to be related to improvement in respiratory muscle function and decreased pulmonary resistance. Reviews on the prophylactic administration of methylxanthines for the extubation of preterm infants reported data from seven trials with a total of 172 infants (four trials with theophylline and two with caffeine).[73] Methylxanthine treatment results in a reduction in the failure of extubation within 1 week [summary *RR*, 0.48; 95% confidence interval (CI), 0.32 to 0.71]. There was a wide variation in baseline rates in the control groups (range, 20% to 100%) in the different studies. The CAP trial enrolled the largest number of infants, but did not report extubation rates. In the caffeine-treated group, postmenstrual ages at the time of discontinuing PPV and endotracheal intubation (ETT) were lower, compared with controls.[64] The number of infants in each study was small, and only a large difference in the outcomes could reliably be detected. A randomized, double-blind clinical trial of three dosing regimens of caffeine citrate (3, 15, and 30 mg per kg) for peri-extubation management of 127 ventilated preterm infants younger than 32 weeks of gestation showed no statistically significant difference in the incidence of extubation failure between the dosing groups.[74] The infants in the two higher dosing groups did have statistically significant less documented apnea in the immediate peri-extubation period. A larger trial involving 234 neonates younger than 30 weeks of gestation reported a significant reduction in failure to extubate in infants receiving 20 mg per kg per day caffeine citrate compared with 5 mg per kg per day (15% vs. 29.8%; *RR*, 0.51; 95% CI, 0.31 to 0.85).[75] A significant difference in the duration of mechanical ventilation was observed in infants younger than 28 weeks of gestation who received the higher dose. No differences were noted in short-term adverse effects or at 12-month follow-up. Based on these data, a recent meta-analysis recommended the routine use of caffeine to improve rates of successful extubation in preterm infants, although an earlier international survey found that only 54% of neonatal units followed this practice for infants below 28 weeks of gestation.[76,77]

EFFECT ON LUNG FUNCTION

In an immature baboon model treated with surfactant, early caffeine treatment was associated with better lung function, higher compliance, and significant decreases in ventilator support.[78] In a rat pup model that received neonatal caffeine, there was a 22% higher minute ventilation response to hypercapnia in males in the juvenile stage, which persisted until adulthood.[79] This reported long-term effect on respiratory control was speculated to be owing to a persistent change in adenosinergic neurotransmission. Small studies in infants with bronchopulmonary dysplasia (BPD) have shown a decrease in airway resistance and improved lung mechanics within 1 hour of caffeine therapy.[80] In another study, improvements in forced vital capacity and forced expiratory volume z-Scores at 0.5 seconds and with caffeine were noted in preterm (less than 31 weeks of gestation) infants without BPD.[81] An increase in mean sensitivity to carbon dioxide of 15.3 (95% CI, 1 to 30) mL per kg per minute with caffeine administration was found in 26 infants born at a median gestation of 32 (range, 31 to 33) weeks.[82] An improvement in respiratory system compliance after caffeine has also been reported in preterm infants with resolving respiratory distress syndrome.[83] Among 30 spontaneously breathing preterm infants (mean gestational age, 29.1 ± 1.3 weeks), a loading dose of caffeine was associated with a 43% median increase in diaphragmatic activity by transcutaneous electromyography at 5 minutes and 30% increase in median tidal volume, sustained until 120 minutes.[84] In the multicenter, randomized, controlled CAP trial, the rates of BPD defined as an oxygen need at 36 weeks of postconceptional age were 36.3% in the caffeine group compared with 46.9% in the placebo group, a statistically significant difference.[64] A subset of 142 trial participants were evaluated at 11 years of age. Children in the caffeine group had better expiratory flows by approximately 0.5 standard deviation (SD), and fewer had forced vital capacity below the fifth centile [11% vs. 28%; odds ratio (*OR*), 0.31; 95% CI, 0.12 to 0.77; $p = 0.012$].[85] When adjusted for BPD, the difference in flow rates between the groups decreased.

EFFECT ON PATENT DUCTUS ARTERIOSUS

There were initial concerns regarding the relaxant effect of the methylxanthines on the ductus arteriosus, presumably because of increased 3′,5′-cyclic AMP caused by phosphodiesterase blockade. The concentration of xanthine required to produce relaxation in vitro (540 to 1,620 mg per L) is far higher than the plasma concentrations achieved in the newborn infant (about 10 mg per L). Caffeine has been shown to be a prostaglandin antagonist at concentrations achieved in plasma.[24] In a preterm sheep model of ductus arteriosus, caffeine (0.003 to 0.3 mM) showed no direct effect on ductus arteriosus tension nor the contractile response to increasing oxygen concentrations.[86] In 25 preterm infants with PDA, left ventricular output decreased progressively during 4 hours after intravenous caffeine citrate loading dose of 20 mg per kg. Superior vena cava flow decreased and ductal shunting flow increased at 1 hour but returned to baseline values at 4 hours. Constriction of PDA was noted at 4 hours after caffeine loading.[87] The CAP trial involving infants weighing less than 1,250 g at birth showed a statistically significant decrease in the incidence of PDA (30% vs. 40%) and in the rates of surgical ligation (4.5% vs. 12.6%) in the group treated with caffeine citrate.[64]

EFFECT ON CARDIAC FUNCTION

Augmentations of cardiac inotropy and chronotropy are reported effects of methylxanthines, although data from systematic human observations are scarce. In an observational study involving 31 premature infants, cardiac index increased by a mean of 14.6% ± 16.3% (SD), stroke volume increased in 24 of 31 trials by 7.8% ± 12.2%, heart rate increased in 28 of 31 trials by 7.7 ± 7.2 beats per minute, and blood pressure increased in 25 of 31 trials by 4.1 ± 5.8 mmHg (all $p < 0.001$) following an intravenous dose of caffeine.[88] Previously, Hoecker et al. reported no change in left ventricular cardiac output (LVCO), heart rate, or blood pressure following caffeine loading.[89,90] In 21 premature newborns, no effects of caffeine administration were demonstrated on heart rate variability.[91] Walther et al. demonstrated an increase in LVCO and heart rate in 11 infants treated with aminophylline and an increase in stroke volume by 15% in the first 3 days of treatment, which returned to baseline by the seventh day of treatment.[92] An increase in LVCO, stroke volume, and heart rate was also shown in a study of theophylline effect on 15 infants by Fesslova et al.[93]

OTHER PHARMACOLOGIC EFFECTS

Besides effects on respirogenesis, lung and cardiac function, caffeine and theophylline exhibit a variety of pharmacologic actions, including CNS stimulation, smooth muscle relaxation, systemic blood vessel dilation, cerebral vessel vasoconstriction, diuresis, and augmentation of metabolic rate, among others[18,19,94,95] (see Table 15.5). Bronchodilation has been demonstrated in premature infants with BPD after the administration of both caffeine and theophylline.[80] Diuresis caused by increased renal blood flow and increased glomerular filtration rate has not been shown to be significant in premature neonates treated with theophylline in some studies.[94] Neonates given theophylline and control infants not given theophylline were similar with respect to urine volume, serum osmolality and electrolytes, and urinary electrolyte excretion. In other studies, though, a marked diuresis was noted immediately after the administration of theophylline.[96] Caffeine is a much weaker diuretic and appears to have no effect on serum sodium, potassium, calcium, and phosphorus levels, while urinary calcium excretion increases and serum creatinine decreases significantly in premature neonates.[97]

Caffeine can shorten the blood coagulation time resulting from increased clotting factors such as factor V, prothrombin, and fibrinogen. A relatively important effect of the methylxanthines pertains to metabolic homeostasis. In experimental animals, adult volunteers and patients, and pancreatic islet cell cultures, caffeine can stimulate insulin and glucagon release and can increase catecholamine release, blood glucose, cortisol secretion, and plasma free fatty acid levels. The increased

TABLE 15.5 Major Pharmacologic Effects of Methylxanthines

Central nervous system: stimulation of all levels
Heart: augmentation of inotropy and chronotropy
Vascular system: pulmonary, dilation, systemic, dilation; cerebral, constriction (in adults)
Smooth muscles: relaxation
Skeletal muscles: stimulation
Kidney: increased renal blood flow and diuresis
Gastrointestinal system: stimulation of gastric acid and fluid secretion
Endocrine system: multiple effects
Hematologic: mild increased clotting and shortened coagulation time
Basal metabolic rate: augmentation

plasma free fatty acid could potentially compete with bilirubin at albumin-binding sites. Studies suggest that there is a transient hyperglycemia following an intravenous infusion of caffeine in the premature infant, with a delayed increase or no change in plasma insulin levels.

Caffeine and theophylline constrict cerebral vessels, increase cerebrovascular resistance, and decrease cerebral blood flow in adults.[98,99] Systematic studies in newborn humans and experimental animals (i.e., newborn piglets) to determine the effect of caffeine and theophylline on cerebral blood flow suggest that cerebral blood flow alteration is not a prime concern.[18,100,101] In contrast, a significant decrease in blood flow velocities in the internal carotid and anterior cerebral arteries has been reported in 16 preterm infants following a 25 mg per kg dose of oral caffeine.[90] No increase in the incidence of cicatricial retrolental fibroplasia was observed in babies treated with caffeine compared with controls. In a subset of CAP trial participants alive at a postmenstrual age of 36 weeks, caffeine was associated with a significant adjusted reduction in the incidence of severe retinopathy of prematurity (ROP).[102] The mechanism of this effect remains unclear, but may involve effects on regulators of angiogenesis such as vascular endothelial growth factor, sonic hedgehog matrix metalloproteinases, and oxidative stress.[103,104] In addition, in the neonatal rat model of intermittent hypoxia, caffeine produced normalization of the retinal proteomic profile that was abnormal in oxygen-induced retinopathy.[105]

Caffeine causes a slight increase in basal metabolic rate, which can be observed in the adult habitual coffee drinker. The ingestion of 0.5 g of caffeine may increase the basal metabolic rate to an average of 10% and occasionally to 25%. In the neonate, a mean increase in oxygen consumption of 25% has been observed following the administration of theophylline. Similarly, an increase in oxygen consumption and energy expenditure has been reported after 48 hours of caffeine therapy, which persisted through 4 weeks.[95] The CAP trial found that the caffeine-treated group of infants had a reduced weight gain, with the greatest difference noted after 2 weeks (mean difference, −23 g).[64] This effect could be of potential significance, especially in the tiny premature infant with limited calorie intake.

A reduction in mesenteric blood flow velocities in response to a loading dose of caffeine has been reported.[90,106] A small trial involving 85 infants had suggested an association between the use of methylxanthines and necrotizing enterocolitis (NEC).[61] In the larger CAP trial, there was no significant difference in the incidence of NEC in the caffeine-treated and placebo groups.[64] Besides, apnea with hypoxemic episodes can, by itself, be a risk factor for the development of NEC.[2,107]

HIGH- VERSUS LOW-DOSE CAFFEINE THERAPY

A meta-analysis designed to compare the efficacy and safety of high (greater than 10 to 20 mg per kg per day) versus low (5 to 10 mg per kg daily) maintenance doses of caffeine citrate for the treatment of apnea in premature infants included 13 randomized controlled trials with 1,515 patients.[108] Compared with the low-dose group, the high-dose group had higher rates of effective treatment and ventilator removal and lower extubation failure, BPD rates, and frequency and duration of apnea. The high-dose group had a higher incidence of tachycardia; adverse events such as hypertension, hyperglycemia, and feeding intolerance and morbidities such as ROP, intracranial hemorrhage, NEC, and in-hospital death were comparable between groups.[108] Other reviews confirmed a reduction in BPD rate in the high-dose group,[109,110] and there was no difference in the rates of neurodevelopmental impairment at 12 and 24 months corrected age, although the quality of evidence was deemed to be low or very low.[110] One randomized controlled trial compared loading doses of 80 versus 20 mg per kg in 74 preterm infants and reported a significantly higher incidence of cerebellar hemorrhage (36% vs. 10%), hypertonicity, and deviant neurologic signs at term equivalent age.[111] There was no difference in magnetic resonance imaging diffusion measures and neurodevelopment at 2 years of age.[111]

EARLY VERSUS LATE CAFFEINE THERAPY

A post hoc analysis of the large randomized controlled CAP trial demonstrated that infants treated with caffeine at or before 3 days of age had a greater reduction in the duration of respiratory support than those in whom it was initiated at 4 to 10 days of age.[68] Since then, a large propensity score–matched cohort study showed that infants treated in the initial 2 days of age had significantly lower rates of death or BPD, BPD alone, PDA with treatment, and a 6-day mean decrease in the duration of mechanical ventilation, compared with those who were treated at or after 3 days of age.[112] The mortality rate was slightly higher (4.5% vs. 3.7%), probably due to survival bias.[112,113] Data from the Canadian Neonatal Network confirmed the lower rates of death or BPD and PDA but reported similar rates of death, NEC, severe neurologic injury, or severe ROP.[114] A beneficial effect of early caffeine on BPD was also found in a meta-analysis, although the quality of evidence was found to be low.[109] Others found a significantly reduced need for mechanical ventilation, total duration of mechanical ventilation, intraventricular hemorrhage, and PDA but comparable rates of death and BPD in groups of infants who received caffeine starting at Day 1 and propensity-matched infants who received later therapy.[115] In a multicenter cohort of preterm infants below 33 weeks of gestational age, incidence and severity of acute kidney injury in the initial week of age were significantly reduced (*OR*, 0.20; 95% CI, 0.11 to 0.34) with caffeine administration.[116] In a study of very low-birth-weight infants maintained on continuous positive airway pressure (CPAP), early (day of birth) caffeine did not have a significant impact on the rate of CPAP failure in the initial week.[117] Most recently, from the follow-up data of the Canadian Neonatal Network, it was found that, among infants born below 29 weeks of gestation, early (2 days or earlier) caffeine was associated with a reduction in the risk of severe neurodevelopmental impairment (*OR*, 0.68; 95% CI, 0.50 to 0.94) and a cognitive score below 85 (0.67; 95% CI, 0.47 to 0.95). A propensity-matched analysis also showed reductions in cerebral palsy and hearing impairment.[118]

LONG-TERM EFFECTS OF METHYLXANTHINES

The methylated xanthines are some of the most psychoactive agents in the human diet and exert significant CNS excitation and other neuronal effects at a very critical time in human development. Caffeine has been demonstrated to induce neuronal death in neonatal rat brain and cortical cell cultures and theophylline to decrease the rate of anoxic survival in vivo.[119,120] In rat pups treated with daily caffeine, transient impairment in motor skills and changes in locomotor activity were observed, depending on the developmental stage.[121] In a newborn mouse model, caffeine did not worsen excitotoxic periventricular white matter lesions.[122] In human infants, data suggest that there is no independent adverse effect of caffeine on the long-term outcome. Gunn et al. followed a group of 21 very low-birth-weight premature neonates treated with caffeine and compared them to a similar group (n = 21) not treated with caffeine.[123] No differences in growth and development were noted at a 12-month follow-up. Similarly, Ment et al. showed no differences in the neurodevelopmental outcome and in Bayley scores at 18 months in 73 infants weighing less than 1,250 g at birth with respect to the presence or absence of intraventricular hemorrhage and with or without treatment with methylxanthines.[124] In fact, infants who received methylxanthine therapy scored better at 18 months, regardless of hemorrhage status. In the CAP trial, which is the largest follow-up study so far, of the 937 infants in the caffeine group, 377 (40.2%) died or survived with a neurodevelopmental disability, as compared with 431 of the 932 infants (46.2%) in the placebo group (*OR* adjusted for center, 0.77; 95% CI, 0.64 to 0.93; p = 0.008).[102] Treatment with caffeine as compared with placebo reduced the incidence of cerebral palsy (4.4% vs. 7.3%; adjusted *OR*, 0.58; 95% CI, 0.39 to 0.87; p = 0.009) and of cognitive delay (33.8% vs. 38.3%; adjusted *OR*, 0.81; 95% CI, 0.66 to 0.99; p = 0.04). The rates of death, deafness, and blindness and the mean percentiles for height, weight, and head circumference at the follow-up did not differ significantly between the two groups.[102] In further analyses, the investigators reported that the size and direction of the caffeine effect on death or disability differed depending on PPV at randomization (p = 0.03).[98] *ORs* (95% CI) were as follows: no support, 1.32 (0.81 to 2.14); noninvasive support, 0.73 (0.52 to 1.03); and ETT, 0.73 (0.57 to 0.94). Adjustment for baseline factors strengthened this effect (p = 0.02). The follow-up of 1,640 trial participants at 5 years of age showed that there were no significant differences between the two groups in death or disability, defined as motor impairment, cognitive impairment, behavior problems, poor general health, deafness, or blindness.[125] Among a subgroup of 1,433 infants who underwent the Movement Assessment Battery for Children test, developmental coordination disorder incidence was found to be lower (*OR*, 0.71; 95% CI, 0.52 to 0.97) in the caffeine-treated group.[126] At 11 years of age, among 920 infants, functional impairment, defined as poor academic performance, motor impairment, or behavioral problems, was comparable between the two groups.[127] The caffeine-treated group did have lower motor impairment. Neurobehavioral outcomes were also comparable between groups.[128] The caffeine-treated group had improved fine motor coordination, visuomotor integration, visual perception, and visuospatial organization. There is a substantial placental transfer of caffeine, and significant numbers of neonates are born with therapeutic concentrations of caffeine in their cord blood. Any follow-up studies must account for antenatal and postnatal exposure to the methylated xanthines because these are pervasive components of dietary, including beverage, intake.

DOXAPRAM

Doxapram, an analeptic and respiratory stimulant in adults used clinically since 1962, has been given to neonates with apnea and those resistant to methylated xanthines. Gupta and Moore used doxapram to produce respiratory stimulation in 83 full-term infants born to mothers who received narcotic analgesics or general anesthesia causing respiratory depression.[129] The doses varied from 0.5 to 3 mg per kg (as a single dose) immediately after birth. A randomized trial by Peliowski and Finer in 1990 including 11 infants given intravenous doxapram and 10 infants given placebo showed less treatment failures with doxapram compared with placebo (4/11 vs. 8/10).[60] This study was reviewed by Henderson-Smart and Steer who suggested that intravenous doxapram might reduce apnea within the first 48 hours of treatment, but there are insufficient data to evaluate the precision of this result or to assess potential adverse effects.[130] A more recent study of 203 preterm infants with a median gestational age of 26.1 (interquartile range, 25.1 to 27.4) weeks who received oral or intravenous doxapram showed that 157 (77%) patients did not need ETT over the initial 48 hours and 127 (63%) patients avoided ETT over the entire treatment course.[131] In contrast, a systematic review included a randomized controlled trial comparing doxapram and standard treatment with standard treatment alone in 29 preterm infants and found no significant difference in extubation failure (*RR*, 0.80; 95% CI, 0.22 to 2.97; *RD*, −0.05; 95% CI, −0.36 to 0.26).[76,132] Data on long-term outcomes related to doxapram therapy are limited. Preterm infants with a gestational age less than 30 weeks and/or a birth weight less than 1,250 g treated with doxapram (n = 142) were compared with a nontreated control group (n = 284).[133] While the proportion of infants with a mental or psychomotor score below 1 SD at 24 months corrected age was not different between the groups, the risk of death or neurodevelopmental delay was significantly lower in the doxapram group after adjustment (*OR*, 0.54; 95% CI, 0.37, 0.78). A previous smaller case–control study in infants less than 1,250 g at birth revealed that isolated mental delay (mental development index < 70) at 18 months corrected age was associated with the total dosage and duration of doxapram therapy for severe apnea.[134]

Henderson-Smart and Steer analyzed data comparing doxapram and methylxanthine and concluded that intravenous doxapram and intravenous methylxanthine appear to be similar in their short-term effects for treating apnea in preterm infants.[135] However, the trials performed are too small to exclude an important difference between the two treatments or to exclude the possibility of less common adverse effects. Longer-term outcome of infants treated in these trials has not been reported. In addition to apnea of prematurity, doxapram has also been used in central hypoventilation, weaning from mechanical ventilation, and in obstructive apnea. In a more recent appraisal of the evidence, randomized controlled trials showed less apnea during doxapram treatment when compared to placebo, but no difference in treatment effect when compared to theophylline.[136] No serious adverse effects were reported. The identified 28 observational studies mostly reported a beneficial effect of doxapram on apnea rate, conflicting and more limited data on long-term outcomes and a range of short-term adverse effects.[136] Because of the known safety and efficacy of the methylated xanthines, doxapram is used only in cases where methylxanthines are not effective and only before considering a more aggressive form of treatment such as mechanical ventilation.

DOSAGE

The dosage regimen of 2.5 mg per kg per hour was basically derived from adult data. A dose–response relationship has been suggested. Barrington et al. showed that incremental doses of continuous intravenous infusion were associated with increased response.[137] In 18 premature infants given doxapram, 47% responded at 0.5 mg per kg per hour and up to 89% responded at 2.5 mg per kg per hour. Hayakawa et al., in a study of 12 premature infants, reported a good correlation between dose and serum concentration and a success rate of 75% with infusion of 1.0 to 1.5 mg per kg per hour.[138] The ideal dosage and route of administration remain to be defined; a regimen of a loading dose of 2.5 to 3 mg per kg administered over 15 to 30 minutes followed by a continuous infusion of 1 mg per kg per hour with careful surveillance of blood pressure changes has been used. This maintenance dosage may be increased if necessary by 0.5 mg per kg per hour up to a maximum of 2.5 mg per kg per hour. Caution must be observed in the use of doxapram as there are various formulations available containing different excipients. Some pharmaceutical preparations may contain benzyl alcohol, chlorobutanol, or sodium benzoate, and extreme caution should be exercised to monitor possible adverse effects of these preservatives.

MODE OF ADMINISTRATION

Doxapram is poorly absorbed enterally and has a short duration of action, despite a relatively apparent long half-life. An intermittent intravenous bolus regimen has been proposed, although continuous intravenous infusion is often used.

THERAPEUTIC PLASMA LEVEL

The ideal plasma therapeutic concentrations need to be defined, but data suggest a possible therapeutic window. Those babies who responded to doxapram all had a serum level of at least 1.5 mg per L; the mean serum concentration related to this response was 2.9 mg per L, with the therapeutic threshold proposed being greater than 2 mg per L. Adverse drug effects become more frequent at plasma levels above 5 mg per L.

PHARMACOKINETICS, PHARMACODYNAMICS, AND METABOLISM

Doxapram is metabolized by the CYP3A4/5 in neonatal human liver[139] to give at least three metabolites. The oxidation pathway that yields metabolites AHR-5955 (ketodoxapram) and AHR-5904 seems more active than the deethylation pathway producing AHR-0914. Ketodoxapram is also a strong respiratory stimulant, without the side effects reported with doxapram (i.e., increase in blood pressure and excitability). Pharmacokinetic studies in newborn infants indicate prolonged elimination in infants compared with adults.[140] The plasma half-life ranges from 6.6 to 8.2 hours, plasma clearance is 0.44 to 0.7 L per kg per hour, and apparent value of distribution is 4.0 to 7.3 L per kg. Beaudry et al.[141] also determined the pharmacokinetics of doxapram in 13 infants with a mean gestational age of 29.4 weeks who received a constant infusion rate of doxapram of 2 to 2.5 mg per kg per hour for 72 to 96 hours. The steady-state plasma doxapram levels were an average of 5.8 ± 1.8 mg/L with a plasma half-life of 6.6 ± 5.7 hour and a plasma clearance of 0.44 ± 0.1 L per kg per hour. Doxapram controlled apnea successfully with a significant fall in P_aCO_2 and a reduction in the rate of apnea corresponding to doxapram levels of 3.7 ± 1.8 mg per L. The pharmacokinetic profile suggests a first-order kinetics in premature infants, with substantial interpatient variability and a decreasing plasma half-life with advancing age. Little doxapram is excreted in the urine, and ketodoxapram is usually detected in every patient receiving doxapram.

SIDE EFFECTS

Adverse reactions to doxapram that have been reported include the following:

- Adverse drug reaction (ADR) definitely related to doxapram: increase in blood pressure, mainly at infusion greater than 1.5 mg per kg per hour or at a level greater than 5 mg per L.
- ADR probably or possibly related to doxapram: regurgitation, excessive salivation, increased agitation, excessive crying, disturbed sleep, jitteriness, increase in gastric residuals, vomiting, and irritability and cardiac conduction blocks; blood in stool, abdominal distension, hyperglycemia, glycosuria, and premature teeth buds (lower central incisors).
- Hypokalemia has been reported in about half of doxapram-treated infants, even at low doses.[142,143] Potassium monitoring during therapy is recommended.
- A potentially dangerous side effect is a potential decrease in cerebral oxygenation and blood flow velocity. This might result in decreased cerebral perfusion and damage to the developing brain leading to long-term developmental delay.[133,144]

MECHANISMS OF ACTION

The exact mechanism of action of doxapram is probably via the stimulation of the peripheral chemoreceptors, mainly at low doses (less than 0.5 mg per kg), and the central respiratory and nonrespiratory neurons, mainly at a higher dose. Doxapram also increases respiratory center output. In human infants, doxapram causes a significant fall in P_aCO_2 and an increase in minute ventilation, tidal volume, and occlusion pressure but no change in respiratory rate, inspiratory, or expiratory time.

CONCLUSION

Available data suggest that doxapram is an effective drug to treat apnea in the premature infant and can be used as a second-line drug in case of failure with methylxanthine and prior to a much more aggressive form of therapy such as ETT and mechanical ventilation. Complications from the latter therapy are significant, particularly in the very small premature infant. Doxapram is used off label, and caution should be exercised when using in newborn infants.

GENERAL CONSIDERATIONS FOR APNEA MANAGEMENT

Although drug therapy is a major component of neonatal apnea management, the multicausal (including metabolic, infectious, neurologic, and other pathophysiologic states) nature of neonatal and infantile apnea should be recognized. Treatment should be directed at those physiologic and biochemical perturbations illustrated in Figure 15.1. In this figure, apnea appears as a common pathway by which various noxious or other stimuli exert their effect on an immature respiratory control system not yet ready for the complex integration of various neural inputs. Whatever the mechanism involved in the pathogenesis of neonatal and infantile apnea, correctable factors associated with the occurrence of apnea should be treated. As the survival of

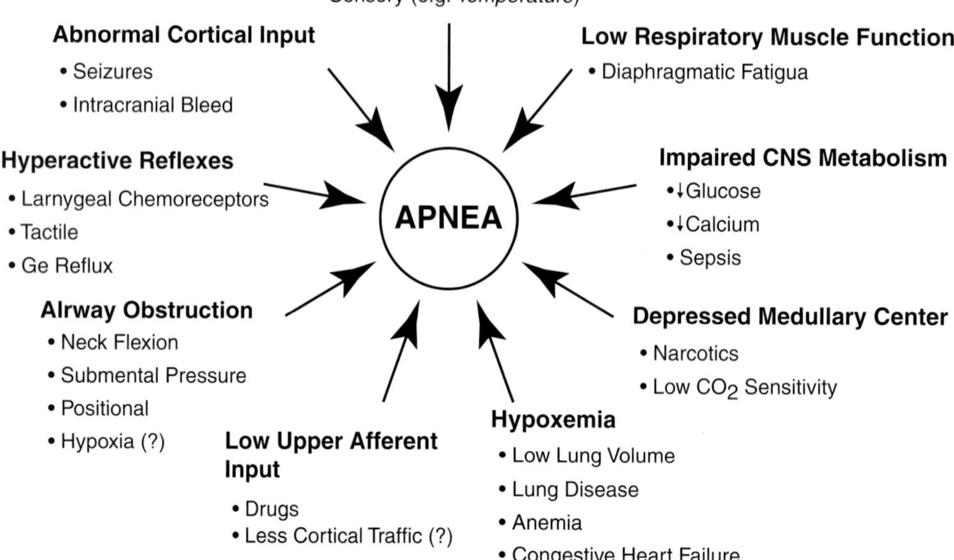

Figure 15.1 Factors associated with the genesis of neonatal apnea. Therapy should be directed toward the correction of etiologic factors. CNS, central nervous system; GE, gastroenteric.

the very low-birth-weight infants at the greatest risk for apnea increases with medical advances, the challenge for safe and effective treatment of apnea remains a primary investigative and clinical concern.

REFERENCES

1. Kuzemko JA, Paala J. Apnoeic attacks in the newborn treated with aminophylline. *Arch Dis Child* 1973;48(5):404–406.
2. Davi MJ, Sankaran K, Simons KJ, et al. Physiologic changes induced by theophylline in the treatment of apnea in preterm infants. *J Pediatr* 1978;92:91–95.
3. Gerhardt T, McCarthy J, Bancalari E. Effect of aminophylline on respiratory center activity and metabolic rate in premature infants with idiopathic apnea. *Pediatrics* 1979;63:537–542.
4. Aranda JV, Gorman W, Bergsteinsson H, et al. Efficacy of caffeine in treatment of apnea in the low-birth-weight infant. *J Pediatr* 1977;90:467–472.
5. Mazzarelli M, Jaspan N, Zin WA, et al. Dose effect of caffeine on control of breathing and respiratory response to CO_2 in cats. *J Appl Physiol* 1986;60:52–59.
6. Aranda JV, Forman W, Cook C, et al. Pharmacokinetic profile of caffeine in the premature newborn infant with apnea. *J Pediatr* 1977;50:467–472.
7. Bellville JW, Escarrage LA, Wallenstein SL, et al. Antagonism by caffeine of the respiratory effects of codeine and morphine. *J Pharmacol Exp Ther* 1962;136:8727.
8. Lambertson CJ. Drugs and respiration. *Annu Rev Pharmacol* 1966;6:327–345.
9. Stroud MW III, Lambertson CJ, Ewing JH, et al. The effects of aminophylline and meperidine alone and in combination on the respiratory response to CO_2 inhalation. *J Pharmacol Exp Ther* 1955;114:461–465.
10. Huidobro F, Amenbar L. Effectiveness of caffeine (1,3,7 trimethylxanthines) against fatigue. *J Pharmacol Exp Ther* 1945;84:82–87.
11. Aubier M, Detroyer A, MacKelem PT, et al. Aminophylline improves diaphragmatic contractility. *N Engl J Med* 1981;305:249–252.
12. Aubier M, Murciano D, Lecocgnic Y, et al. Diaphragmatic contractility enhanced by aminophylline: role of extracellular calcium. *J Appl Physiol* 1983;54:460–464.
13. Lopes JM, LeSoeuf PN, Heather MH, et al. The effects of theophylline on diaphragmatic fatigue in the newborn. *Pediatr Res* 1982;16:355A.
14. Nassar-Gentina J, Passonneau JV, Rapoport SI. Fatigue and metabolism of frog muscle fibers during stimulation and in response to caffeine. *Am J Physiol* 1981;241:C160–C166.
15. Heyman E, Ohlsson A, Heyman Z, et al. The effect of aminophylline on the excursions of the diaphragm in preterm neonates. A randomized double-blind controlled study. *Acta Paediatr Scand* 1991;80:308–315.
16. Meyers RF, Milnap RL, Krauss AN, et al. Low dose theophylline therapy in idiopathic apnea of prematurity. *J Pediatr* 1980;5:99–104.
17. Davis GM, Bureau MA. Pulmonary and chest wall mechanics in the control of respiration in the newborn. *Clin Perinatol* 1987;14:552–579.
18. Dani C, Bertini G, Reali MF, et al. Brain hemodynamic changes in preterm infants after maintenance dose caffeine and aminophylline treatment. *Biol Neonate* 2000;78:27–32.
19. Ritchie JM. Central nervous stimulants. 11. The xanthines. In: Goodman LS, Gilman A, eds. *The pharmacological basis of therapeutics*, 5th ed. London, UK: Cassell & Collier Macmillan, 1975:367–378.
20. Curzi-Dascalova L, Aujard Y, Gaultier C, et al. Sleep organization is unaffected by caffeine in premature infants. *J Pediatr* 2002;140:766–771.
21. Fredholm BB. On the mechanism of action of theophylline and caffeine. *Acta Med Scand* 1985;217:149–153.
22. Aldridge FL, Millhorm DE, Waltrop TG, et al. Mechanisms of respiratory effects of methylxanthines. *Respir Physiol* 1979;53:239–261.
23. Lopes J, Muller N, Bryan AC, et al. Importance of inspiratory muscle tone in maintenance of FRC in the newborn. *J Appl Physiol* 1981;51:830–834.
24. Manku MS, Horrobin DF. Chloroquine, quinine, procaine, quinidine, tricyclic antidepressants and methylxanthines as prostaglandin agonists and antagonists. *Lancet* 1976;2:1115–1117.
25. Clifford E, Miller M, Chakravarti S, et al. Caffeine and hypoxia have opposing effects on GABA A receptor subunit expression in the neonatal rat brainstem. *Pediatr Res* 2005;403:5466A.
26. Phillis JW, Wu PH. The role of adenosine and its nucleotides in central synaptic transmission. *Prog Neurol* 1981;16:287–289.
27. Runold M, Lagercrantz H, Fredholm BB. Ventilatory effect of an adenosine analogue in unanesthetized rabbits during development. *J Appl Physiol* 1986;61:255–259.
28. Winn HR, Rubio R, Berne RM. Brain adenosine concentration during hypoxia in rats. *Am J Physiol* 1981;241:H235–H242.
29. Darnall RA. Aminophylline reduces hypoxic ventilatory depression: possible role of adenosine. *Pediatr Res* 1985;19:206–210.
30. Lopes JM, Davis GM, Mullahoo K, et al. Role of adenosine in the hypoxic ventilatory depression of the newborn piglet. *Pediatr Pulmonol* 1994;17:50–55.
31. Aranda JV, Grondin D, Sasyniuk B. Pharmacologic considerations in the therapy of neonatal apnea. *Pediatr Clin North Am* 1981;28:113–133.
32. Aranda JV. Maturational changes in theophylline and caffeine metabolism and disposition: clinical implications. In: Proceedings of 2nd World Congress, Clinical Pharmacology and Therapeutics. Rockville, MD: American Society for Pharmacology and Experimental Therapeutics, 1984:868–877.
33. De Carolis MP, Romagnoli C, Muzii U, et al. Pharmacokinetic aspects of caffeine in premature infants. *Dev Pharmacol Ther* 1991;16:117–122.
34. Le Guennec JC, Billon B, Pare C. Maturational changes of caffeine concentrations and disposition in infancy during maintenance therapy for apnea of prematurity: influence of gestational age, hepatic disease and breast feeding. *Pediatrics* 1985;76:834–840.
35. Lee TC, Charles BG, Steer PA, et al. Saliva as a valid alternative to serum in monitoring intravenous caffeine treatment for apnea of prematurity. *Ther Drug Monit* 1996;18:288–293.
36. de Wildt SN, Kerkvliet KT, Wezenberg MG, et al. Use of saliva in therapeutic drug monitoring of caffeine in preterm infants. *Ther Drug Monit* 2001;23:250–254.
37. Bory C, Baltassat P, Porthault M, et al. Metabolism of theophylline to caffeine in premature infants. *J Pediatr* 1979;94:988–993.
38. Aranda JV, Louridas AT, Vitullo B, et al. Metabolism of theophylline to caffeine in human fetal liver. *Science* 1979;206:1319–1321.
39. Yazdani M, Kissling GE, Tran TH, et al. Phenobarbital increases theophylline requirement of premature infants being treated for apnea. *Am J Dis Child* 1987;141:97–99.
40. Brouard C, Moriette G, Murat I, et al. Comparative efficacy of theophylline and caffeine in the treatment of idiopathic apnea in premature infants. *Am J Dis Child* 1985;139:698–700.
41. Bairam A, Boutroy MJ, Badonnel Y, et al. Theophylline versus caffeine: comparative effects in treatment of idiopathic apnea in the preterm infants. *J Pediatr* 1987;110:636–639.
42. Scanlon JE, Chin KC, Morgan ME, et al. Caffeine or theophylline for neonatal apnoea? *Arch Dis Child* 1992;67(4 spec no.):425–428.

43. Shivakumar M, Jayashree P, Najih M, et al. Comparative efficacy and safety of caffeine and aminophylline for apnea of prematurity in preterm (≤34 weeks) neonates: a randomized controlled trial. *Indian Pediatr* 2017;54(4):279–283.
44. Henderson-Smart DJ, Steer PA. Caffeine versus theophylline for apnea in preterm infants. *Cochrane Database Syst Rev* 2010;(1):CD000273.
45. Kumar SP, Metha PN, Bradley BS, et al. Documented monitoring show theophylline to be more effective than caffeine in prematurity apnea. *Pediatr Res* 1992;31:208A.
46. Bairam A, Boutroy MJ, Badonnel Y, et al. The choice between theophylline and caffeine in the treatment of apnea in premature infants. *Arch Fr Pediatr* 1990;47:461–465.
47. Larsen PB, Brendstrup L, Skov L, et al. Aminophylline versus caffeine citrate for apnea and bradycardia prophylaxis in premature neonates. *Acta Paediatr* 1995;84:360–364.
48. Fuglsang G, Nielsen K, Kjaer Nielsen L, et al. The effect of caffeine compared with theophylline in the treatment of idiopathic apnea in premature infants. *Acta Paediatr Scand* 1989;78:786–788.
49. Natarajan G, Botica ML, Thomas R, et al. Therapeutic drug monitoring of caffeine in preterm neonates: an unnecessary exercise? *Pediatrics* 2007;119(5):936–940.
50. Pesce AJ, Rakhkin M, Kotagal U. Standards of laboratory practice: theophylline and caffeine monitoring. *Clin Chem* 1998;44:1124–1128.
51. Charles BG, Townsend SR, Steer PA, et al. Caffeine citrate treatment for extremely premature infants with apnea: population pharmacokinetics, absolute bioavailability, and implications for therapeutic drug monitoring. *Ther Drug Monit* 2008;30(6):709–716.
52. Yu T, Balch AH, Ward RM, et al. Incorporating pharmacodynamic considerations into caffeine therapeutic drug monitoring in preterm neonates. *BMC Pharmacol Toxicol* 2016;17(1):22.
53. Kuzemko JA, Paala J. Apnoeic attacks in the newborn treated with aminophylline. *Arch Dis Child* 1973;48(5):404–406.
54. Shannon DC, Gotay F, Stein M, et al. Prevention of apnea and bradycardia in low-birth-weight infants. *Pediatrics* 1975;55:589.
55. Uauy R, Shapiro DL, Smith B, et al. Treatment of severe apnea in prematures with orally administered theophylline. *Pediatrics* 1975;55:595–598.
56. Peabody J, Neese AL, Phillip AG, et al. Transcutaneous oxygen monitoring in aminophylline-treated apnoeic infants. *Pediatrics* 1978;62:698.
57. Murat I, Moriwette G, Blin MC, et al. The efficacy of caffeine in the treatment of recurrent apnea in premature infants. *J Pediatr* 1981;99:984–999.
58. Roberts JL, Mathew OP, Thach BT. The efficacy of theophylline in premature infants with mixed and obstructive apnea associated with pulmonary and neurologic disease. *J Pediatr* 1982;100:968–970.
59. Sims ME, Yau G, Rambhatla S, et al. Limitations of theophylline in the treatment of apnea of prematurity. *Am J Dis Child* 1985;139:567–570.
60. Peliowski A, Finer NN. A blinded, randomized, placebo controlled trial to compare theophylline and doxapram for the treatment of apnea of prematurity. *J Pediatr* 1990;116(4):648–653.
61. Erenberg A, Leff RD, Haack DG, et al. Caffeine citrate for the treatment of apnea of prematurity: a double-blind, placebo-controlled study. *Pharmacotherapy* 2000;20(6):644–652.
62. Eichenwald EC, Howell GR, Leszczynski LE, et al. Theophylline improves coordination of laryngeal abduction and inspiratory effort in premature infants. *Pediatr Res* 1989;25:308A.
63. Henderson-Smart DJ, De Paoli AG. Methylxanthine treatment for apnea in preterm infants. *Cochrane Database Syst Rev* 2010;(12):CD000140.
64. Schmidt B, Roberts RS, Davis P, et al. Caffeine therapy for apnea of prematurity. *N Engl J Med* 2006;354:2112–2121.
65. Muttitt SC, Tierney AJ, Finer NN. The dose response of theophylline in the treatment of apnea of prematurity. *J Pediatr* 1988;112:115–121.
66. Henderson-Smart DJ, De Paoli AG. Prophylactic methylxanthine for prevention of apnea in preterm infants. *Cochrane Database Syst Rev* 2010;(12):CD000432.
67. Bucher HU, Duc G. Does caffeine prevent hypoxaemic episodes in premature infants? A randomized controlled trial. *Eur J Pediatr* 1988;147(3):288–291.
68. Davis PG, Schmidt B, Roberts RS, et al Caffeine for Apnea of Prematurity Trial Group. Caffeine for apnea of prematurity trial: benefits may vary in subgroups. *J Pediatr* 2010;156(3):382–387.
69. Harris MC, Baumgart S, Rocklin AR, et al. Successful extubation of infants with respiratory distress syndrome using aminophylline. *J Pediatr* 1983;103:303–305.
70. Viscardi RM, Faix RG, Nicks JJ, et al. Efficacy of theophylline for prevention of post-extubation respiratory failure in very low birth weight infants. *J Pediatr* 1985;107:469–472.
71. Barrington KJ, Finer NN. A randomized, controlled trial of aminophylline in ventilatory weaning of premature infants. *Crit Care Med* 1993;21:846–850.
72. Sims ME, Rangasamy R, Lee S, et al. Comparative evaluation of caffeine and theophylline for weaning premature infants from the ventilator. *Am J Perinatol* 1989;6:72–75.
73. Henderson-Smart DJ, Davis PG. Prophylactic methylxanthines for endotracheal extubation in preterm infants. *Cochrane Database Syst Rev* 2010;(12):CD000139.
74. Steer PA, Flenady VJ, Shearman A, et al. Periextubation caffeine in preterm neonates: a randomized dose response trial. *J Paediatr Child Health* 2003;39(7):511–514.
75. Steer P, Flenady V, Shearman A, et al. High dose caffeine citrate for extubation of preterm infants: a randomized controlled trial. *Arch Dis Child Fetal Neonatal Ed* 2004;89:499–503.
76. Ferguson KN, Roberts CT, Manley BJ, et al. Interventions to improve rates of successful extubation in preterm infants: a systematic review and meta-analysis. *JAMA Pediatr* 2017;171(2):165–174.
77. Al-Mandari H, Shalish W, Dempsey E, et al. International survey on periextubation practices in extremely preterm infants. *Arch Dis Child Fetal Neonatal Ed* 2015;100(5):F428–F431.
78. Yoder B, Thomson M, Coalson J. Lung function in immature baboons with respiratory distress syndrome receiving early caffeine therapy: a pilot study. *Acta Paediatr* 2005;94:92–98.
79. Montandon G, Bairam A, Kinkead R. Long term consequences of neonatal caffeine on ventilation, occurrence of apneas and hypercapnic chemoreflex in male and female rats. *Pediatr Res* 2006;59:519–524.
80. Davis JM, Bhutani VK, Stefano JL, et al. Changes in pulmonary mechanics following caffeine administration in infants with bronchopulmonary dysplasia. *Pediatr Pulmonol* 1989;6:49–52.
81. Sanchez-Solis M, Garcia-Marcos PW, Aguera-Arenas J, et al. Impact of early caffeine therapy in preterm newborns on infant lung function. *Pediatr Pulmonol* 2020;55(1):102–107. doi:10.1002/ppul.24540.
82. Rossor T, Bhat R, Ali K, et al. The effect of caffeine on the ventilatory response to hypercarbia in preterm infants. *Pediatr Res* 2018;83(6):1152–1157.
83. Laubscher B, Greenough A, Dimitriou G. Comparative effects of theophylline and caffeine on respiratory function of prematurely born infants. *Early Hum Dev* 1998;50:185–192.
84. Kraaijenga JV, Hutten GJ, de Jongh FH, et al. The effect of caffeine on diaphragmatic activity and tidal volume in preterm infants. *J Pediatr* 2015;167(1):70–75.
85. Doyle LW, Ranganathan S, Cheong JLY. Neonatal caffeine treatment and respiratory function at 11 years in children under 1,251 g at birth. *Am J Respir Crit Care Med* 2017;196(10):1318–1324.
86. Clyman RI, Roman C. The effects of caffeine on the preterm sheep ductus arteriosus. *Pediatr Res* 2007;62(62):167–169.
87. Hwang J, Kim YS, Shin JH, et al. Hemodynamic effects on systemic blood flow and ductal shunting flow after loading dose of intravenous caffeine in preterm infants according to the patency of ductus arteriosus. *J Korean Med Sci* 2018;33(4):e25.
88. Soloveychik V, Bin Nun A, Ionchev A, et al. Acute hemodynamic effects of caffeine administration in premature infants. *J Perinatol* 2009;29(3):205–208.
89. Hoecker C, Nelle M, Beedgen B, et al. Effects of a divided high loading dose of caffeine on circulatory variables in preterm infants. *Arch Dis Child Fetal Neonatal Ed* 2006;91(1):F61–F64.
90. Hoecker C, Nelle M, Poeschl J, et al. Caffeine impairs cerebral and intestinal blood flow velocity in preterm infants. *Pediatrics* 2002;109(5):784–787.
91. Ulanovsky I, Haleluya NS, Blazer S, et al. The effects of caffeine on heart rate variability in newborns with apnea of prematurity. *J Perinatol* 2014;34(8):620–623.
92. Walther FJ, Sims ME, Siassi B, et al. Cardiac output changes secondary to theophylline therapy in preterm infants. *J Pediatr* 1986;109(5):874–876.
93. Fesslova V, Caccamo ML, Salice P, et al. Assessment of cardiovascular effects to theophylline in premature newborns by means of serial echocardiography. *Acta Paediatr Scand* 1984;73(3):404–405.
94. Shannon DC, Gotay F. Effects of theophylline on serum and urine electrolytes in preterm infants with apnea. *J Pediatr* 1979;94:963–965.
95. Bauer J, Maier K, Linderkamp O, et al. Effect of caffeine on oxygen consumption and metabolic rate in very low birth weight infants with idiopathic apnea. *Pediatrics* 2001;107:660–663.
96. Pacifici GM. Clinical pharmacology of theophylline in preterm infants: effects, metabolism and pharmacokinetics. *Curr Pediatr Rev* 2014;10(4):297–303.
97. Zanardo V, Dani C, Trevisanuto D, et al. Methylxanthines increase renal calcium excretion in preterm infants. *Biol Neonate* 1995;68:169–174.
98. Lundstrom KE, Larsen PB, Brendstrup L, et al. Cerebral blood flow and left ventricular output in spontaneously breathing, newborn preterm infants treated with caffeine or aminophylline. *Acta Paediatr* 1995;84:6–9.
99. Wechsler RL, Kleiss LM, Kety SS. Effect of intravenously administered aminophylline on cerebral circulation and metabolism in man. *J Clin Invest* 1954;29:28–33.
100. Saliba E, Autret E, Gold F, et al. Effect of caffeine on cerebral blood flow velocity in preterm infants. *Biol Neonate* 1989;56:198–203.
101. Van Bel F, Van de Bor M, Stijnen T, et al. Does caffeine affect cerebral blood flow in the preterm infant? *Acta Paediatr Scand* 1989;78:205–209.
102. Schmidt B, Roberts RS, Davis P, et al. Caffeine for Apnea of Prematurity Trial Group. Long-term effects of caffeine therapy for apnea of prematurity. *N Engl J Med* 2007;357(19):1893–1902.
103. Beharry KD, Valencia GB, Lazzaro DR, et al. Pharmacologic interventions for the prevention and treatment of retinopathy of prematurity. *Semin Perinatol* 2016;40(3):189–202.
104. Varma SD, Hegde KR, Kovtun S. Oxidative stress in lens in vivo: inhibitory effect of caffeine. A preliminary report. *Mol Vis* 2010;16:501–505.
105. Tu C, Beharry KD, Shen X, et al. Proteomic profiling of the retinas in a neonatal rat model of oxygen-induced retinopathy with a reproducible ion-current-based MS1 approach. *J Proteome Res* 2015;14(5):2109–2120.
106. Lane AJ, Coombs RC, Evans DH, et al. Effect of caffeine on neonatal splanchnic blood flow. *Arch Dis Child Fetal Neonatal Ed* 1999;80:F128–F129.
107. Davis JM, Abbasi S, Spitzer AR, et al. Role of theophylline in pathogenesis of necrotizing enterocolitis. *J Pediatr* 1986;109:344–347.
108. Chen J, Jin L, Chen X. Efficacy and safety of different maintenance doses of caffeine citrate for treatment of apnea in premature infants: a systematic review and meta-analysis. *Biomed Res Int* 2018;2018:9061234.
109. Pakvasa MA, Saroha V, Patel RM. Optimizing caffeine use and risk of bronchopulmonary dysplasia in preterm infants: a systematic review, meta-analysis, and application of grading of recommendations assessment, development, and evaluation methodology. *Clin Perinatol* 2018;45(2):273–291.
110. Vliegenthart R, Miedema M, Hutten GJ, et al. High versus standard dose caffeine for apnoea: a systematic review. *Arch Dis Child Fetal Neonatal Ed* 2018;103(6):F523–F529.
111. McPherson C, Neil JJ, Tjoeng TH, et al. A pilot randomized trial of high-dose caffeine therapy in preterm infants. *Pediatr Res* 2015;78(2):198–204.
112. Dobson NR, Patel RM, Smith PB, et al. Trends in caffeine use and association between clinical outcomes and timing of therapy in very low birth weight infants. *J Pediatr* 2014;164(5):992–998.e3.
113. Schmidt B, Davis PG, Roberts RS. Timing of caffeine therapy in very low birth weight infants. *J Pediatr* 2014;164(5):957–958.
114. Lodha A, Seshia M, McMillan DD, et al. Canadian Neonatal Network. Association of early caffeine administration and neonatal outcomes in very preterm neonates. *JAMA Pediatr* 2015;169(1):33–38.

115. Borszewska-Kornacka MK, Hożejowski R, Rutkowska M, et al. Shifting the boundaries for early caffeine initiation in neonatal practice: Results of a prospective, multicenter study on very preterm infants with respiratory distress syndrome. *PLoS One* 2017;12(12):e0189152.
116. Harer MW, Askenazi DJ, Boohaker LJ, et al. Neonatal Kidney Collaborative (NKC). Association between early caffeine citrate administration and risk of acute kidney injury in preterm neonates: results from the AWAKEN study. *JAMA Pediatr* 2018;172(6):e180322.
117. Patel RM, Zimmerman K, Carlton DP, et al. Early caffeine prophylaxis and risk of failure of initial continuous positive airway pressure in very low birth weight infants. *J Pediatr* 2017;190:108.e1–111.e1.
118. Lodha A, Entz R, Synnes A, et al. Investigators of the Canadian Neonatal Network (CNN) and the Canadian Neonatal Follow-up Network (CNFUN). Early Caffeine Administration and Neurodevelopmental Outcomes in Preterm Infants. *Pediatrics* 2019;143(1):pii :e20181348.
119. Kang SH, Lee YA, Won SJ, et al. Caffeine-induced neuronal death in neonatal rat brain and cortical cell cultures. *Neuroreport* 2002;13:1945–1950.
120. Thurston JH, Hauhart RE, Dirgo JA. Aminophylline increases cerebral metabolic rate and decreases anoxic survival in young mice. *Science* 1978;201:649–651.
121. Tchekalarova J, Kubova H, Mares P. Postnatal caffeine exposure: effects on motor skills and locomotor activity during ontogenesis. *Behav Brain Res* 2005;160:99–106.
122. Bahi N, Nehlig A, Evrard P, et al. Caffeine does not affect excitotoxic brain lesions in newborn mice. *Eur J Paediatr Neurol* 2001;5:161–165.
123. Gunn TR, Metrakos K, Riley PS, et al. Sequelae of caffeine treatment in preterm infants with apnea. J Pediatr 1979;94:106–110.
124. Ment LR, Scott DT, Ehrenkranz RA, et al. Early childhood developmental follow-up of infants with GMH/IVH: effect of methylxanthine therapy. *Am J Perinatol* 1985;2:223–227.
125. Schmidt B, Anderson PJ, Doyle LW, et al; Caffeine for Apnea of Prematurity (CAP) Trial Investigators. Survival without disability to age 5 years after neonatal caffeine therapy for apnea of prematurity. *JAMA* 2012;307(3):275–282.
126. Doyle LW, Schmidt B, Anderson PJ, et al. Caffeine for apnea of prematurity trial investigators. Reduction in developmental coordination disorder with neonatal caffeine therapy. *J Pediatr* 2014;165(2):356–359.e2.
127. Schmidt B, Roberts RS, Anderson PJ, et al.; Caffeine for Apnea of Prematurity (CAP) Trial Group. academic performance, motor function, and behavior 11 years after neonatal caffeine citrate therapy for apnea of prematurity: an 11-year follow-up of the CAP randomized clinical trial. *JAMA Pediatr* 2017;171(6):564–572.
128. Mürner-Lavanchy IM, Doyle LW, Schmidt B, et al.; Caffeine for Apnea of Prematurity (CAP) Trial Group. Neurobehavioral outcomes 11 years after neonatal caffeine therapy for apnea of prematurity. *Pediatrics* 2018;141(5).
129. Gupta PK, Moore J. The use of doxapram in the newborn. *J Obstet Gynaecol Br Commonw* 1973;80(11):1002–1006.
130. Henderson-Smart DJ, Steer PA. *Doxapram treatment for apnea in preterm infants Cochrane Database Syst Rev* 2004;(4):CD000074.
131. Flint R, Halbmeijer N, Meesters N, et al. Retrospective study shows that doxapram therapy avoided the need for endotracheal intubation in most premature neonates. *Acta Paediatr* 2017;106(5):733–739.
132. Huon C, Rey E, Mussat P, et al. Low-dose doxapram for treatment of apnoea following early weaning in very low birthweight infants: a randomized, double-blind study. *Acta Paediatr* 1998;87(11):1180–1184.
133. Ten Hove CH, Vliegenthart RJ, Te Pas AB, et al. Long-term neurodevelopmental outcome after doxapram for apnea of prematurity. *Neonatology* 2016;110(1):21–26.
134. Sreenan C, Etches PC, Demianczuk N, et al. Isolated mental developmental delay in very low birth weight infants: association with prolonged doxapram therapy for apnea. *J Pediatr* 2001;139(6):832–837.
135. Henderson-Smart DJ, Steer PA. Doxapram versus methylxanthine for apnea in preterm infants. *Cochrane Database Syst Rev* 2000;(4):CD000075.
136. Vliegenthart RJ, Ten Hove CH, Onland W, et al. Doxapram treatment for apnea of prematurity: a systematic review. *Neonatology* 2017;111(2):162–171.
137. Barrington KJ, Finer NN, Torok-Both G, et al. Dose–response relationship of doxapram in the therapy for refractory idiopathic apnea of prematurity. *Pediatrics* 1987;80(1):22–27.
138. Hayakawa F, Hakamada S, Kuno K, et al. Doxapram in the treatment of idiopathic apnea of prematurity: desirable dosage and serum concentrations. *J Pediatr* 1986;109(1):138–140.
139. Ogawa Y, Irikura M, Kobaru Y, et al. Population pharmacokinetics of doxapram in low-birth-weight Japanese infants with apnea. *Eur J Pediatr* 2015;174(4):509–518.
140. Jamali F, Barrington KJ, Finer NN, et al. Doxapram dosage regimen in apnea of prematurity based on pharmacokinetic data. *Dev Pharmacol Ther* 1988;11(5):253–257.
141. Beaudry MA, Bradley JM, Gramlich LM, et al. Pharmacokinetics of doxapram in idiopathic apnea of prematurity. *Dev Pharmacol Ther* 1988;11(2):65–72.
142. Fischer C, Ferdynus C, Gouyon JB, et al. Doxapram and hypokalaemia in very preterm infants. *Arch Dis Child Fetal Neonatal Ed* 2013;98(5):F416–F418.
143. Shimokaze T, Toyoshima K, Shibasaki J, et al. Blood potassium and urine aldosterone after doxapram therapy for preterm infants. *J Perinatol* 2018;38(6):702–707.
144. Dani C, Bertini G, Pezzati M, et al. Brain hemodynamic effects of doxapram in preterm infants. *Biol Neonate* 2006;89(2):69–74.
145. Bednarek FJ, Roloff DW. Treatment of Apnea of Prematurity with Aminophylline. *Pediatrics* 1975;58:335-339

SECTION

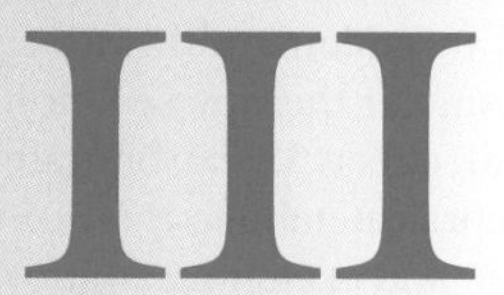

Pharmacology in Special Settings and Population

CHAPTER 16

Ashok P. Sarnaik
Zahraa H. Al-Lawati
Tageldin M. Ahmed
Mary W. Lieh-Lai

Therapeutic Applications in Pediatric Intensive Care

INTRODUCTION

> The worst thing about medicine is that one kind makes another necessary.
>
> Elbert Hubbard

Management of a critically ill child poses a special challenge to the clinician. Most children admitted to an intensive care unit (ICU) have multisystem involvement. The clinician must not only be aware of age-related changes in pharmacokinetics and pharmacodynamics but must also be cognizant of various drug–drug and drug–disease interactions. Because of the ongoing pathophysiologic changes, the physician must also deal with changes in volume of distribution and elimination kinetics during the clinical course. A critically ill child is often exposed to 20 or more medications during their hospital stay. Practically, every organ system and disease entity is represented in the pathophysiologic derangements of the patients in the ICU. A comprehensive discussion of management of an individual disease entity is beyond the scope of this chapter. Instead, we offer a working outline of management of most commonly encountered disease processes in critically ill children.

CENTRAL NERVOUS SYSTEM INJURY AND INCREASED INTRACRANIAL PRESSURE

Children with intracranial hypertension are often seen in the ICU, primarily those with trauma, infection, metabolic derangements, or ischemic brain injury. Secondary brain injury results from pathophysiologic alterations in response to the primary insult. Prolonged increase in intracranial pressure (ICP) can further aggravate brain damage and worsen patient outcome.

OSMOTHERAPY

Osmotherapy takes advantage of the unique nature of the blood–brain barrier (BBB), which freely allows the transport of water across the capillary endothelium while remaining relatively impermeable in varying degrees to osmotic agents.[1] It is most effective in situations where water accumulation is mainly intracellular and the BBB is well preserved. However, disruption of the BBB is neither absolute nor uniform even in conditions such as trauma and infection. Therefore, osmotherapy is still effective to varying degrees in decreasing total brain water in such situations.

The two types of osmotherapeutic agents used are mannitol and hypertonic saline, both of which have been shown to decrease ICP in traumatic brain injuries and subarachnoid hemorrhage (SAH).[2] Superiority of one agent over the other has not been established. However, in patients with diabetic ketoacidosis (DKA) and secondary cerebral edema, the use of mannitol was associated with decreased mortality when compared to the use of hypertonic saline.[3]

Mannitol

The effects of mannitol are due to the temporary increase in plasma osmolality, thereby causing a gradual movement of water from brain parenchyma to the systemic circulation. The increased intravascular water induced by the administration of mannitol is eliminated through osmotic diuresis. Adequate renal function is necessary for mannitol to be effective. It is important for serum osmolality to return to normal before the next dose is administered. Mannitol also decreases blood viscosity and improves rheology.[4] The dose is 0.25 to 1g per kg; the osmotic effects occur within 15 to 30 minutes and persist for up to 6 hours. Because the effectiveness of an osmotic agent depends on the steepness of the osmolal gradient it creates, intermittent administration of a bolus of mannitol over 10 to 15 minutes is preferred to continuous infusion. The dose often needs to be repeated based on clinical response and/or ICP measurement. In addition to its osmotic effects, mannitol may have other salutary effects on cerebral metabolism because of its rheologic and free radical scavenging and anti-inflammatory effects.[5]

The aim of osmotherapy is to decrease brain bulk without causing total body dehydration and hypovolemia. It is important to monitor serum electrolytes, osmolality, and indicators of circulation. Inadequate excretion of mannitol and persistent hyperosmolality are associated with acute tubular necrosis and renal failure.[6] Inadequate renal function may result in hypervolemia and hyperosmolality that are poorly tolerated by patients requiring osmotherapy.

Hypertonic Saline

In recent years, hypertonic saline has been used with increasing frequency in brain-injured patients.[7] Several studies have compared hypertonic saline and mannitol and found that both are effective in reducing ICP, though there is debate in terms of which agent is more efficacious.[8] The effects of hypertonic saline are similar to mannitol in terms of its osmolality and rheology; it shifts water from the brain tissue into the intravascular space by altering the serum osmolality, thereby reducing cerebral edema.[9] Hypertonic saline also has anti-inflammatory effects similar to mannitol,[10] and it decreases apoptosis following neurotrauma.[5]

The recommended single dose of hypertonic saline (3% saline) is 2 to 5 mL per kg administered over 10 to 20 minutes.[11] Continuous intravenous (IV) infusions of hypertonic saline have also been used for control of ICP. The dose of hypertonic saline should be adjusted to maintain the minimum serum osmolality needed to result in the desired ICP control. It would be reasonable to maintain serum sodium less than 160 mEq per L and osmolality below 330 mOsm per kg. Hypertonic saline has been shown to be safe and effective for the use in the treatment of symptomatic hyponatremia and hyponatremic seizures from water intoxication and the syndrome of inappropriate antidiuretic hormone (SIADH). A small (3 to 4 mEq per L) but rapid rise in serum sodium is most desirable for this purpose.[12] With an apparent volume of distribution for sodium being 0.6 L per kg, administration of 4 to 5 mL per kg of 3% saline given over 10 to 15 minutes will raise serum sodium by approximately 3 to 4 mEq per L. For hyponatremia associated with SIADH, IV furosemide (1 mg per kg per dose) given before hypertonic saline is effective in eliminating free water in addition to raising serum sodium.

With administration of mannitol, the increase in osmolality is transient since mannitol is readily excreted by the kidneys. Conversely, the increase in osmolality with hypertonic saline is sustained as most of the administered sodium is retained within the circulation. If a sustained increase in serum osmolality is desired, hypertonic saline is preferable. If the therapeutic aim is to expose the brain to elevated serum osmolality on an intermittent basis, mannitol is the preferred agent.

BARBITURATES

Barbiturate therapy may be used in patients with intracranial hypertension refractory to hyperosmolar therapy, sedation, and surgical treatment. The beneficial effects of barbiturates are likely due to the decrease in cerebral metabolic rate, cerebral vasoconstriction, decrease in lactate and excitatory amino acids, and inhibition of free radical–mediated lipid peroxidation.[13–15] However, the use of barbiturates in this patient population has not been shown to improve long-term outcomes.[16]

Pentobarbital is by far the most commonly used agent for the control of ICP. This can be accomplished by administering an IV bolus of 5 mg per kg followed by continuous infusion of 1 to 2 mg per kg per hour. The infusion rate may be increased and titrated to achieve the desired ICP control. In refractory status epilepticus, a higher infusion rate may be needed to achieve burst suppression or seizure control. Generally, pentobarbital concentrations of 20 to 40 mCg per mL are required for the desired effect. Barbiturate therapy is associated with significant hypotension and myocardial depression; many patients require administration of inotropic agents for hemodynamic stability when high-dose barbiturate therapy is used.

CORTICOSTEROIDS

High-dose steroid therapy in traumatic spinal cord injury is controversial and, more recently, not recommended.[17,18] In addition, steroids have been noted to increase mortality in patients with head injury and, therefore, are not administered in this population.[11] However, corticosteroids have been shown to reduce morbidity and mortality in patients with tuberculosis meningitis.[19]

STATUS EPILEPTICUS

Status epilepticus is one of the most common disorders in children requiring ICU admission; it is defined as continuous or repeated convulsive or nonconvulsive seizures lasting 30 minutes or longer.[20] Within the first 30 minutes of status epilepticus, sympathetic overactivity results in hypertension, tachycardia, and increased cardiac output. Increased catecholamine activity produces hyperglycemia. Combined respiratory and metabolic acidosis is a result of lactic acidosis and CO_2 retention. The increase in cerebral metabolism often outstrips cerebral blood flow, and eventually, this discrepancy leads to depletion of brain glucose and oxygen. Status epilepticus should be considered an emergency (Fig. 16.1), and treatment and determination of the etiology should be instituted immediately (Table 16.1).

In children, the causes of status epilepticus include infection, trauma, toxic ingestion, and metabolic disturbances (e.g., hyponatremia, hypoglycemia, hypocalcemia), brain tumors, epilepsy, and subtherapeutic levels of antiepileptic medications.

INITIAL SURVEY

Complications of status epilepticus may include vomiting and aspiration, apnea, and hypoxia. The initial assessment should ascertain that the airway is adequate. If there is any concern that airway and breathing are compromised, the patient should be intubated and mechanically ventilated. Blood pressure measurement is important to determine the presence of hypertension

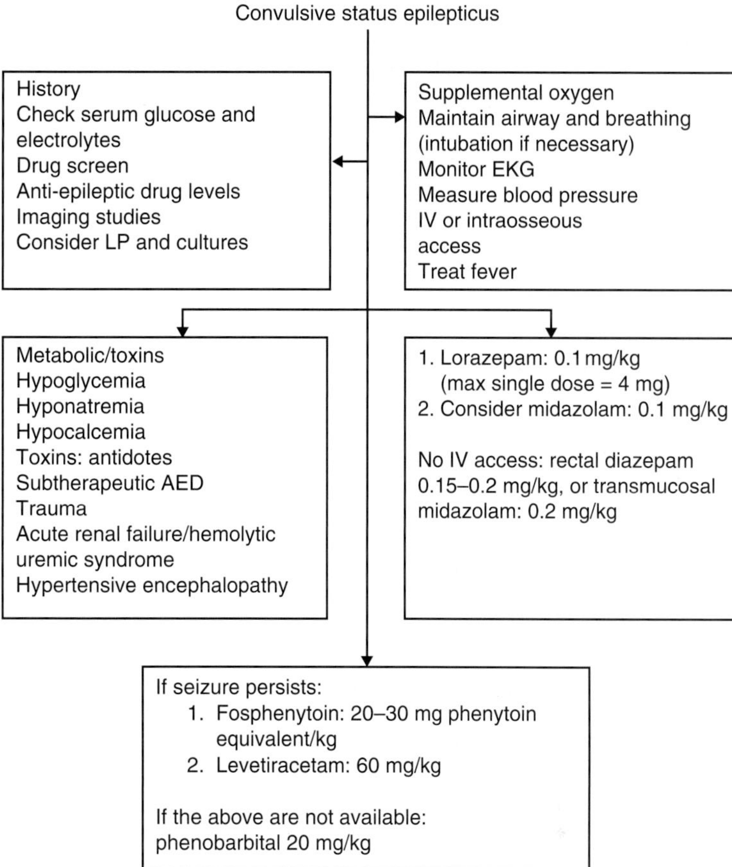

Figure 16.1 **Convulsive status epilepticus.** AED, antiepileptic drug; EKG, electrocardiogram; IV, intravenous; LP, lumbar puncture.

as the cause of seizures. If imaging studies are needed, patients should first have their airway and hemodynamic status stabilized before imaging studies are obtained. A lumbar puncture can be performed as long as the patient has a stable airway and hemodynamic status, and if there are no other contraindications such as an infection at the puncture site, coagulopathy, and increased ICP with evidence of focal neurologic findings.

Hyponatremia resulting from excessive water supplementation or improper mixing of formula can be a common cause of seizures in infants and should be suspected in an infant presenting with status epilepticus who appears otherwise healthy. A proper history should be elicited immediately, and once improper formula mixing or if excessive water administration is confirmed, 3% sodium chloride should be administered pending the results of serum electrolyte determination. Accidental ingestion of toxins should be suspected in toddlers, while intentional overdose should be suspected in older children and adolescents. In addition to removal of the toxin, an appropriate antidote should be administered if available.

TABLE 16.1 Antiepileptic Medications

	Dose	*Comments*
Levetiracetam	Bolus: 60 mg/kg Maintenance: 20 mg/kg/day	PO and IV dosing are equivalent (however administer IV in status epilepticus)
Fosphenytoin	Bolus: 20 mg/kg of PE	Need to monitor levels for titration
	Maintenance: 4–8 mg/kg/day	Should switch to PO phenytoin when able
Phenobarbital	Bolus: 20 mg/kg Maintenance: 5 mg/kg/day	Monitor levels
Lorazepam	Bolus: 0.1 mg/kg	Mixed in polyethylene glycol
Midazolam	Bolus: 0.1 mg/kg Infusion: 0.05–0.5 mg/kg/h	Can be administered intranasally (0.2 mg/kg)
Pentobarbital	Bolus: 2–4 mg/kg Infusion: 1–3 mg/kg/h	Monitor hemodynamics closely

IV, intravenous; PE, phenytoin equivalent; PO, orally.

BENZODIAZEPINES

Benzodiazepine is a group of drugs that bind to the neuronal γ-aminobutyric acid (GABA) receptors and facilitate the inhibitory action of GABA on neuronal transmission. This class of medication is recommended as the initial therapy of choice in status epilepticus.[20]

Lorazepam is the currently recommended first-line drug of choice for the treatment of status epilepticus (0.1 mg per kg per dose) because it can be injected rapidly and has a rapid onset of action of 2 to 3 minutes. Respiratory depression is an important side effect and should be monitored for. Lorazepam is insoluble in water and needs the addition of polyethylene glycol as a solvent. With prolonged and high-dose infusions, lactic acidosis and hyperosmolar coma have been reported.[21]

Midazolam has been successfully used in the treatment of status epilepticus by both IV (0.1 mg per kg per dose) and transmucosal (intranasal or buccal; 0.2 mg per kg per dose with a maximum of 10 mg) routes. The continuous IV infusion of midazolam (0.05 to 0.5 mg per kg per hour) has been used for the treatment of intractable status epilepticus, while the patient is being supported with mechanical ventilation. Close hemodynamic and electroencephalogram (EEG) monitoring are necessary.

Diazepam is highly lipophilic, and it rapidly penetrates the BBB. Although it has been replaced by lorazepam as the first-line drug of choice, 0.15 to 0.2 mg per kg (maximum of 10 mg) rectal diazepam has its place in the treatment of status epilepticus in patients without IV access and is a drug that caregivers can use at home for children known to have frequent seizures.

PHENYTOIN/FOSPHENYTOIN

Fosphenytoin is a prodrug of phenytoin that is water soluble and can be injected more rapidly compared to phenytoin; 1.5 mg of fosphenytoin is equivalent to 1 mg of phenytoin. Dosing for fosphenytoin is referred to as phenytoin equivalent (PE). Phenytoin precipitates when injected rapidly and causes tissue necrosis, arrhythmias, and cardiovascular collapse; thus, fosphenytoin is preferred. When using phenytoin, the dose should be infused no faster than 0.5 mg per kg per min in children younger than 1 month and no faster than 1 mg per kg per min in older patients. Fosphenytoin is used a second-line therapy (along with levetiracetam) for status epilepticus and can be administered intravascularly at a dose of 20 mg PE per kg (half-life of 60 minutes). Serum concentrations should be monitored because of the variability in phenytoin metabolism in infants. Fosphenytoin can also be administered intramuscularly (IM) at the same dose (20 mg PE per kg).

LEVETIRACETAM

Levetiracetam can also be used as a second-line therapy for status epilepticus.[20] When compared to phenytoin, it was noted to be a safer alternative.[22] The suggested dose is 60 mg per kg, followed by 10 mg per kg maintenance dose twice daily (BID). Levetiracetam has been shown to be efficacious, with a good safety profile, and does not have the respiratory depressive effects seen with benzodiazepines and barbiturates. The mechanism of action of the drug is unclear, but may be due to the prevention of hypersynchronization of epileptiform burst firing and propagation of seizure activity. Levetiracetam has linear pharmacokinetics with a predictable dose–serum concentration relationship and a broad therapeutic index.[23] Monitoring of serum concentration is not recommended in most cases. Approximately 66% of the drug is eliminated by the kidneys unchanged. Therefore, dose adjustment is necessary with renal insufficiency.

BARBITURATES

These drugs bind to the GABA-receptor complex, producing sedation, hypnosis, anesthesia, and suppression of epileptiform activity. They are known to decrease cerebral metabolic oxygen demand and ICP. Adverse effects include suppression of myocardial contractility and peripheral vasodilation that can lead to hypotension. With prolonged infusion and use of high doses, patients often require inotropic drug support. With repeated doses, barbiturates can cause respiratory depression and apnea.

Phenobarbital can also be used as initial therapy, but because of its slower rate of action compared to benzodiazepines, phenobarbital is considered more as an alternative rather than a primary treatment for status epilepticus.[20] A loading dose of 20 mg per kg is recommended, with a maintenance dose of 5 mg per kg per day. In the management of status epilepticus, serum levels should be monitored and maintained at 20 to 30 mCg per mL. Higher therapeutic levels may be necessary for the treatment of prolonged status epilepticus resistant to lower levels and/or other antiepileptic drugs.

Pentobarbital is used for the treatment of status epilepticus that is unresponsive to initial and second lines of therapy. It has a rapid onset of action. It is administered as a loading dose of 2 to 4 mg per kg, followed by a continuous infusion of 1 to 3 mg per kg per hour. Dose increases can be titrated based on EEG findings of burst suppression. All patients who require continuous pentobarbital therapy will need intubation and mechanical ventilation.

PROPOFOL

Propofol is a short-acting IV anesthetic agent that is effective in terminating status epilepticus in adults but has not been studied in children. Long-term infusion has been reported to cause severe metabolic acidosis (propofol infusion syndrome).[24]

VALPROIC ACID

Valproic acid by IV injection has been evaluated in adults with status epilepticus as second-line therapy and has no adverse cardiorespiratory effects.[20,25]

PARALDEHYDE

Paraldehyde is a cyclic polymer of acetaldehyde that is rapidly absorbed into the brain. It has been used successfully for over a century in the treatment of seizures. It is no longer available in the United States but is still used in other parts of the world.

MYASTHENIA GRAVIS

Myasthenia gravis (MG) is a chronic, often progressive humoral autoimmune disease caused by autoantibodies directed against the nicotinic receptors in the neuromuscular junction. Myasthenic crisis is a life-threatening exacerbation of MG characterized by weakness of respiratory and oropharyngeal muscles. Medical therapy of MG consists of improving neuromuscular transmission with acetyl cholinesterase inhibitors (e.g., pyridostigmine), immune suppression and immune modulation, or monoclonal antibodies. Treatment of acute exacerbations includes the use of intravenous immunoglobulins (IVIGs), plasmapheresis, and immunoadsorption. Thymectomy may be required.

The anticholinesterase inhibitors used in the diagnosis and management of MG are of the class of quaternary ammonium compounds which do not cross the BBB and, therefore, exert their effects on peripheral nicotinic cholinergic receptors.

Edrophonium is used mainly to establish the diagnosis and also for distinguishing between myasthenic crisis and cholinergic crisis in children receiving anticholinesterase therapy. An IV dose of 0.04 mg per kg is given over 1 minute; if no response is observed to the first dose within 45 seconds, an additional 0.16 mg per kg (maximum 10 mg) is given. The onset of action is within seconds, and duration of action is a few minutes. Objective evidence of improvement of motor function, such as muscle strength and forced vital capacity, should be documented. As with other anticholinesterase agents, severe bradycardia, hypotension, muscle cramps, and other cholinergic effects can occur with the use of edrophonium. Atropine (0.01 mg per kg IV, minimum 0.1 mg, maximum 2 mg) should be immediately available to counteract serious cholinergic effects should they occur.

Neostigmine is used both as a diagnostic agent and for ongoing therapy. It can be given by IM injection at 0.025 to 0.04 mg per kg as a diagnostic tool. For ongoing therapy, 0.04 mg per kg can be given IM every 3 to 4 hours. *Neostigmine* bromide is an oral preparation that can be given at 0.4 mg per kg every 4 to 6 hours. It is given 30 minutes before meals for patients with significant dysphagia. *Pyridostigmine* bromide is the most commonly used acetylcholinesterase inhibitor in the treatment of MG. It has a rapid onset of action (15 to 30 minutes) which lasts for 3 to 4 hours. It is administered orally (PO) in a dose of 5 mg per kg per day in four to six divided doses. The doses of both pyridostigmine and neostigmine may have to be adjusted every 48 hours. In addition to treatment with anticholinesterases, patients will require immunosuppression.

The most commonly used immunosuppressive agent for the treatment of MG is the *corticosteroid* prednisone. Observational studies, clinical experience, and limited controlled trials suggest that prednisone usage leads to remission or marked improvement in 70% to 80% of patients with ocular or generalized MG.[26,27]

Azathioprine is the first choice for long-term immunosuppressive therapy. The starting dose of azathioprine is 50 mg daily, followed by an increase every 2 weeks up to a typical maintenance dose of 2 to 3 mg per kg per day. Its main disadvantage is the delayed onset of action. The combination of steroids and azathioprine is the preferred approach with eventual weaning of steroids over 6 to 8 weeks, thus minimizing their side effects. Other immunosuppressants recommended for use include cyclophosphamide, methotrexate, mycophenolate mofetil, cyclosporine, and tacrolimus.

Rituximab (anti-CD20 antibody) is a monoclonal immunoglobulin therapy that has shown efficacy in severe refractory MG. It reduces the need for other immunosuppressive therapies, improves quality of life, and decreases health care costs.[28]

Thymectomy should be considered for patients with high titers of anti–ACh-receptor antibodies.

Plasmapheresis, immunoadsorption, and the administration of IVIG are considered interventions for management of acute myasthenic exacerbation or crises. IVIG is administered as 2 g per kg as a single dose over 10 to 12 hours or 400 mg per kg daily for 4 days. Relative benefits of immune modulation are still unconfirmed by randomized controlled studies.

NEUROMUSCULAR BLOCKING AGENTS

In addition to sedative agents, critically ill children may require neuromuscular blocking agents (NMBAs) to facilitate mechanical ventilation and invasive procedures and to minimize movements in patients with unstable airways or extensive facial injuries. The addition of NMBAs may help improve respiratory system compliance and reduce barotrauma by preventing the patient from "fighting" the ventilator. When using NMBAs, it is important to ascertain adequacy of sedation to prevent the frightening consequence of paralyzing a child who has total awareness.

DEPOLARIZING AGENTS

Succinylcholine is a depolarizing agent that has a rapid onset of action and a short half-life.[29] It acts similarly to acetylcholine (ACh) and induces membrane depolarization, but is resistant to degradation by acetylcholinesterase and results in persistent depolarization. Administration of succinylcholine produces initial fasciculations resulting from repetitive excitation, which is then followed by flaccid paralysis. The recommended dose in children is 1 mg per kg per dose IV. The onset of paralysis occurs within 1 minute after injection. Effects dissipate quickly as the drug is metabolized by plasma pseudocholinesterase.

Potassium is released during depolarization; therefore, succinylcholine is contraindicated in conditions that can potentiate hyperkalemia, including crush injuries, renal failure, burns, and rhabdomyolysis. It is also contraindicated in patients with increased ICP and intraocular pressure, spinal cord injuries, muscular dystrophies, and known or family history of malignant hyperthermia (MH).[30] Clinical features of MH include hypercarbia, muscle rigidity, hyperthermia, acidosis, hyperkalemia, and rhabdomyolysis. When it occurs, the trigger should be immediately discontinued, the patient cooled, and dantrolene (1.5 mg per kg) administered.[31]

NONDEPOLARIZING AGENTS

Nondepolarizing agents include rocuronium, pancuronium, vecuronium, atracurium, and cisatracurium. These drugs block ACh binding to receptors on the motor endplate, thereby inhibiting depolarization. Elimination of nondepolarizing NMBAs varies, and this characteristic should be taken into account when using these drugs (Table 16.2).

There are a number of drugs frequently used in critically ill children that can potentiate the effects of NMBAs and result in prolonged paralysis. These include antibiotics such as aminoglycosides, antiarrhythmic agents such as β-adrenergic blockers, and other drugs such as furosemide, magnesium, and cyclosporine. Electrolyte abnormalities and hypothermia can also prolong paralysis. A persistent muscle weakness as a manifestation of neuromyopathy can occur with prolonged use of NMBAs, especially when used in combination with corticosteroids.[32,33]

In patients requiring continuous neuromuscular blockade, monitoring the train of four is useful in judging their response to therapy. Train of four uses a series of four electrical impulses (2 Hz) that are usually delivered to the ulnar nerve, evoking a response of the adductor pollicis.[34] If three twitches are observed, approximately 75% to 80% of receptors are occupied; and if one twitch is observed, 90% to 95% of receptors are occupied. One to two twitches indicate approximately 75% to 90% receptor occupancy and are indicative of an optimum level of neuromuscular relaxation. Monitoring of the train of four in patients who are receiving frequent or continuous dosing of NMBAs helps prevent overdosing and prolonged paralysis.

Rapid reversal of neuromuscular blockade is sometimes necessary in patients in the ICU who have received nondepolarizing agents. Neostigmine, 0.05 to 0.07 mg per kg IV (maximum of 5 mg), can be used for this purpose and has a peak action within 5 to 8 minutes. Atropine may have to be administered in conjunction

TABLE 16.2 Nondepolarizing Blocking Agents

Drug	*Dose*	*Duration of Action*	*Route of Elimination*	*Comments*
Pancuronium	0.1–0.15 mg/kg/dose q30–60 min PRN	40–60 min	Kidneys (10% by liver)	• Has an active metabolite • Causes catecholamine and histamine release
Vecuronium	0.1 mg/kg/dose q60 min PRN	30–40 min	Kidneys and liver	• More potent and shorter acting than pancuronium • Has an active metabolite that is cleared by the kidneys
Atracurium	0.3–0.5 mg/kg/dose q45 min PRN	50–60 min	Hoffman elimination—produces Laudanosine which is hepatically and renally excreted	• Causes histamine release with hypotension and bronchospasm • Laudanosine can precipitate seizures
Cisatracurium	0.15–0.2 mg/kg/dose q40–65 min PRN	35–45 min	Hoffman elimination	• Ideal NMB to use in renal and hepatic failure
Rocuronium	0.6 mg/kg/dose initial dose, then 0.075–0.125 q20–30 min PRN	26–40 min	70% by biliary excretion; 30% unchanged via kidneys	• Fast onset of action

NMB, neuromuscular blocking, PRN, as needed; q, every.

with neostigmine in order to counteract excessive muscarinic effects of bradycardia, increased secretions, and bronchospasm.

Sugammadex is a medication that encapsulates rocuronium and vecuronium, thereby directly preventing their pharmacologic actions. It is a noncompetitive antagonist used for reversal of these NMBAs.[35,36] Studies have shown that sugammadex is effective and safe in adults,[37] but it has not received Food and Drug Administration (FDA) approval for use in children.

SEDATION IN INTENSIVE CARE UNIT

Patients in the ICU are subjected to many stressors that provoke anxiety, agitation, and disruption of normal sleep cycle. These include being in an unfamiliar environment, inability to communicate when intubated, mechanical ventilation, inadequate analgesia, and excessive stimulation (light, noise, and tactile). Pain, anxiety, hypoxia, hypoglycemia, hypotension, delirium, and drug withdrawal are some common causes of patient agitation. Left untreated, an agitated patient would be at risk of ventilator dyssynchrony, loss of life-sustaining therapeutic and monitoring devices, and increased metabolic demands.

Sedatives are frequently used in the ICU to combat anxiety, agitation, and their consequences. An optimally sedated patient is calm, lucid, pain free, interactive, and cooperative with care and supporting devices. Some children may need deeper levels of sedation. For example, patients with acute intracranial hypertension, critical airways, severe respiratory failure, and those who need paralytic agents.

The desired level of sedation and patient's response to sedatives varies according to patients and the time during the course of the illness. It is, therefore, imperative that care providers monitor and assess adequacy of sedation. Oversedation can precipitate hemodynamic instability and hinder neurologic assessment of the patient. Prolonged sedation, on the other hand, is associated with difficulties in weaning patients off mechanical ventilation, longer ICU and hospital stays, physical and psychological drug dependence, withdrawal syndromes, development of delirium, and reported long-term cognitive deficits.[38–40]

A number of scales have been devised to assess the level of sedation in children. The validity, reliability, and ease of use are the most important factors in deciding which scale to adopt. Scales commonly in use are the Ramsay Scale, Richmond Agitation-Sedation Scale (RASS), COMFORT Scale, and Penn State Children's Hospital Sedation Algorithm. Shortcomings of the Ramsay Scale in younger patients include children having difficulty understanding commands and the lack of cooperation with the assessor. The RASS is an observational scale that provides scores for sedation and agitation, ranging between overtly combative and violent (4 points) to not responding to voice or physical stimulation (–5 points).[41] The COMFORT Scale was specifically designed for children with endotracheal tubes. It provides scores for eight physiologic and behavioral parameters each between 1 and 5 points to a total ranging from 8 to 40 points. The advantage of this scale is that it is applicable to children of all ages and developmental stages.[42] The Penn State Children's Hospital Sedation Algorithm is devised to reduce the incidence of unplanned extubation in mechanically ventilated children. Here the goal of sedation is determined by the physician, and the medication is prescribed accordingly for the nurse to provide the appropriate regimen for the individual patient. The scale ranges from level 1 (awake and interactive child) to level 6 (continuously asleep and muscle relaxed using paralytic drugs).[43] There are devices used to monitor levels of sedation, including the use of the bispectral index which utilizes EEG signals and provides information regarding the depth of anesthesia and sedation.[44,45] This index has been validated for use in children and proven to be the most sensitive scale in identifying and preventing oversedation in children. While the device is used intraoperatively, its routine use in the ICU has not been widely adopted because of difficulties in equipment and training.[46] Commonly used sedative agents include benzodiazepines, dexmedetomidine, clonidine, propofol, ketamine, barbiturates, and etomidate.

BENZODIAZEPINES

This group of compounds enhances the effect of the neurotransmitter GABA at the $GABA_A$ receptor, resulting in sedative, hypnotic, anxiolytic, anticonvulsant, amnestic, and muscle-relaxant properties. Midazolam and lorazepam are the most commonly used drugs in this group. Respiratory depression and hemodynamic instability are the most important side effects of this class of medications. There are reports of patients developing paradoxical reactions, such as worsened agitation or panic, aggression, or behavioral disinhibition.

Midazolam is a water-soluble compound that becomes lipid soluble in physiologic pH, allowing for rapid BBB penetration. It is metabolized by hepatic microsomal oxidation and eliminated by renal excretion. The latter property necessitates dose adjustment in patients with renal impairment. A dose range between 0.05 and 2 mg per kg per hour results in adequate sedation. Abrupt cessation of long-term infusion of midazolam (over 5 days) can precipitate acute benzodiazepine–withdrawal syndrome. Gradual weaning of the medication should be considered for patients receiving long-term infusions of the drug.

Lorazepam penetrates the BBB more slowly than other benzodiazepines, and this characteristic results in a longer duration of its amnestic effect. It is metabolized by the hepatic glucuronidation to inactive metabolites that are eliminated through the kidneys. Due to the relative longer half-life, it is more suited for intermittent oral or IV dosing. The use of lorazepam is associated with a risk of metabolic acidosis and propylene glycol poisoning with high doses or with prolonged IV use. Dose range of 0.05 to 2 mg per kg per dose given intermittently generally helps in achieving sedation. Oral lorazepam is use as an adjunct medication to avoid benzodiazepine-withdrawal syndromes.

DEXMEDETOMIDINE

Dexmedetomidine is an α-2 agonist agent. It has hypnotic, sedative, and weak analgesic effects with minimal respiratory depression. Effects are mediated centrally at the locus coeruleus of the pons and the spinal cord. Dexmedetomidine has a rapid onset of action and a short half-life, hence the need for the administration of a loading dose prior to continuous infusion. The loading dose is 1 mCg per kg over 10 minutes, followed by an infusion of 0.2 to 1.2 mCg per kg per hour. It is utilized as a sedative for procedural sedation as well as an adjunct for maintenance of sedation. The undesirable side effects of dexmedetomidine are sinus bradycardia and hypotension that tend to occur at high infusion rates and in patients with hypovolemia. These side effects are easily mitigated by reducing the infusion rate or temporarily discontinuing the infusion. For patients with hypovolemia, an IV fluid bolus infusion is needed. It has been recently proposed that the use of dexmedetomidine prior to and during cardiopulmonary bypass in repair of ventricular septal defects (VSDs) may reduce the incidence of junctional ectopic tachycardia (JET), a common dysrhythmia associated with VSD surgical repair.[47] A dexmedetomidine-withdrawal syndrome has been described. Symptoms include tachycardia and hypertension that are often observed after abrupt cessation of dexmedetomidine after prolonged infusion.[48,49] Clonidine has been used to facilitate weaning of dexmedetomidine.

PROPOFOL

Propofol is an IV alkylphenol agent that induces anesthetic effects through GABA-receptor stimulation. It has a rapid onset of action and a short half-life, making it more suitable for induction of anesthesia and procedural sedation. Other uses for propofol include status epilepticus resistant to other therapies. Respiratory depression and hypotension are frequent side effects of propofol infusion, particularly during a loading bolus. The hypotension results from systemic vasodilatory and myocardial depressive effects of the drug, which are exacerbated in patients with intravascular volume depletion and preexisting cardiac dysfunction. Close monitoring of patients during propofol infusion is mandatory, and many institutions restrict propofol use to operating rooms and critical care units. A rare but potentially fatal complication of the drug is the propofol infusion syndrome. It is believed to result from direct inhibition of the mitochondrial respiratory chain or mitochondrial fatty acids metabolism. The syndrome manifests as cardiac and renal failure, hepatic dysfunction, rhabdomyolysis, lactic acidosis, hyperkalemia, and hypertriglyceridemia. It is associated with high doses and long-term use (>4 mg per kg per hour for more than 24 hours). It occurs more commonly in children and critically ill patients. No antidote is available. Management consists of supportive care.[50]

KETAMINE

Ketamine is a derivative of phencyclidine and is an *N*-methyl-D-aspartate (NMDA)–receptor antagonist. It is mainly used for initiating and maintaining anesthesia. Its sedative, analgesic, and minimal respiratory depressive effects make it especially suited for procedural sedation in children. Ketamine increases sympathetic discharge–releasing catecholamines, which result in bronchodilation, tachycardia, and elevated blood pressure. The bronchodilatory effect makes ketamine an ideal agent for sedation of children with status asthmaticus who require intubation. Other characteristics of ketamine include dissociative analgesia, an abnormal state of wakefulness in which a person is not self-aware and is unresponsive to external stimuli.

The main drawbacks of ketamine are the emergence phenomenon, sialagogue effect, and increased myocardial oxygen demand. The use of benzodiazepines in conjunction with ketamine ameliorates the emergence phenomenon. The increase in myocardial oxygen demand induced by ketamine is of particular concern in patients with congestive heart failure.

Ketamine has a rapid onset of action and relatively short half-life. An initial IV dose of 1 to 2 mg per kg can be administered. In the absence of IV access, ketamine can be administered by IM injection of 2 to 4 mg per kg. It is occasionally used as short-term IV infusion of 0.3 to 1.2 mg per kg per hour.

Ketamine and GABA agonist medications, such as benzodiazepines and barbiturates, are some of the drugs implicated in neuroapoptosis and consequent neurocognitive defects in infants and very young children.[51,52]

ETOMIDATE

Etomidate is an imidazole derivative. It has a rapid onset of action and short half-life, hence well suited for rapid sequence intubation and induction of anesthesia. It is a sedative with good hemodynamic profile, but no analgesic property. A potentially serious side effect of etomidate is adrenal gland suppression through the inhibition of adrenocortical hydroxylation enzymes. The drug is generally not recommended for children less than 10 years. The IV dose is 0.3 to 0.6 mg per kg per dose, which may be repeated if necessary.[53,54]

BARBITURATES

This group of GABA agonist medications was the mainstay of sedation before the era of benzodiazepines. With the exception of thiopental—which has been withdrawn from the American drug market, barbiturates generally have a long elimination half-life and a dose-related myocardial depression, respiratory depression, laryngospasm, and bronchospasm. *Pentobarbital* is used for

TABLE 16.3 Continuum of Depth of Sedation

	Minimal Sedation Anxiolysis	*Moderate Sedation Conscious Sedation*	*Deep Sedation/Analgesia*	*General Anesthesia*
Responsiveness	Normal response to verbal stimulation	Purposeful response to verbal or tactile stimulation	Purposeful response following repeated or painful stimulation	Unarousable even with painful stimulus
Airway	Unaffected	No intervention required	Intervention may be required	Intervention often required
Spontaneous ventilation	Unaffected	Adequate	May be adequate	Frequently inadequate
Cardiovascular function	Unaffected	Usually maintained	Usually maintained	May be impaired

NMB, neuromuscular blocking, PRN, as needed; q, every.

inducing barbiturate coma in patients with intractable status epilepticus and patients with traumatic brain injury and intracranial hypertension. The loading dose for pentobarbital is 10 mg per kg IV given over 30 minutes followed by an IV infusion of 1 mg per kg per hour with a gradual increase to 3 mg per kg per hour to achieve burst suppression on the EEG. Patients on pentobarbital infusion require ventilatory support and inotropic support.

PROCEDURAL SEDATION

Uncomfortable and often painful interventions requiring sedation and analgesia are frequently necessary for patient care in the ICU. The American Society of Anesthesiologists (ASA) defines sedation as a continuum ranging from minimal, moderate, deep sedation to anesthesia. Monitoring of patients is crucial as they can easily move from the intended level of sedation to the next level[55] (Table 16.3). The physical status of the patient must be evaluated prior to procedural sedation. The ASA has devised a physical status classification to guide practitioners regarding the suitability of the patient for sedation (Table 16.4). A relatively new sedation scale has been developed and validated: the Pediatric Sedation State Scale (PSSS). It is intended to specifically meet the needs of pediatric procedural sedation to measure effectiveness. It includes behaviors and adverse events that accompany procedural sedation[56] (Table 16.5).

PAIN AND ANALGESIA

The assessment of pain is complex as it is both a sensory and an emotional experience. The consequences of unrelieved pain include agitation, inadequate sleep, acute stress responses, and prolonged hospital stay. Acute stress responses manifest as tachycardia, increased myocardial O_2 consumption, hypercoagulability, immune suppression, and a catabolic state. Post-traumatic stress disorder is a well-established long-term complication of ICU stay where pain is the experience that stands out to many patients months after discharge.

Often, children are too young or may not have achieved the developmental level to articulate the intensity of pain. A number of scoring systems have been devised to assess pain. Two of these scoring systems are well validated: The Children's Hospital of East Ontario Pain Scale (CHEOPS)[57] and the Oucher Scale.[58] CHEOPS is a behavioral scale designed to measure acute pain in children aged 0 to 5 years. The Oucher Scale is a self-report of pain for children. It consists of a series of six pictures of one child face arranged to show increasing levels of pain from "no hurt" to "worst hurt." The Oucher Analogue Scale is recommended for older children. The Face, Leg, Activity, Cry and Consolability (FLACC) tool is designed for pain assessment in children who are unable to verbalize or those who are cognitively impaired.[59]

OPIOIDS

Opioids are the mainstay for pain management in the ICU. Opioid receptors are a group of inhibitory G-protein–coupled structures. They are widely distributed throughout the brain, spinal cord, peripheral neurons, gastrointestinal (GI) tract, and other organs. Major subtypes are mu, kappa, delta, and nociceptin receptors. The most common adverse effects of opioid analgesics include nausea, vomiting, sedation, pruritus, and constipation. Serious adverse effects include respiratory depression, urinary retention, hypotension, delirium, and chest wall rigidity. Tachyphylaxis and physical dependence occur with prolonged use of

TABLE 16.4 The American Society of Anesthesiologists Physical Status Classification

ASA Classes	*Example*	*Suitability for Sedation*
Healthy child	No past medical history	Excellent
Mild systemic disease, no functional limitation	Mild asthma, controlled seizures, controlled diabetes	Generally good
Severe systemic disease, definite functional limitation	Moderate/severe asthma, poorly controlled diabetes, seizures, obesity, pneumonia	Intermediate to poor. Consider benefit versus risks
Severe systemic disease that is a constant threat to life	Severe bronchopulmonary dysplasia, sepsis, advanced cardiac, renal, pulmonary hepatic or endocrine insufficiency	Poor, benefit rarely outweighs the risk
Moribund patient who is not expected to survive with/without procedure	Septic shock, severe trauma	Extremely poor

TABLE 16.5 The Pediatric Sedation State Scale

State	*Behavior*
5	Patient is moving in a manner that impedes the operator and require forceful immobilization; crying or shouting
4	Moving during the procedure (awake or sedated) that requires gentle immobilization for positioning; may verbalize discomfort or stress
3	Facial expression of pain or anxiety, but not moving or impeding completion of procedure; does not require restraint
2	Quiet (asleep or awake) not moving during the procedure; no expression of pain or anxiety; no verbalization of any complaint
1	Deeply asleep with normal vital signs but requiring airway intervention or assistance; for example: central or obstructive sleep apnea
0	Sedation associated with abnormal physiologic parameters that require acute intervention: hypoxia, hypotension, or bradycardia

opioids, and withdrawal syndromes occur if opioids are discontinued abruptly.

Morphine, a naturally occurring opiate, is considered the standard against which other opioids are compared with regard to analgesic potency. It is available in IV, IM, intrathecal, epidural, and enteral formulations. IV and enteral routes are the most commonly utilized in the ICU. An IV bolus of 0.1 mg per kg and infusion rate of 0.01 to 0.02 mg per kg per hour are generally recommended. The infusion rate can be adjusted according to patient's response. Pruritus from histamine release and hypotension are common side effects of morphine.

Fentanyl, a synthetic opioid compound, has a relatively shorter half-life and is commonly used for continuous sedation and analgesia in the ICU. An infusion rate of 0.5 to 2 mCg per kg per hour is recommended. A rare but serious complication of fentanyl is the rigid chest phenomenon. It is seen mostly when an IV bolus dose is given rapidly. To overcome the chest rigidity, a neuromuscular blocker needs to be administered. An antidote (naloxone) will occasionally be required.

Hydromorphone is a semisynthetic opioid. It is six to ten times more potent than morphine. It is best utilized in postoperative patients as intermittent boluses or patient-controlled analgesia (PCA). A bolus dose of 0.05 mg per kg or infusion rate of 2 to 5 mCg per kg per hour is generally recommended.

Weaker opioids or a combination of weaker opioids and acetaminophen are increasingly used for moderate to moderately severe pain management and are mostly given by the oral route. Examples include hydrocodone/acetaminophen and codeine/acetaminophen.

NONSTEROIDAL ANTI-INFLAMMATORY DRUGS

Prostaglandins are eicosanoid compounds derived from lipids by the action of cyclooxygenase enzyme. They are widely distributed in organs and tissues and have diverse hormone-like and pain-modulating properties. Nonsteroidal anti-inflammatory drugs (NSAIDs) inhibit cyclooxygenase enzyme, thereby providing analgesia. Bleeding is a known complication of NSAIDs due to the inhibition of platelet aggregation secondary to inhibited production of thromboxane A. In addition, GI bleeding can be induced by inhibition of prostaglandin E_2 (PGE_2) and prostaglandin I_2 (PGI_2), both of which are known protectors of gastric mucosal integrity. NSAIDs have also been implicated in acute renal failure, particularly in patients who are either dehydrated or have decreased cardiac output. It is believed that NSAIDs prevent local release of PGE_2 in the renal vascular bed, decreasing renal blood flow and leading to renal failure.

Higher potency NSAIDs, such as ketorolac, are utilized for analgesia in children following a variety of surgical procedures, such as spinal fusion, open heart surgery, and craniotomy. The recommended IV dose for ketorolac is 0.25 to 0.5 mg kg every 6 to 8 hours and enteral dose 1 to 2 mg per kg every 4 to 6 hours.

ACETAMINOPHEN

Acetaminophen is a non-NSAID medication with analgesic and antipyretic properties. It is indicated for the management of mild-to-moderate pain and is an adjunct to opioid analgesics for moderate-to-severe pain. It is available in oral, rectal, and IV formulations. IV acetaminophen is indicated for patient who cannot utilize the oral or rectal routes. The recommended dose is 12.5 mg per kg IV every 4 hours or 15 mg per kg IV every 6 hours; not to exceed 75 mg per kg per day. Some degree of hypotension has been reported in critically ill patients given IV acetaminophen.[60]

DISORDERS OF THE RESPIRATORY SYSTEM

LARYNGOTRACHEOBRONCHITIS AND POSTEXTUBATION STRIDOR

Viral laryngotracheobronchitis (croup) is a common childhood disease mostly caused by parainfluenza virus. Occasionally, the severity of the disease requires ICU admission. There is no specific antiviral therapy, and treatment is primarily symptomatic (Table 16.6).

Dexamethasone

Dexamethasone is known to reduce airway edema and inflammation and is recommended as first-line therapy.[61] Budesonide is a form of inhaled corticosteroid and can be used as second-line therapy. Nebulized aerosol of either L-epinephrine (1:1,000) or racemic epinephrine (2.25%) is useful for a child with moderately severe to severe symptoms. Both medications have a rapid onset of action with effects that can last up to 2 to 3 hours.

Studies have shown that dexamethasone or nebulized budesonide is effective in ameliorating airway obstruction associated with viral laryngotracheobronchitis.[62]

Postextubation stridor is often seen following prolonged endotracheal intubation particularly in infants and young children. In a randomized controlled study, it has been shown that four to six doses of 0.15 mg per kg IV dexamethasone administered every 6 hours prior to extubation significantly reduces the incidence of postextubation stridor.[63]

Helium Oxygen Therapy

Children have smaller airways than adults and are more commonly affected by diseases that cause extrathoracic airway obstruction.

TABLE 16.6 Medications for Croup

Medication	*Usual Dose*	*Onset*	*Duration*	*Comments*
Dexamethasone	0.6 mg/kg (max 15 mg) PO, IM, IV	30 min	24–72 h	Repeat doses are not recommended (ref)
Budesonide	2 mg nebulized one time	1–2 h		Second line. Repeat dose not recommended (ref)
Racemic Epinephrine 2.25%	0.5 mL in 2 mL of NS Neb q20 min PRN	10–30 min	2–3 h	Monitor HR and BP
L-Epinephrine 1:1,000	0.5 mL/kg (max 5 mL). Mix in 2 mL of NS q20 min PRN	10–30 min	2–3 h	Alternative to racemic epinephrine. Monitor HR and BP

BP, blood pressure; HR, heart rate; IM, intramuscular; IV, intravenous; NS: 0.9% saline; PRN, as needed; PO, orally; q, every.

This increases the turbulence of airflow which requires a greater driving pressure to move the gas. The Reynolds number (*Re*) describes the relationship between the density and viscosity of a gas in determining whether flow is laminar or turbulent. This number is derived from the formula: $Re = [p \times d \times v]/[u]$, where p is gas density, d is tube diameter, v is gas velocity, and u is gas viscosity. Low *Re* (<2,000) is associated with laminar gas flow and high *Re* (>4,000) with more turbulent flow. Helium is an inert, low-density gas. HeliOx is a mixture of helium and oxygen (70/30 or 60/40). The mix results in a low *Re* and helps create a laminar gas flow in the extrathoracic airway, thereby decreasing the work of breathing in patients with airway obstructive disease. In patients with severe croup, who are at risk for respiratory failure, it may be used to help avoid the need for intubation. The use of HeliOx is limited in patients requiring greater than 40% O_2 to treat hypoxia since at least 60% helium is generally required to reduce the *Re* sufficiently. A clinical trial found a reduction in respiratory distress with HeliOx; however, large clinical trials have been lacking.[64–66]

STATUS ASTHMATICUS

Status asthmaticus is one of the most common causes of admission to the pediatric ICU (PICU). The airway in patients with asthma is characterized by inflammation, bronchoreactivity, and increased mucous production.[67] Pharmacotherapy is directed at maintaining adequate oxygenation, amelioration of mucosal inflammation, and prompt reversal of airway obstruction. IV fluid administration is often necessary due to dehydration and increased insensible losses resulting from increased work of breathing and decreased oral intake. Supplemental oxygen should be administered to maintain SpO_2 above 90% to 95%. Monitoring mental status, respiratory status, and work of breathing is important in these patients; early initiation of noninvasive ventilation such as bimodal positive-airway pressure (BiPAP) and high-flow nasal cannula oxygen for respiratory support should be considered to decrease work of breathing and potentially avoid invasive mechanical ventilation. For patients who require sedation for endotracheal intubation, ketamine has bronchodilatory effects and may, therefore, be preferred.

β-2 Agonists

β-2 *Agonists* are the primary agents used for bronchodilation. Activation of β-2 receptors causes relaxation of the airway smooth muscle. Albuterol is the preferred agent. Continuous nebulization of albuterol via facemask is administered at 0.15 to 0.5 mg per kg per hour with a maximum of 15 mg per hour. The most common side effects are tachycardia and tremors. As the patient improves, continuous albuterol nebulization can be weaned off and switched to intermittent dosing.

Ipratropium Bromide

Ipratropium bromide is a local anticholinergic muscarinic antagonist that can be administered by inhalation and results in bronchodilation.[68] It is known to provide additional bronchodilation when combined with albuterol and should be considered as adjuvant therapy.

Corticosteroids

The predominant pathophysiologic process in asthma is airway inflammation. Corticosteroids are recommended for children with status asthmaticus, and there is evidence that early administration is beneficial.[69] Corticosteroids should be given IV to patients requiring ICU admission at a dose of 1 mg per kg every 6 to 12 hours of methylprednisolone (maximum dose of 60 mg per day) for 5 to 7 days; tapering of steroids has not been shown to have any additional benefit.[69]

Magnesium Sulfate

Magnesium antagonizes calcium channels, resulting in smooth muscle relaxation. In addition, it is known to inhibit mast cell degranulation.[70] Some studies have shown benefit of IV administration of magnesium sulfate at a dose of 25 to 50 mg per kg (maximum of 2 g) over 15 to 20 minutes and repeated if necessary. Repeated dosing necessitates measurement of serum magnesium levels.

Terbutaline

Terbutaline is a selective β-2 agonist used IV in patients with status asthmaticus with worsening respiratory status despite other treatments. In a retrospective study, Doymaz et al. showed that early continuous infusion of terbutaline was associated with a decrease in acute respiratory failure and need for mechanical support.[71] Initial starting dose is 5 mCg per kg bolus, followed by a continuous infusion of 0.2 to 0.3 mCg per kg per min (maximum of 5 mCg per kg per min). Side effects include tachycardia, jitteriness, and chest pain.

Methylxanthines

Methylxanthines are nonspecific phosphodiesterase (PDE) inhibitors that cause relaxation of the smooth muscles by increasing cyclic adenosine monophosphate (cAMP).[72] The most common medication used in this class is aminophylline. A bolus dose of 5 mg per kg is followed by continuous infusion. Aminophylline elimination varies by age. Initial continuous infusion should be at 0.5 mg per kg per hour for children aged 6 weeks to 6 months, 0.6 to 0.7 mg per kg per hour for ages 6 to 12 months, 1 to 1.2 mg per kg per hour for ages 1 to 9 years, 0.9 mg per kg per hour for ages 9 to 12 years, and 0.7 mg per kg per hour for 12 to 16 years of age and nonsmoking adults. The infusion rate should be adjusted to maintain serum concentrations between 10 and 18 mCg per mL. Aminophylline is metabolized in the liver, and its half-life is prolonged in patients with hepatic dysfunction and heart failure necessitating dosage adjustments. Side effects include tachycardia, nausea, and seizures. Close monitoring of serum levels is imperative. The most recent Global Initiative for Asthma guidelines recommend against using methylxanthines in favor of using β agonists due to the narrow therapeutic index.[69]

Helium Oxygen Therapy

HeliOx has been used for patients with asthma to allow for a more laminar flow of air in the airway (as discussed in the section on croup and postextubation stridor). Studies have not shown consistent results in terms of HeliOx in terms of shortening length of ICU and hospital stay. HeliOx should be reserved for patients not responding to standard therapy.[69,72,73]

Inhaled Anesthetics

In a patient with respiratory failure not responding to therapy, inhaled anesthetics may be used to provide further bronchodilation. Sevoflurane and isoflurane are the most common anesthetics used because of fewer side effects.[72,74] Hemodynamic monitoring is important as side effects include myocardial depression along with arrhythmias.[75] Inhaled anesthetics should be delivered with the assistance of an anesthesiologist, to ensure appropriate delivery and scavenging.

PULMONARY HYPERTENSION

Pulmonary hypertension (PH) in children can be idiopathic (primary) or secondary. Secondary PH is more common and can be found in patients with congenital heart disease due to increased pulmonary blood flow, causing increased pulmonary artery pressure. Other causes of secondary PH include medications, pulmonary venous abnormalities, collagen vascular disease, and chronic pulmonary disease. Primary PH is characterized by smooth muscle hypertrophy of the pulmonary arterial wall, intimal proliferation of the pulmonary arterioles, and in situ thrombosis with small-vessel occlusion.[76] Therapeutic options for PH include nitric oxide, prostacyclin, and endothelin antagonism (Fig. 16.2).

Nitric Oxide Pathway

Nitric oxide (NO) is reported to be decreased in patients with PH. It stimulates the formation of cyclic guanosine monophosphate (cGMP) by activating guanylate cyclase, resulting in potent vasodilatory effects.[76] When administered by inhalation, it relaxes vascular smooth muscle and has been shown to improve oxygenation[77] and decrease pulmonary vascular resistance.[78,79] The recommended dose for NO is 20 ppm. The main side effect of NO is occurrence of methemoglobinemia.

Sildenafil works via a pathway similar to NO by inhibiting phosphodiesterase 5 (PDE-5) and preventing the breakdown of cGMP, thus increasing cGMP-mediated vasodilation by nitric oxide. It is frequently used to sustain pulmonary vasodilatation as inhaled nitric oxide (iNO) is being weaned off.[80]

Several studies in children show improvement in oxygenation and hemodynamic parameters with the use of sildenafil.[81,82] The dose is 0.5 mg per kg every 8 hours and can be titrated to a maximum of 1 mg per kg every 6 to 8 hours.

Prostacyclin Pathway

Prostacyclin (PGI_2) is produced in the vascular endothelium and causes vasodilation by the cAMP pathway by activating

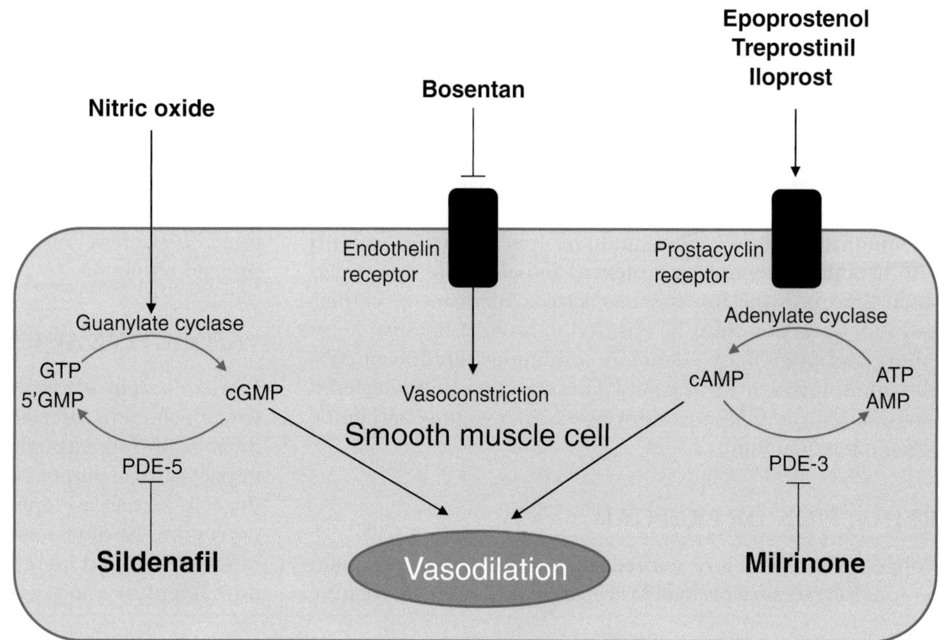

Figure 16.2 **Pulmonary hypertension medications and mechanism of action**. AMP, adenosine monophosphate; ATP, adenosine triphosphate; cAMP, cyclic adenosine monophosphate; cGMP, cyclic guanosine monophosphate; GTP, guanosine triphosphate.

adenylate cyclase. It is a potent vasodilator and inhibitor of platelet aggregation.[83]

Several prostanoid drugs are available, such as *epoprostenol* and *treprostinil* that require a continuous infusion and inhaled *iloprost.* Prostacyclins have been shown to decrease pulmonary pressure and improve cardiac output and oxygenation. Studies show the benefits of long-term continuous PGI_2 infusion for the treatment of PH.[84–86] The disadvantages of prostacyclin infusion include the need for prolonged IV access, life-threatening rebound effects if the drug is discontinued abruptly, systemic vasodilation, jaw pain, and diarrhea. The starting dose for an epoprostenol infusion is 2 ng per kg per min.

Endothelin Pathway

Endothelin pathway antagonists block the activation of the pathway and, therefore, inhibit vasoconstriction. *Bosentan* is a competitive endothelin-receptor antagonist that acts as a vasodilator. It has been shown to slow progression of pediatric PH,[87] improves left ventricular function, and diminishes cardiac remodeling in patients with PH due to congenital heart disease.[88] Its main side effect is elevation of liver transaminases. The dose is 1 mg per kg BID and can be increased to 2 mg per kg BID.

ACUTE CIRCULATORY FAILURE

Disease states characterized by low cardiac output are often encountered in the ICU. Pharmacologic manipulation of the components of cardiac output is necessary in a variety of disorders, such as hypovolemia, hypervolemia, myocardial dysfunction, and septic shock.

AUGMENTATION OF PRELOAD

Crystalloids such as 0.9% saline or lactated Ringer solution are satisfactory, for rapid intravascular expansion (20 mL per kg) is indicated when hypovolemic state accompanied by an overall depletion of the extracellular fluid compartment is suspected. Such a bolus can be repeated as required based on the hemodynamic response. Five percent albumin is often the plasma expander of choice for managing hypovolemia with either normal or expanded interstitial fluid space as in sepsis or after surgery. Because of its colloid oncotic pressure, 5% albumin of 10 to 20 mL per kg bolus is expected to preferentially expand the intravascular space. Despite many studies, superiority of colloids over crystalloids has not been established in management of septic shock.

Administration of 25% albumin is often utilized in patients with hypoproteinemia, hypovolemia, and edema to draw interstitial fluid into the intravascular space. Adequacy of cardiac and renal function must be ensured to avoid congestive heart failure and pulmonary edema. A continuous infusion of 25% albumin solution at 1 to 2 g per kg per day can be administered along with furosemide for restoring vascular volume and mobilizing interstitial fluid.

REDUCTION OF PRELOAD

Congestive heart failure and renal insufficiency are frequent reasons for excessive preload in critically ill children. Decreasing the extracellular fluid space without causing undesirable hypovolemia is the goal in such patients.

Loop Diuretics

Furosemide at 1 mg per kg per dose is the most commonly employed diuretic in these situations. The dose can be repeated every 6 to 8 hours as necessary. It has been shown that continuous infusion of furosemide (0.1 mg per kg per hour) is as effective as intermittent dosing with regard to increasing urine output. Additional benefits include reduction of the total dose and less hemodynamic instability.[89]

Bumetanide (0.015 to 0.1 mg per kg per day IV or PO) is an alternative loop diuretic. Bumetanide has a shorter duration of action (4 to 6 hours vs. 6 to 8 hours) and is 40 times more potent than furosemide. Using equivalent doses, bumetanide and furosemide have the same clinical efficacy and side effects, except in patients with renal disease. These patients seem to respond better to bumetanide.[90] Bumetanide is used less frequently than furosemide in children.

Thiazide Diuretics

Chlorothiazide (10 to 20 mg per kg every 12 hours PO, 1 to 4 mg per kg every 12 hours IV), *hydrochlorothiazide* (1 to 2mg per kg per day as single or divided in to two doses), and *metolazone* (0.1 to 0.2 mg per kg every 12 hours) can be combined with furosemide for greater effect. These thiazide diuretics inhibit sodium transport in the distal convoluted tubule, with minor action in the proximal tubule and cortical-collecting ducts.[91] Metolazone is a thiazide-like diuretic that acts primarily to inhibit sodium reabsorption at the cortical-diluting site and, to a lesser extent, in the proximal convoluted tubule. Sodium and chloride ions are excreted in approximately equivalent amounts. The increased delivery of sodium to the distal tubular exchange site results in increased potassium excretion.

Potassium-Sparing Diuretics

Spironolactone (1 to 3mg per kg per day PO) acts in the principal cells in the connecting and collecting tubules. Sodium entry in these segments occurs through aldosterone-sensitive sodium channels. The reabsorption of cationic sodium without an anion creates a lumen-negative electrical gradient that then favors the secretion of potassium through selective potassium channels (and hydrogen ions). The inhibition of sodium reabsorption at this site can lead to concurrent reduction in potassium excretion.[92] It is often combined with loop or thiazide diuretics for preload reduction.

VASOACTIVE AGENTS

Cardiac output is a product of stroke volume and heart rate; stroke volume is affected by preload, afterload, and contractility. Inotropic agents enhance myocardial contractility and thus impact cardiac output. The inotropic agents commonly used in the ICU setting are epinephrine, milrinone, dobutamine, and dopamine. Vasopressors are agents that cause vasoconstriction of the vessels and increase afterload; the main agents used are norepinephrine and vasopressin.

Inotropic Agents

Epinephrine

When used in low doses of 0.02 to 0.03 mCg per kg per min, epinephrine acts predominantly on β-adrenergic receptors, increasing contractility. It also enhances coronary blood flow and produces vasodilation, resulting in decreased afterload. At higher doses, epinephrine has α-1 adrenergic effects, resulting in vasoconstriction, increased afterload, and tachycardia. In murine models, epinephrine has been shown to have a significantly higher inotropic effect compared to dobutamine and dopamine.[93]

Milrinone

As a PDE-3 inhibitor, milrinone prevents the breakdown of cAMP to AMP, resulting in the increase in cAMP levels, leading to improved myocardial contractility and improved diastolic relaxation of the myocardium (lusitropy).[94] The presence of PDE-3 in vascular smooth muscle results in vasodilation and afterload reduction as well. PDE-3 inhibitors do not increase myocardial oxygen consumption to the same extent as β agonists. Milrinone was shown to decrease the risk of low cardiac output syndrome in infants and young children after repair of congenital heart defects.[95] In this study, a dose of 75 mCg per kg IV bolus followed by 0.75 mCg per kg per min infusion was found to be superior to placebo. Milrinone is also effective for improving cardiac output in patients with cardiogenic shock from other conditions such as myocarditis and cardiomyopathy. A significant side effect of milrinone is vasodilation-related hypotension. In addition, it undergoes renal clearance and, therefore, should be used with caution in patients with oliguria and acute kidney injury (AKI).[96] The recommended starting dose is 0.375 mCg per kg per min, titrated to 0.75 mCg per kg per min. The half-life of milrinone is about 2 hours. Unlike β-agonist agents, the effects of milrinone may last for a longer time (1 to 2 hours vs. minutes) after discontinuation of the infusion.

Dopamine

Dopamine has direct stimulating effects on α- and β-adrenergic and dopaminergic receptors and indirect effects on norepinephrine release from presynaptic sympathetic terminals. Stimulation of the dopamine (DA_1) receptors results in relaxation of renal, cerebral, coronary, mesenteric, and pulmonary vasculature. Stimulation of DA_2 receptors results in renal and mesenteric vasodilation. The effects of dopamine on various receptors are dose dependent. At a low dose of 2 to 5 mCg per kg per min, dopamine stimulates the dopaminergic receptors, resulting in increased renal, mesenteric, and coronary blood flow without significantly increasing myocardial oxygen consumption. At moderate doses of 5 to 10 mCg per kg per min, β-adrenergic receptors are stimulated, resulting in an increase in myocardial contractility, heart rate, and norepinephrine release. At a high dose of 10 to 20 mCg per kg per min, dopamine causes α-adrenergic stimulation, resulting in peripheral vasoconstriction, increases in systemic and pulmonary vascular resistance, and increases in blood pressure.

Dobutamine

Dobutamine is a synthetic catecholamine that acts predominantly on β_1 receptors, increasing myocardial contractility. It also causes β_2-mediated vasodilation. Dobutamine causes greater augmentation of myocardial blood flow for the same increase in myocardial oxygen demand when compared to dopamine.[97] The dosing range is 2.5 to 20 mCg per kg per min.

Vasopressors

Norepinephrine is a potent vasoconstrictor; it acts on the α-adrenergic receptors, with β inotropic and chronotropic effects. It increases systolic and diastolic blood pressures as well as pulse pressure and coronary blood flow. It is one of the preferred agents in vasodilatory (warm) shock.[98] The dose range is 0.03 to 0.3 mCg per kg per min.

Vasopressin has been used for vasodilatory shock as it is a potent systemic vasoconstrictor. It acts on the V1 receptors in the vascular smooth muscles, mediating vasoconstriction. It also increases vascular sensitivity to norepinephrine effects, further enhancing its vasoactive property.[94] Vasopressin has predominant systemic vasoconstrictor effects while causing pulmonary, cerebral, and coronary vasodilation.[99] This medication should be used in caution in patients with heart failure as it increases afterload without inotropicity.

Afterload Reduction

Decreasing the afterload by venous or arterial dilation augments cardiac output by reducing ventricular wall stress and improving stroke volume. Vasodilators are used in critically ill children with myocardial dysfunction after cardiac surgery, myocarditis, myocardial ischemia, dilated cardiomyopathy, and systemic or PH. Commonly used agents include nitroglycerin, sodium nitroprusside, angiotensin-converting enzyme (ACE) inhibitors, calcium channel blockers (CCBs), angiotensin receptor blockers (ARBs), and PDE-3 inhibitors.

Nitroglycerin

Nitroglycerin is a potent venous dilator and relaxes the systemic and pulmonary arterial musculature. Clinically significant effects of nitroglycerin are decreased afterload and preload, decreased myocardial oxygen consumption, increased cardiac output, and increased myocardial blood flow. Excessive vasodilation may result in hypotension, necessitating volume augmentation or dose reduction. Nitroglycerin is infused IV at a rate of 0.5 to 5 mCg per kg per min titrated to effect. The usefulness of nitroglycerin may be limited by the development of tachyphylaxis with prolonged use. It is best suited for use in the immediate postoperative period in patients with surgeries involving coronary circulation [e.g., left coronary artery from the pulmonary artery (ALCAPA) and transposition of great arteries (TGA) repairs].

Sodium Nitroprusside

Sodium nitroprusside stimulates guanylate cyclase, resulting in the increase in intracellular concentrations of cGMP. Desirable pharmacologic effects result from arterial and venous dilation. Nitroprusside causes greater reduction in systemic and pulmonary arterial pressure than nitroglycerin. When used to augment cardiac output, both nitroprusside and nitroglycerin should be used in conjunction with an inotropic agent. Sodium nitroprusside is especially effective in hypertensive emergencies and after coarctectomy. It is used as a continuous infusion titrated to effect in a dose of 0.5 to 10 mCg per kg per min. With prolonged usage, cyanide and thiocyanate toxicity are a concern, especially in those with impaired renal clearance. Significant toxicity is not commonly encountered in children with normal hepatic and renal function. In order to avoid the adverse effects of cyanide toxicity, some institutions routinely add sodium thiosulfate in a ratio of 10:1 nitroprusside to thiosulfate. Thiosulfate provides the sulfur donor that allows the combination of cyanide with thiosulfate to form less toxic sodium thiocyanate, which is then excreted.[100]

Angiotensin-Converting Enzyme Inhibitors

ACE inhibitors inhibit the conversion of angiotensin I to angiotensin II. In addition to its vasoconstrictive properties, angiotensin II releases aldosterone from the adrenal cortex, resulting in sodium and water retention. ACE inhibitors are often used when there is a need for prolonged afterload reduction. ACE inhibitors are particularly helpful after heart surgery, dilated cardiomyopathy, and congestive heart failure from left to right shunts and mitral and aortic regurgitation. In children, enalapril is the most commonly used agent for this purpose. Enalapril is available as IV and oral formulation. The oral route is preferred. The initial oral dose is 0.05 mg per kg every 12 hours, titrated to effect with a maximum dose of 0.25 mg per kg every 12 hours. The IV dose of enalapril is 0.01 to 0.02 mg per kg per day divided every 12 hours. Hyperkalemia and AKI are the main complications of ACE inhibitors, particularly in neonates and when used over a long duration. The combination of ACE inhibitors and diuretics tends to worsen AKI.[101] A study of 63 children with congestive heart failure by Leversha et al. showed improved myocardial function in 58% of patients.[102] However, eight (12%) patients required discontinuation of the drug because of renal failure that developed within 5 days of institution of enalapril. Because ACE inhibitors abolish vasoconstriction in the renal efferent arterioles necessary for maintaining glomerular filtration pressure, they should not be used in patients with renal artery stenosis.

Calcium Channel Blockers

By blocking calcium entry into the cell, administration of CCBs results in vascular smooth muscle relaxation and vasodilation, decreased myocardial force generation (negative inotropy), decreased heart rate (negative chronotropy), and decreased conduction velocity within the heart (negative dromotropy).[103] Nicardipine is a dihydropyridine CCB. It is administered as an infusion of 0.5 to 3 mCg per kg per min for hypertension, particularly in children who do not have an adequate response to nitroprusside.

Angiotensin Receptor Blockers

ARBs are newer medications for afterload reduction. ARBs are receptor antagonists that block type 1 angiotensin II (AT_1) receptors on blood vessels and other tissues such as the myocardium. These receptors are coupled to the Gq protein and IP_3 signal transduction pathway that stimulate vascular smooth muscle contraction. The most commonly used agent in this group is losartan. It is generally used in children aged 6 years and older. The initial dose is 0.7 mg per kg per day, with a maximum of 1.4 mg per kg per day.[104]

Miscellaneous Agents

Prostaglandin E1

PGE_1 (alprostadil) is a temporizing pharmacologic measure to keep the ductus arteriosus open in ductal-dependent congenital heart defects. In neonates with left-sided obstructive lesions such as hypoplastic left heart syndrome, coarctation, and interrupted aortic arch, patency of ductus arteriosus is necessary to maintain blood flow through the descending aorta. Similarly, blood flow across the ductus is essential to maintain pulmonary blood flow in neonates with cyanotic heart defects, such as pulmonary and tricuspid atresia. Alprostadil is administered as a continuous IV infusion of 0.05 to 0.2 mCg per kg per min. Side effects include hypotension resulting from vasodilatory effects, apnea, fever, and seizures. Prolonged therapy for more than 5 days is associated with gastric antral mucosal hyperplasia, cortical hyperostosis, and soft-tissue swelling.

β-Blocking Agents

β-Blocking agents may be used as continuous IV infusions for the management of hypertensive emergencies and tachyarrhythmias. The advantages of continuous infusion of short-acting β-blockers are the rapid onset of action with a relative brief duration of effects after discontinuation of therapy. Side effects include hypotension, negative inotropy, bradycardia, hypoglycemia, and bronchospasm. Patients require electrocardiographic and blood pressure monitoring.

Esmolol has selective β_1-adrenergic blocking properties. It is used as a class II antiarrhythmic agent and to alleviate dynamic left or right outflow tract obstruction, such as in hypertrophic cardiomyopathy and cyanotic spells of tetralogy of Fallot. An initial bolus of 100 to 500 mCg per kg over 1 minute is followed by a continuous infusion of 25 mCg per kg per min as the starting dose and can be increased in increments of 25 to 50 mCg per kg per min depending on the response.

Labetalol has both α- and β-adrenergic blocking properties. *Carvedilol* is a nonselective β-adrenoreceptor and α_1-adrenoreceptor antagonist. *Propranolol* is a β-adrenergic blocking agent. The use of β-blockers, such as carvedilol, can help inhibit sympathetic activity and may reduce progression of congestive heart failure. Carvedilol is the first β-blocker approved by the FDA for the treatment of mild-to-moderate congestive heart failure. The benefits of this drug in patients with congestive heart failure have been shown in several adult[105–107] and pediatric studies.[108,109]

ANTICOAGULATION AND THROMBOLYTICS

Thromboembolic disease is increasingly recognized in pediatric population. Early detection, prompt treatment, and appropriate prophylaxis help avoid long-term consequences. Many risk factors are associated with venous thrombosis in children, including indwelling central venous catheter (CVC) (most common), surgery, trauma, infection, immobilization, malignancy, use of estrogen-containing oral contraceptive pills, inflammatory conditions (e.g., systemic lupus erythematosus), structural venous abnormalities, and inherited thrombophilia. Spontaneous venous thrombosis is rare in children. The approach to treatment of thromboembolic disease in children is largely extrapolated from adult guidelines.[110,111]

Prophylactic treatment should be performed for patients with the following:

- CVCs
- Prosthetic heart valves
- Blalock–Taussig shunt
- Endovascular stents
- Fontan procedure
- Atrial fibrillation
- Continuous arteriovenous hemofiltration
- Hemodialysis
- Extracorporeal membrane oxygenation (ECMO)
- Kawasaki disease

Therapy should be initiated for patients with the following:

- Deep vein thrombosis (DVT)
- Pulmonary embolism
- Arterial thromboembolism
- Venous thromboembolism
- Nonhemorrhagic stroke

HEPARIN

Unfractionated Heparin

Unfractionated heparin is a naturally occurring mucoitin polysulfuric acid stored in mast cells. Heparin activity is standardized by a U.S. Pharmacopeia reference that is measured as the amount of heparin needed to prevent clotting of citrated sheep plasma with calcium. Heparin is ineffective when given PO and must be administered by IV or IM injection. Heparin inhibits coagulation by acting in conjunction with antithrombin to inhibit activated coagulation factors (Table 16.7).

The three major complications associated with the use of heparin include bleeding, osteoporosis with long-term use, and heparin-induced thrombocytopenia (HIT). If immediate reversal of heparin effect is needed, protamine sulfate can be given (Table 16.8).

TABLE 16.7 Protocol for Systemic Heparin Administration and Adjustment for Children

aPTT	*Bolus, units/kg*	*Hold (min)*	*Rate Change (%)*	*Repeat aPTT*
<50	50	0	+10	4 h
50–59	0	0	+10	4 h
60–85	0	0	0	Next day
86–95	0	0	−10	4 h
96–120	0	30	−10	4 h
>120	0	60	−15	4 h

aPTT, activated partial thromboplastin time; IV, intravenous.
Loading dose: Heparin 75 units/kg IV over 10 minutes.
Initial maintenance dose: 28 units/kg/h for infants < 1year, 20 units/kg/h for children older than 1 year.
Adjust heparin to maintain aPTT 60–85 seconds.
Adapted from Michelson AD, Bovill E, Andrew M. Antithrombotic therapy in children. *Chest* 1995;108:506S–522S.

TABLE 16.8 Reversal of Heparin Therapy

Time Since Last Heparin Dose (min)	*Protamine Dose, mg/100 units Heparin*
<30	1
30–60	0.5–0.75
60–120	0.375–0.5
>120	0.25–0.375

Maximum dose = 50 mg. Infusion rate 10 mg/mL solution should not exceed 5 mg/min.
Adapted from Monagle P, Michelson AD, Bovill E, et al. Antithrombotic therapy in children. *Chest* 2001;119:344S–370S.

Low-Molecular Weight Heparin

Low-molecular weight heparin (LMWH) has several advantages over unfractionated heparin that include predictability of effects and lessening the need for frequent monitoring. In addition, the subcutaneous route obviates the need for IV access and lower incidence of HIT. The action of LMWH is similar to heparin. Therapeutic level of LMWH is indicated by a factor Xa level of 0.50 to 1 unit per mL 4 to 6 hours following subcutaneous injection. A study of 900 adults with symptomatic lower extremity DVT showed that once- or twice-daily enoxaparin was as safe and efficacious as continuously infused unfractionated heparin.[112]

Heparin-Induced Thrombocytopenia

Type I HIT is a condition where mild thrombocytopenia develops soon after exposure to heparin and is due to the proaggregating effects of heparin. There is no need to discontinue heparin use with type I HIT. Type II HIT is more severe and is an immune-mediated condition resulting from the development of antibodies to heparin/platelet factor 4 (HPF4) complexes. The complex then binds and cross-links to the platelet Fc ⊠-receptor IIA, resulting in platelet activation, leading to thrombosis and thrombocytopenia. In addition, the antibody activates endothelial cells, increasing expression of tissue factor and thrombin generation.[113,114] Type II HIT generally occurs 7 to 10 days after exposure to heparin. Heparin use should be discontinued immediately. Approximately 1% to 5% of adults who receive heparin develop HIT.[115–117] The incidence of HIT in children is unclear. Schmugge et al. performed a retrospective cohort study in children admitted to the PICU over a 3-year period and found that HIT-associated thrombosis occurred in 2.3% of children who were exposed to heparin.[118]

WARFARIN

Warfarin exerts it anticoagulant effect by inhibiting the synthesis of vitamin K–dependent coagulation factors II, VII, IX, and X. It also inhibits the anticoagulant vitamin K–dependent proteins, protein C and protein S. The overall effect of warfarin depends on the balance of inhibition of procoagulant versus anticoagulant factors. The depletion of vitamin K–dependent factors follows the sequence depending on their half-life. Protein C, protein S, and factor VII have a half-life of approximately 6 hours, whereas other vitamin K–dependent factors have a half-life lasting 2 to 3 days. Therefore, early in the course of warfarin treatment, a procoagulant state may be prevalent, followed by an anticoagulant state a few days later. The early procoagulant state should be managed by the addition of heparin at the initiation of warfarin therapy. Heparin should be discontinued after the warfarin effect is evident [International Normalized Ratio (INR) ≥ 2].[119–121]

Warfarin has a narrow therapeutic window that requires close monitoring of the prothrombin time (PT) and INR to determine the degree of anticoagulation and to guide dose adjustments. Because of the use of different tissue thromboplastins around the world, there is variation in PT values. For example, rabbit brain thromboplastin, which is widely used in North America, is not as sensitive as human brain thromboplastin, which is used in Europe, accounting for a marked difference in PT. To provide standardization, the World Health Organization (WHO) recommends an INR. INR is a dimensionless number used for expressing the patient's PT as a ratio to a reference sample provided by the WHO. The INR measured in this manner provides consistent values across all laboratories.

Currently, the INR is the standard for monitoring adequacy of warfarin anticoagulation. The desired range of INR depends on the clinical condition being addressed. For example, for patients with DVT, an INR of 2 to 3 would generally be targeted, whereas for a mechanical heart valve, an INR range of 2.5 to 3.5 is recommended. A starting dose of 0.1 to 0.2 mg per kg per day is given for 2 days while monitoring INR before gradually increasing the daily dose to achieve the desired therapeutic range, usually over 5 to 7 days.[122] Once maintenance dose of warfarin is established, INR monitoring can be extended to longer intervals depending on the clinical condition and the patient's compliance with treatment (Table 16.9).

Dosing of warfarin is affected by genetic factors, other medications, diet, and intercurrent illness. If indicated (e.g., need for major surgical intervention), the effect of warfarin can be rapidly reversed with vitamin K, fresh-frozen plasma, or prothrombin complex concentrates.

DIRECT THROMBIN INHIBITORS

Direct thrombin inhibitors (DTIs) prevent thrombin from cleaving fibrinogen to fibrin by directly binding thrombin. Bivalirudin and argatroban are parenteral DTIs that are often utilized as an alternative to heparin in patients with severe HIT. Bivalirudin is eliminated via nonenzymatic proteolysis, whereas argatroban is eliminated via the hepatobiliary system. Both medications require monitoring of activated partial thromboplastin time (aPTT), hemoglobin, platelets, and signs and symptoms of bleeding.[123] Dabigatran etexilate is the only oral DTI.

Direct factor Xa inhibitors prevent factor Xa from cleaving prothrombin to thrombin. They bind directly to factor Xa. Examples of direct Xa inhibitors include rivaroxaban, apixaban, edoxaban, and betrixaban. The safety and efficacy of most of these agents has not been established in children.[124,125]

TABLE 16.9 Protocol for Oral Anticoagulation Therapy to Maintain an INR between 2 and 3 in Children

INR	*Action*
I. Day 1	
1–1.3	0.2 mg/kg orally
II. Loading days 2–4	
1.1–1.3	Repeat initial loading dose
1.4–1.9	50% of initial loading dose
2–3	50% of initial loading dose
3.1–3.5	25% of initial loading dose
>3.5	Hold until INR <3.5, then restart at 50% less than previous dose
III. Maintenance oral anticoagulation dose guidelines	
1.1–1.4	Increase by 20% of dose
1.5–1.9	Increase by 10% of dose
2–3	No change
3.1–3.5	Decrease by 10% of dose
>3.5	Hold until INR <3.5, then restart at 20% less than previous dose

INR, International Normalized Ratio.
Adapted from Michelson AD, Bovill E, Andrew M. Antithrombotic therapy in children. *Chest* 1995;108:506S–522S.

THROMBOLYTIC AGENTS

Thrombolytic agents such as streptokinase, urokinase, and tissue plasminogen factor (recombinant tissue plasminogen activator, rtPA) exert their therapeutic effects by converting plasminogen to plasmin. Streptokinase and urokinase are no longer used. Because of the thrombolytic ability of these agents, they are contraindicated in patients with strokes, other neurologic diseases such as traumatic brain injury, and recent surgery.

Recombinant Tissue Plasminogen Activator

Currently, rtPA is the thrombolytic agent of choice. The advantages of rtPA include a short half-life, minimal antigenicity, lack of inhibition by ⊠2 antitrypsin, and a local and specific action on plasminogen-bound fibrin. The experience with rtPA for the treatment of myocardial infarction in adults is well described. In the PICU, it is most commonly used for clot lysis in CVCs (Table 16.10). In a study of 14 neonates with catheter-related thrombus, infusion of rtPA resulted in complete clot dissolution in 11 patients and partial clot lysis in two patients.[126] Complications such as intracranial hemorrhage or allergic reactions were not observed in patients in this study.

More recently, continuous IV infusion of rtPA has also been used for lysis of intracardiac or large-vessel thrombus. A bolus of 0.7 mg per kg is followed by continuous IV infusion of 0.1 to 0.3 mg per kg per hour with a continuous heparin infusion of 4 to 10 International Units per kg per hour. The concomitant use of low-dose heparin prevents reoccurrence of the thrombus.

TABLE 16.10 Guidelines for Local Instillation of Recombinant Tissue Plasminogen Activator

Treatment	*Single-Lumen CVC*	*Double-Lumen CVC*	*SC Port*
rtPA ≤10 kg	0.5 mg diluted in 0.9% NaCl to volume required to fill line	0.5 mg per lumen diluted in 0.9% NaCl to fill volume of line. Treat 1 lumen at a time	0.5 mg diluted with 0.9% NaCl to 3 mL
rtPA ≥10 kg	1 mg in 1 mL 0.9% NaCl. Use amount required to fill volume of line to maximum of 2 mL in 2 mg	1 mg/mL. Use amount required to fill volume of line, to a maximum of 2 mL (2 mg/lumen). Treat 1 lumen at a time.	2 mg diluted with 0.9% NaCl to 3 mL

CVC, central venous catheter; rtPA, recombinant tissue plasminogen activator; SC: subcutaneos.
Adapted from Monagle P, Michelson AD, Bovill E, et al. Antithrombotic therapy in children. *Chest* 2001;119:344S–370S.

GASTROINTESTINAL HEMORRHAGE

Upper GI bleeding is defined as bleeding proximal to the ligament of Treitz and is usually characterized by bright red or coffee-ground emesis and black-tarry stools.[127] The causes of upper GI bleeding include esophageal varices, esophagitis, Mallory–Weiss tears, and peptic ulcer disease.[127]

Lower GI bleeding occurs distal to the ligament of Treitz and is characterized by frank blood from the rectum.[128] The causes include anal fissure, polyps, allergic or infectious colitis, Meckel diverticulum, necrotizing enterocolitis, and intussusception.[128]

Severe GI bleeding results in hemodynamic instability and shock. Initial management includes stabilization of the patient, followed by endoscopy or surgical intervention.[127,128] Specific medical management includes treatment of nonvariceal bleeding with a pantoprazole infusion, while nonsurgical treatment of esophageal varices can be attempted with an octreotide infusion.

Proton Pump Inhibitors (PPIs) decrease secretion of hydrogen protons by blocking the gastric hydrogen potassium ATPase pump and decreasing the acidity of the gastric lumen and, therefore, are used for nonvariceal upper GI bleeding.[129] Patients with upper GI bleeding who received omeprazole prior to undergoing endoscopy have been shown to have less active bleeding and shorter hospital stays.[130] PPI infusions following endoscopy improve patient outcomes compared to endoscopy alone.[131] Pantoprazole is currently the preferred PPI. The patient should first receive a bolus of 1 mg per kg followed by an infusion of 0.1 mg per kg per hour which can be increased as needed.

Octreotide is a somatostatin analog that decreases azygos and variceal blood flow and can be used for the treatment of variceal bleeding.[132–134] Side effects include hyperglycemia, bradycardia, and nausea. The half-life is 1 to 2 hours. A bolus dose of 1 mCg per kg is followed by an infusion of 0.5 mCg per kg per hour with dose adjustments as necessary.

ENDOCRINOPATHIES

SYNDROME OF INAPPROPRIATE ANTIDIURETIC HORMONE SECRETION

The feature of the SIADH secretion is characterized as euvolemic hyponatremia. This results in water retention and, if left untreated, eventually leads to hyponatremia, hypo-osmolality, and cerebral edema. SIADH has been observed with severe pulmonary disease, the use of drugs such as vincristine, traumatic brain injury, meningitis, and surgical procedures such as spinal fusion and craniotomies.[135]

Asymptomatic SIADH can be treated by fluid restriction and monitoring of serum electrolytes. Symptomatic SIADH with a degree of hyponatremia severe enough to cause seizures or encephalopathy requires emergent treatment. Upon documentation of low serum sodium, 5 mL per kg of 3% NaCl should be administered IV. This will increase the serum sodium level by 4 mEq per L. Administration of furosemide is often needed to induce diuresis and elimination of water. We have shown that relatively rapid correction of acute hyponatremia is not likely to lead to central pontine myelinolysis.[12] Following the administration of 3% NaCl and furosemide, further treatment of patients with SIADH should include fluid restriction.

Demeclocycline is a tetracycline derivative that induces nephrogenic diabetes insipidus (DI), resulting in decrease in free water reabsorption.[136] It has been used for adults with SIADH. Side effects include nephrotoxicity, rashes, and hepatic dysfunction.[135]

Conivaptan is a vasopressin receptor antagonists that inhibits the effects of antidiuretic hormone on receptors in the kidney, resulting in aquaresis or the excretion of water without solutes, leading to increased serum sodium and osmolality. IV conivaptan (20 to 40 mg per day) is approved by the FDA for the treatment of adults with euvolemic or hypervolemic hyponatremia such as SIADH.[137]

DIABETIC KETOACIDOSIS

Patients with DKA present with dehydration, hyperglycemia, ketonuria, and electrolyte disturbances. Altered mental status may be present on admission, and cerebral edema is a known complication of treatment. Hemodynamic and airway stability should be ascertained in patients with DKA. Laboratory determinations should include a blood gas, serum electrolytes, urinalysis, β-hydroxybutyrate level, and a point-of-care glucose level. After obtaining IV access, isotonic fluids should be administered at 10 mL per kg. Patients should be reassessed for the need for additional 10 mL per kg fluid bolus based on their degree of dehydration.

Patients with DKA present due to insulin deficiency, leading to a catabolic state, ketone formation and secondary ketonuria, gluconeogenesis, glycogenolysis, and secondary glucosuria. Following rehydration, *insulin* infusion should be started at 0.1 unit per kg per hour. Close monitoring of glucose levels is important to prevent an excessive decline in the glucose concentration or hypoglycemia. Potassium in both potassium chloride and potassium phosphate forms should be added to the IV solution as these patients are overall potassium and phosphate depleted. However, in order to avoid hyperkalemia, potassium should only be added when it is ascertained that the patient has adequate renal function.

THYROID DISEASE

Thyroid hormone is important in the regulation of energy, development, and growth. Patients can present to the ICU with myxedema coma and thyroid storm.

T4

In patients with myxedema, IV dose of T4 of 4 mCg per kg (maximum 200 to 500 mCg) should be administered followed by 1 to 2 mCg per kg per day. Stress dose hydrocortisone (see below) should be administered in these patients as severe hypothyroidism often blunts the cortisol response.[138]

Methimazole

In patients with thyroid storm, methimazole blocks synthesis of thyroid hormone, but it does not inhibit conversion of T4 to T3. The dose is 4 mg per kg per day divided into three doses daily. After stabilization of the patient, maintenance dose can be initiated at 0.2 mg per kg per day divided into three doses daily.[139]

Propylthiouracil

Propylthiouracil (PTU) inhibits thyroid hormone synthesis and conversion of T4 to T3. Side effects include hepatotoxicity.[139] The dose is age dependent, and limited data are available for dosing in children. Patients older than 6 years can receive 150 mg per day divided in three doses.

β-Blocking Agents

β-Blocking agents will help decrease tachycardia and hypertension often associated with thyroid storm and should be added. Propranolol is the most commonly used agent. The added benefit of its use is the inhibition of the conversion of T4 to T3.[139]

ADRENAL CRISIS

Patients with adrenal insufficiency present with anorexia, fatigue, lethargy, and hypotension. Those with shock can present with circulatory collapse and altered mental status. This is a medical emergency and prompt fluid resuscitation, and administration of hydrocortisone is imperative.[140]

Hydrocortisone should be administered at a dose of 100 mg per M^2 per day, followed by 100 mg per M^2 per day divided into doses given every 6 hours. Once the crisis has resolved, the hydrocortisone dose can be slowly weaned every 2 to 3 days. Maintenance dose for patients with adrenal insufficiency is 12.5 mg per M^2 per day.

CENTRAL DIABETES INSIPIDUS

Central DI can occur in critically ill children following surgery for removal of suprasellar or intrasellar tumors, after traumatic brain injuries, and intracranial infections. It is also observed in children with significant intracranial hypertension with or without herniation. The decreased level of ADH leads to uncontrolled excretion of water, producing dilute urine, hypernatremia, dehydration, and hypovolemic shock. During the acute phase, a continuous infusion of vasopressin provides much better therapeutic control and is preferred to intranasal or oral deamino-8-D-arginine-vasopressin (DDAVP). We recommend mixing 10 units of vasopressin in 1,000 mL of D5 water with an infusion rate of 1 to 3 mU per kg per hour, increasing as needed. An initial infusion rate of 0.5 mU per kg per hour can be gradually titrated to a maximum of 10 mU per kg per hour based on serum sodium and osmolality, fluid balance, and urine output. Once intravascular volume and serum electrolytes are under better control, the vasopressin infusion can be discontinued, and the patient started on intranasal (5 to 30 mCg per day, in one or two doses), or oral (0.05 mg BID) desmopressin (DDAVP).

INBORN ERRORS OF METABOLISM

Inborn errors of metabolism are due to enzymatic deficiencies; they are a common presentation of patients in the ICU and need urgent management as early detection and treatment may affect outcome. These patients present in various ways, including failure to thrive, acute encephalopathy, metabolic acidosis, seizures, and shock. Addressing every inherited error of metabolism is beyond the scope of this chapter. Selected group of disorders are addressed in Table 16.11. Three major presentations are discussed:

1. Hyperammonemia
2. Anion gap metabolic acidosis with or without lactic acidosis
3. Hypoglycemia.

HYPERAMMONEMIA

Disorders with hyperammonemia include urea cycle disorders, organic acidemias (i.e., isovaleric acidemia, methylmalonic acidemia), and fatty acid oxidation disorders. These patients present with hypotonia, lethargy, and altered mental status. Hyperammonemia is a medical emergency as ammonia can cross the BBB and produce cerebral edema due to cellular swelling.[141] Diagnosis can be facilitated by testing for urine ketones and measurement of serum amino acid and urine orotic acid levels.

Management of patients with hyperammonemia is directed at reversing catabolism (administration of glucose), promoting anabolism (administration of insulin and lipids), and reducing the plasma ammonia level (reducing the generation and increasing removal of ammonia). Ammonia levels can be reduced with pharmacologic agents and dialysis.

Sodium phenylacetate and sodium phenylbutyrate (Ammonul) bind to glutamine to form phenylacetylglutamine, which is excreted in the urine. The dose used is 250 mg per kg bolus over 2 hours followed by a continuous infusion of 250 to 500 mg per kg per day.[141]

Sodium benzoate binds with glycine (a source of ammonia) to form hippurate, which is excreted in the urine; the dose used is 250 mg per kg bolus over 2 hours followed by an infusion of 250 to 500 mg per kg per day.[141]

Lactulose acidifies the colon lumen, making it a hostile environment for urease-producing bacteria.[141,142] It is frequently used for patients with acute hepatic failure. The starting dose

TABLE 16.11 Inborn Errors of Metabolism Therapy

Suspected Diagnosis	Therapy	Dose
Urea cycle defects	Arginine	250 mg/kg/d
	Sodium benzoate	250 mg/kg bolus followed by infusion of 250 mg/kg/d
	Sodium phenylacetate/sodium phenylbutyrate (Ammonul)	250 mg/kg bolus followed by infusion of 250 mg/kg/d
Glycogen storage disease[147]	Corn starch to maintain glucose overnight	Young children: 1.6 g/kg every 3–4 h Older children/adolescents: 1.7–2.5 g/kg every 4–6 h
Methylmalonic acidemia	Hydroxycobalamin	1 mg IM injection daily
	L-Carnitine	50–100 mg/kg/d
Propionic academia	L-Carnitine	50–100 mg/kg/d
Mitochondrial disorders	L-Carnitine	25–50 mg/kg four times daily
	Coenzyme Q10	Young children: 5 mg/kg/d Older children/adolescents: 400 mg daily

IM, intramuscular.

depends on age (~2 g per day for infants and 25 g per day for adolescents) with the aim of inducing three bowel movements daily.

Rifaximin is an oral antibiotic that inhibits enteral ammonia-producing bacteria[142] and is also used in patients with acute hepatic failure. The dose is age dependent and varies from 100 to 500 mg BID.

In patients with urea cycle defects, *arginine* is an essential amino acid. It can promote ammonia excretion through the urea cycle, but should not be administered in patients with arginase deficiency.[141] The dose is 250 mg per kg bolus followed by 250 mg per kg per day.

METABOLIC ACIDOSIS

Disorders in this category include organic acidemias (propionic academia, methylmalonic acidemia), which all present with slightly elevated or normal lactic acid levels, or mitochondrial disorders, which present with elevated lactic acid levels. Symptoms include vomiting, lethargy, and mental status changes. Patients with organic acidemias are generally dehydrated and require hydration. Specific treatment is based on the diagnosis.[143]

Patients with mitochondrial disorders have a defect in oxidative phosphorylation. A muscle biopsy looking for ragged red fibers helps establish the diagnosis. Mitochondrial sequencing as well as genetic testing may be helpful for the diagnosis of specific disorders [mitochondrial encephalomyopathy, lactic acidosis, and stroke-like episodes (MELAS) and myoclonic epilepsy with ragged red fibers (MERRF)]. Treatment is geared toward improving nutrition and reducing acidosis by providing sodium bicarbonate in addition to other therapeutic agents (see Table 16.11).

TABLE 16.12 Drugs Associated with Neuroleptic Malignant Syndrome

Neuroleptic Agents	Antiemetic Agents
Chlorpromazine	Promethazine
Clozapine	Metoclopramide
Haloperidol	Prochlorperazine
Olanzapine	Domperidone
Quetiapine	
Risperidone	

HYPOGLYCEMIA

Disorders presenting with hypoglycemia include disorders of gluconeogenesis, fatty acid oxidation disorders, glycogen storage diseases, and endocrinopathies such as cortisol deficiency or hyperinsulinism. Patients present with diaphoresis, irritability, lethargy, seizures, and altered sensorium. Initial treatment needs to aim at correcting the hypoglycemia by administering a bolus of IV dextrose of 2 to 4 mL per kg of D25% solution, followed by a dextrose infusion.

SPECIAL CONDITIONS

MH is an autosomal dominant pharmacogenetic disorder that tends to manifest clinically when susceptible patients are exposed to volatile anesthetic gases or succinylcholine. Two genes are associated with MH and result in MH causative mutations (*RYR1* and *CACNA1S*). Patients with central core disease (CCD) and inherited myopathies are susceptible to MH. The uncontrolled passage of cytosolic calcium results in a hypermetabolic state that is manifested as mixed metabolic and respiratory acidosis, muscle rigidity, rhabdomyolysis, cardiac arrhythmia, and hyperthermia.[144]

Dantrolene is the only known antidote for MH. When MH is suspected, dantrolene should be administered immediately as a loading bolus of 2.5 mg per kg IV, with subsequent bolus doses of 1 mg per kg IV until the signs of acute MH have resolved.[145]

Neuroleptic malignant syndrome (NMS) is a life-threatening neurologic emergency associated with the use of neuroleptic and some antiemetic agents. It manifests as mental status changes, rigidity, fever, and dysautonomia (Table 16.12).

Treatment of NMS consists of immediate discontinuation of the offending medication and aggressive support depending on the presenting symptoms. The recommendation for medical therapy is based on case reports and clinical experience as no data from clinical trials exist so far. Benzodiazepines such as lorazepam and diazepam are used to control agitation. For severe cases of NMS, dantrolene, bromocriptine, and amantadine have been used. Dantrolene can be given in a dose of 1 to 2.5 mg per kg IV and repeated to a maximum of 10 mg per kg per day. Bromocriptine is a dopamine agonist used to restore dopaminergic tone. Amantadine has a dopaminergic and an anticholinergic effect. It is used as an alternative to bromocriptine.[146]

REFERENCES

1. Paczynski RP. Osmotherapy. Basic concepts and controversies. *Crit Care Clin* 1997;13(1):105–129.
2. Pasarikovski CR, Alotaibi NM, Al-Mufti F, et al. Hypertonic saline for increased intracranial pressure after aneurysmal subarachnoid hemorrhage: a systematic review. *World Neurosurg* 2017;105:1–6.
3. Decourcey DD, Steil GM, Wypij D, et al. Increasing use of hypertonic saline over mannitol in the treatment of symptomatic cerebral edema in pediatric diabetic ketoacidosis: an 11-year retrospective analysis of mortality. *Pediatr Crit Care Med* 2013;14(7):694–700.
4. Donato T, Shapira Y, Artru A, et al. Effect of mannitol on cerebrospinal fluid dynamics and brain tissue edema. *Anesth Analg* 1994;78(1):58–66.
5. Soustiel JF, Vlodavsky E, Zaaroor M. Relative effects of mannitol and hypertonic saline on calpain activity, apoptosis and polymorphonuclear infiltration in traumatic focal brain injury. *Brain Res* 2006;1101(1):136–144.
6. Dorman HR, Sondheimer JH, Cadnapaphornchai P. Mannitol-induced acute renal failure. *Medicine (Baltimore)* 1990;69(3):153–159.
7. Piper BJ, Harrigan PW. Hypertonic saline in paediatric traumatic brain injury: a review of nine years' experience with 23.4% hypertonic saline as standard hyperosmolar therapy. *Anaesth Intensive Care* 2015;43(2):204–210.
8. Boone MD, Oren-Grinberg A, Robinson TM, et al. Mannitol or hypertonic saline in the setting of traumatic brain injury: what have we learned? *Surg Neurol Int* 2015;6:177.
9. Kheirbek T, Pascual JL. Hypertonic saline for the treatment of intracranial hypertension. *Curr Neurol Neurosci Rep* 2014;14(9):482.
10. Marks JA, Li S, Gong W, et al. Similar effects of hypertonic saline and mannitol on the inflammation of the blood-brain barrier microcirculation after brain injury in a mouse model. *J Trauma Acute Care Surg* 2012;73(2):351–357; discussion 357.
11. Kochanek PM, Tasker RC, Bell MJ, et al. Management of pediatric severe traumatic brain injury: 2019 consensus and guidelines-based algorithm for first and second tier therapies. *Pediatr Crit Care Med* 2019;20(3):269–279.
12. Sarnaik AP, Meert K, Hackbarth R, et al. Management of hyponatremic seizures in children with hypertonic saline: a safe and effective strategy. *Crit Care Med* 1991;19(6):758–762.
13. Kassell NF, Hitchon PW, Gerk MK, et al. Alterations in cerebral blood flow, oxygen metabolism, and electrical activity produced by high dose sodium thiopental. *Neurosurgery* 1980;7(6):598–603.
14. Demopoulos HB, Flamm ES, Pietronigro DD, et al. The free radical pathology and the microcirculation in the major central nervous system disorders. *Acta Physiol Scand Suppl* 1980;492:91–119.
15. Goodman JC, Valadka AB, Gopinath SP, et al. Lactate and excitatory amino acids measured by microdialysis are decreased by pentobarbital coma in head-injured patients. *J Neurotrauma* 1996;13(10):549–556.
16. Abraham P, Rennert RC, Gabel BC, et al. ICP management in patients suffering from traumatic brain injury: a systematic review of randomized controlled trials. *Acta Neurochir (Wien)* 2017;159(12):2279–2287.
17. Eckert MJ, Martin MJ. Trauma: spinal cord injury. *Surg Clin North Am* 2017;97(5):1031–1045.
18. Evaniew N, Dvorak M. Cochrane in CORR1: steroids for acute spinal cord injury (review). *Clin Orthop Relat Res* 2016;474(1):19–24.
19. Prasad K, Singh MB, Ryan H. Corticosteroids for managing tuberculous meningitis. *Cochrane Database Syst Rev* 2016;4:CD002244.
20. Glauser T, Shinnar S, Gloss D, et al. Evidence-based guideline: treatment of convulsive status epilepticus in children and adults: report of the Guideline Committee of the American Epilepsy Society. *Epilepsy Curr* 2016;16(1):48–61.
21. Laine GA, Hossain SM, Solis RT, et al. Polyethylene glycol nephrotoxicity secondary to prolonged high-dose intravenous lorazepam. *Ann Pharmacother* 1995;29(11):1110–1114.
22. Lyttle MD, Rainford NEA, Gamble C, et al. Levetiracetam versus phenytoin for second-line treatment of paediatric convulsive status epilepticus (EcLiPSE): a multicentre, open-label, randomised trial. *Lancet* 2019;393(10186):2125–2134.
23. Tan J, Paquette V, Levine M, et al. Levetiracetam clinical pharmacokinetic monitoring in pediatric patients with epilepsy. *Clin Pharmacokinet* 2017;56(11):1267–1285.
24. Chidambaran V, Costandi A, D'Mello A. Propofol: a review of its role in pediatric anesthesia and sedation. *CNS Drugs* 2015;29(7):543–563.
25. Trinka E, Hofler J, Zerbs A, et al. Efficacy and safety of intravenous valproate for status epilepticus: a systematic review. *CNS Drugs* 2014;28(7):623–639.
26. Palace J, Newsom-Davis J, Lecky B. A randomized double-blind trial of prednisolone alone or with azathioprine in myasthenia gravis. Myasthenia Gravis Study Group. *Neurology* 1998;50(6):1778–1783.
27. Pascuzzi RM, Coslett HB, Johns TR. Long-term corticosteroid treatment of myasthenia gravis: report of 116 patients. *Ann Neurol* 1984;15(3):291–298.
28. Anderson D, Phan C, Johnston WS, et al. Rituximab in refractory myasthenia gravis: a prospective, open-label study with long-term follow-up. *Ann Clin Transl Neurol* 2016;3(7):552–555.
29. Zuppa AF, Curley MAQ. Sedation analgesia and neuromuscular blockade in pediatric critical care: overview and current landscape. *Pediatr Clin North Am* 2017;64(5):1103–1116.
30. Power BM, Forbes AM, van Heerden PV, et al. Pharmacokinetics of drugs used in critically ill adults. *Clin Pharmacokinet* 1998;34(1):25–56.
31. Rosenberg H, Pollock N, Schiemann A, et al. Malignant hyperthermia: a review. *Orphanet J Rare Dis* 2015;10:93.
32. Watling SM, Dasta JF, Seidl EC. Sedatives, analgesics, and paralytics in the ICU. *Ann Pharmacother* 1997;31(2):148–153.
33. Wilcox SR. Corticosteroids and neuromuscular blockers in development of critical illness neuromuscular abnormalities: a historical review. *J Crit Care* 2017;37:149–155.
34. deBacker J, Hart N, Fan E. Neuromuscular blockade in the 21st century management of the critically ill patient. *Chest* 2017;151(3):697–706.
35. Keating GM. Sugammadex: a review of neuromuscular blockade reversal. *Drugs* 2016;76(10):1041–1052.
36. Tobias JD. Current evidence for the use of sugammadex in children. *Paediatr Anaesth* 2017;27(2):118–125.
37. Vanacker BF, Vermeyen KM, Struys MM, et al. Reversal of rocuronium-induced neuromuscular block with the novel drug sugammadex is equally effective under maintenance anesthesia with propofol or sevoflurane. *Anesth Analg* 2007;104(3):563–568.
38. Duerden EG, Guo T, Dodbiba L, et al. Midazolam dose correlates with abnormal hippocampal growth and neurodevelopmental outcome in preterm infants. *Ann Neurol* 2016;79(4):548–559.
39. Tobias JD. Sedation and analgesia in paediatric intensive care units: a guide to drug selection and use. *Paediatr Drugs* 1999;1(2):109–126.
40. Tobias JD. Tolerance, withdrawal, and physical dependency after long-term sedation and analgesia of children in the pediatric intensive care unit. *Crit Care Med* 2000;28(6):2122–2132.
41. Ely EW, Truman B, Shintani A, et al. Monitoring sedation status over time in ICU patients: reliability and validity of the Richmond Agitation-Sedation Scale (RASS). *JAMA* 2003;289(22):2983–2991.
42. Ambuel B, Hamlett KW, Marx CM, et al. Assessing distress in pediatric intensive care environments: the COMFORT scale. *J Pediatr Psychol* 1992;17(1):95–109.
43. Popernack ML, Thomas NJ, Lucking SE. Decreasing unplanned extubations: utilization of the Penn State Children's Hospital Sedation Algorithm. *Pediatr Crit Care Med* 2004;5(1):58–62.
44. De Deyne C, Struys M, Decruyenaere J, et al. Use of continuous bispectral EEG monitoring to assess depth of sedation in ICU patients. *Intensive Care Med* 1998;24(12):1294–1298.
45. Mondello E, Siliotti R, Noto G, et al. Bispectral index in ICU: correlation with Ramsay Score on assessment of sedation level. *J Clin Monit Comput* 2002;17(5):271–277.
46. Vender JS, Szokol JW, Murphy GS, et al. Sedation, analgesia, and neuromuscular blockade in sepsis: an evidence-based review. *Crit Care Med* 2004;32(11 Suppl):S554–S561.
47. Gautam NK, Turiy Y, Srinivasan C. Preincision initiation of dexmedetomidine maximally reduces the risk of junctional ectopic tachycardia in children undergoing ventricular septal defect repairs. *J Cardiothorac Vasc Anesth* 2017;31(6):1960–1965.
48. Haenecour AS, Seto W, Urbain CM, et al. Prolonged dexmedetomidine infusion and drug withdrawal in critically ill children. *J Pediatr Pharmacol Ther* 2017;22(6):453–460.
49. Whalen LD, Di Gennaro JL, Irby GA, et al. Long-term dexmedetomidine use and safety profile among critically ill children and neonates. *Pediatr Crit Care Med* 2014;15(8):706–714.
50. Ahlen K, Buckley CJ, Goodale DB, et al. The 'propofol infusion syndrome': the facts, their interpretation and implications for patient care. *Eur J Anaesthesiol* 2006;23(12):990–998.
51. Jiang S, Li X, Jin W, et al. Ketamine-induced neurotoxicity blocked by N-methyl-d-aspartate is mediated through activation of PKC/ERK pathway in developing hippocampal neurons. *Neurosci Lett* 2018;673:122–131.
52. Olney JW, Wozniak DF, Jevtovic-Todorovic V, et al. Drug-induced apoptotic neurodegeneration in the developing brain. *Brain Pathol* 2002;12(4):488–498.
53. Kaushal RP, Vatal A, Pathak R. Effect of etomidate and propofol induction on hemodynamic and endocrine response in patients undergoing coronary artery bypass grafting/mitral valve and aortic valve replacement surgery on cardiopulmonary bypass. *Ann Card Anaesth* 2015;18(2):172–178.
54. Tobias JD. Etomidate in pediatric anesthesiology: where are we now? *Saudi J Anaesth* 2015;9(4):451–456.
55. Campbell K, Torres L, Stayer S. Anesthesia and sedation outside the operating room. *Anesthesiol Clin* 2014;32(1):25–43.
56. Cravero JP, Askins N, Sriswasdi P, et al. Validation of the pediatric sedation state scale. *Pediatrics* 2017;139(5):e20162897.
57. McGrath PJ, Johnson G, Goodman JT, et al. CHEOPS: A behavioral scale for rating postoperative pain in children. In: Fiels HL, Dubner R, Ververo F, eds. *Advances in pain research and therapy.* New York, NY: Raven Press, 1985;9:395–402.
58. Beyer J. *The Oucher: A user's manual and technical report.* Evanston, IL, Judson Press.
59. Merkel S, Voepel-Lewis T, Malviya S. Pain assessment in infants and young children: the FLACC scale. *Am J Nurs* 2002;102(10):55–58.
60. Ray S, Brick T, Raman S, et al. Haemodynamic changes with paracetamol in critically-ill children. *J Crit Care* 2017;40:108–112.
61. Petrocheilou A, Tanou K, Kalampouka E, et al. Viral croup: diagnosis and a treatment algorithm. *Pediatr Pulmonol* 2014;49(5):421–429.
62. Ausejo M, Saenz A, Pham B, et al. The effectiveness of glucocorticoids in treating croup: meta-analysis. *West J Med* 1999;171(4):227–232.
63. Anene O, Meert KL, Uy H, et al. Dexamethasone for the prevention of postextubation airway obstruction: a prospective, randomized, double-blind, placebo-controlled trial. *Crit Care Med* 1996;24(10):1666–1669.
64. Connolly KM, McGuirt WF Jr. Avoiding intubation in the injured subglottis: the role of heliox therapy. *Ann Otol Rhinol Laryngol* 2001;110(8):713–717.
65. Grosz AH, Jacobs IN, Cho C, et al. Use of helium-oxygen mixtures to relieve upper airway obstruction in a pediatric population. *Laryngoscope* 2001;111(9):1512–1514.
66. Tobias JD. Heliox in children with airway obstruction. *Pediatr Emerg Care* 1997;13(1):29–32.
67. Carroll CL, Sala KA. Pediatric status asthmaticus. *Crit Care Clin* 2013;29(2):153–166.
68. Maselli DJ, Peters JI. Medication regimens for managing acute asthma. *Respir Care* 2018;63(6):783–796.

69. Tamaoki J. Asthma prevention and management guideline 2018. *Arerugi* 2018;67(9):1263–1268.
70. Baker AK, Carroll CL. High-dose magnesium infusions for acute severe asthma in children: if a little is good, is more even better? *Pediatr Crit Care Med* 2016;17(2):177–178.
71. Doymaz S, Schneider J, Sagy M. Early administration of terbutaline in severe pediatric asthma may reduce incidence of acute respiratory failure. *Ann Allergy Asthma Immunol* 2014;112(3):207–210.
72. Rehder KJ. Adjunct therapies for refractory status asthmaticus in children. *Respir Care* 2017;62(6):849–865.
73. Rodrigo G, Pollack C, Rodrigo C, et al. Heliox for nonintubated acute asthma patients. *Cochrane Database Syst Rev* 2006(4):CD002884.
74. Mondonedo JR, McNeil JS, Amin SD, et al. Volatile anesthetics and the treatment of severe bronchospasm: a concept of targeted delivery. *Drug Discov Today Dis Models* 2015;15:43–50.
75. Carrie S, Anderson TA. Volatile anesthetics for status asthmaticus in pediatric patients: a comprehensive review and case series. *Paediatr Anaesth* 2015;25(5):460–467.
76. Lan NSH, Massam BD, Kulkarni SS, et al. Pulmonary arterial hypertension: pathophysiology and treatment. *Diseases* 2018;6(2):38.
77. Adhikari NK, Burns KE, Friedrich JO, et al. Effect of nitric oxide on oxygenation and mortality in acute lung injury: systematic review and meta-analysis. *BMJ* 2007;334(7597):779.
78. Tarry D, Powell M. Hypoxic pulmonary vasoconstriction. *BJA Educ* 2017;17(6):208–213.
79. Coggins MP, Bloch KD. Nitric oxide in the pulmonary vasculature. *Arterioscler Thromb Vasc Biol* 2007;27(9):1877–1885.
80. Lee JE, Hillier SC, Knoderer CA. Use of sildenafil to facilitate weaning from inhaled nitric oxide in children with pulmonary hypertension following surgery for congenital heart disease. *J Intensive Care Med* 2008;23(5):329–334.
81. Abrams D, Schulze-Neick I, Magee AG. Sildenafil as a selective pulmonary vasodilator in childhood primary pulmonary hypertension. *Heart* 2000;84(2):E4.
82. Baquero H, Soliz A, Neira F, et al. Oral sildenafil in infants with persistent pulmonary hypertension of the newborn: a pilot randomized blinded study. *Pediatrics* 2006;117(4):1077–1083.
83. Steinhorn RH. Pharmacotherapy for pulmonary hypertension. *Pediatr Clin North Am* 2012;59(5):1129–1146.
84. Barst RJ, Maislin G, Fishman AP. Vasodilator therapy for primary pulmonary hypertension in children. *Circulation* 1999;99(9):1197–1208.
85. Rosenzweig EB, Kerstein D, Barst RJ. Long-term prostacyclin for pulmonary hypertension with associated congenital heart defects. *Circulation* 1999;99(14):1858–1865.
86. Wax D, Garofano R, Barst RJ. Effects of long-term infusion of prostacyclin on exercise performance in patients with primary pulmonary hypertension. *Chest* 1999;116(4):914–920.
87. Hislop AA, Moledina S, Foster H, et al. Long-term efficacy of bosentan in treatment of pulmonary arterial hypertension in children. *Eur Respir J* 2011;38(1):70–77.
88. Apostolopoulou SC, Manginas A, Cokkinos DV, et al. Long-term oral bosentan treatment in patients with pulmonary arterial hypertension related to congenital heart disease: a 2-year study. *Heart* 2007;93(3):350–354.
89. Luciani GB, Nichani S, Chang AC, et al. Continuous versus intermittent furosemide infusion in critically ill infants after open heart operations. *Ann Thorac Surg* 1997;64(4):1133–1139.
90. Ward A, Heel RC. Bumetanide. A review of its pharmacodynamic and pharmacokinetic properties and therapeutic use. *Drugs* 1984;28(5):426–464.
91. Kunau RT, Jr., Weller DR, Webb HL. Clarification of the site of action of chlorothiazide in the rat nephron. *J Clin Invest* 1975;56(2):401–407.
92. Horisberger JD, Giebisch G. Potassium-sparing diuretics. *Ren Physiol* 1987;10(3–4):198–220.
93. Zausig YA, Geilfus D, Missler G, et al. Direct cardiac effects of dobutamine, dopamine, epinephrine, and levosimendan in isolated septic rat hearts. *Shock* 2010;34(3):269–274.
94. Overgaard CB, Dzavik V. Inotropes and vasopressors: review of physiology and clinical use in cardiovascular disease. *Circulation* 2008;118(10):1047–1056.
95. Hoffman TM, Wernovsky G, Atz AM, et al. Efficacy and safety of milrinone in preventing low cardiac output syndrome in infants and children after corrective surgery for congenital heart disease. *Circulation* 2003;107(7):996–1002.
96. Gist KM, Mizuno T, Goldstein SL, et al. Retrospective evaluation of milrinone pharmacokinetics in children with kidney injury. *Ther Drug Monit* 2015;37(6):792–796.
97. Fowler MB, Alderman EL, Oesterle SN, et al. Dobutamine and dopamine after cardiac surgery: greater augmentation of myocardial blood flow with dobutamine. *Circulation* 1984;70(3 Pt 2):I103–111.
98. Davis AL, Carcillo JA, Aneja RK, et al. The American College of Critical Care Medicine clinical practice parameters for hemodynamic support of pediatric and neonatal septic shock: executive summary. *Pediatr Crit Care Med* 2017;18(9):884–890.
99. Holmes CL, Landry DW, Granton JT. Science review: vasopressin and the cardiovascular system part 1—receptor physiology. *Crit Care* 2003;7(6):427–434.
100. Schulz V. Clinical pharmacokinetics of nitroprusside, cyanide, thiosulphate and thiocyanate. *Clin Pharmacokinet* 1984;9(3):239–251.
101. Ku LC, Zimmerman K, Benjamin DK, et al. Safety of enalapril in infants admitted to the neonatal intensive care unit. *Pediatr Cardiol* 2017;38(1):155–161.
102. Leversha AM, Wilson NJ, Clarkson PM, et al. Efficacy and dosage of enalapril in congenital and acquired heart disease. *Arch Dis Child* 1994;70(1):35–39.
103. Flynn JT, Mottes TA, Brophy PD, et al. Intravenous nicardipine for treatment of severe hypertension in children. *J Pediatr* 2001;139(1):38–43.
104. Shahinfar S, Cano F, Soffer BA, et al. A double-blind, dose-response study of losartan in hypertensive children. *Am J Hypertens* 2005;18(2 Pt 1):183–190.
105. Olsen SL, Gilbert EM, Renlund DG, et al. Carvedilol improves left ventricular function and symptoms in chronic heart failure: a double-blind randomized study. *J Am Coll Cardiol* 1995;25(6):1225–1231.
106. Metra M, Nardi M, Giubbini R, et al. Effects of short-and long-term carvedilol administration on rest and exercise hemodynamic variables, exercise capacity and clinical conditions in patients with idiopathic dilated cardiomyopathy. *J Am Coll Cardiol* 1994;24(7):1678–1687.
107. Packer M, Colucci WS, Sackner-Bernstein JD, et al. Double-blind, placebo-controlled study of the effects of carvedilol in patients with moderate to severe heart failure. The PRECISE Trial. Prospective Randomized Evaluation of Carvedilol on Symptoms and Exercise. *Circulation* 1996;94(11):2793–2799.
108. Price JF. Congestive heart failure in children. *Pediatr Rev* 2019;40(2):60–70.
109. Nishiyama M, Park IS, Yoshikawa T, et al. Efficacy and safety of carvedilol for heart failure in children and patients with congenital heart disease. *Heart Vessels* 2009;24(3):187–192.
110. Monagle P, Michelson AD, Bovill E, et al. Antithrombotic therapy in children. *Chest* 2001;119(1 Suppl):344S–370S.
111. Tuckuviene R, Christensen AL, Helgestad J, et al. Pediatric venous and arterial noncerebral thromboembolism in Denmark: a nationwide population-based study. *J Pediatr* 2011;159(4):663–669.
112. Merli G, Spiro TE, Olsson CG, et al. Subcutaneous enoxaparin once or twice daily compared with intravenous unfractionated heparin for treatment of venous thromboembolic disease. *Ann Intern Med* 2001;134(3):191–202.
113. Amiral J, Bridey F, Dreyfus M, et al. Platelet factor 4 complexed to heparin is the target for antibodies generated in heparin-induced thrombocytopenia. *Thromb Haemost* 1992;68(1):95–96.
114. Visentin GP, Ford SE, Scott JP, et al. Antibodies from patients with heparin-induced thrombocytopenia/thrombosis are specific for platelet factor 4 complexed with heparin or bound to endothelial cells. *J Clin Invest* 1994;93(1):81–88.
115. Warkentin TE, Kelton JG. A 14-year study of heparin-induced thrombocytopenia. *Am J Med* 1996;101(5):502–507.
116. Warkentin TE, Levine MN, Hirsh J, et al. Heparin-induced thrombocytopenia in patients treated with low-molecular-weight heparin or unfractionated heparin. *N Engl J Med* 1995;332(20):1330–1335.
117. Warkentin TE, Sheppard JA, Horsewood P, et al. Impact of the patient population on the risk for heparin-induced thrombocytopenia. *Blood* 2000;96(5):1703–1708.
118. Schmugge M, Risch L, Huber AR, et al. Heparin-induced thrombocytopenia-associated thrombosis in pediatric intensive care patients. *Pediatrics* 2002;109(1):E10.
119. Binymin KA, Nasher M, Patel D. Warfarin-induced deep vein thrombosis. *Int Med Case Rep J* 2014;7:123–125.
120. Brandjes DP, Heijboer H, Buller HR, et al. Acenocoumarol and heparin compared with acenocoumarol alone in the initial treatment of proximal-vein thrombosis. *N Engl J Med* 1992;327(21):1485–1489.
121. Esmon CT, Vigano-D'Angelo S, D'Angelo A, et al. Anticoagulation proteins C and S. *Adv Exp Med Biol* 1987;214:47–54.
122. Harrison L, Johnston M, Massicotte MP, et al. Comparison of 5-mg and 10-mg loading doses in initiation of warfarin therapy. *Ann Intern Med* 1997;126(2):133–136.
123. Warkentin TE, Greinacher A, Koster A, et al. Treatment and prevention of heparin-induced thrombocytopenia: American College of Chest Physicians Evidence-Based Clinical Practice Guidelines, 8th ed. *Chest* 2008;133(6 Suppl):340S–380S.
124. Baglin T, Hillarp A, Tripodi A, et al. Measuring Oral Direct Inhibitors (ODIs) of thrombin and factor Xa: a recommendation from the Subcommittee on Control of Anticoagulation of the Scientific and Standardisation Committee of the International Society on Thrombosis and Haemostasis. *J Thromb Haemost* 2013.
125. Di Nisio M, Middeldorp S, Buller HR. Direct thrombin inhibitors. *N Engl J Med* 2005;353(10):1028–1040.
126. Hartmann J, Hussein A, Trowitzsch E, et al. Treatment of neonatal thrombus formation with recombinant tissue plasminogen activator: six years experience and review of the literature. *Arch Dis Child Fetal Neonatal Ed* 2001;85(1):F18–F22.
127. Lirio RA. Management of upper gastrointestinal bleeding in children: variceal and nonvariceal. *Gastrointest Endosc Clin N Am* 2016;26(1):63–73.
128. Sahn B, Bitton S. Lower gastrointestinal bleeding in children. *Gastrointest Endosc Clin N Am* 2016;26(1):75–98.
129. Worden JC, Hanna KS. Optimizing proton pump inhibitor therapy for treatment of nonvariceal upper gastrointestinal bleeding. *Am J Health Syst Pharm* 2017;74(3):109–116.
130. Lau JY, Leung WK, Wu JC, et al. Omeprazole before endoscopy in patients with gastrointestinal bleeding. *N Engl J Med* 2007;356(16):1631–1640.
131. Laine L, McQuaid KR. Endoscopic therapy for bleeding ulcers: an evidence-based approach based on meta-analyses of randomized controlled trials. *Clin Gastroenterol Hepatol* 2009;7(1):33–47, quiz 31–32.
132. Eroglu Y, Emerick KM, Whitingon PF, et al. Octreotide therapy for control of acute gastrointestinal bleeding in children. *J Pediatr Gastroenterol Nutr* 2004;38(1):41–47.
133. Heikenen JB, Pohl JF, Werlin SL, et al. Octreotide in pediatric patients. *J Pediatr Gastroenterol Nutr* 2002;35(5):600–609.
134. Pai AK, Fox VL. Gastrointestinal bleeding and management. *Pediatr Clin North Am* 2017;64(3):543–561.
135. Cuesta M, Garrahy A, Thompson CJ. SIAD: practical recommendations for diagnosis and management. *J Endocrinol Invest* 2016;39(9):991–1001.
136. Miell J, Dhanjal P, Jamookeeah C. Evidence for the use of demeclocycline in the treatment of hyponatraemia secondary to SIADH: a systematic review. *Int J Clin Pract* 2015;69(12):1396–1417.

137. Cuesta M, Thompson CJ. The syndrome of inappropriate antidiuresis (SIAD). *Best Pract Res Clin Endocrinol Metab* 2016;30(2):175–187.
138. Kwaku MP, Burman KD. Myxedema coma. *J Intensive Care Med* 2007;22(4):224–231.
139. Chiha M, Samarasinghe S, Kabaker AS. Thyroid storm: an updated review. *J Intensive Care Med* 2015;30(3):131–140.
140. Puar TH, Stikkelbroeck NM, Smans LC, et al. Adrenal crisis: still a deadly event in the 21st century. *Am J Med* 2016;129(3):339, e331–339.
141. Savy N, Brossier D, Brunel-Guitton C, et al. Acute pediatric hyperammonemia: current diagnosis and management strategies. *Hepat Med* 2018;10:105–115.
142. Matoori S, Leroux JC. Recent advances in the treatment of hyperammonemia. *Adv Drug Deliv Rev* 2015;90:55–68.
143. Knerr I, Weinhold N, Vockley J, et al. Advances and challenges in the treatment of branched-chain amino/keto acid metabolic defects. *J Inherit Metab Dis* 2012;35(1):29–40.
144. Wappler F. Malignant hyperthermia. *Eur J Anaesthesiol* 2001;18(10):632–652.
145. Denborough M. Malignant hyperthermia. *Lancet* 1998;352(9134):1131–1136.
146. Velamoor R. Neuroleptic malignant syndrome: a neuro-psychiatric emergency: Recognition, prevention, and management. *Asian J Psychiatr* 2017;29:106–109.
147. Kishnani PS, Austin SL, Abdenur JE, et al. Diagnosis and management of glycogen storage disease type I: a practice guideline of the American College of Medical Genetics and Genomics. *Genet Med* 2014;16(11):e1.

CHAPTER

17

Maryann E. Mazer-Amirshahi
James M. Chamberlain

Drug Therapy in the Pediatric Emergency Department

INTRODUCTION

Pharmacotherapy is an essential part of pediatric emergency medicine. Although few data are available, an estimated 70% to 85% of emergency department (ED) encounters result in the prescription of a medication. The spectrum of illness ranges from minor respiratory infections to cardiorespiratory arrest, and the majority of these conditions have the administration of medications as a critical intervention. In addition, a significant percentage of children who come to EDs have a chronic or preexisting condition requiring routine medications (e.g., asthma, seizure disorder, cystic fibrosis, sickle cell anemia). One study in an urban pediatric ED documented one-quarter of patients presenting for care had a preexisting diagnosis of a chronic condition.[1] One study demonstrated a significant increase in the prevalence of prescriptions across multiple therapeutic classes, including antidiabetic drugs, asthma medications, psychiatric medications, and antihyperlipidemic drugs in children between the ages of 5 and 19 years.[2] An understanding of the scope of pediatric drug therapy, including the pharmacology of the drugs commonly prescribed in the pediatric ED setting, is crucial.

Weighted data estimate that 25% of ED visits involve children, accounting for 28 to 32 million visits annually. More importantly, the number of pediatric ED visits has grown at a greater rate than the population, and the complexity of these visits has increased.[3]

Although not exhaustive, this chapter reviews the more common complaints and associated drug therapies in pediatric ED visits. Attention to airway, breathing, and circulation (ABC) is always the first priority in managing all ED patients. The following discussion describes the "D" in the ABCD algorithm, that is, drug therapy.

ANAPHYLAXIS AND ALLERGIC REACTIONS

Anaphylaxis is a life-threatening emergency in children, requiring urgent intervention. Usually precipitated by an identifiable antigen, anaphylaxis is a systemic allergic response mediated by immunoglobulin E (IgE) and subsequent inflammatory processes.[4] Signs and symptoms of anaphylaxis include bronchospasm, urticaria, angioedema, and hypotension. Anaphylactoid reactions present with similar signs and symptoms to anaphylaxis; however, the mechanism is felt to be a direct release of inflammatory components of the cells and not mediated by IgE. For the purposes of this chapter, the term "anaphylaxis" refers to both true anaphylactic and anaphylactoid reactions.

TREATMENT

The drug of choice for the initial treatment of anaphylaxis is epinephrine. Epinephrine is a potent sympathomimetic agent and stimulates both α- and β-adrenergic receptors. Producing vasoconstriction via α-receptor agonism, epinephrine increases blood pressure (BP) and decreases capillary leakage.[5] As a bronchodilator (acting via β_2-receptor agonism-induced relaxation of the bronchial muscle), epinephrine improves ventilation in the bronchioles and concomitantly increases tidal volume.[5] The β_1-receptor agonism results in greater myocardial contraction.

The ideal route of administration of epinephrine in anaphylaxis is intramuscular (IM). Until recently, in the United States, many practitioners historically administered epinephrine subcutaneously (SC). Although it is effective via this route, when given SC, epinephrine induces a local vasoconstriction, resulting in slow and erratic absorption.[6] In Canada, Europe, and the United Kingdom, the majority of practitioners prefer the IM route, citing better blood flow and greater predictability of absorption.[6–8] This has now been adopted by leading experts in the United States as well.[9] Intravenous (IV) epinephrine is used in advanced anaphylactic shock, when blood flow to the extremities is compromised and SC and IM epinephrine is less effective. Caution should be exercised when calculating and infusing IV epinephrine. The administration of epinephrine should not be delayed by placement of an IV line.

Practitioners need to be aware of the correct dosing for epinephrine and potential errors associated with the availability of multiple concentrations. Epinephrine exists as 1:10,000 (0.1 mg per mL) and 1:1,000 (1 mg per mL) concentrations. For IM administration in anaphylaxis, 0.01 mg per kg (0.01 mL per kg, max. 0.5 mL per dose) of the 1:1,000 concentration is used to minimize the volume injected. If the IV route is used, epinephrine 0.005 mg per kg (0.05 mL per kg) of the 1:10,000 concentration is given. Common adverse reactions include tachycardia and dysrhythmia, hypertension, tremor, and headache.

All patients who have experienced an anaphylactic reaction should be given a prescription for an epinephrine autoinjector along with proper instruction for use at discharge.[4,6] Autoinjectors are available in 0.15-mg strength for children younger than 8 years (weighing <30 kg) and 0.3 mg for those 8 years or older (weighing at least 30 kg).

Other agents used in the mitigation of anaphylaxis include H_1-antagonists. H_1-antagonists block the binding of histamine to the receptors on effector cells in the gastrointestinal (GI) tract, blood vessels, and respiratory tract and inhibit vasodilation and increased capillary permeability and edema formation.[10] Diphenhydramine is the most commonly used agent for allergic reactions and is available in both injectable and oral (PO) preparations. Dosing is 1.25 mg per kg per dose (max. 50 mg per dose) IV/PO every 6 hours around the clock for 24 to 48 hours. The onset of the IV preparation occurs within 1 hour, and the duration of action is approximately 6 hours. Adverse effects include sedation, hypotension, and tachycardia.

Corticosteroids are also useful in the treatment of allergic reactions and anaphylaxis, although it is important to note that the peak of action is delayed, approximately 4 to 6 hours following an IV dose.[6,11] Corticosteroids mitigate both immediate and delayed phases of hypersensitivity reaction. Chemotaxis of white blood cells (WBCs) and circulating inflammatory mediators such as histamine, kinins, prostaglandins, and leukotrienes are decreased following the administration of a corticosteroid.[11] Corticosteroids also decrease both vasodilation and vessel permeability, leading to a reduction in edema. For anaphylaxis, methylprednisolone sodium succinate injection is usually initiated at 2 mg per kg and then continued at a dose of 0.5 to 1 mg per kg per dose (max. 80 mg per dose) IV every 6 hours for 24 hours. Methylprednisolone can be converted to PO prednisone or prednisolone when the patient is able to tolerate PO medications at a dose of 1 mg per kg per dose (max. 80 mg per dose) PO every 6 to 12 hours. PO corticosteroids can be given for mild-to-moderate allergic reactions. Given the potentially biphasic nature of anaphylaxis, corticosteroids are generally continued for 24 to 48 hours, although their efficacy in preventing a resurgence of symptoms has been questioned.[12] Side effects include mood changes, electrolyte alterations, and hypertension.

H_2-antagonists are adjuvant medications that may also be added to the patient's regimen. These agents competitively antagonize the histamine (predominantly H_2) receptors primarily in the GI tract and include ranitidine, famotidine, nizatidine, and cimetidine. They are available as injectable and PO preparations. Ranitidine injection is dosed at 1 mg per kg per dose (max. 50 mg per dose) IV every 8 hours; it can be converted to PO dosing at 2 mg per kg per dose (max. 150 mg per dose) PO every 12 hours. Famotidine injection and PO preparations are dosed at 0.5 mg per kg per dose (max. 40 mg per dose) IV/PO every 12 hours. The dose of IV and PO cimetidine is 5 mg per kg per dose IV/PO divided every 6 to 12 hours depending on age. Because cimetidine is a potent inhibitor of several cytochrome (CYP) isozymes, including CYP1A2, CYP2D6, CYP2E1, CYP2C19, and CYP3A3/4, there is potential for significant drug interactions if it is used.[13] Adverse effects of the H_2-antagonists are similar and include headache, dizziness, GI intolerance, and, rarely, thrombocytopenia.

More often, allergic reactions of a less severe nature are seen in the ED. These may include food, drug, and environmental allergen exposures that result in rash, rhinorrhea, and/or itchy, watery eyes. Often, these allergic reactions can be treated with discontinuation or avoidance of the offending agent. In some cases, a traditional antihistamine, such as diphenhydramine, or a nonsedating antihistamine, such as loratadine, fexofenadine, or cetirizine, may be needed. Intranasal steroids and ophthalmic antihistamine preparations may also be helpful.

INFECTION

SEPSIS AND MENINGITIS

Sepsis is defined as the systemic inflammatory response to infection.[14] Elevated temperature, tachycardia, hypotension or shock, tachypnea, and elevated WBC count are common findings in a patient with sepsis. Septic infants and children can become seriously ill in a rapid manner. Infants in particular may present with nonspecific signs and symptoms, such as fever and lethargy. Therefore, febrile infants younger than 4 weeks generally require a full "sepsis workup," consisting of a lumbar puncture and the collection of blood and urine cultures.[15]

Sepsis can progress quite rapidly to septic shock. The resultant hypotension leads to decreased organ perfusion, with altered mental status reflecting the lack of oxygen and nutrients reaching the brain.[14] The incidence of pediatric sepsis has increased, but mortality has decreased from 10.3% to 8.9%.[16] Treatment should begin with fluid resuscitation and vasopressors (see later discussion of shock), with the early administration of broad-spectrum antibiotics. Acyclovir should be added if the diagnosis of herpes simplex virus (HSV) sepsis is suspected.[17] The most recent Surviving Sepsis Campaign update advocates the use of steroids only in children who do not respond to fluids and vasopressors and have suspected or proven adrenal insufficiency.[18]

Meningitis may have a presentation similar to sepsis in infants and young children. Nonspecific signs and symptoms include irritability, vomiting, decreased PO intake, lethargy, inconsolable crying, and fever. Seizures and a bulging fontanel are late signs of meningitis. Older patients may complain of nuchal rigidity, headache, photophobia, and fever. Meningitis may be bacterial, partially treated bacterial, or aseptic in origin. Aseptic meningitis includes viral, fungal, mycoplasma, and drug-induced causes.

Bacterial colonization of mucosal surfaces with subsequent mucosal invasion leads to bacteremia.[19] After crossing the blood–brain barrier (BBB), the bacteria enter the central nervous system (CNS) and induce cytokine production.[19] Leukocytes accumulate in the cerebrospinal fluid (CSF), and albumin begins to pass through the intercellular junctions of the meninges. Brain edema ensues, increasing intracranial pressure (ICP) and compromising cerebral blood flow.[20] Cranial nerve injury, seizures, ischemic injury, and brain herniation can result if the infection is left untreated. Treatment consists of early administration of IV antibiotics.

Treatment of Sepsis and Meningitis

Detailed discussion of the anti-infective agents can be found in Chapters 20 to 26. A brief overview of the anti-infective agents used for the treatment of sepsis and meningitis follows. Penicillins and cephalosporins, the most commonly prescribed antibiotics, are classified as β-lactam agents based on their essential chemical structure. The β-lactam antibiotics destroy cell wall–containing bacteria by inactivating the enzyme peptidoglycan transpeptidase.[21] By binding irreversibly to the penicillin-binding proteins, β-lactam antibiotics interrupt the synthesis of the cell wall and subsequently cause the bacteria to rupture.

A major mechanism of penicillin resistance is bacterial production of a β-lactamase enzyme, usually occurring secondary to gene transfer. The β-lactamase enzyme hydrolyzes the β-lactam ring, destroying the structure of the antibiotic.[21] To circumvent β-lactamase production as a means of resistance, a β-lactamase inhibitor such as clavulanic acid, sulbactam, or tazobactam is added to β-lactam antibiotics. Although these inhibitors possess weak or no intrinsic antimicrobial activity, they protect the β-lactam antibiotic from hydrolysis and thus expand the spectrum of activity.[22] Examples include amoxicillin-clavulanic acid, ampicillin-sulbactam, and piperacillin-tazobactam.

Aminoglycoside antibiotics exert their antimicrobial effect by binding to the 30S ribosome, subsequently inhibiting bacterial protein synthesis.[23] The primary target of aminoglycoside antibiotics is Gram-negative organisms, although they are often used synergistically with β-lactam antibiotics for certain Gram-positive infections. Aminoglycosides are widely distributed in extracellular fluid and have relatively poor tissue penetration. Dosing for obese patients should be based on adjusted body weight. Aminoglycosides are concentration-dependent bactericidal antibiotics, and extended-interval dosing (i.e., "once daily") has become more prevalent in the pediatric population. Although trials were small, it appears once-daily dosing of aminoglycosides decreases costs and may have improved efficacy with fewer adverse effects.[24] The elimination of aminoglycosides is dependent on renal function; therefore, patients with reduced creatinine clearance (calculated creatinine clearance of <60 mL per minute per 1.73 m^2) should not receive extended-interval dosed aminoglycosides. Aminoglycosides can be inactivated by penicillin derivatives, possibly from the formation of an inactive amide with the open β-lactam ring.[25] Coadministration should be separated by at least 30 minutes.

Vancomycin is a glycopeptide antibiotic primarily effective against Gram-positive organisms. Similar to β-lactam antibiotics, vancomycin inhibits synthesis of the cell wall. However, vancomycin binds at the D-alanyl-D-alanine terminus and inhibits the release of building blocks necessary for cell wall synthesis.[26] Vancomycin is a large molecule with poor distribution into the CNS, although greater penetration occurs when the meninges are inflamed. The elimination of vancomycin is also dependent on renal function and requires dosage adjustment in patients with calculated creatinine clearances of less than 70 mL per minute per 1.73 m^2.

Age-specific bacterial pathogen patterns for sepsis and meningitis must be appreciated to choose the most appropriate empiric antibiotic therapy. Neonates and infants should receive antimicrobial agents that cover organisms acquired during birth.[27] Immunocompromised hosts presenting with fever should be treated with an agent that provides adequate Gram-negative antibiotic coverage as well, including activity against *Pseudomonas aeruginosa*. Vancomycin should be added if there is concern for *Staphylococcus aureus* infection[28] (Table 17.1).

As with sepsis, age-specific bacterial pathogen patterns for meningitis must be appreciated to choose the most appropriate antibiotic therapy. Neonates and infants younger than 1 month are most likely to develop meningitis secondary to vaginal flora acquired during birth. Group B streptococcus and *Escherichia coli* are common causes of neonatal meningitis.[27,29] *Listeria monocytogenes* is less commonly implicated. Infants between the ages of 1 and 3 months require coverage for the same pathogens as neonates; however, *Streptococcus pneumoniae* and *Neisseria meningitidis* must also be considered.[30] Infants older than 3 months and children are most likely to present with meningitis caused by *S. pneumoniae* and *N. meningitidis*.[20] Immunocompromised patients may present with atypical organisms such as *L. monocytogenes* or Gram-negative bacilli.[30] Cochlear implants have been associated with an increased risk of meningitis, predominantly with *S. pneumoniae*.[31,32] Patients with ventriculoperitoneal shunts or other hardware may present with staphylococcal meningitis. All patients with suspected *S. pneumoniae* or staphylococcal meningitis should receive vancomycin until susceptibility results are available. Once again, acyclovir should be added if the diagnosis of HSV is suspected.[17]

With meningitis, several factors affect drug penetration into the CNS. Inflammation of the meninges allows larger and more polar drug molecules to penetrate into the CSF.[30] The degree of

TABLE 17.1 Empiric Treatment of Sepsis

Population	*Empiric Antibiotic(s) of Choice*	*Dosage*	*Comments*
Neonates (<30 d)	Ampicillin + gentamicin	Ampicillin 300 mg/kg/d Gentamicin 4 mg/kg/d	Add acyclovir 60 mg/kg/d if HSV suspected Add vancomycin if concern for *Staphylococcus aureus*
Infants 1–3 mo	Ampicillin + gentamicin or ampicillin + cefotaxime or ceftriaxone	Ampicillin 200–300 mg/kg/d Gentamicin 6–7.5 mg/kg/d Ceftriaxone 50–100 mg/kg/d	Add aminoglycoside if Gram-negative organism suspected Add vancomycin if concern for. *S. aureus* Cefotaxime 150 mg/kg/d may be used in place of ceftriaxone
Infants 3 mo–18 y	Ceftriaxone + vancomycin	Ceftriaxone 50–100 mg/kg/d Vancomycin 40 mg/kg/d	Cefotaxime 150 mg/kg/d may be used in place of ceftriaxone
Immuno-compromised	Ceftazidime or piperacillin/tazobactam + gentamicin + vancomycin	Ceftazidime 150 mg/kg/d Piperacillin/tazobactam 300 mg/kg/d (as piperacillin) Gentamicin 6–7.5 mg/kg/d Vancomycin 40 mg/kg/d	Cefepime 100 mg/kg/d can be used as an alternative

CVL, central venous line; HSV, herpes simplex virus.

ionization, lipid solubility, and protein binding are all characteristics that influence the efficacy of antibiotics chosen to treat meningitis. High doses of β-lactam antibiotics and vancomycin are required to achieve necessary CSF concentration to minimum inhibitory concentration ratios for bactericidal activity. The lower pH of the CSF in meningitis decreases the activity of aminoglycoside and macrolide antibiotics[30] (Table 17.2).

Steroid use in childhood meningitis continues to be a controversial topic, reignited in part by recent studies in adults indicating a possible benefit in patients who receive dexamethasone prior to or just at the time of antibiotic administration.[33,34] The greatest benefit of dexamethasone in pediatric patients has been demonstrated in *Haemophilus influenzae* meningitis, a disease that is now rarely seen following the widespread immunization of children.[34–36] Dexamethasone use for *S. pneumoniae* meningitis remains controversial, although the causative organism is often not known at the time of steroid administration. A possible explanation for the positive outcomes in patients receiving dexamethasone is depression of inflammatory response that follows the antibiotic-induced lysis of bacteria. Bacterial cell wall breakdown leads to the release of cytokines such as tumor necrosis factor, interleukin-6 (IL-6), and IL-1 into the subarachnoid space, increasing leukocyte accumulation and inflammation.[29,30,33,37] By decreasing inflammation, corticosteroids may mitigate or prevent sequelae, such as hearing loss, and, therefore, should be considered in *S. pneumoniae* and *N. meningitidis* meningitis.[29,30] Other experts have cautioned against the use of corticosteroids in children with presumed meningitis who have been vaccinated against *H. influenzae.*[38] Concerns around the use of steroids in meningitis include masking of clinical response, GI hemorrhage, and decreases in the CNS penetration of antibiotics with large molecular weights, such as vancomycin.[33,37] However, one study in pediatric patients and another adult study demonstrated no reduction in cephalosporin or vancomycin CSF penetration with concomitant steroid therapy.[39,40]

Acyclovir is an antiviral agent that is incorporated into the viral DNA and competes for DNA polymerase, inhibiting viral replication. Acyclovir should be added in all children in whom the diagnosis of HSV meningoencephalitis is suspected, and particularly in infants younger than 30 days.[41,42] Lack of prompt treatment can have devastating consequences, including permanent neurologic sequelae. Dosing for IV acyclovir is doubled to 60 mg per kg per day IV divided every 8 hours when HSV encephalitis/meningitis is suspected. Acyclovir is widely distributed into body tissues, with CSF concentrations reaching 50% of the serum concentrations. Renal excretion accounts for up to 90% of acyclovir elimination; therefore, the dose must be adjusted for renal insufficiency.[43] Slow infusions and adequate hydration are necessary to prevent drug crystallization into the renal tubules and subsequent renal injury.

Prophylaxis of day care and household contacts may be necessary when a patient is diagnosed with meningococcal meningitis.[44] In addition, persons directly exposed to secretions (e.g., during endotracheal intubation) may also require postexposure prophylaxis (PEP).[45] In outbreaks caused by a serotype contained in the vaccine (A, C, Y, and W-135), immunization of the exposed groups may be recommended by public health authorities (Table 17.3).

CELLULITIS

Cellulitis is a localized bacterial infection of the skin and soft tissue, most often caused by staphylococcal and streptococcal

TABLE 17.2 Empiric Treatment of Meningitis

Population	*Empiric Antibiotic(s) of Choice*	*Dosage*	*Comments*
Neonatal (<30 d)	Ampicillin + gentamicin or ampicillin + cefotaxime	Ampicillin 300 mg/kg/d Gentamicin 4 mg/kg/d Cefotaxime 200 mg/kg/d	If Gram-negative meningitis suspected: ampicillin and gentamicin as shown + cefotaxime 200 mg/kg/d Acyclovir 60 mg/kg/d should be added if HSV suspected
Infants 1–3 mo	Ampicillin + ceftriaxone + vancomycin	Ampicillin 400 mg/kg/d Ceftriaxone 100 mg/kg/d Vancomycin 60 mg/kg/d	Cefotaxime 300 mg/kg/d may be used in place of ceftriaxone
Infants 3 mo–18 y[a]	Ceftriaxone + vancomycin	Ceftriaxone 100 mg/kg/d (max. 4 g/d) Vancomycin 60 mg/kg/d (max. 4 g/d, adjust as needed based on serum concentrations)	Cefotaxime 300 mg/kg/d (max. 12 g/d) may be used in place of ceftriaxone
Cancer and neutropenia	Ceftriaxone + vancomycin + an aminoglycoside	Ampicillin 400 mg/kg/d (max. 12 g/d) Gentamicin 7.5 mg/kg/d	Cefotaxime can be used in place of ceftriaxone Amikacin 15 mg/kg/d may be used instead of gentamicin If concern for resistant organism, can substitute meropenem 120 mg/kg/d for ceftriaxone or cefotaxime
Ventriculoperitoneal shunt, neurosurgery, hardware	Ceftazidime + vancomycin	Ceftazidime 150 mg/kg/d (max. 6 g/d) Vancomycin 60 mg/kg/d (max. 4 g/d, adjust as needed based on serum concentrations)	May substitute cefepime 150 mg/kg/d or meropenem 120 mg/kg

[a]Add ampicillin 300 mg/kg/d in patients with T-cell deficiency.
HSV, herpes simplex virus.

TABLE 17.3 Postexposure Prophylaxis for *Neisseria meningitidis*

Regimen (Choose One)	*Age*	*Medication and Dosage (Choose One)*
1	<1 mo	Rifampin 5 mg/kg p.o. every 12 h for 2 d
	>1 mo	Rifampin 10 mg/kg (max. 600 mg) p.o. every 12 h for 2 d
2	≤15 y	Ceftriaxone 125 mg i.m. × 1 dose
	>15 y	Ceftriaxone 250 mg i.m. × 1 dose
3	>18 y	Ciprofloxacin 500 mg p.o. × 1 dose

i.m., intramuscular; p.o., oral.
Centers for Disease Control and Prevention. Antimicrobial prophylaxis. *MMWR* 2013;62:23–24.

species.[46] The incidence of community-acquired methicillin-resistant *Staphylococcus aureus* (CA-MRSA) has been increasing significantly in recent years. One study demonstrated a rate increase from 9% in 2004 to 21% in 2006, necessitating a shift in empiric treatment.[47] Emergent cellulitis infections include orbital and periorbital cellulitis and necrotizing fasciitis (NF). Cellulitis secondary to human or animal bites is covered later in this chapter.

Cellulitis can follow minor trauma, such as a cut or a scratch. Because skin flora are likely to be the causative agents, empiric antibiotic therapy should have adequate staphylococcal and streptococcal coverage. If a mixed anaerobic infection is suspected, ampicillin-sulbactam or clindamycin provides additional coverage. Children with mild-to-moderate cellulitis can be successfully treated with PO agents on an outpatient basis.[46] First-line antibiotics for cellulitis include PO penicillinase-resistant β-lactams such as dicloxacillin or a first-generation cephalosporin such as cephalexin.[46] If CA-MRSA is suspected, first-line agents may include clindamycin or trimethoprim-sulfamethoxazole depending on local resistance patterns. Cellulitis with purulent drainage, children with significant systemic signs and symptoms, those who have failed outpatient therapy, and immunocompromised children may require hospitalization and parenteral antibiotics.

Periorbital cellulitis usually occurs secondary to trauma, although it can also be the result of contiguous microbial spread from the sinuses or be hematogenous in origin. The affected eye is red with significant eyelid swelling. Seventy-five percent of patients with periorbital cellulitis have fever.[47] If bacteremia is present, the child may have a temperature of more than 39°C and a WBC count of more than 15,000 cells per mm^3.[47] Prior to the introduction of the vaccine, *H. influenzae* was one of the most common pathogens implicated in periorbital and orbital cellulitis. Since 1990, when universal vaccination began, the number of cases of *H. influenzae* periorbital and orbital cellulitis and the overall number of cases have declined.[48] Currently, staphylococcal and streptococcal species are responsible for the majority of periorbital cellulitis. Periorbital cellulitis can be treated with a β-lactam (IM ceftriaxone, PO cefpodoxime, cefdinir, amoxicillin, or amoxicillin-clavulanate), plus clindamycin or trimethoprim-sulfamethoxazole on an outpatient basis if there is no retrobulbar involvement.[48]

Orbital cellulitis is typically a complication of sinusitis.[47] With these infections, eyelid tissue becomes edematous, and a periorbital purple discoloration may ensue. Proptosis, ophthalmoplegia, pain on movement of the eye, and decreased visual acuity necessitate rapid imaging and ophthalmologic consultation. Orbital cellulitis requires hospitalization and treatment with parenteral antibiotics, primarily ceftriaxone or cefotaxime plus vancomycin.[49] Infectious organisms generally include *S. aureus*, *Streptococcus pyogenes*, and *S. pneumoniae*. If there is concern for anaerobic infection, metronidazole can be added.[50]

NF is an infection of the skin and SC soft tissue, resulting in necrosis, often caused by invasive group A β-hemolytic streptococcus (GABHS). Superantigens, in the form of exotoxins, are released by GABHS and induce massive cytokine release.[51] Local inflammation produces extensive tissue damage and shock. Despite a high mortality rate for adults of 30% to 80%, childhood mortality from invasive GABHS infections has a rate of 5% to 10%.[51] The highest risk factor in children for the development of invasive GABHS is intercurrent varicella infection.[51,52]

Treatment of NF

Treatment of NF includes early surgical debridement and administration of parenteral antibiotics. IV penicillin is the drug of choice for GABHS, dosed at 400,000 units per kg per day IV divided every 4 hours. Clindamycin is advocated by many experts as an adjuvant therapy following reports of improved survival in animal trials.[53] Theoretically, clindamycin may be synergistic in overcoming the large inoculum of organisms owing to slow replication and decreased number of penicillin-binding proteins, which may inhibit β-lactam antimicrobial efficacy.[51] Clindamycin also inhibits exotoxin production via inhibition of protein synthesis by binding to the 50S subunit on bacterial ribosomes.[26,53,54] Because of the increasing incidence of bacterial resistance and the bacteriostatic properties (dependent on concentration) of clindamycin, it should not be used as the sole agent.[51] Clindamycin is dosed at 40 mg per kg per day IV divided every 6 hours (max. 4.8 g per day). Although rare, pseudomembranous colitis with severe, persistent diarrhea can occur with clindamycin administration and may be fatal. In cases of NF where a non-GABHS organism is suspected, a combination of clindamycin with a third-generation cephalosporin, or a combination of ampicillin, gentamicin, and metronidazole should be used.[55]

PNEUMONIA

Community-acquired pneumonia is common in children, especially those younger than 5 years.[56–59] Signs and symptoms include fever and acute respiratory distress, which may be accompanied by infiltrates on chest radiograph. The prevalent bacterial organisms vary based on age, and therefore, the most appropriate empiric antibiotics vary.[56,60] The resistance patterns of *S. pneumoniae* in pneumonia are similar to that in meningitis, although the serum concentrations of β-lactam antibiotics in the serum generally exceed the minimum inhibitory concentration several fold.[36] Recently, there has been an estimated 35% reduction in the incidence of *S. pneumoniae* pneumonia following the release of the heptavalent pneumococcal vaccine (Prevnar).[56]

Atypical organisms such as *Chlamydia pneumoniae* and *Mycoplasma pneumoniae* are increasingly common pathogens found in children older than 4 months, particularly those older than

TABLE 17.4 Empiric Treatment of Community-Acquired Pneumonia

Age Group	*Likely Infecting Organism*	*Empiric Antibiotic Recommendations*	*Dosage*	*Comments*
Neonatal[a] (<3 wk)	Perinatal: GBS, enteric Gram-negative bacteria, *Listeria*	**Inpatient:** ampicillin + gentamicin or ampicillin + gentamicin + cefotaxime	Ampicillin 200–300 mg/kg/d Gentamicin 4 mg/kg/d Cefotaxime 200 mg/kg/d	
Infant 3 wk–3 mo	*Chlamydia trachomatis, Bordetella pertussis, Streptococcus pneumoniae*	**Inpatient:** macrolide + cefotaxime or macrolide + cefuroxime **Influenza-associated pneumonia:** oseltamivir: <12 mo: 3 mg/kg b.i.d.	Azithromycin 10 mg/kg × 1 dose, then 5 mg/kg/d Erythromycin 30–40 mg/kg/d Cefotaxime 200 mg/kg/d Cefuroxime i.v. 75–150 mg/kg/d	Azithromycin should be considered in infants <6 wk in light of reports of pyloric stenosis with erythromycin Ceftriaxone may be used in place of cefotaxime
Child 4 mo–4 y	*C. trachomatis, Mycoplasma pneumoniae, Chlamydia pneumoniae, S. pneumoniae*	**Presumed bacterial outpatient:** amoxicillin or amoxicillin-clavulanate **Inpatient:** ampicillin or cefotaxime or ceftriaxone **Presumed atypical pneumonia:** azithromycin **Influenza-associated pneumonia:** oseltamivir: <12 mo: 3 mg/kg b.i.d. >12 mo: <15 kg 30 mg b.i.d. 16–23 kg 45 mg b.i.d.	Amoxicillin 90 mg/kg/d Ampicillin 200 mg/kg/d Cefotaxime 200 mg/kg/d Ceftriaxone 50–100 mg/kg/d Azithromycin 10 g/kg on day 1, then 5 mg/kg/d days 2–5	Viral pneumonia is most common in this age group and requires no antimicrobial therapy Cephalosporin preferred in unvaccinated children Add clindamycin or vancomycin if MRSA is suspected Clarithromycin or erythromycin can be used in place of azithromycin
Child 5–15 y	*M. pneumoniae, C. pneumoniae, S. pneumoniae*	**Presumed bacterial outpatient:** amoxicillin or amoxicillin-clavulanate + azithromycin **Inpatient:** ampicillin or cefotaxime or ceftriaxone + azithromycin **Influenza-associated pneumonia:** oseltamivir 16–23 kg 45 mg b.i.d. 23–45 kg 60 mg b.i.d. >45 kg 75 mg b.i.d.	Amoxicillin 90 mg/kg/d Ampicillin 200 mg/kg/d Cefotaxime 200 mg/kg/d Ceftriaxone 50–100 mg/kg/d Azithromycin 10 g/kg on day 1, then 5 mg/kg/d days 2–5	Cephalosporin preferred in unvaccinated children Add clindamycin or vancomycin if MRSA is suspected Clarithromycin or erythromycin or doxycycline (>8 y) can be used in place of azithromycin

[a]Ceftriaxone directly displaces bilirubin from albumin-binding sites.
b.i.d., twice daily; GBS, group B streptococcus; i.v., intravenous; MRSA, methicillin-resistant *Staphylococcus aureus*.

4 years.[56,59] Concomitant infection with mixed bacterial organisms or bacterial with viral infection can occur in up to 25% of children with pneumonia, most frequently *S. pneumoniae* with respiratory syncytial virus (RSV) or *M. pneumoniae*.[60,61] In cases of severe necrotizing pneumonia, addition of antimicrobial agents with activity against *S. aureus* is warranted,[56,57] Vancomycin should be added if the child is at risk for infection with MRSA.[60]

Viral and bacterial pneumonia may have similar appearance on chest radiograph. Clinically, pneumonia accompanied by wheezing is more likely to be viral in origin, whereas chest pain as a result of pleural irritation is likely to be bacterial.[56] RSV is discussed further in section "Respiratory Distress Syndromes" of this chapter. In children with influenza-associated pneumonia, oseltamivir should be added.[60]

Treatment

Empiric treatment of community-acquired pneumonia in children includes penicillins, cephalosporins, macrolides, and doxycycline. Aminoglycosides and antistaphylococcal agents are added for severe pneumonia.[60] The pharmacology of penicillins, cephalosporins, vancomycin, and aminoglycosides has been discussed previously.

The most common macrolide used for the treatment of community-acquired pneumonia in children is azithromycin. Macrolides are bacteriostatic antibiotics that bind to the 50S ribosome in susceptible organisms, inhibiting protein synthesis.[26] Azithromycin displays extensive tissue distribution, resulting in high intracellular concentrations and subsequent long half-life. Erythromycin is widely distributed in body fluids except the CNS, although it has less tissue binding than azithromycin. Both azithromycin and erythromycin are available in IV and PO preparations. Erythromycin is acid sensitive and is, therefore, administered in enteric-coated formulations to improve stability.[62] Azithromycin and erythromycin are metabolized in the liver. Erythromycin inhibits drug-metabolizing enzymes CYP1A2 and CYP3A3/4, resulting in multiple reported drug interactions.[62] Azithromycin is a mild inhibitor of CYP3A3/4 and demonstrates few clinically significant drug–drug interactions.[63] Common adverse effects include crampy abdominal pain, nausea, vomiting, and diarrhea, especially with erythromycin. Studies recently published describe pyloric stenosis occurring in neonates who have received erythromycin and suggest that it is not a class effect seen with all macrolides.[64,65] Therefore, azithromycin may be a better option for infants requiring a macrolide antibiotic.

Doxycycline is a tetracycline antibiotic, binding to the 30S ribosome in susceptible organisms and inhibiting protein synthesis.[26] Doxycycline has a broad spectrum of activity, including Gram-positive, Gram-negative, and atypical organisms. Distribution is extensive and tissue penetration is excellent, although CNS penetration is poor. Doxycycline is partially chelated in the GI tract and minimally excreted via the kidneys. Adverse effects include GI distress, photosensitivity, hepatotoxicity, and teeth staining in children younger than 8 years (Table 17.4).

A lower hospital admission rate has been demonstrated in children with pneumococcal pneumonia with associated bacteremia when treated with an initial parenteral dose of antibiotics prior to outpatient PO therapy as compared with those who receive PO antibiotics alone.[61] Parenteral antibiotics may achieve higher concentrations in sites of consolidation, resulting in more rapid improvement.

Aspiration pneumonia, especially in children with chronic airway problems or severe reflux, can present in the ED. If antibiotic therapy is necessary, antimicrobial coverage should cover oral anaerobes. Empiric therapy with ampicillin-sulbactam is recommended. Despite concerns over penicillin-resistant *Bacteroides* species, one study has shown equivalent efficacy between IV penicillin G and IV clindamycin.[66]

OSTEOMYELITIS AND SEPTIC ARTHRITIS

Bacterial infections of bone (osteomyelitis) and joint (septic arthritis) are a significant cause of morbidity in children.[67–69] Presentation may vary from unwillingness to move an extremity, to limp, to pseudoparalysis, to local swelling. Fever, pain, and elevated erythrocyte sedimentation rate and C-reactive protein are common features of both infections, although neonates may present with nonspecific signs, such as lethargy and decreased PO intake. Delay in treatment, particularly with septic arthritis, can result in irreversible damage to the articular cartilage.[67] As with other infectious processes, *H. influenzae* was the dominant pathogen prior to widespread vaccination against it. Currently, the most common causes of osteomyelitis and septic arthritis are *S. aureus* and *Streptococcus* species.[68,69] Neonates and immunocompromised hosts can present with infection by Gram-negative organisms; empiric antimicrobial coverage should reflect this possibility. Sickle cell patients demonstrate higher rates of *Salmonella* osteomyelitis than the general population.[70]

Treatment

In infants less than 3 months of age, oxacillin and gentamicin are recommended for empiric therapy.[70] For children older than 3 months of age, antistaphylococcal β-lactam antibiotics are recommended as first-line agents for the treatment of both osteomyelitis and septic arthritis. If there is concern for MRSA infection, clindamycin or vancomycin is recommended.[68–70] Resistant infections may require treatment with alternative agents, such as linezolid or daptomycin. Agents chosen must possess good bone and synovial fluid penetration. Initial IV therapy can be transitioned to PO antibiotics, such as trimethoprim-sulfamethoxazole. Length of IV and subsequent PO therapy is patient specific. Cultures and sensitivities will guide in tailoring antibiotic regimens. Traditionally, 6 to 8 weeks of antibiotic treatment was thought to be necessary, although recent studies have shown similar outcomes with shorter, 3-week courses of antibiotics, with earlier transition to PO antibiotics. There is still controversy over the optimal time to transition to PO therapy and duration of therapy.[70–72]

Patients with sickle cell disease and suspected osteomyelitis should receive coverage for both *Salmonella* and *S. aureus* until culture results are available. Empiric choices include a third-generation cephalosporin or a fluoroquinolone plus an antistaphylococcal β-lactam.[68] Puncture wounds with resulting osteomyelitis may require pseudomonal coverage. Four to 6 weeks of therapy is suggested to prevent relapse.[73]

OTITIS MEDIA

Otitis media is defined as an inflammation of the middle ear and is classified as either acute otitis media (AOM) or otitis media with effusion.[74] AOM is more commonly encountered in the ED and is discussed here. AOM is characterized by fever, pain in the affected ear(s), otorrhea, or a bulging tympanic membrane. It has been well established that up to 80% of AOM episodes will spontaneously resolve if left untreated, although identifying those cases not requiring therapy may be difficult.[36] The most common bacterial causes of AOM include *S. pneumoniae, H. influenzae,* and *Moraxella catarrhalis.*[21,75] Given current resistance patterns of penicillin resistance in *S. pneumoniae* AOM, it is important to achieve adequate antibiotic levels in the middle ear fluid. Pneumococci and other organisms develop resistance through development of penicillin-binding protein mutations. High-dose amoxicillin is usually efficacious when otitis media secondary to penicillin-resistant organisms.

TREATMENT

In children aged 6 months and older, nonsevere, unilateral AOM can usually be treated symptomatically with analgesic agents alone, with reevaluation in 48 to 72 hours. In cases of severe AOM, bilateral AOM, and those that fail to respond to analgesics alone, antibiotic treatment is warranted.[76] The drug of choice for otitis media is high-dose amoxicillin at 80 to 100 mg per kg per day PO divided into two or three doses daily.[75–77] The higher dosing range of amoxicillin should provide adequate coverage against penicillin-nonsusceptible *S. pneumoniae.*[77] Patients who have been treated with amoxicillin within the previous 30 days should be treated with a second-line agent. For patients allergic to penicillins, alternative agents include cefdinir, cefpodoxime, cefuroxime, and ceftriaxone.[76] Azithromycin and other macrolides have high rates of resistance and are no longer recommended as first-line agents. The recommended treatment duration in children less than 2 years of age is 10 days. Children aged 2 to 5 years may be treated for 7 to 10 days, and 5 to 7 days of therapy may be adequate for children aged 6 years and older.[76]

Treatment failures following high-dose amoxicillin may be due to resistant *S. pneumoniae* or β-lactamase–producing *H. influenzae* and may respond to amoxicillin-clavulanic acid, or IM ceftriaxone with or without clindamycin.[76] Amoxicillin-clavulanic acid distributes well into middle ear effusions, achieving bactericidal concentrations.[21] High-dose amoxicillin-clavulanic acid contains 90 mg per kg per day of the amoxicillin component and may be necessary in cases of penicillin-resistant *S.*

pneumoniae. Twice-daily administration of the high-dose amoxicillin-clavulanic acid has produced similar response rates as three divided doses per day, with a better adverse effect profile.[21] Patients at risk for treatment failure tend to be younger than 18 to 24 months, have a history of recurrent AOM, or have underlying immunologic or anatomic abnormalities.[36] These patients should receive 10 days of treatment. Common side effects of amoxicillin-clavulanic acid include diarrhea, vomiting, and rash.

STREPTOCOCCAL PHARYNGITIS

Symptoms of pharyngitis include sore throat, headache, and fever. Viral pharyngitis can be virtually indistinguishable from bacterial pharyngitis on physical examination. However, the presence of rhinorrhea, conjunctivitis, or cough is more suggestive of a viral etiology. GABHS is the most common causative organism of bacterial pharyngitis and can have serious sequelae, including poststreptococcal glomerulonephritis and acute rheumatic fever/carditis.[78,79] Glomerulonephritis is not preventable by treatment. Other bacterial causes of pharyngitis do not require treatment, as no benefit from antimicrobial therapy has been demonstrated.[78] Therefore, a rapid strep antigen detection test and/or throat culture is necessary to make the diagnosis. A positive result is the criterion for antibiotic therapy.[36] The main goal of antibiotic therapy is the prevention of rheumatic fever. This complication can be averted if treatment is instituted within 9 days of the onset of symptoms.[79]

TREATMENT

First-line treatment with penicillin is recommended because of its efficacy and safety profile, narrow spectrum, and low cost.[78,79] Amoxicillin is often substituted because of better tolerability of the PO suspension. Alternatively, benzathine penicillin G can be given IM to patients who are unlikely to be compliant with therapy. Benzathine penicillin G should never be given via the IV route, as fatalities have occurred.[80] Peak serum levels are achieved within 12 to 24 hours following IM administration and remain detectable for 1 to 4 weeks. Pain on injection is common and can be ameliorated by warming the injection to room temperature prior to administration.

Macrolides are acceptable alternatives in children with severe penicillin allergy.[79] For patients who are penicillin allergic, but do not exhibit type I hypersensitivity to penicillin, first-generation cephalosporins may be used. Patients who fail therapy may have a chronic carrier state or have become reinfected[78] (Table 17.5).

The course of therapy is traditionally 10 days to eradication of the organism. Shorter courses have been recommended, although concerns regarding equivalence to standard therapy have been raised.[78]

TABLE 17.5 Empiric Therapy for Group A β-Hemolytic Streptococcus (GABHS) Pharyngitis

Patient Characteristics	*Drug and Dosage*
Children <12 y, no allergy to penicillin	Penicillin VK 250 mg p.o. b.i.d.–t.i.d. for 10 d Or Amoxicillin 25 mg/kg (max. 500 mg) b.i.d. for 10 d
Children >12 y, no allergy to penicillin	Penicillin VK 250 mg p.o. q.i.d. or 500 mg b.i.d. for 10 d or Amoxicillin 250 mg/kg (max. 500 mg) p.o. b.i.d. for 10 d
Children <27 kg, noncompliance suspected	Benzathine penicillin G 600,000 units i.m. × 1 dose
Children >27 kg, noncompliance suspected	Benzathine penicillin G 1,200,000 units i.m. × 1 dose
Penicillin allergy (non–type I hypersensitivity)	First-generation cephalosporin for 10 d such as cephalexin 20 mg/kg (max. 500 mg) p.o. b.i.d. for 10 d
Penicillin allergy (true type I hypersensitivity)	Azithromycin 12 mg/kg daily for 5 d or Clarithromycin 7.5 mg/kg (max. 250 mg) p.o. b.i.d. for 10 d Clindamycin 7 mg/kg (max. 300 mg) p.o. t.i.d. for 10 d or
Recurrent GABHS pharyngitis	Amoxicillin-clavulanic acid 40 mg/kg/d p.o. divided t.i.d. (max. 1 g/d) for 10 d

b.i.d., twice daily; i.m., intramuscular; p.o., oral; q.i.d., four times daily; t.i.d., thrice daily.

PAIN

Acute pain is one of the most common adverse experiences among pediatric patients.[81] Pain in children presenting to the ED has varied etiologies. Common causes include fractures and sprains, sickle cell disease, and migraine headaches. The goal of pain management is early, effective control with appropriate monitoring.[81,82] Pain medication options include opioids, nonsteroidal anti-inflammatory drugs (NSAIDs), acetaminophen, and adjuvant agents such as topical anesthetics. Each drug used for pain has a unique profile and different benefits and risks. Distraction techniques, relaxation, and physical therapy are also important components of effective pain management.[81]

Traditionally, practitioners have been reluctant to utilize appropriate doses of pain medications, particularly opioids, for fear of causing respiratory depression and creating addiction from prolonged use.[75,82] Although drug-seeking behavior does occasionally occur in those who take opioids regularly, the vast majority of patients who come to the ED reporting pain are truly in distress and require analgesia.

Opioids are classified as centrally acting receptor agonists, partial agonists, or mixed agonist–antagonists.[83] The opioid receptors are categorized as mu (μ), kappa (κ), delta (δ), and sigma (σ).[84] Mu-receptor activation results in analgesia, respiratory depression, miosis, decreased GI motility, and euphoria. The κ and σ receptors are responsible for analgesia, dysphoria, and psychomimetic reactions, primarily acting in the spinal cord.[85] The δ receptors may be responsible for some analgesic responses to thermal stimuli.

Adverse reactions are similar within the class and include respiratory depression, sedation, nausea and vomiting, and constipation. Histamine release more commonly occurs with morphine, meperidine, and codeine, resulting in urticaria, generalized pruritus, and hypotension.[85]

Morphine is the most commonly used parenteral opioid.[83,85] As a μ-receptor agonist, morphine is a potent pain reliever. Onset occurs within 15 to 30 minutes following IV administration and within 30 to 60 minutes following IM administration.[85] Duration is usually 3 to 5 hours after IV, IM, or SC administration. The parenteral dose of morphine is commonly 0.05 to 0.1 mg per kg per dose IV/IM/SC. Hypotension, respiratory depression, miosis, bronchospasm, and decreased GI motility are adverse effects of morphine administration.[83,85]

Parenteral hydromorphone is a powerful opioid, approximately seven times as potent as morphine. Onset time is similar to morphine, occurring within 15 to 30 minutes following an IV dose. Dosing references have recently revised initial dose recommendations because of reports of adverse effects from clinical experts.[86] The initial IV dose in an opioid-naive patient should start at 0.015 mg per kg per dose, and the usual maximum first dose range from 0.2 to 0.6 mg. Duration is approximately 4 to 5 hours. Common adverse reactions include hypotension, bradycardia, sedation, and GI disturbances.

Fentanyl is potent lipophilic opioid available in parenteral, transdermal, and PO lozenge forms. As a μ-receptor agonist, fentanyl is 100 times more potent than morphine.[87] In the ED, fentanyl injection is commonly used for pain relief and procedural sedation and analgesia (PSA). Fentanyl does not release histamine and thus results in negligible changes in hemodynamic status.[87] Therefore, it is the agent of choice for patients with mild hypotension who require pain control. The onset of action is rapid, approximately 30 seconds, following IV administration.[85] The duration of action is approximately 30 to 60 minutes when given at a dose of 1 to 2 μg per kg IV. Hypoxemia and apnea occur more frequently when fentanyl is combined with a sedative, such as midazolam.[85,88] Chest wall and tongue rigidity, marked by muscle rigidity, respiratory distress, hypercapnia, hypoxia, and difficult intubation, can occur with rapid administration of fentanyl.[89] If it does occur, naloxone at 10 μg per kg per dose can effectively reverse chest wall rigidity.[90,91] Neuromuscular blocking agents such as succinylcholine or pancuronium have also been successfully used to reverse chest wall rigidity but will mandate endotracheal intubation.[90]

Meperidine is generally no longer used in childhood acute pain management. Nausea and vomiting are common side effects, and the drug is difficult to titrate.[85] Neurotoxicity may occur with meperidine as a result of the formation of its primary metabolite, normeperidine, which can cause tremors, irritability, and seizures.[88] Meperidine is a potent inhibitor of serotonin reuptake into presynaptic neurons and, therefore, can interact with other medications that also affect serotonin, resulting in potentially fatal drug interactions.[92]

Codeine was once commonly used for analgesia in the ED; however, its use has fallen out of favor in recent years because of serious safety concerns. Codeine is metabolized by CYP2D6 to the active metabolite, morphine.[93] Reports of adverse drug events, including death, in patients with CYP2D6 polymorphisms prompted the U.S. Food and Drug Administration (FDA) to issue medication safety warnings regarding codeine.[94] Adverse events have been primarily reported in postoperative tonsillectomy and adenoidectomy patients, but given limited data on the scope of toxicity, codeine is no longer recommended for routine use in pediatric patients.[93]

The current opioid epidemic in the United States has also impacted the adolescent population, with increasing rates of misuse, abuse, addiction, and overdose. It is recommended that opioid analgesics be used only when indicated and short courses of immediate-release agents be prescribed. Parents and patients should be cautioned regarding the risks of opioid analgesics as well as proper storage and disposal techniques.[95]

The PO opioids frequently used in the ED are summarized in Table 17.6.

Acetaminophen is the most commonly used nonopioid analgesic in children. Its mechanism of action involves the inhibition of cyclooxygenase and prostaglandin synthetase in the CNS in a greater proportion than the periphery, therefore accounting for acetaminophen's antipyretic effect and apparent lack of anti-inflammatory effects.[83,96] Dosing is 10 to 15 mg per kg per dose PO/PR every 4 to 6 hours as needed. Single-dose protocols for 30 mg per kg PO loading doses have been shown to decrease fever more quickly than the traditional 15 mg per

TABLE 17.6 Oral Opioid Agents

Drug	*Equivalent Oral Dose (Immediate Release Only)*	*Onset (min)*	*Duration (h)*	*Available Forms*	*Commonly Available Strengths*
Morphine	0.2–0.5 mg/kg/dose (max. 30 mg/dose)	60	3–5	Tablet Solution	15 mg, 30 mg 10 mg/5 mL, 20 mg/5 mL, 100 mg/5 mL
Hydromorphone	0.03–0.08 mg/kg/dose (max. 6 mg/dose[a])	15–30	4–5	Tablet Solution	2 mg, 4 mg, 8 mg 1 mg/mL
Oxycodone	0.2 mg/kg/dose (max. 10 mg/dose)	15–30	4–5	Tablet Solution	5 mg, 15 mg 5 mg/mL, concentrated solution 20 mg/mL
Oxycodone/ acetaminophen[b]	0.2 mg/kg/dose (max. 10 mg/dose) based on oxycodone	10–15	3–6	Tablet Solution	2.5/325, 5/325, 7.5/325, 10/325 5 mg oxycodone and 325 mg acetaminophen per 5 mL
Hydrocodone/ acetaminophen[b]	0.2 mg/kg/dose (max. 10 mg/dose) based on hydrocodone	10–20	3–6	Tablet Elixir	Many 2.5 mg hydrocodone and 167 mg acetaminophen per 5 mL

[a]Maximum dose for opiate-naive patients is 6 mg.

[b]Do not exceed 90 mg/kg or 4 g, whichever is less of acetaminophen from all sources per 24-h period.

kg dose with no increase in adverse effects.[97] Maximum daily dose should not exceed 90 mg per kg per day or 4 g per day, whichever is less. Acetaminophen is metabolized in the liver, primarily via the sulfation pathway in children.[96] In overdose settings, a greater amount of acetaminophen is metabolized outside the major pathways of sulfation and glucuronidation, via the CYP450 isozyme system.[98] The resultant metabolite is toxic to the hepatocytes. Adverse effects are minimal at therapeutic doses, but hepatotoxicity leading to liver failure and death can occur with overdose.

NSAIDs can be used for pain control instead of or in conjunction with acetaminophen or opioid analgesics. NSAIDs are cyclooxygenase inhibitors and prevent the formation of prostaglandins. Prostaglandins, particularly PGE_2, are released when cells are damaged or when the level of circulating cytokine increases.[83] Therefore, NSAIDs are excellent choices for the treatment of pain associated with inflammation. Ibuprofen is widely used, dosed at 10 mg per kg per dose (max. 600 to 800 mg per dose) PO every 6 to 8 hours as needed. Onset occurs in approximately 60 minutes, and the duration is usually 6 to 8 hours. Adverse effects include GI irritation and ulceration, GI hemorrhage, impaired platelet function, and allergic reactions. The chance of causing GI hemorrhage is greater with ketorolac compared to ibuprofen.[88]

Ketorolac is the most commonly used injectable nonspecific NSAID in the United States; although not approved by the FDA for use in children younger than 17 years, ketorolac is commonly used in pediatric patients older than 1 year.[85,99] Pain control with 30 mg of IV ketorolac has been demonstrated comparable with 4 mg of IV morphine.[100] Single-dose treatment doses range from 0.4 to 1 mg per kg IV/IM to a maximum of 30 mg in children weighing less than 50 kg and 60 mg in children weighing more than 50 kg. However, it should be noted that recent data in adult patients suggest that there is an analgesic ceiling for ketorolac at 10 mg IV, and higher dosages may not be more efficacious but may place patients at increased risk of adverse effects.[100] Multiple dosing should be no greater than 0.5 mg per kg per dose (max. 30 mg per dose) IV/IM every 6 hours not to exceed 20 doses.[85] The onset of action occurs 10 minutes after administration, peak effect occurs within 40 to 60 minutes, and the duration of action is approximately 6 hours.[85] The risk for GI hemorrhage increases exponentially after day 5 of therapy and is the subject of a "black box" warning for ketorolac.[99] Additional adverse effects include hemorrhage outside the GI tract, nausea, diarrhea, headache, and drowsiness.

Local anesthetic agents will be covered later in the chapter during the discussion of laceration management.

PROCEDURAL SEDATION

PSA, also erroneously termed conscious sedation, refers to the process of inducing sedation in a patient for the purpose of obtaining stillness for imaging or for completion of a painful procedure, such as laceration repair or fracture reduction. Opioids, benzodiazepines, ketamine, and propofol are the most common medications use to facilitate PSA in children. A concern with using procedural sedation is the need for appropriate monitoring of adverse events both during and following the procedure.[101–103] Death, permanent neurologic injury, and prolonged hospitalization are potential adverse outcomes of procedural sedation.[103] Prolonged recovery effects can include ataxia, agitation, GI effects, and restlessness.[102] Medication errors and drug interactions can contribute to an increased rate of adverse side effects associated with procedural sedation.[102] However, one study demonstrated a low incidence of adverse events (2.3%) associated with procedural sedation in more than 1,000 patients in a pediatric ED.[104]

TREATMENT

Fentanyl is the most commonly used opioid for PSA. Fentanyl is frequently used in conjunction with benzodiazepines, primarily midazolam, for procedural sedation. See section "Pain" for a discussion of fentanyl pharmacology.

Midazolam is a relatively short-acting benzodiazepine, which exerts a sedative effect by binding to the benzodiazepine receptor on the γ-aminobutyric acid (GABA) complex.[105] This action enhances GABA binding to the receptor and increases chloride currents into the cell, thus inhibiting action potential generation.[89] Hypnotic effect is usually seen at doses lower than those producing respiratory depression. Midazolam is dosed at 0.05 to 0.1 mg per kg per dose (max. 2.5 mg per dose) IV every 3 to 5 minutes as needed to obtain adequate sedation. It is important to note that adolescents and adults do not require as high a dose of midazolam to achieve sedation as do younger children. The onset of sedation occurs within 1 to 5 minutes after IV administration and within 5 minutes following IM administration. Duration is commonly 20 to 30 minutes after IV administration. IM administration results in a significantly longer duration of action, ranging from 2 to 6 hours in some cases. Adverse effects include prolonged sedation, hypotension, bradycardia, paradoxical reactions, muscle tremors, and respiratory depression. Because midazolam is a sedative hypnotic and does not possess analgesic effects, fentanyl is often used in conjunction for painful procedures. Fentanyl and midazolam combinations result in greater respiratory depression than midazolam alone.[89]

Ketamine is a phencyclidine derivative and produces a dissociative anesthetic state with analgesia; patients often have involuntary movements, spontaneous respirations, and eye opening.[105,106] The respiratory drive is not compromised with normal procedural sedative dosing, making ketamine a valuable agent in pediatric sedation.[85] Ketamine can be given PO, IV, or IM. The PO dose of ketamine is 6 to 10 mg per kg × 1 dose 30 minutes prior to the procedure. Palatability is improved if ketamine is mixed with cola or other beverage. IV dosing is usually 1 to 1.5 mg per kg with additional 0.5 mg per kg aliquots as needed to maintain sedation. If the IM route is to be used, the dose is 3 to 4 mg per kg. The onset of action occurs within 60 seconds of IV administration and within 5 to 10 minutes following IM administration.[85] The duration of action lasts for 10 to 15 minutes when given IV and 15 to 30 minutes when given IM. Adverse effects from ketamine include laryngospasm, involuntary movements, vomiting, and emergence reactions. Emergence reactions have been reported to occur in up to 34% of patients older than 16 years but occur in less than 10% of patients younger than 10 years.[108] Practice differences exist over the prophylactic use of low-dose midazolam to prevent emergence reactions, because convincing evidence of efficacy is lacking.[109]

Propofol is a relative newcomer to the procedural sedation armamentarium for children. It is an ultra–short-acting nonopioid, nonbarbiturate hypnotic agent with no analgesic property. Structurally unrelated to other general anesthetics, propofol increases the response of $GABA_A$ receptor to GABA, enhancing inhibitory neurotransmission and potentiating glycine-activated currents. Glycine receptors may play a role in mediating response to noxious stimuli. Propofol is insoluble in aqueous solutions, formulated in 10% soybean oil base that also contains glycerol, purified egg phospholipids, and a preservative. Therefore, propofol is contraindicated in patients with egg, soy, lipid, albumin, or metabisulfite allergies. Propofol is attractive in the ED setting because of favorable pharmacokinetic parameters, with an onset of action within 30 seconds, peak within 60 seconds, and a duration of action of 3 to 10 minutes. Because of the short-acting nature of propofol, a continuous infusion is often necessary. As propofol can induce apnea and significant hypotension, a protocol outlining its use is highly recommended.[101,110]

Reversal agents should be readily available during all procedural sedations involving opioids or benzodiazepines.[111,112] Naloxone and nalmefene are opioid-receptor antagonists, reversing the sedative and analgesic effects. Naloxone can be titrated to the degree of reversal desired, depending on the dose used. Doses between 1 and 10 μg per kg can alleviate respiratory depression without fully reversing the analgesic effect of the opioid.[111] Doses of 100 μg per kg are used for full reversal in cases of apnea and overdose. The onset of action occurs within 2 minutes, and the effect lasts for 20 to 60 minutes. It is important to realize that the duration of reversal is shorter than the duration of action of most opioids and will likely result in rebound respiratory depression requiring additional doses.[112] Rare but serious adverse effects of naloxone administration include ventricular arrhythmia and cardiac arrest, primarily in patients with underlying cardiovascular disease or those receiving cardiotoxic drugs.[112] This is believed to be secondary to opioid-reversal–induced catecholamine surge, which can result in hypertension, myocardial infarction, and precipitation of withdrawal. Pulmonary edema has been reported with both low-dose (<100 μg) and high-dose (>100 μg) naloxone administration.[113]

Flumazenil reverses benzodiazepine effects at the GABA receptor and is useful when reversal of benzodiazepine sedation is desired, for example, after excess sedation. It is dosed at 0.01 mg per kg every minute to a cumulative maximum of 0.05 mg per kg or 1 mg, whichever is less.[114] Flumazenil has been shown to safely and effectively reverse benzodiazepine-induced sedation in children following procedural sedation, with no significant adverse effects.[114] The onset of action generally occurs within 1 to 3 minutes. Resedation can occur because the half-life of flumazenil is shorter than the half-life of most benzodiazepines, and therefore, patients should be monitored for the need for additional dosing.[112] Adverse effects are rare and may include dysrhythmias, hypertension, and seizures, primarily in patients dependent on benzodiazepines or who are receiving tricyclic antidepressants (TCAs). Caution should be used when considering the use of flumazenil in a patient dependent on benzodiazepines for seizure control because of the risk of precipitating seizures or status epilepticus (SE).

LACERATIONS

Lacerations are a common injury presenting to the pediatric ED. Several pharmacologic tools are available for wound management. These include analgesics, anxiolytics, local anesthetics, topical anesthetics, topical antimicrobials, tissue adhesives, and tetanus immunization.

TREATMENT

Local anesthetics are used to decrease the pain associated with repair of the laceration. Commonly used local anesthetics include lidocaine and bupivacaine, with or without epinephrine. Distractive techniques; warming the solution to body temperature; use of a long, fine-gauge needle; and the rate of infiltration are important factors in the success of a local anesthetic.[115] In addition, buffering lidocaine with sodium bicarbonate 8.4% in a 10:1 dilution decreases the pH of the local anesthetic and may decrease the pain associated with infiltration.[116] Pretreatment with topical lidocaine–epinephrine–tetracaine (LET) may also reduce the pain of infiltration and, in some cases, may be sufficient as the sole anesthetic (see section on topical anesthetics).

Lidocaine and bupivacaine act by blocking nerve impulse generation and conduction by decreasing the cell membrane permeability to sodium.[117] Toxicity is uncommon in routine clinical use and is related to the amount of free anesthetic released into the circulation. The duration of action is directly related to the contact time with the nerve.[117,118] Adverse reactions to local anesthetics are generally related to toxic levels and include seizures, cardiac arrhythmias, and decreased GI motility. Hypersensitivity is rare and occurs more frequently with the ester-type anesthetics such as procaine and tetracaine as compared with the amide-type anesthetics such as lidocaine and bupivacaine.[119,120] Hypersensitivity reactions are believed to occur to the metabolite *p*-aminobenzoic acid formed from the ester-type anesthetics.[118,121] The preservative methylparaben, which can be found in the amide-type anesthetics, also may be responsible for hypersensitivity reactions.[121] If hypersensitivity occurs with the amide-type anesthetics, most patients will tolerate subsequent skin testing, and the reaction may be shown to be due to the preservative.[116,122]

Lidocaine has a duration of action of approximately 1 to 2 hours (without epinephrine) and is the most commonly used local anesthetic.[117] Lidocaine injection is available in 0.5%, 1%, and 2% solutions. The total amount of lidocaine a patient receives for wound management, including topical and local infiltration, should be kept lower than the toxic range (i.e., no greater than 4.5 mg per kg).[123]

Bupivacaine has a duration of action that is four to six times the duration of lidocaine, but it also has an increased risk of cardiovascular side effects.[117] This effect is likely due to the slower dissociation from the sodium channels. Bupivacaine for simple laceration repair is generally not warranted, although it remains a good option for peripheral nerve blocks in prolonged repairs.[115]

Most local anesthetics are available with and without low-concentration epinephrine (1:200,000).[116] Epinephrine acts primarily as a local vasoconstrictor, slowing down the rate of absorption of the local anesthetic into the systemic circulation and prolonging the action of the anesthetic.[118,124] Concern exists for local tissue damage when using epinephrine as a vasoconstrictor in areas with limited collateral circulation, leading to hypoxic tissue damage, necrosis, and gangrene.[117] Therefore, areas such as the pinna of the ear, the nasal alae, the penis, and skin flaps should not be treated with a local anesthetic containing a vasoconstrictor.[124] The use of epinephrine is safe for digital nerve block.[125,126] Phentolamine may be used to reverse unintended vasoconstriction if necessary. Vasoconstriction in contaminated wounds may increase the likelihood of infection secondary to hindrance of blood flow.[124]

Diphenhydramine injection infiltrated locally can be used as an effective alternative to the ester- and amide-type anesthetics when an allergy truly exists. The structure of the antihistamines is closely related to the structure of local anesthetics.[127] Diphenhydramine diluted to a 1% solution is painful on injection but provides anesthesia similar to 1% lidocaine.[127,128] Skin necrosis is a potential serious side effect of diphenhydramine injection and may be dose related.

Topical anesthetic agents are used either alone or in conjunction with infiltrated local anesthetics. Prior to the introduction of LET, a solution of tetracaine, epinephrine (adrenaline), and cocaine (TAC) was shown to be efficacious in reducing pain associated with laceration repair.[129] However, TAC solutions are associated with significant adverse effects such as seizures and death secondary to cocaine absorption when misapplied, especially when contact with mucous membranes occurred.[115,130] TAC solutions are costlier and subject to regulatory control because of the cocaine component.

Comparison of LET solution with placebo has demonstrated significant reduction in pain associated with repair when applied to lacerations prior to lidocaine infiltration.[131] A direct comparison of LET with TAC solutions showed equivalent efficacy in pediatric patients.[132,133] Subsequent studies demonstrated LET in a gel formulation was at least as effective as the solution and was less likely to drip into the eyes of children with forehead or scalp lacerations.[134]

Topical antibiotic ointments are frequently applied to clean and repaired lacerations prior to dressing coverage. Common topical ointments include bacitracin, a combination of bacitracin/neomycin/polymyxin B, and silver sulfadiazine. When compared with plain petrolatum, the antibiotic ointments resulted in significantly lower infection rates.[135] Several experts recommend bacitracin-only ointments over the triple-antibiotic or silver sulfadiazine ointments because of lower allergic reaction rates with bacitracin alone.

Cyanoacrylates, commonly known as tissue adhesives, are used frequently for wound closure. Primary use in children has been closure of lacerations in the ED.[136] The adhesives form a strong bond when exposed to a fluid or basic medium, creating an exothermic reaction resulting in a polymer.[136] Dermabond, 2-octyl cyanoacrylate, is approved for use in the United States and is available over the counter. Comparable efficacy to sutures under low tension has been demonstrated with acceptable cosmetic results.[136,137] Advantages include ease of application, decreased time of repair, and elimination of needle-induced anxiety and pain of suturing. Dermabond is not recommended for use on nonimmobilized joints, wounds under high tension, or wounds with high risk of infection (e.g., bites). Anecdotally, and based on the author's personal experience, dermabond can be painful when it gets into the wound, so one should prepare the patient/caregiver appropriately.

All patients presenting with puncture wounds should be assessed for tetanus vaccination status.

BITE WOUNDS

Animal bites and/or exposures to saliva of a possibly infected animal are relatively common presentations to the ED. The first concern is the potential rabies status, particularly in wild animals known to be carriers. Bats and carnivores, primarily raccoons, skunks, foxes, and coyotes, transmit rabies to humans.[138,139] The rabies virus enters the system via a bite or secretion exposure and travels to the CNS, eventually causing a fatal encephalomyelitis.

The Advisory Committee for Immunization Practices has set forth guidelines for PEP.[140] Because human rabies is uniformly fatal once symptoms appear, prophylaxis with rabies immunoglobulin (RIG) and vaccination is imperative if exposure to rabies is suspected. Domesticated animals such as dogs and cats may carry rabies, but the incidence varies by region. Therefore, determining the need for PEP may require assistance from state health department resources (Table 17.7).

TABLE 17.7 Rabies Postexposure Prophylaxis

Animal Type	*Evaluation and Disposition of Animal*	*Postexposure Prophylaxis Recommendations*
Dogs, cats, and ferrets	Healthy and available for 10 d of observation	Prophylaxis only if animal develops signs of rabies[a]
	Rabid or suspected of being rabid[b]	Immediate immunization and RIG
	Unknown (escaped)	Consult public health officials for advice
Bats, skunks, raccoons, coyotes, foxes, mongooses, and most other carnivores; woodchucks	Regarded as rabid unless geographic area is known to be free of rabies or until animal proven negative by laboratory tests[b]	Immediate immunization and RIG
Livestock, rodents, and lagomorphs (rabbits, hares, and pikas)	Consider individually	Consult public health officials. Bites of squirrels, hamsters, guinea pigs, gerbils, chipmunks, rats, mice and other rodents, rabbits, hares, and pikas almost never require rabies postexposure prophylaxis

RIG, rabies immunoglobulin.

[a]During the 10-d observation period, at the first sign of rabies in the biting dog, cat, or ferret, prophylaxis of the exposed person with RIG (human) and vaccine should be initiated. The animal should be euthanized immediately and tested.

[b]The animal should be euthanized and tested as soon as possible. Holding for observation is not recommended. Immunization is discontinued if immunofluorescent test result for the animal is negative.

Adapted from Committee on Infectious Diseases, American Academy of Pediatrics, et al. Rabies. In: *Red Book® 2018*. AAP Point-of-Care-Solutions, 2018 [cited April 14, 2020]. https://redbook.solutions.aap.org/chapter.aspx?sectionid=189640168&bookid=2205.

TREATMENT

Rabies vaccine is available as human diploid cell vaccine (HDCV) and purified chick embryo cell-derived vaccine (PCECV). The postexposure treatment schedule consists of 1-mL IM vaccinations on days 0, 3, 7, 14, and 28.[140] Injection site should be the deltoid muscle in children and adults; infants may require injection in the midlateral aspect of the thigh.[140] Side effects occur in 5% to 40% of recipients and include pain and erythema at the injection site, headache, nausea, muscle ache, and dizziness.[140]

RIG provides immediate passive immunity to protect the patient until active immunity is conferred from the vaccine. The immunoglobulin is dosed at 20 units per kg IM × 1 dose, ideally within 72 hours of the bite/wound.[140] However, the incubation of human rabies has been reported at more than 1 year, so postexposure presentation should be treated with RIG as well as the vaccine, no matter the length of delay in seeking treatment.[140] If possible, the entire dose should be used to infiltrate into and around the wound (if present); any remainder is given IM in the opposite arm from the vaccine. Side effects include local muscle soreness and tenderness at the injection site.[140] Individuals who have been previously immunized against rabies should not receive RIG as part of the postexposure treatment because it may interfere with the vaccine efficacy in these individuals.[140]

Antibiotics are not indicated in every animal bite/wound but are strongly encouraged where there is an increased risk of infection, such as when there is extensive tissue damage or a bite to the hand or foot. Cat bites are particularly prone to infection because of the deep-puncture wounds inflicted.[141] Treatment of choice for cat bites includes a β-lactamase–resistant antibiotics to cover *Pasteurella multocida* and *S. aureus*. Commonly, amoxicillin-clavulanic acid is used as first-line therapy because there is a high failure rate for cephalexin against *P. multocida*.[142] Dog bites have a lower infection rate and do not generally require prophylactic treatment unless severe crush injury exists or there is bone, joint, tendon, or ligament involvement.[141] Immunocompromised patients, patients prone to infectious endocarditis, and highly contaminated wounds are indications for prophylactic antibiotic therapy.[142]

Human bites in children are usually minor, often inflicted by another child. However, human bites to an area that is not well vascularized, such as the hand, are highly prone to infection and should be considered for antibiotic prophylaxis.[142] Staphylococcal and streptococcal species in addition to PO anaerobes are the focus of antimicrobial coverage for human bites requiring prophylaxis. A β-lactamase–resistant antibiotic such as amoxicillin-clavulanic acid is usually the treatment of choice.[142] For penicillin-allergic patients, clindamycin can be used in combination with trimethoprim/sulfamethoxazole. Human bites should also prompt an assessment of the risk of transmission of hepatitis B virus and HIV.

RESPIRATORY DISTRESS SYNDROMES

STATUS ASTHMATICUS

Status asthmaticus is an acute severe asthma exacerbation requiring emergency treatment. Patients present with significant wheezing, increased work of breathing, and progressive respiratory failure. All attempts to avoid intubation and mechanical ventilation are undertaken because positive-pressure ventilation will only worsen the underlying hyperinflation of the lungs.[143] Therefore, many pharmacologic agents are used in an effort to avoid intubation.

Treatment

Inhaled β_2-adrenergic agonists, generally in the form of inhaled albuterol, are first-line bronchodilating agents in acute asthma exacerbations. Albuterol exhibits significant activity within 15 minutes of inhalation, with no demonstrable difference in efficacy between nebulization or metered-dose inhaler with spacer administration.[144,145] Initial dosing in status asthmaticus of the undiluted albuterol (0.5%) solution is 0.03 mL per kg (0.15 mg per kg) to a maximum of 1 mL per dose for three doses or 0.5 puffs per kg to maximum of 10 puffs (90-μg spray) with spacer. For patients presenting with acute asthma exacerbations, common regimens consist of three back-to-back treatments together with ipratropium. Continuous nebulized albuterol dosed at 0.5 mg per kg per hour is sometimes required in status asthmaticus. The main adverse effect of albuterol treatment is tachycardia from stimulation of β_1-receptors in the heart. Tremors, hypokalemia, and hyperglycemia can also occur. Levalbuterol, the R-isomer of albuterol, has not been shown to be more effective in children with status asthmaticus.[146]

Additional bronchodilation is achieved by adding ipratropium, an anticholinergic agent, to albuterol. Ipratropium antagonizes the muscarinic receptors in the airway, decreasing parasympathetic tone by blocking further release of acetylcholine and producing resistance to bronchoconstriction.[143,147] A systematic review demonstrates a reduction in hospital admissions for children with acute asthma exacerbations receiving multiple dose ipratropium in addition to standard β_2-agonists and corticosteroids.[147] The dose of ipratropium is 0.25 to 0.5 mg inhaled, and it has an onset of 1 to 3 minutes and a duration of action of up to 4 to 6 hours.

Terbutaline, an injectable selective β_2-receptor agonist, has been used successfully in status asthmaticus.[143,148] Terbutaline is used by many centers as a continuous IV infusion for continued bronchodilation when decreased airflow reduces the amount of nebulized albuterol actually reaching the alveoli. Dosing usually begins with a bolus of 5 to 10 μg per kg given either SC or IV. If response is not adequate, a continuous infusion of 0.05 to 0.1 μg per kg per minute is begun, titrated to a maximum of 10 μg per kg per minute.[143,148] Tachycardia is the most common dose-limiting adverse effect. Hypotension generally occurs between 0.4 and 2 μg per kg per minute, disappearing at doses more than 2 μg per kg per minute, perhaps due to downregulation of the β_2-receptors with higher doses.[148] Cardiac arrhythmias and seizures are possible although rare. Increased troponin and creatine phosphokinase (CPK) serum levels have been reported, although one study failed to find a relationship between CPK-myocardial band and the dose of terbutaline used.[148] Additive β-agonist doses (albuterol and terbutaline) as high as 40 to 45 mg per hour have been used, although most patients will not tolerate more than 20 mg per hour.

Corticosteroids are additional first-line agents in the treatment of asthma exacerbation and exert their effect primarily on the inflammatory response. Several mechanisms, including decreased cytokine and eicosanoid production; reduced accumulation of eosinophils, basophils, and leukocytes in lung tissue; and decreased vascular permeability, contribute to the usefulness of corticosteroids in asthma. Systemic administration is preferred for acute asthma exacerbations.

PO prednisone/prednisolone is generally dosed at 2 mg per kg initially, followed by PO prednisone/prednisolone at 2 mg per kg per day divided every 12 hours. Dexamethasone is also effective when administered PO and may be better tolerated, with less vomiting.[149] Dexamethasone also has a longer duration of action, so dosing is either one dose or two doses 24 hours apart, a simpler regimen than 5 days of twice-daily prednisone/prednisolone. For patients who cannot tolerate PO therapy, IV methylprednisolone dosed at 2 mg per kg or IV dexamethasone dosed at 0.4 mg per kg can be given for the bolus dose. Relatively few adverse side effects occur with short-course steroids given for asthma exacerbations; these include GI disturbances, mood changes, and serum electrolyte alterations.

IM epinephrine is an effective bronchodilator (see discussion of anaphylaxis) but has become less frequently used because of its short duration of action and cardiac side effects.[143] However, it is still used in some centers as a first-line agent in children with severe status asthmaticus with poor air exchange.

Magnesium sulfate has bronchodilator effects, presumably related to smooth muscle relaxation caused by inhibition of calcium uptake.[143] IV magnesium sulfate, usually dosed at 25 to 50 mg per kg (max. 2 g) given over 20 minutes, improves pulmonary function in children with status asthmaticus[150] and reduces the risk of hospitalization.[151] Toxicity should be monitored by continuous electrocardiograph and assessment of reflexes. Common, less serious side effects include hypotension, flushing, and nausea.

CROUP

Laryngotracheobronchitis, commonly known as croup, is a viral infection frequently seen in the ED. Patients with croup are generally younger than 3 years and present with stridor and a barking cough.

Treatment

First-line therapy for croup has traditionally been inhaled racemic epinephrine to reduce airway edema and obstruction. When given by inhalation, racemic epinephrine is largely confined to the airways, although, in large doses, systemic absorption and resulting tachycardia may occur. The peak effect occurs approximately 30 minutes after inhalation, and the duration is 120 minutes.[152] L-Epinephrine can be used in place of racemic epinephrine at an equivalent dose; racemic epinephrine 10 mg = L-epinephrine 5 mg.[153]

Corticosteroid therapy, primarily in the form of dexamethasone, reduces the severity and duration of croup.[152] PO and parenteral dexamethasone are equally efficacious and are dosed at 0.6 mg per kg IM/PO to a maximum of 10 mg per dose.[152]

Inhaled budesonide is as effective as PO or IM dexamethasone.[154,155] Inhaled budesonide has demonstrated favorable results in decreasing hospital admission rates in children with croup.[154] The dose is 1 mg inhaled followed by another 1 mg dose in 30 minutes. Beneficial effects for both dexamethasone and inhaled budesonide were seen as early as 6 hours after treatment.[156]

BRONCHIOLITIS

Bronchiolitis is an inflammation of the lower airways and occurs primarily in children younger than 2 years infected with RSV or other viruses. Primary manifestations include fever, coryza, wheezing, and respiratory distress.[157] Apnea, lethargy, and irritability are common in young infants with this infection.[157]

Treatment

The initial management of bronchiolitis is supportive, with a focus on supportive care. Corticosteroids and antibiotics are not indicated.[158,159]

Bronchiolitis is characterized by airway edema and generally does not have a bronchospastic component.[160] Bronchodilators such as albuterol are of limited benefit in bronchiolitis and are not routinely recommended.[160,161] However, when the distinction between reactive airway disease and bronchiolitis is difficult, some infants may benefit, and albuterol should be given to these patients if a trial dose or doses improve the clinical examination. As in croup, racemic epinephrine appears to offer benefit in bronchiolitis, decreasing respiratory rate and pulmonary resistance.[152] High-flow nasal cannula oxygen may provide noninvasive ventilatory support.[162]

Ribavirin has largely fallen out of favor as a treatment for RSV bronchiolitis. An antiviral agent given as an inhalation treatment, ribavirin carries theoretical risks of teratogenicity to pregnant health care workers.[163] Studies have shown a benefit of ribavirin therapy for children with underlying bronchopulmonary disease, congenital heart disease, or immunodeficiency with RSV infection. However, in light of the preventive and potential treatment measures available with RSV-IG and palivizumab, ribavirin is rarely used.

SEXUAL ASSAULT

There are several pharmacologic interventions to consider for a patient who has been sexually assaulted. Important considerations include the age of the victim and whether the assailant was known to the victim. For example, routine prophylaxis for sexually transmitted infections (STIs) is not indicated for prepubertal victims because they are less likely to become infected, infections are less likely to ascend the female reproductive tract, and follow-up can be better assured.[164]

TREATMENT

Treatment of the patient with sexual assault is aimed at preventing gonorrhea, chlamydia, and trichomonas; pregnancy; hepatitis B; human papilloma virus; and HIV.[164] For the prevention of STIs, the Centers for Disease Control and Prevention (CDC) recommends ceftriaxone 250 mg IM in a single dose plus azithromycin 1 g PO in a single dose plus either metronidazole 2 g PO in a single dose or tinidazole 2 g PO in a single dose.[164] Common side effects of metronidazole include metallic taste, GI disturbances, and disulfiram reaction if combined with alcohol. Pelvic inflammatory disease (PID) may occur in patients who delay seeking treatment for sexual assault. PID requires longer duration of therapy and higher doses for treatment.[165,166]

Hepatitis B prophylaxis should be considered if the patient has not been previously immunized. The initial immunization with hepatitis B vaccine 1 mL (10 µg per mL formulation) IM is given at the acute visit, with follow-up vaccinations at 1 and 6 months.[167] Hepatitis B immunoglobulin is reserved for victims exposed within 14 days with a high-risk exposure.[167]

PEP for HIV infection is considered effective when administered within 72 hours of assault. The risk of HIV transmission is low, but is not zero. Risk is substantially increased when the perpetrator of sexual assault is HIV positive, but this is often unknown, so decisions about PEP must rely on a patient's risk tolerance and the specifics of the assault.[164] For otherwise healthy adolescents, the preferred PEP regimen is tenofovir disoproxil fumarate (tenofovir DF or TDF) (300 mg) with emtricitabine (FTC) (200 mg) once daily plus raltegravir (RAL) 400 mg twice daily or dolutegravir (DTG) 50 mg daily for 28 days. An alternative regimen for otherwise healthy adults and adolescents is tenofovir DF (300 mg) with FTC (200 mg) once daily plus darunavir (DRV) (800 mg) and ritonavir (RTV) (100 mg) once daily. For children aged 2 to 12 years, tenofovir DF, FTC, and RAL for 28 days, with each drug dosed to age and weight. Alternative regimens include zidovudine and lamivudine with RAL or lopinavir/ritonavir, with RAL and lopinavir/ritonavir dosed to age and weight. Another alternative is tenofovir DF and FTC and lopinavir/ritonavir, with each drug dosed to age and weight.[168]

Emergency contraception prophylaxis may also be indicated after sexual assault. The most effective PO agent is ulipristal, which delays or prevents ovulation and is effective within 5 days of unprotected sex.[169] Ulipristal is administered as a single dose of 30 mg. Other options include levonorgestrel (Plan B) and the Yuzpe method. Plan B is available over the counter in many pharmacies and is also administered as a single dose of 1.5 mg. Plan B pregnancy prophylaxis is thought to be effective for at least 72 hours after unprotected intercourse, although efficacy decreases with increasing time. Prior to the introduction of levonorgestrel, high-dose estrogen (Yuzpe method) was commonly used.[170] High-dose estrogen was provided with ethinyl estradiol 50 μg (two tablets, Ovral) PO, given immediately and then repeated after 12 hours.[171]

Other variants of this method are also available[169] (Table 17.8).

STATUS EPILEPTICUS

This section discusses convulsive SE, that is, generalized tonic–clonic seizures. The definition of and treatment recommendations for SE have evolved over the past decade and now involve the concept of time point 1 (t_1), the point at which seizures should be considered continuous, and t_2, the time at which irreversible neuronal damage occurs. The best estimates available for these times are 5 and 30 minutes, respectively.[172] Thus, SE is defined operationally as seizure activity lasting for more than 5 minutes of continuous convulsive seizures, two seizures without return of consciousness between, or three discrete seizures within 1 hour.[173] Five minutes of continuous seizures defines SE because most children will stop within 5 minutes and seizures become more difficult to treat over time[174]; thus, 5 minutes reflects a balance to avoid overtreatment while aborting seizures as soon as possible to prevent morbidity.

There are many potential causes of SE, including fever, electrolyte abnormalities (most commonly hyponatremia and hypoglycemia), toxin exposures, CNS infection, underlying epilepsy, and trauma.[175] Terminating seizure activity and correcting any underlying disorder is the primary goal of therapy. Delays in initiating therapy are associated with increased mortality.[176]

TREATMENT

Benzodiazepines are the first-line medications used for the treatment of SE.[173] Seizure activity is halted when the drug binds to the benzodiazepine site on the GABA-receptor complex in the brain. Injectable preparations of lorazepam, diazepam, and midazolam are available in the United States. The effectiveness (68% to 73%) and safety (intubation rates of 8% to 16%) of these three agents are similar, so the choice of agent should depend on other considerations.[177,178] For example, diazepam can be administered rectally by parents and may provide early abortive therapy. Midazolam has a unique ring structure that allows it to be rapidly absorbed when administered IM, intranasally, or buccally. After absorption, midazolam becomes highly lipophilic at physiologic pH because of changes in the ring structure, thus speeding distribution to the brain.[179] Therefore, midazolam has advantages for use in the prehospital setting and in patients for whom IV access has not been obtained.[178] Although neurologists often prefer lorazepam because of its longer duration of action, lorazepam is more likely to cause deep sedation than diazepam, and sedative effects last for several hours.[177] Because midazolam is shorter acting,[179] it may be preferable for ED patients, for whom more rapid recovery to baseline mental status is important to assess for meningitis and other treatable causes of seizures. Midazolam is administered in doses of 0.2 mg per kg IM or 0.1 mg per kg IV to a maximum of 10 mg. Lorazepam is administered at 0.1 mg per kg IV to a maximum of 4 mg. Diazepam is administered at 0.2 to 0.3 mg per kg to a maximum of 10 mg IV and 0.5 mg per kg rectally. These doses should be repeated in 5 minutes if SE does not terminate. Respiratory depression is the most common side effect of the benzodiazepines, but respiratory depression was more common in adults treated with placebo than with either diazepam or lorazepam.[180]

Optimal second-line therapy for SE refractory to benzodiazepines is unknown. Phenytoin, previously recommended for second-line therapy, has been replaced in many sites in the United States by its prodrug, fosphenytoin, because it can be administered more rapidly. The mechanism of action of fosphenytoin is the same as that of phenytoin, stabilizing the neuronal membranes by blockage of the sodium-dependent voltage channels during depolarization.[181] Side effects of fosphenytoin include hypotension during infusion, which can be ameliorated by slowing the infusion rate. Fosphenytoin should not be infused faster than 3 mg phenytoin equivalents (PE) per kg per minute to a maximum of 150 mg PE per minute. This is approximately three times as fast as the recommended maximum rate for phenytoin. Other side effects are similar to those seen with phenytoin and include nystagmus, ataxia, drowsiness, and hypersensitivity. Because the drug is highly protein bound, unbound concentrations can be higher than expected if hypoalbuminemia is present and may result in toxicity.

Other second-line agents for SE include levetiracetam and valproic acid. Two recent studies in children indicate approximate equivalence in both efficacy and safety when comparing levetiracetam to phenytoin.[182,183] A third study, involving both children and adults, compared levetiracetam, fosphenytoin, and valproic acid and found that all three medications were successful in approximately 50% of patients, with similar safety profiles.[184] The exact mechanism of action of levetiracetam is unknown, although it has been demonstrated to inhibit burst firing without altering normal neuronal functioning. Levetiracetam is minimally metabolized and primarily eliminated by

TABLE 17.8 Postexposure Prophylaxis for Sexual Assault

Chlamydia, gonorrhea, and trichomonas	Ceftriaxone 250 mg i.m. × 1 dose PLUS Azithromycin 1 g p.o. × 1 dose PLUS Metronidazole 2 g p.o. × 1 dose OR Tinidazole 2 g p.o. × 1 dose
Hepatitis B	Hepatitis B vaccine 1 mL i.m. × 1 dose In high-risk situations: Hepatitis B immunoglobulin 0.06 mL (max. 5 mL) i.m. × 1 dose
HIV (<13 y old)	Tenofovir disoproxil fumarate Oral powder: 10 to <12 kg: 80 mg (2 scoops) once daily 12 to <14 kg: 100 mg (2.5 scoops) once daily 14 to <17 kg: 120 mg (3 scoops) once daily 17 to <19 kg: 140 mg (3.5 scoops) once daily 19 to <22 kg: 160 mg (4 scoops) once daily 22 to <24 kg: 180 mg (4.5 scoops) once daily 24 to <27 kg: 200 mg (5 scoops) once daily 27 to <29 kg: 220 mg (5.5 scoops) once daily 29 to <32 kg: 240 mg (6 scoops) once daily 32 to <34 kg: 260 mg (6.5 scoops) once daily 34 to <35 kg: 280 mg (7 scoops) once daily ≥35 kg: 300 mg (7.5 scoops) once daily Oral tablets: 17 to <22 kg: 150 mg once daily 22 to <28 kg: 200 mg once daily 28 to <35 kg: 250 mg once daily ≥35 kg: 300 mg once daily PLUS Emtricitabine Infants 1 to <3 mo: Oral solution: 3 mg/kg/dose once daily Infants ≥3 mo and children: Oral solution: 6 mg/kg/dose once daily; maximum daily dose: 240 mg/d Capsules: Patient weight >33 kg and able to swallow capsule whole: 200 mg once daily PLUS Raltegravir Infants and children <2 y: Oral: oral suspension (10 mg/mL): 6 mg/kg/dose twice daily Children ≥2 y: Oral: Chewable tablets: 11 to <14 kg: 75 mg twice daily 14 to <20 kg: 100 mg twice daily 20 to <28 kg: 150 mg twice daily 28 to <40 kg: 200 mg twice daily ≥40 kg: 300 mg twice daily Film-coated tablet: Isentress 400 mg tablet: Children ≥6 y weighing >25 kg who are able to swallow a tablet whole: 400 mg twice daily
HIV (>13 y old)	Tenofovir disoproxil fumarate 300 mg with emtricitabine 200 mg once daily PLUS Raltegravir 400 mg twice daily OR Dolutegravir 50 mg daily See reference 168 for alternative regimen
Pregnancy	Preferred: Ulipristal 30 mg p.o. × 1 dose Other options: Levonorgestrel 1.5 mg p.o. × 1 dose nelfinavir 1,250 mg p.o. b.i.d. OR Yuzpe method. Ovral 2 tablets p.o. × 1 immediately and repeat in 12 h. See reference 169 for other variants of this method with different oral contraceptives. Levonorgestrel 0.75 μg p.o. × 1 dose immediately, then repeat 0.75 μg p.o. 12 h later

b.i.d., twice daily; i.m., intramuscular; p.o., oral; t.i.d., three times daily.

From CDC. Sexual assault and abuse and STDs—2015 STD treatment guidelines. 2019 [cited May 27, 2019]. https://www.cdc.gov/std/tg2015/sexual-assault.htm; CDC. Chlamydial infections—2015 STD treatment guidelines. 2019 [cited May 27, 2019]. https://www.cdc.gov/std/tg2015/chlamydia.htm; CDC. Gonococcal infections—2015 STD treatment guidelines. 2019 [cited May 27, 2019]. https://www.cdc.gov/std/tg2015/gonorrhea.htm; CDC. Viral hepatitis—2015 STD treatment guidelines. 2019 [cited May 27, 2019]. https://www.cdc.gov/std/tg2015/hepatitis.htm; CDC Stacks. Updated guidelines for antiretroviral postexposure prophylaxis after sexual, injection drug use, or other nonoccupational exposure to HIV—United States, 2016. [cited May 19, 2019]. https://stacks.cdc.gov/view/cdc/38856; ACOG. Emergency contraception—ACOG. 2019 [cited April 14, 2020]. https://www.acog.org/patient-resources/faqs/contraception/emergency-contraception.

the kidney, necessitating dose reduction in renal insufficiency. Optimal dosing during SE is still undetermined, but many experts recommend 40 to 60 mg per kg as the initial loading dose. Ataxia and mood changes are the most common side effects with long-term use, but their relevance to acute therapy for SE is doubtful. Valproic acid acts on both sodium channel recovery time and the GABA receptor, either by increasing the activity of GABA in the brain or by binding directly to the site.[181] The loading dose is 20 to 40 mg per kg IV and is given at a rate no faster than 5 mg per kg per minute.[185] Although valproic acid is not recommended in patients younger than 2 years because of an increased risk of hepatotoxicity, some case reports document successful cessation of refractory SE in patients younger than 24 months.[186] Acute side effects include somnolence, ataxia, nausea, and vomiting.

For SE refractory to the foregoing interventions, there is no convincing evidence to define optimal therapy. Treatment options include repeating a second-line agent or crossing over to another second-line agent, or anesthetic doses of midazolam, a barbiturate, or propofol.[173] Ketamine has also been used for refractory SE. Endotracheal intubation and intensive care monitoring with continuous electroencephalogram (EEG) will be necessary for patients requiring continuous infusions.

SHOCK

Shock is defined as inadequate perfusion of tissues and may result from hypovolemia (including hemorrhage), maldistribution (e.g., sepsis), and poor cardiac output. Primary therapy of shock begins with fluid resuscitation. Vasopressor infusions are instituted in cases of severe hypotension refractory to fluid resuscitation.

TREATMENT OF SHOCK

Fluid resuscitation is accomplished initially with crystalloid infusions such as normal saline or lactated Ringer's solution. Initial bolus is given at 20 mL per kg and repeated up to two times (usual total max. of 60 mL per kg) if no effect is seen. If the patient's hemodynamic status worsens with fluids, then one should consider a poor cardiac output state such as myocarditis. In the case of hemorrhagic shock, early replacement of lost blood products is preferable to multiple boluses of crystalloids.

Vasopressor therapy is instituted if fluid resuscitation alone is not adequate to maintain the patient's perfusion of vital organs. Dopamine, dobutamine, epinephrine, norepinephrine, and vasopressin each have slightly different mechanisms of action and side effects. It is important to obtain central access as soon as possible once the decision is made to begin vasopressor therapy. Although central access should not delay the initiation of vasopressors, inadvertent infiltration of soft tissue with dopamine, epinephrine, vasopressin, and norepinephrine can cause significant local tissue damage and necrosis. Phentolamine, an α-receptor antagonist, should be available for inadvertent infiltrations and injected around the site of extravasation as soon as possible.

Dopamine is usually the first vasopressor begun in a patient who has persistent hypotension after adequate fluid resuscitation. A central neurotransmitter, dopamine activates adenylyl cyclase and thus increases cyclic adenosine monophosphate (AMP) in cells. Dopamine acts on α, β, and dopaminergic receptors in a dose-related response. Dopaminergic D_1 receptors are primarily affected at low doses of 1 to 5 μg per kg per minute. At this dose, renal perfusion is increased, with minimal effect on the systemic circulation. This may also be secondary to an effect on the β_1 receptors, increasing cardiac output enough to improve circulation to the kidneys, thus improving urine output. At a dose of 5 to 10 μg per kg per minute, β_1 receptors are activated in the myocardium, with resultant increase in cardiac output and stroke volume. When the dose is increased to 10 to 20 μg per kg per minute, dopamine activates the α_1 receptors in the peripheral vasculature, producing peripheral vasoconstriction and a rise in systemic BP. For shock states, dopamine should be initiated at a dose that will support the patient's BP. Therefore, a common starting dose is 10 μg per kg per minute and is titrated to effect. Nausea and vomiting, tachycardia, arrhythmias, and hypertension are adverse effects that can occur during dopamine infusions and are secondary to the sympathomimetic effects.

Dobutamine is structurally related to dopamine and acts on the α- and β-adrenergic receptors, although the clinical effect is primarily seen on the heart secondary to the increased inotropy. Dobutamine exists as a racemic mixture, with the (−) isomer exerting α_1-receptor agonism and the (+) isomer exerting α_1-receptor antagonism and potent β-receptor agonism. Peripheral resistance is not greatly affected owing to counterbalancing of the α_1-mediated vasoconstriction and β_2-mediated vasodilation.[7] Dobutamine is frequently chosen for patients requiring greater inotropic support. In addition, dobutamine may be added to vasoconstrictor therapy, such as epinephrine following volume resuscitation. The dose must be individually titrated; usual range is 5 to 20 μg per kg per minute. Side effects may include severe hypertension, myocardial ischemia, tachycardia, and arrhythmias.

Epinephrine is a potent stimulant of both α- and β-adrenergic receptors. Dose-related clinical effects include increased BP and increased cardiac output. BP increases secondary to vasoconstriction by α_1-receptor activation in the systemic vasculature. In addition, β_1-receptor activation in the myocardial tissue increases inotropy and chronotropy. Small doses may produce vasodilation secondary to the greater sensitivity of the β_2 receptors over the α receptors. Use in pediatric shock is reserved for severe hypotension unresponsive to fluid resuscitation and dopamine. The dose range is generally 0.1 to 1 μg per kg per minute. Adverse effects include tachycardia, arrhythmias, myocardial infarction, and severe hypertension, especially in patients receiving β-blocking therapies.

Norepinephrine is structurally related to epinephrine, although the primary action is on the α receptors, with little effect on β receptors. Peripheral resistance is significantly increased without an increase in cardiac output. Norepinephrine is usually the drug of choice in septic or neurogenic shock with fluid-unresponsive severe hypotension. Severe hypertension and ischemia are the principal adverse reactions.

Vasopressin has been used with success as an adjuvant agent in adults with vasodilatory shock.[187] A potent vasoconstrictor, vasopressin activates the V_1 receptors in the vascular smooth muscle.[187,188] Vasopressin may find a place in the treatment of pediatric shock requiring high-dose catecholamines, but it is still controversial and requires more study.[189] Adverse effects include myocardial infarction, arrhythmias, water intoxication, anaphylaxis, and severe hypertension.

MULTIPLE TRAUMA

Trauma is the leading cause of death in children and adolescents.[190] Mortality rates have improved over time.[191,192] Children with initial poor neurologic presentation fare better than adults, emphasizing the need for timely and appropriate care.[193] Children with nonaccidental trauma (NAT) have higher mortality rates than those with accidental trauma, and recognition of NAT can be delayed.[194] As with all other presentations to the ED, attention to the ABCs is paramount. Establishing a patent airway and obtaining vascular access are primary goals. See discussion on rapid sequence intubation (RSI) for intubating medications.

TREATMENT OF MULTIPLE TRAUMATIC INJURIES

Patients with multiple traumatic injuries will likely require pain management and sedation (see sections "Procedural Sedation" and "Pain"). Care must be taken not to compound hypotension in the presence of hemorrhage or shock. Fentanyl is often the drug of choice for pain management because of the relative absence of effects on hemodynamic status.[88] Antibiotics are usually given for prophylaxis of open fractures and should include staphylococcal and streptococcal coverage. The need for tetanus immunization should be assessed for open wounds or burns.

CLOSED HEAD INJURY

Closed head injury with elevated ICP presents a challenge for initial emergency management. Cerebral perfusion depends on the gradient between systemic BP and ICP, so either decreased BP or increased ICP can decrease cerebral perfusion. With decreased perfusion, the brain does not receive necessary oxygen and ischemia with cell death occurs, resulting in further edema. Without initial intracranial monitoring, the degree of elevation is unknown; suspected intracranial hypertension must be managed in all cases with suggestive clinical manifestations.

Treatment

A recent consensus guideline encapsulates the care of pediatric patients with head injury and increased ICP.[195] Baseline care includes adequate systemic BP to maintain cerebral perfusion pressure, adequate oxygenation and hemoglobin levels, elevation of the head of the bed with the head in midline, prevention of hyperthermia, adequate pain control and sedation, and maintenance of ventilation to a PCO_2 of 35 to 40 mmHg. First-line treatments include hyperosmolar therapy with hypertonic (3%) saline or mannitol, increased sedation and neuromuscular blockade, and vasopressors to support cerebral perfusion pressure. Second-line treatments may include barbiturate infusions, moderate hypothermia, additional hyperosmolar therapy, hyperventilation, and advanced monitoring (e.g., EEG). For initial therapy, hypertonic saline is administered at a dose of 5 to 10 mL per kg over 20 minutes and is repeated as needed every 30 minutes. Hypertonic saline can also be administered as a continuous infusion of 0.1 to 1 mL per kg per hour titrated to ICP. Mannitol is administered at a dose of 0.5 to 1 g per kg and must be administered with a filter needle. Mannitol is incompatible with KCl and sodium bicarbonate. The duration of reduction in ICP is dose related and ranges from 2 to 4 hours.

RAPID SEQUENCE INTUBATION

RSI is used when children are unable to maintain adequate ventilation or a patent airway. Medications used for RSI include a combination of premedications, sedatives, and neuromuscular blockade agents given concurrently to achieve a loss of consciousness and paralysis, providing ideal intubating conditions (Table 17.9). The agents of choice depend on the presentation and age of the patient. This method of intubating pediatric patients in an emergency setting has been shown to be effective with minimal side effects.[196,197] Patients presenting in full cardiopulmonary arrest are intubated immediately without medication.

Atropine may be considered as a premedication for patients younger than 7 years who require intubation. The vagolytic properties of atropine may mitigate the effects of vagal stimulation on the heart rate caused by endotracheal tube placement, but the evidence supporting this practice is weak. Atropine may be more important when repeat doses of succinylcholine are required. A minimum dose is no longer recommended; atropine should be administered at a dose of 0.02 mg per kg to a maximum dose of 5 mg.[198]

Etomidate is an ultra–short-acting, nonbarbiturate hypnotic that anesthetizes the patient within 30 seconds. The duration of action ranges from 4 to 8 minutes. Etomidate is especially useful in hypotensive patients, as minimal decreases in BP are seen following administration. Pain on injection, likely due to the propylene glycol solvent, and involuntary muscle movements are common side effects. If used in nonhypotensive patients, pretreatment with low-dose fentanyl (1 to 2 μg per kg IV) may be protective against the hypertensive effect produced by sympathetic stimulation during intubation, because etomidate does not have analgesic properties. Long-term administration of etomidate in the intensive care unit setting has been associated with decreased adrenal function and increased mortality.[199] Clinically significant depressions in serum cortisol have not been demonstrated with

TABLE 17.9 Indications and Medications for Rapid Sequence Intubation[a]

Indication	*Medications*
Nonhead trauma, normotensive	Atropine if <7 y old Midazolam ± fentanyl, rocuronium, or succinylcholine
Head trauma/elevated ICP, normotensive	Atropine if <7 y old Midazolam ± fentanyl, rocuronium, or succinylcholine
Head trauma/elevated ICP, hypotensive	Atropine if <7 y old Etomidate Rocuronium or succinylcholine
Hypotension/hypovolemia	Atropine if <7 y old Etomidate (or ketamine) Rocuronium or succinylcholine
Status asthmaticus	Atropine if <7 y old Ketamine Rocuronium or succinylcholine

ICP, intracranial pressure.

single injections of etomidate for pediatric RSI.[200] Etomidate dosing for RSI is 0.3 mg per kg IV for children. Additional adverse effects include small increases in heart rate, nausea, and vomiting.

Another common medication combination used for endotracheal intubation is midazolam and fentanyl. Midazolam (0.1 mg per kg) provides sedation, and fentanyl can effectively block the increase in BP associated with endotracheal intubation at a dose of 1.5 to 3 μg per kg IV × 1 dose. Fentanyl should not be administered rapidly because of the risk of chest wall rigidity and apnea. See discussion of midazolam and fentanyl in section "Procedural Sedation."

Ketamine is an alternative to etomidate for patients with sepsis because it does not suppress the adrenal cortex[200] and should also be considered for the intubation of a patient in status asthmaticus.[201] Ketamine is a phencyclidine derivative and may block *N*-methyl-D-aspartic acid receptors that mediate airway tone.[202] It is also a potent bronchodilator and provides adrenergic stimulation owing to blockade of norepinephrine reuptake and may inhibit vagal outflow. By increasing secretions, ketamine may also improve the pulmonary toilet and decrease mucus plugging in children with asthma. The intubating dose of ketamine is 1 to 2 mg per kg given IV. The onset of action occurs within 60 seconds, and the duration of action is 10 to 15 minutes. Adverse reactions can include emergence reactions, laryngospasm, and hypertension. Ketamine was thought to increase ICP based on case reports and small case series, but more recent data challenge this.[203]

Neuromuscular blockading agents (NMBAs) that are effective for RSI must have a very short onset time. Three NMBAs are recommended for RSI in pediatrics. Succinylcholine, rocuronium, and high-dose vecuronium (0.3 mg per kg) are all useful agents, having onset times of less than 1 minute.

Composed of two acetylcholine molecules, succinylcholine is a depolarizing paralytic agent that opens the receptor channels on the motor end plate of skeletal muscle and remains in place, causing initial fasciculations and then ultimate skeletal muscle paralysis. Onset occurs within 60 seconds, and the duration of action is a maximum of 5 to 8 minutes due to hydrolysis by plasma cholinesterases.[204] Succinylcholine is commonly dosed at 1 mg per kg IV, although infants younger than 1 year may require 2 mg per kg IV. IM administration is possible with succinylcholine and should be given at a dose of 3 to 4 mg per kg to a maximum of 150 mg. A black box warning issued by the FDA cautions against the use of succinylcholine in children because of the risk of rhabdomyolysis and hyperkalemia, resulting in cardiac arrest.[205] Contraindications include use in patients with chronic myopathies or denervating neuromuscular diseases, a history of malignant hyperthermia, hyperkalemia, or after 24 hours of crush injuries, burns, or denervating injuries. The author is also aware of a case of fatal hyperkalemia in a patient with SE of approximately 1 hour duration; another agent should be strongly considered for patients with prolonged SE. Despite the limitations, succinylcholine remains an important paralytic agent, particularly in patients with difficult or anticipated difficult airways in the emergency setting.[206] The ultra-short onset and duration of action enables the patient to regain respiratory control if the intubation attempt is unsuccessful. The short duration of action can be extremely useful in patients in whom a complete neurologic examination is important for reassessing extension of injury and clinical status, particularly with head trauma.

Adverse events include prolonged paralysis in those with congenital absence of cholinesterases, malignant hyperthermia, masseter muscle spasm, and hyperkalemic cardiac arrest secondary to rapid release of potassium from the cells. Bradycardia can occur in children following repeat succinylcholine doses secondary to an acetylcholine-like effect the drug has on the cardiac postganglionic muscarinic receptors.[106] Histamine release may occur with rapid administration of succinylcholine.[205]

A defasciculating dose of a nondepolarizing paralytic such as pancuronium or vecuronium can be used to minimize the depolarization of the skeletal muscle following succinylcholine administration.[204] The dose is one-tenth of the dose used for induction of paralysis given 1 to 3 minutes prior to succinylcholine. Some paralysis may occur at this dose and may require positive-pressure ventilation until the succinylcholine is given.

Rocuronium is a short-acting, nondepolarizing paralytic agent and has been used successfully in pediatric patients for RSI.[196] As a nondepolarizing paralytic, rocuronium competitively binds to the nicotinic acetylcholinergic receptor on the motor end plate of the skeletal muscle, inhibiting transmission of impulses.[204,207] Rocuronium is an attractive alternative for pediatric RSI because of the relatively short onset of less than 60 seconds with a dose of 1.2 mg per kg and intermediate duration of 30 to 60 minutes.[208] In addition, rocuronium can be given IM if IV access cannot be obtained. Dosing for RSI is 1 to 1.2 mg per kg IV or 1 to 1.8 mg per kg IM × 1 dose. Adverse effects include prolonged paralysis when given with other drugs known to prolong neuromuscular blockade and rare allergic reactions.

Vecuronium is structurally related to rocuronium and can be used for RSI but must be given at three times the normal dose (0.25 to 0.3 mg per kg vs. 0.1 mg per kg) to achieve an adequate onset time.[196,209] By increasing the dose, the duration of action is also increased to as much as 2 hours in some cases. Vecuronium demonstrates an age-related time to recovery from neuromuscular block that is greater in infants than in children and not seen with rocuronium.[204] Histamine release is less likely with vecuronium and rocuronium as compared with succinylcholine.

RESUSCITATION MEDICATIONS

Pediatric advanced life support (PALS) recommendations published by the American Heart Association provide guidelines for the resuscitation of children, with an emphasis on pharmacologic therapies.[210] Current treatment algorithms are given as follows (Table 17.10).

ASYSTOLE/PULSELESS ELECTRICAL ACTIVITY

Unfortunately, the outcome in children presenting in asystole from an out-of-hospital arrest is very poor. However, rapid intervention may improve the chances of successful resuscitation. Initial management of asystole includes assessment of the airway and provision of adequate ventilation with effective and timely chest compressions. Epinephrine is the primary pharmacologic agent used in asystole. Epinephrine may be given via IV/intraosseous (IO) routes or endotracheally. Dosing of epinephrine for IV or IO administration begins at 0.1 mL per kg of a 1:10,000 solution (equivalent to 0.01 mg per kg). If the endotracheal route must be utilized, the higher concentration of epinephrine 1:1,000 is dosed at 0.1 mL per kg (equivalent to 0.1 mg per

TABLE 17.10 Pediatric Advanced Life Support Recommendations

Indication	*Recommendations*
Asystole/pulseless electrical activity	Epinephrine
Ventricular fibrillation/ pulseless ventricular tachycardia	Defibrillation Epinephrine + defibrillation Amiodarone OR lidocaine + defibrillation Magnesium sulfate if torsade des pointes
Bradycardia	Epinephrine Atropine Transcutaneous pacing
Supraventricular tachycardia	
Stable	Vagal maneuvers Adenosine Amiodarone, lidocaine, or procainamide Alternative agents
Unstable	Synchronized cardioversion

kg). To ensure adequate dispersal and absorption in the lungs, the epinephrine dose should be diluted in 3 to 5 mL of normal saline prior to administration; installation should be followed by five positive-pressure breaths. Epinephrine doses should be repeated every 3 to 5 minutes. Despite years of empiric practice, "high-dose epinephrine" (0.1 mg per kg IV) does not appear to improve outcome unless the underlying cause of the arrest is a condition in which the body becomes relatively resistant to exogenous catecholamines (i.e., β-blocker overdose).[211]

Vasopressin dosed at 40 units IV is advocated for cardiac arrest in adults, but there are insufficient data to recommend routine use of vasopressin in pediatric arrest.

Pulseless electrical activity (PEA) may result from several treatable causes, including hypoxia, cardiac tamponade, tension pneumothorax, and hyperkalemia.[208] If any of these conditions exist, it is essential to recognize and correct them immediately. The drug of choice for PEA is epinephrine, as discussed in the preceding paragraph.

PULSELESS VENTRICULAR TACHYCARDIA AND VENTRICULAR FIBRILLATION

The first and foremost treatment for ventricular fibrillation (VF)/pulseless ventricular tachycardia (VT) is defibrillation, followed by immediate cardiopulmonary resuscitation (CPR). In the treatment of VF/pulseless VT, a single "shock" is given with immediate resumption of CPR. The amount of electricity delivered is dependent upon the type of defibrillator available, either monophasic or biphasic. Following subsequent shocks, circulation is reassessed. Initial settings for the monophasic defibrillator begin at 2 joules per kg (max. 300 joules) with the second defibrillation; the second and all subsequent defibrillations are given at 4 joules per kg (max. 360 joules). Adolescent and adult patients should receive the initial and all subsequent shocks at 360 joules. The energy settings on the biphasic defibrillators are reduced and for adults will be set at 150 joules for the initial shock and 200 joules for subsequent shocks.

Secondary treatment of VF/pulseless VT includes epinephrine as dosed for PEA. Each dose of medication given in VF/ pulseless VT should be followed by a defibrillating shock. If no response is seen following the initial dose of epinephrine, the PALS algorithm directs the practitioner to use an antiarrhythmic medication, specifically either amiodarone or lidocaine.[210]

Amiodarone is a class III antiarrhythmic that prolongs the action potential and refractory period in the myocardial tissue primarily via sodium and potassium channel blockade.[212] Additional effects include calcium channel blockade and downregulation of β receptors.[213] Conduction through the atrioventricular node is slowed because of the delay in repolarization. Dosing begins at 5 mg per kg (max. 300 mg per dose) given as a rapid IV/IO bolus. In stable VT, amiodarone is infused over 20 to 60 minutes. Amiodarone must be diluted in 10 to 15 mL of dextrose 5% in water (D5W) prior to administration. Onset time is rapid after IV bolus. Amiodarone is very lipophilic and possesses an extended half-life; in cases of chronic PO administration, the elimination half-life may be several months. Adverse side effects are common and can include complete heart block, hypotension, and the development of torsades de pointes if hypomagnesemia or hypokalemia exists. Amiodarone should not be given if the patient is receiving procainamide or other class I antiarrhythmic agents because of its propensity to prolong the QT interval.

Lidocaine is a class Ib antiarrhythmic agent that suppresses the automaticity of ventricles and the His-Purkinje system by directly blocking the conduction of impulses in the myocardial tissues, thereby decreasing sodium ion permeability of the membranes.[213] Dosing of lidocaine is recommended at 1 to 1.5 mg per kg via IV/IO as a rapid bolus. Fifty percent of the dose (0.5 to 0.75 mg per kg) can be repeated every 3 to 5 minutes until a maximum of 3 mg per kg is reached. A continuous infusion of lidocaine may be necessary to maintain sinus rhythm.

There is insufficient evidence to support the choice of lidocaine versus amiodarone for pediatric VF/pulseless VT; lidocaine was associated with increased rates of return of spontaneous circulation and 24-hour survival, but not survival to hospital discharge.[210,214] If torsades de pointes is present, the drug of choice is magnesium sulfate 25 to 50 mg per kg (max. 2,000 mg per dose).[211] Magnesium sulfate acts as a calcium channel blocker and influences the Na–K-ATPase activity in the heart, terminating the malignant rhythm. Magnesium sulfate is diluted and run over 10 to 20 minutes in torsades de pointes. The onset of action is nearly immediate.

In cases of acute VF secondary to TCA toxicity, sodium bicarbonate is the drug of choice. Sodium bicarbonate in doses of 1 mEq per kg boluses overcome the fast sodium channel blockade produced by the TCAs. The standard 8.4% solution of sodium bicarbonate is extremely hyperosmolar and should not be used in infants because of the risk of intraventricular hemorrhage.[211] The 4.2% solution of sodium bicarbonate (Neut) should be used in infants requiring sodium bicarbonate. A continuous infusion of sodium bicarbonate, 75 to 150 mEq per L, in D5W may be necessary to control the arrhythmia.

BRADYCARDIA

Early correction of possible underlying factors in bradycardia, such as hypoxia and hypothermia, among others, is essential.

The first-line pharmacologic agent for bradycardia is epinephrine, as discussed earlier; the second-line medication is atropine. As a vagolytic agent, atropine decreases the depressive vagal influence on the heart, thus increasing cardiac output. Atropine is dosed at 0.02 mg per kg (min. dose 0.1 mg, max. dose 1 mg) given IV/IO. If the endotracheal route is used, the dose of atropine should be 2 to 10 times the IV/IO dose. As with epinephrine, the dose of atropine should be diluted with 3 to 5 mL of normal saline; administration should be followed by five positive-pressure breaths. Atropine may be repeated once, 3 to 5 minutes after the initial dose. The onset of action occurs within 2 to 4 minutes. It is important to note that atropine's dilating effects on the pupils may last several hours, making pupillary examination more difficult to interpret.

Cardiac pacing may be necessary to maintain perfusion for patients with a bradycardic rhythm. Special situations such as calcium channel blocker induced bradycardia may require the administration of calcium or insulin and dextrose. It is also important to note that calcium should not be given to patients also receiving digoxin, as a worsening of the arrhythmia may be seen. Calcium chloride 10% solution is given at a dose of 20 mg per kg (max. 1,000 mg per dose) IV; it must be further diluted before administration and is ideally infused via a central line. Calcium gluconate 10% solution is dosed at 100 mg per kg (max. 3,000 mg per dose) and may be infused peripherally, although central administration is preferred wherever possible. Calcium administration may also be required in cases of hyperkalemia, hypocalcemia, and magnesium toxicity.

SUPRAVENTRICULAR TACHYCARDIA

The most common cause of malignant tachycardia in children is supraventricular tachycardia (SVT). If signs of poor perfusion, such as altered mental status or hypotension, are present, the patient is considered to be unstable and should immediately proceed to synchronized cardioversion.[211] In the stable patient, vagal maneuvers are initially attempted to interrupt the abnormal conduction, while an IV line is being placed. Vagal maneuvers may include placing ice on the face directly covering the mouth and nose, blowing through an occluded straw, or bearing down as if having a bowel movement.

The first-line pharmacologic agent for the treatment of SVT is adenosine.[211] Because of the ultra-short half-life of adenosine in vivo, all doses must be given as centrally as possible and are immediately followed by a saline flush. Three-way stopcocks are often used to facilitate this process. The dose of adenosine is 0.1 mg per kg to a maximum of 6 mg via rapid IV push for the first dose, followed by 0.2 mg per kg (max. 12 mg) via rapid IV push if the initial dose was unsuccessful at converting the patient to normal sinus rhythm. It is important to realize that a few seconds of asystole follow each dose of adenosine. This short period of asystole allows the heart to resume normal sinus rhythm by interrupting the conduction through the atrioventricular node. The onset is nearly immediate, and the duration of action is generally less than 2 minutes.

Amiodarone, lidocaine, and procainamide may also be useful in perfusing SVT. Amiodarone and lidocaine are described earlier, although the infusion times lengthen to avoid severe hypotension when these drugs are given for SVT. As a class Ia antiarrhythmic agent, procainamide has a similar mechanism of action as lidocaine. The dose of procainamide is 15 mg per kg run over 30 to 60 minutes. Adverse effects requiring cessation of infusion include hypotension and prolongation of the QT interval. Continuous infusion of procainamide may also be necessary to control the arrhythmia.

Synchronized cardioversion is employed as the next intervention if the drugs are ineffective or if the patient becomes unstable at any time. Different from defibrillation, cardioversion energy settings begin at 0.5 joules per kg (max. 50 to 100 joules) and increase incrementally to 2 joules per kg (max. 200 joules). As with defibrillation, the energy settings may vary between monophasic and biphasic machines, so it is important to become familiar with the equipment available to you. Sedation and analgesia with agents such as midazolam and fentanyl (see previous section) are preferable when time allows, as cardioversion is extremely unpleasant.

In conclusion, drug therapy in the ED is complex and varied. Conditions can range from a simple otitis media to CPR. Pharmacotherapy plays an important role in the treatment of children in the ED.

REFERENCES

1. Reynolds S, Desquin B, Uyeda A, et al. Children with chronic conditions in a pediatric emergency department. *Pediatr Emerg Care* 1996;12:166–169.
2. Cox ER, Halloran DR, Homan SM, et al. Trends in the prevalence of chronic medication use in children: 2002–2005. *Pediatrics* 2008;122:e1053–e1061.
3. Rasooly I, Mullins PM, Alpern ER, et al. US emergency department use by children, 2001-2010. *Pediatr Emerg Care* 2014; 30:602–607.
4. Dibs SD, Baker MD. Anaphylaxis in children: a 5-year experience. *Pediatrics* 1997;99:E7.
5. Hoffman BB. Catecholamines, sympathomimetic drugs, and adrenergic receptor antagonists. In: Hardman JG, Limbird LE, eds. *Goodman & Gilman's the pharmacological basis of therapeutics,* 10th ed. New York, NY: McGraw-Hill, 2001:215–268.
6. Simons FE, Roberts JR, Gu X, et al. Epinephrine absorption in children with a history of anaphylaxis. *J Allergy Clin Immunol* 1998;101:33–37.
7. Project Team of the Resuscitation Council (UK). The emergency medical treatment of anaphylactic reactions. *J Accid Emerg Med* 1999;16:243–247.
8. Muraro A, Roberts G, Clark A, et al. The management of anaphylaxis in childhood; position paper on European Academy of Allergology and Clinical Immunology. *Allergy* 2007;62:857–871.
9. Pongracic JA, Kim JS. Update on epinephrine for the treatment anaphylaxis. *Curr Opin Pediatr* 2007;19:94–98.
10. Brown N, Roberts LJ. Histamine, bradykinin and their antagonists. In: Hardman JG, Limbird LE, eds. *Goodman & Gilman's the pharmacological basis of therapeutics,* 10th ed. New York, NY: McGraw-Hill, 2001:651–657.
11. Schimmer BP, Parker KL. Adrenocorticotropic hormone; adrenocortical steroids and their synthetic analogs; inhibitors of the synthesis and actions of adrenocortical hormones. In: Hardman JG, Limbird LE, eds. *Goodman & Gilman's the pharmacological basis of therapeutics,* 10th ed. New York, NY: McGraw-Hill, 2001:1649–1677.
12. Pourmand A, Robinson C, Syed W, et al. Biphasic reaction: a review of the literature and implications for emergency medicine. *Am J Emerg Med* 2018;36:1480–1485.
13. Rendiae S. Drug interactions of H_2-receptor antagonists involving cytochrome P450 (CYPs) enzymes: from the laboratory to the clinic. *Croat Med J* 1999;40(3):357–367.
14. Singer M, Deutschman CS, Seymour CW, et al. The third international consensus definitions for sepsis and septic shock (Sepsis-3). *JAMA* 2016;315:801–810.
15. Kadish HA, Loveridge B, Tobey J, et al. Applying outpatient protocols in febrile infants 1–28 days of age: can the threshold be lowered? *Clin Pediatr (Phila)* 2000;39(2):81–88.
16. Hartman ME, Linde-Zwirble WT, Angus DC, et al. Trends in the epidemiology of pediatric severe sepsis. *Pediatr Crit Care Med* 2013;14:686–693.
17. D'Andrea CC, Ferrera PC. Disseminated herpes simplex virus infection in a neonate. *Am J Emerg Med* 1998;16:376–378.
18. Rhodes A, Evans LE, Alhazzani W et al. Surviving sepsis campaign: international guidelines for the management of severe sepsis and septic shock 2016. *Intensive Care Med* 2017;43(1):304–377.
19. Lipton JD, Schafermeyer RW. Evolving concepts in pediatric bacterial meningitis—Part I: Pathophysiology and diagnosis. *Ann Emerg Med* 1993;22:1602–1615.
20. Wubbel L, McCracken GH. Management of bacterial meningitis: 1998. *Pediatr Rev* 1998;19:78–84.
21. Silverman RB. Enzyme inhibition and inactivation. In: *The organic chemistry of drug design and drug action.* San Diego, CA: Academic Press, 1992:181–185.
22. Easton J, Noble S, Perry CM. Amoxicillin/clavulanic acid: a review of its use in the management of paediatric patients with acute otitis media. *Drugs* 2003;63:311–340.
23. Chopra I, Hesse L, O'Neill AJ. Exploiting current understanding of antibiotic action for discovery of new drugs. *J Appl Microbiol Symp* 2002;92(Suppl):4S–15S.
24. Contopoulos-Ioannidis DG, Giotis ND, Baliatsa DV, et al. Extended-interval aminoglycoside administration for children: a meta-analysis. *Pediatrics* 2004;114:e111—e118.
25. Konishi H, Goto M, Nakamoto Y, et al. Tobramycin inactivation by carbenicillin, ticarcillin and piperacillin. *Antimicrob Agents Chemother* 1983;23:653–657.
26. Chambers HF. Antimicrobial agents: protein synthesis inhibitors and miscellaneous antibacterial agents. In: Hardman JG, Limbird LE, eds. *Goodman & Gilman's the pharmacological basis of therapeutics,* 10th ed. New York, NY: McGraw-Hill, 2001:1239–1271.
27. Bonadio WA, Jeruc W, Anderson Y, et al. Systemic infection due to group B beta-hemolytic streptococcus in children. A review of 75 outpatient-evaluated cases during 13 years. *Clin Pediatr (Phila)* 1992;31:230–234.

28. IDSA Practice Guidelines Committee. 1997 guidelines for the use of antimicrobial agents in neutropenic patients with unexplained fever. *Clin Infect Dis* 1997;25:551–573.
29. Lipton JD, Schafermeyer RW. Evolving concepts in pediatric bacterial meningitis—Part II: current management and therapeutic research. *Ann Emerg Med* 1993;22:1616–1629.
30. Quagliarello VJ, Scheld WM. Treatment of bacterial meningitis. *N Engl J Med* 1997;336:708–716.
31. Wooltorton E. Cochlear implant recipients at risk for meningitis. *Can Med Assoc J* 2002;167:670.
32. Food and Drug Administration. *FDA Public Health Web Notification: cochlear implant recipients may be at greater risk for meningitis.* Originally issued July 24, 2002—Updated October 17, 2002. Rockville, MD: Author, 2002.
33. De Gans J, Van De Beek D. Dexamethasone in adults with bacterial meningitis. *N Engl J Med* 2002;347(20):1549–1556.
34. Wald ER, Kaplan SL, Mason EO Jr, et al. Dexamethasone therapy for children with bacterial meningitis. *Pediatrics* 1995;95(1):21–28.
35. Schaad UB, Lips U, Gnehm HE, et al. Dexamethasone therapy for bacterial meningitis in children. *Lancet* 1993;342:457–461.
36. Swanson D. Meningitis. *Pediatr Rev* 2015;36:514–524.
37. American Academy of Pediatrics. Therapy for children with invasive pneumococcal infections (RE9709). *Pediatrics* 1997;99:289–299.
38. Prober CG. The role of steroids in the management of children with bacterial meningitis. *Pediatrics* 1995;95:29–31.
39. Klugman K, Friedland IR, Bradley JS. Bactericidal activity against cephalosporin-resistant *Streptococcus pneumoniae* in cerebrospinal fluid of children with acute bacterial meningitis. *Antimicrob Agents Chemother* 1995;39:1988–1992.
40. Ricard JD, Wolff M, Lacherade JC, et al. Levels of vancomycin in cerebrospinal fluid of adult patients receiving adjunctive corticosteroids to treat pneumococcal meningitis: a prospective multicenter observational study. *Clin Infect Dis* 2007;44:250–255.
41. Kohl S, James AR. Herpes simplex virus encephalitis during childhood: importance of brain biopsy diagnosis. *J Pediatr* 1985;107:212–215.
42. Whitley RJ. Herpes simplex virus infection. *Semin Pediatr Infect Dis* 2002;1:6–11.
43. *Acyclovir sodium package insert.* Los Angeles, CA: American Pharmaceutical Partners, Inc. 2002.
44. Kimberlin DW, Lin CY, Jacobs RF, et al. Safety and efficacy of high-dose intravenous acyclovir in the management of neonatal herpes simplex virus infections. *Pediatrics* 2001;108:230–238.
45. American Academy of Pediatrics. Meningococcal infections. In: Pickering LK, ed. *2000 red book: report of the Committee on Infectious Diseases,* 25th ed. Elk Grove Village, IL: American Academy of Pediatrics, 2000:396–401.
46. Powers RD. Soft tissue infections in the emergency department: the case for the use of 'simple' antibiotics. *South Med J* 1991; 84:1313–1315.
47. Gupta K, MacIntyre A, Vannasse G, et al. Trends in prescribing beta-lactam antibiotics for treatment of community-associated methicillin resistant *Staphylococcus aureus* infections. *J Clin Microbiol* 2007;45:3930–3934.
48. Howe L, Jones NS. Guidelines for the management of periorbital cellulitis/abscess. *Clin Otolaryngol Allied Sci* 2004;29:725.
49. Ambati BK, Ambati J, Azar N, et al. Periorbital and orbital cellulitis before and after the advent of *Haemophilus influenzae* type B vaccination. *Ophthalmology* 2000;107:1590–1593.
50. Starkey CR, Steele RW. Medical management of orbital cellulitis. *Pediatr Infect Dis J* 2001;20:1002–1005.
51. American Academy of Pediatrics. Severe invasive group a streptococcal infections: a subject review (RE9804). *Pediatrics* 1998;101:136–140.
52. Doctor A, Harper MB, Fleisher GR. Group A beta-hemolytic streptococcal bacteremia: historical overview, changing incidence, and recent association with varicella. *Pediatrics* 1995;96:428–433.
53. Norrby SR, Norrby-Teglund A. Infections due to group A streptococcus: new concepts and potential treatment strategies. *Ann Acad Med Singapore* 1997;26(5):691–693.
54. American Academy of Pediatrics. Toxic shock syndrome. In: Pickering LK, ed. *2000 red book: report of the Committee on Infectious Diseases,* 25th ed. Elk Grove Village, IL: American Academy of Pediatrics, 2000:580–581.
55. Leung AK, Eneli I, Davies HD. Necrotizing fasciitis in children. *Pediatr Ann* 2008;37:704–710.
56. McIntosh K. Community-acquired pneumonia in children. *N Engl J Med* 2002;346(6):429–437.
57. Dellinger RP, Carlet JM, Masur H, et al. Surviving sepsis campaign guidelines for management of severe sepsis and shock. *Crit Care Med* 2004;32(3):853–873.
58. Bradley JS. Management of community-acquired pediatric pneumonia in an era of increasing antibiotic resistance and conjugate vaccines. *Pediatr Infect Dis J* 2002;21(6):592–598.
59. Chumpa A, Bachur RG, Harper MB. Bacteremia-associated pneumococcal pneumonia and the benefit of initial parenteral antimicrobial therapy. *Pediatr Infect Dis J* 1999;18(12):1981–1985.
60. McCracken GH. Etiology and treatment of pneumonia. *Pediatr Infect Dis J* 2000;19(4):373–377.
61. Bradley JS, Byington CL, Shah SS. The management of community-acquired pneumonia in infants and children older than 3 months of age: clinical practice guidelines by the Pediatric Infectious Diseases Society and the Infectious Diseases Society of America. *Clin Infect Dis* 2011;53:e25—e75.
62. Esposito S, Bosis S, Cavagna R, et al. Characteristics of *Streptococcus pneumoniae* and atypical bacterial infections in children 2–5 years of age with community acquired pneumonia. *Clin Infect Dis* 2002;35:1345–1352.
63. *Erythromycin base film-tab package insert.* Abbott Park, IL: Abbott Laboratories, 2000.
64. *Zithromax (azithromycin) package insert.* New York, NY: Pfizer, 2002.
65. Hauben M, Amsden GW. The association of erythromycin and infantile hypertrophic pyloric stenosis: causal or coincidental? *Drug Saf* 2002;25:929–942.
66. Cooper WO, Griffin MR, Arbogast P, et al. Very early exposure to erythromycin and infantile hypertrophic pyloric stenosis. *Arch Pediatr Adolesc Med* 2002;156:647–650.
67. Jacobson SJ, Griffiths K, Diamond S, et al. A randomized controlled trial of penicillin vs clindamycin for the treatment of aspiration pneumonia in children. *Arch Pediatr Adolesc Med* 1997;158:701–704.
68. Kim MK, Karpas A. Orthopedic emergencies: the limping child. *Clin Pediatr Emerg Med* 2002;3(2):129–137.
69. Perron AD, Brady WJ, Miller MD. Orthopedic pitfalls in the ED: osteomyelitis. *Am J Emerg Med* 2003;21:61–67.
70. Castellazzi L, Mantero M, Esposito S. Update on the management of pediatric acute osteomyelitis and septic arthritis. *Int J Mol Sci* 2016;17:pii:e855.
71. Chambers JB, Forsythe DA, Bertrand SL, et al. Retrospective review of osteoarticular infections in a pediatric sickle cell age group. *J Pediatr Orthop* 2000;20:682–685.
72. Vinod MB. Duration of antibiotics in children with osteomyelitis and septic arthritis. *J Paediatr Child Health* 2002;38:363–367.
73. Jaberi FM, Shahcheraghi GH, Ahadzadeh M. Short-term intravenous antibiotic treatment of acute hematogenous bone and joint infection in children: a prospective randomized trial. *J Pediatr Orthop* 2002;22:317–320.
74. American Academy of Pediatrics. *Salmonella* infections. In: Pickering LK, ed. *2000 red book: report of the Committee on Infectious Diseases,* 25th ed. Elk Grove Village, IL: American Academy of Pediatrics, 2000:501–503.
75. American Academy of Pediatrics. Judicious use of antimicrobial agents. In: Pickering LK, ed. *2000 red book: report of the Committee on Infectious Diseases,* 25th ed. Elk Grove Village, IL: American Academy of Pediatrics, 2000:647–648.
76. Lieberthal AS, Carroll AE, Chonmaitree T, et al. The diagnosis and management of acute otitis media. *Pediatrics* 2013;131:e964—e999.
77. American Academy of Pediatrics. *Pneumococcal infections.* In: Pickering LK, ed. *2000 red book: report of the Committee on Infectious Diseases,* 25th ed. Elk Grove Village, IL: American Academy of Pediatrics, 2000:452–460.
78. Dowell SF, Butler JC, Giebink GS, et al. Acute otitis media: management and surveillance in an era of pneumococcal resistance—a report from the Drug-Resistant *Streptococcus pneumoniae* Therapeutic Working Group. *Pediatr Infect Dis J* 1999;18:1–9.
79. Shulman ST, Bisno AL, Clegg HW, et al. Clinical practice guideline for the diagnosis and management of group A streptococcal pharyngitis: 2012 update by the Infectious Diseases Society of America. *Clin Infect Dis* 2012;55:e86—e102.
80. American Academy of Pediatrics. Group A streptococcal infections. In: Pickering LK, ed. *2000 red book: report of the Committee on Infectious Diseases,* 25th ed. Elk Grove Village, IL: American Academy of Pediatrics, 2000:526–536.
81. *Bicillin LA (penicillin G benzathine) package insert.* Bristol, TN: Monarch Pharmaceuticals, 2001.
82. AAP/APS. Policy Statement. The assessment and management of acute pain in infants, children, and adolescents (0793). *Pediatrics* 2001;108:793–797.
83. Read JV. Perceptions of nurses and physicians regarding pain management of pediatric emergency room patients. *Pediatr Nurs* 1994;20:314–318.
84. Roberts LJ, Morrow JD. Analgesic-antipyretic and antiinflammatory agents. In: Hardman JG, Limbird LE, eds. *Goodman & Gilman's the pharmacological basis of therapeutics,* 10th ed. New York, NY: McGraw-Hill, 2001:687–719.
85. Curtis SM, Curtis RL. Somatosensory function and pain. In: Porth CM, ed. *Pathophysiology: concepts of altered health states,* 3rd ed. Philadelphia, PA: Lippincott Williams & Wilkins, 1990:839–872.
86. Rodriquez E, Jordan R. Contemporary trends in pediatric sedation and analgesia. *Emerg Med Clin North Am* 2002;20:199–222.
87. Institute for Safe Medication Practices. ISMP Medication Safety Alert! 2002; October 30, 7(22).
88. Gutstein HB, Akil H. Opioid analgesics. In: Hardman JG, Limbird LE, eds. *Goodman & Gilman's The pharmacological basis of therapeutics,* 10th ed. New York, NY: McGraw-Hill, 2001:595–596.
89. Blackburn P, Vissers R. Pharmacologic advances in emergency medicine: pharmacology of emergency department pain management and conscious sedation. *Emerg Med Clin North Am* 2000;18:803–827.
90. Müller P, Vogtmann C. Three cases with different presentation of fentanyl-induced muscle rigidity—a rare problem in intensive care of neonates. *Am J Perinatol* 2000;17:23–26.
91. Fahnenstich H, Steffan J, Ku N, et al. Fentanyl-induced chest wall rigidity and laryngospasm in preterm and term infants. *Crit Care Med* 2000;28:836–839.
92. Weiner AL. Meperidine as a potential cause of serotonin syndrome in the emergency department. *Acad Emerg Med* 1999; 6(2):156–158.
93. Ciszkowski C, Madadi P, Phillips MS, et al. Codeine, ultrarapid-metabolism genotype, and postoperative death. *N Engl J Med* 2009;361:827Y828
94. US Food and Drug Administration. FDA Drug safety communication: codeine use in certain children after tonsillectomy and/or adenoidectomy may lead to rare, but life-threatening adverse events or death. 2007. https://www.fda.gov/media/85072/download. Accessed April 14, 2020.
95. Mazer-Amirshahi M, Mullins P, Rassoly I, et al. Trends in prescription opioid use in pediatric emergency department patients. *Pediatr Emerg Care* 2014;30:1–6.
96. Tréluyer JM, Tonnelier S, d'Athis P, et al. Antipyretic efficacy of an initial 30-mg/kg loading dose of acetaminophen versus a 15-mg/kg maintenance dose. *Pediatrics* 2001;108(4):e73.
97. Gladtke E. Use of antipyretic analgesics in the pediatric patient. *Am J Med* 1983;75(5A):121–126.
98. Pierce MC, Fuchs S. Evaluation of ketorolac in children with forearm fractures. *Ann Emerg Med* 1997;4:22–26.
99. *Ketorolac tromethamine package insert.* Bedford, OH: Bedford Laboratories, 1999.
100. Motov S, Yasavolian M, Likourezos A, et al. Comparison of intravenous ketorolac at three single-dose regimens for treating acute pain in the emergency department: a randomized controlled trial. *Ann Emerg Med* 2017;70:177–184.
101. Bassett KE, Anderson JL, Pribble CG, et al. Propofol for procedural sedation in children in emergency departments. *Ann Emerg Med* 2003;42:773–782.

102. Malviya S, Voepel-Lewis T, Prochaska G, et al. Prolonged recovery and delayed side effects of sedation for diagnostic imaging studies in children. *Pediatrics* 2000;105:e42.
103. Coté CJ, Karl HW, Notterman DA, et al. Adverse sedation events in pediatrics: analysis of medications used for sedation. *Pediatrics* 2000;106:633–644.
104. Peña B, Krauss B. Adverse events of procedural sedation and analgesia in a pediatric emergency department. *Ann Emerg Med* 1999;34:483–491.
105. Charney DS, Mihic SJ, Harris RA. Hypnotics and sedatives. In: Hardman JG, Limbird LE, eds. *Goodman & Gilman's the pharmacological basis of therapeutics,* 10th ed. New York, NY: McGraw-Hill, 2001:399–427.
106. Wadbrook PS. Pharmacologic advances in emergency medicine—advances in airway pharmacology. *Emerg Med Clin North Am* 2000;18:767–788.
107. Evers AS, Crowder CM. General anesthetics. In: Hardman JG, Limbird LE, eds. *Goodman & Gilman's the pharmacological basis of therapeutics,* 10th ed. New York, NY: McGraw-Hill, 2001: 337–365.
108. Rock MJ, De La Rocha SR, L'Hommedieu CS, et al. Use of ketamine in asthmatic children to treat respiratory failure refractory to conventional therapy. *Crit Care Med* 1986;14:514–516.
109. Wathen JE, Roback MG, Mackenzie T, et al. Does midazolam alter the clinical effects of intravenous ketamine sedation in children? A double-blind, randomized, controlled, emergency department trial. *Ann Emerg Med* 2000;36:579–588.
110. Task Force on Sedation and Analgesia by Non-Anesthesiologists. Practice guidelines for sedation and analgesia by non-anesthesiologists. *Anesthesiology* 1996;84:459–471.
111. Brent AS. Acute pain in children: the management of pain in the emergency department. *Pediatr Clin North Am* 2000;47(3):651–679.
112. *Naloxone hydrochloride package insert.* Abbott Park, IL: Abbott Laboratories, 1999.
113. Johnson C, Mayer P, Grosz D. Pulmonary edema following naloxone administration in a healthy orthopedic patient [Letter]. *J Clin Anesth* 1995;7:356–357.
114. Shannon M, Albers G, Burkhart K, et al. Safety and efficacy of flumazenil in the reversal of benzodiazepine-induced conscious sedation. *J Pediatr* 1997;131:582–586.
115. Knapp JF. Updates in wound management for the pediatrician. *Pediatr Clin North Am* 1999;46(6):1201–1213.
116. Hollander JE, Singer AJ. Laceration management. *Ann Emerg Med* 1999;34(3):56–67.
117. Catterall W, Mackie K. Local anesthetics. In: Hardman JG, Limbird LE, eds. *Goodman & Gilman's the pharmacological basis of therapeutics,* 10th ed. New York, NY: McGraw-Hill, 2001:367–384.
118. Covino BG. Pharmacology of local anaesthetic agents. *Br J Anaesth* 1986;58:701–716.
119. Ball IA. Allergic reactions to lignocaine. *Br Dent J* 1999;186(5):224–226.
120. Gall H, Kaufmann R, Kalveram CM. Adverse reactions to local anesthetics: analysis of 197 cases. *J Allergy Clin Immunol* 1996;97(4):933–937.
121. Eggleston ST, Lush LW. Understanding allergic reactions to local anesthetics. *Ann Pharmacother* 1996;30(7):851–857.
122. Troise C, Voltolini S, Minale P, et al. Management of patients at risk for adverse reactions to local anesthetics: analysis of 386 cases. *J Invest Allergol Clin Immunol* 1998;8(3):172–175.
123. *Xylocaine (lidocaine hydrochloride) package insert.* Wilmington, DE: AstraZeneca, 2000.
124. Emslander HC. Local and topical anesthesia for pediatric wound repair: a review of selected aspects. *Pediatr Emerg Care* 1998;14(2):123–129.
125. Ilicki J. Safety of epinephrine in digital nerve blocks: a literature review. *J Emerg Med* 2015;49(5):799–809.
126. Lalonde D. *Wide awake hand surgery.* New Brunswick, Canada: CRC Press, 2016.
127. Green SM, Rothrock SG, Gorchynski J. Validation of diphenhydramine as a dermal local anesthetic. *Ann Emerg Med* 1994;23(6):1284–1289.
128. Ernst AA, Anand P, Nick T, et al. Lidocaine versus diphenhydramine for local anesthesia minor laceration repair. *J Trauma* 1993;34:354–357.
129. Smith GA, Strausbaugh SD, Harbeck-Weber C, et al. Comparison of topical anesthetics with lidocaine infiltration during laceration repair in children. *Clin Pediatr (Phila)* 1997; 36(1):17–23.
130. Smith GA, Strausbaugh SD, Harbeck-Weber C, et al. Prilocaine–phenylephrine and bupivacaine–phenylephrine topical anesthetics compared with tetracaine–adrenaline–cocaine during repair of lacerations. *Am J Emerg Med* 1998;16:121–124.
131. Singer AJ, Stark MJ. Pretreatment of lacerations with lidocaine, epinephrine and tetracaine at triage: a randomized double-blind trial. *Acad Emerg Med* 2000;7:751–756.
132. Schilling CG, Bank DE, Borchert BA, et al. Tetracaine, epinephrine (adrenaline) and cocaine (TAC) versus lidocaine, epinephrine and tetracaine (LET) for anesthesia of lacerations in children. *Ann Emerg Med* 1995;25:203–208.
133. Ernst AA, Marvez-Valls E, Nick TG, et al. LAT (lidocaine–adrenaline–tetracaine) versus TAC (tetracaine–adrenaline–cocaine) for topical anesthesia in face and scalp lacerations. *Am J Emerg Med* 1995;13:158–154.
134. Resch K, Schilling C, Borchert BD, et al. Topical anesthesia for pediatric lacerations: a randomized trial of lidocaine–epinephrine–tetracaine solution versus gel. *Ann Emerg Med* 1998;36(6):693–697.
135. Dire DJ, Coppola M, Dwyer DA, et al. Prospective evaluation of topical antibiotics for preventing infections in uncomplicated soft-tissue wound repairs in the ED. *Acad Emerg Med* 1995;2:4–10.
136. Bernard L, Doyle J, Friedlander SF, et al. A prospective comparison of octyl cyanoacrylate tissue adhesive (Dermabond) and suture for the closure of excisional wounds in children and adolescents. *Arch Dermatol* 2001;137:1177–1180.
137. Bruns TB, Robinson BS, Smith RJ, et al. A new tissue adhesive for laceration repair in children. *J Pediatr* 1998;132(6):1067–1070.
138. CDC. *Rabies.* 2019 [cited May 27, 2019]. https://www.cdc.gov/rabies/index.html.
139. CDC. *Human rabies prevention – United States, 2008 recommendations of the Advisory Committee on Immunization Practices.* 2008 [cited 2019 May 27]. https://www.cdc.gov/mmwr/preview/mmwrhtml/rr5703a1.htm.
140. Committee on Infectious Diseases, American Academy of Pediatrics, et al. Rabies. In: *Red Book® 2018.* AAP Point-of-Care-Solutions, 2018 [cited May 27, 2019]. https://redbook.solutions.aap.org/chapter.aspx?sectionid=189640168&bookid=2205.
141. Lewis KT, Stiles M. Management of cat and dog bites. *Am Fam Physician* 1995;52(2):479–485.
142. Committee on Infectious Diseases, American Academy of Pediatrics, et al. Bite wounds. In: *Red Book® 2018.* AAP Point-of-Care-Solutions, 2018 [cited December 31, 2019]. https://redbook.solutions.aap.org/chapter.aspx?sectionId=189641714&bookId=2205&resultClick=24.
143. Werner HA. Status asthmaticus in children. *Chest* 2001;119(6):1913–1929.
144. Ploin D, Chapuis FR, Stamm D, et al. High-dose albuterol by metered-dose inhaler plus a spacer device versus nebulization in preschool children with recurrent wheezing: a double-blind, randomized equivalence trial. *Pediatrics* 2000;106(2 Pt 1):311.
145. Castro-Rodriguez JA, Rodrigo GJ. Beta-agonists through metered-dose inhaler with valved holding chamber versus nebulizer for acute exacerbation of wheezing or asthma in children under 5 years of age: a systematic review with meta-analysis. *J Pediatr* 2004;145(2):172.
146. Qureshi F, Zaritsky A, Welch C, et al. Clinical efficacy of racemic albuterol versus levalbuterol for the treatment of acute pediatric asthma. *Ann Emerg Med* 2005;46(1):29.
147. Griffiths B, Ducharme FM. Combined inhaled anticholinergics and short-acting beta2-agonists for initial treatment of acute asthma in children. *Cochrane Database Syst Rev* 2013;(8): CD000060. https://www.cochranelibrary.com/cdsr/doi/10.1002/14651858.CD000060.pub2/abstract.
148. Stephanopoulos DE, Monge R, Schell KH, et al. Continuous intravenous terbutaline for pediatric status asthmaticus. *Crit Care Med* 1998;26(10):1744–1748.
149. Keeney GE, Gray MP, Morrison AK, et al. Dexamethasone for acute asthma exacerbations in children: a meta-analysis. *Pediatrics* 2014;133(3):493–499.
150. Ciarallo L, Sauer AH, Shannon MW. Intravenous magnesium therapy for moderate to severe pediatric asthma: results of a randomized, placebo-controlled trial. *J Pediatr* 1996;129:809–814.
151. Cheuk DKL, Chau TCH, Lee SL. A meta-analysis on intravenous magnesium sulphate for treating acute asthma. *Arch Dis Child* 2005;90(1):74–77.
152. Klassen TP. Recent advances in the treatment of bronchiolitis and laryngitis. *Pediatr Clin North Am* 1997;44(1):249–261.
153. Waisman Y, Klein BL, Boenning DA, et al. A prospective randomized double-blind study comparing L-epinephrine and racemic epinephrine aerosols in the treatment of laryngotracheitis (croup). *Pediatrics* 1992;89:302–306.
154. Hvizdos KM, Jarvis B. Budesonide inhalation suspension: a review of its use in infants, children and adults with inflammatory respiratory disorders. *Drugs* 2000;60(5):1141–1178.
155. Geelhoed GC, Macdonald WBG. Oral and inhaled steroids in croup: a randomized, placebo-controlled trial. *Pediatr Pulmonol* 1995;20:355–361.
156. Russell KF, Liang Y, O'Gorman K, et al. Glucocorticoids for croup. *Cochrane Database Syst Rev* 2011;(1):CD001955. https://www.cochranelibrary.com/cdsr/doi/10.1002/14651858.CD001955.pub3/abstract.
157. Committee on Infectious Diseases, American Academy of Pediatrics, et al. Respiratory syncytial virus. In: *Red Book® 2018.* AAP Point-of-Care-Solutions, 2018 [cited May 27, 2019]. https://redbook.solutions.aap.org/chapter.aspx?sectionid=189640170&bookid=2205.
158. Farley R, Spurling GK, Eriksson L, et al. Antibiotics for bronchiolitis in children under two years of age. *Cochrane Database Syst Rev* 2014;(10):CD005189. https://www.cochranelibrary.com/cdsr/doi/10.1002/14651858.CD005189.pub4/full.
159. Corneli HM, Zorc JJ, Mahajan P, et al. A multicenter, randomized, controlled trial of dexamethasone for bronchiolitis. *N Engl J Med* 2007;357(4):331–339.
160. Perlstein PH, Kotagal UR, Bolling C, et al. Evaluation of an evidence-based guideline for bronchiolitis. *Pediatrics* 1999;104(6):1334–1341.
161. Gadomski AM, Scribani MB. Bronchodilators for bronchiolitis. *Cochrane Database Syst Rev* 2014;(6):CD001266. https://www.cochranelibrary.com/cdsr/doi/10.1002/14651858.CD001266.pub4/full.
162. Dysart K, Miller TL, Wolfson MR, et al. Research in high flow therapy: mechanisms of action. *Respir Med* 2009;103(10):1400–1405.
163. Rakshi K, Couriel JM. Management of acute bronchiolitis. *Arch Dis Child* 1994;71:463–469.
164. CDC. *Sexual assault and abuse and STDs—2015 STD treatment guidelines.* 2019 [cited May 27, 2019]. https://www.cdc.gov/std/tg2015/sexual-assault.htm.
165. CDC. *Chlamydial infections—2015 STD treatment guidelines.* 2019 [cited May 27, 2019]. https://www.cdc.gov/std/tg2015/chlamydia.htm.
166. CDC. *Gonococcal infections—2015 STD treatment guidelines.* 2019 [cited May 27, 2019]. https://www.cdc.gov/std/tg2015/gonorrhea.htm.
167. CDC. *Viral hepatitis—2015 STD treatment guidelines.* 2019 [cited May 27, 2019]. https://www.cdc.gov/std/tg2015/hepatitis.htm.
168. CDC Stacks. *Updated guidelines for antiretroviral postexposure prophylaxis after sexual, injection drug use, or other nonoccupational exposure to HIV—United States, 2016.* [cited May 19, 2019]. https://stacks.cdc.gov/view/cdc/38856.
169. ACOG. *Emergency contraception—ACOG.* 2019 [cited May 28, 2019]. https://www.acog.org/Patients/FAQs/Emergency-Contraception.
170. Wanner MS, Couchenour RL. Hormonal emergency contraception. *Pharmacotherapy* 2002;22(1):43–53.
171. Grimes DA, Raymond EG. Emergency contraception. *Ann Intern Med* 2002;137:180–189.
172. Trinka E, Cock H, Hesdorffer D, et al. A definition and classification of status epilepticus – Report of the ILAE Task Force on Classification of Status Epilepticus. *Epilepsia* 2015;56(10):1515–1523.
173. Glauser T, Shinnar S, Gloss D, et al. Evidence-based guideline: treatment of convulsive status epilepticus in children and adults: report of the Guideline Committee of the American Epilepsy Society. *Epilepsy Curr* 2016;16(1):48–61.
174. Goodkin HP, Sun C, Yeh J-L, et al. GABAA receptor internalization during seizures. *Epilepsia* 2007;48(s5):109–113.
175. LaCroix J, Deal C, Gauthier M, et al. Admissions to a pediatric intensive care unit for status epilepticus: a 10-year experience. *Crit Care Med* 1994;22(5):827–832.
176. Gaínza-Lein M, Fernβndez IS, Jackson M, et al. Association of time to treatment with short-term outcomes for pediatric patients with refractory convulsive status epilepticus. *JAMA Neurol* 2018;75(4):410–418.
177. Chamberlain JM, Okada P, Holsti M, et al. Lorazepam vs diazepam for pediatric status epilepticus: a randomized clinical trial. *JAMA* 2014;311(16):1652–1660.

178. Silbergleit R, Durkalski V, Lowenstein D, et al. Intramuscular versus intravenous therapy for prehospital status epilepticus. *N Engl J Med* 2012;366(7):591–600.
179. Towne AR, DeLorenzo RJ. Use of intramuscular midazolam for status epilepticus. *J Emerg Med* 1999;17(2):323–328.
180. Alldredge BK, Gelb AM, Isaacs SM, et al. A comparison of lorazepam, diazepam, and placebo for the treatment of out-of-hospital status epilepticus. *N Engl J Med* 2001;345:631–637.
181. McNamara O. Drugs effective in the therapy of the epilepsies. In: Hardman JG, Limbird LE, eds. *Goodman & Gilman's the pharmacological basis of therapeutics*, 10th ed. New York, NY: McGraw-Hill, 2001:521–548.
182. Dalziel SR, Borland ML, Furyk J, et al. Levetiracetam versus phenytoin for second-line treatment of convulsive status epilepticus in children (ConSEPT): an open-label, multicentre, randomised controlled trial. *Lancet*. 2019;393:2135–2145. http://www.sciencedirect.com/science/article/pii/S0140673619307226.
183. Lyttle MD, Rainford NEA, Gamble C, et al. Levetiracetam versus phenytoin for second-line treatment of paediatric convulsive status epilepticus (EcLiPSE): a multicentre, open-label, randomised trial. *Lancet*. 2019;393:2125–2134. http://www.sciencedirect.com/science/article/pii/SChildren's National Medical Center
184. Kapur J, Elm J, Chamberlain JM, et al. Randomized trial of three anticonvulsant medications for status epilepticus. *N Engl J Med* 2019;381(22):2103–2113.
185. Venkataraman V, Wheless JW. Safety of rapid intravenous infusion of valproate loading doses in epilepsy patients. *Epilepsy Res* 1999;35(2):154–153.
186. Chez MG, Hammer MS, Loeffel M, et al. Clinical experience of three pediatric and one adult case of spike-and-wave status epilepticus treated with injectable valproic acid. *J Child Neurol* 1999;14(4):239–242.
187. Meyer S, Gortner L, McGuire W, et al. Vasopressin in catecholamine-refractory shock in children. *Anaesthesia* 2008;63(3):288–234.
188. Baldasso E, Ramos Garcia PC, Piva JP, et al. Hemodynamic and metabolic effects of vasopressin infusion in children with shock. *J Pediatr (Rio J)* 2007;83(Suppl 5):S137–S145.
189. Masarwa R, Paret G, Perlman A, et al. Role of vasopressin and terlipressin in refractory shock compared to conventional therapy in the neonatal and pediatric population: a systematic review, meta-analysis, and trial sequential analysis. *Crit Care* 2017;21(1):1.
190. CDC. *WISQARS*. 2019 [cited May 29, 2019]. https://www.cdc.gov/injury/wisqars/index.html.
191. Thurman DJ. The epidemiology of traumatic brain injury in children and youths: a review of research since 1990. *J Child Neurol* 2016;31(1):20–27.
192. Oliver J, Avraham J, Frangos S, et al. The epidemiology of inpatient pediatric trauma in United States hospitals 2000 to 2011. *J Pediatr Surg* 2018;53(4):758–764.
193. Emami P, Czorlich P, Fritzsche FS, et al. Impact of Glasgow Coma Scale score and pupil parameters on mortality rate and outcome in pediatric and adult severe traumatic brain injury: a retrospective, multicenter cohort study. *J Neurosurg* 2017;126(3):760–767.
194. Estroff JM, Foglia RP, Fuchs JR. A comparison of accidental and nonaccidental trauma: it is worse than you think. *J Emerg Med* 2015;48(3):274–279.
195. Kochanek PM, Tasker RC, Bell MJ, et al. Management of pediatric severe traumatic brain injury: 2019 consensus and guidelines-based algorithm for first and second tier therapies. *Pediatr Crit Care Med* 2019;20(3):269–279.
196. Sagarin MJ, Chiang V, Sakles JC, et al. Rapid sequence intubation for pediatric emergency airway management. *Pediatr Emerg Care* 2002;18(6):417–423.
197. Marvez-Valls E, Houry D, Ernst AA, et al. Protocol for rapid sequence intubation in pediatric patients—a four year study. *Med Sci Monit* 2002;8(4):CR229–CR234.
198. de Caen AR, Berg MD, Leon C, et al. Part 12: pediatric advanced life support. *Circulation* 2015;132(18 Suppl 2):S526–S542.
199. Fellows IW, Bastow MD, Byrne AJ, et al. Adrenocortical suppression in multiply injured patients: a complication of etomidate treatment. *Br Med J* 1983;287:1835–1837.
200. Jabre P, Combes X, Lapostolle F, et al. Etomidate versus ketamine for rapid sequence intubation in acutely ill patients: a multicentre randomised controlled trial. *Lancet* 2009;374(9686):293–300.
201. L'Hommedieu CS. The use of ketamine for the emergency intubation of patients with status asthmaticus. *Ann Emerg Med* 1987;16(5):568–571.
202. Undem BJ, Lichtenstein LM. Drugs used in the treatment of asthma. In: Hardman JG, Limbird LE, eds. *Goodman & Gilman's the pharmacological basis of therapeutics*, 10th ed. New York, NY: McGraw-Hill, 2001:738–747.
203. Filanovsky Y, Miller P, Kao J. Myth: Ketamine should not be used as an induction agent for intubation in patients with head injury. *Can J Emerg Med* 2010;12(2):154–157.
204. Taylor P. Agents acting at the neuromuscular junction and autonomic ganglia. In: Hardman JG, Limbird LE, eds. *Goodman & Gilman's the pharmacological basis of therapeutics*, 10th ed. New York, NY: McGraw-Hill, 2001:193–213.
205. *Anectine (succinylcholine chloride) package insert*. Princeton, NJ: Sandoz, Inc, 2010.
206. McAllister JD, Gnauck KA. Emergency medicine—rapid sequence intubation of the pediatric patient. *Pediatr Clin North Am* 1999;46(6):1249–1284.
207. Mazurek AJ, Rae B, Hann S, et al. Rocuronium versus succinylcholine: are they equally effective during rapid-sequence induction of anesthesia? *Anesth Analg* 1998;87:1259–1262.
208. Beun L, Yersin B, Osterwalder J, et al. Pulseless electrical activity cardiac arrest: time to amend the mnemonic "4H&4T"? *Swiss Med Wkly* 2015;145:w14178. http://doi.emh.ch/smw.2015.14178.
209. Brandon BW, Fine GF. Neuromuscular blocking drugs in pediatric anesthesia. *Anesth Clin North Am* 2002;20(1):45–58.
210. Duff JP., Topjian A, Berg MD, et al. 2018 American Heart Association focused update on pediatric advanced life support: an update to the American Heart Association Guidelines for cardiopulmonary resuscitation and emergency cardiovascular care. *Circulation* 2018;138(23):e731–e739.
211. American Heart Association and American Academy of Pediatrics. *PALS provider manual*. Dallas, TX: American Heart Association, 2013.
212. Dorian P, Cass D, Schwartz B, et al. Amiodarone as compared with lidocaine for shock-resistant ventricular fibrillation. *N Engl J Med* 2002;346(12):884–890.
213. Roden D. Antiarrhythmic drugs. In: Hardman JG, Limbird LE, eds. *Goodman & Gilman's the pharmacological basis of therapeutics*, 10th ed. New York, NY: McGraw-Hill, 2001:651–657.
214. Valdes SO, Donoghue AJ, Hoyme DB, et al. Outcomes associated with amiodarone and lidocaine in the treatment of in-hospital pediatric cardiac arrest with pulseless ventricular tachycardia or ventricular fibrillation. *Resuscitation* 2014;85(3):381–386.

SUGGESTED READINGS

1. Anonymous. Pharmacological therapy after acute cervical spinal cord injury. *Neurosurgery* 2002;50(3 Suppl):S63–S72.
2. Bracken MB. Steroids for acute spinal cord injury. *Cochrane Database Syst Rev* 2002(3):CD001046.
3. Bracken MB, Shepard MJ, Holford TR, et al. Administration of methylprednisolone for 24 or 48 hours or tirilazad mesylate for 48 hours in the treatment of acute spinal cord injury—results of the Third National Acute Spinal Cord Injury Randomized Controlled Trial. *J Am Med Assoc* 1997;277(20):1597–1604.
4. Buck ML. Clinical experience with ketorolac in children. *Ann Pharmacother* 1994;28:1009–1013.
5. Burstein GR, Berman SM, Blumer JL, et al. Ciprofloxacin for the treatment of uncomplicated gonorrhea infection in adolescents: does the benefit outweigh the risk? *Clin Infect Dis* 2002;35(Suppl 2):S191–S199.
6. Ciarallo L, Sauer AH, Shannon MW. Intravenous magnesium therapy for moderate to severe pediatric asthma: results of a randomized, placebo-controlled trial. *J Pediatr* 1996;129:809–814.
7. Hugenholtz H, Cass DE, Dvorak MF, et al. High-dose methylprednisolone for acute closed spinal cord injury—only a treatment option. *Can J Neurol Sci* 2002;29(3):227–235.
8. Hurlbert RJ, Moulton R. Why do you prescribe methylprednisolone for acute spinal cord injury? A Canadian perspective and a position statement. *Can J Neurol Sci* 2002;29(3):236–239.
9. Mahabee-Gittens EM. Respiratory emergencies: pediatric pneumonia. *Clin Pediatr Emerg Med* 2002;3(3):200–214.
10. Mandelberg A, Tsehori S, Houri S, et al. Is nebulized aerosol treatment necessary in the pediatric emergency department? *Chest* 2000;117(5):1309–1313.
11. *Orapred (prednisolone sodium phosphate) oral solution package insert*. Wilmington, MA: Ascent Pediatrics, Inc., 2000.
12. Petri WA. Antimicrobial agents: sulfonamides, trimethoprim–sulfamethoxazole, quinolones and agents for urinary tract infections. In: Hardman JG, Limbird LE, eds. *Goodman & Gilman's the pharmacological basis of therapeutics*, 10th ed. New York, NY: McGraw-Hill, 2001:1171–1188.
13. Roberts JS, Bratton SL, Brogan TV. Acute severe asthma: differences in therapies and outcomes among pediatric intensive care units. *Crit Care Med* 2002;30(3):581–585.
14. Rowe BH, Travers AH, Holroyd BR, et al. Nebulized ipratropium bromide in acute pediatric asthma: does it reduce hospital admissions among children presenting to the emergency department? *Ann Emerg Med* 1999;34:75–85.
15. Streetman DD, Bhatt-Mehta V, Johnson CE. Management of acute, severe asthma in children. *Ann Pharmacother* 2002;36:1249–1260.
16. Williams JR, Bothner JP, Swanton RD. Delivery of albuterol in a pediatric emergency department. *Pediatr Emerg Care* 1996;12(4):263–267.
17. *Zemuron (rocuronium) package insert*. West Orange, NJ: Organon, Inc., 2002.

CHAPTER

18

Victoria Tutag Lehr
Geoffrey A. Potts
Mirjana Lulic-Botica

Topical Medications

INTRODUCTION

Topical administration represents an important method of delivery of medications for infants and children. Clinicians must inquire about topical medications or transdermal "patch" delivery systems during a medication history as parents and caregivers may overlook these agents.

Topically applied medications may undergo percutaneous absorption, resulting in systemic effects, particularly in infants, young children, and those with impaired skin barrier.[1–3]

DEVELOPMENTAL CHANGES IN SKIN

Skin development throughout infancy and childhood influences the rate and extent of absorption, metabolism, and bioavailability of topically administered medications.[1] Skin composes up to 13% of an infant's total body weight compared with only 3% of an average adult's body weight.[2] This greater total body surface area to body mass ratio results in a greater proportion of drug absorbed for infants compared with adults.[1–5] Infants are at increased risk for toxic drug serum concentrations with topical administration of anesthetics, corticosteroids, antihistamines, and antiseptics.[5,6]

Human skin is composed of two morphologically distinct layers (epithelial and mesenchymal) originating from two different germ layers during development.[2] Epithelial structures derived from the ectoderm are the epidermis, pilosebaceous–apocrine unit, eccrine unit, and nails. The ectoderm also generates hair and teeth. The mesoderm generates the mesenchymal structures: collagen, reticular and elastic fibers, blood vessels, muscles, and fat. These form the three layers of human skin: the epidermis, dermis, and subcutaneous tissue, which influence the absorption and metabolism of topically administered medications.[3]

Epidermal development is markedly influenced by gestation.[7] Before 30 weeks' gestation, the epidermis is thin and has few cell layers and a poorly formed stratum corneum.[7,8] This functional superficial layer acts as a barrier, composed of closely packed cornified keratinocytes undergoing constant exfoliation. The epidermis matures around 34 weeks' gestation. A profound postnatal effect on epidermal development occurs in preterm infants; therefore, histologically, the epidermis of the most immature infant resembles that of a term infant by 2 weeks of age.[9,10] Preterm infants younger than 35 weeks' gestation have less well-developed stratum corneum and thinner skin than older children and adults. There is no difference in thickness between the stratum corneum of term infants, children, or adults.[8]

The dermis beneath the epidermis has a rich supply of vascular beds, connective tissue, and lymphatics.[8,11] The disorderly horizontal, capillary network at birth organizes into the adult papillary loop pattern during the first 2 weeks of life.[11] Fatty connective tissue starts accumulating around week 14 of gestation and continues until birth.[9,12] The dermis and subcutaneous layer contain sebaceous and sweat glands. Sebaceous glands are not fully functional until puberty, while the sweat glands are mature at day 5 of life.[12]

FACTORS INFLUENCING PERCUTANEOUS DRUG ABSORPTION

Percutaneous absorption of a drug requires transfer from skin surface through the stratum corneum to the underlying epidermis and dermis.[3,13] Factors contributing to percutaneous absorption include physiochemical properties of the drug, concentration of drug in the vehicle, chemical and physical properties of the vehicle, thickness and hydration of the epidermis, occlusion, and the presence of inflamed, diseased, or damaged skin.[14]

Passage through the stratum corneum, a barrier of keratinized corneocytes surrounded by a lipid matrix, is rate limiting for percutaneous absorption of an exogenous substance.[14,15] Major steps in percutaneous absorption include concentration gradient, release of drug from the vehicle into the skin (partition coefficient), and drug diffusion through the epidermis (diffusion coefficient).[15] The thicker stratum corneum on the palms and soles decreases absorption, whereas the thinner skin of the eyelids, face, axillae, and genitals enhances absorption.[16]

PERCUTANEOUS ABSORPTION IN PRETERM AND TERM INFANTS

Percutaneous absorption of topically administered medications in infants differs from that in adults in several clinically significant aspects. Preterm infants have greater cutaneous perfusion and epidermal hydration compared with older infants, children, and adults, which predisposes to enhanced percutaneous absorption of topical medications risking systemic toxicity.[2,17–19]

Hydration enhances permeability of hydrophilic drugs by increasing the diffusion constant.[14–16] Although skin thickness is similar in infants and adults, infants have greater skin hydration and perfusion compared with adults, enhancing skin permeability.[20] Hydration of the stratum corneum is greatest in the axillae, genitals including the diaper area, and the antecubital and popliteal fossae.

DRUG-RELATED FACTORS

Molecular weight and size of drug significantly affect percutaneous absorption.[14–16] Solubility of drug in the vehicle and tissue is also integral to drug absorption. Generally, the more lipophilic the molecule, the more readily it penetrates the skin.[16] The stratum corneum determines the rate of diffusion through the epidermis. Drug may diffuse down along a concentration gradient, bind to sites in the tissue, and undergo vasculature resorption or metabolism by mixed function monooxygenases and other enzymes.[21]

OCCLUSION AND SKIN CONDITION

Occlusion with plastic wrap during application of a topical medication increases percutaneous absorption and risk of toxic serum concentrations of active ingredients or incipients, particularly in infants and young children.[10,17] Infected, broken, or abraded skin allows increased absorption of topical medications.[6,22] Caution is required when applying topical medications to these areas on young infants and children for a prolonged duration. Monitoring for toxicity optimizes the safe use of topical medications on an altered skin barrier.

VEHICLE AND FORMULATIONS

The type of vehicle affects percutaneous absorption and patient compliance. Vehicle pharmacokinetics is reviewed elsewhere.[15,16] *Ointments* are composed of a lipophilic drug in a base of petrolatum, mineral oil, waxes, or organic alcohols.[16,23] Ointments impart a relatively high partition coefficient (relative solubility of a drug in the stratum corneum and vehicle) and are the most efficient vehicle for topical drug delivery.[23] *Emulsions* are mixtures of two immiscible substances. *Creams* are classified as emulsions of oil in water or water in oil, depending on whether or not they can be washed off with water.[23] An oil-in-water emulsion is more cosmetically acceptable, whereas a water-in-oil emulsion is more occlusive. *Foams*, emulsions of liquid and gas, are easy to apply to hair-bearing areas. Liquid preparations consist of monophasic solutions (including *lotions*, *gels*, and *oils*), emulsions, and suspensions.[24]

TRANSDERMAL DRUG DELIVERY SYSTEMS

Transdermal drug delivery (TDD) systems or patches are medicated adhesive patches worn on the skin to deliver a drug dose into the skin to be absorbed into the systemic circulation.[25] Transdermal patches deliver a variety of drugs, including clonidine, estradiol, methylphenidate, nicotine, opioids, oxybutynin, scopolamine, testosterone, and topical anesthetics.[26–28]

Detailed reviews of TDD medications are available.[26,29–32] Application of heat, alcohol, emollients, cutting the patch, cachexia, and febrile illness may affect bioavailability of active ingredients, causing increased therapeutic effect or toxicity.[30,31] The nonadhesive backing of TDD may contain aluminum or other metals, become heated during a magnetic resonance imaging (MRI).[33] Remove any medicated patch prior to MRI and apply a new patch after the scan is complete.

Lidocaine transdermal 4% and 5% transdermal systems are safely and effectively used for older children and adolescents with chronic localized neuropathic scar pain.[32] The 5% patch is indicated for adults with peripheral herpetic neuralgia; therefore, insurers may require authorization for use in younger patients. The 4% lidocaine patch, available without a prescription, is indicated for patients aged 12 years and older.[34] Cut the patch to fit and apply to the painful area for 8 to 12 hours daily and remove for 12 hours. Onset of analgesia is gradual; therefore, use consistently for at least 3 weeks before declaring treatment failure. Common reactions to lidocaine patches are mild or transient erythema or edema, which resolves within minutes or hours after removing the patch.[34] Transdermal lidocaine therapy may significantly improve pain and function, with some patients experiencing complete relief.[32]

INSTRUCTIONS FOR PARENTS AND CAREGIVERS

Instructions for safe and effective application of topical creams and ointments include a description of the area and range of application as well as frequency and duration of use.

Limit product quantity and number of refills according to expected duration of therapy. Indicate whether the product requires rubbing into the skin or applied in a layer of specific thickness. Specify amount of product in terms of fingertip unit (FTU) if possible.[35] Caregivers must wear a sterile, disposable glove when applying creams or ointments to avoid absorbing the drug. Topical medication sharing results in cross-contamination.

Avoid covering the site of application with an occlusive dressing unless the goal is increased absorption. Plastic film occlusive dressings have been associated with bacterial infection in preterm infants.[2] Include information on whether TDD products may be cut, covered, and proper disposal.[26,36] Cautions about exposure to sunlight may be appropriate, as phototoxic reactions are possible with a variety of topical medications.[37] Provide a list of signs and symptoms indicating possible toxicities and provider contact information.

COMMON TOPICAL MEDICATIONS

TOPICAL CORTICOSTEROIDS

Indications and Clinical Use

Topical corticosteroids (TCSs) are the cornerstone of therapy for *pediatric atopic dermatitis (eczema)* as demonstrated by a comparison of international guidelines.[38] Dermatologic conditions responsive to TCS include seborrheic dermatitis, contact dermatitis, nummular dermatitis, psoriasis, lichen simplex chronicus, and arthropod bites.[39]

Selection of the specific corticosteroid strength and vehicle depends on location, extent of the skin condition, patient's age, and anticipated duration of treatment.

Corticosteroids are available as creams, ointment, lotions, gels, solutions, and shampoo and vary in cost.[40] Products are grouped according to relative vasoconstrictive and anti-inflammatory activity being approximately equivalent (Table 18.1).[40] Relative potency of a steroid product depends

TABLE 18.1	Corticosteroid Preparations			
Corticosteroid	*Strength (%)*	*Form*	*Indication and Directions*	*Cost*
VERY POTENT				
Betamethasone dipropionate augmented (Diprolene AF) (Diprosone)	0.05	C, U	Localized area, resistant thick lesion, palms, soles, scalp	$$$
Clobetasol propionate (Temovate)	0.05	C, U, G, S	High-potency indications: alopecia areata, atopic dermatitis (resistant), discoid lupus, hyperkeratotic eczema, lichen planus, lichen sclerosus, lichen simplex chronicus, nummular eczema, psoriasis, severe hand eczema	$$$
Halobetasol propionate (Ultravate)	0.05	C, U		$$$$
Halcinonide (Halog)	0.1	C, U		$$$$
Diflorasone diacetate (Psorcon)	0.05	C, U		$$$$
POTENT				
Amcinonide (Cyclocort)	0.1	C, U, L	Localized area, thick lesion, palms, soles, scalp	$$$$
Betamethasone dipropionate (Diprolene)	0.05	C, U		$$$
Betamethasone valerate (Valisone)	0.1	C, U, L		$$
Desoximetasone (Topicort)	0.25	C, U		$$$
	0.05	G		$$$
Fluocinolone acetonide (Synalar, Derma-Smoothe/FS, Capex)	0.01	C, SO, P		$$$$
	0.025	C, U		$$$
Fluocinonide (Lidex)	0.05	C, UG, S		$$
Fluticasone propionate (Cutivate)	0.05	C, L		$$$
	0.005	U		$$$
Triamcinolone acetonide (Aristocort)	0.5	C, U		$$
MODERATELY POTENT				
Betamethasone dipropionate (Diprosone)	0.05	C, U, L	Moderate-potency indications: anal inflammation, asteatotic eczema, atopic dermatitis, lichen sclerosus, nummular eczema, scabies, seborrheic dermatitis, severe dermatitis, severe intertrigo, stasis dermatitis	$$$
Betamethasone valerate (Valisone)	0.1	C, UL		$$
	0.05	C		$$
	0.01	C		$$
Clobetasone butyrate (Eumovate)	0.05	C, U		$$$
Clocortolone pivalate (Cloderm)	0.1	C		$$$
Desoximetasone (Topicort)	0.05	C, G		$$$
Fluocinolone acetonide (Lidex)	0.025	C, U		$$
Flurandrenolide (Cordran)	0.025	C, U		$$$
	0.05	C, UL		$$$
	0.005	U		$$$
	4 μg/cm²	Tape	Eczema, psoriasis	$$$
Hydrocortisone buteprate (Pandel)	0.1	C		$$
Hydrocortisone butyrate (Locoid)	0.1	C, U, S		$$$
Hydrocortisone valerate (Westcort)	0.2	C, U		$$
Mometasone furoate (Elocon)	0.1	C, U, L		$$
Prednicarbate (Dermatop)	0.1	C		$$$
Triamcinolone acetonide (Kenalog, Aristocort)	0.1, 0.25	C, U		$$
	0.025	C, U, L		$$
Mild				
Alclometasone dipropionate (Aclovate, Aqua Glycolic HC)	0.05	C, U	Face, folds, genitals, extensive areas of skin	$$$
Desonide (DesOwen, Tridesilon)	0.05	C, U, L	Mild potency indications: dermatitis (diaper, face, eyelids), intertrigo, perianal inflammation[11]	$$
Hydrocortisone (Hytone, Hycort)	0.5, 1, 2.5	C, U, L, G	Strengths ≤ 1% available OTC; limit self-treatment to <7 d	$
Hydrocortisone acetate (Cortef, Cortaid)	0.5, 1	C, U	OTC; for limited self-treatment	$

$ = <25.00 USD; $$ = 25.00 to <100.00 USD; $$$ = 100.00 to <400.00 USD; $$$$ = ≥400.00 USD.
C, cream; F, foam; G, gel; L, lotion; O, oil; OTC, over the counter; P, shampoo; Q, powder; S, solution; U, ointment.
Average wholesale price (AWP) data from Cardinal Health, Harvard Drug Group, and AmerisourceBergen; 2019.

on drug characteristics and concentration and vehicle. Generally, ointments and gels may be preferred for thick, lichenified, or excoriated lesions and are more potent than creams or lotions, with some products formulated to yield comparable potency.[39–41] Creams are preferred for acute and subacute dermatoses. Use solutions, lotions, oils, gels, or foams for hair-bearing areas where a non–oil-based vehicle is required.

Mechanism of Action

TCSs are absorbed into skin cells to exert anti-inflammatory, antimitotic, and immunosuppressive effects[42,43]:

- *Anti-inflammatory:* vasoconstriction of blood vessels decreasing inflammatory mediators at affected site; promotes lipocortin synthesis, a glucocorticoid regulated protein, inhibiting phospholipase A2, which ultimately decreases production of prostaglandins and leukotrienes
- *Antimitotic:* decrease epidermal mitosis by promoting lipocortin synthesis; inhibits cell proliferation and collagen synthesis in the dermis
- *Immunosuppressive:* inhibition of humoral factors mediating immune response and suppresses maturation, differentiation, and proliferation of immune cells

Pharmacokinetics

Corticosteroid potency, vehicle, and the skin at site of application determine the pharmacokinetics of a TCS.[42] *Corticosteroid potency* is determined in part by its *chemical structure* and by *manipulation of the steroid molecule* to produce compounds with greater lipophilicity, fewer mineralocorticoid properties, and higher potency.[43]

There are two corticosteroid classes: *fluorinated and nonfluorinated.*[42,43] Fluorinated steroids undergo chemical alteration, such as halogenation, to increase potency. Halogenation also increases mineralocorticoid properties, enhancing systemic side effects. Other chemical modifications include hydroxylation, addition of double bonds, alteration of functional groups (esterification and methylation), and addition of ketone groups. The altered structure and resulting greater potency may be due to increased lipophilicity, percutaneous absorption, and/or glucocorticoid receptor–binding activity.[41–43]

The *vehicle* indirectly affects TCS potency by influencing the environment in which the corticosteroid is absorbed. Ointments help hydrate the stratum corneum, enhancing corticosteroid penetration through occlusion.[44] Solvents such as propylene glycol and ethanol affect solubility of corticosteroids, enhancing percutaneous absorption. Finally, *thickness and integrity of the stratum corneum* are inversely proportional to absorption of TCS.[42–44] Penetration into eyelid skin is better than into palmar skin, and inflamed or diseased skin is more readily penetrated than intact skin.

Adverse Effects

Common side effects of TCS are *atrophy and striae,* which may be irreversible.[45–48] Cutaneous side effects include hypopigmentation, telangiectasias, purpura, tinea and scabies incognito, granuloma gluteale infantum, acneiform eruptions, perioral dermatitis, and steroid rosacea. These side effects are more common with inappropriate prolonged use of high-potency fluorinated TCS applied on the face and intertriginous areas. Applied periocular, there is a risk for development of *glaucoma or cataracts. Allergic contact dermatitis to TCS* should be considered if a patient's condition is unresponsive or worsens with treatment.[49] A combination of corticosteroid–antifungal preparations for treatment of dermatophytosis is associated with persistent and recurrent infections or atrophy.[17] *Tachyphylaxis*—diminished response to prolonged application—may develop with prolonged TCS use.[39]

More serious complications of TCS use are systemic side effects, which have been associated with use of both high- and low-potency formulations.[46] Such effects are identical to those of systemically administered corticosteroids and include suppression of the hypothalamic–pituitary–adrenal (HPA) axis, Cushing syndrome, failure to thrive, poor linear growth, hyperglycemia, and glycosuria. Factors augmenting systemic absorption include more potent steroids, use over large surface areas, application on skin folds, prolonged use, occlusive dressings, younger age, and liver or renal disease.[50] Consider laboratory tests for adrenal suppression after prolonged treatment, particularly over large areas of skin.

Monitoring Parameters for Patients and Caregivers

Patients and caregivers require education prior to initiating TCS therapy to minimize the risk of adverse effects and improve adherence.[46,51–53] *TCS phobia* is a phenomenon of negative feelings and beliefs related to TCS by patients and caregivers that contributes to treatment failure in atopic dermatitis.[53] Consistent information from evidence-based sources regarding TCS adverse effects and monitoring is required from the health care team.

Burning, stinging, itching, and redness often occur in the affected area with initial application but dissipate over time once the skin barrier returns to normal. Closely monitor for atrophy or discoloration. Do not apply TCS on the eyelids or near the eyes long term, especially in patients with a history of glaucoma. Treatment beyond 2 to 3 weeks in any one area with very potent TCS is discouraged. The child's provider should be consulted immediately if vision problems, persistent headaches, increased thirst or urination, unusual weakness or weight loss, and dizziness occur, as these symptoms may indicate HPA suppression from systemic steroid absorption.[47,54]

TOPICAL CALCINEURIN INHIBITORS: TACROLIMUS AND PIMECROLIMUS

Indications and Clinical Use

Topical calcineurin inhibitors (TCIs), tacrolimus (Protopic) and pimecrolimus (Elidel), are macrolides that penetrate the skin, causing local immunosuppression.[55–57] Their development followed failure of topical cyclosporine as an alternative treatment for atopic dermatitis without the corticosteroid side effects. Cyclosporine is ineffective topically due to large molecular size and poor dermal penetration. Tacrolimus and pimecrolimus are currently Food and Drug Administration (FDA) approved for the management of moderate-to-severe atopic dermatitis in patients aged 2 years and older.[56] Tacrolimus ointment was more effective in children with moderate-to-severe atopic dermatitis, with a faster onset of action and similar safety profile compared with pimecrolimus cream.[58] Use in children less than 2 years of age is not FDA approved; children aged 2 to 15 years should only use the 0.03% ointment. Tacrolimus and pimecrolimus products are included in Table 18.2.

TABLE 18.2 Topical Calcineurin Inhibitor Preparations

Topical Calcineurin Inhibitor	*Strength (%)*	*Form*	*Indication and Directions*	*Cost*
Pimecrolimus (Elidel)	1	C	Moderate-severe atopic dermatitis; second-line therapy Apply thin layer to affected skin twice daily <2 y of age (off label) May be preferred for facial skin	$$$$ 60 g cream
Tacrolimus (Protopic)	0.03, 0.1	C, O	Moderate-severe atopic dermatitis; second-line therapy Apply thin layer to affected skin twice daily Children ≥2 y of age (0.03%); adults (0.03, 0.1%) <2 y of age (off label) Ointment preferred for severe disease, elbows or nighttime use	$$$$ 60 g cream, ointment

$ = <25.00 USD; $$ = 25.00 to <100.00 USD; $$$ = 100.00 to <400.00 USD; $$$$ = ≥400.00 USD.
C, cream; O, oil.
Average wholesale price (AWP) data from Cardinal Health, Harvard Drug Group, and AmerisourceBergen; 2019.

Off-label use of tacrolimus and pimecrolimus has been increasing for dermatitis in infants, psoriasis, lichen planus, seborrheic dermatitis, allergic contact dermatitis, and vitiligo.[59–61]

International guidelines for the management of *atopic dermatitis* universally recommended TCI for as second-line therapy.[38] Some guidelines designate TCI as first-line management for skin areas prone to TCS atrophy.[62] TCIs combined with TCS decrease steroid dependency and frequency of disease flare.[63] TCI can be alternated with TCSs for disease flares.[57,64] Apply the TCI at the first sign of itch or rash, then taper and replace with a moisturizer for maintenance when symptoms clear.[55]

Advantages over TCS therapy include patients having inadequate response to TCS, or "steroid phobia" interfering with adherence despite evidence-based education, for dermatitis of head and neck resistant to low-potency TCS.[57] TCIs have a slightly delayed onset of action with longer duration of response.

Mechanism of Action

Topical *tacrolimus* binds to specific T-cell receptors, resulting in inhibition of T-lymphocyte activation.[59] Tacrolimus forms a complex with FKBP-12, calcium, calmodulin, and calcineurin, inactivating the phosphatase activity of calcineurin.[64] This results in the prevention of dephosphorylation and translocation of the nuclear factor of activated T cells (NF-ATs). NF-AT is a nuclear component responsible for initiation of gene transcription for lymphokines, such as interleukin 2 (IL-2) and interferon γ (IFN-γ). These reactions inhibit the transcription of the genes involved in lymphokine formation.[34] Tacrolimus also inhibits transcription of genes encoding for the markers involved in early stages of T-cell activation, such as IL-3, IL-4, IL-5, granulocyte-macrophage colony-stimulating factor, and tumor necrosis factor α (TNF-α). Release of mediators from skin mast cells and basophils are inhibited by tacrolimus.[64,65]

Similar to tacrolimus, *pimecrolimus* binds with increased affinity to macrophilin-12 (FKBP-12) and inhibits T-cell activation by preventing transcription of early cytokines, such as IL-2 and IFN-γ (Th1-type), IL-4, and IL-10 (Th2-type) synthesis from T cells.[64,66]

Pimecrolimus also prevents release of inflammatory cytokines and mediators from mast cells with antigen/immunoglobulin E complex.[64] Studies demonstrate that pimecrolimus, unlike corticosteroids, interferes with the inflammatory cascade, with no effect on keratinocytes, fibroblasts, endothelial cells, Langerhans cells, the hypothalamus, or adrenals.[66–68]

Pharmacokinetics

Tacrolimus, when ingested orally, undergoes hepatic metabolism, with very little drug systemically absorbed from topical application.[59] *Pimecrolimus* is skin selective, being more lipophilic than tacrolimus and corticosteroids, and has higher molecular weight compared with corticosteroids.[65] *Tacrolimus* and *pimecrolimus* do not undergo dermal-mediated drug metabolism.[65] These TCIs show good dermal penetration with minimal systemic absorption as demonstrated by low serum concentrations, useful for applying to thinner and more sensitive skin of children.[69]

With regard to systemic absorption, *tacrolimus* is a relatively large molecule with limited dermal penetration; damaged skin has a sevenfold increased absorption rate.[59,68] Blood concentrations from topical tacrolimus are typically undetectable or subtherapeutic; therapeutic range for organ transplant recipients is 5 to 15 ng/mL. Patients using tacrolimus for moderate-to-severe atopic dermatitis (80%) had tacrolimus serum concentrations below the detectable concentration.[70]

Pimecrolimus has a favorable skin penetration–permeation profile, imparting a low degree of dermal absorption, which may explain why pimecrolimus is less likely than tacrolimus to induce immunosuppression in animal models.[58] However, normal antibody titers were documented after vaccination in children treated with tacrolimus, alleviating systemic immunosuppression concerns.[71] Pimecrolimus has a high affinity to the dermis, making this an ideal therapeutic agent for atopic dermatitis without systemic side effects.[68] A study with 22 infants between the ages of 3 and 23 months, even with the application of pimecrolimus on up to 92% of body surface area, resulted in blood concentrations ranging from 0.1 to 2.6 ng/mL.[72] Blood concentrations from topical pimecrolimus are typically less than 2 ng/mL.[68,70]

Adverse Effects

Tacrolimus is well tolerated, with application-site irritation (pruritus and burning sensation) the most frequently reported adverse event, particularly early in therapy.[55,56,69]

Pimecrolimus causes less burning sensation than tacrolimus.[55] These effects resolve within 2 hours and subside as dermatitis improves.[70,73] Tacrolimus may be preferred for more severe disease and use on elbows or knees or at nighttime secondary to the ointment base.[58]

Cutaneous infections should be treated and cleared prior to TCI as these agents may have a localized immunosuppressive effect.[56]

Significant adverse events, noted more than in vehicle-control groups, include herpes simplex infection, varicella, and non–application-site vesiculobullous eruptions.[63,72] Interestingly, incidence of cutaneous and noncutaneous infections in patients treated with tacrolimus is lower than that in children with atopic diathesis.[55,70] There are case reports of patients with lamellar ichthyosis and Netherton syndrome (triad of trichorrhexis invaginata, ichthyosis linearis circumflexa, and atopic dermatitis) with elevated whole-blood tacrolimus concentrations, but without systemic toxicity.[55,74]

Consider monitoring *serum tacrolimus concentrations* in patients with congenital abnormalities affecting epidermal barrier function. Lymphadenopathy (0.8%) was reported during clinical trials of tacrolimus, usually related to skin infection.[55,68] *Rare adverse events* include pyrexia and diarrhea. Use an effective method of contraception during therapy with TCIs as there are insufficient data on pregnancy outcomes.[75]

In 2006, the FDA issued an advisory based on animal studies, case reports, and mechanism of action about a *potential risk for malignancy* associated with TCI use:

TCIs have been associated with rare cases of malignancy (including skin and lymphoma); therefore, the FDA boxed warning recommends limiting use to short term and intermittent treatment using the minimum amount necessary for symptom control and limit to involved areas.[76]

Reports of TCI-related skin cancer or lymphoma following use of TCI were later demonstrated to be related to severe atopic dermatitis, preexisting malignancy, with no relationship to TCI use.[77] During the past 15 years, studies of pediatric patients treated with tacrolimus ointment 0.03% for atopic dermatitis demonstrated no malignancies.[55,58,78,79,80]

An international database of over 13,000 patients includes safety and efficacy data on up to 4 years of tacrolimus use.[81] Pimecrolimus has been studied extensively in children with atopic dermatitis in large multicenter controlled trials with application twice daily for up to 1 year.[82] Currently, there is no direct evidence to support the association between TCI use and increased risk for malignancy. Debate exists regarding the clinical relevance of this advisory.[82]

Monitoring Parameters for Patients and Caregivers

Counsel patients to expect a slower onset of symptom relief with TCI compared with TCS therapy.[56,68,69] If signs and symptoms of atopic dermatitis do not improve after 6 weeks of TCI therapy, contact provider because cutaneous T-cell lymphoma may present as clinically eczematous dermatitis.[77,83,84] Monitor area of application for infection. If diagnosed with infection, call provider to discontinue TCI application until clinically resolved.[85]

Tacrolimus and *pimecrolimus* should be applied in a thin layer twice daily, rubbing in gently and completely.[84] Wash hands thoroughly after application. Do not swim, shower, or bathe immediately after applying TCI. Continue treatment for 1 week after symptoms clear. Do not apply *tacrolimus ointment* to wet skin. *Pimecrolimus cream* is safe to use on head, neck, and intertriginous areas, applied under clothing and washed off with soap and water.[56,69]

Minimize *burning sensation* on application by chilling medication prior to application. May apply moisturizers after applying TCI and avoid occlusive dressings. Sunlight and ultraviolet A/ultraviolet B (UVA/UVB) rays may cause phototoxic reactions.[84]

Rare adverse events include blistering rash, lymph node swelling, fever, and diarrhea-inform provider. Use an effective method of birth control during TCI therapy.[59,84] Inform your provider if you become pregnant or are breastfeeding.[84]

VITAMIN D3 ANALOGS

Indications and Clinical Use

Since the 1930s, large oral doses of vitamin D were used to control psoriatic lesions, yet limited by efficacy and hypercalcemia.[86] Vitamin D effects include decreased epidermal proliferation and inhibition of inflammatory cytokines IL-12/23 p-40, IL-α, IL-1β, and TNF-α.[87,88] Topical administration of vitamin D3 analogs, including *calcipotriene* and *calcitriol*, provides "nonsteroidal" alternatives for this challenging condition.[89–92] Vitamin D3 analogs may be monotherapy or prescribed combined with TCSs, for example, calcipotriene and betamethasone dipropionate ointment (Taclonex) or foam (Enstilar) for synergy and steroid sparing.[89,93–96]

Calcipotriene is a synthetic vitamin D3 analog approved for the treatment of plaque psoriasis for adults in the United States since 1994.[94,97] Pediatric use is "off label"; trials in children aged 2 to 14 years with mild-to-moderate plaque psoriasis involving less than 30% body surface area show the agent to be effective and well tolerated with mild skin irritation at doses up to 50 g/week.[96,98] However, careful monitoring for hypercalciuria and hypercalcemia is prudent.[93] Recently, the FDA approved calcipotriene foam, 0.005% (Sorilux), for the treatment of plaque psoriasis of the scalp and body in adolescents aged 12 years or older.[97]

Calcipotriene is an effective alternative to TCSs for managing plaque-type psoriasis.[94,99] Improvement usually occurs after 2 weeks of therapy.[94] Topical vitamin D analogs usually have a slower onset of action compared with TCSs in the management of psoriasis, yet tend to provide a longer disease-free interval and greater reduction in disease severity index score.[89,98] When compared with anthralin or 15% of coal tar, calcipotriene was more effective in reducing psoriasis area and severity index score.[96,100]

Although calcipotriene is effective as monotherapy, combined therapy has proven effective for more resistant psoriasis.[99,100] Calcipotriene enhances efficacy of phototherapy, though should be applied after light exposure, both UVB and psoralen UVA.[101] Formulations of topical vitamin D3 analogs are listed in Table 18.3.

Mechanism of Action

The skin converts vitamin D analog to vitamin D3, which undergoes hepatic and renal metabolism into the active form, calcitriol.[88] Calcitriol regulates intestinal calcium and phosphate absorption, promoting bone formation and mineralization.[88] As a synthetic vitamin D3 analog, calcipotriene binds the vitamin D cytoplasmic receptor, subsequently enters the nucleus, and activates gene transcription.[88,102] Although calcipotriene binds the vitamin D receptor with the same affinity as calcitriol, it is 100 times less active on calcium metabolism.[102]

Calcipotriene inhibits keratinocyte proliferation and differentiation, reversing the abnormal keratinocyte change in psoriasis.[102] In addition, calcipotriene acts on cytokines involved

TABLE 18.3 Topical Vitamin D3 Analogs

Vitamin D3 Analog	*Strength*	*Form*	*Indication and Directions*	*Cost*
Calcipotriene (Dovonex)	0.005%	O, S	Plaque psoriasis Children ≥2 y of age: twice daily for up to 8 wk—effective and well tolerated—up to 50 g/wk Adults: apply thin layer to affected area(s) once daily in the morning or twice daily for up to 8 wk. Do not exceed 100 g/wk.	$$$$ 60 g ointment
Calcipotriene/betamethasone (Taclonex)			Increased efficacy when combined with corticosteroids	
Calcipotriene (Sorilux)	0.005	F	Plaque psoriasis of scalp and body in adolescents aged 12 y or older (nongreasy, for hair-bearing areas)	$$$$ 60 g
Calcitriol (Vectical)	3 μg/g	O	Psoriasis, atopic dermatitis Children (off label) May be better tolerated on sensitive skin vs. calcipotriene	$$$$ 100 g

$ = <25.00 USD; $$ = 25.00 to <100.00 USD; $$$ = 100.00 to <400.00 USD; $$$$ = ≥400.00 USD.
F, foam; O, oil; S, solution.
Average wholesale price (AWP) data from Cardinal Health, Harvard Drug Group, and AmerisourceBergen; 2019.

in immune function. Specifically, decreasing pro-inflammatory cytokine IL-8 and increasing IL-10, thereby promoting a Th2 response (humoral) and inhibiting the Th1 response (cell mediated), implicated in psoriasis.[102]

Pharmacokinetics

Systemic absorption of calcipotriene ointment is greater than the cream.[103] Applying the drug in an ointment base to psoriatic lesions results in systemic absorption of up to 6% of the topically applied dose (label). Absorption of calcipotriene scalp solution can be 1% of the applied dose.

Following systemic absorption, the majority of calcipotriene undergoes hepatic metabolism to inactive compounds, with less than 1% of parent drug recovered in urine and feces. Calcipotriene is chemically unstable and degraded in the presence of UV light, hydrocortisone valerate, ammonium lactate, or salicylic acid.[104] Consult a pharmacist for compatibility.

Adverse Effects

Minor adverse effects include transient skin irritation, photosensitivity, allergic contact dermatitis, and exacerbation of psoriasis lesions.[98] Burning sensation has occurred with cream application to face and flexures.[89,93] Combining calcipotriene with betamethasone may decrease local irritating effects of the drug.[93,99,101] Hyperpigmentation is associated with calcipotriene cream, but not the solution.[97] Skin atrophy and folliculitis have occurred.[97,103] Calcitriol (Vectical) is expensive but may be equally effective and, possibly, less irritating than calcipotriene (Dovonex).[105] Topical vitamin D analogs may irritate skin lesions associated with atopic dermatitis.[106]

Serious risks are hypercalcemia and hypercalciuria, which usually do not develop with application of less than 100 g of calcipotriene per week for adults or with doses less than 30% of body surface area or 50 g/week for children.[98,107–109] Consider 24-hour urine collection for elevated ratios of calcium to creatinine to monitor for hypercalciuria in children and infants having calcipotriene applied to extensive body surface areas.[108,109]

Draw serum calcium concentrations and discontinue topical medication to rule out hypercalcemia. Do not use calcipotriene for patients with calcium metabolism disorders or at risk for vitamin D toxicity.[93,109]

Monitoring Parameters for Patients and Their Caregivers

Apply calcipotriene cream in a thin layer to the affected area and rub in gently.[96,109] Wash hands thoroughly after applying product to avoid spreading active drug to other areas or risking systemic absorption. Do not apply to face or skin folds as these areas are more prone to irritation. Avoid exposing areas of application to sun to prevent drug inactivation and phototoxicity reactions due to photosensitizing dermal thinning.[96,109]

Monitor for signs and symptoms of hypercalcemia, including fatigue, confusion, loss of appetite, headache, nausea, vomiting, constipation, and increased urination.[88,107] If these symptoms develop, discontinue calcipotriene and contact prescriber immediately. Hypercalcemia associated with calcipotriene reverses upon discontinuation of therapy.[107]

TOPICAL PHOSPHODIESTERASE-4 INHIBITORS: CRISABOROLE

Crisaborole is a second-line treatment option for mild-to-moderate atopic dermatitis due to cost and limited time on the market.[57,110,111] The 2014 American Academy of Dermatology guidelines include hydration with emollients, moisturizers, and TCSs as first-line treatment for atopic dermatitis.[38] Crisaborole became available in the United States until late 2016.[110,112] See Table 18.4 for crisaborole products. Clinical trials in atopic dermatitis compared with vehicle control showed significant improvement in investigator global assessment and in pruritis.[110–112] An advantage of crisaborole is facial and intertriginous skin tolerability.[57,112] Crisaborole is approved for children older than 2 years and for adults with mild-to-moderate atopic dermatitis and relief of associated symptoms.[113]

Mechanism of Action

Crisaborole is a benzoxaborole that inhibits phosphodiesterase-4 (PDE-4) by binding to the bimetal center of the PDE4 enzyme.[114]

TABLE 18.4 Topical Phosphodiesterase-4 Inhibitors

Phosodiesterase-4 Inhibitor	*Strength*	*Form*	*Indication and Directions*	*Cost*
Crisaborole (Eucrisa)	2%	O	Mild-moderate atopic dermatitis: children aged 2–15 y and adults ≥3 mo (off label) Apply thin layer to affected skin twice daily	$$$$ 60 g

$ = <25.00 USD; $$ = 25.00 to <100.00 USD; $$$ = 100.00 to <400.00 USD; $$$$ = ≥400.00 USD.
O, oil.
Average wholesale price (AWP) data from Cardinal Health, Harvard Drug Group, and AmerisourceBergen; 2019.

Inhibition of normal PDE4 activity suppresses cytokine production and reactive oxygen species production.[114] This is the same enzyme target of oral apremilast (Otezla) for psoriasis, proving the enzyme is active in multiple inflammatory cascades for different dermatologic diseases.[114]

Pharmacokinetics

Crisaborole is absorbed systemically and is highly protein bound (97%). The two inactive metabolites undergo renal elimination.[110,115]

Adverse Effects

The most common adverse effect reported with crisaborole use is application-site burning/pain of mild-to-moderate intensity, especially on the lips. This can be mitigated by applying petroleum jelly first, followed by crisaborole.[111,112] Application-site reactions usually resolve within day of application.[112] Contact urticaria and other hypersensitivity reactions have been associated with crisaborole.[116] Data are accumulating on long-term use and demonstrate use over 1 year with minimal adverse effects.[117]

Monitoring Parameters for Patients and Caregivers

Apply crisaborole ointment in a thin layer to the affected areas twice daily.[116] Mild-to-moderate burning or pain at application site may occur and will subside within 24 hours. If severe pruritus, swelling, and erythema occur, discontinue crisaborole and contact provider as this may indicate a hypersensitivity reaction.[116]

TOPICAL ANTIBACTERIALS

Indications and Clinical Use

Primitive societies derived crude antimicrobials from animals, minerals, and plants to treat infections, promote healing, reduce pain and inflammation, debride damaged tissue, and mask foul smells.[118,119] Discovery of chemical preservatives and disinfectants limited wound infections.[120,121] Modern topical antibacterials prevent infection in abrasions, cuts, burns, and wounds and treat superficial wounds.[122,123]

Mild-to-Moderate Acne Vulgaris

Topical antimicrobials may have decreased efficacy for this indication secondary to resistant strains of *Propionibacterium* bacteria.[124,125] To decrease the number of inflammatory and noninflammatory lesions, a combination of topical agents is recommended over monotherapy.[125]

Pediatric Burns

Microbial proliferation in burn wounds may significantly delay healing.[126] Within 48 hours of burn injury, *Staphylococcus aureus, Corynebacterium,* and *Streptococcus* species colonize the wound.[123] Topically applied antimicrobial products may interfere with wound healing by impairing epithelialization; therefore, a balance is the goal.[123,127,128] First-degree burns are not at risk for infection and do not require antimicrobial therapy.[123] For second-degree (partial-thickness) burns, bacitracin, polymyxin B sulfate, or a combination of ointment or hydrocolloid and hydrofiber nanocrystalline silver dressings are effective.[123] For deep second- and third-degree (full-thickness) burns, silver sulfadiazine or mafenide acetate cream applied once or twice daily, nanocrystalline silver dressings, and hypochlorous antiseptic solutions prior to early excision and wound closure are recommended.[123,129] Selection of a topical antimicrobial agent for burn wounds varies among clinicians and health systems. There are limited data on the efficacy of antimicrobials in preventing burn wound infection, despite their continued use in clinical practice.[122,123,130]

Impetigo

This common skin infection among children and adolescents, usually caused by *S. aureus* and/or *Streptococcus pyogenes,* has two main clinical forms: nonbullous impetigo and bullous or blistering impetigo.[122,131] The nonbullous form usually occurs around the mouth and nose in children aged 2 to 5 years and is treated with topical or systemic antibiotics to avoid spread and decrease symptom duration.[132] Mupirocin, fusidic acid, and retapamulin (Altabax) are the main topical antibiotics for treating minor cases of impetigo with limited, smaller lesions.[122,131,133] Prescribe topical therapy for the shortest possible duration and in context of local resistance patterns.[131]

Topical Antimicrobial Formulations

Antimicrobials are available as over-the-counter (OTC) and prescription products in a variety of topical forms (bars, liquids, creams, ointments, gels, shampoos, solutions, wipes, and gauzes).[122,123,134] Appropriate use may prevent further emergence of antibiotic-resistant strains as well as avoidance of contact dermatitis.[122,135] Selection of an antimicrobial product can be complex as the numerous formulations vary in indication, adverse effects, and cost.[122] Prolonged use of any topical antimicrobial as monotherapy may result in decreased efficacy and antibiotic resistance[136,137]; therefore, alternate antimicrobial agents use is suggested. Combination products are generally more effective than when used alone and may inhibit development of antibiotic resistance.[138] Topical antimicrobial agents frequently used for infants and children are listed in Table 18.5.

TOPICAL ANTIFUNGAL AGENTS

Indications and Clinical Use

Fungi often infect the skin surface, invading the stratum corneum and commonly cause of superficial skin infections in infants and children.[139–141] The three species of aerobic fungi,

TABLE 18.5 Topical Antimicrobial Preparations

Antimicrobial Agent	*Class*	*Mechanism of Action*	*Spectrum of Activity*	*Clinical Use/Therapeutic Guidelines*	*Adverse Effects*	*Cost*
Azelaic acid (20%) (Azelex)	Dietary constituent of whole grain cereals and animal products	Exact mechanism is unknown	*Staphylococcus epidermidis, Propionibacterium acnes*	Acne vulgaris, rosacea[138]	Pruritus, dry skin, dermatitis, hypopigmentation, hypertrichosis, worsening of asthma	$$$
Bacitracin	Isolated in 1943 from a *Bacillus subtilis* strain cultured from an open wound	Inhibits cell wall synthesis by complexing with C55-prenol pyrophosphatase, involved in transfer of polysaccharides, liposaccharides, and peptidoglycans to the cell wall	Bactericidal and has a narrow spectrum of activity directed predominantly against the gram-positive organisms: *Staphylococcus aureus, Streptococcus pneumoniae,* and *Clostridium difficile.* Other susceptible organisms include *Neisseria, Haemophilus influenzae, Treponema pallidum, Actinomyces,* and *Fusobacterium*	To give a broader spectrum of antibacterial coverage, bacitracin is also available in combination with polymyxin and neomycin (Neosporin or triple antibiotic) or with polymyxin alone (Polysporin)	Pruritus and burning at application site *Delayed-type hypersensitivity or anaphylaxis in patients with chronic stasis dermatitis, conjunctivitis, keratoconjunctivitis*	$
Benzoyl peroxide (2.5%–20%)	Derived from chlorohydroxyquinoline, a byproduct of coal tar	Release of active or free-radical oxygen capable of oxidizing bacterial proteins, removal of excess sebum and mild desquamation	*P. acnes*	Acne vulgaris and oily skin Reduces resistance to other antimicrobials[125]	Excessive drying, peeling, erythema, edema	$
Clindamycin (1%) gel	Derivative of lincomycin, an antibiotic derived from *Streptomyces* species	Binds the 50S subunit of bacterial ribosomes and inhibits protein synthesis Both bacteriostatic and bactericidal in susceptible organisms	Aerobic gram-positive cocci (*Streptococcus* and most *S. aureus,* both of which cause folliculitis) and anaerobic gram-positive and gram-negative organisms, including *P. acnes*	Acne vulgaris, folliculitis, erythrasma, rosacea, and Fox–Fordyce disease[204]	Pruritus, burning, erythema, excessive dryness, peeling, and oily skin Rresistance[138]	$$
Erythromycin (2%)	Fermentation product of *Streptomyces erythreus*	Macrolide antibiotic that irreversibly binds the 50S subunit of bacterial ribosomes, thereby inhibiting protein synthesis	Erythromycin is effective against gram-positive cocci, *Corynebacterium diphtheriae, H. influenzae, Legionella pneumophila, Chlamydia* organisms, *T. pallidum, Mycoplasma pneumoniae, Ureaplasma urealyticum,* and *P. acnes* through resistance building	Acne vulgaris	Erythema, scaling, tenderness, burning, itching, oiliness, and dryness	$$
Fusidic acid (2%)	Derived from the fungus *Fusidium coccineum*	Inhibits ribosomal translocation, which blocks protein synthesis	*Staphylococcal* species, limited activity against *Streptococcal* sp., no activity against gram-negative organisms	Acne vulgaris, dermatitis, pyoderma, furuncle, impetigo, eczema, burns[122]	Rash, pruritus Resistance	$$
Gentamicin (0.1%)	Aminoglycoside derived from *Micromonospora purpurea*	Inhibits the 30S ribosomal subunit, thereby inhibiting protein synthesis	*S. aureus* and gram-negative bacteria such as *Escherichia coli, Proteus* organisms, and *Pseudomonas aeruginosa*	Primary skin infections: impetigo contagiosa, superficial folliculitis, ecthyma, furunculosis, sycosis barbae, and pyoderma gangrenosum Secondary skin infections: infectious eczematoid dermatitis, pustular acne, pustular psoriasis, infected seborrheic dermatitis, infected contact dermatitis	Burning, stinging, redness, lacrimation with ophthalmic use, rash, pruritus, erythema with topical use	$

(*continued*)

TABLE 18.5 Topical Antimicrobial Preparations (*continued*)

Antimicrobial Agent	*Class*	*Mechanism of Action*	*Spectrum of Activity*	*Clinical Use/Therapeutic Guidelines*	*Adverse Effects*	*Cost*
Metronidazole (0.75%–1%)	Synthetic nitroimidazole derivative	Exact mechanism is unknown Exhibits anti-inflammatory actions	*Bacillus fragilis, Bacteroides melaninogenicus, Fusobacterium* organisms, *Veillonella* organisms, *Clostridium* organisms, *Peptococcus* organisms, *Peptostreptococcus* organisms, *Entamoeba histolytica, Trichomonas vaginalis, Giardia lamblia,* and *Balantidium coli*	Acne rosacea Decreases number of papules and pustules but has no effect on erythema or telangiectasias[208]	Dryness, stinging, burning Contact allergy	$
Mupirocin (Bactroban)	Mupirocin is a metabolite of *Pseudomonas fluorescens*	Mupirocin (pseudomonic acid) inhibits bacterial isoleucyl-tRNA synthetase, which, in turn, leads to impaired synthesis of bacterial RNA, proteins, and cell wall. The concentrations present in topical formulations allow for bactericidal activity	Mupirocin is bactericidal against *S. aureus, S. epidermidis,* and *S. pyogenes.* Mupirocin is also active against methicillin-resistant *S. aureus* (MRSA). However, MRSA resistance to mupirocin is gradually increasing. Mupirocin is ineffective against *P. aeruginosa, Streptococcus faecalis, Streptococcus faecium, Streptococcus bovis,* and fungi	Mupirocin is used for treatment of skin infections secondary to staphylococci and streptococci, including impetigo, folliculitis, impetiginized atopic dermatitis, burns, lacerations, and leg ulcers. Intranasal mupirocin is used to eliminate staphylococci, including MRSA[122,209]	Adverse events include application-site burning, pain, and itching. Contact allergy is extremely rare; only two cases reported[133]	$$
Neomycin	Neomycin is a bactericidal aminoglycoside first isolated from *Streptomyces fradiae*	Neomycin exerts its effect by binding bacterial 30S ribosomal subunit and inhibiting protein synthesis	Broad gram-negative coverage including *E. coli, Enterobacter aerogenes, Klebsiella pneumoniae,* and *Proteus vulgaris.* Susceptible gram-positive organisms include *S. aureus, Enterobacter faecalis,* and *Mycobacterium tuberculosis.* Neomycin is not active against *P. aeruginosa* and has poor activity against streptococci.	Widely used for infections of skin and mucous membranes. Used in combination with other topical antibiotics because of resistance to neomycin along with its limited spectrum of activity. Specifically, polymyxin B is added to provide anti-*Pseudomonas* activity, and bacitracin may be added to broaden the gram-positive coverage to include antistreptococcal activity	Contact dermatitis, erythema, rash, urticaria	$
Polymyxin B	Isolated from the aerobic gram-positive rod *Bacillus polymyxa*	Cationic-free amino groups of polymyxin function as a deterrent to disrupt the phospholipid bacterial membranes	Polymyxin B is bactericidal in vitro against gram-negative bacteria, including *Proteus mirabilis, P. aeruginosa,* and *Serratia marcescens.*	Open wounds, in combination with other topical antibiotics to broaden antibiotic coverage. Bacitracin + polymyxin B is available OTC as Polysporin cream. Neomycin + polymyxin B + bacitracin is available OTC as Neosporin ointment		$
Retapamulin (Altabax) 1%	Semisynthetic derivative of pleuromutilin from fungus (approved 2007)	Inhibits bacterial protein synthesis on 50S ribosomal unit	Bacteriostatic against *Streptococcus pyogenes* or methicillin-sensitive *S. aureus*	Treatment of impetigo in ages ≥ 9 mo	Burning upon application Not intended for mucosal area	$$$

TABLE 18.5 Topical Antimicrobial Preparations (*continued*)

Antimicrobial Agent	*Class*	*Mechanism of Action*	*Spectrum of Activity*	*Clinical Use/Therapeutic Guidelines*	*Adverse Effects*	*Cost*
Silver sulfadiazine (SSD, Silvadene)	Derived from dual mechanisms of silver and sulfa moieties	Silver ions bind to negatively charged components in proteins and nucleic acids, thereby effecting structural changes in bacterial cell walls, membranes and nucleic acids that affect binding to DNA	Broad-spectrum antimicrobial coverage, including gram-positive bacteria, most gram-negative bacteria, and some yeast forms	Adjunct in prevention and treatment of infection in second- and third- degree burns[210,211]	Significant percutaneous absorption of sulfadiazine can occur especially when applied to extensive burns Do not use in premature neonates and infants aged <2 mo as sulfas may displace bilirubin from protein-binding sites and cause kernicterus	$
Sulfacetamide sodium (Sebizon)	Sulfa derivative	Interferes with bacterial growth; inhibits bacterial folic acid synthesis by a competitive antagonism of *para*-aminobenzoic acid (PABA)	Bacteriostatic effect against gram-positive and gram-negative bacteria	Seborrheic dermatitis, secondary cutaneous bacterial infections	Rare cases of drug-induced systemic lupus erythematous and Stevens–Johnson syndrome reported, exfoliative dermatitis, toxic epidermal necrolysis, rash, erythema	$$
Tetracyclines (Topicycline, Achromycin)	First isolated from the *Streptomyces* species in late 1940s	Reversibly bind to 30S ribosome and inhibit binding of aminoacyl-tRNA to acceptor site on 70S ribosome Mechanism unknown for acne vulgaris. Systemic tetracyclines decrease free fatty acids in acne lesions	Broad spectrum of activity against gram-positive, gram-negative, rickettsiae, mycobacterium, and protozoa.	Treatment of acne vulgaris[138]	Yellowing of skin (may be removed by washing off tetracycline)	$$

$ = <25.00 USD; $$ = 25.00 to <100.00 USD; $$$ = 100.00 to <400.00 USD; $$$$ = ≥400.00 USD.
C, cream; F, foam; G, gel; L, lotion; NA, not available; O, oil; OTC, over the counter; P, shampoo; Q, powder; S, solution; U, ointment.
Average wholesale price (AWP) data from Cardinal Health, Harvard Drug Group, and AmerisourceBergen; 2019.

collectively known as dermatophytes, include *Trichophyton, Microsporum,* and *Epidermophyton,* which require keratin for growth.[141]

Tinea Infections

These superficial fungal infections are caused by three species of fungi and named for affected body part, including tinea capitis (scalp), tinea corporis (general skin), tinea cruris (groin), tinea pedis (feet), and tinea unguium (nails).[139,141,142] Tinea infections are from direct contact with infected humans (anthropophilic organisms), animals (zoophilic organisms), or from exposure to contaminated soil or fomites (geophilic organisms). Diagnosis is via a detailed history and physical examination and potassium hydroxide microscopy. Culture or histologic examination is rarely required, except for tinea capitis.[142]

Most tinea infections can be managed with topical therapies; oral treatment is, however, reserved for tinea capitis, severe tinea pedis, and tinea unguium.[139–142] Topical therapy with fungicidal allylamines may have slightly higher cure rates and shorter treatment courses than with fungistatic azoles.[142–144] Onychomycosis is difficult to treat with topical therapies because the nail bed is difficult to penetrate and, therefore, requires prolonged systemic treatment.[145]

Antifungal agents for application to skin are available as creams, ointments, lotions, shampoos, solutions, sprays, foams, powders, and gels, which readily penetrate the stratum corneum.[141,146] Butenafine (Lotrimin Ultra) and terbinafine are available OTC and in many generic inexpensive forms. Topical antifungal agents used in pediatric practice with mechanism of action, spectrum of activity, indications, and common adverse effects are listed in Table 18.6.

Mechanism of Action

Classification of antifungals depends on site of action: *azoles,* which inhibit the synthesis of ergosterol (the main fungal sterol); *polyenes,* which physically and chemically interact with fungal membrane sterols; and *5-fluorocytosine,* which inhibits macromolecular

TABLE 18.6 Topical Antifungal Preparations

Agent	*Strength*	*Dosage Form*	*Spectrum of Activity*	*Clinical Use/Indications*	*Adverse Effects*	*Cost*
Class	Azoles					
Clotrimazole (Lotrimin AF, Gyne-Lotrimin)	1% 2%	C, U, L, S, Q	Broad-spectrum: *Candida* spp., *Trichophyton tonsurans, Trichophyton rubrum, Trichophyton mentagrophytes, Epidermophyton floccosum, Microsporum canis*	Apply twice daily for tinea cruris (treat for 2 wk), tinea corporis, tinea pedis (treat for 4 wk) Approved for ages ≥2 y Vulvovaginal candidiasis ages ≥12 y: 100 mg/d for 7 d; 200 mg/d intravaginal daily for 3 d at bedtime	Mild skin irritation, burning, itching, dryness May contain benzyl alcohol *Caution: neonates*	$ 30 g cream (generic)
Econazole (Spectazole)	1%	C, F	*T. rubrum, T. mentagrophytes, T. tonsurans, M. canis, Microsporum audouinii, Microsporum gypseum, E. floccosum, C. albicans, Malassezia furfur*	Apply daily for 14 d for tinea corporis, tinea cruris; 30 d for tinea pedis, tinea versicolor Cutaneous candida including diaper dermatitis apply twice daily (limited data)	Burning, itching, stinging Reconsider diagnosis if no improvement after 2 wk	$$ 30 g cream
Efinaconazole (Jublia)	10%	S	*T. rubrum* and *T. mentagrophytes*	Apply daily for 48 wk for toenail onychomycosis for *T. rubrum* and *T. mentagrophytes* Off label for children and adolescents	Burning, vesicle formation on surrounding skin, *flammable liquid*	$$$$ 4 mL
Ketoconazole (Nizoral, Xolegel, Extina)	2% 1%	C, D, G, F, P	*T. rubrum, T. mentagrophytes, E. floccosum, M. furfur, Candida* sp.	Adults: Apply cream once to twice daily for tinea pityriasis versicolor, tinea pedis (6 wk), tinea corporis, tinea cruris (2 wk) ≥12 y: seborrheic dermatitis: apply foam twice daily for 2 wk, or gel once daily Dandruff: 1% shampoo every 3–4 d for 8 wk *(Discontinued 2020)*	Burning, stinging, itching, reaction to sulfite in vehicle *Foam and gel are flammable* *Cream/gel contain propylene glycol: caution in neonates*	$$ 60 g cream
Luliconazole (Luzu)	1%	C	*T. rubrum, T. mentagrophytes, T. tonsurans, Trichophyton* spp., *Candida albicans*	Apply a thin layer to affected areas, and approximately 1 inch of immediate surrounding areas, once daily for 2 wk for tinea pedis, tinea cruris, tinea corporis, *T. rubrum, E. floccosum* Approved for ages ≥12 y	Itching and pain at application site, rare hypersensitivity reactions	$$$ 60 g
Miconazole (Monistat, Monistat-Derm, Micatin, Zeasorb AF) (+zinc oxide/white petrolatum Vusion)	2%	C, G, L, S, U, R	*T. rubrum, T. mentagrophytes, E. floccosum, C. albicans*	Infants, children, adults: apply twice daily for 2–4 wk Diaper dermatitis, tinea corporis, tinea cruris, tinea pedis, tinea corporis, tinea versicolor, cutaneous candidiasis *Adolescents and adults:* vulvovaginal candidiasis	Contact dermatitis, burning, local irritation *Products may contain benzyl alcohol: caution in neonates* *OTC products not for self-care in ages <2 y*	$ 60 g cream
Oxiconazole (Oxistat) 1%	1%	C, L	*T. rubrum, T. mentagrophytes, E. floccosum, M. furfur*	Apply once to twice daily for 2–4 wk Tinea pedis, tinea cruris, tinea corporis, tinea versicolor	Pruritus, burning, stinging	$$$ 60 g cream
Sertaconazole (Ertaczo)	2%	C	*T. rubrum*	Apply twice daily for 4 wk Tinea pedis		$$$$ 60 g
Sulconazole (Exelderm)	1%	C, S	*T. rubrum, T. mentagrophytes, E. floccosum, M. furfur*	Apply daily to twice daily for 3 wk, 4 wk for tinea pedis, tinea cruris, tinea corporis	Itching, burning stinging, redness	$$$ 60 g cream
Terconazole (Terazol)	0.4%, 0.8%	C	*Candida* sp.	Postmenarchal females Intravaginal use for vaginal yeast infections	Burning upon application, itching	$$ 20 g cream

TABLE 18.6 Topical Antifungal Preparations (*continued*)

Agent	*Strength*	*Dosage Form*	*Spectrum of Activity*	*Clinical Use/Indications*	*Adverse Effects*	*Cost*
Class	Allylamines					
Naftifine (Naftin)	1%, 2%	C, G	*T. rubrum, T. mentagrophytes, T. tonsurans, E. floccosum, M. canis, M. audouinii, M. gypseum, Candida* sp.	Tinea pedis, tinea cruris, tinea corporis Response may take up to 4 wk	Burning, stinging, dryness	$$ 2% cream 30 g
Terbinafine (Lamisil)	1%	G, C, R	*E. floccosum, T. mentagrophytes, T. rubrum*	Tinea pedis, tinea cruris, tinea corporis	Local irritation, burning, itching, dryness	$ 30 g cream
Class	Benzylamine					
Butenafine (Mentax, Lotrimin Ultra OTC)	1%	C, G, R	*M. furfur, E. floccosum, T. mentagrophytes, T. rubrum, Trichophyton tonsurans*	Apply twice daily for 1 wk or daily for 4 wk May have better response with 4-wk treatment Tinea corporis, tinea pedis, tinea cruris		$ 30 g cream
Class	Other					
Amphotericin B (Fungizone)	3%	C, L *Not currently available in the United States*	*Candida monilia* spp.	Cutaneous and mucocutaneous mycotic infections	Erythema, burning sensation, drying effect	$
Ciclopirox (Loprox, Penlac)	0.77%, 8%		*T. rubrum, T. mentagrophytes, E. floccosum, M. canis,* cutaneous candidiasis due to *C. albicans,* tinea pityriasis due to *M. furfur*	Tinea pedis, tinea cruris, tinea corporis, onychomycosis of fingernails and toenails	Burning, edema	$ 6.6 mL
Gentian violet	1%, 2%	S	*Candida, Cryptococcus, Epidermophyton, Trichophyton*	Antifungal dye: superficial fungus "thrush" infections of the skin Available OTC in the United States	Allergic contact dermatitis; necrosis of intertriginous areas; avoid using on ulcerated skin or eczema areas Avoid eye contact or internal use Stains skin and clothing	$
Iodochlorhydroxyquin (Clioquinol) (Alaquin) with hydrocortisone 0.5%	3%	C	*T. mentagrophytes, T. rubrum*	Chloroquine derivative use for tinea pedis, tinea cruris in ages >2 y	Burning, skin irritation, skin stain, potential cross-sensitivity with select antimalarials	$$$$ 30 g
Nystatin (Mycostatin)	100,000 U/g	C, S, U, Q	*C. albicans, Candida parapsilosis, Candida krusei,* and *Candida tropicalis* Ineffective against dermatophytes	Polyene antimycotic from *Streptomyces noursei* used for treating *Candida* infections of skin (intertrigo) and mucous membranes (thrush, vaginal candidiasis), diaper dermatitis	Contact dermatitis, rash	$ 30 g cream
Tolnaftate (Tinactin)	1%	C, S, Q Available OTC in the United States	*E. floccosum, T. mentagrophytes, T. rubrum, M. furfur*	Tinea pedis, tinea cruris, tinea corporis, and tinea versicolor infections	Mild irritation, stinging, burning May contain propylene glycol: caution in neonates	$ 60 g cream
Undecylenic acid (Fungi-Nail)	25%	C, S Available OTC in the United States	Natural fatty acid derivative of castor oil *E. floccosum, T. mentagrophytes, T. rubrum*	Tinea pedis, tinea cruris Apply twice daily for 2–4 wk Not for self- medication in ages <2 y	Rash, local irritation, stinging	$ 60 g cream

$ = <25.00 USD; $$ = 25.00 to <100.00 USD; $$$ = 100.00 to <400.00 USD; $$$$ = ≥400.00 USD).
C, cream; F, foam; G, gel; L, lotion; NA, not available; O, oil; OTC, over the counter or available without a prescription in the United States; P, shampoo; Q powder; S, solution; U, ointment.
Average wholesale price (AWP) data from Cardinal Health, Harvard Drug Group, and AmerisourceBergen; 2019.

synthesis.[147,148] A variety of mechanisms contributes to the development of resistance to antifungals.[147] These mechanisms include alteration in drug target, alteration in sterol biosynthesis, reduction in the intercellular concentration of target enzyme, and overexpression of the antifungal drug target. *Azole drugs* such as miconazole, clotrimazole, and ketoconazole are *fungistatic*, limiting fungal growth, depending on epidermal turnover to shed still-living fungus from skin surface.[149] *Allylamines* and *benzylamines* such as terbinafine, naftifine, and butenafine are *fungicidal*.[148,149] Cure rates are higher with shorter treatment courses using topical fungicidal allylamines compared with fungistatic azoles.[148]

PEDICULICIDES

Indications and Clinical Use

Pediculosis and scabies are caused by ectoparasites and affect children worldwide. Head lice infestation is one of the most prevalent communicable conditions in the United States, with over 12 million cases annually.[150] Pruritus is a common presenting symptom.[151] Clinicians caring for infants and children must consider safe, easy to use, and effective treatments for lice or scabies infestations. *Resistance to pediculicides* is increasing worldwide as multiple pediculicides are used over time.[152–154] Studies conducted in the Southern United States, Canada, and the United Kingdom demonstrate increasing resistance to commonly prescribed pediculicides, including pyrethrins, permethrins, and lindane.[151,152,155–157] Clinicians are advised to review local resistance patterns.[150]

Nonpharmacologic Treatments

Treatment with occlusive agents (petroleum jelly) lacks consistent efficacy data.[158] Gentle cleansers lotions have been successful.[159] Alternative or home therapies including neem or tea tree oil, hydrogen peroxide, sodium borate, phenol-based disinfectants, bleach, olive oil and lemon, isopropyl alcohol, apple cider vinegar, and clove oil are not recommended secondary to lack of efficacy data.[160] Keeping finger nails short and clean and shampooing hair regularly to remove any mites or eggs are recommended.[150]

Pharmacologic Treatments

Careful selection of pediculicides minimizes potential toxicities associated with systemic absorption.[5,161] Pyrethrins are natural insecticides found in the pyrethrum flower, *Chrysanthemum cinerariaefolium*, which have been used for centuries in Iran as an insecticide.[162] Permethrin, the generic name for 3-phenoxybenzyl (±)-*cis–trans*-3-(2,2-dichlorovinyl)-2,2-dimethylcyclopropanecarboxylate, is manufactured as a racemic mixture of *cis* and *trans* isomers in a 1:3 ratio for human use.[162] Permethrin is a photostable synthetic pyrethroid modeled after the naturally occurring insecticide.[162]

Permethrin is also available OTC in the United States as a 1% cream rinse for treatment of head lice in children as young as 2 months and is considered first-line treatment secondary to efficacy and safety.[151,162] Permethrin is safe for use in pregnant women. There is no known cross-reactivity with other pyrethrins. The 5% cream formulation is safe and effective for treatment of scabies and is the treatment of choice in children older than 2 years and pregnant women.[163,164] A double-blind, randomized study comparing crotamiton 10% cream with permethrin 5% cream was conducted in children aged 2 months to 5 years, some of whom were lindane treatment failures.[165] Four weeks after treatment, 89% of the permethrin-treated group versus 60% of the crotamiton-treated group was cured. Another study compared 5% permethrin cream with 1% lindane lotion for treatment of scabies in patients aged 2 months to 75 years.[166] The study demonstrated 91% and 86% cure rates approximately 4 weeks after treatment with permethrin and lindane, respectively. Although permethrin is not FDA approved for treatment in infants younger than 2 months, it was used successfully without side effects in a 23-day-old infant.[167] Permethrin 5% cream has been used off label for treating head lice, yet is not FDA approved for this indication.[168]

Pyrethrin is available in combination with piperonyl butoxide without a prescription in the United States for treatment of head lice in children older than 2 years.[162,169] As the pyrethrins are not ovicidal, retreatment is necessary to kill any newly hatched nymphs.

Malathion is an organophosphate acetylcholinesterase inhibitor insecticide indicated for treatment of head lice in children older than 6 years.[170] Trials using malathion lotion have included children aged 2 to 11 years.[153,157] The product was withdrawn from the U.S. market in 1995 and reintroduced in 1999 when more effective pediculicides were needed.[171] Disadvantages of malathion include flammable vehicle, chemical odor, prolonged application time of 8 to 12 hours, and cholinesterase depletion with respiratory depression if accidentally ingested.[172,173] Malathion is available by prescription in the United States and is an effective pediculicide.[169]

Sulfur 5% to 10% compounded in cream or ointment has been used for over 150 years in treating scabies.[174–176] Mechanism of action is unknown. An open-label study used 5% to 10% sulfur in petrolatum to treat scabies in patients aged 2 months to 6 years, with a 71% cure rate at 4 weeks post-treatment.[176] Mild facial edema was the only significant adverse event. Overall, compounded sulfur preparations are safe, with use limited by messiness and offensive odor.

Lindane is an organochlorine insecticide that inhibits neurotransmission, resulting in respiratory and muscular paralysis in arthropods via noncompetitive inhibition of γ-aminobutyric acid (GABA) receptor.[161,177] Resistance is due to GABA-receptor mutations.[178] Lindane toxicity is common, which may result in potentially serious and irreversible central nervous system effects, ranging from headaches to seizures, aplastic anemia, and even death.[161] The FDA has specific instructions for use.[178] Lindane is not recommended for use in children younger than 2 years, pregnant or lactating women, patients weighing less than 50 kg, or patients with extensive dermatitis.[5,161,178] Lindane is no longer used because of resistance and risk for serious toxicity.[179] Commonly prescribed pediculicides are reviewed in Table 18.7.

Mechanism of Action

Pyrethrin and *permethrin* act on the parasite cell membrane ATPases, disrupting sodium transport and causing neurotoxicity and paralysis.[180] Malathion is an acetylcholinesterase inhibitor insecticide, and the action of sulfur is unknown.[174,179]

Pharmacokinetics

Both *pyrethrin* and *permethrin* demonstrate low dermal absorption.[162,170] After application of 5% permethrin cream, mean absorption was less than 1%, and maximum amount absorbed was 2% of the applied dose.[162] Pyrethrin and permethrin are metabolized in the skin via ester cleavage, which subsequently

TABLE 18.7 Summary of Topical Treatments for Head Lice and Scabies

Agent	*Brand Name(s)*	*Formulation*	*Indication(s)*	*Directions*	*Adverse Effects*
Benzyl alcohol	Ulesfia	5% lotion	Head lice May be effective for cases of permethrin and pyrethrins resistance. *Most likely safe during pregnancy; do not exceed recommended dose*	Apply to dry hair and scalp, leave on 10 min, rinse. Dose depends on hair length; refer to labeling. Repeat after 7 d.	Eye irritant; local pain, redness, pruritus; wash hands after applying *Do not use on infants aged <6 mo: respiratory distress risk*
Dimethicone	LiceMD	Gel	Lice: kills via suffocation and disruption of water regulation	Apply to hair; use comb to remove lice, nits, and eggs. Shampoo to remove. Repeat in 10 d.	Burning, stinging; irritation
Ivermectin	Sklice	0.5% lotion	Head lice for ages >6 mo Prescription *Avoid during pregnancy: may cause fetal harm*	Apply to dry hair and scalp; leave on 10 min; rinse Single use only	Conjunctivitis, local burning, irritation *Do not use on infants aged <6 mo*
Lindane	Generic formulas; Kwell brand (NA; withdrawn)	1% shampoo	*Second line:* Resistant head and pubic lice; not for prophylaxis of Norwegian scabies No longer recommended by the American Academy of Pediatrics *Teratogenic: do not use if pregnant*	Apply to dry hear wearing nonlatex gloves; leave on 4 min; rinse *No retreatment* *Hazardous agent disposal precautions*	Contact dermatitis, burning, hair loss, CNS toxicity *U.S. Boxed Warning: severe neurologic toxicities; seizures; death* *Contraindicated: uncontrolled seizure disorders, premature infants* *Caution: infants, elderly, skin conditions, patients weighing <50 kg*
Malathion	Ovide	0.5% lotion	Head lice Ages ≥ 6 y *Most likely safe during pregnancy if do not exceed recommended dose, use aqueous-base product*	Apply to dry hair, leave on 8–12 h, rinse. Repeat once after 7–9 d.	*Flammable vehicle,* scalp irritation
Permethrin	Nix, Elimite, Acticin	1% cream rinse (OTC) 5% cream (prescription in the United States)	1%: head lice 5%: scabies ages >2 mo Pregnancy B: *considered safe for use during pregnancy*	Head lice: apply after shampooing, leave on 10 min, rinse, Scabies: apply cream once; repeat in 14 d if needed	Local irritation, burning, tingling at application site
Pyrethrins extract (with piperonyl butoxide)	A-200, Licide, Pronto, RID, Triple X, and R&C	Shampoo, lotion OTC	Head lice Pregnancy C: *safety during pregnancy unknown*	Apply to dry hair, lather, leave on 10 min, rinse. Repeat in 7–10 d	Local irritation, possible cross-reaction with Compositae (*Chrysanthemum,* ragweed) plants, asthma exacerbations
Sulfur (precipitated)	Compounded in petrolatum	5%–10% ointment	Scabies in patients as young as 2 mo of age *Limited use in pregnancy; likely safe*	For scabies: apply at night for 3 d to clean skin	Offensive odor, messy application

CNS, central nervous system; NA, not available; OTC, over the counter.

allows for rapid urinary excretion of inactive metabolites. Less than 2% of permethrin cream or cream rinse is absorbed into the circulation.[162] Permethrin can be detected on hair for up to 10 days after application, which may contribute to resistance.

Adverse Events

Common complaints associated with *pyrethrin* and *permethrin* are application-site burning, irritation, and tingling sensation.[162,181] Despite permethrin being preserved with formaldehyde, reports of allergic contact dermatitis are rare. Patients allergic to ragweed, *Chrysanthemum* flowers, or plants of the Compositae family, may experience contact sensitivity to pyrethrin.[162,182] Children with a history of asthma may experience asthma exacerbations or breathing difficulties during application of pyrethrin.[183]

Monitoring Parameters for Patients and Caregivers

Pediculicides must be used according to instructions because of the potential for toxicity, particularly in infants and young children.[5,153,182–186] Parents and caregivers require clear education on the use of these agents.

Treatment of scabies involves application of permethrin 5% cream from neck to toes for 8 to 12 hours, with particular attention to postauricular areas, web spaces, genitals, and finger nails.[179,187,188] Treatment of scalp and face is recommended for infants younger than 2 years.[167,169] Close contacts should also be treated. Pruritus may persist for up to 3 weeks after treatment. A second treatment at 1 week is particularly important if there is involvement of palms and soles.

Treatment of *pediculosis (head lice)* involves application of permethrin 1% cream rinse for 10 minutes before washing off.[150,156,169]

General instructions include avoid scratching and keep any open sores clean.[156,158,189]

Appropriate doses of oral antihistamine medications can manage itching. Avoid taking baths or applying calamine lotion to reduce itching while using the prescription cream as these interventions may remove or act as a barrier to the pediculicide.

Environmental management includes washing all clothing, towels, and bed linens in hot water (or isolated) that were used in the past 3 days to minimize reinfection.[150,160,189] Dry at high heat rather than air-drying. Mites can survive on fomites for several days, such as store objects that are not machine washable into a bag for a week. Dry-cleaning will kill the mites. Thoroughly vacuum carpets, furniture, bedding, and car interiors, and discard the vacuum-cleaner bag.

RETINOID THERAPY FOR ACNE

Indications and Clinical Use

Retinoids are composed of natural compounds and synthetic derivatives with vitamin A activity.[190] The era of retinoid therapy for acne vulgaris began in the 1970s with tretinoin (all-*trans*-retinoic acid).[191] New retinoids are compared with tretinoin efficacy. Newer synthetic retinoids may be more advantageous than tretinoin because of their more specific mechanism of action.[125,136] Adapalene, a derivative of naphthoic acid, and tazarotene have retinoid and anti-inflammatory properties.[192,193]

Topical retinoids used in combination with topical or oral antibiotics have been shown to be more effective than either therapy alone.[125,136,194] Antibiotics reduce the *P. acnes* population and have direct anti-inflammatory effects, which make them effective in treating inflammatory lesions. Resistance is increasing; therefore, use of antibiotic monotherapy is discouraged.[135,195] Overall, topical retinoids will reduce the number of acne lesions by 40% to 70%.[196,197] Retinoids are applied at bedtime to the entire surface of skin prone to development of mild-to-moderate acne rather than spot treatment of individual acne lesions.[198,199] The topical retinoids with anti-inflammatory comedolytic actions are recommended as a foundation in acne therapy, except for patients with severe disease (nodular/conglobata types requiring oral therapy).[200]

Product Selection

Tretinoin, adapalene, and tazarotene are all effective for the treatment of comedonal acne.[196,199] All-*trans*-retinoic acid (*tretinoin*), vitamin A acid, is marketed as Retin-A, Retin-A-Micro (0.1% sustained-release gel, less irritating vehicle), and Avita cream.[194,200,201]

Tazarotene (Tazorac) has been shown to be most efficacious, yet may be more expensive than other retinoids.[194] Topical steroids are sometimes combined with tazarotene to decrease irritation.[200] Adapalene (Differin) is not photolabile, allowing daytime application with less skin irritation compared with tretinoin or tazarotene.[200]

Other Indications

Retinoids may also be helpful in treating postinflammatory hyperpigmentation.[190] Retinoids normalize proliferation and differentiation of keratinocytes, giving them usefulness in diseases with abnormal keratinization, such as ichthyosis and palmoplantar keratodermas. Other diseases that may be responsive to topical retinoids include Darier disease, verruca plana, pityriasis rubra pilaris, and oral lichen planus. Tretinoin has demonstrated effectiveness for cosmetic treatment of photoaging and, therefore, may require prior authorization for some prescription plans.[190] Tazarotene is effective in psoriasis.[92] Bexarotene (Targretin) 1% gel is a synthetic retinoid used for treatment of stage I cutaneous T-cell lymphoma.[194] Alitretinoin 0.1% gel, a naturally occurring endogenous retinoid, is effective for Kaposi sarcoma lesions.[194] Commonly prescribed topical retinoid agents are listed in Table 18.8.

Mechanism of Action

Acne lesions are produced by a combination of four primary pathogenic conditions: (a) sebum production by the sebaceous gland, (b) *P. acnes* follicular colonization, (c) alteration in the keratinization process, and (d) release of inflammatory mediators into the skin.[43,196] Topical retinoids act on follicular epithelium and loosen comedo, permitting flow of sebum to skin surface.[6] Inflammatory changes may also precede hyperkeratinization.[202]

Appreciation of *retinoid function* requires an understanding of two retinoid receptor families. These two nuclear receptor families include retinoic acid receptors (RARs) and retinoid X receptors (RXRs).[203] Each family is composed of α, β, and γ subtypes. Predominant subtypes in human skin are RAR-α, RAR-γ, RXR-α, and RXR-β. RARs and RXRs always exist as dimers in vivo, RARs exist as heterodimers complexed with RXR, and RXRs exist as either heterodimers or homodimers. These receptors are bound by their ligands, and the receptor–ligand complex binds promoter regions to initiate transcription. Altered gene transcription affects epidermal and follicular keratinocyte growth and differentiation.[203] The resulting effect may partly explain the *comedolytic* actions of retinoids. All-*trans*-retinoic acid (tretinoin) is a nonspecific ligand that binds all RAR receptors with high affinity.[203]

Adapalene, a naphthoic acid retinoid, is a synthetic molecule that binds more specifically RAR-β and RAR-γ.[192] *Tazarotene*, an acetylenic retinoid, is also a synthetic molecule that selectively binds RAR-β and RAR-γ and has no affinity for RXRs.[193]

Monitoring Parameters for Patients and Caregivers

Advise patients that response to treatment occurs after 6 to 8 weeks of therapy and that symptoms may worsen during the first 2 to 4 weeks.[199,204] Informing patients that side effects improve with increased duration of treatment may help improve adherence.[205] Several months of treatment may be necessary to achieve desired response. Teratogenic and embryotoxic effects have been demonstrated in animals receiving oral retinoids or topical applications greatly exceeding the normal human dose.[206,207] There is a paucity of large, well-controlled trials in women, but increased spontaneous abortions and major congenital abnormalities have occurred in pregnant women on other retinoids.[207] *Counsel patients to use an effective form of contraception while using topical retinoids.*

TABLE 18.8 Topical Retinoid Therapy

Agent	*Brand Name(s)*	*Formulation*	*Directions*	*Adverse Effects*
Adapalene	Differin ProActiv	0.1% gel, cream, pledgets, and solution; 0.3% gel (0.1% gel OTC in the United States, 2016)	Apply gel in thin film once daily at bedtime after cleansing skin Avoid lips, eyes and mucous membranes	Burning sensation, flushing, scaling *Less skin irritation than tretinoin and tazarotene; may apply during day* May interact with other topical agents (salicylic acid) to dry skin Avoid sulfa products and sun exposure Potential pregnancy risk; discontinue, avoid during pregnancy
Alitretinoin	PanRetin	0.1% gel	Apply a generous coat of gel to lesions four times daily without rubbing Allow to dry 3–5 min before covering with clothing Do not cover with occlusive dressing	Rash, pruritus, paresthesia, exfoliative dermatitis Harmful to fetus, *avoid pregnancy during treatment* Breast milk transfer unknown
Bexarotene	Targretin	1% gel	For stage I cutaneous T-cell lymphoma (mycosis fungoides)	Erythema, scaling, pruritus, burning, stinging, dryness, increased photosensitivity, and irritation Teratogenic: *avoid during pregnancy*
Tazarotene	Tazorac	0.05%, 0.1% gel (may be more expensive than other retinoids)	Most efficacious retinoid for comedonal acne	Erythema, scaling, pruritus, burning, stinging, dryness, increased photosensitivity, and irritation Combine with high-potency topical steroids, for example, betamethasone dipropionate or halobetasol to reduce irritation Teratogenic: *avoid during pregnancy*
Tretinoin	Retin-A, Retin-A-Micro, Avita cream	0.025%, 0.05%, and 0.1% cream; 0.01%, 0.025%, 0.04%, 0.1% gel; 0.05% solution; 0.05% lotion	For comedonal acne treatment, apply thin layer to affected area at bedtime for 7 wk Irritation may require spacing applications to every other day or less frequently Also used for reversal of photoaging effects.	All retinoids: Erythema, scaling, pruritus, burning, stinging, dryness, increased photosensitivity, and irritation Try 0.1% sustained-release gel for less irritation or 0.05% lotion is better tolerated. Potential pregnancy risk, discontinue, avoid during pregnancy

OTC, over the counter.

REFERENCES

1. Kearns GL, Abdel-Rahman SM, Alander SW, et al. Developmental pharmacology—drug disposition, action, and therapy in infants and children. *N Engl J Med* 2003;349(12):1157–1167.
2. Rutter N. The immature skin. *Br Med Bull* 1988;44(4)1:957–970.
3. Yosipovitch G, Maayan-Metzger A, Merlob P, et al. Skin barrier properties in different body areas in neonates. *Pediatrics* 2000;106:105–108.
4. Visscher M, Geiss S. Emollient therapy for newborn infants—a global perspective. *Newborn Infant Nurs Rev* 2014;14(4):153–159.
5. Callelo VJ, Curtin P, Eggleston W, et al. Drops, ointments, gels, and patches: the dangers of topical medications. *Emerg Med* 2017;49(4):152–160.
6. Ponnusamy V, Venkatesh V, Clarke P. Skin antisepsis in the neonate: what should we use? *Curr Opin Infect Dis* 2014;27(03):244–250.
7. Visscher M, Narendran V. The ontogeny of skin. *Adv Wound Care* 2013;3:291–303.
8. Fairley JA, Rasmussen JE. Comparison of stratum corneum thickness in children and adults. *J Am Acad Dermatol* 1983;8(5):652–654.
9. Hoath SB, Shah KN. Physiologic development of the skin. In: *Fetal and neonatal physiology*. Philadelphia, PA: Elsevier; 2017:498.e4–514.e4.
10. Hoath SB, Narendran V. Adhesives and emollients in the preterm infant. *Semin Neonatol* 2000;5(4):289–296.
11. Genzel-Boroviczény O, Strötgen JS, Harris AG, et al. Orthogonal polarization spectral imaging (OPS): a novel method to measure the microcirculation in term and preterm infants transcutaneously. *Pediatr Res* 2002;51(3):386–391.
12. Visscher M, Narendran V. Neonatal infant skin: development, structure and function. *Newborn Infant Nurs Rev* 2014;14(4):135–141.
13. Roberts M, Pellett M, Cross ES. Skin transport. In: *Dermatological and transdermal formulations*. New York, NY: Marcel Dekker, 2009:88–194.
14. Wester RC, Maibach HI. Percutaneous absorption of drugs. *Clin Pharmacokinet* 1992;23(4):253–266.
15. Wester RC, Maibach HI. Cutaneous pharmacokinetics: 10 steps to percutaneous absorption. *Drug Metab Rev* 1983;14(2):169–205.
16. Abraham MH, Chadha HS, Mitchell RC. The factors that influence skin penetration of solutes. *J Pharm Pharmacol* 1995;47:8–16.
17. Blume-Peytavi U, Tan J, Tennstedt D, et al. Fragility of epidermis in newborns, children and adolescents. *J Eur Acad Dermatol Venereol* 2016;30(Suppl 4):3–56.
18. Barrett DA, Rutter N. Transdermal delivery and the premature neonate. *Crit Rev Ther Drug Carr Syst* 1994;11:1–30.
19. Blume-Petavi U, Stamatas GN, Hauser M, et al. Skin care practices for newborns and infants: review of the clinical evidence for best practices. *Pediatr Dermatol* 2011;29(1):1–14.
20. Harpin VA, Rutter N. Barrier properties of the newborn infant's skin. *J Pediatr* 1983;102(3):419–442.
21. Tibbitt MW, Dahlman JE, Langer R. Emerging frontiers in drug delivery. *J Am Chem Soc* 2016;138:704–717.
22. Weinberger B, Hanna N, Gropper CA, et al. Transdermal xenobiotics in newborn skin. *J Toxicol Cutaneous Ocul Toxicol* 2003;22(1–2):51–67.
23. Ricciatti-Sibbald D, Sibbald RG. Dermatologic vehicles. *Clin Dermatol* 1989;7(3):11–24.
24. Eaglstein WH, Cash KR, Corcoran GR. Challenges encountered in dermatologic drug development. *Acta Dermosifiliogr* 2009;100(Suppl 1):86–91.
25. Durand C, Alhammad A, Willett KC. Practical considerations for optimal transdermal drug delivery. *Am J Heal Pharm* 2012;69:116–124.
26. Delgado-Charro MB, Guy RH. Effective use of transdermal drug delivery in children. *Adv Drug Deliv Rev* 2014;73:63–82.
27. Ruggiero A, Coccia P, Arena R, et al. Efficacy and safety of transdermal buprenorphine in the management of children with cancer-related pain. *Pediatr Blood Cancer* 2013;60(3):433–437.
28. Findling RL, Dinh S. Transdermal therapy for attention-deficit hyperactivity disorder with the methylphenidate patch (MTS). *CNS Drugs* 2014;28(3):217–218.
29. Zernikow B, Michel E, Anderson B. Transdermal fentanyl in childhood and adolescence: a comprehensive literature review. *J Pain* 2007;8(3):187–207.
30. Hemanth Kumar G. Transdermal drug delivery system: an overview. *Int J Res Pharm Sci* 2012;3(3):451–457.

31. Kadam AS, Ratnaparkhi MP, Chaudhary SP. Transdermal drug delivery: an overview. *Int J Res Dev Pharm Life Sci* 2014;3:1042–1053.
32. Nayak S, Cunliffe M. Lidocaine 5% patch for localized chronic neuropathic pain in adolescents: report of five cases. *Paediatr Anaesth* 2008;18(6):554–558.
33. ISMP. Burns in MRI patients wearing transdermal patches. *Acute Care Inst Safe Medicat Pract* 2004. https://www.pharmacytimes.com/publications/issue/2005/2005-07/2005-07-9732. Accessed May 29, 2019.
34. Lidocare 03-4% lidocaine patch. Nutrition & Fitness, Inc. DBA NFI Consumer Products, Inc. February 2019.
35. Mishra AK, Saraswat D. Topical corticosteroid abuse in dermatology. *IOSR J Dent Med Sci* 2016;15(7):110–114.
36. Lampert A, Haefeli WE, Seidling HM. Information gaps in package inserts cause insufficient patient information on correct handling of transdermal patches. *Dtsch Medizinische Wochenschrift* 2019;144(05):e36–e41.
37. Paller AS, Hawk JLM, Honig P, et al. New insights about infant and toddler skin: implications for sun protection. *Pediatrics* 2011;128(1):92–102.
38. LePoidevin LM, Lee DE, Shi VY. A comparison of international management guidelines for atopic dermatitis. *Pediatr Dermatol* 2019;36(1):36–65.
39. Mehta A, Nadkarni N, Patil S, et al. Topical corticosteroids in dermatology. *Indian J Dermatol Venereol Leprol* 2016;82:371–378.
40. Hengge UR. Topical corticosteroids. In: Gaspari A, Tyring S, Kaplan D, eds. *Clinical and basic immunodermatology: second edition.* Cham, Switzerland: Springer, 2017.
41. Jackson DB, Thompson C, McCormack JR, et al. Bioequivalence (bioavailability) of generic topical corticosteroids. *J Am Acad Dermatol* 1989;20(5)Pt 1:791–796.
42. Goa KL. Clinical pharmacology and pharmacokinetic properties of topically applied corticosteroids: a review. *Drugs* 1988;36(Suppl 5):51–61.
43. Li VC, Chowdhury MM. Dermatological pharmacology: topical agents. *Med (United Kingdom)* 2017;3(12):1941–2166.
44. Kwatra G, Mukhopadhyay S. Topical corticosteroids: pharmacology. In: Lahiri K, eds. *A treatise on topical corticosteroids in dermatology: use, misuse and abuse.* Singapore, Singapore: Springer, 2017:11–22.
45. Barnes L, Kaya G, Rollason V. Topical corticosteroid-induced skin atrophy: a comprehensive review. *Drug Saf* 2015;38(5):493–509.
46. Hengge UR, Ruzicka T, Schwartz RA, et al. Adverse effects of topical glucocorticosteroids. *J Am Acad Dermatol* 2006;54(1):1–15.
47. Sahni D, Darley CR, Hawk JLM. Glaucoma induced by periorbital topical steroid use—a rare complication. *Clin Exp Dermatol* 2004;29:617–619.
48. Schoepe S, Schäcke H, May E, et al. Glucocorticoid therapy-induced skin atrophy. *Exp Dermatol* 2006;15(6):406–420.
49. Butani L. Corticosteroid-induced hypersensitivity reactions. *Ann Allergy Asthma Immunol* 2002;89(5):439–444.
50. Coureau B, Bussières JF, Tremblay S. Cushing's syndrome induced by misuse of moderate-to high-potency topical corticosteroids. *Ann Pharmacother* 2008;42(12):1903–1907.
51. Feldman SR, Camacho FT, Krejci-Manwaring J, et al. Adherence to topical therapy increases around the time of office visits. *J Am Acad Dermatol* 2007;57(1):81–83.
52. Ference JD, Last AR. Choosing topical corticosteroids. *Am Fam Physician* 2009;79(2):135–140.
53. Smith SD, Fischer G. Understanding parent fears associated with the use of topical corticosteroids in paediatric dermatology. *Australas J Dermatol* 2009;57(3):199–204.
54. Levin C, Maibach HI. Topical corticosteroid-induced adrenocortical insufficiency: clinical implications. *Am J Clin Dermatol* 2002;3:141–147.
55. Ohtsuki M, Morimoto H, Nakagawa H. Tacrolimus ointment for the treatment of adult and pediatric atopic dermatitis: review on safety and benefits. *J Dermatol* 2018;45(8):936–942.
56. Carr WW. Topical calcineurin inhibitors for atopic dermatitis: review and treatment recommendations. *Pediatr Drugs* 2013;15(4):303–310.
57. Papier A, Strowd LC. Atopic dermatitis: a review of topical nonsteroid therapy. *Drugs Context* 2018;7:212521.
58. Paller AS, Lebwohl M, Fleischer AB, et al. Tacrolimus ointment is more effective than pimecrolimus cream with a similar safety profile in the treatment of atopic dermatitis: results from 3 randomized, comparative studies. *J Am Acad Dermatol* 2005;52:810–822.
59. Sehgal VN, Srivastava G, Dogra S. Tacrolimus in dermatology—pharmacokinetics, mechanism of action, drug interactions, dosages, and side effects: part I. *Skinmed* 2008;23(10):1218–1219.
60. Shah K, Cortina S, Ernst M, et al. Psoriasis in childhood: effective strategies to improve treatment adherence. *Psoriasis Targets Ther* 2015;5:43–54.
61. Wong R, Lin AN. Efficacy of topical calcineurin inhibitors in vitiligo. *Int J Dermatol* 2013;52:491–496.
62. Tay YK, Chan YC, Chandran NS, et al. Guidelines for the management of atopic dermatitis in Singapore. *Ann Acad Med Singapore* 2016;45(10):439–450.
63. Furue M, Terao H, Moroi Y, et al. Dosage and adverse effects of topical tacrolimus and steroids in daily management of atopic dermatitis. *J Dermatol* 2004;31(4):277–283.
64. Lee JH, Kwon HS, Jung HM, et al. Treatment outcomes of topical calcineurin inhibitor therapy for patients with vitiligo: a systematic review and meta-analysis. *JAMA Dermatol* 2019. doi:10.1001/jamadermatol.2019.0696.
65. Reynolds NJ, Al-Daraji WI. Calcineurin inhibitors and sirolimus: mechanisms of action and applications in dermatology. *Clin Exp Dermatol* 2002;27(7):555–561.
66. Hoetzenecker W, Ecker R, Kopp T, et al. Pimecrolimus leads to an apoptosis-induced depletion of T cells but not Langerhans cells in patients with atopic dermatitis. *J Allergy Clin Immunol* 2005;115(6):1276–1283.
67. Grassberger M, Steinhoff M, Schneider D, et al. Pimecrolimus—an anti-inflammatory drug targeting the skin. *Exp Dermatol* 2004;13(12):721–730.
68. Pariser DJ. Topical corticosteroids and topical calcineurin inhibitors in the treatment of atopic dermatitis: focus on percutaneous absorption. *Am J Ther* 2009;16(3):264–273.
69. Draelos ZD. Use of topical corticosteroids and topical calcineurin inhibitors for the treatment of atopic dermatitis in thin and sensitive skin areas. *Curr Med Res Opin* 2008;24(4):985–994.
70. Boguniewicz M, Fiedler V, Raimer S, et al. A randomized, vehicle-controlled trial of tacrolimus ointment for treatment of atopic dermatitis in children. *J Allergy Clin Immunol* 1998;102:637–644.
71. Hofman T, Cranswick N, Kuna P, et al. Tacrolimus ointment does not affect the immediate response to vaccination, the generation of immune memory, or humoral and cell-mediated immunity in children. *Arch Dis Child* 2006;91:905–910.
72. Chapman MS, Schachner LA, Breneman M, et al. Tacrolimus ointment 0.03% shows efficacy and safety for treatment of mild to moderate atopic dermatitis in children and adults. *J Am Acad Dermatol* 2005;53(2 Suppl 2):S177–S185.
73. Sigurgeirsson B, Boznanski A, Todd G, et al. Safety and efficacy of pimecrolimus in atopic dermatitis: a 5-year randomized trial. *Pediatrics* 2015;135(4):597–606.
74. Olson KA, West K, McCarthy PL. Toxic tacrolimus levels after application of topical tacrolimus and use of occlusive dressings in two bone marrow transplant recipients with cutaneous graft-versus-host disease. *Pharmacotherapy* 2014;34(6):e60–e64.
75. Lin HC, Hunnicutt JN, Moustafa FA, et al. Pharmacological treatments in pregnant women with psoriasis in the U.S.A. *Br J Dermatol* 2015;172(3):807–810.
76. Ring J, Möhrenschlager M, Henkel V. The US FDA "black box" warning for topical calcineurin inhibitors: an ongoing controversy. *Drug Saf* 2008;31(3):185–198.
77. Margolis DJ, Abuabara K, Hoffstad OJ, et al. Association between malignancy and topical use of pimecrolimus. *JAMA Dermatol* 2015;151:594–599.
78. Ashcroft DM, Dimmock P, Garside R, et al. Efficacy and tolerability of pimecrolimus and tacrolimus in the treatment of atopic dermatitis: meta-analysis of randomised controlled trials. *BMJ* 2005;330:516–524.
79. Hanifin JM, Paller AS, Eichenfield L, et al. Efficacy and safety of tacrolimus ointment treatment for up to 4 years in patients with atopic dermatitis. *J Am Acad Dermatol* 2005;53:S186–S194.
80. Reitamo S, Rustin M, Harper J, et al. A 4-year follow-up study of atopic dermatitis therapy with 0.1% tacrolimus ointment in children and adult patients. *Br J Dermatol* 2008;159:942–951.
81. Kuiper JG, van Herk-Sukel MPP, Castellsague J, et al. Use of topical tacrolimus and topical pimecrolimus in four European countries: a multicentre database cohort study. *Drugs Real World Outcomes* 2018;5(2):109–116.
82. Luger T, Boguniewicz M, Carr W, et al. Pimecrolimus in atopic dermatitis: consensus on safety and the need to allow use in infants. *Pediatr Allergy Immunol* 2015;26(4):306–315.
83. Elidel (Pimecrolimus) cream 1% package labeling NDA 21-302/S-011, Hanover, NJ: Novartis Pharmaceuticals, January 2006.
84. Patient Medication guide Pimecrolimus cream 1% Teva Pharmaceuticals USA, Inc. North Wales, PA 19454, May 2018.
85. Yang LPH, Curran MP. Topical pimecrolimus: a review of its use in the management of pediatric atopic dermatitis. *Pediatr Drugs* 2009;11(6):407–426.
86. Ulmar M, Sastry KS, Al Ali F, et al. Vitamin D and the pathophysiology of inflammatory skin diseases. *Skin Pharmacol Physiol* 2018;31(2):74–86.
87. Toniato E, Spinas E, Saggini A, et al. Immunomodulatory effects of vitamin D on skin inflammation. *J Biol Regul Homeost Agents* 2015;29(3):563–567.
88. Nagpal S, Lu J, Boehm MF. Vitamin D analogs: mechanism of action and therapeutic applications. *Curr Med Chem* 2001;8:1679–1697.
89. Ramsay CA. Management of psoriasis with calcipotriol used as monotherapy. *J Am Acad Dermatol* 1997;189(3):260–264.
90. Trémezaygues L, Reichrath J. Vitamin D analogs in the treatment of psoriasis: where are we standing and where will we be going? *Dermatoendocrinology* 2011;3:180–186.
91. Soleymani T, Hung T, Soung J. The role of vitamin D in psoriasis: a review. *Int J Dermatol* 2015;54:383–392.
92. Thomas J, Parimalam K. Treating pediatric plaque psoriasis: challenges and solutions. *Pediatr Heal Med Ther* 2016;7:25–38.
93. Devaux S, Castela A, Archier E, et al. Topical vitamin D analogues alone or in association with topical steroids for psoriasis: a systematic review. *J Eur Acad Dermatol Venereol* 2012;26:52–60.
94. White S, Vender R, Tachi D, et al. Use of calcipotriene cream (Dovonex cream) following acute treatment of psoriasis vulgaris with the calcipotriene/betamethasone dipropionate two-compound product (Taclonex): a randomized, parallel-group clinical trial. *Am J Clin Dermatol* 2006;7(3):177–184.
95. Gerdes S, Krakor M, Anger T, et al. Prospective, observational, non-interventional, multicentre study on the efficacy and tolerability of a new calcipotriol/betamethasone aerosol foam (Enstilar) in patients with plaque psoriasis under daily practice conditions. *Dermatology* 2018;32(10):1710–1727.
96. Segaert S, Duvold LB. Calcipotriol cream: a review of its use in the management of psoriasis. *J Dermatol Treat* 2006;17(6):327–337.
97. West CE, Narahari S, Feldman SR. Calcipotriene foam, 0.005% in mild-to-moderate plaque psoriasis. *Expert Rev Dermatol* 2014;7:17–26.
98. Darley CR, Cunliffe WJ, Green CM, et al. Safety and efficacy of calcipotriol ointment (Dovonex) in treating children with psoriasis vulgaris. *Br J Dermatol* 1996;135:390–393.
99. Frieder J, Kivelevitch D, Mentor A. Calcipotriene betamethasone dipropionate aerosol foam in the treatment of plaque psoriasis: a review of the literature. *Ther Deliv* 2017;8(9):737–746.
100. Alora-Palli MB, Perkins AC, Van Cott A, et al. Efficacy and tolerability of a cosmetically acceptable coal tar solution in the treatment of moderate plaque psoriasis: a controlled comparison with calcipotriene (calcipotriol) cream. *Am J Clin Dermatol* 2010;135:390–393.
101. Del Rosso JQ. Calcipotriene—betamethasone dipropionate topical suspension in the management of psoriasis: a status report on available data with an overview of practical clinical application. *Drug Ther Top* 2014;94(3):127–134.
102. Kang S, Yi S, Griffiths CE, et al. Calcipotriene-induced improvement in psoriasis is associated with reduced interleukin-8 and increased interleukin-10 levels within lesions. *Br J Dermatol* 1998;138:77–83.
103. Highton A, Quell J. Calcipotriene ointment 0.005% for psoriasis: a safety and efficacy study. *J Am Acad Dermatol* 1995;32(1):67–72.

104. Patel B, Siskin S, Krazmien R, et al. Compatibility of calcipotriene with other topical medications. *J Am Acad Dermatol* 1998;6(16):100–101.
105. Abramovits W. Calcitriol 3 microg/g ointment: an effective and safe addition to the armamentarium in topical psoriasis therapy. *J Drugs Dermatol* 2009;83:205–212.
106. Lara-Corrales I, Gomez GR, De Los Rios CP, et al. Vitamin D in patients with atopic dermatitis: a randomized, double-blinded, placebo-controlled study preliminary analysis. *Pediatr Dermatol* 2013;11(5):638.
107. Braun GS, Witt M, Mayer V, et al. Hypercalcemia caused by vitamin D3 analogs in psoriasis treatment. *Int J Dermatol* 2007;46(12):1315–1317.
108. Silverberg NB. Psoriasis in infancy: therapy with calcipotriene ointment. *Cutis* 2001;68(5):341–344.
109. Calcipotriene Cream 0.005% Dovonex product information Leo Pharma NJ 2015.
110. Tom WL, Van Syoc M, Chanda S, et al. Pharmacokinetic profile, safety, and tolerability of crisaborole topical ointment, 2% in adolescents with atopic dermatitis: an open-label phase 2a study. *Pediatr Dermatol* 2016;33(2):150–159.
111. Eichenfield LF, Call RS, Forsha DW, et al. Long-term safety of crisaborole ointment 2% in children and adults with mild to moderate atopic dermatitis. *J Am Acad Dermatol* 2017;75(3):494–503.
112. Zane LT, Hughes MH, Shakib S. Tolerability of crisaborole ointment for application on sensitive skin areas: a randomized, double-blind, vehicle-controlled study in healthy volunteers. *Am J Clin Dermatol* 2016;17(5):519–526.
113. Kailas A. Crisaborole: a new and effective nonsteroidal topical drug for atopic dermatitis. *Dermatol Ther* 2017;30(5).
114. Kitzen JM, Pergolizzi JV Jr, Taylor R Jr, et al. Crisaborole and Apremilast: PDE4 inhibitors with similar mechanism of action, different indications for management of inflammatory skin conditions. *Pharmacol Pharm* 2018;09(09):357–381.
115. Zane LT, Kircik L, Call R, et al. Crisaborole topical ointment, 2% in patients ages 2 to 17 years with atopic dermatitis: a phase 1b, open-label, maximal-use systemic exposure study. *Pediatr Dermatol* 2016;33(4):380–387.
116. Eucrisa package labeling, Anacor Pharmaceuticals, CA. December, 2016.
117. Draelos ZD, Feldman SR, Berman B, et al. Tolerability of topical treatments for atopic dermatitis. *Dermatol Ther (Heidelb)* 2019;9:71–102.
118. Forrest RD. Early history of wound treatment. *J R Soc Med* 1982;75(3):198–205.
119. Klasen HJ. Historical review of the use of silver in the treatment of burns. I. Early uses. *Burns* 2000;26:117–130.
120. Hugo WB. Phenols: a review of their history and development as antimicrobial agents. *Microbios* 1978;23:83–85.
121. Thurston AJ. Of blood, inflammation and gunshot wounds: the history of the control of sepsis. *Aust N Z J Surg* 2008;70(12):855–861.
122. Williamson DA, Carter GP, Howden BP. Current and emerging topical antibacterials and antiseptics: agents, action, and resistance patterns. *Clin Microbiol Rev* 2017;30(3):827–860.
123. Cartotto R. Topical antimicrobial agents for pediatric burns. *Burn Trauma* 2017;5(33):1–8.
124. Noguchi N, Kawashima M, Hayashi N, et al. Relationship between the severity of acne vulgaris and antimicrobial resistance of bacteria isolated from acne lesions in a hospital in Japan. *J Med Microbiol* 2014;63:721–728.
125. Kosmadaki M, Katsambas A. Topical treatments for acne. *Clin Dermatol* 2017;35(2):173–178.
126. Rowan MP, Cancio LC, Elster EA, et al. Burn wound healing and treatment: review and advancements. *Crit Care* 2015;19:243–248.
127. Cambiaso-Daniel J, Boukovalas S, Bitz GH, et al. Topical antimicrobials in burn care. *Ann Plast Surg* 2018. doi:10.1097/SAP.0000000000001297.
128. Atiyeh BS, Costagliola M, Hayek SN, et al. Effect of silver on burn wound infection control and healing: review of the literature. *Burns* 2007;33(2):139–148.
129. Church DL, Slaba I, Winston BW, et al. Burn infections. In: *The prokaryotes: human microbiology*. 2013:353–374.
130. Barajas-Nava LA, López-Alcalde J, Roquéi Figuls M, et al. Antibiotic prophylaxis for preventing burn wound infection. *Cochrane Database Syst Rev* 2013;6(6):CD008738.
131. Hartman-Adams H, Banvard C, Juckett G. Impetigo: diagnosis and treatment. *Am Fam Physician* 2014;90(4):229–235.
132. Bowen AC, Mahé A, Hay RJ, et al. The global epidemiology of impetigo: a systematic review of the population prevalence of impetigo and pyoderma. *PLoS One* 2015;10(8):e0136789.
133. Koning S, van der Sande R, Verhagen AP, et al. Interventions for impetigo. *Cochrane Database Syst Rev* 2012;(1):CD003261.
134. Safety and Effectiveness of Consumer Antiseptics. Topical antimicrobial drug products for over-the-counter human use. Final rule. *Fed Regist* 2016;81(172):61106–61130.
135. Dessinioti C, Katsambas A. Propionibacterium acnes and antimicrobial resistance in acne. *Clin Dermatol* 2017;35(2):163–167.
136. Simonart T. Newer approaches to the treatment of acne vulgaris. *Am J Clin Dermatol* 2012;13(6):357–364.
137. Thielitz A, Gollnick H. Recent therapeutic developments for acne. *Expert Rev Dermatol* 2013;4(1):55–65.
138. Sardana K, Gupta T, Garg VK, et al. Antibiotic resistance to Propionibacterium acnes: worldwide scenario, diagnosis and management. *Expert Rev Anti Infect Ther* 2015;13(7):883–896.
139. Hawkins DM, Smidt AC. Superficial fungal infections in children. *Pediatr Clin North Am* 2014;61(2):443–455.
140. Smolinski KN, Shah SS, Honig PJ, et al. Neonatal cutaneous fungal infections. *Curr Opin Pediatr* 2005;17(4):486–493.
141. Alter SJ, McDonald MB, Schloemer J, et al. Common child and adolescent cutaneous infestations and fungal infections. *Curr Probl Pediatr Adolesc Health Care* 2018;48(1):3–25.
142. Hayette MP, Sacheli R. Dermatophytosis, trends in epidemiology and diagnostic approach. *Curr Fungal Infect Rep* 2015;9(3):164–179.
143. Memißolu H, Erboz S, Akkaya S, et al. Comparative study of the efficacy and tolerability of 4 weeks of terbinafine therapy with 8 weeks of griseofulvin therapy in children with tinea capitis. *J Dermatol Treat* 1999;59(1):41–54.
144. Gupta AK, Nolting S, De Prost Y, et al. The use of itraconazole to treat cutaneous fungal infections in children. *Dermatology* 1999;199(3):248–252.
145. Vander Straten MR, Hossain MA, Ghannoum MA. Cutaneous infections dermatophytosis, onychomycosis, and tinea versicolor. *Infect Dis Clin North Am* 2003;17(1):87–112.
146. Gupta AK, Foley KA, Versteeg SG. New antifungal agents and new formulations against dermatophytes. *Mycopathologia* 2017;182(1–2):127–141.
147. Mukherjee PK, Chandra J, Kuhn DM, et al. Mechanism of fluconazole resistance in Candida albicans biofilms: phase-specific role of efflux pumps and membrane sterols. *Infect Immun* 2003;71:4333–4340.
148. Prasad R, Shah AH, Rawal MK. Antifungals: mechanism of action and drug resistance. *Adv in Exp Med and Biol.* 2016;892:327–349.
149. Kreijkamp-Kaspers S, Hawke K, Guo L, et al. Oral antifungal medication for toenail onychomycosis. *Cochrane Database Syst Rev* 2017;(7). doi:10.1002/14651858.CD010031.pub2.
150. Devore CD, Schutze GE. Clinical report: guidance for the clinician in rendering pediatric care head lice. *Pediatrics* 2015;135(5):e1355–e1365.
151. Sangaré AK, Doumbo OK, Raoult D. Management and treatment of human lice. *Biomed Res Int* 2016;2016:8962685.
152. Marcoux D, Palma KG, Kaul N, et al. Pyrethroid pediculicide resistance of head lice in Canada evaluated by serial invasive signal amplification reaction. *J Cutan Med Surg* 2010;14(3):115–118.
153. Burkhart CG, Burkhart GN. Safety and efficacy of pediculicides for head lice. *Expert Opin Drug Saf* 2006;5(1):169–179.
154. Yoon KS, Gao JR, Lee SH, et al. Permethrin-resistant human head lice, *Pediculus capitis*, and their treatment. *Arch Dermatol* 2003;139(8):994–1000.
155. Jahangiri F. Case report: a new method for treatment of permethrin-resistant head lice. *Clin Case Rep* 2017;5(5):601–604.
156. Frankowski BL, Bocchini JA Jr; Council on School Health and Committee on Infectious Diseases. Clinical report-head lice. *Pediatrics* 2010;126:392–400.
157. Downs AM, Stafford KA, Harvey I, et al. Evidence for double resistance to permethrin and malathion in head lice. *Br J Dermatol* 1999;141(3):508–511.
158. Takano-Lee M, Edman JD, Mullens BA, et al. Home remedies to control head lice: assessment of home remedies to control the human head louse, *Pediculus humanus capitis* (Anoplura: Pediculidae). *J Pediatr Nurs* 2004;19(6):393–398.
159. Pearlman D. Cetaphil cleanser (Nuvo Lotion) cures head lice. *Pediatrics* 2005;116(6):1612.
160. Burgess IF, Kay K, Burgess NA, et al. Soya oil-based shampoo superior to 0.5% permethrin lotion for head louse infestation. *Med Devices Evid Res* 2011;4(1):35–42.
161. Nolan K, Kamrath J, Levitt J. Lindane toxicity: a comprehensive review of the medical literature. *Pediatr Dermatol* 2012;29(2):141–146.
162. Taplin D. Pyrethrins and pyrethroids in dermatology. *Arch Dermatol* 2011;126(2):213–221.
163. Mytton OT, McGready R, Lee SJ, et al. Safety of benzyl benzoate lotion and permethrin in pregnancy: a retrospective matched cohort study. *BJOG* 2007;114(5):582–587.
164. Rosumeck S, Nast A, Dressler C. Ivermectin and permethrin for treating scabies. *Cochrane Database Syst Rev* 2018;(4):CD012994. doi:10.1002/14651858.CD012994.
165. Schultz MW, Gomez M, Hansen RC, et al. Comparative study of 5% permethrin cream and 1% lindane lotion for the treatment of scabies. *Arch Dermatol* 1990;126(2):167–170.
166. Taplin PD, Meinking TL, Porcelain SL, et al. Permethrin 5% dermal cream: a new treatment for scabies. *J Am Acad Dermatol* 1986;15(5):995–1001.
167. Quarterman MJ, Lesher JL. Neonatal scabies treated with permethrin 5% cream. *Pediatr Dermatol* 1994;11(3):264–266.
168. Burkhart FG, Burkhart CN, Burkhart KM. An assessment of topical and oral prescription and over-the-counter treatments for head lice. *J Am Acad Dermatol* 1998;38(6):979–982.
169. Gunning K, Pippitt K, Kiraly B, et al. Pediculosis and scabies: a treatment update. *Am Fam Physician* 2012;86(6):535–541.
170. Koch E, Clark JM, Cohen B, et al. Management of head louse infestations in the United States—a literature review. *Pediatr Dermatol* 2016;33(5):466–472.
171. Bouvresse S, Berdjane Z, Durand R, et al. Permethrin and malathion resistance in head lice: results of ex vivo and molecular assays. *J Am Acad Dermatol* 2012;67(6):1143–1150.
172. Frankowski BL. American Academy of Pediatrics guidelines for the prevention and treatment of head lice infestation. *Am J Manag Care* 2004;10(9 Suppl):S269–S272.
173. Reed NR, Rubin AL. Malathion. In: *Encyclopedia of toxicology: third edition*. San Diego, California: Elsevier Science & Technology, 2014.
174. Scheinfeld N. Controlling Scabies in institutional settings: a review of medications, treatment models, and implementation. *Am J Clin Dermatol* 2004;5(1):31–37.
175. Sharquie KE, Al-Rawi JR, Noaimi AA, et al. Treatment of scabies using 8% and 10% topical sulfur ointment in different regimens of application. *J Drugs Dermatol.* 2012;11(3):357–364.
176. Pruksachatkunakorn C, Damrongsak M, Sinthupuan S. Sulfur for scabies outbreaks in orphanages. *Pediatr Dermatol* 2002;19:448–453.
177. Sharma H, Zhang P, Barber DS, et al. Organochlorine pesticides dieldrin and lindane induce cooperative toxicity in dopaminergic neurons: role of oxidative stress. *Neurotoxicology* 2010;31(2):215–222.
178. Nakao T. Mechanisms of resistance to insecticides targeting RDL GABA receptors in planthoppers. *Neurotoxicology* 2017;60:293–298.
179. Lebwohl M, Clark L, Levitt J. Therapy for head lice based on life cycle, resistance, and safety considerations. *Pediatrics* 2007;119(5):965–974.
180. Kakko I, Toimela T, Tähti H. The synaptosomal membrane bound ATPase as a target for the neurotoxic effects of pyrethroids, permethrin and cypermethrin. *Chemosphere* 2003;51(2003):475–480.
181. Albakri L, Goldman RD. Child health update: permethrin for scabies in children. *Can Fam Physician* 2010;56(10):1005–1006.
182. Culver CA, Malina JJ, Talbert RL. Probable anaphylactoid reaction to a pyrethrin pediculocide shampoo. *Clin Pharm* 1988;7(11):846–849.
183. Proudfoot AT. Poisoning due to pyrethrins. *Toxicol Rev* 2005;24:107–113.
184. Idriss S, Levitt J. Malathion for head lice and scabies: treatment and safety considerations. *J Drugs Dermatol* 2009;8(8):715–720.
185. Patel VM, Lambert WC, Schwartz RA. Safety of topical medications for scabies and lice in pregnancy. *Indian J Dermatol* 2016;61(6):583–587.
186. Choudhary S. Burns due to anti-lice lotion. *Burns* 1999;25(2):184–185.

187. Strong M, Johnstone PW. Interventions for treating scabies. *Cochrane Database Syst Rev* 2007;(3)CD000320.
188. Modi K, Patel D, Shwayder T. Scalp-to-toes application of permethrin for patients with scabies. *Dermatol Online J* 2018;24.
189. Wadowski L, Balasuriya L, Price HN, et al. Lice update: new solutions to an old problem. *Clin Dermatol* 2015;33(3):347–354.
190. Kang S. The mechanism of action of topical retinoids. *Cutis* 2005;75(2 Suppl):10–13.
191. Leyden JJ. Retinoids and acne. *J Am Acad Dermatol* 1988;1(1)Pt 2:164–168.
192. Michel S, Jomard A, Demarchez M. Pharmacology of adapalene. *Br J Dermatol.* 1998;139(Suppl 52):3–7.
193. Tang-Liu DD, Matsumoto RM, Usansky JI. Clinical pharmacokinetics and drug metabolism of tazarotene: a novel topical treatment for acne and psoriasis. *Clin Pharmacokinet* 1999;37(4):273–287.
194. Webster GF. Evidence-based review: fixed-combination therapy and topical retinoids in the treatment of acne. *J Drugs Dermatol* 2011;10(6):636–644.
195. Adler BL, Kornmehl H, Armstrong AW. Antibiotic resistance in acne treatment. *JAMA Dermatol* 2017;153(8):810–811.
196. Leyden J, Stein-Gold L, Weiss J. Why topical retinoids are mainstay of therapy for acne. *Dermatol Ther (Heidelb)* 2017;7(3):293–304.
197. Feldstein S, Afshar M, Krakowski AC, et al. Filling in pediatric acne practice gaps: a prospective multicenter study of case-based education. *J Adolesc Heal* 2016;131:S163–S186.
198. Titus S, Hodge J. Diagnosis and treatment of acne. *Am Fam Physician* 2012;86(8):734–740.
199. Zaenglein AL, Pathy AL, Schlosser BJ, et al. Guidelines of care for the management of acne vulgaris. *J Am Acad Dermatol* 2016;74(5):945–973.
200. Cline A, Kolli SS, Pecone D, et al. Topical retinoids in acne vulgaris: a systematic review. *Am J Clin Dermatol* 2019;20(3):345–365.
201. Dréno B, Bissonnette R, Gagné-Henley A, et al. Long-term effectiveness and safety of up to 48 weeks' treatment with topical adapalene 0.3%/ benzoyl peroxide 2.5% gel in the prevention and reduction of atrophic acne scars in moderate and severe facial acne. *Am J Clin Dermatol* 2019;17. doi:10.1007/s40257-019-00454-6.
202. Jeremy AHT, Holland DB, Roberts SG, et al. Inflammatory events are involved in acne lesion initiation. *J Invest Dermatol* 2003;121:20–27.
203. Fisher GJ, Voorhees JJ. Molecular mechanisms of retinoid actions in skin. *FASEB J* 2018;10(9):1002–1013.
204. Maiti R, Sirka CS, Ashique Rahman MA, et al. Efficacy and safety of Tazarotene 0.1% plus Clindamycin 1% Gel versus Adapalene 0.1% plus Clindamycin 1% Gel in facial acne vulgaris: a randomized, controlled clinical trial. *Clin Drug Investig* 2017;37(11):1083–1091.
205. Han A, Kusari A, Borok J, et al. 600 Improving treatment of acne vulgaris by primary care pediatricians. *J Invest Dermatol* 2018;138(5 Suppl):S102.
206. Chien AL, Qi J, Rainer B, et al. Treatment of acne in pregnancy. *J Am Board Fam Med* 2016;29(2):254–262.
207. Kaplan YC, Ozsarfati J, Etwel F, et al. Pregnancy outcomes following first-trimester exposure to topical retinoids: a systematic review and meta-analysis. *Br J Dermatol* 2015;173(5):1132–1141.
208. Zip CM. Innovative use of topical metronidazole. *Dermatol Clin* 2010;28:525–534.
209. Punjataewakupt A, Napavichayanun S, Aramwit P. The downside of antimicrobial agents for wound healing. *Eur J Clin Microbiol Infect Dis* 2019;38(1):39–54.
210. Lloyd EC, Rodgers BC, Michener M, et al. Outpatient burns: prevention and care. *Am Fam Physician* 2012;85(1):25–32.
211. Rashaan ZM, Krijnen P, Klamer RRM, et al. Nonsilver treatment vs. silver sulfadiazine in treatment of partial-thickness burn wounds in children: a systematic review and meta-analysis. *Wound Repair Regen* 2014;22(4):473–482.

CHAPTER

19

John D. Roarty

Ophthalmologic Drugs in Infants and Children

INTRODUCTION

The study of ocular pharmacology in the pediatric population is often limited to case reports and small clinical series. This problem has occurred in many areas of pediatrics. From 1984 through 1989, the U.S. Food and Drug Administration (FDA) approved 80% of the drugs without pediatric guidelines.[1] The need for inclusion of the child in pharmacologic evaluation has been emphasized by the American Academy of Pediatrics.[2]

Written descriptions of the treatment of eye disorders date to the Egyptians.[3] Greek and Roman literature describe topical therapy with *collyria*, a substance dissolved in egg white, milk, or water. Up to World War II, few ophthalmic medications were commercially available. The 1950 US Pharmacopeia XIV listed three ophthalmic ointments. The FDA suggested sterility for eye preparations in 1953, with a legal requirement in 1955.

PHARMACOKINETICS

TOPICAL MEDICATIONS

The normal tear volume is 8 to 10 µL. The median **tear volume** (interquartile range) is 0.5 µL (0.6 to 2 µL) for newborn infants, 2.5 µL (1.4 to 7.75 µL) for these infants at an older age, and 6 µL (2.73 to 12.75 µL) in adults ($p < 0.001$). Evaporation accounts for 25% of tear film loss, with 75% discharged into the lacrimal system. The tear turnover rate is about 16%. The volume of most topical preparations is 10 to 25 µL. Excess drug often spills in the nasolacrimal system. It is estimated that only 40% of the medication retained within the lids is present after 1 minute.[4] Given the limited amount of drug retained after drop placement and the high washout rate, it is estimated that only 8% of the original medication in the drop is retained after 5 minutes.[4]

There are several natural barriers to topically applied drug penetration. The tear film has natural buffers in proteins and bicarbonates. Tears contain approximately 0.7% protein, mostly albumin. The mean pH of the tear films is 7.5, and tears are most effective against acidic compounds.[5] The corneal epithelium is five cell layers thick. Cell lipid membranes are hydrophobic. The corneal stroma has a lipid content of about 1% and is hydrophilic. The endothelium is only one cell layer thick and is less significant as a barrier.

Lipophilic drugs are absorbed more readily by the nasal mucosa. Up to 80% of the drug may diffuse into the systemic circulation if it drains into the lacrimal system.[6] Methods for decreasing the systemic absorption include punctal occlusion, dilution of drops, and use of microdrops.[7] Punctal plugs have improved the efficacy of glaucoma drops in patients with lacrimal insufficiency.[8] Local tolerance of topical medication is variable. Ocular concerns include pain on instillation, allergic reactions, delayed healing, punctate keratopathy, disturbances of lacrimal secretion, and disturbances of accommodation.[9] Patient comfort is best at a pH of 7.4 (tear film pH). Stability for many topical drugs is a pH as low as 5.0. Thus, choice of the proper pH and buffer capacity is a compromise between drug stability and patient comfort.[3]

PERIOCULAR INJECTION

Periocular injection allows for greater intraocular penetration. This is especially true for penetration into the vitreous and the retina. In rabbits, the intraocular concentration was 41 times greater with a retrobulbar application compared with systemic administration. This ratio doubled if the eye was inflamed.[10] The eye is supplied by the retinal and choroidal circulation. Systemic access to the vitreous and the retina is restricted by a blood–retina barrier with endothelial tight junctions. The vessels of the choroid allow larger molecules to pass into the choroidal space, but the retinal pigment epithelium, under the retina, and the ciliary nonpigmented epithelium have tight junctions.

DIAGNOSTIC DROPS

Pupil size is determined by sympathetic and parasympathetic influence. The pupil dilator is sympathetic, and the constrictor is parasympathetic. The primary sympathetic mydriatic agent is phenylephrine. Phenylephrine is fast acting and of short duration. The 10% solution can cause hypertension, tachycardia, cerebral vascular accidents, and ruptured aneurysms.[11,12] The use of topical phenylephrine intraoperatively to effect pupil dilation for surgery has been associated with the development of pulmonary edema.[13] A 2.5% preparation is considered safe in the pediatric age group.

Anticholinergic agents such as tropicamide, atropine, and cyclopentolate induce dilation by inhibiting the parasympathetic constrictor muscle and inducing cycloplegia. Tropicamide 0.5% or 1.0% is a short-acting agent with little adverse effect.[14] Atropine and cyclopentolate directly inhibit the action of acetylcholine on the smooth muscles in the iris and the ciliary body. They are used to dilate the pupil and to block the accommodative effect of the ciliary muscle. This allows an intraocular examination without pupillary constriction. It also allows determination of the refractive state of the eye without interference from accommodation.

Reported side effects to anticholinergics include angle-closure glaucoma, cardiopulmonary problems, and central nervous system effects. Premature infants and those with neurologic impairments and seizure disorders have a higher risk of systemic side effects. Premature infants are prone to apnea and bradycardia with cyclopentolate. Judicious use in neonates and infants has been recommended. Women, fair children, and children with Down syndrome may be prone to atropine toxicity.[15] Systemic anticholinergic toxicity includes dry mouth, decreased sweating, hyperthermia, rash, tachycardia, urinary retention, and behavioral changes. Fatal complications have been reported, with topical doses no longer available.[16] The risk of an adverse effect is higher with the 2% cyclopentolate solution.[17] However, a seizure was reported in a 4.5-year-old boy with cerebral palsy and no seizure history with a standard topical instillation of cyclopentolate 1%.[18] Topical use of atropine 1% increased the frequency of seizures in a 3-year-old boy.[19] A survey of 57 pediatric ophthalmology facilities estimated the risk of severe (monitored in the office a few hours) or very severe (hospital admission) as 2 to 10 episodes per 1.6 million exposures.[20]

PRESERVATIVES

Preservatives have been added to drops to prevent microbial contamination. Benzalkonium chloride is the most common. The preservative destabilizes the lipid layer of the tear film and increases the evaporation of the tear film.[21] Ocular signs of toxicity can be twice as common with preservative compared with without preservative.[22] Ocular signs include stinging, foreign-body sensation, tearing, and itching. Superficial punctate keratitis can occur indicative of epithelial damage. There have been no specific reports of pediatric sensitivity. Chronic drop use such as with glaucoma therapy results in decreased tear breakup time and increased punctate staining compared to controls. Benzalkonium chloride, the most common preservative, increased the Ocular Surface Disease Index by threefold.[23]

OCULAR CONDITIONS

MYOPIA

Myopia is a refractive condition of the eye, affecting 80 million children worldwide. Atropine 1% has been suggested to decrease progression of myopia but with significant side effects of hypoaccommodation and photosensitivity. Pirenzepine is an M1-receptor antagonist used to treat dyspepsia in Europe. In the United States, a 2-year study of 174 children aged 8 to 12 years treated with topical pirenzepine against placebo showed a 40% reduction in the progression of myopia.[24] Lower dose atropine has been found effective at reducing the progression of myopia. The Low-concentration Atropine for Myopia Progression (LAMP) study found atropine 0.05% to have the best effect with lowest side effects.[25]

Atropine 0.01% is also effective but demonstrates regression once off of drops.[26]

OCULAR ALLERGY

Ocular allergy can be treated with vasoconstrictors, antihistamines, mast cell stabilizers, nonsteroidal preparations, and steroids. Routine allergic conjunctivitis can be treated with over-the-counter preparations. Over-the-counter eye drops contain sympathomimetic agents for α-adrenergic vasoconstriction. Accidental oral ingestion of 2 to 3 mL of imidazole in a 2-year-old child resulted in hypothermia, hypoglycemia, central nervous system depression, and respiratory depression.[27,28] Toxicity has been limited to surface discomfort with topical use similar to adults.[29]

Many topical agents are multimodal in effect. Ketotifen fumarate 0.025% (Zaditor) and olopatadine HCl 0.1% (Patanol) combine an antihistamine and a mast cell stabilizer effect. Many of these are approved by the FDA for children aged 3 years and older. The primary complication is surface irritation. No other systemic complications have been reported in the pediatric age group. Finally, topical steroids are used for short times in conjunction with a nonsteroidal anti-inflammatory, antihistamine, or mast cell stabilizer. Long-term use of steroids is problematic, as described in the next subsection.

Vernal conjunctivitis is a less common form of ocular allergy in children and young adults requiring prescription therapy. It presents with severe itching, photophobia, injection of the conjunctiva, and corneal foreign-body sensation. Obliteration of the ductules of the lacrimal gland can lead to severe keratitis sicca and corneal ulcer. However, Pucci reported that the most common cause of loss of sight was steroid related in a small series.[30] Twenty-five percent of patients had steroid-induced cataracts, and 12% had steroid-induced glaucoma. Topical cyclosporine 2% has been used effectively in pediatric patients with vernal conjunctivitis without complication.[31] Tacrolimus 0.03% and 0.1% have also been effective in lieu of steroids.[32]

Steroids

In the pediatric population, steroids may be used topically for the treatment of external disorders, such as allergic conjunctivitis and keratitis. Intraocular indications include uveitis and postsurgical inflammation. Ocular hypertension secondary to steroid use is well described. Some conditions, such as uveitis and hemangiomas, may require periocular injection of steroids. Systemic Cushingoid toxicity can occur with periocular injection of steroids. An 11-year-old boy with severe uveitis was treated with a periocular injection of 80 mg of methylprednisolone every 6 weeks for 6 months. He developed ocular hypertension and a Cushingoid habitus.[33] Adrenal growth suppression[34] and retinal artery occlusion have occurred after periocular injection for capillary hemangiomas of infancy. Adrenal suppression occurred in 67% of infants under 2 years of age treated with corticosteroids undergoing cataract surgery.[34]

Ocular hypertensive effects have long been described with all methods of delivery. These include oral,[35] inhalation,[36] nasal, intravenous,[37] topical dermatologic,[38] periocular,[39] and topical drops. Glucocorticoids appear to increase outflow resistance in the trabecular meshwork, with no effect on aqueous humor production. Morphologic changes include deposition of amorphous extracellular and fibrillar material in the trabecular beams with long-term use.[40]

Steroid-induced ocular hypertension with topical application occurs in up to 30% of patients. A significant pressure rise of 16 mmHg or more can occur in 5% of a normal population.[41] In adults, intraocular pressure rises occur after 4 to 6 weeks of steroid use. Intraocular pressures may rise to 50 mmHg (normal 10 to 21 mmHg) and is reversible with cessation of the steroids. In children, reports of ocular hypertensive response with topical therapy vary from 11%[42] to 56%.[43] The peak response occurs earlier than in adults, as early as 4 days of continuous use. The younger the patient, the higher is the risk of ocular hypertension.[44] The greater sensitivity has been postulated to be secondary to an immature trabecular meshwork and decreased outflow capacity in children as compared with adults.[44] Glaucoma and buphthalmos occurred in a 3-week-old infant after only 7 days of topical steroids.[45]

Steroid-induced glaucoma may mimic congenital glaucoma with corneal edema, rupture of Descemet's membrane, elevated intraocular pressure, and increased cupping of the optic nerve. This was noted in 73% of 55 eyes in 33 children, with a mean age of 7 years.[46] Cessation of steroids normalized pressure in only four eyes. Trabeculotomy, an angle-opening surgery, was effective in normalizing intraocular pressures in all eyes requiring surgery.

Secondary glaucoma associated with juvenile rheumatoid arthritis and uveitis is particularly difficult to control. Contributing factors are generous steroid use and trabecular changes secondary to the chronic intraocular inflammation. Foster et al.[47] reported an incidence of glaucoma of 42% in their series of 69 patients with juvenile rheumatoid arthritis. Only 17% of the patients were controlled with topical therapy. One cause of failure is poor compliance with chronic use of eye drops. Intravitreal steroid inserts have been found effective in reducing steroids or systemic treatment. However, cataracts are a significant problem.[48]

The response varies with the type of steroid and method of delivery. Ohji et al.[49] reported a higher risk of ocular hypertension with topical dexamethasone compared with topical fluorometholone. Fluorometholone generated an ocular hypertensive response in one patient. The glucocorticoid receptor is encoded by the *GR* gene with 24 polymorphisms described. Efforts to delineate the pharmacogenomics have been unsuccessful to date.[50]

INFECTION

The etiologic agents of pediatric conjunctivitis are viral and bacterial in 85% of the patients. The primary bacterial agents are *Streptococcus pneumoniae* and *Haemophilus influenzae.*[51] A large number of antibiotics are available for the treatment of bacterial conjunctivitis. All of the antibiotics are well tolerated as topical therapy with a few exceptions. Surface irritation is not uncommon, but no more frequent than in the adult population. The antimicrobial spectrum of the antibiotics is the same as in the adult population. Sulfacetamide and neomycin have a particularly high incidence of topical toxicity and hypersensitivity reactions. Antibiotic resistance is becoming a serious problem. Methicillin-resistant *Staphylococcus aureus* has been reported in 42% of cultures[52] and 52% were moxifloxacin-resistant *Pseudomonas aeruginosa.*[53]

Aminoglycosides

Aminoglycosides are effective against a wide range of Gram-negative and some Gram-positive organisms. They inhibit protein synthesis and interfere with messenger RNA (mRNA) in the ribosome. There is no systemic toxicity related to topical use. Burning and stinging are common. Hypersensitivity reactions occur in up to 8% of patients using neomycin. The risk of hypersensitivity is less with the other aminoglycosides.

Intraocular and subconjunctival injection of aminoglycosides is used for the treatment of endophthalmitis. Aminoglycosides for prophylaxis after cataract surgery or traumatic ruptured globe repair had been the standard. Gram-negative organisms are common causative agents with endophthalmitis. However, gentamicin, tobramycin, and amikacin have caused macular infarcts with intravitreal or subconjunctival delivery.[54] Although a macular infarct is infrequent, it is recommended that aminoglycosides not be used for prophylaxis. It may still be considered if a Gram-negative agent is suspected with endophthalmitis. The etiology of the macula infarct is unknown. Infarct may be related to inadvertent perforation of the globe with subconjunctival delivery, sudden changes in the intraocular pressure with injection, or a direct toxic effect due to concentration.

Chloramphenicol

Chloramphenicol is effective against Gram-negative and Gram-positive aerobic organisms causing conjunctivitis but carries risk for aplastic anemia. The first death from aplastic anemia from eye drops was reported in 1955.[55] Chloramphenicol has been reported to cause aplastic anemia after the administration of an ophthalmic ointment in a male adult and recently with drops.[56] With systemic application, the risk of aplastic anemia is from 1 in 30,000 to 1 in 50,000.[9] The risk with topical application is estimated at 1 in 100,000.[57]

Tetracycline

Tetracycline has a wide range of antimicrobial activity against Gram-negative and Gram-positive organisms. It inhibits protein synthesis in the ribosome. Tetracycline may be used orally for ocular complications of rosacea. It can cause permanent discoloration of the teeth and depress bone growth by binding with calcium. Enamel dysplasia can occur with exposure from the second trimester to 8 years of age.[58]

Quinolones

Nalidixic acid, a quinolone, has been used for Gram-negative infections. It inhibits bacterial DNA replication by inhibiting DNA gyrase. Nalidixic acid–induced arthropathy with necrosis of chondrocytes and loss of collagen has been reported in young animals.[59] The present generation of the quinolones is considered safer. Systemic administration of fluoroquinolones in adults and children has rarely caused a reversible arthralgia but never arthropathy. Rare adverse events to systemic therapy reported in children include gastrointestinal disturbances, skin rash, green discoloration of the teeth, and anaphylaxis.[60] In a large series, topical ophthalmic use for pediatric conjunctivitis has not caused any serious adverse events.[61]

Rifabutin

Rifabutin is a semisynthetic antimycobacterial agent similar to rifampin. Uveitis is a known complication in adults. Rifabutin can induce uveitis in the pediatric patient.[62] The uveitis may mimic endophthalmitis.[55] It may be related to serum levels above therapeutic range. It is recommended that the dosage not exceed 10 mg per kg per day.[63]

GLAUCOMA

β-Blockers

Adrenergic blockade may be nonselective, β_1, or β_2. Systemic β-blockers may reduce cardiac output and increase airway resistance in the bronchioles. Topical application results in a reduction in the intraocular pressure. Aqueous production by the ciliary body is decreased. The exact mechanism of this intraocular pressure reduction is unknown. The exacerbation of reactive airway disease has been described with topical application.[64] Apnea was induced by topical instillation of timolol 0.25% in an 18-month-old girl.[65] The resting heart rate can be reduced with topical instillation, but the inotropic cardiac effect is less. Patients with reactive airway disease and cardiac failure should avoid this class. Cardioselective formulations, such as betaxolol and levobetaxolol, are β_1-blockers. The pressure reduction is similar with less risk of bronchospasm.[66]

Oral and topical β-blockers are commonly used for periorbital hemangiomas. Multiple studies have found oral propranolol 2 mg per kg per day is a safe, effective dose to cause hemangioma involution. Bradycardia and hypoglycemia have been reported when the children are ill.[67]

Prostaglandin Analogs

Latanoprost 0.005% is a 17-phenyl-substituted prostaglandin analog for the topical therapy of glaucoma. It works by increasing the uveoscleral outflow. The mechanism is unknown. Associated adult problems include conjunctival hyperemia, punctate keratopathy, increased iris pigmentation, increased eyelash growth, and cystoid macular edema. The pigmentation effect on the iris and eyelashes has been seen in children. The increase pigmentation is due to increase in the size of mature melanin granules.[68] A child with aniridia and glaucoma developed diaphoresis 1 hour after dosing with latanoprost.[69] Although latanoprost seems to have few side effects reported in adults or children, Enyedi and Freedman[70] reported little effect on the intraocular pressure in their pediatric population.

α-Agonists

Brimonidine is a selective α-agonist that reduces aqueous production and increases uveoscleral outflow to control intraocular pressure in glaucoma. In children, it produced a 7% reduction in the pressure. However, Enyedi and Freedman reported that 2 of 32 children, average ages 2.4 and 3.7 years old, respectively, were unarousable and that 5 of 32 children demonstrated extreme fatigue secondary to central nervous system depression after topical application.[71] Apnea and bradycardia have been reported in the neonatal period.

Apraclonidine hydrochloride is a selective α_2-agonist. It decreases aqueous production by decreasing Na–K ATPase activity in the ciliary body epithelium. As an analog of clonidine, it has a systemic hypotensive effect. This effect is limited because apraclonidine is hydrophilic. Local side effects include burning and stinging. In adults, systemic and local side effects were significant enough to stop the medication in 23% of patients. Only 2% had severe systemic reactions to topical therapy.[72]

Apraclonidine has been used in the diagnosis of Horner syndrome. Cocaine and hydroxyamphetamine drops have been traditionally used to differentiate a preganglionic lesion from postganglionic lesion. Apraclonidine can be used in lieu of cocaine. However, hypoxia, apnea, and bradycardia have been reported in a 5-month-old infant.[73]

Carbonic Anhydrase Inhibitors

Carbonic anhydrase is present in the ciliary body of the eye. Inhibitors suppress aqueous production whether given topically or orally. Limited side effects include burning and stinging. There are no significant systemic effects topically.[74]

STRABISMUS

Phospholine iodide 0.125% is a long-acting anticholinesterase that increases tissue acetylcholine. Effects include miosis, increase in outflow of aqueous, decrease in intraocular pressure, and enhanced accommodation. Treatment of glaucoma was the primary indication before development of better medications. Phospholine iodide was used in the past for the treatment of accommodative esotropia in children. It is currently used for short-term treatment of consecutive esotropia after surgery for an exotropia. Short-term effects include burning, lacrimation, and headaches. Retinal detachment has been associated with its use. Long-term use may result in the formation of iris cysts, lens opacities, and depression of plasma cholinesterase activity. An acute cholinergic crisis was reported in a 5-year-old girl with unsuspected myasthenia gravis.[75]

RETINOPATHY OF PREMATURITY

Anti–Vascular Endothelial Growth Factor

In adults, macular degeneration, diabetic retinopathy, sickle cell retinopathy, and vascular occlusion can result in significant abnormal retinal neovascularization. Effective vascular involution has been obtained with intravitreal injection use of anti–vascular endothelial growth factor (VEGF) pharmacotherapies. The majority of the safety and efficacy studies have been for macular degeneration.[76] The use for other ocular disorders such as glaucoma is being explored.[77] Pegaptanib, a selective VEGF-A antagonist, was approved for intraocular use in 2004. Ranibizumab, a recombinant immunoglobulin G1 isotype antibody fragment, inhibits all isoforms of human VEGF-A. It was approved in 2006. Bevacizumab, a full-length monoclonal antibody, inhibits all forms of VEGF. This agent is FDA approved for colorectal, breast, and lung cancer, but not for the eye. These agents have been found to be very effective with the most significant complications related to the delivery. Intraocular inflammation has been reported.[78]

However, it is being used in advanced retinopathy of prematurity (ROP). Intravitreal use as an adjunct to surgical therapy has been useful in the face of vitreous hemorrhage and early retinal traction in a few reported cases.[79,80] Hintz-Minter first published intravitreal Avastin as a primary treatment for ROP in 2008. Since then, parameters for intravitreal treatment have been established; however, the proper dose is still being studied. Of concern is the effect on the long-term development of the eye. Poor foveal development, avascular peripheral retina, and global development are concerns.[81–83]

Erythropoietin

Erythropoietin, a renal hormone, stimulates red blood cell production. It has been used to treat neonatal anemia of prematurity with good effect since 1990. Brown et al.[84] demonstrated an increase in active ROP in patients treated with recombinant human erythropoietin (rhEPO). Suk et al.[85] found that the effect on ROP may be related to the gestational age and the dose. Early rhEPO dosing may result in retinal vessel stability, while later dosing may add to the angiogenic drive.

OPHTHALMOLOGIC EFFECTS WITH SYSTEMIC NONOPHTHALMOLOGIC MEDICATIONS

Transdermal scopolamine has been used to treat nausea and emesis associated with chemotherapy. Unilateral mydriasis with a fixed and dilated pupil occurred with a scopolamine patch in an 11-year-old child with lymphocytic leukemia. Concern for central nervous system disease prompted imaging studies, which were negative.[86] Transdermal scopolamine was used to control excessive drooling in a 4-year-old child with neurodevelopmental issues. This resulted in a reversible esotropia mimicking a sixth nerve palsy.

Cytosine arabinoside may act by interfering with DNA polymerase and disrupting the S-phase of the cell cycle. It may also be incorporated into DNA and RNA to induce chromosomal breaks. General adverse reactions include fever, bone pain, myalgias, rash, and malaise. There are other rare multisystem effects also. Hemorrhagic conjunctivitis and keratitis are common. This results in severe photophobia, which can be treated with artificial tears and topical steroids.[87]

Hydroxychloroquine and *chloroquine sulfate* are used as antimalarial and as anti-inflammatory agents in lupus erythematosus and rheumatoid arthritis. General adverse reactions include headache, gastrointestinal complaints, dermatologic problems, and blood dyscrasias. Ophthalmic effects reported include extraocular muscle palsy, keratitis, corneal deposits, macular edema with a "bull's-eye" maculopathy, pigmentary retinopathy resembling retinitis pigmentosa, and visual field defects. Chloroquine, and less so hydroxychloroquine, damages lysosomes. This may interfere with phospholipid metabolism and disrupt cell membranes. Degenerative changes are seen in the ganglion cells and photoreceptors. The quinines are metabolized slowly, leading to continued cell damage after the medication is stopped. Adverse effects are dose related, with a cumulative effect.

The reversible corneal deposits can occur within the first 3 weeks of therapy. They clear with cessation of the medication. The retinopathy may persist long term. If discovered early, the retinopathy may be reversed. Late damage to the retinal pigment epithelium results in pigment dispersion peripherally and a "bull's-eye" maculopathy that is not reversible. The risk of vision-threatening changes is lowest at a daily hydroxychloroquine dose of 5 mg per kg of real weight, with an estimated risk of 2% at 10 years of use. Screening should be with a Humphrey visual field 10-2 and an SD-OCT of the macula.[88]

Vigabatrin increases γ-aminobutyric acid (GABA) concentration in the brain by inhibiting GABA transaminase. It has been used for infantile spasm, complex partial seizure, and generalized seizures.[89] Color perception was compromised in 32% of adult patients.[90] Peripheral visual field loss has been documented in up to 30% of adult patients. The effect was irreversible 6 months after cessation of the drug in one patient. Electroretinogram (ERG) response is reduced to photopic and scotopic stimulation.[91] This implies that rod and cone functions are affected. GABA may be involved in phototransduction. It is an inhibitory neurotransmitter in retinal bipolar and amacrine cells. The exact mechanism is unknown. No pediatric visual loss has been reported. However, obtaining visual fields and ERGs is problematic in children.

Topiramate is used in children with generalized and localized seizures. It is a sulfamated monosaccharide D-fructose derivative and inhibits Na^+ and Ca^{2+} channels, excitatory amino acid receptors, and carbonic anhydrase isozymes. It potentiates GABA-evoked channels.[92] In children, adverse central nervous system effects, such as somnolence, behavioral changes, and poor concentration, and weight loss appear similar to effects in the adult population. Nephrolithiasis and hepatic toxicity appear less frequently.[93] Unusual ocular effects have been reported. Multiple adult case reports of unilateral and bilateral angle-closure glaucoma and induced myopia have been reported. Uveal effusion with anterior displacement of the iris-lens diaphragm has been documented with ultrasound.[94,95] A 15-year-old boy developed bilateral retinal striae and myopia with a marked decrease in vision. The visual acuity returned to baseline with cessation of the drug.[96] The mechanism of the uveal effusion and retinal edema is unknown. However, uveal effusions have been reported with other sulfa-derived drugs.[97]

NOVEL DELIVERY SYSTEMS FOR OPHTHALMIC MEDICATIONS

Compliance with eye drops varies with technique, missed instillation, and bottle design. Medication reservoirs inserted into the anterior chamber of the eye for steroid and glaucoma medication delivery have been developed. These are biodegradable but require entering the eye. Biodegradable lacrimal plugs and fornix rings have been useful for sustained medication delivery. Finally, phase 3 trials for a microdose delivery at the micron level relying on electrostatic droplet charging for high adhesive coating would significantly reduce waste.[98]

REFERENCES

1. Center for Drug Evaluation and Research, Food and Drug Administration, Public Health Service. Offices of Drug Evaluation statistical report. *Publication no 89-233530*. Rockville, MD: US Department of Health and Human Services, 1989.
2. Guidelines for the ethical conduct of studies to evaluate drugs in pediatric populations. Committee on Drugs. *Pediatrics* 1995;95:286–294.
3. Mullins JD. Ophthalmic preparations. In: Genaro AR, ed. *Remington's pharmaceutical sciences*, 17th ed. Easton, PA: Mack, 1985:1553–1566.

4. Mindel JS. Pharmacokinetics. In: Tasman W, Jaeger EA, eds. *Duane's foundations of clinical ophthalmology*, Vol. 3, 6th ed. Philadelphia, PA: Lippincott Williams & Wilkins, 1993:1–17.
5. Carney LG, Mauger TF, Hill RM. Buffering in human tears: pH responses to acid and base challenge. *Invest Ophthalmol Vis Sci* 1989;30:747–754.
6. Hugues FC, le Jeunne C. Systemic and local tolerability of ophthalmic drug formulations. *Drug Saf* 1995;8:365–380.
7. Bhatia SS, Vidyashankar C, Sharma RK, et al. Systemic toxicity with cyclopentolate eye drops. *Indian Pediatr* 2000;37:329–331.
8. Huang TC, Lee DA. Punctal occlusion and topical medications for glaucoma. *Am J Ophthalmol* 1989;107:151–155.
9. Polak BCP. Drugs used in ocular treatment. In: Dukes MNG, Aronson JK, eds. *Meyeler's side effects of drugs. An encyclopedia of adverse reactions and interactions*, 14th ed. Amsterdam, The Netherlands: Elsevier, 2000:1636–1648.
10. Levine ND, Aronson SB. Orbital infusion of steroids in the rabbit. *Arch Ophthalmol* 1970;83:599–607.
11. Fraunfelder FW, Fraunfelder FT, Jensvold B. Adverse systemic effect from pledgets of topical ocular phenylephrine 10%. *Am J Ophthalmol* 2002;134:624–625.
12. Apt L. Pharmacology. In: Isenberg SJ, ed. *The eye in infancy*. Chicago, IL: Year Book, 1989:91–99.
13. Baldwin FJ, Morley AP. Intraoperative pulmonary oedema in a child following systemic absorption of phenylephrine eyedrops. *Br J Anaesth* 2002;88:440–442.
14. Chiaviello CT, Bond GR. Dilating the pupil in the pediatric emergency department. *Pediatr Emerg Care* 1994;10:216–218.
15. Lyndon WJ, Hodes T. Possible allergic reactions to cyclopentolate hydrochloride: case reports with literature review of uses and adverse reactions. *Ophthalmic Physiol Opt* 1991;11:16–21.
16. Rengstorff RH, Doughty CB. Mydriatic and cycloplegic drugs: a review of ocular and systemic complications. *Am J Optom Physiol Opt* 1982;59:162–177.
17. Adcock EW. Adverse systemic reactions of topical cyclopentolate hydrochloride. *Ann Ophthalmol* 1976;8:695–698.
18. Fitzgerald DA, Hanson RM, West C, et al. Seizures associated with 1% cyclopentolate eyedrops. *J Paediatr Child Health* 1990;26:106–107.
19. Wright BD. Exacerbation of akinetic seizures by atropine eye drops. *Br J Ophthalmol* 1992;76:179–180.
20. Loewen N, Barry JC. Symposium proceedings. Part I: the use of cycloplegic agents. Results of a 1999 survey of German-speaking centers for pediatric ophthalmology and strabology. *Strabismus* 2000;8:91–99.
21. Willson WS, Duncan AJ, Jay JL. Effect of benzalkonium chloride on the stability of the precorneal tear film in rabbit and man. *Br J Ophthalmol* 1975;59:1083–1088.
22. Pisella PJ, Pouliquen P, Baudouin C. Prevalence of ocular symptoms and sign with preserved and preservative free glaucoma medication. *Br J Ophthalmol* 2002;86:418–423.
23. Ramli N, Supramanian G, Smasudin A, et al. Ocular surface disease in Glaucoma: effect of polypharmacy and preservatives. *Optom Vis Science* 2015;92(2):e222–e226.
24. Siatkowski RM, Cotter SA, Crockett RS, et al. Two-year multicenter, randomized, double-masked, placebo controlled, parallel safety and efficacy study of 2% pirenzepine ophthalmic gel in children with myopia. *J AAPOS* 2008;12:332–339.
25. Yam JC, Jiang Y, Tang SM, et al. Low-concentration Atropine for Myopia Progression (LAMP) Study: a randomized, double-blinded, placebo-controlled trial of 0.05%, 0.025%, and 0.01% Atropine eye drops in myopia control. *Ophthalmology* 2019;126(1):113–124.
26. Pineles SL, Kraker RT, VanderVeen DK, et al. Atropine for the prevention of myopia progression in children: a report from the American Academy of Ophthalmology. *Ophthalmology* 2017;124:1857–1866.
27. Tobias JD. Central nervous system depression following accidental ingestion of Visine eye drops. *Clin Pediatr (Phila)* 1996;35:539–540.
28. Mahieu LM, Rooman RP, Goossens E. Imidazoline intoxication in children. *Eur J Pediatr* 1993;152:944–946.
29. Tabbara KF. Ocular complications of vernal keratoconjunctivitis. *Can J Ophthalmol* 1999;34:88–92.
30. Pucci N, Novembre E, Cianferoni A, et al. Efficacy and safety of cyclosporine eyedrops in vernal keratoconjunctivitis. *Ann Allergy Asthma Immunol* 2002;89:298–303.
31. Al Rajhi AA, American Academy of Ophthalmology, Preferred Practice Patterns Committee, et al. *Conjunctivitis preferred practice pattern*. Elsevier, 2018:94–169.
32. Ozerdem U, Levi L, Cheng L, et al. Systemic toxicity of topical and periocular corticosteroid therapy in an 11-year-old male with posterior uveitis. *Am J Ophthalmol* 2000;130:240–241.
33. Steelman J, Kappy M. Adrenal suppression and growth retardation from ocular corticosteroids. *J Pediatr Ophthalmol Strabismus* 2001;38:177–178.
34. Bangsgaard R, Main KM, Bobberg-Ans G, et al. Adrenal suppression in infants treated with topical ocular glucocorticoids. *Ophthalmology* 2018;125:1638–1643.
35. Covell LL. Glaucoma induced by systemic steroid therapy. *Am J Ophthalmol* 1958;45:108–109.
36. Abuekteish F, Kirkpatrick JN, Russell G. Posterior subcapsular cataract and inhaled corticosteroid therapy. *Thorax* 1995;50:674–676.
37. Alfano JE. Changes in the intraocular pressure associated with systemic steroid therapy. *Am J Ophthalmol* 1963;56:245–247.
38. Cubey RB. Glaucoma following the application of corticosteroid to the skin of the eyelids. *Br J Dermatol* 1976;95:207–208.
39. Herschler J. Intractable intraocular hypertension induced by repository triamcinolone acetonide. *Am J Ophthalmol* 1972;74:501–504.
40. Rohen JW, Linner E, Witmer R. Electron microscopic studies on the trabecular meshwork in two cases of corticosteroid-glaucoma. *Exp Eye Res* 1973;17:19–31.
41. Armaly MF. Statistical attributes of the steroid hypertensive response in the clinically normal eye. I. The demonstration of three levels of response. *Invest Ophthalmol* 1963;70:482–491.
42. Biedner BZ, David R, Grudsky A, et al. Intraocular pressure response to corticosteroids in children. *Br J Ophthalmol* 1980;4:198–205.
43. Kwok AK, Lam DS, Ng JS, et al. Ocular-hypertensive response to topical steroids in children. *Ophthalmology* 1997;12:2112–2116.
44. Lam DS, Kwok AD, Chew S. Accelerated ocular hypertensive response to topical steroids in children. *Br J Ophthalmol* 1997;81:422–423.
45. Hutcheson KA. Steroid-induced glaucoma in an infant. *J AAPOS* 2007;11:522–523.
46. Calixto N, Silva SM, Cronemberger S, et al. Corticosteroid-induced pseudocongenital glaucoma. *Rev Bras Oftal* 2000;59:179–190.
47. Foster CS, Havrlikova K, Baltatzis S, et al. Secondary glaucoma in patients with juvenile rheumatoid arthritis-associated iridocyclitis. *Acta Ophthalmol Scand* 2000;78:576–579.
48. Jaffe GJ, Foster CS, Pavesio CE, et al. Effect of an injectable fluocinolone acetonide insert on recurrence rates in chronic noninfectious uveitis affecting the posterior segment. *Ophthalmology* 2019;126:601–610.
49. Ohji M, Kinoshita S, Ohmi E, et al. Marked intraocular pressure response to instillation of corticosteroids in children. *Am J Ophthalmol* 1991;112:450–454.
50. Gerzenstein SM, Pletcher MT, Cervino ACL, et al. Glucocorticoid receptor polymorphisms and intraocular pressure response to intravitreal triamcinolone acetonide. *Ophthalmic Genet* 2008;29:166–170.
51. Weiss A, Brinser JH, Nazar-Stewart V. Acute conjunctivitis in children. *J Pediatr* 1993;122:10–14.
52. Asbell PA, Sanfilippo CM, Pillar CM, et al. Antibiotic resistance among ocular pathogens in the United States: five-year results from the antibiotic resistance monitoring in ocular microorganisms surveillance study. *Ophthalmology* 2015;133(12):1445–1454.
53. Oldenburg CE, Lalitha P, Srinivasan M, et al. Emerging moxifloxacin resistance in *Pseudomonas aeruginosa* keratitis isolates in South India. *Ophthalmic Epidemiol* 2013;20(3):155–158.
54. Compochiaro PA, Conway BP. Aminoglycoside toxicity—a survey of retinal specialists. Implications for ocular use. *Arch Ophthalmol* 1991;109:946–950.
55. Rosenthal RL, Blackman A. Bone marrow hypoplasia following the use of chloramphenicol eye drops. *J Am Med Assoc* 1955;191:36–37.
56. Wiholm BE, Kelly JP, Kaufman D, et al. Relation of aplastic anaemia to use of choloramphenicol eye drops in two international case reports. *Br Med J* 1998;316:666.
57. Lancaster T, Swart AM, Jick H. Risk of serious hematological toxicity with use of chloramphenicol eye drops in a British general practice database. *Br Med J* 1998;316:667.
58. Witkop CJ, Wolf RO. Hypoplasia and intrinsic staining of enamel following tetracycline therapy. *J Am Med Assoc* 1963;185:100.
59. Burkhardt JE, Hill MA, Carlton WW, et al. Histologic and histochemical changes in articular cartilages of immature beagle dogs dosed with difloxicin, a fluoroquinolone. *Vet Pathol* 1990;27:162–170.
60. Sabella C, Goldfarb J. Fluoroquinolone therapy in pediatrics: where we stand [editorial]. *Clin Pediatr (Phila)* 1997;36:445–448.
61. Gross RD, Hoffman RO, Lindsay RN. A comparison of ciprofloxacin and tobramycin in bacterial conjunctivitis in children. *Clin Pediatr (Phila)* 1997;36:435–444.
62. Dunn AM, Tizer K, Cervia JS. Rifabutin-associated uveitis in a pediatric patient. *Pediatr Infect Dis J* 1995;14:246–247.
63. Le Saux N, MacDonald N, Dayneka N. Rifabutin ocular toxicity mimicking endophthalmitis. *Pediatr Infect J* 1997;16:716–718.
64. Jewelewicz DA, Schiff WM, Brown S, et al. Rifabutin-associated uveitis in an immunosuppressed pediatric patient without acquired immunodeficiency syndrome. *Am J Ophthalmol* 1998;125:872–873.
65. Jones FL, Ekberg NL. Exacerbation of asthma by timolol. *N Engl J Med* 1979;301:270.
66. Williams T, Ginther WH. Hazard of ophthalmic timolol. *N Engl J Med* 1982;306:1485–1486.
67. Hutchinson AD, Kraker RT, Pineles SL, et al. The use of B blockers for the treatment of periocular hemangioma in infants. *Ophthalmology* 2019;126:146–155.
68. Cracknell KPB, Grierson I, Hogg P. Morphometric effects of long-term exposure to latanoprost. *Ophthalmology* 2006;114:938–948.
69. Schmidtborn F. Systemic side-effects of latanoprost in a child with aniridia and glaucoma. *Ophthalmologe* 1998;95:633–634.
70. Enyedi LB, Freedman SF. Latanoprost for the treatment of pediatric glaucoma. *Surv Ophthalmol* 2002;47:S129–S132.
71. Enyedi LB, Freedman SF. Safety and efficacy of brimonidine in children with glaucoma. *J AAPOS* 2001;5:281–284.
72. Araujo SV, Bond JB, Wilson RP, et al. Long-term effect of apraclonidine. *Br J Ophthalmol* 1995;79:1098–1101.
73. Watts P, Satterfield D, Lim MK. Adverse effects of apraclonidine used in the diagnosis of Horner syndrome in infants. *J AAPOS* 2007;11:282–283.
74. Whitson JT, Roarty JD, Vijaya L, et al. Efficacy of brinzolamide and levobetaxolol in pediatric glaucomas: a randomized clinical trial. *J AAPOS* 2008;12:239–246.
75. Giles CL, Finkel HP, Nigro MA. Cholinergic crisis induced by phospholine iodide. *Am Orthop J* 1990;40:68–71.
76. Ip MS, Scott IU, Brown GC, et al. Anti-vascular endothelial growth factor pharmacotherapy for age-related macular degeneration: a report by the American Academy of Ophthalmology. *Ophthalmology* 2008;115(10):1837–1846.
77. Grewal DS, Jain R, Kumar H. Evaluation of subconjunctival bevacizumab as an adjunct to trabeculectomy. *Ophthalmology* 2008;115:2141–2145.
78. Wickremasinghe SS, Michalova K, Gilhotra J, et al. Acute intraocular inflammation after injections of bevacizumab for treatment of age-related macular degeneration. *Ophthalmology* 2008;115:1911–1915.
79. Lalwani GA, Berrocal AM, Murray TG, et al. Off-label use of intravitreal bevacizumab for salvage treatment in progressive threshold retinopathy of prematurity. *Retina* 2008;28(3):S13–S18.
80. Quiroz-Mercado H, Martinez-Castellanos MA, Hernandez-Rojas ML. Anti-angiotherapy with intravitreal bevacizumab for retinopathy of prematurity. *Retina* 2008;28(3):S19–S25.
81. Vogel RN, Strampe M, Fagbemi OE, et al. Foveal development in infants treated with bevacizumab or laser photocoagulation for retinopathy of prematurity. *Ophthalmology* 2018;125:444–452.

82. Lepore D, Quinn GE, Molle F. Follow-up to age 4 years of treatment of type 1 retinopathy of prematurity intravitreal injection versus laser: fluorescein angiographic findings. *Ophthalmology* 2018;125:218–226.
83. Kennedy KA, Mintz-Hittner HA, for the BEAT ROP Cooperative Group. Medical and developmental outcomes for bevacizumab versus laser for retinopathy of prematurity. *J AAPOS* 2018;22:61–65.
84. Brown MS, Baron AE, France ED, et al. Association between higher cumulative doses of recombinant erythropoietin and risk for retinopathy of prematurity. *J AAPOS* 2006;10:143–149.
85. Suk KK, Dunbar JA, Liu A, et al. Human recombinant erythropoietin and the incidence of retinopathy of prematurity. *J AAPOS* 2008;12:233–238.
86. Swartz M. Other diseases: drug toxicity and metabolic and nutritional conditions. In: Ryan SJ, ed. *Retina*, Vol. 2. St. Louis, MO: Mosby, 1989:742–744.
87. Itoh M, Aoyama T, Yamamura Y, et al. Effects of the rational use of corticosteroid eye drops for the prevention of ocular toxicity in high dose cytosine arabinoside therapy. *Yakugaku Zasshi* 1999;119:229–235.
88. Marmor MF, Kellner U, Lai TYY, et al. Recommendations on screening for chloroquine and hydroxychloroquine retinopathy. *Ophthalmology* 2016;123:1386–1394.
89. Marson AG, Kadir ZA, Hutton JL, et al. The new antiepileptic drugs: a systemic review of their efficacy and tolerability. *Epilepsia* 1997;38:859–880.
90. Nousiainen I, Kalviainen R, Mantyjarvi M. Color vision in epilepsy patients treated with vigabatrin or carbamazepine monotherapy. *Ophthalmology* 2000;107:884–888.
91. Daneshvar H, Racette L, Coupland SG, et al. Symptomatic and asymptomatic visual loss in patients taking vigabatrin. *Ophthalmology* 1999;106:1792–1798.
92. Bourgeois BFD. Pharmacokinetics and pharmacodynamics of topiramate. *J Child Neurol* 2000;15:S27–S30.
93. Levisohn PM. Safety and tolerability of topiramate in children. *J Child Neurol* 2000;15:S22–S26.
94. Rhee DJ, Goldberg MJ, Parrish RK. Bilateral angle-closure glaucoma and ciliary body swelling from topiramate. *Arch Ophthalmol* 2001;119:1721–1723.
95. Sankar PS, Pasquale LR, Grosskreutz CL. Uveal effusion and secondary angle-closure glaucoma associated with topiramate use. *Arch Ophthalmol* 2001;119:1210–1211.
96. Sen HA, O'Halloran HS, Lee WB. Topiramate-induced acute myopia and retinal striae. *Arch Ophthalmol* 2001;119:775–777.
97. Medeiros FA, Zhang XY, Bernd AS, et al. Angle-closure glaucoma associated with ciliary body detachment in patients using topiramate. *Arch Ophthalmol* 2003;121:282–285.
98. Baker-Schena L. Novel drug delivery systems. *EyeNet* 2019;23(4):47–52.

SECTION

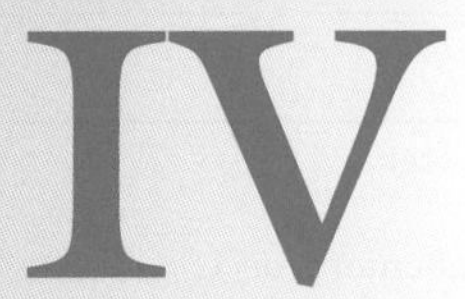

Antimicrobial Pharmacology

CHAPTER

20

Roopali Sharma
Margaret R. Hammerschlag

Penicillins, Cephalosporins, and Other β-Lactams

THE PENICILLINS

INTRODUCTION

Alexander Fleming discovered penicillin in 1928.[1] In the 1940s, penicillin became available for use in clinical practice. Batchelor and coworkers[2] isolated the 6-aminopenicillanic acid nucleus from *Penicillium chrysogenum*, which served as the basis for the development of semisynthetic penicillins. Subsequently, penicillins with expanded spectrum of activity including some gram-negative organisms were developed (Table 20.1).

NATURAL PENICILLINS

Structure–Activity Relationship

All penicillins contain the 6-aminopenicillanic acid nucleus, which is composed of a β-lactam ring and a five-member thiazolidine ring to which is attached a side chain. The penicillin nucleus is the chief structural requirement for biologic activity. The side chain determines many of the antibacterial and pharmacologic characteristics of a particular type of penicillin.[3] Penicillins generally exist as sodium or potassium salts.

Mechanism of Action

Penicillins exert bactericidal action against penicillin-susceptible microorganisms during the stage of active replication. Penicillin interferes with bacterial cell wall synthesis by reacting with one or more penicillin-binding proteins (PBPs). The PBPs, such as transpeptidases, carboxypeptidases, and endopeptidases, are bacterial enzymes involved in cell wall synthesis. Bacteria produce four types of PBPs, and they structurally resemble serine proteases.[4] The transpeptidase activity of PBPs is essential for cross-linking adjacent peptidoglycan, and the carboxypeptidases are important for the modification of peptidoglycan. PBPs account for approximately 1% of membrane proteins. They vary in the amounts present, in their role in cell wall assembly, and in their affinity for binding to β-lactam antibiotics.[5]

TABLE 20.1 Types of Penicillins

Natural Penicillins	*Aminopenicillins*	*Penicillinase-Resistant Penicillins*	*Extended-Spectrum Penicillins*
Penicillin G	Amoxicillin	Cloxacillin	Piperacillin
Penicillin V	Ampicillin	Dicloxacillin	
Penicillin G procaine		Oxacillin	
Penicillin G benzathine		Nafcillin	
		Methicillin	

TABLE 20.2 Spectrum of Activity for Penicillins

Classification of Organism	*Examples*
Gram-positive cocci	Most streptococci; susceptible strains of staphylococci, enterococci, and pneumococci Tolerance to penicillin among group B streptococcal isolates has been reported[6,7] Penicillin acts synergistically with gentamicin or tobramycin against many strains of enterococci
Gram-positive bacilli	*Corynebacterium diphtheriae, Bacillus anthracis, Actinomyces, Erysipelothrix rhusiopathiae,* and *Listeria monocytogenes*
Gram-negative bacteria	Non–β-lactamase–producing strains of *Neisseria gonorrhoeae,* and *Haemophilus influenzae, Neisseria meningitidis, Streptobacillus moniliformis,* and *Pasteurella multocida*
Anaerobic bacteria	*Clostridia* spp., *Peptostreptococcus,* and *Propionibacteria*
Spirochetes	*Treponema pallidum, Borrelia burgdorferi,* and *Spirillum minus*

Resistance

Penicillin resistance is mediated mainly through production of β-lactamase, which covalently binds to the β-lactam bond to form an acyl enzyme intermediate, which undergoes rapid hydrolysis, thus destroying the activity of the drug. Gram-positive β-lactamases, such as the staphylococcal penicillinase, are exoenzymes that destroy penicillins before they reach the target PBPs. The β-lactamases of gram-negative bacteria are cell associated and are located in the periplasmic space between the cytoplasmic membrane and the lipopolysaccharide outer membrane. Alteration of PBPs accounts for penicillin resistance among pneumococci, some strains of *Haemophilus influenzae,* and some *Neisseria* spp.

Pharmacokinetics

Metabolism and disposition vary significantly among the various penicillins and also vary with the age of the patients. They are not well absorbed from the gastrointestinal tract, with the exception of phenoxymethyl penicillin (penicillin V) and amoxicillin. Penicillin V is acid stable and is available only for oral use. Penicillin G is not acid stable and hence is generally used parenterally. Penicillins bind to serum proteins, mainly albumin. Penicillins are primarily excreted in the urine in the unchanged form. Tubular secretion accounts for most of the urinary penicillin, and glomerular filtration accounts for only a small fraction. Penicillin does not penetrate well into the cerebrospinal fluid (CSF) in the absence of meningeal inflammation. Repository penicillins such as procaine penicillin or benzathine penicillin provide tissue depots. Procaine penicillin is absorbed over several hours and benzathine penicillin over several days.

Spectrum of Activity

Penicillins act on gram-positive cocci, gram-positive bacilli, gram-negative bacteria, anaerobic bacteria, and spirochetes (Table 20.2).

Clinical Uses

Penicillin is effective in the treatment of infections caused by group A streptococci, group B streptococci, meningococci, *Actinomyces,* and *Treponema pallidum* (Tables 20.3 to 20.5).[8,9] It is also the treatment of choice for infections due to susceptible *Streptococcus pneumoniae,* enterococci, and gonococci. Infections other than meningitis that are due to penicillin-resistant *S. pneumoniae* may not be associated with a less favorable clinical outcome or increased mortality compared with those for penicillin-susceptible infections when treated with high-dose penicillin.[10] The breakpoints for penicillin in the treatment of pneumococcal pneumonia were recently updated, whereas the breakpoint for meningitis remains unchanged.[11] Infections due to anaerobic mouth flora are generally susceptible to penicillin G. Penicillin V is the drug of choice for prophylaxis against rheumatic carditis and against infections in patients with anatomic or functional asplenia. In patients with poor compliance, intramuscular benzathine penicillin can be used every 3 to 4 weeks. Benzathine penicillin is the drug of choice for primary, secondary, and early or late latent syphilis (except

TABLE 20.3 Pharmacokinetic Properties of Selected Penicillins

Generic Name	*Half-Life (h)*	*Protein Binding (%)*	*Route of Excretion*
Penicillin G	0.5–1.2	55–65	Renal
Penicillin V	1	80	Renal
Oxacillin	0.5–1.2	90–95	Renal, hepatic
Cloxacillin	0.5	90–95	Renal, hepatic
Dicloxacillin	0.8–1	96–98	Renal, hepatic
Nafcillin	0.5	87–90	Hepatic, renal
Ampicillin	1	15–25	Renal
Amoxicillin	1	17–20	Renal
Piperacillin	0.5–1.3	22	Renal

Data from Chambers HF. Penicillins. In: Mandell GL, Bennett JE, Dolin R, eds. *Mandell, Douglas, and Bennett's principles and practice of infectious diseases,* 5th ed. Philadelphia, PA: Churchill Livingstone, 2000:261–274; Reed MD, Blumer JL. Anti-infective therapy. In: Jenson HB, Baltimore RS, eds. *Pediatric infectious diseases,* 2nd ed. Philadelphia, PA: WB Saunders, 2002:147–211.

TABLE 20.4 Penicillin Dosing Recommendations: Neonates (mg/kg/dose or U/kg/dose)

		Infants 0–4 wk of Age	*Infants <1 wk of Age*		*Infants ≥1 wk of Age*	
Antibiotic	*Route*	*BW < 1,200 g*	*BW 1,200–2,000 g*	*BW > 2,000 g*	*BW 1,200–2,000 g*	*BW > 2,000 g*
Penicillin G,[a] aqueous	i.v., i.m.	25,000–50,000 q12 h	25,000–50,000 q12 h	25,000–50,000 q8 h	25,000–50,000 q8 h	25,000–50,000 q6 h
Ampicillin (mg/kg)[a]	i.v., i.m.	25–50 q12 h	25–50 q12 h	25–50 q8 h	25–50 q8 h	25–50 q6 h
Procaine penicillin (U)	i.m.	–	50,000 q24 h	50,000 q24 h	50,000 q24 h	50,000 q24 h
Nafcillin (mg/kg)	i.v., i.m.	25 q12 h	25 q12 h	25 q8 h	25 q8 h	25–35 q6 h
Oxacillin (mg/kg)	i.v., i.m.	25 q12 h	25–50 q12 h	25–50 q8 h	25–50 q8 h	25–50 q6 h

[a]For meningitis, larger dosage is recommended.
BW, body weight; i.m., intramuscular; i.v., intravenous; q6 h, every 6 hours; q8 h, every 8 hours; q12 h, every 12 hours; q24 h, every 24 hours.
Data from American Academy of Pediatrics. Tables of antibacterial drug doses. In: Pickering LK, ed. *2006 Red book: report of the Committee on Infectious Diseases,* 27th ed. Elk Grove Village, IL: American Academy of Pediatrics, 2006:750–765.

neurosyphilis). For infants with congenital syphilis, penicillin G or procaine penicillin is recommended.[12]

Adverse Reactions

Allergic reactions are the major side effects associated with the penicillins. Severe and, occasionally, fatal anaphylaxis has also occurred. This relates to the ability of penicillins to act as haptens and combine with proteins. The most important antigenic component of the penicillins is the penicilloyl determinant produced by opening of the β-lactam ring. Anaphylactic reactions are estimated to occur in 0.01% to 0.05% of persons receiving penicillins. In patients with a history of life-threatening reactions to penicillin, it may be prudent to avoid other β-lactam agents. However, if no other options are available, a trial of desensitization may be attempted. The following hypersensitivity reactions have been described: skin rashes ranging from maculopapular eruptions to exfoliative dermatitis, urticaria, and reactions

TABLE 20.5 Penicillin Dosing Recommendations: Pediatric Patients Excluding Neonates (mg/kg/d or U/kg/d)

		Daily Dose		
Antibiotic	*Route*	*Mild–Moderate Infections*	*Severe Infections*	*Frequency of Administration (i.e., in Divided Doses)*
Penicillin G	i.m., i.v.	25,000–50,000 U	250,000–400,000 U	q4–6 h
Penicillin V	p.o.	25,000–50,000 U	Inappropriate	q6–8 h
Penicillin G, benzathine	i.m.	<27.3 kg (60 lb): 600,000 U		
		≥27.3 kg: 1,200,000 U	Inappropriate	q1–3 wk
Penicillin G, procaine	i.m.	25,000–50,000 U (max. adult dose 48,000,000 U/24 h)	Inappropriate	q12–24 h
Oxacillin	i.m., i.v.	100–150 mg/kg	150–200 mg/kg	q4–6 h
Dicloxacillin	p.o.	25–50 mg/kg	Inappropriate	q6 h
Nafcillin	i.m., i.v.	50–100 mg/kg	100–150 mg/kg	q6 h
Ampicillin	i.m., i.v.	100–150 mg/kg	200–400 mg/kg	q6 h
	p.o.	50–100 mg/kg	Inappropriate	q4–6 h
Amoxicillin	p.o.	25–50 mg/kg	Inappropriate	q8 h
Piperacillin	i.m., i.v.	100–150 mg/kg	200–300 mg/kg	q4–6 h
Amoxicillin–clavulanic acid[a]	p.o.	90 mg/kg	Inappropriate	q12 h
Piperacillin–tazobactam[b]	i.m., i.v.	100 mg piperacillin/12.5 mg tazobactam/kg[c]	240 mg	q8 h
Ampicillin–sulbactam[b]	i.m., i.v.	100–150 mg/kg	200–400 mg/kg	q6 h

[a]Amoxicillin:clavulanate 14:1, approved for infants and children ≥3 months of age.
[b]Based on the penicillin component.
[c]For 2- to 9-month old, 80 mg piperacillin per 10 mg tazobactam per kg per day in three divided doses (product label, https://dailymed.nlm.nih.gov/dailymed/index.cfm).
i.m., intramuscular; i.v., intravenous; p.o., oral; q1–3 wk, every 1 to 3 weeks; q4–6 h, every 4 to 6 hours; q6 h, every 6 hours; q6–8 h, every 6 to 8 hours; q8 h, every 8 hours; q12 h, every 12 hours; q12–24 h, every 12 to 24 hours.
Data from American Academy of Pediatrics. Tables of antibacterial drug doses. In: Pickering LK, ed. 2006 *Red book: report of the Committee on Infectious Diseases,* 27th ed. Elk Grove Village, IL: American Academy of Pediatrics, 2006:750–765.

resembling serum sickness, including chills, fever, edema, arthralgia, and prostration. The Jarisch–Herxheimer reaction has been reported in patients treated for syphilis.

Hematologic toxicity including Coombs-positive hemolytic anemia, leukopenia, and thrombocytopenia has been reported with penicillin use. Penicillins bind to the adenosine diphosphate–receptor site in platelets and thereby interfere with platelet aggregation. Clinically significant bleeding is not common.

Sodium overload and hypokalemia can occur with massive doses of penicillin secondary to the large dose of nonreabsorbable anion in the distal renal tubules. Patients given continuous intravenous (IV) therapy with penicillin G potassium in high dosage (10 to 100 MU daily) may suffer severe or even fatal potassium poisoning, particularly if renal insufficiency is present.

Neurologic toxicity in the form of seizures has been reported following the use of massive doses of penicillin.

Drug Interactions

Concurrent administration of bacteriostatic antibiotics (e.g., erythromycin and tetracycline) may diminish the bactericidal effects of penicillins by slowing the rate of bacterial growth. The clinical significance of this interaction is not well documented. Penicillin blood levels may be prolonged by concurrent administration of probenecid, which blocks the renal tubular secretion of penicillins. Penicillins can interact with oral contraceptives.[13,14]

AMINOPENICILLINS

Structure–Activity Relationship

Aminopenicillins have a free amino group at the α position on the β-lactam ring of the penicillin nucleus, thereby increasing their ability to penetrate the outer membranes of gram-negative organisms.

Mechanism of Action

The mechanism of action is similar to that of penicillins.

Resistance

Aminopenicillins are inactivated by the β-lactamases produced by either gram-positive or gram-negative bacteria.

Pharmacokinetics

Aminopenicillins are cleared by the kidney. Ampicillin achieves therapeutic concentrations in most body fluids, including CSF pleural, joint, and peritoneal fluids, after parenteral administration. Amoxicillin has better absorption and bioavailability and hence is the preferred oral aminopenicillin. The absorption of amoxicillin is not affected by food.

Spectrum

Compared with penicillin G, ampicillin has increased in vitro efficacy against most strains of enterococci and *Listeria monocytogenes* as well as against some gram-negative pathogens, such as non–β-lactamase–producing strains of *H. influenzae* and *Neisseria gonorrhoeae*. Some strains of *Escherichia coli*, *Shigella sonnei*, and *Salmonella* including strains of *Salmonella typhi* are resistant.

Clinical Uses

Amoxicillin is the drug of choice for acute otitis media[15,16] (see Tables 20.3 to 20.5). Oral amoxicillin is also the drug of choice for the treatment of some clinical manifestations of Lyme disease such as erythema migrans, isolated facial palsy, and arthritis.[17] Parenteral ampicillin is widely used in neonates with sepsis because of its activity against *Listeria*. Amoxicillin is used in combination with clarithromycin and a proton-pump inhibitor like omeprazole or lansoprazole for the treatment of *Helicobacter pylori* infections.[18,19] A report from the Food and Drug Administration (FDA) provides information on the pharmacokinetics (PK) and dosing of amoxicillin for use in the prophylaxis of postexposure inhalational anthrax (15 mg per kg per dose given every 8 hours).[20]

Adverse Events

The incidence of hypersensitivity reactions with aminopenicillins is similar to that of natural penicillins. There is a slightly higher incidence of maculopapular rash associated with ampicillin use in patients with intercurrent viral illnesses, especially due to Epstein–Barr virus.

ANTISTAPHYLOCOCCAL PENICILLINS

Structure–Activity Relationship

These are semisynthetic penicillin derivatives synthesized by the acylation of 6-aminopenicillanic acid to prevent the attachment of staphylococcal penicillinases to the β-lactam ring. Methicillin contains a dimethoxyphenyl group on the penicillin nucleus, and nafcillin is a naphthyl analog of methicillin. Cloxacillin and dicloxacillin contain chlorine atoms, which increase gastrointestinal absorption and antibacterial activity as well as serum half-life and protein binding.

Mechanism

The penicillinase-resistant penicillins also act by binding to PBPs and preventing cell wall synthesis. They are resistant to the action of bacterial penicillinases by steric hindrance of the acyl side chain, thereby preventing opening of the β-lactam ring.

Resistance

Resistance to semisynthetic penicillins among staphylococci is related to the presence of the *mecA* gene, which results in the synthesis of a unique PBP, PBP2a, which has low affinity for methicillin and other β-lactam antibiotics.

Spectrum

This group of penicillins is effective against β-lactamase–producing isolates of *Staphylococcus aureus* and coagulase-negative staphylococci. They retain most of the activity of the penicillins but are much less active compared with penicillin G against penicillin-susceptible organisms, including non–penicillinase-producing staphylococci and streptococci. Enterococci, gram-negative cocci, *L. monocytogenes*, and anaerobes are resistant to these penicillins.

Pharmacokinetics

Unlike the natural penicillins, nafcillin is predominantly excreted through the biliary system, and, hence, accumulation can occur in jaundiced neonates. Although nafcillin is available in oral formulations, absorption is erratic. The isoxazolyl penicillins oxacillin, cloxacillin, and dicloxacillin are absorbed after oral administration but adversely affected by food. Serum levels after absorption are higher with cloxacillin and dicloxacillin than with oxacillin. They are excreted primarily by the kidneys with some biliary excretion. Cloxacillin and dicloxacillin are highly protein bound.

Clinical Indications

Methicillin is acid labile, is the least active member of this group of penicillins, and is most likely to cause interstitial nephritis, and hence is no longer used. Semisynthetic penicillins are commonly used in the empiric treatment of skin and skin structure infections and bone and joint infections where *S. aureus* is a likely pathogen (see Tables 20.3 to 20.5).

Adverse Events

Interstitial nephritis manifesting clinically as fever, rash, eosinophilia, proteinuria, eosinophiluria, and hematuria is more commonly reported with methicillin use. Elevated aspartate aminotransferase levels and cholestasis usually without jaundice have been reported with oxacillin use. Liver enzymes usually return to normal after discontinuation of therapy.

Drug Interactions

Drug interactions involving nafcillin with cyclosporine and warfarin have been reported.[21–24]

EXTENDED-SPECTRUM PENICILLINS

Structure–Activity Relationship

The only extended penicillin currently available is piperacillin. Piperacillin is a piperazine analog of ampicillin. Piperacillin is most frequently used today in a formulation with the β-lactamases inhibitor tazobactam.

Resistance

Piperacillin is susceptible to hydrolysis by β-lactamases of both gram-positive and gram-negative bacteria.

Spectrum

Piperacillin has a broader spectrum of activity than natural penicillins and aminopenicillins. Piperacillin is similar to ampicillin in activity against gram-positive species, including good activity against anaerobic cocci and bacilli. It also has activity against members of the Enterobacteriaceae family and *Pseudomonas aeruginosa*. Piperacillin also has activity against enterococci.

Pharmacokinetics

Piperacillin is administered parenterally. It has minimal CSF penetration. Primary route of elimination is renal via glomerular filtration and tubular secretion. The ureidopenicillins show dose-related nonlinear kinetics.

Clinical Indications

Piperacillin is effective against a variety of gram-negative organisms and, in combination with aminoglycosides, is synergistic against many gram-negative bacilli (see Tables 20.3 to 20.5). They are generally used clinically in combination with a β-lactamase inhibitor.

Adverse Events

Hypersensitivity reactions occur similar to those with natural penicillins. Because these agents are negatively charged ions, hypokalemia can result from leaching of anions in the distal renal tubule. Platelet dysfunction and prolonged bleeding times have been observed with the use of extended-spectrum penicillins. They can inhibit platelet aggregation by binding to the adenosine diphosphate receptor on platelets.

Drug Interactions

Piperacillin can interact with warfarin, thereby decreasing its anticoagulant effects. Piperacillin can potentiate the action of nondepolarizing-blocking agents. Some extended-spectrum penicillins have been shown to interact in solution with aminoglycosides, causing degradation of the aminoglycosides. It is recommended that these drugs not be mixed in solution and their administration be separated by 30 to 60 minutes.

β-LACTAMASE INHIBITORS

The β-lactamase inhibitors are compounds that inhibit many β-lactamases and additionally have weak antibacterial activity. They are available as fixed-combination preparations with a β-lactam antibiotic. Clavulanic acid is produced by the fermentation of *Streptomyces clavuligerus.* It is a β-lactam structurally related to the penicillins and cephalosporins. It contains a β-lactam ring attached to an oxazolidine ring. Sulbactam is a synthetic penicillinate sulfone derived from 6-aminopenicillanic acid and contains a β-lactam ring. Tazobactam is a synthetic penicillanic acid sulfone. Avibactam is a new β-lactamase inhibitor that has been FDA approved in combination with ceftazidime. The chemical structure of avibactam consists of a diazabicyclooctane ring rather than a β-lactam ring which is found in clavulanic acid, sulbactam, and tazobactam and thus is the first non–β-lactam β-lactamase inhibitor.[25]

MECHANISM OF ACTION

Clavulanic acid, sulbactam, and tazobactam possess the ability to inactivate a wide variety of β-lactamases by irreversibly binding to the active sites of these enzymes. Clavulanic acid is particularly active against the clinically important plasmid-mediated β-lactamases frequently responsible for transferred drug resistance to penicillins and cephalosporins. Clavulanic acid acts by both transient reversible complex formation and irreversible inactivation. Against *E. coli*–derived β-lactamase, reversible complex formation has been shown to proceed at a faster rate than terminal inactivation. In the presence of excess clavulanic acid, all enzymes will accumulate into one of several irreversibly inactivated forms.[26,27] The mechanism of action of sulbactam and tazobactam is similar to that of clavulanic acid.[28,29]

Clavulanic acid is the most efficient inhibitor of staphylococcal β-lactamase and is also an effective inhibitor of chromosomally mediated β-lactamase liberated by *Klebsiella pneumoniae*, *Proteus mirabilis*, *Proteus vulgaris*, *Moraxella catarrhalis*, *Bacteroides fragilis*, and TEM plasmid-mediated β-lactamase. It less readily inhibits chromosomally mediated β-lactamase of *Citrobacter* species, *Enterobacter* species, indole-positive *Proteus* species, and *Serratia marcescens*.[30] Overall, sulbactam is the least active of the three agents.[31] No significant difference in activity between the inhibitors exists with respect to anaerobes; therefore, they should be considered comparable with respect to extending anaerobic coverage to their partner antibiotic in treating mixed infections.[32]

β-Lactamase inhibitors can act as inducers of certain β-lactamases, thus rendering organisms that produce the enzyme less susceptible to the partner antibiotic.[33] This effect is most pronounced with clavulanic acid and occurs at concentrations at or above those achievable in vivo.[23] Tazobactam does not induce chromosomally mediated β-lactamases at tazobactam levels achieved with the recommended dosage regimen.[34] β-Lactamase inhibitors also have some intrinsic antibacterial activity. Clavulanic acid demonstrates good activity against *B. fragilis*, *Acinetobacter* species, and *Legionella pneumophila*.[35] Tazobactam has very low-level binding to PBPs and has the least intrinsic antibacterial activity.[31]

Avibactam prevents hydrolysis by covalently binding and acetylating β-lactamase active site on ceftazidime, preventing inactivation. The addition of avibactam extends ceftazidime's activity against many β-lactamases that would normally in activate ceftazidime. However, avibactam does not have activity against metallo–β-lactamases including IMP, New Delhi, VIM, and OXA carbapenemases. Avibactam is eliminated in the urine as unchanged drug, 97% with minimum metabolism,[25] and thus requires dose adjustment in patients with renal dysfunction.

PHARMACOKINETICS

Clavulanic acid is well absorbed orally and provides adequate inhibitory activity in most body fluids, except CSF and sputum.[36,37] Sulbactam is available in oral and parenteral formulations. In the United States, it is available only for parenteral use. Tazobactam is also available only in a parenteral formulation.

PENICILLINS AND β-LACTAMASE INHIBITOR COMBINATIONS

Penicillins and β-lactamase inhibitor combinations used clinically include ampicillin + sulbactam, amoxicillin + clavulanic acid, and piperacillin + tazobactam.

PHARMACOKINETICS

Amoxicillin serum concentrations achieved with amoxicillin + clavulanic acid are similar to those produced by the oral administration of equivalent doses of amoxicillin alone. Amoxicillin and clavulanate potassium are well absorbed from the gastrointestinal tract after oral administration. Dosing in the fasted or fed state has minimal effect on the PK of amoxicillin. Ticarcillin can be detected in tissues and interstitial fluid following parenteral administration. Penetration of ticarcillin into bile and pleural fluid has been demonstrated. Penetration of both ampicillin and sulbactam into CSF in the presence of inflamed meninges has been demonstrated after IV administration of ampicillin and sulbactam. Piperacillin and tazobactam are widely distributed into tissues and body fluids, including intestinal mucosa, gallbladder, lung, female reproductive tissues (uterus, ovary, and fallopian tube), interstitial fluid, and bile. Mean tissue concentrations are generally 50% to 100% of those in plasma. Distribution of piperacillin and tazobactam into CSF is low in individuals with noninflamed meninges, as with other penicillins.[34] The protein binding of either piperacillin or tazobactam is unaffected by the presence of the other compound.

CLINICAL USES

Amoxicillin–Clavulanic Acid

Amoxicillin + clavulanic acid is useful in children with acute otitis media and other respiratory tract infections caused by β-lactamase–producing strains of *H. influenzae* and *M. catarrhalis*. It can be used to treat animal or human bites. Various formulations of this combination are available, with the ratio of amoxicillin to clavulanate varying (4:1, 7:1, and 14:1). The 12-hourly regimen is associated with significantly less diarrhea.

It is approved by the FDA for use in pediatric patients for the following infections: lower respiratory tract infections, otitis media, sinusitis, skin and skin structure infections, and urinary tract infections (UTIs). A different dosing regimen is recommended for patients younger than 3 months of age.

Ampicillin–Sulbactam

The safety and effectiveness of ampicillin + sulbactam have been established for pediatric patients aged 1 year and older for skin and skin structure infections. The safety and effectiveness have not been established for pediatric patients for intra-abdominal infections (IAIs).

Piperacillin–Tazobactam

Piperacillin + tazobactam is approved for use in pediatric patients aged 2 months or older with appendicitis and/or peritonitis. The dosing regimens vary for children aged 9 months or older, weighing up to 40 kg, and with normal renal function and for those between the ages of 2 and 9 months (see Table 20.5). Pediatric patients weighing more than 40 kg and with normal renal function should receive the adult dose. There are no dosage recommendations for pediatric patients with impaired renal function.

CEPHALOSPORINS

The first source of cephalosporins was *Cephalosporium acremonium*, a fungus isolated in 1948 by G. Brotzu from the sea near a sewer outlet off the Sardinian coast.

STRUCTURE–ACTIVITY RELATIONSHIP

All cephalosporins are semisynthetic derivatives of a 7-aminocephalosporanic acid nucleus. Like penicillins, cephalosporins possess a β-lactam ring. Modifications of the carbon-3 and carbon-7 positions of the 7-aminocephalosporanic acid nucleus have yielded the three generations. Modifications around this nucleus have stabilized the β-lactam ring to hydrolysis by penicillinases. Modifications around the carbon-3 position are associated with changes in the metabolism or improved PK, and modifications around the carbon-7 position affect β-lactamase stability and antimicrobial activity.[38–41] The cephamycins are similar to cephalosporins, but have a methoxy group at position 7 of the β-lactam ring of the 7-aminocephalosporanic acid nucleus. The cephamycins are discussed along with the second-generation cephalosporins in this chapter.

MECHANISM OF ACTION

Cephalosporins and cephamycins interfere with synthesis of peptidoglycan in the bacterial cell wall. They bind to and inactivate PBPs, which are enzymes responsible for the synthesis of the bacterial cell wall and include transpeptidases, carboxypeptidases, and endopeptidases.

CLASSIFICATION

Cephalosporins are classified into generations on the basis of their spectrum of microbiologic activity (Table 20.6). This classification reflects increasing stability of the higher generations to various bacterial β-lactamases. None of the cephalosporins are effective against organisms like methicillin-resistant *S. aureus* (MRSA), enterococci, *L. monocytogenes, L. pneumophila, Stenotrophomonas maltophilia, Clostridium difficile,* and *Campylobacter jejuni.* Their microbiologic activity is summarized in Table 20.7.

TABLE 20.6 Classification of Cephalosporins

	Route of Administration	*Drug Name*
First generation	Oral	Cephalexin
	Parenteral	Cefazolin Cephalothin
Second generation	Oral	Cefuroxime axetil Cefaclor
	Parenteral	Cefoxitin Cefotetan
Third generation	Oral	Cefixime Cefdinir Cefpodoxime
	Parenteral	Ceftriaxone Ceftazidime
Fourth generation	Parenteral	Cefepime

The first-generation cephalosporins have good activity against gram-positive cocci and relatively modest activity against many gram-negative bacteria. Most gram-positive cocci excluding MRSA, enterococci, and *Staphylococcus epidermidis* are susceptible. Most oral anaerobes are susceptible, excluding *B. fragilis.*

The second-generation cephalosporins are more active against gram-negative bacteria, though less so when compared with the third-generation cephalosporins. They have variable activity against gram-positive cocci. They have improved activity against *H. influenzae, M. catarrhalis, Neisseria meningitidis,* and *N. gonorrhoeae.* The cephamycins have inferior activity against staphylococci but are active against some Enterobacteriaceae and *B. fragilis.*

Third-generation cephalosporins are more active against the Enterobacteriaceae, including the β-lactamase–producing strains. They are also active against *S. pneumoniae* (including those with relative penicillin resistance), *Streptococcus pyogenes,* and, with the exception of ceftazidime, have clinically useful activity against methicillin-sensitive strains of *S. aureus.* They also have excellent activity against *H. influenzae, M. catarrhalis, N. meningitidis,* and *N. gonorrhoeae.* Ceftazidime is the only extended-spectrum cephalosporin with good antipseudomonal activity.

Fourth-generation cephalosporins have a greater spectrum of activity than the third-generation agents. They are stable against the chromosomally mediated AmpC β-lactamases.[42] They are active against the Enterobacteriaceae, *P. aeruginosa, H. influenzae,* and *Neisseria* species.[43] They are also effective against gram-positive cocci, including methicillin-susceptible *S. aureus, S. pneumoniae,* and other streptococci.

BACTERIAL RESISTANCE

Three mechanisms of resistance to cephalosporins that have been described include inactivation by bacterial β-lactamases, alteration of PBPs, and alteration of bacterial permeability to cephalosporins.

Production of β-lactamases is the most common mechanism of resistance among the gram-negative bacteria. These enzymes are encoded either chromosomally or extrachromosomally through plasmids or transposons. The susceptibility to β-lactamases, however, varies among the different agents. Cefoxitin, cefuroxime, and the third-generation cephalosporins

TABLE 20.7 Microbiologic Activity of Cephalosporins

	Gram-Positive Cocci[a]	Gram-Negative Cocci	*Haemophilus influenzae*	*Pseudomonas*	*Enterobacteriaceae*	*Bacteroides fragilis*
First generation	3–4[b]	1	0–2	0	2	0
Second generation	2–3	2	2	0	2–3	0–3[c]
Third generation	0–3	4	4	1–3	4	0–2
Fourth generation	3–4	4	4	4[d]	4	2–3

[a]Excludes methicillin-resistant *Staphylococcus aureus.*
[b]Not effective against penicillin-resistant *Streptococcus pneumoniae.*
[c]The cephamycins have good activity against *Bacteroides* spp.
[d]Ceftazidime has antipseudomonal activity.

are more resistant to hydrolysis by the β-lactamases produced by gram-negative bacteria than the first-generation agents. The third-generation agents are susceptible to hydrolysis by the inducible, chromosomally encoded β-lactamases and the plasmid extended-spectrum β-lactamases (ESBLs). The fourth-generation agents are poor inducers of type I β-lactamases and less susceptible to hydrolysis by these enzymes compared with the third-generation agents. Altered permeability is more important among gram-negative bacteria than gram-positive bacteria due to the differences in the nature of their cell walls. However, it is unlikely that altered porin permeability alone accounts for resistance among gram-negative bacteria.[44] Decreased affinity of PBPs for cephalosporins is the mechanism by which some strains of *N. gonorrhoeae*, *H. influenzae*, and *S. pneumoniae* have developed resistance to cephalosporins.

PHARMACOKINETICS

Cephalosporins are primarily excreted via the kidneys mainly by glomerular filtration. Dosage should be adjusted in patients with renal insufficiency. Ceftriaxone also has biliary excretion. Protein binding varies from 10% for cephalexin to 90% for ceftriaxone. Table 20.8 provides the important PK features of some of the more commonly used cephalosporins.

Most cephalosporins have good penetration into tissues and fluid compartments. Cephalosporins that can achieve adequate levels in the CSF include cefuroxime, ceftriaxone, and cefepime. Cefuroxime is not recommended for treatment of meningitis as it has been associated with delayed CSF sterilization.[45] Use of ceftriaxone in the first month of life is avoided because of the high degree of protein binding and hence likelihood of bilirubin displacement. Oral first- and second-generation agents are well absorbed from the gastrointestinal tract. Some cephalosporins, such as cefuroxime and cefpodoxime, are formulated as esters to facilitate absorption. After oral administration, they are rapidly hydrolyzed by nonspecific esterases in the intestinal mucosa and blood. The oral third-generation cephalosporins, such as cefixime, are not as well absorbed but achieve adequate systemic concentration to treat the respiratory tract infections and UTIs. Coadministration with lidocaine can reduce the discomfort associated with intramuscular cephalosporin administration.

CLINICAL USE

First- and second-generation cephalosporins are used in the treatment of a variety of infections in pediatrics. They are used commonly for the treatment of skin and respiratory tract infections. Third-generation cephalosporins are commonly used for the empiric treatment of hospitalized infants and children. The fourth-generation agents, such as cefepime, are used more commonly in the treatment of patients with febrile neutropenia and nosocomial infections.

First-Generation Agents

Members of this class are widely used in the treatment of skin and soft-tissue infections. Cefazolin is used commonly for preoperative prophylaxis for surgical procedures involving foreign-body implantation and clean and clean-contaminated procedures in which there is a high risk of infection.[46,47] The general dosing schedules for oral and parenteral preparations published in the literature are listed in Tables 20.9 to 20.11.[9,48,49]

TABLE 20.8 Pharmacokinetic Properties of Cephalosporins

Generic Name	*Half-Life (h)*	*Protein Binding (%)*	*Route of Excretion*
First generation			
Cefazolin	1.4	86	Renal
Cephalexin	1.2	14	Renal
Cefadroxil	1.3	15	Renal
Second generation			
Cefuroxime axetil	1.4	33	Renal
Cefoxitin	0.8	73	Renal
Cefotetan	3.5	88	Renal
Third generation			
Ceftriaxone	6–8	90	Renal 65%; biliary 35%
Ceftazidime	1.9	20	Renal
Cefixime	3.8	69	Renal 50%; ? other
Cefpodoxime	2.2	40	Renal
Fourth generation			
Cefepime	1.5–1.7	19	Renal

TABLE 20.9 Dosing of Oral Cephalosporins (Excluding Neonates)

Generic Name	*Dose (mg/kg/d)*	*Frequency*[a]
First generation		
Cephalexin	25–50	q6 h
Cefadroxil	30	q12 h
Second generation		
Cefuroxime axetil	20–40	q12 h
Cefprozil	15–30	q12 h
Cefaclor	20–40	q8–12 h
Third generation		
Cefixime	8	q12 h/24 h
Cefpodoxime proxetil	10	q12 h
Cefdinir	14	q12–24 h

[a]q6 h, every 6 hour; q8–12 h, every 8 to 12 hours; q12 h, every 12 hour; q12 h/24 h, every 12 hours/24 hours; q12–24 h, every 12 to 24 hours; q24 h, every 24 hours.
Data from American Academy of Pediatrics. Tables of antibacterial drug doses. In: Pickering LK, ed. 2006 *Red book: report of the Committee on Infectious Diseases*, 27th ed. Elk Grove Village, IL: American Academy of Pediatrics, 2006:750–765; Philips JL, Abdel-Rahman S, Farrar HC, et al. Antimicrobial agents. In: Long SS, Pickering LK, Prober CG, eds. *Principles and practice of pediatric infectious diseases*, 2nd ed. New York, NY: Churchill Livingstone, 2003:1458–1510.

TABLE 20.10 Dosing of Parenteral Cephalosporins (Excluding Neonates)

	Dose (mg/kg/d)		
Generic Name	*Mild–Moderate Infections*	*Severe Infections*	*Frequency*
First generation			
Cefazolin	25–50	50–100	q8 h
Cephalothin	80–100	100–150	q4–6 h
Second generation			
Cefuroxime	75–100	100–150	q8 h
Cefoxitin	80–100	80–160	q4–6 h
Cefotetan		40–80[a]	q12 h
Third generation			
Cefotaxime	75–100	150–200	q6–8 h[b,c]
Ceftriaxone	50–75	80–100	q12–24 h
Ceftazidime	75–100	125–150	q8 h
Fourth generation			
Cefepime[d]	100–150	150	q8 h
Fifth generation			
Ceftaroline	6–8	12	q8 h

q4–6 h, every 4 to 6 hours; q6–8 h, every 6 to 8 hours; q8 h, every 8 hours; q8–12 h, every 8 to 12 hour; q12 h, every 12 hours; q12–24 h, every 12 to 24 hours.

[a]Not approved for pediatric use.

[b]75 mg/kg every 6 hours for treatment of meningitis.

[c]Dosing as high as 300 mg per kg per day divided into three to four doses has been recommended for meningitis.[9]

[d]Not approved for meningitis.

Data from American Academy of Pediatrics. Tables of antibacterial drug doses. In: Pickering LK, ed. 2006 *Red book: report of the Committee on Infectious Diseases*, 27th ed. Elk Grove Village, IL: American Academy of Pediatrics, 2006:750–765; Philips JL, Abdel-Rahman S, Farrar HC, et al. Antimicrobial agents. In: Long SS, Pickering LK, Prober CG, eds. *Principles and practice of pediatric infectious diseases*, 2nd ed. New York, NY: Churchill Livingstone, 2003:1458–1510.

Second-Generation Agents

Oral second-generation agents were commonly used for the treatment of respiratory infections, including community-acquired pneumonia (CAP), sinusitis, and otitis media, but have largely been supplanted by amoxicillin clavulanate.

Cephamycins, such as cefoxitin and cefotetan, are used frequently in the treatment of IAIs, pelvic inflammatory disease, infected decubitus ulcers, and mixed aerobic–anaerobic soft-tissue infections where gram-negative bacteria and anaerobes are likely to be involved. They have been largely supplanted by piperacillin–tazobactam and meropenem. They should not be used for the treatment of life-threatening *B. fragilis* infections in the absence of susceptibility information, as up to 15% of *B. fragilis* may be resistant to cephamycins.[50]

Third-Generation Agents

The only currently available expanded-spectrum cephalosporins are ceftriaxone and ceftazidime. Cefotaxime is no longer manufactured in the United States. Because of its protein binding, ceftriaxone can be used once daily for most infections, except meningitis, which should be treated with a 12-hourly regimen. Ceftriaxone has been used for the outpatient management of infants with fever without a known source. Ceftriaxone is effective in the treatment of bacterial meningitis caused by *S. pneumoniae, H. influenzae* type b, and *N. meningitidis.* Vancomycin is given in addition to ceftriaxone for the empiric therapy of meningitis in children to cover for pneumococci with penicillin resistance [minimum inhibitory concentration (*MIC*) ≤2 µg per mL].[51,52] Incidence of meningitis and other invasive infections due to *H. influenzae* type b and *S. pneumoniae* have dropped dramatically in the United States since the introduction of conjugate vaccines, starting with *H. influenzae* type b vaccine in 1990. Third-generation cephalosporins are also useful in the treatment of nosocomial infections caused by susceptible gram-negative bacilli, including pneumonia, wound infections, and complicated UTIs (cUTIs).[53,54] Ceftriaxone is the recommended first-line therapy for all forms of gonococcal infection.[55] Ceftriaxone is also effective for treatment of Lyme disease.[17,56] Because

TABLE 20.11 Dosing of Cephalosporins in Neonates

		Dosage (mg/kg/d) and Frequency of Administration				
		0–4 wk	*<1 wk*		*≥1 wk*	
Antibiotic	Route	<1,200 g	1,200–2,000 g	>2,000 g	1,200–2,000 g	>2,000 g
Cefazolin	i.v., i.m.	20 q12 h	20 q12 h	20 q12 h	20 q12 h	20 q8 h
Ceftazidime	i.v., i.m.	50 q12 h	50 q12 h	50 q8–12 h	50 q8 h	50 q8 h
Ceftriaxone[a]	i.v., i.m.	50 q24 h	50 q24 h	50 q24 h	50 q24 h	50–75 q24 h

[a]Should not be used in hyperbilirubinemic neonates, especially preterm.

i.m., intramuscular; i.v., intravenous; q6–8 h, every 6 to 8 hours; q8 h, every 8 hours; q8–12 h, every 8 to 12 hours; q12 h, every 12 hours; q24 h, every 24 hours.

Data from American Academy of Pediatrics. Tables of antibacterial drug doses. In: Pickering LK, ed. 2006 *Red book: report of the Committee on Infectious Diseases*, 27th ed. Elk Grove Village, IL: American Academy of Pediatrics, 2006:750–765; and Saez-llorens X, McCracken GH Jr. Clinical pharmacology of antibacterial agents. In: Remington JS, Klein JO, eds. *Infectious diseases of the fetus and newborn infant*, 5th ed. Philadelphia, PA: WB Saunders, 2001:1419–1466.

of its antipseudomonal activity, use of ceftazidime should be restricted to the treatment of infections due to *P. aeruginosa*.[57] As cefotaxime is no longer manufactured in the United States, it is also being used for the treatment of early- and late-onset sepsis in infants less than 1 month of age, including premature infants.

Fourth-Generation Agents

The safety and effectiveness of cefepime have been established in the age group 2 months to 16 years in the treatment of uncomplicated UTIs and cUTIs, uncomplicated skin and skin structure infections, and pneumonia, and as empiric therapy for febrile neutropenic patients. Safety and effectiveness in pediatric patients younger than 2 months have not been established. Comparative clinical trials have shown that cefepime is comparable to some of the third-generation cephalosporins, including ceftazidime, cefotaxime, and ceftriaxone.[58,59] In the treatment of febrile neutropenia, cefepime was comparable to piperacillin–gentamicin.[60] In the treatment of acute bacterial meningitis in children, cefepime and cefotaxime were comparable.[61] The use of fourth-generation cephalosporins should be limited to the empiric treatment of nosocomial infections in which an increased frequency of AmpC β-lactamase–producing organisms is the likely pathogen.[62] Cefepime is used for the treatment of nosocomial infections when ESBL or chromosomally induced β-lactamase resistance is present. *Enterobacter* species with reduced susceptibility or resistance to ceftazidime has shown a favorable response to cefepime.[63]

ADVERSE REACTIONS

Maculopapular or morbilliform skin eruptions, drug fever, and a positive Coombs test are common adverse reactions to cephalosporins.[64] The frequency of cephalosporin-induced skin rashes varies from 1% to 3%.[65] In children treated with cefaclor, a serum sickness–like reaction manifesting as rash and arthritis has been described.[66] Reactions like anaphylaxis have been reported. Frequency of anaphylactic reactions to cephalosporins varies from 0.0001% to 0.1%.[67,68] Patients who are allergic to penicillins may develop allergic reactions when they receive cephalosporins. The risk in such patients may be up to eight times as for those with no history of penicillin allergy. Patients with a history of allergy to penicillin but with negative skin tests are not at increased risk for cephalosporin allergy.[64] Granulocytopenia has also been reported with cephalosporin use. Cephalosporins can inhibit adenosine diphosphate–induced platelet aggregation. This effect is slowly reversible after discontinuation of drug.[69] Immune-mediated thrombocytopenia has been associated with the administration of cephalothin, cefazolin, cefoxitin, and cefaclor.[70] Renal toxicity can occur with cephalosporin use. Interstitial nephritis and acute tubular necrosis can occur rarely in association with cephalosporin use. Based on reports of fatal cases in neonates, there has been some recent concern about a potential interaction when ceftriaxone and calcium are coadministered.[71] Several cephalosporins have been implicated in triggering seizures, particularly in patients with renal impairment when the dosage was not reduced.[34]

NEWER CEPHALOSPORINS

CEFTAROLINE

Chemistry and Pharmacology

Ceftaroline fosamil is water soluble, an *N*-phosphono type prodrug of a cephalosporin class of β-lactam antibacterial drugs, rapidly converted to the active form, ceftaroline.[72] Ceftaroline was synthesized with specific manipulations of the side chains to provide enhanced activity against MRSA and multidrug-resistant *S. pneumoniae* isolates, making it the first available β-lactam with this ability.[73] One of the mechanisms of resistance to β-lactam agents is through mutations of the PBPs. MRSA and penicillin-resistant *S. pneumoniae* produce PBP2a and PBP2x variant, respectively.[74]

Similar to other cephalosporins, ceftaroline binds to PBPs, inhibiting transpeptidation. This interaction blocks the final stage of peptidoglycan synthesis and inhibits bacterial cell wall synthesis. Ceftaroline binds to PBP1 to PBP4 and has a high affinity to PBP2a, the protein responsible for conferring methicillin resistance in *S. aureus*.[75] Ceftaroline also has activity against penicillin-resistant *S. pneumoniae* due to binding affinity to PBP2x.[75]

Pharmacokinetics and Pharmacodynamics

Limited PK studies on ceftaroline exist for pediatric patients. Phase I study open-label, noncomparative; single-dose examined the PK in nine subjects aged 12 to 17 years.[76] Single 1-hour infusion of ceftaroline 8 mg per kg was to hospitalized patients for suspected infection who weighed less than 75 kg or 600 mg for those who weighed greater than or equal to 75 kg was administered. Patients were excluded if they were allergic to β-lactam agents, have a history of seizures, or were critically ill. The peak plasma concentration (C_{max}) reported in these patients was 15 ± 6 μg per mL, which is comparable to what is reported in adults.[76] This study did not include patients who were obese or critically ill. PK study of ceftaroline was conducted in 53 children less than 12 years of age who were hospitalized with an infection.[77] It was open-label, single-dose, phase IV study. Patients were excluded from the study if they had hypersensitivity to β-lactam agents, renal insufficiency, or history of seizures. The patients received various does of ceftaroline based on their age. The results of this study are not published. In this study, some patients received ceftaroline dose of 15 mg per kg, which is more than the FDA recommended dose of 8 to 12 mg per kg for this age group. Ge et al. conducted a population PK modeling and target simulations by combining the results of five pediatric studies that included 305 children from birth to age 18 years to investigate the dosing of ceftaroline in patients who had acute bacterial skin and skin structure infections (ABSSSIs) and CAP.[78] The studies utilized dosing of 8 mg per kg every 8 hours for children aged 2 months and older and less than 2 years. Children older than 2 years received a dose of 12 mg per kg every 8 hours up to a weight of 33 kg. Older children weighing greater than 33 kg received 400 mg every 8 hours, or an adult dose weighing 600 mg every 12 hours. The objective of the study was to estimate ceftaroline exposures and percentage of time that free drug concentrations of ceftaroline were above the *MIC* (*%fT* > *MIC*) for pediatric dose regimens. The various dosing regimens in pediatric patients maintained a concentration greater than an *MIC* of 1 μg per mL more than 75% of the time. Greater than 90% of children were predicted to achieve a target of 36% *fT* > *MIC* at an *MIC* of 2 μg per mL, and greater than 97% were predicted to achieve 44% *fT* > *MIC* at an *MIC* of 1 μg per mL. The 12-hour dosing alternative for older children maintained concentrations above the *MIC* of 1 μg per mL 44% of the time in 97% of children and above *MIC* of 2 μg per mL for 36% of the time in greater than 90% of children. Elimination half-life was not calculated for the pediatric patients. The authors of this study concluded that the tested dosing regimen would produce similar drug exposures to adult dosing. One of the limitations of this study was that the authors did not study the impact of renal function on dosing of ceftaroline. PK data are lacking in special population of children, such as patients with cystic fibrosis (CF), burn patients, or pediatric patients with central nervous system (CNS) infections. There is one case report published by Molloy and colleagues that describes PK dosing in a 6-year-old male CF patient with MRSA infection.[79] The MRSA isolate had a ceftaroline *MIC* of 1 μg per mL, and the dose given to this patient was 200 mg every 8 hours (32.4 mg per kg per day). Serum ceftaroline concentrations remained above the *MIC* for only 21% of the dosage interval; however, the patient improved clinically.[79] Ceftaroline, like most other β-lactam agents, is a time-dependent (concentration-dependent) antibiotic. The pharmacodynamic (PD) parameter that best predicts ceftaroline efficacy is %*t* > *MIC*.[80] A Monte Carlo simulation of ceftaroline 600 mg every 12 hours given to healthy adults predicted *fT* > *MIC* of 71% and 51% for organisms with *MIC*s of 1 and 2 μg per mL, respectively. Probability of target attainment of 40% *fT* > *MIC* was 100% at an *MIC* of 1 μg per mL and 90% at an *MIC* of 2 μg per mL.[81,82]

Adverse Events and Drug Interactions

Ceftaroline was approved in May 2016 for the treatment of ABSSSIs and community-acquired bacterial pneumonia (CABP) in children aged 2 months and older based on three studies.[83] To date, safety of ceftaroline has been evaluated in three active control studies and two single-dose PK studies in a total of 319 pediatric subjects.[73,79–81] These two randomized controlled studies evaluated the safety of ceftaroline in children.[80,81] Adverse events in both studies were similar between ceftaroline and comparative agents (22% vs. 23% in the ABSSSI and 45% vs. 46% in the CABP studies). Most common side effects experienced in these patients were diarrhea, rash, nausea, vomiting, and fever. Ceftaroline should be used with caution in patients with previous history of hypersensitivity to β-lactam antibiotics and is contraindicated in patients where anaphylaxis has occurred. Direct Coombs test seroconversion is a known side effect of ceftaroline and is listed in the warning section of the package insert for adult patients.[82] In pediatric subjects, the ceftaroline arm experienced higher incidence of Direct Coombs seroconversion as compared to comparators.[80,81] Hemolytic anemia or hemolysis was not documented in any of the patients receiving ceftaroline. This warning is also added for the pediatric patients. Ceftaroline is hydrolyzed into its inactive metabolite, ceftaroline M-1. It undergoes little hepatic metabolism and is not a substrate, inhibitor, or inducer of the CYP450 enzyme system and, therefore, is not likely to cause CYP450-related drug–drug interactions.[83]

Dosing and Administration

Dosing of ceftaroline is based on both age and weight (Table 20.12). According to the package insert, children between the ages of 2 months and less than 2 years should receive a lower dose at 8 mg per kg every 8 hours. Patients aged 2 years and older should be given 12 mg per kg every 8 hours, with a maximum dose of 400 mg per dose in patients weighing greater than 33 kg.[82] Alternatively, a 600-mg dose may be given every 12 hours. The length of therapy of ceftaroline depends on the type of infection being treated. Typical duration is 5 to 14 days. Ceftaroline is excreted by the kidneys, and the elimination of ceftaroline is altered in patients with renal insufficiency. Dosing adjustments are recommended in adult patients with creatinine clearance less than 50 mL per minute and who are on hemodialysis (HD). Intermittent HD removes approximately 21% of ceftaroline.[84] Dosing recommendations in pediatric patients with renal insufficiency or HD are lacking; therefore, children should not receive ceftaroline until further studies are conducted to ensure optimal dosing regimen.

Ceftaroline is only available as an IV agent. Ceftaroline should be reconstituted to be used within 6 hours at room temperature and within 24 hours if refrigerated. The IV infusion time has been approved between 5 and 60 minutes; as ceftaroline is a time-dependent antibiotic, it is best to administer the agent over 60 minutes.[82]

CEPHALOSPORIN–β-LACTAMASE INHIBITOR COMBINATIONS

Two new cephalosporin–β-lactamase inhibitor combinations have recently been approved by the FDA: ceftazidime–avibactam and ceftolozane–tazobactam.[25] Ceftazidime–avibactam also received pediatric approval in March 2019 for the treatment of

TABLE 20.12 Approved and Suggested Ceftaroline Dosing Strategies

	FDA-Approved Dose for CABP and ABSSSI	*Suggested[a] Dose for cCABP, CF, MRSA, Bacteremia/Endocarditis*
2 mo to <2 y	24 mg/kg/d divided every 8 h	Age <6 mo: 30 mg/kg/d divided every 8 h Age 6 mo to <2 y: 45 mg/kg/d divided every 8 h
2 to <18 y	36 mg/kg/d divided every 8 h Maximum 1,200 mg/d, divided every 8–12 h	45 mg/kg/d divided every 8 h Maximum 1,800 mg/d, divided every 8 h

[a]Limited data, not prospectively evaluated for safety outside cCABP.
ABSSSI, acute bacterial skin and skin structure infection; CABP, community-acquired bacterial pneumonia; cCABP, complicated community-acquired bacterial pneumonia; CF, cystic fibrosis.

cUTIs and IAIs (in combination with metronidazole) in children aged 3 months and older to 18 years.[85] Published clinical data on the use of ceftazidime–avibactam in children are limited to two phase 2 randomized controlled trials; one comparing ceftazidime–avibactam plus metronidazole to meropenem for the treatment of complicated IAIs (cIAIs), and the other comparing treatment of cUTI to cefepime.[86,87] Both trials included children aged 3 months and older to 18 years. Isofidis et al.[88] reported a single-center retrospective case series of eight children, age 13 days to 4.5 years, with infections due to extensively resistant or pan-resistant *K. pneumoniae*. All patients received at least 2 days (six doses) of ceftazidime–avibactam. Diagnoses included bloodstream infection, meningitis, and UTI. All patients were clinical and microbiologic cures.

CEFTAZIDIME–AVIBACTAM

Spectrum of Activity

Ceftazidime is an extended-spectrum antipseudomonal cephalosporin that was first approved in 1985 for the treatment of complicated infections in adults, with approval for children shortly thereafter.[18] With widespread β-lactamase–mediated resistance has greatly reduced cephalosporin effectiveness, there have been reports of an increasing trend toward antibiotic resistance among Enterobacteriaceae isolated from children.[89–91] The combination of ceftazidime with avibactam, a novel non–β-lactam β-lactamase inhibitor, represents an important new option for the treatment of serious gram-negative infections.[92] Avibactam has been shown in vitro to inactivate Ambler classes A and C (including *K. pneumoniae* carbapenemases) and some class D β-lactamases, which restores the bactericidal activity of ceftazidime against otherwise ceftazidime-resistant pathogens carrying these β-lactamases. However, avibactam does not inhibit metallo–β-lactamases.[85]

A recent study of 8,461 gram-negative bacterial isolates from pediatric patients less than 17 years tested ceftazidime–avibactam (avibactam at fixed concentration of 4 μg per mL) and comparators including piperacillin–tazobactam, meropenem, levofloxacin, and colistin.[89] Ceftazidime–avibactam inhibited greater than 99.9% of all Enterobacteriaceae at the less than 8 μg per mL susceptibility breakpoint. The combination was active against ESBL-producing *E. coli* and *K. pneumoniae*, whereas meropenem was active against 83.6% ESBL-producing *K. pneumoniae*. Only one (0.02%) of 4,724 Enterobacteriaceae isolates was resistant to ceftazidime–avibactam, *Enterobacter aerogenes*, with an *MIC* of 16 μg per mL. The combination also inhibited 99.1% of *P. aeruginosa* isolates tested compared to 89.6% for ceftazidime alone.

Ceftazidime–avibactam also has in vitro activity against *Burkholderia cepacia* complex, which is of importance in patients with CF. However, ceftazidime–avibactam does not have significant activity against anaerobic bacteria, including *Bacteroides* spp., thus needs to be used in combination with metronidazole for the treatment of IAIs.[85]

Pharmacokinetics and Pharmacodynamics

A phase I study was conducted to characterize the PK profile of a single dose of ceftazidime–avibactam in hospitalized infants and children.[93] Safety and tolerability were evaluated as secondary objectives. Hospitalized male and female patients aged 3 months and older to less than 18 years who were expected to require hospitalization for at least 24 to 48 hours and were receiving systemic antibiotic therapy for the treatment of a suspected or confirmed infection were included in the study. Patients were stratified in four groups based on age, and each group had at least eight evaluable patients, group 1, 12 years and older to less than 18 years; group 2, 6 years and older to less than 12 years; group 3, 2 years and older to less than 6 years; and group 4, 3 years and older months to less than 2 years. Infants born prior to 37 weeks of gestation were excluded. All doses were administered as a 2-hour continuous IV infusion to maximize the PD exposure for β-lactam antibiotics. Patients received a single 2-hour IV infusion of ceftazidime–avibactam [group 1, 2,000 to 500 mg; group 2, 2,000 to 500 mg (≥40 kg) or 50 to 12.5 mg per kg (<40 kg); groups 3 and 4, 50 to 12.5 mg per kg]. Blood samples were collected to describe individual PK characteristics for ceftazidime and avibactam. Population PK modeling was used to describe characteristics of ceftazidime and avibactam PK across all age groups. Thirty-two patients received the study drug. Mean maximum plasma ceftazidime concentrations (C_{max}) for the four cohorts were 79.8, 81.3, 80.1, and 91.7 mg per L, respectively. Additional parameters were only evaluated in the two older groups. Area under the concentration–time curve (*AUC*) results were also similar to adult values, with a mean of 230.6 hour·mg per L in group 1 and 221.2 hour·mg per L in group 2. Mean elimination half-lives for the two groups were 1.7 (range 0.9 to 2.8 hours) and 1.6 hours (0.9 to 1.8 hours). Similarly, avibactam C_{max} was similar across all four groups: 15.1, 14.1, 13.7, and 16.3 mg per L, respectively. Values for avibactam *AUC* in groups 1 and 2 were 36.4 and 34.8 hour mg per L, and half-lives for groups 1 and 2 were 2.0 (2.9 to 2.6 hours) and 2.1 hours (1.9 to 2.4), respectively. Mean plasma concentration–time curves, geometric mean maximum concentration (C_{max}), and $AUC_{0-\infty}$ were similar across all groups for both drugs and comparable with previously observed data in adults. This phase I study led to the dose selection for the two phase II studies of ceftazidime–avibactam in pediatric patients.[86,87]

Bradley et al. studied the safety and efficacy of ceftazidime–avibactam plus metronidazole in the treatment of children aged 3 months and older to less than 18 years with cIAI in a phase II study.[86] Eighty-three patients were randomized in a 3:1 ratio to receive either ceftazidime–avibactam plus metronidazole or meropenem. Randomization was stratified by age across four groups: group 1, 2 to less than 18 years; group 2, 6 to less than 12 years; group 3, 2 to less than 6 years; and group 4, 3 months to less than 2 years. Children and adolescents aged 2 to 18 years received a ceftazidime–avibactam dose of 62.5 mg per kg (50 mg per kg ceftazidime and 12.5 mg per kg of avibactam) up to a maximum of 2.5 g, while infants aged 3 to 6 months were given a dose of 50 mg per kg (40 mg per kg ceftazidime and 10 mg per kg avibactam), infused over 2 hours every 8 hours in combination with metronidazole 20 mg per kg IV every 8 hours. Patients were treated for 72 hours with their assigned study drug but could then be switched to oral therapy to complete 7 to 15 days of treatment. There were no infants in the ceftazidime–avibactam group. Children with creatinine clearance less than 30 mL per minute per 1.73 m^2 were not included in the study. Blood samples for determination of plasma concentrations of ceftazidime and avibactam were collected on day 3 from ceftazidime–avibactam plus metronidazole-treated patients. Mean age of the study patients was 11 years, with a range of 3 to 17 years. Sixty patients were analyzed for the PK study. Median plasma concentrations for ceftazidime and avibactam were similar across age groups 1 to 3. No patients from group 4 received ceftazidime–avibactam; therefore, no PK data were available for this age group. The median plasma concentration of ceftazidime was 62.30 mg per L anytime within 15 minutes before or after stopping ceftazidime–avibactam infusion, 39.45 mg per L anytime between 30 and 90 minutes after stopping ceftazidime–avibactam infusion, and 4.42 mg per L anytime between 300 (5 hours) and 360 minutes (6 hours) after stopping ceftazidime–avibactam infusion. The median plasma concentration of avibactam was 12.40, 7.33, and 0.67 mg per L, respectively. Mean plasma concentrations for ceftazidime and avibactam were consistent across groups 1 to 3, suggesting that the age- and/or weight-based dose adjustments for ceftazidime–avibactam used in this study were appropriate for the population studied. Further population PK modeling for estimation of PK parameters and probability of PK/PD target attainment is ongoing and is planned to be reported separately.[88]

Bradly et al.[87] conducted a multicenter, single-blind, active-comparator safety and tolerability study, which was a phase II study in 95 infants, children, and adolescents from 3 months to less than 18 years of age with cUTI. Patients were randomized to either ceftazidime–avibactam in 3:1 ratio to receive IV or cefepime for greater than or equal to 72 hours, with subsequent optional oral switch. The doses of ceftazidime–avibactam were the same as in the cIAI study, and cefepime was given at the standard recommended dose based on age and weight. Children with creatinine clearance less than 30 mL per minute per 1.73 m^2 were not included in the study. Total treatment duration was 7 to 14 days. The primary objective was to evaluate the safety and tolerability of ceftazidime–avibactam versus cefepime in hospitalized children. Secondary objectives were to evaluate the efficacy and PK of ceftazidime–avibactam. Ninety-seven patients were randomized to the study drugs: 68 patients in the ceftazidime–avibactam group and 29 patients in the cefepime group. PK analysis of ceftazidime–avibactam was done in 64 patients. The median patient age was 4.2 years, with a range of 3.5 to 18 years. Most of the patients had been diagnosed with pyelonephritis. Blood samples were collected from patients randomized to ceftazidime–avibactam treatment on day 3 following a dose administration. Like the cIAI study, median plasma concentrations for ceftazidime and avibactam were similar across age groups, suggesting that the age- and/or weight-based dose adjustments for ceftazidime–avibactam used in this study were appropriate for the population studied. The median plasma concentration of ceftazidime was 78.35 mg per L anytime within 15 minutes before or after stopping ceftazidime–avibactam infusion, 47.10 mg per L anytime between 30 and 90 minutes after stopping ceftazidime–avibactam infusion, and 6.91 mg per L anytime between 300 (5 hours) and 360 minutes (6 hours) after stopping ceftazidime–avibactam infusion. The median plasma concentration of avibactam was 13.2, 6.88, and 0.88 mg per L, respectively. More comprehensive PK modeling for the estimation of PK parameters and probability of PK/PD target attainment from this study is ongoing and will be reported separately.[87]

Adverse Reactions

In phase I study, six (18.8%) patients experienced mild or moderate adverse event. No deaths or serious adverse events were reported.[93] In the children from 3 months up to 6 years of age participating in the PK, safety, and tolerability study described earlier, constipation, diarrhea, vomiting, a local infusion site reaction, increased serum transaminases, an elevated triglyceride level, and an increased γ-glutamyl transferase level were each reported in one patient (3.1% for each reaction). No adverse effects were reported in the patients aged 6 years or older. Ceftazidime–avibactam seems to be well tolerated, with a safety profile similar to ceftazidime alone.[87]

CEFTOLOZANE–TAZOBACTAM

This combination consists of a new cephalosporin, ceftolozane, in combination with tazobactam. Ceftolozane is not available as a stand-alone drug. Like ceftazidime, ceftolozane also contains the same dimethylacetic acid group that is associated with antipseudomonal activity and an aminothiadiazole ring that increases activity against Enterobacteriaceae.[25] Unlike ceftazidime, it has activity against anaerobic bacteria. It is not active against *Acinetobacter* spp. and *S. maltophilia.* The addition of tazobactam extends ceftolozane's spectrum against some of the β-lactamases that inactivate ceftolozane. Ceftolozane–tazobactam does not have approval for use in children. Published data on the use of ceftolozane are limited to two case reports and a single-dose study of 37 children aged 7 days through less than 18 years who were being treated for suspected or proven gram-negative infection.[25,94,95] PK was generally comparable for children aged 3 months to less than 18 years; however, young infants (7 days to 3 months of age) have lower clearance than older children. To determine doses likely to be safe and efficacious in pediatric patients with cUTIs and IAIs, a population PK analysis was conducted to assess each regimen's plasma exposure and the probability of PK/PD target attainment.

Two-compartment linear models with first-order elimination described the concentration–time profiles of ceftolozane and tazobactam in pediatric patients well. Renal function and body weight were identified to be significant predictors of ceftolozane–tazobactam. Based on these simulations, the following doses are recommended for further clinical evaluation in phase 2 pediatric trials for cUTI and cIAI (in patients with an estimated glomerular filtration rate of greater than or equal to 50 mL per minute per 1.73 m^2 only): for children aged 12 years and older, 1.5 g ceftolozane–tazobactam (1 g ceftolozane with 0.5 g tazobactam), and for neonates/very young infants, infants, and children less than 12 years of age, 20 per 10 mg per kg of body weight ceftolozane–tazobactam, both via a 1-hour IV infusion every 8 hours.[95]

CARBAPENEMS

The carbapenems are derivatives of thienamycin, a compound produced by the soil organism *Streptomyces cattleya.* The basic structure of the carbapenems is similar to that of penicillins and cephalosporins. The five-member ring system in the carbapenems is unsaturated and contains a carbon atom instead of a sulfur atom at position 1.[3,96] Carbapenems are stable to most β-lactamases, including AmpC β-lactamases and ESBLs. Resistance to carbapenems develops when bacteria acquire or develop structural changes within their PBPs, when they acquire metallo–β-lactamases, or when loss of specific outer membrane porins causes changes in membrane permeability.[96]

IMIPENEM

Structure

Imipenem is the *N*-formimidoyl derivative of thienamycin. In addition to the structural characteristics of carbapenems, the side chain of imipenem is different from that of penicillins and cephalosporins. Instead of the acylamino side chain, imipenem has a hydroxyethyl side chain, and unlike the other β-lactams, where the side chain is in a *cis* configuration, the side chain of imipenem is in a *trans* configuration. The *trans* conformation is responsible for the stability of imipenem against β-lactamases.[97]

Spectrum of Activity

Gram-Positive Organisms

Streptococci including penicillin-resistant *S. pneumoniae*, methicillin-susceptible *S. aureus*, and penicillin-susceptible strains of *Enterococcus faecalis* are susceptible to imipenem. Like penicillins, imipenem is bacteriostatic and not bactericidal against enterococci. *Listeria* and *Bacillus* species are also susceptible to imipenem. *Enterococcus faecium* and non–β-lactamase–producing strains of enterococci are resistant to imipenem.

Gram-Negative Organisms

Members of the Enterobacteriaceae family including the ESBL producers are susceptible to imipenem. β-Lactamase–producing strains of *H. influenzae* and *N. gonorrhoeae* are also susceptible to imipenem. *P. aeruginosa*, including strains resistant to antipseudomonal penicillins and cephalosporins, and most strains of *Acinetobacter* are susceptible to imipenem. *S. maltophilia* and some strains of *B. cepacia* are resistant.

Anaerobes

Most anaerobes, including *Peptococcus*, *Peptostreptococcus*, *B. fragilis*, *Fusobacterium*, *Actinomyces*, and *Clostridium* species excluding *C. difficile*, are susceptible to imipenem.

Others

Nocardia asteroides, some *Legionella* species, and *Mycobacterium avium-intracellulare* are inhibited by imipenem.

Mechanism of Action

Imipenem binds with high affinity to PBPs of both gram-positive and gram-negative organisms. Unlike penicillins and cephalosporins, imipenem binds with high affinity to PBP2 and less avidly to PBP1 in gram-negative bacteria. It is not hydrolyzed by most β-lactamases, penicillinases, cephalosporinases (plasmid or chromosomal) of *S. aureus*, several enteric gram-negative organisms, *P. aeruginosa*, *B. cepacia*, and *B. fragilis*. It is hydrolyzed by a *S. maltophilia* β-lactamase, as well as some *Bacillus* and *Bacteroides* enzymes. Carbapenems show a postantibiotic effect, which varies by organism and species.[98]

Resistance

S. maltophilia and some strains of *B. cepacia* produce β-lactamases that hydrolyze imipenem and other carbapenems. Resistance in *P. aeruginosa* is due to the absence or loss of an outer membrane protein or due to the presence of efflux pump systems.[99]

Pharmacokinetics

In the kidney, it is hydrolyzed by the renal peptidase, dehydropeptidase-1 located on the brush border of the proximal renal tubules.[100] Thus, imipenem is combined with cilastatin, a dehydropeptidase inhibitor. Cilastatin has no antibacterial activity and does not interfere with the activity of imipenem. Combination with cilastatin also reduces the nephrotoxicity of imipenem.[100] Imipenem is widely distributed to different body tissues. In the absence of meningeal inflammation, levels in the CSF are low.

Adverse Reactions

Nausea and vomiting are the two most common adverse events reported. Elevation of liver enzymes and leukopenia has also been reported. Imipenem can cause seizures, especially in patients with underlying CNS defects and in those with decreased renal function when dose adjustment has not been made.[101,102] Treatment of infants with bacterial meningitis with imipenem has been associated with drug-related seizure activity.[103] Patients who are allergic to other β-lactam antibiotics can have hypersensitivity reactions to imipenem.

Clinical Use

Imipenem is useful in the treatment of infections due to cephalosporin-resistant Enterobacteriaceae, particularly *Citrobacter freundii* and *Enterobacter* species, and in the empiric therapy of serious infections in patients who have previously received multiple antibiotics. Imipenem is effective as a single agent in the therapy of febrile neutropenia.[104] Imipenem has also been used as a single agent for the treatment of acute pulmonary exacerbations in patients with CF. *P. aeruginosa* can develop resistance during therapy.

Imipenem is approved by the FDA for treatment of the following infections: lower respiratory tract infections, UTIs (complicated and uncomplicated), IAIs, gynecologic infections, bacterial septicemia, bone and joint infections, skin and skin structure infections, endocarditis (*S. aureus*), and polymicrobial infections. It is not indicated in patients with meningitis because safety and efficacy have not been established. Imipenem is approved for use in patients from birth through 16 years of age.

Dosage

For patients aged 3 months or older, the recommended regimen for non-CNS infections is 15 to 25 mg per kg per dose administered every 6 hours. Imipenem is not approved in children with CNS infections or in children with impaired renal function who weighed less than 30 kg. For patients aged 3 months or younger who weighed at least 1,500 g, the following dosage schedule is recommended for non-CNS infections[34]:

- Less than 1 week of age: 25 mg per kg every 12 hours
- One to 4 weeks of age: 25 mg per kg every 8 hours
- Four weeks to 3 months of age: 25 mg per kg every 6 hours

MEROPENEM

Structure

Meropenem has a dimethylcarbamoyl pyrolidiolidyn derivative on position 2 of the ring, unlike the *N*-formidyl group in imipenem. This makes it stable to dehydropeptidase-1.

Mechanism of Action

Meropenem acts by binding to the PBPs of bacteria, thereby interfering with cell wall synthesis. Its strongest affinities are toward PBP2, PBP3, and PBP4 of *E. coli* and *P. aeruginosa* and PBP1, PBP2, and PBP4 of *S. aureus.*

Spectrum of Activity

Meropenem is slightly less active against gram-positive bacteria than imipenem and more active against gram-negative bacteria, including some *P. aeruginosa* resistant to imipenem.[105] It penetrates membranes of gram-negative organisms better than imipenem.[106] Meropenem has a postantibiotic effect similar to that of imipenem.

Resistance

Like imipenem, meropenem is not hydrolyzed by most β-lactamases, penicillinases, or cephalosporinases. Meropenem is hydrolyzed by the β-lactamases of *S. maltophilia.* Meropenem does not bind to the PBPs of *E. faecium.* Because it is more rapidly transported through the porins of gram-negative organisms, resistance due to decreased permeability is uncommon.

Pharmacokinetics

Unlike imipenem, meropenem is not hydrolyzed by the renal dehydropeptidase. Its pharmacology is similar to that of imipenem in other respects.

Clinical Use

Meropenem has been shown to be safe and effective in the treatment of meningitis in children with no increase in drug-related seizure activity.[107,108] Studies suggest that meropenem is therapeutically equivalent to imipenem.[109,110] Meropenem has been used as a single agent in the treatment of pulmonary exacerbations in patients with CF. Development of resistance has been uncommon.[48] Meropenem is currently approved by the FDA for pediatric patients aged 3 months or older for the treatment of IAIs like complicated appendicitis and peritonitis and for the treatment of bacterial meningitis in children aged 3 months or older.

Adverse Events

Seizures and other CNS adverse experiences have been reported during treatment with meropenem. These experiences have occurred most commonly in patients with CNS disorders or with bacterial meningitis and/or compromised renal function. Meropenem may be less epileptogenic than imipenem.[110–113] In the pediatric clinical trials in patients without meningitis, the most common adverse events reported were diarrhea, rash, nausea, and vomiting. In clinical trials in patients with meningitis, the most common adverse events reported included diarrhea, moniliasis, and glossitis.

Dosage

For pediatric patients aged 3 months or older, the recommended dosage is as follows[112–114]:

- 10 mg per kg every 8 hours (complicated skin and skin structure infections)
- 20 mg per kg every 8 hours (IAIs)
- 40 mg per kg every 8 hours (meningitis)

There is no experience in pediatric patients with renal impairment.

ERTAPENEM

Ertapenem has broad-spectrum in vitro activity against most commonly encountered gram-positive and gram-negative bacterial pathogens, with the notable exceptions of enterococci, MRSA, *P. aeruginosa,* and *Acinetobacter.*[115,116] Its high level of protein binding and serum half-life of 4 hours allow it to be dosed once daily. Ertapenem may be administered IV or intramuscularly. Ertapenem is approved by the FDA for the treatment of adults with cIAIs, cUTIs and complicated skin and skin structure infections, acute pelvic infections, and CAP. Dosage adjustment is needed in patients with renal impairment. It is also approved for use in children aged 3 months to 17 years for the same indications as in adults. The dose in patients aged 13 years and older is 1 g given once a day. The dose in patients aged 3 months to 12 years is 15 mg per kg twice daily (not to exceed 1 g per day). The product label also states that ertapenem is not recommended for the treatment of meningitis in the pediatric population due to lack of sufficient CSF penetration.[117]

DORIPENEM

Doripenem is a new carbapenem that was approved by the FDA in October 2007. It is approved for use in adults with cUTIs and cIAIs. It is not approved for use in children, except for treatment of anthrax.

MONOBACTAMS

AZTREONAM

Aztreonam is a monocyclic β-lactam compound originally isolated from *Chromobacterium violaceum.*[118] It differs from other β-lactams structurally in its unique monocyclic β-lactam nucleus. Aztreonam is the only available synthetic monobactam antibiotic.

Mechanism of Action

The bactericidal action of aztreonam results from the inhibition of bacterial cell wall synthesis due to a high affinity of aztreonam for PBP3 present in gram-negative bacteria.

Spectrum of Activity

Aztreonam exhibits potent and specific activity in vitro against a wide spectrum of gram-negative pathogens, including members of the Enterobacteriaceae family and *P. aeruginosa.* It is, however, less active than ceftazidime or imipenem against most strains of *P. aeruginosa.*[119,120] Limited activity has been noted against *Acinetobacter* species, *Alcaligenes* species, *B. cepacia,* and *S. maltophilia.* Aztreonam acts synergistically with aminoglycosides against gram-negative bacilli.[119] Aztreonam has no significant antibacterial activity against gram-positive organisms or anaerobes.

Resistance

Unlike the majority of β-lactam antibiotics, aztreonam does not induce β-lactamase activity. Its molecular structure confers a high degree of resistance to hydrolysis by β-lactamases produced by most gram-negative and gram-positive pathogens, although it is affected by some β-lactamases produced by *Klebsiella* species and some pseudomonads, resulting in aztreonam resistance.[120] Aztreonam resistance may also be related to alterations in outer membrane porin proteins.

Pharmacokinetics

In healthy subjects, aztreonam is removed from the body primarily by the kidney, by both active tubular secretion and glomerular filtration. In patients with impaired renal function, the serum half-life and serum concentration of aztreonam are prolonged. The half-life is only slightly prolonged in patients with hepatic impairment. Aztreonam is distributed readily to most body tissues and fluids.[121] It enters the CSF after IV administration.[122] Aztreonam is removed by HD.[123,124]

Clinical Use

Patients who are allergic to penicillins or cephalosporins appear not to react to aztreonam.[125] Aztreonam can be used in the treatment of a variety of gram-negative infections, including UTI, lower respiratory tract, skin and skin structure, IAI, and gynecologic infections, including endometritis and pelvic cellulitis. Aztreonam has been used in the treatment of gram-negative meningitis.[126] As its spectrum of activity is limited to gram-negative organisms, aztreonam should not be used as a single agent for empiric therapy in seriously ill patients if gram-positive or anaerobic infections are a possibility. Aztreonam has been used in combination with clindamycin, erythromycin, metronidazole, penicillins, and vancomycin. Inhaled aztreonam is FDA approved for use in CF patients with *P. aeruginosa.*[127]

The FDA has approved aztreonam for the following indications: cUTIs and uncomplicated UTIs, lower respiratory tract infections, septicemia, skin and skin structure infections, IAIs, and gynecologic infections, including endometritis and pelvic cellulitis. The FDA has approved aztreonam for use in children aged 9 months to 16 years. Sufficient data are not available for pediatric patients less than 9 months of age or for the following treatment indications/pathogens: septicemia and skin and skin structure infections (where the skin infection is believed or known to be due to *H. influenzae* type b).

Dosage

Dosage for aztreonam is as follows:

- Mild-to-moderate infections: 30 mg per kg every 8 hours.
- Moderate-to-severe infections: 30 mg per kg every 6 to 8 hours.
- Maximum recommended dose: 120 mg per kg per day. In pediatric patients with CF, higher doses may be needed.

Insufficient data are available regarding dosing in pediatric patients with renal impairment.[34]

Adverse Reactions

Adverse reactions described in adults include skin rashes, nausea, and diarrhea. In pediatric clinical trials, the common adverse events included rash, diarrhea, and fever. The following laboratory adverse events were noted during clinical trials: increased eosinophils, increased platelets, neutropenia, increased aspartate aminotransferase, increased alanine aminotransferase, and increased serum creatinine. Aztreonam contains 780 mg of arginine per gram of antibiotic; hence, arginine-induced hypoglycemia has been raised as a possible adverse effect.[128]

REFERENCES

1. Fleming A. On the antibacterial action of cultures of a penicillium, with special reference to their use in the isolation of *B. influenzae. Br J Exp Pathol* 1929;10:226.
2. Batchelor FR, Doyle FP, Naylor JHC, et al. Synthesis of penicillin: 6-aminopenicillanic acid in penicillin fermentations. *Nature* 1959;183:257–258.
3. Petri WA Jr. Antimicrobial agents penicillins, cephalosporins, and other lactam antibiotics. In: Hardman JG, Limbird LE, Gilman AG, eds. *Goodman and Gillman's the pharmacological basis of therapeutics,* 10th ed. New York, NY: McGraw-Hill, 2001:1189–1218.
4. Ghuysen JM. Serine beta lactamases and penicillin-binding proteins. *Annu Rev Microbiol* 1991;45:37–67.
5. Chambers HF. Penicillins. In: Mandell GL, Bennett JE, Dolin R, eds. *Mandell, Douglas, and Bennett's principles and practice of infectious diseases,* 5th ed. Philadelphia, PA: Churchill Livingstone, 2000:261–274.
6. Siegel JD, Shannon KM, DePasse BM. Recurrent infection associated with penicillin tolerant group B streptococci: a report of two cases. *J Pediatr* 1981;99(6):920–924.
7. Betriu C, Gomez M, Sanchez A, et al. Antibiotic resistance and penicillin tolerance in clinical isolates of group B streptococci. *Antimicrob Agents Chemother* 1994;38(9):2183–2186.
8. Reed MD, Blumer JL. Anti-infective therapy. In: Jenson HB, Baltimore RS, eds. *Pediatric infectious diseases,* 2nd ed. Philadelphia, PA: WB Saunders, 2002:147–211.
9. American Academy of Pediatrics. Tables of antibacterial drug doses. In: Pickering LK, ed. *2006 Red book: report of the Committee on Infectious Diseases,* 27th ed. Elk Grove Village, IL: American Academy of Pediatrics, 2006:750–765.
10. Choi EH, Lee NJ. Clinical outcome of invasive infections caused by penicillin-resistant *Streptococcus pneumoniae* in Korean children. *Clin Infect Dis* 1998;26:1346–1354.
11. Penicillin G Potassium. Deerfield, IL: Baxter International Inc. 2008. http://www.accessdata.fda.gov/drugsatfda_docs/label/2008/050638s012lbl.pdf. Accessed March 30, 2010.
12. American Academy of Pediatrics. Syphilis. In: Pickering LK, ed. *2000 Red book: report of the Committee on Infectious Diseases,* 25th ed. Elk Grove Village, IL: American Academy of Pediatrics, 2000:547–559.
13. True RJ. Interactions between antibiotics and oral contraceptives. *J Am Med Assoc* 1982;247:1408.
14. Dickinson BD, Altman RD, Nielsen NH, et al. Drug interactions between oral contraceptives and antibiotics. *Obstet Gynecol* 2001;98:853–860.
15. Dowell SF, Butler JC, Giebink GS, et al. Acute otitis media: management and surveillance in an era of pneumococcal resistance—a report from the Drug-resistant *Streptococcus pneumoniae* Therapeutic Working Group. *Pediatr Infect Dis J* 1999;18(1):1–9.
16. American Academy of Pediatrics and American Academy of Family Physicians Clinical Practice Guideline. Subcommittee on Management of Acute Otitis Media.

Diagnosis and management of acute otitis media. https://pediatrics.aappublications.org/content/113/5/1451. Accessed August 5, 2008.
17. American Academy of Pediatrics. Lyme disease. In: Pickering LK, ed. *2006 Red book: report of the Committee on Infectious Diseases*, 27th ed. Elk Grove Village, IL: American Academy of Pediatrics, 2006:428–433.
18. Hassall E. Peptic ulcer disease and current approaches to *Helicobacter pylori*. *J Pediatr* 2001;138(4):462–468.
19. Malaty HM. *Helicobacter pylori* infection and eradication in paediatric patients. *Paediatr Drugs* 2000;2(5):357–365.
20. U.S. Food and Drug Administration. Commentary on non-labeled dosing of oral amoxicillin in adults and pediatrics for post-exposure inhalational anthrax. http://www.fda.gov/Drugs/EmergencyPreparedness/BioterrorismandDrugPreparedness/ucm072106.htm. Accessed March 30, 2010.
21. Jahansouz F, Kriett JM, Smith CM, et al. Potentiation of cyclosporine nephrotoxicity by nafcillin in lung transplant recipients. *Transplantation* 1993;55(5):1045–1048.
22. Veremis SA, Maddux MS, Pollak R, et al. Subtherapeutic cyclosporine concentrations during nafcillin therapy. *Transplantation* 1987;43(6):913–915.
23. Taylor AT, Pritchard DC, Goldstein AO, et al. Continuation of warfarin–nafcillin interaction during dicloxacillin therapy. *J Fam Pract* 1994;39(2):182–185.
24. Davis RL, Berman W Jr, Wernly JA, et al. Warfarin–nafcillin interaction. *J Pediatr* 1991;118(2):300–303.
25. Rodriguez BA, Girotto JF, Nicolau DP. Ceftazidime/avibactam and ceftolozane/tazobactam: novel therapy for multidrug resistant Gram-negative infections in children. *Curr Pediatr Rev* 2018;14:97–109.
26. Fisher J, Charnas RL, Knowles JR. Kinetic studies on the inactivation of *Escherichia coli* RTEM beta-lactamase by clavulanic acid. *Biochemistry* 1978;17:2180–2184.
27. Charnas RL, Fisher J, Knowles JR. Chemical studies on the inactivation of *Escherichia coli* RTEM beta-lactamase by clavulanic acid. *Biochemistry* 1978;17:2185–2189.
28. Labia R, Morand A, Lelievre V, et al. Sulbactam: biochemical factors involved in its synergy with ampicillin. *Rev Infect Dis* 1986;8(Suppl 5):S496–S502.
29. Fu KP, Neu HC. Comparative inhibition of beta-lactamases by novel beta-lactam compounds. *Antimicrob Agents Chemother* 1979;15:171–176.
30. Sutherland R. Beta-lactamase inhibitors and reversal of antibiotic resistance. *Trends Pharmacol Sci* 1991;12:227–232.
31. Abdel-Rahman SM, Gregory LK. The beta-lactamase inhibitors: clinical pharmacology and rational application to combination antibiotic therapy. *Pediatr Infect Dis* 1998;17:1185–1194.
32. Appelbaum PC, Jacobs MR, Spangler SK, et al. Comparative activity of beta-lactamase inhibitors YTR 830, clavulanate, and sulbactam combined with beta-lactams against beta-lactamase-producing anaerobes. *Antimicrob Agents Chemother* 1986;30:789–791.
33. Rolinson GH. Evolution of beta-lactamase inhibitors. *Rev Infect Dis* 1991;13(Suppl 9):S727–S732.
34. Primaxin® product label. https://www.accessdata.fda.gov/drugsatfda_docs/label/2009/050587s072,050630s035lbl.pdf. Accessed August 5, 2008.
35. Williams JD. Beta-lactamase inhibition and *in vitro* activity of sulbactam and sulbactam/cefoperazone. *Clin Infect Dis* 1997;24:494–497.
36. Hampel B, Lode H, Bruckner G, et al. Comparative pharmacokinetics of sulbactam/ampicillin and clavulanic acid/amoxycillin in human volunteers. *Drugs* 1988;35(Suppl 7):29–33.
37. Hoffken G, Tetzel P, Lode H. The pharmacokinetics of ticarcillin, clavulanic acid and their combination. *J Antimicrob Chemother* 1986;17(Suppl C):45–55.
38. Abraham EP, Loder PB. Cephalosporin C. In: Flynn A, ed. *Cephalosporins and penicillin chemistry and biology*. New York, NY: Academic Press, 1972:2–26.
39. Neu HC. Structural relationships affecting *in vitro* activity and pharmacologic properties. *Rev Infect Dis* 1986;8:237–259.
40. Neu HC. Relations of structural properties of beta-lactam antibiotics to antibacterial activity. *Am J Med* 1985;79:2–13.
41. Thornsberry C. Review of *in vitro* activity of third-generation cephalosporins and other newer beta-lactam antibiotics against clinically important bacteria. *Am J Med* 1985;79:14–20.
42. Sanders CC. Cefepime. *Clin Infect Dis* 1993;17:369–379.
43. Garau J, Wilson W, Wood M, et al. Fourth generation cephalosporins: a review of in vitro activity, pharmacokinetics, pharmacodynamics, and clinical utility. *Clin Microbiol Infect* 1997;3(Suppl 1):S87–S101.
44. Nikaido H. Outer membrane barrier as a mechanism of antimicrobial resistance. *Antimicrob Agents Chemother* 1989;33(11):1831–1836.
45. Schaad UB, Suter S, Gianella-Borradori A, et al. A comparison of ceftriaxone and cefuroxime for the treatment of bacterial meningitis in children. *N Engl J Med* 1990;322:141–147.
46. Kaiser AB. Antimicrobial prophylaxis in surgery. *N Engl J Med* 1986;315:1129–1138.
47. Antimicrobial prophylaxis in surgery. *Med Lett* 1993;35:91–94.
48. Philips JL, Abdel-Rahman S, Farrar HC, et al. Antimicrobial agents. In: Long SS, Pickering LK, Prober CG, eds. *Principles and practice of pediatric infectious diseases*, 2nd ed. New York, NY: Churchill Livingstone, 2003:1458–1510.
49. Saez-llorens X, McCracken GH Jr. Clinical pharmacology of antibacterial agents. In: Remington JS, Klein JO, eds. *Infectious diseases of the fetus and newborn infant*, 5th ed. Philadelphia, PA: WB Saunders, 2001:1419–1466.
50. Cuchural GH Jr, Tally FP, Jacobus NV, et al. Comparative activities of newer β-lactam agents against members of the *Bacteroides fragilis* group. *Antimicrob Agents Chemother* 1990;34:479–48
51. Quagliarello VJ, Scheld WM. Treatment of bacterial meningitis. *N Engl J Med* 1997;336:708–716.
52. Committee on Infectious Diseases. Therapy for children with invasive pneumococcal infections. *Pediatrics* 1997;99:289–299.
53. Young JP, Husson JM, Bruch K, et al. The evaluation of efficacy and safety of cefotaxime: a review of 2500 cases. *J Antimicrob Chemother* 1980;6(Suppl A):293–300.
54. Eron LJ, Park CH, Goldenberg RI, et al. Ceftriaxone therapy of serious bacterial infections. *J Antimicrob Chemother* 1983;12:65–78.
55. Centers for Disease Control and Prevention. Sexually transmitted disease treatment guidelines for 2015. *Morb Mortal Wkly Rep* 2015;64(RR-03):1–140.
56. Dattwyler RJ, Halperin JJ, Volkman DJ, et al. Treatment of late Lyme borreliosis—randomized comparison of ceftriaxone and penicillin. *Lancet* 1988;1:1191–1194.
57. Padoan R, Cambisano W, Costantini D, et al. Ceftazidime monotherapy vs. combined therapy in *Pseudomonas* pulmonary infections in cystic fibrosis. *Pediatr Infect Dis J* 1987;6(7):648–653.
58. Hoepelman AI, Kieft H, Aoun M, et al. International comparative study of cefepime and ceftazidime in the treatment of serious bacterial infections. *J Antimicrob Chemother* 1993;32(Suppl B):175–186.
59. Zervos M, Nelson M. Cefepime Study Group. Cefepime versus ceftriaxone for empiric treatment of hospitalized patients with community-acquired pneumonia. *Antimicrob Agents Chemother* 1998;42:729–733.
60. Yamamura D, Gucalp R, Carlisle P, et al. Open randomized study of cefepime versus piperacillin–gentamicin for treatment of febrile neutropenic cancer patients. *Antimicrob Agents Chemother* 1997;41:1704–1708.
61. Saez-Llorens X, Castano E, Garcia R, et al. Prospective randomized treatment of cefepime and cefotaxime for treatment of bacterial meningitis in infants and children. *Antimicrob Agents Chemother* 1995;39:937–940.
62. Karchmer AW. Cephalosporins. In: Mandell GL, Douglas JE, Dolin R, eds. *Mandell, Douglas, and Bennett's principles and practice of infectious diseases*, 5th ed. Philadelphia, PA: Churchill Livingstone, 2000:274–291.
63. Sanders WE Jr, Tenney JH, Kessler RE. Efficacy of cefepime in the treatment of infections due to multiply resistant *Enterobacter* species. *Clin Infect Dis* 1996;23:454–461.
64. Kelkar SP, Li JT. Cephalosporin allergy. *N Engl J Med* 2001;345(11):804–809.
65. Norrby SR. Side effects of cephalosporins. *Drugs* 1987;34(Suppl 2):105–120.
66. Murray DL, Singer DA, Singer AB, et al. Cefaclor—a cluster of adverse reactions. *N Engl J Med* 1980;303:1003.
67. Meyers BR. Comparative toxicities of third-generation cephalosporins. *Am J Med* 1985;79:96–103.
68. Lin RY. A perspective on penicillin allergy. *Arch Intern Med* 1992;152:930–937.
69. Johnson GJ. Antibiotic-induced hemostatic abnormalities. In: Peterson PK, Verhoef J, eds. *The antimicrobial agents annual*. Amsterdam, The Netherlands: Elsevier, 1986:408–419.
70. Bang NU, Kammer RB. Hematologic complications associated with β-lactam antibiotics. *Rev Infect Dis* 1982;4:S546–S554.
71. U.S. Food and Drug Administration. http://www.fda.gov/Drugs/DrugSafety/PostmarketDrugSafetyInformationforPatientsandProviders/ucm109103.htm. Accessed March 30, 2010.
72. Sharma R, Francois D, Hammerschlag MR. New antimicrobial agents for the treatment of staphylococcal infections in children. *Pediatr Clin North Am* 2017; 64:1369–1387.
73. Forest Laboratories. Study of blood levels of ceftaroline fosamil in children who are receiving antibiotic therapy in hospital (NLM Identifier: NCT01298843). In ClinicalTrials.gov [Internet]. Bethesda, MD: National Library of Medicine. 2000. https:// clinicaltrials.gov/show/NCT01298843. Accessed April 28, 2017.
74. Riccobene TA, Rekeda L, Rank D, Llorens L. Evaluation of the effect of a supratherapeutic dose of intravenous ceftaroline fosamil on the corrected QT interval. *Antimicrob Agents Chemother* 2013;57(4):1777–1783.
75. Molloy L, Snyder AH, Srivastava R, et al. Ceftaroline fosamil for methicillin-resistant *Staphylococcus aureus* pulmonary exacerbation in a pediatric cystic fibrosis patient. *J Pediatr Pharmacol Ther* 2014;19(2):135–140.
76. Andes D, Craig WA. Pharmacodynamics of a new cephalosporin, PPI-0903 (TAK-599), activity against methicillin-resistant *Staphylococcus aureus* in murine thigh and lung infection models: identification of an in vivo pharmacokinetic-pharmacodynamic target. *Antimicrob Agents Chemother* 2006;50:1376–1383.
77. Ge Y, Liao S, Thye DA, et al. Ceftaroline (CPT) dose adjustment recommendations for subjects with mild or moderate renal impairment (RI). *Abstracts of the 47th Interscience Conference on antimicrobial agents and chemotherapy* [Abstract A-35]. Chicago, IL. Washington, DC: American Society for Microbiology, 2007.
78. Ge Y, Liao S, Talbot GH. Population pharmacokinetics (PK) analysis of ceftaroline (CPT) in volunteers and patients with complicated skin and skin structure infection (cSSSI). *Abstracts of the 47th Interscience Conference on antimicrobial agents and chemotherapy* [Abstract A-34]. Chicago, IL. Washington, DC: American Society for Microbiology, 2007.
79. Cannavino C, Nemeth A, Korczowski B, et al. A randomized, prospective study of pediatric patients with community-acquired pneumonia treated with ceftaroline versus ceftriaxone. *Pediatr Infect Dis J* 2016;35:752–759.
80. Blumer J, Ghonghadze T, Cannavino C, et al. A multicenter, randomized, observer-blinded, active-controlled study evaluating the safety and effectiveness of ceftaroline compared with ceftriaxone plus vancomycin in pediatric patients with complicated community-acquired bacterial pneumonia. *Pediatr Infect Dis J* 2016;35:760–766.
81. Korczowski B, Antadze T, Giorgobiani M, et al. A multicenter, randomized, observer-blinded, active-controlled study to evaluate the safety and efficacy of ceftaroline versus comparator in pediatric patients with acute bacterial skin and skin structure infection. *Pediatr Infect Dis J* 2016;35:e239–e247.
82. Teflaro® (ceftaroline fosamil) package insert. St. Louis, MO: Forest Pharmaceuticals, Inc. 2016.
83. Riccobene T, Khariton T, Knebel W, et al. Population PK modeling and target attainment simulations to support dosing of ceftaroline fosamil in pediatric patients with acute bacterial skin and skin structure infections and community-acquired bacterial pneumonia. *J Clin Pharmacol* 2017;57(3):345–355.
84. Shirley D, Heil E, Johnson J. Ceftaroline fosamil: a brief clinical review. *Infect Dis Ther* 2013;2:95–119.
85. Avycaz Label. Prescribing information. https://www.accessdata.fda.gov/drugsatfda_docs/label/2019/206494s005,s006lbl.pdf. Accessed November 25, 2019.

86. Bradley JS, Broadhurst H, Cheng K, et al. Safety and efficacy of ceftazidime-avibactam plus metronidazole in the treatment of children ≥3 months to <18 years with complicated intra-abdominal infection: results from a phase 2 randomized, controlled trial. *Pediatr Infect Dis J* 2019;38:816–824.
87. Bradley JS, Roilides E, Broadhurst H, et al. Safety and efficacy of ceftazidime-avibactam in the treatment of children ≥3 months to <18 years with complicated urinary tract infection: results from a phase 2 randomized, controlled trial. *Pediatr Infect Dis J* 2019;38:920–928.
88. Isofidis E, Chorafa E, Agakidou E, et al. Use of ceftazidime-avibactam for the treatment of extensively resistant or pan-resistant *Klebsiella pneumoniae* in neonates and children <5 years of age. *Pediatr Infect Dis J* 2019;38:812–815.
89. Sader HS, Huband MD, Duncan LR, et al. Ceftazidime-avibactam antimicrobial activity and spectrum when tested against Gram-negative organisms from pediatric patients. Results from the INFORM surveillance program (United States, 2011–2015). *Pediatr Infect Dis J* 2018;3:549–554.
90. Pannaraj PS, Bard JD, Cerini C, et al. Pediatric carbapenem-resistant Enterobacteriaceae in Los Angeles, California, a high-prevalence region in the United States. *Pediatr Infect Dis J* 2015;34:11–16.
91. Logan LK, Braykov NP, Weinstein RA, et al. Extended-spectrum β-lactamase-producing and third-generation cephalosporin-resistant Enterobacteriaceae in children: trends in the United States, 1999–2011. *J Pediatr Infect Dis* 2014;3:320–328.
92. Bradley JS, Ang JY, Arrieta AC, et al. Pharmacokinetics and safety of single intravenous doses of ceftolozane-tazobactam in children with proven or suspected Gram-negative infection. *Pediatr Infect Dis J* 2018;37:1130–1136.
93. Zasowski EJ, Rybak JM, Rybak MJ. The β-lactams strike back: ceftazidime-avibactam. *Pharmacotherapy* 2015;35:755–770.
94. Bradley JS, Armstrong J, Arrieta A, et al. Phase I study assessing the pharmacokinetic profile, safety, and tolerability of a single dose of ceftazidime-avibactam in hospitalized pediatric patients. *Antimicrob Agents Chemother* 2016;60:6252–6259.
95. Larson KB, Patel YT, Willavize S, et al. Ceftolozane-tazobactam population pharmacokinetics and dose selection for further clinical evaluation in pediatric patients with complicated urinary tract or complicated intra-abdominal infections. *Antimicrob Agents Chemother* 2019;63:8–14.
96. Zhanel GG, Wiebe R, Dilay L, et al. Comparative review of the carbapenems. *Drugs* 2007;67(7):1027–1052.
97. Kahan FM, Kropp H, Sundelof JG, et al. Thienamycin: development of imipenem–cilastatin. *J Antimicrob Chemother* 1983;12(Suppl D):1–35.
98. Nadler HL, Pitkin DH, Sheikh W. The postantibiotic effect of meropenem and imipenem on selected bacteria. *J Antimicrob Chemother* 1989;24(Suppl A):225–231.
99. Okamoto K, Gotoh N, Nishino T. *Pseudomonas aeruginosa* reveals high intrinsic resistance to penem antibiotics: penem resistance mechanisms and their interplay. *Antimicrob Agents Chemother* 2001;45(7):1964–1971.
100. Kropp H, Sundelof JG, Hajdu R, et al. Metabolism of thienamycin and related carbapenem antibiotics by the renal dipeptidase, dehydropeptidase. *Antimicrob Agents Chemother* 1982;22(1):62–70.
101. Calandra G, Lydick E, Carrigan J, et al. Factors predisposing to seizures in seriously ill infected patients receiving antibiotics: experience with imipenem/cilastatin. *Am J Med* 1988;84(5):911–918.
102. Calandra GB, Brown KR, Grad LC, et al. Review of adverse experiences and tolerability in the first 2,516 patients treated with imipenem/cilastatin. *Am J Med* 1985;78(6A):73–78.
103. Wong VK, Wright HT Jr, Ross LA, et al. Imipenem/cilastatin treatment of bacterial meningitis in children. *Pediatr Infect Dis J* 1991;10(2):122–125.
104. Bodey GP, Alvarez ME, Jones PG, et al. Imipenem/cilastatin as initial therapy for febrile cancer patients. *Antmicrob Agents Chemother* 1986;30:211–214.
105. Iaconis JP, Pitkin DH, Sheikh W, et al. Comparison of antibacterial activities of meropenem and six other antimicrobials against *Pseudomonas aeruginosa* isolates from North American studies and clinical trials. *Clin Infect Dis* 1997;24(Suppl 2):S191–S196.
106. Satake S, Yoshihara E, Nakae T. Diffusion of beta-lactam antibiotics through liposome membranes reconstituted from purified porins of the outer membrane of *Pseudomonas aeruginosa*. *Antimicrob Agents Chemother* 1990;34(5):685–690.
107. Klugman KP, Dagan R, Meropenem Meningitis Study Group. Randomized comparison of meropenem with cefotaxime for treatment of bacterial meningitis. *Antimicrob Agents Chemother* 1995;39:1140–1146.
108. Odio CM, Puig JR, Feris JM, et al. Prospective, randomized, investigator-blinded study of the efficacy and safety of meropenem vs. cefotaxime therapy in bacterial meningitis in children. Meropenem Meningitis Study Group. *Pediatr Infect Dis J* 1999;18(7):581–590.
109. Bradley JS. Meropenem: a new, extremely broad-spectrum beta-lactam antibiotic for serious infections in pediatrics. *Pediatr Infect Dis J* 1997;16(3):263–268.
110. Garau J, Blanquer J, Cobo L, et al. Prospective, randomised, multicentre study of meropenem versus imipenem/cilastatin as empiric monotherapy in severe nosocomial infections. *Eur J Clin Microbiol Infect Dis* 1997;16(11):789–796.
111. Colardyn F, Faulkner KL. Intravenous meropenem versus imipenem/cilastatin in the treatment of serious bacterial infections in hospitalized patients. Meropenem Serious Infection Study Group. *J Antimicrob Chemother* 1996;38(3):523–537.
112. Norrby SR. Neurotoxicity of carbapenem antibacterials. *Drug Saf* 1996;15:87–90.
113. Fujii R, Pediatric Study Group of Meropenem. Pharmacokinetic and clinical studies with meropenem in the pediatric field. *Jpn J Antibiot* 1992;45:697–717.
114. Merrem Product Label. http://www.accessdata.fda.gov/drugsatfda_docs/label/2009/050706s025lbl.pdf. Accessed March 30, 2010.
115. Fuchs PC, Barry AL, Brown SD. *In vitro* activities of ertapenem (MK-0826) against clinical bacterial isolates from 11 North American medical centers. *Antimicrob Agents Chemother* 2001;45:1915–1918.
116. Kohler J, Dorso KL, Young K, et al. *In vitro* activities of the potent, broad-spectrum carbapenem MK-0826 (L-749,345) against broad-spectrum beta-lactamase-and extended-spectrum beta-lactamase producing *Klebsiella pneumoniae* and *Escherichia coli* clinical isolates. *Antimicrob Agents Chemother* 1999;43(5):1170–1176.
117. Product label for Invanz. Whitehouse Station, NJ: Merck. http://www.accessdata.fda.gov/drugsatfda_docs/label/2009/021337s030lbl.pdf. Accessed March 30, 2010.
118. Sykes RB, Cimarusti CM, Bonner DP, et al. Monocyclic beta-lactam antibiotics produced by bacteria. *Nature* 1981;291:489–491.
119. Giamarellou H. Aminoglycosides plus beta-lactams against gram-negative organisms. Evaluation of *in vitro* synergy and chemical interactions. *Am J Med* 1986;80(6B):126–137.
120. Johnson DH, Cunha BA. Aztreonam. *Med Clin North Am* 1995;79:733–743.
121. Swabb EA. Review of the clinical pharmacology of the monobactam antibiotic aztreonam. *Am J Med* 1985;78:11–18.
122. Duma RJ, Berry AJ, Smith SM, et al. Penetration of aztreonam into the cerebrospinal fluid of patients with and without inflamed meninges. *Antimicrob Agents Chemother* 1984;26:730–733.
123. Fillastre JP, Leroy A, Baudoin C, et al. Pharmacokinetics in patients with chronic renal failure. *Clin Pharmacokinet* 1985;10:91–100.
124. Gerig JS, Bolton ND, Swabb EA, et al. Effect of hemodialysis and peritoneal dialysis on aztreonam pharmacokinetics. *Kidney Int* 1984;26:308–318.
125. Saxon A, Hassner A, Swabb EA, et al. Lack of cross-reactivity between aztreonam, a monobactam antibiotic, and penicillin in penicillin-allergic subjects. *J Infect Dis* 1984;149:16–22.
126. Kilpatrick M, Girgis N, Farid Z, et al. Aztreonam for treating meningitis caused by gram-negative rods. *Scand J Infect Dis* 1991;23(1):125–126.
127. Retsch-Bogart GZ, Burns JL, Otto KL, et al., AZLI Phase II Study Group. A phase 2 study of aztreonam lysine for inhalation to treat patients with cystic fibrosis and Pseudomonas aeruginosa infection. *Pediatr Pulmonol* 2008;43(1):47–58.
128. Uauy R, Mize C, Argyle C, et al. Metabolic tolerance to arginine: implications for the safe use of arginine salt–aztreonam combination in the neonatal period. *J Pediatr* 1991;118(6):965–970.

Roopali Sharma
Margaret R. Hammerschlag

CHAPTER 21

Glycopeptides, Lipoglycopeptides, and Lipopeptides

GENERAL ASPECTS OF GLYCOPEPTIDE AND LIPOPEPTIDES ANTIBIOTICS

The clinically important compounds in the glycopeptide group are vancomycin and teicoplanin. Telavancin, dalbavancin, and oritavancin belong to the lipoglycopeptide group. In the mid-1950s, vancomycin was first utilized for the treatment of gram-positive infections in adults and children, but with the advent of extended-spectrum penicillins (PCNs) and cephalosporins, vancomycin was not used widely until 1980s for the treatment of methicillin-resistant *Staphylococcus aureus* (MRSA) strains.[1] In the 2000s, vancomycin became a forefront of concern due to documented decreased susceptibility to vancomycin in MRSA,[2,3] decreased efficacy,[4,5] and increased toxicity with higher doses and in combination therapy with piperacillin–tazobactam.[6–12] Teicoplanin was obtained from *Actinoplanes teichomyceticus* recovered from a soil sample in India in 1978. This glycopeptide antibiotic was introduced in 1982 and is currently available in many countries in Europe, Asia, and South America, but not in the United States. Semisynthetic lipoglycopeptides (telavancin, dalbavancin, and oritavancin) have a similar spectrum of activity to that of glycopeptides, but their additional chemical modifications seem to increase their potency. These lipoglycopeptides are not yet approved by the Food and Drug Administration (FDA) for use in pediatric population, although phase 1 and 2 studies have been completed.[13–16]

STRUCTURE AND CHEMICAL PROPERTIES

Vancomycin and teicoplanin are the commonly used glycopeptide antibiotics and are unrelated to other antibiotics. They are complex soluble glycopeptides, consisting of a seven-membered peptide chain, in the form of three large rings. Five of the seven amino acid residues are common to all glycopeptides.[17–19] A disaccharide, composed of glucose and vancosamine, is also present, but is not part of the cyclic structure. The molecular weight of vancomycin is 1,448 Da.[20] Vancomycin is hydrophobic but less so than teicoplanin.[19] It has a moderate protein binding in adults (10% to 55%) and exerts its activity over a wide pH range of 6.5 to 8.[21,22] Protein binding in neonates is higher (72% to 81%), but binding to bilirubin is not concentration dependent, indicating a low possibility of an increase in free bilirubin.[23] Vancomycin can be inactivated by heparin in high concentrations.[24] Teicoplanin can be added to parenteral solutions.[25]

Telavancin is a semisynthetic derivative of vancomycin with a hydrophobic decylaminoethyl side chain and a hydrophilic phosphonomethylaminomethyl group. The addition of a hydrophobic side chain strengthens the bond with bacterial cell membranes and D-alanyl-D-alanine (D-ala-D-ala) targets, thus improving activity against MRSA phenotypes and vanB enterococci.[26] In addition, binding to the cell membrane disrupts membrane potential and increases permeability, thus enhancing activity.[27]

Dalbavancin is a semisynthetic lipoglycopeptide derived from a teicoplanin-like antimicrobial.[28] Modification to the heptapeptide core includes the addition of a dimethylaminopropylamide group, resulting in enhanced gram-positive activity. The removal of an acetylglucosamine group and the addition of an acylglucosamine on ring 4 result in extended terminal half-life and improved binding characteristics to the D-ala-D-ala terminus.[26] Unlike telavancin and oritavancin, dalbavancin does not appear to destabilize cell membranes.

Oritavancin, a vancomycin analog, is a synthetic derivative of the naturally occurring glycopeptide chloroeremomycin. It differs from vancomycin by the presence of a 4-epivancosamine monosaccharide attached to the amino acid residue in ring 6, the addition of a 4′-chlorobiphenylmethyl substituent on the disaccharide sugar, and a lipophilic side chain.[28] Addition of the first two modifications results in enhanced target site binding with greater activity against vancomycin-susceptible and vancomycin-resistant organisms. The addition of the 4′-chlorobiphenylmethyl and lipid side chain further enhances target site binding by augmenting dimerization, facilitates membrane anchoring (improves activity against vancomycin-resistant enterococci [VRE]), and prolongs half-life.[27]

PHARMACOKINETICS, PHARMACODYNAMICS, AND DOSING

Vancomycin is a time-dependent antibiotic and is administered intravenously (IV) and has poor gastrointestinal absorption. Over 90% of the drug is eliminated by renal excretion, and in patients with reduced creatinine clearance, there is marked accumulation of vancomycin. It is imperative to conduct therapeutic drug monitoring (TDM) of vancomycin for efficacy and toxicity. It is 25% to 50% protein bound, mainly to albumin, and is almost exclusively eliminated by the renal route. The pharmacokinetics (PK) of vancomycin has markedly large interindividual variability, primarily attributed to the patient's age, clinical condition, and disease.

PHARMACOKINETICS OF GLYCOPEPTIDES IN NEONATES

PK parameters of vancomycin in neonates are different from those in adults. These differences are largely determined by the change in amount of body water and maturation of renal function in the first weeks of life, both in term and preterm newborn infants. This means that neonates, especially premature infants, have a larger volume of distribution (V_d) and decreased *CL* than do infants, children, and adults. These changes also result in higher interindividual differences in neonates than in adults.

Distribution or α half-life ($t_{1/2}$) of vancomycin is approximately 0.5 to 1 hour in adults.[29] In neonates and infants, it ranges from 0.05 to 0.49 hour but has only been determined explicitly in one study in which data for infants and neonates were pooled.[30] Others have suggested that $t_{1/2}$ might be longer, even up to 4 hours.[31–33] Average V_d in the steady state (V_{ss}) in term neonates for vancomycin as well as teicoplanin ranges from 0.57 to 0.69 L per kg, although very few studies, totaling only 31 patients, have specifically looked at this age group. For neonates of various gestational ages (GAs), V_{ss} ranges from 0.38 to 0.97 L per kg. Surprisingly, for very low-birth-weight (VLBW) on teicoplanin, a low V_d was found in one study (0.25 to 0.31 L per kg).[34] In special subgroups, especially neonates on extracorporeal membrane oxygenation (ECMO), V_{ss} is even higher. The overall V_{ss} range is comparable to values described in adults. As mentioned by Rodvold et al.,[35] V_d studied after a single dose or calculated with the elimination $t_{1/2}$ was often larger than V_{ss}.

Because meningitis often accompanies sepsis in neonates, penetration of vancomycin in cerebrospinal fluid (CSF) is of possible concern. Vancomycin dosing leads to CSF concentrations of 7% to 21% of the serum concentration in adults.[36] The initial study in infants found a similar percentage.[29] Later reports mentioned CSF concentrations ranging from 0.2 to 17.3 mg per L, with vancomycin CSF penetration ranging from 7.1% to 68%.[37–40] No clear relationship between CSF concentration and serum concentration was found. As in adults, there is a significant correlation between CSF concentration and biomarkers of meningeal inflammation.[21,37] Data on this subject are scarce, however, and vancomycin cannot be relied on to adequately treat gram-positive meningitis when given as a single antibiotic.

There are no published data on PK of intraventricular administration of vancomycin in neonates.

In neonates, 44% of vancomycin was recovered unchanged in urine after 8 hours.[41] Factors that have to be considered in excretion are *CL*, mainly determined by renal function, and serum half-life, which is dependent on the elimination rate constant (K_e). There are several important clinical features, discussed in what follows, that influence PK behavior in neonates.

Mean *CL* of vancomycin in adults (0.71 to 1.31 mL per kg per minute) is often higher than that reported in neonates and infants, although ranges are similar.[42–45]

In neonates, vancomycin *CL* ranges from 0.63 to 1.5 mL per kg per minute, depending on GA and/or postconceptional age (PCA). Teicoplanin *CL* is lower, at 0.26 mL per kg per minute. Vancomycin $t_{1/2}$ in adults ranges from 4 to 8 hours in patients with normal renal function. Mean $t_{1/2}$ in neonates of varying GA and PCA ranges from 3.5 to 10 hours.[41,46–53] for vancomycin and 29.2 to 43.2 hours for teicoplanin[34,54]

Given the route of elimination, an association between glomerular filtration rate (GFR) and excretion is predictable. Serum creatinine and creatinine *CL* in neonates correlated with vancomycin *CL* in several studies.[33,55–60] In population pharmacokinetic (PopPK) studies, the importance of creatinine *CL* as a covariate differs. Three studies found creatinine and creatinine *CL* to be an important covariate,[61–63] but two others did not.[31,60,] One study did not include creatinine or creatinine *CL* as a covariate in the model.[31] In the case of terminal renal failure, vancomycin *CL* by way of hemodialysis and/or peritoneal dialysis is slow, with a single dose of 15 mg per kg leading to trough serum concentrations of greater than 4 to 5 mg per L after 7 days in adults.[64] In neonates with terminal renal failure, a dosing regimen of 15 mg per kg once a week seems justified. In neonates with renal failure, vancomycin *CL* can be significantly increased by using veno-venous hemodiafiltration with a high-flux membrane.[65]

Taken together, the published data strongly favor a clear relationship between renal function in terms of serum creatinine or creatinine *CL* and the *CL* of vancomycin.

Several clinical features are important for PK behavior in neonates. GA, postnatal age (PNA), and PCA can all be expected to alter PK of vancomycin, and all three age-related factors are determinants of vancomycin PK and, therefore, dosing in neonates.

The apparent V_d of most drugs is larger in neonates than in adults, especially in premature infants, and is primarily due to a higher percentage of extracellular water.[66,67] Creatinine *CL* (mL per minute) shows a positive correlation with GA.[68,69] On the basis of GA, premature neonates are expected to have a longer $t_{1/2}$ due to both a larger V_d and a decreased *CL*. In most studies, both unstandardized vancomycin *CL* and V_{ss} demonstrate a relation to GA, but significance disappears when these parameters are normalized for weight.[51,59,60] This implies that if weight is incorporated in the model description, GA is not an important determinant of vancomycin V_{ss} or *CL*.

The postnatal increase in GFR seen in neonates and the reduction of extracellular fluid[70–72] imply that $t_{1/2}$ for vancomycin should decrease with increasing PNA. This is an inconsistent finding in studies.[33,41,50–53,59,60,73,74] V_{ss} (L), but not standardized V_{ss} (L per kg), has been related to PNA.[51,59] PCA has been well described in relation to PK parameters for vancomycin. As might be expected on the basis of the influence of both GA and PNA, there is also a positive relation between PCA and development of renal function.[68] Clearance (mL per minute) as well as standardized *CL* (mL per kg per minute) has been related to PCA with a concomitant change in $t_{1/2}$.[33,41,50–53,55,57–60,62,73,74] PCA is strongly correlated with weight, partly explaining the relation of weight to PK parameters in several studies.[31,33,60–63,74]

As with PNA, only unstandardized V_{ss} (L) has a significant correlation with PCA.[41,51,59,73,74]

Overall, PCA has a stronger influence on vancomycin PK than GA or PNA. The diminished influence of GA and PNA can be explained by several factors. The combined effects of GA and PNA are integrated in PCA. Also, prenatal exposure to corticosteroids seems to increase maturation of renal function prenatally and, therefore, limit the effect of GA on *CL*.[71] Furthermore, postnatal increase in GFR seems to be higher than intrauterine increase.[75] At the same PCA, this might imply that the effect of slower maturation of kidney function in prematures is canceled out by the difference in intrauterine and extrauterine development of GFR. A third and may be more important factor is that vancomycin is seldom given in the first week of life. Because a large increase in kidney function in neonates takes place in this period, the dynamics of these changes and their influence on vancomycin PK are not seen in the studies mentioned here. These data suggest that *CL* in relation to PCA is the main determinant in the PK profile of vancomycin in neonates.

Drug–drug interactions may alter PK profiles of vancomycin. Prenatal and/or postnatal exposure to indomethacin has been shown to negatively affect increase in kidney function in neonates.[71,76,77] A patent ductus arteriosus (PDA) can increase V_{ss} and decrease *CL* in neonates.[75,78] Several studies have addressed the effect of indomethacin or ibuprofen treatment of PDA on vancomycin PK in newborns.[56,60,74,79] Published data suggest that indomethacin treatment of PDA leads to an increase in V_d and a decrease in *CL*, warranting extra TDM and dose readjustments in these patients.

ECMO influences PK behavior of drugs in neonates. Clearance of vancomycin is decreased, V_d is higher, and serum half-life is longer in most studies.[80–83] Although these studies were relatively small and results were somewhat obscured by differences in renal function, a longer serum half-life in vancomycin-treated neonates on ECMO is likely.

PHARMACOKINETICS OF GLYCOPEPTIDES IN INFANTS AND CHILDREN

Distribution (α-phase) half-life ($t_{1/2}$) in pediatric studies ranges from 0.04 to 1.11 hours for vancomycin and 0.79 to 2.0 hours for teicoplanin.[30,84–86] V_d of vancomycin as well as teicoplanin appears to be smaller than that in adults. Teicoplanin is distributed mainly to a third compartment in neonates; in children, a bicompartmental model may suffice.[41,86] Surprisingly, in children younger than 1 year, V_d and *CL* are threefold lower than in children older than 1 year, leading to a larger percentage of expected subtherapeutic serum concentrations in older children.[86]

Continuous intraperitoneal treatment of peritonitis in children on dialysis with either vancomycin 30 mg per L or teicoplanin 20 mg per L of dialysate leads to serum concentrations of approximately 20 mg per L after 1 week for both antibiotics.[87] The bioavailability of vancomycin during intraperitoneal administration is 70%.[88] Intermittent (once a week treatment) with vancomycin (30 mg per kg) or teicoplanin (15 mg per kg) results in trough serum concentrations after 1 week of 8 to 10 mg per L.[98] As in neonates, distribution to CSF is of interest. IV administration of vancomycin leads to an average vancomycin CSF concentration of 10% of the serum concentration, without a significant correlation in individual patients with ventricular shunt infections.[37] In children, Spears and Koch[89] reported CSF concentrations of less than 0.8 mg per L in seven samples 1 to 12 hours after the vancomycin dose. In pediatric patients with meningitis, a CSF-to-serum ratio of 0.14 to 0.28 was found.[90] However, penetration is only 0.77% to 18% in patients without meningeal or ventricular inflammation.[91,92]

Daily intrathecal administration of 10 mg of teicoplanin or 20 mg of vancomycin led to trough CSF concentrations of 3.3 to 4.8 and 14.5 to 193 mg per L, respectively, in single patient and showed wide variability in patients exposed to combined IV and intrathecal treatment, warranting TDM.[93–96]

Vancomycin showed prolonged elimination from CSF in an accidental case of intraventricular administration.[95] Teicoplanin concentrations in pus range from 37% to 110% of serum concentrations.[97]

On cardiopulmonary bypass, vancomycin and teicoplanin concentrations decreased by 77% and 53%, respectively.[98]

Vancomycin and teicoplanin *CL* depends mainly on renal function. Clearance of glycopeptide antibiotics is more rapid in children than in adults, though reasons for this phenomenon are not clear.[30,99] As with distribution, age-related differences in *CL* are not well known, though *CL* of vancomycin seems to peak at 1 year and then decrease.[74] For teicoplanin, there is no age-related difference in elimination half-life.[100] Clearance in pediatric oncology as well as pediatric intensive care patients is higher.[88,99,,101,102] Initiation of cardiopulmonary bypass abruptly decreases vancomycin concentrations by 44.5%.[103] Clearance on ECMO is dependent on the duration of use of the membrane.[104] Clearance with peritoneal dialysis depends on the time of indwelling fluid and accounts for 25% to 32% of total-body clearance.[88]

PHARMACOKINETICS OF LIPOGLYCOPEPTIDES IN NEONATES, INFANTS, AND CHILDREN

Telavancin, oritavancin, and dalbavancin have demonstrated efficacy in the treatment of multidrug-resistant gram-positive infections but have had limited exposure in the pediatric population. The PK, safety, and efficacy of telavancin have not been studied in children or infants. Telavancin is being studied in the pediatric population. There is one planned study examining the single-dose PK of the drug given at 10 mg per kg in pediatric subjects aged 1 to 17 years.[13]

Dalbavancin has interesting PK characteristics, including a long half-life and good tissue distribution mainly due to its high reversible protein binding to serum albumin.[27,28] Dalbavancin has renal and nonrenal clearance via feces. Approximately 30% of dalbavancin is excreted unchanged via the kidney. Hepatic metabolism does not appear to affect dalbavancin clearance, and dose modifications may not be needed in patients with hepatic impairment, although data are limited in patients with moderate-to-severe hepatic impairment.[27,28]

The disposition of dalbavancin in children has been published in two phase 1, open-label, multicenter studies.[14,15] Bradley and colleagues studied the PK of IV dalbavancin in children aged 12 to 17 years.[14] A single dose of 1,000 mg of dalbavancin was administered to children weighing greater than or equal to 60 kg and 15 mg per kg for children weighing less than 60 kg. PK parameters were determined using noncompartmental analysis. There were total of 10 subjects, five in dalbavancin 1,000 mg and five in dalbavancin 15 mg per kg. The peak plasma concentration (C_{max}) and area under the curve (AUC_{inf}) in either 1,000 mg for those who weighed more than 60 kg or 15 mg per kg for those weighing less than 60 kg was similar. The terminal half-life was approximately 9 days in both dosing groups compared to 15 days in adult patients in published studies, highlighting that this PK difference in half-life may be due to age[14] In this study, the *AUC* was 30% less than those documented in adult studies, which probably can be explained by enhanced hepatic/renal clearance in healthy adolescents compared to adults. Nine of the 10 subjects had detectable plasma levels of dalbavancin 55 days after the administration.

The second pediatric study examined the PK of IV dalbavancin following administration of single dose in hospitalized pediatric patients aged 3 months to 11 years.[15] The authors of this study utilized published data from Bradley et al.'s study to further categorize disposition characteristics of dalbavancin in pediatric subjects' age greater than 3 months and perform population PK analysis to identify optimal dalbavancin dosing in children. Three hundred and eleven dalbavancin serum concentrations from 43 subjects were analyzed. Thirty-one patient were males, the median age and weight from the pooled data were 5.9 years (range 0.3 to 16.9 years) and 18.9 kg (range 5.7 to 105.2), respectively. The median dose in both studies was 15 mg per kg (range 9.5 to 25.7). The optimal pediatric age-dependent dosing of dalbavancin based on the population PK model was as follows: age 6 to less than 18 years, 12 mg per kg (1,000 mg maximum) on day 1 and 6 mg per kg (500 mg maximum) on day 8; age 3 months to less than 6 years, 15 mg per kg (1,000 mg maximum) on day 1 and 7.5 mg per kg (500 mg maximum) on day 8. This dosing regimen in children would achieve similar dalbavancin exposure compared to that in adults administered a two-dose regimen (1,000 mg on day 1 plus 500 mg on day 8). Similarly, the following age-dependent regimen was found to match adult exposure after a single dose (1,500 mg): age 6 to less than 18 years, 18 mg per kg (1,500 mg maximum) on day 1; and age 3 months to less than 6 years, 22.5 mg per kg (1,500 mg maximum) on day 1. The data on PK in children are limited to these two studies. There is no dosage defined for neonates, and further studies are needed to define an optimum dose of dalbavancin for maximum efficacy and limited toxicity in pediatric population.

There is currently no published article available for the use of oritavancin in the pediatric population. In 2018, an abstract of phase 1, open-label, sequential, dose-finding study evaluating the PK, safety, and tolerability of a single-dose 15 mg per kg (maximum 1,200 mg) IV infusion of oritavancin in children under 18 years is published.[16] The first three age cohorts (12 to <18 years, 6 to <12 years, and 2 to <6 years) with eight subjects in each cohort thus far has completed the study. Subjects had a suspected or confirmed gram-positive bacterial infection for which they received standard-of-care antibiotic therapy. Following a single dose of oritavancin, PK samples were obtained at 3, 4, 9, 24, 48, 72, and 336 hours after the start of the 3-hour infusion. Plasma concentrations were analyzed by noncompartmental methods. Subjects were evaluated for safety through day 60. In subjects aged 6 to less than 18 years, a single 15 mg per kg dose of oritavancin appeared to be well tolerated and provided a PK profile similar to a single 1,200 mg dose in adults. The mean $AUC_{0\text{-inf}}$ and C_{max} in subjects aged 2 to less than 6 years was lower, 1,963 μg.h/mL and 84 μg per mL, respectively, than the targeted exposure range in adults. A higher dose of oritavancin is currently being studied in this cohort.[16]

GLYCOPEPTIDE PHARMACODYNAMICS, DOSING, AND TOXICITY

To reduce nephrotoxicity and optimize efficacy, serum trough concentrations are monitored. Due to the lack of data for vancomycin dosing and monitoring in pediatric patients, guidelines developed for adults are utilized as a reference. Historically, vancomycin in pediatric patients has been dosed at 40 mg per kg per day for empiric treatment. Previously, serum trough concentrations were targeted to 5 to 10 mg per L in most situations or 10 to 15 mg per L for the treatment of central nervous system infections.[105] Because of an increase in MRSA infections in pediatric patients, increased inhibitory minimum inhibitory concentration (*MIC*), antibiotic penetration issues, and unique metabolic differences between children and adults, it has been shown that higher doses of vancomycin may be required in some pediatric patients. The maximum recommended dose for adult or pediatric patients is 100 mg per kg per day or 6 g per day.[106] To minimize the development of resistant strains, improve tissue penetration, and optimize vancomycin pharmacodynamics (PD), the 2011 Infectious Diseases Society of America (IDSA) guidelines suggested targeting these higher trough concentrations and its effectiveness is more correlated with *AUC:MIC* ratio. The guideline suggests that trough concentrations of 15 to 20 mg per L should achieve an AUC_{24}/MIC greater than 400 in adults if the vancomycin *MIC* is less than or equal to 1 mg per L.[107] In addition, the guidelines state that there are limited data to guide vancomycin dosing in children with MRSA. Although the vancomycin AUC_{24}/MIC ratio greater than 400 has been shown to predict clinical efficacy in adults, this relationship has not been documented very well between vancomycin AUC_{24}/MIC and treatment outcomes in MRSA infections in children. Most of the pediatric studies conducted to date have evaluated dosing that would achieve similar *AUC:MIC* goals. No pediatric outcome data have supported specific *AUC:MIC* concentrations; a recent study demonstrates a correlation between troughs in pediatric patients and outcomes.[108] In a multicenter retrospective study, the optimal vancomycin trough concentration was determined that would impact the duration of MRSA bacteremia in children. It was reported that a median vancomycin trough concentration of less than 10 mg per L within the first 72 hours may be associated with a longer duration of bacteremia compared with a median trough concentration of greater than or equal to 10 mg per L.[108] It remains unclear if vancomycin trough concentrations of greater than or equal to 15 mg per L are needed in children with MRSA bacteremia. This question is important because children have enhanced renal elimination, which makes it challenging for them to obtain a trough concentration of greater than or equal to 15 mg per L, and attempts to reach this goal often require higher doses and an increased frequency of administration. Pediatric patients often clear vancomycin much faster than adults. Analysis of vancomycin clearance has demonstrated a median clearance of 0.12 to 0.04 L per kg per h in patients aged 2.2 to 13.4 years, 2.5 times higher than the reported average renal clearance in adults of 0.048 L per kg per h.[109] Due to increased clearance in pediatric patients, much higher and more frequent mg per kg dosing is needed to achieve similar trough concentrations as adults. PD data suggest that higher dosages 60 mg per kg per day) are required to achieve AUC_{24}/MIC greater than 400 for isolates with a vancomycin *MIC* less than 1 g per mL, and guidelines suggest considering targeting trough concentrations of 15 to 20 μg per mL in children with serious infections.[110] Following adoption of the new target trough levels for vancomycin, typical pediatric starting doses of 40 to 60 mg per kg daily (usually divided for administration every 6 to 8 hour) have remained the same at many institutions. Several studies have shown that such doses are frequently insufficient to achieve the new target trough levels, and recent studies have shown that significantly higher doses than those in current use are required to achieve these higher trough levels; however, more data are needed to support starting doses above 60 mg per kg daily in pediatrics[109,111–115] Several studies have shown low rates of achieving therapeutic vancomycin trough levels in pediatric patients with current starting doses.[111–115] The delay in achieving the target trough level not only impedes early treatment of the infection but also promotes the development of resistant strains. A recent PK evaluation modeled a dose of 15 mg per kg every 6 hour and showed that estimated troughs of 7 to 10 mg per L were predicted to correlate to achieving an *AUC:MIC* goal of more than 400 mg h per L for more than 90%, and 1% to 17% at *MICs* of 1 and 2 mg per L, respectively.[116] Similarly, another published model on 300 pediatric patients aged 3 months and older showed troughs of 8 to 9 mg per L corresponded to *AUC:MIC* goals, but even with doses of 60 to 70 mg per kg per day, trough goals were only obtained in 45% of children.[109] Hwang et al. studied vancomycin dosing and target attainment in 304 Taiwanese children. The mean age was 6.0 ± 5.1 years, and the mean body weight was 20 ± 11.7 kg. Vancomycin trough concentrations were moderately correlated with *AUC* values ($p < 0.01$). Dosing of 15 mg per kg per dose q6h produced significantly higher *AUC* values ($p < 0.001$) and vancomycin trough concentrations ($p < 0.001$) compared with dosing of 10 mg per kg per dose q6h. In children receiving a 10 mg per kg per dose q6h, 5.6% (5/90) achieved the target trough concentrations of 15 to 20 mg per mL, and 9.5% (5/90) achieved the goal *AUC/MIC* greater than or equal to 400. In children receiving a 15 mg per kg per dose q6h, 13% (6/46) achieved the target trough concentrations of 15 to 20 mg per mL, whereas 54.3% (25/46) achieved the goal *AUC/MIC* greater than or equal to 400.[117] Chhim and colleagues evaluated vancomycin dosing practices for suspected invasive staphylococcal infections and found that 40 mg per kg per day did not result in therapeutic trough concentrations or predicted AUC_{24} greater than 400 in the majority of patients. Even 60 mg per kg per day did not routinely achieve these target ranges in children.[118] In addition a meta-analysis of 20 studies revealed that doses lower than 60 mg/kg/day were not enough to achieve desirable vancomycin plasma concentrations "area under the curve in 24 h/minimum inhibitory concentration >400 (AUC0-24/MIC>400) or trough 10–20 mg/L" to control bacterial infections in pediatric patients.[119] Further, some data suggest that young patients between the ages of 1 and 6 years are more likely to require 80 to 85 mg per kg per day divided every 6 hour to achieve troughs of 15 to 20 mg per L.[115] Eighty to 90% of vancomycin is cleared through the kidneys, the half-life of the drug in a patient's body depends heavily on renal function. Given age-related differences in renal function and vancomycin clearance, it seems that vancomycin dosing strategies should be adjusted according to age in pediatric patients, and a few have suggested alternative starting doses, for example, starting dose of 60 mg per kg daily for patients aged 1 to 5 months and those 13 to 18 years and a starting dose of 70 mg per kg daily for patients aged 6 months to 12 years.[120] Although targeting troughs of 15 to 20 mg per L may provide a simplistic means of assurance of PD target attainment in complicated infections, concern has arisen that it may also unnecessarily increase nephrotoxicity risk in some patients. The results of a study showed that although adult patients with trough levels greater than 10 mg per L were more likely to achieve the PD AUC_{24}:*MIC* target than those with trough levels less than 10 mg per L, pushing trough levels greater than 15 mg per L was not associated with a statistically significant increase in AUC_{24}:*MIC* target attainment. In addition, the study results showed that the mean trough in those patients who developed vancomycin-induced nephrotoxicity (**VIN**) was 19.5 mg per L versus 14.5 mg per L in those who did not develop VIN.[121] Thus, targeting a higher trough goal increased the risk for the development of VIN, but did not increase the proportion of patients achieving the PD target. Kishk et al.[122] examined vancomycin *AUC/MIC* and corresponding troughs in pediatrics. Their retrospective study concluded that the probability of achieving an *AUC/MIC* greater than 400 using only a trough serum concentration and an *MIC* with patients receiving 15 mg per kg every 6 hours is variable, based on the method used to calculate the *AUC*. An *AUC/MIC* of 400 in children may be correlated with a trough concentration of 11 mg per L using a trapezoidal method to calculate *AUC*.[122] Recently, a meta-analysis published by Fiorito and colleagues reported that the rate of VIN is increased in pediatrics patients with higher vancomycin troughs along with contributing factors, such an intensive care unit admission, hypovolemia, and concurrent use of nephrotoxic agents.[123]

Overall, specific conclusions on predictors of vancomycin-associated nephrotoxicity in pediatric patients are hampered by much variability in inclusion and exclusion criteria, leading to uncertainties in data interpretation. PD studies to assess *AUC/MIC* ratios in pediatrics may help clarify monitoring recommendations and requirements. It is suggested that Bayesian PK dosing approach based on a single vancomycin level to determine vancomycin exposure may provide a clearer indication of vancomycin efficacy and toxicity and that the risk of nephrotoxicity may be increased by additional risk factors besides vancomycin trough levels.[124]

LIPOGLYCOPEPTIDES PHARMACODYNAMICS AND DOSING

PD parameters of dalbavancin have not been established in children. Based on in vitro and in animal studies, the AUC_{24}/*MIC* parameter and the C_{max}/*MIC* are highly associated with in vivo activity.[125] These PD parameters endorse the infrequent administration of large doses, and the PD parameter most likely to predict efficacy of dalbavancin is *AUC/MIC*. In adults, a regimen of 1,500 mg given on day 1 and then again on day 8 is expected to achieve an *AUC* similar to that for a 1,000-mg initial dose, followed by four subsequent 500-mg weekly doses. Although the same total *AUC* should provide similar outcomes, experimental data suggest that the efficacy of drugs with a long half-life, such as dalbavancin, is enhanced by providing higher doses earlier in the course of therapy.[125] This finding has been observed in animal studies with dalbavancin in which better outcomes were observed when the same total dose was delivered in larger amounts earlier and less frequently.[126]

Dose-fractionation studies in animal models suggested the peak concentration was the major index for efficacy of oritavancin.[127] PD studies in mice have indicated that the surrogate marker that best correlates with the antimicrobial effect of telavancin is the *AUC/MIC* ratio.[127]

There are no dosing recommendations available for dalbavancin, oritavancin, and telavancin in pediatric patients at this time.

MECHANISM OF ACTION OF GLYCOPEPTIDES AND LIPOGLYCOPEPTIDES

The bactericidal activity of glycopeptide and lipoglycopeptide antibiotics is based on the inhibition of bacterial cell wall synthesis, by binding to the D-ala-D-ala portion of peptides found only in bacterial cell walls and disrupting cross-linking and polymerization, resulting in cell wall destabilization and death.[128] Lipoglycopeptide activity is enhanced through the addition of a lipid side chain. The lipophilic tail assists in dimer formation, membrane anchoring, and stabilizing interactions with lipid II. This process enhances target site binding and improves activity against gram-positive organisms, including vancomycin-resistant strains.[128] In addition, side chains on telavancin and oritavancin increase bactericidal activity by disrupting bacterial membrane potential and increasing membrane permeability. Oritavancin interferes with peptidic cross-linking in other portions of the *S. aureus* cell wall.[128] These actions may impart further activity against vancomycin-resistant strains through peptide bridge binding.[128]

IN VITRO ANTIMICROBIAL ACTIVITY

Glycopeptides and lipoglycopeptides are bactericidal for a host of aerobic and anaerobic gram-positive bacteria. Strains of *Staphylococcus epidermidis* and *S. aureus* are susceptible, although emergence of vancomycin-intermediate–resistant strains is a growing concern.[26–28]

In the mid-1950s, vancomycin was first utilized for the treatment of gram-positive infections in adults and children, but with the advent of extended-spectrum PCNs and cephalosporins, vancomycin was not used widely until 1980s.[109] for the treatment of MRSA strains.[4] In the 2000s, vancomycin became a major concern due to documented decreased susceptibility to vancomycin in MRSA,[5–7] decreased efficacy,[8,9] and increased toxicity with higher doses and in combination therapy with piperacillin–tazobactam.[10–12] Resistance to vancomycin in MRSA (*MIC* >2 mg per L) is infrequent, but there is increasing evidence in the literature[5] that vancomycin may be ineffective against increasing proportion of isolates with *MICs* between 1 and 2 mg per L. Recently, several studies and meta-analyses have demonstrated that strains with high vancomycin *MICs* are associated with poor outcomes, especially in patients with bacteremia and deep tissue infections (osteomyelitis, necrotizing pneumonia) due to MRSA.[4,129,130] This gradual increase in the value of vancomycin *MIC* for *S. aureus* has been reported as *MIC* creep or vancomycin heteroresistance (subpopulations of resistant *S. aureus* within a larger population of vancomycin-susceptible bacteria), and patients infected with MRSA isolates who exhibit *MIC* creep might experience poorer clinical outcomes, including delayed treatment response, increased mortality, increase rate of relapse, extended hospitalization, or overall increased cost of hospitalization.[131] This phenomenon of *MIC* creep and vancomycin therapy failure with *S. aureus* infections with an *MIC* greater than or equal to 4 mg per L led the Clinical and Laboratory Standards Institute (CLSI) in 2016 to reduce vancomycin breakpoints for susceptible *S. aureus* from less than or equal to 4 to less than or equal to 2 mg per L, and from greater than or equal to 32 to greater than or equal to 16 mg per L for resistant *S. aureus*.[132] These changes aimed to increase the sensitivity of the detection of nonsusceptible isolates. It has been debated that the *MIC* creep phenomenon may not be real as it has been reported inconsistently and it may be influenced by the type of microbiologic susceptibility test used [Etest, broth microdilution (BMD), or automated systems] or type of *S. aureus* strain or storage of the isolates or type of patient population evaluated. The reference standard for measuring *MIC* remains BMD. Studies have documented vancomycin *MIC* creep with using BMD and Etest methods, and other studies have documented no vancomycin *MIC* creep when using the same methods.[133,134] A recent meta-analysis that included 55 studies and mean values of vancomycin *MICs* of *S. aureus* isolates documented no evidence of *MIC* creep.[135] Goldman and colleagues evaluated vancomycin MIC creep or heteroresistance in 208 pediatric S. aureus blood isolates using three methods (BMD, Etest, and Vitek2).[136] They reported that vancomycin MICs did not increase nor were heteroresistance identified. Vancomycin MIC results did vary across testing methods, with the standard Etest resulting in a higher value 94% of the time when compared with BMD. No MIC was greater than 2 mg per L by any testing method.[136] This can be problematic, as a falsely elevated vancomycin *MIC* may lead the clinician to utilize another agent besides vancomycin. It is important for clinicians to be aware of the testing method utilized for susceptibility testing and consider *MIC* results based on the method utilized and not deter the utilization of vancomycin. This suggests that vancomycin continues to be the standard option in the treatment of MRSA infections when *MIC* is determined with Etest or BMD methods. Current guidelines from the IDSA for the treatment of MRSA infections recommend that for isolates susceptible to vancomycin (*MIC*, 2 mg per L), "the patient's clinical response should determine the continued use of vancomycin, independent of the *MIC*".[137] Despite these recommendations, the literature describing the association between high vancomycin *MICs* and worsened outcomes may likely influence changes in clinical practice for some practitioners solely on the basis of vancomycin *MIC* results, independently of the patient's clinical status. Perhaps, based on these conflicting results and inconsistency, CLSI categorical breakpoint interpretations (S, I, R) should be reported, and *MIC* values should be suppressed in order to prevent misinterpretation and bias from *MIC* values.

Vancomycin remains active against most *Enterococcus faecalis*, but is bacteriostatic.[21] It has variable activity for *Enterococcus faecium* but is not bactericidal even against susceptible isolates; however, as with other cell wall agents, the addition of an aminoglycoside (if the strain is not highly aminoglycoside resistant) increases the bactericidal activity. All strains of *Streptococcus pneumoniae* and *Streptococcus pyogenes* are susceptible to vancomycin, as are virtually all *Streptococcus agalactiae* and group C and group G streptococci, although rare isolates of streptococci have acquired *vanB* genes typical of vanB type enterococci. Vancomycin also shows good in vitro activity against nutritionally variant streptococci.[128] The MIC_{90} is 4 to 6 mg per L for *S. epidermidis*.[21]

Teicoplanin is active against vancomycin-resistant *S. aureus* and *Enterococcus* species harboring vanB resistance. However, it has as poor activity against *Enterococcus* species harboring vanA.[128]

Telavancin

Telavancin exhibits potent activity against methicillin-susceptible *S. aureus* (MSSA), MRSA, and coagulase-negative *Staphylococcus* (CoNS). It is approximately four times more potent than vancomycin against these organisms and equipotent to dalbavancin and oritavancin.[26–28] Telavancin has been found in vitro to have MIC_{90} values of 0.5, 0.03 to 0.06, and 16 µg per mL against MRSA, streptococci, and VRE, respectively (Table 21.1).[138] A study of a total of 9,610 *S. aureus* clinical isolates collected from 28 U.S. sites were analyzed. MRSA with elevated *MIC* values for vancomycin (2 to 4 µg per mL) or daptomycin (1 to 2 µg per mL) had telavancin MIC_{50} (0.06 µg per mL) values twofold higher than those of isolates with lower *MIC* results (MIC_{50} 0.03 µg per mL). However, telavancin had MIC_{90} and MIC_{100} results of 0.06 and 0.12 µg per mL (100% susceptible), respectively, regardless of the MRSA subset.[139]

Oritavancin

Oritavancin also exhibits excellent in vitro activity against many gram-positive aerobic and anaerobic bacteria. It has excellent activity against *Staphylococcus* species, regardless of susceptibility to vancomycin.[26–28] Despite limited clinical data available, in vitro time–kill studies reveal rapid concentration-dependent bactericidal activity against vancomycin-intermediate *S. aureus* (VISA) (*MIC* = 1 mg per mL), suggesting potential use of oritavancin against these pathogens, even though they are classified as nonsusceptible by CLSI.[140] Not specifically in children, an analysis of activity against 13,262 isolates causing acute bacterial skin and skin structure infections (ABSSSIs), collected between 2010 and 2013, demonstrated its activity against *S. aureus* ($MIC_{50/90}$ 0.03/0.06 mg per L, with 98.8% of all isolates being susceptible) and CoNS (MIC_{50} 0.015 and 0.03 mg per L in isolates from the United States and Europe, respectively). Isolates of *E. faecalis* were all susceptible at less than or equal to 0.5 mg per L, although vancomycin-resistant isolates were 16-fold less susceptible ($MIC_{50/90}$ 0.25/0.5 mg per L) than vancomycin-susceptible isolates ($MIC_{50/90}$ 0.015/0.03 mg per L, with 99.2% to 99.8% susceptible). Higher *MICs* ($MIC_{50/90}$ 0.03/0.12 mg per L) were exhibited by vanA-containing strains of *E. faecium*, while vanB-containing and vancomycin-susceptible strains showed identical *MICs* ($MIC_{50/90}$ 0.004/0.008 mg per L). Strong activity was also seen against *S. pyogenes* ($MIC_{50/90}$ 0.03/0.12 mg per L, with 98.4% to 98.6% susceptible), while activity was slightly lower against *Streptococcus dysgalactiae* ($MIC_{50/90}$ 0.06/0.25 mg per L, with ≥98.3% susceptible).[27]

Dalbavancin

Its activity against gram-positive clinical isolates that cause ABSSSIs has been extensively documented, although mostly in adults.[26–28] The first study, which evaluated its activity against 81,673 global gram-positive isolates collected between 2002 and 2007, revealed its activity against oxacillin-susceptible and oxacillin-resistant strains of *S. aureus* ($MIC_{50/90}$ 0.06/0.06 mg per L for both) and against CoNS ($MIC_{50/90}$ ≤0.03/0.06 mg per L). An analysis of dalbavancin's activity against 1,555 isolates, collected in 2011 in the United States, revealed its activity against both MSSA and MRSA ($MIC_{50/90}$ 0.06/0.06 mg per L for both).[141] An evaluation of its activity against 1,600 gram-positive isolates, collected in the United States in 2012, documented its stable activity over time since the initial evaluations [$MIC_{50/90}$ 0.06/0.06 mg per L against MSSA, MRSA, and CoNS; ≤0.03/≤0.03 mg per L against β-hemolytic streptococci; and ≤0.03/0.06 against viridans group streptococci (VGS)].[142] An analysis of dalbavancin's activity against 8,527 gram-positive isolates responsible for SSSIs in the United States and Europe, collected between 2011 and 2013, revealed $MIC_{50/90}$ values of 0.06/0.06 mg per L against *S. aureus* isolates and less than or equal to 0.03/less than or equal to 0.03 against VGS and β-hemolytic streptococci isolates from both regions.[143] Dalbavancin also has in vitro activity against clinically significant gram-positive organisms, including MSSA, MRSA, CoNS, and *Enterococcus* species. Consistent with telavancin and oritavancin, the *MICs* of dalbavancin are significantly lower than vancomycin, with *S. aureus* MIC_{90} of 0.0 6 mg per mL.[26–28] Dalbavancin has activity against heterogeneous VISA (hVISA) and VISA but poor activity against vancomycin-intermediate *S. aureus* (VRSA).[26–28] It has potent activity against *Enterococcus* species, including isolates harboring vancomycin-resistance genes *vanB* and *vanC*. In contrast, it has poor activity against the vanA phenotype.[26–28]

ADVERSE EVENTS AND DRUG INTERACTIONS WITH GLYCOPEPTIDES AND LIPOGLYCOPEPTIDES

Toxicity related to glycopeptides, mainly vancomycin use, has been the subject of numerous reports. Toxicity can be divided into (1) infusion-related adverse effects and (2) drug-related toxicity. The most frequent problem encountered was the "red man" syndrome, a histamine-mediated rash of the face, neck, upper trunk, back, and arms. This phenomenon, extremely uncommon with teicoplanin, is associated with pruritus, tingling,

TABLE 21.1 In Vitro Activity of Vancomycin, Dalbavancin, and Telavancin Compared to New Antibiotics against MSSA and MRSA

	MSSA	*MRSA*
Antibiotic	*MIC range* (µg/mL)	*MIC range* (µg/mL)
Vancomycin	0.5–1.0	0.5–2.0
Telavancin	0.03–0.06	0.03–0.12
Dalbavancin	0.03–0.06	0.03–0.06

MIC, minimum inhibitory concentration; MRSA, methicillin-resistant *S. aureus*; MSSA, methicillin-sensitive *S. aureus*.
Data from references 167, 169, 183–185.

flushing, tachycardia, and shock and is related to the rate of infusion.[28] It has been described in neonates and children, related to an infusion duration of less than 1 hour, and in 7 of 20 patients with infusion duration of 1 hour or more.[30,38] Three cases of cardiac arrest (two fatal) associated with rapid infusion of vancomycin have been described.[89,144,145]

The incidence of most of these side effects decreased enormously with the removal of impurities from early preparations in the 1960s. Reported drug-related toxicity includes neutropenia, thrombocytopenia, eosinophilia, thrombophlebitis, chills, fever, rash, nephrotoxicity, and ototoxicity. The nephrotoxicity of vancomycin is discussed in detail under vancomycin dosing. Glycopeptide-related hearing loss in infants and children is sporadic, and no clear relation to serum concentrations or patterns of underlying illness can be detected.[146]

Dalbavancin seems to be well tolerated, with most of the adverse events being mild. Studies conducted in adult patients with dalbavancin using an IV two-dose scheme of 1,000 mg on day 1 followed by 500-mg 1 week later or one-time 1,100 mg dose have consistently demonstrated that the drug is well tolerated, no dose-limiting toxicities, or relevant laboratory values alterations.[141] One study in adult patients using a similar dosing strategy reported patients having oral candidiasis, diarrhea, constipation, and fever; however, no patients required discontinuation of the drug.[147] Safety data from phase 2 and 3 studies of dalbavancin in adults revealed that 52% of patients had at least one adverse event, which was comparable to 56.9% in the comparator arms of these studies. Approximately 3.5% of patients in the dalbavancin group discontinued the study medication compared to 3.8% in the comparator arm.[148]

Single dose of dalbavancin seems to be well tolerated in children. No severe or serious adverse events have been related to this agent, including ototoxicity, nephrotoxicity, and hepatotoxicity. Despite lack of reported toxicities, additional data are necessary to confirm dalbavancin safety in pediatric population.[14,15]

It is interesting that anaphylactoid reaction such as flushing, hypotension, and rash, which are commonly seen with other glycopeptides, have not been reported with dalbavancin. It is important to note that dalbavancin has not been widely utilized in children, and maximum tolerated dose of dalbavancin has not been established. Given dalbavancin PK profile of a prolonged half-life, if an adverse event did occur, reversing the adverse event may take an extended period of time. Dalbavancin does not have significant drug–drug interactions as it is not a substrate, inhibitor, or inducer of the cytochrome P450 system.[26–28]

LIPOPEPTIDES: DAPTOMYCIN

CHEMISTRY AND PHARMACOLOGY

Daptomycin, a fermentation product derived from *Streptomyces roseosporus*, is the first member of a novel class of antibiotics called the cyclic lipopeptides and presents an attractive option for the treatment of invasive infections due to gram-positive organisms. The mechanism of daptomycin is calcium dependent because to exert its antimicrobial effect, it must first bind to calcium-forming micelles that enhance its affinity for the bacterial cytoplasmic membrane.[149,150] The daptomycin–calcium complex then inserts deep in to the membrane, causing rapid depolarization of the membrane potential, arrest of DNA and RNA synthesis, and cell death without lysis and release of inflammatory mediators.[150]

Daptomycin is structurally and functionally related to cationic antimicrobial peptides produced by the innate immune system. The daptomycin molecule consists of a cyclic polypeptide core of 13 amino acids, in which 10 C-terminal residues form a ring closed by an ester bond and a three-amino acid exocyclic side chain with a terminal tryptophan attached to a fatty acyl residue (decanoic acid). Several of the amino acid residues that make up daptomycin are nonstandard, including three D-amino acids, ornithine, 3-methyl-glutamic acid, and kynurenine.[151,152]

PHARMACOKINETICS/PHARMACODYNAMICS

Daptomycin is a concentration dependent, bactericidal agent that follows first-order linear PK. In adults, it is 90% protein bound, distributes into the extracellular fluid, and is eliminated renally as intact drug with an average $t_{1/2}$ of about 8 hours. An adult given a dose of 4 to 6 mg per kg IV daily yields the PK parameters that are associated with efficacy: C_{max} 50 to 90 µg per mL and *AUC* 400 to 600 mg·L per h.[153–156] Children have several developmental PK differences compared to adults, including higher total-body water content with an increased extracellular fluid proportion and decreased protein binding. Renal function is impaired at birth, with improvement up to and beyond adult values throughout childhood. Such PK changes would theoretically result in an increased V_d, lower peak concentrations, and more rapid clearance of daptomycin.[153] Several small cases series have been conducted evaluating the PK of daptomycin in newborns to adolescents. PK parameters and corresponding current dosing recommendations from these studies are detailed in Table 21.2.

Pharmacokinetic/Pharmacodynamic Data in Children 2 to 17 Years Old

In 2008, Abdel-Rahman et al. conducted a single-dose PK study in 2- to 17-year-olds receiving daptomycin at a dose of 4 mg per kg daily for proven or suspected gram-positive infections.[156] PK analyses resulted in suboptimal daptomycin *AUC* and C_{max} levels in children less than 12 years of age with appropriate levels in those greater than 12 years of age compared to adults.[156] Abdel-Rahman et al. then conducted a second study specifically in children 2 to 6 years old, stratifying the patient population into two dosing groups: 8 and 10 mg per kg daily.[157] PK parameters achieved in this study were similar to those targeted in adults. Average half-life was between 5 and 7 hours in both studies. Current recommended dosing is detailed in Table 21.2.

Pharmacokinetic/pharmacodynamic Data in Children less than 2 Years Old

Cohen-Wolkowiez et al. conducted a single-dose PK study in children less than 120 days receiving daptomycin at a dose of 6 mg per kg for a suspected systemic infection.[158] *AUC* and C_{max} values were reportedly lower than target adult exposure values. Therefore, young infants appear to require a higher dose requirement similarly to children aged 2 to 6 years to achieve typical adult PK parameters. The second study was performed in children aged 3 to 24 months compared to those 2 to 12

TABLE 21.2 Daptomycin Pharmacokinetic/Pharmacodynamic Data and Dosing Recommendations in Children

Author	*Age, n*	*Daily Dose*	*In-study Evaluations*	*AUC (mg·L/h)*	$t_{1/2}$ *(h)*	*Current Recommended Dosing*
Children 2–17 years old						
Abdel-Rahman et al.[154]	2–17 y, n = 22	4 mg/kg	12–17 y	374	6.7	**>12 y**: 4–6 mg/kg daily
			7–11 y	271[a]	5.6	**6–11 y**: 7 mg/kg daily
			2–6 y	215[a]	5.3	**2–5 y**: 10 mg/kg daily
Abdel-Rahman et al.[157]	2–6 y, n = 12	8 mg/kg, 10 mg/kg	8 mg/kg	429.1	5.4	
			10 mg/kg	549.1	5.7	
Children <2 years old						
Cohen-Wolkowiez et al.[158]	<120 d, n = 20	6 mg/kg	NA	262.4[a]	6.2	**<2 y**: 10 mg/kg daily
Bradley et al.[159]	3–24 mo n = 23	4 mg/kg	2–12 mo	217[a]	NR	**Neonates**: 6 mg/kg q12h
		6 mg/kg	13–24 mo	281[a]	NR	

[a]Suboptimal *AUC* based on the levels of 400–600 mg·L/h normally achieved in adults.
Data from references 154, 157–159.

months old receiving 4 mg per kg and those 13 to 24 months old receiving 6 mg per kg. PK parameters were proportionally higher in the children receiving 6 mg per kg compared to those receiving 4 mg per kg.[159] Average half-life was between 5 and 7 hours in both studies. Three published case reports describing four neonates with gram-positive bacteremia utilized a dosing regimen of 6 mg per kg per dose given every 12 hours and attained PK parameters similar to those associated with efficacy in adults.[160–163]

DRUG INTERACTIONS

Due to the potential for creatinine phosphokinase (CPK) elevations with daptomycin therapy, theoretically, there is a concern for the use of HMG-CoA reductase inhibitors with daptomycin and the development of myopathy. Current experience with concomitant therapy is limited; however, in a study evaluating daptomycin use for *S. aureus* endocarditis, 4 of the 11 patients who experienced CPK elevations were also on an HMG-CoA reductase inhibitor.[164] There have also been reports for daptomycin causing a significant concentration-dependent false elevation of prothrombin time and international normalized ratio. This interaction potential can be reduced by drawing these levels at the time of daptomycin trough concentrations. Lastly, increased daptomycin and decreased tobramycin concentrations have been reported with concomitant use, although this interaction has not been clinically evaluated.[155]

ADVERSE REACTIONS

The limited studies in children report similar side effects in adults. A large retrospective review of hospitalized children during a 9-year period evaluated 1,035 different hospitalizations with a least one administration of daptomycin in 794 children. About half (47.3%) of children were less than 10 years of age. Adverse events were reported in eight children, seven had rhabdomyolysis, and one had pulmonary eosinophilia.[165] In a systematic review of 29 studies performed in children, 10 studies reported no side effects, and 93% of the reported adverse effects were considered unrelated to daptomycin. The most common side effects related to daptomycin included increased liver function tests, headache, phlebitis, and infusion site reactions, with one serious side effect of anaphylaxis reported.[166]

IN VITRO ANTIMICROBIAL ACTIVITY

As a result of its unique mechanism of action in targeting the cell membrane, daptomycin has several advantageous microbiologic characteristics, including efficacy against a majority of gram-positive organisms, including *Staphylococcus* and *Enterococcus* species resistant to vancomycin, linezolid, and quinupristin/dalfopristin; rapid bactericidal activity; and antimicrobial effect at all growth phases of the bacterial cell (Table 21.3).[22,23] Daptomycin has rapid in vitro bactericidal activity against a wide spectrum of gram-positive organisms, including VRE, MRSA, and PCN-resistant streptococci, for which there are very few therapeutic alternatives,[23] and is approved for the treatment of complicated SSSIs caused by susceptible strains of *S. aureus* (both methicillin susceptible and resistant), vancomycin-susceptible *E. faecalis, S. pyogenes, S. agalactiae,* and *S. dysgalactiae.*[23] The bactericidal effect of daptomycin is rapid with more than 99.9% of both MRSA and MSSA bacteria dead in less than 1 hour. Daptomycin also remains bactericidal (99.9% kill within 24 hours) against stationary-phase cultures of both MSSA and MRSA present at high density (10^9 CFU) in a simulated endocardial vegetation model.[167–170]

Despite lacking FDA approval for VRE infections, daptomycin has become a first-line agent to treat severe VRE infections. Although robust clinical evidence for the use of daptomycin for this indication is lacking, its in vitro profile and perceived clinical success has made daptomycin attractive for clinicians.[21,25,50] However, the use of daptomycin for these infections has several caveats, including emergence of resistance during therapy, presence of mutations associated with daptomycin resistance in isolates and optimal daptomycin dosing for VRE infections having not been established, with some in vitro data suggesting that doses of 10 to 12 mg per kg should be used to prevent

TABLE 21.3 In Vitro Activity of Daptomycin against Selected Bacteria

		Daptomycin	
Bacteria	*MIC* range	$MIC_{50/90}$ (μg/mL)	*MIC* range
Staphylococcus Aureus			
MSSA	0.06–1.0	0.25/0.25	0.25
MRSA	<0.06–4.0	0.25/0.5	0.06–2.0
Coagulase-negative *Staphylococcus*			
MS	<0.06–0.5	0.25/1.0	0.06–4.0
MR	<0.06–2.0	0.5/0.5	0.06–2.0
Streptococcus pneumonia			
PCN sens	≤0.015–1.0	–	–
PCN res	0.06–1.0	–	–
CTX res	0.25–1.0	–	–

CTX, ceftriaxone; $MIC_{50/90}$, minimum inhibitory concentration for 50% and 90% of isolates; MR, MRSA, methicillin-resistant; MRSA, methicillin-resistant *S. aureus*; MS, methicillin-sensitive; MSSA, methicillin-sensitive *S. aureus*; PCN, penicillin.
Data from references 180–182.

development of resistance.[171] One limitation to daptomycin use is its interaction with pulmonary surfactant, which inactivates daptomycin and reduces its efficacy in the treatment of alveolar pneumonia.[23] Daptomycin is currently FDA approved in adults for the treatment of complicated skin and soft-tissue infections, *S. aureus* bacteremia, and right-sided endocarditis associated with *S. aureus* bacteremia.

Although daptomycin is active against *S. pneumoniae*, the drug cannot be used to treat pneumonia because it is inactivated by surfactant. Resistance to daptomycin developing during treatment of infections owing to MRSA in patients with endocarditis and osteomyelitis has been well documented in adults.[150,151,167] Many of these patients received prior treatment with vancomycin.[169] The occurrence of vancomycin *MIC* creep can influence susceptibility not only to vancomycin but also to daptomycin.[169,170] Reduced susceptibility to vancomycin in VISA isolates is due to the synthesis of an unusually thickened cell wall containing dipeptides (D-ala-D-ala) capable of binding vancomycin, thereby reducing the availability of the drug for intracellular target molecules.[172,173] The altered cell wall results in a reduced diffusion coefficient of vancomycin and sequestration of vancomycin within the cell wall by these false targets. *S. aureus* strains with higher vancomycin *MICs* also tend to have higher daptomycin *MICs*.[150,171,172] Daptomycin resistance in these strains has been linked to polymorphisms in the *mprF* gene, leading to altered membrane phospholipid profiles and cell wall thickening. Jacobson and colleagues[170] reported on a 15-year-old boy with MRSA bacteremia after sustaining 90% body surface area flame burns, where the MRSA became resistant to daptomycin within 5 days of the initiation of therapy.

The patient had not received prior vancomycin. The daptomycin *MIC*, by Etest, increased from 1 to 4 mg per mL. It was also confirmed as nonsusceptible by BMD, with an *MIC* of 2 mg per mL. The patient was switched to vancomycin, and, although the initial MRSA isolate had a vancomycin *MIC* of 1 mg per mL, the *MIC* on day 5 had increased to 2 mg per mL, also by microdilution.

USE OF DAPTOMYCIN IN CHILDREN

Daptomycin was approved for treatment of ABSSSIs in children aged 1 year and older in March 2017. It has been approved for use in adults since 2003. Safety and effectiveness in pediatric patients below the age of 1 year have not been established. Use of daptomycin in pediatric patients younger than 1 year should be avoided due to the risk of potential effects on muscular, neuromuscular, and/or nervous systems observed in neonatal dogs.[151] Daptomycin is not indicated in pediatric patients with renal impairment because dosage has not been established in these patients.[151] Overall, the safety profile in pediatric patients was similar to that observed in adult patients. There are a number of case reports, retrospective, and prospective phase 1 studies of use of daptomycin in children published since 2008.[165,166,172–178] Conditions included cellulitis and abscesses, bacteremia (MSSA, MRSA, enterococci), catheter-related bloodstream infections (CoNS, *Enterococcus*, MSSA, MRSA), endocarditis (MRSA), osteomyelitis and septic arthritis (MRSA), and ventricular peritoneal shunt infection (vancomycin-intermediate *Staphylococcus haemolyticus*, VRE). Overall response rates in terms of clinical cure and bacterial eradication were excellent. Side effects were also similar to those reported in adults. Elevations of CPK were less than 5%. As of this writing, there is only one published randomized controlled trial in children aged 1 to 17 years for the treatment of ABSSSI, which compared daptomycin to local standard of care for skin and soft-tissue infections.[179] Local standard of care included IV vancomycin, clindamycin, or a semisynthetic PCN. A total of 257 patients received daptomycin and 132 standard of care, which was primarily clindamycin or vancomycin. Thirty-five percent of the patients had confirmed MRSA infection. The overall therapeutic success rate was comparable in both groups: 97% for those patients who were treated with daptomycin compared to 98.7% of those who received standard of care. Use of daptomycin was not associated with increased muscular or neurologic toxicity. There were also no instances of emergence of resistance to daptomycin during therapy, in contrast to the experience with adults.

REFERENCES

1. Spagnolo AM, Panatto OD, Amicizia D. Staphylococcus aureus with reduced susceptibility to vancomycin in healthcare settings. *J Prev Med Hyg* 2014;55:137–144.
2. Howden BP, Davies JK, Johnson PD. Reduced vancomycin susceptibility in Staphylococcus aureus, including vancomycin-intermediate and heterogeneous vancomycin-intermediate strains: resistance mechanisms, laboratory detection, and clinical implications. *Clin Microbiol Rev* 2010;23(1):99–139.
3. Cosgrove SE, Carroll KC, Perl TM. Staphylococcus aureus with reduced susceptibility to vancomycin. *Clin Infect Dis* 2004;39(4):539–545.
4. Kalil AC, Van Schooneveld TC, Fey PD, et al. Association between vancomycin minimum inhibitory concentration and mortality among patients with Staphylococcus aureus bloodstream infections: a systematic review and meta-analysis. *JAMA* 2014;312:1552–1564.
5. Murray KP, Zhao JJ, Davis SL, et al. Early use of daptomycin versus vancomycin for methicillin-resistant Staphylococcus aureus bacteremia with vancomycin minimum inhibitory concentration >1 mg/L: a matched cohort study. *Clin Infect Dis* 2013;56:1562–1569.
6. Wong-Beringer A, Joo J, Tse E, et al. Vancomycin-associated nephrotoxicity: a critical appraisal of risk with high-dose therapy. *Int. J. Antimicrob Agents* 2011;37:95–101.
7. Van Hal SJ, Paterson DL, Lodise TP. Systematic review and meta-analysis of vancomycin-induced nephrotoxicity associated with dosing schedules that maintain troughs between 15 and 20 milligrams per liter. *Antimicrob Agents Chemother* 2013;57:734–744.
8. Filippone EJ, Kraft WK, Farber JL. The nephrotoxicity of vancomycin. *Clin Pharmacol Ther* 2017;102(3):459–469.
9. Gomes DM, Smotherman C, Birch A, et al. Comparison of acute kidney injury during treatment with vancomycin in combination with piperacillin-tazobactam or cefepime. *Pharmacotherapy* 2014;4:662–669.
10. Moenster RP, Linneman TW, Finnegan PM, et al. Acute renal failure associated with vancomycin and β–lactams for the treatment of osteomyelitis in diabetics: piperacillin-tazobactam as compared with cefepime. *Clin Microbiol Infect* 2014;20:O384–O388.
11. Hammond DA Smith MN, Painter JT, et al. Comparative incidence of acute kidney injury in critically ill patients receiving vancomycin with concomitant piperacillin-tazobactam or cefepime: a retrospective cohort study. *Pharmacotherapy* 2016;36:463–471.
12. Giuliano C, Patel CR, Kale-Pradhan PB. Is the combination of piperacillin-tazobactam and vancomycin associated with development of acute kidney injury? a meta-analysis. *Pharmacotherapy* 2016;36(12):1217–1228. doi:10.1002/phar.1851.
13. ClinicalTrials.gov. *An open-label study of the pharmacokinetics of a single dose of telavancin in pediatric subjects aged 3 months to 17 years.* Bethesda, MD: National Library of Medicine, 2013, https://clinicaltrials.gov/
14. Bradley JS, Puttagunta S, Rubino CM, et al. Pharmacokinetics, safety and tolerability of single dose dalbavancin in children 12–17 years of age. *Pediatr Infect Dis J* 2015;34(7):748–752.
15. Gonzalez D, Bradley JS, Blumer J, et al. Dalbavancin pharmacokinetics and safety in children 3 months to 11 years of age. *Pediatr Infect Dis J* 2017;36(7):645–653.
16. Bradly JS, Arrieta A, Loutit JS. Pharmacokinetics (PK) of oritavancin in children: the ORKIDS trial. *Open Forum Infect Dis* 2018;5(Suppl 1):S52.
17. Barna JC, Williams DH. The structure and mode of action of glycopeptide antibiotics of the vancomycin group. *Annu Rev Microbiol* 1984;38:339–357.
18. Perkins HR, Nieto M. The chemical basis for the action of the vancomycin group of antibiotics. *Ann NY Acad Sci* 1974;235:348–363.
19. Reynolds PE. Structure, biochemistry and mechanism of action of glycopeptide antibiotics. *Eur J Clin Microbiol Infect Dis* 1989;8(11):943–950.
20. Pfeiffer RR. Structural features of vancomycin. *Rev Infect Dis* 1981;3(Suppl):S205–S209.
21. Fekety R. Vancomycin, teicoplanin and the streptogramins: quinupristin and dalfopristin. In: Mandell GL, Bennet JE, Dolin R, eds. *Mandell, Douglas, and Bennett's principles & practice of infectious diseases*, 5th ed. Philadelphia, PA: Churchill Livingstone, 2000:382–392.
22. Geraci JE, Heilman FR, Nichols DR. Antibiotic therapy of bacterial endocarditis. Vancomycin for acute micrococcal endocarditis. *Proc Staff Meet Mayo Clin* 1958;33:172–181.
23. Sando M, Sato Y, Iwata S, et al. In vitro protein binding of teicoplanin to neonatal serum. *J Infect Chemother* 2004;10(5):280–283.
24. Barg NL, Supena RB, Fekety R. Persistent staphylococcal bacteremia in an intravenous drug abuser. *Antimicrob Agents Chemother* 1986;29(2):209–211.
25. Tounian P, Jehl F, Pauliat S, et al. Stability and compatibility of teicoplanin in parenteral nutrition solutions used in pediatrics. *Clin Nutr* 1999;18(3):159–165.
26. Guskey MT, Tsuji BT. A comparative review of lipoglycopeptides: oritavancin, dalbavancin, and telavancin. *Pharmacotherapy* 2010;30(1):80–94. doi:10.1592/phco.30.1.80.
27. Zhanel GG, Calic D, Schweizer F, et al. New lipoglycopeptides: a comparative review of dalbavancin, oritavancin and telavancin. *Drugs* 2010;70(7):859–886. doi:10.2165/11534440-000000000-00000.
28. Klinker KP, Borgert SJ. Beyond vancomycin: the tail of the lipoglycopeptides. *Clin Ther* 2015;37(12):2619–2636. doi:10.1016/j.clinthera.2015.11.007.
29. Matzke GR, Zhanel GG, Guay DR. Clinical pharmacokinetics of vancomycin. *Clin Pharmacokinet* 1986;11(4):257–282.
30. Schaad UB, McCracken GH Jr, Nelson JD. Clinical pharmacology and efficacy of vancomycin in pediatric patients. *J Pediatr* 1980;96(1):119–126.
31. Seay RE, Brundage RC, Jensen PD, et al. Population pharmacokinetics of vancomycin in neonates. *Clin Pharmacol Ther* 1994;56(2):169–175.
32. Burstein AH, Gal P, Forrest A. Evaluation of a sparse sampling strategy for determining vancomycin pharmacokinetics in preterm neonates: application of optimal sampling theory. *Ann Pharmacother* 1997;31(9):980–983.
33. Schaible DH, Rocci ML Jr, Alpert GA, et al. Vancomycin pharmacokinetics in infants: relationships to indices of maturation. *Pediatr Infect Dis* 1986;5(3):304–308.
34. Moller JC, Nelskamp I, Jensen R, et al. Teicoplanin pharmacology in prophylaxis for coagulase-negative staphylococcal sepsis of very low birthweight infants. *Acta Paediatr* 1996;85(5):638–639.
35. Rodvold KA, Everett JA, Pryka RD, et al. Pharmacokinetics and administration regimens of vancomycin in neonates, infants and children. *Clin Pharmacokinet* 1997;33(1):32–51.
36. Lundstrom TS, Sobel JD. Antibiotics for gram-positive bacterial infections. Vancomycin, teicoplanin, quinupristin/dalfopristin, and linezolid. *Infect Dis Clin North Am* 2000;14(2):463–474.
37. McGee SM, Kaplan SL, Mason EO Jr. Ventricular fluid concentrations of vancomycin in children after intravenous and intraventricular administration. *Pediatr Infect Dis J* 1990;9(2):138–139.
38. Odio C, Mohs E, Sklar FH, et al. Adverse reactions to vancomycin used as prophylaxis for CSF shunt procedures. *Am J Dis Child* 1984;138(1):17–19.
39. Reiter PD, Doron MW. Vancomycin cerebrospinal fluid concentrations after intravenous administration in premature infants. *J Perinatol* 1996;16(5):331–335.
40. Schaad UB, Nelson JD, McCracken GH Jr. Pharmacology and efficacy of vancomycin for staphylococcal infections in children. *Rev Infect Dis* 1981;3(Suppl):S282–S288.
41. Reed MD, Kliegman RM, Weiner JS, et al. The clinical pharmacology of vancomycin in seriously ill preterm infants. *Pediatr Res* 1987;22(3):360–363.
42. Guay DR, Vance-Bryan K, Gilliland S, et al. Comparison of vancomycin pharmacokinetics in hospitalized elderly and young patients using a Bayesian forecaster. *J Clin Pharmacol* 1993;33(10):918–922.
43. Le Normand Y, Milpied N, Kergueris MF, et al. Pharmacokinetic parameters of vancomycin for therapeutic regimens in neutropenic adult patients. *Int J Biomed Comput* 1994;36(1–2):121–125.
44. Pou L, Rosell M, Lopez R, et al. Changes in vancomycin pharmacokinetics during treatment. *Ther Drug Monit* 1996;18(2):149–153.
45. Rodvold KA, Blum RA, Fischer JH, et al. Vancomycin pharmacokinetics in patients with various degrees of renal function. *Antimicrob Agents Chemother* 1988;32(6):848–852.
46. de Hoog M, Schoemaker RC, Mouton JW, et al. Vancomycin population pharmacokinetics in neonates. *Clin Pharmacol Ther* 2000;67(4):360–367.
47. Fofah OO, Karmen A, Piscitelli J, et al. Failure of prediction of peak serum vancomycin concentrations from trough values in neonates. *Pediatr Infect Dis J* 1999;18(3):299–300.
48. Gous AG, Dance MD, Lipman J, et al. Changes in vancomycin pharmacokinetics in critically ill infants. *Anaesth Intensive Care* 1995;23(6):678–682.
49. Gross JR, Kaplan SL, Kramer WG, et al. Vancomycin pharmacokinetics in premature infants. *Pediatr Pharmacol (New York)* 1985;5(1):17–22.
50. Jarrett RV, Marinkovich GA, Gayle EL, et al. Individualized pharmacokinetic profiles to compute vancomycin dosage and dosing interval in preterm infants. *Pediatr Infect Dis J* 1993; 12(2):156–157.
51. Kildoo CW, Lin LM, Gabriel MH, et al. Vancomycin pharmacokinetics in infants: relationship to postconceptional age and serum creatinine. *Dev Pharmacol Ther* 1989;14(2):77–83.
52. Lisby-Sutch SM, Nahata MC. Dosage guidelines for the use of vancomycin based on its pharmacokinetics in infants. *Eur J Clin Pharmacol* 1988;35(6):637–642.
53. Naqvi SH, Keenan WJ, Reichley RM, et al. Vancomycin pharmacokinetics in small, seriously ill infants. *Am J Dis Child* 1986;140(2):107–110.
54. Tarral E, Jehl F, Tarral A, et al. Pharmacokinetics of teicoplanin in children. *J Antimicrob Chemother* 1988;21(Suppl A):47–51.
55. Echeverria P, Siber GR, Paisley J, et al. Age-dependent dose response to gentamicin. *J Pediatr* 1975;87(5):805–808.
56. Spivey JM, Gal P. Vancomycin pharmacokinetics in neonates. *Am J Dis Child* 1986;140(9):859.
57. James A, Koren G, Milliken J, et al. Vancomycin pharmacokinetic and dose recommendations for preterm infants. *Antimicrob Agents Chemother* 1987;31(1):52–54.
58. Leonard MB, Koren G, Stevenson DK, et al. Vancomycin pharmacokinetics in very low birth weight neonates. *Pediatr Infect Dis J* 1989;8(5):282–286.
59. Rodvold KA, Gentry CA, Plank GS, et al. Bayesian forecasting of serum vancomycin concentrations in neonates and infants. *Ther Drug Monit* 1995;17(3):239–246.
60. Silva R, Reis E, Bispo MA, et al. The kinetic profile of vancomycin in neonates. *J Pharm Pharmacol* 1998;50(11):1255–1260.
61. Grimsley C, Thomson AH. Pharmacokinetics and dose requirements of vancomycin in neonates. *Arch Dis Child Fetal Neonatal Ed* 1999;81(3):F221–F227.
62. Kimura T, Sunakawa K, Matsuura N, et al. Population pharmacokinetics of arbekacin, vancomycin, and panipenem in neonates. *Antimicrob Agents Chemother* 2004;48(4):1159–1167.
63. Capparelli EV, Lane JR, Romanowski GL, et al. The influences of renal function and maturation on vancomycin elimination in newborns and infants. *J Clin Pharmacol* 2001;41(9):927–934.
64. Cantu TG, Yamanaka-Yuen NA, Lietman PS. Serum vancomycin concentrations: reappraisal of their clinical value. *Clin Infect Dis* 1994;18(4):533–543.
65. Goebel J, Ananth M, Lewy JE. Hemodiafiltration for vancomycin overdose in a neonate with end-stage renal failure. *Pediatr Nephrol* 1999;13(5):423–425.
66. Miranda JC, Schimmel MM, James LS, et al. Gentamicin kinetics in the neonate. *Pediatr Pharmacol (New York)* 1985;5(1):57–61.
67. van den Anker JN. Pharmacokinetics and renal function in preterm infants. *Acta Paediatr* 1996;85:1393–1399.
68. Leake RD, Trygstad CW, Oh W. Inulin clearance in the newborn infant: relationship to gestational and postnatal age. *Pediatr Res* 1976;10(8):759–762.
69. van den Anker JN, de Groot R, Broerse HM, et al. Assessment of glomerular filtration rate in preterm infants by serum creatinine: comparison with inulin clearance. *Pediatrics* 1995;96(6):1156–1158.
70. Bueva A, Guignard JP. Renal function in preterm neonates. *Pediatr Res* 1994;36:572–577.
71. van den Anker JN, Hop WC, de Groot R, et al. Effects of prenatal exposure to betamethasone and indomethacin on the glomerular filtration rate in the preterm infant. *Pediatr Res* 1994;36(5):578–581.
72. Bidiwala KS, Lorenz JM, Kleinman LI. Renal function correlates of postnatal diuresis in preterm infants. *Pediatrics* 1988;82:50–58.
73. McDougal A, Ling EW, Levine M. Vancomycin pharmacokinetics and dosing in premature neonates. *Ther Drug Monit* 1995;17(4):319–326.
74. Asbury WH, Darsey EH, Rose WB, et al. Vancomycin pharmacokinetics in neonates and infants: a retrospective evaluation. *Ann Pharmacother* 1993;27(4):490–496.
75. van den Anker JN, Hop WC, Schoemaker RC, et al. Ceftazidime pharmacokinetics in preterm infants: effect of postnatal age and postnatal exposure to indomethacin. *Br J Clin Pharmacol* 1995;40(5):439–443.

76. Gleason CA. Prostaglandins and the developing kidney. *Semin Perinatol* 1987;11(1): 12–21.
77. Guignard JP, Gouyon JB. Adverse effects of drugs on the immature kidney. *Biol Neonate* 1988;53(4):243–252.
78. Gal P, Gilman JT. Drug disposition in neonates with patent ductus arteriosus. *Ann Pharmacother* 1993;27(11):1383–1388.
79. Anderson BJ, Allegaert K, Van den Anker JN, et al. Vancomycin pharmacokinetics in preterm neonates and the prediction of adult clearance. *Br J Clin Pharmacol* 2007;63(1):75–84.
80. Mulla H, Pooboni S. Population pharmacokinetics of vancomycin in patients receiving extracorporeal membrane oxygenation. *Br J Clin Pharmacol* 2005;60(3):265–275.
81. Amaker RD, DiPiro JT, Bhatia J. Pharmacokinetics of vancomycin in critically ill infants undergoing extracorporeal membrane oxygenation. *Antimicrob Agents Chemother* 1996;40(5):1139–1142.
82. Buck ML. Vancomycin pharmacokinetics in neonates receiving extracorporeal membrane oxygenation. *Pharmacotherapy* 1998;18(5):1082–1086.
83. Hoie EB, Swigart SA, Leuschen MP, et al. Vancomycin pharmacokinetics in infants undergoing extracorporeal membrane oxygenation. *Clin Pharm* 1990;9(9):711–715.
84. Sanchez A, Lopez-Herce J, Cueto E, et al. Teicoplanin pharmacokinetics in critically ill paediatric patients. *J Antimicrob Chemother* 1999;44(3):407–409.
85. Wrishko RE, Levine M, Khoo D, et al. Vancomycin pharmacokinetic and Bayesian estimation in pediatric patients. *Ther Drug Monit* 2000;22(5):522–531.
86. Lukas JC, Karikas G, Gazouli M, et al. Pharmacokinetics of teicoplanin in an ICU population of children and infants. *Pharm Res* 2004;21(11):2064–2071.
87. Schaefer F, Klaus G, Muller-Wiefel DE, et al. Intermittent versus continuous intraperitoneal glycopeptide/ceftazidime treatment in children with peritoneal dialysis-associated peritonitis. The Mid-European Pediatric Peritoneal Dialysis Study Group (MEPPS). *J Am Soc Nephrol* 1999;10(1):136–145.
88. Blowey DL, Warady BA, Abdel-Rahman S, et al. Vancomycin disposition following intraperitoneal administration in children receiving peritoneal dialysis. *Perit Dial Int* 2007;27(1):79–85.
89. Spears RL, Koch R. The use of vancomycin in pediatrics. *Antibiot Annu* 1959–1960;7:798–803.
90. Klugman KP, Friedland IR, Bradley JS. Bactericidal activity against cephalosporin-resistant Streptococcus pneumoniae in cerebrospinal fluid of children with acute bacterial meningitis. *Antimicrob Agents Chemother* 1995;39(9):1988–1992.
91. Fan-Havard P, Nahata MC, Bartkowski MH, et al. Pharmacokinetics and cerebrospinal fluid (CSF) concentrations of vancomycin in pediatric patients undergoing CSF shunt placement. *Chemotherapy* 1990;36(2):103–108.
92. Jorgenson L, Reiter PD, Freeman JE, et al. Vancomycin disposition and penetration into ventricular fluid of the central nervous system following intravenous therapy in patients with cerebrospinal devices. *Pediatr Neurosurg* 2007;43(6):449–455.
93. Jacobs F, Deleluse F, Raftopoulos C, et al. Intraventricular vancomycin in CSF shunt infections. *Neurosurgery* 1987;21(1):112–113.
94. Losonsky GA, Wolf A, Schwalbe RS, et al. Successful treatment of meningitis due to multiply resistant Enterococcus faecium with a combination of intrathecal teicoplanin and intravenous antimicrobial agents. *Clin Infect Dis* 1994;19(1):163–165.
95. Pau AK, Smego RA Jr, Fisher MA. Intraventricular vancomycin observations of tolerance and pharmacokinetics in two infants with ventricular shunt infections. *Pediatr Infect Dis* 1986;5(1):93–96.
96. Bafeltowska JJ, Buszman E, Mandat KM, et al. Therapeutic vancomycin monitoring in children with hydrocephalus during treatment of shunt infections. *Surg Neurol* 2004;62(2):142–150; discussion 150.
97. Dagan R, Einhorn M, Howard C, et al. Outpatient and inpatient teicoplanin treatment for serious Gram-positive infections in children. *Pediatr Infect Dis J* 1993;12(6):S17–S20.
98. Shime N, Kato Y, Kosaka T, et al. Glycopeptide pharmacokinetics in current paediatric cardiac surgery practice. *Eur J Cardiothorac Surg* 2007;32(4):577–581.
99. Reed MD, Yamashita TS, Myers CM, et al. The pharmacokinetics of teicoplanin in infants and children. *J Antimicrob Chemother* 1997;39(6):789–796.
100. Terragna A, Ferrea G, Loy A, et al. Pharmacokinetics of teicoplanin in pediatric patients. *Antimicrob Agents Chemother* 1988;32(8):1223–1226.
101. Chang D. Influence of malignancy on the pharmacokinetics of vancomycin in infants and children. *Pediatr Infect Dis J* 1995;14(8):667–673.
102. Krivoy N, Peleg S, Postovsky S, et al. Pharmacokinetic analysis of vancomycin in steady state in pediatric cancer patients. *Pediatr Hematol Oncol* 1998;15(4):333–338.
103. Hatzopoulos FK, Stile-Calligaro IL, Rodvold KA, et al. Pharmacokinetics of intravenous vancomycin in pediatric cardiopulmonary bypass surgery. *Pediatr Infect Dis J* 1993;12(4):300–304.
104. Dagan O, Klein J, Gruenwald C, et al. Preliminary studies of the effects of extracorporeal membrane oxygenator on the disposition of common pediatric drugs. *Ther Drug Monit* 1993;15(4):263–266.
105. Rybak M, Lomaestro B, Rotschafer JC, et al. Therapeutic monitoring of vancomycin in adult patients: a consensus review of the American Society of Health-System Pharmacists, the Infectious Diseases Society of America, and the Society of Infectious Diseases Pharmacists. *Am J Health-Syst Pharm* 2009;66:82–98.
106. Frymoyer A, Hersh AL, Benet LZ, et al. Current recommended dosing of vancomycin for children with invasive methicillin-resistant Staphylococcus aureus infections is inadequate. *Pediatr Infect Dis J* 2009;28(5):398–402.
107. Liu C, Bayer A, Cosgrove SE, et al. Clinical practice guidelines by the Infectious Diseases Society of America for the treatment of methicillin-resistant Staphylococcus aureus infections in adults and children. *Clin Infect Dis* 2011;52:e18–e55.
108. Hsu AJ, Hamdy RF, Huang Y, et al. Vancomycin trough concentrations and duration of methicillin-resistant Staphylococcus aureus bacteremia in children. *J Pediatr Infect Dis Soc* 2018;7(4):338–341. doi:10.1093/jpids/pix068.
109. Le J, Bradley JS, Murray W. Improved vancomycin dosing in children using area-under-the-curve exposure. *Pediatr Infect Dis J* 2013;32(4):e155–e163.
110. Hoang J, Dersch-Mills D, Bresee L. Achieving therapeutic vancomycin levels in pediatric patients. *Can J Hosp Pharm* 2014;67(6):416–422.
111. Benner KW, Worthington MA, Kimberlin DW, et al. Correlation of vancomycin dosing to serum concentrations in pediatric patients: a retrospective database review. *J Pediatr Pharmacol Ther* 2009;14(2):86–93.
112. Glover ML, Cole E, Wolfsdorf J. Vancomycin dosage requirements among pediatric intensive care unit patients with normal renal function. *J Crit Care* 2000;15(1):1–4.
113. Frymoyer A, Hersh AL, Coralic Z, et al. Prediction of vancomycin pharmacodynamics in children with invasive methicillin-resistant Staphylococcus aureus infections: a Monte Carlo simulation. *Clin Ther* 2010;32(3):534–542.
114. Geerlof LM, Boucher J. Evaluation of vancomycin dosing and corresponding drug concentrations in pediatric patients. *Hosp Pediatr* 2014;4;342. doi:10.1542/hpeds.2014-0019.
115. Durham SH, Simmons ML, Mulherin DW, et al. An evaluation of vancomycin dosing for complicated infections in pediatric patients. *Hosp Pediatr* 2015;5;276. doi:10.1542/hpeds.2014-0081.
116. Frymoyer A, Guglielmo BJ, Hersh AL. Desired vancomycin trough serum concentration for treating invasive methicillin-resistant Staphylococcal infections. *Pediatr Infect Dis J* 2013;32(10):1077–1079.
117. Hwang D, Chang-Nan C, Chang L, et al. Vancomycin dosing and target attainment in children. *J Microbiol Immunol Infect* 2017;50(4):494–499.
118. Chhim RF, Arnold SR, Lee KR. Vancomycin dosing practices, trough concentrations, and predicted area under the curve in children with suspected invasive staphylococcal infections. *J Pediatr Infect Dis Soc* 2013;2(3):259–262.
119. Silva Alves GC, Dutra da Silva S, Ftade VP, et al. Determining the optimal vancomycin daily dose for pediatrics: a meta-analysis. *Eur J Clin Pharmacol* 2017;73(11):1341–1353.
120. David MZ, Daum RS. Community-associated methicillin-resistant Staphylococcus aureus: epidemiology and clinical consequences of an emerging epidemic. *Clin Microbiol Rev* 2010;23(3):616–687.
121. Hale CM, Seabury RW, Steele JM, et al. Are vancomycin trough concentrations of 15 to 20 mg/L associated with increased attainment of an AUC/MIC ≥400 in patients with presumed MRSA infection? *J Pharm Pract* 2017;30(3):329–335. doi:10.1177/0897190016642692.
122. Kishk OA, Lardieri AB, Heil EL, et al. Vancomycin AUC/MIC and corresponding troughs in a pediatric population. *J Pediatr Pharmacol Ther* 2017;22(1):41–47.
123. Fiorito TM, Luther MK, Dennehy PH, et al. Nephrotoxicity with vancomycin in the pediatric population: a systematic review and meta-analysis. *Pediatr Infect Dis J* 2018;37(7):654–661.
124. Turner RB, Kojiro K, Shephard EA, et al. Review and validation of Bayesian dose-optimizing software and equations for calculation of vancomycin area under the curve in critically ill patients. *Pharmacotherapy* 2018;38(12):1174–1183.
125. Carrothers TJ, Chittenden JT, Critchley I. Dalbavancin population pharmacokinetic modeling and target attainment analysis. *Clin Pharmacol Drug Dev* 2020;9(1):21–31.
126. Andes D, Craig W. In vivo pharmacodynamic activity of the glycopeptide dalbavancin. *Antimicrob Agents Chemother* 2007;51(5):1633–1642. doi:10.1128/AAC.01264-06.
127. Ambrose P, Drusano GL, Craig WA. In vivo activity of oritavancin in animal infection models and rationale for a new dosing regimen in humans. *Clin Infect Dis* 2012;54(Suppl 3): S220–S228. doi:10.1093/cid/cis001.
128. Butler MS, Hansford KA, Blaskovich MA. Glycopeptide antibiotics: back to the future. *J Antibiot* 2014;67:631–644.
129. van Hal SJ, Lodise TP, Paterson DL. The clinical significance of vancomycin minimum inhibitory concentration in Staphylococcus aureus infections: a systematic review and meta-analysis. *Clin Infect Dis* 2012;54:755–771.
130. Song KH, Kim M, Kim JC. Impact of vancomycin MIC on treatment outcomes in invasive Staphylococcus aureus infections. *Antimicrob Agents Chemother* 2017;61(3):e01845–16.
131. Soriano A, Marco F, Martinez JA, et al. Influence of vancomycin minimum inhibitory concentration on the treatment of methicillin-resistant Staphylococcus aureus bacteremia. *Clin Infect Dis* 2008;46:193–200.
132. Clinical and Laboratory Standards Institute (CLSI). *Performance standards for antimicrobial susceptibility testing*, 26th ed. Wayne, PA: CLSI supplement M100S. CLSI, 2016.
133. Kehrmann J, Kaase M, Szabados F, et al. Vancomycin MIC creep in MRSA blood culture isolates from Germany: a regional problem? *Eur J Clin Microbiol Infect Dis* 2011;30:677–683
134. Jones RN. Microbiological features of vancomycin in the 21st century: minimum inhibitory concentration creep, bactericidal/static activity, and applied breakpoints to predict clinical outcomes or detect resistant strains. *Clin Infect Dis* 2006;42(Suppl 1):S13–S24.
135. Hawser SP, Bouchillon SK, Hoban DJ. Rising incidence of Staphylococcus aureus with reduced susceptibility to vancomycin and susceptibility to antibiotics: a global analysis 2004–2009. *Int J Antimicrob Agents* 2011;37:219–224.
136. Goldman JL, Harrison CJ, Myers AL, et al. No evidence of vancomycin minimal inhibitory concentration creep or heteroresistance identified in pediatric Staphylococcus aureus blood isolates. *Pediatr Infect Dis J* 2014;33(2):216–218.
137. Edwards B, Milne K, Lawes T. Is vancomycin MIC "creep" method dependent? Analysis of methicillin-resistant Staphylococcus aureus susceptibility trends in blood isolates from North East Scotland from 2006 to 2010. *J Clin Microbiol* 2012;50(2):318–325.
138. Vibativ, telavancin for injection package insert. South San Francisco, CA: Theravance Biopharma US, Inc., 2014.
139. Mendes RE, helio SS, Flamm RK. Telavancin in vitro activity against a collection of methicillin-resistant Staphylococcus aureus isolates, including resistant subsets, from the United States. *Antimicrob Agents Chemother* 2015;59(3):1811–1814.
140. Saravolatz LD, Stein GE. Oritavancin: a long-half-life lipoglycopeptide. *Clin Infect Dis* 2015;61(4):627–632.
141. Dalvance, dalbavancin for injection package insert. Chicago, IL: Durata Therapeutics US Ltd., 2018.

142. Biedenbach DJ, Bell JM, Sader HS, et al. Activities of dalbavancin against a worldwide collection of 81,673 Gram-positive bacterial isolates. *Antimicrob Agents Chemother* 2009;53(3):1260–1263.
143. McCurdy SP, Jones RN, Mendes RE, et al. In vitro activity of dalbavancin against drug-resistant Staphylococcus aureus isolates from a global surveillance program. *Antimicrob Agents Chemother* 2015;59(8):5007–5009.
144. Best CJ, Ewart M, Sumner E. Perioperative complications following the use of vancomycin in children: a report of two cases. *Br J Anaesth* 1989;62(5):576–577.
145. Boussemart T, Cardona J, Berthier M, et al. Cardiac arrest associated with vancomycin in a neonate. *Arch Dis Child Fetal Neonatal Ed* 1995;73(2):F123.
146. Brummett RE. Ototoxicity of vancomycin and analogues. *Otolaryngol Clin North Am* 1993;26(5):821–828.
147. Boucher HW, Wilcox M, Talbot GH, et al. Once-weekly dalbavancin versus daily conventional therapy for skin infection. *N Engl J Med* 2014;370(23):2169–2179.
148. Dunne MW, Puttagunta S, Giordano P, et al. A randomized clinical trial of single-dose versus weekly dalbavancin for treatment of acute bacterial skin and skin structure infection. *Clin Infect Dis* 2016;62(5):545–551
149. Hancock RE. Mechanisms of action of newer antibiotics for Gram-positive pathogens. *Lancet Infect Dis* 2005;5(4):209–218.
150. Miller WR, Bayer AS, Arias CA, et al. Mechanism of action and resistance to daptomycin in Staphylococcus aureus and Enterococci. *Cold Spring Harb Perspect Med* 2016;6:a026997.
151. Cubicin, daptomycin for injection package insert. Whitehouse Station, NJ: Merck and Co, Inc., 2017.
152. Durand C, Brueckner A, Sampadian C, et al. Daptomycin use in pediatric patients. *Am J Health Syst Pharm* 2014;71(14):1177–1182.
153. Principi N, Caironi M, Venturini F, et al. Daptomycin in paediatrics: current knowledge and the need for future research. *J Antimicrob Chemother* 2015;70(3):643–648.
154. Abdel-Rahman SM, Benziger DP, Jacobs RF, et al. Single-dose pharmacokinetics of daptomycin in children with suspected or proved gram-positive infections. *Pediatr Infect Dis J* 2008;27(4):330–334.
155. Daptomycin for injection. *Full prescribing reference. Monograph: Cubicin.* Lexington, MA: Cubist Pharmaceuticals, 2011.
156. Arbeit RD, Maki D, Tally FP, et al. The safety and efficacy of daptomycin for the treatment of complicated skin and skin-structure infections. *Clin Infect Dis* 2004;38(12):1673–1681.
157. Abdel-Rahman SM, Chandorkar G, Akins RL, et al. Single-dose pharmacokinetics and tolerability of daptomycin 8 to 10 mg/kg in children aged 2 to 6 years with suspected or proved gram-positive infections. *Pediatr Infect Dis J* 2011;30(8):712–714.
158. Cohen-Wolkowiez M, Watt KM, Hornik CP, et al. Pharmacokinetics and tolerability of single-dose daptomycin in young infants. *Pediatr Infect Dis J* 2012;31(9):935–937.
159. Bradley JS, Benziger D, Bokesch P, et al. Single-dose pharmacokinetics of daptomycin in pediatric patients 3–24 months of age. *Pediatr Infect Dis J* 2014;33(9):936–939.
160. Sarafidis K, Iosifidis E, Gikas E, et al. Daptomycin use in a neonate: serum level monitoring and outcome. *Am J Perinatol* 2010;27(5):421–424.
161. Cohen-Wolkowiez M, Smith PB, Benjamin DK Jr, et al. Daptomycin use in infants: report of two cases with peak and trough drug concentrations. *J Perinatol* 2008;28(3):233–234.
162. Gawronski KM. Successful use of daptomycin in a preterm neonate with persistent methicillin-resistant Staphylococcus epidermidis bacteremia. *J Pediatr Pharmacol Ther* 2015;20(1):61–65.
163. Bradley JS, Nelson JD, Barnett E, et al. *Nelson's pediatric antimicrobial therapy*, 22nd ed. American Academy of Pediatrics, 2016.
164. Fowler VG Jr, Boucher HW, Corey GR, et al. Daptomycin versus standard therapy for bacteremia and endocarditis caused by Staphylococcus aureus. *N Engl J Med* 2006;355(7):653–665.
165. Larru B, Cowden CL, Zaoutis TE, et al. Daptomycin use in United States children's hospitals. *J Pediatric Infect Dis Soc* 2015;4(1):60–62.
166. Karageorgos SA, Miligkos M, Dakoutrou M, et al. Clinical effectiveness, safety profile, and pharmacokinetics of daptomycin in pediatric patients: a systematic review. *J Pediatric Infect Dis Soc* 2016;5(4):446–457.
167. Huband MD, Castanheira M, Farrell DJ, et al. In vitro activity of dalbavancin against multidrug-resistant Staphylococcus aureus and streptococci from patients with documented infections in Europe and surrounding regions (2011–2013). *Int J Antimicrob Agents* 2016;47:495–499.
168. Gonzalez-Ruiz A, Seaton RA, Hamed K. Daptomycin: an evidence-based review of its role in the treatment of gram-positive infections. *Infect Drug Resist* 2016;9:47–58.
169. Atkas G, Derbentli S. In vitro activity of daptomycin combined with dalbavancin and linezolid and dalbavancin with linezolid against MRSA strains. *J Antimicrob Chemother* 2017;72:441–443.
170. Jacobson LM, Milstone AM, Zenilman J, et al. Daptomycin therapy failure in an adolescent with methicillin-resistant Staphylococcus aureus bacteremia. *Pediatr Infect Dis J* 2009;28(5):445–447.
171. Smith JR, Claeys K, Ryback M. High dose daptomycin therapy for staphylococcal endocarditis and when to apply it. *Curr Infect Dis Rep* 2014;16(10):429. doi:10.1007/s11908-014-0429-6.
172. Sakoulas G, Alder J, Thauvin-Eliopoulos C, et al. Induction of daptomycin heterogeneous susceptibility in *Staphylococcus aureus* by exposure to vancomycin. *Antimicrob Agents Chemother* 2006, 50:1581–1585.
173. Sieradzki K, Tomasz A. Alterations of cell wall structure and metabolism accompany reduced susceptibility to vancomycin in an isogenic series of clinical isolates of Staphylococcus aureus. *J Bacteriol* 2003;185:7103–7110.
174. Namtu KC, Crain JC, Messina AF, et al. Clinical experience with daptomycin in pediatrics. *Pharmacotherapy* 2017;3(1):105–108.
175. Tedeschi S, Tumietto F, Conti M, et al. Use of daptomycin in critically ill children with bloodstream infections and complicated skin and soft-tissue infections. *Pediatr Infect Dis J* 2016;35(2):180–182.
176. Syriopoulou V, Dailiana Z, Dmitriy N, et al. Clinical experience with daptomycin for the treatment of Gram-positive infections in children and adolescents. *Pediatr Infect Dis J* 2016;35(5):511–516.
177. Garazzino S, Castagnola E, Di Gangi M, et al. Daptomycin for children in clinical practice experience. *Pediatr Infect Dis J* 2016;35(6):639–641.
178. Ardura MI, Mejías A, Katz KS, et al. Daptomycin therapy for invasive Gram-positive bacterial infections in children. *Pediatr Infect Dis J* 2007;26(12):1128–1132.
179. Bradley J, Glasser C, Patino H, et al. Daptomycin for complicated skin infections: a randomized trial. *Pediatrics* 2017;139(3):e20162477.
180. Pfaller MA, Mendes RE, Castanheira M, et al. Ceftaroline activity tested against bacterial isolates causing community-acquired respiratory tract infections and skin and skin structure infections in pediatric patients from United States Hospitals: 2012–2014. *Pediatr Infect Dis J* 2017;36(5):486–490.
181. Rolston KVI, Jamal MA, Nesher L, et al. In vitro activity of ceftaroline and comparator agents against Gram-positive and Gram-negative clinical isolates from cancer patients. *Int J Antimicrob Agents* 2017;49:416–421.
182. Zhang H, Xiao M, Kon F, et al. A multicentre study of methicillin-resistant Staphylococcus aureus in acute bacterial skin and skin structure infections in China: susceptibility to ceftaroline and molecular epidemiology. *Int J Antimicrob Agents* 2015;45:347–350.
183. Malabarba A, Goldstein BP. Origin, structure, and activity in vitro and in vivo of dalbavancin. *J Antimicrob Chemother* 2005;55:ii15–ii20.
184. Sweeny D, Shinabarger DL, Arhin FF, et al. Comparative in vitro activity of oritavancin and other agents against methicillin-susceptible and methicillin-resistant Staphylococcus aureus. *Diagn Microbiol Infect Dis* 2017;87:121–128.
185. Jones RN, Flamm RK, Castanheira M, et al. Activity of telavancin against Gram-positive pathogens isolated from bone and joint infections in North American, Latin American, European and Asia-Pacific nations. *Diagn Microbiol Infect Dis* 2017;88(2):184–187.

CHAPTER

22

Karel Allegaert
Anne Smits
Johannes N. van den Anker

Aminoglycosides

GENERAL ASPECTS OF AMINOGLYCOSIDES

Aminoglycosides have played a major role in antimicrobial therapy since their discovery in the 1940s.[1] Their bactericidal efficacy in Gram-negative infections, synergism with β-lactam antibiotics, limited bacterial resistance, and low costs have given these agents a firm place in current antimicrobial treatment regimens. However, streptomycin (1944), gentamicin (1963), tobramycin (1967), amikacin (1972), and netilmicin (1976) prescriptions have been complicated by nephrotoxicity and ototoxicity in a significant number of patients.

STRUCTURE AND CHEMICAL PROPERTIES

Aminoglycosides are amino-modified glycosides (molecular weight 445 to 600 Da), further divided into chemical families with related structures. Aminoglycosides are water soluble, are cationic at normal pH, distribute in plasma water with minimal protein binding, and have a stable structure over a wide range of temperature and pH.[2,3] The relation between the structure and activity of aminoglycosides is not fully understood.

Aminoglycosides—as cations—bind passively but rapidly to the negatively charged parts of phospholipids and other proteins in the bacterial cell membrane with subsequent cytosol uptake.[4] This cytosol uptake is likely in part passive (porin), in part energy-consuming. This uptake process relates to the aminoglycoside (peak) concentration and can be inhibited by low pH, anaerobic conditions, or hyperosmolarity. This explains the concentration-dependent bacterial killing effect of aminoglycosides. The synergism with β-lactam antibiotics is in part explained by the increased permeability of the bacterial cell membrane (β-lactam target).[5,6] Aminoglycosides subsequently act by disturbing and inhibiting protein synthesis (Fig. 22.1). Once in the cytosol, aminoglycosides interact with the 30S ribosomal subunit, resulting in inaccurate messenger RNA (mRNA) translation (like misreading, premature termination) and subsequent disturbed protein synthesis (quantity or quality). The disturbed protein synthesis disrupts the normal homeostasis in the bacterial cell and alters the bacterial cell membrane integrity, resulting in synergism with β-lactams.[7,8] Protein synthesis interference plays a major part in bacterial cell death, but is likely not the only mechanism for the bactericidal effect. The disruptive mechanism of protein synthesis interference also explains the "postantibiotic" effect (PAE) of aminoglycosides. PAE is hereby defined as persistent suppression of bacterial (re)growth following short exposure (a few hours) to an antibiotic of bacteria, even in the absence of host defense–related mechanisms.

ANTIMICROBIAL ACTIVITY

Aminoglycosides have a concentration-dependent bactericidal spectrum encompassing aerobic and Gram-negative bacteria like Enterobacteriaceae, *Escherichia coli*, *Pseudomonas* species, and *Haemophilus* species. The susceptibility of most Gram-negative bacteria to gentamicin, tobramycin, netilmicin, and amikacin is relatively similar when the compound-specific efficacy/toxicity balance is considered.[9] The amikacin susceptibility is three- to fourfold less, compensated by its lower toxicity and, therefore, higher allowable dose. Gentamicin and tobramycin are comparable in activity, although tobramycin is slightly more active against *Pseudomonas aeruginosa*. They are susceptible to the same modifying enzymes, and resistance rates are, therefore, very similar. In contrast, amikacin is resistant to many of these enzymes and, therefore, is often an alternative if strains are resistant to tobramycin or gentamicin. Netilmicin susceptibility is comparable to that of gentamicin and tobramycin, although netilmicin is resistant to some of the gentamicin-inactivating enzymes and thus, in some cases, is a good alternative.

The antimicrobial activity of aminoglycosides has four distinct and clinically important aspects: (a) *concentration-dependent killing*, (b) a PAE, (c) *adaptive resistance*, and (d) *synergism with other antibiotics*. The aminoglycoside-induced rate of bacterial killing as well as induction of resistance is peak concentration dependent.[10–13] Other in vitro investigations, mimicking in vivo fluctuations of drug concentrations, have shown a single bolus of aminoglycoside to be superior in rate and total amount of bacterial killing to the same dose in a multiple daily dosing (MDD) regimen in non-neutropenic animals.[13–15]

Aminoglycosides have a PAE, meaning that there is suppression of bacterial growth for several hours after antibiotic serum concentrations have dropped below the minimal inhibitory concentration (*MIC*).[13,16,17] There are discrepancies between in vivo and in vitro studies on this effect, and studies have indicated that PAE is partly determined by diminished regrowth of bacteria at sub-*MICs*.[13,16] The clinical relevance of

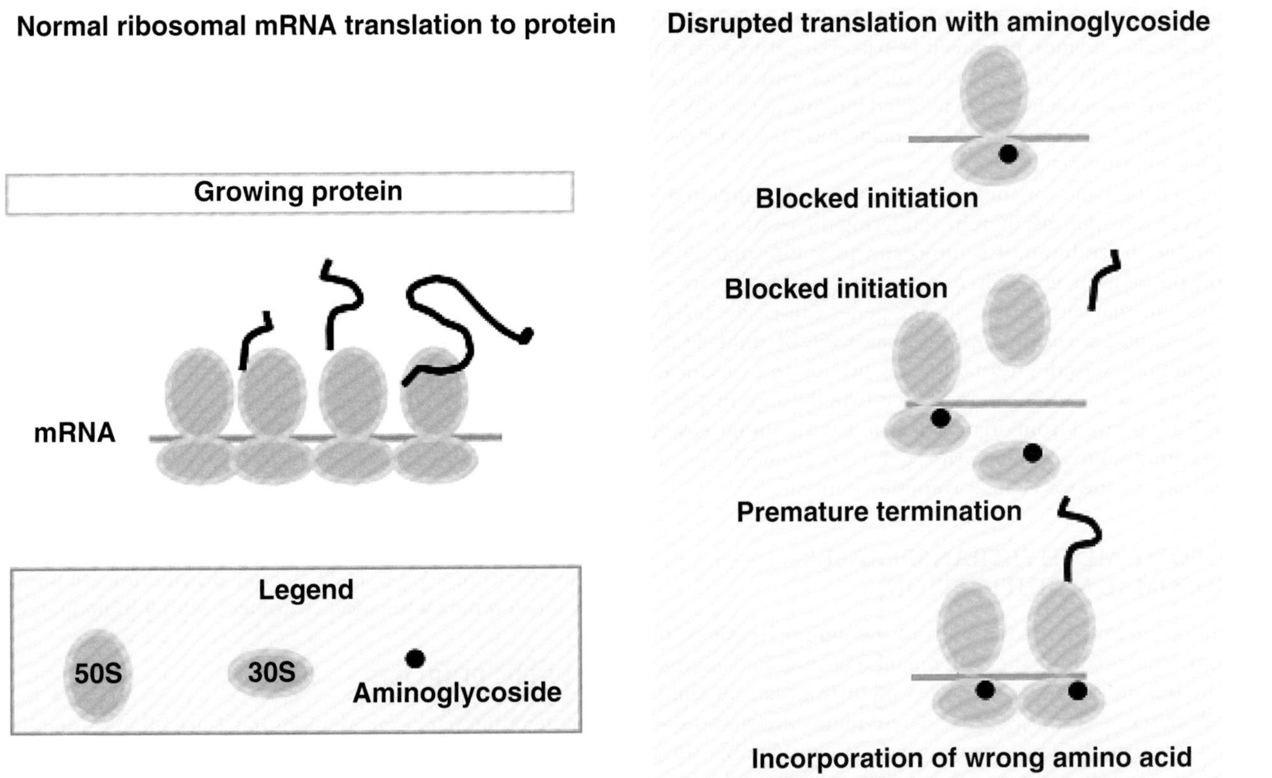

Figure 22.1 Mechanisms of interference with normal ribosomal messenger RNA (mRNA) translation to proteins by aminoglycosides. Following binding to the 30S ribosome subunit, disrupted translation relates to either blocked initiation (no protein), premature termination (too short protein), or incorporation of the wrong amino acid (dysfunction of the protein).

the PAE is unclear, and the emphasis on this effect in discussions on extended-interval dosing of aminoglycosides—even more relevant in (pre)term neonates—is questionable. Synergy of aminoglycosides with other cell-wall–active antibiotics, such as penicillins and cephalosporins, has been established.[18] This synergy is the basis of the clinical choice for combination therapy of aminoglycosides with penicillins or cephalosporins. Their concentration-dependent killing, the PAE, and adaptive resistance, combined with the mechanisms related to toxicity, constitute the rationale for the shift to extended-interval dosing of aminoglycosides.

DRUG RESISTANCE AND SUSCEPTIBILITY

With the exception of *P. aeruginosa* and *Enterococcus* spp., the incidence of aminoglycoside resistance remains low. Resistance occurs by three different mechanisms: (a) ribosomal resistance, (b) decreased uptake and accumulation, or (c) enzymatic modification. Ribosomal resistance is the result of mutations at the ribosomal aminoglycoside–binding site. This ribosomal resistance mechanism will not be further discussed because it is only clinically relevant for streptomycin. In contrast, the growing clinical importance is resistance caused by ribosome methyltransferases (ribosomal modification).[19]

DECREASED UPTAKE AND ACCUMULATION

The bacterial cell wall serves as a natural barrier for small molecules, such as aminoglycosides, and may be further fortified via acquired mutation. Decreased drug uptake or enhanced efflux is a clinically significant aspect of aminoglycoside resistance. This covers both alteration of the outermost lipopolysaccharides (altered negative charge) or downregulation of porins (*decreased uptake*), as well as active transport efflux (*enhanced efflux*) pumps.[19] The underlying mechanism, though probably related to membrane impermeability by cell membrane modification, is not really known.[19] The mechanism is likely chromosomally mediated and results in cross-reactivity to all aminoglycosides. The level of observed resistance is moderate, consequently resulting in intermediate susceptibility.[19,20]

In part related to decreased uptake and accumulation, another important phenomenon in aerobic Gram-negative bacteria is *adaptive resistance*, defined as a reduced antimicrobial killing in originally susceptible bacterial populations after initial incubation with an aminoglycoside.[13,21] It has clinical relevance especially for immunocompromised patients and in serious infections with Gram-negative bacteria. Adaptive resistance is probably related to membrane protein changes and altered expression of regulatory genes of the anaerobic respiratory pathway.[22] It is a pharmacodynamic process characterized by reversible refractoriness to bactericidal action as demonstrated by in vitro and in vivo studies and can be overcome by higher peak serum concentrations of aminoglycosides, which underscores the need for extended-interval dosing.

ENZYMATIC MODIFICATION

Enzymatic modification is the most common type of aminoglycoside resistance, and over 50 different enzymes have been identified.[19] By far, the most widespread mechanism of aminoglycoside resistance is the inactivation of these antibiotics by aminoglycoside-modifying enzymes, produced by bacterial pathogens. This will result in modification of aminoglycosides with subsequent loss of antimicrobial activity due to failed binding at the 30S bacterial ribosomal–binding site.[18] Enzymatic modifications result in high-level resistance.

The genetic code for these enzymes is largely contained in plasmids or transposons, thereby rendering the resistance easily transferable. In addition, it is important to realize that all susceptible positions in aminoglycosides can be modified by several enzymes and that several inactivating genes can easily develop from a common ancestor, implying that it will be unlikely that making aminoglycosides resistant to inactivation by a specific enzyme will be a worthwhile effort.[19,20] It is hypothesized that these enzymes are derived from organisms that make aminoglycosides (initial natural source = *Streptomyces* genus) or from genetic mutations that encode for cellular respiratory enzymes.

RIBOSOME METHYLTRANSFERASES (RIBOSOMAL MODIFICATION)

Instead of enzymatic modification of the aminoglycosides, the aminoglycoside-binding site itself may also be modified enzymatically by 16S ribosomal RNA (rRNA) methyltransferases (initial natural source = *Actinomycetes*).[19] These methyltransferases are located in plasmids. This mechanism is of considerable threat because it results in resistance to clinically relevant aminoglycosides, including amikacin.

Resistance patterns are difficult to predict without advance microbiology laboratory methods. Clinical integration of such methods is relevant when selecting aminoglycosides for either empiric use (gentamicin or tobramycin vs. "semi"-synthetic derivatives like netilmicin or amikacin) or targeted, culture, and susceptibility-driven (antibiogram) pharmacotherapy.

INDICATIONS

Aminoglycosides are used to treat many Gram-negative and some Gram-positive infections and, importantly, multidrug-resistant tuberculosis. At present, aminoglycosides are mainly used for treating serious Gram-negative infections caused by enteric bacilli. Aminoglycosides are synergistic with cephalosporins and penicillins in the setting of Gram-negative infections and are thus often combined with these cell-wall–active antibiotics.[18] They are also used in combination treatment with vancomycin for *Staphylococcus aureus* (both methicillin-sensitive and methicillin-resistant strains), *Staphylococcus epidermidis,* and enterococcal infections.[23,24] In case of empiric treatment with aminoglycosides, local susceptibility patterns have to be taken into account. There are many indications for use of aminoglycosides, but we focus on three conditions: neonatal sepsis, pulmonary infectious exacerbations in cystic fibrosis (CF), and urinary tract infections.

NEONATAL SEPSIS

Among major pathogens responsible for bacterial infections during the first month of life, Gram-negative bacteria like *E. coli, Klebsiella* species, *Enterobacter* species, *Citrobacter* species, and *Pseudomonas* species play an increasing important role, possibly related to the increased prenatal administration of antibiotics and use of percutaneous central venous catheters in the neonatal intensive care unit (NICU).[25–27] Aminoglycosides are effective against most nosocomial-acquired Gram-negative infections in term and preterm infants and are synergistic with β-lactam antibiotics in treating group B streptococcal and coagulase-negative staphylococcal infections. They play an important role in the initial empiric treatment of neonatal septicemia.[25–27] Initial treatment combining amoxicillin (or penicillin in setting where *Listeria* is very rare) with gentamicin (or any other aminoglycoside) may be more effective than a combination with cefotaxime.[28] In general, emergence of aminoglycoside-resistant strains other than coagulase-negative streptococci is relatively slow, which is a definite advantage over third-generation cephalosporins.[29] Consequently, aminoglycosides are among the most common antibiotics used in the neonatal period. In the most recent Pediatrix list (U.S. background) of the 100 most commonly prescribed drugs in the NICU, gentamicin (2nd), tobramycin (15th), and amikacin (48th) are present.[30] However, as aminoglycosides are water soluble (distribution, C_{max}) and are subsequently cleared by glomerular filtration (renal, C_{trough}), this results in a CATCH-22 [higher distribution volume (V_d) + reduced renal elimination clearance] setting in neonates.[26]

CYSTIC FIBROSIS

Acute pulmonary exacerbations in CF are often caused by pseudomonal microorganisms.[31] Standard treatment consists of a combination of an aminoglycoside with a β-lactam antibiotic (e.g., ticarcillin) or a quinolone antibiotic and leads to a longer clinical remission than the use of a β-lactam alone.[31] Sequential intravenous/oral ciprofloxacin monotherapy offers a safe and efficacious alternative.[32] Higher doses, up to 9 mg per kg per day of tobramycin, are needed because of a higher aminoglycoside clearance in patients with CF.[33–35] The safety and efficacy of aerosolized tobramycin maintenance therapy for patients with CF colonized with *P. aeruginosa* has been suggested, but meta-analytical evidence remains limited.[36] Dose advice for inhaled tobramycin is 300 mg twice daily for a period of 28 days.[36] Systemic bioavailability is approximately 12%, and monitoring serum concentrations in patients with renal failure is indicated.[37] Once-daily dosing (ODD) compared to three times daily dosing in pediatric patients with CF is less nephrotoxic.[38]

URINARY TRACT INFECTIONS

Aminoglycosides are excreted by glomerular filtration and are partly actively reabsorbed at the level of the renal tubulus, leading to both high parenchymal and urine concentrations. This makes these drugs useful in treating cystitis and pyelonephritis. Even a single dose results in a prolonged time interval of adequate concentrations in urine for uncomplicated cystitis.[39,40] ODD of aminoglycosides is effective in treating urinary tract infections in children, but there is accumulated evidence that oral antibiotic for 10 to 14 days is as effective.[41]

PHARMACOKINETICS

Aminoglycosides display a pharmacokinetic (PK) profile of rapid distribution ($t_{1/2\alpha}$), with a subsequent elimination phase ($t_{1/2\beta}$) and a second much slower elimination phase ($t_{1/2\gamma}$). This γ phase can only be determined after discontinuation of the drug. Anyhow, the observed PK profile obviously also depends on the sampling

TABLE 22.1 Results of Pharmacokinetic Studies of Aminoglycosides in Neonates

Aminoglycoside (Reference)	*N*	*GA (wk)*	*PNA (d)*	*Weight (g)*	*CL (mL/min/kg)*	V_d *(L/kg)*	$t_{1/2}$ *(h)*
Amikacin (44)	32	32 ± 3.6		1,740 ± 810	1.08 ± 0.51	0.655 ± 0.414	7.6 ± 4.4
Amikacin (45)	28	30.5 ± 2.86		1,380 ± 170	0.83 ± 0.28	0.57 ± 0.11	8.4
Amikacin (45)	6	32–40	1–3	1,500–3,400	1.05 ± 0.30	0.70 ± 0.27	2
	5	36–40	5–8	2,100–3,600	1.08 ± 0.42	0.49 ± 0.11	5.6
	11	32–38	>8	1,900–4,600	1.78 ± 0.53	0.73 ± 0.13	5.1
Amikacin (43)	43	25–41	1–29	865–3,860	1.50[a] ± 8.6[b]	1.07[c] ± 5.9[b]	
Gentamicin (46)	19		1	<1,500	0.75 ± 0.60	0.72 ± 0.45	13
	18		1	≥1,500	0.97 ± 0.23	0.78 ± 0.39	13.8
	20		4	<1,500	0.50 ± 0.18	0.60 ± 0.26	10.9
	28		4	≥1,500	0.72 ± 0.10	0.50 ± 0.18	8.1
Gentamicin (47)	15	<33	<7	<1,500	0.38 ± 0.15	0.53 ± 0.10	11.1
	15	<33	8–30	<1,500	0.45 ± 0.17	0.50 ± 0.11	10.8
	6	<33	>31	<1,500	1.18 ± 0.45	0.50 ± 0.11	4.4
Gentamicin (48)	12		1.8	<1,000	0.52 ± 0.08	0.35 ± 0.07	7.9
	36		1.8	≥1,000	0.65 ± 0.13	0.38 ± 0.13	6.5
	20	≤30	1.8		0.58 ± 0.12		7.4
	28	>30	1.8		0.63 ± 0.13		6.5
Gentamicin (49)	11	28–33	2–30		1.00	0.597	6.53
		35–38	2–30		1.22	0.538	4.95
	55	39–43	2–30		1.15	0.542	5.17
Gentamicin (50)	216	32.39 ± 2.83	?	1,850 ± 670	0.75 ± 0.25	0.54 ± 0.13	8.98 ± 2.86
	106 (PDA)	29.02 ± 2.92	?	1,160 ± 530	0.67 ± 0.28	0.61 ± 0.15	12.24 ± 7.43
Gentamicin (51)	24 (PDA)	?	<1,500	0.93 ± 0.33	0.64 ± 0.20	8.49 ± 2.69	
	16		?	<1,500	0.83 ± 0.4	0.41 ± 0.08	6.23 ± 1.92
Gentamicin (52)	11	26–33	1–10				13
	6	34–40	1–10				6
Gentamicin (53)							
Control	16	30.6 ± 0.86	<12 h	1,600 ± 154		0.57 ± 0.03	10.2 ± 0.89
Loading	18	29.2 ± 0.81	<12 h	1,294 ± 145		0.58 ± 0.02	12.0 ± 0.84
Gentamicin (54)	10 ECMO	36–43	<7		2.78 ± 1.55	0.51 ± 0.11	9.55 ± 4.38
Gentamicin (55)	113	>34 + AS5 ≥ 7	0–50	500–4,500	0.88	0.47	
		≤34 + AS5 < 7			0.73		
		≤34 + AS5 ≥ 7			0.6		
Gentamicin (56)	165	37 ± 4.5	7.8 ± 11.7	2,432 ± 952		0.64 ± 0.22	8.2 ± 4.8
Gentamicin (57)	15	<37	0–2		1.03 ± 0.37		
	27	≥37	0–2		1.40 ± 0.47		
	8	<37	3–7		1.78 ± 0.63		
	16	≥37	3–7		1.78 ± 0.38		
	1	<37	8–28		1.67		
	14	≥37	8–28		1.97 ± 0.43		

(continued)

TABLE 22.1 Results of Pharmacokinetic Studies of Aminoglycosides in Neonates (*continued*)

Aminoglycoside (Reference)	*N*	*GA (wk)*	*PNA (d)*	*Weight (g)*	*CL (mL/min/kg)*	V_d *(L/kg)*	$t_{1/2}$ *(h)*
Gentamicin (58)	79	27–40	3–7	920–3,550	0.7 (0.68–0.72)[d]	0.47 (0.43–0.52)	8 (7.7–8.3)[d]
Netilmicin (59)	22	27–40	<16	800–3,400	1.07 ± 0.28	0.34 ± 0.11	9.6
Netilmicin (60)	12	28–33	<28	770–2,050	0.83 ± 0.27	0.63 ± 0.24	8.6
Netilmicin (61)	16		<7	<2,000		0.609	4.7
3 mg/kg	8		≥7	<2,000		0.599	4.1
	9		<7	>2,000		0.472	3.4
	23		<7	>2,000		0.617	4.4
4 mg/kg	4		≥7	>2,000		0.510	3.8
Tobramycin (62)	19	29–40	2–4	1,000–3,555	1.15 (0.70–1.83)	0.82 (0.54–1.76)	8.6 (3.5–14.1)
	8		4–7	1,000–3,555	1.14 (0.62–1.56)	0.68 (0.40–1.06)	7.1 (4.6–11.6)
			2–4	1,000–1,500	1.09 (0.74–1.15)	1.04 (0.64–1.36)	11.1 (6.6–14.1)
			4–7	1,000–1,500	1.02 (0.62–1.55)	0.73 (0.46–1.06)	8.7 (5.7–11.6)
Tobramycin (63)	9	28–30	2–6		1.04 ± 0.22	0.84 ± 0.31	9.3 ± 2.8
	11	30–34	2–6		1.13 ± 0.35	0.81 ± 0.20	8.9 ± 3.0
	6	34–40	2–6		1.28 ± 0.31	0.61 ± 0.14	5.6 ± 1.2
	7		2–6	1,000–1,250	1.05 ± 0.20	1.02 ± 0.27	11.3 ± 3.0
	6		2–6	1,260–1,500	1.12 ± 0.39	0.74 ± 0.16	8.2 ± 2.0
	7		2–6	1,500–2,000	1.10 ± 0.32	0.69 ±0.16	7.5 ± 1.6
	6		2–6	2,100–3,500	1.28 ± 0.31	0.61 ± 0.14	5.6 ± 1.2
Tobramycin (64)	8	24–30	3–5	<1,000	0.69 ± 0.10	0.59 ± 0.10	9.9 ± 1.5

[a]mL/min.
[b]Standard error of estimate.
[c]L.
[d]95% confidence interval.
AS5, 5′ Apgar score; *CL*, total body clearance; ECMO, extracorporeal membrane oxygenation; GA, gestational age; *N*, number of patients in study; PDA, patent ductus arteriosus; PNA, postnatal age; $t_{1/2}$, serum half-life; V_d, volume of distribution; ?, data unknown/unavailable/not reported.

strategy taken. Distribution half-life is 5 to 10 minutes in adults but has never been measured in newborns. The γ phase in infants is long. Netilmicin was detectable in blood and urine 11 and 14 days after discontinuation, with a $t_{1/2\gamma}$ of 62.4 hours, while the tissue half-life in renal cortical tissue is 4 to 5 days.[42] There is only limited penetration in the cerebrospinal fluid compartment.[43] In general, the serum concentrations and PK data determined in most studies are derived from the elimination phase, adequately described by a one-compartment model. There are, however, some studies that have shown a two-compartment model to be superior in predicting serum $t_{1/2\beta}$ and serum concentrations, but this largely depends on the sampling strategy taken (Tables 22.1 and 22.2).

Because aminoglycosides are distributed over extracellular water, there are age-related changes in V_d related to the maturational proportional decrease in extracellular water with age (see Tables 22.1 and 22.2), further affected by morbidity or disease-related changes such as edema, hydrops fetalis, extracorporeal membrane oxygenation (ECMO), or dehydration. This results in the highest V_d (L per kg) in extreme preterm neonates (see Tables 22.1 and 22.2). Since subsequent elimination is exclusively driven by glomerular filtration, clearance will also display maturational changes with the lowest clearance in these extreme preterm neonates (see Tables 22.1 and 22.2). Similarly, aminoglycoside clearance will be further affected by morbidity or disease-related glomerular filtration rate (GFR) changes such as coadministration of ibuprofen or indomethacin, whole-body hypothermia to treat perinatal asphyxia, and renal impairment or failure, but also disease-related hyperfiltration, like in intensive care or in children with CF, cancer, or burns.[33–35,73–75]

PHARMACOKINETICS IN NEONATES

Since aminoglycosides are frequently prescribed in neonates[30] and therapeutic drug monitoring (TDM) is commonly performed, there is a wealth of retrospective studies, combining these TDM data with clinical characteristics in population PK models.[73,76–78] Many studies in neonates have been performed; however, only larger or specific studies are reported in this chapter. In essence, the elimination half-life ($t_{1/2\beta}$) of aminoglycosides is prolonged in neonates, reflecting both an *increased* V_d and *decreased CL* in this population. Table 22.1 illustrates the patterns and relevant PK covariates in neonates.[43–64]

Distribution Volume

The V_d of aminoglycosides is larger in neonates, most pronounced in preterm neonates, primarily due to their higher percentage of extracellular water.[26,79] As presented in Table 22.1, this is reflected in aminoglycoside V_d. There is a consistently higher V_d for preterm infants, especially in the group with very low birth weight (VLBW) or gestational age (GA) less than 30 weeks. Most authors have found birth weight (BW) to be the best predictor of V_d, although some have found V_d to be independent of GA. V_d of gentamicin ranges from 0.70 L per kg in neonates of a GA less than 32 weeks to 0.32 L per kg in children aged 11 to 18 years.[50,80,81] Similar, amikacin V_d at birth was significantly higher [0.7, standard deviation [*SD*] 0.15 vs. 0.52, *SD* 0.02 L per kg) in preterm infants with a GA less than 28 weeks when compared to term neonates.[79] Nonmaturational covariates of V_d described in neonates are the use of ECMO[82] and the presence of a patent ductus arteriosus[50,51] and sepsis.[81]

Clearance

Aminoglycoside clearance reflects glomerular filtration[83] and, therefore, is associated with GA, weight, and/or postnatal age (PNA).[76,77] This maturational pattern of changes in *CL* has been shown for amikacin, gentamicin, netilmicin, and tobramycin. This and other studies suggest that, though there is a relation, serum creatinine in the first week of life cannot be accurately used to predict aminoglycoside clearance.[73]

Clinically relevant nonmaturational covariates of aminoglycoside *CL* are whole-body hypothermia following perinatal asphyxia,[84,85] co-exposure to ibuprofen[86,87] or indomethacin,[88] and ECMO.[82] Prenatal exposure to corticosteroids ("maternal lung maturation") commonly administered when delivery is imminent up to 34 weeks potentially affect renal clearance, but this could not be confirmed to be a relevant covariate of amikacin clearance[89,90] (see Table 22.1).

Using population PK modeling approaches, substantial effort has been put into developing equations, since this holds the promise to result in better prediction (*targeted, individualized therapy*) of serum concentrations in individual neonates.[76,77] In practice, these equations can only in part explain the observed variability and subsequent serum concentrations in an individual patient.[77,87] This predictability is in part also depending on the PNA.[91] The extensive variability in amikacin clearance is illustrated in Figure 22.2.[91] The clinical relevance of these findings (V_d, clearance, covariates, limited explained variability) is further discussed in the subsection on therapeutic drug monitoring.

PHARMACOKINETICS IN INFANTS AND CHILDREN

The earlier described (patho)physiologic covariates of aminoglycoside PK in neonates (extracellular water and GFR) will also drive the aminoglycoside PK in infants and children. Table 22.2 presents the patterns and relevant PK covariates in infants and children, covering both maturational and disease-related covariates. Figure 22.3 shows that V_d (for amikacin) decreases with increasing PNA, while clearance increases with advancing PNA over the first 2 years of life.[92] Changes in both V_d (see Tables 22.1 and 22.2) and clearance are most pronounced in the first 2 years of life. V_d decreases by one-third when comparing patients either younger or older than 3 months of age.[93] A concomitant increase in peak serum concentrations with age is seen. Similarly, the increase in clearance will result in lower trough concentrations. It is questionable whether maturational changes are of clinical relevance for dose or dose-interval adaptations in pediatric patients beyond the first 2 years of life.

Besides the maturational (age or weight driven) changes, nonmaturational covariates also affect aminoglycoside PK. A relation between GFR and aminoglycoside clearance in pediatric patients has been established, and aminoglycoside dosing has to be adjusted according to GFR, commonly reflected in the creatinine clearance.[94] Consequently, renal impairment will affect clearance, but it is important to realize that the hyperdynamic status during disease may also result in increased clearance. Both V_d and aminoglycoside clearance are increased in patients with CF, necessitating larger doses in this patient group.[33–35] Similar patterns with increased clearance (+55%) and a higher V_d (+17%) were described for children with burns compared to neutropenic children treated for cancer when exposed to amikacin.[75] This reflects the concept and relevance of glomerular hyperfiltration in children.[74]

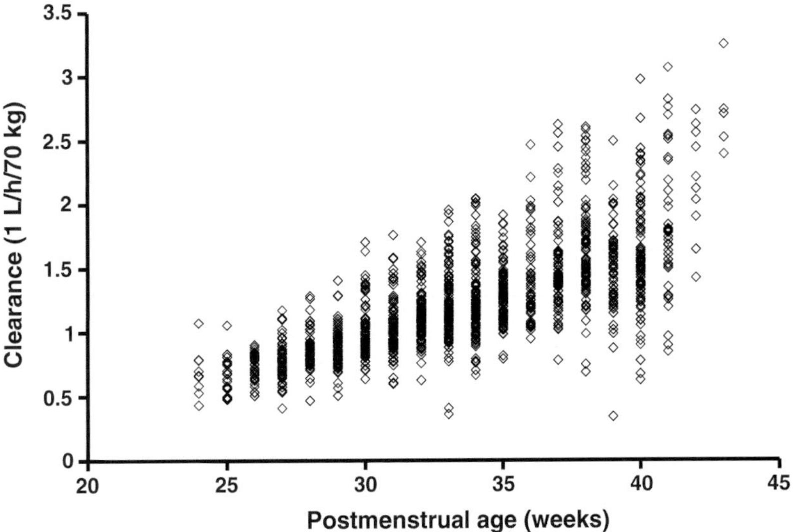

Figure 22.2 Amikacin clearance as estimated in 715 neonates (24 to 43 weeks; weight 0.385 to 4.780 kg), based on 1.862 amikacin time–concentration points, illustrates the extensive variability in amikacin clearance on postmenstrual age. (Data from Allegaert K, Scheers I, Cossey V, et al. Covariates of amikacin clearance in neonates: the impact of postnatal age on predictability. *Drug Metab Lett* 2008;2(4):286–289.)

TABLE 22.2 Results of Pharmacokinetic Studies of Aminoglycosides in Infants and Children

Aminoglycoside (Reference)	*Patient Group*	*N*	*Age*	*CL (mL/min/kg)*	*V_d (L/kg)*	*$t_{1/2}$ (h)*
Amikacin (65)			<3 y		0.40 ± 0.07	
Amikacin (66)	PICU patients	13	6.8 y			2.02 ± 0.64
Amikacin (67)		30	6–12 mo	1.13 (0.3–2.15)	0.50 (0.22–0.73)[a]	2.86 (0.63–6.28)
Amikacin (68)		30	<6 mo	1.05 (0.6–1.8)	0.58 (0.32–0.98)	5.02 (1.46–11.89)
Tobramycin (68)		19	2–8 y	123.5 ± 10.2[b]	0.49 ± 0.06	2 ± 0.17
Tobramycin (68)		22	11–18 y	195.0 ± 16[b]	0.40 ± 0.04	1.4 ± 0.10
Gentamicin (69)		44	2.2 ± 3.5 y	2.05 ± 068	0.424 ± 0.116	2.6 ± 1.0
Gentamicin (70)		8	0.5–4 y		0.43 ± 0.02	0.31 ± 0.01[c]
(ODD)						
		11	5–10 y		0.35 ± 0.01	0.37 ± 0.01
		12	11–18 y		0.32 ± 0.01	0.37 ± 0.01
Gentamicin/tobramycin (71)	Bone marrow transplants	33	9 mo–15 y	1.71 ± 0.53	0.32 ± 0.07	2.32 ± 0.65
Amikacin (72)	Normal renal function	8	3–11 y	3.0 ± 1.25	0.208 ± 0.11	1.19 ± 0.19

CL, total body clearance; ODD, once-daily dosing; PICU, pediatric intensive care unit; $t_{1/2}$, serum half-life; V_d, volume of distribution.
[a]V_d = total V_d.
[b]mL/min/1.73 m^2.
[c]Elimination rate constant K_e.

PHARMACODYNAMICS

EFFICACY

Efficacy of aminoglycosides mainly relates to the peak serum concentration/*MIC* (peak/*MIC*) ratio, with occasionally also the use of the area under the time-versus-concentration curve ($AUC_{0\text{-}24}$/*MIC*) as target, while the trough level is the commonly used marker for toxicity.[13,95,96]

Targets

Peak/*MIC* ratios aimed for vary between 5 and 10. In recent papers on gentamicin and tobramycin in children, targets aimed for were C_{max}/*MIC* greater than 8 (general pediatrics),[97] C_{max}/*MIC* greater than 10 (pediatric oncology),[98] or neonates C_{max}/*MIC* greater than 10 or an $AUC_{0\text{-}24}$/*MIC* of 80 to 100[99] for different populations exposed to gentamicin, while CF patients exposed to tobramycin aimed for C_{max}/*MIC* greater than 10 and $AUC_{0\text{-}24}$/*MIC* 80 to 100.[100] For amikacin, targets reported were C_{max}/*MIC* greater than 4 (general pediatrics),[101] C_{max}/*MIC* greater than 8 (pediatric cancer patients),[102] C_{max}/*MIC* greater than or equal to 8 (burned children),[103] or C_{max}/*MIC* greater than 6 to 8 (neonates).[87]

Efficacy Assessment

A meta-analysis of 20 studies on safety and efficacy of aminoglycosides [netilmicin (n = 11), amikacin (n = 7), gentamicin

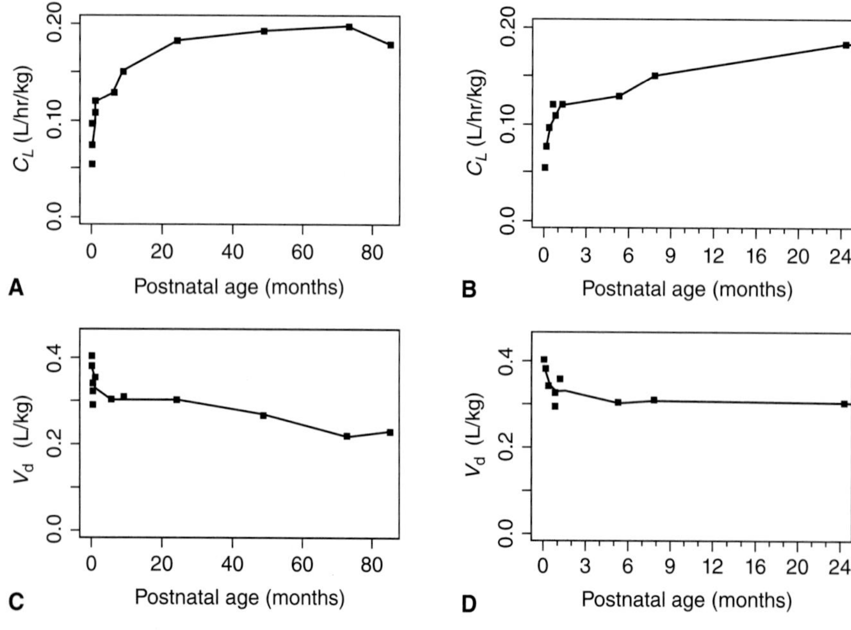

Figure 22.3 Age-dependent differences in amikacin pharmacokinetics in children. Change of mean clearance (*CL*) with increasing postnatal age for all children (**A**) and for neonates and infants only (**B**). Change of volume of distribution (V_d) with increasing postnatal age for all children (**C**) and for neonates and infants only (**D**). In every plot, each dot represents a point estimate of the mean clearance or V_d for a given value of postnatal age. Solid lines correspond to the smoothed data. (Adapted from Tréluyer JM, Merlé Y, Tonnelier S, et al. Nonparametric population pharmacokinetic analysis of amikacin in neonates, infants, and children. *Antimicrob Agents Chemother* 2002;46(5):1381–1387.)

($n = 2$)] given as either an ODD or MDD in adults showed a small statistically significant difference in *clinical efficacy* of 3.5% [95% confidence interval [CI] 0.5%–6.5%) in favor of an ODD approach.[104] In contrast, there is only indirect evidence on the benefits (efficacy and safety) of an extended-interval dosing for aminoglycosides in neonates and children.

Assessment of aminoglycoside efficacy in neonates is difficult, since aminoglycosides are routinely administered in combination treatment of *suspected* neonatal sepsis.[26] Culture-proven early-onset sepsis is rather rare and only occurs in approximately 2% of VLBW infants, but there are limitations to blood cultures (volume and sensitivity) in neonates, while single-blood cultures can be false negative.[27,105] Moreover, maternal–fetal exposure to antibiotics further obscures culture results in newborns. Finally, besides dosing, uncertainties still remain when aiming for rational antibiotic use in neonates. Decisions to prescribe (*when?*) antibiotics are still not based on robust decisions tools, choices (*what?*) on empiric antibiotic regimens should depend on the anticipated pathogens and the available information on efficacy and safety of aminoglycosides.[26,76] As a consequence, there is only meta-analytical evidence that ODD—or more accurate in neonates—extended-interval dosing—does result in better achievement of the generally accepted C_{max} and C_{trough} targets in neonates, but without robust arguments on efficacy (treating culture-proven infection) or toxicity.[106]

In children, the pooled observations support the general adoption of ODD of aminoglycosides in pediatric clinical practice, since it minimizes cost, simplifies administration, and provides similar to potentially improved efficacy and safety. While there is no significant difference between ODD and MDD in the rate of clinical and/or microbiologic failure, trends consistently favored ODD.[107]

TOXICITY

The major specific side effects of aminoglycosides are nephrotoxicity and ototoxicity. Neurotoxicity by blockade of neuromuscular synapses with prolonged muscle weakness after the use of muscle relaxants has not been described in infants, but neonatal myasthenia gravis is a relative contraindication for aminoglycosides. To put things into some perspective, the latest meta-analysis on ODD versus MDD for gentamicin in neonates suggests (pooled, all dosing regimens) that there were no cases ($n = 0/348$, eight studies) of nephrotoxicity (raised creatinine or decreased renal clearance), while the incidence of ototoxicity was 1.4% ($n = 3/214$, five studies).[106] Nestaas et al. also reported (all aminoglycosides, pooled analysis) on nephrotoxicity (increased creatinine, urinary aminopeptidase, 50/589 events, 8.4%) and ototoxicity (1/210 events, 0.5%) in neonates.[108]

For both nephrotoxicity and ototoxicity, intracellular accumulation is the underlying mechanism. Aminoglycosides bind to the negatively charged cell membranes (acidic phospholipids). Binding is much more pronounced at the surface of renal tubular or cochlear hair cells, because of expression of megalin and cubilin as specific ligands. Maturational expression of these ligands may protect neonates to a certain extent to this accumulation.[73,109] Intracellular aminoglycoside accumulation subsequently occurs in the endosomal compartment, the Golgi and endoplasmic reticulum.[110] This accumulation induces a protein unfolding response and cellular stress. At a given threshold concentration, this destabilizes intracellular membranes with redistribution of aminoglycosides to the cytosol and induction of apoptosis. Specific mutations in the mitochondrial 12S rRNA gene in a rRNA base pair (*MT-RNR1* genotype) result in a binding site similar to the aminoglycoside-binding site (bacterial 30S ribosomal subunit) and protein synthesis inhibition, resulting in a specific pharmacogenetic toxicity.[111] Because of differences in repair mechanisms between renal tubular and hair cells, hearing impairment is rather permanent, while renal toxicity is rather transient.

Nephrotoxicity

The mechanism of aminoglycoside nephrotoxicity mainly occurs at the level of the proximal renal tubulus, leading to cell necrosis. The mechanisms of toxicity have been mostly studied in animals, where it was shown to induce glomerular and tubular damage both prenatally and postnatally.[73,109,112] Less than 5% of filtered aminoglycosides binds to the brush-border membrane of proximal tubular cells and is actively reabsorbed, finally causing cell death. The degree of nephrotoxicity is determined by the quantity of aminoglycosides stored in the proximal tubular cell and the intrinsic potency of the drug to damage subcellular structures.[110] In several large meta-analytical studies, toxicity seems to be related to high trough concentrations, indicating that these concentrations are not low long enough over time to prevent renal accumulation. Nephrotoxicity related to ODD as compared with MDD was found to be equal or less in these studies in favor of ODD. A prospective study in 74 adults showed that the probability of nephrotoxicity (6/39 vs. 0/35, overall 8%) is negatively influenced by MDD.[113]

The incidence of aminoglycoside nephrotoxicity in neonates seems to be considerably lower than in adults. The latest meta-analysis on ODD versus MDD for gentamicin in neonates suggests (pooled, all dosing regimens) that there were no cases ($n = 0/348$, 8 studies) of nephrotoxicity (raised creatinine or decreased renal clearance).[106] Nestaas et al. also reported (all aminoglycosides, pooled analysis) on the incidence of nephrotoxicity (increased creatinine, urinary aminopeptidase, 50/589 events, 8.4%) associated with aminoglycoside exposure.[108]

Reversible tubular dysfunction has been shown in many studies involving neonates[109,112,114–118] and is more pronounced in term infants than in preterm newborns.[115,116,118] In infants with a GA greater than 34 weeks, no difference in proximal tubular damage was found between ODD and MDD of amikacin.[115] Urinary electrolyte loss is higher at peak serum concentrations.[114] In the ill-term and especially preterm infant, who is already at risk for electrolyte disturbances, the increased loss during aminoglycoside therapy might be clinically relevant and warrants extra monitoring.[109,112,119] Incidence of nephrotoxicity in children is not well known, but also seems less common than in adults. No difference in nephrotoxicity between ODD and MDD has been demonstrated in most studies in children, except for CF. In this specific population, ODD showed less toxicity (−4.5% vs. +3.7% in creatinine throughout treatment, adjusted mean difference 8%) in children.[38]

Ototoxicity

Aminoglycosides are potentially cochleotoxic and vestibulotoxic. They accumulate in the lymphatic fluid of the inner ear, from which they are only slowly eliminated (24 to 36 hours).[110,120] Sequentially, outer hair cells, inner hair cells, and spiral ganglional neurons are damaged. Hearing loss is usually bilateral, symmetrical, and permanent and can also have a delayed onset of months.[110,120] Most authors suggest that ototoxicity is related to total dose and duration of therapy rather than to serum aminoglycoside serum concentrations, but the relation to aminoglycoside serum concentrations remains unclear.[73,109] This form of toxicity usually occurs in patients who have received either long or repeated courses of aminoglycosides.[121] No difference in incidence between ODD and MDD could be demonstrated.[113,122] In experimental studies, amikacin appears to be more cochleotoxic than gentamicin and tobramycin. Netilmicin is probably the least ototoxic aminoglycoside.[123] Although vestibulotoxicity is a disabling side effect in adults, this side effect is almost impossible to assess in neonates.

There are many pitfalls to assess a causal link between aminoglycosides to hearing loss in infants. The incidence of hearing impairment (>35 to 40 dB) is estimated to be 0.1% to 0.3% in neonates, with a higher incidence in NICU graduates (1% to 3%), most pronounced in extremely preterm infants.[120] The incidence of ototoxicity was 1.4% (n = 3/214) and 0.5% (n = 1/210).[106,108] In some studies, delayed onset of hearing loss has been described.[124,125] Several studies found a transient hearing loss.[126,127] Some studies found a relation with duration or total dose.[128,129] The relation between exposure to tobramycin and the risk of detecting hearing loss with hearing screening was studied.[130] Exposure to tobramycin in terms of treatment duration, total dose, or serum concentrations was not related to a failure to pass hearing screening. Co-treatment with vancomycin or loop diuretics was not associated with an increased chance of hearing loss in this study as in other studies.[115,130] The results lead us to conclude that aminoglycoside-related hearing loss in infants is infrequent, possibly transient, and might be late in appearing. To the very best of our knowledge, the Mitogent (UKCRN ID12004) study is still ongoing.[131] This is a U.K.-based, case–control study to explore the impact of one specific gene variant (m.1555A>G) on hearing impairment in former preterm neonates (survivors, <31 weeks) exposed to gentamicin. In contrast, hearing loss was demonstrated in pediatric patients with CF, with a suggested cumulative effect of intravenous antibiotics (aminoglycosides + glycopeptides).[132]

AMINOGLYCOSIDE THERAPEUTIC DRUG MONITORING AND DOSING

As for any drug, dose and dosing interval are determined by the desired therapeutic range and PK as well as pharmacodynamic properties of a given compound. TDM hereby aims to integrate drug measurements in a clinical decision. It is difficult to define the desired therapeutic range for aminoglycosides. Efficacy of aminoglycosides is related to the ratio of peak serum concentration to the *MIC* of the infecting microorganism and the *AUC*. In vitro ratio of 10:1 prevents the emergence of aminoglycoside-resistant pathogens.[13,95] As discussed earlier in this chapter, efficacy of aminoglycosides mainly relates to peak/*MIC* ratio, with occasionally also the use of $AUC_{0\text{-}24}/MIC$ as target, while the trough level is the commonly used marker for toxicity.[13,95,96] As mentioned previously, peak/*MIC* ratios aimed for vary between 5 and 10. To subsequent avoid toxicity, a reasonable target range for neonates would, therefore, be peak serum concentrations of 5 to 10 mg per L for gentamicin, netilmicin, and tobramycin and 15 to 30 mg per L for amikacin. Trough concentration goals are less than 2 mg per L when dosing thrice daily and less than 0.5 to 1.0 mg per L for ODD in gentamicin, netilmicin, and tobramycin and 1.5 to 3 mg per L for amikacin.

NEONATES

The basic rules to assess TDM obviously also apply to neonates, and as a consequence, TDM for aminoglycosides is commonly used in neonates. However, TDM in neonates warrants focused attention. Similar to the approach taken in adults and children, aminoglycoside dosing in newborns has been revised toward larger doses at extended intervals.[106,108] Most relevant, there is extensive between observation variability, and this variability can only to a certain extent be explained, resulting in uncertainties about target attainment for both efficacy as well as safety.[76,133,134] For the different aminoglycosides, dosing charts for neonates with varying GA, PNA, or weight have been developed with additional adaptations when ibuprofen or indomethacin is coadministered or in the setting of perinatal asphyxia.[84,85,99] Moreover, the time to reach "steady state" is prolonged (V_d related). Consequently, TDM sampling timing matters more in neonates. Finally, in the majority of neonates exposed to aminoglycosides immediately after delivery, this treatment can be stopped within 36 to 48 hours since the suspected infection is commonly not confirmed.[26] Once dosing regimens have been validated (e.g., tobramycin, amikacin), a restrictive sampling, targeted TDM becomes a very reasonable option.[135] This means that only in specific settings, such as prolonged administration, renal impairment, perinatal asphyxia, or ECMO), TDM is recommended.[133,134]

Integration of online available software tools may hereby be very supportive to guide clinical decisions on dose selection, both at initiation as well as after TDM. In a *first step*, validated dosing regimens can be used, either based on clinical characteristics, or applying software programs like NeoGent[136–138] that allows individualized dosing based on demographics, serum creatinine, and *MIC* value for gentamicin to result in probabilistic dosing. Even when this first step is used, the correlation between dose and concentration in neonates remains rather poor. With subsequent integration of a TDM observation (irrespective of the time of sampling), a Bayesian dosing prediction can be provided in a *second step*, again based on datasets and models earlier described and validated in neonates.

INFANTS AND CHILDREN

Aminoglycoside dosing in infants and children has also shifted toward ODD. A number of studies have evaluated ODD versus MDD. While there is no significant difference between ODD and MDD in the rate of clinical and/or microbiologic failure, trends have consistently favored ODD.[107] A similar approach as discussed for neonates can also be applied to children, with initial dosing based on dosing regimens, with subsequent TDM performed around the third or fourth dose. Predicting future serum concentrations in a pediatric population with the help of Bayesian feedback is possible, like for pediatric oncology cases.[138] However, the necessity of routine TDM in pediatric patients with normal renal function and receiving short courses (<10 days) remains questionable.[139,140]

SUMMARY

Aminoglycosides play a major role in antimicrobial therapy in pediatrics with a bactericidal efficacy against Gram-negative pathogens, synergism with β-lactam antibiotics, and limited bacterial resistance. The shift from MDD to ODD or extended-dose intervals has resulted in a more effective and better tolerated therapy, but necessitates more sophisticated dosing practices and TDM in special populations or during prolonged administration.

REFERENCES

1. Waksman SA, Bugie E, Schatz A. Isolation of antibiotic substances from soil microorganisms with special reference to streptothricin and streptomycin. *Proc Staff Meet Mayo Clin* 1944;19:537–548.
2. Gilbert DN, Kohlhepp SJ. New sodium hydroxide digestion method for measurement of renal tobramycin concentrations. *Antimicrob Agents Chemother* 1986;30(3):361–365.
3. Weinstein MJ, Wagman GH, Oden EM, et al. Biological activity of the antibiotic components of the gentamicin complex. *J Bacteriol* 1967;94(3):789–790.
4. Taber HW, Mueller JP, Miller PF, et al. Bacterial uptake of aminoglycoside antibiotics. *Microbiol Rev* 1987;51(4):439–457.
5. Damper PD, Epstein W. Role of the membrane potential in bacterial resistance to aminoglycoside antibiotics. *Antimicrob Agents Chemother* 1981;20(6):803–808.
6. Mates SM, Patel L, Kaback HR, et al. Membrane potential in anaerobically growing *Staphylococcus aureus* and its relationship to gentamicin uptake. *Antimicrob Agents Chemother* 1983;23(4):526–530.
7. Hancock RE. Aminoglycoside uptake and mode of action–with special reference to streptomycin and gentamicin. I. Antagonists and mutants. *J Antimicrob Chemother* 1981;8(4):249–276.
8. Hancock RE, Farmer SW, Li ZS, et al. Interaction of aminoglycosides with the outer membranes and purified lipopolysaccharide and OmpF porin of *Escherichia coli*. *Antimicrob Agents Chemother* 1991;35(7):1309–1314.
9. Sanders CC, Sanders WE Jr, Goering RV. In vitro studies with Sch 21420 and Sch 22591: activity in comparison with six other aminoglycosides and synergy with penicillin against enterococci. *Antimicrob Agents Chemother* 1978;14:171–184.
10. Blaser J, Stone BB, Groner MC, et al. Comparative study with enoxacin and netilmicin in a pharmacodynamic model to determine importance of ratio of antibiotic peak concentration to MIC for bactericidal activity and emergence of resistance. *Antimicrob Agents Chemother* 1987;31(7):1054–1060.
11. Gerber AU, Feller-Segessenmann C. In-vivo assessment of in-vitro killing patterns of *Pseudomonas aeruginosa*. *J Antimicrob Chemother* 1985;15(Suppl A):201–206.
12. Kapusnik JE, Hackbarth CJ, Chambers HF, et al. Single, large, daily dosing versus intermittent dosing of tobramycin for treating experimental pseudomonas pneumonia *J Infect Dis* 1988;158(1):7–12 [published erratum appears in *J Infect Dis* 1988;158(4):911].
13. Mohamed AF, Nielsen EI, Cars O, et al. Pharmacokinetic-pharmacodynamic model for gentamicin and its adaptive resistance with predictions of dosing scheduled in newborn infants. *Antimicrob Agents Chemother* 2012;56(1):179–188.
14. Blaser J, Stone BB, Zinner SH. Efficacy of intermittent versus continuous administration of netilmicin in a two-compartment in vitro model. *Antimicrob Agents Chemother* 1985;27(3):343–349.
15. Dudley MN, Zinner SH. Single daily dosing of amikacin in an in-vitro model. *J Antimicrob Chemother* 1991;27(Suppl C):15–19.
16. Fantin B, Ebert S, Leggett J, et al. Factors affecting duration of in-vivo postantibiotic effect for aminoglycosides against Gram-negative bacilli. *J Antimicrob Chemother* 1991;27(6):829–836.
17. Schlaeffer F, Blaser J, Laxon J, et al. Enhancement of leucocyte killing of resistant bacteria selected during exposure to aminoglycosides or quinolones. *J Antimicrob Chemother* 1990;25(6):941–948.
18. Giamarellou H. Aminoglycosides plus beta-lactams against Gram-negative organisms. Evaluation of in vitro synergy and chemical interactions. *Am J Med* 1986;80(6B):126–137.
19. Garneau-Tsodikova S, Labby KJ. Mechanisms of resistance to aminoglycoside antibiotics: overview and perspectives. *Medchemcomm* 2016;7(1):11–27.
20. Mingeot-Leclercq MP, Glupczynski Y, Tulkens PM. Aminoglycosides: activity and resistance. *Antimicrob Agents Chemother* 1999;43(4):727–737.
21. Karlowsky JA, Zelenitsky SA, Zhanel GG. Aminoglycoside adaptive resistance. *Pharmacotherapy* 1997;17(3):549–555.
22. Karlowsky JA, Hoban DJ, Zelenitsky SA, et al. Altered denA and anr gene expression in aminoglycoside adaptive resistance in *Pseudomonas aeruginosa*. *J Antimicrob Chemother* 1997;40(3):371–376.
23. Karchmer AW, Archer GL, Dismukes WE. *Staphylococcus epidermidis* causing prosthetic valve endocarditis: microbiologic and clinical observations as guides to therapy. *Ann Intern Med* 1983;98(4):447–455.
24. Watanakunakorn C, Tisone JC. Synergism between vancomycin and gentamicin or tobramycin for methicillin-susceptible and methicillin-resistant *Staphylococcus aureus* strains. *Antimicrob Agents Chemother* 1982;22(5):903–905.
25. Litz JE, Goedicke-Fritz S, Härtel C, et al. Management of early- and late-onset sepsis: results from a survey in 80 German NICUs. *Infection* 2019;47(4):557–564. doi:10.1007/s15010-018-1263-9.
26. van den Anker J, Allegaert K. Rational use of antibiotics in neonates: still in search of tailored tools. *Healthcare* 2019;7(1):pii:E28.
27. van Donge T, Bielicki JA, van den Anker J, et al. Key components for antibiotic dose optimization of sepsis in neonates and infants. *Front Pediatr* 2018;6:325.
28. Clark RH, Bloom BT, Spitzer AR, et al. Empiric use of ampicillin and cefotaxime, compared with ampicillin and gentamicin, for neonates at risk for sepsis is associated with an increased risk of neonatal death. *Pediatrics* 2006;117(1):67–74.
29. de Man P, Verhoeven BA, Verbrugh HA, et al. An antibiotic policy to prevent emergence of resistant bacilli. *Lancet* 2000;355(9208):973–978.
30. Hsieh EM, Hornik CP, Clark RH, et al; Best pharmaceuticals for children act-pediatric trials network. Medication use in the neonatal intensive care unit. *Am J Perinatol* 2014;31(9):811–821.
31. Langton Hewer SC, Smyth AR. Antibiotic strategies for eradicating *Pseudomonas aeruginosa* in people with cystic fibrosis. *Cochrane Database Syst Rev* 2017;(4):CD004197.
32. Church DA, Kanga JF, Kuhn RJ, et al. Sequential ciprofloxacin therapy in pediatric cystic fibrosis: comparative study vs. ceftazidime/tobramycin in the treatment of acute pulmonary exacerbations. The Cystic Fibrosis Study Group. *Pediatr Infect Dis J* 1997;16(1):97–105; discussion 123–126.
33. Kearns GL, Hilman BC, Wilson JT. Dosing implications of altered gentamicin disposition in patients with cystic fibrosis. *J Pediatr* 1982;100(2):312–318.
34. Touw DJ, Knox AJ, Smyth A. Population pharmacokinetics of tobramycin administered thrice daily and once daily in children and adults with cystic fibrosis. *J Cyst Fibros* 2007;6(5):327–333.
35. Lam W, Tjon J, Seto W, et al. Pharmacokinetic modelling of a once-daily dosing regimen for intravenous tobramycin in paediatric cystic fibrosis patients. *J Antimicrob Chemother* 2007;59(6):1135–1140.
36. Smith S, Rowbotham NJ, Charbek E. Inhaled antibiotics for pulmonary exacerbations in cystic fibrosis. *Cochrane Database Syst Rev* 2018;(10):CD008319.
37. Patatanian L. Inhaled tobramycin-associated hearing loss in an adolescent with renal failure. *Pediatr Infect Dis J* 2006;25(3):276–278.
38. Smyth AR, Bhatt J, Nevitt SJ. Once-daily versus multiple-daily dosing with intravenous aminoglycosides for cystic fibrosis. *Cochrane Database Syst Rev* 2017;(3):CD002009.
39. Khan AJ, Kumar K, Evans HE. Single-dose gentamicin therapy of recurrent urinary tract infection in patients with normal urinary tracts. *J Pediatr* 1987;110(1):131–135.
40. Wallen L, Zeller WP, Goessler M, et al. Single-dose amikacin treatment of first childhood *E. coli* lower urinary tract infections. *J Pediatr* 1983;103(2):316–319.
41. Strohmeier Y, Hodson EM, Willis NS, et al. Antibiotics for acute pyelonephritis in children. *Cochrane Database Syst Rev* 2014;(7):CD003772.
42. Swan SK. Aminoglycoside nephrotoxicity. *Semin Nephrol* 1997;17(1):27–33.
43. Allegaert K, Scheers I, Adams E, et al. Cerebrospinal fluid compartmental pharmacokinetics of amikacin in neonates. *Antimicrob Agents Chemother* 2008;52(6):1934–1939.
44. Padovani EM, Pistolesi C, Fanos V, et al. Pharmacokinetics of amikacin in neonates. *Dev Pharmacol Ther* 1993;20(3–4):167–173.
45. Kenyon CF, Knoppert DC, Lee SK, et al. Amikacin pharmacokinetics and suggested dosage modifications for the preterm infant. *Antimicrob Agents Chemother* 1990;34(2):265–268.
46. Nakae S, Yamada M, Ito T, et al. Gentamicin dosing and pharmacokinetics in low birth weight infants. *Tohoku J Exp Med* 1988;155(3):213–223.
47. Kildoo C, Modanlou HD, Komatsu G, et al. Developmental pattern of gentamicin kinetics in very low birth weight (VLBW) sick infants. *Dev Pharmacol Ther* 1984;7(6):345–356.
48. Koren G, Leeder S, Harding E, et al. Optimization of gentamicin therapy in very low birth weight infants. *Pediatr Pharmacol (New York)* 1985;5(1):79–87.
49. Izquierdo M, Lanao JM, Cervero L, et al. Population pharmacokinetics of gentamicin in premature infants. *Ther Drug Monit* 1992;14(3):177–183.
50. Williams BS, Ransom JL, Gal P, et al. Gentamicin pharmacokinetics in neonates with patent ductus arteriosus. *Crit Care Med* 1997;25(2):273–275.
51. Watterberg KL, Kelly HW, Johnson JD, et al. Effect of patent ductus arteriosus on gentamicin pharmacokinetics in very low birth weight (less than 1,500 g) babies. *Dev Pharmacol Ther* 1987;10(2):107–117.
52. Dahl LB, Melby K, Gutteberg TJ, et al. Serum levels of ampicillin and gentamicin in neonates of varying gestational age. *Eur J Pediatr* 1986;145(3):218–221.
53. Isemann BT, Kotagal UR, Mashni SM, et al. Optimal gentamicin therapy in preterm neonates includes loading doses and early monitoring. *Ther Drug Monit* 1996;18(5):549–555.
54. Southgate WM, DiPiro JT, Robertson AF. Pharmacokinetics of gentamicin in neonates on extracorporeal membrane oxygenation. *Antimicrob Agents Chemother* 1989;33(6):817–819.
55. Thomson AH, Way S, Bryson SM, et al. Population pharmacokinetics of gentamicin in neonates. *Dev Pharmacol Ther* 1988;11(3):173–179.
56. Faura CC, Feret MA, Horga JF. Monitoring serum levels of gentamicin to develop a new regimen for gentamicin dosage in newborns. *Ther Drug Monit* 1991;13(3):268–276.
57. Pons G, d'Athis P, Rey E, et al. Gentamicin monitoring in neonates. *Ther Drug Monit* 1988;10(4):421–427.
58. Botha JH, du Preez MJ, Adhikari M. Population pharmacokinetics of gentamicin in South African newborns. *Eur J Clin Pharmacol* 2003;59(10):755–759.
59. Granati B, Assael BM, Chung M, et al. Clinical pharmacology of netilmicin in preterm and term newborn infants. *J Pediatr* 1985;106(4):664–669.
60. Kuhn RJ, Nahata MC, Powell DA, et al. Pharmacokinetics of netilmicin in premature infants. *Eur J Clin Pharmacol* 1986;29:635–637.
61. Siegel JD, McCracken GH Jr, Thomas ML, et al. Pharmacokinetic properties of netilmicin in newborn infants. *Antimicrob Agents Chemother* 1979;15(2):246–253.
62. Nahata MC, Powell DA, Durrell DE, et al. Intrapatient variation in tobramycin kinetics in low birth weight infants during first postnatal week. *Eur J Clin Pharmacol* 1984;26(5):647–649.
63. Nahata MC, Powell DA, Durrell DE, et al. Effect of gestational age and birth weight on tobramycin kinetics in newborn infants. *J Antimicrob Chemother* 1984;14(1):59–65.
64. Nahata MC, Powell DA, Gregoire RP, et al. Tobramycin kinetics in newborn infants. *J Pediatr* 1983;103(1):136–138.
65. Bressolle F, Gouby A, Martinez JM, et al. Population pharmacokinetics of amikacin in critically ill patients. *Antimicrob Agents Chemother* 1996;40(7):1682–1689.
66. Kafetzis DA, Sianidou L, Vlachos E, et al. Clinical and pharmacokinetic study of a single daily dose of amikacin in paediatric patients with severe gram-negative infections. *J Antimicrob Chemother* 1991;27(Suppl C):105–112.
67. Marik PE, Havlik I, Monteagudo FS, et al. The pharmacokinetic of amikacin in critically ill adult and paediatric patients: comparison of once- versus twice-daily dosing regimens. *J Antimicrob Chemother* 1991;27(Suppl C):81–89.
68. Hoecker JL, Pickering LK, Swaney J, et al. Clinical pharmacology of tobramycin in children. *J Infect Dis* 1978;137(5):592–596.

69. Kraus DM, Dusik CM, Rodvold KA, et al. Bayesian forecasting of gentamicin pharmacokinetics in pediatric intensive care unit patients. *Pediatr Infect Dis J* 1993;12(9):713–718.
70. Bass KD, Larkin SE, Paap C, et al. Pharmacokinetics of once-daily gentamicin dosing in pediatric patients. *J Pediatr Surg* 1998; 33(7):1104–1107.
71. Jacobson PA, West NJ, Price J, et al. Gentamicin and tobramycin pharmacokinetics in pediatric bone marrow transplant patients. *Ann Pharmacother* 1997;31(10):1127–1131.
72. Lanao JM, Berrocal A, Calvo MV, et al. Population pharmacokinetic study of gentamicin and a Bayesian approach in patients with renal impairment. *J Clin Pharm Ther* 1989;14(3):213–223.
73. Smits A, Kulo A, van den Anker J, et al. The amikacin research program: a stepwise approach to validate dosing regimens in neonates. *Expert Opin Drug Metab Toxicol* 2017;13(2):157–166.
74. Van Der Heggen T, Dhont E, Peperstraete H, et al. Augmented renal clearance: a common condition in critically ill children. *Pediatr Nephrol* 2019;34(6):1099–1106.
75. Liu X, Smits A, Wang Y, et al. Impact of disease on amikacin pharmacokinetics and dosing in children. *Ther Drug Monit* 2019;41(1):44–52.
76. Roberts JK, Stockmann C, Constance JE, et al. Pharmacokinetics and pharmacodynamics of antibacterials, antifungals, and antivirals used most frequently in neonates and infants. *Clin Pharmacokinet* 2014;53(7):581–610.
77. De Cock RF, Allegaert K, Sherwin CM, et al. A neonatal amikacin covariate model can be used to predict ontogeny of other drugs eliminated through glomerular filtration in neonates. *Pharm Res* 2014;31(3):754–767.
78. Allegaert K, van den Anker J. Neonates are not just little children and need more finesse in dosing of antibiotics. *Acta Clin Belg* 2019;74(3):157–163.
79. Langhendries JP, Battisti O, Bertrand JM, et al. Adaptation in neonatology of the once-daily concept of aminoglycoside administration: evaluation of a dosing chart for amikacin in an intensive care unit. *Biol Neonate* 1998;74(5):351–362.
80. de Hoog M, Mouton JW, Schoemaker RC, et al. Extended-interval dosing of tobramycin in neonates: implications for therapeutic drug monitoring. *Clin Pharmacol Ther* 2002;71(5):349–358.
81. Lingvall M, Reith D, Broadbent R. The effect of sepsis upon gentamicin pharmacokinetics in neonates. *Br J Clin Pharmacol* 2005;59(1):54–61.
82. Dodge WF, Jelliffe RW, Zwischenberger JB, et al. Population pharmacokinetic models: effect of explicit versus assumed constant serum concentration assay error patterns upon parameter values of gentamicin in infants on and off extracorporeal membrane oxygenation. *Ther Drug Monit* 1994;16(6):552–559.
83. Koren G, James A, Perlman M. A simple method for the estimation of glomerular filtration rate by gentamicin pharmacokinetics during routine drug monitoring in the newborn. *Clin Pharmacol Ther* 1985;38(6):680–685.
84. Bijleveld YA, de Haan TR, van der Lee HJ, et al. Altered gentamicin pharmacokinetics in term neonates undergoing controlled hypothermia. *Br J Clin Pharmacol* 2016;81(6):1067–1077.
85. Cristea S, Smits A, Kulo A, et al. Amikacin pharmacokinetics to optimize dosing in neonates with perinatal asphyxia treated with hypothermia. *Antimicrob Agents Chemother* 2017;61(12):pii: e01282-17.
86. Allegaert K, Cossey V, Langhendries JP, et al. Effects of co-administration of ibuprofen-lysine on the pharmacokinetics of amikacin in preterm infants during the first days of life. *Biol Neonate* 2004;86(3):207–211.
87. De Cock RF, Allegaert K, Schreuder MF, et al. Maturation of the glomerular filtration rate in neonates, as reflected by amikacin clearance. *Clin Pharmacokinet* 2012;51(2):105–117.
88. König K, Lim A, Miller A, et al. Gentamicin trough levels using a simplified extended-interval dosing regimen in preterm and term newborns. *Eur J Pediatr* 2015;174(5):669–673.
89. van den Anker JN, Hop WC, de Groot R, et al. Effects of prenatal exposure to betamethasone and indomethacin on the glomerular filtration rate in the preterm infant. *Pediatr Res* 1994;36(5):578–581.
90. Allegaert K, Anderson B. Antenatal steroids and neonatal renal function. *Arch Dis Child* 2006;91(5):451.
91. Allegaert K, Scheers I, Cossey V, et al. Covariates of amikacin clearance in neonates: the impact of postnatal age on predictability. *Drug Metab Lett* 2008;2(4):286–289.
92. Tréluyer JM, Merlé Y, Tonnelier S, et al. Nonparametric population pharmacokinetic analysis of amikacin in neonates, infants, and children. *Antimicrob Agents Chemother* 2002;46(5):1381–1387.
93. Kelman AW, Thomson AH, Whiting B, et al. Estimation of gentamicin clearance and volume of distribution in neonates and young children. *Br J Clin Pharmacol* 1984;18(5):685–692.
94. Lanao JM, Dominguez-Gil AA, Dominguez-Gil A, et al. Pharmacokinetics of amikacin in children with normal and impaired renal function. *Kidney Int* 1981;20(1):115–121.
95. Moore RD, Lietman PS, Smith CR. Clinical response to aminoglycoside therapy: importance of the ratio of peak concentration to minimal inhibitory concentration. *J Infect Dis* 1987;155(1):93–99.
96. Craig WA, Redington J, Ebert SC. Pharmacodynamics of amikacin in vitro and in mouse thigh and lung infections. *J Antimicrob Chemother* 1991;27(Suppl C):29–40.
97. Alsultan A, Abouelkheir M, Elsharawy Y, et al. Optimizing gentamicin dosing in pediatrics using Monte Carlo simulations. *Pediatr Infect Dis J* 2019;38(4):390–395.
98. Llanos-Paez CC, Staatz CE, Lawson R, et al. A population pharmacokinetic model of gentamicin in pediatric oncology patients to facilitate personalized dosing. *Antimicrob Agents Chemother* 2017;61(8):pii: e00205-17.
99. Bijleveld YA, van den Heuvel ME, Hodiamont CJ, et al. Population pharmacokinetics and dosing considerations for gentamicin in newborns with suspected or proven sepsis caused by Gram-negative bacteria. *Antimicrob Agents Chemother* 2016;61(1):pii:e01304-16.
100. Gao Y, Barras M, Hennig S. Bayesian estimation of tobramycin exposure in patients with cystic fibrosis: an update. *Antimicrob Agents Chemother* 2018;62(3):pii:e01972-17.
101. Alqahtani S, Abouelkheir M, Alsultan A, et al. Optimizing amikacin dosage in pediatrics based on population pharmacokinetic/pharmacodynamics modeling. *Paediatr Drugs* 2018;20(3):265–272.
102. Alhadab AA, Ahmed MA, Brundage RC. Amikacin pharmacokinetic-pharmacodynamic analysis in pediatric cancer patients. *Antimicrob Agents Chemother* 2018;62(4):pii:e01781-17.
103. Yu T, Stockmann C, Healy DP, et al. Determination of optimal amikacin dosing regimens for pediatric patients with burn wound sepsis. *J Burn Care Res* 2015;36(4):e244–e252.
104. Munckhof WJ, Grayson ML, Turnidge JD. A meta-analysis of studies on the safety and efficacy of aminoglycosides given either once daily or as divided doses. *J Antimicrob Chemother* 1996;37:645–663.
105. Schelonka RL, Chai MK, Yoder BA, et al. Volume of blood required to detect common neonatal pathogens. *J Pediatr* 1996;129(2):275–278.
106. Rao SC, Srinivasjois R, Moon K. One dose per day compared to multiple doses per day of gentamicin for treatment of suspected or proven sepsis in neonates. *Cochrane Database Syst Rev* 2016;(12):CD005091.
107. Contopoulos-Ioannidis DG, Giotis ND, Baliatsa DV, et al. Extended-interval aminoglycoside administration for children: a meta-analysis. *Pediatrics* 2004;114(1):e111–e118.
108. Nestaas E, Bangstad HJ, Sandvik L, et al. Aminoglycoside extended interval dosing in neonates is safe and effective: a meta-analysis. *Arch Dis Child Fetal Neonatal Ed* 2005;90(4):F294–F300.
109. Kent A, Turner MA, Sharland M, et al. Aminoglycoside toxicity in neonates: something to worry about? *Expert Rev Anti Infect Ther* 2014;12(3):319–331.
110. Nagai J, Takano M. Entry of aminoglycosides into renal tubular epithelial cells via endocytosis-dependent and endocytosis-independent pathways. *Biochem Pharmacol* 2014;90(4):331–337.
111. Barbarino JM, McGregor TL, Altman RB, et al. PharmGKB summary: very important pharmacogene information for MT-RNR1. *Pharmacogenet Genomics* 2016;26(12):558–567.
112. McWilliam SJ, Antoine DJ, Smyth RL, et al. Aminoglycoside-induced nephrotoxicity in children. *Pediatr Nephrol* 2017;32(11):2015–2025.
113. Rybak MJ, Abate BJ, Kang SL, et al. Prospective evaluation of the effect of an aminoglycoside dosing regimen on rates of observed nephrotoxicity and ototoxicity. *Antimicrob Agents Chemother* 1999;43(7):1549–1555.
114. Giapros VI, Andronikou S, Cholevas VI, et al. Renal function in premature infants during aminoglycoside therapy. *Pediatr Nephrol* 1995;9(2):163–166.
115. Langhendries JP, Battisti O, Bertrand JM, et al. Once-a-day administration of amikacin in neonates: assessment of nephrotoxicity and ototoxicity. *Dev Pharmacol Ther* 1993;20(3-4):220–230.
116. Parini R, Rusconi F, Cavanna G, et al. Evaluation of the renal and auditory function of neonates treated with amikacin. *Dev Pharmacol Ther* 1982;5(1-2):33–46.
117. Andronikou S, Giapros VI, Cholevas VI, et al. Effect of aminoglycoside therapy on renal function in full-term infants. *Pediatr Nephrol* 1996;10(6):766–768.
118. Gouyon JB, Aujard Y, Abisror A, et al. Urinary excretion of N-acetyl-glucosaminidase and beta-2-microglobulin as early markers of gentamicin nephrotoxicity in neonates. *Dev Pharmacol Ther* 1987;10(2):145–152.
119. Chiruvolu A, Engle WD, Sendelbach D, et al. Serum calcium values in term and late-preterm neonates receiving gentamicin. *Pediatr Nephrol* 2008;23(4):569–574.
120. Zimmerman E, Lahav A. Ototoxicity in preterm infants: effects of genetics, aminoglycosides, and loud environmental noise. *J Perinatol* 2013;33(1):3–8.
121. McCormack JP, Jewesson PJ. A critical reevaluation of the "therapeutic range" of aminoglycosides. *Clin Infect Dis* 1992;14(1):320–339.
122. Ali MZ, Goetz MB. A meta-analysis of the relative efficacy and toxicity of single daily dosing versus multiple daily dosing of aminoglycosides. *Clin Infect Dis* 1997;24(5):796–809.
123. McCracken GH Jr. Aminoglycoside toxicity in infants and children. *Am J Med* 1986;80(6B):172–178.
124. Kawashiro N, Tsuchihashi N, Koga K, et al. Delayed post-neonatal intensive care unit hearing disturbance. *Int J Pediatr Otorhinolaryngol* 1996;34(1-2):35–43.
125. Nield TA, Schrier S, Ramos AD, et al. Unexpected hearing loss in high-risk infants. *Pediatrics* 1986;78(3):417–422.
126. Finitzo-Hieber T, McCracken GH Jr, Brown KC. Prospective controlled evaluation of auditory function in neonates given netilmicin or amikacin. *J Pediatr* 1985;106(1):129–136.
127. Tsai CH, Tsai FJ. Auditory brainstem responses in term neonates treated with gentamicin. *Acta Paediatr Sin* 1992;33(6):417–422.
128. Borradori C, Fawer CL, Buclin T, et al. Risk factors of sensorineural hearing loss in preterm infants. *Biol Neonate* 1997;71(1):1–10.
129. Bernard PA. Freedom from ototoxicity in aminoglycoside treated neonates: a mistaken notion. *Laryngoscope* 1981;91(12):1985–1994.
130. de Hoog M, van Zanten BA, Hop WC, et al. Newborn hearing screening: tobramycin and vancomycin are not risk factors for hearing loss. *J Pediatr* 2003;142(1):41–46.
131. University College London. Mitogent. 2013. www.ucl.ac.uk/mitogent. Accessed April 25, 2019.
132. Garinis AC, Cross CP, Srikanth P, et al. The cumulative effects of intravenous antibiotic treatments on hearing in patients with cystic fibrosis. *J Cyst Fibros* 2017;16(3):401–409.
133. Pauwels S, Allegaert K. Therapeutic drug monitoring in neonates. *Arch Dis Child* 2016;101(4):377–381.
134. Young TE. Therapeutic drug monitoring–the appropriate use of drug level measurement in the care of the neonate. *Clin Perinatol* 2012;39(1):25–31.
135. Fonzo-Christe C, Guignard B, Zaugg C, et al. Impact of clinical decision support guidelines on therapeutic drug monitoring of gentamicin in newborns. *Ther Drug Monit* 2014;36(5):656–662.
136. Rivera-Chaparro ND, Cohen-Wolkowiez M, Greenberg RG. Dosing antibiotics in neonates: review of the pharmacokinetic data. *Future Microbiol* 2017;12:1001–1016.
137. Germovsek E, Kent A, Metsvaht T, et al. Development and evaluation of a gentamicin pharmacokinetic model that facilitates opportunistic gentamicin therapeutic drug monitoring in neonates and infants. *Antimicrob Agents Chemother* 2016;60(8):4869–4877.
138. TDMx. Launch pad. www.tdmx.eu/Launch-TDMx. Accessed April 25, 2019.
139. Logsdon BA, Phelps SJ. Routine monitoring of gentamicin serum concentrations in pediatric patients with normal renal function is unnecessary. *Ann Pharmacother* 1997;31(12):1514–1518.
140. Massey KL, Hendeles L, Neims A. Identification of children for whom routine monitoring of aminoglycoside serum concentrations is not cost effective. *J Pediatr* 1986;109(5):897–901.

CHAPTER 23

Jennifer Le
John S. Bradley

Macrolides, Clindamycin, and Oxazolidinones

MACROLIDES

ERYTHROMYCIN

Erythromycin was the first in the macrolide class of antibiotics that was approved for use in 1952.[1] Erythromycin was derived from *Streptomyces erythreus*, originally obtained from a soil sample in the Philippines,[2] with a spectrum of activity against Gram-positive and limited activity against respiratory Gram-negative pathogens, primarily used to treat skin and soft-tissue infections (SSTIs) in children. However, owing to poor gastrointestinal (GI) tract tolerability, oral erythromycin underwent multiple changes in formulation. Now, it is rarely prescribed and has been replaced by newer, better tolerated oral and parenteral macrolides. Erythromycin is primarily used to treat children who are allergic to penicillins and/or cephalosporins or are infected by penicillin-resistant organisms.

Chemical Structure

Erythromycin consists of a 14-membered macrocyclic lactone ring with two appended deoxy sugar moieties, deconamine and cladinose, at positions 5 and 3 of the ring. Erythromycin base is poorly soluble in water and easily degraded by gastric acid. Because it is a large molecule, erythromycin diffuses through membranes slowly. This results in unpredictable erythromycin levels in serum and tissue following oral administration[3] (Fig. 23.1).

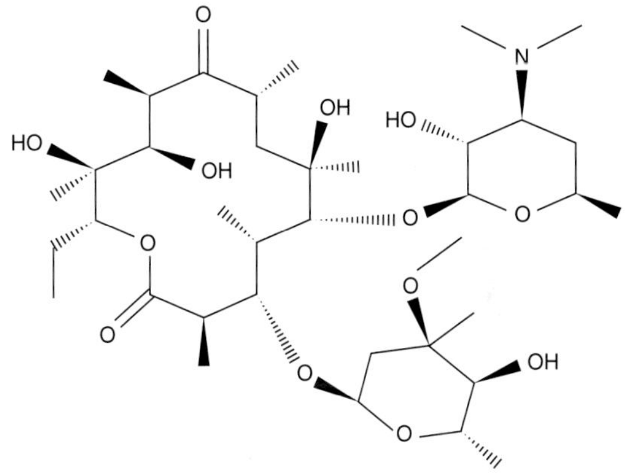

Figure 23.1 Structure of erythromycin.

Mechanism of Action/Mechanism of Antibacterial Resistance

Erythromycin and other macrolides inhibit bacterial pathogens by binding close to the peptidyl transferase region of the 50S subunit of bacterial 70S ribosomes causing inhibition of bacterial protein synthesis. Macrolides are bacteriostatic. Erythromycin and other macrolides do not actually block peptidyl transferase activity, but they bind in the tunnel through which newly forming peptides must travel to exit the ribosome (nascent peptide exit tunnel, NPET), thereby preventing the nascent peptides from forming mature and complete proteins.[4,5] Recent data suggest that binding of the macrolide to the NPET in a ribosome that is actively translating may alter the conformation of the peptidyl transfer center (PTC) site to prevent efficient translation, and the nascent protein can itself cause conformational changes at the PTC.[6]

Acquired bacterial resistance to macrolides involves one of three mechanisms: (a) alteration of the ribosomal binding site, (b) decreased accumulation of the drug due to an active efflux pump, or (c) macrolide inactivation by esterases or by phosphorylation or glycosylation at 2′-position.[7] Modification of the ribosomal binding site by methylation is the most common clinically significant resistance mechanism in both *Streptococcal* and *Staphylococcal* spp. Methylase enzyme activity, if genes are present in the organism, may be either inducible or constitutive and is mediated by *erm* genes (*ermA*, *ermB*, and *ermC*). The MLSB (macrolide/lincosamide/streptogramin B) phenotype is conferred by *erm* methylation, creating a barrier to binding and resistance to macrolides, lincosamides (clindamycin), and type B streptogramins, which share a similar ribosomal binding site. MLSB resistance is due to methylation of the 23S rRNA binding site at adenine 2058.[8,9] Resistance to the 14- or 15-membered macrolides may also be the result of efflux pumps encoded by genes such as *mefE* in *Streptococcus pneumoniae*, *mrsA* in *Staphylococcus aureus*, and *mefA* in group A beta-hemolytic *Streptococcus* (GABHS).[10–12] Chromosomal mutation involving the 50S ribosomal protein is yet another mechanism of resistance to macrolides in Gram-positive cocci.[8]

In Vitro Efficacy

In vitro activity of erythromycin and other macrolides varies based on the structure of the macrolide and may include both Gram-positive and Gram-negative pathogens. The in vitro spectrum of activity of erythromycin, in particular, primarily includes Gram-positive cocci such as *S. pneumoniae*, *Streptococcus pyogenes*, and *S. aureus* as well as Gram-positive bacilli such as *Bacillus anthracis*, *Clostridium* species, and *Corynebacterium* species. Erythromycin also has excellent activity against *Legionella pneumophila*, *Bordetella pertussis*, and *Campylobacter jejuni*. Erythromycin and the macrolides demonstrate activity against intracellular pathogens that lack a formal bacterial cell wall such as *Chlamydia pneumoniae*, *Chlamydia trachomatis*, *Mycoplasma pneumoniae*, and *Ureaplasma urealyticum*.[13,14] Erythromycin is active in vitro against, but has limited clinical use for, infections caused by *Eikenella*, *Haemophilus influenzae*, *Pasteurella*, and *Brucella*. Most *Treponema* species, *Rickettsia rickettsiae*, and to a lesser extent *Borrelia burgdorferi* and *Helicobacter pylori* are inhibited by erythromycin.[15,16]

Clinical Indications

Erythromycin is considered the drug of choice for very few pediatric infections, having been replaced by other macrolides that are better tolerated. It has been considered an alternative to penicillin in patients with penicillin allergy. Erythromycin is still the drug of choice for diphtheria infections, as little data are published for other macrolides. Erythromycin is active against *B. pertussis*, although azithromycin is preferred, particularly for very young infants, for whom the rate of pyloric stenosis following treatment is decreased, compared with erythromycin.[17] In addition to eradicating nasopharyngeal carriage and preventing infection with *B. pertussis* following exposure (prophylaxis), macrolides may shorten the clinical course of illness if started during the catarrhal or early paroxysmal phase of pertussis.[18] Following identification of *M. pneumoniae* as a frequent cause of pneumonia in school-age children, adolescents, and young adults, macrolides have become an important component of antibiotic treatment of pneumonia among these patients.[19]

Erythromycin has been shown to shorten the duration of clinical illness and time to radiologic clearance in adolescents with *Mycoplasma* pneumonia.[20] In the 1970s, *C. trachomatis* was identified as an important cause of neonatal conjunctivitis in infants younger than 30 days, as well as the cause of the interstitial pneumonia syndrome of early infancy. Treatment with oral macrolides has been shown to eradicate nasopharyngeal carriage of the organism, hasten recovery of conjunctivitis and pneumonia, and prevent pneumonia in infants who present initially with conjunctivitis.[21] In addition, nongonococcal urethritis caused by *C. trachomatis* can be treated with macrolides. The role of ureaplasma as a pathogen for normal children, including neonates, is controversial. Although it may be cultured from mucosal surfaces, or sterile sites, the benefit from treatment is uncertain.[22] Ureaplasma may cause symptomatic urethritis in sexually active individuals and is usually susceptible to macrolides as well as other agents. Erythromycin and other macrolides are effective in the treatment of pneumonia caused by *Chlamydophila pneumoniae*, *L. pneumophila*, and *Legionella micdadei* (Legionnaires disease).[23,24]

Erythromycin is an alternative for the treatment of diarrhea caused by *C. jejuni* when clinically indicated, with azithromycin being preferred.[25] Erythromycin may also represent an option for the treatment of cholera, although other antibiotics have been shown to be more effective.[26]

Erythromycin is an alternative to penicillin for the treatment of GABHS pharyngitis in patients who are allergic to penicillin. However, increased rates of infection with macrolide-resistant GABHS have been reported in areas of the world where macrolides are frequently used resulting in treatment failures.[27] Macrolides represent alternatives to penicillin G for the treatment of pneumococcal upper and lower respiratory tract infections, although many strains of pneumococcus remain resistant to macrolides, even in the era of protein-conjugated pneumococcal vaccines and decreasing resistance to penicillins. Similarly, erythromycin may be used as an alternative treatment for infections caused by susceptible strains of *B. anthracis* and *Eikenella corrodens*. Erythromycin is considered an alternative treatment to amoxicillin for early-localized Lyme disease in children younger than 8 years who are allergic to penicillin.[28]

Nontuberculous mycobacterial pathogens (notably Mycobacterium avium-intracellulare) may be susceptible to azithromycin and clindamycin and may represent treatment options. Treatment courses are often prolonged, for up to 6 to 12 weeks, even for normal hosts, with extended courses for children who are immunocompromised.

Pharmacokinetic Properties

Degradation of erythromycin base by gastric acid results in reduced oral bioavailability. Food increases GI acidity and may delay absorption. Esters of the erythromycin base (stearate, estolate, and ethylsuccinate) have been formulated to improve acid stability and facilitate absorption. Erythromycin stearate is less readily destroyed in the stomach and is dissociated in the duodenum liberating erythromycin, which is then absorbed. Erythromycin estolate is absorbed mainly as ester and then hydrolyzed in serum to active erythromycin. Its bioavailability is not affected by food. Erythromycin ethylsuccinate is also well absorbed after oral administration, with food increasing its bioavailability.[29] After absorption, erythromycin ethyl succinate is hydrolyzed into active erythromycin.

Satisfactory serum concentrations are achieved following intravenous administration of erythromycin. Peak concentrations attained 1 hour after intravenous infusion are usually fourfold to tenfold greater than those attained after oral erythromycin.[30] After intravenous administration of erythromycin lactobionate to preterm neonates at either 25 or 40 mg per kg per day divided into four doses every 6 hours, peak serum levels were 3.05 to 3.69 μg per mL and 1.92 to 2.9 μg per mL for the 40 and 25 mg per kg per day groups, respectively.[31] Erythromycin diffuses well into intracellular fluids and body tissues except the cerebrospinal fluid (CSF) and the central nervous system (CNS). Middle ear fluid (MEF) concentration is about 50% of serum concentration. This concentration may be sufficient to inhibit the highly sensitive *S. pyogenes* and *S. pneumoniae* but may be too low for the treatment of otitis media caused by *H. influenzae*.[32] Tonsillar concentrations are adequate after oral administration.[33] Children with chlamydial conjunctivitis treated with erythromycin have tear fluid concentration of erythromycin approximately equal to simultaneous serum concentration. Erythromycin is concentrated in human polymorphonuclear leukocytes.[34] Significant intracellular penetration occurs, resulting in activity against intracellular pathogens.[35]

Studies of single 10 mg per kg oral doses of erythromycin estolate and ethylsuccinate in infants younger than 4 months with *C. trachomatis* infection have shown similar peak serum concentrations (C_{max}) of erythromycin.[36] Similar findings were noted after repeat dosing at a steady state. Single-dose studies also showed similar time to C_{max} (T_{max}) for both formulations. However, multiple-dose studies in infants aged 3 to 48 months showed that T_{max} was longer for the estolate formulation, resulting in larger area of activity under the curve (AUC) at steady state.[36] In neonates, absorption of erythromycin appears to be delayed and bioavailability is not influenced by feeding.[37]

Most macrolides including erythromycin are eliminated via hepatic metabolism and/or biliary excretion. Erythromycin is excreted as the active form in the bile. Macrolides are substrates of the hepatic enzyme cytochrome P450 3A4. Reduction in the activity of this enzyme secondary to disease or immaturity can result in elevated levels of macrolides. At therapeutic concentrations, 80% to 90% of erythromycin in the blood is protein bound. Erythromycin crosses the placenta, but fetal plasma drug concentrations are considerably lower and less predictable than those in the mother.[38] Erythromycin is partly excreted in the urine: about 2.5% of orally administered dose and 15% of parenterally administered dose. A considerable proportion of erythromycin is excreted in the bile. In general, renal or hepatic dysfunction has little effect on the pharmacokinetics of macrolides including erythromycin, and dosage adjustment is not necessary in most occasions.[39,40]

Dose/Regimens

The usual dosage of erythromycin (including base form, stearate, ethyl succinate, and estolate preparations) in children is 30 to 50 mg per kg per day administered in two to four equally divided doses. The maximum daily dose is 2 g (up to 4 g in adults). In severe infections, erythromycin may be administered by the intravenous route at a dosage of 15 to 50 mg per kg per day in four equally divided doses. The intravenous dose should be given by slow infusion over at least 1 hour to minimize the risk of cardiac arrhythmias. For newborns, oral erythromycin is administered at a dose of 10 mg per kg given every 12 hours for those younger than 1 week and every 8 hours for those aged 1 week and older.

Adverse Effects/Toxicity/Precautions

Erythromycin is the least tolerated antibiotic among the macrolides. The most common adverse effects of erythromycin are GI disturbances such as abdominal pain or discomfort and nausea.[41,42] An association between very early exposure to erythromycin and infantile hypertrophic pyloric stenosis was demonstrated, with nearly eightfold increased risk of pyloric stenosis in neonates 3 to 13 days of life.[43]

The GI side effects are possibly related to the prokinetic action of erythromycin on the gut mediated by its motilin-receptor-stimulating activity.[44] Reported allergic reactions include fever, rashes, joint pain, generalized pruritus, and Stevens–Johnson syndrome. Reversible hepatic dysfunction and liver enzyme abnormalities have been reported 10 to 14 days following erythromycin use. These include colicky abdominal pain, cholestasis, elevated transaminase levels, jaundice, and eosinophilia.[41,42] Cholestatic hepatitis has been reported with the estolate formulation, likely representing a hypersensitivity reaction to the estolate ester and only rarely with the other derivatives.[42] Reversible neurosensory hearing loss affecting all hearing frequencies has been reported mostly in association with the use of high doses in patients with impaired renal function.[45] Thrombophlebitis and venous irritation have been reported with intravenous erythromycin infusions. The incidence and severity of these infusion reactions can be reduced by slowing of the rate of infusion and/or by reducing the concentration of erythromycin in the infusate.[42] Intravenous administration of erythromycin to infants and children has been associated with cardiotoxicity manifested by bradycardia, hypotension, Torsades de Pointes (polymorphous ventricular tachycardia), and cardiac arrest.[30]

Drug Interactions

Macrolides interact with many drugs by inhibiting the metabolism of the drugs via the cytochrome P450 (CYP) hepatic microsomal enzymes.[46] Through this inhibition to increase exposure and toxicity of other drugs caused by erythromycin, coadministration is contraindicated for β-hydroxy β-methylglutaryl-coenzyme A reductase (HMG-CoA) reductase inhibitors (e.g., lovastatin and simvastatin), posaconazole, drugs that prolong QT interval (e.g., fluconazole, posaconazole, cisapride, and astemizole), and ergot derivatives. Significant drug interactions also occur with concomitant administration of erythromycin with antihistamines, cisapride, carbamazepine, valproate, theophylline, cyclosporine, digoxin, warfarin, and benzodiazepines.[46–50] The interaction occurs via the induction of the CYP enzymes, which subsequently convert the macrolide to a nitrosoalkane metabolite forming an inactive complex with the iron of CYP. The complete list of drugs should be reviewed to ascertain all potential drug interactions with erythromycin.

Concomitant administration of erythromycin and theophylline can result in increased concentrations of theophylline, likely due to decreased clearance of theophylline. The reduction in clearance is variable (5% to 40%) and is related to the type of erythromycin formulation, type of patient, and dose and duration of erythromycin therapy.[40] Concomitant administration of erythromycin and cyclosporine results in increased exposure of cyclosporine, ranging from 75% to 215% in cyclosporine AUC that is possibly due to decreased cyclosporine clearance, increased bioavailability, or both.[49] The interaction with digoxin is also believed to be via increasing the bioavailability of digoxin secondary to the inhibition of the metabolizing bacteria, particularly *Eubacterium lentum*, in the large bowel. This interaction occurs in a small percentage of patients (10%) and is less likely to occur with the capsule preparations of digoxin.[50]

AZITHROMYCIN

Azithromycin is considered the macrolide of choice for most pediatric infections, with better tolerability and an increased spectrum of activity, as well as dosing once daily for a much shorter treatment course with improved compliance, compared with erythromycin.

Chemical Structure

Azithromycin is synthesized by the incorporation of a 6-methyl-substituted nitrogen atom into position 9a of the

14-member macrolide ring (Fig. 23.2). This results in the expansion of the ring to 15 members, and accordingly, azithromycin is classified as an azalide rather than a macrolide. The modification at position 9a also results in a compound with more stability to degradation by gastric acid, improved oral absorption, and decreased GI distress compared with erythromycin.[51]

Mechanism of Action/Mechanism of Antibacterial Resistance

Similar to other macrolide antibiotics, azithromycin inhibits protein synthesis by binding to the 50S ribosomal subunit within the NPET, resulting in early termination of peptide formation.[6] Azithromycin has been shown to exhibit postantibiotic effect that may reflect high intracellular concentrations[52] and possibly prolonged obstruction of the NPET by aborted, short peptides that remain in the tunnel.[6] The mechanisms of resistance to azithromycin are similar to those of erythromycin and other macrolides.

In Vitro Efficacy

In general, azithromycin is more active than erythromycin against Gram-negative organisms but provides no advantage over erythromycin in activity against Gram-positive organisms.[53] Importantly, the organisms that are resistant to erythromycin are almost uniformly also resistant to azithromycin.[54] Improved in vitro activity compared with that of erythromycin has been shown against *Haemophilus* species, *M. catarrhalis*, *Legionella* species, *Pasteurella multocida*, *B. burgdorferi*, *Mycoplasma* species, *Neisseria gonorrhea*, *C. trachomatis*, and *Campylobacter* species. Azithromycin has appreciable activity against *Mycobacterium avium* complex (MAC) and *Bartonella henselae*.[55,56]

Azithromycin is active against macrolide-susceptible strains of *S. pneumoniae*, *S. pyogenes*, and *S. aureus*.[57] Macrolide resistance is common among staphylococci (*S. aureus* and coagulase-negative staphylococci).[58,59] Penicillin-resistant *S. pneumoniae* strains are often resistant to azithromycin. The prevalence of resistance to macrolides is related to antibiotic usage patterns, often observed in specific geographical regions.

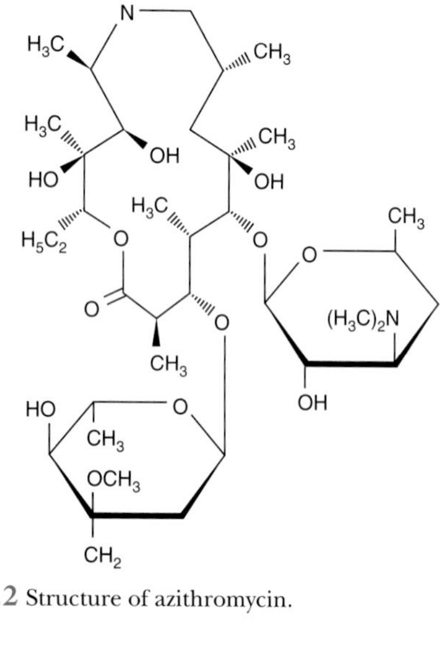

Figure 23.2 Structure of azithromycin.

Azithromycin has similar in vitro activity to erythromycin against *C. pneumoniae* and *B. pertussis*.[60,61] Azithromycin is also active in vitro against *Toxoplasma gondii*.

Clinical Indications

Although oral penicillin V remains the drug of choice for streptococcal pharyngitis, azithromycin given at a dose of 12 mg per kg once a day for 5 days demonstrated similar efficacy.[62] Acute otitis media (AOM) was an important clinical indication for azithromycin prior to the emergence of macrolide resistance in *S. pneumoniae*,[63] given the additional activity against nontypeable strains of *H. influenzae* over that of erythromycin. Children with AOM who demonstrate penicillin allergy and are infected by macrolide-susceptible strains of *S. pneumonia* may still benefit from the treatment (10 mg per kg on Day 1 followed by 5 mg per kg on Days 2 through 5). Azithromycin may also be considered for the treatment of community-acquired pneumonia (CAP) caused by susceptible strains of *S. pneumoniae* in all ages of children. For children older than 5 years and adolescents who are more likely to be infected by *M. pneumoniae*, azithromycin may be added to ampicillin or amoxicillin if needed.[64] Azithromycin may be considered first-line treatment for respiratory tract infections caused by "atypical pneumonia" pathogens *M. pneumoniae*, *C. pneumoniae*, and *L. pneumophila* as well as the treatment for *C. trachomatis* conjunctivitis and pneumonia in young infants.[65]

The treatment for skin and skin structure infections (SSTIs) with azithromycin depends on the local rate of macrolide resistance among *S. pyogenes* and *S. aureus* strains. The efficacy of azithromycin in the treatment of susceptible bacteria causing SSTIs has been shown in adults and children.[66] In areas where the prevalence of macrolide-resistant *S. aureus* is high, a child with SSTI may be treated with azithromycin if the infecting strains are documented to be susceptible. Azithromycin is recommended for the treatment and prevention of pertussis.[67] Azithromycin given at 10 mg per kg on Day 1 followed by 5 mg per kg daily for 4 days was as effective as 10 mg per kg daily for 3 days in eradicating *B. pertussis* from the upper respiratory tract in infants and young children.[68] Because of concerns for the erythromycin adverse drug reaction of pyloric stenosis in young infants, azithromycin is the recommended macrolide for the prevention and treatment of pertussis in infants younger than 1 month.[67]

MAC has been identified as a cause of cervical lymphadenitis in children.[69,70] The definitive treatment of nontuberculous mycobacterial lymphadenitis is surgical excision. However, if the patient is at a high risk of surgical complications or if complete surgical excision is difficult, azithromycin or clarithromycin can be given as an alternative treatment.[71] Azithromycin and clarithromycin have also been used in the treatment and prophylaxis of MAC infections. Patients with acquired immunodeficiency syndrome (AIDS) are at a risk of disseminated MAC. Prophylaxis with either azithromycin or clarithromycin should be offered to children with human immunodeficiency virus (HIV) infection who have advanced immunosuppression, with low CD4 cell counts that vary by age from less than 750 cells/mm^3 for those under 1 year to less than 50 cells per /mm^3 for those older than or equal to 6 years.[72]

Azithromycin has been used in the treatment of lymphadenitis caused by *B. henselae*, the agent causing cat scratch disease (CSD). In a double-blind study, Bass et al. found that azithromycin given as a 5-day course (10 mg per kg on Day 1 followed by 5 mg per kg for 4 consecutive days) accelerated the resolution of lymphadenitis caused by typical, uncomplicated CSD within the first month of treatment.[73] The efficacy of azithromycin in the treatment of other or atypical manifestations of CSD is not clear but is usually assumed. However, in normal children, most clinical manifestations of CSD are benign and self-limited, and many children do not require antibiotic therapy.[74]

Erythromycin has historically been the most commonly used drug for the treatment of Legionnaires disease. However, azithromycin has become the oral drug of choice for the treatment of Legionnaires disease.[75] In critically ill adults with legionellosis, intravenous azithromycin has been recommended.[76] Although limited pharmacokinetics is available for children,[77] the U.S. Food and Drug Administration (FDA) has not reviewed systematically collected data and has not approved the parenteral formulation for use in children.

For the treatment of uncomplicated chlamydia cervicitis and nongonococcal urethritis, a single 2-g dose of azithromycin has been shown to be as effective as the traditional 7-day course of oral doxycycline.[78]

Azithromycin is the treatment of choice for trachoma, an infectious keratoconjunctivitis caused by *C. trachomatis.* It is considered the most common cause of preventable blindness worldwide.[79] Azithromycin has also been shown to have activity against enteric pathogens including pathogenic strains of *Escherichia coli, Campylobacter, Shigella, Cholera,* and *Salmonella typhi* as well as nontyphoidal strains of *Salmonella* sp.[80] Preliminary studies have shown that azithromycin is effective in treating uncomplicated typhoid fever in adults and children.[81,82] A study of 64 Egyptian children aged 4 to 17 years compared azithromycin suspension given at 10 mg per kg per day for 7 days with intramuscular ceftriaxone given at 75 mg per kg per day for 7 days. Cure was achieved in 91% of the azithromycin group and 97% of the ceftriaxone group.[82] None of the children in the azithromycin group had relapses, compared with 14% of those in the ceftriaxone group. Larger studies are needed particularly for those with bacteremic *S. typhi* infection.

Azithromycin is used, in conjunction with ceftriaxone, to treat gonococcal infections in children, although resistance to azithromycin is increasing worldwide.[83]

Azithromycin is used in children with cystic fibrosis as adjunctive therapy, primarily for those colonized with *Pseudomonas aeruginosa.*[84] An anti-inflammatory effect of azithromycin is the most likely mechanism of improvement, but some in vitro studies suggest that, when tested in cell culture media, azithromycin displays antibacterial activity against Pseudomonas.[85]

Azithromycin (20 mg per kg as a single dose) can be used for prophylaxis to prevent endocarditis at the time of dental procedures in high-risk children who are allergic to penicillin.[86]

Azithromycin has been used to treat *Cryptosporidium parvum* infections in immunocompromised adults and children. *C. parvum* causes an asymptomatic or self-limited gastroenteritis in otherwise healthy people. However, in immunocompromised patients, *C. parvum* may cause severe intestinal fluid losses with dehydration or chronic diarrhea and wasting. Different antimicrobial regimens have been used in adults with inconsistent results.[87,88] The role of azithromycin in clinical resolution of cryptosporidiosis remains to be clarified.

Pharmacokinetic Properties

When administered to children at the regimen of 10 mg per kg once followed by 5 mg per kg per day on Days 2 through 5, azithromycin exhibits pharmacokinetic properties similar to those in adults.[89] Food intake significantly decreases the bioavailability of the capsule and the powdered suspension of azithromycin. Therefore, azithromycin should be administered 1 hour before or 2 hours after the intake of food or antacid. However, the tablet form of azithromycin may be taken without regard to food.[90] Peak plasma concentrations are achieved 2 hours after a dose.[89]

Azithromycin distributes well into tissues, including tonsils and adenoid tissues, and into MEF.[91,92] Clinically effective levels are achieved in these tissues and MEF long after the last dose of azithromycin is administered.[91] Tissue concentrations as high as twice the serum concentrations may be achieved. Good intracellular penetration of azithromycin contributes to its efficacy in the management of infections caused by intracellular organisms such as *Chlamydia* species and MAC. Tissue delivery is further enhanced by neutrophil and macrophage uptake of azithromycin to sites of infection.[93]

Despite its fairly rapid absorption and high tissue bioavailability, when azithromycin is given at the recommended dosage regimen, achievable serum concentrations are detected far below the minimum inhibitory concentration (MIC) of some pediatric pathogens (0.026 to 0.043 μg per mL). This should be taken into consideration during the management of potentially bacteremic organisms such as *S. pneumoniae, H. influenzae,* and *S. pyogenes.*[29]

Azithromycin is slowly eliminated. With an elimination half-life of azithromycin in children aged 32 to 64 hours, azithromycin can be administered once daily.[54] Therapeutically significant concentrations of azithromycin may persist in tissues for additional 5 days after a 5-day course. Plasma protein binding of azithromycin is saturable, ranging from 50% at a concentration of 20 to 50 μg per L to 7% at 1,000 μg per L.[57] Azithromycin is largely eliminated unchanged in the urine and stools.[90] Significant renal impairment (creatinine clearance of less than 30 mL per min) reduces the rate of urinary clearance of azithromycin.[90] Azithromycin, like erythromycin, increases the rate of gastric emptying and thus may alter the absorption of azithromycin or other drugs.[94]

An extended-release oral suspension of azithromycin is available for use in pediatrics. Compared with the administration of 1.5 g of azithromycin for 3 or 5 days, a single 2 g dose of the extended-release suspension formulation reaches maximum peak concentration in 5 hours (vs. 2.2 to 4 hours), has a similar serum half-life, and reaches higher drug exposure (which is expected owing to the higher total dose).

Dose/Regimens

For most pediatric infections including otitis media and pneumonia in those 6 months and older, azithromycin is administered in single daily doses at 10 mg per kg on the first day of treatment followed by 5 mg per kg per day on Days 2 through 5. The maximum daily dose is 500 mg. Azithromycin may be administered as a 3-day course of 10 mg per kg per day or as a single dose of 30 mg per kg for AOM or CAP. These clinical indications are approved for pediatric use. For adolescents and adults with uncomplicated *C. trachomatis* genital tract infection, azithromycin may be administered as a single 1-g oral dose.[65]

The recommended dose of the azithromycin extended-release oral suspension for the treatment of CAP is a single oral dose of 60 mg per kg, with a maximum dose of 2 g. This formulation should be taken on an empty stomach (at least 1 hour before or 2 hours following a meal).

For the treatment and postexposure prophylaxis of pertussis in children younger than 6 months including neonates, the recommended dose is 10 mg per kg once daily for 5 days. For children aged 6 months or older, the dose is 10 mg per kg on the first day followed by 5 mg per kg once daily for the next 4 days.[67] Other oral dosing regimens for azithromycin include 12 mg per kg daily over 5 days for GABHS pharyngitis; 250 to 500 mg orally three times per week for children aged 6 years or older with cystic fibrosis; and 20 mg per kg once weekly (maximum 1,200 mg per week) or 5 mg per kg once daily (maximum 250 mg per day) for MAC prevention in children with HIV.

Intravenous azithromycin is given to adults at a dose of 500 mg once daily. There are no current approved indications for the use of intravenous azithromycin in children owing to lack of sufficient data. However, a single-daily dose of 10 mg per kg (maximum 500) given to children aged 6 months to 16 years was tolerated with no serious adverse events and showed comparable pharmacokinetic properties among study patients.[77]

Adverse Effects/Toxicity/Precautions

Azithromycin is more tolerable than erythromycin. Azithromycin oral suspension has demonstrated an excellent safety and tolerability profile in children treated for different infections. Comparative trials with pooled tolerability results have shown overall better tolerability of azithromycin than other oral comparator agents. Adverse events with azithromycin are usually mild, infrequent, of short duration, and reversible. In children, adverse events also appear to be dose-related. They were reported in 7.6% of patients receiving 30 mg per kg and 16.6% of those receiving 60 mg per kg total dose (both given once daily for 5 days). The most prevalent adverse events were GI events such as diarrhea (3.1%), vomiting (2.5%), abdominal pain (1.9%), and loose stools (1.0%). Transient elevation of hepatic transaminases has been reported. Dermatologic complications (mainly rash) occurred in 1.5% of patients, and neurologic side effects (mainly headache) occurred in 0.6% of patients.[95] Children allergic to erythromycin may have cross-hypersensitivity reactions to azithromycin. Azithromycin is contraindicated in children who are allergic to erythromycin or any other macrolide antibiotics.

Drug Interactions

Food, antacids, and H_2-blockers reduce the absorption of azithromycin by 50%. Azithromycin reportedly has no significant interactions with carbamazepine, cimetidine, methylprednisolone, terfenadine, or midazolam. Known or potential interactions with other drugs such as cyclosporine, digoxin, theophylline, and warfarin may occur. Levels of these medications should be monitored with concomitant azithromycin use. Azithromycin should not be administered with ergot alkaloids.[96]

CLARITHROMYCIN

Clarithromycin is a broad-spectrum macrolide, similar to azithromycin in its extended activity beyond erythromycin, with activity against pathogens causing respiratory tract, Helicobacter, and mycobacterial infections in children. Although it has a longer half-life than erythromycin and achieves high intracellular concentrations, it has largely been replaced by azithromycin.[97]

Chemical Structure

Clarithromycin is a 6-methoxy-erythromycin. The addition of a methoxy group at the sixth position of the macrolide ring results in a compound that is less resistant to acid hydrolysis with fewer GI side effects than erythromycin[98–100] (Fig. 23.3).

Mechanism of Action/Mechanism of Antibacterial Resistance

Similar to other macrolide antibiotics, clarithromycin inhibits protein synthesis by binding to the 50S ribosomal subunit and inhibiting peptide formation.[4–6] Like other macrolides, the most clinically significant acquired resistance to clarithromycin is due to methylation of the ribosomal binding site mediated by *erm* genes and indicates cross-resistance to other macrolides.[8]

In Vitro Efficacy

Clarithromycin has a spectrum of activity that is very similar to azithromycin, as noted above. It is active against many Gram-positive and Gram-negative bacteria as well as some mycobacteria and protozoa. Clarithromycin has similar activity to azithromycin against *S. pneumoniae, S. pyogenes, S. aureus, H. influenzae,* and *M. catarrhalis.* Streptococci and staphylococci that are resistant to erythromycin are also resistant to clarithromycin. Penicillin-resistant *S. pneumoniae* strains are usually resistant to clarithromycin. Clarithromycin is more active in vitro than erythromycin against *C. trachomatis, C. pneumoniae, M. pneumoniae, L. pneumophila, B. burgdorferi,* and *B. pertussis.*[61,98,100] Clarithromycin is ineffective against Gram-negative enteric bacteria.[29,101] Clarithromycin has excellent activity against *Haemophilus ducreyi* (causing chancroid). Clarithromycin is more active than azithromycin against certain nontuberculous mycobacteria, particularly MAC, and has activity against other mycobacteria such as *Mycobacterium chelonae* and some subspecies of *Mycobacterium fortuitum.* Clarithromycin is also effective against *Mycobacterium leprae.*[29,102] Clarithromycin has been shown to have inhibitory activity against *T. gondii.*[103]

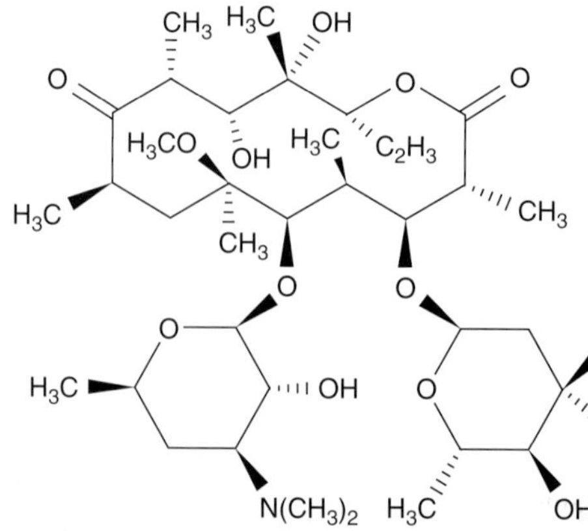

CH_3 H_3C OH O O O H_3CO OH H_3C C_2H_3 H_3C CH_3 CH_3 O O O OCH_3 H_3C OH O CH_3 $N(CH_3)_2$ H_3C OH

Figure 23.3 Structure of clarithromycin.

Clinical Indications

Clarithromycin has been shown to be an effective alternative to penicillin for who are penicillin-allergic, in the treatment of GABHS pharyngitis.[104] Clarithromycin has also been shown to be an effective alternative treatment for AOM and CAP in children, although high rates of macrolide resistance in *S. pneumoniae* limit its efficacy.[105–108] However, clarithromycin has been found to be effective in the treatment of pneumonia caused by atypical organisms such as *M. pneumoniae* and *C. pneumoniae*.[109]

Clarithromycin is part of the combination therapy for *H. pylori*-induced peptic ulcer disease.[110] Clarithromycin, in combination with other antibiotics, is also used for the treatment of nontuberculous mycobacterial infections, including disseminated MAC infection in immunocompromised children.[111]

Pharmacokinetic Properties

Clarithromycin is well absorbed from the GI tract, with an oral bioavailability of 52% to 55%; absorption is not affected by food intake. First-pass metabolism results in the appearance of the active 14-hydroxy metabolite.[100] Clarithromycin is not extensively protein bound. The major route of elimination is biliary excretion. Approximately 30% to 40% of the administered dose is excreted in urine. Elimination half-life of clarithromycin and its 14-hydroxy metabolite is 5 and 7 hours, respectively.[100] Dosage adjustments are required for patients with severe renal failure (creatinine clearance less than 30 mL per min). Clarithromycin's long half-life allows for twice-daily administration. Clarithromycin is concentrated in cells and tissues including lungs, nasal mucosa, and tonsils and in MEF. Clarithromycin and its metabolite concentrate in lungs and MEF at higher levels than in plasma.[91] Clarithromycin concentration in respiratory tract exceeds that of plasma by ratios of up to 8.82:1 in MEF, 3.1:1 in bronchial secretions, and 28.7:1 in lung tissue.[112–114]

Dose/Regimens

The usual dose of clarithromycin in children is 7.5 mg per kg (up to 500 mg per dose) given twice daily. The duration of treatment of AOM and pneumonia in children is generally 10 days.

Adverse Effects/Toxicity/Precautions

Clarithromycin has fewer GI adverse events than erythromycin. The most frequently reported adverse events among children receiving clarithromycin suspension were diarrhea (6.6%), vomiting (6.3%), abdominal pain (2.4%), and headache (1.6%). Adverse events requiring withdrawal of clarithromycin occurred in less than 2% of treated children.[29,115] Hypersensitivity reactions range from mild skin rashes and urticaria to anaphylactic reactions and Stevens–Johnson syndrome. Other adverse events include stomatitis, glossitis, oral candidiasis, and dizziness. Unusual reactions reported among adults with underlying conditions include hepatic failure, cholestatic hepatitis, leukocytoclastic vasculitis, thrombocytopenic purpura, and visual hallucinations. Reversible hearing loss has been reported rarely among adults receiving clarithromycin 1,000 mg twice daily for MAC infection.[116] The risk of long-term hearing impairment among children taking long-term clarithromycin therapy is unclear.

Drug Interactions

Clarithromycin interacts with other drugs via the inhibition of the cytochrome P450 enzyme system, particularly CYP3A.[117] In general, clarithromycin exhibits fewer drug interactions than erythromycin. However, clinically significant interactions have been reported with theophylline, digoxin, carbamazepine, cyclosporine, and tacrolimus. These agents require drug level monitoring and appropriate dose adjustment when used concomitantly with clarithromycin. Significant interactions also occur when clarithromycin is concomitantly used with rifampin and rifabutin. Both rifampin and rifabutin induce the metabolism of clarithromycin.[118]

CLINDAMYCIN

Clindamycin is a semisynthetic lincosamide, a protein synthesis inhibitor first approved by the FDA in 1968. Lincosamides are naturally occurring antibiotic compounds derived from *Streptomyces* spp.

CHEMICAL STRUCTURE

Clindamycin consists of two linked components (Fig. 23.4): an amino acid (trans-methyl-L-proline) linked by a peptide bond with the sugar (6-amino-6,8-dideoxy-1-thio-D-threo-α-D-galacto-pyranoside).

MECHANISM OF ACTION/MECHANISM OF ANTIBACTERIAL RESISTANCE

Clindamycin binds to the 50S ribosomal subunit at a site that prevents the docking of tRNAs and their movement through the peptidyl transferase center, preventing the formation of nascent peptides.[119] The site of attachment of lincosamides to the ribosomal RNA is adjacent to that for the macrolides explaining both the competitive inhibition of binding between the two classes of antibiotics and the resistance that may occur to both classes. Resistance to the lincosamides occurs primarily for Gram-positive bacteria constitutively producing the methyltransferase that mono- or dimethylates, an rRNA adenine residue present at the outlet of the peptidyl transferase center. This inducible enzyme is most often only activated in the presence of the appropriate substrate, most effectively induced by a macrolide. In contrast, the lincosamides are poor inducers of the methylase enzyme.

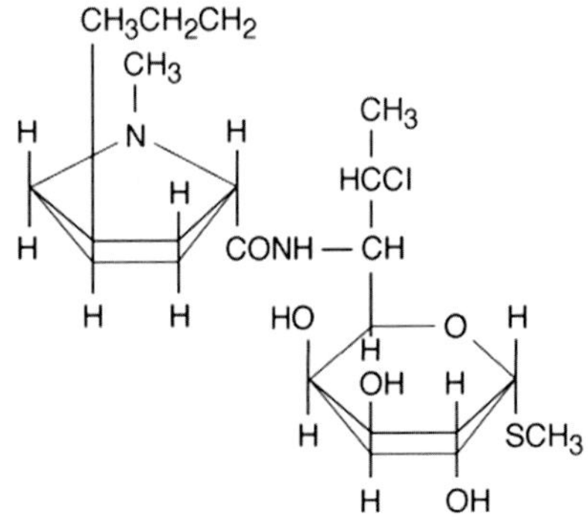

$CH_3CH_2CH_2$ CH_3 H N H CH_3 HCCl H H CONH — CH H H HO O H H OH H H SCH_3 H OH

Figure 23.4 Structure of clindamycin. (Reprinted with permission from Hauser AR. *Antibiotic basics for clinicians*. Philadelphia, PA: Wolters Kluwer Health, 2018. Fig. 6.8.)

Staphylococci that have inducible resistance may remain susceptible to clindamycin, even following exposure to the antibiotic. However, in every population of *S aureus*, approximately one in 10^7 organisms is an unregulated, constitutive producer of methylase, and the selection of constitutive mutants may occur during therapy with subsequent treatment failure. This situation is most likely to occur in serious, deep infections that involve greater than 10^7 organisms, or with prolonged therapy, but is unlikely to occur with mild-to-moderate skin infections or cutaneous and soft-tissue abscesses infections that can be incised and drained. Pathogens that are macrolide-resistant based on the presence of efflux pumps remain susceptible to clindamycin, which is not transported out of the organisms by this mechanism.

Clindamycin is usually considered to be bacteriostatic in activity against susceptible bacteria, although bactericidal activity can be demonstrated against certain organisms in a concentration-dependent manner at antibiotic concentrations 2 to 4 times the MIC.[119]

IN VITRO EFFICACY

Clindamycin has clinically useful activity across a broad range of Gram-positive and anaerobic pathogens. Most clinical use is directed against susceptible Gram-positive aerobic pathogens: *S. aureus*, *S. pyogenes*, and *S. pneumoniae*. Excellent anaerobic activity has been documented for both most oral flora and lower GI tract flora, including many strains of *Bacteroides fragilis*, *Prevotella melaninogenica*, *Fusobacteria* sp., and anaerobic streptococci as well as *Clostridium perfringens* and other *Clostridia* sp. However, increasing resistance in *Bacteroides* spp. has limited its empiric use for intra-abdominal infections.[120]

In addition, clindamycin is often active against *Actinomyces* sp. Based on activity against many strains of *Propionibacterium acnes*, topical clindamycin therapy of acne is widely used. Activity can also be demonstrated against most strains of *B. anthracis*, although anthrax is infrequent in the North America and Europe.

CLINICAL INDICATIONS

Since the mid-1990s, with the dramatic emergence of community-acquired methicillin-resistant *S. aureus* (CA-MRSA), the use of clindamycin for deep SSTIs, as well as pulmonary and osteoarticular infections, has also increased substantially.[121] Data on the efficacy of clindamycin in the treatment of MRSA are both prospective and retrospective and document clinical and microbiologic efficacy that is comparable to other active agents.[122] Although some regions of the United States in which MRSA is prevalent have documented decreasing resistance to clindamycin owing to spread in the community of certain clindamycin-susceptible clones, other areas may experience increasing clindamycin resistance, particularly with methylase-harboring organisms that may confer resistance to both clindamycin and macrolides.[123] Susceptibility of MRSA should be assessed locally to determine appropriate empiric therapy with clindamycin for serious infections.

Clindamycin continues to be used commonly for deep head and neck space infections, dental abscesses, and aspiration pneumonia (with or without empyema), also caused primarily by anaerobes and Gram-positive cocci. In the past, it was extensively used for the treatment of intra-abdominal infections such as complicated appendicitis, but the percentage of strains of *B. fragilis* resistant to clindamycin is increasing, and it is no longer recommended as the anaerobic agent of choice.[124]

Less common uses continue for the treatment of Gram-positive cocci, such as failures of penicillin in group A streptococcal pharyngitis and for the treatment of *S. aureus* infections in children who could not tolerate beta-lactam antibiotics. Although no formal, randomized prospective comparative studies were performed for clindamycin in the treatment of AOM, sinusitis, and pneumonia, clindamycin was recommended for the treatment of penicillin-resistant pneumococci in these situations. Clindamycin can also be used as one of the alternative therapies for *Pneumocystis jiroveci*, in combination with primaquine. Activity has also been demonstrated for the treatment of malaria and toxoplasmosis when other, better studied agents cannot be used.

Apart from the ability of clindamycin to inhibit and kill pathogens, the ability to target ribosomes and protein production has led investigators to consider its use in the treatment of toxin-mediated infections caused by *S. aureus* (toxic shock syndrome) and *S. pyogenes* (toxic shock-like illness), either alone or in combination with cell wall–active antibiotic agents. In vitro data and retrospectively analyzed human data suggest some benefit of combined therapy.[125]

PHARMACOKINETIC PROPERTIES

Routes of administration for clindamycin include oral, parenteral, topical, and vaginal. Peak concentrations occur within 60 min following the administration of the intravenous, intramuscular, and oral (both palmitate and phosphate) formulations.[126] Oral absorption is as high as 90%, and food delays the rate but does not affect the extent of absorption. For other routes of administration, peak concentrations occur within 10 to 30 min after intravenous, 1 hour after intramuscular, 10 to 14 hours after vaginal cream, and 5 hours after vaginal suppository (ovules). Vaginal systemic absorption varies between formulations, with 30% absorption for ovules and 5% for vaginal cream.

DISTRIBUTION

For the oral or parenteral routes, clindamycin distributes extensively into most fluid and body tissues, including bone, bile, pleural fluid, sputum, placenta, and urine.[38,126] However, penetration into the CSF is poor even when meninges are inflamed; thus, clindamycin is not indicated for the treatment of brain infections, except for situations in which the blood–brain barrier is not intact, including brain abscess and toxoplasma encephalitis. The volume of distribution ranges from 0.6 to 1.2 L per kg (i.e., 43 to 74 L).[127] It highly binds (i.e., 80% to 95%) primarily to alpha-1-acid glycoprotein protein.[126]

METABOLISM AND ELIMINATION

Clindamycin is metabolized primarily by CYP3A4 and, to a lesser extent, by CYP3A5, in the liver and intestine to form two bioactive metabolites, clindamycin sulfoxide and N-desmethyl clindamycin. As such, drugs that inhibit or induce these enzymes may interact with clindamycin. Clindamycin moderately inhibits CYP3A4.[126] The plasma half-life in pediatrics with normal renal function is 2 to 3 hours. Approximately 10% of drug is excreted in the urine as active drug and metabolites, 3.6% in the feces, and the remainder as inactive metabolites. Hemodialysis does not remove clindamycin from the serum.

DOSAGE/REGIMEN

The dosing of clindamycin varies by clinical indication, ranging from 15 to 20 mg per kg per day divided every 6 to 8 hours for neonates, 20 to 40 mg per kg per day (or 350 to 450 mg per m^2 per day) divided every 6 to 8 hours for those aged 1 month to 16 years, and 150 to 600 mg divided three times daily in adults.[126] Additional dosing recommendations for special populations and topical preparations can be found in the FDA package labels. Often, then larger doses are used for the treatment of MRSA[121] and anthrax.[128] Dosing between oral and intravenous formulations is comparable owing to its high oral bioavailability. Although hepatic and renal impairment slightly increases the half-life of clindamycin, dosing adjustment is not recommended by the manufacturer's labeling, including for patients end-stage renal disease on dialysis. In patients with severe liver disease, the use of clindamycin should be cautioned, and monitoring liver enzymes periodically during therapy is recommended.

ADVERSE EFFECTS/TOXICITY/PRECAUTIONS

Most adverse drug effects occur with systemic clindamycin therapy, albeit they may occur with topical and vaginal routes if absorption occurs. The most common adverse effect is GI events, with a report of diarrhea in up to 20% of patients, especially in those receiving oral formulation. Diarrhea associated with clindamycin is a direct function of its activity against normal anaerobic GI flora. Clindamycin has been associated with severe, potentially fatal pseudomembranous colitis; hence, this is a black box warning (see the "Pseudomembranous Colitis" section). Other GI-related adverse events include esophagitis (oral only), constipation, abdominal pain/cramps, halitosis, nausea, vomiting, dyspepsia, flatulence, and GI disorder. Administration of oral formulations with food can reduce minor gastric distress. A full glass of water and food are recommended with oral administration to reduce esophageal irritation and gastric distress, respectively.

Other adverse effects associated with systemic clindamycin are rashes, including maculopapular, vesicular, or bullous, and urticaria. Severe skin reactions (such as toxic epidermal necrolysis and Stevens–Johnson syndrome) and hypersensitivity reactions have been reported. Acute generalized exanthematous pustulosis (AGEP), angioedema, drug reaction with eosinophilia and systemic symptoms (DRESS), erythema multiforme, and exfoliative dermatitis have also been reported with systemic clindamycin. Other skin reactions have been reported with topical application, including burning, xerosis, erythema, oiliness/oily skin, peeling, seborrhea, application site rash, folliculitis, and application site pain. Patients with an allergy to tartrazine dye should be treated cautiously as some oral capsule preparations contain this dye.

A metallic or unpleasant taste (dysgeusia) has been reported with the intravenous and oral clindamycin products. Other adverse effects reported during clindamycin therapy include jaundice, elevated hepatic enzymes, headache, dizziness, and vertigo. Although rare and no direct relationship with clindamycin use has been shown, hematologic effects may occur, including transient neutropenia (leukopenia), eosinophilia, agranulocytosis, and thrombocytopenia.

Adverse effects associated specifically with vaginal preparations are hematochezia, vaginitis, vaginal irritation, vulvovaginitis, vaginal pain, vulvovaginal pruritus, vaginal discharge, vaginal swelling, and vaginal bleeding.

PSEUDOMEMBRANOUS COLITIS

Clostridium difficile-associated diarrhea has been reported at a rate of 0.01% to 10%, which may occur during or after discontinuation of therapy (especially systemic ones) with resultant minor diarrhea or fatal pseudomembranous colitis. *C. difficile*-mediated pseudomembranous colitis is a potential complication of virtually any broad-spectrum antibiotic, including clindamycin.[129] Accurate, prospectively collected data on the incidence of *C. difficile-positive* enterocolitis for populations of clindamycin-treated children in different geographic regions and for children who are otherwise healthy versus those with comorbid conditions have not been published, but reports of high attack rates of *C. difficile* enterocolitis have not occurred commensurate with the increased use of clindamycin for staphylococcal infections, in contrast to adult populations. Discontinuation of clindamycin (and all antibiotic therapy, if possible) should occur, with supportive fluid and electrolyte management, *C. difficile* antibiotic treatment, and surgical evaluation as clinically indicated.

DRUG INTERACTIONS

Clindamycin interacts with a few drugs by inhibiting the metabolism of the drugs via CYP3A4. Although the interactions are not as significant as erythromycin, moderate drug interactions may occur with the concurrent administration of clindamycin with muscle relaxants (e.g., atracurium, pancuronium, tubocurarine, and vecuronium) to cause excessive neuromuscular blockade. In addition, clindamycin may decrease cyclosporine bioavailability; therefore, close monitoring of cyclosporine concentrations is recommended.[130] Coadministration with rifampicin significantly decreases clindamycin trough concentrations.[131] Lastly, as some antibiotics, including clindamycin, with activity against *Vibrio cholerae* may interfere with the immunological response to the live cholera vaccine, the vaccine should not be administered to patients who receive antibiotics within 14 days prior to vaccination.

OXAZOLIDINONES

This class of antibiotics is unique in that members are not natural products, but were discovered as one of a number of compounds created as potential monoamine oxidase (MAO)-inhibiting agents. However, some of these compounds also demonstrated antibacterial activity, and subsequent chemical modifications led to the development of linezolid, which demonstrated a reasonable balance between antimicrobial activity, clinical efficacy, and acceptable clinical toxicity.

LINEZOLID

Linezolid is the first antibiotic in the oxazolidinone class to be approved and used in children. Although it was initially developed to treat *S. pneumoniae* infections prior to the widespread use of the protein-conjugated pneumococcal vaccines, the treatment of MRSA infections now represents the overwhelming clinical use of this antibiotic in children. Tedizolid, a second-generation oxazolidinone, is more active against MRSA, with a better safety profile than linezolid, and is currently under investigation in neonates, infants, and children.

Chemical Structure of Linezolid

The chemical structure of linezolid is shown in Figure 23.5.

Mechanism of Action/Mechanism of Antibacterial Resistance

Compared with other agents that target the ribosome, the oxazolidinones have a unique binding site and mechanism of action. The antibiotic binds to an area close to the ribosomal peptidyl transferase center and inhibits the initiation of protein synthesis by preventing the formation of the initiation complex at the peptidyl transferase center. The movement of the complex from the ribosome's "A site" of tRNA attachment to the peptidyl "P site" is blocked, and coupling of amino acids and lengthening of the peptide chain cannot occur.[132]

Resistance to linezolid has been described and consists of structural changes within the ribosome at the linezolid binding site, by both mutational and transferable methylation resistance through conjugative transposons.[133,134] These relatively infrequent changes tend to occur more often with more prolonged therapy and are primarily single-base changes in the rRNA occurring around the peptidyl transferase site.

In Vitro Efficacy

Linezolid is active against numerous clinically relevant Gram-positive bacterial species, including coagulase-positive and coagulase-negative staphylococci (methicillin-susceptible and methicillin-resistant), enterococci (vancomycin-susceptible and vancomycin-resistant), beta- and alpha-hemolytic streptococci (including *S. pneumoniae*), and *Corynebacterium* spp.[134] Activity is primarily limited to Gram-positive bacteria owing to the presence of an effective efflux pump present in many Gram-negative organisms, with the exception of in vitro activity against *P. multocida*. Activity has also been demonstrated against *Mycobacterium tuberculosis*, but the narrow therapeutic index has limited its use for the treatment of tuberculosis. Linezolid is not active against *Mycoplasma* or *Ureaplasma*.

Clinical Indications

Linezolid has been studied clinically for nosocomial and CAP and for complicated and uncomplicated SSTIs.[135,136] The clinical and microbiologic response rates for each of these tissue-specific infections in children were equivalent to comparator agents, usually vancomycin. Linezolid demonstrates bactericidal activity against *S. pneumoniae*, but bacteriostatic activity against *S. aureus* and *Enterococcus* species, although the need for bactericidal activity in infections other than those in neutropenic patients, meningitis, and endocarditis is not clear.[137] Limited studies in adults comparing vancomycin, a bactericidal agent, with linezolid in the treatment of nosocomial pneumonia caused by MRSA documented superior clinical outcomes with linezolid.[138]

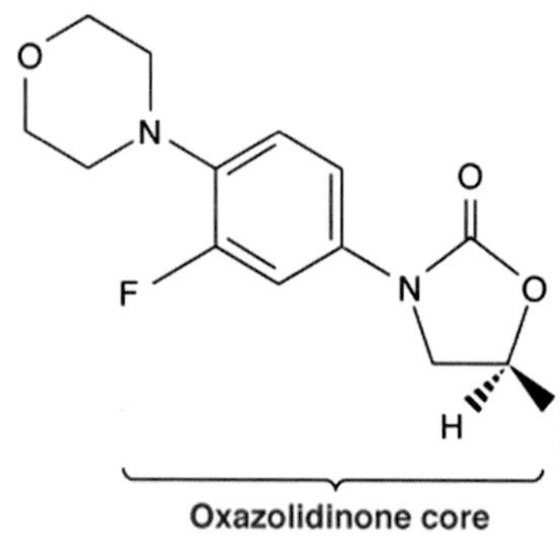

The in vitro activity and clinical efficacy of linezolid in the treatment of infections caused by penicillin- and macrolide-resistant pneumococci, vancomycin-resistant enterococci (VRE), MRSA, and vancomycin-resistant *S. aureus* (VRSA) support a role for linezolid when other, better studied agents are not available or are not tolerated. The most common current clinical use of linezolid in children is for the treatment of MRSA causing skin or respiratory tract infections.[139] Little data other than case reports are available for the use of linezolid in the treatment of bone and joint infections.[140]

Figure 23.5 Structure of linezolid. (Reprinted with permission from Hauser AR. *Antibiotic basics for clinicians*. Philadelphia, PA: Wolters Kluwer Health, 2018. Fig. 6.10.)

Pharmacokinetic Properties

Data on the pharmacokinetics for both parenterally and orally administered linezolid are available in children, including premature neonates.[141] Linezolid is virtually 100% absorbed by the oral route, allowing equivalent mg/kg dosing interchange between intravenous and oral formulations. Linezolid is widely distributed to well-perfused tissues, including skin, bones, muscles, adipose tissues, extracellular lung fluid, and CSF.[142] In fact, linezolid achieves CSF exposure similar to plasma in children, independent of the degree of inflammation.[143] Plasma protein binding is low (i.e., roughly 31%). In healthy adults, the volume of distribution is 40 to 50 L. Pharmacokinetic studies in children suggest similar volume of distribution (0.61 to 0.81 L per kg) and maximum concentration (11 to 16.7 μg per mL).[144]

Linezolid is metabolized via oxidation of the morpholine ring, which results in two inactive carboxylic acid metabolites: aminoethoxy acetic acid (metabolite A) and hydroxyethyl glycine (metabolite B).[144] Metabolite A is presumed to be formed via an enzymatic pathway, whereas the formation of metabolite B is mediated by a nonenzymatic chemical oxidation mechanism in vitro. Approximately 30% of the dose appears unchanged in the urine, 40% as metabolite B, and 10% as metabolite A. The net renal clearance of linezolid is low and is suggestive of net renal tubular reabsorption. Virtually no linezolid appears in the feces as unchanged drug, and the metabolites present in the feces account for only 9% of the total dose.

Unlike volume of distribution, clearance of linezolid is dependent on age.[141] The clearance in preterm neonates ranges from 2 to 5.1 mL per min per kg.[144] The highest clearance of linezolid occurs in infants and children aged greater than 1 week to 11 years, leading to lower drug exposure (AUC) and a shorter elimination half-life in children compared with adults. In fact, reported clearances in infants (aged 28 days to 3 months) and children (aged 3 months to 11 years) are 5.4 and 3.8 L per min per kg, with elimination half-lives of 1.8 and 2.9 hours, respectively.[142] In adolescents, clearance decreases to 2.1 mL per min per kg, which is similar to adults. The half-life of linezolid in children ranges from 1.5 to 5.6 hours compared with 4.26 to 5.4 hours in adults.[144]

The pharmacokinetics of linezolid in patients with hepatic (excluding severe cases where data are unavailable) or renal impairment are unaltered.[144] However, accumulation of the two primary metabolites of linezolid may occur in patients with renal impairment, but the clinical significance is unclear.

Dose/Regimens

The dosing regimen recommended for infants to children up to 11 years old is 10 mg per kg intravenously or orally every 8 hours, with a maximum of 600 mg per dose.[19,121] For children aged 12 years and older, 600 mg every 12 hours is recommended. Although the dosing regimen does not change for most clinical indications, the duration varies from 10 to 14 days for pneumonia and SSTIs, up to 4 weeks for bone and joint infections.

Adverse Effects/Toxicity/Precautions

As a mild, nonselective MAO inhibitor, linezolid may induce hypertensive crisis. In adults, the concomitant use of MAO inhibitors or linezolid use within 2 weeks of taking an MAO inhibitor is contraindicated. In the early pediatric clinical trials of linezolid, there was a concern for hypertension owing to the effects of the antibiotic's MAO inhibiting mild activity. However, side effects of MAO inhibitor were not noted in any phase I to III pediatric trials, permitting children to remain on usual diets while receiving treatment.[145]

Prolonged use of linezolid has been associated with significant side effects, including hyperlactatemia, lactic and metabolic acidosis, reversible myelosuppression leading to thrombocytopenia and anemia, and optic or peripheral neuropathy.[146] As such, linezolid drug has a restricted use for up to 28 consecutive days by the FDA and the European Medicines Agency. Most of these adverse events may be related to linezolid's inhibition with mitochondrial function by reducing mitochondrial protein levels, activity, and mass as well as by potentially increasing the rate of apoptosis.[146,147]

In addition to the duration of therapy, myelosuppression (including neutropenia and thrombocytopenia) has been shown to be dose-dependent.[148] For linezolid-induced thrombocytopenia, it appears mechanistically to originate from the inhibition of the platelet formation and unlikely exacerbated by renal impairment.[149] As such, monitoring complete blood count (including platelets) should be considered before starting and during linezolid treatment, especially if the anticipated duration of therapy exceeds 14 days. In addition, pyridoxine (vitamin B_6) 50 mg orally once a day may reverse linezolid-associated cytopenias but not peripheral neuropathy.[150] Notably, prospective, comparative data in the pediatric FDA registration studies failed to demonstrate a significant difference in toxicity compared with other agents, including cefadroxil and vancomycin.

Peripheral neuropathy and optic neuritis with possible visual loss have been reported in children receiving linezolid, especially when the duration exceeded 28 days.[151] As such, excessively prolonged duration of linezolid use should be avoided, and signs of peripheral neuropathy (including pain, numbness, weakness, and paresthesias) and visual function should be monitored.

Linezolid should be used cautiously in patients with a history of a seizure disorder and those with diabetes mellitus on insulin or oral hypoglycemic therapy as linezolid may cause seizures and hypoglycemia, respectively. As linezolid oral suspension contains approximately 20 mg of phenylalanine per 5 mL of suspension, it (not reported with other formulations) should be used with caution in patients with phenylketonuria.[144]

Drug Interactions

Linezolid is not metabolized by the cytochrome P-450 system and does not induce this enzyme or compete with other drugs in P-450-mediated metabolism. However, as linezolid is a nonselective MAO inhibitor, concurrent use with another MAO inhibitor (e.g., phenelzine, selegiline, and rasagiline) and certain drugs (e.g., methylphenidate and pseudoephedrine) should be avoided to prevent a hypertensive crisis that is characterized by headache, hyperpyrexia, and hypertension. Furthermore, linezolid's MAO-A inhibitory activity increases the risk of serotonin syndrome (which is marked by hypertension, tachycardia, hyperthermia, myoclonus, and mental status changes) when used concurrently with serotonergic drugs (e.g., selective serotonin reuptake inhibitors-escitalopram and fluoxetine; tricyclic antidepressants, atomoxetine, codeine, sumatriptan, venlafaxine, and mirtazapine). These drugs should not be taken with linezolid or within 2 weeks after discontinuing linezolid.

Patients receiving linezolid should be advised to avoid foods containing a high tyramine content, including cheese, meat, fish, beans, avocados, and bitter orange. Tyramine is metabolized by MAO in the gut and may reach excessive systemic levels during the ingestion of MAO inhibitors, potentially leading to hypertensive crisis.

REFERENCES

1. McGuire J, Bunch RL, Anderson RC, et al. Ilotycin, a new antibiotic. *Antibiot Chemother (Northfield)* 1952;2:281–283.
2. Weber JM, Wierman CK, Hutchinson CR. Genetic analysis of erythromycin production in Streptomyces erythreus. *J Bacteriol* 1985;164:425–433.
3. Klein JO. History of macrolide use in pediatrics. *Pediatr Infect Dis J* 1997;16:427–431.
4. Schlunzen F, Zarivach R, Harms J, et al. Structural basis for the interaction of antibiotics with the peptidyl transferase centre in eubacteria. *Nature* 2001;413:814–821.
5. Tenson T, Lovmar M, Ehrenberg M. The mechanism of action of macrolides, lincosamides and streptogramin B reveals the nascent peptide exit path in the ribosome. *J Mol Biol* 2003;330:1005–1014.
6. Vazquez-Laslop N, Mankin AS. How macrolide antibiotics work. *Trends Biochem Sci* 2018;43:668–684.
7. Leclercq R. Mechanisms of resistance to macrolides and lincosamides: nature of the resistance elements and their clinical implications. *Clin Infect Dis* 2002;34:482–492.
8. Horaud T, Le Bouguenec C, Pepper K. Molecular genetics of resistance to macrolides, lincosamides and streptogramin B (MLS) in streptococci. *J Antimicrob Chemother* 1985;16:111–135.
9. Novick RP, Murphy E. MLS-resistance determinants in *Staphylococcus aureus* and their molecular evolution. *J Antimicrob Chemother* 1985;16:101–110.
10. Tait-Kamradt A, Clancy J, Cronan M, et al. mefE is necessary for the erythromycin-resistant M phenotype in *Streptococcus pneumoniae. Antimicrob Agents Chemother* 1997;41:2251–2255.
11. Eady EA, Ross JI, Tipper JL, et al. Distribution of genes encoding erythromycin ribosomal methylases and an erythromycin efflux pump in epidemiologically distinct groups of staphylococci. *J Antimicrob Chemother* 1993;31:211–217.
12. Clancy J, Petitpas J, Dib-Hajj F, et al. Molecular cloning and functional analysis of a novel macrolide-resistance determinant, mefA, from *Streptococcus pyogenes. Mol Microbiol* 1996;22:867–879.
13. Washington JA, Wilson WR. Erythromycin: a microbial and clinical perspective after 30 years of clinical use (first of two parts). *Mayo Clin Proc* 1985;60:189–203.
14. Roblin PM, Montalban G, Hammerschlag MR. Susceptibilities to clarithromycin and erythromycin of isolates of *Chlamydia pneumoniae* from children with pneumonia. *Antimicrob Agents Chemother* 1994;38:1588–1589.
15. Kirst HA. New macrolides: expanded horizons for an old class of antibiotics. *J Antimicrob Chemother* 1991;28:787–790.
16. Shendurnikar N. Erythromycin. *Indian Pediatr* 1988;25:780–783.
17. Eberly MD, Eide MB, Thompson JL, et al. Azithromycin in early infancy and pyloric stenosis. *Pediatrics* 2015;135:483–488.
18. American Academy of Pediatrics. Pertussis. In: Pickering LK, ed. *Red book: 2003 report of the committee on infectious diseases*, 26th ed. Elk Grove, IL: American Academy of Pediatrics, 2003:472–486.
19. Bradley JS, Byington CL, Shah SS, et al. The management of community-acquired pneumonia in infants and children older than 3 months of age: clinical practice guidelines by the Pediatric Infectious Diseases Society and the Infectious Diseases Society of America. *Clin Infect Dis* 2011;53:e25–e76.
20. Atmar RL, Greenberg SB. Pneumonia caused by *Mycoplasma pneumoniae* and the TWAR agent. *Semin Respir Infect* 1989;4:19–31.

21. Bell TA. *Chlamydia trachomatis, Mycoplasma hominis,* and *Ureaplasma urealyticum* infections of infants. *Semin Perinatol* 1985;9:29–37.
22. American Academy of Pediatrics. *Ureaplasma urealyticum* and *Ureaplasma parvum* Infections. In: Kimberlin DW, Brady MT, Jackson MA, Long SS, eds. *Red book: 2018 report of the committee on infectious diseases.* Elk Grove, IL: American Academy of Pediatrics, 2018: 867–869.
23. Rettig PJ. Chlamydial infections in pediatrics. *Pediatr Infect Dis J* 1986;5:158–162.
24. Keys TF. Therapeutic considerations in the treatment of Legionella infections. *Semin Respir Infect* 1987;2:270–273.
25. Kirkpatrick BD, Tribble DR. Update on human *Campylobacter jejuni* infections. *Curr Opin Gastroenterol* 2011;27:1–7.
26. Leibovici-Weissman Y, Neuberger A, Bitterman R, et al. Antimicrobial drugs for treating cholera. *Cochrane Database Syst Rev* 2014:CD008625.
27. Gerber MA. Antibiotic resistance in group a streptococci. *Pediatr Clin North Am* 1995;42:539–551.
28. Berger BW. Lyme disease. *Semin Dermatol* 1993;12:357–362.
29. Guay DR. Macrolide antibiotics in paediatric infectious diseases. *Drugs* 1996;51:515–536.
30. Farrar HC, Walsh-Sukys MC, Kyllonen K, et al. Cardiac toxicity associated with intravenous erythromycin lactobionate. *Pediatr Infect Dis J* 1993;12:688–691.
31. Waites KB, Sims PJ, Crouse DT, et al. Serum concentrations of erythromycin after intravenous infusion in preterm neonates treated for Ureaplasma urealyticum infection. *Pediatr Infect Dis J* 1994;13:287–293.
32. Bass JW, Steele RW, Wiebe RA, et al. Erythromycin concentrations in middle ear exudates. *Pediatrics* 1971;48:417–422.
33. Ginsburg CM, McCracken GH Jr, Culbertson MC Jr. Concentrations of erythromycin in serum and tonsil: comparison of the estolate and ethyl succinate suspensions. *J Pediatr* 1976;89:1011–1013.
34. Ishiguro M, Koga H, Kohno S, et al. Penetration of macrolides into human polymorphonuclear leucocytes. *J Antimicrob Chemother* 1989;24:719–729.
35. van den Broek PJ. Antimicrobial drugs, microorganisms, and phagocytes. *Clin Infect Dis* 1989;11:213–245.
36. Butler DR, Kuhn RJ, Chandler MH. Pharmacokinetics of anti-infective agents in paediatric patients. *Clin Pharmacokinet* 1994;26:374–395.
37. Paap CM, Nahata MC. Clinical pharmacokinetics of antibacterial drugs in neonates. *Clin Pharmacokinet* 1990;19:280–318.
38. Philipson A, Sabath LD, Charles D. Transplacental passage of erythromycin and clindamycin. *N Engl J Med* 1973;288:1219–1221.
39. Kirst HA, Sides GD. New directions for macrolide antibiotics: pharmacokinetics and clinical efficacy. *Antimicrob Agents Chemother* 1989;33:1419–1422.
40. Nilsen OG. Comparative pharmacokinetics of macrolides. *J Antimicrob Chemother* 1987;20:81–88.
41. Eichenwald HF. Adverse reactions to erythromycin. *Pediatr Infect Dis J* 1986;5:147–150.
42. Periti P, Mazzei T, Mini E, et al. Adverse effects of macrolide antibacterials. *Drug Saf* 1993;9:346–364.
43. Cooper WO, Griffin MR, Arbogast P, et al. Very early exposure to erythromycin and infantile hypertrophic pyloric stenosis. *Arch Pediatr Adolesc Med* 2002;156:647.
44. Itoh Z. Motilin and clinical application. *Peptides* 1997;18:593–608.
45. Brummett RE. Ototoxic liability of erythromycin and analogues. *Otolaryngol Clin North Am* 1993;26:811–819.
46. Ludden TM. Pharmacokinetic interactions of the macrolide antibiotics. *Clin Pharmacokinet* 1985;10:63–79.
47. Honig PK, Smith JE, Wortham DC, et al. Population variability in the pharmacokinetics of terfenadine: the case for a pseudo-polymorphism with clinical implications. *Drug Metabol Drug Interact* 1994;11:161–168.
48. Upton RA. Pharmacokinetic interactions between theophylline and other medication (Part I). *Clin Pharmacokinet* 1991;20:66–80.
49. Yee GC, McGuire TR. Pharmacokinetic drug interactions with cyclosporin (Part I). *Clin Pharmacokinet* 1990;19:319–332.
50. Rodin SM, Johnson BF. Pharmacokinetic interactions with digoxin. *Clin Pharmacokinet* 1988;15:227–244.
51. Rodvold KA, Piscitelli SC. New oral macrolide and fluoroquinolone antibiotics: an overview of pharmacokinetics, interactions, and safety. *Clin Infect Dis* 1993;17:S192–S199.
52. Matzneller P, Krasniqi S, Kinzig M, et al. Blood, tissue, and intracellular concentrations of azithromycin during and after end of therapy. *Antimicrob Agents Chemother* 2013;57:1736–1742.
53. Hammerschlag MR. Azithromycin and clarithromycin. *Pediatr Ann* 1993;22:160–166.
54. Langtry HD, Balfour JA. Azithromycin. *Drugs* 1998;56:273–297.
55. Peters DH, Friedel HA, McTavish D. Azithromycin. *Drugs* 1992;44:750–799.
56. Hatzenbuehler LA, Starke JR. Common presentations of nontuberculous mycobacterial infections. *Pediatr Infect Dis J* 2014;33:89–91.
57. Alos JI. Significant increase in the prevalence of erythromycin-resistant, clindamycin-and miocamycin-susceptible (M phenotype) *Streptococcus pyogenes* in Spain. *J Antimicrob Chemother* 2003;51:333–337.
58. Neu HC. Clinical microbiology of azithromycin. *Am J Med* 1991;91:S12–S18.
59. Hammerschlag MR, Qumei KK, Roblin PM. In vitro activities of azithromycin, clarithromycin, L-ofloxacin, and other antibiotics against *Chlamydia pneumoniae. Antimicrob Agents Chemother* 1992;36:1573–1574.
60. Brown BA, Wallace RJ, Onyi GO, et al. Activities of four macrolides, including clarithromycin, against *Mycobacterium fortuitum, Mycobacterium chelonae,* and *M. chelonae*-like organisms. *Antimicrob Agents Chemother* 1992;36:180–184.
61. Wolfson C, Branley J, Gottlieb T. The Etest for antimicrobial susceptibility testing of *Bartonella henselae. J Antimicrob Chemother* 1996;38:963–968.
62. Still JG. Management of pediatric patients with group A beta-hemolytic Streptococcus pharyngitis. *Pediatr Infect Dis J* 1995;14:S57–S61.
63. Dagan R, Johnson CE, McLinn S, et al. Bacteriologic and clinical efficacy of amoxicillin/clavulanate vs. azithromycin in acute otitis media. *Pediatr Infect Dis J* 2000;19:95–104.
64. Harris JA, Kolokathis A, Campbell M, et al. Safety and efficacy of azithromycin in the treatment of community-acquired pneumonia in children. *Pediatr Infect Dis J* 1998;17:865–871.
65. American Academy of Pediatrics. Safety and efficacy of azithromycin in the treatment of community-acquired pneumonia in children. In: Pickering LK, ed. *Red book: 2009 report of the committee on infectious diseases,* 28th ed. Elk Grove, IL: American Academy of Pediatrics, 2009:255–259.
66. Montero L. A comparative study of the efficacy, safety and tolerability of azithromycin and cefaclor in the treatment of children with acute skin and/or soft tissue infections. *J Antimicrob Chemother* 1996;37:125–131.
67. American Academy of Pediatrics. Pertussis (whooping cough). In: Pickering LK, ed. *Red book: 2009 report of the committee on infectious diseases,* 28th ed. Elk Grove, IL: American Academy of Pediatrics, 2009:504–519.
68. Baće A, Zrnić T, Begovac J, et al. Short-term treatment of pertussis with azithromycin in infants and young children. *Eur J Clin Microbiol Infect Dis* 1999;18:296–298.
69. Griffith DE. Risk-benefit assessment of therapies for *Mycobacterium avium* complex infections. *Drug Saf* 1999;21:137–152.
70. Wolinsky E. Mycobacterial lymphadenitis in children: a prospective study of 105 nontuberculous cases with long-term follow-up. *Clin Infect Dis* 1995;20:954–963.
71. Pacifico L, Chiesa C. Azithromycin in children: a critical review of the evidence. *Curr Ther Res* 2002;63:54–76.
72. Panel on Opportunistic Infections in HIV-Exposed and HIV-Infected Children. Guidelines for the prevention and treatment of opportunistic infections in HIV-exposed and HIV-infected children. Department of Health and Human Services. http://aidsinfo.nih.gov/contentfiles/lvguidelines/oi_guidelines_pediatrics.pdf. Accessed May 31, 2019.
73. Bass JW, Freitas BC, Freitas AD, et al. Prospective randomized double blind placebo-controlled evaluation of azithromycin for treatment of cat-scratch disease. *Pediatr Infect Dis J* 1998;17:447–452.
74. Conrad DA. Treatment of cat-scratch disease. *Curr Opin Pediatr* 2001;13:56–59.
75. Edelstein PH. Antimicrobial chemotherapy for legionnaires' disease: a review. *Clin Infect Dis* 1995;21:S265–S276.
76. Klein NC, Cunha BA. Treatment of legionnaires' disease. *Semin Respir Infect* 1998;13:140–146.
77. Jacobs RF, Maples HD, Aranda JV, et al. Pharmacokinetics of intravenously administered azithromycin in pediatric patients. *Pediatr Infect Dis J* 2005;24:34–39.
78. Martin DH, Mroczkowski TF, Dalu ZA, et al. A controlled trial of a single dose of azithromycin for the treatment of chlamydial urethritis and cervicitis. *N Engl J Med* 1992;327: 921–925.
79. Thylefors B, Negrel AD, Pararajasegaram R, et al. Global data on blindness. *Bull World Health Organ* 1995;73:115–121.
80. Shane AL, Mody RK, Crump JA, et al. 2017 Infectious Diseases Society of America clinical practice guidelines for the diagnosis and management of infectious diarrhea. *Clin Infect Dis* 2017;65:1963–1973.
81. Girgis NI, Butler T, Frenck RW, et al. Azithromycin versus ciprofloxacin for treatment of uncomplicated typhoid fever in a randomized trial in Egypt that included patients with multidrug resistance. *Antimicrob Agents Chemother* 1999;43:1441–1444.
82. Frenck RW, Nakhla I, Sultan Y, et al. Azithromycin versus ceftriaxone for the treatment of uncomplicated typhoid fever in children. *Clin Infect Dis* 2000;31:1134–1138.
83. Workowski KA. Centers for disease control and prevention sexually transmitted diseases treatment guidelines. *Clin Infect Dis* 2015;61(Suppl 8):S759–S762.
84. Mogayzel PJ Jr, Naureckas ET, Robinson KA, et al. Cystic fibrosis pulmonary guidelines. Chronic medications for maintenance of lung health. *Am J Respir Crit Care Med* 2013;187:680–689.
85. Buyck JM, Plesiat P, Traore H, et al. Increased susceptibility of Pseudomonas aeruginosa to macrolides and ketolides in eukaryotic cell culture media and biological fluids due to decreased expression of oprM and increased outer-membrane permeability. *Clin Infect Dis* 2012;55:534–542.
86. Wilson W, Taubert KA, Gewitz M, et al. Prevention of infective endocarditis: guidelines from the American Heart Association: a guideline from the American Heart Association Rheumatic Fever, Endocarditis, and Kawasaki Disease Committee, Council on Cardiovascular Disease in the Young, and the Council on Clinical Cardiology, Council on Cardiovascular Surgery and Anesthesia, and the Quality of Care and Outcomes Research Interdisciplinary Working Group. *Circulation* 2007;116:1736–1754.
87. Dionisio D, Orsi A, Sterrantino G, et al. Chronic cryptosporidiosis in patients with AIDS: stable remission and possible eradication after long-term, low dose azithromycin. *J Clin Pathol* 1998;51:138–142.
88. Blanshard C, Shanson DC, Gazzard BG. Pilot studies of azithromycin, letrazuril and paromomycin in the treatment of cryptosporidiosis. *Int J STD AIDS* 1997;8:124–129.
89. Nahata MC, Koranyi KI, Luke DR, et al. Pharmacokinetics of azithromycin in pediatric patients with acute otitis media. *Antimicrob Agents Chemother* 1995;39:1875–1877.
90. Nightingale CH. Pharmacokinetics and pharmacodynamics of newer macrolides. *Pediatr Infect Dis J* 1997;16:438–443.
91. Pukander J, Rautianen M. Penetration of azithromycin into middle ear effusions in acute and secretory otitis media in children. *J Antimicrob Chemother* 1996;37:53–61.
92. Vaudaux BP, Cherpillod J, Dayer P. Concentrations of azithromycin in tonsilar and/or adenoid tissue from paediatric patients. *J Antimicrob Chemother* 1996;37(Suppl C):45–51.
93. Gladue RP, Bright GM, Isaacson RE, et al. In vitro and in vivo uptake of azithromycin (CP-62,993) by phagocytic cells: possible mechanism of delivery and release at sites of infection. *Antimicrob Agents Chemother* 1989;33:277–282.
94. Sifrim D, Matsuo H, Janssens J, et al. Comparison of the effects of midecamycin acetate and azithromycin on gastrointestinal motility in man. *Drugs Exp Clin Res* 1994;20:121–126.
95. Treadway G, Pontani D. Paediatric safety of azithromycin: worldwide experience. *J Antimicrob Chemother* 1996;37:143–149.
96. Wondrack L, Massa M, Yang BV, et al. Clinical strain of *Staphylococcus aureus* inactivates and causes efflux of macrolides. *Antimicrob Agents Chemother* 1996;40:992–998.

97. Wiedermann BL. Macrolides: clarithromycin and azithromycin. *Pediatr Rev* 1998;19:238–239.
98. Neu HC. The development of macrolides: clarithromycin in perspective. *J Antimicrob Chemother* 1991;27:1–9.
99. McCracken GH Jr. Microbiologic activity of the newer macrolide antibiotics. *Pediatr Infect Dis J* 1997;16:432–437.
100. Ferrero JL, Bopp BA, Marsh KC, et al. Metabolism and disposition of clarithromycin in man. *Drug Metab Dispos* 1990;18:441–446.
101. Peters DH, Clissold SP. Clarithromycin. *Drugs* 1992;44:117–164.
102. Gunawan H, Sasmojo M, Putri HE, et al. Clinical pilot study: clarithromycin efficacy in multibacillary leprosy therapy. *Int J Mycobacteriol* 2018;7:152–155.
103. Derouin F, Chastang C. Activity in vitro against *Toxoplasma gondii* of azithromycin and clarithromycin alone and with pyrimethamine. *J Antimicrob Chemother* 1990;25:708–711.
104. Still GJ, Hubbard WC, Poole JM, et al. Comparison of clarithromycin and penicillin VK suspensions in the treatment of children with streptococcal pharyngitis and review of currently available alternative antibiotic therapies. *Pediatr Infect Dis J* 1993;12:S134–S141.
105. Pukander JS, Jero JP, Kaprio EA, et al. Clarithromycin vs. amoxicillin suspensions in the treatment of pediatric patients with acute otitis media. *Pediatr Infect Dis J* 1993;12:S118–S121.
106. Aspin MM, Hoberman A, McCarty J, et al. Comparative study of the safety and efficacy of clarithromycin and amoxicillin-clavulanate in the treatment of acute otitis media in children. *J Pediatr* 1994;125:136–141.
107. Arguedas A, Loaiza C, Rodriguez F, et al. Comparative trial of 3 days of azithromycin versus 10 days of clarithromycin in the treatment of children with acute otitis media with effusion. *J Chemother* 1997;9:44–50.
108. Gooch MW, Gan VN, Corder TW, et al. Clarithromycin and cefaclor suspensions in the treatment of acute otitis media in children. *Pediatr Infect Dis J* 1993;12:S128–S133.
109. Block S, Hedrick J, Hammerschlag MR, et al. Mycoplasma pneumoniae and Chlamydia pneumoniae in pediatric community-acquired pneumonia. *Pediatr Infect Dis J* 1995;14:471–477.
110. Jones NL, Koletzko S, Goodman K, et al. Joint ESPGHAN/NASPGHAN guidelines for the management of Helicobacter pylori in children and adolescents (update 2016). *J Pediatr Gastroenterol Nutr* 2017;64:991–1003.
111. Zimmermann P, Curtis N, Tebruegge M. Nontuberculous mycobacterial disease in childhood - update on diagnostic approaches and treatment. *J Infect* 2017;74(Suppl 1):S136–S142.
112. Gan VN, McCarty JM, Chu S-Y, et al. Penetration of clarithromycin into middle ear fluid of children with acute otitis media. *Pediatr Infect Dis J* 1997;16:39–43.
113. Fraschini F, Scaglione F, Pintucci G, et al. The diffusion of clarithromycin and roxithromycin into nasal mucosa, tonsil and lung in humans. *J Antimicrob Chemother* 1991;27:61–65.
114. Fish DN, Gotfried MH, Danziger LH, et al. Penetration of clarithromycin into lung tissues from patients undergoing lung resection. *Antimicrob Agents Chemother* 1994;38:876–878.
115. Craft CJ, Siepman N. Overview of the safety profile of clarithromycin suspension in pediatric patients. *Pediatr Infect Dis J* 1993;12:S142–S147.
116. Dautzenberg B, Truffot C, Legris S, et al. Activity of clarithromycin against *Mycobacterium avium* infection in patients with the acquired immune deficiency syndrome: a controlled clinical trial. *Am Rev Respir Dis* 1991;144:564–569.
117. Tinel M, Descatoire V, Larrey D, et al. Effects of clarithromycin on cytochrome P-450. Comparison with other macrolides. *J Pharmacol Exp Ther* 1989;250:746–751.
118. Wallace RJ, Brown BA, Griffith DE, et al. Reduced serum levels of clarithromycin in patients treated with multi-drug regimens including rifampin or rifabutin for *Mycobacterium avium*-M. Intracellulare infection. *J Infect Dis* 1995;171:747–750.
119. Spizek J, Rezanka T. Lincosamides: chemical structure, biosynthesis, mechanism of action, resistance, and applications. *Biochem Pharmacol* 2017;133:20–28.
120. Snydman DR, Jacobus NV, McDermott LA, et al. Trends in antimicrobial resistance among Bacteroides species and Parabacteroides species in the United States from 2010–2012 with comparison to 2008–2009. *Anaerobe* 2017;43:21–26.
121. Liu C, Bayer A, Cosgrove SE, et al. Clinical practice guidelines by the infectious diseases society of america for the treatment of methicillin-resistant *Staphylococcus aureus* infections in adults and children. *Clin Infect Dis* 2011;52:e18–e55.
122. Miller LG, Daum RS, Creech CB, et al. Clindamycin versus trimethoprim-sulfamethoxazole for uncomplicated skin infections. *N Engl J Med* 2015;372:1093–1103.
123. Hulten KG, Kaplan SL, Gonzalez BE, et al. Three-year surveillance of community onset health care-associated *Staphylococcus aureus* infections in children. *Pediatr Infect Dis J* 2006;25:349–353.
124. Solomkin JS, Mazuski JE, Bradley JS, et al. Diagnosis and management of complicated intra-abdominal infection in adults and children: guidelines by the Surgical Infection Society and the Infectious Diseases Society of America. *Clin Infect Dis* 2010;50:133–164.
125. Stevens DL, Bisno AL, Chambers HF, et al. Practice guidelines for the diagnosis and management of skin and soft tissue infections: 2014 update by the infectious diseases society of America. *Clin Infect Dis* 2014;59:147–159.
126. Cleocin (clindamycin) package insert. New York, NY: Pharmacia and Upjohn Co, 2019.
127. DeHaan RM, Metzler CM, Schellenberg D, et al. Pharmacokinetic studies of clindamycin phosphate. *J Clin Pharmacol* 1973;13:190–209.
128. Bradley JS, Peacock G, Krug SE, et al. Pediatric anthrax clinical management: executive summary. *Pediatrics* 2014;133:940–942.
129. Adams DJ, Eberly MD, Rajnik M, et al. Risk factors for community-associated clostridium difficile infection in children. *J Pediatr* 2017;186:105–109.
130. Thurnheer R, Laube I, Speich R. Possible interaction between clindamycin and cyclosporin. *BMJ* 1999;319:163.
131. Curis E, Pestre V, Jullien V, et al. Pharmacokinetic variability of clindamycin and influence of rifampicin on clindamycin concentration in patients with bone and joint infections. *Infection* 2015;43:473–481.
132. Wilson DN. On the specificity of antibiotics targeting the large ribosomal subunit. *Ann N Y Acad Sci* 2011;1241:1–16.
133. Long KS, Vester B. Resistance to linezolid caused by modifications at its binding site on the ribosome. *Antimicrob Agents Chemother* 2012;56:603–612.
134. Mendes RE, Deshpande LM, Jones RN. Linezolid update: stable in vitro activity following more than a decade of clinical use and summary of associated resistance mechanisms. *Drug Resist Updat* 2014;17:1–12.
135. Kaplan SL. Use of linezolid in children. *Pediatr Infect Dis J* 2002;21:870–872.
136. Leach KL, Brickner SJ, Noe MC, et al. Linezolid, the first oxazolidinone antibacterial agent. *Ann N Y Acad Sci* 2011;1222:49–54.
137. Nemeth J, Oesch G, Kuster SP. Bacteriostatic versus bactericidal antibiotics for patients with serious bacterial infections: systematic review and meta-analysis. *J Antimicrob Chemother* 2015;70:382–395.
138. Wunderink RG. How important is methicillin-resistant Staphylococcus aureus as a cause of community-acquired pneumonia and what is best antimicrobial therapy? *Infect Dis Clin North Am* 2013;27:177–188.
139. Dotis J, Iosifidis E, Ioannidou M, et al. Use of linezolid in pediatrics: a critical review. *Int J Infect Dis* 2010;14:e638–e648.
140. Chen CJ, Chiu CH, Lin TY, et al. Experience with linezolid therapy in children with osteoarticular infections. *Pediatr Infect Dis J* 2007;26:985–988.
141. Jungbluth GL, Welshman IR, Hopkins NK. Linezolid pharmacokinetics in pediatric patients: an overview. *Pediatr Infect Dis J* 2003;22:S153–S157.
142. Velissariou IM. Use of linezolid in children: an overview of recent advances. *Expert Rev Anti Infect Ther* 2006;4:947–952.
143. Yogev R, Damle B, Levy G, et al. Pharmacokinetics and distribution of linezolid in cerebrospinal fluid in children and adolescents. *Pediatr Infect Dis J* 2010;29:827–830.
144. Zyvox (linezolid) package insert. New York, NY: Pharmacia & Upjohn Company, 2019.
145. Saiman L, Goldfarb J, Kaplan SA, et al. Safety and tolerability of linezolid in children. *Pediatr Infect Dis J* 2003;22:S193–S200.
146. Su E, Crowley K, Carcillo JA, et al. Linezolid and lactic acidosis: a role for lactate monitoring with long-term linezolid use in children. *Pediatr Infect Dis J* 2011;30:804–806.
147. Garrabou G, Soriano A, Pinos T, et al. Influence of mitochondrial genetics on the mitochondrial toxicity of linezolid in blood cells and skin nerve fibers. *Antimicrob Agents Chemother* 2017;61.
148. Moellering RC. Linezolid: the first oxazolidinone antimicrobial. *Ann Intern Med* 2003;138:135–142.
149. Tsuji Y, Holford NHG, Kasai H, et al. Population pharmacokinetics and pharmacodynamics of linezolid-induced thrombocytopenia in hospitalized patients. *Br J Clin Pharmacol* 2017;83:1758–1772.
150. Spellberg B, Yoo T, Bayer AS. Reversal of linezolid-associated cytopenias, but not peripheral neuropathy, by administration of vitamin B6. *J Antimicrob Chemother* 2004;54:832–835.
151. Nambiar S, Rellosa N, Wassel RT, et al. Linezolid-associated peripheral and optic neuropathy in children. *Pediatrics* 2011;127:e1528–e1532.

CHAPTER

24

Stephan A. Kohlhoff

Fluoroquinolones

BACKGROUND

Since the introduction of the first quinolone nalidixic acid in 1964, which is no longer available, there has been a long history of safety concerns due to early experimental toxicities with hesitation to use drugs of this class in neonates and children. These concerns have limited the implementation of clinical trials evaluating older and newer drugs in the class. However, owing to the broad-spectrum antibacterial activity and favorable pharmacokinetics of fluoroquinolones, the derivatives of nalidixic acid, ciprofloxacin in particular, and other newer fluoroquinolones have been used for decades in the pediatric and neonatal population for some indications despite the lack of prospective studies in these age groups. The fluoroquinolones are rapidly bactericidal, and many have an extended antimicrobial spectrum that includes *Pseudomonas*, Gram-positive cocci, and intracellular pathogens. Their pharmacokinetic properties include good absorption from the gastrointestinal tract, excellent penetration into many tissues, and good intracellular diffusion.

The use of fluoroquinolones in children has been limited because of their potential to induce arthropathy in juvenile animals.[1–4] This extraordinary form of age-related drug toxicity has been shown with all the fluoroquinolones tested so far and has led to important restrictions: For a long time, their use has been considered to be contraindicated in children, in growing adolescents, and in women during pregnancy and lactation.

However, the experience over several decades of fluoroquinolone use in pediatric patients demonstrated their effectiveness and did not reveal evidence of arthropathy, bone abnormalities, or other serious adverse events.[5] In the United States, the two fluoroquinolones currently approved for use in children by the U.S. Food and Drug Administration (FDA) are ciprofloxacin and levofloxacin.[6,7] Since the initial approval for these drugs, despite some rare adverse events, drug safety monitoring confirmed that they are generally well tolerated; the most frequent adverse events during treatment are gastrointestinal disturbances, reactions of the central nervous system, and skin reactions.[1,8]

Neither one of the fluoroquinolones approved for pediatric patients has an indication for neonates, but for the abovementioned reasons their use in this age group becomes necessary in certain situations. Owing to the lack of human studies, the early use in neonates was based on extrapolation from data in older children and adults or data from case studies. Surveys of neonatal intensive care units in Europe demonstrated that while quinolones were widely prescribed, there was also variability in frequency of use, indications for usage, and the specific dosing for premature neonates.[9,10] This variability in the use of the drug in neonates can be explained by the lack of dosing recommendations in national guidelines due to limited pharmacokinetic and clinical data. Moreover, a major concern regarding the use of fluoroquinolones in neonates and children is the potential impact on bacterial resistance development.[5]

MECHANISM OF ACTION AND ANTIBACTERIAL SPECTRUM

Quinolones inhibit bacterial cell replication, transcription, and DNA repair by targeting the enzymatic activities of DNA gyrase and topoisomerase IV.[11] By binding to the enzyme–DNA complex, fluoroquinolones cause a conformational change in the enzyme, which leads to cleavage of the DNA and inhibition of DNA synthesis. All quinolones have excellent activity against Gram-negative bacteria, particularly Enterobacteriaceae, *Haemophilus* spp., *Moraxella catarrhalis*, and *Neisseria* spp. They also have activity against many strains of *Pseudomonas aeruginosa* and methicillin-susceptible *Staphylococcus aureus*, but weak activity against methicillin-resistant *S. aureus* and coagulase-negative staphylococci. Ciprofloxacin is the most potent available fluoroquinolone against Gram-negative pathogens. Levofloxacin, gatifloxacin, moxifloxacin, and gemifloxacin are more active against Gram-positive organisms, including *Streptococcus pneumoniae*. Atypical pathogens, including *Mycoplasma* spp., *Chlamydia* spp., *Legionella* spp., and *Ureaplasma urealyticum*, are susceptible to fluoroquinolones. The early fluoroquinolones had limited activity against anaerobes; however, the new compounds (e.g., moxifloxacin and gatifloxacin) have improved anaerobic activity. Of the two fluoroquinolones approved for pediatric patients, levofloxacin has better anaerobic activity compared with ciprofloxacin with many pathogens recovered from intra-abdominal infections inhibited by the drug at achievable levels.[12] They also have activity against mycobacteria and excellent intracellular penetration.

The author would like to acknowledge Dr. Urs B. Schaad's contributions to the previous edition.

MECHANISMS OF RESISTANCE

As mentioned above, there is a great concern regarding the potential impact of widespread fluoroquinolone use in children on the development of bacterial resistance.[13–16] Historically, antimicrobial use led to the development of drug resistance. The relevant drivers are overuse (volume of antibiotic used in humans and in animals), misuse (inappropriate use), clonal spread (global travel, hygiene, hospital, daycare, family, and switch of serotypes), and type of antibiotic. Overuse (e.g., for viral infection, as prophylaxis, many veterinarian indications) reflects inadequate knowledge of the prescribing physician and unavailability of diagnostic methods. Appropriate use (avoidance of misuse) includes not only the selection of an optimal antibiotic but also the individual optimization of dosage and duration of therapy based on clinical diagnosis and identified pathogen. Well-defined antibiotic policies, good hygiene measures, and strong infection control programs represent key points for limiting the spread of antibiotic resistance.

Bacterial resistance to fluoroquinolones is multifactorial and may result from a combination of mechanisms.[17] These include mutations in the target molecules (gyrase protein, topoisomerase), removal of drug by active drug efflux, and alteration of membrane porins.[18] With regard to quinolone resistance, great variations exist among bacterial species, clinical settings, and local epidemiology. In some cases, multidrug resistance occurs. *S. pneumoniae* is one of the most important respiratory pathogens, playing a major role in upper and lower respiratory tract infections in pediatric patients. Pneumococcal resistance to antimicrobials may be acquired by horizontal transfer followed by homologous recombination of genetic material from the normal flora of the human oral cavity or by means of mutation. Resistance of pneumococci to penicillins and macrolides has been increasing for some time, but more recently, fluoroquinolone resistance has become more prevalent as well with the increasing use of this drug class.[19,20] Fluoroquinolone resistance has been documented in many other pathogens, including Gram-negative and Gram-positive bacteria responsible for urinary, respiratory, gastrointestinal tract, and bloodstream infections; skin and soft-tissue infections and bone and joint infections; and sexually transmitted infections.[13,14]

Evidence is accumulating that multidrug resistance in pneumococci is related to the prescription of antimicrobial agents to a crucial reservoir of these organisms—children. This multidrug resistance likely occurs because children, more often than adults, are colonized with high-density populations of pneumococci in the nasopharynx, which increases the potential for resistance development.[13] Overcrowding facilitates the transmission of resistance strains from colonized to susceptible infants and children, who serve as a source for further transmission to family members and ultimately to the general population.[21] However, in a pediatric study of levofloxacin for acute otitis media, there was no emergence of levofloxacin-resistant pneumococci seen at the end of treatment.[22] Larger pediatric and neonatal studies are needed to fully understand the emergence and epidemiology of fluoroquinolone-induced resistance in these populations. A new concern about the widespread use of fluoroquinolones to treat children and adults is the recognition of horizontal transfer of fluoroquinolone resistance from viridans group streptococci (e.g., *Streptococcus oralis* and *Streptococcus mitis*) to *S. pneumoniae*.[23,24] The dangerous triad of antibiotic overuse and misuse, a reservoir of resistant genes, and a closed-space infection could result from the widespread, uncontrolled use of fluoroquinolones in the pediatric population.

PHARMACOLOGY

The pharmacokinetic data on fluoroquinolones in neonatal and pediatric patients are limited. The results of early studies, many of which were conducted in cystic fibrosis patients, indicate that systemic clearance is increased in young children; this has led to recommendations for relatively high doses.[25–29] In general, fluoroquinolones are absorbed rapidly from the gastrointestinal tract. The range for bioavailability is vast, however, with norfloxacin being 10% to 30%, ciprofloxacin 60% to 80%, and levofloxacin 99%. All of the newer compounds except norfloxacin have excellent tissue and intracellular penetration at the recommended therapeutic doses. Concentrations of fluoroquinolones in bile, lung, and urine are higher than in serum, whereas concentrations in saliva, bone, and cerebrospinal fluid (CSF) are usually lower than in serum. However, CSF concentrations are sufficient and clinically useful for the treatment of meningitis caused by many highly resistant Gram-negative organisms. Fluoroquinolones generally are excreted either predominantly in the urine (often as a parent compound) or through the bile, in which some undergo enterohepatic recirculation. They are not highly protein-bound, and drug–drug interactions are not a major concern for their use. Two important, clinically relevant drug interactions are the potential for subtherapeutic fluoroquinolone levels with coadministration of antacids and concomitant use with warfarin leading to supratherapeutic levels.[30]

Fluoroquinolones kill via concentration-dependent killing and postantibiotic effect. The ratio of the 24-hour area under the curve (AUC24) over the minimum inhibitory concentration (MIC) seems to be the most appropriate pharmacodynamic parameter for ciprofloxacin to predict good microbiologic and clinical outcomes.[31]

The difficulty in carrying out pharmacokinetic studies in neonates including premature infants combined with safety concerns is part of the reason for the lack of guidance for quinolone dosing in this age group. Early studies of ciprofloxacin in neonates were limited by study designs (case reports), by small sample size, and by not addressing the current understanding of the ciprofloxacin pharmacokinetic–pharmacodynamic relationship. In a study by Aggarwal et al. using 10 mg per kg per dose twice daily for premature infants with sepsis, no differences in peak levels in relation to birth weight were observed with trough levels exceeding the MIC of the most common pathogens.[32]

Recently, the use of opportunistic blood samples has enabled or helped population pharmacokinetic studies.[33] A pharmacokinetic study using both planned and scavenged blood samples[34] from 60 newborns identified a two-compartment model with first-order elimination. In this study, Monte Carlo simulation demonstrated a dose of 7.5 mg per kg twice daily for newborns with a postmenstrual age (PMA) of less than 34 weeks and a dose of 12.5 mg per kg twice daily for those with a PMA of greater than or equal to 34 weeks.[34] Reduced renal clearance in neonates, especially in those with renal injury and decreased creatinine clearance, may result in higher systemic exposure.

Ciprofloxacin concentrations in CSF of neonates were determined only in case reports and deemed to be adequate for the treatment of select Gram-negative bacilli.[35,36] Based on the experience with treating tuberculous meningitis, fluoroquinolones particularly levofloxacin are considered effective drugs for the treatment of central nervous system infection owing to their excellent CSF penetration.[37]

ADVERSE EFFECTS AND TOXICITY

QUINOLONE ARTHROPATHY

Soon after the marketing of nalidixic acid in 1962, a child with soreness in one wrist during therapy for urinary tract infection was described.[38] Nalidixic acid was not initially contraindicated in children but was approved for use in children with urinary tract infections in March 1964. Eight years later, another report described a 22-year-old woman who developed severe polyarthritis during a second course of nalidixic acid.[39] These "incapacitating" cases of arthralgia/arthritis were considered as allergic manifestations. Data on file of the manufacturers were cited to contain "about a dozen such reports." These clinical observations with nalidixic acid prompted experimental exposure of laboratory animals to quinolone compounds. The first observations of quinolone-induced cartilage toxicity made with nalidixic, oxolinic, and pipemidic acid administration to young beagle dogs were reported by Ingham et al.,[40] Tatsumi et al.,[41] and Gough et al.[2] Four groups performed retrospective matched control search for cartilage toxicity in pediatric patients who had received nalidixic acid therapy, in most cases for acute or recurrent urinary tract infections.[42–45] History for symptoms and clinical/radiologic examinations compatible with possible arthropathies were recorded, and at follow-up, examination growth curves and functional and radiologic joint findings were obtained. The results were similar in the index and control cases. All reports concluded that nalidixic acid does not cause arthropathy in children, even after long-term and high-dose therapy.

ANIMAL EXPERIMENTS

All quinolones tested, including the older compounds and the newer derivatives, have been shown to induce changes in immature cartilage of weight-bearing joints in all laboratory animals tested (mice, rats, dogs, marmosets, guinea pigs, rabbits, and ferrets).[2,4,16,43,46,47] Quinolone-induced arthropathy is limited to juvenile animals, except when pefloxacin has been used. Juvenile dogs are generally more sensitive to the arthropathic effects of quinolones than are other species. Healing of quinolone-induced arthropathy is incomplete even after complete clinical recovery; structural changes are at least in part irreversible. Typical histopathologic lesions after quinolone exposure include fluid-filled blisters, fissures, erosions, and clustering of chondrocytes, usually accompanied by noninflammatory joint effusion. Under the electron microscope, necrosis of the chondrocytes and swelling of the mitochondria are observed initially, followed by the disruption of extracellular matrix.[46] Loss of collagen and glycosaminoglycan is an early sequela to the degeneration of chondrocytes.[47] When clinically manifested, the quinolone-induced joint lesions present as acute arthritis, including limping and swelling. The specific mechanism responsible for the initiation of quinolone-induced arthropathy has not been determined. At present, the inhibition of mitochondrial DNA replication[48] and the role of magnesium deficiency[49] are the most discussed hypotheses. There is no clear effect of the molecular structure of the given compound regarding its cartilage toxicity (e.g., quinolones that are fluorinated versus quinolones that are not fluorinated).

REVIEW OF PUBLISHED SAFETY DATA IN PEDIATRIC PATIENTS

A comprehensive review of published reports including monitoring for quinolone-induced cartilage toxicity in patients was performed.[8,50–63] The reviewed studies included all case reports of suspected quinolone-associated arthralgia/arthropathy in children and adolescents and all multipatient studies on the use of quinolone compounds in skeletally immature patients (open-label and controlled trials) in which there were data on safety, especially regarding potential arthropathy. Most of the data were based on clinical findings—musculoskeletal complaints and joint examination. Such findings do not allow one to distinguish between coincidental joint problems and quinolone-induced arthropathy. Only rarely have magnetic resonance imaging (MRI), ultrasonography, and growth curve been used for either short-term or long-term evaluation. With the exception of the findings in two cystic fibrosis patients,[63] the gold standard parameter "histopathology" is lacking in human studies. The few studies using radiologic methods to determine the effects on cartilage and bone have not identified any changes in fluoroquinolone-treated patients.[60–62] In a large long-term follow-up study of 2,233 children enrolled in levofloxacin treatment studies using clinical outcomes, in particular bone- and joint-related findings, there was no clinically detectable difference between levofloxacin- and comparator-treated children in musculoskeletal adverse events (MSAEs) at 5 years posttreatment.[8]

There are four conclusions: (1) To date, there is no unequivocal documentation of quinolone-induced arthropathy in patients as described in juvenile animals; quinolone arthropathy remains an experimental laboratory phenomenon in juvenile animals. (2) Clinical observations temporally related to quinolone use are reversible episodes of arthralgia, with and without effusions that do not lead to long-term sequelae when the treatment with the agents is discontinued. (3) Most joint complaints associated with quinolone use are coincidental and do not represent adverse effects. Possible coincidental conditions include arthropathy and hypertrophic pulmonary osteoarthropathy associated with cystic fibrosis and reactive, traumatic, and rheumatic joint diseases. (4) It is postulated that the so-called allergic arthritis initially described in nalidixic acid-treated patients does exist but is not the same as the quinolone-induced arthropathy in animals. These adverse events are always transient arthralgic or arthritic manifestations, usually involving large joints and occurring during the first and second weeks of therapy. The overall incidence is 1% to 3% (−18%) depending on the studied patient group and quinolone compound.

Other musculoskeletal adverse effects of quinolones are tendinitis and tendon rupture. Review of the literature on fluoroquinolone-associated tendinopathy[64–67] reveals the following. The incidence in a healthy population is very low, especially in children.[65] In most cases, the Achilles tendon is affected with symptoms compatible with painful tendinitis or with rupture—usually occurring during the second week of treatment.

Fluoroquinolone-associated tendinopathy increases in patients who have renal dysfunction (hemodialysis, after renal transplantation). There is a correlation between long-term cortical steroid therapy and age of 60 years or older; the male-to-female ratio is approximately 2:1.[66,67]

Although the side effects for the vast majority of patients are nonsevere and reversible, the postmarketing reports of cases with significant adverse events led to a change in the labeling of the fluoroquinolones. Both, the FDA and the European Medicines Agency (EMA) recommended restricting the use of fluoroquinolone and quinolone antibiotics (used by mouth, injection, or inhalation) following a review of disabling and potentially long-lasting side effects involving tendons, muscles, joints, nerves, and the central nervous system.[68,69] The fluoroquinolones should be reserved for use in patients with non-life-threatening infections who have no alternative treatment options.

NEONATAL SAFETY STUDIES

Several studies dedicated to studying the safety of ciprofloxacin in neonates specifically have been published, and a systematic review of ciprofloxacin use in neonates summarized outcomes of five observational cohort studies.[70] The combined analysis of 1,000 included neonates with a total of 308 receiving ciprofloxacin and 692 receiving other antibiotics as controls found no serious side effects and one adverse event, greenish discoloration of teeth in the first year of life, which occurred in one neonate receiving ciprofloxacin and one control; dosing schedule ranged from 10 to 20 mg per kg per day divided in twice daily doses.[54,56–59,70] All studies included a clinical evaluation as part of the follow-up, but only one performed radiologic studies. In the study using ultrasound, there was no correlation between cartilage size of the knee and ciprofloxacin exposure at the age of 12 months.[57] There was no effect of ciprofloxacin use on linear growth at the age of 12 months in another study.[58] A 2-year follow-up study of a cohort of 48 patients treated with ciprofloxacin during the neonatal period who were matched with controls treated with other antibiotics did not show any difference in growth and development between the groups.[56]

Although it is reassuring that no osteoarticular toxicity was reported in neonatal studies to date, it is important to emphasize that these studies were observational, indications for fluoroquinolone use were not specified, and long-term follow-up to monitor for adverse events was not standardized. There are no long-term follow-up studies beyond 2 years following exposure. In particular, radiologic studies were not performed in most patients with ciprofloxacin. Finally, case numbers were too small to capture rare adverse events.

CLINICAL INDICATIONS

Since the mid-1980s, fluoroquinolones have been used in pediatric patients primarily in circumstances in which they were the only antimicrobial choice for infections caused by multiple-resistant organisms.[5,16,31] These included pseudomonas infections in children with cystic fibrosis,[61,62,71] complicated urinary tract infections,[72] enteric infections in developing countries,[73,74] and chronic ear infections.[75] Results of controlled clinical trials in patients with these four indications have shown comparable efficacy of the fluoroquinolones and conventional regimens.

The existing experience in pediatric patients also indicates that the fluoroquinolones are effective and safe for the prevention or therapy for infections in neutropenic cancer patients and for the eradication of nasopharyngeal carriage of meningococci.[76–78]

In the United Stated, FDA has approved the following drugs and their usages: The indications for systemic use of ciprofloxacin in children are inhalation anthrax, plague, complicated urinary tract infections, and pyelonephritis.[6] Levofloxacin is FDA-approved for inhalation anthrax and plague in children.[7] Fluoroquinolones are not indicated as a first-line systemic therapy in children due to the concern about safety and lack of studies supporting their use. However, in cases where there are no reasonable alternatives due to multidrug-resistant pathogens, drug allergies, or when an oral antibiotic is deemed optimal, there is consensus that fluoroquinolones may be considered as treatment in pediatric patients.[79] When an alternative antibiotic is unavailable based on bacterial resistance or formulation options, ciprofloxacin is also an option for treating infections due to *Salmonella* or *Shigella* if alternative antibiotics are not available due to bacterial resistance or formulation options.[79] However, owing to rising fluoroquinolone resistance among enteric pathogens, antimicrobial susceptibilities should be confirmed.

The use of a fluoroquinolone for the first-line treatment of complicated urinary tract infections or pyelonephritis caused by a multidrug-resistant Gram-negative pathogen is indicated in children older than 1 year of age if a nonfluoroquinolone agent cannot be used based on susceptibility data or allergy history.

Fluoroquinolones have also been used successfully when severe infections, including sepsis and meningitis during the neonatal period, are due to enterobacteria resistance to standard treatment.[54,56,80] In particular, levofloxacin is considered the drug of choice for children (greater than or equal to 6 months of age) with respiratory infections documented to be caused by highly penicillin-resistant pneumococci.[79] Similarly, pneumococcal meningitis may be an indication when bacterial resistance or contraindications limit the use of beta-lactams, thereby making the use of levofloxacin necessary. The use of fluoroquinolones such as ciprofloxacin or levofloxacin for multidrug-resistant Gram-negative meningitis has been endorsed for older infants and children in particular if it represents the only treatment option.[79] Reports of good clinical outcomes and demonstration of adequate penetration into the CSF in neonates would support a similar practice in that age group.[36]

In addition to numerous case reports, the outcomes of neonates treated with ciprofloxacin have been reported by observational cohort studies. Favorable outcomes in those treated with ciprofloxacin were reported to be at least as good as those in neonates treated with other antibiotics.[54,56,70] Similar to the use of ciprofloxacin in pediatric patients, the fluoroquinolone with the most available evidence supporting its use may be considered in neonates where there are no reasonable alternatives caused by multidrug-resistant pathogens, site of infection, or when an oral antibiotic is deemed optimal. Currently, it is impossible to comprehensively evaluate the efficacy for specific clinical indications of fluoroquinolones compared with other antibiotics in neonates in the absence of prospective clinical trials.

Research on chemical modifications of the quinolones has been aimed at (a) more potent derivatives, (b) less frequent resistance, (c) better penetration into CSF, and (d) improved patient tolerability. Some of the newer compounds have achieved many of these goals. However, although future trials of existing or new fluoroquinolone compounds are warranted in pediatric and neonatal patients, they will be difficult to conduct in view of the risk of rare side effects.

There are clinical studies of newer fluoroquinolone compounds such as gatifloxacin for childhood otitis media,[81,82] but an application for gatifloxacin licensure for pediatric use was withdrawn, because the FDA proposed risk management procedures that precluded reasonable pediatric use.[83] The current warnings against the use of fluoroquinolones for non-life-threatening infections, such as upper respiratory tract infections in older patients, will make it even less likely that clinical studies for existing or novel fluoroquinolones will be conducted in neonates for such indications.

SUMMARY

The two major concerns regarding the use of fluoroquinolones in children are the development of bacterial resistance and cartilage toxicity as described in juvenile animals. The risk for rapid emergence of resistance among pneumococci and other common bacterial pathogens, associated with the widespread, uncontrolled use of fluoroquinolones in pediatric patients, is a realistic threat.

Cartilage toxicity with fluoroquinolones is a laboratory phenomenon in juvenile animals, and no arthropathy has been documented unequivocally in the large numbers of children treated with these agents. This includes the few existing studies in neonates, which have not identified short- or long-term osteoarticular side effects and adverse events. However, neonatal studies are limited by small numbers and lack of consistent follow-up methods. Expectant observation is warranted for any new quinolone use in pediatrics and should be supported by additional studies. Based on available data showing the safety and efficacy of the fluoroquinolones in all age groups, selected pediatric and neonatal patients should not be deprived of the therapeutic advantages that these agents have to offer under certain circumstances outlined above. Although there are FDA-approved indications for patients less than 18 years of age, these do not include the neonatal age group. Therefore, the quinolones should not be used in neonates for routine treatment unless there are no alternative safe and effective antimicrobials.

Regulatory approvals for broader use of new fluoroquinolones in neonates and children must combine the efforts of experts in microbiology and infectious diseases, regulatory authorities, and pharmaceutical manufacturers. Postmarketing surveillance must include an adequate risk management plan feasible for patients, parents, and drug companies. Will fluoroquinolone ever be recommended for common infections in children[84]? The triad of feared arthrotoxicity, potential resistance explosion, and enormous requirements regarding adequate study and postmarketing control suggests that the answer is no. Therefore, fluoroquinolones will continue to serve mainly for second-line use in neonates, only after failure of an earlier treatment and when there are unique circumstances that would indicate clear benefits over other antibiotics approved for pediatric and neonatal use.

REFERENCES

1. Stahlmann R. Safety profile of the quinolones. *J Antimicrob Chemother* 1990;26(Suppl D):31–44.
2. Gough A, Barsoum NJ, Mitchell L, et al. Juvenile canine drug-induced arthropathy: clinicopathological studies on articular lesions caused by oxolinic and pipemidic acids. *Toxicol Appl Pharmacol* 1979;51:177–187.
3. Christ W, Lehnert T, Ulbrich B. Specific toxicologic aspects of the quinolones. *Rev Infect Dis* 1988;10(Suppl 1):141–146.
4. Schluter G. Ciprofloxacin: toxicologic evaluation of additional safety data. *Am J Med* 1989;87(Suppl 5A):37–39.
5. Schaad UB, Salam MA, Aujard Y, et al. Use of fluoroquinolones in pediatrics: consensus report of an International Society of Chemotherapy commission. *Pediatr Infect Dis J* 1995;14:1–9.
6. Department of Health & Human Services. https://www.accessdata.fda.gov/drugsatfda_docs/appletter/2004/19537s049,19857s031,19847s027,20780s013ltr.pdf. Accessed September 3, 2020.
7. FDA. Levaquin (levofloxacin): Highlights of prescribing information. https://www.accessdata.fda.gov/drugsatfda_docs/label/2013/020634s065,020635s071,021721s032lbl.pdf. Accessed September 3, 2020.
8. Bradley JS, Kauffman RE, Balis DA, et al. Assessment of musculoskeletal toxicity 5 years after therapy with levofloxacin. *Pediatrics* 2014;134;(1):e146–e153.
9. Pandolfini C, Marco S, Paolo M, et al. The use of ciprofloxacin and fluconazole in Italian neonatal intensive care units: a nationwide survey. *BMC Pediatr* 2013;13:5
10. Pandolfini C, Kaguelidou F, Sequi M, et al. Wide intra-and inter-country variability in drug use and dosage in very-low-birth-weight newborns with severe infections. *Eur J Clin Pharmacol* 2013;69:1031–1036.
11. Gootz TD, Brighty KE. Fluoroquinolone antibacterials: SAR, mechanism of action, resistance and clinical aspects. *Med Res Rev* 1996;16:433–486.
12. Stein GE, Goldstein EJ. Fluoroquinolones and anaerobes. *Clin Infect Dis* 2006;42(11):1598–1607.
13. Mandell LA, Peterson LR, Wise R, et al. The battle against emerging antibiotic resistance: should fluoroquinolones be used to treat children? *Clin Infect Dis* 2002;35:721–727.
14. Hooper DC. New uses for new and old quinolones and the challenge of resistance. *Clin Infect Dis* 2000;30:243–254.
15. Schaad UB. Use of the quinolones in pediatrics. In: Andriole VT, ed. *The quinolones*, 3rd ed. San Diego, CA: Academic Press, 2000:455–475.
16. Gendrel D, Chalumeau M, Moulin F, et al. Fluoroquinolones in paediatrics: a risk for the patient or for the community? *Lancet Infect Dis* 2003;3:537–546.
17. Redgrave LS, Sutton SB, Webber MA, et al. Fluoroquinolone resistance: mechanisms, impact on bacteria, and role in evolutionary success. *Trends Microbiol* 2014;22(8):438–445. doi:10.1016/j.tim.2014.04.007.
18. Hooper DC. Mechanisms of quinolone resistance. In: Hooper DC, Rubenstein E, eds. *Quinolone antimicrobial agents*, 3rd ed. Washington, DC: American Society for Microbiology Press, 2003:41–67.
19. Chen DK, McGeer A, De Azavedo JC, et al. Decreased susceptibility of *Streptococcus pneumoniae* to fluoroquinolones in Canada. *N Engl J Med* 1999;341:233–239.
20. Ho PL, Yung RW, Tsang DN, et al. Increasing resistance of *Streptococcus pneumoniae* to fluoroquinolones: results of a Hong Kong multicentre study in 2000. *J Antimicrob Chemother* 2001;48:659–665.
21. Mannheimer SB, Riley LW, Roberts RB. Association of penicillin-resistant pneumococci with residence in a pediatric chronic care facility. *J Infect Dis* 1996;174:513–519.
22. Davies TA, Leibovitz E, Noel GJ, et al Characterization and dynamics of middle ear fluid and nasopharyngeal isolates of *Streptococcus pneumoniae* from 12 children treated with levofloxacin. *Antimicrob Agents Chemother* 2008;52(1):378–381.
23. Gonzales J, Georgiou M, Alcaide F, et al. Fluoroquinolone resistance mutations in the parC, parE, and gyrA genes of clinical isolates of viridans group streptococci. *Antimicrob Agents Chemother* 1998;42:2792–2798.
24. Ferrandiz MJ, Fernoll A, Linares J, et al. Horizontal transfer of parC and gyrA in fluoroquinolone-resistant clinical isolates of *Streptococcus pneumoniae*. *Antimicrob Agents Chemother* 2000;44:840–847.
25. Blumer JL, Stern RC, Myers CM, et al. Pharmacokinetics and pharmacodynamics of ciprofloxacin in cystic fibrosis. In: Abstracts of 14th International Congress on Chemotherapy, Kyoto, Japan, 1985:112.
26. Stutman HR, Shalit I, Marks MI, et al. Pharmacokinetics of two dosage regimens of ciprofloxacin during a two-week-therapeutic trial in patients with cystic fibrosis. *Am J Med* 1987;82(Suppl 4A):142–145.
27. Peltola H, Vaarala M, Renkonen O, et al. Pharmacokinetics of single dose of oral ciprofloxacin in infants and small children. *Antimicrob Agents Chemother* 1992;36:1086–1090.
28. Schaeffer HG, Strass H, Wedgwood J, et al. Pharmacokinetics of ciprofloxacin in pediatric cystic fibrosis patients. *Antimicrob Agents Chemother* 1996;40:29–34.
29. Rubio TT, Miles MV, Lettiere JT, et al. Pharmacokinetic disposition of sequential intravenous/oral ciprofloxacin in pediatric cystic fibrosis patients with acute pulmonary exacerbation. *Pediatr Infect Dis J* 1997;16:112–117.
30. Douros A, Grabowski K, Stahlmann R. Safety issues and drug-drug interactions with commonly used quinolones. *Expert Opin Drug Metabol Toxicol* 2015;11:25–39.
31. Forrest A, Nix DE, Ballow CH, et al. Pharmacodynamics of intravenous ciprofloxacin in seriously ill patients. *Antimicrob Agents Chemother* 1993;37:1073–1081.
32. Aggarwal P, Dutta S, Garg SK, et al. Multiple dose pharmacokinetics of ciprofloxacin in preterm babies. *Indian Pediatr* 2004;41(10):1001–1007.
33. Leroux S, Turner MA, Guellec CB, et al.; TINN (Treat Infections in NeoNates) and GRiP (Global Research in Paediatrics) consortiums. Pharmacokinetic studies in neonates: the utility of an opportunistic sampling design. *Clin Pharmacokinet* 2015;54(12):1273–1285. doi:10.1007/s40262-015-0291-1.

34. Zhao W, Hill H, Le Guellec C, et al.; TINN consortium. Population pharmacokinetics of ciprofloxacin in neonates and young infants less than three months of age. *Antimicrob Agents Chemother* 2014;58(11):6572–6580. doi:10.1128/AAC.03568-14.
35. van den Oever HL, Versteegh FG, Thewessen EA, et al. Ciprofloxacin in preterm neonates: case report and review of the literature. *Eur J Pediatr* 1998;157(10):843–845.
36. Green SD, Ilunga F, Cheesbrough JS, et al. The treatment of neonatal meningitis due to Gram-negative bacilli with ciprofloxacin: evidence of satisfactory penetration into the cerebrospinal fluid. *J Infect* 1993;26:253–256.
37. Thwaites GE, Bhavnani SM, Chau TT, et al. Randomized pharmacokinetic and pharmacodynamic comparison of fluoroquinolones for tuberculous meningitis. *Antimicrob Agents Chemother* 2011;55(7):3244–3253. doi:10.1128/AAC.00064-11.
38. McDonald DF, Short HB. Usefulness of nalidixic acid in treatment of urinary tract infections. *Antimicrob Agents Chemother* 1964;64:628–631.
39. Bailey RR, Natale R, Linton AL. Nalidixic acid arthralgia. *Can Med Assoc J* 1972;107:604–607.
40. Ingham B, Brentnall DW, Dale EA, et al. Arthropathy induced by anti-bacterial fused n-alkyl-4-pyrodoine-3-carboxylic acids. *Toxicol Lett* 1977;1:21–26.
41. Tatsumi H, Senda H, Yatera S, et al. Toxicological studies on pipemidic acid. V. Effect on diarthrodial joints of experimental animals. *J Toxicol Sci* 1978;3:357–367.
42. Schaad UB, Wedgwood-Krucko J. Nalidixic acid in children: retrospective matched controlled study for cartilage toxicity. *Infection* 1987;15:165–168.
43. Rumler W, von Rodhden L. Does nalidixic acid produce joint toxicity in childhood? In: Book of abstracts of the 15th International Congress of Chemotherapy, Istanbul, Turkey, 1987:1029–1031.
44. Adam D. Use of quinolone in pediatric patients. *Rev Infect Dis* 1989;11(Suppl 5):S1113–S1116.
45. Nuutinen M, Turtinen J, Uhari M. Growth and joint symptoms in children treated with nalidixic acid. *Pediatr Infect Dis J* 1994;13:798–800.
46. Stahlmann R, Merker HJ, Hinz N, et al. Ofloxacin in juvenile non-human primates and rats: arthropathia and drug plasma concentrations. *Arch Toxicol* 1990;64:193–204.
47. Burkhardt JE, Hill MA, Carlton WW. Morphologic and biochemical changes in articular cartilages of immature beagle dogs dosed with difloxacin. *Toxicol Pathol* 1992;20:246–252.
48. Kato M, Takada S, Ogawara S, et al. Effect of levofloxacin on glycosaminoglycan and DNA synthesis of cultured rabbit chondrocytes at concentrations inducing cartilage lesions in vivo. *Antimicrob Agents Chemother* 1995;39:1979–1983.
49. Forster C, Kociok K, Shakibaei M, et al. Integrins on joint cartilage chondrocytes and alterations by ofloxacin or magnesium deficiency in immature rats. *Arch Toxicol* 1996;70:261–270.
50. Pradhan KM, Arora NK, Jena A, et al. Safety of ciprofloxacin therapy in children: magnetic resonance images, body fluid levels of fluoride and linear growth. *Acta Paediatr* 1995;84:555–560.
51. Bethell DB, Hien TT, Phi LT, et al. Effects on growth of single short courses of fluoroquinolones. *Arch Dis Child* 1996;74:44–46.
52. Burkhardt JE, Walterspiel JN, Schaad UB. Quinolone arthropathy in animals versus children. *Clin Infect Dis* 1997;25:1196–1204.
53. Chalumeau M, Tonnelier S, D'Athis P, et al. Fluoroquinolone safety in pediatric patients: a prospective, multicenter, comparative cohort study in France. *Pediatrics* 2003;111:e714–e719.
54. Drossou-Agakidou V, Roilides E, Papakyriakidou-Koliouska P, et al. Use of ciprofloxacin in neonatal sepsis: lack of adverse effects up to one year. *Pediatr Infect Dis J* 2004;23:346–349.
55. Noel GJ, Bradley JS, Kauffmann RE, et al. Comparative safety profile of levofloxacin in 2523 children with a focus on four musculoskeletal disorders. *Pediatr Infect Dis J* 2007;26:879–891.
56. Ahmed AN, Khan NZ, Saha SK, et al. Ciprofloxacin treatment in preterm neonates in Bangladesh: lack of effected on growth and development. *Pediatric Infect Dis J* 2006;25:1137–1141.
57. Chaudri S, Suryawanshi P, Anbardekar S, et al. Safety profile of ciprofloxacin used for neonatal septicemia. *Indian Pediatr* 2004;41:1246–1251.
58. Dutta S, Chowdhary G, Kumar P, et al. Ciprofloxacin administration to very low birth weight babies has no effect on linear growth in infancy. *J Trop Pediatr* 2006;52:103–106.
59. Gurpinar AN, Balkan E, Kilic N, et al. The effects of a fluoroquinolone on the growth and development of infants. *J Int Med Res* 1997;25:302–306.
60. Schaad UB, Stoupis C, Wedgwood J, et al. Clinical, radiologic and magnetic resonance monitoring for skeletal toxicity in pediatric patients with cystic fibrosis receiving a three-month course of ciprofloxacin. *Pediatr Infect Dis J* 1991;10:723–729.
61. Richard DA, Nousia-Arvanitakis S, Sollich V, et al.; Cystic Fibrosis Study Group. Oral ciprofloxacin versus intravenous ceftazidime plus tobramycin in pediatric cystic fibrosis patients: comparison of antipseudomonas efficacy and assessment of safety using ultrasonography and magnetic resonance imaging. *Pediatr Infect Dis J* 1997;16:572–578.
62. Arico M, Bossi G, Caselli D, et al. Long-term magnetic resonance survey of cartilage damage in leukemic children treated with fluoroquinolones. *Pediatr Infect Dis J* 1995;14:713–714.
63. Schaad UB, Sander E, Wedgwood J, et al. Morphologic studies for skeletal toxicity after prolonged ciprofloxacin therapy in two juvenile cystic fibrosis patients. *Pediatr Infect Dis J* 1992;11:1047–1049.
64. van der Linden PD, Sturkenboom MCJM, Herings RMC, et al. Fluoroquinolones and risk of Achilles tendon disorders: case-control study. *BMJ* 2002;324:1306–1307.
65. Yee CL, Duffy C, Gerbino PG, et al. Tendon or joint disorders in children after treatment with fluoroquinolones or azithromycin. *Pediatr Infect Dis J* 2002;21:525–529.
66. Khaliq Y, Zhanel GG. Fluoroquinolone-associated tendinopathy: a critical review of the literature. *Clin Infect Dis* 2003;36:1404–1410.
67. Arabyat RM, Raisch DW, McKoy JM, et al. Fluoroquinolone-associated tendon rupture: a summary of reports in the Food and Drug Administration's adverse event reporting system. *Expert Opin Drug Saf* 2015;14:1653–1660.
68. European Medicines Agency. Quinolone- and fluoroquinolone-containing medicinal products. https://www.ema.europa.eu/en/medicines/human/referrals/quinolone-fluoroquinolone-containing-medicinal-products. Accessed May 6, 2020.
69. U.S. Food and Drug Administration. FDA Drug Safety Communication: FDA updates warnings for oral and injectable fluoroquinolone antibiotics due to disabling side effects. https://www.fda.gov/drugs/drug-safety-and-availability/fda-drug-safety-communication-fda-updates-warnings-oral-and-injectable-fluoroquinolone-antibiotics. Accessed September 3, 2020.
70. Kaguelidou F, Turner MA, Choonara I, et al. Coprofloxacin use in neonates. *Pediatric Infect Dis J* 2011;30:e29–e37.
71. Schaad UB, Wedgwood J, Ruedeberg A, et al. Ciprofloxacin as antipseudomonal treatment in patients with cystic fibrosis. *Pediatr Infect Dis J* 1997;16:106–111.
72. Koyle MA, Barqawi A, Wild J, et al. Pediatric urinary tract infections: the role of fluoroquinolones. *Pediatr Infect Dis J* 2003;22:1133–1137.
73. Green S, Tillotson G. Use of ciprofloxacin in developing countries. *Pediatr Infect Dis J* 1997;16:150–159.
74. Salam MA, Dhar U, Khan WA, et al. Randomised comparison of ciprofloxacin suspension and pivmecillinam for childhood shigellosis. *Lancet* 1998;352:522–527.
75. Lang R, Goshen S, Raas-Rothschild A. Oral ciprofloxacin in the management of chronic suppurative otitis media without cholesteatoma in children. *Pediatr Infect Dis J* 1992;11:925–929.
76. Freifeld A, Pizzo P. Use of fluoroquinolones for empirical management of febrile neutropenia in pediatric cancer patients. *Pediatr Infect Dis J* 1997;16:140–146.
77. Patrick CC. Use of fluoroquinolones as prophylaxis agents in patients with neutropenia. *Pediatr Infect Dis J* 1997;16:135–139.
78. Cuevas LE, Kazembe P, Mughogho GK, et al. Eradication of nasopharyngeal carriage of Neisseria meningitidis in children and adult in rural Africa: a comparison of ciprofloxacin and rifampicin. *J Infect Dis* 1995;171:728–731.
79. Jackson MA, Schutze GE; Committee on Infectious Diseases. The use of systemic and topical fluoroquinolones. *Pediatrics* 2016;138; doi:10.1542/peds.2016-2706.
80. Krcmery V, Filka J, Uher J, et al. Ciprofloxacin in treatment of nosocomial meningitis in neonates and in infants: report of 12 cases and review. *Diagn Microbiol Infect Dis* 1999;35:75–80.
81. Dagan R, Arguedas A, Schaad UB. Potential role of fluoroquinolone therapy in childhood otitis media. *Pediatr Infect Dis J* 2004;23:390–398.
82. Pichichero ME, Arguedas A, Dagan R, et al. Safety and efficacy of gatifloxacin therapy for children with recurrent acute otitis media (AOM) and/or AOM treatment failure. *Clin Infect Dis* 2005;41:470–478.
83. Marchant CD. Gatifloxacin therapy for children. *Clin Infect Dis* 2005;41:479–480.
84. Schaad UB. Will fluoroquinolones ever be recommended for common infections in children? *Pediatr Infect Dis J* 2007;26:865–867.

CHAPTER

25

Nynke G.L. Jager
David M. Burger

Sulfonamides, Dihydrofolate Reductase Inhibitors, and Dapsone

INTRODUCTION

Sulfonamides, sulfamethoxazole (SMZ), sulfasalazine, and sulfadiazine, and dihydrofolate reductase inhibitors, trimethoprim (TMP) and pyrimethamine (PM), are some of the oldest antimicrobial agents used in children. Their mode of action, efficacy, safety, and pharmacologic properties are well known, and these drugs remain to be a substantial component of antimicrobial therapies in infants beyond the immediate newborn period and in older children.

SULFONAMIDES

Sulfonamides have a wide range of antimicrobial activity against both Gram-positive and Gram-negative organisms. Unfortunately, bacterial resistance to sulfonamides is now common, and their use has decreased with the introduction of more potent classes of antibiotics. However, sulfonamides are still used in combination with dihydrofolate reductase inhibitors, especially for the treatment or prevention of urinary tract infections or parasitic (toxoplasmosis, *Pneumocystis jirovecii*) infections.

In the past, sulfonamides were successfully used for the prevention of meningococcal disease in contacts and for the eradication of the chronic meningococcal carrier state. However, because sulfonamide-resistant meningococci are now common, these drugs are usually no longer suitable for these clinical situations. Rifampin, ceftriaxone, or ciprofloxacin is currently recommended as the chemoprophylactic agents for meningococcal infections in the United States. In localized epidemics of sulfonamide-sensitive meningococcal disease, chemoprophylaxis with sulfonamides can be used.[1]

MECHANISM OF ACTION

Sulfonamides contain a benzene ring, with a sulfonamide group and a primary amino group next to the sulfur side chain of the sulfonamide group. They are synthetic analogs of *para*-aminobenzoic acid (PABA), which is essential for bacterial folic acid biosynthesis. Sulfonamides act by competing with PABA as a substrate for the enzyme dihydropteroate synthase, which incorporates PABA into dihydropteroic acid, the immediate precursor of folic acid. Therefore, those microorganisms that must synthesize their own folic acid (i.e., bacteria) are vulnerable to the effect of sulfonamide, and those that can utilize preformed folic acid (i.e., mammalian cells) are not affected by these drugs. The bacteriostatic effects of sulfonamides can be counteracted by the use of PABA. The sulfonamides are commonly used together with dihydrofolate reductase inhibitors.

SULFAMETHOXAZOLE

SMZ is an intermediate-acting antibacterial sulfonamide. It is nowadays only being used as a component of the trimethoprim–sulfamethoxazole (TMP-SMZ) 5:1 fixed ratio combination product.

Clinical Use

SMZ is indicated for uncomplicated acute and recurrent urinary tract infections caused by susceptible organisms, including *Escherichia coli, Klebsiella, Enterobacter,* and *Proteus mirabilis.* Currently, the increasing frequency of resistant organisms limits the usefulness of several antibacterial agents, including the sulfonamides for the treatment of chronic and recurrent urinary tract infections. Therefore, the fixed combination TMP-SMZ is preferred over SMZ (see "Trimethoprim–Sulfamethoxazole" section).

Pharmacokinetics

SMZ is rapidly absorbed following oral administration. About 80% is metabolized in the liver, where it undergoes N^4-acetylation and N^4-glucuronide. Approximately 70% of SMZ is bound to plasma proteins.[2]

SMZ is widely distributed into most body tissues. It diffuses into cerebrospinal fluid (CSF) with a peak concentration at 8 hours, reaching about 12% to 30% of the simultaneous plasma concentration in inflamed meninges.[3] The drug diffuses into aqueous humor, vaginal fluid, and middle ear fluid. SMZ crosses the placental barrier and is excreted into breast milk.[2]

SMZ and its metabolites are excreted primarily in the urine. The elimination half-life is approximately 10 hours. The unconjugated forms are excreted by tubular secretion, whereas the acetylated drug is excreted by glomerular filtration. In urine, approximately 20% of SMZ is present as unchanged drug, 50% to 70% is acetylated derivative, and 15% to 20% is the glucuronide conjugate. The half-life of SMZ is prolonged in patients with renal insufficiency (creatinine clearance <20 to 30 mL per minute), and reduced doses should be administered in these patients.[2]

Adverse Reactions

SMZ exhibits the toxic potentials of the other sulfonamides. Hemolytic effects include agranulocytosis, aplastic anemia, leukopenia, thrombocytopenia, hemolytic anemia, eosinophilia, and methemoglobinemia. Any sulfonamide may cause hemolysis in patients with glucose-6-phosphate dehydrogenase (G6PD) deficiency. Allergic reactions include anaphylaxis, serum sickness, and conjunctival and scleral injection. Nephrotoxic effects, mainly caused by the major metabolite acetylsulfamethoxazole, include crystalluria that may cause pain and hematuria. These nephrotoxic effects are mainly observed in patients with impaired renal function, and therapeutic drug monitoring (TDM) is advised. See also "Trimethoprim–Sulfamethoxazole" section. Anuria can occur if the renal pelvis or the ureter becomes completely occluded. Alkalinization of the urine increases solubility as well as enhances the urinary excretion of SMZ and should be used when high doses of SMZ are given. Dermatologic effects include erythema multiforme, Stevens-Johnson syndrome, exfoliative dermatitis, photosensitivity, pruritus, urticaria, and generalized skin eruptions. Gastrointestinal (GI) adverse effects include hepatitis, hepatocellular necrosis, pseudomembranous colitis, pancreatitis, nausea, vomiting, diarrhea, anorexia, and abdominal pain. Neurologic complications may include peripheral neuritis, ataxia, vertigo, tinnitus, and headache.

Drug Interactions

SMZ inhibits CYP2C9; via this pathway, the serum concentrations of warfarin and phenytoin are increased when used concomitantly with SMZ. This may result in clinically significant exaggeration of anticoagulant effect and central nervous system (CNS) toxicity of phenytoin.[4]

Pediatric Dosage

See "Trimethoprim–Sulfamethoxazole" section.

SULFASALAZINE

Sulfasalazine is an anti-inflammatory agent structurally composed of a sulfonamide (sulfapyridine) and 5-aminosalicylic acid (5-ASA) joined by an azo bond.

Clinical Use

Sulfasalazine is indicated for the treatment of mild-to-moderate ulcerative colitis and is effective in maintaining disease remission. In addition, it is used as adjunctive therapy with corticosteroids for the treatment of severe ulcerative colitis.[5] Historically, sulfasalazine was used as an induction agent for mild to moderately active Crohn disease, although it has fallen out of favor with meta-analyses reporting lack of effectiveness.[6]

Sulfasalazine is considered a disease-modifying antirheumatic drug for rheumatoid arthritis[7] and juvenile chronic arthritis.[8]

In children younger than 2 years of age, the safety and efficacy of sulfasalazine have not been established.

Pharmacokinetics

Following oral administration, small intestinal absorption accounts for an absolute sulfasalazine bioavailability of approximately 10% to 30%. This fraction is highly protein bound and is subsequently excreted in the urine. However, the majority of an orally administered sulfasalazine dose reaches the colon, where it is cleaved by bacterial azoreductases, thus releasing sulfapyridine and 5-ASA (mesalazine).[9,10] Plasma concentrations of sulfapyridine and 5-ASA show a peak at about 10 hours after dosing. The long time to peak concentrations is a function of the transit time to more distal intestine. Sulfapyridine is relatively well absorbed from the colon with a bioavailability of 60%. Absorbed sulfapyridine undergoes extensive metabolism in the liver via acetylation, hydroxylation, and glucuronidation. Peak concentrations of sulfapyridine depend on the acetylator status of the patient, with slow acetylators having higher concentrations and increased likelihood of adverse events.[10] In contrast, 5-ASA is less well absorbed with a bioavailability of 10% to 30%. 5-ASA is metabolized by the liver and the intestine to *N*-acetyl-5-aminosalicylic acid (acetyl-5-ASA). Acetylation is phenotype independent. Sulfapyridine and 5-ASA and their metabolites are excreted in the urine.[9] However, because the majority of 5-ASA stays in the colon, excretion is primarily in the feces as unchanged 5-ASA or as acetyl-5-ASA.[11]

Adverse Reactions

The adverse effects are more likely to be due to the sulfapyridine moiety and are similar to those of other sulfonamides. These effects are likely to occur among patients who are slow acetylators and when serum concentrations exceed 50 µg per mL. The most frequent adverse effects are GI symptoms, such as abdominal pain, nausea, and vomiting as well as headache, fever, and skin rash. Other adverse events associated with sulfasalazine include hematologic disturbances, for example, leukopenia, neutropenia, aplastic anemia, and thrombocytopenia.

Cardiovascular side effects of sulfasalazine include case reports of Raynaud phenomenon and myocarditis.[12,13] Other rarely reported adverse effects of sulfasalazine include exacerbation of episodes of ulcerative colitis, metallic mouth taste, intestinal villous atrophy, pancreatitis, and hair loss.[14–16] Rare renal side effects include nephritic syndrome and interstitial nephritis.[17] Pulmonary complications have been reported rarely among patients receiving sulfasalazine. Most of these complications are reversible and include cough, dyspnea, fever, pulmonary infiltrates, and eosinophilia. Rarely, fibrosing alveolitis has been reported with sulfasalazine use.[18]

Sulfasalazine-induced lupus has been reported among patients who have a slow acetylator genotype or human leukocyte antigen (HLA) haplotype associated with idiopathic systemic lupus erythematosus.[19] Drug-induced lupus has also been reported with 5-ASA (mesalazine).[20] Sulfasalazine may provoke acute porphyric attacks and should not be used in porphyric patients.[21] Sulfasalazine may provoke hemolysis in patients with G6PD deficiency.[22] Sulfasalazine may cause reversible yellow-orange discoloration of the urine or skin.

Sulfasalazine use in children with inflammatory bowel disease has been rarely associated with immune-mediated hepatitis and fulminant hepatic failure. The sulfapyridine moiety is believed to be the cause of the reaction.[23] Hepatitis has also been reported with 5-ASA use.[24] Sulfasalazine is contraindicated in patients with hypersensitivity to sulfonamides. It is also contraindicated in children younger than 2 months of age because of the risk of kernicterus.

Drug Interactions

Sulfasalazine is converted to active metabolites by the colonic bacterial flora. Concomitant administration of cholestyramine and iron may reduce the efficacy of sulfasalazine by reducing the production of active metabolites. Sulfasalazine may decrease the bioavailability of digoxin and folic acid.[25] Sulfasalazine may increase the toxicity of thiopurine antineoplastic agents by inhibition of their metabolism.[26]

Pediatric Dosage

Sulfasalazine is administered to children with ulcerative colitis who are 2 years and older at a dose of 40 to 70 mg per kg per day divided into two doses. Following clinical improvement, the dose may be reduced to 30 mg per kg per day divided into two doses.[5] In children with polyarticular juvenile rheumatoid arthritis, sulfasalazine is administered at a dose of 25 to 50 mg per kg per day into two evenly divided doses. The maximum daily dose is 2 g. Because of the increased frequency of GI side effects associated with sulfasalazine, it is advisable to start with one-quarter of the maintenance dose with weekly increases to the full maintenance dose in 1 month.[8]

SULFADIAZINE

Clinical Use

Nowadays, the use of sulfadiazine is limited to the treatment of toxoplasmosis, caused by the parasite *Toxoplasma gondii.* Most cases of acquired toxoplasmosis do not require specific antimicrobial therapy, although treatment of toxoplasmosis in HIV patients is advised. When indicated (e.g., chorioretinitis or significant organ damage) for symptomatic and asymptomatic congenital toxoplasmosis, sulfadiazine combined with PM (supplemented with folic acid) is recommended. The combination is synergistic against *T. gondii* and is a widely accepted regimen for the treatment of children and adults with acute symptomatic toxoplasmosis.[27]

Pharmacokinetics

Sulfadiazine is well absorbed from the GI tract. Peak blood concentration is attained 3 to 6 hours after an oral dose. Sulfadiazine is metabolized in the liver to the acetylated form. Approximately 10% to 40% of the drug in plasma is in the acetylated form. Plasma protein binding is 38% to 48%. Sulfadiazine is distributed into most body tissues and diffuses into the CSF. CSF concentrations are approximately 30% of those in the blood and are achieved within 4 hours of administration.[3]

Sulfadiazine is eliminated primarily through the kidneys. Drug urine concentration is 10 to 25 times greater than serum levels. Approximately 30% to 44% of the drug is excreted unchanged in the urine, and 15% to 40% is eliminated as the acetylated form. The half-life of sulfadiazine ranges from 7 to 12 hours and that of the acetylated metabolite from 8 to 12 hours. Sulfadiazine is excreted in breast milk.

Adverse Reactions

Most frequently observed adverse reactions include GI effects such as headache and dizziness. Adverse GI effects that have been reported with sulfadiazine use include nausea, vomiting, anorexia, diarrhea and abdominal pain, stomatitis, hepatitis, and pancreatitis.

Allergic rashes are fairly frequent complications of sulfonamide therapy. Usually, these occur after 1 to 2 weeks of treatment but may appear earlier with prior sensitization. Maculopapular and urticarial rashes are the most common, but erythema nodosum, exfoliative dermatitis, and rarely Stevens-Johnson syndrome may occur. Photosensitivity and serum sickness–like illness may also occur.

Crystalluria and acute renal failure have been described with the use of high-dose sulfadiazine for a number of conditions, including the treatment of toxoplasma encephalitis in patients with AIDS.[28] Crystalluria occurs because the drug and its acetyl conjugate are excreted in the urine in high concentrations and are highly insoluble. Crystalluria may cause pain and hematuria, and anuria can occur if the renal pelvis or the ureter becomes completely occluded.

Hemolytic effects are rare and include leukopenia, thrombocytopenia, hemolytic anemia, agranulocytosis, and aplastic anemia.[29] Acute hemolytic anemia, a rare complication, can occur as a result of prior sensitization with sulfonamides.[28] Sulfonamides can induce hemolysis in patients with G6PD-deficient red blood cells, producing intravascular hemolysis and hemoglobinuria. Agranulocytosis is rare with the currently used sulfonamides.

Pediatric Dosage

For toxoplasmosis, the recommended dose is 100 to 150 mg per kg per day, divided in four doses with a maximum of 8 mg per day.

SILVER SULFADIAZINE CREAM

Silver sulfadiazine (SSD) 1% cream is a topical antimicrobial agent. SSD is formed by combining the weak acid sulfadiazine with silver nitrate to form a white, slightly soluble complex silver salt. SSD complex does not precipitate chlorides in the body fluids as silver nitrate does. SSD is nonstaining and odorless, and its use is painless.

SSD exerts its antibacterial effect by binding to cell membranes and, to a lesser extent, the bacterial cell wall rather than by interacting with cellular DNA. It has bactericidal activity against many Gram-positive and Gram-negative organisms, including *Pseudomonas aeruginosa, E. coli, Proteus* species, staphylococci, streptococci, and yeast. The topical use of SSD has been effective for the prevention and treatment of sepsis in burn wounds.[30]

Clinical Use

Nowadays, SSD is only recommended for the treatment of infections in burn wounds, although newer dressings are suggested to show better results than SSD.[30]

After burn wounds are cleansed and debrided, SSD cream is applied under sterile conditions. It should be applied with a sterile, gloved hand to the burn surface once daily to a thickness approximately 1/16th of an inch. Treatment should be continued until satisfactory healing has occurred or until the burn site is ready for grafting.

Pharmacokinetics

Although silver is not appreciably absorbed systemically, sulfadiazine may be absorbed into the blood, especially when the drug is applied to large areas and/or over prolonged periods of time. During prolonged treatment of wounds involving extensive areas of the body, serum sulfonamide concentrations of 8 to 12 μg per mL are observed. If renal function is sufficiently impaired, accumulation of sulfadiazine may occur, particularly if the patient is dehydrated. In patients with extensive burns, it is recommended that serum concentrations are monitored during prolonged use of the drug.[31]

Adverse Reactions

Absorption of SSD varies and depends on the percentage and extent of tissue damage. Adverse reactions that are reported include skin necrosis, erythema multiforme skin discoloration, burning sensation, and rashes. Because absorption of SSD varies depending on body-surface area, it is possible that adverse reactions may occur, such as associated thrombocytopenia, dermatologic reactions including Stevens-Johnson syndrome, and exfoliative dermatitis as well as hepatitis and toxic nephrosis.[31]

Transient leukopenia has been reported in patients receiving SSD therapy.[29] White blood cell depression occurs within 2 to 4 days of initiation of therapy. Rebound to normal counts follows onset within 2 to 3 days. Recovery is not influenced by continuation of SSD therapy.

DIHYDROFOLATE REDUCTASE INHIBITORS

Just like sulfonamides, dihydrofolate reductase inhibitors act by affecting the folic acid synthesis pathway. They inhibit dihydrofolate reductase, which is necessary for the conversion of dihydrofolic acid to tetrahydrofolic acid.

TRIMETHOPRIM

Clinical Use

In general, susceptible pathogens are *Staphylococcus aureus* (methicillin-susceptible *Staphylococcus aureus* or MSSA) and *Enterococcus faecalis.* TMP is used for the treatment and prophylaxis of uncomplicated urinal tract infections, although increasing resistance of commonly encountered pathogens in urinary tract infections limit its empiric use. Also, TMP is used for the treatment of upper respiratory tract infections.

Pharmacokinetics

TMP is rapidly and well absorbed from the GI tract and is for approximately 45% protein bound. It distributes well to tissues, and tissue concentrations are usually higher than serum concentrations.[32] TMP is mainly (50% to 60%) eliminated via the renal system, by glomerular filtration as well as tubular secretion, with a half-life of approximately 4 to 5.5 hours in children, increasing with age.[33]

Adverse Reactions

Commonly encountered adverse reactions include nausea and vomiting and skin rashes. Other adverse reactions are allergic reactions such as angioedema, anaphylactic reactions, and Stevens-Johnson syndrome. Hematologic disturbances, as a result of folic acid deficiency, such as thrombocytopenia, agranulocytosis, and megaloblastic anemia, are observed. Also, hemolytic anemia is observed in patients with G6PD deficiency.[34]

Drug Interactions

The effect of TMP can decrease when it is used concomitantly with folic acid. TMP increases the half-life of phenytoin, resulting in increased phenytoin blood concentrations. Monitoring of phenytoin concentrations is recommended. In addition, TMP can increase the toxicity, especially the hematologic toxicity, of methotrexate; thus, concomitant use should be avoided. Hyperkalemia is reported when TMP is used concomitantly with renin–angiotensin–aldosterone system inhibitors. Combination of drugs that are positively charged at physiologic pH and that are actively renally excreted (e.g., procainamide and amantadine), blood concentrations of the drugs can increase.[34] TMP may decrease the tubular secretion of creatinine and cause a mild elevation of serum creatinine at standard doses without decreasing the glomerular filtration rate. This is reversible with drug discontinuation.[4]

Pediatric Dosage

For children between the ages of 3 months and 12 years, treated for uncomplicated urinary tract infections or respiratory tract infections, the recommended daily dose is 6 to 9 mg per kg, divided in two doses. From 5 years and older, the dose can be administered once daily.[33] For children older than 12 years, the recommended daily dose is 300 mg for uncomplicated urinary tract infections and 400 mg per day, divided in two doses, for respiratory tract infections.[34]

PYRIMETHAMINE

Clinical Use

PM is, together with sulfadiazine and folic acid, used to treat toxoplasmosis caused by *T. gondii.* It is also registered for the treatment of malaria; however, resistance has become a big problem and, therefore, other drugs are usually used for this indication.[35,36]

Pharmacokinetics

PM is rapidly and well absorbed from the GI tract. Its protein binding is 80% to 90%, and PM gets metabolized in the liver. The metabolites are excreted renally. PM has a long half-life of approximately 85 hours.[36] Its penetration in CSF is moderate, with concentrations of 10% to 20% compared to those in serum.[3]

Adverse Reactions

Adverse reactions are suggested to differ between the different manifestations of toxoplasmosis, where in congenital toxoplasmosis and toxoplasmic encephalitis bone marrow is most frequently reported. Dermatologic reactions have the highest prevalence in toxoplasmic encephalitis, and GI tract reactions are most commonly observed in ocular toxoplasmosis.[35]

Drug Interactions

The concomitant use of PM and other antifolic drugs, such as sulfonamides or TMP-SMZ, may increase the risk of bone marrow suppression. Mild hepatotoxicity has been reported in some patients when lorazepam and PM were administered concomitantly.[36]

Pediatric Dosage

Pediatric dosage for the treatment of toxoplasmosis is 1 mg per kg per day divided into two equal daily doses; after 2 to 4 days, this dose may be reduced to one-half and continued for approximately 1 month.[36]

TRIMETHOPRIM–SULFAMETHOXAZOLE (CO-TRIMOXAZOLE)

Available preparations are manufactured in a 1:5 fixed ratio of TMP and SMZ. The combination of TMP-SMZ is usually synergistic and bactericidal. Both drugs affect bacterial folic acid synthesis, as described in the sections for the separate drugs. By inhibiting tetrahydrofolic acid formation, the active form of folic acid, TMP-SMZ inhibits bacterial thymidine synthesis and results in a bactericidal action.[2] Although these steps follow one another and cause a sequential blockade, this does not necessarily explain the aforementioned synergy. A combination of two drugs that have slightly different bacterial spectrums and different resistance profiles among pathogenic bacteria improves the usefulness of the drug combination.

CLINICAL USE

In general, many Enterobacteriaceae, including *E. coli*, *Klebsiella pneumoniae*, and *P. mirabilis*, are susceptible to TMP-SMZ. *Salmonella* and *Shigella* species were previously susceptible to TMP-SMZ. However, the resistant strains have rapidly increased recently worldwide.[37,38] TMP-SMZ is active against *Stenotrophomonas maltophilia*, which is typically resistant to other classes of broad-spectrum antibiotics.[39] Other nonfermentative organisms, including *Burkholderia cepacia*, *Acinetobacter*, and *Alcaligenes*, which often cause nosocomial infections, are frequently susceptible to TMP-SMZ. *S. aureus*, the most common skin pathogen, is also susceptible to TMP-SMZ. TMP-SMZ is also active against *P. jirovecii* (formerly known as *Pneumocystis carinii*), *Tropheryma whipplei*, *Isospora* species, *Cyclospora* species, and *T. gondii*.

TMP-SMZ is used as empiric treatment and prophylaxis for urinary tract infection in children. However, the recent use of antibiotics, hospitalization, and immunosuppression has been implicated as factors contributing to increasing TMP-SMZ resistance among urinary tract isolates in adults.[40,41] The prevalence of TMP-SMZ resistance among urinary tract isolates in children varies depending on geographic locations. However, limited data indicated an increasing trend of TMP-SMZ resistance up to more than 30% in children with community-acquired urinary tract infection.[42–44]

Previously, TMP-SMZ was an effective treatment for otitis media, sinusitis, and community-acquired pneumonia. Emerging resistance among respiratory pathogens, especially *S. pneumoniae*, has raised serious concerns regarding the use of TMP-SMZ in respiratory tract infections.[45] Thus, the use of TMP-SMZ for respiratory tract infections in children requires consideration of local resistance patterns and individual patient factors such as the severity of disease and risk for resistance.

TMP-SMZ is useful in the treatment of traveler's diarrhea due to enterotoxigenic *E. coli*.[2] However, it may not be effective in some parts of the world where resistant strains of these organisms are common.

TMP-SMZ is the agent of choice for the treatment and prophylaxis for *P. jirovecii* infection in children with malignancy, defects in cell-mediated immunity, and HIV infection. Mutations in the *P. jirovecii* dihydropteroate synthase gene have been identified in patients taking TMP-SMZ prophylaxis, and this may play a major role in TMP-SMZ treatment failure.[46]

Prophylactic use of TMP-SMZ to prevent recurrent bacterial infections in patients with chronic granulomatous disease and other neutrophil-associated immunodeficiencies has been well documented in children.[47,48] Selected patients with Wegener granulomatosis may benefit from TMP-SMZ, although the mechanism of action and degree of clinical efficacy in these patients are uncertain.[49,50]

Bacteria may become resistant to TMP-SMZ by several mechanisms, including the development of permeability barriers, efflux pumps, naturally insensitive target enzymes, and genetic alterations in the genes encoding target enzymes. Resistance is transferable. Resistance to SMZ in Gram-negative organisms is usually plasmid mediated. Resistance to TMP has been shown to occur by several mechanisms, most often chromosomally mediated, but also involving mutations of bacteria to thymidine-dependent strains, or plasmid-mediated resistance involving altered production or sensitivity of bacterial dihydrofolate reductase. Marked geographic variation in resistance has been demonstrated, with higher incidence typically found in developing countries.[51]

CLINICAL PHARMACOKINETICS

The pharmacokinetics of the individual compounds is described in the separate sections. Reference peak serum concentrations range from 1.5 to 2.5 mg per L for TMP and from 40 to 60 mg per L for SMZ. For *P. jirovecii*, reference peak serum concentrations range from 5 to 8 mg per L for TMP and from 100 to 200 mg per L for SMZ.[52]

ADVERSE REACTIONS

The most frequent adverse effects are GI intolerance and cutaneous reactions.[2] Multiple skin reactions have been described, including a maculopapular rash, urticaria, diffuse erythema, morbilliform rash, erythema multiforme, purpura, and photosensitivity.[53,54] These reactions tend to be mild, dose related, and reversible and can occasionally be obviated by reduction in dosage without discontinuation of therapy. Fatal hypersensitivity reaction, including Stevens-Johnson syndrome and toxic epidermal necrolysis, rarely occurs. A drug fever with delayed (1 to 2 weeks) onset, often accompanied by a morbilliform rash, may occur. The more severe form of this with multisystem involvement has sometimes been termed the DRESS (drug rash with eosinophilia and systemic symptoms) syndrome. The frequency of adverse effects is substantially higher in immunocompromised patients, particularly in HIV-infected individuals. The rate of adverse reactions to TMP-SMZ in HIV-infected children is approximately 15%.[4,55] Although this is higher than the rate seen in uninfected children, it is substantially lower than the rate seen in HIV-infected adults. The exact mechanisms of increased risk for adverse reactions in this population have not been determined.

TMP-SMZ has only rarely been associated with direct nephrotoxicity. Hyperkalemia has been observed in patients taking high-dose TMP-SMZ or in patients with preexisting renal insufficiency taking standard TMP-SMZ dosages.[2,4] Hematologic adverse events including anemia, granulocytopenia, megaloblastosis, agranulocytosis, and thrombocytopenia have been reported in children.[56,57] In G6PD-deficient patients, hemolysis can occur.[2]

DRUG INTERACTIONS

The effect of TMP-SMZ can decrease when it is used concomitantly with folic acid. SMZ inhibits CYP2C9; via this pathway, the serum concentrations of warfarin and oral hypoglycemic drugs are increased when used concomitantly with SMZ. This results in clinically significant exaggeration of anticoagulant effect, hypoglycemia, and[4] both SMZ and TMP increase phenytoin serum concentrations, resulting in increased CNS toxicity of phenytoin. Hyperkalemia is reported when TMP is used concomitantly with renin–angiotensin–aldosterone system inhibitors. Combination of drugs that are positively charged at physiologic pH and that are actively renally excreted (e.g., procainamide and amantadine), blood concentrations of the drugs can increase.[34]

In children receiving methotrexate, treatment with TMP-SMZ decreases organic anion transporter–mediated renal clearance of methotrexate by 40% increasing the risk of methotrexate toxicity, including cytopenia, mucositis, hepatotoxicity, and GI symptoms.[4] TMP-SMZ use is associated with increased nephrotoxicity of cyclosporin.

SMZ use is associated with the increased nephrotoxicity of cyclosporin despite reduction of serum cyclosporin concentrations. SMZ increases the free serum methotrexate fraction. TMP increases serum levels and increases elimination half-life of phenytoin and digoxin.

PEDIATRIC DOSAGE

The recommended pediatric dose is 6 to 10 mg per kg per day of TMP component, or 30 to 50 mg per kg per day of SMZ component, in two divided doses.[2] For *P. jirovecii* treatment, the dose should be increased to 20 mg per kg per day of TMP component and 100 mg per kg per day of SMZ component, in four doses intravenously for 21 days.[2] For prophylaxis against *P. jirovecii*, the recommended regimen is 150 mg per m^2 per day of TMP with 750 mg per m^2 per day of SMZ orally, in two divided doses, three times per week on consecutive days.[2,58]

For prophylaxis of recurrent urinary tract infections, the recommended dose is 2 mg of TMP and 10 mg of SMZ per kg per day.[59]

DAPSONE (4,4′-DIAMINODIPHENYLSULFONE)

Dapsone, a sulfonamide-related drug, was previously used for the treatment of several infectious diseases, including bacterial, yeast, and protozoa infections. Nowadays, it is used for the therapy of leprosy and dermatitis herpetiformis.[60] Its bacteriostatic effect originates from inhibition of the folic acid synthesis, just like sulfonamides and dihydrofolate reductase inhibitors. Dapsone inhibits the enzyme dihydropteroate synthetase by competing with PABA.[61]

CLINICAL USE

Dapsone is active in vitro against *Mycobacterium leprae* and several other species of *Mycobacterium*. It is also active against *P. jirovecii* and *Plasmodium* species. The treatment of choice for *Pneumocystis carinii* pneumonia (PCP) remains TMP-SMX. Dapsone, as well as a clindamycin–primaquine regimen, is an alternative drug for PCP prophylaxis in both adults and children intolerant to TMP-SMX or when TMP-SMX is contraindicated.[62] Dapsone is also used to treat *Mycobacterium avium* complex infection, in combination with azithromycin and other active antimicrobial agents. Dapsone is also used in combination with other active agents to treat children with leprosy and in some cases of multidrug-resistant tuberculosis. In addition, dapsone has been used as an antimalarial agent, in combination with chlorproguanil.[63]

CLINICAL PHARMACOKINETICS

Dapsone has an excellent oral bioavailability and, despite plasma protein binding of 50% to 90%, penetrates well into various tissues. Dapsone is extensively metabolized by both oxidative and conjugative processes, forming dapsone hydroxylamine and the *N*-acetylated metabolites MADDS and hydroxy-monoacetyldapsone, respectively.[64] N-hydroxylation, mediated by enzymes of the cytochrome P-450 3A4 subfamily, plays a central role in dapsone elimination. Increased cytochrome P-450 3A4 activity in young children explains the more rapid clearance in the patients younger than 2 years of age compared to older children. The predominant route of elimination of dapsone is metabolism, with only 5% to 15% of an administered dose found in urine as unchanged drug. The half-life of dapsone is approximately 28 hours.[61,62]

ADVERSE REACTIONS

Most frequently observed adverse reactions include nausea, vomiting, and abdominal pains. Fatal agranulocytosis has occurred rarely when dapsone is administered in combination with PM. Less severe granulocytopenia has occurred with dapsone in combination with chloroquine and primaquine. Severe hemolytic anemia can occur in association with large doses of dapsone (300 to 400 mg daily) or in patients with G6PD deficiency. Overdose of dapsone may result in methemoglobinemia; its usual features include dyspnea, fatigue, cyanosis, deceptively high pulse oximetry, and chocolate-colored blood. Dapsone also exhibits neurotoxicity, including peripheral neuropathy. Hypersensitivity reaction can occur 3 to 6 weeks after initiating dapsone. It is more likely to occur in patients with similar adverse reaction to other sulfonamides.[61,62] A rare adverse effect of dapsone is the sulfone syndrome. This is a non–dose-related adverse reaction, occurring within 2 months after starting dapsone therapy. It consists of fever, malaise, exfoliative dermatitis, hepatic necrosis, lymphadenopathy, anemia, and methemoglobinemia.[65]

DRUG INTERACTIONS

Dapsone is a substrate of cytochrome P-450 3A4. Therefore, cytochrome P-450 3A4 inducers, including rifampicin, will increase the hepatic biotransformation of dapsone and thus decrease dapsone blood concentrations. Concomitant use of dapsone with folic acid antagonists, such as PM and sulfonamides, can increase the risk of hematologic disturbances, such as agranulocytosis.[61]

PEDIATRIC DOSAGE

The recommended dosage in pediatrics is 1 to 1.5 mg per kg per day, in one dose.[61]

ACKNOWLEDGMENTS

We would like to acknowledge the authors of the previous edition of this chapter: Chokechai Rongkavilit, Nahed Abdel-Haq, Jocelyn Y. Ang, and Basim I. Asmar.

REFERENCES

1. Jacobson JA, Chester TJ, Fraser DW. An epidemic of disease due to serogroup B *Neisseria meningitidis* in Alabama: report of an investigation and community-wide prophylaxis with a sulfonamide. *J Infect Dis* 1977;136:104–108.
2. AR Scientific Inc. Bactrim (sulfamethoxazole and trimethoprim) package insert. 2013:17. www.accessdata.fda.gov.
3. Nau R, Sorgel F, Eiffert H. Penetration of drugs through the blood-cerebrospinal fluid/blood-brain barrier for treatment of central nervous system infections. *Clin Microbiol Rev* 2010;23:858–883.
4. Ho JM, Juurlink DN. Considerations when prescribing trimethoprim-sulfamethoxazole. *CMAJ* 2011;183:1851–1858.
5. Turner D, Levine A, Escher JC, et al, European Society for Paediatric Gastroenterology, Hepatology, and Nutrition. Management of pediatric ulcerative colitis: joint ECCO and ESPGHAN evidence-based consensus guidelines. *J Pediatr Gastroenterol Nutr* 2012;55:340–361.
6. Coward S, Kuenzig M, Hazlewood G, et al. Comparative effectiveness of mesalamine, sulfasalazine, corticosteroids, and budesonide for the induction of remission in Crohn's disease: a Bayesian network meta-analysis: republished. *Inflamm Bowel Dis* 2017;23:12.
7. 7.Plosker G, Kroom, K. Sulfasalazine: a review of its use in the management of rheumatoid arthritis. *Drugs* 2005;65:25.
8. van Rossum MA, Fiselier TJ, Franssen MJ, et al. Sulfasalazine in the treatment of juvenile chronic arthritis: a randomized, double-blind, placebo-controlled, multicenter study. Dutch Juvenile Chronic Arthritis Study Group. *Arthritis Rheum* 1998;41:808–816.
9. Klotz U. Clinical pharmacokinetics of sulphasalazine, its metabolites and other prodrugs of 5-aminosalicylic acid. *Clin Pharmacokinet* 1985;10:285–302.
10. Das KM, Dubin R. Clinical pharmacokinetics of sulphasalazine. *Clin Pharmacokinet* 1976;1:406–425.
11. Rijk MC, van Schaik A, van Tongeren JH. Disposition of 5-aminosalicylic acid by 5-aminosalicylic acid-delivering compounds. *Scand J Gastroenterol* 1988;23:107–112.
12. Reid J, Holt S, Housley E, et al. Raynaud's phenomenon induced by sulphasalazine. *Postgrad Med J* 1980;56:106–107.
13. Kristensen KS, Hoegholm A, Bohr L, et al. Fatal myocarditis associated with mesalazine. *Lancet* 1990;335:605.
14. Schwartz AG, Targan SR, Saxon A, et al. Sulfasalazine-induced exacerbation of ulcerative colitis. *N Engl J Med* 1982;306:409–412.
15. Garau P, Orenstein SR, Neigut DA, et al. Pancreatitis associated with olsalazine and sulfasalazine in children with ulcerative colitis. *J Pediatr Gastroenterol Nutr* 1994;18:481–485.
16. Fich A, Eliakim R. Does sulfasalazine induce alopecia? *J Clin Gastroenterol* 1988;10:466.
17. Corrigan G, Stevens PE. Review article: interstitial nephritis associated with the use of mesalazine in inflammatory bowel disease. *Aliment Pharmacol Ther* 2000;14:1–6.
18. Wang KK, Bowyer BA, Fleming CR, et al. Pulmonary infiltrates and eosinophilia associated with sulfasalazine. *Mayo Clin Proc* 1984;59:343–346.
19. Gunnarsson I, Kanerud L, Pettersson E, et al. Predisposing factors in sulphasalazine-induced systemic lupus erythematosus. *Br J Rheumatol* 1997;36:1089–1094.
20. Kirkpatrick AW, Bookman AA, Habal F. Lupus-like syndrome caused by 5-aminosalicylic acid in patients with inflammatory bowel disease. *Can J Gastroenterol* 1999;13:159–162.
21. Sieg I, Beckh K, Kersten U, et al. Manifestation of acute intermittent porphyria in patients with chronic inflammatory bowel disease. *Z Gastroenterol* 1991;29:602–605.
22. Peppercorn MA. Sulfasalazine. Pharmacology, clinical use, toxicity, and related new drug development. *Ann Intern Med* 1984;101:377–386.
23. Boyer DL, Li BU, Fyda JN, et al. Sulfasalazine-induced hepatotoxicity in children with inflammatory bowel disease. *J Pediatr Gastroenterol Nutr* 1989;8:528–532.
24. Deltenre P, Berson A, Marcellin P, et al. Mesalazine (5-aminosalicylic acid) induced chronic hepatitis. *Gut* 1999;44:886–888.
25. Shaffer JL, Houston JB. The effect of rifampicin on sulphapyridine plasma concentrations following sulphasalazine administration. *Br J Clin Pharmacol* 1985;19:526–528.
26. Lennard L. Clinical implications of thiopurine methyltransferase – optimization of drug dosage and potential drug interactions. *Ther Drug Monit* 1998;20:527–531.
27. Petersen E, Schmidt DR. Sulfadiazine and pyrimethamine in the postnatal treatment of congenital toxoplasmosis: what are the options? *Expert Rev Anti Infect Ther* 2003;1:175–182.
28. Simon DI, Brosius FC 3rd, Rothstein DM. Sulfadiazine crystalluria revisited. The treatment of toxoplasma encephalitis in patients with acquired immunodeficiency syndrome *Arch Intern Med* 1990;150:2379–2384.
29. Fraser GL, Beaulieu JT. Leukopenia secondary to sulfadiazine silver. *JAMA* 1979;241:1928–1929.
30. Nimia HH, Carvalho VF, Isaac C, et al. Comparative study of silver sulfadiazine with other materials for healing and infection prevention in burns: a systematic review and meta-analysis. *Burns* 2019;45:282–292.
31. King Pharmaceuticals. Silvadene cream 1% (silver sulfadiazine) package insert. 2012. www.accessdata.fda.gov.
32. Jager NGL, van Hest RM, Lipman J, et al. Antibiotic exposure at the site of infection: principles and assessment of tissue penetration. *Expert Rev Clin Pharmacol* 2019;12:623–634.
33. Hoppu K. Age differences in trimethoprim pharmacokinetics: need for revised dosing in children? *Clin Pharmacol Ther* 1987;41:336–343.
34. TEVA. Summary of product characteristics—Trimethoprim, Haarlem, The Netherlands, 2017.
35. Ben-Harari RR, Goodwin E, Casoy J. Adverse event profile of pyrimethamine-based therapy in toxoplasmosis: a systematic review. *Drugs R D* 2017;17:523–544.
36. GlaxoWellcome. Daraprim (Pyrimethamine). 2000. www.accessdata.fda.gov.
37. Parry CM. Antimicrobial drug resistance in *Salmonella enterica*. *Curr Opin Infect Dis* 2003;16:467–472.
38. Puzari M, Sharma M, Chetia P. Emergence of antibiotic resistant *Shigella* species: a matter of concern. *J Infect Public Health* 2018;11:451–454.
39. Tokatly Latzer I, Paret G, Rubinstein M, et al. Management of *Stenotrophomonas maltophilia* infections in critically ill children. *Pediatr Infect Dis J* 2018;37:981–986.
40. Lepelletier D, Caroff N, Reynaud A, et al. *Escherichia coli*: epidemiology and analysis of risk factors for infections caused by resistant strains. *Clin Infect Dis* 1999;29:548–552.
41. Wright SW, Wrenn KD, Haynes ML. Trimethoprim-sulfamethoxazole resistance among urinary coliform isolates. *J Gen Intern Med* 1999;14:606–609.
42. Ladhani S, Gransden W. Increasing antibiotic resistance among urinary tract isolates. *Arch Dis Child* 2003;88:444–445.
43. Prais D, Straussberg R, Avitzur Y, et al. Bacterial susceptibility to oral antibiotics in community acquired urinary tract infection. *Arch Dis Child* 2003;88:215–218.
44. McLoughlin TG Jr, Joseph MM. Antibiotic resistance patterns of uropathogens in pediatric emergency department patients. *Acad Emerg Med* 2003;10:347–351.
45. Hoban DJ, Doern GV, Fluit AC, et al. Worldwide prevalence of antimicrobial resistance in *Streptococcus pneumoniae, Haemophilus influenzae,* and *Moraxella catarrhalis* in the SENTRY Antimicrobial Surveillance Program, 1997-1999. *Clin Infect Dis* 2001;32(Suppl 2):S81–S93.
46. Kazanjian P, Locke AB, Hossler PA, et al. *Pneumocystis carinii* mutations associated with sulfa and sulfone prophylaxis failures in AIDS patients. *AIDS* 1998;12:873–878.
47. Weening RS, Kabel P, Pijman P. Continuous therapy with sulfamethoxazole-trimethoprim in patients with chronic granulomatous disease. *J Pediatr* 1983;103:127–130.
48. Mouy R, Fischer A, Vilmer E, et al. Incidence, severity, and prevention of infections in chronic granulomatous disease. *J Pediatr* 1989;114:555–560.
49. Stegeman CA, Tervaert JW, de Jong PE, et al. Trimethoprim-sulfamethoxazole (co-trimoxazole) for the prevention of relapses of Wegener's granulomatosis. Dutch Co-Trimoxazole Wegener Study Group. *N Engl J Med* 1996;335:16–20.
50. Lynch JP 3rd, Tazelaar H. Wegener granulomatosis (granulomatosis with polyangiitis): evolving concepts in treatment. *Semin Respir Crit Care Med* 2011;32:274–297.
51. Huovinen P, Sundstrom L, Swedberg G, et al. Trimethoprim and sulfonamide resistance. *Antimicrob Agents Chemother* 1995;39:279–289.
52. Brown G. Cotrimoxazole – optimal dosing in the critically ill. *Ann Intensive Care* 2014;4:9.
53. Goldman JL, Jackson MA, Herigon JC, et al. Trends in adverse reactions to trimethoprim-sulfamethoxazole. *Pediatrics* 2013;131:e103–e108.
54. Sattler FR, Cowan R, Nielsen DM, et al. Trimethoprim-sulfamethoxazole compared with pentamidine for treatment of *Pneumocystis carinii* pneumonia in the acquired immunodeficiency syndrome. *Ann Intern Med* 1988;109:7.
55. Hunter JM, Cooper DM, Colin AA. *Pneumocystis carinii* pneumonia: a pediatric perspective. *Pediatr AIDS HIV Infect* 1995;6:262–270.
56. Bose W, Karama A, Linzenmeier G, et al. Controlled trial of co-trimoxazole in children with urinary-tract infection. Bacteriological efficacy and haematological toxicity. *Lancet* 1974;2:614–616.
57. Asmar BI, Maqbool S, Dajani AS. Hematologic abnormalities after oral trimethoprim-sulfamethoxazole therapy in children. *Am J Dis Child* 1981;135:1100–1103.
58. Boast A, Osowicki J, Cole T, et al. Question 1: Co-trimoxazole dosing dilemma: what is the right dose? *Arch Dis Child* 2015;100:1089–1093.
59. Williams G, Craig JC. Long-term antibiotics for preventing recurrent urinary tract infection in children. *Cochrane Database Syst Rev* 2019;4:CD001534.
60. Wolf R, Matz H, Orion E, et al. Dapsone. *Dermatol Online J* 2002;8:2.
61. Holding M. Dapsone – summary of product characteristics, Abcoude, the Netherlands, 2013.
62. Molinelli E, Paolinelli M, Campanati A, et al. Metabolic, pharmacokinetic, and toxicological issues surrounding dapsone. *Expert Opin Drug Metab Toxicol* 2019;15:367–379.
63. Mutabingwa T, Nzila A, Mberu E, et al. Chlorproguanil-dapsone for treatment of drug-resistant falciparum malaria in Tanzania. *Lancet* 2001;358:1218–1223.
64. May DG, Porter JA, Uetrecht JP, et al. The contribution of N-hydroxylation and acetylation to dapsone pharmacokinetics in normal subjects. *Clin Pharmacol Ther* 1990;48:619–627.
65. Lee KB, Nashed TB. Dapsone-induced sulfone syndrome. *Ann Pharmacother* 2003;37:1044–1046.

CHAPTER 26

Basim I. Asmar
Nahed Abdel-Haq

Tetracyclines, Chloramphenicol, and Metronidazole

TETRACYCLINES

Tetracyclines were introduced soon after penicillin G and the sulfonamides. They were discovered by screening soil specimens for antibiotic-producing microorganisms. The first compound, chlortetracycline, was introduced in 1948,[1] and subsequently, many tetracyclines have been developed. Tetracyclines were known as "broad-spectrum" antibiotics because of their activity against a number of Gram-positive and Gram-negative bacteria as well as rickettsiae and chlamydiae. As a result of their broad in vitro activity and proven clinical effectiveness, they became widely used therapeutic agents.

Chlortetracycline was the first natural tetracycline, isolated from *Streptomyces aureofaciens* in 1948, and oxytetracycline was later derived from *Streptomyces rimosus* in 1950. Tetracycline was first produced semisynthetically from chlortetracycline in 1953. Demeclocycline was derived from a mutant strain of *S. aureofaciens*. The two long-acting compounds doxycycline and minocycline were derived semisynthetically in 1966 and 1967, respectively. Those currently marketed include tetracycline, oxytetracycline, and demeclocycline and the newer semisynthetic compounds doxycycline and minocycline. Currently, the most used agents include doxycycline, minocycline, and tetracycline.

CHEMICAL STRUCTURE

The basic tetracycline structure consists of a hydronaphthacene nucleus with four fused rings. Tetracycline analogs differ from each other by substituent variations at carbon 5, 6, or 7 of the basic structure (Fig. 26.1).

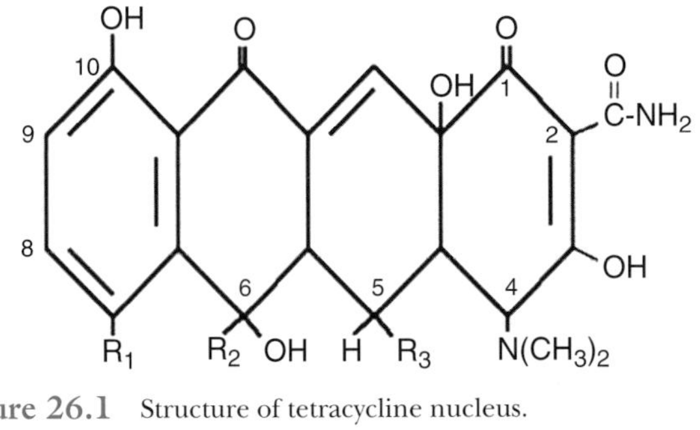

OH O O O OH C-NH2 10 9 8 1 2 4 5 6 OH R1 R2 OH H R3 N(CH3)2

Figure 26.1 Structure of tetracycline nucleus.

MECHANISM OF ACTION/MECHANISM OF BACTERIAL RESISTANCE

Tetracyclines are bacteriostatic agents that inhibit bacterial protein synthesis. They reversibly bind to the 30S subunits of bacterial ribosomes. Tetracyclines inhibit the binding of the enzyme aminoacyl-tRNA to the ribosomal acceptor site on the messenger RNA (mRNA)–ribosome complex.[2,3] This prevents the addition of new amino acids into the growing peptide chain. Studies of tetracycline in *Escherichia coli* show that tetracycline passively diffuses through outer membrane porins and then traverses the cytoplasmic membrane by energy-independent and energy-dependent mechanisms.[4] In higher concentrations, tetracyclines also inhibit mammalian protein synthesis, particularly in mitochondrial ribosomes.[5] Although these ribosomes are not present in sufficient concentration within these structures to produce severe toxicity, this antianabolic effect can aggravate preexisting renal function impairment.[6]

Resistance to tetracyclines occurred quickly following their availability, mainly based on efflux pumps and, to a lesser extent, on the presence of ribosomal protection proteins and tetracycline-inactivating enzymes. The genes encoding for resistance are called tet, or tetracycline resistance determinants. They are most often carried on plasmids but can be chromosomal. Resistance is achieved by increasing ability of the cell to efflux the antibiotic.[7] The *tet* genes encode for membrane proteins that mediate energy-dependent efflux. Efflux has been demonstrated in Enterobacteriaceae, enterococci, staphylococci, *Vibrio cholerae*, and *Bacteroides*. More than 200 different efflux pumps have been characterized. Resistance to one tetracycline usually implies resistance to all tetracyclines. However, partial cross-resistance occurs, and many tetracycline-resistant bacteria are susceptible to doxycycline and minocycline. A second but less common mechanism of resistance is due to altered ribosomal targets (encoded by different *tet* genes). Ribosomal protection proteins bind to the ribosome, causing changes in the conformation at the tetracycline site. This results in the inability of tetracyclines to prevent the attachment of aminoacyl-tRNA to the ribosomal receptor site. This has been described in some organisms, including *Neisseria gonorrhoeae* and *Mycoplasma*. A third mechanism of resistance, enzymatic inactivation of tetracyclines, encoded for by another *tet* gene, has been demonstrated in vitro in *E. coli*, but its clinical significance is not known.[8]

EVIDENCE OF EFFICACY/THERAPEUTIC USES

Tetracyclines have a broad spectrum of activity, which includes aerobic and anaerobic Gram-positive and Gram-negative bacteria, chlamydiae, rickettsiae, mycoplasma, ureaplasma, and spirochetes. In general, the lipophilic analogs have better antibacterial activity by weight than the more hydrophilic ones. Therefore, it follows that minocycline and doxycycline are more active at lower concentration against susceptible organisms than the other tetracyclines. Despite these differences, for cost reasons, it is recommended that tetracycline be used in the clinical microbiology laboratory to determine susceptibility for all analogs.[9] Organisms inhibited by 1 μg per mL or less are considered highly susceptible, those inhibited by 1 to 5 μg per mL are intermediately susceptible, whereas those not inhibited by 5 μg per mL are resistant. Bacterial resistance to any one member of the class usually results in cross-resistance to the other tetracyclines.

Tetracyclines are in general active against Gram-positive microorganisms; however, problems of resistance and the availability of more effective agents limit their use for treatment of infections caused by many Gram-positive bacteria. Tetracyclines are active against staphylococci; however, many strains, especially those recovered in hospitals, readily develop resistance. Both doxycycline and minocycline are more active against *Staphylococcus aureus* than tetracycline. Therefore, in vitro susceptibility testing should be performed if these drugs are to be used for treatment of staphylococcal infections.[10,11]

Resistance to tetracyclines among group A streptococci has varied from 5% to 35% in Europe and in the United States.[12,13] Group B streptococci are frequently resistant to tetracyclines.[14]

Most *Streptococcus pneumoniae* strains are susceptible to tetracycline and doxycycline; however, penicillin-resistant strains are often resistant to them.[15] Tetracycline- and penicillin-resistant pneumococci are very prevalent in some European countries.[16] In the United States, some penicillin-resistant pneumococci are also tetracycline resistant.[17] Most enterococci are resistant to tetracycline.

Minocycline has excellent activity against *Nocardia* species, especially *Nocardia asteroides*. Other tetracyclines are less active.[18]

Tetracyclines are considered effective against several Gram-negative bacteria; however, their activity has been limited by the emergence of resistant strains.

Most *Pseudomonas aeruginosa* and many *Salmonella* and *Shigella* strains are resistant. *Serratia marcescens* and *Proteus* species are usually resistant.

Gonococci and meningococci are very susceptible; however, gonococci resistant to penicillin tend to be resistant to tetracycline.[19]

Most strains of Campylobacter *jejuni* and *Campylobacter fetus* are susceptible to tetracyclines.[20] *Helicobacter pylori* is susceptible to tetracyclines and also to penicillins, erythromycin, cephalosporins, clindamycin, and rifampicin and usually metronidazole.[21] Tetracyclines are active against *Aeromonas hydrophila* and *Plesiomonas shigelloides*.[22] *Brucella* species are uniformly susceptible to tetracycline.[23,24]

V. cholerae, both classical and El Tor biotypes, which cause gastroenteritis, *Vibrio vulnificus*, which is associated with septicemia or cellulites, and other vibrios (*Vibrio parahaemolyticus, Vibrio alginolyticus*), which cause foodborne gastroenteritis, are susceptible to tetracyclines.[25,26] Some strains of enterotoxigenic *E. coli* are also susceptible.[27] Most *Yersinia enterocolitica* and *Yersinia pseudotuberculosis* are susceptible to tetracycline, aminoglycosides, third-generation cephalosporins, trimethoprim–sulfamethoxazole, and chloramphenicol.[28] *Yersinia pestis*, the etiologic agent of plague, is susceptible in vitro to tetracycline, streptomycin, gentamicin, and chloramphenicol.[29]

Bartonella henselae, the etiologic agent of cat-scratch disease (CSD), and *Bartonella quintana*, which causes louse trench fever, are susceptible to tetracycline.[30,31] *Legionella pneumophila* is quite susceptible to doxycycline and minocycline.[32] *Burkholderia (Pseudomonas) pseudomallei* (melioidosis) is usually susceptible to tetracycline and minocycline.[33]

Tetracyclines are active against many anaerobic bacteria.[34] Of the Gram-negative anaerobes, *Fusobacterium* and *Prevotella* are frequently susceptible. A variable number of *Bacteroides* species are susceptible to doxycycline; however, clindamycin, chloramphenicol, and metronidazole are more active and are the preferred drugs for treatment of infections caused by *Bacteroides fragilis*. Gram-positive anaerobes also have variable susceptibility. The activity of tetracyclines against *Actinomyces* is especially clinically relevant. *Propionibacterium* is frequently susceptible, whereas *Peptococcus* is frequently resistant.

Mycoplasma pneumoniae is susceptible to all tetracyclines.[35,36] *Mycoplasma hominis* is usually susceptible, but some resistant strains have been recently noted.[37]

Tetracyclines are effective against *Ureaplasma urealyticum*; however, resistant strains have been reported to naturally exist[38,39] and shown to be induced in vitro.[34]

Chlamydia trachomatis, the cause of trachoma, genital infections, and perinatally acquired respiratory infections in young infants, is susceptible to tetracyclines, especially doxycycline and minocycline. The minimum inhibitory concentration (*MIC*) of doxycycline against this organism is 0.06 μg per mL or less.[40] Occasional resistant strains have been encountered.[41,42] *Chlamydia pneumoniae* (respiratory pathogen) is susceptible to tetracyclines.[43,44] *Chlamydia psittaci*, which causes psittacosis, is also susceptible to tetracyclines.[45]

Many pathogenic spirochetes are susceptible to tetracyclines. *Borrelia burgdorferi*, the etiologic agent of Lyme disease, is highly susceptible to tetracyclines and is also susceptible to ampicillin, ceftriaxone, and imipenem.[46] *Treponema pallidum* is susceptible to tetracycline; however, its *MIC* (0.2 μg per mL) against this organism is much higher than that of penicillin G (0.0005 μg per mL).[47] The leptospira are susceptible to tetracycline.

Tetracyclines are very effective against the rickettsiae, which cause a variety of spotted fevers and typhus fevers. Rocky Mountain spotted fever is caused by *Rickettsia rickettsiae* and Mediterranean spotted fever by *Rickettsia conorii*. Murine typhus is caused by *Rickettsia typhi*, epidemic typhus by *Rickettsia prowazekii*, and scrub typhus by *Rickettsia tsutsugamushi*. Tetracyclines are active against all these rickettsiae (*MIC* = 0.25 μg per mL), with doxycycline being the most active (*MIC* = 0.1 μg per mL).[48] *Coxiella burnetii*, the etiologic agent of Q fever, is also susceptible.[48]

Ehrlichia species, which are obligate intracellular bacteria, are susceptible to tetracyclines.[49] Tetracyclines, especially doxycycline, are effective against malarial parasites, including chloroquine-resistant *Plasmodium falciparum*.[50,51]

THERAPEUTIC USES

The extensive use of tetracyclines for treatment of infections and as an additive to animal feeds (to facilitate growth) has led to a dramatic increase in bacterial resistance, and as a result, their use has declined. However, tetracyclines remain the drugs of choice or are the effective alternative therapy for a variety of bacterial infections. They are especially useful for the treatment of infections caused by rickettsiae, mycoplasma, and chlamydiae.

The use of tetracyclines during tooth development, during infancy and childhood to age 8 years, may cause permanent discoloration of the teeth. The degree of staining is directly proportional to the number of tetracycline courses prescribed. Therefore, tetracycline drugs should not be used in this age group, unless other treatment is not likely to be effective or if alternative therapy is contraindicated. Tetracyclines cross the placenta to expose the fetus; skeletal embryopathy in experimental animals has been reported. Doxycycline binds less readily to calcium compared with other members of the tetracycline class. Recent comparative data in younger children suggest that doxycycline is not likely to cause visible teeth staining or enamel hypoplasia in children younger than 8 years. These reassuring data support the revised recommendation of the American Academy of Pediatrics that doxycycline can be administered for a short duration (21 days or less) without regard to patient age.[52]

Rickettsial Infections

Tetracyclines are very effective in the treatment of rickettsial infections, including Rocky Mountain spotted fever, Q fever, rickettsial pox, epidemic typhus (Brill disease), murine typhus, and scrub typhus.[53,54] In almost all clinical situations, doxycycline is the drug of choice. Chloramphenicol is also effective for these diseases and is sometimes preferred for very severe infections. For adults and children weighing more than 45 kg, the recommended doxycycline treatment is 100 mg orally every 12 hours. For children weighing less than 45 kg, doxycycline 2.2 mg per kg per day is given every 12 hours for 7 to 10 days. Patients with severe disease who require hospitalization, are vomiting, or are comatose should receive parenteral therapy at a dose of 100 mg intravenously (IV) every 12 hours.[55]

Mycoplasma pneumoniae *Infections*

The drugs of choice in pneumonia due to *M. pneumoniae* are either a macrolide (azithromycin, clarithromycin, and erythromycin) or a tetracycline like doxycycline. Both drugs are equally effective in shortening the duration of illness.[35] A macrolide is the drug of choice in children because of the adverse effects of tetracyclines on teeth. The regimen of tetracycline in children with *M. pneumoniae* pneumonia is 40 to 50 mg per kg per 24 hour administered every 6 hours for 10 days. For adolescents and adults, the dose is 2 g per 24 hour divided every 6 hours. The regimen of doxycycline for children weighing less than 45 kg is 2.2 mg per kg per day given every 12 hours for 7 to 10 days. For adults and children weighing more than 45 kg, the recommended doxycycline treatment is 100 mg orally every 12 hours.

Mycoplasma hominis *Infections*

M. hominis is an inhabitant of the genitourinary tract and has been implicated as a cause of salpingitis and postpartum septicemia. Illness due to *M. hominis* infection is rare in children. This organism should be considered as an etiologic possibility in neonates with meningitis and with abscesses in whom routine cultures are negative.[56,57] *M. hominis* is usually resistant to erythromycin and azithromycin. Therapy with doxycycline is usually successful.[58]

Ureaplasma urealyticum

U. urealyticum and *Chlamydia* species are the major cause of nongonococcal urethritis. Tetracyclines are usually effective against infections caused by both organisms.[59] However, resistant strains have been reported.[60] Patients with nongonococcal urethritis should be treated with tetracycline 40 mg per kg per 24 hour every 6 hours; patients weighing more than 50 kg should receive 500 mg every 6 hours for 10 days.[61] *Ureaplasma* and *Chlamydia* are also susceptible to erythromycin, which is a useful alternative for patients in whom tetracycline is contraindicated.

Chlamydia Infections

Tetracyclines are effective for the treatment of *Chlamydia* infections. Lymphogranuloma venereum, caused by *C. trachomatis* serovars L1, L2, and L3, responds to tetracycline treatment.[62] Recommended treatment is doxycycline 100 mg twice daily for 3 weeks. Alternative treatment is erythromycin.

For uncomplicated *C. trachomatis* genital tract infection in adolescents and adults, oral doxycycline 100 mg twice daily for 7 days is effective; however, azithromycin 1 g given as a single dose is also effective and preferred because of better compliance.[63] Because coinfection with *N. gonorrhoeae* and *C. trachomatis* is common, doxycycline or azithromycin should be administered empirically in addition to the other agent used for treatment of gonorrhea.[64]

C. trachomatis frequently is a coexistent pathogen in acute pelvic inflammatory disease. Recommended treatment is doxycycline, 100 mg IV twice daily, for at least 48 hours after clinical improvement followed by oral therapy at the same dosage to complete 14 days.[64]

Respiratory infections due to *C. pneumoniae* in older children and adults are commonly treated with doxycycline 100 mg twice daily for 14 to 21 days. Erythromycin, azithromycin, and clarithromycin are also effective. For children, either erythromycin (for 10 to 14 days) or clarithromycin (for 10 days) can be used.[44]

The most widely used therapy for trachoma is topical treatment with tetracycline, erythromycin, or sulfacetamide ointment twice a day for 2 months or oral erythromycin or doxycycline for 40 days if the infection is severe. Azithromycin 20 mg per kg (maximum 1 g once per week) for 3 weeks is also effective.[63]

Penicillin G is the best drug for treatment of syphilis. Nonpregnant, penicillin-allergic patients who have primary, secondary, or latent syphilis can be treated with a tetracycline (500 mg four times daily for 14 days) or doxycycline (100 mg orally twice daily for 2 weeks). However, pregnant patients, children and adults with neurosyphilis, and patients allergic to penicillin should be treated whenever possible with penicillin G after desensitization.[64]

Ehrlichiosis and Anaplasmosis

These are tick-borne infections caused by obligate intracellular bacteria that belong to the two genera *Ehrlichia* and *Anaplasma*. Infection causes undifferentiated fever with leukopenia, thrombocytopenia, and elevations in serum aminotransferase levels. Rash is an infrequent sign. The treatment of choice for human ehrlichiosis (*Ehrlichia chaffeensis*), also known as human monocytic ehrlichiosis, and anaplasmosis (*Anaplasma phagocytophilum*), also known as granulocytic anaplasmosis, is doxycycline usually administered for 7 days.[49,65] The recommended pediatric dosage of doxycycline is 4.4 mg per kg per day divided every 12 hours, IV or orally (maximum 100 mg per dose).

Lyme Disease

B. burgdorferi, the etiologic agent of Lyme disease, is highly sensitive to tetracycline.[66] It is also susceptible to ampicillin, ceftriaxone, and imipenem. Erythromycin appears to be active in vitro but may be less so in vivo. Tetracycline is considered the most effective treatment for early manifestations, such as erythema migrans, of this disease. Recommendation for treatment of early disease is tetracycline orally four times per day, or doxycycline 100 mg twice daily for 20 to 30 days for adults and children older than 8 years. In younger children, amoxicillin or cefuroxime is alternative agent. Lyme arthritis can also be treated successfully with a 1-month course of oral doxycycline.[67] Although doxycycline has been successful in treatment of Lyme meningitis in some patients, ceftriaxone is superior.[68] Guidelines for the assessment, treatment, and prevention of Lyme disease have been published by the Infectious Diseases Society of America.[69]

Brucellosis

Tetracyclines are effective in the treatment of acute and chronic infections caused by *Brucella melitensis*, *Brucella suis*, and *Brucella abortus*. Because brucellae are intracellular pathogens, it is believed that penetration into the cells is a requirement for effective therapy. Tetracyclines are very effective agents for treating brucellosis and have a mean *MIC* of less than 1 µg per mL. The regimen of choice is tetracycline 30 to 40 mg per kg per 24 hour, maximum daily dose 2 g per 24 hour, divided into four oral doses for 4 to 6 weeks (or doxycycline 5 mg per kg per 24 hour, maximum daily dose 200 mg, divided twice a day) in combination with streptomycin 15 to 30 mg per kg per 24 hour, maximum daily dose 1 g, divided into two intramuscular doses for 2 to 3 weeks (or gentamicin 5 mg per kg per 24 hour divided twice daily for 5 days).[70] For children younger than 8 years, recommended treatment is a combination of trimethoprim and sulfamethoxazole (10/50 mg per kg per 24 hour) given twice daily for 3 weeks plus gentamicin (5 mg per kg per 24 hour) twice daily for the first 5 days[71] or trimethoprim–sulfamethoxazole plus rifampin (20 mg per kg per 24 hour) for 8 to 12 weeks.[72]

Cholera

Correction of dehydration associated with cholera is the most important treatment measure. Oral tetracyclines have been shown to be effective in eradicating *Vibrio* organisms from stools and shortening the volume and duration of diarrhea. Tetracycline-resistant strains of *V. cholerae* are uncommon. Oral tetracycline is given as 50 mg per kg per 24 hour, divided into four doses every 6 hours for 3 days (maximum dose 2 g per day) or as a single dose of 25 mg per kg (maximum dose 1 g). Oral doxycycline is given as two doses of 2 mg per kg on day 1 followed by single dose of 2 mg per kg on days 2 and 3 (maximum single dose 100 mg) or a single dose of 7 mg per kg (maximum dose 300 mg).[73] Because tetracyclines can cause discoloration of deciduous and permanent teeth, they have not been routinely used to treat children, even though the risk is small with such relatively short courses. Furazolidone has been the agent used routinely in children to treat cholera (5 mg per kg per day divided into four doses for 3 days, maximum dose 400 mg; or a single dose of 7 mg per kg, maximum dose 300 mg).[74]

Malaria

Tetracyclines have been used for treatment of chloroquine-resistant *Malaria falciparum*. The response to tetracycline alone is slow, and a regimen of quinine sulfate combined with tetracycline is more successful. Tetracycline 6.25 mg per kg every 6 hours (maximum 250 mg daily) or doxycycline 2 mg per kg every 12 hours (maximum 100 mg every 12 hours) is given for 7 days, in addition to a full course of quinine sulfate 25 mg per kg per 24 hour orally in divided doses every 8 hours (maximum 650 mg every 8 hours) for 3 to 7 days. For prevention of chloroquine-resistant *M. falciparum* infection, doxycycline 2 mg per kg daily, up to 100 mg, is given (beginning 1 to 2 days before travel, continuing for the duration of stay, and for 4 weeks after leaving).[75]

Acne

Topical keratolytic agents may be effective for mild disease; however, for severe acne, the addition of antibiotics may be of benefit. Tetracyclines often given in an oral dose of 250 mg twice daily may be continued for months or even years. Tetracyclines may act by inhibiting the anaerobic *Propionibacterium acnes* organisms that colonize the sebaceous follicles. These organisms metabolize lipids into free fatty acids, which cause inflammation in the follicular wall. They also produce chemotactic agents that attract polymorphonuclear cells into the follicular wall. Long-term use of tetracyclines seems to be well tolerated with few side effects because of the low dose used and the age of the patients. Erythromycin or trimethoprim–sulfamethoxazole was also shown to be effective oral agent.

PHARMACOKINETIC PROPERTIES: ABSORPTION, METABOLISM, AND ELIMINATION

Tetracycline compounds can be divided into three groups according to their different half-lives. The short-acting group includes chlortetracycline, oxytetracycline, and tetracycline; demeclocycline is an intermediate-acting compound; and long-acting agents include doxycycline and minocycline. Some pharmacokinetic properties of these compounds are given in Table 26.1.

Oral administration is the preferred route because of thrombophlebitis associated with the IV route and pain with the intramuscular injection. Absorption of most tetracyclines from the gastrointestinal tract, primarily in the proximal small bowel, is incomplete. Tetracyclines form insoluble complexes with aluminum, calcium, iron, magnesium, zinc, and other bivalent and trivalent cations. Therefore, concurrent ingestion of milk and other dairy products, antacids, calcium or iron supplements, bismuth subsalicylate, and other agents can impair tetracycline absorption.

Plasma concentrations of tetracyclines achieved following oral administration vary among individuals due to the variability of their absorption. Oxytetracycline and tetracycline are incompletely absorbed (58% to 77%). Their peak plasma concentration is achieved 2 to 4 hours after an oral dose. Their

TABLE 26.1 Pharmacokinetic Properties of Tetracyclines

Antibiotic	*Gastrointestinal Absorption (%)*	*Half-Life (h)*	*Protein Binding (%)*
Short acting			
Oxytetracycline	58	9	35
Tetracycline	77	8	65
Intermediate acting			
Demeclocycline	66	12	91
Long acting			
Doxycycline	93	18	93
Minocycline	95	16	76

half-lives range from 8 to 9 hours. These drugs are given every 6 hours. Peak plasma concentrations of 2 to 2.5 μg per mL are achieved after 250 mg oral dose. Demeclocycline is also incompletely absorbed (66%) and has a half-life of about 12 hours, resulting in effective plasma concentration for 24 to 48 hours. Therefore, this drug is administered in lower daily doses than oxytetracycline and tetracycline.

Doxycycline and minocycline are absorbed almost completely (93% to 95%) and have the longest half-lives, 16 to 18 hours. Thus, high serum levels are achieved with relatively small doses. Because of its long half-life, therapeutic plasma levels of doxycycline can be maintained with a single-daily dose, although twice-daily dosing is usually recommended.[76]

Following an oral dose of 200 mg of doxycycline, a plasma concentration of 3 μg per mL is achieved at 2 hours and a sustained concentration of 1 μg per mL for 8 to 12 hours. The plasma concentrations of doxycycline are equivalent following oral and parenteral routes. The absorption of doxycycline or minocycline is not affected by food. The half-lives of these compounds are mainly determined by their rate of renal excretion. Chlortetracycline is an exception; it has a short half-life despite having a slow rate of renal clearance due to its instability both in vitro and in vivo.[77] Adequate therapeutic concentrations in the urine are achieved by all tetracyclines, with the exception of chlortetracycline and minocycline, for the treatment of urinary tract infections by susceptible bacteria. Serum protein binding of these compounds varies but tends to be higher for the intermediate- and long-acting compounds (Table 32.1).[9,78,79] This is a possible contributing factor to their slow rate of renal excretion.

Tetracyclines are distributed widely throughout the body. They can be found in many tissues and body fluids, including the lung, liver, kidney, brain, sputum, and mucosal secretions. They accumulate in the liver, spleen, bone marrow, bone, dentine, and the enamel, including the enamel of nonerupted teeth. Levels of tetracycline in cerebrospinal fluid (CSF) are about 10% to 26% of blood levels.[80,81] Inflammation of the meninges is not a requirement for penetration into CSF. Concentrations in synovial fluid and sinus mucosa approach that in blood.[82,83] Tetracyclines concentrate in bile at levels 5 to 20 times those in serum. Minocycline and, to a lesser extent, doxycycline are more lipophilic than the other tetracyclines. This is the likely reason why these two agents attain higher concentrations in saliva and tears.[84] Tetracyclines cross the placenta and enter fetal circulation and amniotic fluid. They accumulate in fetal bone and teeth and, therefore, should not be given during pregnancy.[85] Relatively high concentrations of tetracyclines are detected in breast milk.[86] Most tetracyclines, with the exception of doxycycline, are eliminated primarily by the kidneys. Although they are concentrated in the liver and then excreted by way of bile into the intestines, they are partially reabsorbed via the enterohepatic circulation. Even when given parenterally, these drugs are excreted into the intestinal tract as a result of excretion into bile. Clearance of these drugs in the kidneys is by glomerular filtration. Therefore, their renal excretion is significantly affected by the renal function status of the patient. The tetracyclines should not be used in patients with renal failure. Doxycycline is the only exception, because it is excreted in the gastrointestinal tract mostly as an inactive conjugate and does not accumulate significantly in patients with renal failure. Decreased hepatic function or biliary tract obstruction decreases biliary excretion of these drugs and results in higher plasma concentration and longer half-life. Minocycline is significantly metabolized in the liver and is recovered in much lower concentration from both urine and feces than the other tetracyclines. Its renal clearance is also low, and it persists in the body after its administration is stopped because of its retention in fatty tissues. Minocycline half-life is not prolonged in patients with hepatic failure. All tetracyclines are slowly removed from blood by hemodialysis, but the rate of removal by peritoneal dialysis is poor.[87,88]

DOSES AND ROUTES

Tetracyclines are available in different forms for oral, parenteral, and topical administration. For oral administration, the recommended oral dose of tetracyclines varies with the severity and nature of the infection being treated. Oral tetracycline dose ranges from 1 to 2 g per day in adults; for children older than 8 years, the regimen is 25 to 50 mg per kg daily in four divided doses. The regimen of doxycycline for adults is 100 mg every 12 hours for the first 24 hours, followed by 100 mg once a day, or twice daily when severe infection is present. For children older than 8 years, the doxycycline regimen is 4 to 5 mg per kg per day divided into two doses given every 12 hours for the first day, followed by 2 to 2.5 mg per day given as a single-daily dose.

The regimen of minocycline for adults is 200 mg on day 1, then 100 mg every 12 hours after that; for children older than 8 years, minocycline is given at 4 mg per kg on the first day, then 2 mg per kg every 12 hours.

Parenteral Administration

The preferred parenteral tetracycline is doxycycline. It is used for treatment of severe infections, or in patients who cannot ingest the oral preparation or have associated nausea or vomiting. For adults, the IV regimen of doxycycline is 200 mg given in one or two doses on the first day, followed by 100 to 200 mg daily thereafter. The dosage for children is 4 mg per kg given in two equal doses on the first day, followed by 2.2 mg per kg single-daily maintenance dose. Minocycline IV dosing for adults is an initial loading dose of 200 mg, followed by 100 mg every 12 hours. In children older than 8 years, the initial dose is 4 mg per kg, followed by 2 mg per kg every 12 hours.

Parenteral preparations of tetracycline are no longer available in the United States. Where available, the usual adult daily dose is 500 mg to 1 g, administered in equally divided doses every 6 to 12 hours. In severe infections, a maximum dose of 2 g per day may be given.

Local Application

Topical use of tetracyclines is not recommended, except for local use in the eye. Ophthalmic ointments and suspensions of tetracycline hydrochloride, chlortetracycline hydrochloride, and oxytetracycline hydrochloride are available.

ADVERSE EFFECTS

Gastrointestinal Effects

All tetracyclines may produce gastrointestinal irritation to varying degrees, especially when given orally. Gastric distress, abdominal discomfort, nausea, and vomiting may occur. Gastrointestinal symptoms usually subside quickly when the tetracycline is stopped. Tetracyclines may also cause antibiotic-associated colitis. Gastric distress can be reduced by administering the drug with food. However, tetracyclines should not be given with dairy products.

Hepatic Toxicity

Rarely, hepatitis-like illness may develop during oral treatment with tetracycline, doxycycline, or minocycline or following IV administration of doxycycline. The hepatitis can occasionally be severe but usually resolves after discontinuation of the drug. The risk of such complication has been estimated to be 1.56 cases per 1 million.[89] Overdosing of IV tetracycline can be particularly dangerous during pregnancy and has been associated with symptoms of nausea, fever, and vomiting, followed by jaundice. In severe cases, the disease can be associated with hematemesis, renal failure with acidosis, and, in fatal cases, coma and terminal hypotension.[90]

Hypersensitivity Reactions

These are uncommon and usually manifest as urticaria, facial swelling, or bronchospasm. Rarely, anaphylaxis may occur. The Jarisch–Herxheimer reaction may occur when tetracyclines are used to treat a spirochetal infection such as *B. burgdorferi* infection (Lyme disease) or other infections such as brucellosis or tularemia.

Photosensitivity

Patients treated with doxycycline, and less often other tetracyclines, may develop mild-to-severe photosensitivity reactions when exposed to sunlight.[91] Minocycline is less likely to cause this side effect.

Effects on Teeth

Tetracyclines are deposited in calcifying areas of bones and teeth and may cause permanent yellow or brown discoloration of the teeth. This is purely a cosmetic disadvantage of these agents. Tetracyclines may deposit in the deciduous teeth if administered to children early in life or given to their mother during pregnancy because they cross the placenta.[92] Risk is highest when tetracycline is given to neonates and babies prior to first dentition. Pigmentation of permanent teeth may occur if the drug is given between 2 months and 5 years of age when the teeth are being calcified. However, children up to 8 years may be susceptible to this complication. The type of discoloration may vary according to the particular tetracycline used. Chlortetracycline produces gray-brown teeth, whereas tetracycline and oxytetracycline cause yellow discoloration. The degree of discoloration depends on the amount of tetracycline administered. Discoloration becomes obvious in children who have several courses of the drug.

Nephrotoxicity

Tetracyclines may cause further rise in blood urea and serum creatinine in patients with renal disease. This is probably due to inhibition of protein synthesis by the drug, which results in a catabolic effect.[93]

Neurotoxic Effects

An uncommon complication of bulging anterior fontanel may occur in infants receiving usual doses of tetracycline. The condition is characterized by irritability, vomiting, and tense bulging fontanel associated with elevated CSF pressure, normal number of cells, and normal glucose and protein content. Rapid resolution occurs when the drug is discontinued.[94] Benign increased intracranial hypertension caused by tetracycline and minocycline has been reported in both adults and children.[95,96] Clinical manifestations include severe headache and blurring of vision associated with papilledema. Most cases have occurred in young adults and some children, and the majority had been taking tetracycline for acne for periods of days to months.

Minocycline, but not other tetracyclines, has been associated with reversible vestibular disturbance manifesting as dizziness, ataxia, vertigo, tinnitus with weakness, nausea, and vomiting. Minocycline has also been associated with lightheadedness and feeling of dissociation.[97]

DRUG INTERACTIONS

Tetracyclines form insoluble complexes with bivalent and trivalent cations, including aluminum, calcium, iron, magnesium, and zinc. Therefore, concurrent ingestion of antacids, calcium, iron supplements, or bismuth subsalicylate as well as milk and other dairy products can impair tetracycline absorption. Therefore, administration of the drugs should be spaced by 2 hours.[98,99]

Carbamazepine, diphenylhydantoin, and barbiturates increase the hepatic metabolism of doxycycline, causing a decrease in the normal half-life of the drug by almost one-half.[100,101] Digoxin is inactivated by gastrointestinal bacteria in some patients, and a course of tetracycline might reduce that. Therefore, antibiotic administration to such patients may cause a rise in serum digoxin level.[102]

CHLORAMPHENICOL

Chloramphenicol is an antibiotic that was first isolated in 1947 from the soil bacterium *Streptomyces venezuelae*.[103] After its relatively simple structure was determined, it was prepared synthetically, and by 1948, chloramphenicol became available for general use. Chloramphenicol was considered the first "broad-spectrum" antibiotic because of its activity against many Gram-positive and Gram-negative bacteria, anaerobic bacteria, as well as rickettsiae.

By 1950, chloramphenicol was incriminated as a cause of serious and fatal blood dyscrasias. In 1958, a unique toxic effect of chloramphenicol on the newborn infants known as "gray baby syndrome" was recognized, which resulted in further uncertainty regarding chloramphenicol use. For these reasons, chloramphenicol is reserved as alternative therapy in patients with serious infections such as meningitis, typhoid fever, and typhus who cannot be treated with other, safer drugs because of resistance or allergy.

CHEMICAL STRUCTURE

The chloramphenicol molecule contains a nitrobenzene moiety and is a derivative of dichloroacetic acid. Its structural formula is shown in Figure 26.2.

MECHANISM OF ACTION/MECHANISM OF ANTIBACTERIAL RESISTANCE

Chloramphenicol inhibits bacterial protein synthesis by binding reversibly to the 50S ribosomal subunit. This prevents the attachment of the amino acid–containing end of the aminoacyl-tRNA to the acceptor site on the 50S ribosomal subunit. As a result, the interaction between peptidyltransferase and its amino acid substrate cannot occur, and the peptide bond formation is prevented.[7] This results in the block of protein synthesis, producing static inhibition of most sensitive microorganisms. Mammalian mitochondria contain 70S ribosomes that also bind chloramphenicol, leading to inhibition of mitochondrial protein synthesis in mammalian cells. The effect of chloramphenicol against these cells has been suggested as the cause of the dose-related bone marrow suppression of the drug.[104]

Resistance to chloramphenicol is primarily due to production of the enzyme acetyltransferase, which acetylates the antibiotic to an inactive diacetyl derivative.[105] The acetylated derivative fails to bind to bacterial ribosomes. The production of acetyltransferase is plasmid (R factor) mediated and has been responsible for epidemics of chloramphenicol-resistant typhoid fever and Shigella dysentery.[106–108] The unrestricted over-the-counter sales of chloramphenicol in certain developing countries may have contributed to the emergence of resistant *Salmonella* strains.[108,109] In the United States, chloramphenicol resistance in *Salmonella* has been linked to the use of chloramphenicol in dairy farms.[110]

Nonenzymatic resistance to chloramphenicol, either due to reduced drug uptake mediated by chromosomal mutation or by acquired genetic genes and mutation in the bacterial 50S ribosome, has been described but is rare.

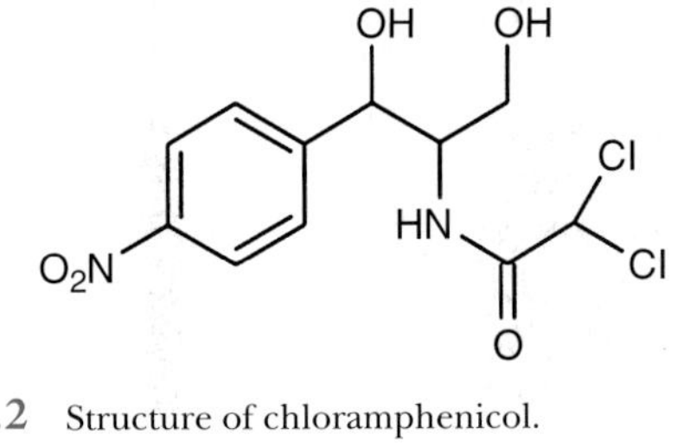

Figure 26.2 Structure of chloramphenicol.

INDICATIONS/THERAPEUTIC USES

Chloramphenicol has a wide spectrum of antimicrobial activity, which includes aerobic and anaerobic bacteria, rickettsiae, mycoplasma, and chlamydiae. Bacterial strains are considered susceptible if they are inhibited by concentration of 8 μg per mL or less. Most of the susceptible Gram-positive and Gram-negative bacteria are inhibited by concentrations easily achievable in serum. However, more active or less toxic therapeutic agents are available for treatment of infections caused by these pathogens.

Although chloramphenicol is classified as a bacteriostatic agent, it may be bactericidal against certain species such as *Haemophilus influenzae, Neisseria meningitidis,* and *S. pneumoniae.*

Gram-Negative Aerobic Bacteria

Most *E. coli* and *Klebsiella pneumoniae* strains and many *Proteus* species are usually susceptible to chloramphenicol. However, resistant strains have emerged as a result of the clinical use of chloramphenicol. For example, the routine use of chloramphenicol for treating neonatal sepsis resulted in the emergence of chloramphenicol resistance in up to 50% of *E. coli* or *Klebsiella* in one neonatal unit.[111] The combination of chloramphenicol and gentamicin may exhibit an antagonistic effect against some enteric Gram-negative organisms, such as *E. coli* and *Klebsiella.* Chloramphenicol appears to suppress the bactericidal action of gentamicin against these organisms.[112] In vitro studies have also shown that chloramphenicol antagonizes cefotaxime and ceftriaxone bactericidal activity against *E. coli* and group B streptococci.[113]

Salmonella strains including *Salmonella typhi* are generally susceptible to chloramphenicol. Resistant *Salmonella* strains have been occasionally recovered in the United States, but imported *Salmonella* strains may be highly resistant. Chloramphenicol-resistant *S. typhi* isolates have been detected in several countries. In India, occasional strains of *S. typhi* resistant to chloramphenicol have been isolated since 1962, but since 1972, multiple antibiotic-resistant strains of *S. typhi* and of other salmonellae have been encountered increasingly.[114] Of 241 *S. typhi* isolates recovered in Peru during 1981 to 1983, 71 (29.9%) were resistant to chloramphenicol. These strains were susceptible to ceftriaxone, imipenem, ampicillin–clavulanate, norfloxacin, and ciprofloxacin. More recently, in Pakistan, 20% of cases of typhoid fever were caused by strains of *S. typhi* resistant to ampicillin, chloramphenicol, and co-trimoxazole.[115] Other reports of multiresistant *Salmonella* were from India[116] and Bangladesh.[117] Acquired resistance of *S. typhi* can occur during treatment by acquisition of resistance gene(s) on a plasmid or transposon from other intestinal organisms.[118]

Most other Gram-negative bacteria are susceptible to chloramphenicol. *Neisseria meningitides* and *N. gonorrhoeae* are very sensitive. Resistant strains of *N. meningitides* have been reported but are rare. *N. gonorrhoeae* strains including β-lactamase producers are almost always susceptible to chloramphenicol. *H. influenzae* and *Haemophilus parainfluenzae* are also very sensitive. Chloramphenicol-resistant but ampicillin-susceptible strains of *H. influenzae b* have been isolated in the United States[119] and England[120] from children with meningitis. Strains of *H. influenzae b* resistant to chloramphenicol and ampicillin were also isolated from patients with meningitis or bacteremia in the United States,[121,122] England,[123–125] Australia,[126,127] Spain,[128] and the Dominican Republic.[129] Three children who died of meningitis due to *H. influenzae b* resistant to chloramphenicol and ampicillin in Bangkok were reported in 1980.[130] On the other hand, in a study from Pakistan, 47.5% of *H. influenzae* strains were resistant to co-trimoxazole, 5.1% to ampicillin, but none to chloramphenicol.[131] Nonencapsulated *H. influenzae* resistant to chloramphenicol and ampicillin has also been reported from Holland[132] and the United Kingdom.[133,134] Overall, chloramphenicol-resistant *Haemophilus* species remain relatively rare in developed countries. In the United States, the resistance rate of *H. influenzae b* is less than 1%.[129,135] Similar results of surveys in the United Kingdom have been reported. Data from developing countries are not available.

Brucella species, *Bordetella pertussis, Pasteurella multocida, V. cholerae*, and *V. parahaemolyticus* are susceptible to chloramphenicol. Rare resistant strains of *V. cholerae* have been detected.[136] The *Moraxella* species are susceptible, as is *H. pylori*,[137] and most strains of *Aeromonas* species[22] are also sensitive. *P. aeruginosa* has always been completely resistant, and this is due to an active efflux pump, which removes chloramphenicol from the bacterial cell.[138] *Burkholderia cepacia*[139] and *Flavobacteria*[140] are also resistant.

Gram-Positive Cocci

S. pneumoniae, Streptococcus *pyogenes*, group B streptococci, and α-hemolytic streptococci (viridans streptococci) are usually sensitive to chloramphenicol. *S. aureus* strains tend to be less susceptible, with *MIC* greater than 8 μg per mL. Methicillin-resistant strains of *S. aureus* are usually resistant to chloramphenicol, and this is due to inactivation of the drug by plasmid-mediated chloramphenicol acetyltransferase.[141] Chloramphenicol-resistant *S. pyogenes* have been detected in Japan[142] but appear to be rare elsewhere. Although chloramphenicol-resistant pneumococci have been detected in several countries, including France, Britain, West Africa, Australia, and the United States, they are also considered to be rare. Resistance in these strains is due to plasmid-mediated chloramphenicol acetyltransferase. Pneumococci resistant to multiple drugs including penicillin G and chloramphenicol detected in South Africa were associated with serious infections.[143,144] Pneumococci resistant to penicillin and chloramphenicol have also been reported in Spain, Pakistan,[131] and Korea.[145] Chloramphenicol-resistant *Enterococcus faecalis* strains are not uncommon.

Anaerobic Bacteria

Anaerobic Gram-positive cocci including *Peptococcus* and *Peptostreptococcus* species are susceptible to chloramphenicol.[146] Among the anaerobic Gram-positive bacilli, most *Clostridium* species including *Clostridium tetani* and *Clostridium perfringens* are susceptible. However, many strains of *Clostridium difficile* are resistant.[147] The Gram-negative anaerobic bacilli *Bacteroides*, including *B. fragilis*,[112] *Fusobacterium, Prevotella*, and *Veillona* species, are very susceptible to chloramphenicol.[148] Chloramphenicol is also active against mycoplasmas, leptospira, and *T. pallidum. Chlamydia* species including those that cause pneumonia, conjunctivitis, psittacosis, and lymphogranuloma venereum are sensitive. Rickettsiae that cause Rocky Mountain spotted fever and various typhus fevers are susceptible to chloramphenicol. Chloramphenicol is also active against *C. burnetii*, the agent that causes Q fever.

Historically, chloramphenicol had a prominent role in the treatment of children with serious infections, including meningitis. Factors that favored its use included its excellent diffusion into all body fluids, such as CSF, vitreous humor, and joint fluid. This made it useful in the treatment of meningitis, bacterial ophthalmitis, and septic arthritis. Chloramphenicol concentrations in CSF average 0.5 to 0.66 of serum concentration.[149] Chloramphenicol also penetrates into leukocytes and tissues, making it useful in the treatment of typhoid fever and infections in patients with chronic granulomatous disease. The diffusion of chloramphenicol into the central nervous system (CNS) tissue fluid is superior to that of any other antibiotic because of its high lipid solubility. Brain tissue levels are about nine times the simultaneous serum level.[150] This and the knowledge that anaerobic bacteria are almost always present in brain abscesses made chloramphenicol an ideal antimicrobial for the treatment of brain abscesses.

INDICATIONS FOR USE

Chloramphenicol is no longer the drug of choice for any specific infection, except for typhoid fever in areas where cost and availability make it the drug of choice for infections due to susceptible strains of *S. typhi.* Therapy with chloramphenicol must be limited to conditions where the benefit of the drug outweighs the risks of the potential toxicities.

Typhoid Fever

Chloramphenicol remains an excellent drug for treatment of typhoid fever and other types of systemic *Salmonella* infections; however, safer drugs are available, including ampicillin, co-trimoxazole, and third-generation cephalosporins. Third-generation cephalosporins are the drugs of choice for treatment of such infections.

Typhoid fever is usually treated by chloramphenicol for a period of 2 weeks.[151] Chloramphenicol is of no value for the eradication of *Salmonella* carrier state. In addition, treatment of patients with acute Salmonella gastroenteritis with chloramphenicol usually prolongs the period of excretion of *Salmonella* after clinical recovery.[152]

Bacterial Meningitis

Chloramphenicol is very effective for the treatment of meningitis due to *H. influenzae type b.*[153] Following the widespread occurrence of strains of *H. influenzae* resistant to ampicillin, chloramphenicol became the preferred drug for serious infections due to this organism. However, the third-generation cephalosporin ceftriaxone is used by clinicians in developed countries for both the initial and continuation treatment of *H. influenzae* meningitis. Chloramphenicol remains an alternative effective drug for treatment of meningitis in patients who have severe allergy to β-lactams. Chloramphenicol is a good alternative agent for treatment of meningococcal meningitis.[154] Treatment of *S. pneumoniae* meningitis with chloramphenicol may be unsatisfactory at times because some strains are inhibited, but not killed. In addition, penicillin-resistant *S. pneumoniae* strains are frequently resistant to chloramphenicol. Third-generation cephalosporins are very effective for the treatment of these infections. The use of chloramphenicol in Gram-negative bacillary meningitis has been disappointing both in neonates and in adults.[155] This is probably due to lack of bactericidal activity against Gram-negative bacilli at concentrations achieved in the CSF.

Anaerobic Infections

Chloramphenicol is very active against most anaerobic bacteria, including *B. fragilis.* The drug is effective for the treatment of brain abscesses and intra-abdominal infections, which are frequently caused by anaerobic organisms. However, other equally effective and less toxic drugs are available for treatment of such infections, including metronidazole for brain abscesses and clindamycin, cefoxitin, cefotetan, and ampicillin/sulbactam for intra-abdominal infections.

Rickettsial Infections

Chloramphenicol is effective in the treatment of Rocky Mountain spotted fever, epidemic typhus, scrub typhus, murine typhus, and Mediterranean fever.[48,156] Tetracyclines are equally effective and less toxic and are usually used in moderate cases. Chloramphenicol is preferred by some when parenteral therapy is required for very ill patients, during pregnancy, and for young children younger than 8 years. Moreover, tetracycline cannot be used in the presence of renal failure.

Gram-Negative Aerobic Enteric Infections

Chloramphenicol is effective in many infections caused by these organisms, except *P. aeruginosa.* However, aminoglycosides such as gentamicin or tobramycin or a third-generation cephalosporin are usually preferred. Chloramphenicol should not be used for treatment of urinary tract infections because other effective and safer drugs are available.

Enterococcal Infections

Strains of *Enterococcus faecium* have become resistant to penicillin, ampicillin, and vancomycin. Some of these strains may be susceptible to chloramphenicol, and the drug has been shown to be effective in the treatment of some serious vancomycin-resistant enterococcal infections.[157] Other effective and less toxic agents are available for treatment of these infections, such as linezolid and quinupristin–dalfopristin.[158]

PHARMACOKINETIC PROPERTIES

Chloramphenicol is very lipid soluble but is minimally water soluble. Water solubility is achieved by attaching a polar group to the chloramphenicol molecule by an ester linkage. The palmitate ester is available in liquid preparation for oral use, and the succinate ester is provided for IV use. Both ester forms are biologically inactive and must be hydrolyzed after administration to release the active free chloramphenicol. Chloramphenicol palmitate, taken orally, is hydrolyzed in the proximal small intestine by pancreatic enzymes, which results in the release of free chloramphenicol, which is absorbed as the active compound. The crystalline form of chloramphenicol (in capsule form) is well absorbed from the gastrointestinal tract after oral administration.

Chloramphenicol succinate is rapidly hydrolyzed within the body following IV administration into the biologically active chloramphenicol. The mechanism of in vivo hydrolysis is not clear, but esterases of the liver, kidneys, and lungs may be involved. The disappearance of chloramphenicol succinate from serum of infants and children is highly variable and unpredictable. In 14 infants younger than 1 month, the mean unhydrolyzed serum chloramphenicol succinate measured at 6 hours after administration was 11% compared with a mean of 1.4% in 11 children aged 1 to 16 years.[159] Therefore, infants during the first month of life appear to hydrolyze the succinate ester less efficiently than older infants. Chloramphenicol succinate also is subject to renal elimination from plasma before hydrolysis. The renal clearance of the "prodrug" in infants and children is highly variable and, therefore, affects the bioavailability of chloramphenicol. In 45 hospitalized infants and children aged 3 days to 16 years who were receiving chloramphenicol succinate, only 51% of peak serum concentrations were within the "therapeutic" range, defined as 10 to 25 μg per mL. Seven of 45 had "subtherapeutic" concentrations, and 15 of 45 had chloramphenicol concentrations above 25 μg per mL. A substantial but variable fraction of chloramphenicol succinate was excreted unchanged in urine. A mean of 33% (range 6% to 60%) of the administered dose was recovered unhydrolyzed in the urine. A mean of 18% of the dose was excreted as chloramphenicol glucuronide and 14% as free chloramphenicol.[159]

The variation in the hydrolysis rate and the variable renal elimination of chloramphenicol succinate following IV administration markedly influence the achievable serum concentrations of active chloramphenicol. The succinate ester that persists in the body also acts as "prodrug" reservoir, which releases chloramphenicol continuously and results in lower and delayed serum peaks.

Nonesterified active chloramphenicol is metabolized primarily in the liver, where it is conjugated into water-soluble glucuronide and then is excreted in this inactive form by the kidneys. Eighty-five to 90% of the dose is excreted as glucuronide and 10% to 15% as chloramphenicol base. The partial renal elimination of unhydrolyzed chloramphenicol succinate results in an unusual bioavailability problem because this excreted fraction of the drug is quite variable, and it is impossible to compensate for it by increasing the dose by a predetermined percentage.

The high variation in hydrolysis and renal excretion of chloramphenicol succinate contributes substantially to the wide variability in its apparent half-life and body clearance. Reported apparent half-lives range from 2.1 to 8.3 hours (mean 3.98 hours)[160] and 1.7 to 12 hours (mean 5.1 hours).[159] Body clearance of chloramphenicol also ranges from 0.122 to 0.429 L per kg per hour.[160]

Chloramphenicol palmitate taken orally is hydrolyzed in the small intestine by pancreatic esterases, yielding free chloramphenicol. The bioavailability of chloramphenicol is approximately 80% when administered as a suspension of chloramphenicol palmitate. Peak serum chloramphenicol concentrations are generally observed between 2 and 3 hours following oral administration.[161,162]

Distribution

Chloramphenicol is extensively distributed to many tissues and body fluids. Various concentrations have been detected in the brain, heart, lung, kidney, liver, and spleen. Chloramphenicol also diffuses into vitreous humor,[163] CSF,[149,161,162,164,165] pleural fluid, synovial fluid,[166] and saliva[167] and crosses the placenta. Chloramphenicol crosses the blood–brain barrier into CSF in children and adults with normal and inflamed meninges. CSF concentration is approximately 50% of simultaneous serum concentration but may range from 20% to 99% of serum concentration.[161,162,164,165] Only minor fluctuations were noted during a dosing interval, in contrast to the respective serum concentration.

Protein Binding

Protein binding of chloramphenicol is about 53% in serum and 66% in plasma of adults.[168] Binding occurs primarily with albumin. Bilirubin does not appear to displace chloramphenicol from bilirubin-binding sites and does not alter serum protein binding of chloramphenicol.[167] In general, the unbound drug is considered to be the active entity. The percentage of unbound chloramphenicol increases as serum albumin concentration decreases.[168] The percentage of unbound chloramphenicol may increase in other body fluids with less protein content than plasma, such as CSF.[168]

DOSAGE

Most chloramphenicol-susceptible organisms are inhibited by a concentration of 10 μg per mL or less. Chloramphenicol dose-dependent toxicity is very unlikely at serum concentration less than 25 μg per mL. Therefore, a dose of chloramphenicol that provides serum concentration of 10 to 25 μg per mL would be generally effective and safe for treatment of serious infections. A calculated dose that can theoretically provide a serum concentration within this therapeutic range is not always feasible because of the wide variability in the metabolism and excretion of chloramphenicol.

Chloramphenicol palmitate suspension given orally produces more predictable serum levels than those obtained after the succinate ester is given IV. Oral doses of 60 to 75 mg per kg per day result in serum concentrations between 15 and 25 μg per mL.[169] A dose of 75 mg per kg per day is recommended as a starting dose for most patients beyond the newborn period. The total daily dose is administered in four daily doses given every 6 hours. This dose may subsequently be adjusted contingent on serum concentrations.

Recommended doses for the IV chloramphenicol succinate are 25 mg per kg per day for premature infants and term infants younger than 2 weeks and 50 mg per kg per day for older-term infants and children. For serious infections, 75 to 100 mg per kg per day is suggested for infants older than 2 weeks and for older children. The total daily dose is given in four daily doses every 6 hours. These doses, however, frequently result in serum concentrations outside the therapeutic range. In one study of 107 infants receiving recommended doses of chloramphenicol, 33% had serum concentrations between 10 and 20 μg per mL, 50% above 20 μg per mL, and 11% below 10 μg per mL.[170] In another study of 45 infants and children receiving IV chloramphenicol succinate, only 51% of peak serum concentration was within the "therapeutic" range of 10 to 25 μg per mL. Seven of 45 had "subtherapeutic" levels, and 15 of 45 had chloramphenicol concentration above 25 μg per mL.[159]

Because of the narrow therapeutic range of chloramphenicol concentrations and the lack of correlation between dose and serum concentration, it is recommended that serum concentrations be monitored during therapy if at all possible.[149,159,164,171] Active chloramphenicol does not accumulate in patients with renal failure; therefore, the drug may be given in the usual recommended dose. Inactive chloramphenicol metabolites accumulate in the serum of patients with renal failure but have not been associated with known toxicity.

Because chloramphenicol is metabolized in the liver, its body clearance is reduced in patients with liver dysfunction. When used in these patients, chloramphenicol serum levels should be monitored.

TOXICITY

The most important toxic effects of chloramphenicol occur in the bone marrow. These effects are of two types. The first is a reversible erythroid suppression of the bone marrow probably due to chloramphenicol inhibition of mitochondrial protein synthesis, which, in turn, impairs iron incorporation into heme. Suppression of erythropoiesis occurs if excessive concentrations of the drug are maintained for a sufficient length of time.[172] This effect is dose related and usually reversible. Bone marrow suppression tends to occur when peak chloramphenicol concentrations consistently exceed 25 μg per mL or concentrations at 6 hours after a dose that exceed 15 μg per mL.[173] Early signs reflect arrest of erythropoiesis and include reticulocytopenia, increased serum iron, and, eventually, a decrease in erythrocyte count. With continued use of the drug at sufficient doses, thrombocytopenia and neutropenia may occur within 2 to 3 weeks. The risk of this dose-related toxicity can be minimized by maintaining serum chloramphenicol concentration less than 25 μg per mL and by limiting the duration of drug administration to the minimum required for adequate treatment.

The second type of toxicity is a rare, but usually fatal, idiosyncratic response frequently manifested as aplastic anemia. It is not dose related, and a genetic predisposition is suggested by the occurrence of pancytopenia in identical twins. It is rare and is estimated to occur once in every 24,500 to 40,000 patients (0.004% to 0.0025%) who receive the antibiotic.[174] All blood cell lines are affected, resulting in pancytopenia, which is frequently irreversible. This toxicity most commonly occurs after therapy is discontinued. The fatality rate is high when bone marrow aplasia is complete. Although several theories have been advanced, the mechanism of this aplastic anemia associated with chloramphenicol administration is unknown. Although most cases have been reported after oral therapy, a number of cases of aplastic anemia from parenteral chloramphenicol and even after the administration of eye drops have also been reported.[175,176]

Gray Baby Syndrome

Fatal chloramphenicol toxicity may develop in neonates, especially premature babies, when they are exposed to high doses of chloramphenicol. The illness, the gray baby syndrome, has been reported in infants who were receiving chloramphenicol doses of 100 to 200 mg per kg per day and had serum chloramphenicol serum concentrations of 70 to 250 μg per mL, which are 10 times the therapeutic blood concentrations.[170,171] The illness usually begins 2 to 9 days after treatment is started and manifests as vomiting, refusal to suck, irregular and rapid breathing, abdominal distention, and periods of cyanosis and passage of loose green stools. In the subsequent 24 hours, affected infants become flaccid, turn ashen gray in color, and become hypothermic. Death can occur within 2 days of onset of symptoms. Chloramphenicol toxicity in neonates results from (a) failure of drug conjugation because of inadequate hepatic glucuronosyltransferase activity during the first 3 to 4 weeks of life and (b) inadequate renal excretion of unconjugated chloramphenicol in the newborn.[177] In premature infants and neonates, chloramphenicol should be reduced to 25 mg per kg per day, and antibiotic blood levels should be monitored. This syndrome has also been reported in toddlers[178] and after accidental overdoses in adults.[179] Impaired myocardial contractility due to interference in myocardial tissue respiration and oxidative phosphorylation contributes to the clinical picture.[180] It is generally associated with serum chloramphenicol of greater than 50 μg per mL and unexplained acidosis.[181]

Chloramphenicol is removed to a small extent by peritoneal dialysis or hemodialysis. Exchange transfusion or charcoal hemoperfusion has been used to accelerate drug removal.[182,183]

Decreased visual acuity due to optic neuritis has been described in patients who received prolonged chloramphenicol treatment. Although this effect is generally reversible, loss of vision has occurred in some cases.[184] Other neurologic sequelae that have been described include peripheral neuritis, headache, depression, and mental confusion. Adverse effects involving the gastrointestinal tract include nausea, vomiting and diarrhea, and stomatitis. Prolonged chloramphenicol administration can result in bleeding due to decreased vitamin K synthesis.

Drug Interactions

Chloramphenicol inhibits hepatic microsomal cytochrome P450 enzymes, which results in prolongation of half-lives of drugs metabolized by this system.[185] This includes tolbutamide, phenytoin, dicoumarol, chlorpropamide, antiretroviral protease inhibitors, and rifabutin. Toxicity due to these drugs may occur if they are given in their usual doses to patients who are receiving chloramphenicol.[186,187] Conversely, concurrent administration of phenytoin and chloramphenicol succinate results in elevated chloramphenicol peak and trough serum levels. This may be the result of competition for binding sites rather than induction of hepatic enzymes. Concurrent administration of chloramphenicol succinate and phenobarbital shortens the half-life of the antibiotic, causing reduction of the peak and trough serum levels of chloramphenicol.[188] Chloramphenicol is primarily bacteriostatic and will antagonize the bactericidal activity of penicillins, cephalosporins, and aminoglycosides. In vitro growth kinetic assays have demonstrated inhibition of the early bactericidal activity of ampicillin against group B streptococci by chloramphenicol.[189] In vitro time–kill curves have also shown the antagonistic effect of chloramphenicol on the bactericidal activity of cefotaxime and ceftriaxone against *E. coli* and group B streptococci.[113] Chloramphenicol also appears to suppress the bactericidal action of gentamicin against *E. coli* and *Klebsiella*.[112]

METRONIDAZOLE

CHEMICAL STRUCTURE

Metronidazole [1-(2-hydroyethyl)-2-methyl-5-nitroimidazole] is the prototype of the nitroimidazole group of antibiotics that has been used in clinical practice for decades (Figure 26.3). It was first discovered in the 1950s in France from a *Streptomyces* species while researchers were attempting to synthesize a product with activity against *Trichomonas vaginalis*. Since then, metronidazole has been used to treat a variety of anaerobic bacterial and parasitic infections.[190]

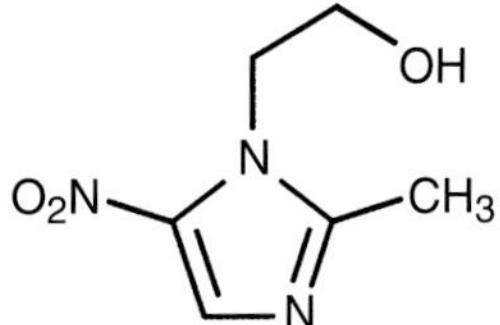

Figure 26.3 Structure of metronidazole.

MECHANISM OF ACTION/MECHANISM OF RESISTANCE

The mechanism of bactericidal action of metronidazole and other nitroimidazole compounds is believed to be through a four-phase process. This includes entry of the compound into the bacterial cell followed by nitro group reduction. The reduced intermediates exhibit cytotoxic activity that is essential in the killing of the microorganism. However, metronidazole's main action is DNA breakage and inhibition of repair, inhibition of transcription, and, ultimately, cellular death. In the last phase, liberation of end products that are inactive will occur.[191,192]

Resistance to metronidazole can develop in vivo and in vitro by different mechanisms, including reduced drug uptake, increased efflux from bacterial cell, or by reduced activation inside anaerobes.[193] Certain genes have been associated with metronidazole resistance, such as (*nim*) genes. These genes code for an alternative set of enzymes that coverts activated forms of metronidazole into inactivated no-toxic compounds.[194,195] Alteration of the DNA repair system is another mechanism of drug resistance. Overexpression of enzymes involved in DNA repair such as recA protein has been correlated with reduced metronidazole susceptibility.[195] In *Bacteroides* species, inducible resistance has been reported with exposure to subinhibitory concentrations of metronidazole.[194]

IN VITRO EFFICACY

Susceptibility testing for anaerobic bacteria is not routinely performed due to technical difficulties and lack of standardization. The clinical relevance of susceptibility testing of anaerobes to metronidazole is unclear, especially in the setting of mixed infection. Treatment outcome may be related to other factors, such as surgical drainage, comorbid conditions, and the immune status of the host. However, susceptibility testing is recommended in certain serious infections, such as endocarditis, brain abscess, osteomyelitis, or prosthetic device infections. Testing may also be useful when there is a persistent infection and when antibiotic therapy is the mainstay of treatment due to limited surgical options.[196] A susceptibility breakpoint of 8 μg per mL has been established by the Clinical Laboratory Standards Institute, with 16 μg per mL for intermediate susceptibility and >32 μg per mL for resistance to metronidazole.[197]

Metronidazole is active against a wide range of anaerobic organisms, microaerophilic bacteria and parasites. *B. fragilis* and other members of the genus *Bacteroides* have been historically susceptible to metronidazole. Metronidazole has retained its notorious anaerobic activity for decades primarily due to its rapid killing of *Bacteroides* species. Metronidazole is also bactericidal against *Prevotella* species, *Fusobacterium* species, and *Porphyromonas* species.[198,199] *Clostridium* spp. are usually susceptible, but *Clostridium ramosum* may require higher concentrations of metronidazole than others.[200] Anaerobic cocci such as *Peptostreptococcus* and *Veillonella* species are also susceptible to metronidazole. *Capnocytophaga* species is usually susceptible, but *H. pylori* susceptibility can be variable.[201–203] Resistance to metronidazole has been reported among Gram-positive anaerobic and facultative bacilli such as *Actinomyces* spp., *Propionibacterium* spp., and *Lactobacillus* species.[199,204] *Gardrenella vaginalis* and *Actinobacillus actinomycetemcomitans* are usually susceptible to metronidazole, although the hydroxy metabolite is two to eight times more active. Metronidazole is active against multiple parasites, including *Entamoeba histolytica, T. vaginalis, Giardia lamblia, Balantidium coli,* and *Blastocystis hominis.*[64,205–208]

CLINICAL INDICATIONS

Metronidazole is effective in treatment of anaerobic infections, including intra-abdominal infections, gynecologic infections, endocarditis, sepsis, CNS infections, respiratory tract infections, oral and dental infections, skin soft-tissue infections as well as musculoskeletal infection. Metronidazole is also given in preoperative prophylactic regimens for abdominal and gynecologic surgical procedures. In cases of mixed bacterial infections, metronidazole should be given in combination with an antibiotic that is effective against aerobes.[209] Although metronidazole is not Food and Drug Administration (FDA) approved for use in infants and children, it is used extensively off-label for different infections in pediatric patients. Metronidazole is used in treatment of giardiasis, trichomoniasis, as well as bacterial vaginosis caused by *G. vaginalis.* Metronidazole may also be a component of multidrug regimen used in treatment of *H. pylori* infections.[191,209]

In adults, topical metronidazole is used for treatment of moderate-to-severe rosacea.[210] Metronidazole gel has also been used as adjunctive therapy with debridement for adult patients with periodontitis.[211]

Gardnerella vaginalis

G. vaginalis has long been implicated as the main cause of bacterial vaginosis. This is based on the consistent isolation of *G. vaginalis* from women with bacterial vaginosis. However, this association is complicated by the high rates of isolation of *G. vaginalis* from healthy women.[212] The pathogenesis of *G. vaginalis* is unclear; however, the ability of organism to adhere to the epithelium cells in the genital and urinary tract may be an important factor.[213] In addition, factors that impair the balance between *G. vaginalis* and *Lactobacillus* species, allowing *Gardnerella* and anaerobes to proliferate, may be another factor.[214] *G. vaginalis* is mainly sexually transmitted, although colonization of the genital tract may occur due to transfer from the gastrointestinal tract.[215] The isolation of *G. vaginalis* from vaginal specimens of prepubertal girls or from asymptomatic prepubertal boys should raise suspicion of sexual abuse.[216,217] In pregnant women, bacterial vaginosis has been associated with adverse outcomes, including premature delivery and chorioamnionitis. *G. vaginalis* has been associated with cases of sepsis, meningitis, cellulitis, conjunctivitis, and pneumonia in infected neonates.[218–221] It has also been reported to cause urinary tract infections.[222]

Metronidazole is the drug of choice for treatment of bacterial vaginosis, with a cure rate of 90% or greater.[223] For non-pregnant females, the recommended dose is 1 g orally in two divided dose for 7 days. Other options include intravaginally applied metronidazole gel 0.75% (one full 5-g applicator once daily for 5 days), metronidazole gel 1.3% (administered intravaginally once daily at bedtime for 5 days), or clindamycin cream 2% for 7 days once daily.[224] Alternative treatment options include tinidazole (2 g, orally, once daily for 2 days, or 1 g, orally, once daily for 5 days) or orally administered clindamycin (600 mg per day in two divided doses for 7 days).[224]

Symptomatic pregnant females should be treated. This can be accomplished with either of the oral or vaginal metronidazole or with oral clindamycin regimens recommended for non-pregnant females. Metronidazole crosses the placenta but has not been shown to have teratogenic effects.[225] However, tinidazole should be avoided during pregnancy as animal studies suggest it has teratogenic potential.[226] Treatment of symptomatic breastfeeding mother is also recommended. Topical metronidazole is preferred to oral metronidazole as metronidazole is secreted in breast milk, although no adverse effects were reported in babies.[224] If a mother receives a 2-g dose of metronidazole, cessation of breastfeeding for 12 to 24 hours may be advised.[224,227] For females with multiple recurrences, metronidazole gel 0.75%, twice weekly for 4 to 6 months, has been suggested.[64] Treatment of sexual partners or women with bacterial vaginosis has not been shown to prevent recurrence of infection.[228,229]

Anaerobic Infections

Anaerobic infections are frequently mixed infections in association with other aerobes and facultative bacteria and are frequently associated with formation of abscesses and necrotizing infections. Surgical management including drainage of abscesses and debridement of devitalized tissues is very essential. Although the mechanism of resistance to antibiotics in anaerobic bacteria varies, production of β-lactamase is the most common as has been demonstrated in many clinical isolates of *Prevotella, Fusobacterium, Porphyromonas,* and *Bacteroides* species to render these organisms resistant to penicillin.[230,231] Antibiotic treatment options for anaerobic Gram-negative organisms include metronidazole, clindamycin, imipenem/meropenem, and penicillin/β-lactamase inhibitor combinations. Metronidazole remains active against these anaerobes despite increasing resistance to other antibiotics such as clindamycin. For example, resistance rate to clindamycin in *B. fragilis* group in the United States and Europe is 35% compared to less than 1% to metronidazole.[230,232] *Prevotella, Fusobacterium,* and *Porphyromonas* species isolates are more likely than *B. fragilis* group to be susceptible to clindamycin. However, a study showed the rate of resistance to clindamycin is increasing to 10% among some *Prevotella* species, such as *Prevotella melaninogenica* and *Prevotella intermedia,* with all tested isolates remain susceptible to metronidazole.[232] Resistance to metronidazole in *Fusobacterium* species such as *Fusobacterium necrophorum* and *Fusobacterium nucleatum* has not been reported.[233] Infections associated with Fusobacteria such as Lemierre disease can be polymicrobial and associated with serious complications. Most experts recommend a regimen of metronidazole in combination with a penicillin or cephalosporin, with or without clindamycin for treatment of severe infections.[233–235]

Intra-abdominal Infections

Intra-abdominal infections are potentially serious and require early diagnosis, timely control of source of infection as well as prompt start of effective antibiotic therapy. The most common organisms encountered in community-acquired infections are *E. coli* and *Bacteroides* species. Additional pathogens include other Enterobacteriaceae, *Streptococcus* species as well as *Clostridium* species. In hospital-acquired, severe or complicated infections, additional pathogens such as *P. aeruginosa, Enterococcus* species, and, rarely, *S. aureus* should be considered.[236–238] Surgical drainage of infected fluid, debridement of necrotic tissue, and restoration of anatomy of the gastrointestinal tract are crucial. Acceptable antibiotic regimens for treatment of complicated intra-abdominal infection include an advanced generation cephalosporin (ceftriaxone, ceftazidime, cefepime) plus metronidazole, piperacillin/tazobactam, or a carbapenem (ertapenem, meropenem, imipenem). In patients with severe β-lactam allergy, ciprofloxacin plus metronidazole or an aminoglycoside-based regimen: gentamicin or tobramycin with metronidazole or clindamycin, with or without ampicillin, is recommended.[239,240] Metronidazole is given at 30 to 40 mg per kg per day in three divided doses.

Antimicrobial therapy for enterococci is given when these organisms are recovered in culture. Empirical coverage for enterococci is given in health care–associated intra-abdominal infections, patients who received prior therapy with cephalosporins, immunocompromised patients, and those who have underlying heart disease or prosthetic material.[240] Empiric methicillin-resistant *Staphylococcus aureus* (MRSA) coverage is not indicated in community-acquired infections. However, vancomycin should be provided to patients with health care–associated infections who are known to have prior MRSA colonization or those with increased risk of MRSA infection, such as patients who failed prior antibiotic treatment.[240]

Necrotizing enterocolitis (NEC) is a potentially serious intra-abdominal infection in premature neonates. NEC is typically managed with fluid resuscitation, board-spectrum antibiotics, and bowel decompression. It may be complicated by bowel perforation that requires urgent operative intervention, including laparotomy or percutaneous drainage. Intraoperative Gram stain and culture should be obtained to guide appropriate antimicrobial therapy. Appropriate antibiotic therapy in neonates with NEC includes ampicillin, gentamicin, and metronidazole; ampicillin, cefotaxime, and metronidazole or meropenem. Ampicillin may be replaced by vancomycin if MRSA or ampicillin-resistant enterococcal infection is suspected.[240]

Amebiasis

Invasive intestinal amebiasis caused by *E. histolytica* is treated with metronidazole and a luminal agent such as paromomycin, iodoquinol, or diloxanide furoate. The dose of metronidazole is 30 to 50 mg per kg per day in three divided doses (maximum daily dose is 750 mg). Therapy should be given for a minimum of 10 days. A shorter course may be associated with relapse of invasive infections months later.[208,241] Metronidazole should not be used as a single agent to treat asymptomatic amebiasis.

Entamoeba gingivalis is another *Entamoeba* species that is found in the mouth and has been reported to cause periodontal disease in HIV-infected patients, although a causal relationship has not been established.[242] *E. gingivalis* has occasionally been isolated form needle aspirates of neck nodules and from the female genital tract.[243,244] Treatment with metronidazole is effective.[242(p471)]

Metronidazole has been effective in treatment of other protozoan such as *B. coli, B. hominis,* and *Entamoeba polecki.*[205,206,245]

Trichomoniasis

The only agents approved in the United States for treatment of trichomoniasis are metronidazole and tinidazole. Sexually transmitted disease guidelines published by the Centers for Disease Control and Prevention (CDC) recommend the use of 2-g dose of either metronidazole or tinidazole. For recurrent or persistent infections, additional doses may be given.[64] Treatment of all sexual partners is recommended to prevent recurrences in index patient and reduce transmission in the community. Most strains of *T. vaginalis* are susceptible to metronidazole. Low-level in vitro resistance has been reported in 4.3% of tested isolates from different geographical sites in the United States.[246] Reinfection should be distinguished from antimicrobial resistance in patients with trichomoniasis who fail metronidazole therapy.[64]

Giardiasis

Children with acute and chronic diarrhea, malabsorption, failure to thrive, or other gastrointestinal symptoms who are found to have giardia in stool or duodenal samples should receive antimicrobial treatment. Metronidazole, tinidazole, and nitazoxanide are the drugs of choice. Although not FDA approved for giardiasis, metronidazole is the least expensive of these medications.[207] A 5- to 7-day course is 80% to 100% effective in children.[207] The recommended dose is 15 mg per kg per day in three divided doses. Poor palatability of the metronidazole oral suspension may be a limitation of use in children.

Clostridium difficile *Infections*

C. difficile is the most common infectious cause of health care–associated diarrhea. Similar to adult findings, the incidence of *C. difficile* infections (CDIs) has increased in children since 2000. Among children with CDI, 71% were identified as community acquired.[247] Guidelines for treatment of CDIs in adults by the Infectious Diseases Society of America in 2018 recommend the use of oral vancomycin or fidaxomicin over metronidazole.[248] However, for children, either metronidazole or oral vancomycin is recommended for the treatment of initial episode or first recurrence of CDI. Oral metronidazole (30 mg per kg per day in four divided doses, maximum 2 g per day) is given in mild-to-moderate CDIs, including those with first episode and first recurrence. Oral vancomycin is recommended for children with severe CDIs, such as those requiring intensive care, children or unresponsive to metronidazole, because of modestly superior activity of vancomycin to that of metronidazole.[249] Similarly, for children with a second or greater recurrence of CDI, vancomycin is recommended over metronidazole due to vancomycin efficacy and the potential cumulative neurotoxicity of metronidazole.[250] For children with severe *C. difficile* disease and complications such as ileus, toxic megacolon, or shock, IV metronidazole is recommended to be given along with vancomycin administered orally or by enema.[248] IV vancomycin is ineffective in treatment of CDI. Nitazoxanide is another alternative therapy for CDI. Adults with recurrent CDI have been treated with fecal microbiota transplantation.[251]

Helicobacter pylori *infections*

Clinical practice guidelines for treatment of *H. pylori* infection in children have been published.[252] Children with *H. pylori*–positive peptic ulcer disease should receive antimicrobial therapy to eradicate infection. Treatment may be considered in children when *H. pylori* is detected by biopsy in the absence of peptic ulcer disease. A test and treat strategy is not recommended in children. Treatment may be offered to infected children whose first-degree relative has gastric cancer.[252] Triple therapy is given taking into the account cost, compliance, and adverse effects when choosing antibiotic regimen. The most effective regimen in children is a 14-day course of triple therapy that includes a proton pump inhibitor (PPI), such as lansoprazole or omeprazole, clarithromycin, and amoxicillin. A triple regimen that includes a PPI, amoxicillin, and metronidazole (20 mg per kg per day) may be used as a first-line regimen. An alternative regimen may include a bismuth salt, such as subsalicylate or citrate, amoxicillin, and metronidazole.[253] Antibiotic susceptibility testing is advisable to monitor resistance and guide treatment failure. Treatment regimen should be guided by local susceptibility patterns that may vary in different geographic locations. In the United States and Europe, resistance to metronidazole occurs at a rate of 34% to 46% compared to 21% to 41% for clarithromycin and 5% resistance rate for amoxicillin.[201–203] In developing countries, resistance rate to metronidazole can be as high as 60% to 80%.[254–256]

PHARMACOKINETIC/PHARMACODYNAMIC PROPERTIES

Oral absorption of metronidazole is excellent with more than 90% reported bioavailability. The peak plasma concentration (C_{max}) after a single dose of 500 mg is approximately 8 to 13 mg per L, with time to C_{max} (T_{max}) of 0.25 to 4 hours.[257] Oral bioavailability of a suspension formulation of benzoylmetronidazole has been reported to be 20% less bioavailable than metronidazole.[258] Protein binding is less than 20%. Metronidazole is metabolized by the liver by hydroxylation into its active metabolite hydroxyl-metronidazole. Metronidazole is eliminated via renal excretion as well as hepatic glucuronidation and oxidation.[259] Metronidazole has a long half-life of 6 to 10 hours. It exhibits concentration-dependent killing and has postantibiotic effect of at least 3 hours.[260] The volume of distribution is 0.76 to 0.87 L per kg, and the clearance is 0.056 to 0.064 L per hour per kg.[257(p353)] In infants, a study that used plasma and dried spot samples has shown that metronidazole clearance increased and half-life decreased with increasing postnatal age.[261]

The pharmacokinetic and pharmacodynamic properties of metronidazole suggest that modeling for plasma concentration–time area under the curve (*AUC*) to *MIC* is most appropriate. A predicted *AUC/MIC* ratio of at least 70:1 is needed for effective killing of anaerobic bacteria, including *B. fragilis.* Metronidazole is dosed every 6 to 8 hours for most clinical indications. However, recent studies suggest less frequent dosing including once daily[257,262,263] may be appropriate in certain infections, such as appendicitis. In pediatric patients with acute appendicitis, once-daily dosing at 30 mg per kg has been shown to meet target *AUC/MIC* ratio of ≥70% for *B. fragilis* strains with *MIC* of 2 or less.[262] In the United States, 90% of *B. fragilis* isolates have *MIC* ≤2.[264] Metronidazole is usually used in combination with ceftriaxone for the prevention of infection or treatment of complicated acute appendicitis.

Metronidazole has good penetration and diffusion into tissues and body fluids. The concentration of metronidazole in polymorphonuclear has been reported to be equal to that in extracellular fluid.[265] Metronidazole penetrates well into the CSF and CNS.[266,267] Concentration of metronidazole in CSF, saliva, and breast milk are similar to those in plasma.[257] The pharmacokinetics of metronidazole is not significantly changed with altered renal function. In patients with impaired renal function, the half-life of metronidazole is similar to those with normal renal function. However, decreased renal clearance of metronidazole metabolites such as hydroxyl-metronidazole has been reported in patients with impaired renal function. The accumulation of metabolites requires monitoring metabolite concentration and monitoring for metronidazole adverse events in patients with creatinine clearance less than 30 mL per min and avoiding metronidazole when creatinine clearance is less than 10 mL per minute.[268]

The effect of hemodialysis and continuous ambulatory peritoneal dialysis (CAPD) on metronidazole and its metabolites has been studied in adult patients with end-stage renal disease (ESRD).[269,270] Metronidazole and its hydroxyl metabolites are extensively removed by hemodialysis. The efficiency of clearance depends on the type of dialyzer membrane used and the duration of dialysis.[271] A hemodialysis session lasting 4 to 8 hours was associated with clearance of 40% to 65% of the dose. Thus, if metronidazole dose administration cannot be separated from hemodialysis session, dosage supplementation should be considered. In contrast to hemodialysis, CAPD contributed less than 9% of total body clearance of metronidazole and its metabolites. Dose adjustment is not routinely recommended in patients with ESRD who require CAPD.[272]

Because metronidazole is extensively metabolized by the liver, hepatic dysfunction is expected to affect its clearance. Studies have demonstrated that rates of clearance depend on the degree of hepatic impairment.[273] Although patients with mild-to-moderate hepatic impairment do not require adjustment of the metronidazole dosing, they need to be watched closely for adverse effects. Patients with severe hepatic impairment require 50% reduction in dosage.

Metronidazole pharmacokinetics may be altered in children with severe malnutrition. Clearance of metronidazole has been found to be reduced in children with severe protein malnutrition compared to those who had recovered from severe malnutrition.[274] It is unclear if such patients require dosage adjustment.

DOSAGE/REGIMENS

In infants, a loading dose of 15 mg per kg is given, followed by 7.5 mg per kg for subsequent dosing. The frequency of metronidazole varies with postmenstrual age (PMA). Metronidazole is given every 12 hours in infants with PMA less than 34 weeks, every 8 hours in those with PMA 34 to 40 weeks and every 6 hours in infants with PMA greater than 40 weeks. Metronidazole in infants may also be given according weight and postnatal age. For infants who weigh 2 kg or less, metronidazole is given at a dose of 7.5 mg per kg per dose every 12 hours for those who are ≤28 days of postnatal age and at a dose of 10 mg per kg per dose every 8 hours for infants 29 to 60 days. For infants who weigh more than 2 kg, metronidazole is given at a dose of 7.5 mg per kg per dose every 8 hours if the baby is ≤7 days of postnatal age and at a dose of 10 mg per kg per dose every 8 hours if the infant is 8 to 60 days of postnatal age.[275,276]

For most infections, the oral dose of metronidazole in children is 15 to 50 mg per kg per day in divided doses three times daily; maximum daily dose: 2,250 mg per day. For IV dosing, metronidazole is given at 22.5 to 40 mg per kg per day in divided doses three or four times daily; maximum daily dose: 4,000 mg per day.[276]

ADVERSE EFFECTS/TOXICITY/PRECAUTIONS

The most common side effects related to metronidazole use are gastrointestinal.[277] These include nausea, metallic or bitter taste, anorexia, and epigastric pain and vomiting. Stomatitis and glossitis have also been reported with metronidazole use and are associated with overgrowth of *Candida* species. Transient darkening of the urine may occur during metronidazole treatment. Other less common side effects include thrombophlebitis, joint pain, and paresthesia. Long-term systemic therapy or use of high doses has been associated with hematologic side effects, such as reversible leukopenia, neutropenia, and thrombocytopenia as well neurologic side effects such as peripheral neuropathy and CNS toxicities.[278,279] Rare side effects include autoimmune hepatitis, pancreatitis, dysuria, and polyuria.[280,281]

Neurologic adverse effects of metronidazole are rare and are associated with the use of high doses; the most common is polyneuropathy.[282] Metronidazole can cause CNS side effects, including metronidazole-induced encephalopathy. CNS involvement is characterized by cerebellar and brain involvement, encephalopathy, and, occasionally, seizures.[279] Patients may present with altered mental status, dysarthria, limb incoordination, and gait instability. Other symptoms include seizures, vertigo, ataxia, weakness, insomnia, headache, and tremors.[283,284] Polyneuropathy is a common associated finding. Liver disease is also commonly present. Magnetic resonance imaging (MRI) typically shows symmetric T2-hyperintense lesions of the dentate nuclei. Most patients improve after discontinuation of metronidazole.[279,284] However, patients with preexisting conditions may develop serious complications, including death or persistent neurologic deficits.[279]

Cockayne syndrome is a rare genetic disorder characterized by intellectual disability, short stature, and accelerated aging. Acute hepatic failure has been reported after metronidazole IV administration, including cases with fatal outcome in both adults and children with Cockayne syndrome. In fatal cases, death was reported 3 to 11 days after administration. Concomitant neurotoxicity was also reported in these patients. Metronidazole is generally contraindicated in patients diagnosed with Cockayne syndrome, unless no other alternative therapy can be used.[285] If metronidazole is used in a patient with Cockayne syndrome, careful monitoring of liver enzymes is recommended. Metronidazole should be stopped if liver enzymes are elevated, and levels should be followed to baseline values.

Prolongation of QT interval has been described in few reports raising concern with metronidazole use with other drugs that prolong the QT interval or in patients who have underlying medical conditions associated with QT prolongation.[286] Hypersensitivity reactions have been reported with metronidazole use, including erythematous rash, urticaria, flushing, serum sickness, and bronchospasm.[287] Metronidazole has been associated with cancer in animal studies, but no clear association was noted in humans.[288]

DRUG INTERACTIONS

Metronidazole has low incidence of drug interactions. Historically, metronidazole is known to have propensity for a disulfiram-like reaction when given with alcohol. This reaction is characterized by nausea, vomiting, skin flushing, difficulty breathing, tachycardia, and reports of sudden death.[289] Patients are advised not to drink alcohol during metronidazole treatment and until 48 hours after last dose. The mechanism of this reaction is not clear, and a possible central toxic serotonin reaction has been postulated.[290] Ethanol-containing medications as well as elixirs may also lead to disulfiram-like reaction. Because metronidazole inhibits liver metabolism of propylene alcohol, which is found in some food and medications, a similar reaction may occur when both are taken together.

Metronidazole is metabolized by the liver. Metronidazole inhibits CYP2C9; thus, drug interactions are expected when medications that metabolized by this enzyme are given concomitantly.[291,292] Metronidazole has been reported to potentiate the anticoagulant properties of warfarin and other coumarin-type anticoagulants. When given concurrently, prothrombin time and international normalized ratio (INR) should be monitored closely. Metronidazole decreases the clearance of phenytoin by about 15%, with resultant increase in phenytoin levels.[293] Potential drug interaction with potential carbamazepine toxicity may also occur with concomitant administration of carbamazepine and metronidazole.[294]

Cardiac arrhythmias including torsades de pointes have been rarely reported when metronidazole is administered concomitantly with amiodarone. This may be related to cytochrome P4503A4 inhibition by metronidazole that may lead to increase serum concentration of metronidazole and marked prolongation of the QTc interval.[295]

In patients receiving lithium, metronidazole can cause renal retention and may cause elevation of serum lithium levels.[296] Patients need to be monitored for lithium toxicity.

A study of patients who received concomitant metronidazole and omeprazole for treatment of *H. pylori* infection has demonstrated that omeprazole had no influence on the plasma pharmacokinetics of metronidazole.[297]

Drugs that induce hepatic enzymes, such as phenytoin, barbiturates, and rifampin, can reduce plasma concentrations of metronidazole due to increase in its hepatic clearance.[298] This may lead to loss of clinical efficacy of metronidazole therapy. Similar effect may occur with concomitant administration of prednisone and metronidazole.[298] Oral bioavailability of metronidazole may decrease when it is given with aluminum- and magnesium-containing antacids or with cholestyramine.[299] This occurs due to gastrointestinal binding of these compounds to metronidazole in the gastrointestinal tract.

REFERENCES

1. Finland M. Twenty-fifth anniversary of the discovery of Aureomycin: the place of the tetracyclines in antimicrobial therapy. *Clin Pharmacol Ther* 1974;15(1):3–8.
2. Cundliffe E, McQuillen K. Bacterial protein synthesis: the effects of antibiotics. *J Mol Biol* 1967;30(1):137–146.
3. Craven GR, Gavin R, Fanning T. The transfer RNA binding site of the 30 S ribosome and the site of tetracycline inhibition. *Cold Spring Harb Symp Quant Biol* 1969;34:129–137.
4. Chopra I, Hawkey PM, Hinton M. Tetracyclines, molecular and clinical aspects. *J Antimicrob Chemother* 1992;29(3):245–277.
5. Bread NS Jr, Armentrout SA, Weisberger AS. Inhibition of mammalian protein synthesis by antibiotics. *Pharmacol Rev* 1969;21(3):213–245.
6. Shils ME. Renal disease and the metabolic effects of tetracycline. *Ann Intern Med* 1963;58:389–408.
7. Yamaguchi A, Ohmori H, Kaneko-Ohdera M, et al. Delta pH-dependent accumulation of tetracycline in *Escherichia coli*. *Antimicrob Agents Chemother* 1991;35(1):53–56.
8. Benveniste R, Davies J. Mechanisms of antibiotic resistance in bacteria. *Ann Rev Biochem* 1973;42:471–506.
9. Clinical and Laboratory Standards Institute. *Methods for dilution antimicrobial susceptibility tests for bacteria that grow aerobically M07*, 11th ed. Wayne, PA: Clinical laboratory Standards Institute, 2018.

10. Han LL, McDougal LK, Gorwitz RJ, et al. High frequencies of clindamycin and tetracycline resistance in methicillin-resistant *Staphylococcus aureus* pulsed-field type USA300 isolates collected at a Boston ambulatory health center. *J Clin Microbiol* 2007;45(4):1350–1352.
11. Ayliffe GA, Lilly HA, Lowbury EJ. Decline of the hospital *Staphylococcus*? Incidence of multiresistant *Staph. aureus* in three Birmingham hospitals. *Lancet* 1979;1(8115):538–541.
12. Tetracycline resistance in pneumococci and group A streptococci. Report of an ad-hoc study group on antibiotic resistance. *Br Med J* 1977;1(6054):131–133.
13. Bourbeau P, Campos JM. Current antibiotic susceptibility of group A beta-hemolytic streptococci. *J Infect Dis* 1982;145(6):916.
14. Baker CJ, Webb BJ, Barrett FF. Antimicrobial susceptibility of group B streptococci isolated from a variety of clinical sources. *Antimicrob Agents Chemother* 1976;10(1):128–131.
15. Doern GV, Pfaller MA, Kugler K, et al. Prevalence of antimicrobial resistance among respiratory tract isolates of *Streptococcus pneumoniae* in North America: 1997 results from the SENTRY antimicrobial surveillance program. *Clin Infect Dis* 1998;27(4):764–770.
16. Hryniewicz W. Bacterial resistance in eastern Europe—selected problems. *Scand J Infect Dis Suppl* 1994;93:33–39.
17. Moreno F, Crisp C, Jorgensen JH, et al. The clinical and molecular epidemiology of bacteremias at a university hospital caused by pneumococci not susceptible to penicillin. *J Infect Dis* 1995;172(2):427–432.
18. Gutmann L, Goldstein FW, Kitzis MD, et al. Susceptibility of *Nocardia asteroides* to 46 antibiotics, including 22 beta-lactams. *Antimicrob Agents Chemother* 1983;23(2):248–251.
19. Unemo M, Shafer WM. Antimicrobial resistance in *Neisseria gonorrhoeae* in the 21st century: past, evolution, and future. *Clin Microbiol Rev* 2014;27(3):587–613.
20. Vanhoof R, Vanderlinden MP, Dierickx R, et al. Susceptibility of *Campylobacter fetus* subsp. *jejuni* to twenty-nine antimicrobial agents. *Antimicrob Agents Chemother* 1978;14(4):553–556.
21. Fennerty MB. *Helicobacter pylori. Arch Intern Med* 1994;154(7):721–727.
22. Janda JM, Guthertz LS, Kokka RP, et al. *Aeromonas* species in septicemia: laboratory characteristics and clinical observations. *Clin Infect Dis* 1994;19(1):77–83.
23. Farrell ID, Hinchliffe PM, Robertson L. Sensitivity of *Brucella* spp to tetracycline and its analogues. *J Clin Pathol* 1976;29(12):1097–1100.
24. Rubinstein E, Lang R, Shasha B, et al. In vitro susceptibility of *Brucella melitensis* to antibiotics. *Antimicrob Agents Chemother* 1991;35(9):1925–1927.
25. Morris JG Jr, Black RE. Cholera and other vibrioses in the United States. *N Engl J Med* 1985;312(6):343–350.
26. Midani S, Rathore MH. *Vibrio* species infection of a catfish spine puncture wound. *Pediatr Infect Dis J* 1994;13(4):333–334.
27. Sack DA, Kaminsky DC, Sack RB, et al. Prophylactic doxycycline for travelers' diarrhea. Results of a prospective double-blind study of Peace Corps volunteers in Kenya. *N Engl J Med* 1978;298(14):758–763.
28. Abdel-Haq NM, Asmar BI, Abuhammour WM, et al. *Yersinia enterocolitica* infection in children. *Pediatr Infect Dis J* 2000;19(10):954–958.
29. Wong JD, Barash JR, Sandfort RF, et al. Susceptibilities of *Yersinia pestis* strains to 12 antimicrobial agents. *Antimicrob Agents Chemother* 2000;44(7):1995–1996.
30. Regnery R, Tappero J. Unraveling mysteries associated with cat-scratch disease, bacillary angiomatosis, and related syndromes. *Emerg Infect Dis* 1995;1(1):16–21.
31. Maurin M, Gasquet S, Ducco C, et al. MICs of 28 antibiotic compounds for 14 *Bartonella* (formerly *Rochalimaea*) isolates. *Antimicrob Agents Chemother* 1995;39(11):2387–2391.
32. Thornsberry C, Baker CN, Kirven LA. In vitro activity of antimicrobial agents on Legionnaires disease bacterium. *Antimicrob Agents Chemother* 1978;13(1):78–80.
33. Eickhoff TC, Bennett JV, Hayes PS, et al. *Pseudomonas pseudomallei*: susceptibility to chemotherapeutic agents. *J Infect Dis* 1970;121(2):95–102.
34. Sutter VL, Finegold SM. Susceptibility of anaerobic bacteria to 23 antimicrobial agents. *Antimicrob Agents Chemother* 1976;10(4):736–752.
35. McCormack WM. Susceptibility of mycoplasmas to antimicrobial agents: clinical implications. *Clin Infect Dis* 1993;17(Suppl 1):S200–S201.
36. Rylander M, Hallander HO. In vitro comparison of the activity of doxycycline, tetracycline, erythromycin and a new macrolide, CP 62993, against *Mycoplasma pneumoniae, Mycoplasma hominis* and *Ureaplasma urealyticum. Scand J Infect Dis Suppl* 1988;53:12–17.
37. Roberts MC, Koutsky LA, Holmes KK, et al. Tetracycline-resistant *Mycoplasma hominis* strains contain streptococcal tetM sequences. *Antimicrob Agents Chemother* 1985;28(1):141–143.
38. Taylor-Robinson D, Furr PM. Clinical antibiotic resistance of *Ureaplasma urealyticum. Pediatr Infect Dis* 1986;5(6, Suppl):S335–S337.
39. Robertson JA, Stemke GW, Maclellan SG, et al. Characterization of tetracycline-resistant strains of *Ureaplasma urealyticum. J Antimicrob Chemother* 1988;21(3):319–332.
40. Rice RJ, Bhullar V, Mitchell SH, et al. Susceptibilities of *Chlamydia trachomatis* isolates causing uncomplicated female genital tract infections and pelvic inflammatory disease. *Antimicrob Agents Chemother* 1995;39(3):760–762.
41. Stimson JB, Hale J, Bowie WR, et al. Tetracycline-resistant *Ureaplasma urealyticum*: a cause of persistent nongonococcal urethritis. *Ann Intern Med* 1981;94(2):192–194.
42. Jones RB, Van der Pol B, Martin DH, et al. Partial characterization of *Chlamydia trachomatis* isolates resistant to multiple antibiotics. *J Infect Dis* 1990;162(6):1309–1315.
43. Grayston JT, Campbell LA, Kuo CC, et al. A new respiratory tract pathogen: *Chlamydia pneumoniae* strain TWAR. *J Infect Dis* 1990;161(4):618–625.
44. Hammerschlag MR. Antimicrobial susceptibility and therapy of infections caused by *Chlamydia pneumoniae. Antimicrob Agents Chemother* 1994;38(9):1873–1878.
45. Khatib R, Thirumoorthi MC, Kelly B, et al. Severe psittacosis during pregnancy and suppression of antibody response with early therapy. *Scand J Infect Dis* 1995;27(5):519–521.
46. Johnson SE, Klein GC, Schmid GP, et al. Susceptibility of the Lyme disease spirochete to seven antimicrobial agents. *Yale J Biol Med* 1984;57(4):549–553.
47. Norris SJ, Edmondson DG. In vitro culture system to determine MICs and MBCs of antimicrobial agents against *Treponema pallidum* subsp. pallidum (Nichols strain). *Antimicrob Agents Chemother* 1988;32(1):68–74.
48. Raoult D, Drancourt M. Antimicrobial therapy of rickettsial diseases. *Antimicrob Agents Chemother* 1991;35(12):2457–2462.
49. Dumler JS, Bakken JS. Ehrlichial diseases of humans: emerging tick-borne infections. *Clin Infect Dis* 1995;20(5):1102–1110.
50. Clyde DF, Miller RM, DuPont HL, et al. Antimalarial effects of tetracyclines in man. *J Trop Med Hyg* 1971;74(11):238–242.
51. Colwell EJ, Hickman RL, Kosakal S. Tetracycline treatment of chloroquine-resistant falciparum malaria in Thailand. *JAMA* 1972;220(5):684–686.
52. American Academy of Pediatrics. Tetracyclines. In: Kimberlin D, Brady M, Long S, eds. *Red Book: 2018-2021 Report of the Committee of Infectious Diseases*, 31st ed. Itasca, IL: American Academy of Pediatrics, 2018:905–906.
53. Fan MY, Walker DH, Yu SR, et al. Epidemiology and ecology of rickettsial diseases in the People's Republic of China. *Rev Infect Dis* 1987;9(4):823–840.
54. Perine PL, Chandler BP, Krause DK, et al. A clinico-epidemiological study of epidemic typhus in Africa. *Clin Infect Dis* 1992;14(5):1149–1158.
55. American Academy of Pediatrics. Rocky Mountain spotted fever In: Kimberlin D, Brady M, Long S, eds. *Red Book: 2018-2021 Report of the Committee of Infectious Diseases*, 31st ed. Itasca, IL: American Academy of Pediatrics, 2018:697–700.
56. Valencia GB, Banzon F, Cummings M, et al. *Mycoplasma hominis* and *Ureaplasma urealyticum* in neonates with suspected infection. *Pediatr Infect Dis J* 1993;12(7):571–573.
57. Abdel-Haq N, Asmar B, Brown W. *Mycoplasma hominis* scalp abscess in the newborn. *Pediatr Infect Dis J* 2002;21(12):1171–1173.
58. Spencer RC, Brown CB. Septicaemia in a renal transplant patient due to *Mycoplasma hominis. J Infect* 1983;6(3):267–268.
59. Bowie WR, Alexander ER, Stimson JB, et al. Therapy for nongonococcal urethritis: double-blind randomized comparison of two doses and two durations of minocycline. *Ann Intern Med* 1981;95(3):306–311.
60. Prentice MJ, Taylor-Robinson D, Csonka GW. Non-specific urethritis. A placebo-controlled trial of minocycline in conjunction with laboratory investigations. *Br J Vener Dis* 1976;52(4): 269–275.
61. Handsfield HH. Gonorrhea and nongonococcal urethritis. Recent advances. *Med Clin North Am* 1978;62(5):925–943.
62. Jawetz E. Chemotherapy of chlamydial infections. *Adv Pharmacol Chemother* 1969;7:253–282.
63. American Academy of Pediatrics. *Chlamydia trachomatis* infections. In: Kimberlin D, Brady M, Long S, eds. *Red Book: 2018-2021 Report of the Committee of Infectious Diseases*, 31st ed. Itasca, IL American Academy of Pediatrics, 2018:276–283.
64. Workowski KA, Bolan GA. Sexually transmitted diseases treatment guidelines, 2015. MMWR Recommendations and reports. *MMWR Recomm Rep* 2015;64(Rr-03):1–137.
65. American Academy of Pediatrics. Ehrlichia, anaplasma, and related infections. In: Kimberlin D, Brady M, Long S, eds. *Red Book: 2018-2021 Report of the Committee of Infectious Diseases*, 31st ed. Itasca, IL: American Academy of Pediatrics, 2018:323–328.
66. Johnson RC, Kodner C, Russell M. In vitro and in vivo susceptibility of the Lyme disease spirochete, *Borrelia burgdorferi*, to four antimicrobial agents. *Antimicrob Agents Chemother* 1987;31(2):164–167.
67. Steere AC. Musculoskeletal manifestations of Lyme disease. *Am J Med* 1995;98(4a): 44S–48S; discussion 8S–51S.
68. Pachner AR. Early disseminated Lyme disease: Lyme meningitis. *Am J Med* 1995;98(4a): 30S–37S; discussion 7S–43S.
69. Lantos PM, Charini WA, Medoff G, et al. Final report of the Lyme disease review panel of the Infectious Diseases Society of America. *Clin Infect Dis* 2010;51(1):1–5.
70. Hall WH. Modern chemotherapy for brucellosis in humans. *Rev Infect Dis* 1990;12(6):1060–1099.
71. Lubani MM, Dudin KI, Sharda DC, et al. A multicenter therapeutic study of 1100 children with brucellosis. *Pediatr Infect Dis J* 1989;8(2):75–78.
72. al-Eissa YA, Kambal AM, al-Nasser MN, et al. Childhood brucellosis: a study of 102 cases. *Pediatr Infect Dis J* 1990;9(2):74–79.
73. Cholera in 1994. Part I [in French]. *Releve Epidemiologique Hebdomadaire* 1995;70(28):201–208.
74. Rabbani GH, Butler T, Shahrier M, et al. Efficacy of a single dose of furazolidone for treatment of cholera in children. *Antimicrob Agents Chemother* 1991;35(9):1864–1867.
75. American Academy of Pediatrics. Malaria. In: Kimberlin D, Brady M, Long S, eds. *Red Book: 2018-2021 Report of the Committee of Infectious Diseases.* Itasca, IL: American Academy of Pediatrics, 2018:527–537.
76. Fabre J, Milek E, Kalfopoulos P, et al. Tetracycline kinetics in man. Digestive absorption and serum concentration [in French]. *Schweiz Med Wochenschr* 1971;101(17):593–598.
77. Kunin CM, Dornbush AC, Finland M. Distribution and excretion of four tetracycline analogues in normal young men. *J Clin Invest* 1959;38:1950–1963.
78. Bennett JV, Mickelwait JS, Barrett JE, et al. Comparative serum binding of four tetracyclines under simulated in vivo conditions. *Antimicrob Agents Chemother* 1965;5:180–182.
79. Macdonald H, Kelly RG, Allen ES, et al. Pharmacokinetic studies on minocycline in man. *Clin Pharmacol Ther* 1973;14(5):852–861.
80. Karlsson M, Hammers S, Nilsson-Ehle I, et al. Concentrations of doxycycline and penicillin G in sera and cerebrospinal fluid of patients treated for neuroborreliosis. *Antimicrob Agents Chemother* 1996;40(5):1104–1107.
81. Yim CW, Flynn NM, Fitzgerald FT. Penetration of oral doxycycline into the cerebrospinal fluid of patients with latent or neurosyphilis. *Antimicrob Agents Chemother* 1985;28(2):347–348.
82. Parker RH, Schmid FR. Antibacterial activity of synovial fluid during therapy of septic arthritis. *Arthritis Rheum* 1971;14(1):96–104.
83. Lundberg C, Malmborg AS, Ivemark BI. Antibiotic concentrations in relation to structural changes in maxillary sinus mucosa following intramuscular or peroral treatment. *Scand J Infect Dis* 1974;6(2):187–195.
84. Hoeprich PD, Warshauer DM. Entry of four tetracyclines into saliva and tears. *Antimicrob Agents Chemother* 1974;5(3):330–336.
85. Leblanc AL, Perry JE. Transfer of tetracycline across the human placenta. *Texas Rep Biol Med* 1967;25(4):541–545.
86. Matsuda S. Transfer of antibiotics into maternal milk. *Biol Res Pregnancy Perinatol* 1984;5(2):57–60.

87. Greenberg PA, Sanford JP. Removal and absorption of antibiotics in patients with renal failure undergoing peritoneal dialysis. Tetracycline, chloramphenicol, kanamycin, and colistimethate. *Ann Intern Med* 1967;66(3):465–470.
88. Whelton A, von Wittenau MS, Twomey TM, et al. Doxycycline pharmacokinetics in the absence of renal function. *Kidney Int* 1974;5(5):365–371.
89. Carson JL, Strom BL, Duff A, et al. Acute liver disease associated with erythromycins, sulfonamides, and tetracyclines. *Ann Intern Med* 1993;119(7, Pt 1):576–583.
90. Schultz JC, Adamson JS Jr, Workman WW, et al. Fatal liver disease after intravenous administration of tetracycline in high dosage. *N Engl J Med* 1963;269:999–1004.
91. Glette J, Sandberg S, Haneberg B, et al. Effect of tetracyclines and UV light on oxygen consumption by human leukocytes. *Antimicrob Agents Chemother* 1984;26(4):489–492.
92. Kline AH, Blattner RJ, Lunin M. Transplacental effect of tetracyclines on teeth. *JAMA* 1964;188:178–180.
93. Lew HT, French SW. Tetracycline nephrotoxicity and nonoliguric acute renal failure. *Arch Int Med* 1966;118(2):123–128.
94. Mull MM. The tetracyclines. A critical reappraisal. *Am J Dis Child* 1966;112(5):483–493.
95. Maroon JC, Mealy J Jr. Benign intracranial hypertension. Sequel to tetracycline therapy in a child. *JAMA* 1971;216(9):1479–1480.
96. Walters BN, Gubbay SS. Tetracycline and benign intracranial hypertension: report of five cases. *Br Med J (Clin Res Ed)* 1981;282(6257):19–20.
97. Fanning WL, Gump DW, Sofferman RA. Side effects of minocycline: a double-blind study. *Antimicrob Agents Chemother* 1977;11(4):712–717.
98. Neuvonen PJ, Gothoni G, Hackman R, et al. Interference of iron with the absorption of tetracyclines in man. *Br Med J* 1970;4(5734):532–534.
99. Gugler R, Allgayer H. Effects of antacids on the clinical pharmacokinetics of drugs. An update. *Clin Pharmacokinet* 1990;18(3):210–219.
100. Penttila O, Neuvonen PJ, Aho K, et al. Interaction between doxycycline and some antiepileptic drugs. *Br Med J* 1974;2(5917):470–472.
101. Neuvonen PJ, Penttila O. Interaction between doxycycline and barbiturates. *Br Med J* 1974;1(5907):535–536.
102. Lindenbaum J, Rund DG, Butler VP Jr, et al. Inactivation of digoxin by the gut flora: reversal by antibiotic therapy. *N Engl J Med* 1981;305(14):789–794.
103. Bartz QR. Isolation and characterization of chloromycetin. *J Biol Chem* 1948;172(2):445–450.
104. Yunis AA, Manyan DR, Arimura GK. Comparative effect of chloramphenicol and thiamphenicol on DNA and mitochondrial protein synthesis in mammalian cells. *J Lab Clin Med* 1973;81(5):713–718.
105. Okamoto S, Mizuno D. Mechanism of chloramphenicol and tetracycline resistance in *Escherichia coli*. *J Gen Microbiol* 1964;35:125–133.
106. Gangarosa EJ, Bennett JV, Wyatt C, et al. An epidemic-associated episome? *J Infect Dis* 1972;126(2):215–218.
107. Butler T, Linh NN, Arnold K, et al. Chloramphenicol-resistant typhoid fever in Vietnam associated with R factor. *Lancet* 1973;302(7836):983–985.
108. Halder KK, Dalal BS, Ghose E, et al. Chloramphenicol resistant *Salmonella typhi*: the cause of recent out-break of enteric fever in Calcutta. *Indian J Pathol Microbiol* 1992;35(1):11–17.
109. Drug resistance in salmonellas. *Lancet* 1982;1(8286):1391–1392.
110. Spika JS, Waterman SH, Hoo GW, et al. Chloramphenicol-resistant *Salmonella* newport traced through hamburger to dairy farms. A major persisting source of human salmonellosis in California. *N Engl J Med* 1987;316(10):565–570.
111. Prober CG, Rajchgot P, Bannatyne RM, et al. Impact of chloramphenicol use on bacterial resistance in a neonatal intensive care unit. *Lancet* 1983;2(8342):158.
112. Klastersky J, Husson M. Bactericidal activity of the combinations of gentamicin with clindamycin or chloramphenicol against species of *Escherichia coli* and *Bacteroides fragilis*. *Antimicrob Agents Chemother* 1977;12(2):135–138.
113. Asmar BI, Prainito M, Dajani AS. Antagonistic effect of chloramphenicol in combination with cefotaxime or ceftriaxone. *Antimicrob Agents Chemother* 1988;32(9):1375–1378.
114. Sharma KB, Bhat MB, Pasricha A, et al. Multiple antibiotic resistance among salmonellae in India. *J Antimicrob Chemother* 1979;5(1):15–21.
115. Bhutta ZA, Naqvi SH, Razzaq RA, et al. Multidrug-resistant typhoid in children: presentation and clinical features. *Rev Infect Dis* 1991;13(5):832–836.
116. Multiresistant *Salmonella typhi* in India. *Lancet* 1990;336(8709):252.
117. Albert MJ, Haider K, Nahar S, et al. Multiresistant *Salmonella typhi* in Bangladesh. *J Antimicrob Chemother* 1991;27(4):554–555.
118. Datta N, Richards H, Datta C. *Salmonella typhi* in vivo acquires resistance to both chloramphenicol and co-trimoxazole. *Lancet* 1981;1(8231):1181–1183.
119. Barrett FF, Taber LH, Morris CR, et al. A 12 year review of the antibiotic management of *Hemophilus influenzae* meningitis. Comparison of ampicillin and conventional therapy including chloramphenicol. *J Pediatr* 1972;81(2):370–377.
120. Kinmonth AL, Storrs CN, Mitchell RG. Meningitis due to chloramphenicol-resistant *Haemophilus influenzae* type b. *Br Med J* 1978;1(6114):694.
121. Mendelman PM, Doroshow CA, Gandy SL, et al. Plasmid-mediated resistance in multiply resistant *Haemophilus influenzae* type b causing meningitis: molecular characterization of one strain and review of the literature. *J Infect Dis* 1984;150(1):30–39.
122. Doern GV, Jorgensen JH, Thornsberry C, et al. National collaborative study of the prevalence of antimicrobial resistance among clinical isolates of *Haemophilus influenzae*. *Antimicrob Agents Chemother* 1988;32(2):180–185.
123. Garvey RJ, McMullin GP. Meningitis due to beta lactamase producing type b *Haemophilus influenzae* resistant to chloramphenicol. *Br Med J (Clin Res Ed)* 1983;287(6400):1183–1184.
124. Powell M, Price EH. Invasive infections due to *Haemophilus influenzae* type b resistant to ampicillin and chloramphenicol. *J Antimicrob Chemother* 1990;26(1):149–151.
125. Dimopoulou ID, Kraak WA, Anderson EC, et al. Molecular epidemiology of unrelated clusters of multiresistant strains of *Haemophilus influenzae*. *J Infect Dis* 1992;165(6):1069–1075.
126. Wild BE, Pearman JW, Richardson CJ, et al. Multiply-antibiotic-resistant *Haemophilus influenzae* type b meningitis in Western Australia. *Med J Aust* 1986;144(12):666–667.
127. Collignon PJ, Bell JM, MacInnes SJ, et al. A national collaborative study of resistance to antimicrobial agents in *Haemophilus influenzae* in Australian hospitals. The Australian Group for Antimicrobial Resistance (AGAR). *J Antimicrob Chemother* 1992;30(2):153–163.
128. Catry MA, Vaz Pato MV. *Haemophilus influenzae* type b resistant to ampicillin and chloramphenicol. *Br Med J (Clin Res Ed)* 1983;287(6403):1471.
129. Centers for Disease Control. Ampicillin and chloramphenicol resistance in systemic *Haemophilus influenzae* disease. *MMWR Morb Mortal Wkly Rep* 1984;33(3):35–37.
130. Simasathien S, Duangmani C, Echeverria P. *Haemophilus influenzae* type B resistant to ampicillin and chloramphenicol in an orphanage in Thailand. *Lancet* 1980;2(8206): 1214–1217.
131. Mastro TD, Nomani NK, Ishaq Z, et al. Use of nasopharyngeal isolates of *Streptococcus pneumoniae* and *Haemophilus influenzae* from children in Pakistan for surveillance for antimicrobial resistance. *Pediatr Infect Dis J* 1993;12(10):824–830.
132. Manten A, van Klingeren B, Dessens-Kroon M. Chloramphenicol resistance in *Haemophilus influenzae*. *Lancet* 1976;1(7961):702.
133. Campos J, Seuba T, Trujillo G, et al. Multiple antibiotic resistance in *Haemophilus influenzae* [in Spanish]. *Enferm Infecc Microbiol Clin* 1981;1(8219):553–554.
134. Sills JA, MacMahon P, Hall E, et al. *Haemophilus influenzae* type b resistant to chloramphenicol and ampicillin. *Br Med J (Clin Res Ed)* 1983;286(6366):722.
135. Jorgensen JH. Update on mechanisms and prevalence of antimicrobial resistance in *Haemophilus influenzae*. *Clin Infect Dis* 1992;14(5):1119–1123.
136. Mhalu FS, Mmari PW, Ijumba J. Rapid emergence of El Tor *Vibrio cholerae* resistant to antimicrobial agents during first six months of fourth cholera epidemic in Tanzania. *Lancet* 1979;1(8112):345–347.
137. Goodwin CS, Blake P, Blincow E. The minimum inhibitory and bactericidal concentrations of antibiotics and anti-ulcer agents against *Campylobacter pyloridis*. *J Antimicrob Chemother* 1986;17(3):309–314.
138. Li XZ, Ma D, Livermore DM, et al. Role of efflux pump(s) in intrinsic resistance of *Pseudomonas aeruginosa*: active efflux as a contributing factor to beta-lactam resistance. *Antimicrob Agents Chemother* 1994;38(8):1742–1752.
139. Burns JL, Hedin LA, Lien DM. Chloramphenicol resistance in *Pseudomonas cepacia* because of decreased permeability. *Antimicrob Agents Chemother* 1989;33(2):136–141.
140. Aber RC, Wennersten C, Moellering RC Jr. Antimicrobial susceptibility of flavobacteria. *Antimicrob Agents Chemother* 1978;14(3):483–487.
141. Schwarz S, Cardoso M. Nucleotide sequence and phylogeny of a chloramphenicol acetyltransferase encoded by the plasmid pSCS7 from *Staphylococcus aureus*. *Antimicrob Agents Chemother* 1991;35(8):1551–1556.
142. Nakae M, Murai T, Kaneko Y, et al. Drug resistance in *Streptococcus pyogenes* isolated in Japan. *Antimicrob Agents Chemother* 1977;12(3):427–428.
143. Oppenheim B, Koornhof HJ, Austrian R. Antibiotic-resistant pneumococcal disease in children at Baragwanath Hospital, Johannesburg. *Pediatr Infect Dis* 1986;5(5):520–524.
144. Klugman KP, Koornhof HJ. Drug resistance patterns and serogroups or serotypes of pneumococcal isolates from cerebrospinal fluid or blood, 1979-1986. *J Infect Dis* 1988;158(5):956–964.
145. Lee HJ, Park JY, Jang SH, et al. High incidence of resistance to multiple antimicrobials in clinical isolates of *Streptococcus pneumoniae* from a university hospital in Korea. *Clin Infect Dis* 1995;20(4):826–835.
146. Ohm-Smith MJ, Hadley WK, Sweet RL. In vitro activity of new beta-lactam antibiotics and other antimicrobial drugs against anaerobic isolates from obstetric and gynecological infections. *Antimicrob Agents Chemother* 1982;22(4):711–714.
147. Delmee M, Avesani V. Correlation between serogroup and susceptibility to chloramphenicol, clindamycin, erythromycin, rifampicin and tetracycline among 308 isolates of *Clostridium difficile*. *J Antimicrob Chemother* 1988;22(3):325–331.
148. George WL, Kirby BD, Sutter VL, et al. Gram-negative anaerobic bacilli: Their role in infection and patterns of susceptibility to antimicrobial agents. II. Little-known *Fusobacterium* species and miscellaneous genera. *Rev Infect Dis* 1981;3(3):599–626.
149. Friedman CA, Lovejoy FC, Smith AL. Chloramphenicol disposition in infants and children. *J Pediatr* 1979;95(6):1071–1077.
150. Kramer PW, Griffith RS, Campbell RL. Antibiotic penetration of the brain. A comparative study. *J Neurosurg* 1969;31(3):295–302.
151. Snyder MJ, Gonzalez O, Palomino C, et al. Comparative efficacy of chloramphenicol, ampicillin, and co-trimoxazole in the treatment of typhoid fever. *Lancet* 1976;2(7996):1155–1157.
152. Aserkoff B, Bennett JV. Effect of antibiotic therapy in acute salmonellosis on the fecal excretion of salmonellae. N Engl J Med 1969;281(12):636–640.
153. Koskiniemi M, Pettay O, Raivio M, et al. *Haemophilus influenzae* meningitis. A comparison between chloramphenicol and ampicillin therapy with special reference to impaired hearing. *Acta Paediatr Scand* 1978;67(1):17–24.
154. Halstensen A, Vollset SE, Haneberg B, et al. Antimicrobial therapy and case fatality in meningococcal disease. *Scand J Infect Dis* 1987;19(4):403–407.
155. Cherubin CE, Corrado ML, Nair SR, et al. Treatment of gram-negative bacillary meningitis: role of the new cephalosporin antibiotics. *Rev Infect Dis* 1982;4(Suppl):S453–S464.
156. Snyder MJ, Woodward TE. The clinical use of chloramphenicol. *Med Clin North Am* 1970;54(5):1187–1197.
157. Norris AH, Reilly JP, Edelstein PH, et al. Chloramphenicol for the treatment of vancomycin-resistant enterococcal infections. *Clin Infect Dis* 1995;20(5):1137–1144.
158. Shrestha NK, Chua JD, Tuohy MJ, et al. Antimicrobial susceptibility of vancomycin-resistant *Enterococcus faecium*: potential utility of fosfomycin. *Scand J Infect Dis* 2003;35(1):12–14.
159. Kauffman RE, Miceli JN, Strebel L, et al. Pharmacokinetics of chloramphenicol and chloramphenicol succinate in infants and children. *J Pediatr* 1981;98(2):315–320.
160. Sack CM, Koup JR, Smith AL. Chloramphenicol pharmacokinetics in infants and young children. *Pediatrics* 1980;66(4):579–584.
161. Pickering LK, Hoecker JL, Kramer WG, et al. Clinical pharmacology of two chloramphenicol preparations in children: sodium succinate (iv) and palmitate (oral) esters. *J Pediatr* 1980;96(4):757–761.

162. Yogev R, Kolling WM, Williams T. Pharmacokinetic comparison of intravenous and oral chloramphenicol in patients with *Haemophilus influenzae* meningitis. *Pediatrics* 1981;67(5):656–660.
163. Abraham RK, Burnett HH. Tetracycline and chloramphenicol studies on rabbit and human eyes. *AMA Arch Ophthalmol* 1955;54(5):641–659.
164. Black SB, Levine P, Shinefield HR. The necessity for monitoring chloramphenicol levels when treating neonatal meningitis. *J Pediatr* 1978;92(2):235–236.
165. Dunkle LM. Central nervous system chloramphenicol concentration in premature infants. *Antimicrob Agents Chemother* 1978;13(3):427–429.
166. Rapp GF, Griffith RS, Hebble WM. The permeability of traumatically inflamed synovial membrane to commonly used antibiotics. *J Bone Joint Surg Am* 1966;48(8):1534–1540.
167. Koup JR, Lau AH, Brodsky B, et al. Relationship between serum and saliva chloramphenicol concentrations. *Antimicrob Agents Chemother* 1979;15(5):658–661.
168. Kurz H, Mauser-Ganshorn A, Stickel HH. Differences in the binding of drugs to plasma proteins from newborn and adult man. I. European *J Clin Pharmacol* 1977;11(6):463–467.
169. Kauffman RE, Thirumoorthi MC, Buckley JA, et al. Relative bioavailability of intravenous chloramphenicol succinate and oral chloramphenicol palmitate in infants and children. *J Pediatr* 1981;99(6):963–967.
170. Lietman PS. Chloramphenicol and the neonate—1979 view. *Clin Perinatol* 1979;6(1):151–162.
171. Lietman PS, White TJ, Shaw WV. Chloramphenicol: an enzymological microassay. *Antimicrob Agents Chemother* 1976;10(2):347–353.
172. Oski FA. Hematologic consequences of chloramphenicol therapy. *J Pediatr* 1979;94(3):515–516.
173. O'Gorman Hughes DW. Studies on chloramphenicol. II. Possible determinants and progress of haemopoietic toxicity during chloramphenicol therapy. *Med J Aust* 1973;2(26):1142–1146.
174. Wallerstein RO, Condit PK, Kasper CK, et al. Statewide study of chloramphenicol therapy and fatal aplastic anemia. *JAMA* 1969;208(11):2045–2050.
175. Plaut ME, Best WR. Aplastic anemia after parenteral chloramphenicol: warning renewed. *N Engl J Med* 1982;306(24):1486.
176. Daum RS, Cohen DL, Smith AL. Fatal aplastic anemia following apparent "dose-related" chloramphenicol toxicity. *J Pediatr* 1979;94(3):403–406.
177. Burns LE, Hodgman JE, Cass AB. Fatal circulatory collapse in premature infants receiving chloramphenicol. *N Engl J Med* 1959;261:1318–1321.
178. Craft AW, Brocklebank JT, Hey EN, et al. The 'grey toddler'. Chloramphenicol toxicity. *Arch Dis Child* 1974;49(3):235–237.
179. Thompson WL, Anderson SE, Lipsky JJ, et al. Letter: Overdoses of chloramphenicol. *JAMA* 1975;234(2):149–150.
180. Fripp RR, Carter MC, Werner JC, et al. Cardiac function and acute chloramphenicol toxicity. *J Pediatr* 1983;103(3):487–490.
181. Evans LS, Kleiman MB. Acidosis as a presenting feature of chloramphenicol toxicity. *J Pediatr* 1986;108(3):475–477.
182. Freundlich M, Cynamon H, Tamer A, et al. Management of chloramphenicol intoxication in infancy by charcoal hemoperfusion. *J Pediatr* 1983;103(3):485–487.
183. Stevens DC, Kleiman MB, Lietman PS, et al. Exchange transfusion in acute chloramphenicol toxicity. *J Pediatr* 1981;99(4):651–653.
184. Woolf DL. Chloramphenicol blindness. *Br Med J* 1965;1(5449):1511.
185. Halpert J. Further studies of the suicide inactivation of purified rat liver cytochrome P-450 by chloramphenicol. *Mol Pharmacol* 1982;21(1):166–172.
186. Christensen LK, Skovsted L. Inhibition of drug metabolism by chloramphenicol. *Lancet* 1969;2(7635):1397–1399.
187. Rose JQ, Choi HK, Schentag JJ, et al. Intoxication caused by interaction of chloramphenicol and phenytoin. *JAMA* 1977;237(24):2630–2631.
188. Krasinski K, Kusmiesz H, Nelson JD. Pharmacologic interactions among chloramphenicol, phenytoin and phenobarbital. *Pediatr Infect Dis* 1982;1(4):232–235.
189. Weeks JL, Mason EO Jr, Baker CJ. Antagonism of ampicillin and chloramphenicol for meningeal isolates of group B streptococci. *Antimicrob Agents Chemother* 1981;20(3): 281–285.
190. Cosar C, Julou L. The activity of 1-(2-hydroxyethyl)-2-methyl-5-nitroimidazole (R. P. 8823) against experimental *Trichomonas vaginalis* infections [in French]. *Ann Inst Pasteur* 1959;96(2):238–241.
191. Freeman CD, Klutman NE, Lamp KC. Metronidazole. A therapeutic review and update. *Drugs* 1997;54(5):679–708.
192. Muller M. Mode of action of metronidazole on anaerobic bacteria and protozoa. *Surgery* 1983;93(1, Pt 2):165–171.
193. Smith A. Metronidazole resistance: a hidden epidemic? *Br Dent J* 2018;224(6):403–404.
194. Lofmark S, Fang H, Hedberg M, et al. Inducible metronidazole resistance and nim genes in clinical *Bacteroides fragilis* group isolates. *Antimicrob Agents Chemother* 2005;49(3):1253–1256.
195. Leiros HK, Kozielski-Stuhrmann S, Kapp U, et al. Structural basis of 5-nitroimidazole antibiotic resistance: the crystal structure of NimA from *Deinococcus radiodurans*. *J Biol Chem* 2004;279(53):55840–55849.
196. Schuetz AN. Antimicrobial resistance and susceptibility testing of anaerobic bacteria. *Clin Infect Dis* 2014;59(5):698–705.
197. Clinical and Laboratory Standards Institute. *Performance standards for antimicrobial susceptibility testing M100*, 28th ed. Wayne, PA: Clinical and Laboratory Standards Institute, 2018.
198. Pankuch GA, Jacobs MR, Appelbaum PC. Susceptibilities of 428 gram-positive and-negative anaerobic bacteria to Bay y3118 compared with their susceptibilities to ciprofloxacin, clindamycin, metronidazole, piperacillin, piperacillin-tazobactam, and cefoxitin. *Antimicrob Agents Chemother* 1993;37(8):1649–1654.
199. Sheikh W, Pitkin DH, Nadler H. Antibacterial activity of meropenem and selected comparative agents against anaerobic bacteria at seven North American centers. *Clin Infect Dis* 1993;16(Suppl 4):S361—S366.
200. Alexander CJ, Citron DM, Brazier JS, et al. Identification and antimicrobial resistance patterns of clinical isolates of *Clostridium clostridioforme, Clostridium innocuum*, and *Clostridium ramosum* compared with those of clinical isolates of *Clostridium* perfringens. *J Clin Microbiol* 1995;33(12):3209–3215.
201. Bourke B, Ceponis P, Chiba N, et al. Canadian *Helicobacter* Study Group Consensus Conference: Update on the approach to *Helicobacter pylori* infection in children and adolescents—an evidence-based evaluation. *Can J Gastroenterol* 2005;19(7):399–408.
202. Koletzko S, Richy F, Bontems P, et al. Prospective multicentre study on antibiotic resistance of *Helicobacter pylori* strains obtained from children living in Europe. *Gut* 2006;55(12):1711–1716.
203. Tolia V, Brown W, El-Baba M, et al. *Helicobacter pylori* culture and antimicrobial susceptibility from pediatric patients in Michigan. *Pediatr Infect Dis J* 2000;19(12):1167–1171.
204. Goldstein EJ, Citron DM, Cherubin CE, et al. Comparative susceptibility of the *Bacteroides fragilis* group species and other anaerobic bacteria to meropenem, imipenem, piperacillin, cefoxitin, ampicillin/sulbactam, clindamycin and metronidazole. *J Antimicrob Chemother* 1993;31(3):363–372.
205. Nasirudeen AM, Hian YE, Singh M, et al. Metronidazole induces programmed cell death in the protozoan parasite *Blastocystis hominis*. *Microbiology* 2004;150(Pt 1):33–43.
206. Schuster FL, Ramirez-Avila L. Current world status of *Balantidium coli*. *Clin Microbiol Rev* 2008;21(4):626–638.
207. American Academy of Pediatrics. *Giardia intestinalis* infections. In: Kimberlin D, Brady M, Long S, eds. *Red Book: 2018-2021 Report of the Committee of Infectious Diseases*, 31st ed. Itasca, IL: American Academy of Pediatrics, 2018:352–355.
208. Bassily S, Farid Z, el-Masry NA, et al. Treatment of intestinal *E. histolytica* and *G. lamblia* with metronidazole, tinidazole and ornidazole: a comparative study. *J Trop Med Hyg* 1987;90(1):9–12.
209. Lofmark S, Edlund C, Nord CE. Metronidazole is still the drug of choice for treatment of anaerobic infections. *Clin Infect Dis* 2010;50(Suppl 1):S16–S23.
210. Dahl MV, Katz HI, Krueger GG, et al. Topical metronidazole maintains remissions of rosacea. *Arch Dermatol* 1998;134(6):679–683.
211. Sato S, Fonseca MJ, Ciampo JO, et al. Metronidazole-containing gel for the treatment of periodontitis: an in vivo evaluation. *Braz Oral Res* 2008;22(2):145–150.
212. Totten PA, Amsel R, Hale J, et al. Selective differential human blood bilayer media for isolation of *Gardnerella* (*Haemophilus*) *vaginalis*. *J Clin Microbiol* 1982;15(1):141–147.
213. Peeters M, Piot P. Adhesion of *Gardnerella vaginalis* to vaginal epithelial cells: variables affecting adhesion and inhibition by metronidazole. *Genitourin Med* 1985;61(6):391–395.
214. Eschenbach DA, Davick PR, Williams BL, et al. Prevalence of hydrogen peroxide-producing *Lactobacillus* species in normal women and women with bacterial vaginosis. *J Clin Microbiol* 1989;27(2):251–256.
215. Holst E. Reservoir of four organisms associated with bacterial vaginosis suggests lack of sexual transmission. *J Clin Microbiol* 1990;28(9):2035–2039.
216. Ingram DL, White ST, Lyna PR, et al. *Gardnerella vaginalis* infection and sexual contact in female children. *Child Abuse Negl* 1992;16(6):847–853.
217. Wahl NG, Castilla MA, Lewis-Abney K. Prevalence of *Gardnerella vaginalis* in prepubertal males. *Arch Pediatr Adolesc Med* 1998;152(11):1095–1099.
218. Berardi-Grassias L, Roy O, Berardi JC, et al. Neonatal meningitis due to *Gardnerella vaginalis*. *Eur J Clin Microbiol Infect Dis* 1988;7(3):406–407.
219. Leighton PM, Bulleid B, Taylor R. Neonatal cellulitis due to *Gardnerella vaginalis*. *Pediatr Infect Dis* 1982;1(5):339–340.
220. Chowdhury MN, Kambal AM. A case of conjunctivitis in a neonate due to *Gardnerella vaginalis*. *Trop Geogr Med* 1985;37(4):365–366.
221. Amaya RA, Al-Dossary F, Demmler GJ. *Gardnerella vaginalis* bacteremia in a premature neonate. *J Perinatol* 2002;22(7):585–587.
222. Petit PL, Mouton RP. *Gardnerella vaginalis* in urinary tract infections of immunocompromised patients. *Eur J Clin Microbiol* 1985;4(3):357.
223. Catlin BW. *Gardnerella vaginalis*: characteristics, clinical considerations, and controversies. *Clin Microbiol Rev* 1992;5(3):213–237.
224. American Academy of Pediatrics. Bacterial vaginosis. In: Kimberlin D, Brady M, Long S, eds. *Red Book: 2018-2021 Report of the Committee of Infectious Diseases*, 31st ed. Itasca, IL: American Academy of Pediatrics, 2018:239–244.
225. Koss CA, Baras DC, Lane SD, et al. Investigation of metronidazole use during pregnancy and adverse birth outcomes. *Antimicrob Agents Chemother* 2012;56(9):4800–4805.
226. Czeizel AE, Kazy Z, Vargha P. Oral tinidazole treatment during pregnancy and teratogenesis. *Int J Gynaecol Obstet* 2003;83(3):305–306.
227. Spencer JP, Gonzalez LS III, Barnhart DJ. Medications in the breast-feeding mother. *Am Fam Phys* 2001;64(1):119–126.
228. Moi H, Erkkola R, Jerve F, et al. Should male consorts of women with bacterial vaginosis be treated? *Genitourin Med* 1989;65(4):263–268.
229. Vejtorp M, Bollerup AC, Vejtorp L, et al. Bacterial vaginosis: a double-blind randomized trial of the effect of treatment of the sexual partner. *Br J Obstet Gynaecol* 1988;95(9):920–926.
230. Nagy E, Urban E, Nord CE. Antimicrobial susceptibility of *Bacteroides fragilis* group isolates in Europe: 20 years of experience. *Clin Microbiol Infect* 2011;17(3):371–379.
231. Snydman DR, Jacobus NV, McDermott LA, et al. Lessons learned from the anaerobe survey: historical perspective and review of the most recent data (2005-2007). *Clin Infect Dis* 2010;50(Suppl 1):S26–S33.
232. Boyanova L, Kolarov R, Gergova G, et al. Trends in antibiotic resistance in *Prevotella* species from patients of the University Hospital of Maxillofacial Surgery, Sofia, Bulgaria, in 2003-2009. *Anaerobe* 2010;16(5):489–492.
233. Brook I. Microbiology and principles of antimicrobial therapy for head and neck infections. *Infect Dis Clin North Am* 2007;21(2):355–391, vi.
234. Brazier JS. Human infections with *Fusobacterium necrophorum*. *Anaerobe* 2006;12(4):165–172.
235. Riordan T. Human infection with *Fusobacterium necrophorum* (necrobacillosis), with a focus on Lemierre's syndrome. *Clin Microbiol Rev* 2007;20(4):622–659.
236. Montravers P, Lepape A, Dubreuil L, et al. Clinical and microbiological profiles of community-acquired and nosocomial intra-abdominal infections: results of the French prospective, observational EBIIA study. *J Antimicrob Chemother* 2009;63(4):785–794.

237. Montravers P, Gauzit R, Muller C, et al. Emergence of antibiotic-resistant bacteria in cases of peritonitis after intraabdominal surgery affects the efficacy of empirical antimicrobial therapy. *Clin Infect Dis* 1996;23(3):486–494.
238. Goldstein EJ, Citron DM, Warren YA, et al. In vitro activity of moxifloxacin against 923 anaerobes isolated from human intra-abdominal infections. *Antimicrob Agents Chemother* 2006;50(1):148–155.
239. Solomkin JS, Dellinger EP, Bohnen JM, et al. The role of oral antimicrobials for the management of intra-abdominal infections. *New Horiz* 1998;6(2, Suppl):S46–S52.
240. Solomkin JS, Mazuski JE, Bradley JS, et al. Diagnosis and management of complicated intra-abdominal infection in adults and children: guidelines by the Surgical Infection Society and the Infectious Diseases Society of America. *Clin Infect Dis* 2010;50(2):133–164.
241. Simjee AE, Gathiram V, Jackson TF, et al. A comparative trial of metronidazole v. tinidazole in the treatment of amoebic liver abscess. *S Afr Med J* 1985;68(13):923–924.
242. Lucht E, Evengard B, Skott J, et al. *Entamoeba gingivalis* in human immunodeficiency virus type 1-infected patients with periodontal disease. *Clin Infect Dis* 1998;27(3):471–473.
243. Perez-Jaffe L, Katz R, Gupta PK. *Entamoeba gingivalis* identified in a left upper neck nodule by fine-needle aspiration: a case report. *Diagn Cytopathol* 1998;18(6):458–461.
244. Foda AA, El-Malky MM. Prevalence of genital tract infection with *Entamoeba gingivalis* among copper T 380A intrauterine device users in Egypt. *Contraception* 2012;85(1):108–112.
245. Chacin-Bonilla L. Successful treatment of human *Entamoeba polecki* infection with metronidazole. *Am J Trop Med Hyg* 1980;29(4):521–523.
246. Kirkcaldy RD, Augostini P, Asbel LE, et al. *Trichomonas vaginalis* antimicrobial drug resistance in 6 US cities, STD Surveillance Network, 2009-2010. *Emerg Infect Dis* 2012;18(6):939–943.
247. Wendt JM, Cohen JA, Mu Y, et al. *Clostridium difficile* infection among children across diverse US geographic locations. *Pediatrics* 2014;133(4):651–658.
248. McDonald LC, Gerding DN, Johnson S, et al. Clinical practice guidelines for *Clostridium difficile* infection in adults and children: 2017 update by the Infectious Diseases Society of America (IDSA) and Society for Healthcare Epidemiology of America (SHEA). *Clin Infect Dis* 2018;66(7):e1–e48.
249. Bartlett JG. The case for vancomycin as the preferred drug for treatment of *Clostridium difficile* infection. *Clin Infect Dis* 2008;46(10):1489–1492.
250. Kapoor K, Chandra M, Nag D, et al. Evaluation of metronidazole toxicity: a prospective study. *Int J Clin Pharmacol Res* 1999;19(3):83–88.
251. Drekonja D, Reich J, Gezahegn S, et al. Fecal microbiota transplantation for *Clostridium difficile* infection: a systematic review. *Ann Intern Med* 2015;162(9):630–638.
252. Koletzko S, Jones NL, Goodman KJ, et al. Evidence-based guidelines from ESPGHAN and NASPGHAN for *Helicobacter pylori* infection in children. *J Pediatric Gastroenterol Nutr* 2011;53(2):230–243.
253. Nijevitch AA, Farztdinov KM, Sataev VU, et al. *Helicobacter pylori* infection in childhood: results of management with ranitidine bismuth citrate plus amoxicillin and tinidazole. *J Gastroenterol Hepatol* 2000;15(11):1243–1250.
254. Ghotaslou R, Leylabadlo HE, Asl YM. Prevalence of antibiotic resistance in *Helicobacter pylori*: A recent literature review. *World J Methodol* 2015;5(3):164–174.
255. Hunt RH, Xiao SD, Megraud F, et al. *Helicobacter pylori* in developing countries. World Gastroenterology Organisation Global Guideline. *J Gastrointest Liver Dis* 2011;20(3):299–304.
256. Jaka H, Rhee JA, Ostlundh L, et al. The magnitude of antibiotic resistance to *Helicobacter pylori* in Africa and identified mutations which confer resistance to antibiotics: systematic review and meta-analysis. *BMC Infect Dis* 2018;18(1):193.
257. Lamp KC, Freeman CD, Klutman NE, et al. Pharmacokinetics and pharmacodynamics of the nitroimidazole antimicrobials. *Clin Pharmacokinet* 1999;36(5):353–373.
258. Houghton GW, Hundt HK, Muller FO, et al. A comparison of the pharmacokinetics of metronidazole in man after oral administration of single doses of benzoylmetronidazole and metronidazole. *Br J Clin Pharmacol* 1982;14(2):201–206.
259. Loft S, Dossing M, Poulsen HE, et al. Influence of dose and route of administration on disposition of metronidazole and its major metabolites. *Eur J Clin Pharmacol* 1986;30(4):467–473.
260. Nix DE, Tyrrell R, Muller M. Pharmacodynamics of metronidazole determined by a time-kill assay for *Trichomonas vaginalis*. *Antimicrob Agents Chemother* 1995;39(8):1848–1852.
261. Cohen-Wolkowiez M, Sampson M, Bloom BT, et al. Determining population and developmental pharmacokinetics of metronidazole using plasma and dried blood spot samples from premature infants. *Pediatr Infect Dis J* 2013;32(9):956–961.
262. Child J, Chen X, Mistry RD, et al. Pharmacokinetic and pharmacodynamic properties of metronidazole in pediatric patients with acute appendicitis: a prospective study. *J Pediatr Infect Dis Soc* 2019; 8(4):297–302.
263. Ibrahim KH, Gunderson BW, Hermsen ED, et al. Pharmacodynamics of pulse dosing versus standard dosing: in vitro metronidazole activity against *Bacteroides fragilis* and *Bacteroides thetaiotaomicron*. *Antimicrob Agents Chemother* 2004;48(11):4195–4199.
264. Koeth LM, Good CE, Appelbaum PC, et al. Surveillance of susceptibility patterns in 1297 European and US anaerobic and capnophilic isolates to co-amoxiclav and five other antimicrobial agents. *J Antimicrob Chemother* 2004;53(6):1039–1044.
265. Hand WL, King-Thompson N, Holman JW. Entry of roxithromycin (RU 965), imipenem, cefotaxime, trimethoprim, and metronidazole into human polymorphonuclear leukocytes. *Antimicrob Agents Chemother* 1987;31(10):1553–1557.
266. Feldman WE. *Bacteroides fragilis* ventriculitis and meningitis. Report of two cases. *Am J Dis Child* 1976;130(8):880–883.
267. Soriano F, Aguado JM, Tornero J, et al. *Bacteroides fragilis* meningitis successfully treated with metronidazole after a previous failure with thiamphenicol. *J Clin Microbiol* 1986;24(3):472–473.
268. Bergan T, Thorsteinsson SB. Pharmacokinetics of metronidazole and its metabolites in reduced renal function. *Chemotherapy* 1986;32(4):305–318.
269. Kreeft JH, Ogilvie RI, Dufresne LR. Metronidazole kinetics in dialysis patients. *Surgery* 1983;93(1, Pt 2):149–153.
270. Cassey JG, Clark DA, Merrick P, et al. Pharmacokinetics of metronidazole in patients undergoing peritoneal dialysis. *Antimicrob Agents Chemother* 1983;24(6):950–951.
271. Lau AH, Chang CW, Sabatini S. Hemodialysis clearance of metronidazole and its metabolites. *Antimicrob Agents Chemother* 1986;29(2):235–238.
272. Guay DR, Meatherall RC, Baxter H, et al. Pharmacokinetics of metronidazole in patients undergoing continuous ambulatory peritoneal dialysis. *Antimicrob Agents Chemother* 1984;25(3):306–310.
273. Muscara MN, Pedrazzoli J Jr, Miranda EL, et al. Plasma hydroxy-metronidazole/metronidazole ratio in patients with liver disease and in healthy volunteers. *Br J Clin Pharmacol* 1995;40(5):477–480.
274. Lares-Asseff I, Cravioto J, Santiago P, et al. Pharmacokinetics of metronidazole in severely malnourished and nutritionally rehabilitated children. *Clin Pharmacol Ther* 1992;51(1):42–50.
275. Johnson JK, Laughon MM. Antimicrobial agent dosing in infants. *Clin Ther* 2016;38(9):1948–1960.
276. American Academy of Pediatrics. Antimicrobial agents and related therapy. In: Kimberlin D, Brady M, Long S, eds. *Red Book: 2018-2021 Report of the Committee of Infectious Diseases*, 31st ed. Itasca, IL: American Academy of Pediatrics, 2018:915–932.
277. Urtasun RC, Rabin HR, Partington J. Human pharmacokinetics and toxicity of high-dose metronidazole administered orally and intravenously. *Surgery* 1983;93(1, Pt 2):145–148.
278. Smith JA. Neutropenia associated with metronidazole therapy. *Can Med Assoc J* 1980;123(3):202.
279. Sorensen CG, Karlsson WK, Amin FM, et al. Metronidazole-induced encephalopathy: a systematic review. *J Neurol* 2020; 267: 1–13.
280. Kancherla D, Gajendran M, Vallabhaneni P, et al. Metronidazole induced liver injury: a rare immune mediated drug reaction. *Case Rep Gastrointest Med* 2013;2013:568193.
281. Celifarco A, Warschauer C, Burakoff R. Metronidazole-induced pancreatitis. *Am J Gastroenterol* 1989;84(8):958–960.
282. Goolsby TA, Jakeman B, Gaynes RP. Clinical relevance of metronidazole and peripheral neuropathy: a systematic review of the literature. *Int J Antimicrob Agents* 2018;51(3):319–325.
283. Kafadar I, Moustafa F, Yalcin K, et al. A rare adverse effect of metronidazole: nervous system symptoms. *Pediatr Emerg Care* 2013;29(6):751–752.
284. Lefkowitz A, Shadowitz S. Reversible cerebellar neurotoxicity induced by metronidazole. *CMAJ* 2018;190(32):E961.
285. Wilson BT, Strong A, O'Kelly S, et al. Metronidazole toxicity in Cockayne syndrome: a case series. *Pediatrics* 2015;136(3):e706–e708.
286. Cohen O, Saar N, Swartzon M, et al. First report of metronidazole-induced QT interval prolongation. *Int J Antimicrob Agents* 2008;31(2):180–181.
287. Knowles S, Choudhury T, Shear NH. Metronidazole hypersensitivity. *Ann Pharmacother* 1994;28(3):325–326.
288. Falagas ME, Walker AM, Jick H, et al. Late incidence of cancer after metronidazole use: a matched metronidazole user/nonuser study. *Clin Infect Dis* 1998;26(2):384–388.
289. Cina SJ, Russell RA, Conradi SE. Sudden death due to metronidazole/ethanol interaction. *Am J Forensic Med Pathol* 1996;17(4):343–346.
290. Karamanakos PN, Pappas P, Boumba VA, et al. Pharmaceutical agents known to produce disulfiram-like reaction: effects on hepatic ethanol metabolism and brain monoamines. *Int J Toxicol* 2007;26(5):423–432.
291. Lynch T, Price A. The effect of cytochrome P450 metabolism on drug response, interactions, and adverse effects. *Am Fam Phys* 2007;76(3):391–396.
292. Kudo T, Endo Y, Taguchi R, et al. Metronidazole reduces the expression of cytochrome P450 enzymes in HepaRG cells and cryopreserved human hepatocytes. *Xenobiotica* 2015;45(5):413–419.
293. Blyden GT, Scavone JM, Greenblatt DJ. Metronidazole impairs clearance of phenytoin but not of alprazolam or lorazepam. *J Clin Pharmacol* 1988;28(3):240–245.
294. Patterson BD. Possible interaction between metronidazole and carbamazepine. *Ann Pharmacother* 1994;28(11):1303–1304.
295. Kounas SP, Letsas KP, Sideris A, et al. QT interval prolongation and torsades de pointes due to a coadministration of metronidazole and amiodarone. *Pacing Clin Electrophysiol* 2005;28(5):472–473.
296. Teicher MH, Altesman RI, Cole JO, et al. Possible nephrotoxic interaction of lithium and metronidazole. *JAMA* 1987;257(24):3365–3366.
297. Jessa MJ, Goddard AF, Barrett DA, et al. The effect of omeprazole on the pharmacokinetics of metronidazole and hydroxymetronidazole in human plasma, saliva and gastric juice. *Br J Clin Pharmacol* 1997;44(3):245–253.
298. Eradiri O, Jamali F, Thomson AB. Interaction of metronidazole with phenobarbital, cimetidine, prednisone, and sulfasalazine in Crohn's disease. *Biopharm Drug Dispos* 1988;9(2):219–227.
299. Miljkovic V, Arsic B, Bojanic Z, et al. Interactions of metronidazole with other medicines: a brief review. *Pharmazie* 2014;69(8):571–577.

CHAPTER

27

Elizabeth A. Ashley
Sir Nicholas J. White

Antimalarials

The majority of the almost half a million deaths from malaria that occur each year are in children.[1] Most of these deaths are the result of severe falciparum malaria and take place in sub-Saharan Africa. The other common human malarias are caused by *Plasmodium vivax*, *Plasmodium ovale* (*curtisi* and *wallikeri*), *Plasmodium malariae*, and *Plasmodium knowlesi*, which are usually not associated with a fatal outcome. *P. vivax* is a major cause of malaria in Asia, the Americas, and the Horn of Africa. Although severe malaria and death following an acute episode of vivax malaria are infrequent, recurrent episodes may lead to significant morbidity from severe anemia, particularly in the very young.[2] In 2018, there were an estimated 228 million cases of malaria worldwide and 405,000 deaths.[1] Frequent malaria results in an imperfect immunity, so the burden of disease and death in malaria-endemic areas falls on young children. Progress in controlling malaria has stalled in the last 5 years and worsening antimalarial and insecticide resistance threaten to derail ambitions of eradicating malaria from the world.

There are three main clinical presentations of malaria in children: congenital malaria (malaria acquired from the mother at birth), uncomplicated malaria, and severe malaria. Congenital and severe malaria are treated initially with parenteral antimalarial drugs (artesunate, artemether, or quinine) and uncomplicated disease with oral drugs. The artemisinin-based combination therapies (ACTs) have been recommended as first-line treatment of falciparum malaria everywhere in the world since the mid-2000s.[3] This strategy was employed first in Southeast Asia in the early 1990s to combat the sequential loss of antimalarial monotherapies to resistance (i.e., chloroquine, sulfadoxine–pyrimethamine [SP], mefloquine). The ACTs were highly effective and well tolerated, but in 2009 the first confirmed reports of artemisinin resistance emerged from Cambodia.[4] This soon led to increasing ACT failure rates. The situation in Southeast Asia is evolving rapidly as artemisinin and piperaquine resistance sweeps across the region (Table 27.1).

Artesunate–mefloquine was redeployed in Cambodia as mefloquine susceptibility had returned. The window to eliminate drug-resistant malaria in the region is closing.

Prevention of malaria in children relies on insecticide-treated bed nets and, in the sub-Sahel region, the use of seasonal malaria chemoprevention. In 2015, after years of research, the RTS,S/AS01 malaria vaccine received a positive scientific opinion from the European Medicines Agency. Protective efficacy is partial and short-lived. The strategy for future deployment of the vaccine is undecided while further large-scale pilot studies are conducted.

Although children are most at risk from dying from malaria, they are typically not well represented in clinical drug development studies.[5] This has led to the belated discovery that dosing recommendations for several antimalarial drugs in children were suboptimal.[6] The pooling of individual patient data from antimalarial drug efficacy and pharmacokinetic (PK) studies and the conduct of meta-analyses have led to revised dosing guidelines in children for two important antimalarials from different drug classes: parenteral artesunate (for severe malaria) and dihydroartemisinin–piperaquine (for uncomplicated malaria).

Pediatric dosing guidelines for amodiaquine, SP, and artemether–lumefantrine may also need revising.[7–10] Most of the PK–PD (pharmacodynamic) data in children have been generated in field trials using a population PK approach with drug assays adapted and validated for small blood volumes.[11] The PD properties of the antimalarials are relatively straightforward to assess because parasite clearance from the circulation can be documented easily by microscopy examination of stained blood smears, but there are two caveats:

1. In falciparum malaria, parasitized erythrocytes are sequestered in the microcirculation, so peripheral parasite densities do not reflect total parasite biomass (of particular relevance to severe malaria).
2. The microscopy level of detection for malaria parasitemia is approximately 50,000 per mL (corresponding to ~10^8 in the body of an adult), so a negative blood smear does not mean all of the parasites have been killed or removed from the blood and recrudescence may still occur.

In severe malaria, it is essential that therapeutic drug concentrations are reached quickly to maximize parasite killing and prevent a fatal outcome. Drug classes with a broader stage specificity of action, such as the artemisinin derivatives, which kill the younger ring trophozoites as well as more mature parasites, reduce parasite densities more rapidly than the other classes in use.

The approach to selecting the optimum dose for new antimalarials is changing. Controlled human malaria infection (CHMI) models enable more accurate early prediction of the PK–PD of new drugs.[12,13] The CHMI approach is not perfect because volunteers are not symptomatic of the disease, thus the impact of the disease state on oral bioavailability and splenic function may be underestimated. Malaria alters the PK properties of most antimalarial drugs. It has been proposed that the

TABLE 27.1 Molecular Markers Associated with Antimalarial Drug Resistance in *Plasmodium falciparum*

Antimalarial	*Resistance Marker*	*Notes*	*Geographical Distribution*
Amodiaquine	*pfcrt pfmdr1*	SVMNT haplotype including K76T N86Y	East Africa, Southeast Asia
Artemisinin	*kelch13*	Single mutations: F446I, P553L, N458Y, R561H, M476I, Y493H, R539T, I543T C580Y dominates in areas of high-level resistance	Southeast Asia
Atovaquone	*CytB*	Y268S/C/N	Deployment of atovaquone–proguanil in Cambodia in 2014 was followed by rapid emergence of atovaquone resistance
Chloroquine	*pfcrt pfmdr1*	"CVIET" haplotype including K76T N86Y (augments resistance)	Worldwide
Lumefantrine	*pfmdr1*	Gene amplification (associated with low-grade resistance in Southeast Asia). Selection of pfmdr1 86N allele after treatment observed in Africa	High failure rates of artemether–lumefantrine documented in Cambodia (2000–2005). Not reevaluated since
Mefloquine	*pfmdr1*	Gene amplification	Thailand, Myanmar although susceptibility may return after discontinuation (cf. Cambodia)
Piperaquine	*plasmepsin2*	Gene amplification	Cambodia, Thailand, Laos, Vietnam
Pyrimethamine	*dhfr pfgch1*	N51I, C59R, S108N, I164L compensatory GTP-cyclohydrolase amplification	Worldwide
Sulfadoxine	*Dhps*	S436A/F, A437G, K540E, A581G, A613S/T	Worldwide

in vivo minimum inhibitory concentration (MIC) of new antimalarials should be estimated to determine the optimal dose, by studying the drug effects in malaria patients and tracking parasite densities below the microscopy level of detection using ultrasensitive PCR-based methods (Fig. 27.1).[6,14] In children, age-based dosing is more convenient than weight-based or surface area–based dosing, and a reference database of age and weight data for children from low- and middle-income countries has been compiled and used to create both age and weight dosing bands for some antimalarials.[15]

The majority of antimalarials in use are well tolerated and safe. Safety concerns have emerged after registration for some of the drugs, for example, fatal tachycardias following halofantrine ultimately leading to its withdrawal, and agranulocytosis following amodiaquine,[16,17] hepatotoxicity and severe skin reactions following SP when these drugs were used as chemoprophylaxis in travelers in the 1980s, and more recently post artesunate delayed hemolysis in returned travelers with high parasite densities.[18]

In this chapter, we summarize the PK and PD of the antimalarial drugs in children organized by indication for use, with an emphasis on clinically relevant findings.

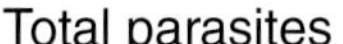

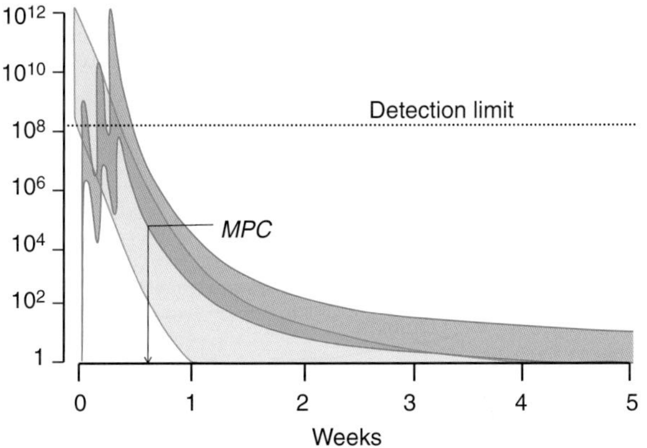

Figure 27.1 Population PK–PD responses following a 3-day antimalarial treatment with a slowly eliminated drug. The light blue shading represents the total parasite biomass in a range of hypothetical patients with pretreatment parasite densities of 50 to 200,000 per μL with the detection level by microscopy shown as a dotted line. The dark blue shaded area represents a range of drug concentration profiles. The minimum parasiticidal concentration (MPC) is the lowest drug concentration (free, or in blood or plasma) producing the maximum parasiticidal effect.

DRUGS USED IN THE TREATMENT OF MALARIA

Evidence-based treatment guidelines for malaria are produced and updated regularly by the World Health Organization (WHO).[19] The choice of drug depends on the infecting malaria species, clinical presentation, and the latest information on drug susceptibility from the area where malaria was acquired (Table 27.2).

TREATMENT OF SEVERE OR CONGENITAL MALARIA

Initial treatment of severe or congenital malaria is with parenteral drugs. The treatment of choice is intravenous artesunate because this has been shown unequivocally to reduce mortality substantially (Fig. 27.2); however, unfortunately, several countries are still reliant on less effective medicines such as intramuscular (IM) artemether and parenteral quinine. The significantly more toxic quinidine was recommended for the treatment of severe malaria in the United States until 2019 when manufacturing was discontinued and it was finally replaced with artesunate, despite lack of U.S. Food and Drug Administration (FDA) approval.

TABLE 27.2 Drugs Used in the Treatment of Malaria in Children

Treatment	*Notes*
SEVERE OR CONGENITAL MALARIA	
Initial Treatment	
Intravenous artesunate Children with body weight <25 kg: 3.0 mg/kg h 0, 12, and 24; then 24-hourly Children with body weight ≥25 kg: dose is 2.4 mg/kg	Artesunate may be given by intramuscular injection Post artesunate delayed hemolytic anemia has been described in nonimmune returned travelers
Alternatives	
Intramuscular artemether injection: 3.2 mg/kg initial dose, then 1.6 mg/kg at 24 hour intervals	Artemether absorption may be slow and erratic in shocked patients
OR	
Intravenous quinine infusion; loading dose of 20 mg quinine dihydrochloride salt/kg (given over 4 h) then 10 mg/kg (given over 2 h) every 8 h. Reduce dose by one-third in severe malaria after 48 h if no clinical improvement	Bolus intravenous injections of quinine are associated with lethal hypotension GTP-cyclohydrolase and should never be given
ONCE ABLE TO EAT AND DRINK	
Oral treatment with an ACT for 3 d	Avoid mefloquine as follow-on treatment owing to increased risk of post-malaria neurological syndrome
UNCOMPLICATED MALARIA	
Uncomplicated Plasmodium falciparum or Plasmodium knowlesi malaria	
Artemether–lumefantrine 1.4–4 mg/kg of artemether and 10–16 mg/kg of lumefantrine twice daily for 3 d	Artemether–lumefantrine should be given with food containing fat to increase absorption
OR	
Dihydroartemisinin–piperaquine 4 mg/kg of dihydroartemisinin and 18 mg/kg of piperaquine once daily for 3 d (children with body weight <25 kg should receive at least 2.5 mg/kg/d of dihydroartemisinin and 20 mg/kg/d piperaquine)	
OR	
Artesunate 4 mg/kg/d with mefloquine 8 mg/kg/d for 3 d	
OR	
Artesunate 4 mg/kg/d with amodiaquine 10 mg base/kg/d for 3 d	
OR	
Artesunate 4 mg/kg/d for 3 d with single-dose sulfadoxine–pyrimethamine (25 mg/kg–1.25 mg/kg)	
Chloroquine-sensitive Plasmodium vivax, Plasmodium ovale, Plasmodium malariae	
Chloroquine 10 mg base/kg at hour 0 and hour 24 followed by 5 mg base/kg at hour 48 or 10mg base/kg initial dose followed by 5mg base/kg at 12, 24, and 36 hours.	If chloroquine resistance is suspected treat with an ACT, or quinine plus either clindamycin or doxycycline (children >8 y)

Notes: Always seek up-to-date information on antimalarial drug susceptibility in the area malaria was acquired before selecting which ACT to use. ACT, artemisinin-based combination therapy.

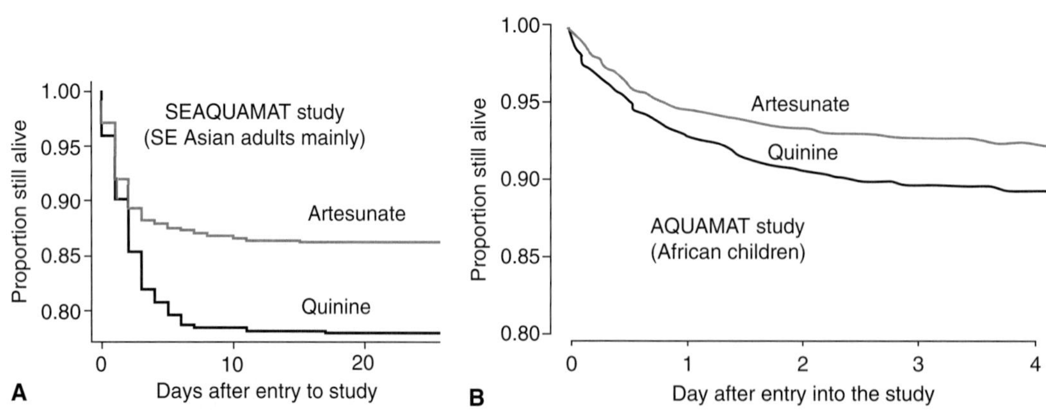

Figure 27.2 Survival of children and adults with severe malaria treated with parenteral artesunate compared to quinine. Two very large trials (SEAQUAMAT [**A**] and AQUAMAT [**B**]) unequivocally demonstrated improved survival from severe malaria following artesunate treatment compared to quinine. The mortality reduction in African children was lower (22.5%; 95% confidence interval [CI], 8.1–36.9; $p = 0.0022$) than in the Southeast Asian study conducted mainly in adults (absolute reduction, 34.7%; 95% CI, 18.5%–47.6%; $p = 0.0002$). Plausible explanations for this observation are (i) incidental parasitemia in some of the children in the AQUAMAT study with an alternative diagnosis (likely sepsis) causing their symptoms and (ii) more children presenting with severe malarial anemia rather than cerebral malaria.

ARTEMISININ AND ITS DERIVATIVES

Artemisinin (qinghaosu) is a sesquiterpene lactone endoperoxide[20] extracted from the sweet wormwood plant, *Artemisia annua* L. The first description of its use as a febrifuge was recorded in China by Ge Hong in the *Handbook of Emergency Prescriptions* between 317 and 400 AD.[21] The mechanism of action of the artemisinin derivatives dihydroartemisinin, artesunate, and artemether is unclear, but a key step is thought to be oxidant damage from the peroxide moiety. Artesunate is a hemisuccinate derivative of artemisinin. Artesunate for parenteral use is an unstable compound and it is supplied currently as a freeze-dried powder that needs to be reconstituted by mixing with sodium bicarbonate before intravenous (bolus) or IM injection (a formulation that avoids this step is under development). Artesunate is effectively a prodrug, as following intravenous injection it is hydrolyzed rapidly to dihydroartemisinin. Following IM injection, peak plasma concentrations are reached within 30 minutes. Time above the MIC is thought to be the principal determinant of cure for most antimalarials. Given the short half-life of the artemisinin derivatives, it was once postulated that increasing the dose frequency should increase the parasiticidal effect but this has not been observed in practice and, in studies, increasing the dose frequency of artesunate does not improve efficacy.[22] Artesunate is given once daily, but for patients with severe malaria, an interval parenteral dose (at 12 hours) is recommended on the first day of treatment. This is likely to benefit those few patients with a highly synchronous infection in which mature schizonts are the predominant parasite stage at the time of the initial dose.

A rectal formulation of artesunate has been developed for use as a prereferral treatment for children with severe malaria in remote areas. Peak concentrations are reached after approximately 3 hours (Table 27.3).[23]

Plasma concentrations after an oral dose of artesunate are very variable. Peak mean time to peak plasma bioactivity was 1.7 hours (95% confidence interval [95% CI], 0.8–2.6) in Vietnamese children with moderately severe falciparum malaria.[24] In adult malaria patients, 2 mg per kg was the average lower limit of the maximally effective dose.[22,25]

Artemether is a methyl ethyl derivative of dihydroartemisinin and a less effective alternative treatment for severe malaria, administered as an oil-based IM injection. PK studies in Vietnamese adults and Kenyan children with severe malaria showed slow and unpredictable absorption in some patients.[26,27] Time to peak concentration is typically less than 2 hours but was as long as 8 hours in children with cerebral malaria in one study.[28] A crossover study in healthy adults showed similarly erratic absorption of rectal artemether, with mean (95% CI) rectal bioavailability in the 6 hours following administration (0 to 6 hours) of 35% (10% to 60%) compared to the drug given orally.[29] Oral artemether is well absorbed, reaching peak concentrations in 1 hour.[30] Bioavailability is increased by coadministration with grapefruit juice (which inhibits intestinal CYP3A4).[31] A sublingual spray formulation of artemether has also been developed and evaluated in African children, with early evidence suggesting it is well absorbed.[32]

Distribution

In a PK study of 70 children with severe malaria treated with IM artesunate (2.4 mg per kg), clearance and apparent volume of distribution were affected by body weight, resulting in lower artesunate and DHA exposures in younger children.[33] This has led to a higher dose (3 mg per kg) being recommended for children weighing less than 25 kg.[34] Following intravenous artesunate, CSF concentrations of DHA are less than 10% of that in plasma in severe malaria.[35]

Metabolism and Elimination

The artemisinin derivatives are eliminated rapidly. Both artesunate and artemether are converted rapidly to DHA in vivo. Plasma esterases hydrolyze artesunate and metabolic conversion is mediated by CYP2A6 (predominant enzyme for artesunate) or CYP3A4 (artemether). DHA is converted to inactive glucuronide conjugates by phase II UDP-glucuronosyltransferases.[36] There is substantial variation in the reported values of the PK parameters of the artemisinin derivatives in the literature.[37] Estimates of elimination of half-life of DHA are generally between 0.75 and 3 hours. Following an IM dose, clearance of artemether is reduced and elimination is reportedly slower in patients with acute renal failure.[38]

QUININE

The first description of the use of the cinchona bark to treat fever and agues by the Spanish in Peru dates back to 1630.[39] After 1800, quinine was purified and found to be the predominant of the four alkaloids extracted from the cinchona bark. Eventually a quinine dose of 10 mg (salt) per kg body weight three times daily was adopted; however, it was shown that not all patients with severe falciparum malaria achieved adequate serum concentrations above the MIC during the first 8 hours of treatment. With the objective of achieving therapeutic concentrations in patients with severe malaria as quickly as possible, a loading dose of 20 mg per kg body weight has been advocated since the early 1980s.[40,41] Like the other arylamino alcohol drugs, quinine acts by inhibiting heme detoxification. The dose–response relationship between quinine and parasite clearance and clinical recovery has been characterized in several studies, although there has never been a trial large enough to show an impact of dose on mortality outcomes.[42] Dangerous hypotension can occur if quinine is infused too quickly. IM injection is a practical alternative to IV administration, although there have been occasional reports of suboptimal plasma concentrations in children with severe malaria.[43,44] The widely used dihydrochloride salt is acidic (pH 2) and painful when injected intramuscularly, so the initial loading dose in severe malaria (20 mg per kg salt) is split in half. Complications of sterile abscesses, muscle necrosis, tetanus, and sciatic nerve injury have been reported,[45,46] and the anterior thigh has become the preferred site for injection. IM injectate concentrations of 60 to 100 mg per mL are preferable to higher concentrations. Buffered formulations are less painful. In the late 1990s and early 2000s, a rectal formulation of quinine (20 mg per kg 8 to 12 hourly) was evaluated in children with malaria in a series of small studies in Madagascar and Niger. Clinical outcomes were similar, but bioavailability was 40% to 60% relative to IM or intravenous injection.[47–49]

Quinine is well absorbed orally (bioavailability ~89% in healthy volunteers),[50] reaching peak concentrations at around 4 hours.[51,52]

Distribution

Quinine is highly (>90%) bound to plasma proteins (mainly to α-1-acid glycoprotein) with increased binding in proportion to disease severity. Quinine has a large apparent volume of distribution, but this contracts with increasing disease severity. Systemic

TABLE 27.3 Summary of Pharmacokinetic Properties of Antimalarials in Pediatric Studies

Antimalarial Drug	*Route*	*Unit dose (total dose)*	*Malaria Disease Severity*	T_{max}	C_{max}	*AUC*	*CL/F*	*V/F*	*Elimination HL*
Artemether[30,31]	IM	3.2 mg/kg then 1.6 mg/kg/d	Severe	1–3 h	33–41 ng/mL	194–490 ng·h/L (0–12 h)	14 L/h	382 L	19 h[a]
Artemisinin[67,68]	PO	3–20 mg/kg/d (100 mg/kg)	Uncomp.	—	—	1,652 µg·h/L	1.8–14 L/kg/h	8.4–38 L/kg	2–7 h
Artesunate (converted rapidly in vivo to DHA)[24,26,154,155]	PO	4 mg/kg (12 mg/kg)	Moderate	2 h	664 ng/mL	1,286 ng·h/mL	—	—	1 h
	IM	2.4–3.0 mg/kg	Severe	7 min (AS) 35 min (DHA)	943 ng/mL (AS) 547 ng/mL (DHA)	570 ng·h/mL (0–12 h) (AS) 890 ng·h/mL (0–12 h) (DHA)	3–4 L/h/kg (AS) 2 L/kg/h (DHA)	3 L/kg (AS) 1 L/kg (DHA)	25–42 min (AS) 26 min (DHA)
	IV	2.4–3.0 mg/kg	Severe	1 h (DHA)	—	—	3 L/kg/h	—	3 min
	PR	1.8–19 mg/kg	Uncomp.	1–2 h	242–973 ng/mL	1,153 ng·h/mL	—	—	—
	PR	9–20 mg/kg	Moderate to Severe	1–2 h	923–1,495 ng/mL	3,844–4,997 ng·h/mL	—	—	—
Amodiaquine[90,156–158]	PO	~10 mg AQ base/kg/d ± artesunate (30 mg/kg)	Uncomp.	47–48 h	—	39 ng·h/mL	—	—	3 h
Desethylamodiaqui ne (principal metabolite of amodiaquine)					537 ng/mL to 1,185 ng/mL	40,339–55,000 ng·h/mL	0.6 L/kg/h	35 L/kg	3–9 d
Atovaquone[119]	PO	17 mg/kg with proguanil (51 mg/kg)	Uncomp.	6 h	3 µg/mL	162 mg·h/mL	162 mL/h/kg	8 L/kg	32 h
Chloroquine[101,159]	PO	~10 mg/kg/dose (25 mg base/kg)	Uncomp.	7 h	1 µg/mL	39 or 78 µg·h/mL (0-336h)	1 L/kg/h	32–154 L/kg	108–233 h
Lumefantrine[79,160,161]	PO	8–12 mg/kg with artemether (48–72 mg/kg)	Uncomp.	—	5–9 µg/mL	441–460 µg·h/mL	77–100 mL/h/kg	3–9 L/kg	3–6 d
Mefloquine[73,162]	PO	8–15 mg/kg base (25 mg/kg)	Uncomp.	—	1,377–2,031 ng/mL	906–1,194 ng·h/mL	0.5–1 mL/min/kg	18–19 L/kg	12–14 d
Piperaquine[10,94,97,163]	PO	20 mg/kg base with DHA (60 mg/kg)	Uncomp.	3–4 h	146–730 ng/mL	42–71 µg·h/L	2 L/h/kg	614 L/kg	13–31 d
Primaquine[135]	PO	0.25–0.5 mg/kg radical cure (3.5–7 mg/kg)	Uncomp.	2 h	50–89 ng/mL	450–731 ng·h/mL	—	2 L/kg	3.5–8 h
Proguanil[119,120]	PO	7 mg/kg (21 mg/kg)	Uncomp.	—	244 ng/mL	4,646 ng·h/mL	1,600 mL/h/kg to 2.82 L/h	33–36 L/kg	12–15 h
Pyrimethamine[104,105]	PO	1.25 mg/kg with sulfadoxine	Uncomp.	4 h	193–342 ng/mL	25,248–72,254 ng·h/mL	22–42 mL/kg/h	4 L/kg	3–5 d
Pyronaridine[115,117]	PO	6–12 mg/kg	Uncomp.	3 h	88–339 mg/mL	17,623–35,360 ng·h/mL	—	—	12.3 d
Quinine[42–44,62,164–166]	PO	8.3 mg base/kg tds	Uncomp.	—	—	—	0.5 L/h/kg	57 L/kg	9 h
	IM	16.7 mg base (equivalent to 20 mg dihydrochloride salt)/kg followed by 8.3 mg/kg 8 hourly	Uncomp.	1 h	9 µg/mL	297 µg·h/mL	—	—	—
	IM		Severe	1–2 h	13–16 mg/L	332–358 mg·h/L	1 mL/min/kg	1 L/kg	12–19 h
	IV		Severe	2–3 h	10–17 mg/L	145–354 mg·h/L	0.5–1 mL/min/kg	0.5–1 L/kg	9–16 h
Sulfadoxine[104,105]	PO	25 mg/kg with pyrimethamine	Uncomp.	8 h	58–218 µg/mL	19–20,756 µg·h/mL	1–24 mL/kg/h	274–372 mL/kg	5–9 d

Notes: Data shown are ranges of summary statistics (lowest and highest) reported from studies in children with malaria. Units were harmonized for comparability with other studies where possible. *AUC* is zero to infinity unless otherwise stated.

[a]The elimination of IM artemether and artemotil is determined by their (slow) absorption.

AUC, area under the concentration–time curve; *CL/F*, apparent clearance; C_{max}, peak concentration; HL, half-life; IM, intramuscular; IV, intravenous; NG, nasogastric; PO, per os (oral); PR, per rectum (rectal); T_{max}, time to peak concentration; Uncomp., uncomplicated; *V/F*, apparent volume of distribution. CSF, cerebrospinal fluid; CNS, central nervous system; DHA, dihydroartemisinin; ECG, electrocardiogram; HIV, human immunodeficiency virus; TB, tuberculosis.

clearance of quinine is also reduced in malaria.[53] Protein binding was observed to be higher in patients with cerebral malaria compared to uncomplicated disease. The ratio of cerebrospinal fluid to free (unbound) plasma quinine was 0.55 ± 0.33.[54]

Metabolism and Elimination

Quinine undergoes hepatic biotransformation to 3-hydroxyquinine and dihydroquinine. Unchanged drug is excreted via the kidney (20% of total clearance). Metabolism to the biologically active 3-hydroxyquinine increases with recovery from acute malaria.[55] Plasma concentrations of 3-hydroxyquinine increase in renal failure, which is common in adults but rare in children with severe malaria.[56] Elimination half-life in children with malaria is between 9 and 18 hours,[41,43,52,57] depending on disease severity. If severe malaria does not respond rapidly to treatment (i.e., the patient remains unconscious or renal function continues to deteriorate), the dose should be reduced after at least 2 full days of treatment (i.e. to 12 hourly rather than 8 hourly).

Drug–Drug Interactions

Rifampicin increases metabolic clearance of quinine with an associated reduction in efficacy (Table 27.4).[58]

Adverse Drug Reactions and Special Groups of Patients

Quinine stimulates pancreatic β-cell secretion and may cause hyperinsulinemic hypoglycemia.[59,60] In a very large trial comparing artesunate to quinine for the treatment of severe malaria in more than 5,000 African children, hypoglycemia was more common in the quinine-treated group (2.8% vs. 1.8%; $p = 0.013$).[61] Quinine also delays ventricular depolarization (ECG QRS widening) slightly and prolongs repolarization (QT lengthening), although there is no evidence that it is proarrhythmic.[62,63]

In malnourished children, quinine exposure is higher, clearance is reduced, and elimination is prolonged.[64,65]

In severe malaria, once the patient is stable, has received at least three doses of parenteral therapy, and can swallow reliably, then treatment is completed with one of the oral regimens used for treating uncomplicated malaria (see below). None of the treatments is licensed for use in infants weighing less than 4.5 kg; however, the WHO recommends they still be given, targeting the same mg per kg dose.

TREATMENT OF UNCOMPLICATED FALCIPARUM MALARIA

ACTs recommended for the treatment of uncomplicated falciparum malaria combine the highly potent, short-acting artemisinin or one of its derivatives (artesunate, dihydroartemisinin, or artemether) with a longer acting partner drug with a different mechanism of action. ACTs are also the treatment of choice for uncomplicated malaria caused by *P. knowlesi* because of the propensity for high parasite densities and severe malaria to develop, and they are used increasingly to treat vivax malaria. The ACTs in current use are artemether–lumefantrine, dihydroartemisinin–piperaquine, artesunate–mefloquine, artesunate–amodiaquine, and artesunate–SP. Artesunate–pyronaridine has been registered recently. Most are developed as fixed-dose combinations and typical course length is 3 days. Newer ACTs that have not been deployed on a large scale are artemisinin–naphthoquine and artemisinin–piperaquine. In endemic countries, a single low (0.25 mg per kg) dose of primaquine is given with the ACT

TABLE 27.4 Important Drug–Drug Interactions with Antimalarials

Antimalarial	*Other Drug(s)*	*Description of Interaction*
Amodiaquine	Efavirenz	Hepatotoxicity[167]
	Zidovudine	Neutropenia
Artemether–lumefantrine	Rifampicin	Decreases lumefantrine (and artemether) exposure (CYP3A4 induction)
	Efavirenz	Reduces artemether and dihydroartemisinin exposure[168–170]
	Nevirapine	Reduces artemether and dihydroartemisinin exposure[168–170] Conflicting results for changes in lumefantrine exposure when coadministered with nevirapine have been reported[168,171]
	Lopinavir–ritonavir	Increases lumefantrine exposure[172,173]
	Darunavir–ritonavir	Increases lumefantrine exposure[172,173]
	Etravirine	Reduces artemether, DHA, and lumefantrine exposure[173]
	Mefloquine	Coadministration with mefloquine has been shown to result in lower lumefantrine concentrations[174]
Atovaquone–proguanil	Efavirenz	Atovaquone exposure is reduced[175]
	Lopinavir/ritonavir	
	Atazanavir/ritonavir	
Dihydroartemisinin–piperaquine	Efavirenz	Decreased piperaquine exposure
Primaquine	Chloroquine, DHA–piperaquine, Artesunate–pyronaridine	Coadministration increases primaquine exposure[118,131,176]
Quinine	Rifampicin	Increases metabolic clearance of quinine
Sulfadoxine–pyrimethamine	Other antifols, e.g., trimethoprim	Increased risk of toxicity

course for *Plasmodium falciparum* malaria because it rapidly sterilizes stage V gametocytes, which reduces transmissibility of the treated infection.

ORAL ARTEMISININ AND ITS DERIVATIVES

The WHO called for a ban on monotherapies of the oral artemisinin derivatives (artesunate, artemether, dihydroartemisinin) in 2007 as a measure to reduce the risk of resistance emerging, but these drugs are still sometimes available in the private sector, driven by consumer demand.[66] There is typically a high degree of interindividual variation in the oral absorption of artemisinin and its derivatives. The PK properties of oral artemether and artesunate are described above. Artemisinin is well absorbed orally, with peak concentrations reached in 2 to 3 hours and a reduction in bioavailability observed on repeated dosing because it induces its own metabolism.[67,68] Unlike its derivatives, artemisinin is not metabolized to DHA. It is also eliminated rapidly ($t_{1/2}$ ~2 hours).

ARYLAMINO ALCOHOL PARTNER DRUGS

Mefloquine

Mefloquine, a fluorinated 4-quinoline methanol compound, is only available as an oral formulation, either alone or coformulated with artesunate. It is manufactured as a racemic mixture of the (*R,S*)- and (*S,R*)-enantiomers. The PK of mefloquine has been studied after different dosing regimens and either alone or coadministered with SP or artesunate. Bioavailability in patients with malaria is improved by splitting the dose and giving it over 2 or preferably 3 days.[69,70] This has the added advantage of reducing the frequency of early vomiting in young children. Peak concentrations in pediatric studies were reached in 7 to 13 hours (see Table 27.3). The PK of mefloquine is stereoselective with higher maximum plasma concentrations and exposure and longer elimination of the (−) enantiomer and a larger apparent volume of distribution and increased clearance of the (+) enantiomer.[71]

Distribution

Mefloquine is extensively (>95%) protein bound.[72] Clearance is faster in children than in adults.[73]

Metabolism and Elimination

Mefloquine is metabolized mainly to 2,8-bis-trifluoromethyl-4-quinoline carboxylic acid, which is mainly excreted in the bile and thus feces. The drug is eliminated slowly with a half-life of approximately 10 days in children with malaria, making it a good candidate for chemoprophylaxis (see later).[74]

Adverse Drug Reactions and Contraindications

Mefloquine may cause nausea and sometimes vomiting and dysphoria. The main adverse effect is neuropsychiatric toxicity (nightmares and, rarely, seizures or psychosis), for which there is some evidence for dose dependence, although this is uncommon in children.[75] Repeated treatment within 2 months of administration is not recommended. Mefloquine is a risk factor for the development of postmalaria neurological syndrome and so should not be given as follow-on treatment for severe malaria.[76]

Lumefantrine

Lumefantrine (formerly benflumetol) is a racemic 2,4,7,9-substituted fluorene derivative coformulated with artemether and also under evaluation in combination with a newer imidazolopiperazine antimalarial (KAF156 or ganaplacide) in phase 2 development. The new formulation has substantially improved oral bioavailability. Absorption of lumefantrine from the current artemether–lumefantrine formulations is highly variable and dose limited, necessitating twice-daily dosing. Absorption is enhanced by coadministration with a small amount of fat (~1.2 g) and by recovery from the acute symptoms of malaria.[77–79] There is a delay of approximately 2 hours between drug administration and absorption, which takes 18 hours to complete.[80] Lumefantrine exposure correlates with treatment response, and a day 7 plasma or blood concentration of 200 ng per mL or more the initial dose of is associated with greater than 98% cure rates in drug-sensitive infections (if parasite density is <135,000 per µL).[80,81] A pooled analysis of individual patient data found that children aged 3 to 5 years receive lower median lumefantrine doses compared to older children and adults.[9] In multivariable analyses, children aged 1 to 5 years were at increased risk of recrudescence, with underweight children aged 1 to 3 years at greatest risk compared to those weighing within the normal range. Mathematical modeling to determine how the regimen could be optimized in this age group suggests that the treatment course would need to be prolonged to restore full efficacy, an unpopular move with policy-makers.[82] A pediatric dispersible formulation of artemether–lumefantrine (Coartem) is available. Its lumefantrine absorption kinetics are similar to crushed tablets. In a study of 625 children, mean (standard deviation [SD]) maximum plasma lumefantrine concentrations were 6.3 (4.6) and 7.7 (5.9) mg per L after treatment with dispersed or crushed tablets, respectively, and the corresponding areas under the concentration–time curves were 574 and 636 mg per hour per L. As of December 2018, more than 385 million treatments of a dispersible formulation of artemether-lumefantrine had been delivered to over 50 countries.[83] Total usage (all products) is estimated at over 500 million treatments annually. The new solid dispersion formulation of lumefantrine with enhanced oral bioavailability that is under development will permit once-daily dosing.[84]

Distribution

Lumefantrine is highly plasma protein bound (>99%) mainly to lipoproteins. Because of high variability in absorption, estimates of apparent volume of distribution are unreliable.[80]

Metabolism and Elimination

Lumefantrine is converted in vivo to the active metabolite desbutyl-lumefantrine, and plasma concentrations of the metabolite are correlated with treatment efficacy.[85] Metabolism is by the liver with excretion in bile and thus feces. There is no significant renal excretion in humans.[86] The terminal elimination half-life is 3 to 4 days in malaria patients.[87]

Drug–Drug Interactions

Artemether–lumefantrine interacts with rifampicin and a number of antiretroviral drugs (see Table 27.4).

QUINOLINE PARTNER DRUGS

Amodiaquine

Amodiaquine is a 4-aminoquinoline combined with artesunate in a fixed-dose combination for treatment or combined with SP for prevention during the malaria season in the Sahel (seasonal malaria chemoprevention; see later). Amodiaquine PK is relatively understudied compared to other antimalarials. The drug is well absorbed orally,[88,89] but undergoes very rapid first-pass hepatic metabolism to the biologically active metabolite desethylamodiaquine (DEAQ) mediated by cytochrome P450 (CYP2C8). Peak concentrations in whole blood or plasma occur within 2 to 3 hours.

Distribution

Both amodiaquine and its metabolite DeAQ are greater than 90% protein bound. In a population PK study of children with falciparum malaria treated with artesunate plus amodiaquine in Burkina Faso,[90] the PK properties of the coformulated product (Coarsucam) were similar to the loose drugs (see Table 27.3).

Metabolism and Elimination

DeAQ is further metabolized to an inactive compound, bis-DeAQ. The terminal elimination half-life of DeAQ was estimated as 9 days in the Burkina Faso study.[90] Pooled individual patient data from 261 patients (median age 8 years) with falciparum or vivax malaria were used to generate a population PK model for amodiaquine, published in 2018.[8] Data simulations suggested that current doses for children may be too low.

CYP2C8 polymorphisms are common in Africa and affect amodiaquine metabolism (Table 27.5). There is some evidence that patients with these polymorphisms may have more adverse events with amodiaquine, but no definite link with efficacy or serious toxicity has been established to date.[91] Coadministration with zidovudine is associated with high rates of neutropenia,[92] whereas nevirapine-containing regimens are associated with reduced amodiaquine and DeAQ exposure (see Table 27.4).[93] Efavirenz coadministered with amodiaquine has been associated with hepatotoxicity.

Piperaquine

Piperaquine is a bisquinoline given as part of a fixed-dose combination with dihydroartemisinin, artemisinin, or the newer synthetic trioxolane peroxide arterolane maleate. The most widely used piperaquine-containing combination is DHA–piperaquine. Post-registration, it became apparent that the risk of treatment failure was higher in young children, related to their larger apparent volumes of distribution and higher clearances. As a result, dosing recommendations have changed such that children weighing less than 25 kg should receive 2.5 mg per kg DHA and 20 mg per kg piperaquine daily for 3 days (Fig. 27.3).[94,95] Piperaquine is well absorbed orally in both fed and fasted states, although high-fat meals may enhance absorption.[96] Time to reach peak concentrations is around 5 hours.

Distribution

Piperaquine is highly bound to plasma proteins and has a very large apparent volume of distribution. It is cleared more rapidly in children than in adults.[97] Clearance has been shown to be influenced by body weight,[98] and children weighing less than 25 kg have lower piperaquine exposures than heavier children.

Metabolism and Elimination

A number of piperaquine metabolites have been identified.[99,100] The carboxylic acid metabolite has been well characterized and is biologically active. The elimination half-life of the parent compound in children with malaria is around 14 days.[97,101]

Drug–Drug Interactions

Efavirenz-containing antiretroviral treatment is associated with decreased piperaquine exposure.[102]

Toxicity Concerns

DHA–piperaquine administration is associated with QT prolongation (a common finding with quinoline antimalarials). This led to heightened concerns about the proarrythmogenic potential of the combination, but very large studies show no evidence for an increased risk of sudden death.[103]

SULFADOXINE–PYRIMETHAMINE

SP is a combination of two synergistic inhibitors of folate biosynthesis: sulfadoxine, an inhibitor of dihydropteroate synthase, and pyrimethamine, an inhibitor of dihydrofolate reductase. As an ACT, SP is combined with 3 days of artesunate treatment. After oral administration, sulfadoxine and pyrimethamine are well absorbed and peak concentrations are reached in approximately 8 and 4 hours, respectively.[104] In a PK study of SP treatment of patients with malaria in Mozambique and South Africa,[105] exposure to sulfadoxine and pyrimethamine was lower in children aged 2 to 5 years than in older age groups, whereas in children aged 6 to 12 years, only the *AUC* for sulfadoxine was lower. This was not observed in a study in Malawi.[104] An analysis of pooled data from four studies using a population PK nonlinear mixed-effects model suggests that SP bioavailability is lower in children who are underweight for age.[7]

A parenteral formulation of SP was manufactured but is no longer recommended.[106]

Distribution

Both sulfadoxine and pyrimethamine are extensively (~90%) protein bound. Pyrimethamine has a large volume of distribution compared to sulfadoxine (see Table 27.3). In a study of infants receiving pyrimethamine to treat congenital toxoplasmosis, CNS concentrations were approximately 10% to 25% of serum concentrations.[107]

Metabolism and Elimination

Sulfadoxine is partially metabolized to both N-acetyl sulfadoxine and sulfadoxine glucuronide. Pyrimethamine is metabolized by the liver, although the metabolites have not been well characterized. Both drugs are excreted via the kidneys. Elimination half-lives in children with malaria were estimated as 8.6 and 4.7 days for sulfadoxine in children aged 1 to less than 2 years (n = 11) and 2 to 5 years (n = 63), respectively. Corresponding numbers for pyrimethamine were 3.3 (n = 11) and 2.8 (n = 62) days.[105]

Adverse Drug Reactions

Passive surveillance data from Malawi have estimated the rate of severe skin reactions (Stevens–Johnson syndrome or toxic epidermal necrolysis) following SP treatment in children less than 15 years as 0.3 per 100,000 exposures.[108] The high rate of hepatotoxicity observed when used in weekly prophylaxis has not been observed in treatment or in intermittent preventive treatments (monthly).

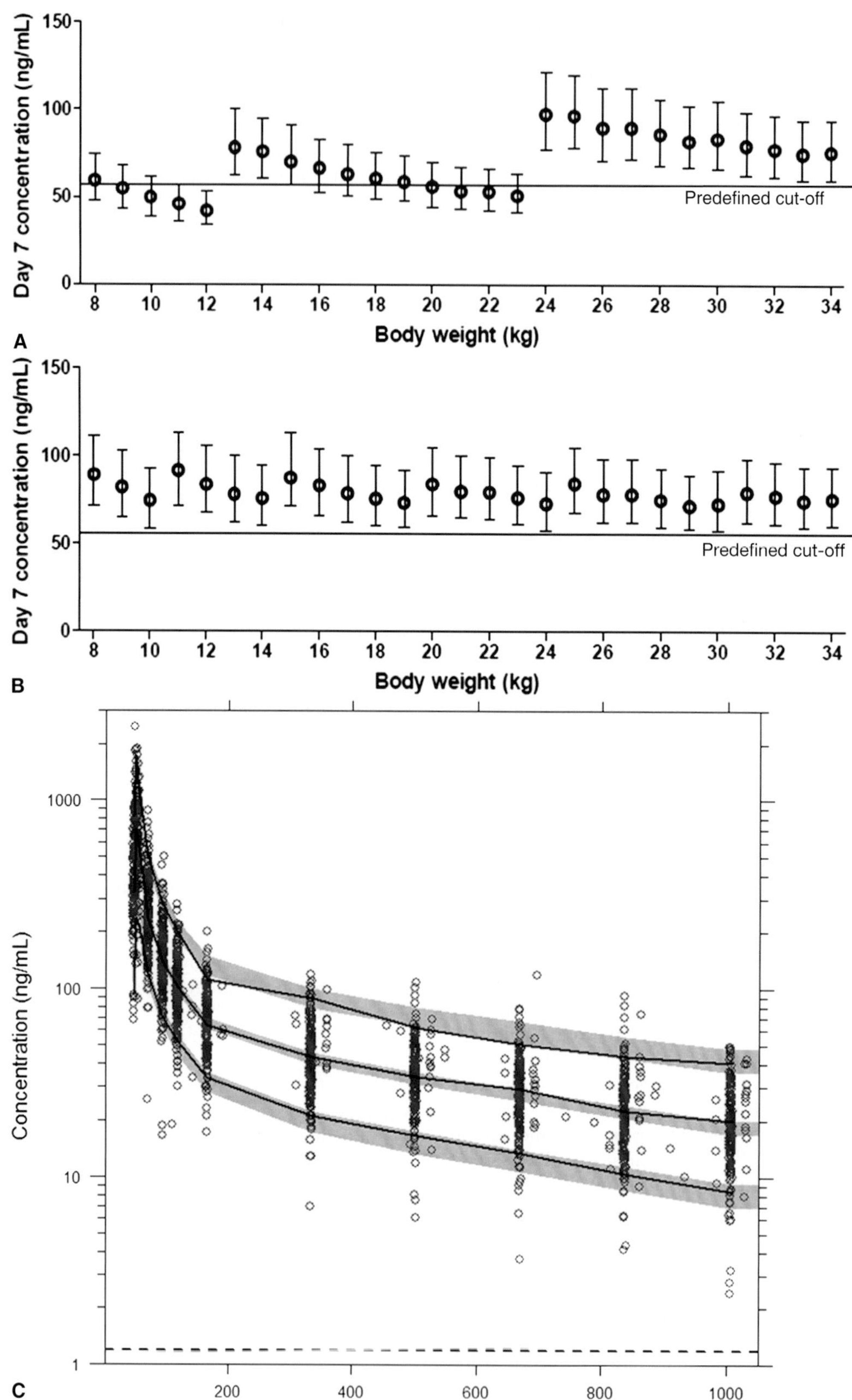

Figure 27.3 Predicted day 7 capillary piperaquine concentrations following a new dosing regimen of DHA–piperaquine in children. Observed and simulated median ± interquartile range day 7 capillary piperaquine concentrations stratified for body weight (1,000 simulated patients at each body weight) after **(A)** original and **(B)** revised dosing regimens of DHA–piperaquine.[94] **(C)** Population PK model showing observed data points (open circles) and 5th, 50th, and 95th percentiles (solid lines) from children with uncomplicated falciparum malaria in Burkina Faso. The shaded area represents 95% confidence interval of simulated (n = 2,000) 5th, 50th, and 95th percentiles. Capillary plasma piperaquine concentrations were transformed into their logarithms (base 10).

Drug–Drug Interactions

SP has no effect on mefloquine, quinine, or chloroquine PK.[109–111] Combining SP with amodiaquine was associated with a reduction in apparent volume of distribution and elimination half-life of pyrimethamine.[112] SP should be avoided in children receiving other antifol drugs; for example, trimethoprim–sulfamethoxazole, methotrexate. Large doses of folic acid antagonize the antimalarial activity of pyrimethamine.

PYRONARIDINE

Pyronaridine is a benzonaphthyridine derivative, structurally related to amodiaquine, first synthesized in 1970.[113] It is combined with artesunate for malaria treatment and a pediatric granule coformulation has been developed. There was some evidence of hepatotoxicity in early studies; however, concerns have been partially assuaged following a large repeated dosing study in Mali.[114] Results of a full safety review are pending. Following oral administration of artesunate–pyronaridine, peak concentrations in children with malaria are reached in 2 to 3 hours.[115]

Distribution

Pyronaridine is a lipophilic compound with a large volume of distribution.

Metabolism and Elimination

Thirteen metabolites of pyronaridine have been identified from human blood, urine, and feces, as well as the pyronaridine itself.[116] The drug has a long terminal elimination half-life of between 6.6 and 12.3 days (see Table 27.3).[115,117]

Drug–Drug Interactions

Given together with primaquine to healthy Thai adults, primaquine concentrations increased but there was no clinically relevant effect on pyronaridine PK.[118]

NONARTEMISININ-BASED TREATMENT OF UNCOMPLICATED FALCIPARUM MALARIA

There are a small number of non-artemisinin-containing treatment options for malaria.

ATOVAQUONE–PROGUANIL

Atovaquone–proguanil is rarely used to treat malaria in endemic areas but can be a useful option for treatment of returned travelers. Readers may be more familiar with its use for chemoprevention. Pediatric tablets contain 62.5 mg of atovaquone (*trans*-2-[4-(4-chlorophenyl)cyclohexyl]-3-hydroxy-1,4-naphthalenedione) and 25 mg of proguanil hydrochloride [1-(4-chlor ophenyl)-5-isopropyl-biguanide hydrochloride]. Atovaquone should be taken with food or milk to increase absorption. Time to peak absorption for both constituents is approximately 6 hours.[119] Atovaquone acts by inhibiting parasite mitochondrial cytochrome electron transport and cellular respiration. Proguanil is metabolized via cytochrome P450 2C19 to the antifol triazine metabolite cycloguanil, but it is the parent compound proguanil that synergizes with atovaquone through an action on the mitochondrion, and not the metabolite. As a result, CYP2C19 loss-of-function polymorphisms (which are common in Asia) affect proguanil metabolism but clinical outcomes with atovaquone–proguanil are not affected.[91]

Distribution

Both atovaquone and proguanil are highly protein bound. Atovaquone has a small apparent volume of distribution, whereas that of proguanil is very large. Apparent clearance of both drugs is affected by body weight.[120]

Metabolism and Elimination

In a study of Thai children with falciparum malaria, mean (SD) terminal elimination half-lives of atovaquone, proguanil, and cycloguanil were estimated as 31.8 (8.9), 14.9 (3.3), and 14.6 (2.6) hours, respectively.[119] Proguanil and cycloguanil accumulate in renal impairment and dose modification may be needed.

Drug–Drug Interactions

Combining atovaquone–proguanil with artesunate does not affect the PK of the drugs.[121] Atovaquone–proguanil should be prescribed with caution to patients on antiretroviral therapy (see Table 27.4). Rifampicin reduces atovaquone concentrations.

QUININE

If ACTs are not available, oral quinine is a common alternative treatment. Disadvantages are the thrice-daily regimen for 5 to 7 days, extremely bitter taste, and poor tolerability and side-effect profile compared to the ACTs. To improve efficacy, quinine should be given with a second agent, and it is typically paired with antibiotics with antimalarial activity such as doxycycline or clindamycin (children <8 years).

Distribution

Quinine is well absorbed orally and can be given by IM injection to the anterior thigh or by carefully rate-controlled intravenous infusion (see Treatment of Severe or Congenital Malaria section). The apparent volume of distribution is contracted in proportion to disease severity. Quinine binds principally to α-1-acid glycoprotein in plasma, so binding is increased in malaria.

Metabolism and Elimination

Quinine is cleared principally (~80%) by hepatic metabolism through CYP3A4, first to the bioactive 3-OH quinine and then to inactive metabolites, and 20% is eliminated in the urine unchanged. Clearance is reduced in proportion to disease severity, so plasma concentrations typically decline after the first 2 to 3 days of treatment as the patient recovers; V_d expands and clearance increases.

Drug–Drug Interactions

Quinine clearance is increased by CYP inducers.

TREATMENT OF UNCOMPLICATED VIVAX MALARIA

Chloroquine remains the first-line treatment for uncomplicated malaria caused by *P. vivax* (and *P. ovale* or *P. malariae*) in most endemic countries except for Indonesia where dihydroartemisinin–piperaquine is used because of unacceptably high levels of chloroquine resistance.[122] ACTs (except AS-SP) or, if unavailable, quinine are alternative treatments.

CHLOROQUINE

Chloroquine is a 4-aminoquinoline, first synthesized in 1934 and probably the most used antimalarial drug of all time. Despite this, the PK of chloroquine monotherapy in children with malaria has not been studied extensively. Treatment courses are typically 25 to 30 mg base equivalent per kg body weight given over 3 days, although shorter (36 hours) courses have been evaluated with 10 mg per kg followed by 5 mg per kg at 6 and 12 hours.[123] Chloroquine concentrates within the parasite food vacuole and inhibits heme detoxification. Chloroquine is administered orally as the phosphate, sulfate or sometimes hydrochloride salt and is well absorbed with bioavailability of 80% to 90% in healthy adult volunteers without malaria.[124] Given parenterally, chloroquine has a narrow therapeutic ratio. It may be given by carefully rate-controlled intravenous infusion (never injection) or by IM or subcutaneous injection. Parenteral doses of 5 mg of base per kilogram every 12 hours to treat severe falciparum malaria in Gambian children were associated with significant hypotension, leading to recommendations for adapted dosing regimens (giving smaller doses more frequently) to avoid high peak concentrations; however, because of worsening resistance in *P. falciparum*, parenteral chloroquine was superseded by parenteral quinine before this occurred.[125]

Distribution

Chloroquine has a very large total apparent volume of distribution of more than 100 L per kg[51,124]; thus, distribution rather than elimination determines the blood concentration profile and therefore safety and efficacy. It is extensively tissue bound with moderate (~60%) binding to plasma proteins.[126] In the study of 18 Gambian children with severe falciparum malaria treated with chloroquine either parenterally or via a nasogastric tube, median CSF concentrations were low at 12 μg per L.[125]

Metabolism and Elimination

N-desethylchloroquine is the major metabolite of chloroquine. Both chloroquine and the metabolite are excreted via the renal tract. Chloroquine is a very slowly eliminated drug with a terminal elimination half-life of approximately 1 month. This is further prolonged in renal failure.[51]

Relapse Prevention

Malaria infections caused by *P. vivax* and *P. ovale* may relapse because of activation of dormant forms or hypnozoites in the liver. Chloroquine and the ACTs do not have hypnozoiticidal activity. To prevent relapse, patients with vivax or ovale malaria require treatment with the 8-aminoquinoline drug primaquine. The exceptions to this are congenital vivax or ovale malaria when blood stage infection occurs directly from the mother, or transfusion acquired malaria; thus, there are no dormant hypnozoites in the liver and radical cure is not indicated.

PRIMAQUINE

Primaquine (phosphate) is an 8-aminoquinoline synthesized first in the 1940s. The standard dosing regimen for vivax malaria relapse prevention is 0.25 to 0.5 mg base equivalent per kg per day for 14 days. However, there is evidence that equivalent total doses given over 7 days to adults or children have similar effects.[127,128] Early studies of primaquine and observations of drug-induced hemolysis in African American prison volunteers led to the discovery of the most common human enzymopathy: X-linked glucose-6-phosphate dehydrogenase (G6PD) deficiency.[129] G6PD deficiency is common (gene frequencies 3% to 30%) in malaria-endemic regions. Ready access to G6PD deficiency testing is unusual in tropical countries and thus concerns about the risks of dangerous hemolysis following primaquine treatment have curtailed its use. Primaquine is currently not recommended for use in children less than 6 months old. Primaquine is administered as the phosphate that is a racemic (50:50) mixture and its PK are enantioselective.[130]

After oral administration in patients with malaria or in healthy adults, the drug is very well absorbed, and peak concentrations are reached in about 2 to 3 hours.[131–133]

Distribution

Primaquine has a large apparent volume of distribution, suggesting extensive tissue binding.

Metabolism and Elimination

Primaquine is biotransformed rapidly by two discrete routes: one via monoamine oxidase to the principal plasma metabolite, carboxyprimaquine, that appears to be biologically inactive[134] and the other via cytochrome P450 2D6 to reactive metabolites (which have not been well characterized), which mediate its antiparasitic and hemolytic effects. Exposure to primaquine and carboxyprimaquine was shown to correlate with body weight (and age) in a study of African children.[135] Less than 5% of a primaquine dose can be detected in urine.[134]

Drug–Drug Interactions

Primaquine exposure increases when coadministered with several other antimalarials (see Table 27.4).

TAFENOQUINE

Tafenoquine is a longer acting slowly eliminated 8-aminoquinoline antimalarial structurally related to primaquine that has been developed for single-dose relapse prevention in vivax malaria. It is not approved for use in children because there is insufficient evidence of safety and efficacy in younger age groups. A PK, efficacy, and safety study in pediatric subjects is recruiting (NCT02563496). In healthy adults, peak concentrations in blood and plasma are reached in approximately 14 hours.[136]

Distribution

Tafenoquine has a large apparent volume of distribution that is reduced in malaria.[137]

Metabolism and Elimination

Tafenoquine is metabolized slowly with an elimination half-life of around 2 weeks.[137] The impact of CYP2D6 polymorphisms on tafenoquine metabolism in humans is unclear.[138]

Drug–Drug Interactions

Coadministration of tafenoquine with DHA–piperaquine and artemether–lumefantrine has been studied in healthy adults with no clinically relevant interaction detected.[139]

DRUGS USED FOR MALARIA PREVENTION

Prevention of malaria in children is with the same drugs as those used for treatment. In high transmission areas, there are two main preventive strategies targeting children: intermittent preventive treatment for infants (IPTi), which is given with the WHO's Expanded Program on Immunization schedule (10 weeks, 14 weeks, and 9 months of age), and seasonal malaria chemoprevention (SMC) that targets children aged 3 to 59 months living in the Sahel, where transmission is very high but confined to the 3- to 4-month rainy season. SP is used for IPTi provided resistance is low to moderate (<50% prevalence of *Pfdhps* 540 mutation). To date, this approach has not been deployed widely. For SMC, single-dose SP plus 3 days of amodiaquine are given monthly for a maximum of four cycles. DHA–piperaquine has been evaluated as a potential alternative agent. Its protective effect is strongly associated with piperaquine exposure.[140,141] Data from Burkina Faso findings of a PK–PD modeling study suggest younger children should receive the new higher DP dose recommended for treatment (see Table 27.2) and that four rounds should be given to maximize the effect of malaria prevention.[142] Other modeling outputs suggest that weekly administration would be preferable to the current monthly schedule.

For pediatric travelers from nonendemic countries, the choice lies between daily atovaquone–proguanil or weekly mefloquine for children weighing more than 5 kg or doxycycline in children older than 8 years.[75,143] Primaquine terminal prophylaxis is not recommended.

EXCRETION OF ANTIMALARIAL DRUGS IN BREAST MILK

Many antimalarials are present in small amounts in human breast milk. These include quinine, chloroquine, piperaquine, mefloquine, artemether–lumefantrine, pyrimethamine, and primaquine.[144–152] The main clinical concern regarding continuing breastfeeding when taking primaquine has been concern over the possibility of causing acute hemolytic anemia in G6PD-deficient infants. In a study of 20 mother–infant pairs without G6PD deficiency where the mothers received 0.5 mg per kg primaquine daily for 14 days, primaquine was detectable in capillary plasma in only one infant at a concentration of 2.6 ng per mL, suggesting the risk is extremely low after the neonatal period.[147]

TABLE 27.5 Pharmacogenetic Considerations in Antimalarial Prescribing

Antimalarial	*Gene*	*Description*
Amodiaquine	*CYP 2C8*	Affects amodiaquine metabolism. Relationship to toxicity unclear
Artesunate	*CYP 2A6*	Malaysian volunteers with CYP 2A6*1B variants responsible for very rapid metabolism of artesunate experienced more adverse effects after artesunate–amodiaquine administration[177]
Lumefantrine	*ABCB1*	ABCB1 c.3435CC genotype associated with reduced risk malaria recurrence[178]
Primaquine	*G6PD, CYP 2D6*	G6PD deficiency associated with hemolytic anemia. CYP 2D6 implicated in primaquine metabolism and possibly hypnozoiticidal activity
Proguanil	*CYP 2C19*	Affects metabolism to cycloguanil
Tafenoquine	*G6PD*	G6PD deficiency associated with hemolytic anemia

NEW ANTIMALARIAL DRUGS

The focus of drug developers for the last 10 years has been on identifying drugs that might provide single-exposure radical cure and prophylaxis (SERCaP) and single-exposure chemoprotection (SEC). Although this is an ideal objective, it is uncertain whether it can be achieved. Nevertheless, there are a number of promising new candidate antimalarials in the pipeline (e.g., artefenomel, cipargamin, ganaplacide) but limited experience of their use in children.[5] In a PK study of artefenomel–piperaquine that included children, it was observed that geometric mean artefenomel exposure following an 800 mg dose given with piperaquine was lowest in African children aged 6 months to 2 years.[153] Some older drugs are being resurrected for use in new combinations (e.g., methylene blue, fosmidomycin, azithromycin).

THE FUTURE OF ANTIMALARIAL TREATMENT IN CHILDREN

The main threat to antimalarial drug efficacy in the future is worsening antimalarial drug resistance. In the absence of suitable candidate treatments to take their place, the consequences of losing ACTs to resistance across Africa would be so devastating that there are calls to take preventive action now. The leading strategy that has been put forward is to increase the number of antimalarials in first-line combination therapies to a minimum of three drugs (as it is in the treatment of TB and HIV infections). Increasing understanding of the pharmacogenetics of the antimalarials may improve prediction of efficacy and toxicity in individual patients in the future (see Table 27.5). Dose optimization for children earlier in the development process should be prioritized.

ACKNOWLEDGMENT

The MORU Tropical Health Network is funded by the Wellcome Trust.

REFERENCES

1. World Health Organization. *World malaria report 2019*. Geneva, Switzerland: World Health Organization, 2019.
2. Pava Z, Burdam FH, Handayuni I, et al. Submicroscopic and asymptomatic *Plasmodium* parasitaemia associated with significant risk of anaemia in Papua, Indonesia. *PLoS One* 2016;11:e0165340.
3. White N. Antimalarial drug resistance and combination chemotherapy. *Philos Trans R Soc Lond B Biol Sci* 1999;354:739–749.
4. Dondorp AM, Nosten F, Yi P, et al. Artemisinin resistance in *Plasmodium falciparum* malaria. *N Engl J Med* 2009;361:455–467.
5. Ashley EA, Phyo AP. Drugs in development for malaria. *Drugs* 2018;78:861–879.
6. White NJ. Pharmacokinetic and pharmacodynamic considerations in antimalarial dose optimization. *Antimicrob Agents Chemother* 2013;57:5792–5807.
7. de Kock M, Tarning J, Workman L, et al. Population pharmacokinetic properties of sulfadoxine and pyrimethamine: a pooled analysis to inform optimal dosing in African children with uncomplicated malaria. *Antimicrob Agents Chemother* 2018;62:e01370-17.
8. Ali AM, Penny MA, Smith TA, et al. Population pharmacokinetics of the antimalarial amodiaquine: a pooled analysis to optimize dosing. *Antimicrob Agents Chemother* 2018;62:e02193-17.
9. Worldwide Antimalarial Resistance Network ALDISG. The effect of dose on the antimalarial efficacy of artemether-lumefantrine: a systematic review and pooled analysis of individual patient data. *Lancet Infect Dis* 2015;15:692–702.
10. Sambol NC, Yan L, Creek DJ, et al. Population pharmacokinetics of piperaquine in young Ugandan children treated with dihydroartemisinin-piperaquine for uncomplicated malaria. *Clin Pharmacol Ther* 2015;98:87–95.
11. Simpson JA, Aarons L, White NJ. How can we do pharmacokinetic studies in the tropics? *Trans R Soc Trop Med Hyg* 2001;95:347–351.
12. Stanisic DI, McCarthy JS, Good MF. Controlled human malaria infection: applications, advances, and challenges. *Infect Immun* 2017;86.pii: e00479-17.
13. McCarthy JS, Lotharius J, Ruckle T, et al. Safety, tolerability, pharmacokinetics, and activity of the novel long-acting antimalarial DSM265: a two-part first-in-human phase 1a/1b randomised study. *Lancet Infect Dis* 2017;17:626–635.
14. Hien TT, White NJ, Thuy-Nhien NT, et al. Estimation of the *in vivo* MIC of cipargamin in uncomplicated *Plasmodium falciparum* malaria. *Antimicrob Agents Chemother* 2017;61.pii: e01940-16.
15. Taylor W, Terlouw DJ, Olliaro PL, et al. Use of weight-for-age data to optimize tablet strength and dosing regimens for a new fixed-dose artesunate–amodiaquine combination for treating falciparum malaria. *Bull World Health Organ* 2006;84:956–964.
16. Hatton CS, Peto TE, Bunch C, et al. Frequency of severe neutropenia associated with amodiaquine prophylaxis against malaria. *Lancet* 1986;1:411–414.
17. Neftel KA, Woodtly W, Schmid M, et al. Amodiaquine induced agranulocytosis and liver damage. *Br Med J (Clin Res Ed)* 1986;292:721–723.
18. Jaureguiberry S, Ndour PA, Roussel C, et al. Post artesunate delayed hemolysis is a predictable event related to the lifesaving effect of artemisinins. *Blood* 2014;124:167–175.
19. World Health Organization. *Guidelines for the treatment of Malaria*. 3rd ed. Geneva, Switzerland: World Health Organization; 2015.
20. White NJ. Clinical pharmacokinetics and pharmacodynamics of artemisinin and derivatives. *Trans R Soc Trop Med Hyg* 1994; 88(Suppl 1):S41–S43.
21. Klayman DL. Qinghaosu (artemisinin): an antimalarial drug from China. *Science* 1985;228:1049–1055.
22. White NJ, Watson J, Ashley EA. Split dosing of artemisinins does not improve antimalarial therapeutic efficacy. *Sci Rep* 2017;7:12132.
23. Simpson JA, Agbenyega T, Barnes KI, et al. Population pharmacokinetics of artesunate and dihydroartemisinin following intra-rectal dosing of artesunate in malaria patients. *PLoS Med* 2006;3:e444.
24. Bethell DB, Teja-Isavadharm P, Cao XT, et al. Pharmacokinetics of oral artesunate in children with moderately severe *Plasmodium falciparum* malaria. *Trans R Soc Trop Med Hyg* 1997;91:195–198.
25. Angus BJ, Thaiaporn I, Chanthapadith K, et al. Oral artesunate dose-response relationship in acute falciparum malaria. *Antimicrob Agents Chemother* 2002; 46:778–782.
26. Hien TT, Davis TM, Chuong LV, et al. Comparative pharmacokinetics of intramuscular artesunate and artemether in patients with severe falciparum malaria. *Antimicrob Agents Chemother* 2004; 48:4234–4239.
27. Mithwani S, Aarons L, Kokwaro GO, et al. Population pharmacokinetics of artemether and dihydroartemisinin following single intramuscular dosing of artemether in African children with severe falciparum malaria. *Br J Clin Pharmacol* 2004;57:146–152.
28. Murphy SA, Mberu E, Muhia D, et al. The disposition of intramuscular artemether in children with cerebral malaria; a preliminary study. *Trans R Soc Trop Med Hyg* 1997;91:331–334.
29. Teja-Isavadharm P, Nosten F, Kyle DE, et al. Comparative bioavailability of oral, rectal, and intramuscular artemether in healthy subjects: use of simultaneous measurement by high performance liquid chromatography and bioassay. *Br J Clin Pharmacol* 1996;42:599–604.
30. Silamut K, Newton PN, Teja-Isavadharm P, et al. Artemether bioavailability after oral or intramuscular administration in uncomplicated falciparum malaria. *Antimicrob Agents Chemother* 2003;47:3795–3798.
31. van Agtmael MA, Gupta V, van der Wosten TH, et al. Grapefruit juice increases the bioavailability of artemether. *Eur J Clin Pharmacol* 1999;55:405–410.
32. Salman S, Bendel D, Lee TC, et al. Pharmacokinetics of a novel sublingual spray formulation of the antimalarial drug artemether in African children with malaria. *Antimicrob Agents Chemother* 2015;59:3208–3215.
33. Hendriksen IC, Mtove G, Kent A, et al. Population pharmacokinetics of intramuscular artesunate in African children with severe malaria: implications for a practical dosing regimen. *Clin Pharmacol Ther* 2013;93:443–450.
34. Zaloumis SG, Tarning J, Krishna S, et al. Population pharmacokinetics of intravenous artesunate: a pooled analysis of individual data from patients with severe malaria. *CPT Pharmacometrics Syst Pharmacol* 2014;3:e145.
35. Davis TM, Binh TQ, Ilett KF, et al. Penetration of dihydroartemisinin into cerebrospinal fluid after administration of intravenous artesunate in severe falciparum malaria. *Antimicrob Agents Chemother* 2003;47:368–370.
36. Piedade R, Gil JP. The pharmacogenetics of antimalaria artemisinin combination therapy. *Expert Opin Drug Metab Toxicol* 2011;7:1185–1200.
37. Morris CA, Duparc S, Borghini-Fuhrer I, et al. Review of the clinical pharmacokinetics of artesunate and its active metabolite dihydroartemisinin following intravenous, intramuscular, oral or rectal administration. *Malar J* 2011;10:263.
38. Karbwang J, Na-Bangchang K, Tin T, et al. Pharmacokinetics of intramuscular artemether in patients with severe falciparum malaria with or without acute renal failure. *Br J Clin Pharmacol* 1998;45:597–600.
39. Gachelin G, Garner P, Ferroni E, et al. Evaluating *Cinchona* bark and quinine for treating and preventing malaria. *J R Soc Med* 2017;110:31–40.
40. White NJ, Looareesuwan S, Warrell DA, et al. Quinine loading dose in cerebral malaria. *Am J Trop Med Hyg* 1983;32:1–5.
41. Shann F, Stace J, Edstein M. Pharmacokinetics of quinine in children. *J Pediatr* 1985;106:506–510.
42. Pasvol G, Newton CR, Winstanley PA, et al. Quinine treatment of severe falciparum malaria in African children: a randomized comparison of three regimens. *Am J Trop Med Hyg* 1991;45:702–713.
43. Waller D, Krishna S, Craddock C, et al. The pharmacokinetic properties of intramuscular quinine in Gambian children with severe falciparum malaria. *Trans R Soc Trop Med Hyg* 1990;84:488–491.
44. Krishna S, Nagaraja NV, Planche T, et al. Population pharmacokinetics of intramuscular quinine in children with severe malaria. *Antimicrob Agents Chemother* 2001;45:1803–1809.
45. Viswanathan A. Intramuscular quinine injections in malaria. *Ind Med Gaz* 1926;61:398.
46. Yen LM, Dao LM, Day NP, et al. Role of quinine in the high mortality of intramuscular injection tetanus. *Lancet* 1994;344:786–787.
47. Barennes H, Kahiatani F, Pussard E, et al. Intrarectal Quinimax (an association of Cinchona alkaloids) for the treatment of *Plasmodium falciparum* malaria in children in Niger: efficacy and pharmacokinetics. *Trans R Soc Trop Med Hyg* 1995;89:418–421.
48. Eisenhut M, Omari AA. Intrarectal quinine versus intravenous or intramuscular quinine for treating *Plasmodium falciparum* malaria. *Cochrane Database Syst Rev* 2009:Cd004009.
49. Barennes H, Sterlingot H, Nagot N, et al. Intrarectal pharmacokinetics of two formulations of quinine in children with falciparum malaria. *Eur J Clin Pharmacol* 2003;58:649–652.
50. Paintaud G, Alvan G, Ericsson O. The reproducibility of quinine bioavailability. *Br J Clin Pharmacol* 1993;35:305–307.
51. Krishna S, White NJ. Pharmacokinetics of quinine, chloroquine and amodiaquine. Clinical implications. *Clin Pharmacokinet* 1996;30:263–299.
52. Sabchareon A, Chongsuphajaisiddhi T, Attanath P. Serum quinine concentrations following the initial dose in children with falciparum malaria. *Southeast Asian J Trop Med Public Health* 1982;13:556–562.
53. Supanaranond W, Davis TM, Pukrittayakamee S, et al. Disposition of oral quinine in acute falciparum malaria. *Eur J Clin Pharmacol* 1991;40:49–52.
54. Silamut K, White NJ, Looareesuwan S, et al. Binding of quinine to plasma proteins in falciparum malaria. *Am J Trop Med Hyg* 1985;34:681–686.
55. Pukrittayakamee S, Looareesuwan S, Keeratithakul D, et al. A study of the factors affecting the metabolic clearance of quinine in malaria. *Eur J Clin Pharmacol* 1997;52:487–493.
56. Newton P, Keeratithakul D, Teja-Isavadharm P, et al. Pharmacokinetics of quinine and 3-hydroxyquinine in severe falciparum malaria with acute renal failure. *Trans R Soc Trop Med Hyg* 1999;93:69–72.
57. Le Jouan M, Jullien V, Tetanye E, et al. Quinine pharmacokinetics and pharmacodynamics in children with malaria caused by *Plasmodium falciparum*. *Antimicrob Agents Chemother* 2005;49:3658–3662.
58. Pukrittayakamee S, Prakongpan S, Wanwimolruk S, et al. Adverse effect of rifampin on quinine efficacy in uncomplicated falciparum malaria. *Antimicrob Agents Chemother* 2003;47:1509–1513.
59. Taylor TE, Molyneux ME, Wirima JJ, et al. Blood glucose levels in Malawian children before and during the administration of intravenous quinine for severe falciparum malaria. *N Engl J Med* 1988;319:1040–1047.
60. Ogetii GN, Akech S, Jemutai J, et al. Hypoglycaemia in severe malaria, clinical associations and relationship to quinine dosage. *BMC Infect Dis* 2010;10:334.
61. Dondorp AM, Fanello CI, Hendriksen IC, et al. Artesunate versus quinine in the treatment of severe falciparum malaria in African children (AQUAMAT): an open-label, randomised trial. *Lancet* 2010;376:1647–1657.
62. van Hensbroek MB, Kwiatkowski D, van den Berg B, et al. Quinine pharmacokinetics in young children with severe malaria. *Am J Trop Med Hyg* 1996;54:237–242.
63. Roggelin L, Pelletier D, Hill JN, et al. Disease-associated QT-shortage versus quinine associated QT-prolongation: age dependent ECG-effects in Ghanaian children with severe malaria. *Malar J* 2014;13:219.
64. Salako LA, Sowunmi A, Akinbami FO. Pharmacokinetics of quinine in African children suffering from kwashiorkor. *Br J Clin Pharmacol* 1989;28:197–201.
65. Pussard E, Barennes H, Daouda H, et al. Quinine disposition in globally malnourished children with cerebral malaria. *Clin Pharmacol Ther* 1999;65:500–510.

66. Thein ST, Khin HSS, Thi A. Insights into the availability and distribution of oral artemisinin monotherapy in Myanmar: evidence from a nationally representative outlet survey. *Malar J* 2017;16:170.
67. Salman S, Page-Sharp M, Batty KT, et al. Pharmacokinetic comparison of two piperaquine-containing artemisinin combination therapies in Papua New Guinean children with uncomplicated malaria. *Antimicrob Agents Chemother* 2012;56:3288–3297.
68. Sidhu JS, Ashton M, Huong NV, et al. Artemisinin population pharmacokinetics in children and adults with uncomplicated falciparum malaria. *Br J Clin Pharmacol* 1998;45:347–354.
69. Simpson JA, Price R, ter Kuile F, et al. Population pharmacokinetics of mefloquine in patients with acute falciparum malaria. *Clin Pharmacol Ther* 1999;66:472–484.
70. Ashley EA, Stepniewska K, Lindegardh N, et al. Population pharmacokinetic assessment of a new regimen of mefloquine used in combination treatment of uncomplicated falciparum malaria. *Antimicrob Agents Chemother* 2006;50:2281–2285.
71. Bourahla A, Martin C, Gimenez F, et al. Stereoselective pharmacokinetics of mefloquine in young children. *Eur J Clin Pharmacol* 1996;50:241–244.
72. Karbwang J, White NJ. Clinical pharmacokinetics of mefloquine. *Clin Pharmacokinet* 1990;19:264–279.
73. Nosten F, ter Kuile F, Chongsuphajaisiddhi T, et al. Mefloquine pharmacokinetics and resistance in children with acute falciparum malaria. *Br J Clin Pharmacol* 1991;31:556–559.
74. Singhasivanon V, Chongsuphajaisiddhi T, Sabchareon A, et al. Pharmacokinetic study of mefloquine in Thai children aged 5-12 years suffering from uncomplicated falciparum malaria treated with MSP or MSP plus primaquine. *Eur J Drug Metab Pharmacokinet* 1994;19:27–32.
75. Schlagenhauf P, Adamcova M, Regep L, et al. Use of mefloquine in children: a review of dosage, pharmacokinetics and tolerability data. *Malar J* 2011;10:292.
76. Nguyen TH, Day NP, Ly VC, et al. Post-malaria neurological syndrome. *Lancet* 1996;348:917–921.
77. Ashley EA, Stepniewska K, Lindegardh N, et al. How much fat is necessary to optimize lumefantrine oral bioavailability? *Trop Med Int Health* 2007;12:195–200.
78. Ashley EA, Stepniewska K, Lindegardh N, et al. Pharmacokinetic study of artemether-lumefantrine given once daily for the treatment of uncomplicated multidrug-resistant falciparum malaria. *Trop Med Int Health* 2007;12:201–208.
79. Djimde AA, Tekete M, Abdulla S, et al. Pharmacokinetic and pharmacodynamic characteristics of a new pediatric formulation of artemether-lumefantrine in African children with uncomplicated *Plasmodium falciparum* malaria. *Antimicrob Agents Chemother* 2011;55:3994–3999.
80. White NJ, van Vugt M, Ezzet F. Clinical pharmacokinetics and pharmacodynamics and pharmacodynamics of artemether-lumefantrine. *Clin Pharmacokinet* 1999;37:105–125.
81. Worldwide Antimalarial Resistance Network, Lumefantrine PK/PD Study Group. Artemether-lumefantrine treatment of uncomplicated *Plasmodium falciparum* malaria: a systematic review and meta-analysis of day 7 lumefantrine concentrations and therapeutic response using individual patient data. *BMC Med* 2015;13:227.
82. Kloprogge F, Workman L, Borrmann S, et al. Artemether-lumefantrine dosing for malaria treatment in young children and pregnant women: a pharmacokinetic-pharmacodynamic meta-analysis. *PLoS Med* 2018;15:e1002579.
83. Medicines for Malaria Venture. 390 million treatments of Coartem® Dispersible delivered to over 50 countries. https://www.mmv.org/our-impact/achievements/390-million-treatments-coartem-dispersible-delivered-over-50-countries. Accessed April 19, 2020.
84. Jain JP, Leong FJ, Chen L, et al. Bioavailability of lumefantrine is significantly enhanced with a novel formulation approach, an outcome from a randomized, open-label pharmacokinetic study in healthy volunteers. *Antimicrob Agents Chemother* 2017;61.pii: e00868-17.
85. Wong RP, Salman S, Ilett KF, et al. Desbutyl-lumefantrine is a metabolite of lumefantrine with potent *in vitro* antimalarial activity that may influence artemether-lumefantrine treatment outcome. *Antimicrob Agents Chemother* 2011;55:1194–1198.
86. Djimde A, Lefevre G. Understanding the pharmacokinetics of Coartem. *Malar J* 2009;8(Suppl 1):S4.
87. Ezzet F, Mull R, Karbwang J. Population pharmacokinetics and therapeutic response of CGP 56697 (artemether + benflumetol) in malaria patients. *Br J Clin Pharmacol* 1998;46:553–561.
88. Orrell C, Little F, Smith P, et al. Pharmacokinetics and tolerability of artesunate and amodiaquine alone and in combination in healthy volunteers. *Eur J Clin Pharmacol* 2008;64:683–690.
89. Winstanley P, Edwards G, Orme M, et al. The disposition of amodiaquine in man after oral administration. *Br J Clin Pharmacol* 1987;23:1–7.
90. Stepniewska K, Taylor W, Sirima SB, et al. Population pharmacokinetics of artesunate and amodiaquine in African children. *Malar J* 2009;8:200.
91. Elewa H, Wilby KJ. A review of pharmacogenetics of antimalarials and associated clinical implications. *Eur J Drug Metab Pharmacokinet* 2017;42:745–756.
92. Gasasira AF, Kamya MR, Achan J, et al. High risk of neutropenia in HIV-infected children following treatment with artesunate plus amodiaquine for uncomplicated malaria in Uganda. *Clin Infect Dis* 2008;46:985–991.
93. Scarsi KK, Fehintola FA, Ma Q, et al. Disposition of amodiaquine and desethylamodiaquine in HIV-infected Nigerian subjects on nevirapine-containing antiretroviral therapy. *J Antimicrob Chemother* 2014;69:1370–1376.
94. Tarning J, Zongo I, Some FA, et al. Population pharmacokinetics and pharmacodynamics of piperaquine in children with uncomplicated falciparum malaria. *Clin Pharmacol Ther* 2012;91:497–505.
95. Worldwide Antimalarial Resistance Network DPSG. The effect of dosing regimens on the antimalarial efficacy of dihydroartemisinin-piperaquine: a pooled analysis of individual patient data. *PLoS Med* 2013;10:e1001564; discussion e.
96. Annerberg A, Lwin KM, Lindegardh N, et al. A small amount of fat does not affect piperaquine exposure in patients with malaria. *Antimicrob Agents Chemother* 2011;55:3971–3976.
97. Hung TY, Davis TM, Ilett KF, et al. Population pharmacokinetics of piperaquine in adults and children with uncomplicated falciparum or vivax malaria. *Br J Clin Pharmacol* 2004;57:253–262.
98. Hoglund RM, Workman L, Edstein MD, et al. Population pharmacokinetic properties of piperaquine in falciparum malaria: an individual participant data meta-analysis. *PLoS Med* 2017;14:e1002212.
99. Tarning J, Bergqvist Y, Day NP, et al. Characterization of human urinary metabolites of the antimalarial piperaquine. *Drug Metab Dispos* 2006;34:2011–2019.
100. Liu H, Zhou H, Cai T, et al. Metabolism of piperaquine to its antiplasmodial metabolites and their pharmacokinetic profiles in healthy volunteers. *Antimicrob Agents Chemother* 2018;62. pii: e00260-18.
101. Karunajeewa HA, Ilett KF, Mueller I, et al. Pharmacokinetics and efficacy of piperaquine and chloroquine in Melanesian children with uncomplicated malaria. *Antimicrob Agents Chemother* 2008;52:237–243.
102. Banda CG, Dzinjalamala F, Mukaka M, et al. Pharmacokinetics of piperaquine and safety profile of dihydroartemisinin-piperaquine coadministered with antiretroviral therapy in malaria-uninfected HIV-positive Malawian adults. *Antimicrob Agents Chemother* 2018;62. pii: e00634-18.
103. Chan XHS, Win YN, Mawer LJ, et al. Risk of sudden unexplained death after use of dihydroartemisinin-piperaquine for malaria: a systematic review and Bayesian meta-analysis. *Lancet Infect Dis* 2018;18:913–923.
104. Bell DJ, Nyirongo SK, Mukaka M, et al. Population pharmacokinetics of sulfadoxine and pyrimethamine in Malawian children with malaria. *Clin Pharmacol Ther* 2011;89:268–275.
105. Barnes KI, Little F, Smith PJ, et al. Sulfadoxinepyrimethamine pharmacokinetics in malaria: pediatric dosing implications. *Clin Pharmacol Ther* 2006;80:582–596.
106. Winstanley PA, Watkins WM, Newton CR, et al. The disposition of oral and intramuscular pyrimethamine/sulphadoxine in Kenyan children with high parasitaemia but clinically non-severe falciparum malaria. *Br J Clin Pharmacol* 1992;33:143–148.
107. McLeod R, Mack D, Foss R, et al. Levels of pyrimethamine in sera and cerebrospinal and ventricular fluids from infants treated for congenital toxoplasmosis. Toxoplasmosis Study Group. *Antimicrob Agents Chemother* 1992;36:1040–1048.
108. Gimnig JE, MacArthur JR, M'Bang'ombe M, et al. Severe cutaneous reactions to sulfadoxine-pyrimethamine and trimethoprim-sulfamethoxazole in Blantyre District, Malawi. *Am J Trop Med Hyg* 2006;74:738–743.
109. Mansor SM, Navaratnam V, Mohamad M, et al. Single dose kinetic study of the triple combination mefloquine/sulphadoxine/pyrimethamine (Fansimef) in healthy male volunteers. *Br J Clin Pharmacol* 1989;27:381–386.
110. Newton CR, Winstanley PA, Watkins WM, et al. A single dose of intramuscular sulfadoxine-pyrimethamine as an adjunct to quinine in the treatment of severe malaria: pharmacokinetics and efficacy. *Trans R Soc Trop Med Hyg* 1993;87:207–210.
111. Bustos DG, Lazaro JE, Gay F, et al. Pharmacokinetics of sequential and simultaneous treatment with the combination chloroquine and sulfadoxine-pyrimethamine in acute uncomplicated *Plasmodium falciparum* malaria in the Philippines. *Trop Med Int Health* 2002;7:584–591.
112. Tekete MM, Toure S, Fredericks A, et al. Effects of amodiaquine and artesunate on sulphadoxine-pyrimethamine pharmacokinetic parameters in children under five in Mali. *Malar J* 2011;10:275.
113. Chang C, Lin-Hua T, Jantanavivat C. Studies on a new antimalarial compound: pyronaridine. *Trans R Soc Trop Med Hyg* 1992;86:7–10.
114. Sagara I, Beavogui AH, Zongo I, et al. Safety and efficacy of re-treatments with pyronaridine-artesunate in African patients with malaria: a substudy of the WANECAM randomised trial. *Lancet Infect Dis* 2016;16:189–198.
115. Ramharter M, Kurth F, Schreier AC, et al. Fixed-dose pyronaridine-artesunate combination for treatment of uncomplicated falciparum malaria in pediatric patients in Gabon. *J Infect Dis* 2008;198:911–919.
116. Morris CA, Dueker SR, Lohstroh PN, et al. Mass balance and metabolism of the antimalarial pyronaridine in healthy volunteers. *Eur J Drug Metab Pharmacokinet* 2015;40:75–86.
117. Ayyoub A, Methaneethorn J, Ramharter M, et al. Population pharmacokinetics of pyronaridine in pediatric malaria patients. *Antimicrob Agents Chemother* 2015;60:1450–1458.
118. Jittamala P, Pukrittayakamee S, Ashley EA, et al. Pharmacokinetic interactions between primaquine and pyronaridine-artesunate in healthy adult Thai subjects. *Antimicrob Agents Chemother* 2015;59:505–513.
119. Sabchareon A, Attanath P, Phanuaksook P, et al. Efficacy and pharmacokinetics of atovaquone and proguanil in children with multidrug-resistant *Plasmodium falciparum* malaria. *Trans R Soc Trop Med Hyg* 1998;92:201–206.
120. Hussein Z, Eaves CJ, Hutchinson DB, et al. Population pharmacokinetics of proguanil in patients with acute *P. falciparum* malaria after combined therapy with atovaquone. *Br J Clin Pharmacol* 1996;42:589–597.
121. van Vugt M, Edstein MD, Proux S, et al. Absence of an interaction between artesunate and atovaquone–proguanil. *Eur J Clin Pharmacol* 1999;55:469–474.
122. Price RN, von Seidlein L, Valecha N, Nosten F, et al. Global extent of chloroquine-resistant Plasmodium vivax: a systematic review and meta-analysis. *Lancet Infect Dis 2014*;14(10):982–991.
123. Pussard E, Lepers JP, Clavier F, et al. Efficacy of a loading dose of oral chloroquine in a 36-hour treatment schedule for uncomplicated *Plasmodium falciparum* malaria. *Antimicrob Agents Chemother* 1991;35:406–409.
124. Gustafsson LL, Walker O, Alvan G, et al. Disposition of chloroquine in man after single intravenous and oral doses. *Br J Clin Pharmacol* 1983;15:471–479.
125. White NJ, Miller KD, Churchill FC, et al. Chloroquine treatment of severe malaria in children. Pharmacokinetics, toxicity, and new dosage recommendations. *N Engl J Med* 1988;319:1493–1500.
126. Walker O, Birkett DJ, Alvan G, et al. Characterization of chloroquine plasma protein binding in man. *Br J Clin Pharmacol* 1983;15:375–357.
127. Clyde DF, McCarthy VC. Radical cure of Chesson strain vivax malaria in man by 7, not 14, days of treatment with primaquine. *Am J Trop Med Hyg* 1977; 26:562–563.
128. Chu CS, Phyo AP, Turner C, et al. Chloroquine versus dihydroartemisinin-piperaquine with standard high-dose primaquine given either for 7 days or 14 days in *Plasmodium vivax* malaria. *Clin Infect Dis* 2019;68:1311–1319.

129. Beutler E. Study of glucose-6-phosphate dehydrogenase: history and molecular biology. *Am J Hematol* 1993;42:53–58.
130. Chairat K, Jittamala P, Hanboonkunupakarn B, et al. Enantiospecific pharmacokinetics and drug-drug interactions of primaquine and blood-stage antimalarial drugs. *J Antimicrob Chemother* 2018;73:3102–3113.
131. Pukrittayakamee S, Tarning J, Jittamala P, et al. Pharmacokinetic interactions between primaquine and chloroquine. *Antimicrob Agents Chemother* 2014;58:3354–3359.
132. Bangchang KN, Songsaeng W, Thanavibul A, et al. Pharmacokinetics of primaquine in G6PD deficient and G6PD normal patients with vivax malaria. *Trans R Soc Trop Med Hyg* 1994;88:220–222.
133. Mihaly GW, Ward SA, Edwards G, et al. Pharmacokinetics of primaquine in man. I. Studies of the absolute bioavailability and effects of dose size. *Br J Clin Pharmacol* 1985;19:745–750.
134. Mihaly GW, Ward SA, Edwards G, et al. Pharmacokinetics of primaquine in man: identification of the carboxylic acid derivative as a major plasma metabolite. *Br J Clin Pharmacol* 1984;17:441–446.
135. Goncalves BP, Pett H, Tiono AB, et al. Age, weight, and CYP2D6 genotype are major determinants of primaquine pharmacokinetics in African children. *Antimicrob Agents Chemother* 2017;61. pii: e02590-16.
136. Brueckner RP, Lasseter KC, Lin ET, et al. First-time-in-humans safety and pharmacokinetics of WR 238605, a new antimalarial. *Am J Trop Med Hyg* 1998;58:645–649.
137. Thakkar N, Green JA, Koh G, et al. Population pharmacokinetics of tafenoquine, a novel antimalarial. *Antimicrob Agents Chemother* 2018;62. pii: e00711-18.
138. St Jean PL, Xue Z, Carter N, et al. Tafenoquine treatment of *Plasmodium vivax* malaria: suggestive evidence that CYP2D6 reduced metabolism is not associated with relapse in the Phase 2b DETECTIVE trial. *Malar J* 2016;15:97.
139. Green JA, Mohamed K, Goyal N, et al. Pharmacokinetic interactions between tafenoquine and dihydroartemisinin-piperaquine or artemether-lumefantrine in healthy adult subjects. *Antimicrob Agents Chemother* 2016;60:7321–7332.
140. Zongo I, Milligan P, Compaore YD, et al. Randomized noninferiority trial of dihydroartemisinin-piperaquine compared with sulfadoxine-pyrimethamine plus amodiaquine for seasonal malaria chemoprevention in Burkina Faso. *Antimicrob Agents Chemother* 2015;59:4387–4396.
141. Sundell K, Jagannathan P, Huang L, et al. Variable piperaquine exposure significantly impacts protective efficacy of monthly dihydroartemisinin-piperaquine for the prevention of malaria in Ugandan children. *Malar J* 2015;14:368.
142. Chotsiri P, Zongo I, Milligan P, et al. Optimal dosing of dihydroartemisinin-piperaquine for seasonal malaria chemoprevention in young children. *Nat Commun* 2019;10:480.
143. Schlagenhauf P, Petersen E. Malaria chemoprophylaxis: strategies for risk groups. *Clin Microbiol Rev* 2008;21:466–472.
144. Akintonwa A, Gbajumo SA, Mabadeje AF. Placental and milk transfer of chloroquine in humans. *Ther Drug Monit* 1988;10:147–149.
145. Edstein MD, Veenendaal JR, Hyslop R. Excretion of mefloquine in human breast milk. *Chemotherapy* 1988;34:165–169.
146. Fulton B, Moore LL. Antiinfectives in breastmilk. Part II: sulfonamides, tetracyclines, macrolides, aminoglycosides and antimalarials. *J Hum Lact* 1992;8:221–223.
147. Gilder ME, Hanpithakphong W, Hoglund RM, et al. Primaquine pharmacokinetics in lactating women and breastfed infant exposures. *Clin Infect Dis* 2018;67:1000–1007.
148. Jain JP, Ganesan S, Lefèvre G, et al . Estimation of the amount of artemether and lumefantrine excreted through breast milk. *Trop Med Int Health* 2015;20(Suppl s1):184–185.
149. Law I, Ilett KF, Hackett LP, et al. Transfer of chloroquine and desethylchloroquine across the placenta and into milk in Melanesian mothers. *Br J Clin Pharmacol* 2008;65:674–679.
150. Moore BR, Salman S, Benjamin J, et al. Pharmacokinetics of piperaquine transfer into the breast milk of Melanesian mothers. *Antimicrob Agents Chemother* 2015;59:4272–4278.
151. Ogunbona FA, Onyeji CO, Bolaji OO, et al. Excretion of chloroquine and desethylchloroquine in human milk. *Br J Clin Pharmacol* 1987;23:473–476.
152. Parke AL. Antimalarial drugs, pregnancy and lactation. *Lupus* 1993;2(Suppl 1):S21–S23.
153. Macintyre F, Adoke Y, Tiono AB, et al. A randomised, double-blind clinical phase II trial of the efficacy, safety, tolerability and pharmacokinetics of a single dose combination treatment with artefenomel and piperaquine in adults and children with uncomplicated *Plasmodium falciparum* malaria. *BMC Med* 2017;15:181.
154. Nealon C, Dzeing A, Muller-Romer U, et al. Intramuscular bioavailability and clinical efficacy of artesunate in Gabonese children with severe malaria. *Antimicrob Agents Chemother* 2002;46:3933–3999.
155. Karunajeewa HA, Manning L, Mueller I, et al. Rectal administration of artemisinin derivatives for the treatment of malaria. *JAMA* 2007;297:2381–2390.
156. Mwesigwa J, Parikh S, McGee B, et al. Pharmacokinetics of artemether-lumefantrine and artesunate-amodiaquine in children in Kampala, Uganda. *Antimicrob Agents Chemother* 2010;54:52–59.
157. Adjei GO, Amponsah SK, Goka BQ, et al. Population pharmacokinetic estimates suggest elevated clearance and distribution volume of desethylamodiaquine in pediatric patients with sickle cell disease treated with artesunate-amodiaquine. *Curr Ther Res Clin Exp* 2019;90:9–15.
158. Adjei GO, Kristensen K, Goka BQ, et al. Effect of concomitant artesunate administration and cytochrome P4502C8 polymorphisms on the pharmacokinetics of amodiaquine in Ghanaian children with uncomplicated malaria. *Antimicrob Agents Chemother* 2008;52:4400–4406.
159. Obua C, Hellgren U, Ntale M, et al. Population pharmacokinetics of chloroquine and sulfadoxine and treatment response in children with malaria: suggestions for an improved dose regimen. *Br J Clin Pharmacol* 2008;65:493–501.
160. Salman S, Page-Sharp M, Griffin S, et al. Population pharmacokinetics of artemether, lumefantrine, and their respective metabolites in Papua New Guinean children with uncomplicated malaria. *Antimicrob Agents Chemother* 2011;55:5306–5313.
161. Hietala SF, Martensson A, Ngasala B, et al. Population pharmacokinetics and pharmacodynamics of artemether and lumefantrine during combination treatment in children with uncomplicated falciparum malaria in Tanzania. *Antimicrob Agents Chemother* 2010;54:4780–4788.
162. Price R, Simpson JA, Teja-Isavatharm P, et al. Pharmacokinetics of mefloquine combined with artesunate in children with acute falciparum malaria. *Antimicrob Agents Chemother* 1999;43:341–346.
163. Moore BR, Benjamin JM, Salman S, et al. Effect of coadministered fat on the tolerability, safety, and pharmacokinetic properties of dihydroartemisinin-piperaquine in Papua New Guinean children with uncomplicated malaria. *Antimicrob Agents Chemother* 2014;58:5784–5794.
164. Hendriksen IC, Maiga D, Lemnge MM, et al. Population pharmacokinetic and pharmacodynamic properties of intramuscular quinine in Tanzanian children with severe falciparum malaria. *Antimicrob Agents Chemother* 2013;57:775–783.
165. Mansor SM, Taylor TE, McGrath CS, et al. The safety and kinetics of intramuscular quinine in Malawian children with moderately severe falciparum malaria. *Trans R Soc Trop Med Hyg* 1990;84:482–487.
166. Winstanley PA, Mberu EK, Watkins WM, et al. Towards optimal regimens of parenteral quinine for young African children with cerebral malaria: unbound quinine concentrations following a simple loading dose regimen. *Trans R Soc Trop Med Hyg* 1994;88:577–580.
167. German P, Greenhouse B, Coates C, et al. Hepatotoxicity due to a drug interaction between amodiaquine plus artesunate and efavirenz. *Clin Infect Dis* 2007;44:889–891.
168. Hoglund RM, Byakika-Kibwika P, Lamorde M, et al. Artemether-lumefantrine co-administration with antiretrovirals: population pharmacokinetics and dosing implications. *Br J Clin Pharmacol* 2015;79:636–649.
169. Byakika-Kibwika P, Lamorde M, Mayito J, et al. Significant pharmacokinetic interactions between artemether/lumefantrine and efavirenz or nevirapine in HIV-infected Ugandan adults. *J Antimicrob Chemother* 2012;67:2213–2221.
170. Zakaria Z, Badhan RKS. The impact of CYP2B6 polymorphisms on the interactions of efavirenz with lumefantrine: implications for paediatric antimalarial therapy. *Eur J Pharm Sci* 2018;119:90–101.
171. Huang L, Carey V, Lindsey JC, et al. Concomitant nevirapine impacts pharmacokinetic exposure to the antimalarial artemether-lumefantrine in African children. *PLoS One* 2017;12:e0186589.
172. German P, Parikh S, Lawrence J, et al. Lopinavir/ritonavir affects pharmacokinetic exposure of artemether/lumefantrine in HIV-uninfected healthy volunteers. *J Acquir Immune Defic Syndr* 2009;51:424–429.
173. Kakuda TN, DeMasi R, van Delft Y, et al. Pharmacokinetic interaction between etravirine or darunavir/ritonavir and artemether/lumefantrine in healthy volunteers: a two-panel, two-way, two-period, randomized trial. *HIV Med* 2013;14:421–429.
174. Lefevre G, Bindschedler M, Ezzet F, et al. Pharmacokinetic interaction trial between co-artemether and mefloquine. *Eur J Pharm Sci* 2000;10:141–151.
175. van Luin M, Van der Ende ME, Richter C, et al. Lower atovaquone/proguanil concentrations in patients taking efavirenz, lopinavir/ritonavir or atazanavir/ritonavir. *AIDS* 2010;24:1223–1226.
176. Hanboonkunupakarn B, Ashley EA, Jittamala P, et al. Open-label crossover study of primaquine and dihydroartemisinin-piperaquine pharmacokinetics in healthy adult Thai subjects. *Antimicrob Agents Chemother* 2014;58:7340–7346.
177. Yusof W, Hua GS. Gene, ethnic and gender influences predisposition of adverse drug reactions to artesunate among Malaysians. *Toxicol Mech Methods* 2012;22:184–192.
178. Kiaco K, Rodrigues AS, do Rosario V, et al. The drug transporter ABCB1 c.3435C>T SNP influences artemether-lumefantrine treatment outcome. *Malar J* 2017;16:383.

CHAPTER

28

David J. Diemert

Anthelminthics Drugs in Children

INTRODUCTION

Worldwide, some of the most common childhood infections are caused by helminths. Of these, schistosomiasis and the soil-transmitted helminths (STHs), which include roundworm (*Ascaris lumbricoides*), whipworm (*Trichuris trichiura*), and the hookworms *Ancylostoma duodenale* and *Necator americanus*, are the most prevalent. According to the World Health Organization (WHO), approximately 300 million preschool-aged children (ages 1 to 4 years) and 600 million school-aged children (ages 5 to 14 years) live in areas that put them at risk of being infected with one or more of the STHs or schistosomes.[1] School-aged children living in the rural, resource-limited areas of the tropics are at particular risk of helminth infections due to the STHs and schistosomes.[2,3] This age group often suffers from the highest worm burdens and, in turn, the related complications such as iron deficiency anemia due to hookworm, intestinal or biliary tract obstruction due to *A. lumbricoides*, dysentery or rectal prolapse due to *T. trichiura*, and hepatobiliary or urinary schistosomiasis.[4] However, considerably greater numbers of children develop more insidious disease due to chronic infections with these parasites, such as malnutrition and impaired physical fitness and development.[5,6] Additionally, chronic infection with STHs and schistosomes impairs childhood intellectual and cognitive development, thus adversely affecting both learning capacity and school attendance.[7,8]

Due to the negative impact on childhood growth and development of the STHs and schistosomiasis, the WHO, the World Bank, governments, nongovernmental development organizations, industry, and other funders have committed to and funded programs to provide anthelminthic medications to children living in endemic areas through periodic mass administration (MDA) campaigns in school-aged and preschool-aged children.[9] In these MDA programs, children receive a single dose of a benzimidazole drug such as albendazole or mebendazole once or twice a year in regions of high STH prevalence. Additionally, those living in areas endemic for schistosomiasis receive a single dose of praziquantel at the same interval. Both drugs are administered simultaneously in areas such as many parts of sub-Saharan Africa and Brazil, where the infections are co-endemic.

Although the challenges of administering hundreds of millions of doses of anthelminthic drugs annually throughout the developing world are significant, the potential benefits are evident. However, a major drawback to this approach is that children remain susceptible to STH and schistosome infections following treatment, and in areas of intense transmission, reinfection can occur rapidly within months.[10,11] Therefore, in many parts of the developing world, administration of anthelminthics would have to be conducted on a twice- or thrice-yearly basis to have a substantial impact, which is difficult to sustain.[12] Furthermore, although school-aged children typically experience the highest *Ascaris*, *Trichuris*, and schistosome worm burdens, adults can also be infected, particularly with hookworm; so, school-based interventions might miss an important reservoir and, therefore, not interrupt the transmission cycle within a community.[13] Another potentially critical problem with current MDA programs is that benzimidazole drug resistance might develop in STHs that infect humans, as has already been documented in intestinal nematodes that infect sheep and cattle, in which these drugs have been used indiscriminately.[14] Widespread use of the benzimidazoles in humans could similarly lead to the development of resistance in the STHs.[15] The same concern exists for praziquantel in the case of schistosomiasis.[16] Given the lack of alternative medications that are effective against the major STHs or schistosomiasis, such a scenario could be potentially devastating.

Unfortunately, the situation is exacerbated by the fact that there are only few new anthelminthic medications that are currently under development. Interestingly, some drugs that have been developed for nonhelminth infections have been found to have effects on some widespread helminth infections and could potentially make up for the dearth of alternative anthelminthics to the current first-line therapies. For example, the artemisinins such as artesunate and artemether, although originally developed as antimalarials, have been shown to be active against the early liver stages of schistosomes.[17] Although not beneficial as monotherapy due to stage-specific activity, combination with existing drugs such as praziquantel is being explored to improve efficacy. Similarly, the antibacterial doxycycline has been shown to be effective in the control of lymphatic filariasis and onchocerciasis,[18] by targeting the *Wolbachia* endosymbionts present in most human filariae, except *Loa loa* that are essential for worm fertility and survival. Treatment with several weeks of doxycycline has been shown to sterilize or kill adult female filarial worms; amelioration of symptomatic disease has also been observed in clinical trials.[19] The use of the artemisinins and doxycycline in the treatment of schistosomiasis and filariasis, respectively, represents exciting new developments in the field of anthelminthic drug research; however, these drugs are covered in separate chapters of this book, given that their primary indications are for microbial and bacterial infections other than helminths.

This chapter gives special attention to the benzimidazoles and praziquantel due to their widespread use throughout the world to treat the STHs and schistosomiasis, respectively. In the United States, these helminthiases are seen predominantly in children who have immigrated from endemic areas. Of the endemically transmitted helminths, infections caused by the dog roundworm, *Toxocara canis*, has emerged as one of the most common helminthiases in the United States as estimated by seroprevalence data, especially in socioeconomically disadvantaged children living in urban areas.[20,21] Albendazole is the treatment of choice for toxocariasis. Finally, cysticercosis caused by infection with the larval stage of the pork tapeworm *Taenia solium* is a leading cause of childhood seizures in the southern states of the United States, particularly in those who have immigrated from Mexico and Central and South America.[22] Both albendazole and praziquantel are first-line agents for treating active cysticercal lesions. Table 28.1 lists the recommended drugs for treating helminthic infections in pediatric patients.

BENZIMIDAZOLE COMPOUNDS

This class of drugs includes some of the most commonly used anthelminthics in the world, such as albendazole, mebendazole, and triclabendazole. Thiabendazole, although previously a widely used benzimidazole, is no longer licensed or available in many countries due to its unfavorable side-effect profile. Albendazole and mebendazole, in particular, are widely used and

TABLE 28.1 Recommended Drugs for Treatment of Pediatric Helminthic Infections

Helminth	*Drug of Choice*
NEMATODES	
Ascaris lumbricoides (roundworm)	Albendazole 400 mg × 1
	Mebendazole 500 mg × 1 or 100 mg b.i.d. × 3 d
	Pyrantel pamoate 11 mg/kg base × 1 (not to exceed 1 g)
	Ivermectin 150–200 µg/kg × 1
	Levamisole 2.5 mg/kg × 1
Trichuris trichiura (whipworm)	Mebendazole 100 mg b.i.d. × 3 d
	Albendazole 400 mg/d × 3 d
Hookworm	
Necator americanus, Ancylostoma duodenale	Albendazole 400 mg × 1
	Mebendazole 500 mg × 1 or 100 mg b.i.d. × 3 d
	Pyrantel pamoate 11 mg/kg/d base × 3 d (not to exceed 1 g/d)
Cutaneous larva migrans (dog and cat hookworm)	Ivermectin 200 µg/kg/d × 1–2 d
	Albendazole 400 mg q.d. × 3–7 d
Enterobius vermicularis (pinworm)	Pyrantel pamoate 11 mg/kg base × 1 (not to exceed 1 g); repeat treatment in 2 wk
	Albendazole 400 mg × 1, repeat in 2 wk
	Mebendazole 100 mg × 1, repeat in 2 wk
	(All family members or persons in close contact with the patient should also be treated)
Strongyloides stercoralis	Ivermectin 200 µg/kg/d × 2 d
	Thiabendazole 50 mg/kg/d divided into two doses × 2–7 d
	(Longer treatment may be required in hyperinfection or disseminated disease)
Capillaria philippinensis	Albendazole 400 mg q.d. × 10 d
	Mebendazole 200 mg b.i.d. × 20 d
Toxocara canis (visceral/ocular larva migrans)	Albendazole 400 mg b.i.d. × 5 d
	Mebendazole 200 mg b.i.d. × 5 d
	(Optimal duration of treatment unknown. For severe disease or ocular involvement, consider corticosteroids)
Trichinella spiralis	Albendazole 400 mg b.i.d. × 8–14 d
	Mebendazole 500 mg t.i.d. × 10 d
	(Consider corticosteroids for severe disease)

TABLE 28.1 Recommended Drugs for Treatment of Pediatric Helminthic Infections (*continued*)

Helminth	*Drug of Choice*
Trichostrongylus spp.	Pyrantel pamoate 11 mg/kg base × 1 (not to exceed 1g)
	Albendazole 400 mg/d × 10 d
	Mebendazole 500 mg/d × 10 d
Gnathostoma spinigerum	Albendazole 400 mg b.i.d. × 21 d
	Ivermectin 200 μg/kg/d × 2 d
FILARIAL NEMATODES	
Lymphatic filariasis (*Wuchereria bancrofti, Brugia malayi, Brugia timori*)	Diethylcarbamazine[a] 6 mg/kg/d × 1–12 d; if high microfilaremia, start at 1 mg/kg × 1 on day 1, 3 mg/kg/d divided into three doses on day 2, 3–6 mg/kg/d divided into three doses on day 3, then 6 mg/kg/d divided into three doses on days 4–12
Tropical pulmonary eosinophilia	Diethylcarbamazine 6 mg/kg/d × 21 d
Loa loa	
Microfilaremia < 2,500/mL	Diethylcarbamazine 9 mg/kg/d divided into three doses × 21 days; may start at start at 50 mg × 1 on day 1, 150 mg divided into three doses on day 2, 300 mg divided into three doses on day 3, then 9 mg/kg/d divided into three doses
Microfilaremia > 2,500/mL	Pretreatment with apheresis or albendazole may be attempted in consultation with an expert.
Onchocerca volvulus	Ivermectin 150 μg/kg × 1 every 6–12 mo[b]
	Moxidectin 8 mg × 1[b]
Mansonella ozzardi	Ivermectin 200 μg/kg × 1[b]
Mansonella perstans	Albendazole 400 mg b.i.d. × 10 d
	Doxycycline 200 mg/d × 1 or 100 mg b.i.d. × 6 wk
Mansonella streptocerca	Diethylcarbamazine 6 mg/kg/d × 12 d
	Ivermectin 150 μg/kg × 1[b]
CESTODES	
Taenia saginata, Taenia solium, Diphyllobothrium latum, Dipylidium caninum	Praziquantel 10 mg/kg × 1
Hymenolepis nana	Praziquantel 25 mg/kg × 1
Taenia solium (neurocysticercosis)	Albendazole 15 mg/kg/d divided into two doses for 7–14 d[c]
	>2 viable parenchymal cysts: add praziquantel 50 mg/kg/d × 10–14 d
	(Consider corticosteroids and anticonvulsants during administration of larvicidal therapy)
Echinococcus granulosus (hydatid disease)	Albendazole 15 mg/kg/d (maximum 800 mg) b.i.d. × 1–6 mo
	(Chemotherapy is usually an adjunct to surgery or percutaneous cyst drainage)
TREMATODES	
Schistosoma haematobium, Schistosoma mansoni, Schistosoma intercalatum	Praziquantel 40 mg/kg/d in 1–2 doses × 1 d
Schistosoma japonicum, Schistosoma mekongi	Praziquantel 60 mg/kg/d in 2–3 doses × 1 d
Fasciola hepatica	Triclabendazole 10 mg/kg × 1
Clonorchis sinensis, Opisthorchis viverrini, Metorchis conjunctus	Praziquantel 75 mg/kg/d divided into 3 three doses × 2 d
Fasciolopsis buski, Heterophyes heterophyes, Metagonimus yokogawai, Echinostoma sp.	Praziquantel 75 mg/kg/d divided into three doses × 1 d
Paragonimus westermani (lung fluke)	Praziquantel 75 mg/kg/d divided into three doses × 2 d
	Triclabendazole 10 mg/kg (may divide dose)

[a]Coadminister with doxycycline 200 mg/d × 6 wk.
[b]Not macrofilaricidal but temporarily decreases blood or skin microfilaria count.
[c]Single-enhancing lesion, maximum dose = 800 mg/d × 7–14 d; viable parenchymal lesion(s) = maximum dose = 1,200 mg/d × 10–14 d.
b.i.d., twice daily; q.d., daily; t.i.d., thrice daily.

have been proven to be extremely effective in the WHO's global deworming programs. Due to their broad spectrum of activities, albendazole and mebendazole are the cornerstone medications for treating intestinal nematode helminth infections. Globally, they are the two major drugs used to treat the pediatric STH infections trichuriasis, ascariasis, and hookworm, which together are estimated to affect over one billion children worldwide.[4] In addition, albendazole is used in combination with diethylcarbamazine (DEC) or ivermectin for the control of lymphatic filariasis in MDA programs in endemic regions.[23]

MECHANISM OF ACTION

The benzimidazoles act by binding irreversibly to intracellular tubulin in nematodes and platyhelminths, thereby inhibiting its polymerization and assembly into microtubules. The loss of cytoplasmic microtubule formation results in impaired uptake of glucose by the adult and larval stages of susceptible helminths,[24] leading to depletion of glycogen stores and reduced production of adenosine triphosphate.[25] Death of the helminth is likely achieved due to this disruption of energy production, which results in starvation of the parasite.[24,26]

ALBENDAZOLE

Albendazole is a broad-spectrum, synthetic, oral benzimidazole-derivative anthelminthic agent. It was originally introduced in Australia in 1977 as an anthelminthic for sheep, and in the early 1980s, it was licensed for human use. Albendazole is comparable in efficacy to mebendazole, but offers two distinct advantages over it. First, for most intestinal nematode infections, albendazole requires only a single administration to be effective. This offers an obvious advantage in ensuring patient compliance, especially in the pediatric population. For MDA programs in endemic regions, albendazole is often preferred over mebendazole due to its greater efficacy and ease of use. Another advantage offered by albendazole is that it has an active metabolite, albendazole sulfoxide, which undergoes slower elimination than the parent drug and likely accounts for most of the activity. For systemic helminth infections such as cysticercosis, albendazole can be administered in moderate doses to achieve the same effect as high doses of mebendazole. Along with mebendazole, albendazole is currently one of the main drugs used to treat intestinal nematode infections, although it should be noted that in the United States, albendazole is not licensed for this indication.

Indications

Albendazole is currently licensed in the United States for the treatment of cystic hydatid disease (echinococcosis) of the liver, lung, and peritoneum caused by the larval form of the dog tapeworm *Echinococcus granulosus*.[27] However, for this disease, albendazole is most often used as an adjunct to surgical excision or percutaneous drainage of hydatid cysts, both preoperatively and postoperatively, to reduce the risk of recurrence due to spillage of scolices during surgery.[28–33] Although the efficacy of albendazole in the treatment of alveolar hydatid disease due to *Echinococcus multilocularis* is less clear than for cystic echinococcosis, it is nevertheless recommended in unresectable cases as well as for 2 years postresection.[31,32,34]

The other label indication for albendazole is for treatment of parenchymal neurocysticercosis due to active lesions caused by the larval forms of the pork tapeworm *T. solium*. In neurocysticercosis, *T. solium* larvae localize to the brain of the human intermediate host where it can remain encysted for years before dying. Albendazole, along with praziquantel, is one of the chemotherapeutic agents used as part of the medical management of this clinical syndrome.[35–40] The role of larvicidal medications such as albendazole in the treatment of neurocysticercosis is complicated and far from straightforward. Albendazole appears to be most effective in symptomatic patients with viable cysts within the cerebral parenchyma and in the rapidly progressive form of cysticercosis.[39] Recent guidelines issued by the Infectious Diseases Society of America and the American Society of Tropical Medicine and Hygiene recommend monotherapy with albendazole for one to two viable cysts but albendazole combined with praziquantel therapy for patients with more than two viable cysts.[39] Cysts that appear calcified on imaging represent old cysticerci that have died, patients with these will not benefit from treatment with albendazole. Evidence from clinical trials indicates that even patients with only a single-ring–enhancing lesion, likely representing a dying cyst, benefit from albendazole therapy in terms of long-term seizure outcome.

Patients with intraventricular or meningeal cysts may be treated with albendazole as part of a multidisciplinary approach that often involves measures to reduce intracranial pressure, and surgery. It is extremely important to note that the use of larvicidal chemotherapy in neurocysticercosis may result in an intense inflammatory response that can induce seizures and life-threatening increases in intracranial pressure. Therefore, concurrent administration of systemic corticosteroids, together with careful monitoring for intracranial hypertension, is recommended in neurocysticercosis patients who receive albendazole, as well as anticonvulsants in patients with seizures.[39,40] Additionally, before initiating albendazole therapy for neurocysticercosis, patients should be examined for ocular cysticerci. If retinal lesions are visualized, the benefits of larvicidal drugs should be weighed against the possibility of permanent visual loss caused by retinal damage due to the inflammatory response to dying larvae.[27]

Besides these approved indications, the most common use of albendazole worldwide is to treat intestinal STH infections due to *A. lumbricoides*, *T. trichiura*, and hookworm. Furthermore, although also not listed on the product label, albendazole has been used to successfully treat cutaneous larva migrans caused by *Ancylostoma braziliense* or *Ancylostoma caninum* (dog and cat hookworm) and enterobiasis.[41,42] When used to treat pinworm infection due to *Enterobius vermicularis*, single-dose treatment should be repeated 2 weeks later to kill worms that have developed from eggs that were not affected by the initial treatment; also, since this infection is highly contagious and other family members are frequently infected, treatment of the entire household is recommended.[42]

Other off-label uses of albendazole include as an alternative agent for treating infection with *Strongyloides stercoralis*, *Capillaria philippinensis*, and *Trichostrongylus*. Albendazole is also used as an alternative treatment for taeniasis caused by adult *T. solium* or *Taenia saginata* (beef tapeworm).[43,44] Even though praziquantel is superior for the treatment of taeniasis, albendazole is often used in endemic countries because it is cheaper and has a broader spectrum of anthelminthic activity.

In visceral larva migrans due to infection with *T. canis* or *Toxocara cati*, the use of chemotherapy is only warranted when the disease is severe or when there is ocular involvement; as with neurocysticercosis, treatment is usually combined with a corticosteroid to reduce the inflammatory response to dying parasites.[45] Albendazole is also used in the treatment of trichinosis (trichinellosis) caused by *Trichinella spiralis*.[46] Administration of the drug is most effective if given early in the course of infection and works by acting on adult worms within the intestinal mucosa before they produce larvae that then penetrate muscle. Systemic corticosteroids are commonly used concurrently, especially in patients with severe symptoms, to minimize potential inflammatory reactions to dying larvae.

Finally, albendazole has recently been used in combination with either DEC or ivermectin for the control of filarial infections.[23] MDA programs for the reduction of morbidity due to *Wuchereria bancrofti* or *Brugia malayi* (lymphatic filariasis) and *Onchocerca volvulus* (river blindness) are the current strategies for these diseases; annual or biannual administration of the drug combinations leads to reduction in microfilaremia, which both reduces the clinical manifestations of infection but also transmission within affected communities.

Pharmacokinetics

Albendazole is poorly and erratically absorbed from the gastrointestinal tract due to its low aqueous solubility.[24,27] However, absorption of albendazole is greatly increased (up to fivefold) if the medication is taken with food containing relatively high-fat content.[24] Albendazole is rapidly metabolized by the liver mostly to its active metabolite albendazole sulfoxide, which undergoes slower elimination than the parent drug, which is, therefore, detectable in only negligible amounts in the plasma. Albendazole sulfoxide is mostly protein bound and is widely distributed throughout the body (as opposed to mebendazole) and can be detected in cerebrospinal fluid (CSF), urine, bile, hydatid cyst fluid, cyst wall, and liver.[24,27,47,48] Urinary excretion of albendazole sulfoxide is minimal, whereas concentrations in bile are similar to those achieved in plasma. Albendazole sulfoxide is also further metabolized to albendazole sulfone and other oxidative metabolites.

Pediatric Considerations

Albendazole has been found to be teratogenic (embryotoxicity and skeletal malformations) in pregnant rats and rabbits.[24,27,49,50] Teratogenicity occurred in rats given oral daily doses of 10 and 30 mg per kg during gestation days 6 to 15 and in rabbits given oral doses of 30 mg per kg daily during gestation days 7 to 19. In the rabbit study, maternal toxicity (33% mortality) was noted at 30 mg per kg daily. Teratogenicity in humans has not been observed, and a study of over 800 women treated with albendazole during the second and third trimesters demonstrated no adverse effects.[51] Use in the first trimester, however, is still not recommended.

Limited studies on the relationship of age to the effects of albendazole have been performed in children younger than 6 years of age. Although hydatid disease is uncommon in infants and young children, no pediatric-specific problems have been documented in infants and young children who were treated with albendazole for this infection. In addition, five studies involving children as young as 1 year of age treated with albendazole for neurocysticercosis, which occurs more frequently than hydatid disease in children, did not document pediatric-specific problems.[27] Given the limited available safety information, albendazole use in children younger than 2 years of age, like that of mebendazole, is not recommended in the prescribing information given by the manufacturer.

Since the 1990s, however, albendazole has been used safely in treating populations of entire communities irrespective of age, sex, or infection status as part of MDA programs. As the result of albendazole's widespread use and the lack of observed pediatric-specific problems, the WHO has developed a different recommendation than the manufacturer's and recommends that it can be used safely in a single, reduced dose of 200 mg in children older than 12 months and less than 24 months of age.[52]

Drug–drug Interactions

Cimetidine

Cimetidine decreases the oral bioavailability of albendazole, either by reducing gastric acid production or inhibiting cytochrome P (CYP) 450-mediated metabolism of albendazole to its active metabolite.[53]

Corticosteroids

Coadministration of albendazole with high-dose corticosteroids (such as in the treatment of neurocysticercosis) has been shown to increase the steady-state plasma concentration of albendazole sulfoxide, possibly by reducing the rate of elimination.[27,54,55] However, no modification of the dose of albendazole is recommended in this situation.

Praziquantel

Praziquantel increases the mean maximum plasma concentration and area under the plasma concentration–time curve of albendazole sulfoxide by approximately 50%, but does not require modification of albendazole dosing.[27]

Theophylline

Although the pharmacodynamics of theophylline was unchanged after a single dose of albendazole when tested in six healthy subjects, this drug has been shown to induce CYP1A activity in human hepatoma cells in vitro.[27] Since theophylline is a substrate for this enzyme, plasma concentrations should be monitored during and following treatment with albendazole.

Precautions

Patients with Biliary Obstruction

Patients with extrahepatic biliary obstruction have reduced elimination of albendazole and increased plasma concentrations of albendazole sulfoxide, potentially increasing the incidence of toxicities such as bone marrow suppression, although no specific dosing modification is recommended by the manufacturer.[27]

Side Effects

Albendazole is generally very well tolerated. The most common reported side effects include abdominal pain, nausea, vomiting, and headache.[26,27,34,55–58] Much less common are hypersensitivity reactions, including rash, urticaria, reversible alopecia, and leukopenia.[27,59] Rarely, agranulocytosis and aplastic anemia can occur. With prolonged therapy such as for hydatid disease, mild-to-moderate elevations of hepatic enzymes can occur that resolve upon discontinuation of the drug, although acute hepatic failure and hepatitis have been reported.[60] Hepatic transaminases should be measured at regular intervals while on extended therapy.

Pediatric Dosage

Albendazole is available only as an oral tablet: for younger children, tablets should be crushed or chewed and swallowed. Information on the use of albendazole in children less than 12 months old is limited. If used for extended periods at high doses such as for hydatid disease, complete blood counts with leukocyte differential and hepatic transaminases should be performed regularly due to the risk of blood dyscrasias and hepatitis, respectively.

- *Ascariasis, trichuriasis, hookworm*: 400 mg as a single dose. For trichuriasis, three daily doses may be required.
- *Cystic hydatid disease*: 15 mg per kg per day (maximum 800 mg) in two divided doses for 3 to 6 months when only medical management is attempted. Given in 28-day cycles with 14-day albendazole-free intervals. When used as an adjunct to surgery or percutaneous drainage, it should be started at least 1 week prior to drainage and for up to 1 to 2 months after.
- *Neurocysticercosis:*
    - Single-enhancing lesion: 15 mg per kg per day (maximum 800 mg) in two divided doses for 7 to 14 days
    - Viable parenchymal lesion(s): 15 mg per kg per day (maximum 1,200 mg) in two divided doses for 10 to 14 days. Retreatment should be considered for lesions persisting for 6 months after the end of the initial course of therapy.
- *Cutaneous larva migrans*: 400 mg daily for 3 to 7 days
- *Toxocariasis (visceral and ocular larval migrans)*: 400 mg twice daily for 5 days
- *Capillariasis*: 400 mg daily for 10 days
- *Enterobiasis*: 400 mg as a single dose; repeat in 2 weeks
- *Trichinosis*: 400 mg twice daily for 8 to 14 days
- *Trichostrongyliasis*: 400 mg daily for 10 days

WHO Recommendation

In community MDA programs for intestinal helminthiases, a single 200-mg dose of albendazole has been shown to be both safe and effective in children older than 12 months and younger than 24 months.[23] Children older than 24 months should receive the full 400-mg dose during MDA programs.

MEBENDAZOLE

Mebendazole is an orally administered, synthetic benzimidazole that has a broad spectrum of anthelminthic activity and a low incidence of adverse effects. It was originally licensed in the United States by the Food and Drug Administration (FDA) in 1974, but it was unavailable for several years until 2015, when a marketing application was approved. It is structurally similar to albendazole, and, like albendazole, it is particularly effective against susceptible intestinal nematodes, such as *A. lumbricoides*, *T. trichiura*, *E. vermicularis*, and hookworm. Together with pyrantel pamoate, albendazole, and levamisole, mebendazole is one of the four essential broad-spectrum anthelminthics recommended by the WHO for the treatment of intestinal nematode infections.

Indications

Mebendazole is used to treat the most common intestinal nematodes, such as ascariasis, enterobiasis, trichuriasis, and hookworm infections (*A. duodenale* and *N. americanus*).[61–63] It is one of the most commonly used drugs in MDA programs worldwide for the control of intestinal nematode infections, although single-dose mebendazole has been shown in several studies to be less effective against these helminths than single-dose albendazole.[61] Although not specifically licensed for these indications, mebendazole is also used to treat infections caused by *C. philippinensis* and *Gnathostoma spinigerum*.[25,64]

Since mebendazole is poorly adsorbed from the gastrointestinal tract, it is not a recommended first-line treatment for tissue-dwelling helminth infections, such as cysticercosis or hydatid disease. Although mebendazole has been used in the past as an adjunct treatment for hydatid and alveolar echinococcosis, it has since been replaced by albendazole for these infections due to its superior systemic absorption from the gastrointestinal tract.

Mebendazole is also used as an alternative to albendazole in the treatment of trichinosis.[46] As with albendazole, treatment is most effective if given early in the course of infection and concomitant administration of systemic corticosteroids reduces the likelihood of complications due to inflammatory reactions to dying parasites.

Pharmacokinetics

Mebendazole has limited solubility in water; therefore, only 5% to 10% is absorbed from the gastrointestinal tract.[65] However, absorption is increased when it is ingested with fatty foods, although even then the amount absorbed shows remarkable interindividual variability.[24] Given its poor absorption, mebendazole is poorly effective in treating systemic helminth infections. Whatever is absorbed undergoes rapid first-pass metabolism in the liver to multiple different protein-bound metabolites. Clearance is predominantly as metabolites in urine and bile, although the majority is found unchanged in the feces due to lack of absorption.[24]

Pediatric Considerations

Mebendazole crosses the placenta, and studies in rats given single oral doses as low as 10 mg per kg have shown it to be teratogenic and embryotoxic. However, a study in pregnant women who inadvertently took mebendazole during the first trimester did not show an incidence of spontaneous abortion or malformation greater than that of the general population.[62] Additionally, studies in which pregnant women were specifically treated with mebendazole have shown no increase in spontaneous abortions or congenital defects.[66] Due to the important impact of hookworm infection and other STHs during pregnancy, the WHO recommends the use of mebendazole during the second and third trimesters of pregnancy.

Although the use of mebendazole in children younger than 2 years has traditionally not been recommended, this was solely on the basis of a lack of adequate safety information in this age group. However, several large studies have shown the anthelminthic efficacy of this drug in this age group without significant adverse effects.[67] Accordingly, the WHO recommends that mebendazole can be safely used in children between the ages of 12 and 24 months, in addition to use in older children.[52]

Drug–drug Interactions

Carbamazepine

Carbamazepine lowers mebendazole plasma concentrations by inducing hepatic microsomal enzymes, thereby impairing the therapeutic response. Adjustment of dosage may be required.[68]

Metronidazole

Stevens–Johnson syndrome and toxic epidermal necrolysis have been reported when mebendazole was used in combination with metronidazole.[69] Therefore, this combination should be avoided.

Precautions

Patients with Inflammatory Bowel Disease

Patients with inflammatory bowel disease (Crohn disease or ulcerative colitis) may experience increased absorption and toxicity of mebendazole, especially if given in high doses.[70]

Patients with Hepatic Impairment

Patients with impaired hepatic function may experience increased incidence of side effects because of reduced metabolism of the drug. Accordingly, the dose may need to be decreased.

Side Effects

Mebendazole is very well tolerated, likely due to its poor absorption, so systemic side effects are rare. Reported side effects include gastrointestinal disturbances such as abdominal pain, diarrhea, nausea, and vomiting; headache and dizziness; hypersensitivity reactions such as fever, skin rash, and pruritis; and seizures in infants.[24,47,62] Transient increases in serum levels of hepatic transaminases, alkaline phosphatase, and blood urea nitrogen may be seen following prolonged periods of use.[47] Similarly, although not commonly used now for this indication, high-dose therapy for hydatid disease has been associated with development of alopecia and reversible neutropenia and lymphopenia.[47]

Pediatric Dosage

Mebendazole is supplied as a chewable tablet or suspension for oral administration. Due to the lack of safety information and postmarketing reports of seizures in children younger than 12 months, use of mebendazole in the age group should be avoided.

- *Ascariasis, hookworm*: 500 mg as a single dose or 100 mg twice daily for 3 days
- *Trichuriasis:* 100 mg twice daily for 3 days
- *Enterobiasis*: 100 mg as a single dose. Repeat in 2 weeks
- *Capillariasis*: 200 mg twice daily for 20 days
- *Trichinosis*: 500 mg three times daily for 10 days

WHO Recommendation

For the treatment of intestinal nematodes, mebendazole can be safely used in children between the ages of 12 and 24 months when given at the same dose as for older children.[52]

TRICLABENDAZOLE

Triclabendazole is a benzimidazole compound that differs from others in this class, in that it lacks activity against nematodes. However, it has been widely used since coming onto the market in 1983 for the treatment of fascioliasis in livestock, for which it is very effective. The first reported use of triclabendazole to treat fascioliasis in humans was in 1986.[71] It has been on the WHO's list of essential medicines since 1997 and was licensed for the treatment of fascioliasis in the United States in 2019.

Fascioliasis is an infection of livestock, such as cattle and sheep, but humans can be infected by eating raw or undercooked aquatic vegetables such as watercress that are contaminated with encysted larvae. Fascioliasis has become a foodborne infection of significant importance in several areas of the world, such as the Andean Highlands of Bolivia, Ecuador, and Peru, the Nile Delta of Egypt, and northern Iran. Because praziquantel is not generally efficacious for the treatment of fascioliasis, triclabendazole is an important drug in the treatment and control of this infection.

Indications

Triclabendazole is the first-line treatment for infections caused by *Fasciola hepatica* (sheep liver fluke) and *Fasciola gigantica* (giant liver fluke). It is active against both adult *Fasciola* worms present in the biliary ducts and also against the immature larval stages that migrate through the hepatic parenchyma.[71–73] Triclabendazole is also used as an alternative agent in the treatment of infections caused by *Paragonimus westermani* (lung fluke).[74,75]

Pharmacokinetics

Following oral administration, absorption of triclabendazole from the gastrointestinal tract is increased two- to threefold when taken after a fatty meal.[73,74] The drug undergoes extensive first-pass metabolism in the liver, where it is oxidized to active sulfoxide and sulfone metabolites that are highly protein bound.[76] Triclabendazole and its metabolites are further hydroxylated by the liver and secreted into the biliary tract. Approximately 95% of orally administered triclabendazole (unchanged or as metabolites) is secreted in bile.

Pediatric Considerations

Safety data on the use of triclabendazole in children are limited.[73,74] However, children in fascioliasis- and paragonimiasis-endemic regions have been successfully treated with triclabendazole, without pediatric-specific adverse reactions being reported. In the United States, this drug is only approved for children aged 6 years and older due to inadequate safety information in younger children.

Side Effects

Treatment with triclabendazole is generally well tolerated. Mild and transient abdominal pain, biliary colic, nausea, vomiting, fever, and hepatomegaly, as well as transient increases in hepatic enzymes, are likely related to self-limited biliary obstruction caused by the dying liver flukes.[71,73,74,77]

Pediatric Usage

Triclabendazole is supplied as chewable tablets.

- *Fascioliasis:* 10 mg per kg as a single dose. Treatment may be repeated after 2 weeks or 6 months if necessary. The WHO recommends 20 mg per kg in two doses given 12 hours apart for severe cases of fascioliasis.
- *Paragonimiasis:* 10 mg per kg as a single dose or twice in one day

THIABENDAZOLE

Thiabendazole was the first benzimidazole anthelminthic to be developed and was licensed for human use by the FDA in 1967. Although it is one of the most potent anthelminthic drugs, thiabendazole is also one of the least tolerated, given its association with a high incidence of side effects such as gastrointestinal upset. Accordingly, thiabendazole has largely been replaced by the newer benzimidazoles, such as albendazole and mebendazole, and marketing approval in the United States has been discontinued by the manufacturer.

Indications

With the development of less toxic anthelminthics such as mebendazole, albendazole, and ivermectin, oral thiabendazole is now uncommonly used in areas of the world where it is still registered for the treatment of helminth infections. These include infection with *S. stercoralis* and *T. spiralis*, as well as for cutaneous and visceral larva migrans. Because of the toxicity associated with oral administration, off-label topical application of the oral suspension has been used in treating localized cutaneous larva migrans, although this is not an approved use of the drug.

In the past, a topical formulation of thiabendazole was marketed for the treatment of cutaneous larva migrans. This form of the drug is no longer commercially available in North America, although off-label topical application of the oral suspension has been used for this indication.[73]

Oral thiabendazole may be used to treat infections with *S. stercoralis*, including the hyperinfection syndrome, in both immunosuppressed and immunocompetent patients. However, ivermectin has effectively supplanted its use for this indication due to possible greater efficacy (although results of comparative studies are mixed) and lower incidence of side effects.[78,79] Combination therapy with ivermectin has been suggested by some experts, especially for disseminated strongyloidiasis, although results from clinical trials are lacking.[80] Thiabendazole is also indicated for the treatment of visceral larva migrans and trichinosis; when used during the invasion stage of infection with *T. spiralis*, thiabendazole has been associated with improvement in symptoms and fever as well as reduction in eosinophilia.[81] Although not listed on the product label, thiabendazole has also been successfully used to treat capillariasis and trichostrongyliasis.

Given its relatively higher toxicity and lower effectiveness, thiabendazole should not be considered a first-line treatment for ascariasis, enterobiasis, trichuriasis, or hookworm infection, although it may be used if more effective and less toxic drugs are unavailable or their use is contraindicated.

Pharmacokinetics

Thiabendazole is rapidly and well absorbed from the gastrointestinal tract and reaches peak plasma concentrations within 1 to 2 hours. Thiabendazole differs from both mebendazole and albendazole, in that it undergoes both hepatic and renal elimination. Following absorption, it is rapidly metabolized by the liver to inactive 5-hydroxythiabendazole, which is further metabolized into glucuronide and sulfate conjugates that are eliminated in the urine within 48 hours after an oral dose.

Pediatric Considerations

Since data on the safety and effectiveness of thiabendazole in children weighing less than 13.6 kg (30 lb) are limited, the use of this medication in such children is not recommended by the manufacturer. Reproduction studies in rabbits given doses of up to 15 times the usual human dose and in rats given doses equivalent to the usual human have not resulted in teratogenic effects. However, in another study in mice given 10 times the usual human dose in olive oil (but not in aqueous suspension), cleft palate and axial skeletal defects were observed. Because of this, use of thiabendazole is not recommended during pregnancy. Furthermore, since it is not known if thiabendazole is excreted in breast milk, the drug should not be administered to nursing mothers.

Drug–drug Interactions

Theophylline

Thiabendazole may compete with theophylline for sites of hepatic metabolism and reduce its clearance by more than 50%, raising its serum levels to potentially toxic concentrations.[82,83] Blood levels of theophylline should, therefore, be monitored carefully when these drugs are administered together.

Precautions

Hepatic and Renal Impairment

Thiabendazole levels can be increased in patients with renal or hepatic impairment, and dosage may need to be adjusted.[84]

Side Effects

Thiabendazole is one of the more poorly tolerated anthelminthics. Among the more common side effects are gastrointestinal reactions such as anorexia, diarrhea, nausea, abdominal pain, and vomiting which may sometimes be severe, and neurologic reactions such as dizziness, fatigue, headache, irritability, and numbness or tingling of the hands and feet. Less commonly, hypersensitivity reactions may be observed, including skin rashes, erythema multiforme, and, rarely, fatal Stevens–Johnson syndrome.[85] Intrahepatic cholestasis, jaundice, and parenchymal liver damage have been reported in patients treated with thiabendazole, and in some cases, hepatic damage has been severe and irreversible.

Rarely, ocular symptoms (blurred vision and abnormal sensation in the eyes), drying of the mucous membranes, and sicca syndrome have been reported, sometimes lasting for prolonged periods after use of thiabendazole.[86] In some patients, neuropsychiatric toxicity can be severe and includes seizures, tinnitus, delirium, confusion, and hallucinations. An interesting yet harmless effect has been reported by some patients who excrete a metabolite that imparts an asparagus-like or other unusual odor to the urine.

Pediatric Usage

Where available, thiabendazole is supplied as chewable tablets or an oral suspension (100 mg per mL). Experience with thiabendazole in children weighing less than 13.6 kg (30 lb) is limited.

- *Strongyloidiasis*: 50 mg per kg daily divided into two doses, for 2 days. For hyperinfection syndrome: 50 mg per kg daily divided into two doses, for 5 to 7 days. May be repeated if required
- *Cutaneous larva migrans*: 50 mg per kg daily divided into two doses for 2 to 4 days
- *Visceral larva migrans, trichinosis*: 50 mg per kg daily divided into two doses for 2 to 4 days

OTHER ANTINEMATODE AGENTS

PYRANTEL PAMOATE

Pyrantel pamoate is a tetrahydropyrimidine-derived anthelminthic agent first developed for veterinarian use in 1966. In 1971, it was approved by the FDA for the treatment of pinworm (*E. vermicularis*) infections, but it is now sold over the counter for this indication and is no longer a regulated product. It is listed by the WHO as one of the four essential broad-spectrum drugs for intestinal helminth infections and has been extensively used in helminth control programs, especially in Latin America and South-East Asia.

Indications

In the United States, pyrantel has been primarily used for the treatment of pinworm. However, it is also very effective against the intestinal nematodes *A. lumbricoides* and *Trichostrongylus*.[61,42,87] It is only moderately effective against both species of hookworm, *N. americanus* than *A. duodenale*.[61] It is not very effective in treating either trichuriasis or strongyloidiasis.

Mechanism of Action

Pyrantel pamoate binds to an ion channel that forms a nicotinic acetylcholine receptor on the body muscle of nematodes.[88] Binding to the recognition site of this excitatory receptor induces entry of calcium, which, in turn, leads to depolarization and spastic paralysis of the nematode muscle that can result in passive expulsion of the worm from the host's gastrointestinal tract.[89] Because pyrantel causes paralysis of the worms prior to expulsion, they are typically expelled intact, which makes it useful as a tool for identifying the morphologic features of adult parasites.

Pharmacokinetics

Pyrantel is poorly and incompletely absorbed from the gastrointestinal tract, with a time to peak concentration of between 1 and 3 hours.[42,87] The drug is partially metabolized in the liver, and a small percentage is excreted in the urine, while the majority is eliminated unchanged in the feces.

Pediatric Considerations

Studies in animals have not shown that pyrantel causes adverse effects in the fetus. Adequate and well-controlled studies in humans have not been done. The use of pyrantel in the first trimester of pregnancy is not recommended.

As with albendazole and mebendazole, children younger than 2 years who are infected with helminths are excluded from treatment with pyrantel on the basis of the information given by the manufacturers of the drugs. However, this recommendation is made solely on the basis of a lack of information on the treatment of this age group, rather than studies documenting adverse effects. Furthermore, the WHO has been using pyrantel as a single dose for the treatment of STH infections in endemic communities for years, and no age-specific adverse effects have been reported.

Precautions

Two cases have been reported of patients with myasthenia gravis with worsening of symptoms after use of pyrantel.[90,91] Although a cause-and-effect relationship was not clearly established in either care, caution should be exercised when prescribing pyrantel to patients with this autoimmune disorder.

Side Effects

Side effects of pyrantel are generally mild and transient and include diarrhea, abdominal cramps, nausea, vomiting, and headache. Less common neurologic effects, such as dizziness, drowsiness, irritability, and insomnia, may also occur. In some individuals, skin hypersensitivity reactions, such as rash and pruritis, have been reported.[42,87] Transient mild elevations in serum hepatic transaminases have been detected in up to 2% of patients after a single dose.[87]

Pediatric Dosage

Pyrantel pamoate is supplied as either chewable tablets or an oral suspension (50 mg per mL). Children younger than 2 years and those weighing less than 11 kg (24.2 lb) should not be treated with pyrantel pamoate. For children older than 2 years, the maximum dosage should not exceed 1 g.

- *Ascariasis, trichostrongyliasis, enterobiasis:* 11 mg per kg base as a single dose. For enterobiasis, repeat in 2 weeks.

WHO Recommendation

Pyrantel pamoate is one of the four drugs recommended by the WHO as essential medications for the treatment of soil-transmitted helminthiases. For the treatment of *Ascaris*, *Trichuris*, and hookworm infections in MDA programs, pyrantel pamoate is given as a single 10 mg per kg dose, regardless of age.

LEVAMISOLE

Levamisole hydrochloride is a synthetic imidazothiazole derivative with both broad-spectrum anthelminthic and immunomodulating activities. It was first marketed as a veterinary anthelminthic in Belgium in 1965 but was licensed for human use in Brazil in 1966. However, the drug was never approved in the United States as an anthelminthic, but rather as an adjunct therapy with 5-fluorouracil after surgical resection in patients with Dukes stage C colon cancer. Since it was withdrawn from the market by the manufacturer in 2001, the drug is no longer commercially available in the United States or in many other countries. Nonetheless, it remains one of the four broad-spectrum anthelminthics recommended by the WHO for the treatment of intestinal nematodes together with albendazole, mebendazole, and pyrantel pamoate.

Indications

Although not available in the United States, levamisole is still used in helminth control programs in parts of the world. In several clinical trials conducted in endemic areas, levamisole has been shown to be very effective in treating *A. lumbricoides* and *Trichostrongylus*, although it has shown considerably less activity against hookworm, *T. trichiura*, *S. stercoralis*, and *E. vermicularis*.[61]

Mechanism of Action

Levamisole binds to an ion channel that forms a nicotinic acetylcholine receptor on the body muscle of nematodes.[88] Binding to the recognition site of this excitatory receptor induces entry of calcium, which, in turn, leads to depolarization and spastic paralysis of the nematode muscle that can result in passive expulsion of the worm from the host's gastrointestinal tract.[89]

Pharmacokinetics

The drug is rapidly and almost completely absorbed from the gastrointestinal tract, after which it is metabolized in the liver and then eliminated in the urine largely as metabolites within 2 days of ingestion.[92,93]

Pediatric Considerations

Levamisole has been widely administered as single-dose treatments in global helminth control programs. No specific adverse effects in children have been reported. Levamisole is excreted in breast milk, and treatment of nursing mothers is not recommended.

Side Effects

When used as a single-dose treatment for nematode infections, levamisole is generally well tolerated. Although blood dyscrasias, including agranulocytosis and leukopenia, have been reported following prolonged high-dose adjuvant treatment for colon cancer, these have not been observed when used as an anthelminthic. Mostly mild and transient side effects have been reported, including nausea, vomiting, abdominal pain, dizziness, and headache.[94]

Pediatric Dosage

Levamisole is supplied as chewable tablets for oral administration.

- *Ascariasis, Trichostrongylus*: 2.5 mg per kg as a single dose

ANTIFILARIAL ANTHELMINTHICS

The medications ivermectin and DEC have traditionally formed this class of anthelminthics, although albendazole also has antifilarial activity and is used in combination with both of these drugs as part of MDA programs in endemic areas. In 2018, the U.S. FDA approved moxidectin, a milbemycin-class macrocyclic lactone, for the management of onchocerciasis.

IVERMECTIN

Ivermectin is a semisynthetic, oral macrocyclic lactone derived from the avermectins, a class of broad-spectrum antiparasitic agents produced naturally by *Streptomyces avermitilis*. The drug was originally developed as a veterinary product but was approved for human use by the FDA in 1996. Worldwide, it has been used primarily for the treatment of filarial infections: the WHO lists ivermectin as a core essential antifilarial drug and recommends its use for the treatment of onchocerciasis, or river blindness. In the United States, the drug is also licensed for the treatment of *S. stercoralis* intestinal infections.

Mechanism of Action

The specific mechanism by which ivermectin exerts its microfilaricidal effect is unclear.[95] However, it binds selectively and with high affinity to glutamate-gated chloride ion channels in invertebrate muscle and nerve cells of microfilaria, and it is postulated that this binding causes an increase in the permeability of the cell membrane to chloride ions, resulting in hyperpolarization of the cell that leads to paralysis and death of the parasite. It is also believed to act as an agonist of the neurotransmitter γ-aminobutyric acid (GABA), thereby disrupting GABA-mediated neurosynaptic transmission in the central nervous system (CNS).[95–97]

Although not macrofilaricidal (i.e., does not kill adult worms), ivermectin may also impair normal intrauterine development of *O. volvulus* microfilariae and inhibit their release from the uteri of gravid female worms.

Indications

Ivermectin is licensed in the United States for the treatment of onchocerciasis and intestinal strongyloidiasis. For the management and control of river blindness caused by *O. volvulus*, it is the drug of choice.[18,96,98] The drug has no effect on adult *O. volvulus* worms; rather, the microfilariae are targeted. Since it is the host reaction to microfilaria that results in most of the pathology due to this infection, repeated episodic treatment with ivermectin has been shown to reduce levels of microfilaria in the skin and cornea and thus prevent morbidity.[99] In endemic regions, annual treatment with 150 μg per kg effectively and drastically reduces transmission of *O. volvulus* and the incidence of river blindness.[99,100] Although not licensed for this use, ivermectin is also used for the treatment of several other filarial parasites, including *W. bancrofti*, *B. malayi*, *Mansonella ozzardi*, and *L. loa*.[18,98,101,102] Furthermore, global elimination programs targeting lymphatic filariasis incorporate ivermectin as a component of MDA regimens in combination with DEC or albendazole,[101,102] although a recent randomized controlled trial demonstrated the superiority of coadministering all three microfilaricidal drugs over two-drug combinations in sustained reduction in microfilaremia.[103]

Besides onchocerciasis, the other primary indication for ivermectin is in the treatment of strongyloidiasis. Ivermectin is the treatment of choice for both intestinal and disseminated strongyloidiasis because of its favorable side-effect profile compared to thiabendazole, although the manufacturer only lists the intestinal, no disseminated form of the infection as an approved indication.[79,80,96,104,105] For uncomplicated intestinal disease, treatment for 2 days is recommended; in the case of immunocompromised patients, treatment should be repeated 2 to 3 weeks after the first course to ensure eradication of the infection. For hyperinfection and/or disseminated infection, daily treatment should be continued until resolution of symptoms and larvae has not been detected in the feces or sputum for at least 2 weeks (i.e., the duration of one autoinfection cycle). Some authors recommend continuing ivermectin in individuals with a history of hyperinfection for prolonged periods, given the possibility of relapse that has been documented following treatment and apparent clearance of the parasite, especially if a state of immunocompromise continues.[106]

Ivermectin has been shown to be highly effective in treating cutaneous larva migrans and is generally considered to be the treatment of choice for this condition.[107,108] Single-dose treatment is usually effective, although, in some cases, one or two additional doses may be necessary. Although not usually used for treating ascariasis, ivermectin does have good activity against this nematode infection, although its efficacy for treating hookworm or *T. trichiura* is much poorer.[109]

Besides being an effective anthelminthic, single-dose ivermectin is also very effective in treating scabies.

Pharmacokinetics

Ivermectin is absorbed from the gastrointestinal tract into the blood following oral administration and reaches peak plasma levels in 4 hours.[96,97,110] It is metabolized by the liver and is excreted in the feces over an estimated period of 12 days, with less than 1% of the dose excreted in the urine. The drug does not cross the blood–brain barrier.

Pediatric Considerations

Given the lack of well-controlled safety and efficacy studies in young children, the use of ivermectin is not recommended in children weighing less than 15 kg (33 lb).[97] Similarly, adequate studies have not been conducted in pregnant women. Although some studies of mothers who had been inadvertently treated with ivermectin during pregnancy have reported no significant increase in the rate of spontaneous abortion, stillbirth, or major congenital malformations, a recent meta-analysis of available data concluded that there is insufficient evidence to assess the safety profile of ivermectin in pregnancy.[111,112]

Precautions

Patients who are coinfected with *O. volvulus* and *L. loa* and who receive ivermectin as part of MDA programs targeting the former may suffer from serious encephalopathy following treatment.[113,114] The etiology of this adverse effect is not well understood, but it has been shown to correlate with the level of *L. loa* microfilaremia.[114]

Side Effects

Ivermectin is generally well tolerated. The most common side effects are mild abdominal pain, abdominal distention, nausea, diarrhea, dizziness, and pruritis. When used in the treatment of onchocerciasis, multiple adverse reactions have been reported, although most of these are likely due to the body's reaction to the dying microfilaria than to direct effects of the drug. These are more common in patients with advanced disease and high microfilariae counts in the eye. They include limbitis, punctate opacity, conjunctivitis, and eyelid edema (eye or eyelid irritation, pain, redness, or swelling). These side effects usually resolve without corticosteroid treatment. Other side effects reported during the treatment of onchocerciasis include arthralgia, myalgia, facial and peripheral edema, headache, fever, lymphadenopathy, pruritis, and tachycardia. Many of these side effects can be effectively treated. For instance, systemic corticosteroids may be administered concurrently either with ivermectin or with the onset of severe reactions. Antihistamines and analgesics may also be used to alleviate some of the side effects, which usually peak around the second or third day following ivermectin administration.

Patients taking ivermectin for the treatment of strongyloidiasis and other helminthiases report a different set of side effects, including diarrhea, dizziness, skin rash, postural hypotension, anorexia, somnolence, and tremor.[96]

Pediatric Dosage

Ivermectin is only indicated for children weighing 15 kg (33 lb) or more due to a lack of safety information in smaller children. The drug is supplied as oral tablets that should be taken on an empty stomach with liquids.

- *Onchocerciasis*: 150 μg per kg as a single dose; may be repeated every 6 to 12 months, depending on the recurrence of symptoms and/or microfilariae in the skin
- *Strongyloidiasis*: 200 μg per kg daily for 2 days. In general, additional doses are not necessary, except in select patients with hyperinfection syndrome or disseminated disease. Follow-up fecal examination should be performed to verify clearance of infection.
- *Cutaneous larva migrans*: 200 μg per kg daily for 1 to 2 days

WHO Recommendation

The WHO recommends community-wide annual or biannual treatment with a single-oral dose of 150 μg per kg ivermectin in regions where onchocerciasis is endemic.[23] In areas where lymphatic filariasis is co-endemic with onchocerciasis (and therefore DEC is contraindicated), ivermectin should be administered in combination with a single dose of albendazole.[23] In regions of Central and West Africa where onchocerciasis and *L. loa* are coexist, the WHO recommends use of ivermectin if onchocerciasis is hyperendemic given because the potential benefits are thought to outweigh the risk of encephalopathy; however, in areas where loiasis is endemic but onchocerciasis is hypoendemic, use of ivermectin is not recommended, although alternative strategies such as "test and not treat" using new point-of-care tests for *L. loa* are being evaluated.[115]

MOXIDECTIN

Moxidectin is an oral macrocyclic lactone of the milbemycin subfamily that is produced by the actinomycete *Streptomyces cyanogriseus*. Like ivermectin, the drug has been used extensively in veterinary medicine but was approved for human use by the FDA in 2018 as a treatment option for onchocerciasis. However, it is not yet widely commercially available.

Mechanism of Action

The mechanism by which moxidectin exerts its microfilaricidal effect is unknown, but is assumed to be similar to that of ivermectin. Like ivermectin, moxidectin binds with high affinity to glutamate-gated chloride ion channels in microfilaria, causing increased cell membrane permeability to chloride ions that can result in paralysis and death of the parasite.[116] Moxidectin has no effect on the macrofilarial stage of *O. volvulus*.

Indications

Although used for decades as an anthelminthic by veterinarians, moxidectin was licensed for use in humans only in 2018 and only for the treatment of onchocerciasis.[117] The drug is microfilaricidal and has no effect on adult *O. volvulus* worms. Treatment with a single dose of moxidectin has been shown to dramatically and sustainably reduce levels of microfilaremia in endemic regions.[118] Given moxidectin's rapid microfilaricidal effect and its considerably longer half-life compared to ivermectin, it has the potential to have a greater impact on transmission of *O. volvulus* and the incidence of river blindness than ivermectin. However, it has not yet been incorporated into MDA programs in endemic areas since clinical trials in children have yet to be completed and registration in many affected countries is pending.

Besides being effective against *O. volvulus* microfilariae, single-dose moxidectin also appears to effective in treating soil-transmitted intestinal nematode infections including *T. trichiura*, although these indications are still being evaluated in clinical trials and have not been added to the drug's label.[119]

Pharmacokinetics

Moxidectin is absorbed from the gastrointestinal tract into the blood following oral administration and reaches peak plasma levels in 3 hours.[120,121] It is minimally metabolized in the liver and has a plasma half-life of between 20 and 43 days.

Pediatric Considerations

Given the lack of well-controlled safety and efficacy studies in children younger than 12 years, the use of moxidectin is not recommended in this age group.[117] Similarly, adequate studies have not been conducted in pregnant women.

Precautions

Patients who are coinfected with *O. volvulus* and *L. loa* may develop potentially fatal encephalopathy following treatment with moxidectin, especially at high levels of *L. loa* microfilaremia.[117]

Side Effects

The most common side effects (seen in >10%) of moxidectin are pruritus, myalgias, arthralgias, headache, lymphopenia, rash, nausea, diarrhea, leukocytosis, fever, cough, dizziness, lymph node pain, and peripheral edema.[117,120,122] As with ivermectin, many of these reactions may be secondary to the inflammatory response to dying microfilaria rather directly related to the drug.

When used in the treatment of onchocerciasis, multiple adverse reactions of varying severity have been reported and are thought to be due to inflammatory and allergic host responses to dying microfilaria, termed the Mazzotti reaction.[122] These are more common in patients with high microfilariae counts. They include pruritus, rash, fever, chills, urticaria, hypotension (including symptomatic orthostatic hypotension), peripheral edema and worsening onchodermatitis, and ophthalmologic reactions (ocular discomfort or pain, blurred vision, photophobia, conjunctivitis, and eyelid edema). These side effects usually resolve within the first week following treatment. Treatment with antihistamines and/or analgesics is usually sufficient for mild-to-moderate reactions, whereas parenteral corticosteroids have been used to manage more severe reactions.

Pediatric Dosage

Ivermectin is only indicated for children older than 12 years due to a lack of safety information in younger children. The drug is supplied as oral tablets that should be taken on an empty stomach with liquids.

- *Onchocerciasis*: 8 mg as a single dose (with or without food)

DIETHYLCARBAMAZINE

Diethylcarbamazine (DEC), a synthetic derivative of piperazine, is a highly effective antifilarial drug that has been in use since the 1940s. It is the drug of choice in the treatment of lymphatic filariasis, including tropical pulmonary eosinophilia, and loiasis. In contrast to ivermectin, DEC has both macrofilaricidal (against the adult worm) and microfilaricidal (against the larvae) properties.[123] Unfortunately, manufacturing and marketing of DEC was discontinued in the United States in 2007 due to the paucity of filariasis cases in this country, in addition to its decreasing use in the veterinary field due to the availability of newer drugs. Although it is not commercially available in the United States, the drug can still be obtained from the Drug Service of the Centers for Disease Control and Prevention (CDC) on an investigational use basis.

However, in regions of the world where lymphatic filariasis is endemic such as India, sub-Saharan Africa, and South-East Asia, DEC is available through the auspices of the WHO for control programs in which annual community-wide single-dose administration has been shown to drastically reduce transmission and, over time, the number of infected individuals in the community. In China, for example, where during the 1950s there were more than 30 million cases of lymphatic filariasis, the widespread use of DEC has resulted in the elimination of transmission.

Indications

DEC remains a mainstay for both the curative and suppressive therapy of systemic lymphatic filariasis caused by *W. bancrofti*, *B. malayi*, and *Brugia timori* and loiasis caused by *L. loa*.[18,123,124] Although administration of multiday courses of DEC can be curative for lymphatic filariasis and loiasis, worldwide, the most common use of DEC is in community-wide filariasis control programs in endemic regions, where the goal is suppression of microfilaremia to interrupt the transmission cycle. Once-yearly single-dose administration of the drug, either alone or in combination with albendazole or ivermectin, reduces blood microfilaria levels by greater than 90% for a full year and is highly effective in reducing the number of new infections in these communities over time.[125] Some studies have shown an improved effect on microfilaremia when DEC is administered in combination with albendazole over DEC alone, although a recent systematic review did not significantly improve clearance of microfilaremia or adult filarial worms.[126] Nevertheless, WHO still recommends this strategy as part of lymphatic filariasis elimination programs. Interestingly, in the past, DEC-fortified salt has been used in areas such as parts of China to eliminate lymphatic filariasis, although currently, this strategy is not being pursued.[127]

Mechanism of Action

DEC has primarily microfilaricidal actions, but it also has some activity against adult *W. bancrofti*, *B. malayi*, and *B. timori* worms.[128] Despite more than 70 years of use, the mechanism of action remains unclear, although it likely involves both direct effects against the worm and indirect effects on the host. Pharmacologic studies have shown that DEC inhibits the synthesis of cyclooxygenase products such as prostacyclin and prostaglandin-E2 by microfilariae.[129] DEC can also induce fragmentation of nuclear DNA in microfilariae, leading to induction of apoptosis. Additionally, DEC may alter the host–parasite interface at the level of the immune system by inducing host mechanisms that lead to the degeneration of the parasite.[130]

Pharmacokinetics

DEC is rapidly absorbed following oral administration and widely distributed in nonfatty tissues. It undergoes primarily hepatic metabolism to DEC *N*-oxide.[131] Peak serum concentrations are reached in 1 to 2 hours, and it is excreted, largely as urinary metabolites, within 48 hours.

Pediatric Considerations

Although no specific safety studies of DEC have been performed in children, experience from many years of use in filariasis eradication programs in endemic areas has not indicated any pediatric-specific problems.[132,133] Accordingly, the WHO recommends the use of DEC as part of lymphatic filariasis control programs in endemic areas in all children older than 2 years.[23] In the United States, the CDC recommends against the use of DEC in children younger than 18 months.

Drug–drug Interactions

Any substance that alkalinizes the urine, such as sodium bicarbonate, may reduce renal clearance of the drug and its metabolites and, therefore, increase the incidence of side effects.

Precautions

Renal Impairment

In instances of significant renal impairment (e.g., glomerular filtration rate <50 mL per minute), dose reduction should be considered, although no specific recommendations exist.

Side Effects

DEC is generally well tolerated, although arthralgia, headache, malaise, dizziness, nausea, and vomiting have all been reported.[18] In individuals who are heavily infected, more severe reactions may be observed, which are most likely due to a host immunologic reaction to disintegrating worms.[134] In the case of lymphatic filariasis, these effects may include fever, myalgia, transient hematuria, urticaria, bronchospasm, transient lymphangitis and lymphadenitis, scrotal pain, and exacerbation of lymphedema.[18] In patients with high levels of microfilaremia due to *L. loa*, encephalopathy and retinal hemorrhage may occur following treatment with DEC.

Severe Mazzotti reactions may occur following a single dose of DEC in patients coinfected with *O. volvulus*, characterized by fever, hypotension, and an ocular reaction that results from the death of microfilariae and can be fatal or cause permanent vision loss. For this reason, treatment with DEC in coinfected patients or in regions endemic for onchocerciasis is contraindicated.

Pediatric Dosage

DEC is supplied as tablets for oral administration. Use in children less than 18 months is not recommended.

- *Lymphatic filariasis*: 6 mg per kg as a single dose or daily for 12 days. If high microfilaremia, scale up starting at 1 mg per kg as a single dose on the first day, 3 mg per kg divided into three doses on the second day, 3 to 6 mg per kg divided into three doses on the third day, and then 6 mg per kg per day divided into three doses on days 4 through 12.
- *Tropical pulmonary eosinophilia*: 6 mg per kg per day for 21 days
- *Loiasis:* in patients with microfilaremia below 2,500 per mL of blood, 9 mg per kg per day divided into three doses for 21 days. May scale up dosage as for lymphatic filariasis. For higher levels of microfilaremia, pretreatment with apheresis or albendazole may be attempted in consultation with an expert.

WHO Recommendation

For suppression of microfilaremia in MDA programs in regions where lymphatic filariasis is endemic but onchocerciasis is not co-endemic, the WHO recommends community-wide annual treatment with a single dose of 6 mg per kg DEC orally, in combination with a single dose of albendazole.[23]

ANTICESTODE AND ANTITREMATODE ANTHELMINTHICS

PRAZIQUANTEL

Praziquantel is a synthetic isoquinoline–pyrazine derivative that has broad anthelminthic activity. It is effective in the treatment of infections due to all species of *Schistosoma*, as well as most other trematodes (flukes) and the cestodes (tapeworms). Its safety and effectiveness when administered as a single oral dose have also lent it to easy incorporation into MDA programs for control of several infections but, most importantly, for schistosomiasis.[23] Because praziquantel is the only currently available medication that is effective against all species of *Schistosoma*, there is concern that resistance to praziquantel may develop, given its increasing usage.[135] Of concern, there have been reports of reduced cure rates using praziquantel to treat schistosomiasis in regions of Africa,[136,137] although this finding has been attributed by some authors to the intense transmission that leads to rapid reinfection with the parasite in these regions.[138]

Indications

Praziquantel is highly effective in treating most cestode and trematode infections. In the United States, it is licensed for the treatment of infections due to all species of *Schistosoma*, including *Schistosoma mansoni*, *Schistosoma haematobium*, *Schistosoma mekongi*, *Schistosoma japonicum*, and *Schistosoma intercalatum*, as well as infections due to the liver flukes *Clonorchis sinensis* (Chinese or Oriental liver fluke) and *Opisthorchis viverrini*.[139,140] Importantly, however, it is not effective in treating acute schistosomiasis that is an immune-mediated reaction to eggs and/or immature stages of the helminth.

Although not listed on the manufacturer's label, there is also wide experience in using praziquantel in the treatment of *Diphyllobothrium latum*, *Dipylidium caninum*, *Hymenolepis nana* (dwarf tapeworm), *Metagonimus yokogawai* (intestinal fluke), *P. westermani* (oriental lung fluke) and other *Paragonimus* species, and taeniasis caused by *T. solium* (pork tapeworm) or *T. saginata* (beef tapeworm).[139,141]

Praziquantel is also one of the two recommended cysticidal treatments for neurocysticercosis.[38] For patients with more than two viable parenchymal cysts, the addition of praziquantel to first-line albendazole has been shown in randomized studies to result in faster radiologic resolution of lesions.[142] As with albendazole, corticosteroids should be administered concurrently in most cases to control inflammation, edema, and/or other reactions due to dying cysticerci.

Despite its otherwise broad-spectrum anthelminthic effects, praziquantel is not effective in treating infections caused by *Echinococcus* species or *F. hepatica* (sheep liver fluke).

Mechanism of Action

Although the precise mechanism of action for praziquantel is unknown, studies suggest that the drug increases cell membrane permeability in susceptible worms, which leads to tegumental damage and paralytic muscular contraction, leading to worm death and elimination.[143,144] The muscular contraction and paralysis may be due to a specific action on calcium ion channels, leading to an influx into the parasite. After exposure to praziquantel, the tegument in the neck region of adult schistosomes develops blebs as well as intense vacuolization at several sites that ultimately results in its disintegration, leading to exposure or release of concealed antigens that serve as targets for the host immune system. This is followed by attachment of phagocytes to the parasite and, ultimately, death of the worm.[143] A functioning host immune system is, therefore, critical in inducing parasite death.

Praziquantel is manufactured as a 1:1 racemic mixture, with only the levo-enantiomer having antischistosomal properties.[144] Therefore, half of a praziquantel tablet consists of an inactive ingredient, which is responsible for the drug's bitter taste.[145] To develop suitable pediatric praziquantel formulations for treating schistosomiasis, the Pediatric Praziquantel Consortium was formed in 2012. It has prioritized the low-cost production of pure levo-praziquantel, which is currently being tested in a phase 3 clinical trial in Africa.

Pharmacokinetics

Praziquantel is rapidly absorbed (>80%) from the gastrointestinal tract following oral administration, particularly if ingested with a carbohydrate-rich meal.[144,146] Maximum serum concentrations are achieved between 1 and 3 hours following an oral dose.[146,147] It undergoes extensive first-pass hepatic metabolism mostly into monohydroxylated and dihydroxylated derivatives that lack anthelminthic activity, with only a small amount of active drug reaching the systemic circulation.[139,140] Concentrations of the drug in CSF are between 15% and 20% those in serum. Praziquantel and its metabolites are also found in breast milk, at levels approximately 25% those of maternal serum. Elimination is through the kidneys and occurs rapidly, with greater than 70% excreted within 24 hours; small amounts are eliminated in the feces.[139]

Pediatric Considerations

Praziquantel has not been found to have adverse effects on fertility or to be teratogenic in animal reproductive toxicity studies conducted in rats and rabbits given up to 300 mg per kg per day.[52] Although the manufacturer recommends the use of praziquantel during pregnancy only if clearly needed, two randomized controlled trials demonstrated no significant effect on birth weight, apparently safe use, and causation of minimal side effects that were similar to those seen in treated nonpregnant subjects.[148,149] Accordingly, the WHO recommends that, given the morbidity related to schistosomiasis and the beneficial effect of praziquantel treatment, pregnant women with schistosomiasis should be offered treatment.[150] In particular, they should not be excluded from MDA programs in regions of high prevalence of schistosomiasis.

Similarly, although the manufacturer recommends withholding breastfeeding on the day of praziquantel treatment and for the subsequent 72 hours because the drug is excreted in breast milk in miniscule amounts, the WHO regards the use of praziquantel during lactation as safe.[150]

Finally, adequate safety studies of praziquantel have not been performed in children younger than 1 year, so use of the drug in this pediatric population is not recommended.[150]

Drug–drug Interactions

Anticonvulsants

Antiseizure medications such as carbamazepine, phenobarbital, and phenytoin that are CYP450 inducers may reduce plasma concentrations of praziquantel. In a small controlled study, it was found that patients taking carbamazepine or phenytoin chronically for seizure disorders achieved significantly lower plasma concentrations following a single dose of praziquantel (7.9% and 24% of the control group, respectively).[151] Accordingly, patients on carbamazepine or phenytoin may require a larger dose of praziquantel.

Rifampin

Coadministration with rifampin, a potent CYP450 inducer, has been shown to decrease plasma levels of praziquantel by over 50%.[152] If treatment with praziquantel is necessary, rifampin should be held for at least 4 weeks before administration of praziquantel.[140]

CYP450 Inhibitors

CYP450 inhibitors such as cimetidine, ketoconazole, itraconazole, and erythromycin may increase plasma concentrations of praziquantel.[153,154] For example, cimetidine has been shown to increase the plasma concentration of praziquantel by twofold when these medications are taken together.[153]

Corticosteroids

Concurrent administration of dexamethasone with praziquantel reduces praziquantel plasma concentrations by approximately half.[155] However, the clinical implications of this finding have not been determined, and an increase in the dose of praziquantel when used with corticosteroids to treat neurocysticercosis is not recommended.

Precautions

Hepatic Dysfunction

In patients with moderate or severe hepatic impairment due to chronic *S. mansoni* infection (Child-Pugh class B or C), significant increases in praziquantel half-life and maximum plasma concentrations have been observed due to reduced hepatic metabolism.[156] Use of praziquantel in this population should be exercised with caution.

Neurocysticercosis

For parenchymal neurocysticercosis with more than two viable cysts, coadministration of praziquantel with albendazole is recommended.[38] Just as with albendazole, if praziquantel is used in the treatment of neurocysticercosis, concurrent administration of a systemic corticosteroid is recommended, especially if there are multiple cysts, to reduce the inflammatory reaction to dying cysts that may result in seizures or raised intracranial pressure. The use of praziquantel is absolutely contraindicated in the presence of retinal cysticercosis because the destruction of parasites in the eye may result in irreversible loss of vision. A thorough ophthalmologic examination for ocular cysticerci should be conducted prior to treatment with praziquantel.

Side Effects

Praziquantel is generally considered to be a very safe drug. Side effects are usually mild and transient and may include dizziness, fatigue, headache, and malaise, as well as gastrointestinal effects such as abdominal cramps or pain and loss of appetite, although all of these can also be associated with schistosomiasis, the most common indication for its use.[140] These side effects are more common and may be more severe in patients with heavy worm burdens and likely result from the body's response to the dying worms. Less common side effects include nausea, vomiting, diarrhea, urticaria, arthralgia, myalgia, and low-grade fever. The drug has an unpleasant, bitter taste, which can make it unpalatable especially to younger children.

Pediatric Dosage

The use of praziquantel is not recommended in children younger than 1 year due to a lack of adequate safety information.[140] The WHO has developed and validated a "dose pole" that calculates the amount of drug to be administered by measurement of a child's height (by having them stand next to it).[23,157] Tablets of praziquantel should be washed down unchewed with liquids during a meal, as the bitter taste may cause vomiting. To prevent choking in children below the age of 6 years, tablets may be crushed and mixed with liquid or semisolid food (administered within 1 hour of mixing). If administered in divided doses, intervals of not less than 4 hours and not more than 6 hours should be used.

- *Schistosomiasis:*
  - *S. haematobium, S. intercalatum,* and *S. mansoni:* 40 mg per kg per day in a single or divided dose, for 1 day
  - *S. japonicum* and *S. mekongi:* 60 mg per kg per day in a single or divided dose, for 1 day
- *Clonorchiasis, opisthorchiasis, Metorchis conjunctus*: 75 mg per kg per day in three divided doses, for 2 days
- *Neurocysticercosis* (>2 viable parenchymal lesions): 50 mg per kg per day for 10 to 14 days, in combination with albendazole
- *Fasciolopsis buski, Heterophyes heterophyes, Echinostoma* sp., *M. yokogawai*: 75 mg per kg per day in three divided doses, for 1 day
- *Paragonimiasis*: 75 mg per kg per day in three divided doses, for 2 days
- *Tapeworms*:
  - *D. latum, T. saginata, T. solium,* and *D. caninum*: 10 mg per kg as a single dose
  - *H. nana*: 25 mg per kg as a single dose. Heavy infections may require a repeat dose after 10 days.

FUTURE DEVELOPMENTS

Unfortunately, given the fact that helminth infections affect predominantly the rural poor living in the tropics and subtropics,[158] investment in developing new anthelminthic medications has been limited, and in fact, several of the existing medications have significant availability problems. Should widespread resistance develop to the currently used medications such as the benzimidazoles in the case of nematode infections or praziquantel in the case of schistosomiasis, the consequences in terms of global health would be devastating, given the lack of alternative medications that are active against these parasites. Drug resistance may develop via various mechanisms, including reduced binding affinity of the drugs to targets such as β-tubulin in the case of the benzimidazoles, or calcium ion channels in the case of praziquantel. Interference with these mechanisms of resistance might also serve as strategies for future drug development.

Several strategies are being developed to either delay or deal with the likelihood of drug resistance developing in helminths. First, although small in number, there are some new drugs that are being developed for use in humans. For the intestinal nematodes, the anthelminthic tribendimidine is most likely to be licensed in the near future. Although first developed in the early 1980s in China, where it is currently licensed for human use, it has not yet been licensed elsewhere, and further clinical trials will likely be required before registration can occur outside China. Tribendimidine is a synthetic derivative of amidantel and has been shown in both animal models and human studies to be highly active against *A. lumbricoides* and hookworm infections due to either *N. americanus* or *A. duodenale*; activity against *T. trichiura* and *E. vermicularis* appears to be less impressive.[159]

Second, the option of using anthelminthics in combination—similar to the current strategies targeting treatment of malaria, *Mycobacterium tuberculosis*, and human immunodeficiency virus infections—is being tested as a strategy for reducing the likelihood of resistance developing to any single anthelminthic drug. MDA programs are already administering the combination of DEC or ivermectin with albendazole for the control of lymphatic filariasis.[23] Clinical trials conducted so far indicate that combinations of oxantel pamoate, a pyrimidine derivate developed from pyrantel, and either albendazole or tribendimidine are significantly more effective than either drug alone against hookworm and *T. trichiura* infections.[10,160] Similarly, the combination of ivermectin and albendazole has been shown to increase the cure rate of *T. trichiura* infections over that of either drug.[160,161] For schistosomiasis, the combination of praziquantel with artemisinins, such as artesunate or artemether that have activity against the early liver stage of infection, is currently being studied, although the evidence so far is inconclusive.[162]

Lastly, for several reasons, including the possibility of drug resistance developing in existing anthelminthics, the lack of alternative anthelminthics, and the fact that in highly endemic areas, reinfection following treatment occurs frequently and rapidly for several of the helminth infections described in this chapter such as the STHs and schistosomiasis, control measures other than anthelminthic medications are being developed. High on the list of such alternative control tools are new vaccines targeting infections, such as hookworm, schistosomiasis, and onchocerciasis.[163–165] Hopefully, if widespread drug resistance in these parasites does develop, new vaccines will be ready by the time this occurs.

REFERENCES

1. World Health Organization. Schistosomiasis and soil-transmitted helminthiases: numbers of people treated in 2017. *Wkly Epidemiol Rec* 2018;93(50):681–692.
2. Jourdan PM, Lamberton PHL, Fenwick A, et al. Soil-transmitted helminth infections. *Lancet* 2018;391(10117):252–265.
3. Colley DG, Bustinduy AL, Secor WE, et al. Human schistosomiasis. *Lancet* 2014;383(9936):2253–2264.
4. Bethony J, Brooker S, Albonico M, et al. Soil-transmitted helminth infections: ascariasis, trichuriasis, and hookworm. *Lancet* 2006;367(9521):1521–1532.
5. Pabalan N, Singian E, Tabangay L, et al. Soil-transmitted helminth infection, loss of education and cognitive impairment in school-aged children: a systematic review and meta-analysis. *PLoS Negl Trop Dis* 2018;12(1):e0005523.
6. Ezeamama AE, Bustinduy AL, Nkwata AK, et al. Cognitive deficits and educational loss in children with schistosome infection-A systematic review and meta-analysis. *PLoS Negl Trop Dis* 2018;12(1):e0005524.
7. Drake LJ, Jukes MCH, Sternberg RJ, et al. Geohelminth infections (ascariasis, trichuriasis, and hookworms): cognitive and developmental impacts. *Semin Pediatr Infect Dis* 2000;11:245–251.
8. Jardim-Botelho A, Raff S, Rodrigues R, et al. Hookworm, *Ascaris. lumbricoides* infection and polyparasitism associated with poor cognitive performance in Brazilian schoolchildren. *Trop Med Int Health* 2008;13(8):994–1004.
9. Molyneux DH. The London declaration on neglected tropical diseases: 5 years on. *Trans R Soc Trop Med Hyg* 2016;110(11):623–625.
10. Albonico M, Bickle Q, Ramsan M, et al. Efficacy of mebendazole and levamisole alone or in combination against intestinal nematode infections after repeated targeted mebendazole treatment in Zanzibar. *Bull World Health Organ* 2003;81(5):343–352.
11. Favre TC, Pereira AP, Beck LC, et al. School-based and community-based actions for scaling-up diagnosis and treatment of schistosomiasis toward its elimination in an endemic area of Brazil. *Acta Trop* 2015;149:155–162.
12. Albonico M, Smith PG, Ercole E, et al. Rate of reinfection with intestinal nematodes after treatment of children with mebendazole or albendazole in a highly endemic area. *Trans R Soc Trop Med Hyg* 1995;89:538–541.
13. Cundill B, Alexander N, Bethony JM, et al. Rates and intensity of re-infection with human helminths after treatment and the influence of individual, household, and environmental factors in a Brazilian community. *Parasitology* 2011;138(11):1406–1416.
14. Jaeger LH, Carvalho-Costa FA. Status of benzimidazole resistance in intestinal nematode populations of livestock in Brazil: a systematic review. *BMC Vet Res* 2017;13(1):358.
15. Orr AR, Quagraine JE, Suwondo P, et al. Genetic markers of benzimidazole resistance among human hookworms (*Necator americanus*) in Kintampo North Municipality, Ghana. *Am J Trop Med Hyg* 2019;100(2):351–356.
16. Wang W, Wang L, Liang YS. Susceptibility or resistance of praziquantel in human schistosomiasis: a review. *Parasitol Res* 2012;111(5):1871–1877.
17. Pérez del Villar L, Burguillo FJ, López-Abán J, et al. Systematic review and meta-analysis of artemisinin based therapies for the treatment and prevention of schistosomiasis. *PLoS One* 2012;7(9):e45867.
18. Taylor MJ, Hoerauf A, Bockarie M. Lymphatic filariasis and onchocerciasis. *Lancet* 2010;376(9747):1175–1185.
19. Mand S, Pfarr K, Sahoo PK, et al. Macrofilaricidal activity and amelioration of lymphatic pathology in bancroftian filariasis after 3 weeks of doxycycline followed by single-dose diethylcarbamazine. *Am J Trop Med Hyg* 2009;81(4):702–711.
20. Ma G, Holland CV, Wang T, et al. Human toxocariasis. *Lancet Infect Dis* 2018;18(1):e14–e24.
21. Won KY, Kruszon-Moran D, Schantz PM, et al. National seroprevalence and risk factors for zoonotic *Toxocara* spp. infection. *Am J Trop Med Hyg* 2008;79(4):552–557.
22. O'Keefe KA, Eberhard ML, Shafir SC, et al. Cysticercosis-related hospitalizations in the United States, 1998-2011. *Am J Trop Med Hyg* 2015;92(2):354–359.
23. World Health Organization. Preventive chemotherapy in human helminthiasis. Geneva, Switzerland: World Health Organization, 2006.
24. Dayan AD. Albendazole, mebendazole and praziquantel. Review of non-clinical toxicity and pharmacokinetics. *Acta Trop* 2003;86:141–159.
25. Keystone JS, Murdoch JK. Mebendazole. *Ann Intern Med* 1979;91(4):582–586.
26. Horton J. Albendazole: a broad spectrum anthelminthic for treatment of individuals and populations. *Curr Opin Infect Dis* 2002;15(6):599–608.
27. Albenza (albendazole) prescribing information. Hayward, CA: Impax Specialty Pharma, 2019.
28. Dehkordi AB, Sanei B, Yousefi M, et al. Albendazole and treatment of hydatid cyst: review of the literature. *Infect Disord Drug Targets* 2019;19(2):101–104.
29. Aygun E, Sahin M, Odev K, et al. The management of liver hydatid cysts by percutaneous drainage. *Can J Surg* 2001;44(3):203–209.
30. Vuitton DA. Benzimidazoles for the treatment of cystic and alveolar echinococcosis: what is the consensus? *Expert Rev Anti Infect Ther* 2009;7:145–149.
31. Brunetti E, Kern P, Vuitton DA; Writing Panel for the WHO-IWGE. Expert consensus for the diagnosis and treatment of cystic and alveolar echinococcosis in humans. *Acta Trop* 2010;114:1–16.
32. Wen H, Vuitton L, Tuxun T, et al. Echinococcosis: advances in the 21st century. *Clin Microbiol Rev* 2019;32(2).
33. Junghanss T, da Silva AM, Horton J, et al. Clinical management of cystic echinococcosis: state of the art, problems, and perspectives. *Am J Trop Med Hyg* 2008;79(3):301–311.
34. Vuitton DA, Azizi A, Richou C, et al. Current interventional strategy for the treatment of hepatic alveolar echinococcosis. *Expert Rev Anti Infect Ther* 2016;14(12):1179–1194.
35. Garcia HH. Neurocysticercosis. *Neurol Clin* 2018;36(4):851–864.
36. Del Brutto OH, Sotelo J, Aguirre R, et al. Albendazole therapy for giant subarachnoid cysticerci. *Arch Neurol* 1992;49(5):535–538.
37. Cruz M, Cruz I, Horton J. Clinical evaluation of albendazole and praziquantel in the treatment of cerebral cysticercosis. *Trans R Soc Trop Med Hyg* 1991;85:244–247.
38. Botero D, Uribe CS, Sanchez JL, et al. Short course albendazole treatment for neurocysticercosis in Colombia. *Trans R Soc Trop Med Hyg* 1993;87(5):576–577.
39. White AC, Coyle CM, Rajshekhar V, et al. Diagnosis and treatment of neurocysticercosis: 2017 clinical practice guidelines by the Infectious Diseases Society of America (IDSA) and the American Society of Tropical Medicine and Hygiene (ASTMH). *Am J Trop Med Hyg* 2018; 98:945–966.
40. Garcia HH, Del Brutto OH; Cysticercosis Working Group in Peru. Neurocysticercosis: updated concepts about an old disease. *Lancet Neurol* 2005;4:653–661.
41. Purdy KS, Langley RG, Webb AN, et al. Cutaneous larva migrans. *Lancet* 2011; 377(9781):1948.
42. St Georgiev V. Chemotherapy of enterobiasis (oxyuriasis). *Expert Opin Pharmacother* 2001;2(2):267–275.
43. Haby MM, Sosa Leon LA, Luciañez A, et al. Systematic review of the effectiveness of selected drugs for preventive chemotherapy for *Taenia solium* taeniasis. *PLoS Negl Trop Dis* 2020;14(1):e0007873.
44. de Kaminsky RG. Albendazole treatment in human taeniasis. *Trans R Soc Trop Med Hyg* 1991;85:648–650.
45. Despommier D. Toxocariasis: clinical aspects, epidemiology, medical ecology, and molecular aspects. *Clin Microbiol Rev* 2003;16(2):265–272.
46. Gottstein B, Pozio E, Nöckler K. Epidemiology, diagnosis, treatment, and control of trichinellosis. *Clin Microbiol Rev* 2009;22(1):127–145.
47. Reynolds JEF, ed. Martindale, the extra pharmacopeia, 29th ed. London, England: Pharmaceutical Press, 1989:47–48, 57–59.
48. De Rosa F, Teggi A. Treatment of *Echinococcus granulosus* hydatid disease with albendazole. *Ann Trop Med Parasitol* 1990;84(5):467–472.
49. Liu YH, Wang XG, Gao P, et al. Experimental and clinical trial of albendazole in the treatment of clonorchis sinensis. *Chin Med J (Engl)* 1991;104(1):27–31.
50. Ramalingam S, Sinniah B, Krishnan U. Albendazole, an effective single dose, broad spectrum anthelminthic drug. *Am J Trop Med Hyg* 1982;31(2):263–266.
51. Ndyomugyenyi R, Kabatereine N, Olsen A, et al. Efficacy of ivermectin and albendazole alone and in combination for treatment of soil-transmitted helminths in pregnancy and adverse events: a randomized open label controlled intervention trial in Masindi district, western Uganda. *Am J Trop Med Hyg* 2008;79(6):856–863.
52. World Health Organization. Report of the WHO informal consultation on the use of praziquantel during pregnancy/lactation and albendazole/mebendazole in children under 24 months. Geneva, Switzerland: World Health Organization, 2002.
53. Nagy J, Schipper HG, Koopmans RP, et al. Effect of grapefruit juice or cimetidine coadministration on albendazole bioavailability. *Am J Trop Med Hyg* 2002;66(3):260–263.
54. Takayanagui OM, Lanchote VL, Marques MP, et al. Therapy for neurocysticercosis: pharmacokinetic interaction of albendazole sulfoxide with dexamethasone. *Ther Drug Monit* 1997;19(1):51–55.

55. Jung H, Hurtado M, Medina MT, et al. Dexamethasone increases plasma levels of albendazole. *J Neurol* 1990;237:279–280.
56. Pene P, Mojon M, Garin JP, et al. Albendazole: a new broad spectrum anthelminthic. Double-blind multi-center clinical trial. *Am J Trop Med Hyg* 1982;31(2):263–266.
57. Macedo NA, Pineyro MI, Carmona C. Contact urticaria and contact dermatitis from albendazole. *Contact Dermatitis* 1991;25(1):73–75.
58. Rossignol JF, Maisonneuve H. Albendazole: placebo-controlled study in 870 patients with intestinal helminthiasis. *Trans R Soc Trop Med Hyg* 1983;77(5):707–711.
59. Steiger U, Cotting J, Reichen J. Albendazole treatment of echinococcosis in humans: effects on microsomal metabolism and drug tolerance. *Clin Pharmacol Ther* 1990;47(3):347–353.
60. Ben Fredj N, Chaabane A, Chadly Z, et al. Albendazole-induced associated acute hepatitis and bicytopenia. *Scand J Infect Dis* 2014;46(2):149–151.
61. Moser W, Schindler C, Keiser J. Efficacy of recommended drugs against soil transmitted helminths: systematic review and network meta-analysis. *BMJ* 2017;358:j4307.
62. Emverm (mebendazole) prescribing information. Bridgewater, NJ: Amneal Pharmaceuticals, 2019.
63. Mrus J, Baeten B, Engelen M, et al. Efficacy of single-dose 500 mg mebendazole in soil-transmitted helminth infections: a review. *J Helminthol* 2018;92(3):269–278.
64. Sadaow L, Sanpool O, Intapan PM, et al. A hospital-based study of intestinal capillariasis in Thailand: clinical features, potential clues for diagnosis, and epidemiological characteristics of 85 patients. *Am J Trop Med Hyg* 2018;98(1):27–31.
65. Dollery CT. Mebendazole. In: Therapeutic drugs, Vol. 2, 2nd ed. Edinburgh, Scotland: Churchill Livingstone, 1999:M12–M15.
66. Gyorkos TW, Larocque R, Casapia M, et al. Lack of risk of adverse outcomes after deworming in pregnant women. *Pediatr Infect Dis J* 2006;25:791–794.
67. Montresor A, Awasthi S, Crompton DW. Use of benzimidazoles in children younger than 24 months for the treatment of soil-transmitted helminthiasis. *Acta Trop* 2003;86:223–232.
68. Luder PJ, Siffert B, Witassek F, et al. Treatment of hydatid disease with high oral doses of mebendazole. *Eur J Clin Pharmacol* 1986;31(4):443–448.
69. Chen KT, Twu SJ, Chang HJ, et al. Outbreak of Stevens-Johnson syndrome/toxic epidermal necrolysis associated with mebendazole and metronidazole use among Filipino laborers in Taiwan. *Am J Public Health* 2003;93(3):489–492.
70. Braithwaite PA, Roberts MS, Allan RJ, et al. Clinical pharmacokinetics of high dose mebendazole in patients treated for cystic hydatid disease. *Eur J Clin Pharmacol* 1982;22:161–169.
71. Keiser J, Utzinger J. Food-borne trematodiasis: current chemotherapy and advances with artemisinins and synthetic trioxolanes. *Trends Parasitol* 2007;23(11):555–562.
72. Bennett JL, Kohler P. *Fasciola hepatica*: action in vitro of triclabendazole on immature and adult stages. *Exp Parasitol* 1987;63(1):49–57.
73. Apt W, Aguilera X, Vega F, et al. Treatment of human chronic fascioliasis with triclabendazole: drug efficacy and serologic response. *Am J Trop Med Hyg* 1995;52(6):532–535.
74. Triclabendazole and trematode worm infections. *Drugs Q* 1997;1(1):38–39.
75. Calvopiña M, Guderian RH, Paredes W, et al. Comparison of two single-day regimens of triclabendazole for the treatment of human pulmonary paragonimiasis. *Trans R Soc Trop Med Hyg* 2003;97(4):451–454.
76. Fairweather I. Triclabendazole: new skills to unravel an old(ish) enigma. *J Helminthol* 2005;79(3):227–234.
77. Belgraier AH. Common bile duct obstruction due to *Fasciola hepatica*. *N Y State J Med* 1976;76:936–937.
78. Igual-Adell R, Oltra-Alcaraz C, Soler-Company E, et al. Efficacy and safety of ivermectin and thiabendazole in the treatment of strongyloidiasis. *Expert Opin Pharmacother* 2004;5(12):2615–2619.
79. Gann PH, Neva FA, Gam AA. A randomized trial of single- and two-dose ivermectin versus thiabendazole for treatment of strongyloidiasis. *J Infect Dis* 1994;169(5):1076–1079.
80. Lim S, Katz K, Krajden S, et al. Complicated and fatal *Strongyloides* infection in Canadians: risk factors, diagnosis and management. *CMAJ* 2004;171(5):479–484.
81. Watt G, Saisorn S, Jongsakul K, et al. Blinded, placebo-controlled trial of antiparasitic drugs for trichinosis myositis. *J Infect Dis* 2000;182(1):371–374.
82. Sugar AM, Kearns PJ Jr, Haulk AA, et al. Possible thiabendazole-induced theophylline toxicity. *Am Rev Respir Dis* 1980;122(3):501–503.
83. Lew G, Murray WE, Lane JR, et al. Theophylline–thiabendazole drug interaction. *Clin Pharm* 1989;8:225–227.
84. Bauer LA, Raisys VA, Watts MT, et al. The pharmacokinetics of thiabendazole and its metabolites in an anephric patient undergoing hemodialysis and hemoperfusion. *J Clin Pharmacol* 1982;22:276–280.
85. Johnson-Reagan L, Bahna SL. Severe drug rashes in three siblings simultaneously. *Allergy* 2003;58(5):445–447.
86. Bion E, Pariente EA, Maitre F. Severe cholestasis and sicca syndrome after thiabendazole. *J Hepatol* 1995;23(6):762–763.
87. Pitts NE, Migliardi JR. Antiminth (pyrantel pamoate). *Clin Pediatr (Phila)* 1974;13(1):87–94.
88. Köhler P. The biochemical basis of anthelmintic action and resistance. *Int J Parasitol* 2001;31(4):336–345.
89. Martin RJ, Robertson AP. Mode of action of levamisole and pyrantel, anthelmintic resistance, E153 and Q57. *Parasitology* 2007;134(Pt 8):1093–1104.
90. Bescansa E, Nicolas M, Aguado C, et al. Myasthenia gravis aggravated by pyrantel pamoate. *J Neurol Neurosurg Psychiatry* 1991;54(6):563.
91. Shen C, Li M, Zhao X, et al. An ocular myasthenia gravis attack after oral pyrantel pamoate: an unusual case report. *Medicine (Baltimore)* 2019;98(27):e16321.
92. Renoux G. The general immunopharmacology of levamisole. *Drugs* 1980;19:89–99.
93. Kouassi E, Caillé G, Léry L, et al. Novel assay and pharmacokinetics of levamisole and p-hydroxylevamisole in human plasma and urine. *Biopharm Drug Dispos* 1986;7(1):71–89.
94. Awadzi K, Edwards G, Opoku NO, et al. The safety, tolerability and pharmacokinetics of levamisole alone, levamisole plus ivermectin, and levamisole plus albendazole, and their efficacy against *Onchocerca volvulus*. *Ann Trop Med Parasitol* 2004;98(6):595–614.
95. Laing R, Gillan V, Devaney E. Ivermectin - old drug, new tricks? *Trends Parasitol* 2017;33(6):463–472.
96. Stromectol (ivermectin) package insert. Whitehouse Station, NJ: Merck and Co, Inc., 2009.
97. Gyatt H, de Silva N, Bundy D. Anthelminthics: a comparative review of their clinical pharmacology. *Drugs* 1997;53(5):769–788.
98. Udall DN. Recent updates on onchocerciasis: diagnosis and treatment. *Clin Infect Dis* 2007;44(1):53–60.
99. Boussinesq M, Chippaux JP, Ernould JC, et al. Effect of repeated treatments with ivermectin on the incidence of onchocerciasis in northern Cameroon. *Am J Trop Med Hyg* 1995;53:63–67.
100. Diawara L, Traore MO, Badji A, et al. Feasibility of onchocerciasis elimination with ivermectin treatment in endemic foci in Africa: first evidence from studies in Mali and Senegal. *PLoS Negl Trop Dis* 2009;3:e497.
101. Tisch DJ, Michael E, Kazura JW. Mass chemotherapy options to control lymphatic filariasis: a systematic review. *Lancet Infect Dis* 2005;5(8):514–523.
102. Ottesen EA, Vijayasekaran V, Kumaraswami V, et al. A controlled trial of ivermectin and diethylcarbamazine in lymphatic filariasis. *N Engl J Med* 1990;322(16):1113–1117.
103. King CL, Suamani J, Sanuku N, et al. A trial of a triple-drug treatment for lymphatic filariasis. *N Engl J Med* 2018;379(19):1801–1810.
104. Marti H, Haji HJ, Savioli L, et al. A comparative trial of a single-dose ivermectin versus three days of albendazole for treatment of *Strongyloides stercoralis* and other soil-transmitted helminth infections in children. *Am J Trop Med Hyg* 1996;55(5):477–481.
105. Henriquez-Camacho C, Gotuzzo E, Echevarria J, et al. Ivermectin versus albendazole or thiabendazole for *Strongyloides stercoralis* infection. *Cochrane Database Syst Rev* 2016;(1):CD007745.
106. Keiser PB, Nutman TB. *Strongyloides stercoralis* in the immunocompromised population. *Clin Microbiol Rev* 2004;17(1):208–217.
107. Heukelbach J, Feldmeier H. Epidemiological and clinical characteristics of hookworm-related cutaneous larva migrans. *Lancet Infect Dis* 2008;8(5):302–309.
108. Caumes E, Carriere J, Datry A, et al. A randomized trial of ivermectin versus albendazole for the treatment of cutaneous larva migrans. *Am J Trop Med Hyg* 1993;49(5):641–644.
109. Wen LY, Yan XL, Sun FH, et al. A randomized, double-blind, multicenter clinical trial on the efficacy of ivermectin against intestinal nematode infections in China. *Acta Trop* 2008;106(3):190–194.
110. Edwards G, Dingsdale A, Helsby N, et al. The relative systemic availability of ivermectin after administration as capsule, tablet, and oral solution. *Eur J Clin Pharmacol* 1988;35:681–684.
111. Gyapong JO, Chinbuah MA, Gyapong M. Inadvertent exposure of pregnant women to ivermectin and albendazole during mass drug administration for lymphatic filariasis. *Trop Med Int Health* 2003;8(12):1093–1101.
112. Nicolas P, Maia MF, Bassat Q, et al. Safety of oral ivermectin during pregnancy: a systematic review and meta-analysis. *Lancet Glob Health* 2020;8(1):e92–e100.
113. Scientific Working Group on Serious Adverse Events in *Loa loa* endemic areas. Report of a Scientific Working Group on Serious Adverse Events following Mectizan® treatment of onchocerciasis in *Loa* endemic areas. *Filaria J* 2003;2(Suppl 1):S2.
114. Boussinesq M, Gardon J, Gardon-Wendel N, et al. Clinical picture, epidemiology and outcome of Loa-associated serious adverse events related to mass ivermectin treatment of onchocerciasis in Cameroon. *Filaria J* 2003;2(Suppl 1):S4.
115. Kamgno J, Pion SD, Chesnais CB, et al. A test-and-not-treat strategy for onchocerciasis in Loa loa-endemic areas. *N Engl J Med* 2017;377(21):2044–2052.
116. Prichard R, Ménez C, Lespine A. Moxidectin and the avermectins: consanguinity but not identity. *Int J Parasitol Drugs Drug Resist* 2012;2:134–153.
117. Moxidectin package insert. Melbourne, Australia: Medicines Development for Global Health, 2018.
118. Opoku NO, Bakajika DK, Kanza EM, et al. Single dose moxidectin versus ivermectin for *Onchocerca volvulus* infection in Ghana, Liberia, and the Democratic Republic of the Congo: a randomised, controlled, double-blind phase 3 trial. *Lancet* 2018;392(10154):1207–1216.
119. Barda B, Ame SM, Ali SM, et al. Efficacy and tolerability of moxidectin alone and in co-administration with albendazole and tribendimidine versus albendazole plus oxantel pamoate against *Trichuris trichiura* infections: a randomised, non-inferiority, single-blind trial. *Lancet Infect Dis* 2018;18(8):864–873.
120. Cotreau MM, Warren S, Ryan JL, et al. The antiparasitic moxidectin: safety, tolerability, and pharmacokinetics in humans. *J Clin Pharmacol* 2003;43(10):1108–1115.
121. Korth-Bradley JM, Parks V, Patat A, et al. Relative bioavailability of liquid and tablet formulations of the antiparasitic moxidectin. *Clin Pharmacol Drug Dev* 2012;1(1):32–37.
122. Awadzi K, Opoku NO, Attah SK, et al. A randomized, single-ascending-dose, ivermectin-controlled, double-blind study of moxidectin in *Onchocerca volvulus* infection. *PLoS Negl Trop Dis* 2014;8(6):e2953.
123. Ottesen EA. Lymphatic filariasis: treatment, control and elimination. *Adv Parasitol* 2006;61:395–441.
124. Ramaiah KD, Das PK, Vanamail P, et al. Impact of 10 years of diethylcarbamazine and ivermectin mass administration on infection and transmission of lymphatic filariasis. *Trans R Soc Trop Med Hyg* 2007;101(6):555–563.
125. Rebollo MP, Bockarie MJ. Can lymphatic filariasis be eliminated by 2020? *Trends Parasitol* 2017;33(2):83–92.
126. Macfarlane CL, Budhathoki SS, Johnson S, et al. Albendazole alone or in combination with microfilaricidal drugs for lymphatic filariasis. *Cochrane Database Syst Rev* 2019;1:CD003753.
127. Lammie P, Milner T, Houston R. Unfulfilled potential: using diethylcarbamazine-fortified salt to eliminate lymphatic filariasis. *Bull World Health Organ* 2007;85(7):545–549.
128. Norões J, Dreyer G, Santos A, et al. Assessment of the efficacy of diethylcarbamazine on adult *Wuchereria bancrofti* in vivo. *Trans R Soc Trop Med Hyg* 1997;9(1):78–81.
129. McGarry HF, Plant LD, Taylor MJ. Diethylcarbamazine activity against *Brugia malayi* microfilariae is dependent on inducible nitric oxide synthase and the cyclooxygenase pathway. *Filaria J* 2005;4:4.
130. Maizels RM, Denham DA. Diethylcarbamazine (DEC): immunopharmacological interactions of an anti-filarial drug. *Parasitology* 1992;105 Suppl:S49–S60.

131. Edwards G, Awadzi K, Breckenridge AM, et al. Diethylcarbamazine disposition in patients with onchocerciasis. *Clin Pharmacol Ther* 1981;30(4):551–557.
132. Pani S, Subramanyam Reddy G, Das L, et al. Tolerability and efficacy of single dose albendazole, diethylcarbamazine citrate (DEC) or co-administration of albendazole with DEC in the clearance of *Wuchereria bancrofti* in asymptomatic microfilaraemic volunteers in Pondicherry, South India: a hospital-based study. *Filaria J* 2002;1(1):1.
133. Fox LM, Furness BW, Haser JK, et al. Tolerance and efficacy of combined diethylcarbamazine and albendazole for treatment of *Wuchereria bancrofti* and intestinal helminth infections in Haitian children. *Am J Trop Med Hyg* 2005;73(1):115–121.
134. Addiss D, Dreyer G. Treatment of lymphatic filariasis. In: Nutman BT, ed. Lymphatic filariasis. London, England: Imperial College Press, 2000:151–199.
135. Doenhoff MJ, Cioli D, Utzinger J. Praziquantel: mechanisms of action, resistance and new derivatives for schistosomiasis. *Curr Opin Infect Dis* 2008;21(6):659–667.
136. Gryseels B, Mbaye A, De Vlas SJ, et al. Are poor responses to praziquantel for the treatment of *Schistosoma mansoni* infections in Senegal due to resistance? An overview of the evidence. *Trop Med Int Health* 2001;6(11):864–873.
137. Crellen T, Walker M, Lamberton PH, et al. Reduced efficacy of praziquantel against *Schistosoma mansoni* is associated with multiple rounds of mass drug administration. *Clin Infect Dis* 2016;63(9):1151–1159.
138. King CH, Muchiri EM, Ouma JH. Evidence against rapid emergence of praziquantel resistance in *Schistosoma haematobium*, Kenya. *Emerg Infect Dis* 2001;7(6):1069–1070.
139. King CH, Mahmoud AA. Drugs five years later: praziquantel. *Ann Intern Med* 1989;110(4):290–296.
140. Biltricide (praziquantel) package insert. Whippany, NJ: Bayer HealthCare Pharmaceuticals, Inc., 2019.
141. The Medical Letter, Inc. Tapeworm infection. In: Abramowicz M, ed. Drugs for parasitic infections, 1st ed. New Rochelle, NY: Medical Letter, 2007:53–54.
142. Garcia HH, Gonzales I, Lescano AG, et al; Cysticercosis Working Group in Peru. Efficacy of combined antiparasitic therapy with praziquantel and albendazole for neurocysticercosis: a double-blind, randomised controlled trial. *Lancet Infect Dis* 2014;14(8):687–695.
143. Brindley PJ, Sher A. The chemotherapeutic effect of praziquantel against *Schistosoma mansoni* is dependent on host antibody response. *J Immunol* 1987;139:215–220.
144. Vale N, Gouveia MJ, Rinaldi G, et al. Praziquantel for schistosomiasis: single-drug metabolism revisited, mode of action, and resistance. *Antimicrob Agents Chemother* 2017;61(5).
145. Meyer T, Sekljic H, Fuchs S, et al. Taste, a new incentive to switch to (R)-praziquantel in schistosomiasis treatment. *PLoS Negl Trop Dis* 2009;3(1):e357.
146. Mandour ME, el Turabi H, Homeida MM, et al. Pharmacokinetics of praziquantel in healthy volunteers and patients with schistosomiasis. *Trans R Soc Trop Med Hyg* 1990;84(3):389–393.
147. Kovač J, Meister I, Neodo A, et al. Pharmacokinetics of praziquantel in *Schistosoma mansoni*- and *Schistosoma haematobium*-infected school- and preschool-aged children. *Antimicrob Agents Chemother* 2018;62(8): e02253-17.
148. Ndibazza J, Muhangi L, Akishule D, et al. Effects of deworming during pregnancy on maternal and perinatal outcomes in Entebbe, Uganda: a randomized controlled trial. *Clin Infect Dis* 2010;50(4):531–540.
149. Olveda RM, Acosta LP, Tallo V, et al. Efficacy and safety of praziquantel for the treatment of human schistosomiasis during pregnancy: a phase 2, randomised, double-blind, placebo-controlled trial. *Lancet Infect Dis* 2016;16(2):199–208.
150. Friedman JF, Olveda RM, Mirochnick MH, et al. Praziquantel for the treatment of schistosomiasis during human pregnancy. *Bull World Health Organ* 2018;96(1):59–65.
151. Bittencourt PR, Gracia CM, Martins R, et al. Phenytoin and carbamazepine decrease oral bioavailability of praziquantel. *Neurology* 1992;42:492–496.
152. Ridtitid W, Wongnawa M, Mahatthanatrakul W, et al. Rifampin markedly decreases plasma concentrations of praziquantel in healthy volunteers. *Clin Pharmacol Ther* 2002;72(5):505–513.
153. Jung H, Medina R, Castro N, et al. Pharmacokinetic study of praziquantel administered alone and in combination with cimetidine in a single-day therapeutic regimen. *Antimicrob Agents Chemother* 1997;41:1256–1259.
154. Ridtitid W, Ratsamemonthon K, Mahatthanatrakul W, et al. Pharmacokinetic interaction between ketoconazole and praziquantel in healthy volunteers. *J Clin Pharm Ther* 2007;32(6):585–593.
155. Romo ML, Carpio A, Kelvin EA. Routine drug and food interactions during antihelminthic treatment of neurocysticercosis: a reason for the variable efficacy of albendazole and praziquantel? *J Clin Pharmacol* 2014;54(4):361–367.
156. el Guiniady MA, el Touny MA, Abdel-Bary MA, et al. Clinical and pharmacokinetic study of praziquantel in Egyptian schistosomiasis patients with and without liver cell failure. *Am J Trop Med Hyg* 1994;51(6):809–818.
157. Montresor A, Odermatt P, Muth S, et al. The WHO dose pole for the administration of praziquantel is also accurate in non-African populations. *Trans R Soc Trop Med Hyg* 2005;99(1):78–81.
158. Hotez PJ, Fenwick A, Savioli L, et al. Rescuing the bottom billion through control of neglected tropical diseases. *Lancet* 2009;373(9674):1570–1575.
159. Bergquist R. Tribendimidine: great expectations. *Lancet Infect Dis* 2016;16(10):1089–1091.
160. Clarke NE, Doi SAR, Wangdi K, et al. Efficacy of anthelminthic drugs and drug combinations against soil-transmitted helminths: a systematic review and network meta-analysis. *Clin Infect Dis* 2019;68(1):96–105.
161. Olsen A. Efficacy and safety of drug combinations in the treatment of schistosomiasis, soil-transmitted helminthiasis, lymphatic filariasis and onchocerciasis. *Trans R Soc Trop Med Hyg* 2007;101(8):747–758.
162. Danso-Appiah A, Utzinger J, Liu J, et al. Drugs for treating urinary schistosomiasis. *Cochrane Database Syst Rev* 2008;(3):CD000053.
163. Diemert DJ, Bottazzi ME, Plieskatt J, et al. Lessons along the critical path: developing vaccines against human helminths. *Trends Parasitol* 2018;34(9):747–758.
164. Hotez PJ, Bottazzi ME, Bethony J, et al. Advancing the development of a human schistosomiasis vaccine. *Trends Parasitol* 2019;35(2):104–108.
165. Lustigman S, Makepeace BL, Klei TR, et al. *Onchocerca volvulus*: the road from basic biology to a vaccine. *Trends Parasitol* 2018;34(1):64–79.

Charles A. Peloquin
Wael A. Alghamdi
Mohammad H. Al-Shaer

CHAPTER 29

Antimycobacterial Drugs (*Mycobacterium tuberculosis* and Atypical Mycobacteria)

MYCOBACTERIUM TUBERCULOSIS

Tuberculosis (TB) remains a major global health problem, though the incidence per capita, prevalence, and death rates for TB are falling. Current challenges include the difficulty in correctly prescribing and adhering to complex and lengthy treatment protocols, emergence of *Mycobacterium tuberculosis* (MTB) strains resistant to multiple drugs, and human immunodeficiency virus (HIV) infection.[1] An estimated 1.6 million died due to TB in 2017. Of an estimated 10 million new cases in the same year, 9% were HIV positive, and about 10% occur in children younger than 15 years. The World Health Organization (WHO) estimated that 234,000 children died because of TB in 2018, which represented 15% of all TB deaths.[2]

Children are commonly infected through exposure to an infectious adult. The majority of infected children remain well, and the only evidence of infection may be a positive tuberculin skin test, termed latent tuberculosis infection (LTBI). Progression to disease usually occurs within 2 to 12 months following exposure and infection. Infants and children younger than 5 years and the immunocompromised are at particular risk of developing disease. A small proportion of children, who are generally older, develop postprimary TB either due to reactivation or by reinfection within 1 to 2 years of initial infection.[3,4]

Severe and disseminated TB, such as tuberculous meningitis and miliary TB, may occasionally occur especially in children younger than 3 years.[5] It is commonly primary, which has a much smaller bacterial load than adult-type TB with cavitation and sputum production. Bacterial confirmation of TB, therefore, will be difficult in children, and the choice of drugs will usually depend on results from the index case. On the other hand, failure, relapse, and development of resistance to anti-TB drugs are of lesser concern when treatment is started promptly.[6]

Management guidelines are available (Table 29.1) for both resource-poor and affluent areas.[6,7] Central to these recommendations are short-course drug regimens administered by directly observed therapy (DOT), which involves providing the anti-TB drugs directly to the patient and watching as he or she swallows the medications. While bacillary load and the type of disease may influence the effectiveness of treatment regimens, treatment outcomes in children are generally good, even in young and immunocompromised children, provided that treatment starts promptly. There is a low risk of adverse events associated with the use of the recommended treatment regimens.[7–9]

For LTBI in children, historically, isoniazid administered for 6 to 12 months has been the preferred treatment. It also has been shown to be effective as prophylaxis,[10] but poor adherence is observed, especially with unsupervised treatment.[10–12] An alternative treatment regimen of 3 to 4 months isoniazid plus rifampin for the treatment of LTBI showed similar efficacy to 9 months isoniazid treatment with improved adherence.[12–14] Rifapentine plus isoniazid once weekly for 12 weeks has been studied in children.[15,16] On the other hand, preventive therapy with rifampin plus pyrazinamide causes severe hepatotoxicity and should generally not be offered to treat LTBI.[17–20]

For an asymptomatic infant born into a household with an infectious TB patient, daily isoniazid is administered for 6 months and should be followed up every 2 months until treatment completion.[7] Other LTBI regimens that can be used in children are isoniazid and rifapentine for 3 months, rifampin for 4 months, and isoniazid for 9 months.[21]

The principles of treatment of TB disease in infants and children are similar to those in adults, while keeping in mind pharmacokinetic differences and possibility of adverse effects.[6,7,22–25] Published studies of treatment of children with TB[26–37] caused by organisms known or presumed to be susceptible to the first-line drugs have shown excellent results for pulmonary and lymph node TB, but less so for meningitis. For tuberculous meningitis, the higher end of the daily doses is recommended.[36,38,39] Also, recent pharmacokinetic studies of isoniazid, pyrazinamide, and ethambutol have shown lower plasma drug concentrations in children than in adults, suggesting that dosages per kilogram body weight need to be higher for children.[25,40–43]

Short-course treatments are administered in two phases. An initial intensive phase, typically 2 months, employs a combination of drugs that is effective in rapidly eliminating the

TABLE 29.1 Recommended Treatment Regimens for Drug-Susceptible Tuberculosis in Children

	WHO[7]		*ATS/CDC/IDSA*[6]	
Clinical Presentation	Intensive Phase	Continuation Phase	Intensive Phase	Continuation Phase
HIV (−)	2HRZE	4HR	2HRZE or 2(HRZE)5	4HR or 4(HR)5
			2HRZE or 2(HRZE)5	4(HR)3
			2(HRZE)3	4(HR)3
			2 wk(HRZE) then 6 wk(HRZE)2	4(HR)2
HIV (+)	2HRZE	4HR	2HRZE	4HR[a]
TB meningitis or osteoarticular TB	2HRZE	10HR	2HRZE	7–10HR

Note: The number before a phase is the duration in months. A number after a letter is the number of doses per week. If there is no number after a letter, then treatment with that drug is daily. Daily dosing appears to be the most effective.
[a]Continuation phase therapy should be extended to 7 months if HIV-infected patient is not on antiretroviral therapy.
ATS, American Thoracic Society; CDC, Centers for Disease Control and Prevention; E, ethambutol; H, isoniazid; HIV, human immunodeficiency virus; IDSA, Infectious Diseases Society of America; R, rifampin; S, streptomycin; TB, tuberculosis; WHO, World Health Organization; Z, pyrazinamide.

organism and in minimizing the chance for the development of resistance. Four drugs, usually isoniazid, rifampin, pyrazinamide, and ethambutol, are recommended when there is risk of resistance, or when children and adolescents develop adult-type pulmonary TB. However, when the infecting strain is fully susceptible to isoniazid, rifampin, and pyrazinamide, the prevalence of HIV is low, or the likelihood of failure is low as in primary TB commonly seen in children, an initial phase combination of isoniazid, rifampin, and pyrazinamide may be used. In the subsequent continuation phase, less number of drugs are administered but for at least 4 months to ensure that the patient is completely cured and does not relapse after completion of therapy.[6,7,24,44]

Children with HIV infection and confirmed or presumptive TB disease are treated with the 6-month regimen if on antiretroviral therapy. In patients who are not receiving antiretroviral therapy, the continuation phase should be extended to 7 months, which will result in a total treatment duration of 9 months. Co-trimoxazole as prophylaxis for other infections is administered, and antiretroviral therapy should be initiated in patients with CD4 count 500 cells per mm^3 or less. TB treatment failure can be due to noncompliance with therapy, poor drug absorption, drug resistance, and alternative diagnoses.[6,7]

Resistance to isoniazid and/or rifampin is the most important, as these two drugs form the mainstay of current chemotherapy. For cases with monoresistance to isoniazid, the patient should receive rifampin, pyrazinamide, ethambutol, and levofloxacin for 6 months.[45]

Multidrug-resistant tuberculosis (MDR-TB) is resistant to at least both isoniazid and rifampin and accounts for 4.6% of all TB cases.[2] Mainly transmitted from an adult-source case with MDR-TB, it is often not suspected unless a history of contact with an adult case is known. Children with MDR-TB should be treated with at least five drugs to which the bacterial strain, or that of its source case, is susceptible. Treatment should be given daily and preferably under DOT. Duration of treatment is usually 18 months or more. With correct drug exposure, few long-term adverse events are seen with any of the more toxic second-line drugs in children. Treatment, however, is difficult, and referral to a specialist and therapeutic drug monitoring are advised.[46,47]

ISONIAZID

Isoniazid, a hydrazide derivative of isonicotinic acid, is the most widely used first-line drug for TB. Isoniazid inhibits synthesis of long-chain mycolic acids, which are constituents of mycobacterial cell walls. It has the most potent early bactericidal activity against actively dividing MTB[22] but has limited activity against nondividing tubercle bacilli. Some isoniazid-resistant strains demonstrate a reduced catalase-peroxidase activity, which has been associated with deletions or point mutations in the *katG* gene.[48–50]

Isoniazid as single-drug therapy is indicated only for the prophylaxis of contacts of sputum smear-positive or culture-positive TB cases and for the treatment of LTBI. It must be used in combination with other drugs for active disease (see Table 29.1). In both, susceptibility of the bacilli to isoniazid should be established (active disease) or reasonably estimated based on exposure history (LTBI). Isoniazid is administered orally at 10 mg per kg (range 7 to 15 mg per kg) daily, with doses trending upward in recent years,[6,46] or 20 to 30 mg per kg twice weekly, targeting low-level isoniazid-resistant organisms.[51] Isoniazid may be administered intramuscularly or intravenously, the latter as a slow bolus over 5 minutes, diluted in normal saline.

Pharmacokinetics in Children

Absorption of isoniazid is rapid and complete but is slowed and modestly reduced by food. The effect of antacids on absorption is less clear.[52–54] Typical peak plasma concentrations of 3 to 5 μg per mL are reached in 1 to 2 hours after a 300-mg dose.[23,52–54] Isoniazid is distributed in all body fluids and tissues,[23,55] with excellent penetration into the cerebrospinal fluid (CSF).[56–58] The apparent volume of distribution is 0.62 to 0.83 L per kg, with no significant difference between slow and rapid acetylators.[59,60]

Isoniazid undergoes extensive presystemic metabolism. Isoniazid is acetylated by the liver to several metabolites, most of which are excreted in the urine. Acetylisoniazid is further hydrolyzed to isonicotinic acid and monoacetylhydrazine. Isonicotinic acid is conjugated with glycine to form isonicotinylglycine, whereas monoacetylhydrazine is further acetylated to diacetylhydrazine. All metabolites are devoid of anti-TB activity. Hepatotoxicity is associated with an incompletely acetylated hydrazide group found in monoacetylhydrazine and isoniazid.[61] However, a clear association between isoniazid dose and liver toxicity has not been proven.

The pharmacokinetic profile is dependent on N-acetylation capacity, which is trimodally distributed into slow, intermediate, or rapid phenotypes in accordance with the genotype of the polymorphic *N*-acetyltransferase-2.[62,63] People of European origin are about 50% slow acetylators, whereas many Asian populations are about 80% rapid acetylators.[61,64] The lower plasma concentration seen in rapid acetylators has been shown to be less effective in once-weekly dosing regimens, and there is a trend in that direction even with more frequent dosing, since area under the plasma concentration versus time curve divided by minimal inhibitory concentration (AUC/MIC) is the main driver of efficacy.[61,65]

Half-life in adults is 0.7 to 2 hours for rapid acetylators and 2.3 to 3.5 hours for slow acetylators.[54,61,66] The typical categories are fast (<2 hours) and slow (≥2 hours). Isoniazid is largely excreted in the urine within 24 hours, mostly as inactive metabolites. Renal excretion is independent of acetylator status.

Isoniazid concentrations expected in children are similar to adults. Excellent penetration into the CSF of children with tuberculous meningitis has been demonstrated.[58,67] A trimodal pharmacokinetic profile also is evident in children. Clearance is 3.83 and 6.88 mL per minute per kg, and half-life is 2.91 and 1.36 hours in slow and rapid acetylators, respectively. Apparent volume of distribution is 0.83 L per kg and, as in adults, is not affected by acetylator phenotype.[59,68] Younger children eliminate isoniazid faster than older children in all three genotypes. As a group, children eliminate isoniazid faster and achieve significantly lower serum concentrations than adults who receive the same milligram per kilogram body weight dose. An isoniazid dose of at least 10 mg per kg might be more appropriate for rapid acetylators to achieve the recommended serum concentration of 1.5 mg per L.[40,43]

In children who received isoniazid prophylaxis for 6 months, only 1.9% developed active TB within a 10-year follow-up period.[69] In another study, development of active disease was low among tuberculin-positive children who received isoniazid. A morbidity rate of 4.2 per 1,000 children was observed after a mean observation period of 6.1 years.[70] Efficacy studies of isoniazid combined with other first-line drugs in short-course treatments in children with active TB showed excellent results, approaching at least 95% efficacy in pulmonary and lymph node TB.[26–33,71] The efficacy against tuberculous meningitis, however, is less, with increased mortality and sequelae for survivors.[34–36]

Isoniazid inhibits cytochromes (CYP) P450 2C19, CYP3A4, CYP2A6, and CYP2E1.[72,73] Metabolism may be impaired, leading to increased serum concentrations and potentiation of the effects of warfarin, theophylline, triazolam,[22] diazepam,[74] and antiepileptics such as carbamazepine,[75] phenytoin,[76,77] and valproic acid.[78] On the other hand, concomitant administration of isoniazid leads to decreased effectiveness of methoxyflurane, isoflurane, sevoflurane, and enflurane.[79]

Concentrations of isoniazid increase with concomitant administration of aminosalicylic acid[22] or ethionamide,[52] which, in theory, may lead to toxic manifestations. In practice, these combinations are uncommon. On the other hand, isoniazid concentrations may decrease with antacids,[53] prednisone, and prednisolone.[22] Isoniazid may act as a monoamine oxidase inhibitor and may lead to excessive responses to pressor amines.[22,80] Increased risk of hepatotoxicity has been observed with administration of isoniazid with paracetamol[22] and rifampin, but with the latter, benefits far outweigh the risks.

Isoniazid is readily transported across the placenta, but is not associated with a detectable increase in birth defects.[81] It is excreted in breast milk, but the reported relative infant dose, about 1.2% of the weight-adjusted maternal dose, is below the 10% notional level of concern for nursing infants.[55,82]

Safety in Children

Genetically, slow acetylators are more at risk for various isoniazid-related toxicities. Acute poisoning is associated with significant toxicity and mortality, with slow acetylators at risk. Nausea, vomiting, hypotension, leukocytosis, hyperpyrexia, respiratory distress, seizures, and coma are seen in children. Metabolic acidosis, ketonuria, hyperglycemia, mild hyperkalemia, increased urinary excretion of pyridoxine, impaired liver function, and rhabdomyolysis have been observed.[83–87] Therefore, isoniazid must be stored safely in the home, away from children.

The induction of seizures by isoniazid has been attributed to its lowering effect on pyridoxine concentrations, which may affect formation and catabolism of γ-aminobutyric acid. Gram-for-gram treatment with vitamin B_6 (pyridoxine) is recommended, and high-dose intravenous pyridoxine terminates seizures and may wake patients from coma.[84,88] Niacinamide also has been shown to be effective in reversing isoniazid-induced hyperkinesis, suggesting interference by isoniazid of nicotinamide adenine dinucleotide–catalyzed reactions.[83]

Dose-dependent peripheral neuropathies occur more often in slow acetylators.[89] It is uncommon and rare in children, except in malnourished patients whose vitamin B_6 deficiency may result from or be aggravated by loss of pyridoxal hydrazone of isoniazid. Symptoms include tingling, numbness, tenderness, weakness, and stiffness in the extremities. It can be prevented by daily administration of supplementary vitamin B_6.[23,90] Additionally, isoniazid may increase pyridoxine requirements in children.[90,91] Serum vitamin D concentrations are low when isoniazid is taken but rise to normal after discontinuation of isoniazid.[92,93]

Asymptomatic liver dysfunction to frank liver disease can occur with isoniazid administration in children. Risk factors include severe tuberculous disease, higher isoniazid doses, and coadministration with rifampin. With isoniazid alone, the occurrence is 0.18% to 0.5%, which is much less common than in adults.[94–97] There is an appreciable but low risk of hepatotoxicity with isoniazid at current recommended dosing regimens. Elevations of liver enzymes are usually transient and normalize with continued therapy. Slow acetylators possibly are at increased risk.[64] Caution must be observed in the presence of liver disease, and regular monitoring of liver enzymes is recommended. A full dose may still be given in impaired renal function.[98]

Reported hematologic adverse effects include agranulocytosis, hemolytic anemia, sideroblastic anemia, aplastic anemia, thrombocytopenia, eosinophilia, red cell aplasia, and disseminated intravascular coagulation,[99–101] although they are not common. Anorexia and nausea,[100] gynecomastia,[102] hyperthermia,[103] pancreatitis,[104,105] rheumatoid-like and lupus-like arthritis,[100] and rhabdomyolysis[86,87] have been reported. Dermatologic side effects and hypersensitivity are uncommon.[30,100]

RIFAMPIN

Rifampin (rifampin) is a semisynthetic derivative of the natural antibiotic rifamycin B and belongs to the class of naphthalenic rifamycins.[22,106] It has a wide spectrum of activity against bacteria, including some strains of atypical mycobacteria.

Rifampin binds to the β-subunit of bacterial RNA polymerase, thereby inhibiting transcription of DNA to RNA. It specifically inhibits the transition from synthesis of short oligoribonucleotides to full-length transcripts. Rifampin is bactericidal for both intracellular and extracellular mycobacteria and against "nonreplicating persisters."[23] Bacilli dormant much of the time but occasionally metabolizing for short periods are killed more rapidly by rifampin than by isoniazid during short-course chemotherapy. [107] Most resistant isolates have missense mutations, deletions, or insertions within the region of the RNA polymerase β-subunit gene (*rpoB*).[108,109]

Rifampin is an essential drug in the treatment of TB with susceptible bacilli (see Table 29.1 for use in treatment regimens). It should be given by DOT combined with other effective antimycobacterial agents to avoid the emergence of resistance. Rifampin is administered orally at 15 mg per kg (range 10 to 20 mg per kg, maximum 600 mg) daily, with a trend toward higher doses.[6,7] It may be administered intravenously over 30 minutes.

Pharmacokinetics in Children

Rifampin is rapidly but variably absorbed from the gastrointestinal tract. The suspension may be only 50% absorbed by pediatric patients[110] and is subject to degradation. Food may delay and reduce peak serum concentrations.[106,111] The bentonite excipient in certain older *p*-aminosalicylic acid preparations may impede gastrointestinal absorption of rifampin.[106,112] Peak concentrations of 8 to 24 μg per mL are reached in 1 to 4 hours.[113]

Rifampin distributes widely, including exudates in tuberculous lung cavities, bronchial secretions, and alveolar macrophages.[106,114] Protein binding is 72% to 91%, and the volume of distribution is 55 L.[52,115] CSF penetration is slow,[56] but therapeutic concentrations may be achieved with inflamed meninges.[57,116] Higher doses are being studied for central nervous system (CNS) disease. There is little presystemic metabolism, but repeated administration induces intestinal and hepatic transporters (efflux pumps), with consequent reduction in serum half-life and AUC.[106,117]

Rifampin is deacetylated to a partially active metabolite, 25-*O*-desacetylrifampin, and hydrolyzed to 3-formylrifamycin. Part of rifampin may be conjugated with glucuronic acid during hepatic metabolism. Desacetylrifampin is a more polar compound with increased capacity for biliary excretion. Unchanged rifampin is reabsorbed, creating enterohepatic circulation, whereas 25-*O*-desacetylrifampin is poorly absorbed, facilitating elimination. Transporter induction increases the metabolism of rifampin and the biliary excretion of desacetylrifampin.[106,118]

It was thought that rifampin had a dose-dependent half-life (2.3 to 5.1 hours), although this is more likely due to prolonged absorption mixed with temporary saturation of clearance (nonlinear pharmacokinetics).[119] At steady-state, half-life may be as short as 1 to 2 hours.[52,106,120,121] The principal excretion pathway is bile, with urine as secondary pathway. Urinary concentration increases with doses above 450 mg, when biliary excretion is more saturated. Impaired hepatic function or biliary excretion, but not impaired renal function, may require modification of dosage and careful monitoring.

In children older than 1 year, metabolism of rifampin is similar to that in adults. Peak serum concentrations of 1.9 to 21.9 μg per mL were reached 2 to 4 hours after preprandial administration of 5 to 20 mg per kg body weight of rifampin.[122] In general, concentrations above 8 μg per mL are preferred, since rifampin has profound concentration-dependent activity (AUC/MIC).[123] Doses up to 40 mg per kg are being studied.[119] Half-life and urinary excretion are the same as in adults. In infants, serum peak concentrations are delayed, and elimination is comparatively slow. Furthermore, because hepatic mechanisms and biliary excretion are less fully developed, more rifampin is excreted in the urine, and there is less change with time because induction is low at this age.[106]

Rifampin profoundly induces hepatic microsomal enzymes, especially but not exclusively CYP3A4.[124] Serum concentrations of drugs metabolized by these liver enzymes may be decreased by the coadministration of rifampin. Examples of drugs relevant to children include corticosteroids,[125] diazepam,[126] digoxin,[127] midazolam,[128] narcotics and analgesics (methadone, morphine, phenobarbitone),[100] theophylline,[129] and vitamin D.[92,130] Some reports suggest that rifampin concentrations may be decreased by ethambutol, *p*-aminosalicylic acid, ketoconazole, and phenobarbital, although this does not appear to be a common clinical problem.[131]

Serum concentrations at birth range from 12% to 33% of maternal serum.[81,106] While rifampin is dysmorphogenic in rats and mice, there has been no evidence of teratogenicity in infants.[100,132,133] It is excreted in breast milk, but not in amounts likely to cause harm.[55]

Safety in Children

Gastrointestinal adverse reactions include anorexia, nausea, vomiting, and abdominal discomfort. Diarrhea is less frequently reported.[100] Severe adverse effects are not common but are usually related to sensitization or to its effects on other drugs through enzyme induction. Sensitivity is more common with intermittent therapy, which may result in the flu-like syndrome, shock, hemolytic anemia, and renal failure.[100,134] If thrombocytopenia, purpura, or renal failure occurs, permanent discontinuation of rifampin is recommended.

Hepatic reactions occur with rifampin in chronic liver disease, and patients need careful monitoring. Combination with drugs such as isoniazid and pyrazinamide may aggravate the situation.[135,136] In children treated with rifampin and isoniazid, 3.3% developed jaundice in the first 10 weeks of treatment. Some suggest limiting the dose of isoniazid to 10 mg per kg and rifampin to 15 mg per kg in order to limit hepatotoxicity, but this toxicity has not been proven to be dose or concentration related.[96,137] The rise in liver enzymes is usually transient.[138] Unless liver function tests continue to deteriorate, these changes are not an indication for discontinuing treatment. The TB treatment guidelines describe the process of treatment interruption and resumption in detail.[6]

Other uncommon adverse effects reported include cutaneous pigmentation, or the red man syndrome,[139] cutaneous vasculitis,[140] hyperglycemia, which is probably due to increased glucose absorption,[141] thrombocytopenia,[142] lupus syndrome,[143] ulcerative colitis,[144] and venous thrombosis.[145] Urine becomes highly colored (red, orange, pink), and tears turn pink.[100]

PYRAZINAMIDE

Pyrazinamide is a synthetic pyrazine analog of nicotinamide. It is an essential drug and one of the cornerstones of short-course TB therapy. Pyrazinamide is bactericidal to MTB at acidic pH values. To be bactericidal, it requires an enzyme, pyrazinamidase, to produce active pyrazinoic acid.[146] Like rifampin, pyrazinamide kills the slowly or intermittently metabolizing semidormant bacilli.[147] It may act by disruption of membrane transport and energy depletion, although debate continues regarding the exact mechanism of action.[148] Importantly, due to its selective targeting of subpopulations of MTB, pyrazinamide does not protect other drugs from the selection of drug-resistant isolates.

Pyrazinamide increases the efficacy of other anti-TB drugs. Its use in combination with other drugs as part of short-course regimens has shown excellent results. Resistance is rapid if used solely. Table 29.1 presents recommended treatment regimens with pyrazinamide. It is administered orally at 35 mg per kg (range 30 to 40 mg per kg) daily, or intermittently at 50 mg per kg twice to thrice weekly.[6,7]

Pharmacokinetics in Children

Absorption of pyrazinamide after oral administration is rapid and nearly complete.[52] Peak plasma concentrations are observed within 1 to 2 hours.[149–151] Pyrazinamide is widely distributed in tissues and fluids, including CSF,[57] although its activity in normal pH areas may be reduced. The volume of distribution is 0.75 to 1.65 L per kg.[150] Pyrazinamide is hydrolyzed in the liver to the major active metabolite, pyrazinoic acid, by a microsomal deamidase. Pyrazinoic acid is hydroxylated to the main excretory product, 5-hydroxypyrazinoic acid, by xanthine oxidase.[151,152] Alternatively, pyrazinamide may be converted to 5-hydroxypyrazinamide by xanthine oxidase and further to 5-hydroxypyrazinoic acid by deamidase. Of the dose, 30% to 40% is excreted in urine as pyrazinoic acid and 2% to 4% as unchanged pyrazinamide.[52,149,150,152] Half-life is 9 hours (typically 6 to 10 hours) and prolonged with impaired hepatic and renal function.[149–151,153] Clearance is 61 mL per minute.[151]

Estimates of pyrazinamide concentrations indicate linear pharmacokinetics in children with TB. After administration of pyrazinamide, incomplete or delayed absorption and greater volume of distribution are seen in children compared with adults. However, reported half-life and clearance estimates in children have been varied.[41] Based on a recent review, the reported maximum concentration range in studies on children was 21.1 to 49.4 μg per mL after 15 to 35 mg per kg dose.[154]

Safety in Children

The principal adverse effect appears to be dose-related liver toxicity, which is usually asymptomatic but may appear anytime during therapy. Rapid elevation of liver enzymes occurs but does resolve over time. Clinical observations suggest that isoniazid- and rifampin-induced increases in serum concentrations of liver enzymes resolve more rapidly than pyrazinamide-induced elevations. Hyperuricemia occurs but is usually asymptomatic.[100] Monitoring of liver enzymes and uric acid is recommended. Pyrazinamide should be promptly discontinued with rising liver enzymes, evidence of clinical hepatotoxicity, or significant joint pains. Other common adverse effects include flushing, mild anorexia, nausea, and myalgia.[100,155] Hypersensitivity, photosensitization, and rash are rarely observed.[156] Sideroblastic anemia is rare and reversible.[100]

In 114 children with pulmonary TB, clinical adverse effects to pyrazinamide were uncommon and mild. Slight elevation in liver enzymes was observed in 20%, with none exhibiting clinical hepatitis. Serum uric acid increased above normal in 10% of children, but none had signs of gout or arthralgia. Abdominal pain was seen in 1.8%, and vomiting with anorexia in 2.6%. In no case was treatment interrupted.[32]

There are no data on safety and teratogenicity in pregnancy.[157] There is minimal transfer in breast milk.[55]

ETHAMBUTOL

Ethambutol is the dextrorotatory isomer of the synthetic compound 2,2′-ethylenediimino-di-1-butanol dihydrochloride. It is bacteriostatic against MTB. At higher doses of 50 mg per kg, it exhibits bactericidal activity, but such doses are not tolerated on a daily basis.[158] Ethambutol produces detrimental alteration of cell wall structure by inhibiting the biosynthesis of the arabinan of arabinogalactan and lipoarabinomannan.[159,160] Missense changes in *embB* codon 306 are associated with resistance in MTB isolates.[161,162]

Ethambutol is used primarily to prevent the emergence of resistance to first-line drugs. In the treatment of MDR-TB, ethambutol becomes a first-line agent (see Table 29.1). Because pyrazinamide does not protect other drugs from the selection of drug-resistant isolates, and because preexisting isoniazid resistance is common, the primary role of ethambutol is to protect rifampin until susceptibility data are available. It may demonstrate synergism by enhancing penetration of the other drugs, especially ciprofloxacin.[163]

Pharmacokinetics in Children

Oral absorption of ethambutol is approximately 80%.[52] Peak concentrations are reached in 2 to 4 hours[23] but are lower following a meal than when fasting.[164] Protein binding is 12% (up to 24%), and the volume of distribution is 18.9 to 21.2 L.[52,115] Ethambutol concentrates in erythrocytes, which act as a depot from which the drug slowly reenters plasma.

Tissue concentrations are higher than in serum or plasma, except for the CNS[164] where it penetrates poorly. CSF concentrations rise with meningeal inflammation, but only to levels below inhibitory concentration.[23,52] About 10% to 20% of the drug undergoes hepatic metabolism. The metabolite ethambutol aldehyde is inactive.[52] Approximately 50% to 70% of an oral dose is excreted and unchanged in the urine. The α half-life for most of the dose is 3.5 to 4.6 hours, followed by slow release of a small amount of drug from red blood cells and other tissues over many hours. In impaired renal function, the dose must be reduced.[23,52,100,165]

Slow and incomplete absorption of ethambutol is common in children.[42] Ethambutol serum concentrations reached after oral administration increase with age, with serum concentrations lower in younger children than in older children.[166] Children with TB showed faster elimination and shorter half-lives than adults. Furthermore, apparent volume of distribution and clearance are lower, though weight-normalized clearance is higher. Studies of ethambutol in children have found plasma drug concentrations lower than typical minimum inhibitory concentration values. In almost all cases, maximal serum concentrations failed to reach MICs, and higher dosages per kilogram body weight compared with those for adults have been suggested for children.[42,167] Children appear to have shortened periods of serum concentrations above the MIC as compared with adults.[168]

Table 29.1 presents recommended regimens using ethambutol. Ethambutol sometimes is avoided in children too young to undergo visual acuity testing, unless it is used to treat drug-resistant TB. However, there are no reports of ocular toxicity in this population, and they tend to rapidly eliminate ethambutol. Some clinicians are perfectly comfortably using ethambutol in younger patients. Based on recent studies that raised concern on low drug concentrations achieved in children, a daily dose of 20 mg per kg 15 to 25 mg per kg is recommended. At this dose, effective therapeutic concentration (defined as >2 μg per mL) is approached and balances compensation for deficiency of serum concentration and risk of ocular toxicity.[164,169] A dose of 50 mg per kg is recommended when given twice weekly.[6] Higher doses may be preferred in HIV-positive patients, who tend to have lower ethambutol concentrations and in patients to whom ethambutol is especially important to the regimen as when isoniazid- or rifampin-resistant MTB isolates are documented or suspected.[42]

Ethambutol has been used successfully in pregnancy. Transplacental transfer has been documented to be at least 75% of that of maternal serum concentrations. This was associated with a normal infant.[81] Ethambutol is excreted in trace amounts in breast milk, which should be safely ingested by an infant.[55]

Safety in Children

Ethambutol generally is well tolerated. Mild hyperuricemia and gouty arthritis have been reported infrequently.[100] Rare adverse effects include hypersensitivity, hepatitis,[100] thrombocytopenia,[170] neutropenia, and eosinophilia.[171] The most serious adverse effect is retrobulbar optic neuritis,[100,172] which can lead to decrease in visual acuity and even loss of ability to discriminate colors red and green. It is fairly common with high doses of 50 mg per kg per day and is also related to duration of treatment and renal insufficiency. However, a review of the literature did not reveal major ocular side effects among children treated with ethambutol. Only 2 (0.05%) of 3,811 children who received ethambutol developed possible ocular toxicity.[173] However, it has been suggested that the rare ethambutol toxicity is due to the considerably lower serum concentrations reached in children.[164]

SECOND-LINE DRUGS

Second-line drugs are mainly used for the treatment of MDR-TB (see Table 29.2). Resistant cases are difficult to treat; thus, a referral to a specialist is required. The current classifications for the drugs used in MDR-TB consist of three groups. Group A includes levofloxacin or moxifloxacin, bedaquiline, and linezolid; group B includes clofazimine and cycloserine (or terizidone); and group C includes ethambutol, delamanid, pyrazinamide, imipenem-cilastatin, meropenem, amikacin (or streptomycin), ethionamide (or prothionamide), and *p*-aminosalicylic acid.[174] When drug susceptibility tests are available, they should be utilized to direct the therapy. In treating these cases, a minimum of four drugs which are likely to be effective should be administered. Daily dosing, rather than intermittent dosing, is preferred, and DOT is necessary.[7] The duration of the conventional regimen is typically 18 to 20 months.[174] A shorter regimen (the Bangladesh regimen), lasting 9 to 12 months, can also be considered in patients who were not previously treated with second-line agents and resistance to fluoroquinolones or injectable agents is highly unlikely. The use of second-line drugs in children has not been thoroughly explored. Clinical trials are underway to evaluate the pharmacokinetics and the safety of several second-line drugs in children, including the novel drugs delamanid and bedaquiline.[175]

Table 29.2 presents the key points of the second-line drugs used for RR/MDR-TB. Aminoglycosides, fluoroquinolones, and linezolid are primarily used for nonmycobacterial infections; hence, their pharmacology in children is discussed in Chapters 22, 23, and 24. The recent WHO guidelines promote injectable-free regimens. In children with a mild type of the disease (e.g., clinically diagnosed TB), the use of aminoglycosides is discouraged, as the harms may outweigh the benefits. In addition, there were no significant differences in treatment success between patients treated with or without an injectable agent.[47] Nonetheless, two aminoglycosides can be used for MDR-TB: amikacin and streptomycin. Ototoxicity and nephrotoxicity are the most frequent adverse effects associated with the use of aminoglycosides.[174,176] The consequences of ototoxicity can be profound in children, as it may affect their progress in language acquisition and formal education. On the other hand, the later-generation fluoroquinolones and linezolid have demonstrated remarkable improvements in treatment outcomes. In fact, fluoroquinolones are considered the cornerstone of the MDR-TB regimen. In young children, moxifloxacin is available in tablet dosage form, and splitting or crushing them results in highly unpleasant taste. On the other hand, levofloxacin is available in oral solution (pediatric-friendly dosage form). Linezolid has also been associated with treatment success, even in patients with extensively drug-resistant TB.[47,177] Thus, it has been prioritized to group A. Its use may be affected by the severity of the side effects, such as myelosuppression, optic neuropathy, and peripheral neuropathy; hence, close monitoring is needed.

Among the drugs that are no longer recommended are kanamycin and capreomycin, which is an injectable that acts similar to aminoglycosides. The recent guidelines specifically recommend against their use, as they have been associated with increased risk of relapse and treatment failure.[174] Also, thioacetazone, a derivative of thiosemicarbazone, has fallen out of favor due to its high rates of adverse events, limited efficacy, and low available in a quality-assured formulation. Gastrointestinal (weight loss, nausea, vomiting) and neurologic (headache, blurred vision, perioral numbness, mental symptoms, and peripheral nerve symptoms) adverse events are most frequent, followed by serious cutaneous adverse events. Idiosyncratic toxic epidermolysis may occur in HIV-infected patients, and it is contraindicated in this population.[22]

Clofazimine

The primary indication for clofazimine is leprosy, largely due to its high lipophilicity and anti-inflammatory properties.[178–180] Early in vitro studies showed excellent activity for clofazimine against MTB; however, later animal studies did not show improved survival outcomes. With the emergence of extensively drug-resistant TB (i.e., resistant to rifampin, isoniazid, aminoglycosides, and fluoroquinolones), there has been a renewed interest in clofazimine. In fact, the WHO has recently prioritized

TABLE 29.2	Second-Line Drugs for the Treatment of Drug-Resistant Tuberculosis in Children					
Drug, Route	*Mechanism of Action*	*Target Site*	*Daily Dose (mg/kg)*	*Pharmacology*	*Adverse Effects*	*Precautions*
Aminoglycosides, IV, IM	Inhibition of protein synthesis	16S rRNA		Bactericidal; low CSF concentrations; kanamycin and amikacin cross-resistance; resistant to amikacin may be susceptible to capreomycin	Ototoxic, nephrotoxic, neuromuscular blockade	Avoid in pregnancy; renal dosing[a]
Amikacin			15-20			
Streptomycin			20–40			
Bedaquiline, PO	Interfering with mycobacterial energy production	Mycobacterial ATP synthase	15–29 kg: 200 mg QD for 2 wk, then 100 mg TIW for 22 wk >29 kg: 400 mg QD for 2 wk, then 200 mg TIW for 22 wk	Bactericidal; limited data on CSF penetration; extremely long half-life	Nausea, headache, hepatotoxicity, QT prolongation	Not recommended in pregnancy (can be considered when effective regimen cannot be constructed using safer agents; FDA category B)
Clofazimine, PO	Disruption of membrane and intracellular redox cycling[b]	-	2–5	Bacteriostatic (late bactericidal activity); limited data on CSF penetration; extremely long half-life	Reddish-orange discoloration of skin, conjunctivae, and body fluids, QT prolongation, GI irritation	Not recommended in pregnancy (limited data; infant pigmentation)
Cycloserine or terizidone, PO	Inhibition of peptidoglycan synthesis	Alanine racemase, D-alanine ligase	15–20 (usually divided into 2 doses)	Bacteriostatic; excellent CSF penetration; no cross-resistance with other agents	Psychiatric, neurologic; pyridoxine used for prevention	Avoid in pregnancy; renal dosing[a]
Delamanid, PO	Inhibition of mycolic acid synthesis	Methoxy-mycolic and keto-mycolic acid synthesis	3–5 y old: 25 mg BID 6–11 y old: 50 mg BID 12–17 y old: 100 mg BID	Bactericidal; limited data on CSF penetration	Nausea, headache, QT prolongation	Not recommended in pregnancy (limited data); avoid in patients with hypoalbuminemia (<2.8 g/dL)
Ethionamide or prothionamide, PO	Inhibition of mycolic acid synthesis	Enoyl-acyl carrier protein reductase	15–20 (usually divided into 2–3 doses)	Bactericidal; excellent CSF penetration; hepatic metabolism	Vomiting, GI irritation, hypothyroidism, elevated liver transaminases	Teratogenic; contraindicated in pregnancy
Fluoroquinolones, PO, IV	Inhibition of DNA synthesis	DNA gyrase		Bactericidal; poor to moderate CSF penetration; cross-resistance within the class	GI irritation, concern with arthropathy and arthritis in children	Avoid in pregnancy; renal dosing[a]
Levofloxacin			15–20			
Moxifloxacin			10–15			
Linezolid, PO, IV	Inhibition of protein synthesis	50S bacterial ribosomal subunit	15 (<16 kg) 10–12 (>15 kg)	Bactericidal; excellent CSF penetration avoid use with serotonergic agents	Myelosuppression, lactic acidosis, optic and peripheral neuropathy; pyridoxine used for prevention	Not recommended in pregnancy (limited data)
Para-aminosalicylic acid, PO, IV	Disruption of folate pathway	Dihydrofolate reductase	200–300 (divided into 2–4 doses)	Bacteriostatic; low CSF concentrations; acetylated in the liver	Vomiting, GI irritation, hypothyroidism, hypersensitivity reactions	Teratogenic in animals; avoid in pregnancy; renal dosing[a]

[a]Adjust dose in renal impairment.
[b]The exact mechanism of clofazimine is not fully understood.
BID, twice daily; CSF, cerebrospinal fluid; FDA, U.S. Food and Drug Administration; GI, gastrointestinal; IM, intramuscular; IV, intravenous; PO, oral; QD, once daily; TIW, three times per week.
Data from references 51, 148, 183, 188, 206, 231, 232.

clofazimine to group B, given the current clinical evidence.[174,177] Although the exact mechanism of action for clofazimine is not fully understood, several mechanisms have been proposed, including membrane disruption, intracellular redox cycling, and the generation of antimicrobial reactive oxygen species.[179,180] It is believed that clofazimine exerts its effect via several mechanisms, which possibly contributes to its low frequency of resistance.

Clofazimine is lipophilic and accumulates in the skin and tissues; hence, it has a very long half-life, approximately 70 days. Administering clofazimine with high-fat food significantly improves its bioavailability, while antacids and orange juice decrease the drug's bioavailability.[181] Clofazimine is not removed by hemodialysis.[182] Limited pharmacokinetic data are available on clofazimine in both adults and children. Clofazimine has no pediatric formulations, and dividing the capsules may not be practical.[174,183] Therefore, if the weight-based calculated dose is smaller than the available strength, dosing every other day may be considered as an alternative approach due to its long half-life.

Gastrointestinal intolerance, including nausea, vomiting, and abdominal pain, has been reported with the use of clofazimine.[176] It also causes reddish-brown or orange discoloration of the skin, conjunctivae, and body fluids. Clofazimine can cause QT prolongation.[183] Therefore, close monitoring is recommended, especially when it is coadministered with other drugs known to prolong the QT interval.

Cycloserine or Terizidone

Cycloserine was discovered in 1954. It is a cyclic analog of D-alanine that inhibits two sequential enzymes, alanine racemase and D-alanine D-alanine ligase, resulting in the inhibition of peptidoglycan synthesis.[184,185] Cycloserine is classified as group B in the most recent WHO guidelines.[174] Since terizidone contains two molecules of cycloserine, higher cycloserine concentrations were observed with terizidone, compared to cycloserine formulations given at the same dose.[186–188] This difference, however, was significantly less than proportional to the presence of two cycloserine molecules in the terizidone formulation. Compared to cycloserine, less data are available for terizidone.[188]

Cycloserine has a relatively long half-life in adult patients with TB, with an average of 17 hours.[189,190] In children, the average half-life was approximately 11 hours.[191] Cycloserine is primarily cleared renally; therefore, drug concentration monitoring is recommended in patients with reduced renal function. Cycloserine has good penetration to the CSF.[192] Administering cycloserine with high-fat food delays absorption and reduces peak concentration, while antacids and orange juice have no effect on drug absorption.[193] A significant amount of cycloserine is removed by hemodialysis; hence, administering it after hemodialysis is recommended.[182]

Cycloserine can cause neuropsychiatric side effects, including anxiety, depression, psychosis, and, in rare cases, seizures. This is likely due to its binding to *N*-methyl-D-aspartate receptors.[194–196] Psychiatric and neurologic side effects have been reported in 5.7% and 1.1% of patients receiving cycloserine, respectively.[197] It is thought that these side effects are concentration dependent, although no studies have examined this relationship. The typical dose is 250 to 500 mg, given once or twice daily. It is preferable to divide the daily dose to reduce the peak concentration, which may potentially reduce the neuropsychiatric side effects while preserving its microbial kill.[189]

Ethionamide/Prothionamide

Ethionamide and prothionamide are considered interchangeable prodrugs and are structurally similar to isoniazid.[198,199] The active form of ethionamide and prothionamide adducts with nicotinamide adenine dinucleotide, resulting in the inhibition of the enoyl-acyl carrier protein reductase (inhA) and ultimately the inhibition of mycolic acid biosynthesis. Ethionamide and prothionamide possess bactericidal activity against MTB, along with other mycobacteria.

Ethionamide shows linear pharmacokinetics with dose increase from 250 to 1,000 mg in adults.[200] The current pediatric dosing, 15 to 20 mg per kg, seems sufficient to produce concentrations corresponding to the recommended range for adults.[201] Ethionamide has an average half-life ranging from 1 to 3 hours in older children (>2years).[191,201] In a study of 31 children, younger children (<2years) achieved lower plasma concentrations and had a shorter half-life of less than 1 hour; hence, they may need higher doses.[201] Ethionamide absorption is nearly complete and is not affected by high-fat food, orange juice, or antacids.[202] Therefore, ethionamide can be administered with food to improve tolerance. Ethionamide has good CSF penetration, and a negligible amount is removed by hemodialysis.[182,192]

Ethionamide is metabolized in the liver into active and inactive metabolites.[198,203,204] The ethionamide sulfoxide, an active metabolite, has demonstrated antimicrobial activity. It is also thought that the sulfoxide metabolite is responsible for the drug-related hepatotoxicity. Ethionamide and prothionamide often cause asymptomatic elevation of liver transaminases. Hepatotoxicity, however, is rare, affecting only about 2% of the patients receiving ethionamide or prothionamide.[137,198] Ethionamide is notorious for its dose-related gastrointestinal intolerance, causing nausea, vomiting, and abdominal discomfort.[198] The gastrointestinal intolerance usually improves within 2 to 4 weeks if initiating treatment. Dividing the dose and administering it with food can help patients tolerate the drug. Patients may also develop hypothyroidism and experience neurologic side effects.[198,205] In children taking ethionamide or prothionamide, monitoring thyroid function is important, and thyroxine supplementation should be considered.

Para-aminosalicylic Acid

Para-aminosalicylic acid (PAS) may compete with its structural analog, para-aminobenzoic acid, in a reaction catalyzed by dihydropteroate synthase and subsequently processed by dihydrofolate synthase.[206] This results in the formation of hydroxyl dihydrofolate, which inhibits dihydrofolate reductase and results in blocking the folate pathway in MTB.

PAS is metabolized in the liver to form acetyl-PAS, along with other metabolites.[207] PAS and its metabolites are excreted renally. Therefore, a dosing adjustment may be considered in patients with significantly reduced renal function. A dose of 150 mg per kg PASER (extended-release granules) given once or divided to twice daily in children was found to produce drug concentrations similar to adults receiving 4 g twice daily.[208] The American Thoracic Society recommends a pediatric daily dose of 200 to 300 mg per kg (divided into 2 to 4 doses per day).[6] Coadministering PAS with high-fat food increases the peak concentration by 1.5 times and the extent of absorption by 1.7 times, compared to giving the drug on empty stomach.[209] Antacids and orange juice have minimal effects on drug absorption. PAS has low CSF penetration and is not significantly removed by hemodialysis.[182,192]

One of the common side effects for PAS is gastrointestinal intolerance, including nausea, vomiting, and abdominal cramps.[176] The formulation containing enteric-coated granules seems to alleviate some of this effect.[210] PAS can also cause hypothyroidism, especially when it is coadministered with ethionamide or prothionamide.[46,198] Hypothyroidism is reversible when PAS (or ethionamide) is discontinued. Hypothyroidism may affect the neurodevelopment of children; therefore, monitoring thyroid function is essential. Thyroxine supplementation should be considered in these cases. Hypersensitivity reactions and hepatotoxicity were also reported with the use of PAS.[137,176,211] However, the reported frequency rate of hepatotoxicity was low (0.3%).

Novel Agents

Two novel TB drugs have been approved recently, after nearly four decades since the last new treatment for active TB was introduced to the market.[212] Bedaquiline was the first drug to be approved specifically for MDR-TB by the U.S. Food and Drug Administration in 2012, and later in Europe and other countries.[213] Two years later, delamanid was also approved for MDR-TB by Europe and Japan, but has not yet been approved by the United States.[214] They were approved for use in combination along with other TB drugs.

Bedaquiline

Bedaquiline is a diarylquinoline that has a novel mechanism of action. It exhibits its bactericidal activity against MTB by inhibiting the mycobacterial adenosine triphosphate (ATP) synthase in the replicating and dormant bacteria.[215] Bedaquiline can be used in children aged 6 years or older, although additional safety data are still needed.[174] The WHO dose recommendation for children weighing 15 to 29 kg is 200 mg daily for 2 weeks, then 100 mg thrice weekly for 22 weeks. For children weighing greater than 29 kg, the dose is 400 mg daily for 2 weeks, then 200 mg thrice weekly for 22 weeks.

Bedaquiline has a very long half-life (5.5 months) and has been characterized by three- and four-compartment models, indicating a large tissue distribution.[216–218] It exhibits linear pharmacokinetics, meaning that plasma concentration increases proportionally with the administered dose. Since bedaquiline exposure increases twofold when given with food compared to fasting, it is recommended that bedaquiline be administered after meals. It is primarily metabolized by CYP3A4 to form its *N*-desmethyl metabolite (M2), which is three to six times less active than the parent drug.[219] To a lesser extent, CYP2C8 and CYP2C19 also contribute to its metabolism. Therefore, it bedaquiline exposure might be affected by CYP inducers or inhibitors.

The adverse effects associated with the use of bedaquiline include nausea, headache, arthralgia, and hepatotoxicity.[220,221] Bedaquiline also causes QT prolongation.[220] Although the QT interval prolongation may be minimal, some cases were observed with a greater than 60-millisecond increase from baseline, and this led to drug discontinuation. Therefore, caution and close monitoring are needed, especially when bedaquiline is coadministered with drugs, causing QT prolongation.

Delamanid

Delamanid is a prodrug from the nitroimidazole class. In part, it disrupts the mycobacterial cell wall synthesis by inhibiting the formation of methoxy-mycolic and keto-mycolic acid.[222,223] The recommended dose for delamanid is 50 mg twice daily for 6- to 11-year olds, and 100 mg twice daily for 12- to 17-year olds.[174] Delamanid is currently approved for a treatment duration of 6 months. These dosage regimens were well tolerated in pediatric cases and resulted in plasma concentrations similar to adults.[223] The WHO also recommends delamanid 25 mg twice daily for children aged 3 to 5 years; however, the 25-mg formulation used in the trial is not yet available.[174] Delamanid may be considered when an MDR-TB regimen cannot be fully composed of drugs in groups A and B.

Delamanid exhibits nonlinear pharmacokinetics and has a long half-life of 30 to 38 hours.[223] Its absorption increases by approximately twofold when administered with food; hence, it should be administered after a meal.[223,224] Delamanid is primarily metabolized by serum albumin, so CYP-mediated drug–drug interactions are unlikely.[223,225] A minimal amount is excreted in urine. The majority of the parent drug and its metabolites are excreted in feces.

Delamanid may cause nausea, vomiting, and headache. It has also been associated with QT prolongation. Although no clinical cardiac event has been reported, patients need to be monitored, especially if delamanid is being coadministered with another drug known to cause QT prolongation.[224]

ATYPICAL MYCOBACTERIA

Atypical mycobacteria, or more commonly nontuberculous mycobacteria (NTM), encompass more than 200 bacterial species. Only a small number of them are known to cause disease in humans, including *Mycobacterium avium* complex (MAC), *Mycobacterium kansasii,* and *Mycobacterium abscessus.* Having a doubling time of about 1 day, *M. kansasii* and MAC are considered slow-growing mycobacteria.[226] On the other hand, *M. abscessus, Mycobacterium chelonae,* and *Mycobacterium fortuitum* are consider rapidly growing mycobacteria, with doubling times closer to 4 hours.[227] The drugs used to treat rapid- and slow-growing mycobacteria are often not the same. None of the agents were designed specifically to treat NTM. In some cases, treatment has been extrapolated from TB, but there remain significant differences. Increasingly, patients with cystic fibrosis are being diagnosed with NTM infections. Expert consultation is highly recommended, since the decision to start treatment is complex, and discordance between in vitro susceptibilities and in vivo treatment responses for NTM is common.

NTM infections may occur in people who have age- or disease-related changes in their pharmacokinetics, and this can affect the efficacy and toxicity profiles of the drugs.[228] Additionally, long treatment durations may lead to more adverse events, drug interactions, and nonadherence.

For MAC, treatment usually includes rifampin, ethambutol, and a macrolide (either clarithromycin or, increasingly, azithromycin), the latter drugs being the key to success. For cases of macrolide-resistant MAC, clarithromycin and azithromycin should be replaced, and the choices vary. Treatment outcomes for macrolide-resistant MAC are significantly worse. For cases of *M. kansasii*, rifampin, ethambutol, plus isoniazid, moxifloxacin, or a macrolide are typically used. For *Mycobacterium malmoense*, the patient may receive rifampin, ethambutol, and a macrolide. *Mycobacterium xenopi* is usually treated with rifampin, ethambutol, plus at least one of the following: macrolide or moxifloxacin. The treatment duration should be for a minimum of 12 months following conversion to culture-negative sputum. Clinicians may consider adding amikacin for 3 months in case of severe disease, especially cavitary disease, caused by the strains above.[229,230]

M. abscessus regimens often consist of an intensive initial phase, followed by a continuation phase. Clinicians must know the subspecies they are treating (subsp. *abscessus*, *massiliense*, or *bolletii*), and if an active *erm* gene is present, which leads to macrolide resistance. Expert laboratory and clinical advice should be sought. In the initial phase, the patients may receive combinations including intravenous amikacin, tigecycline, imipenem, or cefoxitin. A macrolide may be used if the isolate is susceptible. In the continuation phase, the patient may receive nebulized amikacin, a macrolide, plus more than one of the following antibiotics: clofazimine, linezolid, minocycline, moxifloxacin, and/or trimethoprim/sulfamethoxazole.[229] Given the complexity of these conditions, please refer to the references provided. Also, excellent reviews are provided in two recent publications:

1. Nontuberculous Mycobacteria, edited by Gwen A. Huitt and Charles L. Daley, Clinics in Chest Medicine, March 2015, and
2. Nontuberculous Mycobacterial Disease. A Comprehensive Approach to Diagnosis and Management, edited by David E. Griffith, Humana Press, 2019.

REFERENCES

3. Laurenzi M, Ginsberg A, Spigelman M. Challenges associated with current and future TB treatment. *Infect Disord Drug Targets* 2007;7(2):105–119.
4. World Health Organization. *Global tuberculosis report 2018*. Geneva, Switzerland: WHO, 2018.
5. Cruz AT, Starke JR. Pediatric tuberculosis. *Pediatr Rev* 2010;31(1):13–25; quiz-6.
6. Cruz AT, Starke JR. Clinical manifestations of tuberculosis in children. *Paediatr Respir Rev* 2007;8(2):107–117.
7. Marais BJ, Gie RP, Schaaf HS, et al. The natural history of childhood intra-thoracic tuberculosis: a critical review of literature from the pre-chemotherapy era. *Int J Tuberc Lung Dis* 2004;8(4):392–402.
8. Nahid P, Dorman SE, Alipanah N, et al. Official American Thoracic Society/Centers for Disease Control and Prevention/Infectious Diseases Society of America Clinical Practice Guidelines: treatment of drug-susceptible tuberculosis. *Clin Infect Dis* 2016;63(7):e147–e195.
9. World Health Organization. *Guidance for national tuberculosis programmes on the management of tuberculosis in children*, 2nd ed. Geneva, Switzerland: WHO, 2014.
10. Osman M, Lee K, Du Preez K, et al. Excellent treatment outcomes in children treated for tuberculosis under routine operational conditions in Cape Town, South Africa. *Clin Infect Dis* 2017;65(9):1444–1452.
11. Diallo T, Adjobimey M, Ruslami R, et al. Safety and Side effects of rifampin versus isoniazid in children. *N Engl J Med* 2018;379(5):454–463.
12. Smieja MJ, Marchetti CA, Cook DJ, et al. Isoniazid for preventing tuberculosis in non-HIV infected persons. *Cochrane Database Syst Rev* 2000(2):CD001363.
13. Marais BJ, van Zyl S, Schaaf HS, et al. Adherence to isoniazid preventive chemotherapy: a prospective community based study. *Arch Dis Child* 2006;91(9):762–765.
14. van Zyl S, Marais BJ, Hesseling AC, et al. Adherence to anti-tuberculosis chemoprophylaxis and treatment in children. *Int J Tuberc Lung Dis* 2006;10(1):13–18.
15. Spyridis NP, Spyridis PG, Gelesme A, et al. The effectiveness of a 9-month regimen of isoniazid alone versus 3-and 4-month regimens of isoniazid plus rifampin for treatment of latent tuberculosis infection in children: results of an 11-year randomized study. *Clin Infect Dis* 2007;45(6):715–722.
16. Zenner D, Beer N, Harris RJ, et al. Treatment of latent tuberculosis infection: an updated network meta-analysis. *Ann Intern Med* 2017;167(4):248–255.
17. Sun HY, Huang YW, Huang WC, et al. Twelve-dose weekly rifapentine plus isoniazid for latent tuberculosis infection: a multicentre randomised controlled trial in Taiwan. *Tuberculosis (Edinb)* 2018;111:121–126.
18. Sterling TR, Scott NA, Miro JM, et al. Three months of weekly rifapentine and isoniazid for treatment of *Mycobacterium tuberculosis* infection in HIV-coinfected persons. *AIDS* 2016;30(10):1607–1615.
19. van Hest R, Baars H, Kik S, et al. Hepatotoxicity of rifampin-pyrazinamide and isoniazid preventive therapy and tuberculosis treatment. *Clin Infect Dis* 2004;39(4):488–496.
20. Centers for Disease Control and Prevention (CDC). Update: adverse event data and revised American Thoracic Society/CDC recommendations against the use of rifampin and pyrazinamide for treatment of latent tuberculosis infection–United States, 2003. *MMWR Morb Mortal Wkly Rep* 2003;52(31):735–739.
21. Jasmer RM, Saukkonen JJ, Blumberg HM, et al. Short-course rifampin and pyrazinamide compared with isoniazid for latent tuberculosis infection: a multicenter clinical trial. *Ann Intern Med* 2002;137(8):640–647.
22. McNeill L, Allen M, Estrada C, et al. Pyrazinamide and rifampin vs isoniazid for the treatment of latent tuberculosis: improved completion rates but more hepatotoxicity. *Chest* 2003;123(1):102–106.
23. Centers for Disease Control and Prevention. Latent tuberculosis infection: a guide for primary health care providers. https://www.cdc.gov/tb/publications/ltbi/default.htm. Accessed March 15, 2019.
24. Rieder HL. *Interventions for tuberculosis control and elimination*. Paris, France: International Union Against Tuberculosis and Lung Disease, 2002.
25. Bass JB, Farer LS, Hopewell PC, et al. Treatment of tuberculosis and tuberculosis infection in adults and children. American Thoracic Society and The Centers for Disease Control and Prevention. *Am J Respir Crit Care Med* 1994;149(5):1359–1374.
26. Schaaf HS, Garcia-Prats AJ, Donald PR. Antituberculosis drugs in children. *Clin Pharmacol Ther* 2015;98(3):252–265.
27. Thee S, Seddon JA, Donald PR, et al. Pharmacokinetics of isoniazid, rifampin, and pyrazinamide in children younger than two years of age with tuberculosis: evidence for implementation of revised World Health Organization recommendations. *Antimicrob Agents Chemother* 2011;55(12):5560–5567.
28. Reis FJ, Bedran MB, Moura JA, et al. Six-month isoniazid-rifampin treatment for pulmonary tuberculosis in children. *Am Rev Respir Dis* 1990;142(5):996–999.
29. Abernathy RS, Dutt AK, Stead WW, et al. Short-course chemotherapy for tuberculosis in children. *Pediatrics* 1983;72(6):801–806.
30. Al-Dossary FS, Ong LT, Correa AG, et al. Treatment of childhood tuberculosis with a six month directly observed regimen of only two weeks of daily therapy. *Pediatr Infect Dis J* 2002;21(2):91–97.
31. Tsakalidis D, Pratsidou P, Hitoglou-Makedou A, et al. Intensive short course chemotherapy for treatment of Greek children with tuberculosis. *Pediatr Infect Dis J* 1992;11(12):1036–1042.
32. Biddulph J. Short course chemotherapy for childhood tuberculosis. *Pediatr Infect Dis J* 1990;9(11):794–801.
33. Te Water Naude JM, Donald PR, Hussey GD, et al. Twice weekly vs. daily chemotherapy for childhood tuberculosis. *Pediatr Infect Dis J* 2000;19(5):405–410.
34. Kumar L, Dhand R, Singhi PD, et al. A randomized trial of fully intermittent vs. daily followed by intermittent short course chemotherapy for childhood tuberculosis. *Pediatr Infect Dis J* 1990;9(11):802–806.
35. Sánchez-Albisua I, Vidal ML, Joya-Verde G, et al. Tolerance of pyrazinamide in short course chemotherapy for pulmonary tuberculosis in children. *Pediatr Infect Dis J* 1997;16(8):760–763.
36. Jawahar MS, Sivasubramanian S, Vijayan VK, et al. Short course chemotherapy for tuberculous lymphadenitis in children. *BMJ* 1990;301(6748):359–362.
37. Visudhiphan P, Chiemchanya S. Evaluation of rifampicin in the treatment of tuberculous meningitis in children. *J Pediatr* 1975;87(6 Pt 1):983–986.
38. Ramachandran P, Duraipandian M, Nagarajan M, et al. Three chemotherapy studies of tuberculous meningitis in children. *Tubercle* 1986;67(1):17–29.
39. Cruz AT, Starke JR. Safety and adherence for 12 weekly doses of isoniazid and rifapentine for pediatric tuberculosis infection. *Pediatr Infect Dis J* 2016;35(7):811–813.
40. Thwaites G, Fisher M, Hemingway C, et al. British Infection Society guidelines for the diagnosis and treatment of tuberculosis of the central nervous system in adults and children. *J Infect* 2009;59(3):167–187.
41. Donald PR. The chemotherapy of tuberculous meningitis in children and adults. *Tuberculosis (Edinb)* 2010;90(6):375–392.
42. Schaaf HS, Parkin DP, Seifart HI, et al. Isoniazid pharmacokinetics in children treated for respiratory tuberculosis. *Arch Dis Child* 2005;90(6):614–618.
43. Zhu M, Starke JR, Burman WJ, et al. Population pharmacokinetic modeling of pyrazinamide in children and adults with tuberculosis. *Pharmacotherapy* 2002;22(6):686–695.
44. Zhu M, Burman WJ, Starke JR, et al. Pharmacokinetics of ethambutol in children and adults with tuberculosis. *Int J Tuberc Lung Dis* 2004;8(11):1360–1367.
45. McIlleron H, Willemse M, Werely CJ, et al. Isoniazid plasma concentrations in a cohort of South African children with tuberculosis: implications for international pediatric dosing guidelines. *Clin Infect Dis* 2009;48(11):1547–1553.
46. Rieder HL, Arnadottir T, Trébucq A, et al. Tuberculosis treatment: dangerous regimens? *Int J Tuberc Lung Dis* 2001;5(1):1–3.
47. World Health Organization. *WHO treatment guidelines for isoniazid-resistant tuberculosis*. Geneva, Switzerland: WHO, 2018.
48. World Health Organization. *WHO treatment guidelines for drug-resistant tuberculosis - 2016 update*. Geneva, Switzerland: WHO, 2016.
49. World Health Organization. *Rapid communication: Key changes to treatment of multidrug-and rifampicin-resistant tuberculosis (MDR/RR-TB)*. Geneva, Switzerland: WHO, 2018.
50. van Soolingen D, de Haas PE, van Doorn HR, et al. Mutations at amino acid position 315 of the katG gene are associated with high-level resistance to isoniazid, other drug resistance, and successful transmission of *Mycobacterium tuberculosis* in the Netherlands. *J Infect Dis* 2000;182(6):1788–1790.

51. Wengenack NL, Uhl JR, St Amand AL, et al. Recombinant *Mycobacterium tuberculosis* KatG(S315T) is a competent catalase-peroxidase with reduced activity toward isoniazid. *J Infect Dis* 1997;176(3):722–727.
52. Ramaswamy S, Musser JM. Molecular genetic basis of antimicrobial agent resistance in *Mycobacterium tuberculosis*: 1998 update. *Tuber Lung Dis* 1998;79(1):3–29.
53. Blumberg HM, Burman WJ, Chaisson RE, et al. American Thoracic Society/Centers for Disease Control and Prevention/Infectious Diseases Society of America: treatment of tuberculosis. *Am J Respir Crit Care Med* 2003;167(4):603–662.
54. Holdiness MR. Clinical pharmacokinetics of the antituberculosis drugs. *Clin Pharmacokinet* 1984;9(6):511–544.
55. Hurwitz A, Schlozman DL. Effects of antacids on gastrointestinal absorption of isoniazid in rat and man. *Am Rev Respir Dis* 1974;109(1):41–47.
56. Peloquin CA, Namdar R, Dodge AA, et al. Pharmacokinetics of isoniazid under fasting conditions, with food, and with antacids. *Int J Tuberc Lung Dis* 1999;3(8):703–710.
57. Snider DE, Powell KE. Should women taking antituberculosis drugs breast-feed? *Arch Intern Med* 1984;144(3):589–590.
58. Ellard GA, Humphries MJ, Allen BW. Cerebrospinal fluid drug concentrations and the treatment of tuberculous meningitis. *Am Rev Respir Dis* 1993;148(3):650–655.
59. Holdiness MR. Cerebrospinal fluid pharmacokinetics of the antituberculosis drugs. *Clin Pharmacokinet* 1985;10(6):532–534.
60. Donald PR, Gent WL, Seifart HI, et al. Cerebrospinal fluid isoniazid concentrations in children with tuberculous meningitis: the influence of dosage and acetylation status. *Pediatrics* 1992;89(2):247–250.
61. Kergueris MF, Bourin M, Larousse C. Pharmacokinetics of isoniazid: influence of age. *Eur J Clin Pharmacol* 1986;30(3):335–340.
62. Dompreh A, Tang X, Zhou J, et al. Effect of genetic variation of NAT2 on isoniazid and SLCO1B1 and CES2 on rifampin pharmacokinetics in Ghanaian children with tuberculosis. *Antimicrob Agents Chemother* 2018;62(3).
63. Ellard GA. The potential clinical significance of the isoniazid acetylator phenotype in the treatment of pulmonary tuberculosis. *Tubercle* 1984;65(3):211–227.
64. Deguchi T, Mashimo M, Suzuki T. Correlation between acetylator phenotypes and genotypes of polymorphic arylamine N-acetyltransferase in human liver. *J Biol Chem* 1990;265(22):12757–12760.
65. Parkin DP, Vandenplas S, Botha FJ, et al. Trimodality of isoniazid elimination: phenotype and genotype in patients with tuberculosis. *Am J Respir Crit Care Med* 1997;155(5):1717–1722.
66. Weber WW, Hein DW. N-acetylation pharmacogenetics. *Pharmacol Rev* 1985;37(1):25–79.
67. Gumbo T, Louie A, Liu W, et al. Isoniazid bactericidal activity and resistance emergence: integrating pharmacodynamics and pharmacogenomics to predict efficacy in different ethnic populations. *Antimicrob Agents Chemother* 2007;51(7):2329–2336.
68. Acocella G, Bonollo L, Garimoldi M, et al. Kinetics of rifampicin and isoniazid administered alone and in combination to normal subjects and patients with liver disease. *Gut* 1972;13(1):47–53.
69. Pouplin T, Bang ND, Toi PV, et al. Naïve-pooled pharmacokinetic analysis of pyrazinamide, isoniazid and rifampicin in plasma and cerebrospinal fluid of Vietnamese children with tuberculous meningitis. *BMC Infect Dis* 2016;16:144.
70. Horita Y, Alsultan A, Kwara A, et al. Evaluation of the adequacy of WHO revised dosages of the first-line antituberculosis drugs in children with tuberculosis using population pharmacokinetic modeling and simulations. *Antimicrob Agents Chemother* 2018;62(9).
71. Comstock GW, Hammes LM, Pio A. Isoniazid prophylaxis in Alaskan Boarding schools. A comparison of two doses. *Am Rev Respir Dis* 1969;100(6):773–779.
72. Hsu KH. Thirty years after isoniazid. Its impact on tuberculosis in children and adolescents. *JAMA* 1984;251(10):1283–1285.
73. Göçmen A, Ozçelic U, Kiper N, et al. Short course intermittent chemotherapy in childhood tuberculosis. *Infection* 1993;21(5):324–327.
74. Zand R, Nelson SD, Slattery JT, et al. Inhibition and induction of cytochrome P4502E1-catalyzed oxidation by isoniazid in humans. *Clin Pharmacol Ther* 1993;54(2):142–149.
75. Desta Z, Soukhova NV, Flockhart DA. Inhibition of cytochrome P450 (CYP450) isoforms by isoniazid: potent inhibition of CYP2C19 and CYP3A. *Antimicrob Agents Chemother* 2001;45(2):382–392.
76. Ochs HR, Greenblatt DJ, Roberts GM, et al. Diazepam interaction with antituberculosis drugs. *Clin Pharmacol Ther* 1981;29(5):671–678.
77. Block SH. Carbamazepine-isoniazid interaction. *Pediatrics* 1982;69(4):494–495.
78. Miller RR, Porter J, Greenblatt DJ. Clinical importance of the interaction of phenytoin and isoniazid: a report from the Boston Collaborative Drug Surveillance Program. *Chest* 1979;75(3):356–358.
79. Kutt H, Brennan R, Dehejia H, et al. Diphenylhydantoin intoxication. A complication of isoniazid therapy. *Am Rev Respir Dis* 1970;101(3):377–384.
80. Dockweiler U. Isoniazid-induced valproic-acid toxicity, or vice versa. *Lancet* 1987;2(8551):152.
81. Mazze RI, Woodruff RE, Heerdt ME. Isoniazid-induced enflurane defluorination in humans. *Anesthesiology* 1982;57(1):5–8.
82. Gannon R, Pearsall W, Rowley R. Isoniazid, meperidine, and hypotension. *Ann Intern Med* 1983;99(3):415.
83. Holdiness MR. Transplacental pharmacokinetics of the antituberculosis drugs. *Clin Pharmacokinet* 1987;13(2):125–129.
84. Singh N, Golani A, Patel Z, et al. Transfer of isoniazid from circulation to breast milk in lactating women on chronic therapy for tuberculosis. *Br J Clin Pharmacol* 2008;65(3):418–422.
85. Brown CV. Acute isoniazid poisoning. *Am Rev Respir Dis* 1972;105(2):206–216.
86. Miller J, Robinson A, Percy AK. Acute isoniazid poisoning in childhood. *Am J Dis Child* 1980;134(3):290–292.
87. Shah BR, Santucci K, Sinert R, et al. Acute isoniazid neurotoxicity in an urban hospital. *Pediatrics* 1995;95(5):700–704.
88. Blowey DL, Johnson D, Verjee Z. Isoniazid-associated rhabdomyolysis. *Am J Emerg Med* 1995;13(5):543–544.
89. Panganiban LR, Makalinao IR, Corte-Maramba NP. Rhabdomyolysis in isoniazid poisoning. *J Toxicol Clin Toxicol* 2001;39(2):143–151.
90. Brent J, Vo N, Kulig K, et al. Reversal of prolonged isoniazid-induced coma by pyridoxine. *Arch Intern Med* 1990;150(8):1751–1753.
91. Tuberculosis Chemotherapy Centre. The prevention and treatment of isoniazid toxicity in the therapy of pulmonary tuberculosis: 1. An assessment of two vitamin B preparations and glutamic acid. *Bull World Health Organ* 1963;28(4):455–475.
92. Krishnamurthy DV, Selkon JB, Ramachandran K, et al. Effect of pyridoxine on vitamin B6 concentrations and glutamic-oxaloacetic transaminase activity in whole blood of tuberculous patients receiving high-dosage isoniazid. *Bull World Health Organ* 1967;36(5):853–870.
93. Pellock JM, Howell J, Kendig EL, et al. Pyridoxine deficiency in children treated with isoniazid. *Chest* 1985;87(5):658–661.
94. Davies PD, Brown RC, Church HA, et al. The effect of anti-tuberculosis chemotherapy on vitamin D and calcium metabolism. *Tubercle* 1987;68(4):261–266.
95. Naik AL, Rajan MG, Manjrekar PA, et al. Effect of DOTS treatment on vitamin D levels in pulmonary tuberculosis. *J Clin Diagn Res* 2017;11(4):BC18–BC22.
96. Beaudry PH, Brickman HF, Wise MB, et al. Liver enzyme disturbances during isoniazid chemoprophylaxis in children. *Am Rev Respir Dis* 1974;110(5):581–584.
97. Bailey WC, Weill H, DeRouen TA, et al. The effect of isoniazid on transaminase levels. *Ann Intern Med* 1974;81(2):200–202.
98. O'Brien RJ, Long MW, Cross FS, et al. Hepatotoxicity from isoniazid and rifampin among children treated for tuberculosis. *Pediatrics* 1983;72(4):491–499.
99. Nakajo MM, Rao M, Steiner P. Incidence of hepatotoxicity in children receiving isoniazid chemoprophylaxis. *Pediatr Infect Dis J* 1989;8(9):649–650.
100. Bowersox DW, Wintebauer RH, Stewart GL, et al. Isoniazid dosage in patients with renal failure. *N Engl J Med* 1973;289(2):84–87.
101. Stuart JJ, Roberts HR. Letter: Isoniazid and disseminated intravascular coagulation. *Ann Intern Med* 1976;84(4):490–491.
102. Girling DJ. Adverse effects of antituberculosis drugs. *Drugs* 1982;23(1-2):56–74.
103. Veale KS, Huff ES, Nelson BK, et al. Pure red cell aplasia and hepatitis in a child receiving isoniazid therapy. *J Pediatr* 1992;120(1):146–148.
104. Braunstein GD. Gynecomastia. *N Engl J Med* 1993;328(7):490–495.
105. Lopez-Contreras J, Ruiz D, Domingo P. Isoniazid-induced toxic fever. *Rev Infect Dis* 1991;13(4):775.
106. Rabassa AA, Trey G, Shukla U, et al. Isoniazid-induced acute pancreatitis. *Ann Intern Med* 1994;121(6):433–434.
107. Chan KL, Chan HS, Lui SF, et al. Recurrent acute pancreatitis induced by isoniazid. *Tuber Lung Dis* 1994;75(5):383–385.
108. Kenny MT, Strates B. Metabolism and pharmacokinetics of the antibiotic rifampin. *Drug Metab Rev* 1981;12(1):159–218.
109. Dickinson JM, Mitchison DA. Experimental models to explain the high sterilizing activity of rifampin in the chemotherapy of tuberculosis. *Am Rev Respir Dis* 1981;123(4 Pt 1):367–371.
110. Telenti A, Imboden P, Marchesi F, et al. Detection of rifampicin-resistance mutations in *Mycobacterium tuberculosis*. *Lancet* 1993;341(8846):647–650.
111. Donnabella V, Martiniuk F, Kinney D, et al. Isolation of the gene for the beta subunit of RNA polymerase from rifampicin-resistant *Mycobacterium tuberculosis* and identification of new mutations. *Am J Respir Cell Mol Biol* 1994;11(6):639–643.
112. Koup JR, Williams-Warren J, Viswanathan CT, et al. Pharmacokinetics of rifampin in children. II. Oral bioavailability. *Ther Drug Monit* 1986;8(1):17–22.
113. Siegler DI, Bryant M, Burley DM, et al. Effect of meals on rifampicin absorption. *Lancet* 1974;2(7874):197–198.
114. Boman G, Hanngren A, Malmborg A, et al. Drug interaction: decreased serum concentrations of rifampicin when given with P.A.S. *Lancet* 1971;1(7703):800.
115. Abulfathi AA, Decloedt EH, Svensson EM, et al. Clinical pharmacokinetics and pharmacodynamics of rifampicin in human tuberculosis. *Clin Pharmacokinet* 2019;58(9):1103–1129.
116. Braga PC. Antibiotic penetrability into bronchial mucus: pharmacokinetics and clinical considerations. *Curr Ther Res* 1991;49(2):300–327.
117. Alghamdi WA, Al-Shaer MH, Peloquin CA. Protein binding of first-line antituberculosis drugs. *Antimicrob Agents Chemother* 2018;62(7).
118. D'Oliveira JJ. Cerebrospinal fluid concentrations of rifampin in meningeal tuberculosis. *Am Rev Respir Dis* 1972;106(3):432–437.
119. Acocella G, Nonis A, Perna G, et al. Comparative bioavailability of isoniazid, rifampin, and pyrazinamide administered in free combination and in a fixed triple formulation designed for daily use in antituberculosis chemotherapy. II. Two-month, daily administration study. *Am Rev Respir Dis* 1988;138(4):886–890.
120. Strolin Benedetti M, Dostert P. Induction and autoinduction properties of rifamycin derivatives: a review of animal and human studies. *Environ Health Perspect* 1994;102(Suppl 9):101–105.
121. Boeree MJ, Diacon AH, Dawson R, et al. A dose-ranging trial to optimize the dose of rifampin in the treatment of tuberculosis. *Am J Respir Crit Care Med* 2015;191(9):1058–1065.
122. Peloquin CA, Namdar R, Singleton MD, et al. Pharmacokinetics of rifampin under fasting conditions, with food, and with antacids. *Chest* 1999;115(1):12–18.
123. Douglas JG, McLeod MJ. Pharmacokinetic factors in the modern drug treatment of tuberculosis. *Clin Pharmacokinet* 1999;37(2):127–146.
124. Donald PR, Maritz JS, Diacon AH. The pharmacokinetics and pharmacodynamics of rifampicin in adults and children in relation to the dosage recommended for children. *Tuberculosis (Edinb)* 2011;91(3):196–207.
125. Jayaram R, Gaonkar S, Kaur P, et al. Pharmacokinetics-pharmacodynamics of rifampin in an aerosol infection model of tuberculosis. *Antimicrob Agents Chemother* 2003;47(7):2118–2124.
126. Adedoyin A, Mauro K, Kubisty C, et al. Chronic modulation of CYP2D6 and CYP3A4 activities by quinidine and rifampicin respectively [abstract]. *Clin Pharmacol Ther* 1995;57(2):210.

127. Lee KH, Shin JG, Chong WS, et al. Time course of the changes in prednisolone pharmacokinetics after co-administration or discontinuation of rifampin. *Eur J Clin Pharmacol* 1993;45(3):287–289.
128. Ohnhaus EE, Brockmeyer N, Dylewicz P, Habicht H. The effect of antipyrine and rifampin on the metabolism of diazepam. *Clin Pharmacol Ther* 1987;42(2):148–156.
129. Rodin SM, Johnson BF. Pharmacokinetic interactions with digoxin. *Clin Pharmacokinet* 1988;15(4):227–244.
130. Backman JT, Olkkola KT, Neuvonen PJ. Rifampin drastically reduces plasma concentrations and effects of oral midazolam. *Clin Pharmacol Ther* 1996;59(1):7–13.
131. Powell-Jackson PR, Jamieson AP, Gray BJ, et al. Effect of rifampicin administration on theophylline pharmacokinetics in humans. *Am Rev Respir Dis* 1985;131(6):939–940.
132. Brodie MJ, Boobis AR, Hillyard CJ, et al. Effect of rifampicin and isoniazid on vitamin D metabolism. *Clin Pharmacol Ther* 1982;32(4):525–530.
133. Venkatesan K. Pharmacokinetic drug interactions with rifampicin. *Clin Pharmacokinet* 1992;22(1):47–65.
134. Steen JS, Stainton-Ellis DM. Rifampicin in pregnancy. *Lancet* 1977;2(8038):604–605.
135. Nguyen HT, Pandolfini C, Chiodini P, et al Tuberculosis care for pregnant women: a systematic review. *BMC Infect Dis* 2014;14:617.
136. Cohn JR, Fye DL, Sills JM, et al. Rifampicin-induced renal failure. *Tubercle* 1985;66(4):289–293.
137. Girling DJ. The hepatic toxicity of antituberculosis regimens containing isoniazid, rifampicin and pyrazinamide. *Tubercle* 1978;59(1):13–32.
138. Lees AW, Allan GW, Smith J, et al. Toxicity form rifampicin plus isoniazid and rifampicin plus ethambutol therapy. *Tubercle* 1971;52(3):182–190.
139. Saukkonen JJ, Cohn DL, Jasmer RM, et al. An official ATS statement: hepatotoxicity of antituberculosis therapy. *Am J Respir Crit Care Med* 2006;174(8):935–952.
140. Baron DN, Bell JL. Serum enzyme changes in patients receiving antituberculosis therapy with rifampicin or p-aminosalicylic acid, plus isoniazid and streptomycin. *Tubercle* 1974;55(2):115–120.
141. Holdiness MR. A review of the Redman syndrome and rifampicin overdosage. *Med Toxicol Adverse Drug Exp* 1989;4(6):444–451.
142. Iredale JP, Sankaran R, Wathen CG. Cutaneous vasculitis associated with rifampin therapy. *Chest* 1989;96(1):215–216.
143. Takasu N, Yamada T, Miura H, et al. Rifampicin-induced early phase hyperglycemia in humans. *Am Rev Respir Dis* 1982;125(1):23–27.
144. Blajchman MA, Lowry RC, Pettit JE, et al. Rifampicin-induced immune thrombocytopenia. *Br Med J* 1970;3(5713):24–26.
145. Berning SE, Iseman MD. Rifamycin-induced lupus syndrome. *Lancet* 1997;349(9064):1521–1522.
146. Tajima A, Mine T, Ogata E. Rifampicin-associated ulcerative colitis. *Ann Intern Med* 1992;116(9):778–779.
147. White NW. Venous thrombosis and rifampicin. *Lancet* 1989;2(8660):434–435.
148. Konno K, Feldmann FM, McDermott W. Pyrazinamide susceptibility and amidase activity of tubercle bacilli. *Am Rev Respir Dis* 1967;95(3):461–469.
149. Crowle AJ, Sbarbaro JA, May MH. Inhibition by pyrazinamide of tubercle bacilli within cultured human macrophages. *Am Rev Respir Dis* 1986;134(5):1052–1055.
150. Zhang Y. The magic bullets and tuberculosis drug targets. *Annu Rev Pharmacol Toxicol* 2005;45:529–564.
151. Ellard GA. Absorption, metabolism and excretion of pyrazinamide in man. *Tubercle* 1969;50(2):144–158.
152. Bareggi SR, Cerutti R, Pirola R, et al. Clinical pharmacokinetics and metabolism of pyrazinamide in healthy volunteers. *Arzneimittelforschung* 1987;37(7):849–854.
153. Lacroix C, Hoang TP, Nouveau J, et al. Pharmacokinetics of pyrazinamide and its metabolites in healthy subjects. *Eur J Clin Pharmacol* 1989;36(4):395–400.
154. Ellard GA, Haslam RM. Observations on the reduction of the renal elimination of urate in man caused by the administration of pyrazinamide. *Tubercle* 1976;57(2):97–103.
155. Peloquin CA, Bulpitt AE, Jaresko GS, et al. Pharmacokinetics of pyrazinamide under fasting conditions, with food, and with antacids. *Pharmacotherapy* 1998;18(6):1205–1211.
156. Mukherjee A, Lodha R, Kabra SK. Pharmacokinetics of first-line anti-tubercular drugs. *Indian J Pediatr* 2019;86(5):468–478.
157. Zierski M, Bek E. Side-effects of drug regimens used in short-course chemotherapy for pulmonary tuberculosis. A controlled clinical study. *Tubercle* 1980;61(1):41–49.
158. Maurya V, Panjabi C, Shah A. Pyrazinamide induced photoallergy. *Int J Tuberc Lung Dis* 2001;5(11):1075–1076.
159. Snider DE, Layde PM, Johnson MW, et al. Treatment of tuberculosis during pregnancy. *Am Rev Respir Dis* 1980;122(1):65–79.
160. Jindani A, Aber VR, Edwards EA, et al. The early bactericidal activity of drugs in patients with pulmonary tuberculosis. *Am Rev Respir Dis* 1980;121(6):939–949.
161. Deng L, Mikusová K, Robuck KG, et al. Recognition of multiple effects of ethambutol on metabolism of mycobacterial cell envelope. *Antimicrob Agents Chemother* 1995;39(3):694–701.
162. Mikusova K, Slayden RA, Besra GS, et al. Biogenesis of the mycobacterial cell wall and the site of action of ethambutol. *Antimicrob Agents Chemother* 1995;39(11):2484–2489.
163. Telenti A, Philipp WJ, Sreevatsan S, et al. The emb operon, a gene cluster of *Mycobacterium tuberculosis* involved in resistance to ethambutol. *Nat Med* 1997;3(5):567–570.
164. Sreevatsan S, Stockbauer KE, Pan X, et al. Ethambutol resistance in *Mycobacterium tuberculosis*: critical role of embB mutations. *Antimicrob Agents Chemother* 1997;41(8):1677–1681.
165. Hoffner SE, Kratz M, Olsson-Liljequist B, et al. In-vitro synergistic activity between ethambutol and fluorinated quinolones against Mycobacterium avium complex. *J Antimicrob Chemother* 1989;24(3):317–324.
166. Donald PR, Maher D, Maritz JS, et al. Ethambutol dosage for the treatment of children: literature review and recommendations. *Int J Tuberc Lung Dis* 2006;10(12):1318–1330.
167. Jenne JW, Beggs WH. Correlation of in vitro and in vivo kinetics with clinical use of isoniazid, ethambutol, and rifampin. *Am Rev Respir Dis* 1973;107(6):1013–1021.
168. Hussels H, Kroening U, Magdorf K. Ethambutol and rifampicin serum levels in children: second report on the combined administration of ethambutol and rifampicin. *Pneumonologie* 1973;149(1):31–38.
169. Graham SM, Bell DJ, Nyirongo S, et al. Low levels of pyrazinamide and ethambutol in children with tuberculosis and impact of age, nutritional status, and human immunodeficiency virus infection. *Antimicrob Agents Chemother* 2006;50(2):407–413.
170. Thee S, Detjen A, Quarcoo D, et al. Ethambutol in paediatric tuberculosis: aspects of ethambutol serum concentration, efficacy and toxicity in children. *Int J Tuberc Lung Dis* 2007;11(9):965–971.
171. World Health Organization. *Implementing the WHO stop TB strategy: a handbook for national tuberculosis programmes*. Geneva, Switzerland: WHO, 2008.
172. Rabinovitz M, Pitlik SD, Halevy J, et al. Ethambutol-induced thrombocytopenia. *Chest* 1982;81(6):765–766.
173. Wong CF, Yew WW. Ethambutol-induced neutropenia and eosinophilia. *Chest* 1994;106(5):1638–1639.
174. Kahana LM. Toxic ocular effects of ethambutol. *CMAJ* 1987;137(3):213–216.
175. Trebucq A. Should ethambutol be recommended for routine treatment of tuberculosis in children? A review of the literature. *Int J Tuberc Lung Dis* 1997;1(1):12–15.
176. World Health Organization. *WHO consolidated guidelines on drug-resistant tuberculosis treatment*. Geneva, Switzerland: WHO, 2019.
177. McAnaw SE, Hesseling AC, Seddon JA, et al. Pediatric multidrug-resistant tuberculosis clinical trials: challenges and opportunities. *Int J Infect Dis* 2017;56:194–199.
178. Ramachandran G, Swaminathan S. Safety and tolerability profile of second-line anti-tuberculosis medications. *Drug Saf* 2015;38(3):253–269.
179. Ahmad N, Ahuja SD, Akkerman OW, et al. Treatment correlates of successful outcomes in pulmonary multidrug-resistant tuberculosis: an individual patient data meta-analysis. *Lancet* 2018;392(10150):821–834.
180. Arbiser JL, Moschella SL. Clofazimine: a review of its medical uses and mechanisms of action. *J Am Acad Dermatol* 1995;32(2 Pt 1):241–247.
181. Cholo MC, Mothiba MT, Fourie B, et al. Mechanisms of action and therapeutic efficacies of the lipophilic antimycobacterial agents clofazimine and bedaquiline. *J Antimicrob Chemother* 2017;72(2):338–353.
182. Cholo MC, Steel HC, Fourie PB, et al. Clofazimine: current status and future prospects. *J Antimicrob Chemother* 2012;67(2):290–298.
183. Nix DE, Adam RD, Auclair B, et al. Pharmacokinetics and relative bioavailability of clofazimine in relation to food, orange juice and antacid. *Tuberculosis (Edinb)* 2004;84(6):365–373.
184. Malone RS, Fish DN, Spiegel DM, et al. The effect of hemodialysis on cycloserine, ethionamide, para-aminosalicylate, and clofazimine. *Chest* 1999;116(4):984–990.
185. Harausz EP, Garcia-Prats AJ, Seddon JA, et al. New and repurposed drugs for pediatric multidrug-resistant tuberculosis. practice-based recommendations. *Am J Respir Crit Care Med* 2017;195(10):1300–1310.
186. Bankier RG. Psychosis associated with cycloserine. *Can Med Assoc J* 1965;93:35–37.
187. Azam MA, Jayaram U. Inhibitors of alanine racemase enzyme: a review. *J Enzyme Inhib Med Chem* 2016;31(4):517–526.
188. Zítková L, Tousek J. Pharmacokinetics of cycloserine and terizidone. A comparative study. *Chemotherapy* 1974;20(1):18–28.
189. Court R, Wiesner L, Stewart A, et al. Steady state pharmacokinetics of cycloserine in patients on terizidone for multidrug-resistant tuberculosis. *Int J Tuberc Lung Dis* 2018;22(1):30–33.
190. World Health Organization. *Companion handbook to the WHO guidelines for the programmatic management of drug-resistant tuberculosis*. Geneva, Switzerland: WHO, 2014.
191. Alghamdi WA, Alsultan A, Al-Shaer MH, et al. Cycloserine population pharmacokinetics and pharmacodynamics in patients with tuberculosis. *Antimicrob Agents Chemother* 2019;63(5).
192. Deshpande D, Alffenaar JC, Köser CU, et al. D-cycloserine pharmacokinetics/pharmacodynamics, susceptibility, and dosing implications in multidrug-resistant tuberculosis: a Faustian deal. *Clin Infect Dis* 2018;67(Suppl_3):S308–S316.
193. Hemanth Kumar AK, Kumar A, Kannan T, et al. Pharmacokinetics of second-line antituberculosis drugs in children with multidrug-resistant tuberculosis in India. *Antimicrob Agents Chemother* 2018;62(5).
194. Donald PR. Cerebrospinal fluid concentrations of antituberculosis agents in adults and children. *Tuberculosis (Edinb)* 2010;90(5):279–292.
195. Zhu M, Nix DE, Adam RD, et al. Pharmacokinetics of cycloserine under fasting conditions and with high-fat meal, orange juice, and antacids. *Pharmacotherapy* 2001;21(8):891–897.
196. Kass JS, Shandera WX. Nervous system effects of antituberculosis therapy. *CNS Drugs* 2010;24(8):655–667.
197. Carroll MW, Lee M, Cai Y, Hallahan CW, et al. Frequency of adverse reactions to first-and second-line anti-tuberculosis chemotherapy in a Korean cohort. *Int J Tuberc Lung Dis* 2012;16(7):961–966.
198. Mataix-Cols D, Fernández de la Cruz L, Monzani B, et al. D-cycloserine augmentation of exposure-based cognitive behavior therapy for anxiety, obsessive-compulsive, and post-traumatic stress disorders: a systematic review and meta-analysis of individual participant data. *JAMA Psychiatry* 2017;74(5):501–510.
199. Hwang TJ, Wares DF, Jafarov A, et al. Safety of cycloserine and terizidone for the treatment of drug-resistant tuberculosis: a meta-analysis. *Int J Tuberc Lung Dis* 2013;17(10):1257–1266.
200. Thee S, Garcia-Prats AJ, Donald PR, et al. A review of the use of ethionamide and prothionamide in childhood tuberculosis. *Tuberculosis (Edinb)* 2016;97:126–136.
201. Wang F, Langley R, Gulten G, et al. Mechanism of thioamide drug action against tuberculosis and leprosy. *J Exp Med* 2007;204(1):73–78.
202. Zhu M, Namdar R, Stambaugh JJ, et al. Population pharmacokinetics of ethionamide in patients with tuberculosis. *Tuberculosis (Edinb)* 2002;82(2-3):91–96.

203. Thee S, Seifart HI, Rosenkranz B, et al. Pharmacokinetics of ethionamide in children. *Antimicrob Agents Chemother* 2011;55(10):4594–4600.
204. Auclair B, Nix DE, Adam RD, et al. Pharmacokinetics of ethionamide administered under fasting conditions or with orange juice, food, or antacids. *Antimicrob Agents Chemother* 2001;45(3):810–804.
205. DeBarber AE, Mdluli K, Bosman M, et al. Ethionamide activation and sensitivity in multidrug-resistant *Mycobacterium tuberculosis*. *Proc Natl Acad Sci U S A* 2000;97(17):9677–9682.
206. Henderson MC, Siddens LK, Morré JT, et al. Metabolism of the anti-tuberculosis drug ethionamide by mouse and human FMO1, FMO2 and FMO3 and mouse and human lung microsomes. *Toxicol Appl Pharmacol* 2008;233(3):420–427.
207. McDonnell ME, Braverman LE, Bernardo J. Hypothyroidism due to ethionamide. *N Engl J Med* 2005;352(26):2757–2759.
208. Zheng J, Rubin EJ, Bifani P, et al. para-Aminosalicylic acid is a prodrug targeting dihydrofolate reductase in *Mycobacterium tuberculosis*. *J Biol Chem* 2013;288(32):23447–23456.
209. Donald PR, Diacon AH. Para-aminosalicylic acid: the return of an old friend. *Lancet Infect Dis* 2015;15(9):1091–1099.
210. Liwa AC, Schaaf HS, Rosenkranz B, et al. Para-aminosalicylic acid plasma concentrations in children in comparison with adults after receiving a granular slow-release preparation. *J Trop Pediatr* 2013;59(2):90–94.
211. Peloquin CA, Zhu M, Adam RD, et al. Pharmacokinetics of para-aminosalicylic acid granules under four dosing conditions. *Ann Pharmacother* 2001;35(11):1332–1338.
212. Peloquin CA, Berning SE, Huitt GA, et al. Once-daily and twice-daily dosing of p-aminosalicylic acid granules. *Am J Respir Crit Care Med* 1999;159(3):932–934.
213. Matsaniotis N, Jacobs J, Smith MH. Hypersensitivity reactions associated with sodium para-aminosalicylate therapy; four case reports and review of the literature. *Pediatrics* 1958;21(5):781–792.
214. Zumla A, Nahid P, Cole ST. Advances in the development of new tuberculosis drugs and treatment regimens. *Nat Rev Drug Discov* 2013;12(5):388–404.
215. Cox E, Laessig K. FDA approval of bedaquiline—the benefit-risk balance for drug-resistant tuberculosis. *N Engl J Med* 2014;371(8):689–691.
216. Ryan NJ, Lo JH. Delamanid: first global approval. *Drugs* 2014;74(9):1041–1045.
217. Koul A, Vranckx L, Dendouga N, et al. Diarylquinolines are bactericidal for dormant mycobacteria as a result of disturbed ATP homeostasis. *J Biol Chem* 2008;283(37):25273–25280.
218. Svensson EM, Dosne AG, Karlsson MO. Population pharmacokinetics of bedaquiline and metabolite M2 in patients with drug-resistant tuberculosis: the effect of time-varying weight and albumin. *CPT Pharmacometrics Syst Pharmacol* 2016;5(12):682–691.
219. McLeay SC, Vis P, van Heeswijk RP, et al. Population pharmacokinetics of bedaquiline (TMC207), a novel antituberculosis drug. *Antimicrob Agents Chemother* 2014;58(9):5315–5324.
220. van Heeswijk RP, Dannemann B, Hoetelmans RM. Bedaquiline: a review of human pharmacokinetics and drug-drug interactions. *J Antimicrob Chemother* 2014;69(9):2310–2318.
221. Liu K, Li F, Lu J, et al. Bedaquiline metabolism: enzymes and novel metabolites. *Drug Metab Dispos* 2014;42(5):863–866.
222. Schaaf HS, Thee S, van der Laan L, et al. Adverse effects of oral second-line antituberculosis drugs in children. *Expert Opin Drug Saf* 2016;15(10):1369–1381.
223. Nguyen TV, Cao TB, Akkerman OW, et al. Bedaquiline as part of combination therapy in adults with pulmonary multi-drug resistant tuberculosis. *Expert Rev Clin Pharmacol* 2016;9(8):1025–1037.
224. Matsumoto M, Hashizume H, Tomishige T, et al. OPC-67683, a nitro-dihydro-imidazooxazole derivative with promising action against tuberculosis in vitro and in mice. *PLoS Med* 2006;3(11):e466.
225. Liu Y, Matsumoto M, Ishida H, et al. Delamanid: From discovery to its use for pulmonary multidrug-resistant tuberculosis (MDR-TB). *Tuberculosis (Edinb)* 2018;111:20–30.
226. World Health Organization. *The use of delamanid in the treatment of multidrug-resistant tuberculosis in children and adolescents - Interim policy guidance.* Geneva, Switzerland: WHO, 2016.
227. Sasahara K, Shimokawa Y, Hirao Y, et al. Pharmacokinetics and metabolism of delamanid, a novel anti-tuberculosis drug, in animals and humans: importance of albumin metabolism in vivo. *Drug Metab Dispos* 2015;43(8):1267–1276.
228. Runyon EH. Identification of mycobacterial pathogens utilizing colony characteristics. *Am J Clin Pathol* 1970;54(4):578–586.
229. Nie W, Duan H, Huang H, et al. Species identification of Mycobacterium abscessus subsp. abscessus and Mycobacterium abscessus subsp. bolletii using rpoB and hsp65, and susceptibility testing to eight antibiotics. *Int J Infect Dis* 2014;25:170–174.
230. Mangoni AA, Jackson SH. Age-related changes in pharmacokinetics and pharmacodynamics: basic principles and practical applications. *Br J Clin Pharmacol* 2004;57(1):6–14.
231. Haworth CS, Banks J, Capstick T, et al. British Thoracic Society guidelines for the management of non-tuberculous mycobacterial pulmonary disease (NTM-PD). *Thorax* 2017;72(Suppl 2):ii1–ii64.
232. Griffith DE, Aksamit T, Brown-Elliott BA, et al. An official ATS/IDSA statement: diagnosis, treatment, and prevention of nontuberculous mycobacterial diseases. *Am J Respir Crit Care Med* 2007;175(4):367–416.
233. Brunton L, Lazo J, Parker K. *Goodman & Gilman's the pharmacological basis of therapeutics*, 11th ed. New York, NY: The McGraw-Hill Companies, 2006.
234. Dietze R, Hadad DJ, McGee B, et al. Early and extended early bactericidal activity of linezolid in pulmonary tuberculosis. *Am J Respir Crit Care Med* 2008;178(11):1180–1185.

CHAPTER

30

Michael J. Smith
William J. Steinbach
Daniel K. Benjamin, Jr.
Michael Cohen-Wolkowiez

Antifungal Agents

Because of advances in aggressive chemotherapeutic agents and frequent use of organ transplantation, fungal pathogens are an expanding complication in immunocompromised patients.[1] Fortunately, the therapeutic armamentarium for invasive fungal infections has markedly increased in the past decade, and more importantly, both regulatory agencies and the industry have worked cohesively to evaluate the use of these agents in the pediatric population. In the past decade, the use of the echinocandins and mold-active triazoles largely replaced amphotericin B as agents of choice for invasive fungal infection.[2] However, fluconazole remains the most commonly prescribed antifungal agent in hospitalized children due to its prophylactic use in neonates and children with cancer. We will review the major systemic antifungal agents in clinical use (Table 30.1), including their activity against clinically relevant fungal pathogens (Table 30.2). This review excludes those antifungal agents that presently remain in the earlier stages of development (i.e., sordarins, pradimicins, or benanomycins).

TABLE 30.1 Formulations of Selected Systemic Antifungal Agents

Drug Class	*Drug Name (Brand/Investigational Name)*	*Formulation*
Pyrimidine analog	5-Fluorocytosine (Ancoban)	p.o.
Polyene	Amphotericin B deoxycholate (Fungizone)	i.v.
	Amphotericin B lipid complex (Abelcet)	i.v.
	Liposomal amphotericin B (AmBisome)	i.v.
Triazole	Fluconazole (Diflucan)	p.o., i.v.
	Itraconazole (Sporanox)	p.o., i.v.
	Voriconazole (VFend)	p.o., i.v.
	Posaconazole (Noxafil)	p.o., i.v.
	Isavuconazole (Cresemba)	p.o., i.v.
Echinocandin	Caspofungin (Cancidas)	i.v.
	Anidulafungin (Eraxis)	i.v.
	Micafungin (Mycamine)	i.v.

i.v., intravenous; p.o., oral.

TABLE 30.2 Spectrum of Activity of Selected Antifungal Agents

Drug	*Important Clinical Uses*
Amphotericin B	*Blastomyces dermatitidis, Coccidioides immitis, Cryptococcus neoformans, Histoplasma capsulatum, Paracoccidioides brasiliensis, Sporothrix schenckii,* most *Candida* species, *Aspergillus, Mucormycetes* (Not: *Candida lusitaniae, Scedosporium, Fusarium, Trichosporon*)
5-Fluorocytosine	Only in combination therapy for *Candida, Candida neoformans,* dematiaceous molds
Fluconazole	Most *Candida, C. neoformans, B. dermatitidis, H. capsulatum, C. immitis, P. brasiliensis* (Not: *Candida krusei, Candida glabrata, Aspergillus*)
Itraconazole	*Candida, Aspergillus, B. dermatitidis, H. capsulatum, C. immitis, P. brasiliensis*
Voriconazole	*Candida, Aspergillus, Fusarium, B. dermatitidis, H. capsulatum, C. immitis, Malassezia* species, *Scedosporium,* dematiaceous molds (Not: *Mucormycetes*)
Posaconazole	*Candida, Aspergillus, Fusarium, H. capsulatum, C. immitis, Mucormycetes,* dematiaceous molds
Isavuconazole	*Aspergillus, Mucormycetes*
Caspofungin	*Candida, Aspergillus* (Not: *C. neoformans, Fusarium, Mucormycetes*)
Micafungin	*Candida, Aspergillus* (Not: *C. neoformans, Fusarium, Mucormycetes*)
Anidulafungin	*Candida, Aspergillus* (Not: *C. neoformans, Fusarium, Mucormycetes*)

POLYENES

AMPHOTERICIN B

Mechanism of Action

The oldest antifungal class is the polyene macrolides, amphotericin B and nystatin. Initially approved for use in 1958, amphotericin B initially served as the "gold standard" for invasive fungal infection treatment as well as the standard of comparison for all newer antifungal agents. However, the fact that amphotericin B remained at such a post was not solely by virtue of its effectiveness but rather due to the lack of alternatives until recent studies.[3] Given the favorable efficacy and safety profiles of the echinocandins and triazoles, the use of amphotericin B has decreased substantially in pediatric clinical practice. Amphotericins A and B are natural fermentation products of a soil actinomycete collected in Venezuela in 1953, but although each has antifungal properties, amphotericin A was not developed.[4] Amphotericin B is so named because it is amphoteric, forming soluble salts in both acidic and basic environments.[5] However, because of its insolubility in water, amphotericin B for clinical use is actually amphotericin B mixed with the detergent deoxycholate in a 3:7 ratio.[5,6]

The polyenes bind to ergosterol, the major sterol found in fungal cytoplasmic membranes. The lipophilic amphotericin B acts by preferential binding to fungal membrane ergosterols, and classically, it was thought they created transmembrane channels, which result in an increased permeability to monovalent cations. The fungicidal activity is believed to be due to a damaged barrier and subsequent cell death through leakage of essential nutrients from the fungal cell. Amphotericin B also has oxidant activity that disrupts cellular metabolism,[7] inhibits proton adenosine triphosphatase (ATPase) pumps, depletes cellular energy reserves, and promotes lipid peroxidation to result in an increase in membrane fragility and ionized calcium leakage.[6,8,9] Newer molecular mechanistic studies suggest that channel formation may instead be a complementary mechanism and amphotericin B simply binds ergosterol for its main cytocidal effect.[10]

Pharmacology

Amphotericin B is released from its carrier and distributes very efficiently (>90%) with lipoproteins, taken up preferentially by organs of the reticuloendothelial system, and follows a three-compartment distribution model. There is an initial 24- to 48-hour distributional half-life, reflecting uptake by host lipids, very slow release and excretion into urine and bile, and a subsequent terminal elimination half-life of up to 15 days.[10] In a small series ($n = 13$) evaluating the pharmacokinetics (PK) of amphotericin B among premature infants (27.4 ± 5 weeks), nine subjects showed elimination of amphotericin B at steady state, with an estimated elimination half-life of 14.8 hours (5/82). The rest of the infants, however, showed minimal drug elimination during the dosing interval, suggesting substantial drug accumulation and interindividual variability.[11]

Experimental in vitro and in vivo studies support concentration-dependent killing with a prolonged post-antifungal effect, suggesting that large daily doses will be most effective and that achieving optimal peak concentrations is important.[12] Peak levels are achieved 1 hour after a 4-hour infusion and reach a plateau at the third consecutive day of a constant dose.[5] There is a relationship between total dose administered and tissue concentrations, suggesting a progressive accumulation with continued drug administration.[13] However, there is no evidence of a clinical dose effect[14] to support higher doses (>1 mg per kg per day) of amphotericin B.[15] In adults, cerebrospinal fluid (CSF) values are only 2% to 4% of serum concentrations and sometimes difficult to detect.[16] In a small series of premature infants born at 27.4 (±5) weeks' gestational age ($n = 5$), however, CSF amphotericin B concentrations were 40% to 90% of the serum concentrations obtained simultaneously.[11]

In addition to conventional amphotericin B deoxycholate, three fundamentally different lipid-associated formulations have been developed that offer the advantage of an increased daily dose of the parent drug, better delivery to the primary reticuloendothelial organs (lungs, liver, spleen),[17,18] and reduced toxicity. The U.S. Food and Drug Administration (FDA) approved amphotericin B lipid complex (ABLC) in December 1995, amphotericin B colloidal dispersion (ABCD) in December 1996, and liposomal amphotericin B (L-amphotericin B) in August 1997.[17]

ABLC (Abelcet, Leadiant Biosciences, Gaithersburg, MD) is a tightly packed ribbon-like structure of a bilayered membrane formed by combining dimyristoyl phosphatidylcholine, dimyristoyl phosphatidylglycerol, and amphotericin B in a ratio of 7:3:3. L-Amphotericin B (AmBisome, Astellas, Northbrook, IL), the only "true liposomal" product, consists of small uniformly sized unilamellar vesicles of a lipid bilayer of hydrogenated soy phosphatidylcholine–distcaryl phosphatidylglycerol–cholesterol–amphotericin B in the ratio 2:0.8:1:0.4.[19,20]

Lipid formulations of amphotericin B generally have a slower onset of action and are less active than amphotericin B in time–kill studies, presumably due to the required disassociation of free amphotericin B from the lipid vehicle.[21] It is postulated that activated monocytes/macrophages take up drug-laden lipid formulations and transport them to the site of infection where phospholipases release the free drug.[22,23] The different PK and toxicities of the lipid formulations are reflected in the dosing recommendations: ABLC is recommended at 5 mg per kg per day, and L-amphotericin B at 1 to 5 mg per kg per day. However, most clinical data have been obtained with the use of these preparations at 5 mg per kg per day. Animal studies indicate that on a similar dosing schedule, the lipid products are not as potent as amphotericin B, but that the ability to safely administer higher daily doses of the parent drug improves their efficacy[16] and the lipid products compare favorably with amphotericin B deoxycholate with less toxicity. A multicenter maximum tolerated dose study of L-amphotericin B using doses from 7.5 to 15 mg per kg per day found a nonlinear plasma PK profile with a maximal concentration at 10 mg per kg per day and no demonstrable dose-limiting nephrotoxicity or infusion-related toxicity.[24] A recent phase I–II dose-escalation study of L-amphotericin B in children aged 1 to 17 years compared doses of 2.5, 5, 7.5, and 10 mg per kg administered once daily for at least 3 days and found similar nonlinear pharmokinetics.[25]

Lipid formulations have the added benefit of increased tissue concentration compared with conventional amphotericin B, specifically in the liver, lungs, and spleen. However, it is not entirely clear whether these higher concentrations in tissue are truly available to the microfoci of infection. L-Amphotericin B has a comparatively higher peak plasma level and prolonged circulation in plasma.[19]

Several reviews have focused on amphotericin B PK in children. In one study of five premature infants and five older children, the volume of distribution was smaller, and the elimination clearance more rapid than previously reported in adults. Serum levels were approximately half of those in adults with comparable doses, and interpatient variability was marked in the premature infants.[26] Other studies have confirmed interpatient variability in pediatric patients including lower serum levels in smaller children with higher total clearance, indicating perhaps that they received too low of a dose. In addition, older, heavier children with a relatively higher exposure to amphotericin B may be overdosed and at higher risk for toxicity.[27,28] One study examined ABLC in six children with hepatosplenic candidiasis and showed that steady state was reached in 7 days with continued resolution of lesions even after drug discontinuation.[29] A population PK analysis of 39 pediatric patients with cancer aged an average of 6.5 years (0.17 to 17) weighing an average of 21.1 kg (6.1 to 84.1) and receiving 0.8 to 5.9 mg per kg of body weight per day of L-amphotericin B found that body weight exhibits a significant influence on its PK parameters. The estimated clearance and volume of distribution in the central compartment in this population was 0.44 L per hour and 3.12 L, respectively. Through simulations of doses ranging from 1 to 12.5 mg per kg per day, it was found that infants weighing less than 20 kg may require higher doses than heavier children.[30] Weight was also the most influential predictor of population PK parameters among neonates [median weight 1.06 kg (0.48 to 4.9); median gestational age, 27 weeks (24 to 41)] with invasive candidiasis treated with ABLC at 2.5 to 5 mg per kg of body weight for a median of 21 days (4 to 47 days). In this population, postnatal and gestational age did not influence clearance or volume of distribution of ABLC.[31]

Toxicities, Side Effects, and Drug Interactions

Tolerance to amphotericin B deoxycholate is limited by its acute and chronic toxicities. In addition to fungal ergosterol, the drug also interacts with cholesterol in human cell membranes, which likely accounts for its toxicity.[32] Up to 80% of patients receiving amphotericin B develop either infusion-related toxicity or nephrotoxicity,[4] especially with concomitant therapy with nephrotoxic drugs such as aminoglycosides, vancomycin, cyclosporine, or tacrolimus.[33,34] Amphotericin B also has a constrictive effect on the afferent and efferent renal arterioles, leading to a reduction in the glomerular filtration rate.[35]

Renal function usually returns to normal after cessation of amphotericin B, although permanent renal impairment is common after larger doses.[3] Amphotericin B nephrotoxicity is generally less severe in infants and children than in adults, likely due to the more rapid clearance of the drug in children. In practice, this limits the use of amphotericin B deoxycholate largely to the neonatal population. Lipid formulations appear to stabilize amphotericin B in a self-associated state so that it is not available to interact with the cholesterol of human cellular membranes.[19,36] Another theory for the decreased nephrotoxicity of lipid formulations is the preferential binding of its amphotericin B to serum high-density lipoproteins compared with binding of amphotericin B to low-density lipoproteins.[37] The high-density lipoprotein-bound amphotericin B appears to be released to the kidney more slowly, or to a lesser degree. For infusion-related toxicity, there is a general agreement that L-amphotericin B has less toxicity than ABLC, whereas ABCD appears closer in toxicity to conventional amphotericin B.[38,39] In the 2017 pediatric dose-escalation study, there were 63 (11%) episodes of infusion-related reactions with no association between dosage group and frequency of infusion reaction or discontinuation.[25]

Clinical Studies

The recommended dose of amphotericin B deoxycholate is 1.0 to 1.5 mg per kg per day, and optimal duration of therapy is unknown but largely dependent on underlying disease, extent of the patient's fungal infection, resolution of any neutropenia, lessening immunosuppression, and the return of graft function following bone marrow or organ transplantation.[40,41] There is no total dose of amphotericin B recommended, and the key to success has been giving high doses in the initial phase of therapy and reducing the dose if toxicity develops.[42] According to the FDA, the lipid formulation is currently indicated for patients with systemic mycoses, primarily invasive aspergillosis, who are intolerant of or refractory to conventional amphotericin B. In addition, L-amphotericin B is approved as empiric therapy for the neutropenic patient with persistent fever, despite broad-spectrum antibiotic therapy.[18]

Pediatric Clinical Studies

Because amphotericin B is the oldest commonly used systemic antifungal, there are the most pediatric data for this agent. The first review of pediatric antifungal therapy was in 1969[43] and covered the nephrotoxicity of amphotericin B in 39 pediatric patients. An open-label study of 111 treatment episodes with ABLC in pediatric patients revealed a well-tolerated drug with generally stable renal function over 6 weeks of therapy. There was a complete or partial therapeutic response in 70% of patients, including 56% for aspergillosis and 81% for candidiasis.[44] A retrospective study of 46 pediatric patients who received ABLC confirmed the minimal decline in renal function and reported an overall response rate of 83%, including 78% against aspergillosis and 89% against candidiasis.[45]

In a prospective, randomized controlled trial of 49 children who received ABCD versus amphotericin B, there was significantly less renal toxicity in the ABCD group (12%) versus the amphotericin B group (52.4%). Although not statistically significant, a greater proportion of children who received ABCD (69%) versus amphotericin B (41%) also had a successful outcome.[46] A retrospective analysis of 30 children found that a short course of 7 to 14 days of amphotericin B after the last positive blood culture for *Candida* species was adequate for treatment in children.[47] Prophylactic L-amphotericin B administered for the first 100 days post–allogeneic stem cell transplantation in children reduced the incidence of invasive mold infections in a retrospective single-center study.[48] From 1996 to 2000, the safety and efficacy of ABLC injection was assessed in 548 children with cancer (0 to 20 years of age) who were enrolled in the Collaborative Exchange of Antifungal Research registry. Response data for 89% (255/285) of patients with documented pathogens showed that a complete or partial response was achieved in 54.9% of patients. Among patients with proven *Aspergillus* infection, the response rates were 37.5% to 40.5%. In this report, elevations in serum creatinine of more than 1.5 and more than 2.5 times the baseline values were seen in 24.8% and 8.8% of all patients, respectively. The use of ABLC in pediatric patients with cancer intolerant of or refractory to conventional antifungal therapy is recommended.[49]

Although amphotericin B products have been extensively used in neonates, there are limited published data to compare the safety, tolerability, and effectiveness of the various formulations. Several small retrospective studies have demonstrated better safety profiles of L-amphotericin B as compared to amphotericin B deoxycholate, but the two have not been compared in a randomized manner. One large retrospective cohort study including 730 infants with candidiasis at 192 neonatal intensive care units found higher mortality rates among infants treated with amphotericin B lipid products (29%) as compared to amphotericin B deoxycholate (18%).[50]

PYRIMIDINE ANALOGS

5-FLUOROCYTOSINE

Mechanism of Action

5-Fluorocytosine (5-FC; Ancoban, ICN Pharmaceuticals, Costa Mesa, CA) is a fluorinated analog of cytosine first synthesized in 1957 as a potential antitumor agent,[51] first used to treat human disease in 1968,[52] and initially approved for use in 1972.[16] Unfortunately, 5-FC has little inherent anti-*Aspergillus* activity[53] and most reports detail clinical failure with monotherapy for yeast infections.[54] Its antimycotic activity results from the rapid conversion of 5-FC into 5-fluorouracil (5-FU) within susceptible fungal cells.[55,56] The two mechanisms of action of 5-FU are incorporation into fungal RNA in place of uridylic acid to inhibit fungal protein synthesis and inhibition of thymidylate synthase to inhibit fungal DNA synthesis.[55] The latter appears to be the dominant mechanism. Clinical and microbiologic antifungal resistance appears to develop quickly to 5-FC monotherapy, so clinicians have reserved it for combination approaches to augment other more potent antifungals.

Pharmacology

Fungistatic 5-FC is thought to enhance the antifungal activity of amphotericin B, especially in anatomic sites where amphotericin B penetration is often suboptimal, such as CSF, heart valves, and the vitreal body.[14] 5-FC penetrates well into most body sites because it is small, highly water soluble, and not bound by serum proteins to any great extent.[55] One explanation for the synergism detected with amphotericin B + 5-FC is that the membrane-permeabilizing effects of low concentrations of amphotericin B facilitate penetration of 5-FC to the cell interior.[4] Using a *Candida albicans* model, Beggs and Sarosi suggested that synergism actually results from sequential and not combined action, with amphotericin B acting alone until its gradual oxidation results in its depletion, at which point 5-FC acts on surviving fungal cells' RNA and DNA synthesis.[4,57] 5-FC is available only as an oral formulation in the United States, and the correct dose is 150 mg per kg per day in four divided doses.

Toxicities, Side Effects, and Drug Interactions

The toxicity of 5-FC is hypothesized to be due to its conversion to 5-FU, with reports of patients receiving 5-FC for antifungal treatment having serum 5-FU levels in the range found after chemotherapeutic doses.[58] However, a pilot study of six patients found undetectable levels of 5-FU in patients receiving 5-FC therapy, suggesting it unlikely that 5-FC toxicity is indeed caused by 5-FU exposure, as originally hypothesized. However, the patients in this study received 5-FC intravenously (IV) and thereby bypassed the conversion of oral 5-FC to 5-FU by the human intestinal microflora.[59]

5-FC may exacerbate myelosuppression in patients with neutropenia, and toxic levels may develop when used in combination with amphotericin B due to nephrotoxicity of the amphotericin B and the decreased renal clearance of 5-FC.[60] Routine serum 5-FC level monitoring is warranted in high-risk patients, since peak serum concentrations of 100 μg per mL or greater (2 hours postdose) are associated with bone marrow aplasia. In a review of a multicenter trial of 194 patients who received amphotericin B + 5-FC for cryptococcal meningitis, one or more toxic drug reactions (including azotemia, renal tubular acidosis, leukopenia, and thrombocytopenia) developed in 103 patients.[61] Toxicity appeared in the first 2 weeks of therapy in 56% of patients and in the first 4 weeks of therapy in 87% of patients. In a study involving 33 neonates in the United Kingdom treated with IV or oral 5-FC who underwent therapeutic drug monitoring, drug concentrations were low (trough, <20 mg per L or peak, <50 mg per L) in 40.5%; undetectable in 5.1%; high (trough level > 40 mg per L or peak > 80 mg per L) in 38.9%; and potentially toxic (>100 mg per L) in 9.9%.[62] Given the narrow therapeutic range, the need for therapeutic drug monitoring and oral administration in the United States, this drug is seldom used in neonates.

Clinical Studies

Nearly all clinical studies involving 5-FC are combination antifungal protocols for cryptococcal meningitis, due to the inherently rather weak antifungal activity of 5-FC monotherapy. The first comparative clinical cryptococcal meningitis study with amphotericin B + 5-FC was in 1979[63] and found a benefit to the combination over amphotericin B alone. One multicenter study of 194 patients with cryptococcal meningitis concluded that 4 weeks of amphotericin B + 5-FC should be reserved for patients without neurologic complications or immunosuppressive therapy, but in a more high-risk population, 6 weeks of combination therapy resulted in less relapses.[64] Further studies included a multicenter trial that found similar results with consolidation therapy using either itraconazole or fluconazole for 8 weeks after 2 weeks of initial amphotericin B + 5-FC therapy.[65]

While other studies have evaluated different combinations for cryptococcal meningitis,[65–68] amphotericin B + 5-FC is currently recommended as initial therapy for cryptococcal meningitis after substantial study, and it is also suggested for use in candidal meningitis.[68] 5-FC fills an important role in conjunction with amphotericin B, as 5-FC will penetrate into the CSF much better compared with amphotericin B's poor penetration and 5-FC–treated patients had less relapses compared with those receiving only amphotericin B.

Pediatric Clinical Studies

The use of 5-FC in premature neonates is discouraged. A study evaluating risk factors and mortality of neonatal candidiasis among extremely premature infants showed that infants with *Candida* meningitis who received amphotericin B in combination with 5-FC had a prolonged time to sterilize the CSF compared with those receiving amphotericin B monotherapy (median of 17.5 days vs. 6 days).[69] The Infectious Diseases Society of America (IDSA) recommends the addition of 5-FC only for cases of refractory central nervous system (CNS) candidiasis.[68]

AZOLES

The azoles are subdivided into imidazoles and triazoles on the basis of the number of nitrogens in the azole ring,[8] with the structural differences resulting in different binding affinities for the cytochrome P450 (CYP) enzyme system. With the exception of ketoconazole, the imidazoles have been limited to treatment of superficial mycoses and none, including ketoconazole, have activity against the mold *Aspergillus.* Of the older first-generation triazoles, fluconazole is also ineffective against *Aspergillus*, but itraconazole does possess activity against *Aspergillus.* Newer second-generation triazoles (voriconazole, posaconazole, and isavuconazole) are modifications of prior triazoles with an expanded antifungal spectrum of activity and generally lower minimum inhibitory concentration values compared to the older compounds.[70]

MECHANISM OF ACTION

The azole antifungals are heterocyclic synthetic compounds that inhibit the fungal cytochrome $P450_{14DM}$ (also known as lanosterol 14α-demethylase), which catalyzes a late step in ergosterol biosynthesis. The drugs bind to the heme group in the target protein and block demethylation of the C-14 of lanosterol, leading to substitution of methylated sterols in the membrane and depletion of ergosterol. The result is an accumulation of precursors with abnormalities in fungal membrane permeability, membrane-bound enzyme activity, and lack of coordination of chitin synthesis.[71,72]

FLUCONAZOLE

Pharmacology

Fluconazole (Diflucan, Pfizer Inc., New York, NY) is a bis-triazole that was discovered in 1982 and approved by the FDA for use in treating cryptococcosis and *Candida* infections in 1990. An in vitro time–kill study showed that the rate of fluconazole fungistatic activity was not influenced by concentration once the maximal fungistatic concentration was surpassed (concentration independent), which is in contrast to the concentration-dependent fungicidal activity of amphotericin B[71] or caspofungin.[73] Fluconazole is well absorbed from the gastrointestinal (GI) tract and is cleared predominantly by the renal route as unchanged drug, whereas metabolism accounts for only a minor proportion of fluconazole clearance.[74] Binding to plasma proteins is low (12%).[75] Gastric absorption of oral fluconazole is virtually unaffected by pH or the presence of food in the stomach.

Fluconazole is available as either an oral or an IV form, and oral fluconazole has a high bioavailability of approximately 90% relative to its IV administration. Fluconazole passes into tissues and fluids very rapidly, probably due to its relatively low lipophilicity and limited degree of binding to plasma proteins. Concentrations of fluconazole are 10- to 20-fold higher in the urine than in blood, and drug concentrations in the CSF and vitreous humor of the eye are approximately 80% of those found simultaneously in blood.[75] The concentrations of fluconazole in body fluids such as vaginal secretions, breast milk, saliva, and sputum are also similar to those in blood, and the fluid-to-blood ratio remains stable after multiple doses. There is a linear plasma concentration–dose relationship.

It is clear that simple conversion of the corresponding adult dosage of fluconazole on a weight basis is inappropriate for pediatric patients. A review of five separate fluconazole PK studies in 113 pediatric patients, including 12 premature neonates,[74] showed that with the exception of neonates, fluconazole clearance is generally more rapid in children than in adults, with a mean plasma half-life of approximately 20 hours compared with approximately 30 hours in adult patients. Therefore, to achieve comparable exposure in pediatric patients, the daily fluconazole dose needs to be essentially doubled for children older than 3 months. Correct pediatric fluconazole doses should be proportionately higher than adult doses, generally 10 to 12 mg per kg per day.

In neonates, the volume of distribution is significantly greater and more variable than in infants and children, and doubling the dose for neonatal patients is necessary to achieve comparable plasma concentrations. The increased volume of distribution is thought to be due to the larger amount of body water found in the total body volume of neonates. However, there is also a slow elimination of fluconazole, with a mean half-life of 88.6 hours at birth, decreasing to approximately 55 hours at 2 weeks of age. This is due to the reduced activity of hepatic enzymes for biotransformation as well as reduced glomerular filtration for the first month of life. As renal function continues to develop, the fluconazole plasma half-life decreases[74]; however, a recent population PK study in premature infants suggests that maintenance fluconazole doses of 12 mg per kg per day are necessary to achieve exposures similar to older children and adults.[76] In addition, a loading dose of 25 mg per kg would achieve steady-state concentrations sooner than the traditional dosing scheme.[77] This strategy was confirmed in a phase I clinical trial that included 10 infants at risk for invasive fungal infection.[78] Even higher loading doses are needed in children supported by extracorporeal membrane oxygenation (ECMO), which is associated with increases in volume of distribution. A population PK study found that children on ECMO require loading doses of 12 mg per kg for prophylaxis and 35 mg per kg for treatment of candidiasis to achieve exposure similar to children not on ECMO.[79] Children with human immunodeficiency virus (HIV) infection who receive oral fluconazole achieve similar serum concentrations to IV dosing, and this indicates a nearly complete degree of absorption.[80] In fact, there have also been comparable concentrations after either oral or IV administration in children younger than 3 months.[81] The bioavailability of enteral fluconazole is adequate in even critically ill surgical patients.[81] The peritoneal bioavailability of fluconazole is also excellent for treating dialysis patients with peritonitis. A prospective study of 17 children on dialysis found that fluconazole was excreted almost solely through the dialysate and that the terminal half-life was significantly longer in the children requiring peritoneal dialysis.[82] Finally, there is a theoretical advantage to the oral suspension of fluconazole over capsules for oral thrush, as in one study of healthy volunteers, the peak saliva levels of fluconazole were higher in those flushing their mouth for 2 minutes with the oral suspension than in those who swallowed the capsule.[83]

Toxicities, Side Effects, and Drug Interactions

Side effects of fluconazole are uncommon. In one study of 24 immunocompromised children, elevated transaminases were observed in only two cases.[84] A large review of 78 reports that used fluconazole in a total of 726 children younger than 1 year showed that it was generally well tolerated and reaffirmed the guidelines to increase the interval between doses due to the prolonged elimination during the first month of life.[85] Another review of 562 children from 12 clinical studies confirmed that pediatric results mirror the excellent safety profile seen in adults. The most common side effects were GI upset (7.7%) (vomiting, diarrhea, nausea) and a skin rash (1.2%).[86] Fluconazole affects the metabolism of cyclosporine, leading to its increased concentration when used together.[76]

Clinical Studies

A review of two randomized clinical trials showed that patients who received fluconazole versus placebo for prophylaxis against candidiasis while undergoing allogeneic bone marrow transplantation had lower rates of candidal infection and gut graft-versus-host disease.[87] Additional studies revealed that neither fluconazole (200 mg per day) versus low-dose amphotericin B (0.2 mg per kg per day) nor high-dose (400 mg per day) versus low-dose (200 mg per day) fluconazole prophylaxis showed any difference in incidence of fungal infections or survival.[88,89]

For treatment of invasive candidiasis, a multicenter trial of 236 patients found that those treated with fluconazole + amphotericin B versus fluconazole alone trended toward better success and more rapid resolution of *Candida* fungemia.[90] In another randomized trial for treatment of fungal infections using medical and surgical intensive care unit patients, there was a significant decrease in *Candida* species infections in the group that received fluconazole versus placebo.[91]

Unlike itraconazole or ketoconazole, fluconazole is particularly appropriate for urinary tract infections due to its concentrating effect in the bladder. Fluconazole is also effective for superficial skin infections, since the stratum corneum-to-serum ratio is 37.[92]

Pediatric Clinical Studies

An open, prospective, randomized pilot study in 50 children undergoing remission induction or consolidation chemotherapy showed that those patients who received either fluconazole or nystatin prophylaxis for *Candida* infections had similar rates of success.[93] A study of 40 young infants (aged 2 days to 3 months) with either nonresponse or contraindication to standard antifungal therapy treated with fluconazole showed a 97% clinical and mycologic response rate.[94] In a prospective, randomized, double-blind trial over a 30-month period of 100 infants with birth weight less than 1,000 g, those infants who received fluconazole for 6 weeks had a decrease in fungal colonization (22% vs. 60%) as well as a decrease in the development of invasive fungal infection compared with placebo (0% vs. 20%).[95] A larger prospective, randomized, double-blind, controlled trial conducted in nine neonatal intensive care units in Italy among 322 infants with birth weight less than 1,500 g showed that a fluconazole prophylaxis regimen of 3 to 6 mg per kg several times per week for 4 to 6 weeks reduced the incidence of *Candida* colonization (9.8% in the 6 mg group, 7.7% in the 3 mg group, and 29.2% in the placebo group; $p < 0.001$) and invasive fungal infections (2.7% in the 6 mg group, $p = 0.005$; 3.8% in the 3 mg group, $p = 0.02$; and 13.2% in the placebo group).[96] A randomized, placebo-controlled trial of fluconazole prophylaxis (6 mg per kg twice weekly over 6 weeks) administered to infants with birth weight less than 750 g in low-incidence centers did not find any difference in a composite outcome of death or invasive candidiasis between the fluconazole and placebo groups.[97] Although the primary outcome of this study was a composite outcome, rates of invasive candidiasis and death were also reported separately. As compared to placebo, fluconazole was associated with a decreased incidence (3% vs. 9%) of definite or probable candidiasis; this was not associated with any differences in mortality. This study also provided reassuring 2-year follow-up data for safety and neurodevelopmental outcomes.

ITRACONAZOLE

First publicly described in 1983[98,99] and available for clinical use in 1990, itraconazole (Sporanox, Janssen Pharmaceuticals, Titusville, NJ) adopted a triazole nucleus with higher specificity for the fungal CYP enzyme system than the older imidazoles.[100] Itraconazole's fungicidal activity is not as efficient as that of amphotericin B because inhibition of sterol synthesis takes longer than directly creating channels within the cell membrane.[101]

Pharmacology

Itraconazole has a high volume of distribution and accumulates in tissues, and the tissue-bound levels are probably more clinically relevant to infection treatment than serum levels.[72] Itraconazole is poorly water soluble, not reliably absorbed from the GI tract in its capsule formulation, and has high-protein binding.[12] It has a relatively long half-life of 25 to 50 hours, which allows for once-daily dosing.[102]

Dissolution and absorption of itraconazole are affected by gastric pH. Patients with achlorhydria or H_2-receptor antagonist use may demonstrate impaired absorption, whereas coadministration of the capsule with acidic beverages such as colas or cranberry juice may enhance its absorption.[103] Administering a dose with food significantly increases the absorption of the capsule formulation, but the new oral suspension with a cyclodextrin base is better absorbed on an empty stomach.[16] Elimination of itraconazole is primarily hepatic, so there is no need for dosage adjustment in renal failure.[72]

To overcome problems with variable absorption, itraconazole has been solubilized in cyclodextrin, with substantial improvement in absorption of drug as an oral solution.[71,104] This allows itraconazole to be available as an oral capsule, oral solution, and IV formulation. Cyclodextrins are naturally occurring doughnut-shaped glucose oligomers produced by enzymatic degradation of starch that have been chemically modified for medical use. The external face of the molecule is hydrophilic to facilitate solubilization of the complex in water and shield a lipophilic guest molecule.[105] Once itraconazole is released from the host cyclodextrin, it follows its standard PK, with steady-state concentration reached in the second week of daily dosing.

An IV formulation of itraconazole was approved by the FDA for pulmonary and extrapulmonary aspergillosis in patients who are intolerant of or refractory to amphotericin B.[106] The IV formulation can rapidly achieve high steady-state plasma concentrations[107,108] as opposed to the 7- to 10-day period needed for the capsule or oral formulation.[109] In children, itraconazole oral solution produces a maximum concentration lower than in adults, which could potentially justify higher dosing in younger children, whereas other PK properties such as half-life are similar to values in adults.[110] The IV preparation is not recommended for patients with reduced renal clearance because the impact or toxicity of the cyclodextrin is not known. In a single-dose (2.5 mg per kg) PK study of itraconazole in children aged 7 months to 17 years ($n = 33$), PK parameters of itraconazole were highly variable across age groups, and, therefore, no age dependence was observed in drug disposition. Overall, the estimated C_{max} was 1,015 (±692) ng per mL, systemic clearance was 702.8 (±499.4) mL per hour per kg, and half-life was 20.2 (±12.8) hours.[111] Pediatric dosing for itraconazole is not exact, but generally felt to be higher than adult doses and approximately 3 to 10 mg per kg per day.

In 2018, the FDA approved a new formulation designed to increase bioavailability. Tolsura (Mayne Pharma, Salisbury, Australia) is labeled for use in adults with invasive aspergillosis, histoplasmosis, and blastomycosis.

Toxicities, Side Effects, and Drug Interactions

Side effects are relatively few and include nausea and vomiting (10%), elevated transaminases (5%),[112] and peripheral edema. Although it has not been shown in children, there have been reports of development of cardiomyopathy while receiving this azole. As a potent inhibitor of the fungal CYP3A4 enzyme, itraconazole also has affinity for the human enzyme, and this produces important drug interactions. Prior or concurrent use of rifampin, phenytoin, carbamazepine, and phenobarbital should be avoided. Any drug handled by this cytochrome pathway with normally low bioavailability, extensive first-pass metabolism, or a narrow therapeutic window may be especially vulnerable.[113]

Patients receiving cyclosporine who are treated with a triazole should have an immediate-dose reduction of cyclosporine, followed by frequent monitoring of serum levels. In one study, there was an increase in tacrolimus or cyclosporine levels 48 hours after completing an IV itraconazole loading dose, so a 50% tacrolimus or cyclosporine dose reduction is recommended after an IV itraconazole loading dose.[114] Furthermore, the azoles may also increase serum levels and intracellular levels of cytotoxic drugs such as vincristine and anthracyclines[32] or protease inhibitors.[115] Azole–drug interactions may also lead to decreased plasma concentration of the azole, related to either decreased absorption or increased metabolism.[18]

Although the theoretical concern of polyene–azole antagonism due to ergosterol mechanisms of action exists, combination with amphotericin B does appear safe in a recent survey of clinical practice of 93 invasive aspergillosis patients treated with this sequential therapy.[116]

Clinical Studies

Itraconazole has roles in the therapy of numerous fungal infections. A multicenter, open-label study was performed in 31 patients with pulmonary invasive aspergillosis who received 14 days of IV itraconazole followed by 12 weeks of capsules. The IV form was well tolerated, and target therapeutic concentrations were obtained within 2 days in 91% of patients and in all patients within 1 week of IV treatment. These levels were also maintained after switching to oral therapy, and a complete or partial response was seen in 48% (15/31) of patients.[107]

A randomized controlled trial comparing itraconazole oral solution versus fluconazole suspension for prevention of fungal infections in 445 hematologic malignancy patients revealed that more proven fungal infections occurred in the fluconazole arm, and more of these were fatal.[117] In addition, there were no cases of invasive aspergillosis in the itraconazole arm, there were significantly more cases of aspergillosis in the fluconazole arm, and most were fatal. This study reinforces that while itraconazole and fluconazole provide effective prophylaxis against *Candida* infections, itraconazole offers additional protection against aspergillosis. Similarly, in a randomized trial of liver transplant recipients, those patients treated with oral itraconazole developed less proven fungal infections than did those receiving fluconazole for the same time period.[118]

A double-blind trial of 63 patients with HIV infection in Thailand with itraconazole versus placebo showed that development of systemic fungal infection decreased from 16.7% of patients given placebo versus 1.6% taking itraconazole, with only one infection with *Penicillium marneffei* in the itraconazole treatment arm.[119]

Pediatric Clinical Studies

A phase I study in 26 HIV-infected children showed that the cyclodextrin itraconazole solution was well tolerated and efficacious against oropharyngeal candidiasis, including responses in all patients with fluconazole-resistant isolates.[120] Although not standardized, a commonly used dose of itraconazole for pediatric patients is 3 to 5 mg per kg per day once daily, with doses used up to 10 mg per kg per day. Itraconazole (10 mg per kg per day loading dose and 5 mg per kg per day maintenance dose) administered to 53 pediatric patients for 100 days following hematologic stem cell transplantation to prevent invasive fungal infections was well tolerated. In this cohort, one patient suffered from invasive candidiasis, 21% (11/53) discontinued the medication mostly due to prolonged fever ($n = 7$), and 19% (10/53) had doubling of aspartate aminotransferase baseline values.[121] The use of itraconazole over fluconazole in this population is attractive because of its antimold properties; however, given the metabolic profile of itraconazole, high potential for drug interactions, and high exposure variability in pediatric patients, newer triazole agents (i.e., voriconazole) continue to be the first line of therapy against invasive mold infections. However, itraconazole remains a mainstay of treatment for the endemic mycosis *Histoplasma capsulatum*.[122]

VORICONAZOLE

Voriconazole (VFend; Pfizer Inc., New York, NY) is a second-generation triazole and a synthetic derivative of fluconazole. First introduced in 1995, it was developed as part of a program to enhance the potency and antifungal spectrum of fluconazole largely through the addition of a methyl group to fluconazole's propyl backbone and the substitution of a triazole moiety with a fluoropyrimidine group.[123] Voriconazole generally has the spectrum of activity of itraconazole, yet the bioavailability of fluconazole. Importantly, it has both fungicidal and fungistatic activity against *Aspergillus* and is recommended by the IDSA as first-line therapy for aspergillosis.[40,123–125]

Pharmacology

Voriconazole is extensively metabolized by the liver and shows approximately 90% oral bioavailability. It appears that CYP2C19 plays a major role in the metabolism of voriconazole, and this enzyme exhibits genetic polymorphism, dividing the population into poor and extensive metabolizers as a result of a point mutation in the gene encoding the protein of CYP2C19.[126] About 5% to 7% of the white population has a deficiency in expressing this enzyme, so genotype plays a key role in the PK of voriconazole.[127] As many as 20% of non–Indian Asians have low CYP2C19 activity and can achieve voriconazole levels as much as fourfold greater than those homozygous subjects who metabolize the drug more extensively.[128] Even though most of the voriconazole metabolism occurs through the cytochrome P450 enzymatic system, animal models suggest that 25% of the remaining metabolism is mediated by the flavin-containing monooxygenase pathway.[129]

Voriconazole is available as an oral tablet or an IV solution. Voriconazole is 44% to 67% plasma bound; in adults, it exhibits nonlinear PK, has a variable half-life of approximately 6 hours[130] with large interpatient variation in blood levels,[131] and has good CSF penetration.[69,100,132–135] Time–kill studies against *Candida* species and *Cryptococcus neoformans* revealed in vitro nonconcentration-dependent fungistatic activity, similar to that of fluconazole.[136]

Oral absorption is nonlinear and rapid, with an approximately fivefold accumulation over 14 days in one study of hematologic malignancy patients.[135] In a study assessing voriconazole levels after IV -to-oral switching, mean voriconazole levels did fall following oral administration compared to IV administration, but most subjects achieved steady state 4 days after dosing began. Maximum plasma voriconazole levels occurred at the end of the 1-hour IV infusion and between 1.4 and 1.8 hours after oral administration.[127] A PK study in six patients with cirrhosis demonstrated that hepatic-impaired patients should receive the same oral loading dose, but half the maintenance dose.[137] A multicenter safety, population PK study of single (3 to 4 mg per kg) and multiple (12 mg per kg per day loading dose, 6 to 8 mg per kg per day maintenance dose) IV voriconazole doses in immunocompromised pediatric patients (n = 35, 2 to 11 years of age) showed that body weight was more influential than age in accounting for the observed variability in voriconazole PK and elimination capacity correlated with CYP2C19 genotype. Exposures were similar at 4 mg per kg every 12 hours in children (median area under the concentration–time curve 14,227 ng per hour per mL) and 3 mg per kg in adults [median area under the curve (*AUC*), 13,855 ng per hour per mL]. Visual disturbances occurred in 13% of the patients.[138]

Higher doses (in mg per kg) of voriconazole are needed in children to achieve similar exposures to the 6 mg per kg loading dose recommended for adults with invasive aspergillosis. An open-label study of immunocompromised children found that exposures after a 7 mg per kg dose were lower than adults receiving 6 mg per kg.[139] At steady state, the 7 mg per kg per dose every 12 hours achieved lower median *AUC* than adults receiving 4 mg per kg per dose. A subsequent population PK study included data from 112 immunocompromised children (2 to <12 years), 26 immunocompromised adolescents (12 to <17 years), and 35 healthy adults.[140] Pediatric exposure after 9 mg per kg dose was similar to adults receiving 6 mg per kg. Exposures in adolescents were weight dependent; children 12 to 14 years of age weighing less than 50 kg should receive the pediatric dose; children weighing greater or equal to 50 kg and anyone aged 15 years or older should receive adult dosing.

Toxicities, Side Effects, and Drug Interactions

The main side effects of voriconazole include reversible dose-dependent visual disturbances (increased brightness, blurred vision)[141] in as many as one-third of treated patients; elevated hepatic transaminases with increasing doses[142,143]; and occasional skin reactions likely due to photosensitization.[100,122,144]

As with other azoles, the potential exists to modify the metabolism of other drugs, including a contraindication for concomitant use with sirolimus. In one study, coadministration of voriconazole and tacrolimus elevated trough tacrolimus levels in one liver transplant patient nearly 10-fold,[145] and in another study, tacrolimus levels were significantly increased 2.2-fold when coadministered with voriconazole.[146] In a study of renal transplant patients, concomitant administration of voriconazole with cyclosporine also resulted in a 1.7-fold increase in the geometric mean for cyclosporine area under the plasma concentration–time curve, so it is recommended that the cyclosporine dose be halved and levels monitored frequently.[147] However, voriconazole does not affect mycophenolic acid.[148]

Clinical Studies

The largest prospective clinical trial of voriconazole as primary therapy for invasive aspergillosis involved 392 patients at 92 centers in 19 countries over 3 years and compared initial randomized therapy with voriconazole versus amphotericin B followed by conventional therapy. Patients who initially received voriconazole had statistically significantly better complete or partial response (53%) versus those initially receiving amphotericin B (32%). Survival also improved to 71% for voriconazole versus 58% for those initially receiving amphotericin B.[149] Analysis in an open, noncomparative multicenter study of 116 patients, treated with voriconazole as primary therapy (60 patients) or salvage therapy (56 patients) also yielded encouraging results: 14% had a complete, 34% had a partial, and 21% had a stable response to voriconazole, whereas 31% failed to respond to therapy.[131] These data forged the way for FDA approval of voriconazole for initial therapy for invasive aspergillosis in May 2002.

A multicenter trial of voriconazole versus fluconazole in treating esophageal candidiasis in 391 immunocompromised patients showed similar success rates with voriconazole (98.3%) and fluconazole (95.1%).[150] Although overall safety and tolerability of both antifungals was acceptable, fewer patients discontinued voriconazole due to poor clinical response, but more patients discontinued voriconazole than fluconazole because of laboratory abnormalities or adverse events (AEs).

Pediatric Clinical Studies

Voriconazole has been studied in an open-label evaluation of 58 children with a proven or probable invasive fungal infection who received voriconazole on a compassionate basis if they were refractory or intolerant of conventional antifungal therapy.[151] Most patients (72%) had aspergillosis, but the group also included scedosporiosis (14%), candidiasis (7%), and others. At the end of therapy (median duration 93 days), a total of 45% of children had a complete or partial response, and only 7% were discontinued from voriconazole because of intolerance. Stratifying outcome by pathogen revealed a complete or partial response of 43% against aspergillosis, 50% against candidemia, and 63% against scedosporiosis. The most commonly reported AEs in these children included elevation in hepatic transaminases, skin rash and photosensitivity reaction, and abnormal vision. Dosing in neonates and children younger than 3 years is challenging. A retrospective review of clinically obtained drug levels from 10 infants aged 2 weeks to 35 months found that weight-based dosing did not reliably predict plasma levels, suggesting that therapeutic drug monitoring should be routinely used in this population.[152]

POSACONAZOLE

In September 2006, the FDA approved posaconazole (Noxafil, Merck & Co., Whitehouse Station, NJ) for the prophylaxis and treatment of disseminated candidiasis and aspergillosis in severely immunocompromised patients and for the treatment of oropharyngeal candidiasis. Posaconazole is a second-generation triazole antifungal agent available as a suspension for oral administration, as an extended-release tablet, or as IV injection. The oral formulations are FDA approved for individuals aged 13 years or greater; the injection is only approved for those 18 years and older. The antimicrobial spectrum of posaconazole is similar to that of voriconazole; however, the former is active against mucoromycetes.

Pharmacology

Oral posaconazole reaches maximum plasma concentrations 3 to 5 hours after ingestion. Dose-proportional increases in plasma exposure (*AUC*) to posaconazole were observed following single oral doses from 50 to 800 mg and following multiple-dose administration from 50 to 400 mg twice per day (BID). Steady-state plasma concentrations are attained at 7 to 10 days following multiple-dose administration.[153] When administered with a nonfat and high-fat diet, posaconazole exposure and maximum concentration are three to four times higher than the fasting state.[154] In addition, posaconazole exposure is maximized with acidic beverages, administration in divided doses, and absence of proton pump inhibitors.[155] Posaconazole distributes well into tissues, is 98% protein bound, and is not a substrate for the cytochrome P450 enzymatic system. However, about 20% of the parent drug is glucuronidated by phase 2 enzymes. Posaconazole is eliminated with a mean half-life of 25 hours (19 to 31 hours) and with a total body clearance (*CL/F*) of 4.1 to 6.6 mL per minute per kg[156]; it is predominantly eliminated in the feces, with renal clearance playing a minor role. Therefore, no dose adjustment is necessary in mild-to-moderate renal insufficiency. Posaconazole is fungicidal in vitro, with likely time-dependent killing.[157] IV posaconazole also demonstrates dose-proportional increases in plasma exposure. A phase I trial in adults compared exposure after infusions of 200 and 300 mg daily, after an initial twice-daily loading dose. A dose of 300 mg IV achieved exposure comparable to oral doses known to be efficacious in adults and was chosen as the dose for the subsequent phase III trial.[158]

Toxicities, Side Effects, and Drug Interactions

Posaconazole is primarily metabolized via uridine diphosphate (UDP) glucuronidation (phase 2 enzymes) and is a substrate for P-glycoprotein (P-gp) efflux. Therefore, inhibitors or inducers (i.e., rifabutin, phenytoin) of these clearance pathways may affect posaconazole plasma concentrations.[159] Posaconazole is also a CYP34A inhibitor, and therefore, coadministration results in increased plasma concentrations of the following products: cyclosporine (75% dose reduction required),[159] tacrolimus (60% dose reduction required), rifabutin, midazolam, and phenytoin.[159] Posaconazole causes transient hepatic reactions, including mild-to-moderate elevations in alanine aminotransferase, aspartate aminotransferase, alkaline phosphatase, and total bilirubin.[159] In a juvenile dog model, administration of IV posaconazole was associated with the development of lateral ventricle enlargement in five of eight dogs as compared to placebo.[160] The clinical significance of this finding is uncertain, but for this reason, the IV formulation of posaconazole has not been approved for use in children younger than 18 years.

Clinical Studies

In a multicenter, randomized, single-blinded study of posaconazole (n = 304) versus fluconazole or itraconazole (n = 298) in neutropenic patients undergoing chemotherapy for acute myelogenous leukemia or myelodysplastic syndromes, posaconazole was superior in preventing invasive fungal infections.[161] Proven or probable invasive fungal infections were reported in 2% in the posaconazole group versus 8% in the fluconazole or itraconazole group [absolute reduction in the posaconazole group, −6%; 95% confidence interval (CI), −9.7% to −2.5%; $p < 0.001$]. Fewer patients in the posaconazole group had invasive aspergillosis (1% vs. 7%, $p < 0.001$), and survival was significantly longer among recipients of posaconazole than among recipients of fluconazole or itraconazole ($p = 0.04$). Serious AEs (i.e., torsades de pointes) possibly or probably related to posaconazole were higher when compared with fluconazole or itraconazole (6% vs. 2%, $p = 0.01$).[161] Another multiple site, randomized, double-blinded study in patients with allogeneic hematopoietic stem cell transplantation (HSCT) and graft-versus-host disease showed that posaconazole was not inferior to fluconazole in the prevention of invasive fungal infections.[162] Posaconazole has also been used successfully in the treatment of six adult patients who received salvage treatment (800 mg per day) for 6 to 34 weeks for severe forms of histoplasmosis (n = 1, pulmonary; n = 5, disseminated disease).[163]

Pediatric Clinical Studies

In a study of eight patients (seven pediatric patients aged 9 to 18 years) with chronic granulomatous disease and proven invasive mold infection refractory to standard therapy, posaconazole (n = 6,400 mg orally BID; n = 1,200 mg orally three times per day) was well tolerated.[164] Another report including data from 24 patients with active zygomycosis who were enrolled in two open-label, nonrandomized, multicentered compassionate trials that evaluated oral posaconazole as salvage therapy for invasive fungal infections showed that two children aged 7 and 17 years had partial response to posaconazole.[165]

A recent prospective open-label study assessed the PK of the oral suspension in children aged 3 months to 18 years with documented or anticipated neutropenia.[166] The target exposure was mean steady-state C_{avg} of 1,200 ng per mL, based on efficacious dosing in clinical trials in adults.[167] However, none of the proposed doses achieved this exposure. A population PK study using retrospective data from therapeutic drug monitoring also concluded that the oral suspension is not reliably absorbed in young children.[168] A newer oral formulation of posaconazole has recently completed phase I studies for children.

ISAVUCONAZOLE

Isavuconazole (Cresemba, Merck & Co., Whitehouse Station, NJ) is an extended-spectrum azole FDA approved in 2015 for the treatment of invasive aspergillosis and invasive mucormycosis in adults. It is available in both IV and oral formulations. Isavuconazonium, the prodrug, is water soluble; therefore, the IV formulation does not require cyclodextrin.

Pharmacology

Isavuconazonium sulfate is rapidly hydrolyzed to isavuconazole. Isavuconazole reaches maximum plasma concentrations 2 to 3 hours after ingestion and almost immediately after IV administration. Unlike posaconazole, isavuconazole may be administered with or without food. It is well distributed and highly protein bound, with a mean steady-state volume of distribution of 450 L. Isavuconazole is cleared hepatically, with a mean half-life of 130 hours with little to no renal excretion. Therefore, no dose adjustment is needed in patients with renal insufficiency.

Toxicities, Side Effects, and Drug Interactions

Similar to the other azoles, isavuconazole is a substrate for CYP3A4, and levels may be impacted by inhibitors or inducers of these clearance pathways. Coadministration of strong CYP3A4 inhibitors and inducers—specifically ketoconazole, lopinavir/ritonavir, and rifampin—are contraindicated. Isavuconazole itself is a mild inhibitor of CYP3A4.[169]

In clinical trials, isavuconazole was comparable to voriconazole in its side-effect profile.[170] GI disturbances (most commonly nausea, vomiting, and diarrhea) predominated in 68% of isavuconazole recipients and 69% of voriconazole recipients. Notably, skin and subcutaneous disorders (33% vs. 42%), eye disorders (15% vs. 27%), and hepatobiliary disorders (9% vs. 16%) were less common in the isavuconazole group. Isavuconazole has been associated with shortening (as compared to the other azoles) of QT interval and is contraindicated in patients with familial short QT syndrome.

Clinical Studies

Isavuconazole was compared to voriconazole in a randomized, multicenter noninferiority trial of 527 adults with suspected invasive mold disease.[170] Noninferiority was met in the intention-to-treat analyses for the primary outcome, all-cause mortality at 6 weeks, with 45 (17%) deaths in the isavuconazole group as compared to 50 (19%) in the voriconazole group.[170] A prospective study of 37 adult patients with mucormycosis compared outcomes among patients prospectively treated with isavuconazole to matched patients from a fungal disease registry who had been treated with amphotericin B.[171] Subjects were matched on disease severity, type of malignancy, and the presence of surgical treatment within 7 days. All-cause mortality did not differ between treatment groups in crude (33% vs. 39%) or weighted (33% vs. 41%) analyses.

A phase III trial randomized 450 with candidemia or invasive candidiasis to either isavuconazole or caspofungin.[172] The primary efficacy outcome was overall response to therapy (mycologic eradication and clinical cure or improvement) at the end of IV therapy. Isavuconazole did not meet noninferiority criteria, with rates of overall response 60% in the isavuconazole group as compared to 71% in the caspofungin group. Despite in vitro activity against *Candida,* isavuconazole is not labeled for this indication.

Pediatric Clinical Studies

A phase I trial of isavuconazole in pediatric patients with hematologic malignancy has recently been completed (NCT03241550), and phase II studies for efficacy in invasive mold infections are underway.

ECHINOCANDINS

MECHANISM OF ACTION

For years, most development of new systemic antifungals focused on chemically modifying existing classes.[173] An entirely new class of antifungals, the echinocandins and the amino-containing pneumocandin analogs, are cyclic hexapeptide agents that interfere with cell wall biosynthesis by noncompetitive inhibition of 1,3-β-D-glucan synthase, an enzyme present in fungi but absent in mammalian cells.[69,100] This 1,3-β-D-glucan, an essential cell wall polysaccharide, forms a fibril of three helically entwined linear polysaccharides and provides structural integrity for the fungal cell wall.[174,175]

Echinocandins inhibit hyphal tip growth, converting the mycelium to small clumps of cells, but the older septated cells with little glucan synthesis are not killed.[173] Therefore, the echinocandin activity end point is morphologic change, not in vitro medium clearing. Echinocandins are generally fungicidal in vitro against *Candida* species, although not as rapidly as amphotericin B,[100,157] but appear to be fungistatic against *Aspergillus.*[39] As a class these agents are not metabolized through the CYP enzyme system but through a presumed *O*-methyl-transferase, lessening some of the drug interactions and side effects seen with the azole class. The echinocandins appear to have a prolonged and dose-dependent fungicidal antifungal effect on *C. albicans,* compared with the fungistatic fluconazole.[176]

Although echinocandin B was first described in 1974 as a natural product of *Aspergillus nidulans,*[177] drug development in this class has only recently expanded. Cilofungin, the first echinocandin B, was developed for *Candida* infections, but clinical investigation was discontinued due to possible toxicity of the vehicle, polyethylene glycol.[178] Three compounds in this class (caspofungin, micafungin, and anidulafungin) are FDA approved for use in adults; only micafungin and caspofungin are FDA approved for pediatric patients. Labeled indications for micafungin include treatment of candidiasis and candidemia in 4 months and older and prophylaxis of candidal infections in children undergoing stem cell transplant. Caspofungin is labeled in pediatric patients aged 3 months to 17 years for empiric therapy in febrile neutropenia, treatment of candidemia, treatment of esophageal candidiasis, and treatment of invasive aspergillosis in patients refractory to or intolerant of other therapies.

Because neonates with candidemia often suffer from disseminated disease in the CNS, which is associated with neurodevelopmental impairment, dosing of antifungal agents in this population should target the CNS.

An experimental rabbit model of hematogenous *Candida* meningoencephalitis in which micafungin was used as a prototype echinocandin suggests that doses of 8 mg per kg per day are necessary to achieve maximal microbicidal activity in the CNS parenchyma of rabbits.[179] When these data are extrapolated to the neonatal population using simulation techniques, the lowest fungal burden in the neonatal CNS parenchyma is achieved with micafungin doses of 10 to 15 mg per kg per day.[179]

CASPOFUNGIN

Pharmacology

Caspofungin (Cancidas; Merck & Co., Whitehouse Station, NJ) is a fungicidal, water-soluble semisynthetic derivative of the natural product pneumocandin B_0.[180] It has linear PK,[181] is hepatically excreted with a β-phase half-life of 9 to 10 hours,[182] and has uncommon AEs.[183–185] Parenteral administration is preferred due to the low bioavailability when administered orally.[184,185] It is not metabolized by the CYP isoenzyme system,[186] and the rate of killing for caspofungin in time–kill studies is greater than that of amphotericin B, which does not require cell growth for activity.[175]

The usual course is to begin with a loading dose followed by a daily maintenance dose,[173] usually 70 mg followed by 50 mg daily in adults. PK in healthy volunteers revealed linear PK and dose-proportional *AUC* concentration data. Much of the dose accumulation is achieved in the first week of dosing, and renal insufficiency has little effect on the PK of caspofungin.[187,188] Caspofungin has been evaluated at double the recommended dose (100 mg in adults), with an approximately 2.5-fold *AUC*.[189] Two PK studies of mild-to-moderate hepatic insufficiency resulted in elevations of caspofungin plasma concentrations observed in patients with mild hepatic insufficiency, and a dose reduction from 50 to 35 mg daily following the standard 70-mg loading dose was recommended in this setting.[187]

PK is different in children: levels are lower in smaller children, and the half-life is reduced. A study evaluated the PK of caspofungin in 39 children (2 to 17 years) with neutropenia and showed that in patients receiving 50 mg per m^2 per day (maximum, 70 mg per day), the AUC_{0-24} was similar to that for the exposure in adults receiving 50 mg per day and was consistent across age ranges. In this study, weight-based dosing (1 mg per kg per day) was suboptimal when compared with body surface area regimens and adult dosing.[190] A subsequent study including children aged 3 to 24 months found that the 50 mg per m^2 per day resulted in similar exposure for younger children.[191] Infants have lower clearance of caspofungin. A study of 18 patients younger than 3 months with documented or confirmed *Candida* infection found that doses of 25 mg per m^2 per day achieved exposure comparable to adults receiving 50 mg per day.[192]

Toxicities, Side Effects, and Drug Interactions

1,3-β-Glucan is a selective target present only in fungal cell walls and not in mammalian cells; therefore, the drug mechanism–based toxicity for the echinocandins is limited.[175] Plasma concentrations of tacrolimus are reduced by about 20% with coadministration of caspofungin, necessitating the close monitoring of tacrolimus levels, but tacrolimus does not alter the PK of caspofungin.[143] Cyclosporine increased the *AUC* of caspofungin by about 35%, although plasma concentrations of cyclosporine were not altered by coadministration of caspofungin.[193] Mycophenolate and caspofungin have no relevant interactions.[188] There appears to be no apparent myelotoxicity or nephrotoxicity with the agent.[188]

Clinical Studies

Caspofungin was approved by the FDA in February 2001 for refractory aspergillosis or intolerance to other therapies, and in January 2003, it was approved for candidemia and various other sites of invasive *Candida* infections. In the pivotal clinical study leading to FDA approval, 83 patients with acute invasive aspergillosis underwent "salvage" therapy after failing (71 patients) primary therapy for more than a week or developing significant nephrotoxicity (12 patients). Recipients had a 45% (37/83) favorable response with caspofungin.[194] A Spanish study before licensure revealed a 67% (8/12) favorable response rate among patients with proven or probable invasive aspergillosis.[195]

There have been several clinical trials evaluating caspofungin in esophageal candidiasis. One study of 128 patients found an 89% clinical success rate, compared with 63% in those patients receiving amphotericin B. In addition, therapy was stopped only in 7% of caspofungin patients, compared with 24% of amphotericin B patients.[196,197] A study comparing daily caspofungin with fluconazole showed favorable similar response rates (81% vs. 85%), but symptoms recurred 4 weeks after stopping therapy in 28% of patients who received caspofungin versus 17% of those who received fluconazole.[198] Another study evaluated patients with clinically fluconazole-resistant esophageal candidiasis and found that 7 (64%) of 11 patients had favorable responses to caspofungin, including patients with isolates showing in vitro fluconazole resistance.[199]

In a multicenter trial of 239 patients with invasive candidiasis, 73.4% of patients who received caspofungin had a favorable response at the end of therapy, compared with 61.7% in the amphotericin B group.[200] There was a comparable outcome for both candidemia and intra-abdominal candidiasis. Mortality was similar in both groups, and the proportion of patients with drug-related AEs was significantly higher in the amphotericin B group. Caspofungin was evaluated against L-amphotericin B in the empirical treatment of patients with persistent fever and neutropenia. Caspofungin was not inferior to L-amphotericin B in 1,095 subjects (including 11 children), with overall success rates of 34% for caspofungin and for L-amphotericin B (95.2% CI for the difference, −5.6% to 6.0%). Among patients with baseline fungal infections, a higher proportion of those treated with caspofungin had a successful outcome (52% vs. 26%, $p = 0.04$). Patients who received caspofungin sustained fewer renal and infusion-related events than those treated with the comparator.[201] Caspofungin also had similar success rates as itraconazole in an open-label, randomized study of antifungal prophylaxis in patients undergoing induction chemotherapy for acute myelogenous leukemia or myelodysplastic syndrome.[202]

Pediatric Clinical Studies

A single-center, retrospective review of 56 children (median age, 8 years; range 1 to 17 years) who received caspofungin as empirical therapy for fever and neutropenia during 2005 to 2006 showed that 79% of caspofungin courses resulted in an overall favorable response; 15% of courses experienced a drug-related AE that was probably or possibly attributable to caspofungin; and 1 of 19 children receiving caspofungin and cyclosporine concurrently developed hepatotoxicity, possibly related to caspofungin.[203] A multicenter, open-label study of caspofungin in 49 children aged 6 months to 17 years with proven aspergillosis ($n = 10$) or candidiasis ($n = 39$) found favorable response in 50% of all aspergillosis cases and 81% of all candidiasis cases; 13 (27%) patients had at least one clinical AE potentially related to therapy.[204] The most common clinical AEs were fever (6%) and rash (4%). Seventeen (35%) participants experienced a laboratory AE, most commonly transaminitis. None of these resulted in discontinuation of therapy.

Additional studies of caspofungin in the pediatric population are necessary to assess its efficacy. In addition, additional

PK studies in neonates are needed prior to the widespread use of this antifungal agent in the nursery.

MICAFUNGIN

Pharmacology

Micafungin (Astellas, Northbrook, IL) is an echinocandin lipopeptide compound[100,205,206] with a half-life of approximately 12 hours and, similar to other echinocandins, is fungistatic in vitro versus *Aspergillus*.[207] A population PK analysis of micafungin administered to adults after stem cell transplantation revealed that a two-compartment model with zero-order input and first-order elimination best described micafungin disposition. Estimated population PK parameters included volume of distribution at the central compartment of 10.4 L (±5.60) and systemic clearance of 1.165 L per hour (±0.38). Weight was a significant predictor of micafungin clearance, suggesting that patients weighing 66.3 kg or more require higher micafungin doses (150 mg daily) to achieve similar exposures as in patients of lower body weight receiving 100 mg daily of micafungin.[208]

There are dose-independent linear plasma PK with the highest drug concentrations detected in the lung, followed by the liver, spleen, and kidney. Micafungin was undetectable in the CSF,[209] but levels were detected in the brain tissue, choroidal layer, meninges, and cerebellum in an experimental rabbit animal model.[179] Time–kill study of micafungin against *Candida* species demonstrated potent fungicidal activity against most isolates, including a concentration-dependent postantifungal effect.[210]

The PK of micafungin has been evaluated in children and young infants. A phase I, dose-escalation study evaluated the PK of micafungin in 77 children (2 to 17 years of age) with fever and neutropenia. Within the dosing range of 0.5 to 4 mg per kg per day, micafungin demonstrated linear PK; clearance, volume of distribution, and half-life remained relatively constant over the dose range and did not change with repeated administration; and an inverse relation between age and clearance was observed. Mean systemic clearance (0.385 ± 0.15 mL per minute per kg for 2 to 8 years vs. 0.285 ± 0.12 mL per minute per kg for 9 to 17 years) was significantly greater and mean half-life (11.6 ± 2.8 hours vs. 13.3 ± 4.3 hours) was significantly shorter in patients aged 2 to 8 years compared with those of 9 to 17 years.[211] A follow-up population PK study using the same data showed that weight was a significant predictor of micafungin clearance in pediatric patients. To achieve micafungin exposures equivalent to adults receiving 100, 150, and 200 mg daily, as evidenced by simulation profiles, children require dosages higher than 3 mg per kg.[212] Another population PK study of micafungin administered to a Japanese population (including children) also showed that weight was the most significant predictor of micafungin clearance in pediatric patients.[213]

A phase I, sequential and single-dose (0.75, 1.5, and 3.0 mg per kg) study of IV micafungin in 18 premature infants (mean gestational age 26.4 ± 2.4 weeks) weighing more than 1,000 g showed that micafungin PK in preterm infants was linear; premature infants displayed a shorter half-life (8 hours) and a more rapid rate of clearance (~39 mL per hour per kg) compared with published data in older children and adults.[214] In this study, an additional four infants weighing less than 1,000 g received 0.75 mg per kg per day of micafungin and demonstrated shorter mean half-life (5.5 hours) and more rapid mean clearance per body weight (79.3 ± 12.5 mL per hour per kg) when compared with the heavier infants.[214] These results suggest that young infants may require higher micafungin doses when compared with older children and adults. Preliminary data in 12 premature infants (mean birth weight and gestational age 851 g and 27 weeks, respectively) suggest that a micafungin dose of 15 mg per kg per day achieves similar exposures [mean *AUC* 437.5 (±99.4) mg per hour per L] to adults receiving 5 mg per kg per day.[215] Micafungin doses of 7 to 10 mg per kg per day administered to 13 premature infants [mean birth weight and gestational age 1,449 (±1,211) g and 27.3 (±4.68) weeks, respectively] provided adequate exposure (median *AUC* of 258.1 to 291.2 mg per hour per L) to achieve levels thought to be needed to treat CNS candidiasis.[216]

Toxicities, Side Effects, and Drug Interactions

The safety profile of micafungin is optimal when compared with other antifungal agents. In clinical trials including those of micafungin used for treatment of localized and invasive candidiasis as well as prophylaxis studies in patients post–stem cell transplantation have demonstrated fewer AEs than L-amphotericin B and fluconazole. Overall, the safety of micafungin was assessed in 3,083 patients and 501 volunteers in 41 clinical studies, who received single or multiple doses of the drug, ranging from 12.5 mg to 150 or more mg per day. The most common AEs experienced by these patients were related to the GI tract (i.e., nausea, diarrhea). Hypersensitivity reactions associated with micafungin have been reported, and 5% of patients receiving the product may develop liver enzyme elevation.[217] Hyperbilirubinemia, renal impairment, and hemolytic anemia related to micafungin use have also been identified in postmarketing surveillance of the drug. The most common AEs in a phase I micafungin study of 77 children (2 to 17 years of age) with fever and neutropenia were diarrhea (19.5%), epistaxis (18.2%), abdominal pain (16.9%), and headache (16.9%).[211] Micafungin has very few drug interactions; however, when administered simultaneously, it increases overall exposure (*AUC*) of sirolimus (21%), nifedipine (18%), and itraconazole (22%).[217]

Clinical Studies

In a study of 20 patients, micafungin was well tolerated with no severe AEs, and a maximum tolerated dose was not reached at 4 mg per kg per day.[218] In an open-label, multicenter study of micafungin monotherapy against invasive fungal infections, overall clinical response was 60% with no safety-related issues.[219] A recent study of micafungin combined with an existing antifungal agent in pediatric and adult bone marrow transplant patients with invasive aspergillosis revealed an overall complete or partial response of 39%, including 40% specifically in allogeneic transplant patients.[220] A study comparing prophylaxis of 882 stem cell transplant patients found that micafungin had greater success for preventing yeast and mold infections (80%) versus fluconazole prophylaxis (73.5%), with a comparable safety profile.[221] An open-label, noncomparative, multinational study in adult and pediatric patients with a variety of diagnoses (i.e., HSCT, hematologic malignancies) conducted from 1998 to 2002 evaluated the use of micafungin monotherapy and combination therapy in 225 patients with invasive aspergillosis.[222] A favorable response at the end of therapy was seen in 36% of patients. Of those treated only with micafungin, favorable responses were seen in 50% of the primary and 41% of the salvage therapy group.[222]

Micafungin has been evaluated in the treatment of immunocompromised patients with candidiasis. A randomized, double-blind, dose–response study of 245 patients with acquired immunodeficiency syndrome/HIV infection and esophageal candidiasis showed that the endoscopic cure rate was dose dependent, with 50 mg [16.3 (±4.2) days duration], 100 mg [13.4 (±4.5) days duration], and 150 mg [14.0 (±3.5) days duration] of micafungin per day at 68.8%, 77.4%, and 89.8%, respectively.[223] The endoscopic cure rate for 100 and 150 mg of micafungin per day (83.5%) was comparable to that for 200 mg of fluconazole [14.0 (±3.3) days duration] per day (86.7%; 95% CI for the difference in endoscopic cure rate, −14.0% to 7.7%). Clinical and severity secondary end points were also comparable between the two products; however, after discontinuation of therapy, nine patients receiving micafungin had a worsening of severity score or had relapsed disease versus none of the patients in the fluconazole group.[223] More recently, micafungin (100 mg per day, n = 202) was evaluated in a phase III, randomized, double-blind study against L-amphotericin B (3 mg per kg per day, n = 190) for candidemia and invasive candidiasis. Treatment success was observed for 89.6% of patients treated with micafungin versus 89.5% of patients treated with L-amphotericin B, meeting noninferiority criteria.[224] There were fewer treatment-related AEs with micafungin than there were with L-amphotericin B.[224] Micafungin at doses of 100 and 150 mg daily was also noninferior to caspofungin in an international, randomized, double-blinded study of adults (n = 595) with candidemia or invasive candidiasis,[225] and in a phase III randomized study, it was found to be superior to fluconazole in the prevention of invasive fungal infections among adults (n = 882) undergoing HSCT.[226]

Pediatric Studies

Of the three drugs within the echinocandin class, micafungin has been the one most extensively studied in children, including several PK studies in neonates. A pediatric substudy (n = 106, ages 0 to 16 years including 14 neonates) was conducted between 2003 and 2005 as part of a double-blind, randomized, multinational trial comparing micafungin (2 mg per kg per day) with L-amphotericin B (3 mg per kg per day) as first-line treatment for invasive candidiasis.[227] Treatment success was defined as clinical and mycologic response at the end of therapy. The median duration of study drug administration was 15 days for micafungin (range, 3 to 42 days) and 14.5 days for L-amphotericin B (range, 2 to 34 days). In a modified intent-to-treat analysis, the rate of overall treatment success was similar for micafungin (72.9%, 35/48) when compared with L-amphotericin B (76.0%, 38/50), with an adjusted difference between treatment groups of −2.4 (95% CI, 20.1 to 15.3) when stratified by neutropenic status. However, when stratified by age group, L-amphotericin B outperformed micafungin in all age groups, except for the neonatal group.[227] This observation could be related to the low micafungin dose used in this trial. In general, micafungin was better tolerated than L-amphotericin B as evidenced by the fewer AEs that led to discontinuation of therapy.[227]

A phase III trial micafungin 10 mg per kg per day versus Amb-D 1 mg per kg per day in infants older than 2 to 120 days with invasive candidiasis was performed at 71 sites.[228] Although it was closed early due to slow recruitment, this study provides the best evidence for the relative efficacy of micafungin for invasive candidiasis in infants. Participants were randomized 2:1, and 30 infants (micafungin = 20, amphotericin = 10) were enrolled in the study. The primary efficacy outcome, fungal-free survival, was achieved by 12 (60%) infants in the micafungin group and 7 (70%) infants in the amphotericin group. There were no differences (90% both groups) in treatment emergent adverse events (TEAEs) or drug-related TEAEs (55% micafungin vs. 50% Amb-D).

ANIDULAFUNGIN

Pharmacology

Anidulafungin (Eraxis; Pfizer Inc., New York, NY) is a semisynthetic terphenyl-substituted antifungal derived from echinocandin B, a lipopeptide fungal product.[229] It has linear PK with the longest half-life of all the echinocandins (~18 hours)[230] and has shown fungistatic or fungicidal activity in different settings.[231] PK analysis in healthy rabbits revealed linear PK with dose-proportional increases in AUC.[232] Neither end-stage renal impairment, dialysis, nor mild-to-moderate hepatic failure changes the PK of anidulafungin in patients.[233]

Anidulafungin fits a three-compartment open PK model, with a terminal elimination half-life of up to 30 hours.[232] Tissue concentrations after multiple dosing were highest in the lung and liver, followed by the spleen and kidney, with measurable concentrations in the brain tissue. The PK showed approximately sixfold lower mean peak concentrations in plasma and twofold lower AUC values compared to values with similar doses of caspofungin and micafungin.

There are few studies evaluating the PK of anidulafungin in pediatric patients.[234] Twenty-five children aged 2 to 17 years with neutropenia were given anidulafungin (1.5 to 3 mg per kg loading dose, 0.75 to 1.5 mg per kg per day maintenance dose), with a mean duration of 8.7 days (range, 1 to 23 days). Exposure to anidulafungin increased in a manner consistent with dose proportionality within all age cohorts. Maximum anidulafungin plasma concentrations occurred immediately after administration, and steady-state plasma concentrations were achieved after administration of the loading dose. At steady state, the mean half-life, systemic clearance, and AUC within a dosing interval were 23.1 (±9.0) and 19.9 (±4.3) hours, 0.0175 (±0.0077) and 0.0159 (±0.0063) L per hour per kg, and 48.6 (±15.7) and 99.5 (±33.5) mg per hour per L for children receiving 0.75 and 1.5 mg per kg per day, respectively.[232] The concentration profiles at those maintenance doses of anidulafungin in pediatric patients aged 2 to 17 years were similar to those of adult patients receiving 50 or 100 mg per day, respectively. A single-center, multi-dose PK study that included 15 neonates and infants less than 2 years of age found that a loading dose of 3 mg per kg followed by 1.5 mg per kg per day achieved concentrations similar to older children enrolled in the previous trial and to adults receiving 100 mg per day.[235]

Toxicities, Side Effects, and Drug Interactions

A phase I study reported anidulafungin to be well tolerated in 29 healthy volunteers, with the highest dose cohort experiencing transient liver function test elevations that exceeded twice the upper limit of normal.[236] In a separate study, 12 subjects with mild or moderate hepatic impairment did not cause clinically significant changes in the PK parameters of anidulafungin.[237] However, in patients with severe hepatic impairment, the plasma concentrations of anidulafungin are decreased, and plasma clearance increased.[238] In vitro testing in human hepatic microsomes showed that anidulafungin did not affect cyclosporine[239] nor tacrolimus,[240] but there was a small (21%) increase in anidulafungin concentration when coadministered with cyclosporine.[241] In a study of 25 neutropenic children receiving anidulafungin as empirical therapy, four patients in the group receiving 0.75 mg per kg per day experienced AEs considered by the investigator to be possibly or probably related to anidulafungin. These events included feeling abnormal, facial erythema and rash, elevation in serum blood urea nitrogen, and fever and hypotension.[234]

Clinical Studies

In a phase II, open-label, dose range study, adult patients (n = 120) with candidemia and/or candidiasis were randomized to receive 50, 75, or 100 mg of IV anidulafungin daily (after a loading dose on day 1) until 2 weeks after clinical cure or improvement (and eradication or presumed eradication of *Candida*). Of the 68 patients available at follow-up, eradication showed a dose-related trend with 74%, 85%, and 89% success at 50, 75, and 100 mg per day of anidulafungin, respectively.[242] In this study, no correlation was found between in vitro *Candida* minimum inhibitory concentration and anidulafungin eradication. Another phase II study showed clinical and endoscopic success in 95% and 92% of patients, respectively, with azole-refractory mucosal candidiasis and sustained clinical success in 47% of patients after discontinuation of anidulafungin (100 mg loading, 50 mg maintenance dose) therapy.[243]

A phase III, randomized, double-blind study in adult patients (n = 245, 97% without neutropenia) with invasive candidiasis (89% with candidemia) showed that anidulafungin was not inferior to fluconazole in the treatment of invasive candidiasis.[244] In this study, the frequency and types of AEs were similar in the two groups, and all-cause mortality was 31% in the fluconazole group and 23% in the anidulafungin group (p = 0.13).[244]

Pediatric Studies

An open-label study of 49 pediatric patients aged 2 to less than 18 years assessed the safety, tolerability, and efficacy of anidulafungin in children with invasive candidiasis.[245] Subjects received 3 mg per kg on day 1, followed by 1.5 mg per kg maintenance dosing for a minimum of 10 days of therapy. Vomiting (24.5%) and diarrhea (22.4%) were the most commonly reported TEAEs. The overall mortality rate was 14% at the end of 6 weeks; none of the deaths were attributable to anidulafungin.

ALLYLAMINES

The allylamine class of antifungals,[246] which includes terbinafine, inhibits the enzyme squalene epoxidase in the fungal biosynthesis of ergosterol and is currently indicated for the treatment of superficial dermatophyte and yeast infections. Since its introduction into clinical practice in 1991, clinicians have used oral terbinafine (Lamisil; Novartis Research Institute, Vienna, Austria) mainly for dermatophyte infections of the skin and nails.[247] There is no available IV formulation. Terbinafine is well tolerated,[248] has a bioavailability after oral administration of 70% to 80%, and is highly lipophilic with a terminal half-life of up to 3 weeks.[249] The metabolism of terbinafine is not dependent on the CYP system, but metabolism takes place extensively in the liver,[14] with subsequent excretion in the urine.[247] Terbinafine is rapidly absorbed following oral administration in humans.[250]

The lipophilic terbinafine concentrates highest in the sebum and hair with quantifiable concentrations 56 to 90 days after a final oral dose and a slow redistribution from the peripheral sites back to the central plasma compartment. Tissue distribution in rats using high-performance liquid chromatography after a 6 mg per kg IV dose revealed a slow uptake and efflux of terbinafine in the skin, with an estimated redistribution half-life from the skin of 1.6 days. Approximately 60% and 28% of the apparent volume of distribution of terbinafine was to the skin and adipose tissue, respectively.[251] Further analysis of terbinafine distribution in human blood shows a higher affinity for plasma proteins than blood cells in a concentration-independent manner.[252] There have been reports of side effects with terbinafine, including hepatitis,[253,254] pancytopenia,[253,255] hair loss,[256] and drug interaction with tricyclic antidepressants.[257,258] PK modeling indicated that at steady state, almost all of the terbinafine (94%) in the human body resides in adipose and skin tissues, with only 0.4% in the lung,[259] which might theoretically lead to difficulty in treating systemic fungal infections with terbinafine.[260]

FUTURE DIRECTIONS

Amphotericin B deoxycholate has historically been the preferred antifungal agent used in children and adults; however, its clinical use was hampered by the nephrotoxicity and infusion-related toxicity. Lipid formulations of amphotericin B improved its side-effects profile, but over the past decade, newer therapies, including second-generation triazoles and the echinocandins, have overtaken amphotericin B in routine pediatric clinical practice. These agents have excellent safety profiles and, in adults, have proven efficacious in phase II and III studies. Of all these agents, micafungin is the best studied in the pediatric population. However, the echinocandins lack activity against the mucormycetes, which are developing pathogens in pediatric cancer patients. The newer triazoles, posaconazole and isavuconazole, are active against mucormycetes, but there are limited data to support safe and effective dosing in children.

The number of antifungal studies conducted in children is limited and is mainly related to phase I-II safety and PK studies. While there have been many phase III antifungal clinical trials in adults, there only been one large phase III antifungal clinical trial dedicated to children. Consequently, most information for the pediatrician has been extrapolated from adults.

REFERENCES

1. Groll AH, Shah PM, Mentzel C, et al. Trends in postmortem epidemiology of invasive fungal infections at a university hospital. *J Infect* 1996;33:23–32.
2. Downes KJ, Ellis D, Lavigne S, et al. The use of echinocandins in hospitalized children in the United States. *Med Mycol* 2018;57:534.
3. Kullberg BJ, de Pauw BE. Therapy of invasive fungal infections. *Neth J Med* 1999;55:118–127.
4. Warnock DW. Amphotericin B: an introduction. *J Antimicrob Chemother* 1991;28:27–38.
5. Gallis HA, Drew RH, Pickard WW. Amphotericin B: 30 years of clinical experience. *Rev Infect Dis* 1990;12:308–329.
6. Latge JP. *Aspergillus fumigatus* and aspergillosis. *Clin Microbiol Rev* 1999;12:310–350.

7. Brajtburg J, Powderly WG, Kobayashi GS, et al. Amphotericin B: current understanding of mechanisms of action. *Antimicrob Agents Chemother* 1990;34:183–188.
8. Meis JF, Verweij PE. Current management of fungal infections. *Drugs* 2001;61:13–25.
9. Manavathu EK, Dimmock JR, Vashishtha SC, et al. In-vitro and in-vivo susceptibility of *Aspergillus fumigatus* to a novel conjugated styryl ketone. *J Antimicrob Chemother* 1998;42:585–590.
10. Gray KC, Palacios DS, Dailey I, et al. Amphotericin primarily kills yeast by simply binding ergosterol. *Proc Natl Acad Sci U S A* 2012;109:2234–2239.
11. Baley JE, Meyers C, Kliegman RM, et al. Pharmacokinetics, outcome of treatment, and toxic effects of amphotericin B and 5-fluorocytosine in neonates. *J Pediatr* 1990;116:791–797.
12. Groll AH, Piscitelli SC, Walsh TJ. Antifungal pharmacodynamics: concentration-effect relationships in vitro and in vivo. *Pharmacotherapy* 2001;21:133S–148S.
13. Christensen KJ, Bernard EM, Gold JW, et al. Distribution and activity of amphotericin B in humans. *J Infect Dis* 1985;152:1037–1043.
14. Denning DW, Stevens DA. Antifungal and surgical treatment of invasive aspergillosis: review of 2,121 published cases. *Rev Infect Dis* 1990;12:1147–1200.
15. Ellis M. Amphotericin B preparations: a maximum tolerated dose in severe invasive fungal infections? *Transpl Infect Dis* 2000;2:51–61.
16. Luna B, Drew RH, Perfect JR. Agents for treatment of invasive fungal infections. *Otolaryngol Clin North Am* 2000;33:277–299.
17. Proffitt RT, Satorius A, Chiang SM, et al. Pharmacology and toxicology of a liposomal formulation of amphotericin B (AmBisome) in rodents. *J Antimicrob Chemother* 1991;28:49–61.
18. Dismukes WE. Introduction to antifungal agents. *Clin Infect Dis* 2000;30:653–657.
19. Hiemenz JW, Walsh TJ. Lipid formulations of amphotericin B: recent progress and future directions. *Clin Infect Dis* 1996;22:S133–S144.
20. Brajtburg J, Bolard J. Carrier effects on biological activity of amphotericin B. *Clin Microbiol Rev* 1996;9:512–531.
21. Ralph ED, Khazindar AM, Barber KR, et al. Comparative in vitro effects of liposomal amphotericin B, amphotericin B-deoxycholate, and free amphotericin B against fungal strains determined by using MIC and minimal lethal concentration susceptibility studies and time–kill curves. *Antimicrob Agents Chemother* 1991;35:188–191.
22. Wong-Beringer A, Jacobs RA, Guglielmo BJ. Lipid formulations of amphotericin B: clinical efficacy and toxicities. *Clin Infect Dis* 1998;27:603–618.
23. Luke RG, Boyle JA. Renal effects of amphotericin B lipid complex. *Am J Kidney Dis* 1998;31:780–785.
24. Walsh TJ, Goodman JL, Pappas P, et al. Safety, tolerance, and pharmacokinetics of high-dose liposomal amphotericin B (AmBisome) in patients infected with *Aspergillus* species and other filamentous fungi: maximum tolerate dose study. *Antimicrob Agents Chemother* 2001;45:3487–3496.
25. Seibel NL, Shad AT, Bekersky I, et al. Safety, tolerability, and pharmacokinetics of liposomal amphotericin B in immunocompromised pediatric patients. *Antimicrob Agents Chemother* 2017;61:e01477-16.
26. Starke JR, Mason EOJ, Kramer WG, et al. Pharmacokinetics of amphotericin B in infants and children. *J Infect Dis* 1987;155:766–774.
27. Nath CE, McLachlan AJ, Shaw PJ, et al. Population pharmacokinetics of amphotericin B in children with malignant diseases. *Br J Clin Pharmacol* 2001;52:671–680.
28. Benson JM, Nahata MC. Pharmacokinetics of amphotericin B in children. *Antimicrob Agents Chemother* 1989;33:1989–1993.
29. Walsh TJ, Whitcomb T, Piscitelli S, et al. Safety, tolerance, and pharmacokinetics of amphotericin B lipid complex in children with hepatosplenic candidiasis. *Antimicrob Agents Chemother* 1997;41:1944–1948.
30. Hong Y, Shaw PJ, Nath CE, et al. Population pharmacokinetics of liposomal amphotericin B in pediatric patients with malignant diseases. *Antimicrob Agents Chemother* 2006;50:935–942.
31. Wurthwein G, Groll AH, Hempel G, et al. Population pharmacokinetics of amphotericin B lipid complex in neonates. *Antimicrob Agents Chemother* 2005;49:5092–5098.
32. de Pauw BE. New antifungal agents and preparations. *Int J Antimicrob Agents* 2000;16:147–150.
33. Patterson DL, Singh N. Interactions between tacrolimus and antimicrobial agents. *Clin Infect Dis* 1997;21:430–435.
34. Finquelievich JL, Odds FC, Queiroz-Telles F, et al. New advances in antifungal treatment. *Med Mycol* 2000;38:317–322.
35. Walsh TJ, Hiemenz JW, Seibel NL, et al. Amphotericin B lipid complex for invasive fungal infections: analysis of safety and efficacy in 556 cases. *Clin Infect Dis* 1998;26:1383–1396.
36. Schmitt HJ. New methods of delivery of amphotericin B. *Clin Infect Dis* 1993;17:S501–S506.
37. Wasan KM, Rosenblum MG, Cheung L, et al. Influence of lipoproteins on renal cytotoxicity and antifungal activity of amphotericin B. *Antimicrob Agents Chemother* 1994;38:223–227.
38. Ringden O, Jonsson V, Hansen M, et al. Severe and common side-effects of amphotericin B lipid complex (Abelcet). *Bone Marrow Transplant* 1998;22:733–734.
39. Graybill JR, Tollemar J, Torres-Rodriguez JM, et al. Antifungal compounds: controversies, queries and conclusions. *Med Mycol* 2000;38:323–333.
40. Patterson TF, Thompson GR, Denning DW, et al. Practice guidelines for the diagnosis and management of *Aspergillus*: 2016 update by the Infectious Diseases Society of America. *Clin Infect Dis* 2016;63:e1–e60.
41. Kontoyiannis DP. A clinical perspective for the management of invasive fungal infections: focus on IDSA guidelines. *Pharmacotherapy* 2001;21:175S–187S.
42. Denning DW. Invasive aspergillosis. *Clin Infect Dis* 1998;26:781–805.
43. Cherry JD, Lloyd CA, Quilty JF, et al. Amphotericin B therapy in children. A review of the literature and a case report. *J Pediatr* 1969;75:1063–1069.
44. Walsh TJ, Seibel NL, Arndt C, et al. Amphotericin B lipid complex in pediatric patients with invasive fungal infections. *Pediatr Infect Dis J* 1998;18:702–708.
45. Herbrecht R, Auvrignon A, Andres E, et al. Efficacy of amphotericin B lipid complex in the treatment of invasive fungal infections in immunocompromised paediatric patients. *Eur J Clin Microbiol Infect Dis* 2001;20:77–82.
46. Sandler ES, Mustafa MM, Tkaczewski I, et al. Use of amphotericin B colloidal dispersion in children. *J Pediatr Hematol Oncol* 2000;22:242–246.
47. Donowitz LG, Hendley JO. Short-course amphotericin B therapy for candidemia in pediatric patients. *Pediatrics* 1995;95:888–891.
48. Roman E, Osunkwo I, Militano O, et al. Liposomal amphotericin B prophylaxis of invasive mold infections in children post allogeneic stem cell transplantation. *Pediatr Blood Cancer* 2008;50:325–330.
49. Wiley JM, Seibel NL, Walsh TJ. Efficacy and safety of amphotericin B lipid complex in 548 children and adolescents with invasive fungal infections. *Pediatr Infect Dis J* 2005;24:167–174.
50. Ascher SB, Smith PB, Watt K, et al. Antifungal therapy and outcomes in infants with invasive *Candida* infections. *Pediatr Infect Dis J* 2012;31:439–443.
51. Duschinsky R, Pleven E, Heidelberger C. The synthesis of 5-fluoropyrimidines. *J Am Chem Soc* 1957;79:4559–4560.
52. Benson JM, Nahata MC. Clinical use of systemic antifungal agents. *Clin Pharm* 1988;7:424–438.
53. Firkin FC. Therapy of deep-seated fungal infections with 5-fluorocytosine. *Aust N Z J Med* 1974;4:462–467.
54. Young RC, Bennett JE, Vogel CL, et al. Aspergillosis: the spectrum of the disease in 98 patients. *Medicine* 1970;49:147–173.
55. Vermes A, Guchelaar HJ, Dankert J. Flucytosine: a review of its pharmacology, clinical indications, pharmacokinetics, toxicity and drug interactions. *J Antimicrob Chemother* 2000;46:171–179.
56. Bennett JE. Flucytosine. *Ann Intern Med* 1977;86:319–321.
57. Beggs WH, Sarosi GA. Further evidence for sequential action of amphotericin B and 5-fluorocytosine against *C. albicans*. *Chemotherapy* 1982;28:341–344.
58. Diasio RB, Lakings DE, Bennett JE. Evidence for conversion of 5-fluorocytosine to 5-fluorouracil in humans: possible factor in 5-fluorocytosine clinical toxicity. *Antimicrob Agents Chemother* 1978;14:903–908.
59. Vermes A, Guchelaar HJ, van Kuilenburg AB, et al. 5-fluorocytosine-related bone-marrow depression and conversion to fluorouracil: a pilot study. *Fundam Clin Pharmacol* 2002;16:39–47.
60. Pasqualotto AC, Howard SJ, Moore CB, et al. Flucytosine therapeutic monitoring: 15 years experience from the UK. *J Antimicrob Chemother* 2007;59:791–793.
61. Stamm AM, Diasio RB, Dismukes WE, et al. Toxicity of amphotericin B plus flucytosine in 194 patients with cryptococcal meningitis. *Am J Med* 1987;83:236–242.
62. Bennett JE, Dismukes WE, Duma RJ, et al. A comparison of amphotericin B alone and combined with flucytosine in the treatment of cryptococcal meningitis. *N Engl J Med* 1979;301:126–128.
63. Dismukes WE, Cloud G, Gallis HA, et al. Treatment of cryptococcal meningitis with combination amphotericin B and flucytosine for four as compared with six weeks. *N Engl J Med* 1987;317:334–341.
64. van der Horst CM, Saag MS, Cloud GA, et al. Treatment of cryptococcal meningitis associated with the acquired immunodeficiency syndrome. National Institute of Allergy and Infectious Diseases Mycoses Study Group and AIDS Clinical Trials Group. *N Engl J Med* 1997;337:15–21.
65. Mayanja-Kizza H, Oishi K, Mitarai S, et al. Combination therapy with fluconazole and flucytosine for cryptococcal meningitis in Ugandan patients with AIDS. *Clin Infect Dis* 1998;26:1362–1366.
66. Larsen RA, Bozzette SA, Jones BE, et al. Fluconazole combined with flucytosine for treatment of cryptococcal meningitis in patients with AIDS. *Clin Infect Dis* 1994;19:741–745.
67. Chotmongkol V, Sukeepaisarncharoen W, Thavornpitak Y. Comparison of amphotericin B, flucytosine and itraconazole with amphotericin B and flucytosine in the treatment of cryptococcal meningitis in AIDS. *J Med Assoc Thai* 1997;80:416–425.
68. Pappas PG, Kauffman CA, Andes DR, et al. Practice guidelines for the management of candidiasis: 2016 update by the Infectious Diseases Society of America. *Clin Infect Dis* 2015;62:e1–e50.
69. Benjamin DK Jr, Stoll BJ, Fanaroff AA, et al. Neonatal candidiasis among extremely low birth weight infants: risk factors, mortality rates, and neurodevelopmental outcomes at 18 to 22 months. *Pediatrics* 2006;117:84–92.
70. Ernst EJ. Investigational antifungal agents. *Pharmacotherapy* 2001; 21:165S–175S.
71. Klepser ME, Wolfe EJ, Jones RN, et al. Antifungal pharmacodynamic characteristics of fluconazole and amphotericin B tested against *Candida albicans*. *Antimicrob Agents Chemother* 1997;41:1392–1395.
72. De Beule K, Van Gestel J. Pharmacology of itraconazole. *Drugs* 2001;61:27–37.
73. Ernst EJ, Klepser ME, Ernst ME, et al. In vitro pharmacodynamic properties of MK-0991 determined by time–kill methods. *Diagn Microbiol Infect Dis* 1999;33:75–80.
74. Brammer KW, Coates PE. Pharmacokinetics of fluconazole in pediatric patients. *Eur J Clin Microbiol Infect Dis* 1994;13:325–329.
75. Wildfeuer A, Laufen H, Schmalreck AF, et al. Fluconazole: comparison of pharmacokinetics, therapy, and in vitro susceptibility. *Mycoses* 1997;40:259–265.
76. Wade KC, Wu D, Kaufman DA, et al. Population pharmacokinetics of fluconazole in young infants. *Antimicrob Agents Chemother* 2008;52:4043–4049.
77. Debruyne D. Clinical pharmacokinetics of fluconazole in superficial and systemic mycoses. *Clin Pharmacokinet* 1997;33:52–77.
78. Piper L, Smith PB, Hornik CP, et al. Fluconazole loading dose pharmacokinetics and safety in infants. *Pediatr Infect Dis J* 2011;30:375–378.
79. Watt KM, Gonzalez D, Benjamik DK, et al. Fluconazole population pharmacokinetics and dosing for prevention and treatment of invasive candidiasis in children supported with extracorporeal membrane oxygenation. *Antimicrob Agents Chemother* 2015;59:3935–3943.
80. Nahata MC, Brady MT. Pharmacokinetics of fluconazole after oral administration in children with human immunodeficiency virus infection. *Eur J Clin Pharmacol* 1995;48:291–293.
81. Buijk SL, Gyssens IC, Mouton JW, et al. Pharmacokinetics of sequential intravenous and enteral fluconazole in critically ill surgical patients with invasive mycoses and compromised gastro-intestinal function. *Intensive Care Med* 2001;27:115–121.
82. Wong S-F, Leung MP, Chan MY. Pharmacokinetics of fluconazole in children requiring peritoneal dialysis. *Clin Ther* 1997;19:1039–1047.

83. Koks CH, Meenhorst PL, Hillebrand MJ, et al. Pharmacokinetics of fluconazole in saliva and plasma after administration of an oral suspension and capsules. *Antimicrob Agents Chemother* 1996;40:1935–1937.
84. Vscoli CE, Castagnola M, Fioredda B, et al. Fluconazole in the treatment of candidiasis in immunocompromised children. *Antimicrob Agents Chemother* 1991;35:365–367.
85. Schwarze R, Penk A, Pittrow L. Administration of fluconazole in children below 1 year of age. *Mycoses* 1999;42:3–16.
86. Novelli V, Holzel H. Safety and tolerability of fluconazole in children. *Antimicrob Agents Chemother* 1999;43:1955–1960.
87. Marr KA, Seidel K, Slavin MA, et al. Prolonged fluconazole prophylaxis is associated with persistent protection against candidiasis-related death in allogeneic marrow transplant recipients: long-term follow-up of a randomized, placebo-controlled trial. *Blood* 2000;96:2055–2061.
88. MacMillan ML, Goodman JL, DeFor TE, et al. Fluconazole to prevent yeast infections in bone marrow transplantation patients: a randomized trial of high versus reduced dose, and determination of the value of maintenance therapy. *Am J Med* 2002;112:369–379.
89. Koh LP, Kurup A, Goh YT, et al. Randomized trial of fluconazole versus low-dose amphotericin B in prophylaxis against fungal infections in patients undergoing hematopoietic stem cell transplantation. *Am J Hematol* 2002;71:260–267.
90. Rex JH, Pappas PG, Karchmer AW, et al. A randomized and blinded multicenter trial of high-dose fluconazole plus placebo vs. fluconazole plus amphotericin B as therapy for candidemia and its consequences in non-neutropenic patients. *Clin Infect Dis.* 2003;36(10):1221–1228.
91. Garbino J, Lew DP, Romand JA, et al. Prevention of severe *Candida* infections in nonneutropenic, high-risk, critically ill patients: a randomized, double-blind, placebo-controlled trial in patients treated by selective digestive decontamination. *Intensive Care Med* 2002;28:1708–1717.
92. Faergemann J, Laufen H. Levels of fluconazole in serum, stratum corneum, epidermis-dermis (without stratum corneum) and eccrine sweat. *Clin Exp Dermatol* 1993;18:102–106.
93. Groll AH, Just-Nuebling G, Kurz M, et al. Fluconazole versus nystatin in the prevention of *Candida* infections in children and adolescents undergoing remission induction or consolidation chemotherapy for cancer. *J Antimicrob Chemother* 1997;40:855–862.
94. Fasano C, O'Keeffe J, Gibbs D. Fluconazole treatment of neonates and infants with severe fungal infections not treatable with conventional agents. *Eur J Clin Microbiol Infect Dis* 1994;13:325–354.
95. Kaufman D, Boyle R, Hazen KC, et al. Fluconazole prophylaxis against fungal colonization and infection in preterm infants. *N Engl J Med* 2001;345:1660–1666.
96. Manzoni P, Stolfi I, Pugni L, et al. A multicenter, randomized trial of prophylactic fluconazole in preterm neonates. *N Engl J Med* 2007;356:2483–2495.
97. Benjamin DK Jr, Hudak ML, Duara S, et al. Effect of fluconazole prophylaxis on candidiasis and mortality in premature infants: a randomized clinical trial. *JAMA* 2014;311:1742–1749.
98. Van Cutsem J, Van Gerven F, Van de Ven MA, et al. Itraconazole, a new triazole that is orally active against *Aspergillus*. *Antimicrob Agents Chemother* 1984;26:527–534.
99. Borgers M, Van de Ven MA, Willemsens G, et al. *Morphologic evaluation of R 51211, a new antimycotic.* Presented at Program and abstracts of the 13th Annual International Congress on Chemotherapy Proceedings part 61, SE 48/2–13, Vienna, Austria, 1983.
100. Walsh TJ, Viviani MA, Arathoon E, et al. New targets and delivery systems for antifungal therapy. *Med Mycol* 2000;38:335–347.
101. Manavathu EK, Cutright JL, Chandrasekar PH. Organism-dependent fungicidal activity of azoles. *Antimicrob Agents Chemother* 1998;42:3018–3021.
102. Heykants J, Van de Valde V, Van Rooy P. The clinical pharmacokinetics of itraconazole: an overview. *Mycoses* 1989;32:67–87.
103. Anonymous. Itraconazole. *Med Lett Drugs Ther* 1993;35:7–9.
104. Barone JA, Moskovitz BL, Guarnieri J, et al. Enhanced bioavailability of itraconazole in hydroxypropyl-beta-cyclodextrin solution versus capsules in healthy volunteers. *Antimicrob Agents Chemother* 1998;42:1862–1865.
105. Stevens DA. Itraconazole in cyclodextrin solution. *Pharmacotherapy* 1999;19:603–611.
106. Slain D, Rogers PD, Cleary JD, et al. Intravenous itraconazole. *Ann Pharmacother* 2001;35:720–729.
107. Caillot D, Bassaris H, McGeer A, et al. Intravenous itraconazole followed by oral itraconazole in the treatment of invasive pulmonary aspergillosis in patients with hematologic malignancies, chronic granulomatous disease, or AIDS. *Clin Infect Dis* 2001;33:e83–e90.
108. Boogaerts M, Maertens J. Clinical experience with itraconazole in systemic fungal infections. *Drugs* 2001;61:39–47.
109. Chiller TM, Stevens DA. Treatment strategies for *Aspergillus* infections. *Drug Resist Updat* 2000;3:89–97.
110. de Repentigny L, Ratelle J, Leclerc JM, et al. Repeated-dose pharmacokinetic of an oral solution of itraconazole in infants and children. *Antimicrob Agents Chemother* 1998;42:404–408.
111. Abdel-Rahman SM, Jacobs RF, Massarella J, et al. Single-dose pharmacokinetics of intravenous itraconazole and hydroxypropyl-beta-cyclodextrin in infants, children, and adolescents. *Antimicrob Agents Chemother* 2007;51:2668–2673.
112. Tucker RM, Haq Y, Denning DW, et al. Adverse events associated with itraconazole in 189 patients on chronic therapy. *J Antimicrob Chemother* 1990;26:561–566.
113. Katz HI. Drug interactions of the newer oral antifungal agents. *Br J Dermatol* 1999;141:26–32.
114. Leather HL, Boyette RM, Tian L, et al. Pharmacokinetic evaluation of the drug interaction between intravenous itraconazole and intravenous tacrolimus or intravenous cyclosporine A in allogeneic bone marrow transplant patients. *Biol Blood Marrow Transplant.* 2006;12:325–334.
115. MacKenzie-Wood AR, Whitfield MJ, Ray JE. Itraconazole and HIV protease inhibitors: an important interaction. *Med J Aust* 1999;170:46–47.
116. Patterson TF, Kirkpatrick WR, White M, et al. Invasive aspergillosis: disease spectrum, treatment practices, and outcomes. *Medicine* 2000;79:250–260.
117. Morgenstern GR, Prentice AG, Prentice HG, et al. A randomized controlled trial of itraconazole versus fluconazole for the prevention of fungal infections in patients with haematological malignancies. *Br J Haematol* 1999;105:901–911.
118. Winston DJ, Busuttil RW. Randomized controlled trial of oral itraconazole solution versus intravenous/oral fluconazole for prevention of fungal infections in liver transplant recipients. *Transplantation* 2002;74:688–694.
119. Chariyalertsak S, Supparatpinyo K, Sirisanthana T, et al. A controlled trial of itraconazole as primary prophylaxis for systemic fungal infections in patients with advanced human immunodeficiency virus infection in Thailand. *Clin Infect Dis* 2002;34:277–284.
120. Groll AH, Wood L, Roden M, et al. Safety, pharmacokinetics, and pharmacodynamics of cyclodextrin itraconazole in pediatric patients with oropharyngeal candidiasis. *Antimicrob Agents Chemother* 2002;46:2554–2563.
121. Grigull L, Kuehlke O, Beilken A, et al. Intravenous and oral sequential itraconazole antifungal prophylaxis in paediatric stem cell transplantation recipients: a pilot study for evaluation of safety and efficacy. *Pediatr Transplant* 2007;11:261–266.
122. Wheat LJ, Freifield AG, Kleiman MB, et al. Clinical practice guidelines for the management of patients with histoplasmosis: 2007 update by the Infectious Diseases Society of America. *Clin Infect Dis* 2007;45:807–825.
123. Sabo JA, Abdel-Rahman SM. Voriconazole: a new triazole antifungal. *Ann Pharmacother* 2000;34:1032–1043.
124. Manavathu EK, Cutright JL, Chandrasekar PH. In vitro susceptibility of itraconazole-resistant isolates of *Aspergillus fumigatus* to voriconazole. *Clin Microbiol Infect* 1997;3:81.
125. Johnson EM, Szekely A, Warnock DW. In-vitro activity of voriconazole, itraconazole and amphotericin B against filamentous fungi. *J Antimicrob Chemother* 1998;42:741–745.
126. Goldstein JA, deMorais SMF. Biochemistry and molecular biology of the human CYP2 C subfamily. *Pharmacogenetics* 1994;4:285–299.
127. Purkins L, Wood N, Ghahramani P, et al. Pharmacokinetics and safety of voriconazole following intravenous- to oral-dose escalation regimens. *Antimicrob Agents Chemother* 2002;46:2546–2553.
128. Johnson LB, Kauffman CA. Voriconazole: a new triazole antifungal agent. *Clin Infect Dis* 2003;36:630–637.
129. Yanni SB, Annaert PP, Augustijns P, et al. Role of flavin-containing monooxygenase in oxidative metabolism of voriconazole by human liver microsomes. *Drug Metab Dispos* 2008;36:1119–1125.
130. Ghannoum MA, Kuhn DM. Voriconazole—better chances for patients with invasive mycoses. *Eur J Med Res* 2002;7:242–256.
131. Denning DW, Ribaud P, Milpied N, et al. Efficacy and safety of voriconazole in the treatment of acute invasive aspergillosis. *Clin Infect Dis* 2002;34:563–571.
132. Sheehan DJ, Hitchcock CA, Sibley CM. Current and emerging azole antifungal agents. *Clin Microbiol Rev* 1999;12:40–79.
133. Clancy C, Nguyen N. In vitro efficacy and fungicidal activity of voriconazole against *Aspergillus* and *Fusarium* species. *Eur J Clin Microbiol Infect Dis* 1998;17:573–575.
134. Chiou CC, Groll AH, Walsh TJ. New drugs and novel targets for treatment of invasive fungal infections in patients with cancer. *Oncologist* 2000;5:120–135.
135. Lazarus HM, Blumer JL, Yanovich S, et al. Pharmacokinetics and safety of oral voriconazole in patients at risk of fungal infections: a dose escalation study. *J Clin Pharmacol.* 2002;42:395-402.
136. Klepser ME, Malone D, Lewis RE, et al. Evaluation of voriconazole pharmacodynamics using time-kill methodology. *Antimicrob Agents Chemother* 2000;44:1917–1920.
137. Tan KKC, Wood N, Weil A. Multiple-dose pharmacokinetics of voriconazole in chronic hepatic impairment. In: *Program and Abstracts of the 41st Interscience Conference on Antimicrobial Agents and Chemotherapy, Chicago, IL, December 16–19, 2001.* Washington, DC: American Society for Microbiology, 2001.
138. Walsh TJ, Karlsson MO, Driscoll T, et al. Pharmacokinetics and safety of intravenous voriconazole in children after single- or multiple-dose administration. *Antimicrob Agents Chemother* 2004;48:2166–2172.
139. Driscoll TA, Frangoul H, Nemecek ER, et al. Comparison of pharmacokinetics and safety of voriconazole intravenous-to-oral switch in immunocompromised adolescents and healthy adults. *Antimicrob Agents Chemother* 2011;55:6780–6789.
140. Friberg LE, Ravva P, Karlsson MO, Liu P. Integrated population pharmacokinetic analysis of voriconazole in children, adolescents, and adults. *Antimicrob Agents Chemother* 2012;56:3032–3042.
141. Lazarus HM, Blummer JL, Yanovich S, et al. Safety and pharmacokinetics of oral voriconazole in patients at risk of fungal infection: a dose escalation study. *J Clin Pharmacol* 2002;42:395–402.
142. Tan KKC, Brayshaw N, Oakes M. Investigation of the relationship between plasma voriconazole concentrations and liver function test abnormalities in therapeutic trials. In: *Program and Abstracts of the 41st Annual Interscience Conference on Antimicrobial Agents and Chemotherapy, Chicago, IL, December 16–19, 2001.* Washington, DC: American Society for Microbiology, 2001.
143. Stone J, Holland S, Wickersham P, et al. Drug interactions between caspofungin and tacrolimus. In: *Program and abstracts of the 41st Interscience Conference on Antimicrobial Agents and Chemotherapy, Chicago, IL, 2001.* Washington, DC: American Society for Microbiology, 2001.
144. Denning DW, Griffiths CE. Muco-cutaneous retinoid-effects and facial erythema related to the novel triazole antifungal agent voriconazole. *Clin Dermatol* 2001;26:648–653.
145. Venkataramanan R, Zang S, Gayowski T, et al. Voriconazole inhibition of the metabolism of tacrolimus in a liver transplant recipient and in human liver microsomes. *Antimicrob Agents Chemother* 2002;46:3091–3093.
146. Wood N, Tan K, Allan R, et al. Effect of voriconazole on pharmacokinetics of tacrolimus. In: *Program and Abstracts of the 41st Interscience Conference on Antimicrobial Agents and Chemotherapy, Chicago, IL, 2001.* Washington, DC: American Society for Microbiology, 2001.
147. Romero A, Le Pogamp P, Nilsson LG, et al. Effect of voriconazole on the pharmacokinetics of cyclosporine in renal transplant patients. *Clin Pharmacol Ther* 2002;71:226–234.
148. Wood N, Abel S, Fielding A, et al. Voriconazole does not affect the pharmacokinetics of mycophenolic acid. In: *Program and Abstracts of the 41st Interscience Conference on*

Antimicrobial Agents and Chemotherapy, Chicago, IL, 2001. Washington, DC: American Society for Microbiology, 2001.
149. Herbrecht R, Denning DW, Patterson TF, et al. Voriconazole versus amphotericin B for primary therapy of invasive aspergillosis. *N Engl J Med* 2002;347:408–415.
150. Ally R, Schurmann D, Kreisel W, et al. A randomized, double-blind, double-dummy, multicenter trial of voriconazole and fluconazole in the treatment of esophageal candidiasis in immunocompromised patients. *Clin Infect Dis* 2001;33:1447–1454.
151. Walsh TJ, Lutsar I, Driscoll T, et al. Voriconazole in the treatment of aspergillosis, scedosporiosis and other invasive fungal infections in children. *Pediatr Infect Dis J* 2002;21:240–248.
152. Doby EH, Benjamin DK Jr, Blaschke AJ, et al. Therapeutic monitoring of voriconazole in children less than three years of age: a case report and summary of voriconazole concentrations for ten children. *Pediatr Infect Dis J* 2012;31:632–635.
153. Courtney R, Pai S, Laughlin M, et al. Pharmacokinetics, safety, and tolerability of oral posaconazole administered in single and multiple doses in healthy adults. *Antimicrob Agents Chemother* 2003;47:2788–2795.
154. Courtney R, Wexler D, Radwanski E, et al. Effect of food on the relative bioavailability of two oral formulations of posaconazole in healthy adults. *Br J Clin Pharmacol* 2004;57:218–222.
155. Krishna G, Moton A, Ma L, et al. The pharmacokinetics and absorption of posaconazole oral suspension under various gastric conditions in healthy volunteers. *Antimicrob Agents Chemother* 2009;53(3):958–966.
156. Courtney R, Sansone A, Smith W, et al. Posaconazole pharmacokinetics, safety, and tolerability in subjects with varying degrees of chronic renal disease. *J Clin Pharmacol* 2005;45:185–192.
157. Atkinson AJ Jr, Bennett JE. Amphotericin B pharmacokinetics in humans. *Antimicrob Agents Chemother* 1978;13:271–276.
158. Maertens J, Cornely O, Ullmann AJ, et al. Phase 1B study of the pharmacokinetics and safety or posaconazole intravenous solution in patients at risk for invasive fungal disease. *Antimicrob Agents Chemother* 2014;58:3610–3617.
159. Schiller DS, Fung HB. Posaconazole: an extended-spectrum triazole antifungal agent. *Clin Ther* 2007;29:1862–1886.
160. Food and Drug Administration. Current Noxafil label. 2019. https://www.accessdata.fda.gov/drugsatfda_docs/label/2019/022003s024,205053s008,205596s007lbl.pdf.
161. Cornely OA, Maertens J, Winston DJ, et al. Posaconazole vs. fluconazole or itraconazole prophylaxis in patients with neutropenia. *N Engl J Med* 2007;356:348–359.
162. Ullmann AJ, Lipton JH, Vesole DH, et al. Posaconazole or fluconazole for prophylaxis in severe graft-versus-host disease. *N Engl J Med* 2007;356:335–347.
163. Restrepo A, Tobon A, Clark B, et al. Salvage treatment of histoplasmosis with posaconazole. *J Infect* 2007;54:319–327.
164. Segal BH, Barnhart LA, Anderson VL, et al. Posaconazole as salvage therapy in patients with chronic granulomatous disease and invasive filamentous fungal infection. *Clin Infect Dis* 2005;40:1684–1688.
165. Greenberg RN, Mullane K, van Burik JA, et al. Posaconazole as salvage therapy for zygomycosis. *Antimicrob Agents Chemother* 2006;50:126–133.
166. Arrieta AC, Sung L, Bradley JS, et al. A non-randomized trial to assess the safety, tolerability, and pharmacokinetics of posaconazole oral suspension in immunocompromised children with neutropenia. *PLoS One* 2019;14;e0212837.
167. Walsh TJ, Raad I, Patterson TF, et al. Treatment of invasive aspergillosis with posaconazole in patients who are refractory or intolerant of conventional therapy: an externally controlled trial. *Clin Infect Dis* 2007;44:2–12.
168. Boonsathorn S, Cheng I, Kloprogge F, et al. Clinical pharmacokinetics and dose recommendations for posaconazole in infants and children. *Clin Pharmacokinet* 2019;58:53–61.
169. Food and Drug Administration. Current Isavuconazole label. 2019. https://www.accessdata.fda.gov/drugsatfda_docs/label/2019/207500s005,207501s004lbl.pdf.
170. Maertens JA, Raad II, Marr, KA, et al. Isavuconazole versus voriconazole for primary treatment of invasive mould disease caused by *Aspergillus* and other filamentous fungi (SECURE): a phase 3, randomized-controlled, non-inferiority trial. *Lancet* 2016;387:760–769.
171. Marty FM, Ostrosky-Zeichner L, Corenly OA, et al. Isavuconazole treatment for mucormycosis: a single-arm open-label trial and case-control analysis. *Lancet Infect Dis* 2016;16:828–837.
172. Kullberg BJ, Viscoli C, Pappas PG, et al. Isavuconazole versus caspofungin in the treatment of candidemia and other invasive Candida infections: the ACTIVE trial. *Clin Infect Dis* 2019;68:1981–1989.
173. Graybill JR. The echinocandins, first novel class of antifungals in two decades: will they live up to their promise? *Int J Clin Pract* 2001;55:633–638.
174. Kurtz MB, Douglas CM. Lipopeptide inhibitors of fungal glucan synthase. *J Med Vet Mycol* 1997;35:79–86.
175. Bartizal K, Gill CJ, Abruzzo GK, et al. In vitro preclinical evaluation studies with the echinocandin antifungal MK-0991 (L-743,872). *Antimicrob Agents Chemother* 1997;41:2326–2332.
176. Ernst EJ, Klepser ME, Pfaller MA. Postantifungal effects of echinocandin, azole, and polyene antifungal agents against *Candida albicans* and *Cryptococcus neoformans*. *Antimicrob Agents Chemother* 2000;44:1108–1111.
177. Benz F, Knuessel F, Nuesch J, et al. Echinocandin B, ein neuartiges polypeptid antibioticum aus *Aspergillus nidulans* var echinulatus: isolierung and baudsteine. *Helv Chim Acta* 1974;57:2459–2477.
178. Arathoon E. Clinical efficacy of echinocandin antifungals. *Curr Opin Infect Dis* 2001;14:685–691.
179. Hope WW, Mickiene D, Petraitis V, et al. The pharmacokinetics and pharmacodynamics of micafungin in experimental hematogenous Candida meningoencephalitis: implications for echinocandin therapy in neonates. *J Infect Dis* 2008;197:163–171.
180. Chiller T, Farrokhshad K, Brummer E, et al. Influence of human sera on the *in vitro* activity of the echinocandin caspofungin (MK-0991) against *Aspergillus fumigatus*. *Antimicrob Agents Chemother* 2000;44(12):3302–3305.
181. Groll AH, Gullick BM, Petraitiene R, et al. Compartmental pharmacokinetics of the antifungal echinocandin caspofungin (MK-0991) in rabbits. *Antimicrob Agents Chemother* 2001;45:596–600.
182. Stone JA, Holland SD, Wickersham PJ, et al. Single- and multiple-dose pharmacokinetics of caspofungin in healthy men. *Antimicrob Agents Chemother* 2002;46:739–745.
183. Stone EA, Fung HB, Kirschenbaum HL. Caspofungin: an echinocandin antifungal agent. *Clin Ther* 2002;24:351–377.
184. Hajdu R, Thompson R, Sundelof JG, et al. Preliminary animal pharmacokinetics of the parenteral antifungal agent MK-0991 (L-743,872). *Antimicrob Agents Chemother* 1997;41:2339–2344.
185. Abruzzo GK, Flattery AM, Gill CJ, et al. Evaluation of the echinocandin antifungal MK-0991 (L-743,872): efficacies in mouse models of disseminated aspergillosis, candidiasis, and cryptococcosis. *Antimicrob Agents Chemother* 1997;41:2333–2338.
186. Hoang A. Caspofungin acetate: an antifungal agent. *Am J Health Syst Pharm* 2001;58:1206–1214.
187. Stone J, Holland S, Li S, et al. Effect of hepatic insufficiency on the pharmacokinetics of caspofungin. In: *Program and Abstracts of the 41st Interscience Conference on Antimicrobial Agents and Chemotherapy, Chicago, IL, December 16–19, 2001.* Washington, DC: American Society for Microbiology, 2001.
188. Sable CA, Nguyen BY, Chodakewitz JA, et al. Safety and tolerability of caspofungin acetate in the treatment of fungal infections. *Transpl Infect Dis* 2002;4:25–30.
189. Migoya EM, Mistry GC, Stone J, et al. Safety and pharmacokinetics of higher doses of caspofungin in healthy adult patients. *J Clin Pharmacol.* 2011;51:202–211.
190. Walsh TJ, Adamson PC, Seibel NL, et al. Pharmacokinetics, safety, and tolerability of caspofungin in children and adolescents. *Antimicrob Agents Chemother* 2005;49:4536–4545.
191. Neely M, Jafri HS, Seibel N, et al. Pharmacokinetics and safety of caspofungin in older infants and toddlers. *Antimicrob Agents Chemother* 2009;53:1450–1456.
192. Saez-Llorens X, Macias M, Maiya P, et al. Pharmacokinetics and safety of caspofungin in neonates and infants less than 3 months of age. *Antimicrob Agents Chemother* 2009;53:869–875.
193. Keating GM, Jarvis B. Caspofungin. *Drugs* 2001;61:1121–1129.
194. Maertens J, Raad I, Petrikkos G, et al. Efficacy and safety of caspofungin for treatment of invasive aspergillosis in patients refractory to or intolerant of conventional antifungal therapy. *Clin Infect Dis.* 2004;39(11):1563–1571.
195. Sanz-Rodriguez C, Aguado JM, Cisneros JM, et al. Caspofungin therapy in documented fungal infections: Spanish experience before licensure of the drug. In: *Program and Abstracts of the 42nd Interscience Conference on Antimicrobial Agents and Chemotherapy, San Diego, CA, September 27–30, 2002.* Washington, DC: American Society for Microbiology, 2002.
196. Villaneuva A, Arathoon EG, Gotuzzo E, et al. A randomized double-blind study of caspofungin versus amphotericin for the treatment of candidal esophagitis. *Clin Infect Dis* 2001;33:1529–1535.
197. Arathoon E, Gotuzzo E, Noriega LM, et al. Randomized, double-blind multicenter study of caspofungin versus amphotericin B for treatment of oropharyngeal and esophageal candidiasis. *Antimicrob Agents Chemother* 2002;46:451–457.
198. Villaneuva A, Gotuzzo E, Arathoon E, et al. A randomized double-blind study of caspofungin versus fluconazole for the treatment of esophageal candidiasis. *Am J Med* 2002;113:294–299.
199. Kartsonis N, DiNubile MJ, Bartizal K, et al. Efficacy of caspofungin in the treatment of esophageal candidiasis resistant to fluconazole. *J Acquir Immune Defic Syndr* 2002;31:183–187.
200. Mora-Duarte J, Betts R, Rotstein C, et al. Comparison of caspofungin and amphotericin B for invasive candidiasis. *N Engl J Med* 2002;347:2020–2029.
201. Walsh TJ, Teppler H, Donowitz GR, et al. Caspofungin versus liposomal amphotericin B for empirical antifungal therapy in patients with persistent fever and neutropenia. *N Engl J Med* 2004;351:1391–1402.
202. Mattiuzzi GN, Alvarado G, Giles FJ, et al. Open-label, randomized comparison of itraconazole versus caspofungin for prophylaxis in patients with hematologic malignancies. *Antimicrob Agents Chemother* 2006;50:143–147.
203. Koo A, Sung L, Allen U, et al. Efficacy and safety of caspofungin for the empiric management of fever in neutropenic children. *Pediatr Infect Dis J* 2007;26:854–856.
204. Zaoutis T, Lehrnbecher T, Groll AH, et al. Safety experience with caspofungin in pediatric patients. *Pediatr Infect Dis J* 2009;28:1132–1135.
205. Mikamo H, Sato Y, Tamaya T. In vitro antifungal activity of FK463, a new water-soluble echinocandin-like lipopeptide. *J Antimicrob Chemother* 2000;46:485–487.
206. Hatano K, Morishita Y, Nakai T, et al. Antifungal mechanism of FK463 against *Candida albicans* and *Aspergillus fumigatus*. *J Antibiot (Tokyo)* 2002;55:219–222.
207. Tawara S, Ikeda F, Maki K, et al. In vitro activities of a new lipopeptide antifungal agent, FK463, against a variety of clinically important fungi. *Antimicrob Agents Chemother* 2000;44:57–62.
208. Gumbo T, Hiemenz J, Ma L, et al. Population pharmacokinetics of micafungin in adult patients. *Diagn Microbiol Infect Dis* 2008;60:329–331.
209. Okugawa S, Ota Y, Tatsuno K, et al. A case of invasive central nervous system aspergillosis treated with micafungin with monitoring of micafungin concentrations in the cerebrospinal fluid. *Scand J Infect Dis* 2007;39:344–346.
210. Ernst EJ, Roling EE, Petzold CR, et al. In vitro activity of micafungin (FK-463) against *Candida* spp.: microdilution, time–kill, and postantifungal-effect studies. *Antimicrob Agents Chemother* 2002;46:3846–3853.
211. Seibel NL, Schwartz C, Arrieta A, et al. Safety, tolerability, and pharmacokinetics of micafungin (FK463) in febrile neutropenic pediatric patients. *Antimicrob Agents Chemother* 2005;49:3317–3324.
212. Hope WW, Seibel NL, Schwartz CL, et al. Population pharmacokinetics of micafungin in pediatric patients and implications for antifungal dosing. *Antimicrob Agents Chemother* 2007;51:3714–3719.
213. Tabata K, Katashima M, Kawamura A, et al. Linear pharmacokinetics of micafungin and its active metabolites in Japanese pediatric patients with fungal infections. *Biol Pharm Bull* 2006;29:1706–1711.

214. Heresi GP, Gerstmann DR, Reed MD, et al. The pharmacokinetics and safety of micafungin, a novel echinocandin, in premature infants. *Pediatr Infect Dis J* 2006;25:1110–1115.
215. Smith P, Walsh T, Hope W, et al. Pharmacokinetics of an elevated dosage of micafungin in premature neonates. *Pediatr Infect Dis J.* 2009;28:412–415.
216. Benjamin DK Jr, Smith P, Arrieta A, et al. Safety and pharmacokinetics of repeat-dose micafungin in neonates. *Clin Pharmacol Ther.* 2010;87:93–99.
217. Food and Drug Administration. Current micafungin label. 2019. https://www.accessdata.fda.gov/drugsatfda_docs/label/2019/021506s023lbl.pdf.
218. Powles R, Sirohi B, Chopra R, et al. A study to determine the safety profile and maximum tolerated dose of micafungin (FK463) in patients undergoing haematopoietic stem cell transplantation. *Bone Marrow Transplant.* 2006;38:47–51.
219. Kohno S, Masaoka T, Yamaguchi H, et al. A multicenter, open-label clinical study of micafungin (FK463) in the treatment of deep mycosis in Japan. *Scand J Infect Dis* 2004;36:372–379.
220. Ratanatharathorn V, Flynn P, Van Burik JA, et al. Micafungin in combination with systemic antifungal agents in the treatment of refractory aspergillosis in bone marrow transplant patients. In: *Program and Abstracts of the American Society of Hematology 44th Annual Meeting, Philadelphia, PA, December 6–10, 2002.* Washington, DC: American Society of Hematology, 2002.
221. Van Burik J, Ratanatharathorn V, Stepan DE, et al. Randomized, double-blind trial of micafungin versus fluconazole for prophylaxis of invasive fungal infections in patients undergoing hematopoietic stem cell transplant. *Clin Infect Dis.* 2004;39:1407–1416.
222. Denning DW, Marr KA, Lau WM, et al. Micafungin (FK463), alone or in combination with other systemic antifungal agents, for the treatment of acute invasive aspergillosis. *J Infect* 2006;53:337–349.
223. de Wet N, Llanos-Cuentas A, Suleiman J, et al. A randomized, double-blind, parallel-group, dose-response study of micafungin compared with fluconazole for the treatment of esophageal candidiasis in HIV-positive patients. *Clin Infect Dis* 2004;39:842–849.
224. Kuse ER, Chetchotisakd P, da Cunha CA, et al. Micafungin versus liposomal amphotericin B for candidaemia and invasive candidosis: a phase III randomised double-blind trial. *Lancet* 2007;369:1519–1527.
225. Pappas PG, Rotstein CM, Betts RF, et al. Micafungin versus caspofungin for treatment of candidemia and other forms of invasive candidiasis. *Clin Infect Dis* 2007;45:883–893.
226. van Burik JA, Ratanatharathorn V, Stepan DE, et al. Micafungin versus fluconazole for prophylaxis against invasive fungal infections during neutropenia in patients undergoing hematopoietic stem cell transplantation. *Clin Infect Dis* 2004;39:1407–1416.
227. Queiroz-Telles F, Berezin E, Leverger G, et al. Micafungin versus liposomal amphotericin B for pediatric patients with invasive candidiasis: substudy of a randomized double-blind trial. *Pediatr Infect Dis J* 2008;27:820–826.
228. Benjamin DK Jr, Kaufman DA, Hope WW, et al. A phase 3 study of micafungin versus amphotericin B deoxycholate in infants with invasive candidiasis. *Pediatr Infect Dis J* 2018;37:992–998.
229. Zhanel GG, Karlowsky JA, Harding GA, et al. *In vitro* activity of a new semisynthetic echinocandin, LY-303366, against systemic isolates of *Candida* species, *Cryptococcus neoformans, Blastomyces dermatitidis,* and *Aspergillus* species. *Antimicrob Agents Chemother* 1997;41: 863–865.
230. Lucas R, De Sante K, Hatcher B, et al. LY303366 single dose pharmacokinetics and safety in healthy volunteers. In: *Program and Abstracts of the 36th Annual Interscience Conference on Antimicrobial Agents and Chemotherapy, New Orleans, LA, 1996.* Washington, DC: American Society for Microbiology, 1996.
231. Petraitis V, Petraitiene R, Groll AH, et al. Antifungal efficacy, safety, and single-dose pharmacokinetics of LY303366, a novel echinocandin B, in experimental pulmonary aspergillosis in persistently neutropenic rabbits. *Antimicrob Agents Chemother* 1998;42:2898–2905.
232. Groll AH, Mickiene D, Petraitiene R, et al. Pharmacokinetic and pharmacodynamic modeling of anidulafungin (LY303366): reappraisal of its efficacy in neutropenic animal models of opportunistic mycoses using optimal plasma sampling. *Antimicrob Agents Chemother* 2001;45:2845–2855.
233. Dowell JA, Stogniew M, Krause D, et al. Anidulafungin does not require dosage adjustment in subjects with varying degrees of hepatic or renal impairment. *J Clin Pharmacol* 2007;47:461–470.
234. Benjamin DKJ, Driscoll T, Seibel NL, et al. Safety and pharmacokinetics of intravenous anidulafungin in children with neutropenia at high risk for invasive fungal infections. *Antimicrob Agents Chemother* 2006;50:632–638.
235. Cohen-Wolkowiez M, Benjamin DK Jr, Piper L. Safety and pharmacokinetics of multiple-dose anidulafungin in infants and neonates. *Clin Pharmacol Ther* 2011;89:702–707.
236. Thye D, Shepherd B, White RJ, et al. Anidulafungin: a phase 1 study to identify the maximum tolerated dose in healthy volunteers. In: *Program and Abstracts of the 41st Interscience Conference on Antimicrobial Agents and Chemotherapy, Chicago, IL, December 16–19, 2001.* Washington, DC: American Society for Microbiology, 2001.
237. Thye D, Kilfoil T, White RJ, et al. Anidulafungin: pharmacokinetics in subjects with mild and moderate hepatic impairment. In: *Program and Abstracts of the 41st Interscience Conference on Antimicrobial Agents and Chemotherapy, Chicago, IL, December 16–19, 2001.* Washington, DC: American Society for Microbiology, 2001.
238. Thye D, Kilfoil T, Kilfoil G, et al. Anidulafungin: pharmacokinetics in subjects with severe hepatic impairment. In: *Program and Abstracts of the 42nd Annual Interscience Conference on Antimicrobial Agents and Chemotherapy, San Diego, CA, 2002.* Washington, DC: American Society for Microbiology, 2002.
239. White RJ, Thye D. Anidulafungin does not affect the metabolism of cyclosporine by human hepatic microsomes. In: *Program and Abstracts of the 41st Interscience Conference on Antimicrobial Agents and Chemotherapy, Chicago, IL, 2001.* Washington, DC: American Society for Microbiology, 2001.
240. Dowell JA, Stogniew M, Krause D, et al. Lack of pharmacokinetic interaction between anidulafungin and tacrolimus. *J Clin Pharmacol* 2007;47:305–314.
241. Thye D, Kilfoil T, Kilfoil G, et al. Anidulafungin: safety and pharmacokinetics in subjects receiving concomitant cyclosporine. In: *Program and abstracts of the 42nd Annual Interscience Conference on Antimicrobial Agents and Chemotherapy, San Diego, CA, 2002.* Washington, DC: American Society for Microbiology, 2002.
242. Pfaller MA, Diekema DJ, Boyken L, et al. Effectiveness of anidulafungin in eradicating Candida species in invasive candidiasis. *Antimicrob Agents Chemother* 2005;49:4795–4797.
243. Vazquez JA, Schranz JA, Clark K, et al. A phase 2, open-label study of the safety and efficacy of intravenous anidulafungin as a treatment for azole-refractory mucosal candidiasis. *J Acquir Immune Defic Syndr* 2008;48:304–309.
244. Reboli AC, Rotstein C, Pappas PG, et al. Anidulafungin versus fluconazole for invasive candidiasis. *N Engl J Med* 2007;356:2472–2482.
245. Roilides E, Carlesse F, Leister-Tebbe H, et al. A prospective open-label study to assess the safety, tolerability and efficacy of anidulafungin in the treatment of invasive candidiasis in children 2 to <18 years of age. *Pediatr Infect Dis J* 2019;38:275–279.
246. Petranyi G, Ryder NS, Stutz A. Allylamine derivatives: new class of synthetic antifungal agents inhibiting fungal squalene epoxidase. *Science* 1984;224:1239–1241.
247. Perez A. Terbinafine: broad new spectrum of indications in several subcutaneous and systemic and parasitic diseases. *Mycoses* 1999;42:111–114.
248. Harrari S. Current strategies in the treatment of invasive *Aspergillus* infections in immunocompromised patients. *Drugs* 1999;58:621–631.
249. Balfour JA, Faulds D. Terbinafine, a review of its pharmacodynamic and pharmacokinetic properties, and therapeutic potential in superficial mycoses. *Drugs* 1992;43:259–284.
250. Kovarik JM, Kirkessell S, Humbert H, et al. Dose-proportional pharmacokinetics of terbinafine and its N-demethylated metabolite in healthy volunteers. *Br J Dermatol* 1992;126:8–13.
251. Hosseini-Yeganeh M, McLachlan AJ. Tissue distribution of terbinafine in rats. *J Pharm Sci* 2001;90:1817–1828.
252. Hosseini-Yeganeh M, McLachlan AJ. In-vitro distribution of terbinafine in rat and human blood. *J Pharm Pharmacol* 2002;54:277–281.
253. Conjeevaram G, Vongthavaravat V, Sumner R, et al. Terbinafine-induced hepatitis and pancytopenia. *Dig Dis Sci* 2001;46:1714–1716.
254. Anania FA, Rabin L. Terbinafine hepatotoxicity resulting in chronic biliary ductopenia and portal fibrosis. *Am J Med* 2002;112:741–742.
255. Aguilar C, Mueller KK. Reversible agranulocytosis associated with oral terbinafine in a pediatric patient. *J Am Acad Dermatol* 2001;45:632–634.
256. Richert B, Uhoda I, De la Brassinne M. Hair loss after terbinafine treatment. *Br J Dermatol* 2001;145:842.
257. Teitelbaum ML, Pearson VE. Imipramine toxicity and terbinafine. *Am J Psychiatry 2001*;158:2086.
258. O'Reardon JP, Hetznecker JM, Rynn MA, et al. Desipramine toxicity with terbinafine. *Am J Psychiatry* 2002;159:492.
259. Hosseini-Yeganeh M, McLachlan AJ. Physiologically based pharmacokinetic model for terbinafine in rats and humans. *Antimicrob Agents Chemother* 2002;46:2219–2228.
260. Kovarik JM, Mueller EA, Zehender H, et al. Multiple-dose pharmacokinetics and distribution in tissue of terbinafine and metabolites. *Antimicrob Agents Chemother* 1995;39:2738–2741.

CHAPTER

31

Claudette L. Poole
David W. Kimberlin
Richard J. Whitley

Antivirals in Newborns and Children

INTRODUCTION

There are several viral infections for which safe and effective antiviral drugs exist. These include influenza, several human herpes viruses, hepatitis B and C, and, to a lesser extent, respiratory syncytial virus (RSV). Through the work of the Collaborative Antiviral Study Group, evidence-based recommendations have been developed for the treatment of neonatal herpes simplex virus (HSV)[1,2] and congenital cytomegalovirus (CMV) infections.[3] Dosing recommendations have been established for infants for the treatment of influenza,[4] and a new agent with a completely novel mechanism of action has recently been licensed for the treatment of influenza in children aged 12 years and older.[5] Several safe and effective treatment options are now available for chronic hepatitis B and C infections in children. With advances in transplant medicine, the need for novel approaches to overcome the development of viral resistance in immunocompromised patients receiving prolonged antiviral courses has increased. This chapter reviews the main viral infections affecting newborns and children for which effective antiviral medications are currently in use.

THERAPY OF HERPES SIMPLEX VIRUS INFECTIONS

HSVs rarely cross the placenta to cause congenital infection, and instead are more commonly acquired perinatally by the newborn at the time of delivery. Neonatal HSV disease presents as three clinical categories: (1) confined to the skin, eyes, or mucous membranes (SEM disease); (2) widely disseminated with evidence of multiorgan involvement (disseminated disease); or (3) involving the central nervous system (CNS disease). Since the introduction of early acyclovir therapy, there has been a shift to a greater proportion of HSV-infected neonates having SEM disease, which has the best prognosis, and fewer having disseminated disease, which has the highest mortality.[6] Although the mortality has substantially improved in the era of acyclovir therapy, up to 30% of neonates with disseminated disease will die.[1,7] Among the survivors of CNS disease, approximately 30% will have significant neurologic sequelae even with optimal therapy with 21 days of intravenous (IV) acyclovir[1] followed by 6 months of oral acyclovir.[2]

Neonatal HSV disease has a higher incidence rate than historically estimated, with more recent data suggesting an incident rate of between 50 and 60 cases per 100,000 live births.[8,9] In the 1970s and early 1980s, vidarabine was the first agent to demonstrate efficacy in the treatment of neonatal HSV disease.[10,11] By the mid-1980s, this drug was replaced by IV acyclovir, which is safer and more easily administered than vidarabine.[12] In the 1990s, higher doses of parenteral acyclovir administered for longer durations[1] improved mortality outcomes. And in the 2000s, the use of 6 months of oral acyclovir suppression following the parenteral treatment with IV acyclovir improved morbidity outcomes.[2] Beyond the neonatal period, infants and older children will commonly present with primary gingivostomatitis due to HSV-1. Limited data are available on the effects of systemic acyclovir on the course of primary or recurrent nongenital mucocutaneous HSV infections in immunocompetent hosts, but topical acyclovir is ineffective. It is, however, recommended that mucocutaneous disease in immunocompromised hosts be treated with parenteral acyclovir, in spite of the lack of unequivocal efficacy data from clinical trials.

Herpes simplex encephalitis (HSE) is a rare occurrence of CNS disease occurring beyond the neonatal period and is virtually always caused by HSV-1. Patients with HSE should be treated with at least 21 days of IV acyclovir, and treatment should not be stopped until documented negative polymerase chain reaction (PCR) on the cerebrospinal fluid (CSF).

Ocular HSV: Topical agents include 1% trifluridine and 0.15% ganciclovir. For children with recurrent ocular lesions, oral suppressive therapy with acyclovir or valacyclovir may be indicated for months or even years.

Genital infections may be due to either HSV-1 or HSV-2. Several agents are available with equivocal efficacy in shortening the duration of illness and viral shedding. These include acyclovir, valacyclovir, and famciclovir. IV acyclovir is indicated for patients with severe disease, immunocompromised patients, and pregnant women with severe disease.

THERAPY OF VARICELLA ZOSTER VIRUS INFECTIONS

Antiviral therapy is generally not recommended for otherwise healthy children less than 12 years of age with chickenpox. Oral valacyclovir is recommended for those deemed at higher risk for severe disease, such as those who are older than 12 years, have chronic cutaneous or pulmonary diseases, are secondary household contacts, are on long-term salicylates, or are receiving short-term courses of corticosteroids. IV acyclovir therapy is recommended for immunocompromised patients, including neonates.[13]

THERAPY OF CONGENITAL CYTOMEGALOVIRUS INFECTION

CMV commonly infects humans worldwide, with a seroprevalence of approximately 40% in adolescents and approaching 90% in adults of poor socioeconomic status.[14,15] Congenital CMV infection is the most common congenital infection in the developed world and occurs in about 0.5% of live born infants in the United States.[16] Of all infants born with congenital CMV infection, approximately 7% to 10% have clinically evident disease at birth.[17] Mortality for symptomatic infants is estimated around 5% to 10%.[18] Death is usually due to non-CNS manifestations of the infection, such as hepatic dysfunction or bleeding. An estimated 40% to 58% of infants with symptomatic congenital CMV infection have permanent sequelae, most notably sensorineural hearing loss and developmental delay, whereas infants who are asymptomatic at birth suffer permanent sequelae nearly 14% of the time.[19] In contrast with congenital infection, perinatally acquired CMV infections are not typically associated with long-term sequelae, though acute illness has been reported in premature very low-birth-weight infants.[20] In full-term infants, perinatal infections are commonly asymptomatic but may present with pneumonitis within the first few months of life.[21]

IV ganciclovir therapy in neonates with symptomatic congenital CMV disease has been assessed in a phase 3 randomized controlled trial, in which 6 weeks of therapy improved hearing outcomes until at least around 2 years of age and may have improved neurologic outcomes; however, significant neutropenia developed in roughly two-thirds of the patients necessitating dose adjustments.[3,22] A subsequent phase 3 randomized controlled study using oral valganciclovir comparing 6 weeks of therapy with 6 months of therapy further improved audiologic and neurodevelopmental outcomes out to 2 years of age, with significantly lower rates of neutropenia compared with IV ganciclovir.[23]

Currently, 6 months of oral valganciclovir for neonates with moderate-to-severe symptomatic congenital CMV disease is recommended.[24,25]

THERAPY OF CYTOMEGALOVIRUS IN IMMUNOSUPPRESSED CHILDREN

CMV poses a significant disease burden in children undergoing both solid organ and stem cell transplantation. The incidence of CMV viremia is reportedly between 40% and 80% in CMV-seropositive allogeneic hematopoietic stem cell transplant (allo-HCT) recipients not receiving antiviral prophylaxis. This viremia is linked to several negative outcomes, including increased mortality due to CMV disease, an increased incidence of graft-versus-host disease (GVHD), an increased risk of post-transplant malignancy relapse, and mortality linked to the side effects of currently approved antiviral agents, notably myelosuppression and renal failure.[26]

IV ganciclovir therapy is indicated for the treatment of CMV infections in immunosuppressed patients with systemic or ocular CMV disease. Valganciclovir is used for the suppression of CMV retinitis and prevention of CMV disease in transplant patients.[27] Foscarnet or cidofovir is indicated for the treatment of ganciclovir-resistant CMV disease. Letermovir is a recently approved, highly effective agent for the prevention of CMV in adult transplant patients, and pediatric studies of letermovir are ongoing.

AVAILABLE THERAPIES FOR HERPES SIMPLEX VIRUS, VARICELLA ZOSTER VIRUS, AND CYTOMEGALOVIRUS INFECTIONS

ACYCLOVIR (ACYCLOGUANOSINE, ZOVIRAX, ACV) AND VALACYCLOVIR (VALTREX)

Acyclovir is the most frequently prescribed antiviral agent for the management of HSV and varicella zoster virus (VZV) infections and has demonstrated remarkable safety and efficacy.

Chemistry and Mechanism of Action

Acyclovir is a deoxyguanosine analog, with preferential uptake by viral-infected cells, undergoing initial phosphorylation by virus-encoded thymidine kinase (TK). Subsequent diphosphorylation and triphosphorylation events are catalyzed by host cell enzymes. Acyclovir triphosphate exhibits enhanced affinity for viral DNA polymerase over cellular polymerase, and its incorporation into the growing viral chain results in chain termination.[28,29]

Valacyclovir is the L-valyl ester of acyclovir that markedly improves oral absorption. It is rapidly converted to acyclovir after oral administration by first-pass metabolism in the liver.[30]

Spectrum and Resistance

Acyclovir is most active against HSV; activity against VZV is also substantial, but approximately 10-fold less. Epstein-Barr virus (EBV) is only moderately susceptible to acyclovir because EBV has minimal TK activity. Acyclovir activity against CMV is poor because of the absence of TK.[31]

Resistance of HSV and VZV to acyclovir has become an important clinical problem in select populations due mostly to mutations in the *TK* gene and less frequently in the viral DNA polymerase gene. Acyclovir resistance occurs most frequently in immunocompromised patients[32–34] but has been reported uncommonly in immunocompetent hosts on chronic suppressive acyclovir therapy for genital herpes[35] and in neonates.[36,37] Acyclovir-resistant VZV strains have been isolated from profoundly immunosuppressed patients with HIV[38] as well as patients with hematologic malignancies or following bone marrow transplantation.[39] Foscarnet is the drug of choice for acyclovir-resistant strains of VZV and HSV.[36]

Indications

Acyclovir is effective for the treatment of infections caused by HSV and VZV. Higher dosing at 20 mg per kg every 8 hours IV is indicated for neonatal disease. Importantly, following neonatal HSV infections, oral suppressive acyclovir therapy at 300 mg per m^2 per dose administered three times per day for 6 months has been shown to improve neurologic outcome.[2]

Pharmacokinetics

After IV doses of 2.5 to 15 mg per kg, steady-state concentrations of acyclovir range from 6.7 to 20.6 μg per mL. Acyclovir is widely distributed; high concentrations are attained in the kidneys, lung, liver, heart, and skin vesicles; concentrations in the CSF are about 50% of those in the plasma.[40] Acyclovir crosses the placenta and accumulates in breast milk. Protein binding ranges from 9% to 33%, and less than 20% of drug is metabolized to biologically inactive metabolites. The half-life of acyclovir is 2 to 3 hours in older children and adults and 2.5 to 5 hours in neonates with normal creatinine clearance. More than 60% of administered drug is excreted in the urine.[40] Elimination is prolonged in patients with renal dysfunction; the half-life is approximately 20 hours in persons with end-stage renal disease, necessitating dose modifications for those with creatinine clearance less than 50 mL per minute per 1.73 m^2.[41] Acyclovir is effectively removed by hemodialysis, but not by continuous ambulatory peritoneal dialysis.[42]

Oral acyclovir has poor bioavailability, with only 15% to 30 % of the dose being absorbed. The development of the prodrug valacyclovir has overcome this limitation, though, with over 50% of the dose being absorbed in adults and achieving acyclovir plasma levels similar to the IV administration of acyclovir. Peak serum concentrations ranging from 0.8 to 8.5 μg per mL following doses of 100 to 2,000 mg are attained about 1.5 hours after a dose.[43] The bioavailability of valacyclovir suspension (only available as a compounded medication, with the recipe provided in the package insert) in children is somewhat reduced, being less than 50%, but still better than oral acyclovir.[44,45] All other pharmacokinetic (PK) characteristics are similar to those of acyclovir.[46]

There are insufficient PK data for valacyclovir in neonates and young infants, and oral acyclovir is still the recommended drug of choice for oral suppressive therapy following neonatal HSV disease.

Adverse Effects

Oral acyclovir sometimes causes mild gastrointestinal upset, rash, and headache. If it extravasates, IV acyclovir can cause severe inflammation, phlebitis, and sometimes a vesicular eruption, leading to cutaneous necrosis at the injection site.

Nephrotoxicity has been described in all age groups and for the most part is reversible on cessation of drug administration. A well-described obstructive nephropathy can result from the formation of acyclovir crystals that precipitate in renal tubules, with the risk increased if the drug is given by rapid IV infusion or if the patient is dehydrated or has preexisting renal compromise.[47] The risk of nephrotoxicity appears to be increased with the use of higher dosing beyond the neonatal period. Acute kidney injury has been described in children receiving doses of acyclovir greater than 15 mg per kg per dose, with a higher incidence in children with baseline renal compromise and those receiving concomitant administration of other nephrotoxic agents. Acute kidney injury typically occurs within the first 48 hours of initiation of therapy but has been described up to 2 weeks into therapy.[48,49]

Neutropenia occurs in approximately 20% neonates being treated with high-dose IV acyclovir (60 mg per kg per day), as well as in approximately the same percentage of infants during the 6 months of oral suppressive therapy. Neutropenia resolves on cessation of therapy.[1,2] Absolute neutrophil counts should be checked at 2 and 4 weeks after initiating suppressive therapy and then monthly during the suppressive treatment period.[50]

The most serious side effect of acyclovir is neurotoxicity, which occurs rarely and has only been reported postlicensure.[47] This results in lethargy, confusion, hallucinations, tremors, myoclonus, seizures, extrapyramidal signs, and changes in state of consciousness that develop within the first few days of starting therapy. Risk factors predisposing a patient to developing neurotoxicity are compromised renal function and concurrent administration of interferon or intrathecal methotrexate.[51] These neurotoxic manifestations usually resolve with discontinuation of the drug within several days, but hemodialysis may be useful in severe cases associated with high serum concentrations.

Other reported side effects of IV acyclovir include rash, sweating, nausea, headache, hematuria, and hypotension. The profiles of adverse effects and potential drug interactions observed with valacyclovir therapy are the same as those observed with acyclovir therapy. Neurotoxicity has not been reported in humans to date, although it has been observed in animal models.[43] Although acyclovir is mutagenic at high concentrations in some in vitro assays, it is not teratogenic in animals. Limited human data suggest that acyclovir use in pregnant women is not associated with congenital defects or other adverse pregnancy outcomes.

FAMCICLOVIR (FAMVIR)

Chemistry and Mechanism of Action

Famciclovir is the prodrug of penciclovir, which is a guanosine analog requiring initial phosphorylation by viral TK and then diphosphorylation and triphosphorylation by cellular enzymes to its active form, penciclovir triphosphate. Penciclovir triphosphate is a competitive inhibitor of DNA polymerase but, in contrast to acyclovir, does not cause chain termination.

Spectrum and Resistance

The spectrum of activity of penciclovir is identical to acyclovir with activity against HSV-1, HSV-2, and VZV. Resistance occurs in a way identical to that of acyclovir as well, with mutation of the viral TK being the most common.[31]

Indications

Famciclovir is indicated for treatment of herpes zoster infections as well as genital herpes in adults and has similar efficacy to valacyclovir. Studies of the PK and safety of famciclovir in children aged 1 month and older have been conducted, but there are insufficient efficacy data to recommend routine use in children.

Pharmacokinetics

Penciclovir has minimal oral bioavailability. Famciclovir is the diacetyl ester prodrug of penciclovir and confers 70% bioavailability.[31] Famciclovir is excreted by the kidney and, therefore, requires dose adjustment in patients with renal insufficiency.[31] The systemic exposure of penciclovir is similar in children aged 6 to 12 years and slightly reduced in children aged 1 to 6 years,[52] but systemic exposure is significantly lower in children less than 6 months of age.[53]

Adverse Effects

Famciclovir is well tolerated with minimal side effects, with headache and gastrointestinal upset being most common.

GANCICLOVIR (DHPG, CYTOVENE, GCV) AND VALGANCICLOVIR (VALCYTE, VGCV)

Chemistry and Mechanism of Action

Ganciclovir is structurally similar to acyclovir, except for a hydroxymethyl group on its acyclic side chain. The initial phosphorylation step is carried out by the serine/threonine kinase expressed by human CMV from gene *UL97*. Cellular kinases then phosphorylate the drug two additional times to convert it into its active triphosphate moiety, which inhibits the CMV DNA polymerase through incorporation into and termination of viral DNA.[54] Ganciclovir is preferentially taken up by CMV-infected cells, and the intracellular half-life is more than 24 hours. It does have some activity against cellular DNA and can be incorporated into host cellular DNA, resulting in toxicity.[55] Valganciclovir is the L-valine ester prodrug of ganciclovir and as such has the same mechanism of action, antiviral spectrum, and potential for development of resistance as ganciclovir.[31]

Spectrum and Resistance

Ganciclovir has similar activity to acyclovir against HSV-1, HSV-2, and VZV, but, in contrast with acyclovir, its greatest activity is against CMV.[56,57] Resistance of CMV isolates usually results from mutations in the *UL97* gene or less frequently in the DNA polymerase gene.[54]

Indications

Ganciclovir is indicated for the treatment of CMV infections in immunosuppressed patients with systemic or ocular CMV disease. It is also used for the suppression of CMV retinitis and prevention of CMV disease in transplant patients.[27]

Six weeks of IV ganciclovir improves hearing outcomes to approximately 2 years of age and may improve neurologic outcomes; however, significant neutropenia develops in roughly two-thirds of the patients necessitating dose adjustments.[3,22] Six months of oral valganciclovir further improves audiologic and neurodevelopmental outcomes at 2 years of age, with significantly less neutropenia than with IV ganciclovir.[23] As a result, 6 months of oral valganciclovir is recommended for neonates with moderate and severe symptomatic congenital CMV disease.[24,25] Trials are currently ongoing to evaluate the efficacy of valganciclovir for infants with asymptomatic congenital CMV infection (https://clinicaltrials.gov/ct2/show/NCT03107871 and https://clinicaltrials.gov/ct2/show/NCT03301415).

Pharmacokinetics

Less than 10% of ganciclovir is absorbed following oral administration,[58] and since the availability of valganciclovir the oral formulation of ganciclovir is no longer marketed. Peak serum concentrations of ganciclovir after 6 mg per kg (newborn dose) of IV administered drug range from 8 to 11 μg per mL, with concentrations sufficient to inhibit sensitive strains of CMV in aqueous humor, subretinal fluid, CSF, and brain tissue.[31] The elimination half-life of ganciclovir is 2 to 3 hours, and most of the drug is eliminated unchanged in the urine. The PK of ganciclovir in the neonatal population is similar to that of adults.[59,60] Dose reduction, proportional to the degree of reduction in creatinine clearance, is necessary for persons with impaired renal function. A supplemental dose is recommended after dialysis because it is efficiently removed by hemodialysis.[61]

Valganciclovir is the L-valine ester prodrug of ganciclovir, with markedly improved oral bioavailability exceeding 60% that is enhanced further by concomitant administration of food.[62,63] Valganciclovir is rapidly converted to ganciclovir, with a mean plasma half-life of about 30 minutes.[64] The area under the curve of ganciclovir after oral administration of valganciclovir is one-third to one-half of that attained after IV administration of ganciclovir.[65] Patients with impaired renal function require dosage reduction that is roughly proportional to their reduction in creatinine clearance.

The PK of valganciclovir in the newborn is different from older children and adults. Following an average single dose of 16 mg per kg valganciclovir in 19 neonates, mean ganciclovir clearance was 9.3 mL per minute per kg, and distribution volume was 2.2 L per kg.[66] In a healthy adult population receiving a single 900-mg valganciclovir dose (n = 12), these same ganciclovir parameters were 5.4 mL per minute per kg and 1.6 L per kg, respectively.[67] Other PK parameters were similar, but the decreased neonatal clearance is consistent with age-related changes in ganciclovir disposition.

Adverse Effects

Ganciclovir has some activity against cellular DNA polymerases and the potential for incorporation into host cellular DNA, which accounts for its toxicity. The main toxicity of ganciclovir is myelosuppression, with a dose-dependent neutropenia being the most common. About 40% of patients will develop neutropenia during a 2-week course, which can be dose limiting in up to 15% of courses. The neutropenia is reversible on cessation of the medication.[27] Thrombocytopenia is seen in about 20% of patients receiving ganciclovir, and anemia occurs in about 2%. Approximately 5% of patients receiving IV ganciclovir experience some combination of headache, confusion, altered mental status, hallucinations, nightmares, anxiety, ataxia, tremors, and seizure. About 2% of recipients develop fever, rash, and abnormal levels of serum hepatic enzymes.

The most common side effects reported with valganciclovir therapy include diarrhea (41%), nausea (30%), neutropenia (27%), anemia (26%), and headache (22%).[64] Neutropenia was the most common side effect reported in infants, occurring in two-thirds treated with IV ganciclovir[3] and one-fifth treated with oral valganciclovir.[23] It is recommended to check the neutrophil count weekly during the first 6 weeks of therapy, then at week 8 of therapy and monthly thereafter. Additionally, serum aminotransferase concentration should be measured monthly throughout duration of therapy.[68]

Preclinical tests demonstrate that ganciclovir is mutagenic, carcinogenic, and teratogenic and has been shown to cause irreversible reproductive toxicity in animals. None of these effects have been demonstrated in humans; however, the long-term safety in infants and children treated with either ganciclovir or valganciclovir has not been established.[3,23,57]

FOSCARNET (PFA, FOSCAVIR)

Chemistry and Mechanism of Action

Foscarnet is an inorganic pyrophosphate analog that directly inhibits DNA polymerase by blocking the pyrophosphate-binding site and preventing cleavage of pyrophosphate from deoxynucleotide triphosphates.[69] It is a noncompetitive inhibitor of viral DNA polymerase or human immunodeficiency virus (HIV) reverse transcriptase and is not incorporated into the growing viral DNA chain. It is approximately 100-fold more active against viral enzymes than host cell enzymes.[69]

Spectrum and Resistance

Foscarnet has demonstrated activity against all known human herpes viruses, including most acyclovir-resistant HSV and VZV strains and ganciclovir-resistant CMV isolates, as well as HIV.[70] Resistance occurs as a result of DNA polymerase mutations. Strains of CMV, HSV, and VZV with reduced sensitivity to foscarnet have been reported. These isolates may respond to treatment with acyclovir or cidofovir.[71,72]

Indications

Currently, foscarnet is approved by the U.S. Food and Drug Administration (FDA) for the treatment of ganciclovir-resistant CMV retinitis in patients with AIDS,[73] and in refractory cases, foscarnet and ganciclovir therapy have been given in combination.[74] Foscarnet is recommended for treatment of both resistant CMV and HSV disease in neonates; however, data on safety and efficacy are sparse, and PK is lacking. There are only case reports published on the use of foscarnet in neonates, with dosages ranging from 100 to 180 mg per kg per day divided 8 to 12 hourly.[75–78]

Pharmacokinetics

Foscarnet is only administered as an IV medication. Maximum serum concentration attained after an IV dose of 60 mg per kg is approximately 500 μmol per L.[70] CSF concentrations are about two-thirds of those in serum.[79] The half-life of foscarnet is about 48 hours, and 80% of an administered dose is eliminated unchanged in the urine. Dose reduction, proportional to reduction in creatinine clearance, is necessary. Hemodialysis efficiently eliminates foscarnet; therefore, a supplemental dose is recommended after dialysis.[80]

Adverse Effects

The most common adverse effects of foscarnet are nephrotoxicity and metabolic derangements. Evidence of nephrotoxicity includes azotemia, proteinuria, acute tubular necrosis, crystalluria, and interstitial nephritis. Serum creatinine concentrations increase in up to 50% of patients, but usually returns to normal within 2 to 4 weeks after discontinuing therapy. Preexisting renal disease, concurrent use of other nephrotoxic drugs, dehydration, rapid injection, and/or continuous IV infusion of drug are risk factors for developing renal dysfunction.[81,82] Metabolic disturbances associated with foscarnet therapy include hypocalcemia and hypercalcemia and hypophosphatemia and hyperphosphatemia. Hypocalcemia can be associated with paresthesia, tetany, seizures, and arrhythmias.[83] Metabolic disturbances are minimized if foscarnet is administered by slow infusion. CNS symptoms associated with foscarnet therapy include headache, tremor, irritability, seizures, and hallucinations. Fever, nausea, vomiting, abnormal serum hepatic enzymes, anemia, granulocytopenia, and genital ulcerations have also been reported.[84]

CIDOFOVIR (HPMPC, VISTIDE)

Chemistry and Mechanism of Action

Cidofovir is an acyclic phosphonate nucleotide analog with a mechanism of action similar to that of nucleoside analogs. In contrast to acyclovir, viral enzymes are not required for initial phosphorylation because native cidofovir has a single phosphate group already attached. Following diphosphorylation by cellular kinases, cidofovir competitively inhibits DNA polymerase. The active form of cidofovir exhibits a 25- to 50-fold greater affinity for viral DNA polymerase compared with the cellular DNA polymerase.[85,86]

Spectrum and Resistance

Cidofovir is active against HSV and CMV, including acyclovir- and foscarnet-resistant HSV isolates and ganciclovir- and foscarnet-resistant CMV mutants.[87] It is also active in vitro against VZV, EBV, human herpes virus-6, human herpes virus-8, polyomaviruses, adenovirus, and human HPV. A small number of cidofovir-resistant CMV isolates that are also resistant to ganciclovir on the basis of mutations within the DNA polymerase gene have been described.[88] A CMV mutant resistant to ganciclovir, foscarnet, and cidofovir has also been reported.[89,90]

Indications

Cidofovir is indicated for the treatment of HSV and CMV infections in immunocompromised hosts that have developed resistance to acyclovir, ganciclovir, and foscarnet.[91,92] Additionally, cidofovir has shown efficacy in treating adenovirus[93–95] and BK virus[96,97] in immunocompromised hosts. Data on cidofovir use in neonates are anecdotal.[98]

Pharmacokinetics

Cidofovir is administered IV and has a plasma half-life of 2.6 hours, but an intracellular half-life of 17 to 48 hours. Approximately 90% of the drug is excreted in the urine primarily by renal tubular secretion.[86,99–101] Importantly, the drug does not cross the blood–brain barrier and, therefore, should not be used to treat CNS infections.

Adverse Effects

Because cidofovir concentrates in renal cells in amounts 100 times greater than in other tissues, nephrotoxicity is the main adverse effect, especially if hydration is not well maintained.[100,101] Manifestations of renal toxicity include proteinuria and glycosuria. Aggressive IV prehydration, coadministration of probenecid, and avoidance of other nephrotoxic agents reduce the likelihood of toxicity.[102] Cidofovir is contraindicated in patients with a serum creatinine of more than 1.5 mg per dL, a calculated creatinine clearance of 55 mL per minute or less, or a urine protein of 100 mg per dL, and drug should be discontinued if serum creatinine increases to 0.5 mg per dL or more above baseline.

LETERMOVIR (PREVYMIS)

Chemistry and Mechanism of Action

Letermovir targets the terminase enzyme complex utilized by CMV in the terminal phase of the replication life cycle. This enzyme complex cuts the CMV genome units, which are generated in tandem before being packaged into preformed virus capsids.[103]

Spectrum and Resistance

Letermovir is highly specific to CMV and currently is the most active molecule against CMV. Emergence of resistance has been demonstrated in vitro[104] and in clinical use, mostly due to mutations in the *UL59* gene of the terminase complex.[105]

Indications

Letermovir was licensed in the United States in November 2017, in both oral and IV formulations, for the prophylaxis of CMV infection in adult CMV-seropositive recipients of an allo-HCT.[106] There is a phase 2 trial ongoing to determine the PK, safety, and efficacy of letermovir in children (https://clinicaltrials.gov/ct2/show/NCT03940586).

Pharmacokinetics

Letermovir has good bioavailability following oral administration, with a median time to peak serum concentration of 1.5 to 3 hours. It is highly protein bound to human plasma proteins. The main route of elimination is via the biliary–fecal route with 93% of the dose excreted in the feces, of which 70% is unchanged drug and the remainder are the hepatic metabolites. The mean terminal half-life was around 12 hours after a single dose of 480 mg IV in healthy adult subjects. Due to hepatic metabolism, there are several drug interactions that may result, the full list of which can be found in the package insert. No dosage adjustment is required for patients with moderate renal impairment; however, the safety in patients with end-stage renal disease including those on dialysis is unknown. No dosage adjustment is required for patients with mild or moderate hepatic impairment, and it is not recommended for use in patients with severe hepatic impairment. The dosage, however, should be decreased if administered with cyclosporine.[107]

Adverse Effects

In clinical trials, letermovir was generally well tolerated, with the most frequently reported side effect being nausea. Time to engraftment following bone marrow transplantation was the same in the letermovir compared to placebo group.[107]

INFLUENZA

There are three influenza viruses (A, B, and C), which are members of the orthomyxovirus family. These viruses have segmented negative-sense RNA genomes, an envelope derived from the host cell, and characteristic surface glycoproteins that are involved in the entry and release of the virus from host cells. Influenza C causes only minor illness that does not usually require therapy. Influenza A and B, however, can both cause seasonal epidemics with significant morbidity and mortality, particularly in the young child less than 1 year of age. Influenza A is also the source of occasional pandemics.

AGENTS APPROVED TO TREAT INFLUENZA IN CHILDREN

Recognizing that vaccination is most effective to prevent influenza, several antiviral agents are effective for both the prevention and treatment of influenza. Three separate targets for the action of antiviral agents against influenza exist. These include M2 protein, which is an ion channel in the viral membrane of influenza A; neuraminidase, which is a surface glycoprotein common to both influenza A and B; and cap-dependent endonuclease. Circulating influenza viruses are virtually uniformly resistant to M2-ion channel inhibitors (amantadine and rimantadine), rendering these agents obsolete.

The neuraminidase inhibitors (oseltamivir, zanamivir, and peramivir) are the most commonly prescribed agents; however, emergence of antiviral resistance is an ongoing threat. A novel agent targeting the influenza polymerase, baloxavir marboxil, was FDA approved in 2018 for use in patients aged 12 years and older; phase 3 clinical trials in children less than 12 years are ongoing. Importantly, following its use during one season, polymerase mutations have been reported.[5]

OSELTAMIVIR PHOSPHATE (TAMIFLU)

Chemistry and Mechanism of Action

Oseltamivir is an ethyl ester prodrug, hydrolyzed by hepatic esterases to biologically active oseltamivir carboxylate. Its biologic action results from inhibition of influenza neuraminidase. Inhibition of neuraminidase prevents penetration of the virus to the cell surface, and because neuraminidase is required for optimal release of progeny virus from infected cells, inhibition of this enzyme decreases the spread of virus and intensity of infection.[108]

Spectrum and Resistance

Because neuraminidase is a highly conserved enzyme in influenza viruses, oseltamivir is active against all strains of influenza type-A and influenza type-B viruses. Resistance occurs due to mutations in viral neuraminidase or hemagglutinin or both.[109–111] Resistance in adult populations has been documented around 1.5%[112] and is significantly higher in pediatric populations at between 4.4%[4] and 8.6%.[113] In spite of these resistance mutations, disease resolution does not appear prolonged.[114] Seasonal data on oseltamivir resistance are reported in near real time by the Centers for Disease Control and Prevention on their website.

Indications

Dosing recommendations have been established for preterm infants and older children with weight-based dosing adjusted by age.[4] The earlier the initiation of therapy in the course of illness, the greater is the observed benefit.[108,115]

Oseltamivir can be given to asymptomatic patients who have been exposed and are at high risk of becoming ill with influenza. Chemoprophylaxis is not recommended for patients less than 3 months of age due to unfavorable PK and limited safety and efficacy data in this age group.

Pharmacokinetics

The bioavailability of oseltamivir is about 75%; coadministration with food does not affect absorption. More than 90% of oseltamivir (prodrug) is metabolized to oseltamivir carboxylate, the active metabolite. Peak plasma concentration of active compound following multiple 75-mg doses administered twice a day is approximately 350 ng per mL. The half-life of oseltamivir carboxylate is 6 to 10 hours; it is eliminated by glomerular filtration and tubular secretion.[116] Dose adjustment is recommended for patients with a creatinine clearance of less than 30 mL per minute, as oseltamivir carboxylate exposure is inversely proportional to declining renal function.[116] The PK of oseltamivir in pediatric patients older than 12 years is similar to that in adult patients, but younger patients (3 to 12 years) have more rapid clearance of the prodrug and carboxylate, resulting in lower exposures. As age increases, oral clearance of the carboxylate decreases in a linear manner. Carboxylate exposure in older patients (65 to 78 years) is 25% to 35% higher compared with younger adults, but no dose change is recommended in this population.

Adverse Effects

The drug was well tolerated in clinical testing, and there was no relationship between drug exposure and adverse events or laboratory abnormalities at dosages up to 1,000 mg per day.[117] The most common adverse effect reported is nausea with or without vomiting. Insomnia and vertigo have been rarely reported. There have been no drug interactions described to date.[118] Concern had been raised regarding neuropsychiatric events related to oseltamivir use in children. In response, the FDA conducted a comprehensive review and posted their findings and recommendations in 2007. The analysis to date is inconclusive to determine causality of neuropsychiatric events to oseltamivir, as these events are seen in children with influenza not taking oseltamivir. The FDA determined that there was insufficient evidence to restrict the use of oseltamivir but recommended a highlighted precaution to closely monitor for unusual behavior in children, especially on the first day initiating treatment.[119]

ZANAMIVIR (RELENZA)

Chemistry and Mechanism of Action

Zanamivir is structurally similar to oseltamivir, and it also interferes with the function of the influenza neuraminidase enzyme. It can be administered either as a powder for inhalation or IV.

Spectrum and Resistance

Zanamivir has demonstrated antiviral activity against influenza A and B viruses. Zanamivir retains activity against influenza viruses that have developed the most common resistance substitution, H275Y, which confers high-level resistance to oseltamivir and reduced susceptibility to peramivir in N1 viruses.[120] Resistance to zanamivir has been described in an immunocompromised child receiving IV zanamivir; the resistant isolate was demonstrated to have mutations in both the viral neuraminidase and the viral hemagglutinin.[121]

Indications

Zanamivir is FDA approved as an inhaled powder for treatment of influenza A and B in children aged 7 years and older, and for prophylaxis in children aged 5 years and older. It is not recommended for people with breathing ailments like asthma or chronic obstructive pulmonary disease (COPD).

Inhaled zanamivir demonstrated efficacy for prophylaxis both in community exposure to influenza[122,123] and within households.[124] Inhaled zanamivir has demonstrated efficacy for the treatment of both adults[125] and children[126] with influenza A or B. Results of a phase 3 trial comparing IV zanamivir to oral oseltamivir for hospitalized patients aged 16 years and older with influenza showed similar outcomes and adverse events.[127] Additionally, the results of a phase 2 study of IV zanamivir in pediatric patients aged 6 months and older with influenza have been reported, and overall, the PK parameters were similar to those in adults.[128] However, there are no plans currently to bring IV zanamivir to the US market, and it is not available through emergency Investigational New Drug (IND) at this time.

Pharmacokinetics

Zanamivir has very poor oral bioavailability. With inhalation, about 13% of the administered dose distributes to the airways and lungs, providing local drug concentrations that greatly exceed the inhibitory concentrations for influenza A and B viruses. The IV administration is distributed in extracellular body fluids with a volume of distribution of 16 L. High concentrations of the drug are detectable in respiratory secretions after IV infusion. Between 4% and 17% of the inhaled dose is systemically absorbed, with the peak serum concentration of 17 to 142 ng per mL occurring within 1 to 2 hours following a 10-mg dose. The serum half-life following oral inhalation ranges from 2.5 to 5.1 hours, and total clearance ranges from 2.5 to 10.9 L per hour. In contrast, the serum half-life with IV administration is approximately 2 hours, with a total clearance of 5.7 L per hour. Zanamivir has limited plasma protein binding, is not metabolized, and is excreted unchanged in the urine. Unabsorbed drug is excreted in the feces.[129] Due to the low systemic bioavailability following oral inhalation, no dose adjustments are necessary in patients with renal insufficiency.[129,130] With IV administration, 90% of the drug is excreted unchanged in the urine, and dosage adjustment is required for renal insufficiency. Steady state is reached by day 3.[128]

Adverse Effects

Patients with underlying airway disease have an increased risk of developing bronchospasm or decline in pulmonary function; therefore, it is not recommended for use in patients with underlying pulmonary disease, including asthma.[131] The drug-related adverse events reported in the pediatric phase 2 study of IV zanamivir that comprised a cohort of 71 patients included neutropenia in 2 patients and elevation in aspartate aminotransferase, delirium, eosinophilia, insomnia, left ventricular hypertrophy, elevation in troponin I, and vomiting each in 1 patient, respectively.[128]

PERAMIVIR (RAPIVAB)

Chemistry and Mechanism of Action

Peramivir has the same mechanism of action as oseltamivir targeting influenza neuraminidase.

Spectrum and Resistance

Peramivir has demonstrated antiviral activity against both influenza A and B viruses. Resistance occurs due to amino acid substitutions in viral neuraminidase and hemagglutinin proteins. Isolates with substitutions associated with reduced susceptibility to peramivir have been observed both in clinical trials with peramivir and during community surveillance studies.[111,132]

Indications

Results of a phase 3 study demonstrating the safety and efficacy of a single dose of IV peramivir resulted in FDA approval in 2014 for the treatment of uncomplicated influenza in children aged 2 years and older.[133] Efficacy was not demonstrated in clinical trials in patients with serious influenza requiring hospitalization.[134]

Pharmacokinetics

After the IV administration of peramivir, there is a linear relationship between dose and exposure parameters. Following an infusion over 30 minutes of a single 600 mg dose in adults and adolescents, a maximum serum concentration of 46.8 μg per mL is reached at the end of the infusion. Binding to plasma proteins is less than 30%, and the volume of distribution is 12.56 L. Peramivir is not significantly metabolized, and 90% is excreted unchanged in the urine. The elimination half-life following a single 600-mg IV dose is approximately 20 hours. Dose adjustment is recommended for patients with creatinine clearance below 50 mL per minute. The PK of peramivir in children is comparable to adults.[133,135]

Adverse Effects

The drug is very well tolerated, with the most commonly reported adverse reaction being diarrhea, reported in 8% compared with 7% on placebo in clinical trials. Laboratory abnormalities reported in clinical trials included moderate neutropenia in 8%, hyperglycemia in 5%, elevation in creatinine phosphokinase in 4%, and an elevation of alanine aminotransferase in 3%.[133]

BALOXAVIR MARBOXIL (XOFLUZA)

Chemistry and Mechanism of Action

Baloxavir marboxil has a novel mechanism of action as an inhibitor of influenza cap-dependent endonuclease. The influenza virus polymerase complex is composed of three protein subunits, namely, polymerase basic protein 1 (PB1), polymerase basic protein 2 (PB2), and polymerase acidic protein (PA). The PB2 subunit binds to the cap of host cellular pre–messenger RNA, which is subsequently cleaved by the cap-dependent endonuclease in the PA subunit. This process is described as "cap-snatching" and provides an RNA primer for transcription of viral messenger RNA by the RNA-dependent RNA polymerase function of PB1.[5]

Spectrum and Resistance

Baloxavir has demonstrated activity against both influenza A and B viruses, including those resistant to neuraminidases. Unfortunately, emergence of PA variants conferring resistance was seen during the phase 3 trial in close to 10% of adults,[5] and in the phase 3 trials in children aged 6 months to 12 years in Japan during the 2016/2017 influenza season, 23.5% of influenza A (H3N2) isolates contained variants resistant to baloxavir.[136]

Indications

Baloxavir is FDA approved in pill formulation and is given as a single dose for the treatment of influenza aged 12 years and older. The liquid formulation for the treatment of children less than 12 years of age is currently in phase 3 clinical trials.

In the randomized, double-blind, placebo compared to oseltamivir-controlled trial, baloxavir had a similar time to alleviation of symptoms compared to oseltamivir, was associated with a greater reduction in viral load 1 day after initiation of treatment compared with oseltamivir, and had fewer adverse events reported.[5]

Pharmacokinetics

Baloxavir marboxil is taken orally as a single dose at 40 mg if weight between 40 and 80 kg and 80 mg if 80 kg or greater. It can be taken with or without food. Baloxavir marboxil is a prodrug with good oral bioavailability and, after absorption, is almost completely converted to its active metabolite, baloxavir. Serum concentration peaks around 4 hours. Baloxavir is largely metabolized by the UGT1A3, one of the uridine diphosphate–glucuronosyl transferase enzymes, with 80% of the dose excreted in feces and an elimination half-life of 79 hours.

Adverse Effects

The most commonly reported adverse effects considered related to baloxavir are diarrhea and nausea. Coadministration with polyvalent cation-containing products such as antacids and oral calcium may reduce the plasma concentration. Animal data showed no mutagenic or teratogenic effects, or effects on infertility.

RIBAVIRIN (VIRAZOLE; REBETRON COMBINATION THERAPY: RIBAVIRIN PLUS PEGYLATED INTERFERON-α)

Ribavirin is available for inhaled use for the therapy of severe lower respiratory tract infection due to RSV, and in oral form coadministered with pegylated interferon for the treatment of hepatitis C. It is also available as an oral and IV formulation (compassionate plea release from the FDA) for the treatment of Lassa fever.

Chemistry and Mechanism of Action

Ribavirin is a synthetic nucleoside analog and most closely resembles guanosine in structure. The 5′-phosphate derivatives and the deribosylated base of ribavirin interfere with the capping and elongation of messenger RNA.[137]

Spectrum and Resistance

Ribavirin is active against a wide range of both RNA and DNA viruses, including myxo-, paramyxo-, arena-, bunya-, herpes-, adeno-, pox-, and retroviruses.[138] Activity against RNA viruses is greater than that against DNA viruses,[139] and viral resistance to ribavirin has not been observed.

Indications

The role of ribavirin therapy for the treatment of RSV disease is controversial. Ribavirin aerosol was approved for the therapy of lower respiratory tract infections caused by RSV in children; however, efficacy for the treatment of otherwise healthy infants hospitalized with RSV bronchiolitis is lacking,[140–145] and as such, it is currently not recommended by the American Academy of Pediatrics. There are both limited and conflicting data on efficacy of ribavirin for the treatment of RSV in children with profound immunocompromising conditions, such as hematologic malignancies and post-transplantation. There appears to be a benefit for the use of either aerosolized or oral ribavirin for the treatment of upper respiratory tract infections in adults post-HCT[146,147]; however, this benefit has not been demonstrated to date in children.[148–150]

Implementation of well-designed studies to answer these questions is hampered by the prohibitive cost of aerosolized ribavirin and by the need for specialized delivery equipment. IV administered ribavirin is effective in the management of life-threatening infections caused by Lassa fever and hemorrhagic fever with renal syndrome.[151] Oral ribavirin has been recommended for prophylaxis against Lassa fever in exposed contacts.[152] Although there are many anecdotal reports of ribavirin therapy for other infections, including those caused by influenza, parainfluenza, and measles virus, efficacy against these infections is not established. As noted above, ribavirin in combination with interferon-α (Rebetron) is useful in the management of infections caused by hepatitis C virus (HCV).[153,154]

Pharmacokinetics

The aerosolized formulation of ribavirin (Virazole) and the oral formulation in combination with pegylated interferon-α (Rebetron) are approved for use in the United States. Aerosolized delivery of ribavirin is accomplished with a small particle aerosol generator (SPAG), which delivers a steady flow of small particles (median mass diameter of 1.3 mm). When 20 mg per mL of drug is instilled into the SPAG reservoir, an estimated 1.8 mg per kg per hour of ribavirin is deposited in the respiratory tract; the precise amount of drug delivered to the respiratory tract depends on the child's ventilation and lung pathology.[155] A small amount of ribavirin is absorbed systemically following aerosolized delivery, but the concentration of drug in the respiratory tract is much higher than that in plasma. Levels in respiratory secretions often exceed 1,000 µg per mL, and mean plasma concentration is 1.10 µg per mL after 8 hours of aerosolization.[156] The half-life of ribavirin in tracheal secretions ranges from 1.4 to 2.5 hours.

The oral bioavailability of ribavirin is about 40%; peak plasma concentrations range from 1.3 to 3.2 µg per mL after doses of 600 to 2,400 mg.[157] Peak concentrations following IV therapy are approximately 10-fold greater. Levels of ribavirin in CSF are approximately 70% of plasma concentrations of the drug.[158] The half-life of ribavirin is 18 to 36 hours; less than one-third of systemically administered drug is recovered unchanged in the urine, and an additional one-third is excreted as metabolites.[157]

Adverse Effects

Ribavirin is concentrated in red blood cells, and high concentrations of the drug are associated with reversible anemia.[157] Increases in serum bilirubin, iron, and uric acid may also result from systemic therapy. Aerosolized ribavirin occasionally is associated with mild conjunctival irritation and rash. Transient wheezing may accompany therapy. Unless careful attention is paid to modifying the circuitry and frequently changing in line filters, ribavirin can precipitate, plugging the ventilator valves and tubing when used in mechanically ventilated infants.[159] Health care personnel caring for children receiving aerosolized ribavirin may be exposed inadvertently to the drug, and as such, it is recommended to deliver with a scavenging system or in a negative-pressure environment.[160,161]

HEPATITIS B AND HEPATITIS C VIRUS INFECTIONS IN CHILDREN

Both hepatitis B and C can be acquired through vertical transmission from mother to child and result in chronic infection with increased risk of liver cirrhosis and hepatocellular carcinoma.[162] Although the incidence of hepatitis B infection has dramatically declined since the implementation of universal immunization campaigns, approximately 350 million persons worldwide are still infected with hepatitis B.[162] In the United States, approximately 1% of infants born to hepatitis B surface antigen–positive mothers acquire infection despite provision of both hepatitis B immunoglobulin and hepatitis B vaccine within 12 hours of birth.[163] Without postexposure prophylaxis, the risk of the infant acquiring hepatitis B virus (HBV) as a result of perinatal exposure is up to 90% for infants born to mothers who are hepatitis B surface antigen and hepatitis B e-antigen positive. Chronic disease will develop in approximately 90% of perinatally infected infants.[163] During childhood, 3% to 5% of chronic carriers develop cirrhosis, and 0.01% to 0.03% develop hepatocellular carcinoma.[162]

The goal of treatment in chronic HBV infection is to prevent progression to cirrhosis, hepatic failure, and hepatocellular carcinoma. Current indications for treatment include evidence of ongoing HBV viral replication together with elevated serum alanine transaminase (ALT) or evidence of chronic hepatitis on liver biopsy. Treatment of pregnant women with a high viral load has been shown to reduce perinatal transmission.[164]

It is estimated that approximately 5 million children are infected with chronic hepatitis C worldwide.[165] In the United States, approximately 0.2% of children aged 6 to 11 years and 0.4% of children aged 12 to 16 years are chronically infected with HCV.[166]

The rate of mother-to-child transmission of HCV infection is approximately 5%, although rates are higher among women with inadequately controlled HIV coinfection and women with higher HCV RNA levels.[167–169] It is estimated that between 25% and 50% of infected infants spontaneously resolve HCV infection by 3 years of age.[170] The progression of liver disease is slow, and as such, development of advanced liver disease in children is infrequent.[171–173] The current guidelines for the treatment of chronic HCV infection by the Infectious Disease Society of America (IDSA) is to defer treatment in children less than 12 years of age until interferon-free regimens are available if no evidence of advanced fibrosis or the presence of extrahepatic manifestations, such as cryoglobulinemia, rashes, and glomerulonephritis. None of the direct-acting HCV drugs currently have been approved for use in children less than 12 years of age; however, clinical trials are ongoing. Sofosbuvir (Sovaldi), sofosbuvir in a fixed-dose combination tab with ledipasvir (Harvoni), and glecaprevir/pibrentasvir (Mavyret) are now approved for patients aged 12 years or older. Treatment with approved direct-acting antiviral regimens is recommended for all children aged 12 years and older with chronic HCV infection.[174]

THERAPIES FOR THE TREATMENT OF CHRONIC HEPATITIS B INFECTION

LAMIVUDINE (EPIVIR, 3TC)

Chemistry and Mechanism of Action

Lamivudine is a nucleoside analog that is phosphorylated by cellular kinases. In its triphosphate form, it inhibits the reverse transcriptase of both HBV and HIV, resulting in DNA chain termination.[175,176]

Activity and Resistance

Lamivudine has activity against both HBV and HIV.[177] In patients who are HBeAg positive, about 20% will achieve seroconversion and undetectable serum HBV DNA at the end of 1 year of therapy, with around 50% showing improvement of liver disease on biopsy.[176,178,179] Unfortunately, lamivudine-resistant HBV mutants frequently emerge during treatment, with mutations occurring in the HBV polymerase gene. Up to two-thirds of patients develop recurrence of their HBV viremia within 3 years of therapy, which is manifest by the reappearance of HBV DNA in serum after its initial disappearance. Additionally, most patients, including children, will have an increase in their HBV viremia on discontinuing therapy.[176,180,181]

Indications

Lamivudine is indicated for the treatment of HIV in children aged 3 months and older as part of a combined antiretroviral regimen and for the treatment of chronic HBV infection in children aged 2 years and older with evidence of active viral replication and either evidence of persistent elevations in serum aminotransferases or histologically active disease. The dose used is lower than that to treat HIV.

Pharmacokinetics

After oral administration, lamivudine is rapidly absorbed with peak serum concentrations occurring between 0.5 to 2 hours. It can be administered as either a tablet or oral solution, and absorption is the same. Absolute bioavailability is above 80%, and volume of distribution suggests distribution into the extravascular spaces, and plasma protein binding is less than 36%. It has a half-life of less than 2 hours in children and 3.5 hours in adults.[175] The majority of lamivudine is eliminated unchanged in the urine by tubular secretion, and dosage needs to be adjusted for renal impairment.

Adverse Effects

Lamivudine is generally well tolerated with few reported toxicities. In a prospective study for the treatment in children with chronic HBV infection, there were no reported adverse effects.[176] Rare side effects that have been attributed to lamivudine include pancreatitis, paresthesia, peripheral neuropathy, neutropenia, anemia, rashes, nausea, vomiting, and hair loss. A rare but potentially fatal side effect is lactic acidosis with severe hepatomegaly with steatosis. Most of these cases have been reported in adults, and lamivudine should immediately be discontinued in any patient who develops clinical or laboratory findings suggestive of lactic acidosis or pronounced hepatotoxicity. Patients should be monitored regularly during treatment by a physician experienced in the management of chronic HBV infection.[177]

ENTECAVIR (BARACLUDE)

Chemistry and Mechanism of Action

Entecavir is a guanosine nucleoside analog, which, after uptake by the cell, undergoes phosphorylation by cellular kinases to its active triphosphate form. Entecavir triphosphate inhibits HBV polymerase base priming, reverse transcription of the negative strand from the pregenomic messenger RNA, and synthesis of positive-strand HBV DNA. It is a weak inhibitor of cellular DNA polymerases. Entecavir is the most potent anti-HBV treatment currently available.[182–184]

Spectrum and Resistance

Entecavir triphosphate has demonstrated antiviral activity against both adefovir- and lamivudineresistant HBV strains. In vitro and in vivo data suggest that emergence of entecavir-resistant strains are rare in nucleoside-naïve patients. Five-year resistance rates are 1.2% in nucleoside-naïve and 51% in lamivudine-refractory patients. Several mutations have been identified in the HBV polymerase gene. Emergence of entecavir-resistant mutations is usually associated with virologic rebound during therapy.[185]

Indications

Entecavir has been licensed for the treatment of chronic HBV infection in children aged 16 years and older since 2005[185] and has since been FDA approved in March 2014 in children aged 2 years and older who weigh at least 10 kg.[186]

Pharmacokinetics

Entecavir is orally administered with good oral bioavailability; however, it needs to be given on an empty stomach as absorption is decreased by food.[187] Peak plasma concentrations occur between 0.5 to 1.5 hours after an oral dose, and steady state is achieved following 6 to 10 days of once-daily dosing. The intracellular half-life is around 15 hours. Approximately two-thirds to three-quarters of the drug are excreted unchanged in the urine and require dose adjustment in renal compromise.[185]

Adverse Effects

Entecavir is well tolerated with minimally reported side effects. In the phase 3 study of the safety and efficacy of entecavir in children, there have been no adverse events or abnormalities in growth parameters in those treated with the drug over placebo,[186] and there have been no significant adverse events reported in children in the postlicensure surveillance.

ADEFOVIR DIPIVOXIL (HEPSERA)

Chemistry and Mechanism of Action

Adefovir is an acyclic nucleotide analog of deoxyadenosine-5′-monophosphate. This compound is converted to the active adefovir diphosphate by host cellular adenylate kinase. Adefovir diphosphate then acts as a competitive inhibitor of deoxyadenosine triphosphate for viral DNA polymerase, resulting in DNA chain termination following its incorporation in HBV DNA.[188,189] Adefovir diphosphate also competitively inhibits deoxyadenosine triphosphate as a substrate for HIV-1 reverse transcriptase, resulting in chain termination following its incorporation in HIV DNA.

Activity and Resistance

Adefovir has demonstrated activity against both HBV and HIV-1. Resistance to adefovir is a limiting factor with prolonged use. Several mutations have been identified in the HBV polymerase, which confer in vitro and in vivo resistance. Rates of HBV resistance to adefovir at 1, 2, 4, and 5 years are 0%, 3%, 18%, and 29%, respectively.[190,191]

Indications

Adefovir has been studied in children with chronic HBV infection and was approved by the FDA for the treatment of chronic HBV infection in children aged 12 years and older in 2010.[192]

Pharmacokinetics

Adefovir dipivoxil is absorbed rapidly following orally administration and is not affected by food. Following absorption, adefovir dipivoxil is cleaved to adefovir by extracellular esterases. The plasma half-life at steady state is 7 hours, and the intracellular half-life of adefovir diphosphate is estimated to be 16 to 18 hours. Adefovir is excreted renally as unchanged drug, and dosing needs to be adjusted in patients with reduced renal function.[193]

Adverse Effects

In randomized clinical trials, the drug was well tolerated, with diarrhea, headache, and abdominal pain occurring only slightly more frequently in adefovir dipivoxil–treated patients compared to placebo.[191,194–196] Long-term administration can result in nephrotoxicity, but the risk is considered low in patients with normal baseline renal function.[191,197] There have been no serious adverse events reported in children in postlicensing surveillance.

TENOFOVIR DISOPROXIL FUMARATE (VIREAD)/TENOFOVIR ALAFENAMIDE FUMARATE (VEMLIDY)

Chemistry and Mechanism of Action

Tenofovir is an acyclic nucleotide analog with activity against both HBV and HIV. Tenofovir disoproxil fumarate (TDF) and tenofovir alafenamide fumarate (TAF) are both prodrugs of tenofovir. After oral absorption, the promoieties are cleaved, releasing tenofovir into systemic circulation. After cellular uptake, it undergoes phosphorylation by cellular enzymes to its active diphosphate form, which acts as a competitive inhibitor to viral reverse transcriptase.[198]

Spectrum and Resistance

Tenofovir is a potent inhibitor of HIV and HBV reverse transcriptase. The results of a longitudinal study of TDF treatment for chronic HBV demonstrated no development of resistance,[199] and although rare, a few case reports of resistance mutations in the HBV reverse transcriptase gene have since been reported.[200]

Indications

TDF is FDA approved for the treatment of chronic HBV infection in patients aged 2 years and older weighing at least 10 kg. It is also indicated for the treatment of HIV as part of a combined antiretroviral treatment protocol. Administration of TDF during pregnancy has demonstrated a reduction in perinatal transmission of HBV in women with high viral loads.[164] TAF is currently only approved for the treatment of adults, but clinical trials in pediatrics are ongoing (https://clinicaltrials.gov/ct2/show/NCT02932150).

Pharmacokinetics

Approximately 25% of an orally administered dose of TDF is absorbed, which is increased up to 40% with a high-fat meal. Binding to human plasma protein is less than 0.7% and serum proteins less than 7%, with a volume of distribution at steady state of 1.3 L per kg and 1.2 L per kg following IV administration of tenofovir of 1 mg per kg and 3 mg per kg, respectively. Tenofovir is not a substrate of CYP450 enzymes. Tenofovir is renally excreted, with 70% to 80% of an IV administered dose being recovered unchanged in the urine within 72 hours of dosing. It is recommended that the dosing interval of tenofovir be modified in patients with creatinine clearance less than 50 mL per minute, and it is efficiently removed by hemodialysis.[201]

TAF is more stable in plasma than TDF, provides higher intracellular levels of the active phosphorylated metabolite TFV-DP to target cells (HBV-infected hepatocytes and HIV-infected lymphoid cells), and is associated with approximately 90% lower circulating tenofovir levels relative to TDF at therapeutically active doses. As such, it offers the potential for a better safety profile, with fewer adverse effects on renal function and bone mineral density due to lower systemic tenofovir exposure.[202–204]

Adverse Effects

Renal impairment, including cases of acute renal failure and Fanconi syndrome, has been reported with TDF. The risk is increased with the concomitant administration of other nephrotoxic agents. In clinical trials, TDF was associated with a decrease in bone mineral density and increases in biochemical markers of bone metabolism, suggesting increased bone turnover. These findings were also demonstrated in pediatric studies, both for HIV and chronic HBV.

Lactic acidosis and severe hepatomegaly with steatosis, including fatal cases, have been reported with TDF. Given the lower systemic exposure to tenofovir with TAF, the renal impairments and bone metabolism effects are greatly reduced.[204]

TELBIVUDINE (TYZEKA)

Chemistry and Mechanism of Action

Telbivudine is the unmodified L-enantiomer of the naturally occurring nucleoside D-thymidine. After uptake into the cell, host cell kinases phosphorylate telbivudine to telbivudine-5′-triphosphate, which then is incorporated into HBV DNA resulting in viral DNA chain termination.[205]

Spectrum and Resistance

Telbivudine is active only against hepadnaviruses. Telbivudine resistance mutations have been demonstrated. The principle mutations conferring in vivo lamivudine resistance do not produce cross-resistance to telbivudine. Telbivudine retains activity in vitro against adefovir-resistant HBV strains.[206]

Indications

Telbivudine was FDA approved in October 2006 for the treatment of chronic HBV in adolescents and adults aged 16 years and older.[207,208] A phase 3 clinical trial to evaluate the safety and efficacy of telbivudine in the treatment of chronic HBV infection in children aged 2 years and older was completed in January 2019, with results pending at this time (https://clinicaltrials.gov/ct2/show/NCT02058108).

Pharmacokinetics

Telbivudine is administered orally and is rapidly absorbed. Absorption is not influenced by food. The plasma half-life of telbivudine is about 40 hours. Approximately 40% of the dose is excreted unchanged by the kidneys requiring dose adjustment in renal impairment. Dosage adjustment is not required for patients with impaired hepatic function.[207,208]

Adverse Effects

Side effects reported include fatigue, abdominal pain, cough, and elevated creatinine phosphokinase. Significant myopathy can occur, which should be monitored for and prompt discontinuation of the drug.[207,208]

THERAPIES FOR THE TREATMENT OF CHRONIC HEPATITIS C INFECTION

The early antiviral regimens were based on pegylated interferons with and without ribavirin. These regimens were complicated and poorly tolerated. Progress in understanding the biology of HCV has led to the development of direct-acting antiviral agents that target specific steps in the viral replication cycle, allowing for interferon-free regimens. The major classes of direct-acting antivirals include protease inhibitors, nucleotide polymerase inhibitors, non-nucleoside polymerase inhibitors, and the nonstructural 5A protein (NS5A)–directed inhibitors. These agents if given together have synergistic effects with each other, possibly by modulating different viral proteins to help suppress the emergence of resistant viruses.[209]

SOFOSBUVIR (SOVALDI)/LEDIPASVIR-SOFOSBUVIR (HARVONI)

Chemistry and Mechanism of Action

Sofosbuvir is a nucleotide analog inhibitor of HCV NS5B polymerase, which is the key enzyme mediating HCV RNA replication. After uptake by hepatocytes, sofosbuvir undergoes phosphorylation by cellular kinases to its active triphosphate form, which then competes with uridine to be incorporated by the HCV RNA polymerase into the elongating RNA primer strand, resulting in chain termination.[210] Ledipasvir is a potent inhibitor of HCV NS5A, a viral phosphoprotein that plays an important role in viral replication, assembly, and secretion.[211]

Spectrum and Resistance

Sofosbuvir was initially approved for treatment of HCV genotypes 2 and 3 in combination with ribavirin and for genotypes 1 and 4 in combination with pegylated interferon plus ribavirin regimens. Resistance occurs due to mutations in the RNA-dependent RNA polymerase; however, these mutations are poorly tolerated and tend to not persist on cessation of the drug.[212] Due to the conserved structural feature of domain 1 of NS5A, ledipasvir is highly effective against all HCV genotypes, but if given alone has a low genetic barrier to resistance with rapid selection of resistant mutants. Development of resistance is overcome by the administration of a combination of sofosbuvir with ledipasvir, providing antiviral activity against all genotypes of HCV.[212,213]

Indications

These drugs are indicated for the treatment of chronic HCV infection[214] and, as a combination, were approved in April 2017 for the treatment of chronic HCV in children and adolescents aged 12 years and older or weighing at least 35 kg with HCV genotype 1, 4, 5, or 6 infection without cirrhosis or with compensated cirrhosis. A phase 2, multicenter open-label study of ledipasvir-sofosbuvir in children aged 12 to 17 years demonstrated the drug was well tolerated with sustained virologic response 12 weeks post-treatment.[215] Additionally, ongoing studies in younger children are indicating that ledipasvir-sofosbuvir is both safe and effective.[216,217]

Pharmacokinetics

Both these drugs are orally absorbed, can be administered without regard to food, and do not require dose adjustment in patients with any degree of hepatic impairment or mild-to-moderate renal impairment. Following oral administration of Harvoni, ledipasvir median peak concentrations occur approximately 4 to

4.5 hours postdose, and sofosbuvir is absorbed quickly, with a median peak concentration occurring within 1 hour postdose. Approximately 65% of sofosbuvir is bound to human plasma proteins, and virtually, all ledipasvir is plasma protein bound. Sofosbuvir is extensively metabolized in the liver to form the pharmacologically active nucleoside analog triphosphate as well as an inactive dephosphorylated metabolite, which accounts for more than 90% of the total systemic exposure and is predominantly renally excreted. The median terminal half-life of sofosbuvir is 0.5 hours, and 27 hours for the inactive dephosphorylated metabolite. In comparison, ledipasvir does not undergo hepatic metabolism, and more than 98% of systemic exposure is due to the parent drug and is mostly recovered unchanged in the feces, with biliary excretion being the major route of elimination. The median terminal half-life is 47 hours.[218]

Adverse Effects

A serious risk of hepatitis flare due to reactivation of untreated HBV in coinfected patients can occur if the patient is not on HBV-specific therapy. Serious symptomatic bradycardia has been reported in patients if administering sofosbuvir with amiodarone.[219] Other reported side effects include headache, diarrhea, and fatigue.[213,218]

GLECAPREVIR/PIBRENTASVIR (MAVYRET)

Chemistry and Mechanism of Action

Glecaprevir is an NS3/4A protease inhibitor that prevents the cleavage of the HCV polyprotein. Pibrentasvir is an NS5A inhibitor, a nonstructural viral phosphoprotein involved in viral replication, assembly, and secretion.

Spectrum and Resistance

Glecaprevir and pibrentasvir have demonstrated potent antiviral activity across all HCV genotypes, including common HCV genotype 1 variants that are resistant to older-generation HCV protease inhibitors. Selection of resistance mutations, usually due to individual amino acid substitutions in both the NS3 and NS5A proteins, has been demonstrated in both cell culture and clinical trials.[220]

Indications

Glecaprevir/pibrentasvir is indicated for the treatment of chronic HCV infection of all genotypes in patients aged 12 years and older. Based on clinical trials demonstrating high cure rates in adults, it was FDA approved for adults in 2017.[221] These findings were demonstrated in adolescents,[222] leading to FDA approval in 2019 for children aged 12 years and older, and clinical trials in children aged 3 to 11 years are ongoing (https://clinicaltrials.gov/ct2/show/NCT03067129).

Pharmacokinetics

Oral absorption is improved when administered with a meal for both agents with a peak serum concentration around 5 hours. Both are highly protein bound, in excess of 95%. Both agents are metabolized in the liver, and mode of excretion is via the biliary–fecal route. The elimination half-life for glecaprevir is approximately 6 hours, and pibrentasvir is 13 hours. Only 0.7% of the dose of glecaprevir is recovered in the urine, and there is no renal excretion of pibrentasvir. As such, these agents can be administered without dose adjustment in patients with renal impairment, including those on dialysis. No dosage adjustment is required for mild hepatic impairment, but their use is contraindicated in patients with moderate-to-severe hepatic impairment.[220,223]

Adverse Effects

The main reported side effects include headache, nausea, and diarrhea. A major risk is reactivation of HBV in coinfected patients not receiving HBV antiviral therapy, which can lead to fulminant hepatitis and death. Elevations of total bilirubin at least twice the upper limit of normal occurred in 3.5% of patients treated in the clinical trials, compared to placebo, possibly due to Mavyret being an inhibitor of OATP1B1/3 as well as a weak inhibitor of UGT1A1. Levels returned to normal on cessation of the drug. As Mavyret is metabolized in the liver, there are several known interactions with other hepatically metabolized medications requiring careful attention to coadministration, monitoring of drug levels, and dosage adjustments. A full list of known and potential interactions is found in the package insert.[220]

INTERFERONS AND PEGYLATED INTERFERONS

These are nonspecific regulatory proteins with antiviral, antiproliferative, and immunomodulating properties. Interferons do not have direct antiviral properties, but rather exert their effects through immune mediation. These agents have been administered in conjunction with other antiviral agents for the treatment of chronic HBV and HCV. A barrier to their use is they are administered by either subcutaneous or intramuscular injection and they have a wide range of side effects. As orally available effective and safe antivirals against HBV and HCV become available for use in children, they will replace the current regimens that rely on interferons.

ACKNOWLEDGMENT

Dr. Richard Whitley serves on the Board of Directors of Gilead Sciences Inc.

REFERENCES

1. Kimberlin DW, Lin CY, Jacobs RF, et al. Safety and efficacy of high-dose intravenous acyclovir in the management of neonatal herpes simplex virus infections. *Pediatrics* 2001;108(2):230–238.
2. Kimberlin DW, Whitley RJ, Wan W, et al. Oral acyclovir suppression and neurodevelopment after neonatal herpes. *N Engl J Med* 2011;365(14):1284–1292.
3. Kimberlin DW, Lin CY, Sanchez PJ, et al. Effect of ganciclovir therapy on hearing in symptomatic congenital cytomegalovirus disease involving the central nervous system: a randomized, controlled trial. *J Pediatr* 2003;143(1):16–25.
4. Kimberlin DW, Acosta EP, Prichard MN, et al. Oseltamivir pharmacokinetics, dosing, and resistance among children aged <2 years with influenza. *J Infect Dis* 2013;207(5):709–720.
5. Hayden FG, Sugaya N, Hirotsu N, et al. Baloxavir marboxil for uncomplicated influenza in adults and adolescents. *N Engl J Med* 2018;379(10):913–923.
6. Whitley RJ, Corey L, Arvin A, et al. Changing presentation of herpes simplex virus infection in neonates. *J Infect Dis* 1988;158(1):109–116.
7. Kimberlin DW, Lin CY, Jacobs RF, et al. Natural history of neonatal herpes simplex virus infections in the acyclovir era. *Pediatrics* 2001;108(2):223–229.
8. Whitley R, Davis EA, Suppapanya N. Incidence of neonatal herpes simplex virus infections in a managed-care population. *Sex Transm Dis* 2007;34(9):704–708.

9. Shah SS, Hall M, Schondelmeyer AC, et al. *Trends in neonatal herpes simplex virus infection in the United States, 2000-2012* [Abstract A195]. Presented at the Pediatric Hospital Medicine, Nashville, TN, July 20–23, 2017.
10. Whitley RJ, Nahmias AJ, Soong SJ, et al. Vidarabine therapy of neonatal herpes simplex virus infection. *Pediatrics* 1980;66(4):495–501.
11. Whitley RJ, Yeager A, Kartus P, et al. Neonatal herpes simplex virus infection: follow-up evaluation of vidarabine therapy. *Pediatrics* 1983;72(6):778–785.
12. Whitley R, Arvin A, Prober C, et al. A controlled trial comparing vidarabine with acyclovir in neonatal herpes simplex virus infection. Infectious Diseases Collaborative Antiviral Study Group. *N Engl J Med* 1991;324(7):444–449.
13. American Academy of Pediatrics. Varicella-zoster virus infections. In: Kimberlin DW, Brady MT, Jackson MA, eds. *Red book: 2018 report of the Committee on Infectious Diseases*, 31st ed. Itasca, IL: American Academy of Pediatrics, 2018:869–883.
14. Griffiths PD, Reeves M. Cytomegalovirus. In: Richman D, Whitley R, Hayden FG, eds. *Clinical virology*. Washington DC: ASM Press, 2017:481–510.
15. Colugnati FA, Staras SA, Dollard SC, et al. Incidence of cytomegalovirus infection among the general population and pregnant women in the United States. *BMC Infect Dis* 2007;7:71.
16. Demmler GJ. Infectious Diseases Society of America and Centers for Disease Control. Summary of a workshop on surveillance for congenital cytomegalovirus disease. *Rev Infect Dis* 1991;13(2):315–329.
17. Conboy TJ, Pass RF, Stagno S, et al. Early clinical manifestations and intellectual outcome in children with symptomatic congenital cytomegalovirus infection. *J Pediatr* 1987;111(3):343–348.
18. Ross SA, Boppana SB. Congenital cytomegalovirus infection: outcome and diagnosis. *Semin Pediatr Infect Dis* 2005;16(1):44–49.
19. Dollard SC, Grosse SD, Ross DS. New estimates of the prevalence of neurological and sensory sequelae and mortality associated with congenital cytomegalovirus infection. *Rev Med Virol* 2007;17(5):355–363.
20. Maschmann J, Hamprecht K, Dietz K, et al. Cytomegalovirus infection of extremely low-birth weight infants via breast milk. *Clin Infect Dis* 2001;33(12):1998–2003.
21. Brasfield DM, Stagno S, Whitley RJ, et al. Infant pneumonitis associated with cytomegalovirus, chlamydia, pneumocystis, and urea plasma: follow-up. *Pediatrics* 1987;79(1):76–83.
22. Oliver SE, Cloud GA, Sanchez PJ, et al. Neurodevelopmental outcomes following ganciclovir therapy in symptomatic congenital cytomegalovirus infections involving the central nervous system. *J Clin Virol* 2009;46 (Suppl 4):S22–S26.
23. Kimberlin DW, Jester PM, Sanchez PJ, et al. Valganciclovir for symptomatic congenital cytomegalovirus disease. *N Engl J Med* 2015;372(10):933–943.
24. American Academy of Pediatrics. Cytomegalovirus infection. In: Kimberlin DW, Brady MT, Jackson MA, eds. *Red book: 2018 report of the Committee on Infectious Diseases*, 31st ed. Itasca IL: American Academy of Pediatrics, 2018:310–316.
25. Rawlinson WD, Boppana SB, Fowler KB, et al. Congenital cytomegalovirus infection in pregnancy and the neonate: consensus recommendations for prevention, diagnosis, and therapy. *Lancet Infect Dis* 2017;17(6):e177–e188.
26. Chan ST, Logan AC. The clinical impact of cytomegalovirus infection following allogeneic hematopoietic cell transplantation: why the quest for meaningful prophylaxis still matters. *Blood Rev* 2017;31(3):173–183.
27. Markham A, Faulds D. Ganciclovir. An update of its therapeutic use in cytomegalovirus infection. *Drugs* 1994;48(3):455–484.
28. Elion GB. Mechanism of action and selectivity of acyclovir. *Am J Med* 1982;73(1A):7–13.
29. Reardon JE, Spector T. Herpes simplex virus type 1 DNA polymerase. Mechanism of inhibition by acyclovir triphosphate. *J Biol Chem* 1989;264(13):7405–7411.
30. Lai L, Xu Z, Zhou J, et al. Molecular basis of prodrug activation by human valacyclovirase, an alpha-amino acid ester hydrolase. *J Biol Chem* 2008;283(14):9318–9327.
31. Kimberlin DW. Antiviral agents. In: Long SS, Pickering LK, Prober CG, eds. *Principles and practice of pediatric infectious diseases*. Philadelphia, PA: Churchill Livingstone Elsevier, 2008:1470–1488.
32. Field AK, Biron KK. "The end of innocence" revisited: resistance of herpesviruses to antiviral drugs. *Clin Microbiol Rev* 1994;7(1):1–13.
33. Gateley A, Gander RM, Johnson PC, et al. Herpes simplex virus type 2 meningoencephalitis resistant to acyclovir in a patient with AIDS. *J Infect Dis* 1990;161(4):711–715.
34. Kakiuchi S, Tsuji M, Nishimura H, et al. Association of the emergence of acyclovir-resistant herpes simplex virus type 1 with prognosis in hematopoietic stem cell transplantation patients. *J Infect Dis* 2017;215(6):865–873.
35. Kost RG, Hill EL, Tigges M, et al. Brief report: recurrent acyclovir-resistant genital herpes in an immunocompetent patient. *N Engl J Med* 1993;329(24):1777–1782.
36. Laufer DS, Starr SE. Resistance to antivirals. *Pediatr Clin North Am* 1995;42(3):583–599.
37. Kimberlin D, Powell D, Gruber W, et al. Administration of oral acyclovir suppressive therapy after neonatal herpes simplex virus disease limited to the skin, eyes and mouth: results of a phase I/II trial. *Pediatr Infect Dis J* 1996;15(3):247–254.
38. Lyall EG, Ogilvie MM, Smith NM, et al. Acyclovir resistant varicella zoster and HIV infection. *Arch Dis Child* 1994;70(2):133–135.
39. Sauerbrei A, Taut J, Zell R, et al. Resistance testing of clinical varicella-zoster virus strains. *Antiviral Res* 2011;90(3):242–247.
40. Wagstaff AJ, Faulds D, Goa KL. Aciclovir. A reappraisal of its antiviral activity, pharmacokinetic properties and therapeutic efficacy. *Drugs* 1994;47(1):153–205.
41. Laskin OL, Longstreth JA, Whelton A, et al. Effect of renal failure on the pharmacokinetics of acyclovir. *Am J Med* 1982;73(1A):197–201.
42. Krasny HC, Liao SH, de Miranda P, et al. Influence of hemodialysis on acyclovir pharmacokinetics in patients with chronic renal failure. *Am J Med* 1982;73(1A):202–204.
43. Jacobson MA. Valaciclovir (BW256U87): the L-valyl ester of acyclovir. *J Med Virol* 1993; Suppl 1:150–153.
44. Nadal D, Leverger G, Sokal EM, et al. An investigation of the steady-state pharmacokinetics of oral valacyclovir in immunocompromised children. *J Infect Dis* 2002;186(Suppl 1):S123–S130.
45. Kimberlin DW, Jacobs RF, Weller S, et al. Pharmacokinetics and safety of extemporaneously compounded valacyclovir oral suspension in pediatric patients from 1 month through 11 years of age. *Clin Infect Dis* 2010;50(2):221–228.
46. Soul-Lawton J, Seaber E, On N, et al. Absolute bioavailability and metabolic disposition of valaciclovir, the L-valyl ester of acyclovir, following oral administration to humans. *Antimicrob Agents Chemother* 1995. 39(12):2759–2764.
47. Tilson HH. Monitoring the safety of antivirals. The example of the acyclovir experience. *Am J Med* 1988;85(2A):116–122.
48. Rao S, Abzug MJ, Carosone-Link P, et al. Intravenous acyclovir and renal dysfunction in children: a matched case control study. *J Pediatr* 2015;166(6):1462–1468.e1–4.
49. Steinberg I, Kimberlin DW. Acyclovir dosing and acute kidney injury: deviations and direction. *J Pediatr* 2015;166(6):1341–1344.
50. American Academy of Pediatrics. Herpes simplex. In: Kimberlin DW, Brady MT, Jackson MA, eds. *Red book: 2018 report of the Committee on Infectious Diseases*, 31st ed. Itasca, IL: American Academy of Pediatrics, 2018:437–449.
51. Revankar SG, Applegate AL, Markovitz DM. Delirium associated with acyclovir treatment in a patient with renal failure. *Clin Infect Dis* 1995;21(2):435–436.
52. Saez-Llorens X, Yogev R, Arguedas A, et al. Pharmacokinetics and safety of famciclovir in children with herpes simplex or varicella-zoster virus infection. *Antimicrob Agents Chemother* 2009;53(5):1912–1920.
53. Blumer J, Rodriguez A, Sanchez PJ, et al. Single-dose pharmacokinetics of famciclovir in infants and population pharmacokinetic analysis in infants and children. *Antimicrob Agents Chemother* 2010;54(5):2032–2041.
54. Littler E, Stuart AD, Chee MS. Human cytomegalovirus UL97 open reading frame encodes a protein that phosphorylates the antiviral nucleoside analogue ganciclovir. *Nature* 1992;358(6382):160–162.
55. Faulds D, Heel RC. Ganciclovir. A review of its antiviral activity, pharmacokinetic properties and therapeutic efficacy in cytomegalovirus infections. *Drugs* 1990;39(4):597–638.
56. Smee DF, Martin JC, Verheyden JP, et al. Anti-herpesvirus activity of the acyclic nucleoside 9-(1,3-dihydroxy-2-propoxymethyl)guanine. *Antimicrob Agents Chemother* 1983;23(5):676–682.
57. Wald A. New therapies and prevention strategies for genital herpes. *Clin Infect Dis* 1999;28(Suppl 1):S4–S13.
58. Reddy V, Hao Y, Lipton J, et al. Management of allogeneic bone marrow transplant recipients at risk for cytomegalovirus disease using a surveillance bronchoscopy and prolonged pre-emptive ganciclovir therapy. *J Clin Virol* 1999;13(3):149–159.
59. Frenkel LM, Capparelli EV, Dankner WM, et al. Oral ganciclovir in children: pharmacokinetics, safety, tolerance, and antiviral effects. *J Infect Dis* 2000;182(6):1616–1624.
60. Trang JM, Kidd L, Gruber W, et al. Linear single-dose pharmacokinetics of ganciclovir in newborns with congenital cytomegalovirus infections. *Clin Pharmacol Ther* 1993;53(1):15–21.
61. Swan SK, Munar MY, Wigger MA, et al. Pharmacokinetics of ganciclovir in a patient undergoing hemodialysis. *Am J Kidney Dis* 1991;17(1):69–72.
62. Jung D, Dorr A. Single-dose pharmacokinetics of valganciclovir in HIV-and CMV-seropositive subjects. *J Clin Pharmacol* 1999;39(8):800–804.
63. Brown F, Banken L, Saywell K, et al. Pharmacokinetics of valganciclovir and ganciclovir following multiple oral dosages of valganciclovir in HIV-and CMV-seropositive volunteers. *Clin Pharmacokinet* 1999;37(2):167–176.
64. Cocohoba JM, McNicholl IR. Valganciclovir: an advance in cytomegalovirus therapeutics. *Ann Pharmacother* 2002;36(6):1075–1079.
65. Wiltshire H, Hirankarn S, Farrell C, et al. Pharmacokinetic profile of ganciclovir after its oral administration and from its prodrug, valganciclovir, in solid organ transplant recipients. *Clin Pharmacokinet* 2005;44(5):495–507.
66. Kimberlin DW, Acosta EP, Sanchez PJ, et al. Pharmacokinetic and pharmacodynamic assessment of oral valganciclovir in the treatment of symptomatic congenital cytomegalovirus disease. *J Infect Dis* 2008;197(6):836–845.
67. Czock D, Scholle C, Rasche FM, et al. Pharmacokinetics of valganciclovir and ganciclovir in renal impairment. *Clin Pharmacol Ther* 2002;72(2):142–150.
68. Kimberlin DW, Brady MT, Jackson MA, et al., eds. Red *book: 2015 report* of the Committee on Infectious Diseases, 30th ed. Elk Grove Village, IL: American Academy of Pediatrics, 2015.
69. Crumpacker CS. Mechanism of action of foscarnet against viral polymerases. *Am J Med* 1992;92(2A):3S–7S.
70. Wagstaff AJ, Bryson H.M. Foscarnet. A reappraisal of its antiviral activity, pharmacokinetic properties and therapeutic use in immunocompromised patients with viral infections. *Drugs* 1994;48(2):199–226.
71. Safrin S, Kemmerly S, Plotkin B, et al. Foscarnet-resistant herpes simplex virus infection in patients with AIDS. *J Infect Dis* 1994;169(1):193–196.
72. Snoeck R, Andrei G, Gerard M, et al. Successful treatment of progressive mucocutaneous infection due to acyclovir-and foscarnet-resistant herpes simplex virus with (S)-1-(3-hydroxy-2-phosphonylmethoxypropyl)cytosine (HPMPC). *Clin Infect Dis* 1994;18(4):570–578.
73. Jacobson MA, Drew WL, Feinberg J, et al. Foscarnet therapy for ganciclovir-resistant cytomegalovirus retinitis in patients with AIDS. *J Infect Dis* 1991;163(6):1348–1351.
74. Dieterich DT, Poles MA, Lew EA, et al. Concurrent use of ganciclovir and foscarnet to treat cytomegalovirus infection in AIDS patients. *J Infect Dis* 1993;167(5):1184–1188.
75. Vora SB, Brothers AW, Waghmare A, et al. Antiviral combination therapy for cytomegalovirus infection in high-risk infants. *Antivir Ther* 2018;23(6):505–511.
76. Knorr B, Kessler U, Poschl J, et al. A haemophagocytic lymphohistiocytosis (HLH)-like picture following breastmilk transmitted cytomegalovirus infection in a preterm infant. *Scand J Infect Dis* 2007;39(2):173–176.
77. Levin MJ, Weinberg A, Leary JJ, et al. Development of acyclovir-resistant herpes simplex virus early during the treatment of herpes neonatorum. *Pediatr Infect Dis J* 2001;20(11):1094–1097.
78. Nyquist AC, Rotbart HA, Cotton M, et al. Acyclovir-resistant neonatal herpes simplex virus infection of the larynx. *J Pediatr* 1994;124(6):967–971.

79. Hengge UR, Brockmeyer NH, Malessa R, et al. Foscarnet penetrates the blood-brain barrier: rationale for therapy of cytomegalovirus encephalitis. *Antimicrob Agents Chemother* 1993;37(5):1010–1014.
80. Safrin S, Berger TG, Gilson I, et al. Foscarnet therapy in five patients with AIDS and acyclovir-resistant varicella-zoster virus infection. *Ann Intern Med* 1991;115(1):19–21.
81. MacGregor RR, Graziani AL, Weiss R, et al. Successful foscarnet therapy for cytomegalovirus retinitis in an AIDS patient undergoing hemodialysis: rationale for empiric dosing and plasma level monitoring. *J Infect Dis* 1991;164(4):785–787.
82. Deray G, Martinez F, Katlama C, et al. Foscarnet nephrotoxicity: mechanism, incidence and prevention. *Am J Nephrol* 1989;9(4):316–321.
83. Jacobson MA, Gambertoglio JG, Aweeka FT, et al. Foscarnet-induced hypocalcemia and effects of foscarnet on calcium metabolism. *J Clin Endocrinol Metab* 1991;72(5):1130–1135.
84. Palestine AG, Polis MA, De Smet MD, et al. A randomized, controlled trial of foscarnet in the treatment of cytomegalovirus retinitis in patients with AIDS. *Ann Intern Med* 1991;115(9):665–673.
85. Ho HT, Woods KL, Bronson JJ, et al. Intracellular metabolism of the antiherpes agent (S)-1-[3-hydroxy-2-(phosphonylmethoxy)propyl]cytosine. *Mol Pharmacol* 1992;41(1):197–202.
86. Yang H, Datema R. Prolonged and potent therapeutic and prophylactic effects of (S)-1-[(3-hydroxy-2-phosphonylmethoxy)propyl]cytosine against herpes simplex virus type 2 infections in mice. *Antimicrob Agents Chemother* 1991;35(8):1596–1600.
87. Safrin S, Cherrington J, Jaffe HS. Cidofovir. Review of current and potential clinical uses. *Adv Exp Med Biol* 1999;458:111–120.
88. Lurain NS, Thompson KD, Holmes EW, et al. Point mutations in the DNA polymerase gene of human cytomegalovirus that result in resistance to antiviral agents. *J Virol* 1992;66(12):7146–7152.
89. Cherrington JM, Miner R, Allen SJW, et al. *Sensitivities of human cytomegalovirus (HCMV) clinical isolates to cidofovir.* Presented at the 8th International Conference on Antiviral Research, Sante Fe, NM, April 23–28, 1995.
90. Sullivan V, Biron KK, Talarico C, et al. A point mutation in the human cytomegalovirus DNA polymerase gene confers resistance to ganciclovir and phosphonylmethoxyalkyl derivatives. *Antimicrob Agents Chemother* 1993;37(1):19–25.
91. Parenteral cidofovir for cytomegalovirus retinitis in patients with AIDS: the HPMPC peripheral cytomegalovirus retinitis trial. A randomized, controlled trial. Studies of Ocular Complications of AIDS Research Group in collaboration with the AIDS Clinical Trials Group. *Ann Intern Med* 1997;126(4):264–274.
92. Lalezari JP, Stagg RJ, Kuppermann BD, et al. Intravenous cidofovir for peripheral cytomegalovirus retinitis in patients with AIDS. A randomized, controlled trial. *Ann Intern Med* 1997;126(4):257–263.
93. Fanourgiakis P, Georgala A, Vekemans M, et al. Intravesical instillation of cidofovir in the treatment of hemorrhagic cystitis caused by adenovirus type 11 in a bone marrow transplant recipient. *Clin Infect Dis* 2005;40(1):199–201.
94. Hatakeyama N, Suzuki N, Kudoh T, et al. Successful cidofovir treatment of adenovirus-associated hemorrhagic cystitis and renal dysfunction after allogenic bone marrow transplant. *Pediatr Infect Dis J* 2003;22(10):928–929.
95. Carter BA, Karpen SJ, Quiros-Tejeira RE, et al. Intravenous cidofovir therapy for disseminated adenovirus in a pediatric liver transplant recipient. *Transplantation* 2002;74(7):1050–1052.
96. Kadambi PV, Josephson MA, Williams J, et al. Treatment of refractory BK virus-associated nephropathy with cidofovir. *Am J Transplant* 2003;3(2):186–191.
97. Vats A, Shapiro R, Singh Randhawa P, et al. Quantitative viral load monitoring and cidofovir therapy for the management of BK virus-associated nephropathy in children and adults. *Transplantation* 2003;75(1):105–112.
98. Ronchi A, Doern C, Brock E, et al. Neonatal adenoviral infection: a seventeen year experience and review of the literature. *J Pediatr* 2014;164(3):529–535.e1–4.
99. Bronson JJ, Ferrara LM, Hitchcock MJ, et al. (S)-1-(3-hydroxy-2-(phosphonylmethoxy)propyl)cytosine (HPMPC): a potent antiherpesvirus agent. *Adv Exp Med Biol* 1990;278:277–283.
100. Cundy KC, Petty BG, Flaherty J, et al. Clinical pharmacokinetics of cidofovir in human immunodeficiency virus-infected patients. *Antimicrob Agents Chemother* 1995;39(6): 1247–1252.
101. Lalezari JP, Drew WL, Glutzer E, et al. (S)-1-[3-hydroxy-2-(phosphonylmethoxy)propyl] cytosine (cidofovir): results of a phase I/II study of a novel antiviral nucleotide analogue. *J Infect Dis* 1995;171(4):788–796.
102. Lalezari JP, Drew WL, Glutzer E, et al. Treatment with intravenous (S)-1-[3-hydroxy-2-(phosphonylmethoxy)propyl]-cytosine of acyclovir-resistant mucocutaneous infection with herpes simplex virus in a patient with AIDS. *J Infect Dis* 1994;170(3):570–572.
103. Goldner T, Hewlett G, Ettischer N, et al. The novel anticytomegalovirus compound AIC246 (Letermovir) inhibits human cytomegalovirus replication through a specific antiviral mechanism that involves the viral terminase. *J Virol* 2011;85(20):10884–10893.
104. Ligat G, Cazal R, Hantz S, et al. The human cytomegalovirus terminase complex as an antiviral target: a close-up view. *FEMS Microbiol Rev* 2018;42(2):137–145.
105. Jung S, Michel M, Stamminger T, et al. Fast breakthrough of resistant cytomegalovirus during secondary letermovir prophylaxis in a hematopoietic stem cell transplant recipient. *BMC Infect Dis* 2019;19(1):388.
106. Marty FM, Ljungman P, Chemaly RF, et al. Letermovir prophylaxis for cytomegalovirus in hematopoietic-cell transplantation. *N Engl J Med* 2017;377(25):2433–2444.
107. Prevymis package insert. Whitehouse Station, NJ: Merck and Co. Inc., 2017. https://www.fda.gov/drugs/drug-approvals-and-databases/drug-trials-snapshots-prevymis.
108. Treanor JJ, Hayden FG, Vrooman PS, et al. Efficacy and safety of the oral neuraminidase inhibitor oseltamivir in treating acute influenza: a randomized controlled trial. US Oral Neuraminidase Study Group. *JAMA* 2000;283(8):1016–1024.
109. Gubareva LV. Molecular mechanisms of influenza virus resistance to neuraminidase inhibitors. *Virus Res* 2004;103(1–2):199–203.
110. Kiso M, Mitamura K, Sakai-Tagawa Y, et al. Resistant influenza A viruses in children treated with oseltamivir: descriptive study. *Lancet* 2004;364(9436):759–765.
111. Takashita E, Kiso M, Fujisaki S, et al. Characterization of a large cluster of influenza A(H1N1)pdm09 viruses cross-resistant to oseltamivir and peramivir during the 2013-2014 influenza season in Japan. *Antimicrob Agents Chemother* 2015;59(5):2607–2617. doi:10.1128/AAC.04836-14. Epub February 17, 2015.
112. Covington E, Mendel DB, Escarpe PA, et al. *Phenotypic and genotypic assay of influenza virus neuraminidase indicates a low incidence of viral drug resistance during treatment with oseltamivir.* Presented at the 11th International Symposium on Influenza and other Respiratory Viruses, Grand Cayman, 1999.
113. Tamiflu (oseltamivir phosphate) package insert. Foster City, CA: Gilead Sciences, Inc., 2008. https://www.fda.gov/downloads/drugs/drugsafety/informationbydrugclass/ucm147992.pdf.
114. Treanor JJ, Hayden FG, Vrooman PS, et al. Efficacy and safety of the oral neuraminidase inhibitor oseltamivir in treating acute influenza: a randomized controlled trial. US Oral Neuraminidase Study Group. *JAMA* 2000;283(8):1016–1024.
115. Nicholson KG, Aoki FY, Osterhaus AD, et al. Efficacy and safety of oseltamivir in treatment of acute influenza: a randomised controlled trial. Neuraminidase Inhibitor Flu Treatment Investigator Group. *Lancet* 2000;355(9218):1845–1850.
116. Wood ND, Aitken M, Sharp S, et al. *Tolerability and pharmacokinetics of the influenza neuraminidase inhibitor Ro-64-0802 (GS4071) following oral administration of the prodrug Ro-64-0796 (GS4104) to healthy male volunteers.* Presented at the 37th Interscience Conference on Antimicrobial Agents and Chemotherapy (ICAAC), Toronto, 1997.
117. He G, Massarella J, Ward P. Clinical pharmacokinetics of the prodrug oseltamivir and its active metabolite Ro 64-0802. *Clin Pharmacokinet* 1999;37(6):471–484.
118. Hayden FG, Treanor JJ, Fritz RS, et al. Use of the oral neuraminidase inhibitor oseltamivir in experimental human influenza: randomized controlled trials for prevention and treatment. *JAMA* 1999;282(13):1240–1246.
119. Tamiflu (oseltamivir) – Safety Update on Neuropsychiatric Events; Review of Neuropsychiatric Events with other antiviral products. 2007. https://www.drugs.com/fda/tamiflu-oseltamivir-phosphate-mar-3-2008-12350.html.
120. Nguyen HT, Sheu TG, Mishin VP, et al. Assessment of pandemic and seasonal influenza A (H1N1) virus susceptibility to neuraminidase inhibitors in three enzyme activity inhibition assays. *Antimicrob Agents Chemother* 2010;54(9):3671–3677.
121. Gubareva LV, Matrosovich MN, Brenner MK, et al. Evidence for zanamivir resistance in an immunocompromised child infected with influenza B virus. *J Infect Dis* 1998;178(5):1257–1262.
122. Monto AS, Robinson DP, Herlocher ML, et al. Zanamivir in the prevention of influenza among healthy adults: a randomized controlled trial. *JAMA* 1999;282(1):31–35.
123. Kaiser L, Henry D, Flack NP, et al. Short-term treatment with zanamivir to prevent influenza: results of a placebo-controlled study. *Clin Infect Dis* 2000;30(3):587–589.
124. Hayden FG, Gubareva LV, Monto AS, et al. Inhaled zanamivir for the prevention of influenza in families. Zanamivir Family Study Group. *N Engl J Med* 2000;343(18):1282–1289.
125. Monto AS, Webster A, Keene O. Randomized, placebo-controlled studies of inhaled zanamivir in the treatment of influenza A and B: pooled efficacy analysis. *J Antimicrob Chemother* 1999;44:23–29.
126. Hedrick JA, Barzilai A, Behre U, et al. Zanamivir for treatment of symptomatic influenza A and B infection in children five to twelve years of age: a randomized controlled trial. *Pediatr Infect Dis J* 2000;19(5):410–417.
127. Marty FM, Vidal-Puigserver J, Clark C, et al. Intravenous zanamivir or oral oseltamivir for hospitalised patients with influenza: an international, randomised, double-blind, double-dummy, phase 3 trial. *Lancet Respir Med* 2017;5(2):135–146.
128. Bradley JS, Blumer JL, Romero JR, et al. Intravenous zanamivir in hospitalized patients with influenza. *Pediatrics* 2017;140(5).
129. Cass LM, Efthymiopoulos C, Marsh J, et al. Effect of renal impairment on the pharmacokinetics of intravenous zanamivir. *Clin Pharmacokinet* 1999;1:13–19.
130. Bergstrom M, Cass LM, Valind S, et al. Deposition and disposition of [11C]zanamivir following administration as an intranasal spray. Evaluation with positron emission tomography. *Clin Pharmacokinet* 1999;1:33–39.
131. Cass LM, Gunawardena KA, Macmahon MM, et al. Pulmonary function and airway responsiveness in mild to moderate asthmatics given repeated inhaled doses of zanamivir. *Respir Med* 2000;94(2):166–173.
132. Takashita E, Ejima M, Itoh R, et al. A community cluster of influenza A(H1N1)pdm09 virus exhibiting cross-resistance to oseltamivir and peramivir in Japan, November to December 2013. *Euro Surveill* 2014;19(1).(pii):20666.
133. Vanchiere J, Plunkett S, Annamalai R, et al. Single dose IV peramivir is safe and effective in the treatment of pediatric influenza. *Open Forum Infect Dis* 2017;4(Suppl 1): S694–S694.
134. de Jong MD, Ison MG, Monto AS, et al. Evaluation of intravenous peramivir for treatment of influenza in hospitalized patients. *Clin Infect Dis* 2014;59(12): e172–e185. doi:10.1093/cid/ciu632. Epub August 12, 2014.
135. Sugaya N, Kohno S, Ishibashi T, et al. Efficacy, safety, and pharmacokinetics of intravenous peramivir in children with 2009 pandemic H1N1 influenza A virus infection. *Antimicrob Agents Chemother* 2012;56(1):369–377. doi:10.1128/AAC.00132-11. Epub October 24, 2011.
136. Takashita E, Kawakami C, Morita H, et al. Detection of influenza A(H3N2) viruses exhibiting reduced susceptibility to the novel cap-dependent endonuclease inhibitor baloxavir in Japan, December 2018. *Euro Surveill* 2019;24(3).
137. Sidwell RW, Robins RK, Hillyard, IW. Ribavirin: an antiviral agent. *Pharmacol Ther* 1979;6(1):123–146.
138. Huggins JW. Prospects for treatment of viral hemorrhagic fevers with ribavirin, a broad-spectrum antiviral drug. *Rev Infect Dis* 1989;11(Suppl 4):S750–S761.
139. Gilbert BE, Knight V. Biochemistry and clinical applications of ribavirin. *Antimicrob Agents Chemother* 1986;30(2):201–205.

140. Hall CB, McBride JT, Walsh EE, et al. Aerosolized ribavirin treatment of infants with respiratory syncytial viral infection. A randomized double-blind study. *N Engl J Med* 1983;308(24):1443–1447.
141. Groothuis JR, Woodin KA, Katz R, et al. Early ribavirin treatment of respiratory syncytial viral infection in high-risk children. *J Pediatr* 1990;117(5):792–798.
142. Conrad DA, Christenson JC, Waner JL, et al. Aerosolized ribavirin treatment of respiratory syncytial virus infection in infants hospitalized during an epidemic. *Pediatr Infect Dis J* 1987;6(2):152–158.
143. Smith DW, Frankel LR, Mathers LH, et al. A controlled trial of aerosolized ribavirin in infants receiving mechanical ventilation for severe respiratory syncytial virus infection. *N Engl J Med* 1991;325(1):24–29.
144. Moler FW, Steinhart CM, Ohmit SE, et al. Effectiveness of ribavirin in otherwise well infants with respiratory syncytial virus-associated respiratory failure. Pediatric Critical Study Group. *J Pediatr* 1996;128(3):422–428.
145. Law BJ, Wang EE, MacDonald N, et al. Does ribavirin impact on the hospital course of children with respiratory syncytial virus (RSV) infection? An analysis using the pediatric investigators collaborative network on infections in Canada (PICNIC) RSV database. *Pediatrics* 1997;99(3):E7.
146. Shah DP, Ghantoji SS, Shah JN, et al. Impact of aerosolized ribavirin on mortality in 280 allogeneic haematopoietic stem cell transplant recipients with respiratory syncytial virus infections. *J Antimicrob Chemother* 2013;68(8):1872–1880.
147. Foolad F, Aitken SL, Shigle TL, et al. Oral versus aerosolized ribavirin for the treatment of respiratory syncytial virus infections in hematopoietic cell transplant recipients. *Clin Infect Dis* 2019;68(10):1641–1649.
148. Chavez-Bueno S, Mejias A, Merryman RA, et al. Intravenous palivizumab and ribavirin combination for respiratory syncytial virus disease in high-risk pediatric patients. *Pediatr Infect Dis J* 2007;26(12):1089–1093.
149. El-Bietar J, Nelson A, Wallace G, et al. RSV infection without ribavirin treatment in pediatric hematopoietic stem cell transplantation. *Bone Marrow Transplant* 2016;51(10):1382–1384.
150. Chemaly RF, Ghantoji SS, Shah DP, et al. Respiratory syncytial virus infections in children with cancer. *J Pediatr Hematol Oncol* 2014;36(6):e376–e381.
151. McCormick JB, King IJ, Webb PA, et al. Lassa fever. Effective therapy with ribavirin. *N Engl J Med* 1986;314(1):20–26.
152. Holmes GP, McCormick JB, Trock SC, et al. Lassa fever in the United States. Investigation of a case and new guidelines for management. *N Engl J Med* 1990;323(16):1120–1123.
153. McHutchison JG, Gordon SC, Schiff ER, et al. Interferon alfa-2b alone or in combination with ribavirin as initial treatment for chronic hepatitis C. Hepatitis Interventional Therapy Group. *N Engl J Med* 1998;339(21):1485–1492.
154. Poynard T, Marcellin P, Lee SS, et al. Randomised trial of interferon alpha2b plus ribavirin for 48 weeks or for 24 weeks versus interferon alpha2b plus placebo for 48 weeks for treatment of chronic infection with hepatitis C virus. International Hepatitis Interventional Therapy Group (IHIT). *Lancet* 1998;352(9138):1426–1432.
155. Knight V, Yu CP, Gilbert BE, et al. Estimating the dosage of ribavirin aerosol according to age and other variables. *J Infect Dis* 1988;158(2):443–448.
156. Connor JD, Hintz M, Van Dyke R, et al. Ribavirin pharmacokinetics in children and adults during therapeutic trials, In: Smith RA, Knight V, Smith JAD, eds. *Clinical applications of ribavirin*, New York, NY: Academic Press, 1984:107–230.
157. Laskin OL, Longstreth JA, Hart CC, et al. Ribavirin disposition in high-risk patients for acquired immunodeficiency syndrome. *Clin Pharmacol Ther* 1987;41(5):546–555.
158. Connor E, Morrison S, Lane J, et al. Safety, tolerance, and pharmacokinetics of systemic ribavirin in children with human immunodeficiency virus infection. *Antimicrob Agents Chemother* 1993;37(3):532–539.
159. Frankel LR, Wilson CW, Demers RR, et al. A technique for the administration of ribavirin to mechanically ventilated infants with severe respiratory syncytial virus infection. *Crit Care Med* 1987;15(11):1051–1054.
160. Shults RA, Baron S, Decker J, et al. Health care worker exposure to aerosolized ribavirin: biological and air monitoring. *J Occup Environ Med* 1996;38(3):257–263.
161. Bradley JS, Connor JD, Compogiannis LS, et al. Exposure of health care workers to ribavirin during therapy for respiratory syncytial virus infections. *Antimicrob Agents Chemother* 1990;34(4):668–670.
162. El-Shabrawi M, Hassanin F. Treatment of hepatitis B and C in children. *BMC Infect Dis* 2014;14(Suppl 6):S5. doi:10.1186/1471-2334-14-S6-S5. Epub September 19, 2014.
163. Schillie S, Walker T, Veselsky S, et al. Outcomes of infants born to women infected with hepatitis B. *Pediatrics* 2015;135(5):e1141–e1147.
164. Pan CQ, Duan Z, Dai E, et al. Tenofovir to prevent hepatitis b transmission in mothers with high viral load. *N Engl J Med* 2016;374(24):2324–2334.
165. Gower E, Estes C, Blach S, et al. Global epidemiology and genotype distribution of the hepatitis C virus infection. *J Hepatol* 2014;61(1 Suppl):S45–S57.
166. Denniston MM, Jiles RB, Drobeniuc J, et al. Chronic hepatitis C virus infection in the United States, National Health and Nutrition Examination Survey 2003 to 2010. *Ann Intern Med* 2014;160(5):293–300.
167. Benova L, Mohamoud YA, Calvert C, et al. Vertical transmission of hepatitis C virus: systematic review and meta-analysis. *Clin Infect Dis* 2014;59(6):65–773.
168. Delotte J, Barjoan EM, Berrebi A, et al. Obstetric management does not influence vertical transmission of HCV infection: results of the ALHICE group study. *J Matern Fetal Neonatal Med* 2014;27(7):664–670.
169. Cottrell EB, Chou R, Wasson N, et al. Reducing risk for mother-to-infant transmission of hepatitis C virus: a systematic review for the U.S. Preventive Services Task Force. *Ann Intern Med* 2013;158(2):109–113.
170. European Paediatric Hepatitis C Virus Network. A significant sex–but not elective cesarean section–effect on mother-to-child transmission of hepatitis C virus infection. *J Infect Dis* 2005;192(11):1872–1879.
171. Jhaveri R. Diagnosis and management of hepatitis C virus-infected children. *Pediatr Infect Dis J* 2011;30(11):983–985.
172. Goodman ZD, Makhlouf HR, Liu L, et al. Pathology of chronic hepatitis C in children: liver biopsy findings in the Peds-C Trial. *Hepatology* 2008;47(3):836–843.
173. Minola E, Prati D, Suter F, et al. Age at infection affects the long-term outcome of transfusion-associated chronic hepatitis C. *Blood* 2002;99(12):4588–4591.
174. American Association for the Study of Liver Diseases and the Infectious Diseases Society of America. HCV guidance: recommendations for testing, managing, and treating hepatitis C. HCV in children. 2019. https://www.hcvguidelines.org/unique-populations/children.
175. Lewis LL, Venzon D, Church J, et al. Lamivudine in children with human immunodeficiency virus infection: a phase I/II study. The National Cancer Institute Pediatric Branch-Human Immunodeficiency Virus Working Group. *J Infect Dis* 1996;174(1):16–25.
176. Hartman C, Berkowitz D, Shouval D, et al. Lamivudine treatment for chronic hepatitis B infection in children unresponsive to interferon. *Pediatr Infect Dis J* 2003;22(3):224–229.
177. Jennings R, Smith TL, Myhren F, et al. Evaluation of a novel, anti-herpes simplex virus compound, acyclovir elaidate (P-4010), in the female guinea pig model of genital herpes. *Antimicrob Agents Chemother* 1999;43(1):53–61.
178. Dienstag JL, Schiff ER, Wright TL, et al. Lamivudine as initial treatment for chronic hepatitis B in the United States. *N Engl J Med* 1999;341(17):1256–1263.
179. Lai CL, Chien RN, Leung NW, et al. A one-year trial of lamivudine for chronic hepatitis B. Asia Hepatitis Lamivudine Study Group. *N Engl J Med* 1998;339(2):61–68.
180. Liaw YF. Therapy of chronic hepatitis B: current challenges and opportunities. *J Viral Hepat* 2002;9(6):393–399.
181. Bain VG, Kneteman NM, Ma MM, et al. Efficacy of lamivudine in chronic hepatitis B patients with active viral replication and decompensated cirrhosis undergoing liver transplantation. *Transplantation* 1996;62(10):1456–1462.
182. Opio CK, Lee W.M, Kirkpatrick P. Entecavir. *Nat Rev Drug Discov* 2005;4(7):535–536.
183. Marion PL, Salazar FH, Winters MA, et al. Potent efficacy of entecavir (BMS200475) in a duck model of hepatitis B virus replication. *Antimicrob Agents Chemother* 2002;46(1):82–88.
184. Levine S, Hernandez D, Yamanaka G, et al. Efficacies of entecavir against lamivudine-resistant hepatitis B virus replication and recombinant polymerases in vitro. *Antimicrob Agents Chemother* 2002;46(8):2525–2532.
185. Baraclude (entecavir) package insert. Princeton, NJ: Bristol-Myers Squibb Company, 2015. https://packageinserts.bms.com/pi/pi_baraclude.pdf.
186. Jonas MM, Chang MH, Sokal E, et al. Randomized, controlled trial of entecavir versus placebo in children with hepatitis B envelope antigen-positive chronic hepatitis B. *Hepatology* 2016;63(2):377–387.
187. Shaw T, Locarnini S. Entecavir for the treatment of chronic hepatitis B. *Expert Rev Anti Infect Ther* 2004;2(6):853–871.
188. Torresi J, Locarnini SA. New therapeutic strategies in the treatment of hepatitis B virus infection. *Expert Opin Investig Drugs* 1999;8(3):289–305.
189. Torresi J, Locarnini S. Antiviral chemotherapy for the treatment of hepatitis B virus infections. *Gastroenterology* 2000;118(2 Suppl 1):S83–S103.
190. Yang H, Westland CE, Delaney WE, et al. Resistance surveillance in chronic hepatitis B patients treated with adefovir dipivoxil for up to 60 weeks. *Hepatology* 2002;36(2):464–473.
191. Hadziyannis SJ, Tassopoulos NC, Heathcote EJ, et al. Long-term therapy with adefovir dipivoxil for HBeAg-negative chronic hepatitis B for up to 5 years. *Gastroenterology* 2006;131(6):1743–1751.
192. Hepsera (adefovir dipivoxil) package insert. Foster City, CA: Gilead Sciences, Inc., 2012. https://www.accessdata.fda.gov/drugsatfda_docs/label/2012/021449s020lbl.pdf.
193. Adefovir package insert. Foster City, CA: Gilead Sciences, Inc., 2007. http://www.accessdata.fda.gov/drugsatfda_docs/label/2007/021449s011lbl.pdf.
194. Hadziyannis SJ, Tassopoulos NC, Heathcote EJ, et al. Long-term therapy with adefovir dipivoxil for HBeAg-negative chronic hepatitis B. *N Engl J Med* 2005;352(26):2673–2681.
195. Hadziyannis SJ, Tassopoulos NC, Heathcote EJ, et al. Adefovir dipivoxil for the treatment of hepatitis B e antigen-negative chronic hepatitis B. *N Engl J Med* 2003;348(9):800–807.
196. Marcellin P, Chang TT, Lim SG, et al. Adefovir dipivoxil for the treatment of hepatitis B e antigen-positive chronic hepatitis B. *N Engl J Med* 2003;348(9):808–816.
197. Perrillo R, Hann HW, Mutimer D, et al. Adefovir dipivoxil added to ongoing lamivudine in chronic hepatitis B with YMDD mutant hepatitis B virus. *Gastroenterology* 2004;126(1):81–90.
198. Delaney WE, Ray AS, Yang H, et al. Intracellular metabolism and in vitro activity of tenofovir against hepatitis B virus. *Antimicrob Agents Chemother* 2006;50(7):2471–2477.
199. Liu Y, Corsa AC, Buti M, et al. No detectable resistance to tenofovir disoproxil fumarate in HBeAg+ and HBeAg− patients with chronic hepatitis B after 8 years of treatment. *J Viral Hepat* 2017;24(1):68–74.
200. Cho WH, Lee HJ, Bang KB, et al. Development of tenofovir disoproxil fumarate resistance after complete viral suppression in a patient with treatment-naive chronic hepatitis B: a case report and review of the literature. *World J Gastroenterol* 2018;24(17):1919–1924.
201. Viread package insert. Foster City, CA: Gilead Sciences, Inc., 2008. https://www.viread.com/.
202. Vemlidy package insert. Foster City, CA: Gilead Sciences, Inc., 2019. https://www.gilead.com/-/media/files/pdfs/medicines/liver-disease/vemlidy/vemlidy_pi.
203. Chan HL, Fung S, Seto WK, et al. Tenofovir alafenamide versus tenofovir disoproxil fumarate for the treatment of HBeAg-positive chronic hepatitis B virus infection: a randomised, double-blind, phase 3, non-inferiority trial. *Lancet Gastroenterol Hepatol* 2016;1(3):185–195.
204. Buti M, Gane E, Seto WK, et al. Tenofovir alafenamide versus tenofovir disoproxil fumarate for the treatment of patients with HBeAg-negative chronic hepatitis B virus infection: a randomised, double-blind, phase 3, non-inferiority trial. *Lancet Gastroenterol Hepatol* 2016;1(3):196–206.
205. Keam SJ. Telbivudine. *Drugs* 2007;67(13):1917–1929.
206. Seifer M, Patty A, Serra I, et al. Telbivudine, a nucleoside analog inhibitor of HBV polymerase, has a different in vitro cross-resistance profile than the nucleotide analog inhibitors adefovir and tenofovir. *Antiviral Res* 2009;81(2):147–155.

207. Zhou XJ, Lim SG, Lloyd DM, et al. Pharmacokinetics of telbivudine following oral administration of escalating single and multiple doses in patients with chronic hepatitis B virus infection: pharmacodynamic implications. *Antimicrob Agents Chemother* 2006;50(3):874–879.
208. Stein DS, Ke J, Uy G, et al. Phase I, open-label, single-dose study to evaluate the pharmacokinetics and safety of telbivudine in children and adolescents with chronic hepatitis B. *Antimicrob Agents Chemother* 2013;57(9):4128–4133. doi:10.1128/AAC.00117-13.
209. Kohler JJ, Nettles JH, Amblard F, et al. Approaches to hepatitis C treatment and cure using NS5A inhibitors. *Infect Drug Resist* 2014;7:41–56.
210. Membreno FE, Lawitz EJ. The HCV NS5B nucleoside and non-nucleoside inhibitors. *J Org Chem* 2011;76(20):8311–8319. doi:10.1021/jo201492m. Epub September 26, 2011.
211. Pawlotsky JM. NS5A inhibitors in the treatment of hepatitis C. *Antimicrob Agents Chemother* 2013;57(12):6333–6340. doi:10.1128/AAC.02193-12. Epub July 22, 2013.
212. Kayali Z, Schmidt WN. Finally sofosbuvir: an oral anti-HCV drug with wide performance capability. *Pharmgenomics Pers Med* 2014;7:387–398.
213. German P, Mathias A, Brainard D, et al. Clinical pharmacokinetics and pharmacodynamics of ledipasvir/sofosbuvir, a fixed-dose combination tablet for the treatment of hepatitis C. *Clin Pharmacokinet* 2016;55(11):1337–1351.
214. Reddy KR, Bourliere M, Sulkowski M, et al. Ledipasvir and sofosbuvir in patients with genotype 1 hepatitis C virus infection and compensated cirrhosis: an integrated safety and efficacy analysis. *Hepatology* 2015;4(10):27826.
215. Balistreri WF, Murray KF, Rosenthal P, et al. The safety and effectiveness of ledipasvir-sofosbuvir in adolescents 12 to 17 years old with hepatitis C virus genotype 1 infection. *Hepatology* 2017;66(2):371–378.
216. Murray KF, Balistreri W, Bansal S, et al. *Ledipasvir/sofosbuvir ± ribavirin for 12 or 24 weeks is safe and effective in children 6–11 years old with chronic hepatitis C infection.* Presented at the International Liver Congress, Amsterdam, The Netherlands, April 19–23, 2017.
217. Schwartz K, Rosenthal P, Murray K, et al. *Ledipasvir/sofosbuvir for 12 weeks is safe and effective in children 3 to <6 years old with chronic hepatitis C virus infections.* Presented at the Annual Meeting of the American Association for the Study of Liver Disease, San Francisco, CA, November 9–13, 2018.
218. Harvoni package insert. Foster City, CA: Gilead Sciences, Inc., 2017. https://www.accessdata.fda.gov/drugsatfda_docs/label/2014/205834s000lbl.pdf.
219. Sovaldi package insert. Foster City, CA: Gilead Sciences, Inc., 2017. https://www.accessdata.fda.gov/drugsatfda_docs/label/2015/204671s002lbl.pdf.
220. Mavyret package insert. North Chicago, IL: AbbVie Inc., 2017. https://www.accessdata.fda.gov/drugsatfda_docs/label/2017/209394s000lbl.pdf.
221. Lamb YN. Glecaprevir/pibrentasvir: first global approval. *Drugs* 2017;77(16):1797–1804.
222. Jonas MM, Squires RH, Rhee SM, et al. Pharmacokinetics, safety, and efficacy of glecaprevir/pibrentasvir in adolescents with chronic HCV: part 1 of the DORA study. *Hepatology* 2020;71(2):456–462.
223. University of Washington. Hepatitis C Online. https://www.hepatitisc.uw.edu/page/treatment/drugs. Accessed 2019.

Rachel K. Scott
Mark Mirochnick
Brookie M. Best
Natella Rakhmanina

CHAPTER 32

Pharmacology of Antiretroviral Drugs in Pregnant and Breastfeeding Women and Their Newborns

INTRODUCTION

Currently, more than 30 antiretroviral (ARV) drugs in five classes are available in the United States, and several novel agents are in development (Table 32.1). The use of combination regimens of three or more ARVs, referred to as combination antiretroviral treatment (ART), has resulted in a dramatic improvement in HIV morbidity and mortality globally. However, while ART continues to prolong the lives of people living with HIV and to improve their health, it is unable to fully eradicate the virus and permanently cure the infection and, therefore, has to be continued for life. Current global, United States (U.S.), and European HIV treatment guidelines recommend universal initiation of lifelong ART following HIV diagnosis in all patients, including women of childbearing potential, pregnant, and breastfeeding women.[1–3] Studies of long-acting formulations of ARVs for both prevention and treatment of HIV are currently underway in adults and adolescents, including breastfeeding women, but pregnant women typically remain excluded from these clinical trials.[4]

HIV can be passed vertically from the mother to the child in three pathways: (a) across the placenta during pregnancy (transplacental), (b) through maternal blood and other bodily fluids during labor and delivery (intrapartum), and (c) through breast milk during nursing. In the absence of treatment, 15% to 45% of pregnant women living with HIV will transmit HIV to their infants, with 5% to 10% of infants born infected across the placenta, 10% to 20% infected from exposure at or around the time of delivery, and 10% to 20% infected from breast milk.[5] In the absence of maternal and infant ART, breastfed infants continue to have a risk of transmission of 0.6% to 0.9% for every month of breastfeeding, and the risk of transmission of HIV infection from breast milk is increased when infants received mixed feeding combining breastfeeding with formula, water, juice, and other liquids or solids.[6,7]

Despite significant progress in the reduction of AIDS-related deaths and new HIV infections during the first two decades of the third millennium, global targets for elimination of the HIV epidemic remain currently unreachable. A staggering 18.8 million women are living with HIV worldwide, mostly women of childbearing potential living in resource-limited settings.[8] The worldwide scale-up of universal HIV testing in pregnancy, provision of ART to pregnant and breastfeeding women, and infant prophylaxis has had a substantial impact, leading to a 60% reduction in new pediatric HIV infections in 21 high-burden resource-limited countries in sub-Saharan Africa, the region most heavily affected by the HIV epidemic.[9,10] In resource-rich settings, including the U.S. and European countries, the rate of perinatal HIV transmission has diminished to less than 2%.[11,12] Despite the overall decrease in perinatal transmission of HIV worldwide, new pediatric infections continue to occur, and the dynamics of infection of infants with HIV have recently shifted toward an increase in infection from breastfeeding during the postnatal period.[13–16] Currently, 1.7 million children younger than 15 years are estimated to be living with HIV globally, and 160,000 new pediatric infections, mostly driven by vertical transmission, occurred in 2018.[8]

GLOBAL RECOMMENDATIONS FOR USING ANTIRETROVIRAL DRUGS IN PREGNANT AND POSTPARTUM WOMEN AND THEIR NEONATES

THERAPEUTIC ANTIRETROVIRAL TREATMENT FOR WOMEN LIVING WITH HIV

In 1994, the National Institutes of Health (NIH)-sponsored PACTG 076 study demonstrated that a nucleoside/tide reverse transcriptase inhibitor (NRTI) zidovudine (ZDV) regimen comprised of oral dosing initiated at 14 to 34 weeks of gestation, continuous intravenous (IV) infusion during labor, and 6 weeks of oral dosing to the newborn, reduced vertical HIV transmission by 67% (transmission rate of 7.6% with ZDV vs. 22.6% with placebo).[17] In the next 25 years, multiple studies have explored different modalities of maternal and neonatal ART, including abbreviated courses of dual and triple ARV combinations during the third trimester of pregnancy, in labor, and during a limited postpartum period.[18–24] Administration of combination triple

TABLE 32.1 Dosing and Safety Considerations for Antiretroviral Drugs during Pregnancy

ARV Drug	*Pregnancy Dosing Recommendations*[a,b]	*Evidence of Human Teratogenicity and Relevant Comments*
	Nucleoside/Tide Reverse Transcriptase Inhibitors	
Abacavir (ABC)	Standard adult once-daily or twice-daily dosing	No
Emtricitabine (FTC)	Standard adult once-daily dosing for treatment and PrEP	No
Lamivudine (3TC)	Standard adult twice-daily or once-daily dosing	No
Tenofovir disoproxil fumarate (TDF)	Standard adult once-daily dosing for treatment and PrEP	No
Tenofovir alafenamide fumarate (TAF)	Standard adult once-daily dosing[c]	Insufficient data to assess teratogenicity in humans
Zidovudine (ZDV, AZT)	Standard adult oral-daily or twice-daily dosing Dosed IV throughout labor for high vertical transmission risk	No
	Non-Nucleoside Reverse Transcriptase Inhibitors	
Doravirine (DOR)	Insufficient data to make dosing recommendation	Insufficient data to assess teratogenicity in humans
Efavirenz (EFV)	Standard adult dosing 600 or 400 mg[c]	Limited data on first-trimester EFV exposure suggest possibility of a twofold to threefold increased incidence of neural tube defect (NTD) Observational human cohort studies suggest no significant (10-fold) increase in the NTD risk with first-trimester exposure FDA advises avoiding EFV during conception and the first trimester of pregnancy EFV can be continued in virologically suppressed women on EFV-based regimen
Etravirine (ETR)	Standard adult twice daily dosing	Insufficient data to assess for teratogenicity in humans
Nevirapine (NVP)	Standard adult once-daily or twice-daily dosing NVP should be initiated in pregnant women with CD4 cell counts ≥250 cells/mm^3 only when benefit clearly outweighs risk because of potential increased risk of life-threatening hepatotoxicity with high CD4 cell counts.	No
Rilpivirine (RPV)	Standard adult once-daily dosing[c] While RPV plasma concentration is reduced during pregnancy, higher-than-standard doses have not been studied. Insufficient data are available to recommend a dosing change in pregnancy. With standard dosing, viral loads should be monitored more frequently.	No
	Protease inhibitors	
Atazanavir (ATV)	ATV without RTV boosting is not recommended in pregnancy Use of ATV is not recommended for ARV-experienced pregnant women taking TDF *and* an H_2-receptor antagonist.	No Effect of in utero ATV exposure on infant indirect bilirubin levels is unclear. Nonpathologic ranges of neonatal hyperbilirubinemia have been observed in some clinical trials.
ATV/RTV	Standard once-daily adult dosing[c] Low concentrations reported with standard dosing during pregnancy. Some experts recommend increased ATV dosing in all women during the second and third trimesters. Consider increased dose in second and third trimesters, especially in ARV-experienced pregnant women taking TDF *and* an H_2-receptor antagonist.	Insufficient data to assess for teratogenicity in humans
ATV/COBI	Because of low exposures, use of ATV/COBI during pregnancy is not recommended.	
Darunavir (DRV)	DRV without RTV boosting is not recommended in pregnancy.	No

TABLE 32.1 Dosing and Safety Considerations for Antiretroviral Drugs During Pregnancy (*continued*)

ARV Drug	*Pregnancy Dosing Recommendations*[a,b]	*Evidence of Human Teratogenicity and Relevant Comments*
DRV/RTV	Standard twice-daily DRV/RTV (600 mg/100 mg) adult dosing[c] Low concentrations reported with standard dosing during pregnancy. Once-daily dosing with DRV/r during pregnancy Increased twice-daily DRV dose (DRV 800 mg/RTV 100 mg with food) during pregnancy does not result in an increase in DRV exposure and is not recommended.	Insufficient data to assess for teratogenicity in humans
DRV/COBI	Because of low exposures, use of DRV/COBI during pregnancy is not recommended	Insufficient data to assess for teratogenicity in humans
Lopinavir/ritonavir (LPV/RTV)	Standard adult twice-daily dosing Once-daily dosing is not recommended during pregnancy. Low LPV concentrations with standard dosing during second and third trimesters. Some experts recommend an increased dose LPV/RTV (600 mg/150 mg) twice daily or LPV/RTV (500 mg/125 mg) twice daily in the second and third trimesters, especially in PI experienced and women who start treatment during pregnancy with a baseline viral load >50 copies/mL.	No
Ritonavir (RTV)	Only used as a low-dose PK booster with PIs LPV (co-formulated), ATV, and DRV	No
	Viral entry and fusion inhibitors	
Enfuvirtide (T-20)	Insufficient data to make dosing recommendation	Insufficient data to assess teratogenicity in humans
Maraviroc (MVC)	Insufficient data to make dosing recommendation	Insufficient data to assess for teratogenicity in humans
	Integrase inhibitors	
Dolutegravir (DTG)	Standard adult once-daily or twice-daily dosing DTG *AUC* may be decreased during the third trimester compared with postpartum.	Possible increased risk of NTD in infants born to women who were receiving DTG at time of conception DTG is not recommended during the early first trimester of pregnancy prior to closure of the neural tube.
Elvitegravir (EVG) EVG/COBI	EVG/COBI is not recommended for use in pregnancy. Significant reduction in EVG plasma exposure during pregnancy	Insufficient data to assess for teratogenicity in humans
Raltegravir (RAL)	Standard twice-daily dosing Once-daily dosing of two RAL 600-mg film-coated tablets is not recommended until more information is available	No

[a]Dosing confirmed in PK studies among pregnant women, except when indicted differently in the table.
[b]Doses of individual ARVs and Fixed Dose Combinations (FDCs) may need to be adjusted with renal or hepatic impairment or when coadministered with other drugs.
[c]For food interactions: all TAF formulations are recommended to be dosed with food. EFV needs to be taken on empty stomach (without food) to decrease potential side effects. RPV needs to be taken with food.
AUC, area under the curve; IV, intravenous; PK, pharmacokinetics; PrEP, preexposure prophylaxis.
From Panel on Treatment of Pregnant Women with HIV Infection and Prevention of Perinatal Transmission. Recommendations for use of antiretroviral drugs in transmission in the United States. http://aidsinfo.nih.gov/contentfiles/lvguidelines/PerinatalGL.pdf. Accessed December 26, 2019.

ARV regimens before or early in pregnancy has been associated with maximal reductions in the rate of vertical transmissions (≤1.5% or less) in women who did not breastfeed their infants.[18,19] The introduction of the cesarean delivery prior to the onset of labor in women with higher levels of HIV viremia and elimination of breastfeeding led to further decreases in vertical transmission rates in resource-rich settings.[25–27] However, due to high infant morbidity and mortality associated with formula feeding in resource-limited settings with restricted access to safe water for formula reconstitution, breastfeeding is critical to infant survival and remains the recommended feeding mode in such settings, with the use of postpartum maternal and/or infant ARV regimens to minimize breast milk transmission of HIV.[2,3,28]

Due to multiple logistical and financial constraints, the applicability of the most comprehensive prevention of vertical transmission interventions has been limited in resource-limited settings. Until 2013, the majority of pregnant women living with HIV were only provided with short courses of ARVs in late pregnancy, loading maternal ARV dosing during delivery, such as single-dose non-nucleoside/tide reverse transcriptase inhibitor (NNRTI) nevirapine (NVP), and short courses of ARVs during early breastfeeding focusing primarily on the goal of prevention of vertical transmission, rather than long-term maternal health outcomes. For women living with HIV in resource-limited settings, this approach meant repeat treatment interruptions between pregnancies, rebound HIV viremia, and development of viral resistance. Only recently, maternal ART during pregnancy, labor and delivery, and breastfeeding has been viewed as advantageous not only from the prospective of prevention of vertical transmission, but rather from the perspective of tri-fold benefits, including (a) treatment of maternal HIV; (b) prevention of transmission to the fetus, unborn child, newborn, and nursing infant; and (c) prevention of horizontal transmission to sexual partners.[29] This change in the approach to maternal ART has led to the harmonization of the ART regimens between pregnant and breastfeeding women with other adult populations, except for the circumstances where pregnancy-related changes in the pharmacokinetic (PK) properties of the ARVs or fetal/child toxicity considerations restrict the use of certain ARVs during the conception of pregnancy or data are lacking on certain ART approaches during pregnancy, such as dual regimens. Novel dual ART regimens are currently recommended for treatment-naïve and treatment-experienced virally suppressed adults living with HIV. However, there are currently no data on the use of dual ART regimens during pregnancy and no dual ARV combinations are currently recommended for use in pregnant and breastfeeding women.

In 2013 the World Health Organization (WHO) introduced Option B+ in perinatal HIV management guidelines, recommending lifelong universal ART for all pregnant women diagnosed with HIV.[30] In the following years, a significantly higher number of women of reproductive potential living with HIV have been initiated on preferred combination ART regimens with NNRTI efavirenz (EFV) combined with two NRTIs as a backbone.[31] Most recently, the integrase strand transferase inhibitor (INSTI) dolutegravir (DTG) in combination with two NRTIs has become a preferred ART regimen in pregnancy and postpartum in WHO, U.S., and European ART guidelines.[1,2,16] The integrase inhibitor raltegravir (RAL) and protease inhibitors (PIs) atazanavir/ritonavir (ATV/RTV) and darunavir/ritonavir (DRV/RTV) in combination with two NRTIs are also recommended as preferred[1] or alternative ART regimens during pregnancy.[1,2,16] The NNRTI rilpivirine (RPV) and PI lopinavir/ritonavir (LPV/RTV) in combination with two NRTIs are considered alternative ART regimens during pregnancy.[1,2,16]

Along with the changes in maternal ART, the approach to the intrapartum and preventive neonatal ART for low and high vertical transmission risk deliveries also has evolved. Parenteral use of IV ZDV during labor and delivery is now restricted to high-risk prenatal exposure when maternal viral load is high or unknown.[1,16] For low vertical transmission risk deliveries, the postnatal course of oral ZDV in the newborn has been shortened to 2 to 4 weeks or completely eliminated in resource-rich settings.[1–3,16,32] For high vertical transmission risk deliveries with unknown or unsuppressed maternal HIV RNA viral load, newborns may receive an enhanced dual regimen (ZDV plus NVP) or empiric triple ART with full-treatment doses of all three ARVs [ZDV plus lamivudine (3TC) plus RAL or NVP], as recommended by WHO, U.S., and European perinatal guidelines.[1,2,16,33,34] The use of the empiric therapy approach is based on the evidence that early initiation of ART in infants with vertically transmitted HIV infection is beneficial for short- and long-term neonatal outcomes, including smaller size of the viral reservoir and higher potential for ARV-free remission or functional cure in the future.[35–38]

Maternal ART regimens during pregnancy and breastfeeding are not only relevant to the virologic suppression during these time periods but also have implications on the future maternal and neonatal ART choices. Adherence to ART during pregnancy and breastfeeding is frequently suboptimal[39–41] and may lead to ongoing viral replication and development of the genetic mutations for drug-resistant HIV variants, which can be passed to newborns and infants.[42,43] In the U.S., national Health and Human Services (HHS) guidelines recommend genotype resistance testing before starting ART in women who are ARV naïve or ARV experienced and before modifying ART regimens in women whose HIV RNA levels are above the threshold for resistance testing (i.e., >500 to 1,000 copies/mL).[1]

Neonatal ARV prophylaxis is also frequently challenged by adherence and may generate viral resistance in those infants who become HIV infected. This is particularly relevant to the first-generation NNRTI NVP which only requires a single mutation of the HIV genome for resistance to develop.[44] NVP has a long half-life and can be detected in plasma up to 3 weeks after administration, especially in slow metabolizers, causing suboptimal plasma concentrations and creating conditions for the development of viral resistance.[45] Among women exposed to a single dose of NVP during labor (used for prevention of vertical transmission prior to 2013 WHO guidelines), NVP-resistant HIV isolates were detected 6 weeks after delivery in 20% of women receiving no other ARVs and in 15% of women receiving three-drug ART regimens.[46,47] In women who received a second or third course of single-dose intrapartum NVP in subsequent pregnancies, resistant virus was detected in 38% within 1 year after delivery.[48] Recent studies have identified widespread pretreatment NNRTI resistance in young infants with a history of perinatal exposure to NVP and have prompted the 2018 WHO HIV treatment guidelines and 2019 policy brief update to introduce DTG as a first-line choice ART during pregnancy and RAL as a first-line choice for neonatal ART and recommend switching to PI-based ART in children who cannot be placed on DTG.[2,49,50] Resistance to NRTIs, except 3TC and emtricitabine (FTC), and PIs requires multiple mutations and develops more slowly compared to the resistance to the first-generation NNRTIs.[51–53] Development of resistance to the NRTIs 3TC and FTC requires only a single mutation and is encountered significantly more frequently among women and children globally.[54]

PREVENTIVE ANTIRETROVIRAL TREATMENT FOR WOMEN AT RISK FOR ACQUIRING HIV

Introduction of preexposure prophylaxis (PrEP) for use in adult and adolescent populations by the global, U.S., and European guidelines opens the door for use of ARV as prevention in women at risk for HIV infection throughout pregnancy and breastfeeding.[1,2,16,55] While global and national HIV prevention and management guidelines highlight limited data on PrEP during pregnancy,[56–59] they do not explicitly recommend PrEP during pregnancy and breastfeeding.[1,2,16] They do, however, acknowledge that pregnancy is associated with a higher risk of acquiring HIV and an increased risk of HIV transmission to the infant[60] and, therefore, include pregnant and breastfeeding women within the PrEP-eligible populations. Currently, the combination of two NRTIs, tenofovir disoproxil fumarate (TDF) with FTC, is used without sufficient data or understanding of pregnancy and lactation-specific risks/benefits for PrEP globally among childbearing and lactating women and rely on the known PK, efficacy, and safety data from the use of TDF and FTC in pregnant women living with HIV and/or hepatitis B, and their neonates.[61–63]

EFFECT OF PREGNANCY ON DRUG DISPOSITION

For multiple logistical and ethical reasons, PK studies are challenging to conduct in pregnant women. Maternal physiologic changes associated with pregnancy may have a considerable impact on absorption, distribution, metabolism, and excretion of ARVs and may affect their dosing (Fig. 32.1).[64–67] These effects have been evaluated in a rigorous manner for a significant number of ARVs, but for many novel HIV drugs, the PK changes during pregnancy remain currently understudied.[4,68]

Published data on several ARVs highlight the significance of PK and pharmacodynamics (PD) changes during pregnancy. Pregnancy results in significant changes in gastrointestinal function, including nausea and vomiting, which is especially pronounced in early pregnancy, capable of decreasing drug intake and absorption. Plasma progesterone increase during pregnancy is associated with a 30% to 50% decrease in intestinal motility and increases in gastric emptying and intestinal transit times.[69] The ionization and absorption of weak acids and bases may be affected by increased gastric pH due to a 40% reduction in acid secretion.[64] These physiologic changes could potentially result in delayed drug absorption and reduced peak maternal blood concentrations.[69]

During an average pregnancy, total body water content increases by 8 L, plasma volume expands by 50%, and body fat stores increase, changing volume of distribution of both hydrophilic and lipophilic drugs.[66,67] The dilutional decrease in serum albumin as well as competitive inhibition from steroid hormones results in decreased protein binding,[70] leading to an increase in volume of distribution and decrease in peak drug concentrations. The decrease in protein binding also results in an increase in the free fraction, or unbound pharmacologically active drug moiety, available for binding to sites of action and for biotransformation and elimination for some drugs. For other highly bound drugs, however, having more unbound drug means more active drug moiety is available for elimination from the body, and elimination may increase, leading to no meaningful difference in the free fraction during pregnancy. The free fraction of several drugs, including diazepam, salicylates, and some β-lactam antibiotics, has been shown to increase during pregnancy as a result of changes in protein binding.[66] Routine laboratory therapeutic monitoring drug assays, therefore, must be interpreted with caution during pregnancy, as they measure total drug concentration, not the free fraction, and therapeutic and toxic effects may occur at lower total concentrations in the face of decreased protein binding of highly protein-bound drugs.

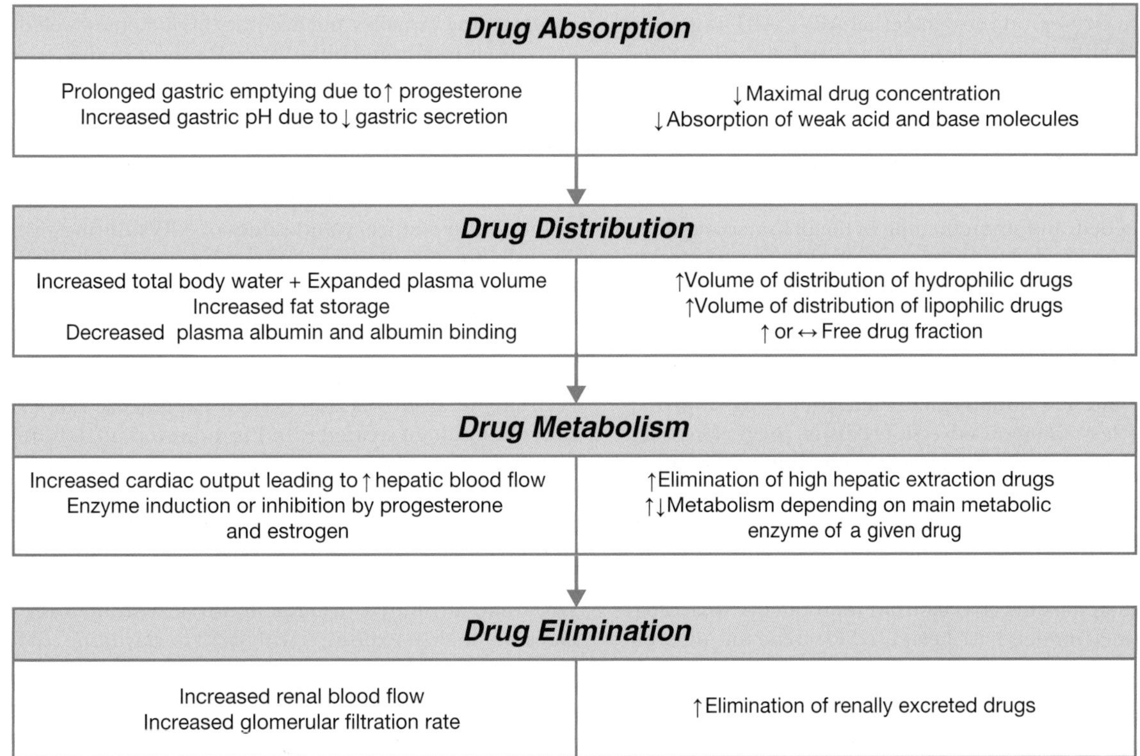

Figure 32.1 Major physiologic changes during pregnancy and potential impact on drug disposition. (Modified from Hodel EM, Marzolini C, Waitt C, et al. Pharmacokinetics, placental and breast milk transfer of antiretroviral drugs in pregnant and lactating women living with HIV. *Curr Pharm Des* 2019;25(5):556–576.)

The activity of several important drug-metabolizing enzymes such as cytochrome (CYP) P450 CYP2B6, CYP2C8, CYP2C9, CYP2D6, CYP2E1, CYP3A4, and uridine diphosphate glucuronosyltransferases (UGTs), all critically important in the metabolism of ARVs, is induced during pregnancy through activation of nuclear receptors by progesterone, which leads to suboptimal drug exposure of certain drugs.[71–73] In contrast, the activity of CYP1A2 and CYP2C19 is inhibited, resulting in higher exposure of drugs metabolized by these enzymes.[68] Renal function increases during pregnancy, with 25% to 50% increases in renal plasma flow and glomerular filtration rate (GFR), leading to increases in clearance of renally excreted drugs and their metabolites during pregnancy.[67]

Although the disposition of most drugs is measurably changed by the physiologic changes of pregnancy, the need for actual dosing adjustment is determined by the magnitude and complexity of these changes and the PK and PD parameters for each drug. Studying the PK of ARVs in pregnant women and understanding their interactions with other commonly used drugs or supplements are necessary to ensure adequate maternal drug exposure during pregnancy and to assess the possible transfer of drugs across the placenta and into breast milk.[4]

SAFETY OF ANTIRETROVIRAL DRUGS DURING PREGNANCY

The scale-up of ART use among millions of pregnant and breastfeeding women living with HIV globally has made the safety of the ARVs for the fetus, infant, breastfeeding child, and mother of paramount importance. Despite being considered generally safe for use during pregnancy, a series of studies have found an association between diverse maternal ARVs, ART regimens, and maternal HIV (both with nonsuppressed and suppressed viral load), with adverse pregnancy outcomes such as prematurity, small size for gestational age, stillbirths, and neonatal death.[74–76] The biologic mechanisms that underlie the observed associations between antenatal ART and adverse outcomes in pregnancy and birth are not completely understood; further research are needed and strengthening of the pharmacovigilance (PV) systems are needed to assess safety of ARVs for the mother and HIV-exposed children with ART and HIV exposure in utero and during breastfeeding.[77]

The safety of drug use in pregnancy is difficult to assess as evaluations of new drugs in pregnancy are often limited to small safety and PK studies conducted after drug approval. Detection of less common adverse events in pregnancy, such as birth defects, requires evaluation of large numbers of exposures, which only occurs when the ARVs are introduced among women of reproductive potential.[74,78] As with other drugs, preclinical novel ARV evaluations include *in vitro* and animal *in vivo* studies for carcinogenicity, mutagenicity, and reproductive and teratogenic effects. Data from reproductive toxicology studies in animal models have been used to screen for potential developmental and reproductive hazards of new drugs.[78] While negative preclinical reproductive toxicology results are reassuring, they cannot definitively predict the lack of teratogenic effects in humans.[79] Similarly, teratogenicity in animal studies is not always confirmed by the teratogenic effects in humans. In fact, among multiple known animal teratogens, only a few have been shown to be teratogenic in humans. The best example of this discrepancy among ARVs is represented by NNRTI EFV. In cynomolgus monkeys, in utero EFV exposure at plasma concentrations 1.3 times systemic human therapeutic exposure was associated with fetal central nervous system (CNS) malformations; however, prospective human pregnancy outcome data did not support this teratogenic effect of EFV exposure in human pregnancy.[75,78,80,81]

Pregnant women are generally excluded from the drug development process leading to licensure of novel ARVs.[4,78] Moreover, preclinical perinatal phase I, II, and III ARV studies are too small and of limited duration to adequately assess for adverse effects, especially those effects that are uncommon or first appear outside of infancy. Monitoring of pregnancy and postnatal outcomes associated with ART use during pregnancy is essential and is currently carried on by international postmarketing surveillances systems, such as the U.S.-based Antiretroviral Pregnancy Registry (APR) (http://www.apregistry.com/) and the European Pregnancy and Pediatric HIV Cohort Collaboration (EPPICC) (http://penta-id.org/hiv/eppicc/). These systems depend on voluntary reporting and, therefore, have relatively low numbers of events. They also gather data primarily from high- and middle-income countries and do not reflect data with ART combinations and populations from regions most heavily affected by the HIV epidemic. Observational cohort studies of pregnant and breastfeeding women living with HIV from low- and middle-income countries, where most HIV-positive women of reproductive age reside and exposures of concern occur, have shown to be of great value for global strategies on using ARVs at conception and during pregnancy and need to continue being funded and expanded. Despite the fact that these studies can be limited by ethnic, social, and clinical differences in the relevant populations, lack of randomized comparator groups, and restricted capacity to evaluate multiple confounding variables and accuracy of outcomes, well-designed and closely monitored observational cohort studies, such as Botswana Tsepamo study,[82] have demonstrated the ability to collect high-quality perinatal safety data and support rolling out similar prospective cohort studies of pregnant and breastfeeding women in other countries.[78]

The health of the mother must not be forgotten when evaluating the efficacy and safety of ARVs during pregnancy. The physiologic changes of pregnancy may make the mother more susceptible to toxicities described in nonpregnant adults. Abnormalities in carbohydrate metabolism are common side effects in nonpregnant adults receiving combined ART regimens, especially those including PIs, raising concerns about an increase in gestational glucose intolerance in pregnant women treated with PIs; however, no definitive association between ART and gestational diabetes has been found to date.[83,84] Pregnancy may also predispose to mitochondrial dysfunction associated with exposure to NRTIs. Lactic acidosis, hepatic steatosis, acute fatty liver, and development of the HELLP (hemolysis, elevated liver enzymes, and low platelets) syndrome attributed to mitochondrial dysfunction from nucleoside analog exposure with NRTIs stavudine (d4T) and didanosine (ddI) have led to the recommendations against using these agents in pregnant women, much earlier than their discontinuation in nonpregnant adults and children.[85] Recent signals of the weight gain and increase in body mass index (BMI) associated with the use of DTG[86] prompts consideration of the significance of these bodily changes on the pregnancy and call for the studies of short- and long-term neonatal outcomes.

PHARMACOLOGY AND SAFETY OF DIFFERENT CLASSES AND INDIVIDUAL ANTIRETROVIRAL DRUGS IN PREGNANT WOMEN AND NEONATES

PK/PD and major safety considerations of individual ARVs by each drug class during pregnancy, labor, and postpartum in mothers and newborns are reviewed below. The following older ARVs are no longer recommended by the global, U.S., and European HIV treatment guidelines and are not included in the review: NRTIs stavudine (d4T) and didanosine (ddI), NNRTI delavirdine(DKV), and PIs fosamprenavir (f-AMP), indinavir (IDV), nelfinavir (NFV), saquinavir (SQV), and tipranavir (TPV).

NUCLEOSIDE/TIDE REVERSE TRANSCRIPTASE INHIBITORS

NRTIs were the first ARV agents developed to treat HIV infection. Structurally similar to endogenous deoxynucleosides, nucleoside analogs are inactive prodrugs that require three phosphorylation steps to form a triphosphate nucleoside, the active drug moiety, which inhibits HIV reverse transcriptase and viral DNA replication.[87] Quantification of the intracellular concentrations of these active triphosphorylated forms is difficult, requiring large blood samples and sophisticated assay techniques.[88,89] The half-life of these active intracellular metabolites generally exceeds that of the parent drug in plasma.[87] Extracellular plasma NRTI concentrations do not correlate well with concentrations of the active intracellular forms, and the plasma NRTIs PK does not generally correlate with therapeutic effect.[90] Tenofovir, the first nucleotide to be approved for use against HIV, is an acyclic analog of adenosine monophosphate that requires only *two* phosphorylation steps to reach its active form, tenofovir diphosphate.[91]

NRTIs are recommended as an integral part of ART, most commonly two NRTIs forming the dual-NRTI backbone of first-line ART, in combination with a PI, INSTI, or an NNRTI.[1] Clinical trials PK and safety data on NRTIs in pregnancy are available for ZDV, abacavir (ABC), 3TC, FTC, and the NRTIs TDF and tenofovir alafenamide fumarate (TAF). NRTIs are known to inhibit mitochondrial function, and their use has been linked to the potential long-term toxicity associated with depletion of mitochondrial DNA.[92–95]

Abacavir

ABC is an oral, synthetic, guanosine analog NRTI used in pregnancy with potent activity against HIV-1.

Maternal Pharmacokinetics

In nonpregnant adults, ABC is predictably and extensively absorbed with a mean absolute bioavailability of 83%.[96] Protein binding is approximately 50%, and the mean volume of distribution is 0.86 L/kg. ABC is metabolized primarily by alcohol dehydrogenase and glucuronosyltransferase to inactive metabolites, with no significant metabolism by the cytochrome P450 enzyme system. Plasma *Cl/F* is 0.8 L per hour per kg, and $t_{1/2}$ is 1.5 hours.[97,98] ABC is metabolized inside cells to its active moiety, carbovir triphosphate, which has a median intracellular half-life of 18 hours.[99] The limited published literature on the ABC PK in pregnancy does not indicate significant changes in pregnancy. A phase I study of 25 women showed decreased maximum plasma ABC concentrations in pregnancy with similar overall plasma exposure (*AUC*) in the third trimester compared with 6 to 12 weeks' postpartum and compared with nonpregnant individuals.[100] Similarly, a PK study of ABC 600 mg daily concluded that the PK in pregnancy was equivalent to the PK observed in the postpartum period.[101] Lastly, a population PK study of 150 women during pregnancy found no effect of any covariates (age, body weight, pregnancy, or gestational age) on ABC plasma exposures.[102] Standard adult dosing of ABC 300 mg orally twice daily or 600 mg once daily is recommended in pregnancy.

Placental transfer of ABC is high, with cord blood concentrations equivalent to maternal concentrations at delivery.[100,103] ABC is excreted in breast milk. A study of 15 breastfeeding women in Botswana found that median breast milk-to-plasma ratio was 0.85 at 1 month postpartum; ABC was detected in plasma of one of nine breastfeeding infants.[104]

Infant Pharmacokinetics

ABC PK data for use in neonates are currently not available, and the U.S. pediatric HIV management guidelines do not recommended ABC to be used in infants less than 3 months of age.[105] The WHO guidelines do allow ABC in infants who weigh ≥3 kg starting at 4 weeks of age, based on the use of nonthymidine analogs in first-line regimens and thymidine analogs in second-line regimens in this weight range.[50]

Safety and Outcome Data

Sufficient numbers of exposures to ABC in humans have been monitored in the APR to be able to determine that first-trimester ABC exposure is not associated with a 1.5-fold increase in the risk of overall birth defects.[106] ABC-associated birth defect prevalence in the U.S. is commensurate with levels reported by the Centers for Disease Control (CDC) for the general population. Similarly, first-trimester exposure to ABC has not been associated with birth defects in several longitudinal studies.[93,107–109]

Serious, sometimes fatal, hypersensitivity reactions to ABC have occurred in nonpregnant adults. Carriage of the HLA-B*5701 allele is associated with a significantly increased risk of a hypersensitivity reaction to ABC, and screening for this allele is recommended to all patients prior to initiating treatment with ABC.[96]

Emtricitabine

FTC is an oral synthetic cytidine analog NRTI frequently used as part of the dual-NRTI backbone of first-line ART in pregnancy with potent activity against HIV-1. FTC is also commonly used in combination with TDF for PrEP.

Pharmacokinetics

In nonpregnant adults, FTC is well absorbed and has low protein binding; the standard dose of 200 mg once daily results in an average *AUC* of 10 μg × hour per mL.[110] Less than 15% of FTC is metabolized, primarily by oxidation of the thiol moiety to form the 3′-sulfoxide diastereomers and conjugation with glucuronic acid to form 2′-*O*-glucuronide, with no significant metabolism by the CYP450 enzyme system. Most is eliminated unchanged in the urine, and its clearance is proportional to renal function. Plasma $t_{1/2}$ is 8 hours, and intracellular FTC triphosphate $t_{1/2}$ is 20 to 39 hours.[111–113]

Several studies have demonstrated lower FTC exposure in the third trimester compared to postpartum and nonpregnant populations, specifically higher apparent clearance and lower trough (24-hour postdose) concentrations.[114–117] Increased FTC clearance in pregnancy is correlated with the normal pregnancy-related increase in GFR. The changes in exposure in pregnancy are not believed to be significant enough to warrant dose adjustment.[116]

FTC has high placental transfer.[117] A study of 15 women who received FTC during pregnancy demonstrated a mean cord blood to maternal blood ratio of 1.2 [90% confidence interval (CI), 1.0 to 1.5].

FTC is excreted into breast milk. A study of women taking an ART regimen containing FTC found that concentrations in breast milk peaked later than in maternal plasma (at 4 to 8 hours vs. 2 to 4 hours) and were threefold higher than maternal plasma concentrations. FTC was detectable in 3 (19%) infants.[118] In a study of 50 women without HIV who received 200 mg FTC per 300 mg TDF orally daily as PrEP, median peak and trough breast milk concentrations of FTC were 212.5 ng per mL [interquartile range (IQR) 140.0 to 405.0] and 183.0 ng per mL (IQR 113.0 to 250.0), respectively. FTC was detectable in 47 of 49 infants at a median (IQR) concentration of 13.2 ng per mL (9.3 to 16.7), corresponding to estimated daily infant ingestion of a 31.9 μg per kg FTC dose (IQR 21.0 to 60.8), or 0.5% of the daily dose for treating infants.[119]

Infant Pharmacokinetics

FTC PK in the first 3 months of life was studied in 20 infants at doses of 3 mg per kg once daily for 4 days, with two 4-day courses administered at least 2 weeks apart.[32] Oral clearance increased with age, with mean values of 13, 22, and 29 mL per min at postnatal days 0 to 21, 22 to 42, and 43 to 90, respectively. Mean *AUCs* ranged from 8.55 to 13.44 μg × hour per mL, similar to values seen in older children taking 6 mg per kg once daily and adults taking 200 mg once daily.

Safety

The Partners Demonstration study as well as two studies of FTC for HIV treatment demonstrated no associated increase in birth defects. In the APR, there are sufficient reports of first-trimester exposures to FTC to be able to detect at least a 1.5-fold increased risk of overall birth defects and a twofold increase in cardiovascular and genitourinary defects (the most common classes); no such increase in birth defects has been observed. Among cases of first-trimester FTC exposure reported to the APR, the prevalence of birth defects was 2.44% (77/3,158 births; 95% CI, 1.93% to 3.04%), compared with a 2.72% total prevalence in the U.S. population, based on CDC surveillance.[120] The PHACS/SMARTT cohort has also not identified any additional increased risk of adverse outcomes.[109]

Lamivudine

3TC is a deoxycytidine analog used as part of combination ART in pregnancy and, in combination with ZDV and NVP, as neonatal prophylaxis in infants at higher risk of perinatal HIV transmission. 3TC can also be used to treat hepatitis B.

Maternal Pharmacokinetics

In nonpregnant adults, 3TC is rapidly absorbed with bioavailability averaging 85%. Protein binding is low (10% to 50%), and the volume of distribution (V/F) is large (1.3 L per kg).[121,122] 3TC is rapidly eliminated via renal excretion as unchanged drug with a $t_{1/2}$ of around 6 hours.[122,123] The median intracellular $t_{1/2}$ of 3TC triphosphate is 15 hours.[124] In a study of women receiving ZDV plus 3TC, no drug–drug interactions were reported, and no significant differences were found in 3TC PK during pregnancy and the first week after delivery.[125] A subsequent study of 114 pregnant women, 123 parturient women, and 47 nonpregnant women found 3TC clearance to be 22% higher in pregnancy, but did not conclude that increased clearance resulted in subtherapeutic exposure or necessitated dose adjustment.[126]

3TC crosses the placenta by simple diffusion, and the ratio of 3TC concentration in maternal plasma at the time of delivery and cord blood is around 1.0.[127,128] In the abovementioned study of 123 mother–infant pairs, the placental 3TC transfer (expressed as fetal-to-maternal *AUC* ratio) was 0.86.[126] Infant 3TC clearance is prolonged immediately after birth, with the elimination $t_{1/2}$ of transplacentally acquired 3TC averaging around 14 hours.[129]

3TC is excreted into human breast milk. A study of 67 nursing mothers in Kenya on combination ZDV, 3TC, and NVP demonstrated median breast milk 3TC concentration at 1,214 ng per mL and a median ratio of 3TC concentration in breast milk to that in plasma of 2.56.[130] In infants solely exposed to 3TC via breast milk, median plasma 3TC concentration was 23 ng per mL [50% inhibitory concentration (IC_{50}) of 3TC against wild-type HIV = 0.6 to 21 ng per mL]. A study of breastfeeding women in Malawi receiving 3TC, TDF, and EFV demonstrated concentrations of 3TC in breast milk to be higher than those in maternal plasma at 1 month (3.29-fold higher) and 12 months (2.35-fold higher) postpartum. Infant median 3TC concentrations, however, were found to be only 2.5 ng per mL at 6 months of life (with an IQR of 2.5 to 7.6) and 0 ng per mL at 12 months of life (with an IQR of 0 to 2.5).[131]

Infant Pharmacokinetics

3TC elimination increases as renal function improves after birth, with clearance averaging 0.25 L per kg per hour on day 1 after birth and 0.40 L per kg per hour after 1 week of life, compared to 0.53 L per kg per hour in older children.[125,129,132] The recommended 3TC dose for neonates less than 1 month of age is 2 mg per kg every 12 hours, compared with the standard dose in infants up to 3 months of 4 mg per kg every 12 hours (up to a maximum of 150 mg per12 hours).[105] In infants at higher risk of perinatal HIV transmission, treatment dose 3TC is recommended up to 6 weeks of life.[105]

Safety

3TC is known to depress bone marrow function, and hematologic toxicity is the most common toxicity reported with perinatal exposure. The only safety data for perinatal 3TC monotherapy come from a small phase I study from South Africa where 3TC monotherapy was given to 10 pregnant women starting at 38 weeks gestation and to their infants for 1 week after birth; the only toxicities noted were mild anemia in one mother and one infant.[125] The French Perinatal Cohort study found an association between 3TC exposure in the first trimester and an increased risk of overall birth defects [adjusted odds ratio (aOR) = 1.37; 95% CI, 1.06 to 1.73], but there was no specific affected organ system or birth defect that predominated.[133] A large U.S. cohort study of HIV-exposed uninfected infants found that 3TC exposure during pregnancy was not associated with increased risk of adverse infant outcomes.[109] Sufficient numbers of exposures to 3TC in humans have been monitored in the APR to be able to determine that first-trimester 3TC exposure is not associated with a 1.5-fold or greater increase in the risk of overall birth defects or with a twofold or greater increase in the risk of cardiovascular or genitourinary system defects.[106] Among reported cases of first-trimester 3TC exposure, the prevalence of birth defects was 3.0% (151/5,008 births; 95% CI, 2.6% to 3.5%) compared to 2.7% prevalence among the U.S. general population. An analysis of APR data demonstrated a lower risk of spontaneous and induced abortions and preterm births with use of 3TC-containing regimens compared to non–3TC-containing regimens.[134]

Tenofovir

Tenofovir, the first nucleotide approved for use against HIV, is now available as TDF and TAF. Tenofovir is also effective treatment for hepatitis B.

Tenofovir Disoproxil Fumarate

Maternal Pharmacokinetics. In nonpregnant adults, the bioavailability of tenofovir, when administered as the TDF prodrug, is 25%, with maximum tenofovir concentrations of 200 to 300 ng per mL reached 1 to 2 hours postdose.[111,135–137] Protein binding is low, and tenofovir is not a substrate for the cytochrome P450 enzyme system. Tenofovir has a plasma half-life of 15 hours, and the active moiety, tenofovir diphosphate, has a long intracellular half-life of 60 hours or more.[112]

A retrospective population PK study of 46 pregnant women and 156 nonpregnant women on combination TDF regimens demonstrated a 39% higher tenofovir apparent clearance in pregnancy; apparent clearance decreased significantly with increasing age.[138] The International Maternal Pediatric Adolescent AIDS Clinical Trials Network (IMPAACT) P1026s prospective PK study of 37 pregnant women on TDF-based combination ART at 30 to 36 weeks' gestation and at 6 to 12 weeks' postpartum found that the proportion of women with tenofovir *AUC* greater than the target of 1.99 μg×h per mL (10th percentile in nonpregnant adults) was lower in the third trimester (73%, 27/37 women) than postpartum (84%, 27/32 women). Trough levels and *AUCs* were also 17% to 20% lower during the third trimester versus postpartum. Of note, the median weight of women below the target exposure (97.9 kg) was significantly higher than the median weight of women who met the target exposure (74.2 kg).[139] Another study of 34 women who were on TDF plus FTC in the third trimester and postpartum, tenofovir *AUC*, peak, and trough were all approximately 25% lower in pregnancy. These decreased exposures were not associated with virologic failure.[114] Standard adult TDF dosing continues to be recommended in pregnancy.

In the Partners Demonstration study of women without HIV using TDF plus FTC for PrEP, intracellular concentrations of tenofovir diphosphate in pregnant women were found to be approximately 70% of levels in nonpregnant women.[56] There is no established tenofovir concentration threshold for HIV prevention. However, limited data on PrEP use in pregnancy do not indicate an increased risk of HIV acquisition secondary to inadequate TDF dosing.[57,59]

There is high placental transfer of tenofovir; the cord blood to maternal blood ratio of tenofovir ranges from 0.60 to 1.03 with chronic TDF use in pregnancy.[115,139,140,141] After a single maternal dose of TDF 600 mg with FTC 400 mg, intracellular tenofovir concentrations were detected in the cord blood peripheral blood mononuclear cells (PBMCs) in (36/36) neonates. However, intracellular tenofovir diphosphate was detectable in only two (5.5%) of 36 infants, suggesting a lag in the appearance of tenofovir diphosphate.[142]

Tenofovir is excreted in breast milk, although infant plasma concentrations are low. Data are from studies of women without HIV on a TDF-based PrEP regimen or from African studies, where breastfeeding is recommended in women living with HIV. In a study of 50 breastfeeding women who received TDF plus FTC for HIV PrEP, median peak and trough time-averaged tenofovir breast milk concentrations were similar: 3.2 ng per mL (IQR 2.3 to 4.7) versus 3.3 ng per mL (IQR 2.3 to 4.4).[119] Infant plasma tenofovir concentration was unquantifiable (<0.31 ng per mL) in 94% of infants and very low in the three infants with detectable tenofovir: 0.9 ng per mL in two and 17.4 ng per mL in one. This study estimated that the median tenofovir dose ingested through breast milk was 0.47 μg per kg, or less than 0.01% of the proposed daily 6 mg per kg pediatric TDF dose.[119] In a study of 59 breastfeeding women living with HIV on TDF/3TC/EFV, no infants had detectable tenofovir plasma levels.[118]

Infant Pharmacokinetics. No PK data are available describing tenofovir use in neonates, and TDF is currently not recommended for use in children under age 2 years.

Safety. Despite safety signals in animal studies and in preliminary analysis of some human studies, in multiple prospective cohort studies, TDF is not associated with increased teratogenicity, whether given for treatment in women living with HIV or for prevention (PrEP).[59,107,133,143,144] In the APR, sufficient numbers of first-trimester exposures to TDF have been monitored to be able to detect at least a 1.5-fold increased risk of overall birth defects and a twofold increase in risk of birth defects in the cardiovascular and genitourinary systems. Among the cases of first-trimester TDF exposure reported to the APR, the prevalence of overall birth defects was 2.4% (91/3,851 births; 95% CI, 1.9% to 2.9%), similar to the national prevalence of 2.7% in the U.S. general population.[106] Concern remains for a potential link between maternal antenatal TDF use and preterm birth or low birth weight, but the data are conflicting and necessitate further research.[12,145–149] There is inconsistent evidence that maternal antenatal TDF use may be associated with transient growth delays of uncertain clinical significance in the first year of life.[150–153]

Tenofovir Alafenamide

Tenofovir alafenamide is a newer, orally bioavailable form of tenofovir. Much less is known about TAF than TDF in pregnancy, and there are insufficient data to assess TAF-associated risk for birth defects or miscarriage. TAF is a prodrug of tenofovir and, like TDF, is hydrolyzed to tenofovir in plasma and converted to tenofovir diphosphate intracellularly, where it exerts its activity as an NRTI.

Maternal Pharmacokinetics. Unlike TDF, which readily converts to tenofovir in plasma after oral absorption, TAF remains relatively stable in plasma, resulting in lower plasma and higher intracellular tenofovir concentrations. After oral administration, TAF 25 mg resulted in plasma tenofovir concentrations that were 90% lower than those seen with TDF

300 mg. Intracellular tenofovir diphosphate concentrations, however, were substantially higher with TAF.[154,155]

As a relatively new ARV, there are limited TAF PK data available in pregnancy. Most pregnancy data come from one clinical trial of 31 women receiving TAF 25 mg without a pharmacoenhancer, and 27 receiving TAF 10 mg with cobicistat (COBI) boosting. In this study, there were no significant differences in PK between pregnant and postpartum women on COBI-boosted TAF. Among women taking unboosted TAF, there were significantly different plasma exposures during pregnancy and postpartum, driven by higher exposures in the postpartum period.[156] A subsequent report described the PK of TAF in 17 women taking TAF 25 mg boosted with either COBI or RTV without differences in plasma exposures between pregnancy and postpartum.[157]

Little is known about TAF placental transfer and excretion in breast milk. In the above referenced study, TAF was below the assay limit of quantification (<3.9 ng per mL) in all 15 cord blood samples tested.[156]

Infant Pharmacokinetics. TAF is not currently approved for children under age 18 years, and there are no data on the PK in children younger than 6 years.[105]

Safety and Outcome Data. There are not a sufficient number of reported cases in the APR to draw any conclusions about risk of birth defects.

Zidovudine

ZDV, the first drug developed for treatment of HIV, was also the first ARV shown to prevent perinatal transmission.[5] Currently, ZDV remains a component of combination ART to treat HIV infection and, most commonly, of maternal and neonatal prophylactic regimens to prevent perinatal transmission at the time of delivery.[1]

Maternal Pharmacokinetics. Following oral dosing, ZDV absorption is rapid and complete. In nonpregnant adults receiving ZDV oral doses of 200 mg, the average maximum concentration (C_{max}) of 1.0 µg per mL is reached at an average time to maximum concentration (T_{max}) of 0.65 hours.[158] ZDV is largely metabolized by the liver through glucuronidation and undergoes extensive first-pass metabolism; bioavailability averages 63% despite nearly complete absorption.[159] ZDV is eliminated primarily by renal excretion as glucuronide[160] and has a half-life ($t_{1/2}$) of around 1.1 hours and oral clearance (Cl/F) of approximately 1.3 L per kg per h in nonpregnant adults.[161] Like the other NRTIs, ZDV is a prodrug that requires intracellular metabolism by cellular enzymes to the active triphosphorylated nucleotide form.[90] The rate-limiting step in ZDV activation is the conversion of ZDV monophosphate to diphosphate, catalyzed by cellular thymidylate kinase.[162,163] This enzyme is saturated at relatively low substrate concentrations, so that intracellular concentrations of ZDV monophosphate greatly exceed those of ZDV diphosphate and triphosphate, and plasma ZDV concentrations do not correlate with intracellular concentrations of ZDV triphosphate.[162,163] The half-life of intracellular ZDV triphosphate exceeds that of ZDV in plasma, averaging 3 to 4 hours.[164,165] As a result, ZDV dose and plasma concentration do not directly correlate with the concentration of intracellular phosphorylated metabolites or clinical effects.[90,166]

In early studies, ZDV C_{max}, T_{max}, bioavailability, and $t_{1/2}$ in pregnancy appeared no different from historical values in nonpregnant adults.[167,168] In two subsequent studies, ZDV PK was compared during pregnancy and at 1 to 4 weeks' postpartum; average Cl/F significantly increased during pregnancy by 47% to 65%, while average AUC decreased by 34% to 39%.[125,169] The clinical significance of the decrease in ZDV plasma exposure during pregnancy is not known. Current standard adult ZDV oral doses of either 200 mg every 8 hours or 300 mg every 12 hours are recommended as a second-line NRTI backbone, as part of a multi-ARV regimen during pregnancy.[1]

IV ZDV infusion during labor was part of the original regimen used in the PACTG 076 protocol, the first study to demonstrate the efficacy of ARVs in preventing perinatal HIV transmission.[17] Although IV ZDV infusion is no longer indicated in labor for women with well-controlled HIV, it remains standard clinical practice for high risk for transmission pregnant women with unknown or elevated HIV viral load at the time of delivery in resource-rich settings (in addition to the oral combination ART, cesarean delivery, and the extended multidrug neonatal ARV prophylaxis).[1] Continuous IV ZDV dosing is recommended rather than intermittent dosing, because with noncontinuous dosing ZDV concentrations in umbilical cord and neonatal plasma at the time of delivery are highly variable and dependent on the length of time separating delivery and the previous dose.[168] Current continuous IV infusion recommend dosing is a 2 mg per kg loading dose followed by 1 mg per kg per hour until delivery, which usually produces ZDV plasma concentration at the time of birth of 0.82 µg per mL in the mother and 0.75 µg per mL in the neonate.[1,168] IV ZDV is not available in many resource-limited settings where the majority of women living with HIV reside. Although less intensive oral ZDV regimens to reduce perinatal transmission have been developed,[20,170] oral maternal perinatal prophylaxis has largely been replaced by more potent combination ART (initiated at time of presentation to prenatal care or/and time of HIV diagnosis).

Primate and human studies suggest that ZDV moves across the placenta by simple diffusion, achieving cord blood to maternal blood ratio of approximately 0.80.[103,171–174] The human placenta phosphorylates ZDV to its active metabolite; the intracellular mechanisms needed to phosphorylate ZDV are also present in the developing fetus.[87] Intracellular concentrations of phosphorylated ZDV metabolites in maternal and cord blood have been studied following administration of continuous infusions during labor; as in nonpregnant populations, intracellular ZDV triphosphate concentrations do not appear to vary with plasma levels.[175] Median levels of ZDV monophosphate (1,556 and 67 fmol per 10^6 cells) and triphosphate (1,464 and 70 fmol per 10^6 cells) have been found to be similar in maternal and cord blood, respectively; however, considerable variability was observed among study subjects.[176] These values are two to three times higher than those reported in adults living with HIV receiving oral ZDV and, assuming uniform intracellular distribution of ZDV triphosphate, around five times the ZDV triphosphate IC_{50}) for HIV reverse transcriptase (~0.05 µM).[176] Although continuous IV infusion of ZDV during labor provides maternal and cord blood intracellular ZDV triphosphate levels consistent with high antiviral activity, the relative contributions of maternal, placental, and fetal ZDV triphosphate in preventing intrapartum and early postpartum perinatal transmission are unknown. A population PK analysis of intrapartum IV dosing demonstrated high fetal exposure to ZDV with recommended dosing; simulations from this modeling suggest that reduced intrapartum ZDV dosing regimens may provide lower but adequate fetal exposures.[177] Both hepatic glucuronidation and renal function are depressed in infants immediately after birth, and the washout $t_{1/2}$ of transplacentally acquired ZDV is extremely prolonged, averaging 13 hours.[178]

ZDV is excreted into human breast milk. Breast milk to maternal plasma ZDV concentration ratios range from 0.44 to 1.35; however, plasma ZDV levels have not been detectable in infants receiving ZDV only via breast milk.[130,131,179]

Infant Pharmacokinetics

ZDV elimination increases rapidly during the first days of life, with $t_{1/2}$ averaging 3 hours during days 3 to 10.[178] A population analysis combining ZDV PK data from six studies demonstrated a further increase in ZDV clearance over the first 2 months of life, reaching adult levels by 4 to 8 weeks of life (Fig. 32.2).[180] The developmental pattern of the increase in ZDV clearance in the infant parallels that of bilirubin, whose primary route of elimination is also via hepatic glucuronidation.[181] However, although bilirubin and ZDV clearance mature in parallel, they are metabolized by different isoenzymes of the UGT family, with ZDV metabolized primarily by UGT 2B7 and bilirubin by UGT 1A1.[182,183]

The current U.S. Food and Drug Administration (FDA)–approved dosing recommendation for ZDV in infants from birth (starting at ≥35 weeks' gestation) to 4 weeks of age is 4 mg per kg orally every 12 hours and 12 mg per kg after 4 weeks of age. ZDV clearance is decreased in premature infants, (Fig. 32.2) and a dosing reduction is needed to avoid the accumulation of

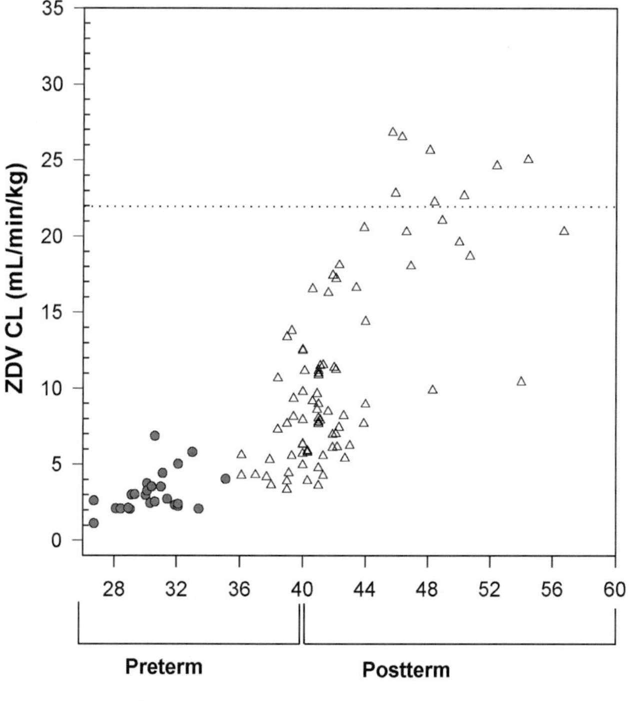

Figure 32.2 Zidovudine clearance plotted against postconceptional age (gestational age at birth plus postnatal age) for infants from birth to age 5 months. *Open triangles*, term infants; *solid circles*, preterm infants; *broken line*, average adult clearance. (Adapted from Mirochnick M, Capparelli E, Connor J. Pharmacokinetics of zidovudine in infants: a population analysis across studies. *Clin Pharmacol Ther* 1999;66(1):16–24.)

potentially toxic serum ZDV concentrations.[184,185] Infants born before 35 weeks' gestation are prescribed initial doses of 2 mg per kg orally or 1.5 mg per kg IV every 12 hours. Due to maturation in glucuronidation processes after birth, ZDV dosing frequency needs to increase at 2 weeks of age if gestational age at birth is above 30 weeks or at 4 weeks of age if gestational age at birth is less than 30 weeks.[105,186] ZDV prophylaxis is recommended for the first 4 weeks of life in neonates at low risk of perinatal HIV transmission and for 6 weeks in combination with RAL or NVP (with or without 3TC) in neonates at increased risk of perinatal HIV transmission.[105]

Safety

ZDV has the longest history of use during pregnancy and the most safety information; ZDV use in pregnancy does not appear to be associated with increased risk of maternal or fetal adverse outcomes.[187] Bone marrow depression is a common toxicity of ZDV, and mild, transient depression of hematologic parameters has been observed in the newborn after exposure to the full PACTG 076 regimen and to less intensive regimens.[17,188] Hemoglobin was decreased by an average of 1 mg per dL at 3 weeks of age in newborns exposed to ZDV in PACTG 076 compared with those exposed to placebo; however, by 12 weeks of age, no differences were seen in hemoglobin between the two groups.[17] No long-term adverse effects of ZDV exposure have been detected in exposed infants to date.[189,190] There is, however, a concern for potential cardiotoxicity with a case report of ZDV-exposed female infants with higher left ventricular shortening fraction at 1 month of life and increased posterior wall thickness at 1 year, suggestive of myocardial remodeling.[93] A subsequent study also showed that perinatal ZDV exposure was associated with thicker neonatal myocardial walls and smaller left ventricular cavities.[191] Despite potential safety signals, the APR has found no evidence of cardiotoxicity when comparing ZDV-exposed and ZDV-unexposed infants born to mothers living with HIV by trimester of exposure.[192,193] The Women and Infants Transmission Study (WITS) documented a 10-fold increased risk of hypospadias with first-trimester ZDV use in their preliminary data; however, this was not substantiated in the full analysis.[192,194] Sufficient numbers of exposures to ZDV in humans have been monitored in the APR to be able to determine that first-trimester ZDV exposure is not associated with a 1.5-fold or greater increase in the risk of overall birth defects or with a twofold or greater increase in the risk of cardiovascular or genitourinary system defects.[106] Two large longitudinal studies further found no association between first-trimester ZDV exposure and birth defects.[108,195]

NON-NUCLEOSIDE/TIDE REVERSE TRANSCRIPTASE INHIBITORS

NNRTIs bind directly and noncompetitively to HIV reverse transcriptase without intracellular phosphorylation or activation.[196] Five drugs in this class are approved for clinical use in the U.S., including first-generation NNRTIs (NVP, EFV) and second-generation NNRTIs etravirine (ETR), doravirine (DOR), and RPV. There are currently limited PK and safety data in pregnancy for ETR and RPV and no pregnancy data for DOR. There are no neonatal PK and safety data on second-generation NNRTIs in neonates. ETR and DOR are recommended only as part of second- or third-line combination ART regimens in pregnant and nonpregnant adults. Because of the lack of the pregnancy and neonatal data, DOR is not discussed below.

Efavirenz

Despite reassuring observational data, the FDA cautions against using EFV in the first trimester of pregnancy secondary to concerns for increased neural tube defects (NTDs) observed in both human and animal studies.[197] Based on updated clinical trials and observational data, the U.S. HHS perinatal guidelines, WHO, and the British HIV Association guidelines no longer recommend against EFV in pregnancy or in women planning to conceive.[1,3,198] EFV is commonly used in combination with NRTIs.

Maternal Pharmacokinetics

The primary route of EFV metabolism is to 8-hydroxyefavirenz (8-hydroxy-EFV), formed predominately by CYP2B6, and excretion is predominantly as glucuronides (8-hydroxy-EFV-glucuronide) in the urine.[32,199–201] A pharmacogenomics study found that nonpregnant women with the CYP2B6 516 TT genotype had greater than threefold increases in both short-term and long-term EFV exposure, as measured by plasma and hair drug levels. Significant variation in EFV plasma concentrations has been observed in patients with diverse CYP2B6 polymorphisms.[202] The frequency of this allele varies significantly between different ethnic populations and may explain ethnic differences in drug concentrations noted in African, European, and Asian studies.

In a third-trimester intensive sampling PK study of 25 women receiving EFV, clearance was slightly increased and trough levels were decreased compared with postpartum levels.[203] Differences were not of sufficient magnitude to warrant dose adjustment during pregnancy. A subsequent intensive PK study in the second and third trimesters of pregnancy found that *AUC* in pregnancy was similar to 6 to 12 weeks' postpartum values.[204] A systematic review that included the former study, and four additional studies that measured EFV concentrations in pregnancy, concluded that EFV concentrations were not significantly affected by pregnancy and that high rates of HIV RNA suppression at delivery were achieved with EFV-based regimens.[205]

Placental transfer of EFV was evaluated in three studies. A study of 56 mother–infant pairs in which the mothers received EFV-based combination ART during pregnancy and breastfeeding, neonatal plasma drug concentration levels at delivery and hair drug concentration levels at age 12 weeks suggested moderate in utero transfer of EFV during pregnancy, with approximately one-third of transfer occurring postpartum (40% cumulative transfer, with 15% of transfer occurring during breastfeeding).[206] These data are consistent with two studies of 25 and of 40 mother–infant pairs, which found the median EFV cord blood to maternal blood concentration ratio was 0.49 (range 0.37 to 0.74)[203] and 0.67 (0.36 to 0.95), respectively.[204]

EFV is excreted in breast milk. A study of 13 mother–infant pairs in Rwanda found that EFV concentration was significantly higher in maternal plasma than that in breast milk (with a mean breast milk to mean maternal plasma concentration ratio of 0.54) and higher in breast milk than in infant plasma (with a mean breast milk to mean newborn plasma concentration ratio of 4.08). Mean infant plasma EFV concentrations were 13.1% (860 ng per mL) of maternal plasma concentrations. All infants had detectable plasma concentrations of EFV; 8 of 13 had concentrations below the minimum target therapeutic concentration of 1,000 ng per mL recommended for treatment of adults with HIV.[207] A study of breastfeeding mother–infant pairs in Mali found that the median ratios of infant plasma to maternal plasma were 0.057 at month 1, 0.072 at month 3, and 0.048 at month 6 postpartum. During the study period, the median breast milk to maternal plasma ratio was 1.16 (IQR, 0.96 to 20.62), which corresponds to a relative infant dose of 2.46% of the recommended weight-adjusted pediatric EFV dose at 6 months of age.[208] Similarly, additional studies have found that most breastfed infants are exposed to less than 10% of the weight-adjusted therapeutic pediatric EFV dose, the safety threshold for exposure to maternal drugs from breast milk.[209,210]

Infant Pharmacokinetics

No data currently are available about the PK of EFV in neonates, and EFV is not recommended for use in infants younger than 3 months.

Safety

Studies of EFV in pregnant cynomolgus monkeys demonstrated severe NTD,[211] and small numbers of overlapping cases in early human studies led to concern for the potential teratogenicity in periconception and early first-trimester use in humans.[143,144,212–215] Subsequently, sufficient numbers of exposures to EFV in humans have been prospectively monitored in the APR to be able to determine that first-trimester EFV exposure is not associated with a 1.5 or greater increase in the risk of overall birth defects; the rate of birth defects among prospectively reported pregnancies with first-trimester EFV exposure is not increased (2.4%) compared to the general population in the U.S.[106] A meta-analysis of 23 studies (including the APR data) found 44 birth defects among 2,026 live births to women who received EFV during the first trimester (1.63%, 95% CI, 0.78% to 2.48%), similar to the rate among women who received non–EFV-containing regimens in the first trimester.[80] Additional studies of pregnancies with first-trimester EFV exposure have similarly not identified an associated increased risk of NTD.[107,133,216,217] Given the low incidence of NTD in the general population, however, a greater number of exposures are still needed to definitively rule out an increased risk. The FDA advises women to avoid becoming pregnant while taking EFV and advises health care providers to avoid administration during the first trimester of pregnancy, as fetal harm may occur.[197] Although the limited data on first-trimester EFV exposure cannot rule out a twofold or threefold increased incidence of a rare outcome, such as NTDs, the available data suggest that there is no large increase in the risk of NTDs with first-trimester exposure (e.g., a 10-fold increase to a rate of 1%). As a result, the current U.S. HHS perinatal guidelines, British HIV Association guidelines, and WHO guidelines do not restrict the use of EFV in pregnancy or in women who are planning to become pregnant.[1,3,198]

Etravirine

ETR is a second-generation NNRTI with activity against HIV strains resistant to EFV and NVP.[218] There are limited data on the PK and safety of ETR in pregnancy, and it is not recommended as first-line therapy.[1]

Maternal Pharmacokinetics

The ETR PK in pregnant women has been reported in two small studies; both found significantly increased *AUC*, C_{min}, and C_{max}

in the second and third trimesters compared to postpartum (1.1- to 1.4-fold and 1.3- to 1.9-fold, respectively). ETR was well tolerated without adverse outcomes in both studies.[219,220]

Placental transfer of ETR has been reported in the same two studies, reporting median ratios of cord blood to maternal plasma ETR concentration at delivery of 0.32 (with a range of 0.19 to 0.63) and 0.52 (with a range of 0.19 to 4.25).[219,220] There is scanty published literature on ETR secretion in breast milk. A study of eight women who initiated ETR postpartum concluded that ETR penetrates well and may accumulate in breast milk.[221]

Infant Pharmacokinetics

There are no data currently available about the PK and safety of ETR in neonates, and it is not recommended in children under 2 years of age.[105]

Safety

In the limited published data on ETR in pregnancy, there is no evidence of maternal, fetal, or neonatal adverse outcomes.[106,222,223] Given the low numbers of reported cases, no definitive conclusions can be made about the safety of ETR or associated teratogenicity.

Nevirapine

NVP, a dipyridodiazepinone, a potent first-generation NNRTI, has been replaced by newer, safer ARVs as a first-line drug in pregnancy, secondary to its potential for serious side effects in pregnancy. NVP remains highly relevant, however, for neonatal prophylaxis and, along with ZDV, forms the first-line neonatal prophylaxis for infants at high risk of perinatal HIV transmission.

Maternal Pharmacokinetics

NVP absorption is rapid and complete, with bioavailability exceeding 90% following oral administration in tablet or liquid form.[224,225] NVP is highly lipophilic at physiologic pH and is rapidly and widely distributed throughout the body.[226] Mean apparent volume of distribution exceeds total body water and is significantly higher in adult women than in men (1.54 L per kg vs. 1.38 L per kg, $p = 0.001$).[227] The protein-bound fraction of NVP in plasma is approximately 60%.[226] The main route of NVP elimination is hepatic metabolism by enzymes of the cytochrome P450 family, primarily CYP3A4 and CYP2B6, followed by renal excretion.[226] Elimination following initial doses is slow, with a mean elimination half-life of 40 hours (range: 22 to 84 hours).[224] With chronic therapy, metabolic autoinduction of the elimination pathway occurs, so that after 2 weeks of treatment, NVP clearance increases 1.5-fold to twofold and mean elimination half-life decreases to 20 to 30 hours.[228,229] To avoid elevated NVP concentrations and minimize toxicity during this autoinduction phase, the recommended dosing schedule for NVP as part of combination ART in HIV-infected adults is 200 mg once daily for the first 2 weeks, followed by an increase to 200 mg twice daily.[230] The literature is divided between studies that found steady-state NVP concentrations to be equivalent to those in nonpregnant adults[231] and without significant alteration to PK parameters,[232] and studies which identified trends toward lower steady-state concentrations and increased clearance with associated lower AUC and C_{max}.[233–235]

NVP crosses the placenta well; the ratio of the NVP concentrations in cord blood and maternal blood at the time of delivery averages approximately 80%.[236,237] Average cord blood concentration doubles to over 2,000 ng per mL with chronic maternal dosing during the last trimester of pregnancy.[238] NVP is also excreted in breast milk; multiple African studies have documented biologically significant detectable plasma NVP concentrations in breastfeeding infants, but without sufficient data to draw conclusions on adverse outcomes of neonatal exposure or potential resistance.[104,130,131,239]

Infant Pharmacokinetics

Chronic maternal NVP dosing prior to delivery appears to accelerate NVP elimination in the infant after birth, presumably due to in utero autoinduction of NVP elimination. Following administration of a 2 mg per kg oral dose of NVP to infants at 48 to 72 hours after birth, median $t_{1/2}$ was 43.6 hours (range: 23.6 to 81.6 hours), and median Cl/F was 36.1 mL per kg per hour (range: 22.0 to 40.0 mL per kg per hour). Absorption was variable and prolonged in the newborns, with a median T_{max} of 8.2 hours (range: 2.0 to 26.1 hours).[237] NVP is most commonly used in combination with ZDV (with or without 3TC) as neonatal prophylaxis in infants at higher risk of HIV transmission and greater than 32 weeks' gestation. For prophylaxis, doses within 48 hours of birth, 48 hours after the first dose, and 96 hours after the second dose are used by two weight bands: 1.5 to 2 kg (8 mg NVP) and greater than 2 kg (12 mg NVP). Alternatively, in these higher risk neonates, empiric treatment NVP dose is recommended for 2 to 6 weeks. Treatment doses in infants born greater than 37 weeks gestation is 6 mg per kg twice daily up to 4 weeks of life. For infants born between 34 and 37 weeks, 4 mg per kg twice daily is recommended for the first week of life.[105]

Safety

In the APR, sufficient numbers of first-trimester exposures to NVP in humans have been reported to detect at least a 1.5-fold increase in risk of overall birth defects and a twofold increase in cardiovascular and genitourinary defects; no increase has been noted with first-trimester NVP exposure. Among cases of first-trimester NVP exposure reported to the APR, the prevalence of birth defects was 2.80% (32/1,153 births; 95% CI, 1.9% to 3.9%) commensurate with a total prevalence in the general U.S. population of (2.72%), based on CDC surveillance.[106] The French Perinatal Cohort similarly found no association with NVP and birth defects.[133]

NVP, however, is associated with rare but significant toxicities. Severe, life-threatening hypersensitivity skin reactions, including Stevens–Johnson syndrome, and severe, life-threatening, and in some cases, fatal hepatotoxicity, including fulminant and cholestatic hepatitis, hepatic necrosis, and hepatic failure, have been reported in patients receiving NVP in combination with other ARVs and in a small number of individuals receiving NVP as part of postexposure prophylaxis (PEP) to prevent HIV transmission.[240] The highest risk of severe rash and hepatic morbidity occurs in the first 6 to 18 weeks of NVP therapy, although the risk of NVP toxicity continues past this period, and monitoring should continue for the duration of therapy. In clinical trials, clinical hepatic morbidity occurred in 4.0% (range 0% to 11.0%) of patients who received NVP, with NVP-associated liver failure or hepatic mortality from 0.04% to 0.40%.[241,242]

The development of severe NVP-associated skin rash is 5.5 to 7.3 times more common in women and is associated with higher CD4 cell counts.[243–245] NVP-associated hepatic toxicity with systemic symptoms is also more common in women than men (3.4-fold higher), and associated with CD4 cell counts greater than 250 cells per mm^3.[242,246,247] Both severe NVP-associated skin rash and hepatotoxicity have been reported in pregnancy. Although fatal cases of hepatic failure have been reported in pregnant women with HIV receiving NVP as part of ART, it is unclear if pregnancy potentiates the risk of hepatotoxicity.[247–251] The U.S. HHS perinatal guidelines suggest that NVP (as a component of a combination ART) should be initiated in pregnant women with CD4 cell counts ≥250 cells per mm^3 only if the benefit clearly outweighs the risk. Women with CD4 cell counts less than 250 cells per mm^3 can receive NVP-based regimens, and women who become pregnant while taking NVP and who are tolerating their regimens well can continue therapy, regardless of CD4 cell count.[1] Pregnancy can mimic early symptoms of hepatotoxicity (i.e., pregnancy-related nausea and vomiting), and it is important to monitor for clinical symptoms and with serial hepatic transaminases (i.e., alanine aminotransferase [ALT] and aspartate aminotransferase [AST]) in pregnant women on NVP-based ART, particularly during the first 18 weeks of therapy.[1]

There are reports of rash and hyperbilirubinemia in infants exposed to NVP through breast milk.[241]

Rilpivirine

RPV is a second-generation NNRTI recommended for use as an alternative component of the first-line ART only in women with pretreatment HIV RNA less than 100,000 copies per mL or CD4 cell counts greater than 200 cells per mm^3. Recently, RPV has been co-formulated with the INSTI cabotegravir (CAB) as a parenteral long-acting formulation for intramuscular injection. No data are currently available on the PK and safety of this formulation in pregnant and breastfeeding women.

Maternal Pharmacokinetics

Three PK studies have found that RPV exposure is 20% to 50% lower in pregnancy than postpartum and highly variable.[252–254] While RPV plasma concentration is reduced during pregnancy, increased doses have not been studied, and standard adult dosing continues to be recommended in pregnancy. Given lower RPV exposure in pregnancy, viral loads should be monitored more frequently.[1]

Placental passage of RPV has been evaluated in three PK studies which have demonstrated similar cord blood to maternal plasma ratios of 0.5 to 0.55.[252–254] An ex vivo human cotyledon perfusion model also demonstrated that placental transfer of RPV with fetal transfer rates ranges from 17% to 37%.[255,256] There are no data on RPV excretion in breast milk.

Infant Pharmacokinetics

No PK or safety data are available for RPV in neonates or infants.

Safety

Among cases of first-trimester exposures to RPV reported to the APR, there was no increased risk of birth defects compared to the general U.S. population. Sufficient numbers of exposures to RPV in humans have been prospectively monitored in the APR to be able to determine that first-trimester exposure is not associated with a twofold or greater increase in the risk of overall birth defects.[106]

PROTEASE INHIBITORS

PIs are potent ARVs used as components of ART regimens for the first-, second-, and third-line ART. Inhibition of HIV protease, the enzyme responsible for cleavage of large polypeptide chains into the smaller proteins needed for production of functional HIV virions, leads to the release of structurally disorganized and noninfectious viral particles. PI-based regimens produce a sustained suppression of HIV replication and have been historically the preferred first-line ART choice in pregnancy in resource-rich settings and an alternative first-line ART component globally. Gastrointestinal symptoms (e.g., nausea, vomiting, abdominal pain, diarrhea) are common with all PIs, including PI PK enhancer RTV. Following the introduction of better-tolerated and less toxic INSTIs, PIs are currently considered as alternative to the first-line ART in resource-rich settings and are used mostly for the second- and third-line ART in HIV-infected pregnant and breastfeeding women globally.[1–3]

PIs are metabolized by cytochrome P450 enzyme system, especially enzymes of the CYP3A family, with lesser contributions by CYP2C9 and CYP2D6, and many PIs have the capacity to alter the activity of these enzymes, leading to complex interactions among drugs of this class acting as inducers, competitive inhibitors, and substrates. PI RTV and non-PI drug COBI act as PK enhancers, and both are potent cytochrome P450 enzyme inhibitors, increasing concentrations of PIs when administered together.

PIs cross the placenta poorly with only low or undetectable concentrations found in cord blood, suggesting that the primary mechanism of action of PIs in preventing mother-to-child HIV transmission is by decreasing maternal HIV RNA viral load.[257,258]

An association between PI-based ART and preterm delivery has been reported in multiple studies from Europe, North America, and Africa, with risk ranging from 1.14 to 3.4.[74,195,259–263]

A summary of 4,646 live birth outcomes from the Surveillance Monitoring for ART Toxicities (SMARTT) study and four IMPAACT studies reported that rates of preterm delivery and low birth weight were 19% among women taking PI-based regimens.[150]

Atazanavir

Maternal Pharmacokinetics

ATV is a first-line PI that can be administered to adults as 300 mg once daily in combination with PK enhancer 100 mg RTV or 150 mg COBI, although treatment-naïve adults may receive 400 mg once daily without RTV or COBI.[264] ATV inhibits activity of the enzyme uridine 5′-diphospho-glucuronosyltransferase (UGT) 1A1, which is responsible for glucuronidation of bilirubin, and mild reversible unconjugated hyperbilirubinemia with clinical symptoms of jaundice is often seen with ATV use.[264]

ATV when administered during pregnancy once daily with RTV has been shown to achieve adult therapeutic PK targets, and most pregnant women achieved undetectable HIV RNA at the time of delivery.[265–270] In a retrospective study of 19 pregnant women, trough ATV concentrations were measured at a median of 30 weeks' gestation. The majority of women had a mean ATV plasma trough concentration above 100 ng per mL.[271] In studies that evaluated full ATV PK profiles (administered daily as 300 mg ATV per 100 mg RTV), ATV *AUC* was lower during pregnancy than the *AUC* reported in other studies of nonpregnant adults living with HIV.[267,269,270,272,273] In some studies, ATV *AUC* was lower during pregnancy than it was in the same patients postpartum and in nonpregnant control populations.[266,267,269,272,273] Intracellular ATV levels in women taking 300 mg ATV per 100 mg RTV appear to be stable throughout pregnancy.[274]

As with nonpregnant adults, administration of ATV/RTV in combination with TDF appears to affect the PK of ATV during pregnancy. ATV *AUC* of pregnant women in the third trimester who received concomitant TDF was 30% lower than the ATV *AUC* of women who were not receiving concomitant TDF, an effect similar to that seen in nonpregnant adults.[269,273] The increase in ATV *AUC* postpartum relative to that in the third trimester was similar for women taking concomitant TDF and for those not taking concomitant TDF.[269] A couple of PK studies, however, have contradicting findings where concomitant TDF did not result in lower ATV *AUC* or lower ATV trough concentrations in pregnant women in their third trimester.[268,275]

In studies of ATV 400 mg per 100 mg RTV once daily during pregnancy, pregnant women receiving the increased dose without TDF had ATV *AUC* equivalent to that seen in historic nonpregnant controls with HIV infection who received standard-dose ATV without TDF.[266,267] Although some experts recommend an increased dose of ATV for all women during the second and third trimesters, the use of an increased dose of ATV in the second and third trimesters is generally recommended only for ART-experienced pregnant women who are also receiving either TDF or an H_2-receptor antagonist.[264]

Limited data from studies of COBI as a pharmacoenhancer for other ARVs in pregnant women suggest that COBI exposure is substantially reduced in pregnancy (see "Pharmacokinetic Enhancers" section).[276–278] Based on these studies, ATV/COBI is not recommended for use in pregnant women because of substantially lower exposures of DRV and COBI during pregnancy.[1]

In studies of women receiving ATV/RTV combination therapy during pregnancy, cord blood ATV concentration averaged 13% to 21% of maternal serum levels at delivery.[264,269,270] In a study of three women, the median ratio of ATV breast milk to plasma concentration was 13%.[279]

Infant Pharmacokinetics

No PK or safety data are available for ATV in newborns and young infants.

Safety

The prevalence of birth defects reported in the APR with first-trimester ATV exposure was 2.2% (28/1,279 births; 95% CI, 1.5% to 3.2%) compared with a 2.7% total prevalence in the U.S. population, based on CDC surveillance.[120] In a U.S. cohort of HIV-negative children exposed to HIV in utero, first-trimester ATV exposure was associated with increased odds of congenital anomalies of the skin (aOR = 5.24; $p = 0.02$) and the musculoskeletal system (aOR = 2.55; $p = 0.007$).[107] These findings were not confirmed in the study of a French cohort, with lower (<50%) power to detect an aOR of 1.5.[93]

Due to the ATV-related inhibition of hepatic UGT enzyme, elevation in indirect (unconjugated) bilirubin can occur with ATV use, including use during pregnancy.[280] It remains unknown whether ATV-associated elevated maternal indirect bilirubin throughout pregnancy has any effects on the fetus. Serious postnatal elevations in bilirubin have not been reported in infants born to mothers who received ATV during pregnancy.[264,266,269,270,281–283] In selected studies, neonatal bilirubin elevations requiring treatment with phototherapy have been reported to occur more frequently after prenatal ATV exposure.[281,282] Elevated neonatal bilirubin in neonates with in utero ATV exposure has not been associated with slower metabolizer UGT-1 genotypes.[283]

Darunavir

Maternal Pharmacokinetics

DRV is a second-generation PI that can be administered to treatment-naïve and treatment-experienced adults as 800 mg once daily in combination with PK enhancer 100 mg RTV or 150 mg COBI, although treatment-experienced adults with DRV resistance-associated mutations or unknown baseline resistance need to be dosed twice daily with DRV 600 mg boosted with 100 mg RTV.[284] Several studies of the DRV/RTV PK during pregnancy have been completed.[285–289] DRV *AUC* during the third trimester was reduced by 17% to 26% with DRV 600 mg per RTV 100 mg twice-daily dosing and by 33% to 39% with DRV 800 mg per RTV 100 mg once-daily dosing.[285–287,289] Compared to the postpartum DRV trough concentrations, third-trimester DRV trough plasma concentrations were reduced by 8% to 12% with DRV 600 mg per RTV 100 mg twice-daily dosing and by 42% to 58% with DRV 800 mg per RTV 100 mg once-daily dosing.[286,287,289] Increased 800 mg DRV dose administered twice daily did not increase DRV exposure in pregnant women.[288] Among three studies that measured DRV protein binding during pregnancy, two studies reported decreased unbound DRV concentrations during pregnancy that were not considered clinically significant.[285,286,289] Because of low DRV plasma trough levels with once-daily dosing, twice-daily DRV dosing is recommended during pregnancy, especially for treatment-experienced women.[1,264] Once-daily DRV 800 mg per RTV 100 mg can be used only in pregnant women who are virally suppressed on a stable once-daily DRV/RTV regimen prior to pregnancy and whose adherence or ability to tolerate a regimen may be compromised by a switch to twice-daily DRV/RTV.[264]

Two studies evaluated the PK and safety of once-daily DRV 800 mg per COBI 150 mg during pregnancy.[277,290] In a study of seven pregnant women, total DRV *AUC* was reduced by 56% and 50%, and plasma trough DRV concentration was reduced by 92% and 89%, with DRV/COBI. Unbound DRV concentrations were also decreased during pregnancy, with *AUC* 45% and 40% lower and trough concentration 92% and 88% lower during the second and third trimesters than postpartum. COBI exposures were lower during pregnancy (see "Pharmacokinetic Enhancers" section).[283] Despite lower exposure, six of seven participants remained virally suppressed during pregnancy, and none of the infants were infected with HIV. In a larger study of 29 pregnant women treated with DRV/COBI, total DRV *AUC* was reduced by 33% and 48% and DRV trough concentrations were reduced by 71% and 75% during second and third trimesters compared to postpartum PK.[290] Based on these studies, DRV/COBI is not recommended for use in pregnant women because of substantially lower exposures of DRV and COBI during pregnancy.[284]

In an ex vivo human perfusion model, the mean fetal transfer rate of DRV was 15%.[291] In five studies that reported data from 6 to 14 subjects each, the median of the ratio of DRV concentrations in cord blood to maternal delivery plasma concentration ranged from 13% to 24%.[283,285–287,292] No data are available that describe the breast milk passage of DRV in humans.

Infant Pharmacokinetics

No PK or safety data are available on DRV in newborns and young infants.

Safety

Among cases of first-trimester DRV exposure reported to the APR, the prevalence of birth defects was 2.4% (11/456 births; 95% CI, 1.2% to 4.3%), which is a sufficient number of first-trimester exposures to conclude that there is no two-fold increase in the risk of overall birth defects compared to control populations.

Lopinavir

Maternal Pharmacokinetics

LPV, a potent first-generation PI, is available only in a fixed-dose combination with RTV. In treatment-experienced adults, LPV 400 mg per RTV 100 mg is dosed twice daily, and in treatment-naïve adults, it can be dosed once daily at double dose of LPV 800 mg per RTV 200 mg. LPV/RTV has poor gastrointestinal palatability and frequently causes nausea, vomiting, and diarrhea.[293]

Until the introduction of once-daily ATV/RTV and INSTIs, LPV/RTV has been used extensively in the U.S. and globally during pregnancy. The older capsule formulation has been replaced with the tablet and is not discussed here.

PK studies of LPV 400 mg/RTV 100 mg twice daily in pregnant women have demonstrated a reduction in LPV plasma concentrations during pregnancy of around 30% compared with those seen in nonpregnant adults.[294–296] Increasing the dose of LPV/r during pregnancy to LPV 600 mg/RTV 150 mg results in LPV plasma concentrations equivalent to those seen in nonpregnant adults receiving standard doses.[297,298] A population PK study of LPV/RTV in 154 pregnant women demonstrated that increased body weight influences LPV clearance and volume, with heavier women (>100 kg) being at higher risk for subtherapeutic trough concentrations when taking the standard dose during pregnancy.[299] LPV plasma protein binding was shown to be reduced during pregnancy; however, the resulting increase in free (unbound) drug might be insufficient to make up for the reduction in total plasma LPV concentration during pregnancy.[300,301] Population PK modeling of the total and unbound PK data, however, suggests that standard dosing should be effective during pregnancy with susceptible virus.[301–303] The LPV/RTV pregnancy PK data have led some experts to support the use of an increased dose of LPV/RTV in pregnant women with HIV during the second and third trimesters, especially in women who are PI experienced and women who start treatment during pregnancy with a baseline viral load greater than 50 copies per mL.[1] Once-daily dosing of LPV/RTV is not recommended in pregnancy because no data support reaching therapeutic drug concentrations.

LPV poorly crosses the human placenta, and the average ratio of LPV concentration in cord blood to maternal plasma at delivery was 0.20±0.13. However, in a study among 51 mother–infant pairs in Uganda treated with LPV/RTV during pregnancy and breastfeeding, 41% of infants had detectable plasma LPV concentrations at birth, and mean LPV infant hair to maternal hair concentration at 12 weeks postpartum was 0.87.[211] There was no transfer during breastfeeding observed, and no infant had detectable plasma LPV concentrations at 12 weeks. LPV concentrations in human breast milk are very low to undetectable, and LPV concentrations in breastfeeding infants whose mothers received LPV/RTV are not clinically significant.[104,131,183,211,304]

Infant Pharmacokinetics

There are no data on the appropriate dose of LPV/RTV for neonates and no data on the safety of using this drug combination in this age group. The PK of the oral LPV/RTV solution at approximately LPV/RTV 300 mg per 75 mg per m^2 of body surface area per dose twice daily was evaluated in infants younger than 6 weeks.[305] Even at this higher dose, LPV plasma trough concentrations were highly variable but were lower in younger infants aged less than 6 months compared to older infants and children.

Safety

In the United Kingdom/Ireland National Study of HIV in Pregnancy and Childhood, LPV/RTV use was significantly associated with preterm delivery after adjustment for other factors when compared to other boosted-PI regimens or to NNRTI-based regimens.[263] In the PROMISE study, LPV/RTV-based ART regimens were associated with an increased incidence of low birth weight (<2,500 g) and increased rates of preterm delivery (<37 weeks).[12]

The French Perinatal Cohort found no association between birth defects and LPV or RTV, with 85% power to detect a 1.5-fold increase.[133] The Pediatric HIV/AIDS Cohort Study (PHACS)also found no association between LPV and congenital anomalies.[25] Surveillance data from the United Kingdom and Ireland over a 10-year period showed a 2.9% incidence of congenital abnormalities (134 children of 4,609 LPV-exposed pregnancies), comparable to rates of congenital abnormalities in populations without HIV.[306] In the APR, sufficient numbers of first-trimester exposures to LPV/RTV did not detect an increase in risk of overall birth defects and the cardiovascular and genitourinary system defects with LPV/RTV.[120] Among cases of first-trimester exposure to LPV/r reported to the APR, the prevalence of birth defects was 2.1% (30/1,418 births; 95% CI, 1.4% to 3.0%) compared with a prevalence of either 2.7% when using data from the Metropolitan Atlanta Congenital Defects Program (MACDP) or 4.2% when using data from the Texas Birth Defects Registry (TBDR).[120]

Pediatric LPV/RTV oral solution contains 42.4% (vol./vol.) alcohol and 15.3% (wt./vol.) propylene glycol. Reduced hepatic metabolic and kidney excretory function in newborns can lead to accumulation of LPV as well as alcohol and propylene glycol, resulting in adverse events (e.g., serious cardiac, renal, metabolic, or respiratory problems). Preterm babies are at increased risk for this toxicity because their metabolism and elimination of LPV, propylene glycol, and alcohol are reduced. Postmarketing surveillance has identified 10 LPV/RTV-treated neonates less than 4 weeks of age, 9 of whom were born prematurely, who experienced life-threatening events.[307] In a separate report comparing 50 newborns exposed to HIV and treated with LPV/RTV after birth to 108 neonates exposed to HIV and treated with ZDV alone, elevated concentrations of 17-hydroxyprogesterone and dehydroepiandrosterone sulfate, consistent with impairment of 21α-hydroxylase activity, were seen only in the infants with LPV exposure. All full-term infants were asymptomatic, but three of eight preterm infants had life-threatening symptoms, including hyponatremia, hyperkalemia, and cardiogenic shock, consistent with adrenal insufficiency.[308] As a result of these reports, LPV/RTV oral solution is contraindicated in neonates younger than a postmenstrual age (first day of the mother's last menstrual period to birth, plus the time elapsed after birth) of 42 weeks, and a postnatal age of at least 14 days has been attained. The novel LPV/RTV formulations of pellets and granules recently approved for use in infants in resource-limited settings do not contain propylene glycol and alcohol and might be studied in neonates in the future.

INTEGRASE STRAND TRANSFERASE INHIBITORS

INSTIs are a newer class of ARVs that inhibit integrase, the viral enzyme that catalyzes the two-step process of insertion of HIV DNA into the genome of the human cell. Integrase is responsible for the stable maintenance of the viral genome as well as for efficient viral gene expression and replication. HIV integrase is a distinct therapeutic target from other ARV drug classes; thus, INSTIs maintain activity against HIV that is resistant to other classes of ART, allowing for the potential for viral suppression in treatment-experienced populations.[1,309,310] INSTIs are recommended as first-line ART therapy in the U.S. and globally.[3,230] RAL is a first-generation INSTI, while DTG, bictegravir (BIC), and CAB are second-generation integrase inhibitors. There are no data on BIC or CAB in pregnancy. Available data on integrase inhibitors are reviewed below.

Dolutegravir

DTG is a well-tolerated, potent second-generation INSTI that rapidly became a first-line ARV drug in global ART guidelines after approval. DTG, however, has garnered international concern for a possible increased risk of NTD when used during periconception and in the early first trimester. DTG was rolled out in Botswana as first-line ART (in combination with TDF/FTC) for adults in 2016, replacing EFV-based ART.[311] The ongoing Botswana Tsepamo birth outcome study collected data on ART exposure from eight government hospitals and was focused on identifying congenital anomalies secondary to concern for increased risk of NTD with EFV exposure in the early first trimester. The Tsepamo study detected a safety signal for increased risk of NTD with DTG in an analysis of preliminary data in 2018.[311] That signal prompted significant global response and changes in the WHO, U.S., and other national guidelines, which restricted use of DTG during periconception period and early first trimester (prior to closure of the neural tube). Since that time, there has been only one additional case of NTD associated with periconception DTG use in Botswana, and the associated risk become smaller with the addition of more good-quality data.[82] An additional year of data has not, however, totally refuted the safety signal. This same increased risk has not been demonstrated in countries with folate supplementation, other than one case in the APR, but the studies in folate-supplementing countries are notably limited by lack of internal comparators, prospective evaluation, and ascertainment of NTD among spontaneous and induced abortions. In light of the still present but decreased safety signal and advantages of DTG, namely, the minimal drug–drug interactions, overall good safety and side-effect profile, low cost, and low annual discontinuation rate, the WHO updated their guidelines in summer of 2019 recommending use of DTG for all adults living with HIV, including women in the periconception period. Guidelines in resource-rich settings, however, continue to advise more caution restricting use of DTG during preconception and in the early first trimester of pregnancy.

Maternal Pharmacokinetics

DTG is primarily metabolized through hepatic glucuronidation by UDP-glucuronosyltransferase 1A.[312,313] It has a half-life ($t_{½}$) of 13 to 14 hours and shows a predictable PK profile and a well-defined exposure–response relationship.[312] DTG absorption is not affected by meals, but can be affected by coadministered cation-containing antacids or laxatives, sucralfate, oral iron supplements, oral calcium supplements, or buffered medications. Ideally, DTG should not be administered within 2 hours of intake containing minerals or buffers.[314]

DTG PK in pregnancy has been evaluated in several studies, as well as in several case reports, and appears to have adequate plasma exposures throughout pregnancy The largest of these studies included 29 women in the U.S. and demonstrated a 21% lower *AUC* in pregnancy; trough concentrations were 34% lower in the third trimester compared to postpartum, although trough concentrations in pregnancy were greater than 0.064 μg per mL, the 90% effective DTG concentrations. DTG was well tolerated in pregnancy and in the third trimester, HIV RNA was undetectable in 27 of 29 participants, with no cases of perinatal transmission to infants.[315]

High placental transfer of DTG has been demonstrated both *in vivo* and ex vivo.[315,316] The largest *in vivo* PK study demonstrated median cord blood to maternal blood ratio for DTG concentration was 1.25.[315] Infant washout of DTG received across the placenta during pregnancy is slow, with median (IQR) half-life of 32.8 hours (25.9 to 35.9).[315] There are limited data that DTG is secreted in breast milk.[317]

Infant Pharmacokinetics

There are not data on DTG PK and safety, and DTG is not approved in neonates and infants.[105]

Safety

In the PK study referenced above, birth abnormalities were reported in 7 of 29 infants, although three anomalies are considered normal variants, and in the other four cases, DTG was initiated after the completion of organogenesis.[219] Among live births with first-trimester DTG exposure logged with the APR as January 2019, the overall birth defect rate for infants with first-trimester exposure to DTG was 3.6% (11 infants of 306 live births).[106] A review of the APR and the European cohort found that birth defects occurred in 7 (2.7%) of 255 live births, 5 (3.1%) of 162 with conception/first-trimester DTG exposure.[318] Previous smaller observational studies found no birth defects in infants born to 280 women with first-trimester exposure to DTG in Botswana[75] and two in infants born to women in the U.S.[319]

A preliminary report from an observational surveillance study of birth outcomes among pregnant women on ART in Botswana indicated a potential increase in the incidence of NTD in infants born to women who initiated a DTG-containing regimen that they were receiving at the time of conception [4 (0.94%) cases of 426 women on DTG at time of conception].[311] This finding was surprising, given that there were no previous safety signals. Further, the pathophysiology of this increased risk is poorly understood, as DTG appears to only partially inhibit folate metabolism[320] (or only at very high concentrations) and has not been shown to cause NTDs in several animal models. This safety signal has diminished with the addition of subsequent birth data in Botswana, but has not been refuted; the associated risk of NTD remains very low (0.3%), but higher compared to women on non-DTG ART (0.1%).[82,321,322] Further, this safety signal has not been registered in countries with folate supplementation, although one U.S. case was recently reported to the APR.[323] Currently, though, the U.S. guidelines still caution against use in the periconception and first-trimester period, while the WHO does not restrict its use in women throughout conception and pregnancy.[1,2]

Elvitegravir

Elvitegravir (EVG) is a second-generation INSTI that can only be used with the pharmacoenhancer COBI as a first-line ARV drug in adults, except for pregnant women.

Maternal Pharmacokinetics

EVG is primarily metabolized by hepatic and intestinal cytochrome P450 (CYP3A).[324,325] In clinical practice, EVG is coadministered with the PK enhancer COBI, a potent inhibitor of CYP3A, in order to increase EVG exposure and allow for once-daily dosing.[325,326] Compared to RAL, COBI-boosted EVG has an improved PK profile, with less intrapatient and interpatient variability and a longer half-life allowing for once-daily dosing.[325]

Two PK studies and several case reports have found that standard EVG dosing in pregnancy results in significantly lower exposure in the second and third trimesters. The largest study of EVG PK and safety included 30 pregnant women on a fixed-dose combination of EVG and COBI. EVG *AUC* was 24% lower in the second trimester and 44% lower in the third trimester compared to postpartum values. EVG trough plasma concentration (C_{24}) was 81% lower in the second trimester and 89% lower in the third trimester. EVG *AUC* failed to reach the exposure target of 23 µg×hour per mL (the 10th percentile for nonpregnant adults) in 50% of women during the second trimester and 55% during the third trimester, compared to 12% of women postpartum. Plasma HIV RNA at delivery was undetectable in 19 (76%) of 25 women.[326] A smaller PK EVG/COBI study in seven pregnant women found 33% reduction in *AUC* and 65% reductions in C_{trough} during the third trimester compared to postpartum. One in seven participants had detectable HIV viral load at the time of delivery.[327] Two case reports of EVG/COBI in pregnancy have demonstrated similar findings.[73,328] EVG is best absorbed when taken with a meal and should not be administered within 2 hours of intake containing minerals, such as iron or calcium, including prenatal vitamins.[329]

Placental EVG transfer has been evaluated in two PK studies. In the larger PK study, EVG crossed the placenta well with a median ratio of cord to maternal plasma of 0.91. Median maternal EVG elimination half-life in neonates was 7.6 hours, similar to nonpregnant adults.[326–328] Smaller case series and case reports demonstrated similar results.[73,328] There are no published data on the excretion of EVG into breast milk.

Infant Pharmacokinetics

There are no data on EVG PK or safety in neonates or infants.

Safety

There are insufficient cases of first-trimester exposures to EVG in humans to determine the risk of birth defects and adverse outcomes.[106] A small study reported congenital anomalies in 2 infants of 26 live-born infants: one infant with amniotic band syndrome, microcephaly, and intrauterine growth restriction, and one infant with ulnar postaxial polydactyly.[326] An additional small study found no birth defects in the 10 infants born to the women on EVG-based ART.[327]

Raltegravir

RAL was the first INSTI developed and introduced to clinical practice.

Maternal Pharmacokinetics

RAL is primarily metabolized by glucuronidation by uridine glucuronosyltransferase and has limited drug interactions.[325,330] Caution is advised when coadministered with the PI ATV, a UGT inhibitor, as this drug combination results in elevated levels of RAL in healthy, nonpregnant adult women.[331] Compared to the newer INSTIs, RAL has a higher PK variability within and between patients.[1,325] RAL's large therapeutic window and mild side-effect profile make the drug's PK variability less clinically relevant.[325]

Similar to the nonpregnant population, the PK in pregnancy from the IMPAACT 1026s and PANNA networks studies demonstrates extensive variability. In the IMPAACT 1026s study of 42 women on RAL, the median area under the curve was decreased by approximately 50% during pregnancy. There was no significant difference between third-trimester and postpartum trough concentrations. Plasma HIV RNA viral load was undetectable in 92% of women at the time of delivery.[332] A PANNA network study of 22 women with paired third-trimester and postpartum data similarly demonstrated decreases in RAL concentrations during third-trimester exposure. The geometric mean ratios of third trimester to postpartum values were $AUC_{0-12\,h}$ 0.71 (0.53 to 0.96), C_{max} 0.82 (0.55 to 1.253), and $C_{12\,h}$ 0.64 (0.34 to 1.22). One patient was reported to be below the target $C_{12\,h}$ in the third trimester; none were below the threshold postpartum.[333] Neither study concluded a change in dosing in pregnancy was indicated, largely secondary to high rates of virologic suppression and the lack of a clear relationship between RAL concentration and virologic effect in nonpregnant adults.[332]

Both *in vivo* and ex vivo studies have demonstrated high placental transfer of RAL. Three network trials found the *in vivo* maternal cord blood to maternal plasma RAL concentration to be between 1.2 and 1.5.[332–334] An ex vivo study of full-term placentas from pregnancies without HIV infection found high bidirectional transfer of RAL across the placenta.[335] In a study of washout PK in 21 neonates of mothers who received chronic RAL during pregnancy, elimination was highly variable and prolonged in some infants (median $t_{1/2}$ 26.6 hours; range 9.3 to 184 hours).[334]

There are currently no data on RAL secretion in breast milk.

Infant Pharmacokinetics

RAL is approved for use in combination ART in newborns weighting 2 kg or more based on the PK and safety data from 42 full-term neonates (with or without in utero RAL exposure) treated for up to 6 weeks starting from birth and followed for a total of 24 weeks within the phase 1 multicenter trial IMPAACT

P1110 clinical trial.[366] In this trial, RAL-exposed neonates born to mothers who received an RAL dose within 2 to 24 hours of delivery received the initial RAL dose at 12 to 60 hours after delivery. The study enrolled two cohorts: cohort 1 infants received two RAL doses administered 1 week apart, and cohort 2 infants received daily RAL doses for the first 6 weeks of life. PK data from cohort 1 and from older infants and children were combined in a population PK model, and simulations were used to select the final RAL dosing regimen for evaluation in 26 RAL-naïve and 10 in utero RAL-exposed infants (to maternal RAL) in cohort 2 to meet RAL PK targets for $AUC_{0-24\ h}$ 12 mg×hour per L to 40 mg×h per L, $AUC_{0-12\ h}$ 6 mg×h per L to 20 mg×h per L, and $C_{12\ h}$ or $C_{24\ h}$ greater than 33 ng per mL, and all these targets were met among both RAL-naïve and RAL-experienced infants.[337,338] Results from P1110 confirmed the PK modeling and simulation and were used by the FDA to approve dosing of RAL granules formulation to be reconstituted to the suspension for neonates and infants. Neonates born to mothers who received RAL 2 to 24 hours prior to delivery should have their first dose of RAL delayed until 24 to 48 hours after birth.[336]

Based on weight bands, the newborn infants are dosed at approximately 1.5 mg per kg per dose twice daily the first week of life and 3 mg per kg per dose twice daily starting second week through 4 weeks of life.[336] Premature neonates have prolonged RAL elimination due to immaturity of RAL glucuronidation and may accumulate RAL to potentially toxic concentrations if they receive the term-infant dosing regimen.[339–342] RAL use should be avoided in premature infants until studies have been completed that allow determination of a safe RAL dosing regimen.

Safety

As of January 2019, nine cases of birth defects have been reported among the 327 infants with first-trimester exposure to RAL in the APR. The prevalence of birth defects among exposed infants was 2.9%, similar to the prevalence in the general U.S. population.[106] The French Perinatal Cohort included 497 women who received RAL during pregnancy with similar rates of birth defects among infants born to mothers on RAL in the first trimester and infants of mothers who initiated RAL after the first trimester (5.7% vs. 3.5%, $p = 0.29$).[133]

In both the P1026s and the PANNA study, RAL was well tolerated, and there were no drug-related serious adverse events. There is one case report of a transient elevation of maternal liver transaminases after initiation of RAL that resolved with discontinuation of the drug.[332,333] Additionally, there was one case of a drug reaction with eosinophilia and systemic symptoms syndrome with extensive pulmonary involvement in a postpartum woman; the drug reaction resolved with discontinuation of RAL.[343] Similar reactions have been reported in nonpregnant adults receiving RAL, and drug reactions should be considered in the differential diagnosis of fever in women on RAL during pregnancy or the postpartum period.[344]

Daily RAL was safe and well tolerated in all infants during the first 6 weeks of life. Three laboratory adverse reactions were reported among the RAL-naïve infants and included grade 4 transient neutropenia occurring in one infant receiving a ZDV-containing regimen; two bilirubin elevations (grades 1 and 2) were considered nonserious.[336] Among the RAL-exposed infants, four infants had grade 3 and 4 toxicities, including anemia, neutropenia, and hyperbilirubinemia.

FUSION AND ENTRY INHIBITORS

Entry and fusion inhibitors inhibit viral binding or fusion of HIV to host target cells. Enfuvirtide (T-20) requires subcutaneous administration, binds to the HR1 region, preventing the HR1–HR2 interaction and the correct folding of gp41 into its secondary structure, thereby inhibiting virus–cell fusion. Maraviroc (MVC) is a CCR5 co-receptor antagonist that interferes with viral entry at the chemokine co-receptor level. Ibalizumab-uiyk (IBA), a recombinant humanized monoclonal antibody, is a CD4-directed postattachment HIV-1 inhibitor. IBA blocks HIV from infecting CD4+ T cells by binding to domain 2 of CD4, thereby interfering with postattachment steps required for viral entry and preventing viral transmission that occurs via cell–cell fusion. No data are available on the IBA PK and safety in pregnant women and newborns.

Enfuvirtide

Maternal Pharmacokinetics

For enfuvirtide (T-20), several reports have described its use during pregnancy to successfully prevent vertical transmission of multidrug-resistant HIV-1.[228,345–349] In a single case, however, perinatal transmission was reported despite maternal viral suppression on the T-20 regimen.[350] Placental transfer of T-20 is low, with mean cord blood concentrations of 83 ng per mL in 12 women with mean plasma concentrations of 1,008 ng per mL.[345] Minimal placental passage of T-20 was confirmed in other human studies and was supported by data from an ex vivo human placental perfusion model.[345,351,352]

Infant Pharmacokinetics

No PK or safety data are available for T-20 in newborns.

Safety

Insufficient numbers of first-trimester exposures to T-20 in humans have been reported to be able to make a risk determination.[1,120]

Maraviroc

Maternal Pharmacokinetics

MVC PK was studied in the third trimester among 18 women (67% took MVC 150 mg twice daily with a PI, 11% took MVC 300 mg twice daily, and 22% took MVC with an alternative ART).[353] The geometric mean ratios for third-trimester MVC *AUC* versus postpartum *AUC* were 0.72 and 0.70 for maximum MVC concentration. Despite an overall 30% decrease in MVC *AUC* during pregnancy and a 15% decrease in C_{trough}, C_{trough} exceeded the minimum target concentration of 50 ng per mL in all participants, except for one woman who had a C_{trough} below 50 ng per mL during both pregnancy and postpartum. Based on these data, the standard adult dose adjusted for concomitant ARVs was recommended in pregnancy.[1]

An ex vivo human placental perfusion model demonstrated minimal placental passage of MVC.[354] In a study of six mother and infant pairs, the median ratio of cord blood to maternal plasma drug concentrations was 0.33 (0.03 to 0.56).[353,355] Whether MVC is secreted into human milk is currently unknown.

Infant Pharmacokinetics

MVC PK has been evaluated in an ongoing multicenter, open-label phase I IMPAACT 2007 study of MVC safety and PK in HIV-exposed neonates on standard ARV prophylaxis.[4] Data from 47 MVC-naïve, HIV-exposed neonates have confirmed safety of MVC during the first 6 weeks of life. Target MVC plasma concentrations ($C_{avg} \geq$ 75ng per mL from adult treatment studies) were met in most infants receiving 8 mg per kg twice daily, but with considerable variability in exposure.[4] The final neonatal MVC dose recommendation will be determined accounting for patient variability.

Safety

A retrospective study from a cohort of 857 pregnant women in Europe showed an increased rate of hepatotoxicity among the 492 women who started ART, including MVC during pregnancy.[251] MVC is one of three ARVs that was associated with an increased risk of liver enzyme elevation during pregnancy, with an adjusted hazard ratio of 4.19 (1.34 to 13.1, $p = 0.01$), along with EFV and NVP. In a model using human placental cells, MVC inhibited transplacental passage of two fluorescent organic cations, suggesting that it might influence placental drug transfer and cause drug–drug interactions.[356] The limited data available on the use of MVC during pregnancy are not sufficient to assess any potential drug-associated risk of birth defects.[120]

PHARMACOKINETIC ENHANCERS

RTV and COBI are used as PK enhancers slowing down the metabolism of concomitantly administered and frequently co-formulated drugs to achieve higher plasma concentrations.

Booster Ritonavir

Booster RTV is the first-generation PI which is no longer used for its ARV effect and is used solely as a PK enhancer of other PIs (ATV, DRV, and LPV).

Maternal Pharmacokinetics

RTV concentrations are reduced during pregnancy versus postpartum when the drug is used at 100 mg dose to boost the concentrations of other PIs.[268,297] PK of booster RTV dose in a group of 26 pregnant women receiving LPV has shown that RTV *AUC* and plasma trough concentrations were decreased by 40% to 50% during pregnancy compared to 2 weeks' postpartum.[298]

RTV transport across the placenta is poor, with cord blood RTV concentrations averaging 5.3% of maternal plasma concentration at delivery.[68,298] In a human placental perfusion model, the clearance of RTV was very low, with little accumulation in the fetal compartment and no accumulation in placental tissue.[357] In a study of cord blood samples from six women treated with RTV during pregnancy, the cord blood concentration was less than the assay limit of detection in five of the women and was only 0.38 μg per mL in the remaining woman.[257] In contrast, in a study of plasma and hair drug concentrations in 51 mother–infant pairs in Uganda receiving LPV/RTV-based ART during pregnancy and breastfeeding, infant plasma levels at delivery and hair levels at age 12 weeks suggested in utero RTV transfer.[211] However, transfer during breastfeeding was not observed, and no infant had detectable RTV plasma levels at 12 weeks of age.

Infant Pharmacokinetics

RTV is administered to newborns only as a PK booster to LPV starting at a postmenstrual age (first day of the mother's last menstrual period to birth, plus the time elapsed after birth) of 42 weeks and a postnatal age of at least 14 days. There are no data on the appropriate dose of LPV/RTV for neonates and no data on the safety of using this drug combination in this age group. The PK of the oral LPV/RTV solution at approximately LPV/RTV 300 mg per 75 mg per m^2 of body surface area per dose twice daily was evaluated in infants younger than 6 weeks, but did not report any data on RTV PK.[305]

Safety

In the APR, sufficient numbers of first-trimester exposures to RTV have been monitored and did not detect a significant (at least 1.5-fold) increase in risk of overall birth defects. Among cases of first-trimester RTV exposure reported to the APR, the prevalence of birth defects was 2.2% (70/3,155 births; 95% CI, 1.7% to 2.8%) compared with a total prevalence of 2.7% in the U.S. population, based on CDC surveillance.[120] PI-based ART regimens boosted with RTV have been associated with preterm delivery compared to nonboosted PI regimens.

Cobicistat

COBI does not possess any ARV activity and is used as a PK enhancer for PIs (ATV and DRV), INSTI EVG, and NRTI TAF.

Maternal Pharmacokinetics

COBI PK had been described in pregnant and postpartum women who were taking concomitant EVG and DRV.[278,283,336] In a study of 30 pregnant women who were receiving EVG/COBI, *AUC* of COBI was 44% and 59% lower in the second trimester and third trimester than during the postpartum period, respectively.[336] COBI plasma trough concentrations were 60% and 76% lower in the second trimester and third trimester than during the postpartum period, respectively. COBI plasma trough concentrations were below the assay quantitation limit (<10 ng per mL) in 65% of women during the second trimester, 73% of women during the third trimester, and 24% of postpartum women. The pharmacoenhancing effect of COBI on EVG was impacted during pregnancy, leading to significant decreases in EVG plasma concentrations (see "Elvitegravir" section).[336] Study results reported in two conference abstracts have described decreases of similar magnitudes in COBI, ATV, and DRV exposures among pregnant women.[283,290] PK of COBI was reported in the study of seven women dosed with once-daily DRV 800 mg per COBI 150 mg during pregnancy.[277,290] Along with decreased DRV plasma concentrations (see "darunavir" section), COBI exposures were lower during pregnancy, with reductions of 63% and 49% for *AUC* and 83% and 83% for trough concentration during the second and third trimesters, respectively, compared to postpartum.[283]

Because of the substantial reductions in COBI and enhanced ARVs drug exposures during pregnancy, the use of EVG/COBI or DRV/COBI is not recommended during pregnancy.[291,329]

A study in 10 pregnant women receiving EVG/COBI found a median cord blood to maternal delivery plasma COBI concentration ratio of 0.09 and measurable concentrations of COBI in placental tissue and cord blood PBMCs, with a cord to maternal PBMC ratio of 0.49.[31] In another study with seven pregnant women treated with EVG/COBI, the median ratio for cord blood to maternal delivery plasma COBI concentration was 0.09. In 27 neonates born to mothers who were receiving EVG/COBI, COBI was below the assay quantitation limit of 10 ng per mL in all washout PK samples taken between 2 hours and 9 days postdelivery.[336] No data are available on breast milk passage of COBI in humans.

Infant Pharmacokinetics

No PK or safety COBI data are available in newborns.

Safety

In the APR, five birth defects have been reported out of 204 live births to mothers with first-trimester exposure to COBI. The number of first-trimester exposures to COBI in humans is insufficient to be able to make a risk determination.[120]

SUMMARY

Introduction and scale-up of ART among pregnant women and their newborns has contributed to dramatic changes in the epidemiology of pediatric HIV infection and led to a significant decrease in maternal morbidity and mortality. Millions of women receive ARVs from conception through pregnancy, delivery, and breastfeeding. Fewer of their children become HIV infected, but they all are exposed to ARVs (in utero and many during breastfeeding as well). Currently, our knowledge about the short- and long-term health outcomes and perinatal ART exposure remains limited.

The use of ARVs in pregnant women and newborns is complicated by dynamic differences in PK and safety profiles compared with nonpregnant adults and older children. Compared to other morbidities, significant knowledge has been gained about PK of the drugs during pregnancy and neonatal period through remarkable commitment of experts in the field combined with strong voices from the community and advocacy. PK and safety data, crucial for the safe and effective use of these drugs during pregnancy and the first months of life, remain incomplete for most currently approved ARVs, as well as for newer agents now in development. Traditional phase 1 studies are difficult to perform during pregnancy for ethical and practical reasons. Dedicated clinical pharmacology studies in pregnant and breastfeeding women should be initiated once initial phase 2 safety and efficacy data have been demonstrated in nonpregnant adults.[355] Ethically acceptable strategies for conducting research on HIV treatment and prevention during pregnancy need to be further studied.[358] Basic and clinical research exploring the mechanisms (i.e., enzyme/transporter expression) of the pregnancy effect on maternal drug exposure, as well as the mechanisms behind transfer of drugs across the placenta and into breast milk, is needed and will allow development of more robust physiologically based PK models of pregnancy. Finally, global PV with postmarketing pregnancy surveillance of ARV studies is critical to identify low-frequency adverse pregnancy outcomes.

REFERENCES

1. Panel on Treatment of Pregnant Women with HIV Infection and Prevention of Perinatal Transmission. *Recommendations for use of antiretroviral drugs in transmission in the United States.* http://aidsinfo.nih.gov/contentfiles/lvguidelines/PerinatalGL.pdf. Accessed on December 26, 2019.
2. World Health Organization. *Updated guidance on first-line and second-line antiretroviral regimens.* July 2019. https://apps.who.int/iris/bitstream/handle/10665/325892/WHO-CDS-HIV-19.15-eng.pdf?ua=1. Accessed July 27, 2019.
3. World Health Organization (WHO). *Consolidated guidelines on the use of antiretroviral drugs for treating and preventing HIV infection. Recommendations for a public health approach.* 2nd ed. Geneva: World Health Organization. 2016. http://apps.who.int/iris/bitstream/handle/10665/208825/9789241549684_eng.pdf?sequence=1. Accessed July 27, 2019.
4. Colbers A, Mirochnick M, Schalkwijk S, et al. Importance of prospective studies in pregnant and breastfeeding women living with HIV. *Clin Infect Dis* 2019;69(7):1254–1258.
5. De Cock KM, Fowler MG, Mercier E, et al. Prevention of mother-to-child HIV transmission in resource-poor countries: translating research into policy and practice. *JAMA* 2000;283(9):1175–1182.
6. Coovadia HM, Rollins NC, Bland RM, et al. Mother-to-child transmission of HIV-1 infection during exclusive breastfeeding in the first 6 months of life: an intervention cohort study. *Lancet* 2007;369(9567):1107–1116.
7. Nduati R, John G, Mbori-Ngacha D, et al. Effect of breastfeeding and formula feeding on transmission of HIV-1: a randomized clinical trial. *JAMA* 2000;283(9):1167–1174.
8. Joint United Nations Programme on HIV and AIDS (UNAIDS). *UNAIDS Data* 2019. https://www.unaids.org/sites/default/files/media_asset/2019-UNAIDS-data_en.pdf. Accessed July 27, 2019.
9. Joint United Nations Programme on HIV and AIDS (UNAIDS). *UNAIDS. On the Fast-track to an AIDS-Free Generation.* Geneva: UNAIDS. 2016.
10. Joint United Nations Programme on HIV and AIDS (UNAIDS). *UNAIDS. Global Plan towards the elimination of new HIV infections among children by 2015 and keeping their mothers alive.* Geneva: UNAIDS. 2016.
11. Townsend CL, Byrne L, Cortina-Borja M, et al. Earlier initiation of ART and further decline in mother-to-child HIV transmission rates, 2000-2011. *AIDS* 28(7):1049–1057.
12. Fowler MG, Qin M, Fiscus SA, et al. Benefits and risks of antiretroviral therapy for perinatal HIV prevention. *N Engl J Med* 2016;375(18):1726–1737.
13. Joint United Nations Programme on HIV and AIDS (UNAIDS). *UNAIDS. Start free Stay Free AIDS free: 2017 progress report.* Geneva: UNAIDS; 2017.
14. Penazzato M, Lule F, Essajee S. Paediatric HIV: the unfinished business. *Lancet HIV* 2017;4(10):e425–e427.
15. Joint United Nations Programme on HIV and AIDS (UNAIDS). *Ending AIDS—progress towards the 90-90-90 targets. Global AIDS update 2017.* 2017. http://www.unaids.org/sites/default/files/media_asset/Global_AIDS_update_2017_en.pdf. Accessed July 21, 2019.
16. European AIDS Clinical Society (EACS). *Guidelines Version 9.1.* 2018. http://www.eacsociety.org/guidelines/eacs-guidelines/eacs-guidelines.html. Accessed July 11, 2019.
17. Connor EM, Sperling RS, Gelber R, et al. Reduction of maternal-infant transmission of human immunodeficiency virus type 1 with zidovudine treatment. Pediatric AIDS Clinical Trials Group Protocol 076 Study Group. *N Engl J Med* 1994;331(18):1173–1180.
18. Dorenbaum A, Cunningham CK, Gelber RD, et al. Two-dose intrapartum/newborn nevirapine and standard antiretroviral therapy to reduce perinatal HIV transmission: a randomized trial. *JAMA* 2002;288(2):189–198.
19. Cooper ER, Charurat M, Mofenson L, et al. Combination antiretroviral strategies for the treatment of pregnant HIV-1-infected women and prevention of perinatal HIV-1 transmission. *J Acquir Immune Defic Syndr* 2002;29(5):484–494.
20. Shaffer N, Chuachoowong R, Mock PA, et al. Short-course zidovudine for perinatal HIV-1 transmission in Bangkok, Thailand: a randomised controlled trial. Bangkok Collaborative Perinatal HIV Transmission Study Group. *Lancet* 1999;353(9155):773–780.
21. Dabis F, Msellati P, Meda N, et al. 6-month efficacy, tolerance, and acceptability of a short regimen of oral zidovudine to reduce vertical transmission of HIV in breastfed children in Cote d'Ivoire and Burkina Faso: a double-blind placebo-controlled multicentre trial. DITRAME Study Group. DIminution de la Transmission Mere-Enfant. *Lancet* 1999;353(9155):786–792.
22. Wiktor SZ, Ekpini E, Karon JM, et al. Short-course oral zidovudine for prevention of mother-to-child transmission of HIV-1 in Abidjan, Cote d'Ivoire: a randomised trial. *Lancet* 1999;353(9155):781–785.
23. Petra Study Team Efficacy of three short-course regimens of zidovudine and lamivudine in preventing early and late transmission of HIV-1 from mother to child in Tanzania, South Africa, and Uganda (Petra study): a randomised, double-blind, placebo-controlled trial. *Lancet* 2002;359(9313):1178–1186.
24. Jackson JB, Musoke P, Fleming T, et al. Intrapartum and neonatal single-dose nevirapine compared with zidovudine for prevention of mother-to-child transmission of HIV-1 in Kampala, Uganda: 18-month follow-up of the HIVNET 012 randomised trial. *Lancet* 2003;362(9387):859–868.
25. International Perinatal HIV Group, Andiman W, Bryson Y, et al. The mode of delivery and the risk of vertical transmission of human immunodeficiency virus type 1—a meta-analysis of 15 prospective cohort studies. *N Engl J Med* 1999;340(13):977–987.
26. European Mode of Delivery Collaboration. Elective caesarean-section versus vaginal delivery in prevention of vertical HIV-1 transmission: a randomised clinical trial. *Lancet* 1999;353(9158):1035–1039.
27. Townsend CL, Cortina-Borja M, Peckham CS, et al. Low rates of mother-to-child transmission of HIV following effective pregnancy interventions in the United Kingdom and Ireland, 2000-2006. *AIDS* 2008;22(8):973–981.
28. Effect of breastfeeding on infant and child mortality due to infectious diseases in less developed countries: a pooled analysis. WHO Collaborative Study Team on the Role of Breastfeeding on the Prevention of Infant Mortality. *Lancet* 2000;355(9202):451–455.
29. Giuliano M, Guidotti G, Andreotti M, et al. Triple antiretroviral prophylaxis administered during pregnancy and after delivery significantly reduces breast milk viral load: a study within the Drug Resource Enhancement Against AIDS and Malnutrition Program. *J Acquir Immune Defic Syndr* 2007;44(3):286–291.
30. World Health Organization (WHO). *Consolidated guidelines on general HIV care and the use of antiretroviral drugs for treating and preventing HIV infection: recommendations for a public health approach.* Geneva: World Health Organization; 2013:269.
31. Rimawi BH, Johnson E, Rajakumar A, et al. Pharmacokinetics and placental transfer of elvitegravir, dolutegravir, and other antiretrovirals during pregnancy. *Antimicrob Agents Chemother* 2017;61(6):e02213-16.
32. *Recommandations de la Commission fédérale pour la santé sexuelle (CFSS) concernant la prise en charge des mères infectées par le VIH et de leur enfant. Maladies Transmissibles. OFSP-Bulletin* 50 du 10 décembre 2018.
33. Hoffman RM, Mofenson LM. Decision-making in a time of uncertainty: Dolutegravir for reproductive-age women. *Ann Intern Med* 2019;170(9):658–659.

34. British HIV Association. *BHIVA guidelines for the management of HIV in pregnancy and postpartum 2018 (2019 interim update)*. 2019. https://www.bhiva.org/pregnancy-guidelines. Accessed July 27, 2019.
35. Nielsen-Saines K, Watts DH, Veloso VG, et al. Three postpartum antiretroviral regimens to prevent intrapartum HIV infection. *N Engl J Med* 2012;366(25):2368–2379.
36. Persaud D, Gay H, Ziemniak C, et al. Absence of detectable HIV-1 viremia after treatment cessation in an infant. *N Engl J Med* 2013;369(19):1828–1835.
37. Klein N, Palma P, Luzuriaga K, et al. Early antiretroviral therapy in children perinatally infected with HIV: a unique opportunity to implement immunotherapeutic approaches to prolong viral remission. *Lancet Infect Dis* 2015;15(9):1108–1114.
38. Martinez-Bonet M, Puertas MC, Fortuny C, et al. Establishment and replenishment of the viral reservoir in perinatally HIV-1-infected children initiating very early antiretroviral therapy. *Clin Infect Dis* 2015;61(7):1169–1178.
39. Bardeguez AD, Lindsey JC, Shannon M, et al. Adherence to antiretrovirals among US women during and after pregnancy. *J Acquir Immune Defic Syndr* 2008;48(4):408–417.
40. Erlwanger AS, Joseph J, Gotora T, et al. Patterns of HIV care clinic attendance and adherence to antiretroviral therapy among pregnant and breastfeeding women living with HIV in the context of option B+ in Zimbabwe. *J Acquir Immune Defic Syndr* 2017;75 (Suppl 2):S198–S206.
41. Tesfaye DJ, Hibistu DT, Abebo TA, et al. Option B plus antiretroviral therapy adherence and associated factors among HIV positive pregnant women in Southern Ethiopia. *BMC Pregnancy Childbirth* 2019;19(1):82.
42. Tobin NH, Frenkel LM. Human immunodeficiency virus drug susceptibility and resistance testing. *Pediatr Infect Dis J* 2002;21(7):681–683.
43. Parker MM, Wade N, Lloyd RM, Jr, et al. Prevalence of genotypic drug resistance among a cohort of HIV-infected newborns. *J Acquir Immune Defic Syndr* 2003;32(3):292–297.
44. Witvrouw M, Pannecouque C, Van Laethem K, et al. Activity of non-nucleoside reverse transcriptase inhibitors against HIV-2 and SIV. *AIDS* 1999;13(12):1477–1483.
45. Cressey TR, Jourdain G, Lallemant MJ, et al. Persistence of nevirapine exposure during the postpartum period after intrapartum single-dose nevirapine in addition to zidovudine prophylaxis for the prevention of mother-to-child transmission of HIV-1. *J Acquir Immune Defic Syndr* 2005;38(3):283–288.
46. Jackson JB, Becker-Pergola G, Guay LA, et al. Identification of the K103N resistance mutation in Ugandan women receiving nevirapine to prevent HIV-1 vertical transmission. *AIDS* 2000;14(11):F111–F115.
47. Cunningham CK, Chaix ML, Rekacewicz C, et al. Development of resistance mutations in women receiving standard antiretroviral therapy who received intrapartum nevirapine to prevent perinatal human immunodeficiency virus type 1 transmission: a substudy of pediatric AIDS clinical trials group protocol 316. *J Infect Dis* 2002;186(2):181–188.
48. Flys TS, McConnell MS, Matovu F, et al. Nevirapine resistance in women and infants after first versus repeated use of single-dose nevirapine for prevention of HIV-1 vertical transmission. *J Infect Dis* 2008;198(4):465–469.
49. Jordan MR, Penazzato M, Cournil A, et al. Human immunodeficiency virus (HIV) drug resistance in African infants and young children newly diagnosed with HIV: a multicountry analysis. *Clin Infect Dis* 2017;65(12):2018–2025.
50. WHO. *HIV diagnosis and ARV use in HIV-exposed infants: a programmatic update.* July 2018. https://apps.who.int/iris/bitstream/handle/10665/273155/WHO-CDS-HIV-18.17-eng.pdf?ua=1. Accessed July 27, 2019.
51. Hirsch MS, Conway B, D'Aquila RT, et al. Antiretroviral drug resistance testing in adults with HIV infection: implications for clinical management. International AIDS Society—USA Panel. *JAMA* 1998;279(24):1984–1991.
52. Eastman PS, Shapiro DE, Coombs RW, et al. Maternal viral genotypic zidovudine resistance and infrequent failure of zidovudine therapy to prevent perinatal transmission of human immunodeficiency virus type 1 in pediatric AIDS Clinical Trials Group Protocol 076. *J Infect Dis* 1998;177(3):557–564.
53. Bardeguez AD, Shapiro DE, Mofenson LM, et al. Effect of cessation of zidovudine prophylaxis to reduce vertical transmission on maternal HIV disease progression and survival. *J Acquir Immune Defic Syndr* 2003;32(2):170–181.
54. Mandelbrot L, Landreau-Mascaro A, Rekacewicz C, et al. Lamivudine-zidovudine combination for prevention of maternal-infant transmission of HIV-1. *JAMA* 2001;285(16):2083–2093.
55. Eke AC, McCormack SA, Best BM, et al. Pharmacokinetics of increased nelfinavir plasma concentrations in women during pregnancy and postpartum. *J Clin Pharmacol* 2019;59(3):386–393.
56. Pyra M, Anderson PL, Hendrix CW, et al. Tenofovir and tenofovir-diphosphate concentrations during pregnancy among HIV-uninfected women using oral preexposure prophylaxis. *AIDS* 2018;32(13):1891–1898.
57. Heffron R, Mugo N, Hong T, et al. Pregnancy outcomes and infant growth among babies with in utero exposure to tenofovir-based pre-exposure prophylaxis for HIV prevention. *AIDS* 2018;32(12):1707–1713.
58. Seidman DL, Weber S, Timoney MT, et al. Use of HIV pre-exposure prophylaxis during the preconception, antepartum and postpartum periods at two United States medical centers. *Am J Obstet Gynecol* 2016;215(5):632.e1–632.e7.
59. Mugo NR, Hong T, Celum C, et al. Pregnancy incidence and outcomes among women receiving preexposure prophylaxis for HIV prevention: a randomized clinical trial. *JAMA* 2014;312(4):362–371.
60. Mugo NR, Heffron R, Donnell D, et al. Increased risk of HIV-1 transmission in pregnancy: a prospective study among African HIV-1-serodiscordant couples. *AIDS* 2011;25(15):1887–1895.
61. Siberry GK, Williams PL, Mendez H, et al. Safety of tenofovir use during pregnancy: early growth outcomes in HIV-exposed uninfected infants. *AIDS* 2012;26(9):1151–1159.
62. Gibb DM, Kizito H, Russell EC, et al. Pregnancy and infant outcomes among HIV-infected women taking long-term ART with and without tenofovir in the DART trial. *PLoS Med* 2012;9(5):e1001217.
63. Mirochnick M, Best BM, Clarke DF. Antiretroviral pharmacology: special issues regarding pregnant women and neonates. *Clin Perinatol* 2010;37(4):907–927, xi.
64. Rakhmanina NY, Dirajlal-Fargo S, Capparelli EV, et al. Pharmacokinetic considerations of perinatal antiretroviral therapy. *Curr Drug Metab* 2012;13(6):744–759.
65. Loebstein R, Lalkin A, Koren G. Pharmacokinetic changes during pregnancy and their clinical relevance. *Clin Pharmacokinet* 1997;33(5):328–343.
66. Koren G, Pariente G. Pregnancy-associated changes in pharmacokinetics and their clinical implications. *Pharm Res* 2018;35(3):61.
67. Pariente G, Leibson T, Carls A, et al. Pregnancy-associated changes in pharmacokinetics: a systematic review. *PLoS Med* 2016;13(11):e1002160.
68. Hodel EM, Marzolini C, Waitt C, et al. Pharmacokinetics, placental and breast milk transfer of antiretroviral drugs in pregnant and lactating women living with HIV. *Curr Pharm Des* 2019;25(5):556–576.
69. Morgan DJ. Drug disposition in mother and foetus. *Clin Exp Pharmacol Physiol* 1997;24(11):869–873.
70. Krauer B, Dayer P, Anner R. Changes in serum albumin and alpha 1-acid glycoprotein concentrations during pregnancy: an analysis of fetal-maternal pairs. *Br J Obstet Gynaecol* 1984;91(9):875–881.
71. Aweeka FT, Hu C, Huang L, et al. Alteration in cytochrome P450 3A4 activity as measured by a urine cortisol assay in HIV-1-infected pregnant women and relationship to antiretroviral pharmacokinetics. *HIV Med* 2015;16(3):176–183.
72. Jeong H, Choi S, Song JW, et al. Regulation of UDP-glucuronosyltransferase (UGT) 1A1 by progesterone and its impact on labetalol elimination. *Xenobiotica* 2008;38(1):62–75.
73. Marzolini C, Decosterd L, Winterfeld U, et al. Free and total plasma concentrations of elvitegravir/cobicistat during pregnancy and postpartum: a case report. *Br J Clin Pharmacol* 2017;83(12):2835–2838.
74. Zash R, Jacobson DL, Diseko M, et al. Comparative safety of antiretroviral treatment regimens in pregnancy. *JAMA Pediatr* 2017;171(10):e172222.
75. Zash R, Jacobson DL, Diseko M, et al. Comparative safety of dolutegravir-based or efavirenz-based antiretroviral treatment started during pregnancy in Botswana: an observational study. *Lancet Glob Health* 2018;6(7):e804–e810.
76. Sibiude J, Warszawski J, Tubiana R, et al. Premature delivery in HIV-infected women starting protease inhibitor therapy during pregnancy: role of the ritonavir boost? *Clin Infect Dis* 2012;54(9):1348–1360.
77. Bailey H, Zash R, Rasi V, et al. HIV treatment in pregnancy. *Lancet HIV* 2018;5(8):e457–e467.
78. Mofenson LM, Pozniak AL, Wambui J, et al. Optimizing responses to drug safety signals in pregnancy: the example of dolutegravir and neural tube defects. *J Int AIDS Soc* 2019;22(7):e25352.
79. Carney EW, Ellis AL, Tyl RW, et al. Critical evaluation of current developmental toxicity testing strategies: a case of babies and their bathwater. *Birth Defects Res B Dev Reprod Toxicol* 2011;92(5):395–403.
80. Ford N, Mofenson L, Shubber Z, et al. Safety of efavirenz in the first trimester of pregnancy: an updated systematic review and meta-analysis. *AIDS* 2014;28 (Suppl 2):S123–S131.
81. Chetty T, Thorne C, Coutsoudis A. Preterm delivery and small-for-gestation outcomes in HIV-infected pregnant women on antiretroviral therapy in rural South Africa: Results from a cohort study, 2010-2015. *PLoS One* 2018;13(2):e0192805.
82. Zash R, Holmes L, Diseko M, et al. Neural-tube defects and antiretroviral treatment regimens in Botswana. *N Engl J Med* 2019;381(9):827–840.
83. Watts DH, Balasubramanian R, Maupin RT, Jr, et al. Maternal toxicity and pregnancy complications in human immunodeficiency virus-infected women receiving antiretroviral therapy: PACTG 316. *Am J Obstet Gynecol* 2004;190(2):506–516.
84. Hitti J, Andersen J, McComsey G, et al. Protease inhibitor-based antiretroviral therapy and glucose tolerance in pregnancy: AIDS Clinical Trials Group A5084. *Am J Obstet Gynecol* 2007;196(4):331.e1–331.e7.
85. Food and Drug Administration. *Important drug warning: retyped text of a letter from Bristol-Myers Squibb*, January 5, 2001. http://www.fda.gov/medwatch/safety/2001/zerit&videx_letter.htm. Accessed July 25, 2019.
86. Venter WDF, Moorhouse M, Sokhela S, et al. Dolutegravir plus two different prodrugs of tenofovir to treat HIV. *N Engl J Med* 2019;381(9):803–815.
87. Sandberg JA, Slikker W. Developmental pharmacology and toxicology of anti-HIV therapeutic agents: dideoxynucleosides. *FASEB J* 1995;9(12):1157–1163.
88. Robbins BL, Waibel BH, Fridland A. Quantitation of intracellular zidovudine phosphates by use of combined cartridge-radioimmunoassay methodology. *Antimicrob Agents Chemother* 1996;40(11):2651–2654.
89. Rodriguez JF, Rodriguez JL, Santana J, et al. Simultaneous quantitation of intracellular zidovudine and lamivudine triphosphates in human immunodeficiency virus-infected individuals. *Antimicrob Agents Chemother* 2000;44(11):3097–3100.
90. Barry MG, Khoo SH, Veal GJ, et al. The effect of zidovudine dose on the formation of intracellular phosphorylated metabolites. *AIDS* 1996;10(12):1361–1367.
91. Grim SA, Romanelli F. Tenofovir disoproxil fumarate. *Ann Pharmacother* 2003;37(6):849–859.
92. Kirmse B, Baumgart S, Rakhmanina N. Metabolic and mitochondrial effects of antiretroviral drug exposure in pregnancy and postpartum: implications for fetal and future health. *Semin Fetal Neonatal Med* 2013;18(1):48–55.
93. Sibiude J, Le Chenadec J, Bonnet D, et al. In utero exposure to zidovudine and heart anomalies in the ANRS French perinatal cohort and the nested PRIMEVA randomized trial. *Clin Infect Dis* 2015;61(2):270–280.
94. Martin JL, Brown CE, Matthews-Davis N, et al. Effects of antiviral nucleoside analogs on human DNA polymerases and mitochondrial DNA synthesis. *Antimicrob Agents Chemother* 1994;38(12):2743–2749.
95. Brogly SB, Ylitalo N, Mofenson LM, et al. In utero nucleoside reverse transcriptase inhibitor exposure and signs of possible mitochondrial dysfunction in HIV-uninfected children. *AIDS* 2007;21(8):929–938.
96. Ziagen package insert. Research Triangle Park, NC: GlaxoSmithKline, 2008.
97. Kumar PN, Sweet DE, McDowell JA, et al. Safety and pharmacokinetics of abacavir (1592U89) following oral administration of escalating single doses in human immunodeficiency virus type 1-infected adults. *Antimicrob Agents Chemother* 1999;43(3):603–608.

98. McDowell JA, Lou Y, Symonds WS, et al. Multiple-dose pharmacokinetics and pharmacodynamics of abacavir alone and in combination with zidovudine in human immunodeficiency virus-infected adults. *Antimicrob Agents Chemother* 2000;44(8):2061–2067.
99. Hawkins T, Veikley W, St Claire RL, et al. Intracellular pharmacokinetics of tenofovir diphosphate, carbovir triphosphate, and lamivudine triphosphate in patients receiving triple-nucleoside regimens. *J Acquir Immune Defic Syndr* 2005;39(4):406–411.
100. Best BM, Mirochnick M, Capparelli EV, et al. Impact of pregnancy on abacavir pharmacokinetics. *AIDS* 2006;20(4):553–560.
101. Schalkwijk S, Colbers A, Konopnicki D, et al. The pharmacokinetics of abacavir 600 mg once daily in HIV-1-positive pregnant women. *AIDS* 2016;30(8):1239–1244.
102. Fauchet F, Treluyer JM, Préta LH, et al. Population pharmacokinetics of abacavir in pregnant women. *Antimicrob Agents Chemother* 2014;58(10):6287–6289.
103. Chappuy H, Tréluyer JM, Jullien V, et al. Maternal-fetal transfer and amniotic fluid accumulation of nucleoside analogue reverse transcriptase inhibitors in human immunodeficiency virus-infected pregnant women. *Antimicrob Agents Chemother* 2004;48(11):4332–4336.
104. Shapiro RL, Rossi S, Ogwu A, et al. Therapeutic levels of lopinavir in late pregnancy and abacavir passage into breast milk in the Mma Bana Study, Botswana. *Antivir Ther* 2013;18(4):585–590.
105. Panel on Antiretroviral Therapy and Medical Management of Children Living with HIV. *Guidelines for the use of antiretroviral agents in pediatric HIV infection.* http://aidsinfo.nih.gov/contentfiles/lvguidelines/pediatricguidelines.pdf. Accessed December 28, 2019.
106. Antiretroviral Pregnancy Registry Steering Committee. *Antiretroviral pregnancy registry international interim report for 1 January 1989–31 January 2019.* Wilmington, NC: Registry Coordinating Center. 2019.
107. Williams PL, Crain MJ, Yildirim C, et al. Congenital anomalies and in utero antiretroviral exposure in human immunodeficiency virus-exposed uninfected infants. *JAMA Pediatr* 2015;169(1):48–55.
108. Prieto LM, González-Tomé MI, Muñoz E, et al. Birth defects in a cohort of infants born to HIV-infected women in Spain, 2000-2009. *BMC Infect Dis* 2014;14:700.
109. Williams PL, Hazra R, Van Dyke RB, et al. Antiretroviral exposure during pregnancy and adverse outcomes in HIV-exposed uninfected infants and children using a trigger-based design. *AIDS* 2016;30(1):133–144.
110. Emtriva package insert. Foster City, CA: Gilead Sciences, 2008.
111. Ramanathan S, Shen G, Cheng A, et al. Pharmacokinetics of emtricitabine, tenofovir, and GS-9137 following coadministration of emtricitabine/tenofovir disoproxil fumarate and ritonavir-boosted GS-9137. *J Acquir Immune Defic Syndr* 2007;45(3):274–279.
112. Stevens RC, Blum MR, Rousseau FS, et al. Intracellular pharmacology of emtricitabine and tenofovir. *Clin Infect Dis* 2004;39(6):877–878; author reply 878–879.
113. Wang LH, Begley J, St Claire RL, et al. Pharmacokinetic and pharmacodynamic characteristics of emtricitabine support its once daily dosing for the treatment of HIV infection. *AIDS Res Hum Retroviruses* 2004;20(11):1173–1182.
114. Colbers AP, Hawkins DA, Gingelmaier A, et al. The pharmacokinetics, safety and efficacy of tenofovir and emtricitabine in HIV-1-infected pregnant women. *AIDS* 2013;27(5):739–748.
115. Colbers A, Greupink R, Burger D. Pharmacological considerations on the use of antiretrovirals in pregnancy. *Curr Opin Infect Dis* 2013;26(6):575–588.
116. Valade E, Tréluyer JM, Dabis F, et al. Modified renal function in pregnancy: impact on emtricitabine pharmacokinetics. *Br J Clin Pharmacol* 2014;78(6):1378–1386.
117. Stek AM, Best BM, Luo W, et al. Effect of pregnancy on emtricitabine pharmacokinetics. *HIV Med* 2012;13(4):226–235.
118. Waitt C, Olagunju A, Nakalema S, et al. Plasma and breast milk pharmacokinetics of emtricitabine, tenofovir and lamivudine using dried blood and breast milk spots in nursing African mother-infant pairs. *J Antimicrob Chemother* 2018;73(4):1013–1019.
119. Mugwanya KK, Hendrix CW, Mugo NR, et al. Pre-exposure prophylaxis use by breastfeeding HIV-uninfected women: a prospective short-term study of antiretroviral excretion in breast milk and infant absorption. *PLoS Med* 2016;13(9):e1002132.
120. Antiretroviral Pregnancy Registry Steering Committee. *Antiretroviral pregnancy registry international interim report for 1 January 1989 through 31 July 2018.* 2018. Wilmington, NC: Registry Coordinating Center. www.APRegistry.com. Accessed December 26, 2019.
121. Perry CM, Faulds D. Lamivudine. A review of its antiviral activity, pharmacokinetic properties and therapeutic efficacy in the management of HIV infection. *Drugs* 1997;53(4):657–680.
122. Barry M, Mulcahy F, Merry C, et al. Pharmacokinetics and potential interactions amongst antiretroviral agents used to treat patients with HIV infection. *Clin Pharmacokinet* 1999;36(4):289–304.
123. Moore KH, Yuen GJ, Raasch RH, et al. Pharmacokinetics of lamivudine administered alone and with trimethoprim-sulfamethoxazole. *Clin Pharmacol Ther* 1996;59(5):550–558.
124. Moore KH, Barrett JE, Shaw S, et al. The pharmacokinetics of lamivudine phosphorylation in peripheral blood mononuclear cells from patients infected with HIV-1. *AIDS* 1999;13(16):2239–2250.
125. Moodley J, Moodley D, Pillay K, et al. Pharmacokinetics and antiretroviral activity of lamivudine alone or when coadministered with zidovudine in human immunodeficiency virus type 1-infected pregnant women and their offspring. *J Infect Dis* 1998;178(5):1327–1333.
126. Benaboud S, Tréluyer JM, Urien S, et al. Pregnancy-related effects on lamivudine pharmacokinetics in a population study with 228 women. *Antimicrob Agents Chemother* 2012;56(2):776–782.
127. Bloom SL, Dias KM, Bawdon RE, et al. The maternal-fetal transfer of lamivudine in the ex vivo human placenta. *Am J Obstet Gynecol* 1997;176(2):291–293.
128. Mandelbrot L, Peytavin G, Firtion G, et al. Maternal-fetal transfer and amniotic fluid accumulation of lamivudine in human immunodeficiency virus-infected pregnant women. *Am J Obstet Gynecol* 2001;184(2):153–158.
129. Moodley D, Pillay K, Naidoo K, et al. Pharmacokinetics of zidovudine and lamivudine in neonates following coadministration of oral doses every 12 hours. *J Clin Pharmacol* 2001;41(7):732–741.
130. Mirochnick M, Thomas T, Capparelli E, et al. Antiretroviral concentrations in breast-feeding infants of mothers receiving highly active antiretroviral therapy. *Antimicrob Agents Chemother* 2009;53(3):1170–1176.
131. Palombi L, Pirillo MF, Andreotti M, et al. Antiretroviral prophylaxis for breastfeeding transmission in Malawi: drug concentrations, virological efficacy and safety. *Antivir Ther* 2012;17(8):1511–1519.
132. Mueller BU, Lewis LL, Yuen GJ, et al. Serum and cerebrospinal fluid pharmacokinetics of intravenous and oral lamivudine in human immunodeficiency virus-infected children. *Antimicrob Agents Chemother* 1998;42(12):3187–3192.
133. Sibiude J, Mandelbrot L, Blanche S, et al. Association between prenatal exposure to antiretroviral therapy and birth defects: an analysis of the French perinatal cohort study (ANRS CO1/CO11). *PLoS Med* 2014;11(4):e1001635.
134. Vannappagari V, Koram N, Albano J, et al. Abacavir and lamivudine exposures during pregnancy and non-defect adverse pregnancy outcomes: data from the antiretroviral pregnancy registry. *J Acquir Immune Defic Syndr* 2015;68(3):359–364.
135. Viread package insert. Foster City, CA: Gilead Sciences, 2008.
136. Blum MR, Chittick GE, Begley JA, et al. Steady-state pharmacokinetics of emtricitabine and tenofovir disoproxil fumarate administered alone and in combination in healthy volunteers. *J Clin Pharmacol* 2007;47(6):751–759.
137. Parks DA, Jennings HC, Taylor CW, et al. Pharmacokinetics of once-daily tenofovir, emtricitabine, ritonavir and fosamprenavir in HIV-infected subjects. *AIDS* 2007;21(10):1373–1375.
138. Benaboud S, Hirt D, Launay O, et al. Pregnancy-related effects on tenofovir pharmacokinetics: a population study with 186 women. *Antimicrob Agents Chemother* 2012;56(2):857–862.
139. Best BM, Burchett S, Li H, et al. Pharmacokinetics of tenofovir during pregnancy and postpartum. *HIV Med* 2015;16(8):502–511.
140. Bonora S, Gonzalez De Requena D, Chiesa E, et al. Transplacental passage of tenofovir (TDF) and other antiretrovirals (ARVs) at delivery. Presented at: 14th Conference on Retroviruses and Opportunistic Infections; February 25-28, 2010; Los Angeles, CA. Abstract 738a.
141. Hirt D, Urien S, Ekouévi DK, et al. Population pharmacokinetics of tenofovir in HIV-1-infected pregnant women and their neonates (ANRS 12109). *Clin Pharmacol Ther* 2009;85(2):182–189.
142. Hirt D, Ekouévi DK, Pruvost A, et al. Plasma and intracellular tenofovir pharmacokinetics in the neonate (ANRS 12109 trial, step 2). *Antimicrob Agents Chemother* 2011;55(6):2961–2967.
143. Brogly SB, Abzug MJ, Watts DH, et al. Birth defects among children born to human immunodeficiency virus-infected women: pediatric AIDS clinical trials protocols 219 and 219C. *Pediatr Infect Dis J* 2010;29(8):721–727.
144. Knapp KM, Brogly SB, Muenz DG, et al. Prevalence of congenital anomalies in infants with in utero exposure to antiretrovirals. *Pediatr Infect Dis J* 2012;31(2):164–170.
145. Zash R, Jacobson D, Mayondi G, et al. eds. Dolutegravir/tenofovir/emtricitabine (DTG/TDF/FTC) started in pregnancy is as safe as efavirenz/tenofovir/emtricitabine (EFV/TDF/FTC) in nationwide birth outcomes surveillance in Botswana. *J Int AIDS Soc.* 2017. Geneva. Switzerland.
146. Rough K, Seage GR, Williams PL, et al. Birth Outcomes for Pregnant Women with HIV Using Tenofovir-Emtricitabine. *N Engl J Med* 2018;378(17):1593–1603.
147. Jourdain G, Ngo-Giang-Huong N, Harrison L, et al. Tenofovir versus placebo to prevent perinatal transmission of hepatitis B. *N Engl J Med* 2018;378(10):911–923.
148. Brophy J, Lee T, Bitnun A, et al. eds. Is tenofovir use in pregnancy associated with preterm delivery? A Canadian perinatal HIV surveillance program analysis. Presented at: 9th IAS Conference on HIV Science; 2017; Paris, France.
149. Denneman L, Cohen S, Godfried MH, et al. In-utero exposure to tenofovir is associated with impaired fetal and infant growth: need for follow-up studies in combination antiretroviral therapy/HIV-exposed infants. *AIDS* 2016;30(13):2135–2137.
150. Liotta G, Floridia M, Andreotti M, et al. Growth indices in breastfed infants pre and postnatally exposed to tenofovir compared with tenofovir-unexposed infants. *AIDS* 2016;30(3):525–527.
151. Ransom CE, Huo Y, Patel K, et al. Infant growth outcomes after maternal tenofovir disoproxil fumarate use during pregnancy. *J Acquir Immune Defic Syndr* 2013;64(4):374–381.
152. M le Roux S, Jao J, Brittain K, et al. Tenofovir exposure in utero and linear growth in HIV-exposed, uninfected infants. *AIDS* 2017;31(1):97–104.
153. Pintye J, Langat A, Singa B, et al. Maternal tenofovir disoproxil fumarate use in pregnancy and growth outcomes among HIV-exposed uninfected infants in Kenya. *Infect Dis Obstet Gynecol* 2015:276851.
154. De Clercq E. Tenofovir alafenamide (TAF) as the successor of tenofovir disoproxil fumarate (TDF). *Biochem Pharmacol* 2016;119:1–7.
155. Sax PE, Zolopa A, Brar I, et al. Tenofovir alafenamide vs. tenofovir disoproxil fumarate in single tablet regimens for initial HIV-1 therapy: a randomized phase 2 study. *J Acquir Immune Defic Syndr* 2014;67(1):52–58.
156. Momper J, Best B, Wang J, et al., eds. Tenofovir alafenamide pharmacokinetics with and without cobicistat in pregnancy. Presented at: 22nd International AIDS Conference (AIDS 2018); July 23–27, 2018; Amsterdam, The Netherlands.
157. Brooks K, Pinilla M, Shapiro D, et al. Pharmacokinetics of tenofovir alafenamide 25 mg with PK boosters during pregnancy and postpartum. Presented at: Workshop on Clinical Pharmacology of HIV, Hepatitis, and Other Antiviral Drugs; May 14–16, 2019; Noordwijk, The Netherlands.
158. Singlas E, Pioger JC, Taburet AM, et al. Comparative pharmacokinetics of zidovudine (AZT) and its metabolite (G.AZT) in healthy subjects and HIV seropositive patients. *Eur J Clin Pharmacol* 1989;36(6):639–640.
159. Klecker RW, Collins JM, Yarchoan R, et al. Plasma and cerebrospinal fluid pharmacokinetics of 3′-azido-3′-deoxythymidine: a novel pyrimidine analog with potential application for the treatment of patients with AIDS and related diseases. *Clin Pharmacol Ther* 1987;41(4):407–412.

160. Yarchoan R, Mitsuya H, Myers CE, et al. Clinical pharmacology of 3′-azido-2′,3′-dideoxythymidine (zidovudine) and related dideoxynucleosides. *N Engl J Med* 1989;321(11):726–738.
161. Collins JM, Unadkat JD. Clinical pharmacokinetics of zidovudine. an overview of current data. *Clin Pharmacokinet* 1989;17(1):1–9.
162. Furman PA, Fyfe JA, St Clair MH, et al. Phosphorylation of 3′-azido-3′-deoxythymidine and selective interaction of the 5-triphosphate with human immunodeficiency virus reverse transcriptase. *Proc Natl Acad Sci U S A* 1986;83(21):8333–8337.
163. Wattanagoon Y, Na Bangchang K, Hoggard PG, et al. Pharmacokinetics of zidovudine phosphorylation in human immunodeficiency virus-positive Thai patients and healthy volunteers. *Antimicrob Agents Chemother* 2000;44(7):1986–1989.
164. Stretcher BN, Pesce AJ, Frame PT, et al. Pharmacokinetics of zidovudine phosphorylation in peripheral blood mononuclear cells from patients infected with human immunodeficiency virus. *Antimicrob Agents Chemother* 1994;38(7):1541–1547.
165. Ho HT, Hitchcock MJ. Cellular pharmacology of 2′,3′-dideoxy-2′,3′-didehydrothymidine, a nucleoside analog active against human immunodeficiency virus. *Antimicrob Agents Chemother* 1989;33(6):844–849.
166. Sale M, Sheiner LB, Volberding P, et al. Zidovudine response relationships in early human immunodeficiency virus infection. *Clin Pharmacol Ther* 1993;54(5):556–566.
167. Sperling RS, Roboz J, Dische R, et al. Zidovudine pharmacokinetics during pregnancy. *Am J Perinatol* 1992;9(4):247–249.
168. O'Sullivan MJ, Boyer PJ, Scott GB, et al. The pharmacokinetics and safety of zidovudine in the third trimester of pregnancy for women infected with human immunodeficiency virus and their infants: phase I acquired immunodeficiency syndrome clinical trials group study (protocol 082). Zidovudine Collaborative Working Group. *Am J Obstet Gynecol* 1993;168(5):1510–1516.
169. Watts DH, Brown ZA, Tartaglione T, et al. Pharmacokinetic disposition of zidovudine during pregnancy. *J Infect Dis* 1991;163(2):226–232.
170. Lallemant M, Jourdain G, Le Coeur S, et al. A trial of shortened zidovudine regimens to prevent mother-to-child transmission of human immunodeficiency virus type 1. Perinatal HIV Prevention Trial (Thailand) Investigators. *N Engl J Med* 2000;343(14):982–991.
171. Bennetto-Hood C, Bryson YJ, Stek A, et al. Zidovudine, lamivudine, and nelfinavir concentrations in amniotic fluid and maternal serum. *HIV Clin Trials* 2009;10(1):41–47.
172. Schenker S, Johnson RF, King TS, et al. Azidothymidine (zidovudine) transport by the human placenta. *Am J Med Sci* 1990;299(1):16–20.
173. Patterson TA, Binienda ZK, Lipe GW, et al. Transplacental pharmacokinetics and fetal distribution of azidothymidine, its glucuronide, and phosphorylated metabolites in late-term rhesus macaques after maternal infusion. *Drug Metab Dispos* 1997;25(4):453–459.
174. Dancis J, Lee J, Mendoza S, et al. Nucleoside transport by perfused human placenta. *Placenta* 1993;14(5):547–554.
175. Kinai E, Kato S, Hosokawa S, et al. High plasma concentrations of zidovudine (AZT) do not parallel intracellular concentrations of AZT-triphosphates in infants during prevention of mother-to-child HIV-1 transmission. *J Acquir Immune Defic Syndr* 2016;72(3):246–253.
176. Rodman JH, Flynn PM, Robbins B, et al. Systemic pharmacokinetics and cellular pharmacology of zidovudine in human immunodeficiency virus type 1-infected women and newborn infants. *J Infect Dis* 1999;180(6):1844–1850.
177. Fauchet F, Treluyer JM, Valade E, et al. Maternal and fetal zidovudine pharmacokinetics during pregnancy and labour: too high dose infused at labour? *Br J Clin Pharmacol* 2014;78(6):1387–1396.
178. Boucher FD, Modlin JF, Weller S, et al. Phase I evaluation of zidovudine administered to infants exposed at birth to the human immunodeficiency virus. *J Pediatr* 1993;122(1):137–144.
179. Corbett AH, Kayira D, White NR, et al. Antiretroviral pharmacokinetics in mothers and breastfeeding infants from 6 to 24 weeks post-partum: results of the BAN Study. *Antivir Ther* 2014;19(6):587–595.
180. Mirochnick M, Capparelli E, Connor J. Pharmacokinetics of zidovudine in infants: a population analysis across studies. *Clin Pharmacol Ther* 1999;66(1):16–24.
181. Kawade N, Onishi S. The prenatal and postnatal development of UDP-glucuronosyltransferase activity towards bilirubin and the effect of premature birth on this activity in the human liver. *Biochem J* 1981;196(1):257–260.
182. Rajaonarison JF, Lacarelle B, De Sousa G, et al. In vitro glucuronidation of 3′-azido-3′-deoxythymidine by human liver. Role of UDP-glucuronosyltransferase 2 form. *Drug Metab Dispos* 1991;19(4):809–815.
183. Herber R, Magdalou J, Haumont M, et al. Glucuronidation of 3 -azido-3 -deoxythymidine in human liver microsomes: enzyme inhibition by drugs and steroid hormones. *Biochim Biophys Acta* 1992;1139(1–2):20–24.
184. Mirochnick M, Capparelli E, Dankner W, et al. Zidovudine pharmacokinetics in premature infants exposed to human immunodeficiency virus. *Antimicrob Agents Chemother* 1998;42(4):808–812.
185. Balis FM, Pizzo PA, Murphy RF, et al. The pharmacokinetics of zidovudine administered by continuous infusion in children. *Ann Intern Med* 1989;110(4):279–285.
186. Capparelli EV, Mirochnick M, Dankner WM, et al. Pharmacokinetics and tolerance of zidovudine in preterm infants. *J Pediatr* 2003;142(1):47–52.
187. Zidovudine package insert. Food and Drug Administration. 2017. https://www.accessdata.fda.gov/drugsatfda_docs/label/2008/019910s033lbl.pdf. Accessed December 10, 2019.
188. Taha TE, Kumwenda N, Gibbons A, et al. Effect of HIV-1 antiretroviral prophylaxis on hepatic and hematological parameters of African infants. *AIDS* 2002;16(6):851–858.
189. Chotpitayasunondh T, Vanprapar N, Simonds RJ, et al. Safety of late in utero exposure to zidovudine in infants born to human immunodeficiency virus-infected mothers: Bangkok. Bangkok Collaborative Perinatal HIV Transmission Study Group. *Pediatrics* 2001;107(1):E5.
190. Culnane M, Fowler M, Lee SS, et al. Lack of long-term effects of in utero exposure to zidovudine among uninfected children born to HIV-infected women. Pediatric AIDS Clinical Trials Group Protocol 219/076 Teams. *JAMA* 1999;281(2):151–157.
191. García-Otero L, López M, Gómez O, et al. Zidovudine treatment in HIV-infected pregnant women is associated with fetal cardiac remodelling. *AIDS* 2016;30(9):1393–1401.
192. Vannappagari V, Albano JD, Koram N, et al. Prenatal exposure to zidovudine and risk for ventricular septal defects and congenital heart defects: data from the Antiretroviral Pregnancy Registry. *Eur J Obstet Gynecol Reprod Biol* 2016;197:6–10.
193. Lipshultz SE, Easley KA, Orav EJ, et al. Absence of cardiac toxicity of zidovudine in infants. Pediatric pulmonary and cardiac complications of vertically transmitted HIV infection study group. *N Engl J Med* 2000;343(11):759–766.
194. Watts DH, Li D, Handelsman E, et al. Assessment of birth defects according to maternal therapy among infants in the Women and Infants Transmission Study. *J Acquir Immune Defic Syndr* 2007;44(3):299–305.
195. Van Dyke RB, Chadwick EG, Hazra R, et al. The PHACS SMARTT study: assessment of the safety of in utero exposure to antiretroviral drugs. *Front Immunol* 2016;7:199.
196. Temesgen Z, Wright AJ. Antiretrovirals. *Mayo Clin Proc* 1999;74(12):1284–1301.
197. Efavirenz package insert. Food and Drug Administration. 2017.
198. de Ruiter A, Taylor GP, Clayden P, et al. British HIV Association guidelines for the management of HIV infection in pregnant women 2012 (2014 interim review). *HIV Med* 2014;15 (Suppl 4):1–77.
199. McDonagh EM, Lau JL, Alvarellos ML, et al. PharmGKB summary: efavirenz pathway, pharmacokinetics. *Pharmacogenet Genomics* 2015;25(7):363–376.
200. Pfister M, Labbé L, Hammer SM, et al. Population pharmacokinetics and pharmacodynamics of efavirenz, nelfinavir, and indinavir: adult AIDS Clinical Trial Group Study 398. *Antimicrob Agents Chemother* 2003;47(1):130.
201. Ward BA, Gorski JC, Jones DR, et al. The cytochrome P450 2B6 (CYP2B6) is the main catalyst of efavirenz primary and secondary metabolism: implication for HIV/AIDS therapy and utility of efavirenz as a substrate marker of CYP2B6 catalytic activity. *J Pharmacol Exp Ther* 2003;306(1):287–300.
202. Gandhi M, Greenblatt RM, Bacchetti P, et al. A single-nucleotide polymorphism in CYP2B6 leads to >3-fold increases in efavirenz concentrations in plasma and hair among HIV-infected women. *J Infect Dis* 2012;206(9):1453–1461.
203. Cressey TR, Stek A, Capparelli E, et al. Efavirenz pharmacokinetics during the third trimester of pregnancy and postpartum. *J Acquir Immune Defic Syndr* 2012;59(3):245–252.
204. Kreitchmann R, Schalkwijk S, Best B, et al. Efavirenz pharmacokinetics during pregnancy and infant washout. *Antivir Ther* 2019;24(2):95–103.
205. Hill A, Ford N, Boffito M, et al. Does pregnancy affect the pharmacokinetics of efavirenz? *AIDS* 2014;28(10):1542–1543.
206. Gandhi M, Mwesigwa J, Aweeka F, et al. Hair and plasma data show that lopinavir, ritonavir, and efavirenz all transfer from mother to infant in utero, but only efavirenz transfers via breastfeeding. *J Acquir Immune Defic Syndr* 2013;63(5):578–584.
207. Schneider S, Peltier A, Gras A, et al. Efavirenz in human breast milk, mothers', and newborns' plasma. *J Acquir Immune Defic Syndr* 2008;48:450–454.
208. Oumar AA, Bagayoko-Maiga K, Bahachimi A, et al. Efavirenz and lopinavir levels in HIV-infected women and their nursing infants, in Mali. *J Pharmacol Exp Ther* 2018;366(3):479–484.
209. Olagunju A, Bolaji O, Amara A, et al. Breast milk pharmacokinetics of efavirenz and breastfed infants' exposure in genetically defined subgroups of mother-infant pairs: an observational study. *Clin Infect Dis* 2015;61(3):453–463.
210. Palombi L, Pirillo MF, Marchei E, et al. Concentrations of tenofovir, lamivudine and efavirenz in mothers and children enrolled under the Option B-Plus approach in Malawi. *J Antimicrob Chemother* 2016;71(4):1027–1030.
211. Sustiva package insert. Wilmington, DE: Dupont Pharmaceuticals Company. 2000.
212. Ford N, Calmy A. Efavirenz is not a known teratogen. *Pediatr Infect Dis J* 2012;31(9):999; author reply 1000.
213. De Santis M, Carducci B, De Santis L, et al. Periconceptional exposure to efavirenz and neural tube defects. *Arch Intern Med* 2002;162(3):355.
214. Saitoh A, Hull AD, Franklin P, et al. Myelomeningocele in an infant with intrauterine exposure to efavirenz. *J Perinatol* 2005;25(8):555–556.
215. Fundarò C, Genovese O, Rendeli C, et al. Myelomeningocele in a child with intrauterine exposure to efavirenz. *AIDS* 2002;16(2):299–300.
216. Mofenson LM, Watts DH. Safety of pediatric HIV elimination: the growing population of HIV-a nd antiretroviral-exposed but uninfected infants. *PLoS Med* 2014;11(4):e1001636.
217. Floridia M, Mastroiacovo P, Tamburrini E, et al. Birth defects in a national cohort of pregnant women with HIV infection in Italy, 2001-2011. *BJOG* 2013;120(12):1466–1475.
218. Intelence package insert. Raritan, NJ: Tibotec, Inc., 2008.
219. Mulligan N, Schalkwijk S, Best BM, et al. Etravirine pharmacokinetics in HIV-infected pregnant women. *Front Pharmacol* 2016;7:239.
220. Ramgopal M, Osiyemi O, Zorrilla C, et al. Pharmacokinetics of total and unbound etravirine in HIV-1-infected pregnant women. *J Acquir Immune Defic Syndr* 2016;73(3): 268–274.
221. Spencer L, Liu S, Wang C, eds. Intensive etravirine PK and HIV-1 viral load in breast milk and plasma in HIV+ women receiving HAART. Poster 891 presented at: Conference on Retroviruses and Opportunistic Infections; March 3-6, 2014; Boston, MA.
222. Calcagno A, Trentini L, Marinaro L, et al. Transplacental passage of etravirine and maraviroc in a multidrug-experienced HIV-infected woman failing on darunavir-based HAART in late pregnancy. *J Antimicrob Chemother* 2013;68(8):1938–1939.
223. Furco A, Gosrani B, Nicholas S, et al. Successful use of darunavir, etravirine, enfuvirtide and tenofovir/emtricitabine in pregnant woman with multiclass HIV resistance. *AIDS* 2009;23(3):434–435.
224. Cheeseman SH, Hattox SE, McLaughlin MM, et al. Pharmacokinetics of nevirapine: initial single-rising-dose study in humans. *Antimicrob Agents Chemother* 1993;37(2):178–182.
225. Lamson MJ, Sabo JP, MacGregor TR, et al. Single dose pharmacokinetics and bioavailability of nevirapine in healthy volunteers. *Biopharm Drug Dispos* 1999;20(6):285–291.
226. Murphy RL, Montaner J. Drug evaluations anti-infectives: nevirapine: a review of its development, pharmacological profile and potential for clinical use. *Expert Opin Investig Drugs* 1996;5(9):1183–1199.
227. Little BB. Pharmacokinetics during pregnancy: evidence-based maternal dose formulation. *Obstet Gynecol* 1999;93(5 Pt 2):858–868.

228. Cheeseman SH, Havlir D, McLaughlin MM, et al. Phase I/II evaluation of nevirapine alone and in combination with zidovudine for infection with human immunodeficiency virus. *J Acquir Immune Defic Syndr Hum Retrovirol* 1995;8(2):141–151.
229. Havlir D, Cheeseman SH, McLaughlin M, et al. High-dose nevirapine: safety, pharmacokinetics, and antiviral effect in patients with human immunodeficiency virus infection. *J Infect Dis* 1995;171(3):537–545.
230. Panel on Antiretroviral Guidelines for Adults and Adolescents. *Guidelines for the use of antiretroviral agents in adults and adolescents with HIV.* Department of Health and Human Services. http://aidsinfo.nih.gov/contentfiles/lvguidelines/AdultandAdolescentGL.pdf. Accessed December 10, 2019.
231. Taylor GP, Lyall EG, Back D, et al. Pharmacological implications of lengthened in-utero exposure to nevirapine. *Lancet* 2000;355(9221):2134–2135.
232. Capparelli EV, Aweeka F, Hitti J, et al. Chronic administration of nevirapine during pregnancy: impact of pregnancy on pharmacokinetics. *HIV Med* 2008;9(4):214–220.
233. Nellen JF, Damming M, Godfried MH, et al. Steady-state nevirapine plasma concentrations are influenced by pregnancy. *HIV Med* 2008;9(4):234–238.
234. Lamorde M, Byakika-Kibwika P, Okaba-Kayom V, et al. Suboptimal nevirapine steady-state pharmacokinetics during intrapartum compared with postpartum in HIV-1-seropositive Ugandan women. *J Acquir Immune Defic Syndr* 2010;55(3):345–350.
235. von Hentig N, Carlebach A, Gute P, et al. A comparison of the steady-state pharmacokinetics of nevirapine in men, nonpregnant women and women in late pregnancy. *Br J Clin Pharmacol* 2006;62(5):552–559.
236. Mirochnick M, Fenton T, Gagnier P, et al. Pharmacokinetics of nevirapine in human immunodeficiency virus type 1-infected pregnant women and their neonates. Pediatric AIDS Clinical Trials Group Protocol 250 Team. *J Infect Dis* 1998;178(2):368–374.
237. Musoke P, Guay LA, Bagenda D, et al. A phase I/II study of the safety and pharmacokinetics of nevirapine in HIV-1-infected pregnant Ugandan women and their neonates (HIVNET 006). *AIDS* 1999;13(4):479–486.
238. Mirochnick M, Siminski S, Fenton T, et al. Nevirapine pharmacokinetics in pregnant women and in their infants after in utero exposure. *Pediatr Infect Dis J* 2001;20(8):803–805.
239. Olagunju A, Bolaji O, Neary M, et al. Pregnancy affects nevirapine pharmacokinetics: evidence from a CYP2B6 genotype-guided observational study. *Pharmacogenet Genomics* 2016;26(8):381–389.
240. Patel SM, Johnson S, Belknap SM, et al. Serious adverse cutaneous and hepatic toxicities associated with nevirapine use by non-HIV-infected individuals. *J Acquir Immune Defic Syndr* 2004;35(2):120–125.
241. Viramune (nevirapine) package insert. Food and Drug Administration. 2017. https://www.accessdata.fda.gov/drugsatfda_docs/label/2011/020636s039_020933s030lbl.pdf. Accessed December 10, 2019.
242. Stern JO, Robinson PA, Love J, et al. A comprehensive hepatic safety analysis of nevirapine in different populations of HIV infected patients. *J Acquir Immune Defic Syndr* 2003;34 (Suppl 1):S21–S33.
243. Knudtson E, Para M, Boswell H, et al. Drug rash with eosinophilia and systemic symptoms syndrome and renal toxicity with a nevirapine-containing regimen in a pregnant patient with human immunodeficiency virus. *Obstet Gynecol* 2003;101(5 Pt 2):1094–1097.
244. Bersoff-Matcha SJ, Miller WC, Aberg JA, et al. Sex differences in nevirapine rash. *Clin Infect Dis* 2001;32(1):124–129.
245. Mazhude C, Jones S, Murad S, et al. Female sex but not ethnicity is a strong predictor of non-nucleoside reverse transcriptase inhibitor-induced rash. *AIDS* 2002;16(11):1566–1568.
246. Hitti J, Frenkel LM, Stek AM, et al. Maternal toxicity with continuous nevirapine in pregnancy: results from PACTG 1022. *J Acquir Immune Defic Syndr* 2004;36(3):772–776.
247. Lyons F, Hopkins S, Kelleher B, et al. Maternal hepatotoxicity with nevirapine as part of combination antiretroviral therapy in pregnancy. *HIV Med* 2006;7(4):255–260.
248. Ouyang DW, Shapiro DE, Lu M, et al. Increased risk of hepatotoxicity in HIV-infected pregnant women receiving antiretroviral therapy independent of nevirapine exposure. *AIDS* 2009;23(18):2425–2430.
249. Ouyang DW, Brogly SB, Lu M, et al. Lack of increased hepatotoxicity in HIV-infected pregnant women receiving nevirapine compared with other antiretrovirals. *AIDS* 2010;24(1):109–114.
250. Ford N, Calmy A, Andrieux-Meyer I, et al. Adverse events associated with nevirapine use in pregnancy: a systematic review and meta-analysis. *AIDS* 2013;27(7):1135–1143.
251. Huntington S, Thorne C, Anderson J, et al. Does pregnancy increase the risk of ART-induced hepatotoxicity among HIV-positive women? *J Int AIDS Soc* 2014;17(4 Suppl 3):19486.
252. Tran AH, Best BM, Stek A, et al. Pharmacokinetics of rilpivirine in HIV-infected pregnant women. *J Acquir Immune Defic Syndr* 2016;72(3):289–296.
253. Osiyemi O, Yasin S, Zorrilla C, et al. Pharmacokinetics, antiviral activity, and safety of rilpivirine in pregnant women with HIV-1 infection: results of a phase 3b, multicenter, open-label study. *Infect Dis Ther* 2018;7(1):147–159.
254. Schalkwijk S, Colbers A, Konopnicki D, et al. Lowered rilpivirine exposure during the third trimester of pregnancy in human immunodeficiency virus type 1-infected women. *Clin Infect Dis* 2017;65(8):1335–1341.
255. Mandelbrot L, Duro D, Belissa E, et al. Erratum for Mandelbrot et al., placental transfer of rilpivirine in an ex vivo human cotyledon perfusion model. *Antimicrob Agents Chemother* 2015;59(9):5869.
256. Mandelbrot L, Duro D, Belissa E, et al. Placental transfer of rilpivirine in an ex vivo human cotyledon perfusion model. *Antimicrob Agents Chemother* 2015;59(5):2901–2903.
257. Mirochnick M, Dorenbaum A, Holland D, et al. Concentrations of protease inhibitors in cord blood after in utero exposure. *Pediatr Infect Dis J* 2002;21(9):835–838.
258. Marzolini C, Rudin C, Decosterd LA, et al. Transplacental passage of protease inhibitors at delivery. *AIDS* 2002;16(6):889–893.
259. European Collaborative Study, Swiss Mother and Child HIV Cohort Study. Combination antiretroviral therapy and duration of pregnancy. *AIDS* 2000;14(18):2913–2920.
260. Cotter AM, Garcia AG, Duthely ML, et al. Is antiretroviral therapy during pregnancy associated with an increased risk of preterm delivery, low birth weight, or stillbirth? *J Infect Dis* 2006;193(9):1195–1201.
261. Kourtis AP, Schmid CH, Jamieson DJ, et al. Use of antiretroviral therapy in pregnant HIV-infected women and the risk of premature delivery: a meta-analysis. *AIDS* 2007;21(5):607–615.
262. Ravizza M, Martinelli P, Bucceri A, et al. Treatment with protease inhibitors and coinfection with hepatitis C virus are independent predictors of preterm delivery in HIV-infected pregnant women. *J Infect Dis* 2007;195(6):913–914; author reply 916–917.
263. Favarato G, Townsend CL, Bailey H, et al. Protease inhibitors and preterm delivery: another piece in the puzzle. *AIDS* 2018;32(2):243–252.
264. Atazanavir package insert. Food and Drug Administration. 2017. https://www.accessdata.fda.gov/drugsatfda_docs/label/2011/021567s026lbl.pdf. Accessed December 19, 2019.
265. Eley T, Bertz R, Hardy H, et al. Atazanavir pharmacokinetics, efficacy and safety in pregnancy: a systematic review. *Antivir Ther* 2013;18(3):361–375.
266. Conradie F, Zorrilla C, Josipovic D, et al. Safety and exposure of once-daily ritonavir-boosted atazanavir in HIV-infected pregnant women. *HIV Med* 2011;12(9):570–579.
267. Kreitchmann R, Best BM, Wang J, et al. Pharmacokinetics of an increased atazanavir dose with and without tenofovir during the third trimester of pregnancy. *J Acquir Immune Defic Syndr* 2013;63(1):59–66.
268. Le MP, Mandelbrot L, Descamps D, et al. Pharmacokinetics, safety and efficacy of ritonavir-boosted atazanavir (300/100 mg once daily) in HIV-1-infected pregnant women. *Antivir Ther* 2015;20(5):507–513.
269. Mirochnick M, Best BM, Stek AM, et al. Atazanavir pharmacokinetics with and without tenofovir during pregnancy. *J Acquir Immune Defic Syndr* 2011;56(5):412–419.
270. Ripamonti D, Cattaneo D, Maggiolo F, et al. Atazanavir plus low-dose ritonavir in pregnancy: pharmacokinetics and placental transfer. *AIDS* 2007;21(18):2409–2415.
271. Natha M, Hay P, Taylor G, et al. Atazanavir use in pregnancy: a report of 33 cases. Presented at: 14th Conference on Retroviruses and Opportunistic Infections; 2007; Los Angeles, CA.7.
272. Colbers A, Molto J, Ivanovic J, et al. A comparison of the pharmacokinetics of darunavir, atazanavir and ritonavir during pregnancy and post-partum. Presented at: 19th Conference on Retroviruses and Opportunistic Infections; 2012; Seattle, WA. Abstract 1013.2.
273. Taburet AM, Piketty C, Chazallon C, et al. Interactions between atazanavir-ritonavir and tenofovir in heavily pretreated human immunodeficiency virus-infected patients. *Antimicrob Agents Chemother* 2004;48(6):2091–2096.
274. Foca E, Calcagno A, Bonito A, et al. Atazanavir intracellular concentrations remain stable during pregnancy in HIV-infected patients. *J Antimicrob Chemother* 2017;72(11):3163–3166.
275. Colbers A, Hawkins D, Hidalgo-Tenorio C, et al. Atazanavir exposure is effective during pregnancy regardless of tenofovir use. *Antivir Ther* 2015;20(1):57–64.
276. Best B, Caparelli E, Stek A, et al. Elvitegravir/cobicistat pharmacokinetics in pregnancy and postpartum. Presented at: Conference on Retroviruses and Opportunistic Infections; 2017; Seattle, WA.7.
277. Crauwels HM, Osiyemi O, Zorilla C, et al. Pharmacokinetics of total and unbound darunavir in HIV-1–infected pregnant women receiving a darunavir/cobicistat-based regimen. Presented at: 8th International Workshop on HIV & Women; 2018; Boston, MA.8.
278. Momper JD, Stek A, Wang J, et al; IMPAACT P1026s Protocol Team. Pharmacokinetics of atazanavir boosted with cobicistat during pregnancy and postpartum. Presented at: 20th International Workshop on Clinical Pharmacology of HIV, Hepatitis & Other Antiviral Drugs; May 14–16, 2019; Noordwijk, The Netherlands.9.
279. Spencer L, Neely M, Mordwinkin N, et al. Intensive pharmacokinetics of zidovudine, lamivudine, and atazanavir and HIV-1 viral load in breast milk and plasma in HIV+ women receiving HAART. Presented at: 16th Conference on Retroviruses and Opportunistic Infections; 2009; Montreal, Canada.
280. Floridia M, Ravizza M, Masuelli G, et al. Atazanavir and lopinavir profile in pregnant women with HIV: tolerability, activity and pregnancy outcomes in an observational national study. *J Antimicrob Chemother* 2014;69(5):1377–1384.
281. Mandelbrot L, Mazy F, Floch-Tudal C, et al. Atazanavir in pregnancy: impact on neonatal hyperbilirubinemia. *Eur J Obstet Gynecol Reprod Biol* 2011;157(1):18–21.
282. Atrio JM, Sperling RS, Posada R, et al. Maternal atazanavir usage in HIV-infected pregnant women and the risk of maternal and neonatal hyperbilirubinemia. *J Acquir Immune Defic Syndr* 2013;63(5):e158–e159.
283. Eley T, Huang SP, Conradie F, et al. Clinical and pharmacogenetic factors affecting neonatal bilirubinemia following atazanavir treatment of mothers during pregnancy. *AIDS Res Hum Retroviruses* 2013;29(10):1287–1292.
284. Darunavir/cobicistat (Prezcobix) package insert. Food and Drug Administration. 2018 https://www.accessdata.fda.gov/drugsatfda_docs/label/2018/205395s009lbl.pdf. Accessed December 10, 2019.
285. Zorrilla CD, Wright R, Osiyemi OO, et al. Total and unbound darunavir pharmacokinetics in pregnant women infected with HIV-1: results of a study of darunavir/ritonavir 600/100 mg administered twice daily. *HIV Med* 2014;15(1):50–56.
286. Colbers A, Molto J, Ivanovic J, et al. Pharmacokinetics of total and unbound darunavir in HIV-1-infected pregnant women. *J Antimicrob Chemother* 2015;70(2):534–542.
287. Stek A, Best BM, Wang J, et al. Pharmacokinetics of once versus twice daily darunavir in pregnant HIV-infected women. *J Acquir Immune Defic Syndr* 2015;70(1):33–41.
288. Stek A, Best B, Capparelli E, et al. Pharmacokinetics of increased dose darunavir during late pregnancy and postpartum. Presented at: 23rd Conference on Retroviruses and Opportunistic Infections; 2016; Boston, MA.
289. Crauwels HM, Kakuda TN, Ryan B, et al. Pharmacokinetics of once-daily darunavir/ritonavir in HIV-1-infected pregnant women. *HIV Med* 2016;17(9):643–652.
290. Momper J, Best B, Wang J, et al. Pharmacokinetics of darunavir boosted with cobicistat during pregnancy and postpartum. Presented at: International AIDS Conference; 2018; Amsterdam, The Netherlands.
291. Mandelbrot L, Duro D, Belissa E, et al. Placental transfer of darunavir in an ex vivo human cotyledon perfusion model. *Antimicrob Agents Chemother* 2014;58(9):5617–5620.

292. Courbon E, Matheron S, Mandelbrot L. *Safety, efficacy, and pharmacokinetic of darunavir/ritonavir-containing regimen in pregnant HIV+ women. Presented at: 19th Conference on Retroviruses and Opportunistic Infections; 2012; Seattle, WA.*2.
293. Lopinavir/ritonavir (Kaletra) package insert. Food and Drug Administration. 2017.
294. Stek AM, Mirochnick M, Capparelli E, et al. Reduced lopinavir exposure during pregnancy. *AIDS* 2006;20(15):1931–1939.
295. Ramautarsing RA, van der Lugt J, Gorowara M, et al. Thai HIV-1-infected women do not require a dose increase of lopinavir/ritonavir during the third trimester of pregnancy. *AIDS* 2011;25(10):1299–1303.
296. Bouillon-Pichault M, Jullien V, Azria E, et al. Population analysis of the pregnancy-related modifications in lopinavir pharmacokinetics and their possible consequences for dose adjustment. *J Antimicrob Chemother* 2009;63(6):1223–1232.
297. Best BM, Stek AM, Mirochnick M, et al. Lopinavir tablet pharmacokinetics with an increased dose during pregnancy. *J Acquir Immune Defic Syndr* 2010;54(4):381–388.
298. Mirochnick M, Best BM, Stek AM, et al. Lopinavir exposure with an increased dose during pregnancy. *J Acquir Immune Defic Syndr* 2008;49(5):485–491.
299. Cressey TR, Urien S, Capparelli EV, et al. Impact of body weight and missed doses on lopinavir concentrations with standard and increased lopinavir/ritonavir doses during late pregnancy. *J Antimicrob Chemother* 2015;70(1):217–224.
300. Aweeka FT, Stek A, Best BM, et al. Lopinavir protein binding in HIV-1-infected pregnant women. *HIV Med* 2010;11(4):232–238.
301. Patterson KB, Dumond JB, Prince HA, et al. Protein binding of lopinavir and ritonavir during 4 phases of pregnancy: implications for treatment guidelines. *J Acquir Immune Defic Syndr* 2013;63(1):51–58.
302. Chen J, Malone S, Prince HM, et al. Model-based analysis of unbound lopinavir pharmacokinetics in HIV-infected pregnant women supports standard dosing in the third trimester. *CPT Pharmacometrics Syst Pharmacol* 2016;5(3):147–157.
303. Fauchet F, Treluyer JM, Illamola SM, et al. Population approach to analyze the pharmacokinetics of free and total lopinavir in HIV-infected pregnant women and consequences for dose adjustment. *Antimicrob Agents Chemother* 2015;59(9):5727–5735.
304. Rezk NL, White N, Bridges AS, et al. Studies on antiretroviral drug concentrations in breast milk: validation of a liquid chromatography-tandem mass spectrometric method for the determination of 7 anti-human immunodeficiency virus medications. *Ther Drug Monit* 2008;30(5):611–619.
305. Chadwick EG, Pinto J, Yogev R, et al. Early initiation of lopinavir/ritonavir in infants less than 6 weeks of age: pharmacokinetics and 24-week safety and efficacy. *Pediatr Infect Dis J* 2009;28(3):215–219.
306. Tookey PA, Thorne C, van Wyk J, et al. Maternal and foetal outcomes among 4118 women with HIV infection treated with lopinavir/ritonavir during pregnancy: analysis of population-based surveillance data from the national study of HIV in pregnancy and childhood in the United Kingdom and Ireland. *BMC Infect Dis* 2016;16:65.
307. Boxwell D, Cao K, Lewis L, et al. Neonatal toxicity of Kaletra oral solution: LPV, ethanol or propylene glycol? Presented at: 18th Conference on Retroviruses and Opportunistic Infections; 2011; Boston, MA.
308. Simon A, Warszawski J, Kariyawasam D, et al. Association of prenatal and postnatal exposure to lopinavir-ritonavir and adrenal dysfunction among uninfected infants of HIV-infected mothers. *JAMA* 2011;306(1):70–78.
309. Pommier Y, Johnson AA, Marchand C. Integrase inhibitors to treat HIV/AIDS. *Nat Rev Drug Discov* 2005;4(3):236.
310. Messiaen P, Wensing AM, Fun A, et al. Clinical use of HIV integrase inhibitors: a systematic review and meta-analysis. *PLoS One* 2013;8(1):e52562.
311. Zash R, Makhema J, Shapiro RL. Neural-tube defects with dolutegravir treatment from the time of conception. *N Engl J Med* 2018;379(10):979–981.
312. Cottrell ML, Hadzic T, Kashuba AD. Clinical pharmacokinetic, pharmacodynamic and drug-interaction profile of the integrase inhibitor dolutegravir. *Clin Pharmacokinet* 2013;52(11):981–994.
313. Castellino S, Moss L, Wagner D, et al. Metabolism, excretion, and mass balance of the HIV-1 integrase inhibitor dolutegravir in humans. *Antimicrob Agents Chemother* 2013;57(8):3536–3546.
314. Tivicay (dolutegravir) package insert. Food and Drug Administration. 2016. https://www.accessdata.fda.gov/drugsatfda_docs/label/2013/204790lbl.pdf. Accessed December 10, 2019.
315. Mulligan N, Best BM, Wang J, et al. Dolutegravir pharmacokinetics in pregnant and postpartum women living with HIV. *AIDS* 2018;32(6):729–737.
316. Schalkwijk S, Greupink R, Colbers AP, et al. Placental transfer of the HIV integrase inhibitor dolutegravir in an ex vivo human cotyledon perfusion model. *J Antimicrob Chemother* 2016;71(2):480–483.
317. Kobbe R, Schalkwijk S, Dunay G, et al. Dolutegravir in breast milk and maternal and infant plasma during breastfeeding. *AIDS* 2016;30(17):2731–2733.
318. Vannappagari V, Thorne C, for APR, EPPICC. Pregnancy and neonatal outcomes following prenatal exposure to dolutegravir. *J Acquir Immune Defic Syndr* 2019;81(4):371–378.
319. Grayhack C, Sheth A, Kirby O, et al. Evaluating outcomes of mother-infant pairs using dolutegravir for HIV treatment during pregnancy. *AIDS* 2018;32(14):2017–2021.
320. Cabrera RM, Souder JP, Steele JW, et al. The antagonism of folate receptor by dolutegravir: developmental toxicity reduction by supplemental folic acid. *AIDS* 2019;33(13):1967–1976.
321. Zash R, Holmes L, Diseko M, et al. Neural tube defects by antiretroviral and HIV exposure in the Tsepamo Study, Botswana. Presented at: AIDS Conference; July 2019; Mexico City, Mexico. Abstract MOAX0105LB.
322. Raesima MM, Forhan S, Thomas V, et al. Addressing the safety signal with dolutegravir use at conception: additional surveillance data from Botswana. Presented at: AIDS Conference; July 2019; Mexico City, Mexico. Abstract MOAX0106LB.
323. Mofenson LM, Vannappagari V, Scheuerle AE, et al. Periconceptional antiretroviral exposure and central nervous system (CNS) and neural tube birth defects data from Antiretroviral PregnancyRegistry (APR). Presented at: AIDS Conference; July 2019; Mexico City, Mexico. Abstract TUAB0101.
324. Ramanathan S, Mathias AA, German P, et al. Clinical pharmacokinetic and pharmacodynamic profile of the HIV integrase inhibitor elvitegravir. *Clin Pharmacokinet* 2011;50(4):229–244.
325. Adams JL, Greener BN, Kashuba AD. Pharmacology of HIV integrase inhibitors. *Curr Opin HIV AIDS* 2012;7(5):390–400.
326. Momper JD, Best BM, Wang J, et al. Elvitegravir/cobicistat pharmacokinetics in pregnant and postpartum women with HIV. *AIDS* 2018;32(17):2507–2516.
327. Colbers A, Schalkwijk S, Konopnicki D, et al. eds. Elvitegravir pharmacokinetics during pregnancy and postpartum. Presented at: 19th International Workshop on Clinical Pharmacology of Antiviral Therapy; 2018; Baltimore, MD. Abstract 17.
328. Schalkwijk S, Colbers A, Konopnicki D, et al. First reported use of elvitegravir and cobicistat during pregnancy. *AIDS* 2016;30(5):807–808.
329. Genvoya package insert. Food and Drug Administration. 2017. https://www.accessdata.fda.gov/drugsatfda_docs/label/2017/207561s014lbl.pdf. Accessed December 10, 2019.
330. Kassahun K, McIntosh I, Cui D, et al. Metabolism and disposition in humans of raltegravir (MK-0518), an anti-AIDS drug targeting the human immunodeficiency virus 1 integrase enzyme. *Drug Metab Dispos* 2007;35(9):1657–1663.
331. Krishna R, East L, Larson P, et al. Atazanavir increases the plasma concentrations of 1200 mg raltegravir dose. *Biopharm Drug Dispos* 2016;37(9):533–541.
332. Watts DH, Stek A, Best BM, et al. Raltegravir pharmacokinetics during pregnancy. *J Acquir Immune Defic Syndr* 2014;67(4):375–381.
333. Blonk MI, Colbers AP, Hidalgo-Tenorio C, et al. Raltegravir in HIV-1-infected pregnant women: pharmacokinetics, safety, and efficacy. *Clin Infect Dis* 2015;61(5):809–816.
334. Clarke DF, Acosta EP, Rizk ML, et al. Raltegravir pharmacokinetics in neonates following maternal dosing. *J Acquir Immune Defic Syndr* 2014;67(3):310–315.
335. Vinot C, Tréluyer JM, Giraud C, et al. Bidirectional transfer of raltegravir in an ex vivo human cotyledon perfusion model. *Antimicrob Agents Chemother* 2016;60(5):3112–3114.
336. Raltegravir package insert. Food and Drug Administration. 2018. https://www.accessdata.fda.gov/drugsatfda_docs/label/2018/022145s038,205786s007,0203045s015lbl.pdf. Accessed December 10, 2019.
337. Rockstroh JK, DeJesus E, Lennox JL, et al. Durable efficacy and safety of raltegravir versus efavirenz when combined with tenofovir/emtricitabine in treatment-naive HIV-1-infected patients: final 5-year results from STARTMRK. *J Acquir Immune Defic Syndr* 2013;63(1):77–85.
338. Lommerse J, Clarke DF, Chain A. Use of allometry and maturation in PK modeling to develop a daily dosing regimen for investigation during the first weeks of life. Presented at: Population Approach Group Europe Conference; 2015; Hersonissos, Crete, Greece.
339. Hegazi A, Mc Keown D, Doerholt K, et al. Raltegravir in the prevention of mother-to-child transmission of HIV-1: effective transplacental transfer and delayed plasma clearance observed in preterm neonates. *AIDS* 2012;26(18):2421–2423.
340. Clarke DF, Wong RJ, Wenning L, et al. Raltegravir in vitro effect on bilirubin binding. *Pediatr Infect Dis J* 2013;32(9):978–980.
341. Clavel-Osorio C, Cazassus F, Stegmann S, et al. One-month transplacental pharmacokinetics of raltegravir in a premature newborn after short-course treatment of the HIV-1-infected mother. *Antimicrob Agents Chemother* 2013;57(12):6393–6394.
342. Kreutzwiser D, Sheehan N, Dayneka N, et al. Therapeutic drug monitoring guided raltegravir dosing for prevention of vertical transmission in a premature neonate born to a woman living with perinatally acquired HIV. *Antivir Ther* 2017;22(6):545–549.
343. Renet S, Closon A, Brochet MS, et al. Increase in transaminase levels following the use of raltegravir in a woman with a high HIV viral load at 35 weeks of pregnancy. *J Obstet Gynaecol Can* 2013;35(1):68–72.
344. Yee BE, Nguyen NH, Lee D. Extensive pulmonary involvement with raltegravir-induced DRESS syndrome in a postpartum woman with HIV. *BMJ Case Rep* 2014;2014.
345. Brennan-Benson P, Pakianathan M, Rice P, et al. Enfurvitide prevents vertical transmission of multidrug-resistant HIV-1 in pregnancy but does not cross the placenta. *AIDS* 2006;20(2):297–299.
346. Meyohas MC, Lacombe K, Carbonne B, et al. Enfuvirtide prescription at the end of pregnancy to a multi-treated HIV-infected woman with virological breakthrough. *AIDS* 2004;18(14):1966–1968.
347. Sued O, Lattner J, Gun A, et al. Use of darunavir and enfuvirtide in a pregnant woman. *Int J STD AIDS* 2008;19(12):866–867.
348. Madeddu G, Calia GM, Campus ML, et al. Successful prevention of multidrug resistant HIV mother-to-child transmission with enfuvirtide use in late pregnancy. *Int J STD AIDS* 2008;19(9):644–645.
349. Shust GF, Jao J, Rodriguez-Caprio G, et al. Salvage regimens containing darunavir, etravirine, raltegravir, or enfuvirtide in highly treatment-experienced perinatally infected pregnant women. *J Pediatr Infect Dis Soc* 2014;3(3):246–250.
350. Chohan BH, Tapia K, Benki-Nugent S, et al. Nevirapine resistance in previously nevirapine-unexposed HIV-1-infected Kenyan infants initiating early antiretroviral therapy. *AIDS Res Hum Retroviruses* 2015;31(8):783–791.
351. Weizsaecker K, Kurowski M, Hoffmeister B, et al. Pharmacokinetic profile in late pregnancy and cord blood concentration of tipranavir and enfuvirtide. *Int J STD AIDS* 2011;22(5):294–295.
352. Ceccaldi PF, Ferreira C, Gavard L, et al. Placental transfer of enfuvirtide in the ex vivo human placenta perfusion model. *Am J Obstet Gynecol* 2008;198(4):433.e1–433.e2.
353. Colbers A, Best B, Schalkwijk S, et al. Maraviroc pharmacokinetics in HIV-1-infected pregnant women. *Clin Infect Dis* 2015;61(10):1582–1589.
354. Vinot C, Gavard L, Treluyer JM, et al. Placental transfer of maraviroc in an ex vivo human cotyledon perfusion model and influence of ABC transporter expression. *Antimicrob Agents Chemother* 2013;57(3):1415–1420.
355. Colbers A, Mirochnick M, Schalkwijk S, et al. Importance of prospective studies in pregnant and breastfeeding women living with human immunodeficiency virus. *Clin Infect Dis* 2019;69(7):1254–1258.
356. Nabekura T, Kawasaki T, Kamiya Y, et al. Effects of antiviral drugs on organic anion transport in human placental BeWo cells. *Antimicrob Agents Chemother* 2015;59(12):7666–7670.
357. Casey BM, Bawdon RE. Placental transfer of ritonavir with zidovudine in the ex vivo placental perfusion model. *Am J Obstet Gynecol* 1998;179(3 Pt 1):758–76.
358. Pregnancy and HIV/AIDS: Seeking Equitable Study (PHASES). Pregnancy and HIV/AIDS: seeking equitable study. 2019. http://www.hivpregnancyethics.org/. Accessed October 10, 2019.

SECTION

V

Neuropharmacology

CHAPTER

33

Victoria Tutag Lehr
Mitchel T. Williams

Anticonvulsants

INTRODUCTION

Epilepsy during infancy and childhood is a therapeutic challenge because more than 30% of children continue to have seizures refractory to treatment.[1] Antiepileptic drugs (AEDs) remain the primary treatment modality for seizures.[2–5] Multidrug regimens are often necessary to maximize seizure control and minimize adverse effects. During the past 30 years, several second- and third-generation AEDs were approved in the United States.[6–9] Newly approved AEDs include brivaracetam (BRV), cannabidiol (CBD) oral solution, clobazam (CLB), eslicarbazepine acetate (ESL), perampanel, and stiripentol (STP).[7,8,10] Overall, third-generation AEDs have broader or novel mechanism of actions, fewer drug–drug interactions, and improved bioavailability and tolerability compared with older AEDs.[11,12] Clinicians may be slow to adopt and prescribe new AEDs due to familiarity with older agents, insufficient postmarketing experience in infants and children, and higher relative cost.[13]

DEVELOPMENTAL CONSIDERATIONS FOR ANTICONVULSANT THERAPY

Data from well-designed clinical trials of the newer AEDs in infants and children are required. [14,15] Extrapolation of data from trials in adults to pediatric patients is questionable, given age-related differences in pharmacokinetics (PK), seizure types, and seizure etiology.[16] In addition, children with epilepsy commonly have developmental delay and behavioral disorders, adding another dimension of complexity when selecting an appropriate AED.[17] Adverse medication effects and variable developmental influences on PK, pharmacodynamics (PD), and pharmacogenomics, combined with comorbidities, complicate anticonvulsant therapy.[5,18,19] PK differences contribute to age-related differences in AED adverse effects.[16]

Interactions of AEDs with other agents are common; therefore, it is important to minimize the risks of interactions to avoid loss of seizure control or development of toxicity.[20] Agents such as lacosamide, levetiracetam (LEV), and topiramate (TPM) do not extensively induce metabolism of other AEDs, offering an advantage over older agents.[8,12,20] Clinicians are encouraged to consult with pharmacists and review current literature and labeling when prescribing AEDs to avoid precipitating a drug or drug–disease state interaction.

In January 2008, the U.S. Food and Drug Administration (FDA) issued an alert about a possible increased risk for suicidality associated with the use of AEDs for epilepsy.[21] The relationship between suicidality and epilepsy is a complex, multifactorial issue.[22,23] The contribution of AEDs to suicidality is unclear in view of confounders, such as concomitant drug therapy, mental health diagnoses, and effects of severity and chronicity of epilepsy. Parents, caregivers, and patients must be reassured and counseled about risks of discontinuing AED therapy without clinician supervision. Routine evaluation for depression, anxiety, and suicidality, especially during AED dosage adjustment, is recommended for all patients with epilepsy.[24]

INITIATION OF ANTICONVULSANT THERAPY

Initial anticonvulsant therapy depends upon seizure type and electroencephalogram (EEG) findings.[25] In 2017, seizure types were reclassified from the 1981 classification system.[26] While the expanded classification accurately describes more seizure types, many clinicians continue to use the old classification.

Additional factors influencing AED selection include patient age, gender, drug reaction history, concomitant diseases and medications, ease of administration, cost, and clinician familiarity with the individual AED. Genetic factors may be important in predicting response or toxicity to certain AEDs.[19,27–29] A well-known example is the HLA-B*15:02 allele association with increased risk of Stevens–Johnson syndrome/toxic epidermal necrolysis (SJS/TEN) after exposure to phenytoin and lamotrigine.[30]

FIRST-GENERATION AGENTS

PHENYTOIN

Indications and Clinical Use

Phenytoin continues to be used in pediatrics for status epilepticus, generalized tonic–clonic seizures, and partial seizures with or without secondary generalization.[3,31] This hydantoin is a second-line agent for status epilepticus after failure of benzodiazepines.[31,32]

Phenytoin is considered second-line therapy for managing neonatal seizures after failure of phenobarbital.[33] However, in a randomized clinical trial by Painter et al., in 59 neonates with seizures, phenytoin and phenobarbital were equally, but incompletely, effective in controlling neonatal seizures.[34] When either of these medications was administered as monotherapy, fewer than half of the babies had control of their seizures. Phenytoin and phenobarbital may be used for neonatal seizures, although LEV is gaining popularity secondary to efficacy and less potential for drug interactions and cognitive effects.[35]

Mechanism of Action

Phenytoin's primary anticonvulsant effect at therapeutic concentrations is use-dependent blockade of voltage-sensitive sodium channels, inhibiting repetitive neuronal firing.[36] Additional actions include alteration of Na^+, K^+, and Ca^{2+} conduction; membrane potentials; and concentrations of amino acids, norepinephrine, acetylcholine, and γ-aminobutyric acid (GABA).

Pharmacokinetics

The major route of phenytoin metabolism is hepatic oxidation by cytochrome P450 (CYP450) enzymes CYP2C9 and CYP2C19 to the inactive metabolite 5-(*p*-hydroxyphenyl)-5-phenylhydantoin.[28] This metabolic pathway is capacity limited and saturable.[37,38] As phenytoin serum concentrations increase, the fraction of drug eliminated per unit time decreases. Small increases in dose can cause disproportionately large increases in phenytoin serum concentration. These nonlinear kinetics occur in patients of all ages and are described by Michaelis–Menten equations.[39] Therefore, smaller incremental dose increases are recommended, as therapeutic phenytoin serum concentrations are approached.

Initial phenytoin dosing for neonates is 15 to 20 mg per kg intravenous (IV) or oral as a loading dose, followed by 4 to 7 mg per kg per day in divided doses every 12 hours as a maintenance dose.[25,40] To avoid cardiotoxicity, bradyarrhythmias, and hypotension associated with the propylene glycol and ethanol constituents of parenteral formulations, the maximum rate of phenytoin IV infusion is 0.5 mg per kg per minute. Phenytoin injection is compatible only with normal saline. Oral phenytoin-loading doses must be divided into two to three doses and administered every 12 hours to optimize absorption. Initiate the maintenance dose 12 hours after administration of the loading dose.[41]

Phenytoin dosage must be *slowly adjusted* according to individual patient's requirements, clinical response, and serum concentrations.[38,39] Because of nonlinear kinetics, it is prudent to initiate therapy at the lower end of the dosing range, increasing incrementally to clinical response while assessing for toxicity.[39] Initial maintenance dosages are based on age and weight: neonates (<4 weeks), 3 to 5 mg per kg per day; infants (4 weeks to <1 year), 4 to 8 mg per kg per day; children (1 to <12 years), 4 to 10 mg per kg per day; adolescents (12 to <18 years), 4 to 8 mg per kg per day; adults (18 years and older), 4 to 7 mg per kg per day.[41]

Use caution when changing dosage forms of phenytoin, as these vary in phenytoin content. The parenteral form, phenytoin sodium, contains 92% phenytoin, and the oral suspension is free phenytoin acid. As the phenytoin dose is increased and the therapeutic range is approached, the difference in phenytoin content between dose formulations becomes critical to avoid toxicity secondary to a disproportionate increase in serum concentration.[39]

Therapeutic Range

Phenytoin has a narrow therapeutic range for the general population of 10 to 20 µg per mL for *total drug concentration* and 1 to 2 µg per mL for *unbound or free drug*.[42] Free phenytoin serum determinations are essential in cases of hypoalbuminemia, azotemia, or reduced binding because the free fraction determines therapeutic effect and toxicity. A lower therapeutic range of 8 to 15 µg per mL because of reduced plasma protein binding and decreased metabolic capacity.[43] Phenytoin binding approaches adult values at approximately 3 months of age.

Infants exposed to phenytoin in utero or to phenobarbital therapy before phenytoin will have increased phenytoin elimination secondary to hepatic enzyme induction.[44] Considerable variability in correlating clinical response with serum concentration is due to decreased plasma protein binding, hypoalbuminemia, uremia, renal dysfunction, and hyperbilirubinemia. During the first 2 weeks of life, the infant's metabolic capacity increases significantly, resulting in increased phenytoin dose requirements. In general, infants have the highest phenytoin metabolic capacity, generally resulting in dose requirements up to four times that of adults. During childhood, phenytoin metabolism decreases, approaching that of adults at around 10 years of age.[38,45] Polymorphisms of CYP2C9 affect rate of phenytoin metabolism.[19,46] For example, individuals carrying CYP2C9*3 [rs1057910(C)] alleles are predisposed to concentration-dependent neurotoxicity due to slower phenytoin elimination.[46]

Therapeutic Drug Monitoring

Therapeutic drug monitoring (TDM) is recommended for phenytoin to optimize therapeutic effect and minimize risk of toxicity.[47] Frequency of phenytoin serum sampling depends on the clinical situation. After administration of a phenytoin-loading dose, serum sampling is often performed to verify therapeutic serum concentrations. Avoid drawing samples within 1 hour after the end of phenytoin infusion to allow for drug distribution.

During oral and IV maintenance therapy, trough serum concentrations are usually drawn just before the morning dose. Phenytoin concentrations are drawn within 3 to 4 days of starting maintenance therapy. While not at steady state, subtherapeutic or supratherapeutic concentrations may be detected, avoiding breakthrough seizures or toxicity.

Once a stable phenytoin regimen is achieved, serum sampling is performed every 1 to 2 weeks in hospital or every 1 to 6 months in outpatients. Sampling is indicated when a change in clinical status occurs, when a adding or deleting a drug with potential phenytoin interaction, when changing phenytoin dosage forms or dosage, or to verify dose absorption or adherence. Significant variations in PK occur during the neonatal period with IV and oral phenytoin therapy.[45] Controversy exists regarding neonates' ability to absorb oral formulations of phenytoin. Oral phenytoin therapy achieved predicted serum concentrations in a study of premature infants.[34] In addition to rapidly changing elimination kinetics, concomitant therapy with potent enzyme inducers, such as phenobarbital and carbamazepine (CBZ), may cause unpredictable fluctuations in phenytoin serum concentration.[48]

Drug Interactions

Numerous clinically significant PK and PD drug interactions involving phenytoin are possible.[49–52] Potential phenytoin drug interactions are too numerous to list here as new drugs are developed and introduced into practice. Clinicians are encouraged to consult pharmacists and review the current drug interaction literature when prescribing phenytoin therapy. Phenytoin serum concentrations may be increased by zidovudine and reduced by continuous nasogastric feedings.[53,54] Concomitant therapy with valproic acid (VPA) significantly increases phenytoin free fraction.[49] Phenytoin interactions with other AEDs are common and potentially significant.[55] Phenytoin may decrease serum concentrations and effectiveness of lamotrigine, VPA, felbamate, ethosuximide, and primidone, potentially causing loss of seizure control. Adolescents receiving phenytoin with oral contraceptives may have lower estrogen and progestin serum concentrations, causing contraceptive failure.[50] Higher dose oral contraceptives in addition to barrier methods are recommended for these patients. Evaluate the potential for precipitating drug interactions whenever making changes to a regimen containing phenytoin.

FOSPHENYTOIN

Indications and Clinical Use

Advantages of fosphenytoin over phenytoin include an aqueous solution without propylene glycol and a more neutral pH of 8.6.[56] Fosphenytoin is compatible with dextrose 5% water or normal saline and may be administered via intramuscular injection. Cardiotoxicity during IV infusion and local reactions at the infusion site are less frequent with fosphenytoin compared with phenytoin. Transient paresthesia, burning, and pruritus can occur during IV infusion of fosphenytoin, but the rate of infusion is three times faster than phenytoin, allowing for rapid loading in status epilepticus.[57]

Fosphenytoin is approximately two to five times the cost of phenytoin injection.[58] Restricting fosphenytoin use to patients without IV access or with prior local reactions to phenytoin administration, or for status epilepticus is common.[59] Infants and children in status epilepticus are at high risk for site reactions from phenytoin IV infusions. There is no apparent therapeutic benefit in using fosphenytoin over phenytoin, justifying the higher cost in other situations.[60] There is a paucity of data on the comparative efficacy of phenytoin and fosphenytoin, although fosphenytoin is better tolerated compared with phenytoin (Level B evidence). Therefore, fosphenytoin is preferred, and phenytoin is an acceptable alternative.[40]

Data are increasing on use of fosphenytoin in the newborn.[59] Fosphenytoin was administered to two extremely low birth weight infants with apparent adequate conversion to phenytoin and no adverse effects.[61] Seizure control was reported in four infants ranging in age from 34 weeks to 1 year treated with fosphenytoin; however, doses of up to 10 mg phenytoin equivalent (PE) per kg per day were required to maintain therapeutic phenytoin serum concentrations.[62] Three infants had been receiving phenobarbital at the time of fosphenytoin administration. In addition to probable induction of CYP450 by phenobarbital, the investigators suggested that the infants may have had an enhanced phenytoin rate of elimination.

Mechanism of Action

Fosphenytoin sodium (Cerebyx, Fosphenytoin Sodium Injection USP), 5,5-diphenyl-3-(phosphonooxy)methyl-2,4-imidazolidine-dione disodium, is the phosphorylated prodrug of phenytoin.[63] Fosphenytoin is available as a 75-mg per mL parenteral injection, equivalent to 50 mg phenytoin sodium per mL. Fosphenytoin must be prescribed in terms of PEs, with 1 mg PE equal to 1.5 mg fosphenytoin. Phenytoin toxicity and overdose can occur if fosphenytoin dosage is misinterpreted.

Pharmacokinetics

Fosphenytoin is cleaved to phenytoin by nonspecific phosphatases in red blood cells, and hepatic and other tissues. Conversion half-life is 8 to 15 minutes and prolonged in renal or hepatic insufficiency.[63] Fosphenytoin displaces phenytoin from plasma proteins, increasing free phenytoin concentrations until conversion is complete.

There was no significant difference in conversion rate of fosphenytoin to phenytoin in two multicenter studies of 78 patients ranging in age from 1 day to 16 years.[64] Subjects received fosphenytoin-loading doses of 18 to 20 mg PE per kg per minute via IV infusion (62/78) or 12 to 20 mg PE per kg per minute via intramuscular injection (16/78). Mean fosphenytoin-to-phenytoin conversion half-life was 8.3 minutes (2.5 to 18.5 minutes), similar to adult values (7.9 minutes). There was no significant difference in conversion half-life across age groups. Total and free phenytoin serum concentrations were similar to those in adults. There were no documented cases of toxicity or serious adverse effects.

Therapeutic Drug Monitoring

Phenytoin serum concentrations should not be drawn until after 2 hours after the end of IV infusion of fosphenytoin or 4 hours after intramuscular administration to allow for conversion to phenytoin.[5] The increased free fraction during conversion of fosphenytoin to phenytoin may be cleared rapidly by infants, making it difficult to maintain therapeutic phenytoin serum concentrations.

Drug Interactions

Fosphenytoin provides an effective, well-tolerated alternative to phenytoin in infants and children where venous access is not available and/or rapid loading is desirable, including neonatal seizures or status epilepticus.[59]

PHENOBARBITAL

Indications and Clinical Use

Phenobarbital remains first-line management for neonatal seizures.[33] However, it is often ineffective in achieving complete seizure control in neonatal seizures.[34] A multicenter retrospective study of infants with neonatal seizures (n = 146) showed no benefit of phenobarbital treatment after discharge home in preventing seizure recurrence or long-term disability compared with no treatment.[34] Experience with newer agents for neonatal seizures such as LEV is increasing.[35]

Other indications are generalized tonic–clonic seizures, partial seizures, and prolonged febrile convulsions. Advantages of phenobarbital include treatment of a wide spectrum of seizure activity, wide therapeutic range, availability of parenteral and oral dose forms, low cost, and extensive experience of use in pediatrics. Disadvantages include respiratory depression, sedation, physical dependence, negative cognitive effects, hyperactivity, and potential adverse effects on developing neuronal cells.[65]

Mechanism of Action

Phenobarbital is a 5-ethyl-5-phenyl–substituted barbiturate with an anticonvulsant effect related to potentiation of inhibitory neurotransmission by prolonging the open state of GABA-mediated sodium channels. Glutamate-induced excitatory transmission is decreased, and neurotransmitter release from nerve terminals is diminished via blocking of L-type and N-type calcium currents. Selective suppression of abnormal neurons may also contribute to its therapeutic effect.[66]

Pharmacokinetics

Phenobarbital has a large volume of distribution (V_d), distributing into all tissues, with approximately 50% bound to plasma protein. V_d decreases with increasing gestational age as total body water decreases and body fat increases. These changes in V_d may result in high (interpatient) variability in phenobarbital serum concentrations achieved after standard loading doses. In general, initial dosing recommendations for 10 to 20 mg per kg assume a V_d of 1.0 L per kg to achieve serum concentrations of 15 to 20 mg per mL. Therapeutic phenobarbital serum concentrations are 10 to 30 mg per mL. Reduced binding on the order of 20% to 25% has been demonstrated in neonates.[67] Because phenobarbital is a weak acid, lower serum pH will enhance tissue penetration. Distribution across the blood–brain barrier is relatively slow (15 to 20 minutes after peak serum concentrations); therefore, allow for equilibration after administration. Wide interindividual variability in V_d and elimination among neonates makes it necessary to measure phenobarbital serum concentrations.[67]

The primary route of elimination for phenobarbital is metabolism via hepatic microsomal CYP450 enzymes and NADPH–cytochrome c reductase. Dosing reduction is advised in hepatic insufficiency. Phenobarbital clearance does not appear to undergo significant changes due to autoinduction, although it is a potent inducer of other hepatic metabolized agents, such as theophylline, CBZ, phenytoin, cimetidine, and digoxin.[49]

Phenobarbital has a long elimination half-life, with newborns having the slowest clearance (average 100 to 200 hours). Premature neonates may have unexpectedly increased clearance of phenobarbital, possibly secondary to increased liver size compared to body weight. Touw et al. reported increasing total body clearance of phenobarbital per kilogram of body weight with increasing fetal maturity.[68] Therefore, extremely premature infants would have not yet undergone the decrease in liver size relative to increasing body weight during the final weeks of gestation. During the first weeks of life, considerable variability occurs in phenobarbital elimination as hepatic enzymes mature or as a result of enzyme induction from exposure to other drugs.[69] Phenobarbital clearance rapidly increases during the first 2 weeks of life, peaking between the ages of 6 and 12 months.

The IV loading dose of phenobarbital for neonatal seizures is 20 mg per kg.[70] The goal is a phenobarbital serum concentration of 15 to 40 µg per mL. Serum concentrations above 40 to 50 µg per mL may produce respiratory depression and coma, with 80 µg per mL associated with respiratory depression and death. There are reports of neonates tolerating phenobarbital serum concentrations of 60 to 80 µg per mL with respiratory support; however, bradycardia is frequently associated with serum concentrations greater than 50 µg per mL.

Additional doses of 5 to 10 mg per kg administered at 30-minute to 1-hour intervals may be required if seizures persist. Maintenance doses of 6 mg per kg per day are administered every 12 hours in divided doses. The long half-life of phenobarbital precludes need for continuous infusions. However, continuous administration of daily doses of 5 mg per kg per day or more cause phenobarbital accumulation during the first weeks of life; therefore, doses of 2 to 4 mg per kg per day may be more appropriate for neonates younger than 2 weeks.

Studies have demonstrated that infants may require up to 40 mg per kg total loading dose.[69,71] Effective seizure control has been related to phenobarbital dose, with 70% control with doses of 40 mg per kg.[70] Neonates receiving extracorporeal membrane oxygenation may require larger phenobarbital doses to achieve effective serum concentrations secondary to a larger V_d.[72]

Children aged 1 to 18 years usually require phenobarbital-loading doses of 10 to 20 mg per kg. The rate of administration is 2 mg per kg per minute for children weighing less than 40 kg and not more than 100 mg per minute for children weighing more than 40 kg; the rate is 60 mg per minute for adults. Maintenance doses are 3 to 5 mg per kg per day for children aged 1 to 15 years and 2 mg per kg per day for adults.

Therapeutic Drug Monitoring

An initial phenobarbital serum concentration may be drawn 2 to 3 hours after administration of a loading dose to verify serum concentration.[71] Secondary to a long half-life, steady-state serum concentrations may not be achieved for 2 to 4 weeks in neonates and infants. Serum concentration sampling may be repeated after 3 to 4 days of maintenance dosing to determine whether dose titration is needed; however, this does not reflect steady-state phenobarbital serum concentration. Steady-state serum concentration should be documented after 3 to 4 weeks of therapy. Indications for phenobarbital serum concentration sampling include loss of seizure control, possible toxicity, dosage changes, and addition or deletion of interacting agents.

Drug Interactions

Phenobarbital serum concentrations may be increased by VPA or, in some instances, phenytoin. Serum concentration monitoring of phenobarbital is indicated when potentially interacting agents are added to or removed from therapeutic regimens.[49]

ETHOSUXIMIDE

Indications and Clinical Use

Ethosuximide (2-ethyl-2-methyl succinimide) is a drug of choice for absence seizures.[13] However, this agent is ineffective for partial seizures or tonic–clonic seizures. In patients with tonic–clonic seizures, ethosuximide is administered in combination with wider spectrum AEDs such as phenobarbital or phenytoin for management of absence seizures to avoid exacerbating generalized tonic–clonic seizures. Overall, generalized tonic–clonic seizures were demonstrated to be rare in children with absence seizures receiving ethosuximide.[3,73] This retrospective study (n = 238) reported that children receiving valproate and ethosuximide monotherapy had the same low risk of generalized tonic–clonic seizures.[73] Prospective trials are necessary to further evaluate the role of ethosuximide in this seizure type. Dosage forms are 250-mg capsules (Zarontin) and 250 mg per 5 mL oral solution. The oral solution may contain sodium benzoate, which displaces bilirubin and is a metabolite of benzyl alcohol; therefore, use cautious monitoring if administering to neonates.

Initial pediatric ethosuximide dosing is 20 to 30 mg per kg per day.[74] To improve tolerance and avoid gastrointestinal adverse effects of nausea, vomiting, and diarrhea, it is best to administer one-third of the total daily dose after evening meal for 5 days, then administer one-third after lunch for 5 days, and finally add the remaining one-third after breakfast.[74] Side effects and adverse reactions include headaches, sedation, fatigue, insomnia, ataxia, or extrapyramidal reactions and rare reports of drug-induced lupus.[74] Behavioral effects may include anxiety, irritability, depression, hallucinations, and psychosis.

Mechanism of Action

Ethosuximide reduces low-threshold T-type calcium currents, blocking synchronized firing of pacemaker neurons responsible for generating an absence seizure. During a trial of Childhood Absence Epilepsy, the presence of genetic variants encoding T-type calcium channel subunits, *CACNA1H* missense variant (rs61734410/P640L), rather than a disease variant, was associated with ethosuximide nonresponse.[75]

Pharmacokinetics

Ethosuximide is rapidly absorbed and is not plasma protein bound.[76] Metabolism is hepatic hydroxylation to inactive metabolites, with 10% to 20% of dose excreted unchanged in the urine. Clearance is increased in children, with half-lives of 30 hours compared with 40 to 60 hours in adults. Steady-state serum concentrations are not achieved until 7 to 10 days.

Therapeutic Drug Monitoring

The therapeutic range for ethosuximide is 40 to 100 mg per L.[76] Recent recommendations updated the range to 39 to 99 mg per L.[77]. Wide variability due to apparent nonlinearity in the relationship between dose per kilogram and respective plasma concentration makes PK adjustment difficult. Serum ethosuximide concentrations can verify therapeutic range when initiating therapy, rule out toxicity, noncompliance, or identify high-dose requirements. Rare blood dyscrasias have been reported with ethosuximide use. Complete blood counts are often used in monitoring despite no evidence that this is sufficient to identify these serious reactions.

Drug Interactions

Numerous medications interact significantly with ethosuximide. For example, ethosuximide serum concentrations can be increased by CYP3A4 inhibitors and decreased by CYP3A4 inducers (e.g., rifampin, CBZ, phenytoin, phenobarbital), central nervous system (CNS) depressants, selective serotonin reuptake inhibitor (SSRI) antidepressants, and amphetamines may decrease ethosuximide effects.[76,78] Metabolism of ethosuximide is inhibited by VPA, which may provide a synergistic anticonvulsant effect.[78]

CARBAMAZEPINE

Indications and Clinical Use

CBZ an iminodibenzyl derivative (iminostilbene) with a tricyclic antidepressant structure, has been used in adults and children as anticonvulsant for over 30 years.[79] CBZ is a first-line treatment for partial motor, partial complex, and secondarily generalized tonic–clonic seizures. CBZ is not recommended for first-line management of primary generalized seizures due to possible seizure exacerbation.[80] Advantages over other older AEDs include less sedation and a mood stabilization effect.[81]

CBZ has been used for controlling neonatal seizures as primary or second- or third-line therapy after phenobarbital and phenytoin.[82,83] Loading doses of 10 mg per kg via nasogastric tube followed by maintenance doses of 7 to 23 mg per kg daily in two to three divided doses are reported to be safe and effective in neonates, including preterm infants (gestational age <30 weeks, weight <1,000 g). Apparent adequate absorption of CBZ occurs in the smallest, critically ill neonates. This agent offers another therapeutic option for the management of refractory neonatal seizures; however, this is limited by lack of a parenteral dosage form and low neonatal CYP3A4 activity.[82] Neonatal CBZ dosages are 5 to 20 mg per kg loading dose and 5 to 8 mg per kg given every 8 to 12 hours as maintenance.[82–84]

CBZ is available as an oral liquid suspension (Tegretol, 50 mg per mL), chewable tablets (Tegretol, 100 mg per mL), regular tablets (Tegretol and generic, 200 mg), sustained-release granules (Carbitrol, 200, 400 mg), and controlled-release formulation (Tegretol XR, 100, 200, 400 mg). Considerable variability exists in rate of absorption of generic CBZ formulations compared with Tegretol; therefore, change products with caution and close monitoring.[85]

Serious, although rare, aplastic anemia and agranulocytosis have been associated with CBZ therapy.[86] Leukopenia and thrombocytopenia may occur, requiring hematologic monitoring.[86] Rash; hypersensitivity reactions, including SJS; and TEN are possible.[29] CBZ is also associated with significant weight gain.[87]

CBZ clinical use in pediatric seizure management over the past 20 years has been decreasing in favor of utilizing oxcarbazepine (OXC) due to it having an overlapping mechanism of action but with less significant drug–drug interaction, lack of autoinduction, and more favorable side-effect profile.

Mechanism of Action

The mechanism of action for CBZ is similar to that of phenytoin, use-dependent blockade of voltage-sensitive sodium channels, resulting in neuronal membrane stabilization and inhibition of repetitive firing of neurons.[36] Anticonvulsant effects include presynaptic decrease in synaptic transmission and, possibly, potentiation of postsynaptic effects of GABA.

Pharmacokinetics

The primary elimination pathway of CBZ is metabolism via the CYP3A4 and CYP1A2/2C8 isozymes.[39] Half-lives of CBZ in adults are 12 to 17 hours, with shorter values in children and infants.[88] Neonates exposed to CBZ in utero have half-lives of 8.2 to 48.0 hours.[89] An active metabolite, CBZ-10,11-epoxide, is formed in a 0.1:0.2 ratio and is inactivated via epoxide hydrolysis.[39] CBZ induces its own metabolism (autoinduction) in a dose-dependent manner, resulting in decreased half-life and increased dose requirements several weeks after initiating or adjusting dosing.

Therapeutic Drug Monitoring

CBZ requires serum concentration monitoring for optimal therapeutic benefit because of interpatient variability in PK and narrow therapeutic range.[77] Serum *total CBZ* therapeutic range is 4 to 12 μg per mL, with toxic level greater than 15 μg per mL, and *free CBZ* therapeutic range is to 1 to 3 μg per mL with toxicity usually occurring at greater than 3.8 μg per mL.[77] Free CBZ is generally 8% to 35% of the total concentration.

Drug Interactions

CBZ is prone to interactions with other drugs metabolized by the CYP450 enzyme system.[49,51] Common drug interactions between CBZ and drugs used in the newborn include phenytoin (variable effect, phenytoin serum concentrations may increase, decrease, or remain unchanged, or CBZ concentrations may decrease) and phenobarbital (decreased CBZ serum concentrations).[51] As CBZ is approximately 75% bound to albumin (and CBZ-10,11-epoxide is ~50% albumin bound), there is potential for drug interactions involving binding.[88] Valproate will increase the unbound fraction of CBZ-10,11-epoxide, possibly resulting in increased neurotoxicity; however, this interaction may not be clinically significant.[49] Concomitant therapy with LEV may potentiate adverse CNS effects of CBZ.[90]

VALPROIC ACID AND SODIUM VALPROATE

Indications and Clinical Use

VPA is effective for many seizure types, including myoclonic, tonic, atonic, absence, generalized tonic–clonic seizures, and partial-onset seizures.[91,92] Many clinicians consider VPA to be the drug of choice for absence or atypical absence seizures.[93] VPA has been used in the management of neonatal seizures, usually as a second- or third-line alternative after failure with phenobarbital and phenytoin.[94,95] There is evidence that VPA may be effective for Lennox–Gastaut syndrome (LGS) and infantile spasms (IS).[96,97] VPA can be a management strategy for IS resistant to adrenocorticotropic hormone (ACTH), vigabatrin (VGB), or prednisone.[98]

VPA (2-propylvaleric dipropyl acetic acid), the free acid form of sodium valproate, has been approved for anticonvulsant use in the United States for over 40 years as oral and IV formulations.[99] The active form in plasma is the valproate ion; therefore, we will refer to all dosage forms as VPA.

Dosage forms are valproate sodium for IV injection, 100 mg (of VPA) per mL (Depacon), and valproate sodium oral solution (Depakene) 250 mg per 5 mL.[100] Other formulations are VPA liquid-filled capsules (Depakene) 250 mg; divalproex sodium capsules containing coated particles to mix with food (Depakote Sprinkle) 125 mg VPA equivalent; enteric-coated delayed-release tablets (Depakote) containing 125-, 250-, and 500-mg VPA equivalent; and extended-release tablets (Depakote ER) containing 250- and 500-mg VPA equivalent. Parenteral valproate sodium is indicated for situations when therapeutic serum concentrations need to be rapidly achieved, such as in status epilepticus, neonatal seizures, following surgery, or other illness when the patient cannot tolerate oral medications.

Initial oral doses of VPA are 20 to 30 mg per kg per day for premature infants, 40 mg per kg per day for term neonates younger than 10 days, and 50 mg per kg for infants older than 10 days. Initial doses in children are 10 to 20 mg per kg per day, but they may require 30 to 100 mg per kg per day to achieve adequate serum concentrations. For neonatal seizures, the oral dose is 20 mg per kg, followed by 10 mg per kg every 12 hours.[95]

Hepatotoxicity and embryotoxicity are associated with the active 4-ene VPA metabolite and have a *U.S. boxed warning.*[101–103] These serious adverse effects of VPA are more frequent in children younger than 2 years of age and those receiving anticonvulsant polytherapy.[104] Side effects frequently encountered during VPA therapy include weight gain, nausea, easy bruising secondary to thrombocytopenia, and tremor.[104] Weight gain secondary to VPA therapy is often a major concern among clinicians, parents, and patients.[105,106] A retrospective review of 94 patients aged 2 to 20 years taking VPA suggests children may be less likely to gain significant amounts of weight while taking this medication compared with adult patients.[106] The longer acting VPA preparations are associated with less weight gain when administered once daily.[107]

Mechanism of Action

The broad spectrum of anticonvulsant activity of VPA has not been fully elucidated. Mechanisms of action include (a) use-dependent blockade of voltage-sensitive sodium channels, resulting in neuronal membrane stabilization and inhibition of repetitive firing of neurons; (b) increased brain concentrations of GABA, possibly secondary to increased synthesis via glutamic acid decarboxylase; (c) increasing GABA concentrations by inhibition of GABA transporter GAT-1, therefore blocking conversion of GABA to succinic semialdehyde; and (d) increased membrane potassium conduction.[99]

Pharmacokinetics

The rate of gastric absorption of VPA is dose-form dependent; overall bioavailability is 80% to 90%.[76] Food slows down the rate, but not the extent of absorption. Peak serum VPA concentrations are achieved approximately 2 hours after oral administration of syrup or uncoated tablets, 3 to 5 hours after single-dose administration of the enteric-coated divalproex sodium tablet, and 7 to 13 hours after multiple dosing. VPA is highly plasma protein bound in a concentration-dependent manner, with the free fraction increasing with increasing serum concentration. Binding is reduced in renal or hepatic disease, uremia, or in the presence of other highly plasma protein–bound drugs.

VPA undergoes hepatic biotransformation via glucuronidation, β and ω oxidation, hydroxylation, ketone formation, and desaturation.[76] Glucuronidation with urinary excretion of the β glucuronide conjugate is the most important pathway. There are two metabolites with anticonvulsant activity, 2-ene VPA and 4-ene VPA.

Clearance of VPA follows first-order kinetics, with half-lives ranging from 5 to 20 hours in adults and 9 hours in adults receiving multiple AEDs.[76] Wide interpatient differences in clearance have been reported. Variables affecting VPA clearance include age, VPA serum concentration, treatment duration, dose, free fraction, and current enzyme-inducing AED polytherapy. Age is one of the most important variables affecting intrapatient variability of VPA elimination, and polytherapy has greatest effect on interpatient variability.[76,95] Premature newborns have the slowest clearance, but gestational age does not appear to influence clearance after 10 days of age. Neonates have VPA half-lives of 15 to 65 hours.[95] Clearance increases over the first months of life, with adult values achieved at around 14 years of age.

Therapeutic Drug Monitoring

TDM is of limited use for VPA therapy because of the wide therapeutic index, high intrapatient variability, poor correlation between clinical response and serum concentration, serum concentration-dependent binding, and short half-life.[77] The clinical effect of VPA can lag behind therapeutic concentrations. In addition, there is a nonlinear relationship between dose and plasma concentration. Thus, free serum concentrations can increase without increase in total concentration.

Serum monitoring of VPA concentrations can be valuable; however, it requires cautious interpretation. Therapeutic range is 40 to 100 µg per mL.[77] Toxicity usually occurs at serum concentrations more than 80 to 100 µg per mL, although some patients may tolerate VPA serum concentrations up to 150 µg per mL. Serum concentrations are drawn prior to the morning dose (trough concentration). Because of diurnal variation in VPA serum concentration, sampling times relative to dose administration must be consistent when comparing serum concentrations for useful interpretation.[77]

Drug Interactions

The metabolism of VPA is sensitive to enzyme induction and inhibits the metabolism of other drugs.[108] Therefore, patients receiving phenobarbital, CBZ, or primidone may have increased VPA dose requirements.[55] Doses of phenobarbital or primidone may need to be reduced by 20% to 40% when VPA is added to a regimen containing these agents. VPA also inhibits the metabolism of ethosuximide and lamotrigine.[49] Phenytoin serum concentrations may be decreased by adding VPA, or free fractions of phenytoin may be increased by binding displacement as described previously.[49] It is prudent to monitor serum concentrations of concomitantly administered anticonvulsants with clinical signs and symptoms of toxicity whenever VPA therapy is initiated or discontinued.

SECOND-GENERATION AGENTS

GABAPENTIN

Indications and Clinical Use

Gabapentin (GBP; Neurontin) is an amino acid analog of GABA developed during a search for a spasmolytic,[109] approved in the United States in 1994. Indications include add-on management of partial seizures with or without secondary generalization in adults and children aged 12 years and older and partial seizures in children aged 3 to 12 years.[110] GBP is not effective for myoclonic or absence seizures. GBP is also used for neuropathic pain management in children and adults.

Dosage forms of GBP (Neurontin; generic) are capsules 100, 300, and 400 mg; solution 250 mg per 5 mL; and tablets 100, 300, 400, 600, and 800 mg.[110] As of 2019, several states have classified GBP as a controlled substance or a monitored drug because of misuse primarily in combination with opioids predisposing to respiratory depression.[111] In December 2019, the FDA warned of possible serious breathing difficulties when gabapentinoids (GBP and pregabalin) are used by patients with preexisting respiratory risk factors.[112–114] Animal studies have demonstrated a respiratory depressant effect of GBP.[112] Overall, GBP is well tolerated, with frequent adverse effects consisting of somnolence, dizziness, ataxia, fatigue, tremor, and headache. In children aged 3 to 12 years, viral infection, fever, nausea, somnolence, and behavioral disturbances have been associated with GBP therapy.[115] Behavioral disturbances and exacerbation of preexisting conditions (developmental delays, attention deficit hyperactivity disorder) may be dose related.[116]

The regimen of GBP as an add-on therapy for managing partial seizures in adults and children older than 12 years is 900 to 1,800 mg daily, initiating with 300 mg three times daily. Some patients have tolerated daily GBP doses of 3,600 mg.[110] Discontinuation or addition of GBP to an established AED regimen should conducted over a minimum of 7 days to avoid withdrawal and allow tolerance to common sedating adverse effects.

The short half-life of GBP requires administering doses three times daily, not exceeding 12 hours between doses.[110] For children aged 3 to 4 years, 40 mg per kg daily administered in three divided doses is the usual recommendation, with therapy initiated at 10 to 15 mg per kg per day, increasing in weekly increments. Children aged 5 years and older usually require 25 to 35 mg per kg per day. Children aged 3 to 12 years have tolerated daily doses up to 50 mg per kg. There are no data on GBP dosing in premature infants.

Mechanism of Action

The exact mechanism of action for GBP is unknown. Contrary to the GABA-like structure, GBP is not a GABA mimetic. However, GBP modifies the synaptic or nonsynaptic release of GABA in the brain, as patients receiving GBP show increased concentrations of brain GABA.[117] GBP may modulate neurotransmission through binding with the α_2-δ voltage-dependent calcium subunit.[117] GBP decreases the glutamate release on reduced presynaptic entry on calcium via voltage-activated channels.

Pharmacokinetics

GBP demonstrates dose-related, saturable, oral bioavailability, which is not significant with the three-times-daily administration regimen at usual doses. Doses greater than 4,800 mg daily and four-times-daily dosing may increase bioavailability.[118] GBP is water soluble, widely distributed, and binds minimally (<3%) to plasma protein. GBP is not metabolized, therefore does not induce hepatic metabolism, and is primarily excreted unchanged by the kidneys. Clearance correlates with creatinine clearance (*CrCl*).[119] Half-life in adults with normal renal function is 5 to 7 hours. Higher clearances are observed in children younger than 5 years, with variable clearances in infants. Infants younger than 1 year may require up to 30% higher daily doses of GBP than older children. Guidelines for GBP dosage adjustment for patients with renal insufficiency are established.[110]

Therapeutic Drug Monitoring

Serum concentration monitoring is not routinely performed for GBP. Linear kinetics and clinical response suggest the therapeutic range is 2 to 20 μg per mL. Doses are adjusted on basis of clinical response and adverse effects.[77]

Drug Interactions

Significant drug interactions do not occur with GBP.[49] Aluminum hydroxide and magnesium salts reduce the oral bioavailability of GBP by 20% and, therefore, recommend separating doses of GBP and these agents by more than 2 hours.[51] The lack of effect on hepatic enzymes and protein binding enhance GBP's role as add-on therapy with other AEDs.[119]

OXCARBAZEPINE

Indications and Clinical Use

OXC was approved for use in the United States in 2000, but it was prescribed for decades in Denmark and European countries.[120] A review of European practice reveals OXC initial monotherapy as a treatment of choice for complex partial seizures in children.[121] Indications include monotherapy of partial seizures in children aged 4 years or older or as add-on therapy in partial seizures with or without secondary generalization for children aged 2 years or older with partial seizures.[9]

In a blinded, randomized, parallel-group study of infants and young children (1 month to <4 years of age, $n = 128$), with inadequately controlled partial seizures, OXC oral suspension was administered in low-dose (10 mg per kg per day) or high-dose (60 mg per kg per day) regimens as add-on therapy.[122] Overall, high-dose OXC was significantly ($p < 0.05$) more effective than low dose in controlling partial seizures as measured by during continuous video-EEG monitoring. Adverse effects associated with OXC treatment (>10% patients) were primarily mild somnolence and temperature elevation.

There are limited data on OXC in neonates, with exception of reports of OXC PK-PD in newborns acquiring the drug transplacentally.[123,124] Further investigation is needed to define the role and dosage of this agent in the management of seizures in the neonate and young infant.

Dosage forms are an oral suspension, Trileptal, 300 mg per 5 mL (of OXC), and 150-, 300-, and 600-mg tablets.[125] The oral tablets and suspension are interchangeable on a milligram-to-milligram equivalent basis. This is an important consideration when converting from one dosage form to another as a child matures and prefers a tablet form.

Oxtellar XR is the brand of extended-release OXC tablets recently approved in the United States (150-, 300-, and 600-mg strengths) for adjunctive and monotherapy for partial-onset seizures in adults and in children aged 6 to 17 years.[125]

Mechanism of Action

OXC (Trileptal) is the 10-ketocogener of CBZ and requires hepatic metabolism to 10-monohydroxy-carbamazepine, which is primarily responsible for its pharmacologic effects.[126]

OXC is a "cleaner" version of CBZ due to lack of autoinduction and less CNS and hematologic adverse effects.[127] However, there is an increased potential for hyponatremia with OXC compared with CBZ. This may be significant, as a serum sodium less than 125 mEq per L has been reported in 2.5% of patients receiving OXC.[128] Skin rashes and serious dermatologic manifestations, such as SJS and TEN, have developed during therapy with OXC.[129,130] Cross-reactivity with CBZ is possible; therefore, switching between these agents requires close monitoring in the event of a potential adverse reaction.[129]

Pharmacokinetics

Monohydroxy-CBZ is eliminated 96% by the kidneys.[126] There is a lower potential for drug interactions due to reduced plasma protein binding and less potent induction of hepatic enzymes as compared to CBZ.[126]

Therapeutic Drug Monitoring

Serum concentrations of the primary anticonvulsant metabolite of OXC, 10-monohydroxy-CBZ of 12 to 35 μg per mL, are clinically effective, with toxicity and side effects more common at greater than 35 mg per L.[77] Overall, TDM is useful for patients with conditions for reduced OXC clearance (renal insufficiency, pregnancy) and to verify drug–drug interactions.

Drug Interactions

As an inducer of hepatic microsomal enzymes, OXC is prone to drug interactions, although to a lesser extent than CBZ.[20,50] OXC may inhibit hepatic metabolism of phenytoin and phenobarbital, resulting in supratherapeutic concentrations of these agents.[131] When adding or removing OXC from a patient's drug regimen, recommend monitoring for potential drug–drug interactions.[132] Strong CYP3A4 inducers or UGT inducers (e.g., rifampin, CBZ, phenytoin, phenobarbital) may increase the metabolism of OXC requiring close monitoring and careful adjustment if these drugs are added or discontinued from the patient's regimen.[20,133] As with CBZ, OXC may decrease effectiveness of hormonal contraceptives, an important counseling point for adolescents and young adults.[50]

LAMOTRIGINE

Indications and Clinical Use

Lamotrigine, 3,5-diamino-6-(2,3-dichlorapenyl)-1,2,4-triazine, was FDA approved in 1994. This broad-spectrum AED is indicated as adjunctive therapy for management of partial seizures in adults and as monotherapy in patients converting from VPA or a hepatic enzyme-inducing AED (CBZ, phenytoin, phenobarbital, or primidone).[134] Lamotrigine is also effective as adjunctive therapy for generalized seizures in LGS in adults and children.[135]

Lamotrigine has become widely used in children for typical and atypical absence; atonic, myoclonic, and tonic seizures; Rett syndrome; and IS.[136] Advantages over CBZ and phenytoin include minimal cognitive side effects and improved behavior.[137]

Lamotrigine (Lamictal; generic) is available as oral tablets in 25-, 100-, 150-, and 200-mg forms. Chewable/dispersible tablets are available in 2-, 5-, and 25-mg strengths.[134] Dispersible tablets can be dissolved in a small amount of water or juice, by waiting 1 minute, swirling to disperse the drug, and immediately administering. Extemporaneous oral preparations of 1 mg per mL with short-term stability may be compounded from tablets by a pharmacist.[138]

Mechanism of Action

The complete mechanism of action for lamotrigine has not been fully described. The inhibition of voltage- and use-dependent sodium channels in a manner similar to CBZ and phenytoin does not explain the efficacy of lamotrigine in absence seizures or in other generalized seizures.[139] Proposed mechanisms of action include modulation of excitatory amino acid neurotransmission and voltage-activated Ca^{2+} channels.[134]

Pharmacokinetics

Lamotrigine is metabolized via glucuronidation to 2-*N*-glucuronide.[134] Average lamotrigine half-life in adults was 24.1 to 35 hours in patients receiving lamotrigine monotherapy and was decreased to 14 hours (6.4 to 32.2 hours) by concurrent treatment with enzyme-inducing AEDs.[140] Increased clearance of lamotrigine in infants younger than 2 months was reported by Mikati et al.[140] Age-related decreases in clearance occur during the first year of life.[141] Children aged 5 to 11 years have significantly longer lamotrigine half-lives than younger children; however, concurrent therapy with enzyme-inducing agents decreases apparent clearance of lamotrigine at any age. Considerable intraindividual variation in lamotrigine half-life occurs in all age groups.[142]

Concurrent VPA therapy may reduce clearance of lamotrigine by 40% to 60% via inhibition of glucuronidation independent of enzyme-inducing agents[143] and increases risk for lamotrigine rash.[144] Rash is the most severe adverse effect associated with lamotrigine therapy and is more frequent in children compared with adults. Rash usually occurs within the first 8 weeks of therapy and may progress to life-threatening SJS or TEN. The rash is considered to be a generalized hypersensitivity reaction, and risk may be minimized by slow dose titration during initiation of lamotrigine therapy. The estimated risk of developing a potentially life-threatening rash with lamotrigine is 1 in 1,000 for adults and from 1 in 100 to 1 in 200 for children.[144,145] The risk of rash is described in a U.S. boxed warning for lamotrigine.

Lamotrigine dosage depends on the patient's concomitant medications, such as VPA and the enzyme-inducing AEDs (phenytoin, phenobarbital, CBZ, or primidone).[145] Clinicians are advised to consult current package labeling and literature for stepwise dosing guidelines when initiating lamotrigine therapy for their patients.[141] Current recommendations include the following:

1. Patients older than 16 years receiving enzyme-inducing AEDs without VPA should receive 50 mg once daily for 2 weeks, increasing to 100 mg daily divided into two doses for 2 weeks, titrating by 100 mg daily every 1 to 2 weeks to an effective maintenance dose of 300 to 500 mg per day.
2. For patients taking VPA, the initial lamotrigine dose is 25 mg every other day for 2 weeks, then 25 mg daily for 2 weeks, then titrating upward by 25 to 50 mg daily every 1 to 2 weeks until effective response is achieved (usually 100 to 150 mg per day in two divided doses).
3. For children aged 2 to 12 years receiving enzyme-inducing AEDs without VPA, the regimen is 0.6 mg per kg per day in two divided doses, increasing by 1.2 mg per kg per day every 1 to 2 weeks to effective response, usually at 5 to 15 mg per kg per day. Younger children may require three daily doses due to increased apparent clearances.
4. For children aged 2 to 12 years receiving VPA, the regimen is 0.2 per mg per kg per day for 2 weeks, increasing to 0.5 mg per kg per day and 1 mg per kg per day at 2-week intervals (maximum recommended dose of 5 mg per kg per day). Because of tablet size, dose should be rounded down to the nearest whole tablet size.
5. Limited experience exists with lamotrigine dosing in the newborn; however, doses of 2 to 10 mg per kg per day have been used in infants ranging in age from 2 weeks to 1 year for the management of intractable partial seizures (IS and/or partial seizures).[146]

Therapeutic Drug Monitoring

Serum lamotrigine concentrations are not routinely monitored due to lack of reliable concentration response data. Reported serum concentrations associated with efficacy are 2 to 4 μg per mL and 1 to 5 μg per mL.[77] A suggested reference range is 3 to 15 μg per mL, with higher rate of mild-to-moderate toxicities occurring at greater than 15 μg per mL.[147] Some patients achieve effective seizure control without adverse effects at these concentrations, underscoring need for individual therapeutic target concentrations.

Drug Interactions

Patients taking lamotrigine should be instructed to inform all clinicians involved in their care when adding or stopping medications as this agent participates in many drug interactions, especially with oral contraceptives.[50] Lamotrigine may cause photosensitivity reactions; therefore, it is imperative to instruct the patient about the use of physical sunscreen protection methods and sunblock.[148]

FELBAMATE

Indications and Clinical Use

Felbamate, a derivative of the sedative meprobamate, was approved in the United States in 1993 for partial seizures, with or without secondary generalization, in adults and in children with LGS.[149,150] This agent has demonstrated effectiveness in treatment of refractory IS.[151] Felbamate is administered orally as Felbatol suspension 600 mg per 5 mL and scored tablets 400 and 600 mg.[152]

Felbamate use is limited only to cases of severe seizures refractory to alternative AEDs due to severe toxicities of aplastic anemia and acute hepatic failure.[153] Risk of aplastic anemia with felbamate is estimated to be 1 in 2,000 with female gender, age greater than 17 years, prior AED hypersensitivity, AED polytherapy, and prior immune disease or cytopenia as risk factors.[153,154]

Dosage recommendations for felbamate in children aged 2 to 14 years are 15 mg per kg per day in three to four divided doses, increasing at weekly intervals to a maximum of 45 mg per kg per day in divided doses or 3,600 mg per day whichever is less.[152] For children older than 14 years and adults, initial dose is 1.2 g daily in divided doses, increasing in 1.2 g daily increments at weekly intervals to a maximum daily dose of 3.6 g in three to four divided doses. Data are limited on use of felbamate in children younger than 2 years.

Monitoring for toxicities consists of complete blood cell count with differential, platelet count, and hepatic function tests at baseline and regularly during therapy and immediately after discontinuation.[155] Patients and caregivers must receive self-monitoring instruction for signs and symptoms of rash, bruising, bleeding, sore throat, yellow tinged skin, gastrointestinal symptoms, unusual fatigue, loss of appetite, and dark urine. Instruct patient to contact their physician immediately if these signs of possible felbamate toxicity occur.

Mechanism of Action

Proposed mechanisms of action for felbamate are via *N*-methyl-D-aspartate receptor antagonism at glycine-binding sites and, possibly, a direct effect on ion channels.[156]

Pharmacokinetics

The primary route of elimination is hepatic hydroxylation (<20%) via CYP3A4/2E1, 10% glucuronidation, and 25% hydrolysis, with approximately 50% eliminated unchanged in the urine.[141] A reactive metabolite, atropaldehyde, may be related to cytotoxicity.[153] Felbamate clearance is inversely correlated with age; therefore, children (half-life 16 hours) require higher doses per kilogram compared with adults (half-life 16 to 23 hours).[141]

Therapeutic Drug Monitoring

Serum felbamate monitoring has not been established for routine use.[141] Dose is titrated to clinical efficacy; however, the International League Against Epilepsy (ILAE) reference range is 30 to 60 µg per mL.[77,157] Concentrations greater than 60 µg per mL are associated not only with better therapeutic response but also with significantly higher incidence of adverse effects.[158]

Drug Interactions

As felbamate participates in some clinically important interactions with other AEDs, it is imperative to review the patient's medications prior to prescribing.[159] Caution must be used when adding felbamate to regimens of enzyme-inducing AEDs, in which case doses of the other agents must be decreased by 20% to 30% to prevent related toxicities.[55] For example, felbamate increases serum concentrations of phenytoin in a dose-dependent manner; therefore, recommend decrease phenytoin dosage by 20% to 30% when adding felbamate to the regimen.[132] Effectiveness of oral contraceptives may be decreased via induction of metabolism by felbamate.[160]

TOPIRAMATE

Indications and Clinical Use

TPM was approved in 1996 as initial monotherapy for primary generalized tonic–clonic seizures or partial-onset seizures in children aged 10 years or older through adulthood. TPM is used as adjunctive treatment of primary generalized tonic–clonic seizures or partial-onset seizures in children aged 2 to 16 years and in adults.[9,135,161] TPM is considered first-line therapy in myoclonic and generalized tonic–clonic seizures after VPA and first-line monotherapy in symptomatic generalized tonic–clonic seizures in healthy infants. Efficacy has been demonstrated in LGS in combination with other AEDs in children and adults and for IS.[98,135]

Formulations of TPM are Topamax Sprinkle capsules 15 and 25 mg, and tablets 25, 50, 100, and 200 mg.[162] Generic formulations are available at a lower cost. Newer extended release formulations are Qudexy XR 25-mg sprinkle capsules and Trokendi XR 50-mg tablets. An extemporaneous TPM oral 6 mg per mL suspension can be prepared using 100-mg tablets.[163] In late 2019, a commercially available oral suspension received FDA approval replacing the compounded formulation.[162]

The use of TPM is limited primarily by CNS-related adverse effects.[164] A slower initial dose titration schedule improves tolerability and reduces likelihood of discontinuation. Initial TPM dosage as add-on therapy for partial seizures with or without secondary generalization, primary generalized tonic–clonic seizures, or seizures associated with LGS in children aged 2 to 16 years is 5 to 9 mg per kg per day in two divided doses (initial dose should be 25 mg or less, using a range of 1 to 3 mg per kg per day) administered at night for 1 week.[162] On the basis of clinical response and tolerability, dose is increased every 1 to 2 weeks by 1 to 3 mg per kg in two divided doses. Initial daily doses of 0.5 to 1 mg per kg may be followed by increases of 0.5 to 1 mg weekly or 1 to 3 mg every other week. Young children (<5 years of age) may require daily doses of 15 to 20 mg per kg, and infants may require up to 30 mg per kg per day divided into three daily doses. The usual adult (17 years and older) dose for TPM is 400 mg daily divided into two daily doses.[162]

Frequent adverse effects associated with TPM are somnolence, fatigue, concentration difficulty, word-finding disturbance, nervousness, headache, ataxia, and anorexia, with or without weight loss. Somnolence and fatigue occur early in therapy and affect up to 30% of patients receiving TPM, particularly at higher doses. Weight loss associated with appetite decrease may be a concern for young children undergoing rapid growth and development. Language problems, speech disorders, and aggressive behavior have been reported.[165]

An increased incidence of nephrolithiasis, metabolic acidosis,[166] and acute myopia associated with secondary angle-closure glaucoma was reported in children and adults receiving TPM.[167] The ocular syndrome usually develops within 1 month of initiating TPM therapy with symptoms of a sudden decrease in visual acuity with or without eye pain. Risk factors for metabolic acidosis and nephrolithiasis are concomitant use of another carbonic anhydrase inhibitor and co-treatment with the ketogenic diet. Maintenance of adequate fluid intake and acid–base monitoring are recommended for patients receiving TPM. Serum bicarbonate concentrations should be obtained at baseline prior to initiation of therapy and periodically throughout treatment to detect hyperchloremic metabolic acidosis prior to signs and symptoms of hyperventilation, arrhythmias, fatigue, and altered consciousness.

Oligohydrosis and hyperthermia have been observed in patients, primarily children, during TPM therapy.[168,169] Cases were associated with warm environments and/or vigorous activity. The mechanism for this adverse effect is unknown.

Mechanism of Action

TPM, 2,3:4,5-bis-*O*-(1-methylethylidene)-(β)-D-fructopyranose sulfamate, was originally synthesized during an effort to develop a gluconeogenesis-blocking agent.[170,171] TPM has several mechanisms of anticonvulsant activity: (a) blockade of neuronal membrane sodium channels, (b) enhancement of GABA inhibition via modulation of a nonbenzodiazepine-type receptor, (c) blockade of kainate-evoked currents at the glutamate receptor, and (d) selective inhibition of central carbonic anhydrase isozymes II and IV.[172] This AED is also a weak carbonic anhydrase inhibitor.

Pharmacokinetics

The primary route of elimination for TPM is renal, with minimal hepatic oxidation via CYP3A. In absence of hepatic enzyme induction, 50% to 80% of a dose is excreted unchanged in the urine.[172] Age significantly correlates with TPM clearance.[173] Mean elimination half-life is 19 to 23 hours in adults and 15.4 hours in children, and TPM serum concentrations are usually 33% lower in children than in adults. In the presence of concomitant therapy with enzyme-inducing AEDs, TPM clearance is increased, and half-life is reduced to 12 to 15 hours in adults and 7.5 hours in children. There are limited data on the clearance of TPM in the newborn. Infants receiving TPM therapy for management of refractory IS demonstrated slightly higher mean clearances than children and adolescents.[174]

Therapeutic Drug Monitoring

TDM of TPM is not routinely performed secondary to wide interpatient variability in dose–serum concentration relationship, and overlap of serum concentrations related to toxicity and nonresponse. The reference serum concentration range is 2 to 10 μg per mL, which reflects 80% of patients receiving maintenance steady-state therapy.[77]

Drug Interactions

When combined with phenytoin, CBZ, phenobarbital, and OXC, TPM serum concentrations are significantly lower compared with TPM monotherapy.[49] VPA and lamotrigine have no significant effect on TPM metabolism.[132] TPM may decrease the effectiveness of hormonal contraceptives, reducing serum concentrations of ethinylestradiol by up to 50%.[50] As with other AEDs, caution and a careful review of the patient's current medications is warranted when prescribing or discontinuing TPM from a therapeutic regimen.

LEVETIRACETAM

Indications and Clinical Use

LEV (Keppra; generic), (*S*)-α-ethyl-2-oxo-1-pyrrolidine acetamide, was approved in 1999 as add-on therapy for partial-onset seizures in adult and adolescents (16 years and older).[175–177] LEV is used as an alternative to phenobarbital for neonatal seizures.[178] Dosage forms are scored tablets (Keppra); 250-, 500-, 750-, or 1,000-mg tablets; oral solution 100 mg per mL, or solution for IV infusion 100 mg per mL.[179] The parenteral form must be diluted with 100 mL of an appropriate IV solution prior to injection and administered via *IV infusion* only, *not direct IV or intramuscular injection.*

The dose of LEV for adolescents aged 16 years and older and adults as adjunct therapy for management of partial seizures is 500 mg twice daily, increasing by 1,000 mg daily at weekly intervals based on response, to a maximum of 3,000 mg daily.[179] Data on LEV dosage for younger children and infants are limited.[180,181] Daily doses of 20 and 60 mg per kg have been reported in children.[179,182] Initial doses are 10 to 15 mg per kg per day in two divided doses, increasing by 10 to 20 mg per kg per day every 1 to 2 weeks to effective response, or a maximum dose of 60 mg per kg per day. A rapid titration schedule over a mean period of 10 days in a small number of patients (n = 8) has been used.[183] Dosage must be adjusted in renal insufficiency.[142]

LEV was administered in doses of 8 to 10 mg per day to children (n = 200), aged 0.3 to 19 years (median age 9 years), for intractable epilepsy.[180] A small (n = 28) retrospective study of children younger than 2 years (mean age 12.5 months, range 2 weeks to 22 months) showed that LEV was associated with seizure reduction in 54% of patients. Efficacy was highest in patients with generalized epilepsy compared with focal epilepsy. Overall adverse events were minimal.[181]

Adverse effects with LEV therapy are dose related and include somnolence, fatigue, ataxia, headache, and behavioral changes (agitation, hostility, aggression, irritability).[176] Overall, adverse effects associated with LEV have been mild to moderate, dose related, and primarily occur within the first month of therapy.[184,185]

Behavioral effects including depression, emotional liability, nervousness, and agitation usually appear within the first months of therapy.[184] Cases of suicidal ideation and rage reactions have been reported in adolescents and young adults taking LEV.[186]

Mechanism of Action

The mechanism of action for LEV may be counteraction of kindling acquisition evoked by $GABA_A$-receptor antagonism.[187] LEV binds to synaptic vesicle protein, affecting neuronal GABA and glycine-gated currents, as well as voltage-dependent potassium currents.[182]

Pharmacokinetics

Oral absorption of LEV is rapid and complete. LEV undergoes minimal metabolism, with approximately 24% undergoing hydrolysis of the acetamide group to an inactive carboxylic acid metabolite, independent of CYP450 isozymes.[182] Plasma protein binding is only 10%, and as a low-affinity substrate for inhibitor of isozymes, significant drug interactions are rare.[20,188] The remainder of the dose is excreted unchanged in the urine. PK is linear, with apparent clearance correlating with glomerular filtration. The half-life of LEV in adults is 7 to 8 hours, compared with 6 hours in children. Children may require higher LEV doses on a milligram per kilogram per day basis compared with adults.[182] Increased renal clearance for LEV in children compared with adults has been documented.[182]

Therapeutic Drug Monitoring

The role of TDM for LEV therapy is not well established. A therapeutic range of 5 to 41 µg per mL is used in Norway, which is lower than previously published ILAE range of 12 to 46 µg per mL, which was based on highest doses from a retrospective database.[77]

Drug Interactions

LEV may increase adverse effects of CBZ or TPM requiring a dosage reduction in these drugs.[49]

PREGABALIN

Indications and Clinical Use

Pregabalin (Lyrica; generic) was the first AED with controlled substance status (Schedule V) in the United States related to side effects of euphoria and somnolence.[189] Pregabalin is approved as adjunctive therapy in patients aged 1 month and older for partial-onset seizures.[190,191] Pregabalin is available as 25-, 50-, 75-, 100-, 150-, 200-, 225-, and 300-mg capsules and 20 mg per mL oral solution.[192]

Pregabalin dosage regimens for adjunctive therapy for partial-onset seizures in patients aged 1 month and older are established[192]:

1. *Patients aged greater than 1 month and weighing less than 30 kg:* Initiate 3.5 mg per kg per day divided in two to three doses; titrate weekly based on response and tolerability to 14 mg per kg per day. For aged 1 month to 4 years, administer in three daily doses.
2. *Patients aged greater than 1 month and weighing greater than 30 kg:* Initiate 2.5 mg per kg per day divided in two to three doses; titrate weekly based on response and tolerability to 10 mg per kg per day (maximum daily dose 600 mg per day).
3. Adult patients: Initiate 150 mg per day given in two to three divided doses; titrate weekly based on clinical response and tolerability to a maximum dose of 600 mg per day.
4. Dosage adjustments for renal insufficiency: *CrCl* less than or equal to 60 mL per minute are available.[192]

A small (n = 19) open-label study in children aged 4 to 15 years with resistant seizures used 150 to 300 mg per day with good results and minimal adverse effects.[190] Common adverse effects were somnolence, weight gain, and worsening of myoclonic seizures. Pregabalin is approved for neuropathic pain in adults and is used off-label in children for this indication.[193]

Mechanism of Action

Pregabalin is similar to GBP as it is a structural, not a functional, analog of the neurotransmitter GABA.[194] Pregabalin is a specific ligand that potently binds to the α2-δ type 1 and 2 subunits, a protein associated with voltage-gated calcium channels in the CNS. This agent is hydrophilic but readily crosses the blood–brain barrier, decreasing depolarization-induced calcium influx in nerve terminals. The reduction in the inward calcium currents reduces the release of glutamate, noradrenaline, and substance P in the brain. Although structurally related to GABA, pregabalin does not affect GABA uptake or degradation and is not active at $GABA_A$- and $GABA_B$-receptor sites.[190,194]

Pharmacokinetics

Absorption from the gut is rapid, with approximately 90% bioavailability and peak plasma concentration is achieved in 1 hour.[190] Elimination follows linear PK. Half-life ranges from 5.8 to 6.3 hours. Pregabalin undergoes minimal hepatic metabolism (<2%) and is not protein bound. Similar to GBP, approximately 98% of pregabalin is eliminated unchanged through renal excretion and requires dosage adjustment for renal insufficiency. Pregabalin does not induce or inhibit hepatic enzyme activity.

Therapeutic Drug Monitoring

Anticonvulsant therapeutic ranges for pregabalin of 2.8 to 8.3 µg per mL are established; however due to variability in correlation of response for a wide range of patients, serum concentrations are not routinely monitored.[77] Role of TDM is limited to patients with renal failure or verification of adherence.

Drug Interactions

Pregabalin and AED combinations are generally well tolerated and may be used concomitantly with VPA, lamotrigine, phenytoin, TPM, and CBZ without concern for drug–drug interactions because of minimal pregabalin metabolism and lack of protein binding.[49,159] The 2019 FDA warning regarding respiratory depression risk of gabapentinoids in patients with respiratory conditions and in combination with opioids includes pregabalin.[113] PD interactions include additive effects on cognitive and gross motor function with concomitant use of pregabalin with benzodiazepines, alcohol, and opioids.[195]

Indications and Clinical Use

Tiagabine (TIG; Gabitril; generic), a GABA reuptake inhibitor, was approved in 1997 for adjunctive treatment of partial seizures in adolescents and adults.[196,197] Efficacy was demonstrated in young children with refractory complex partial seizures, with poor response reported for myoclonic seizures and IS.[198] There is insufficient evidence to recommend TIG as first-line therapy for partial seizures in pediatric patients. Formulations of TIG (Gabitril) are 2-, 4-, 12-, and 16-mg tablets. Extemporaneously prepared oral solutions can be compounded for young children unable to swallow tablets.[199]

The adult regimen of TIG for adjunctive therapy with enzyme-inducing AEDs in the management of partial seizures is 4 mg once daily for the first week, increased by 4 to 8 mg (administered as two to four daily doses) at weekly intervals to reach a daily dose of 32 to 56 mg.[196] For adolescents aged 12 to 18 years, initial TIG dosing is 4 mg once daily for the first week of therapy, followed by 4 mg twice daily, increasing by 4 to 8 mg daily (in two to four divided doses) weekly, until a maximum daily dose is reached if necessary. TIG dose needs to be reduced in hepatic insufficiency, but there are no data on specific recommendations. Dose-related adverse effects of TIG are dizziness, difficulty with concentration, irritability, and paresthesia.[200] Moderately severe to incapacitating generalized weakness may occur, resolving after dose reduction or discontinuation of TIG. Less common are ataxia and depression. Overall, TIG has been well tolerated in children.

Mechanism of Action

TIG preferentially inhibits GABA transporter isoform-1 (GAT-1) in neurons and glia and increases extracellular GABA concentrations in the forebrain and hippocampus, thus prolonging inhibitory effects on receptors of postsynaptic cells.[201]

Pharmacokinetics

TIG is highly (96%) plasma protein bound and undergoes extensive metabolism via CYP3A4 isozymes, with less than 2% of a dose is excreted unchanged in the urine.[202] TIG does not appear to induce or inhibit hepatic microsomal enzymes; however, concomitant therapy with enzyme-inducing AEDs will decrease its elimination half-life from 7 to 9 hours to 4 to 7 hours.[55] In children aged 3 to 10 years, TIG half-life is 3 hours with concomitant enzyme-inducing AED therapy.[203] Dosage does not need to be adjusted in renal impairment; however, hepatic impairment requires lower doses administered at longer intervals as clearance of unbound drug may be decreased by as much as 60%.

Therapeutic Drug Monitoring

TDM is useful for TIG because of the drug's high protein binding and variable PK.[77] The anticonvulsant reference range is 0.02 to 0.2 μg per mL.[77]

Drug Interactions

Clinically important drug interactions with TIG increase dose requirements secondary to increased clearance with concomitant therapy with enzyme-inducing AEDs.[20,204] Concomitant therapy with CBZ, phenytoin, primidone, and phenobarbital may increase TIG clearance up to 60%. TIG dose reductions may be necessary when the concomitant AED is discontinued or dose is decreased. Because macrolides are inhibitors of CYP3A4, concomitant therapy with erythromycin, troleandomycin, or clarithromycin may increase TIG plasma concentrations. Displacement from plasma proteins of TIG by other highly bound agents such as VPA, salicylates, and naproxen can result in increased free TIG concentrations.[205]

ZONISAMIDE

Indications and Clinical Use

Zonisamide (ZNS) was approved in the United States in 2000 for adjunctive therapy in the management of partial-onset epilepsy in patients aged 16 years and older.[206] Presently, ZNS lacks an indication for general pediatric use in the United States, although the drug was available in Japan and South Korea since 1989 as Excegran.[207] A sulfonamide derivative, ZNS is contraindicated in patients with sulfonamide hypersensitivity.[208] Dosage forms are Zonegran capsules 100 mg (United States) and Excegran tablets 100 mg, 200 mg per g powder formulation (Japan).[209]

Clinical experience and open-label trials suggest efficacy in children with partial- and generalized-onset epilepsies, IS, and West syndrome.[98,210–212] In a randomized multicenter trial of pediatric patients with newly diagnosed epilepsy, low-dose (3 to 4 mg per kg per day) versus high-dose (6 to 8 mg per kg per day) ZNS was evaluated.[213] Of the 90 of 125 patients who completed the trial, 49 of 65 were enrolled in the low-dose group, and 41 of 60 were enrolled in the high-dose group. The seizure free rate at 6 months was reported to be 63.1% (41/65) in the low-dose group and 57.6% (34/60) in the high-dose group.[213] In practice, ZNS is used off-label as adjunctive therapy for many types of intractable seizures, including primary generalized epilepsy.[213]

Initial ZNS dose for adults and adolescents older than 16 years as adjunctive therapy for partial seizures is 100 mg daily, increasing after 2 weeks to 200 mg daily for 2 weeks.[214] ZNS may be administered as a single-daily dose secondary to a long half-life. Dose may be further increased to 300 and 400 mg daily at 2-week intervals, allowing serum concentrations to reach steady state at each dose level. Because of long half-life (63 hours), steady state may not be achieved for 2 to 3 weeks. Increasing the ZNS dose at 3-week intervals may allow for improved tolerance of drug-related drowsiness, headache, or mental slowing. Usual adult dose range is 100 to 600 mg daily, with increased adverse effects at doses above 300 mg daily. Doses may be given with or without food.

ZNS dosing for infants and children is 1 to 2 mg per kg per day administered in two to three divided doses, increasing on response and tolerance of adverse effects by increments of 1 to 2 mg per kg per day every 2 weeks to a maximum of 12 mg per kg per day or total maximum dose of 1 g per day.[215] Effective dose ranges are reported to be 2 to 12 mg per kg per day. Low-dose ZNS monotherapy (3 to 5 mg per kg per day) was reported to be effective and well tolerated in infants with IS.[216] Dosage reduction is indicated in renal and hepatic disease.[216] ZNS should not be used in patients with *CrCl* less than 50 mL per minute.

Mechanism of Action

The anticonvulsant action of ZNS (Zonegran), 1,2-benzisoxazole-3-methanesulfonamide, involves blocking of sodium channel recovery and T-type calcium channel currents and binding to GABA-receptor chloride channels. Inhibition of dopamine turnover and increased dopamine synthesis may contribute to anticonvulsant activity.[217] ZNS, like TPM, is a weak inhibitor of carbonic anhydrase, predisposing to oligohydrosis.[215,218]

Oligohydrosis and hyperthermia, similar to effects with TPM, have been reported in children receiving ZNS therapy.[218] Cases of ZNS-associated oligohydrosis and/or fever, the majority in children, have been reported in the United States.[218] Parents and caregivers must be instructed to maintain adequate hydration and avoid overheated conditions for children receiving ZNS, particularly in hot climates or during warm weather. However, in comparison with other newer AEDs, ZNS appears to be well tolerated. Clinical trials comparing ZNS to other AEDs in children and infants are needed.

Adverse effects associated with ZNS include fatigue, somnolence, dizziness, ataxia, headache, nystagmus, paresthesia, confusion, difficulty concentrating, impaired memory, mental slowing, loss of spontaneity, agitation, irritability, depression, anorexia, diarrhea, abdominal pain, anorexia, and rash.[207,219] Mania in children and psychosis in adults have been associated with ZNS.[220] The true incidence of adverse effects related to ZNS monotherapy is difficult to ascertain because this drug is frequently administered with other AEDs. Postmarketing surveillance in Japan showed that children less than 12 years of age had a significantly lower rate of adverse effects than adults (24.3% vs. 40.1%).[221,222]

Pharmacokinetics

ZNS is well absorbed after oral administration with 85% bioavailability and has been administered as a rectal suppository.[207] Approximately 40% to 60% is plasma protein bound. Similar to other sulfonamide derivatives, ZNS demonstrates saturable binding to erythrocytes, achieving concentrations two to eight times higher than in plasma.

Metabolism involves hepatic acetylation to *N*-acetyl ZNS and reduction primarily via CYP3A4 to inactive 2-sulfamoylacetyl phenol and subsequent glucuronide formation. Approximately 15% of a dose is eliminated unchanged in the urine. Elimination half-life is 24 to 60 hours. Clearance of ZNS is linear and follows first-order kinetics in children at daily doses greater than 10 mg per kg.[207] A meta-analysis from Japan suggests increased clearance in children compared with adults.[223]

Therapeutic Drug Monitoring

Overall, TDM is useful for ZNS as efficacy is associated with serum concentrations of 10 to 40 μg per mL.[77] Adverse CNS effects are more frequent at serum concentrations greater than 30 μg per mL.

Drug Interactions

ZNS does not appear to inhibit P450 isoenzymes and has no significant effect on steady-state serum concentrations of phenytoin, VPA, phenobarbital, or CBZ. However, ZNS inhibits metabolism of CBZ to 10,11-epoxide.[224] Metabolism of ZNS is subject to induction by other AEDs.[224] Plasma concentrations of ZNS may be decreased by phenytoin, phenobarbital, and CBZ, possibly increasing ZNS dose requirements. Use caution when adding or removing ZNS from a patient's regimen.

THIRD-GENERATION AGENTS

BRIVARACETAM

Indications and Clinical Use

BRV (Briviact), the *n*-propyl analog of LEV, received initial FDA approval in 2016 for adjunctive management of partial-onset (focal) seizures in patients aged 16 years and older.[225] BRV is a Schedule V–controlled substance due to CNS effects. During the next 3 years, international indications expanded to include patients aged 1 month and older (adjunctive therapy for focal seizures). Additional indications include adjunctive therapy of idiopathic generalized seizures (ages 12 years and older) and monotherapy for focal seizures.[226] Dosage forms are tablets (10, 25, 50, 75, and 100 mg), an oral solution 10 mg per mL, and an IV injection 50 mg per 5 mL.[227] All dosage forms of BRV may be used interchangeably because of high oral bioavailability. BRV may be taken with or without food.

There is a paucity of controlled trials comparing BRV and LEV. A meta-analysis of randomized controlled trials with LEV and BRV (n = 1,876 patients) concluded that LEV had slightly higher efficacy and a lower incidence of dizziness compared with BRV.[228] Patients with previous LEV exposure had less than or equal to 50% response to BRV. There is no additional therapeutic benefit to concurrent administration of LEV and BRV.[229] Therefore, BRV has restricted or criteria monitored status on many health system and insurer formularies secondary to high cost and lack of evidence regarding benefit over LEV.

No dosage adjustment is needed for impaired renal function does not require dose adjustments of BRV, and dosage recommendations are lacking for end-stage renal disease with dialysis.[230,231] For patients with any stage of hepatic impairment, the recommended initial BRV dose is 25 mg twice daily with a maximum of 75 mg twice daily.[230,232]

Mechanism of Action

BRV acts as a selective, high-affinity ligand for synaptic vesicle protein 2A (SV2A), a glycoprotein involved in modulation of synaptic vesicle exocytosis and neurotransmitter release.[233] SV2A protein deficiency predisposes to seizure activity. BRV has a 15- to 30-fold higher affinity than LEV, the first AED with SV2A activity. These drugs may bind or interact at different SV2A protein sites. BRV appears to produce a frequency-dependent decrease of synaptic transmission at 100-fold concentrations than LEV.[234]

Pharmacokinetics

BRV demonstrates linear and time-independent PK at therapeutic doses.[235,236] Absorption is nearly complete after oral administration, with minimal plasma protein binding. V_d is 0.5 L per kg, with rapid distribution and absorption into majority of tissues. The amide moiety of the drug is hydrolyzed via hepatic (CYP2C19) and extrahepatic amidase to a carboxylic acid metabolite.[235,237] Polymorphisms of CYP2C19 may decrease production of the metabolite.[238] Patients who are poor CYP2C19 metabolizers or those taking concurrent CYP2C19 inhibitors may require a reduced BRV dose. BRV is excreted in the urine within 72 hours of administration.[239]

Therapeutic Drug Monitoring

A steady-state reference range established for BRV is 0.2 to 2 mg per L.[157] The role of TDM for BRV is currently limited to patients receiving enzyme-inducing medications and to verify adherence.

Drug Interactions

Rifampin with the potential for CYP2C19 induction decreases BRV plasma concentrations, causing increased BRV dose requirements (consider doubling the dose) in patients receiving concomitant treatment.[240] Administration with CBZ may increase exposure to its active metabolite, carbamazepine-epoxide. No safety concerns in patients receiving concomitant treatment with CBZ have been documented, the CBZ may need to be reduced if tolerability issues arise during therapy. Because BRV may increase the phenytoin plasma concentrations, monitor phenytoin serum concentrations when adding or removing BRV from phenytoin therapy.[240]

VIGABATRIN

Indications and Clinical Use

VGB (Sabril; generic), a structural GABA analog, has efficacy in adults and children as adjunctive therapy for the management of refractory partial seizures, with or without generalization, and as monotherapy for the treatment of IS.[198,241] VGB appears to be very effective in reducing seizures caused by tuberous sclerosis.[198] VGB may be used as monotherapy for IS for infants aged 1 month to 2 years. It may also be used as combination therapy for refractory partial complex seizures in patients aged 10 years and older.

VGB exacerbates typical absence and myoclonic seizures; therefore, it should not be used for idiopathic generalized seizures.[242] Experience with VGB in treating LGS is limited, particularly in cases with predominately myoclonic type seizures. VGB has been used in many countries since 1989, but was approved in the United States in 2009.[243]

VGB is administered as the racemic mixture, although only the *S*(+)-enantiomer is active. Dosage formulations of VGB are 500-mg tablets and 500-mg powder sachets for dissolution in 10 mL of water, juice, milk, or infant formula.[243]

Peripheral visual field defects are found to occur in up to 40% of patients receiving VGB.[244] Since 1997 when visual field defects from VGB exposure were published, observational studies have investigated the prevalence.[245,246] VGB affects vision by causing permanent bilateral concentric visual field constriction, including tunnel vision.[247] Ophthalmic evaluation is recommended prior to initiating VGB due to risk of peripheral visual field deficit and irreversible vision loss.[248] Guidelines for visual screening for VGB adverse effects are included in the VGB risk evaluation and mitigation strategy (REMS).[243] Ophthalmic evaluation can be challenging for young children and infants. For certification in the REMS, prescribers must agree to ensure conducting periodic visual monitoring as described in the VGB labeling.[243]

Adverse effects of VGB are fatigue, somnolence, dizziness, blurred vision, nystagmus, ataxia, weight gain, abdominal pain, diarrhea, depression, mania, and psychosis.[249] Infants and young children may also exhibit hypotonia or hypertonia, hyperexcitability, and insomnia. Intramyelinic edema was reported in postmortem examination of infants being treated for IS with VGB, resulting in 2019 warning in the package labeling.[243]

Initial VGB dosing for children with refractory epilepsy is 40 mg per day administered in one or two doses, titrating, based on response, to 100 mg per kg per day.[243] Efficacy in children is similar to that observed in adults. For infants with IS, initial dose of VGB is 50 to 100 mg per kg per day, administered in two divided doses, titrating up to 150 mg per kg per day. VGB doses of up to 400 mg per kg daily have been reported.[250] Variable efficacy has been reported in studies comparing VGB and ACTH for IS; however, VGB is better tolerated than ACTH.[251,252]

The initial adult daily dose of VGB is 1,000 mg divided in one to two doses, increasing by 250- to 500-mg increments weekly to total daily dose of 2,000 to 4,000 mg.[243] Slow titration may improve tolerance of somnolence and mood effects. Considerable variation in response has been demonstrated with some patients between doses of 1 and 4 g. A ceiling effect and tachyphylaxis may also occur.[253] Responses from placebo-controlled clinical trials of VGB 2 and 3 g daily as add-on therapy in adults with refractory partial seizures demonstrated a 50% or greater reduction in seizure frequency.[254] VGB is not effective as monotherapy in adults.

Petroff and Rothman, using magnetic resonance spectroscopy, measured the increase in GABA associated with VGB in the human brain and cerebrospinal fluid.[255] A plateau in GABA concentrations was achieved with a daily VGB dose of 3,000 mg. This dose–response curve demonstrates there is no need to increase VGB dose above 3,000 mg daily. Doses of up to 6,000 mg daily have been used; however, higher doses may be associated with more adverse effects without therapeutic benefit.

Mechanism of Action

As with TIG, VGB exerts anticonvulsive activity by decreasing the inactivation of GABA. VGB increases brain concentrations of GABA by acting as a surrogate substrate for GABA-transaminase (GABA-T).[256] VGB binds irreversibly to GABA-T, permanently inactivating the enzyme. Upon withdrawal of VGB, normal GABA-T activity takes several days to be restored. A ceiling effect demonstrated with VGB dosing beyond which there is no more therapeutic effect, only more adverse effects may be related to a negative feedback inhibition of GABA synthesis, secondary to high GABA concentrations. Therefore, PD effect does not correlate with VGB half-life.

Pharmacokinetics

VGB is primarily eliminated via the kidneys, with up to 70% of drug eliminated unchanged in the urine. Elimination half-life for adults is 5 to 7 hours, and oral absorption is rapid and complete, with minimal plasma protein binding. VGB does not appear to induce CYP450 enzymes, but concomitant therapy with enzyme-inducing agents decreases its elimination half-life.[257] There have been no significant differences in PK parameters of the biologically active enantiomer between young children

(5 months to 2 years) and older children (4 to 14 years), and therefore a weight-based dose adjustment is not recommended for these age ranges.[258]

Therapeutic Drug Monitoring

Because VGB acts as an irreversible inactivator of GABA-T, there is no correlation with plasma/serum concentrations and drug at the site of action. A wide range of trough serum/plasma concentrations of 0.8 to 36 μg per mL is associated with effective VGB treatment; therefore, TDM may be limited to excluding toxicity, malabsorption, or nonadherence in specific cases.[77]

Drug Interactions

Drug interactions with VGB include an increased clearance of phenytoin.[205,259] When VGB is added to a regimen with phenytoin, monitoring of patient response and serum concentrations of the other AED is recommended.

LACOSAMIDE

Indications and Clinical Use

Lacosamide (Vimpat) was approved in the United States in 2008 as add-on treatment for partial seizures in adults.[260] The indication was expanded in 2017 to include treatment of partial-onset seizures in children aged 4 years and older as monotherapy or add-on therapy.[261] Lacosamide is used off-label for refractory seizures in children.[262,263] Data from lacosamide use in infants are accumulating; however, controlled clinical trials are needed. Data from head to head with lacosamide and other newer AEDs are needed for pediatric patients. No clear advantage of lacosamide over LEV has been observed.[13]

Lacosamide (Vimpat) is available in 20 mg per mL IV solution, tablets (50, 100, 150, and 200 mg), and oral solution (10 mg per mL), with a generic formulation targeted for 2022.[264] Dosage formulations may contain propylene glycol which can induce metabolic acidosis in neonates. Secondary to high oral bioavailability, there is no advantage to using the IV lacosamide in patients with intact oral routes.[265]

Lacosamide dosing by age and indication is as follows[264]:

1. Infants aged 6 months and older and adolescents aged 17 years and younger for severe refractory seizures: Oral: 1 to 2 mg per kg per day divided twice daily (maximum initial dose 50 mg per day), titrate weekly by 1 mg per kg per day based on response and tolerability.[266]
2. Pediatric patients aged 4 years and older and weighing 11 to less than 30 kg for partial-onset seizures: 2 mg per kg per day divided twice daily; increase by 2 mg per kg per day every week to a maintenance of 4 to 8 mg per kg per day divided twice daily.
3. Pediatric patients aged 4 years and older and weighing 30 to less than 50 kg for partial-onset seizures: 2 mg per kg per day divided twice daily; increase by 2 mg per kg per day every week to a maintenance of 6 to 12 mg per kg per day divided twice daily.
4. Pediatric patients weighing greater than or equal to 50 kg for partial-onset seizures: 50 mg twice daily; increase by 100 mg per day given twice daily every week to a maintenance of 300 to 400 mg per day (monotherapy) or 200 to 400 mg per day (adjunctive therapy).
5. Adult patients: 100 mg twice daily (monotherapy); increase by 100 mg per day weekly to a maintenance of 300 to 400 mg per day (adjunctive therapy) or 200 to 400 mg per day. Alternate initial regimen: Loading dose 200 mg followed 12 hours later by 100 mg twice daily.[267]

Patients already receiving a single AED and converting to lacosamide monotherapy should not have the concomitant AED withdrawn until taking the therapeutic lacosamide dosage for at least 3 days. Withdrawal of concomitant AED over at least 6 weeks is recommended.

Side effects include dizziness, headache, double vision, ataxia, multiorgan hypersensitivity reaction, PR interval prolongation, and heart block. Euphoria associated with lacosamide administration designated its Schedule V–controlled substance status in the United States. A caution for pediatric use of lacosamide has been made as possible adverse neurodevelopmental effects secondary to interference with CRMP-2 protein, and neuronal differentiation has been postulated.[268,269]

Mechanism of Action

Lacosamide's anticonvulsant effect involves interaction with slow sodium channel inactivation without affecting fast inactivation.[267] In contrast to AEDs, such as phenytoin and lamotrigine that block sodium channels when activated, lacosamide facilitates slow inactivation of sodium channels in terms of kinetics and voltage dependency.[267] The effect may be selective for those neurons participating in seizure activity. Repeatedly depolarized neurons have persistent sodium activity, which promotes neuronal excitation.

Pharmacokinetics

Lacosamide is completely absorbed after oral administration, with minimal first-pass effect giving approximately 100% absolute bioavailability, unaffected by food.[261] The V_d is approximately 0.6 L per kg, and the drug is less than 15% bound to plasma proteins. PK is predictable across all ages and is cleared almost equally by the liver and kidney. The major metabolite (*O*-desmethyl-lacosamide) formed by CYP3A4, CYP2C9, and CYP2C19 is inactive. The elimination half-life of unchanged drug is approximately 13 hours and unaffected by dose, multiple dosing, or IV administration. Moderate hepatic impairment (Child-Pugh B) resulted in approximately 50% to 60% higher lacosamide area under the curve (*AUC*) compared to healthy volunteers.

Therapeutic Drug Monitoring

A lacosamide therapeutic serum concentration ranging from 3 to 10 μg per mL was developed from studies in Italy ($n = 75$) and Norway ($n = 344$).[77,270] TDM has low utility for lacosamide, except in patients with severe hepatic and/or renal failure.

Drug Interactions

Drug interactions to date include drugs that prolong the PR interval, such as calcium channel blockers and β-blockers causing bradycardia.[267,268] Clinically significant drug–drug interactions involving lacosamide are uncommon; however, potential exists because of weak inhibition of CYP2C19, CYP2C9, and CYP3A4. Because lacosamide is a substrate of CYP3A4, CYP2C9, and

CYP2C19, patients with renal or hepatic impairment who are taking strong inhibitors of these isoenzymes may have increased lacosamide concentrations. Population lacosamide PK from patients with partial-onset seizures showed a 15% to 20% decrease in lacosamide plasma concentrations when administered with CBZ, phenobarbital or fosphenytoin, and phenytoin.[267]

RUFINAMIDE

Indications and Clinical Use

Rufinamide (Banzel), a triazole derivative (1-[2,6-difluorobenzyl]-1H-1,2,3-triazole-4-carboxamide), received FDA approval in 2008 for adjunctive treatment of seizures associated with LGS in patients aged 1 year and older.[271] Dosage forms are 200- and 400-mg tablets, and an oral suspension (contains propylene glycol) 40 mg per mL. A generic product is expected to be marketed in 2022.

Approval was based on the results of a single, multicenter, double-blind study of 138 male and females with refractory seizures between the ages of 4 and 30 years, which compared rufinamide with placebo.[272] Study patients had 90 or more seizures per months while receiving three AEDs, and severity of seizures decreased in 53.4% of patients.

In a 2009 study aimed to explore the effectiveness and tolerability of rufinamide in 45 children and 15 adults (age range 1 to 50 years), the highest response rate was observed in patients with LGS (54.8%), while the lowest was observed in patients with partial epilepsy (23.5%). Rufinamide was well tolerated, with most frequently occurring adverse events being fatigue (18.3%), vomiting (13.3%), and loss of appetite (10.0%).[272]

Risk of adverse effects with rufinamide is concentration related[273] and includes shortening of the QT interval and CNS-related adverse effects (ataxia, dizziness, gait disturbance). A serious, potentially fatal multiorgan hypersensitivity reaction (drug rash with eosinophilia and systemic symptoms [DRESS] syndrome), including severe hepatitis, has been reported in children under 12 years of age during first 4 weeks of rufinamide therapy.[274]

Rufinamide doses for children aged 1 year and older: 10 mg per kg per day by mouth divided twice daily, increasing 10 mg per kg per day every other day to a maximum dose of 45 mg per kg per day.[275] *Adult rufinamide dose:* 400 to 800 mg by mouth per day in two equally divided doses, increasing every other day by 400 to 800 mg to a daily maximum dose of 3,200 mg. Overall, rufinamide provides an additional AED option for add-on therapy in refractory condition and is easily titrated with manageable drug–drug interactions; however, it may be expensive than other comparable AEDs as there is currently no generic product.

Mechanism of Action

Rufinamide exhibits its anticonvulsant effects through limiting neuronal sodium-dependent action potential firing. The drug may prolong the recovery phase of the inactivated neuronal sodium channel and exert a membrane stabilizing effect.[276]

Pharmacokinetics

Rufinamide is well absorbed, greater than 85%, and, in the lower dosage range, is better absorbed in the fed state, doses should be administered with food. Rufinamide is not a CYP450 substrate but is extensively metabolized by the liver through hydrolysis by carboxylesterases to carboxylic acid derivative (pharmacologically inactive), which is then excreted in the urine. Impaired renal function does not affect rufinamide PK.[277,278] Steady-state serum concentrations are achieved in 2 days, which is consistent with the elimination half-life of 6 to 10 hours.[278] Plasma protein binding of rufinamide is minimal, with apparent V_d and apparent oral clearance related to body surface area. Population modeling shows a positive correlation between a reduction in seizure frequency and steady-state plasma rufinamide concentrations using data from placebo-controlled trials. In the absence of interacting concomitant medication, population PK modeling indicates the oral clearance of rufinamide may be higher in children than in adults.[278]

Therapeutic Drug Monitoring

Serum rufinamide concentrations can help guide clinical decision-making for a given patient as population PK studies show a positive correlation between reduction in seizure numbers and plasma rufinamide concentrations.[270] Rufinamide concentrations of up to 50 µg per mL may be required for LGS, which is higher than most patients achieve in practice. The mean plasma rufinamide concentration to reduce seizure frequency by 25% or 50% was predicted to be 15 and 30 µg per mL, respectively.[270] A range of 4 to 31 µg per mL correlates well with seizure control.[77,270] Monitoring serum concentrations can be helpful in patients taking concomitant liver enzyme inducers or undergoing hemodialysis.

Drug Interactions

A general precaution is electrocardiogram (ECG) monitoring with drugs that prolong the QT interval. There are no known significant drug interactions involving rufinamide with requiring avoiding concomitant use; therefore, rufinamide dosage modification may be required when administered with select AEDs.[278] Rufinamide is a weak inhibitor of CYP2E1, causing additive sedation and CNS depression when administered with alcohol. Rufinamide is a mild inducer of CYP3A4; however, drug interactions are not entirely explained by CYP isoenzymes.[278] Because rufinamide is metabolized by carboxylesterases, drugs that induce carboxylesterase activity may increase rufinamide clearance. Broad-spectrum inducers, such as CBZ and phenobarbital, may have minor effects on rufinamide metabolism via this mechanism. Drugs that inhibit carboxylesterases may decrease metabolism of rufinamide.

Population PK modeling suggests that rufinamide does not alter the oral clearance of TPM or VPA, but may increase the oral clearance of CBZ and lamotrigine with small decreases (<20%) in the clearance of phenobarbital and phenytoin.[273] With the exception of phenytoin, in which a dosage reduction may be required with concomitant rufinamide, adjustment in the other AEDs described earlier appears unnecessary. Lamotrigine, TPM, or benzodiazepines do not affect rufinamide PK based on population-based PK modeling.

However, VPA may *increase* plasma rufinamide concentrations up to 70%.[275] Patients stabilized rufinamide before being started on VPA should begin VPA therapy at a lower dose. Similarly, patients on VPA should begin at a rufinamide dose lower than 10 mg per kg per day (pediatric patients) or 400 mg per day (adults).[275] Conversely, concomitant use of CBZ, VGB, phenytoin, phenobarbital, and primidone was associated with a −13.7% to −46.3% range decrease in plasma rufinamide concentrations. The minimum of 13.7% decrease was seen in female children co-medicated with VGB, and the maximum of 46.3% decrease was seen in female adults who were concomitantly taking phenytoin, phenobarbital, or primidone.[273]

CLOBAZAM

Indications and Clinical Use

CLB (Onfi, Sympazan, Frisium; generic) is a benzodiazepine, Schedule IV–controlled substance, with a slightly different chemical structure, associated with less sedation.[279] Strong anticonvulsant properties were discovered during its use as an anxiolytic in Europe since 1975. CLB was finally FDA approved in 2011 for LGS in patients aged 2 years and older.[280] Off-label use includes monotherapy and adjunctive treatment for refractory epilepsy and anxiety. Dosage forms are Onfi 10- and 20-mg tablets and a 2.5 mg per mL oral suspension (contains propylene glycol); Sympazan, 5, 10, and 20 mg soluble oral filmstrip.[281]

Adverse effects of CLB are generally mild and usually disappear with time or dosage reduction.[280,282] Adverse effects most frequently reported include drowsiness, dizziness, ataxia, drooling, restlessness, and aggressive behavior. Paradoxical or aggressive behavior can be precipitated by CLB therapy, particularly in children and adolescents with psychiatric conditions. As expected with benzodiazepines, monitor for dose-related sedation with high doses and avoid acute withdrawal to avoid seizures.

A *serious adverse effect of CLB is rare cases of SJS and TEN, primarily in combination with other AED medications lamotrigine and VPA.*[283,284] A Medication Guide describes FDA warnings and precautions on risk of serious skin reactions occurring at any time during treatment, but are more likely within the first 2 months of therapy, or when CLB is discontinued and restarted.[285] Patients and caregivers must be cautioned to seek immediate medical treatment if rash, blistering, skin peeling, hives, or mouth sores occur while taking CLB.[286]

The long-term safety and efficacy of CLB for pediatric patients with LGS, a chronic condition requiring lifelong treatment, is supported by randomized clinical trials[287] and a 6-year open-label study.[288] The majority of patients in the CLB extension study (n = 267, mean age 11.3 years) did not show tolerance to antiepileptic effects over 5 years of treatment.[287] The adjunctive CLB mean modal daily dose, 0.90 mg per kg per day at year 1 and 0.97 mg per kg per day at year 5, sustained seizure free and substantial seizure improvements. Median percentage decrease from baseline in average weekly rate of drop seizures (85% to 91%) was maintained through year 5. There was an 85% reduction in median percentage decrease in total seizures from baseline. Patients reaching year 5 maintained reduction in total seizures. Adverse events were experienced by 60% of patients, most frequently upper respiratory tract infection (28%) and pyrexia (19%), which were attributed to the long study duration in a primarily pediatric population.

CLB oral dosing for LGS[289]:

1. *Patients aged 2 years and older and adolescents weighing less than or equal to 30 kg:* Initial 5 mg once daily for at least a week, then increase to 5 mg twice daily for 1 week, then increase to 10 mg twice daily thereafter, maximum daily dose is 20 mg.
2. *Patients aged 2 years and older and adolescents weighing greater than or equal to 30 kg:* Initial 5 mg once daily for at least a week, then increase to 10 mg twice daily for 1 week, then increase to 20 mg twice daily thereafter, maximum daily dose is 40 mg.
3. *Dosage adjustment in renal failure: CrCl* less than 30 mL per minute, use with caution, no data available.
4. *Dosage adjustment in hepatic failure undergoes extensive hepatic metabolism, Child-Pugh score 5 to 9:*
   a. *Patients aged 2 years and older and adolescents weighing less than or equal to 30 kg:* Initial 5 mg once daily for at least a week, then increase to 5 mg twice daily for 1 week, then increase to 10 mg twice daily thereafter, maximum daily dose is 20 mg.
   b. *Patients aged 2 years and older and adolescents weighing greater than or equal to 30 kg:* Initial 5 mg once daily for at least a week, then increase to 10 mg twice daily for 1 week, then increase to 20 mg twice daily thereafter, maximum daily dose is 40 mg.

Mechanism of Action

CLB, 1,5-benzodiazepine, modulates GABAergic neurotransmission by positive allosteric modulation of $GABA_A$ receptors and increases expression of transporters for both GABA and glutamate.[290] The active metabolite *n*-desmethylclobazam (*n*-DCLB; norclobazam) also modulates $GABA_A$ receptors, contributing to seizure control.

Pharmacokinetics

Oral absorption of CLB is rapid and complete and not affected by food or crushing the tablets, with a high bioavailability (87%).[291] CLB is lipophilic, distributing throughout the body, and is moderately plasma protein bound (80%). The drug undergoes extensive hepatic metabolism primarily by CYP3A4, CYP2C19, and CYP2B6, with renal excretion of metabolites. Active metabolite concentrations can be three to five times higher in poor CYP2C19 metabolizers compared with extensive metabolizers, requiring CLB dosage adjustment.

Therapeutic Drug Monitoring

Reference ranges (0.03 to 0.3 mg per L) for the parent drug CLB and for the active metabolite DCLB (0.3 to 3 mg per L) are established.[77] Analysis of DCLB metabolite is useful due to more changes in concentration than the parent drug and, at steady state, can indicate genetic mutations in CYP2C19.[292] Steady-state serum DCLB/CLB ratio greater than 25 in the absence of inhibitors can be useful to identify poor CYP2C19 metabolizers. The CLB concentration-to-dose ratio can measure CYP3A4 activity, contributing to CLB clearance. The (CLB + DCLB)/dose ratio is a good indicator of CLB clearance.[291]

Drug Interactions

The majority of CLB drug–drug interactions have been documented in small numbers of patients, primarily adults; therefore, vigilant monitoring is recommended when CLB is added to drug regimens for young children and adolescents. Significant drug–drug interactions with CLB and drugs metabolized by

CYP3A4, CYP2C19, CYP1A2, or CYP2D6 are possible.[293] Drugs inhibiting CYP3A4 (e.g., ketoconazole-strong inhibitor) or CYP2C19 (e.g., omeprazole-moderate inhibitor) have potential to decrease the clearance of CLB and NCLB.[294] Closely observe patients receiving strong or moderate CYP2C19 inhibitors with CLB for signs and symptoms of CLB toxicity. Concurrent use of CLB and CBD (a CYP3A4 and CYP2C19 inhibitor) is common in LGS and Dravet syndrome and should be closely monitored (discussed further under "Cannabidiol Oral Solution" section). Phenytoin toxicity was reported when CLB was added to the regimen and saturated CYP2C19 metabolism, decreasing phenytoin clearance.[293] Concomitant use of CLB with drugs metabolized by CYP2D6 (e.g., oxycodone, STP, serotonin reuptake inhibitors) may require dosage adjustment. Concomitant administration of benzodiazepines with opioids and/or alcohol has an increased risk of respiratory depression.[295]

Add CLB with caution to regimens containing VPA or lamotrigine and monitor serum concentrations.[296] Increased serum concentrations of VPA and lamotrigine by CLB may risk development of SJS.[284] Inform patient and caregivers of the increased risk of SJS/TEN when CLB is combined with VPA and lamotrigine.

ESLICARBAZEPINE ACETATE

Indications and Clinical Use

ESL (Aptiom, Stedesa, United States; Zebinix, Exalief, Europe), a dibenzazepine related to CBZ and OXC, approval was expanded in 2017 for monotherapy or adjunctive management of partial-onset seizures in patients aged 4 years and older.[297] ESL was FDA approved for adults in 2013. Pediatric approval was obtained on data extrapolation from multicenter, randomized controlled efficacy and safety trials in adults.[298] Dosage forms are 200-, 400-, 600-, and 800-mg tablets, no generic formulations are available in the United States.[297]

ESL provides a once-daily option for partial-onset seizures that has been effective and well tolerated in clinical trials.[297] Efficacy outcomes showed benefit of treatment, with 10% of patients remaining seizure free and 46% of patients experiencing greater than or equal to 50% reduction from baseline in standardized seizure frequency during monotherapy trial periods. ESL monotherapy was well tolerated, most treatment-emergent adverse events were mild to moderate and consistent with adjunctive therapy.

Common adverse effects (i.e., >10%) of ESL include dizziness, somnolence, nausea, headache, and diplopia. The drug is contraindicated in patients with hypersensitivity or adverse reactions to OXC. Severe reactions include allergic reactions, such as angioedema and bronchospasm, and severe skin reactions including SJS and TEN. ESL can also induce clinically significant hyponatremia (sodium < 125 mEq per L) similar to CBZ and OXC. Patients with hypersensitivity or adverse reactions to these AEDs should not receive ESL therapy because of cross-reactivity.[299,300]

Dosage regimens for children aged 4 to 17 years are based on body weight and administered orally once daily, increased at weekly intervals to maximum ranges[301]:

1. 11 to 21 kg: Initial daily dose: 200 mg; maintenance daily dose: 400 to 600 mg
2. 22 to 31 kg: Initial daily dose: 300 mg; maintenance daily dose: 500 to 800 mg
3. 32 to 38 kg: Initial daily dose: 300 mg; maintenance daily dose: 600 to 900 mg
4. Greater than 38 kg: Initial daily dose: 400 mg; maintenance daily dose: 800 to 1,200 mg

Reduce initial and maintenance ESL dosages by 50% in patients with moderate and severe renal impairment (*CrCl* < 50 mL per minute). Use is not recommended in severe hepatic impairment as data are lacking.[301]

Mechanism of Action

The primary anticonvulsant mechanism of action for eslicarbazepine is blocking the voltage-gated sodium channel.[302]

Pharmacokinetics

ESL is an oral prodrug that is rapidly and extensively metabolized by the liver via a hydrolytic first-pass metabolism into S-licarbazepine, the major active metabolite of OXC, the biologically active drug with peak plasma concentrations reached at 1 to 4 hours postdose.[303] The drug demonstrates linear and dose-proportional kinetics, with half-life of 13 to 20 hours (adult data).

Therapeutic Drug Monitoring

A trough steady-state serum concentration range for eslicarbazepine of 3 to 26 mg per L was determined based on PK/PD modeling.[77]

Drug Interactions

Eslicarbazepine has an overall favorable drug–drug interaction profile because of low protein binding and minimal effects on cytochrome P450 enzymes.[303] ESL may inhibit CYP2C19, increasing plasma concentrations of phenytoin, CLB, omeprazole, and other drugs metabolized by CYP2C19.[20] ESL is a CYP3A4 inducer, potentially decreasing plasma concentrations of drugs metabolized by this isoenzyme. Concurrent use of ESL and ethinylestradiol and levonorgestrel is associated with lower plasma concentrations of these oral contraceptive hormones.

PERAMPANEL

Indications and Clinical Use

Perampanel (Fycompa) is FDA approved for monotherapy and adjunctive therapy for partial-onset seizures, with or without secondarily generalized seizures, in children aged 4 years and older.[304] This AED may be used as adjunctive therapy to treat primary generalized tonic–clonic seizures in children aged 12 years and older.[305] Perampanel may be useful in refractory partial-onset seizures, but less effective for drug-resistant patients.[306]

Fycompa is available as 2-, 4-, 6-, 8-, 10-, and 12-mg tablets and an oral suspension 0.5 mg per 1 mL and is a Schedule III–controlled substance because of potential for misuse and dependence.[307] Perampanel may benefit from formulary monitoring criteria to ensure appropriate use and titration in view of potential side effects and high cost. No generic currently is available in the United States.

Dosage recommendations[307]: Initial oral dose of perampanel for adults and for children aged 4 years and older with partial-onset or primary generalized tonic–clonic seizures and *not receiving* an enzyme-inducing AED is 2 mg daily at bedtime, titrating by 2 mg daily at weekly intervals. Recommended maintenance dosage range is 8 to 12 mg daily for partial-onset seizures (without enzyme-inducing AEDs) and for primary generalized tonic–clonic seizures is 8 mg at bedtime.

If the patient is *concomitantly taking an enzyme-inducer* (e.g., phenytoin, CBZ, OXC), the recommended initial perampanel oral dose is 4 mg once a day at bedtime, titrating by 2 mg daily at weekly intervals. Dose requirements are individualized upon patient's clinical response and tolerability. The maximum daily recommended perampanel dose is 12 mg at bedtime irrespective of concomitant medications.

For patients with mild-to-moderate hepatic impairment, start perampanel at 2 mg daily, then titrate by no more than 2 mg every 2 weeks to a maximum of 4 to 6 mg daily. The manufacturer does not recommend using in severe hepatic impairment. No specific recommendations are available for perampanel dosing in patients with moderate renal impairment other than close monitoring and slower dosage increases. Avoid use in severe renal impairment or ongoing hemodialysis.[307]

Mechanism of Action

Perampanel (2-[2-oxo-1-phenyl-5-pyridin-2-yl-1,2 dihydropyridin-3-yl]benzonitrile hydrate) is a noncompetitive selective antagonist at the postsynaptic ionotropic α-amino-3-hydroxy-5-methyl-4-isoxazolepropionic acid (AMPA) glutamate receptor.[304] Antagonizing AMPA receptors may reduce overstimulation and inhibit seizure generation and spread while preventing neuronal death. This mechanism of action is similar to TPM; however, perampanel may be preferred for patients with a history of renal stones, narrow angle glaucoma, or metabolic acidosis.

Pharmacokinetics

Oral administration is rapid and complete with minimal first-pass metabolism. Food delays time to reach peak concentration, but not the extent of absorption.[308] Plasma protein binding is approximately 95%. Metabolism is by CYP3A4/5, CYP1A2, and CYP2B6 followed by glucuronidation. Approximately 30% and 70% of metabolites are eliminated via the urine and feces, respectively.[308] Half-life is approximately 105 hours in the absence of concomitant enzyme-inducing drugs; therefore, steady-state serum concentrations will not be achieved for up to 30 days.[309] Long half-life is useful in that a missed dose will not affect the steady-state perampanel serum concentration. Age does not appear to affect clearance rates.

Therapeutic Drug Monitoring

A serum concentration reference range of 0.1 to 1 mg per L is used for perampanel, pending increased clinical data.[77]

Drug Interactions

Perampanel doses of 12 mg per day reduce levonorgestrel serum concentrations by 40%, decreasing effectiveness of these contraceptives.[20,310] CYP3A4 enzyme inducers (e.g., CBZ, phenytoin, OXC) can decrease serum perampanel concentrations by 67%.[310] Close monitoring and careful adjustment of perampanel dosage is needed when giving the drug concomitantly with a CYP3A4 enzyme-inducing agent.

STIRIPENTOL

Indications and Clinical Use

STP (Diacomit), an aromatic allylic alcohol, first demonstrated anticonvulsant effectiveness in the 1970s and received Orphan Drug status in 2008.[311] In 2018, STP was approved for seizures associated with Dravet syndrome in patients aged 2 years and older who are taking CLB.[312] There is no evidence supporting STP monotherapy for Dravet syndrome seizures. STP is available as oral 250- and 500-mg capsules and as oral suspension powder packets of 250 and 500 mg.

Oral dosage of STP is 50 mg per kg per day, given in two or three divided doses, given during a meal, gradually reducing dose or discontinuing the drug. Maximum recommended total dose is 3,000 mg per day.[312] There are limited data on STP dosage adjustments for moderate-to-severe hepatic and renal impairment, and extreme caution is advised as the drug undergoes extensive hepatic metabolism and renal elimination.[188]

Adverse effects observed in greater than or equal to 10% patients during STP therapy are sedation, decreased appetite, agitation, ataxia, weight loss, hypotonia, nausea, tremor, dysarthria, and insomnia.[313] As with other AEDs, risks include suicidality, agitation, new or worsening depression, aggression, and panic attacks. Significant declines in neutrophil and platelet counts may occur, requiring hematologic monitoring at baseline and every 6 months during STP therapy.[313]

Two multicenter, placebo-controlled, double-blind randomized studies demonstrated effectiveness of STP for Dravet syndrome seizures.[314] Response rate was significantly greater for STP compared with placebo in both studies. STP was superior in reducing mean frequency of generalized clonic or tonic–clonic seizures, with 43% and 25% of patients reporting no generalized clonic or tonic–clonic seizures during the study, with greatest benefit in seizure reduction in children starting STP before 15 years of age.

A longitudinal study (n = 40) reported children who started STP before the age of 15 years. Participants were followed until a median age of 23 years (18 to 40 years) and were receiving concomitant CLB (n = 40), VPA (n = 39), and TPM (n = 21).[315] At study end, no patients had episodes of status epilepticus despite continuing generalized tonic–clonic seizures.

Mechanism of Action

STP is an allosteric modulator of the $GABA_A$ receptor.[316] Direct anticonvulsant activity is via enhancement of inhibitory, GABAergic neurotransmission. STP increases activity of neuronal and recombinant $GABA_A$ receptors. At recombinant receptors, STP acts through a unique site in a subunit-dependent manner. Positive modulation by STP was most effective at $GABA_A$ receptors containing α3 subunits. Expression of α3 subunits is developmentally regulated, and highest in the immature brain, accounting for greater clinical efficacy of STP in childhood-onset seizures, such as Dravet syndrome.

Pharmacokinetics

After oral administration, peak STP serum concentrations are achieved in 2 to 3 hours (median). The drug is 99% protein bound and undergoes dose dependent, nonlinear saturation kinetics.[316] Elimination half-life of STP ranges from 4.5 to 13 hours, with metabolism by CYP1A2, CYP2C19, and CYP3A4 isoenzymes. In children (median age 7.3 years) with Dravet syndrome treated with STP, VPA, and CLB, apparent clearance and V_d of STP were related to weight, with elimination half-life of 8.5 and 23.5 hours for patients weighing 10 and 60 kg, respectively.[317]

Therapeutic Drug Monitoring

A serum concentration range for STP supported by clinical data is 4 to 22 mg per L.[77]

Drug Interactions

STP is a potent cytochrome P450 inhibitor, which decreases metabolism, and increasing serum concentrations of drugs such as CLB increased concentrations twofold and the active norclobazam metabolite fivefold, requiring a CLB dosage reduction if adverse effects develop.[318] Various drug interactions between STP and CYP1A2, CYP2B6, CYP3A4, CYP2C8, CYP2C19 (diazepam, clopidogrel), P-glycoprotein (CBZ), and breast cancer resistance protein (BCRP) substrate medications (methotrexate, prazosin, glyburide) are possible.[319]

CANNABIDIOL ORAL SOLUTION

Indications and Clinical Use

CBD oral solution (Epidiolex), the nonpsychoactive ingredient in cannabis, was FDA approved in 2018 for treating seizures associated with LGS or Dravet syndrome in patients aged 2 years and older.[320,321] Epidiolex is a highly purified prescription CBD 100 mg per mL oral solution in 100 mL bottles. This product was given the least restrictive controlled substance status, Schedule V, due to the low (<0.1%) THC) concentration. To preserve potency, store product in original bottle, and use within 12 weeks of opening. Stability of drug when dispensed in an oral syringe is 24 hours.

An advantage to using the prescription product is assurance of labeling accuracy. A recent analysis showed 70% of CBD extracts sold online were mislabeled and varied widely in THC concentrations.[322]

Epidiolex dosing: Initiate at 2.5 mg per kg by mouth twice daily and increase by 2.5 mg per kg per dose weekly as needed to a maximum dose of 10 mg per kg twice daily. Dose adjustment is required for hepatic impairment: moderate hepatic disease 1.25 mg per kg twice daily with a maximum 5 mg per kg twice daily. Severe hepatic impairment: 0.5 mg per kg twice daily with a maximum of 2 mg per kg twice daily.

Frequent adverse reactions associated with CBD oil include somnolence; decreased appetite; diarrhea; elevated hepatic enzymes; fatigue, malaise, and asthenia; rash; insomnia, sleep disorder; and infections.[323] Recommended monitoring includes baseline aspartate transaminase (AST), alanine transaminase (ALT), and total bilirubin concentrations. Repeat laboratory monitoring at 1, 3, and 6 months after starting therapy and 1 month after dosage change or adding other potentially hepatotoxic drugs.

The efficacy and safety of CBD 10 or 20 mg per kg per day as an adjunct to AEDs in treating several types of epilepsy has been investigated in numerous clinical trials.[324] In the GWPCARE3 randomized, double-blind, placebo-controlled trial of patients ($n = 225$; ages 2 to 55 years) with treatment-resistant LGS randomly assigned received 20 mg per kg per day CBD or placebo for 14 weeks.[325] Primary outcome was percentage change from baseline in monthly frequency of drop seizures. Median reduction in monthly drop seizure frequency was 43.9% in CBD group versus 21.8% in placebo group. Difference between groups was −17.21 [95% confidence interval (CI), −30.32 to −4, $p = 0.013$]. There were higher adverse drug events and study withdrawal with CBD.

A randomized, double-blind, placebo-controlled study of 120 children and young adults with Dravet syndrome and drug-resistant seizures received either CBD 20 mg per kg per day or placebo in addition to standard AED treatment.[326] Change in convulsive seizure frequency over a 14-week treatment period versus a 4-week baseline period was analyzed between groups. Median frequency of convulsive seizure per month decreased from 12.4 to 5.9 in CBD group and 14.9 to 14.1 in placebo group, with the median difference between groups was −22.8% (95% CI, −41 to −5.4, $p = 0.01$).[326] Long-term CBD administration in open-label studies (up to 48 weeks) showed sustained improvement in seizure frequency and mild-to-moderate adverse effects.[327]

Mechanism of Action

The anticonvulsant mechanism of CBD is not well defined. CBD may reduce neuronal excitability and neuronal transmission by modulating intracellular calcium by interaction with TRP channels, GPR55 or VDAC1.[328] The anti-inflammatory effects involving modulation of tumor necrosis factor-α release and inhibition of adenosine reuptake may contribute to anticonvulsant activity.[329]

Pharmacokinetics

Oral bioavailability of CBD is very low (13% to 19%)[330] due to extensive first-past metabolism. Protein binding is high (>94%). CBD is highly lipophilic, with a large V_d (~32 L per kg) with rapid distribution into the brain, adipose tissue, and other organs. The plasma half-life was 56 to 61 hours (healthy volunteers). The C_{max} and *AUC* appear to be dose dependent, with a saturation effect reported at higher oral doses of 400 and 800 mg in adults.[331] Metabolism is primarily hepatic by CYP2C19 and CYP3A4, and UGT1A7, UGT1A9, and UGT2B7 into an active metabolite with anticonvulsant activity, 7-OH-CBD. Metabolites undergo renal elimination.

Therapeutic Drug Monitoring

A relationship with serum concentration and clinical efficacy has not been established for CBD anticonvulsant therapy.

Drug Interactions

A CBD dose *reduction* should be considered when concomitantly prescribed with moderate or strong inhibitors of CYP3A4 or CYP2C19 to avoid adverse effects of increased CBD plasma concentrations.[321,324] When coadministered with strong inducers of CYP3A4 or CYP2C19, consider *increasing* dose of CBD oil to avoid reduced clinical anticonvulsant effect. Consider reducing dose of UGT1A9, UGT2B7, CYP2C8, CYP2C9, and CYP2C19 (e.g., diazepam, CBZ) substrate drugs when concurrently prescribed with CBD oil. Drugs that are substrates of CYP1A2 and CYP2B6 may also require dose adjustment when coadministered with CBD oil.[321] Use with VPA increases risk of transaminase elevations. Use of alcohol and other sedatives enhances the CNS effects of CBD.[321,323]

POTENTIAL ANTIEPILEPTIC DRUGS IN CLINICAL DEVELOPMENT

Ongoing AED developments are imperative as current regimens provide adequate seizure control only in approximately 30% to 50% of patients.[332–334] Efforts continue to develop more effective and less toxic AEDs for drug-refractory seizures and disease modification.[334] Agents under development include the glucose analog 2-dexoy-D-glucose (2DG).[332] It is imperative to include infants and children in well-designed, controlled trials of AEDs that include outcomes of behavior and cognitive development. Age and developmental PD, PK, pharmacogenomic, and safety data assist in optimizing management of AED therapy in this vulnerable population.

REFERENCES

1. Sillanpää M, Schmidt D. Natural history of treated childhood-onset epilepsy: Prospective, long-term population-based study. *Brain* 2006;129(Pt 3):617–624. doi:10.1093/brain/awh726.
2. Sillanpää M, Schmidt D. Predicting antiepileptic drug response in children with epilepsy. *Expert Rev Neurother* 2011;11(6):877–885. doi:10.1586/ern.11.11.
3. Glauser T, Ben-Menachem E, Bourgeois B, et al. Updated ILAE evidence review of antiepileptic drug efficacy and effectiveness as initial monotherapy for epileptic seizures and syndromes. *Epilepsia* 2013;54(3):551–563. doi:10.1111/epi.12074.
4. Rosati A, De Masi S, Guerrini R. Antiepileptic drug treatment in children with epilepsy. *CNS Drugs* 2015;29(10):847–863. doi:10.1007/s40263-015-0281-8.
5. Dang LT, Silverstein FS. Drug treatment of seizures and epilepsy in newborns and children. *Pediatr Clin North Am* 2017;64(6):1291–1308. doi:10.1016/j.pcl.2017.08.007.
6. Moavero R, Santarone ME, Galasso C, et al. Cognitive and behavioral effects of new antiepileptic drugs in pediatric epilepsy. *Brain Dev* 2017;39(6):464–469. doi:10.1016/j.braindev.2017.01.006.
7. Younus I, Reddy DS. A resurging boom in new drugs for epilepsy and brain disorders. *Expert Rev Clin Pharmacol* 2018;11(1):27–45. doi:10.1080/17512433.2018.1386553.
8. Łuszczki JJ. Third-generation antiepileptic drugs: mechanisms of action, pharmacokinetics and interactions. *Pharmacol Rep* 2009;61(2):197–216. doi:10.1016/S1734-1140(09)70024-6.
9. Chung AM, Eiland LS. Use of second-generation antiepileptic drugs in the pediatric population. *Pediatr Drugs* 2008;10(4):217–254. doi:10.2165/00148581-200810040-00003.
10. Mudigoudar B, Weatherspoon S, Wheless JW. Emerging antiepileptic drugs for severe pediatric epilepsies. *Semin Pediatr Neurol* 2016;23(2):167–179. doi:10.1016/j.spen.2016.06.003.
11. Patsalos PN, Berry DJ. Pharmacotherapy of the third-generation AEDs: lacosamide, retigabine and eslicarbazepine acetate. *Expert Opin Pharmacother* 2012;13(5):699–715. doi:10.1517/14656566.2012.667803.
12. LaPenna P, Tormoehlen LM. The pharmacology and toxicology of third-generation anticonvulsant drugs. *J Med Toxicol* 2017;13(4):329–342. doi:10.1007/s13181-017-0626-4.
13. Kanner AM, Ashman E, Gloss D, et al. Practice guideline update summary: efficacy and tolerability of the new antiepileptic drugs I: treatment of new-onset epilepsy. *Epilepsy Curr* 2018;18(4):260–268. doi:10.5698/1535-7597.18.4.260.
14. Arzimanoglou A, D'Cruz ON, Nordli D, et al. A review of the new antiepileptic drugs for focal-onset seizures in pediatrics: role of extrapolation. *Pediatr Drugs* 2018;20(3):249–264. doi:10.1007/s40272-018-0286-0.
15. Walker MC, Sander J. Difficulties in extrapolating from clinical trial data to clinical practice: the case of antiepileptic drugs. *Neurology* 1997;49(2):333–337. doi:10.1212/WNL.49.2.333.
16. van den Anker J, Reed MD, Allegaert K, et al. Developmental changes in pharmacokinetics and pharmacodynamics. *J Clin Pharmacol* 2018;58(Suppl 10):S10–S25. doi:10.1002/jcph.1284.
17. Russ SA, Larson K, Halfon N. A national profile of childhood epilepsy and seizure disorder. *Pediatrics* 2012;129(2):256–264. doi:10.1542/peds.2010-1371.
18. Cross JH. Neurodevelopmental effects of anti-epileptic drugs. *Epilepsy Res* 2010;88(1):1–10. doi:10.1016/j.eplepsyres.2009.08.015.
19. López-García MA, Feria-Romero IA, Serrano H, et al. Influence of genetic variants of CYP2D6, CYP2C9, CYP2C19 and CYP3A4 on antiepileptic drug metabolism in pediatric patients with refractory epilepsy. *Pharmacol Rep* 2017;69(3):504–511. doi:10.1016/j.pharep.2017.01.007.
20. Patsalos PN. Drug interactions with the newer antiepileptic drugs (AEDs) - Part 2: pharmacokinetic and pharmacodynamic interactions between AEDs and drugs used to treat non-epilepsy disorders. *Clin Pharmacokinet* 2013;52(12):1045–1061. doi:10.1007/s40262-013-0088-z.
21. Hesdorffer DC, Kanner AM. The FDA alert on suicidality and antiepileptic drugs: fire or false alarm? *Epilepsia* 2009;50(5):978–986. doi:10.1111/j.1528-1167.2009.02012.x.
22. Britton JW, Shih JJ. Antiepileptic drugs and suicidality. *Drug Healthc Patient Saf* 2010;2:181–189. doi:10.2147/DHPS.S13225.
23. Arana A, Wentworth CE, Ayuso-Mateos JL, et al. Suicide-related events in patients treated with antiepileptic drugs. *N Engl J Med* 2010;363(6):542–551. doi:10.1056/NEJMoa0909801.
24. Mason S, Doss R. Screening for depression and suicidality in an epilepsy clinic. *Epilepsy Curr* 2011;11(Suppl 1).
25. Ravat S, Gupta R. Antiepileptic drugs in pediatric epilepsy. *J Pediatr Neurosci.* 2008;3(1):5–17.
26. Fisher RS, Cross JH, D'Souza C, et al. Instruction manual for the ILAE 2017 operational classification of seizure types. *Epilepsia* 2017;58(4):531–542. doi:10.1111/epi.13671.
27. French JA. Refractory epilepsy: clinical overview. *Epilepsia* 2007;48(Suppl 1):3–7. doi:10.1111/j.1528-1167.2007.00992.x.
28. Gambardella A, Labate A, Mumoli L, et al. Role of pharmacogenomics in antiepileptic drug therapy: current status and future perspectives. *Curr Pharm Des* 2017;23(37):5760–5765. doi:10.2174/1381612823666170911111536.
29. Hsu DY, Brieva J, Silverberg NB, et al. Pediatric Stevens-Johnson syndrome and toxic epidermal necrolysis in the United States. *J Am Acad Dermatol* 2017;76(5):811–817.e4. doi.org/10.1016/j.jaad.2016.12.024.
30. Li X, Yu K, Mei S, et al. HLA-B* 1502 increases the risk of phenytoin or lamotrigine induced Stevens-Johnson syndrome/toxic epidermal necrolysis: evidence from a meta-analysis of nine case-control studies. *Drug Res (Stuttg)* 2014;65(2):107–111. doi:10.1055/s-0034-1375684.
31. Abend NS, Loddenkemper T. Management of pediatric status epilepticus. *Curr Treat Options Neurol* 2014;16(7):301. doi:10.1007/s11940-014-0301-x.
32. Lyttle MD, Rainford NEA, Gamble C, et al. Levetiracetam versus phenytoin for second-line treatment of paediatric convulsive status epilepticus (EcLiPSE): a multicentre, open-label, randomised trial. *Lancet* 2019;393(10186):2125–2134. doi:10.1016/S0140-6736(19)30724-X.
33. El-Dib M, Soul JS. The use of phenobarbital and other anti-seizure drugs in newborns. *Semin Fetal Neonatal Med* 2017;22(5):321–327. doi:10.1016/j.siny.2017.07.008.
34. Painter MJ, Scher MS, Stein AD, et al. Phenobarbital compared with phenytoin for the treatment of neonatal seizures. *N Engl J Med* 1999; 341(7):485–489. doi:10.1056/NEJM199908123410704.
35. Khan O, Cipriani C, Wright C, et al. Role of intravenous levetiracetam for acute seizure management in preterm neonates. *Pediatr Neurol* 2013;49(5):340–343. doi:10.1016/j.pediatrneurol.2013.05.008.
36. Ferrendelli JA. Pharmacology of antiepileptic drugs. *Epilepsia* 1987;28(Suppl 3):S14–S16. doi:10.1111/j.1528-1157.1987.tb05772.x.
37. Gugler R, Manion CV, Azarnoff DL. Phenytoin: pharmacokinetics and bioavailability. *Clin Pharmacol Ther* 1976;19(2):135–142. doi:10.1002/cpt1976192135.
38. Blain P, Mucklow J, Bacon C, et al. Pharmacokinetics of phenytoin in children. *Br J Clin Pharmacol* 1981;12(5):659–661. doi:10.1111/j.1365-2125.1981.tb01285.x.
39. Ludden TM. Nonlinear pharmacokinetics. *Clin Pharmacokinet* 1991;20(6):429–446. doi:10.2165/00003088-199120060-00001.
40. Lawton B, Davis T, Goldstein H, et al. An update in the initial management of paediatric status epilepticus. *Curr Opin Pediatr* 2018;30(3):359–363. doi:10.1097/MOP.0000000000000616.
41. Phenytoin in Lexi-Comp Online™, Pediatric & Neonatal Lexi-Drugs Online™. Hudson, OH: Lexi-Comp, Inc., 2020.
42. Wolf GK, McClain CD, Zurakowski D, et al. Total phenytoin concentrations do not accurately predict free phenytoin concentrations in critically ill children. *Pediatr Crit Care Med* 2006;7(5):434–439. doi:10.1097/01.PCC.0000235252.43921.DE.
43. Cheng A, Banwell B, Levin S, et al. Oral dosing requirements for phenytoin in the first three months of life. *Can J Clin Pharmacol* 2010;17(2):e256–e261.
44. Johnson TN, Rostami-Hodjegan A, Tucker GT. Prediction of the clearance of eleven drugs and associated variability in neonates, infants and children. *Clin Pharmacokinet* 2006;45(9):931–956. doi:10.2165/00003088-200645090-00005.
45. Leff RD, Fischer LJ, Roberts RJ. Phenytoin metabolism in infants following intravenous and oral administration. *Dev Pharmacol Ther* 1986;9(4):217–223. doi:10.1159/000457096.
46. Van der Weide J, Steijns LS, Van Weelden MJ, et al. The effect of genetic polymorphism of cytochrome P450 CYP2C9 on phenytoin dose requirement. *Pharmacogenetics* 2001;11(4):287–291. doi:10.1097/00008571-200106000-00002.
47. Patsalos PN, Berry DJ, Bourgeois BF, et al. Antiepileptic drugs - best practice guidelines for therapeutic drug monitoring: a position paper by the subcommission on therapeutic drug monitoring, ILAE Commission on Therapeutic Strategies. *Epilepsia* 2008;49(7):1239–1276. doi:10.1111/j.1528-1167.2008.01561.x.
48. Levy RH. Cytochrome P450 isozymes and antiepileptic drug interactions. *Epilepsia* 1995;36(Suppl 5):S8–S13. doi:10.1111/j.1528-1157.1995.tb06007.x.
49. Patsalos PN. Antiepileptic drug interactions. In: Miller JW, Goodkin HP, eds. *Epilepsy.* Chichester, England: Wiley, 2014:91–101. doi:10.1002/9781118456989.ch13.
50. Sabers A. Pharmacokinetic interactions between contraceptives and antiepileptic drugs. *Seizure* 2008;17(2):141–144. doi:10.1016/j.seizure.2007.11.012.
51. Spina E, Pisani F, Perucca E. Clinically significant pharmacokinetic drug interactions with carbamazepine. *Clin Pharmacokinet* 1996;31(3):198–214. doi:10.2165/00003088-199631030-00004.

52. Stöllberger C, Finsterer J. Interactions between non-vitamin K oral anticoagulants and antiepileptic drugs. *Epilepsy Res* 2016;126:98–101. doi:10.1016/j.eplepsyres.2016.06.003.
53. Barry M, Gibbons S, Back D, et al. Protease inhibitors in patients with HIV disease. clinically important pharmacokinetic considerations. *Clin Pharmacokinet* 1997;32(3):194–209. doi:10.2165/00003088-199732030-00003.
54. Phelps N. Management of phenytoin with enteral tube feeding. *Ment Heal Clin* 2012;2(5):108–109. doi:10.9740/mhc.n126907.
55. Perucca E. Clinically relevant drug interactions with antiepileptic drugs. *Br J Clin Pharmacol* 2006;61(3):246–255. doi:10.1111/j.1365-2125.2005.02529.x.
56. Mueller EW, Boucher BA. Fosphenytoin: current place in therapy. *J Pediatr Pharmacol Ther* 2004;9(4):265–273. doi:10.5863/1551-6776-9.4.265.
57. Aaronson PM, Belgado BS, Spillane JP, et al. Evaluation of intramuscular fosphenytoin vs intravenous phenytoin loading in the ED. *Am J Emerg Med* 2011;29(9):983–988. doi:10.1016/j.ajem.2010.05.005.
58. Kai E, Tapani K, Reetta K. Fosphenytoin. *Expert Opin Drug Metab Toxicol* 2009;5(6)695–701. doi:10.1517/17425250902997975.
59. Glauser T, Shinnar S, Gloss D, et al. Evidence-based guideline: treatment of convulsive status epilepticus in children and adults. *Epilepsy Curr* 2016;16(1):48–61. doi:10.5698/1535-7597-16.1.48.
60. Johnson J, Wrenn K. Inappropriate fosphenytoin use in the ED. *Am J Emerg Med.* 2001;19(4)July 1:293–294. doi:10.1053/ajem.2001.24471.
61. Prasad AN, Seshia SS. Status epilepticus in pediatric practice: neonate to adolescent. *Adv Neurol* 2006;97:229–243.
62. Takeoka M, Krishnamoorthy KS, Soman TB, et al. Fosphenytoin in infants. *J Child Neurol* 1998;13(11):537–540. doi:10.1177/088307389801301102.
63. Browne TR, Kugler AR, Eldon MA. Pharmacology and pharmacokinetics of fosphenytoin. *Neurology* 1996;46(6 Suppl 1):S3–S7. doi:10.1212/wnl.46.6_suppl_1.3s.
64. Morton LD. Clinical experience with fosphenytoin in children. *J Child Neurol* 1998;13(Suppl 1):S19–S22. doi:10.1177/0883073898013001061.
65. Wallace SJ. A comparative review of the adverse effects of anticonvulsants in children with epilepsy. *Drug Saf* 1996;15(6):378–393. doi:10.2165/00002018-199615060-00003.
66. Pacifici GM. Clinical pharmacology of phenobarbital in neonates: effects, metabolism and pharmacokinetics. *Curr Pediatr Rev* 2016;12(1):48–54. doi:10.2174/1573397111666615102 6223914.
67. Yukawa M, Yukawa E, Suematsu F, et al. Population pharmacokinetics of phenobarbital by mixed effect modelling using routine clinical pharmacokinetic data in Japanese neonates and infants: an update. *J Clin Pharm Ther* 2011;36(6):704–710. doi:10.1111/j.1365-2710.2010.01220.x.
68. Touw DJ, Graafland O, Cranendonk A, et al. Clinical pharmacokinetics of phenobarbital in neonates. *Eur J Pharm Sci* 2000;12(2):111–116. doi:10.1016/S0928-0987(00)00145-7.
69. Fischer JH, Lockman LA, Zaske D, et al. Phenobarbital maintenance dose requirements in treating neonatal seizures. *Neurology* 1981;31(8):1042–1044. doi:10.1212/wnl.31.8.1042.
70. Evans D, Levene M. Neonatal seizures. *Arch Dis Child Fetal Neonatal Ed* 1998;78(1):F70–F75. doi:10.1136/fn.78.1.F70.
71. Gilman ME, Toback JW, Gal P, et al. Individualizing phenobarbital dosing in neonates. *Clin Pharm* 1983;2(3):258–262.
72. Elliott ES, Buck ML. Phenobarbital dosing and pharmacokinetics in a neonate receiving extracorporeal membrane oxygenation. *Ann Pharmacother* 1999;33(4):419–422. doi:10.1345/aph.18248.
73. Schmitt B, Kovacevic-Preradovic T, Critelli H, et al. Is ethosuximide a risk factor for generalised tonic-clonic seizures in absence epilepsy? *Neuropediatrics* 2007;38(2):83–87. doi:10.1055/s-2007-984446.
74. Kessler SK, McGinnis E. A practical guide to treatment of childhood absence epilepsy. *Pediatr Drugs* 2019;21(1):15–24. doi:10.1007/s40272-019-00325-x.
75. Glauser TA, Holland K, O'Brien VP, et al. Pharmacogenetics of antiepileptic drug efficacy in childhood absence epilepsy. *Ann Neurol* 2017;81(3):444–453. doi:10.1002/ana.24886.
76. Battino D, Estienne M, Avanzini G. Clinical pharmacokinetics of antiepileptic drugs in paediatric patients: part I: phenobarbital, primidone, valproic acid, ethosuximide and mesuximide. *Clin Pharmacokinet* 1995;29(4):257–286. doi:10.2165/00003088-199529040-00005.
77. Patsalos PN, Spencer EP, Berry DJ. Therapeutic drug monitoring of antiepileptic drugs in epilepsy: a 2018 update. *Ther Drug Monit* 2018;40(5):526–548. doi:10.1097/FTD.0000000000000546.
78. Bourgeois BF. Combination of valproate and ethosuximide: antiepileptic and neurotoxic interaction. *J Pharmacol Exp Ther* 1988;247(3):1128–1132.
79. Rosati A, Ilvento L, Lucenteforte E, et al. Comparative efficacy of antiepileptic drugs in children and adolescents: a network meta-analysis. *Epilepsia* 2018;59(2):297–314. doi:10.1111/epi.13981.
80. Osorio I, Reed RC, Peltzer JN. Refractory idiopathic absence status epilepticus: a probable paradoxical effect of phenytoin and carbamazepine. *Epilepsia* 2000;41(7):887–894. doi:10.1111/j.1528-1157.2000.tb00258.x.
81. Amann B, Grunze H, Vieta E, et al. Antiepileptic drugs and mood stability. *Clin EEG Neurosci* 2007;38(2):116–123. doi:10.1177/155005940703800214.
82. Singh B, Singh P, Al Hifzi I, et al. Treatment of neonatal seizures with carbamazepine. *J Child Neurol* 1996;11(5):378–382. doi:10.1177/088307389601100506.
83. Hoppen T, Elger CE, Bartmann P. Carbamazepine in phenobarbital-nonresponders: Experience with ten preterm infants. *Eur J Pediatr* 2001;160(7):444–447. doi:10.1007/s004310100760.
84. Sands TT, Balestri M, Bellini G, et al. Rapid and safe response to low-dose carbamazepine in neonatal epilepsy. *Epilepsia* 2016;57(12):2019–2030. doi:10.1111/epi.13596.
85. Tothfalusi L, Endrenyi L. Approvable generic carbamazepine formulations may not be bioequivalent in target patient populations. *Int J Clin Pharmacol Ther* 2013;51(6):525–528. doi:10.5414/CP201845.
86. Sobotka JL, Alexander B, Cook BL. A review of carbamazepine's hematologic reactions and monitoring recommendations. *DICP* 1990;24(12):1214–1219. doi:10.1177/106002809002401214.
87. Post RM, Ketter TA, Uhde T, et al. Thirty years of clinical experience with carbamazepine in the treatment of bipolar illness: principles and practice. *CNS Drugs* 2007;21(1):47–71. doi:10.2165/00023210-200721010-00005.
88. Djordjevic N, Jankovic SM, Milovanovic JR. Pharmacokinetics and pharmacogenetics of carbamazepine in children. *Eur J Drug Metab Pharmacokinet* 2017;42(5):729–744. doi:10.1007/s13318-016-0397-3.
89. Nau H, Kuhnz W, Egger HJ, et al. Anticonvulsants during pregnancy and lactation transplacental, maternal and neonatal pharmacokinetics. *Clin Pharmacokinet* 1982;7(6):508–543. doi:10.2165/00003088-198207060-00003.
90. Sisodiya SM, Sander JW, Patsalos PN. Carbamazepine toxicity during combination therapy with levetiracetam: a pharmacodynamic interaction. *Epilepsy Res* 2002;48(3):217–219. doi:10.1016/S0920-1211(01)00309-6.
91. Owens MJ, Nemeroff CB. Pharmacology of valproate. *Psychopharmacol Bull* 2003;37(Suppl 2):17–24. doi:10.2165/00023210-200216100-00003.
92. Cook AM, Bensalem-Owen MK. Mechanisms of action of antiepileptic drugs. *Therapy* 2011;8(3):307–313. doi:10.2217/thy.11.19.
93. Guerrini R. Valproate as a mainstay of therapy for pediatric epilepsy. *Pediatr Drugs* 2006;8(2):113–129. doi:10.2165/00148581-200608020-00004.
94. Bassan H, Bental Y, Shany E, et al. Neonatal seizures: dilemmas in workup and management. *Pediatr Neurol* 2008;38(6):415–421. doi:10.1016/j.pediatrneurol.2008.03.003.
95. Gal P, Oles KS, Gilman JT, et al. Valproic acid efficacy, toxicity, and pharmacokinetics in neonates with intractable seizures. *Neurology* 1988;38(3):467–471. doi:10.1212/wnl.38.3.467.
96. Bachman DS. Use of valproic acid in treatment of infantile spasms. *Arch Neurol* 1982;39(1):49–52. doi:10.1001/archneur.1982.00510130051013.
97. Verrotti A, Striano P, Iapadre G, et al. The pharmacological management of Lennox-Gastaut syndrome and critical literature review. *Seizure* 2018;63:17–25. doi:10.1016/j.seizure.2018.10.016.
98. Mikati MA, Lepejian GA, Holmes GL. Medical treatment of patients with infantile spasms. *Clin Neuropharmacol* 2002;25(2):61–70. doi:10.1097/00002826-200203000-00001.
99. Löscher W. Basic pharmacology of valproate: a review after 35 years of clinical use for the treatment of epilepsy. *CNS Drugs* 2002;16(10):669–694. doi:10.2165/00023210-200216100-00003.
100. Taketomo CK, Hodding JH, Kraus DM. Vaproic acid. In: *Pediatric & neonatal dosage handbook*, 26th ed. Hudson, OH: Lexi-Comp, 2019.
101. Star K, Edwards IR, Choonara I. Valproic acid and fatalities in children: a review of individual case safety reports in VigiBase. *PLoS One* 2014;9(10):e108970. doi:10.1371/journal.pone.0108970.
102. Ornoy A. Valproic acid in pregnancy: how much are we endangering the embryo and fetus? *Reprod Toxicol* 2009;28(1):1–10. doi:10.1016/j.reprotox.2009.02.014.
103. Tanoshima M, Kobayashi T, Tanoshima R, et al. Risks of congenital malformations in offspring exposed to valproic acid in utero: a systematic review and cumulative meta-analysis. *Clin Pharmacol Ther* 2015;98(4):417–441. doi:10.1002/cpt.158.
104. Nanau RM, Neuman MG. Adverse drug reactions induced by valproic acid. *Clin Biochem* 2013;46(15):1323–1338. doi:10.1016/j.clinbiochem.2013.06.012.
105. Wirrell EC. Valproic acid-associated weight gain in older children and teens with epilepsy. *Pediatr Neurol* 2003;28(2):126–129. doi:10.1016/S0887-8994(02)00505-2.
106. Sharpe C, Wolfson T, Trauner DA. Weight gain in children treated with valproate. *J Child Neurol* 2009;24(3):338–341. doi:10.1177/0883073808323023.
107. Smith MC, Centorrino F, Welge JA, et al. Clinical comparison of extended-release divalproex versus delayed-release divalproex: pooled data analyses from nine trials. *Epilepsy Behav* 2004;5(5):746–751. doi:10.1016/j.yebeh.2004.07.007.
108. Granneman GR, Wang SI, Machinist JM, et al. Aspects of the metabolism of valproic acid. *Xenobiotica* 1984;14(5):375–387. doi:10.3109/00498258409151426.
109. Chadwick DW, Anhut H, Greiner MJ, et al. A double-blind trial of gabapentin monotherapy for newly diagnosed partial seizures. International Gabapentin Monotherapy Study Group 945-77. *Neurology* 1998;51(5):1282–1288.
110. Taketomo CK, Hodding JH, Kraus DM. Gabapentin. In: *Pediatric & neonatal dosage handbook*, 26th ed. Hudson, OH: Lexi-Comp, 2019.
111. Peckham AM, Ananickal MJ, Sclar DA. Gabapentin use, abuse, and the US opioid epidemic: the case for reclassification as a controlled substance and the need for pharmacovigilance. *Risk Manag Healthc Policy* 2018;11:109–116. doi:10.2147/RMHP.S168504.
112. Quintero GC. Review about gabapentin misuse, interactions, contraindications and side effects. *J Exp Pharmacol* 2017;9:13–21. doi:10.2147/JEP.S124391.
113. Savelloni J, Gunter H, Lee KC, et al. Risk of respiratory depression with opioids and concomitant gabapentinoids. *J Pain Res* 2017;10:2635–2641. doi:10.2147/JPR.S144963.
114. Finlayson G, Chavarria M, Chang S, et al. Gabapentin in mixed drug fatalities: does this frequent analyte deserve more attention? *Acad Forensic Pathol* 2017;7(1):99–111. doi:10.23907/2017.012.
115. Panebianco M, Al-Bachari S, Weston J, et al. Gabapentin add-on treatment for drug-resistant focal epilepsy. *Cochrane Database Syst Rev* 2018;10:CD001415. doi:10.1002/14651858.CD001415.pub3.
116. Lee DO, Steingard RJ, Cesena M, et al. Behavioral side effects of gabapentin in children. *Epilepsia* 1996;37(1):87–90. doi:10.1111/j.1528-1157.1996.tb00517.x.
117. Maneuf YP, Gonzalez MI, Sutton KS, et al. Cellular and molecular action of the putative GABA-mimetic, gabapentin. *Cell Mol Life Sci* 2003;60(4):742–750. doi:10.1007/s00018-003-2108-x.
118. Gidal BE, DeCerce J, Bockbrader HN, et al. Gabapentin bioavailability: effect of dose and frequency of administration in adult patients with epilepsy. *Epilepsy Res* 1998;31(2):91–99. doi:10.1016/S0920-1211(98)00020-5.
119. Ouellet D, Bockbrader HN, Wesche DL, et al. Population pharmacokinetics of gabapentin in infants and children. *Epilepsy Res* 2001;47(3):229–241. doi:10.1016/S0920-1211(01)00311-4.
120. Wellington K, Goa KL. Oxcarbazepine: an update of its efficacy in the management of epilepsy. *CNS Drugs* 2001;15(2):137–163. doi:10.2165/00023210-200115020-00005.
121. Wheless JW, Clarke DF, Arzimanoglou A, et al. Treatment of pediatric epilepsy: European expert opinion, 2007. *Epileptic Disord* 2007;9(4):353–412. doi:10.1684/epd.2007.0144.

122. Piña-Garza JE, Espinoza R, Nordli D, et al. Oxcarbazepine adjunctive therapy in infants and young children with partial seizures. *Neurology* 2005;65(9):1370–1375. doi:10.1212/01.wnl.0000186800.18456.72.
123. Bülau P, Paar WD, von Unruh GE. Pharmacokinetics of oxcarbazepine and 10-hydroxy-carbazepine in the newborn child of an oxcarbazepine-treated mother. *Eur J Clin Pharmacol* 1988;34(3):311–313. doi:10.1007/BF00540963.
124. Rolnitsky A, Merlob P, Klinger G. In utero oxcarbazepine and a withdrawal syndrome, anomalies, and hyponatremia. *Pediatr Neurol* 2013;48(6):466–468. doi:10.1016/j.pediatrneurol.2013.02.012.
125. Taketomo CK, Hodding JH, Kraus DM. Oxcarbazepine. In: *Pediatric & neonatal dosage handbook*, 26th ed. Hudson, OH: Lexi-Comp, 2019.
126. May TW, Korn-Merker E, Rambeck B. Clinical pharmacokinetics of oxcarbazepine. *Clin Pharmacokinet* 2003;42(12):1023–1042. doi:10.2165/00003088-200342120-00002.
127. Dam M, Ekberg R, Løyning Y, et al. A double-blind study comparing oxcarbazepine and carbamazepine in patients with newly diagnosed, previously untreated epilepsy. *Epilepsy Res* 1989;3(1):70–76. doi:10.1016/0920-1211(89)90070-3.
128. Berghuis B, van der Palen J, de Haan GJ, et al. Carbamazepine- and oxcarbazepine-induced hyponatremia in people with epilepsy. *Epilepsia* 2017;58(7):1227–1233. doi:10.1111/epi.13777.
129. Beran RG. Cross-reactive skin eruption with both carbamazepine and oxcarbazepine. *Epilepsia* 1993;34(1):163–165. doi:10.1111/j.1528-1157.1993.tb02392.x.
130. Błaszczyk B, Lasoń W, Czuczwar SJ. Antiepileptic drugs and adverse skin reactions: an update. *Pharmacol Rep* 2015;67(3):426–434. doi:10.1016/j.pharep.2014.11.009.
131. Sallas WM, Milosavljev S, D'Souza J, et al. Pharmacokinetic drug interactions in children taking oxcarbazepine. *Clin Pharmacol Ther* 2003;74(2):138–149. doi:10.1016/S0009-9236(03)00124-3.
132. Zaccara G, Perucca E. Interactions between antiepileptic drugs, and between antiepileptic drugs and other drugs. *Epileptic Disord* 2014;16(4):409–431. doi:10.1684/epd.2014.0714
133. Flesch G. Overview of the clinical pharmacokinetics of oxcarbazepine. *Clin Drug Investig* 2004;24(4):185–203. doi:10.2165/00044011-200424040-00001.
134. Yasam VR, Jakki SL, Senthil V, et al. A pharmacological overview of lamotrigine for the treatment of epilepsy. *Expert Rev Clin Pharmacol* 2016;9(12):1533–1546. doi:10.1080/17512433.2016.1254041.
135. Mastrangelo M. Lennox-Gastaut syndrome: a state of the art review. *Neuropediatrics* 2017;48(3):143–151. doi:10.1055/s-0037-1601324.
136. Shih JJ, Whitlock JB, Chimato N, et al. Epilepsy treatment in adults and adolescents: expert opinion, 2016. *Epilepsy Behav* 2017;69:186–222. doi:10.1016/j.yebeh.2016.11.018.
137. Brodie MJ, Richens A, Yuen A. Double-blind comparison of lamotrigine and carbamazepine in newly diagnosed epilepsy. UK Lamotrigine/Carbamazepine Monotherapy Trial Group. *Lancet* 1995;345(8948):476–479. doi:10.1016/S0140-6736(95)90581-2.
138. Nahata MC, Morosco RS, Hipple TF. Stability of lamotrigine in two extemporaneously prepared oral suspensions at 4 and 25 degrees C. *Am J Heal Pharm* 1999;56(3):240–242. doi:10.1093/ajhp/56.3.240.
139. Walton NY, Jaing Q, Hyun B, et al. Lamotrigine vs. phenytoin for treatment of status epilepticus: comparison in an experimental model. *Epilepsy Res* 1996;24(1):19–28. doi:10.1016/0920-1211(96)00007-1.
140. Mikati MA, Fayad M, Koleilat M, et al. Efficacy, tolerability, and kinetics of lamotrigine in infants. *J Pediatr* 2002;141(1):31–35. doi:10.1067/mpd.2002.125256.
141. Battino D, Estienne A, Avanzini G. Clinical pharmacokinetics of antiepileptic drugs in paediatric patients. Part II. Phenytoin, carbamazepine, sulthiame, lamotrigine, vigabatrin, oxcarbazepine and felbamate. *Clin Pharmacokinet* 1995;29(5):341–369.
142. Messenheimer J. Efficacy and safety of lamotrigine in pediatric patients. *J Child Neurol* 2002;17(Suppl 2):2S34–2S42. doi:10.1177/08830738020170021001.
143. Martin AC, Besag FM, Berry DJ, et al. The effect of lamotrigine on valproic acid concentrations. *Curr Drug Saf* 2011;6(1):23–29. doi:10.2174/157488611794480061.
144. Vázquez M, Maldonado C, Guevara N, et al. Lamotrigine-valproic acid interaction leading to Stevens-Johnson syndrome. *Case Rep Med* 2018;2018:5371854. doi:10.1155/2018/5371854.
145. Eriksson AS, Hoppu K, Nergårdh A, et al. Pharmacokinetic interactions between lamotrigine and other antiepileptic drugs in children with intractable epilepsy. *Epilepsia* 1996;37(8):769–773. doi:10.1111/j.1528-1157.1996.tb00650.x.
146. Tsao CY. Current trends in the treatment of infantile spasms. *Neuropsychiatr Dis Treat* 2009;5:289–299. doi:10.2147/ndt.s4488.
147. Søndergaard Khinchi M, Nielsen KA, Dahl M, et al. Lamotrigine therapeutic thresholds. *Seizure* 2008;17(5):391–395. doi:10.1016/j.seizure.2007.11.023.
148. Huang HT, Chang CL, Tzeng DS. Toxic epidermal necrolysis after sun-exposure probably due to lamotrigine and chlorpromazine. *Asian J Psychiatr* 2010;3(4):240–242.
149. Pellock JM, Faught E, Leppik IE, et al. Felbamate: consensus of current clinical experience. *Epilepsy Res* 2006;71(2–3):89–101. doi:10.1016/j.eplepsyres.2006.06.020.
150. Shi LL, Dong J, Ni H, et al. Felbamate as an add-on therapy for refractory partial epilepsy. *Cochrane Database Syst Rev* 2017;7:CD008295. doi:10.1002/14651858.CD008295.pub4.
151. Hosain S, Nagarajan L, Carson D, et al. Felbamate for refractory infantile spasms. *J Child Neurol* 1997;12(7):466–468. doi:10.1177/088307389701200711.
152. Taketomo CK, Hodding JH, Kraus DM. Felbamate. In: *Pediatric & neonatal dosage handbook*, 26th ed. Hudson, OH: Lexi-Comp, 2019.
153. Pellock JM. Felbamate in epilepsy therapy: evaluating the risks. *Drug Saf* 1999;21(3):225–239. doi:10.2165/00002018-199921030-00006.
154. Shah YD, Singh K, Friedman D, et al. Evaluating the safety and efficacy of felbamate in the context of a black box warning: a single center experience. *Epilepsy Behav* 2016;56:50–33. doi:10.1016/j.yebeh.2016.01.006.
155. Heyman E, Levin N, Lahat E, Epstein O, Gandelman-Marton R. Efficacy and safety of felbamate in children with refractory epilepsy. *Eur J Paediatr Neurol* 2014;18(6):658–62.
156. Rho JM, Donevan SD, Rogawski MA. Mechanism of action of the anticonvulsant felbamate: opposing effects on N-methyl-D-aspartate and γ-aminobutyric acid A receptors. *Ann Neurol* 1994;35(2):229–234. doi:10.1002/ana.410350216.
157. Reimers A, Berg JA, Burns ML, et al. Reference ranges for antiepileptic drugs revisited: a practical approach to establish national guidelines. *Drug Des Devel Ther* 2018;12:271–280. doi:10.2147/DDDT.S154388.
158. Harden CL, Trifiletti R, Kutt H. Felbamate levels in patients with epilepsy. *Epilepsia* 1996;37(3):280–283. doi:10.1111/j.1528-1157.1996.tb00026.x.
159. Patsalos PN. Drug interactions with the newer antiepileptic drugs (AEDs) - Part 1: pharmacokinetic and pharmacodynamic interactions between AEDs. *Clin Pharmacokinet* 2013;52(11):927–966. doi:10.1007/s40262-013-0087-0.
160. Wilbur K, Ensom MH. Pharmacokinetic drug interactions between oral contraceptives and second-generation anticonvulsants. *Clin Pharmacokinet* 2000;38(4):355–365. doi:10.2165/00003088-200038040-00004.
161. Faught E. Topiramate in the treatment of partial and generalized epilepsy. *Neuropsychiatr Dis Treat* 2007;3(6):811–821 doi:10.2147/ndt.s512.
162. Topiramate in Lexi-Comp Online™, Pediatric & Neonatal Lexi-Drugs Online™. Hudson, OH: Lexi-Comp, Inc., 2020.
163. Topiramate. In: Nahata MC, Pi VB, Hipple TF, eds. *Pediatric drug formulations*. Cincinnati, OH: Harvey Whitney Books, 2004:1–7.
164. Kennedy GM, Lhatoo SD. CNS adverse events associated with antiepileptic drugs. *CNS Drugs* 2008;22(9):739–760. doi:10.2165/00023210-200822090-00003.
165. Lee S, Sziklas V, Andermann F, et al. The effects of adjunctive topiramate on cognitive function in patients with epilepsy. *Epilepsia* 2003;44(3):339–347. doi:10.1046/j.1528-1157.2003.27402.x.
166. Mirza N, Marson AG, Pirmohamed M. Effect of topiramate on acid-base balance: extent, mechanism and effects. *Br J Clin Pharmacol* 2009;68(5):655–661. doi:10.1111/j.1365-2125.2009.03521.x.
167. Etminan M, Maberley D, Mikelberg FS. Use of topiramate and risk of glaucoma: a case-control study. *Am J Ophthalmol* 2012;153(5):827–830. doi:10.1016/j.ajo.2011.10.018.
168. Fung EL, Nelson EA. Oligohydrosis and topiramate. *Pediatr Neurol* 2006;34(5):392–394. doi:10.1016/j.pediatrneurol.2006.08.012.
169. Ben-Zeev B, Watemberg N, Augarten A, et al. Oligohydrosis and hyperthermia: pilot study of a novel topiramate adverse effect. *J Child Neurol* 2003;18(4):254–257. doi:10.1177/08830738030180041001.
170. Hottinger A, Sutter R, Marsch S, et al. Topiramate as an adjunctive treatment in patients with refractory status epilepticus: an observational cohort study. *CNS Drugs* 2012;26(9):761–772. doi:10.2165/11633090-000000000-00000.
171. Patsalos PN. The mechanism of action of topiramate. *Rev Contemp Pharmacother* 1999;10:147–153.
172. Shank RP, Gardocki JF, Streeter AJ, et al. An overview of the preclinical aspects of topiramate: pharmacology, pharmacokinetics, and mechanism of action. *Epilepsia* 2000;41(Suppl 1):S3–S9. doi:10.1111/j.1528-1157.2000.tb02163.x.
173. Glauser TA, Miles MV, Tang P, et al. Topiramate pharmacokinetics in infants. *Epilepsia* 1999;40(6):788–791. doi:10.1111/j.1528-1157.1999.tb00780.x.
174. May TW, Rambeck B, Jürgens U. Serum concentrations of topiramate in patients with epilepsy: Influence of dose, age, and comedication. *Ther Drug Monit* 2002;24(3):366–374. doi:10.1097/00007691-200206000-00007.
175. Deshpande LS, DeLorenzo RJ. Mechanisms of levetiracetam in the control of status epilepticus and epilepsy. *Front Neurol* 2014;5:11. doi:10.3389/fneur.2014.00011.
176. Lyseng-Williamson KA. Levetiracetam: a review of its use in epilepsy. *Drugs* 2011;71(4):489–514. doi:10.2165/11204490-000000000-00000.
177. Gorji A, Höhling JM, Madeja M, et al. Effect of levetiracetam on epileptiform discharges in human neocortical slices. *Epilepsia* 2002;43(12):1480–1487. doi:10.1046/j.1528-1157.2002.23702.x.
178. Han JY, Moon CJ, Youn YA, et al. Efficacy of levetiracetam for neonatal seizures in preterm infants. *BMC Pediatr* 2018;18(1):131. doi:10.1186/s12887-018-1103-1.
179. Levetiracetam in Lexi-Comp Online™, Pediatric & Neonatal Lexi-Drugs Online™. Hudson, OH: Lexi-Comp, Inc., 2020.
180. Perry MS, Benatar M. Efficacy and tolerability of levetiracetam in children younger than 4 years: a retrospective review. *Epilepsia* 2007;48(6):1123–1127. doi:10.1111/j.1528-1167.2007.01003.x.
181. Krief P, Kan L, Maytal J. Efficacy of levetiracetam in children with epilepsy younger than 2 years of age. *J Child Neurol* 2008;23(5):582–584. doi:10.1177/0883073807309781.
182. Pellock JM, Glauser TA, Bebin EM, et al. Pharmacokinetic study of levetiracetam in children. *Epilepsia* 2001;42(12):1574–1579. doi:10.1046/j.1528-1157.2001.41300.x.
183. Vaisleib II, Neft RA. Rapid dosage titration of levetiracetam in children. *Pharmacotherapy* 2008;28(3):393–396. doi:10.1592/phco.28.3.393.
184. Halma E, de Louw AJ, Klinkenberg S, et al. Behavioral side-effects of levetiracetam in children with epilepsy: a systematic review. *Seizure* 2014;23(9):685–691. doi:10.1016/j.seizure.2014.06.004.
185. Chen B, Detyniecki K, Choi H, et al. Psychiatric and behavioral side effects of anti-epileptic drugs in adolescents and children with epilepsy. *Eur J Paediatr Neurol* 2017;21(3):441–449. doi:10.1016/j.ejpn.2017.02.003.
186. Bektaş G, Tekin U, Özkan MU, et al. The influence of levetiracetam on psychosocial and behavioral functioning in children: a case–control and follow-up study. *Epilepsy Behav* 2017;72:39–42. doi:10.1016/j.yebeh.2017.04.042.
187. Stratton SC, Large CH, Cox B, et al. Effects of lamotrigine and levetiracetam on seizure development in a rat amygdala kindling model. *Epilepsy Res* 2003;53(1–2):95–106. doi:10.1016/S0920-1211(02)00254-1.
188. Italiano D, Perucca E. Clinical pharmacokinetics of new-generation antiepileptic drugs at the extremes of age: an update. *Clin Pharmacokinet* 2013;52(8):627–645. doi:10.1007/s40262-013-0067-4.
189. Uthman BM, Bazil CW, Beydoun A, et al. Long-term add-on pregabalin treatment in patients with partial-onset epilepsy: pooled analysis of open-label clinical trials. *Epilepsia* 2010;51(6):968–978. doi:10.1111/j.1528-1167.2010.02532.x.
190. Ben-Menachem E. Pregabalin pharmacology and its relevance to clinical practice. *Epilepsia* 2004;45(Suppl 6):13–18. doi:10.1111/j.0013-9580.2004.455003.x.
191. Jan MM, Zuberi SA, Alsaihati BA. Pregabalin: preliminary experience in intractable childhood epilepsy. *Pediatr Neurol* 2009;40(5):347–350. doi:10.1016/j.pediatrneurol.2008.12.016.
192. Lyrica CIV (Pregabalin) medical information. New York, NY: Pfizer Inc., 2019.
193. Derry S, Bell RF, Straube S, et al. Pregabalin for neuropathic pain in adults. *Cochrane Database Syst Rev* 2019;2019(1):CD007076. doi:10.1002/14651858.CD007076.pub3.

194. Sills GJ. The mechanisms of action of gabapentin and pregabalin. *Curr Opin Pharmacol* 2006;6(1):108–113. doi:10.1016/j.coph.2005.11.003.
195. Elliott SP, Burke T, Smith C. Determining the toxicological significance of pregabalin in fatalities. *J Forensic Sci* 2017;62(1):169–173. doi:10.1111/1556-4029.13263.
196. Tiagabine in Lexi-Comp Online™, Pediatric & Neonatal Lexi-Drugs Online™. Hudson, OH: Lexi-Comp, Inc., 2020.
197. Genton P, Guerrini R, Perucca E. Tiagabine in clinical practice. *Epilepsia* 2001;42(Suppl 3):42–45. doi:10.1046/j.1528-1157.2001.042suppl.3042.x.
198. van der Poest Clement EA, Sahin M, Peters JM. Vigabatrin for epileptic spasms and tonic seizures in tuberous sclerosis complex. *J Child Neurol* 2018;33(8):519–524.
199. Nahata MC, Morosco RS. Stability of tiagabine in two oral liquid vehicles. *Am J Heal Pharm* 2003;60(1):75–77. doi:10.1093/ajhp/60.1.75.
200. Kälviäinen R. Long-term safety of tiagabine. *Epilepsia* 2001;42(Suppl 3):46–48. doi:10.1046/j.1528-1157.2001.042suppl.3046.x.
201. Sills GJ. Pre-clinical studies with the GABAergic compounds vigabatrin and tiagabine. *Epileptic Disord* 2003;5(1):51–56.
202. Perucca E, Bialer M. The clinical pharmacokinetics of the newer antiepileptic drugs. Focus on topiramate, zonisamide and tiagabine. *Clin Pharmacokinet* 1996;31(1):29–46. doi:10.2165/00003088-199631010-00003.
203. Pellock JM. Tiagabine (Gabitril) experience in children. *Epilepsia* 2001;42(Suppl 3):49–51. doi:10.1046/j.1528-1157.2001.042suppl.3049.x.
204. Dudra-Jastrzebska M, Andres-Mach MM, Sielski M, et al. Pharmacodynamic and pharmacokinetic interaction profiles of levetiracetam in combination with gabapentin, tiagabine and vigabatrin in the mouse pentylenetetrazole-induced seizure model: an isobolographic analysis. *Eur J Pharmacol* 2009;605(1–3):87–94. doi:10.1016/j.ejphar.2008.12.046.
205. Johannessen LC, Patsalos PN. Drug interactions involving the new second and third-generation antiepileptic drugs. *Expert Rev Neurother* 2010;10(1):119–140. doi:10.1586/ern.09.136.
206. Arzimanoglou A, Rahbani A. Zonisamide for the treatment of epilepsy. *Expert Rev Neurother* 2006;6(9):1283–1292. doi:10.1586/14737175.6.9.1283.
207. Wallander KM, Ohman I, Dahlin M. Zonisamide: pharmacokinetics, efficacy, and adverse events in children with epilepsy. *Neuropediatrics* 2014;45(6):362–370. doi:10.1055/s-0034-1387815.
208. Vivar KL, Mancl K, Seminario-Vidal L. Stevens-Johnson syndrome/toxic epidermal necrolysis associated with zonisamide. *Clin Case Rep* 2018;6(2):258–261. doi:10.1002/ccr3.1288.
209. Zonisamide (Zonegran) in Lexi-Comp Online™, Pediatric & Neonatal Lexi-Drugs Online™. Hudson, OH: Lexi-Comp, Inc., 2020.
210. Lotze TE, Wilfong AA. Zonisamide treatment for symptomatic infantile spasms. *Neurology* 2004;62(2):296–298. doi:10.1212/01.WNL.0000103284.73495.35.
211. Song JM, Hahn J, Kim SH, et al. Efficacy of treatments for infantile spasms. *Clin Neuropharmacol* 2017;40(2):63–84. doi:10.1097/wnf.0000000000000200.
212. Wilfong A, Wilmorei LJ. Zonisamide - a review of experience and use in partial seizures. *Neuropsychiatr Dis Treat* 2006;2(3):269–280. doi:10.2147/nedt.2006.2.3.269.
213. Eun SH, Kim HD, Eun BL, et al. Comparative trial of low and high-dose zonisamide as monotherapy for childhood epilepsy. *Seizure* 2011;20(7):558–563. doi:10.1016/j.seizure.2011.04.005.
214. Mimaki T. Clinical pharmacology and therapeutic drug monitoring of zonisamide. *Ther Drug Monit* 1998;20(6):593–597. doi:10.1097/00007691-199812000-00001.
215. Low PA, James S, Peschel T, et al. Zonisamide and associated oligohydrosis and hyperthermia. *Epilepsy Res* 2004;62(1):27–34. doi:10.1016/j.eplepsyres.2004.06.009.
216. Zonegran (Zonisamide) product labeling. Woodcliff Lake, NJ: Eisai Inc., 2016.
217. Okada M, Kaneko S, Hirano T, et al. Effects of zonisamide on dopaminergic system. *Epilepsy Res* 1995;22(3):193–205. doi:10.1016/0920-1211(95)00078-X.
218. Knudsen JF, Thambi LR, Kapcala LP, et al. Oligohydrosis and fever in pediatric patients treated with zonisamide. *Pediatr Neurol* 2003;28(3):184–189. doi:10.1016/S0887-8994(02)00511-8.
219. Liava A, Bonanni P. Efficacy of ZNS in highly refractory epilepsy in children: A monocentre clinical experience. *Epilepsia* 2009;50(Suppl 4). doi:10.1111/j.1528-1167.2009.02063.x.
220. Zaccara G, Tramacere L, Cincotta M. Drug safety evaluation of zonisamide for the treatment of epilepsy. *Expert Opin Drug Saf* 2011;10(4):623–631. doi:10.1517/14740338.2011.571201.
221. Ohtahara S, Yamatogi Y. Safety of zonisamide therapy: prospective follow-up survey. *Seizure* 2004;13(Suppl 1):S50–S55. doi:10.1016/j.seizure.2004.04.006.
222. Ohtahara S, Yamatogi Y. Erratum to Safety of zonisamide therapy: prospective follow-up survey. *Seizure* 2007;16(1):87–93. doi:10.1016/j.seizure.2006.01.005.
223. Ohtahara S. Zonisamide in the management of epilepsy - Japanese experience. *Epilepsy Res* 2006;68(Suppl 2):S25–S33. doi:10.1016/j.eplepsyres.2005.11.007.
224. Sills GJ, Brodie MJ. Pharmacokinetics and drug interactions with zonisamide. *Epilepsia* 2007;48(3):435–441. doi:10.1111/j.1528-1167.2007.00983.x.
225. Kappes JA, Hayes WJ, Strain JD, et al. Brivaracetam: an adjunctive treatment for partial-onset seizures. *J Clin Pharmacol* 2017;57(7):811–817. doi:10.1002/jcph.900.
226. Kwan P, Trinka E, Van Paesschen W, et al. Adjunctive brivaracetam for uncontrolled focal and generalized epilepsies: results of a phase III, double-blind, randomized, placebo-controlled, flexible-dose trial. *Epilepsia* 2014;55(1):38–46. doi:10.1111/epi.12391.
227. Brivaracetam in Lexi-Comp Online™, Pediatric & Neonatal Lexi-Drugs Online™. Hudson, OH: Lexi-Comp, Inc., 2020.
228. Zhang L, Li S, Li H, et al. Levetiracetam vs. brivaracetam for adults with refractory focal seizures: a meta-analysis and indirect comparison. *Seizure* 2016;39:28–33. doi:10.1016/j.seizure.2016.05.004.
229. Khaleghi F, Nemec EC. Brivaracetam (Briviact): a novel adjunctive therapy for partial-onset seizures. *P T* 2017;42(2):92–96.
230. Briviact (brivaracetam) product labeling. Smyrna, GA: UCB Inc., 2016.
231. Sargentini-Maier ML, Sokalski A, Boulanger P, et al. Brivaracetam disposition in renal impairment. *J Clin Pharmacol* 2012;52(12):1927–1933. doi:10.1177/0091270011431457.
232. Stockis A, Sargentini-Maier ML, Horsmans Y. Brivaracetam disposition in mild to severe hepatic impairment. *J Clin Pharmacol* 2013;53(6):633–641. doi:10.1002/jcph.82.
233. Klitgaard H, Matagne A, Nicolas JM, et al. Brivaracetam: rationale for discovery and preclinical profile of a selective SV2A ligand for epilepsy treatment. *Epilepsia* 2016;57(4):538–548. doi:10.1111/epi.13340.
234. Matagne A, Margineanu DG, Kenda B, et al. Anti-convulsive and anti-epileptic properties of brivaracetam (ucb 34714), a high-affinity ligand for the synaptic vesicle protein, SV2A. *Br J Pharmacol* 2008;154(8):1662–1671. doi:10.1038/bjp.2008.198.
235. Sargentini-Maier ML, Espié P, Coquette A, et al. Pharmacokinetics and metabolism of 14C-brivaracetam, a novel SV2A ligand, in healthy subjects. *Drug Metab Dispos* 2008;36(1):36–45. doi:10.1124/dmd.107.017129.
236. Stephen LJ, Brodie MJ. Brivaracetam: a novel antiepileptic drug for focal-onset seizures. *Ther Adv Neurol Disord* 2017;11:1756285617742081. doi:10.1177/1756285617742081.
237. Stockis A, Watanabe S, Rouits E, et al. Brivaracetam single and multiple rising oral dose study in healthy Japanese participants: influence of CYP2C19 genotype. *Drug Metab Pharmacokinet* 2014;29(5):394–399. doi:10.2133/dmpk.DMPK-14-RG-010.
238. Dean L. Brivaracetam therapy and CYP2C19 genotype. In: Pratt VM, McLeod HL, Rubinstein WS, et al., eds. *Medical genetics summaries.* Bethesda, MD: National Center for Biotechnology Information, 2012.
239. Schoemaker R, Wade JR, Stockis A. Extrapolation of a brivaracetam exposure–response model from adults to children with focal seizures. *Clin Pharmacokinet* 2018;57(7):843–854. doi:10.1007/s40262-017-0597-2.
240. Moseley BD, Kervyn S, Nicolas JM, et al. A review of the drug-drug interactions of the new antiepileptic drug brivaracetam. *Epilepsia* 2016;57(S2). doi:10.1111/epi.13609.
241. Hemming K, Maguire MJ, Hutton JL, et al. Vigabatrin for refractory partial epilepsy. *Cochrane Database Syst Rev* 2013;(1):CD007302. doi:10.1002/14651858.CD007302.pub2.
242. Perucca E, Gram L, Avanzini G, et al. Antiepileptic drugs as a cause of worsening seizures. *Epilepsia* 1998;39(1):5–17. doi:10.1111/j.1528-1157.1998.tb01268.x.
243. Taketomo CK, Hodding JH, Kraus DM. Vigabatrin. In: *Pediatric & neonatal dosage handbook*, 26th ed. Hudson, OH: Lexi-Comp, 2019.
244. Kälviäinen R, Nousiainen I, Mäntyjärvi M, et al. Vigabatrin, a GABAergic antiepileptic drug, causes concentric visual field defects. *Neurology* 1999;53(5):922–926. doi:10.1212/wnl.53.5.922.
245. Manuchehri K, Goodman S, Siviter L, et al. A controlled study of vigabatrin and visual abnormalities. *Br J Ophthalmol* 2000;84(5):499–505. doi:10.1136/bjo.84.5.499.
246. Spencer EL, Harding GF. Examining visual field defects in the paediatric population exposed to vigabatrin. *Doc Ophthalmol* 2003;107(3):281–287. doi:10.1023/B:DOOP.0000005337.39947.83.
247. Heim MK, Gidal BE. Vigabatrin-associated retinal damage - potential biochemical mechanisms. *Acta Neurol Scand* 2012;126(4):219–228. doi:10.1111/j.1600-0404.2012.01684.x.
248. Appleton R, Baxter P, Calver D, et al. Guideline for prescribing vigabatrin in children has been revised. *Br Med J* 2001;322(7280):236–237. doi:10.1136/bmj.320.7246.1404.
249. Walker SD, Kälviäinen R. Non-vision adverse events with vigabatrin therapy. *Acta Neurol Scand* 2011;192:72–82. doi:10.1111/j.1600-0404.2011.01602.x.
250. Carmant L. Vigabatrin therapy for infantile spasms: review of major trials in Europe, Canada, and the United States; and recommendations for dosing. *Acta Neurol Scand* 2011;192:36–47. doi:10.1111/j.1600-0404.2011.01599.x.
251. Vigevano F, Cilio MR. Vigabatrin versus ACTH as first-line treatment for infantile spasms: a randomized, prospective study. *Epilepsia* 1997;38(12):1270–1274. doi:10.1111/j.1528-1157.1997.tb00063.x.
252. Knupp KG, Coryell J, Nickels KC, et al. Response to treatment in a prospective national infantile spasms cohort. *Ann Neurol* 2016;79(3):475–484. doi:10.1002/ana.24594.
253. Herranz JL, Arteaga R, Farr IN, et al. Dose-response study of vigabatrin in children with refractory epilepsy. *J Child Neurol* 1991;(Suppl 2):S45–S51. doi:10.1177/0883073891006002091.
254. Ben-Menachem E, Sander JW. Vigabatrin therapy for refractory complex partial seizures: review of major European trials. *Acta Neurol Scand Suppl* 2011;192:16–28. doi:10.1111/j.1600-0404.2011.01597.x.
255. Petroff OA, Rothman DL. Measuring human brain GABA in vivo - Effects of GABA-transaminase inhibition with vigabatrin. *Mol Neurobiol* 1998;16(1):97–121. doi:10.1007/BF02740605.
256. Schechter P. Clinical pharmacology of vigabatrin. *Br J Clin Pharmacol* 1989;27(Suppl 1):19S–22S. doi:10.1111/j.1365-2125.1989.tb03456.x.
257. Rey E, Pons G, Olive G. Vigabatrin: clinical pharmacokinetics. *Clin Pharmacokinet* 1992;23(4):267–278. doi:10.2165/00003088-199223040-00003
258. Nielsen JC, Kowalski KG, Karim A, et al. Population pharmacokinetics analysis of vigabatrin in adults and children with epilepsy and children with infantile spasms. *Clin Pharmacokinet* 2014;53(11):1019–1031. doi:10.1007/s40262-014-0172-z.
259. Lundbeck Canada Inc., Saint-Laurent QH 0A9. Vigabatrin product monograph (Sabril).
260. Perucca E, Yasothan U, Clincke G, et al. Lacosamide. *Nat Rev Drug Discov* 2008;7(12):973–974. doi:10.1038/nrd2764.
261. de Biase S, Valente M, Gigli GL, et al. Pharmacokinetic drug evaluation of lacosamide for the treatment of partial-onset seizures. *Expert Opin Drug Metab Toxicol* 2017;13(9):997–1005. doi:10.1080/17425255.2017.1360278.
262. Grosso S, Parisi P, Spalice A, et al. Efficacy and safety of lacosamide in infants and young children with refractory focal epilepsy. *Eur J Paediatr Neurol* 2014;18(1):55–59. doi:10.1016/j.ejpn.2013.08.006.
263. Sanmartí-Vilaplana F, Díaz-Gómez A. The effectiveness and safety of lacosamide in children with epilepsy in a clinical practice setting. *Epilepsy Behav* 2018;79:130–137. doi:10.1016/j.yebeh.2017.11.024.
264. Taketomo CK, Hodding JH, Kraus DM. Lacosamide. In: *Pediatric & neonatal dosage handbook*, 26th ed. Hudson, OH: Lexi-Comp, 2019.
265. Cawello W, Stockis A, Andreas JO, et al. Advances in epilepsy treatment: lacosamide pharmacokinetic profile. *Ann N Y Acad Sci* 2014;1329:18–32. doi:10.1111/nyas.12513.
266. Fernandez A, Claassen J. Refractory status epilepticus. *Curr Opin Crit Care* 2012;18(2):127–131. doi:10.1097/MCC.0b013e32835132cc.

267. Cross SA, Curran MP. Lacosamide: in partial-onset seizures. *Drugs* 2009;69(4):449–459. doi:10.2165/00003495-200969040-00005.
268. Curia G, Biagini G, Perucca E, et al. Lacosamide: a new approach to target voltage-gated sodium currents in epileptic disorders. *CNS Drugs* 2009;23(7):555–568. doi:10.2165/00023210-200923070-00002.
269. Verrotti A, Loiacono G, Pizzolorusso A, et al. Corrigendum to "lacosamide in pediatric and adult patients: comparison of efficacy and safety" *[Seizure* 22 (2013) 210–216]. *Seizure* 2014;23(4)325. doi:10.1016/j.seizure.2013.10.007.
270. Jacob S, Nair AB. An updated overview on therapeutic drug monitoring of recent antiepileptic drugs. *Drugs R D* 2016;16(4):303–316. doi:10.1007/s40268-016-0148-6.
271. Besag FM. Rufinamide for the treatment of Lennox-Gastaut syndrome. *Expert Opin Pharmacother* 2011;12(5):801–806. doi:10.1517/14656566.2011.560836.
272. Saneto RP, Anderson GD. Onset of action and seizure control in Lennox-Gastaut syndrome: focus on rufinamide. *Ther Clin Risk Manag* 2009;5:271–280. doi:10.2147/tcrm.s4282.
273. Hakimian S, Hakimian AC, Anderson GD, et al. Rufinamide: a new anti-epileptic medication. *Expert Opin Pharmacother* 2007;8(12):1931–1940.
274. Miller-Horn J, Spiegel R, Bello L, et al. Clinical experience with rufinamide in an academic medical center. *Epilepsia* 2009;50(Suppl 11):253. doi:10.1111/j.1528-1167.2009.02377.x.
275. Glauser T, Kluger G, Sachdeo R, et al. Rufinamide for generalized seizures associated with Lennox-Gastaut syndrome. *Neurology* 2008;70(21):1950–1958. doi:10.1212/01.wnl.0000303813.95800.0d.
276. Rufinamide: CGP 33101, E 2080, RUF 331, Xilep. *Drugs R D* 2005;6(4):249–252. doi:10.2165/00126839-200506040-00010.
277. Deeks ED, Scott LJ. Rufinamide. *CNS Drugs* 2006;20(9):751–760. doi:10.2165/00023210-200620090-00007.
278. Perucca E, Cloyd J, Critchley D, et al. Rufinamide: clinical pharmacokinetics and concentration-response relationships in patients with epilepsy. *Epilepsia* 2008;49(7):1123–1141. doi:10.1111/j.1528-1167.2008.01665.x.
279. Klehm J, Thome-Souza S, Sánchez Fernández I, et al. Clobazam: effect on frequency of seizures and safety profile in different subgroups of children with epilepsy. *Pediatr Neurol* 2014;51(1):60–66.
280. Yang LP, Scott LJ. Clobazam: in patients with Lennox-Gastaut syndrome. *CNS Drugs* 2012;26(11):983–991. doi:10.1007/s40263-012-0007-0.
281. Mahmoud SH, Rans C. Systematic review of clobazam use in patients with status epilepticus. *Epilepsia Open* 2018;3(3):323–330. doi:10.1002/epi4.12230.
282. Paolicchi JM, Ross G, Lee D, et al. Clobazam and aggression-related adverse events in pediatric patients with Lennox-Gastaut syndrome. *Pediatr Neurol* 2015;53(4):338–342. doi:10.1016/j.pediatrneurol.2015.06.021.
283. Dang CD, Beets-Shay L, Kahn EC. Toxic epidermal necrolysis triggered by clobazam: a case report in a 13-year-old girl. *Pediatr Dermatol* 2015;32(3):e102–e103. doi:10.1111/pde.12527.
284. Yapici AK, Fidanci MK, Kilic S, et al. Stevens-Johnson syndrome triggered by a combination of clobazam, lamotrigine and valproic acid in a 7-year-old child. *Ann Burns Fire Disasters.* 2014;27(3):121–125.
285. ONFI® (clobazam) tablets, for oral use, CIV None (4) ONFI® (clobazam) oral suspension, CIV. Deerfield, IL: Lundbeck, 2013.
286. Capecitabine, clobazam: risk of SJS/TEN. *React Wkly* 2013;1482:5. doi:10.1007/s40278-013-7687-1.
287. Conry JA, Ng YT, Paolicchi JM, et al. Clobazam in the treatment of Lennox-Gastaut syndrome. *Epilepsia* 2009;50(5):1158–1166. doi:10.1111/j.1528-1167.2008.01935.x.
288. Ng YT, Conry J, Paolicchi J, et al. Long-term safety and efficacy of clobazam for Lennox-Gastaut syndrome: interim results of an open-label extension study. *Epilepsy Behav* 2012;25(4):687–694. doi:10.1016/j.yebeh.2012.09.039.
289. Taketomo CK, Hodding JH, Kraus DM. Clobazam. In: *Pediatric & neonatal dosage handbook*, 26th ed. Hudson, OH: Lexi-Comp, 2019.
290. Gauthier AC, Mattson RH. Clobazam: a safe, efficacious, and newly rediscovered therapeutic for epilepsy. *CNS Neurosci Ther* 2015;21(7):543–548. doi:10.1111/cns.12399.
291. Tolbert D, Larsen F. A comprehensive overview of the clinical pharmacokinetics of clobazam. *J Clin Pharmacol* 2019;59(1):7–19. doi:10.1002/jcph.1313.
292. Burns ML, Baftiu A, Opdal MS, et al. Therapeutic drug monitoring of clobazam and its metabolite-impact of age and comedication on pharmacokinetic variability. *Ther Drug Monit* 2016;38(3):350–357. doi:10.1097/FTD.0000000000000272.
293. Walzer M, Bekersky I, Blum RA, et al. Pharmacokinetic drug interactions between clobazam and drugs metabolized by cytochrome P450 isoenzymes. *Pharmacotherapy* 2012;32(4):340–353. doi:10.1002/j.1875-9114.2012.01028.x.
294. Tolbert D, Bekersky I, Chu HM, et al. Drug-metabolism mechanism: knowledge-based population pharmacokinetic approach for characterizing clobazam drug-drug interactions. *J Clin Pharmacol* 2016;56(3):365–374. doi:10.1002/jcph.603.
295. Taeuber K, Badian M, Brettel H, et al. Kinetic and dynamic interaction of clobazam and alcohol. *Br J Clin Pharmacol* 1979;7(Suppl 1):91S–97S. doi:10.1111/j.1365-2125.1979.tb04672.x.
296. Theis JG, Koren G, Daneman R, et al. Interactions of clobazam with conventional antiepileptics in children. *J Child Neurol* 1997;12(3):208–213. doi:10.1177/088307389701200311.
297. Galiana GL, Gauthier AC, Mattson RH. Eslicarbazepine acetate: a new improvement on a classic drug family for the treatment of partial-onset seizures. *Drugs R D* 2017;17(3):329–339. doi:10.1007/s40268-017-0197-5.
298. Lattanzi S, Brigo F, Grillo E, et al. Adjunctive eslicarbazepine acetate in pediatric patients with focal epilepsy: a systematic review and meta-analysis. *CNS Drugs* 2018;32(3):189–196. doi:10.1007/s40263-018-0504-x.
299. Kay L, Willems LM, Zöllner JP, et al. Eslicarbazepine acetate as a therapeutic option in a patient with carbamazepine-induced rash and HLA-A*31:01. *Seizure* 2017;47:81–82. doi:10.1016/j.seizure.2017.02.019.
300. Zaccara G, Giovannelli F, Maratea D, et al. Neurological adverse events of new generation sodium blocker antiepileptic drugs. Meta-analysis of randomized, double-blinded studies with eslicarbazepine acetate, lacosamide and oxcarbazepine. *Seizure* 2013;22(7):528–536. doi:10.1016/j.seizure.2013.03.016.
301. Taketomo CK, Hodding JH, Kraus DM. Eslicarbazepine acetate. In: *Pediatric & neonatal dosage handbook*, 26th ed. Hudson, OH: Lexi-Comp, 2019.
302. Soares-da-Silva P, Pires N, Bonifácio MJ, et al. Eslicarbazepine acetate for the treatment of focal epilepsy: an update on its proposed mechanisms of action. *Pharmacol Res Perspect* 2015;3(2):e00124. doi:10.1002/prp2.124.
303. Almeida L, Minciu I, Nunes T, et al. Pharmacokinetics, efficacy, and tolerability of eslicarbazepine acetate in children and adolescents with epilepsy. *J Clin Pharmacol* 2008;48(8):966–977. doi:10.1177/0091270008319706.
304. Shvarts V, Chung S. Perampanel: newly approved, novel antiepileptic medication for partial-onset seizures. *Expert Rev Neurother* 2013;13(2):131–134. doi:10.1586/ern.12.154.
305. Cokley J, Kotagal P, Hoover J. Perampanel (Fycompa) use in the treatment of pediatric epilepsy P5.234. *Neurology* 2017;88(16 Suppl). http://www.neurology.org/cgi/content/short/88/16_Supplement/P5.234?rss=1.
306. Dougherty ML. Epilepsy essentials. Perampanel: novel mechanism for the management of epilepsy an epilepsy specialist reviews the role of a new AMPA receptor agonist for epilepsy. 2014 https://practicalneurology.com/articles/2014-julyaug/perampanel-novel-mechanism-for-the-management-of-epilepsy. .
307. Fycompa (Perampanel) prescribing information. Woodcliff Lake, NJ: Eisai R&D Management, 2016.
308. Franco V, Crema F, Iudice A, et al. Novel treatment options for epilepsy: focus on perampanel. *Pharmacol Res* 2013;70(1):35–40. doi:10.1016/j.phrs.2012.12.006.
309. Hussein Z, Critchley D, Ferry J, et al. Population pharmacokinetics of perampanel, a selective, noncompetitive AMPA receptor antagonist, in patients with refractory partial-onset seizures participating in a randomized, double-blind, placebo-controlled phase III study. *Epilepsia* 2011;52(Suppl 6):248–249. doi:10.1111/j.1528-1167.2011.03207.x.
310. Bialer M, Soares-Da-Silva P. Pharmacokinetics and drug interactions of eslicarbazepine acetate. *Epilepsia* 2012;53(6):935–946. doi:10.1111/j.1528-1167.2012.03519.x.
311. Nickels KC, Wirrell EC. Stiripentol in the management of epilepsy. *CNS Drugs* 2017;31(5):405–416. doi:10.1007/s40263-017-0432-1.
312. Taketomo CK, Hodding JH, Kraus DM. Stiripentol. In: *Pediatric & neonatal dosage handbook*, 26th ed. Hudson, OH: Lexi-Comp, 2019:2004–2006.
313. Diacomit® (Stiripentol) prescribing information. Beauvais, France: Laboratoires Biocodex, 2018.
314. Chiron C, Marchand MC, Tran A, et al. Stiripentol in severe myoclonic epilepsy in infancy: a randomised placebo-controlled syndrome-dedicated trial. *Lancet* 2000;356(9242):1638–1642. doi:10.1016/S0140-6736(00)03157-3.
315. Chiron C, Helias M, Kaminska A, et al. Do children with Dravet syndrome continue to benefit from stiripentol for long through adulthood? *Epilepsia* 2018;59(9):1705–1717. doi:10.1111/epi.14536.
316. Levy RH, Lin HS, Blehaut HM, et al. Pharmacokinetics of stiripentol in normal man: evidence of nonlinearity. *J Clin Pharmacol* 1983;23(11–12):523–533. doi:10.1002/j.1552-4604.1983.tb01799.x.
317. Peigné S, Chhun S, Tod M, et al. Population pharmacokinetics of stiripentol in paediatric patients with Dravet syndrome treated with stiripentol, valproate and clobazam combination therapy. *Clin Pharmacokinet* 2018;57(6):739–748. doi:10.1007/s40262-017-0592-7.
318. Giraud C, Treluyer JM, Rey E, et al. In vitro and in vivo inhibitory effect of stiripentol on clobazam metabolism. *Drug Metab Dispos* 2006;34(4):608–611. doi:10.1124/dmd.105.007237.
319. Patsalos PN, Zugman M, Lake C, et al. Serum protein binding of 25 antiepileptic drugs in a routine clinical setting: a comparison of free non–protein-bound concentrations. *Epilepsia* 2017;58(7):1234–1243. doi:10.1111/epi.13802.
320. Szaflarski JP, Bebin EM, Cutter G, et al. Cannabidiol improves frequency and severity of seizures and reduces adverse events in an open-label add-on prospective study. *Epilepsy Behav* 2018;87:131–136. doi:10.1016/j.yebeh.2018.07.020.
321. Taketomo CK, Hodding JH, Kraus DM. Cannabidiol. In: *Pediatric & neonatal dosage handbook*, 26th ed. Hudson, OH: Lexi-Comp, 2019:378–380.
322. Bonn-Miller MO, Loflin MJE, Thomas BF, Marcu JP, Hyke T, Vandrey R. Labeling Accuracy of Cannabidiol Extracts Sold Online. *JAMA.* 2017;318(17):1708–1709. doi:10.1001/jama.2017.11909.
323. EPIDIOLEX® (cannabidiol) oral solution package insert. Carlsbad, CA: Greenwich Biosciences, 2018.
324. Samanta D. Cannabidiol: a review of clinical efficacy and safety in epilepsy. *Pediatr Neurol* 2019;96:24–29. doi:10.1016/j.pediatrneurol.2019.03.014.
325. Devinsky O, Patel AD, Cross JH, et al. Effect of cannabidiol on drop seizures in the Lennox–Gastaut syndrome. *N Engl J Med* 2018;378(20):1888–1897. doi:10.1056/NEJMoa1714631.
326. Devinsky O, Nabbout R, Miller I, et al. Maintenance of long-term safety and efficacy of cannabidiol (CBD) treatment in Dravet syndrome (DS): results of the open-label extension (OLE) trial (GWPCARE 5). *Dev Med Child Neurol* 2017. doi:10.1111/dmcn.13623.
327. Devinsky O, Nabbout R, Miller I, et al. Long-term cannabidiol treatment in patients with Dravet syndrome: an open-label extension trial. *Epilepsia* 2019;60(2):294–302. doi:10.1111/epi.14628.
328. Rimmerman N, Ben-Hail D, Porat Z, et al. Direct modulation of the outer mitochondrial membrane channel, voltage-dependent anion channel 1 (VDAC1) by cannabidiol: A novel mechanism for cannabinoid-induced cell death. *Cell Death Dis* 2013;4:e949. doi:10.1038/cddis.2013.471.
329. Vezzani A, French J, Bartfai T, et al. The role of inflammation in epilepsy. *Nat Rev Neurol* 2011;7(1):31–40. doi:10.1038/nrneurol.2010.178.
330. Wheless JW, Dlugos D, Miller I, et al. Pharmacokinetics and tolerability of multiple doses of pharmaceutical-grade synthetic cannabidiol in pediatric patients with treatment-resistant epilepsy. *CNS Drugs* 2019;33(6):593–604. doi:10.1007/s40263-019-00624-4.
331. Millar SA, Stone NL, Yates AS, et al. A systematic review on the pharmacokinetics of cannabidiol in humans. *Front Pharmacol* 2018;9:1365. doi:10.3389/fphar.2018.01365.
332. Stafstrom CE, Ockuly JC, Murphree L, et al. Anticonvulsant and antiepileptic actions of 2-deoxy-D-glucose in epilepsy models. *Ann Neurol* 2009;65(4):435–447. doi:10.1002/ana.21603.
333. Bialer M, White HS. Key factors in the discovery and development of new antiepileptic drugs. *Nat Rev Drug Discov* 2010;9(1):68–82. doi:10.1038/nrd2997.
334. Depondt C, Godard P, Espel RS, et al. A candidate gene study of antiepileptic drug tolerability and efficacy identifies an association of CYP2C9 variants with phenytoin toxicity. *Eur J Neurol* 2011;18(9):1159–1164. doi:10.1111/j.1468-1331.2011.03361.x.

Ayman Saleh
Gabrielle Sky Cardwell
Robert L. Findling
Adelaide S. Robb

CHAPTER 34

Antidepressants and Mood Stabilizers

Antidepressants and mood stabilizers are important treatment options for pediatric mood and anxiety disorders and should be used as part of a comprehensive treatment plan including psychotherapy and appropriate educational placement. Clinicians should complete a detailed psychiatric and family history from the patient, parent, and collateral sources and identify target symptoms for treatment with medication. This chapter covers the major antidepressant classes and mood stabilizers used to treat major depressive disorder (MDD), anxiety disorders, and bipolar disorder (BD) in children and adolescents.

Presenting psychiatric and somatic complaints should be well documented, may be measured by standard scales, and compared after a sufficient trial of the medication. Baseline parameters, including laboratories, electrocardiogram for tricyclic antidepressants (TCAs), vital signs, weight, and height, should be obtained and followed throughout the treatment period. All medications should be initiated at the labeled starting dose and titrated to reach the recommended therapeutic level or dose. This titration process should be clearly explained to patients and families. Side effects, including boxed warnings (BWs), should be monitored closely, especially in the first few weeks after initiating or titrating the medication.

The evidence base of positive trials for the use of antidepressants and mood stabilizers in pediatric populations is smaller than that in adults. Therefore, some medications are prescribed off-label in certain diagnoses and age ranges.

BOXED WARNING

Following the completion of a safety review of the use of nine antidepressants in pediatric populations, the U.S. Food and Drug Administration (FDA) issued a BW to indicate an increased risk of suicidal ideation and suicidal attempts in children and adolescents treated with certain antidepressants.[1] The safety review included fluoxetine, sertraline, paroxetine, fluvoxamine, citalopram, bupropion, venlafaxine, and nefazodone. The results indicated a 3.8% increase in suicidal ideation/attempts in the medication group, compared to 2.1% in the placebo group.[1] The increase in suicidal ideation was most significant in the paroxetine group, so the FDA added a contraindication warning for the use of paroxetine in children.[1] It is important to note that none of the 4,400 trial participants in the FDA database completed suicide.[1] The BW was extended to young adults (ages 18 to 24 years) in 2006, after a second review of adult data showed a similar trend of increased suicidal ideation/attempts with the use of antidepressants in the young adult age group.[2] The FDA, in consultation with the American Academy of Child and Adolescent Psychiatry (AACAP), issued guidelines for monitoring children and adolescents using antidepressants. The guidelines recommend weekly face-to-face monitoring after initiating or increasing the dose of an antidepressant. The monitoring frequency can be decreased to biweekly or monthly in the follow-up period.[3,4]

SELECTIVE SEROTONIN REUPTAKE INHIBITORS

Selective serotonin reuptake inhibitors (SSRIs) are the most commonly used antidepressants in pediatric populations due to their low side effect profile and good tolerability. SSRIs are reported to be helpful in a variety of mood and anxiety disorders including, but not limited to, MDD, generalized anxiety disorder (GAD), and obsessive-compulsive disorder (OCD). The six main SSRIs are fluoxetine, sertraline, fluvoxamine, citalopram, escitalopram, and paroxetine (Table 34.1).

Fluoxetine is the most studied SSRI in pediatric populations. Fluoxetine has the longest half-life (16 days after long-term use) in the SSRI group. The long half-life decreases the withdrawal symptoms and improves tolerability.[5] Fluoxetine was the first antidepressant to show superiority to placebo (56% improved vs. 33% improved) in a double-blind trial for child and adolescent MDD in 96 youth at a dose of 20 mg daily.[6] A second multisite trial of 20 mg fluoxetine versus placebo confirmed these findings with a significantly greater decrease in depression scores on medication than placebo.[7] These two positive MDD trials led to the FDA labeling of fluoxetine for MDD in youth ages 8 to 17 years. Fluoxetine is effective in treating pediatric OCD and is FDA approved for OCD treatment in children ages 8 to 17 years. Two randomized controlled trials (RCTs) in children with OCD showed a 40% to 49% response rate using the Children's Yale-Brown Obsessive-Compulsive Scale (CY-BOCS) after being treated with fluoxetine (20 to 60 mg daily) for 8 weeks.[8,9] Fluoxetine was found to be effective in treating several additional anxiety disorders. Birmaher et al. compared fluoxetine to placebo in an RCT for 12 weeks in 74 children with anxiety disorders: social anxiety disorder (SAD), GAD, and separation anxiety disorder (SepD). Sixty-one percent of the fluoxetine group showed a reduction in Clinical Global Impression (CGI)

TABLE 34.1 SSRI and SNRI FDA Indications and Positive Trials in Pediatric Population

Medication	*FDA Indication*	*Other Positive Trials*	*Daily Dose*	*Schedule*
SSRIs				
Fluoxetine	MDD (ages 8–17) OCD (ages 8–17)	SAD, GAD, SepD	10–60 mg[5–10]	Qday
Sertraline	OCD (ages 6–17)	SAD, GAD, SepD	25–200 mg[12–16,19–21]	Qday
Citalopram		MDD	10–40 mg[31]	Qday
Escitalopram	MDD (ages 12–17)	SAD	5–20 mg[28–32]	Qday
Fluvoxamine	OCD (ages 8–17)	MDD, SAD, GAD, SepD	25–300 mg[34–36]	Qday
SNRIs				
Venlafaxine		MDD, SAD	37.5–300 mg[37,38,40]	Qday
Desvenlafaxine			25–100 mg[39,41]	Qday
Duloxetine	GAD (ages 7–17)	Chronic pain	30–120 mg[42–45]	Qday
TCAs				
Clomipramine	OCD (ages 10–17)		25–200 mg[50]	Qday or BID

BID, twice a day; FDA, U.S. Food and Drug Administration; GAD, generalized anxiety disorder; MDD, major depressive disorder; OCD, obsessive-compulsive disorder; Qday, once a day; SAD, social anxiety disorder; SepD, separation anxiety disorder; SNRIs, serotonin norepinephrine reuptake inhibitors; SSRIs, selective serotonin reuptake inhibitors; TCAs, tricyclic antidepressants.

scale score to subclinical level.[10] Long-term use of fluoxetine showed progressive improvement in anxiety symptoms and CGI score even after 6 months, compared to placebo.[11]

Sertraline has been widely studied in pediatric anxiety and MDD trials funded by federal and industry sponsors. Several studies showed consistent benefits of sertraline in treating children with OCD and OCD with comorbid tic disorder.[12–15] Long-term use of sertraline showed persistent reduction of OCD symptoms and good tolerability in a study that lasted for 52 weeks.[16] The National Institutes of Health (NIH) POTS (pediatric OCD treatment study) compared placebo, sertraline, cognitive behavioral therapy (CBT), and combination therapy (sertraline plus CBT). Combination treatment was more effective and long-lasting in treating OCD, compared to sertraline alone.[17–19] Based on these trials sertraline was FDA approved for the treatment of pediatric OCD in children aged 6 to 17 years.[12,20] Additional RCTs showed significant effects of sertraline in treating MDD and GAD compared to placebo.[21,22] The MDD trials were two separate multisite studies that only showed separation from placebo when combined into one large trial, so the medication was not approved for the treatment of pediatric MDD (two positive trials are necessary for FDA approval in MDD). The Child/Adolescent Anxiety Multimodal Study (CAMS) compared the effectiveness of placebo, sertraline, CBT, and combination treatment (sertraline plus CBT) in three common pediatric anxiety disorders—SAD, GAD, and SepD—in 488 participants. Combination therapy had an 81% response rate (CGI score ≤ 2), followed by 60% response rate for CBT, 55% response rate in sertraline, and finally 28% response rate in placebo.[23] Robb et al. studied the effect of sertraline in treating posttraumatic stress disorder (PTSD) in 131 participants for 10 weeks. Sertraline did not demonstrate efficacy in treating PTSD compared to placebo.[24]

Citalopram was found to be effective in treating MDD in a double-blind RCT with 174 children and adolescents with a maximum dose of 40 mg per day.[25] Citalopram was also found to be effective in treating anxiety-induced recurrent abdominal pain in children.[26,27] Escitalopram is a highly selective inhibitor for serotonin transporter and is the active *S*-enantiomer of citalopram.[28] It shows a rapid onset of symptom improvement and has a predictable tolerability profile of mild adverse events.[28] Escitalopram is approved for the treatment of MDD in children between ages 12 and 17 years based on several large trials of children and adolescents.[29–32] An open-label trial of escitalopram for SAD in 20 children (age 10 to 17 years) showed significant response (CGI score ≤ 2) in 65% of the population after 12 weeks.[33]

Fluvoxamine received FDA approval for the treatment of pediatric OCD in children ages 8 to 17 years after showing significant efficacy compared to placebo in a 10-week RCT. Patients were provided a dose ranging between 50 and 200 mg daily (the dose was divided into twice a day). Thirty-nine percent of those treated with fluvoxamine showed a significant reduction in CY-BOCS ratings compared to 28% of those treated with placebo.[34] A large NIH trial of 128 youth with SAD, GAD, or SepD compared fluvoxamine up to 300 mg daily with placebo and had a statistically significant reduction in anxiety symptoms compared with placebo and had 76% responders versus 29% responders on placebo.[35] Fluvoxamine showed low evidence of benefit in the treatment of GAD and MDD in a combination trial.[36]

SELECTIVE NOREPINEPHRINE REUPTAKE INHIBITORS

Selective norepinephrine reuptake inhibitors (SNRIs) are the second antidepressant group extensively studied in pediatric MDD and anxiety disorders. The SNRI group includes venlafaxine, desvenlafaxine, duloxetine, and levomilnacipran. None of the SNRIs are FDA approved for the treatment of pediatric MDD, but duloxetine is FDA approved for the treatment of pediatric GAD. Levomilnacipran is currently under investigation in Phase III trials for the treatment of pediatric MDD (see Table 34.1).

Venlafaxine was found to be effective in treating adolescents with MDD ages 12 to 17 years, but not in children younger than

12 years based on two large randomized trials.[37] The TORDIA (treatment of resistant depression in adolescents) study examined teenagers who had already failed a trial of an antidepressant by switching them to venlafaxine or a second SSRI with or without add-on CBT. TORDIA demonstrated that venlafaxine was equal to other SSRI antidepressants in treating teens with resistant MDD.[38] However, venlafaxine was associated with a higher rate of secondary hypertension compared to SSRIs, as two patients on venlafaxine and none on SSRI were withdrawn from the study for the development of hypertension.[39] In a study that was conducted in 48 academic centers with 293 participants ages 8 to 17 years, venlafaxine (37.5 to 225 mg) was compared to placebo in 293 youth with SAD, and 56% of those on venlafaxine were responders on the clinical global improvement scale compared to 37% on placebo.[40] There are only two RCTs that have investigated desvenlafaxine in pediatric MDD. Both studies failed to prove its effectiveness in treating pediatric MDD compared to placebo.[39,41] In an RCT examining duloxetine as a treatment for GAD in 272 participants ages 7 to 17 years, duloxetine was found to be superior to placebo on both the pediatric anxiety rating scale and on measures of remission and response. This finding led to the FDA approval of duloxetine to treat GAD.[42] Duloxetine was also found to be effective in treating chronic pain disorder (see Table 34.1).[43,44] However, duloxetine was not effective in treating pediatric MDD.[45]

TRICYCLIC ANTIDEPRESSANTS

TCAs are known to be effective in treating adults with mood and anxiety disorder; however, they are used as a second-line treatment due to the risk of severe side effects, most significantly cardiovascular.[46–48] TCAs commonly used in pediatric populations are clomipramine and imipramine. Clomipramine was the first FDA-approved treatment for pediatric OCD.[49] A recent meta-analysis found that clomipramine was more effective than SSRIs including fluoxetine, fluvoxamine, paroxetine, and sertraline in treating pediatric OCD.[50] Imipramine is FDA approved for the treatment of nocturnal enuresis for children older than 6 years. Results from controlled trials evaluating the effectiveness of imipramine to treat pediatric anxiety and mood disorders, however, have yielded mixed results. In an early double-blind, placebo-controlled study of 35 children with school-related phobia, imipramine was more effective than placebo in reducing anxiety, and children who received imipramine were more likely to return to school.[51] Another study found that imipramine plus CBT is more effective than placebo plus CBT in improving symptoms of depression and inducing greater school attendance in school-refusing adolescents.[52] However, a double-blind, placebo-controlled study in 20 children (ages 6 to 15 years) with separation anxiety found that imipramine was not superior to placebo.[53] Therefore, imipramine may be an effective treatment for some pediatric anxiety–related disorders, such as school phobias, but not for others, such as separation anxiety.

OTHER ANTIDEPRESSANTS INCLUDING SELEGILINE, BUPROPION, MIRTAZAPINE, AND BUSPIRONE

Selegiline is the only monoamine oxidase inhibitor (MAOI) antidepressant medication studied in the pediatric population. Transdermal selegiline failed to separate from placebo in a double-blind RCT of adolescents with MDD.[54] Bupropion has a unique mechanism of action in which it blocks dopamine and norepinephrine reuptake[55] and antagonizes nicotinic receptors.[56] Although there are no available double-blind, placebo-controlled studies examining its effects in treating children with mood disorders, an open-label trial in 24 adolescents found bupropion to be effective in treating comorbid MDD and Attention-Deficit/Hyperactivity Disorder (ADHD).[57] Further studies are needed to determine if bupropion is an effective treatment for pediatric mood disorders. Mirtazapine enhances noradrenergic and serotonergic neurotransmission by blocking α2-adrenergic and postsynaptic 5-HT2 and 5-HT3 receptors.[49] Mirtazapine showed marked effect in treating MDD in an open-label trial with 24 adolescents.[58] However, it was not an effective treatment for adolescents with SAD due to severe side effects including sedation, irritability, and weight gain.[59] Buspirone is a nonhypnotic anxiolytic medication. Two RCTs examining the use of buspirone to treat pediatric GAD reported null results.[60]

MOOD STABILIZERS

The main psychiatric use of mood stabilizers in children is to treat pediatric BD. Prevalence rates of pediatric BD diagnosis have markedly increased in the United States (40-fold between 1994 and 2003).[61] BD diagnosis and treatment in children are complicated by overlapping comorbid disorders and developmental symptom presentation.[62] The BD course in children often presents with rapidly fluctuating spontaneous mood episodes and higher rates of psychotic symptoms compared to the classic adult presentation.[63] The treatment of pediatric BD should include close monitoring of the symptoms, providing psychoeducation to the patients and families, and providing support in multiple settings, including home and school. Mood stabilizers are the key psychopharmacologic intervention and include lithium, antiepileptic drugs (AEDs), and antipsychotic medications (Table 34.2). Antipsychotics will be discussed in another chapter.

Lithium is the oldest and most studied mood stabilizer for the treatment of BD and was recently FDA approved for BD treatment in children ages 7 to 17 years based on the National Institute of Child Health and Human Development (NICHD) Collaborative Lithium Trial (CoLT) that examined appropriate weight-based dosing and titration in CoLT I and then blinded comparison to placebo in CoLT II.[63,64] In CoLT II Findling et al. showed the efficacy and safety of using lithium compared to placebo in children ($n = 53$) ages 7 to 17 years with acute manic or mixed episodes.[63] The NICHD-sponsored CoLT studied the short- and long-term effect of lithium use in children and found a positive effect on mood at 8 weeks.[63,64] Appropriate starting lithium dosing is 300 mg BID in youth under 30 kg and 300 TID in youth over 30 kg. The target serum trough level is 1.0 mEq per L and the mean daily dose was approximately 1,500 mg. Lithium has been used alone or in combination with antipsychotic medications to treat acute mania.[65] Further studies, such as the National Institute of Mental Health (NIMH)-sponsored TEAM study, have shown that antipsychotics like risperidone may be more effective than lithium in treating acute mania.[66]

Before starting lithium, a baseline measure of thyroid and kidney functions, urinalysis, pregnancy test, and electrocardiogram should be performed for patients with high risk of cardiovascular disease.[67] Thyroid function, creatinine level, and urinalysis should be repeated every 6 months thereafter.[67]

TABLE 34.2 Lithium and AED FDA Indications and Positive Trials in Pediatric Population

Medication	*FDA Indication*	*Other Positive Trials*	*Daily Dose*	*Schedule*
Lithium	BD (ages 7–17)		Initiate 600–900 mg daily Titrate to trough target level of 1.0 mEq/L Max dose: 40 mg/k/d[63,64]	BID-TID
Valproic acid		BD	Initiate 125 mg BID and titrate up to max trough level of 125 µg/mL[63,64]	BID
Lamotrigine		BD (add-on)	Initiate at 25 mg daily Max dose: 152–240 mg daily[77]	BID
Carbamazepine		BD	Initiate 200 mg QPM May titrate up to 1,200 mg per day in divided doses[76]	QPM
Topiramate		BD (showed possible benefit in post hoc analyses)	25–300 mg[81]	Qday

AED, antiepileptic drugs; BD, bipolar disorder; BID, twice a day; FDA, U.S. Food and Drug Administration; Qday, once a day; QPM, once a day in the evening; TID, three times a day.

Lithium blood levels have a therapeutic window between 0.6 and 1.2 mEq per L and should be checked after 5 half-lives (3 days).[67] Lithium toxicity may develop with excessive blood levels and can be fatal if not recognized. Mild lithium toxicity may develop at blood level of 1.5 mEq per L; and blood levels of 2.5 mEq per L or more constitute a medical emergency.[68] Lithium toxicity often develops after excessive ingestion of the medication, development of renal insufficiency, or as a result of drug interaction with medications that change the renal function, salt balance, or water balance.[68]

None of the AEDs are FDA approved for treating children with BD. Studies examining valproic acid (VA) to treat pediatric BD have yielded mixed results. Two RCTs, including the TEAM trial, showed smaller effect of VA in treating BD manic or mixed episodes compared to risperidone or lithium.[66,69] In two double-blind, placebo-controlled studies comparing VA and risperidone in children ages 4 to 7 years and 8 to 17 years, risperidone was more effective in treating pediatric BD.[70,71] Further, in two trials, VA failed to show superior efficacy compared to placebo in youth (ages 4 to 7 years and ages 10 to 17 years) with BP manic or mixed episode.[70,72] Carbamazepine was found to be effective and safe in treating children with BD in open-label trials.[73–75] Oxcarbazepine was not effective in treating children ($n = 116$) with BD manic or mixed episode compared to placebo in a double-blind RCT.[76] A double-blind discontinuation trial of 173 children ages 10 to 17 years diagnosed with BD examined lamotrigine as an add-on mood stabilizer.[77] Although the treatment effect of lamotrigine was not significant in primary study analyses, post hoc analyses found that lamotrigine may be an effective add-on to treat pediatric BD in the 12- to 17-year age group.[77] Moreover, in a small open-label study, lamotrigine was found to be effective in treating children with BD depression ages 12 to 17 years ($n = 20$) as an adjunctive medication.[78] After noncontrolled studies indicated that topiramate may be a beneficial treatment for pediatric BD,[79,80] a double-blind, placebo-controlled study was performed to examine effectiveness of topiramate in children ages 6 to 17 years with pediatric BD.[81] Although topiramate was well tolerated, the trial was discontinued due to lack of efficacy in adult trials. In post hoc analyses, topiramate showed potential benefit over placebo in general measures of psychopathology, but not on measures specifically related to mania.[81] Therefore, it is unclear if topiramate is an effective treatment for pediatric BD.

SUMMARY

The last 20 years in pediatric mood and anxiety disorder pharmacology research has shown that many medications are effective in treating youth with these disorders and these agents are frequently FDA approved for use. In pediatric MDD, first-line medication choices are fluoxetine and escitalopram followed by the other agents shown in Table 34.1. For OCD, options include sertraline, fluvoxamine, fluoxetine, and clomipramine. Youth with GAD can be effectively treated with duloxetine. For those with GAD, SAD, and SepD, the NIH studies demonstrated benefits with fluvoxamine and sertraline.

In pediatric BD the mood-stabilizing medication lithium is an effective agent to treat mixed and manic episodes. Studies have indicated that lamotrigine may be an effective add-on medication for pediatric BD.

REFERENCES

1. Richmond TK, Rosen DS. The treatment of adolescent depression in the era of the black box warning. *Curr Opin Pediatr* 2005;17(4):466–472.
2. Friedman RA, Leon AC. Expanding the black box—depression, antidepressants, and the risk of suicide. *N Engl J Med* 2007;356(23):2343–2346.
3. Dopheide JA. Recognizing and treating depression in children and adolescents. *Am J Health Syst Pharm* 2006;63(3):233–243.
4. Cheung A, Sacks D, Dewa CS, et al. Pediatric prescribing practices and the FDA black-box warning on antidepressants. *J Dev Behav Pediatr* 2008;29(3):213–215.
5. Lemberger L, Bergstrom RF, Wolen RL, et al. Fluoxetine: clinical pharmacology and physiologic disposition. *J Clin Psychiatry* 1985;46(3 Pt 2):14–19.
6. Emslie GJ, Rush AJ, Weinberg WA, et al. A double-blind, randomized, placebo-controlled trial of fluoxetine in children and adolescents with depression. *Arch Gen Psychiatry* 1997;54(11):1031–1037.
7. Emslie GJ, Heiligenstein JH, Wagner KD, et al. Fluoxetine for acute treatment of depression in children and adolescents: a placebo-controlled, randomized clinical trial. *J Am Acad Child Adolesc Psychiatry* 2002;41(10):1205–1215.
8. Riddle MA, Scahill L, King RA, et al. Double-blind, crossover trial of fluoxetine and placebo in children and adolescents with obsessive-compulsive disorder. *J Am Acad Child Adolesc Psychiatry* 1992;31(6):1062–1069.
9. Geller DA, Hoog SL, Heiligenstein JH, et al. Fluoxetine treatment for obsessive-compulsive disorder in children and adolescents: a placebo-controlled clinical trial. *J Am Acad Child Adolesc Psychiatry* 2001;40(7):773–779.
10. Birmaher B, Axelson DA, Monk K, et al. Fluoxetine for the treatment of childhood anxiety disorders. *J Am Acad Child Adolesc Psychiatry* 2003;42(4):415–423.
11. Clark DB, Birmaher B, Axelson D, et al. Fluoxetine for the treatment of childhood anxiety disorders: open-label, long-term extension to a controlled trial. *J Am Acad Child Adolesc Psychiatry* 2005;44(12):1263–1270.
12. Alderman J, Wolkow R, ChungM, et al. Sertraline treatment of children and adolescents with obsessive-compulsive disorder or depression: pharmacokinetics, tolerability, and efficacy. *J Am Acad Child Adolesc Psychiatry* 1998;37(4):386–394.

13. Wagner KD, Cook EH, Chung H, et al. Remission status after long-term sertraline treatment of pediatric obsessive-compulsive disorder. *J Child Adolesc Psychopharmacol* 2003;13(2 Suppl 1):53–60.
14. Skarphedinsson G, Compton S, Thomsen PH, et al. Tics moderate sertraline, but not cognitive-behavior therapy response in pediatric obsessive-compulsive disorder patients who do not respond to cognitive-behavior therapy. *J Child Adolesc Psychopharmacol* 2015;25(5):432–439.
15. March JS, Franklin ME, Leonard H, et al. Tics moderate treatment outcome with sertraline but not cognitive-behavior therapy in pediatric obsessive-compulsive disorder. *Biol Psychiatry* 2007;61(3):344–347.
16. Cook EH, Wagner KD, March JS, et al. Long-term sertraline treatment of children and adolescents with obsessive-compulsive disorder. *J Am Acad Child Adolesc Psychiatry* 2001;40(10):1175–1181.
17. The Pediatric OCD Treatment Study POTS Team Cognitive-behavior therapy, sertraline, and their combination for children and adolescents with obsessive-compulsive disorder: the Pediatric OCD Treatment Study (POTS) randomized controlled trial. *JAMA* 2004;292(16):1969–1976. doi:10.1001/jama.292.16.1969.
18. Garcia AM, Sapyta JJ, Moore PS, et al. Predictors and moderators of treatment outcome in the Pediatric Obsessive Compulsive Treatment Study (POTS I). *J Am Acad Child Adolesc Psychiatry* 2010;49(10):1024–1033.
19. Storch EA, Bussing R, Small BJ, et al. Randomized, placebo-controlled trial of cognitive-behavioral therapy alone or combined with sertraline in the treatment of pediatric obsessive–compulsive disorder. *Behav Res Ther* 2013;51(12):823–829.
20. March JS, Biederman J, Wolkow R, et al. Sertraline in children and adolescents with obsessive-compulsive disorder: a multicenter randomized controlled trial. *JAMA* 1998;280(20):1752–1756.
21. Wagner KD, Ambrosini P, Rynn M, et al. Efficacy of sertraline in the treatment of children and adolescents with major depressive disorder: two randomized controlled trials. *JAMA* 2003;290(8):1033–1041.
22. Rynn MA, Siqueland L, Rickels K. Placebo-controlled trial of sertraline in the treatment of children with generalized anxiety disorder. *Am J Psychiatry* 2001;158(12):2008–2014.
23. Compton SN, Walkup JT, Albano AM, et al. Child/adolescent anxiety multimodal study (CAMS): Rationale, design, and methods. *Child Adol Psych Men* 2010;4(1):1.
24. Robb AS, Cueva JE, Sporn J, et al. Sertraline treatment of children and adolescents with posttraumatic stress disorder: a double-blind, placebo-controlled trial. *J Child Adolesc Psychopharmacol* 2010;20(6):463–471.
25. Wagner KD, Robb AS, Findling RL, et al. A randomized, placebo-controlled trial of citalopram for the treatment of major depression in children and adolescents. *Am J Psychiatry* 2004;161(6):1079–1083.
26. Roohafza H, Pourmoghaddas Z, Saneian H, et al. Citalopram for pediatric functional abdominal pain: a randomized, placebo-controlled trial. *Neurogastroenterol Motil* 2014;26(11):1642–1650.
27. Campo JV, Perel J, Lucas A, et al. Citalopram treatment of pediatric recurrent abdominal pain and comorbid internalizing disorders: an exploratory study. *J Am Acad Child Adolesc Psychiatry* 2004;43(10):1234–1242.
28. Waugh J, Goa KL. Escitalopram. *CNS Drugs* 2003;17(5):343–362.
29. Emslie GJ, Ventura D, Korotzer A, et al. Escitalopram in the treatment of adolescent depression: a randomized placebo-controlled multisite trial. *J Am Acad Child Adolesc Psychiatry* 2009;48(7):721–729.
30. Wagner KD, Jonas J, Findling RL, et al. A double-blind, randomized, placebo-controlled trial of escitalopram in the treatment of pediatric depression. *J Am Acad Child Adolesc Psychiatry* 2006;45(3):280–288.
31. Von Knorring AL, Olsson GI, Thomsen PH, et al. A randomized, double-blind, placebo-controlled study of citalopram in adolescents with major depressive disorder. *J Clin Psychopharmacol* 2006;26(3):311–315.
32. Findling RL, Robb A, Bose A. Escitalopram in the treatment of adolescent depression: a randomized, double-blind, placebo-controlled extension trial. *J Child Adolesc Psychopharmacol* 2013;23(7):468–480.
33. Isolan L, Pheula G, Salum GA Jr, et al. An open-label trial of escitalopram in children and adolescents with social anxiety disorder. *J Child Adolesc Psychopharmacol* 2007;17(6):751–760.
34. Riddle MA, Reeve EA, Yaryura-Tobias JA, et al. Fluvoxamine for children and adolescents with obsessive-compulsive disorder: a randomized, controlled, multicenter trial. *J Am Acad Child Adolesc Psychiatry* 2001;40(2):222–229.
35. Walkup JT, Labellarte MJ, Riddle MA, et al. Fluvoxamine for the treatment of anxiety disorders in children and adolescents. *N Engl J Med* 2001;344(17):1279–1285.
36. Gothelf D, Rubinstein M, Shemesh E, et al. Pilot study: fluvoxamine treatment for depression and anxiety disorders in children and adolescents with cancer. *J Am Acad Child Adolesc Psychiatry* 2005;44(12):1258–1262.
37. Emslie GJ, Findling RL, Yeung PP, et al. Venlafaxine ER for the treatment of pediatric subjects with depression: results of two placebo-controlled trials. *J Am Acad Child Adolesc Psychiatry* 2007;46(4):479–488.
38. Brent D, Emslie G, Clarke G, et al. Switching to another SSRI or to venlafaxine with or without cognitive behavioral therapy for adolescents with SSRI-resistant depression: the TORDIA randomized controlled trial. *JAMA* 2008;299(8):901–913.
39. Weihs KL, Murphy W, Abbas R, et al. Desvenlafaxine versus placebo in a fluoxetine-referenced study of children and adolescents with major depressive disorder. *J Child Adolesc Psychopharmacol* 2018;28(1):36–46.
40. March JS, Entusah AR, Rynn M, et al. A randomized controlled trial of venlafaxine ER versus placebo in pediatric social anxiety disorder. *Biol Psychiatry* 2007;62(10):1149–1154.
41. Atkinson S, Lubaczewski S, Ramaker S, et al. Desvenlafaxine versus placebo in the treatment of children and adolescents with major depressive disorder. *J Child Adolesc Psychopharmacol* 2018;28(1):55–65.
42. Strawn JR, Prakash A, Zhang Q, et al. A randomized, placebo-controlled study of duloxetine for the treatment of children and adolescents with generalized anxiety disorder. *J Am Acad Child Adolesc Psychiatry* 2015;54(4):283–293.
43. Meighen KG. Duloxetine treatment of pediatric chronic pain and co-morbid major depressive disorder. *J Child Adolesc Psychopharmacol* 2007;17(1):121–127.
44. Kachko L, Ben Ami S, Liberman A, et al. Duloxetine contributing to a successful multimodal treatment program for peripheral femoral neuropathy and comorbid 'reactive depression' in an adolescent. *Pain Res Manag* 2011;16(6):457–459.
45. Atkinson SD, Prakash A, Zhang Q, et al. A double-blind efficacy and safety study of duloxetine flexible dosing in children and adolescents with major depressive disorder. *J Child Adolesc Psychopharmacol* 2014;24(4):180–189.
46. Anderson IM. Selective serotonin reuptake inhibitors versus tricyclic antidepressants: a meta-analysis of efficacy and tolerability. *J Affect Disord* 2000;58(1):19–36.
47. Bartels MG, Varley CK, Mitchell J, et al. Pediatric cardiovascular effects of imipramine and desipramine. *J Am Acad Child Adolesc Psychiatry* 1991;30(1):100–103.
48. Watson HJ, Rees CS. Meta-analysis of randomized, controlled treatment trials for pediatric obsessive-compulsive disorder. *J Child Psychol Psychiatry* 2008;49(5):489–498.
49. Varigonda AL, Jakubovski E, Bloch MH. Systematic review and meta-analysis: early treatment responses of selective serotonin reuptake inhibitors and clomipramine in pediatric obsessive-compulsive disorder. *J Am Acad Child Adolesc Psychiatry* 2016;55(10):851–859.
50. Holm KJ, Markham A. Mirtazapine. *Drugs* 1999;57(4):607–631.
51. Gittelman-Klein R, Klein DF. Controlled imipramine treatment of school phobia. *Arch Gen Psychiatry* 1971;25(3):204–207.
52. Bernstein GA, Borchardt CM, Perwien AR, et al. Imipramine plus cognitive-behavioral therapy in the treatment of school refusal. *J Am Acad Child Adolesc Psychiatry* 2000;39(3):276–283.
53. Klein RG, Koplewicz HS, Kanner A. Imipramine treatment of children with separation anxiety disorder. *J Am Acad Child Adolesc Psychiatry* 1992;31(1):21–28.
54. DelBello MP, Hochadel TJ, Portland KB, et al. A double-blind, placebo-controlled study of selegiline transdermal system in depressed adolescents. *J Child Adolesc Psychopharmacol* 2014;24(6):311–317.
55. Horst WD, Preskorn SH. Mechanisms of action and clinical characteristics of three atypical antidepressants: venlafaxine, nefazodone, bupropion. *J Affect Disord* 1998;51(3):237–254.
56. Slemmer JE, Martin BR, Damaj MI. Bupropion is a nicotinic antagonist. *J Pharmacol Exp Ther* 2000;295(1):321–327.
57. Daviss WB, Bentivoglio P, Racusin R, et al. Bupropion sustained release in adolescents with comorbid attention-deficit/hyperactivity disorder and depression. *J Am Acad Child Adolesc Psychiatry* 2001;40(3):307–314.
58. Haapasalo-Pesu KM, Vuola T, Lahelma L, et al. Mirtazapine in the treatment of adolescents with major depression: an open-label, multicenter pilot study. *J Child Adolesc Psychopharmacol* 2004;14(2):175–184.
59. Mrakotsky C, Masek B, Biederman J, et al. Prospective open-label pilot trial of mirtazapine in children and adolescents with social phobia. *J Anxiety Disord* 2008;22(1):88–97.
60. Strawn JR, Mills JA, Cornwall GJ, et al. Buspirone in children and adolescents with anxiety: a review and Bayesian analysis of abandoned randomized controlled trials. *J Child Adolesc Psychopharmacol* 2018;28(1):2–9.
61. Holtmann M, Duketis E, Poustka L, et al. Bipolar disorder in children and adolescents in Germany: national trends in the rates of inpatients, 2000–2007. *Bipolar Disord* 2010;12(2):155–163.
62. McClellan J, Kowatch R, Findling RL. Practice parameter for the assessment and treatment of children and adolescents with bipolar disorder. *J Am Acad Child Adolesc Psychiatry* 2007;46(1):107–125.
63. Findling RL, Robb A, McNamara NK, et al. Lithium in the acute treatment of bipolar I disorder: a double-blind, placebo-controlled study. *Pediatrics* 2015;136(5):885.
64. Findling RL, Frazier JA, Kafantaris V, et al. The Collaborative Lithium Trials (CoLT): specific aims, methods, and implementation. *Child Adol Psych Men* 2008;2(1):21.
65. Pavuluri MN, Henry DB, Carbray JA, et al. Open-label prospective trial of risperidone in combination with lithium or divalproex sodium in pediatric mania. *J Affect Disord* 2004;82:S103–S111.
66. Geller B, Luby JL, Joshi P, et al. A randomized controlled trial of risperidone, lithium, or divalproex sodium for initial treatment of bipolar I disorder, manic or mixed phase, in children and adolescents. *Arch Gen Psychiatry* 2012;69(5):515–528.
67. Malhi GS, Gessler D, Outhred T. The use of lithium for the treatment of bipolar disorder: recommendations from clinical practice guidelines. *J Affect Disord* 2017;217:266–280.
68. Schou M, Amdisen A, Trap-Jensen JENS. Lithium poisoning. *Am J Psychiatry* 1968;125(4):520–527.
69. Pavuluri MN, Henry DB, Findling RL, et al. Double-blind randomized trial of risperidone versus divalproex in pediatric bipolar disorder. *Bipolar Disord* 2010;12(6):593–605.
70. Kowatch RA, Scheffer RE, Monroe E, et al. Placebo-controlled trial of valproic acid versus risperidone in children 3–7 years of age with bipolar I disorder. *J Child Adolesc Psychopharmacol* 2015;25(4):306–313.
71. West AE, Weinstein SM, Celio CI, et al. Co-morbid disruptive behavior disorder and aggression predict functional outcomes and differential response to risperidone versus divalproex in pharmacotherapy for pediatric bipolar disorder. *J Child Adolesc Psychopharmacol* 2011;21(6):545–553.
72. Wagner KD, Redden L, Kowatch RA, et al. A double-blind, randomized, placebo-controlled trial of divalproex extended-release in the treatment of bipolar disorder in children and adolescents. *J Am Acad Child Adolesc Psychiatry* 2009;48(5):519–532.
73. Kowatch RA, Suppes T, Carmody TJ, et al. Effect size of lithium, divalproex sodium, and carbamazepine in children and adolescents with bipolar disorder. *J Am Acad Child Adolesc Psychiatry* 2000;39(6):713–720.
74. Joshi G, Wozniak J, Mick E, et al. A prospective open-label trial of extended-release carbamazepine monotherapy in children with bipolar disorder. *J Child Adolesc Psychopharmacol* 2010;20(1):7–14.
75. Wagner KD, Kowatch RA, Emslie GJ, et al. A double-blind, randomized, placebo-controlled trial of oxcarbazepine in the treatment of bipolar disorder in children and adolescents. *Am J Psychiatry* 2006;163(7):1179–1186.
76. Findling RL, Ginsberg LD. The safety and effectiveness of open-label extended-release carbamazepine in the treatment of children and adolescents with bipolar I disorder suffering from a manic or mixed episode. *Neuropsychiatr Dis Treat* 2014;10:1589.

77. Findling RL, Chang K, Robb A, et al. Adjunctive maintenance lamotrigine for pediatric bipolar I disorder: a placebo-controlled, randomized withdrawal study. *J Am Acad Child Adolesc Psychiatry* 2015;54(12):1020–1031.
78. Chang K, Saxena K, Howe M. An open-label study of lamotrigine adjunct or monotherapy for the treatment of adolescents with bipolar depression. *J Am Acad Child Adolesc Psychiatry* 2006;45(3):298–304.
79. DelBello MP, Kowatch RA, Warner J, et al. Adjunctive topiramate treatment for pediatric bipolar disorder: a retrospective chart review. *J Child Adolesc Psychopharmacol* 2002;12(4):323–330.
80. Barzman DH, DelBello MP, Kowatch RA, et al. Adjunctive topiramate in hospitalized children and adolescents with bipolar disorders. *J Child Adolesc Psychopharmacol* 2005;15(6):931–937.
81. Delbello MP, Findling RL, Kushner S, et al. A pilot controlled trial of topiramate for mania in children and adolescents with bipolar disorder. *J Am Acad Child Adolesc Psychiatry* 2005;44(6):539–547.

Ekaterina Stepanova
Bradley Grant
Adelaide S. Robb
Robert L. Findling

CHAPTER 35

Stimulants, ADHD Treatments, and Antipsychotics

STIMULANTS

Attention-deficit hyperactivity disorder (ADHD) is a neurodevelopmental disorder characterized by impairments in attention and concentration with or without hyperactivity and impulsivity.[1] For pediatric patients, the *DSM-5* requires six or more persistent (at least 6 months in duration) symptoms of inattention and/or six or more persistent symptoms of hyperactivity-impulsivity that begin prior to age 12 and impair functioning in two of three settings—home, school, and social.[2]

A recent meta-analysis suggests a child and adolescent ADHD prevalence of 7.2% that has remained stable since the 1980s.[3] In childhood, ADHD seems to be more common in boys, but as one passes through adolescence and into adulthood, the ratio becomes closer to 1:1.[1,4] Long-term consequences of ADHD include school and occupational failure, substance abuse, divorce, car accidents, legal problems, and a variety of comorbid psychiatric disorders.[5–7] Despite these disheartening statistics, young men with ADHD treated with stimulants have reduced rates of comorbid psychiatric disorders and grade retention at 10-year follow-up as compared to those without stimulant treatment, suggesting that treatment had short- and long-term consequences on quality of life and psychiatric sequelae.[8]

According to the most recent CDC National Prevalence of ADHD and Treatment parent-report data, 1 in 20 children in the United States currently takes medication for ADHD,[9] and 66.9% of children with ADHD receive medication as part of their treatment plan, which may also include psychosocial interventions and academic accommodations.[10] Long-acting agents are now available in both stimulant and nonstimulant categories.[1] Positive trials for a variety of methylphenidate (MPH) and amphetamine (AMP) preparations and the norepinephrine reuptake inhibitor atomoxetine have led to labeling for pediatric and adolescent use, and all three medications can be used as first-line treatment.[11]

Stimulants remain the most frequently used medications for the treatment of ADHD in children and adolescents[12] (Table 35.1). Both MPH- and AMP-based products can improve core symptoms of inattention, hyperactivity, and impulsivity within 30 minutes of administration. The benefits of racemic AMP on behavior and school performance were first noted by Bradley in 1937.[13] Clinical trials conducted by Eisenberg and Conners[14,15] demonstrated the effects of AMP and the more potent D-isomer in treating core symptoms of ADHD in children. Currently available AMP formulations vary by dose, ratios of stereoisomers, and delivery. Clinicians can choose from short- and long-acting AMP, as well as a pro-drug formulation (lisdexamfetamine). MPH is also available in a range of doses, short- and long-duration forms, racemic and D-enantiomer preparations, and capsule, tablet, suspension, chewable and transdermal products. Both classes of stimulant medications yield comparable levels of clinically significant side effects.[16] The most frequent side effects of stimulant medication include appetite suppression, sleep difficulties, transient headache, and increased heart rate or blood pressure. Less frequent side effects may include nausea, irritability, and rarely, psychosis.[17]

OTHER ADHD TREATMENTS

When children and adolescents fail to respond adequately to stimulant medication or experience significant side effects that cannot be mitigated with changes in preparation, there are several nonstimulant medications that have been proven effective for ADHD (Table 35.2).

The selective norepinephrine reuptake inhibitor atomoxetine has demonstrated efficacy for ADHD in double-blind, placebo-controlled trials with a target dose range of approximately 1.2 to 1.5 mg per kg.[47,48] The overall effect size of atomoxetine is modestly smaller compared to stimulant treatments.[49] The most common side effects are abdominal pain (16.1%), headache (15.8%), and decreased appetite (15.4%).[48] It should be noted that atomoxetine carries a Food and Drug Administration (FDA)-required boxed warning for suicidality—though at rates lower than those seen in the antidepressants.[44] Atomoxetine requires a gradual titration and can be given once a day in the evenings. The dose should be decreased by approximately 50% in patients with hepatic dysfunction.[44]

Clonidine and guanfacine are α-2 adrenergic agents that were initially developed as antihypertensive agents but have shown efficacy in the treatment of pediatric ADHD.[50,51] Both medications are available in short- and long-acting forms and can be used either alone or in conjunction with a stimulant.[52,53] The most common treatment-related adverse events (AEs) include upper abdominal pain, fatigue, headache, and

TABLE 35.1 FDA-Approved Stimulant Medications Used in the Treatment of Attention-Deficit/Hyperactivity Disorder in Children and Adolescents

Medication (Brand Name)	*Formulation*	*Duration of Action*	*Starting Dose*	*Typical Dose Range*
Dexmethylphenidate (Focalin)	Tablet containing D-*threo*-enantiomer of racemic methylphenidate[18]	4 h	2.5 mg twice daily or half current dose of methylphenidate	2.5–10 mg twice daily
Dexmethylphenidate (Focalin XR)	Capsule containing extended-release (ER) D-*threo*-enantiomer of racemic methylphenidate; capsules may be swallowed whole or opened and the entire contents sprinkled on applesauce[19]	6–8 h; dual pulse	5 mg once daily	5–30 mg once daily
Methylphenidate (Methylin Chewable tablets)	Chewable tablet; grape flavor[20]	3–5 h	5 mg twice daily	5–10 mg twice or trice daily
Methylphenidate (Methylin Solution)	Oral solution available in 5 mg/5 mL or 10 mg/5 mL; grape flavor[21]	3–5 h	5 mg twice daily	5–10 mg twice or thrice daily
Methylphenidate (Ritalin)	Tablet[22]	3–5 h	5 mg twice daily	5–10 mg twice or thrice daily
Methylphenidate (Ritalin SR)	ER tablets (swallow whole, do not crush); 20 mg only[22]	6–8 h	Titrate to 20 mg/d of immediate-release, then switch to 20 mg once daily of Ritalin SR	20–40 mg once daily
Methylphenidate (Metadate ER)	ER tablets (swallow whole, do not crush); 20 mg only[23]	6–8 h	Titrate to 20 mg/d of immediate-release, then switch to 20 mg once daily of Metadate ER	20–40 mg once daily
Methylphenidate (Metadate CD)	ER capsules containing 30% immediate-release and 70% ER beads[24]	8–10 h	10–20 mg once a day	20–60 mg once per day
Methylphenidate (Ritalin LA)	ER capsules; may be swallowed whole, or opened and the entire contents sprinkled on applesauce[25]	8–10 h	10–20 mg once a day	20–60 mg once per day
Methylphenidate (Concerta)	ER tablets; swallow whole, do not crush[26]	8–12 h	18 mg once a day	Children: 18–54 mg once daily Adolescents: 18–72 mg once daily
Methylphenidate (Quillivant XR)	ER oral suspension 5 mg/mL; banana flavor. Before administering the dose, vigorously shake bottle for at least 10 s[27]	10–12 h	20 mg once a day	20–60 mg once daily
Methylphenidate (Quillichew ER)	Chewable ER tablet; cherry flavor[28]	10–12 h	20 mg once a day	20–60 mg once daily
Methylphenidate (Contempla XR-ODT)	ER oral disintegrating tablets (25% immediate release, 75% extended release); grape flavor[29]	10–12 h	17.3 mg once a day	17.3–51.8 mg once daily
Methylphenidate (Aptensio XR)	ER capsules; may be swallowed whole or opened and the entire contents sprinkled on applesauce[30]	10–12 h	10 mg once daily	10–60 mg once daily
Methylphenidate (Adhansia XR)	ER capsules; may be swallowed whole or opened and the entire contents sprinkled on applesauce[31]	12–13 h	25 mg once daily Do not substitute for other methylphenidate products on a milligram-per-milligram basis	25–70 mg once daily
Methylphenidate (Jornay PM)	Delayed-release and ER capsule; may be swallowed whole or opened and the entire contents sprinkled onto applesauce[32]	10–12 h	20 mg daily in the evening	20–100 mg once daily in the evening
Methylphenidate (Daytrana)	Transdermal patch; applied to the hip area (using alternating sites) 2 h before an effect is needed and removed 9 h after application. Effects persist approximately 3 h after patch is removed[33]	10–12 h	10 mg patch for 9 h	10–30 mg patch for 9 h

TABLE 35.1 FDA-Approved Stimulant Medications Used in the Treatment of Attention-Deficit/Hyperactivity Disorder in Children and Adolescents (*continued*)

Medication (Brand Name)	*Formulation*	*Duration of Action*	*Starting Dose*	*Typical Dose Range*
Amphetamine mixed salts (Adderall)	Tablet[34]	4–6 h	Children 3–5 y old: 2.5 mg once daily Children ≥6 y old and adolescents: 5 mg once or twice daily	5–20 mg twice daily
Amphetamine mixed salts (Adderall XR)	ER capsule[35]	8–10 h	5–10 mg once daily	5–30 mg once daily
Amphetamine mixed salts (Mydayis)	ER capsule (immediate and two types of delayed-release beads)[36]	12–14 h	Not for children under 13 y old. Adolescents: 12.5 mg once daily	Not for children under 13 y old. Adolescents: 12.5–25 mg once daily
D- and L-Amphetamine (Adzenys XR-ODT)	ER oral disintegrating tablet; orange flavor[37]	8–10 h	6.3 mg once daily	Children (6–12 y old): 6.3–18.8 mg once daily Adolescents: 6.3–12.5 mg once daily
D- and L-Amphetamine (Adzenys ER)	Oral solution 1.25 mg/mL; orange flavor[38]	8–10 h	6.3 mg once daily	Children (6–12 y old): 6.3–18.8 mg once daily Adolescents: 6.3–12.5 mg once daily
D- & L-Amphetamine (Dyanavel)	Oral solution 2.5 mg/mL; bubblegum flavor[39]	10–12 h	2.5–5 mg once daily	2.5–20 mg once daily
D-Amphetamine (Zenzedi)	Tablet[40]	4–6 h	Children 3–5 y old: 2.5 mg once daily Children ≥6 y old and adolescents: 5 mg twice daily	5–15 mg twice daily
D-Amphetamine (Dexedrine Spansule)	ER capsule[41]	6–8 h	5 mg once daily	5–15 mg once daily
D-Amphetamine (ProCentra)	Oral suspension 5 mg/5 mL; bubblegum flavor[42]	4–6 h	Children 3–5 y old: 2.5 mg once daily Children ≥6 y old and adolescents: 5 mg twice daily: 5–15 mg twice daily	5–15 mg twice daily
Lisdexamfetamine (Vyvanse)	Capsules or chewable tablets containing pro-drug converted into D-amphetamine after ingestion[43]	10–12 h	30 mg once daily	30–70 mg once daily

TABLE 35.2 FDA-Approved Nonstimulant Medications Used in the Treatment of Attention-Deficit/Hyperactivity Disorder in Children and Adolescents

Medication	*Formulation*	*Duration of Action*	*Starting Dose*	*Dose Range*
SELECTIVE NOREPINEPHRINE REUPTAKE INHIBITORS				
Atomoxetine (Strattera)	Capsule[44]	24 h	0.5 mg/kg/d in divided doses (twice daily)	18–100 mg (1.4 mg/kg/d given either once daily or in divided doses)
α-2 AGONISTS				
Clonidine (Kapvay)	Extended-release (ER) tablets (cannot be crushed, broken, or chewed)[45]	24 h	0.1 mg at bedtime	0.1–0.2 mg twice daily
Guanfacine (Intuniv ER)	ER tablets (cannot be crushed, broken, or chewed)[46]	24 h	1 mg	1–4 mg once daily (0.05–0.12 mg/kg/d)

somnolence.[52,53] Doses are titrated gradually and blood pressure and pulse should be monitored during treatment. Clonidine is used off-label for insomnia[54] and conduct problems,[55] while long-acting guanfacine may be helpful for oppositional behaviors[56] and posttraumatic stress disorder (PTSD).[57]

This selection of agents—stimulants, norepinephrine reuptake inhibitors, and α-2 agonists—and the option to combine treatments makes it unlikely that clinicians would need to try off-label medications. In these uncommon cases, clinicians may need to balance efficacy reported in clinical trials to important safety concerns, such as modafinil and Stevens–Johnson syndrome,[58] bupropion and seizures,[59] or tricyclic antidepressants and cardiac toxicity.[60]

ANTIPSYCHOTICS

Antipsychotic medications are generally divided into two major classes: first-generation or "typical" antipsychotics and second-generation or "atypical" antipsychotics. First-generation antipsychotics (FGA), such as haloperidol, molindone, and pimozide, have less evidence for their use in the pediatric population, compared to the second-generation antipsychotics (SGA), including risperidone, quetiapine, olanzapine, and others.[61] Over the past two decades, the use of antipsychotic medications, especially SGAs, in children and adolescents has been increasing significantly.[62] The FDA approved several antipsychotics for the treatment or schizophrenia, bipolar disorder (BPD), Tourette disorder (TD), and irritability associated with autism spectrum disorder (ASD) (Table 35.3).

SCHIZOPHRENIA

Schizophrenia is a severe and chronic disorder affecting reality testing.[63] Early-onset schizophrenia (EOS) occurs prior to age 17 and is associated with increased morbidity and functional impairment when compared to the adult-onset form of this disorder.[64] According to the most recent American Academy of Child and Adolescent Psychiatry practice parameters for the management of EOS, the primary treatment focuses on psychopharmacotherapy.[65] However, psychosocial interventions are an important adjunct to the medication management and should include cognitive behavior therapy, social skills training and family involvement.

Several SGAs are currently approved by the FDA for the treatment of schizophrenia in youth, including risperidone, olanzapine, quetiapine, and paliperidone. Some of the older FGAs are also approved for this indication. However, the regulatory approval for these older drugs is not the result of methodologically stringent research. Very few randomized placebo-controlled trials of FGAs are available in the pediatric population.

While most of the trials in adolescents with schizophrenia compared active treatment to placebo, the Treatment of Early Onset Schizophrenia Spectrum Disorders Study (TEOSS) evaluated the efficacy of olanzapine, risperidone, and molindone in youth with EOS.[66] The reduction in psychotic symptoms was similar between the groups. However, the side effects did differ across the different medicines. Additionally, participants that showed improvement during the first 8 weeks of treatment did not demonstrate additional reduction in psychotic symptoms with longer time in treatment.[67]

Another trial compared the efficacy of paliperidone extended release and aripiprazole in adolescents with schizophrenia.[68] Both medications were effective in reducing psychotic symptoms with no significance difference in efficacy between the groups.

Clozapine is considered superior to other antipsychotics for treatment-resistant schizophrenia.[69,70] However, due to the requirements for monitoring and side effect profile, it is not used as a first-line agent.

Generally when treating EOS the recommendation is to start with one of the FDA-approved SGAs.[63] It is recommended that

TABLE 35.3 FDA-Approved Uses of Second-Generation Antipsychotics in Children and Adolescents

Medication	*FDA-Approved Indication*	*Age Range, y*	*Recommended Dose Range, mg*
Risperidone	Schizophrenia	13–17	1–6
	BPD (mixed/manic episode)	10–17	1–6
	Irritability, associated with ASD	5–18	0.5–3
Aripiprazole	Schizophrenia	13–17	10–30
	BPD (mixed/manic episode)	10–17	10–30
	Irritability, associated with ASD	6–17	5–15
	TD	6–18	<50 kg: 5–10 ≥50 kg: 10–20
Olanzapine	Schizophrenia	13–17	10
	BPD (mixed/manic episode)	13–17	10
Asenapine	BPD (mixed/manic episode)	10–17	2.5–10 twice daily
Quetiapine	Schizophrenia	13–17	400–800
	BPD (mixed/manic episode)	10–17	400–600
Lurasidone	Schizophrenia	13–17	40–80
	BPD (depressive episode)	10–17	20–80
Paliperidone	Schizophrenia	12–17	<51 kg: 3–6 ≥51 kg: 3–12
Olanzapine/fluoxetine combination	BPD (depressive episode)	10–17	3/25–12/50

ASD, autism spectrum disorder; BPD, bipolar disorder; TD, Tourette disorder.

olanzapine should not be the first option due to the increased risk for metabolic AEs. Clozapine may be considered after failure of several other antipsychotic medications.

BIPOLAR DISORDER

BPD is a chronic and debilitating illness, characterized by the presence of mixed/manic and/or depressive episodes.[2] The comprehensive treatment of pediatric BPD includes psychosocial interventions and psychopharmacological therapy.[71] Based on randomized placebo-controlled trials, the FDA approved several antipsychotic medications for the management of acute mixed and manic episodes of BPD, including aripiprazole, asenapine, risperidone, olanzapine, and quetiapine.[72] While no SGAs are approved by the FDA for maintenance treatment of pediatric BPD, two trials of aripiprazole suggest long-term efficacy.[73,74] The only two medications that are approved by the FDA for the treatment of bipolar depression are lurasidone and olanzapine/fluoxetine combination.[75] Additionally, a trial of ziprasidone in the management of acute mixed/manic episodes in youth showed reduction of manic symptoms.[76] Quetiapine was not effective for treatment of bipolar depression in youth.[77,78]

TOURETTE DISORDER

TD is characterized by the presence of both vocal and motor tics at some time during the course of the illness, although not necessarily at the same time.[2] Chronic tics are burdensome to patients and their families and can cause social and emotional impairment.[79] The first-line intervention for TD is usually behavior management, such as habit reversal training.[80] Medication management is recommended in severe and impairing cases. Haloperidol, pimozide, and aripiprazole are currently approved by the FDA for management of TD in youth. Trials of risperidone suggest efficacy in reducing the tic severity in patients with chronic tic disorders.[81]

AUTISM SPECTRUM DISORDER

ASD is a pervasive developmental disorder characterized by persistent deficits in social interactions and restricted, repetitive patterns of behavior or interests.[2] In addition to these core symptoms of ASD, many children suffer from emotional and behavioral disturbances, including irritability, aggression, mood lability, and others.[82] These associated symptoms are often disruptive to youth and their caregivers, leading to difficulties in the school setting and a risk of out of home placement. While there is no psychopharmacological intervention for the management of core symptoms of ASD, the FDA approved two medications (risperidone and aripiprazole) for the management of irritability associated with ASD.[83] Additionally, a head-to-head comparison of aripiprazole and risperidone showed similar reduction of irritability scores in children with ASD; however, the response was achieved faster with aripiprazole.[81] Several small open-label trials of olanzapine[84,85] and one trial of paliperidone[86] suggest effectiveness in reduction of irritability associated with ASD. The trials of quetiapine showed mixed results,[87,88] while lurasidone was not superior to placebo for the management of irritability in children with ASD.[89]

DISRUPTIVE BEHAVIOR DISORDERS

Disruptive behavior disorders (DBDs) is a group of externalizing disorders, including ADHD, oppositional defiant disorder (ODD), and conduct disorder (CD). Psychosocial treatments can be effective in managing some disruptive behaviors. Aggressive behaviors in children with ADHD are usually responsive to stimulant medications; however, the presence of comorbid ODD or CD frequently necessitates treatment with additional psychotropic agents.[90] Risperidone was shown to be effective in the Treatment of Severe Childhood Aggression Study (TOSCA) when added to a stimulant medication for the treatment of children with ADHD and aggressive behaviors.[91,92] A similarly designed trial of risperidone used as an adjunct to the stimulant in youth diagnosed with ADHD and ODD showed improvement in ADHD symptoms over time with the addition of risperidone versus placebo.[93] A recent meta-analysis of both aripiprazole and risperidone reported efficacy in reducing irritability and aggression in children regardless of the diagnosis.[90]

Antipsychotics agents carry a risk of AEs that requires monitoring. Both FGAs and SGA may cause weight gain and increase the rates of extrapyramidal symptoms, including tardive dyskinesia, which can occur months or even years after initiation of treatment. SGAs have been associated with higher rates of metabolic abnormalities, and some have contributed to elevated prolactin levels. Therefore, it is recommended to monitor fasting lipid panel, liver function tests, weight, and body mass index (BMI) in patients receiving antipsychotics. A more detailed AE profile is detailed elsewhere.[75]

REFERENCES

1. Pliszka S, AACAP Work Group on Quality Issues. Practice parameter for the assessment and treatment of children and adolescents with attention-deficit/hyperactivity disorder. *J Am Acad Child Adolesc Psychiatry* 2007;46(7):894–921.
2. American Psychiatric Association. *Diagnostic and Statistical Manual of Mental Disorders*, 5th ed. Washington, DC: American Psychiatric Association, 2013.
3. Thomas R, Sanders S, Doust J, et al. Prevalence of attention-deficit/hyperactivity disorder: a systematic review and meta-analysis. *Pediatrics* 2015;135(4):e994–e1001.
4. Kessler RC, Chiu WT, Demler O, et al. Prevalence, severity, and comorbidity of 12-month DSM-IV disorders in the National Comorbidity Survey Replication. *Arch Gen Psychiatry* 2005;62(6):617–627.
5. Hansen C, Weiss D, Last CG. ADHD boys in young adulthood: psychosocial adjustment. *J Am Acad Child Adolesc Psychiatry* 1999;38(2):165–171.
6. Mannuzza S, Klein RG, Bessler A, et al. Educational and occupational outcome of hyperactive boys grown up. *J Am Acad Child Adolesc Psychiatry* 1997;36(9):1222–1227.
7. Mohr-Jensen C, Muller Bisgaard C, Boldsen SK, et al. Attention-deficit/hyperactivity disorder in childhood and adolescence and the risk of crime in young adulthood in a Danish nationwide study. *J Am Acad Child Adolesc Psychiatry* 2019;58(4):443–452.
8. Biederman J, Monuteaux MC, Spencer T, et al. Do stimulants protect against psychiatric disorders in youth with ADHD? A 10-year follow-up study. *Pediatrics* 2009;124(1):71–78.
9. Danielson ML, Bitsko RH, Ghandour RM, et al. Prevalence of parent-reported ADHD diagnosis and associated treatment among U.S. children and adolescents, 2016. *J Clinical Child Adolesc Psychol* 2018;47(2):199–212.
10. Danielson ML, Visser SN, Chronis-Tuscano A, et al. A national description of treatment among United States children and adolescents with attention-deficit/hyperactivity disorder. *J Pediatr* 2018;192:240.e1–246.e1.
11. Pliszka SR, Crismon ML, Hughes CW, et al. The Texas Children's Medication Algorithm Project: revision of the algorithm for pharmacotherapy of attention-deficit/hyperactivity disorder. *J Am Acad Child Adolesc Psychiatry* 2006;45(6):642–657.
12. National Institute of Mental Health. Attention-deficit/hyperactivity disorder. 2016. https://www.nimh.nih.gov/health/topics/attention-deficit-hyperactivity-disorder-adhd/index.shtml. Accessed June, 2020.
13. Bradley C. Behaviour of children receiving benzedrine. *Am J Psychiatr* 1937;94:577–585.
14. Conners CK, Rothschild G, Eisenberg L, et al. Dextroamphetamine sulfate in children with learning disorders. Effects on perception, learning, and achievement. *Arch Gen Psychiatry* 1969;21(2):182–190.
15. Conners CK, Eisenberg L, Barcai A. Effect of dextroamphetamine on children. Studies on subjects with learning disabilities and school behavior problems. *Arch Gen Psychiatry* 1967;17(4):478–485.
16. Pelham WE, Aronoff HR, Midlam JK, et al. A comparison of ritalin and adderall: efficacy and time-course in children with attention-deficit/hyperactivity disorder. *Pediatrics* 1999;103(4):e43.
17. Brown KA, Samuel S, Patel DR. Pharmacologic management of attention deficit hyperactivity disorder in children and adolescents: a review for practitioners. *Transl Pediatr* 2018;7(1):36–47.
18. Focalin [product information]. East Hanover, NJ: Novartis Pharmaceuticals Corporation, 2019.
19. Focalin XR [product information]. East Hanover, NJ: Novartis Pharmaceuticals Corporation, 2019.

20. Methylin® chewable tablets [product information]. Florham Park, NJ: Shionogi Inc., 2013.
21. Methylin oral solution [product information]. Florham Park, NJ: Shionogi Inc., 2013.
22. Ritalin and Ritalin SR [product information]. East Hanover, NJ: Novartis Pharmaceuticals Corporation, 2019.
23. METADATE ER [product information]. Smyrna, GA: Unither Manufacturing LLC, 2014.
24. Metadate CD [product information]. Smyrna, GA: UCB Inc., 2007.
25. Ritalin LA [product information]. East Hanover, NJ: Novartis Pharmaceuticals Corporation, 2019.
26. Concerta [product information]. Titusville, NJ: Janssen Pharmaceuticals Inc., 2013.
27. Quillivant XR (product information). NextWave Pharmaceuticals Inc. New York, NY, 2017.
28. Quillichew ER [product information]. Monmouth Junction, NJ: NextWave Pharmaceuticals Inc., 2018.
29. Contempla XR-ODT [product information]. Grand Prarie, TX: Neos Therapeutics Inc., 2018.
30. Aptensio XR [product information]. Coventry, RI: Rhodes Pharmaceuticals LP, 2017.
31. Adransia XR [product information]. Wilson, NC: Purdue Pharmaceuticals LP, 2019.
32. Jornay PM [product information]. Camana Bay, Cayman Islands: Ironshore Pharmaceuticals & Development Inc., 2018.
33. Daytrana [product information]. Miami, FL: Noven Therapeutics LLC, 2017.
34. Adderall [product information]. Pomona, NY: DSM Pharmaceuticals Inc., 2007.
35. Adderall XR [product information]. Lexington, MA: Shire US Inc., 2018.
36. Mydayis [product information]. Lexington, MA: Shire US Inc., 2017.
37. Adzenys XR-ODT [product information]. Grand Prarie, TX: Neos Therapeutics Inc., 2017.
38. Adzenys ER [product information]. Grand Prarie, TX: Neos Therapeutics Inc., 2017.
39. Dynavel [product information]. Monmouth, NJ: Tris Pharma Inc., 2017.
40. Zenzedi (product information). Arbor Pharmaceuticals LLC. Atlanta, GA, 2017.
41. Dexedrine and Dexedrine Spansule [product information]. Research Triangle Park, NC: GlaxoSmithKline, 2007.
42. ProCentra [product information]. Newport, KY: Independent Pharmaceuticals LLC, 2017.
43. Vyvanse [product information]. Lexington, MA: Shire US Inc., 2017.
44. Strattera [product information]. Indianapolis, IN: Lilly USA LLC, 2017.
45. Kapvay [product inormation]. Atlanta, GA: Shionogi Inc., 2010.
46. Intuniv ER [product information]. Wayne, PA: Shire US Inc., 2013.
47. Cheng JY, Chen RY, Ko JS, et al. Efficacy and safety of atomoxetine for attention-deficit/hyperactivity disorder in children and adolescents-meta-analysis and meta-regression analysis. *Psychopharmacology* 2007;194(2):197–209.
48. Kratochvil CJ, Milton DR, Vaughan BS, et al. Acute atomoxetine treatment of younger and older children with ADHD: a meta-analysis of tolerability and efficacy. *Child Adolesc Psychiatry Ment Health* 2008;2(1):25.
49. Faraone SV, Glatt SJ. A comparison of the efficacy of medications for adult attention-deficit/hyperactivity disorder using meta-analysis of effect sizes. *J Clin Psychiatry* 2010;71(6):754–763.
50. Sallee FR, Lyne A, Wigal T, et al. Long-term safety and efficacy of guanfacine extended release in children and adolescents with attention-deficit/hyperactivity disorder. *J Child Adolesc Psychopharmacol* 2009;19(3):215–226.
51. Palumbo DR, Sallee FR, Pelham WE Jr, et al. Clonidine for attention-deficit/hyperactivity disorder: I. Efficacy and tolerability outcomes. *J Am Acad Child Adolesc Psychiatry* 2008;47(2):180–188.
52. Spencer TJ, Greenbaum M, Ginsberg LD, et al. Safety and effectiveness of coadministration of guanfacine extended release and psychostimulants in children and adolescents with attention-deficit/hyperactivity disorder. *J Child Adolesc Psychopharmacol* 2009;19(5):501–510.
53. Kollins SH, Jain R, Brams M, et al. Clonidine extended-release tablets as add-on therapy to psychostimulants in children and adolescents with ADHD. *Pediatrics* 2011;127(6): e1406–e1413.
54. Pelayo R, Yuen K. Pediatric sleep pharmacology. *Child Adolesc Psychiatr Clin N Am* 2012;21(4):861–883.
55. Pringsheim T, Hirsch L, Gardner D, et al. The pharmacological management of oppositional behaviour, conduct problems, and aggression in children and adolescents with attention-deficit hyperactivity disorder, oppositional defiant disorder, and conduct disorder: a systematic review and meta-analysis. Part 1: psychostimulants, alpha-2 agonists, and atomoxetine. *Can J Psychiatry* 2015;60(2):42–51.
56. Connor DF, Findling RL, Kollins SH, et al. Effects of guanfacine extended release on oppositional symptoms in children aged 6-12 years with attention-deficit hyperactivity disorder and oppositional symptoms: a randomized, double-blind, placebo-controlled trial. *CNS Drugs* 2010;24(9):755–768.
57. Connor DF, Grasso DJ, Slivinsky MD, et al. An open-label study of guanfacine extended release for traumatic stress related symptoms in children and adolescents. *J Child Adolesc Psychopharmacol* 2013;23(4):244–251.
58. Biederman J, Pliszka SR. Modafinil improves symptoms of attention-deficit/hyperactivity disorder across subtypes in children and adolescents. *J Pediatr* 2008;152(3):394–399.
59. Beyens MN, Guy C, Mounier G, et al. Serious adverse reactions of bupropion for smoking cessation: analysis of the French Pharmacovigilance Database from 2001 to 2004. *Drug Saf* 2008;31(11):1017–1026.
60. Ghanizadeh A. A systematic review of the efficacy and safety of desipramine for treating ADHD. *Curr Drug Saf* 2013;8(3):169–174.
61. Ben Amor L. Antipsychotics in pediatric and adolescent patients: a review of comparative safety data. *J Affect Disord* 2012;138(Suppl):S22–S30.
62. Olfson M, Blanco C, Liu SM, et al. National trends in the office-based treatment of children, adolescents, and adults with antipsychotics. *Arch Gen Psychiatry* 2012;69(12):1247–1256.
63. McClellan J. Psychosis in children and adolescents. *J Am Acad Child Adolesc Psychiatry* 2018;57(5):308–312.
64. Gillberg C. *Epidemiology of early onset schizophrenia*. Cambridge, UK: Cambridge University Press, 2001.
65. McClellan J, Stock S, American Academy of Child and Adolescent Psychiatry (AACAP) Committee on Quality Issues (CQI). Practice parameter for the assessment and treatment of children and adolescents with schizophrenia. *J Am Acad Child Adolesc Psychiatry* 2013;52(9):976–990.
66. Sikich L, Frazier JA, McClellan J, et al. Double-blind comparison of first- and second-generation antipsychotics in early-onset schizophrenia and schizo-affective disorder: findings from the treatment of early-onset schizophrenia spectrum disorders (TEOSS) study. *Am J Psychiatry* 2008;165(11):1420–1431.
67. Findling RL, Johnson JL, McClellan J, et al. Double-blind maintenance safety and effectiveness findings from the Treatment of Early-Onset Schizophrenia Spectrum (TEOSS) study. *J Am Acad Child Adolesc Psychiatry* 2010;49(6):583–594; quiz 632.
68. Savitz AJ, Lane R, Nuamah I, et al. Efficacy and safety of paliperidone extended release in adolescents with schizophrenia: a randomized, double-blind study. *J Am Acad Child Adolesc Psychiatry* 2015;54(2):126–137.e1.
69. Shaw P, Sporn A, Gogtay N, et al. Childhood-onset schizophrenia: a double-blind, randomized clozapine-olanzapine comparison. *Arch Gen Psychiatry* 2006;63(7):721–730.
70. Siskind D, McCartney L, Goldschlager R, et al. First- and second-generation antipsychotics in treatment-refractory schizophrenia: systematic review and meta-analysis. *Br J Psychiatry* 2016;209(5):385–392.
71. Findling RL, Frazier JA, Kafantaris V, et al. The Collaborative Lithium Trials (CoLT): specific aims, methods, and implementation. *Child Adolesc Psychiatry Ment Health* 2008;2(1):21.
72. Stepanova E, Findling RL. Psychopharmacology of bipolar disorders in children and adolescents. *Pediatr Clin North Am* 2017;64(6):1209–1222.
73. Findling RL, Correll CU, Nyilas M, et al. Aripiprazole for the treatment of pediatric bipolar I disorder: a 30-week, randomized, placebo-controlled study. *Bipolar Disord* 2013;15(2):138–149.
74. Findling RL, Youngstrom EA, McNamara NK, et al. Double-blind, randomized, placebo-controlled long-term maintenance study of aripiprazole in children with bipolar disorder. *J Clin Psychiatry* 2012;73(1):57–63.
75. Lee ES, Vidal C, Findling RL. A focused review on the treatment of pediatric patients with atypical antipsychotics. *J Child Adolesc Psychopharmacol* 2018;28(9):582–605.
76. Findling RL, Cavu⊠ I, Pappadopulos E, et al. Efficacy, long-term safety, and tolerability of ziprasidone in children and adolescents with bipolar disorder. *J Child Adolesc Psychopharmacol* 2013;23(8):545–557.
77. DelBello MP, Chang K, Welge JA, et al. A double-blind, placebo-controlled pilot study of quetiapine for depressed adolescents with bipolar disorder. *Bipolar Disord* 2009;11(5):483–493.
78. Findling RL, Pathak S, Earley WR, et al. Efficacy and safety of extended-release quetiapine fumarate in youth with bipolar depression: an 8 week, double-blind, placebo-controlled trial. *J Child Adolesc Psychopharmacol* 2014;24(6):325–335.
79. Whittington C, Pennant M, Kendall T, et al. Practitioner review: treatments for Tourette syndrome in children and young people—a systematic review. *J Child Psychol Psychiatry* 2016;57(9):988–1004.
80. Piacentini J, Woods DW, Scahill L, et al. Behavior therapy for children with Tourette disorder: a randomized controlled trial. *JAMA* 2010;303(19):1929–1937.
81. Ghanizadeh A, Sahraeizadeh A, Berk M. A head-to-head comparison of aripiprazole and risperidone for safety and treating autistic disorders, a randomized double blind clinical trial. *Child Psychiatry Hum Dev* 2014;45(2):185–192.
82. Simonoff E, Pickles A, Charman T, et al. Psychiatric disorders in children with autism spectrum disorders: prevalence, comorbidity, and associated factors in a population-derived sample. *J Am Acad Child Adolesc Psychiatry* 2008;47(8):921–929.
83. Stepanova E, Dowling S, Phelps M, et al. Pharmacotherapy of emotional and behavioral symptoms associated with autism spectrum disorder in children and adolescents. *Dialogues Clin Neurosci* 2017;19(4):395–402.
84. Kemner C, Willemsen-Swinkels SH, de Jonge M, et al. Open-label study of olanzapine in children with pervasive developmental disorder. *J Clin Psychopharmacol* 2002;22(5):455–460.
85. Hollander E, Wasserman S, Swanson EN, et al. A double-blind placebo-controlled pilot study of olanzapine in childhood/adolescent pervasive developmental disorder. *J Child Adolesc Psychopharmacol* 2006;16(5):541–548.
86. Stigler KA, Mullett JE, Erickson CA, et al. Paliperidone for irritability in adolescents and young adults with autistic disorder. *Psychopharmacology* 2012;223(2):237–245.
87. Findling RL, McNamara NK, Gracious BL, et al. Quetiapine in nine youths with autistic disorder. *J Child Adolesc Psychopharmacol* 2004;14(2):287–294.
88. Golubchik P, Sever J, Weizman A. Low-dose quetiapine for adolescents with autistic spectrum disorder and aggressive behavior: open-label trial. *Clin Neuropharmacol* 2011;34(6):216–219.
89. Loebel A, Brams M, Goldman RS, et al. Lurasidone for the treatment of irritability associated with autistic disorder. *J Autism Dev Disord* 2016;46(4):1153–1163.
90. Connor DF, Glatt SJ, Lopez ID, et al. Psychopharmacology and aggression. I: a meta-analysis of stimulant effects on overt/covert aggression-related behaviors in ADHD. *J Am Acad Child Adolesc Psychiatry* 2002;41(3):253–261.
91. Aman MG, Bukstein OG, Gadow KD, et al. What does risperidone add to parent training and stimulant for severe aggression in child attention-deficit/hyperactivity disorder? *J Am Acad Child Adolesc Psychiatry* 2014;53(1):47.e1–60.e1.
92. Findling RL, Townsend L, Brown NV, et al. The treatment of severe childhood aggression study: 12 weeks of extended, blinded treatment in clinical responders. *J Child Adolesc Psychopharmacol* 2017;27(1):52–65.
93. Jahangard L, Akbarian S, Haghighi M, et al. Children with ADHD and symptoms of oppositional defiant disorder improved in behavior when treated with methylphenidate and adjuvant risperidone, though weight gain was also observed - Results from a randomized, double-blind, placebo-controlled clinical trial. *Psychiatry Res* 2017;251:182–191.

CHAPTER

36

Sinno H. P. Simons
Gerbrich E. van den Bosch
Dick Tibboel

Analgesics and Sedatives

PAIN AND DISTRESS

Pain is an "unpleasant sensory and emotional experience associated with actual or potential tissue damage, or described in terms of such damage," as defined by the International Association for the Study of Pain (IASP).[1] With the important note that "pain is always subjective and each individual learns the application of the word pain through experiences related to injury in early life."[1] However, some children experience substantially more pain than others in their early life. Besides the fact that pain should always be prevented because it is very uncomfortable, it should also be prevented due to negative short- and long-term consequences. Pain and related distress have short-term negative consequences, such as a higher morbidity rate.[2] With regard to the long term, we know that the development of pain pathways extends beyond the neonatal period and structural and functional fine-tuning of the nociceptive system and spinal circuit is activity dependent.[3] It could, therefore, be affected by noxious stimuli received in the neonatal period, inducing potential long-term negative effects.[4,5] The use of preemptive analgesia during the neonatal phase is thought to play an important role in the prevention of the long-term side effects of pain. This is based on animal studies, which have shown more negative effects of neonatal pain when pain experiments were conducted in the absence of adequate analgesic therapy.[6] So, treating pain is in the first place important to guarantee comfort and avoid distress but also in order to prevent those short-term and potential long-term consequences.

Hence, experiencing pain is always uncomfortable and causes distress. However, pediatric patients are also exposed to experiences that might not be painful but are considered to be stressful. For example, diaper changes in critically ill neonates and infants, gavage feeding, and medical examinations are not painful but can be very stressful for children. In response to stress, the hypothalamic–pituitary axis (HPA) produces corticotrophin-releasing hormones (CRHs) in the hippocampus, followed by adrenocorticotrophic hormones (ACTHs) in the anterior pituitary gland and glucocorticoids, including the steroid hormone cortisol in the adrenal cortex. Those steroid hormones are multifunctional and have immunomodulating properties, for example. The HPA undergoes major developmental changes after birth and is sensitive to a variety of stressors during infancy. Therefore, alterations in steroid hormone levels, which are influenced by stress, could be held responsible for neonatal morbidity. From the landmark study of Anand et al., we learned that stress caused by untreated pain due to surgery in preterm-born children resulted in greater hormonal and metabolic changes in plasma adrenaline, noradrenaline, glucagon, aldosterone, corticosterone, 11-deoxycorticosterone, and 11-deoxycortisol levels, in the insulin/glucagon, molar ratio, and in glucose, lactate, and pyruvate concentrations. Those changes were significantly greater in the children not treated with fentanyl compared to children treated with fentanyl. The children who were not treated with fentanyl suffered more respiratory, circulatory, and metabolic complications.[2] Interestingly, different fentanyl dosing regimens (administered as a continuous infusion or with bolus technique) with or without the addition of midazolam to large-dose fentanyl did not result in less stress hormone release compared to large-dose fentanyl alone after cardiac surgery in infants. Moreover, no adverse postoperative outcome was found in the different groups.[7] This implies that the need for stress reducing therapy is well known and important, but the choice of the agent is variable and might be less important. The importance of antinociceptive and sedative therapy in newborns, infants, children, and adolescents has, therefore, been increasingly acknowledged over the past decades, leading to a burst of research and increased use of analgesic agents in children of all ages. Research has concentrated on the development of pain assessment instruments, nonpharmacologic interventions, and clinical trials investigating the effectiveness and safety of analgesics and opioids, in particular in infants.

NONPHARMACOLOGIC INTERVENTIONS

To reduce distress and treat pain, the first step should always be nonpharmacologic therapy. Nonpharmacologic treatment in newborns includes facilitated tucking, non-nutritive sucking, massage, and sucrose.[8,9] The administration of oral sucrose significantly reduces procedural pain expression from heel lances, venipunctures, and intramuscular injections and especially when combined with non-nutritive sucking.[10] Sucrose also reduces distress during medical examinations, such as echocardiography.[11] Massage has shown to be effective to reduce procedural pain in preterm-born infants.[12] Moreover, massage therapy combined to skin-to-skin care also improved long-term neurodevelopmental outcome in very low birth weight neonates.[13] To reduce distress and procedural pain in older children, nonpharmacologic interventions such as a preparation and distraction protocol are effective as well.[14] When nonpharmacologic treatment is not sufficient, pharmacologic interventions are needed in addition. In the following parts of this chapter, we discuss various pharmacologic analgesic options to treat pain and several sedative agents to reduce distress.

PHARMACOLOGIC INTERVENTIONS

ANALGESICS

Knowledge about analgesic effects has been enlarged using a number of validated pain assessment tools in randomized trials comparing different dose regimens and different agents.[15–17] Several trials have gained more insight into the specific pharmacokinetics (PK) and pharmacodynamics (PD) of analgesics in children.[18,19] Pediatric PK alters with age through developmental changes such as the maturation of enzyme systems and physiologic processes responsible for absorption and elimination.[20–23] Moreover, changes in body composition alter disposition. PD changes from neonatal life through adolescence are poorly documented. Although it is thought that PD is commonly similar in children and adults after the first years of life.[24] In the near future, the application of physiology-based PK dosing will certainly bring new insights in optimal dosages.[25]

Analgesics in pediatric patients can be broadly divided into opioids and nonopioids. A good understanding of the nociceptive system is necessary to improve pain assessment and, most importantly, to treat pain adequately in neonates and older children and eventually prevent pain using the concept of preemptive analgesia. We have to bear in mind that differences exist between different indications for analgesic therapy. For example, a different analgesic agent is needed for pain due to tissue damage because of surgical procedures and procedural pain such as heel lances. This will have consequences for the choice of analgesic therapy since intravenous (IV) acetaminophen (also known as paracetamol) and morphine are recommended after major surgery, while acetaminophen and morphine are not recommended for procedural pain, for example.[26,27] The World Health Organization (WHO) developed a three-step ladder for analgesic therapy (Fig. 36.1).[28] Interestingly, this ladder was designed to treat cancer pain in adults but is very often used in children. The first step of the ladder consists of a nonopioid. In newborns, acetaminophen is often used as this first step. For infants older than 3 months, a nonsteroidal anti-inflammatory drug (NSAID) such as ibuprofen can be added (see Chapter 39 for more information on NSAIDs). Next, a weak opioid such as tramadol can be added. The last step consists of strong opioids such as fentanyl of morphine. Both fentanyl and morphine are commonly used in the intensive care units (ICUs).[29] See also Figure 36.2 for an overview of commonly used analgesics in children.

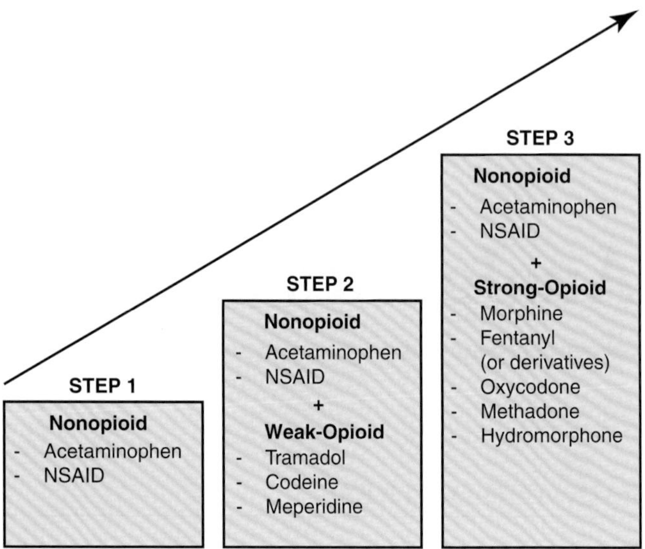

Figure 36.1 World Health Organization Pain Ladder. NSAID, nonsteroidal anti-inflammatory drug.

Acetaminophen

Indications and Clinical Use

The nonopioid analgesic agent *N*-acetyl-para-aminophenol, better known as acetaminophen in the United States and paracetamol in Europe, or by its brand name Tylenol, is the most commonly used drug for pain relief worldwide. Acetanilid, the parent compound of acetaminophen, was introduced in 1886. Toxicity-related problems with acetanilid led to the introduction of acetaminophen in 1893. The popularity of acetaminophen over the NSAID agents rose after the reported association between Reye syndrome and aspirin in the 1980s.[30] Acetaminophen is widely used to treat mild-to-moderate pain and is also commonly used as an antipyretic agent in children and adults. In contrast to NSAIDs, it has no anti-inflammatory effects.

Major differences exist regarding the labeling of acetaminophen under the age of 1 year. When dosed adequately, acetaminophen is a poor procedural analgesic, but it is very effective for mild-to-moderate pain with its additional morphine-sparing effects.[31] It has been shown that the use of IV acetaminophen reduces the use of morphine after surgery in neonates and infants and is, therefore, the analgesic of first choice after surgery in these patients.[26] In preterm-born children, a single dose during painful procedures showed no analgesic benefit,[32] and it is generally believed that acetaminophen is not an appropriate drug to treat the acute pain related to procedures.[33] Interestingly,

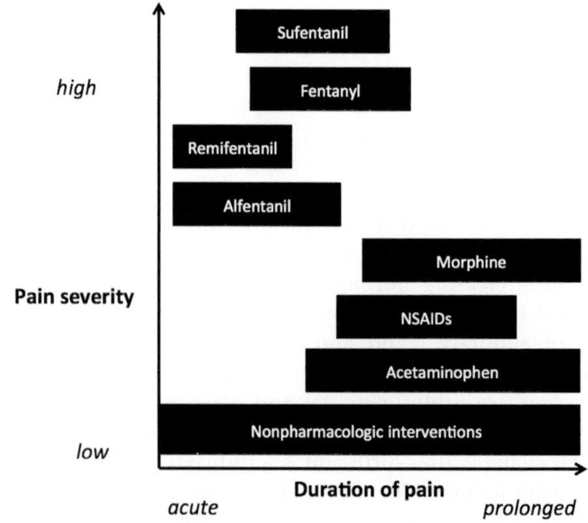

Figure 36.2 Overview of analgesics. NSAIDs, nonsteroidal anti-inflammatory drugs.

preemptive rectal acetaminophen after assisted vaginal delivery was even associated with increased pain responses 2 to 3 days later during procedural pain.[34]

Mechanism of Action

The mechanism of action is complex and includes the effects of both the peripheral [cyclooxygenase (COX) inhibition] and central antinociception processes and the so-called redox mechanism.[35] Debate exists about the primary site of action of acetaminophen, which may be inhibition of prostaglandin synthesis or through an active metabolite influencing cannabinoid receptors.[36] Acetaminophen prevents peripheral sensitization and has an important central analgesic effect that is mediated through this activation of descending serotonergic pathways. However, in newborn children, the serotonergic system is more facilitatory instead of inhibitory.[37] The selectivity of serotonergic control of spinal somatosensation changes with postnatal age. Preclinical studies showed that in young animals, the descending serotonergic control is nonselective and amplifies the saliency of low- and high-threshold mechanical sensory inputs in the spinal cord.[37] This occurs both by increasing neuronal activity and spatial receptive field sizes of dorsal horn neurons. The antipyretic effect of acetaminophen is likely attributed to the effect on the heat-regulating centers in the brain, resulting in vasodilation, sweating, and loss of body heat.

Pharmacokinetics

Acetaminophen has a low first-pass metabolism. The relative bioavailability of rectal compared with oral acetaminophen formulations ($F_{rectal/oral}$) has been reported as 0.52 (range 0.24 to 0.98).[38] The relative bioavailability is higher in neonates, where it is possible suppository insertion height may result in a different rectal venous drainage pattern. Previous studies showed that the area under the curve (AUC) in neonates after suppository administration was significantly greater than that in infants and older children. Thus, the relative bioavailability of rectal formulations appears to be age related.

Absorption from the duodenum to the systemic circulation is rapid with a $T_{1/2,abs}$ of 2.7 to 6.8 minutes.[39,40] Absorption in children under the age of 3 months is delayed by a factor of 3.68[41] because absorption depends on gastric emptying, and gastric emptying is slow and erratic in the neonate.[42] Moreover, oral absorption is considerably delayed in premature neonates in the first few days of life.[43] Absorption through the rectal route is slow and unpredictable with large variability. The absorption half-life for rectal formulations was prolonged in infants younger than 3 months (1.51 times greater) compared to values in older children.[43,44]

With the availability of IV acetaminophen, these issues can nowadays be bypassed if necessary. The metabolism of acetaminophen changes with age. In newborns, the largest part is metabolized by sulfation and with increasing age glucuronidation rapidly becomes more important.[45] Thus, the AUC ratio of glucuronide to acetaminophen increases with gestational age, that of sulfate decreases, and the ratio of cysteine and mercapturate remains unchanged in preterm-born children.[45] Approximately 4% of acetaminophen is excreted in urine unchanged, and the amount is dependent on urine flow.[46] Clearance increased from 27 weeks patient-controlled analgesia (PCA) (1.87 L per hour per 70 kg) to reach 84% of the mature value by 1 year of age.[47] Approximately 5% to 10% of acetaminophen is metabolized by cytochrome P-450 (CYP) and especially by the CYP2E1 enzyme,[48–50] to the toxic metabolite *N*-acetyl-*p*-benzoquinone imine (NAPQI)[45] (see "Adverse Effects and Toxicity" section).

Pharmacodynamics

A study showed that acetaminophen resulted in a dose-related reduction in the number of children who required postoperative rescue opioids, with significance reached with 40 or 60 mg per kg doses.[51] Calculated dose of acetaminophen at which 50% of the children did not require a rescue opioid was 35 mg per kg. Neither the antipyretic nor the analgesic effect of acetaminophen is directly related to plasma concentration. A delay of approximately 1 hour between peak concentration and peak effect is reported.[52,53] However, fluctuations in pain, type of pain, and the placebo effect complicate interpretation of clinical studies.[54] Anderson et al.[55] reported PD population parameter estimates (population variability *CV*) in children after tonsillectomy. An E_{max} model in which the greatest possible pain relief (visual analog scale 0 to 10) equates to an E_{max} of 10 were E_{max} = 5.17 (64%) and EC_{50} = 9.98 (107%) mg per L. The equilibration half-time (T_{eq}) of the analgesic effect compartment was 53 (217%) minutes. A target effect compartment concentration of 10 mg per L is associated with a pain reduction of 2.6/10. Effect site concentrations associated with analgesia for the pains experienced as a neonate are unknown. The use of an IV acetaminophen formulation allows greater dosing accuracy, less PK variability attributable to absorption, and more rapid speed of effect onset.[54]

Adverse Effects and Toxicity

Acetaminophen overdose results in increased production of highly reactive electrophilic metabolites by the hepatic cytochrome P-450–dependent mixed-function oxidase enzyme system.[56] The toxic metabolite of acetaminophen, NAPQI, is formed by the CYP2E1, CYP1A2, and CYP3A4.[57] This metabolite binds to intracellular hepatic macromolecules to produce cell necrosis and damage. Acetaminophen concentrations may increase in pediatric patients with low clearance after regular doses of 15 mg per kg every 4 hours.[58] There is evidence of glutathione depletion in adult volunteers, given doses of 0.5 and 3 g acetaminophen separated by 4 to 10 days.[59] Penna and Buchanan[60] reported 7 deaths and 11 cases of hepatotoxicity associated with acetaminophen in children. Mortality due to hepatotoxicity was associated with doses greater than 300 mg per day per kg for 1 to 6 days. Survival was usually seen in those children suffering hepatotoxicity due to acetaminophen greater than 150 mg per day per kg for 2 to 8 days. Subsequent guidelines[61,62] recommend that doses should not exceed 90 mg per day per kg. Significant hepatic and renal disease, malnutrition, and dehydration increase the propensity for toxicity. Medications that induce the hepatic CYP2E1, CYP1A2, and CYP3A4 systems (e.g., phenobarbitone, phenytoin, rifampicin) may also increase the risk of hepatotoxicity. It has been speculated that ingestion of acetaminophen increases the potential for liver injury by another cause, such as a viral agent.[63] Hepatotoxicity causing death or requiring liver transplantation has been reported, with doses above 75 mg per kg per day in children and 90 mg per kg per day in infants.[64–67] It is possible that even these regimens may cause hepatotoxicity if used for longer than 2 to 3 days.[64] It is unknown whether there is a difference in the propensity to toxicity between children given acetaminophen for fever and those given acetaminophen for postoperative analgesia.

Opioids

Mechanism of Action

The analgesic effects of opioids occur by activation of μ, κ, and/or δ receptors in the central nervous system (CNS).[68] Each class of receptors is divided into subtypes that have different clinical effects. Analgesia is obtained by spinal or supraspinal activation of opioid receptors, leading to decreased neurotransmitter release from nociceptive neurons, inhibiting the ascending neuronal pain pathways, and altering perception and response to pain.[69] Endogenous opioids β-endorphin and enkephalins (met-enkephalin and leu-enkephalin) or analgesic drugs such as morphine or fentanyl can produce powerful analgesia by inhibiting the firing of nociceptive neurons in the dorsal horn of the spinal cord.[70] The μ-opioid receptor (OPRM1), the most potent target for analgesia, is distributed throughout the CNS with a high density in the dorsal horn. Opioids activate the descending pathway from the brainstem by suppressing the inhibitory control of local GABAergic interneurons in the rostral ventromedial medulla and periaqueductal gray, thereby activating projection neurons that, in turn, inhibit nociceptive transmission at the pain gate.[70]

Indications and Clinical Use

Opioids in neonates, infants, children, and adolescents are reserved for moderate-to-severe types of pain, such as postoperative pain and palliative care,[71] or as an additive to acetaminophen or NSAIDs if pain is moderate, as recommended by the WHO Analgesic Ladder (Fig. 36.1). Opioids are often used at the ICU to treat pain or distress. The most frequently used opioids are fentanyl and morphine, but also oxycodone, methadone, hydromorphone, and meperidine are used in children, as well as fentanyl derivatives such as alfentanil and sufentanil. Codeine and tramadol are contraindicated in children younger than 12 years because of serious side effects. Therefore, acetaminophen, NSAIDs, and other opioids are recommended (see also Fig. 36.1).

Adverse Effects

Opioids have adverse effects that may be minimized by appropriate drug selection and adequate dosing. From studies in children with neonatal abstinence syndrome (NAS), we know that different polymorphisms in the μ-opioid receptor affect the incidence and severity of NAS.[72] Moreover, we know that severe adverse effects can occur after use of tramadol or codeine in patients who are genetically CYP2D6 ultra-rapid extensive metabolizers. So there is an interindividual variability in opioid sensitivity. Moreover, ontogeny plays an important role in the need for different dosing regimens of opioids.[73,74] Well-known adverse effects of opioids are respiratory depression, hypotension, glottic and chest wall rigidity, constipation, urinary retention, seizures, sedation, and bradycardia. Continuous monitoring and frequent assessment of vital signs should be conducted during opioid administration, especially in those under 3 months of age and in former preterm infants under 60 weeks postmenstrual age (PMA). Naloxone is a competitive opioid receptor agonist that reverses many of these side effects but that also antagonizes the effects of endorphins.

Codeine

Indication and Clinical Use

Codeine, or methylmorphine, is a morphine-like opioid with one-tenth the potency of morphine. Codeine has been used in neonates and infants and neonates after major surgery as an adjunct to acetaminophen or NSAIDs (optimal oral codeine dosage 1 to 1.5 mg per kg every 4 to 6 hours, oral acetaminophen 20 mg per kg every 6 hours in infants older than 3 months).[75] Combinations of codeine and NSAIDs or acetaminophen are available and produce additive analgesic effects because of different mechanisms of action.

Mechanism of Action

Codeine is mainly metabolized by glucuronidation, but minor pathways are N-demethylation to norcodeine and O-demethylation to morphine. Around 10% of codeine is metabolized to morphine. As codeine's affinity for opioid receptors is very low, the analgesic effect of codeine is mainly due to its metabolite, morphine.[76] The CYP enzyme CYP2D6 catalyzes the metabolism of codeine to morphine. A genetic polymorphism of this enzyme causes distinct phenotypes responsible for the presence of ultra-rapid extensive, extensive, and slow codeine metabolizers in the population.[77,78] Between 7% and 10% of the population are believed to be slow metabolizers of codeine,[78–80] but this percentage has been reported to be much higher.[78,79] Other medications competing for the CYP2D6 enzyme (e.g., quinidine) may decrease the analgesic effect of codeine. Case reports of pediatric patients with overactive CYP2D6 enzymes have been reported. These ultra-rapid metabolizers (UMs) experience an increase in the production of active metabolites of codeine and tramadol, which can lead to oversedation, respiratory depression, and death. With this knowledge, it is problematic that the genotype of most patients is unknown.

Pharmacokinetics

The plasma half-life of codeine is 3 to 4 hours. Codeine can be given intramuscularly, orally, and rectally. IV codeine is not recommended because of hypotensive side effects.[81] Rectal codeine achieves lower concentrations than intramuscular codeine because of incomplete, slower, more variable absorption.[82] In children, it is generally given in doses of 1 to 3 mg per kg per day.

Peak plasma concentration (C_{max}) occurs after 1 hour (T_{max}) after oral administration. The plasma half-life is 3 to 3.5 hours. The C_{max} is reached 30 minutes after intramuscular injection.[76] A volume of distribution (V) of 3.6 L per kg and a clearance (CL) of 0.85 L per hour have been described in adults, but there are few data detailing pediatric PK developmental changes. The neonatal half-life is longer due to immature clearance (e.g., 4.5 hours), while that of an infant is shorter (e.g., 2.6 hours).[83] The PK of codeine is poorly described in children despite use over decades.

Adverse Effects

The adverse effects of codeine are broadly similar to those of other opioids. Although codeine has been shown to cause no analgesic effect in the poor metabolizers, side effects persist.[80] Importantly, high incidences of adverse effects might be expected in patients who have an ultra-rapid extensive metabolism, as described above. These patients achieve higher morphine concentrations. Cautiousness is also needed when codeine is used during breastfeeding since a newborn once died from morphine poisoning when his mother used codeine while breastfeeding. The mother, a UM, produced much more morphine when taking codeine than most people do.[84,85] In 2017, the U.S. Food and Drug Administration (FDA) updated their warnings regarding codeine and tramadol use in the pediatric population, making their use contraindicated in patients under the age of 12 years.[86,87] Moreover, the FDA also warns against the use of codeine and tramadol in case of a medical history of obesity, sleep apnea, severe lung disease, or after surgical removal of tonsils or adenoids.[87,88] For this reason, acetaminophen and NSAIDs or, if insufficient, other opioids are recommended.

Tramadol

Indications and Clinical Use

Tramadol is a weak opioid and is involved in the third step of the WHO Analgesic Ladder. It is used to treat moderate to moderately severe acute and chronic pain. Evidence for the use of tramadol for postoperative pain in children is low.[89] Combinations of tramadol and acetaminophen are available. In line with codeine, the FDA contraindicates the use of tramadol in patients under the age of 12 years as well, because of the genetic heterogeneity in CYP2D6 with the risk of side effects, such as oversedation, respiratory depression, and death in UMs.[86]

Mechanism of Action

Tramadol ((1RS,2RS)-2-[(dimethylamino)methyl]-1-(3-methoxyphenyl)-cyclo-hexanol) is a synthetic opioid with opioid agonist properties that act on the neurotransmission of noradrenalin and serotonin. It is converted in the liver into either the active metabolite *O*-desmethyltramadol, an opioid with stronger binding to the μ-opioid receptor, catalyzed by CYP2D6, or into the inactive *N*-desmethyltramadol by CYP3A4.[90]

Pharmacokinetics

Besides CYP2D6 polymorphisms, extensive between-individual variability in tramadol disposition has been linked to size, age, comedication, and comorbidity. Total tramadol clearance has been estimated for adults (28 L per hour), children aged 1 to 7 years (8.86 L per hour per 70 kg), and full-term gestation neonates and infants (17.1 L per hour per 70 kg).[91,92] Maturation and size are key predictors of PK variability. Maturation of tramadol elimination occurs in early development, with 50% of adult value reached at term gestation.

Adverse Effects

The adverse effects are comparable to those of codeine, and the use is contraindicated in children younger than 12 years as well. The FDA also warns against the use of tramadol in breastfeeding women because of possible harm to infants. In children and adolescents between the ages 12 and 18 years, the FDA warns against its use when there is a history of obesity, obstructive sleep apnea, severe lung disease, or after surgery to remove the tonsils or adenoids.[87] In children older than 12 years requiring chronic pain treatment with tramadol, a personalized approach is needed to sustain safe use, with dose adaptation according to CYP2D6 activity.[93]

Morphine

Indications and Clinical Use

Historically, the most common opioid used for pediatric pain is morphine. However, morphine is not a suitable drug for short painful procedures, because of its pharmacologic properties with a slow onset of action and a long half-life. IV morphine is administered to pediatric patients with prolonged pain such as after surgery, to uncomfortable ventilated premature newborns, or to those suffering from necrotizing enterocolitis. Though two large randomized controlled trials in preterm-born–ventilated children showed no positive effects of routine administration of IV morphine.[94,95] Moreover, it is not recommended to administer oral morphine to nonventilated premature infants for procedural pain because of respiratory side effects without analgesic efficacy.[27] Morphine can also be administered by other routes, such as rectally or intramuscularly. Administration in premature newborns is limited to the IV route. The painful administration of intramuscular morphine injections is not acceptable. Subcutaneous intermittent boluses through an indwelling catheter offer an alternative route.[96] The large variability observed after rectal administration is a major disadvantage of this route, although clinically frequently used.[97] Oral morphine, either as elixir or slow-release formulations, offers a good alternative despite a high first-pass effect. Epidural or intrathecal administration may cause delayed respiratory depression due to slow rostral migration within the cerebrospinal fluid (CSF).[98] PCA is possible in some children aged as young as 6 years, and nurse-controlled analgesia (NCA) can be used effectively in younger children.[99]

Mechanism of Action/Metabolism

The analgesic effect of morphine is mainly caused by an activation of μ receptors, as confirmed by a lack of analgesic effect of morphine in murine studies using μ-receptor knockout mice.[100–102] The most important positions on the morphine molecule, next to the nitrogen atom (probably responsible for the analgesic activity, as modifications reduce penetration into the CNS), are the phenolic hydroxyl at position 3 and the alcoholic hydroxyl at position 6. Morphine is mainly metabolized by the enzyme UDP–glucuronosyltransferase 2B7 (UGT2B7) into morphine-3-glucuronide (M3G) and morphine-6-glucuronide (M6G).[103] Contributions to both the desired effect (analgesia) and the undesired effects (nausea, respiratory depression) of M6G are the subject of clinical controversy.[104–110] M3G has been suggested to antagonize the antinociceptive and respiratory depressive effects of morphine and M6G[111,112] and contribute to the development of tolerance. The enzyme responsible for morphine glucuronidation, UGT2B7,[20] is mainly found in the liver, but also exists in the intestines and kidneys.[113] Sulfation is a minor pathway.[114,115] The metabolites are cleared by the kidneys and partly by biliary excretion. Some recirculation of morphine occurs due to β-glucuronidase activity in the gut.[116] Impaired renal function leads to accumulation of M3G and M6G.[117]

Pharmacokinetics

Morphine clearance matures with postconceptual age[20,118] and reaches adult rates at 6 to 12 months. In premature newborns, morphine clearance increases with gestation and postnatal age.[119] Morphine plasma concentrations show large interindividual variability.[120] Clinical circumstances, such as type of surgery, concurrent illness, whole-body cooling after perinatal asphyxia, and infants requiring extracorporeal membrane oxygenation (ECMO),[121,122] also have reduced morphine clearance.[123] Protein binding of morphine is low, from 20% in premature neonates[124] to 35% in adults,[125] and has no impact on disposition changes with age.[126]

Pharmacodynamics

There is a delay between analgesic effect and plasma concentration. The effect compartment equilibration half-time (T_{eq}) for morphine is approximately 17 minutes in adults,[127] but is anticipated to be shortened with decreasing age. A concentration–response relationship for morphine analgesia in children has not been described, although adverse effect relationships for both vomiting[128] and respiratory depression are reported.[129] The effectiveness of IV morphine in infants using validated pain assessment tools has been studied in different age groups. After major surgery, continuous morphine doses of 10 to 40 µg per kg have been shown to be effective in alleviating pain in infants and children aged 0 to 14 years.[130] No difference in analgesic effect was found between continuous and intermittent dosing. Randomized controlled trials showed different PD effects of IV morphine in premature neonates requiring artificial ventilation with continuous doses of 10 to 30 µg per kg.[94,95] Morphine did not reduce pain responses during endotracheal suctioning.[119] As a consequence, the routine use is not advocated during artificial ventilation. Another study reported mean morphine concentrations required to produce adequate sedation in 50% of neonates to be 125 ng per mL,[131] but analgesic target plasma concentrations for postoperative morphine analgesia are generally believed to be around 15 to 20 ng per mL.[118,132] For preterm infants who suffer from necrotizing enterocolitis, high plasma levels might be needed.[133] The large PK and PD variability means that morphine is often titrated to effect using small incremental doses (0.02 mg per kg) in children suffering postoperative pain.[134] Evidence-based morphine dosing algorithms for postoperative neonatal patients corrected for PK differences have shown to be effective and prevent overdosing.[26,135] As morphine should not be routinely prescribed for ventilated newborns, morphine should only be used in those newborns who have increased pain scores and doses again should be titrated to the individual needs of each neonate.[94,95]

Adverse Effects

Respiratory depression may occur at concentrations of 20 ng per mL.[132] Respiratory depression, as measured by carbon dioxide response curves or by arterial oxygen tension, is similar in children aged 2 to 570 days at the same morphine concentration.[129] Hypotension, bradycardia, and flushing are part of the histamine response to morphine and are associated with a rapid IV bolus administration. Morphine in preterm newborns has only small effects on blood pressure, but the effect might be more significant in extreme premature infants and dependent of the morphine doses.[136,137] The incidence of vomiting in children after tonsillectomy is related to morphine dose. Doses above 0.1 mg per kg were associated with a greater than 50% incidence of vomiting.[128] Regarding the potential and suggested long-term negative effects in the human, no such effects could be found in 5- and 8-year-old former preterm infants representing well-defined cohorts.[138,139]

Fentanyl

Indications and Clinical Use

Fentanyl may be the preferred analgesic agent for critically ill patients with hemodynamic instability, patients with symptoms related to histamine release during morphine infusion, or patients with morphine tolerance. Because of its relatively rapid onset of action and short duration of effect, fentanyl efficiently alleviates procedural pain.[140] It has been used in neonates on artificial ventilation[141] with bronchopulmonary dysplasia, pulmonary hypertension, and/or diaphragmatic hernia. One study showed a need to escalate dose during ECMO, indicating a rapid development of tolerance.[142] Overall, the use of synthetic opioids shows a more rapid tolerance (3 to 5 days) than that of morphine (2 weeks) and heroin (weeks).[143,144] A plasma concentration of greater than 20 ng per mL is required to provide total IV anesthesia.[145] This is probably due to the relative increased lipid solubility and molecular conformation, enabling efficient penetration of the blood–brain barrier. Fentanyl has been shown to effectively prevent preterm neonates from surgical stress responses and to improve postoperative outcome.[2] Single fentanyl doses (3 µg per kg) and infusion (1.1 µg per kg per hour) reduced physiologic and behavioral measures of pain and stress during mechanical ventilation in preterm neonates[146,147] as effectively as morphine.[141] International recommended starting doses are, however, smaller, as is presented in Table 36.1. In older infants and children, fentanyl has been shown to be effective for the management of perioperative and postoperative pain[148] and for the management of procedural pain. Transdermal fentanyl can be used for severe cancer-related pain[149] or in palliative pediatric care.[71]

Mechanism of Action

Fentanyl is a synthetic opioid that acts as a "morphine-like agonist." Its potency is about 100- to 300-fold that of morphine, with a large postulated effect on the µ receptor.[145] Fentanyl metabolism is related to the activity of the hepatic cytochrome P-450 system (CYP3A4) and is metabolized by oxidative N-dealkylation into nor-fentanyl and hydroxylized.[150,151] All metabolites are inactive, and a small amount of fentanyl is renally eliminated unchanged.[152]

Pharmacokinetics

Fentanyl has a relatively rapid onset of 1.5 minutes and a short duration of action of approximately 60 to 120 minutes, with a peak effect of 20 to 30 minutes (see Table 36.1).[145] Following removal, serum fentanyl concentrations decline gradually and fall to 50% in approximately 16 hours. This prolonged apparent elimination half-life occurs because fentanyl continues to be absorbed from the skin, where a fentanyl depot concentrates.[153] The systemic availability of fentanyl by this route is approximately 30% of that found using the IV route.[154] Oral transmucosal fentanyl provides consistent analgesia for brief painful procedures.[155] Transdermal and transmucosal fentanyl have not been studied in newborns. Because fentanyl has very high lipid solubility, it is widely distributed in tissues. Its short duration of effect is due to redistribution to deep, lipid-rich compartments. Accumulation of fentanyl in lipid-rich tissues may redistribute slowly after discontinuation of therapy, resulting in prolonged periods of sedation and respiratory depression after an extended period of use.[156] The context-sensitive half-time after an infusion of 1 hour is approximately 20 minutes, but it is 270 minutes after an 8-hour infusion.[157] The clearance of fentanyl appears to be immature at birth, especially in very preterm infants,[158] but increases dramatically after birth. Fentanyl clearance is 70% to 80% of adult values in term neonates and, standardized to a 70-kg person, appears to reach adult levels within the first 2 weeks of life.[156,159] The volume of distribution of fentanyl at steady state is around 5.9 L per kg in term-born neonates and decreases with age to 4.5 L per kg during infancy, 3.1 L per kg during childhood, and 1.6 L per kg in adults.[160] Initial plasma concentrations in pediatric patients are lower than in adults due to larger distribution volumes. Fentanyl, alfentanil, and sufentanil are metabolized by CYP3A4, and other drugs that also use this enzyme (e.g.,

TABLE 36.1 Overview of Pharmacologic Properties of Morphine, Fentanyl, and Derivatives of Fentanyl

	Morphine	*Fentanyl*	*Sufentanil*	*Alfentanil*	*Remifentanil*
Potency compared with morphine	NA	100–300	800–1,000	40–50	100–200
IV induction dose (μg/kg)	50–100	2–6	0.25–2.0	25–100	1–2
IV infusion rate (μg/kg/h)	5–30	0.5–5	0.5–1.5	30–120	0.1–1.0
Routes of administration other than IV	Oral, rectal	Transdermal, transmucosal (buccal, nasal, sublingual), epidural	Epidural, sublingual		
Time to onset (min)	15	1.5	1	0.75	<1
Time to peak effect (min)	20	4.5–8	2.5–5	1.5	1.5
Duration of peak effect (min)	60	20–30	30	15	
Duration of analgesic effect (min)	240–420	60–120	100–150	30–60	5–10
Analgesic plasma concentration (ng/mL)	15–20	0.6–3.0	0.5–2.5	50–300	0.3–3
Plasma concentration associated with loss of consciousness (ng/mL)	>125	>20.0	>2.5	>400	>4
Metabolism	UGT2B7	CYP3A	CYP3A	CYP3A	Plasma and tissue esterases

Adapted from Ziesenitz VC, Vaughns JD, Koch G, et al. Correction to: pharmacokinetics of fentanyl and its derivatives in children: a comprehensive review. *Clin Pharmacokinet* 2018;57:393–417.
IV, intravenous.

cyclosporine, erythromycin) may decrease clearance, leading to increased fentanyl plasma concentrations.[161,162] Acetaminophen has been shown to interact with fentanyl metabolism in vitro,[163] although the clinical importance of this interaction is probably unimportant.

Adverse Effects

Fentanyl has a wide margin of safety and beneficial effects on hemodynamic stability.[164,165] Fentanyl has a propensity for muscular rigidity.[166] With regard to respiratory depression, fentanyl has similar side effects in infants and adults when plasma concentrations are similar.[167] The intraoperative use of high-dose (3 μg per kg) fentanyl in infants did not result in respiratory depression or hypoxemia in a placebo-controlled trial.[148] Only 3 of 2,000 nonintubated infants and children experienced short apneic episodes after a low dose of fentanyl for the repair of facial lacerations.[168]

Alfentanil

Indications and Clinical Use

Alfentanil is a synthetic opioid that is chemically a derivate of fentanyl. It has a rapid onset of 0.75 minute, a brief duration of action of 30 to 60 minutes with a peak analgesic effect of 15 minutes, and its potency is about 40- to 50-fold that of morphine.[145] It is used as a procedural analgesic for pediatric patients.[169]

Pharmacokinetics

Phase 1 metabolism goes via oxidative N-dealkylation by CYP3A4 and O-dealkylation and then phase 2 conjugation to renally excreted end products.[170] Alfentanil plasma protein binding increases from 65% in preterm neonates and 79% in term infants to around 90% in adults.[171,172] The volume of distribution is smaller in infants than in adults.[173] Clearances of alfentanil, standardized to a 70-kg person, are similar at different ages (250 to 500 mL per min per 70 kg), except for the neonatal age group, in which clearances are decreased (20 to 60 mL per min per 70 kg). Consequently, elimination half-life in children (40 to 68 minutes) is higher in the neonatal period. In premature neonates, the half-life is as long as 6 to 9 hours.[174,175]

Pharmacodynamics

Alfentanil has lower lipid solubility and causes less histamine release[176] than fentanyl. Sufficient analgesia during endotracheal intubation and suctioning has been found using 10 to 20 μg per kg alfentanil in preterm neonates.[169,177,178] A target plasma concentration of 400 ng per mL is used in anesthesia.[145]

Adverse Effects

Alfentanil cannot be used without neuromuscular blocking drugs in newborns because of a very high incidence of rigidity.[169,179]

Sufentanil

Indications and Clinical Use

Sufentanil is a most potent opioid analgesic and is 800 to 1,000 times more potent than morphine, with an onset of 1 minute, an analgesic effect of 100 to 150 minutes and a peak analgesic effect of 30 minutes.[145] A plasma concentration of greater than 2.5 ng per mL is required for total IV anesthesia and 0.5 to 2.5 ng per mL for analgesia.[145]

Pharmacokinetics

Like fentanyl and alfentanil, the P-450 CYP3A4 enzyme is responsible for the N-dealkylation.[150] The amount of free sufentanil decreases with age (neonates 19%; infants 11%; children/adults 8%) and is strongly correlated with the α-1-acid glycoprotein plasma concentration.[171] The lower concentration of α-1-acid glycoprotein in newborns and infants contributes to the increased free fraction of sufentanil in these age groups. Although sufentanil, fentanyl, alfentanil, and remifentanil have high protein binding (>70%) and have high hepatic (or nonhepatic for remifentanil) extraction ratios, protein-binding changes are probably clinically unimportant[126] because dose is titrated to effect and clearance variability has greater impact.

Remifentanil

Indications and Clinical Use

Remifentanil resembles fentanyl, sufentanil, and alfentanil in chemical structure. It is a selective μ-receptor agonist with a higher potency than alfentanil. Its potency is about 100- to 200-fold that of morphine.[145] Remifentanil works fast with a time to onset of less than a minute and has a short duration of analgesic effect of 5 to 10 minutes.[145] Therefore, it is often given as a continuous infusion. Because the inhibitory neurotransmitter glycine is used as a carrier for remifentanil, it should not be used for spinal or epidural applications.[180] A concentration of greater than 4 ng per mL supplements anesthesia for major surgery. Analgesic concentrations are 0.3 to 3 ng per mL.[145] Because of its short duration, remifentanil seems to be ideally suited for pediatric neurosurgical patients who may require neurologic assessment at completion of surgery.[181] Administration of 1 μg per kg IV followed by 0.1 to 1.0 μg per kg per min results in sufficient analgesia during surgery in children.[182–185]

Pharmacokinetics

Remifentanil is metabolized to carbonic acid. The metabolism is independent of liver and renal function. Remifentanil reacts with nonspecific esterase in tissue and erythrocytes.[186,187] Clearances decreases with age, with rates of 90 mL per kg per min in infants less than 2 years, 60 mL per kg per min between the ages of 2 and 12 years, and 40 mL per kg per min in adults.[188–190] Volume of distribution in children is lower (200 to 300 mL per kg) than with adults (400 mL per kg) but might be increased in young infants (450 mL per kg). Elimination half-life seems to be constant, around 3 to 6 minutes.[98,191]

Adverse Effects

The use of remifentanil is accompanied by a high incidence of life-threatening respiratory depression at subtherapeutic concentrations.[192] As a result of a rapid development of μ-receptor tolerance with remifentanil use, higher subsequent opioid doses are required. IV remifentanil doses of 0.25 μg per kg per min appear to be safe and effective in neonates,[193,194] but data concerning the use of remifentanil in this group are scarce. For mechanically ventilated preterm infants, the use of remifentanil at 0.25 μg per kg per min as an analgesic for short procedures represents a therapeutic option.[195] Fast infusion is related to life-threatening thorax rigidity in preterm newborns, and loading doses should be discouraged, especially in this group of patients.[196]

Oxycodone

Indications and Clinical Use

Oxycodone is a semisynthetic analgesic that is available as an immediate-release product (oral solution and capsule) as well as a controlled-release tablet for 12-hourly administration. Immediate- and controlled-release preparations of oxycodone have similar efficacy and comparable side-effect profiles in adults.[197]

Pharmacokinetics

The relative bioavailability of intranasal, oral, and rectal formulations was approximately 50% that of IV in adults. The buccal and sublingual absorption of oxycodone is similar in young children.[198] Intramuscular administration provides relatively constant drug absorption, while buccal and gastric administration is associated with large interindividual variation in the rate of absorption.[199] Mean values of drug clearance and volume of distribution (V_d) were 15.2 [standard deviation (SD) 4.2] mL per min per kg and 2.1 (SD 0.8) L per kg, respectively, in children after ophthalmic surgery.[200]

Adverse Effects

Olkkola et al. showed that oxycodone (0.1 mg per kg) in children after ophthalmic surgery caused greater ventilatory depression compared to other opioids.[200]

Methadone

Indications and Clinical Use

Methadone is a synthetic opioid with an analgesic potency similar to that of morphine but with a more rapid distribution and a slower elimination. Methadone might have beneficial effects because it is a long-acting synthetic opioid with a very high bioavailability by the enteral route. Methadone is used as a maintenance drug in opioid-addicted adults to prevent withdrawal effects. Although only few data on the efficacy and safety of methadone are available, methadone is also widely used for the treatment of opioid withdrawal in neonates and children.[201,202] Moreover, IV methadone has been shown to be an effective analgesic for postoperative pain relief,[203] and oral administration has been recommended as the first-line opioid for severe and persistent pain in children.[204] Although a predominant role for methadone in the management of prolonged pain in neonates has been suggested, the use still needs to be evaluated in a clinical research setting.[144]

Mechanism of Action

Methadone activates the opioid receptor similar to morphine, but it also blocks the *N*-methyl-*D*-aspartate (NMDA) receptor. NMDA blockade is hypothesized to produce acute upregulation of the NMDA receptor, discontinuation of the NMDA receptor blocker is hypothesized to lead to excitotoxic neurotoxicity.[205] Not all NMDA antagonists induce apoptosis, however; and cell death can also occur during the NMDA blockade.[205] Therefore, the exact underlying mechanisms are not yet unraveled.

Pharmacokinetics

Methadone PK shows a slow elimination half-life with large interindividual variability (3.8 to 62 hours).[144] Recent studies have shown that CYP2B6 is the most important metabolizing enzyme and CYP3A4 is of less importance.[206] Clearance increases with gestational age and within the first year of life. Based on simulated exposure using new PK data, simplified and shortened dosing schedules have been shown to be suitable to treat NAS.[207] The lipid solubility of methadone is greater than that of morphine.[208] The increased lipid solubility and longer duration of effect give this drug potential for single-shot epidural use.

Adverse Effects

The effect of maternal methadone on the newborn infant might partially be explained by the CYP2B6 genotype.[209] In the near future, genomic tests might be used to predict the expected severity of NAS. Methadone seems to be a safe enteral alternative for IV opioids in palliative pediatric oncologic patients.[210] Reported common adverse effects include sedation, nausea, and constipation.[211]

Hydromorphone

Indications and Clinical Use

Hydromorphone is a semisynthetic congener of morphine, with a potency of around 5 to 7.5 times that of morphine.[212] Hydromorphone is used for chronic cancer pain and postoperative analgesia.

Pharmacokinetics

Hydromorphone is metabolized to hydromorphone-3-glucuronide and also, to a lesser extent, to dihydroisomorphine and dihydromorphine.[213] The IV versus oral dose ratio is 1:5, as there is high first-pass metabolism.[214] A clearance of 51.7 (range, 28.6 to 98.2) mL per min per kg is reported in children.[215] Time to peak concentration is 4 to 6 hours, and clearance is 51.7 mL per min per kg in children.[212,215]

Adverse Effects

The side-effect profile is comparable to that of other strong opioids, and hydromorphone does not convincingly demonstrate clinical superiority in adults over other strong opioid analgesics.[216]

Goodarzi showed that epidural hydromorphone caused fewer side effects than morphine and fentanyl in children undergoing orthopedic procedures.[217] PCA with hydromorphone seems to result in similar analgesia and side effects compared to morphine in children for the management of mucositis pain after bone marrow transplantation.[212]

Meperidine (Pethidine)

Indications and Clinical Use

Meperidine is a weak opioid, primarily μ-receptor, agonist with a potency of one-tenth that of morphine. The analgesic effects are detectable within 5 minutes of IV administration, and peak effect is reached within 10 minutes.[116,218] Meperidine was initially synthesized as an anticholinergic agent, but was soon discovered to have analgesic properties. Although meperidine's anticholinergic effects were demonstrated in vivo, the anticholinergic effects on the biliary and renal tracts have not been demonstrated in vivo. Studies have clearly demonstrated that meperidine is no more efficacious in treating biliary or renal tract spasm than comparative μ opioids. And because morphine results in better analgesia with fewer side effects, there are no particular advantages of meperidine as an analgesic.[219]

Pharmacokinetics

In adults, meperidine is metabolized to meperidinic acid and normeperidine. Meperidine clearance in infants and children is approximately 10 mL per min per kg.[220,221] Elimination in neonates is greatly reduced, and elimination half-time in neonates, who have received pethidine by placental transfer, may be two to seven times longer than that in adults.[222]

Adverse Effects

Accumulation of the metabolite normeperidine results in seizures and dysphoria.[18] Intramuscular administration of meperidine was frequently used in pediatric patients, but this route of administration is unfavorable because it is painful.

Sedation

Besides suitable analgesia, adequate sedation during intensive care treatment and for procedures is very important as well. The aim is to reduce distress and anxiety. Sedation is not analgesia, although both may have the same aim and off course show an important overlap. Nonpharmacologic interventions, supporting and providing comfort by nurses and parents, are of course needed in every pediatric patient, even to prevent stress. Analgesia is needed in case of pain, where sedation might be needed in case of scary, unpleasant procedures, or in very uncomfortable procedures or situations that are not painful per se, but do cause stress. Opioids also have sedative effects, next to their analgesic properties. Anticonvulsive agents, by inhibiting the seizure and "making the neurons asleep," often also induct sedation.

We can divide sedatives broadly into benzodiazepines, α-2-adrenergic receptor agonists, NMDA receptor antagonists, barbiturates, and other sedatives such as propofol. In this paragraph, we discuss the agents that primarily have sedative properties. During the past years, the numbers of studies on the "old school" benzodiazepine sedative agents in newborns and infants was limited, but "newer" sedatives including dexmedetomidine and ketamine gained popularity. See Table 36.2.[223]

SEDATIVES

Benzodiazepines

Benzodiazepines are psychoactive drugs that enhance the effect of the neurotransmitter γ-aminobutyric acid (GABA) at the GABA-A receptor. In this way, benzodiazepines can be used for different indications and reduce anxiety, induce sleep, can treat seizures, and have muscle relaxant properties. In pediatric patients, they are frequently used to sedate patients, as is discussed here, and to treat withdrawal. Benzodiazepines can be categorized based on their PK and PD properties as short-, intermediary-, or long acting.

Next to opioids, benzodiazepines are very frequently used in critically ill pediatric patients. The use of benzodiazepines is, however, not without danger. As everyone knows, there is a high risk for tolerability and abstinence. Sedation with benzodiazepines should, unless for palliative care, always be done with close monitoring patients in a hospital setting with qualified personal and equipment to provide necessary intensive care treatment if needed.

TABLE 36.2 Sedative Pharmacokinetic/Pharmacodynamic Properties

	Elimination Half-Life	*Metabolism*	*Recommended Dose*	*Advantages*	*Caveats*
BENZODIAZEPINES					
Midazolam	3–4 h	CYP3A4/CYP3A5, glucuronidation of phase 1 metabolite	IV: Bolus of 0.1–0.2 mg/kg, followed by 0.1–0.6 mg/kg/h CI	Fast-acting	Accumulation in hepatic/renal failure
Lorazepam	10–20 h	Glucuronidation	IV: 0.02–0.1 mg/kg q4–8 h or 0.025 mg/kg/h CI	Metabolism independent of liver and kidney function	Propylene glycol toxicity
BARBITURATES					
Pentobarbital	15–50 h	Hepatic microsomal enzyme system	IV: 0.5–5 mg/kg/h	Decreases intracranial pressure, profound sedation	Not suitable for hemodynamically unstable patients
Thiopental	6–15 h	Oxidation (CYP2C19) and hydroxylation	IV: Bolus of 4–6 mg/kg followed by 5 mg/kg/h up to a maximum of 10 mg/kg/h	Decreases intracranial pressure, profound sedation	Not suitable for hemodynamically unstable patients
α-2-ADRENERGIC RECEPTOR AGONISTS					
Clonidine	7–17 h	60% kidney excretion, metabolism by CYP2D6	IV: Bolus of 2 μg/kg, followed by 0.1–2 μg/kg/h CI	Preserves respiratory drive and has analgesic properties	Bradycardia and rebound hypertension
Dexmedetomidine	2–4 h	CYP2A6 and glucuronidation	IV: 0.2–2.5 μg/kg/h CI	Short half-life	Rebound hypertension
OTHER					
Propofol	30–60 min	CYP2B6/CYP2C9, glucuronidation	3–15 mg/kg/h	Fast-acting, short half-life	Associated with PRIS at higher doses or prolonged use
Ketamine	2–3 h	CYP3A4/CYP2B6/CYP2A9	IV: Bolus of 1 mg/kg followed by 16 μg/kg/min (1 mg/kg/h) CI	Preserves respiratory drive and has analgesic properties	Hypertension, raised intracranial pressure
Chloral hydrate	8–35 h	Glucuronidation	PO or RC: 25–75 mg/kg q4–6 h	Does not interfere with EEG results	No IV solution available

CI, continuous infusion; EEG, electroencephalogram; IV, intravenous; PO, orally; PRIS, propofol infusion syndrome; q, every; RC, rectal.
Baarslag MA, Allegaert K, Knibbe CA, et al. Pharmacological sedation management in the paediatric intensive care unit. *J Pharm Pharmacol.* 2017;69:498–513.

Midazolam

Indications and Clinical Use

Midazolam is known as a relatively short-acting benzodiazepine with rapid onset of action. Midazolam is a widely used sedative in the pediatric and neonatal ICU.[29]

Mechanism of Action

The sedative and anticonvulsant effects of midazolam are related to GABA accumulation and occupation of benzodiazepine receptors, whereas antianxiety effects are related to increasing the glycine inhibitory neurotransmitter.

Pharmacokinetics

PK of midazolam shows important changes with age. In adults, the half-life of midazolam is 1.9 hours. This is much shorter than that of diazepam. Bioavailability of midazolam is about 50% when absorbed after oral or gastroenteral administration.[224] Midazolam is metabolized in the liver. Midazolam is hydroxylated into the active metabolite 1-hydroxymidazolam by CYP3A4 and CYP3A5 enzymes. The metabolite is glucuronidated before excretion into the urine. The clearance of midazolam is highly dependent on the ontogeny of the P-450 system, with an almost absent CYP3A4 activity directly after birth. Within the first weeks of life, the clearance rapidly increases.[225] Total body clearance of 1.8 (0.7 to 6.7) mL per kg per min was found in preterm neonates.[225] As a consequence, much lower dosing of midazolam is needed in the youngest infants, and doses need to be adapted with (postnatal) age.[226] If a midazolam sedation target concentration of 0.1 mg per L is aimed for, similar to that given to adults, then infusion rates of about 0.01 to 0.02 mg per kg per hour in neonates and 0.05 mg per kg per hour in a 1-year-old, 0.06 mg per kg per hour in a 5-year-old, and 0.05 mg per kg per hour in a 12-year-old child have been suggested based on a population PK model.[227] For preterm neonates, this could be further specified, where the dosage would have to be further reduced in children weighing 1 kg or less and would have to be increased in children weighing 1.75 kg or more.[226] It is important, however, to realize that midazolam PK also depends on the severity of illness[228] and genotype and may be importantly altered by renal function and comedication. Consequently, large interindividual variability warrants individual titration of midazolam in neonates and young children. In the next years, a further optimization of individually based dosages might become available.[229]

Pharmacodynamics

Data on the PD of midazolam in newborns are relatively scarce. Especially in preterm newborns, the results are controversial, with a potential risk for severe side effects. A few studies investigated the sedative effect compared to morphine and placebo.[230–232] In a meta-analyses of these studies, a higher incidence of adverse neurologic events at 28 days postnatal age were reported when midazolam is compared with morphine.[233] Nowadays, midazolam sedation for mechanical ventilation in the neonatal ICU is, therefore, not recommended. Many preterm newborns seem to be comfortable even without any sedation.[94,95,234] On the other hand, the effect on sedation scores of midazolam is difficult to measure.[224] In mechanically ventilated critically ill term-born newborns and infants, sedation is needed to enhance their comfort and to facilitate synchronization with mechanical ventilation. Studies that compared continuous infusion with daily sedation interruption are partly inconclusive. Although sedation interruption seems an interesting method to reduce oversedation risks and to improve sedation management that might also lead to a reduced duration of mechanical ventilation,[235] a large trial in infants was not able to show these benefits.[236] For unclear reasons, daily sedation interruption in addition to protocolized sedation did not improve clinical outcome and was associated with increased mortality in critically ill children compared with protocolized sedation only.

Lorazepam

Indications and Clinical Use

Lorazepam is a rapid-onset benzodiazepine with anxiolytic and sedative properties. Oral lorazepam is commonly used off-label for anxiety management among pediatric patients. Lorazepam effectively reduces preoperative anxiety in children aged 6 to 18 years undergoing reconstructive burn surgery.[237] Although lorazepam showed no effect on the stress experienced before a stressful procedure, it potentially increases the success rate of comfortable procedures, such as endoscopies.[238] Lorazepam might also be used to prevent iatrogenic withdrawal syndrome.

Pharmacokinetics

Oral lorazepam has a relatively long half-life in children, which prevents large fluctuations in plasma concentrations, and also has a lack of active metabolites. This off-label use as a substitute for IV midazolam seems effective and safe.[239] Lorazepam is metabolized by glucuronidation to an inactive glucuronide metabolite, which is then excreted in the urine. The involved enzymes UGT2B4, UGT2B7, and UGT2B15 have been shown in vitro to be important for the glucuronidation of the R- and S-lorazepam enantiomers, whereas R-lorazepam is also metabolized by the extrahepatic enzymes UGT1A7 and UGT1A10.[240] In adult studies, the average lorazepam *CL* ranges from 0.75 to 1.28 mL per min per kg, and the half-life ranges from 9 to 22 hours. Lorazepam is a lipophilic drug that has a large volume of distribution of approximately 1.3 L per kg in adults. In a pediatric population with patients who suffered from a status epilepticus, lorazepam clearance was 1.2 mL per min per kg, with a half-life of 16.8 hours and volume of distribution of 1.5 L per kg.[241] Another study showed a maturation-age effect when size was allometrically scaled (0.75 L per hour per kg), weight-normalized clearance was 0.058 L per hour per kg in younger patients (<13 years) compared with 0.048 L per hour per kg in adolescents. Very limited data in newborns are available. The few newborns studied showed a smaller V_d of 0.76 L per kg, consistent with the lower percentage of adipose tissue in the neonatal population that would probably be even lower in preterm neonates. Lorazepam clearance and half-life are decreased by less UGT activity in neonates studied with a mean half-life reported of 40.2 hours.[242] Attention should be given to the propylene glycol that is added during formulation of lorazepam to improve its solubility. In a pediatric study, propylene glycol accumulated significantly in patients who received continuous lorazepam infusion.[243] Although no direct adverse effect was observed, prolonged use of lorazepam might not be preferred.

Temazepam

Temazepam is a longer acting benzodiazepine that is only registered for insomnia in adult patients. Because of its high risk for tolerance and abstinence, it is advised to only use the drug for short periods of time of around 7 to 10 days. In children, temazepam is used as premedication before anesthesia and as sedative for dental procedures and magnetic resonance imaging (MRI) scans. Only limited studies are available, most of them preformed more than 30 years ago. No PK study is published. Temazepam, mostly used as an elixir in children, has been compared to chloral hydrate before MRI scans. It seems to provide adequate sedation in a relatively high proportion of children, if adequate support with trained nurses is provided.[244] No data are available for neonates and infants.

Oxazepam

Oxazepam, known in adults as a relatively short-acting benzodiazepine, can be used for pathologic anxiety and stress. Although no PK studies have been published in infants and children, the use in this population might be considered. It is probably reserved for children older than 12 years. Data from trials are almost completely absent and use under the age of 6 years should be reluctant.

Barbiturates

Barbiturates are CNS depressant drugs that can be used for anesthesia and sedation and to treat convulsions. Barbiturates show superior CNS depressant effects because they potentiate inhibitory GABA-A receptors but also inhibit excitatory glutamate receptors. Because high and/or continuous dosages can lead to death, the relatively high rate of side effects, abstinence, and tolerance, the use of barbiturates in medicine has been reduced, and for sedation, they have been largely replaced for other sedatives. Pentobarbital, phenobarbital, and thiopental still might be considered for procedural sedation, for treatment of convulsions, or for sedation in those patients who remain uncomfortable with other sedatives.

Pentobarbital

Pentobarbital has a potent effect on GABA-sensitive chloride channels and is a potent CNS depressant. Pentobarbital enters the brain rapidly and also is a very potent antiepileptic drug. Pentobarbital is an ideal drug when sedation is the primary goal, but its use is restricted because of side effects. It has respiratory depressant and hypotensive side effects in some patients. Pentobarbital has been recommended as a sedative agent for diagnostic imaging studies such as MRI,[245] although sedation might be prolonged if dosages are too high.

Although pentobarbital pharmacology has been well studied in adults, limited pediatric PK and PD data are available to guide therapy, particularly in neonates, infants, and children. After cardiac surgery, pentobarbital clearance showed to be related to body weight and age in infants who received pentobarbital postoperatively in a dose that ranged from 0.8 to 14 mg per kg.[246]

Phenobarbital

Phenobarbital, although largely abandoned from medical care, still is one of the first choice off-label treatments for neonatal seizures. Consequently, the knowledge about PK, PD, and safety of the drug is much better than of many other sedatives in newborns[233] and infants.[247] Prolonged use of phenobarbital in newborns is associated with impaired neurodevelopmental outcome, but incidental use seems relatively safe. Dosages advised for neonatal sedation (5 to 10 mg per kg) are not validated, but often lower than the dosages needed to treat neonatal convulsions. During ECMO, phenobarbital dosages for optimal sedation are a bit higher, with a suggested loading dose of 15 mg per kg and maintenance of 4 mg per kg per day. As plasma concentrations show high interindividual variability, TDM might be indicated.[247] The volume of distribution is highest in the smallest infants, and for seizures, a loading dose of 30 mg per kg is currently recommended.[233,248] Clearance is very slow and importantly predicted by birth weight and postnatal age in the neonatal period. Clearance increases by 36.7% per kg bodyweight and with 5.3% per postnatal day of living.[233]

Thiopental

Thiopental is a rapid-onset, short-acting barbiturate that is mostly used for induction of anesthesia and rapid-sequence intubation. Data from clinical trials are limited. Short use is indicated because of slow elimination. For radiologic procedures, rectal thiopental seems safe and effective. Young children who received 15 to 50 mg rectal thiopental showed successful sedation for computed tomography (CT) imaging[249] and MRI scans.[250] Rectal thiopental administration in sedation for pediatric echocardiographic examination was also very effective when a dose of 50 mg per kg was used in patients younger than 6 months, 35 mg per kg in infants ranging from 6 months to 2 years of age, and 25 mg per kg in children above 2 years of age. The induction time was mostly less than 20 minutes, and sedation mostly lasted for more than 30 minutes.[251] Thiopental has also been studied for endotracheal intubation in preterm newborns, where, in combination with suxamethonium and remifentanil, it forms an effective strategy.[252] In neonates, thiopental clearance at 26 weeks PMA was 0.015 L per min per 70 kg and increased to 0.119 L per min per 70 kg by 42 weeks PMA after a single dose of 4 mg per kg. The maximum rate of elimination (V_{max}) at 26 weeks PMA was 0.22 mg per min per 70 kg and increased to 4.13 mg per min per 70 kg by 42 weeks PMA.[253] These parameter estimates are approximately 40% adult values at term gestation.

α-2-Adrenergic Receptor Agonists

Agonists of α-2 adrenergic receptor have been used for decades to treat hypertension, but also for psychiatric diseases such as attention-deficit/hyperactivity disorder (ADHD) and panic disorders. However, in recent years, α-2 adrenergic receptor agonists have been used as adjuncts for sedation and to reduce anesthetic requirements. The α-2 receptors constitute a family of G-protein–coupled receptors with three pharmacologic subtypes, α-2A, α-2B, and α-2C. The α-2A and α-2C subtypes are found mainly in the CNS. Stimulation of these receptor subtypes may be responsible for sedation, analgesia, and sympatholytic effects. The α-2B receptors are found more frequently on vascular smooth muscle and have been shown to mediate vasopressor effects.

Clonidine

Indications and Clinical Use

Clonidine, an α-adrenoreceptor agonist, produces sedation without causing respiratory depression, and exerts anxiolytic effects that are comparable with those of benzodiazepines. Clonidine, however, may reduce the requirement for other sedative agents and improve hemodynamic and sympathoadrenal stability. Clonidine has beneficial effects for preoperative sedation and to reduce anxiety, to reduce hemodynamic stress responses related to endotracheal intubation, and can decrease anesthetic requirements. Also during surgery, clonidine can increase hemodynamic stability and analgesia without respiratory depression. Clonidine is being used with increasing frequency as a first-line agent to provide sedation.[254] In critically ill children, clonidine, often in combination with midazolam, provides adequate sedation and remains cardiovascular stability.[254] Clonidine given by continuous IV infusion may be used as an alternative sedative agent to midazolam.[255]

It also has analgesic properties, which are probably mediated through the prevention of substance P release.

Pharmacokinetics

Clonidine is partly metabolized by CYP2D6 and the major metabolite formed is *p*-hydroxy-clonidine. About half of clonidine is excreted unchanged by the kidney. PK data in children are available after neonatal abstinence, oral, rectal, nasal, and IV administrations of clonidine. Potts et al. published a population PK model for clonidine.[256] They showed that clearance at birth was 3.8 L per hour per 70 kg and matured with a half-time of 25.7 weeks to reach 82% adult rate by 1 year of age. Rectal clonidine administration of 2.5 μg per kg in children achieves plasma concentrations within the range known to be clinically effective in adults[257] and if a solution is used, rectal clonidine absorption was rapid with maximum concentrations reached within 30 minutes.[256] Gastroenterally dosed absorption is hampered by a considerable interindividual variability and, more importantly, has a very long T_{max} of median 190 minutes in pediatric patients.[258] If relatively rapid sedation is required, IV or rectal administration is preferred.

Adverse Effects

Adverse effects associated with the use of clonidine include bradycardia and hypotension. Withdrawal of clonidine after prolonged administration has been associated with hypertension and seizures, and abrupt discontinuation should be avoided.

Dexmedetomidine

Indications and Clinical Use

Dexmedetomidine is another α-adrenergic agonist that is increasingly used for procedural sedation, during anesthesia, and at the ICU in pediatric patients. In adult intensive care, dexmedetomidine is most often used for light-to-moderate sedation and is not recommended for long-term sedation. Dexmedetomidine also has analgesic properties in addition to its role as a sedative and, in that way, may reduce the need for opioids. Data for children are still limited, especially in neonates, but it is increasingly used for relatively small procedures such as MRI and CT scans, echocardiography, hearing, or eye examinations. Dexmedetomidine has been successfully used to sedate children for MRI using 2 µg per kg IV dexmedetomidine administered for 10 minutes followed by an infusion of 1 µg per kg per hour. The amount of IV dexmedetomidine was titrated to the deep level of sedation.[259] For sedation during transthoracic echocardiography, intranasally administered dexmedetomidine was comparable to oral chloral hydrate and did not increase the risk of clinically important adverse events.[260] Intranasal dosing was also used to treat anxiety for CT scans,[261] and 2.5 mg per kg dexmedetomidine was beneficial in reducing distress compared to 0.5 mg midazolam.[262] Intranasal dexmedetomidine also improved the success rate of auditory brainstem response (ABR) testing when compared to oral chloral hydrate.[263] During the past years, dexmedetomidine is also finding its way into pediatrics anesthesia. Up till now, most reports are about local anesthesia, where dexmedetomidine with a caudal block, for instance, recently provided a feasible alternative to general anesthesia in infants undergoing inguinal hernia surgery. This technique avoids the need for tracheal intubation, which may be beneficial in neonates, especially in those born preterm and suffering from bronchopulmonary dysplasia.[264] A dexmedetomidine/remifentanil caudal anesthetic was effective in 87.5% of infants who needed lower abdominal or lower extremity surgery.[265] A relatively high rate of hypertension in these patients warrants further and larger studies. Long-term effects in children are unknown. Animal studies suggest a neuroapoptotic protective effect,[266] and dexmedetomidine showed a beneficial effect when administered with another anesthetic.[267]

Pharmacokinetics

Because of a slightly different mechanism of action, not directly increasing GABA neurons, dexmedetomidine provides less amnesia and respiratory depression than other sedatives such as benzodiazepines. IV dexmedetomidine exhibits linear PK, with a rapid distribution half-life of approximately 6 minutes and a terminal elimination half-life of approximately 2 hours in adults. Because dexmedetomidine undergoes almost complete hepatic transformation, clearance of dexmedetomidine in infants is lower within the first year of life. This reflects the decreased hepatic enzyme activity compared to adults, where dexmedetomidine is glucuronidated by UGTs and oxygenated by CYP2D6. Clearance in neonates is approximately one-third of that described in adults[267] and also decreased after cardiac surgery.[268,269] These patients would need lower maintenance doses of dexmedetomidine.

N-METHYL-*D*-ASPARTATE RECEPTOR ANTAGONISTS

Ketamine

Indications and Clinical Use

A relatively new sedative agent is ketamine that has been used for a long time already for by anesthetists, most importantly found its place in the emergency department and as additive treatment for severe postoperative pain. During the past years, it is increasingly used in young patients, but still has a relative contraindication for young infants and newborns. Ketamine is most often used and studied as a single dose for procedural analgesia and sedation. In anesthesia, it is routinely used for induction and maintenance, especially in children with heart diseases or sepsis because of the cardiovascular stability observed with ketamine.[270] The S-enantiomer of ketamine, esketamine, appears to have a favorable cardiovascular profile and neuroprotective effects, with a lower required dose and fewer side effects. Continuous ketamine infusion, next to severe asthma exacerbations, might be effective for sedation in the ICU. A loading dose of 0.5 to 1.0 mg per kg followed by a starting dose of 0.25 mg per kg per hour has been suggested.[271] The optimal dose probably needs to be titrated to the individual patient's needs, because of high variability in PK.[272] In newborns, the use of ketamine remains controversial. Animal studies have shown that ketamine may have neurotoxic effects and may hamper brain development. Yan et al. suggest that the ketamine effects depend on the clinical situation of the patient. Repeated ketamine usage may be neurotoxic to immature brains in the absence of noxious stimuli, whereas it may be neuroprotective in the same brains in the presence of strong painful stimuli.[273] Nasal ketamine administration for endotracheal intubation directly after birth has been studied, but is less effective than nasal midazolam.[274]

Mechanism of Action

Ketamine is an NMDA antagonist. It is well known for its ability to provide conscious sedation. By NMDA antagonism, it disconnects the thalamocortical and limbic areas of the brain and, in that way, provides a functional and electrophysiologic dissociation.[275]

Pharmacokinetics

PK data of ketamine in pediatric patients are sparse and show half-lives of 100 to 125 minutes for IV administration, with a clearance of 16.8 to 22 mL per min per kg.[276,277]

OTHER SEDATIVE AGENTS

Propofol

Indications and Clinical Use

Propofol is a unique anesthetic agent with GABAergic properties as well as anti-NMDA and sodium channel blocking effects. Propofol is not suitable for long-term sedation in the pediatric population, due to the perceived risk of propofol infusion syndrome, a metabolic derangement accompanied by severe metabolic acidosis, hyperkalemia, hyperlipidemia, rhabdomyolysis, and organ failure, associated with an increased risk of mortality.[278] Because of its beneficial clinical properties, being easy to use, showing a fast onset of action, maintaining own respiration, and a relatively fast recovery, propofol has taken an important role in neonatal and pediatric sedation. Next to its use in anesthesia, propofol is used in newborns for sedation of endotracheal intubation[279] and minimally invasive surfactant therapy.[280] In the preterm-born neonatal population, propofol administration might lead to hypotension,[281,282] although cerebral autoregulation remains intact[283] and the hypotension might not harm the cerebral perfusion.[284] Propofol starting dosages of 0.5 to 2.5 mg per kg have been used for neonatal procedural sedation.

Pharmacokinetics

Propofol clearance increases throughout infancy to reach 92% that reported in adults 1.93 L per min per 70 kg by 6 months postnatal age. Recently, a manual dosing regimen for infants was calculated to achieve steady-state plasma concentrations of 3 μg per mL that contains a loading dose and maintenance infusion dosages that depend on age.[285]

Chloral Hydrate

Chloral hydrate is a very old drug that is still commonly used for procedural sedation in children. It shows a comparable effectiveness compared to other sedative agents.[286] It is rapidly absorbed from the gastrointestinal tract and is converted to the active metabolite trichloroethanol. The drug starts to act within 15 to 60 minutes, being metabolized in the liver and other tissues and excreted in the urine and bile. PK data warrant to use chloral hydrate with caution, especially in neonates and young children. After a single oral dose of 50 mg per kg, chloral hydrate remains detectable for several hours in children. The half-life of the active trichloroethanol metabolite was found to be highly age dependent and highest in newborns, with a mean of 39.8 hours.[287]

Melatonin

Melatonin may induce a natural sleepiness and improve predictability of sedation drugs. In a randomized, placebo-controlled trial, melatonin showed only a nonsignificant more rapid closure of the eyes if used next to chloralhydrate or temazepam sedation for an MRI scan in children.[288] Because of its potential as a neuroprotective agent after asphyxia and preterm birth, PK studies have been performed in newborns. The half-life is relatively long, median about 16 hours, making it less suitable for procedural sedation.[289]

DRUG INTERACTIONS

The concomitant use of benzodiazepines and opioids increases the risk of respiratory depression because of actions at different receptor sites in the CNS that control respiration. Benzodiazepines interact at GABA-A sites, and opioids interact primarily at μ receptors. When benzodiazepines and opioids are combined, the potential for benzodiazepines to significantly worsen opioid-related respiratory depression exists. Limit dosage and duration of concomitant use of benzodiazepines and opioids, and follow up patients closely for respiratory depression and sedation.

LONG-TERM EFFECTS OF ACETAMINOPHEN, OPIOIDS, AND SEDATIVES

Although several animal studies show negative histologic and morphologic changes in the CNS with associated functional and behavioral changes in the long term after exposure to analgesics and sedatives, studies in human are scarce.[6] The potential long-term effects of anesthesia have been studied in large prospective trials and showed no differences in IQ scores, cognitive scores, memory/learning ability, motor/processing speed, visuospatial function, attention, executive function, language, or behavior compared to unexposed siblings or local anesthesia.[290,291] While those large prospective studies are conducted with regard to the potential effects of anesthesia, those large studies are lacking with regard to the potential effects of analgesics and sedatives.

ACETAMINOPHEN

Large studies on the preemptive use of acetaminophen or on the potential long-term effects of acetaminophen are needed.[33] Especially since previous studies showed potential associations and causal links between acetaminophen exposure and neurobehavioral issues, increased incidence of atopy, and reduced fertility.[31] With regard to neurodevelopment, concerns have been raised about a higher risk for ADHD, autism spectrum disorders, and neurocognitive deficits following early exposure to acetaminophen. However, most studies are based on prenatal exposure or animal studies; therefore, large prospective studies in human are needed.[292,293]

OPIOIDS

Since opioid receptors are very important for normal brain development, including neuronal migration, differentiation, and maturation, it is plausible that administration of high dosages of opioids during a period of rapid brain development will have adverse effects.[205] There are indications that opioids affect the dendritic architecture, neuronal density, and μ-receptor density based on animal studies.[205] Especially neonates and infants would, therefore, hypothetically be very vulnerable for adverse effects since their brain is rapidly developing.

However, in humans, several studies regarding the potential long-term effects of neonatal opioid exposure have been conducted but show contradictory results. With regard to brain development, no major alterations in brain morphology or in brain activation during pain have not yet been found in children who received opioids and sedatives for extended periods of time as a neonate, generally in the absence of major pain.[294] However, diffusion tensor imaging in this same cohort of children did show lower global fractional anisotropy compared to healthy children.[295] In preterm-born children receiving low doses of morphine as a neonate in the absence of severe pain, no differences in morphology or brain volume at the age of 10 years compared to healthy controls were found.[296] This is in contradiction with the results of a small follow-up study of the NEOPAIN cohort, which showed that preemptive morphine administration in the first weeks of life in preterm-born children was associated with a smaller head circumference during childhood in. However, overall IQ and academic achievement did not differ between the morphine-treated and placebo-treated children.[297] In another study in very preterm-born neonates (24 to 32 weeks of gestational age), morphine exposure was associated with poorer neurodevelopmental outcome at 18 months of corrected age.[298] Yet the question arises whether this observation is causal or caused by confounding, even though the investigators corrected for multiple clinical confounders. In general, sick infants will receive more morphine on clinical grounds, and they will also have an increased risk of impaired neurodevelopmental outcome due to their underlying severity of illness.[299]

Only few studies have addressed specific effects of opioid exposure on pain sensitivity. Those few studies found no abnormal pain sensitivity later in life in ECMO-treated children receiving opioids and sedatives such as midazolam in the absence of severe pain and in prematurely born children receiving low doses of morphine.[294,296] Regarding cognition, a follow-up study among preterm-born mechanically ventilated children found that the scores on one IQ subtest, "visual analysis," measured at the age of 5 years, were significantly negatively related to having received morphine in the first 28 days of life.[138] There were no other statistical differences between preterm-born children exposed to morphine versus placebo with respect to intelligence, visual motor integration, behavior, chronic pain, and health-related quality of life. Interestingly, morphine-treated children in the same cohort had even significantly fewer problems in executive functioning at age 8 or 9 years.[139] Extended neonatal exposure to opioids and sedatives in the absence of severe pain was associated with specific worse verbal memory performance.[294] In conclusion, studies in human show contradictory results, but the very alarming findings as expected form animal studies are not observed in humans.

SEDATIVES

We know from rodent studies that sedatives such as midazolam can trigger neuroapoptosis in the developing brain.[300] In human, studies on the long-term effects of sedatives are scarce. A previous study showed that prolonged continuous administration sedatives in neonates did not negatively affect pain sensitivity, brain morphology, cortical thickness and brain functioning later in life.[294] However, extended neonatal exposure to opioids and sedatives in the absence of severe pain was associated with specific worse verbal memory performance.[294] Interestingly, another study demonstrated a selective negative effect of midazolam on the growth of the hippocampus in preterm-born children.[301] This could be explained by the fact that the hippocampus is vulnerable to cerebral hypoperfusion in particular.[302] More studies are needed regarding the long-term effects of sedatives and in particular with regard to hippocampal growth and memory deficits.[303]

REFERENCES

1. Merskey H, Bogduk N. *Classifications of chronic pain: description of chronic pain syndromes and definitions of pain terms.* Seattle, WA: IASP Press, 1994:209–214.
2. Anand KJ, Sippell WG, Aynsley-Green A. Randomised trial of fentanyl anaesthesia in preterm babies undergoing surgery: effects on the stress response. *Lancet.* 1987;1:62–66.
3. van den Hoogen NJ, de Kort AR, Allegaert KM, et al. Developmental neurobiology as a guide for pharmacological management of pain in neonates. *Semin Fetal Neonatal Med.* 2019;24:101012.
4. Beggs S, Torsney C, Drew LJ, et al. The postnatal reorganization of primary afferent input and dorsal horn cell receptive fields in the rat spinal cord is an activity-dependent process. *Eur J Neurosci.* 2002;16:1249–1258.
5. Knaepen L, Patijn J, van Kleef M, et al. Neonatal repetitive needle pricking: plasticity of the spinal nociceptive circuit and extended postoperative pain in later life. *Dev Neurobiol.* 2013;73:85–97.
6. van den Bosch GE, Dijk MV, Tibboel D, et al. Long-term effects of early exposure to stress, pain, opioids and anaesthetics on pain sensitivity and neurocognition. *Curr Pharm Des.* 2017;23:5879–5886.
7. Gruber EM, Laussen PC, Casta A, et al. Stress response in infants undergoing cardiac surgery: a randomized study of fentanyl bolus, fentanyl infusion, and fentanyl-midazolam infusion. *Anesth Analg.* 2001;92:882–890.
8. Committee on Fetus and Newborn and Section on Anesthesiology and Pain Medicine. Prevention and management of procedural pain in the neonate: an update. *Pediatrics.* 2016;137:e20154271.
9. Hall RW, Anand KJ. Pain management in newborns. *Clin Perinatol.* 2014;41:895–924.
10. Stevens B, Yamada J, Lee GY, et al. Sucrose for analgesia in newborn infants undergoing painful procedures. *Cochrane Database Syst Rev.* 2013:CD001069.
11. Potana NT, Dongara AR, Nimbalkar SM, et al. Oral sucrose for pain in neonates during echocardiography: a randomized controlled trial. *Indian Pediatr.* 2015;52:493–497.
12. Jain S, Kumar P, McMillan DD. Prior leg massage decreases pain responses to heel stick in preterm babies. *J Paediatr Child Health.* 2006;42:505–508.
13. Procianoy RS, Mendes EW, Silveira RC. Massage therapy improves neurodevelopment outcome at two years corrected age for very low birth weight infants. *Early Hum Dev.* 2010;86:7–11.
14. Miller K, Tan X, Hobson AD, et al. A prospective randomized controlled trial of nonpharmacological pain management during intravenous cannulation in a pediatric emergency department. *Pediatr Emerg Care.* 2016;32:444–451.
15. Hummel P, van Dijk M. Pain assessment: current status and challenges. *Semin Fetal Neonatal Med.* 2006;11:237–245.
16. Crellin DJ, Harrison D, Santamaria N, et al. Systematic review of the Face, Legs, Activity, Cry and Consolability scale for assessing pain in infants and children: is it reliable, valid, and feasible for use? *Pain.* 2015;156:2132–2151.
17. Harris J, Ramelet AS, van Dijk M, et al. Clinical recommendations for pain, sedation, withdrawal and delirium assessment in critically ill infants and children: an ESPNIC position statement for healthcare professionals. *Intensive Care Med.* 2016;42:972–986.
18. Berde CB, Sethna N. Analgesics for the treatment of pain in children. *N Engl J Med.* 2002;347:1094–1103.
19. Bellu R, de Waal KA, Zanini R. Opioids for neonates receiving mechanical ventilation. *Cochrane Database Syst Rev.* 2008:CD004212.
20. Faura CC, Collins SL, Moore RA, et al. Systematic review of factors affecting the ratios of morphine and its major metabolites. *Pain.* 1998;74:43–53.
21. de Wildt SN, Kearns GL, Leeder JS, et al. Glucuronidation in humans. Pharmacogenetic and developmental aspects. *Clin Pharmacokinet.* 1999;36:439–452.
22. de Wildt SN, Kearns GL, Leeder JS, et al. Cytochrome P450 3A: ontogeny and drug disposition. *Clin Pharmacokinet.* 1999;37:485–505.
23. Kearns GL, Abdel-Rahman SM, Alander SW, et al. Developmental pharmacology—drug disposition, action, and therapy in infants and children. *N Engl J Med.* 2003;349: 1157–1167.
24. Stephenson T. How children's responses to drugs differ from adults. *Br J Clin Pharmacol.* 2005;59:670–673.
25. Sager JE, Yu J, Ragueneau-Majlessi I, et al. Physiologically based pharmacokinetic (PBPK) modeling and simulation approaches: a systematic review of published models, applications, and model verification. *Drug Metab Dispos.* 2015;43:1823–1837.
26. Ceelie I, de Wildt SN, van Dijk M, et al. Effect of intravenous paracetamol on postoperative morphine requirements in neonates and infants undergoing major noncardiac surgery: a randomized controlled trial. *JAMA.* 2013;309:149–154.
27. Hartley C, Moultrie F, Hoskin A, et al. Analgesic efficacy and safety of morphine in the Procedural Pain in Premature Infants (Poppi) study: randomised placebo-controlled trial. *Lancet.* 2018;392:2595–2605.
28. World Health Organization. *Cancer pain relief.* Geneva, Switzerland: World Health Press; 1986.
29. Carbajal R, Eriksson M, Courtois E, et al. Sedation and analgesia practices in neonatal intensive care units (EUROPAIN): results from a prospective cohort study. *Lancet Respir Med.* 2015;3:796–812.
30. Commitee on Infectious Disease AAoP. Aspirin and Reye's syndrome. *Pediatrics.* 1982;69:810.
31. Allegaert K, van den Anker JN. Perinatal and neonatal use of paracetamol for pain relief. *Semin Fetal Neonatal Med.* 2017;22:308–313.
32. Roofthooft DWE, Simons SHP, van Lingen RA, et al. Randomized controlled trial comparing different single doses of intravenous paracetamol for placement of peripherally inserted central catheters in preterm infants. *Neonatology.* 2017;112:150–158.
33. Ohlsson A, Shah PS. Paracetamol (acetaminophen) for prevention or treatment of pain in newborns. *Cochrane Database Syst Rev.* 2016;10:CD011219.
34. Tinner EM, Hoesli I, Jost K, et al. Rectal paracetamol in newborn infants after assisted vaginal delivery may increase pain response. *J Pediatr.* 2013;162:62–66.
35. Jozwiak-Bebenista M, Nowak JZ. Paracetamol: mechanism of action, applications and safety concern. *Acta Pol Pharm.* 2014;71:11–23.
36. Anderson BJ. Paracetamol (Acetaminophen): mechanisms of action. *Paediatr Anaesth.* 2008;18:915–921.
37. Schwaller F, Kanellopoulos A, Fitzgerald M. The developmental emergence of differential brainstem serotonergic control of the sensory spinal cord. *Sci Rep.* 2017;7:2215.
38. Montgomery CJ, McCormack JP, Reichert CC, et al. Plasma concentrations after high-dose (45 mg.kg-1) rectal acetaminophen in children. *Can J Anaesth.* 1995;42:982–986.
39. Clements JA, Heading RC, Nimmo WS, et al. Kinetics of acetaminophen absorption and gastric emptying in man. *Clin Pharmacol Ther.* 1978;24:420–431.
40. Brown RD, Wilson JT, Kearns GL, et al. Single-dose pharmacokinetics of ibuprofen and acetaminophen in febrile children. *J Clin Pharmacol.* 1992;32:231–241.

41. Anderson BJ, Woollard GA, Holford NH. A model for size and age changes in the pharmacokinetics of paracetamol in neonates, infants and children. *Br J Clin Pharmacol.* 2000;50:125–134.
42. Gupta M, Brans Y. Gastric retention in neonates. *Pediatrics.* 1978;62:26–29.
43. Anderson BJ, van Lingen RA, Hansen TG, et al. Acetaminophen developmental pharmacokinetics in neonates and infants: a pooled population analysis. *Anesthesiology.* 2002;96(6):1336–1345.
44. van Hoogdalem EJ, de Boer AG, Breimer DD. Pharmacokinetics of rectal drug administration, Part II. Clinical applications of peripherally acting drugs, and conclusions. *Clin Pharmacokinet.* 1991;21:110–128.
45. Flint RB, Roofthooft DW, van Rongen A, et al. Exposure to acetaminophen and all its metabolites upon 10, 15, and 20 mg/kg intravenous acetaminophen in very-preterm infants. *Pediatr Res.* 2017;82:678–684.
46. Miners JO, Osborne NJ, Tonkin AL, et al. Perturbation of paracetamol urinary metabolic ratios by urine flow rate. *Br J Clin Pharmacol.* 1992;34:359–362.
47. Anderson BJ, Pons G, Autret-Leca E, et al. Pediatric intravenous paracetamol (propacetamol) pharmacokinetics: a population analysis. *Paediatr Anaesth.* 2005;15:282–292.
48. Rumack BH. Acetaminophen hepatotoxicity: the first 35 years. *J Toxicol Clin Toxicol.* 2002;40:3–20.
49. Park JM, Lin YS, Calamia JC, et al. Transiently altered acetaminophen metabolism after liver transplantation. *Clin Pharmacol Ther.* 2003;73:545–553.
50. Manyike PT, Kharasch ED, Kalhorn TF, et al. Contribution of CYP2E1 and CYP3A to acetaminophen reactive metabolite formation. *Clin Pharmacol Ther.* 2000;67:275–282.
51. Korpela R, Korvenoja P, Meretoja OA. Morphine-sparing effect of acetaminophen in pediatric day-case surgery. *Anesthesiology.* 1999;91:442–447.
52. Arendt Nielsen L, Nielsen JC, Bjerring P. Double-blind, placebo controlled comparison of paracetamol and paracetamol plus codeine—a quantitative evaluation by laser induced pain. *Eur J Clin Pharmacol.* 1991;40:241–247.
53. Nielsen JC, Bjerring P, Arendt Nielsen L, et al. Analgesic efficacy of immediate and sustained release paracetamol and plasma concentration of paracetamol. Double blind, placebo-controlled evaluation using painful laser stimulation. *Eur J Clin Pharmacol.* 1992;42:261–264.
54. Anderson BJ, Gibb IA. Paracetamol (acetaminophen) pharmacodynamics; interpreting the plasma concentration. *Arch Dis Child.* 2008;93:241–247.
55. Anderson BJ, Woollard GA, Holford NHG. Acetaminophen analgesia in children: placebo effect and pain resolution after tonsillectomy. *Eur J Clin Pharmacol.* 2001;57:559–569.
56. Miner DJ, Kissinger PT. Evidence for the involvement of N-acetyl-p-quinoneimine in acetaminophen poisoning. *Ann Rev Pharmacol Toxicol.* 1983;12:251.
57. Slattery JT, Nelson SD, Thummel KE. The complex interaction between ethanol and acetaminophen. *Clin Pharmacol Ther.* 1996;60:241–246.
58. Nahata MC, Powell DA, Durrell DE, et al. Acetaminophen accumulation in pediatric patients after repeated therapeutic doses. *Eur J Clin Pharmacol.* 1984;27:57–59.
59. Slattery JT, Wilson JM, Kalhorn TF, et al. Dose-dependent pharmacokinetics of acetaminophen: evidence of glutathione depletion in humans. *Clin Pharmacol Ther.* 1987;41:413–418.
60. Penna A, Buchanan N. Paracetamol poisoning in children and hepatotoxicity. *Br J Clin Pharmacol.* 1991;32:143–149.
61. Temple AR. Pediatric dosing of acetaminophen. *Pediatr Pharmacol New York.* 1983;3:321–327.
62. Shann F. Paracetamol: when, why and how much. *J Paediatr Child Health.* 1993;29:84–85.
63. Alonso EM, Sokol RJ, Hart J, et al. Fulminant hepatitis associated with centrilobular necrosis in young children. *J Pediatr.* 1995;127:888–894.
64. Kearns GL, Leeder JS, Wasserman GS. Acetaminophen overdose with therapeutic intent. *J Pediatr.* 1998;132:5–8.
65. Heubi JE, Barbacci MB, Zimmerman HJ. Therapeutic misadventures with acetaminophen: hepatoxicity after multiple doses in children. *J Pediatr.* 1998;132:22–27.
66. Heubi JE, Bien JP. Acetaminophen use in children: more is not better. *J Pediatr.* 1997;130:175–177.
67. Rivera Penera T, Gugig R, Davis J, et al. Outcome of acetaminophen overdose in pediatric patients and factors contributing to hepatotoxicity. *J Pediatr.* 1997;130:300–304.
68. Inturrisi CE. Clinical pharmacology of opioids for pain. *Clin J Pain.* 2002;18:S3–S13.
69. Suresh S, Anand KJS. Opioid tolerance in neonates: mechanisms, diagnosis, assessment, and management. *Semin Perinatol.* 1998;22:425–433.
70. Fields H. State-dependent opioid control of pain. *Nat Rev Neurosci.* 2004;5:565–575.
71. Zernikow B, Michel E, Craig F, et al. Pediatric palliative care: use of opioids for the management of pain. *Paediatr Drugs.* 2009;11:129–151.
72. Wachman EM, Hayes MJ, Brown MS, et al. Association of OPRM1 and COMT single-nucleotide polymorphisms with hospital length of stay and treatment of neonatal abstinence syndrome. *JAMA.* 2013;309:1821–1827.
73. Lam J, Baello S, Iqbal M, et al. The ontogeny of P-glycoprotein in the developing human blood-brain barrier: implication for opioid toxicity in neonates. *Pediatr Res.* 2015;78:417–421.
74. Allegaert K, van den Anker J. Ontogeny of phase I metabolism of drugs. *J Clin Pharmacol.* 2019;59 Suppl 1:S33–S41.
75. Cunliffe M. Codeine phosphate in children: time for re-evaluation? *Br J Anaesth.* 2001;86:329–331.
76. William DG, Hatch DJ, Howard RF. Codeine phosphate in paediatric medicine. *Br J Anaesth.* 2001;86:413–421.
77. Chen ZR, Somogyi AA, Bochner F. Polymorphic O-demethylation of codeine. *Lancet.* 1988;2:914–915.
78. Sindrup SH, Brosen K. The pharmacogenetics of codeine hypoalgesia. *Pharmacogenetics.* 1995;5:335–346.
79. Williams DG, Patel A, Howard RF. Pharmacogenetics of codeine metabolism in an urban population of children and its implications for analgesic reliability. *Br J Anaesth.* 2002;89:839–845.
80. Eckhardt K, Li S, Ammon S, et al. Same incidence of adverse drug events after codeine administration irrespective of the genetically determined differences in morphine formation. *Pain.* 1998;76:27–33.
81. Parke TJ, Nandi PR, Bird KJ, et al. Profound hypotension following intravenous codeine phosphate. Three case reports and some recommendations. *Anaesthesia.* 1992;47:852–854.
82. McEwan A, Sigston PE, Andrews KA, et al. A comparison of rectal and intramuscular codeine phosphate in children following neurosurgery. *Paediatr Anaesth.* 2000;10:189–193.
83. Quiding H, Olsson GL, Boreus LO, et al. Infants and young children metabolise codeine to morphine. A study after single and repeated rectal administration. *Br J Clin Pharmacol.* 1992;33:45–49.
84. Ciszkowski C, Madadi P, Phillips MS, et al. Codeine, ultrarapid-metabolism genotype, and postoperative death. *N Engl J Med.* 2009;361:827–828.
85. Madadi P, Shirazi F, Walter FG, et al. Establishing causality of CNS depression in breastfed infants following maternal codeine use. *Paediatr Drugs.* 2008;10:399–404.
86. Fortenberry M, Crowder J, So TY. The use of codeine and tramadol in the pediatric population-what is the verdict now? *J Pediatr Health Care.* 2019;33:117–123.
87. Jin J. Risks of codeine and tramadol in children. *JAMA.* 2017;318:1514.
88. Chidambaran V, Sadhasivam S, Mahmoud M. Codeine and opioid metabolism: implications and alternatives for pediatric pain management. *Curr Opin Anaesthesiol.* 2017;30:349–356.
89. Schnabel A, Reichl SU, Meyer-Friessem C, et al. Tramadol for postoperative pain treatment in children. *Cochrane Database Syst Rev.* 2015:CD009574.
90. Leppert W. Tramadol as an analgesic for mild to moderate cancer pain. *Pharmacol Rep.* 2009;61:978–992.
91. Allegaert K, Anderson BJ, Verbesselt R, et al. Tramadol disposition in the very young: an attempt to assess in vivo cytochrome P-450 2D6 activity. *Br J Anaesth.* 2005;95:231–239.
92. Allegaert K, Holford N, Anderson BJ, et al. Tramadol and O-desmethyl tramadol clearance maturation and disposition in humans: a pooled pharmacokinetic study. *Clin Pharmacokinet.* 2015;54:167–178.
93. Rodieux F, Vutskits L, Posfay-Barbe KM, et al. When the safe alternative is not that safe: tramadol prescribing in children. *Front Pharmacol.* 2018;9:148.
94. Simons SHP, van Dijk M, van Lingen RA, et al. Routine morphine infusion in preterm neonates who received ventilatory support: a randomized controlled trial. *JAMA.* 2003;290:2419–2427.
95. Anand KJ, Hall RW, Desai N, et al. Effects of morphine analgesia in ventilated preterm neonates: primary outcomes from the NEOPAIN randomised trial. *Lancet.* 2004;363:1673–1682.
96. Lamacraft G, Cooper MG, Cavalletto BP. Subcutaneous cannulae for morphine boluses in children: assessment of a technique. *J Pain Symptom Manage.* 1997;13:43–49.
97. Lundeberg S, Beck O, Olsson GL, et al. Rectal administration of morphine in children. Pharmacokinetic evaluation after a single-dose. *Acta Anaesthesiol Scand.* 1996;40:445–451.
98. Reich A, Beland B, van Aken H. Intravenous narcotics and analgesic agents. In: Bissonnette B, Dalens BJ, eds. *Pediatric anesthesia.* New York, NY: McGraw-Hill; 2002.
99. Schiessl C, Gravou C, Zernikow B, et al. Use of patient-controlled analgesia for pain control in dying children. *Support Care Cancer.* 2008;16:531–536.
100. Loh HH, Liu HC, Cavalli A, et al. mu Opioid receptor knockout in mice: effects on ligand-induced analgesia and morphine lethality. *Brain Res Mol Brain Res.* 1998;54:321–326.
101. Matthes HW, Maldonado R, Simonin F, et al. Loss of morphine-induced analgesia, reward effect and withdrawal symptoms in mice lacking the mu-opioid-receptor gene. *Nature.* 1996;383:819–823.
102. Sora I, Takahashi N, Funada M, et al. Opiate receptor knockout mice define mu receptor roles in endogenous nociceptive responses and morphine-induced analgesia. *Proc Natl Acad Sci U S A.* 1997;94:1544–1549.
103. Coffman BL, Rios GR, King CD, et al. Human UGT2B7 catalyzes morphine glucuronidation. *Drug Metab Dispos.* 1997;25:1–4.
104. Wittwer E, Kern SE. Role of morphine's metabolites in analgesia: concepts and controversies. *Aaps J.* 2006;8:E348–E352.
105. Romberg R, Olofsen E, Sarton E, et al. Pharmacokinetic-pharmacodynamic modeling of morphine-6-glucuronide-induced analgesia in healthy volunteers: absence of sex differences. *Anesthesiology.* 2004;100:120–133.
106. van Dorp EL, Romberg R, Sarton E, et al. Morphine-6-glucuronide: morphine's successor for postoperative pain relief? *Anesth Analg.* 2006;102:1789–1797.
107. Osborne PB, Chieng B, Christie MJ. Morphine-6 beta-glucuronide has a higher efficacy than morphine as a mu-opioid receptor agonist in the rat locus coeruleus. *Br J Pharmacol.* 2000;131:1422–1428.
108. Murthy BR, Pollack GM, Brouwer KL. Contribution of morphine-6-glucuronide to antinociception following intravenous administration of morphine to healthy volunteers. *J Clin Pharmacol.* 2002;42:569–576.
109. Osborne R, Thompson P, Joel S, et al. The analgesic activity of morphine-6-glucuronide. *Br J Clin Pharmacol.* 1992;34:130–138.
110. Thompson PI, Joel SP, John L, et al. Respiratory depression following morphine and morphine-6-glucuronide in normal subjects. *Br J Clin Pharmacol.* 1995;40:145–152.
111. Gong QL, Hedner J, Bjorkman R, et al. Morphine-3-glucuronide may functionally antagonize morphine-6-glucuronide induced antinociception and ventilatory depression in the rat. *Pain.* 1992;48:249–255.
112. Smith MT, Watt JA, Cramond T. Morphine-3-glucuronide—a potent antagonist of morphine analgesia. *Life Sci.* 1990;47:579–585.
113. Fisher MB, Vandenbranden M, Findlay K, et al. Tissue distribution and interindividual variation in human UDP-glucuronosyltransferase activity: relationship between UGT1A1 promoter genotype and variability in a liver bank. *Pharmacogenetics.* 2000;10:727–739.
114. Choonara I, Ekbom Y, Lindstrom B, et al. Morphine sulphation in children. *Br J Clin Pharmacol.* 1990;30:897–900.
115. McRorie TI, Lynn AM, Nespeca MK, et al. The maturation of morphine clearance and metabolism. *Am J Dis Child.* 1992;146:972–976.
116. Koren G, Maurice L. Pediatric uses of opioids. *Pediatr Clin North Am.* 1989;36:1141–1156.
117. Choonara IA, McKay P, Hain R, et al. Morphine metabolism in children. *Br J Clin Pharmacol.* 1989;28:599–604.
118. Kart T, Christrup LL, Rasmussen M. Recommended use of morphine in neonates, infants and children based on a literature review: part 2—clinical use. *Paediatr Anaesth.* 1997;7:93–101.

119. Anand KJ, Anderson BJ, Holford NH, et al. Morphine pharmacokinetics and pharmacodynamics in preterm and term neonates: secondary results from the NEOPAIN trial. *Br J Anaesth.* 2008;101:680–689.
120. Knibbe CA, Krekels EH, van den Anker JN, et al. Morphine glucuronidation in preterm neonates, infants and children younger than 3 years. *Clin Pharmacokinet.* 2009;48:371–385.
121. Peters JW, Anderson BJ, Simons SH, et al. Morphine pharmacokinetics during venoarterial extracorporeal membrane oxygenation in neonates. *Intensive Care Med.* 2005;31:257–263.
122. Favie LMA, Groenendaal F, van den Broek MPH, et al. Pharmacokinetics of morphine in encephalopathic neonates treated with therapeutic hypothermia. *PLoS One.* 2019;14:e0211910.
123. Allegaert K, Simons SHP, Tibboel D, et al. Non-maturational covariates for dynamic systems pharmacology models in neonates, infants, and children: Filling the gaps beyond developmental pharmacology. *Eur J Pharm Sci.* 2017;109S:S27–S31.
124. Bhat R, Chari G, Gulati A, et al. Pharmacokinetics of a single dose of morphine in preterm infants during the first week of life. *J Pediatr.* 1990;117:477–481.
125. Olsen GD. Morphine binding to human plasma proteins. *Clin Pharmacol Ther.* 1975;17:31–35.
126. Benet LZ, Hoener BA. Changes in plasma protein binding have little clinical relevance. *Clin Pharmacol Ther.* 2002;71:115–121.
127. Inturrisi CE, Colburn WA. Application of pharmacokinetic-pharmacodynamic modeling to analgesia. In: Foley KM, Inturrisi CE, eds. *Advances in pain research and therapy opioid analgesics in the management of clinical pain.* New York, NY: Raven Press; 1986.
128. Anderson BJ, Ralph CJ, Stewart AW, et al. The dose-effect relationship for morphine and vomiting after day-stay tonsillectomy in children. *Anaesth Intensive Care.* 2000;28:155–160.
129. Lynn AM, Nespeca MK, Opheim KE, et al. Respiratory effects of intravenous morphine infusions in neonates, infants, and children after cardiac surgery. *Anesth Analg.* 1993;77:695–701.
130. van Dijk M, Bouwmeester NJ, Duivenvoorden HJ, et al. Efficacy of continuous versus intermittent morphine administration after major surgery in 0-3-year-old infants; a double-blind randomized controlled trial. *Pain.* 2002;98:305–313.
131. Chay PC, Duffy BJ, Walker JS. Pharmacokinetic-pharmacodynamic relationships of morphine in neonates. *Clin Pharmacol Ther.* 1992;51:334–342.
132. Lynn A, Nespeca MK, Bratton SL, et al. Clearance of morphine in postoperative infants during intravenous infusion: the influence of age and surgery. *Anesth Analg.* 1998;86:958–963.
133. Meesters NJ, van Dijk M, Knibbe CA, et al. Infants operated on for necrotizing enterocolitis: towards evidence-based pain guidelines. *Neonatology.* 2016;110:190–197.
134. Anderson BJ, Persson M, Anderson M. Rationalising intravenous morphine prescriptions in children. *Acute Pain.* 1999;2:59–67.
135. Krekels EH, Tibboel D, de Wildt SN, et al. Evidence-based morphine dosing for postoperative neonates and infants. *Clin Pharmacokinet.* 2014;53:553–563.
136. Hall RW, Kronsberg SS, Barton BA, et al. Morphine, hypotension, and adverse outcomes among preterm neonates: who's to blame? Secondary results from the NEOPAIN trial. *Pediatrics.* 2005;115:1351–1359.
137. Simons SHP, Roofthooft DW, van Dijk M, et al. Morphine in ventilated neonates: its effects on arterial blood pressure. *Arch Dis Child Fetal Neonatal Ed.* 2006;91:F46–F51.
138. de Graaf J, van Lingen RA, Simons SH, et al. Long-term effects of routine morphine infusion in mechanically ventilated neonates on children's functioning: five-year follow-up of a randomized controlled trial. *Pain.* 2011;152:1391–1397.
139. de Graaf J, van Lingen RA, Valkenburg AJ, et al. Does neonatal morphine use affect neuropsychological outcomes at 8 to 9 years of age? *Pain.* 2013;154:449–458.
140. Barrington KJ, Byrne PJ. Premedication for neonatal intubation. *Am J Perinatol.* 1998;15:213–216.
141. Saarenmaa E, Huttunen P, Leppaluoto J, et al. Advantages of fentanyl over morphine in analgesia for ventilated newborn infants after birth: a randomized trial. *J Pediatr.* 1999;134:144–150.
142. Arnold JH, Truog RD, Scavone JM, et al. Changes in the pharmacodynamic response to fentanyl in neonates during continuous infusion. *J Pediatr.* 1991;119:639–643.
143. Franck LS, Vilardi J, Durand D, et al. Opioid withdrawal in neonates after continuous infusions of morphine or fentanyl during extracorporeal membrane oxygenation. *Am J Crit Care.* 1998;7:364–369.
144. Chana SK, Anand KJS. Can we use methadone for analgesia in neonates? *Arch Dis Child Fetal Neonatal Ed.* 2001;85:F79–F81.
145. Ziesenitz VC, Vaughns JD, Koch G, et al. Correction to: pharmacokinetics of fentanyl and its derivatives in children: a comprehensive review. *Clin Pharmacokinet.* 2018;57:393–417.
146. Guinsburg R, Kopelman BI, Anand KJS, et al. Physiological, hormonal, and behavioral responses to a single fentanyl dose in intubated and ventilated preterm neonates. *J Pediatr.* 1998;132:954–959.
147. Lago P, Benini F, Agosto C, et al. Randomised controlled trial of low dose fentanyl infusion in preterm infants with hyaline membrane disease. *Arch Dis Child Fetal Neonatal Ed.* 1998;79:F194–F197.
148. Barrier G, Attia J, Mayer MN, et al. Measurement of post-operative pain and narcotic administration in infants using a new clinical scoring system. *Intensive Care Med.* 1989;15:S37–S39.
149. Collins JJ, Dunkel IJ, Gupta SK, et al. Transdermal fentanyl in children with cancer pain: feasibility, tolerability, and pharmacokinetic correlates. *J Pediatr.* 1999;134:319–323.
150. Tateishi T, Krivoruk Y, Ueng YF, et al. Identification of human liver cytochrome P-450 3A4 as the enzyme responsible for fentanyl and sufentanil N-dealkylation. *Anesth Analg.* 1996;82:167–172.
151. Labroo RB, Paine MF, Thummel KE, et al. Fentanyl metabolism by human hepatic and intestinal cytochrome P450 3A4: implications for interindividual variability in disposition, efficacy, and drug interactions. *Drug Metab Dispos.* 1997;25:1072–1080.
152. Jacqz-Aigrain E, Burtin P. Clinical pharmacokinetics of sedatives in neonates. *Clin Pharmacokinet.* 1996;31:423–443.
153. Grond S, Radbruch L, Lehmann KA. Clinical pharmacokinetics of transdermal opioids: focus on transdermal fentanyl. *Clin Pharmacokinet.* 2000;38:59–89.
154. Sebel PS, Barrett CW, Kirk CJ, et al. Transdermal absorption of fentanyl and sufentanil in man. *Eur J Clin Pharmacol.* 1987;32:529–531.
155. Schechter NL, Weisman SJ, Rosenblum M, et al. The use of oral transmucosal fentanyl citrate for painful procedures in children. *Pediatrics.* 1995;95:335–339.
156. Koehntop DE, Rodman JH, Brundage DM, et al. Pharmacokinetics of fentanyl in neonates. *Anesth Analg.* 1986;65:227–232.
157. Hughes MA, Glass PS, Jacobs JR. Context-sensitive half-time in multicompartment pharmacokinetic models for intravenous anesthetic drugs. *Anesthesiology.* 1992;76:334–341.
158. Voller S, Flint RB, Andriessen P, et al. Rapidly maturing fentanyl clearance in preterm neonates. *Arch Dis Child Fetal Neonatal Ed.* 2019;104:F598–F603.
159. van Lingen R, Simons S, Anderson B, et al. The effects of analgesia in the vulnerable infant during transition from the intrauterine to the extrauterine environment. *Clin Perinatol.* 2002;29.
160. Johnson KL, Erickson JP, Holley FO, et al. Fentanyl pharmacokinetics in the paediatric population. *Anesthesiology.* 1984;61:A441.
161. Touw DJ. Clinical implications of genetic polymorphisms and drug interactions mediated by cytochrome P-450 enzymes. *Drug Metabol Drug Interact.* 1997;14:55–82.
162. Tanaka E. Clinically important pharmacokinetic drug-drug interactions: role of cytochrome P450 enzymes. *J Clin Pharm Ther.* 1998;23:403–416.
163. Feierman DE. The effect of paracetamol (acetaminophen) on fentanyl metabolism in vitro. *Acta Anaesthesiol Scand.* 2000;44:560–563.
164. Yaster M, Koehler RC, Traystman RJ. Effects of fentanyl on peripheral and cerebral hemodynamics in neonatal lambs. *Anesthesiology.* 1987;66:524–530.
165. Hickey PR, Hansen DD, Wessel DL, et al. Blunting of stress responses in the pulmonary circulation of infants by fentanyl. *Anesth Analg.* 1985;64:1137–1142.
166. Taddio A. Opioid analgesia for infants in the neonatal intensive care unit. *Clin Perinatol.* 2002;29:493–509.
167. Hertzka RE, Gauntlett IS, Fisher DM, et al. Fentanyl-induced ventilatory depression: effects of age. *Anesthesiology.* 1989;70:213–218.
168. Billmire DA, Neale HW, Gregory RO. Use of i.v. fentanyl in the outpatient treatment of pediatric facial trauma. *J Trauma.* 1985;25:1079–1080.
169. Saarenmaa E, Huttunen P, Leppaluoto J, et al. Alfentanil as procedural pain relief in newborn infants. *Arch Dis Child Fetal Neonatal Ed.* 1996;75:F103–F107.
170. Davis PJ, Cook DR. Clinical pharmacokinetics of the newer intravenous anaesthetic agents. *Clin Pharmacokinet.* 1986;11:18–35.
171. Meuldermans W, Woestenborghs R, Noorduin H, et al. Protein binding of the analgesics alfentanil and sufentanil in maternal and neonatal plasma. *Eur J Clin Pharmacol.* 1986;30:217–219.
172. Wilson AS, Stiller RL, Davis PJ, et al. Fentanyl and alfentanil plasma protein binding in preterm and term neonates. *Anesth Analg.* 1997;84:315–318.
173. Meistelman C, Saint-Maurice C, Lepaul M, et al. A comparison of alfentanil pharmacokinetics in children and adults. *Anesthesiology.* 1987;66:13–16.
174. Marlow N, Weindling AM, Van Peer A, et al. Alfentanil pharmacokinetics in preterm infants. *Arch Dis Child.* 1990;65:349–351.
175. Killian A, Davis PJ, Stiller RL, et al. Influence of gestational age on pharmacokinetics of alfentanil in neonates. *Dev Pharmacol Ther.* 1990;15:82–85.
176. Olkkola KT, Hamunen K. Pharmacokinetics and pharmacodynamics of analgesic drugs. In: Anand KJ, Stevens B, McGrath P, eds. *Pain in neonates.* 2nd Revised and Enlarged Edition. Amsterdam, Netherlands: Elsevier; 2000.
177. Pokela ML. Effect of opioid-induced analgesia on beta-endorphin, cortisol and glucose responses in neonates with cardiorespiratory problems. *Biol Neonate.* 1993;64:360–367.
178. Pokela ML, Koivisto M. Physiological changes, plasma beta-endorphin and cortisol responses to tracheal intubation in neonates. *Acta Paediatr.* 1994;83:151–156.
179. Pokela ML, Ryhanen PT, Koivisto ME, et al. Alfentanil-induced rigidity in newborn infants. *Anesth Analg.* 1992;75:252–257.
180. Thompson JP, Rowbotham DJ. Remifentanil—an opioid for the 21st century. *Br J Anaesth.* 1996;76:341–343.
181. German JW, Aneja R, Heard C, et al. Continuous remifentanil for pediatric neurosurgery patients. *Pediatr Neurosurg.* 2000;33:227–229.
182. Marsh DF, Hodkinson B. Remifentanil in paediatric anaesthetic practice. *Anaesthesia.* 2009;64:301–308.
183. Davis PJ, Lerman J, Suresh S, et al. A randomized multicenter study of remifentanil compared with alfentanil, isoflurane, or propofol in anesthetized pediatric patients undergoing elective strabismus surgery. *Anesth Analg.* 1997;84:982–989.
184. Prys-Roberts C, Lerman J, Murat I, et al. Comparison of remifentanil versus regional anaesthesia in children anaesthetised with isoflurane/nitrous oxide. International Remifentanil Paediatric Anaesthesia Study group. *Anaesthesia.* 2000;55:870–876.
185. Donmez A, Kizilkan A, Berksun H, et al. One center's experience with remifentanil infusions for pediatric cardiac catheterization. *J Cardiothorac Vasc Anesth.* 2001;15:736–739.
186. Egan TD. Remifentanil pharmacokinetics and pharmacodynamics. A preliminary appraisal. *Clin Pharmacokinet.* 1995;29:80–94.
187. Dershwitz M, Hoke JF, Rosow CE, et al. Pharmacokinetics and pharmacodynamics of remifentanil in volunteer subjects with severe liver disease. *Anesthesiology.* 1996;84:812–820.
188. Rigby-Jones AE, Priston MJ, Sneyd JR, et al. Remifentanil-midazolam sedation for paediatric patients receiving mechanical ventilation after cardiac surgery. *Br J Anaesth.* 2007;99:252–261.
189. Rigby-Jones AE, Priston MJ, Thorne GC, et al. Population pharmacokinetics of remifentanil in critically ill post cardiac neonates, infants and children. *Br J Anaesth.* 2005;95:578P–579P.
190. Davis PJ, Wilson AS, Siewers RD, et al. The effects of cardiopulmonary bypass on remifentanil kinetics in children undergoing atrial septal defect repair. *Anesth Analg.* 1999;89:904–908.
191. Ross AK, Davis PJ, Dear Gd GL, et al. Pharmacokinetics of remifentanil in anesthetized pediatric patients undergoing elective surgery or diagnostic procedures. *Anesth Analg.* 2001;93:1393–1401, table of contents.
192. Litman RS. Conscious sedation with remifentanil during painful medical procedures. *J Pain Symptom Manage.* 2000;19:468–471.

193. Chiaretti A, Pietrini D, Piastra M, et al. Safety and efficacy of remifentanil in craniosynostosis repair in children less than 1 year old. *Pediatr Neurosurg.* 2000;33:83–88.
194. Davis PJ, Galinkin J, McGowan FX, et al. A randomized multicenter study of remifentanil compared with halothane in neonates and infants undergoing pyloromyotomy. I. Emergence and recovery profiles. *Anesth Analg.* 2001;93:1380–1386, table of contents.
195. Shin SH, Kim HS, Lee J, et al. A comparative study of two remifentanil doses for procedural pain in ventilated preterm infants: a randomized, controlled study. Pediatr Crit Care Med. 2014;15:451–455.
196. de Kort EH, Hanff LM, Roofthooft D, et al. Insufficient sedation and severe side effects after fast administration of remifentanil during INSURE in preterm newborns. *Neonatology.* 2017;111:172–176.
197. Rischitelli DG, Karbowicz SH. Safety and efficacy of controlled-release oxycodone: a systematic literature review. *Pharmacotherapy.* 2002;22:898–904.
198. Kokki H, Rasanen I, Lasalmi M, et al. Comparison of oxycodone pharmacokinetics after buccal and sublingual administration in children. *Clin Pharmacokinet.* 2006;45:745–754.
199. Kokki H, Rasanen I, Reinikainen M, et al. Pharmacokinetics of oxycodone after intravenous, buccal, intramuscular and gastric administration in children. *Clin Pharmacokinet.* 2004;43:613–622.
200. Olkkola KT, Hamunen K, Seppala T, et al. Pharmacokinetics and ventilatory effects of intravenous oxycodone in postoperative children. *Br J Clin Pharmacol.* 1994;38:71–76.
201. Suresh S, Anand KJS. Opioid tolerance in neonates: a state of the art review. *Paediatr Anaesth.* 2001;11:511–521.
202. Tobias JD. Tolerance, withdrawal, and physical dependency after long-term sedation and analgesia of children in the pediatric intensive care unit. *Crit Care Med.* 2000;28:2122–2132.
203. Berde CB, Beyer JE, Bournaki MC, et al. Comparison of morphine and methadone for prevention of postoperative pain in 3-to 7-year-old children. *J Pediatr.* 1991;119:136–141.
204. Shir Y, Shenkman Z, Shavelson V, et al. Oral methadone for the treatment of severe pain in hospitalized children: a report of five cases. *Clin J Pain.* 1998;14:350–353.
205. Davidson A, Flick RP. Neurodevelopmental implications of the use of sedation and analgesia in neonates. *Clin Perinatol.* 2013;40:559–573.
206. Kharasch ED. Current concepts in methadone metabolism and transport. *Clin Pharmacol Drug Dev.* 2017;6:125–134.
207. van Donge T, Samiee-Zafarghandy S, Pfister M, et al. Methadone dosing strategies in preterm neonates can be simplified. *Br J Clin Pharmacol.* 2019;85:1348–1356.
208. Berkowitz BA. The relationship of pharmacokinetics to pharmacological activity: morphine, methadone and naloxone. *Clin Pharmacokinet.* 1976;1:219–230.
209. Mactier H, McLaughlin P, Gillis C, et al. Variations in infant CYP2B6 genotype associated with the need for pharmacological treatment for neonatal abstinence syndrome in infants of methadone-maintained opioid-dependent mothers. *Am J Perinatol.* 2017;34:918–921.
210. Davies D, DeVlaming D, Haines C. Methadone analgesia for children with advanced cancer. *Pediatr Blood Cancer.* 2008;51:393–397.
211. Anghelescu DL, Faughnan LG, Hankins GM, et al. Methadone use in children and young adults at a cancer center: a retrospective study. *J Opioid Manag.* 2011;7:353–361.
212. Collins JJ, Geake J, Grier HE, et al. Patient-controlled analgesia for mucositis pain in children: a three-period crossover study comparing morphine and hydromorphone. *J Pediatr.* 1996;129:722–728.
213. Hagen N, Thirlwell MP, Dhaliwal HS, et al. Steady-state pharmacokinetics of hydromorphone and hydromorphone-3-glucuronide in cancer patients after immediate and controlled-release hydromorphone. *J Clin Pharmacol.* 1995;35:37–44.
214. Volles DF, McGory R. Perspectives in pain management: pharmacokinetic considerations: pharmacokinetic considerations. *Crit Care Clin.* 1999;15:55–75.
215. Babul N, Darke AC, Hain R. Hydromorphone and metabolite pharmacokinetics in children. *J Pain Symptom Manage.* 1995;10:335–337.
216. Quigley C. A systematic review of hydromorphone in acute and chronic pain. *J Pain Symptom Manage.* 2003;25:169–178.
217. Goodarzi M. Comparison of epidural morphine, hydromorphone and fentanyl for postoperative pain control in children undergoing orthopaedic surgery. *Paediatr Anaesth.* 1999;9:419–422.
218. Jaffe JH, Martine WR. Opioid analgesics and antagonists. In: Goodman Gilman A, Rall TW, Nies AS, Taylor P, eds. *The pharmacological basis of therapeutics.* New York, NY: Pergamon Press; 1990.
219. Vetter TR. Pediatric patient-controlled analgesia with morphine versus meperidine. *J Pain Symptom Manage.* 1992;7:204–208.
220. Hamunen K, Maunuksela EL, Seppala T, et al. Pharmacokinetics of i.v. and rectal pethidine in children undergoing ophthalmic surgery. *Br J Anaesth.* 1993;71:823–826.
221. Pokela ML, Olkkola KT, Koivisto M, et al. Pharmacokinetics and pharmacodynamics of intravenous meperidine in neonates and infants. *Clin Pharmacol Ther.* 1992;52:342–349.
222. Caldwell J, Wakile LA, Notarianni LJ, et al. Maternal and neonatal disposition of pethidine in childbirth—a study using quantitative gas chromatography-mass spectrometry. *Life Sci.* 1978;22:589–596.
223. Baarslag MA, Allegaert K, Knibbe CA, et al. Pharmacological sedation management in the paediatric intensive care unit. *J Pharm Pharmacol.* 2017;69:498–513.
224. de Wildt SN, Kearns GL, Sie SD, et al. Pharmacodynamics of intravenous and oral midazolam in preterm infants. *Clin Drug Investig.* 2003;23:27–38.
225. de Wildt SN, Kearns GL, Hop WC, et al. Pharmacokinetics and metabolism of intravenous midazolam in preterm infants. *Clin Pharmacol Ther.* 2001;70:525–531.
226. Voller S, Flint RB, Beggah F, et al. Recently registered midazolam doses for preterm neonates do not lead to equal exposure: a population pharmacokinetic model. *J Clin Pharmacol.* 2019;59:1300–1308.
227. Anderson BJ, Larsson P. A maturation model for midazolam clearance. *Paediatr Anaesth.* 2011;21:302–308.
228. Peeters MY, Prins SA, Knibbe CA, et al. Pharmacokinetics and pharmacodynamics of midazolam and metabolites in nonventilated infants after craniofacial surgery. *Anesthesiology.* 2006;105:1135–1146.
229. Zuppa AF, Conrado DJ, Zane NR, et al. Midazolam dose optimization in critically ill pediatric patients with acute respiratory failure: a population pharmacokinetic-pharmacogenomic study. *Crit Care Med.* 2019;47:e301–e309.
230. Jacqz-Aigrain E, Daoud P, Burtin P, et al. Placebo-controlled trial of midazolam sedation in mechanically ventilated newborn babies. *Lancet.* 1994;344:646–650.
231. Anand KJ, Barton BA, McIntosh N, et al. Analgesia and sedation in preterm neonates who require ventilatory support: results from the NOPAIN trial. Neonatal Outcome and Prolonged Analgesia in Neonates. *Arch Pediatr Adolesc Med.* 1999;153:331–338.
232. Arya V, Ramji S. Midazolam sedation in mechanically ventilated newborns: a double blind randomized placebo controlled trial. *Indian Pediatr.* 2001;38:967–972.
233. Ng E, Taddio A, Ohlsson A. Intravenous midazolam infusion for sedation of infants in the neonatal intensive care unit. *Cochrane Database Syst Rev.* 2017;1:CD002052. doi:10.1002/14651858.CD002052.pub.
234. Carbajal R, Lenclen R, Jugie M, et al. Morphine does not provide adequate analgesia for acute procedural pain among preterm neonates. *Pediatrics.* 2005;115:1494–1500.
235. Gupta K, Gupta VK, Jayashree M, et al. Randomized controlled trial of interrupted versus continuous sedative infusions in ventilated children. *Pediatr Crit Care Med.* 2012;13:131–135.
236. Vet NJ, de Wildt SN, Verlaat CW, et al. A randomized controlled trial of daily sedation interruption in critically ill children. *Intensive Care Med.* 2016;42:233–244.
237. McCall JE, Fischer CG, Warden G, et al. Lorazepam given the night before surgery reduces preoperative anxiety in children undergoing reconstructive burn surgery. *J Burn Care Rehabil.* 1999;20:151–154.
238. Chennou F, Bonneau-Fortin A, Portolese O, et al. Oral lorazepam is not superior to placebo for lowering stress in children before digestive endoscopy: a double-blind, randomized, controlled trial. *Paediatr Drugs.* 2019;21:379–387.
239. van der Vossen AC, van Nuland M, Ista EG, et al. Oral lorazepam can be substituted for intravenous midazolam when weaning paediatric intensive care patients off sedation. *Acta Paediatr.* 2018. doi:10.1111/apa.14327.
240. Uchaipichat V, Suthisisang C, Miners JO. The glucuronidation of R-and S-lorazepam: human liver microsomal kinetics, UDP-glucuronosyltransferase enzyme selectivity, and inhibition by drugs. *Drug Metab Dispos.* 2013;41:1273–1284.
241. Chamberlain JM, Capparelli EV, Brown KM, et al. Pharmacokinetics of intravenous lorazepam in pediatric patients with and without status epilepticus. *J Pediatr.* 2012;160:667–672.
242. McDermott CA, Kowalczyk AL, Schnitzler ER, et al. Pharmacokinetics of lorazepam in critically ill neonates with seizures. *J Pediatr.* 1992;120:479–483.
243. Chicella M, Jansen P, Parthiban A, et al. Propylene glycol accumulation associated with continuous infusion of lorazepam in pediatric intensive care patients. *Crit Care Med.* 2002;30:2752–2756.
244. Woodthorpe C, Trigg A, Alison G, et al. Nurse led sedation for paediatric MRI: progress and issues. *Paediatr Nurs.* 2007;19:14–18.
245. Greenberg SB, Adams RC, Aspinall CL. Initial experience with intravenous pentobarbital sedation for children undergoing MRI at a tertiary care pediatric hospital: the learning curve. *Pediatr Radiol.* 2000;30:689–691.
246. Zuppa AF, Nicolson SC, Barrett JS, et al. Population pharmacokinetics of pentobarbital in neonates, infants, and children after open heart surgery. *J Pediatr.* 2011;159:414.e1–419.e3.
247. Pokorna P, Sima M, Vobruba V, et al. Phenobarbital pharmacokinetics in neonates and infants during extracorporeal membrane oxygenation. *Perfusion.* 2018;33:80–86.
248. Moffett BS, Weingarten MM, Galati M, et al. Phenobarbital population pharmacokinetics across the pediatric age spectrum. *Epilepsia.* 2018;59:1327–1333.
249. Akhlaghpoor S, Shabestari AA, Moghdam MS. Low dose of rectal thiopental sodium for pediatric sedation in spiral computed tomography study. *Pediatr Int.* 2007;49:387–391.
250. Beekman RP, Hoorntje TM, Beek FJ, et al. Sedation for children undergoing magnetic resonance imaging: efficacy and safety of rectal thiopental. *Eur J Pediatr.* 1996;155:820–822.
251. Okutan V, Lenk MK, Sarici SU, et al. Efficacy and safety of rectal thiopental sedation in outpatient echocardiographic examination of children. *Acta Paediatr.* 2000;89:1340–1343.
252. Norman E, Wikström S, Hellström-Westas L, et al. Rapid sequence induction is superior to morphine for intubation of preterm infants: a randomized controlled trial. *J Pediatr.* 2011;159(6):893.e1–899.e1. doi:10.1016/j.jpeds.2011.06.003.
253. Larsson P, Anderson BJ, Norman E, et al. Thiopentone elimination in newborn infants: exploring Michaelis-Menten kinetics. *Acta Anaesthesiol Scand.* 2011;55:444–451.
254. Ambrose C, Sale S, Howells R, et al. Intravenous clonidine infusion in critically ill children: dose-dependent sedative effects and cardiovascular stability. *Br J Anaesth.* 2000;84:794–796.
255. Playfor S, Jenkins I, Boyles C, et al. Consensus guidelines on sedation and analgesia in critically ill children. *Intensive Care Med.* 2006;32:1125–1136.
256. Potts AL, Larsson P, Eksborg S, et al. Clonidine disposition in children; a population analysis. *Paediatr Anaesth.* 2007;17:924–933.
257. Lonnqvist PA, Bergendahl HT, Eksborg S. Pharmacokinetics of clonidine after rectal administration in children. *Anesthesiology.* 1994;81:1097–1101.
258. Arenas-Lopez S, Mulla H, Manna S, et al. Enteral absorption and haemodynamic response of clonidine in infants post-cardiac surgery. *Br J Anaesth.* 2014;113:964–969.
259. Ahmed SS, Unland T, Slaven JE, et al. Successful use of intravenous dexmedetomidine for magnetic resonance imaging sedation in autistic children. *South Med J.* 2014;107:559–564.
260. Miller J, Xue B, Hossain M, et al. Comparison of dexmedetomidine and chloral hydrate sedation for transthoracic echocardiography in infants and toddlers: a randomized clinical trial. *Paediatr Anaesth.* 2016;26:266–272.
261. Yuen VM, Li BL, Cheuk DK, et al. A randomised controlled trial of oral chloral hydrate vs. intranasal dexmedetomidine before computerised tomography in children. *Anaesthesia.* 2017;72:1191–1195.
262. Ghai B, Jain K, Saxena AK, et al. Comparison of oral midazolam with intranasal dexmedetomidine premedication for children undergoing CT imaging: a randomized, double-blind, and controlled study. *Paediatr Anaesth.* 2017;27:37–44.

263. Reynolds J, Rogers A, Medellin E, et al. A prospective, randomized, double-blind trial of intranasal dexmedetomidine and oral chloral hydrate for sedated auditory brainstem response (ABR) testing. *Paediatr Anaesth.* 2016;26:286–293.
264. Bong CL, Tan J, Lim S, et al. Randomised controlled trial of dexmedetomidine sedation vs general anaesthesia for inguinal hernia surgery on perioperative outcomes in infants. *Br J Anaesth.* 2019;122:662–670.
265. Szmuk P, Andropoulos D, McGowan F, et al. An open label pilot study of a dexmedetomidine-remifentanil-caudal anesthetic for infant lower abdominal/lower extremity surgery: The T REX pilot study. *Paediatr Anaesth.* 2019;29:59–67.
266. Perez-Zoghbi JF, Zhu W, Grafe MR, et al. Dexmedetomidine-mediated neuroprotection against sevoflurane-induced neurotoxicity extends to several brain regions in neonatal rats. *Br J Anaesth.* 2017;119:506–516.
267. van Hoorn CE, Hoeks SE, Essink H, et al. A systematic review and narrative synthesis on the histological and neurobehavioral long-term effects of dexmedetomidine. *Paediatr Anaesth.* 2019;29:125–136.
268. Potts AL, Warman GR, Anderson BJ. Dexmedetomidine disposition in children: a population analysis. *Paediatr Anaesth.* 2008;18:722–730.
269. Greenberg RG, Wu H, Laughon M, et al. Population pharmacokinetics of dexmedetomidine in infants. *J Clin Pharmacol.* 2017;57:1174–1182.
270. Bhutta AT. Ketamine: a controversial drug for neonates. *Semin Perinatol.* 2007;31:303–308.
271. Golding CL, Miller JL, Gessouroun MR, et al. Ketamine continuous infusions in critically ill infants and children. *Ann Pharmacother.* 2016;50:234–241.
272. Flint RB, Brouwer CNM, Kranzlin ASC, et al. Pharmacokinetics of S-ketamine during prolonged sedation at the pediatric intensive care unit. *Paediatr Anaesth.* 2017;27:1098–1107.
273. Yan J, Li YR, Zhang Y, et al. Repeated exposure to anesthetic ketamine can negatively impact neurodevelopment in infants: a prospective preliminary clinical study. *J Child Neurol.* 2014;29:1333–1338.
274. Milesi C, Baleine J, Mura T, et al. Nasal midazolam vs ketamine for neonatal intubation in the delivery room: a randomised trial. *Arch Dis Child Fetal Neonatal Ed.* 2018;103:F221–F226.
275. Mistry RB, Nahata MC. Ketamine for conscious sedation in pediatric emergency care. *Pharmacotherapy.* 2005;25:1104–1111.
276. Malinovsky JM, Servin F, Cozian A, et al. Ketamine and norketamine plasma concentrations after i.v., nasal and rectal administration in children. *Br J Anaesth.* 1996;77:203–207.
277. Grant IS, Nimmo WS, McNicol LR, et al. Ketamine disposition in children and adults. *Br J Anaesth.* 1983;55:1107–1111.
278. Hemphill S, McMenamin L, Bellamy MC, et al. Propofol infusion syndrome: a structured literature review and analysis of published case reports. *Br J Anaesth.* 2019;122:448–459.
279. Durrmeyer X, Breinig S, Claris O, et al. Effect of atropine with propofol vs atropine with atracurium and sufentanil on oxygen desaturation in neonates requiring nonemergency intubation: a randomized clinical trial. *JAMA.* 2018;319:1790–1801.
280. Dekker J, Lopriore E, van Zanten HA, et al. Sedation during minimal invasive surfactant therapy: a randomised controlled trial. *Arch Dis Child Fetal Neonatal Ed.* 2019;104:F378–F383.
281. Simons SH, van der Lee R, Reiss IK, et al. Clinical evaluation of propofol as sedative for endotracheal intubation in neonates. *Acta Paediatr.* 2013;102:e487–e492.
282. Welzing L, Kribs A, Eifinger F, et al. Propofol as an induction agent for endotracheal intubation can cause significant arterial hypotension in preterm neonates. *Paediatr Anaesth.* 2010;20:605–611.
283. Thewissen L, Caicedo A, Dereymaeker A, et al. Cerebral autoregulation and activity after propofol for endotracheal intubation in preterm neonates. *Pediatr Res.* 2018;84:719–725.
284. Smits A, Thewissen L, Caicedo A, et al. Propofol dose-finding to reach optimal effect for (semi-)elective intubation in neonates. *J Pediatr.* 2016;179:54.e9–60.e9.
285. Morse J, Hannam JA, Cortinez LI, et al. A manual propofol infusion regimen for neonates and infants. *Paediatr Anaesth.* 2019;29:907–914.
286. Fong CY, Tay CG, Ong LC, et al. Chloral hydrate as a sedating agent for neurodiagnostic procedures in children. *Cochrane Database Syst Rev.* 2017;11:CD011786. doi:10.1002/14651858.CD011786.pub2.
287. Mayers DJ, Hindmarsh KW, Sankaran K, et al. Chloral hydrate disposition following single-dose administration to critically ill neonates and children. *Dev Pharmacol Ther.* 1991;16:71–77.
288. Sury MR, Fairweather K. The effect of melatonin on sedation of children undergoing magnetic resonance imaging. *Br J Anaesth.* 2006;97:220–225.
289. Merchant NM, Azzopardi DV, Hawwa AF, et al. Pharmacokinetics of melatonin in preterm infants. *Br J Clin Pharmacol.* 2013;76:725–733.
290. Sun LS, Li G, Miller TL, et al. Association between a single general anesthesia exposure before age 36 months and neurocognitive outcomes in later childhood. *JAMA.* 2016;315:2312–2320.
291. Davidson AJ, Disma N, de Graaff JC, et al. Neurodevelopmental outcome at 2 years of age after general anaesthesia and awake-regional anaesthesia in infancy (GAS): an international multicentre, randomised controlled trial. *Lancet.* 2015;387:239–250.
292. Avella-Garcia CB, Julvez J, Fortuny J, et al. Acetaminophen use in pregnancy and neurodevelopment: attention function and autism spectrum symptoms. *Int J Epidemiol.* 2016;45:1987–1996.
293. de Fays L, Van Malderen K, De Smet K, et al. Use of paracetamol during pregnancy and child neurological development. *Dev Med Child Neurol.* 2015;57:718–724.
294. van den Bosch GE, IJsselstijn H, van der Lugt A, et al. Neuroimaging, pain sensitivity, and neuropsychological functioning in school-age neonatal extracorporeal membrane oxygenation survivors exposed to opioids and sedatives. *Pediatr Crit Care Med.* 2015;16:652–662.
295. Schiller RM, van den Bosch GE, Muetzel RL, et al. Neonatal critical illness and development: white matter and hippocampus alterations in school-age neonatal extracorporeal membrane oxygenation survivors. *Dev Med Child Neurol.* 2017;59:304–310.
296. van den Bosch GE, White T, El Marroun H, et al. Prematurity, opioid exposure and neonatal pain: do they affect the developing brain? *Neonatology.* 2015;108:8–15.
297. Ferguson SA, Ward WL, Paule MG, et al. A pilot study of preemptive morphine analgesia in preterm neonates: effects on head circumference, social behavior, and response latencies in early childhood. *Neurotoxicol Teratol.* 2012;34:47–55.
298. Zwicker JG, Miller SP, Grunau RE, et al. Smaller cerebellar growth and poorer neurodevelopmental outcomes in very preterm infants exposed to neonatal morphine. *J Pediatr.* 2016;172:81.e2–87.e2.
299. van den Anker JN, van Dijk M, Tibboel D. Impaired neurodevelopmental outcomes in very preterm infants: much too easy to blame it just on morphine! *J Pediatr.* 2016;172:7–8.
300. Young C, Jevtovic-Todorovic V, Qin YQ, et al. Potential of ketamine and midazolam, individually or in combination, to induce apoptotic neurodegeneration in the infant mouse brain. *Br J Pharmacol.* 2005;146:189–197.
301. Duerden EG, Guo T, Dodbiba L, et al. Midazolam dose correlates with abnormal hippocampal growth and neurodevelopmental outcome in preterm infants. *Ann Neurol.* 2016;79:548–559.
302. Schmidt-Kastner R. Genomic approach to selective vulnerability of the hippocampus in brain ischemia-hypoxia. *Neuroscience.* 2015;309:259–279.
303. Schiller RM, Allegaert K, Hunfeld M, et al. Analgesics and sedatives in critically ill newborns and infants: the impact on long-term neurodevelopment. *J Clin Pharmacol.* 2018;58 Suppl 10:S140–S150.

CHAPTER

37

Elizabeth Yen
Walter K. Kraft
Jonathan M. Davis

Pharmacologic Management of Neonatal Abstinence Syndrome

BACKGROUND

The opium poppy was first cultivated in Lower Mesopotamia nearly 6,000 years ago. Referred to as the "joy plant" by the Sumerians, opium initially found use as an analgesic. The term *opiate* referred to derivatives of opium with pharmacologic activity, with morphine being the prototypic drug of the class. Semisynthetic opioids such as oxycodone were then developed in the 1930s along with synthetic opioids such as meperidine and methadone. The term *opioid* more broadly describes drugs with similar pharmacologic properties of the opiates, but encompasses both naturally derived and synthetic drugs. The similarity of pharmacologic effects and structural features of opiate and opioid drugs led investigators to propose the existence of an endogenous receptor target in the 1950s.[1] In the 1970s, binding sites for opioids were found to be localized in the brain, including the μ receptor, named for its interaction with the ligand morphine.[2] This receptor is the primary pharmacologic site of action for opioids. Opioids are defined as substances that bind to opioid receptors. Although the δ- and κ-opioid receptors share a G-protein–coupled structure with the μ receptor, the binding affinity to opioid drugs differs between the three. The functions of the δ and κ receptors are less well defined than the μ, with nociception and analgesia among the putative domains. The endogenous ligands for these receptors are the endorphins and enkephalins. Although the clinical use of opioids is primarily for the relief of pain, drugs that are agonists of the μ-opioid receptor can cause a number of acute physiologic effects (Table 37.1). The euphoric effects of morphine and other μ-opioid–binding drugs have led to abuse, with the development of physical dependence as early as 2 weeks in new users. Severe withdrawal symptoms (if the drugs are abruptly stopped) and increasing need for higher doses (e.g., tolerance) lead to continued use despite the negative impact.

TABLE 37.1 Effects of Opioids

Central Nervous System Effects	*Peripheral Effects*
Analgesia	Bronchial relaxation
Euphoria	Cough suppression
Respiratory depression	Decreased gastric motility
Miosis	Histamine release

There have been a number of epidemics of opioid abuse that have caused significant societal disruption, such as the opium epidemic in the 19th century in China. Widespread abuse in the United States eventually led to legislation and policies in the early 1900s that limited access to opioids. Abuse of opioids remained an issue throughout the 20th century, but was significantly reduced in the number and scope of populations affected. Starting in the 1990s, opioid use in clinical practice greatly expanded. The reasons for this are complex, but this was followed by a significant increase in opioid abuse and dependency in users. In 2016, 4.3% of the U.S. population aged 12 years and older reported recent misuse of opioids.[3] Opioid abuse is more common in males than females (57% vs. 43% with prescription opioids, 68% vs. 32% with heroin).[4] Women represent a unique group affected by the opioid epidemic, with the majority using prescribed drugs to treat chronic pain and a variety of other illnesses prior to developing opioid use disorders (OUDs). OUD describes consumption that exceeds the intended amount or duration of treatment as well as continued use despite negative physical, social, and psychological consequences (e.g., tolerance, craving, uncontrolled use).[5] Between 2008 and 2012, approximately 39% of Medicaid recipients and 28% of privately insured women of reproductive age used prescription opioids.[6] Although most prescriptions were given to treat short-term pain and did not lead to abuse, exposure to even short durations of opioids increases the risk of long-term use and abuse. The incidence of pregnant women using opioids parallels the global increase in opioid consumption. Between 1999 and 2014, the number of pregnant women using opioids in the United States increased dramatically from 1.5 to 6.5 per 1,000 deliveries.[7] An estimated one-fourth of pregnant women in the United States fill a prescription for opioids on an annual basis.[8]

The American College of Obstetrics and Gynecologists (ACOG) guidelines recommend universal substance use screening to identify and manage OUD.[9,10] The presence of OUD should prompt clinicians to prescribe or appropriately refer patients to programs using medication-assisted therapy (MAT). The keystone of MAT is the use of the long-acting opioid agonist methadone or the partial agonist buprenorphine to reduce physical withdrawal symptoms. Ideally paired with comprehensive counseling and social services, MAT markedly reduces the use of illicit opioids and other harmful health behaviors and significantly improves neonatal outcome. MAT is preferred to medication-assisted withdrawal, as the latter is often associated with high relapse rates and carries negative consequences for both the mother and the fetus.[10–13] Both methadone and buprenorphine have been demonstrated to be safe and effective in pregnant women and the fetus.[14–17]

SIGNS OF WITHDRAWAL IN NEONATES

In the late 19th century, the first case of a neonate exhibiting signs of withdrawal was reported and termed "congenital morphinism." This was followed by several similar case reports with many neonates dying due to the lack of specific treatments. It was not until the mid-20th century when treatment with morphine was found to improve neonatal survival and outcome. The term "neonatal abstinence syndrome" (NAS) emerged to describe withdrawal from opioids as well as substances such as alcohol, tobacco, and many other psychotropic medications.[18] The term "neonatal opioid-withdrawal syndrome" (NOWS) has been proposed to highlight the key role of opioids in driving the withdrawal complex.[19] The term NAS continues to be used in the context of signs of withdrawal that are likely to be opioid related, but can be impacted by (a) other nonopioid drugs of abuse, (b) other prescription (psychotropic) medications, and (c) cigarette smoking.

As water-soluble, low-molecular weight, and lipophilic drugs, opioids readily cross the placenta. Transfer of opioids increases with gestational age and concurrent use of methadone with heroin or cocaine.[20–22] This is directly related to the number of placental enzymes and transporters that change with gestation. For example, P-glycoprotein expression (a placental efflux transporter) in the placenta has been found to decrease as pregnancy progresses, which can increase drug transfer later in gestation.[23,24]

Opioid receptors are localized in the central nervous system, peripheral nervous system, and gastrointestinal system. Transfer of opioids across the placenta leads to opioid binding to these multisystem receptors (Fig. 37.1). Although the density of μ receptors in the neonatal brain is comparable to adults, there are significantly fewer κ and δ receptors. μ-Opioid receptors are expressed early with localization near germinal zones, suggesting a developmental function.[25–27] In animal models, exogenous opioids suppress receptor binding as well as ligand affinity during this early postnatal period, followed by increased binding later in adult life.[28] The early suppression of μ-opioid receptor binding is associated with altered dendritic length, spine density, myelination, neurotransmitters (acetylcholine, serotonin, dopamine), and postsynaptic activity.[28,29] The clinical correlates of these animal findings in humans are unclear. While infants with in utero opioid exposure have smaller head circumferences and altered brain volumes, the relative weight of exogenous opioids compared to other confounding environmental factors on fetal brain development has not been well defined.[30–32]

As shown in Figure 37.2, ligand binding of μ-opioid receptors in the locus coeruleus decreases adenylyl cyclase activity in

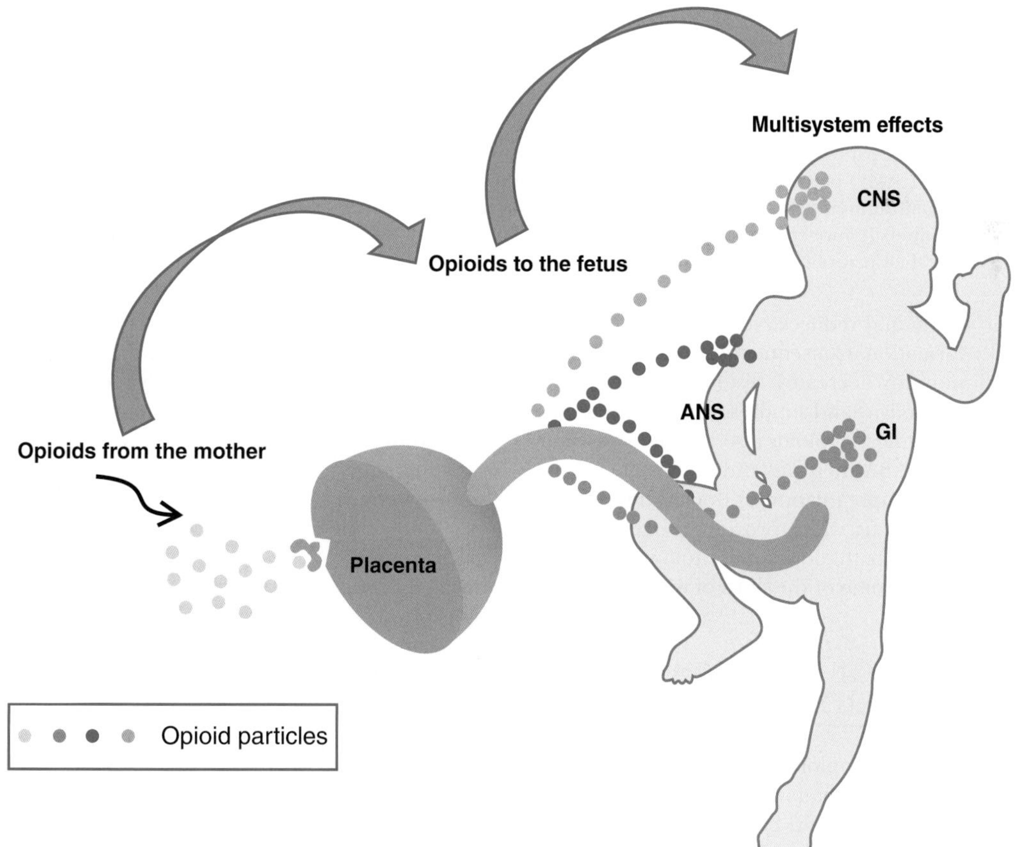

Figure 37.1 Maternal–fetal transmission of opioids across the placenta and binding of opioids to opioid receptors in the central nervous system (CNS), autonomic nervous system (ANS), and gastrointestinal (GI) system, resulting in multisystem effects [figure created using derivatives of "People" by Servier Medical Art (https://smart.servier.com/) under the Creative Commons License (CC BY 3.0)].

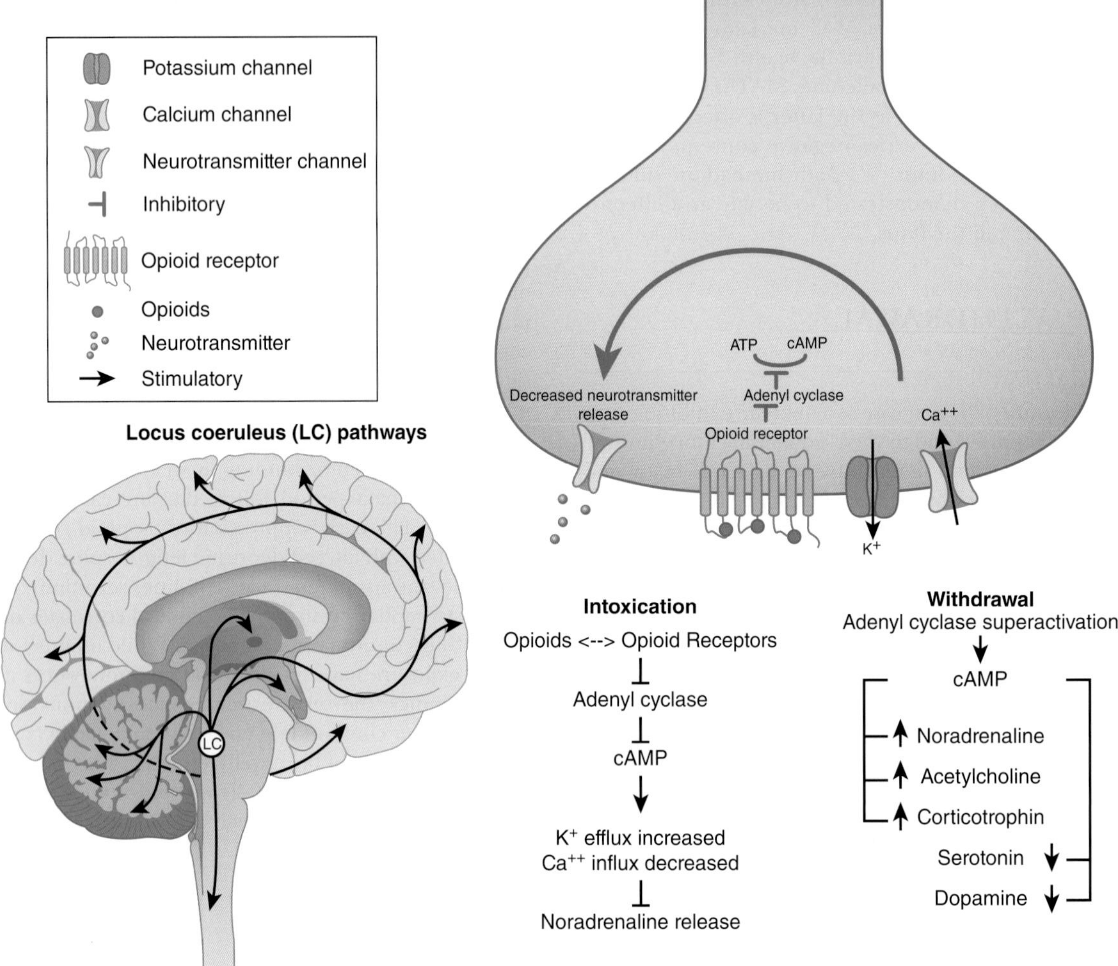

Figure 37.2 Molecular mechanism of opioid binding, intoxication, and withdrawal. A schematic diagram of multicenter opioid activation within the locus coeruleus (LC) pathways in the brain. Opioid binding to opioid receptors inhibits adenylyl cyclase, which further inhibits cyclic adenosine monophosphate (cAMP) production, leading to increased potassium efflux and decreased calcium influx, culminating in inhibition of noradrenaline and other neurotransmitter release. Conversely, a hyperadrenergic state occurs during opioid withdrawal with modulatory effects on numerous neurotransmitters [figure created using derivatives of "Nervous System," "Receptors and Channels" by Servier Medical Art (https://smart.servier.com/) under the Creative Commons License (CC BY3.0)].

the noradrenergic system and reduces cyclic adenosine monophosphate (cAMP) formation. Consequently, potassium efflux increases and calcium influx decreases, resulting in downregulation of noradrenergic activity and suppression of sympathetic and catecholamine signaling.[33] Opioids also activate presynaptic γ-aminobutyric acid (GABA) neurons and inhibit the release of GABA. This permits an upregulation of dopaminergic neurons in the nucleus accumbens, which provides the reward perception.[34] The rebound sympathetic response following opioid cessation is responsible for some of the signs of withdrawal.

MANIFESTATIONS OF NEONATAL ABSTINENCE SYNDROME

When the umbilical cord is cut, opioid concentrations drop precipitously as the neonate's elimination mechanisms eliminate maternally transferred drug. Adenylyl cyclase is then activated, which precipitates the release of multiple neurotransmitters.[35] Signs of withdrawal develop from this over activity in the adrenergic system. Specific findings include high-pitched cry, irritability, jitteriness, tremors, hypertonia, hyperphagia, feeding intolerance, sleep disturbance, and loose stools. Seizures have been described, but are very rarely seen with current treatment regimens. Autonomic nervous system manifestations include increased heart rate and respiratory rate, temperature instability, sweating, sneezing, and mottling. The onset of these signs range from as early as 24 hours after birth for shorter acting substances (e.g., morphine) to several days for longer acting opioids (e.g., methadone).[18,36,37] Most centers will observe neonates in the hospital for up to 5 days prior to discharge to allow for the late signs of withdrawal to appear. Premature neonates have less severe signs of withdrawal relative to term neonates, presumably due to neurodevelopmental immaturity.[38]

THE INCIDENCE AND SEVERITY OF NEONATAL ABSTINENCE SYNDROME

Paralleling the steep increase in the number of pregnant women with OUD is the number of neonates born with NAS. Between 2000 and 2014, there was a several fold increase in the incidence of NAS from 1.2 to 8.0 per 1,000 hospital births, with rates as high as 20.0 per 1,000 hospital births in some areas.[39,40] A critical principle is that NAS as a disease is defined not by the need for pharmacologic treatment, but instead the manifestations of withdrawal in the setting of known exposure. Although all neonates with prolonged in utero opioid exposure will demonstrate signs of withdrawal, these signs exist along a spectrum of severity. The heterogeneity of symptomatic expression has only been partially defined, but it is impacted in part by the type and amount of in utero exposure. Adult withdrawal and addiction syndromes have a high degree of heritability, so it is very likely that genetics has a significant role in explaining some inter-individual variability. Once an in utero exposure has been identified, the core element of treatment is to optimize nonpharmacologic care to reduce signs. This approach is complicated by the wide variety in practice-based management of NAS across hospitals in the United States.[41] When nonpharmacologic interventions are inadequate, pharmacotherapy may be needed in 50% or more of exposed neonates.

There are multiple factors that may modulate the timing and severity of withdrawal. This includes the timing during gestation of prenatal opioid use, types of opioids used (e.g., prescription opioids vs. MAT), cigarette smoking, polysubstance use (e.g., other illicit substances and/or psychotropic medications), sex, and birth weight.[18] Maternal methadone dose as a potential modifiable covariate of NAS severity has been extensively investigated, with varied methodologic quality of studies. Although a meta-analysis did not identify a statistically significant difference in outcomes between high- and low-dose methadone, there is a trend suggestive of a modest interaction between maternal dose and NAS severity.[42] This dose relationship is likely to be loosely associated with the severity of withdrawal and is not relevant in terms of choosing a maternal dose or NAS treatment approaches. Lower maternal methadone doses have been associated with higher rates of illicit drug use. ACOG and others suggest that maternal doses of methadone should not be reduced solely to reduce NAS severity.[10]

Cigarette smoking has been shown to be associated with earlier and more severe withdrawal in several studies.[43,44] In addition, since many women with OUD have psychiatric comorbidities, it is common for pregnant women to be on opioids as well as barbiturates, benzodiazepines, antidepressants, gabapentin, and/or other psychotropic drugs. Huybrechts et al. demonstrated that exposure to a single additional psychotropic medication was associated with a 37% increased risk of neonatal drug withdrawal, with exposure to two or more of these medications associated with a doubling of the risk[45] (Fig. 37.3). Male sex has been linked to higher vulnerability and more severe withdrawal in some studies, but not in others.[46,47] Breastfeeding or use of breast milk is protective and reduces the need for pharmacotherapy and length of hospital stay.[48,49] It is unclear whether this effect of breast milk is due to additional opioids being delivered to the neonate or other protective components.

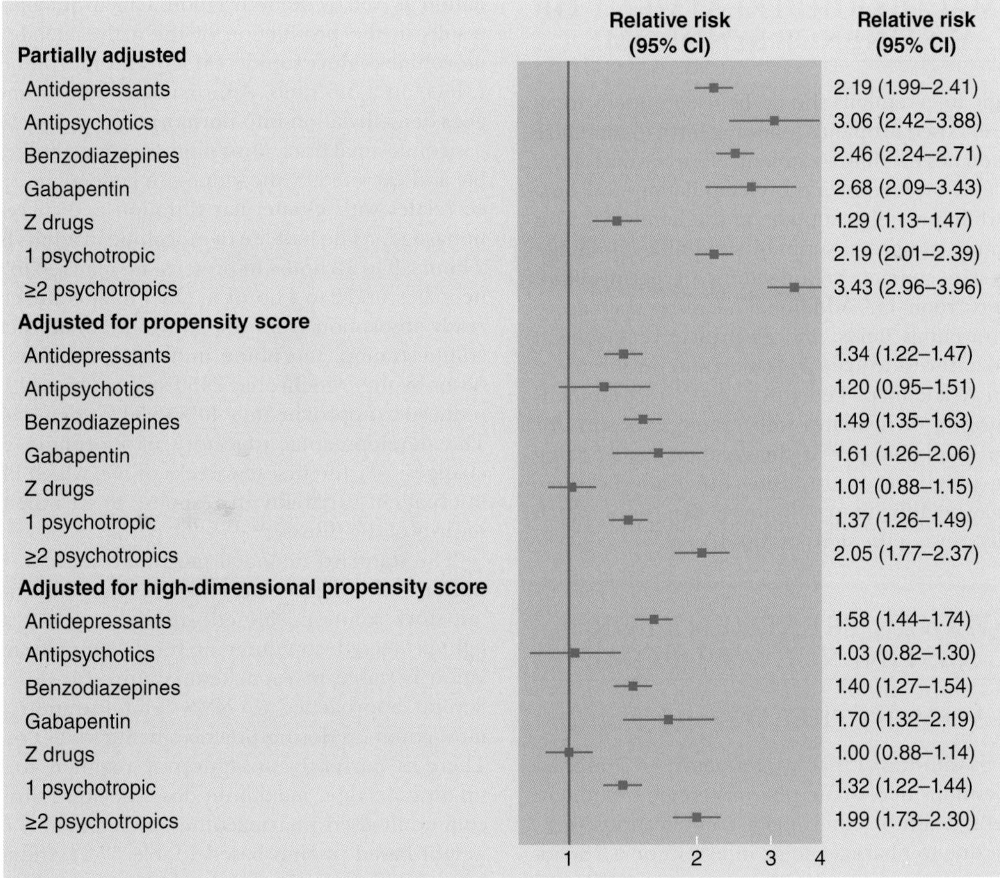

Figure 37.3 Adjusted relative risk of neonatal drug withdrawal after intrauterine coexposure to opioids and psychotropic medications: cohort study. CI, confidence interval. (Reprinted with permission from Huybrechts KF, Bateman BT, Desai RJ, et al. Risk of neonatal drug withdrawal after intrauterine co-exposure to opioids and psychotropic medications: cohort study. *BMJ* 2017;358:j3326.)

SCORING TOOLS FOR NEONATAL ABSTINENCE SYNDROME

Several assessment approaches have been developed to quantify and qualify the signs of withdrawal in term neonates with NAS.[50,51] However, the most common is the Finnegan Neonatal Abstinence Scoring System, which was developed in 1975 with subsequent modification.[52,53] This 21-item scale was designed to quantify signs of withdrawal and guide the need for treatment. A derivative of the score used in the MOTHER trial is also commonly used.[14] While there have been several attempts to modify the Finnegan score, it remains the predominant tool used to assess NAS and direct the comprehensive approach to treatment.[54,55]

Eat, Sleep, Console (ESC) is a more recent approach that focuses on three central signs of withdrawal believed to affect the physiologic functions of neonates (i.e., eating, sleeping, ability to console the neonate).[56] This system has three scored elements compared to 21 in the Finnegan. While the time to administer is shorter for nursing staff, it is not clear if the reduction in a summation of all domains of withdrawal impacts the accuracy of this instrument. The ESC system has not been subject to rigorous evaluation and has generally been implemented along with a number of other interventions, making the utility of this specific intervention difficult to assess.

NONPHARMACOLOGIC TREATMENT OF NEONATAL ABSTINENCE SYNDROME

Nonpharmacologic interventions should be used initially in all neonates who are exposed to opioids following birth to minimize the number of neonates needing treatment. Nonpharmacologic management focuses on minimizing overstimulation and optimizing comfort while providing support to the family.[57,58] This includes positioning (prone vs. supine), swaddling, holding/cuddling, skin-to-skin contact, breastfeeding (if permissible), and having parents "room-in." Additional measures such as gavage feeding, intravenous fluids, and electrolyte replacement may be needed to ensure adequate hydration and nutrition.

The American Academy of Pediatrics (AAP) recommends in-hospital monitoring of neonates with opioid exposure for 5 to 7 days prior to discharge.[59] If the mother was smoking cigarettes during pregnancy or receiving other psychotropic medications, it may be difficult to definitively determine which agents are actually causing the signs of withdrawal.

PHARMACOLOGIC TREATMENT FOR NEONATAL ABSTINENCE SYNDROME

OPIOID REPLACEMENT THERAPY

Significant signs of withdrawal that are refractory to nonpharmacologic interventions necessitate pharmacologic treatment. In the modern era, death or other major complications (e.g., seizures) are rare due to pharmacologic interventions. The rationale for pharmacologic treatment is to promote growth and development and control the signs of withdrawal. Treatment also improves mother–infant bonding and relieves stress and guilt parents experience with severe signs. The ideal threshold for initiation of pharmacologic therapy remains unclear. A higher threshold for treatment may reduce the use of medication and duration of hospitalization, but at the expense of weight gain and poorer control of signs of withdrawal. It is also unclear if there are long-term effects from either under-treatment when indicated or exposure to one or more medications used to treat NAS. First-line pharmacologic therapy involves treatment with an opioid, which includes morphine, methadone, and buprenorphine.[59–61] Consistent with the treatment of adult opioid withdrawal, opioids are consistently superior in clinical trials compared to other drugs used to treat NAS.[62,63] Elevated Finnegan scores trigger the use of pharmacologic treatment with opioid dosing increasing until symptoms stabilize. If withdrawal signs are not controlled with a maximum dose, a nonopioid adjunct medication is added. With stable control of signs, doses are weaned and then discontinued. Regardless of the specific drugs or regimens used, standardization of treatment is a key element in optimizing therapy. Uniform institutional treatment protocols within a health system results in 15% to 50% reduction in length of treatment and duration of hospitalization.[64–68]

Morphine

While the pharmacokinetics (PK) of morphine in neonates has been best characterized in intravenous use for sedation and pain control, a pharmacometric model of drug disposition in NAS has been described.[69] Morphine is metabolized by glucuronidation as well as demethylation. Glucuronidation of morphine results in the production of the active metabolites, including morphine-3 glucuronide (M3G) and morphine-6 glucuronide (M6G) in a 1:6 ratio. Approximately 5% of morphine undergoes demethylation into normorphine and is eliminated via the gastrointestinal tract. Most morphine metabolites are water soluble and excreted by the kidney. In general, morphine clearance correlates with glomerular filtration and increases with gestational age.[70] The half-life of morphine in adults is approximately 2 hours, 9 to 12 hours in preterm neonates, 6 to 9 hours in term neonates, and 2 to 4 hours in older infants and children. With its ready absorption from the gastrointestinal tract following oral administration, morphine undergoes first-pass hepatic metabolism by the cytochrome P450 system. Its oral bioavailability is reduced to approximately 40% to 50% when it reaches the CNS. The developmental trajectory of morphine glucuronidation changes over the first few weeks of life, which likely adds to the interpatient variability in response to treatment based on the severity of the disease.[71]

The standard neonatal morphine solution (NMS) concentration is 0.4 mg per mL, which is prepared from a 2 mg per mL stock solution, diluted with sterile water, and stored in a light-protected container at room temperature. This formulation is stable in room temperature for at least 60 days.[72,73] Several approaches to NMS administration exist, with the most common dosing practices being weight or sign based.[74,75] There is currently no universal regimen for starting dose, up-titration rate, maximum dose, or down-titration rate. Most commonly used pharmacotherapy regimen is based on either weight based or sign based (Table 37.2). Initiation of weight-based NMS dosing is commonly between 0.02 and 0.06 mg per kg per dose given every 3 to 4 hours.[61,76] Weight-based dosing is more common and assumes that the weight of the neonates is the primary source of variability. Sign-based dosing ignores

TABLE 37.2 Representative Morphine Treatment Regimens

Weight Based	*Symptom Based (Doses Are NOT Weight Based)*
Initial dose: For two consecutive scores >8 or one score ≥12, rescore in 1 h to verify. If still elevated: 0.3–0.4 mg/kg/day divided every 4 h **Dose increase:** 20% per day for scores >24 total on three consecutive measurements or a single score ≥12 (primarily related to NAS) **Weaning dose:** After 48 h of clinical stability, reduce dose by 10% of the total initial dose (based on starting weight) every 24 h Reduce dose when the sum of the previous three scores is <18 and scores are not generally >8 Cease therapy when dose is 0.15 mg/kg/day If inadequate control of symptoms when weaning, administer additional morphine. Then can increase the maintenance dose or keep it the same **Adjunctive treatment:** At dose of morphine 1.25 mg/kg/day, initiate second medication[a]	**Initial dose:** For two consecutive scores >8 or one score ≥12, rescore in 1 h to verify. If still elevated: **Single NAS Score** — **Dose Every 4 h (mg)** 9–12: 0.04 13–16: 0.08 17–20: 0.12 21–24: 0.16 ≥25: 0.20 **Dose increase:** **Single NAS Score** — **Increase Dose (mg)** 0–8: None 9–12: 0.02 13–16: 0.04 17–20: 0.06 **Weaning dose:** • After 48 h of clinical stability, reduce dose by 0.02 mg every 24 h if scores generally <8 • Cease therapy when dose is 0.02 mg **Adjunctive treatment:** When morphine 1.6 mg/day, initiate second medication[a]

NAS, neonatal abstinence syndrome.
[a]Phenobarbital loading dose of 20mg/kg followed by 5mg/kg/day OR clonidine.
Reprinted with permission from Kraft WK, Stover MW, Davis JM. Neonatal abstinence syndrome: pharmacologic strategies for the mother and infant. *Sem Perinatol* 2016;40:203–212.

neonatal weight and uses fixed doses based on the severity of signs. These two approaches have not been directly compared, and definitive statements about the superiority of one to the other cannot be made. A hybrid regimen combining the two approaches has been used in the setting of a clinical trial comparing methadone and morphine (Table 37.3). Although this approach resulted in rapid control of signs of withdrawal and a reduced need for dose escalation, this regimen has not been systematically compared to other regimens. It is unclear if the greater complexity of this regimen is offset by clinical gains.[77]

Methadone

Methadone is an established treatment for use in opioid withdrawal as well as MAT.[78,79] Although methadone is a racemate, L-methadone is a μ-opioid agonist, and both the L- and D-enantiomers are noncompetitive antagonists of *N*-methyl-D-aspartate (NMDA) receptors.[80,81] Methadone is lipophilic and has excellent bioavailability (>90% in most patients). The half-life of methadone is longer than morphine, ranging from 13 to 50 hours, which permits once-daily dosing in adults. In neonates and older children, the plasma half-life of methadone is 16 to 25 hours.[82,83] Similar to morphine, methadone is metabolized in the liver by demethylation and cytochrome P450 cyclization.

Methadone has also been used as a treatment for neonates with NAS. A methadone PK study recommended a starting dose of 0.1 mg per kg per dose every 6 hours, followed by a detailed tapering regimen.[83] Retrospective studies and one small single-center prospective clinical trial compared methadone to morphine and found conflicting results (Table 37.4). While some studies showed no significant differences in length of treatment and length of hospital stay between the two drugs, others

TABLE 37.3 Dosing Schedules

Level	*Finnegan Score*	*Starting Dose*
MORPHINE, 0.2 mg/mL		
1	8–10	0.3 mg/kg/day divided every 4 h
2	11–13	0.5 mg/kg/day divided every 4 h
3	14–16	0.7 mg/kg/day divided every 4 h
4	17+	0.9 mg/kg/day divided every 4 h
METHADONE, 0.4 mg/mL		
1	8–10	0.3 mg/kg/day divided every 4 h
2	11–13	0.5 mg/kg/day divided every 4 h
3	14–16	0.7 mg/kg/day divided every 4 h
4	17+	0.9 mg/kg/day divided every 4 h

Starting dose: Pharmacologic treatment initiated when Finnegan scores ≥8 on two consecutive Finnegan scores or ≥12 on one score. The starting dose of the study medication is based on the highest score in the previous 8- to 12-hour period.
Dose escalation: Once the medication is initiated at dosing levels of 1, 2, or 3 and the neonate continues to have scores ≥8 for two consecutive scores or one score ≥12, the dose is increased to the next level.
Medication weaning: When adequate control of symptoms is achieved (e.g., NAS scores generally <8), the same dose is maintained for 12 to 48 hours before weaning initiated. The drugs are then weaned by 10% of the maximum dose. Subsequent weans by 10% occurs every 12 to 48 hours if scores were generally <8. The study drug is discontinued when the dose is 20% of the maximum dose with scoring, then continuing for an additional 48 hours.
Reprinted with permission from Haight SC, Ko JY, Tong VT, et al. Opioid use disorder documented at delivery hospitalization—United States, 1999–2014. *Morb Mortal Wkly Rep* 2018;67:845–849.

TABLE 37.4 Comparison of Morphine versus Methadone

Author (Reference)	*Year*	*Design*	*N*	*Morphine (Days Treated)*	*Methadone (Days Treated)*	*p*
Brown et al.[86]	2015	Prospective (single site)	31	21	14	0.008
Davis et al.[77]	2018	Prospective (multisite)	183	15	11.5	0.02
Hall et al.[65]	2014	Retrospective	383	16	16	NS
Lainwala et al.[85]	2005	Retrospective	46	36	40	NS
Tolia et al.[87]	2018	Retrospective	7,667	23	18	<0.001
Young et al.[128]	2015	Retrospective	26	7	38	0.001

NS, nonsignificant.

demonstrated a shorter length of stay in neonates treated with methadone.[84–86] Davis et al. conducted the first multicenter, randomized controlled trial comparing the safety and efficacy of methadone to morphine in 116 neonates with NAS requiring treatment.[77] Methadone was associated with decreased mean number of days for length of hospital stay by 14% (corresponding to a difference of 2.9 days) and 16% reduction in length of treatment (corresponding to a difference of 2.3 days). All 116 neonates enrolled in the study had better short-term outcomes than 170 nonrandomized infants treated with morphine per standard institutional protocols. The study was conducted using preservative-free methadone (compounded with methadone powder) instead of the commercial methadone which contained 15% alcohol as a preservative. It is likely that commercially available ethanolic preparations of methadone will have similar efficacy outcomes. This presumption is supported by retrospective real-world evidence from 7,667 infants across multiple hospitals using a variety of treatment protocols, which demonstrated a 22% reduction in length of hospitalization for neonates treated with methadone compared to morphine.[87] In all published reports, safety appears to be similar between methadone and other opioids in an inpatient setting. In the Davis trial, preliminary analyses of Bayley III neurodevelopmental assessments at 18 months of age showed no significant differences between the two treatment groups, as well as between treatment groups and the normal reference control group.[88] While there is no widely accepted dosing regimen, a pharmacometric informed dose and exposure response model has been developed with improved outcomes compared to an empirically derived regimen.[89]

Buprenorphine

A long-acting partial μ-opioid receptor agonist and a κ-opioid receptor antagonist, buprenorphine was approved by the Food and Drug Administration (FDA) in 2002 for the treatment of OUD.[90] As a partial agonist, buprenorphine has a more favorable safety profile and ceiling effect against fatal respiratory depression than a full agonist, such as methadone. The benefits of this effect are primarily in the outpatient setting, where almost all opioid overdoses occur. Buprenorphine is metabolized by cytochrome 3A4/5 and, to a much lesser extent, fetal 3A7.[91] The half-life of buprenorphine in adults is 25 hours, while in neonates, it is approximately 11 hours.[92,93]

Maternal use of buprenorphine has a favorable profile relative to methadone for MAT, with a lower incidence and severity of withdrawal in neonates with NAS.[14,17] Buprenorphine is also associated with a lower risk of premature birth, larger head circumference at birth, higher birth weight, and improved neurobehavioral scores compared to methadone.[14,94,95] There is no dose-dependency effect of maternal buprenorphine on (a) the concentration of buprenorphine and its metabolite (e.g., norbuprenorphine) in meconium or (b) the incidence and severity of NAS.[96]

Buprenorphine can also be administered sublingually as a treatment for NAS.[93] Kraft and colleagues studied 63 neonates with NAS at a single center and demonstrated that the median duration of treatment was significantly shorter with buprenorphine than morphine (15 days vs. 28 days), as was the median length of hospital stay (21 days vs. 33 days) ($p < 0.001$ for both comparisons).[97] A similar magnitude of effect relative to methadone- and morphine-based regimens has been demonstrated in retrospective cohorts.[98,99] A pharmacometric model of buprenorphine in NAS identified a clear exposure response relationship driven primarily by clearance of the drug.[100] This model should permit optimization of dosing strategies in future clinical trials. The buprenorphine formulation used in these studies contains 30% ethanol and can be stored in room temperature for at least 30 days.[101] PK evaluation revealed a rapid fall in alcohol concentration between buprenorphine doses, consistent with faster clearance in neonates compared to adults.[102,103] All ethanol concentrations were 70 mg per L, which is less than the AAP suggested limit of less than 250 mg per L after a single dose.[104] Approximately one-third of infants had a concentration above the 2014 European Medicines Agency draft guidance, which suggested a lower limit of 10 mg per L.

NONOPIOID REPLACEMENT/ADJUNCTIVE THERAPY

Phenobarbital and clonidine are nonopioid adjuncts used primarily in conjunction with an opioid. While a few small studies have compared clonidine or phenobarbital to an opioid as a primary treatment of NAS, a much more common approach is to use these agents as an adjunct to an opioid. The rationale behind this adjunctive use is that combination drug therapy will create a synergy that allows for enhanced efficacy than either agent alone. An adjunct is generally given only when signs of NAS are not adequately controlled with an opioid alone. The opioid is most often weaned first, and the adjunct is discontinued later as an inpatient or outpatient. This approach is much more common for phenobarbital than clonidine. The third approach is the parallel opioid-and-clonidine therapy, with a goal of reducing opioid exposure as well as length of treatment. The optimal adjunctive drug for specific populations and the optimized treatment regimen have not been clearly defined.

Clonidine

Clonidine is an α-2-adrenergic agonist used as a treatment for hypertension and opioid withdrawal in adults. Clonidine is an agonist of central presynaptic α-2 receptors, inhibiting norepinephrine release and downregulating sympathetic tone.[105] Oral bioavailability of clonidine is approximately 90%, with a half-life ranging from 17 hours in neonates to 7 hours in older infants.[106] Clonidine is an attractive choice as a primary or adjunctive treatment of NAS due to its safety profile, lack of respiratory depression seen with other opioids, ease of administration, and simple tapering approaches.

In a randomized controlled trial, clonidine given in parallel to morphine (in the form of diluted tincture of opium) was associated with lower doses of morphine and had a significantly shorter duration of treatment compared with morphine alone (11 days vs. 15 days, $p = 0.02$).[107] Another unblinded prospective trial comparing phenobarbital with clonidine as an adjunct to morphine showed that neonates treated with morphine and phenobarbital had a shorter initial hospital stay, but neonates continued to receive phenobarbital as an outpatient for up to 8 months before weaning off.[108] The doses of both clonidine and phenobarbital used in this trial were high. A prospective pilot study of clonidine with morphine as a primary therapy for NAS demonstrated a significantly shorter duration of treatment with the combination treatment approach compared to morphine alone.[109] In addition, early assessments using the neonatal intensive care unit (NICU) neonatal neurobehavioral scale (NNNS) found that neonates receiving clonidine had significantly lower arousal and excitability. At 1-year follow-up, language, cognitive, and motor scores were similar for the two groups. While hypotension, rebound hypertension, atrioventricular block, and bradycardia have been reported, the safety profile of clonidine across clinical trials has been reassuring.[110]

Phenobarbital

Phenobarbital (also known as phenobarbitone) is a $GABA_A$ receptor agonist with a long half-life in neonates, ranging from 67 to 115 hours.[111] Phenobarbital remains the most common adjunctive therapy to opioids in severe NAS. Compared with clonidine, it has a more global sedative effect and is less specific to opioid-driven symptomatology by mechanism of action. Though the hypothesis has not been directly tested, it is thought that phenobarbital may provide additional benefit in cases where the fetus has been exposed to both opioids and other psychotropic medications. Cochrane review has supported the use of phenobarbital as an adjunct to morphine in reducing the severity of withdrawal, maximal morphine dose, and length of hospital stay.[112] Despite AAP recommending the use of an opioid as the first-line agent for NAS, phenobarbital remains the initial choice of agent for many hospitals across the United States.[113] Comparison of phenobarbital with morphine as monotherapy has yielded conflicting results, with some studies demonstrating shorter duration of treatment with morphine while others showed no significant differences.[114–116] More widespread use of phenobarbital has been limited by concerns of adverse neurodevelopmental outcomes associated with this treatment. An examination of phenobarbital as an antiepileptic drug found an association between phenobarbital exposure and major cognitive and motor impairments in early childhood.[117] The issue of potential bias by indication for a population with seizure disorders makes direct comparisons to neonates with NAS difficult. Phenobarbital remains widely used as an antiepileptic and in the treatment of NAS. However, there is no consensus about how to weigh the short-term efficacy with possible longer term adverse effects.

CHOICE OF AGENT

A systematic review and network meta-analysis compared various pharmacotherapies across 18 trials. Sublingual buprenorphine was found to be the optimal treatment with respect to reducing the length of treatment.[118] However, this systematic review had many limitations and warned against universally accepting buprenorphine as standard therapy prior to larger multisite, randomized controlled trials being conducted. Ultimately, the answer to "what is the best opioid for NAS?" is not straightforward. The results of randomized controlled trials are specific to a particular drug and dosing regimen. A treatment protocol defines not only the specific opioid but also the initial dose, rate of up-titration, maximum dose, weaning rate, and a cessation dose. Other differences are the severity score cut-points used to initiate and intensify pharmacologic treatment, as well as the choice and dose of nonpharmacologic adjunct therapy. Up to this point, the end point used to gauge success of a regimen has been the drug dose and not the drug concentration within the neonate. More modern approaches will use pharmacometric modeling to measure drug exposure, identify covariates of NAS severity, and use a disease state model to generate a dose regimen that will more closely link drug dose to desired effect. Future studies must consider how to best design a pharmacologic approach that practitioners are willing to accept while acknowledging that the long-term effects of undertreated NAS and pharmacotherapy have not been fully defined.

Completion of pharmacologic therapy as an outpatient is associated with a shorter hospitalization, but longer total duration of therapy.[119] In a population-based observation of 532 infants treated with phenobarbital in the state of Tennessee, outpatient treatment was associated with higher number of emergency department visits at 6 months. Though not statistically significant, the point estimate odds ratio for emergency visit at 6 weeks, or any hospitalization at 6 or 24 weeks, was approximately 1.5 times higher for outpatient compared to inpatient treatment.[120]

LONGER TERM FOLLOW-UP FOR NEONATAL ABSTINENCE SYNDROME

Although prenatal exposure to opioids and other drugs can predispose neonates to longer term medical and neurodevelopmental abnormalities, it is often difficult to differentiate the impact of the drug exposure from any postnatal environmental effects. In a population-based linkage study in Australia, children with NAS were more likely to be rehospitalized during childhood for maltreatment, trauma, and mental and behavioral disorders.[121] This risk continued into adolescence and reinforced the need for continued follow-up and support of this vulnerable population after treatment for NAS is completed. A meta-analysis of 26 studies by Yeoh et al. found that prenatal opioid exposure correlated with adverse cognitive, mental, and physical/motor performance starting as early as 6 months and again persisting through adolescence.[122] Another large retrospective review in

Australia demonstrated that neonates with prenatal opioid exposure and NAS had poorer school performance in grades 3 to 7 compared to unexposed control neonates.[123] Whether these findings are generalizable to the U.S. population is unclear. There remains a strong association between the diagnosis of NAS and future mental health disorders, with one study reporting approximately 50% of neonates with NAS having evidence of a mental health disorder before age 5 compared with 30% incidence in all other births.[124] Finally, neonates with prenatal opioid exposure are also at high risk to develop eye abnormalities, including delayed visual development, abnormal visual evoked potentials, strabismus, nystagmus, and reduced visual acuity, suggesting the need for careful ophthalmologic follow-up.[125–127] For individual practitioners, data on long-term outcomes may be difficult to assess and provide limited guidance on creating a personalized and optimal treatment approach for NAS. However, on a societal level, these outcome data may support more broad-based interventions for infants and older children.

SUMMARY

Opioids can provide effective short-term pain relief. However, the addictive properties of opioids are strong and have resulted in a public health emergency in many countries around the world. Nonpharmacologic interventions remain the primary approach for all neonates, with the addition of pharmacologic treatment if signs of withdrawal are not well controlled. There is wide practice variation in the treatment of NAS that calls for multisite clinical trials in order to establish more definitive evidence-based treatment approaches. There is still significant uncertainty about when to initiate treatment, how long to maintain it, and the best timing for weaning/tapering the medications. Designing future clinical trials for antenatal and postnatal pharmacologic interventions of NAS should include appropriate physiologic outcome measures in addition to other shorter term outcomes (e.g., duration of treatment) as well as longer term neurobehavioral development.

REFERENCES

1. Beckett AH, Casy AF. Synthetic analgesics: stereochemical considerations. *J Pharm Pharmacol* 1954;6:986–999.
2. Pert CB, Snyder SH. Opiate receptor: demonstration in nervous tissue. *Science* 1973;179:1011–1014.
3. National Survey on Drug Use and Health. *Key substance use and mental health indicators in the United States: results from the 2016.* Rockville, MD: National Survey on Drug Use and Health.
4. Substance Abuse and Mental Health Services Administration. *Behavioral Health Barometer: United States, Volume 4: Indicators as measured through the 2015 National Survey on Drug Use and Health and National Survey of Substance Abuse Treatment Services. HHS Publication No. SMA–17–BaroUS–16.* Rockville, MD: Substance Abuse and Mental Health Services Administration, 2017.
5. American Psychiatric Association. *Diagnostics and statistical manual of mental disorders,* 5th ed. Washington DC: American Psychiatric Association, 2013.
6. Ailes EC, Dawson AL, Lind JN, et al. Opioid prescription claims among women of reproductive age—United States, 2008–2012. Centers for Disease Control and Prevention (CDC). *Morb Mortal Wkly Rep* 2015;64:37–41.
7. Haight SC, Ko JY, Tong VT, et al. Opioid use disorder documented at delivery hospitalization—United States, 1999–2014. *Morb Mortal Wkly Rep* 2018;67:845–849.
8. Bakhireva LN, Holbrook BD, Shrestha S, et al. Association between prenatal opioid exposure, neonatal opioid withdrawal syndrome, and neurodevelopmental and behavioral outcomes at 5–8 months of age. *Early Hum Dev* 2019;128:69–76.
9. Dowell D, Haegerich TM, Chou R. CDC guideline for prescribing opioids for chronic pain—United States, 2016. *JAMA* 2016;315:1624–1645.
10. American College of Obstetricians and Gynecologists; American Society of Addiction Medicine. *ACOG Committee Opinion No. 711: opioid use and opioid use disorder in pregnancy.* Washington, DC: American College of Obstetricians and Gynecologists; Rockville, MD: American Society of Addiction Medicine, 2017. https://www.acog.org/clinical/clinical-guidance/committee-opinion/articles/2017/08/opioid-use-and-opioid-use-disorder-in-pregnancy. Accessed June 8, 2020.
11. Bell J, Towers CV, Hennessy MD, et al. Detoxification from opiate drugs during pregnancy. *Am J Obstet Gynecol* 2016;215:374.e1–374.e6.
12. Saia KA, Schiff D, Wachman EM, et al. Caring for pregnant women with opioid use disorder in the USA: expanding and improving treatment. *Curr Obstet Gynecol Rep* 2016;5:257–263.
13. Hand DJ, Short VL, Abatemarco DJ. Treatments for opioid use disorder among pregnant and reproductive-aged women. *Fertil Steril* 2017;108:222–227.
14. Jones HE, Kaltenbach K, Heil SH, et al. Neonatal abstinence syndrome after methadone or buprenorphine exposure. *N Engl J Med* 2010;363:2320–2331.
15. Kakko J, Heilig M, Sarman I. Buprenorphine and methadone treatment of opiate dependence during pregnancy: comparison of fetal growth and neonatal outcomes in two consecutive case series. *Drug Alcohol Depend* 2008;96:69–78.
16. Lejeune C, Simmat-Durand L, Gourarier L, et al. Prospective multicenter observational study of 260 infants born to 259 opiate-dependent mothers on methadone or high-dose buprenorphine substitution. *Drug Alcohol Depend* 2006;82:250–257.
17. Jansson LM, DiPietro JA, Velez M, et al. Fetal neurobehavioral effects of exposure to methadone or buprenorphine. *Neurotoxicol Teratol* 2011;33:240–243.
18. Kocherlakota P. Neonatal abstinence syndrome. *Pediatrics* 2014;134:e547–e561.
19. U.S. Food and Drug Administration (FDA). Neonatal opioid withdrawal syndrome and medication-assisted treatment with methadone and buprenorphine. https://www.fda.gov/Drugs/DrugSafety/ucm503630.htm. Accessed May 17, 2019.
20. Nanovskaya TN, Nekhayeva IA, Hankins GD, et al. Transfer of methadone across the dually perfused preterm human placental lobule. *Am J Obstet Gynecol* 2008:198:126.e1–126.e4.
21. Szeto HH. Kinetics of drug transfer to the fetus. *Clin Obstet Gynecol* 1993;36(2):246–254.
22. Malek A, Obrist C, Wenzinger S, et al. The impact of cocaine and heroin on the placental transfer of methadone. *Reprod Biol Endocrinol* 2009;7:61.
23. Gil S, Saura R, Forestier F, et al. P-glycoprotein expression of the human placenta during pregnancy. *Placenta* 2005;26:268–270.
24. Nanovskaya T, Nekhayeva I, Karunaratne N, et al. Role of P-glycoprotein in transplacental transfer of methadone. *Biochem Pharmacol* 2005;69:1869–1878.
25. Khachaturian H, Alessi NE, Munfakh N, et al. Ontogeny of opioid and related peptides in the rat CNS and pituitary: an immunocytochemical study. *Life Sci* 1983;33(Suppl 1):61–64.
26. Loh YP, Rius RA, Elkabes S, et al. Prenatal expression of proopiomelanocortin mRNA, POMC-derived peptides, and mu-opiate receptors in the mouse embryo. *NIDA Res Monogr* 1991:111:96–112.
27. Tong Y, Chabot J, Shen S, et al. Ontogenic profile of the expression of the mu opioid receptor gene in the rat telencephalon and diencephalon: an in situ hybridization study. *J Chem Neuroanat* 2000;18:209–222.
28. Byrnes EM, Vassoler FM. Modeling prenatal opioid exposure in animals: current findings and future directions. *Front Neuroendocrinol* 2018;51:1–13.
29. Rehni AK, Jaggi AS, Singh N. Opioid withdrawal syndrome: emerging concepts and novel therapeutic targets. *CNS Neurol Disord Drug Targets* 2013;12:112–125.
30. Towers CV, Hyatt BW, Visconti KC, et al. Neonatal head circumference in newborns with neonatal abstinence syndrome. *Pediatrics* 2019;143:e20180541.
31. Yuan Q, Rubic M, Seah J, et al. Do maternal opioids reduce neonatal regional brain volumes? A pilot study. *J Perinatol* 2014;34:909–913.
32. Monnelly VJ, Anblagan D, Quigley A, et al. Prenatal methadone exposure is associated with altered neonatal brain development. *Neuroimage Clin* 2018;18:9–14.
33. Johnson K, Gerarda C, Greenough A. Treatment of neonatal abstinence syndrome. *Arch Dis Child Fetal Neonatal Ed* 2003;88:F2–F5.
34. Trescot AM, Datta S, Lee M, et al. Opioid pharmacology. *Pain Physician* 2008;11:S133–S153.
35. Mangat AK, Schmölzer GM, Kraft WK. Pharmacological and non-pharmacological treatment for neonatal abstinence syndrome. *Semin Fetal Neonatal Med* 2019;24(2):133–141. doi:10.1016/j.siny.2019.01.009.
36. Seligman NS, Salva N, Hayes EJ, et al. Predicting length of treatment for neonatal abstinence syndrome in methadone exposed neonates. *Am J Obstet Gynecol* 2008;199:396.e1–396.e7.
37. Dryden C, Young D, Hepburn M, et al. Maternal methadone use in pregnancy: factors associated with the development of neonatal abstinence syndrome and implications for healthcare resources. *BJOG* 2009;116:665–671.
38. Ruwanpathirana R, Abdel-Latif ME, Burns L, et al. Prematurity reduces the severity of and need for treatment of neonatal abstinence syndrome. *Acta Paediatr* 2015;104:e188–e194.
39. Winkelman TNA, Villapiano N, Kozhimannil KB, et al. Incidence and costs of neonatal abstinence syndrome among infants with Medicaid: 2004–2014. *Pediatrics* 2018;141:e20173520.
40. Tolia VN, Patrick SW, Bennett MM, et al. Increasing incidence of the neonatal abstinence syndrome in U.S. neonatal ICUs. *N Engl J Med* 2015;372:2118–2126.
41. Coyle MG, Brogly SB, Ahmed MS, et al. Neonatal abstinence syndrome. *Nat Rev Dis Primers* 2018;4:47.
42. Cleary BJ, Donnelly J, Strawbridge J, et al. Methadone dose and neonatal abstinence syndrome-systematic review and meta-analysis. *Addiction* 2010;105:2071–2084.
43. Winklbaur B, Baewert A, Jagsch R, et al. Association between prenatal tobacco exposure and outcome of neonates born to opioid-maintained mothers. Implications for treatment. *Eur Addict Res* 2009;15:150–156.
44. Jones HE, Heil SH, Tuten M, et al. Cigarette smoking in opioid-dependent pregnant women: neonatal and maternal outcomes. *Drug Alcohol Depend* 2013;131:271–277.
45. Huybrechts KF, Bateman BT, Desai RJ, et al. Risk of neonatal drug withdrawal after intrauterine co-exposure to opioids and psychotropic medications: cohort study. *BMJ* 2017;358:j3326.
46. Unger A, Jagsch R, Bäwert A, et al. Are male neonates more vulnerable to neonatal abstinence syndrome than female neonates? *Gend Med* 2011;8:355–364.
47. Gaalema DE, Scott TL, Heil SH, et al. Differences in the profile of neonatal abstinence syndrome signs in methadone-versus buprenorphine-exposed neonates. *Addiction* 2012;107:53–62.

48. Welle-Strand GK, Skurtveit S, Jansson LM, et al. Breastfeeding reduces the need for withdrawal treatment in opioid-exposed infants. *Acta Paediatr* 2013;102:1060–1066.
49. Short VL, Gannon M, Abatemarco DJ. The association between breastfeeding and length of hospital stay among infants diagnosed with neonatal abstinence syndrome: a population-based study of in-hospital births. *Breastfeed Med* 2016;11:343–349.
50. Jansson LM, Velez M, Harrow C. The opioid exposed newborn: assessment and pharmacologic management. *J Opioid Manag* 2009;5:47–55.
51. Raffeli G, Cavallaro G, Allegaert K, et al. Neonatal abstinence syndrome: update on diagnostic and therapeutic strategies. *Pharmacotherapy* 2017;37;814–823.
52. Finnegan LP, Connaughton JF Jr, Kron RE, et al. Neonatal abstinence syndrome: assessment and management. *Addict Dis* 1975;2:141–158.
53. Finnegan LP, Kaltenbach K. Neonatal abstinence syndrome. In: Hoekelman RA, Friedman SB, Nelson N, et al, eds. *Pediatric Primary Care, 2nd Ed.* St. Louis, MO: Mosby, 1992:1367–1378.
54. Jones HE, Harrow C, O'Grady KE, et al. Neonatal abstinence syndrome scores in opioid exposed and non-exposed neonates: a blinded comparison. *J Opioid Man* 2010;6:409–413.
55. Jones HE, Seashore C, Johnson E, et al. Psychometric assessment of the neonatal abstinence scoring system and the MOTHER NAS scale. *Am J Addict* 2016;25:370–373.
56. Grossman MR, Lipshaw MJ, Osborn RR, et al. A novel approach to assessing infants with neonatal abstinence syndrome. *Hosp Pediatr* 2018;8:1–6.
57. Pahl A, Young L, Buus-Frank ME, et al. Non-pharmacological care for opioid withdrawal in newborns. *Cochrane Database Syst Rev* 2018;(12):CD013217.
58. Ryan G, Dooley J, Gerber Finn L, et al. Nonpharmacological management of neonatal abstinence syndrome: a review of the literature. *J Matern Fetal Neonatal Med* 2018;8:1–6.
59. Hudak ML, Tan RC; Committee on Drugs; Committee on Fetus and Newborn, American Academy of Pediatrics Clinical Report. Neonatal drug withdrawal. *Pediatrics* 2012;129:e540–e560.
60. Osborn DA, Jeffrey HE, Cole MJ. Opiate treatment for opiate withdrawal in newborn infants. *Cochrane Database Syst Rev* 2010;(10):CD002059.
61. Kraft WK, Stover MW, Davis JM. Neonatal abstinence syndrome: pharmacologic strategies for the mother and infant. *Semin Perinatol* 2016;40:203–212.
62. Gowing L, Ali R, White JM, et al. Buprenorphine for managing opioid withdrawal. *Cochrane Database Syst Rev* 2017;(2):CD002025.
63. Gowing L, Farrell M, Ali R, et al. Alpha(2)-adrenergic agonists for the management of opioid withdrawal. *Cochrane Database Syst Rev* 2016;(5):CD002024.
64. Burnette T, Chernicky L, Towers CV. The effect of standardizing treatment when managing neonatal abstinence syndrome. *J Matern Fetal Neonatal Med* 2018;14:1–5.
65. Hall ES, Wexelblatt SL, Crowley M, et al. A multicenter cohort study of treatments and hospital outcomes in neonatal abstinence syndrome. *Pediatrics* 2014;134:e527–e534.
66. Hall ES, Wexelblatt SL, Crowley M, et al. Implementation of a neonatal abstinence syndrome weaning protocol: a multicenter cohort study. *Pediatrics* 2015;136:e803–e810.
67. Asti L, Magers JS, Keels E, et al. A quality improvement project to reduce length of stay for neonatal abstinence syndrome. *Pediatrics* 2015;135:e1494–e1500.
68. Patrick SW, Schumacher RE, Horbar JD, et al. Improving care for neonatal abstinence syndrome. *Pediatrics* 2016;137:e20153835.
69. Liu T, Lewis T, Gauda E, et al. Mechanistic population pharmacokinetics of morphine in neonates with abstinence syndrome after oral administration of diluted tincture of opium. *J Clin Pharmacol* 2015;56:1009–1018.
70. Kart C, Christrup LL, Rasmussen M. Recommended use of morphine in neonates, infants and children based on a literature review: part I—pharmacokinetics. *Paediatr Anaesth* 2004;92:208–217.
71. Liu T, Lewis TR, Moore JN, et al. Could postnatal age-related uridine diphosphate glucuronic acid be a rate-limiting factor in the metabolism of morphine during the first week of life? *CPT Pharmacometrics Syst Pharmacol* 2019;8(7):469–477. doi:10.1002/psp4.12407.
72. Colombini N, Elias R, Busuttil M, et al. Hospital morphine preparation for abstinence syndrome in newborns exposed to buprenorphine or methadone. *Pharm World Sci* 2008;30:227–234.
73. Sauberan J, Rossi S, Kim JH. Stability of dilute oral morphine solution for neonatal abstinence syndrome. *J Addict Med* 2013;7:113–115.
74. Kraft WK, van den Anker JN. Pharmacologic management of the opioid neonatal abstinence syndrome. *Pediatr Clin North Am* 2012;59:1147–1165.
75. Mian P, Tibboel D, Wildschut ED, et al. Morphine treatment for neonatal abstinence syndrome: huge dosing variability underscores the need for a better clinical study design. *Minerva Pediatr* 2019;71:263–286.
76. DeAtley HN, Burton A, Fraley MD, et al. Evaluation of the effectiveness of two morphine protocols to treat neonatal abstinence syndrome in a level II nursery in a community hospital. *Pharmacotherapy* 2017;37:856–860.
77. Davis JM, Shenberger J, Terrin N, et al. Comparison of safety and efficacy of methadone vs morphine for treatment of neonatal abstinence syndrome: a randomized clinical trial. *JAMA Pediatr* 2018;172:741–748.
78. Rahimi-Movaghar A, Gholami J, Amato L, et al. Pharmacological therapies for management of opium withdrawal. *Cochrane Database Syst Rev* 2018;(6):CD007522.
79. Mattick RP, Breen C, Kimber J, et al. Methadone maintenance therapy versus no opioid replacement therapy for opioid dependence. *Cochrane Database Syst Rev* 2009;(8): CD002209.
80. Inturrisi CE. Pharmacology of methadone and its isomers. *Minerva Anestesiol* 2005;71:435–437.
81. Chana SK, Anand KJ. Can we use methadone for analgesia in neonates? *Arch Dis Child Fetal Neonatal Ed* 2001;85:F79–F81.
82. Rosen TS, Pippenger CE. Pharmacologic observations on the neonatal withdrawal syndrome. *J Pediatr* 1976;88:1044–1048.
83. Wiles JR, Isemann B, Mizuno T, et al. Pharmacokinetics of oral methadone in the treatment of neonatal abstinence syndrome: a pilot study. *J Pediatr* 2015;167:1214.e3–1220.e3.
84. Burke S, Beckwith AM. Morphine versus methadone treatment for neonatal withdrawal and impact on early infant development. *Glob Pediatr Health* 2017;4:1–6.
85. Lainwala S, Brown ER, Weinschenk NP, et al. A retrospective study of length of hospital stay in infants treated for neonatal abstinence syndrome with methadone versus oral morphine preparations. *Adv Neonatal Care* 2005;5:265–272.
86. Brown MS, Hayes JM, Thornton LM. Methadone versus morphine for treatment of neonatal abstinence syndrome: a prospective randomized clinical trial. *J Perinatol* 2015;35:278–283.
87. Tolia VN, Murthy K, Bennett MM, et al. Morphine vs methadone treatment for infants with neonatal abstinence syndrome. *J Pediatr* 2018;203:185–189.
88. Czynski A, Davis JM, Breeze J, et al. *Neurodevelopmental outcomes of infants treated with either morphine or methadone for neonatal abstinence syndrome.* Baltimore, MD: Society for Pediatric Research, 2019.
89. Hall ES, Meinzen-Derr J, Wexelblatt SL. Cohort analysis of a pharmacokinetic-modeled methadone weaning optimization for neonatal abstinence syndrome. *J Pediatr* 2015;167:1221.e1–1225.e1.
90. Substance Abuse and Mental Health Services Administration (SAMSHA). Buprenorphine. https://www.samhsa.gov/medication-assisted-treatment/treatment/buprenorphine. Accessed June 8, 2020.
91. Chang Y, Moody DE, McCance-Katz EF. Novel metabolites of buprenorphine detected in human liver microsomes and human urine. *Drug Metab Dispos* 2006;34:440–448.
92. Huestis MA, Cone EJ, Pirnay SO, et al. Intravenous buprenorphine and norbuprenorphine pharmacokinetics in humans. *Drug Alcohol Depend* 2013;131:258–262.
93. Kraft WK. Buprenorphine in the neonatal abstinence syndrome. *Clin Pharm Ther* 2018;103:112–119.
94. Zedler BK, Mann AL, Kim MM, et al. Buprenorphine compared with methadone to treat pregnant women with opioid use disorder: a systematic review and meta-analysis of safety in the mother, fetus and child. *Addiction* 2016;111:2115–2128.
95. Coyle MG, Salisbury AL, Lester BM, et al. Neonatal neurobehavior effects following buprenorphine versus methadone exposure. *Addiction* 2012;107:S63–S73.
96. Kacinko SL, Jones HE, Johnson RE, et al. Correlations of maternal buprenorphine dose, buprenorphine, and metabolite concentrations in meconium with neonatal outcomes. *Clin Pharmacol Ther* 2008;84:604–612.
97. Kraft WK, Adeniyi-Jones SC, Chervoneva I. Buprenorphine for the treatment of the neonatal abstinence syndrome. *N Engl J Med* 2017;376:2341–2348.
98. Hall ES, Rice WR, Folger AT, et al. Comparison of neonatal abstinence syndrome treatment with sublingual buprenorphine versus conventional opioids. *Am J Perinatol* 2018;35:405–412.
99. Hall ES, Isemann BT, Wexelblatt SL, et al. A cohort comparison of buprenorphine versus methadone treatment for neonatal abstinence syndrome. *J Pediatr* 2016;170:39.e1–44.e1.
100. Moore JN, Gastonguay MR, Ng CM, et al. The pharmacokinetics and pharmacodynamics of buprenorphine in neonatal abstinence syndrome. *Clin Pharmacol Ther* 2018;103:1029–1037.
101. Anagnostis EA, Sadaka RE, Sailor LA, et al. Formulation of buprenorphine for sublingual use in neonates. *J Pediatr Pharmacol Ther* 2011;16:281–284.
102. Marek E, Adeniyi-Jones SC, Roke L, et al. Ethanol pharmacokinetics in neonates secondary to medication administration. http://jdc.jefferson.edu/petposters/1/. Accessed May 17, 2019.
103. Marek E, Kraft WK. Ethanol pharmacokinetics in neonates and infants. *Curr Ther Res Clin Exp* 2014;76:90–97.
104. American Academy of Pediatrics. Ethanol in liquid preparations intended for children. *Pediatrics* 1984;73:405–407.
105. Esmaeili A, Keinhorst AK, Schuster T. Treatment of neonatal abstinence syndrome with clonidine and chloral hydrate. *Acta Paediatr* 2010;99:209–214.
106. Sheng Y, Standing JF. Pharmacokinetic reason for negative results of clonidine sedation in long-term ventilated neonates and infants. *Pediatr Crit Care Med* 2015;16:92–93.
107. Agthe AG, Kim GR, Mathias KB, et al. Clonidine as an adjunct therapy to opioids for neonatal abstinence syndrome: a randomized, controlled trial. *Pediatrics* 2009;123:e849–e856.
108. Surran B, Visintainer P, Chamberlain S, et al. Efficacy of clonidine versus phenobarbital in reducing neonatal morphine sulfate therapy days for neonatal abstinence syndrome. A prospective randomized clinical trial. *J Perinatol* 2013;33:954–959.
109. Bada HS, Sithisarn T, Gibson J, et al. Morphine versus clonidine for neonatal abstinence syndrome. *Pediatrics* 2015;135:e383–e391.
110. Streetz VN, Gildon BL, Thompson DF. Role of clonidine in neonatal abstinence syndrome: a systematic review. *Ann Pharmacother* 2016;50:301–310.
111. Pitlick W, Painter M, Pippenger C. Phenobarbital pharmacokinetics in neonates. *Clin Pharmacol Ther* 1978;23:346–350.
112. Osborn DA, Jeffrey HE, Cole MJ. Sedatives for opiate withdrawal in newborn infants. *Cochrane Database Syst Rev* 2010;(10):CD002053.
113. Patrick SW, Kaplan HC, Passarella M, et al. Variation in treatment of neonatal abstinence syndrome in US children's hospitals, 2004–2011. *J Perinatol* 2014;867–872.
114. Jackson L, Ting A, McKay S, et al. A randomised controlled trial of morphine versus phenobarbitone for neonatal abstinence syndrome. *Arch Dis Child Fetal Neonatal Ed* 2004;89:F300–F304.
115. Ebner N, Rohrmeister K, Winklbaur B, et al. Management of neonatal abstinence syndrome in neonates born to opioid maintained women. *Drug Alcohol Depend* 2007;87:131–138.
116. Nayeri F, Sheikh M, Kalani M, et al. Phenobarbital versus morphine in the management of neonatal abstinence syndrome, a randomized control trial. *BMC Pediatr* 2015;15:57.
117. Maitre NL, Smolinsky C, Slaughter JC, et al. Adverse neurodevelopmental outcomes after exposure to phenobarbital and levetiracetam for the treatment of neonatal seizures. *J Perinatol* 2013;33:841–846.
118. Disher T, Gullickson C, Singh B, et al. Pharmacological treatments for neonatal abstinence syndrome: a systematic review and network meta-analysis. *JAMA Pediatr* 2019;173(3):234–243. doi:10.1001/jamapediatrics.2018.5044.

119. Murphy-Oikonen J, McQueen K. Outpatient pharmacologic weaning for neonatal abstinence syndrome: a systematic review. *Prim Health Care Res Dev* 2018;20:1–9.
120. Maalouf FI, Cooper WO, Slaughter JC, et al. Outpatient pharmacotherapy for neonatal abstinence syndrome. *J Pediatr* 2018;199:151.e1–157.e1.
121. Uebel H, Wright IM, Burns L, et al. Reasons for re-hospitalization in children who had neonatal abstinence syndrome. *Pediatrics* 2015;136:e811–e820.
122. Yeoh SL, Eastwood J, Wright IM, et al. Cognitive and motor outcomes of children with prenatal opioid exposure: a meta-analysis of 1,455 children. In: Proceedings of the Perinatal Society of Australia and New Zealand meeting, Gold Coast, Queensland, Australia, March 17–21, 2019.
123. Oei JL, Melhuish E, Uebel H, et al. Neonatal abstinence syndrome and high school performance. *Pediatrics* 2017;139:e20162651.
124. Sherman LJ, Ali MM, Mutter R, et al. Mental disorders among children born with neonatal abstinence syndrome. *Psych Serv* 2019;70:151.
125. McGlone L, Mactier H, Weaver LT. Drug misuse in pregnancy: losing sight of the baby? *Arch Dis Child* 2009;94:708–712.
126. McGlone L, Hamilton R, McCulloch DL, et al. Visual outcome in infants born to drug-misusing mothers prescribed methadone in pregnancy. *Br J Ophthalmol* 2014;98:238–245.
127. Walhovd KB, Bjørnebekk A, Haabrekke K, et al. Child neuroanatomical, neurocognitive, and visual acuity outcomes with maternal opioid and polysubstance detoxification. *Pediatr Neurol* 2015;52:326–332.
128. Young ME, Hager SJ, Spurlock D Jr. Retrospective chart review comparing morphine and methadone in neonates treated for neonatal abstinence syndrome. *Am J Health Syst Pharm* 2015;72:S162–S167.

CHAPTER 38

Joseph D. Tobias

Local Anesthetic Agents for Regional and Superficial Anesthesia in Infants, Children, and Adolescents

INTRODUCTION

In pediatric-aged patients, there are various applications for local anesthetic agents (LAAs) including the therapeutic administration for the treatment of cardiac arrhythmias (lidocaine), superficial infiltration to provide analgaesia during minor surgical procedures, and superficial and deep infiltration to augment analgesia following major surgical interventions. Additionally, these agents are being used more commonly to provide surgical anesthesia (spinal anesthesia, epidural anesthesia, and peripheral nerve blockade) or during regional anesthetic techniques for postoperative analgesia.[1,2] To ensure both the safety and effectiveness of such techniques, the practitioner should have a clear understanding of the mechanism of action, potential adverse effects, pharmacology, and dosing guidelines of LAAs. This chapter reviews the basic mechanisms of LAAs, methods to reduce potential toxicity, and directions for resuscitation should local anesthetic systemic toxicity (LAST) or unintended intravenous injection occurs.

MECHANISM OF ACTION OF LOCAL ANESTHETIC AGENTS

Sodium (Na^+) channels are necessary for the propagation and generation of nerve impulses. The generation of the action potential results from the opening of Na^+ channels and the inward movement of the cation. LAAs reversibly bind to Na^+ channels of the nerve and thereby block the inward Na^+ movement, thereby inhibiting the genesis and propagation of nerve impulses. Although individual sensory axons and other parts of the nervous system have different types of Na^+ channels, the general action of the LAAs on these channels is the same.[3,4] Sodium channels can be inhibited in two ways: (a) by a conformational mechanism (where the activation gating is suppressed; mainly neutral anesthetic agents) or (b) by an occlusion mechanism (where the pore or channel is physically blocked; mainly charged LAAs). As most tertiary amine LAAs are in a dynamic equilibrium between charged and neutral forms based on the local pH and the p*Ka* of the solution, they inhibit Na^+ channels through both the mechanisms.

LAAs bind to their target sites on the Na^+ channels in bare nerve membranes rapidly (1 to 10 seconds) at the 50% inhibitory drug concentration (IC50) and dissociate in about the same time. The IC50s are much lower than the clinically injected concentrations. For example, IC50 for Na^+ channel inhibition by lidocaine is 0.2 mmol per L, but a successful block requires an injection of a 1% solution that provides a concentration of approximately 40 mmol per L. Less than one molecule in 20 of the injected dose is found within the nerve during blockade.[3,4] The protonated drug has a pH of 5 to 6, and thus poorly penetrates the perineural area/nerve membrane owing to low lipid solubility, and the extraneural and intraneural vasculature rapidly removes the LAA from the area around the nerve.[4] Hydrophobic (lipid-soluble) LAAs such as bupivacaine cross the fat layer of biologic membranes and penetrate into neural tissue more rapidly than hydrophilic agents (procaine).

The solution in which the LAA is delivered can be manipulated to affect delivery, onset, and potency. The unionized fraction of the LAA penetrates the nerve membrane, whereas the ionized form bins to the Na^+ channel. The onset of action of an LAA is determined primarily by the fraction that is unionized and hence the pK_a of the medication.[3–5] The pK_a of LAAs ranges from 7.6 to 9.1. As the pK_a approaches the physiologic pH of 7.4, the percentage of local anesthetic in the unionized form is greater, promoting the penetration of the nerve membrane. The more rapid penetration of the nerve membrane results in a more rapid onset of action. Lidocaine has a pK_a of 7.7, and at a pH of 7.4, 35% exists in the nonionized base form, yielding a relatively rapid onset of blockade. In contrast, tetracaine has a pK_a of 8.6 with only 5% in the unionized form at a tissue pH of 7.4, resulting in a slower onset of blockade compared with lidocaine. Local factors may significantly affect the onset as local inflammation or infection may lower the tissue pH, thereby delaying the onset of the LAA when it is injected into these tissues.

Two methods to increase the delivery of an LAA to their effect site and hence to speed the onset are to alkalinize the injectate, thereby increasing the fraction of uncharged drug molecules to promote perineural penetration and to add a vasoconstrictor such as epinephrine to decrease the rate of vascular removal.[6] Alkalinization of the LAA is often advocated as a means for improving drug delivery to the nerve tissue; however, if the pH exceeds 7, the solution becomes less soluble, hence leading to precipitation.[7] Therefore, it is crucial not to overneutralize the local anesthetic solution, and the addition of sodium bicarbonate should occur just prior to the injection to avoid precipitation. This is especially true with bupivacaine and ropivacaine where a small amount of bicarbonate (0.1 mEq of sodium bicarbonate or 0.1 mL of a 1 mEq per mL solution per 10 mL of the LAA) may cause precipitation within a matter of minutes.[6–8] Vasoconstrictors (epinephrine and phenylephrine) are effective in prolonging a block only for LAAs that do not have intrinsic vasoconstrictive properties (e.g., bupivacaine, but not ropivacaine) and those that are hydrolyzed by local esterases (e.g., chloroprocaine). Vasoconstrictors should not be added when the LAA is injected near end arteries as vasoconstrictor can lead to ischemia.

Another method to speed the onset, to prolong the duration of local anesthetic action, and to increase the intensity of the block is to increase the concentration of the medication (e.g., 2% vs. 0.5% lidocaine). This should only be done with a strict attention to dosing limits (see below) to avoid toxicity. Conversely, if the intended effect of the local anesthetic injection is primarily to produce analgesia (e.g., pure sensory blockade vs. sensory plus motor blockade), a more dilute concentration of local anesthetic solution generally will preferentially block sensory fibers while sparing motor fibers. These issues become of clinical importance when performing neuraxial and peripheral blocks of the lower extremities in particular as the provision of analgesia when preserving motor function allows for normal ambulation.

LOCAL ANESTHETIC AGENTS: AMIDES

Based on the chemical structure, the LAAs can be classified as amino esters or amino amides. Amino amides used clinically include lidocaine, mepivacaine, prilocaine, bupivacaine, levobupivacaine, and ropivacaine, whereas amino esters include procaine, chloroprocaine, and tetracaine[9] (Table 38.1). These two classes of LAAs differ in their site of metabolism, plasma half-lives, adverse effect profile, potency, and allergic potential. Furthermore, differences exist in potency and half-life (Tables 38.2 and 38.3). An example of a specific clinical difference is that, although rare, allergic reactions may occur with the ester group related to para-aminobenzoic acid (PABA), a metabolite, whereas the amino amides rarely cause allergic reactions. Amino esters are metabolized in the plasma by serum cholinesterases, whereas amino amides are metabolized in the liver. The metabolism of the amino esters by serum cholinesterases generally results in a rapid serum half-life with a decreased potential for toxicity, especially in neonates and infants[10,11] (see below).

The LAAs of the amide group include lidocaine, bupivacaine, ropivacaine, and levobupivacaine. Levobupivacaine is not available for commercial use in North America. These are the most commonly used LAAs in infants and children. These agents are used frequently in the practice of pediatric anesthesiology for neuraxial and peripheral nerve blockade. Their popularity rests primarily in their long duration of action, which can be used to provide a prolonged period of analgesia following a single dose.

TABLE 38.1 Examples of Local Anesthetic Agents: Esters and Amides

Esters	*Amides*
Procaine	Lidocaine
Tetracaine	Mepivacaine
2-chloroprocaine	Bupivacaine
	Ropivacaine
	Levobupivacaine
	Etidocaine
	Prilocaine

BUPIVACAINE

Bupivacaine is the most commonly used LAA in infants and children in North America. The pharmacokinetics and the pharmacodynamics have been well studied and described in infants and children.[12–17] Depending on the site of administration, the average duration of analgesia may vary from 4 to 8 hours.[18,19] Various concentrations are commercially available for clinical use, varying from 0.25% to 0.75% with or without epinephrine 1:200,000. The higher concentrations are rarely used in the pediatric-aged patient as volume requirements generally limit the concentration used to less than or equal to 0.25%. When used to provide postoperative analgesia for lower extremity and subumbilical surgery (herniorrhaphy), concentrations of 0.125% to 0.25% have been shown to be effective. However, in adolescents and older patients, higher concentrations (0.5%) are occasionally used to provide surgical anesthesia.[20]

Bupivacaine is bound to α-1-acid glycoprotein. Lower levels of α-1-acid glycoprotein are presented in infants owing to the delayed maturation of hepatic enzymes, thereby accounting for a higher free fraction of the LAA in young infants. The latter is one of the several factors that increase the risk of LAST in neonates and infants. Bupivacaine is commercially available as a racemic mixture of its two enantiomers (levo or S and dextro or R). Although the levo-enantiomer is the active form that provides the clinical effect of the local anesthetic solution, the dextro-enantiomer is also responsible for adverse effects including cardiac and central nervous system (CNS) toxicity. The isolated levo-enantiomer is available outside of North America for clinical use as levobupivacaine[21] (Chirocaine; see below). Bupivacaine undergoes hepatic metabolism by the P450 cytochrome system, CYP3A4. As with other hepatic microsomal enzymes, CYP3A4 may be immature in neonates and infants less than 6 months of age, thus accounting in part for the delayed clearance compared with older children and the need to reduce total drug exposure.[22,23] The latter is particularly relevant during continuous infusions as accumulation, and increasing concentrations have been documented over time, thereby necessitating the use of even lower concentrations (less than 0.1%) for infusions greater than 24 hours in neonates and infants. Given the need to limit the concentration of the LAA, adjunctive agents (opioids or clonidine) are frequently used to enhance analgesia.

TABLE 38.2 Relative Potency of Local Anesthetic Agents

	Short Duration	*Medium Duration*		*Long Duration*		
Site of Action	*2-Chloroprocaine*	*Lidocaine*	*Mepivacaine*	*Bupivacaine*	*Ropivacaine*	*Tetracaine*
Peripheral nerve	NA	1.0	2.6	3.6	3.6	NA
Spinal	NA	1.0	1.0	9.6	NA	6.3
Epidural	2.0	1.0	1.0	4.0	4.0	NA

NA, data not available.
From Hassan HG, Renck H, Akerman B, et al. On the relative potency of amino-amide local anaesthetics in vivo. *Acta Anaesthesiol Scand* 1994;38:505–509.

TABLE 38.3 Local Anesthetic Agents

Agent	*Onset*	*Relative Potency*	pK_a	*Duration*	*% Protein Binding*	*Maximum Dose (mg/kg)*[a]
ESTERS						
Procaine	Slow	1	8.9	Short	6	7–10
Chloroprocaine	Fast	1	9.1	Short	—	7–10
Tetracaine	Slow	8	8.5	Long	76	—
AMIDES						
Mepivacaine	Fast	2	7.6	Moderate	78	5–7
Prilocaine	Fast	2	7.7	Moderate	55	8–10
Lidocaine	Fast	2	8.1	Moderate	64	5–7
Bupivacaine	Moderate	8	8.1	Long	96	2–3
Ropivacaine	Moderate	6	8.2	Long	94	2–4
Etidocaine	Fast	6	8.1	Long	94	3–4

[a]Upper dose range is for drug combined with epinephrine.

Although the selection of the LAA is related to the clinical need including the onset time and the desired duration of action, attention must be paid to the potential for LAST. The delayed maturation of hepatic microsomal enzymes decreases the hepatic metabolism of the LAA in a neonate or an infant when compared with that of the adult.[24,25] At approximately 3 to 6 months of age, the ability to conjugate drugs achieves adult levels.[25] Another consideration is that older children will absorb LAAs more rapidly than do adults and therefore achieve a higher blood concentration for a similar mg per kg dose. Higher serum concentrations have been reported in children than in adults following intercostal nerve blockade with bupivacaine.[26]

The steady-state volume of distribution (V_{dss}) for amides is increased in children compared with adults although clearance (Cl) is similar.[11–13] As the elimination half-life ($t_{1/2}$) is related to the volume of distribution and clearance as follows $t_{1/2} = (0.693 \times V_{dss})/Cl$, the larger steady-state volume of distribution results in prolongation of the elimination half-life. The clinical significance of this is limited following single-dose injections, but as noted above must be considered when using continuous infusions or repeated injections of bupivacaine in neonates and infants. The risk of toxicity with repeated doses or a continuous infusion is greater in infants and children than in adults.[27,28]

The major adverse effects of bupivacaine include cardiac and CNS toxicity (Table 38.4). As the systemic concentration of the local anesthetic increases, the incidence of complications also increases.[23] LAAs cross the blood–brain barrier and cause alterations in CNS function. CNS toxicity includes initially excitatory signs and symptoms with perioral numbness and tingling, tinnitus and dizziness followed by seizures. As serum concentrations increase CNS depression with depressed mental status and electroencephalogram (EEG) slowing may be seen. Cardiotoxicity relates to the effects of the LAA on sodium channels in the myocardium with alterations of conduction and function. Although it is generally taught that CNS signs occur first, when these agents are administered during general anesthesia as is frequently done in the pediatric-aged patient, there are no premonitory CNS signs with cardiotoxicity occurring without CNS signs.[29–31] Given these concerns, a test dose may be used which contains a small amount of epinephrine as a sign of inadvertent systemic injection (see below).[32,33]

Bupivacaine can be used for most peripheral nerve blocks as well as for epidural and caudal infusions in infants and children. The maximum dosage suggested for bolus injections in the caudal space or epidural space for toddlers and older children is 3 mg per kg, 2 to 2.5 mg per kg for neonates and infants.[32,34] Although toxicity can occur with bolus dosing especially if inadvertent systemic injection occurs, toxicity is more of a concern with prolonged infusions. Strict adherence to dosing guidelines is recommended especially in neonates and infants as accumulation may occur with infusions lasting more than 24 hours.[35] Given these concerns, dosing recommendations for

TABLE 38.4 Systemic Toxicity of Local Anesthetic Agents

1. Central nervous system
   a. Lightheadedness and dizziness
   b. Visual and auditory disturbances
   c. Muscle twitching and tremors
   d. Generalized convulsions
2. Cardiovascular toxicity
   a. Direct cardiac effects
      i. Depresses rapid phase of depolarization of Purkinje fibers leading to cardiac dysrhythmias
      ii. Depresses spontaneous pacemaker activity in the sinus node
      iii. Negative inotropic effect on the heart
      iv. Depresses myocardial contractility by affecting calcium influx and triggered release
   b. Direct peripheral vascular effects
      i. Biphasic effect; low concentrations cause vasoconstriction, and high concentrations cause vasodilation.
      ii. Increased pulmonary vascular resistance (animal studies)
      iii. Acidosis and hypoxia markedly increase the toxicity of local anesthetic solutions.
   c. Ventricular arrhythmias
      i. Ventricular fibrillation
      ii. Reentrant arrhythmias similar to torsades de pointes

continuous infusions are no more than 2.5 to 3 mg per kg per hour in toddlers and older children and 0.15 to 0.2 mg per kg per hour in neonates and infants.[35] A continuous infusion in a 10-kg infant set at 0.2 mg per kg per hour would be delivered 2 mL per hour of a 0.1% (1 mg per mL) solution of bupivacaine. The concentration of the solution used for single-shot caudal epidural is generally 0.2% to 0.25%, whereas higher concentration (0.25% to 0.5%) may be used for peripheral nerve blocks, especially in older patients. As such, when higher concentrations are used, the volume must be appropriately decreased to stay within safe dosing guidelines. A discussion of the volume, concentration, and total dose to be administered (mg per kg or mg per kg per hour) should be included in the preblock time-out to ensure safety.

ROPIVACAINE

Ropivacaine is a levo-enantiomer and one of the newer of the amide LAAs. Originally marketed as a safer alternative to bupivacaine as it may have less of a cardiotoxic effect, subsequent clinical use has also shown it to have less potency than that of equivalent concentrations of bupivacaine.[36,37] The lethal dose in rats is higher than that of bupivacaine (LD_{50}).[38,39] Ropivacaine produces less motor blockade when compared with bupivacaine, especially when a concentration greater than or equal to 0.375% is used. This may offer some advantages in an outpatient setting when preservation or earlier return of motor function is desired.[40] However, these effects must be considered in the context of its potential decreased potency when compared to bupivacaine. Despite these concerns, ropivacaine is commonly used for both single-short and continuous infusions in children. Duration of action following a single-shot technique parallels that of bupivacaine and exceeds that of other amide anesthetic agents such as mepivacaine.[41]

As with bupivacaine, ropivacaine is 95% protein-bound to α-1-acid glycoprotein.[16] As noted, with both bupivacaine and ropivacaine, the lower α-1-acid glycoprotein concentration in neonates and infants increases the potential for LAST. A number of studies have examined the absorption of ropivacaine in children.[42–48] Absorption from deposition sites is slower than a similar dose of bupivacaine, perhaps in part related to its intrinsic vasoconstrictive properties.[48] The cytochrome involved with the metabolism of ropivacaine (CYP1A2) is also immature in neonates and infants, thus necessitating a reduced dose just as with bupivacaine especially when continuous infusions are used.[16] A caudal block with ropivacaine 2 mg per kg (0.1 mL per kg of a 0.2% solution) in children, 1 to 8 years of age, resulted in plasma concentrations of ropivacaine well below toxic levels in adults.[46] This dose was also noted to produce less motor block than bupivacaine, but provided adequate analgesia. The mean C_{max} of total ropivacaine at 2 mg per kg was 0.47 mg per L. A threshold of CNS toxicity was noted at a plasma concentration of 0.6 mg per L. Body-weight-adjusted clearance (*Cl*) was the same as in adults (5 mL per min per kg). Ropivacaine clearance depends on the unbound fraction of ropivacaine rather than the liver blood flow.

Although an improved safety profile of ropivacaine compared with bupivacaine has been demonstrated in animal experiments,[39] ropivacaine is not devoid of these effects as there have been clinical reports of CNS toxicity with ropivacaine with its use for regional anesthesia.[49,50] Hence, it is important to calculate doses and follow dosing guidelines so that excessive dosing of ropivacaine is avoided. Of note, unlike ropivacaine, accumulation has not been noted with continuous infusions for 48 to 72 hours.[48,51] These data have led to an increased used of ropivacaine in place of bupivacaine for postoperative infusions, especially in neonates and infants. When considering single bolus administration, single-shot caudal administration of 1 to

3 mg per kg in children resulted in free ropivacaine concentrations well below the toxic level reported in adults.[52] Our recommended dosing is a bolus dose of 2 mg per kg and infusions of 2 mg per kg per hour.

LEVOBUPIVACAINE

Levobupivacaine is a newer levo-enantiomer that was introduced into clinical practice as an alternative to bupivacaine, given its more favorable cardiovascular (CV) adverse effect profile and its decreased incidence and degree of motor blockade than bupivacaine.[52–57] Although still available outside of the United States, it never gained significant clinical use there and is not commercially available. A population-based pharmacokinetic study in infants younger than 3 months found markedly reduced clearance (approximately half that of adults), which the authors ascribed to the immaturity of CYP3A4 and CYP1A2.[58] Thus, a lower dose would be indicated in this population. Pharmacokinetic studies in older children demonstrate a similar profile as bupivacaine.[58,59] Several pediatric trials have demonstrated its efficacy for a variety of regional anesthetic techniques.[56,60–65]

The available clinical information suggests that levobupivacaine has a better safety profile than bupivacaine.[66] In animal models, when comparing with bupivacaine, levobupivacaine has been shown to have less cardiotoxicity, have less myocardial depression, and be less likely to cause fatal dysrhythmias.[67]

LIDOCAINE

For general clinical use including subcutaneous infiltration, lidocaine remains the most well-known and commonly used of the LAAs. It is a short-acting, but rapid-onset amide local anesthetic. It is used and administered in various concentrations and solutions as a topical anesthetic for airway procedures, for facilitating insertion of intravenous catheters, and for intravenously reducing the pain of intravenous drug administration (e.g., propofol) and may be combined with other agents such as bupivacaine (equal volumes of 1% lidocaine with epinephrine 1:200,000 and 0.2% to 0.5% bupivacaine with epinephrine 1:200,000) to provide a more rapid onset of analgesia for local infiltration of surgical incisions at the end of the case.

As with all of the LAAs, an understanding of absorption and pharmacokinetics is mandatory to allow safe clinical use. Lidocaine is rapidly and nearly completely absorbed from mucosal membranes so that appropriate total dose calculation is important.[68,69] In the emergency room, lidocaine is the most frequently used LAA to provide superficial cutaneous analgesia prior to puncture of the skin for diagnostic or invasive procedures. Dilute concentrations (0.25% to 0.5%) are also being used for intravenous regional anesthesia (Bier block) for forearm fracture reduction.[70–72] When performing a Bier block, a tourniquet is inflated and the lidocaine is injected into a vein that has been cannulated distal to the tourniquet. Because of safety concerns, lidocaine (a maximum dose of 5 mg per kg or 1 mL per kg of a 0.5% solution) is the only LAA with a sufficient safety profile for this technique. Deaths have occurred when bupivacaine was used for intravenous regional anesthesia.[73,74] Regardless of the site of injection, the total dose must be calculated as systemic toxicity and significant absorption may occur.[75–77] Unlike the other agents, lidocaine is frequently used in various preparations for topical administration. Small doses of lidocaine (2% viscous solution) have been used to provide topical analgesia to children with oral mucositis with limited systemic absorption.[78] However, repeated administration may result in toxicity.

Studies of intravenous lidocaine in children under general anesthesia revealed that the distribution half-life (3.2 min), elimination half-life (58 min), volume of distribution (1.1. L per kg), and total plasma clearance (11 mL per min per kg) were similar in adults and in children aged 6 months or older.[79] Similar pharmacokinetic parameters were found following epidural administration.[80] As with all local anesthetics, toxicity is generally manifest as CNS excitation (seizures) and secondarily with cardiac manifestations (hypotension and cardiac arrest). Fortunately, the cardiac toxicity is far less than with the other amide local anesthetics, thereby making successful resuscitation more likely.[81–83]

LOCAL ANESTHETIC AGENTS: ESTERS

LAAs of the ester class are metabolized by plasma cholinesterases. As a result, in populations with lower pseudocholinesterase plasma concentrations,[9,84] there is an increase in the duration of activity. However, because there is no metabolism by the liver or kidney and that metabolism by cholinesterases is generally rapid even in neonates and infants, the safety profile is improved compared with amide LAAs, offering improved safety when used as a bolus dose of a continuous infusion even in concentrations required to provide surgical anesthesia (2% to 3%).[85,86] Chloroprocaine is the only drug of this class that is commonly used in children.

Systemic toxicity parallels that of the other LAAs including effects on the CV system and CNS. However, given to its rapid metabolism, such toxicity is generally short-lived, allowing for effective resuscitation or even spontaneous recovery.[87,88] When compared with bupivacaine, the cardiotoxic effects are less and certainly short-lived. Given these effects, it has seen resurgence in use in pediatric anesthesia, most commonly for intraoperative and postoperative infusions.[89–91] The risk of toxicity owing to delayed metabolism is uncommon except in rare clinical circumstances related to decreased plasma pseudocholinesterase levels caused by comorbid conditions, medications, or therapeutic endeavors (plasmapheresis).

After a bolus dose of 1 mL per kg, a continuous infusion of chloroprocaine at 0.3 mL per kg per hour of a 3% 2-chloroprocaine is recommended to achieve and sustain surgical anesthesia for abdominal procedures such as herniorrhaphy or urological surgery.[85,86,92] For postoperative analgesia, a lower concentration (1% to 2%) may be used.[89,90] These effects have led to its reintroduction into the practice of pediatric anesthesiology for various clinical scenarios.

CLINICAL APPLICATIONS

Outside of the perioperative setting where LAAs are used for regional anesthesia, these agents are used more commonly to provide topical and infiltrative analgesia of the skin prior to invasive procedures. Several local topical anesthetic preparations are now commonly used to reduce procedural pain in neonates, infants, and children.[93–100] The local anesthetic preparations used most commonly for topical and dermal administration include lidocaine, amethocaine, tetracaine, benzocaine, and prilocaine. The latter four are in the commonly used commercially available creams that provide painless cutaneous and dermal analgesia after an application time of 30 to 60 min. When these creams and topical agents are used, application to mucus membranes should be avoided, to prevent absorption and ingestion. Additionally, prolonged application should be avoided and attention should be paid to dosing recommendations to avoid toxicity and even death.[101–105]

The first commercially available topical anesthetic formulation was eutectic mixture of local anesthetic (EMLA) cream that contains a mixture of lidocaine 2.5% and prilocaine 2.5%. This preparation has been used extensively for topical anesthesia prior to commonly performed procedures in the pediatric population including the placement of an intravenous cannula, lumbar puncture, and even circumcision.[106–111] The preparation has to be applied under an occlusive bandage for 45 to 60 min to obtain effective cutaneous analgesia. Although the incidence of methemoglobinemia from prilocaine is not very common in clinical practice, large doses of prolonged exposure may result in this adverse effect, especially in neonates (see below), related to the sensitivity of fetal hemoglobin to oxidizing agents and the limit capacity of the neonatal enzyme system for the reduction of methemoglobin to hemoglobin.[101–103,112] With these caveats in mind, EMLA cream has been shown to provide effective analgesia during circumcision in neonates while avoiding more invasive techniques such as dorsal nerve block.[111]

A newer topical anesthetic solution that offers a faster rate of onset is a 4% or 5% liposomal lidocaine solution (LMX-4 formerly ELA-max 4 and ELA-max 5). With this topical cream, there is no need for an occlusive dressing, and it has the same efficacy as EMLA but with a more rapid onset (30 vs. 60 min).[113–116] Liposome-encapsulated lidocaine and tetracaine have been shown to remain in the epidermis after topical application affording a fast and long-lasting local anesthetic effect.[117,118] Amethocaine 4% (Ametop) is another addition to the topical analgesic local anesthetics also with a slightly fast onset compared with EMLA.[119] It has a clinical efficacy similar to EMLA with a more rapid onset.[120] A Cochrane review concluded that amethocaine was superior to EMLA for venipuncture, whereas another described a more rapid onset.[98] Given the longer onset time of EMLA, many institutions have switched to either the amethocaine or liposomal lidocaine preparations.

In addition to manipulations of the LAAs contained in topical preparations, there have been various devices introduced that have been purported to allow the painless delivery of LAAs for cutaneous analgesia. One such device is a jet-infused local anesthetic administration system called the J-tip.[121] Reports suggest that it provides adequate analgesia without needle insertion with an immediate onset of analgesia. It has been shown to be superior to a 30-min application of LMX-4 or a 60-min application of EMLA.[122,123] Other methods for the topical and local enhancement of LAAs include local heating, the use of ultrasound, iontophoresis, and lidocaine transdermal patches.[124–129]

Topical anesthesia through lacerations or cut skin may be provided by a mixture of tetracaine, epinephrine, and cocaine (known as TAC). TAC is used in pediatric emergency departments for suturing lacerations.[130,131] TAC is provided as tetracaine 0.5%, epinephrine 1:2,000, and cocaine 10% to 11.8%. A more dilute solution of cocaine may be able to provide similar topical anesthesia without the risk of complications. The maximum dose is 0.05 mL per kg in children. TAC is ineffective when applied to intact skin and has to be applied to abraded skin or lacerated skin. There are reports of toxicity associated with the topical absorption of TAC related primarily to the cocaine component.[132–134] Because of the potential for abuse, a newer tetracaine–phenylephrine solution has been shown to be as effective as TAC.

SPECIFIC CLINICAL CONCERNS INCLUDING LOCAL ANESTHETIC SYSTEMIC TOXICITY

Specific Concerns Related to Chloroprocaine

Despite enthusiasm for its use related to its rapid onset and offset, chloroprocaine was replaced by other LAAs related to various concerns regarding its clinical profile including the potential for tachyphylaxis, back pain, and reports of neurotoxicity with spinal/intrathecal administration. Tachyphylaxis is a clinical phenomenon whereby repeated injections of the same dose of local anesthetic solution lead to a decreasing clinical effect. An interesting clinical phenomenon that is related to tachyphylaxis is the dosing intervals. If the dosing intervals are short enough that no pain is perceived, tachyphylaxis is less likely to occur. This is thought to be due to a central sensitization (the so-called "wind-up") phenomenon.[135] Despite lack of specific evidence-based medicine, clinical teaching and discussions regarding chloroprocaine also mention the issue of tachyphylaxis. However, recent years have seen resurgence in the use of chloroprocaine for regional anesthesia in neonates and infants. This practice has been driven by toxicity concerns with prolonged infusions of amide anesthetics. Given the rapid metabolism of chloroprocaine across all age groups, there may be an enhanced safety profile with its use. Recent clinical reports have demonstrated the efficacy of chloroprocaine infusions for epidural and peripheral nerve blockade without concerns of tachyphylaxis or interference with the efficacy of epidural opioids.[90,91,136]

The issue of greater concern that perhaps caused the decrease in the use of chloroprocaine for epidural analgesia was the development of neurotoxicity with inadvertent spinal administration. Previous preparations were considered to be neurotoxic because some patients developed arachnoiditis after accidental subarachnoid injection. These concerns were subsequently demonstrated to be related to the pH of the solution and the presence of various preservatives including ethylenediaminetetraacetic acid (EDTA), metabisulfite, and methylparaben. The parent compound, chloroprocaine, is not considered neurotoxic, and preparations are available that are preservative-free. Although the responsible agents have been eliminated from the solution, thereby eliminating this risk, caution is advised because the former preparations are still commercially available. A minor, secondary effect related to one of the preservatives, EDTA, is back pain. This is related to the chelation of calcium with localized spasm and contraction of the paraspinal muscles.

Methemoglobin Formation

When hemoglobin is exposed to oxidizing agents, methemoglobin is formed where the iron in the hemoglobin is converted from the 2+ to the 3+ state. In this form, hemoglobin is ineffective in carrying oxygen, and when levels exceed 15% to 20% clinical signs of tissue, hypoxia may occur. The potential for such issues is greatest in neonates as fetal hemoglobin is more susceptible to oxidizing agents, and the ability to convert the iron moiety back to the reduced state is limited as there may be a delay in the maturation of the enzymes required for this process. Fortunately, the risk of clinically significant methemoglobin formation is generally limited to two of the LAAs, prilocaine and benzocaine, although reports exist of methemoglobin related to lidocaine, especially in patients receiving other oxidizing medications. Although prilocaine is no longer used for regional anesthesia, it is one of the two agents in the topical anesthetic cream, EMLA. As EMLA is frequently used in the pediatric population including neonates, methemoglobin has been reported. The potential for such problems is higher when EMLA is applied to a large surface area, with prolonged administration or when it is applied to denuded skin. Given these concerns, the package insert contains safety recommendations regarding surface area application, duration of application, and avoidance of denuded skin and mucus membranes. Benzocaine (Hurricaine® Topical Anesthetic Spray) was previously a commonly used agent for topical anesthesia of the airway. It was available as a spray formulation used to anesthetize the mucus membranes for upper airway endoscopy and placement of transesophageal echocardiogram probes. Exact dosing was difficult, and many of the reports were linked to the incorrect use of benzocaine sprays including longer duration or more frequent sprays than recommended.

Local Anesthetic System Toxicity

With the use of LAAs, the greatest risk of morbidity is the potential for the achievement of toxic plasma concentrations of the drug. Local anesthetic-induced systemic toxicity affects the CNS and the CV system. The potential for CNS versus CV effects varies with the specific agents. With most LAAs, CNS toxicity occurs at doses and blood levels below those that produce CV toxicity. The latter provides some degree of safety as the CNS symptoms (seizures) are generally more amenable to treatment than the CV effects (arrhythmias and conduction blockade). CNS toxicity with lidocaine occurs at 8 to 10 mg per mL, whereas CV toxicity occurs at 20 mg per mL.[137,138] The signs and symptoms of CNS toxicity include lightheadedness, dizziness, circumoral numbness, tinnitus, twitching, tremors, and ultimately tonic–clonic seizures. With higher doses, CNS excitation including seizure activity is followed by CNS depression, unconsciousness, and respiratory arrest. Seizures result from the blockade of inhibitory pathways in the cerebral cortex, yielding unopposed activity of facilitatory neurons.[138] CNS depression and unconsciousness result from the inhibition of inhibitory and facilitatory pathways. Hypercarbia and acidosis decrease the convulsive threshold of LAAs as well as potentiating their cardiotoxicity. As children usually receive high-dose local anesthetics while under anesthesia, the vast majority, if not all of the CNS symptoms, are masked. The CNS manifestations of local anesthetic overdose or intravascular injection are readily treated with intravenous anesthetic/sedative agents including benzodiazepines, barbiturates, or propofol. However, these agents do not reverse or prevent the CV effects.

Death from local anesthetic toxicity is most commonly the result of the CV effects of these agents. Local anesthetic toxicity can adversely affect cardiac electrical and mechanical activity.[139–142] Bupivacaine may produce severe cardiac dysrhythmias by inhibiting the fast sodium channels and the slow calcium channels in the cardiac membrane. LAAs depress myocardial contractility, with the most potent drugs (bupivacaine and tetracaine) causing the greatest dose-dependent myocardial depression.[141–143] At toxic plasma concentrations, bupivacaine can cause profound myocardial depression and intractable cardiac arrest. These effects are so profound that resuscitative measures for ventricular tachycardia/fibrillation including standard Algorithms for Advanced Cardiac Life Support (ACLS) protocols may be ineffective. It is only the free fraction and not the local anesthetic that is bound to plasma proteins that has the potential to cause toxicity. In some cases, resuscitation has included the use of extracorporeal circulation. The toxic effects of bupivacaine on the CNS and CV system occur at the same plasma level of 3 to 5 µg per mL. Ropivacaine and levobupivacaine have pharmacological properties similar to bupivacaine, but demonstrate fewer cardio-depressant and arrhythmogenic effects. The signs of local anesthetic CV toxicity include electrocardiographic effects, hypertension, and tachycardia during the CNS excitation phase followed by myocardial depression and mild-to-moderate hypotension, then sinus bradycardia, profound hypotension, ventricular dysrhythmias, and finally circulatory collapse. Hypercarbia, acidosis, and hypoxia potentiate the negative chronotropic and inotropic effects of high plasma concentrations of LAAs. On vascular smooth muscle, most local anesthetics have a biphasic effect producing vasoconstriction at low concentrations and vasodilation at high concentrations.

Toxicity is related to the dose and the site of administration, which affects the rate of absorption into the systemic circulation (Table 38.5). Altered pharmacokinetics with decreased hepatic metabolism can lead to a prolonged half-life, which may be particularly relevant to repeated dosing or a continuous infusion. Absorption is most rapid with interpleural or intercostal administration and then decreases in the following order: caudal › epidural › peripheral nerve blockade › subcutaneous administration. Epinephrine (0.5 µg per mL or a concentration of 1:200,000) may be added to the local anesthetic solution during the performance of a regional anesthetic technique (epidural or peripheral nerve blockade) to decrease the vascular absorption of the drug, thereby increasing the number of anesthetic molecules available to diffuse to the nerve membrane. This results in an increase in the duration of action and an increase in the density of the blockade. However, the ability of epinephrine

TABLE 38.5 Maximum Recommended Doses of Commonly Used Local Anesthetic Agents

Local Anesthetic Agent	*Maximum Dose (mg/kg)*[a]
Procaine	10
2-Chloroprocaine	20
Tetracaine	1.5
Lidocaine	5–7
Mepivacaine	7
Bupivacaine	2.5
Ropivacaine	3

[a]These are maximum doses of local anesthetic agents for a single bolus dose for regional anesthesia. Doses of amides should be decreased by 30% in infants less than 6 months of age.

to prolong the duration of action depends on the local anesthetic used and the site of administration. For peripheral nerve blocks and skin infiltration, epinephrine prolongs the duration of action of all LAAs. For epidural anesthesia, epinephrine added to lidocaine increases the duration of action, but epinephrine added to bupivacaine does not. This relates to the fact that lidocaine causes more vasodilatation than bupivacaine. Therefore, the addition of epinephrine to lidocaine counteracts its vasodilatory effects, which would normally hasten the resolution of the block. As less vasodilatation occurs with bupivacaine, the effect of epinephrine is less pronounced. For spinal anesthesia, epinephrine added to a local anesthetic will prolong the duration of action through decreased vascular absorption and possibly through a direct antinociceptive effect on the spinal cord.

Epinephrine is also used as a marker for inadvertent intravascular injection. This is especially important when large doses of LAAs (epidural or plexus blockade) are administered. For such procedures, gentle aspiration is recommended prior to injection and intermittently when the dose of LAA is administered. However, even with negative aspiration for blood, there is the potential for inadvertent intravascular administration. In an attempt to identify such a problem, a "test dose" is frequently used. This test dose entails the administration of 0.1 mL per kg of the 5 µg per mL epinephrine solution or a total epinephrine dose of 0.5 µg per kg. If this amount of epinephrine is injected intravascular, it can generally be detected by changes in the heart rate, blood pressure, or the ST-T wave segment of the electrocardiogram and thereby alert the practitioner that inadvertent intravascular injection is occurring. Electrocardiographic monitoring can be particularly helpful, as doubling or tripling of the amplitude of the T wave and ST segment elevation often indicate intravascular injection of epinephrine, particularly with bupivacaine[143] (Fig. 38.1). Given the difficulties with resuscitation once LAST has occurred, avoidance is primary with careful calculation of the dose, use of the lowest necessary dose (concentration and volume), use of a test dose with epinephrine to identify inadvertent intravascular injection, intermittent aspiration to identify vascular penetration, and slow incremental injection of the dose.

Although primary resuscitation protocols should be immediately implemented when LAST is identified, during the past several years, the successful use of intralipid has been reported and is now recommended (Table 38.6). The use of intralipid for the resuscitation was originally based on the observation that an adult with carnitine deficiency seemed to be sensitive to cardiac arrhythmias induced by bupivacaine.[144] As carnitine is essential for fatty acid mitochondrial transport to the heart, the authors postulated that bupivacaine may cause further impairment of fatty acid transport. The same investigators performed a laboratory dose escalation experiment with Sprague Dawley rats that were pretreated or received 10%, 20%, or 30% intralipid compared with saline and found a shift in the dose response to bupivacaine-induced cardiac arrest with an increased dose of bupivacaine required in animals treated with intralipid.[145] The authors subsequently demonstrated accelerated removal of bupivacaine and recovery from bupivacaine-induced cardiac toxicity in an isolated rat heart model.[146] There are many proposed mechanisms of action; the most prominent involves the hypothesis that lipid emulsion creates an intravascular lipophilic sink into which lipid-soluble LAAs are partitioned and thereby removed from the active circulation and tissues. Since the publication of these animal experiments, a number of case reports demonstrated the efficacy of intralipid for the management of local anesthetic toxicity.[147–151] An expanded description of the literature and the evolvement of this therapy can be found on www.lipidrescue.org maintained by the University of Illinois in Chicago. Given these reports, guidelines for resuscitation from LAST include the ready available of intralipid in any location where local anesthetic solutions are used.[152–155] The 20% intralipid emulsion should be administered as soon as the local anesthetic toxicity is suspected. As anecdotal reports have noted the recurrence of cardiotoxicity after a single bolus of the intralipid solution, a continuous infusion is recommended for 1 hour following the event.

In summary, the treatment of LAST initially focuses on securing the airway, thus preventing hypoxia, hypercarbia, and acidosis, factors that enhance the severity of LAST and negatively affect resuscitation. Early initiation of effective CPR is important to ensure that coronary perfusion is preserved, thus helping LAAs reduce myocardial concentrations and attain maximum benefit from lipid emulsion therapy. After appropriate resuscitation efforts have been initiated, the first line of management from a pharmacological point of view is lipid

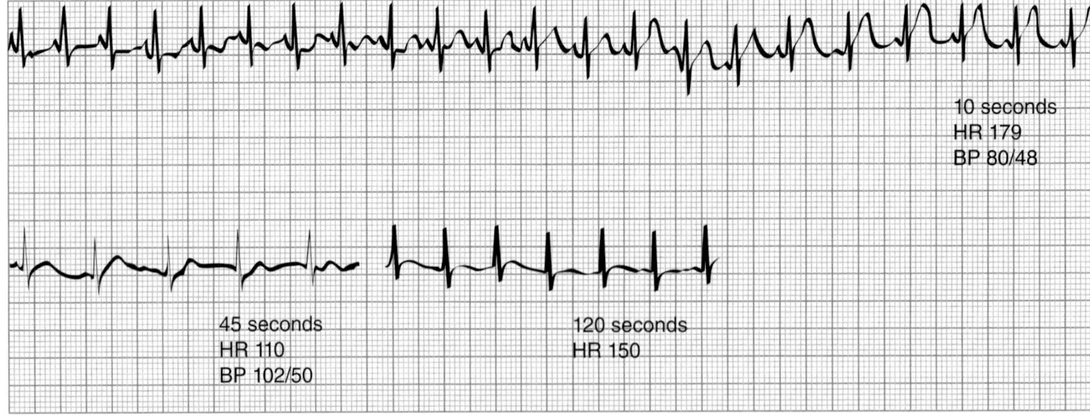

Figure 38.1 Electrocardiographic changes associated with the intravenous injection of bupivacaine and epinephrine 1:200,000. Note the marked increase in the height of the T wave. BP, blood pressure; HR, heart rate. (Reproduced with permission from Freid EB, Bailey AG, Valley RD. Electrocardiographic and hemodynamic changes associated with unintentional intravascular injection of bupivacaine with epinephrine in children. *Anesthesiology* 1993;79:394–398.)

TABLE 38.6 Current Recommendations for the Treatment of LAST

- Airway management to prevent or reverse hypoxia, hypercarbia, and acidosis.
- Standard resuscitation guidelines.
- Lipid emulsion therapy
  - 20% lipid emulsion bolus (initial)
    - 100 mL over 2–3 min if the patient weighs over 70 kg
    - 1.5 mL/kg over 2–3 min if the patient weighs less than 70 kg
  - 20% lipid emulsion infusion
    - 200–250 mL over 15–20 min if the patient weighs more than 70 kg
    - 0.25 mL/kg/min if patient weighs less than 70 kg
  - Continue infusion for a minimum of 10 min after return to spontaneous circulation.
  - 12 mL/kg is recommended as the upper limit for initial dose
  - Avoid using propofol
- Seizure control with benzodiazepines, if seizures persist, use neuromuscular blocking agents (NMBA) to reduce hypoxemia and acidosis
- If cardiac arrest occurs
  - Use epinephrine (less than 1 μg/kg)
  - Avoid calcium channel blockers and β-adrenergic receptor antagonists.
  - Amiodarone is preferable if ventricular arrhythmias develop.
- Failure to respond to all previous efforts should prompt institution of cardiopulmonary bypass or extracorporeal membrane oxygenation (ECMO).

emulsion therapy. The use of epinephrine at doses of 1 μg per kg or less remains fundamental in the management of hemodynamic collapse that does not respond to lipid emulsion therapy. The use of a checklist is suggested to ensure adherence to the current recommendations.

SUMMARY

LAAs are key pharmacologic agents in the management of pain of various causes in the pediatric-aged patient. Applications include superficial infiltration to provide cutaneous and dermal analgesia during minor invasive procedures as well as the performance of neuraxial and peripheral nerve blockade to provide surgical anesthesia and postoperative analgesia. Through their ability to block sodium channels, these agents interrupt a primary pathway in nociception. Despite their efficacy, high plasma concentrations related to rapid systemic administration or excessive dosing can lead to significant morbidity and even mortality. To ensure the safe and effective use of these agents, the practitioner should have a clear understanding of their mechanism of action, potential adverse effects, pharmacology, and dosing guidelines. Toxicity can generally be prevented by adherence to dosing guidelines as well as the use of techniques to avoid inadvertent systemic administration. Should LAST occur, a thorough understanding of current guidelines for resuscitation including the use of intralipid therapy is suggested.

REFERENCES

1. Suresh S, Wheeler M. Practical pediatric regional anesthesia. *Anesthesiol Clin North Am* 2002;20:83–113.
2. Goeller JK, Bhalla T, Tobias JD. Combined use of neuraxial and general anesthesia during major abdominal procedures in neonates and infants. *Paediatr Anaesth* 2014;24:553–560.
3. Butterworth JF, Strichartz GR. Molecular mechanisms of local anesthesia: a review. *Anesthesiology* 1990;72:711–734.
4. Covino BG. Pharmacology of local anaesthetic agents. *Br J Anaesth* 1986;58:701–716.
5. Wildsmith JA, Gissen AJ, Takman B, et al. Differential nerve blockade: esters vs amides and the influence of pKa. *Br J Anaesth* 1987;59:379–384.
6. Kinoshita H, Iranami H, Kimoto Y, et al. Mild alkalinization and acidification differentially modify the effects of lidocaine or mexiletine on vasorelaxation mediated by ATP-sensitive K+ channels. *Anesthesiology* 2001;95:200–206.
7. Fulling PD, Peterfreund RA. Alkalinization and precipitation characteristics of 0.2% ropivacaine. *Reg Anesth Pain Med* 2000;25:518–521.
8. Peterfreund RA, Datta S, Ostheimer GW. pH adjustment of local anesthetic solutions with sodium bicarbonate: laboratory evaluation of alkalinization and precipitation. *Reg Anesth* 1989;14:265–270.
9. Hassan HG, Renck H, Akerman B, et al. On the relative potency of amino-amide local anaesthetics in vivo. *Acta Anaesthesiol Scand* 1994;38:505–509.
10. Raj PP, Ohlweiler D, Hitt BA, et al. Kinetics of local anesthetic esters and the effects of adjuvant drugs on 2-chloroprocaine hydrolysis. *Anesthesiology* 1980;53:307–314.
11. Besunder JB, Reed MD, Blumer JL. Principles of drug biodisposition in the neonate. A critical evaluation of the pharmacokinetic–pharmacodynamic interface (part II). *Clin Pharmacokinet* 1988;14:261–286.
12. Ecoffey C, Desparmet J, Maury M, et al. Bupivacaine in children: pharmacokinetics following caudal anesthesia. *Anesthesiology* 1985;63:447–448.
13. Murat I, Montay G, Delleur MM, et al. Bupivacaine pharmacokinetics during epidural anaesthesia in children. *Eur J Anaesthesiol* 1988;5:113–120.
14. Frawley G, Ragg P, Hack H. Plasma concentrations of bupivacaine after combined spinal epidural anaesthesia in infants and neonates. *Paediatr Anaesth* 2000;10:619–625.
15. Larsson BA, Lonnqvist PA, Olsson GL. Plasma concentrations of bupivacaine in neonates after continuous epidural infusion. *Anesth Analg* 1997;84:501–505.
16. Mazoit JX, Denson DD, Samii K. Pharmacokinetics of bupivacaine following caudal anesthesia in infants. *Anesthesiology* 1988;68:387–391.
17. Meunier JF, Goujard E, Dubousset AM, et al. Pharmacokinetics of bupivacaine after continuous epidural infusion in infants with and without biliary atresia. *Anesthesiology* 2001;95:87–95.
18. Payne KA, Hendrix MR, Wade WJ. Caudal bupivacaine for postoperative analgesia in pediatric lower limb surgery. *J Pediatr Surg* 1993;28:155–157.
19. Fisher QA, McComiskey CM, Hill JL, et al. Postoperative voiding interval and duration of analgesia following peripheral or caudal nerve blocks in children. *Anesth Analg* 1993;75:173–177.
20. Jöhr M. Regional anaesthesia in neonates, infants and children: an educational review. *Eur J Anaesthesiol* 2015;32:289–297.
21. Smith RH, Sanders JC. Safe dose of levobupivacaine (Chirocaine®) in caudal analgesia in children. *Br J Anaesth* 2003;90:400–401.
22. Weston PJ, Bourchier D. The pharmacokinetics of bupivacaine following interpleural nerve block in infants of very low birthweight. *Paediatr Anaesth* 1995;5:219–222.
23. Berde CB. Toxicity of local anesthetics in infants and children. *J Pediatr* 1993;122:S14–S20.
24. Rane A, Sjoqvist F. Drug metabolism in the human fetus and newborn infant. *Pediatr Clin North Am* 1972;19:37–49.
25. Levy G. Pharmacokinetics of fetal and neonatal exposure to drugs. *Obstet Gynecol* 1981;58(Suppl):9S–16S.
26. Rothstein P, Arthur GR, Feldman HS, et al. Bupivacaine for intercostal nerve blocks in children: blood concentrations and pharmacokinetics. *Anesth Analg* 1986;65:625–632.
27. Berde C. Epidural analgesia in children. *Can J Anaesth* 1994;41:555–560.
28. Luz G, Wieser C, Innerhofer P, et al. Free and total bupivacaine plasma concentrations after continuous epidural anaesthesia in infants and children. *Paediatr Anaesth* 1998;8:473–478.
29. Groban L, Deal DD, Vernon JC, et al. Cardiac resuscitation after incremental overdosage with lidocaine, bupivacaine, levobupivacaine, and ropivacaine in anesthetized dogs. *Anesth Analg* 2001;92:37–43.
30. Chang DH, Ladd LA, Copeland S, et al. Direct cardiac effects of intracoronary bupivacaine, levobupivacaine and ropivacaine in the sheep. *Br J Pharmacol* 2001;132:649–658.
31. Badgwell JM, Heavner JE, Kytta J. Bupivacaine toxicity in young pigs is age-dependent and is affected by volatile anesthetics. *Anesthesiology* 1990;73:297–303.
32. Berde CB. Convulsions associated with pediatric regional anesthesia. *Anesth Analg* 1992;75:164–166.

33. Tobias JD. Caudal epidural block: a review of test dosing and recognition of systemic injection in children. *Anesth Analg* 2001;93:1156–1161.
34. Peutrell JM, Hughes DG. A grand mal convulsion in a child in association with a continuous epidural infusion of bupivacaine. *Anaesthesia* 1995;50:563–564.
35. Peutrell JM, Holder K, Gregory M. Plasma bupivacaine concentrations associated with continuous extradural infusions in babies. *Br J Anaesth* 1997;78:160–162.
36. Luz G, Innerhofer P, Häussler B, et al. Comparison of ropivacaine 0.1% and 0.2% with bupivacaine 0.2% for single-shot caudal anaesthesia in children. *Paediatr Anaesth* 2000;10:499–504.
37. Ingelmo PM, Locatelli BG, Sonzogni V, et al. Caudal 0.2% ropivacaine is less effective during surgery than 0.2% levobupivacaine and 0.2% bupivacaine: a double-blind, randomized, controlled trial. *Paediatr Anaesth* 2006;16:955–961.
38. Kohane DS, Sankar WN, Shubina M, et al. Sciatic nerve blockade in infant, adolescent, and adult rats: a comparison of ropivacaine with bupivacaine. *Anesthesiology* 1998;89:1199–1208.
39. Dony P, Dewinde V, Vanderick B, et al. The comparative toxicity of ropivacaine and bupivacaine at equipotent doses in rats. *Anesth Analg* 2000;91:1489–1492.
40. Da Conceicao MJ, Coelho L. Caudal anaesthesia with 0.375% ropivacaine or 0.375% bupivacaine in paediatric patients. *Br J Anaesth* 1998;80:507–508.
41. Fernandez-Guisasola J, Andueza A, Burgos E, et al. A comparison of 0.5% ropivacaine and 1% mepivacaine for sciatic nerve block in the popliteal fossa. *Acta Anaesthesiol Scand* 2001;45:967–970.
42. Koinig H, Krenn CG, Glaser C, et al. The dose-response of caudal ropivacaine in children. *Anesthesiology* 1999;90:1339–1344.
43. Habre W, Bergesio R, Johnson C, et al. Pharmacokinetics of ropivacaine following caudal analgesia in children. *Paediatr Anaesth* 2000;10:143–147.
44. Wulf H, Peters C, Behnke H. The pharmacokinetics of caudal ropivacaine 0.2% in children. A study of infants aged less than 1 year and toddlers aged 1–5 years undergoing inguinal hernia repair. *Anaesthesia* 2000;55:757–760.
45. Hansen TG, Ilett KF, Reid C, et al. Caudal ropivacaine in infants: population pharmacokinetics and plasma concentrations. *Anesthesiology* 2001;94:579–584.
46. Lonnqvist PA, Westrin P, Larsson BA, et al. Ropivacaine pharmacokinetics after caudal block in 1–8 year old children. *Br J Anaesth* 2000;85:506–511.
47. McCann ME, Sethna NF, Mazoit JX, et al. The pharmacokinetics of epidural ropivacaine in infants and young children. *Anesth Analg* 2001;93:893–897.
48. Bösenberg AT, Thomas J, Cronje L, et al. Pharmacokinetics and efficacy of ropivacaine for continuous epidural infusion in neonates and infants. *Paediatr Anaesth* 2005;15:739–749.
49. Abouleish EI, Elias M, Nelson C. Ropivacaine-induced seizure after extradural anaesthesia. *Br J Anaesth* 1998;80:843–844.
50. Eledjam JJ, Gros T, Viel E, et al. Ropivacaine overdose and systemic toxicity. *Anaesth Intensive Care* 2000;28:705–707.
51. Berde CB, Yaster M, Meretoja O, et al. Stable plasma concentrations of unbound ropivacaine during postoperative epidural infusion for 24–72 hours in children. *Eur J Anaesthesiol* 2008;25:410–417.
52. Bosenberg AT, Thomas J, Lopez T, et al. Plasma concentrations of ropivacaine following a single-shot caudal block of 1, 2 or 3 mg/kg in children. *Acta Anaesthesiol Scand* 2001;45:1276–1280.
53. McLeod GA, Burke D. Levobupivacaine. *Anaesthesia* 2001;56:331–341.
54. Foster RH, Markham A. Levobupivacaine: a review of its pharmacology and use as a local anaesthetic. *Drugs* 2000;59:551–579.
55. Ivani G, Borghi B, van Oven H. Levobupivacaine. *Minerva Anestesiol* 2001;67:20–23.
56. Ivani G, De Negri P, Lonnqvist PA, et al. A comparison of three different concentrations of levobupivacaine for caudal block in children. *Anesth Analg* 2003;97:368–371.
57. Locatelli B, Ingelmo P, Sonzogni V, et al. Randomized, double-blind, phase III, controlled trial comparing levobupivacaine 0.25%, ropivacaine 0.25% and bupivacaine 0.25% by the caudal route in children. *Br J Anaesth* 2005;94:366–371.
58. Chalkiadis GA, Eyres RL, Cranswick N, et al. Pharmacokinetics of levobupivacaine 0.25% following caudal administration in children under 2 years of age. *Br J Anaesth* 2004;92:218–222.
59. Cortinez LI, Fuentes R, Solari S, et al. Pharmacokinetics of levobupivacaine (2.5 mg/kg) after caudal administration in children younger than 3 years. *Anesth Analg* 2008;107:1182–1184.
60. Gunter JB, Gregg T, Varughese AM, et al. Levobupivacaine for ilioinguinal/iliohypogastric nerve block in children. *Anesth Analg* 1999;89:647–649.
61. Lerman J, Nolan J, Eyres R, et al. Efficacy, safety, and pharmacokinetics of levobupivacaine with and without fentanyl after continuous epidural infusion in children: a multicenter trial. *Anesthesiology* 2003;99:1166–1174.
62. Astuto M, Disma N, Arena C. Levobupivacaine 0.25% compared with ropivacaine 0.25% by the caudal route in children. *Eur J Anaesthesiol* 2003;20:826–830.
63. Ala-Kokko TI, Raiha E, Karinen J, et al. Pharmacokinetics of 0.5% levobupivacaine following ilioinguinal–iliohypogastric nerve blockade in children. *Acta Anaesthesiol Scand* 2005;49:397–400.
64. Frawley GP, Downie S, Huang GH. Levobupivacaine caudal anesthesia in children: a randomized double-blind comparison with bupivacaine. *Paediatr Anaesth* 2006;16:754–760.
65. Yao YS, Qian B, Chen BZ, et al. The optimum concentration of levobupivacaine for intra-operative caudal analgesia in children undergoing inguinal hernia repair at equal volumes of injectate. *Anaesthesia* 2009;64:23–26.
66. Giaufre E, Dalens B, Gombert A. Epidemiology and morbidity of regional anesthesia in children: a one-year prospective survey of the French-Language Society of Pediatric Anesthesiologists. *Anesth Analg* 1996;83:904–912.
67. Huang YF, Pryor ME, Mather LE, et al. Cardiovascular and central nervous system effects of intravenous levobupivacaine and bupivacaine in sheep. *Anesth Analg* 1998;86:797–804.
68. Amitai Y, Zylber-Katz E, Avital A, et al. Serum lidocaine concentrations in children during bronchoscopy with topical anesthesia. *Chest* 1990;98:1370–1373.
69. Eyres RL, Bishop W, Oppenheim RC, et al. Plasma lignocaine concentrations following topical laryngeal application. *Anaesth Intensive Care* 1983;11:23–26.
70. Werk LN, Lewis M, Armatti-Wiltrout S, et al. Comparing the effectiveness of modified forearm and conventional minidose intravenous regional anesthesia for reduction of distal forearm fractures in children. *J Pediatr Orthop* 2008;28:410–416.
71. Bratt HD, Eyres RL, Cole WG. Randomized double-blind trial of low-and moderate-dose lidocaine regional anesthesia for forearm fractures in childhood. *J Pediatr Orthop* 1996;16:660–663.
72. Colizza WA, Said E. Intravenous regional anesthesia in the treatment of forearm and wrist fractures and dislocations in children. *Can J Surg* 1993;36:225–228.
73. Heath ML. Deaths after intravenous regional anaesthesia. *Br Med J (Clin Res Ed)* 1982;285:913–914.
74. Moore DC. Bupivacaine toxicity and Bier block: the drug, the technique, or the anesthetist. *Anesthesiology* 1984;61:782.
75. Elad S, Cohen G, Zylber-Katz E, et al. Systemic absorption of lidocaine after topical application for the treatment of oral mucositis in bone marrow transplantation patients. *J Oral Pathol Med* 1999;28:170–172.
76. Cassidy SC, Jones PR, Cox S, et al. Serum lidocaine concentrations after subcutaneous administration in patients undergoing cardiac catheterization in a pediatric institution. *J Pediatr* 1996;129:464–466.
77. Ryan CA, Robertson M, Coe JY. Seizures due to lidocaine toxicity in a child during cardiac catheterization. *Pediatr Cardiol* 1993;14:116–118.
78. Gunter JB. Benefit and risks of local anesthetics in infants and children. *Paediatr Drugs* 2002;4:649–672.
79. Finholt DA, Stirt JA, DiFazio CA, et al. Lidocaine pharmacokinetics in children during general anesthesia. *Anesth Analg* 1986;65:279–282.
80. Ecoffey C, Desparmet J, Berdeaux A, et al. Pharmacokinetics of lignocaine in children following caudal anaesthesia. *Br J Anaesth* 1984;56:1399–1402.
81. Mather LE, Copeland SE, Ladd LA. Acute toxicity of local anesthetics: underlying pharmacokinetic and pharmacodynamic concepts. *Reg Anesth Pain Med* 2005;30:553–566.
82. Casati A, Putzu M. Bupivacaine, levobupivacaine and ropivacaine: are they clinically different? *Best Pract Res Clin Anaesthesiol* 2005;19:247–268.
83. Groban L. Central nervous system and cardiac effects from long-acting amide local anesthetic toxicity in the intact animal model. *Reg Anesth Pain Med* 2003;28:3–11.
84. Kuhnert BR, Philipson EH, Pimental R, et al. A prolonged chloroprocaine epidural block in a postpartum patient with abnormal pseudocholinesterase. *Anesthesiology* 1982;56:477–478.
85. Tobias JD, Rasmussen GE, Holcomb GW, et al. Continuous caudal anaesthesia with chloroprocaine as an adjunct to general anaesthesia in neonates. *Can J Anaesth* 1996;43:69–72.
86. Henderson K, Sethna NF, Berde CB. Continuous caudal anesthesia for inguinal hernia repair in former preterm infants. *J Clin Anesth* 1993;5:129–133.
87. Hernandez MA, Boretsky K. Chloroprocaine: local anesthetic systemic toxicity in a 9-month infant with paravertebral catheter. *Paediatr Anaesth* 2016;26:665–666.
88. Cladis FP, Litman RS. Transient cardiovascular toxicity with unintentional intravascular injection of 3% 2-chloroprocaine in a 2-month-old infant. *Anesthesiology* 2004;100:181–183.
89. Veneziano G, Tobias JD. Chloroprocaine for epidural anesthesia in infants and children. *Paediatr Anaesth* 2017;27:581–590.
90. Veneziano G, Iliev P, Tripi J, et al. Continuous chloroprocaine infusion for thoracic and caudal epidurals as a postoperative analgesia modality in neonates, infants, and children. *Paediatr Anaesth* 2016;26:84–91.
91. Bairdain S, Dodson B, Zurakowski D, et al. Paravertebral nerve block catheters using chloroprocaine in infants with prolonged mechanical ventilation for treatment of long-gap esophageal atresia. *Paediatr Anaesth* 2015;25:1151–1157.
92. Trifa M, Tumin D, Whitaker EE, et al. Spinal anesthesia for surgery longer than 60 min in infants: experience from the first 2 years of a spinal anesthesia program. *J Anesth* 2018;32:637–640.
93. Cregin R, Rappaport AS, Montagnino G, et al. Improving pain management for pediatric patients undergoing nonurgent painful procedures. *Am J Health Syst Pharm* 2008;65:723–727.
94. Khan AN, Sachdeva S. Current trends in the management of common painful conditions of preschool children in United States pediatric emergency departments. *Clin Pediatr (Phila)* 2007;46:626–631.
95. Lemyre B, Hogan DL, Gaboury I, et al. How effective is tetracaine 4% gel, before a venipuncture, in reducing procedural pain in infants: a randomized double-blind placebo controlled trial. *BMC Pediatr* 2007;7:7.
96. Eidelman A, Weiss JM, Lau J, et al. Topical anesthetics for dermal instrumentation: a systematic review of randomized, controlled trials. *Ann Emerg Med* 2005;46:343–351.
97. Anand KJ, Johnston CC, Oberlander TF, et al. Analgesia and local anesthesia during invasive procedures in the neonate. *Clin Ther* 2005;27:844–876.
98. O'Brien L, Taddio A, Lyszkiewicz DA, et al. A critical review of the topical local anesthetic amethocaine (Ametop) for pediatric pain. *Paediatr Drugs* 2005;7:41–54.
99. Priestley S, Kelly AM, Chow L, et al. Application of topical local anesthetic at triage reduces treatment time for children with lacerations: a randomized controlled trial. *Ann Emerg Med* 2003;42:34–40.
100. Houck CS, Sethna NF. Transdermal analgesia with local anesthetics in children: review, update and future directions. *Expert Rev Neurother* 2005;5:625–634.
101. American Academy of Pediatrics. Committee on drugs. Alternate routes of drug administration—advantages and disadvantages. *Pediatrics* 1997;100:143–152.
102. Curtis LA, Dolan TS, Seibert HE. Are one or two dangerous? Lidocaine and topical anesthetic exposures in children. *J Emerg Med* 2008;37(1):32–39.
103. Raso SM, Fernandez JB, Beobide EA, et al. Methemoglobinemia and CNS toxicity after topical application of EMLA to a 4-year-old girl with molluscum contagiosum. *Pediatr Dermatol* 2006;23:592–593.
104. Hua YM, Hung CH, Yuh YS. Acute intoxication of lidocaine and chlorpheniramine: report of one case. *Acta Paediatr Taiwan* 2005;46:385–387.

105. Dahshan A, Donovan GK. Severe methemoglobinemia complicating topical benzocaine use during endoscopy in a toddler: a case report and review of the literature. *Pediatrics* 2006;117:e806–e809.
106. Corbett JV. EMLA cream for local anesthesia. *Am J Matern Child Nurs* 1995;20:178.
107. Chang PC, Goresky GV, O'Connor G, et al. A multicentre randomized study of single-unit dose package of EMLA patch vs EMLA 5% cream for venepuncture in children. *Can J Anaesth* 1994;41:59–63.
108. Gourrier E, Karoubi P, el Hanache A, et al. Use of EMLA cream in a department of neonatology. *Pain* 1996;68:431–434.
109. Stevens B, Johnston C, Taddio A, et al. Management of pain from heel lance with lidocaine-prilocaine (EMLA) cream: is it safe and efficacious in preterm infants? *J Dev Behav Pediatr* 1999;20:216–221.
110. Taddio A, Ohlsson K, Ohlsson A. Lidocaine–prilocaine cream for analgesia during circumcision in newborn boys. *Cochrane Database Syst Rev* 2000;(2):CD000496.
111. Lander J, Brady-Fryer B, Metcalfe JB, et al. Comparison of ring block, dorsal penile nerve block, and topical anesthesia for neonatal circumcision: a randomized controlled trial. *JAMA* 1997;278:2157–2162.
112. Brisman M, Ljung BM, Otterbom I, et al. Methaemoglobin formation after the use of EMLA cream in term neonates. *Acta Paediatr* 1998;87:1191–1194.
113. Eichenfield LF, Funk A, Fallon-Friedlander S, et al. A clinical study to evaluate the efficacy of ELA-Max (4% liposomal lidocaine) as compared with eutectic mixture of local anesthetics cream for pain reduction of venipuncture in children. *Pediatrics* 2002;109:1093–1099.
114. Koh JL, Harrison D, Myers R, et al. A randomized, double-blind comparison study of EMLA and ELA-Max for topical anesthesia in children undergoing intravenous insertion. *Paediatr Anaesth* 2004;14:977–982.
115. Smith DP, Gjellum M. The efficacy of LMX versus EMLA for pain relief in boys undergoing office meatotomy. *J Urol* 2004;172:1760–1761.
116. Kleiber C, Sorenson M, Whiteside K, et al. Topical anesthetics for intravenous insertion in children: a randomized equivalency study. *Pediatrics* 2002;110:758–761.
117. Fisher R, Hung O, Mezei M, et al. Topical anaesthesia of intact skin: liposome-encapsulated tetracaine vs EMLA. *Br J Anaesth* 1998;81:972–973.
118. Gesztes A, Mezei M. Topical anesthesia of the skin by liposome-encapsulated tetracaine. *Anesth Analg* 1988;67:1079–1081.
119. O'Brien L, Taddio A, Ipp M, et al. Topical 4% amethocaine gel reduces the pain of subcutaneous measles–mumps–rubella vaccination. *Pediatrics* 2004;114:e720–e724.
120. Arendts G, Stevens M, Fry M. Topical anaesthesia and intravenous cannulation success in paediatric patients: a randomized double-blind trial. *Br J Anaesth* 2008;100:521–524.
121. Cooper JA, Bromley LM, Baranowski AP, et al. Evaluation of a needle-free injection system for local anaesthesia prior to venous cannulation. *Anaesthesia* 2000;55:247–250.
122. Spanos S, Booth R, Koenig H, et al. Jet injection of 1% buffered lidocaine versus topical ELA-Max for anesthesia before peripheral intravenous catheterization in children: a randomized controlled trial. *Pediatr Emerg Care* 2008;24:511–515.
123. Jimenez N, Bradford H, Seidel KD, et al. A comparison of a needle-free injection system for local anesthesia versus EMLA for intravenous catheter insertion in the pediatric patient. *Anesth Analg* 2006;102:411–414.
124. Zempsky WT, Anand KJ, Sullivan KM, et al. Lidocaine iontophoresis for topical anesthesia before intravenous line placement in children. *J Pediatr* 1998;132:1061–1063.
125. Spierings EL, Brevard JA, Katz NP. Two-minute skin anesthesia through ultrasound pretreatment and iontophoretic delivery of a topical anesthetic: a feasibility study. *Pain Med* 2008;9:55–59.
126. Zempsky WT, Robbins B, McKay K. Reduction of topical anesthetic onset time using ultrasound: a randomized controlled trial prior to venipuncture in young children. *Pain Med* 2008;9:795–802.
127. Miller KA, Balakrishnan G, Eichbauer G, et al. 1% lidocaine injection, EMLA cream, or "numby stuff" for topical analgesia associated with peripheral intravenous cannulation. *AANA J* 2001;69:185–187.
128. Squire SJ, Kirchhoff KT, Hissong K. Comparing two methods of topical anesthesia used before intravenous cannulation in pediatric patients. *J Pediatr Health Care* 2000;14:68–72.
129. Leopold A, Wilson S, Weaver JS, et al. Pharmacokinetics of lidocaine delivered from a transmucosal patch in children. *Anesth Prog* 2002;49:82–87.
130. Blackburn PA, Butler KH, Hughes MJ, et al. Comparison of tetracaine–adrenaline–cocaine (TAC) with topical lidocaine–epinephrine (TLE): efficacy and cost. *Am J Emerg Med* 1995;13:315–317.
131. Kuhn M, Rossi SO, Plummer JL, et al. Topical anaesthesia for minor lacerations: MAC versus TAC. *Med J Aust* 1996;164:277–280.
132. Bonadio WA. Safe and effective method for application of tetracaine, adrenaline, and cocaine to oral lacerations. *Ann Emerg Med* 1996;28:396–398.
133. Bonadio WA, Wagner V. TAC (tetracaine, adrenaline, cocaine) for the repair of minor dermal lacerations. *Pediatr Emerg Care* 1988;4:82.
134. Bonadio WA. TAC: a review. *Pediatr Emerg Care* 1989;5:128–130.
135. Wang C, Liu H, Wilder RT, et al. Effects of repeated injection of local anesthetic on sciatic nerve blocks response. *J Huazhong Univ Sci Technol Med Sci* 2004;24:497–499.
136. Ross EL, Reiter PD, Murphy ME, et al. Evaluation of prolonged epidural chloroprocaine for postoperative analgesia in infants. *J Clin Anesth* 2015;27:463–469.
137. Scott DB. Toxic effects of local anaesthetic agents on the central nervous system. *Br J Anaesth* 1986;58:732–735.
138. Wagman IH, DeJong RH, Prince DA. Effects of lidocaine on the central nervous system. *Anesthesiology* 1967;28:155–172.
139. Moller RA, Covino BG. Cardiac electrophysiologic effects of lidocaine and bupivacaine. *Anesth Analg* 1988;67:107–114.
140. Block A, Covino BG. Effect of local anesthetic agents on cardiac conduction and contractility. *Reg Anesth* 1982;6:55.
141. Pitkanen M, Feldman HS, Arthur GR, et al. Chronotropic and inotropic effects of ropivacaine, bupivacaine, and lidocaine in the spontaneously beating and electrically paced isolated, perfused rabbit heart. *Reg Anesth* 1992;17:183–192.
142. Kasten GW. Amide local anesthetic alterations of effective refractory period temporal dispersion: relationship to ventricular arrhythmias. *Anesthesiology* 1986;65:61–66.
143. Freid EB, Bailey AG, Valley RD. Electrocardiographic and hemodynamic changes associated with unintentional intravascular injection of bupivacaine with epinephrine in infants. *Anesthesiology* 1993;79:394–398.
144. Weinberg GL, Laurito CE, Geldner P, et al. Malignant ventricular dysrhythmias in a patient with isovaleric acidemia receiving general and local anesthesia for suction lipectomy. *J Clin Anesth* 1997;9:668–670.
145. Weinberg GL, VadeBoncouer T, Ramaraju GA, et al. Pretreatment or resuscitation with a lipid infusion shifts the dose-response to bupivacaine-induced asystole in rats. *Anesthesiology* 1998;88:1071–1075.
146. Weinberg GL, Ripper R, Murphy P, et al. Lipid infusion accelerates removal of bupivacaine and recovery from bupivacaine toxicity in the isolated rat heart. *Reg Anesth Pain Med* 2006;31:296–303.
147. Spence AG. Lipid reversal of central nervous system symptoms of bupivacaine toxicity. *Anesthesiology* 2007;107:516–517.
148. Whiteside J. Reversal of local anaesthetic induced CNS toxicity with lipid emulsion. *Anaesthesia* 2008;63:203–204.
149. Mathieu S, Cranshaw J. Treatment of severe local anaesthetic toxicity. *Anaesthesia* 2008;63:202–203.
150. McCutchen T, Gerancher JC. Early intralipid therapy may have prevented bupivacaine-associated cardiac arrest. *Reg Anesth Pain Med* 2008;33:178–180.
151. Ludot H, Tharin JY, Belouadah M, et al. Successful resuscitation after ropivacaine and lidocaine-induced ventricular arrhythmia following posterior lumbar plexus block in a child. *Anesth Analg* 2008;106:1572–1574.
152. Gitman M, Barrington MJ, Local anesthetic systemic toxicity: a review of recent case reports and registries. *Reg Anesth Pain Med* 2018;43:124–130.
153. Neil JM, Barrington MJ, Fettiplace MR, et al. The third American society of regional anesthesia and pain medicine practice advisory on local anesthetic systemic toxicity. *Reg Anesth Pain Med* 2018;43:113–123.
154. Brull SJ. Lipid emulsion for the treatment of local anesthetic toxicity: patient safety implications. *Anesth Analg* 2008;106:1337–1339.
155. Picard J, Ward SC, Zumpe R, et al. Guidelines and the adoption of "lipid rescue" therapy for local anaesthetic toxicity. *Anaesthesia* 2009;64:122–125.

SECTION VI

Immunopharmacology, Allergy, and Inflammation

Sylvain Chemtob
John Jeffrey Reese
Anie Lapointe
Mathieu Nadeau-Vallée
Victoria Tutag Lehr

CHAPTER 39

Nonsteroidal Anti-Inflammatory Drugs

INTRODUCTION

Inflammation is among the most important tissue responses to injury; it is observed in all acquired disorders as well as genetic conditions modified by environmental exposures. The outcome of the inflammatory response may be beneficial as is the case in limiting invading organisms. However, the outcome may be deleterious if chronic inflammation ensues, as seen with chronic rheumatic disorders, which lead to pain and destruction of musculoskeletal tissues, resulting in potentially severe disability. Inflammation involves a complex sequence paradigm implicating responses of a number of cell types, such that, upon early activation of endothelium, leukocytes and monocytes are chemoattracted to the site to contain the injury. The elimination of triggering noxious stimulus is associated with the sacrifice of certain cells. Repair involves repopulation of some cells associated with revascularization.

There are numerous mediators of inflammation, and their properties are intertwined with one another. For instance, effects of chemokines, interleukins (ILs), leukotrienes, and histamine are interlinked in lung inflammation associated with asthma; in degenerative arthritis, ILs (especially IL-1 and IL-18) interact with prostanoids. Growth factors such as platelet-derived growth factor and vascular endothelial growth factor participate in these processes, especially during the repair phases. In this chapter, we shall focus on lipid mediators modulated by nonsteroidal anti-inflammatory drugs (NSAIDs); we will also cover some pharmacology of acetaminophen that exerts effects via cyclooxygenases (COXs). A review of prostanoid biochemistry and pharmacology will be presented relevant to the mode of action of NSAIDs. Applications of NSAIDs in three major conditions related to pediatrics and perinatology will be covered herein, notably in pediatric fever, in neonatal patent ductus arteriosus (PDA), and in perinatal preterm labor (PTL). Detailed descriptions of other agents indicated in pain, asthma, and arthritis, some of which also act via prostanoids, will be covered elsewhere in this textbook.

PROSTANOIDS: METABOLISM AND ACTIONS

PROSTANOID SYNTHESIS

The eicosanoid family of oxygenated 18-, 20-, and 22-carbon fatty acids (FAs) are important signaling molecules in most biologic systems. Eicosanoid family members are derivatives of omega-3 and omega-6 polyunsaturated fatty acids (PUFAs) and include (1) prostanoid products of the COX pathway, (2) leukotrienes, lipoxins, eoxins, and other products of the lipoxygenase (LOX) pathway, (3) epoxy and dihydroxy FAs formed by monooxygenase/cytochrome P450 (CYP) enzymes, (4) resolvins, protectins, maresins, and less-well-described anti-inflammatory PUFA derivatives, and (5) isoprostanes, isofurans, isoleukotrienes, and other products that are generated nonenzymatically (Fig. 39.1). The prostanoid subfamily are key biologic mediators of diverse physiologic and pathophysiologic effects in various systems. These involve modulation of neuronal activity, pyrexia and sleep induction, alterations in platelet aggregation, relaxation and contraction of smooth muscle, and

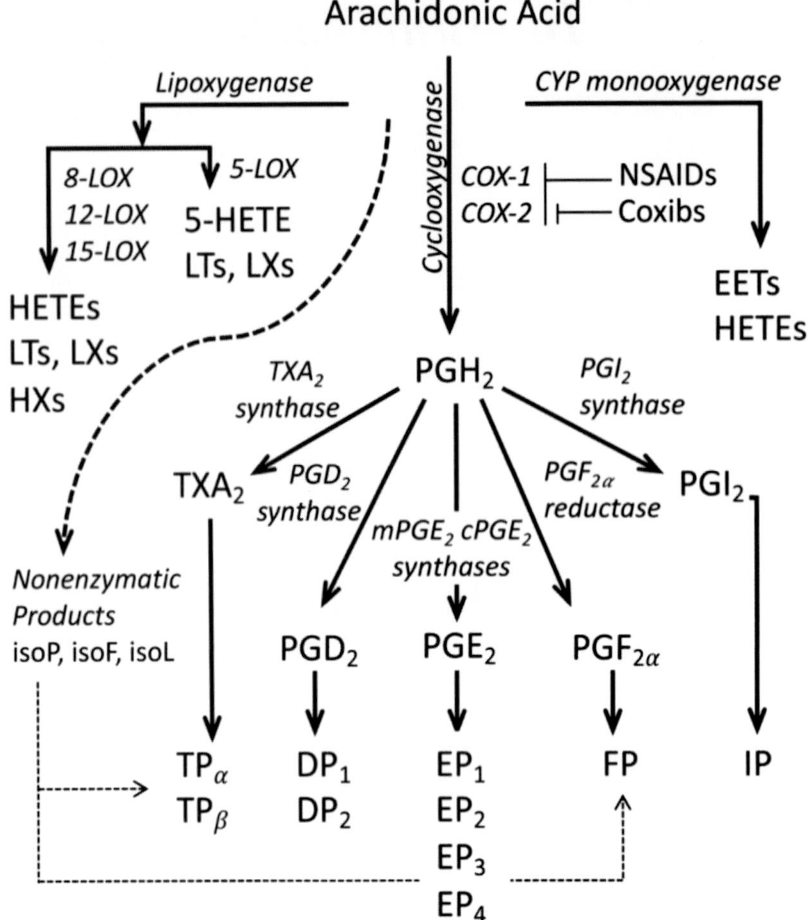

Figure 39.1 Arachidonic acid metabolism. Arachidonic acid is metabolized by lipoxygenase (LOX), cytochrome P450 (CYP), cyclooxygenase (COX), and other pathways. Nonsteroidal anti-inflammatory drugs (NSAIDs) and selective COX-2 inhibitors (Coxibs) block conversion of arachidonic acid into prostaglandin H_2 (PGH_2). Individual synthases convert PGH_2 into PG species which act via their respective receptors.

regulation of ion and water transport in the kidneys as well as of gastrointestinal motility and secretion. The "2-series" prostanoids (indicating the number of carbon–carbon double bonds) are the most abundant and well-characterized physiologic mediators: prostaglandin E_2 (PGE_2), $PGF_{2\alpha}$, PGD_2, PGI_2 (prostacyclin), and thromboxane A_2 (TXA_2). Other prostanoid-like eicosanoid family members (such as isoprostanes and neuroprostanes) also exert biologic effects through receptors and mechanisms that are not yet clearly identified, but will not be covered in this chapter.

PG biosynthesis relies on the mobilization of arachidonic acid (AA) from membrane-bound glycerophospholipids by cytosolic phospholipases or secretory phospholipases ($cPLA_2$, $sPLA_2$). PLA enzymes operate at basal homeostatic levels and in response to intracellular and extracellular stimuli. PLA activity plays a substrate-limiting role in AA availability and thus the regulation of PG synthesis. The PG endoperoxide H synthase enzymes (PGHS1 or COX-1 and PGHS2 or COX-2) are responsible for the committed step in PG synthesis, resulting in the conversion of AA to prostanoids (Fig. 39.2). There are two different genes encoding the COX-1 and COX-2 proteins, with 60% to 65% sequence identity between isoforms and 85% to 90% sequence conservation between different species.[1] An mRNA splice variant that retains intron-1 of COX-1, termed COX-3, and a novel COX-2 variant have also been identified and may have roles in acetaminophen response or the resolution of inflammation, respectively,[2–4] but neither of these variants have been validated clinically.

In general, COX-1 is constitutively expressed in most tissues and is responsible for the maintenance of tissue homeostasis and basal PG production, whereas COX-2 is considered an inducible isoform that is highly and rapidly expressed in response to inflammation and other molecular or environmental triggers. However, the complexity of COX isoform specificity defies simple categorization[5] as COX-1 contributes to PG generation in some inflamed tissues and during tumorigenesis.[6–8] Moreover, COX-2 may be expressed in a number of normal tissues independent of noxious stimuli, particularly during development.[9–11] For instance, COX-2 is highly expressed in kidneys, and disruption of its gene (in mice) leads to fatal renal failure[12,13]; adverse renal effects have also been observed with selective COX-2 inhibitors (coxibs).[14] COX-2 may be normally expressed in perinatal brain, skin, heart, cartilage, placenta, and other tissues, depending on the developmental stage.[11,15] Gene deletion studies in mice also reveal that one COX isoform may be upregulated to compensate for the absence of the other COX isoform in certain tissues.[16–19]

The COX-1 and COX-2 proteins are bifunctional enzymes that catalyze similar oxygenation–reduction reactions by converting AA, two electrons, and two oxygen molecules into PGH_2

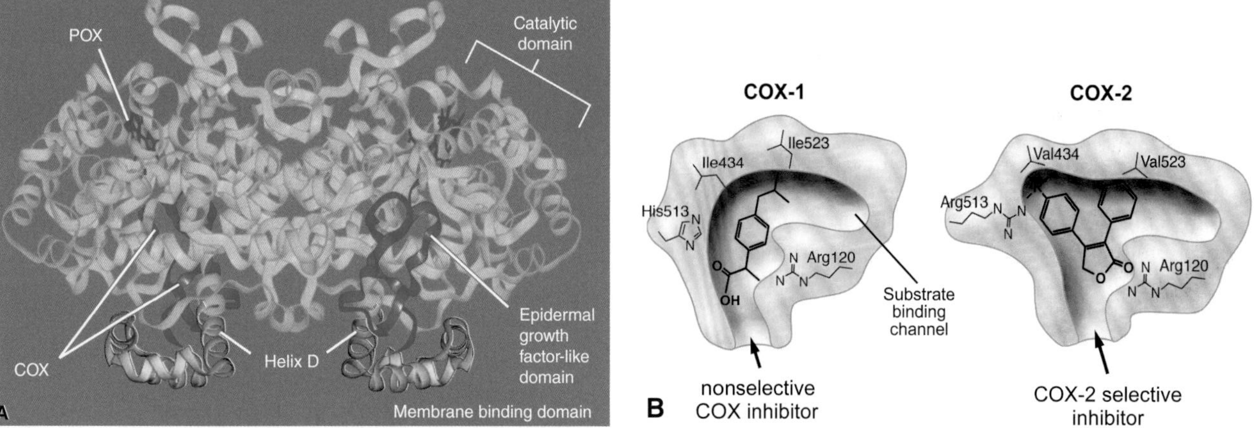

Figure 39.2 Cyclooxygenase structure. **A:** Ribbon diagram representing the COX-2 homodimer and major functional domains. (Adapted with permission from Marnett LJ. The COXIB experience: a look in the rearview mirror. *Annu Rev Pharmacol Toxicol* 2009;49:265.) **B:** Depiction of different COX-1 and COX-2 substrate binding channels illustrating various amino acid residues that create a side pocket that is more accessible in COX-2, whereas residues occupying more space in the COX-1 channel block the bulky side chains of selective COX-2 inhibitors. (Adapted with permission from Grosser T, Fries S, FitzGerald GA. Biological basis for the cardiovascular consequences of COX-2 inhibition: therapeutic challenges and opportunities. *J. Clin Invest* 2006; 116: 4–15.)

in two steps: (1) a bis-dioxygenation (COX) reaction to form PGG_2 as an intermediate PG species and (2) a peroxidation (POX) reaction that reduces the hydroperoxide group of PGG_2 to form PGH_2. The COX and POX reactions are interconnected but occur at different physical locations on the COX enzyme, requiring movement of intermediates from the internal COX catalytic pocket to the superficial POX site[20] (see Fig. 39.2). Despite their biochemical similarities, COX-1 has more limited substrate specificity, preferentially oxygenating AA to form various prostanoids. COX-2 has more liberal substrate specificity, including the ability to oxygenate dihomo-linolenic acid (DHLA), eicosapentaenoic acid (EPA), and neutral derivatives of AA such as 2-arachidonylglycerol (2-AG) and anandamide (AEA).[21,22] 2-AG and AEA are endogenous ligands of the cannabinoid receptor system, which mediates numerous physiologic processes including pain, inflammation, stress, hemodynamic stability, immunomodulation, and cellular homeostasis. Thus, pharmacologic inhibitors of COX enzymes may impact the oxygenation of 2-AG, AEA, and other substrates with important biologic functions.

COX enzymes are hemeproteins that exist as homodimers of two 70-kDa subunits. Their membrane binding domains are anchored to the cell membrane at the cell surface, of the nuclear envelope, endoplasmic reticulum or Golgi, and form a central opening where AA and FAs originating from within the lipid membrane gain access to the COX catalytic site. Evidence suggests that COX monomers within a homodimer may not function independently[23,24] and that COX dimers act as a conformational heterodimer consisting of an allosteric and a catalytic monomer that function cooperatively.[21,25,26] The downstream PGH_2 product derived from homodimers of either COX-1 or COX-2 is converted into specific prostanoids by individual tissue-specific PG isomerases or synthases. PGE_2 formation is catalyzed by at least one cytosolic (cPGES) and two microsomal (mPGES) isoforms[27–29]; PGD_2 by three PGD_2 synthases of which the principal one is lipocalin PGD_2 synthase; and $PGF_{2\alpha}$, PGI_2, and TXA_2 by specific individual enzymes. Synthases for PGI_2 and TXA_2 also exhibit CYP properties and belong to corresponding CYP8 and CYP5 subfamilies, respectively. Tissues typically convert PGH_2 to a subset of these prostanoids, but not all five, based on cell-specific synthase activity. For example, COX-1 activity in platelets results in TXA_2 and PGD_2 production, whereas the endothelium typically makes PGI_2 and PGE_2 based on the predominance of select synthases.

PROSTANOID RECEPTORS

Individual prostanoids exert their effects through their respective G protein–coupled receptors. Distinct receptors were identified for each prostanoid by pharmacologic characterization and were subsequently confirmed biochemically. Prostanoid receptors are designated according to their ligands such that receptors for PGD_2, PGE_2, $PGF_{2\alpha}$, PGI_2, and TXA_2 are classified, respectively, as DP, EP, FP, IP, and TP. The EP receptors are further divided into EP_1, EP_2, EP_3, and EP_4 subtypes.[30,31] The eight known types of prostanoid receptors are each encoded by an individual gene and are highly conserved across mammalian species. Although evidence exists for two DP receptors, DP_1 and DP_2 (CRTh2), DP_2 is more closely related to chemoattractant receptors and shares little homology with other prostanoid receptors. Cloning of the prostanoid receptors identified another degree of heterogeneity related to mRNA splicing. Splice variants have been identified for most prostanoid receptor homologues of various species. There are currently 10 known EP_3 splice variants coding for eight different human EP_3 receptor isoforms: $EP_{3\text{-Ia}}$, $EP_{3\text{-Ib}}$, $EP_{3\text{-Ic}}$, $EP_{3\text{-II}}$, $EP_{3\text{-III}}$, $EP_{3\text{-IV}}$, $EP_{3\text{-V}}$, $EP_{3\text{-VI}}$, $EP_{3\text{-e}}$, and $EP_{3\text{-f}}$[32–36]; subtypes of the EP_3 receptors are distinguished by variation in the tail of the carboxy-terminal portion. Human subtypes also exist for the TP receptor[37] (TP_α and TP_β), which vary in their carboxy terminus, similar to EP_3 subtypes, and the FP receptor (FP-v1 and FP-v2), where FP-v2 forms a truncated protein.[38,39]

Prostanoid receptors are rhodopsin-type receptors containing seven transmembrane domains, an extracellular amino terminus and intracellular carboxy terminus and belong to the superfamily of G protein–coupled receptors. There are 28 amino acid residues conserved within all prostanoid receptor sequences, and eight of these are shared with other G protein–coupled receptors. These conserved regions are particularly important in receptor structure/function and are thought to play fundamental roles in the structure of the prostanoid binding domains. For instance, an arginine in the seventh transmembrane domain conserved between all prostanoid receptors is proposed to be the binding site for the carboxyl moiety of the prostanoids[40,41]; the conserved motif in the second extracellular loop may also function in this regard.[40] In addition, glycosylation is required for ligand binding of certain prostanoid receptors.[42,43] Prostanoid receptors are also known to form heterodimers with other prostanoid receptor subtypes or nonprostanoid receptors. Receptor heterodimerization creates novel binding sites, expands the repertoire of G protein coupling, and provides alternative regulatory control mechanisms for simultaneously released ligands. Notable examples include heterodimerization between IP and TP receptors,[44,45] EP_1 and β_2-adrenergic receptors,[46] and EP_2 and the calcitonin receptor.[47]

The overall sequence homology between different prostanoid receptors within a species is only 20% to 30%, although sequence conservation between specific receptor homologues in mice and humans ranges from 70% to 90%.[48] Receptor homology is mainly based on signaling pathway rather than ligand preference.[49–51] The effects mediated by prostanoid receptors in smooth muscle reflect this relationship. Thus, DP_1, EP_2, EP_4, and IP elicit smooth muscle relaxation and are more closely related to each other than to the other prostanoid receptors. Similarly, EP_1, FP, and TP receptors cause smooth muscle contraction and form another group based on sequence homology.

Three groups of related receptors have been defined based on phylogenetic clustering of their signaling pathways: (i) DP_1, EP_2, EP_4, and IP; (ii) EP_1, FP, and TP; and (iii) EP_3. Prostanoid receptors in Group (i) are linked to heterotrimeric G proteins that are composed of a G_α subunit that generally stimulates adenylate cyclase (designated G_s) to produce cyclic adenosine monophosphate (AMP). Accordingly, its dominant effect on smooth muscle is relaxation. Prostanoid receptors in Group (ii) couple mostly to increases in intracellular free Ca^{2+} through the activation of PLC by G_q, with subsequent inositol phosphate liberation. In smooth muscle, stimulation of this group of receptors leads to contraction. Group (iii), which constitutes the EP_3 subtypes of the prostanoid receptor family, employs as its primary effector pathway inhibition of adenylate cyclase through the G_i family.[52] However, because of the variant molecular nature of EP_3, the latter can couple to a variety of G proteins.

The biologic effects of prostanoids are largely defined by their receptors. For example, the roles of PGE_2 and PGD_2 in inflammation are well established.[53] PGE_2 through its EP_3 receptor is also significantly implicated in pyrexia,[54] whereas PGD_2 via its DP receptor seems to contribute to allergen-evoked bronchoconstriction[55]; moreover, the PGD_2 metabolite 15-deoxy-Δ-PGJ_2[28,56] is a potent immune modulator. The overall importance of prostanoid receptor signaling and their distinct temporal expression and cellular distribution patterns render them attractive targets for selective pharmacologic antagonism.[48,57–59] Corresponding compounds are emerging as alternatives to traditional NSAIDs, but require further study.

NONSTEROIDAL ANTI-INFLAMMATORY DRUGS

NSAIDs are a heterogeneous group of agents, which inhibit COX-mediated PG synthesis (see Fig. 39.1). The NSAID parent compound, salicylic acid, was purified in 1829 and commercially synthesized in the mid-1800s. By 1853, salicylic acid had been successfully acetylated and was marketed as aspirin in 1899. Subsequent NSAID development led to the production of phenacetin (1887), acetaminophen (1888), phenylbutazone (1949), the fenamates (the 1950s), ibuprofen (1961), and indomethacin (1963). NSAIDs can be classified based on their chemical structure. Soon after the identification of the inducible COX-2 isoform,[60,61] aggressive efforts were made to develop compounds with selective COX-2 inhibitory properties ("coxibs").[62] Older NSAIDs with COX-2 preferential inhibitory properties were also identified, including nimesulide, meloxicam, and etodolac[63] (Fig. 39.3). The race to identify compounds with selective COX-2 inhibitory properties was spurred by the adverse gastrointestinal, renal, and other systemic side effects of nonselective NSAIDs (discussed below).

NSAIDs exert antipyretic, anti-inflammatory, and antinociceptive effects. Their long-term use has been associated with reductions in thrombosis, certain cancers, and some

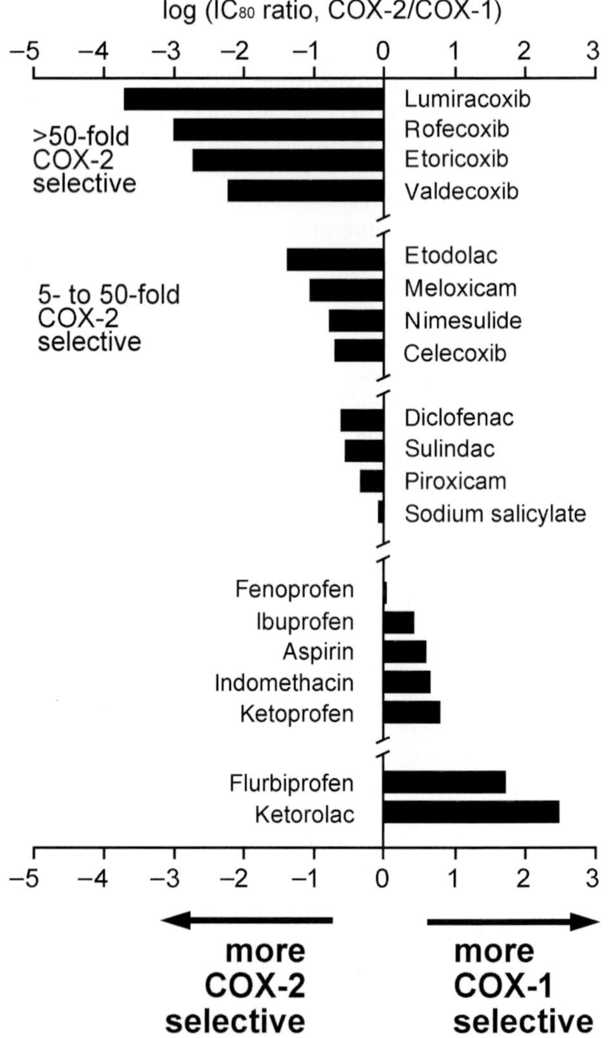

Figure 39.3 Relative selectivity of different nonsteroidal anti-inflammatory drugs (NSAIDs). Values extrapolated from inhibition curves for each compound against COX-1 and COX-2 in a human modified whole blood assay. Bars represent the ratio of IC_{80} plotted logarithmically. (Adapted with permission from Warner TD, Mitchell JA. Cyclooxygenases: new forms, new inhibitors, and lessons from the clinic. *FASEB J* 2004;18;790.)

neuroinflammatory conditions like Alzheimer's disease and possibly Parkinson's disease. The general mechanism of action of NSAIDs is based on competitive inhibition of substrate (AA or other FA) binding at the internal COX catalytic site. One helix of the membrane binding domain of each COX monomer forms an orifice that allows arachidonate or NSAIDs, which are hydrophobic, to gain access to the COX active site from within the lipid bilayer (see Fig. 39.2). NSAID binding involves drug entry into the COX channel, where a positively charged Arg120 residue binds to the negatively charged carboxylate groups of substrates and most NSAIDs.[1] Multiple residues lining the COX channel further orient FA substrates and influence the position of NSAID binding (see Fig. 39.2). The function of COX enzymes as conformational heterodimers results in NSAID binding with higher affinity to either the catalytic or the allosteric monomer to inhibit PG synthesis.[21,25,26,62] Some NSAIDs exert their effects on catalytic enzyme activity by binding to the allosteric subunit (ibuprofen, naproxen, and flurbiprofen). NSAIDs may also act via a novel substrate-selective COX inhibitory mechanism where binding of the inhibitor to a single COX monomer inhibits endocannabinoid, but not arachidonate oxygenation.[64–66] This mechanism may be relevant for neuropsychiatric or other pathophysiologic conditions where the generation of increased endocannabinoid signaling is beneficial.

Most NSAIDs exhibit time-dependent, competitive enzyme inhibition in experimental assays. Thus, in addition to their catalytic or allosteric inhibitory properties, three modes of inhibition have been used to describe the binding of NSAIDs to the COX active site: (1) rapid and reversible (e.g., ibuprofen), (2) rapid, time-dependent, and slowly reversible (e.g., flurbiprofen), or (3) rapid, briefly reversible followed by covalent (irreversible) modification of the serine-530 residue in the COX channel (e.g., the site of COX acetylation by aspirin). In general, COX-1 and COX-2 isoforms have relatively similar COX active sites, catalytic mechanisms, prostanoid products, and enzyme kinetics. Despite these similarities, gene-swapping studies in mice show that COX-1 and COX-2 functions are not fully interchangeable.[67] In addition, the COX-2 catalytic channel is approximately 20% larger and shaped differently than COX-1 owing to the position of one helix in the membrane binding domain of COX-2 and three amino acid differences that help form a larger side pocket for drug and substrate binding in the COX-2 channel[1] (see Fig. 39.2). COX-2 selectivity is thus conferred by less stringent steric and ionic properties, different residues lining the COX-2 channel that favor some compounds, and complex enzyme inhibitor kinetics that are not fully defined.[62] Coxibs take advantage of these properties as selective, time-dependent, pseudo-irreversible inhibitors of the COX-2 isoform.

Despite the pleiotropic nature of PGs in various physiologic and pathologic processes, the effects of NSAIDs cannot be solely attributed to the inhibition of COX. Indeed, COX inhibitors exert a number of COX-independent actions. For instance, doses of aspirin needed to treat chronic inflammatory conditions are much higher than those required to inhibit PG synthesis. A number of cellular mechanisms affected by NSAIDs, such as angiogenesis, apoptosis, and cell cycle progression, have been observed at NSAID concentrations 100- to 1,000-fold greater than those needed to inhibit PG formation. In this process, a number of targets other than COX have been identified that are affected by NSAIDs, including nuclear factor κB (NF-κB), mitogen-activated protein kinase (Erk2), ribosomal S6 kinase 2, signal transducer and activator of transcription-1 (STAT1), peroxisome proliferator-activated receptor γ (PPARγ), and Akt protein kinase.[68–71] However, the effects of NSAIDs on these targets differ between NSAIDs.[72] Moreover, although effects on COX are relatively restricted to the S-stereoisomers, R-stereoisomers act on some of the targets mentioned above.

Notwithstanding these diverse molecular effects, the major mechanism of action of NSAIDs is through the inhibition of PG biosynthesis. This is consistent with the proinflammatory properties of certain PGs,[63] the fever-inducing actions of PGE_2 via its EP_3 receptors, and nociceptive actions of PGI_2. The mechanism of action of acetaminophen is somewhat debatable. Although attempts to explain its main mechanism of action in vivo through the inhibition of COX-3 have been challenged,[73,74] some studies report significant COX-2 inhibition[56] particularly in the physiologic setting when AA levels and peroxide tone are relatively low[74,75]; but at present, increasing evidence points to interference with POX portion of the COX enzyme as acetaminophen's main mode of action.[76] Nonetheless, some nociceptive modulation by acetaminophen may also arise from the activation of descending serotonergic pathways.[77,78]

PHARMACOKINETIC PROPERTIES OF NONSTEROIDAL ANTI-INFLAMMATORY DRUGS

Detailed reviews on the pharmacokinetics of NSAIDs in the pediatric population have been reported.[79–81] The pharmacokinetic properties of NSAIDs in children are notable for interindividual differences. In general, NSAIDs are rapidly absorbed from the intestine to reach maximal plasma concentrations within 1 to 2 hours. They tend to equilibrate in a small volume of distribution and are highly bound to plasma proteins. In children, the apparent volume of distribution is greater than that in adults for diclofenac, ibuprofen, ketorolac, and nimesulide for reasons that are not yet clear. Assuming a comparable concentration–efficacy relationship, children may require higher loading doses; this is readily observed for effective treatment of PDA in neonates where a higher loading dose of NSAIDs increases closure rate.[82–84] NSAIDs are metabolized via Phases I and II biotransformations. Conjugation occurs mostly with glucuronic acid and sulfate producing mostly inactive compounds. Approximately 60% to 70% of metabolized agents are excreted in urine and the rest in feces.

Aspirin is rapidly absorbed enterally with a t_{max} of 2 hours. It is readily deacetylated by intestinal, hepatic, and blood esterases. Distribution is throughout most body tissues, including the central nervous system, and crosses the placental barrier. The volume of distribution for aspirin is approximately 170 mL per kg at normal doses. Protein binding and volume of distribution are dose-dependent.[85] Aspirin is metabolized by liver enzymes mostly into salicyluric acid, salicyl phenolic glucuronide, and salicyl acyl glucuronide and altogether accounts for 90% of metabolites that are inactive and eliminated by the kidneys; because of the ionized form of this acid, its renal elimination is favored in alkaline urine. Interestingly, aspirin metabolism is relatively rapidly saturated, such that its kinetics proceeds from first to zero order; accordingly, the half-life of aspirin changes as a function of dose.

Acetaminophen (paracetamol) is commonly used in the pediatric population. Orally administered acetaminophen is rapidly (t_{max} = 0.5–0.75 hour) and nearly fully absorbed (90% bioavailability). The absorption of rectally administered acetaminophen, however, is variable with a mean bioavailability of 47% in children. In contrast to most NSAIDs, this drug has limited protein binding (10% to 25%). Plasma clearance of acetaminophen was also shown to increase (and thus correspondingly the half-life to decrease) as a function of maturation in preterm infants.[84,86] Accordingly, terminal $t½$ is 3.25 hours in extremely premature neonates versus 2.4 hours in adults.[87] Acetaminophen is principally metabolized in the liver by glucuronidation (50% to 60%) and sulfation (25% to 30%), and less than 10% remains unmodified. Developmental aspects of acetaminophen metabolism are important. In children, sulfate conjugation is the dominant pathway up to 9 years of age, and glucuronidation pathways mature over the first few years of life. A small amount of acetaminophen is oxidized by hepatic CYP2E1 and other CYP enzymes.[88,89] This pathway generates electrophilic compounds that require glutathione for detoxification. In an overdose, this pathway is overutilized, resulting in glutathione depletion and hepatic toxicity caused by the acetaminophen metabolite *N*-acetyl-*p*-benzoquinone imine (NAPQI). Term and preterm newborns may be at lower risk for hepatic injury owing to the relative lack of glucuronidation activity in the neonatal liver, although some exceptions are reported.[90]

In the neonate, indomethacin displays a prolonged half-life (17 to 20 hours) particularly in subjects weighing below 1 kg at birth.[91,92] $t_{½}$ for ibuprofen is even longer especially prior to postnatal day 3 when it is ~43 hours and then decreases to 20 to 27 hours by postnatal day 5 in preterm infants on average at 28 weeks postconceptional age[82,93]; at maturation, ibuprofen $t_{½}$ is ~2 hours. Other than developmental differences in metabolism which participates significantly to the decreased clearance of NSAIDs in newborns, genetic polymorphism also contributes to variability in the disposition of NSAIDs. In this case, *CYP2C9* and carboxylesterase-1 polymorphism affect elimination of indomethacin, whereas *CYP2C8*3* genetic variability affects disposition of ibuprofen.[94]

Selective coxibs were approved by the U.S. Food and Drug Administration (FDA) for a number of inflammatory and nociceptive indications. Coxibs demonstrate 200- to 300-fold selectivity for the inhibition of COX-2 over COX-1 at therapeutic doses.[95] Compounds such as celecoxib, rofecoxib, valdecoxib, and meloxicam (semi-selective coxibs) are readily absorbed enterally within 2 to 3 hours for the coxibs and 5 to 6 hours for meloxicam. Celecoxib, valdecoxib, and meloxicam are mainly metabolized by *CYP2C9* and to some extent by *CYP3A4*[96] and exhibit in the adult $t_{1/2}$ values of 11 to 20 hours. In children, celecoxib is also well absorbed orally but is cleared much faster with a $t_{1/2}$ of approximately 4 hours.[97] Rofecoxib is metabolized by *CYP1A2* and cytosolic liver enzymes[98] and has a $t_{1/2}$ of 17 hours; its disposition in children is reported to be similar to that in adults.[99] Although nonselective and selective coxibs have similar analgesic, anti-inflammatory, and antipyretic efficacy at clinical doses, coxibs have been prescribed with the goal of reducing risk for gastrointestinal toxicity. However, increased cardiovascular morbidity (and mortality) with a number of coxibs limited their availability in adult populations.[100,101] Coxibs are still prescribed for pediatric pain and inflammatory conditions, tempered by cardiovascular concerns.[102] Yet coxib-associated nephrotoxicity and other serious adverse events have also been reported in children.[103,104]

ANTIPYRETIC EFFICACY OF NONSTEROIDAL ANTI-INFLAMMATORY DRUGS

DEFINITION OF FEVER

Fever continues to be one of the most common symptoms why infants and children are brought to a health-care provider or to the emergency department.[105] The treatment of fever often represents a clinical dilemma "to treat or not to treat," a prescribing controversy, and can predispose to adverse effects.[106] Fever is defined herein as established in 1987 by the International Union of Physiological Sciences Thermal Commission, namely, "a state of elevated core temperature, which is often, but not necessarily, part of the defensive responses of multicellular organisms (host) to the invasion of live (microorganisms) or inanimate matter recognized as pathogenic or alien by the host."[107] Fever as a component of the febrile response involves a cytokine-mediated rise in core temperature, generation of acute-phase reactants, and activation of numerous physiologic, endocrinologic, and immunologic systems.[107] It is important to distinguish fever from hyperthermia, an unregulated rise in body temperature that does not involve pyrogenic cytokines and is unresponsive to antipyretics.[107]

PHYSIOLOGY OF FEVER

Fever involves the body's thermoregulatory system, a complex neural network extending from the hypothalamus and limbic system through the lower brain stem and reticular formation into the spinal cord and sympathetic ganglia. Thermosensitive neurons in the preoptic region of the rostral hypothalamus of the thermoregulatory system maintain the body's temperature within a narrow range via a central entity termed the "set point." Deviations from the set point can provoke multiple thermoregulatory responses.[107] When the preoptic temperature rises above its set point, based on circulation-borne neuronal signals from thermosensors throughout the skin and core body areas, physiologic heat loss responses are triggered. If the temperature falls below the set point, heat retention and heat production responses are activated.[107,108] The febrile response is stimulated with endogenous mediators of fever activating a series of responses to decrease heat loss and to increase heat production. This contrasting phenomenon that produces fever is clinically recognized as "a pyrogen-mediated rise in body temperature above the normal range."[107] In this context, fever is regarded to be an adaptive response, potentially beneficial to the patient.

Cytokines are among the more important pyrogens. These pleiotropic, intensely powerful proteins function singly or in groups to convey information from cell to cell within a complex network. The febrile response is mediated by exogenous and endogenous pyrogens. Exogenous pyrogens are of microbial origin inducing host cells, especially macrophages, to produce endogenous pyrogens. The most common endogenous pyrogenic cytokines are IL-1, tumor necrosis factor-α (TNF-α), IL-6, and interferon-γ (IFN-γ). These cytokines interact with receptors in the anterior hypothalamus to activate PLA_2, which in turn liberates plasma AA as a substrate for PGE_2 production, catalyzed by COX. PGE_2 in turn resets the hypothalamic set point and produces fever. Antipyretic drugs interrupt this pathway producing their pharmacologic effect.[107]

NONSTEROIDAL ANTI-INFLAMMATORY DRUGS AS ANTIPYRETIC DRUGS

NSAIDs are efficacious as antipyretic drugs for exogenous or endogenous pyrogen-induced fever, specifically the inhibition of COX to decrease hypothalamic PGE_2 and reduce proinflammatory mediators, among other actions.[109] In general, NSAIDs should be used with caution in patients with asthma, renal or hepatic insufficiency, bleeding disorders, gastrointestinal (GI) disease (particularly bleeding or ulcers), and those receiving anticoagulants. Use of more than one NSAID at the same time is not recommended. Non-aspirin NSAID agents have a possible cross-sensitivity with aspirin. Potential adverse cardiovascular effects of NSAIDs include prothrombotic effects, blood pressure elevation, reduced renal perfusion, fluid retention, and exacerbation of heart failure.[110]

NONSTEROIDAL ANTI-INFLAMMATORY DRUGS FOR NEOPLASTIC FEVER

Fever of nonmicrobial nature may also be responsive to NSAIDs. In this case, it has been suggested that NSAIDs (naproxen, indomethacin, and diclofenac) may be more effective for fever from cancer than from infection.[111] In a meta-analysis, naproxen in various dosages was shown to be highly successful for treating neoplastic fever and fever of unknown origin associated with solid tumors and hematologic malignancies.[112] We are unaware of pediatric studies that have demonstrated this distinction, yet it would be important for drug selection.

PROPERTIES OF NONSTEROIDAL ANTI-INFLAMMATORY DRUGS FOR FEVER

Aspirin

Pharmacokinetic and pharmacodynamic data and plasma concentration range for aspirin toxicity and efficacy were described after 80 years of pediatric dosing.[113] Although effective in treating fever, pain, and inflammatory diseases and as an antiplatelet agent, it causes a number of adverse effects (see below).

Ibuprofen

Ibuprofen, a nonselective COX inhibitor, is a commonly used effective analgesic, anti-inflammatory, and antipyretic drug in children.[114,115] Ibuprofen is approved for infants and children over 3 months of age.[116] Wide nonprescription use of ibuprofen may be responsible for the increased reported adverse effects in children.[117]

For infants greater than or equal to 6 months old, children, and adolescents ibuprofen is administered as 5 to 10 mg per kg per dose by mouth every 6 to 8 hours, maximum single dose of 400 mg, with a daily limit of 40 mg per kg per day, (maximum of 2,400 mg per day for adult-sized patient).[118] A variety of ibuprofen dosage forms include a concentrated infant drop formulation, 50 mg per 1.25 mL and oral liquid 20 mg per mL, in addition to chewable and regular tablets in over-the-counter and prescription strengths. Owing to the lack of over-the-counter labeling for infants less than 6 months old in the United States, clinicians may interpret this as ibuprofen is unsafe for younger infants. However, the British National Formulary provides specific dosing guidance for infants aged 1 to 3 months.[119]

Acetaminophen: Alone or Alternating with Ibuprofen

Controversy persists about whether combined or alternate therapy with ibuprofen and acetaminophen is superior to single-drug therapy, especially in terms of discomfort reduction and adverse effect profile. Pharmacokinetic–pharmacodynamic (PK–PD) analysis provides insights into the use of more than one antipyretic, either alternatingly or concurrently. Ibuprofen, with a longer duration of antipyresis, is expected to cover periods of acetaminophen ineffectiveness. Accordingly, alternating regimens seemed to stem from parents or physicians reacting to a minimal antipyretic efficacy, especially following the first dose of either drug. Despite the lack of scientific evidence that this practice is beneficial, the alternating use of ibuprofen and acetaminophen is commonly recommended by pediatricians. Alternating therapy may complicate a caregiver's dosing instructions, increasing the potential for inaccurate dosing or overdosing. The labeled dosing schedule differs for each drug (i.e., ibuprofen every 6 to 8 hours and acetaminophen every 4 hours) so that time of dosing may prove awkward for parents, caregiver, and nursing staff to follow.

Two studies addressed the antipyretic efficacy and short-term safety of alternating acetaminophen with ibuprofen with varied results.[120,121] The study by Sarrell et al.[120] was a randomized, double-blinded, parallel-group trial, which demonstrated a mean lower temperature, a more rapid reduction in fever, and fewer fever recurrences in the alternating antipyretic group. There were no serious adverse effects of alternating acetaminophen and ibuprofen in this 2-week study. Critiques of this trial include study design (subjects had unusually high temperatures and received a loading dose of an antipyretic prior to maintenance therapy), clinical significance of the fever reduction, and concerns that alternating antipyretic therapy will increase chances of dosing error and promote parental fever phobia.[122] A recent meta-analysis of nine studies of combined or alternating therapy with ibuprofen or acetaminophen demonstrated more effectiveness than monotherapy in reducing body temperature[106]; however, investigators pointed out that this greater efficacy was modest and not clinically relevant. In this context, the American Academy of Pediatrics,[123] the National Institute for Health and Clinical Excellence,[124] and international guidelines[105] support treating fever to reduce the child's discomfort but advise against the routine use of combined and alternating acetaminophen and ibuprofen.

Ketorolac

Ketorolac is the only parenteral NSAID available in the United States that is approved for pain and has been used off-label in the treatment of fever.[125–127] This NSAID is frequently used for analgesia in children for the management of sickle cell pain or for postoperative pain.[125,126] The availability in parenteral dosage form and rapid onset of action would make this agent an ideal antipyretic in situations where an oral route is unavailable, provided there are no contraindications to NSAID use. Randomized, controlled trials are needed to determine antipyretic efficacy and safety of ketorolac in pediatrics.

Overall, it is important to use the same type of thermometer device and the same body site when comparing serial temperature measurements. When prescribing antipyretic therapy, inform caregivers of risks of excessive dosing. Risks from antipyretic drug therapy can be minimized by careful attention to the pediatric label for dose and frequency of administration.

NONSTEROIDAL ANTI-INFLAMMATORY DRUGS FOR PATENT DUCTUS ARTERIOSUS OF THE NEWBORN

Patency of the ductus arteriosus (DA) is essential for fetal well-being because it allows 90% of the right ventricular output to bypass the high-resistance pulmonary vascular bed in utero.[128] It connects the systemic and pulmonary vasculature compartments in utero and remains open owing to the presence of PGs (secreted by the placenta and the ductus itself) and the low arterial content in oxygen.[129] Normally, in term newborns, the PDA closes in the first 72 hours of life. Preterm infants exhibit immaturity in ductal closure mechanisms such that the incidence of spontaneous closure varies according to gestational age; only 35% of preterm infants less than 28 weeks' gestation spontaneously close their PDA.[130] PDA in preterm infants has been associated with increased mortality[131] and worsened outcome to lungs,[132] intestine,[133,134] and brain.[135–137] Its incidence is inversely related to gestational age; 50% to 70% of infants less than 28 weeks of gestation have a moderate-to-large PDA that persists for weeks after birth.[128,138] Sepsis, respiratory distress syndrome, and intrauterine growth restriction are among other clinical risk factors that predispose to PDA.[139] Genetic predispositions to PDA and treatment response also exist.[94] The optimal management of PDA in preterm newborns is controversial and remains debated. The major issue is the choice and timing of treatment if any. NSAIDs were traditionally used to treat the PDA in newborn as it decreases PG (PGE_2 is the most important DA relaxant) production by nonselective inhibition of the COX-1 and COX-2 enzymes.[128] Accordingly, the inhibition of PG formation favors ductal constriction. Other drug factors such as pharmacokinetics, pharmacodynamics, pharmacogenetics, additional confounding medical/physiologic factors, and environmental factors all interplay and contribute to DA patency. The two COX inhibitors approved for the treatment of ductal patency in North America are indomethacin and ibuprofen. Both have a success rate at closing the PDA of approximately 70% to 85%.[140] Lately, acetaminophen has also been shown to close the PDA and may be particularly valuable when contraindications to other NSAIDs are present; but in very immature newborns, acetaminophen seems less effective.[141]

CONSERVATIVE MANAGEMENT OF PDA

In the last decade, a watchful waiting approach on PDA management has emerged. When left untreated, most PDAs close spontaneously by 44 weeks postmenstrual age, providing arguments against pharmacologic closure of the PDA.[142–144] Thirty-four percent of extremely low birth weight (ELBW) infants (<1,000 g) will permanently close their DA by postnatal day 8,[145] and a greater number of PDA will close over the following weeks.[146–149] Two recent large meta-analyses involving greater than 4,000 babies each evaluated different treatment regimens with indomethacin, ibuprofen, and acetaminophen and concluded that there was no evidence to support the treatment of the PDA.[150,151] The recent exploratory randomized controlled trial of treatment of moderate-to-large PDA (PDA-TOLERATE study) showed that early (<7 days of age) routine pharmacologic PDA treatment, compared to conservative management in preterm infants less than 28 weeks of gestation, did not reduce neonatal morbidities (necrotizing enterocolitis, bronchopulmonary dysplasia, and death).[152] Despite evidence against treating all neonates with PDA, there are patients at higher risk of enduring significant blood flow deviation from the aorta to the pulmonary arteries that would benefit from PDA closure[153–155]; a better identification of clinical and/or echocardiographic criteria is thus needed[144] to deliver personalized treatment to infants most likely to benefit from it.[156–159]

TREATMENT OF PDA

In an attempt to potentially avoid complications of prematurity, numerous studies have shown that ductal closure is accelerated with NSAIDs. Nonselective inhibitors of COX (such as indomethacin and ibuprofen) exert comparable closure rates (~75% to 85% after a 3-day treatment course).[160] The following related sections will address prophylactic versus symptomatic management of PDA and the use and comparisons of indomethacin, ibuprofen, and acetaminophen.

Prophylactic versus Symptomatic Approach

The effectiveness of drugs that promote ductal closure is inversely related to the developmental age at the time of treatment.[161] Prophylactic or early pharmacologic PDA closure has been reported to decrease the incidence of several acute neonatal morbidities that occur during the first week after birth, including vasopressor-dependent hypotension,[162] early hemorrhagic pulmonary edema,[163] and the intensity of respiratory support[164]; in the longer term, bronchopulmonary dysplasia and death have been reduced.[165] The large (1,202 subjects) Trial of Indomethacin Prophylaxis in Preterm Infants (TIPP) was a multicenter, randomized, placebo-controlled trial on the use of prophylactic (first 12 hours of life) indomethacin in extremely premature newborns,[166] which confirmed ductal closure in response to treatment and revealed decreased early cerebral bleeding, consistent with prior reports.[167] However, survival without neurosensory impairments at 18 months of corrected age was not improved.[168] Despite the absence of long-term improvement of outcomes, many centers still use prophylactic indomethacin for premature newborns in view of tackling acute complications.[169]

Ibuprofen has also been used prophylactically to close the DA. Trials reveal that compared to placebo or no intervention, prophylactic ibuprofen probably decreases the incidence of PDA, the need for further treatment with cyclooxygenase inhibitors, and the need for surgical closure.[170] In a meta-analysis of nine trials (n = 1,070 infants), ibuprofen was found, as expected, to close the DA, with improved cerebral blood flow autoregulation[171] and reduced severe forms of intraventricular hemorrhage[170]; but the latter diverges from reports by others.[150] Furthermore, compared to placebo (or no treatment), prophylactic ibuprofen did not affect mortality, chronic lung disease, necrotizing enterocolitis, or time to reach full feeds.[170] Consequently, current evidence does not support the use of ibuprofen for the prevention of PDA. The main concern with a prophylactic approach is the wide exposure of subjects to a medication with potential side effects, when in most cases the PDA closes spontaneously in newborns.

Indomethacin for PDA

Indomethacin is the NSAID most studied for PDA in neonates, but exerts several adverse effects, notably renal failure and necrotizing enterocolitis.[172] It is successful in closing 80% to 86%

of DA in infants weighing 1,000 to 1,750 g and 54% of infants weighing less than 1,000 g.[173] This variable response is due to physiologic constraints of the more immature DA[174] and differing volume of distribution,[175] leading to high levels of variability in plasma concentrations for the same weight-based dosing. Accordingly, optimal therapeutic dosing is difficult to establish; acceptable doses range from 0.1 to 0.25 mg per kg administered every 12 to 24 hours. The cumulative closure rate reaches 90% with three courses but potentially increases the risk of periventricular leukomalacia.[176]

Numerous randomized trials (more than 50) have been performed to date to evaluate the efficacy of indomethacin in DA closure. The rate of success in DA closure is irrespective of the age of onset within ages studied. Despite its efficacy in the majority of preterm infants, response to indomethacin seems to be diminished in children of lowest gestational age.[177] In these cases, it has been observed that PGE_2 production resurges within 5 days of indomethacin treatment (~36 hours).[178,179] To circumvent this problem, prolonged treatments (5 to 7 days) with indomethacin were found to minimize ductal reopening.[180–182] Evaluation of longer term morbidities revealed that overall the duration of oxygen therapy, hospital stay, the rate of bronchopulmonary dysplasia, necrotizing enterocolitis, retinopathy of prematurity, and the rate of death, were unaffected by indomethacin treatment.

The TIPP discussed earlier revealed that prophylactic indomethacin reduces the rate of PDA in preterm infants and the rate of pulmonary hemorrhage in the first 72 hours of life, but the rate of bronchopulmonary dysplasia does not seem to be diminished[166,183,184]; this may partly be explained by harmful side effects of indomethacin on oxygenation and edema formation.[183] Prophylactic indomethacin also reduced the rate of severe (Grade 4) intraventricular hemorrhage,[166,167] but did not lead to improved long-term neurodevelopmental outcome,[166,185,186] possibly due to direct cerebral hemodynamic compromising effects of indomethacin.[187,188] When used in high-risk preterm infants (less than 28 weeks), prophylactic indomethacin does not affect the incidence of bronchopulmonary dysplasia but does reduce mortality,[189] and thus may be considered in extreme premature infants. Because bolus injections of indomethacin cause rapid decreases in renal,[54,187] cerebral,[190] and mesenteric blood flow,[187,191] continuous slow rate infusion of indomethacin has been suggested; using a 36-hour infusion of indomethacin, ductal closure rate was found to be similar to that after bolus injection without the cerebral, renal, and mesenteric hemodynamic compromise seen with the latter.[179,187,192]

Ibuprofen for PDA

Several randomized trials on symptomatic patent DA compared intravenous (IV) ibuprofen to indomethacin. Compared to placebo, ibuprofen is safe and effective in ELBW infants.[193] Ibuprofen is comparable to indomethacin in closing the DA (Fig. 39.4), with fewer side effects,[170,194] including minimal changes in cerebral, renal, and mesenteric hemodynamics in the neonate.[190,195,196] Population kinetics in neonates less than 29 weeks of gestation at birth reveal that the efficacy of ibuprofen can be optimized by doubling the dose to 20 mg per kg, followed by 10 mg per kg every 24 hour for 2 days, without increasing side effects.[83,197] Likewise, 24-hour infusion of ibuprofen was found to be more effective for sustained closure of PDA, with fewer gastrointestinal symptoms.[198]

Oliguria is the only physiologic variable found to be consistently observed in ibuprofen-treated infants. Otherwise there was no statistically significant difference between ibuprofen and indomethacin with regards to mortality, surgical ligation, the duration of ventilator support, intraventricular hemorrhage, periventricular leukomalacia, necrotizing enterocolitis, retinopathy of prematurity, sepsis, time to full feeds, gastrointestinal

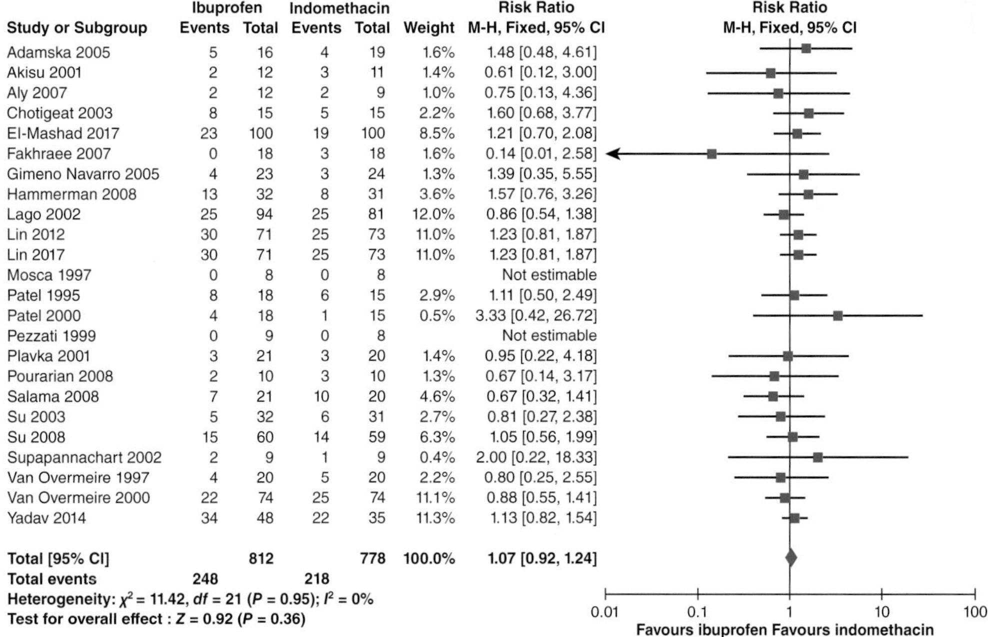

Study or Subgroup	Ibuprofen Events	Ibuprofen Total	Indomethacin Events	Indomethacin Total	Weight	Risk Ratio M-H, Fixed, 95% CI
Adamska 2005	5	16	4	19	1.6%	1.48 [0.48, 4.61]
Akisu 2001	2	12	3	11	1.4%	0.61 [0.12, 3.00]
Aly 2007	2	12	2	9	1.0%	0.75 [0.13, 4.36]
Chotigeat 2003	8	15	5	15	2.2%	1.60 [0.68, 3.77]
El-Mashad 2017	23	100	19	100	8.5%	1.21 [0.70, 2.08]
Fakhraee 2007	0	18	3	18	1.6%	0.14 [0.01, 2.58]
Gimeno Navarro 2005	4	23	3	24	1.3%	1.39 [0.35, 5.55]
Hammerman 2008	13	32	8	31	3.6%	1.57 [0.76, 3.26]
Lago 2002	25	94	25	81	12.0%	0.86 [0.54, 1.38]
Lin 2012	30	71	25	73	11.0%	1.23 [0.81, 1.87]
Lin 2017	30	71	25	73	11.0%	1.23 [0.81, 1.87]
Mosca 1997	0	8	0	8		Not estimable
Patel 1995	8	18	6	15	2.9%	1.11 [0.50, 2.49]
Patel 2000	4	18	1	15	0.5%	3.33 [0.42, 26.72]
Pezzati 1999	0	9	0	8		Not estimable
Plavka 2001	3	21	3	20	1.4%	0.95 [0.22, 4.18]
Pourarian 2008	2	10	3	10	1.3%	0.67 [0.14, 3.17]
Salama 2008	7	21	10	20	4.6%	0.67 [0.32, 1.41]
Su 2003	5	32	6	31	2.7%	0.81 [0.27, 2.38]
Su 2008	15	60	14	59	6.3%	1.05 [0.56, 1.99]
Supapannachart 2002	2	9	1	9	0.4%	2.00 [0.22, 18.33]
Van Overmeire 1997	4	20	5	20	2.2%	0.80 [0.25, 2.55]
Van Overmeire 2000	22	74	25	74	11.1%	0.88 [0.55, 1.41]
Yadav 2014	34	48	22	35	11.3%	1.13 [0.82, 1.54]
Total [95% CI]		**812**		**778**	**100.0%**	**1.07 [0.92, 1.24]**
Total events	**248**		**218**			

Heterogeneity: $\chi^2 = 11.42$, $df = 21$ ($P = 0.95$); $I^2 = 0\%$
Test for overall effect : $Z = 0.92$ ($P = 0.36$)

Figure 39.4 Comparisons of ibuprofen (oral or intravenous, IV) versus indomethacin (oral or IV) for ductus arteriosus closure after a first treatment course, depicted as forest plot. (Adapted with permission from Ohlsson A, Shah PS. Ibuprofen for the treatment of patent ductus arteriosus in preterm or low birth weight (or both) infants. *Cochrane Database Syst Rev* 2018; 9:CD003481.)

bleed, and the duration of hospital stay[199]; yet, a tendency toward decreased periventricular leukomalacia was observed in a large U.S. multicenter trial.[193] Along these lines, in contrast to indomethacin bolus dose of ibuprofen (10 mg per kg) does not compromise cerebral blood flow.[190] Yet, neither IV ibuprofen or indomethacin affects 2-year neurodevelopmental outcomes in preterm infants[200]; similar long-term observations have been made with oral ibuprofen.[201,202]

The relative unavailability of IV ibuprofen in many developing countries has fuelled the assessment of safety and efficacy of oral ibuprofen in the treatment or prophylaxis of PDA. Many studies have reported successful ductal closure with oral ibuprofen. Dosing employed is the same from the IV trials (10 mg per kg, followed by 5 mg per kg every 24 hours for 2 days). Pharmacokinetic studies revealed lower plasma ibuprofen concentration following oral compared with IV administration.[203,204] However, studies have shown that oral ibuprofen leads to higher primary closure rate (83.3% vs. 61.7%) than that of IV ibuprofen.[205,206] To explain this, it has been proposed that a more gradual rise in ibuprofen plasma levels and longer duration of action from the oral administration could potentially lead to a more sustained inhibition of PG synthesis despite the lower plasma levels.[42,203,207] Although none of the studies on oral ibuprofen reported gastrointestinal adverse events, the safety of the osmolarity of oral ibuprofen formulations and its potential impact on the preterm gut have been raised as a concern.[15] Interestingly, rectal ibuprofen was also effective in closing the PDA in very low birth weight infants.[208]

Overall, ibuprofen and indomethacin exert similar efficacy in ductal closure, but the former appears to display slightly fewer adverse effects.

Acetaminophen for PDA

Adverse effects associated with the use of indomethacin and to a lesser extent ibuprofen have encouraged the search for alternative drug treatments for PDA. Paracetamol was first suggested as an alternative in a case report of five preterm infants who failed or had contraindications to treatment with ibuprofen[209]; PDA successfully closed in three of five infants. In a meta-analysis involving eight eligible studies enrolling 916 infants, both oral and IV forms can be used and exhibit similar efficacy to ibuprofen and indomethacin in closing the DA in moderate-to-late preterm infants[210] (Fig. 39.5), without the gastrointestinal complications associated with NSAIDs; creatinine and bilirubin levels were lower in the paracetamol-treated group. In extremely premature infants, acetaminophen seems to be less effective than indomethacin and ibuprofen to achieve PDA closure[141,211]; girls

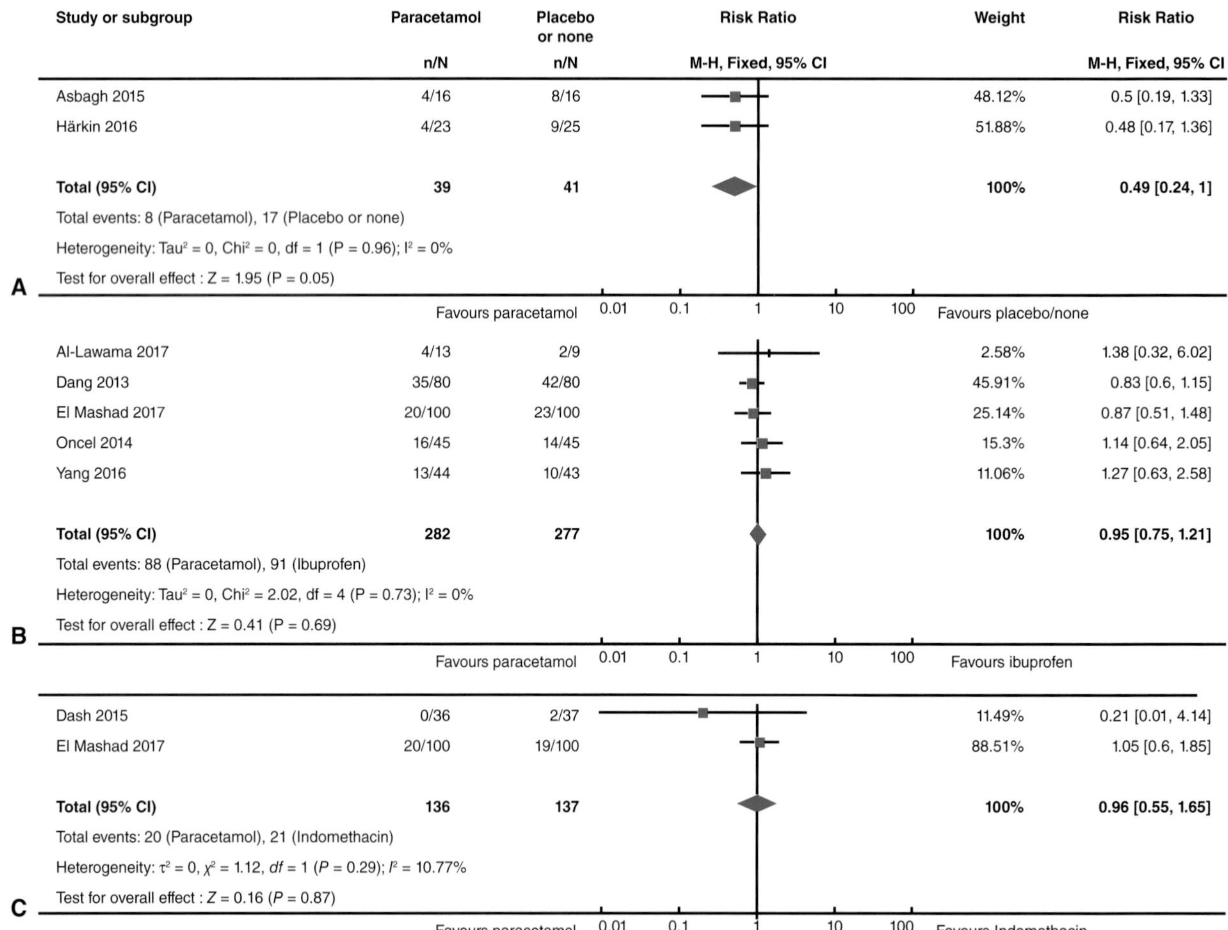

Figure 39.5 Comparisons of paracetamol (acetaminophen) (oral or intravenous, IV) versus placebo/none **(A)**, ibuprofen (oral or IV) **(B)**, or indomethacin (oral or IV) **(C)** for the closure of ductus arteriosus after a first treatment course, depicted as forest plot. (Adapted with permission from Ohlsson A, Shah PS. Paracetamol (acetaminophen) for patent ductus arteriosus in preterm or low birth weight infants. *Cochrane Database Syst Rev.* 2018;4:CD010061.)

also appear to be less responsive to acetaminophen.[212] Overall, acetaminophen causes PDA closure, respectively, in 49% and 76% of subjects after 3 and 6 days of treatment.[213] Combined treatment of ibuprofen and acetaminophen has been proposed, but benefits are unknown.[214,215] An IV dose of 60 mg per kg per day of acetaminophen divided in four doses for a period of 3 days effectively closes the PDA.[216] The same oral dose is effective; but treatment prolongation for 3 to 7 days augments definitive closure rate.[217] The optimal drug concentration for PDA closure is unknown. Acetaminophen is well tolerated in preterm neonates consistent with its safety.[218–220]

Regarding long-term outcomes, only one study reported a follow-up to 18 to 24 months of age following treatment with acetaminophen and ibuprofen for PDA and found no significant difference.[216] Yet, regular exposure (> six times) to acetaminophen (or ibuprofen) in the neonatal period has been reported to increase the risk of abnormal executive function,[221] attention deficit disorders,[222] and autistic behavior later in life,[223,224] but these sequelae have been contested[225,226] consistent with a long-standing safety profile of acetaminophen,[227] as adverse effects are more likely associated with frequent treatments[221]; along these lines, a meta-analysis of studies on single acetaminophen treatment of PDA was not significantly associated with neurodevelopmental disorders.[210] Yet, careful evaluation of long-term effects of acetaminophen needs to be pursued.

COX-1, COX-2, AND PGE_2 RECEPTORS IN THE DA

The fetal DA expresses EP_2, EP_3, and EP_4 receptors of PGE_2.[228–230] Interestingly, stimulation of all three receptors evokes DA relaxation.[229] Ontogenic changes in PGE_2 receptor profile in the DA are still debated. PGE_2 mediates DA relaxation through the EP_4 receptor,[231] and EP_4 is the most important PGE receptor in the DA.[7] Stimulation of EP_4 opens the DA,[232,233] and antagonism of EP_4 closes it.[234,235] Genetic disruption of EP_4 is associated with patent DA,[231] and chronic stimulation of EP_4 promotes hyaluronan-mediated neointimal formation of the DA.[236] Hence, as suggested above for COX-2,[237,238] it may be conceivable that EP_4 participates in triggering the ultimate closure of the DA. Recently, in a research for finding explanation in the PDA closure failure, isoprostanes were described as another potential mechanism for the relaxation of the premature DA that is independent of COX/EP_4.[239]

COX-1 is broadly expressed in the DA, whereas COX-2 is mostly localized on endothelium.[240] Coxibs have been introduced with the claim that they cause fewer adverse effects, but developmental compromise has limited the pursuit of coxibs for the newborn. Animal experiments have revealed in some species expression of COX-2 in the fetal DA,[241,242] which appears to increase with advancing gestation and contributes to most of the local PGE_2 generation.[243] However, selective inhibition of COX-2 (including celecoxib) increases ductal tone to a lesser extent than COX-1 or nonselective COX inhibitors.[241,243] Interestingly, COX-2 deficiency in the DA may interfere with DA closure,[237,238] suggesting that COX-2 may be required for DA closure. Consistent with these observations, a randomized trial for women at a risk of preterm delivery revealed that maternal administration of the selective coxib celecoxib did not cause fetal ductal closure,[97] whereas the semi-selective coxib nimesulide may not be as safe to the fetus as it caused ductal contraction comparable to that seen with indomethacin.[244] More importantly, even if selective coxibs do not close DA in the fetus and may be ineffective in the preterm neonate, adverse renal effects are a serious concern,[245] possibly particularly to the neonate.[246] Hence, along with the current relative moratorium on coxibs because of potential serious adverse effects, the use of coxibs cannot be justified.

Microsomal PGE synthase is the principal generator of PGE_2 in the DA.[247] Genetic deletion and pharmacologic-induced diminished expression of microsomal PGE synthase[248] are associated with increased DA tone; this suggests that microsomal PGE synthase may be a potential target for DA closure.

Certain congenital heart malformations (e.g., transposition of great vessels, tetralogy of Fallot, and coarctation of aorta) require that the DA remains patent via PG infusion (PGE_1) for adequate systemic or pulmonary circulation prior to corrective surgery.[249] PGE^1 infusion is associated with adverse effects such as apnea and peripheral vasodilation.[250] More selective EP stimulation or gene expression target may offer advantages, and the development of DA-specific pharmacologic therapies should be prioritized.

NONSTEROIDAL ANTI-INFLAMMATORY DRUGS IN PRETERM LABOR

Preterm birth (PTB; delivery before 37 weeks of gestation) affects one in 10 newborns and is the second leading cause of infant deaths worldwide.[251,252] The etiology of PTB remains mostly unknown.

As reviewed by the present authors, the onset of labor begins several days before delivery with changes in gestational tissues, culminating in powerful contractions to expulse the conceptus.[253] Term labor and PTL (labor before term) share a common (patho) physiologic process, including activation of the membranes/decidua (detachment of the chorioamniotic membranes from the decidua and rupture of the membrane), uterine contractility (shift from irregular contractions to functional contractions), and cervical ripening (dilatation and effacement of the cervix owing to changes in cervical composition and increasing myometrial contractility).[254] Based on predominant medical condition at presentation, many causes of PTL have been suggested, including infection (causally linked to PTL), fetal growth disorders, ischemia, uterine overdistension, cervical incompetence, fetal and maternal stress, hemorrhage, and several others[255]; yet, PTL in early third trimester is mostly associated with inflammation.[256] Converging lines of evidences suggest that inflammation plays a prominent role in very PTL, regardless of the presence of infection, other etiology, or timing of delivery.[257,258]

Inflammatory Cascade and Activation of COX Leading to PTB

Birth reflects transition from a pro-pregnancy state and immunologic tolerance toward the fetus allograft to a pro-labor, pro-inflammatory state. Notwithstanding the role of hormones, pro-inflammatory cytokines are thought to orchestrate the on-time synchronization of the aforementioned physiologic events characterizing labor through the induction of uterine activation proteins (UAPs; including COX-2, $PGF_{2\alpha}$ receptor, oxytocin receptor, connexin-43, and others).[259–261] Once activated, the uterus produces powerful contractions in response to endogenous uterotonins, mostly $PGF_{2\alpha}$, resulting in labor at term or at preterm.[262–265]

Based on earlier observations that PGs contribute to parturition,[266] including evidence that PGE_2 and $PGF_{2\alpha}$ induce labor,[267] a rationale to lower PG levels had been introduced. The use of nonselective COX inhibitor, indomethacin, was first shown to treat PTL in the early 1970s.[268] This was followed by a study demonstrating the success of indomethacin in treated versus placebo-administered patients[269] and a superiority of indomethacin over betamimetics.[270,271] This preliminary efficacy of COX inhibition led to investigation of inducible coxibs in PTL.[272] The latter potentially promising single-case study was subsequently followed by the documentation of significant adverse effects of coxibs (nimesulide and to a greater extent rofecoxib) on fetal kidney function and development,[273,274] which halted pursuit of investigations using coxibs for PTL.

The above divergent conclusions on the efficacy of COX inhibition in PTL beg the question as to evidence for increased COX expression, as well as the tissue and timing involved. In a recent evaluation of various studies conducted on COX-1 and COX-2 expression,[275] most samples were found to arise from the amnion, which is not the contractile tissue but rather the tissue weakened by specific PGs.[276] A similar argument can be made about the unprecise timing of sampling. Furthermore, an unbiased transcriptomic or proteomic approach has been utilized, but only in four of 12 studies analyzed[275] was COX-2 found to increase during labor; a recent well-conducted microarray study on myometrium failed to show any labor-associated changes in the expression of COX-1 or COX-2[277]; nonetheless, the precise timing, spatial collection from the tissue, and expanded clinical information on the cause of PTL may contribute to such discrepancies.

Nonsteroidal Anti-inflammatory Drugs - Efficacy for Preterm Labor

In a meta-analysis review of 42 studies identified to evaluate the efficacy of NSAIDs in treating PTL and assessing newborn outcome, 20 studies were included and involved 1,509 patients.[271] Fifteen of the 20 studies used indomethacin. A nonstatistically significant modest improvement in pregnancy prolongation was observed compared to placebo, without any advantages to acute/subacute newborn outcome. A slight decrease in the number of infants born within 48 hours of drug trial (seven studies) was observed for indomethacin compared to betamimetics and placebo; but no benefit was observed for births within 7 days of study entry (Fig. 39.6). Also no differences were noted for comparisons with $MgSO_4$ (four studies—508 women) or calcium channel blockers (one study—79 women). Importantly, there were neither data available for very premature births (less than 28 weeks of gestation) nor on longer outcome measures. In addition to negligible effects of NSAIDs in prolonging gestation, these drugs administered antenatally

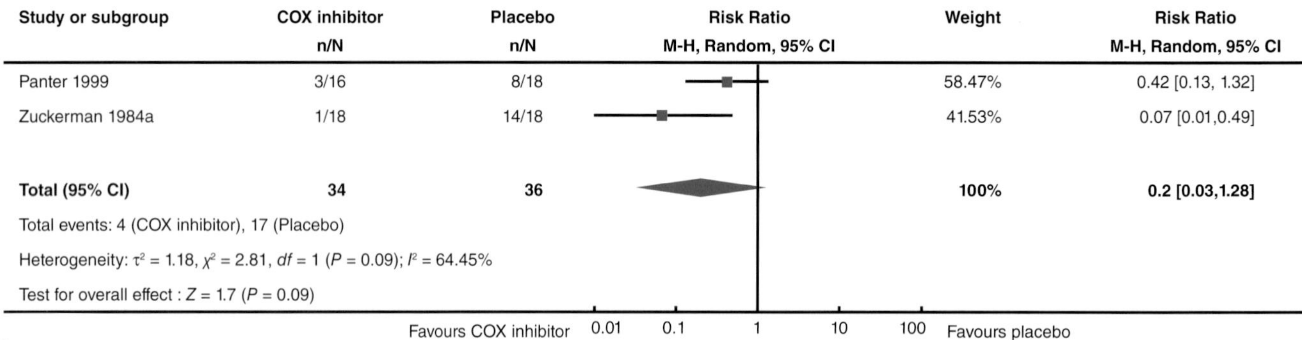

Study or subgroup	COX inhibitor n/N	Placebo n/N	Weight	Risk Ratio M-H, Random, 95% CI
Panter 1999	8/16	12/18	54.89%	0.75 [0.42, 1.35]
Zuckerman 1984a	3/18	15/18	45.11%	0.2 [0.07,0.57]
Total (95% CI)	**34**	**36**	**100%**	**0.41 [0.1, 1.66]**

Total events: 11 (COX inhibitor), 27 (Placebo)

Heterogeneity: $\tau^2 = 0.83$, $\chi^2 = 5.36$, $df = 1$ ($P = 0.02$); $I^2 = 81.34\%$

Test for overall effect : $Z = 1.25$ ($P = 0.21$)

Favours COX inhibitor 0.01 0.1 1 10 100 Favours placebo

B

Figure 39.6 Comparisons of COX inhibitors with placebo on preterm birth. (**A**) Less than 48 hours after starting the treatment; (**B**) less than 7 days after starting the treatment, depicted as forest plot. (Adapted with permission from Reinebrant HE, Pileggi-Castro C, Romero CL, et al. Cyclo-oxygenase (COX) inhibitors for treating preterm labour. *Cochrane Database Syst Rev.* 2015;CD001992.)

have been reported to increase the risk of ductal closure, intraventricular hemorrhage, renal compromise, necrotizing enterocolitis, and death[278]; however, discordances exist in the literature based on the duration and timing of indomethacin administration.[279] Evidence suggests slight efficacy of low-dose aspirin (81 mg per day) in reducing the risk of PTB (as well as improving preeclampsia) as reported in meta-analyses[280] and well-structured randomized trial.[281] Yet, overall, COX inhibitors offer little benefits over placebo or other currently utilized tocolytics considered mostly ineffective.[271,282]

Alternative Approaches to Nonsteroidal Anti-inflammatory Drugs by Using Selective Prostaglandin Receptor Antagonists for Preterm Labor

Based on the evidence that the contractile receptor of $PGF_{2\alpha}$ (FP) reveals increased expression at the onset of labor,[283] that labor can be induced by stimulants of FP,[267] and that conversely FP knockout animals fail to go into labor and do not respond to $PGF_{2\alpha}$ analogs,[284] a rationale was made to design and test specific FP antagonists for PTL. The first attempt was made with a small octapeptide (sequence: ILGHRDYK) labeled THG113.[285] THG113 was found to inhibit myometrial contractility ex vivo and delayed lipopolysaccharide-induced preterm delivery in vivo in animal model. A single amino acid substitution of Arg to Cit (PDC31) resulted in improved potency with comparable efficacy to THG113, and led to subsequent human testing, which substantiated myometrial relaxant efficacy of FP antagonist in a Phase 1 trial.[286] Similar preclinical observations were made with a more potent derivative of THG113, namely PDC113.824[287]; the latter study revealed clear biased signaling causing negative allosteric modulation of Rho/ROCK and positive allosteric modulation of PKC/Erk1/2 signaling. A distinct FP antagonist, OBE022, has also lately been found to exert uterine relaxant properties on human myometrium and prolonged gestation to the same degree (24 hours) as nifedipine in pregnant mice induced with the progesterone receptor antagonist RU-486,[288] without adverse effects on DA or renal function. A Phase 1 trial revealed human safety of oral OBE022[289]; a Phase 2a clinical trial is ongoing. Collectively, FP antagonists provide a potentially improved alternative to NSAIDs with a possibly better safety profile, albeit none of these agents tackle underlying inflammation, which is involved in greater than 70% of very PTBs.[256]

On the whole, tocolytics at best delay labor only to a modest extent, in most part because they act downstream of the inflammatory cascade, leading to PTL, which is undoubtedly too late to halt labor. In addition, the final biologic signaling pathways of labor are redundant, and current tocolysis strategy only targets one of many failure-proof mechanisms. More importantly, tocolytics do not address fetomaternal inflammation, which has marked impact on neonatal outcome.[256] Development of safe and effective tocolytic agents remains important to prolong gestation, but based on current knowledge should be done by concomitantly tackling inflammation. In this context, recent studies reveal superiority of targeting prominent IL-1 using small molecules to prolong gestation, enhance safe maturation of fetus, and improve fetal/neonatal outcome.[290,291]

ADVERSE EFFECTS OF NONSTEROIDAL ANTI-INFLAMMATORY DRUGS

The adverse effects of NSAIDs in children are similar in nature to those described in adults, albeit with lower frequency. Aspirin exerts a number of adverse effects, such as GI bleeding, hypersensitivity, and particularly Reye syndrome, and is thus seldom recommended for fever in children. Ibuprofen is reported to exert a 7.2 per 100,000 risk of GI bleeding.[292] Mild reversible renal impairment is also observed in 8% to 10% of patients[293]; dehydration doubles the risk. Gastric bleeding occurs in 10% to 15% of patients. More rarely, Steven–Johnson Syndrome is reported secondary to ibuprofen. Other potential adverse effects of ibuprofen include aseptic meningitis and increased susceptibility of enhanced infections associated with group A β-hemolytic streptococci in children with varicella.

Oral acetaminophen is safe for children when dosed appropriately. IV acetaminophen was approved for pediatric use by the U.S. FDA in 2010 and is likely to have an equivalent safety profile to oral dosing but may pose greater risks for medication error.[294] Overdose and high chronic doses are associated with hepatotoxicity. Limiting acetaminophen doses to less than 60 mg per kg per day virtually abolishes the risk of hepatotoxicity, unless used with other hepatotoxic agents.[80,295] The overall safety and efficacy profiles for acetaminophen and ibuprofen are generally equivalent in children.[117,296] All in all, NSAIDs have a good tolerance record in pediatrics. Nonetheless, in certain cases, they are contraindicated such as in hepatic failure. In light of the cardiovascular effects associated with long-term coxib use in adults, the dosing, tolerance, and safety of selective coxibs in children require additional scrutiny.[102]

In the newborn, NSAIDs exert a number of adverse effects particularly associated with the administration of indomethacin. Renal function compromise leading to oliguria is the most clearly documented adverse effect of indomethacin.[297] Oliguria is routinely observed in response to indomethacin[151,166]; this effect is less pronounced with ibuprofen[151,170,194] and hardly observed with acetaminophen.[151,210] Other undesirable effects of indomethacin and ibuprofen include spontaneous intestinal perforation particularly when combined with corticosteroids.[298–300] Although an increased risk of necrotizing enterocolitis was linked to the early use of indomethacin in retrospective analyses involving more than 18,000 subjects,[301,302] prospective analyses including the TIPP and an observational population study that together amount to more than 1,800 patients did not show an increased risk of necrotizing enterocolitis with indomethacin.[166,303] Likewise, a large meta-analysis that included 64 randomized trials and 24 observational studies involving 14,568 subjects also did not detect an increase in the rate of necrotizing enterocolitis or intestinal perforation with indomethacin.[151] Yet, upon comparison of indomethacin with ibuprofen, the latter was associated with a lower risk of necrotizing enterocolitis[194]; this trend is further diminished with acetaminophen administration.[151] These observations are consistent with preserved abdominal vascular flow after ibuprofen.[196] In contrast to indomethacin, ibuprofen has been reported in retrospective analyses to elicit pulmonary hypertension in premature infants with severe intrauterine growth retardation.[304–308] Other minor effects of NSAIDs have been reported, such as increasing free bilirubin plasma levels,[309] but their clinical impact appears limited.[310] All in all, indomethacin seems to be the NSAID most associated with adverse effects in newborns particularly as it applies to renal function.

ACKNOWLEDGMENTS

The authors thank the following agencies that contributed to personal works presented: Canadian Institutes of Health Research (CIHR), Fonds de la Recherche du Québec—Santé (FRQS), and Heart & Stroke Foundation of Québec. J. Reese is supported by grants from the U.S. National Institutes of Health (HL128386 and HD081121), and the Mildred T. Stahlman endowed chair in perinatal research. M. Nadeau-Vallée was a Vanier Scholar and a recipient of CIHR and FRQS bursaries. S. Chemtob is a recipient of a Canada Research Chair and the Leopoldine Wolfe Chair in Translational Macula Research.

REFERENCES

1. Smith WL, DeWitt DL, Garavito RM. Cyclooxygenases: structural, cellular, and molecular biology. *Annu Rev Biochem* 2000;69:145–182.
2. Simmons DL, Botting RM, Hla T. Cyclooxygenase isozymes: the biology of prostaglandin synthesis and inhibition. *Pharmacol Rev* 2004;56:387–437.
3. Chandrasekharan NV, Dai H, Roos KL, et al. COX-3, a cyclooxygenase-1 variant inhibited by acetaminophen and other analgesic/antipyretic drugs: cloning, structure, and expression. *Proc Natl Acad Sci U S A* 2002;99:13926–13931.
4. Botting RM. Vane's discovery of the mechanism of action of aspirin changed our understanding of its clinical pharmacology. *Pharmacol Rep* 2010;62:518–525.
5. Zidar N, Odar K, Glavac D, et al. Cyclooxygenase in normal human tissues—is COX-1 really a constitutive isoform, and COX-2 an inducible isoform? *J Cell Mol Med* 2009;13:3753–3763.
6. Gretzer B, Ehrlich K, Maricic N, et al. Selective cyclo-oxygenase-2 inhibitors and their influence on the protective effect of a mild irritant in the rat stomach. *Br J Pharmacol* 1998;123:927–935.
7. Siegle I, Klein T, Backman JT, et al. Expression of cyclooxygenase 1 and cyclooxygenase 2 in human synovial tissue: differential elevation of cyclooxygenase 2 in inflammatory joint diseases. *Arthritis Rheum* 1998;41:122–129.
8. Pannunzio A, Coluccia M. Cyclooxygenase-1 (COX-1) and COX-1 inhibitors in cancer: a review of oncology and medicinal chemistry literature. *Pharmaceuticals (Basel)* 2018;11:101.
9. Burdan F, Szumilo J, Marzec B, et al. Skeletal developmental effects of selective and nonselective cyclooxygenase-2 inhibitors administered through organogenesis and fetogenesis in Wistar CRL:(WI)WUBR rats. *Toxicology* 2005;216:204–223.
10. Slattery P, Frolich S, Schreiber Y, et al. COX-2 gene dosage-dependent defects in kidney development. *Am J Physiol Renal Physiol* 2016;310:F1113–F1122.
11. Stanfield KM, Bell RR, Lisowski AR, et al. Expression of cyclooxygenase-2 in embryonic and fetal tissues during organogenesis and late pregnancy. *Birth Defects Res A Clin Mol Teratol* 2003;67:54–58.
12. Dinchuk JE, Car BD, Focht RJ, et al. Renal abnormalities and an altered inflammatory response in mice lacking cyclooxygenase II. *Nature* 1995;378:406–409.
13. Morham SG, Langenbach R, Loftin CD, et al. Prostaglandin synthase 2 gene disruption causes severe renal pathology in the mouse. *Cell* 1995;83:473–482.
14. Gambaro G, Perazella MA. Adverse renal effects of anti-inflammatory agents: evaluation of selective and nonselective cyclooxygenase inhibitors. *J Intern Med* 2003;253:643–652.
15. Pereira-da-Silva L, Pita A, Virella D, et al. Oral ibuprofen for patent ductus arteriosus closure in preterm infants: does high osmolality matter? *Am J Perinatol* 2008;25:319–320.
16. Islam AB, Dave M, Amin S, et al. Genomic, lipidomic and metabolomic analysis of cyclooxygenase-null cells: eicosanoid storm, cross talk, and compensation by COX-1. *Genomics Proteomics Bioinf* 2016;14:81–93.
17. Li X, Mazaleuskaya LL, Ballantyne LL, et al. Differential compensation of two cyclooxygenases in renal homeostasis is independent of prostaglandin-synthetic capacity under basal conditions. *FASEB J* 2018;32:5326–5337.
18. Li X, Ballantyne LL, Crawford MC, et al. Isoform-specific compensation of cyclooxygenase (Ptgs) genes during implantation and late-stage pregnancy. *Sci Rep* 2018;8:12097.
19. Reese J, Brown N, Paria BC, et al. COX-2 compensation in the uterus of COX-1 deficient mice during the pre-implantation period. *Mol Cell Endocrinol* 1999;150:23–31.
20. Garavito RM, DeWitt DL. The cyclooxygenase isoforms: structural insights into the conversion of arachidonic acid to prostaglandins. *Biochim Biophys Acta* 1999;1441:278–287.
21. Smith WL, Malkowski MG. Interactions of fatty acids, nonsteroidal anti-inflammatory drugs, and coxibs with the catalytic and allosteric subunits of cyclooxygenases-1 and -2. *J Biol Chem* 2019;294:1697–1705.
22. Rouzer CA, Marnett LJ. Endocannabinoid oxygenation by cyclooxygenases, lipoxygenases, and cytochromes P450: cross-talk between the eicosanoid and endocannabinoid signaling pathways. *Chem Rev* 2011;111:5899–5921.
23. Kiefer JR, Pawlitz JL, Moreland KT, et al. Structural insights into the stereochemistry of the cyclooxygenase reaction. *Nature* 2000;405:97–101.
24. Kulmacz RJ, Lands WE. Stoichiometry and kinetics of the interaction of prostaglandin H synthase with anti-inflammatory agents. *J Biol Chem* 1985;260:12572–12578.
25. Dong L, Vecchio AJ, Sharma NP, et al. Human cyclooxygenase-2 is a sequence homodimer that functions as a conformational heterodimer. *J Biol Chem* 2011;286:19035–19046.
26. Yuan C, Rieke CJ, Rimon G, et al. Partnering between monomers of cyclooxygenase-2 homodimers. *Proc Natl Acad Sci U S A* 2006;103:6142–6147.
27. Ogorochi T, Ujihara M, Narumiya S. Purification and properties of prostaglandin H-E isomerase from the cytosol of human brain: identification as anionic forms of glutathione S-transferase. *J Neurochem* 1987;48:900–909.
28. Tanikawa N, Ohmiya Y, Ohkubo H, et al. Identification and characterization of a novel type of membrane-associated prostaglandin E synthase. *Biochem Biophys Res Commun* 2002;291:884–889.
29. Watanabe K, Kurihara K, Tokunaga Y, et al. Two types of microsomal prostaglandin E synthase: glutathione-dependent and-independent prostaglandin E synthases. *Biochem Biophys Res Commun* 1997;235:148–152.
30. Coleman RA, Kennedy I, Sheldrick RL. New evidence with selective agonists and antagonists for the subclassification of PGE2-sensitive (EP) receptors. *Adv Prostaglandin Thromboxane Leukot Res* 1987;17A:467–470.
31. Coleman RA, Smith WL, Narumiya S. International Union of Pharmacology classification of prostanoid receptors: properties, distribution, and structure of the receptors and their subtypes. *Pharmacol Rev* 1994;46:205–229.
32. Adam M, Boie Y, Rushmore TH, et al. Cloning and expression of three isoforms of the human EP3 prostanoid receptor. *FEBS Lett* 1994;338:170–174.
33. Kotani M, Tanaka I, Ogawa Y, et al. Structural organization of the human prostaglandin EP3 receptor subtype gene (PTGER3). *Genomics* 1997;40:425–434.
34. Regan JW, Bailey TJ, Donello JE, et al. Molecular cloning and expression of human EP3 receptors: evidence of three variants with differing carboxyl termini. *Br J Pharmacol* 1994;112:377–385.
35. Schmid A, Thierauch KH, Schleuning WD, et al. Splice variants of the human EP3 receptor for prostaglandin E2. *Eur J Biochem* 1995;228:23–30.
36. Kotelevets L, Foudi N, Louedec L, et al. A new mRNA splice variant coding for the human EP3-I receptor isoform. *Prostaglandins Leukot Essent Fatty Acids* 2007;77:195–201.
37. Raychowdhury MK, Yukawa M, Collins LJ, et al. Alternative splicing produces a divergent cytoplasmic tail in the human endothelial thromboxane A2 receptor. *J Biol Chem* 1994;269:19256–19261.
38. Vielhauer GA, Fujino H, Regan JW. Cloning and localization of hFP(S): a six-transmembrane mRNA splice variant of the human FP prostanoid receptor. *Arch Biochem Biophys* 2004;421:175–185.
39. Hay A, Wood S, Olson D, et al. Labour is associated with decreased expression of the PGF2alpha receptor (PTGFR) and a novel PTGFR splice variant in human myometrium but not decidua. *Mol Hum Reprod* 2010;16:752–760.
40. Audoly L, Breyer RM. The second extracellular loop of the prostaglandin EP3 receptor is an essential determinant of ligand selectivity. *J Biol Chem* 1997;272:13475–13478.
41. Huang C, Tai HH. Expression and site-directed mutagenesis of mouse prostaglandin E2 receptor EP3 subtype in insect cells. *Biochem J* 1995;307(Pt 2):493–498.
42. Chiang N, Tai HH. The role of N-glycosylation of human thromboxane A2 receptor in ligand binding. *Arch Biochem Biophys* 1998;352:207–213.
43. Woodward DF, Jones RL, Narumiya S. International Union of Basic and Clinical Pharmacology. LXXXIII: classification of prostanoid receptors, updating 15 years of progress. *Pharmacol Rev* 2011;63:471–538.
44. Wilson SJ, Roche AM, Kostetskaia E, et al. Dimerization of the human receptors for prostacyclin and thromboxane facilitates thromboxane receptor-mediated cAMP generation. *J Biol Chem* 2004;279:53036–53047.
45. Ibrahim S, McCartney A, Markosyan N, et al. Heterodimerization with the prostacyclin receptor triggers thromboxane receptor relocation to lipid rafts. *Arterioscler Thromb Vasc Biol* 2013;33:60–66.
46. McGraw DW, Mihlbachler KA, Schwarb MR, et al. Airway smooth muscle prostaglandin-EP1 receptors directly modulate beta2-adrenergic receptors within a unique heterodimeric complex. *J Clin Invest* 2006;116:1400–1409.
47. Matsubara S, Shiraishi A, Sakai T, et al. Heterodimerization of the prostaglandin E2 receptor EP2 and the calcitonin receptor CTR. *PLoS One* 2017;12:e0187711.
48. Matsuoka T, Narumiya S. Prostaglandin receptor signaling in disease. *Sci World J* 2007;7:1329–1347.
49. Boardman PL, Hart FD. Clinical measurement of the anti-inflammatory effects of salicylates in rheumatoid arthritis. *Br Med J* 1967;4:264–268.
50. Regan JW, Bailey TJ, Pepperl DJ, et al. Cloning of a novel human prostaglandin receptor with characteristics of the pharmacologically defined EP2 subtype. *Mol Pharmacol* 1994;46:213–220.
51. Toh H, Ichikawa A, Narumiya S. Molecular evolution of receptors for eicosanoids. *FEBS Lett* 1995;361:17–21.
52. Negishi M, Ito S, Yokohama H, et al. Functional reconstitution of prostaglandin E receptor from bovine adrenal medulla with guanine nucleotide binding proteins. *J Biol Chem* 1988;263:6893–6900.
53. Harris SG, Padilla J, Koumas L, et al. Prostaglandins as modulators of immunity. *Trends Immunol* 2002;23:144–150.
54. van Bel F, Guit GL, Schipper J, et al. Indomethacin-induced changes in renal blood flow velocity waveform in premature infants investigated with color Doppler imaging. *J Pediatr* 1991;118:621–626.
55. Matsuoka T, Hirata M, Tanaka H, et al. Prostaglandin D2 as a mediator of allergic asthma. *Science* 2000;287:2013–2017.
56. Hinz B, Cheremina O, Brune K. Acetaminophen (paracetamol) is a selective cyclooxygenase-2 inhibitor in man. *FASEB J* 2008;22:383–390.
57. Jones RL, Giembycz MA, Woodward DF. Prostanoid receptor antagonists: development strategies and therapeutic applications. *Br J Pharmacol* 2009;158:104–145.

58. Sharif NA, Klimko PG. Prostaglandin FP receptor antagonists: discovery, pharmacological characterization and therapeutic utility. *Br J Pharmacol* 2019;176:1059–1078.
59. Olson DM, Ammann C. Role of the prostaglandins in labour and prostaglandin receptor inhibitors in the prevention of preterm labour. *Front Biosci* 2007;12:1329–1343.
60. Kujubu DA, Fletcher BS, Varnum BC, et al. TIS10, a phorbol ester tumor promoter-inducible mRNA from Swiss 3T3 cells, encodes a novel prostaglandin synthase/cyclooxygenase homologue. *J Biol Chem* 1991;266:12866–12872.
61. O'Banion MK, Sadowski HB, Winn V, et al. A serum-and glucocorticoid-regulated 4-kilobase mRNA encodes a cyclooxygenase-related protein. *J Biol Chem* 1991;266:23261–23267.
62. Marnett LJ. The COXIB experience: a look in the rearview mirror. *Annu Rev Pharmacol Toxicol* 2009;49:265–290.
63. Warner TD, Mitchell JA. Cyclooxygenases: new forms, new inhibitors, and lessons from the clinic. *FASEB J* 2004;18:790–804.
64. Duggan KC, Hermanson DJ, Musee J, et al. (R)-Profens are substrate-selective inhibitors of endocannabinoid oxygenation by COX-2. *Nat Chem Biol* 2011;7:803–809.
65. Hermanson DJ, Hartley ND, Gamble-George J, et al. Substrate-selective COX-2 inhibition decreases anxiety via endocannabinoid activation. *Nat Neurosci* 2013;16:1291–1298.
66. Orlando BJ, Malkowski MG. Substrate-selective inhibition of cyclooxygeanse-2 by fenamic acid derivatives is dependent on peroxide tone. *J Biol Chem* 2016;291:15069–15081.
67. Yu Y, Fan J, Hui Y, et al. Targeted cyclooxygenase gene (ptgs) exchange reveals discriminant isoform functionality. *J Biol Chem* 2007;282:1498–1506.
68. Hsu AL, Ching TT, Wang DS, et al. The cyclooxygenase-2 inhibitor celecoxib induces apoptosis by blocking Akt activation in human prostate cancer cells independently of Bcl-2. *J Biol Chem* 2000;275:11397–11403.
69. Jones MK, Wang H, Peskar BM, et al. Inhibition of angiogenesis by nonsteroidal anti-inflammatory drugs: insight into mechanisms and implications for cancer growth and ulcer healing. *Nat Med* 1999;5:1418–1423.
70. Kopp E, Ghosh S. Inhibition of NF-kappa B by sodium salicylate and aspirin. *Science* 1994;265:956–959.
71. Lehmann JM, Lenhard JM, Oliver BB, et al. Peroxisome proliferator-activated receptors alpha and gamma are activated by indomethacin and other non-steroidal anti-inflammatory drugs. *J Biol Chem* 1997;272:3406–3410.
72. Rheinlaender C, Helfenstein D, Walch E, et al. Total serum bilirubin levels during cyclooxygenase inhibitor treatment for patent ductus arteriosus in preterm infants. *Acta Paediatr* 2009;98:36–42.
73. Li S, Dou W, Tang Y, et al. Acetaminophen: antipyretic or hypothermic in mice? In either case, PGHS-1b (COX-3) is irrelevant. *Prostaglandins Other Lipid Mediat* 2008;85:89–99.
74. Boutaud O, Aronoff DM, Richardson JH, et al. Determinants of the cellular specificity of acetaminophen as an inhibitor of prostaglandin H(2) synthases. *Proc Natl Acad Sci U S A* 2002;99:7130–7135.
75. Graham GG, Scott KF. Mechanism of action of paracetamol. *Am J Ther* 2005;12:46–55.
76. Graham GG, Davies MJ, Day RO, et al. The modern pharmacology of paracetamol: therapeutic actions, mechanism of action, metabolism, toxicity and recent pharmacological findings. *Inflammopharmacology* 2013;21:201–232.
77. Pickering G, Esteve V, Loriot MA, et al. Acetaminophen reinforces descending inhibitory pain pathways. *Clin Pharmacol Ther* 2008;84:47–51.
78. Pickering G, Loriot MA, Libert F, et al. Analgesic effect of acetaminophen in humans: first evidence of a central serotonergic mechanism. *Clin Pharmacol Ther* 2006;79:371–378.
79. Litalien C, Jacqz-Aigrain E. Risks and benefits of nonsteroidal anti-inflammatory drugs in children: a comparison with paracetamol. *Paediatr Drugs* 2001;3:817–858.
80. de Martino M, Chiarugi A. Recent advances in pediatric use of oral paracetamol in fever and pain management. *Pain Ther* 2015;4:149–168.
81. de Martino M, Chiarugi A, Boner A, et al. Working towards an appropriate use of ibuprofen in children: an evidence-based appraisal. *Drugs* 2017;77:1295–1311.
82. Hirt D, Van Overmeire B, Treluyer JM, et al. An optimized ibuprofen dosing scheme for preterm neonates with patent ductus arteriosus, based on a population pharmacokinetic and pharmacodynamic study. *Br J Clin Pharmacol* 2008;65:629–636.
83. Dani C, Vangi V, Bertini G, et al. High-dose ibuprofen for patent ductus arteriosus in extremely preterm infants: a randomized controlled study. *Clin Pharmacol Ther* 2012;91:590–596.
84. Anderson BJ, van Lingen RA, Hansen TG, et al. Acetaminophen developmental pharmacokinetics in premature neonates and infants: a pooled population analysis. *Anesthesiology* 2002;96:1336–1345.
85. Levy G, Yaffe SJ. Relationship between dose and apparent volume of distribution of salicylate in children. *Pediatrics* 1974;54:713–717.
86. Cook SF, Stockmann C, Samiee-Zafarghandy S, et al. Neonatal maturation of paracetamol (acetaminophen) glucuronidation, sulfation, and oxidation based on a parent-metabolite population pharmacokinetic model. *Clin Pharmacokinet* 2016;55:1395–1411.
87. Hammer GB, Maxwell LG, Taicher BM, et al. Randomized population pharmacokinetic analysis and safety of intravenous acetaminophen for acute postoperative pain in neonates and infants. *J Clin Pharmacol* 2020;60:16–27.
88. Strassburg CP, Strassburg A, Kneip S, et al. Developmental aspects of human hepatic drug glucuronidation in young children and adults. *Gut* 2002;50:259–265.
89. McGill MR, Jaeschke H. Metabolism and disposition of acetaminophen: recent advances in relation to hepatotoxicity and diagnosis. *Pharm Res* 2013;30:2174–2187.
90. Anderson BJ, Allegaert K. Intravenous neonatal paracetamol dosing: the magic of 10 days. *Paediatr Anaesth* 2009;19:289–295.
91. Yaffe SJ, Friedman WF, Rogers D, et al. The disposition of indomethacin in preterm babies. *J Pediatr* 1980;97:1001–1006.
92. Smyth JM, Collier PS, Darwish M, et al. Intravenous indometacin in preterm infants with symptomatic patent ductus arteriosus. A population pharmacokinetic study. *Br J Clin Pharmacol* 2004;58:249–258.
93. Aranda JV, Varvarigou A, Beharry K, et al. Pharmacokinetics and protein binding of intravenous ibuprofen in the premature newborn infant. *Acta Paediatr* 1997;86:289–293.
94. Lewis TR, Shelton EL, Van Driest SL, et al. Genetics of the patent ductus arteriosus (PDA) and pharmacogenetics of PDA treatment. *Semin Fetal Neonatal Med* 2018;23:232–238.
95. FitzGerald GA, Patrono C. The coxibs, selective inhibitors of cyclooxygenase-2. *N Engl J Med* 2001;345:433–442.
96. Rodrigues AD. Impact of CYP2C9 genotype on pharmacokinetics: are all cyclooxygenase inhibitors the same? *Drug Metab Dispos* 2005;33:1567–1575.
97. Stika CS, Gross GA, Leguizamon G, et al. A prospective randomized safety trial of celecoxib for treatment of preterm labor. *Am J Obstet Gynecol* 2002;187:653–660.
98. Karjalainen MJ, Neuvonen PJ, Backman JT. Rofecoxib is a potent, metabolism-dependent inhibitor of CYP1A2: implications for in vitro prediction of drug interactions. *Drug Metab Dispos* 2006;34:2091–2096.
99. Prescilla RP, Frattarelli DA, Haritos D, et al. Pharmacokinetics of rofecoxib in children with sickle cell hemoglobinopathy. *J Pediatr Hematol Oncol* 2004;26:661–664.
100. Fosbol EL, Gislason GH, Jacobsen S, et al. Risk of myocardial infarction and death associated with the use of nonsteroidal anti-inflammatory drugs (NSAIDs) among healthy individuals: a nationwide cohort study. *Clin Pharmacol Ther* 2009;85:190–197.
101. McGettigan P, Henry D. Cardiovascular risk and inhibition of cyclooxygenase: a systematic review of the observational studies of selective and nonselective inhibitors of cyclooxygenase 2. *JAMA* 2006;296:1633–1644.
102. Levy DM, Imundo LF. Nonsteroidal anti-inflammatory drugs: a survey of practices and concerns of pediatric medical and surgical specialists and a summary of available safety data. *Pediatr Rheumatol Online J* 2010;8:7.
103. Fletcher, JT, Graf N, Scarman A, et al. Nephrotoxicity with cyclooxygenase 2 inhibitor use in children. *Pediatr Nephrol* 2006;21:1893–1897.
104. Eccleston C, Cooper TE, Fisher E, et al. Non-steroidal anti-inflammatory drugs (NSAIDs) for chronic non-cancer pain in children and adolescents. *Cochrane Database Syst Rev* 2017;8:CD012537.
105. Chiappini E, Bortone B, Galli L, et al. Guidelines for the symptomatic management of fever in children: systematic review of the literature and quality appraisal with AGREE II. *BMJ Open* 2017;7:e015404.
106. Trippella G, Ciarcia M, de Martino M, et al. Prescribing controversies: an updated review and meta-analysis on combined/alternating use of ibuprofen and paracetamol in febrile children. *Front Pediatr* 2019;7:217.
107. Mackowiak PA. Physiological rationale for suppression of fever. *Clin Infect Dis* 2000;31(Suppl 5):S185–S189.
108. Dinarello CA, Cannon JG, Wolff SM. New concepts on the pathogenesis of fever. *Rev Infect Dis* 1988;10:168–189.
109. Aronoff DM, Neilson EG. Antipyretics: mechanisms of action and clinical use in fever suppression. *Am J Med* 2001;111:304–315.
110. Schmidt M, Lamberts M, Olsen AM, et al. Cardiovascular safety of non-aspirin non-steroidal anti-inflammatory drugs: review and position paper by the working group for Cardiovascular Pharmacotherapy of the European Society of Cardiology. *Eur Heart J Cardiovasc Pharmacother* 2016;37:1015–1023.
111. Chang JC, Gross HM. Utility of naproxen in the differential diagnosis of fever of undetermined origin in patients with cancer. *Am J Med* 1984;76:597–603.
112. Zhang H, Wu Y, Lin Z, et al. Naproxen for the treatment of neoplastic fever: a PRISMA-compliant systematic review and meta-analysis. *Medicine (Baltimore)* 2019;98:e15840.
113. Wilson JT, Brown RD, Bocchini JA Jr, et al. Efficacy, disposition and pharmacodynamics of aspirin, acetaminophen and choline salicylate in young febrile children. *Ther Drug Monit* 1982;4:147–180.
114. Wilson JT, Brown RD, Kearns GL, et al. Single-dose, placebo-controlled comparative study of ibuprofen and acetaminophen antipyresis in children. *J Pediatr* 1991;119:803–811.
115. Barbagallo M, Sacerdote P. Ibuprofen in the treatment of children's inflammatory pain: a clinical and pharmacological overview. *Minerva Pediatr* 2019;71:82–99.
116. Ziesenitz VC, Zutter A, Erb TO, et al. Efficacy and safety of ibuprofen in infants aged between 3 and 6 months. *Paediatr Drugs* 2017;19:277–290.
117. Kanabar DJ. A clinical and safety review of paracetamol and ibuprofen in children. *Inflammopharmacology* 2017;25:1–9.
118. Lexicomp. Ibuprofen. In: *Pediatric and neonatal lexi-drugs online*. Hudson, OH: Wolters Kluwer Clinical Drug Information, Inc, 2019.
119. Joint Formulatory Committee. *British national formulary for children*. London, UK: British Medical Journal Group Ltd, 2012: 503.
120. Sarrell EM, Wielunsky E, Cohen HA. Antipyretic treatment in young children with fever: acetaminophen, ibuprofen, or both alternating in a randomized, double-blind study. *Arch Pediatr Adolesc Med* 2006;160:197–202.
121. Kramer LC, Richards PA, Thompson AM, et al. Alternating antipyretics: antipyretic efficacy of acetaminophen versus acetaminophen alternated with ibuprofen in children. *Clin Pediatr (Phila)* 2008;47:907–911.
122. Schmitt BD. Concerns over alternating acetaminophen and ibuprofen for fever. *Arch Pediatr Adolesc Med* 2006;160:757.
123. Section on Clinical Pharmacology and Therapeutics, Committee on Drugs, Sullivan JE, et al. Fever and antipyretic use in children. *Pediatrics* 2011;127:580–587.
124. National Collaborating Centre for Women's and Children's Health (UK). Feverish Illness in Children: Assessment and Initial Management in Children Younger Than 5 Years. London: Royal College of Obstetricians & Gynaecologists (UK); 2013.
125. Beiter JL Jr, Simon HK, Chambliss CR, et al. Intravenous ketorolac in the emergency department management of sickle cell pain and predictors of its effectiveness. *Arch Pediatr Adolesc Med* 2001;155:496–500.
126. Munro HM, Walton SR, Malviya S, et al. Low-dose ketorolac improves analgesia and reduces morphine requirements following posterior spinal fusion in adolescents. *Can J Anaesth* 2002;49:461–466.
127. Gerhardt RT, Gerhardt DM. Intravenous ketorolac in the treatment of fever. *Am J Emerg Med* 2000;18:500–501.
128. Clyman RI. Ibuprofen and patent ductus arteriosus. *N Engl J Med* 2000;343:728–730.
129. Coceani F, Olley PM. The response of the ductus arteriosus to prostaglandins. *Can J Physiol Pharmacol* 1973;51:220–225.
130. Clyman RI, Couto J, Murphy GM. Patent ductus arteriosus: are current neonatal treatment options better or worse than no treatment at all? *Semin Perinatol* 2012;36:123–129.

131. Noori S, Seri I. Treatment of the patent ductus arteriosus: when, how, and for how long? *J Pediatr* 2009;155:774–776.
132. Schena F, Francescato G, Cappelleri A, et al. Association between hemodynamically significant patent ductus arteriosus and bronchopulmonary dysplasia. *J Pediatr* 2015;166:1488–1492.
133. Ryder RW, Shelton JD, Guinan ME. Necrotizing enterocolitis: a prospective multicenter investigation. *Am J Epidemiol* 1980;112:113–123.
134. Havranek T, Rahimi M, Hall H, et al. Feeding preterm neonates with patent ductus arteriosus (PDA): intestinal blood flow characteristics and clinical outcomes. *J Matern Fetal Neonatal Med* 2015;28:526–530.
135. Lemmers PM, Benders MJ, D'Ascenzo R, et al. Patent ductus arteriosus and brain volume. *Pediatrics* 2016;137:e20153090.
136. Cohen E, Dix L, Baerts W, et al. Reduction in cerebral oxygenation due to patent ductus arteriosus is pronounced in small-for-gestational-age neonates. *Neonatology* 2017;111:126–132.
137. Dix L, Molenschot M, Breur J, et al. Cerebral oxygenation and echocardiographic parameters in preterm neonates with a patent ductus arteriosus: an observational study. *Arch Dis Child Fetal Neonatal Ed* 2016;101:F520–F526.
138. Sung SI, Chang YS, Kim J, et al. Natural evolution of ductus arteriosus with noninterventional conservative management in extremely preterm infants born at 23-28 weeks of gestation. *PLoS One* 2019;14:e0212256.
139. Reese J, Veldman A, Shah L, et al. Inadvertent relaxation of the ductus arteriosus by pharmacologic agents that are commonly used in the neonatal period. *Semin Perinatol* 2010;34:222–230.
140. Mohanty M, Lawal OD, Skeer M, et al. Medication errors involving intravenous patient-controlled analgesia: results from the 2005–2015 MEDMARX database. *Ther Adv Drug Saf* 2018;9:389–404.
141. Liebowitz M, Kaempf J, Erdeve O, et al. Comparative effectiveness of drugs used to constrict the patent ductus arteriosus: a secondary analysis of the PDA-TOLERATE trial (NCT01958320). *J Perinatol* 2019;39:599–607.
142. Benitz WE. Treatment of persistent patent ductus arteriosus in preterm infants: time to accept the null hypothesis? *J Perinatol* 2010;30:241–252.
143. Hamrick SE, Hansmann G. Patent ductus arteriosus of the preterm infant. *Pediatrics* 2010;125:1020–1030.
144. Slaughter JL, Cua CL, Notestine JL, et al. Early prediction of spontaneous patent ductus arteriosus (PDA) closure and PDA-associated outcomes: a prospective cohort investigation. *BMC Pediatr* 2019;19:333.
145. Koch J, Hensley G, Roy L, et al. Prevalence of spontaneous closure of the ductus arteriosus in neonates at a birth weight of 1000 grams or less. *Pediatrics* 2006;117:1113–1121.
146. Rolland A, Shankar-Aguilera S, Diomande D, et al. Natural evolution of patent ductus arteriosus in the extremely preterm infant. *Arch Dis Child Fetal Neonatal Ed* 2015;100:F55–F58.
147. Nemerofsky SL, Parravicini E, Bateman D, et al. The ductus arteriosus rarely requires treatment in infants >1000 grams. *Am J Perinatol* 2008;25:661–666.
148. Weber SC, Weiss K, Buhrer C, et al. Natural history of patent ductus arteriosus in very low birth weight infants after discharge. *J Pediatr* 2015;167:1149–1151.
149. Herrman K, Bose C, Lewis K, et al. Spontaneous closure of the patent ductus arteriosus in very low birth weight infants following discharge from the neonatal unit. *Arch Dis Child Fetal Neonatal Ed* 2009;94:F48–F50.
150. Mitra S, Florez ID, Tamayo ME, et al. Association of placebo, indomethacin, ibuprofen, and acetaminophen with closure of hemodynamically significant patent ductus arteriosus in preterm infants: a systematic review and meta-analysis. *JAMA* 2018;319:1221–1238.
151. Marconi E, Bettiol A, Ambrosio G, et al. Efficacy and safety of pharmacological treatments for patent ductus arteriosus closure: a systematic review and network meta-analysis of clinical trials and observational studies. *Pharmacol Res* 2019;148:104418.
152. Clyman RI, Liebowitz M, Kaempf J, et al. PDA-TOLERATE trial: an exploratory randomized controlled trial of treatment of moderate-to-large patent ductus arteriosus at 1 week of age. *J Pediatr* 2019;205:41.e6–48.e6.
153. Hagadorn JI, Bennett MV, Brownell EA, et al. Covariation of neonatal intensive care unit-level patent ductus arteriosus management and in-neonatal intensive care unit outcomes following preterm birth. *J Pediatr* 2018;203:225–233.
154. Reese J, Laughon MM. The patent ductus arteriosus problem: infants who still need treatment. *J Pediatr* 2015;167:954–956.
155. Gillam-Krakauer M, Hagadorn JI, Reese J. Pharmacological closure of the patent ductus arteriosus: when treatment still makes sense. *J Perinatol* 2019;39:1439–1441.
156. Benitz WE, Committee on Fetus and Newborn. Patent ductus arteriosus in preterm infants. *Pediatrics* 2016;137:e20153730.
157. El-Khuffash A, Weisz DE, McNamara PJ. Reflections of the changes in patent ductus arteriosus management during the last 10 years. *Arch Dis Child Fetal Neonatal Ed* 2016;101:F474–F478.
158. McNamara PJ, Sehgal A. Towards rational management of the patent ductus arteriosus: the need for disease staging. *Arch Dis Child Fetal Neonatal Ed* 2007;92:F424–F427.
159. Dani C, Mosca F, Cresi F, et al. Patent ductus arteriosus in preterm infants born at 23–24 weeks' gestation: should we pay more attention? *Early Hum Dev* 2019;135:16–22.
160. Neumann R, Schulzke SM, Buhrer C. Oral ibuprofen versus intravenous ibuprofen or intravenous indomethacin for the treatment of patent ductus arteriosus in preterm infants: a systematic review and meta-analysis. *Neonatology* 2012;102:9–15.
161. Shelton EL, Singh GK, Nichols CG. Novel drug targets for ductus arteriosus manipulation: looking beyond prostaglandins. *Semin Perinatol* 2018;42:221–227.
162. Liebowitz M, Koo J, Wickremasinghe A, et al. Effects of prophylactic indomethacin on vasopressor-dependent hypotension in extremely preterm infants. *J Pediatr* 2017;182:21.e2–27.e2.
163. Kluckow M, Jeffery M, Gill A, et al. A randomised placebo-controlled trial of early treatment of the patent ductus arteriosus. *Arch Dis Child Fetal Neonatal Ed* 2014;99:F99–F104.
164. Bancalari E. Patent ductus arteriosus and short-and long-term respiratory outcomes. *Am J Perinatol* 2016;33:1055–1057.
165. Liebowitz M, Katheria A, Sauberan J, et al. Lack of equipoise in the PDA-TOLERATE trial: a comparison of eligible infants enrolled in the trial and those treated outside the trial. *J Pediatr* 2019;213:222.e2–226.e2.
166. Schmidt B, Davis P, Moddemann D, et al. Long-term effects of indomethacin prophylaxis in extremely-low-birth-weight infants. *N Engl J Med* 2001;344:1966–1972.
167. Ment LR, Oh W, Ehrenkranz RA, et al. Low-dose indomethacin and prevention of intraventricular hemorrhage: a multicenter randomized trial. *Pediatrics* 1994;93:543–550.
168. Schmidt B, Asztalos EV, Roberts RS, et al. Impact of bronchopulmonary dysplasia, brain injury, and severe retinopathy on the outcome of extremely low-birth-weight infants at 18 months: results from the trial of indomethacin prophylaxis in preterms. *JAMA* 2003;289:1124–1129.
169. Nelin TD, Pena E, Giacomazzi T, et al. Outcomes following indomethacin prophylaxis in extremely preterm infants in an all-referral NICU. *J Perinatol* 2017;37:932–937.
170. Ohlsson A, Shah SS. Ibuprofen for the prevention of patent ductus arteriosus in preterm and/or low birth weight infants. *Cochrane Database Syst Rev* 2019;6:CD004213.
171. Chemtob S, Beharry K, Rex J, et al. Prostanoids determine the range of cerebral blood flow autoregulation of newborn piglets. *Stroke* 1990;21:777–784.
172. Cooke L, Steer P, Woodgate P. Indomethacin for asymptomatic patent ductus arteriosus in preterm infants. *Cochrane Database Syst Rev* 2003;CD003745.
173. Gersony WM, Peckham GJ, Ellison RC, et al. Effects of indomethacin in premature infants with patent ductus arteriosus: results of a national collaborative study. *J Pediatr* 1983;102:895–906.
174. Clyman RI, Chen YQ, Chemtob S, et al. In utero remodeling of the fetal lamb ductus arteriosus: the role of antenatal indomethacin and avascular zone thickness on vasa vasorum proliferation, neointima formation, and cell death. *Circulation* 2001;103:1806–1812.
175. Gal P, Ransom JL, Weaver RL, et al. Indomethacin pharmacokinetics in neonates: the value of volume of distribution as a marker of permanent patent ductus arteriosus closure. *Ther Drug Monit* 1991;13:42–45.
176. Sangem M, Asthana S, Amin S. Multiple courses of indomethacin and neonatal outcomes in premature infants. *Pediatr Cardiol* 2008;29:878–884.
177. Shaffer CL, Gal P, Ransom JL, et al. Effect of age and birth weight on indomethacin pharmacodynamics in neonates treated for patent ductus arteriosus. *Crit Care Med* 2002;30:343–348.
178. Clyman RI, Campbell D, Heymann MA, et al. Persistent responsiveness of the neonatal ductus arteriosus in immature lambs: a possible cause for reopening of patent ductus arteriosus after indomethacin-induced closure. *Circulation* 1985;71:141–145.
179. Seyberth HW, Muller H, Wille L, et al. Recovery of prostaglandin production associated with reopening of the ductus arteriosus after indomethacin treatment in preterm infants with respiratory distress syndrome. *Pediatr Pharmacol (New York)* 1982;2:127–141.
180. Hammerman C, Aramburo MJ. Prolonged indomethacin therapy for the prevention of recurrences of patent ductus arteriosus. *J Pediatr* 1990;117:771–776.
181. Leonhardt A, Isken V, Kuhl PG, et al. Prolonged indomethacin treatment in preterm infants with symptomatic patent ductus arteriosus: efficacy, drug level monitoring, and patient selection. *Eur J Pediatr* 1987;146:140–144.
182. Rhodes PG, Ferguson MG, Reddy NS, et al. Effects of prolonged versus acute indomethacin therapy in very low birth-weight infants with patent ductus arteriosus. *Eur J Pediatr* 1988;147:481–484.
183. Schmidt B, Roberts RS, Fanaroff A, et al. Indomethacin prophylaxis, patent ductus arteriosus, and the risk of bronchopulmonary dysplasia: further analyses from the Trial of Indomethacin Prophylaxis in Preterms (TIPP). *J Pediatr* 2006;148:730–734.
184. Alfaleh K, Smyth JA, Roberts RS, et al. Prevention and 18-month outcomes of serious pulmonary hemorrhage in extremely low birth weight infants: results from the trial of indomethacin prophylaxis in preterms. *Pediatrics* 2008;121:e233–e238.
185. Ment LR, Vohr B, Allan W, et al. Outcome of children in the indomethacin intraventricular hemorrhage prevention trial. *Pediatrics* 2000;105:485–491.
186. Vohr BR, Allan WC, Westerveld M, et al. School-age outcomes of very low birth weight infants in the indomethacin intraventricular hemorrhage prevention trial. *Pediatrics* 2003;111:e340–e346.
187. Christmann V, Liem KD, Semmekrot BA, et al. Changes in cerebral, renal and mesenteric blood flow velocity during continuous and bolus infusion of indomethacin. *Acta Paediatr* 2002;91:440–446.
188. Ohlsson A, Bottu J, Govan J, et al. Effect of indomethacin on cerebral blood flow velocities in very low birth weight neonates with a patent ductus arteriosus. *Dev Pharmacol Ther* 1993;20:100–106.
189. Jensen EA, Dysart KC, Gantz MG, et al. Association between use of prophylactic indomethacin and the risk for bronchopulmonary dysplasia in extremely preterm infants. *J Pediatr* 2017;186:34.e2–40.e2.
190. Mosca F, Bray M, Lattanzio M, et al. Comparative evaluation of the effects of indomethacin and ibuprofen on cerebral perfusion and oxygenation in preterm infants with patent ductus arteriosus. *J Pediatr* 1997;131:549–554.
191. Van Bel F, Van Zoeren D, Schipper J, et al. Effect of indomethacin on superior mesenteric artery blood flow velocity in preterm infants. *J Pediatr* 1990;116:965–970.
192. Hammerman C, Shchors I, Jacobson S, et al. Ibuprofen versus continuous indomethacin in premature neonates with patent ductus arteriosus: is the difference in the mode of administration? *Pediatr Res* 2008;64:291–297.
193. Aranda JV, Clyman R, Cox B, et al. A randomized, double-blind, placebo-controlled trial on intravenous ibuprofen L-lysine for the early closure of nonsymptomatic patent ductus arteriosus within 72 hours of birth in extremely low-birth-weight infants. *Am J Perinatol* 2009;26:235–245.
194. Ohlsson A, Walia R, Shah SS. Ibuprofen for the treatment of patent ductus arteriosus in preterm or low birth weight (or both) infants. *Cochrane Database Syst Rev* 2018;9:CD003481.
195. Patel J, Roberts I, Azzopardi D, et al. Randomized double-blind controlled trial comparing the effects of ibuprofen with indomethacin on cerebral hemodynamics in preterm infants with patent ductus arteriosus. *Pediatr Res* 2000;47:36–42.

196. Pezzati M, Vangi V, Biagiotti R, et al. Effects of indomethacin and ibuprofen on mesenteric and renal blood flow in preterm infants with patent ductus arteriosus. *J Pediatr* 1999;135:733–738.
197. Pourarian S, Takmil F, Cheriki S, et al. The effect of oral high-dose ibuprofen on patent ductus arteriosus closure in preterm infants. *Am J Perinatol* 2015;32:1158–1163.
198. Lago P, Salvadori S, Opocher F, et al. Continuous infusion of ibuprofen for treatment of patent ductus arteriosus in very low birth weight infants. *Neonatology* 2014;105:46–54.
199. Ohlsson A, Walia R, Shah S. Ibuprofen for the treatment of a patent ductus arteriosus in preterm and/or low birth weight infants. *Cochrane Database Syst Rev* 2003;CD003481.
200. Rheinlaender C, Helfenstein D, Pees C, et al. Neurodevelopmental outcome after COX inhibitor treatment for patent ductus arteriosus. *Early Hum Dev* 2010;86:87–92.
201. Eras Z, Gokmen T, Erdeve O, et al. Impact of oral versus intravenous ibuprofen on neurodevelopmental outcome: a randomized controlled parallel study. *Am J Perinatol* 2013;30:857–862.
202. Oncel MY, Eras Z, Uras N, et al. Neurodevelopmental outcomes of preterm infants treated with oral paracetamol versus ibuprofen for patent ductus arteriosus. *Am J Perinatol* 2017;34:1185–1189.
203. Sangtawesin V, Sangtawesin C, Raksasinborisut C, et al. Oral ibuprofen prophylaxis for symptomatic patent ductus arteriosus of prematurity. *J Med Assoc Thai* 2006;89:314–321.
204. Sharma PK, Garg SK, Narang A. Pharmacokinetics of oral ibuprofen in premature infants. *J Clin Pharmacol* 2003;43:968–973.
205. Gokmen T, Erdeve O, Altug N, et al. Efficacy and safety of oral versus intravenous ibuprofen in very low birth weight preterm infants with patent ductus arteriosus. *J Pediatr* 2011;158:549–554.
206. Erdeve O, Yurttutan S, Ozdemir R, et al. Oral ibuprofen for treatment of patent ductus arteriosus: more than a cheap alternative? *Neonatology* 2012;102:196; author reply 196.
207. Sangtawesin C, Sangtawesin V, Lertsutthiwong W, et al. Prophylaxis of symptomatic patent ductus arteriosus with oral ibuprofen in very low birth weight infants. *J Med Assoc Thai* 2008;91(Suppl 3):S28–S34.
208. Demir N, Peker E, Ece I, et al. Efficacy and safety of rectal ibuprofen for patent ductus arteriosus closure in very low birth weight preterm infants. *J Matern Fetal Neonatal Med* 2017;30:2119–2125.
209. Hammerman C, Bin-Nun A, Markovitch E, et al. Ductal closure with paracetamol: a surprising new approach to patent ductus arteriosus treatment. *Pediatrics* 2011;128:e1618–e1621.
210. Ohlsson A, Shah PS. Paracetamol (acetaminophen) for patent ductus arteriosus in preterm or low birth weight infants. *Cochrane Database Syst Rev* 2018;4:CD010061.
211. Lu J, Li Q, Zhu L, et al. Oral ibuprofen is superior to oral paracetamol for patent ductus arteriosus in very low and extremely low birth weight infants. *Medicine (Baltimore)* 2019;98:e16689.
212. Harkin P, Harma A, Aikio O, et al. Paracetamol accelerates closure of the ductus arteriosus after premature birth: a randomized trial. *J Pediatr* 2016;177:72.e2–77.e2.
213. Terrin G, Conte F, Oncel MY, et al. Paracetamol for the treatment of patent ductus arteriosus in preterm neonates: a systematic review and meta-analysis. *Arch Dis Child Fetal Neonatal Ed* 2016;101:F127–F136.
214. Hochwald O, Mainzer G, Borenstein-Levin L, et al. Adding paracetamol to ibuprofen for the treatment of patent ductus arteriosus in preterm infants: a double-blind, randomized, placebo-controlled pilot study. *Am J Perinatol* 2018;35:1319–1325.
215. Yurttutan S, Bozkaya A, Hudayioglu F, et al. The effect of combined therapy for treatment of monotherapy-resistant PDA in preterm infants. *J Matern Fetal Neonatal Med* 2019;32:3662–3665.
216. Oncel M.Y, Yurttutan S, Erdeve O, et al. Oral paracetamol versus oral ibuprofen in the management of patent ductus arteriosus in preterm infants: a randomized controlled trial. *J Pediatr* 2014;164:510.e1–514.e1.
217. El-Khuffash A, Jain A, Corcoran D, et al. Efficacy of paracetamol on patent ductus arteriosus closure may be dose dependent: evidence from human and murine studies. *Pediatr Res* 2014;76:238–244.
218. Dani C, Poggi C, Mosca F, et al. Efficacy and safety of intravenous paracetamol in comparison to ibuprofen for the treatment of patent ductus arteriosus in preterm infants: study protocol for a randomized control trial. *Trials* 2016;17:182.
219. El-Mashad AE, El-Mahdy H, El Amrousy D, et al. Comparative study of the efficacy and safety of paracetamol, ibuprofen, and indomethacin in closure of patent ductus arteriosus in preterm neonates. *Eur J Pediatr* 2017;176:233–240.
220. Karabulut B, Paytoncu S. Efficacy and safety of oral paracetamol vs. oral ibuprofen in the treatment of symptomatic patent ductus arteriosus in premature infants. *Paediatr Drugs* 2019;21:113–121.
221. Rifas-Shiman SL, Cardenas A, Hivert MF, et al. Associations of prenatal or infant exposure to acetaminophen or ibuprofen with mid-childhood executive function and behaviour. *Paediatr Perinat Epidemiol* 2020;34(3):287–298.
222. Ji Y, Azuine RE, Zhang Y, et al. Association of cord plasma biomarkers of in utero acetaminophen exposure with risk of attention-deficit/hyperactivity disorder and autism spectrum disorder in childhood. *JAMA Psychiatry* 2020;77(2):180–189.
223. Masarwa R, Levine H, Gorelik E, et al. Prenatal exposure to acetaminophen and risk for attention deficit hyperactivity disorder and autistic spectrum disorder: a systematic review, meta-analysis, and meta-regression analysis of Cohort studies. *Am J Epidemiol* 2018;187:1817–1827.
224. Bauer AZ, Kriebel D, Herbert MR, et al. Prenatal paracetamol exposure and child neurodevelopment: a review. *Horm Behav* 2018;101:125–147.
225. Laue H.E, Cassoulet R, Abdelouahab N, et al. Association between meconium acetaminophen and childhood neurocognitive development in GESTE, a Canadian Cohort Study. *Toxicol Sci* 2019;167:138–144.
226. Juujarvi S, Kallankari H, Patsi P, et al. Follow-up study of the early, randomised paracetamol trial to preterm infants, found no adverse reactions at the two-years corrected age. *Acta Paediatr* 2019;108:452–458.
227. Olsen J, Liew Z. Fetal programming of mental health by acetaminophen? Response to the SMFM statement: prenatal acetaminophen use and ADHD. *Expert Opin Drug Saf* 2017;16:1395–1398.
228. Bhattacharya M, Asselin P, Hardy P, et al. Developmental changes in prostaglandin E(2) receptor subtypes in porcine ductus arteriosus. Possible contribution in altered responsiveness to prostaglandin E(2). *Circulation* 1999;100:1751–1756.
229. Bouayad A, Kajino H, Waleh N, et al. Characterization of PGE2 receptors in fetal and newborn lamb ductus arteriosus. *Am J Physiol Heart Circul Physiol* 2001;280: H2342–H2349.
230. Stempak D, Gammon J, Klein J, et al. Single-dose and steady-state pharmacokinetics of celecoxib in children. *Clin Pharmacol Ther* 2002;72:490–497.
231. Nguyen M, Camenisch T, Snouwaert JN, et al. The prostaglandin receptor EP4 triggers remodelling of the cardiovascular system at birth. *Nature* 1997;390:78–81.
232. Kajino H, Taniguchi T, Fujieda K, et al. An EP4 receptor agonist prevents indomethacin-induced closure of rat ductus arteriosus in vivo. *Pediatr Res* 2004;56:586–590.
233. Momma K, Toyoshima K, Takeuchi D, et al. In vivo reopening of the neonatal ductus arteriosus by a prostanoid EP4-receptor agonist in the rat. *Prostaglandins Other Lipid Mediat* 2005;78:117–128.
234. Momma K, Toyoshima K, Takeuchi D, et al. In vivo constriction of the fetal and neonatal ductus arteriosus by a prostanoid EP4-receptor antagonist in rats. *Pediatr Res* 2005;58:971–975.
235. Wright DH, Abran D, Bhattacharya M, et al. Prostanoid receptors: ontogeny and implications in vascular physiology. *Am J Physiol Regul Integr Comp Physiol* 2001;281:R1343–R1360.
236. Yokoyama U, Minamisawa S, Quan H, et al. Chronic activation of the prostaglandin receptor EP4 promotes hyaluronan-mediated neointimal formation in the ductus arteriosus. *J Clin Invest* 2006;116:3026–3034.
237. Loftin CD, Trivedi DB, Tiano HF, et al. Failure of ductus arteriosus closure and remodeling in neonatal mice deficient in cyclooxygenase-1 and cyclooxygenase-2. *Proc Natl Acad Sci U S A* 2001;98:1059–1064.
238. Trivedi DB, Sugimoto Y, Loftin CD. Attenuated cyclooxygenase-2 expression contributes to patent ductus arteriosus in preterm mice. *Pediatr Res* 2006;60:669–674.
239. Chen JX, O'Mara PW, Poole SD, et al. Isoprostanes as physiological mediators of transition to newborn life: novel mechanisms regulating patency of the term and preterm ductus arteriosus. *Pediatr Res* 2012;72:122–128.
240. Basaran A, Gyimadu A, Gucer S, et al. Cyclooxygenase immunohistochemical staining in the human ductus arteriosus after 24 weeks of gestational age. *J Obstet Gynaecol* 2012;32:120–123.
241. Clyman RI, Hardy P, Waleh N, et al. Cyclooxygenase-2 plays a significant role in regulating the tone of the fetal lamb ductus arteriosus. *Am J Physiol* 1999;276:R913–R921.
242. Coceani F, Ackerley C, Seidlitz E, et al. Function of cyclo-oxygenase-1 and cyclo-oxygenase-2 in the ductus arteriosus from foetal lamb: differential development and change by oxygen and endotoxin. *Br J Pharmacol* 2001;132:241–251.
243. Guerguerian AM, Hardy P, Bhattacharya M, et al. Expression of cyclooxygenases in ductus arteriosus of fetal and newborn pigs. *Am J Obstet Gynecol* 1998;179:1618–1626.
244. Sawdy RJ, Lye S, Fisk NM, et al. A double-blind randomized study of fetal side effects during and after the short-term maternal administration of indomethacin, sulindac, and nimesulide for the treatment of preterm labor. *Am J Obstet Gynecol* 2003;188:1046–1051.
245. Giovanni G, Giovanni P. Do non-steroidal anti-inflammatory drugs and COX-2 selective inhibitors have different renal effects? *J Nephrol* 2002;15:480–488.
246. Peruzzi L, Gianoglio B, Porcellini G, et al. Neonatal chronic kidney failure associated with cyclo-oxygenase-2 inhibitors administered during pregnancy. *Minerva Urol Nefrol* 2001;53:113–116.
247. Bouayad A, Fouron JC, Hou X, et al. Developmental regulation of prostaglandin E2 synthase in porcine ductus arteriosus. *Am J Physiol Regul Integr Comp Physiol* 2004;286:R903–R909.
248. Baragatti B, Sodini D, Uematsu S, et al. Role of microsomal prostaglandin E synthase-1 (mPGES1)-derived PGE2 in patency of the ductus arteriosus in the mouse. *Pediatr Res* 2008;64:523–527.
249. Coceani F, Olley PM, Lock JE. Prostaglandins, ductus arteriosus, pulmonary circulation: current concepts and clinical potential. *Eur J Clin Pharmacol* 1980;18:75–81.
250. Talosi G, Katona M, Racz K, et al. Prostaglandin E1 treatment in patent ductus arteriosus dependent congenital heart defects. *J Perinat Med* 2004;32:368–374.
251. Liu L, Johnson HL, Cousens S, et al. Global, regional, and national causes of child mortality: an updated systematic analysis for 2010 with time trends since 2000. *Lancet* 2012;379:2151–2161.
252. Hamilton BE, Hoyert DL, Martin JA, et al. Annual summary of vital statistics: 2010–2011. *Pediatrics* 2013;131:548–558.
253. Nadeau-Vallee M, Obari D, Quiniou C, et al. A critical role of interleukin-1 in preterm labor. *Cytokine Growth Factor Rev* 2016;28:37–51.
254. Smith R. Parturition. *N Engl J Med* 2007;356:271–283.
255. Simhan HN, Caritis SN. Prevention of preterm delivery. *N Engl J Med* 2007;357:477–487.
256. Romero R, Miranda J, Chaiworapongsa T, et al. Prevalence and clinical significance of sterile intra-amniotic inflammation in patients with preterm labor and intact membranes. *Am J Reprod Immunol* 2014;72:458–474.
257. Romero R, Mazor M, Munoz H, et al. The preterm labor syndrome. *Ann NY Acad Sci* 1994;734:414–429.
258. Rinaldi SF, Hutchinson JL, Rossi AG, et al. Anti-inflammatory mediators as physiological and pharmacological regulators of parturition. *Expert Rev Clin Immunol* 2011;7:675–696.
259. Cook JL, Shallow MC, Zaragoza DB, et al. Mouse placental prostaglandins are associated with uterine activation and the timing of birth. *Biol Reprod* 2003;68:579–587.
260. Arthur P, Taggart MJ, Zielnik B, et al. Relationship between gene expression and function of uterotonic systems in the rat during gestation, uterine activation and both term and preterm labour. *J Physiol* 2008;586:6063–6076.
261. Christiaens I, Zaragoza DB, Guilbert L, et al. Inflammatory processes in preterm and term parturition. *J Reprod Immunol* 2008;79:50–57.
262. Hillier SL, Witkin SS, Krohn MA, et al. The relationship of amniotic fluid cytokines and preterm delivery, amniotic fluid infection, histologic chorioamnionitis, and chorioamnion infection. *Obstet Gynecol* 1993;81:941–948.

263. Steinborn A, Gunes H, Roddiger S, et al. Elevated placental cytokine release, a process associated with preterm labor in the absence of intrauterine infection. *Obstet Gynecol* 1996;88:534–539.
264. Gomez R, Romero R, Edwin SS, et al. Pathogenesis of preterm labor and preterm premature rupture of membranes associated with intraamniotic infection. *Infect Dis Clin North Am* 1997;11:135–176.
265. Mazor M, Furman B, Bashiri A. Cytokines in preterm parturition. *Gynecol Endocrinol* 1998;12:421–427.
266. Challis JR, Sloboda DM, Alfaidy N, et al. Prostaglandins and mechanisms of preterm birth. *Reproduction* 2002;124:1–17.
267. Sanchez-Ramos L. Induction of labor. *Obstet Gynecol Clin North Am* 2005;32:181–200.
268. Zuckerman H, Reiss U, Rubinstein I. Inhibition of human premature labor by indomethacin. *Obstet Gynecol* 1974;44:787–792.
269. Niebyl JR, Blake DA, White RD, et al. The inhibition of premature labor with indomethacin. *Am J Obstet Gynecol* 1980;136:1014–1019.
270. Kurki T, Eronen M, Lumme R, et al. A randomized double-dummy comparison between indomethacin and nylidrin in threatened preterm labor. *Obstet Gynecol* 1991;78:1093–1097.
271. Reinebrant HE, Pileggi-Castro C, Romero CL, et al. Cyclo-oxygenase (COX) inhibitors for treating preterm labour. *Cochrane Database Syst Rev* 2015;CD001992.
272. Sawdy R, Slater D, Fisk N, et al. Use of a cyclo-oxygenase type-2-selective non-steroidal anti-inflammatory agent to prevent preterm delivery. *Lancet* 1997;350:265–266.
273. Peruzzi L, Gianoglio B, Porcellini MG, et al. Neonatal end-stage renal failure associated with maternal ingestion of cyclo-oxygenase-type-1 selective inhibitor nimesulide as tocolytic. *Lancet* 1999;354:1615.
274. Groom KM, Shennan AH, Jones BA, et al. TOCOX—a randomised, double-blind, placebo-controlled trial of rofecoxib (a COX-2-specific prostaglandin inhibitor) for the prevention of preterm delivery in women at high risk. *BJOG* 2005;112:725–730.
275. Urrego D, Liwa AC, Cole WC, et al. Cyclooxygenase inhibitors for treating preterm labour: What is the molecular evidence? *Can J Physiol Pharmacol* 2019;97:222–231.
276. Astle S, Newton R, Thornton S, et al. Expression and regulation of prostaglandin E synthase isoforms in human myometrium with labour. *Mol Hum Reprod* 2007;13:69–75.
277. Sharp GC, Hutchinson JL, Hibbert N, et al. Transcription analysis of the myometrium of labouring and non-labouring women. *PLoS One* 2016;11:e0155413.
278. Amin SB, Sinkin RA, Glantz JC. Metaanalysis of the effect of antenatal indomethacin on neonatal outcomes. *Am J Obstet Gynecol* 2007;197:486.e1–486.e10.
279. Rovers JFJ, Thomissen IJC, Janssen LCE, et al. The relationship between antenatal indomethacin as a tocolytic drug and neonatal outcomes: a retrospective cohort study. *J Matern Fetal Neonatal Med* 2019;1.
280. Roberge S, Nicolaides KH, Demers S, et al. Prevention of perinatal death and adverse perinatal outcome using low-dose aspirin: a meta-analysis. *Ultrasound Obstet Gynecol* 2013;41:491–499.
281. Hoffman MK, Goudar SS, Kodkany BS, et al. Low-dose aspirin for the prevention of preterm delivery in nulliparous women with a singleton pregnancy (ASPIRIN): a randomised, double-blind, placebo-controlled trial. *Lancet* 2020;395:285–293.
282. Haram K, Mortensen JH, Morrison JC. Tocolysis for acute preterm labor: does anything work. *J Matern Fetal Neonatal Med* 2015;28:371–378.
283. Olson DM. The role of prostaglandins in the initiation of parturition. *Best Pract Res Clin Obstet Gynaecol* 2003;17:717–730.
284. Sugimoto Y, Yamasaki A, Segi E, et al. Failure of parturition in mice lacking the prostaglandin F receptor. *Science* 1997;277:681–683.
285. Peri KG, Quiniou C, Hou X, et al. THG113: a novel selective FP antagonist that delays preterm labor. *Semin Perinatol* 2002;26:389–397.
286. Bottcher B, Laterza RM, Wildt L, et al. A first-in-human study of PDC31 (prostaglandin F2alpha receptor inhibitor) in primary dysmenorrhea. *Hum Reprod* 2014;29:2465–2473.
287. Goupil E, Tassy D, Bourguet C, et al. A novel biased allosteric compound inhibitor of parturition selectively impedes the prostaglandin F2alpha-mediated Rho/ROCK signaling pathway. *J Biol Chem* 2010;285:25624–25636.
288. Pohl O, Chollet A, Kim SH, et al. OBE022, an oral and selective prostaglandin F2alpha receptor antagonist as an effective and safe modality for the treatment of preterm labor. *J Pharmacol Exp Ther* 2018;366:349–364.
289. Pohl O, Marchand L, Gotteland JP, et al. Pharmacokinetics, safety and tolerability of OBE022, a selective prostaglandin F2alpha receptor antagonist tocolytic: a first-in-human trial in healthy postmenopausal women. *Br J Clin Pharmacol* 2018;84:1839–1855.
290. Nadeau-Vallee M, Chin PY, Belarbi L, et al. Antenatal suppression of IL-1 protects against inflammation-induced fetal injury and improves neonatal and developmental outcomes in mice. *J Immunol* 2017;198:2047–2062.
291. Nadeau-Vallee M, Quiniou C, Palacios J, et al. Novel noncompetitive IL-1 receptor-biased ligand prevents infection-and inflammation-induced preterm birth. *J Immunol* 2015;195:3402–3415.
292. Lesko SM, Mitchell AA. An assessment of the safety of pediatric ibuprofen. A practitioner-based randomized clinical trial. *JAMA* 1995;273:929–933.
293. Lesko SM, Mitchell AA. Renal function after short-term ibuprofen use in infants and children. *Pediatrics* 1997;100:954–957.
294. Shastri N. Intravenous acetaminophen use in pediatrics. *Pediatr Emerg Care* 2015; 31:444–448.
295. Heubi JE, Barbacci MB, Zimmerman HJ. Therapeutic misadventures with acetaminophen: hepatoxicity after multiple doses in children. *J Pediatr* 1998;132:22–27.
296. Pierce CA, Voss B. Efficacy and safety of ibuprofen and acetaminophen in children and adults: a meta-analysis and qualitative review. *Ann Pharmacother* 2010;44:489–506.
297. Mahony L, Carnero V, Brett C, et al. Prophylactic indomethacin therapy for patent ductus arteriosus in very-low-birth-weight infants. *N Engl J Med* 1982;306:506–510.
298. Stark AR, Carlo WA, Tyson JE, et al. Adverse effects of early dexamethasone treatment in extremely-low-birth-weight infants. National Institute of Child Health and Human Development Neonatal Research Network. *N Engl J Med* 2001;344:95–101.
299. Watterberg KL, Gerdes JS, Cole CH, et al. Prophylaxis of early adrenal insufficiency to prevent bronchopulmonary dysplasia: a multicenter trial. *Pediatrics* 2004;114:1649–1657.
300. Peltoniemi O, Kari MA, Heinonen K, et al. Pretreatment cortisol values may predict responses to hydrocortisone administration for the prevention of bronchopulmonary dysplasia in high-risk infants. *J Pediatr* 2005;146:632–637.
301. Grosfeld JL, Chaet M, Molinari F, et al. Increased risk of necrotizing enterocolitis in premature infants with patent ductus arteriosus treated with indomethacin. *Ann Surg* 1996;224:350–357.
302. Sankaran K, Puckett B, Lee DS, et al. Variations in incidence of necrotizing enterocolitis in Canadian neonatal intensive care units. *J Pediatr Gastroenterol Nutr* 2004;39:366–372.
303. Dollberg S, Lusky A, Reichman B. Patent ductus arteriosus, indomethacin and necrotizing enterocolitis in very low birth weight infants: a population-based study. *J Pediatr Gastroenterol Nutr* 2005;40:184–188.
304. Bellini C, Campone F, Serra G. Pulmonary hypertension following L-lysine ibuprofen therapy in a preterm infant with patent ductus arteriosus. *CMAJ* 2006;174:1843–1844.
305. Amendolia B, Lynn M, Bhat V, et al. Severe pulmonary hypertension with therapeutic L-lysine ibuprofen in 2 preterm neonates. *Pediatrics* 2012;129:e1360–e1363.
306. Sehgal A, Kumarshingri PS. Pulmonary hypertension in an infant treated with ibuprofen. *Indian J Pediatr* 2013;80:697–699.
307. Rodriguez-Castano MJ, Aleo E, Arruza L. Oral sildenafil for severe pulmonary hypertension developing after ibuprofen use in a neonate. *Indian Pediatr* 2016;53:349–350.
308. Gournay V, Savagner C, Thiriez G, et al. Pulmonary hypertension after ibuprofen prophylaxis in very preterm infants. *Lancet* 2002;359:1486–1488.
309. Ahlfors CE. Effect of ibuprofen on bilirubin-albumin binding. *J Pediatr* 2004;144:386–388.
310. Desfrere L, Thibaut C, Kibleur Y, et al. Unbound bilirubin does not increase during ibuprofen treatment of patent ductus arteriosus in preterm infants. *J Pediatr* 2012;160:258.e1–264.e1.

CHAPTER 40

Diana Muñoz-Mendoza
Kim Jackson
Sasha A. Alvarado
Sami L. Bahna

Antihistamine Drugs

Antihistamines are among the most frequently used medications worldwide. As a body chemical, histamine has a role in health as well as in a variety of diseases. This chapter describes the physiologic role and the pathologic consequences of histamine release. The histamine receptors and their various functions are reviewed, and the clinical pharmacology and therapeutic uses of H_1 antihistamines are summarized. Antagonists to H_2 and H_3 receptors as well as the H_4 receptors are briefly discussed.

HISTORICAL BACKGROUND

Histamine, initially called β-aminoethylimidazole, was first discovered as a constituent of ergot and then was chemically synthesized in 1907[1] (Fig. 40.1). Soon after, Dale and Laidlaw[2,3] discovered that histamine stimulated a host of smooth muscle cells and had an intense vasodilator action. In their experiments, they found that histamine induced a shock-like syndrome in frogs and mammals. Histamine caused bronchospasm, myocardial contraction, and cardiac and pulmonary vasoconstriction. It also caused a fall in the systemic blood pressure due to capillary dilation, resulting in pooling of blood in the capillary bed and a substantial extravascular loss of plasma.

In 1927, Best and coworkers[4] isolated histamine from fresh samples of liver and lung, establishing that this amine is a natural constituent of the body. Demonstration of its presence in a variety of other tissues soon followed, hence its name after the Greek word "histos" for tissues. In the same year, Lewis[5] further expanded on the vascular effects of histamine, which suggested that this mediator could be released from cells in the skin on stimulation with appropriate trauma, causing the "wheal-and-flare response," which is also known as "the triple wheal-and-flare response." This reaction includes an immediate local reddening due to vasodilatation, a wheal due to increased vascular permeability, and a flare response due to indirect vasodilatation secondary to axonal reflex. In 1952, Riley and West[6] discovered that the mast cell is the major source for histamine. Later, they showed a correlation between the number of mast cells and the histamine content in a variety of animal tissues as well as in urticaria pigmentosa lesions in humans.[7] They also found histamine in the circulating basophils. In 1953, Mongar and Schild[8] published the first series of studies concerning the mechanism of histamine release from mast cells. Subsequent studies focused on the role of calcium in histamine release by antigens and other ligands.[9]

HISTAMINE

SYNTHESIS, STORAGE, AND METABOLISM OF HISTAMINE

Histamine is a hydrophilic molecule comprising an imidazole ring and an amino group connected by two methylene groups.[10] Histamine occurs in plants as well as in animal tissues and is a component of some venoms and a variety of insect secretions. Histamine is formed by the decarboxylation of the amino acid histidine by the enzyme L-histidine decarboxylase, found in every mammalian tissue that contains histamine. The chief site of histamine storage in most tissues is the mast cell; in the blood, it is the basophil. These cells synthesize histamine and store it in secretory granules. Histamine is mostly (70%) metabolized through methylation by *N*-methyltransferase to *N*-methyl histamine and partly (30%) through oxidation by diamine oxidase to imidazole acetic acid.[11] A very small amount of released histamine (2% to 3%) is excreted in the urine unchanged. The turnover of histamine in the mast cell secretory granules is slow (days to weeks). When histamine is depleted from its stores, it may take weeks before its concentration returns to normal levels. Histamine metabolites have little or no activity and are excreted in the urine.

Mast cells are found in the loose connective tissue of all organs, especially around blood vessels, nerves, and lymphatics. It is most abundant in the shock organs of allergic diseases, namely, the skin and the mucosa of the respiratory and the gastrointestinal tracts.[12] The human heart contains large numbers of mast cells, localized primarily in the wall of the right atrium.[13] Non–mast cell sites of histamine formation include the epidermis, enterochromaffin-like cells of the gastric mucosa, neurons within the central nervous system (CNS), and cells in regenerating or rapidly growing tissues. Turnover is rapid at these non–mast cell sites because the histamine is released continuously rather than stored.[10,14]

HISTAMINE RECEPTORS

Histamine exerts its effects through the activation of four distinct histamine receptors (H_1, H_2, H_3, and H_4) that belong to the G-protein–coupled receptor (GPCR) superfamily.[15] The existence of more than one type of histamine receptor was suggested in 1966 by Ash and Schild,[16] who noted that the classic antihistamine mepyramine could block histamine-induced

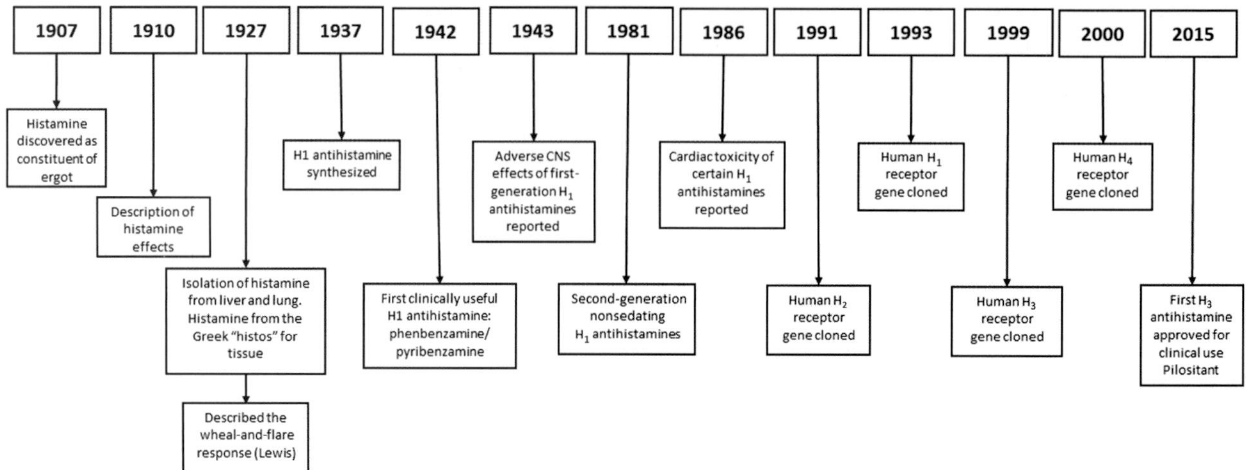

Figure 40.1 Sequential timeline of the discovery of histamine, its receptors, and histamine antagonists. CNS, central nervous system. (Modified from Simons FE, Simons KJ. Histamine and H_1-antihistamines: celebrating a century of progress. *J Allergy Clin Immunol* 2011;128:1139.e1134–1150.e1134.)

contractions of guinea pig ileum, but not histamine-induced gastric acid secretion. The effects of histamine on H_1, H_2, H_3, and H_4 receptors and their distributions in humans are presented in Table 40.1. Human H_1 receptors have approximately 45% homology with muscarinic receptors.[17]

The H_3 and H_4 receptors have a much higher affinity for histamine than H_1 and H_2 receptors.[10] The H_3 receptor was identified in 1983,[18] and its gene was cloned in 1999.[19] It is highly expressed in the CNS and acts as a presynaptic autoreceptor, inhibiting histamine release and modulating the release of other neurotransmitters.[10] It has been shown that H_3 receptors are involved in the blood–brain barrier function and may play a favorable role in neuroinflammation.[20]

H_3 agonists promote sleep, and H_3 antagonists promote wakefulness, attention, and cognition. Among the four histamine receptors, the H_3 receptor has received particular attention as a target for the treatment of neurodegenerative diseases and sleep disorders.[21] Pitolisant (also known as tiprolisant or ciproxidine) was the first H_3-receptor antagonist to progress into clinical development, ultimately being approved for the treatment of narcolepsy.[22]

The H_4 receptor was cloned in 2000 and is mainly expressed on hematopoietic cells such as eosinophils, dendritic cells, mast cells, monocytes, basophils, and T cells, as well as the immune cells in various parts of the gastrointestinal tract, CNS, and primary sensory afferent neurons.[23–25] Its structure showed about 40% similarity to H_3 receptor.[27] It may have a significant role in the inflammatory process in atopic dermatitis and asthma.[28,29] The H_4-receptor gene was mapped to chromosome 18.[30]

EFFECTS OF HISTAMINE

Cardiovascular

Injection of histamine in human causes a decrease in blood pressure and an increase in the heart rate. The blood pressure drops because of the direct vasodilator action on the arterioles and precapillary sphincters. The increase in heart rate results from a direct stimulatory action on the myocardium, mainly through the H_2 receptors, as well as through a reflex-compensatory tachycardia secondary to hypotension.[14] Both H_1 and H_2 receptors seem to be involved in these responses; hence, a combination of H_1 and H_2 antihistamines is often more effective in preventing the cardiovascular effects of histamine than either alone.

Stimulation of H_1 receptors in the atrioventricular node slows down the heart rate by decreasing atrioventricular nodal conduction.[29] Cardiac H_1 receptors are also found in epicardial coronary vessels where they mediate vasoconstriction.[31] H_2 receptors are found in the coronary vasculature, where their vasodilator action opposes that of H_1 receptors.[31] H_2 receptors are also widely distributed throughout the myocardium and nodal tissue where they exert positive inotropic and chronotropic effects, respectively.[29,31] H_3 receptors in the heart are present in the presynaptic postganglionic sympathetic fibers and are autoinhibitory to presynaptic norepinephrine release.[32,33] The widespread distribution of histamine receptors throughout the myocardium, nodal tissue, and coronary vasculature suggests a significant role in the physiologic regulation of the normal healthy heart. Nault and coworkers[34] reported that H_1 antihistamines (loratadine) in young healthy subjects did not alter the autonomic cardiovascular control. However, an H_2 antihistamine (ranitidine) altered cardiac sympathovagal balance when administered alone. Such a finding indicates a shift toward sympathetic predominance in heart rate regulation, with a potential of inducing arrhythmias.

Histamine-induced vasodilation causes transudation of fluid, and even large molecules such as proteins, into the perivascular tissue, resulting in skin hives or mucosal edema associated with allergic reactions. The vasodilator effect of histamine is mediated by both H_1 and H_2 receptors located on different cell types in the vascular bed: H_1 receptors on the endothelium, and both H_1 and H_2 receptors on the smooth muscle cells.[10] Stimulation of H_1 receptors on smooth muscle causes contraction, whereas activation of H_2 receptors on the same smooth muscle will cause relaxation.

Activation of H_1 receptors leads to increased intracellular Ca^{2+}, activation of phospholipase A_2, and the local production of nitric oxide—an endothelium-derived relaxing factor.[35] Nitric oxide diffuses to the vascular smooth muscle, where it causes increase in cyclic guanosine monophosphate (cGMP), which, in turn, results in short-lived vasodilation.

TABLE 40.1 Histamine Receptor Types

	H_1 Receptor	*H_2 Receptor*	*H_3 Receptor*	*H_4 Receptor*
Chromosome	3p25	5q35.2	20q13.33	18q11.2
Amino acids	487	359	445	390
G-protein coupling	$G_{q/11}$	G_s	$G_{i/o}$	$G_{i/o}$
Signal transduction	↑PLC-IP_3-Ca^{2+}, ↑NO, ↑cGMP	↑cAMP	↓cAMP, ↑MAPK	↓cAMP, ↑Ca^{2+}
Tissues/cells	Lung, CNS, CVS, adrenals, epithelial cells, neutrophils, eosinophils, monocytes/macrophages, DC, T cells, B cells, hepatocytes	Heart, stomach, CNS, airway and vascular smooth muscle, endothelial cells, epithelial cells, neutrophils, eosinophils, monocytes	CNS: pre- and postsynaptic neurons, eosinophils, DC, monocytes	Eosinophils, DC, monocytes, T cells, basophils, mast cells, gastrointestinal tract, dermal fibroblasts, neurons
Functions	Pruritus, pain, flushing, headache, cough, sleep/wakefulness, decreased appetite, body temperature, hypotension, tachycardia, vasoconstriction, vasodilation (through NO), vascular permeability, decreased AV node conduction, bronchial smooth muscle constriction, prostaglandin secretion, recruitment of inflammatory cells, release of inflammatory mediators	Flushing, headache, hypotension, gastric acidity, vasodilation, vascular permeability, chronotropic, inotropic, bronchial smooth muscle relaxation, airway mucus secretion, stimulation of T-suppressor cells, decreased neutrophil and basophil chemotaxis, inhibition of natural killer cells, reduced lymphocyte cytotoxicity and proliferation	Sleep, cognition, inhibition of histamine synthesis, and neurotransmitter release (histamine, dopamine, serotonin, norepinephrine, acetylcholine)	Pruritus, bronchoconstriction, chemotaxis

AV node, atrioventricular node; cAMP, cyclic adenosine monophosphate; cGMP, cyclic guanosine monophosphate; CNS, central nervous system; CVS, cardiovascular system; DC, dendritic cells; IP_3, inositol triphosphate; MAPK, mitogen-activated protein kinase; NO, nitric oxide; PLC, phospholipase C; ↓, decrease; ↑, increase.

Adapted from Simons FE. Advances in H_1-antihistamines. *N Engl J Med* 2004;351:2203–2217 and Skidgel RA. Histamine, bradykinin, and their antagonists. In: Brunton LL, Hilal-Dandan R, Knollman BC, eds. *Goodman & Gilman's The pharmacological basis of therapeutics*, 13th ed. New York, NY: McGraw-Hill Companies Inc., 2018.

Nonvascular Smooth Muscle

Histamine-induced bronchospasm has been demonstrated in both humans and guinea pigs. Although some H_2 receptors are present in human bronchial smooth muscle, their dilator effect is much dominated by the spasmogenic influence of H_1 receptors. In asthma, histamine-induced bronchospasm may involve an additional reflex component that arises from irritation of afferent vagal nerve endings.[10]

Histamine has lesser effects on nonbronchial smooth muscle. It causes various degrees of uterine muscle contraction, but such an effect is negligible on the human uterus, gravid or not. The response of the intestinal muscle varies according to the species and region but is primarily contraction. The effect on other smooth muscles (e.g., urinary bladder, ureter, gallbladder, iris) is minimal or inconsistent.

Gastric Acid Secretion

Histamine stimulates gastric acid secretion by the parietal cells through H_2 receptors as well as stimulation of vagal reflex and gastrin release.[36] It also increases the output of pepsin and the intrinsic factor. The activation of H_2 receptors on the parietal cells leads to increase in adenylyl cyclase activity, cyclic adenosine monophosphate (cAMP) concentration, and intracellular Ca^{2+}.

Central Nervous System

Histaminergic neurons have been identified in some areas of the brain. H_1 receptors are found throughout the CNS and are densely concentrated in the hypothalamus. Histamine acts as a neurotransmitter along with the other biogenic amines, serotonin, dopamine, norepinephrine, and acetylcholine.[37] Histamine increases wakefulness and inhibits appetite through H_1 receptors. Neuronal histamine is involved in arousal, learning, memory, locomotor activity, food intake, and other physiologic processes.

Presynaptic H_3 receptors play important role in inhibiting the synthesis and release of histamine in the histaminergic neurons in the CNS. H_3-receptor agonists (e.g., (*R*)-α-methylhistamine, imetit, immepip) reduce the release of several amines in various areas of the brain, including histamine, norepinephrine, dopamine, 5-hydroxytryptamine, and, possibly, acetylcholine.[14]

H_1, H_3, and H_4 receptors have been detected on skin, innervating sensory neurons isolated from dorsal root ganglia.[38] Histamine stimulates cutaneous sensory nerve endings, resulting in pruritus and pain.[10]

Immune System and Inflammatory Response

Many inflammatory cells express H_1, H_2, and H_4 receptors.[39] The H_4 receptor is found more on the dendritic cells, mast cells, eosinophils, monocytes, basophils, and T cells. In general, H_1 receptors stimulate pro-inflammatory activity through increased cell migration to areas of inflammation, whereas H_2 receptors act as a potent suppressor of inflammatory and effector functions. Histamine also facilitates several pro-inflammatory activities through H_4 receptors.[25] Most ligands that target H_1 and H_2 receptors have little affinity for H_4 receptors. The H_4 receptor may play a role in chemotaxis of mast cells, eosinophils, and dendritic cells. The role of the H_4 receptor in inflammatory and pruritic response has been verified in vivo.[40–42]

Allergy Response

Histamine release occurs when allergen binds to the specific immunoglobulin E (IgE) molecule on the mast cells and basophils in previously sensitized individuals. Histamine release from these cells depends on the rise in intracellular Ca^{2+}.[10] Although histamine was the first identified mediator of allergic inflammation, numerous other mediators exist. They are either preformed in the granules (e.g., serotonin, tryptase, chymases, carboxypeptidases, acid hydrolases, oxidative enzymes, chemotactic factors, and proteoglycans, such as heparin and chondroitin sulfate) or newly formed from the mast cell membrane (e.g., prostaglandin D_2 and leukotrienes).

Elevated plasma histamine levels are present in conditions associated with increased mast cell number (e.g., mastocytosis) or activation (e.g., anaphylaxis or other allergic diseases).[43] Increased histamine levels have also been noted in the skin and plasma of patients with atopic dermatitis and in chronic urticaria.[44–46] Recently, it was demonstrated that a special type of dendritic cells (the inflammatory dendritic epidermal cells) express H_4 receptors in skin lesions of atopic dermatitis.[28] Increased levels of histamine have been found in bronchoalveolar lavage fluid in patients with asthma.[47] However, H_1 and H_2 blockers have minimal therapeutic effect in asthma, suggesting a possible role of H_4 receptors.

EXTRINSIC FACTORS CAUSING DIRECT HISTAMINE RELEASE

A large number of agents cause direct histamine release from mast cells without prior sensitization or involvement of specific antibodies. These include peptides that contain basic amino acids (arginine and/or lysine), complement derivatives (C3a, C4a, and C5a), substance P, hymenoptera venom constituents such as melittin, and chemicals and therapeutic agents such as morphine, codeine, dextrans, blood substitutes, polymyxin B, radiocontrast media, quaternary ammonium compounds, pyridinium compounds, piperidines, alkaloids, and plasma expanders. Basically, pathways that result in a decrease in cAMP or pathways that result in an increase in cGMP will cause histamine release. The flushing and hypotension (the red-man syndrome) that often occurs during vancomycin infusion is probably due to direct histamine release.[48] Various degrees of direct histamine release may also occur in certain individuals in response to particular foods (e.g., tomatoes, strawberries) or physical agents (e.g., dermographism).[49]

ANTIHISTAMINE PREPARATIONS

Development of antihistamines for allergy, gastric ulcers, motion sickness, and insomnia has utilized the diverse actions of histamine. These drugs have been so successful and widely used that the term "antihistamine" has become commonplace and mostly refer to H_1 antihistamines. In general, an antihistamine to a particular type of histamine receptor is not effective against the others. Since allergic reactions are primarily mediated through the activation of H_1 receptors, emphasis in this chapter is given to H_1 antihistamines more than to the other types of antihistamines.

For years, it was believed that H_1 antihistamines acted through competition with histamine for the receptors. Research showed that H_1 receptors exist in both active and inactive isoforms that are in equilibrium on the cellular surface and respond to the agonist (histamine) and inverse agonists (antihistamines), respectively.[50] In other words, antihistamines act as inverse agonists that bind and stabilize the inactive form of the receptor, shifting the equilibrium to the inactive state.

H_1 ANTIHISTAMINES

The first H_1 antihistamine, compound F929, was discovered in 1937 by Staub and Bovet.[51] Shortly afterward, Halpern in 1942 developed the first antihistamine for human use, phenbenzamine (*Antergan*).[52] Later, diphenhydramine and numerous other preparations became available. Most H_1 antihistamines are stable, water-soluble salts and have similar pharmacologic actions and therapeutic applications. In general, the molecular structure of H_1 antihistamines comprises a double-aromatic unit linked by a two- or three-atom chain attached to a tertiary amino basic group. The histamine molecule has similar structure but differs from antihistamines (i.e., inverse agonists) in possessing only one aromatic (imidazole) unit and in being levorotatory, whereas antihistamines are dextrorotatory.

H_1 antihistamines have been traditionally classified into six groups: the ethanolamines, ethylenediamines, alkylamines, piperazines, piperidines, and phenothiazines. With the development of newer "nonsedating" preparations, they are generally classified as first- and second-generation antihistamines (Table 40.2). Some of the second-generation preparations are active metabolites of first-generation compounds; for example, fexofenadine, levocetirizine, and desloratadine are active metabolites of terfenadine, cetirizine, and loratadine, respectively.

PHARMACOLOGIC PROPERTIES OF H_1 ANTIHISTAMINES

In general, first-generation H_1 antihistamines are rapidly absorbed and metabolized. Following oral administration, peak plasma concentrations are achieved in 1 to 3 hours, and the effects usually last 4 to 6 hours. Peak concentrations of these drugs in skin may persist long after plasma levels have declined. Thus, inhibition of "wheal-and-flare" responses can last up to 7 days after discontinuation.[10] Their binding to the receptors is readily reversible by spontaneous dissociation or by high levels of histamine. Because of their lipophilicity and low-molecular weight, they easily cross the blood–brain barrier, bind to the H_1 receptors, and create CNS side effects (Table 40.3), primarily sedation, but in certain subjects, CNS stimulation may occur.

The second-generation H_1 antihistamines are lipophobic and have high-molecular weights and thus do not easily cross the blood–brain barrier, with minimal CNS adverse effects.[17,53] They have longer duration of action (12 to 24 hours) because they strongly bind to the receptors and dissociate slowly.[54] To date, at least 11 second-generation anti-H_1 preparations were studied in double-blind, placebo-controlled studies in children.

TABLE 40.2 Chemical and Functional Classifications of H_1 Antihistamines

Drug	*Generation*	*Drug*	*Generation*
ALKYLAMINES		Oxatomide	First
Acrivastine	Second	**Piperidines**	
Brompheniramine	First	Astemizole[a]	Second
Chlorpheniramine	First	Bilastine[b]	Second
Pheniramine	First	Cyproheptadine	First
ETHANOLAMINES		Desloratadine	Second
Carbinoxamine	First	Diphenylpyraline	First
Dimenhydrinate	First	Ebastine	Second
Diphenhydramine	First	Fexofenadine	Second
Doxylamine	First	Ketotifen	First
Phenyltoloxamine	First	Levocabastine	Second
ETHYLENEDIAMINES		Loratadine	Second
Antazoline	First	Mizolastine	Second
Pyrilamine	First	Olopatadine	Second
Tripelennamine	First	Terfenadine[a]	Second
PHENOTHIAZINES		PHENOTHIAZINES	
Methdilazine	First	Methdilazine	First
Promethazine	First	Promethazine	First
PIPERAZINES		OTHERS	
Cetirizine	Second	Azelastine	Second
Hydroxyzine	First	Doxepin[c]	First
Levocetirizine	Second	Emedastine	Second
Meclizine	First	Epinastine	Second

[a]Discontinued due to cardiotoxicity
[b]Unavailable in U.S.
[c]Classified as a tricyclic antidepressant and has H_1- and H_2-antihistamine effects
Data from Simons FE. Advances in H_1-antihistamines. N Engl J Med 2004;351:2203–2217.

Almost all first-generation H_1 preparations have some antimuscarinic effect. Even at usual doses, they often cause dryness of the mucous membranes and sometimes urinary retention or blurred vision. Certain first-generation H_1 antihistamines, particularly promethazine, have α-adrenergic–blocking ability.[14] Others may exhibit antiserotonin activity (e.g., cyproheptadine)[14] or antidopamine effect (e.g., phenothiazines).[55] In high concentrations, some H_1 antihistamines, particularly promethazine, have a local anesthetic effect that can be more potent than procaine.[10] Some CNS effects can be of therapeutic value, for example, dimenhydrinate and diphenhydramine for motion sickness and diphenhydramine in decreasing drug-induced extrapyramidal symptoms. Over the past two decades, some H_1 antihistamines have been found to have antiallergic, anti-inflammatory properties apart from their action on H_1 receptors.[56,57] They downregulate allergic inflammation by direct activation of H_1 receptors and indirectly through nuclear factor-κB (NFκB) by suppressing antigen presentation, expression of pro-inflammatory cytokines and cell adhesion molecules, and chemotaxis. These antiallergic properties are believed to be due to their suppression of mast cell and basophil activity.[58,59]

In addition to variation in their H_1-blocking activity and anti-inflammatory properties, the effect of H_1 antihistamines on various target organs varies widely, probably due to differences in their tissue deposition capacity. Moreover, it seems that the response in terms of clinical efficacy and side effects to any particular anti-H_1 medication varies from one patient to another.[60] Such heterogeneity in response can be due to gene

TABLE 40.3 Mechanism of Common Side Effects of H_1 Antihistamines

THROUGH H_1 RECEPTOR
- Increased sedation
- Decreased cognitive and psychomotor performance
- Increased appetite

THROUGH MUSCARINIC RECEPTOR
- Dry mouth
- Urinary retention
- Sinus tachycardia

THROUGH A-ADRENERGIC RECEPTOR
- Hypotension
- Dizziness
- Reflex tachycardia

THROUGH SEROTONIN RECEPTOR
- Increased appetite

K^+ AND OTHER CARDIAC ION CHANNELS
- Prolonged QT intervals

Adapted from Simons FE. New H_1-receptor antagonists: clinical pharmacology. *Clin Exp Allergy* 1990;20(Suppl 2):19–24.

abnormalities in the synthetic and/or metabolic pathways or in the receptors.[61,62] Polymorphisms of the enzymes in the metabolic pathway could enhance or delay their degradation. For example, one single-nucleotide polymorphism for histamine *N*-methyltransferase, C314 T, results in decrease in enzyme activity and is found in 5% to 10% of the general population.[63] Desloratadine has better pharmacokinetics and lesser drug–drug interactions than its parent drug loratadine. Also, levocetirizine has better receptor affinity and selectivity than cetirizine.

PHARMACOKINETICS AND METABOLISM OF H_1 ANTIHISTAMINES

Comparative pharmacology of H_1 antihistamines has been reviewed.[64] For most first-generation H_1 antihistamines, the pharmacokinetics (absorption, distribution, metabolism, and eliminations) has not been optimally investigated. Pharmacodynamic studies (correlations between drug concentrations and activity) were carried out for only a few preparations. Furthermore, first-generation H_1 antihistamines have not been investigated in young children or in patients with renal or hepatic insufficiency. Also, there are only a few studies regarding drug–drug and drug–food interactions (Table 40.4).

Most antihistamines are well absorbed from the gastrointestinal tract, achieving peak plasma concentration generally in 1 to 3 hours, with a therapeutic effect usually for 4 to 6 hours, and may last up to 24 hours for the newer preparations.[10] The clinical effect persists, even though the serum concentration of the parent compound has declined to the lowest limit of analytical detection, which suggests a continued action by active metabolites in the tissues. For some antihistamines, such as fexofenadine, bioavailability can be affected by the coadministration of foods, such as grapefruit or bitter orange juice,[65] or of other drugs, such as verapamil, probenecid, and cimetidine.[66] Although plasma concentration of fexofenadine can be increased by these agents, significant adverse reactions are rarely noted.[67]

Drug clearance is a measure of elimination. It is the volume of plasma that is completely cleared of the drug within a given period of time and is expressed as volume/time. The total body clearance of H_1 antihistamines is the sum of clearance from all organs and includes both hepatic and renal clearances. The clearance rate and plasma half-life ($t_{1/2}$) vary widely from one preparation to another. The half-life is a measure of the time during which the drug plasma concentration decreases by 50%. H_1 antihistamines have half-life ranging from less than 24 hours up to a few days in children[68,69] and up to several days in adults[70,71] (Table 40.4).

The volume of distribution (V_d) is a proportionality factor that relates the drug plasma concentration to its total amount in the body. Hence, the higher the degree of the drug's tissue distribution and binding, the lower is its concentration in the plasma. The volume of distribution of H_1 antihistamines varies widely, for example, 0.33 L per kg for levocabastine but exceeds 100 L per kg for loratadine and ebastine.[10,14]

All first-generation H_1 antihistamines and most of the second generation are metabolized by the hepatic cytochrome P450 (CYP450) system.[72] Consequently, their metabolism can be affected by competition for the CYP enzymes by other drugs (e.g., ketoconazole and macrolide antibiotics).[68] Certain metabolites of two specific preparations, namely, astemizole and terfenadine, can cause cardiac arrhythmia (torsades de pointes) if administered in high doses or in association with drugs that compete with the CYP system, or in the presence of liver or heart disease. This led to the withdrawal of terfenadine from the U.S. market in 1998 and of astemizole in 1999.[10] Such arrhythmias have not been reported in association with loratadine, cetirizine, azelastine, or fexofenadine (the active metabolite of terfenadine).[14] The latter has slow and limited absorption by the oral route, minimal hepatic metabolism, with bioavailability around 30%, and a half-life around 14.4 hours.[73]

Cetirizine and loratadine are primarily excreted into the urine, whereas fexofenadine and azelastine are mostly excreted in feces[14,74,75] (Table 40.4). It is worth noting that when combined with pseudoephedrine, the pharmacokinetics of loratadine or cetirizine does not change.[76] Unlike other H_1 antihistamines, cetirizine is not metabolized by the CYP system, and 70% of the drug is excreted unchanged in the urine within 72 hours.[69,70] The suppressive effect of antihistamines on the wheal-and-flare response to the percutaneous application of histamine or specific allergens varies from one preparation to another.[72] Before allergy skin testing or bronchial challenge, it is generally recommended to discontinue first-generation H_1 antihistamines for 2 to 3 days and second-generation preparations for 7 to 10 days.[77]

CLINICAL USES OF H_1 ANTIHISTAMINES

H_1 antihistamines are primarily used in the treatment of allergic diseases, particularly of the skin and the upper respiratory tract. First-generation preparations have not been optimally studied in allergic disorders. On the other hand, second-generation preparations have been adequately investigated in seasonal and perennial allergic rhinoconjunctivitis and chronic urticaria, especially in adults. In fact, they are the first choice in the treatment of allergic rhinitis, allergic conjunctivitis, and chronic urticaria.[17,53,78,79] Studies on these drugs in children are limited in number and are mostly for short durations.[80]

In general, H_1 antihistamines are most effective in controlling allergy symptoms when taken on a regular basis rather than as needed[81]; development of tolerance is rare.[82] A study on respiratory allergies demonstrated that during the offending pollen season, the as-needed use of desloratadine was as effective as regular intake in relieving nasal symptoms. However, the lower airway symptoms were better controlled on daily treatment.[83]

Allergic Rhinoconjunctivitis

Histamine is one of the principle mediators released during nasal and ocular allergic inflammation, causing itching, sneezing, rhinorrhea, and lacrimation. Histamine-induced nasal obstruction is due to increased mucosal blood flow, enhanced nasal vascular permeability, and plasma protein exudation from fenestrated superficial capillaries.

The efficacy of H_1 antihistamines in allergic rhinitis has been well documented.[84] Several studies have shown the efficacy and safety of H_1 antihistamines in children aged 4 to 12 years with seasonal allergic rhinitis.[80,84] Using nasal airflow measurement, fexofenadine and desloratadine significantly reduced the nasal airway resistance.[85,86] Antihistamines are most effective if started before the peak of pollination.[71] Studies on children showed that all nasal symptoms and quality of life significantly improved on desloratadine 5 mg daily[87] or fexofenadine 30 mg twice daily.[88] Also, levocetirizine 5 mg per day was highly effective in improving nasal symptoms in school-aged children with seasonal or perennial allergic rhinitis and in adolescents with perennial allergic rhinitis.[89,90] To increase the relief of nasal

TABLE 40.4 Pharmacokinetics, Formulations, and Pediatric Doses of Oral H_1 Antihistamine Preparations

Generic Name	t_{max} *(h) in Children*	$t_{1/2}$ *(h) in Children*	*Metabolism*	*Pediatric Dose*
First Generation				
Brompheniramine maleate	3–3.5	12	Hepatic	2–5 y:1 mg q4–6 h 6–11 y: 2 mg q4 h
Carbinoxamine maleate	1.5–5	17	Hepatic	2–5 y: 0.2–0.4 mg/kg/d divided q6–8 h 6–11 y: 2–4 mg q6–8 h ≥12 y: 4–6 mg q6–8 h
Chlorpheniramine maleate	2.5	13.1	Hepatic	2–5 y: 1 mg q4–6 h 6–11 y: 2 mg q4–6 h ≥12 y: 4 mg q4–6 h
Cyproheptadine hydrochloride	6–9	16	Hepatic	2–6 y: 0.25 mg/kg/d divided q8–12 h 7–14 y: 4 mg/d (q8–12 h)
Dimenhydrinate	Data not available	5–8	Hepatic	2–5 y: 12.5–25 mg q6–8 h 6–11 y: 25 mg q6–8 h ≥12 y: 50–100 mg q4–6 h
Diphenhydramine hydrochloride	2	5	Hepatic	5 mg/kg/d divided q6 h (max dose: 300 mg/d)
Hydroxyzine hydrochloride	2	7.1	Hepatic	<6 y: 12.5 mg q6–8 h ≥6 y: 12.5–25 mg q6–8 h
Promethazine	2.8	16–19	Hepatic	≥2 y: 0.125 mg/kg q6 h (max: 12.5 mg/dose) for antiallergic action ≥2 y: 0.25–1 mg/kg q4–6 h (max: 25 mg/dose) for nausea/vomiting
Second Generation				
Acrivastine[a]	1.1	2–4	Renal	≥12 y: 8 mg q6 h
Cetirizine hydrochloride[a,b]	1	6.2	Renal	6 mo to <2 y: 2.5 mg/d 2–5 y: 2.5–5 mg/d ≥6–11 y: 5–10 mg/d
Desloratadine[c]	3	24	Renal	6 mo to <1 y: 1 mg q24 h 1–5 y: 1.25 mg q24 h 6–11 y: 2.5 mg q24 h ≥12 y: 5 mg q24 h
Fexofenadine[c]	2	14.4	Bile	6 mo to <2 y: 15 mg q12 h 2–11 y: 30 mg q12 h ≥12 y: 60 mg q12 h
Ketotifen[a]	2–4	3–5	Hepatic	6 mo–3 y: 0.05 mg/kg q12–24 h >3 y: 1 mg q12 h
Levocetirizine	1	4–5	Renal	≥6 mo–5 y: 1.25 mg q24 h 6–11 y: 2.5 mg q24 h ≥12 y: 5 mg q24 h
Loratadine[c]	1.3	8.4	Hepatic	2–5 y: 5 mg q24 h ≥6 y: 10 mg q24 h

The proprietary names and formulations of the above preparations may vary from one country to another.
[a]Mild sedative effect.
[b]Dose may be increased for children aged 12 to 23 months to a maximum of 2.5 mg PO q12 h, for children aged 2 to 5 years to a maximum of 5 mg/24 hours.
[c]No sedative effect.
PO, orally; q, every; t_{max}, average time from oral intake to peak plasma drug concentration; $t_{1/2}$, average terminal elimination half-life.

TABLE 40.5 Common Nasal Antihistamine Preparations

Drug	*Action*	*Dosage*	*Side Effects*
Azelastine	H_1 antihistamine	5–11 y: 1 spray per nostril q12 h ≥12 y: 1–2 sprays per nostril q12 h ≥12 y: 1–2 sprays per nostril q12 h	Bitter taste
Olopatadine	H_1 antihistamine	6–12 y: 1 spray per nostril q12 h ≥12 y: 2 sprays per nostril q12 h	Minimal
Azelastine/Fluticasone	H_1 antihistamine combined with corticosteroid	≥6 y: 1 spray per nostril q12 h	Headache, dysgeusia, epistaxis

q, every.

blockage, α-adrenergic agonist decongestants, such as pseudoephedrine or phenylpropanolamine, may be added. In fact, the combination significantly improves other allergic rhinitis symptoms better than either drug alone.[91]

In general, topical H_1 antihistamines have a more rapid onset of action than oral formulations. However, topical formulations require administration more than once a day.[92] For example, both azelastine nasal preparation and levocabastine nasal and ocular preparations have onset of action in 10 to 15 minutes and duration of effect for up to 12 hours.[93,94] Although some systemic absorption of nasal and ocular formulations occurs, no dose adjustments are required in the elderly or other vulnerable populations as the sedative effect is minimal, and no clinically relevant drug–drug, drug–food, or drug–herbal product interactions have been described. In a randomized, controlled study of patients with seasonal allergic rhinitis, nasal H_1 antihistamines (Table 40.5) were reported to be as efficacious or more efficacious than oral H_1 antihistamines, particularly for relief from nasal congestion.[82] However, the choice of oral versus topical antihistamine preparation depends primarily on the patient's preference for route of administration, dose regimen, individual response, and side effects.

Likewise, ophthalmic preparations provide faster and superior relief than systemic antihistamines. Most of the ophthalmic H_1 antihistamines have multiple actions, such as mast cell stabilization, inhibition of eosinophil chemotaxis, and H_2 antihistamine properties.[95] Table 40.6 presents the common preparations, recommended dosage, mechanism of action, and side effects.

Asthma

Histamine is among several mediators of asthma, though not a major one. Clinical studies of antihistamine use in asthma have shown mixed results. Some reported beneficial effects on symptoms or physiologic measures, whereas others did not.[96,97]

The differential effect of H_1 antihistamines on the early-phase versus late-phase bronchial responses is not clear.[98] A prospective large multicenter study showed that cetirizine delays or, in some cases, prevents the development of asthma in infants with atopic dermatitis sensitized to grass pollen and, to a lesser extent, house dust mite during the 18-month treatment period and for the following 18-month duration.[99]

Skin Disorders

H_1 antihistamines are the mainstay in the treatment of urticaria, with more striking benefit in acute than in chronic cases. Their action on the afferent C nerve fibers of the skin reduces the itching, on the axonic reflexes reduces the erythema, and on the endothelium of the postcapillary venules reduces extravasation and wheal formation.[100] In chronic urticaria, fexofenadine in a dose of 120 mg per day was superior to diphenhydramine 50 mg per day,[101] and of 180 mg per day was superior to chlorpheniramine 8 mg per day.[100] Cetirizine 10 mg once daily was as effective as

TABLE 40.6 Common Ocular Antihistamine Preparations

Drug	*Action*	*Dosage*	*Side Effects*
Olopatadine	H_1 antihistamine, mast cell stabilizer	≥2 y: 1–2 drops q6–12 h	Headache
Emedastine	H_1 antihistamine, inhibits eosinophil chemotaxis	≥3 y: 1 drop q6 h	Headache
Ketotifen	H_1 antihistamine, mast cell stabilizer, inhibits PAF, inhibits eosinophils	≥3 y: 1 drop q8–12 h	Conjunctival injection, headache, rhinitis
Azelastine	H_1 antihistamine, mast cell stabilizer	≥3 y: 1 drop q12 h	Ocular burning, headache, bitter taste
Epinastine	H_1 and H_2 antihistamine, mast cell stabilizer, anti-inflammatory	≥2 y: 1 drop q12 h	Upper respiratory tract infection
Bepotastine	H_1 antihistamine, mast cell stabilizer	≥2 y: 1 drop q12 h	Dysgeusia
Alcaftadine	H_1 antihistamine, mast cell stabilizer	≥2 y: 1 drop once daily	Minimal

PAF, platelet-activating factor; q, every.

hydroxyzine 25 mg three times a day in reducing the frequency of exacerbation and average size of skin wheals.[102] In some cases, the combination of H_1 and H_2 antihistamines results in better effect.[103] Doxepin (a strong H_1 and H_2 antihistamine) is frequently used, particularly in severe cases, with good results.[104] Cetirizine has been found to relieve delayed-pressure urticaria.[105] In addition to clinical improvement, ketotifen reduced the plasma histamine levels in some patients with physical urticaria.[106] The regular, long-term intake of levocetirizine, 0.125 mg per kg per day, was effective in preventing and treating urticaria in atopic young children.[107] Treatment guidelines for chronic urticaria now recommend second-generation H_1 antihistamines as the medications of choice, starting with standard doses and increasing up to fourfold as needed to relieve symptoms.[108] This approach has not yet been validated in children.[67]

In atopic dermatitis, histamine acts as a pruritogen. However, other mediators of pruritus in eczema have been identified, including interleukin-31, thymic stromal lymphopoietin, and lysophosphatidic acid.[109] First-generation antihistamines are commonly used in alleviating itching. It is debatable whether such effect is through blocking H_1 receptors in the skin or through inducing central sedation. In a study on children with atopic dermatitis, the antipruritic effect of a single dose of hydroxyzine was maintained for up to 24 hours when the drug's plasma concentration had become negligible.[110] Some studies showed that loratadine and cetirizine can relieve atopic dermatitis symptoms in doses higher than those used for rhinitis.[111,112] In addition, long-term regular treatment with levocetirizine prevented and treated urticaria in young children with atopic dermatitis.[107] However, a recent Cochrane review study revealed no consistency in the efficacy of H_1 antihistamines as add-on therapy for eczema.[109]

In addition to the above conditions, antihistamines are useful in alleviating the symptoms of various cutaneous adverse drug reactions, including serum sickness. They are effective in preventing reactions secondary to direct histamine releasers, such as vancomycin (red-man syndrome).[10] They also induce marked relief of local reactions to insect stings or bites[113] and to various degrees in cases of mastocytosis.[114]

Anaphylaxis

In systemic anaphylaxis, where the initial treatment must include epinephrine, H_1 antihistamines may be useful in limiting cutaneous symptoms. For rapid onset, parenteral administration is preferable over the oral route. A Cochrane systematic review of 2,070 publications on H_1 antihistamines in the treatment of anaphylaxis did not identify any randomized controlled trials that provided satisfactory evidence.[115]

Upper Respiratory Tract Infections

H_1 antihistamines, either alone or in combination with other medications, are commonly used to alleviate the symptoms of upper respiratory tract infections. Such a practice is not well supported by well-controlled studies. In most studies on children with viral upper respiratory infections, the administration of H_1 antihistamines resulted in the same rate of improvement in symptoms as placebo did.[116] A meta-analysis[117] concluded that antihistamines as monotherapy did not significantly alleviate the symptoms of common cold in adults or children. However, when combined with decongestants, a modest beneficial effect was noted in older children and adults, but not in young children. The weak anticholinergic effects of the older antihistamines may decrease rhinorrhea, but this drying effect may do more harm than good, due to their tendency to induce somnolence.[10]

Otitis Media

In otitis media, viral or bacterial, increased histamine levels can be seen in the middle ear fluid.[118] A meta-analysis[119] found that the routine use of antihistamines for treating acute otitis media in children has no significant benefit. No combination of antihistamines and decongestants has been shown to be clinically effective, and there are potential adverse effects. Recent guidelines, which are based on study findings with negative results, recommend against routine use of this combination.[120]

Other

First-generation antihistamines, particularly hydroxyzine and diphenhydramine, are commonly used short term to improve sleep problems in children, particularly in those with comorbid atopic disease.[121]

Certain H_1 antihistamines, such as diphenhydramine, hydroxyzine, and promethazine, are known to have analgesic action. It is possible that this action is not due to histamine receptor binding but rather due to antiserotonin and/or antiadrenergic effects.[122] Combination of a first-generation antihistamine with a cyclooxygenase-1 inhibitor can enhance analgesic effect in mice.

In addition to the above effects, certain antihistamines block the histaminergic signal from the vestibular nucleus to the vomiting center in the medulla and have been used in the prevention of hypersensitivity reactions in patients receiving chemotherapy.[123] Historically, diphenhydramine has been the agent of choice; however, a recent study demonstrated that cetirizine can be a viable substitute for diphenhydramine for the prevention of infusions reactions with cetuximab, paclitaxel, and rituximab infusions in adults. However, prospective studies are needed to determine the efficacy and safety of cetirizine compared with diphenhydramine in the prevention of chemotherapy-related infusion reactions.

H_1 antihistamine premedication is often used in preventing nonsteroidal anti-inflammatory drug–induced urticaria,[124] recurrent reaction to radiocontrast,[125] and infusion-related reactions.[126–128]

ADVERSE EFFECTS OF H_1 ANTIHISTAMINES

The common mechanisms of side effects of H_1 antihistamines are summarized in Table 40.3. Sedation is the most frequently encountered side effect of the first-generation group and varies widely from one preparation to another and from one person to another. However, this effect may be desirable in cases of severe itching, such as in urticaria and atopic dermatitis. Sedation is less with the concomitant use of α-adrenergic decongestants. Concurrent ingestion of alcohol or other CNS suppressants markedly enhances the CNS side effects.[129]

On the other hand, most second-generation H_1 antihistamines have no or minimal sedative effect due to poor binding to the CNS H_1 receptors.[130] They, therefore, can be administered with alcohol, sedatives, hypnotics, antidepressants, or other CNS-active substances.[131,132] The sedative effect of cetirizine is reported by 6% of patients.[133]

First-generation H_1 antihistamines may have paradoxical CNS stimulatory effect in infants and young children, resulting in irritability, nervousness, excitation, insomnia, and even seizures.[17,134,135] There was some concern about apnea in infants and even sudden infant death syndrome related to the administration of first-generation antihistamines.[136] The U.S. Food and Drug Administration (FDA) added a warning black box to the label of promethazine, including a contraindication for use in children younger than 2 years because of reported serious adverse events, such as respiratory depression and CNS reactions, including seizures.[137]

It has been reported that school performance is worsened by the intake of first-generation H_1 antihistamines, but not by the second generation.[138] However, this finding was not confirmed by another study.[139] Elevated pollen counts have been associated with poorer school test performance,[140,141] and this may be an effect independent of antihistamine use. In fact, treatment of allergic rhinitis has been shown to improve attention in children.[142] Although cetirizine causes sedation in a small but significant number of subjects, long-term intake by children with atopic dermatitis showed no adverse effects on learning.[143]

The antimuscarinic effect of first-generation antihistamines can cause dry mouth, dysfunctional urine voiding, and sinus tachycardia. Through α-adrenergic suppression, some antihistamines cause hypotension, dizziness, and reflex tachycardia.[17]

Gastrointestinal adverse effects of antihistamines are seen in 1.4% to 10.1% of patients and include loss of appetite, nausea, vomiting, dyspepsia, and constipation or diarrhea.[133] These can be reduced by taking the drug with meals. Cyproheptadine, however, causes appetite stimulation, which is believed to be secondary to antiserotonin effect.[144] Ketotifen may cause some weight gain as well.[145] Patients taking intranasal azelastine often complain of a bitter taste.

Cardiac arrhythmias have been a main concern in treatment with antihistamines. They are not class effects but rather are related to particular preparations. Terfenadine and astemizole have been abandoned because of their increased risk of causing serious arrhythmias, particularly in patients with heart disease, hypokalemia, or concomitant intake of medications metabolized by the CYP450 system.[146,147] Arrhythmias are very rarely associated with the intake of cyproheptadine, diphenhydramine, hydroxyzine, or tricyclic antidepressants.[148] In the recommended doses, acrivastine, azelastine, cetirizine, ebastine, fexofenadine, loratadine, and mizolastine have not been reported to cause any electrocardiographic changes.[149–151]

Other rare adverse effects include hypersensitivity reactions in the form of drug fever,[10] pruritic exanthema,[152] urticaria,[153] dermatitis,[154] photosensitization,[155] and even anaphylaxis.[156] Hematologic adverse reactions are rare and can be in the form of leukopenia, agranulocytosis, or hemolytic anemia.[10]

OVERDOSAGE

Toxicity usually results from the administration of a quantity several-fold the recommended dose or occurs in patients with renal or hepatic disease. Most reported toxicities have been related to the first-generation antihistamines—brompheniramine, chlorpheniramine, cyproheptadine, dimenhydrinate, diphenhydramine, doxylamine, hydroxyzine, and promethazine. These preparations are also implicated in suicide attempts and in infant homicides.[134,157] Cardiac arrest and death has been reported in a case of intentional overdose of diphenhydramine, with serum concentration 18.7 µg per mL.[158] A recent review of adverse events data found that liquid diphenhydramine had the highest rate of unintentional pediatric ingestion, resulting in emergency department visits (8.1 per 100,000 bottles sold) compared to other common over-the-counter medications.[159]

Symptoms of overdose usually occur within 15 to 30 minutes after ingestion and are mostly related to the CNS. Although adults and older children usually develop drowsiness and lethargy, young children often develop stimulation, such as hallucination, excitation, ataxia, incoordination, athetosis, and convulsions.[10]

The antimuscarinic effect is manifested as dry mouth, flushed face, fever, pupillary dilation, urinary retention, decreased gastrointestinal motility, hypotension, and tachycardia. In patients overdosed with a first-generation antihistamine, dose-dependent cardiac toxicity, including prolonged QTc interval and torsade de pointes, may occur. The patient should be monitored until QTc interval normalizes. Torsade de pointes requires cardioversion and pacing. In such instances, it would be prudent to avoid the antiarrhythmic medications—quinidine, flecainide, amiodarone, and sotalol, as they may further prolong the QTc interval.[148] Severe cases may lead to cardiorespiratory collapse, coma, and even death.[160] Because there are no specific antidotes for H_1 antihistamines, treatment consists of symptomatic and supportive measures. Some cases might need hemodialysis. Activated charcoal is helpful in reducing the absorption of the drug.[161] Because of the CNS suppressive effect of antihistamines, ipecac is usually ineffective in inducing emesis in such patients.

Second-generation H_1 antihistamines rarely cause significant toxicity, and the treatment is primarily supportive and symptomatic because most such preparations are not dialyzable.[162]

USE DURING PREGNANCY AND LACTATION

H_1 antihistamines can cross the placenta to various degrees. Controlled studies of antihistamine use during pregnancy are lacking. Data on safety often conflict, and recommendations can change, as in the case of the H_1 antihistamine doxylamine with vitamin B6.[163] This drug was voluntarily withdrawn from the market in 1983 due to reports of birth defects. However, in April 2013, the FDA approved doxylamine with vitamin B6 as a pregnancy category A drug. In fact, as of 2018, it is considered safe as first-line therapy for nausea and vomiting of pregnancy.[164]

In 2014, the FDA amended the regulations on labeling of drugs with regard to safety in pregnancy due to frequent misinterpretation of the categories and their failure to communicate different degrees of fetal risk.[165] Categories A, B, C, D, and X from the previous classification have been removed and replaced with a summary of risks and data on use in pregnancy for each product. Therefore, the drug labeling for each product should be consulted for specific, detailed information about possible risks to the fetus and mother.

Reports on the relationship between antihistamine use during pregnancy and major congenital anomalies have been inconsistent. For example, chlorpheniramine may be associated with neural tube defects, such as encephalocele, but statistical adjustment for possible confounders negates this finding.[163] The same is true of possible associations of diphenhydramine with transposition of great arteries and doxylamine with cystic kidney disease. A study found that none of the 14 antihistamines taken during early pregnancy by 738 women was linked to any of 26 isolated major birth defects.[166] Another study found no significant difference in the rate of congenital anomalies in the offspring of pregnant women who took loratadine or other antihistamines, compared with those who took nonteratogenic medications.[167] The administration of a large therapeutic dose of a first-generation H_1 antihistamine such as hydroxyzine or diphenhydramine shortly before delivery may be associated with withdrawal symptoms (tremulousness and irritability) in the newborn.[168,169]

LACTMED, a database maintained online by the U.S. National Library of Medicine, can be a useful resource for recommendations for lactating mothers. Irritability or drowsiness has been reported in nursing infants of mothers receiving first-generation H_1 antihistamines.[170] Second-generation H_1 antihistamines are also excreted in breast milk (e.g., 0.03% of the total maternal loratadine dose)[171]; however, they are less often reported to cause symptoms in the nursing neonate.

INTERACTIONS WITH OTHER MEDICATIONS AND FOODS

For H_1 antihistamines that cause sedation, the addition of other drugs that suppress the CNS (e.g., tricyclic antidepressants, barbiturates, hypnotics, sedatives, tranquilizers, alcohol) would impose danger, particularly while the patient is driving or operating machinery. Similarly, the autonomic blocking effects of conventional antihistamines are additional to the antimuscarinic and α-adrenergic–blocking effects. Monoamine oxidase inhibitors were found to prolong and intensify the antimuscarinic effects of antihistamines.[14]

All first-generation H_1 antihistamines and some second-generation preparations such as desloratadine and loratadine are metabolized by CYP450 system in the liver. The activity of this enzyme can be altered by other drugs. Therefore, plasma concentration of H_1 antihistamines decreases with the concomitant intake of drugs that stimulate the CYP450 enzyme system, for example, benzodiazepines. The opposite would occur as a result of coadministration of macrolides, antifungals, or calcium antagonists, which compete for the CYP450 system.

The coadministration of fexofenadine and ketoconazole or erythromycin increases the plasma level of fexofenadine, but does not affect the pharmacokinetics of ketoconazole or erythromycin. The fexofenadine absorption is decreased by approximately 40% if administered within 15 minutes of taking aluminum- and magnesium-containing antacid.[172]

Fexofenadine is absorbed via an active transport system in the intestine. The ingestion of grapefruit juice with fexofenadine lowers the peak plasma drug concentration to 58% and mean area under the curve (plasma drug concentration–time) to 53% by inhibiting an organic anion transporting polypeptide.[65]

H_2 ANTIHISTAMINES

H_2 antihistamines have been widely used in gastric peptic disease (see Chapter 55) and in a variety of conditions that are briefly mentioned below.

CHEMISTRY AND PHARMACOKINETICS OF H_2 ANTIHISTAMINES

In the United States, at present, there are four preparations of H_2 antihistamines: cimetidine, famotidine, nizatidine, and ranitidine. They differ mainly in their pharmacokinetics and propensity to cause drug interactions. H_2 antihistamines do not bind to other histamine-receptor subtypes.

H_2 antihistamines are rapidly absorbed after oral administration, with peak plasma concentrations at 1 to 3 hours. Their volume of distribution ranges from 0.8 to 1.18 L per kg, and binding to plasma proteins from 15% to 35%.[173] Absorption may be enhanced by food or decreased by antacids, but these effects probably are not clinically significant. Therapeutic levels are achieved rapidly after intravenous administration and are maintained for 4 to 5 hours for cimetidine, 6 to 8 hours for ranitidine, and 10 to 12 hours for famotidine. Only small quantities are metabolized by the liver. The half-life of H_2 antihistamines ranges from 1.3 to 4 hours. Their excretion is mainly by the kidney; hence, the dose should be reduced in patients with renal disease.[173,174] Neither hemodialysis nor peritoneal dialysis clears significant amounts.

USES IN ALLERGIC, METABOLIC, AND IMMUNOLOGIC DISORDERS

Allergic Rhinitis and Asthma

H_2 antihistamines have no primary role in the treatment of allergic rhinitis or asthma, but they could be useful in patients with concomitant gastroesophageal reflux.[175]

Skin Disorders

As mentioned earlier, some patients with chronic urticaria or dermographism experience more improvement by adding H_2 antihistamines to anti-H_1 preparations.[103] Some tricyclic antidepressants, such as doxepin, have potent H_1 and H_2 antihistamine properties.[176] As an H_1 antihistamine, doxepin is 800 times more potent than diphenhydramine and 50 times more potent than hydroxyzine, and as an H_2 antihistamine, it is six times more potent than cimetidine.[177]

The combination of oral H_2 antihistamine (ranitidine) and topical corticosteroid was shown to be more effective than the latter alone in atopic dermatitis.[178] Doxepin ointment has shown marked relief of pruritus associated with atopic dermatitis, but in some patients, it causes burning sensation and, occasionally, sensitization.[179] Skin photodamage in children with erythropoietic protoporphyria has been successfully treated with cimetidine, presumably due to its ability to inhibit heme biosynthesis.[180]

Anaphylaxis

In anaphylaxis, increased histamine release results in a variety of responses, including vasodilation and hypotension. However, the rapid intravenous administration of cimetidine can induce hypotension, bradycardia, and even asystole.[181]

Immunomodulation

Some studies have demonstrated a role for H_2 antihistamines as potential immunomodulators. Cimetidine has been reported to resolve molluscum contagiosum.[182] Enhancement of cell-mediated immunity (natural killer cells) is thought to be the mechanism of action. Cimetidine 30 to 40 mg per kg of body weight daily for 3 to 6 months results in resolution of warts in some patients and has been found to be safe in pediatric heart transplant recipients.[183] Cimetidine therapy may also resolve fevers in some children with periodic fever, cervical adenitis, pharyngitis, aphthous stomatitis (PFAPA) syndrome.[184] Lymph node–positive colorectal cancer patients experience longer time for recurrence and longer survival when given perioperative cimetidine at the time of tumor resection.[185] H_2 antihistamines may also have immunomodulatory functions in patients with autoimmune disorders, such as sclerosing panencephalomyelitis or psoriasis.[186,187]

USE DURING PREGNANCY AND LACTATION

The intake of H_2 antihistamines during the first trimester does not seem to have a teratogenic risk.[188] Nevertheless, its use during pregnancy should be limited to cases when the anticipated benefits outweigh the unknown fetal risks. Although H_2 antihistamines are excreted in breast milk,[189] the quantity seems to be too small to constitute a risk to the nursing infant.

ADVERSE EFFECTS OF H_2 ANTIHISTAMINES

Less than 3% of patients receiving cimetidine and less than 1% of those receiving ranitidine, famotidine, or nizatidine develop side effects, mainly gastrointestinal (diarrhea or constipation) or CNS (headache, somnolence, or confusion).[10]

In neonates, particularly those who are very low birth weight, the use of H_2 antihistamines was associated with increased risk of infections, necrotizing enterocolitis, and fatality.[190]

Prolonged (2 years or more) use of H_2-receptor antagonists has been associated with vitamin B_{12} deficiency, especially in younger patients.[191] Prolonged use of cimetidine in high doses may cause reversible gynecomastia, breast tenderness, or impotence in men, possibly because it displaces endogenous androgens from their receptor sites.[10]

INTERACTIONS WITH OTHER MEDICATIONS

Cimetidine reduces the hepatic metabolism of certain drugs, including warfarin, phenytoin, propranolol, nifedipine, chlordiazepoxide, diazepam, certain tricyclic antidepressants, lidocaine, theophylline, and metronidazole,[192] especially in the presence of hepatic dysfunction or in the elderly.[174] Drugs that are best absorbed in acidic environment (e.g., ketoconazole and itraconazole) should be given at least 2 hours before H_2 antihistamines.[193] The gastrointestinal absorption of cimetidine is reduced if administered with certain antacids.[10]

In recommended doses, ranitidine does not inhibit the CYP450 enzymes in the liver, though it may affect the bioavailability of certain drugs (e.g., triazolam). On the other hand, famotidine and nizatidine do not bind to the CYP450 system, and no drug interactions have been identified with these two drugs.[14]

H_3 ANTIHISTAMINES

H_3 receptors are found mainly in the CNS and act as autoreceptors which control the release of histamine via negative feedback and regulate release of other neurotransmitters, such as dopamine, norepinephrine, serotonin, and acetylcholine.[194] Thus, H_3-receptor antagonists increase the release of histamine and have the opposite effect of H_1 antihistamines in the CNS, enhancing attention and wakefulness. Hence, they have potential in the management of certain neurologic disorders, including dementia, attention-deficit/hyperactivity disorder, schizophrenia, epilepsy, narcolepsy, neuropathic pain, and overeating disorders.[82]

TABLE 40.7 H_3-Receptor Antagonist Preparations

Drug	*Clinical Application*
Betahistine	Treatment of Ménière disease
Pitolisant	Treatment of narcolepsy
Thioperamide	Preclinical models of parkinsonism
SAR110894	Preclinical models of tauopathies
DL77	Preclinical models of autism

The H_3-receptor antagonist betahistine, which is also a weak H_1-receptor agonist, reduces histamine-induced excitatory response in vestibular cells and is used for the treatment of Ménière disease and vertigo symptoms.[195] Pitolisant is an H_3-receptor antagonist, which is used for the treatment of narcolepsy.[196]

Other H_3-receptor antagonists including thioperamide, SAR110894, and DL77 have shown promise in preclinical models of parkinsonism,[21] tauopathies,[197] and autism,[198] respectively (Table 40.7).

Because the stimulation of H_3 receptors inhibits norepinephrine release, which is involved in reversing the hypotension in anaphylaxis, blockade of H_3 receptor may have a beneficial effect as demonstrated in canine model of anaphylaxis.[199]

H_4 ANTIHISTAMINES

H_4 receptor has the highest sequence homology with the H_3 receptor and can bind to H_3 antihistamines, though with lower affinity.[61] It is expressed primarily on cells of hematopoietic origin (notably, mast cells, basophils, and eosinophils) and, to a lesser extent, on the intestinal mucosal epithelium,[61,200,201] suggesting a possible pathogenic role in inflammation. The H_4 antihistamine toreforant has been tested in clinical studies in patients with asthma,[202] psoriasis,[203] and rheumatoid arthritis.[204]

ACKNOWLEDGMENTS

The authors thank the contribution of Dr. Yesim Yilmaz-Demirdag and Dr. Sanaa A. Mahmoud to this chapter in the previous third and fourth editions of this textbook.

REFERENCES

1. Windaus A, Vogt W. Synthèse des imidazolyllathylamins. *Ber Deutsch Chem Ges* 1907;3:3691–3695.
2. Dale HH, Laidlaw PP. Further observations on the action of beta-iminazolylethylamine. *J Physiol* 1911;43:182–195.
3. Dale HH, Laidlaw PP. The physiological action of beta-iminazolylethylamine. *J Physiol* 1910;41:318–344.
4. Best CH, Dale HH, Dudley HW, et al. The nature of the vaso-dilator constituents of certain tissue extracts. *J Physiol* 1927;62:397–417.
5. Lewis T. *The blood vessels of human skin and their responses.* London, UK: Shaw & Son, 1927.
6. Riley JF, West GB. Histamine in tissue mast cells. *J Physiol* 1952;117:72–73.
7. Riley JF, West GB. The occurrence of histamine in mast cells. In: Silva RE, ed. *Handbook of experimental pharmacology: histamine and antihistamines*, vol. XVIII, Part I. New York, NY: Springer-Verlag, 1966:116–135.

8. Mongar JL, Schild HO. Quantitative measurement of the histamine-releasing activity of a series of mono-alkyl-amines using minced guinea pig lung. *Br J Pharmacol Chemother* 1953;8:103–109.
9. Foreman J, Mongar JL. The control of secretion from mast cells. In: Pepys J, Edwards AM, eds. *The mast cell in health and disease*. England: Pitman Medical, 1980:30–37.
10. Skidgel RA. Histamine, bradykinin, and their antagonists. In: Brunton LL, Hilal-Dandan R, Knollman BC, eds. *Goodman & Gilman's The pharmacological basis of therapeutics*, 13th ed. New York, NY: McGraw-Hill Companies Inc., 2018.
11. Kapeller-Adler R. Histamine catabolism in vitro and in vivo. *Fed Proc* 1965;24:757–765.
12. Metcalfe DD. Effector cell heterogeneity in immediate hypersensitivity reactions. *Clin Rev Allergy* 1983;1:311–325.
13. McNeill JH. Histamine and the heart. *Can J Physiol Pharmacol* 1984;62:720–726.
14. Katzung BG. Histamine, serotonin, & the ergot alkaloids. In: Katzung BG, ed. *Basic & clinical pharmacology*, 10th ed. New York, NY: McGraw-Hill Companies Inc., 2007.
15. Shimamura T, Shiroishi M, Weyand S, et al. Structure of the human histamine H_1 receptor complex with doxepin. *Nature* 2011;475:65–70.
16. Ash AS, Schild HO. Receptors mediating some actions of histamine. *Br J Pharmacol Chemother* 1966;27:427–439.
17. Simons FE. Advances in H_1-antihistamines. *N Engl J Med* 2004;351:2203–2217.
18. Arrang JM, Garbarg M, Schwartz JC. Auto-inhibition of brain histamine release mediated by a novel class (H_3) of histamine receptor. *Nature* 1983;302:832–837.
19. Lovenberg TW, Roland BL, Wilson SJ, et al. Cloning and functional expression of the human histamine H_3 receptor. *Mol Pharmacol* 1999;55:1101–1107.
20. Teuscher C, Subramanian M, Noubade R, et al. Central histamine H_3 receptor signaling negatively regulates susceptibility to autoimmune inflammatory disease of the CNS. *Proc Natl Acad Sci U S A* 2007;104:10146–10151.
21. Masini D, Lopes-Aguiar C, Bonito-Oliva A, et al. The histamine H_3 receptor antagonist thioperamide rescues circadian rhythm and memory function in experimental parkinsonism. *Transl Psychiatry* 2017;7:e1088.
22. Riddy DM, Cook AE, Shackleford DM, et al. Drug-receptor kinetics and sigma-1 receptor affinity differentiate clinically evaluated histamine H_3 receptor antagonists. *Neuropharmacology* 2019;144:244–255.
23. Venail F, Attali P, Wersinger E, et al. Safety, tolerability, pharmacokinetics and pharmacokinetic-pharmacodynamic modelling of the novel H_4 receptor inhibitor SENS-111 using a modified caloric test in healthy subjects. *Br J Clin Pharmacol* 2018;84:2836–2848.
24. Deiteren A, De Man JG, Pelckmans PA, et al. Histamine H_4 receptors in the gastrointestinal tract. *Br J Pharmacol* 2015;172:1165–1178.
25. Zampeli E, Tiligada E. The role of histamine H_4 receptor in immune and inflammatory disorders. *Br J Pharmacol* 2009;157:24–33.
26. Nakamura T, Itadani H, Hidaka Y, et al. Molecular cloning and characterization of a new human histamine receptor, HH4R. *Biochem Biophys Res Commun* 2000;279:615–620.
27. Dijkstra D, Stark H, Chazot PL, et al. Human inflammatory dendritic epidermal cells express a functional histamine H_4 receptor. *J Invest Dermatol* 2008;128:1696–1703.
28. Hattori Y. Cardiac histamine receptors: their pharmacological consequences and signal transduction pathways. *Methods Find Exp Clin Pharmacol* 1999;21:123–131.
29. Nguyen T, Shapiro DA, George SR, et al. Discovery of a novel member of the histamine receptor family. *Mol Pharmacol* 2001;59:427–433.
30. Bristow MR, Ginsburg R, Harrison DC. Histamine and the human heart: the other receptor system. *Am J Cardiol* 1982;49:249–251.
31. Imamura M, Poli E, Omoniyi AT, et al. Unmasking of activated histamine H_3-receptors in myocardial ischemia: their role as regulators of exocytotic norepinephrine release. *J Pharmacol Exp Ther* 1994;271:1259–1266.
32. Malinowska B, Godlewski G, Schlicker E. Histamine H_3 receptors—general characterization and their function in the cardiovascular system. *J Physiol Pharmacol* 1998;49:191–211.
33. Nault MA, Milne B, Parlow JL. Effects of the selective H_1 and H_2 histamine receptor antagonists loratadine and ranitidine on autonomic control of the heart. *Anesthesiology* 2002;96:336–341.
34. Palmer RM, Ferrige AG, Moncada S. Nitric oxide release accounts for the biological activity of endothelium-derived relaxing factor. *Nature* 1987;327:524–526.
35. Bechi P, Romagnoli P, Panula P, et al. Gastric mucosal histamine storing cells. Evidence for different roles of mast cells and enterochromaffin-like cells in humans. *Dig Dis Sci* 1995;40:2207–2213.
36. Panula P, Airaksinen MS, Pirvola U, et al. A histamine-containing neuronal system in human brain. *Neuroscience* 1990;34:127–132.
37. Rossbach K, Nassenstein C, Gschwandtner M, et al. Histamine H_1, H_3 and H_4 receptors are involved in pruritus. *Neuroscience* 2011;190:89–102.
38. Thurmond RL, Gelfand EW, Dunford PJ. The role of histamine H_1 and H_4 receptors in allergic inflammation: the search for new antihistamines. *Nat Rev Drug Discov* 2008;7:41–53.
39. Varga C, Horvath K, Berko A, et al. Inhibitory effects of histamine H_4 receptor antagonists on experimental colitis in the rat. *Eur J Pharmacol* 2005;522:130–138.
40. Dunford PJ, O'Donnell N, Riley JP, et al. The histamine H_4 receptor mediates allergic airway inflammation by regulating the activation of CD4+ T cells. *J Immunol* 2006;176:7062–7070.
41. Dunford PJ, Williams KN, Desai PJ, et al. Histamine H_4 receptor antagonists are superior to traditional antihistamines in the attenuation of experimental pruritus. *J Allergy Clin Immunol* 2007;119:176–183.
42. Serafin WE, Austen KF. Mediators of immediate hypersensitivity reactions. *N Engl J Med* 1987;317:30–34.
43. Johnson HH Jr, Deoreo GA, Lascheid WP, et al. Skin histamine levels in chronic atopic dermatitis. *J Invest Dermatol* 1960;34:237–238.
44. Juhlin L. Localization and content of histamine in normal and diseased skin. *Acta Derm Venereol* 1967;47:383–391.
45. Kaplan AP, Horakova Z, Katz SI. Assessment of tissue fluid histamine levels in patients with urticaria. *J Allergy Clin Immunol* 1978;61:350–354.
46. Wenzel SE, Fowler AA III, Schwartz LB. Activation of pulmonary mast cells by bronchoalveolar allergen challenge. In vivo release of histamine and tryptase in atopic subjects with and without asthma. *Am Rev Respir Dis* 1988;137:1002–1008.
47. Levy JH, Kettlekamp N, Goertz P, et al. Histamine release by vancomycin: a mechanism for hypotension in man. *Anesthesiology* 1987;67:122–125.
48. de Weck AL. Pathophysiologic mechanisms of allergic and pseudo-allergic reactions to foods, food additives and drugs. *Ann Allergy* 1984;53:583–586.
49. Leurs R, Church MK, Taglialatela M. H_1-antihistamines: inverse agonism, anti-inflammatory actions and cardiac effects. *Clin Exp Allergy* 2002;32:489–498.
50. Staub AM, Bovet D. Action de la thymoxyethyl-diethylamine (929F) et des ethers phenoliques sur le choc anaphylactique du cobaye. *CRS Soc Biol* 1937;125:818.
51. Halpern BN. Les antihistaminiques de synthèse: essai de chimio-thérapie des etas allergiques. *Arch Int Pharmacodyn Ther* 1942;68:339–408.
52. Holgate ST, Canonica GW, Simons FE, et al. Consensus Group on New-Generation Antihistamines (CONGA): present status and recommendations. *Clin Exp Allergy* 2003;33:1305–1324.
53. Simons FE. New H_1-receptor antagonists: clinical pharmacology. *Clin Exp Allergy* 1990;20(Suppl 2):19–24.
54. Campbell M, Bateman DN. Pharmacokinetic optimisation of antiemetic therapy. *Clin Pharmacokinet* 1992;23:147–160.
55. Church MK, Gradidge CF. Inhibition of histamine release from human lung in vitro by antihistamines and related drugs. *Br J Pharmacol* 1980;69:663–667.
56. Vena GA, Cassano N, Buquicchio R, et al. Antiinflammatory effects of H_1-antihistamines: clinical and immunological relevance. *Curr Pharm Des* 2008;14:2902–2911.
57. Agrawal DK. Anti-inflammatory properties of desloratadine. *Clin Exp Allergy* 2004;34:1342–1348.
58. Wu P, Mitchell S, Walsh GM. A new antihistamine levocetirizine inhibits eosinophil adhesion to vascular cell adhesion molecule-1 under flow conditions. *Clin Exp Allergy* 2005;35:1073–1079.
59. Carlsen KH, Kramer J, Fagertun HE, et al. Loratadine and terfenadine in perennial allergic rhinitis. Treatment of nonresponders to the one drug with the other drug. *Allergy* 1993;48:431–436.
60. Hough LB. Genomics meets histamine receptors: new subtypes, new receptors. *Mol Pharmacol* 2001;59:415–419.
61. Tsai YJ, Hoyme HE. Pharmacogenomics: the future of drug therapy. *Clin Genet* 2002;62:257–264.
62. Igaz P, Fitzimons CP, Szalai C, et al. Histamine genomics in silico: polymorphisms of the human genes involved in the synthesis, action and degradation of histamine. *Am J Pharmacogenomics* 2002;2:67–72.
63. Simons FE, Simons KJ. H_1 antihistamines: current status and future directions. *World Allergy Organ J* 2008;1:145–155.
64. Dresser GK, Kim RB, Bailey DG. Effect of grapefruit juice volume on the reduction of fexofenadine bioavailability: possible role of organic anion transporting polypeptides. *Clin Pharmacol Ther* 2005;77:170–177.
65. Yasui-Furukori N, Uno T, Sugawara K, et al. Different effects of three transporting inhibitors, verapamil, cimetidine, and probenecid, on fexofenadine pharmacokinetics. *Clin Pharmacol Ther* 2005;77:17–23.
66. Church MK, Weller K, Stock P, et al. Chronic spontaneous urticaria in children: itching for insight. *Pediatr Allergy Immunol* 2011;22:1–8.
67. Simons FE, Bergman JN, Watson WT, et al. The clinical pharmacology of fexofenadine in children. *J Allergy Clin Immunol* 1996;98:1062–1064.
68. Watson WT, Simons KJ, Chen XY, et al. Cetirizine: a pharmacokinetic and pharmacodynamic evaluation in children with seasonal allergic rhinitis. *J Allergy Clin Immunol* 1989;84:457–464.
69. Simons FE, Simons KJ. H_1 receptor antagonists: clinical pharmacology and use in allergic disease. *Pediatr Clin North Am* 1983;30:899–914.
70. Wood SG, John BA, Chasseaud LF, et al. The metabolism and pharmacokinetics of 14 C-cetirizine in humans. *Ann Allergy* 1987;59:31–34.
71. Simons FE, Simons KJ. The pharmacology and use of H_1-receptor-antagonist drugs. *N Engl J Med* 1994;330:1663–1670.
72. Chen C. Some pharmacokinetic aspects of the lipophilic terfenadine and zwitterionic fexofenadine in humans. *Drugs R D* 2007;8:301–314.
73. Spencer CM, Faulds D, Peters DH. Cetirizine. A reappraisal of its pharmacological properties and therapeutic use in selected allergic disorders. *Drugs* 1993;46:1055–1080.
74. Russell T, Stoltz M, Weir S. Pharmacokinetics, pharmacodynamics, and tolerance of single-and multiple-dose fexofenadine hydrochloride in healthy male volunteers. *Clin Pharmacol Ther* 1998;64:612–621.
75. Wellington K, Jarvis B. Cetirizine/pseudoephedrine. *Drugs* 2001;61:2231–2240; discussion 2241–2242.
76. Bernstein IL, Li JT, Bernstein DI, et al. Allergy diagnostic testing: an updated practice parameter. *Ann Allergy Asthma Immunol* 2008;100:S1–S148.
77. Plaut M, Valentine MD. Clinical practice. Allergic rhinitis. *N Engl J Med* 2005;353:1934–1944.
78. Hair PI, Scott LJ. Levocetirizine: a review of its use in the management of allergic rhinitis and skin allergies. *Drugs* 2006;66:973–996.
79. de Benedictis FM, de Benedictis D, Canonica GW. New oral H_1 antihistamines in children: facts and unmet needs. *Allergy* 2008;63:1395–1404.
80. Ciprandi G, Ricca V, Tosca M, et al. Continuous antihistamine treatment controls allergic inflammation and reduces respiratory morbidity in children with mite allergy. *Allergy* 1999;54:358–365.
81. Simons FE, Simons KJ. Histamine and H_1-antihistamines: celebrating a century of progress. *J Allergy Clin Immunol* 2011;128:1139–1150.e1134.
82. Dizdar EA, Sekerel BE, Keskin O, et al. The effect of regular versus on-demand desloratadine treatment in children with allergic rhinitis. *Int J Pediatr Otorhinolaryngol* 2007;71:843–849.
83. Carr WW. Pediatric allergic rhinitis: current and future state of the art. *Allergy Asthma Proc* 2008;29:14–23.

84. Horak F, Stubner UP, Zieglmayer R, et al. Effect of desloratadine versus placebo on nasal airflow and subjective measures of nasal obstruction in subjects with grass pollen-induced allergic rhinitis in an allergen-exposure unit. *J Allergy Clin Immunol* 2002;109:956–961.
85. Wilson AM, Haggart K, Sims EJ, et al. Effects of fexofenadine and desloratadine on subjective and objective measures of nasal congestion in seasonal allergic rhinitis. *Clin Exp Allergy* 2002;32:1504–1509.
86. Kim K, Sussman G, Hebert J, et al. Desloratadine therapy for symptoms associated with perennial allergic rhinitis. *Ann Allergy Asthma Immunol* 2006;96:460–465.
87. Meltzer EO, Scheinmann P, Rosado Pinto JE, et al. Safety and efficacy of oral fexofenadine in children with seasonal allergic rhinitis—a pooled analysis of three studies. *Pediatr Allergy Immunol* 2004;15:253–260.
88. Potter PC. Levocetirizine is effective for symptom relief including nasal congestion in adolescent and adult (PAR) sensitized to house dust mites. *Allergy* 2003;58:893–899.
89. Potter PC. Efficacy and safety of levocetirizine on symptoms and health-related quality of life of children with perennial allergic rhinitis: a double-blind, placebo-controlled randomized clinical trial. *Ann Allergy Asthma Immunol* 2005;95:175–180.
90. Sussman GL, Mason J, Compton D, et al. The efficacy and safety of fexofenadine HCl and pseudoephedrine, alone and in combination, in seasonal allergic rhinitis. *J Allergy Clin Immunol* 1999;104:100–106.
91. Horak F, Zieglmayer UP, Zieglmayer R, et al. Azelastine nasal spray and desloratadine tablets in pollen-induced seasonal allergic rhinitis: a pharmacodynamic study of onset of action and efficacy. *Curr Med Res Opin* 2006;22:151–157.
92. McTavish D, Sorkin EM. Azelastine. A review of its pharmacodynamic and pharmacokinetic properties, and therapeutic potential. *Drugs* 1989;38:778–800.
93. Dechant KL, Goa KL. Levocabastine. A review of its pharmacological properties and therapeutic potential as a topical antihistamine in allergic rhinitis and conjunctivitis. *Drugs* 1991;41:202–224.
94. Bielory L, Lien KW, Bigelsen S. Efficacy and tolerability of newer antihistamines in the treatment of allergic conjunctivitis. *Drugs* 2005;65:215–228.
95. Nelson HS. Prospects for antihistamines in the treatment of asthma. *J Allergy Clin Immunol* 2003;112:S96–S100.
96. Bachert C, Maspero J. Efficacy of second-generation antihistamines in patients with allergic rhinitis and comorbid asthma. *J Asthma* 2011;48:965–973.
97. Jutel M, Blaser K, Akdis CA. Histamine in allergic inflammation and immune modulation. *Int Arch Allergy Immunol* 2005;137:82–92.
98. Warner JO. A double-blinded, randomized, placebo-controlled trial of cetirizine in preventing the onset of asthma in children with atopic dermatitis: 18 months' treatment and 18 months' posttreatment follow-up. *J Allergy Clin Immunol* 2001;108:929–937.
99. Simons FE, Silver NA, Gu X, et al. Clinical pharmacology of H_1-antihistamines in the skin. *J Allergy Clin Immunol* 2002;110:777–783.
100. Simons FE, Johnston L, Gu X, et al. Suppression of the early and late cutaneous allergic responses using fexofenadine and montelukast. *Ann Allergy Asthma Immunol* 2001;86:44–50.
101. Breneman DL. Cetirizine versus hydroxyzine and placebo in chronic idiopathic urticaria. *Ann Pharmacother* 1996;30:1075–1079.
102. Bleehen SS, Thomas SE, Greaves MW, et al. Cimetidine and chlorpheniramine in the treatment of chronic idiopathic urticaria: a multi-centre randomized double-blind study. *Br J Dermatol* 1987;117:81–88.
103. Greene SL, Reed CE, Schroeter AL. Double-blind crossover study comparing doxepin with diphenhydramine for the treatment of chronic urticaria. *J Am Acad Dermatol* 1985;12:669–675.
104. Kontou-Fili K, Maniatakou G, Demaka P, et al. Therapeutic effects of cetirizine in delayed pressure urticaria: clinicopathologic findings. *J Am Acad Dermatol* 1991;24:1090–1093.
105. Huston DP, Bressler RB, Kaliner M, et al. Prevention of mast-cell degranulation by ketotifen in patients with physical urticarias. *Ann Intern Med* 1986;104:507–510.
106. Simons FE. H_1-antihistamine treatment in young atopic children: effect on urticaria. *Ann Allergy Asthma Immunol* 2007;99:261–266.
107. Maurer M, Weller K, Bindslev-Jensen C, et al. Unmet clinical needs in chronic spontaneous urticaria. A GA²LEN task force report. *Allergy* 2011;66:317–330.
108. Matterne U, Bohmer MM, Weisshaar E, et al. Oral H_1 antihistamines as 'add-on' therapy to topical treatment for eczema. *Cochrane Database Syst Rev* 2019;1:CD012167.
109. Simons FE, Simons KJ, Becker AB, et al. Pharmacokinetics and antipruritic effects of hydroxyzine in children with atopic dermatitis. *J Pediatr* 1984;104:123–127.
110. Juhlin L, Arendt C. Treatment of chronic urticaria with cetirizine dihydrochloride a non-sedating antihistamine. *Br J Dermatol* 1988;119:67–71.
111. Monroe EW. Relative efficacy and safety of loratadine, hydroxyzine, and placebo in chronic idiopathic urticaria and atopic dermatitis. *Clin Ther* 1992;14:17–21.
112. Karppinen A, Kautiainen H, Petman L, et al. Comparison of cetirizine, ebastine and loratadine in the treatment of immediate mosquito-bite allergy. *Allergy* 2002;57:534–537.
113. Friedman BS, Santiago ML, Berkebile C, et al. Comparison of azelastine and chlorpheniramine in the treatment of mastocytosis. *J Allergy Clin Immunol* 1993;92:520–526.
114. Sheikh A, Ten Broek V, Brown SG, et al. H_1-antihistamines for the treatment of anaphylaxis: Cochrane systematic review. *Allergy* 2007;62:830–837.
115. Smith MB, Feldman W. Over-the-counter cold medications. A critical review of clinical trials between 1950 and 1991. *JAMA* 1993;269:2258–2263.
116. Sutter AI, Lemiengre M, Campbell H, et al. Antihistamines for the common cold. *Cochrane Database Syst Rev* 2003:CD001267.
117. Chonmaitree T, Patel JA, Lett-Brown MA, et al. Virus and bacteria enhance histamine production in middle ear fluids of children with acute otitis media. *J Infect Dis* 1994;169:1265–1270.
118. Coleman C, Moore M. Decongestants and antihistamines for acute otitis media in children. *Cochrane Database Syst Rev* 2008:CD001727.
119. Bonney AG, Goldman RD. Antihistamines for children with otitis media. *Can Fam Physician* 2014;60:43–46.
120. Pelayo R, Dubik M. Pediatric sleep pharmacology. *Semin Pediatr Neurol* 2008;15:79–90.
121. Takahashi M, Shima K, Tsuchiya M, et al. Analgesic effects of 1st generation anti-histamines in mice. *Biol Pharm Bull* 2016;39:620–624.
122. Durham CG, Thotakura D, Sager L, et al. Cetirizine versus diphenhydramine in the prevention of chemotherapy-related hypersensitivity reactions. *J Oncol Pharm Pract* 2019;25(6):1396–1401. doi:1078155218811505.
123. Trautmann A, Anders D, Stoevesandt J. H_1-antihistamine premedication in NSAID-associated urticaria. *J Allergy Clin Immunol Pract* 2016;4:1205–1212.
124. Bae YJ, Hwang YW, Yoon SY, et al. The effectiveness of automatic recommending system for premedication in reducing recurrent radiocontrast media hypersensitivity reactions. *PLoS One* 2013;8:e66014.
125. Conte WL, Arndt N, Cipriani VP, et al. Reduction in ocrelizumab-induced infusion reactions by a modified premedication protocol. *Mult Scler Relat Disord* 2019;27:397–399.
126. Bonilla FA. Intravenous immunoglobulin: adverse reactions and management. *J Allergy Clin Immunol* 2008;122:1238–1239.
127. Chung CH. Managing premedications and the risk for reactions to infusional monoclonal antibody therapy. *Oncologist* 2008;13:725–732.
128. Roehrs T, Zwyghuizen-Doorenbos A, Roth T. Sedative effects and plasma concentrations following single doses of triazolam, diphenhydramine, ethanol and placebo. *Sleep* 1993;16:301–305.
129. Hiraoka K, Tashiro M, Grobosch T, et al. Brain histamine H_1 receptor occupancy measured by PET after oral administration of levocetirizine, a non-sedating antihistamine. *Expert Opin Drug Saf* 2015;14:199–206.
130. Patat A, Stubbs D, Dunmore C, et al. Lack of interaction between two antihistamines, mizolastine and cetirizine, and ethanol in psychomotor and driving performance in healthy subjects. *Eur J Clin Pharmacol* 1995;48:143–150.
131. Hindmarch I, Bhatti JZ. Psychomotor effects of astemizole and chlorpheniramine, alone and in combination with alcohol. *Int Clin Psychopharmacol* 1987;2:117–119.
132. Kalivas J, Breneman D, Tharp M, et al. Urticaria: clinical efficacy of cetirizine in comparison with hydroxyzine and placebo. *J Allergy Clin Immunol* 1990;86:1014–1018.
133. Baker AM, Johnson DG, Levisky JA, et al. Fatal diphenhydramine intoxication in infants. *J Forensic Sci* 2003;48:425–428.
134. Wyngaarden JB, Seevers MH. The toxic effects of antihistaminic drugs. *J Am Med Assoc* 1951;145:277–282.
135. Cantu TG. Phenothiazines and sudden infant death syndrome. *DICP* 1989;23:795–796.
136. Starke PR, Weaver J, Chowdhury BA. Boxed warning added to promethazine labeling for pediatric use. *N Engl J Med* 2005;352:2653.
137. Vuurman EF, van Veggel LM, Uiterwijk MM, et al. Seasonal allergic rhinitis and antihistamine effects on children's learning. *Ann Allergy* 1993;71:121–126.
138. Bender BG, McCormick DR, Milgrom H. Children's school performance is not impaired by short-term administration of diphenhydramine or loratadine. *J Pediatr* 2001;138:656–660.
139. Bensnes SS. You sneeze, you lose: the impact of pollen exposure on cognitive performance during high-stakes high school exams. *J Health Econ* 2016;49:1–13.
140. Marcotte DE. Allergy test: seasonal allergens and performance in school. *J Health Econ* 2015;40:132–140.
141. Kim DK, Rhee CS, Han DH, et al. Treatment of allergic rhinitis is associated with improved attention performance in children: the Allergic Rhinitis Cohort Study for Kids (ARCO-Kids). *PLoS One* 2014;9:e109145.
142. Stevenson J, Cornah D, Evrard P, et al. Long-term evaluation of the impact of the h_1-receptor antagonist cetirizine on the behavioral, cognitive, and psychomotor development of very young children with atopic dermatitis. *Pediatr Res* 2002;52:251–257.
143. Arisaka O, Shimura N, Nakayama Y, et al. Cyproheptadine and growth. *Am J Dis Child* 1988;142:914–915.
144. Schwarzer G, Bassler D, Mitra A, et al. Ketotifen alone or as additional medication for long-term control of asthma and wheeze in children. *Cochrane Database Syst Rev* 2004:CD001384.
145. Monahan BP, Ferguson CL, Killeavy ES, et al. Torsades de pointes occurring in association with terfenadine use. *JAMA* 1990;264:2788–2790.
146. Woosley RL, Sale M. QT interval: a measure of drug action. *Am J Cardiol* 1993;72:36B–43B.
147. Woosley RL. Cardiac actions of antihistamines. *Annu Rev Pharmacol Toxicol* 1996;36:233–252.
148. Sale ME, Barbey JT, Woosley RL, et al. The electrocardiographic effects of cetirizine in normal subjects. *Clin Pharmacol Ther* 1994;56:295–301.
149. Craig-McFeely PM, Acharya NV, Shakir SA. Evaluation of the safety of fexofenadine from experience gained in general practice use in England in 1997. *Eur J Clin Pharmacol* 2001;57:313–320.
150. Ten Eick AP, Blumer JL, Reed MD. Safety of antihistamines in children. *Drug Saf* 2001;24:119–147.
151. Demoly P, Messaad D, Benahmed S, et al. Hypersensitivity to H_1-antihistamines. *Allergy* 2000;55:679–680.
152. Tella R, Gaig P, Bartra J, et al. Urticaria to cetirizine. *J Investig Allergol Clin Immunol* 2002;12:136–137.
153. Epstein E. Dermatitis due to antihistaminic agents. *J Invest Dermatol* 1949;12:151.
154. Horio T. Allergic and photoallergic dermatitis from diphenhydramine. *Arch Dermatol* 1976;112:1124–1126.
155. Shakouri AA, Bahna SL. Hypersensitivity to antihistamines. *Allergy Asthma Proc* 2013;34:488–496.
156. Bockholdt B, Klug E, Schneider V. Suicide through doxylamine poisoning. *Forensic Sci Int* 2001;119:138–140.
157. Nishino T, Wakai S, Aoki H, et al. Cardiac arrest caused by diphenhydramine overdose. *Acute Med Surg* 2018;5:380–383.
158. Lovegrove MC, Weidle NJ, Budnitz DS. Ingestion of over-the-counter liquid medications: emergency department visits by children aged less than 6 years, 2012–2015. *Am J Prev Med* 2019;56:288–292.

159. Hestand HE, Teske DW. Diphenhydramine hydrochloride intoxication. *J Pediatr* 1977;90:1017–1018.
160. Guay DR, Meatherall RC, Macaulay PA, et al. Activated charcoal adsorption of diphenhydramine. *Int J Clin Pharmacol Ther Toxicol* 1984;22:395–400.
161. Awni WM, Yeh J, Halstenson CE, et al. Effect of haemodialysis on the pharmacokinetics of cetirizine. *Eur J Clin Pharmacol* 1990;38:67–69.
162. Li Q, Mitchell AA, Werler MM, et al. Assessment of antihistamine use in early pregnancy and birth defects. *J Allergy Clin Immunol Pract* 2013;1:666–674.e661.
163. ACOG Practice Bulletin No. 189: nausea and vomiting of pregnancy. *Obstet Gynecol* 2018;131:e15–e30.
164. Food and Drug Administration. Content and format of labeling for human prescription drug and biological products; requirements for pregnancy and lactation labeling. *Fed Regist* 2014;79:72063–72103.
165. Gilboa SM, Strickland MJ, Olshan AF, et al. Use of antihistamine medications during early pregnancy and isolated major malformations. *Birth Defects Res A Clin Mol Teratol* 2009;85:137–150.
166. Diav-Citrin O, Shechtman S, Aharonovich A, et al. Pregnancy outcome after gestational exposure to loratadine or antihistamines: a prospective controlled cohort study. *J Allergy Clin Immunol* 2003;111:1239–1243.
167. Parkin DE. Probable Benadryl withdrawal manifestations in a newborn infant. *J Pediatr* 1974;85:580.
168. Prenner BM. Neonatal withdrawal syndrome associated with hydroxyzine hydrochloride. *Am J Dis Child* 1977;131:529–530.
169. Ito S, Blajchman A, Stephenson M, et al. Prospective follow-up of adverse reactions in breast-fed infants exposed to maternal medication. *Am J Obstet Gynecol* 1993;168:1393–1399.
170. Hilbert J, Radwanski E, Affrime MB, et al. Excretion of loratadine in human breast milk. *J Clin Pharmacol* 1988;28:234–239.
171. Physicians' desk reference: PDR, 63rd ed. Montvale, NJ, Thomson Reuters; 2009:2684–2687.
172. Lin JH. Pharmacokinetic and pharmacodynamic properties of histamine H_2-receptor antagonists. Relationship between intrinsic potency and effective plasma concentrations. *Clin Pharmacokinet* 1991;20:218–236.
173. Gladziwa U, Koltz U. Pharmacokinetic optimisation of the treatment of peptic ulcer in patients with renal failure. *Clin Pharmacokinet* 1994;27:393–408.
174. Gustafsson PM, Kjellman NI, Tibbling L. A trial of ranitidine in asthmatic children and adolescents with or without pathological gastro-oesophageal reflux. *Eur Respir J* 1992;5:201–206.
175. Goldsobel AB, Rohr AS, Siegel SC, et al. Efficacy of doxepin in the treatment of chronic idiopathic urticaria. *J Allergy Clin Immunol* 1986;78:867–873.
176. Richelson E. Tricyclic antidepressants and histamine H_1 receptors. *Mayo Clin Proc* 1979;54:669–674.
177. Veien NK, Kaaber K, Larsen PO, et al. Ranitidine treatment of hand eczema in patients with atopic dermatitis: a double-blind, placebo-controlled trial. *J Am Acad Dermatol* 1995;32:1056–1057.
178. Shelley WB, Shelley ED, Talanin NY. Self-potentiating allergic contact dermatitis caused by doxepin hydrochloride cream. *J Am Acad Dermatol* 1996;34:143–144.
179. Tu JH, Sheu SL, Teng JM. Novel treatment using cimetidine for erythropoietic protoporphyria in children. *JAMA Dermatol* 2016;152:1258–1261.
180. Coursin DB, Farin-Rusk C, Springman SR, et al. The hemodynamic effects of intravenous cimetidine versus ranitidine in intensive care unit patients: a double-blind, prospective, cross-over study. *Anesthesiology* 1988;69:975–978.
181. Dohil M, Prendiville JS. Treatment of molluscum contagiosum with oral cimetidine: clinical experience in 13 patients. *Pediatr Dermatol* 1996;13:310–312.
182. Das BB, Anton K, Soares N, et al. Cimetidine: a safe treatment option for cutaneous warts in pediatric heart transplant recipients. *Med Sci (Basel)* 2018;6:30.
183. Feder HM, Salazar JC. A clinical review of 105 patients with PFAPA (a periodic fever syndrome). *Acta Paediatr* 2010;99:178–184.
184. Ali AH, Hale L, Yalamanchili B, et al. The effect of perioperative cimetidine administration on time to colorectal cancer recurrence. *Am J Ther* 2018;25:e405–e411.
185. Anlar B, Gucuyener K, Imir T, et al. Cimetidine as an immunomodulator in subacute sclerosing panencephalitis: a double blind, placebo-controlled study. *Pediatr Infect Dis J* 1993;12:578–581.
186. Kristensen JK, Petersen LJ, Hansen U, et al. Systemic high-dose ranitidine in the treatment of psoriasis: an open prospective clinical trial. *Br J Dermatol* 1995;133:905–908.
187. Magee LA, Inocencion G, Kamboj L, et al. Safety of first trimester exposure to histamine H_2 blockers. A prospective cohort study. *Dig Dis Sci* 1996;41:1145–1149.
188. Obermeyer BD, Bergstrom RF, Callaghan JT, et al. Secretion of nizatidine into human breast milk after single and multiple doses. *Clin Pharmacol Ther* 1990;47:724–730.
189. Terrin G, Passariello A, De Curtis M, et al. Ranitidine is associated with infections, necrotizing enterocolitis, and fatal outcome in newborns. *Pediatrics* 2012;129:e40–e45.
190. Lam JR, Schneider JL, Zhao W, et al. Proton pump inhibitor and histamine 2 receptor antagonist use and vitamin B12 deficiency. *JAMA* 2013;310:2435–2442.
191. Shapiro LE, Shear NH. Drug interactions: proteins, pumps, and P-450s. *J Am Acad Dermatol* 2002;47:467–484; quiz 485–468.
192. Bodey GP. Azole antifungal agents. *Clin Infect Dis* 1992;14(Suppl 1):S161–S169.
193. Ghamari N, Zarei O, Reiner D, et al. Histamine H_3 receptor ligands by hybrid virtual screening, docking, molecular dynamics simulations, and investigation of their biological effects. *Chem Biol Drug Des* 2019;93(5):832–843.
194. Parfenov VA, Golyk VA, Matsnev EI, et al. Effectiveness of betahistine (48 mg/day) in patients with vestibular vertigo during routine practice: The VIRTUOSO study. *PLoS One* 2017;12:e0174114.
195. Romigi A, Vitrani G, Lo Giudice T, et al. Profile of pitolisant in the management of narcolepsy: design, development, and place in therapy. *Drug Des Dev Ther* 2018;12:2665–2675.
196. Delay-Goyet P, Blanchard V, Schussler N, et al. SAR110894, a potent histamine H_3-receptor antagonist, displays disease-modifying activity in a transgenic mouse model of tauopathy. *Alzheimers Dement (NY)* 2016;2:267–280.
197. Eissa N, Jayaprakash P, Azimullah S, et al. The histamine H3R antagonist DL77 attenuates autistic behaviors in a prenatal valproic acid-induced mouse model of autism. *Sci Rep* 2018;8:13077.
198. Chrusch C, Sharma S, Unruh H, et al. Histamine H_3 receptor blockade improves cardiac function in canine anaphylaxis. *Am J Respir Crit Care Med* 1999;160:1142–1149.
199. Oda T, Morikawa N, Saito Y, et al. Molecular cloning and characterization of a novel type of histamine receptor preferentially expressed in leukocytes. *J Biol Chem* 2000;275:36781–36786.
200. Hofstra CL, Desai PJ, Thurmond RL, et al. Histamine H_4 receptor mediates chemotaxis and calcium mobilization of mast cells. *J Pharmacol Exp Ther* 2003;305:1212–1221.
201. Kollmeier AP, Barnathan ES, O'Brien C, et al. A phase 2a study of toreforant, a histamine H_4 receptor antagonist, in eosinophilic asthma. *Ann Allergy Asthma Immunol* 2018;121:568–574.
202. Frankel E, Song M, Li S, et al. Efficacy and safety of toreforant, a selective histamine H_4 receptor antagonist, for the treatment of moderate-to-severe plaque psoriasis: results from a phase 2 multicenter, randomized, double-blind, placebo-controlled trial. *J Drugs Dermatol* 2018;17:873–879.
203. Boyle DL, DePrimo SE, Calderon C, et al. Toreforant, an orally active histamine H_4-receptor antagonist, in patients with active rheumatoid arthritis despite methotrexate: mechanism of action results from a phase 2, multicenter, randomized, double-blind, placebo-controlled synovial biopsy study. *Inflamm Res* 2019;68:261–274.

CHAPTER 41

Hengameh H. Raissy
Elissa Abrams
H. William Kelly
Stanley J. Szefler

Antiasthmatics

INTRODUCTION

Asthma is the most common chronic disease among children in the United States, affecting about 6 million children under 18 years of age.[1] The rate of asthma in children increased from 8.7% in 2001 to 9.4% in 2010 and then decreased to 8.3% in 2016.[2] In 2017, 8.4% of children had a current diagnosis of asthma,[2] and an asthma attack was reported by about 3.5 million children in the previous year.[3] Twenty percent of emergency department visits in children less than 15 years was for asthma in 2015[1] and accounted for 21% of the asthma hospitalizations in 2010.[4] The prevalence of asthma is highest in children aged 5 to 17 years at 10%,[2] which resulted in 13.8 million missed schooldays by this age group in 2013.[2] In 2016, the rate of asthma remained greater in boys than girls (9.2% vs. 7.4 %), and in black compared to white children (15.7% vs. 7.1%).[2] In addition, the prevalence of asthma attack, emergency department or urgent care visit, and hospitalization in 2016 was higher among children aged 0 to 4 years compared to the 12–17 years age group; black children have a higher rate of emergency department or urgent care visits (22.5%) compared to white children (12.2%).[2] In children, males and non-Hispanic blacks are more likely to die due to asthma.[5] In 2016, 3,518 asthma-related deaths were reported, of whom 209 were children.[6] Asthma-related death is rare, and 80% to 90% of the asthma deaths are preventable.[7]

Asthma is a multifactorial and complex disease. The National Asthma Education and Prevention Program's Expert Panel Report 3 (EPR3): Guidelines for the Diagnosis and Management of Asthma defines asthma as "a common chronic disorder of the airways that is complex and characterized by variable and recurring symptoms, airflow obstruction, bronchial hyperresponsiveness, and an underlying inflammation." Airway inflammation has been demonstrated in the central and peripheral airways, and it involves activation of all airway cells, including eosinophils, T lymphocytes, macrophages, mast cells, bronchial smooth muscle, epithelial cells, and fibroblasts.[7] These activated cells, further, regulate airway inflammation and release cytokines and growth factors, leading to chronic inflammation, airway remodeling, airflow obstruction, bronchial hyperresponsiveness, and increased risk of asthma exacerbations. Although the exact etiology of the inflammatory process leading to asthma is not well defined, innate immunity (the balance between Th-1 and Th-2 cytokine response), genetics, and environmental factors seem to interact for different asthma phenotypic expressions.[8]

The developing immune system begins in the early weeks of gestation, going through several steps of maturation up until and beyond birth. However, due to this immaturity and continual development of the immune system, asthma per se is not observed in the neonate. Approximately 80% of childhood asthma develops before the age of 6 years[8] and may present differently among children. The asthma phenotype differentiates between transient wheezers and persistent wheezers. Transient wheezers (wheezing only at <3 years old) are not at an increased risk for developing asthma later in life; persistent wheezers or late-onset wheezers (wheezing only between 3 and 6 years old) are at higher risk for development of asthma later in life.[9] Interestingly, longitudinal studies have shown that a decline in lung function growth occurs by the age of 6, with the most deficits in children with the onset of symptoms before age of 3.[9] Recently, a positive asthma predictive index has been developed to identify children younger than 3 years with high risk of developing persistent asthma later in life. The risk factors are either one of the following: parental history of asthma, a physician diagnosis of atopic dermatitis, or evidence of sensitization to aeroallergens, or two of the following: evidence of sensitization to foods, greater than or equal to 4% peripheral blood eosinophilia, or wheezing apart from colds.[7,10] In general, a decline in lung growth has not been noted in children aged 5 to 12 years, with mild or moderate persistent asthma through aged 11 to 17 years, except for a subset of children.[11]

Asthma begins early in life, and what determines the severity of asthma or its persistent versus intermittent characteristics yet remains to be determined. It has consistently been shown that asthma is a chronic inflammatory disease, regardless of its severity, and the therapy has been focused on the prevention and suppression of inflammation. The current therapeutic options are use of long-term controller medications to manage underlying inflammation and use of rescue medications to manage acute exacerbations.[7] The EPR3 provides recommendations for assessment of severity and control, which require assessing both impairment and risk domains in children aged 0 to 4 and 5 to 11 years[7] (Fig. 41.1). The EPR3 also provides guidance on classifying severity based on the level of therapy required to control asthma[7] (Fig. 41.2). The steps of therapy recommended by EPR3 for infants and young children are provided in Figure 41.3.[7] Adolescents are treated as adults and not presented here.[7] This chapter provides the pharmacologic basis for those recommendations.

Components of Severity		Classifying Asthma Severity and Initiating Therapy in Children							
				Persistent					
		Intermittent		Mild		Moderate		Severe	
		Ages 0–4	Ages 5–11	Ages 0–4	Ages 5–11	Ages 0–4	Ages 5–11	Ages 0–4	Ages 5–11
Impairment	Symptoms	≤2 days/week		>2 days/week but not daily		Daily		Throughout the day	
	Nighttime awakenings	0	≤2x/month	1–2x/month	3–4x/month	3–4x/month	>1x/week but not nightly	>1x/week	Often 7x/week
	Short-acting beta$_2$-agonist use for symptom control	≤2 days/week		>2 days/week but not daily		Daily		Several times per day	
	Interference with normal activity	None		Minor limitation		Some limitation		Extremely limited	
	Lung function		Normal FEV_1 between exacerbations						
	• FEV_1 (predicted) or peak flow (personal best)	N/A	>80%	N/A	>80%	N/A	60–80%	N/A	<60%
	• FEV_1/FVC		>85%		>80%		75–80%		<75%
Risk	Exacerbations requiring oral systemic corticosteroids (consider severity and interval since last exacerbations)	0–1/ year (see notes)		≥2 exacerbations in 6 months requiring oral systemic corticosteroids, or >4 wheezing episodes/1 year lasting >1 day AND risk factors for persistent asthma	≥2x/year (see notes) Relative annual risk may be related to FEV1				
Recommended step for Initiating Therapy (See Figure 41.3 for treatment steps) The stepwise approach is meant to assist, not replace, the clinical decisionmaking required to meet individual patient needs		Step 1 (for both age groups)		Step 2 (for both age groups)		Step 3 and consider short course of oral systemic corticosteroids	Step 3: medium-dose ICS option and consider short course of oral systemic corticosteroids	Step 3 and consider short course of oral systemic corticosteroids	Step 3: medium-dose ICS option OR Step 4 and consider short course of oral systemic corticosteroids
		In 2–6 weeks, depending on severity, evaluate level of asthma control that is achieved. • Children 0–4 years old: If no clear benefit is observed in 4–6 weeks, stop treatment and consider alternative diagnoses or adjusting therapy. • Children 5–11 years old: Adjust therapy accordingly.							

Figure 41.1 Classifying asthma severity and initiating therapy in children. Data from National Heart, Lung, and Blood Institute; National Institutes of Health; U.S. Department of Health and Human Services. Full Report of the Expert Panel: Guidelines for the diagnosis and management of asthma (EPR-3) 2007. Available at http://www.nhlbi.nih.gov/guidelines/asthma (Last Accessed April 2019).

Components of Control		Assessing Asthma Control and Adjusting Therapy in Children					
		Well-controlled		**Not well controlled**		**Very poorly controlled**	
		Ages 0–4	**Ages 5–11**	**Ages 0–4**	**Ages 5–11**	**Ages 0–4**	**Ages 5–11**
Impairment	Symptoms	≤2 days/week but not more than once on each day		>2 days/week or multiple times on >2 days/week		Throughout the day	
	Nighttime awakenings	≤1x/month		>1x/month	≥2x/month	>1x/week	≥2x/week
	Interference with normal activity	None		Some limitation		Extremely limited	
	Short-acting beta$_2$-agonist use for symptom control (not prevention of EIB)	≤2 days/week		>2 days/week		Several times per day	
	Lung function FEV$_1$ (predicted) or peak flow (personal best) FEV$_1$/FVC	N/A	>80% >80%	N/A	60–80% 75–80%	N/A	<60% <75%
	Exacerbations requiring oral systemic corticosteroids	0–1x/year		2–3x/year	≥2x/year	>3x/year	≥2x/year
	Reduction in lung growth	N/A	Requires long-term followup	N/A		N/A	
	Treatment-related adverse effects	Medication side-effects can vary from none to very troublesome and worrisome. The level of intensity does not correlate to specific levels of control but should be considered in the overall assessment of risk.					
Recommended Action for Treatment (See Figure 41.3 for treatment steps) The stepwise approach is meant to assist, not replace, the clinical decisionmaking required to meet individual patient needs.		• Maintain current step. • Regular follow up every 1–6 months. • Consider step down if well controlled for at least 3 months		Step up 1 step	Step up at least 1 step	• Consider short course of oral systemic corticosteroids • Step up 1–2 steps	
				• **Before step up:** • Review adherence to medication, inhaler technique, and environmental control. • If alternative treatment was used, discontinue it and use preferred treatment for that step. • **Reevaluate the level of asthma control in 2–6 weeks to achieve control; every 1–6 months to maintain control.** • **Children 0–4 years old:** If no clear benefit is observed in 4–6 weeks, consider alternative diagnosis or adjusting therapy. • **Children 5–11 years old:** Adjust therapy accordingly. • **For side effects,** consider alternative treatment options.			

Figure 41.2 Assessing asthma control and adjusting therapy in children. Data from National Heart, Lung, and Blood Institute; National Institutes of Health; U.S. Department of Health and Human Services. Full Report of the Expert Panel: Guidelines for the diagnosis and management of asthma (EPR-3) 2007. Available at http://www.nhlbi.nih.gov/guidelines/asthma (Last Accessed April 2019).

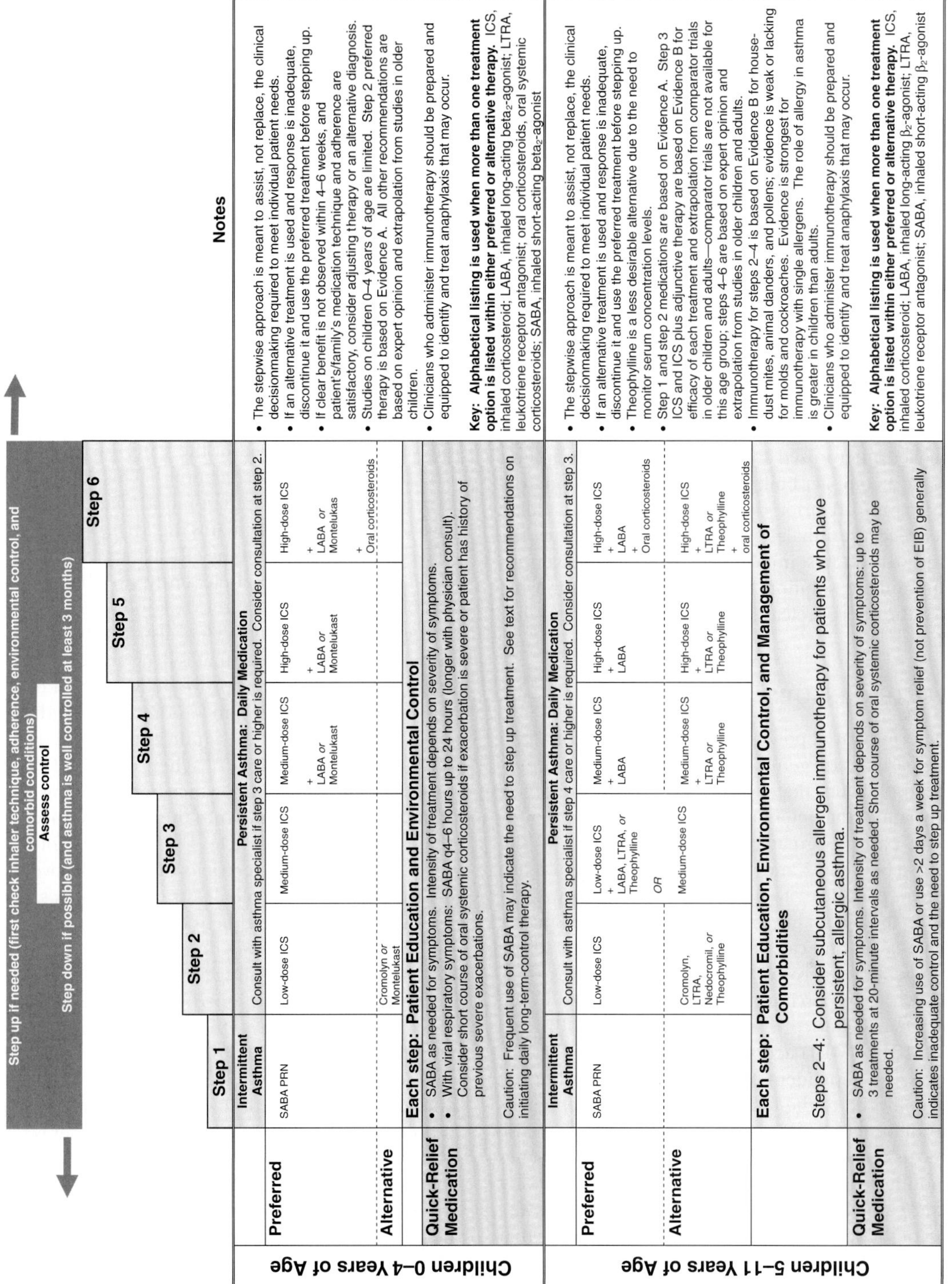

Step up if needed (first check inhaler technique, adherence, environmental control, and comorbid conditions)

Assess control

Step down if possible (and asthma is well controlled at least 3 months)

Children 0–4 Years of Age

	Step 1	Step 2	Step 3	Step 4	Step 5	Step 6
	Intermittent Asthma	Persistent Asthma: Daily Medication Consult with asthma specialist if step 3 care or higher is required. Consider consultation at step 2.				
Preferred	SABA PRN	Low-dose ICS	Medium-dose ICS	Medium-dose ICS + LABA *or* Montelukast	High-dose ICS + LABA *or* Montelukast	High-dose ICS + LABA *or* Montelukas + Oral corticosteroids
Alternative		Cromolyn *or* Montelukast				
	Each step: Patient Education and Environmental Control					
Quick-Relief Medication	• SABA as needed for symptoms. Intensity of treatment depends on severity of symptoms. • With viral respiratory symptoms: SABA q4–6 hours up to 24 hours (longer with physician consult). Consider short course of oral systemic corticosteroids if exacerbation is severe or patient has history of previous severe exacerbations. Caution: Frequent use of SABA may indicate the need to step up treatment. See text for recommendations on initiating daily long-term-control therapy.					

Notes

- The stepwise approach is meant to assist, not replace, the clinical decisionmaking required to meet individual patient needs.
- If an alternative treatment is used and response is inadequate, discontinue it and use the preferred treatment before stepping up.
- If clear benefit is not observed within 4–6 weeks, and patient's/family's medication technique and adherence are satisfactory, consider adjusting therapy or an alternative diagnosis.
- Studies on children 0–4 years of age are limited. Step 2 preferred therapy is based on Evidence A. All other recommendations are based on expert opinion and extrapolation from studies in older children.
- Clinicians who administer immunotherapy should be prepared and equipped to identify and treat anaphylaxis that may occur.

Key: Alphabetical listing is used when more than one treatment option is listed within either preferred or alternative therapy. ICS, inhaled corticosteroid; LABA, inhaled long-acting beta$_2$-agonist; LTRA, leukotriene receptor antagonist; oral corticosteroids, oral systemic corticosteroids; SABA, inhaled short-acting beta$_2$-agonist

Children 5–11 Years of Age

	Step 1	Step 2	Step 3	Step 4	Step 5	Step 6
	Intermittent Asthma	Persistent Asthma: Daily Medication Consult with asthma specialist if step 4 care or higher is required. Consider consultation at step 3.				
Preferred	SABA PRN	Low-dose ICS	Low-dose ICS + LABA, LTRA, *or* Theophylline *OR*	Medium-dose ICS + LABA	High-dose ICS + LABA	High-dose ICS + LABA + Oral corticosteroids
Alternative		Cromolyn, LTRA, Nedocromil, *or* Theophylline	Medium-dose ICS	Medium-dose ICS + LTRA *or* Theophylline	High-dose ICS + LTRA *or* Theophylline	High-dose ICS + LTRA *or* Theophylline + oral corticosteroids
	Each step: Patient Education, Environmental Control, and Management of Comorbidities Steps 2–4: Consider subcutaneous allergen immunotherapy for patients who have persistent, allergic asthma.					
Quick-Relief Medication	• SABA as needed for symptoms. Intensity of treatment depends on severity of symptoms: up to 3 treatments at 20-minute intervals as needed. Short course of oral systemic corticosteroids may be needed. Caution: Increasing use of SABA or use >2 days a week for symptom relief (not prevention of EIB) generally indicates inadequate control and the need to step up treatment.					

Notes

- The stepwise approach is meant to assist, not replace, the clinical decisionmaking required to meet individual patient needs.
- If an alternative treatment is used and response is inadequate, discontinue it and use the preferred treatment before stepping up.
- Theophylline is a less desirable alternative due to the need to monitor serum concentration levels.
- Step 1 and step 2 medications are based on Evidence A. Step 3 ICS and ICS plus adjunctive therapy are based on Evidence B for efficacy of each treatment and extrapolation from comparator trials in older children and adults—comparator trials are not available for this age group; steps 4–6 are based on expert opinion and extrapolation from studies in older children and adults.
- Immunotherapy for steps 2–4 is based on Evidence B for house-dust mites, animal danders, and pollens; evidence is weak or lacking for molds and cockroaches. Evidence is strongest for immunotherapy with single allergens. The role of allergy in asthma is greater in children than adults.
- Clinicians who administer immunotherapy should be prepared and equipped to identify and treat anaphylaxis that may occur.

Key: Alphabetical listing is used when more than one treatment option is listed within either preferred or alternative therapy. ICS, inhaled corticosteroid; LABA, inhaled long-acting β_2-agonist; LTRA, leukotriene receptor antagonist; SABA, inhaled short-acting β_2-agonist

Figure 41.3 The stepwise approach for management of asthma in children. Data from National Heart, Lung, and Blood Institute; National Institutes of Health; U.S. Department of Health and Human Services. Full Report of the Expert Panel: Guidelines for the diagnosis and management of asthma (EPR-3) 2007. Available at http://www.nhlbi.nih.gov/guidelines/asthma (Last Accessed April 2019).

AEROSOL DELIVERY IN CHILDREN

The most effective antiasthmatics are delivered as aerosols, and delivery of the aerosols into the airways of children is the primary determinant of dose, but like all dosage forms, aerosol delivery presents many unique challenges depending on the age of the child.[7] There are three systems of aerosol delivery in clinical practice: (a) nebulizers that generate aerosol clouds by forcing air and fluid up through adjacent open-ended tubes that strike a baffle at high speed, creating the aerosol (jet nebulizer) and ultrasonic nebulizers that produce an aerosol by vibrating liquid above a transducer; (b) metered-dose inhalers (MDIs) that force a propellant and solution or micronized suspension of drug stored in a pressurized canister out through a small orifice by opening a stem valve, creating an aerosol of particles that diminish in size as the propellant evaporates; (c) breath-activated, dry-powder inhalers (DPIs) that contain either individually packed micronized doses of drug plus excipients such as lactose or a compact bulk of drug from which micronized doses are shaven off prior to inhalation (they are called breath activated because inhalation by the patient creates the aerosol)[12,13]; and (d) soft mist inhalers (SMIs) which delivers active drug in an aqueous solution by generating a slow-moving aerosol cloud by the energy released from a coiled spring rather than a propellant.[14,15]

DEVICE-SPECIFIC ISSUES

The primary determinant of potential delivered dose from each of the systems is particle size generated. All devices produce heterodispersed aerosol clouds that are characterized by their mass median aerodynamic diameter (MMAD). In spontaneously breathing adults, particles greater than 10 μm deposit in the oropharynx, those between 5 and 10 μm deposit in the trachea and large bronchi, particles 1 to 5 μm deposit in the lower airways (often called the respirable fraction), and particles smaller than 0.5 μm act as a gas and can be exhaled.[12,13] Very few of the delivery devices generate aerosols with the same MMAD; thus, significant differences in percent of drug dose delivered to the lung occur both across devices (i.e., jet nebulizer vs. DPI) and within devices (MDI vs. MDI) across the manufacturers. The labeling of doses is also dependent on the type of device, but not on actual dose delivered to the lung. The dosing for nebulizers is based on the amount of drug put into the nebulizer. The dose for MDIs and SMIs is based on the amount of drug that reaches the patient's mouth (leaves the actuator/mouthpiece) following actuation in the United States and the amount that exits the canister in most of the rest of the world. The dose of a DPI is that dose that is available for inhalation following activation of the dose (puncturing the blister, breaking the capsule, or shaving off the dose).

The most frequently prescribed delivery device is the MDI due to its portability and convenience. Since 1993, the MDI has undergone significant changes due to the 1989 Montreal Protocol of Substances that Deplete the Ozone Layer and the Clean Air Act of 1990 to eventually end the use of ozone depleting chlorofluorocarbons (CFCs)[7,14]; by December 2013, seven MDIs containing CFC were phased out. The introduction of hydrofluoroalkanes (HFAs) as a propellant has been associated with reformulation of some of the inhaled corticosteroids (ICSs) as solutions instead of micronized suspensions.[12,14] The reformulation in concert with valve stem and actuator redesign has resulted in products with significantly reduced MMADs, markedly improving lower airway delivery. For example, HFA-propelled beclomethasone dipropionate has a lung delivery in adults of 50% to 60% in both children and adults versus 4% to 10% delivery for the older CFC-propelled preparations.[14] However, other HFA-MDIs such as albuterol, fluticasone propionate, and budesonide/formoterol combination are still formulated as micronized suspensions and deliver 10% to 25% of the actuated dose.[14]

The MDI is the most complicated system to use for patients. It requires multiple steps and good coordination of actuation during a slow deep inhalation. Many patients have significant difficulty coordinating actuation and inhalation, reducing lower airway delivery of drug from MDIs.[7,12] Spacer devices, particularly valved holding chambers (VHCs), have been developed to overcome the inability to coordinate actuation and inhalation. The VHCs are attached to the mouthpiece of an MDI, and the valve allows flow out of the VHC during inhalation and not into the VHC during exhalation.[12] This allows young patients to breathe normally through a mouthpiece or a snug-fitting facemask, while an adult actuates the MDI.[16] Although this method of delivery has proven to be efficacious in numerous clinical trials, it is noteworthy that currently, no MDI+VHC combination has been approved by the U.S. Food and Drug Administration (FDA).[7,17] The various VHCs also produce significant differences in delivery of drug that is drug and device dependent. For example, a VHC may improve delivery from one MDI product and decrease delivery from another MDI product, or two different VHCs may result in significantly different deliveries from the same MDI product.[12,18] When using VHCs, it is important to actuate the inhaler only once before taking the inhalation as actuating multiple times into the device reduces delivery due to coalescence of the particles.[12,19] Lastly, the older plastic VHCs could develop static electricity on the walls over time, resulting in attraction of the smaller respirable particles, decreasing drug availability.[19] This could be reduced by rinsing the devices with dilute home dishwashing detergent weekly or using the newer VHCs with antistatic lining.[20]

The DPIs were developed in response to the Montreal Protocol, but the FDA has determined that they are not considered an alternative to CFC MDIs. However, they continue to be developed and are probably the easiest to teach patients to use and are associated with fewer mistakes by patients.[12] The DPIs require a different inhalation technique that is rapid and deep, and most produce optimal delivery at inspiratory flows greater than or equal to 60 L per min.[12] The rapid deep inhalation, while not optimal for delivery of drug into peripheral airways, helps break up the larger drug particle aggregates. The effect of inspiratory flow is dependent on the DPI. For example, the Pulmicort® Flexhaler™, with a higher internal resistance, has a reduction in respirable particles of 50% at an inspiratory flow of 30 L per min compared to that of 60 L per min, whereas with the Asmanex® Twisthaler™ the amount of drug emitted from the device was constant at inspiratory flows of 30 to 70 L per min.[21,22]

SMIs were originally launched in Europe in 2004.[15] Currently, there are four approved products containing either a single or combination of long-acting β_2 agonist (LABA) and long-acting muscarinic antagonists (LAMAs). Similar to MDIs, SMIs require coordination of actuation during a slow deep inhalation. A dose will be loaded with turning the base of the device, which results in delivery of drug solution to the dosing chamber. A soft mist is released via actuation of the device. With most formulations, SMIs can deliver 75% of MMAD of less than or equal to 5.8 µm at a velocity of 0.8 m per sec.[15] A longer spray duration of 1.2 seconds may offer patients a better chance to coordinate their breathing with administration of the inhaler. Use of SMIs is limited to adequate solubility of the agents in the metered volume of 15 µL.

Nebulizers are approved as medical devices and so do not have as stringent criteria for approval as generic drugs. They need only to be as good as any product that is already marketed.[12] Jet nebulizers require a source of compressed air and so are not as portable as either an MDI or DPI. Each nebulizer has optimal operating conditions, but in general, an airflow of 5 to 12 L per min produces aerosol clouds with an MMAD of 4 to 8 µm.[12] Ultrasonic nebulizers produce similar delivery as jet nebulizers, with the exception of micronized suspensions for which they are ineffective.[12] Once nebulizers are set up, they are the simplest for the patient as they require only normal tidal breathing and so are often favored for young infants who use them with a facemask. However, due to the inconsistent and often poor delivery from nebulizers, it has been posited that MDI plus VHC be the preferred delivery method for aerosol drugs in infants and toddlers, particularly the extrafine particle generating HFA-propelled ICSs beclomethasone dipropionate and ciclesonide.[16] Although studies have shown improved delivery from these devices, the recommendation does not consider the possibility of increased adverse systemic effects nor the marked differences in delivery between VHCs.[10,18]

Due to the complex nature of orally inhaled drug products including the interaction between drug propellants, the quantity and nature of excipients such as lactose, the solubility in the lung tissue and distribution and absorption from the lung, as well as the patient–device interface, the development of generic products has been slow. However, research over the past 10 years has resulted in the publication of product-specific guidances for the development of generic albuterol HFA-propelled MDIs and DPIs for combined fluticasone propionate and salmeterol xinafoate in 2013 and 17 additional guidances that will no doubt increase the availability of more generic orally inhaled products.[23] The guidances provide the in vitro and in vivo studies required to show bioequivalence between products.

PATIENT-SPECIFIC ISSUES

Infants and young children clearly have significant differences in airway geometry so that data from normal adults do not necessarily apply, but because of logistical and ethical considerations, radiolabeled aerosol studies are rare in children. However, the adult values for respirable particles are used as a measuring stick for the development of aerosol delivery devices, all of which are designed for adults and then used in children. Many children aged 5 years and younger cannot coordinate inhalation and actuation with MDIs and children aged 4 years and younger often require the use of a facemask for delivery from both nebulizers and MDI+VHC.[12,17,18] The use of a facemask reduces delivery to about one-half that from a mouthpiece as infants are obligate nose breathers and part of the dose is filtered out by the nose.[16,24] Infants also have lower tidal volumes (tidal volume is a relatively constant 7 to 10 mL per kg throughout life). Infants weighing less than 15 kg will not necessarily be able to completely empty the VHC; however, they may receive higher µg per kg doses based on lack of air entrainment on inhalation.[16,25] So, there are a number of factors that can have potentially offsetting effects on aerosol delivery in infants compared to older children. For example, in vitro models of less than or equal to 2-year-old tidal volumes versus those for 4- to 5-year-olds show higher µg per kg doses delivered to those 2 years and younger.[16,26–28] However, a wait time between actuation and inhalation of 5 seconds decreases delivery by 30% to 50%.[19,27] Finally, the child should be breathing quietly and not crying as delivery by both nebulizer and MDI+VHC in the crying infant reduces delivery by as much as 80%.[24] Unfortunately, if infants and young children resist the use of a facemask, parents and caregivers revert to a "blow-by" method where they hold the mask or end of the tube connected to the nebulizer close to the infants' mouth and nose. However, studies have shown that holding the mask 1 cm from the face can reduce delivery 50% to 60% and at 2 cm as much as 85%.[25] In clinical trials superiority has not been established for MDI+VHC over nebulization.[16,17]

Unfortunately, many children aged 5 years and younger cannot attain a peak inspiratory flow of 60 L per min.[12] The internal resistance of the DPI can also affect the ability of children to generate flow through the device. In one study, 78% of 4-year-olds could generate an inspiratory flow of at least 30 L per min through a Diskus®, 89% through an Aerolizer®, but only 56% through a Turbuhaler™.[29] The use of DPIs should be reserved for children aged 4 years and older.

INHALED CORTICOSTEROIDS

MECHANISM OF ACTION

Corticosteroids are the most potent anti-inflammatory agents available for the management of asthma. They have a broad array of anti-inflammatory effects. The glucocorticoid receptor (GR) resides in the cytoplasm of cells and is ubiquitous in tissues and cells throughout the body, explaining its myriad effects. The corticosteroid enters the cell cytoplasm via passive diffusion across the cell membrane and binds with the inactive GR complex, dissociating the GR complex from heat shock proteins and immunophilin.[30] Then, the activated GR translocates into the nucleus where it binds to DNA at specific sequences called glucocorticoid response elements where it promotes the production of anti-inflammatory proteins such as lipocortin-1, β_2-adrenergic receptor (β_2AR), secretory leukocyte inhibitory protein, and IκB-α.[30] In addition, it inhibits transcription activation of many pro-inflammatory cytokines that are activated through tumor necrosis factor-α and nuclear factor-κB (i.e., interleukins 1–6, 8, 11, 12, 13, chemokines, matrix metalloproteinase-9, adhesion molecules, inducible nitric oxide synthase, endothelin-1, etc.).[30] Although there is a single gene encoding the human GR, splice variants have been identified and one, the GRβ isoform, although usually inactive, has been reported to be increased in corticosteroid-resistant patients.[30]

The effects of corticosteroids are cell and tissue specific, which explain many of their clinical effects. Corticosteroids reduce mucus secretion and produce vasoconstriction, reducing airway mucosal blood flow and endothelial cell leaking.[30] These latter effects, along with reduction in nitric oxide production, decrease vascular and tissue edema that contribute to airways obstruction. It has been posited that the vascular effects of corticosteroids contribute to the acute improvement following frequent high doses of ICSs in patients presenting to the emergency department.[30] Corticosteroids inhibit cytokine release from respiratory epithelial cells, macrophages, and T lymphocytes.[30] Corticosteroids increase the number of β_2ARs in airway smooth muscle, attenuating or modulating tolerance due to chronic β_2 agonist stimulation, but not completely reversing it.[30] Corticosteroids decrease the number of dendritic cells and eosinophils in the airways by inducing apoptosis, reduce the number of circulating eosinophils, and reduce the number and activation of T lymphocytes. Corticosteroids do not inhibit the release of soluble mediators from tissue mast cells [histamine and leukotrienes (LTs)] but reduce their number and influx into airway smooth muscle cells.[30] This explains why acute administration of a corticosteroid has no effect on the early asthmatic response to inhaled allergen or exercise but that chronic administration results in significant attenuation of these responses. As the GR is found throughout all cells and tissues, a potential for significant adverse effects listed in Table 41.1 exists.[31] Therefore, corticosteroids with high topical activity with pharmacokinetic properties that limit systemic activity that can be administered by inhalation were developed.

The ICSs are considered the preferred long-term controller medications for all levels of persistent asthma due to their consistent efficacy, resulting in reduction in bronchial hyperresponsiveness and asthma exacerbations and improvement in lung function. The current ICSs approved for use in the United States and their recommended doses for children aged 5 to 11 years are listed in Table 41.2, which is modified from the EPR3.[7,13,32] Chemical modifications of the corticosteroids produce different binding affinities (potency) for the GR (Table 41.3) that can simply be overcome by giving equipotent doses.[13,31–33] Thus, when assessing "clinically comparable doses," lung delivery from various delivery devices as well as potency need to be taken into account. Table 41.2 also presents the clinically comparable doses for children established by comparative clinical trials.[7,13,32] There are relatively little data in children aged 4 years and younger, where delivery issues become even more variable. While it has been postulated that the newer HFA-MDI ICSs formulated to deliver ultrafine particles may have greater efficacy due to penetration into the small airways, clinical trials do not support a difference from that produced by total lung delivery.[13,34,35]

TABLE 41.1	Adverse Effects of Glucocorticoid Administration
Aseptic necrosis of bone	
Cataracts	
Central redistribution of fat	
Glaucoma	
Hypertension	
Hypokalemia	
Hyperglycemia	
Hypothalamus–pituitary–adrenal axis suppression	
Impaired wound healing	
Moon face	
Osteoporosis (bone fracture)	
Pseudotumor cerebri	
Psychiatric disorders	
Pancreatitis	
Skin striae	
Subcutaneous tissue atrophy	
Sodium and water retention	
Myopathy (skeletal muscle)	

Data from Kelly HW. Potential adverse effects of inhaled corticosteroids. *J Allergy Clin Immunol* 2003;112:469–478.

PHARMACOKINETICS

Differences in the molecular structures of ICSs result in altered pharmacokinetics properties of these agents (see Table 41.3), which are the primary determinants of the topical to systemic activity (therapeutic index).[13,32,33] Figure 41.4 provides a schematic of each of the pharmacokinetic variables that can affect the therapeutic index.[7,12,13,31,33] The inhaled route of administration has the advantage of delivering drug to the site of action, but only 5% to 60% of the inhaled dose is delivered to the lung, about 50% to 80% of the drug deposits in the oropharynx and swallowed, while the rest is exhaled or left in the device.[7,12,13] Topical selectivity of the ICSs can be improved by decreasing oral bioavailability, increasing systemic clearance, and prolonging residence time in the lung.[13,31,33] Systemic bioavailability of ICSs depends on the oral bioavailability and the amount of drug which enters the systemic circulation via the lungs. Oral bioavailability can be altered by oral absorption, increased first-pass intestinal wall and hepatic metabolism mediated by the cytochrome P450 3A4 (CYP3A4) isozymes, and decreasing oropharyngeal deposition using a VHC with MDI for compounds with significant oral absorption, such as beclomethasone dipropionate.[13,31,33] However, for compounds with very high first-pass metabolism such as fluticasone propionate, using a VHC with the MDI can actually increase systemic exposure by increasing lung delivery.[18,31] This can adversely affect the therapeutic index.[31,36] Children aged 2 years and younger can receive higher microgram per kilogram doses of ICSs than do older children as discussed above, and this may put them at higher risk for adverse systemic effects, such as growth reduction.[37,38]

Systemic clearance is the primary determinant other than dose for steady-state serum concentrations with chronic dosing. Most of the ICSs undergo unrestrictive hepatic extraction and metabolism by CYP3A4 so that their clearances approach liver blood flow (≈90 L per hour).[13,33] The exceptions are the active metabolites of beclomethasone dipropionate (beclomethasone 17-monopropionate) and ciclesonide (desisobutyryl-ciclesonide) that apparently undergo extrahepatic metabolism, possibly via blood esterases.[13,33] Retention in the lung allows ongoing exposure to the GRs and exposes the systemic circulation to lower concentrations. It occurs with more lipophilic compounds, such as fluticasone propionate, and is evidenced by a longer elimination half-life for inhaled rather than intravenous (IV) administration.[16] Some of the ICSs undergo intracellular fatty acid esterification at the free hydroxyl group at the carbon-21 position (i.e., budesonide and desisobutyryl-ciclesonide), which maintains a depot of drug in the cell.[13,33] However, this property has not been established to confer an improved therapeutic index or prolonged duration of effect over agents that do not undergo esterification.[32]

CLINICAL USE

Table 41.2 presents the current EPR3 recommendations that, regardless of age, ICSs are the preferred agents for persistent asthma and that the dose should be based on the severity and control of the disease. The ICSs are the only agents demonstrated

TABLE 41.2 Current ICS Available for Children and Their Clinically Comparable Doses

Agent	*Low Daily Dose (μg)*	*Medium Daily Dose (μg)*	*High Daily Dose (μg)*
Beclomethasone dipropionate HFA-MDI, Qvar Redihaler (40 and 80 μg/actuation) HFA-MDI, Qvar (40 and 80 μg/actuation)	80–160	>160–320	>320
Budesonide DPI, Flexhaler (90 and 180 μg/dose)	180–360	>360–720	>720
Nebulizer solution, Pulmicort Respules (250, 500, and 1,000 μg/2 mL)	500	1,000	2,000
Dose for children 0–4 years old	250–500	>500	>1,000
Ciclesonide[a] HFA-MDI, Alvesco (80 and 160 μg/actuation)	80–160	>160–320	>320
Flunisolide HFA-MDI, Aerospan (80 μg/actuation)	160	320	>640
Fluticasone furoate DPI, Arnuity Ellipta (50, 100, and 200 μg/dose) Approved dose for children 5–11 years old: 50 μg/dose	50	Not evaluated	Not evaluated
Fluticasone propionate HFA-MDI, Flovent (44, 110, and 220 μg/actuation)	88–176	>176–352	>352
Dose for children 0–4 years old[b]	176	>176–352	>352
DPI, Flovent Diskus (50, 100, and 250 μg/dose)	100–200	>200–400	>400
DPI, ArmonAir RespiClick (55, 113, and 232 μg/dose)[c]	110–226	>226–464	>464
Mometasone furoate HFA, MDI, Asmanex (100 and 200 μg/actuation)[a]	110	220–440	>440
DPI, Asmanex Twisthaler (110 and 220[a] μg delivers 100 and 200 μg/actuation, respectively)	110	220–440	>440

[a] Not approved for children <12 years old.
[b] Not FDA approved for the age group.
[c] BX rated generic product.
DPI, dry-powder inhaler; FDA, Food and Drug Administration; HFA, hydrofluoroalkane; ICS, inhaled corticosteroid; MDI, metered-dose inhaler.
Data from National Institutes of Health, National Heart, Lung, and Blood Institute. National Asthma Education and Prevention Program. Full Report of the Expert Panel: Guidelines for the diagnosis and management of asthma (EPR-3) 2007. http://www.nhlbi.nih.gov/guidelines/asthma. Accessed April 2019; and Dolovich MB, Dhand R. Aerosol drug delivery: developments in device design and clinical use. *Lancet* 2011;377(9770):1032–1045.

TABLE 41.3 Receptor-Binding Affinities and Pharmacokinetic Properties of the Inhaled Corticosteroid

ICS	*Binding Affinity*[a]	*Systemic Clearance (L/h)*	*Oral Bioavailability (%)*	*Lung Delivery (%)*
Beclomethasone dipropionate	0.4	150	20	50–60
Budesonide	9.4	84	11	15–30
Ciclesonide	0.12	152	<1	50
Flunisolide	1.8	58	20	68
Fluticasone propionate	18	66	<1	20
Mometasone furoate	23	53	<1	11
Fluticasone furoate	29	65	<1	15

[a] Receptor-binding affinities of ICS relative to dexamethasone equal to 1.
Data from Dolovich MB, Dhand R. Aerosol drug delivery: developments in device design and clinical use. *Lancet* 2011; 377(9770):1032–1045; and Kelly HW. Potential adverse effects of inhaled corticosteroids. *J Allergy Clin Immunol* 2003;112:469–478.

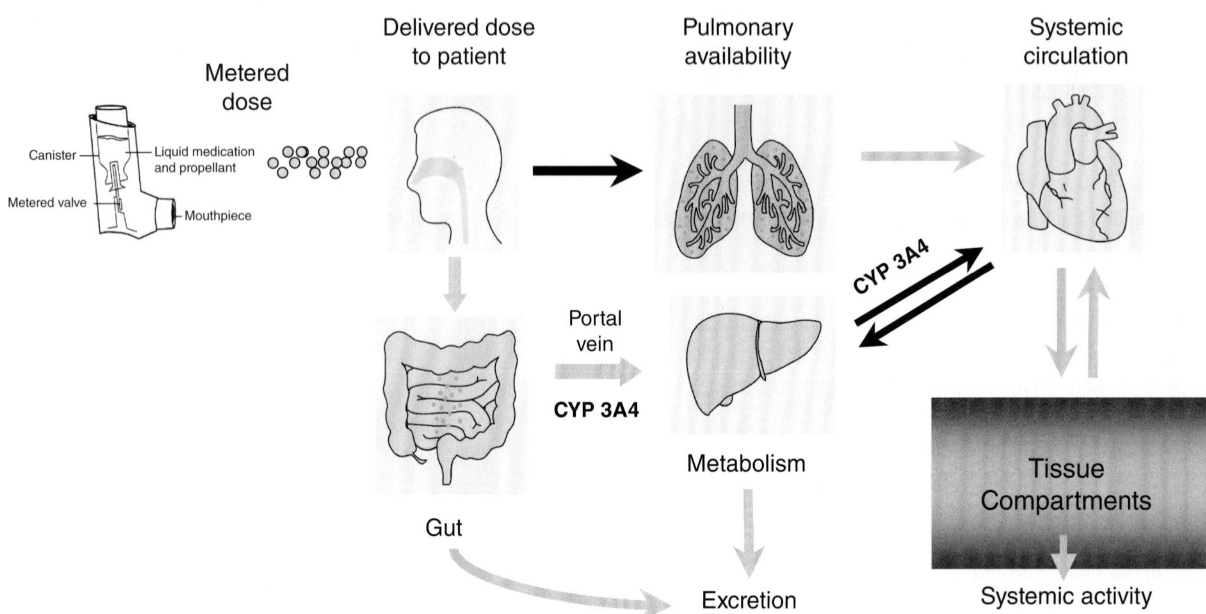

Figure 41.4 Effects of various factors on systemic activity of inhaled corticosteroid. Data from National Institutes of Health, National Heart, Lung, and Blood Institute. National Asthma Education and Prevention Program. Full Report of the Expert Panel: Guidelines for the diagnosis and management of asthma (EPR-3) 2007. http://www.nhlbi.nih.gov/guidelines/asthma. Accessed April 2019.
Kelly HW. Comparison of inhaled corticosteroids: an update. *Ann Pharmacother* 2009;43:519–527.
Kelly HW. Potential adverse effects of inhaled corticosteroids. *J Allergy Clin Immunol* 2003;112:469–478. Derendorf H, Nave R, Drollman A, et al. Relevance of pharmacokinetics and pharmacodynamics of inhaled corticosteroids to asthma. Eur Respir J 2006;28:1042–1050.

to reduce the risk of dying from asthma.[7] Furthermore, low-medium doses of ICSs have consistently been shown to improve lung function, decrease bronchial hyperresponsiveness and asthma exacerbation, and reduce the need for as-needed rescue with short-acting β_2 agonists (SABAs) and oral corticosteroids.[7,32,39,40] In addition, ICSs reduce sputum eosinophils and fraction of exhaled nitric oxide (FeNO), a downstream end product of eosinophilic inflammation.[7] Comparative clinical trials in children aged 5 to 11 years show they are more effective than all alternative long-term controllers.[7,41–43] In addition, studies in children less than 5 years of age have shown fluticasone propionate by MDI+VHC and budesonide nebulization suspension to be more efficacious than cromolyn and budesonide nebulization to be more effective than montelukast.[44,45] Chronic administration of ICSs reduces the degree of bronchial hyperresponsiveness in children, including exercise-induced bronchospasm (EIB).[41,46] They reduce EIB more effectively and consistently than montelukast.[47] Despite their activity in preventing exacerbations and reducing symptoms and airway responsiveness, ICS therapy does not prevent loss of lung function, prevent development of asthma in high-risk infants, nor enhance the lung growth in children with asthma.[10,11,39,48]

The clinical response to ICSs varies among patients, but most asthma symptoms will improve in 1 to 2 weeks, with maximum improvement in 1 to 2 months. Maximum improvement in lung function requires 3 to 6 weeks of treatment and at least 1 to 3 months to improve bronchial hyperresponsiveness, although it may continue to improve over many months.[32] The response for FeNO occurs within a few days so that it has been touted as a means of monitoring ICS therapy for adherence and adjusting doses.[49] In clinical trials, FeNO has been used as an inflammatory biomarker to characterize patients, compare relative potency of ICSs, as well as to compare ICSs to other therapies.[50–52] A chemiluminescence analyzer has been approved by the FDA for use in monitoring ICS therapy, and handheld devices are being developed.[49] However, clinical trials in children assessing the utility of monitoring FeNO in addition to symptoms and lung function have obtained mixed results; although it has been shown to be able to predict future exacerbations, its routine use is uncertain and requires further study.[52,53]

For those patients who have not achieved adequate control on low doses of ICSs, the EPR3 recommends an increase in the dose of ICSs or add-on adjunct therapy such as a leukotriene-receptor antagonist (LTRA) or an inhaled LABA.[7] The preferred recommendations vary with age, primarily because no adjunctive therapy to ICSs has been evaluated in children less than 5 years and minimal studies have compared adjunctive therapy to increased ICS in those aged 5 to 11 years.[54,55] Adjunctive therapies have been directly compared in a recent study for this age group, showing that the addition of an LABA provided a greater improvement in asthma control than the addition of an LTRA or the ICS dose by 2.5-fold.[54] This is consistent with a meta-analysis of 11 studies demonstrating greater improvement in lung function with the addition of an LABA than doubling the dose of ICS in children.[55]

Dose–response studies for ICSs in children are few. The ICSs are considered to have a relatively flat dose–response curve, particularly for lung function improvement. In children aged 4 to 14 years, the response to fluticasone propionate tends to plateau between 100 and 200 μg daily in most patients, with some further benefit in more severe patients obtained at 400 μg daily.[56] A dose–response study of budesonide between

200, 400, and 800 µg daily, which is one-half as potent as fluticasone propionate, confirms these findings.[57] In adults with relatively moderate-to-severe asthma, doubling the dose of ICS does not decrease asthma exacerbations, but quadrupling the dose does despite small improvements.[58,59] Similar studies have not been carried out in children, but in general, doubling the dose of ICS does not significantly increase benefit.[13,56,57] In a recent study in children (ages 5 to 11 years) with mild-moderate asthma, quintupling the dose of ICS at the early signs of loss of asthma control did not reduce the rate of severe asthma exacerbation.[60] In young children and infants, the data are even less clear. One study comparing fluticasone propionate 100 and 200 µg daily by MDI+VHC and facemask in 237 infants aged 12 to 47 months reported a dose response for decreased exacerbations; however, the decrease in exacerbations for the 100 µg daily was not significantly different from placebo.[40] In addition, the pivotal trials for budesonide nebulizer suspension failed to demonstrate a dose response for 500 to 1,000 µg daily after the dose exceeded 250 µg once daily, which was not consistently more effective than placebo across studies.[61]

The issue of once-daily administration of the ICSs to improve compliance is often raised. Budesonide, mometasone furoate, and fluticasone furoate currently have once-daily FDA-approved labeling; most mild persistent patients controlled on low- to medium-dose ICS can be adequately controlled with once-daily administration with all the ICSs. Only fluticasone furoate has specific pharmacokinetic properties, a prolonged lung retention and systemic half-life that allows for once-daily dosing.[62] The other ICSs all work more effectively in moderate-to-severe asthma with twice-daily dosing.[13]

Oral corticosteroids are indicated for asthma exacerbations not responding to inhaled SABAs.[7] They are usually administered as a short course or burst (3 to 10 days) at the equivalent dose of 1 to 2 mg per kg daily prednisolone equivalent once or twice daily. Multiple-daily dosing may provide superior activity and decreased gastrointestinal effects. The number of oral corticosteroid bursts is used to determine both risk and the level of control (see Fig. 41.2).[7] Oral corticosteroids administered in the emergency department and continued for 3 to 7 days reduce the risk of relapse.[7] Use of oral corticosteroid for the management of asthma exacerbation in adolescent and school-aged children is supported by a large body of literature; however, there is a lack of evidence for use of oral corticosteroids in preschool children. A post hoc analysis of two large trials in preschool children showed that oral corticosteroids did not reduce the severity of asthma exacerbation.[63] Although an entrenched practice in preschool children, prospective trials are needed to identify the best treatment approach.[64]

ADVERSE EFFECTS

The adverse effects of ICSs are dose related.[31] The degree of systemic exposure depends on the inhaler design, patient's technique, aerodynamic and physicochemical properties of the particles, and the pharmacokinetics. All of the ICSs have relatively few adverse effects at the low-medium doses and when they are used properly. Although there are potential differences based on pharmacokinetics, patients are at risk of experiencing systemic effects at high doses of the ICSs and should be monitored appropriately.

Deposition of the ICSs in the oropharynx may lead to dysphonia and hoarseness, oral candidiasis, and cough at the time of inhalation. Dysphonia and hoarseness are dose-related side effects, with an incidence of 5% to 50%, and may be due to the myopathy of the laryngeal muscles.[31,65] Oral candidiasis is also dose related, with an incidence of less than 5%, and may be prevented by rinsing the mouth with water after the dose.[65] In infants using either nebulized ICS or MDI+VHC with a facemask, the nose and mouth should be washed off after each treatment. Cough is mainly due to local irritation and may be resolved by changing the delivery device, the rate of inhalation, or using a VHC.

The systemic side effects of the ICSs include suppression of the hypothalamus–pituitary–adrenal (HPA) axis, adrenal insufficiency, Cushing syndrome, osteoporosis, skin thinning and ecchymoses, cataracts, and growth retardation in children. Suppression of HPA axis is a rare event and is usually clinically insignificant.[31,66] Nonetheless, evidence of adrenal insufficiency has been reported in children when high doses have been used.[67,68] A large survey in France found 46 cases of adrenal insufficiency, of which 24 were associated with ICS use, and 14 were children aged 0.3 to 14 years (median 9.5 years).[68] Seven were with fluticasone propionate, five with budesonide, and two with beclomethasone dipropionate. All patients received a daily dose greater than or equal to 500 µg daily beclomethasone equivalent (≥250 µg daily fluticasone propionate). Of the total of 24 cases, 12 were associated with potential drug interactions (six ritonavir and six itraconazole) with fluticasone propionate and budesonide (see discussion below). There are several methods for assessing the integrity of the HPA axis, ranging from testing for basal production of the adrenal glands to reserve capacity. Tests of basal production include spot morning serum cortisol, serial overnight (12-hour) or serum cortisol 24-hour area under the curve (AUC_{0-24}), and 12-hour (overnight) and 24-hour urine-free cortisol (UFC) (corrected for creatinine to normalize data) concentration testing.[31,69,70] Serum cortisol AUC_{0-24} and 24-hour UFC are the most sensitive, and UFC has the advantage of not requiring blood draws in children; however, they do not assess the ability of the HPA axis to respond to stress.[31,69] The gold standards for assessing full integrity of the HPA axis are the insulin tolerance test and metyrapone tests, which are relatively invasive and difficult to perform; therefore, adrenocorticotropic hormone (ACTH) cortisol stimulation test is performed as the standard. Low-dose slow infusion of ACTH is being touted as more sensitive as it gives a dose of ACTH similar to that seen during stress, as opposed to the supraphysiologic doses used with the standard ACTH stimulation that may give false-negative results.[69] However, the results of low-dose ACTH tests have not been completely validated and may produce false-positive results in patients without clinically relevant suppression.[31,69] There does not appear to be a chronic cumulative effect of medium-dose ICSs on the HPA axis as measured over 3 years in children receiving budesonide 400 µg daily.[71] Four or less oral courses of prednisone per year is not associated with adrenal suppression, and significant adrenal suppression does not occur following individual short courses less than 10 days.[7]

High-dose ICSs can reduce bone mineral density and increase the risk of fracture in at-risk older patients; however, the data in children are less clear.[31,72] Bone mineral density does not seem to be altered with low-to-medium doses of the ICSs[39]; however, a prospective study over a median of 7 years in children aged 5 to 12 years reported a decrease in bone mineral accretion, with medium-dose ICS in boys, but not girls, that did not result in an increased risk of osteopenia or fractures.[73]

An epidemiologic study of 97,387 children aged 4 to 17 years receiving ICSs in the United Kingdom reported an increased crude risk of fracture in those receiving greater than 200 μg per day beclomethasone dipropionate equivalent, but when adjusted for measures of asthma severity, the increased risk disappeared.[74] A nested case–control analysis using the same U.K. database also failed to demonstrate a significant increase in fracture risk from current ICS use or current long-term exposure (≥20 prescriptions).[75] However, short courses of oral prednisone have been associated with a dose-dependent decrease in bone mineral accretion and an increased risk of osteopenia (at least two bursts per year) and fractures (four or greater bursts per year).[73,76]

A more relevant potential adverse event and a great concern of some parents is the effect of the ICSs on growth. Long-term prospective studies in prepubertal children on low-medium doses of the ICSs have shown a reduction in growth velocity in the first 6 months to 2 years of therapy that then returns to normal.[10,31,38,39,48,72] The overall effect on height is 1 to 2 cm.[72] Early retrospective studies suggested that most children were expected to achieve their predicted adult height.[31,72,77] However, the only prospective long-term trial that followed children into adulthood found that the initial reduction in height persisted.[78] Differences on growth have been detected between the ICSs as would be predicted by their differences in delivery and pharmacokinetics.[31,72] Fluticasone dipropionate by DPI produced less effect on growth than equivalent doses of either budesonide or beclomethasone dipropionate by DPI,[79,80] but produced similar effect to budesonide when administered by MDI+VHC, which enhances systemic availability of fluticasone propionate.[81] Of note, fluticasone propionate by DPI at 100 and 200 μg daily did not produce a decrease in growth in children down to 4 years of age, but did produce a significant reduction of 1.1 cm over 2 years in infants aged 1 to 3 years receiving 176 μg daily by MDI+VHC and facemask.[10,38] Monitoring the linear growth in all children on ICSs is recommended by the EPR3.[7]

Cataracts are uncommon in children and have not been reported in children on low- to medium-dose long-term ICSs.[31,32,82] Other suspected adverse reactions with ICSs reported from pharmacovigilance reporting systems include psychiatric symptoms and abnormalities of teeth.[83] The association with ICSs is not clear, but various psychiatric symptoms have been reported for systemic corticosteroids.

DRUG INTERACTIONS

Most of the ICSs undergo hepatic and intestinal metabolism by cytochrome (CYP) P450 3A4 isoenzymes.[13,84] As a result, ICSs should be used cautiously with potent inhibitors of CYP3A4, such as protease inhibitors, macrolides, ketoconazole, and itraconazole.[84] Clinically significant Cushing syndrome and adrenal suppression and deaths have been reported.[67,85,86] Systemic corticosteroids will also have decreased clearance and prolonged half-lives when coadministered with CYP3A4 inhibitors.

β_2 AGONISTS

The β_2 agonists are the most effective bronchodilators for asthma and are classified as either SABAs or LABAs. SABAs have about 3 to 8 hours duration of action depending on how it is measured, and they include albuterol, levalbuterol, pirbuterol, terbutaline, and epinephrine, a nonselective catecholamine which is the only one available over the counter. In 2018, FDA approved over-the-counter inhaled epinephrine (Primatene® Mist HFA) for temporary relief of mild symptoms of intermittent asthma in patients aged 12 years or older who have been diagnosed with mild intermittent asthma by a health care professional. Availability of over-the-counter epinephrine remains controversial as it offers a symptomatic management of asthma without necessary assessments by a provider; its use is also not recommended by EPR3.[7] LABAs have a duration of action of 12 to 24 hours and are primarily used in combination with ICSs in asthma. Available LABAs in combination with ICSs for pediatric indication are formoterol and salmeterol. The newer 24-hour LABAs (olodaterol, vilanterol, and indacaterol) have not been approved in children, either alone or in combination with an ICS.

MECHANISM OF ACTION

All of the β_2 agonists work through binding of the β_2AR, a G-protein–coupled receptor on cell surfaces.[87] Infants are born with fully functional airway smooth muscles (both neural network and functional receptors) whose mass relative to airway size is fully developed by 25 weeks' gestation.[88] In the body, the β_2ARs are in a state of equilibrium between the active and inactive isoforms, and binding by an agonist results in a shift of the equilibrium, favoring the activated isoform.[87] Activation results in adenylate cyclase producing cyclic adenosine monophosphate (cAMP) to increase protein kinase A, resulting in a decrease in unbound calcium to produce smooth muscle relaxation.[87] Pharmacologically, β_2 agonists are functional antagonists because they reverse smooth muscle constriction, regardless of the mechanism.[89] As the β_2AR is designed to accommodate endogenous catecholamines (dopamine, L-epinephrine, and norepinephrine), the chemical modifications designed to produce greater selectivity for the β_2AR produce compounds less efficient for shifting the equilibrium.[87] Thus, all synthetic β_2 agonists exhibit less efficacy for increasing cyclic AMP levels and are considered partial agonists. Each drug exhibits a different level of partial agonism, with salmeterol having the most, followed by albuterol, terbutaline, and pirbuterol, with formoterol having greater efficacy, though less than the full agonists epinephrine and isoproterenol.[89] Partial agonism is less important in tissue with large numbers of β_2ARs (bronchial smooth muscle) than tissues with low numbers (cardiac tissue, mast cells, and inflammatory cells). The β_2 agonists are selective by virtue of having even less efficacy for other adrenergic receptors (i.e., α_1, α_2, and β_1). Their relative selectivity for adrenergic receptors is illustrated in Table 41.4, with salmeterol and formoterol equivalent with greater selectivity than albuterol, pirbuterol, and terbutaline that are equivalent.[87,89] Aerosol administration makes them all more bronchoselective, and the selectivity of all these agents diminishes at high doses.

Unlike the endogenously produced catecholamines, the synthetic β_2 agonists have a chiral carbon and exist as a 1:1 racemic mixture of enantiomers, except for levalbuterol and arformoterol.[90] Formoterol has two chiral carbons.[91] As biologic systems are stereoselective, one of the enantiomers provides a better fit and greater efficacy at the β_2AR, and for β_2 agonists, the *R*-enantiomers are the most active component, with higher affinities ranging from 100- to 1,000-fold for the β_2AR (90, 91). Two products are approved: levalbuterol, the single

TABLE 41.4 Relative Selectivity and Potency of β Agonists for Adrenergic Receptors

	β_1 Receptor	β_2	β_2 Potency
Albuterol	+	+++	2
Formoterol	+	++++	0.12
Isoproterenol	++++	++++	1
Metaproterenol	+++	+++	15
Pirbuterol	+	+++	5
Salmeterol	+	++++	0.5
Terbutaline	+	+++	4

Data from Anderson GP. Interactions between corticosteroids and β-adrenergic agonists in asthma disease induction, progression, and exacerbation. *Am J Respir Crit Care Med* 2000;61:S188–S196.

[*R*]-enantiomer of albuterol; and, more recently, arformoterol the [*R,R*]-enantiomer of formoterol.[90,91] Standard bronchodilator dose–response studies have established that all of the bronchodilation and systemic β_2 adrenergic effects reside in the [*R*]-enantiomers so that when administered in equivalent [*R*]-enantiomeric doses, racemic albuterol and formoterol do not differ from levalbuterol and arformoterol, respectively.[91,92] The effect of the [*S*]-enantiomer of albuterol on airway responsiveness in humans has been inconsistent.[90,93] If it does enhance airways responsiveness, the effect is small and easily overcome by the properties of the [*R*]-enantiomer.[93]

The *β_2AR* genes are located on the long arm of chromosome 5q31–q32 coding for a protein containing 413 amino acids.[90] The amino acid sequence of the receptor can be altered by producing polymorphisms. The most common polymorphisms of the β_2AR are single amino acid substitutions called single-nucleotide polymorphisms (SNPs). Genetic variation may explain some of the interindividual differences in response to a β_2 agonist.[90] A total of nine different polymorphisms have been identified, and three common ones have been studied in detail due to functional differences found in vitro: amino acid at position 16, encoding either arginine [Arg] or glycine [Gly]; position 27, encoding either glutamine [Gln] or glutamic acid [Glu]; and position 164, encoding either isoleucine (Ile) or threonine (Thr).[94] Individuals may be heterozygous or homozygous for each polymorphism, and there are differences between races in allele frequency as well as haplotype structure (paired SNPs) that represent linkage disequilibrium (SNP pairs that occur more frequently together in populations than by chance alone, i.e., 94% of Arg/Arg is found with Gln/Gln).[90,94] The homozygous Gly/Gly 16 β_2AR downregulates to a greater extent than Gly/Arg followed by Arg/Arg.[90] The homozygous Glu/Glu at position 27 of the receptor protects against downregulation compared to homozygous Gln/Gln; however, when Glu/Glu and Gly/Gly are combined, the effect of Gly/Gly is more dominant and the protection against downregulation diminishes.[94] Substitution of Ile for Thr in position 164 can decrease the binding affinity of the receptor by as much as four times, and the homozygous Ile appears to be lethal.[94] Clinical studies in asthma have been inconsistent, with some showing greater bronchodilation for Arg/Arg patients with other studies not showing that effect.[90] In addition, tolerance has been demonstrated across all genotypes.[90] Newer investigations are assessing haplotypes as well as expanding haplotypes to include polymorphisms into other areas of the *β_2AR* gene. Additional studies are exploring alternate genes that may determine response, such as the receptors for the signal transduction that activate adenylyl cyclase.[94]

Continuous stimulation of the β_2AR will result in diminished response or tolerance. Tolerance to the β_2 agonists can occur within a week of regular administration as a result of downregulation of the receptors as well as a decrease in binding affinity to the receptors (uncoupling).[86,89] Tolerance levels off after a few weeks and does not worsen over time. Since tolerance develops at the receptor level, cross-tolerance to other β_2 agonists occurs. There is no relationship between potency or efficacy and the induction of tolerance, and clinical trials demonstrate tolerance from all of the β_2 agonists.[87,90] Due to the large number of β_2ARs in bronchial smooth muscle, tolerance is more easily detected in other cells with a lower density of receptors (i.e., cardiac, vascular, mast cells, epithelium, lymphocytes, etc.).[90] Bronchoprovocation studies using bronchoconstriction (exercise, methacholine, or histamine) challenges more readily detect tolerance in patients than do bronchodilation studies.[87,90] Unlike the decreased bronchodilation that can easily be overcome with an additional dose of β_2 agonist, the decrease in bronchoprotection cannot be easily overcome by an increased dose.[90,95,96] Agonist-induced tolerance of the β_2ARs can be at least partially overcome by the administration of systemic corticosteroids and partially prevented by coadministration of ICSs.[89,90,97] Although the time required for a clinical response differs among patients, β_2 receptors density increases within 4 hours after administration of systemic steroid, and response to β_2 agonist occurs within 2 to 12 hours depending on the severity of the acute asthma exacerbation.[89,90]

In addition to tolerance from continuous stimulation, severe airway inflammation, particularly that induced by viral infections, reduces the efficacy of β_2 agonists by producing uncoupling with the receptors.[89,90] Increased concentrations of bronchoconstrictive functional antagonists [i.e., cysteinyl leukotrienes (CysLTs), histamine, acetylcholine, or substance P] produce a right shift and flattening of the dose–response curve, reducing both the apparent potency and efficacy of the β_2 agonists.[87] In theory, the weaker partial agonists would be the most affected but that has not been shown clinically. These factors probably all come into play during severe asthma exacerbations where patients do not respond to the usual low doses of SABAs.[89,90]

PHARMACOKINETICS

The SABAs are hydrophilic and relatively rapidly absorbed orally and from the lung tissue, which limits their duration when taken as aerosols. The SABAs do not partition into the plasmalemma lipid bilayer of airway smooth muscle and so readily diffuse into the microcirculation away from the β_2ARs.[98] Albuterol, pirbuterol, and terbutaline are well absorbed orally, but undergo first-pass sulfate conjugation in the gut and liver, so their systemic bioavailability varies ($\approx$50% albuterol and $\approx$20% terbutaline).[98] The SABAs are eliminated unchanged renally and through hepatic sulfate conjugation and have widely varying elimination half-lives: albuterol 3.2 to 6 hours, pirbuterol 2.5 hours, and terbutaline 20 hours.[98] A study in children aged 8 to 15 years reported a slightly greater clearance and shorter terminal half-life of 12 hours for terbutaline.[98]

LABAs are highly lipophilic, accounting for their longer lung retention and greater duration of action.[87,98] Following inhalation, the LABAs partition into the lipid bilayer where they then slowly leak into the aqueous biophase to attach to the receptor.[87,98] Formoterol has about a 10-fold lower lipophilicity and an amphiphilic component compared to salmeterol so that its onset of action is similar to SABAs.[90,102] On the other hand, salmeterol has a longer duration and slower offset.[87,89] Formoterol is about 50% to 60% orally available and 10% excreted unchanged, and the rest metabolized by glucuronide conjugation and, to a minor extent, O-demethylation, involving CYP2D6, CYP2C19, CYP2C9, and CYP2A6.[99] Pharmacokinetic data on salmeterol are extremely limited due to low systemic concentrations achieved with usual doses. It appears to have 25% oral bioavailability due to extensive first-pass metabolism by gut and hepatic CYP3A4 isozymes, and it is primarily eliminated by CYP3A4 hydroxylation, with an elimination half-life of 5.5 hours.[90] Newer LABAs include olodaterol, vilanterol, and indacaterol, with rapid onset of action and with a bronchodilatory effect lasting over 24 hours that is dose dependent; these medications do not have any approved indications for pediatric asthma.[87,100-103]

CLINICAL USE

The inhaled SABAs are indicated for the management of bronchospasm manifested by cough, dyspnea, shortness of breath, and wheezing on an as-needed basis. Regular use of SABAs is not indicated because it does not improve outcomes.[104,105] Regular use of SABAs can result in an increase in bronchial hyperresponsiveness.[106] Using SABAs only as rescue, their use is also a monitoring tool to assess control of asthma, patients who need to use their rescue medication more than 2 days per week are considered not well controlled and need to be evaluated further.[7] Patients using greater than or equal to two canisters per month are at an increased risk of severe life-threatening asthma exacerbations. The SABAs are the most effective therapy for the prevention of EIB used 5 to 15 minutes before exercise.[7,87,107,108] They provide complete protection against EIB greater than or equal to 95% of patients even if the patients have been taking regular β_2 agonists and have tolerance.[87,108] Although available as syrups for young children, oral SABAs are not recommended due to their poor efficacy, longer duration until effect, greater toxicity and inability to prevent EIB.[7] Other than delivery device, there are no specific age-related issues involving SABAs in children. Infants have fully functional smooth muscle and β_2ARs throughout their bronchioles, and comparisons of MDIs+VHCs versus nebulization show that they are equally effective for acute bronchospasm.[17,109]

The LABAs are currently indicated as an adjunct therapy with ICSs in patients who are not controlled with low-to-medium doses of ICSs[7] (see Fig. 41.3) Currently, LABAs are not approved by FDA in children less than 4 years nor have they been assessed in clinical trials for this age group. The LABAs are also approved for protection against EIB in children aged 5 to 11 years. After single doses, they effectively block EIB for up to 8 to 9 hours postdose; however, regular use leads to tolerance and decreases the duration of protection to 4 to 6 hours and, therefore, not much better than the SABAs.[108]

Early long-term trials in children clearly demonstrated that LABAs were inferior to ICS therapy.[55] Due to the lack of any clinically relevant anti-inflammatory activity, the national guidelines have always stated that LABAs are not indicated for monotherapy.[7] LABAs have been shown to improve lung function and decrease symptoms and the use of rescue medication in children when added to ICSs.[55] However, unlike in adults, combination ICS/LABA therapy has not produced a reduction in risk of exacerbations and was thought to increase risk of severe exacerbations, resulting in hospitalization.[110,111] Indeed, since early 2000s, the use of LABAs even when used in combination with ICSs has been controversial as a result of studies suggesting an increased risk of serious asthma events, including death in patients receiving LABAs.[87,112,113] Although a risk of death was not found in children, there was an increased risk of hospitalizations that was higher in younger children and adolescents than adults.[113] Although highly controversial as a result of design issue of some of the studies, the FDA mandated prospective randomized clinical trials by companies marketing LABAs to compare the safety of ICSs to the combination of ICSs plus LABAs in children and adolescents and adults with asthma. More than 30,000 patients were enrolled in the four adolescent/adult trials, and over 6,000 children aged 4 to 11 years in the pediatric study.[114,115] LABAs plus ICSs compared to ICSs did not result in a significantly higher risk of serious asthma-related events or deaths in adolescents and adults, and the combination resulted in significantly fewer asthma exacerbations compared to ICS alone.[115] Of interest was the post hoc subgroup analysis that found no significant decrease in severe asthma exacerbations requiring systemic corticosteroids in adolescents aged 12 to 17 years. The pediatric study also found similar risks of serious asthma-related events and no deaths with both treatments, but did not find a decrease in asthma exacerbations requiring systemic corticosteroids with the combination.[114] This latter finding and the similar finding in the adolescent subgroup in these studies seem to confirm the results of the previous meta-analysis of no reduction in risk of asthma exacerbations with the addition of LABAs to ICSs in children despite improvements in lung function and symptoms.[55] However, it belies the assertion that LABAs increase exacerbation in children.[110] These findings were likely a result of including studies not using ICSs.

Although chronic use produces tolerance, patients receiving LABAs respond as well to the inhaled SABAs they receive in the emergency department as those who did not receive LABAs.[95,96] The worsening of peak flow and increased exacerbations associated with regular administration of SABAs to patients with Arg/Arg genotype is not seen with LABAs.[116] In fact, increasing bronchial hyperresponsiveness is not seen with regular use of LABAs in adults or children.[117,118] The combination of LABAs added to ICS therapy is superior to the addition of an LTRA in children.[54]

ADVERSE EVENTS

Paradoxical bronchospasm has been reported with use of β_2 agonists, but this is a relatively rare phenomenon. The β_2ARs are ubiquitous throughout the body. In cardiac tissue, they affect conductance to increase heart rate as well as prolong QTc interval and produce ST segment depression, but have not been associated with Torsades de pointes.[90] The vascular effects of β_2 stimulation include vasodilation leading to lower diastolic blood pressure and decreased microvascular leakage, with the former contributing to the reflex increase in heart rate.[117] The metabolic effects include gluconeogenesis, sodium/potassium ATPase stimulation, and increased lactate production, resulting in hypokalemia, hyperglycemia, and lactic acidosis at high doses (87). Potassium and glucose should be monitored in children receiving continuously nebulized albuterol for severe asthma exacerbations.[7] Skeletal muscle and neuromuscular transmission is enhanced, leading to fine tremor that usually disappears with chronic administration. In general, these agents should be used with caution in patients with cardiovascular disorders, convulsive disorders, diabetes mellitus, hyperthyroidism, and hypokalemia, since the adverse events of β_2 agonists may potentiate the underlying disease or they may interact with other medications. As these adverse effects are all mediated by β_2AR stimulation, they occur similarly for the single-enantiomer drugs as for the racemic mixtures when given in equipotent doses.[87,90] Due to their greater retention in the lung, the LABAs produce fewer systemic effects than the SABAs, with a fourfold or greater increase over recommended dose to produce significant changes in heart rate, serum potassium, glucose, or QTc interval.[117,118] In a crossover study of 20 children aged 6 to 11 years with asthma administered cumulative doses of formoterol 45 µg and terbutaline 5,000 µg (equipotent) over a 2.5-hour time period, formoterol produced significantly less hypokalemia, hyperglycemia, QTc prolongation, blood pressure effect, and increased lactate.[119] Values fell out of the normal range more frequently with the terbutaline than formoterol, and the duration of abnormalities was not significantly longer for formoterol. Comparisons of formoterol and salmeterol administered by DPIs in adults and children indicate a four- to fivefold difference in potency for both bronchodilation and systemic activity.[117,120]

DRUG INTERACTIONS

Potential physiologic drug interactions with β_2 agonists include nonselective β antagonists, thiazide and loop diuretics, digoxin, theophylline, and other drugs that prolong QTc interval. The product label for all β_2 agonists includes the statement that coadministration of monoamine oxidase inhibitors or tricyclic antidepressants with β_2 agonists may potentiate the cardiovascular effect of these agents. However, this is a holdover from the potential hypertensive crisis mediated by the coadministration of ephedrine, the indirect-acting drug that causes the release of endogenous catecholamines from nerve terminals as well as administration of epinephrine. The β_2 agonists do not induce the release of endogenous catecholamines nor do they produce vasoconstriction, and there is a paucity of data supporting these interactions.

There are few pharmacokinetic interactions with the β_2 agonists. Serum digoxin has decreased by 16% and 22% after a single dose of IV and oral albuterol, respectively, in patients who have been on digoxin for at least 10 days. Coadministration of salmeterol with strong CYP3A4 inhibitors, such as ketoconazole, ritonavir, atazanavir, clarithromycin, indinavir, itraconazole, nefazodone, nelfinavir, saquinavir, and telithromycin, may increase risk of cardiovascular adverse events due to increased oral bioavailability of salmeterol. Ketoconazole 400 mg daily for 7 days resulted in a 16-fold increase in plasma salmeterol *AUC* in 20 healthy subjects who were withdrawn from the study due to cardiovascular side effects. Coadministration of erythromycin and salmeterol has resulted in a 40% increase in salmeterol serum concentration at steady state.[121]

CHROMONES

MECHANISM OF ACTION

The chromones include cromolyn sodium and nedocromil with mild anti-inflammatory activity used in the treatment of asthma. They are only active by inhalation. The chromones prevent the mast cell activation and degranulation, possibly by inhibiting chloride transport and protein kinase C.[122] Administered just prior to allergen exposure, they prevent both the early and late asthma response, including eosinophil activation and mediator release.[122] They both inhibit EIB administered prior to exercise.[108,123] In addition, they inhibit bronchoconstriction induced by sulfur dioxide and bradykinin, presumably by inhibiting afferent C-fiber stimulation.[122] This mechanism may be responsible for their activity in reducing cough in asthma as well as angiotensin-converting enzyme induced cough.

PHARMACOKINETICS

Both cromolyn and nedocromil are highly ionized water-soluble compounds at physiologic pH and so do not enter cells and cross membranes and are poorly absorbed orally (<1%) and hence only effective by inhalation.[122] They are rapidly eliminated unchanged in the urine or biliary tract. IV cromolyn has a terminal half-life of 11 to 22 minutes; therefore, inhaled cromolyn exhibits an absorption rate limited half-life of less than 2 hours.[122] They are rapidly absorbed from the lung and so require multiple-daily dosing (four times daily for cromolyn and two to four times daily for nedocromil) for optimal benefit. Lack of absorption across cell membranes probably accounts for the lack of significant adverse effects from the chromones.[122]

CLINICAL USE

Cromolyn sodium by nebulizer solution is indicated as an alternative to ICSs for the treatment of mild persistent asthma.[7] Several clinical trials have shown that chromones are not as effective as ICSs for controlling asthma symptoms, improving lung function, and preventing exacerbations.[39,43,44,122] The few comparative trials with other controllers (theophylline and montelukast) have failed to demonstrate significant differences in controlling asthma.[122,124] However, parents preferred once-daily montelukast to three times daily cromolyn.[124] A meta-analysis has suggested that there is insufficient evidence to support the use of cromolyn in young children.[125] However, the study providing the largest population that drove the results of this meta-analysis administered the cromolyn by actuating multiple puffs from an MDI into a VHC with a facemask while the patients breathed for 30 seconds.[126] This dosage and delivery method for patients aged 1 to 4 years is an unproven method (>1 puff in a VHC at a time reduces delivery).[19] In addition, numerous studies in the meta-analysis used different dosage forms and doses and various age ranges; therefore, it is unclear that it was even appropriate to combine the studies. Retrospective studies of large integrated medical/pharmacy databases suggest that dispensing of cromolyn reduces the risk of emergency department visits and hospitalizations at least for children.[127,128]

Pretreatment with the chromones prior to exercise is effective for preventing EIB.[108,122] The chromones are less effective than inhaled SABAs, protecting 73% of patients.[108] They appear to be more effective than LTRAs that generally produce attenuation and only produce complete blocking in 40% to 55% of children.[107]

Except for cough with cromolyn and bad taste with nedocromil, these drugs have a strong safety profile.[122] However, they have been relegated to a secondary role as a result of frequent dosing requirement.

LEUKOTRIENE MODIFIERS

MECHANISM OF ACTION

Leukotrienes (LTs) are eicosanoids derived from arachidonic acid via the 5-lipoxygenase pathway and are produced in eosinophils, mast cells, and alveolar macrophages.[7] The synthesis can lead to the production of LTB_4 that is involved with the chemotaxis of neutrophils and/or to the production of the CysLTs, such as LTC_4, LTD_4, and LTE_4. These stimulate the CysLT1 receptor in airway smooth muscle to cause constriction and the CysLT2 receptor in the vascular smooth muscle to produce constriction and promote chemotaxis.[7] CysLTs produce bronchoconstriction, tissue edema, and increased mucus secretion. The LT modifiers currently consist of a 5-lipoxygenase inhibitor, zileuton, and two selective CystLT1-receptor antagonists (LTRAs), montelukast, and zafirlukast.[129–131] The relative localization of CysLT1 receptors accounts for their selectivity for the lungs and peripheral eosinophils and relative lack of systemic effects so that it is unnecessary to give them as aerosols.

PHARMACOKINETICS

Zileuton is only available as extended-release tablets for twice-daily dosing in children aged 12 years and adults and is recommended to be used with food since food increases its bioavailability.[129] Zileuton is metabolized by hepatic CYP1A2, CYP2C9, and CYP3A4. About 94% of the zileuton dose is excreted in the urine, and the rest in the feces.[129] Zafirlukast is approved for children down to 5 years of age and should be taken 1 hour before or 2 hours after meals since administration with food decreased the bioavailability by 40%.[130] Zafirlukast is extensively metabolized by CYP2C9. Following oral administration, 10% of the dose is excreted renally, and the rest is excreted in the urine. Montelukast has been approved down to 2 years of age and has a mean oral bioavailability of 64%, which is not affected by meals.[131] Montelukast is metabolized by CYP3A4 and CYP2C9.[131] Montelukast and its metabolites are extensively excreted via the biliary tract.

CLINICAL USE

No evidence exists for significant differences in efficacy for the various LT modifiers. Differences in dosing and relative safety (see below) do exist that have made montelukast the de facto preferred LTRA in children. The LT modifiers are often considered anti-inflammatory, and they do result in a decrease in FeNO that is considered a marker of airway inflammation, reduce serum eosinophils, and have decreased sputum eosinophils.[7,108,132] However, they are significantly less effective than low-dose ICSs for improving lung function, controlling asthma symptoms, reducing asthma exacerbations and bronchial hyperresponsiveness, and reducing FeNO.[41,42,45,51,54,133] They have been used as adjunctive therapy with ICS, as studies have demonstrated that LT production may be relatively resistant to ICS therapy but have not provided significant added improvement.[134] Compared to LABAs as adjunctive therapy, the LT modifiers are less effective for reducing the risk of exacerbations requiring corticosteroids, improving daily symptom scores, nighttime awakenings, rescue medication use, and lung function.[134]

In a 24-week comparison of the addition of either theophylline or montelukast to usual therapy in 489 patients with poorly controlled asthma (74% to 79% receiving ICSs across groups), neither theophylline nor montelukast reduced the number of episodes of poor asthma control compared to placebo, although both produced small improvements in lung function.[135] In the subset of patients not receiving ICSs, theophylline was more effective than montelukast and placebo at improving asthma symptoms, and montelukast was not better than placebo. The second study compared the combination of an LTRA and LABA to low-dose ICS and LABA in 192 patients randomized in the 14-week crossover trial with a 4-week washout between treatments.[136] The Data Safety and Monitoring Board terminated the study after only 94 patients completed because of a highly significant greater number of treatment failures, the primary end point, in the LTRA plus LABA combination. In addition, measures of airway inflammation (i.e., FeNO, sputum eosinophils, and sputum eosinophil cationic protein) all worsened on the LT arm of the study. A crossover trial in 24 children aged 5 to 12 years with persistent asthma controlled with ICS therapy, comparing 4 weeks of placebo, 5-mg montelukast, and 50-μg fluticasone by DPI confirmed these results.[51] Both post-bronchodilator forced expiratory volume in 1 second (FEV_1) and FeNO were significantly better on fluticasone than either placebo or montelukast, and montelukast was not better than placebo.

Montelukast is often prescribed for children with persistent asthma because of its lack of adverse effects and ease of administration. However, comparative trials have demonstrated it to be significantly less effective in children aged 6 to 14 years than therapy with low-dose ICSs.[41,45,47,133] Due to the variability in response to various antiasthmatics, a crossover trial in 144 children aged 6 to 17 years with mild-to-moderate asthma was designed to determine which patients may preferentially respond to montelukast versus ICS.[137] Five percent of patients responded to montelukast only, defined as a 7.5% increase in FEV_1 compared to 23% that responded to only ICSs. Overall, 22% of the children had a positive response to montelukast and was associated with higher urinary LTE_4 concentrations. Interestingly, this compares to 58% of adults who achieved that level or greater lung function response in a recent large randomized parallel trial comparing montelukast with beclomethasone dipropionate.[138] Other evidence that the response to LT modifiers may be age dependent is that montelukast was approved based on pharmacokinetics and safety and extrapolated efficacy for all of the dosage forms for children less than 6 years.[131] In children aged 2 to 5 years, montelukast improved some asthma outcomes compared to placebo in reducing daytime and nighttime symptoms, thus increasing asthma-free days and as-needed β_2 agonists.[139] However, no improvement in any of those same outcomes was seen in a placebo-controlled trial in infants aged 6 to 24 months.[140] On the other hand, ICS therapy has been shown to markedly improve the above constellation of symptoms as well as significantly decrease the risk of asthma exacerbations in infants down to 6 months of age.[41,45]

It has been argued that the "real-world" effectiveness of the LTRAs in children is underestimated by randomized clinical trials as the ease of administration (once-daily oral therapy) will improve compliance compared to ICSs and result in similar effectiveness over time.[141] However, adherence with long-term therapy in asthma, as in other chronic diseases, is generally poor (40% to 70% as measured by pharmacy refill rates), and studies have demonstrated only marginally greater adherence to montelukast compared to ICSs in children, and the only independently supported study found no difference in adherence in children aged 3 to 18 years between montelukast and ICSs.[142] In addition, a large retrospective study of a medical/pharmacy-integrated database assessing outcomes over 12 months in 3,647 children prescribed either an ICS or montelukast found significantly more treatment failures, hospitalizations for asthma, and a significantly greater annualized cost for asthma care for those receiving montelukast, despite significantly greater numbers of dispensing of the montelukast than the ICS.[143] These "real-world" effectiveness results are consistent with the differences seen in the randomized clinical trials.

Montelukast has FDA-approved labeling for prevention of EIB in patients aged 15 years and older. LTRAs attenuate but rarely completely protect against EIB. Chronic treatment with montelukast reduces EIB by 20% to 50%; however, up to 50% of patients may not respond.[108] The onset and duration of effect on EIB after one dose of montelukast have been evaluated in children.[144] Children, ages 7 to 13 years, performed an exercise challenge 2, 12, and 24 hours after a single dose of montelukast. Montelukast produced a significant protection against EIB compared to placebo, only at 12 hours postdose.

LTRAs have been studied for the prophylaxis against viral-induced asthma exacerbations in patients who are symptom free between exacerbations as ICSs have not been considered effective for this asthma phenotype in children. However, a Cochrane library review found no evidence of reducing exacerbations requiring rescue with oral corticosteroids, hospitalization or unscheduled physician visits, and minimal evidence for reducing other outcomes, such as days off from school or as-needed bronchodilator use.[145]

Montelukast has not been found to be superior to ICSs in episodic viral wheezing in infants and children.[146]

ADVERSE EVENTS

Elevation of one or more hepatic function enzymes has been reported with zileuton and zafirlukast, which may progress, remain unchanged, or resolve within 3 weeks of therapy.[129,130] Cases of liver failure have been reported with zafirlukast. A baseline alanine transaminase (ALT) measurement followed monthly for the next 3 months and then every 2 to 3 months is recommended for zileuton, whereas signs of liver dysfunction (diarrhea, jaundice) are recommended for zafirlukast with monitoring ALT if these signs occur.

Churg–Strauss syndrome, a vascular inflammation that is accompanied by tissue and blood eosinophilia and severe asthma symptoms, has been reported in patients taking zafirlukast or montelukast.[147,148] Although the frequency of this adverse effect is rare and appears primarily as case reports, it is important to be aware of this possible effect. Although the exact cause of the syndrome is not known, the syndrome has been reported when the dose of oral steroid was reduced, and some have suggested that it is merely an unmasking of a disease that was misdiagnosed as asthma initially. However, cases have occurred in patients not receiving oral corticosteroids. Other adverse events reported with zafirlukast include headache, infection, nausea, diarrhea, abdominal pain, asthenia, fever, myalgia, vomiting, and dizziness. The most common side effects of montelukast include fatigue, fever, pain, dyspepsia, headache, dizziness, rash, nasal congestion, cough, influenza, and elevated aspartate transaminase (AST) and ALT. Recently, FDA required Boxed Warning about serious mental health side effects for montelukast.[131]

DRUG INTERACTION

Zileuton significantly interacts with theophylline, warfarin, and propranolol, resulting in an increase in concentration of these medications. Coadministration of these medications with zileuton requires close monitoring and dose adjustment. Coadministration of zafirlukast and warfarin has also lead to an increase in prothrombin time by 35%. Plasma concentration of zafirlukast was decreased by 30% and 40% when coadministered with theophylline or erythromycin, and the concentration was increased by 45% when it was used with high doses of aspirin. Studies looking at coadministration of montelukast and theophylline, warfarin, or digoxin did not show any significant reaction with these drugs.

METHYLXANTHINES (THEOPHYLLINE)

MECHANISM OF ACTION

Theophylline is a nonselective phosphodiesterase (PDE) inhibitor that prevents degradation of intracellular cyclic AMP and cyclic guanosine monophosphate (GMP).[149] The PDE isoenzymes currently thought to be important for theophylline's clinical effects are PDE-III, predominant in airway smooth muscle, and PDE-IV, involved in regulation of the inflammatory cells, mast cells, neutrophils, eosinophils, and T lymphocytes.[149] In addition, theophylline has been shown to activate histone deacetylase that is involved in the corticosteroid-induced decrease in pro-inflammatory gene expression.[149] Decreased histone deacetylase activity is felt to be involved in the relative resistance to corticosteroids seen in some patients with asthma and in most patients with chronic obstructive pulmonary disease (COPD).[150] However, it would appear that the moderate bronchodilation is primarily responsible for the antiasthmatic effect of theophylline. Selective PDE-IV inhibitors have not demonstrated significant effects in clinical asthma.[149]

PHARMACOKINETICS

The benefit and risks from theophylline relate to serum concentrations. Maximum potential benefit with minimal risk of adverse effects is achieved at peak concentrations of 5 to 15 μg per mL.[7] Since concentrations can vary greatly among children receiving the same dose, because of variable rates of metabolism, serum concentrations must be measured to adjust dosage. Outside the neonatal period, theophylline is principally eliminated by capacity-limited hepatic metabolism that is genetically determined and can be further altered by environmental exposures, such as age, febrile viral infections, smoking, and dietary changes.[151] Theophylline is predominantly metabolized by CYP1A2 and, to a lesser extent, CYP3A3 and CYP2E1 isozymes and is about 35% to 40% protein bound.[151] In general, children aged 1 to 6 years have the greatest systemic clearance and, therefore, require higher milligram per kilogram maintenance dosing. Theophylline is 95% to 100% absorbed orally, and its absorption rate exhibits diurnal variability with slower absorption in the evening.[151] Clinically, it is primarily administered as sustained-release preparations to minimize multiple-daily dosing and serum concentration fluctuations.[151]

CLINICAL USE

Sustained-release theophylline is still considered an alternative, not preferred, maintenance, and adjunctive therapy to the ICSs in children aged 5 to 11 years, but not in children aged 0 to 4 years.[7] Lack of clinical trial data on efficacy and potential for serious adverse effects in young children and infants is the reason why it is no longer recommended in those 0 to 4 years old.[7,152] When using theophylline in those 5 to 11 years old, serum drug concentration monitoring is required to prevent serious toxicity. As a result of the potential for severe toxicity, the moderate bronchodilation is produced by theophylline relative to the β_2 agonists, and questionable anti-inflammatory activity of theophylline has been relegated to second-line adjunctive therapy with ICSs.[7,153] No advantage of montelukast or theophylline has been found when added to usual therapy in adult patients with poorly controlled asthma receiving ICSs.[151] Comparisons of LABAs with theophylline consistently show LABAs to be superior in efficacy.[151] Theophylline has modest dose-related attenuation of EIB.[151]

ADVERSE EFFECTS

Theophylline produces significant dose-related toxicity from mild caffeine-like central nervous stimulation, headache, and nausea at high therapeutic concentrations that can be uncomfortable for some patients to serious vomiting, cardiac arrhythmias, seizures, and cerebral ischemia at high concentrations. Some of these toxicities are due to adenosine antagonistic effects of theophylline. Elderly and young children are at particular risk for serious toxicities due to altered metabolism in young children secondary to acute febrile viral illnesses.[7,151,153]

DRUG INTERACTIONS

Theophylline is associated with a number of drug interactions from drugs that inhibit and induce the hepatic cytochrome P450 enzymes. Only those drugs that produce at least a 20% reduction or 50% increase in clearance are likely to produce clinically significant interactions, but there is a significant interpatient variability and so the clinician should use caution with all potentially interacting drugs. These are listed in Table 41.5.[153]

TABLE 41.5 Factors Affecting Theophylline Clearance

Decreased Clearance	*% Decrease*	*Increased Clearance*
Cimetidine	−25 to −60	Rifampin
Macrolides: erythromycin, TAO, clarithromycin	−25 to −50	Carbamazepine
		Phenobarbital
		Phenytoin
Allopurinol	−20	Charcoal-broiled meat
Propranolol	−30	
Quinolones:	−20 to −50	High-protein diet
Ciprofloxacin, enoxacin, pefloxacin		Smoking
Interferon	−50	Sulfinpyrazone
Thiabendazole	−65	Moricizine
Ticlopidine	−25	Aminoglutethimide
Zileuton	−35	
Systemic viral illness	−10 to −50	

TAO, triacetyloleandomycin.
Data from Edwards DJ, Zarowitz BJ, Slaughter RL. Theophylline. In: Evans WE, Schentag JJ, Jusko WJ, eds. *Applied pharmacokinetics, principles of therapeutic drug monitoring*, 3rd ed. Vancouver, WA: Applied Therapeutics, 1992:131–1338.

LONG-ACTING MUSCARINIC ANTAGONISTS

MECHANISM OF ACTION

Tiotropium is an LAMA in the form of a bronchodilator that works on the acetylcholine pathways, which play a major role in the underlying pathophysiology of asthma.[154] Acetylcholine is involved in the airways in tone, smooth muscle contraction, mucus secretion, and vasodilation through its interaction with the muscarinic receptors.[154] Different muscarinic receptors (M1 to M3) are expressed in different areas of the airways (airway epithelial cells, nerve terminals/fibroblasts/smooth muscle cells, and mucosal glands respectively).[154] While tiotropium binds all three muscarinic receptors, it disengages slower from the M1 and M3 receptors and hence causes a prolonged bronchodilatory effect.[154] Due to its effect on smooth muscle cells and mucosal glands, there may also be an inhibitory effect on airway remodeling.[155]

PHARMACOKINETICS

On average, the bioavailability of tiotropium is 19.5% (DPI) and 33% (SMI). Peak plasma concentrations are observed 5 to 7 minutes after inhalation.[156] The apparent volume of distribution is 32 L per kg. It has an average half-life of approximately 27 to 45 hours, and clearance is renal.[156]

CLINICAL USE

Tiotropium is an SMI that is approved by the FDA for maintenance treatment of asthma in children aged 6 years and older at a dose of 1.25 to 2.5 μg at two inhalations once a day as add-on therapy to ICS and/or other maintenance therapy.[156] In one phase II and one phase III randomized, double-blind, placebo-controlled trials (RDBPCTs) of children aged 6 to 11 years, tiotropium had a higher peak FEV_1 postdose compared to placebo with good safety and tolerability, although the effect in the phase III study was dose dependent.[157,158] A phase III RDBPCT of children aged 1 to 5 years found tiotropium to reduce exacerbations (although not mean daytime asthma scores) with once again a favorable safety profile.[159] Thus far, studies have supported a clinical response independent of atopic phenotype,[160] and adult studies have noted that clinical response is greater in those who have a stronger bronchodilator response to SABA therapy.[161]

ADVERSE EFFECTS

Common side effects with tiotropium include nasopharyngitis and gastrointestinal symptoms.[156] In general, tiotropium is well tolerated. Contraindications to tiotropium (narrow angle glaucoma, urinary retention) would be rare in the pediatric population.[156]

DRUG INTERACTION

Tiotropium may enhance the anticholinergic effects of other medications, diminish the therapeutic effects of prokinetic agents, and decrease the absorption of nitroglycerin.[156]

BIOLOGICS

MECHANISM OF ACTION

Omalizumab is a humanized anti-immunoglobulin (Ig)E monoclonal antibody that binds to the Fc portion of circulating unbound serum IgE, thereby preventing its binding to high-affinity receptors on eosinophils, basophils, mast cells, and neutrophils.[162,163] This results in decreased serum IgE levels and downregulation of IgE receptors, ultimately decreasing the release of inflammatory mediators in response to allergen exposure.[162] Omalizumab only binds serum circulating IgE as the cross-linking of bound IgE would actually increase the inflammatory cascade.164 Studies have also noted omalizumab to increase eosinophil apoptosis,[165] downregulate inflammatory cytokines such as interleukin (IL)2 and IL13,[165] decrease B-lymphocyte counts (thereby downregulating IgE production in vitro),[166] downregulate bronchial smooth muscle proteins,[167] and prevent airway matrix deposition, thereby supporting a role in prevention of airway remodeling. It has recently been shown that omalizumab, through reduction in IgE, restores innate viral immunity in dendritic cells as well.[168]

Mepolizumab is a fully humanized monoclonal antibody against IL5, a cytokine responsible for eosinophil development, function, and longevity.[169] Mepolizumab blocks binding of IL5 to the α chain of the IL5-receptor complex on the eosinophil, which is responsible for signal transduction.[162,163,169] IL5 is the cytokine most selective for eosinophils, and stimulation of its receptor is responsible for growth, proliferation, differentiation, maturation, activation, and survival of eosinophils.[162,163,170–173] Studies have noted mepolizumab to dramatically decrease serum,[174–177] sputum,[173,177–179] and bone marrow eosinophil counts,[175,180] although the greatest reduction is in blood eosinophil levels.[162] Mepolizumab has been shown to reduce eosinophil precursors in the bone marrow, with partial maturational arrest of eosinophil lineage noted and decreases in the number of eosinophil progenitors in the bronchial mucosa.[180] Reslizumab is a monoclonal antibody against IL5, but differs from mepolizumab, as it is a humanized rat antibody instead of a fully humanized antibody. Benralizumab is a fully humanized afucosylated monoclonal antibody against the IL5-receptor α subunit, which results in inhibition of IL5 signaling.181 IL5 receptor is expressed exclusively on eosinophil and basophil progenitors in the bone marrow and on mature eosinophils and basophils.[182] In addition, afucosylation results in a higher affinity to human FcγRIIIa (the main activating receptor expressed on natural killer cells, macrophages, and neutrophils), which increase the antibody-dependent cell-mediated cytotoxicity function of these cells, resulting in increased removal of airway eosinophils and basophils.[182]

Dupilumab is a human monoclonal antibody to the α subunit of the IL4 receptor, thereby blocking the activity of IL4 and IL13 as the IL4 receptor is critical for signal transduction of both interleukins.[163] Both IL4 and IL13 are involved in Ig switching from IgM to IgE, enhance airway smooth muscle contractility, and facilitate airway recruitment of eosinophils (through activation of eotaxin synthesis and upregulation of adhesion molecules).[163,183,184] IL13 stimulates airway mucous production and promotes airway remodeling through multiple mechanisms, including stimulating collagen deposition, proliferation of airway smooth muscle cells, and goblet cell hyperplasia.[184] IL4 is a key mediator in the polarization toward a Th2 response.[183]

PHARMACOKINETICS

On average, the bioavailability of omalizumab is 62%.[185] Peak concentrations are achieved 7 to 8 days after administration.[186] Steady serum concentrations are reached in 14 to 28 days.[187] The apparent volume of distribution is about 78 ± 32 mL per kg.[187] It has an average serum half-life of 26 days, and its clearance is thought to be through the reticuloendothelial system, although the details are unclear.[186,188] Serum-unbound IgE levels reduce within 1 hour after first dose in 95% of patients, although it takes 12 to 16 weeks for maximal clinical effect.[162,186,187,189] Following discontinuation of treatment, serum IgE levels return to baseline within 120 days.[187]

The bioavailability of mepolizumab ranges from 64% to 75% in studies with subcutaneous (SC) injection, and up to 81% with intramuscular (IM) injection, although rates are higher with IV injection.[169] Peak concentrations are achieved in 5 to 7 days with SC dosing, 4 days with IM dosing, and 0.04 to 0.08 days with IV dosing. Steady serum concentrations are reached in 34 to 49 days. The apparent volume of distribution ranges from 49 to 93 mL per kg.[169]

Mepolizumab has a slow elimination, with initial and terminal phase half-lives of approximately 2 and 20 days, respectively; the details of its route of elimination are unclear.[169] Serum eosinophil levels are reduced by up to 73% from baseline in 8 days (and up to 87% by 29 days) in asthmatics.[174] Mepolizumab also attenuated the increase in blood eosinophils noted post allergen challenge, although there was a degree of dose response.[174] A decrease in eosinophil counts has been noted up to 16 weeks after dosing.[169] Mepolizumab has also been shown to decrease induced sputum eosinophil numbers by 1 week after first dose that persists for up to 16 weeks after dosing discontinuation.[169]

Less has been described about the pharmacokinetics and pharmacodynamics of reslizumab. Plasma concentrations of reslizumab are dose proportional.[190] The apparent volume of distribution is approximately 5 L, and half-life is approximately 24 days.[190] Serum eosinophils are reduced by up to 52% from baseline in 48 hours after reslizumab administration.[191] Studies have shown the reduction in serum eosinophil counts to persist throughout treatment, with no evidence of tachyphylaxis.[192]

Within 90 days after completion of therapy, eosinophil levels begin to increase back toward baseline.[192]

The bioavailability of benralizumab is approximately 52% to 59%, with no differences noted based on the site of SC injection.[181,193] The apparent volume of distribution ranges from 65 to 71 mL per kg.[181] Elimination half-life is approximately 7 to 16 days; mechanism of excretion is not well described.[181] Benralizumab has been shown to decrease airway eosinophil counts by up to 96% (by day 84), sputum eosinophil counts by 90% (by day 28), and decrease blood eosinophil counts by 100% (day 84).[194]

On average, the bioavailability of dupilumab is 61% to 64%. Peak concentrations are achieved approximately 7 days after administration.[195] Steady serum concentrations were achieved after approximately 16 weeks. The apparent volume of distribution is approximately 4.8 L.[195] The details of dupilumab metabolic elimination pathways have not been well described. Little is known about the pharmacodynamics of dupilumab.[183,195] Table 41.6 summarizes the dosing and route of administration of these agents.

CLINICAL USE

Omalizumab is approved in children aged 6 and older with moderate-to-severe persistent asthma, although the definition of moderate-to-severe asthma varies by region. Patients must also have a serum IgE level between 30 and 700 IU per mL (to 1,300 IU per mL in children aged 6 to 11 years) and allergic sensitization to perennial aeroallergens.[196] Omalizumab is the only biologic therapy for asthma to be studied in children as young as 5 years of age.[163] There have been two observational studies and four RDBPCTs of omalizumab in the pediatric asthma population which have noted omalizumab to decrease oral corticosteroid requirements,[197] decrease asthma exacerbation and hospitalization rates,[197–201] improve asthma control,[198] and improve quality of life.[197] No significant improvement in FEV_1 has been consistently noted.[197,198]

Predictors of clinical response to omalizumab have been studied in children, but results are mixed and include thus far perennial aeroallergen sensitization, increased asthma severity,[168] and elevated baseline eosinophil counts (>300 per μL).[202] The Composite Asthma Severity Index (CASI) has recently been developed as a means of determining asthma severity and has been demonstrated in post hoc analysis to serve as a useful outcome measure in assessing response with omalizumab.[203] A major concern with the use of omalizumab is its cost (about $1,084.66 per 150 mg vial).[204] A recent Institute for Clinical and Economic Review (ICER) report on cost-effectiveness of biologics notes that no biologics (including omalizumab) met the threshold for cost-effectiveness and recommended a reduction in biologic costs of up to 80% to meet a threshold of cost-effectiveness.[204,205] A recent systematic review (19 studies; 2 included pediatric patients) noted that omalizumab was cost-effective only in patients with difficult-to-treat persistent asthma who demonstrate a clinical response.[206]

Mepolizumab is approved in children aged 12 years and older with eosinophilic asthma.[207] No other prerequisite criteria are required. Mepolizumab has been studied in adolescents in three RDBPCTs that included adolescents in the inclusion criteria: DREAM (Dosing Range Efficacy and safety with Mepolizumab in severe asthma),[179] MENSA (Mepolizumab as Adjunctive Therapy in Patients with Severe Asthma),[208] and SIRIUS (Steroid Reduction with Mepolizumab).[209] These three RDBPCTs found mepolizumab to reduce asthma exacerbations.[179,208,209] asthma symptoms,[208,209] and oral corticosteroid requirements,[209] although no significant improvement in quality of life was noted.[179] It is important to note that while all three of these studies included adolescents as young as age 12 in the inclusion criteria, data on adolescents were not reported separately, and, in at least one of these studies, no adolescents were actually enrolled.[179]

The studies thus far have only enrolled patients with eosinophilic asthma, which is supported by studies noting no benefit with mepolizumab in the absence of eosinophilia.[210] As a result, eosinophilia is the best predictor of clinical response thus far. MENSA noted that the only covariate that influenced mepolizumab efficacy was blood eosinophil count on screening (enhanced response ≥500 cells per μL),[208] but further studies are required to determine an absolute level of eosinophilia that is associated with efficacy. As with omalizumab, a major

TABLE 41.6 Dose and Route of Administration of Biologics

Biologic Agent	*Dosing*	*Route of Administration*	*Pediatric Age of Approval*
Omalizumab	Every 2–4 wk based on weight and serum IgE level[a]	SC	6 years and older
Mepolizumab	100 mg once every 4 wk	SC	12 years and older
Reslizumab	3 mg/kg once every 4 wk as an infusion	IV	NA
Benralizumab	30 mg every 4 wk for first 3 doses, then 30 mg every 8 wk	SC	12 years and older (the United States)
Dupilumab	Either 400 mg first dose (then 200 mg maintenance every 2 wk) or 600 mg first dose (then 300 mg every 2 wk)	SC	12 years and older

[a] Different dosing in different countries; United States guidance: 150–375 mg every 2–4 weeks. Should be administered for the first time in a center prepared to treat anaphylaxis with a 2-hour observation period for the first dose (and 30 minutes thereafter).

IgE, immunoglobulin E; IV, intravenous; NA, not applicable; SC, subcutaneous.

Luu M, Bardou M, Bonniaud P, Goirand F. Pharmacokinetics, pharmacodynamics and clinical efficacy of omalizumab for the treatment of asthma. *Expert Opin Drug Metab Toxicol* 2016;12(12):1503–1511; Omalizumab (XOLAIR) monograph. https://pdfs.semanticscholar.org/38f8/e33927f24312052df35a25fb2e483f2c192c.pdf. Accessed April 12, 2019; Reslizumab product monograph (TEVA). https://www.cinqair.com/globalassets/cinqair/prescribinginformation.pdf. Accessed June 25, 2020; Benralizumab product monograph. https://www.astrazeneca.ca/content/dam/az-ca/downloads/productinformation/fasenra-product-monograph-en.pdf. Accessed April 12, 2019; FDA: Dupilumab. https://www.accessdata.fda.gov/drugsatfda_docs/label/2017/761055lbl.pdf. Accessed April 12, 2019; and FDA: Omalizumab monograph. https://www.gene.com/download/pdf/xolair_prescribing.pdf. Accessed June 25, 2020.

concern with mepolizumab is cost (~$3,500 per 100 mg).[207] A cost-effectiveness analysis of mepolizumab noted that to achieve cost-effectiveness, mepolizumab would require a more than 60% price discount.[205,211]

Reslizumab is only approved in adults over the age of 18 years with eosinophilic asthma (eosinophil counts ≥400 cells per μL at initiation of treatment).[192] While no studies have been limited to the pediatric or adolescent population, two RDB-PCTs have included adolescents and adults with eosinophilic asthma and have noted reslizumab to improve asthma control and reduce asthma exacerbations, although effect on quality of life was less clear.[212,213] In addition, analysis of adolescent-only data paradoxically suggests an increased rate of asthma exacerbations in the reslizumab-treated group.[214] The studies thus far have only enrolled patients with eosinophilic asthma, which is supported by studies noting no benefit with reslizumab in the absence of eosinophilia.[215] However, in one RDBPCT, baseline eosinophil level did not influence the magnitude of clinical benefit, although the number of patients included in analysis was small.[212]

In the United States, benralizumab is approved for adolescents aged 12 years and older with severe eosinophilic asthma; in Canada, there is no pediatric indication for benralizumab as yet.[193,216] Benralizumab has been studied in two RDBPCTs of adolescents aged 12 years and older and adults with severe uncontrolled asthma on high-dose ICS and LABA therapy (SIROCCO and CALIMA).[217,218] These studies noted benralizumab to reduce asthma exacerbation rates and asthma symptoms. In these studies, benralizumab was more effective in patients with blood eosinophil counts greater than or equal to 300 cells per μL; in SIROCCO, some benefit was noted in the patients with lower eosinophil counts as well, although the treatment effect was "smaller." The absolute magnitude of eosinophilia required for optimal effect remains to be seen; a pooled analysis of SIROCCO and CALIMA supported the use of benralizumab in patients with blood eosinophil counts greater than 150 cells per μL,[219] although a recent pooled analysis extends the efficacy irrespective of eosinophil count, again noting a greater benefit with higher eosinophil levels.[220]

Dupilumab is approved in adolescents aged 12 years and older with moderate-to-severe eosinophilic asthma or corticosteroid-dependent asthma (regardless of phenotype).[195] There has been one RDBPCT of adolescents aged 12 years and over and adults with uncontrolled asthma that found dupilumab to significantly reduce asthma exacerbations while also increasing FEV_1 compared to placebo.[221] Predictors of clinical response are not well defined, although recent studies have supported an increased benefit with higher baseline levels of eosinophils and a greater reduction in asthma exacerbation among patients with higher baseline FeNO.[221]

ADVERSE EFFECTS

Common side effects to omalizumab include local injection site reactions (45%) and, less commonly, upper respiratory tract infection, headache, and gastrointestinal side effects (although differences between treatment and placebo groups are small).[187] A recent systematic review and meta-analysis noted an "acceptable" safety profile to omalizumab with similar rates of adverse events between treatment and placebo groups.[222] The concerns with omalizumab are potential anaphylaxis (0.2%)[223] and malignancy. While a 2003 analysis of pooled clinical trial data noted a malignancy risk of 0.5% (compared to 0.2% in controls), a subsequent prospective study of over 7,000 adolescents and adults noted no increased malignancy risk with omalizumab compared to control.[224]

An open-label extension of the DREAM study followed 326 patients over a mean period of 3.5 years found that 94% of patients experienced at least one adverse event while on treatment with mepolizumab, the most common being respiratory tract infection, headache, asthma worsening, and bronchitis.[225] There were six deaths, but none deemed to be medication related. In general, mepolizumab is well tolerated. As mepolizumab decreases eosinophils, which are essential in the immune response to helminth infections, it is recommended that patients with preexisting helminth infection be treated prior to starting mepolizumab.[207]

In general, reslizumab is well tolerated, and the most commonly experienced adverse effects include oropharyngeal pain, increased levels of creatinine phosphokinase (2%), and myalgias.[190] Anaphylaxis (0.3%)[226] is a concern, and, as a result, reslizumab must be given in a facility capable of recognizing and treating anaphylaxis. There was no significant difference in rates of malignancies between reslizumab (<1%) and placebo (<1%) groups.[192] Adverse effects are generally thought to be mild with benralizumab and similar between treatment and placebo arms of studies.[217,218]

Common side effects with dupilumab include nasopharyngitis, injection site reactions, and headaches.[183] In general, dupilumab is well tolerated.

DRUG INTERACTIONS

There are no known significant drug interactions for omalizumab, mepolizumab, reslizumab, benralizumab, or dupilumab.

SUMMARY

Asthma therapy for children has advanced significantly over the past 40 years with a change in approach to management occurring almost every 10 years. This is primarily based on the introduction of new medications at intervals approximating 10 years. As usual, all medications are initially studied in adults and adolescents, then studies are conducted in children aged 5 to 11 years, and finally studies are conducted for those children less than 5 years of age. The steps to studying medications in children have been accelerated in the past 15 years due to FDA directives. For asthma, several long-term control medications including nebulized budesonide and oral montelukast are now approved down to 1 year of age.

With the advances in conducting clinical trials in young children, prompted by studies conducted in the National Institutes of Health (NIH) asthma networks and the National Institute for Child Health and Human Development (NICHD) Pediatric Pharmacology Research Unit Network, it is anticipated that more medications will continue to be evaluated in children to provide specific product labeling for all age groups. The next significant advance in childhood asthma will be to identify medications designed to prevent the onset and progression of asthma. This might even mean developing a medication that is primarily used for the treatment of emerging asthma in young children.

REFERENCES

1. Summary Health Statistics: National Health Interview Survey, 2017. https://www.cdc.gov/nchs/fastats/asthma.htm. Accessed April 2019.
2. Centers for Disease Control. Vital signs: asthma in children—United States, 2001–2016. *Morbid Mortal Wkly Rep* 2018;67:149–155.
3. Centers for Disease Control and Prevention. National Center for Health Statistics. National Health Interview Survey, 2016. Analysis by the American Lung Association Epidemiology and Statistics Unit using SPSS software. https://www.lung.org/lung-health-and-diseases/lung-disease-lookup/asthma/learn-about-asthma/asthma-children-facts-sheet.html. Accessed April 2019.
4. American Lung Association. Monitoring trends in Lung Disease: Data &Statistics. https://www.lung.org/research/trends-in-lung-disease/asthma-trends-brief/trends-and-burden. Accessed June 2020.
5. Center for Disease Control and Prevention. Asthma as the underlying cause of death; https://www.cdc.gov/asthma/asthma_stats/asthma_underlying_death.html. Accessed April 2019.
6. Center for Disease Control and Prevention. Most Recent National Asthma Data. https://www.cdc.gov/asthma/most_recent_national_asthma_data.htm. Accessed April 2019.
7. National Institutes of Health, National Heart, Lung, and Blood Institute. National Asthma Education and Prevention Program. Full Report of the Expert Panel: Guidelines for the diagnosis and management of asthma (EPR-3) 2007. http://www.nhlbi.nih.gov/guidelines/asthma. Accessed April 2019.
8. Busse WW, Lemanske RF Jr. Asthma. *N Engl J Med* 2001:344:350–362.
9. Morgan WJ, Stern DA, Sherrill DL, et al. Outcome of asthma and wheezing in the first 6 years of life: follow-up through adolescence. *Am J Respir Crit Care Med* 2005;172:1253–1258.
10. Guilbert TW, Morgan WJ, Zeiger RS, et al. Long-term inhaled corticosteroids in preschool children at high risk for asthma. *N Engl J Med* 2006;354:1985–1997.
11. Covar RA, Spahn JD, Murphy JR, et al; Childhood Asthma Management Program Research Group. Progression of asthma measured by lung function in the childhood asthma management program. *Am J Respir Crit Care Med* 2004;170:234–241.
12. Dolovich MB, Dhand R. Aerosol drug delivery: developments in device design and clinical use. *Lancet* 2011;377(9770):1032–1045.
13. Kelly HW. Comparison of inhaled corticosteroids: an update. *Ann Pharmacother* 2009;43:519–527.
14. Leach CL. Inhalation aspects of therapeutic aerosols. *Toxicol Pathol* 2007;35:23–26.
15. Dalby RN, Eicher J, Zierenberg B. Development of Respimat® Soft Mist™ Inhaler and its clinical utility in respiratory disorders. *Med Devices (Auckl)* 2011;4:145–155.
16. Amirav I, Newhouse MT, Minocchieri S, et al. Factors that affect the efficacy of inhaled corticosteroids for infants and young children. *J Allergy Clin Immunol* 2010;125:1206–1211.
17. Raissy HH, Kelly HW. MDI versus nebulizers for acute asthma. *J Pediatr Pharmacol Ther* 2004;9:226–234.
18. Liang J, Asmus MJ, Hochaus G, et al. Differences in inhaled fluticasone bioavailability between holding chambers in children with asthma. *Pharmacotherapy* 2002;22:947–953.
19. Wildhaber JH, Devadason SG, Eber E, et al. Effect of electrostatic charge, flow, delay and multiple actuations on the in vitro delivery of salbutamol from different small volume spacers for infants. *Thorax* 1996;51:985–988.
20. Pierart F, Wildhaber JH, Vrancken I, et al. Washing plastic spacers in household detergent reduces electrostatic charge and greatly improves delivery. *Eur Respir J* 1999;13:673–678.
21. Product information: Pulmicort Flexhaler®, (budesonide inhalation powder) for oral inhalation. Wilmington, DE: AstraZeneca LP, 2007.
22. Product information: Asmanex Twisthaler®, (mometasone furoate inhalation powder) for oral inhalation only. Whitehouse Station, NJ: Merck &Co., 2008.
23. U.S. Food and Drug Administration. https://www.fda.gov/Drugs/ResourcesForYou/Consumers/BuyingUsingMedicineSafely/GenericDrugs/ucm592245.htm. Accessed April 2019.
24. Wildhaber JH, Dore ND, Wilson JM, et al. Inhalation therapy in asthma: nebulizer or pressurized metered-dose inhaler with holding chamber? In vivo comparison of lung deposition in children. *J Pediatr* 1999;135:28–33.
25. Everard ML, Clark AR, Milner AD. Drug delivery from jet nebulisers. *Arch Dis Child* 1992;67:586–591.
26. Janssens HM, De Jongste JC, Hop WC, et al. Extra-fine particles improve lung delivery of inhaled steroids in infants: a study in an upper airway model. *Chest* 2003;123:2083–2088.
27. Finlay WH, Zuberbuhler P. In vitro comparison of beclomethasone and salbutamol metered-dose inhaler aerosols inhaled during pediatric tidal breathing from four valved holding chambers. *Chest* 1998;114:1676–1680.
28. Product information: QVAR®, (beclomethasone dipropionate HFA) Inhalation Aerosol. Horsham, PA: Teva Specialty Pharmaceuticals LLC, 2008.
29. Raissy HH, Davies L, Marshik P, et al. Inspiratory flow through dry-powder inhalers (DPIs) in asthmatic children 2 to 12 years old. *Pediatr Asthma Allergy Immunol* 2006;19:223–230.
30. Adcock IM, Chung KF. Glucocorticoids. In: Adkinson N, Bochner B, Bursk AW, et al., eds. *Middleton's allergy principles and practice*, 8th ed. Philadelphia, PA: Elsevier Saunders, 2014:1578–1601.
31. Kelly HW. Potential adverse effects of inhaled corticosteroids. *J Allergy Clin Immunol* 2003;112:469–478.
32. Raissy H, Kelly HW, Harkins M, et al. Inhaled corticosteroids in lung disease. *Am J Respir Crit Care Med* 2013;187(8):798–803.
33. Derendorf H, Nave R, Drollman A, et al. Relevance of pharmacokinetics and pharmacodynamics of inhaled corticosteroids to asthma. *Eur Respir J* 2006;28:1042–1050.
34. van Aalderen WM, Grigg J, Guilbert TW, et al. Small-particle inhaled corticosteroid as first-line or step-up controller therapy in childhood asthma. *J Allergy Clin Immunol Pract* 20153(5):721.e16–731.e16.
35. Kelly HW. Ultrafine-particle inhalers, the holy grail of inhaled corticosteroid therapy, or not! *J Allergy Clin Immunol Pract* 2015;3(5):732–733.
36. Martin RJ, Szefler SJ, Chinchilli VM, et al. Systemic effect comparisons of six inhaled corticosteroid preparations. *Am J Respir Crit Care Med* 2002;165:1377–1383.
37. Elmallah MK, Khan Y, Hochhaus G, et al. Systemic exposure to fluticasone MDI delivered through antistatic chambers. *J Allergy Clin Immunol* 2011;128:1113–1115.
38. Guilbert TW, Mauger DT, Allen DB, et al. Growth of preschool children at high risk for asthma 2 years after discontinuation of fluticasone. *J Allergy Clin Immunol* 2011;128:956–963.
39. Childhood Asthma Management Program Research Group. Long-term effects of budesonide or nedocromil in children with asthma. *N Engl J Med* 2000;343:1054–1063.
40. Bisgaard H, Gillies J, Groenewald M, et al. The effect of inhaled fluticasone propionate in the treatment of young asthmatic children. A dose comparison study. *Am J Respir Crit Care Med* 1999;160:126–131.
41. Garcia Garcia ML, Wahn U, Gilles L, et al. Montelukast, compared with fluticasone, for control of asthma among 6- to 14-year-old patients with mild asthma: the MOSAIC study. *Pediatrics* 2005;116:360–369.
42. Ostrom NK, Decotis BA, Lincourt WR, et al. Comparative efficacy and safety of low-dose fluticasone propionate and montelukast in children with persistent asthma. *J Pediatr* 2005;147:213–220.
43. Guevara JP, Ducharme FM, Keren R, et al. Inhaled corticosteroids versus sodium cromoglycate in children and adults with asthma. *Cochrane Database Syst Rev* 2006;(2):CD003558.
44. Leflein JG, Szefler SJ, Murphy KR, et al. Nebulized budesonide inhalation suspension compared with cromolyn sodium nebulizer solution for asthma in young children: results of a randomized outcomes trial. *Pediatrics* 2002;109:866–872.
45. Castro-Rodriguez JA, Rodriguez-Martinez CE, Ducharme FM. Daily inhaled corticosteroids or montelukast for preschoolers with asthma or recurrent wheezing: a systematic review. *Pediatr Pulmonol* 2018;53(12):1670–1677.
46. Petersen R, Agertoft L, Pedersen S. Treatment of exercise-induced asthma with beclomethasone dipropionate in children with asthma. *Eur Respir J* 2004;24:932–937.
47. Vidal C, Fernández-Ovide E, Piñeiro J, et al. Comparison of montelukast versus budesonide in the treatment of exercise-induced bronchoconstriction. *Ann Allergy Asthma Immunol* 2001;86:655–658.
48. Pauwels RA, Pedersen S, Busse WW, et al. Early intervention with budesonide in mild persistent asthma: a randomized, double-blind trial. *Lancet* 2003;361:1071–1076.
49. Silkoff PE, Carlson M, Burke T, et al. The Aerocrine exhaled nitric oxide monitoring system NIOX is cleared by the US Food and Drug Administration for monitoring therapy in asthma. *J Allergy Clin Immunol* 2004;114:1241–1256.
50. Raissy HH, Cain H, Crowley M, et al. Comparison of the systemic effects of fluticasone propionate and triamcinolone acetonide administered in equipotent doses in children with asthma. *Pediatr Asthma Allergy Immunol* 2003;16:283–293.
51. Caffey LF, Raissy HH, Marshik P, et al. A crossover comparison of fluticasone propionate and montelukast on inflammatory indices in children with asthma. *Pediatr Asthma Allergy Immunol* 2005;18:123–130.
52. Szefler SJ, Mitchell H, Sorkness CA, et al. Management of asthma based on exhaled nitric oxide in addition to guideline-based treatment for inner-city adolescents and young adults: a randomised controlled trial. *Lancet* 2008;372:1065–1072.
53. de Jongste JC, Carraro S, Hop WC, et al. Daily telemonitoring of exhaled nitric oxide and symptoms in the treatment of childhood asthma. *Am J Respir Crit Care Med* 2009;179:93–97.
54. Lemanske RF Jr, Mauger DT, Sorkness CA, et al. Step-up therapy for children with uncontrolled asthma receiving inhaled corticosteroids. *N Engl J Med* 2010;362:975–985.
55. Chauhan BF, Chartrand C, Ni Chroinin M, et al. Addition of long-acting beta2-agonists to inhaled corticosteroids for chronic asthma in children. *Cochrane Database Syst Rev* 2015;(11):CD007949.
56. Masoli M, Weatherall M, Holt S, et al. Systematic review of the dose-response relation of inhaled fluticasone propionate. *Arch Dis Child* 2004;89:902–907.
57. Shapiro G, Bronsky EA, LaForce CF, et al. Dose-related efficacy of budesonide administered via a dry powder inhaler in the treatment of children with moderate to severe persistent asthma. *J Pediatr* 1998;132:976–982.
58. O'Byrne PM, Barnes PJ, Rodriguez-Roisin R, et al. Low dose inhaled budesonide and formoterol in mild persistent asthma: the OPTIMA randomized trial. *Am J Respir Crit Care Med* 2001;164:1392–1397.
59. Pauwels RA, Lofdahl CG, Postma DS, et al. Effect of inhaled formoterol and budesonide on exacerbations of asthma. Formoterol and corticosteroids establishing therapy (FACET) international study group. *N Engl J Med* 1997;337:1405–1411.
60. Jackson DJ, Bacharier LB, Mauger DT, et al. Quintupling inhaled glucocorticoids to prevent childhood asthma exacerbations. *N Engl J Med* 2018;378(10):891–901.
61. Szefler SJ, Eigen H. Budesonide inhalation suspension: a nebulized corticosteroid for persistent asthma. *J Allergy Clin Immunol* 2002;109:730–742.
62. Daley-Yates PT. Inhaled corticosteroids: potency, dose equivalence and therapeutic index. *Br J Clin Pharmacol* 2015;80(3):372–380.
63. Beigelman A, Bacharier LB. Management of preschool children with recurrent wheezing: lessons from the NHLBI's asthma research networks. *J Allergy Clin Immunol Pract* 2016;4(1):1–8.
64. Guilbert TW, Bacharier LB, Mauger DT, et al. Challenges in assessing the efficacy of systemic corticosteroids for severe wheezing episodes in preschool children. *J Allergy Clin Immunol* 2019;143(5):1934.e4–1937.e4. doi:10.1016/j.jaci.2018.10.071.
65. Ronald NJ, Bhalla RK, Earis J. The local side effects of inhaled corticosteroids: current understanding and review of the literature. *Chest* 2004;126:213–219.
66. Zöllner EW. Hypothalamic-pituitary-adrenal axis suppression in asthmatic children on inhaled corticosteroids (Part 2)—the risk as determined by gold standard adrenal function tests: a systematic review. *Pediatr Allergy Immunol* 2007;18:469–474.
67. Cavkaytar O, Vuralli D, Yilmaz EA, et al. Evidence of hypothalamic-pituitary-adrenal axis suppression during moderate-to-high-dose inhaled corticosteroid use. *Eur J Pediatr* 2015;174:1421–1431.
68. Molimard M, Girodet PO, Pollet C, et al. Inhaled corticosteroids and adrenal insufficiency: prevalence and clinical presentation. *Drug Saf* 2008;31:769–774.
69. Zöllner EW. Hypothalamic-pituitary-adrenal axis suppression in asthmatic children on inhaled corticosteroids: Part 1. Which test should be used? *Pediatr Allergy Immunol* 2007;18:401–409.

70. Raissy HH, Marshik PL, Scott S, et al. Urinary free cortisol in hispanic and non-hispanic children with mild asthma and non-asthmatic normals. *Pediatr Asthma Allergy Immunol* 2006;19:100–105.
71. Bacharier LB, Raissy HH, Wilson L, et al. The long-term effect of budesonide on hypothalamic-pituitary-adrenal axis function in children with mild to moderate asthma. *Pediatrics* 2004;113:1693–1699.
72. Fuhlbrigge AL, Kelly HW. Inhaled corticosteroids in children: effects on bone mineral density and growth. *Lancet Respir Med* 2014;2(6):487–496.
73. Kelly HW, Van Natta ML, Covar RA, et al.; CAMP Research Group. Effect of long-term corticosteroid use on bone mineral density in children: a prospective longitudinal assessment in the Childhood Asthma Management Program (CAMP) study. *Pediatrics* 2008;122:e53–e61.
74. van Staa TP, Bishop N, Leufkens HG, et al. Are inhaled corticosteroids associated with an increased risk of fracture in children? *Osteoporos Int* 2004;15:785–791.
75. Schlienger RG, Jick SS, Meier CR. Inhaled corticosteroids and the risk of fractures in children and adolescents. *Pediatrics* 2004;469–473.
76. van Staa TP, Cooper C, Leufkens HG, et al. Children and the risk of fractures caused by oral corticosteroids. *J Bone Miner Res* 2003;18:913–918.
77. Agertoft L, Pedersen S. Effect of long term treatment with budesonide on adult height in children with asthma. *N Engl J Med* 2000;343:1064–1069.
78. Kelly HW, Sternberg AL, Lescher R, et al. Effect of inhaled glucocorticoids in childhood on adult height. *N Engl J Med* 2012;367(10):904–912.
79. Ferguson AC, Van Bever HP, Teper AM, et al. A comparison of the relative growth velocities with budesonide and fluticasone propionate in children with asthma. *Respir Med* 2007;101:118–129.
80. Allen DB. Inhaled corticosteroids and growth: still an issue after all these years. *J Pediatr* 2015;166:463–469.
81. Acun C, Tomac N, Ermis B, et al. Effects of inhaled corticosteroids on growth in asthmatic children: a comparison of fluticasone propionate with budesonide. *Allergy Asthma Proc* 2005;26:204–206.
82. Raissy HH, Sternberg AL, Williams P, et al. Risk of cataracts in the Childhood Asthma Management Program Cohort. *J Allergy Clin Immunol* 2010;126:389–392.
83. De Vries TW, de Langen-Wourste JJ, van Puijenbroek E, et al. Reported adverse drug reactions during use of inhaled steroids in children with asthma in the Netherlands. *Eur J Clin Pharmacol* 2006;62:343–346.
84. Dresser GK, Spence JD, Bailey DG. Pharmacokinetic-pharmacodynamic consequences and clinical relevance of cytochrome P450 3A4 inhibition. *Clin Pharmacokinet* 2000;38:41–57.
85. Samaras K, Pett S, Gowers A, et al. Iatrogenic Cushing's syndrome with osteoporosis and secondary adrenal failure in human immunodeficiency virus-infected patients receiving inhaled corticosteroids and ritonavir-boosted protease inhibitors: six cases. *J Clin Endocrinol Metab* 2005;90:4394–4398.
86. Bolland MJ, Bagg W, Thomas MG, et al. Cushing's syndrome due to interaction between inhaled corticosteroids and itraconazole. *Ann Pharmacother* 2004;38:46–49.
87. O'Byrne PM, Sears MR. Inhaled β2-agonists. In: Adkinson NF, Bochner BS, Burks AW, et al., eds. *Middleton's allergy principles and practice*, 8th ed. Philadelphia, PA: Elsevier Saunders, 2014:1534–1541.
88. Sward-Comunelli SL, Mabry SM, Truog WE, et al. Airway muscle in preterm infants: changes during development. *J Pediatr* 1997;130:570–576.
89. Anderson GP. Interactions between corticosteroids and beta-adrenergic agonists in asthma disease induction, progression, and exacerbation. *Am J Respir Crit Care Med* 2000;61:S188–S196.
90. Kelly HW. What is new with the β2 agonists: issues in the management of asthma. *Ann Pharmacother* 2005;39:931–938.
91. Lötvall J, Palmqvist M, Ankerst J, et al. The effect of formoterol over 24 h in patients with asthma: the role of enantiomers. *Pulm Pharmacol Ther* 2005;18:109–113.
92. Lotvall J, Palmqvist M, Arvidsson P, et al. The therapeutic ratio of R-albuterol is comparable with that of RS-albuterol in asthmatic patients. *J Allergy Clin Immunol* 2001;108:726–731.
93. Raissy HH, Harkins M, Esparham A, et al. Comparison of the dose-response to levalbuterol with and without pretreatment with S-albuterol after methacholine-induced bronchoconstriction. *Pharmacotherapy* 2007;27:1231–1236.
94. Raby BA, Israel E. Pharmacogenomics of asthma therapies. In: Adkinson N, Bochner B, Bursk AW, et al., eds. *Middleton's allergy principles and practice*, 8th ed. Philadelphia, PA: Elsevier Saunders, 2014:1460–1470.
95. Van der Woude HJ, Winter TH, Aalbers R. Decreased bronchodilating effect of salbutamol in relieving methacholine induced moderate bronchoconstriction during high dose treatment with long acting beta2 agonists. *Thorax* 2001;56:529–535.
96. Jones SL, Cowan JO, Flannery EM, et al. Reversing acute bronchoconstriction in asthma: the effect of bronchodilator tolerance after treatment with formoterol. *Eur Respir J* 2001;17:368–373.
97. Lipworth BJ, Aziz I. Bronchodilator response to albuterol after regular formoterol and effects of acute corticosteroid administration. *Chest* 2000;117:156–162.
98. Morgan DJ. Clinical pharmacokinetics of beta-agonists. *Clin Pharmacokinet* 1990;18:270–294.
99. Bartow RA, Brogden RN. Formoterol: an update of its pharmacological properties and therapeutic efficacy in the management of asthma. *Drugs* 1998;56:303–322.
100. LaForce C, Alexander M, Deckelmann R, et al. Indacaterol provides sustained 24 h bronchodilation on once-daily dosing in asthma: a 7-day dose-ranging study. *Allergy* 2008;63:103–111.
101. Pearlman DS, Greos L, LaForce C, et al. Bronchodilator efficacy of indacaterol, a novel once-daily beta2-agonist, in patients with persistent asthma. *Ann Allergy Asthma Immunol* 2008;101:90–95.
102. Product information: BREO ELIPTA,®, (fluticasone furoate and vilanterol inhalation powder), for oral inhalation use, for oral inhalation. GlaxoSmithKline, Research Triangle Park, NC: GlaxoSmithKline, 2013.
103. Product information: STRIVERDI® RESPIMAT® (olodaterol) Inhalation Spray for oral inhalation. Ridgefield, CT: Boehringer Ingelheim Pharmaceuticals Inc., 2014.
104. Dennis SM, Sharp SJ, Vickers MR, et al. Regular inhaled salbutamol and asthma control: the TRUST randomized trial. *Lancet* 2000;355:1675–1679.
105. Drazen JM, Israel E, Boushey HA, et al. Comparison of regularly scheduled with as-needed use of albuterol in mild asthma. *N Engl J Med* 1996;335:841–847.
106. Van Schayck CP, Graafsma SJ, Visch MB, et al. Increased bronchial hyperresponsiveness after inhaling salbutamol during 1 year is not caused by subsensitization to salbutamol. *J Allergy Clin Immunol* 1990;86:793–800.
107. Raissy HH, Kelly F, Harkins M, et al. Pretreatment with albuterol vs. montelukast in exercise induced bronchospasm in children. *Pharmacotherapy* 2008;28:287–294.
108. Weiler JM, Brannan JD, Randolph CC, et al. Exercise-induced bronchoconstriction update—2016. *J Allergy Clin Immunol* 2016;138:1292–1295.
109. Cates CJ, Bara A, Crilley JA, et al. Holding-chambers versus nebulizers for beta-agonist treatment of acute asthma. *Cochrane Database Syst Rev* 2003;(2):CD000052.
110. Malone R, LaForce C, Nimmagadda S, et al. The safety of twice daily treatment with fluticasone propionate and salmeterol in pediatric patients with persistent asthma. *Ann Allergy Asthma Immunol* 2005;95:66–71.
111. Bisgaard H. Effect of long-acting beta2 agonists on exacerbation rates of asthma in children. *Pediatr Pulmonol* 2003;36:391–398.
112. Nelson HS, Weiss ST, Bleecker ER, et al. The Salmeterol Multicenter Asthma Research Trial: a comparison of usual pharmacotherapy for asthma or usual pharmacotherapy plus salmeterol. *Chest* 2006;129:15–26.
113. McMahon AW, Levenson MS, McEvoy BW, et al. Age and risks of FDA-approved long-acting beta(2)-adrenergic receptor agonists. *Pediatrics* 2011;128:e1147–e1154.
114. Stempel DA, Szefler SJ, Pedersen S, et al. Safety of adding salmeterol to fluticasone propionate in children with asthma. *N Engl J Med.*2016;375:840–849.
115. Busse WW, Bateman ED, Caplan AL, et al. Combined analysis of asthma safety trials of long-acting β2-agonists. *N Engl J Med* 2018;378:2497–2505.
116. Bleecker ER, Yancey SW, Baitinger LA, et al. Salmeterol response is not affected by beta2-adrenergic receptor genotype in subjects with persistent asthma. *J Allergy Clin Immunol* 2006;118:809–816.
117. Guhan AR, Cooper S, Oborne J, et al. Systemic effects of formoterol and salmeterol: a dose-response comparison in healthy subjects. *Thorax* 2000;55:650–656.
118. Palmqvist M, Ibsen T, Mellén A, et al. Comparison of the relative efficacy of formoterol and salmeterol in asthmatic patients. *Am J Respir Crit Care Med* 1999;160:244–249.
119. Kaae R, Agertoft L, Pedersen S, et al. Cumulative high doses of inhaled formoterol have less systemic effects in asthmatic children 6–11 years-old than cumulative high doses of inhaled terbutaline. *Br J Clin Pharmacol* 2004;58:411–418.
120. Pohunek P, Matulka M, Rybnícek O, et al. Dose-related efficacy and safety of formoterol (Oxis) Turbuhaler compared with salmeterol Diskhaler in children with asthma. *Pediatr Allergy Immunol* 2004;15:32–39.
121. Product Information. SEREVENT DISKUS (salmeterol xinafoate inhalation powder), for oral inhalation use. Research Triangle Park, NC: GlaxoSmithKline, 2018.
122. Edwards AM, Holgate ST. The chromones: cromolyn sodium and nedocromil sodium. In: Adkinson N, Bochner B, Bursk AW, et al., eds. *Middleton's allergy principles and practice*, 8th ed. Philadelphia, PA: Elsevier Saunders, 2014:1567–1577.
123. Kelly K, Spooner CH, Rowe BH. Nedocromil sodium versus sodium cromoglycate for preventing exercise-induced bronchoconstriction: a systematic review. *Eur Respir J* 2001;17:39–45
124. Bukstein DA, Bratton DL, Firriolo KM, et al. Evaluation of parental preference for the treatment of asthmatic children aged 6 to 11 years with oral montelukast or inhaled cromolyn: a randomized, open-label, crossover study. *J Asthma* 2003;40:475–485.
125. Van der Wouden JC, Tasche MJA, Bernsen RMD, et al. Sodium cromoglycate for asthma in children. *Cochrane Database Syst Rev* 2003;(3):CD002173.
126. Tasche MJA, van der Wouden JC, Uijen JHJM, et al. Randomised, placebo-controlled trial of inhaled sodium cromoglycate in 1–4-year-old children with moderate asthma. *Lancet* 1997;350:1060–1064.
127. Donahue JG, Weiss ST, Livingston JM, et al. Inhaled steroids and the risk of hospitalization for asthma. *JAMA* 1997;277:887–891.
128. Adams RJ, Fuhlbrigge A, Finkelstein JA, et al. Impact of inhaled antiinflammatory therapy on hospitalization and emergency department visits for children with asthma. *Pediatrics* 2001;107:706.
129. Zileuton extended-release oral tablets (Zyflo CR) package insert. Cary, NC: Chiesi USA, Inc.
130. Zafirlukast (Accolate) package insert. Wilmington, DE: Zeneca Pharmaceuticals, 2007.
131. Montelukast sodium (Singulair) package insert. Whitehouse Station, NJ: Merck & Co., Inc., 2008. https://www.merck.com/product/usa/pi_circulars/s/singulair/singulair_pi.pdf. Accessed June 25, 2020.
132. Wenzel SE. Antileukotriene therapy in asthma. In: Adkinson N, Bochner B, Bursk AW, et al., eds. *Middleton's allergy principles and practice*, 8th ed. Philadelphia, PA: Elsevier Saunders, 2014:100, 1602–1615.
133. Chauhan BF, Ducharme FM. Anti-leukotriene agents compared to inhaled corticosteroids in the management of recurrent and/or chronic asthma in adults and children. *Cochrane Database Syst Rev* 2012;(5):CD002314.
134. Ducharme F, Schwartz Z, Kakuma R. Addition of anti-leukotriene agents to inhaled corticosteroids for chronic asthma. *Cochrane Database Syst Rev* 2004;(1):CD003133.
135. The American Lung Association Asthma Clinical Research Centers. Clinical trial of low-dose theophylline and montelukast in patients with poorly controlled asthma. *Am J Respir Crit Care Med* 2007;175:235–242.
136. Deykin A, Wechsler ME, Boushey HA, et al. Combination therapy with a long-acting β-agonist and a leukotriene antagonist in moderate asthma. *Am J Respir Crit Care Med* 2007;175:228–234.
137. Szefler SJ, Phillips BR, Martinez FD, et al. Characterization of within-subject responses to fluticasone and montelukast in childhood asthma. *J Allergy Clin Immunol* 2005;115:233–242.
138. Israel E, Chervinsky PS, Friedman B, et al. Effects of montelukast and beclomethasone on airway function and asthma control. *J Allergy Clin Immunol* 2002;110:847–854.

139. Knorr B, Franchi LM, Bisgaard H, et al. Montelukast, a leukotriene receptor antagonist, for the treatment of persistent asthma in children aged 2 to 5 years. *Pediatrics* 2001;108(3):E48.
140. Van Adelsberg J, Moy J, Wei LX, et al. Safety, tolerability, and exploratory efficacy of montelukast in 6-to 24-month-old patients with asthma. *Curr Med Res Opin* 2005;21:971–979.
141. Bukstein DA, Luskin AT, Bernstein A. "Real world" effectiveness of daily controller medicine in children with mild persistent asthma. *Ann Allergy Asthma Immunol* 2003;90:543–549.
142. Carter ER, Ananthakrishnan M. Adherence to montelukast versus inhaled corticosteroids in children with asthma. *Pediatr Pulmonol* 2003;36:301–304.
143. Stempel DA, Kruzikas DT, Manjunath R. Comparative efficacy and cost of asthma care in children with asthma treated with fluticasone propionate and montelukast. *J Pediatr* 2007;150:162–167.
144. Peroni DG, Piacentini GL, Ress M, et al. Time efficacy of a single dose of montelukast on exercise-induced asthma in children. *Pediatr Allergy Immunol* 2002;13:434–437.
145. Brodlie M, Gupta A, Rodriguez-Martinez CE, et al. Leukotriene receptor antagonists as maintenance and intermittent therapy for episodic viral wheeze in children. *Cochrane Database Syst Rev* 2015;(10):CD008202.
146. Bacharier LB, Phillips BR, Zeiger RS, et al. Episodic use of an inhaled corticosteroid or leukotriene receptor antagonist in preschool children with moderate-to-severe intermittent wheezing. *J Allergy Clin Immunol* 2008;122(6):1127–1135
147. Katz RS, Papernick M. Zafirlukast and Churg-Strauss syndrome. *JAMA* 1998;279:1949.
148. Solans R, Bosch JA, Selva A, et al. Montelukast and Churg-Strauss syndrome. *Thorax* 2002;57:183–185.
149. Barnes PJ. Theophylline: new perspectives for an old drug. *Am J Respir Crit Care Med* 2003;167:813–818.
150. Adcock IM, Barnes PJ. Molecular mechanisms of corticosteroid resistance. *Chest* 2008;134:394–401.
151. Kelly HW. Non-corticosteroid therapy for the long-term control of asthma. *Expert Opin Pharmacother* 2007;8:2077–2087.
152. Suessmuth S, Freihorst J, Gappa M. Low-dose theophylline in childhood asthma: a placebo-controlled, double-blind study. *Pediatr Allergy Immunol* 2003;14:394–400.
153. Edwards DJ, Zarowitz BJ, Slaughter RL. Theophylline. In: Evans WE, Schentag JJ, Jusko WJ, eds. *Applied pharmacokinetics, principles of therapeutic drug monitoring*, 3rd ed. Vancouver, WA: Applied Therapeutics, 1992:1331–1338.
154. Hamelmann E, Szefler SJ. Efficacy and safety of tiotropium in children and adolescents. *Drugs* 2018;78(3):327–338.
155. Halpin DM, Kaplan AG, Russell RK. Why choose tiotropium for my patient? A comprehensive review of actions and outcomes versus other bronchodilators. *Respir Med* 2017;128:28–41.
156. Tiotropium Product Monograph (Spiriva). https://www.boehringer-ingelheim.ca/sites/ca/files/documents/spirivapmen.pdf. Accessed April 16, 2019.
157. Vogelberg C, Moroni-Zentgraf P, Leonaviciute-Klimantaviciene M, et al. A randomised dose-ranging study of tiotropium Respimat® in children with symptomatic asthma despite inhaled corticosteroids. *Respir Res* 2015;16:20. doi:186/s12931-015-0175-9.
158. Szefler SJ, Murphy K, Harper T 3rd, et al. A phase III randomized controlled trial of tiotropium add-on therapy in children with severe symptomatic asthma. *J Allergy Clin Immunol* 2017;140(5):1277–1287.
159. Vrijlandt EJLE, El Azzi G, Vandewalker M, et al. Safety and efficacy of tiotropium in children aged 1–5 years with persistent asthmatic symptoms: a randomised, double-blind, placebo-controlled trial. *Lancet Respir Med* 2018;6(2):127–137.
160. Szefler SJ, Vogelberg C, Bernstein JA, et al. Tiotropium is efficacious in 6–17-year-olds with asthma, independent of T2 phenotype. *J Allergy Clin Immunol Pract* 2019;7(7):2286.e4–2295.e4.
161. Peters SP, Bleecker ER, Kunselman SJ, et al. Predictors of response to tiotropium versus salmeterol in asthmatic adults. *J Allergy Clin Immunol* 2013;132(5):1068–1074.
162. Hoch H, Anderson WC, Szefler SJ. Modern molecular therapies for application in managing childhood asthma. In: Wilmott RW, Deterding R, Li A, et al., eds. *Kendig disorders of the respiratory tract in children*, 9th ed. St. Louis, MO: Elsevier Inc., 2019: 747–755.
163. Abrams EM, Becker AB, Szefler SJ. Current state and future of biologic therapies in the treatment of asthma in children. *Pediatr Allergy Immunol Pulmonol* 2018;31(3):119–131.
164. Holgate S, Smith N, Massanari M, et al. Effects of omalizumab on markers of inflammation in patients with allergic asthma. *Allergy* 2009;64(12):1728–1736.
165. Noga O, Hanf G, Brachmann I, et al. Effect of omalizumab treatment on peripheral eosinophil and T-lymphocyte function in patients with allergic asthma. *J Allergy Clin Immunol* 2006;117(6):1493–1499.
166. Hanf G, Brachmann I, Kleine-Tebbe J, et al. Omalizumab decreased IgE-release and induced changes in cellular immunity in patients with allergic asthma. *Allergy* 2006;61(9):1141–1144.
167. Mauri P, Riccio AM, Rossi R, et al. Proteomics of bronchial biopsies: galectin-3 as a predictive biomarker of airway remodelling modulation in omalizumab-treated severe asthma patients. *Immunol Lett* 2014;162(1 Pt A):2–10.
168. Teach SJ, Gill MA, Togias A, et al. Preseasonal treatment with either omalizumab or an inhaled corticosteroid boost to prevent fall asthma exacerbations. *J Allergy Clin Immunol* 2015;136(6):1476–1485.
169. Smith DA, Minthorn EA, Beerahee M. Pharmacokinetics and pharmacodynamics of mepolizumab, an anti-interleukin-5 monoclonal antibody. *Clin Pharmacokinet* 2011;50(4):215–227.
170. Lopez AF, Sanderson CJ, Gamble JR, et al. Recombinant human interleukin 5 is a selective activator of human eosinophil function. *J Exp Med* 1988;167(1):219–224.
171. Rosenberg HF, Phipps S, Foster PS. Eosinophil trafficking in allergy and asthma. *J Allergy Clin Immunol* 2007;119(6):1302–1303.
172. Berair R, Pavord ID. Rationale and clinical results of inhibiting interleukin-5 for the treatment of severe asthma. *Curr Allergy Asthma Rep* 2013;13(5):469–476.
173. Varricchi G, Bagnasco D, Borriello F, et al. Interleukin-5 pathway inhibition in the treatment of eosinophilic respiratory disorders: evidence and unmet needs. *Curr Opin Allergy Clin Immunol* 2016;16(2):186–200.
174. Leckie MJ, ten Brinke A, Khan J, et al. Effects of an interleukin-5 blocking monoclonal antibody on eosinophils, airway hyper-responsiveness, and the late asthmatic response. *Lancet* 2000;356(9248):2144–2148.
175. Flood-Page PT, Menzies-Gow AN, Kay AB, et al. Eosinophil's role remains uncertain as anti-interleukin-5 only partially depletes numbers in asthmatic airway. *Am J Respir Crit Care Med* 2003;167(2):199–204.
176. Stein ML, Villanueva JM, Buckmeier BK, et al. Anti-IL-5 (mepolizumab) therapy reduces eosinophil activation ex vivo and increases IL-5 and IL-5 receptor levels. *J Allergy Clin Immunol* 2008;121(6):1473–1483.
177. Haldar P, Brightling CE, Hargadon B, et al. Mepolizumab and exacerbations of refractory eosinophilic asthma. *N Engl J Med* 2009;360(10):973–984.
178. Nair P, Pizzichini MMM, Kjarsgaard M, et al. Mepolizumab for prednisone-Dependent Asthma With Sputum Eosinophilia. *N Engl J Med* 2009;5;360(10):985-993.
179. Pavord ID, Korn S, Howarth P, et al. Mepolizumab for severe eosinophilic asthma (DREAM): a multicentre, double-blind, placebo-controlled trial. *Lancet* 2012;380(9842):651–659.
180. Menzies-Gow A, Flood-Page P, Sehmi R, et al. Anti-IL-5 (mepolizumab) therapy induces bone marrow eosinophil maturational arrest and decreases eosinophil progenitors in the bronchial mucosa of atopic asthmatics. *J Allergy Clin Immunol* 2003;111(4):714–719.
181. Matera MG, Calzetta L, Rinaldi B, et al. Pharmacokinetic/pharmacodynamic drug evaluation of benralizumab for the treatment of asthma. *Expert Opin Drug Metab Toxicol* 2017;13(9):1007–1013.
182. Kolbeck R, Kozhich A, Koike M, et al. MEDI-563, a humanized anti-IL-5 receptor alpha mAb with enhanced antibody-dependent cell-mediated cytotoxicity function. *J Allergy Clin Immunol* 2010;125(6):1344–1353.
183. Barranco P, Phillips-Angles E, Dominguez-Ortega J, et al. Dupilumab in the management of moderate-to-severe asthma: the data so far. *Ther Clin Risk Manag* 2017;13:1139–1149.
184. Vatrella A, Fabozzi I, Calabrese C, et al. Dupilumab: a novel treatment for asthma. *J Asthma Allergy* 2014;7:123–130.
185. Hendeles L, Sorkness CA. Anti-immunoglobulin E therapy with omalizumab for asthma. *Ann Pharmacother* 2007;41(9):1397–1410.
186. Luu M, Bardou M, Bonniaud P, et al. Pharmacokinetics, pharmacodynamics and clinical efficacy of omalizumab for the treatment of asthma. *Expert Opin Drug Metab Toxicol* 2016;12(12):1503–1511.
187. Omalizumab (XOLAIR) Monograph. https://pdfs.semanticscholar.org/38f8/e33927f24312052df35a25fb2e483f2c192c.pdf. Accessed April 12, 2019.
188. Onizawa Y, Noguchi E, Okada M, et al. The association of the delayed introduction of cow's milk with IgE-mediated cow's milk allergies. *J Allergy Clin Immunol Pract* 2016;4(3):481.e2–488.e2.
189. Lowe PJ, Tannenbaum S, Gautier A, et al. Relationship between omalizumab pharmacokinetics, IgE pharmacodynamics and symptoms in patients with severe persistent allergic (IgE-mediated) asthma. *Br J Clin Pharmacol* 2009;68(1):61–76.
190. Matera MG, Rogliani P, Calzetta L, et al. Pharmacokinetic/pharmacodynamic profile of reslizumab in asthma. *Expert Opin Drug Metab Toxicol* 2018;14(2):239–245.
191. Kips JC, O'Connor BJ, Langley SJ, et al. Effect of SCH55700, a humanized anti-human interleukin-5 antibody, in severe persistent asthma: a pilot study. *Am J Respir Crit Care Med* 2003;167(12):1655–1659.
192. Reslizumab PRODUCT MONOGRAph (TEVA). https://www.cinqair.com/globalassets/cinqair/prescribinginformation.pdf. Accessed June 25, 2020.
193. Benralizumab Product Monograph. https://www.astrazeneca.ca/content/dam/az-ca/downloads/productinformation/fasenra-product-monograph-en.pdf. Accessed April 12, 2019.
194. Laviolette M, Gossage DL, Gauvreau G, et al. Effects of benralizumab on airway eosinophils in asthmatic patients with sputum eosinophilia. *J Allergy Clin Immunol* 2013;132(5):1086–1096.
195. FDA. Dupilumab. https://www.accessdata.fda.gov/drugsatfda_docs/label/2017/761055lbl.pdf. Accessed April 12, 2019.
196. FDA Omalizumab Monograph. https://www.gene.com/download/pdf/xolair_prescribing.pdf. Accessed June 25, 2020.
197. Brodlie M, McKean MC, Moss S, et al. The oral corticosteroid-sparing effect of omalizumab in children with severe asthma. *Arch Dis Child* 2012;97(7):604–609.
198. Deschildre A, Marguet C, Salleron J, et al. Add-on omalizumab in children with severe allergic asthma: a 1-year real life survey. *Eur Respir J* 2013;42(5):1224–1233.
199. Busse WW, Morgan WJ, Gergen PJ, et al. Randomized trial of omalizumab (anti-IgE) for asthma in inner-city children. *N Engl J Med* 2011;364(11):1005–1015.
200. Lanier B, Bridges T, Kulus M, et al. Omalizumab for the treatment of exacerbations in children with inadequately controlled allergic (IgE-mediated) asthma. *J Allergy Clin Immunol* 2009;124(6):1210–1216.
201. Milgrom H, Berger W, Nayak A, et al. Treatment of childhood asthma with anti-immunoglobulin E antibody (omalizumab). *Pediatrics* 2001;108(2):E36.
202. Hanania NA, Alpan O, Hamilos DL, et al. Omalizumab in severe allergic asthma inadequately controlled with standard therapy: a randomized trial. *Ann Intern Med* 2011;154(9):573–582.
203. Wildfire JJ, Gergen PJ, Sorkness CA, et al. Development and validation of the Composite Asthma Severity Index—an outcome measure for use in children and adolescents. *J Allergy Clin Immunol* 2012;129(3):694–701.
204. (ICER) I for C and ER. Biologic therapies for treatment of asthma associated with type 2 inflammation: effectiveness, value, and value-based price benchmarks. https://icer-review.org/wp-content/uploads/2018/04/ICER_Asthma_Draft_Report_092418v1.pdf. Accessed June 25, 2020.
205. Anderson WC 3rd, Szefler SJ. To biologic or not to biologic?: the question of cost-effectiveness. *Ann Allergy Asthma Immunol* 2019;122(4):367–372. doi:10.1016/j.anai.2019.01.018.
206. McQueen RB, Sheehan DN, Whittington MD, et al. Cost-effectiveness of biological asthma treatments: a systematic review and recommendations for future economic evaluations. *Pharmacoeconomics* 2018;36(8):957–971.

207. Mepolizumab Product Monograph (GSK). https://ca.gsk.com/media/1209435/nucala.pdf. Accessed April 12, 2019.
208. Ortega HG, Liu MC, Pavord ID, et al. Mepolizumab treatment in patients with severe eosinophilic asthma. *N Engl J Med* 2014;371(13):1198–1207.
209. Bel EH, Wenzel SE, Thompson PJ, et al. Oral glucocorticoid-sparing effect of mepolizumab in eosinophilic asthma. *N Engl J Med* 2014;371(13):1189–1197.
210. Flood-Page P, Swenson C, Faiferman I, et al. A study to evaluate safety and efficacy of mepolizumab in patients with moderate persistent asthma. *Am J Respir Crit Care Med* 2007;176(11):1062–1071.
211. Whittington MD, McQueen RB, Ollendorf DA, et al. Assessing the value of mepolizumab for severe eosinophilic asthma: a cost-effectiveness analysis. *Ann Allergy Asthma Immunol* 2017;118(2):220–225.
212. Bjermer L, Lemiere C, Maspero J, et al. Reslizumab for inadequately controlled asthma with elevated blood eosinophil levels: a randomized phase 3 study. *Chest* 2016;150(4):789–798.
213. Castro M, Zangrilli J, Wechsler ME, et al. Reslizumab for inadequately controlled asthma with elevated blood eosinophil counts: results from two multicentre, parallel, double-blind, randomised, placebo-controlled, phase 3 trials. *Lancet Respir Med* 2015;3(5):355–366.
214. FDA. Reslizumab. https://www.fda.gov/downloads/Drugs/DevelopmentApprovalProcess/DevelopmentResources/UCM499687.pdf. Accessed April 12, 2019.
215. Corren J, Weinstein S, Janka L, et al. Phase 3 study of reslizumab in patients with poorly controlled asthma: effects across a broad range of eosinophil counts. *Chest* 2016;150(4):799–810.
216. U.S. Food and Drug Administration. FDA benralizumab. https://www.accessdata.fda.gov/drugsatfda_docs/nda/2017/761070Orig1s000TOC.cfm. Accessed April 12, 2019.
217. Bleecker ER, FitzGerald JM, Chanez P, et al. Efficacy and safety of benralizumab for patients with severe asthma uncontrolled with high-dosage inhaled corticosteroids and long-acting beta2-agonists (SIROCCO): a randomised, multicentre, placebo-controlled phase 3 trial. *Lancet* 2016;388(10056):2115–2127.
218. FitzGerald JM, Bleecker ER, Nair P, et al. Benralizumab, an anti-interleukin-5 receptor alpha monoclonal antibody, as add-on treatment for patients with severe, uncontrolled, eosinophilic asthma (CALIMA): a randomised, double-blind, placebo-controlled phase 3 trial. *Lancet* 2016;388(10056):2128–2141.
219. Goldman M, Hirsch I, Zangrilli JG, et al. The association between blood eosinophil count and benralizumab efficacy for patients with severe, uncontrolled asthma: subanalyses of the Phase III SIROCCO and CALIMA studies. *Curr Med Res Opin* 2017;33(9):1605–1613.
220. FitzGerald JM, Bleecker ER, Menzies-Gow A, et al. Predictors of enhanced response with benralizumab for patients with severe asthma: pooled analysis of the SIROCCO and CALIMA studies. *Lancet Respir Med* 2018;6(1):51–64.
221. Castro M, Corren J, Pavord ID, et al. dupilumab efficacy and safety in moderate-to-severe uncontrolled asthma. *N Engl J Med* 2018;378(26):2486–2496.
222. Lai T, Wang S, Xu Z, et al. Long-term efficacy and safety of omalizumab in patients with persistent uncontrolled allergic asthma: a systematic review and meta-analysis. *Sci Rep* 2015;5:8191. doi:10.1038/srep08191.
223. Limb SL, Starke PR, Lee CE, et al. Delayed onset and protracted progression of anaphylaxis after omalizumab administration in patients with asthma. *J Allergy Clin Immunol* 2007;120(6):1378–1381.
224. Long A, Rahmaoui A, Rothman KJ, et al. Incidence of malignancy in patients with moderate-to-severe asthma treated with or without omalizumab. *J Allergy Clin Immunol* 2014;134(3):560.e4–567.e4.
225. Khatri S, Moore W, Gibson PG, et al. Assessment of the long-term safety of mepolizumab and durability of clinical response in patients with severe eosinophilic asthma. *J Allergy Clin Immunol* 2019;43(5):1742.e7–1751.e7. doi:10.1016/j.jaci.2018.09.033.
226. Hussar DA, Dimaculangan CA. Reslizumab, ixekizumab, and pimavanserin tartrate. *J Am Pharm Assoc (2003)* 2016;56(5):595–598.

CHAPTER

42

Burkhard Tönshoff
Britta Höcker

Immunosuppressive and Immunomodulatory Drugs

INTRODUCTION

Organ transplantation has been performed successfully in infants, children, and adolescents for over five decades and is the standard of care for end-stage organ disease. In many centers across the world, increasing numbers of kidney, heart, liver, and other solid-organ transplants are being performed. The goal of organ transplantation has been to achieve long-term patient and graft survival. This has been possible as a result of major advances in understanding immunobiology, use of novel immunosuppressive and immunomodulatory drug regimens, advancement of operative techniques in transplant surgery, and the development of anti-infective agents for the prevention of infectious complications. To understand the basis of immunosuppressive protocols and rationalize current transplantation practices, a brief history of transplant immunosuppression is provided.

HISTORICAL OVERVIEW

Major advances in immunosuppressive therapy can be related to a surge in the interest in organ transplantation after World War II. Alexis Carrel made the early observation that allografts were quickly destroyed, whereas autotransplants maintained long-term graft function. He surmised that allograft loss was due to biologic phenomena rather than technical problems.[1] Modern transplant immunology developed in the 1940s with Gibson and Medawar's work established an immune basis for graft rejection and the need for immunosuppressive therapy.[2] Initial efforts at immunosuppression with total body irradiation yielded very poor results. In 1954, the first successful live-donor kidney transplant was performed between identical twins by Murray et al.[3]

The era of drug therapy for immunosuppression was launched after Schwartz and Dameshek[4] demonstrated drug-assisted tolerance using 6-mercaptopurine (6-MP) in 1959. Its analog, azathioprine (AZA), in combination with glucocorticoids, formed the mainstay of early immunosuppressive protocols in the 1960s. The addition of polyclonal antibodies in the 1970s marked the introduction of biologic agents.[5] Much of the current success of organ transplantation can be attributed to discovery of the potent immunosuppressive agent cyclosporin A (CsA) by Borel in 1972.[6] The widespread clinical use of CsA in the early 1980s increased 1-year renal graft survival from about 50% to more than 80%. OKT3, the first monoclonal antibody (MAb) to be used in clinical transplantation, gained widespread acceptance despite its side effects in the middle of the 1980s as an adjunct to CsA, AZA, and prednisone (PRED). In the 1990s, the immunosuppressive armamentarium expanded rapidly with addition of mycophenolate mofetil (MMF), tacrolimus (TAC), and murine as well as humanized interleukin-2 receptor (IL-2R) MAbs. In 1999, sirolimus (SRL) was introduced, and in 2003, its analog everolimus (EVR), which has similar effectiveness and side-effect profile as SRL, but different pharmacokinetics (shorter half-life). In the 21st century, both drugs became a rescue agent in patients with calcineurin inhibitor (CNI)–induced nephrotoxicity. Table 42.1 summarizes the

TABLE 42.1 Landmarks in Each Decade in the History of Transplant Immunosuppression

Year in Transplant History	*Milestone in Transplant Immunosuppression*
1950s	Successful live-donor kidney transplant between identical twins
1960s	Introduction of azathioprine and use in combination with corticosteroids
1970s	Availability of antithymocyte globulin (ATG) and antilymphocyte globulin (ALG)
1980s	Cyclosporine introduction
1985	Use of OKT3, first monoclonal antibody
1990s	Tacrolimus, mycophenolate mofetil, daclizumab, and basiliximab availability
1999	Sirolimus introduction
2000s	Introduction of steroid and calcineurin inhibitor-avoidance/sparing protocols
2003	Everolimus introduction
2003	Rituximab introduction
2011	Belatacept introduction

major historical landmarks in transplant immunosuppression over the past several decades.

Advances in the pharmacology of these drugs, along with widespread use of therapeutic drug monitoring (TDM), have resulted in increased antirejection efficacy and reduced toxicity while ensuring high graft survival rates and overall improvements in the quality of life for transplant recipients. The current decade has focused on adding novel biologic agents to achieve improved long-term patient and graft survival. On the other hand, the concept of tolerance or near-tolerance is fast emerging. Current immunosuppressive agents reduce acute rejection, but do not induce tolerance. It is true that a few patients with organ transplants successfully can withdraw their immunosuppression without rejecting their grafts for long periods of time. However, these are rare exceptions, and such patients may eventually reject, even after years. Even though antigen-specific T cells with reactivity to the foreign antigen persist in the host indefinitely, some graft-and-host adaptation must occur, since the level of immunosuppression required long term is very low compared to the levels required within the first weeks. This adaptation makes long-term immunosuppression possible; however, the long-term risk of cancer in the immunosuppressed patient remains increased. Thus, the distinction between immunosuppression and tolerance induction is partly artificial: any immunosuppression involves some apparent antigen-specific adaptation, that is, downregulation of the host response to the graft; and many tolerance protocols involve some nonspecific immunosuppressive therapies. Now, the goal of transplantation is to achieve a state where the graft continues to function well with minimal immunosuppression to avoid side effects of immunosuppressants, such as post-transplant infections, malignancies, and increased cardiovascular risk. Thus, achieving a balance between over- and under-immunosuppression has become an important task in the advancement of organ transplantation.

Pediatric solid-organ transplants constituted only 5.2% of the 36,529 transplants performed in the United States in 2018.[7] The recent U.S. Renal Data System (USRDS) data documents that, as of December 31, 2016, the point prevalence of children and adolescents, 0 to 21 years of age, with end-stage renal disease (ESRD) was 9,721, or 99.1 per million population.[8] Twenty percent of incident and 72% of prevalent children and adolescents with ESRD have kidney transplants, in 2016. Despite this low incidence and prevalence, more data are becoming available on the pharmacology of immunosuppressants in children. For newer therapies, few studies exist, and only limited data are available in the pediatric population. Although many drugs have immunosuppressive properties, this chapter focuses on those agents primarily used as immunosuppressants for organ transplantation in children. A detailed discussion of the pharmacology of other drugs that may also have immunosuppressive and immunomodulatory properties, such as chemotherapeutic agents and biologics, can be found in other sections of this book.

CLASSIFICATION

Immunosuppressive and immunomodulatory drugs can be pharmacologically categorized on the basis of their mechanism of action. The three-signal model of T-cell activation and proliferation is helpful in understanding the molecular mechanisms and site of action of various immunosuppressive drugs.[9,10] Signal 1 features antigen-presenting cells (APCs; macrophages and dendritic cells) presenting the foreign antigen to the T lymphocyte, activating the T-cell receptor (TCR), which further relays the signal through the transduction apparatus known as the CD3 complex. Signal 2 is a nonantigen-specific costimulatory signal which occurs as a result of binding of the B7 molecule on the APC to CD28 on the T cell. Both signal 1 and signal 2 activate signal transduction pathways: the calcium–calcineurin pathway, mitogen-activated protein (MAP) pathway, and the nuclear factor-κB (NF-κB) pathway. This, in turn, leads to increased expression of IL-2, which through its receptor (IL-2R) activates the cell cycle (signal 3). Signal 3 activation requires the enzyme target of rapamycin for translation of messenger RNA (mRNA) and cell proliferation. Thus, various drugs act on different cellular signals and achieve immunosuppression by a number of mechanisms: depleting lymphocytes, diverting lymphocyte traffic, or blocking lymphocyte response pathways. Table 42.2 lists the immunosuppressive drugs and their mechanism of action. Figure 42.1 depicts a schematic representation of the three-signal model along with the site of action of common immunosuppressive drugs.

Immunosuppressive agents are also classified on the basis of the phase of transplantation for which they are used (Table 42.3). Different immunosuppressive drugs are used for induction versus maintenance of immunosuppression, while others may be used for the treatment and reversal of graft rejection. The commonly used agents in immunosuppressive protocols are discussed in greater detail in the following section.

TABLE 42.2 Immunosuppressive Agents Categorized According to Mechanism of Action

Mechanism of Action	*Drugs*
Polyclonal antibodies	Antithymocyte globulin
	Thymoglobulin (rabbit)
	ATGAM (equine)
Monoclonal antibodies	Anti-CD3 antibody: OKT3 (murine)
	Anti-CD52 antibody: Alemtuzumab (human)
	Anti-CD20 antibody: Rituximab
	Anti-CD25 antibody: Daclizumab (human), Basiliximab (chimeric)
	Selective blocker of CD86-CD28 costimulation: Belatacept
Calcineurin inhibitors	Cyclosporine
	Tacrolimus
Target of rapamycin inhibitors	Sirolimus
	Everolimus
Antimetabolites	Azathioprine
Purine synthesis inhibitors	Mycophenolate mofetil
Others	Glucocorticoids
	Intravenous immunoglobulin G

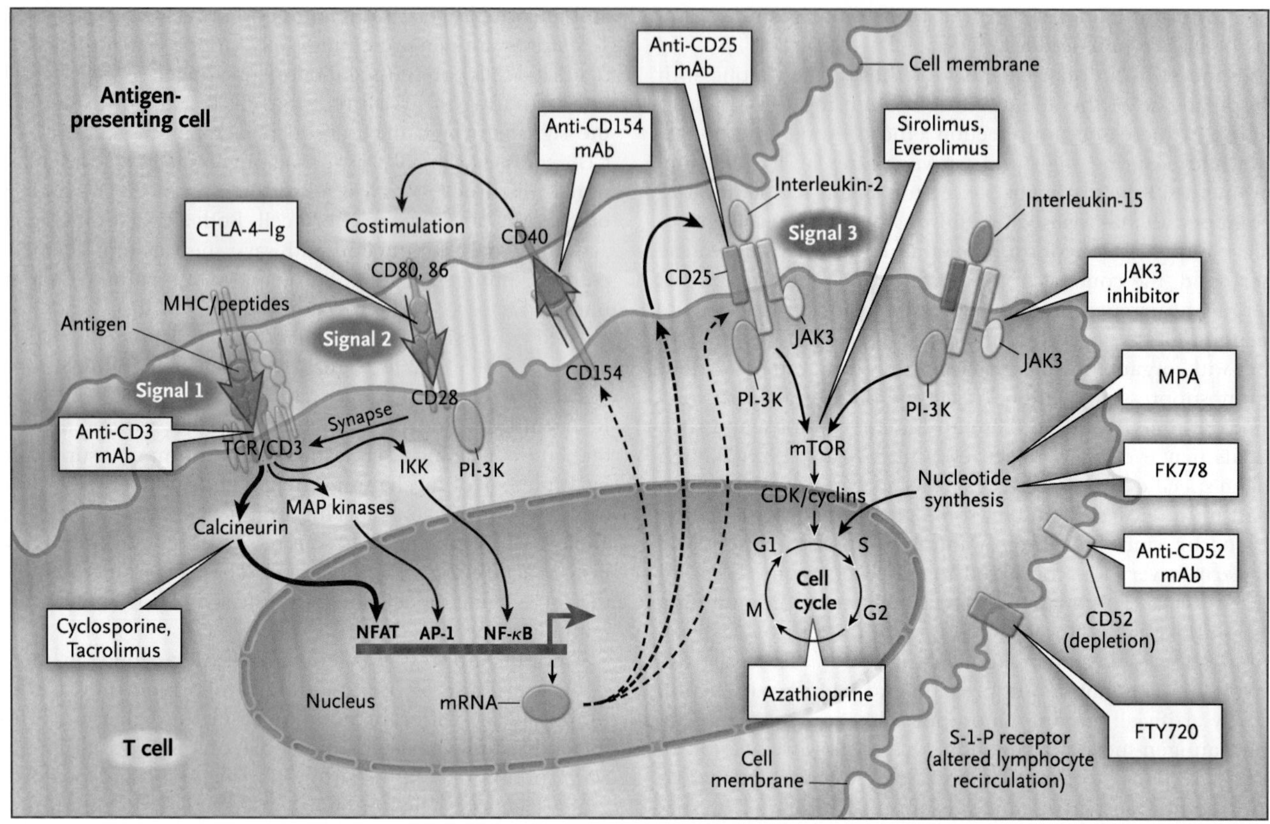

Figure 42.1 Individual immunosuppressive drugs and sites of action in the three-signal model. Anti-CD154 antibody has been withdrawn from clinical trials but remains of interest. FTY720 engagement of sphingosine-1-phosphate (S-1-P) receptors triggers and internalizes the receptors and alters lymphocyte recirculation, causing lymphopenia. Antagonists of chemokine receptors (not shown) are also being developed in preclinical models. MPA, mycophenolic acid. (Modified according to Halloran PF. Immunosuppressive drugs for kidney transplantation. *N Engl J Med* 2004;351:2715–2729.)

TABLE 42.3 Immunosuppressive Agents Categorized According to Phase of Immunosuppression

Phase of Immunosuppression	*Drugs*
Induction phase	Basiliximab
	Thymoglobulin
	Glucocorticoids
Maintenance phase	Tacrolimus
	Cyclosporine
	Mycophenolate mofetil, azathioprine
	Sirolimus, everolimus
	Glucocorticoids
	Belatacept
Treatment of rejection	Glucocorticoids
	Thymoglobulin
	Intravenous immunoglobulin G
	Rituximab

CALCINEURIN INHIBITORS

The two drugs in the class of CNIs, CsA and TAC, form the backbone of current immunosuppressive protocols (Table 42.2). They share a common mechanism of action, although they differ markedly in their biochemical structure and properties. CsA revolutionized immunosuppressive therapy for solid-organ transplantation after the U.S. Food and Drug Administration (FDA) approved it in 1983. Before the introduction of CsA, there was a failure rate of 50% of renal grafts by 1 year as compared with 80% 1-year graft survival following CsA incorporation into most immunosuppressive protocols.[11] TAC, which came into use in the 1990s, is 10 to 100 times more potent on a molar basis and has increased antirejection efficacy. It has a slightly different side-effect profile when compared with CsA.[12] TAC was used initially in liver transplantation and subsequently in renal transplantation. Currently, the vast majority of the renal, liver, and pancreas transplants, and virtually all small bowel transplants, are being performed using TAC-based protocols.

Chemistry

CsA is a nonpolar, hydrophobic, small cyclic polypeptide antibiotic produced by the fungi *Beauveria nivea* (formerly *Tolypocladium inflatum* Gams or *Trichoderma polysporum*) and *Cylindrocarpon lucidum* Booth. It has a molecular weight of 1,203 with 11 amino acids. Amino acids at the 1, 2, 3, and 11 positions form the active site, and its cyclic structure is critical for immunosuppression. TAC is a macrolide antibiotic with limited antimicrobial activity that is derived from the fungus *Streptomyces tsukubaensis*, originally isolated from a soil sample taken from the base of Mount Tsukuba in Japan.

Mechanism of Action and Pharmacologic Effects

T cells are stimulated by binding of an antigen to the TCR–CD3 complex (signal 1; Fig. 42.1). This leads to intracellular release of Ca^{2+} and causes Ca^{2+}/calmodulin-dependent activation of calcineurin, a serine/threonine phosphatase. The phosphatase activity of calcineurin is crucial to the dephosphorylation of a nuclear regulatory protein known as the nuclear factor of activated T cells, which allows it to translocate into the nucleus and activate, directly or indirectly, transcription of genes encoding critical cytokines important in initiating the immune response, including IL-2, IL-4, interferon-γ (IFN-γ), and tumor necrosis factor α (TNF-α).[13,14]

Despite differences in molecular structure, both CsA and TAC bind to ubiquitous cytosolic proteins called "immunophilins." CsA binds to cyclophilin, and TAC, previously known as FK506, binds to the FK-binding protein FKBP12. These drug–immunophilin complexes bind to a calcineurin–calmodulin–calcium complex resulting in noncompetitive inhibition of calcineurin's phosphatase activity, thereby blocking the immune response. IL-2 is the most important T-cell growth factor and acts in an autocrine as well as paracrine manner.[13,14] Thus, as a result of calcineurin inhibition, there is marked decrease in IL-2 production and downstream lymphocyte proliferation. Since T cells contain relatively low levels of calcineurin, CNIs are potent and selective inhibitors of T-cell activation. At therapeutic drug levels, calcineurin activity is reduced by about 50%.[15] Although TAC is 10- to 100-fold more active than CsA on a molecular level, TAC does not inhibit secondary proliferation of activated T cells in response to IL-2.[12,16] It also does not appear to modify mononuclear phagocyte or natural killer cell function.[16]

Other well-described effects of CsA include increased transforming growth factor β (TGF-β) production, sympathetic activation, vasoconstriction, increased plasma endothelin-1 levels, and upregulation of angiotensin-II receptors on vascular smooth muscle. These actions may explain some of the side effects of the drug, such as arterial hypertension. Enhancement of TGF-β expression may contribute not only to immunosuppressive activity but also to renal interstitial fibrosis[17] and development of post-transplant neoplasia.

Pharmacokinetics

The pharmacokinetics of both CsA and TAC is characterized by high interindividual and intraindividual variability and a narrow therapeutic index. Thus, TDM is essential to identify under-immunosuppression resulting in graft failure as well as over-immunosuppression leading to toxicity, infections, and/or malignancy.

Cyclosporin

Absorption

CsA is primarily absorbed from the upper small intestine, with no apparent absorption from the colon.[18] The original oil-based formulation of CsA was approved by the FDA in 1983 and was characterized by wide interpatient and intrapatient variation in its bioavailability, especially in young children. The absorption of oral Sandimmune™ is highly bile dependent; thus, absorption is unpredictable in patients with liver transplant, cholestasis, biliary disorder, diarrhea, and malabsorption. A microemulsion formulation (Neoral™) was approved in 1995 because of its better absorption profile, since it is less dependent on bile, food, or other factors for its dispersion. Food tends to increase the absorption of CsA, and its bioavailability also increases with time post-transplant, possibly because of improved absorption from the nonuremic gut in the post-transplant period. Bowel length, interaction with other drugs, presystemic metabolism in the gut wall, and type of transplant are all contributing factors to the variation of bioavailability patterns in pediatric transplant patients.

Bioavailability of oral preparations averages 30% to 45%; hence, a 1:3 ratio is used to convert intravenous to oral dosing. Time to peak blood concentration (T_{max}) ranges between 1 and 4 hours depending on the formulation, patient age, transplant type, and time after transplant. In general, Neoral™ shows a faster peak and greater area under the curve (AUC) when compared with Sandimmune™.

Distribution

CsA is widely distributed to tissues outside the intravascular space. In the blood, up to 50% of the drug is in erythrocytes, about 40% is in plasma, and the rest is in other cells.[19] Plasma CsA is 90% protein bound, mostly to low-density lipoproteins.[19] The binding of low-density lipoprotein receptor with CsA is implicated as a cause of hyperlipidemia in transplant patients. On the other hand, lipoprotein binding is important for transfer of CsA across plasma membranes, and toxic effects may be reduced by lowering cholesterol levels. The volume of distribution (V_d) of CsA is 3 to 5 L per kg[19] and does not appear to differ between pediatric and adult transplant recipients. However, systemic clearance is comparatively higher in the pediatric population, with the highest clearance in infants.[20] The half-life of parent drug is approximately 8 hours.

Metabolism

CsA is extensively metabolized by the cytochrome P450 3A4 (CYP3A4) system in the liver and, to some extent, in the gastrointestinal tract and kidneys. The intestinal CYP3A4 and P-glycoprotein (P-gp), a drug efflux pump on the luminal surface of the intestinal epithelium, are responsible for first-pass metabolism.[21,22] Marked interindividual and ethnic differences in activity of these enzyme systems, due to genetic polymorphisms, account for reduced and variable oral absorption.[23]

The liver is the primary site of drug metabolism, but gastrointestinal metabolism may contribute up to half of CsA metabolism. CsA may be metabolized to more than 25 compounds, although most of the immunosuppressive activity and toxicity is attributable to the parent drug. Some CsA metabolites may have nephrotoxic and immunosuppressive potential, and one of the metabolites, M17, exhibits plasma levels similar to the parent compound. Excretion is primarily via the biliary route, and only about 6% of the dose is excreted in the urine.[19] In cases of renal dysfunction, the dose does not require modification. Also, CsA is not dialyzable and can be given during dialysis without dose modification. CsA crosses the placenta and is distributed in mother's milk, but it does not cross the blood–brain barrier.

Dosing

The usual initial oral dose of CsA is 8 to 12 mg per kg per day, given in two to three divided doses during the induction phase, with target trough levels of 150 to 300 ng per mL. Higher doses are needed in the immediate post-transplant period to maintain higher blood levels (see later discussion) in the face of decreased absorption, which improves with time. Some authors recommend 300 mg per m^2 body surface area (BSA) as daily dose in children, with whole-blood concentrations within the range of 150 to 250 ng per mL for the first 6 weeks and 100 to 200 ng per mL thereafter.[24] In general, pediatric patients require higher doses of CsA per kilogram of body weight to achieve target whole-blood concentrations of drug equivalent to that used in the adults. Younger patients (<8 years of age) may be managed more effectively with a thrice-daily administration schedule rather than the conventional twice-daily dosing used in the older pediatric and adult transplant populations.[20] The comparatively higher doses and more frequent administration schedule used in pediatric transplant recipients are a consequence of age-related differences in bioavailability and increased metabolic clearance of the drug in younger patients.[20] Several generic formulations of CsA are now available that have been deemed bioequivalent to Neoral by the FDA. However, bioavailability may vary; therefore, switching between different formulations is not recommended.[25]

Tacrolimus

Absorption

TAC shares many pharmacokinetic features with CsA but has its own unique characteristics as well. TAC is rapidly absorbed from the small intestine, when administered orally. Peak levels are reached within 1 to 2 hours.[26] Unlike Sandimmune™, its absorption is bile independent, thus making it the preferred agent in liver transplant patients. In spite of its relative effectiveness and consistency of absorption, the drug has poor oral bioavailability (25% on average). TAC has wide interpatient and intrapatient variability[27,28] due to extensive first-pass metabolism in the gastrointestinal tract and liver similar to that of CsA.[29] Intravenous-to-oral conversion is, therefore, estimated by a 1:4 or 1:5 dose ratio. Pharmacokinetic profiling demonstrates both prolonged T_{max} and low C_{max} values following oral administration, indicating slow and poor absorption.[30] The concomitant presence of food decreases both C_{max} and AUC. Gastric emptying of solids is faster in patients receiving TAC as compared with CsA, an effect that may be beneficial for patients with gastric motility disorders. Also, of interest is the role of transporter proteins, P-gp in the gut wall, which results in up to 50% of drug being excreted back into the lumen.[31] This explains why drug concentrations tend to be higher during episodes of diarrhea, as the injured gut wall loses transporter capacity.

Distribution

In the blood, TAC is highly bound to erythrocytes, partly accounting for its extensive V_d. Indeed, V_d ranges from 2.6 to 2.76 L per kg in pediatric liver transplant patients based on whole-blood levels.[28,29,32] Seventy-two percent to 98% of plasma TAC is bound to plasma proteins.[29] This is unlike CsA, which is more bound to lipoproteins, and hence, TAC causes less hyperlipidemia than CsA.

Metabolism

Genetic polymorphisms in genes encoding TAC-metabolizing enzymes partly explain the interpatient variability in TAC pharmacokinetics.[33] The key enzymes involved in the metabolism of TAC are CYP3A4 and CYP3A5.[34] Individuals are considered expressers of CYP3A5 if they carry at least one CYP3A5*1 allele, whereas individuals homozygous for the CYP3A5*3 allele are classified as CYP3A5 nonexpressers. In addition to CYP3A5*3, the CYP3A5*6 and CYP3A5*7 variant alleles can also lead to nonfunctional CYP3A5 protein.[35] There are also ethnic distribution differences of CYP3A5 variant alleles, with expressers (carriers of the CYP3A5*1 variant allele) being more frequently found among non-Caucasian populations. Approximately 10% to 40% of Caucasians are CYP3A5 expressers, 33% of Asians, and 55% of African Americans.[36] CYP3A5 expressers require a TAC dose that is approximately 1.5- to 2-fold higher than nonexpressers to reach the same exposure.[37,38] This implies that following a standard, body weight–based TAC dose, CYP3A5 expressers are prone to have subtherapeutic TAC concentrations, whereas nonexpressers are expected to have supratherapeutic TAC concentrations.[39]

TAC is primarily metabolized via demethylation and hydroxylation into 10 metabolites or more. Although some metabolites may have biologic activity, most of the immunosuppressive activity and toxicity is due to parent drug. The terminal elimination half-life of TAC ranges between 4 and 41 hours. Clearance is mainly via biliary excretion, whereas urinary excretion is negligible and no dose change is required in patients with renal dysfunction. Temporary elevation of TAC trough concentrations (about twofold and more) has been observed in patients with diarrhea.[40] This may be because intestinal P-gp activity is impaired in patients with persistent diarrhea, leading to increased bioavailability.

Dosing

TAC is usually administered orally at 0.1 to 0.3 mg per kg per day in two divided doses. Most pharmacokinetic studies in children show that the dose required to maintain target blood concentrations is two to three times higher per kilogram of body weight than that in adults.[30,41,42] This is related to the larger V_d and higher clearance of drug in the pediatric population, which are about twice that observed in adults.[29,30,32,43] Pediatric renal transplant recipients may have lower C_{max} and AUC values than liver transplant patients, consistent with decreased hepatic clearance in the latter group.[41] Hepatitis C virus–positive patients may also require lower drug doses based on decreased liver metabolism.[44,45] In general, patients with liver disease and older patients require longer dose intervals as compared with pediatric patients. Patients of African American ethnicity may also require larger doses of TAC at shorter intervals.

TAC granules (Modigraf™) are also available, developed for patients who are unable to swallow capsules, in particular infants.[46] The guidelines for dosing and TDM are the same as for TAC capsules. There is also a prolonged-release TAC formulation available for older children and adolescents (Advagraf™ in Europe, Astagraf™ in the United States). Comparative pharmacokinetic studies have shown that stable pediatric transplant recipients can be converted from immediate-release to prolonged-release-TAC at the same total daily dose, using the same TDM method.[47,48]

Therapeutic Drug Monitoring

The measurement of CsA and TAC levels is a routine practice in the management of all transplant patients because of the wide variability in pharmacokinetics and strong correlation between the level of drug and the incidence of graft rejection and toxicity.[49,50] However, controversy prevails regarding the optimal strategy for monitoring drug concentrations. Interpretation of drug concentration depends on sample matrix, assay methodology, type of organ transplant, and time post-transplant.

CsA concentrations can be measured in whole blood or plasma. Whole-blood measurement is now preferred due to the wide distribution of the drug in red blood cells and the temperature dependence of plasma levels. Clinicians need to emphasize the assay used to detect these levels, since different methods are available. Analysis of CsA in whole blood is performed either by immunoassays or by liquid chromatography–tandem mass spectrometry (LC–MS/MS). The commonly used immunoassays for whole-blood sample measurement of CsA are the fluorescence polarization immunoassay and the enzyme-multiplied immunoassay technique. The commonly used immunoassays cross-react with CsA metabolites to different degrees, and therefore, target blood levels are specific to the assay technique utilized[51]; hence, many transplant centers prefer the LC–MS/MS assay. Clinical outcomes correlate best with AUC, which provides the best estimate of total drug exposure in an individual. Because AUC estimation requires multiple blood draws at specific times, surrogates for drug exposure are utilized. Trough level (C_0) is easier to obtain and is not greatly affected by small inaccuracies in the time of blood collection and, therefore, is most commonly used. However, trough levels correlate poorly with AUC or with calcineurin phosphatase activity in renal or liver transplant patients.[39,40]

Neoral™ has a more consistent initial absorption profile than does Sandimmune™. With the microemulsion formulation, CsA levels at 2 hours postdose (C_2) have been found to correlate better with total drug exposure and immunosuppressive efficacy than C_0 levels.[52,53] A C_2 blood sample also has a higher proportion of parent drug when compared with a C_0 sample; this results in better agreement in C_2 levels measured by different assay methodologies than occurs with C_0 concentrations, which have a greater proportion of metabolites. However, error margins are greater for C_2 levels if the sample is not collected within a narrow (±15 minute) time window. Overall, C_2 monitoring has not been universally adopted.

Similar to CsA, TAC is a drug with a narrow therapeutic index. Because of variable bioavailability and clearance, TDM is mandatory for optimizing clinical outcome.[54] Whole blood is preferred to plasma as the preferred means for measurement of TAC levels because at least 75% to 80% of drug is bound to erythrocytes. Analysis of TAC in whole blood is performed either by immunoassays or by LC–MS/MS, with both techniques being represented in nearly equal proportions at measurement service providers worldwide. Unlike CsA, the 12-hour trough level of TAC correlates well with AUC and clinical outcomes and is the accepted standard for monitoring TAC therapy. Guidelines provided for target levels in adults (8 to 12 ng per mL in the first 3 to 6 months post-transplant) seem applicable to the pediatric age group, but more clinical outcome data are needed.[55,56] Currently, target TAC trough whole-blood level guidelines followed at the University Children's Hospital of Heidelberg, Germany, pediatric renal transplant program are summarized in Table 42.4. It is noteworthy that these target levels are adjusted according to the patient's immunologic risk and the concomitant immunosuppressive medication.

TABLE 42.4 Target Ranges for Tacrolimus Whole-Blood Trough Levels in Pediatric Renal Transplant Recipients at the University Children's Hospital, Heidelberg, Germany

Time Post-Transplant	*Liquid Chromatography–Tandem Mass Spectrometry (ng/mL)*
Week 0–3	10–12
Week 4 to month 5	8–10
Month 6 to 11	5–10
≥ Month 12	5–8

Adverse Effects

CsA and TAC have similarities as well as differences in their toxicity profiles. Renal, metabolic, hematologic, neurologic, gastrointestinal, cosmetic, and other side effects are summarized in Tables 42.5 and 42.6.

Renal Toxicity

The most common dose-limiting side effect of CNIs is nephrotoxicity. CNI-induced acute renal toxicity is due to a decrease in renal blood flow and glomerular filtration rate (GFR) produced by a dose-dependent, reversible vasoconstriction affecting primarily afferent arterioles, resulting in a picture of "prerenal dysfunction" with intact tubular function. Vasoconstriction is the combined effect of increased thromboxane and endothelin production, increased sympathetic activity and nitric oxide synthase inhibition with a decrease in nitric oxide, a preglomerular arteriolar relaxant. This renal vasoconstriction may manifest clinically as a delay in recovery of early graft function in kidney transplant patients, a rise in serum creatinine, or worsening hypertension. Renal vasoconstriction is more prominent with CsA than with TAC, also accounting for increasing sodium retention

TABLE 42.5 Adverse Effects of Calcineurin Inhibitors

Organ System	*Toxicity*
Renal	Acute vasoconstriction—prerenal dysfunction
	Chronic interstitial fibrosis
	Thrombotic microangiopathy—hemolytic–uremic syndrome–like picture
	Salt and water retention, hyperkalemia, hypomagnesemia
Gastrointestinal	Anorexia, nausea, vomiting, abdominal discomfort, diarrhea
Hepatobiliary	Elevated transaminases, cholelithiasis
Neurologic	Tremors, seizures, headache, insomnia, encephalopathy
Metabolic/endocrine	Diabetes mellitus, hyperlipidemia, hyperuricemia
Cosmetic	Gingival hyperplasia, hirsutism, hypertrichosis, alopecia, gynecomastia
Cardiovascular	Hypertension

TABLE 42.6 Semiquantitative Comparison of Safety Profiles of Current Primary Immunosuppressive Compounds

	Tacrolimus	*Cyclosporine*	*Mycophenolate Mofetil*	*Sirolimus/Everolimus*	*Glucocorticoids*
Nephrotoxicity[a]	++(+)	+++	−	+	−
Hyperlipidemia	+(+)	++	−	+++	++
Arterial hypertension	++	+++	−	−	+
Neurotoxicity	+++	+++	−	−	+
Post-transplant diabetes mellitus	+++	++	−	−	++
Bone marrow suppression	−	−	++	++	−
Gastrointestinal adverse effects[b]	+	+	+++	+	−
Hepatotoxicity	+	+	−	+	−
Esthetical changes	+	++	−	−	++
Wound healing problems[c]	−	−	+	++	+
Pulmonary toxicity	−	−	−	+	−
Fetal toxicity	+	+	++	NA	−
Osteoporosis	+	+	−	?	++
Inhibition of longitudinal growth	−	−	−	+	+++

[a]Sirolimus without calcineurin inhibitor; [b]Gastrointestinal disorders: diarrhea, abdominal pain, nausea and vomiting, ileus, rectal disorders, mucosal ulcerations; [c]Wound healing problems including lymphocele formation; − indicates the drug has no effect on this adverse effect; + indicates mild; ++ indicates moderate; +++ indicates severe; ? indicates clinical data available but insufficient to provide conclusions; NA = no information available.

and hypertension. Acute microvascular disease can rarely be caused by either of the CNIs and has been shown to produce thrombotic microangiopathy, resulting in a hemolytic–uremic syndrome (HUS)–like picture due to a direct toxic effect on vascular endothelial cells inhibiting prostacyclin production.

Chronic toxicity from CNIs can lead to characteristic afferent arteriolar hyalinosis and patchy or striped interstitial fibrosis on renal biopsy. These lesions appear to be a result of long-standing renal vasoconstriction along with ischemia. The resulting chronic renal ischemia increases the accumulation of extracellular matrix proteins in the interstitium. Interstitial fibrosis is felt to be the result of a CNI-stimulated increase in TGF-β production, thus resulting in chronic allograft nephropathy and ultimately leading to poor graft survival.

Fluid and Electrolyte Abnormalities

CsA is a more potent renal vasoconstrictor and, as a result, causes more sodium retention, edema, and hypertension when compared with TAC. Other side effects include hyperkalemia and mild hyperchloremic acidosis (a picture of type-IV renal tubular acidosis). Concomitant administration of a β-blocker, angiotensin-converting-enzyme (ACE) inhibitor, and/or angiotensin-receptor blocker may further exaggerate hyperkalemia. Hypomagnesemia is more common with TAC than with CsA. Hyperuricemia is also a common abnormality, although gouty attacks are more common with CsA than with TAC.

Glucose Metabolism Disorders

Post-transplant diabetes mellitus (PTDM) is a serious adverse effect of CsA and TAC therapy. A meta-analysis demonstrated a significantly higher incidence of PTDM among TAC-treated adult renal transplant recipients when compared with CsA recipients.[57] Interestingly, a prospective randomized trial in children showed no differences in the PTDM rate.[58] The proposed mechanism of CNI-induced PTDM includes a direct toxic effect on β islet cells and an increase in peripheral insulin resistance.

Dyslipidemia

CsA has an adverse effect on lipid profile, leading to hypercholesterolemia and hypertriglyceridemia.[59] The binding of low-density lipoprotein receptor with CsA is implicated as a cause of hyperlipidemia in transplant patients and may also be related to abnormal low-density lipoprotein feedback to the liver. The effect is markedly less with TAC, and switching from CsA to TAC improves the lipid profile.

Malignancies

Patients receiving immunosuppressants are at increased risk for development of infections, post-transplant lymphoproliferative disorder (PTLD), and other viral-associated malignancies. This risk is related to the overall intensity of immunosuppression rather than to specific individual agents. Although large studies focusing on the toxicity of these drugs in the pediatric population are not available, their adverse reaction profile in children appears to be similar to that in the adult population. However, the incidence of PTLD is higher in pediatric allograft recipients because these patients tend to be more heavily immunosuppressed (receive antilymphocyte antibody for induction and/or treatment of acute rejection) and are more likely to be Epstein-Barr virus (EBV) seronegative and receive EBV-seropositive donor organs. Although PTLD was initially shown to be more common with TAC, a randomized controlled trial in the pediatric population did not report increased malignancy with TAC when compared with CsA.[58]

Neurotoxicity

Coarse tremors, headaches, and insomnia are dose related and more common with TAC. Seizures and leukoencephalopathy have also been reported.

Hematologic Toxicity

Hemolytic anemia with thrombocytopenia may occur as a part of HUS in transplant patients. Rarely, autoimmune hemolytic anemia requiring multiple transfusions, which improved after withdrawal of CNI and substitution with SRL, may occur.[59]

Cosmetic

Gingival hyperplasia and hypertrichosis are more common with CsA than with TAC. CsA may also cause gynecomastia in men and breast enlargement in women. TAC may produce hair loss and alopecia.

To summarize, although there are similarities in their side-effect profiles, CsA has a greater tendency to produce gingival hyperplasia, hirsutism, hyperlipidemia, and hypertension. TAC is more likely to cause PTDM and neurotoxicity. In a randomized trial of TAC versus CsA microemulsion in pediatric renal transplant recipients, 95% to 100% of patients experienced at least one adverse event,[58] most commonly hypertension, hypomagnesemia, and urinary tract infections. Hypomagnesemia and diarrhea were more common with TAC use, whereas hypertrichosis, flu syndrome, and gingival hyperplasia were more frequently seen with CsA. In this study, no differences were noted in the incidence of post-transplant infections, diabetes mellitus, or lymphoproliferative disorders.

Drug Interactions

Because of the prime importance of the intestinal P-gp and the CYP3A4 and CYP3A5 systems in absorption and metabolism of CNIs, a large number of drugs that affect these systems can cause significant interactions,[22,60] as given in Table 42.7. Additive toxicity may also occur with other drugs, such as hyperkalemia with ACE inhibitors; nephrotoxicity with aminoglycosides, amphotericin B, and nonsteroidal anti-inflammatory drugs; and myopathy and rhabdomyolysis with lipid-lowering statins.

Therapeutic Efficacy and Pharmacoeconomics

The clinician has to balance efficacy and toxicity when choosing a CNI for transplant patients. A meta-analysis of 30 randomized controlled trials in adult renal transplant patients[57] showed TAC to be more effective than the CsA microemulsion formulation in preventing rejection episodes. However, a higher rate of diabetes and PTLD was reported in the TAC study group. In the pediatric population, there is a paucity of studies comparing the

TABLE 42.7 Examples of Common Drug Interactions of Immunosuppressants Used in Solid-Organ Transplantation: Cyclosporine, Tacrolimus, Sirolimus, and Everolimus

Common Types of Drug Interactions	*Examples of Interacting Drugs*
Coadministration of drugs that inhibit CYP3A metabolism and/or P-gp efflux can increase immunosuppressant whole-blood concentrations, leading to significant toxicities.	Amiodarone ART-boosting agents (e.g., ritonavir, cobicistat) Azole antifungals (e.g., fluconazole, posaconazole, voriconazole) HIV protease inhibitors (e.g., atazanavir, nelfinavir, saquinavir) Macrolide antibiotics (except azithromycin) Non–dihydropyridine calcium channel blockers Ombitasvir–paritaprevir–ritonavir with or without dasabuvir (an HCV, direct-acting antiviral regimen) Grapefruit juice
Coadministration of drugs that induce CYP3A metabolism and/or P-gp efflux pumping can decrease immunosuppressant whole-blood concentrations, increasing the risk of organ rejection.	Antiseizure drugs, enzyme inducing (e.g., carbamazepine, fosphenytoin, oxcarbazepine, phenobarbital, phenytoin, primidone) Enzalutamide Nafcillin Rifamycins (e.g., rifabutin, rifampin, rifapentine) St. John's wort
Coadministration of nephrotoxic drugs with cyclosporine or tacrolimus can cause additive or synergistic kidney injury.	Aminoglycosides Amphotericin B Colchicine Nonsteroidal anti-inflammatory drugs (NSAIDs)
Coadministration of drugs that increase serum potassium with cyclosporine or tacrolimus may cause severe hyperkalemia.	ACE inhibitors/ARBs Amiloride Spironolactone Triamterene Trimethoprim, trimethoprim–sulfamethoxazole (co-trimoxazole)
Coadministration of statin drugs with cyclosporine can increase statin levels and risk of myotoxicity.	Atorvastatin Lovastatin Pitavastatin Rosuvastatin Simvastatin

ACE, angiotensin-converting enzyme; ARB, angiotensin-II receptor blocker; ART, antiretroviral therapy; CYP, cytochrome P450 metabolism; HCV, hepatitis C virus; HIV, human immunodeficiency virus; P-gp, P-glycoprotein.

two CNI drugs. A randomized controlled trial in pediatric renal transplants demonstrated that at 4 years, patient survival was similar, but graft survival significantly favored TAC. In children, both PTDM and PTLD were reported to be similar in the TAC and CsA study groups.[58,61] Also, the medication costs were not significantly different over the 4-year post-transplant period.[16] Because graft survival is better with TAC, it has a pharmacoeconomic advantage over CsA as also shown in adult trials.

MYCOPHENOLATE MOFETIL

The prodrug MMF is a 2-morpho-linoethyl ester of mycophenolic acid (MPA), the active immunosuppressive metabolite. MPA was initially isolated as a fermentation product of the fungus *Penicillium* in 1898, but its immunosuppressive properties were not fully recognized until the 1970s. Approved by the FDA in 1995, it is primarily used as an adjunctive agent in combination with CNIs with or without steroids as maintenance therapy for prevention of acute transplant rejection. It has almost completely replaced AZA in this role.

Mechanism of Action

MPA acts by blocking de novo purine synthesis in lymphocytes. Purines can be generated by de novo synthesis or by recycling (salvage pathway), and lymphocytes preferentially use the former. MPA is a selective and noncompetitive inhibitor of inosine monophosphate dehydrogenase 2 (IMPDH2), the rate-limiting enzyme in the de novo purine biosynthetic pathway for converting inosine monophosphate to guanosine monophosphate (GMP). Depletion of GMP by MPA has a relatively selective antiproliferative effect on lymphocytes. In vitro, MMF blocks the proliferation of T and B cells and inhibits clonal expansion. This results in inhibition of antibody production, generation of cytotoxic T cells, and development of delayed-type hypersensitivity. Because of greater dependence of lymphocytes on de novo synthesis of purines as compared to the "salvage" pathway, MPA is a more selective inhibitor of T- and B-cell proliferation than AZA. Furthermore, MPA impairs the ability of dendritic cells to present antigen, suppresses the recruitment of monocyte lineage cells, suppresses the glycosylation of adhesion molecules, inhibits vascular smooth muscle proliferation, improves endothelial function, and inhibits mononuclear cell recruitment into allografts and nephritic kidneys.[62] MPA also decreases cytokine-induced nitric oxide synthesis and prevents the formation of reactive species such as peroxynitrite. Furthermore, MPA exhibits antioxidant effects in experimental nephropathies. These properties of MPA likely augment its immunosuppressive properties by limiting fibrosis and vascular sclerosis after immunologic injury.[63] Hence, MPA may also be beneficial in patients with chronic rejection by delaying and preventing proliferative arteriolopathy.

Pharmacokinetics

The pharmacokinetics of MMF appears to be similar in both the pediatric and adult transplant population. However, pharmacokinetic data in children are less available, with the focus mainly on renal transplant recipients.[64-69]

MMF is rapidly and completely absorbed after oral administration, with the mofetil moiety helping to improve oral bioavailability. It undergoes immediate hydrolysis by esterases into the active compound, MPA. Peak concentrations are noted within 1 to 2 hours postdose, and absorption may be faster in pediatric liver transplant patients than that in adults.[58,63] The presence of food prolongs T_{max} and decreases C_{max} by 40%. MPA undergoes significant enterohepatic recirculation. It is highly bound to serum albumin, but the free drug is pharmacologically active. MPA is primarily metabolized in the liver by β-glucuronidase to MPA glucuronide (MPAG), an inactive metabolite that may undergo enterohepatic recirculation. The excretion of MPAG in the gut may account for a second peak at 5 to 6 hours and may contribute to gastrointestinal side effects. MPAG is finally excreted in the urine. The half-life of the drug is 17 hours.

MMF is available as capsules, tablets, oral suspension, and intravenous solution. An enteric-coated form of MPA (Myfortic™) is also available, but only approved for adults. The recommended dose of MMF in pediatric patients in conjunction with CsA is 1,200 mg per m^2 per day in two divided doses, the recommended MMF dose in conjunction with TAC is 800 mg per m^2 per day in two divided doses. However, data from a large prospective randomized study in both pediatric and adult renal transplant recipients on fixed-dose MMF versus a concentration-controlled regimen, the FDCC study, indicate that a higher initial MMF dose, for example, 1,800 mg MMF/m^2 per day in conjunction with CsA and 1,200 mg MMF/m^2 per day in conjunction with TAC for the first 2 to 4 weeks post-transplant, is required to achieve adequate MPA exposure in the majority of patients.[69-71]

The difference in MMF dosing depending on the concomitant CNI is explained by a pharmacokinetic interaction of CsA with the main MPA metabolite 7-O-MPA glucuronide (7-O-MPAG). CsA inhibits the multidrug resistance protein 2–mediated transport of 7-O-MPAG into the bile. MPAG is subject to enzymatic and nonenzymatic hydrolysis in bile and, more importantly, in the intestine, thereby liberating the unconjugated drug MPA, which is then reabsorbed into the systemic circulation. This enterohepatic circulation is responsible for a secondary MPA peak occurring 6 to 12 hours after administration. The impact of the enterohepatic cycle on the MPA plasma concentration varies within and between individuals due to factors such as meal times or comedication of drugs that interrupt the enterohepatic circulation (e.g., bile acid sequestrants, antibiotics). These factors should be considered when evaluating MPA concentrations (particularly predose concentrations) in clinical practice. Furthermore, genetic polymorphisms and disease can affect enterohepatic cycling and thus the bioavailability of MPA.[72] When using MMF in combination with TAC, lower MMF doses can be used to achieve comparable MPA exposure, guided by TDM, to that seen with CsA.[72] No dose adjustment is necessary in patients with hepatic impairment; however, in the presence of renal insufficiency (GFR $<$ 25 mL per min per 1.73 m^2), dose reduction may be necessary to prevent drug-induced toxicity due to increased MPAG and free MPA levels.[73] Neither MMF nor MPA is dialyzable.

Therapeutic Drug Monitoring

MPA pharmacokinetic profiling demonstrates higher intraindividual variability in the immediate post-transplant period, which decreases over time while interindividual variability persists.[74] Overall, AUC and C_{max} increase with time after transplantation.[74] In pediatric renal transplant patients, MPA-AUC was found to inversely correlate with the development of acute rejection, whereas the free MPA level was a better predictor of adverse effects.[66] A literature review noted that TDM has limitations and has revealed conflicting results. A predose trough level appears less reliable as a predictor of risk of rejection.[75] Although evidence is limited, a total MPA-AUC value between 30 and 60 μg per mL by high-performance liquid chromatography (HPLC) has been suggested for at least the first 6 months after renal or heart transplantation when used in combination with steroids and CsA.[69,76] The steady-state trough MPA concentration is to be maintained between 1.5 and 4 μg per mL for a favorable clinical outcome. One study in adults, for example, showed significantly fewer treatment failures and acute rejection episodes in the monitoring arm compared with the fixed-dose arm, with no significant difference in side effects.[77] In general, monitoring of MPA exposure by MPA predose plasma levels is more popular in clinical practice than monitoring of the area under the concentration–time curve (MPA-AUC), for example, by a limited sampling strategy, but less precise. Such findings in several other studies indicate that routine or selective pharmacokinetic or pharmacodynamic TDM of MMF may be advisable, but the ideal strategy, based on either trough MPA levels, abbreviated pharmacokinetic profiles by a limited sampling strategy, or IMPDH activity, remains debatable.[69,78]

Adverse Effects

MMF commonly produces gastrointestinal side effects, including diarrhea (most prominent), abdominal pain, nausea, vomiting, and enterocolitis. Diarrhea can be seen in up to one-third of patients, especially in infants. Esophagitis and gastritis may also occur, and, rarely, gastrointestinal bleeding or perforation may ensue. The gastrointestinal side effects may be improved after reduction in dosage or splitting among three or four doses. The gastrointestinal side effects of the enteric-coated formulation have not been found to be significantly different from those of MMF. In spite of its more selective action on lymphocytes, MMF can produce severe leukopenia, anemia, and thrombocytopenia as a result of bone marrow suppression. MMF dosing should be discontinued or reduced if the absolute neutrophil count is less than 1,300 per mm^3. An increased incidence of herpes simplex, varicella zoster, and cytomegalovirus (CMV) infections has been noted with MMF use when compared with AZA. The MMF dose should be reduced with active CMV infection. MMF does not have any nephrotoxicity, neurotoxicity, or hepatotoxicity. Finally, MMF should be avoided in conditions of hereditary hypoxanthine–guanine phosphoribosyltransferase deficiency, such as the Lesch-Nyhan and Kelley-Seegmiller syndromes.

Drug Interactions

Concurrent administration of antacids, cholestyramine, or iron should be avoided with MMF because they decrease its bioavailability. Bile sequestrants reduce MPA-AUC by interfering with enterohepatic circulation. MPA levels decrease from baseline requiring an increase in MMF dose by almost 50% when used in combination with CsA as a result of a decrease in enterohepatic circulation. This is in contrast to MMF usage with TAC or SRL, where no effect is seen, and therefore, no MMF dose adjustment is needed.[79] Glucocorticoids have been shown to reduce MPA exposure in adult renal transplant recipients by inducing glucuronosyltransferase expression and thereby increasing MPA metabolism,[80] but the clinical significance of this effect is not clear. MMF and AZA should not be given at the same time, as hematologic toxicity may be additive.

Therapeutic Efficacy

MMF is indicated for prophylaxis of allogeneic kidney, heart, and liver transplant rejection along with CNIs and steroids.[81-83] MMF has been associated with improved graft survival and improved renal function in combination with steroids and CNIs. It has been used to support immunosuppression while withdrawing CNIs in patients with chronic CNI toxicity. There have been studies with CNI avoidance and using SRL and/or MMF instead, but this is not an advisable regimen.[84] Also, the use of MMF with reduction of CNI has a favorable effect on renal function and blood pressure.[85] Its use in primary glomerulopathy, lupus nephritis, rheumatoid arthritis, graft-versus-host disease after bone marrow transplantation, and atopic dermatitis has been gaining popularity based on clinical trials, though it is not FDA approved for these indications.

AZATHIOPRINE

A prodrug for 6-MP, AZA, was responsible for the initial success of renal transplantation when used in combination with glucocorticoids for immunosuppression. After the introduction of CsA, it formed the second component of "standard" triple-drug therapy (CsA, AZA, PRED). Currently, however, its use has virtually been completely replaced by MMF because of the latter's higher lymphocyte selectivity and greater antirejection efficacy.

Mechanism of Action

AZA suppresses the proliferation of B and T cells and decreases the number of monocytes circulating in the blood by arresting the cell cycle of promyelocytes in the bone marrow. Thus, AZA is an S-phase–specific agent that inhibits DNA synthesis by interfering with purine biosynthesis. This antiproliferative effect is a result of its metabolites, which include 6-MP, 6-thiouric acid, 6-methyl-mercaptopurine, and 6-thioguanine. They also block the de novo pathway by formation of thioinosinic acid, accounting for the specificity of action on lymphocytes.

Pharmacokinetics

There are few pharmacokinetic studies in the pediatric population. Data from studies in adults demonstrate that AZA is rapidly absorbed after oral administration and is converted to 6-MP. When administered orally, about 50% of the dose is absorbed. Hence, intravenous-to-oral dose equivalence is 1:2. AZA is primarily metabolized by the liver to 6-MP and further converted to the active metabolite thioinosinic acid by hypoxanthine–guanine phosphoribosyltransferase, and subsequently, the metabolites are excreted by the kidney. About 1% of Caucasians are homozygous for an abnormal allele causing deficiency of thiopurine methyltransferase (TPMT), a key enzyme in AZA metabolism. These individuals are at high risk for developing drug-induced toxicity and can be potentially identified by TPMT genotyping.[86] The drug is not significantly dialyzed, and dose reduction may be needed with renal failure.

Dosing

AZA is administered orally at 2 to 3 mg per kg per day when used as a primary immunosuppressant. However, it is most commonly used in combination with CNIs at a dose of 1 to 2 mg per kg per day. Allopurinol will increase the levels of the metabolite thioinosinic acid, and AZA dose may have to be reduced by two-thirds in patients requiring coadministration. TDM is not performed in patients on AZA, since therapeutic activity and toxicity is related to tissue levels and is independent of blood levels.

Side Effects

Its major toxicity is myelosuppression, predominantly leukopenia. It may also lead to anemia and thrombocytopenia and red cell aplasia in occasional cases. The hematologic side effects are dose related and may occur late in therapy. They are usually reversible on discontinuation or on dose reduction. Other adverse effects include gastrointestinal disturbances, hepatitis (reversible elevation in transaminases and bilirubin levels), and, rarely, pancreatitis. AZA also increases susceptibility to infections and is also associated with skin cancer development.

Therapeutic Efficacy

AZA is still infrequently used as an adjunctive agent in immunosuppressive protocols to prevent allograft rejection. It is also used in other disorders such as rheumatoid arthritis.

SIROLIMUS (RAPAMYCIN) AND EVEROLIMUS

SRL is a lactone macrolide antibiotic derived from the fungus *Streptomyces hygroscopicus*, originally isolated from a soil sample taken from Easter Island (Rapa Nui, hence the name rapamycin) in 1975. Although it was being investigated as an antifungal and antitumor agent, its lymphopenic properties became apparent, which led to its use as an immunosuppressant.[87] The FDA approved it in 1999 for clinical use in preventing renal allograft rejection in adults. It is 100 times more potent than CsA in vitro, and because of different mechanisms of action, it works synergistically with CNIs. EVR is the 40-O-(2-hydroxyethyl) derivative of SRL, a modification that results in some important pharmacokinetic differences between the two drugs. EVR is more hydrophilic than SRL and is absorbed more rapidly from the gut with more systemic clearance than SRL. As a result, the elimination half-life of EVR is shorter than for SRL (mean 28 hours vs. 62 hours).[88-89] The clinical effect is that no loading dose is required for EVR and that is administered twice a day in both adults and children.

Mechanism of Action

SRL and EVR are similar to TAC in its molecular structure and also bind to the cytosolic protein FKBP12.[90] However, TAC acts as a CNI, and SRL and EVR act on signal 3 (Fig. 42.1). Thus, both act on different sites in the signal transduction pathway in spite of competition for the same cellular receptor, resulting in immunosuppressive synergism in vivo.[14,90,91] SRL and EVR primarily inhibit T-cell proliferation in response to various stimuli, such as cytokines, alloantigens, and mitogens. The SRL-FKBP complex binds to the mammalian target of rapamycin protein, a key regulatory kinase, which blocks the activation of the 70-kDa S6 protein kinases necessary for cellular proliferation. The final result is an inhibition of DNA and protein synthesis and eventual arrest of cell-cycle progression in the mid- to late G1 phase.[14,90,91] Unlike CsA or TAC, SRL and EVR block IL-2–mediated signal transduction and cell proliferation and block lymphocyte response to IL-4, IL-7, and other cytokines. SRL and EVR also inhibit antigen- and cytokine-mediated B-cell proliferation independent of its effect on T helper cells. Finally, cytokine-dependent differentiation of B cells into antibody-producing cells is blocked, resulting in decreased immunoglobulin synthesis.[90]

Pharmacokinetics

Similar to CNIs, SRL and EVR also have poor bioavailability, demonstrate wide intra- and interpatient variability, have the potential for drug interactions by virtue of metabolism by CYP3A4, have its own side-effect profile, and require TDM.[91-93] SRL is absorbed from the gastrointestinal tract, absorption being delayed by a fatty meal. The peak concentration is reached in 1 to 2 hours, with excellent penetration in most tissues. Its long half-life (average 62 hours) requires a loading dose but permits convenient once-daily dosing. SRL is a substrate for both CYP3A4 and P-gp. It is extensively metabolized in the liver by O-methylation and/or hydroxylation, and the parent drug accounts for more than 90% of its immunosuppressive activity. The drug is primarily excreted by the biliary system, and renal excretion is minimal. Hence, dose adjustment is required in patients with liver dysfunction and not in patients with kidney dysfunction.

The half-life of SRL increases with age in children,[91] so twice-daily dosing is recommended in young children, in contrast to older recipients. It has not been defined at what age or body weight the switch to twice-daily dosing should take place. One trial used 13 years of age as a cutoff point.[94] In a pharmacokinetic study of 13 children receiving SRL in a CNI-free regimen, with a median age of 15.5 years, the authors concluded that twice-daily dosing was required in this setting due to more rapid metabolism of SRL in the absence of concomitant CNI therapy.[95] High SRL trough concentrations (>10 μg per L) either with or without concomitant CNI appear inadvisable in children in view of the high risk of toxicity and discontinuation. One small prospective study (n = 19) converted pediatric kidney transplant patients to a CNI-free regimen of SRL with MMF using a single SRL loading dose of 5 to 7 mg per m^2 BSA, then a daily dose of 2 to 4 mg per m^2 BSA adjusted to target an SRL trough concentration of 5 to 10 μg per L, and achieved a low rate of rejection with a good renal response.[94]

EVR is the 40-O-(2-hydroxyethyl) derivative of SRL, a modification that results in some important pharmacokinetic differences between the two drugs. EVR is more hydrophilic than SRL and is absorbed more rapidly from the gut with more systemic clearance than SRL.[96] As a result, the elimination half-life of EVR is shorter than for SRL (mean 28 hours vs. 62 hours).[88,89] The clinical effect is that no loading dose is required for EVR. Moreover, EVR is administered twice a day in both adults and children.

Therapeutic Drug Monitoring and Dosing

SRL is available as 1-, 2-, or 5-mg tablets or an oral solution. Whole-blood trough levels correlate well with AUC and are considered adequate for TDM, and a target range of 5 to 15 ng per mL has been recommended in adults.[97,98] Since SRL has a long half-life, once-daily dose adjustments have been made, levels should be checked 5 to 7 days later. Also, once steady state is reached, frequent monitoring of levels may not be required.

EVR is available as tablets and dispersible tablets for administration in water. The current evidence from pediatric kidney transplantation suggests that EVR be administered at an initial dose of 0.8 mg per m^2 BSA twice daily when given in combination with CsA therapy, adjusted to target a trough concentration of 3 μg per L or higher.[99,100] In patients receiving EVR with concomitant TAC or MMF, a dose of 2.0 mg per m^2 BSA twice daily is appropriate.[101]

Drug Interaction

There is a well-documented drug–drug interaction between mTOR inhibitors and CsA,[102] arising from a shared metabolic pathway (via the cytochrome P450 CYP3A4 isoenzyme system) and the fact that both are substrates for the drug transporter P-gp. EVR exposure is increased by up to threefold in patients receiving concomitant CsA,[101,103] although less extensive evidence suggests that TAC may exert only a minimal effect.[103,104] Similarly, SRL bioavailability is higher in the presence of CsA than TAC.[105,106]

Adverse Effects

Clinically relevant adverse effects of SRL and EVR that require a specific therapeutic response or can potentially influence short- and long-term patient morbidity and mortality as well as graft survival include hypercholesterolemia, hypertriglyceridemia, infectious and noninfectious pneumonia, anemia, lymphocele formation, and impaired wound healing (Tables 42.6 and 42.8). These drug-related adverse effects are important determinants in the choice of a tailor-made immunosuppressive drug regimen that complies with the individual patient risk profile. Equally important in the latter decision is the lack of severe intrinsic nephrotoxicity associated with SRL and EVR and its advantageous effects on arterial hypertension, PTDM, and esthetic changes induced by CNIs. Mild and transient thrombocytopenia, leukopenia, gastrointestinal adverse effects, and mucosal ulcerations are all minor complications of SRL and EVR therapy that have less impact on the decision for choosing this drug as the basis for tailor-made immunosuppressive therapy.

An additional side effect in the setting of CNI withdrawal and mTOR inhibitor introduction is aggravation of proteinuria in patients with preexisting proteinuria by a still incompletely defined mechanism. Available data are consistent with the hypothesis that the increase in proteinuria is causally related to CNI withdrawal and not because of initiation of an mTOR inhibitor.[107] On the other hand, it cannot be excluded that SRL and EVR themselves might also affect glomerular permeability in some patients. The potential complication of increased proteinuria, which is an independent risk factor for long-term renal allograft function, should, therefore, be borne in mind when a conversion of the immunosuppressive regimen from a CNI-based to an mTOR-based maintenance therapy is considered.

TABLE 42.8 Common Adverse Effects of Sirolimus and Everolimus

Organ System	*Toxicity*
Renal	Prolonged delayed graft function
	Proteinuria
	Hypokalemia
	Hypophosphatemia
Metabolic	Hypertriglyceridemia
	Hypercholesterolemia
Hematologic	Bone marrow suppression
	Anemia, leucopenia, thrombocytopenia
	Thrombotic microangiopathy
Gastrointestinal	Diarrhea
	Mouth ulcers
Pulmonary	Pneumonitis
Cosmetic	Impaired wound healing
Others	Lymphocele
	Reflex sympathetic dystrophy

Therapeutic Use

The most frequent reason to include an mTOR inhibitor in the immunosuppressive regimen is to facilitate a reduction in CNI exposure or to eliminate CNI therapy entirely. The current evidence suggests that de novo administration of EVR with low-exposure CNI therapy in children undergoing renal transplantation is efficacious and safe.[108] The use of de novo EVR with complete CNI avoidance has not been explored in large trials in pediatric transplant recipients, but is unlikely to be preferable to concomitant reduced-exposure CNI. Switching maintenance patients to an mTOR inhibitor to facilitate CNI minimization can improve renal function or avoid further functional deterioration, particularly when undertaken before irreversible damage has developed. Late switch below an estimated GFR of 40 mL per min per 1.73 m^2, however, may be associated with an increase in preexisting proteinuria due to podocytopenia, favoring early conversion. It remains unresolved whether CNI therapy should be reduced or, indeed, eliminated in maintenance patients, regardless of whether renal dysfunction is believed to be due to CNI-related nephrotoxicity. Currently, many transplant centers use mTOR inhibitors as part of a maintenance immunosuppressive regimen only in the following patient subsets in which this drug class may have particular utility: (a) in patients who have histologically proven CNI nephrotoxicity despite low levels and doses of the CNI; (b) in patients with malignancy (e.g., skin cancers and Kaposi sarcoma), either in remission or being actively treated; (c) after treatment of B-cell PTLD; and (d) in patients with recurrent CMV viremia, because EVR has anti-CMV activity in vitro and is associated with less CMV replication and disease in vivo compared to MMF.[109,110] Notably, the incidence of EBV or BK polyoma virus infection is not lower in EVR-treated patients compared to MMF-treated patients.[108]

ANTILYMPHOCYTE ANTIBODIES

Polyclonal antibodies (antilymphocyte globulins) were among the earliest immunosuppressants used in organ transplantation in the 1960s along with AZA and PRED. Since then, the availability of MAbs, such as OKT3 and anti–IL-2R antibodies, has expanded the spectrum of biologic agents in transplantation. Although mainly used for induction therapy to reduce the incidence of graft rejection in the early post-transplant period or to treat severe or steroid-resistant acute rejection episodes, these agents are also finding wider application in delaying CNI introduction or in permitting steroid avoidance or withdrawal.

Polyclonal Antibodies: ATGAM and Thymoglobulin

Two antithymocyte globulin preparations are commercially available in the United States, ATGAM™ and Thymoglobulin™, prepared by immunizing horses or rabbits, respectively, with human thymic lymphocytes followed by harvesting the immunoglobulin G (IgG) fraction of immune sera. These preparations contain several antibodies that react with many different clones of cells and with a variety of molecules on lymphocytes.

Mechanism of Action

Their immunosuppressive effect is primarily due to lymphocyte depletion resulting from opsonization, leading to complement-mediated lysis or mononuclear phagocytosis and induction of Fas-mediated apoptosis.[111] However, nondepletive actions such as partial T-cell activation due to binding of multiple cell-surface receptors inducing anergy may also be important.[112]

Dosing

In pediatric renal transplant patients, 5 days of Thymoglobulin™ therapy was found to produce equal or greater immunosuppression than 10 days of ATGAM™ treatment.[113] ATGAM at 15 mg per kg per day for 10 days and Thymoglobulin at 2 mg per kg per day for 5 days produced a rapid reduction in CD3, CD4, and CD8 lymphocytes to 2% to 15% of baseline within 24 hours. By day 10, the numbers increased to 14% to 34% with Thymoglobulin and 52% to 56% with ATGAM.[113] In general, Thymoglobulin™ is considered the more potent preparation, may have beneficial effects in reducing the incidence of delayed graft function, and is more widely used.

Thymoglobulin™ is usually administered in a dose of 1.5 mg per kg per day for a 4- to 7-day period. The first dose is administered intraoperatively, when Thymoglobulin is used as an induction agent. It is infused over a 4- to 8-hour period via a central venous catheter. In rare circumstances, it may be infused through a peripheral vein by adding hydrocortisone and heparin to the infusion and increasing the volume to prevent thrombophlebitis. Premedication with steroids, antihistamine, and acetaminophen is used in most centers, especially for the first two doses before ATGAM administration. Dose adjustment according to absolute CD3 (<10 to 20 per μL) or absolute lymphocyte (<250 per μL) count is performed in some centers.

Side Effects

Chills, fever, and arthralgia are the most common side effects; anaphylaxis has occurred in rare instances. This "cytokine-release syndrome" is less common with Thymoglobulin™. Because of polyspecificity, these agents not infrequently produce leukopenia and thrombocytopenia, necessitating dose reduction or occasionally temporary cessation. They also tend to cause increasing susceptibility to viral infections, especially CMV, as a result of prolonged depletion of lymphocytes.

Therapeutic Efficacy

Thymoglobulin™ is used as an induction agent in high-risk patients who have high panel-reactive antibody and are a repeat transplant. Thymoglobulin is also used to treat steroid-resistant rejection and acute humoral rejection.

Monoclonal Antibodies: OKT3, Basiliximab, and Daclizumab

Mouse Monoclonal Anti-CD3 Antibody: OKT3

MAbs have also been produced to different T-cell surface receptors. The first antibody used in clinical transplantation was the anti-CD3 antibody, OKT3, which binds to the δ chain of the TCR and is a potent inhibitor of almost all T-cell functions. OKT3 is extremely effective, but its use is limited in part by serious side effects. Meanwhile, OKT3 has been withdrawn from the market and will, therefore, not be discussed further in this chapter.

Monoclonal Anti-CD25 Antibody: Basiliximab and Daclizumab

The use of polyclonal antibodies for induction has decreased in the past decade and is being replaced by MAbs. The 2014 North American Pediatric Renal Trials and Collaborative Studies (NAPRTCS) report suggests that the use of polyclonal antibodies versus MAbs was 28% versus 22% in 1996 as compared with 26% versus 7% in 2013, respectively[114] (Fig. 42.2). The two

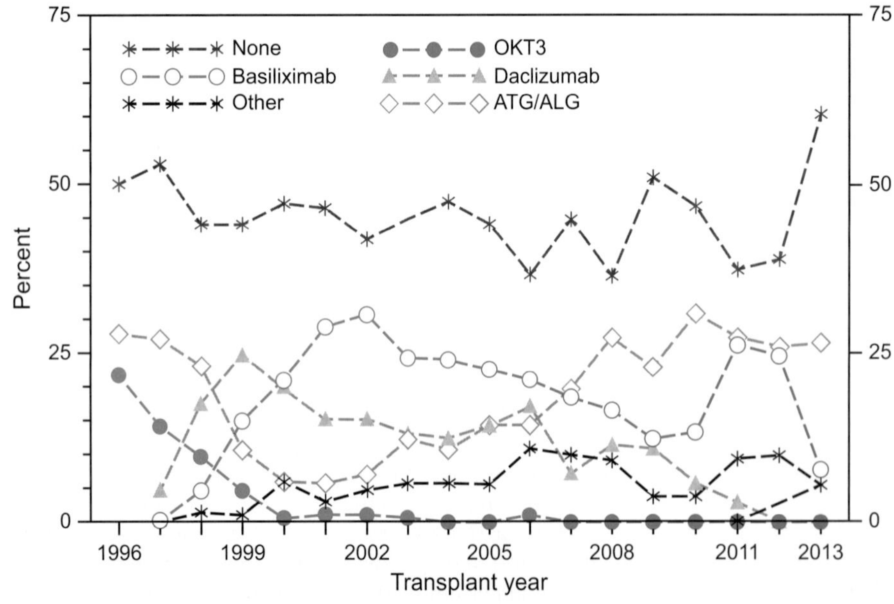

Figure 42.2 Induction antibody use in North American pediatric renal transplant recipients, by year of renal transplantation. (Adapted from The NAPRTCS 2014 Annual Report. https://web.emmes.com/study/ped/index.htm. Accessed August 15, 2019.)

commonly used MAbs were basiliximab (24%) and daclizumab (9.5%)[115]; however, daclizumab is no longer commercially available and will, therefore, not be discussed further in this chapter.

Mechanism of Action. The anti–IL-2R antibodies basiliximab and daclizumab exert their immunosuppressive effect by binding to the α chain of the IL-2R (anti-CD25). The IL-2R consists of three transmembrane protein chains: CD25, CD122, and CD132. CD25 is present on nearly all activated T cells, but not on resting T cells. IL-2 induces clonal expansion of activated T cells. Although CD25 does not transduce the signal, it is responsible for the association of IL-2 with the β and γ chains, which triggers the activated T cell to undergo rapid proliferation. These antibodies bind to activated T cells and render them resistant to IL-2 by blocking, shedding, or internalizing the receptor; they may also deplete and sequester some activated T cells. However, IL-2R functions are partially redundant because other cytokine receptors have overlapping functions, for example, IL-15Rs. Therefore, saturating IL-2Rs produces stable but relatively mild immunosuppression and is only effective in combination with other immunosuppressants.

Dosing and Pharmacokinetics. The dosing schedule for basiliximab is the following: intravenous administration of two 10-mg doses to children weighing less than 35 kg and of two 20-mg doses to children weighing 35 kg or greater, with the first dose given with surgery and the second on post-transplant day 4. In the 14 patients who were evaluated for the pharmacokinetics and pharmacodynamics of basiliximab and received concomitant immunosuppression with CsA and AZA, the mean duration of IL-2R saturation was 42 ± 16 days.[116] In a larger study of 82 patients who received basiliximab in combination with MMF, MMF reduced basiliximab clearance and prolonged CD25 saturation from 5 to 10 weeks.[117] In liver transplant patients, basiliximab has been found to have a shorter half-life of about 4 days and IL-2R blockade lasting 13 to 41 days because of loss of antibody in ascitic fluid and perioperative blood loss. However, satisfactory immunosuppression was achieved despite altered pharmacokinetics.

Therapeutic Efficacy. The effectiveness of IL-2R antibody therapy was best reported in a meta-analysis involving 38 trials that enrolled nearly 5,000 patients that assessed the impact of therapy on allograft loss and rejection.[118] Data were derived from published trials and abstracts of completed and ongoing trials. From these 38 trials, 14 trials enrolling 2,410 patients compared IL-2R antagonists with placebo for at least one outcome. Compared with placebo, IL-2R antagonists reduced acute rejection rates at 6 months (relative risk [RR: 0.66], confidence interval [CI]: 0.59 to 0.74) and 1 year (RR: 0.67, CI: 0.60 to 0.75), but the incidence of graft loss was the same. In pediatric renal transplant recipients, two large prospective randomized controlled trials showed that induction therapy with basiliximab in patients with low-to-standard immunologic risk on maintenance therapy (TAC in conjunction with AZA, or CsA in conjunction with MMF) did not lead to a statistically significant reduction in the incidence of acute rejection episodes.[119,120] As a result, there is presently no consensus among pediatric renal transplantation centers regarding the use and regimen for immunosuppressive induction therapy. Considerations in choosing the appropriate agent include the efficacy in the patient population (e.g., recipients with high or low risk of graft loss), the side-effect profile, and the concomitant immunosuppressive therapy (steroid avoidance, early steroid withdrawal, or conventional steroid therapy).

Side Effects. The safety profile of anti–IL-2R antibodies makes them an attractive choice for induction therapy.[121,122] They do not result in cytokine-release syndrome, thrombocytopenia, or anti-idiotype antibody development, and their use per se has not been associated with an increased incidence of CMV infection and PTLD. However, long-term studies, especially in children, are lacking.

GLUCOCORTICOIDS

Although there is much interest in developing and testing steroid-sparing, steroid-withdrawal, and steroid-avoidance immunosuppressive protocols in solid-organ transplantation,[123,124] glucocorticoids (steroids) continue to be involved in all phases of post-transplant management, including induction and maintenance therapy for prevention of allograft rejection and first-line treatment of acute rejection episodes.

Mechanism of Action

Steroids have an effect on almost all components of the immune and inflammatory response, which contributes to their global immunosuppressive effect. Steroids complex with cytoplasmic glucocorticoid receptors, which translocate into the nucleus and bind to glucocorticoid response elements in the promoter region of critical cytokine genes, thus inhibiting their transcription.[125,126] Steroids also reduce transcription of NF-κB–dependent cytokines by inducing transcription of the *IκBα* gene. IκBα protein then binds to NF-κB and prevents its translocation into the nucleus.[14,127,128] The reduced production of immunoregulatory and pro-inflammatory cytokines, such as TNF-α, IL-1, IL-2, IL-6, IL-8, and IFN-γ, inhibits T-cell proliferation, prevents upregulation of adhesion molecules, and reduces the intensity of the inflammatory response. Glucocorticoids also increase production of Th2 cytokines, such as IL-4, IL-10, and IL-13, which have anti-inflammatory and antiproliferative effect.[124,129]

Pharmacokinetics

Glucocorticoids are primarily metabolized in the liver by cytochrome P450 microsomal enzymes. The hydroxyl derivatives are then conjugated with glucuronic acid, forming water-soluble compounds that are excreted by the kidneys. Because no TDM system is available for glucocorticoids, it is important to keep in mind possible pharmacokinetic interactions with other inducers or inhibitors of the cytochrome P450 system or with drugs metabolized by the same microsomal enzymes.

Dosing

The commonly used formulations are intravenous methylprednisolone and oral PRED or methylprednisolone, which has less mineralocorticoid activity than PRED and, therefore, causes less sodium retention. In many transplant centers, the initial dose of glucocorticoids is administered during surgery as intravenous methylprednisolone, at doses between 2 and 10 mg per kg body weight. The oral dose of glucocorticoids used for maintenance therapy varies between 15 and 60 mg per m^2 per day

(0.5 to 2 mg per kg body weight per day), which is gradually tapered over time to approximately 3 to 5 mg PRED per m^2 BSA, usually taken as a single morning dose. Alternate-day dosing is often administered 6 to 12 months post-transplant to minimize the effect of steroids on growth. When used for acute rejection episodes, methylprednisolone 10 mg per kg is given for 3 to 5 days, followed by a tapering schedule of oral PRED.

Side Effects

Steroid-induced side effects include Cushingoid habitus, hypertension, hyperlipidemia, osteopenia, growth retardation, aseptic necrosis of the femoral head, cataracts, glaucoma hyperglycemia, psychopathologic effects, impaired wound healing, and acne.

Therapeutic Use

Because of the multiple adverse effects of maintenance corticosteroid therapy, attempts have been made to withdraw or minimize steroid therapy in children with a renal allograft.[108,130-141] There are two major approaches in steroid minimization in pediatric renal transplantation: (a) late steroid withdrawal (>1 year post-transplantation) and (b) either complete steroid avoidance or early steroid withdrawal (<7 days post-transplantation). In the late steroid-withdrawal approach, the patients suitable for minimization are identified by stable post-transplant clinical course and renal function. In late steroid withdrawal, there is no need for an antibody induction in the perioperative period.[133,134] In early withdrawal or complete avoidance protocols, the criteria of suitability are predefined before transplantation (e.g., criteria of low immunologic risk), and antibody induction is used in all enrolled patients.[137-140] There is also an "intermediate" approach, combining elements from early and late withdrawal protocols, in which antibody induction is used; however, the decision of steroid withdrawal is delayed until 6 to 9 months, post-transplant, when stable renal graft function (sometimes combined with normal picture of protocol biopsy) allows to identify suitable candidates (as in the late withdrawal approach).[141] Steroid withdrawal has the advantage over steroid avoidance in that immunologically high-risk patients and those with unstable graft function can easily be identified beforehand and be excluded from steroid-free immunosuppression.

Steroid-avoidance protocols have been used successfully in both the United States and Europe. However, many of these protocols have chosen low-risk individuals and utilized intensive induction therapy, with induction therapy with thymoglobulin, TAC, and MMF.[140] Regarding the efficacy and safety of early steroid withdrawal or complete steroid avoidance, a randomized controlled study in 196 pediatric renal transplant recipients, two doses of daclizumab in patients treated with a regimen of TAC and MMF allowed early steroid withdrawal on day 5 post-transplant.[138] There was a comparable rate of biopsy-proven acute rejection rates after 6 months in patients off steroids compared with controls (10.2% vs. 7.1%). In addition, prepubertal patients with early steroid withdrawal showed better growth and lipid and glucose metabolism profiles compared with controls, without increases in graft rejection or loss. These favorable effects were confirmed in a follow-up study over a 2-year observation period.[139] The results of the North American randomized controlled multicenter study with a follow-up of 3 years post-transplant showed that the steroid-free group showed lower systolic blood pressure and lower cholesterol levels.[140] The authors concluded that complete steroid avoidance is safe and effective in nonsensitized children receiving primary kidney transplants.[140]

Nevertheless, steroid withdrawal or avoidance following renal transplantation remains a controversial issue. Although the benefits of using steroid-free protocols in pediatric patients show great promise, further study is needed to determine the impact on long-term allograft function and to identify patients (e.g., low immunologic risk) who can be successfully converted to steroid-free immunosuppression without increasing the risk of acute rejection.

CURRENT DESIGN OF IMMUNOSUPPRESSIVE PROTOCOLS

The incidence of acute rejection is highest in the early post-transplant period, with the majority of acute rejection episodes occurring in the first 3 months. Acute rejection is perhaps the single most important risk factor for subsequent development of chronic allograft nephropathy and graft loss in renal transplant recipients. This concept is incorporated in the typical design of immunosuppressive regimens, which call for intensified immunosuppression within the first week(s) post-transplant, called the induction phase, followed by a long-term maintenance phase.

INDUCTION PHASE

There is at present no consensus for immunosuppressive induction therapy following renal transplantation in children. At the present time, there is no consistent evidence that induction therapy is beneficial or cost-effective in low-risk patients on triple therapy with CNIs in conventional doses, MMF, and glucocorticoids. According to two prospective randomized controlled trials, induction therapy with basiliximab in pediatric patients with low or standard immunologic risk on maintenance therapy with either TAC in conjunction with AZA or CsA in conjunction with MMF did not lead to a statistically significant reduction in the incidence of acute rejection episodes.[119,120] Recent studies in the United States and Europe have investigated the potential of IL-2R antibodies or thymoglobulin in replacement of steroids with promising results. Another potential application is delayed graft function when the use of CNIs should be avoided.

Induction therapy produces the greatest benefits in groups at high risk for allograft rejection. These high-risk groups include African Americans, recipients of kidneys with prolonged cold ischemia time, and those at high immunologic risk, particularly individuals who are presensitized. The sequential induction regimen of thymoglobulin or IL-2R blocking antibodies followed by TAC or CsA is recommended in these high-risk groups.

MAINTENANCE PHASE

The optimal maintenance immunosuppressive therapy in pediatric renal transplantation is not established. The major immunosuppressive agents currently used in various combination regimens are TAC, CsA, MMF, AZA, EVR, SRL, and glucocorticoids (primarily oral PRED or methylprednisolone). We and most transplant centers currently utilize a maintenance regimen consisting of triple immunosuppression therapy with a CNI (TAC or CsA), an antimetabolite (MMF or AZA), and, in some patients, methylprednisolone. EVR or SRL is also used by some transplant centers in triple therapy regimens, sometimes in place of the CNI or the antimetabolite. Within the NAPRTCS registry, marked changes in the type of maintenance immunosuppression and dosing strategies have been observed over time.[142] These are substantially caused by the introduction of newer drugs, such as MMF and TAC (Tables 42.9 and 42.10). In the Cooperative European Paediatric Renal Transplant Initiative (CERTAIN) registry in the transplant era 2010 to 2018, the most popular immunosuppressive regimen at post-transplant day 30, applied in the majority of patients, was triple therapy with TAC, MMF, and PRED (Fig. 42.3).[143]

Thus, increasing utilization of potent induction and maintenance immunosuppressive medications has improved long-term graft survival and also helped in achieving the short-term goal of reduced rejection rates. On the other hand, we have seen an increase in infections and PTLD, and hence, immunosuppression minimization is being studied. The approach is targeted to either avoid or withdraw glucocorticoids or CNIs early on and normalize growth curves with minimal drug nephrotoxicity.

TABLE 42.9 Percent Drug Utilization—Day 30 Post-Transplant (Patients with Functioning Grafts)

	Transplant Era 1996–2001	*Transplant Era 2002–2007*	*Transplant Era 2008–2017*
Prednisone	97.8	82.4	59.7
Cyclosporine	71.8	15.5	3.1
TAC	23.9	78.9	92.7
MMF	52.5	77.0	87.7
AZA	26.6	3.1	4.9
Sirolimus	3.6	13.4	0.5

AZA, azathioprine; CsA, cyclosporin A; MMF, mycophenolate mofetil; TAC, tacrolimus.
From Chua A, Cramer C, Moudgil A, et al. Kidney transplant practice patterns and outcome benchmarks over 30 years: the 2018 report of the North American Pediatric Renal Trials and Collaborative Studies. *Pediatr Transplant.* 2019;23:e13597.

TABLE 42.10 Percent Drug Utilization—Post Transplant (Patients with Functioning Grafts)

	Transplant Era 1996–2001				*Transplant Era 2002–2007*				*Transplant Era 2008–2017*			
	30 d	**1 y**	**3 y**	**5 y**	**30 d**	**1 y**	**3 y**	**5 y**	**30 d**	**1 y**	**3 y**	**5 y**
Prednisone/CsA/MMF	35.4	38.1	30.6	22.4	9.7	8.6	7.9	7.5	1.7	1.9	0.5	0.7
Prednisone/CsA/AZA	23.1	17.7	14.2	8.9	0.8	0.8	0.6	0.7	0.1	0.2	0.3	0.4
Prednisone/CsA	10.7	4.4	3.8	3.5	1.5	0.8	0.3	0.8	0.4	0.3	0.2	0.0
Prednisone/TAC/MMF	14.3	19.6	24.4	30.1	51.3	49.6	44.2	42.1	48.9	41.7	38.6	33.1
Prednisone/TAC/AZA	2.3	4.9	6.5	6.9	1.7	2.4	2.7	3.9	2.0	2.3	4.3	6.3
Prednisone/TAC	4.2	5.0	6.7	6.9	4.1	5.8	6.7	6.2	2.9	8.2	8.0	6.7
TAC/MMF	0.4	1.1	1.7	2.5	10.7	9.4	11.5	13.1	33.8	27.3	26.5	27.5
Other combination	9.5	9.2	12.0	17.3	20.1	22.7	26.0	25.8	10.1	18.1	21.6	25.3

AZA, azathioprine; CsA, cyclosporin A; MMF, mycophenolate mofetil; TAC, tacrolimus.
From Chua A, Cramer C, Moudgil A, et al. Kidney transplant practice patterns and outcome benchmarks over 30 years: the 2018 report of the North American Pediatric Renal Trials and Collaborative Studies. *Pediatr Transplant* 2019;23:e13597.

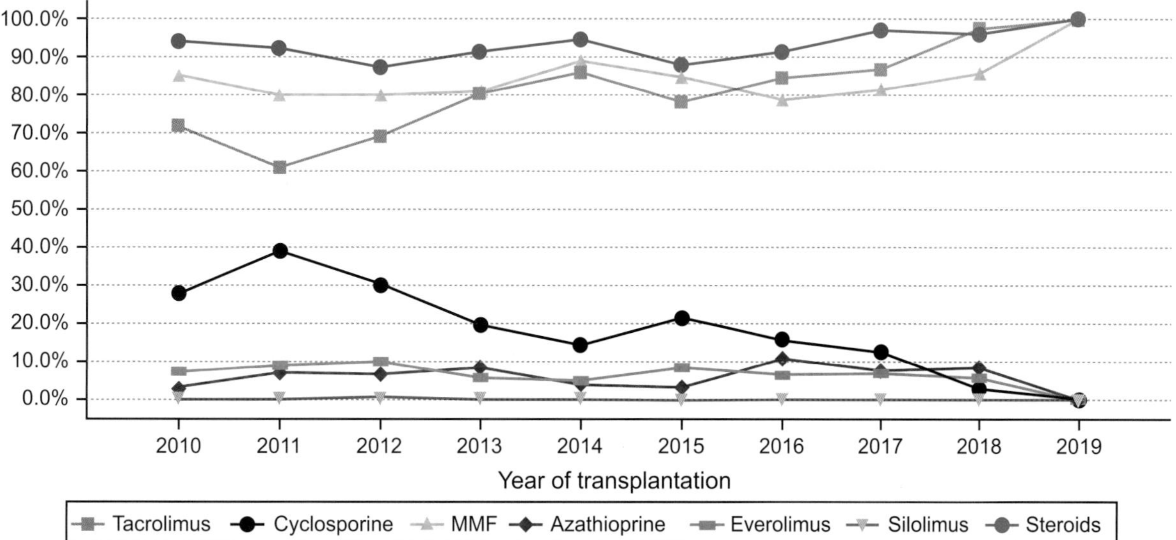

Figure 42.3 Observed drug utilization rates in European pediatric renal transplant recipients among transplanted grafts with ≥30 days function, by year of renal transplantation. (Adapted from Cooperative European Paediatric Renal Transplant Initiative (CERTAIN) registry. www.certain-registry.eu. Accessed August 15, 2019).

ACKNOWLEDGMENTS

The authors are thankful to Dr. Amrish Jain, Dr. Rudolph P. Valentini, Dr. Tej K. Mattoo, and Dr. Scott A. Gruber for their contribution to the previous version of this chapter.

REFERENCES

1. Papalois VE, Najarian JS. Pediatric kidney transplantation: historic hallmarks and a personal perspective. *Pediatr Transplant* 2001;5:239–245.
2. Gibson T, Medawar PB. The behavior of skin homografts in man. *J Anat* 1943;77:299–310.
3. Murray JE, Merrill JP, Harrison JH. Kidney transplantation between seven pairs of identical twins. *Ann Surg* 1958;148:343–359.
4. Schwartz R, Dameshek W. Drug-induced immunological tolerance. *Nature* 1959;183:1682–1683.
5. Starzl TE, Marchioro TL, Porter KA, et al. The use of heterologous antilymphoid agents in canine renal and liver homotransplantation and in human renal homotransplantation. *Surg Gynecol Obstet* 1967;124:301–308.
6. Borel JF, Feurer C, Gubler HU, et al. Biological effects of cyclosporin A: a new antilymphocytic agent. *Agents Actions* 1976;6:468–475.
7. Organ Procurement and Transplant Network. http://optn.transplant.hrsa.gov/latestData/viewDataReports.asp. Accessed September 1, 2019.
8. United States Renal Data System. http://www.usrds.org/2018. Accessed September 1, 2019.
9. Pietra BA. Transplantation immunology 2003: simplified approach. *Pediatr Clin N Am* 2003;50:1233–1259.
10. Halloran PF. Immunosuppressive drugs for kidney transplantation. *N Engl J Med* 2004;351:2715–2729.
11. Kari JA, Trompeter RS. What is the calcineurin inhibitor of choice for pediatric renal transplantation? *Pediatr Transplant* 2004;8:437–444.
12. Scott LJ, McKeage K, Keam SJ, et al. Tacrolimus: a further update of its use in the management of organ transplantation. *Drugs* 2003;63:1247–1297.
13. Hutchinson IV, Bagnall W, Bryce P, et al. Differences in the mode of action of cyclosporine and FK 506. *Transplant Proc* 1998;30:959–960.
14. Suthanthiran M, Strom TB. Immunoregulatory drugs: mechanistic basis for use in organ transplantation. *Pediatr Nephrol* 1997;11:651–657.
15. Batiuk TD, Pazderka F, Halloran PF. Calcineurin activity is only partially inhibited in leukocytes of cyclosporine-treated patients. *Transplantation* 1995;59:1400–1404.
16. Filler G. Calcineurin inhibitors in pediatric renal transplant recipients. *Pediatr Drugs* 2007;9:165–174.
17. Khanna AK, Cairns VR, Becker CG, et al. TGF-beta: a link between immunosuppression, nephrotoxicity, and CsA. *Transplant Proc* 1998;30:944–945.
18. Drewe J, Beglinger C, Kissel T. The absorption site of cyclosporin in the human gastrointestinal tract. *Br J Clin Pharmacol* 1992;33:39–43.
19. Dunn CJ, Wagstaff AJ, Perry CM, et al. Cyclosporin: an updated review of the pharmacokinetic properties, clinical efficacy and tolerability of a microemulsion-based formulation (Neoral) in organ transplantation. *Drugs* 2001;61:1957–2016.
20. Cooney GF, Habucky K, Hoppu K. Cyclosporin pharmacokinetics in paediatric transplant recipients. *Clin Pharmacokinet* 1997;32:481–495.
21. Roberts MS, Magnusson BM, Burczynski FJ, et al. Enterohepatic circulation: physiological, pharmacokinetic and clinical implications. *Clin Pharmacokinet* 2002;41:751–790.
22. van Gelder T. Drug interactions with tacrolimus. *Drug Saf* 2002;25:707–712.
23. Macphee IA, Fredericks S, Tai T, et al. Tacrolimus pharmacogenetics: polymorphisms associated with expression of cytochrome p4503A5 and P-glycoprotein correlate with dose requirement. *Transplantation* 2002;74:1486–1489.
24. Filler G, Trompeter R, Webb NJ, et al. One year glomerular filtration rate predicts graft survival in pediatric renal recipients: a randomized trial of tacrolimus vs cyclosporine microemulsion. *Transplant Proc* 2002;34:1935–1938.
25. van Gelder T. ESOT advisory committee on generic substitution. European Society for Organ Transplantation Advisory Committee recommendations on generic substitution of immunosuppressive drugs. *Transpl Int* 2011; 24:1135–1141.
26. Montini G, Ujka F, Varagnolo C, et al. The pharmacokinetics and immunosuppressive response of tacrolimus in pediatric renal transplant recipients. *Pediatr Nephrol* 2006;21:719–724.
27. Venkataramanan R, Swaminathan A, Prasad T, et al. Clinical pharmacokinetics of tacrolimus. *Clin Pharmacokinet* 1995;29:404–430.
28. Yasuhara M, Hashida T, Toraguchi M, et al. Pharmacokinetics and pharmacodynamics of FK 506 in pediatric patients receiving living-related donor liver transplantations. *Transplant Proc* 1995;27:1108–1110.
29. Wallemacq PE, Verbeeck RK. Comparative clinical pharmacokinetics of tacrolimus in paediatric and adult patients. *Clin Pharmacokinet* 2001;40:283–295.
30. Shishido S, Asanuma H, Tajima E, et al. Pharmacokinetics of tacrolimus in pediatric renal transplant recipients. *Transplant Proc* 2001;33:1066–1068.
31. Christians U, Strom T, Zhang YL, et al. Active drug transport of immunosuppressants: new insights for pharmacokinetics and pharmacodynamics. *Ther Drug Monit* 2006;28:39–44.
32. Wallemacq PE, Furlan V, Moller A, et al. Pharmacokinetics of tacrolimus (FK506) in paediatric liver transplant recipients. *Eur J Drug Metab Pharmacokinet* 1998;23:367–370.
33. Andrews LM, Li Y, De Winter BCM, et al. Pharmacokinetic considerations related to therapeutic drug monitoring of tacrolimus in kidney transplant patients. *Expert Opin Drug Metab Toxicol* 2017;13:1225–1236
34. De Jonge H, De Loor H, Verbeke K, et al. In vivo CYP3A4 activity, CYP3A5 genotype, and hematocrit predict tacrolimus dose requirements and clearance in renal transplant patients. *Clin Pharmacol Ther* 2012;92:366–375.
35. Tang JT, Andrews LM, Van Gelder T, et al. Pharmacogenetic aspects of the use of tacrolimus in renal transplantation: recent developments and ethnic considerations. *Expert Opin Drug Metab Toxicol* 2016;12:555–565.
36. Kuehl P, Zhang J, Lin Y, et al. Sequence diversity in CYP3A promoters and characterization of the genetic basis of polymorphic CYP3A5 expression. *Nat Genet* 2001;27:383–391.
37. Picard N, Bergan S, Marquet P, et al. Pharmacogenetic biomarkers predictive of the pharmacokinetics and pharmacodynamics of immunosuppressive drugs. *Ther Drug Monit* 2016;38(Suppl 1):S57–S69.
38. Billing H, Höcker B, Fichtner A, et al. Single-nucleotide polymorphism of CYP3A5 impacts the exposure to tacrolimus in pediatric renal transplant recipients: a pharmacogenetic substudy of the TWIST trial. *Ther Drug Monit* 2017;39:21–28
39. Andrews LM, De Winter BC, Tang JT, et al. Overweight kidney transplant recipients are at risk of being overdosed following standard bodyweight-based tacrolimus starting dose. *Transplant Direct* 2017;3:e129.
40. Lemahieu W, Maes B, Verbeke K, et al. Cytochrome P450 3A4 and P-glycoprotein activity and assimilation of tacrolimus in transplant patients with persistent diarrhea. *Am J Transplant* 2005;5:1383–1391.
41. Filler G, Grygas R, Mai I, et al. Pharmacokinetics of tacrolimus (FK 506) in children and adolescents with renal transplants. *Nephrol Dial Transplant* 1997;12:1668–1671.
42. McDiarmid SV, Colonna JO, Shaked A, et al. Differences in oral FK506 dose requirements between adult and pediatric liver transplant patients. *Transplantation* 1993;55:1328–1332.
43. Mehta P, Beltz S, Kedar A, et al. Increased clearance of tacrolimus in children: need for higher doses and earlier initiation prior to bone marrow transplantation. *Bone Marrow Transplant* 1999;24:1323–1327.
44. Manzanares C, Moreno M, Castellanos F, et al. Influence of hepatitis C virus infection on FK 506 blood levels in renal transplant patients. *Transplant Proc* 1998;30:1264–1265.
45. Moreno M, Manzanares C, Castellano F, et al. Monitoring of tacrolimus as rescue therapy in pediatric liver transplantation. *Ther Drug Monit* 1998;20:376–379.
46. Webb NJA, Baumann U, Camino M, et al. Pharmacokinetics of tacrolimus granules in pediatric de novo liver, kidney, and heart transplantation: The OPTION study. *Pediatr Transplant* 2019;23:e13328.
47. Rubik J, Debray D, Iserin F, et al. Comparative pharmacokinetics of tacrolimus in stable pediatric allograft recipients converted from immediate-release tacrolimus to prolonged-release tacrolimus formulation. *Pediatr Transplant* 2019;23:e13391.
48. Rubik J, Debray D, Kelly D, et al. Efficacy and safety of prolonged-release tacrolimus in stable pediatric allograft recipients converted from immediate-release tacrolimus – a Phase 2, open-label, single-arm, one-way crossover study. *Transpl Int* 2019;32:1182–1193.
49. Lindholm A, Kahan BD. Influence of cyclosporine pharmacokinetics, trough concentrations, and AUC monitoring on outcome after kidney transplantation. *Clin Pharmacol Ther* 1993;54:205–218.
50. Mahalati K, Belitsky P, Sketris I, et al. Neoral monitoring by simplified sparse sampling area under the concentration–time curve: its relationship to acute rejection and cyclosporine nephrotoxicity early after kidney transplantation. *Transplantation* 1999;68:55–62.
51. Shaw LM, Holt DW, Keown P, et al. Current opinions on therapeutic drug monitoring of immunosuppressive drugs. *Clin Ther* 1999;21:1632–1652.
52. Kahan BD, Keown P, Levy GA, et al. Therapeutic drug monitoring of immunosuppressant drugs in clinical practice. *Clin Ther* 2002;24:330–350.
53. Weber LT, Armstrong VW, Shipkova M, et al. Cyclosporin A absorption profiles in pediatric renal transplant recipients predict the risk of acute rejection. *Ther Drug Monit* 2004;26:415-424
54. Brunet M, van Gelder T, Åsberg A, et al. Therapeutic drug monitoring of tacrolimus-personalized therapy: second consensus report. *Ther Drug Monit* 2019;41:261–307
55. Jusko WJ, Thomson AW, Fung J, et al. Consensus document: therapeutic monitoring of tacrolimus (FK-506). *Ther Drug Monit* 1995;17:606–614.
56. Shapiro R. Tacrolimus in pediatric renal transplantation: a review. *Pediatr Transplant* 1998;2:270–276.
57. Webster A, Woodroffe RC, Taylor RS, et al. Tacrolimus versus cyclosporine as primary immunosuppression for kidney transplant recipients. *Cochrane Database Syst Rev* 2005;4:CD003961.
58. Trompeter R, Filler G, Webb NJ, et al. Randomized trial of tacrolimus versus cyclosporin microemulsion in renal transplantation. *Pediatr Nephrol* 2002;17:141–149.
59. Valentini RP, Imam A, Warrier I, et al. Sirolimus rescue for tacrolimus-associated post-transplant autoimmune hemolytic anemia. *Pediatr Transplant* 2006;10:358–361.
60. Campana C, Regazzi MB, Buggia I, et al. Clinically significant drug interactions with cyclosporin. An update. *Clin Pharmacokinet* 1996;30:141–179.
61. Filler G, Webb NJ, Milford DV, et al. Four-year data after pediatric renal transplantation: a randomized trial of tacrolimus vs cyclosporine microemulsion. *Pediatr Transplant* 2005;9:498–503.
62. Allison AC, Eugui EM. Mechanisms of action of mycophenolate mofetil in preventing acute and chronic allograft rejection. *Transplant* 2005; 80:181–190.
63. van Leuven SI, Kastelein JJ, Allison AC, et al. Mycophenolate mofetil (MMF): firing at the atherosclerotic plaque from different angles? *Cardiovasc Res* 2006; 69:341–347.
64. Jacqz-Aigrain E, Khan SE, Baudouin V, et al. Pharmacokinetics and tolerance of mycophenolate mofetil in renal transplant children. *Pediatr Nephrol* 2000;14:95–99.
65. Weber LT, Shipkova M, Armstrong VW, et al. Comparison of the Emit immunoassay with HPLC for therapeutic drug monitoring of mycophenolic acid in pediatric renal-transplant recipients on mycophenolate mofetil therapy. *Clin Chem* 2002;48:517–525.
66. Weber LT, Shipkova M, Armstrong VW, et al. The pharmacokinetic–pharmacodynamic relationship for total and free mycophenolic acid in pediatric renal transplant recipients: a report of the German study group on mycophenolate mofetil therapy. *J Am Soc Nephrol* 2002;13:759–768.

67. Weber LT, Schutz E, Lamersdorf T, et al. Therapeutic drug monitoring of total and free mycophenolic acid (MPA) and limited sampling strategy for determination of MPA-AUC in paediatric renal transplant recipients. The German Study Group on Mycophenolate Mofetil (MMF) Therapy. *Nephrol Dial Transplant* 1999;14(Suppl 4): 34–35.
68. Weber LT, Schutz E, Lamersdorf T, et al. Pharmacokinetics of mycophenolic acid (MPA) and free MPA in paediatric renal transplant recipients—a multicentre study. The German Study Group on Mycophenolate Mofetil (MMF) Therapy. *Nephrol Dial Transplant* 1999;14(Suppl 4):33–34.
69. Tönshoff B, David-Neto E, Ettenger R, et al. Pediatric aspects of therapeutic drug monitoring of mycophenolic acid in renal transplantation. *Transplant Rev (Orlando)* 2011;25:78–89.
70. van Gelder T, Silva HT, de Fijter JW, et al. Comparing mycophenolate mofetil regimens for de novo renal transplant recipients: the fixed-dose concentration-controlled trial. *Transplantation* 2008 86:1043–1051.
71. Höcker B, van Gelder T, Martin-Govantes J, et al. Comparison of MMF efficacy and safety in paediatric vs. adult renal transplantation: subgroup analysis of the randomised, multicentre FDCC trial. *Nephrol Dial Transplant* 2011 26:1073–1079
72. Shipkova M, Armstrong VW, Oellerich M, et al. Mycophenolate mofetil in organ transplantation: focus on metabolism, safety and tolerability. *Expert Opin Drug Metab Toxicol* 2005;1:505–526
73. Kaplan B, Gruber SA, Nallamathou R, et al. Decreased protein binding of mycophenolic acid associated with leukopenia in a pancreas transplant recipient with renal failure. *Transplantation* 1998;65:1127–1129.
74. Weber LT, Lamersdorf T, Shipkova M, et al. Area under the plasma concentration–time curve for total, but not for free, mycophenolic acid increases in the stable phase after renal transplantation: a longitudinal study in pediatric patients. German Study Group on Mycophenolate Mofetil Therapy in Pediatric Renal Transplant Recipients. *Ther Drug Monit* 1999;21:498–506.
75. Arns W, Cibrik DM, Walker RG, et al. Therapeutic drug monitoring of mycophenolic acid in solid organ transplant patients treated with mycophenolate mofetil: review of the literature. *Transplantation* 2006;82:1004–1012.
76. Shaw LM, Holt DW, Oellerich M, et al. Current issues in therapeutic drug monitoring of mycophenolic acid: report of a roundtable discussion. *Ther Drug Monit* 2001;23:305.
77. Le Meur Y, Büchler M, Thierry A, et al. Individualized mycophenolate mofetil dosing based on drug exposure significantly improves patient outcomes after renal transplantation. *Am J Transplant* 2007; 7:2496–2503
78. Mourad M, Wallemacq P, Konig J, et al. Therapeutic monitoring of mycophenolate mofetil in organ transplant recipients: is it necessary? *Clin Pharmacokinet* 2002;41:319–327.
79. Filler G, Zimmering M, Mai I. Pharmacokinetics of mycophenolate mofetil are influenced by concomitant immunosuppression. *Pediatr Nephrol* 2000;14:100–104.
80. Cattaneo D, Perico N, Gaspari F, et al. Glucocorticoids interfere with mycophenolate mofetil bioavailability in kidney transplantation. *Kidney Int* 2002;62:1060–1067.
81. Zimmerhackl LB, Wiesmayr S, Kirste G, et al. Mycophenolate mofetil (Cellcept) in pediatric renal transplantation. *Transplant Proc* 2006;38:2038–2040.
82. Bunchman T, Navarro M, Broyer M, et al. The use of mycophenolate mofetil suspension in pediatric renal allograft recipients. *Pediatr Nephrol* 2001;16:978–984.
83. Höcker B, Weber LT, Bunchman T, et al. Mycophenolate mofetil suspension in pediatric renal transplantation: three-year data from the tricontinental trial. *Pediatr Transplant* 2005;9:504–511.
84. Höcker B, Tönshoff B. Calcineurin inhibitor-free immunosuppression in pediatric renal transplantation: a viable option? *Paediatr Drugs* 2011;13:49–69.
85. Höcker B, Tönshoff B. Treatment strategies to minimize or prevent chronic allograft dysfunction in pediatric renal transplant recipients: an overview. *Paediatr Drugs* 2009;11:381–396.
86. Yagil Y, Yagil C. Insights into pharmacogenomics and its impact upon immunosuppressive therapy. *Transpl Immunol* 2002;9:203–209.
87. Abraham RT, Wiederrecht GJ. Immunopharmacology of rapamycin. *Annu Rev Immunol* 1996;14:483–510.
88. Rapamune. *Summary of product characteristics*. New York: Pfizer, Last updated 2011
89. Certican. *Basic prescribing information*. Basel, Switzerland: Novartis Pharma AG, 2012
90. Sehgal SN, Rapamune (RAPA, rapamycin, sirolimus): mechanism of action; immunosuppressive effect results from blockade of signal transduction and inhibition of cell cycle progression. *Clin Biochem* 1998;31:335–340.
91. Ettenger RB, Grimm EM. Safety and efficacy of TOR inhibitors in pediatric renal transplant recipients. *Am J Kidney Dis* 2001;38:S22–S28.
92. Gallant-Haidner HL, Trepanier DJ, Freitag DG, et al. Pharmacokinetics and metabolism of sirolimus. *Ther Drug Monit* 2000;22:31–35.
93. Mahalati K, Kahan BD. Clinical pharmacokinetics of sirolimus. *Clin Pharmacokinet* 2001;40:573–585.
94. Höcker B, Feneberg R, Köpf S, et al. SRL-based immunosuppression vs. CNI minimization in pediatric renal transplant recipients with chronic CNI nephrotoxicity. *Pediatr Transplant* 2006 10:593–601.
95. Schachter AD, Meyers KE, Spaneas LD, et al. Short sirolimus half-life in pediatric renal transplant recipients on a calcineurin inhibitor-free protocol. *Pediatr Transplant* 2004;8:171–177.
96. Crowe A, Bruelisauer A, Duerr L, et al. Absorption and intestinal metabolism of SDZ-RAD and rapamycin in rats. *Drug Metab Dispos* 1999;27:627–632.
97. Meier-Kriesche HU, Kaplan B. Toxicity and efficacy of sirolimus: relationship to whole-blood concentrations. *Clin Ther* 2000;22(Suppl B):B93–B100.
98. Kahan BD, Napoli KL, Kelly PA, et al. Therapeutic drug monitoring of sirolimus: correlations with efficacy and toxicity. *Clin Transplant* 2000;14:97–109.
99. Ettenger R, Hoyer PF, Grimm P, et al. Multicenter trial of everolimus in pediatric renal transplant recipients: Results at three year. *Pediatr Transplant* 2008;12: 456–463.
100. Pape L, Ahlenstiel T, Ehrich JH, et al. Reversal of loss of glomerular filtration rate in children with transplant nephropathy after switch to everolimus and low-dose cyclosporine A. *Pediatr Transplant* 2007;11:291–295.
101. Kovarik JM, Curtis JJ, Hricik DE, et al. Differential pharmacokinetic interaction of tacrolimus and cyclosporine on everolimus. *Transplant Proc* 2006;38:3456–3458.
102. Kirchner GI, Meier-Wiedenbach I, Manns MP. Clinical pharmacokinetics of everolimus. *Clin Pharmacokinet* 2004;43:83–95.
103. Kovarik JM, Kalbag J, Figuerredo J, et al. Differential influence of two cyclosporine formulations on everolimus pharmacokinetics: a clinically relevant pharmacokinetic interaction. *J Clin Pharmacol* 2002;42:95–99.
104. Brandhorst G, Tenderich G, Zittermann A, et al. Everolimus exposure in cardiac transplant recipients is influenced by concomitant calcineurin inhibitor. *Ther Drug Monit* 2008;30:113–116.
105. Ciancio G, Burke GW, Gaynor JJ, et al. A randomized long-term trial of tacrolimus and sirolimus versus tacrolimus and mycophenolate mofetil versus cyclosporine (Neoral) and sirolimus in renal transplantation. I. Drug interactions and rejection at one year. *Transplantation* 2004;77:244–251.
106. Wu FL, Tsai MK, Chen RR, et al. Effects of calcineurin inhibitors on sirolimus pharmacokinetics during staggered administration in renal transplant recipients. *Pharmacotherapy* 2005;25:646–653.
107. Ganschow R, Pape L, Sturm E, et al. Growing experience with mTOR inhibitors in pediatric solid organ transplantation. *Pediatr Transplant* 2013;17:694–706
108. Tönshoff B, Ettenger R, Dello Strologo L, et al. Early conversion of pediatric kidney transplant patients to everolimus with reduced tacrolimus and steroid elimination: results of a randomized trial. *Am J Transplant* 2019;19:811–822.
109. Tedesco-Silva H, Felipe C, Ferreira A, et al. Reduced incidence of cytomegalovirus infection in kidney transplant recipients receiving everolimus and reduced tacrolimus doses. *Am J Transplant* 2015;15:2655–2664.
110. Höcker B, Zencke S, Pape L, et al. Impact of everolimus and low-dose cyclosporin on cytomegalovirus replication and disease in pediatric renal transplantation. *Am J Transplant* 2016;16:921–929.
111. Brennan DC. Polyclonal antibodies in immunosuppression. *Transplant Proc* 2001;33:1002–1004.
112. Merion RM, Howell T, Bromberg JS. Partial T-cell activation and anergy induction by polyclonal antithymocyte globulin. *Transplantation* 1998;65:1481–1489.
113. Brophy PD, Thomas SE, McBryde KD, et al. Comparison of polyclonal induction agents in pediatric renal transplantation. *Pediatr Transplant* 2001;5:174–178.
114. The NAPRTCS 2014 Annual Report. https://web.emmes.com/study/ped/index.htm. Accessed August 15, 2019.
115. Pescovitz MD. Use of antibody induction in pediatric renal transplantation. *Curr Opin Organ Transplant* 2008;13:495–499.
116. Sterkers G, Baudouin V, Ansart-Pirenne H, et al. Duration of action of a chimeric interleukin-2 receptor monoclonal antibody, basiliximab, in pediatric kidney transplant recipients. *Transplant Proc* 2000;32:2757–2759.
117. Höcker B, Kovarik JM, Daniel V, et al. Pharmacokinetics and immunodynamics of basiliximab in pediatric renal transplant recipients on mycophenolate mofetil comedication. *Transplantation* 2008;86:1234–1240.
118. Webster AC, Playford EG, Higgins G, et al. Interleukin 2 receptor antagonists for renal transplant recipients: a meta-analysis of randomized trials. *Transplantation* 2004;77:166–176.
119. Grenda R, Watson A, Vondrak K, et al. A prospective, randomized, multicenter trial of tacrolimus-based therapy with or without basiliximab in pediatric renal transplantation. *Am J Transplant* 2006;6:1666–1672.
120. Offner G, Toenshoff B, Höcker B, et al. Efficacy and safety of basiliximab in pediatric renal transplant patients receiving cyclosporine, mycophenolate mofetil, and steroids. *Transplantation* 2008;86:1241–1248.
121. Kelly DA. The use of anti-interleukin-2 receptor antibodies in pediatric liver transplantation. *Pediatr Transplant* 2001;5:386–389.
122. Ettenger RB. Antibody therapy as an induction regimen in pediatric renal transplantation. *Transplant Proc* 1999;31:2677–2678.
123. Ponticelli C, Tarantino A, Montagnino G. Steroid withdrawal in renal transplant recipients. *Transplant Proc* 2001;33:987–988.
124. Ponticelli C. Steroid-free immunosuppression. *Transplant Proc* 2001;33:3259–3260.
125. Almawi WY, Hess DA, Rieder MJ. Multiplicity of glucocorticoid action in inhibiting allograft rejection. *Cell Transplant* 1998;7:511–523.
126. Almawi WY, Abou Jaoude MM, Li XC. Transcriptional and post-transcriptional mechanisms of glucocorticoid antiproliferative effects. *Hematol Oncol* 2002;20:17–32.
127. Almawi WY, Melemedjian OK. Negative regulation of nuclear factor-kappaB activation and function by glucocorticoids. *J Mol Endocrinol* 2002;28:69–78.
128. Tsoulfas G, Geller DA. NF-kappaB in transplantation: friend or foe? *Transpl Infect Dis* 2001;3:212–219.
129. Almawi WY, Melemedjian OK, Rieder MJ. An alternate mechanism of glucocorticoid anti-proliferative effect: promotion of a Th2 cytokine-secreting profile. *Clin Transplant* 1999;13:365–374.
130. Benfield MR, Bartosh S, Ikle D, et al. A randomized double-blind, placebo controlled trial of steroid withdrawal after pediatric renal transplantation. *Am J Transplant* 2010;10:81–88.
131. Sutherland S, Li L, Concepcion W, et al. Steroid-free immunosuppression in pediatric renal transplantation: rationale for and outcomes following conversion to steroid based therapy. *Transplantation* 2009;87:1744–1748.
132. Barletta GM, Kirk E, Gardner JJ, et al. Rapid discontinuation of corticosteroids in pediatric renal transplantation. *Pediatr Transplant* 2009; 13:571–578.
133. Höcker B, Weber LT, Feneberg R, et al. Prospective, randomized trial on late steroid withdrawal in pediatric renal transplant recipients under cyclosporine microemulsion and mycophenolate mofetil. *Transplantation* 2009; 87:934–941.

134. Höcker B, Weber L, Feneberg R, et al. Improved growth and cardiovascular risk after late steroid withdrawal: 2-year results of a prospective, randomized trial in paediatric renal transplantation. *Nephrol Dial Transplant* 2010;25:617–624
135. Sarwal MM, Vidhun JR, Alexander SR, et al. Continued superior outcomes with modification and lengthened follow-up of a steroid-avoidance pilot with extended daclizumab induction in pediatric renal transplantation. *Transplantation* 2003;76:1331–1339.
136. Shapiro R, Ellis D, Tan HP, et al. Antilymphoid antibody preconditioning and tacrolimus monotherapy for pediatric kidney transplantation. *J Pediatr* 2006; 148:813–818.
137. Chavers BM, Chang C, Gillingham KJ, et al. Pediatric kidney transplantation using a novel protocol of rapid (6-day) discontinuation of prednisolone: 2-year results. *Transplantation* 2009;88:237–241.
138. Grenda R, Watson A, Trompeter R, et al. A randomized trial to assess the impact of early steroid withdrawal on growth in pediatric renal transplantation: the TWIST Study. *Am J Transplant* 2010;10:828–836.
139. Webb N, Douglas S, Rajai A, et al. Corticosteroid-free kidney transplantation improves growth: two-year follow-up of the TWIST randomised controlled trial. *Transplantation* 2015;99:1178–1185.
140. Sarwal MM, Ettenger RB, Dharnidharka V, et al. Complete corticosteroid avoidance is effective and safe in children with renal transplants: a multicentre randomized trial with three year follow-up. *Am J Transpl* 2012;12:2719–2729.
141. Pape L, Offner G, Kreuzer M, et al. De novo therapy with everolimus, low-dose cyclosporine A, basiliximab and steroid elimination in pediatric kidney transplantation. *Am J Transplant* 2010;10:2349–2354.
142. Chua A, Cramer C, Moudgil A, et al. Kidney transplant practice patterns and outcome benchmarks over 30 years: the 2018 report of the North American Pediatric Renal Trials and Collaborative Studies. *Pediatr Transplant* 2019;23:e13597
143. Cooperative European Paediatric Renal Transplant Initiative (CERTAIN) registry. www.certain-registry.eu. Accessed August 15, 2019.

SECTION

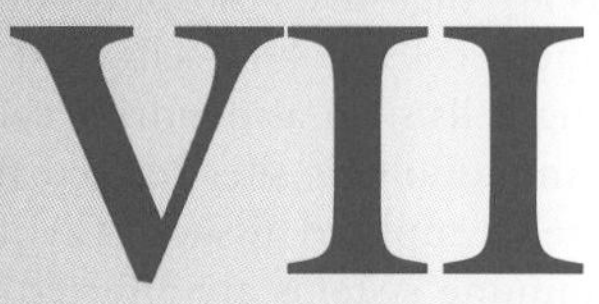

Pharmacology of Biologic Drugs

CHAPTER

43

Desirée Rivera-Nieves
Josef Neu

Microbial Therapeutics: Beyond Probiotics

INTRODUCTION

Trillions of microbes reside within the human gastrointestinal (GI) tract. There is an aboral gradient of microbial concentration, with the lowest in the upper GI tract and the highest in the large intestine, where the concentration of microbes approximates 10^{11} microbes per gram of intestinal content.[1] Culture-based techniques employed to evaluate microbes in complex niches, such as soils, bodies of water, and the GI tract, have been insufficient when attempting to address the "great plate count anomaly," which refers to the barriers to cultivation of the fastidious and, mostly strictly, anaerobic bacteria that reside in these niches.

Nonculture-based technologies using high-throughput microbial DNA sequencing technologies along with sophisticated bioinformatics analyses, algorithms, and pipelines with the ability to handle large amounts of data recently developed have stimulated paradigm shifting advances in the field of microbial analysis, especially when it comes to mining information about the intestinal microbiota. Using 16S ribosomal DNA and whole-genome metagenomics technologies has provided tools for identifying various microbes in a particular niche and also helped predict their function.[2]

With these recently developed novel technologies, investigators are now challenged with answering the following questions:

1. What other microbes exist?
2. Why are they in a particular niche?
3. What roles do different microbes play in the GI tract?
4. How do they interact with nutritional substrates, and what substances do they metabolize?
5. What are the products of microbial metabolism?
6. How do the microbes in a particular region of the intestinal tract respond to environmental pressures such as antibiotics and other drugs?
7. How do these microbes, their components, and their metabolic products interact with the host's immune system?
8. How do these microbial metabolites affect the host metabolic and physiologic responses such as nerve conduction?
9. How do the commensal microbes help protect the human host?
10. Is it possible to manipulate these microbes to further benefit the human host?

In this chapter, we address several of these questions. With the burgeoning thrust toward probiotic use over the past several decades, it will be necessary to address several of the issues associated with probiotic use, but we also address several related areas of microbial therapeutics, including fecal microbial transplantation, the best ways to identify specific cohorts of microbes to perform certain functions, and where this field will be heading in the future. First, it will be important to provide a brief overview of the microbial ecology of the GI tract during development.

THE MICROBIAL ECOLOGY OF THE DEVELOPING INTESTINE

THE FETUS

The GI tract of the newborn infant was at one time thought to be sterile. However, numerous studies have shown that meconium, the first stool of the newborn, often contains microbes.[3–7] As with studies of the placental microbiology, the presence and function of microbes seen in meconium remains controversial,[8] with the collection techniques, adequacy of controls, and possible kit contamination remaining contentious. The presence of live microbes in meconium indicates exposure to microbes in the GI tract prior to birth, with potentially major implications for intestinal development as well as development of the innate and adaptive immune systems. If there are in fact microbes present in the meconium that originate from a nonsterile fetal intestine, then the origin of these microbes is very likely due to entry from one of three potential sites: (1) ascending colonization from the vagina through the choriodecidual plate into the amniotic fluid that is swallowed by the fetus; (2) carriage of microbes that have translocated through the maternal intestine either by simple paracellular translocation directly into the maternal bloodstream or with the help of antigen-presenting (dendritic) cells that carry the bacteria from the maternal GI tract to that of the fetus; and/or (3) hematogenous spread from the maternal skin or the maternal oral cavity.[9–11]

Even if we do not invoke a colonized GI tract in fetus or the newborn infant that is immediately present at birth, it is likely that maternal microbes play a role in the development of the newborn immune system. This is evidenced by studies showing that various cells of the innate immune system are elevated for months when one compares newborn mice from germ-free mothers who had been treated with only one microbe during pregnancy compared to nontreated mothers.[12]

CONTRIBUTION OF MOTHER'S MILK AND DIET

The microbial ecosystems after birth are highly dependent on diet. Babies who are fed their own mother's milk compared to donor milk or formula harbor different microbial ecosystems in their GI tract.[13,14] With the onset of solid food intake, the microbial ecosystems of the developing GI tract become even more complex, and the type of diet plays a large role[15,16] not only in the different types of taxa of microbes that are present in the gut but also metabolic capabilities and immunologic interactions with the host.

ANTIBIOTICS AND H2 BLOCKER EFFECTS ON MICROBIAL DEVELOPMENT

It is clear that various perturbations in the GI tract, such as antibiotic use, use of H2 blocker protein pump inhibitors, and other pharmacologic agents, may have dramatic effects on the GI tract.[17–19] Furthermore as we discuss later, introduction of certain microbe-containing foods and/or probiotics may have profound effects on not only the intestinal microbial ecology but also many downstream effects in terms of metabolite production that can modulate the genomic transcriptional capabilities via epigenetic means that may have significant downstream effects throughout the individual's lifetime.

MICROBIAL–HOST INTERACTIONS

A comprehensive review of diet host–microbe interactions is beyond the scope of this chapter. However, it is critical to note there is an interplay between the intestinal microbiota, diet, other environmental factors such stress, pharmacologic agents, and the several cell types that form the intestinal epithelial surface, which is comprised by one layer of cells separating the intestinal contents from a highly immunoreactive subepithelium. Among the epithelial cells are digestive absorptive intestinal epithelial cells, M-cells, Paneth cells, goblet cells, and in the submucosa antigen-presenting cells such as dendritic cells, macrophages, and a myriad of immunologic sites termed the lamina propria and gut-associated lymphoid tissues (GALT). Both the innate and adaptive immune systems are affected by the intestinal microbiota.

Goblet cells produce a mucus layer that is involved in the protection of the intestinal mucosa. Paneth cells are found in the lowermost crypt regions and secrete defensive peptides that are thought to be critical for protection of the mitotically active stem cells in the crypt region. Dendritic cells are of the monocyte macrophage lineage and are involved in microbial uptake, antigen processing, and interaction with naïve T cells that will differentiate into effector or suppressor T cells depending on the signal that is provided by the dendritic cell. The proximity of the dendritic cell and its appendages to the microbial lumen is of major significance. This appendage consists of dendritic "arms" that have the capability of internalizing antigens and luminal microbial components and processing specific signals to naïve T cells underlying the mucosa, which then may differentiate into effector TH1 or TH17, TH2, or regulatory T cells that produce interleukin 10 (IL-10) or transforming growth factor β (TGF-β). Imbalances of these pathways may lead to autoimmunity or allergy and have been hypothesized to be involved in the development of diseases, such as type 1 diabetes, multiple sclerosis, atopy, and inflammatory bowel diseases.

Dietary substrates provided to the host and microbes undergo metabolic conversions to highly bioactive metabolites that are critical to the host. Among these are the short-chain fatty acids (SCFAs), acetate, propionate, and butyrate. The apical interepithelial paracellular tight junctions are highly responsive to certain microbial metabolic products, such as butyrate.[20] Opening and closing tight junctions are highly responsive butyrate. This four-carbon SCFA acts on tight junctions by its effects on tight junction proteins, such as claudins. It is important to note that these tight junctions control the intercellular permeability of the intestinal surface, and loss of tight junction integrity allows translocation of microbes and microbial products, which may, in turn, act on the mucosal immune system and/or enter the bloodstream and be associated with bacteremia. There are numerous other bioactive roles for these SCFAs that are beyond the scope of this chapter.

Other products of microbial metabolism relate to neurotransmitter function. For example, intestinal microbiota acting through SCFA metabolism are important for serotonin [5-hydroxytryptamine (5-HT)] production via tryptophan.[21] It is thought that intestinal microbial metabolism is one of the major synthetic pathways for production of this neurotransmitter, sometimes called the "happy chemical" because of its effect on mood activation.

MICROBIAL THERAPEUTICS

PROBIOTICS

Probiotics are defined as live microorganisms that, when administered in adequate amounts, confer health benefits to the host. It is common to see advertisements in the popular media that suggest various health benefits of probiotics. Usually, this is limited to a generally healthy population, with no claims being made in the prevention or treatment of a particular disease. When used in this way, the need for regulatory agencies to monitor these agents is minimized. However, probiotic products are also being used in situations where there is a medical claim, such as for the prevention of diarrhea, prevention of preterm birth, and in the prevention of necrotizing enterocolitis (NEC). When used in these situations, regulatory agencies may consider these agents to be a drug and should undergo much more rigorous testing and quality control measures, such as would be the case for pharmaceuticals. The case for and against probiotics in situations where they are considered for the prevention or treatment of disease is somewhat complex.

Mechanisms of action for probiotics remain only partially understood and may vary markedly depending on the agent. They may have several effects on the host, including metabolism of nutrients to improve digestion. Microbes belonging to the genus *Lactobacillus*, for example, are highly efficient in metabolizing the disaccharide lactose into lactic acid. This is not the case for many other microbes being used as probiotics. Other probiotics may be highly active in immunomodulation, but this is not the case for all. Some of these effects could be through the Toll-like receptor–dependent stimulation for the production of various cytokines via NF-κB–mediated mechanisms. These effects require physical contact between the host cell and probiotic for induction of either anti-inflammatory or program inflammatory responses. Very few mechanistic studies have been done in humans.

It has also been suggested that probiotics inhibit pathogen colonization by blocking the capability of the pathogen to adhere to the intestinal epithelial cells area they can regulate the acid–base environment and thus inhibit certain pathogens. They may also disrupt quorum sensing, thereby interfering with pathogen proliferation. Again, there are major differences based on the microbe chosen as a probiotic. In addition to effects on the immune system, probiotics may also affect signaling in the central nervous system. *Lactobacillus rhamnosus* affects mice by altering their expression of messenger RNA for γ-aminobutyric acid (GABA) and attenuate the corticosteroid response to stress- and anxiety-related behavior.[22] However even though some of these effects may be clear in animal models, they may not translate to effect in humans. Recently, a study that may have meta-analyzed the effects of probiotics on anxiety in humans did not demonstrate benefits that could be seen in rodent studies.[23]

Probiotics may also interact with the host intestinal microbiota. In most cases, probiotic microbes do not confer major colonization in healthy adults[24] putatively because of colonization resistance of the indigenous microbes. However, antibiotics significantly perturb intestinal microbial ecology. By doing this, antibiotics may relieve the colonization resistance to probiotics as well as to potentially resistant pathogens. However, this has not been conclusively shown and remains highly debated. The other side of the story is that following antibiotic treatment of human individuals, colonization by probiotic strains may result in a long-term probiotic colonization and delay reconstitution of the normal mucosal microbiota. This may result in significant long-term health effects in terms of increased risk of communicable diseases as well as contributing to the development of the autoimmunity and allergies.

Next, we describe several disease entities for which probiotics have been studied.

INFLAMMATORY BOWEL DISEASE

There are two major subsets of pathology comprising inflammatory bowel disease. The first is ulcerative colitis and the second is Crohn disease. Crohn disease can affect any portion of the GI tract and is characterized by transmural inflammation. Ulcerative colitis is limited to the colon and primarily involves only mucosal inflammation. The composition of the fecal microbiota of ulcerative colitis patients differs from that of healthy individuals: one study found a reduction in *Roseburia hominis* and *Faecalibacterium prausnitzii*, both well-known butyrate-producing bacteria of the Firmicutes phylum.[25] In Crohn disease, there is an overall reduction in microbial diversity with increased abundance of *Bacteroides*.[26]

There have been several reviews relating probiotics to the treatment of both Crohn disease and ulcerative colitis. Studies using animal models suggest the potential of several bacterial strains to modify the natural history of inflammatory bowel disease. There is some evidence for efficacy in ulcerative colitis and pouchitis, whereas in Crohn disease, there has been little indication that probiotics exert any benefit.[27]

IRRITABLE BOWEL DISEASE

Irritable bowel syndrome is quite common, especially in adolescence. It is defined as abdominal pain that also includes improvement of the pain with defecation, onset of pain associated with change in frequency of stooling, or onset of pain associated with a change in stool appearance or texture. The pathophysiology remains poorly understood. It is thought that visceral hypersensitivity may play a major role. Numerous studies have evaluated probiotics with irritable bowel syndrome. A systematic review of studies using probiotics in the treatment of irritable bowel syndrome showed that symptom outcomes for dose-specific probiotics were heterogeneous. Specific probiotic recommendations for irritable bowel syndrome management in adults were not possible using the available studies. It was concluded that "more data from high-quality RCTs treating specific symptom profiles are needed to support probiotic therapy in the management of IBS."[28]

DIARRHEAL ILLNESS AND ACUTE GASTROENTERITIS

Diarrhea, a condition associated with passage of frequent, loose stools, is the second leading cause of death in children under 5 years of age. The clinical presentation may be quite varied depending on the whether the underlying cause is malabsorption, autoimmune, infectious, antibiotic induced, or other etiology. Because of the multifactorial etiology of diarrheal illnesses, the use of probiotics for the prevention and treatment should theoretically be targeted for that specific etiology, with targeted therapies based on mechanistic data. In a recent review, different single- and multi-strain probiotics are described as they pertain to the prevention of antibiotic induced diarrhea. A specific recommendation for the use of *Lactobacillus rhamnosus* GG (LGG) and *Saccharomyces boulardii* (*Sb*) emerged. However, in spite of a demonstrated positive effect of specific strains of probiotics on antibiotic-associated diarrhea, "safety issues still remain among which are the risk of associated severe infections and of antibiotic resistant gene exchange."[29] A recent review of probiotics and prebiotics in the prevention of infectious diarrhea stated that "both pro- and prebiotics have limited to no efficacy in the prevention of acute gastroenteritis."[30]

Clostridium difficile colitis results when colonization resistance is compromised, most frequently after antibiotic treatment for hospitalized patients. This can be a very severe disease. There is some data to suggest that probiotic use may be beneficial in antibiotic-associated diarrheal illness, including *C. difficile* infections (CDIs). In a systematic review using meta-regression analysis, there was evidence that administration of probiotics close to the first dose of antibiotic reduces the risk of CDI by greater than 50% in hospitalized adults.[31] Several questions were raised by this study, including the need for prospective randomized controlled trials to better test this relationship as well as accounting for the timing and type of antibiotic use.[32] Nevertheless, overall, the preventive effects of probiotics against *C. difficile*–associated diarrhea remain weak.

NEONATAL NECROTIZING ENTEROCOLITIS

NEC is a devastating disease affecting primarily premature infants. Even after decades of research, a clear definition of NEC is not yet available, largely based on the number of entities with different pathophysiologies that are being termed necrotizing enterocolitis (NEC). Misleading animal models as well as in vitro systems have not been helpful. Numerous risk factors are implicated in the pathogenesis of NEC. Among these, premature birth is the major risk factor. Various other factors are involved, including intestinal dysbiosis, immature mucosal protective mechanisms, genetic predisposition, immature mucosal development with subsequent increases in permeability, formula feeds, antibiotics, H2 blockers, and poor motility.[33,34]

Numerous statistically underpowered studies have evaluated a myriad of probiotics for the prevention of NEC. Of note is that most of these studies evaluated different probiotic agents. Despite this, meta-analyses were done analyzing probiotics not as single agents, but as a group. In these meta-analyses, it appeared that there was a beneficial effect.[35] However, despite the promising results, most of the studies done at this juncture are highly problematic. While the definition of NEC remains unclear, the meta-analyses themselves remain problematic. For example, no single strain or even combination of strains in a single-blinded prospective randomized study has been shown to be of benefit. The one study that met criteria for a well-designed randomized trial with over 1,300 subjects did not show a benefit, even though it was adequately powered for testing the effect on NEC.[36] There are numerous small reports about sepsis due to the probiotic microorganisms. There is the Centers for Disease Control and Prevention (CDC) warning on the use of a single type of probiotic strain after a neonate died and at autopsy was diagnosed as having mucormycosis, which may have been associated with contamination of the preparation lot (https://www.cdc.gov/fungal/outbreaks/rhizopus-investigation.html). This underlines the importance of quality control and regulatory oversight when utilizing these preparations for vulnerable populations, such as preterm infants. Thus despite the promise provided by the numerous meta-analyses, considerable caution is warranted in terms of strain composition, dose, mode of administration, birth weight of the patient, previous exposure to antibiotics, and quality control of the product. Consideration should also be given to the fact that fresh human milk contains considerable microbes and oligosaccharides that may provide even better benefits than commercially manufactured probiotics.

FECAL TRANSPLANTS

Fecal microbial transplantation over the past few years has been widely performed to manage CDIs. The concept that restoration of a balanced microbial ecosystems in the GI tract in patients with recurrent *C. difficile* has appeared to be a logical solution to this problem. The success rate for fecal microbial transplants for CDI has been high.[37–39] In comparison to drug therapy, several trials have suggested benefit of fecal microbial transplant over pharmacologic therapy, such as vancomycin. Whether these were adequate comparisons has been up to debate. Multiple courses of fecal microbial transplantation were allowed in the studies, whereas multiple courses of the drug therapies were not. In light of this, it appears that the success rate of a single fecal microbial transplant is not as high as some of the studies portrayed it to be. While the randomized controlled trials comparing fecal microbial transplant protocols suggest some benefits and support the need for better preparations and identification of benefits of administration, the current studies are less than optimal to improve the overall efficacy of fecal microbial transplantation. Furthermore, safety matters have come into question. The risk of transmission of infectious diseases, bloodborne pathogens, and enteric infections is of concern.[40] Although these safety concerns have been expressed, there have been patients especially those with immunocompromised systems who have experienced invasive infections with resistant bacteria after fecal microbial transplant. It is clear that this is another area where caution is warranted, and large prospective studies with longer follow-up periods are necessary before widespread institution of this practice.

HUMAN MILK

Studies done over the past decade had demonstrated that the human milk provides beneficial bacteria to the infant GI tract.[41,42] Both culture- and nonculture-based studies have demonstrated the existence of the microorganisms and microbial DNA in human milk. These may play a significant role in the maturation of the digestive and immune function in the infant. Although many studies are still in progress, the role these microbes play in terms of both protecting the mammary gland for the mother and providing protection of the GI tract and contributing to immune development in the GI tract of the infant is highly likely. Proposed mechanisms include colonization of the GI tract in babies of women who have delivered by cesarean section versus vaginal delivery.[43]

In neonatal intensive care, it has become very common practice to use banked donor breast milk if the milk of the baby's mother is not available. Banked donor milk has in most cases previously been exposed to a treatment, such as a pasteurization process with heating at 62.5°C for at least 30 minutes. This inactivates various enzymes in the milk and kills most of the bacteria present in the donor milk samples. Nevertheless, some of the microbial DNA remains, and the relative contribution of killed microbial parts versus live microbes to the developing infant is not fully understood.[44]

It appears that live microbes may have numerous functions that are contributory to the developing physiology of the newborn infant, including a production of metabolites and stimulation of communal responsiveness. Thus, techniques that provide a personalized microbiome to an infant whose mother may not be able to make adequate quantities of milk for her own infant but where donor milk can be provided have been studied.[44] Such refaunation techniques may provide the possibility of providing an adequate quantity of milk to the infant that has been personalized with the baby's own mother's microbes and that may also provide the same or similar metabolic profile in the milk as would be provided by the baby's own mother.

MICROBIAL CONSORTIUM THERAPEUTICS

Bacterial Consortium transplantation refers to the use of a characterized microbial population of specific fecal bacteria developed to provide a functional microbial ecosystem to a host.[45–47] This can be personalized based on different desired levels of bacteria or the type of dysbiosis that it may be intended to treat. It is likely that this would be a safer approach than fecal microbial transplantation.

Approaches are being developed in order to provide defined microbial colonization into subjects with malnutrition and then testing dietary regimens to determine which would best ameliorate the malnutrition.[48,49] These studies in Bangladeshi and Malawi children undergoing severe malnutrition have been shown to exhibit a maturational delay in the development of their intestinal microbes. In studies that better defined interactions within an ecosystem rather than just the microbes themselves, using a set of approximately 15 taxa that exhibit consistent co-variation in healthy children termed an "ecogroup" could potentially be utilized for colonization in severely malnourished children to test the efficacy of the various diets that would be of potentially greatest efficacy in reading nourishing these individuals.

MICROBIAL THERAPEUTICS REGULATORY ISSUES: FOODS OR DRUGS?

According to regulatory agencies, a substance for which a claim is made for treatment or prevention of a disease differs from one that putatively promotes a healthy lifestyle. The latter of these would be considered more food than a drug. Furthermore, biologic drugs differ from therapeutic drugs in terms of their greater complexity and greater difficulty to evaluate. For example, a probiotic meant to treat or prevent a disease can be considered in the category of a drug, but because it is a living system, it may have a different long-term effect on the individual than a drug that is only dosed for a few days. It is thus imperative for regulatory agencies to look upon these agents and proceed carefully with the implementation, especially in highly vulnerable individuals such as immunocompromised hosts and infants who were born prematurely.

THE FUTURE

In this review, we have attempted to summarize some of the issues related to microbial therapies and how they relate to primarily the intestinal tract. There are other areas not covered in this chapter, including the cutaneous microbiology, vaginal microbiology, and lung microbiology, and even another very controversial area such as the in utero microbiome and how these might be affected using microbial therapeutic approaches.

Much of the recent focus in the area of microbial therapeutics has been on probiotics. However, much of the work related to probiotics has been flawed. Administering one or a few members of a limited set of bacteria in order to elicit health-promoting effects is a somewhat haphazard approach. Future studies should include microbial preparations that are devised for certain medical indications after careful consideration of the potential mechanism of action and how this particular agent will interact with the already existing ecosystems to which it will be added. This will include consideration of colonization resistance where the therapeutic agent of choice is not inhibited by commensals.

The attitude that all probiotics may be the same and should be classified as one is simply wrong. Grouping different probiotics into a meta-analysis which may show some benefit does not provide evidence that all the probiotics placed in that meta-analysis are useful for the prevention of the certain disease. Furthermore, the state of the host needs to be taken into consideration. For example, a healthy young adult differs markedly from a preterm infant weighing less than 750 g and also differs markedly from an individual who is immunocompromised secondary to cancer chemotherapy, a burn patient, a patient who has recently had major surgery, or an elderly individual.

Once a good mechanistic basis is established for a particular agent that is targeted for a particular problem, and the scientific rationale is strong, time should not be wasted on small studies other than if they are intended as phase 1 or 2 safety studies. Large-scale studies should be randomized and blinded and, whenever possible, devoid of commercial interests. The end points should be carefully stated a priori with a well-done statistical power analysis. Whenever possible, these trials should be done in more than one center. Regulatory agencies need to work closely with the investigative team, and data should be made available to allow for reproducibility and several different global environments.

However, this area is highly complex, involving multiple "-omic" considerations, which include not just microbial–host interactions but also intermediate factors such as the individual's genomic background, the metabolites that are produced by both the microbes and the host in their interactions, immunologic considerations, and epigenetic considerations. Long-term outcomes should also be considered not just as an individual matures from early life through adulthood but also how these microbial therapeutics may affect the next generation.

REFERENCES

1. Sender R, Fuchs S, Milo R. Revised estimates for the number of human and bacteria cells in the body. *PLoS Biol* 2016;14:e1002533.
2. Morgan XC, Huttenhower C. Meta'omic analytic techniques for studying the intestinal microbiome. *Gastroenterology* 2014;146:1437.e1–1448.e1.
3. Ardissone AN, de la Cruz DM, Davis-Richardson AG, et al. Meconium microbiome analysis identifies bacteria correlated with premature birth. *PLoS One* 2014;9:e90784.
4. Moles L, Gómez M, Heilig H, et al. Bacterial diversity in meconium of preterm neonates and evolution of their fecal microbiota during the first month of life. *PLoS One* 2013;8:e66986.
5. Younge N, McCann JR, Ballard J, et al. Fetal exposure to the maternal microbiota in humans and mice. *JCI Insight* 2019;4(19).
6. Stinson LF, Boyce MC, Payne MS, et al. The not-so-sterile womb: evidence that the human fetus is exposed to bacteria prior to birth. *Front Microbiol* 2019;10:1124.
7. Hu J, Ly J, Zhang W, et al. Microbiota of newborn meconium is associated with maternal anxiety experienced during pregnancy. *Dev Psychobiol* 2019;61:640–649.
8. Malmuthuge N, Griebel PJ. Fetal environment and fetal intestine are sterile during the third trimester of pregnancy. *Vet Immunol Immunopathol* 2018;204:59–64.
9. Chen HJ, Gur TL. Intrauterine microbiota: missing, or the missing link? *Trends Neurosci* 2019;42:402–413.
10. Gomez-Arango LF, Barrett HL, McIntyre HD, et al. Contributions of the maternal oral and gut microbiome to placental microbial colonization in overweight and obese pregnant women. *Sci Rep* 2017;7:2860.
11. Neu J. The microbiome during pregnancy and early postnatal life. *Semin Fetal Neonatal Med* 2016;21:373–379.

12. Gomez de Aguero M, Ganal-Vonarburg SC, Fuhrer T, et al. The maternal microbiota drives early postnatal innate immune development. *Science* 2016;351:1296–1302.
13. Parra-Llorca A, Gormaz M, Alcántara C, et al. Preterm gut microbiome depending on feeding type: significance of donor human milk. *Front Microbiol* 2018;9:1376.
14. Gregory KE, Samuel BS, Houghteling P, et al. Influence of maternal breast milk ingestion on acquisition of the intestinal microbiome in preterm infants. *Microbiome* 2016;4:68.
15. Chong CYL, Bloomfield FH, O'Sullivan JM. Factors affecting gastrointestinal microbiome development in neonates. *Nutrients* 2018;10(3).
16. Cong X, Xu W, Janton S, et al. Gut microbiome developmental patterns in early life of preterm infants: impacts of feeding and gender. *PLoS One* 2016;11:e0152751.
17. Romano-Keeler J, Shilts MH, Tovchigrechko A, et al. Distinct mucosal microbial communities in infants with surgical necrotizing enterocolitis correlate with age and antibiotic exposure. *PLoS One* 2018;13:e0206366.
18. Zou ZH, Liu D, Li HD, et al. Prenatal and postnatal antibiotic exposure influences the gut microbiota of preterm infants in neonatal intensive care units. *Ann Clin Microbiol Antimicrob* 2018;17:9.
19. Gupta RW, Tran L, Norori J, et al. Histamine-2 receptor blockers alter the fecal microbiota in premature infants. *J Pediatr Gastroenterol Nutr* 2013;56:397–400.
20. Zheng L, Kelly CJ, Battista KD, et al. Microbial-derived butyrate promotes epithelial barrier function through IL-10 receptor-dependent repression of claudin-2. *J Immunol* 2017;199:2976–2984.
21. Reigstad CS, Salmonson CE, Rainey JF III, et al. Gut microbes promote colonic serotonin production through an effect of short-chain fatty acids on enterochromaffin cells. *FASEB J* 2015;29:1395–1403.
22. McVey Neufeld KA, Kay S, Bienenstock J. Mouse strain affects behavioral and neuroendocrine stress responses following administration of probiotic *Lactobacillus rhamnosus* JB-1 or traditional antidepressant fluoxetine. *Front Neurosci* 2018;12:294.
23. Reis DJ, Ilardi SS, Punt SEW. The anxiolytic effect of probiotics: a systematic review and meta-analysis of the clinical and preclinical literature. *PLoS One* 2018;13:e0199041.
24. Kristensen NB, Bryrup T, Allin KH, et al. Alterations in fecal microbiota composition by probiotic supplementation in healthy adults: a systematic review of randomized controlled trials. *Genome Med* 2016;8:52.
25. Machiels K, Joossens M, Sabino J, et al. A decrease of the butyrate-producing species *Roseburia hominis* and *Faecalibacterium prausnitzii* defines dysbiosis in patients with ulcerative colitis. *Gut* 2014;63:1275–1283.
26. Khanna S, Raffals LE. The microbiome in Crohn's disease: role in pathogenesis and role of microbiome replacement therapies. *Gastroenterol Clin North Am* 2017;46:481–492.
27. Abraham BP, Quigley EMM. Probiotics in lase. *Gastroenterol Clin North Am* 2017;46:769–782.
28. McKenzie YA, Thompson J, Gulia P, et al. British Dietetic Association systematic review of systematic reviews and evidence-based practice guidelines for the use of probiotics in the management of irritable bowel syndrome in adults (2016 update). *J Hum Nutr Diet* 2016;29:576–592.
29. Mantegazza C, Molinari P, D'Auria E, et al. Probiotics and antibiotic-associated diarrhea in children: a review and new evidence on *Lactobacillus rhamnosus* GG during and after antibiotic treatment. *Pharmacol Res* 2018;128:63–72.
30. Vandenplas Y. Probiotics and prebiotics in infectious gastroenteritis. *Best Pract Res Clin Gastroenterol* 2016;30:49–53.
31. Shen NT, Maw A, Tmanova LL, et al. Timely use of probiotics in hospitalized adults prevents *Clostridium difficile* infection: a systematic review with meta-regression analysis. *Gastroenterology* 2017;152:1889.e9–1900.e9.
32. Rao K, Young VB. Probiotics for prevention of *Clostridium difficile* infection in hospitalized patients: is the jury still out? *Gastroenterology* 2017;152:1817–1819.
33. Neu J, Walker WA. Necrotizing enterocolitis. *N Engl J Med* 2011;364:255–264.
34. Neu J, Modi N, Caplan M. Necrotizing enterocolitis comes in different forms: Historical perspectives and defining the disease. *Semin Fetal Neonatal Med* 2018;23:370–373.
35. Athalye-Jape G, Rao S, Patole S. Effects of probiotics on experimental necrotizing enterocolitis: a systematic review and meta-analysis. *Pediatr Res* 2018;83:16–22.
36. Costeloe K, Hardy P, Juszczak E, et al. Bifidobacterium breve BBG-001 in very preterm infants: a randomised controlled phase 3 trial. *Lancet* 2016;387:649–660.
37. Mullish BH, Quraishi MN, Segal JP, et al. The use of faecal microbiota transplant as treatment for recurrent or refractory *Clostridium difficile* infection and other potential indications: joint British Society of Gastroenterology (BSG) and Healthcare Infection Society (HIS) guidelines. *Gut* 2018;67:1920–1941.
38. Dinleyici M, Vandenplas Y. *Clostridium difficile* colitis prevention and treatment. *Adv Exp Med Biol* 2019;1125:139–146.
39. Madoff SE, Urquiaga M, Alonso CD, et al. Prevention of recurrent Clostridioides difficile infection: a systematic review of randomized controlled trials. *Anaerobe* 2019;61:102098.
40. Daliri EB, Tango CN, Lee BH, et al. Human microbiome restoration and safety. *Int J Med Microbiol* 2018;308:487–497.
41. Gomez-Gallego C, Garcia-Mantrana I, Salminen S, et al. The human milk microbiome and factors influencing its composition and activity. *Semin Fetal Neonatal Med* 2016;21:400–405.
42. Bode L, McGuire M, Rodriguez JM, et al. It's alive: microbes and cells in human milk and their potential benefits to mother and infant. *Adv Nutr* 2014;5:571–573.
43. Azad MB, Konya T, Maughan H, et al. Gut microbiota of healthy Canadian infants: profiles by mode of delivery and infant diet at 4 months. *CMAJ* 2013;185:385–394.
44. Cacho NT, Harrison NA, Parker LA, et al. Personalization of the microbiota of donor human milk with mother's own milk. *Front Microbiol* 2017;8:1470.
45. Gagliardi A, Totino V, Cacciotti F, et al. Rebuilding the gut microbiota ecosystem. *Int J Environ Res Public Health* 2018;15:1679.
46. Li M, Li Z, Wen S, et al. Transplantation of a bacterial consortium ameliorates trinitrobenzenesulfonic acid-induced colitis and intestinal dysbiosis in rats. *Future Microbiol* 2016;11:887–902.
47. Li M, Wang B, Sun X, et al. Upregulation of intestinal barrier function in mice with DSS-induced colitis by a defined bacterial consortium is associated with expansion of IL-17A producing gamma delta T cells. *Front Immunol* 2017;8:824.
48. Raman AS, Gehrig JL, Venkatesh S, et al. A sparse covarying unit that describes healthy and impaired human gut microbiota development. *Science* 2019;365.
49. Gehrig JL, Venkatesh S, Chang HW, et al. Effects of microbiota-directed foods in gnotobiotic animals and undernourished children. *Science* 2019;365.

CHAPTER

44

Zaid H. Temrikar
Satyendra Suryawanshi
Bernd Meibohm

Monoclonal Antibodies

INTRODUCTION

Monoclonal antibodies (mAbs) and their derivatives have developed in the past two decades into the backbone of pharmacotherapeutic interventions in a variety of diseases and are now a mainstay in the armamentarium of contemporary pharmacotherapy for numerous indications.[1,2] MAbs are increasingly also used in pediatric pharmacotherapy, and the number of antibody-based drug products with approved pediatric indications is continuously growing. Table 44.1 provides an overview on currently approved mAbs for pediatric indications. Similar to the majority of small molecule drugs, pediatric use of most mAbs has been pursued after efficacy and safety had first been established in adult indications. Nevertheless, in some rare instances, pediatric indications were the initial target for mAb development programs, for example, for palivizumab for the prevention of respiratory syncytial virus infection in newborns and infants.[3]

Similar to small molecule drugs, the pharmacokinetics (PK) and clinical pharmacology of mAbs are expected to be affected by childhood maturational changes in drug disposition processes that are relevant for this specific set of compounds. In addition, size-specific adjustments for dosing are expected based on the generally accepted relationship between body size measures and determinants of systemic drug exposure, particularly clearance as predictor of steady-state concentrations.[4,5]

STRUCTURE AND ORIGIN

All currently clinically used therapeutic antibodies are immunoglobulin G (IgG) mAbs and possess the same basic structure, which comprises the four subclasses IgG1, IgG2, IgG3, and IgG4.[6] Currently marketed mAbs are predominantly IgG1, with a lesser degree of IgG2 and IgG4.[1] Similar to endogenous IgG, they are large heterodimeric protein molecules with a molecular weight of approximately 150 kDa and are composed of four polypeptide chains, two identical heavy chains, and two light chains. These chains are held together by disulfide bonds to form a Y-shaped structure consisting of constant domains and variable domains. The variable domains contain the complementarity-determining regions, which are highly specific for the target antigen. The two variable regions and the C_{H1} domains of the heavy chains comprise the antigen-binding fragment (Fab), whereas the C_{H2} and C_{H3} domains of the heavy chain make up the Fc (fragment, crystallizable) region of the antibody. While the Fab fragment carries two binding sites for the target of the mAb, the Fc fragment can bind to a variety of cell surface receptors, including the Fcγ receptors and the neonatal Fc receptor (FcRn), as well as components of the complement system.

Similar to other protein-based therapeutics, mAbs are produced batch-wise in genetically modified living cells using biotechnology processes. As such, they are defined by the production process rather than their chemical structure, and batch-to-batch variability in the resulting product is well recognized and needs to be tightly controlled through carefully established critical quality attributes, that are ensured by tightly controlling the conditions during the cell culturing, product processing, and purification steps.[7]

DRUG DISPOSITION OF MONOCLONAL ANTIBODIES IN PEDIATRIC PATIENTS

One overarching principle governing the drug disposition behavior of mAbs is the appreciation that the physicochemical properties of these IgG molecules are determined by their hydrophilic macromolecule nature [molecular weight (MW) ~150 kDa] as proteins consisting of linear amino acid polymer chains. This is further complicated by their highly charged structure in the aqueous environment at physiologic pH. In addition, many mAbs interact with a variety of generalized as well as

TABLE 44.1 Antibodies and Antibody Derivatives Approved for Pediatric Indications

INN	*Trade Name*	*Class*	*Specification/Subclass*	*Therapeutic Area*	*Approved Pediatric Indication*	*Approved Age Group (y)*	*Route of Administration and Dosing for Pediatric Population*
Abatacept	Orencia	Fusion protein	Extracellular domain of human cytotoxic T-lymphocyte–associated antigen 4 linked to IgG1 Fc domain	Autoimmune disease	Juvenile idiopathic arthritis	IV: ≥6	IV: Once weekly BW <75 kg: 10 mg/kg BW ≥75 kg: Adult dosing (750 mg; BW >100: 1,000 mg)
						SC: ≥2	SC: Once weekly BW 10 to <25 kg: 50 mg BW 25 to <50 kg: 87.5 mg BW ≥50 kg: 125 mg
Adalimumab	Humira	Monoclonal antibody	Human IgG1	Autoimmune disease	Juvenile idiopathic arthritis Pediatric uveitis	≥2	SC every other week: BW 10 to <15 kg: 10 mg BW 15 to <30 kg: 20 mg BW ≥30 kg: 40 mg
					Pediatric Crohn disease	≥6	SC every other week: BW 17 to <40 kg: 20 mg (induction dose 80 mg on day 1, 40 mg on day 15) BW ≥40 kg: 40 mg (induction dose 160 mg on day 1, 80 mg on day 15)
					Hidradenitis suppurativa	≥12	BW 30 to <60 kg: 40 mg SC every other week (induction dose 80 mg on day 1, 40 mg on day 8) BW ≥60 kg: 40 mg SC every week (induction dose 160 mg on day 1, 80 mg on day 15, 40 mg on day 29)
Avelumab	Bavencio	Monoclonal antibody	Human IgG1	Oncology	Metastatic Merkel cell carcinoma	≥12	800 mg IV every 2 wk (same as adults)
Basiliximab	Simulect	Monoclonal antibody	Chimeric IgG1	Transplant rejection	Prophylaxis of acute organ rejection in patients receiving renal transplantation	All age groups	BW <35 kg: two IV doses of 10 mg each BW ≥35 kg: two IV doses of 20 mg each The first dose should be given within 2 h prior to transplantation surgery. The second dose should be given 4 d after transplantation.
Benralizumab	Fasenra	Monoclonal antibody	Humanized IgG1	Asthma	Severe asthma with an eosinophilic phenotype	≥12	30 mg SC every 4 wk for the first 3 doses, followed by once every 8 wk thereafter (same as adults)
Canakinumab	Ilaris	Monoclonal antibody	Human IgG1	Autoimmune disease	Cryopyrin-associated periodic syndromes	≥4	SC every 8 wk BW 15 to <40 kg: 2 mg/kg BW >40 kg: 150 mg
					Tumor necrosis factor receptor–associated periodic syndrome Hyperimmunoglobulin D syndrome/mevalonate kinase deficiency Familial Mediterranean fever	All age groups	SC every 4 wk BW ≤40 kg: 2 mg/kg (can be increased to 4 mg/kg) BW >40 kg: 150 mg (can be increased to 300 mg)
					Systemic juvenile idiopathic arthritis	≥2	SC every 4 wk BW ≥7.5 kg: 4 mg/kg (maximum 300 mg)

		antibody			syndrome		BW 5 to <10 kg: 300 mg week 1 and week 2, then 300 mg every 3 wk BW 10 to <20 kg: 600 mg week 1, 300 mg week 2, then 300 mg every 2 wk BW 20 to <30 kg: 600 mg week 1, week 2, and week 3, then 600 mg every 2 wk BW 30 to <40 kg: 600 mg week 1 and week 2, 900 mg week 3, then 900 mg every 2 wk BW ≥40 kg: 900 mg week 1, week 2, week 3, and week 4; 1,200 mg week 5; then 1,200 mg every 2 wk
Emicizumab	Hemlibra	Monoclonal antibody	Bispecific humanized IgG4	Hematology	Hemophilia A	All age groups	Loading dose 3 mg/kg SC once weekly for the first 4 wk, followed by a maintenance dose of 1.5 mg/kg once every week, or 3 mg/kg once every 2 wk, or 6 mg/kg once every 4 wk (same as adults)
Etanercept	Enbrel	Fusion protein	Ligand-binding domain of the human tumor necrosis factor receptor linked to human IgG1 Fc domain	Autoimmune disease	Polyarticular juvenile idiopathic arthritis	≥2	BW < 63 kg: 0.8 mg/kg SC weekly BW ≥ 63 kg: 50 mg SC weekly
					Plaque psoriasis	≥4	BW < 63 kg: 0.8 mg/kg SC weekly BW ≥ 63 kg: 50 mg SC weekly
Gemtuzumab ozogamicin	Mylotarg	Antibody–drug conjugate	IgG4 covalently linked to *N*-acetyl γ calicheamicin	Oncology	Relapsed or refractory CD33-positive acute myeloid leukemia	≥2	3 mg/m^2 on days 1, 4, and 7 given as an IV infusion
Infliximab	Remicade	Monoclonal antibody	Chimeric IgG1	Autoimmune disease	Pediatric Crohn disease Pediatric ulcerative colitis	≥6	All IV doses: 5 mg/kg at 0, 2, and 6 wk, then every 8 wk
Ipilimumab	Yervoy	Monoclonal antibody	Human IgG1	Oncology	Unresectable or metastatic melanoma Microsatellite instability-high or mismatch repair deficient metastatic colorectal cancer	≥12	3 mg/kg IV every 3 wk for a total of four doses
Mepolizumab	Nucala	Monoclonal antibody	Humanized IgG1	Asthma	Severe asthma with an eosinophilic phenotype	≥6	SC every 4 wk: Ages 6–11 y: 40 mg Age ≥12 y: 100 mg
Nivolumab	Opdivo	Monoclonal antibody	Human IgG4	Oncology	Microsatellite instability-high or mismatch repair deficient metastatic colorectal cancer	≥12	BW <40 kg: 3 mg/kg every 2 wk BW ≥40 kg: 240 mg every 2 wk or 480 mg every 4 wk
Obiltoxaximab	Anthim	Monoclonal antibody	Chimeric IgG1	Anti-infective	Prophylaxis and therapy of inhalational anthrax	All age groups	All IV doses: BW ≤15 kg: 32 mg/kg BW >15–40 kg: 24 mg/kg BW >40 kg: 16 mg/kg
Omalizumab	Xolair	Monoclonal antibody	Humanized IgG1	Asthma	Moderate-to-severe persistent asthma	≥6	SC dosing every 2 or 4 wk based on weight strata and pretreatment serum IgE levels according to dosing table; separate dosing tables for ages 6 to <12 and ≥12 y
					Chronic idiopathic urticaria	≥12	150 or 300 mg SC every 4 wk (same as adults)

(*continued*)

TABLE 44.1 Antibodies and Antibody Derivatives Approved for Pediatric Indications (*continued*)

INN	*Trade Name*	*Class*	*Specification/Subclass*	*Therapeutic Area*	*Approved Pediatric Indication*	*Approved Age Group (y)*	*Route of Administration and Dosing for Pediatric Population*
Palivizumab	Synagis	Monoclonal antibody	Humanized IgG1	Anti-infective	Prevention respiratory syncytial virus infection	All age groups	15 mg/kg IM monthly throughout RSV season
Raxibacumab	Abthrax	Monoclonal antibody	Human IgG1	Anti-infective	Prophylaxis and therapy of inhalational anthrax	All age groups	All IV doses: BW ≤15 kg: 80 mg/kg BW >15–50 kg: 60 mg/kg BW >50 kg: 40 mg/kg
Rilonacept	Arcalyst	Fusion protein	Fusion protein consisting of the ligand-binding domains of the human IL-1 receptor component and IL-1 receptor accessory protein linked to human IgG1 Fc domain	Autoimmune disease	Cryopyrin-associated periodic syndromes	≥12	Loading dose: 4.4 mg/kg SC, up to a maximum of 320 mg Maintenance dose: 2.2 mg/kg once weekly, up to a maximum of 160 mg
Tocilizumab	Actemra	Monoclonal antibody	Humanized IgG1	Autoimmune disease	Polyarticular juvenile idiopathic arthritis	≥2	IV: BW <30 kg: 10 mg/kg every 4 wk BW ≥30 kg: 8 mg/kg every 4 wk SC: BW <30 kg: 162 mg every 3 wk BW ≥30 kg: 162 mg every 2 wk
					Systemic juvenile idiopathic arthritis	≥2	IV: BW <30 kg: 12 mg/kg every 2 wk BW ≥30 kg: 8 mg/kg every 2 wk SC: BW <30 kg: 162 mg every 2 wk BW ≥30 kg: 162 mg every week
					Cytokine release syndrome	≥2	IV: BW <30 kg: 12 mg/kg BW ≥30 kg: 8 mg/kg

Based on labeling information at Drugs@FDA (https://www.accessdata.fda.gov/scripts/cder/daf/).

BW, body weight; IL-1, interleukin-1; IM, intramuscular; INN, international nonproprietary name; IV, intravenous; RSV, respiratory syncytial virus; SC, subcutaneous.

specific receptor systems that may further affect their disposition. Age-associated changes in any of these processes and receptor systems as well as the physicochemical properties of the extracellular environment in pediatric patients of different age may thus modulate the disposition behavior of mAbs.

DISTRIBUTION PROCESSES

As large therapeutic proteins, mAbs are, to a large degree, confined to the vascular space, with substantially reduced extravascular relative to the vascular concentrations.[8] Thus, the PK of mAbs can in most cases be described by the two-compartment distribution model, where the volume of distribution of the central compartment is equal to or slightly larger than the plasma volume, and the total volume of distribution is not more than two to three times the initial distribution volume.[9] The limited tissue access of mAbs is reflected by the endogenous IgG concentrations in interstitial fluid of most tissues being only 10% of the concentration in plasma, although some tissues have more "leaky" blood vessels and thus lower concentration differences. On the contrary, tight junctions between endothelial cells of brain capillaries lead to brain tissue concentrations for mAbs that are only 0.1% to 1% relative to plasma.[10]

The extravasation of mAbs, that is, the transfer from the plasma into the interstitial space, can occur via three basic processes: passive diffusion, convective transport, and transcytosis through vascular epithelial cells. Due to the physiochemical properties and large size of mAbs, passive diffusion does not play a significant role in the extravasation process. The main mechanism by which mAbs distribute from the blood into the tissue is through convective transport.[11] Convection is determined by the flux of fluid from the vascular space to the tissue, which is driven by the blood-tissue hydrostatic gradient, as well as by the sieving effect of the paracellular pores in the vascular endothelium.[11–13] The sieving effect is determined by the size, tortuosity, and number of the pores, as well as the size, shape, and charge of the mAb.[11,13] The principle behind convection is that the differential between hydrostatic and colloid osmotic pressures, coupled with the sieving effect, contributes to the net driving force for the extravasation of the mAb[1] (Fig. 44.1). Transcytosis through vascular endothelial cells, mediated via the neonatal FcRn, may also play a role in the extravasation of some mAbs. Lymphatic drainage of the interstitial space facilitates continuous fluid flux from the vascular space to the interstitial space and via lymphatic vessels, ultimately back into the venous vascular system.[8]

Tissue distribution by large proteins such mAbs is further hindered by the extracellular matrix. The interstitial space is filled with extracellular matrix, which has a gel-like consistency with a net negative charge and is predominantly comprised of glycosaminoglycans (e.g., hyaluronic acid) and structural proteins, such as collagen. There is a mutual exclusion between IgG molecules and the structural proteins of the extracellular matrix. The fraction of the extracellular matrix that is not available for distribution has been reported as approximately 50% in muscle and skin tissue.[8]

Although initial assessments reported that distribution behavior of mAbs is likely not affected by childhood development after differences in body size have been taken into account,[3] more recent reports suggest several processes that are affected by age-associated changes and are important for mAb distribution.[14] Most strikingly, there is a well-known difference in tissue water content of newborns and infants relative to older children and adults.[15,16] Thus, the fraction of total body volume available for distribution is higher in children for hydrophilic macromolecules such as mAbs. In addition, the perfusion rate of tissues in newborns and infants has been reported as higher than for the corresponding tissues in adults. Furthermore, infants have larger capillary beds and thus a larger capillary surface area per

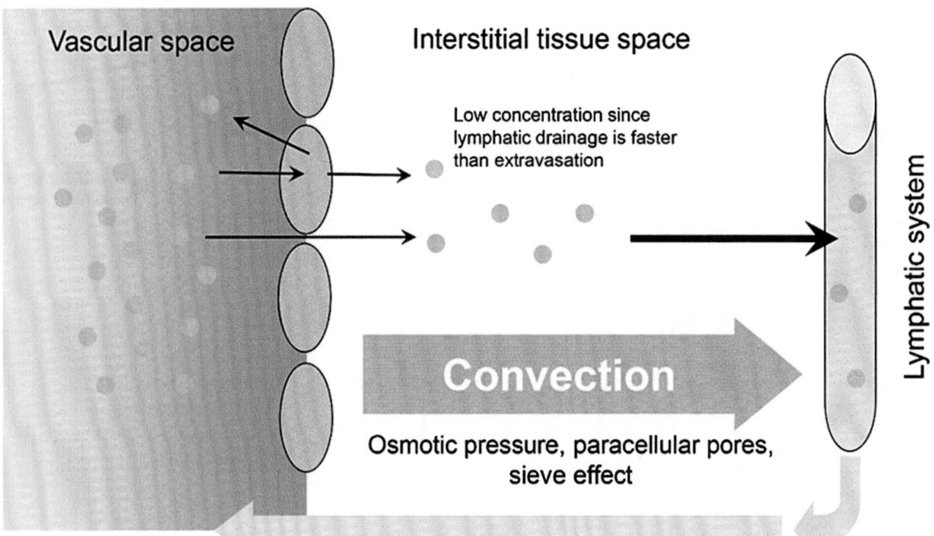

Figure 44.1 Convective extravasation as major distribution process for monoclonal antibodies. (Modified from Ryman JT, Meibohm B. Pharmacokinetics of monoclonal antibodies. *CPT Pharmacometrics Syst Pharmacol* 2017;6:576–588; reproduced with permission.)

unit tissue volume as well as a larger proportion of "leaky" organs and tissues (e.g., liver, kidneys, spleen) with increased capillary permeability relative to their body size.[17] Taken together, extravasation would be expected to be faster and concentration differences between vascular and extravascular space lower in newborns and infants compared to older children and adults.

These considerations are supported by extravasation studies with labeled IgG and albumin molecules. Although the transcapillary escape rate for IgG molecules is typically 40% lower than for albumin, the rate of extravasation for each of these proteins is approximately three times higher in neonates relative to adults.[14,18] Whether this translates into differences in distribution parameters for plasma PK remains to be seen. Further studies will need to assess whether the theoretically expected increase in rate and extent of mAb distribution into young pediatric patients translates into clinically observable differences.

ELIMINATION PROCESSES

The elimination of mAbs from the body is largely facilitated by intracellular catabolism via lysosomal degradation after uptake into cells by either pinocytosis, an unspecific fluid-phase endocytosis, or by a receptor-mediated endocytosis process.[19] Unlike small molecules, mAbs are too large to be filtered by the kidneys and are not eliminated in the urine, except in pathologic conditions.[20]

Pinocytosis is a relatively unspecific fluid-phase endocytosis by endothelial cells lining the blood vessels. Due to the large surface area of endothelial cells in the body, the process efficiently eliminates IgG molecules from the body. Catabolic degradation of IgG following pinocytotic uptake is not limited to a specific organ but occurs throughout the body, particularly in those organs and tissues rich in capillary beds with endothelial cells. Thus, the skin, muscle, and gastrointestinal tract are the major elimination organs for IgG molecules.[21]

Elimination through receptor-mediated endocytosis is facilitated through binding of the Fc domain of an IgG molecule to Fc-γ-receptors (FcγR) expressed on many immune cells, including monocytes, macrophages, and dendritic cells.[22] Binding of mAbs to FcγR triggers the endocytosis of the complex and subsequent intracellular degradation. Studies with FcγR knockout mice suggest that FcγR-mediated elimination plays likely only a minor role (if any) for most mAbs.[23] For those mAbs, however, that form soluble immune complexes, mediate their pharmacology activity through effector functions, such as antibody-dependent cellular cytotoxicity (ADCC), and/or have increased binding affinity to FcγR, receptor-mediated endocytosis via FcγR may constitute an additional elimination pathway that contributes to the overall elimination of the mAb.

Since the intracellular uptake via pinocytosis does not differentiate which proteins in the surrounding of a cell are taken up for degradation, a protective mechanism for IgG molecules is necessary to maintain their concentrations in the plasma in order to support their physiologic function to provide long-term immunity. This salvage pathway is provided by the neonatal FcRn.[24] As illustrated in Figure 44.2, IgG is taken

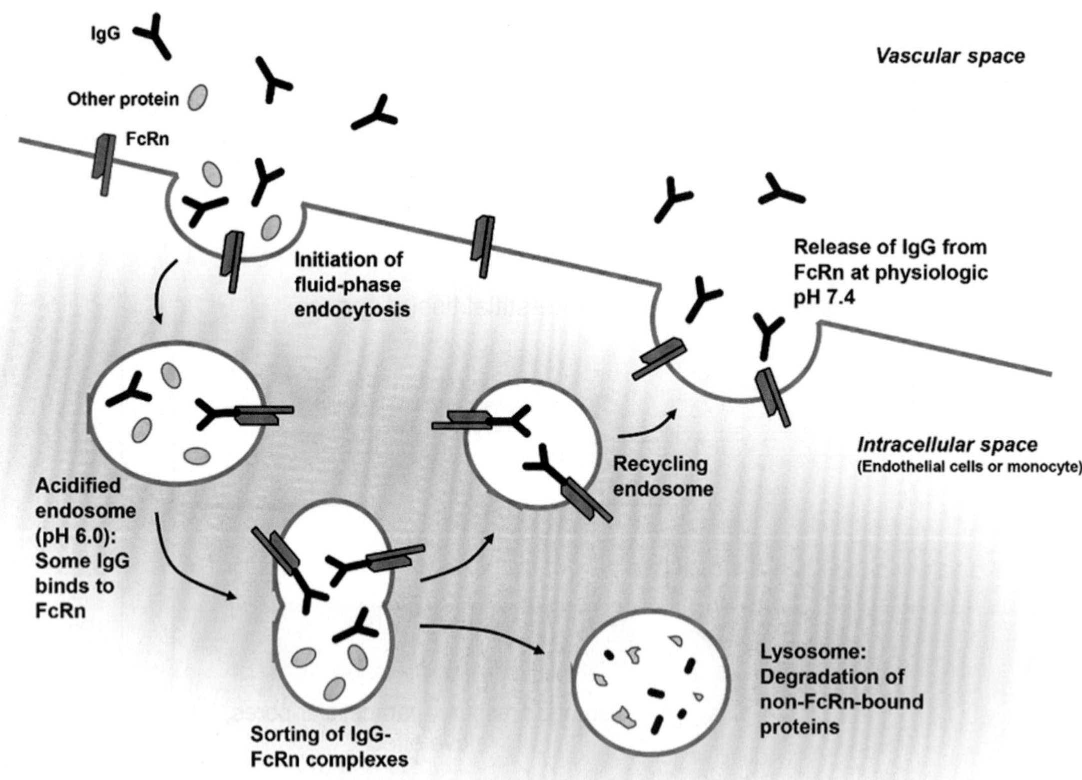

Figure 44.2 Protection of immunoglobulin G (IgG) molecules from lysosomal degradation by the neonatal Fc-receptor (FcRn) salvage pathway. (From Ryman JT, Meibohm B. Pharmacokinetics of monoclonal antibodies. *CPT Pharmacometrics Syst Pharmacol* 2017;6:576–588; reproduced with permission.)

up into endothelial cells by pinocytosis, forming an endosome which includes FcRn. At physiologic pH, FcRn has low affinity for IgG, but as the endosome is acidified, the affinity of FcRn increases and allows the IgG to attach via a specific binding site in the Fc domain. Once bound, the FcRn–IgG complex will be returned to the cell surface and will release the IgG molecule from the binding once physiologic pH has been re-established. Proteins in the endosomes that are not bound to FcRn and recycled undergo proteolytic degradation in the lysosome. The protective effect of FcRn-mediated recycling of IgG molecules thereby prolongs the elimination half-life of IgG, with a more pronounced effect, the stronger the binding of the Fc fragment of the antibody is to the receptor. FcRn recycling is the major reason that IgG1, IgG2, and IgG4 have a half-life in humans of 18 to 21 days, whereas the less strongly bound IgG3 has a half-life of only 7 days.[9]

The efficiency of the FcRn recycling process, including binding affinity to FcRn, protein expression of functional FcRn, and endogenous IgG concentrations competing for FcRn, as well as general age-associated differences in lysosomal protein turnover, could be sources for differences in mAb elimination between children and adults after correction for size differences. Since children of all age groups are able to maintain the homeostasis of immunoglobulins, they also should be able to eliminate therapeutic mAbs through the endosomal clearance pathway.[3] Expression of FcRn is likely not substantially different between children and adults. Although a study investigating messenger RNA (mRNA) expression of the FcRn α chain of FcRn in rats suggested an age-associated increase in mRNA,[25] more recent results on age-associated expression at the protein level in mice suggest no relevant differences in expression from newborn through juvenile animals to adults in skin and spleen tissues,[26] which may be interpreted as more definitive due to the often limited mRNA-to-functional protein correlation for many endogenous proteins.

In addition, infants have substantially lower reference values for endogenous IgG subclasses compared to older children and adults once residual maternal immunoglobulin from placental transfer has been lost several weeks after birth. Those values slowly rise to adult levels over the first months and years of life[27] (Fig. 44.3). Although the FcRn recycling system is efficient, therapeutically used mAbs and endogenous IgG molecules compete for the available recycling capacity. Thus, in young pediatric patients with less competing endogenous IgG present, one would expect a more efficient FcRn recycling and thus a reduced clearance of mAbs in this age group.[28]

Although some differences in the expression and activity of FcγR have been reported in neonatal versus adult immune cells,[29] the overall limited impact of FcγR on the elimination of most mAbs renders this potential source of age-associated differences only relevant for those few mAbs where this pathway may play a larger role.

Protein turnover, that is, catabolism in general, seems to be substantially higher in young pediatric patients compared to adults. For low birth weight infants, protein metabolism has been described as two to three times faster than in adults when normalized for body weight.[30] Whether the effects of pediatric age on these processes related to mAb elimination cancel out, or whether they actually achieve clinically detectable differences in mAb elimination between children and adults remains to be determined in future studies.

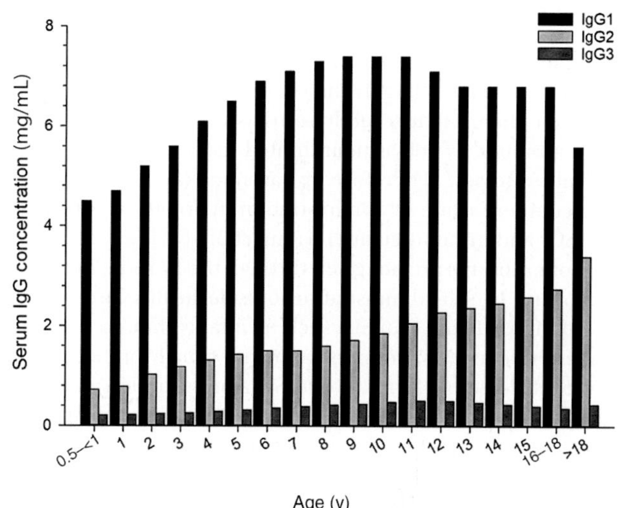

Figure 44.3 Median serum immunoglobulin G (IgG) subclass concentrations in healthy subjects at different ages. (Based on data from Plebani A, Ugazio AG, Avanzini MA, et al. Serum IgG subclass concentrations in healthy subjects at different age: age normal percentile charts. *Eur J Pediatr* 1989;149:164–167.)

TARGET-MEDIATED DRUG DISPOSITION

All therapeutically used mAbs are designed to specifically bind to a target structure, usually a soluble antigen or a membrane-standing receptor. For cell surface receptors, this binding event serves as trigger for the endocytic internalization of the IgG molecule into a vesicle and subsequent lysosomal degradation. Thus, binding of a mAb to its target can constitute an additional elimination pathway.[1] This process has been termed "target-mediated drug disposition" (TMDD).[31]

The rate of elimination of a mAb through TMDD is dependent on the expression of the target receptor, the affinity of the mAb for the receptor, the dose of the mAb, the rate of receptor–mAb complex internalization, and the rate of catabolism within the target cell. MAbs that are primarily cleared by TMDD have dose-dependent nonlinear elimination. Due to the high binding specificity and affinity of the mAb for its target, TMDD is for many mAbs with a membrane-standing target a major route of elimination, especially at low doses and concentrations. At higher doses and concentrations, especially therapeutic doses for mAbs intended to block a cell surface receptor, the TMDD elimination pathway is often saturated due to the limited availability of the target receptors, thereby resulting in a limited or no relevant contribution to overall clearance of the mAb.[8]

TMDD is not only occurring for mAbs targeting membrane-standing receptors but can also be seen for soluble targets if the formed mAb–antigen complex triggers the usual endogenous elimination processes for immune complexes.[32]

Potential differences in the age-associated expression of mAb targets, their turnover kinetics, binding affinity, and internalization rates have so far not been reliably described and would likely be tissue, indication, and target specific. Those potential differences, however, could be a source for additional deviations for the clinical pharmacology of mAbs in children relative to adults.

ROUTES OF ADMINISTRATION

MAbs are not bioavailable after oral administration to any relevant extent. This is largely the consequence of their large size and high charge that severely restricts their ability to transfer biomembranes, as well as their limited stability toward gastrointestinal proteases.[8] Therefore, intravenous (IV) infusion is the most common route of administration, followed by subcutaneous (SC) and intramuscular (IM) injection. SC is used for a majority of mAbs that are not given through the IV route due to the ease of use by self-administration outside health care settings. For young pediatric patients such as infants, however, IV and, to a lesser degree, IM administration are usually preferred. The preferential use of IM relative to SC administration in this patient population is based on the ease of injection to the muscles (vastus lateralis) of the thigh in young children.[14]

Both SC and IM administration of mAbs involve an absorption process from the site of injection that relies significantly on the convective transport of the mAb through the interstitial space into the lymphatic system, draining into the systemic circulation.[34] Similar to the distribution processes for mAbs, uptake of IgG molecules after injection into the interstitial space of subcutaneous tissues is largely driven by convective transport, with only minor contribution from diffusion processes. Since the flow of lymph fluid in lymphatic vessels is very slow compared to the blood flow in capillary vessels (~0.2% of plasma flow rate), the resulting absorption process of mAbs into the systemic circulation after SC administration is also slow, with a corresponding slow increase in plasma concentration and delayed time of the maximum concentration (T_{max}), ranging for mAbs from 1.7 to 13.5 days,[33] with frequent values of T_{max} around 6 to 8 days. A model-based analysis suggests that lymphatic flow rate is the most influential factor to T_{max}.[33]

MAbs administered by the SC or IM route may undergo presystemic elimination. This is thought to be a combination effect of soluble peptidase activity in the interstitial space, endocytosis, and subsequent lysosomal degradation in endothelial cells lining the lymphatic vessels with involvement of the FcRn recycling pathway, as well as interaction with phagocytic immune cells in the lymph nodes. The resulting reported bioavailability for SC-administered mAbs ranges from 52% to 80%.[9] The underlying degree of presystemic degradation has been suggested to be a function of lymphatic residence time and elimination rate during lymphatic transport.[33]

A variety of factors have been identified that affect the rate and extent of absorption after SC and IM administration.[35] This includes the site of injection, which determines the pressure gradients in the local interstitial space,[36] but also body weight, gender, age, activity level, disease state, respiratory rate, and blood pressure.[37] As a consequence of all these factors, there is substantial variability in the rate and extent of absorption between different mAbs and between different individuals for the same mAb.[1,38]

Based on the increased extracellular fluid volume in young pediatric patients compared to older children and adults, as well as the previously discussed higher perfusion rates that are assumed to be equally affected for plasma and lymph, one would expect an increased absorption rate for mAbs in infants and young children. This seems to be confirmed by palivizumab IM administration to infants and adults, with a three times faster absorption rate in children relative to adults.[39]

IMMUNOGENICITY

Administration of therapeutic mAbs to patients may trigger an immune response, leading to the formation of antidrug antibodies (ADA).[40] Immunogenicity is the ability of a substance to elicit an immune response. The immunogenic potential of mAbs is related to a variety of factors, including the fraction of nonhuman sequence in the mAb molecule, the route of administration, as well as dose and duration of therapy.[41] The observed incidence of ADA positivity in a study, however, may also be influenced by other factors, such as sample handling, timing of sample collection, use of concomitant medications, and underlying disease. Predisposition to form an immune response has also been linked to patient genotype, for example, certain human leukocyte antigen (HLA) haplotypes.[42] Thus, there is often substantial variability observed in ADA incidences for the same product in a particular patient group. This makes it challenging to identify patterns and compare ADA occurrence and severity in different populations and to draw reliable conclusions.[43,44]

Immunogenicity resulting in ADA formation is usually a polyclonal response, with multiple ADA species concurrently available and interindividual differences from patient to patient. The formed ADA can either be neutralizing antibodies or nonneutralizing antibodies. Neutralizing ADA obliterate the effect of the mAb by binding to its complementarity-determining regions, that is, its antigen-binding sites. The level of neutralization is often dependent on the titer of ADA. Neutralizing antibodies that are at low titers may not show a clinical effect, but at high titers, there is a greater potential to see a decrease in clinical efficacy.[41] Nonneutralizing ADA do not interfere with the antigen-binding capacity of the mAbs.[1,2]

Independent of whether ADA are neutralizing or nonneutralizing, ADA formation frequently has an effect on the PK and systemic exposure of the affected mAb, although not all ADA formation results in a change in the PK behavior of the mAbs. If there is an effect on PK, it is usually a dramatic increase in the elimination rate of the affected mAb, resulting in a substantially reduced or no appreciable systemic exposure of the mAb.[40] The mechanistic basis for this increased clearance is the formation of circulating ADA–mAb immune complexes that are large enough to trigger uptake and lysosomal degradation by the reticuloendothelial system, mediated via binding of the Fc domain to Fcγ receptors, primarily on platelets, and subsequent internalization by circulating phagocytes. Thus, ADA–mAb complex formation is an additional clearance pathway for the affected mAb.[8]

With over 1,600 genes involved in innate and adaptive immune responses, the human immune system is extraordinarily complex.[45] The transcription of many of these genes changes with age, and the overall immune system undergoes dramatic developmental changes throughout childhood development.[45,46] Age-related alterations that have been shown to cause changes in immune reactivity include, for example, maturation of regulatory T cells and other T-lymphocyte populations,[47,48] and generation of robust memory responses.[49] Although differences in immune reactivity may be expected between pediatric patients and adults based on the maturation of immune system functionality, the detection and magnitude of assessing these differences is complex and has considerable caveats. These are largely related to the fact that the assay technology used to quantify ADA formation relies on semiquantitative assays, with the consequence that the assay results cannot be compared between different mAbs or even the same mAb in different studies when different assays are applied.[44]

ADA formation is a well-recognized impediment to mAb-based therapies in pediatric indications, such as juvenile idiopathic arthritis.[50] Current literature suggests no significant difference in immunogenicity between adults and pediatric populations for most investigated mAbs, including etanercept, infliximab, and tocilizumab. Nevertheless, a careful review considering the noted methodologic limitations reported that notably higher ADA incidence rates were reported for adalimumab, abatacept, and daclizumab in children compared to the respective adult populations.[3] Whether these perceived differences in immunogenicity between children and adults are indeed based in differences in immunoreactivity between different age groups, and whether these ultimately translate into actionable differences in the clinical pharmacology of the affected mAbs remains to be confirmed in more systematic and controlled future investigations.

EXTRAPOLATION OF PEDIATRIC PHARMACOKINETIC AND PHARMACOKINETIC-PHARMACODYNAMIC RELATIONSHIPS

Pediatric drug development and applied pharmacotherapy are often hampered by a lack of experimental data in pediatric populations that may inform dosing regimen selection. To overcome this limitation, a frequently applied approach is to extrapolate the PK and exposure–response relationships from adults to pediatric populations of different age.[5]

For mAbs, body size–based allometric scaling approaches have been shown to be relatively reliable for extrapolating PK parameters between different mammalian species, as long as the disposition processes for the mAb are governed by unspecific proteolytic degradation pathways and do not include interaction with endogenous receptor systems. The reason is probably the similarity in handling proteins, including mAbs, among different mammalian species. Species differences, however, need to be considered once receptor-mediated processes are involved.[8] In analogy to between-species scaling, allometric approaches are frequently also applied to extrapolate adult mAb PK data to pediatric patients. Again, this size-based allometric approach usually works well until a lower age range is reached in which immature and age-specific disposition processes require additional consideration, oftentimes in the age group below 6 months.

The concept of pediatric extrapolation may further facilitate the development of dosing regimens for mAb-based therapeutics if the corresponding exposure–response relationship can be established.[51] Golimumab is an example where a model-based analysis of clinical end points in children (6 to 17 years) with ulcerative colitis indicated that the exposure–response relationship was similar between the pediatric patients and adults. Therefore, dosing recommendations for the pediatric age groups were established by exposure matching of golimumab serum concentrations with the corresponding concentrations observed at the approved dose level in adults.[52]

Pediatric extrapolation becomes more challenging if exposure–response relationships are not identical between children and adults, for example, if the childhood condition is distinctively different from the adult disease. In those instances, more clinical efficacy and exposure data may be necessary to inform pediatric dosing regimen design.

PEDIATRIC DOSING APPROACHES

In order to achieve reproducible mAb exposures across different age groups of pediatric patients, a variety of dosing approaches are used to account for maturation- and size-related differences between children and adults.[53] Table 44.1 illustrates the applied dosing strategies for currently approved pediatric indications of mAb-based therapeutics. In most cases, these approaches try to strike a balance between sufficient granularity to account for age- and size-related differences to ensure comparable systemic exposure, and limited clinical complexity in order to avoid overburdening health care providers and limit dosing errors. It should also be noted that based on therapeutic needs, the same mAb can have different dosing approaches in different pediatric indications.

Flat dosing across different age groups would likely result in large exposure differences among children of different ages for the reasons outlined in the previous paragraphs. Thus, such an approach would only by acceptable for mAbs that are well tolerated and thus can be given at doses resulting in effective and safe plasma concentrations across the pediatric age spectrum or that have flat exposure–response relationships for both, efficacy and safety. The anti–interleukin-5 receptor mAb benralizumab against eosinophilic asthma and the anti–programmed death receptor ligand 1 mAb avelumab for the treatment of metastatic Merkel cell carcinoma seem to fall into this category (Table 44.1).

Body weight–based dosing remains a frequently applied pediatric dosing strategy for mAbs. Examples are the anti–tumor necrosis factor-α mAb infliximab for the treatment of pediatric Crohn disease and pediatric ulcerative colitis, and the anti–interleukin-1β mAb canakinumab in the systemic juvenile idiopathic arthritis indication (Table 44.1). When the approved dosing covers a wide age range, weight-based dosing may not be optimal for all children due to the common nonlinearity of mAb clearance relative to body weight, as discussed earlier.[9] In order to address this shortcoming, several dosing approaches use more than one weight-based dose throughout the pediatric spectrum.

Body-surface area (BSA)-based dosing remains limited to few mAbs, particularly in cancer indications. The major reasons seem to be complexity of estimating BSA from height and weight with its associated inaccuracies,[3] the limited relationship between clearance and BSA for most mAbs,[2] and the lack of a substantial advantage of this dosing strategy relative to the other discussed approaches. At the current time, only gemtuzumab ozogamicin uses BSA-based dosing in children (Table 44.1).

Allometrically adjusted dosing based on theoretical considerations[4,5] as well as practical observations from population PK analyses[9] seems to be the most precise approach when clearance and volume of distribution scaling is performed with the classical allometric exponents of 0.75 and 1, respectively, as long as no other maturation-related processes beyond body weight affect the mAb PK. While dose adjustments based on allometric equations seem attractive as they account for the nonlinearity in the weight versus clearance relationship, they remain impractical in clinical practice and are thus not applied for any of the mAbs approved for pediatric indications.

Tiered-fixed dosing uses one or several body weight or age cutoffs to define patient strata that receive different flat doses. It allows to account for different dosing needs based on body weight and/or age and is highly attractive due to its simplicity of implementation. Since most mAb-based therapeutics have relatively good tolerability, a certain limited variability in drug exposure may be acceptable,[3] making tiered-fixed dosing a viable option despite its theoretically lower dosing precision relative to allometric or body weight–adjusted dosing. The anti–interleukin-6 receptor mAb tocilizumab for the treatment of polyarticular and systemic juvenile idiopathic arthritis uses for its SC dosing the tiered-fixed dosing approach based on body weight, while the anti–interleukin-5 mAb mepolizumab for the treatment of eosinophilic asthma uses fixed doses based on age strata (Table 44.1). To define adequate weight and/or age cutoffs, prior PK data in the covered age group and pharmacometric analyses are usually needed to derive optimal strata sizes through model-based simulations.

Tiered body weight–based dosing is probably the currently most widely applied dosing strategy for mAbs in children. This approach uses one or several body weight or age cutoffs to define patient strata that receive different body weight–adjusted doses. It allows more individualized dosing than the tiered-fixed dosing approach, but still seems very well accepted and manageable in clinical settings. Similar to tired-fixed dosing, weight and/or age strata cutoffs are usually developed based on prior PK data in the covered age groups and model-based pharmacometric simulation exercises. The anti–tumor necrosis factor-α mAb adalimumab in juvenile idiopathic arthritis and pediatric uveitis as well as the anthrax prophylactic mAb raxibacumab are examples for tiered body weight–based dosing (Table 44.1).

Hybrid approaches of tiered-fixed dosing and body weight–based dosing have also successfully been applied, where patients above a certain body weight cutoff receive a flat, fixed dose, while those below receive a body weight–adjusted dose. This approach seems particularly attractive for mAbs with flat dosing in the adult population, but that need dose adjustments below a certain age range. The anti–tumor necrosis factor-α Fc fusion protein etanercept applies the hybrid approach with flat dosing above and body weight–based dosing below a body weight cutoff (see Table 44.1).

Pharmacodynamic (PD) end point approaches have so far only been utilized in rare instances, but can be useful if TMDD affects the disposition of the mAb and the mAb target is easily accessible for quantification. This is, for example, the case for omalizumab, where the dosing strategy in children with allergic asthma is based on the patient's body weight and the baseline level for endogenous IgE, the pharmacologic target of omalizumab.[53]

CONCLUSIONS

With an increasing number of mAbs being approved for pediatric indications, there is a growing knowledgebase on the PK and clinical pharmacology of this class of compounds in pediatric patient populations of different ages. Based on the clinical experiences and theoretical considerations, there are a variety of drug disposition mechanisms that may be affected by age and can thus result in differences in the PK behavior of mAbs in children compared to adults. While these age-based differences can, to a large degree, be addressed by body size–based dosing, especially by adequately considering the nonlinear relationship between clearance and body size according to allometric principles, additional age-related dose adjustments may be necessary in younger pediatric populations, such as neonates and infants. As conceptual clinical pharmacology approaches, mechanistic understanding of relevant drug disposition processes and clinical experience with mAbs in pediatric populations are becoming increasingly available, the fundamental framework for the rationale use of this class of compounds in pediatric pharmacotherapy is rapidly evolving. With the advent of this increasing information on the use of mAbs in children, the extension of newly approached mAb-based therapeutics to pediatric indications will hopefully be streamlined and accelerated, so that all pediatric patient populations will have access to the full benefits of this innovative class of novel medications.

REFERENCES

1. Ryman JT, Meibohm B. Pharmacokinetics of monoclonal antibodies. *CPT Pharmacometrics Syst Pharmacol* 2017;6:576–588.
2. Mould DR, Meibohm B. Drug development of therapeutic monoclonal antibodies. *BioDrugs* 2016;30:275–293.
3. Xu Z, Davis HM, Zhou H. Rational development and utilization of antibody-based therapeutic proteins in pediatrics. *Pharmacol Ther* 2013;137:225–247.
4. Anderson BJ, Holford NH. Mechanism-based concepts of size and maturity in pharmacokinetics. *Annu Rev Pharmacol Toxicol* 2008;48:303–332.
5. Meibohm B, Laer S, Panetta JC, et al. Population pharmacokinetic studies in pediatrics: issues in design and analysis. *AAPS J* 2005;7:E475–E487.
6. Davis JD, Deng R, Boswell CA, et al. Monoclonal antibodies: from structure to therapeutic application. In: Crommelin DJA, Sindelar RD, Meibohm B, eds. *Pharmaceutical biotechnology: fundamentals and applications*, 4th ed. New York, NY: Springer, 2013:143–178.
7. Kadir F, Ives P, Luitjens A, et al. Production and purification of recombinant proteins. In: Crommelin DJA, Sindelar RD, Meibohm B, eds. *Pharmaceutical biotechnology: fundamentals and applications*, 4th ed. New York, NY: Springer, 2013:47–67.
8. Meibohm B. Pharmacokinetics and pharmacodynamics of therapeutic peptides and proteins. In: Crommelin DJA, Sindelar RD, Meibohm B, eds. *Pharmaceutical biotechnology: fundamentals and applications*, 5th ed. New York, NY: Springer, 2019:105–137.
9. Dirks NL, Meibohm B. Population pharmacokinetics of therapeutic monoclonal antibodies. *Clin Pharmacokinet* 2010;49:633–659.
10. Kingwell K. Drug delivery: new targets for drug delivery across the BBB. *Nat Rev Drug Discov* 2016;15:84–85.
11. Baxter LT, Zhu H, Mackensen DG, et al. Physiologically based pharmacokinetic model for specific and nonspecific monoclonal antibodies and fragments in normal tissues and human tumor xenografts in nude mice. *Cancer Res* 1994;54:1517–1528.
12. Flessner MF, Lofthouse J, Zakaria el R. In vivo diffusion of immunoglobulin G in muscle: effects of binding, solute exclusion, and lymphatic removal. *Am J Physiol* 1997;273:H2783–H2793.
13. Covell DG, Barbet J, Holton OD, et al. Pharmacokinetics of monoclonal immunoglobulin G1, F(ab')2, and Fab' in mice. *Cancer Res* 1986;46:3969–3978.
14. Malik P, Edginton A. Pediatric physiology in relation to the pharmacokinetics of monoclonal antibodies. *Expert Opin Drug Metab Toxicol* 2018;14:585–599.
15. Friis-Hansen B. Water distribution in the foetus and newborn infant. *Acta Paediatr Scand Suppl.* 1983;305:7–11.
16. Kearns GL, Abdel-Rahman SM, Alander SW, et al. Developmental pharmacology—drug disposition, action, and therapy in infants and children. *N Engl J Med* 2003;349:1157–1167.
17. Schaefer B, Bartosova M, Macher-Goeppinger S, et al. Quantitative histomorphometry of the healthy peritoneum. *Sci Rep* 2016;6:21344.
18. Malik PRV, Hamadeh A, Phipps C, et al. Population PBPK modelling of trastuzumab: a framework for quantifying and predicting inter-individual variability. *J Pharmacokinet Pharmacodyn* 2017;44:277–290.
19. Waldmann TA, Strober W. Metabolism of immunoglobulins. *Prog Allergy* 1969;13:1–110.
20. Berdeja J, Jagannath S, Zonder J, et al. Pharmacokinetics and safety of elotuzumab combined with lenalidomide and dexamethasone in patients with multiple myeloma and various levels of renal impairment: results of a phase Ib study. *Clin Lymphoma Myeloma Leuk* 2016;16:129–138.
21. Wright A, Sato Y, Okada T, et al. In vivo trafficking and catabolism of IgG1 antibodies with Fc associated carbohydrates of differing structure. *Glycobiology* 2000;10:1347–1355.
22. Gessner JE, Heiken H, Tamm A, et al. The IgG Fc receptor family. *Ann Hematol* 1998;76:231–248.
23. Abuqayyas L, Balthasar JP. Application of knockout mouse models to investigate the influence of FcγR on the tissue distribution and elimination of 8C2, a murine IgG1 monoclonal antibody. *Int J Pharm* 2012;439:8–16.
24. Roopenian DC, Akilesh S. FcRn: the neonatal Fc receptor comes of age. *Nat Rev Immunol* 2007;7:715–725.
25. Tian Z, Sutton BJ, Zhang X. Distribution of rat neonatal Fc receptor in the principal organs of neonatal and pubertal rats. *J Recept Signal Transduct Res* 2014;34:137–142.
26. Limothai W, Meibohm B. *Effect of developmental growth and FcRn expression on the pharmacokinetics of monoclonal antibodies in mice.* Brisbane, Australia: World Conference on Pharmacometrics, 2016.

27. Plebani A, Ugazio AG, Avanzini MA, et al. Serum IgG subclass concentrations in healthy subjects at different age: age normal percentile charts. *Eur J Pediatr* 1989;149:164–167.
28. Morell A, Terry WD, Waldmann TA. Metabolic properties of IgG subclasses in man. *J Clin Invest* 1970;49:673–680.
29. Maeda M, van Schie RC, Yuksel B, et al. Differential expression of Fc receptors for IgG by monocytes and granulocytes from neonates and adults. *Clin Exp Immunol* 1996;103:343–347.
30. Beaufrere B. Protein turnover in low-birth-weight (LBW) infants. *Acta Paediatr Suppl* 1994;405:86–92.
31. Levy G. Pharmacologic target-mediated drug disposition. *Clin Pharmacol Ther* 1994;56:248–252
32. Sutjandra L, Rodriguez RD, Doshi S, et al. Population pharmacokinetic meta-analysis of denosumab in healthy subjects and postmenopausal women with osteopenia or osteoporosis. *Clin Pharmacokinet* 2011;50:793–807.
33. Zhao L, Ji P, Li Z, et al. The antibody drug absorption following subcutaneous or intramuscular administration and its mathematical description by coupling physiologically based absorption process with the conventional compartment pharmacokinetic model. *J Clin Pharmacol* 2013;53:314–325.
34. Porter CJ, Charman SA. Lymphatic transport of proteins after subcutaneous administration. *J Pharm Sci* 2000;89:297–310.
35. Richter WF, Bhansali SG, Morris ME. Mechanistic determinants of biotherapeutics absorption following SC administration. *AAPS J* 2012;14:559–570.
36. Olszewski W, Engeset A, Jaeger PM, et al. Flow and composition of leg lymph in normal men during venous stasis, muscular activity and local hyperthermia. *Acta Physiol Scand* 1977;99:149–155.
37. Chow TW, Wright MR, Hop C, et al. Evaluation of the predictive performance of physiologically based pharmacokinetic models for intramuscular injections of therapeutic proteins. *Xenobiotica* 2019;49:1423–1433.
38. Richter WF, Jacobsen B. Subcutaneous absorption of biotherapeutics: knowns and unknowns. *Drug Metab Dispos* 2014;42:1881–1889.
39. Robbie GJ, Zhao L, Mondick J, et al. Population pharmacokinetics of palivizumab, a humanized anti-respiratory syncytial virus monoclonal antibody, in adults and children. *Antimicrob Agents Chemother* 2012;56:4927–4936.
40. Chirmule N, Jawa V, Meibohm B. Immunogenicity to therapeutic proteins: impact on PK/PD and efficacy. *AAPS J* 2012;14:296–302.
41. Schellekens H. Immunogenicity of therapeutic proteins: clinical implications and future prospects. *Clin Ther* 2002;24:1720–1740; discussion 1719.
42. Sethu S, Govindappa K, Alhaidari M, et al. Immunogenicity to biologics: mechanisms, prediction and reduction. *Arch Immunol Ther Exp (Warsz)* 2012;60:331–344.
43. Gunn GR III, Sealey DC, Jamali F, et al. From the bench to clinical practice: understanding the challenges and uncertainties in immunogenicity testing for biopharmaceuticals. *Clin Exp Immunol* 2016;184:137–146.
44. Shakhnovich V, Meibohm B, Rosenberg A, et al. Immunogenicity in clinical practice and drug development: when is it significant? *Clin Transl Sci* 2020;13:219–223.
45. Simon AK, Hollander GA, McMichael A. Evolution of the immune system in humans from infancy to old age. *Proc Biol Sci* 2015;282.
46. Ygberg S, Nilsson A. The developing immune system—from foetus to toddler. *Acta Paediatr* 2012;101:120–127.
47. Tulic MK, Andrews D, Crook ML, et al. Changes in thymic regulatory T-cell maturation from birth to puberty: differences in atopic children. *J Allergy Clin Immunol* 2012;129:199.e1–206.e4.
48. Wilson CB. The ontogeny of T lymphocyte maturation and function. *J Pediatr* 1991;118:S4–S9.
49. Basha S, Surendran N, Pichichero M. Immune responses in neonates. *Expert Rev Clin Immunol* 2014;10:1171–1184.
50. Doeleman MJH, van Maarseveen EM, Swart JF. Immunogenicity of biologic agents in juvenile idiopathic arthritis: a systematic review and meta-analysis. *Rheumatology* 2019;58:1839–1849.
51. Mehrotra N, Bhattaram A, Earp JC, et al. Role of quantitative clinical pharmacology in pediatric approval and labeling. *Drug Metab Dispos* 2016;44:924–933.
52. Xu Y, Adedokun OJ, Chan D, et al. Population pharmacokinetics and exposure-response modeling analyses of golimumab in children with moderately to severely active ulcerative colitis. *J Clin Pharmacol* 2019;59:590–604.
53. Zhang Y, Wei X, Bajaj G, et al. Challenges and considerations for development of therapeutic proteins in pediatric patients. *J Clin Pharmacol* 2015;55(Suppl 3):S103–S115.

CHAPTER

45

Karen C. Young

Stem Cells

INTRODUCTION

The term "stem cell" was first coined by Ernst Haeckel in 1868 to describe a fertilized egg[1] that gives rise to all cells. But it was Alexander Maximow's work in 1909, entitled "The lymphocyte as a stem cell, common to different blood elements in embryonic development and during postfetal life of mammals" that introduced the concept of multipotency.[2] The scientific field was skeptical about Maximow's findings, and stem cell research did not significantly advance until 50 years later, when McCulloch and Till, while studying the effect of radiation on mice bone marrow, demonstrated the existence of hematopoietic stem cells (HSCs).[3–5] These cells exhibited the ability to proliferate indefinitely and gave rise to specialized cells. By the 1970s, Alexander Friedenstein identified a rare population of plastic adherent bone marrow stromal cells, now known as mesenchymal stem cells (MSCs),[6–10] and in 1998, James Thomson and his team in Wisconsin created the first batch of human embryonic stem cells from early embryos.[11] This opened the door not only for tremendous therapeutic opportunities but also for ethical concerns and controversies. By 2001, the use of federal funds for embryonic stem cell research was restricted to a limited number of existing embryonic stem cell lines. However, in 2006, a major breakthrough occurred when Japanese scientists discovered that mouse skin cells could be reprogrammed to function like embryonic stem cells.[12] These cells named "induced pluripotent stem cells" (iPSCs) provided a novel platform to recapitulate some of the crucial differentiation cues that promote cell lineage commitment, model diseases, engineer new tissues, and test drug efficacy.[13] Discoveries such as these have revolutionized the stem cell field, and the old paradigm that organ replacement is the main clinical use of stem cells is debunked.

Stem cells of varying potency are being isolated from virtually every organ,[14] and they are being investigated as therapeutic delivery vehicles in several developmental disorders. Studies evaluating tissue engineering strategies to manufacture functional tissue ex vivo are also underway.[15] Owing to the abundance of MSCs, their ease of isolation, immunomodulatory properties, and other pleiotropic effects, MSCs are the most widely used cellular population in regenerative medicine.[16] In preterm infants, MSCs are a promising strategy to improve respiratory and neurologic outcomes, and clinical trials are ongoing using MSCs for bronchopulmonary dysplasia (BPD),[17,18] hypoplastic left heart disease,[19] and hypoxic–ischemic encephalopathy (HIE).[20] In pediatric patients, clinical trials are also underway using MSCs to reduce autism symptoms,[21] and in patients with graft-versus-host disease, MSCs in combination with immunosuppressive therapy shows encouraging effects.[22] Alternative cell-free approaches such as stem cell–derived exosomes are promising options as they lack tumorigenicity and allow easier biodistribution.[23]

This chapter reviews the various stem cell populations, their mechanisms of the action, and potential therapeutic applications in neonatal and pediatric diseases.

STEM CELL TYPES AND CHARACTERISTICS

Stem cells are unspecialized cells with two fundamental properties: the ability to divide and make more copies of themselves through a process of self-renewal and the ability to differentiate into various mature specialized progeny depending on their potency (Fig. 45.1).[24]

Totipotent stem cells are capable of differentiating into all adult, embryonic, and extraembryonic tissues, such as placenta and fetal membranes.[25] In mammals, only progeny of the zygote up to the eight-cell stage of the morula are totipotent.[26] ***Pluripotent stem cells*** such as embryonic stem cells are capable of differentiating into derivatives of all three germ layers (ectoderm, mesoderm, and endoderm). They are not able to form extraembryonic tissues, such as the placenta. ***Multipotent stem cells*** are able to differentiate into discrete cell types of one lineage.[27] The most prominent example is the HSC, which is capable of differentiating into all cell types of the hematopoietic system.[28] ***Unipotent stem cells*** have the lowest differentiation potential and are only able to differentiate into a single mature cell line. Epidermal and satellite stem cells are unipotent as they only differentiate into keratinocytes and skeletal muscle, respectively.

Stem cells may also be categorized based on their origin as embryonic, adult, or fetal.

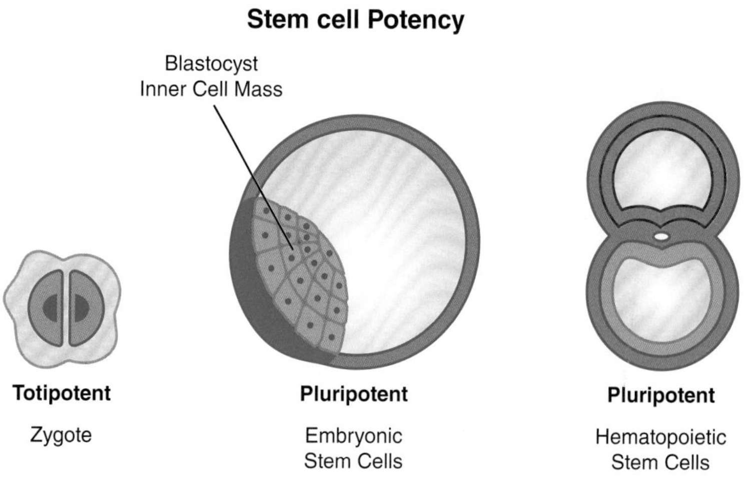

Stem cell Potency
Blastocyst
Inner Cell Mass
Totipotent
Zygote
Pluripotent
Embryonic
Stem Cells
Pluripotent
Hematopoietic
Stem Cells

Figure 45.1 Stem cell potency. Totipotent stem cells can give rise to all cells in the embryo and placenta. In mammals, only the zygote and morula are totipotent. Pluripotent stem cells (e.g., embryonic stem cells) originate from the inner cell mass blastocyst and can rise to all three cell lineages (endoderm, mesoderm, and ectoderm). Trilaminar disc cells give rise to multipotent stem cells. One example is the hematopoietic stem cell. Illustration done by Dr. Andreas Damianos.

EMBRYONIC STEM CELLS

Embryonic stem cells are derived from blastocysts in the developing embryo and have the ability to differentiate into cellular derivatives of all three germ layers.[29] The pluripotency of embryonic stem cells is tightly regulated by several transcription factors, including Nanog,[30] Oct4,[31] and Sox2,[32,33] but because embryonic stem cells have unlimited differentiation potential, they can be guided to differentiate into all cell types, including cardiomyocytes,[34] neurons,[35] pancreatic β cells,[36] and endothelial cells.[37] Not only does this make them an attractive source for tissue regeneration, but it also provides a unique tool to recapitulate the crucial induction cues that lead to cell lineage commitment.[38] For instance, one method for in vitro differentiation removes embryonic stem cells from their feeder layer and cultivates them into three-dimensional (3D) aggregates called embryoid bodies.[38] Exposure of early differentiating embryonic bodies to activin A, a member of the Nodal signaling family, enhances the specification of distal lung epithelium and yields cells with a phenotype most closely resembling that of lung-committed progenitor cells.[39] Multiple preclinical models also demonstrate the therapeutic efficacy of embryonic stem cells for cell replacement. In a genetic cardiomyopathy model, allogeneic embryonic stem cells engraft in the heart, contribute to new cardiac tissue formation, and improve cardiac function and structure.[40] Although there was no evidence of dysregulated growth 1 month following transplantation, the inherent tumorigenesis risks and ethical concerns of embryonic stem cells have limited clinical translation.

An alternative approach to improve the safety of embryonic stem cells is to differentiate them into specific cell types prior to clinical use. In proof of this concept, embryonic stem cell–derived type 2 alveolar cells abrogate bleomycin-induced acute lung injury.[41] The transplanted cells behave as normal primary alveolar type 2 cells, differentiating into cells expressing phenotypic markers of alveolar type I epithelial cells.[41] No tumorigenic side effects were observed, and up to 20% of the total surfactant protein C–expressing cells appeared to be of embryonic stem cell–derived origin.[41] Similarly, human embryonic-derived cardiomyocytes improve left ventricular function in macaque monkeys with myocardial infarction, but a subset of animals experienced graft-associated arrhythmias.[42]

In 2010, the first clinical trial using embryonic stem–derived oligodendrocyte progenitor cells in five patients with spinal cord injury was performed. Results are yet to be published, but preliminary findings suggest that the therapy was safe, although there was no clinical improvement.[43] In 2011, another phase 1 trial using embryonic stem cell–derived retinal pigment epithelium cells for macular degeneration demonstrated that the therapy was safe, with some improvement in vision at medium- to long-term follow-up.[44]

Currently, there are no pediatric trials using embryonic stem cell–based therapies. Obtaining a purified population of embryonic stem cell–derived differentiated cells continues to be challenging. Embryonic stem cells are also not protected against T-lymphocyte–mediated cytotoxicity, and cellular derivatives of embryonic stem cells may be rejected after implantation.[45] Nonetheless, emerging evidence that human embryonic stem cells can been used as a platform to model diseases such as pediatric brain tumors and screen pathways that contribute to tumor maintenance is encouraging.[25]

ADULT STEM CELLS

Mesenchymal Stem Cells

MSCs or mesenchymal stromal cells are a heterogeneous population of multipotent adult stem cells which exhibit the following characteristics: adherence to plastic under standard tissue culture conditions[46] and expression of cell-surface markers, CD105, CD90, and CD73, but not CD79α, CD45, CD34, CD14, CD19, or CD11b. They self-renew and exhibit the capacity to differentiate into osteoblasts, chondroblasts, and adipocytes under appropriate in vitro conditions.[47,48]

MSCs are the most extensively studied stem cell population for cell regenerative therapy as they are easily expanded and readily isolated from accessible sources,[49] such as the bone marrow,[50] adipose tissue,[51] dental pulp,[52] placenta,[53] amniotic fluid,[54] umbilical cord blood,[54] and Wharton jelly[55] (Fig. 45.2).

Bone marrow–derived MSCs are obtained by bone marrow aspiration, but while the procedure is easy in adults, this is a limiting factor for autologous transplantation in neonates and young children. There is also a growing concern of the age-dependent decline in regenerative potential of these

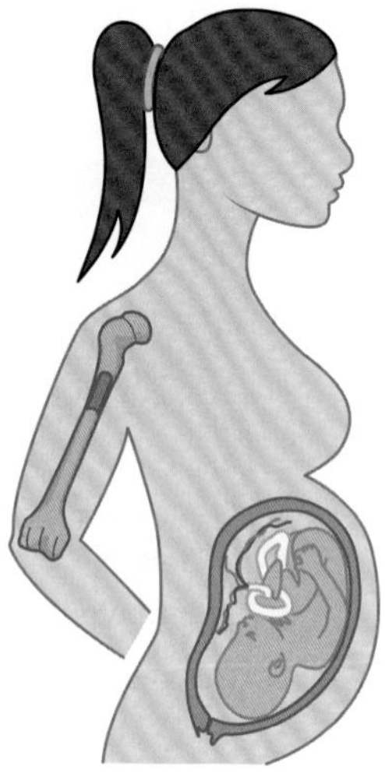

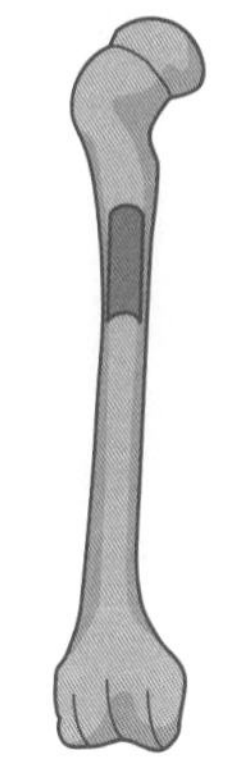

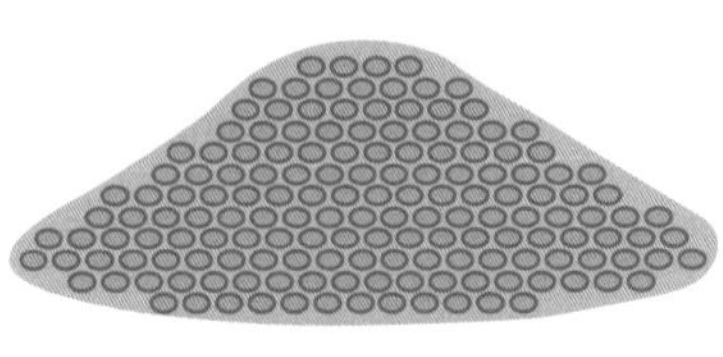

Figure 45.2 Mesenchymal stem cell sources. Mesenchymal stem cells can be isolated from virtually every organ. However, the most common sources for regenerative therapy are derived from perinatal, bone marrow, and adipose tissues. Illustration done by Dr. Andreas Damianos.

cells.[56] *Adipose tissue–derived MSCs* are obtained from liposuction aspirates, have comparable characteristics to bone marrow–derived MSCs, but unlike the bone marrow, the yield of MSCs from adipose tissue is quite high. In a study comparing the proliferative and differentiation capacity of donor-matched adipose tissue and bone marrow–derived MSCs, greater cell proliferation and adipogenic potential was evident with adipose tissue–derived MSCs,[57] but the cells have comparable effects on both innate and adaptive immunity.[58] Adipose tissue may, however, have endocrine effects, and obesity may influence the immunophenotype of adipose tissue–derived MSCs.[59]

MSCs may be transplanted between incompatible patients as they constitutively express low levels of human leukocyte antigen (HLA) class I molecules and do not express either HLA class II molecules or the co-stimulatory molecules CD40, CD80, and CD86, which are essential for activation of T-lymphocyte–mediated immune responses.[60] Although initial studies suggested that MSCs engraft and differentiate, these events are rare. Instead, accumulating evidence suggests that growth factors, nucleotides and mitochondria,[61] mediate MSCs' immunomodulatory, antifibrotic, and proangiogenic regenerative effects through paracrine signaling, direct cell–cell interactions, and microvesicles[62] (Fig. 45.3).

Immunomodulatory Effects

MSCs interact with cells of both the innate and adaptive immune system.[48] These immunomodulatory effects provide the rationale for MSCs use in a myriad of neonatal and pediatric conditions, including BPD,[18] necrotizing enterocolitis,[63] and graft-versus-host disease.[64] MSCs attenuate the respiratory burst in activated neutrophils,[65] suppress natural killer cell proliferation, cytokine production, and cytotoxicity[66]; inhibit dendritic cell maturation and activation[67]; induce changes in macrophage polarization to an M2, anti-inflammatory phenotype[68–70]; suppress T-cell cytokine secretion and cytotoxicity[71–73]; and inhibit B-cell survival, proliferation, and differentiation.[74] This is achieved by direct cell–cell crosstalk and by the secretion of soluble factors including prostaglandin E2 (PGE2),[75] tumor necrosis factor (TNF)–stimulated gene 6 (*TSG-6*),[68] indoleamine 2,3-dioxygenase,[76] interleukin-10,[77] and nitric oxide.[48,78] For instance, in a recent study, TSG-6 knockdown attenuates the anti-inflammatory and regenerative effects of MSCs in neonatal hyperoxia-induced lung injury.[79]

Antifibrotic Effects

In preclinical models, MSCs from varying sources attenuated fibrosis.[80–84] MSC immunomodulatory properties may mediate some of its antifibrotic effects,[85] but MSCs also directly affect myofibroblast accumulation and reduce their differentiation by modulating Wnt signaling.[86] In addition, MSCs decrease transforming growth factor β (TGF-β) levels, a key factor in myofibroblast differentiation.[87] By regulating the production of matrix metalloproteinases and their inhibitors, MSCs also modulate extracellular matrix remodeling.[88]

Though the aforementioned studies support MSC antifibrotic effects, concern remains that MSCs themselves may transform into myofibroblasts, depending on the microenvironment. Some genetic fate mapping studies suggest that bone marrow–derived MSC-like pericytes are a major source of myofibroblasts, but more recent robust lineage tracing studies do not support this hypothesis.[89,90] Indeed, in one study, autocrine production of TGF-β1 drives lung MSCs obtained from the tracheal aspirate of preterm infants with BPD toward myofibroblastic differentiation,[91] but the same is not true for infused bone marrow–derived MSCs.[91] To date, there is no evidence that infused MSCs contribute to fibrosis, but an important consideration is that the antifibrotic properties of MSCs are directly modulated by cell–cell interactions and soluble factors within the infused microenvironment.

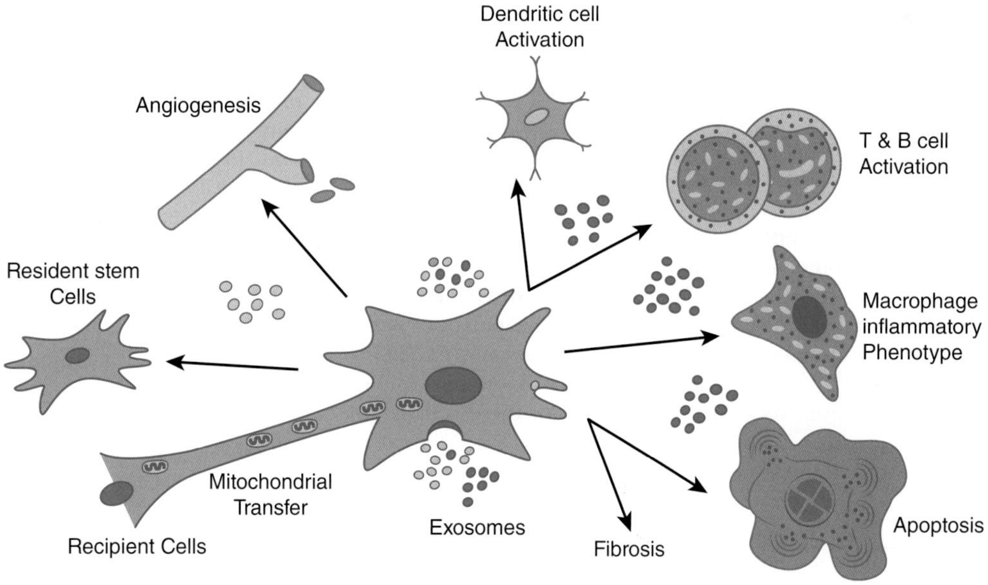

Figure 45.3 Mesenchymal stem cells: Mechanisms of repair. Mesenchymal stem cells augment endogenous repair by secreting exosomes and soluble factors, which modulate angiogenesis, fibrosis, apoptosis, and inflammation. Through complex and dynamic cell–cell interactions, MSCs also replenish the endogenous stem cell niche and transfer mitochondria to damaged cells. Illustration done by Dr. Andreas Damianos.

Proangiogenic Effects

MSCs contribute to neovascularization by secreting several proangiogenic factors.[92] In rodent models of BPD, MSC regenerative effects are, in part, mediated by vascular endothelial growth factor (VEGF)[93] and stromal-derived factor-1.[94] There is also evidence that other growth factors such as angiopoietin-1, keratinocyte growth factor, and hepatocyte growth factor restore endothelial cell integrity.[95–100]

Antibacterial Effects

Another interesting property of MSCs is their ability to improve bacterial clearance by their secretion of antimicrobial peptides, including cathelicidin LL-37,[101] human β-defensin-2,[102] and lipocalin-2.[103] This antimicrobial effect is modulated by the microenvironment.[104] For instance, when MSCs are subjected to toll-like receptor 4 priming conditions, increased secretion of human β-defensin-2 enhances bacterial clearance.[102] In proof of this concept, intratracheally delivered MSCs enhance survival and bacterial clearance in mice with gram-negative pneumonia.[103] In a phase 1 dose-escalation trial of MSCs in nine adult patients with septic shock, MSC delivery was feasible, and no adverse effects were evident.[105] Larger trials are underway, but questions related to dosing, timing, and study end points remain. Nonetheless, for the neonatal population, these results are encouraging as they have potential applicability in very low birth weight preterm infants who are prone to infections.

Mitochondrial Transfer

In preclinical models of lung,[106] heart,[107] and kidney injury,[108] transfer of mitochondria from MSCs to damaged cells restores their bioenergetics.[109] The mechanisms underlying this transfer are not entirely clear, but there is evidence that extracellular vesicles,[61] tunneling nanotubes,[110] and gap junctions containing connexin-43[106,111] are involved. Of interest, upregulation of Miro1, a mitochondrial Rho-GTPase involved in mitochondrial transport, increases the efficiency of MSC mitochondrial transfer,[112] and MSCs overexpressing Miro1 exhibit enhanced reparative effects.[113]

Modulating the Endogenous Stem Niche

Environmental perturbations alter stem cell function and fate, leading to dysfunctional repair and remodeling. For example, lung MSCs are decreased in newborn rodents exposed to hyperoxia,[114] and preterm infants who develop BPD have decreased and dysfunctional endothelial progenitor cells (EPCs).[115,116] By direct cell–cell interactions and paracrine-mediated mechanisms, MSCs reprogram endogenous stem cells and augment repair. In preclinical BPD models, MSCs increase lung epithelial stem cell proliferation[117] and stimulate alveolar differentiation in lung progenitor organoid cultures.[118] Similarly, MSCs implanted into the dentate gyrus of the hippocampus increase Sox2+ endogenous neural stem cell proliferation,[119] and in patients with dilated and ischemic cardiomyopathy, allogeneic MSCs increase the proliferation of functional EPCs and improve vascular reactivity.[120]

Hematopoietic Stem Cells

HSCs are a rare population of multipotent stem cells that have the unique ability to differentiate into all mature blood cells.[121] Most HSCs express CD34, a cell-surface glycoprotein, but exact markers to define HSCs are controversial. In the past, HSCs for transplantation were isolated mainly from the bone marrow, but peripheral and umbilical blood are now the most frequent sources. Umbilical cord–derived HSCs are easy to access, with lower risk of graft-versus-host disease, but immune reconstitution takes long. Historically, HSC transplantation was utilized primarily for malignancies complicated by bone marrow failure, but its use has expanded to nonmalignant conditions, such as genetic, autoimmune, and metabolic disorders.[122] There are, however, significant immunologic barriers, particularly with allogeneic transplantation.

PERINATAL STEM CELLS

Perinatal tissue–derived stem cells derived from umbilical cord blood, Wharton jelly, placenta, and amniotic fluid are also a source of stem cells for organ repair.[123–126] These cells are highly attractive, as they do not cause morbidity to the donor and are easily accessible and free from the ethical concerns of embryonic stem cells. They exhibit less senescence,[127] more anti-inflammatory effects,[128] less immunogenicity,[129] and higher proliferative potential[130,131] as compared to adult sources.[131]

Within the umbilical cord blood, along with HSCs, there is also the added advantage of several non-HSC populations being present, including endothelial colony-forming cells (ECFCs)[132] and MSCs.[55,133,134] The frequency of MSCs in umbilical cord blood is, however, very low, and isolation of these cells is not always successful.[135]

Wharton jelly–derived MSCs are emerging as a potent source for regenerative therapy as these cells are easily expanded and have greater differentiation potential and higher expression of anti-inflammatory and angiogenesis-related growth factors as compared to bone marrow–derived MSCs.[135–138]

Several populations of cells with varying plasticity have also been isolated from the placenta.[139] These include HSCs, human amniotic MSCs, and human chorionic MSCs. Compared to adult MSCs, they appear to be a more primitive population[140] with varying differentiation potential.[141] Of interest, a population of Cdx2 cells, which retain the "stemness" of embryonic stem cells, was recently isolated from the placenta. These cells differentiate into cardiomyocytes and vascular cells and significantly improve cardiac function in mice with myocardial infarction.[142] No tumor formation was evident in the transplanted mice.

Amniotic fluid stem cells are another heterogeneous fetal stem cell population. These cells, including hematopoietic progenitors and MSCs express both adult and embryonic stem cell markers.[143] One subset of amniotic fluid stem cells, which are enriched for the surface antigen c-kit (CD117), have the ability to differentiate into cell types of each embryonic germ layer,[144] but the rarity of these cells limits their clinical applicability. Similar to MSCs, amniotic fluid stem cells have paracrine-mediated reparative effects, and this has been demonstrated in multiple preclinical disease models.[145,146] For instance, in a preclinical model of BPD, a single dose of amniotic fluid stem cells protects the hyperoxia-exposed neonatal lung from injury.[147] Amniotic fluid–derived stem cells are also being investigated as a therapeutic option for congenital disorders, such as spina bifida and congenital diaphragmatic herniation.

ENDOTHELIAL PROGENITOR CELLS

EPCs were first described by Asahara et al. in 1997[148] as a population of peripheral blood mononuclear cells, which could differentiate into endothelial cells.[148] Since then, various markers have been used to identify this population, and though unclear, current data suggest that the original term "endothelial progenitor cells" (EPCs) includes a heterogeneous population of cells.[132,149] One subset appears early in culture, displays a profile more similar to monocytes than endothelial cells, and does not form vessels in vivo.[149,150] These cells, the so-called myeloid angiogenic cells, exert mainly paracrine effects on endothelial cells. Another subset, termed endothelial colony-forming cells (ECFCs),[132] give rise to colonies 7 to 21 days after plating, have robust proliferative potential, and form vessels when transplanted in vivo.[132,149] These potent proangiogenic cells, which can be isolated from umbilical cord blood, are reduced in preterm infants with BPD[151] and, when infused attenuate lung injury, augment angiogenesis and reduce pulmonary hypertension (PH) in preclinical models of BPD.[152]

Several clinical trials have investigated EPCs for peripheral vascular disease,[153] PH,[154] and coronary artery disease[155] with varying efficacy. In one study, EPCs administered to children with idiopathic PH were safe, with some improvement in exercise capacity.[156] Culture times are, however, long to obtain sufficient cells for infusion, and unlike MSCs, EPCs are immunogenic. One possibility to reduce immune rejection and enhance retention is co-transplantation of EPCs with MSCs. In one study, ECFCs primed via MSC contact had improved engraftment and angiogenic potential, and this was mediated through NOTCH signaling.[157]

INDUCED PLURIPOTENT STEM CELLS

iPSCs are derived by directly reprogramming mature somatic cells to an embryonic pluripotent state, unidentifiable from embryonic stem cells.[12,158] In 2006, Yamanaka and colleagues demonstrated that by overexpressing four transcription factors (Oct4, Sox2, Klf4, and c-myc), murine fibroblasts could be transformed into embryonic stem–like pluripotent stem cells, free of the ethical concerns of embryonic stem cells, but capable of differentiating into derivatives of all three germ layers. iPSCs have since been generated from multiple somatic cell sources, and using specific cell differentiation cocktails, iPSCs can be differentiated into any cell of interest (Fig. 45.4).

As iPSCs are abundant and patient specific, they are an attractive autologous source for cell replacement, with little risk of rejection.[159] However, because their pluripotency increases the risk of tumor formation, "iPSCs-derived" cell-based strategies are being evaluated. For instance, airway delivery of iPSC-derived type 2 alveolar epithelial cells or iPSC-derived lung progenitor cells improve lung function and structure in an experimental model of BPD.[160]

Since iPSCs have the genetic makeup and disease susceptibility of the patient from which they are derived, iPSCs are also being used to recapitulate developmental processes, explore novel mechanisms of disease, and test drug efficacy and toxicity. For instance, human iPSCs derived from patients with long QT syndrome were used to generate a cardiac tissue model to evaluate the potency of existing and novel pharmacologic agents that may either aggravate or ameliorate the disease.[161]

iPSCs-derived 3D structures, such as "organoids" and organ-on-chip, are also emerging as an effective platform for disease modeling. For example, iPSC-derived brain organoids generated from patients with autism exhibit an accelerated cell cycle and overproduction of GABAergic inhibitory neurons,[162] providing a potential mechanistic pathway for drug development.

The use of gene-editing technology in combination with iPSC technology is also a promising approach to cure monogenic disorders. For instance, gene correction of iPSCs derived from patients carrying a homozygous surfactant mutation restores surfactant processing in type 2 alveolar epithelial cells.[163]

Though the potential of iPSCs-based therapies is great, much work remains. Cell differentiation efficiency needs improvement as it may take months to get adequate quantities

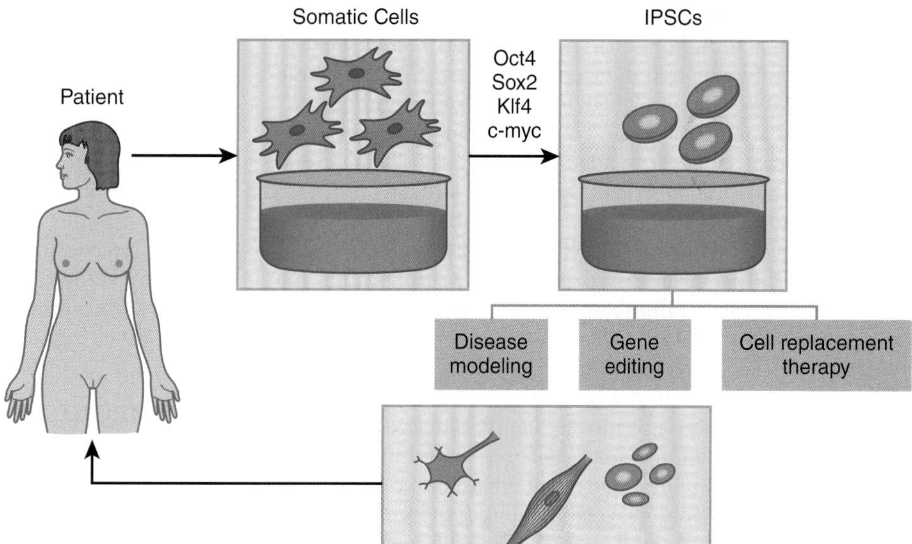

Figure 45.4 Induced pluripotent stem cells (iPSCs): Disease modeling, cell regeneration, and drug screening. Patient-derived somatic cells are reprogrammed into pluripotent stem cells by forced expression of transcription factors (Oct4, Sox2, Klf4, c-myc). These iPSCs can be differentiated into various cell types for regenerative therapy or combined with gene-editing approaches to correct genetic defects. They can also serve as novel platforms to study developmental processes, disease pathophysiology, and screen drugs. Illustration done by Dr. Andreas Damianos.

of differentiated cell populations for transplantation. Another important issue is that some pluripotent cells could potentially remain in the iPSCs-derived differentiated cell population and lead to malignancy in the recipient. There is also evidence that the process used to reprogram somatic cells to iPSCs alters DNA methylation. Whether this is also evident in iPSC cell derivatives needs to be clarified, and screening iPSCs-derived cells for any genetic variants will be crucial in moving this therapy forward.

STEM CELL APPLICATIONS IN PEDIATRIC AND NEONATAL DISEASES

RESPIRATORY DISEASES

Bronchopulmonary Dysplasia

BPD is a multifactorial disease, affecting 20% to 40% of extremely low birth weight preterm infants. Characterized by an arrest of alveolar and vascular development, there are few effective therapeutic strategies. Owing to its pleiotropic effects, MSCs have emerged as a promising option. In preclinical rodent models of BPD, a single intratracheal or intravenous dose of MSCs preserves lung alveolar and vascular structures, reduces PH, improves survival, and prevents cardiac dysfunction.[114,164–175] Lung protective effects were better if the cells were administered earlier than late in the disease course and MSCs limited the inflammatory process, reduced apoptosis, increased angiogenesis, and preserved bronchoalveolar stem cells.[117,165,170] Lung regenerative effects were observed for up to 6 months, and no tumor formation was evident.

Other cell populations such as ECFCs,[152] amniotic fluid stem cells,[176] and bone marrow–derived c-kit+ cells[177] have also been evaluated in preclinical models of BPD with varying beneficial effects. A recent systematic review and meta-analysis of 53 preclinical studies assessing 15 different cell-based therapies for BPD, however, concluded that MSCs were the most effective cell therapy, although there were few head-to-head comparisons and substantial risk of bias was identified.[178]

MSC therapy for BPD has now reached the bedside.[17] Two phase 1 trials using intratracheal allogeneic umbilical cord blood–derived MSCs demonstrate that MSC administered to preterm infants at risk of BPD is safe and feasible. The first dose-escalation study was performed in Korea using intratracheal cord blood–derived MSCs in nine preterm infants, with a mean gestational age and birth weight of 25 weeks and 793 g, respectively.[18] The treatment was well tolerated, without serious adverse effects. Follow-up at 2 years also showed no adverse effects.[179] The second study performed in the United States tested the same cells in 12 extremely low birth weight infants less than 28 weeks of gestation and less than 1,000 g at birth at 5 to 14 days of life.[180] The treatment was well tolerated, safe, and feasible. There is now an ongoing multicenter phase 2 trial with planned enrollment of 60 infants, 23 to 25 weeks' gestation with long-term follow-up (NCT03392467).

Asthma

Asthma is one of the most debilitating diseases of childhood characterized by airway inflammation, hyperresponsiveness, and airflow obstruction. In preclinical models, MSC administration before or after allergen challenge reduces bronchoalveolar lavage fluid inflammatory markers, eosinophilia, Th2 cytokines, and airway hyperresponsiveness.[181] In another study, bone marrow–derived MSCs, adipose tissue–derived MSCs, and lung-derived MSCs reduce lung inflammation and improve lung mechanics and histology in an experimental allergic asthma model, but the beneficial effects are more pronounced with bone marrow–derived MSCs than with either adipose tissue–derived MSCs or lung-derived MSCs.[182] There is currently one ongoing phase 1 trial testing bone marrow–derived MSCs in adult patients with mild asthma (NCT03137199). No pediatric trials are in progress.

Cystic Fibrosis

Cystic fibrosis (CF) is an autosomal recessive disease caused by a mutation in the cystic fibrosis transmembrane conductance regulator (*CFTR*) gene. There is currently no cure. Early studies showed that adult bone marrow cells could be recruited to the airway epithelium and induced to express CFTR, but these events were rare and not likely to be clinically significant.[183] The unique antimicrobial and anti-inflammatory properties of MSCs[184] have, however, yielded promising results in several experimental CF models, and there is an ongoing phase 1 open-label study testing the safety and tolerability of allogeneic MSCs in adult patients with CF (NCT02866721).

iPSCs are a promising strategy for CF as fully differentiated cells such as skin fibroblasts from CF patients can be reprogrammed into iPSCs.[185] Using gene-editing tools, the CF mutation can be corrected in patient-derived iPSCs[186,187] and utilized for development of a bioartificial lung or direct transplantation. While there is evidence that iPSC-derived lung epithelial cells engraft and persist in murine-injured lungs for up to 6 months,[188] obtaining a pure and adequate population of iPSC-derived airway epithelial cells to engraft in human airways is yet to be achieved. Nonetheless, iPSCs could provide an excellent platform for organotypic models of CF and precision drug screening.[189,190]

CARDIOVASCULAR DISEASES

The majority of clinical studies using cell therapies for cardiac diseases have been performed in adults. The exact mechanisms underlying cardiac repair remain unclear, but the limited engraftment and retention of stem cells in the myocardium suggest paracrine-mediated effects similar to other organs.[191,192] In preclinical models, proangiogenic and antifibrotic factors secreted by infused stem cells mediate the cardioprotective effects.[193]

Congenital Heart Diseases

Cell therapies for congenital heart diseases (CHDs) have only advanced in the past decade,[19,194] but there are now several clinical trials evaluating stem cell approaches for structural CHDs and cardiomyopathy.[195–198] In a phase 1 study, autologous transcoronary cardiac progenitor cells in pediatric patients with hypoplastic left heart syndrome were safe, and patients treated with cardiac progenitor cells had significantly greater right ventricular ejection fraction at 18- and 36-month follow-up.[199,200] In a phase 2 randomized controlled study of patients with single ventricle physiology, cardiosphere-derived cells, given early or late after staged palliative surgery, improve ventricular function, somatic growth, and quality of life.[201] There were, however, more patients in the control group who had hypoplastic left heart versus right heart syndrome, potentially biasing these results. Nonetheless, in a systemic review including six clinical studies, cell therapies in the form of either direct transplantation or cell-based tissue engineering in conjunction with surgical palliation provided some benefits over surgery alone in terms of cardiac function, somatic growth, and quality of life.[201]

Moving forward, in order for stem cell therapies to become standard adjunctive therapy for patients with CHD, several important issues need to be addressed. Some data suggest an inverse relationship between the age of the patient and response to cell therapy,[202] implying that treatment for patients with CHD should be implemented earlier than later, but exactly when is the ideal time remains unresolved. Another issue is the ideal cell donor. The cardiac progenitor cell population is nearly threefold higher in neonates as compared to children,[203] and their proliferative and regenerative capacity is greater as compared to adults,[204] suggesting that neonatal stem cells maybe the most effective strategy for heart repair, but obtaining these cells in sufficient quantities may be challenging. Whether autologous or allogeneic stem cells are ideal is also an important issue. Most studies have used autologous cells, but the cost and time for preparation of these cells maybe a limiting factor. The ideal route of injection also needs further evaluation. Intracoronary injections, while efficacious, do carry the risk of occlusion,[205] and intramyocardial injections, while feasible at the time of surgery, may be technically challenging in small neonates.

NEUROLOGIC DISEASES

Stem cell interventions for pediatric and neonatal neurologic conditions, such as HIE, intraventricular hemorrhage (IVH), cerebral palsy, and autism, are also being evaluated. Though endogenous brain repair is superior in neonates and children compared with adults, the developing brain is more susceptible to oxidative stress.[206] In preclinical models of pediatric brain injury, infused stem cells do not remain in the brain, but as previously stated, the stem cells secrete trophic and immunomodulatory growth factors which reduce inflammation, oxidative stress, and apoptosis and promote neurogenesis, angiogenesis, and synaptogenesis.[207–212]

Hypoxic–Ischemic Encephalopathy

Therapeutic hypothermia improves the outcomes of patients with HIE, but a significant number of infants either die or develop cerebral palsy. The degree of neuroprotection conferred by hypothermia is also dependent on the severity of the injury and the timing of hypothermia. In preclinical studies, intra-arterial administration of autologous umbilical cord blood–derived mononuclear cells to newborn lambs with HIE attenuates neuroinflammation and neuronal apoptosis. MSCs from multiple sources,[210,211] neural stem cells[213] and ECFCs,[214] with/without hypothermia also show positive effects on neurobehavioral outcome in HIE preclinical models.[215] Park et al. compared the efficacy of intraventricular umbilical cord–derived MSCs in combination with hypothermia to stand-alone therapy.[216] Whereas neonatal rodents who have severe HIE exhibit progressively increased brain infarction over time, along with more apoptosis, microgliosis, and impaired function in behavioral tests, all of these abnormalities show greater improvement after combined treatment with hypothermia and MSC transplantation than with either therapy alone.[216]

These findings are encouraging, but issues pertaining to ideal timing, cell source, route of delivery, and dosing and safety of cell therapies for HIE remain unresolved. Autologous cord stem cells have less risk of rejection, but not all patients with HIE have their cord cells collected. Intracerebral, intravenous, intra-arterial, intraventricular, and intranasal routes of cell administration have varying efficacy, but direct comparisons have been limited. Intravenous delivery is simple, but cells may become trapped in the lungs.[217] Intra-arterially delivered cells directly reach the brain, but there is a potential risk of cerebral embolism.[218] Intranasal MSC delivery is, however, promising as it is less invasive and cells rapidly distribute to the brain.[219] Early cell infusion appears to be the most efficacious strategy, but Donega et al. demonstrated that MSCs administered up to 10 days after induction of neonatal brain damage improve sensorimotor outcomes,[219] suggesting a therapeutic window potentially equivalent to several months in human patients. In terms of safety, most large animal studies have been short term, but positive neurologic effects and no tumor formation were evident 14 months after MSC administration in a rodent HIE model.[220]

Currently, only one clinical trial using cell-based therapies for HIE has been published. Cotton et al. administered volume and erythrocyte-reduced autologous umbilical cord blood mononuclear cells to 23 patients with HIE and demonstrated that transplantation of the cells was safe, well tolerated, and potentially efficacious.[20] At 1-year follow-up, 72% of patients who received the cell therapy had scores in all three Bayley III domains greater than 85 compared to 41% in the cooled-only group. With the promising preclinical and early clinical evidence, several long-term clinical trials using cell-based therapies for HIE are now ongoing or being planned.

Cerebral Palsy

Stem cell–based therapies in patients with cerebral palsy have also shown some positive effects up to 2 years after cell infusion, but more work is needed to understand the mechanisms of cell repair in patients with cerebral palsy.[221–225] In a recent meta-analysis including five trials testing stem cell therapies with or without rehabilitation in patients with cerebral palsy, stem cells with or without rehabilitation have a small but greater short-term effect on gross motor function than rehabilitation alone.[226] The rate of adverse effects was low (3% stem cells, 2% controls), suggesting an acceptable benefit-to-risk ratio,[226] but the studies had very small sample sizes. Future randomized controlled double-blinded studies with long-term follow-up and clear end points are necessary prior to this intervention becoming the standard of care for cerebral palsy.

Autism

With some evidence of an imbalance in the innate and immune system, and increased pro-inflammatory cytokine production in patients with autism, this formed the rationale for stem cell therapies for autism.[227–230] In rodent autism models, stem cells improve hippocampal neurogenesis and reduce stereotypic behaviors.[231–233] Several clinical trials also demonstrate the safe and feasibility of stem cell therapies for autism.[21,234,235] In a single-arm phase I/II clinical trial of repeated-dose umbilical cord MSCs administration in 20 children diagnosed with autism spectrum disorder (ASD), umbilical cord MSCs infusions were safe, and 40% of children showed improvements of symptoms as measured by standardized autism diagnosis tools.[236] Other studies, however, showed no therapeutic benefits, and larger studies will be required to elucidate the efficacy of stem cell therapies for autism.

Intraventricular Hemorrhage

In preclinical models, injecting blood into the lateral ventricle of postnatal day 4 rats induces severe intraventricular bleed and hydrocephalus. Intraventricular transplantation of umbilical cord blood–derived MSCs significantly attenuates the posthemorrhagic hydrocephalus and brain injury after experimental IVH. Moreover, early (2 days after induction of IVH) but not late MSC treatment (7 days after induction of IVH) attenuates brain injury, and this is potentially mediated by brain-derived neurotropic factor.[237] A single–center, open-label phase 1 dose-escalation study to assess the feasibility of a single intraventricular transplantation of allogeneic MSCs in nine premature infants with mean gestational age of 26 weeks who had grade 4 IVH was well tolerated, and no patients showed serious adverse effects or dose-limiting toxicities attributable to MSC transplantation.[238] There was no mortality in IVH patients receiving MSCs. A phase 2 trial is being planned, but ongoing questions as to the ideal route and timing of cell therapy for IVH and the mechanisms of neuroprotection are yet to be resolved.

GASTROINTESTINAL DISORDERS

Necrotizing Enterocolitis

In preclinical necrotizing enterocolitis (NEC) models, stem cell therapies preserve intestinal epithelial integrity, reduce bacterial translocation, attenuate inflammation, and enhance enterocyte proliferation.[239,240] Varying stem cells sources show efficacy in NEC experimental models, but thus far, none have clear regenerative superiority. Amniotic fluid MSCs administered to rat pups with established NEC improve survival, gut structure, and function, and this is potentially related to cyclooxygenase-2 activity.[145] Though promising, there are no current clinical trials evaluating stem cells for NEC as challenges in optimizing timing of therapy, and patient selection remains. In more advanced cases, intestinal organoids or neointestines formed by reconstituting decellularized intestines with stem cells may provide novel options for short gut syndrome.

OTHER USES

Graft-versus-Host Disease

Graft-versus-host disease is a condition that often occurs in patients who receive allogeneic HSC transplantation. The immunomodulatory effects of MSCs, in particular their ability to suppress proliferation of activated lymphocytes, provide a rationale for their use in graft-versus-host disease patients who are steroid resistant. In 2004, haploidentical MSCs were transplanted in a pediatric patient with severe treatment-resistant grade 4 graft-versus-host disease, and the treatment was successful.[241] This case report provided proof of concept that MSCs could be used for this condition. Since then, multiple studies showing variable efficacy have been reported. In a recent meta-analysis, prophylactic allogeneic MSCs reduce the risk of chronic graft-versus-host disease, but there is no effect on the risk of acute graft-versus-host disease.[64] The quality of evidence was, however, low, and further studies clarifying MSC efficacy in graft-versus-host disease are warranted.

Transamniotic Stem Cell Therapies

Transamniotic stem cell therapy is an emerging strategy to treat congenital malformations, such as spina bifida, congenital diaphragmatic hernia (CDH), and abdominal wall defects.[242] This therapy augments the effects of stem cells naturally present in amniotic fluid and enhances fetal wound healing. In an experimental model of gastroschisis, intra-amniotic injection of amniotic fluid–derived MSCs mitigates bowel damage.[243] Similarly, intra-amniotic injection of amniotic fluid–derived MSCs induces partial coverage of surgically created spina bifida in rabbit fetuses and promotes lung growth in experimental CDH models.[244,245] This therapy is in its infancy, and issues related to ideal gestational age/timing for therapy, dosing, mechanisms of repair, and safety need further investigation.

OPTIMIZING STEM CELL THERAPIES: OPPORTUNITIES AND CHALLENGES

CELL-FREE APPROACHES

The paracrine-mediated effects of stem cells, such as MSCs, provide an opportunity for cell-free approaches. Cell-free approaches are advantageous as compared to cell-based therapeutics as there is less risk of tumorigenesis and rejection. In addition, batch-to-batch variability may be less as compared to the stem cells themselves. In a preclinical severe BPD model, intravenously administered MSC-conditioned media exhibit superior alveolar protective effects as compared to the cells themselves.[164] On the other hand, Sutsko et al. demonstrated that whereas a single dose of MSCs or their conditioned media similarly improve lung structure in the short term, the MSCs themselves have more pronounced lung regenerative effects in the long term.[165] MSC and recipient cell interactions potentially explain these differential effects, but other investigators show at 6-month follow-up, similar lung protective effects of repetitive MSC-conditioned media injections and a single dose of MSC, suggesting that constant release of the MSC cocktail maybe sufficient to confer equivalent benefits.[172]

There is also emerging evidence that exosomes mediate most of the paracrine effects of MSCs. Exosomes are nanosized membrane vesicles of endocytic origin, released extracellularly following fusion of multivesicular bodies with the plasma membrane.[246,247] They carry a cargo of proteins, nucleic acids, and lipids, and following binding to recipient cells, they transfer this cargo and modify the target cells phenotype.[247] MSC-derived exosomes reduce lung inflammation[81] and alter macrophage polarization toward a more anti-inflammatory phenotype in hyperoxia models of BPD, and the therapeutic effects persist long after the hyperoxic injury.[248] In experimental NEC, MSC-derived exosomes reduce the incidence and severity of gut injury as effectively as the MSCs from which they are derived,[249] and intravenous administration of MSC-derived exosomes prevents functional impairment after global hypoxic–ischemia of the preterm brain.[250] Various clinical trials using MSC-derived exosomes for neonatal and pediatric conditions are underway, but one concern is that cell-free approaches lack the ability to respond to microenvironmental cues as the MSCs from which they are derived. Furthermore, issues with standardization of exosome isolation, purification, manufacturing techniques, potency assays, industrial scale up, circulation kinetics, and biodistribution also need optimization.

STEM CELL PRECONDITIONING

Preconditioning of stem cells with physical factors, chemical agents, growth factors, cytokines, hypoxia, and hyperoxia is a potential strategy to augment stem cell therapeutic effects.[251,252] For instance, MSCs express a sialyllactosamine form of the transmembrane protein CD44, and this can be fucosylated to force creation of a potent homing molecule that reprograms the migratory behavior of MSCs.[253] Moreover, culturing MSCs in serum-depleted media just before transplant drives them into a quiescent state, which allows them to withstand glucose deprivation and enhances engraftment rate in vivo.[254] Ischemic preconditioning also increases the tolerance of cells to injurious conditions, and exposure of MSCs to a short duration of hypoxia increases their survival, migration, and chromosome stability.[251,255–257] In preclinical disease models, implantation of hypoxia-conditioned MSCs shows greater proangiogenic, antiapoptotic, and immunomodulatory effects as compared to nonconditioned cells,[257–259] and in BPD models, ex vivo hyperoxia preconditioning increases the beneficial effects of systemically administered MSC-conditioned media.

Pretreatment of recipients is also another strategy. For instance, low-energy shock wave treatment increases cell homing, and targeted cardiac shock pretreatment with subsequent application of bone marrow mononuclear cells in patients with chronic heart failure modestly improves cardiac function as compared to placebo pretreatment.[260]

GENETICALLY ENGINEERED STEM CELLS

Modification of stem cells to replace an abnormal gene or to overexpress a gene is another area of promise. As stem cells are a self-renewing population, this lessens the need for repeated injections as are often required with gene therapy. In patients with diseases such as adenosine deaminase (ADA), severe combined immunodeficiency (SCID), and X-linked SCID, HSCs can be harvested from the patient and a virus used to insert the healthy gene.[261] In an open-label, nonrandomized phase II trial, 10 patients with ADA-deficient SCID received transplantation with autologous hematopoietic CD34+ cells modified with a human ADA complementary DNA (cDNA) γ-retroviral vector. Nine of 10 patients showed sustained benefits and sufficient immune reconstitution to remain free of infections.[262] Autologous hematopoietic stem gene therapy is now a recommended option for a select group of patients with ADA-deficient SCID.[263]

Metachromatic leukodystrophy is a lysosomal storage disease caused by a deficiency of arylsulfatase A. Ad hoc analysis of a nonrandomized, open-label, single-arm phase I/II trial of HSC gene therapy in patients with early-onset metachromatic leukodystrophy revealed that HSC gene therapy is safe, with eight of nine patients receiving the therapy having prevention of disease onset or halted disease progression after a median period of 36 months follow-up.[264]

For hemoglobinopathies such as β-thalassemia in which there is a genetic mutation reducing or abolishing the production of functioning β-globin chains, therapy with autologous CD34+ cells transduced with a β-globin lentiviral vectors also offers promise. In two companion phase I/II studies including 22 patients with severe β-thalassemia, genetically engineered autologous CD34+ cells reduce or eliminate the need for long-term red blood cell transfusions.[265]

In a patient with laminin 5-β3–deficient epidermolysis bullosa, genetically modified epidermal stem cell–derived grafts led to full functional correction of the disease.[266] A phase I/II study investigating the safety and efficacy of autologous cultured epidermal grafts containing epidermal stem cells genetically modified with the aid of a γ-retroviral vector carrying

COL7A1 cDNA in patients with epidermolysis bullosa is now ongoing (NCT02984085).

One of the challenges with genetic engineering of stem cells is the use of viral vectors. Some viruses such as adenoviruses have high immunogenicity that may cause early clearance of the modified stem cells. There is also potential risk of insertional mutagenesis, though the risk appears to be lower with lentiviral vectors and gene silencing may occur during differentiation. Alternative combined approaches using a combination of genome-editing technologies and iPSCs are being investigated, as aforementioned, with encouraging results. There is, however, a risk that editing the genome can result in off-target effects and potentially induce oncogenesis. Several phase 3 trials are now underway, and this should help determine risk-to-benefit ratios.[267]

TISSUE ENGINEERING

Tissue engineering is the creation of living, physiologic 3D tissues, or organs utilizing specific combinations of cells and scaffolds.[268–270] Stem cells are attractive for tissue engineering as they have the ability to expand, differentiate, and secrete growth factors and immunomodulatory cytokines, which create a conducive microenvironment for regeneration.[271] Typically, stem cells are combined with a biomaterial, such as a synthetic scaffold or decellularized tissue. The construct is cultured in a bioreactor and transplanted to the defect site.

Tissue engineering approaches are being used for various conditions, including intestinal repair, tracheal reconstruction, bladder reconstruction, cartilage repair, congenital heart defects, and valve replacement. In one study, decellularized pulmonary allografts seeded with autologous EPCs were used to replace heart valves in two pediatric patients with tetralogy of Fallot. At 3.5-year follow-up, there was no stenosis or regurgitation. Shin'oka et al. seeded autologous bone marrow cells onto a scaffold and created patches and conduits for the treatment of congenital heart defects.[272] The investigators found no evidence of thrombosis, aneurysmal formation, or calcification after a median follow-up of 16.7 months, and the diameter of the grafts increased an average of 10% compared to the implanted size.[272] These findings are encouraging, but further research optimizing biomaterial selection will be crucial in moving this approach forward.

CHALLENGES IN MOVING CELL THERAPIES TO THE BEDSIDE

Culture Conditions and Manufacturing

For clinical use, stem cells must be manufactured in facilities designed and organized according to Good Manufacturing Practice (GMP) for Pharmaceutical Manufacturers. The GMP facility must have strict quality control and assurance programs, ensuring manufacturing of sterile, potent, and uncontaminated products.

One concern is that the expansion of stem cells in media containing fetal bovine serum (FBS) increases the risk of zoonotic infections and immunologic reactions. Platelet concentrates are an alternative, but obtaining sufficient quantities of autologous platelets from children is challenging. Moreover, if donor platelets are used, variability in donor characteristics may modify stem cell function.[273] An emerging possibility is Xeno-free synthetic media as there is evidence of increased viable cell yield as compared to FBS-containing expansion media.[274]

Another important issue is the influence of high passage number, freezing, and thawing on stem cell behavior. There is substantial evidence that extended cell passages may induce senescence and genetic instability,[275] and thus, most clinical trials utilize early passage cells. The effect of cryopreservation on MSC behavior has yielded controversial results. In one animal study, freshly isolated stem cells have a higher therapeutic value than cryopreserved cells as the latter impairs immunosuppressive properties and disrupts the actin cytoskeleton, altering their biodistribution.[276] Other studies, however, report similar efficacy of fresh and cryopreserved cells.[277] Most preclinical and clinical studies to date utilize cryopreserved cells, but some investigators suggest that cryopreserved cells should be recovered in culture prior to administration. Whether this alters stem cell behavior and potency needs to be studied.

Allogeneic Versus Autologous Stem Cells

Another important issue is the choice of cell donor. Autologous stem cells are attractive as there is no risk of rejection. However, generating sufficient cells for therapy takes weeks, and alterations in endogenous stem cell function by comorbidities limit autologous therapy in acute conditions and prematurity-related diseases. On the other hand, allogeneic stem cells, particularly MSCs, are a readily available off-the-shelf source, economical, and feasible. Issues with donor variability, however, present challenges. MSCs from young donors promote more rapid and robust wound repair compared to old MSCs,[278] and female MSCs have more anti-inflammatory effects as compared to male cells.[279] In addition, while most studies using allogeneic MSCs do not evaluate if the cells induce an immune response, or consider donor–host compatibility, there is some evidence of immune rejection and generation of alloantibodies following allogeneic MSC transplantation.[280] In one preclinical study, implanted allogeneic MSCs transition from an immunoprivileged to an immunogenic state after differentiation.[281] Despite this, allogeneic MSCs have been shown to be efficacious in multiple diseases, suggesting that either the cells exert their actions prior to immune recognition or the degree of rejection is minimal or the immunogenicity of MSCs is regulated by the microenvironment.[282] In the POSEIDON-DCM trial, allogeneic MSCs obtained from young healthy donors as compared to autologous MSCs have superior functional and immunomodulatory effects in patients with chronic nonischemic dilated cardiomyopathy, and only one patient developed MHC class 1 alloantibodies.[283]

Stem Cell Route of Administration

Intravenous delivery is the most frequently used approach as it is minimally invasive. There is, however, substantial evidence that stem cells are often trapped in the pulmonary capillaries.[217] Despite this, intravenous delivery of stem cells has shown efficacy in multiple conditions. This may be secondary to the paracrine-mediated effects of the stem cells. But, in one recent study, monocytes engulf MSCs trapped in the lung, and these circulating monocytes mediate MSC anti-inflammatory effects.[284]

Local delivery with approaches such as intratracheal, intracerebral, and intrathecal, though more invasive, may have more beneficial effects with lower cell doses. Plausibly, locally delivered stem cells are able to sense the microenvironment and respond dynamically to mediate repair.

There are no clear answers, but the ideal route of administration for stem cell therapies should be disease and patient dependent, and careful consideration of the risk-to-benefit ratio is necessary. For instance, intramyocardial delivery may not be feasible in a neonate, and intracerebral or intrathecal routes may not be an option in a critically ill infant.

Stem Cell Timing of Administration

The optimal therapeutic window for cell therapies is unclear, but earlier appears to be better in multiple disease models. For instance, whereas MSCs administered immediately after bleomycin exposure reduce collagen deposition and mortality,[84,285,286] administration of MSCs 7 days after bleomycin exposure has no protective effects. Similarly, in models of HIE, early administration of MSCs is beneficial, but no therapeutic effects were evident if the cells were administered 17 days after injury.[287] Of interest, stem cell therapies are being tested in small clinical trials for cerebral palsy, with some positive effects, but no preclinical studies have explored the efficacy of these therapies in animals with the age equivalence of children. Moving forward, it will be important to answer these pertinent timing questions in established diseases.

Stem Cell Potency

Potency assays predicting the therapeutic efficacy of stem cells are mandatory for clinical trials but challenging to develop. Currently, both the U.S. Food and Drug Administration (FDA) and the European Medicines Agency (EMA) have provided guidance for potency testing of cellular products, but uncertainty regarding which assay would be most predictive persists.[288] Ideally, potency testing should evaluate the ability of cell therapy to achieve a specific biologic effect, but since stem cell function is driven by microenvironmental cues, potency assays need to be patient and disease specific. Immune cell inhibition and suppressor cell activation assays are most commonly used, but recent advances in organoid-based assays and organ-on-chip technology provide sophisticated tools to personalize cell therapy.[289] A CLinical Indications Prediction (CLIP) scale predicting how donor-to-donor heterogeneity and culture conditions impact the therapeutic efficacy of MSC populations for different disease indications has been recently developed. This scale, based on TWIST1 levels, is a promising model to build other potency assays, but clear functional end points will be required.[290]

Clinical Trial Design

Preclinical studies for multiple pediatric and neonatal conditions demonstrate variable efficacy of stem cell–based products. Lack of standardization of cell isolation, manufacturing, timing, dose, and route of administration, however, limits interpretation of the data. Some phase 1 and 2 studies demonstrate the safety and feasibility of stem cell–based therapies for diseases such as BPD, IVH, and HIE. But moving forward, larger clinical trials must be designed assessing the effect of co-therapies, the best dosing, route, and timing. There must also be clear end points to assess efficacy. Often, surrogate markers used to assess efficacy in phase 2 studies do not necessarily correlate with clinical outcomes in larger phase 3 studies. Identifying novel markers that link disease pathogenesis, stem cell mechanistic pathways and clinical outcomes will be crucial.[291]

Another key issue, which must be addressed, is long-term safety. A recent meta-analysis demonstrated that infusion of bone marrow–derived MSCs is safe,[292] but there is still concern of carcinogenesis, particularly with iPSC and ESC-derived populations. There is also evidence that MSCs may develop chromosomal aberrations after extended passage. For neonates and children, it will be important to have long-term safety follow-up into adulthood.

CONCLUSION

In conclusion, stem cell–based therapies have remarkable potential for pediatric and neonatal diseases. From organ regeneration to curing genetic and metabolic diseases, encouraging preclinical data provide the rationale for multiple clinical applications. Combining stem technologies with new gene-editing approaches and tissue engineering techniques has tremendous promise. Hurdles, however, remain, and optimizing the true potential of stem cell–based therapies will require that no shortcuts be taken.

Animal models have inherent limitations, and the behavior of stem cells in adults may not predict their effects in neonates and children. In addition, while stem cells have medicinal properties, they are biologics with complex and dynamic behaviors. The ideal stem cell source should be patient and disease specific, but it should be recognized that even the most rigorously sorted stem cell population might be heterogeneous. Deciphering the biologic and functional significance of the variable subpopulations will provide an opportunity to generate targeted therapies. Further mechanistic studies focused on improving understanding of stem cell interactions with the microenvironment will also be required. Judicious optimization and standardization of cell manufacturing techniques is critical, and careful design of clinical trials with well-defined end points is paramount.

ACKNOWLEDGMENT

The authors thank Dr. Andreas Damianos for the illustrations in this chapter.

REFERENCES

1. Natürliche Schöpfungsgeschichte von Dr. Ernst Häckel, Professor in Jena. Berlin bei Georg Reimer. 1868 S. 568. *Arch Pharm* 1869;189:282–283.
2. Konstantinov IE. In search of Alexander A. Maximow: the man behind the unitarian theory of hematopoiesis. *Perspect Biol Med* 2000;43:269–276.
3. Becker AJ, McCulloch EA, Till JE. Cytological demonstration of the clonal nature of spleen colonies derived from transplanted mouse marrow cells. *Nature* 1963;197:452–454.
4. Till JE, McCulloch EA. A direct measurement of the radiation sensitivity of normal mouse bone marrow cells. *Radiat Res* 1961;14:213–222.
5. Till JE, McCulloch EA, Siminovitch L. A stochastic model of stem cell proliferation, based on the growth of spleen colony-forming cells. *Proc Natl Acad Sci U S A* 1964;51:29–36.
6. Friedenstein AJ, Piatetzky S II, Petrakova KV. Osteogenesis in transplants of bone marrow cells. *J Embryol Exp Morphol* 1966;16:381–390.
7. Friedenstein AJ, Chailakhyan RK, Latsinik NV, et al. Stromal cells responsible for transferring the microenvironment of the hemopoietic tissues. Cloning in vitro and retransplantation in vivo. *Transplantation* 1974;17:331–340.
8. Friedenstein AJ, Deriglasova UF, Kulagina NN, et al. Precursors for fibroblasts in different populations of hematopoietic cells as detected by the in vitro colony assay method. *Exp Hematol* 1974;2:83–92.

9. Friedenstein AJ, Gorskaja JF, Kulagina NN. Fibroblast precursors in normal and irradiated mouse hematopoietic organs. *Exp Hematol* 1976;4:267–274.
10. Friedenstein AJ, Ivanov-Smolenski AA, Chajlakjan RK, et al. Origin of bone marrow stromal mechanocytes in radiochimeras and heterotopic transplants. *Exp Hematol* 1978;6:440–444.
11. Thomson JA, Itskovitz-Eldor J, Shapiro SS, et al. Embryonic stem cell lines derived from human blastocysts. *Science* 1998;282:1145–1147.
12. Takahashi K, Yamanaka S. Induction of pluripotent stem cells from mouse embryonic and adult fibroblast cultures by defined factors. *Cell* 2006;126:663–676.
13. Shi Y, Inoue H, Wu JC, et al. Induced pluripotent stem cell technology: a decade of progress. *Nat Rev Drug Discov* 2017;16:115–130.
14. Gele L, David BT, Trawczynski M, et al. Advances in pluripotent stem cells: history, mechanisms, technologies, and applications. *Stem Cell Rev Rep* 2020;16(1):3–32
15. Mao AS, Mooney DJ. Regenerative medicine: current therapies and future directions. *Proc Natl Acad Sci U S A* 2015;112:14452–14459.
16. Williams AR, Hare JM, Dimmeler S, et al. Mesenchymal stem cells. *Circ Res* 2011;109:923–940.
17. Lim R, Malhotra A, Tan J, et al. First-in-human administration of allogeneic amnion cells in premature infants with bronchopulmonary dysplasia: a safety study. *Stem Cells Transl Med* 2018;7:628–635.
18. Chang YS, Ahn SY, Yoo HS, et al. Mesenchymal stem cells for bronchopulmonary dysplasia: phase 1 dose-escalation clinical trial. *J Pediatr* 2014;164:966.e6–972.e6.
19. Bittle GJ, Morales D, Deatrick KB, et al. Stem cell therapy for hypoplastic left heart syndrome: mechanism, clinical application, and future directions. *Circ Res* 2018;123:288–300.
20. Cotten CM, Murtha AP, Goldberg RN, et al. Feasibility of autologous cord blood cells for infants with hypoxic-ischemic encephalopathy. *J Pediatr* 2014;164:973.e1–979.e1.
21. Chez M, Lepage C, Parise C, et al. Safety and observations from a placebo-controlled, crossover study to assess use of autologous umbilical cord blood stem cells to improve symptoms in children with autism. *Stem Cells Transl Med* 2018;7:333–341.
22. Prasad VK, Lucas KG, Kleiner GI, et al. Efficacy and safety of ex vivo cultured adult human mesenchymal stem cells (Prochymal™) in pediatric patients with severe refractory acute graft-versus-host disease in a compassionate use study. *Biol Blood Marrow Transplant* 2011;17:534–541.
23. Willis GR, Kourembanas S, Mitsialis SA. Toward exosome-based therapeutics: isolation, heterogeneity, and fit-for-purpose potency. *Front Cardiovasc Med* 2017;4:63.
24. Zipori D. The nature of stem cells: state rather than entity. *Nat Rev Genet* 2004;5:873–878.
25. Funato K, Major T, Lewis PW, et al. Use of human embryonic stem cells to model pediatric gliomas with H3.3K27M histone mutation. *Science* 2014;346:1529–1533.
26. Modlinski JA. The fate of inner cell mass and trophectoderm nuclei transplanted to fertilized mouse eggs. *Nature* 1981;292:342–343.
27. Ratajczak MZ, Zuba-Surma E, Kucia M, Poniewierska A, Suszynska M, Ratajczak J. Pluripotent and multipotent stem cells in adult tissues. *Adv Med Sci* 2012; 57:1-17.
28. Wu AM, Siminovitch L, Till JE, et al. Evidence for a relationship between mouse hemopoietic stem cells and cells forming colonies in culture. *Proc Natl Acad Sci U S A* 1968;59:1209–1215.
29. Wobus AM, Boheler KR. Embryonic stem cells: prospects for developmental biology and cell therapy. *Physiol Rev* 2005;85:635–678.
30. Mitsui K, Tokuzawa Y, Itoh H, et al. The homeoprotein nanog is required for maintenance of pluripotency in mouse epiblast and ES cells. *Cell* 2003;113:631–642.
31. Niwa H, Miyazaki J-i, Smith AG. Quantitative expression of Oct-3/4 defines differentiation, dedifferentiation or self-renewal of ES cells. *Nat Genet* 2000;24:372–376.
32. Niwa H. How is pluripotency determined and maintained? *Development* 2007;134:635–646.
33. Masui S, Nakatake Y, Toyooka Y, et al. Pluripotency governed by Sox2 via regulation of Oct3/4 expression in mouse embryonic stem cells. *Nat Cell Biol* 2007;9:625–635.
34. Kehat I, Kenyagin-Karsenti D, Snir M, et al. Human embryonic stem cells can differentiate into myocytes with structural and functional properties of cardiomyocytes. *J Clin Invest* 2001;108:407–414.
35. Reubinoff BE, Itsykson P, Turetsky T, et al. Neural progenitors from human embryonic stem cells. *Nat Biotechnol* 2001;19:1134–1140.
36. Assady S, Maor G, Amit M, et al. Insulin production by human embryonic stem cells. *Diabetes* 2001;50:1691–1697.
37. Levenberg S, Golub JS, Amit M, et al. Endothelial cells derived from human embryonic stem cells. *Proc Natl Acad Sci U S A* 2002;99:4391–4396.
38. Gepstein L. Derivation and potential applications of human embryonic stem cells. *Circ Res* 2002;91:866–876.
39. Rippon HJ, Polak JM, Qin M. Derivation of distal lung epithelial progenitors from murine embryonic stem cells using a novel 3-step differentiation protocol. *Stem Cells* 2006;24:1389.
40. Yamada S, Nelson TJ, Crespo-Diaz RJ, et al. Embryonic stem cell therapy of heart failure in genetic cardiomyopathy. *Stem Cells* 2008;26:2644–2653.
41. Wang D, Morales JE, Calame DG, et al. Transplantation of human embryonic stem cell-derived alveolar epithelial type II cells abrogates acute lung injury in mice. *Mol Ther* 2010;18:625–634.
42. Liu Y-W, Chen B, Yang X, et al. Human embryonic stem cell-derived cardiomyocytes restore function in infarcted hearts of non-human primates. *Nat Biotechnol* 2018;36:597–605.
43. Scott CT, Magnus D. Wrongful Termination: lessons from the Geron clinical trial. *Stem Cells Transl Med* 2014;3:1398–1401.
44. Schwartz SD, Regillo CD, Lam BL, et al. Human embryonic stem cell-derived retinal pigment epithelium in patients with age-related macular degeneration and Stargardt's macular dystrophy: follow-up of two open-label phase 1/2 studies. *The Lancet* 2015;385:509–516.
45. Wu DC, Boyd AS, Wood KJ. Embryonic stem cells and their differentiated derivatives have a fragile immune privilege but still represent novel targets of immune attack. *Stem Cells* 2008;26:1939–1950.
46. Friedenstein AJ, Petrakova KV, Kurolesova AI, et al. Heterotopic of bone marrow. Analysis of precursor cells for osteogenic and hematopoietic tissues. *Transplantation* 1968;6:230–247.
47. Dominici M, Le Blanc K, Mueller I, et al. Minimal criteria for defining multipotent mesenchymal stromal cells. The International Society for Cellular Therapy position statement. *Cytotherapy* 2006;8:315–317.
48. Nauta AJ, Fibbe WE. Immunomodulatory properties of mesenchymal stromal cells. *Blood* 2007;110:3499–3506.
49. Young HE, Mancini ML, Wright RP, et al. Mesenchymal stem cells reside within the connective tissues of many organs. *Dev Dyn* 1995;202:137–144.
50. Andrzejewska A, Lukomska B, Janowski M. Concise review: mesenchymal stem cells: from roots to boost. *Stem Cells* 2019;37:855–864.
51. Zuk PA, Zhu M, Mizuno H, et al. Multilineage cells from human adipose tissue: implications for cell-based therapies. *Tissue Eng* 2001;7:211–228.
52. Pierdomenico L, Bonsi L, Calvitti M, et al. Multipotent mesenchymal stem cells with immunosuppressive activity can be easily isolated from dental pulp. *Transplantation* 2005;80:836–842.
53. Zhang Y, Li C, Jiang X, et al. Human placenta-derived mesenchymal progenitor cells support culture expansion of long-term culture-initiating cells from cord blood CD34+ cells. *Exp Hematol* 2004;32:657–664.
54. Kwon A, Kim Y, Kim M, et al. Tissue-specific differentiation potency of mesenchymal stromal cells from perinatal tissues. *Sci Rep* 2016;6:23544.
55. Romanov YA, Svintsitskaya VA, Smirnov VN. Searching for alternative sources of postnatal human mesenchymal stem cells: candidate MSC-like cells from umbilical cord. *Stem Cells* 2003;21:105–110.
56. Yu JM, Wu X, Gimble JM, et al. Age-related changes in mesenchymal stem cells derived from rhesus macaque bone marrow. *Aging Cell* 2011;10:66–79.
57. Mohamed-Ahmed S, Fristad I, Lie SA, et al. Adipose-derived and bone marrow mesenchymal stem cells: a donor-matched comparison. *Stem Cell Res Ther* 2018;9:168.
58. Valencia J, Blanco B, Yáñez R, et al. Comparative analysis of the immunomodulatory capacities of human bone marrow- and adipose tissue-derived mesenchymal stromal cells from the same donor. *Cytotherapy* 2016;18:1297–1311.
59. Pachón-Peña G, Serena C, Ejarque M, et al. Obesity determines the immunophenotypic profile and functional characteristics of human mesenchymal stem cells from adipose tissue. *Stem Cells Transl Med* 2016;5:464–475.
60. Patel SA, Sherman L, Munoz J, et al. Immunological properties of mesenchymal stem cells and clinical implications. *Arch Immunol Ther Exp (Warsz)* 2008;56:1–8.
61. Morrison TJ, Jackson MV, Cunningham EK, et al. Mesenchymal stromal cells modulate macrophages in clinically relevant lung injury models by extracellular vesicle mitochondrial transfer. *Am J Respir Crit Care Med* 2017;196:1275–1286.
62. Hoogduijn MJ, Lombardo E. Mesenchymal stromal cells anno 2019: dawn of the therapeutic era? Concise review. *Stem Cells Transl Med* 2019;8:1126–1134.
63. Tayman C, Uckan D, Kilic E, et al. Mesenchymal stem cell therapy in necrotizing enterocolitis: a rat study. *Pediatr Res* 2011;70:489–494.
64. Fisher SA, Cutler A, Doree C, et al. Mesenchymal stromal cells as treatment or prophylaxis for acute or chronic graft-versus-host disease in haematopoietic stem cell transplant (HSCT) recipients with a haematological condition. *Cochrane Database Syst Rev* 2019;1(1):CD009768.
65. Raffaghello L, Bianchi G, Bertolotto M, et al. Human mesenchymal stem cells inhibit neutrophil apoptosis: a model for neutrophil preservation in the bone marrow niche. *Stem Cells* 2008;26:151–162.
66. Sotiropoulou PA, Perez SA, Gritzapis AD, et al. Interactions between human mesenchymal stem cells and natural killer cells. *Stem Cells* 2006;24:74–85.
67. Nauta AJ, Kruisselbrink AB, Lurvink E, et al. Mesenchymal stem cells inhibit generation and function of both CD34+-derived and monocyte-derived dendritic cells. *J Immunol* 2006;177:2080–2087.
68. Ko JH, Lee HJ, Jeong HJ, et al. Mesenchymal stem/stromal cells precondition lung monocytes/macrophages to produce tolerance against allo- and autoimmunity in the eye. *Proc Natl Acad Sci U S A* 2016;113:158–163.
69. Németh K, Leelahavanichkul A, Yuen PST, et al. Bone marrow stromal cells attenuate sepsis via prostaglandin E(2)-dependent reprogramming of host macrophages to increase their interleukin-10 production. *Nat Med* 2009;15:42–49.
70. Kim J, Hematti P. Mesenchymal stem cell-educated macrophages: a novel type of alternatively activated macrophages. *Exp Hematol* 2009;37:1445–1453.
71. Chiesa S, Morbelli S, Morando S, Massollo M, Marini C, Bertoni A, Frassoni F, Bartolomé ST, Sambuceti G, Traggiai E, Uccelli A. Mesenchymal stem cells impair in vivo T-cell priming by dendritic cells. *PNAS* 2011;108:17384-17389.
72. Zappia E, Casazza S, Pedemonte E, et al. Mesenchymal stem cells ameliorate experimental autoimmune encephalomyelitis inducing T-cell anergy. *Blood* 2005;106:1755–1761.
73. Krampera M, Glennie S, Dyson J, et al. Bone marrow mesenchymal stem cells inhibit the response of naive and memory antigen-specific T cells to their cognate peptide. *Blood* 2003;101:3722–3729.
74. Corcione A, Benvenuto F, Ferretti E, et al. Human mesenchymal stem cells modulate B-cell functions. *Blood* 2006;107:367–372.
75. Aggarwal S, Pittenger MF. Human mesenchymal stem cells modulate allogeneic immune cell responses. *Blood* 2005;105:1815–1822.
76. Meisel R, Zibert A, Laryea M, et al. Human bone marrow stromal cells inhibit allogeneic T-cell responses by indoleamine 2,3-dioxygenase–mediated tryptophan degradation. *Blood* 2004;103:4619–4621.
77. Beyth S, Borovsky Z, Mevorach D, et al. Human mesenchymal stem cells alter antigen-presenting cell maturation and induce T-cell unresponsiveness. *Blood* 2005;105:2214–2219.
78. Sato K, Ozaki K, Oh I, Meguro A, Hatanaka K, Nagai T, Muroi K, Ozawa K. Nitric oxide plays a critical role in suppression of T-cell proliferation by mesenchymal stem cells. *Blood* 2007;109:228-234.
79. Chaubey S, Thueson S, Ponnalagu D, et al. Early gestational mesenchymal stem cell secretome attenuates experimental bronchopulmonary dysplasia in part via exosome-associated factor TSG-6. *Stem Cell Res Ther* 2018;9:173.

80. Usunier B, Benderitter M, Tamarat R, et al. Management of fibrosis: the mesenchymal stromal cells breakthrough. *Stem Cells Int* 2014;2014:340257.
81. Nasir GA, Mohsin S, Khan M, et al. Mesenchymal stem cells and interleukin-6 attenuate liver fibrosis in mice. *J Transl Med* 2013;11:78.
82. Li T, Yan Y, Wang B, et al. Exosomes derived from human umbilical cord mesenchymal stem cells alleviate liver fibrosis. *Stem Cells Dev* 2013;22:845–854.
83. Semedo P, Correa-Costa M, Antonio Cenedeze M, et al. Mesenchymal stem cells attenuate renal fibrosis through immune modulation and remodeling properties in a rat remnant kidney model. *Stem Cells* 2009;27:3063–3073.
84. Ortiz LA, Gambelli F, McBride C, et al. Mesenchymal stem cell engraftment in lung is enhanced in response to bleomycin exposure and ameliorates its fibrotic effects. *Proc Natl Acad Sci U S A* 2003;100:8407–8411.
85. Horton JA, Hudak KE, Chung EJ, et al. Mesenchymal stem cells inhibit cutaneous radiation-induced fibrosis by suppressing chronic inflammation. *Stem Cells* 2013;31:2231–2341.
86. Zhang C, Zhu Y, Zhang Y, et al. Therapeutic potential of umbilical cord mesenchymal stem cells for inhibiting myofibroblastic differentiation of irradiated human lung fibroblasts. *Tohoku J Exp Med* 2015;236:209–217.
87. Dong L-H, Jiang Y-Y, Liu Y-J, et al. The anti-fibrotic effects of mesenchymal stem cells on irradiated lungs via stimulating endogenous secretion of HGF and PGE2. *Sci Rep* 2015;5:8713.
88. Mias C, Lairez O, Trouche E, et al. Mesenchymal stem cells promote matrix metalloproteinase secretion by cardiac fibroblasts and reduce cardiac ventricular fibrosis after myocardial infarction. *Stem Cells* 2009;27:2734–2743.
89. Xie T, Liang J, Liu N, et al. Transcription factor TBX4 regulates myofibroblast accumulation and lung fibrosis. *J Clin Invest* 2016;126:3063–3079.
90. Kramann R, Schneider RK, DiRocco DP, et al. Perivascular Gli1+ progenitors are key contributors to injury-induced organ fibrosis. *Cell Stem Cell* 2015;16:51–66.
91. Popova AP, Bozyk PD, Goldsmith AM, et al. Autocrine production of TGF-B1 promotes myofibroblastic differentiation of neonatal lung mesenchymal stem cells. *Am J Physiol Lung Cell Mol Physiol* 2010;298:L735–L743.
92. Kinnaird T, Stabile E, Burnett MS, et al. Marrow-derived stromal cells express genes encoding a broad spectrum of arteriogenic cytokines and promote in vitro and in vivo arteriogenesis through paracrine mechanisms. *Circ Res* 2004;94:678–685.
93. Chang YS, Ahn SY, Jeon HB, et al. Critical role of vascular endothelial growth factor secreted by mesenchymal stem cells in hyperoxic lung injury. *Am J Respir Crit Care Med* 2014;51:391–399.
94. Reiter J, Drummond S, Sammour I, et al. Stromal derived factor-1 mediates the lung regenerative effects of mesenchymal stem cells in a rodent model of bronchopulmonary dysplasia. *Respir Res* 2017;18:137.
95. Fang X, Neyrinck AP, Matthay MA, et al. Allogeneic human mesenchymal stem cells restore epithelial protein permeability in cultured human alveolar type II cells by secretion of angiopoietin-1. *J Biol Chem* 2010;285:26211–26222.
96. Zhao YD, Ohkawara H, Vogel SM, et al. Bone marrow-derived progenitor cells prevent thrombin-induced increase in lung vascular permeability. *Am J Physiol Lung Cell Mol Physiol* 2010;298:L36–L44.
97. Lee JW, Fang X, Gupta N, et al. Allogeneic human mesenchymal stem cells for treatment of E. coli endotoxin-induced acute lung injury in the ex vivo perfused human lung. *Proc Natl Acad Sci U S A* 2009;106:16357–16362.
98. Mei SHJ, McCarter SD, Deng Y, et al. Prevention of LPS-induced acute lung injury in mice by mesenchymal stem cells overexpressing angiopoietin 1. *PLoS Med* 2007;4:e269.
99. Katsha AM, Ohkouchi S, Xin H, et al. Paracrine factors of multipotent stromal cells ameliorate lung injury in an elastase-induced emphysema model. *Mol Ther* 2007;19: 196–203.
100. Lee JW, Fang X, Krasnodembskaya A, et al. Mesenchymal stem cells for acute lung injury: role of paracrine soluble factors. *Stem Cells* 2011;29(6):913–919.
101. Krasnodembskaya A, Song Y, Fang X, et al. Antibacterial effect of human mesenchymal stem cells is mediated in part from secretion of the antimicrobial peptide LL-37. *Stem Cells (Dayton, Ohio)* 2010;28:2229–2238.
102. Sung DK, Chang YS, Sung SI, et al. Antibacterial effect of mesenchymal stem cells against *Escherichia coli* is mediated by secretion of beta-defensin-2 via toll-like receptor 4 signalling. *Cell Microbiol* 2016;18:424–436.
103. Gupta N, Krasnodembskaya A, Kapetanaki M, et al. Mesenchymal stem cells enhance survival and bacterial clearance in murine *Escherichia coli* pneumonia. *Thorax* 2012;67:533–539.
104. Alcayaga-Miranda F, Cuenca J, Khoury M. Antimicrobial activity of mesenchymal stem cells: current status and new perspectives of antimicrobial peptide-based therapies. *Front Immunol* 2017;8:339.
105. McIntyre LA, Stewart DJ, Mei SHJ, et al. Cellular immunotherapy for septic shock. A phase I clinical trial. *Am J Respir Crit Care Med* 2018;197:337–347.
106. Islam MN, Das SR, Emin MT, et al. Mitochondrial transfer from bone-marrow-derived stromal cells to pulmonary alveoli protects against acute lung injury. *Nat Med* 2012;18:759–765.
107. Acquistapace A, Bru T, Lesault P-F, et al. Human mesenchymal stem cells reprogram adult cardiomyocytes toward a progenitor-like state through partial cell fusion and mitochondria transfer. *Stem Cells (Dayton, Ohio)* 2011;29:812–824.
108. Konari N, Nagaishi K, Kikuchi S, et al. Mitochondria transfer from mesenchymal stem cells structurally and functionally repairs renal proximal tubular epithelial cells in diabetic nephropathy in vivo. *Sci Rep* 2019;9:5184.
109. Spees JL, Olson SD, Whitney MJ, et al. Mitochondrial transfer between cells can rescue aerobic respiration. *Proc Natl Acad Sci U S A* 2006;103:1283–1288.
110. Jackson MV, Morrison TJ, Doherty DF, et al. Mitochondrial transfer via tunneling nanotubes is an important mechanism by which mesenchymal stem cells enhance macrophage phagocytosis in the in vitro and in vivo models of ARDS. *Stem Cells (Dayton, Ohio)* 2016;34:2210–2223.
111. Yao Y, Fan X-L, Jiang D, et al. Connexin 43-mediated mitochondrial transfer of iPSC-MSCS alleviates asthma inflammation. *Stem Cell Rep* 2018;11:1120–1135.
112. Babenko VA, Silachev DN, Popkov VA, et al. Miro1 enhances mitochondria transfer from multipotent mesenchymal stem cells (MMSC) to neural cells and improves the efficacy of cell recovery. *Molecules* 2018;23:687.
113. Ahmad T, Mukherjee S, Pattnaik B, et al. Miro1 regulates intercellular mitochondrial transport & enhances mesenchymal stem cell rescue efficacy. *EMBO J* 2014;33:994–1010.
114. van Haaften T, Byrne R, Bonnet S, et al. Airway delivery of mesenchymal stem cells prevents arrested alveolar growth in neonatal lung injury in rats. *Am J Respir Crit Care Med* 2009;180:1131–1142.
115. Baker CD, Balasubramaniam V, Mourani PM, et al. Cord blood angiogenic progenitor cells are decreased in bronchopulmonary dysplasia. *Eur Resp J* 2012;40:1516.
116. Borghesi A, Massa M, Campanelli R, et al. Circulating endothelial progenitor cells in preterm infants with bronchopulmonary dysplasia. *Am J Respir Crit Care Med* 2009;180:540–546.
117. Tropea KA, Leder E, Aslam M, et al. Bronchioalveolar stem cells increase after mesenchymal stromal cell treatment in a mouse model of bronchopulmonary dysplasia. *Am J Physiol Lung Cell Mol Physiol* 2012;302:L829–L837.
118. Leeman KT, Pessina P, Lee J-H, et al. Mesenchymal stem cells increase alveolar differentiation in lung progenitor organoid cultures. *Sci Rep* 2019;9:6479.
119. Munoz JR, Stoutenger BR, Robinson AP, et al. Human stem/progenitor cells from bone marrow promote neurogenesis of endogenous neural stem cells in the hippocampus of mice. *Proc Natl Acad Sci U S A* 2005;102:18171–18176.
120. Premer C, Blum A, Bellio MA, et al. Allogeneic mesenchymal stem cells restore endothelial function in heart failure by stimulating endothelial progenitor cells. *EBioMedicine* 2015;2:467–475.
121. Wilson A, Trumpp A. Bone-marrow haematopoietic-stem-cell niches. *Nat Rev Immunol* 2006;6:93–106.
122. Duarte RF, Labopin M, Bader P, et al. Indications for haematopoietic stem cell transplantation for haematological diseases, solid tumours and immune disorders: current practice in Europe, 2019. *Bone Marrow Transplant* 2019;54:1525–1552.
123. Broxmeyer HE, Douglas GW, Hangoc G, et al. Human umbilical cord blood as a potential source of transplantable hematopoietic stem/progenitor cells. *Proc Natl Acad Sci U S A* 1989;86:3828.
124. Arien-Zakay H, Lazarovici P, Nagler A. Tissue regeneration potential in human umbilical cord blood. *Best Pract Res Clin Haematol* 2010;23:291–303.
125. Murohara T, Ikeda H, Duan J, et al. Transplanted cord blood-derived endothelial precursor cells augment postnatal neovascularization. *J Clin Invest* 2000;105:1527–1536.
126. Nagano M, Yamashita T, Hamada H, Ohneda K, Kimura K, Nakagawa T, Shibuya M, Yoshikawa H, Ohneda O. Identification of functional endothelial progenitor cells suitable for the treatment of ischemic tissue using human umbilical cord blood. *Blood* 2007;110:151-160..
127. Guillot PV, Gotherstrom C, Chan J, et al. Human first-trimester fetal MSC express pluripotency markers and grow faster and have longer telomeres than adult MSC. *Stem Cells* 2007;25:646–654.
128. Bárcia RN, Santos JM, Filipe M, et al. What makes umbilical cord tissue-derived mesenchymal stromal cells superior immunomodulators when compared to bone marrow derived mesenchymal stromal cells? *Stem Cells Int* 2015;2015:583984.
129. Götherström C, Ringdén O, Tammik C, et al. Immunologic properties of human fetal mesenchymal stem cells. *Am J Obstet Gynecol* 2004;190:239–245.
130. Wyrsch A, dalle Carbonare V, Jansen W, et al. Umbilical cord blood from preterm human fetuses is rich in committed and primitive hematopoietic progenitors with high proliferative and self-renewal capacity. *Exp Hematol* 1999;27:1338–1345.
131. Sagar R, Walther-Jallow L, David AL, et al. Fetal mesenchymal stromal cells: an opportunity for prenatal cellular therapy. *Curr Stem Cell Rep* 2018;4:61–68.
132. Ingram DA, Mead LE, Tanaka H, et al. Identification of a novel hierarchy of endothelial progenitor cells using human peripheral and umbilical cord blood. *Blood* 2004;104:2752–2760.
133. Lee OK, Kuo TK, Chen W-M, et al. Isolation of multipotent mesenchymal stem cells from umbilical cord blood. *Blood* 2004;103:1669–1675.
134. Erices A, Conget P, Minguell JJ. Mesenchymal progenitor cells in human umbilical cord blood. *Br J Haematol* 2000;109:235–242.
135. Kern S, Eichler H, Stoeve J, et al. Comparative analysis of mesenchymal stem cells from bone marrow, umbilical cord blood, or adipose tissue. *Stem Cells* 2006;24:1294–1301.
136. Chen M-Y, Lie P-C, Li Z-L, et al. Endothelial differentiation of Wharton's jelly–derived mesenchymal stem cells in comparison with bone marrow–derived mesenchymal stem cells. *Exp Hematol* 2009;37:629–640.
137. Hsieh J-Y, Wang H-W, Chang S-J, et al. Mesenchymal stem cells from human umbilical cord express preferentially secreted factors related to neuroprotection, neurogenesis, and angiogenesis. *PLoS One* 2013;8:e72604.
138. Li X, Bai J, Ji X, et al. Comprehensive characterization of four different populations of human mesenchymal stem cells as regards their immune properties, proliferation and differentiation. *Int J Mol Med* 2014;34:695–704.
139. In't Anker PS, Scherjon SA, Kleijburg-van der Keur C, et al. Isolation of mesenchymal stem cells of fetal or maternal origin from human placenta. *Stem Cells* 2004;22:1338–1345.
140. Jones GN, Moschidou D, Puga-Iglesias T-I, et al. Ontological differences in first compared to third trimester human fetal placental chorionic stem cells. *PLoS One* 2012;7:e43395.
141. Barlow S, Brooke G, Chatterjee K, et al. Comparison of human placenta-and bone marrow–derived multipotent mesenchymal stem cells. *Stem Cells Dev* 2008;17:1095–1108.
142. Vadakke-Madathil S, LaRocca G, Raedschelders K, et al. Multipotent fetal-derived Cdx2 cells from placenta regenerate the heart. *Proc Natl Acad Sci U S A* 2019;116:11786–11795.
143. Spitzhorn L-S, Rahman MS, Schwindt L, et al. Isolation and molecular characterization of amniotic fluid-derived mesenchymal stem cells obtained from caesarean sections. *Stem Cells Int* 2017;2017:5932706.
144. De Coppi P, Bartsch G, Siddiqui MM, et al. Isolation of amniotic stem cell lines with potential for therapy. *Nat Biotechnol* 2007;25:100–106.

145. Zani A, Cananzi M, Fascetti-Leon F, et al. Amniotic fluid stem cells improve survival and enhance repair of damaged intestine in necrotising enterocolitis via a COX-2 dependent mechanism. *Gut* 2014;63:300–309.
146. Loukogeorgakis SP, De Coppi P. Concise review: amniotic fluid stem cells: the known, the unknown, and potential regenerative medicine applications. *Stem Cells* 2017;35:1663–1673.
147. Grisafi D, Pozzobon M, Dedja A, et al. Human amniotic fluid stem cells protect rat lungs exposed to moderate hyperoxia. *Pediatr Pulmonol* 2013;48:1070–1080.
148. Asahara T, Murohara T, Sullivan A, et al. Isolation of putative progenitor endothelial cells for angiogenesis. *Science* 1997;275:964–966.
149. Medina RJ, Barber CL, Sabatier F, et al. Endothelial progenitors: a consensus statement on nomenclature. *Stem Cells Transl Med* 2017;6:1316–1320.
150. Yoder MC, Mead LE, Prater D, et al. Redefining endothelial progenitor cells via clonal analysis and hematopoietic stem/progenitor cell principals. *Blood* 2007;109:1801.
151. Bertagnolli M, Nuyt AM, Thébaud B, et al. Endothelial progenitor cells as prognostic markers of preterm birth-associated complications. *Stem Cells Transl Med* 2017;6:7–13.
152. Alphonse RS, Vadivel A, Fung M, et al. Existence, functional impairment, and lung repair potential of endothelial colony-forming cells in oxygen-induced arrested alveolar growth. *Circulation* 2014;129:2144–2157.
153. Lara-Hernandez R, Lozano-Vilardell P, Blanes P, et al. Safety and efficacy of therapeutic angiogenesis as a novel treatment in patients with critical limb ischemia. *Ann Vasc Surg* 2010;24:287–294.
154. Wang X-X, Zhang F-R, Shang Y-P, et al. Transplantation of autologous endothelial progenitor cells may be beneficial in patients with idiopathic pulmonary arterial hypertension: a pilot randomized controlled trial. *J Am Coll Cardiol* 2007;49:1566–1571.
155. Jimenez-Quevedo P, Gonzalez-Ferrer JJ, Sabate M, et al. Selected CD133+ progenitor cells to promote angiogenesis in patients with refractory angina. *Circ Res* 2014;115:950–960.
156. Zhu JH, Wang XX, Zhang FR, et al. Safety and efficacy of autologous endothelial progenitor cells transplantation in children with idiopathic pulmonary arterial hypertension: open-label pilot study. *Pediatr Transplant* 2008;12:650–655.
157. Shafiee A, Patel J, Wong HY, et al. Priming of endothelial colony-forming cells in a mesenchymal niche improves engraftment and vasculogenic potential by initiating mesenchymal transition orchestrated by NOTCH signaling. *FASEB J* 2017;31:610–624.
158. Lengner CJ. iPS cell technology in regenerative medicine. *Ann N Y Acad Sci* 2010;1192:38–44.
159. Singh VK, Kalsan M, Kumar N, et al. Induced pluripotent stem cells: applications in regenerative medicine, disease modeling, and drug discovery. *Front Cell Dev Biol* 2015;3:2.
160. Shafa M, Ionescu LI, Vadivel A, et al. Human induced pluripotent stem cell-derived lung progenitor and alveolar epithelial cells attenuate hyperoxia-induced lung injury. *Cytotherapy* 2018;20:108–125.
161. Itzhaki I, Maizels L, Huber I, et al. Modelling the long QT syndrome with induced pluripotent stem cells. *Nature* 2011;471:225–229.
162. Mariani J, Coppola G, Zhang P, et al. FOXG1-dependent dysregulation of GABA/Glutamate neuron differentiation in autism spectrum disorders. *Cell* 2015;162:375–390.
163. Jacob A, Morley M, Hawkins F, et al. Differentiation of human pluripotent stem cells into functional lung alveolar epithelial cells. *Cell Stem Cell* 2017;21:472.e10–488.e10.
164. Aslam M, Baveja R, Liang OD, et al. Bone marrow stromal cells attenuate lung injury in a murine model of neonatal chronic lung disease. *Am J Respir Crit Care Med* 2009;180:1122–1130.
165. Sutsko RP, Young KC, Ribeiro A, et al. Long-term reparative effects of mesenchymal stem cell therapy following neonatal hyperoxia-induced lung injury. *Pediatr Res* 2013;73:46–53.
166. Elmasri H, Ghelfi E, Yu CW, et al. Endothelial cell-fatty acid binding protein 4 promotes angiogenesis: role of stem cell factor/c-kit pathway. *Angiogenesis* 2012;15:457–468.
167. Mesenchymal stem cell-mediated reversal of bronchopulmonary dysplasia and associated pulmonary hypertension. *Pulm Circ* 2012;2:170-181.
168. Simones AA, Beisang DJ, Panoskaltsis-Mortari A, Roberts KD. Mesenchymal stem cells in the pathogenesis and treatment of bronchopulmonary dysplasia: a clinical review. *Pediatric Research* 2018;83:308-317.
169. Moreira A, Winter C, Joy J, Winter L, Jones M, Noronha M, Porter M, Quim K, Corral A, Alayli Y, Seno T, Mustafa S, Hornsby P, Ahuja S. Intranasal delivery of human umbilical cord Wharton's jelly mesenchymal stromal cells restores lung alveolarization and vascularization in experimental bronchopulmonary dysplasia. 2020;9:221-234.
170. Chen C-M, Chou H-C. Human mesenchymal stem cells attenuate hyperoxia-induced lung injury through inhibition of the renin-angiotensin system in newborn rats. *American journal of translational research* 2018;10:2628-2635.
171. Kim YE, Park WS, Ahn SY, Sung DK, Chang YS. Intratracheal transplantation of mesenchymal stem cells attenuates hyperoxia-induced lung injury by down-regulating, but not direct inhibiting formyl peptide receptor 1 in the newborn mice. *PLoS One* 2018;13:e0206311.
172. Pierro M, Ionescu L, Montemurro T, et al. Short-term, long-term and paracrine effect of human umbilical cord-derived stem cells in lung injury prevention and repair in experimental bronchopulmonary dysplasia. *Thorax* 2013;68:475–484.
173. Sung DK, Chang YS, Ahn SY, et al. Optimal route for human umbilical cord blood-derived mesenchymal stem cell transplantation to protect against neonatal hyperoxic lung injury: gene expression profiles and histopathology. *PLoS One* 2015;10:e0135574.
174. Chang YS, Choi SJ, Ahn SY, et al. Timing of umbilical cord blood derived mesenchymal stem cells transplantation determines therapeutic efficacy in the neonatal hyperoxic lung injury. *PLoS One* 2013;8:e52419.
175. Chang YS, Oh W, Choi SJ, et al. Human umbilical cord blood-derived mesenchymal stem cells attenuate hyperoxia-induced lung injury in neonatal rats. *Cell Transplant* 2009;18:869–886.
176. Zhu D, Tan J, Maleken AS, et al. Human amnion cells reverse acute and chronic pulmonary damage in experimental neonatal lung injury. *Stem Cell Res Ther* 2017;8:257.
177. Ramachandran S, Suguihara C, Drummond S, et al. Bone marrow-derived c-kit+ cells attenuate neonatal hyperoxia-induced lung injury. *Cell Transplant* 2015;24:85–95.
178. Augustine S, Cheng W, Avey MT, et al. Are all stem cells equal? Systematic review, evidence map, and meta-analyses of preclinical stem cell-based therapies for bronchopulmonary dysplasia: concise review. *Stem Cells Transl Med* 2020;9(2):158–168.
179. Ahn SY, Chang YS, Kim JH, et al. Two-year follow-up outcomes of premature infants enrolled in the phase I trial of mesenchymal stem cells transplantation for bronchopulmonary dysplasia. *J Pediatr* 2017;185:49.e2–54.e2.
180. Powell SB, Silvestri JM. Safety of intratracheal administration of human umbilical cord blood derived mesenchymal stromal cells in extremely low birth weight preterm infants. *J Pediatr* 2019;210:209.e2–213.e2.
181. Takeda K, Webb TL, Ning F, et al. Mesenchymal stem cells recruit CCR2+ monocytes to suppress allergic airway inflammation. *J Immunol* 2018;200:1261–1269.
182. Abreu SC, Antunes MA, Xisto DG, et al. Bone marrow, adipose, and lung tissue-derived murine mesenchymal stromal cells release different mediators and differentially affect airway and lung parenchyma in experimental asthma. *Stem Cells Transl Med* 2017;6:1557–1567.
183. Loi R, Beckett T, Goncz KK, et al. Limited restoration of cystic fibrosis lung epithelium in vivo with adult bone marrow–derived cells. *Am J Respir Crit Care Med* 2006;173: 171–179.
184. Sutton MT, Fletcher D, Episalla N, et al. Mesenchymal stem cell soluble mediators and cystic fibrosis. *J Stem Cell Res Ther* 2017;7:400.
185. Wong AP, Bear CE, Chin S, et al. Directed differentiation of human pluripotent stem cells into mature airway epithelia expressing functional CFTR protein. *Nat Biotechnol* 2012;30:876–882.
186. Pollard BS, Pollard HB. Induced pluripotent stem cells for treating cystic fibrosis: state of the science. *Pediatr Pulmonol* 2018;53:S12–S29.
187. Crane AM, Kramer P, Bui JH, et al. Targeted correction and restored function of the CFTR gene in cystic fibrosis induced pluripotent stem cells. *Stem Cell Rep* 2015;4:569–577.
188. Miller AJ, Hill DR, Nagy MS, et al. In vitro induction and in vivo engraftment of lung bud tip progenitor cells derived from human pluripotent stem cells. *Stem Cell Rep* 2018;10:101–119.
189. Simsek S, Zhou T, Robinson CL, et al. Modeling cystic fibrosis using pluripotent stem cell-derived human pancreatic ductal epithelial cells. *Stem Cells Transl Med* 2016;5:572–579.
190. Merkert S, Schubert M, Olmer R, et al. High-throughput screening for modulators of CFTR activity based on genetically engineered cystic fibrosis disease-specific iPSCs. *Stem Cell Rep* 2019;12:1389–1403.
191. Lezaic L, Socan A, Peitl PK, et al. Imaging and 1-day kinetics of intracoronary stem cell transplantation in patients with idiopathic dilated cardiomyopathy. *Nucl Med Biol* 2016;43:410–414.
192. Hou D, Youssef Eyas A-S, Brinton TJ, et al. Radiolabeled cell distribution after intramyocardial, intracoronary, and interstitial retrograde coronary venous delivery. *Circulation* 2005;112:150–156.
193. Mirotsou M, Jayawardena TM, Schmeckpeper J, et al. Paracrine mechanisms of stem cell reparative and regenerative actions in the heart. *J Mol Cell Cardiol* 2011;50:280–289.
194. Tsilimigras DI, Oikonomou EK, Moris D, et al. Stem cell therapy for congenital heart disease. *Circulation* 2017;136:2373–2385.
195. Rupp S, Jux C, Bönig H, et al. Intracoronary bone marrow cell application for terminal heart failure in children. *Cardiol Young* 2012;22:558–563.
196. Rupp S, Zeiher AM, Dimmeler S, et al. A regenerative strategy for heart failure in hypoplastic left heart syndrome: intracoronary administration of autologous bone marrow-derived progenitor cells. *J Heart Lung Transplant* 2010;29:574–577.
197. Lacis A, Erglis A. Intramyocardial administration of autologous bone marrow mononuclear cells in a critically ill child with dilated cardiomyopathy. *Cardiol Young* 2010;21:110–112.
198. Burkhart HM, Qureshi MY, Peral SC, et al. Regenerative therapy for hypoplastic left heart syndrome: first report of intraoperative intramyocardial injection of autologous umbilical-cord blood–derived cells. *J Thorac Cardiovasc Surg* 2015;149:e35–e37.
199. Ishigami S, Ohtsuki S, Tarui S, et al. Intracoronary autologous cardiac progenitor cell transfer in patients with hypoplastic left heart syndrome. *Circ Res* 2015;116:653–664.
200. Tarui S, Ishigami S, Ousaka D, et al. Transcoronary infusion of cardiac progenitor cells in hypoplastic left heart syndrome: three-year follow-up of the transcoronary infusion of cardiac progenitor cells in patients with single-ventricle physiology (TICAP) trial. *J Thorac Cardiovasc Surg* 2015;150:1198.e2–1208.e2.
201. Ishigami S, Ohtsuki S, Eitoku T, et al. Intracoronary cardiac progenitor cells in single ventricle physiology. *Circ Res* 2017;120:1162–1173.
202. Bergmann O, Bhardwaj RD, Bernard S, et al. Evidence for cardiomyocyte renewal in humans. *Science* 2009;324:98–102.
203. Mishra R, Vijayan K, Colletti Evan J, et al. Characterization and functionality of cardiac progenitor cells in congenital heart patients. *Circulation* 2011;123:364–373.
204. Sharma S, Mishra R, Bigham GE, et al. A deep proteome analysis identifies the complete secretome as the functional unit of human cardiac progenitor cells. *Circ Res* 2017;120:816–834.
205. Freyman T, Polin G, Osman H, et al. A quantitative, randomized study evaluating three methods of mesenchymal stem cell delivery following myocardial infarction. *Eur Heart J* 2006;27:1114–1122.
206. Lafemina MJ, Sheldon RA, Ferriero DM. Acute hypoxia-ischemia results in hydrogen peroxide accumulation in neonatal but not adult mouse brain. *Pediatr Res* 2006;59:680–683.
207. Rosenkranz K, Kumbruch S, Tenbusch M, et al. Transplantation of human umbilical cord blood cells mediated beneficial effects on apoptosis, angiogenesis and neuronal survival after hypoxic-ischemic brain injury in rats. *Cell Tissue Res* 2012;348:429–438.
208. Taguchi A, Soma T, Tanaka H, et al. Administration of CD34+ cells after stroke enhances neurogenesis via angiogenesis in a mouse model. *J Clin Invest* 2004;114:330–338.
209. Pimentel-Coelho PM, Mendez-Otero R. Cell therapy for neonatal hypoxic-ischemic encephalopathy. *Stem Cells Dev* 2010;19:299–310.
210. van Velthoven CTJ, Kavelaars A, van Bel F, et al. Mesenchymal stem cell treatment after neonatal hypoxic-ischemic brain injury improves behavioral outcome and induces neuronal and oligodendrocyte regeneration. *Brain Behav Immun* 2010;24:387–393.
211. van Velthoven CTJ, Kavelaars A, van Bel F, et al. Repeated mesenchymal stem cell treatment after neonatal hypoxia-ischemia has distinct effects on formation and maturation of new neurons and oligodendrocytes leading to restoration of damage, corticospinal motor tract activity, and sensorimotor function. *J Neurosci* 2010;30:9603–9611.

212. Vaes JEG, Vink MA, de Theije CGM, et al. The potential of stem cell therapy to repair white matter injury in preterm infants: lessons learned from experimental models. *Front Physiol* 2019;10:540.
213. Daadi MM, Davis AS, Arac A, et al. Human neural stem cell grafts modify microglial response and enhance axonal sprouting in neonatal hypoxic–ischemic brain injury. *Stroke* 2010;41:516–523.
214. Grandvuillemin I, Garrigue P, Ramdani A, et al. Long-term recovery after endothelial colony-forming cells or human umbilical cord blood cells administration in a rat model of neonatal hypoxic-ischemic encephalopathy. *Stem Cells Transl Med* 2017;6:1987–1996.
215. Archambault J, Moreira A, McDaniel D, et al. Therapeutic potential of mesenchymal stromal cells for hypoxic ischemic encephalopathy: a systematic review and meta-analysis of preclinical studies. *PLoS One* 2017;12:e0189895.
216. Park WS, Sung SI, Ahn SY, et al. Hypothermia augments neuroprotective activity of mesenchymal stem cells for neonatal hypoxic-ischemic encephalopathy. *PLoS One* 2015;10:e0120893.
217. Fischer UM, Harting MT, Jimenez F, et al. Pulmonary passage is a major obstacle for intravenous stem cell delivery: the pulmonary first-pass effect. *Stem Cells Dev* 2009;18:683–692.
218. Argibay B, Trekker J, Himmelreich U, et al. Intraarterial route increases the risk of cerebral lesions after mesenchymal cell administration in animal model of ischemia. *Sci Rep* 2017;7:40758.
219. Donega V, Nijboer CH, van Tilborg G, et al. Intranasally administered mesenchymal stem cells promote a regenerative niche for repair of neonatal ischemic brain injury. *Exp Neurol* 2014;261:53–64.
220. Donega V, Nijboer CH, van Velthoven CTJ, et al. Assessment of long-term safety and efficacy of intranasal mesenchymal stem cell treatment for neonatal brain injury in the mouse. *Pediatr Res* 2015;78:520–526.
221. Jantzie LL, Scafidi J, Robinson S. Stem cells and cell-based therapies for cerebral palsy: a call for rigor. *Pediatr Res* 2018;83:345–355.
222. Feng M, Lu A, Gao H, et al. Safety of allogeneic umbilical cord blood stem cells therapy in patients with severe cerebral palsy: a retrospective study. *Stem Cells Int* 2015;2015:325652.
223. Liu X, Fu X, Dai G, et al. Comparative analysis of curative effect of bone marrow mesenchymal stem cell and bone marrow mononuclear cell transplantation for spastic cerebral palsy. *J Transl Med* 2017;15:48.
224. Chen G, Wang Y, Xu Z, et al. Neural stem cell-like cells derived from autologous bone mesenchymal stem cells for the treatment of patients with cerebral palsy. *J Transl Med* 2013;11:21.
225. Huang L, Zhang C, Gu J, et al. A randomized, placebo-controlled trial of human umbilical cord blood mesenchymal stem cell infusion for children with cerebral palsy. *Cell Transplant* 2018;27:325–334.
226. Novak I, Walker K, Hunt RW, et al. Concise review: stem cell interventions for people with cerebral palsy: systematic review with meta-analysis. *Stem Cells Transl Med* 2016;5:1014–1025.
227. Siniscalco D, Mijatovic T, Bosmans E, et al. Decreased numbers of CD57+CD3− cells identify potential innate immune differences in patients with autism spectrum disorder. *In Vivo* 2016;30:83–89.
228. Hsiao EY, McBride SW, Chow J, et al. Modeling an autism risk factor in mice leads to permanent immune dysregulation. *Proc Natl Acad Sci U S A* 2012;109:12776–12781.
229. Ashwood P, Krakowiak P, Hertz-Picciotto I, et al. Altered T cell responses in children with autism. *Brain Behav Immun* 2011;25:840–849.
230. Ashwood P, Krakowiak P, Hertz-Picciotto I, et al. Elevated plasma cytokines in autism spectrum disorders provide evidence of immune dysfunction and are associated with impaired behavioral outcome. *Brain Behav Immun* 2011;25:40–45.
231. Segal-Gavish H, Karvat G, Barak N, et al. Mesenchymal stem cell transplantation promotes neurogenesis and ameliorates autism related behaviors in BTBR mice. *Autism Res* 2016;9:17–32.
232. Perets N, Segal-Gavish H, Gothelf Y, et al. Long term beneficial effect of neurotrophic factors-secreting mesenchymal stem cells transplantation in the BTBR mouse model of autism. *Behav Brain Res* 2017;331:254–260.
233. Ha S, Park H, Mahmood U, et al. Human adipose-derived stem cells ameliorate repetitive behavior, social deficit and anxiety in a VPA-induced autism mouse model. *Behav Brain Res* 2017;317:479–484.
234. Dawson G, Sun JM, Davlantis KS, et al. Autologous cord blood infusions are safe and feasible in young children with autism spectrum disorder: results of a single-center phase I open-label trial. *Stem Cells Transl Med* 2017;6:1332–1339.
235. Bradstreet JJ, Sych N, Antonucci N, et al. Efficacy of fetal stem cell transplantation in autism spectrum disorders: an open-labeled pilot study. *Cell Transplant* 2014;23(Suppl 1):S105–S112.
236. Riordan NH, Hincapié ML, Morales I, et al. Allogeneic human umbilical cord mesenchymal stem cells for the treatment of autism spectrum disorder in children: safety profile and effect on cytokine levels. *Stem Cells Transl Med* 2019;8:1008–1016.
237. Park WS, Sung SI, Ahn SY, et al. Optimal timing of mesenchymal stem cell therapy for neonatal intraventricular hemorrhage. *Cell Transplant* 2016;25:1131–1144.
238. Ahn SY, Chang YS, Sung SI, et al. Mesenchymal stem cells for severe intraventricular hemorrhage in preterm infants: phase I dose-escalation clinical trial. *Stem Cells Transl Med* 2018;7:847–856.
239. Drucker NA, McCulloh CJ, Li B, et al. Stem cell therapy in necrotizing enterocolitis: current state and future directions. *Semin Pediatr Surg* 2018;27:57–64.
240. McCulloh CJ, Olson JK, Wang Y, et al. Evaluating the efficacy of different types of stem cells in preserving gut barrier function in necrotizing enterocolitis. *J Surg Res* 2017;214:278–285.
241. Le Blanc K, Rasmusson I, Sundberg B, et al. Treatment of severe acute graft-versus-host disease with third party haploidentical mesenchymal stem cells. *Lancet* 2004;363:1439–1441.
242. Fauza DO. Transamniotic stem cell therapy: a novel strategy for the prenatal management of congenital anomalies. *Pediatr Res* 2018;83:241–248.
243. Feng C, Graham CD, Shieh HF, et al. Transamniotic stem cell therapy (TRASCET) in a leporine model of gastroschisis. *J Pediatr Surg* 2017;52:30–34.
244. Takayama S, Sakai K, Fumino S, et al. An intra-amniotic injection of mesenchymal stem cells promotes lung maturity in a rat congenital diaphragmatic hernia model. *Pediatr Surg Int* 2019;35:1353–1361.
245. Dionigi B, Ahmed A, Brazzo J, III, et al. Partial or complete coverage of experimental spina bifida by simple intra-amniotic injection of concentrated amniotic mesenchymal stem cells. *J Pediatr Surg* 2015;50:69–73.
246. Valadi H, Ekström K, Bossios A, et al. Exosome-mediated transfer of mRNAs and microRNAs is a novel mechanism of genetic exchange between cells. *Nat Cell Biol* 2007;9:654–659.
247. van Niel G, Porto-Carreiro I, Simoes S, et al. Exosomes: a common pathway for a specialized function. *J. Biochem* 2006;140:13–21.
248. Willis GR, Fernandez-Gonzalez A, Anastas J, et al. Mesenchymal stromal cell exosomes ameliorate experimental bronchopulmonary dysplasia and restore lung function through macrophage immunomodulation. *Am J Respir Crit Care Med* 2018;197:104–116.
249. McCulloh CJ, Olson JK, Wang Y, et al. Treatment of experimental necrotizing enterocolitis with stem cell-derived exosomes. *J Pediatr Surg* 2018;53:1215–1220.
250. Ophelders DRMG, Wolfs TGAM, Jellema RK, et al. Mesenchymal stromal cell-derived extracellular vesicles protect the fetal brain after hypoxia-ischemia. *Stem Cells Transl Med* 2016;5:754–763.
251. Hu C, Li L. Preconditioning influences mesenchymal stem cell properties in vitro and in vivo. *J Cell Mol Med* 2018;22:1428–1442.
252. Baldari S, Di Rocco G, Piccoli M, et al. Challenges and strategies for improving the regenerative effects of mesenchymal stromal cell-based therapies. *Int J Mol Sci* 2017;18:2087.
253. Sackstein R, Merzaban JS, Cain DW, et al. Ex vivo glycan engineering of CD44 programs human multipotent mesenchymal stromal cell trafficking to bone. *Nat Med* 2008;14:181–187.
254. Moya A, Larochette N, Paquet J, et al. Quiescence preconditioned human multipotent stromal cells adopt a metabolic profile favorable for enhanced survival under ischemia. *Stem Cells* 2017;35:181–196.
255. Yu SP, Wei Z, Wei L. Preconditioning strategy in stem cell transplantation therapy. *Transl Stroke Res* 2013;4:76–88.
256. Estrada JC, Albo C, Benguría A, et al. Culture of human mesenchymal stem cells at low oxygen tension improves growth and genetic stability by activating glycolysis. *Cell Death Differ* 2012;19:743–755.
257. Saparov A, Ogay V, Nurgozhin T, et al. Preconditioning of human mesenchymal stem cells to enhance their regulation of the immune response. *Stem Cells Int* 2016;2016:1–10.
258. Hu X, Xu Y, Zhong Z, et al. A large-scale investigation of hypoxia-preconditioned allogeneic mesenchymal stem cells for myocardial repair in nonhuman primates: paracrine activity without remuscularization. *Circ Res* 2016;118:970–983.
259. Wang X, Liu C, Li S, et al. Hypoxia precondition promotes adipose-derived mesenchymal stem cells based repair of diabetic erectile dysfunction via augmenting angiogenesis and neuroprotection. *PLoS One* 2015;10:e0118951.
260. Assmus B, Walter DH, Seeger FH, et al. Effect of shock wave–facilitated intracoronary cell therapy on LVEF in patients with chronic heart failure: the cellwave randomized clinical trial. *JAMA* 2013;309:1622–1631.
261. Cavazzana M, Bushman FD, Miccio A, et al. Gene therapy targeting haematopoietic stem cells for inherited diseases: progress and challenges. *Nat Rev Drug Discov* 2019;18:447–462.
262. Shaw KL, Garabedian E, Mishra S, et al. Clinical efficacy of gene-modified stem cells in adenosine deaminase–deficient immunodeficiency. *J Clin Invest* 2017;127:1689–1699.
263. Kohn DB, Hershfield MS, Puck JM, et al. Consensus approach for the management of severe combined immune deficiency caused by adenosine deaminase deficiency. *J Allergy Clin Immunol* 2019;143:852–863.
264. Sessa M, Lorioli L, Fumagalli F, et al. Lentiviral haemopoietic stem-cell gene therapy in early-onset metachromatic leukodystrophy: an ad-hoc analysis of a non-randomised, open-label, phase 1/2 trial. *Lancet* 2016;388:476–487.
265. Thompson AA, Walters MC, Kwiatkowski J, et al. Gene therapy in patients with transfusion-dependent β-thalassemia. *N Engl J Med* 2018;378:1479–1493.
266. Mavilio F, Pellegrini G, Ferrari S, et al. Correction of junctional epidermolysis bullosa by transplantation of genetically modified epidermal stem cells. *Nat Med* 2006;12:1397–1402.
267. Sii-Felice K, Giorgi M, Leboulch P, et al. Hemoglobin disorders: lentiviral gene therapy in the starting blocks to enter clinical practice. *Exp Hematol* 2018;64:12–32.
268. Griffith LG. Emerging design principles in biomaterials and scaffolds for tissue engineering. In: Sipe JD, Kelley CA, McNicol LA, eds. *Reparative medicine: growing tissues and organs.* New York, NY: New York Academy of Sciences, 2002:83–95.
269. Bianco P, Robey PG. Stem cells in tissue engineering. *Nature* 2001;414:118–121.
270. Patel M, Fisher JP. Biomaterial scaffolds in pediatric tissue engineering. *Pediatr Res* 2008;63:497–501.
271. Brown PT, Handorf AM, Jeon WB, et al. Stem cell-based tissue engineering approaches for musculoskeletal regeneration. *Curr Pharm Des* 2013;19:3429–3445.
272. Shin'oka T, Matsumura G, Hibino N, et al. Midterm clinical result of tissue-engineered vascular autografts seeded with autologous bone marrow cells. *J Thorac Cardiovasc Surg* 2005;129:1330–1338.
273. Lohmann M, Walenda G, Hemeda H, et al. Donor age of human platelet lysate affects proliferation and differentiation of mesenchymal stem cells. *PLoS One* 2012;7:e37839.
274. Lensch M, Muise A, White L, et al. Comparison of synthetic media designed for expansion of adipose-derived mesenchymal stromal cells. *Biomedicines* 2018;6:54.
275. Yang Y-HK, Ogando CR, Wang See C, et al. Changes in phenotype and differentiation potential of human mesenchymal stem cells aging in vitro. *Stem Cell Res Ther* 2018;9:131.
276. Chinnadurai R, Garcia MA, Sakurai Y, et al. Actin cytoskeletal disruption following cryopreservation alters the biodistribution of human mesenchymal stromal cells in vivo. *Stem Cell Rep* 2014;3:60–72.
277. Gramlich OW, Burand AJ, Brown AJ, et al. Cryopreserved mesenchymal stromal cells maintain potency in a retinal ischemia/reperfusion injury model: toward an off-the-shelf therapy. *Sci Rep* 2016;6:26463.

278. Khong SML, Lee M, Kosaric N, et al. Single-cell transcriptomics of human mesenchymal stem cells reveal age-related cellular subpopulation depletion and impaired regenerative function. *Stem Cells* 2019;37:240–246.
279. Sammour I, Somashekar S, Huang J, et al. The effect of gender on mesenchymal stem cell (MSC) efficacy in neonatal hyperoxia-induced lung injury. *PLoS One* 2016;11:e0164269.
280. Ankrum JA, Ong JF, Karp JM. Mesenchymal stem cells: immune evasive, not immune privileged. *Nat Biotechnol* 2014;32:252–260.
281. Huang XP, Sun Z, Miyagi Y, et al. Differentiation of allogeneic mesenchymal stem cells induces immunogenicity and limits their long-term benefits for myocardial repair. *Circulation* 2010;122:2419–2429.
282. Berglund AK, Fortier LA, Antczak DF, et al. Immunoprivileged no more: measuring the immunogenicity of allogeneic adult mesenchymal stem cells. *Stem Cell Res Ther* 2017;8:288.
283. Hare JM, DiFede DL, Rieger AC, et al. Randomized comparison of allogeneic versus autologous mesenchymal stem cells for nonischemic dilated cardiomyopathy: POSEIDON-DCM trial. *J Am Coll Cardiol* 2017;69:526–537.
284. de Witte SFH, Luk F, Sierra Parraga JM, et al. Immunomodulation by therapeutic mesenchymal stromal cells (msc) is triggered through phagocytosis of MSC by monocytic cells. *Stem Cells* 2018;36:602–615.
285. Ortiz LA, Dutreil M, Fattman C, et al. Interleukin 1 receptor antagonist mediates the antiinflammatory and antifibrotic effect of mesenchymal stem cells during lung injury. *Proc Natl Acad Sci U S A* 2007;104:11002–11007.
286. Lee SH, Jang AS, Kim YE, et al. Modulation of cytokine and nitric oxide by mesenchymal stem cell transfer in lung injury/fibrosis. *Respir Res* 2010;11:16.
287. Donega V, Nijboer CH, Braccioli L, et al. Intranasal administration of human MSC for ischemic brain injury in the mouse: in vitro and in vivo neuroregenerative functions. *PLoS One* 2014;9:e112339.
288. de Wolf C, van de Bovenkamp M, Hoefnagel M. Regulatory perspective on in vitro potency assays for human mesenchymal stromal cells used in immunotherapy. *Cytotherapy* 2017;19:784–797.
289. Esch EW, Bahinski A, Huh D. Organs-on-chips at the frontiers of drug discovery. *Nat Rev Drug Discov* 2015;14:248–260.
290. Boregowda SV, Krishnappa V, Haga CL, et al. A clinical indications prediction scale based on TWIST1 for human mesenchymal stem cells. *EBioMedicine* 2015;4:62–73.
291. Butler J, Hamo CE, Udelson JE, et al. Reassessing phase II heart failure clinical trials: consensus recommendations. *Circ Heart Fail* 2017;10:e003800.
292. Lalu MM, McIntyre L, Pugliese C, et al. Safety of cell therapy with mesenchymal stromal cells (safecell): a systematic review and meta-analysis of clinical trials. *PLoS One* 2012;7:e47559.

CHAPTER

46

Alan H. Jobe

Drugs, Lung Development, and Pulmonary Surfactant

Lung immaturity and development are the major challenges for the survival of infants born prematurely. Antenatal corticosteroids (ACS) are standard care for women at high risk of preterm delivery to decrease the risk of respiratory distress syndrome (RDS) and increase infant survival.[1] Corticosteroids have pleiotropic effects, which can be both beneficial and potentially harmful to the fetus and newborn. The second unique drug for decreasing RDS and mortality is surfactant, and, together, they are the major advances for drug therapies targeting to preterm infant. This chapter reviews the clinical literature for ACS and surfactant with an emphasis on areas of uncertainty.

THE HISTORY OF ANTENATAL CORTICOSTEROIDS

Liggins observed in 1969 that fetal sheep infused with dexamethasone had lungs that were better aerated than control lungs after preterm delivery.[2] Liggins and Howie[3] reported the first randomized controlled trial of ACS in 1972, which demonstrated decreased RDS and decreased death in preterms, with no increase in complications. Over the next 18 years, multiple trials were reported, which generally supported the benefits of ACS treatments. However, few at-risk pregnancies were treated with ACS in the United States. The trials were controversial because the obstetric community was concerned about adverse effects of "steroids" on human development after the experience with diethylstilbestrol.[4] In 1990, Crowley and colleagues published a meta-analysis of ACS, demonstrating compelling benefits with minimal risk.[5] In 1995, U.S. National Institutes of Health (NIH) Consensus Conference strongly endorsed the use of ACS[6] (Table 46.1), and utilization rates increased to current treatment rates of about 90% for women at risk in high-resource environments. However, a single course of ACS only decreased RDS by about 40%, and repetitive courses of ACS were frequently used. This untested use resulted in a second Consensus Conference in 2000, which recommended against repetitive courses of corticosteroids until further studies were available.[7] Multiple trials of repetitive ACS dosing for gestational ranges of 24- to 34-week gestational age range are now available.[8] Although ACS are the standard care endorsed by obstetric societies worldwide, ACS are not approved by the U.S. Food and Drug Administration (FDA) as the research for ACS was investigator initiated and not sponsored by pharmaceutical companies. The theoretical risks for pregnant women and preterm infants are problematic for pharma.

SINGLE-COURSE TREATMENTS WITH ANTENATAL CORTICOSTEROIDS

Single-course ACS trials were completed by 1993 primarily in high-resource medical locations and with a few trials in low- and middle-resource environments. The 2006 meta-analysis by Roberts and Dalziel included 21 randomized controlled trials that included 3,885 women, primarily to assess outcomes of ACS for 24- to 28-week deliveries.[9] An updated meta-analysis in 2017 includes 30 trials and 7,774 randomized women, with the additional trials primarily for gestations >34 weeks.[1] The core result (Fig. 46.1) is that ACS are highly effective with multiple benefits for the premature newborn. No risks for the mother were identified, even for women with preeclampsia or diabetes, although attention to glycemic control is required after corticosteroids are administered to women with diabetes. The benefits for the newborn are substantial, with large decreases in death, RDS, intraventricular hemorrhage, and necrotizing enterocolitis. The risk of developing bronchopulmonary dysplasia is not decreased.

The primary indication for ACS treatment in most studies was the prevention of RDS. The effect of ACS on RDS is robust, with comparable percent decreases in RDS independent of gestational age for pregnancies more than 28 weeks of gestation. However, the outcomes from meta-analysis for single ACS are very dated relative to current care for women and preterm infants. For example, although the recommendation in 1995 was to treat pregnancies at 24 to 34 weeks, only 102 infants were randomized to ACS and delivered at less than 28 weeks' gestation.[10] Given that trials for at-risk pregnancies at 24- to 34-week were considered unethical after 1994, we have no current information from trials to validate the magnitude of ACS benefits for the very preterm infants that are the primary concern for current management.

There are recent very large epidemiology studies reporting impressive benefits with ACS for very preterm infants,

TABLE 46.1 Indications for ACS

Major events that defined whom to treat	*Outcomes*
The 1994 Consensus Conference[6]	• All fetuses between 24 and 34 weeks of gestation at risk of imminent delivery • The benefits vastly outweigh risks: decreased RDS, intraventricular hemorrhage, and death • Patients eligible for tocolytic should receive ACS • Preterm prolonged rupture of membranes is not a contraindication for ACS
The 2000 Consensus Conference on repeated ACS treatments[7]	• Reaffirmed the 1994 recommendations for single treatments • Insufficient data to support repeated treatments • Repeated courses should be used only in context of trials
The 2015 World Health Organization Recommendation for low-resource environments[14]	ACS should be used for pregnancies at risk of imminent delivery between 24 and 34 wk if • Gestational age can be accurately assessed • Birth is imminent: 1–7 d after treatment • No clinical evidence of maternal infection • Adequate care is available for the mother and premature infant
Periviable pregnancies at risk of delivery at 20^0–26^5 wk' gestational age[16]	2017 statement: Consider ACS with discussion with family
Late preterm pregnancies can be selectively treated	ACS will benefit neonatal adaptation but increase hypoglycemia[22]
Repeat courses of ACS	2016 ACOG Committee Opinion to consider one retreatment once for infants <34 wk and ≥14 d beyond initial treatment who will deliver in next 7 d[39]

ACOG, American College of Obstetricians and Gynecologists; ACS, antenatal corticosteroids; RDS, respiratory distress syndrome.

but these reports need to be interpreted with caution. The primary outcome for the early randomized trials was a decrease in RDS. For very preterm infants, RDS is coded for the majority of infants often for mild respiratory problems, and RDS is not a discriminatory outcome for infants less than 28 weeks' gestational age.[11] The epidemiology reports generally use death as the primary outcome. Carlo and colleagues used the National Institute of Child Health and Human Development (NICHD) Neonatal Research Network data to conclude that ACS decreased death and improved neurodevelopment.[12] Another large study using the Neonatal Research Network database of 11,022 infants 22 to 29 weeks demonstrated a mortality decrease with ACS from 42% to 23%, with 88% of infants exposed to ACS.[13] These reports do not characterize the pregnancies that did not receive ACS. A recent report from the Effective Perinatal Intensive Care in Europe (EPICE) cohort of 4,590 infants demonstrates the striking differences between the ACS treated and the 14% not treated. For the not ACS-treated pregnancies, there were 10% fewer women with preeclampsia, 20% more women with ruptured membranes, 22% more delivered outside a Level 3 unit, and 49% more deliveries on the day of admission than the ACS-exposed infants. The no ACS infants are from more abnormal pregnancies that delivered under more adverse conditions and would be expected to have worse outcomes, independent of ACS.[10] Thus, for the standard care of ACS

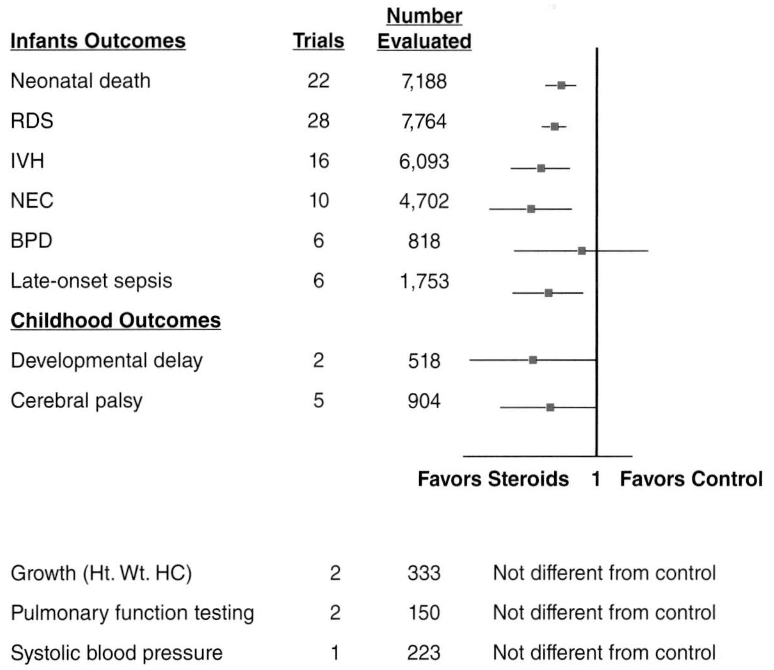

Figure 46.1 Selected outcomes from the 2017 meta-analyses of Roberts et al.[1] summarizing the multiple trials of antenatal corticosteroids (ACS) and demonstrating benefits of ACS for the outcomes other than bronchopulmonary dysplasia.

for pregnancies at risk of preterm delivery at 24- to 34-week gestation, the magnitude of any benefits must be tempered because of the age of the trial data and other large changes in clinical practice.

ANTENATAL CORTICOSTEROIDS: INTERVAL FROM TREATMENT TO BENEFIT

The interval from treatment to benefit remains poorly defined. In the first trial, Liggins and Howie reported in 1972 that benefit occurred only between 48 hours and 7 days after initiation of treatment.[3] The subsequent 2006 meta-analysis identified the efficacy interval as 24 hours to 7 days.[9] The trial data were reanalyzed by the World Health Organization in 2015 to demonstrate a death benefit for 24 to 48 hours that was not significant for 1 day or 4 to 7 days or longer.[14] The outcome of decreased RDS was significant for 1 to 7 days, but not for 24 hours or longer than 7 days, and the only interval of benefit for intraventricular hemorrhage was to 48 hours. These variable times from treatment to benefit result in part from the small number of trials that reported outcomes by time after treatment. There are multiple reports from cohort studies that evaluate treatment to benefit interval with varied results. In general, the studies are of small size, and the large epidemiology studies do not contain the time from treatment to delivery. Only 12% of a recent population-based study of the 707 preterm infants born in Sweden at 22- to 26-week gestation did not receive ACS.[15] Relative to the no ACS group, there was a death benefit of ACS for 24 hours to 7 days. This result is consistent with the efficacy results in sheep models and is probably a reasonable estimate clinically. The question of durability of antenatal steroid (ANS) benefits beyond 7 days is poorly documented but critical for considerations of repeat ACS.

ANTENATAL CORTICOSTEROIDS FOR PERIVIABLE PREGNANCIES

In 1995, the recommendation of the Consensus Conference included treatment of 24- to 26-week pregnancies at risk of preterm delivery, which were periviable pregnancies at that time.[6] There were no trial data to support treatment at those gestations, and there are no trial data even now. As the gestational window for survival has decreased, clinicians now are seeking guidance for gestational ages of 21 to 23 weeks when an attempt at achieving a survival might be considered. In 2017, the Obstetric Care Consensus No. 6 defined periviable as 20^0 to 25^6 weeks and recommended that ACS could be considered with discussion with the family.[16] To emphasize again, there are no trial data to support such early ACS. As with older gestations, there are epidemiology and cohort data, suggesting that ACS have benefit at 22 and 23 weeks' gestational age.[13] These results are problematic as there is likely selection of which pregnancies to treat and for the level of care to be offered.[10] The information to support very early ACS is that primates and explants of human fetal lungs have lung maturation in response to corticosteroids at very early gestational ages.[17,18] Fetal sheep have a partial response to ACS at about 60% gestation.[19] The biology indicates that lung maturation will occur, but there is no randomized information about safety and clinical benefit.

ANTENATAL CORTICOSTEROIDS FOR LATE PRETERM PREGNANCIES

Moderate and late preterm infants are at increased risk for transitional abnormalities and neurodevelopmental problems as children.[20] Pregnancies delivering at less than 38 weeks' gestation have progressively increasing incidences of RDS and transient tachypnea of the newborn that are likely to be responsive to ACS. Although the attack rate is low, these infants represent about 7% of the delivery population and about 60% of the premature population. The large Antenatal Late Preterm Steroids (ALPS) trial randomized 2,831 pregnancies at 34^0 to 36^6 weeks' gestation to ACS and reported that ACS decreased the primary composite outcome (oxygen use, respiratory support, or death) from 14.4% to 11.6% ($p = 0.023$) and decreased respiratory morbidity from 12.1% to 8.1% ($p < 0.001$), but without a death benefit.[21] An unanticipated risk was an increase in hypoglycemia from 15% to 24% ($p < 0.0001$). Other smaller trials have also shown some benefits for ACS in late preterm infants. The Society for Maternal-Fetal Medicine recommended in 2015 that ACS be used for the majority of late preterm pregnancies likely to deliver within 7 days.[22] Some editorials have supported treatment of this population, while others have questioned the magnitude of the benefit for otherwise easily managed problems related to moderate prematurity.[23]

ANTENATAL CORTICOSTEROIDS FOR ELECTIVE CESAREAN DELIVERY AT TERM

Infants delivered by cesarean section at term and without prior labor have adaptation and respiratory problems more frequently than vaginally delivered infants.[24] A large trial from the United Kingdom randomized 998 pregnancies to ACS or no treatment 48 hours prior to elective cesarean section.[25] ACS decreased neonatal intensive care unit (NICU) admissions and qualitatively decreased respiratory abnormalities. Saccone and Berghella included six late preterm and term trials in a meta-analysis that demonstrated decreased RDS and transient tachypnea with ACS in over 5,000 randomized pregnancies[26] (Fig. 46.2). However, attack rates for these outcomes are low, and many women would be treated for a modest benefit. An expansion of ACS to elective cesarean deliveries in parts of the world where such deliveries are the norm would end up in practice, with exposure of the majority of infants to ACS with very little safety information.

OFF-TARGET ANTENATAL CORTICOSTEROIDS TREATMENTS

ACS benefits are thought to occur for the initiation of treatment to delivery interval of 24 hours to 7 days, with no real precision in this estimate. A result of the concerted efforts to treat all women with ACS at risk of delivery at 24 to 34 weeks is that over half of the ACS-treated women will deliver beyond 7 days and many will deliver normally at term.[27] Concerning cohort reports found low global cognition and increased cortisol responses at 6 to 11 years of age after ACS at less than 34 weeks' gestation and delivery at term.[28,29] Adverse effects of ACS may differ for ACS at periviability, at 24 to 34 weeks' gestation or at term, but there

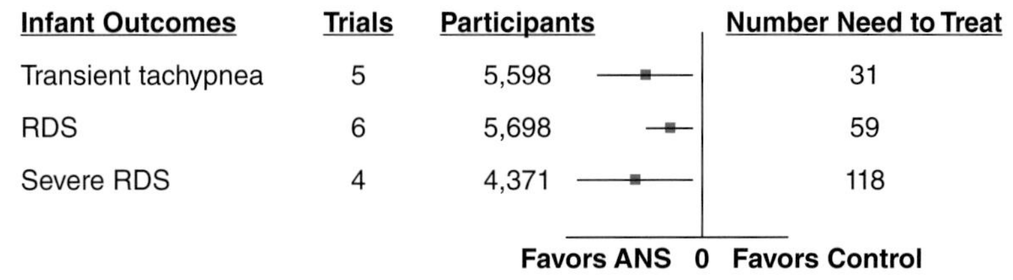

Infant Outcomes	Trials	Participants	Number Need to Treat
Transient tachypnea	5	5,598	31
RDS	6	5,698	59
Severe RDS	4	4,371	118

Favors ANS 0 Favors Control

Figure 46.2 Meta-analysis of trials for antenatal corticosteroids used for late preterm and elective cesarean deliveries demonstrating benefit. Data from Saccone G, Berghella V. Antenatal corticosteroids for maturity of term or near term fetuses: systematic review and meta-analysis of randomized controlled trials. *BMJ* 2016;355:i5044.

is no information about gestation-specific risks in the human. Another large group of off-target ACS treatments is for pregnancies that will not benefit from ACS. As ACS decrease RDS by only 40% in the trials before 1993, a legitimate question is how best to avoid the fetuses who will not respond received any benefit. The reasons that some pregnancies do not respond in the human trials and in animal models of ACS remain enigmatic. Another problem is that a substantial number of fetuses already have lung maturation, particularly for infants greater than 28 weeks' gestational age. It is not known if the fetus who already has mature lungs receives any benefit from ACS. A goal in the future is to identify biomarkers in maternal plasma or to use new technologies such as fetal lung ultrasound to determine whether the pregnancy will benefit from ACS.[30,31] Estimates of patient populations who may receive ACS and also have off-target treatments are listed in Table 46.2.

ANTENATAL CORTICOSTEROIDS IN LOW-RESOURCE ENVIRONMENTS

Although ACS are standard of care worldwide, they are used consistently only in high-resource environments.[32] Nevertheless, ACS in low- and middle-resource environments is the number 1 of 10 interventions recommended by the World Health Organization to decrease preterm infant mortality and improve outcomes.[14] There are a few trials or cohort studies to evaluate the efficacy of ACS in low-resource environments. The challenges are considerable, because gestational age is often unknown, facilities for the delivery and care of the preterm infant are inadequate, and the safety of ACS for women with nutritional, infection, or other health problems is not known. The NICHD Global Health Research Network enrolled almost 100,000 women into the ACT trial in low-resource sites in India, Pakistan, Africa, and Central and South America to test implementation of ACS with an intervention to identify women at risk, initiate treatment, and recommend delivery in an adequate facility.[33] The results of this ACT trial were unanticipated (Table 46.3). ACS did not improve outcomes for infants with birth weights less than the 5th percentile, presumed to be primarily preterm infants, as gestational age information was not reliably available. The surprise was increased perinatal mortality for the larger infants, many of whom were likely term. Secondary analyses identified no process differences between groups, but there were indications of increased maternal and infant infections with ACS.[34] This result changed the World Health Organization recommendations: ACS should be used only if gestational age is known and care is available for a preterm delivery[14] (see Table 46.1). A large cohort study from Brazil also reported worse outcomes for infants exposed to ACS.[35] ACS trials sponsored by the Bill and Melinda Gates Foundation and the World Health Organization to evaluate safety and efficacy of ACS in low-resource environments are ongoing. Much more need to be known about safety and efficacy of ACS in medically limited environments.[36]

REPEAT ANTENATAL CORTICOSTEROIDS TREATMENTS

Repeat ACS treatments were frequently given empirically with the recognition that ACS decreased RDS by about 40% and many at-risk patients had not delivered by 7 days. A second NIH Consensus Conference in 2000 discouraged repeated treatments at 7- to 14-day intervals outside trials[7] (see Table 46.1). A meta-analysis in 2015 included 10 trials of 4,733 women

TABLE 46.2 Estimated Delivery Populations That Could Be Exposed to ACS

Indication	*Population Treated and Delivered in <7 d*	*Off-Target Population Treated and Delivered <7 d to Term*	*Total Treated Population*
Periviable (<24 wk)	0.5%	0.5%	1%
24–34 wk	4%	2%	8%
Late preterm (35–37 wk)	7%	1%	8%
Elective C-section	10%–60%	No off-target for elective C-sections by definition	10%–60%
			25%–75%

ACS, antenatal corticosteroids.

TABLE 46.3 NICHD ACT Trial of Antenatal Steroids

	Implementation of ACS	*Control*	*P value*
Number randomized	48,219	51,523	
Percent given ACS	12	2	
Percent ACS for infants <5th percentile	45	10	
Delivery location			
Hospital	49%	53%	
Clinic	28%	23%	
Home	22%	24%	
Outcomes[a] for infants <5th percentile			
Stillbirths	230	247	0.81
Death before 7 d	181	192	0.30
Perinatal deaths	368	391	0.46
Outcomes,[a] all births			
Stillbirths	21.9	19.1	0.016
Death before 7 d	26.8	24.3	0.018
Perinatal deaths	48.0	42.9	0.003

Steroid treatment: four doses of 6-mg dexamethasone.
[a]Values per 1,000 births.
ACS, antenatal corticosteroids; NICHD, National Institute of Child Health and Human Development.
Data from Althabe F, Belizan JM, McClure EM, et al. A population-based, multifaceted strategy to implement antenatal corticosteroid treatment versus standard care for the reduction of neonatal mortality due to preterm birth in low-income and middle-income countries: the ACT cluster-randomised trial. *Lancet* 2015;385(9968):629–639.

reported no death, intraventricular hemorrhage, or necrotizing enterocolitis benefit for the infants, although there was a modest decrease in RDS.[8] As with single ACS treatments, many women delivered at greater than 34 weeks after receiving multiple ACS treatments. For example, 36% of women in the ACTORDS trial[37] and 66% of women in the MACs trial delivered after 34 weeks.[38] The American College of Obstetricians and Gynecologists (ACOG) Practice Committee Opinion in 2016 considered a single-repeat treatment for infants less than 34 weeks and 14 or above days beyond the initial treatment who will deliver in the next 7 days.[39]

BENEFITS AND RISKS OF ANTENATAL CORTICOSTEROIDS

ACS have substantial benefits for infants born at 24 to 34 weeks' gestational age based on the early single-treatment trials[1] (see Fig. 46.1). The clinical literature supports other benefits, which were also demonstrated in experimental animal models.[40] Fetal exposure to corticosteroids increased blood pressure and myocardial performance after preterm delivery.[41] The blood pressure was higher, despite lower levels of circulating catecholamines in the sheep. Kidney tubular function as measured by an improved ability to handle salt and water loads was also improved by fetal exposure to corticosteroids. A fetal exposure to corticosteroids resulted in an integrated response that made the preterm lamb more tolerant to postnatal asphyxia.[42] The pleiotropic organ maturational effects of corticosteroids result in global adaptive responses that benefit the preterm. Within the context of normal development, these effects can be viewed as replicating the normal fetal adaptations from the increases in cortisol that precedes term birth.

A continuing concern has been the potential for harm from hormones that clearly alter development. Corticosteroids cause dysmorphic changes in rodents and decrease brain and body growth in multiple animal models.[43] A single course of corticosteroids did not decrease birth weight in the preterm human in 11 studies of 3,586 infants [weight difference −17.5 g; 95% confidence interval (CI), −62 to 27 g].[9] When used as a single-treatment course at gestations more than 28 weeks, ACS have been remarkably safe. No acute adverse effects after preterm birth have been reported despite widespread use. The risks of infection in the newborn and postpartum infection in the mother were not increased, except possibly in low-resource environments.[34] Hypoglycemia was increased in late preterm infants in the ALPS trial.[21]

The lingering concern has been the potential for long-term adverse effects of ACS exposure of preterm fetuses. The long-term outcomes that are available are reassuring.[1] Children exposed to a single course of ACS were taller and had better cognitive function than controls at a 14-year follow-up.[44] However, they also had higher blood pressures, although few were in the hypertensive range.[45] In contrast, in 6- and 23-year follow-up reports, the steroid-exposed young adults had lower systolic blood pressures.[46] A 30-year follow-up of the newborns from the original Liggins and Howie trial found some evidence of insulin resistance in the steroid-exposed adults, but no other cardiovascular abnormalities relative to controls.[47] Very long-term adverse effects consistent with the Developmental

Origins of Health and Disease hypothesis have been detected in baboon and sheep models of ACS.[48,49] These potential adverse effects become more relevant as ACS use expands to populations that receive less benefit or receive off-target treatments. A remaining concern is adverse corticosteroid effects of periviable exposures that are not included in any trial-based outcome evaluation.

DRUGS FOR ANTENATAL CORTICOSTEROIDS

The Consensus Conference recommended maternal treatment with betamethasone or dexamethasone rather than cortisol or methylprednisolone because the fluorinated corticosteroids efficiently cross the placenta from the mother to the fetus, have no mineralocorticoid activity, and have a relatively long duration of action.[6] Betamethasone and dexamethasone are equivalent structurally, except for the isomeric position of the 16-methyl group. Betamethasone was given as the suspension of the relatively insoluble acetate and soluble phosphate by Liggins and Howie in the original trial.[3] This two-drug formulation is the only betamethasone preparation available for injection in the United States. Betamethasone-phosphate preparations are available elsewhere. Dexamethasone is given as the soluble sodium phosphate. The soluble phosphates of betamethasone and dexamethasone are prodrugs that are rapidly dephosphorylated to yield high maternal blood levels of betamethasone or dexamethasone after intramuscular (IM) injection. Two dosing schedules were empirically evaluated in the clinical trials and are currently recommended by the World Health Organization.[14] A total dose of 24-mg betamethasone (acetate plus phosphate) is given as a divided dose of 12 mg at the recognition of risk of preterm delivery and 24 hours later. The same total dose of 24 mg of betamethasone sodium phosphate is given as a four-dose treatment, with 6 mg given at the recognition of the risk of preterm delivery and three subsequent doses of 6 mg given at 12-hour intervals. Both agents readily cross the placenta and achieve fetal plasma levels of 30% to 40% of the maternal levels. The pharmacology is complex as both drugs are prodrugs given to the mother to treat the fetus. The resulting corticosteroid exposures for the fetus were modeled by Ballard and Ballard[50] (Fig. 46.3). Multiple other drugs, doses, and dosing schedules are used worldwide without validation.

A maternal drug treatment with potent corticosteroids that are known to be developmental disruptors are designed to achieve fetal responses and should have the characteristics of as low a fetal exposure as possible for the minimal duration to achieve the treatment goals. Surprisingly, ACS therapy has not been critically evaluated, and it is not an approved indication by the FDA in the United States. Corticosteroids given even for short duration have substantial risks in adults of increased sepsis, venous thrombosis, and facture that are proportionate to dose and duration of exposure.[51] The total dose of 24-mg ACS over 48 hours is high relative to routine treatments for anti-inflammation or immunosuppression. Although the half-life of betamethasone or dexamethasone in plasma is only about 4 hours after IM or oral dosing, the pharmacodynamic effect of cortisol suppression can persist for days.[52] The doses of betamethasone or dexamethasone are high and not without risk, although there have been no systemic evaluations related to ACS.

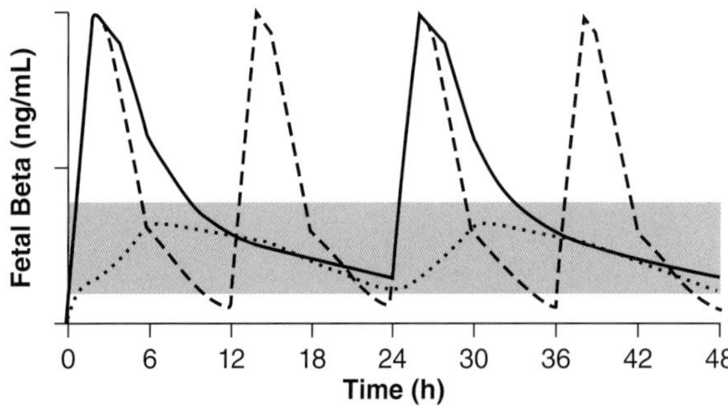

Figure 46.3 Idealized sketch of fetal blood levels following maternal antenatal corticosteroids treatments with two doses of 12-mg betamethasone-phosphate+betamethasone-acetate given at a 24-hour interval (*solid lines*), betamethasone-phosphate or dexamethasone-phosphate given as four doses of 6 mg at 12-hour intervals (*dashed lines*), or two doses of betamethasone-acetate given as 6 mg at 24-hour intervals (*dotted line*). The blue zone is the presumed dose range to minimize fetal exposure and be effective. Drug levels are based on Ballard PL, Ballard RA. Scientific basis and therapeutic regimens for use of antenatal glucocorticoids. *Am J Obstet Gynecol* 1995;173(1):254–262 and our recent pharmacokinetic measurements.[54,55]

We have used fetal sheep and monkey models to learn what fetal exposures are required for efficacy. In sheep models, the fetal exposures from a single maternal IM dose, of betamethasone-phosphate or dexamethasone-phosphate, will not induce fetal lung maturation,[53] but a single dose of 0.125 mg/kg betamethasone-acetate alone (equivalent to about 6 mg for 50-kg woman) will induce comparable lung maturation to the clinical dose of 12-mg betamethasone-phosphate+betamethasone-acetate given twice in fetal sheep.[54] Further, maternal infusions of betamethasone-phosphate to target fetal betamethasone levels of 1 to 4 ng/mL will induce lung maturation.[55] The initial high peak betamethasone levels from maternal IM betamethasone-phosphate or dexamethasone-phosphate are not required for lung maturational effects and simply have a toxicity potential. Empirically, a 48-hour exposure duration is used clinically. In sheep, a 24-hour exposure from betamethasone-acetate or a maternal infusion of betamethasone-phosphate for 26 hours causes fetal lung maturation when assessed at 48 hours.[55] However, the lung maturation response is not durable as it is lost by 7 days. Two doses of betamethasone-acetate cause a durable response to 7 days. We have learned that the fetal exposure to achieve persistent lung maturation needs to be low continuous fetal plasma levels in the range of 1 to 4 ng/mL for 48 hours in sheep. Studies in primates are pending to test this exposure strategy.

There are some fetal cord blood levels reported for preterm infants that delivered within 24 hours of maternal ACS. Figure 46.4 gives values that are above the presumed target fetal blood levels for betamethasone or dexamethasone.[56–58] We suspect that the recommended treatments for ACS expose the fetus to excess drug. Oral dosing to achieve lower fetal exposures may be an attractive option for low- and middle-resource environments as oral betamethasone-phosphate or dexamethasone-phosphate preparations are readily available and very inexpensive. However, oral treatments need to be tested against the accepted treatments.

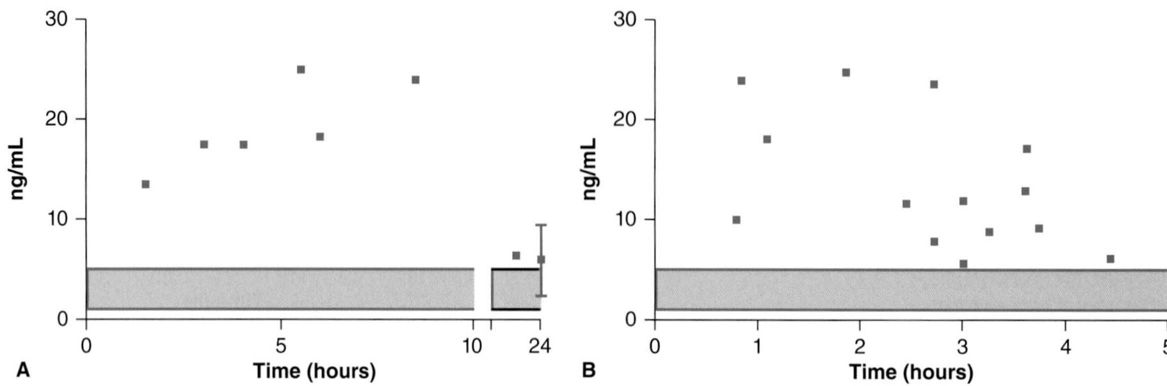

Figure 46.4 **A:** Values for betamethasone in cord blood following 12-mg betamethasone-phosphate+betamethasone-acetate. Cord blood was collected at preterm delivery. Betamethasone levels are above the presumed target range before 10 hours and are close to the target range at 24 hours. Data from Ballabh P, Lo ES, Kumari J, et al. Pharmacokinetics of betamethasone in twin and singleton pregnancy. *Clin Pharmacol Ther* 2002;71(1):39–45; and Gyamfi C, Mele L, Wapner RJ, et al. The effect of plurality and obesity on betamethasone concentrations in women at risk for preterm delivery. *Am J Obstet Gynecol* 2010;203(3):219.E1–219.E5. **B:** Values for dexamethasone following 6 mg of maternal intramuscular dexamethasone-phosphate are above the presumed target range for 4 hours. In clinical practice, a second dose would be given at 12 hours. Data from Tsuei SE, Petersen MC, Ashley JJ, et al. Disporition of synthetic glucocorticoids. II. Dexamethasone in parturient women. *Clin Pharmacol Ther* 1980;28(1):88–98.

SURFACTANTS FOR RESPIRATORY DISTRESS SYNDROME: HISTORY

RDS was a highly fatal disease for preterm infants until the late 1960s when NICUs were developed for preterm infants, initially providing temperature support, nutrition, infection control, and oxygen for respiratory problems. Continuous positive airway pressure (CPAP) followed by infant ventilators provided the first targeted interventions for RDS after 1971.[59] Although Avery and Mead had identified surfactant deficiency in RDS in 1959,[60] no progress was made with surfactant treatments until the 1970s with demonstrations by Enhorning and Robertson that surfactant isolated from lungs could improve the lung mechanics of preterm rabbits.[61] Fujiwara and colleagues demonstrated in 1980 that a lipid extract of cow lungs supplemented with dipalmitoylphosphatidylcholine, the most surface active phospholipid in surfactant, and palmitic acid rapidly improved oxygenation when instilled into the lungs of infants with RDS.[62] In clinical trials, amniotic fluid and animal lung extracts sourced surfactants, and a synthetic surfactant improved lung function, decreased pneumothorax, and decreased death in randomized controlled trials with FDA approval of surfactant for RDS in 1990.[63] At that time, surfactants were the first class of drugs approved for airway instillation in any patient population. Surfactant for RDS is now standard of care for infants with RDS, but with treatment techniques and drugs continue to evolve over almost 30 years.

CHARACTERISTICS OF SURFACTANTS

Surfactants for clinical use were developed empirically to have the biophysical properties of natural surfactants recovered from animal airspaces. Simple lipid extracts of alveolar washes and lipid extracts of lungs were tested for surface activity and for their ability to improve the compliance of saline lavaged rat lungs or ventilated premature rabbit lungs as bioassays for function.[64] Dipalmitoylphosphatidylcholine is the major surface active lipid in all animal source surfactants. When it is combined with other lipids and the highly conserved lipophilic proteins SP-B and SP-C, the mixtures have the biophysical properties of natural surfactant. Although there are synthetic surfactants, the most effective and widely used surfactants continue to be derived from animal lungs or alveolar washes.

Clinical surfactants correct the surfactant deficiency of the immature lungs acutely after administration. The net effects are best illustrated by the static surfactant treatment responses of surfactant-deficient lungs[65] (Fig. 46.5). The surfactant-deficient lung does not begin to inflate until the pressure is greater than 20 cm H_2O, and inflation is primarily of airways as maximal volume at a pressure of 30 cm H_2O is only about 25 mL/kg. The lung completely deflates as pressure is lowered below 10 cm H_2O. In contrast, surfactant permits the lung to begin inflation at 15 cm H_2O pressure, to a maximal volume of 80 mL/kg, and the lung retains 50 mL/kg gas volume on deflation to 5 cm H_2O pressure. Anatomically, surfactant allows the lung to uniformly inflate.[66] The physiologic effects are a rapid increase in oxygenation as fluid filled and/or atelectatic lungs open.[67] Surfactant augments positive end-expiratory pressures to increase functional residual capacity and improve compliance for the initial breaths of ventilated preterm rabbits[68] (Fig. 46.6). The net effects of a surfactant treatment are to increase lung gas volume, improve gas exchange, improve lung mechanics, decrease work of breathing, and normalize alveolar size to decrease over- and under-inflation–mediated injury.

SURFACTANT METABOLISM AND SURFACTANT TREATMENT

The preterm surfactant-deficient lung has inadequate surfactant stored in lamellar bodies in type II cells that can be secreted at birth. In large animal models and infants with RDS, newly synthetized surfactant is processed to lamellar bodies for secretion over 2 to 3 days, as measured with isotope-labeled

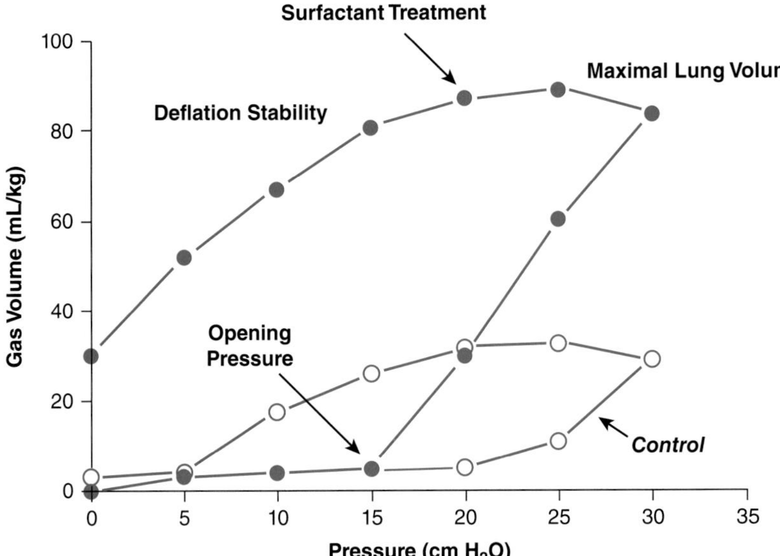

Figure 46.5 Surfactant effects on static pressure–volume curves measured from preterm surfactant-deficient rabbits. The control lungs do not inflate even at a pressure of 30 cm H_2O. In contrast, a surfactant treatment decreased the pressure required for opening, increased total gas capacity, and stabilized the lung on deflation. Adapted and redrawn from Rider ED, Ikegami M, Whitsett JA, et al. Treatment responses to surfactants containing natural surfactant proteins in preterm rabbits. *Am Rev Respir Dis* 1993;147(3):669–676.

precursors.[69,70] This long delay corresponded with the period of increasing respiratory distress and oxygen need for infants before the surfactant treatment era. Isotope labeling of clinical surfactants were used to measure the clearance rates of treatment doses of surfactant.[71] A large fraction of a treatment dose of surfactant quickly becomes associated with the lung tissue, and the lipid and some of the protein components are recycled back into the synthesis and secretion pathways.[72] Thus, surfactant treatments have the remarkable effect of loading the intracellular precursor pools, which the uninjured preterm lung will reprocess to maintain surfactant function. The fraction of the treatment dose that remains in the airspace has a half-life of about 3 days.

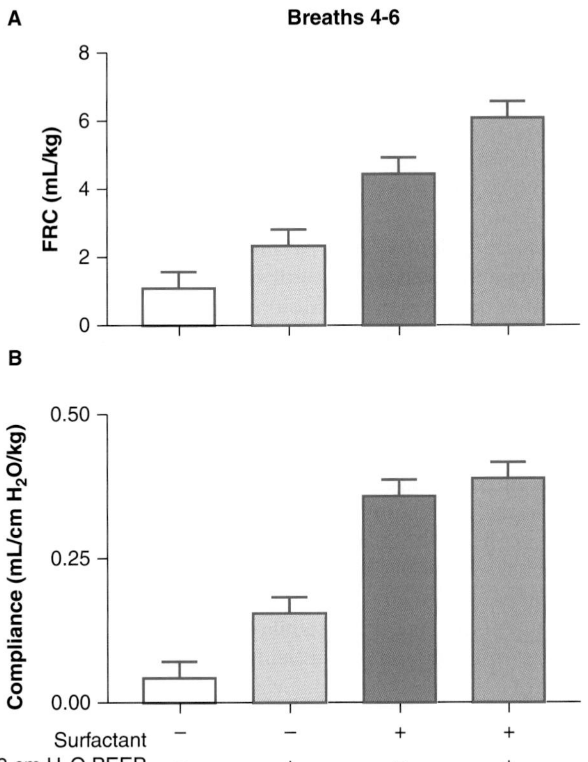

Figure 46.6 Combined effects of positive end-expiratory pressure (PEEP) and surfactant on functional capacity (FRC) (**A**) and compliance (**B**) for preterm-ventilated rabbits. There was a large increase in FRC and compliance over the first four breaths with surfactant, which increased further with PEEP. Data from Siew ML, Te Pas AB, Wallace MJ, et al. Surfactant increases the uniformity of lung aeration at birth in ventilated preterm rabbits. *Pediatr Res* 2011;70(1):50–55.

The potential airspace pool size of surfactant at term is large, probably on the order of 100 mg/kg. In contrast, the infant with RDS has a small pool size of about 2 to 10 mg/kg.[73] The surfactant from the preterm lung has less dipalmitoylphosphatidylcholine and less of the surfactant proteins than surfactant from mature lungs.[74] This immature surfactant is more sensitive to inhibition of its biophysical activity by proteinaceous pulmonary edema, inflammation, and blood components.[75] If the infant has only RDS and not inflammation-associated lung injury, then a single dose of 100 to 200 mg/kg surfactant is sufficient for treatment of acute RDS. However, a lung injured from fetal inflammation or early neonatal ventilation-mediated injury may not respond as well to surfactant treatment and need another treatment, generally because of surfactant inhibition.[76]

SURFACTANT TREATMENT AND COMPLICATIONS

Following approval of surfactant in the 1990s, treatments were given in the delivery room soon after birth to infants thought to be at high risk of RDS—called prophylactic treatments. The other option was surfactant treatment, once RDS was diagnosed, usually within 6 hours of birth—called rescue treatment.[63] For both approaches, the infant was intubated and receiving mechanical ventilation. Surfactant treatment responses were striking in the randomized trials of surfactant versus untreated controls[77] (Fig. 46.7). Surfactant decreased death and pneumothorax but had little effect on other outcomes. Outcomes were better for infants treated soon after delivery than those after the diagnosis of RDS, presumably because ventilation-mediated

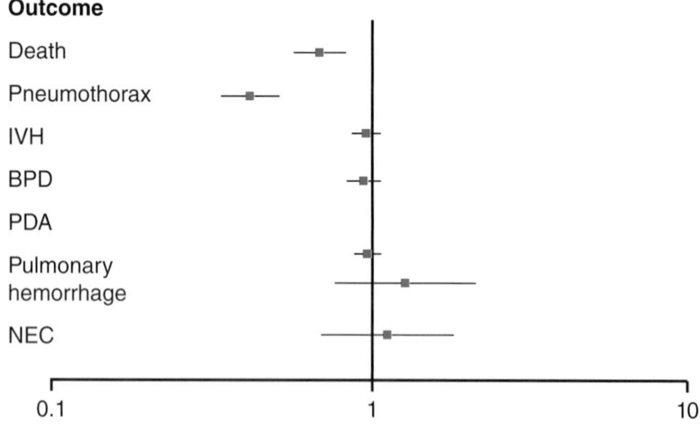

Figure 46.7 Meta-analysis of 13 trials of animal lung–sourced surfactant for treatment of respiratory distress syndrome. Risk ratios and 95% confidence intervals indicate that the significant benefits for decreased death and pneumothorax. Data from Seger N, Soll R. Animal derived surfactant extract for treatment of respiratory distress syndrome. *Cochrane Database Syst Rev* 2009;(2):CD007836.

injury was avoided. Subsequent clinical experiences indicated no clear benefit of prophylactic relative to rescue treatments because in clinical practice, the delays for the diagnosis and treatment decreased.[78]

Initially, surfactant treatments were ritualized by positioning the infant to optimize surfactant distribution, by increasing the ventilator support to avoid airway obstruction from the volume of surfactant, and by increasing oxygen to avoid hypoxemia. These maneuvers were specified by the package inserts, based on the trial designs of the different surfactants for FDA approval. The different maneuvers for surfactant treatments are seldom adhered to today. Consequently, clinicians may not anticipate acute events that can occur with surfactant treatment simply from the volume of 1.5 to 4 mL/kg fluid given into the airways[79] (Table 46.4).

TABLE 46.4 Adverse Events from Surfactant Treatment—Data from 17,641 Treatments[a]

Event	*Percent of Treatments*
Decreased oxygen saturation	16.6
Increased oxygen saturation	3.3
Decreased Pco_2	0.1
Increased Pco_2	0.5
Reflux of surfactant	14.6
Bradycardia	4.2
Other events	2.7
At least one event	30.4

[a]Data abstracted from Zola EM, Overbach AM, Gunkel JH, et al. Treatment Investigational New Drug experience with Survanta (beractant). *Pediatrics* 1993;91(3):546–551.

SURFACTANT DISTRIBUTION IN THE LUNGS

Instillation of saline into the lungs distributes primarily to the large airways very nonhomogeneously based on the physical variables of gravity, the volume being instilled, and the speed of the instillation. In contrast, the highly surface active surfactant quickly spreads to the distal airspaces.[80] This spreading is truly remarkable as the fetal lung has developed by about 18 weeks' gestational age, all of the approximately 17 generations of airways that are in the adult human lung. This number of generations translates to about 250,000 binary airway branches, and any inhomogeneity of distribution at a branch point will be reflected at all branches more distal. Thus, the very low surface tension of surfactant is essential for its distribution to the distal lung and the acute physiologic effects on lung mechanics and gas exchange.

EVOLUTION OF SURFACTANT TREATMENT STRATEGIES

The delivery room care of the very preterm infant has changed from routine intubation and mechanical ventilation to transition of the infants to air breathing to lung protective strategies with CPAP support and without immediate surfactant treatment. Trials of intubation and prophylactic surfactant treatment as compared to CPAP with subsequent surfactant treatment if the infant has RDS favor marginally the CPAP and delayed surfactant approach.[81] A recent population-based report from Denmark demonstrates how CPAP can decrease the need for surfactant treatments.[82] In this clinical experience with initial CPAP support for 6,628 infants, surfactant was subsequently given to 59% of 24- to 27-week preterm, 29% of 28- to 31-week preterm, and 7% of 31- to 33-week preterm infants. For infants who have transitioned on CPAP but have RDS, treatment with intubation and mechanical ventilation is now frequently modified to minimize stress and avoid mechanical ventilation. The INSURE approach is to intubate the infant, give surfactant and extubate back to CPAP to avoid mechanical ventilation.[83] Another approach with the acronym of LISA (less invasive surfactant administration) is to intubate with a fine catheter followed by surfactant treatment and CPAP.[84] A third approach is the MIST strategy for placement of a fine catheter in the airways and for the surfactant treatment, while CPAP is maintained to avoid any lung collapse and any positive-pressure ventilation.[85] These approaches work well for the larger and more mature infants, but controversy remains about how to best give surfactant for the infants at the margins of viability.

Other approaches also are being evaluated. Surfactant can be given to the spontaneously breathing larger premature infants by laryngeal mask to avoid intubation and ventilation.[86] This approach may be useful in low-resource environments where intubation skills are lacking. The ultimate noninvasive approach is to deliver a surfactant aerosol, a dream of neonatologists for years. The substantial limitations to aerosols are that large amounts of surfactant cannot be delivered rapidly, aerosols preferentially go to the ventilated (good) lung rather than to atelectatic or hyperinflated lung regions. Surfactant delivery through nasal prongs for CPAP, high-flow cannula, or masks is very inefficient because of losses before the aerosol reaches the lungs. New devices may overcome the limitations, as suggested by a recent report of nebulized surfactant delivered through a CPAP device to infants with RDS.[87]

THE FUTURE OF SURFACTANTS FOR RESPIRATORY DISTRESS SYNDROME

There is substantial innovation as how to best treat infants with surfactant to minimize stress to the infant. The techniques depend on operator skills and the support environment for the care of the infant. It is worth remembering that gentle intubation, surfactant treatment, and gentle assisted ventilation with extubation to CPAP when the infant has improved works well and has stood the test of time. Very few infants die of RDS in advanced care environments. A major challenge is to provide access to surfactant in low-intensity care setting worldwide. The surfactants used were most widely developed in the 1980s and approved in the 1990s. The animal-sourced surfactants are given in different doses, but overall similarly benefit infants with RDS, and those clinical surfactants are similar to native surfactant. It is unlikely that a new surfactant that has much better response characteristics can be developed. However, surfactants that contain synthetic lipids and synthetic surfactant protein analogs can be made and can be effective.[88]

ANTENATAL STEROIDS AND SURFACTANT

This chapter has focused on two major pharmacologic interventions for preterm infants—ACS and surfactant. In animal models, ACS "prepare" the immature lung for surfactant treatments. Contrary to the general understanding, ACS do not increase surfactant pools within 3 to 4 days of treatment. The short-term effects of the corticosteroids are to shrink the mesenchyme and increase the potential airspaces in the fetal lung. In the fetal sheep, the surfactant increases lung gas volume from a control value of 10 to 36 mL/kg, ANS increase the lung gas exchange volume to 23 mL/kg, and animals exposed to ANS and then treated with surfactant had a mean lung gas volume of 52 mL, which is the sum of the individual effects.[89] There has not been and will not be a trial that randomizes fetuses to ANS, followed by birth and then randomization to surfactant. Not treating with ANS and surfactant would be unethical. The neonatal community is most fortunate to have two effective and complementary therapies that decrease death and improve outcomes.

REFERENCES

1. Roberts D, Brown J, Medley N, et al. Antenatal corticosteroids for accelerating fetal lung maturation for women at risk of preterm birth. *Cochrane Database Syst Rev* 2017;3:CD004454.
2. Liggins GC. Premature delivery of foetal lambs infused with glucocorticoids. *J Endocrinol* 1969;45(4):515–523.
3. Liggins GC, Howie RN. A controlled trial of antepartum glucocorticoid treatment for prevention of the respiratory distress syndrome in premature infants. *Pediatrics* 1972;50(4):515–525.
4. Troisi R, Hatch EE, Titus L. The Diethylstilbestrol Legacy: a powerful case against intervention in uncomplicated pregnancy. *Pediatrics* 2016;138(Suppl 1):S42–S44.
5. Crowley P, Chalmers I, Keirse MJ. The effects of corticosteroid administration before preterm delivery: an overview of the evidence from controlled trials. *Br J Obstet Gynaecol* 1990;97(1):11–25.
6. Effect of corticosteroids for fetal maturation on perinatal outcomes. NIH Consensus Development Panel on the Effect of Corticosteroids for Fetal Maturation on Perinatal Outcomes. *JAMA* 1995;273(5):413–418.
7. National Institutes of Health Consensus Development Panel. Antenatal corticosteroids revisited: repeat courses—National Institutes of Health Consensus Development Conference Statement, August 17–18, 2000. *Obstet Gynecol* 2001;98(1):144–150.
8. Crowther CA, McKinlay CJ, Middleton P, et al. Repeat doses of prenatal corticosteroids for women at risk of preterm birth for improving neonatal health outcomes. *Cochrane Database Syst Rev* 2015;(7):CD003935.
9. Roberts D, Dalziel S. Antenatal corticosteroids for accelerating fetal lung maturation for women at risk of preterm birth. *Cochrane Database Syst Rev* 2006(3):CD004454.
10. Jobe AH, Goldenberg RL. Antenatal corticosteroids: an assessment of anticipated benefits and potential risks. *Am J Obstet Gynecol* 2018;219(1):62–74.
11. Bancalari EH, Jobe AH. The respiratory course of extremely preterm infants: a dilemma for diagnosis and terminology. *J Pediatr* 2012;161(4):585–588.
12. Carlo WA, McDonald SA, Fanaroff AA, et al. Association of antenatal corticosteroids with mortality and neurodevelopmental outcomes among infants born at 22 to 25 weeks' gestation. *JAMA* 2011;306(21):2348–2358.
13. Travers CP, Carlo WA, McDonald SA, et al. Mortality and pulmonary outcomes of extremely preterm infants exposed to antenatal corticosteroids. *Am J Obstet Gynecol* 2018;218(1):130.e1–130.e13.
14. WHO. *WHO recommendations on interventions to improve preterm birth outcomes.* Geneva, Switzerland: WHO Publication, 2015. https://pubmed.ncbi.nlm.nih.gov/26447264/. Accessed July 23, 2020.
15. Norberg H, Kowalski J, Marsal K, et al. Timing of antenatal corticosteroid administration and survival in extremely preterm infants: a national population-based cohort study. *BJOG* 2017;124(10):1567–1574.
16. American College of Obstetricians and Gynecologists, Society for Maternal-Fetal Medicine. Obstetric Care Consensus No. 6: periviable birth. *Obstet Gynecol* 2017;130(4):e187–e199.
17. Karinch AM, Deiter G, Ballard PL, et al. Regulation of expression of human SP-A1 and SP-A2 genes in fetal lung explant culture. *Biochim Biophys Acta* 1998;1398(2):192–202.
18. Bunton TE, Plopper CG. Triamcinolone-induced structural alterations in the development of the lung of the fetal rhesus macaque. *Am J Obstet Gynecol* 1984;148(2):203–215.
19. Visconti K, Senthamaraikannan P, Kemp MW, et al. Extremely preterm fetal sheep lung responses to antenatal steroids and inflammation. *Am J Obstet Gynecol* 2018;218(3):349.e1–349.e10.
20. Raju TNK, Buist AS, Blaisdell CJ, et al. Adults born preterm: a review of general health and system-specific outcomes. *Acta Paediatr* 2017;106(9):1409–1437.
21. Gyamfi-Bannerman C, Thom EA, Blackwell SC, et al. Antenatal betamethasone for women at risk for late preterm delivery. *N Engl J Med* 2016;374(14):1311–1320.
22. American College of Obstetricians and Gynecologists' Committee on Obstetric Practice, Society for Maternal-Fetal Medicine. Committee Opinion No. 677: antenatal corticosteroid therapy for fetal maturation. *Obstet Gynecol* 2016;128(4):e187–e194.
23. Kamath-Rayne BD, Rozance PJ, Goldenberg RL, et al. Antenatal corticosteroids beyond 34 weeks gestation: what do we do now? *Am J Obstet Gynecol* 2016;215(4):423–430.
24. Jain L, Raju TN. Late preterm and early term births. *Clin Perinatol* 2013;40(4):xix–xx.
25. Stutchfield P, Whitaker R, Russell I; Antenatal Steroids for Term Elective Caesarean Section Research Team. Antenatal betamethasone and incidence of neonatal respiratory distress after elective caesarean section: pragmatic randomised trial. *BMJ* 2005;331(7518):662.
26. Saccone G, Berghella V. Antenatal corticosteroids for maturity of term or near term fetuses: systematic review and meta-analysis of randomized controlled trials. *BMJ* 2016;355:i5044.
27. Makhija NK, Tronnes AA, Dunlap BS, et al. Antenatal corticosteroid timing: accuracy after the introduction of a rescue course protocol. *Am J Obstet Gynecol* 2016;214(1):120.E1–120.E6.
28. Paules C, Pueyo V, Marti E, et al. Threatened preterm labor is a risk factor for impaired cognitive development in early childhood. *Am J Obstet Gynecol* 2017;216(2):157.e1–157.e7.
29. Alexander N, Rosenlocher F, Stalder T, et al. Impact of antenatal synthetic glucocorticoid exposure on endocrine stress reactivity in term-born children. *J Clin Endocrinol Metab* 2012;97(10):3538–3544.
30. Palacio M, Bonet-Carne E, Cobo T, et al. Prediction of neonatal respiratory morbidity by quantitative ultrasound lung texture analysis: a multicenter study. *Am J Obstet Gynecol* 2017;217(2):196.e1–196.e14.
31. Kamath-Rayne BD, Du Y, Hughes M, et al. Systems biology evaluation of cell-free amniotic fluid transcriptome of term and preterm infants to detect fetal maturity. *BMC Med Genomics* 2015;8:67.
32. Golding N, Burstein R, Longbottom J, et al. Mapping under-5 and neonatal mortality in Africa, 2000–15: a baseline analysis for the Sustainable Development Goals. *Lancet* 2017;390(10108):2171–2182.
33. Althabe F, Belizan JM, McClure EM, et al. A population-based, multifaceted strategy to implement antenatal corticosteroid treatment versus standard care for the reduction of neonatal mortality due to preterm birth in low-income and middle-income countries: the ACT cluster-randomised trial. *Lancet* 2015;385(9968):629–639.
34. Althabe F, Thorsten V, Klein K, et al. The Antenatal Corticosteroids Trial (ACT)'s explanations for neonatal mortality—a secondary analysis. *Reprod Health* 2016;13(1):62.
35. Dias TZ, Passini R Jr, Tedesco RP, et al. Evaluation of prenatal corticosteroid use in spontaneous preterm labor in the Brazilian Multicenter Study on Preterm Birth (EMIP). *Int J Gynaecol Obstet* 2017;139(2):222–229.
36. Hodgins S. Antenatal corticosteroids: primum non nocere. *Glob Health Sci Pract* 2018;6(4):620–623.
37. Crowther CA, Haslam RR, Hiller JE, et al; Australasian Collaborative Trial of Repeat Doses of Steroids Study Group. Neonatal respiratory distress syndrome after repeat exposure to antenatal corticosteroids: a randomised controlled trial. *Lancet* 2006;367(9526):1913–1919.
38. Murphy KE, Hannah ME, Willan AR, et al. Multiple courses of antenatal corticosteroids for preterm birth (MACS): a randomised controlled trial. *Lancet* 2008;372(9656):2143–2151.
39. Committee Opinion No. 677 Summary: antenatal corticosteroid therapy for fetal maturation. *Obstet Gynecol* 2016;128(4):940–941.
40. Padbury JF, Polk DH, Ervin MG, et al. Postnatal cardiovascular and metabolic responses to a single intramuscular dose of betamethasone in fetal sheep born prematurely by cesarean section. *Pediatr Res* 1995;38(5):709–715.

41. Stein HM, Oyama K, Martinez A, et al. Effects of corticosteroids in preterm sheep on adaptation and sympathoadrenal mechanisms at birth. *Am J Physiol* 1993;264(5 Pt 1): E763–E769.
42. Ervin MG, Padbury JF, Polk DH, et al. Antenatal glucocorticoids alter premature newborn lamb neuroendocrine and endocrine responses to hypoxia. *Am J Physiol Regul Integr Comp Physiol* 2000;279(3):R830–R838.
43. Moisiadis VG, Matthews SG. Glucocorticoids and fetal programming part 1: outcomes. *Nat Rev Endocrinol* 2014;10(7):391–402.
44. Doyle LW, Ford GW, Rickards AL, et al. Antenatal corticosteroids and outcome at 14 years of age in children with birth weight less than 1501 grams. *Pediatrics* 2000;106(1):E2.
45. Doyle LW, Ford GW, Davis NM, et al. Antenatal corticosteroid therapy and blood pressure at 14 years of age in preterm children. *Clin Sci (Lond)* 2000;98(2):137–142.
46. Dessens AB, Haas HS, Koppe JG. Twenty-year follow-up of antenatal corticosteroid treatment. *Pediatrics* 2000;105(6):E77.
47. Dalziel SR, Walker NK, Parag V, et al. Cardiovascular risk factors after antenatal exposure to betamethasone: 30-year follow-up of a randomised controlled trial. *Lancet* 2005;365(9474):1856–1862.
48. Zhang J, Massmann GA, Rose JC, et al. Differential effects of clinical doses of antenatal betamethasone on nephron endowment and glomerular filtration rate in adult sheep. *Reprod Sci* 2010;17(2):186–195.
49. Kuo AH, Li J, Li C, et al. Prenatal steroid administration leads to adult pericardial and hepatic steatosis in male baboons. *Int J Obes (Lond)* 2017;41(8):1299–1302.
50. Ballard PL, Ballard RA. Scientific basis and therapeutic regimens for use of antenatal glucocorticoids. *Am J Obstet Gynecol* 1995;173(1):254–262.
51. Waljee AK, Rogers MA, Lin P, et al. Short term use of oral corticosteroids and related harms among adults in the United States: population based cohort study. *BMJ* 2017;357:j1415.
52. Mager DE, Lin SX, Blum RA, et al. Dose equivalency evaluation of major corticosteroids: pharmacokinetics and cell trafficking and cortisol dynamics. *J Clin Pharmacol* 2003;43(11):1216–1227.
53. Jobe AH, Nitsos I, Pillow JJ, et al. Betamethasone dose and formulation for induced lung maturation in fetal sheep. *Am J Obstet Gynecol* 2009;201(6):611.E1–611.E7.
54. Schmidt AF, Kemp MW, Rittenschober-Bohm J, et al. Low-dose betamethasone-acetate for fetal lung maturation in preterm sheep. *Am J Obstet Gynecol* 2018;218(1):132.e1–132.e9.
55. Kemp MW, Saito M, Usuda H, et al. The efficacy of antenatal steroid therapy is dependent on the duration of low-concentration fetal exposure: evidence from a sheep model of pregnancy. *Am J Obstet Gynecol* 2018;219(3):301.e1–301.e16.
56. Ballabh P, Lo ES, Kumari J, et al. Pharmacokinetics of betamethasone in twin and singleton pregnancy. *Clin Pharmacol Ther* 2002;71(1):39–45.
57. Gyamfi C, Mele L, Wapner RJ, et al. The effect of plurality and obesity on betamethasone concentrations in women at risk for preterm delivery. *Am J Obstet Gynecol* 2010;203(3):219.E1–219.E5.
58. Tsuei SE, Petersen MC, Ashley JJ, et al. Disporition of synthetic glucocorticoids. II. Dexamethasone in parturient women. *Clin Pharmacol Ther* 1980;28(1):88–98.
59. Gregory GA, Kitterman JA, Phibbs RH, et al. Treatment of the idiopathic respiratory-distress syndrome with continuous positive airway pressure. *N Engl J Med* 1971;284(24): 1333–1340.
60. Avery ME, Mead J. Surface properties in relation to atelectasis and hyaline membrane disease. *AMA J Dis Child* 1959;97(5, Part 1):517–523.
61. Enhorning G, Robertson B. Lung expansion in the premature rabbit fetus after tracheal deposition of surfactant. *Pediatrics* 1972;50(1):58–66.
62. Fujiwara T, Maeta H, Chida S, et al. Artificial surfactant therapy in hyaline-membrane disease. *Lancet* 1980;1(8159):55–59.
63. Jobe AH. Pulmonary surfactant therapy. *N Engl J Med* 1993;328(12):861–868.
64. Notter RH, Finkelstein JN. Pulmonary surfactant: an interdisciplinary approach. *J Appl Physiol Respir Environ Exerc Physiol* 1984;57(6):1613–1624.
65. Rider ED, Ikegami M, Whitsett JA, et al. Treatment responses to surfactants containing natural surfactant proteins in preterm rabbits. *Am Rev Respir Dis* 1993;147(3):669–676.
66. Pinkerton KE, Lewis JF, Rider ED, et al. Lung parenchyma and type II cell morphometrics: effect of surfactant treatment on preterm ventilated lamb lungs. *J Appl Physiol (1985)*. 1994;77(4):1953–1960.
67. Jobe AH, Ikegami M. Biology of surfactant. *Clin Perinatol* 2001;28(3):655–669, vii–viii.
68. Siew ML, Te Pas AB, Wallace MJ, et al. Surfactant increases the uniformity of lung aeration at birth in ventilated preterm rabbits. *Pediatr Res* 2011;70(1):50–55.
69. Carnielli VP, Giorgetti C, Simonato M, et al. Neonatal respiratory diseases in the newborn infant: novel insights from stable isotope tracer studies. *Neonatology* 2016;109(4):325–333.
70. Cavicchioli P, Zimmermann LJ, Cogo PE, et al. Endogenous surfactant turnover in preterm infants with respiratory distress syndrome studied with stable isotope lipids. *Am J Respir Crit Care Med* 2001;163(1):55–60.
71. Bunt JE, Carnielli VP, Janssen DJ, et al. Treatment with exogenous surfactant stimulates endogenous surfactant synthesis in premature infants with respiratory distress syndrome. *Crit Care Med* 2000;28(10):3383–3388.
72. Jobe AH, Ikegami M, Seidner SR, et al. Surfactant phosphatidylcholine metabolism and surfactant function in preterm, ventilated lambs. *Am Rev Respir Dis* 1989;139(2):352–359.
73. Rebello CM, Jobe AH, Eisele JW, et al. Alveolar and tissue surfactant pool sizes in humans. *Am J Respir Crit Care Med* 1996;154(3 Pt 1):625–628.
74. Ueda T, Ikegami M, Jobe AH. Developmental changes of sheep surfactant: in vivo function and in vitro subtype conversion. *J Appl Physiol (1985)* 1994;76(6):2701–2706.
75. Ueda T, Ikegami M, Jobe A. Surfactant subtypes. In vitro conversion, in vivo function, and effects of serum proteins. *Am J Respir Crit Care Med* 1994;149(5):1254–1259.
76. Been JV, Rours IG, Kornelisse RF, et al. Chorioamnionitis alters the response to surfactant in preterm infants. *J Pediatr* 2010;156(1):10.e1–15.e1.
77. Seger N, Soll R. Animal derived surfactant extract for treatment of respiratory distress syndrome. *Cochrane Database Syst Rev* 2009;(2):CD007836.
78. Horbar JD, Carpenter JH, Buzas J, et al. Collaborative quality improvement to promote evidence based surfactant for preterm infants: a cluster randomised trial. *BMJ* 2004; 329(7473):1004.
79. Zola EM, Overbach AM, Gunkel JH, et al. Treatment Investigational New Drug experience with Survanta (beractant). *Pediatrics* 1993;91(3):546–551.
80. Ueda T, Ikegami M, Rider ED, et al. Distribution of surfactant and ventilation in surfactant-treated preterm lambs. *J Appl Physiol (1985)* 1994;76(1):45–55.
81. Schmolzer GM, Kumar M, Pichler G, et al. Non-invasive versus invasive respiratory support in preterm infants at birth: systematic review and meta-analysis. *BMJ* 2013;347:f5980.
82. Wiingreen R, Greisen G, Ebbesen F, et al. Surfactant need by gestation for very preterm babies initiated on early nasal CPAP: a Danish Observational Multicentre Study of 6,628 infants born 2000-2013. *Neonatology* 2017;111(4):331–336.
83. Chun J, Sung SI, Ho YH, et al. Prophylactic versus early rescue surfactant treatment in preterm infants born at less than 30 weeks gestation or with birth weight less than or equal 1,250 grams. *J Korean Med Sci* 2017;32(8):1288–1294.
84. Kurepa D, Perveen S, Lipener Y, et al. The use of less invasive surfactant administration (LISA) in the United States with review of the literature. *J Perinatol* 2019;39(3):426–432.
85. Langhammer K, Roth B, Kribs A, et al. Treatment and outcome data of very low birth weight infants treated with less invasive surfactant administration in comparison to intubation and mechanical ventilation in the clinical setting of a cross-sectional observational multicenter study. *Eur J Pediatr* 2018;177(8):1207–1217.
86. Roberts KD, Brown R, Lampland AL, et al. Laryngeal mask airway for surfactant administration in neonates: a randomized, controlled trial. *J Pediatr* 2018;193:40.e41–46.e41.
87. Minocchieri S, Berry CA, Pillow JJ; CureNeb Study Team. Nebulised surfactant to reduce severity of respiratory distress: a blinded, parallel, randomised controlled trial. *Arch Dis Child Fetal Neonatal Ed* 2019;104(3):F313–F319.
88. Sweet DG, Turner MA, Stranak Z, et al. A first-in-human clinical study of a new SP-B and SP-C enriched synthetic surfactant (CHF5633) in preterm babies with respiratory distress syndrome. *Arch Dis Child Fetal Neonatal Ed* 2017;102(6):F497–F503.
89. Ikegami M, Polk D, Tabor B, et al. Corticosteroid and thyrotropin-releasing hormone effects on preterm sheep lung function. *J Appl Physiol* (1985) 1991;70(5):2268–2278.

CHAPTER 47

Jan Bonhoeffer
Ulrich Heininger

Childhood Vaccines

INTRODUCTION

Childhood vaccines are used to prevent infectious diseases and their complications. A brief overview of the milestones in the history of human vaccines is presented in Table 47.1. Opportunities to reduce morbidity and mortality globally vary depending on the regional epidemiology of the target disease. Possibilities to implement national immunization programs largely depend on the countries' health systems and resources. Accordingly, vaccines are produced in many facilities around the globe, resulting in a wide variety of available products. Therefore, neonatal and pediatric pharmacologists will need to familiarize themselves with the local immunization schedules and available products. This chapter aims to provide a comprehensive overview of the basic principles and pharmacologic aspects of vaccines, disease-specific immunization strategies, and a framework for clinical decision-making on indications, contraindications, and safety evaluation of vaccines for the benefit of the individuals receiving them.

GENERAL PRINCIPLES OF VACCINE IMMUNITY

Vaccines are generally given to healthy individuals to induce specific immunity. Healthy neonates are born with some degree of unspecific innate immunity. This is conferred by the skin and mucosal membranes as mechanical barriers, by soluble factors (e.g., lysozyme, complement system, acute-phase proteins), and cells (e.g., phagocytes, natural killer cells). Once an organism has overcome the barriers, proteolytic cascades will aim to wall off the antigen, followed by antigen-presenting cells or dendritic cells engulfing and processing the antigen and presenting them to T-helper cells and B lymphocytes on their surface. As a result of the interaction of these cell types, the adaptive immune system will either mount a humoral or a cellular immune response (Fig. 47.1).

At the core of the humoral immune response, B lymphocytes will develop into plasma cells, producing antigen-specific–neutralizing antibodies. As part of a primary immune response,

TABLE 47.1 Milestones in the History of Human Vaccines

Year	*Live Vaccine*	*Inactivated Vaccine*	*Component Vaccine*	*Genetic Vaccine*
1774/1796	Smallpox			
1885	Rabies			
1896		Typhoid		
1896		Cholera		
1897		Plague		
1923			Diphtheria	
1926		Pertussis		
1927	Tuberculosis			
1935	Yellow fever			
1936	Influenza			
1955		Poliomyelitis		
1960	Poliomyelitis			
1967	Mumps			
1968	Measles			
1969	Rubella			
1971			Influenza (reassortant)	
1971		Tick-borne encephalitis		

(continued)

TABLE 47.1 Milestones in the History of Human Vaccines (*continued*)

Year	*Live Vaccine*	*Inactivated Vaccine*	*Component Vaccine*	*Genetic Vaccine*
1974	Varicella			
1975	Typhus			
1977			Pneumococcal (polysaccharide, 14-valent)	
1980			Tick-borne encephalitis	
1981			Hepatitis B (plasma)	
1981			Pertussis (acellular)	
1982			Meningococcal (polysaccharide, A+C+W135+Y)	
1984			Pneumococcal (polysaccharide, 23-valent)	
1985			*Haemophilus influenzae* (polysaccharide)	
1986			Hepatitis B (inactivated)	Recombinant protein
1987			*H. influenzae* (conjugate)	
1992			Hepatitis A	
1998	Rotavirus			Human-rhesus reassortant
1999			Meningococcal C (conjugate, monovalent)	
2000			Pneumococcal (conjugate, 7-valent)	
2003	Influenza			Cold adapted, intranasal
2005	Measles–mumps–rubella–varicella			
2005	Rotavirus, pentavalent Rotavirus, monovalent			Bovine assorted Human, attenuated
2005			Meningococcal (conjugate, A+C+W135+Y)	
2006			Human papillomavirus (6,-11,-16,-19)	Recombinant protein
2007			Human papillomavirus (-16,-18)	
2007	Herpes zoster			
2009			Pneumococcal (conjugate, 10-valent)	
2005			Meningococcal (conjugate, A+C+W135+Y)	
2010			Pneumococcal (conjugate, 13-valent)	
2012	Influenza (trivalent)			Cold adapted
2013			Influenza (tetravalent)	Reassortant
2013			Meningococcal B (4-component protein)	"Reverse vaccinology"
2015			Human papillomavirus (9-valent)	
2015	Dengue			
2017			Meningococcal B (factor H–binding protein)	
2017			Herpes zoster	Recombinant
2019			Ebola	Recombinant, replication-competent viral vector
2019	Smallpox			
2019			Dengue	

typically, immunoglobulin M (IgM) antibodies with low affinity start appearing after approximately 7 to 10 days. This is followed by a switch to increasingly produced IgG with peak concentrations 2 to 6 weeks after infection or immunization. A subset of B lymphocytes will differentiate into memory cells to allow for recognition of previously identified antigens and to confer duration of immunity. A secondary immune response after re-exposure to the same antigen will typically lead to a strong increase (hence "booster" reaction) of IgG, while IgM response will be minimal or absent. The IgG-booster responses will be fast (4 to 5 days), antigen-binding specificity will be improved, and the strength of molecular affinity of the IgG will be increased, that is, increased antibody avidity. A typical pattern of primary and secondary immune response is shown in Figure 47.2.

Duration of immunity depends on the activation and differentiation of memory B and T cells. This memory is generally long lasting and independent of the circulation and re-exposure to wild-type organisms.[1,2]

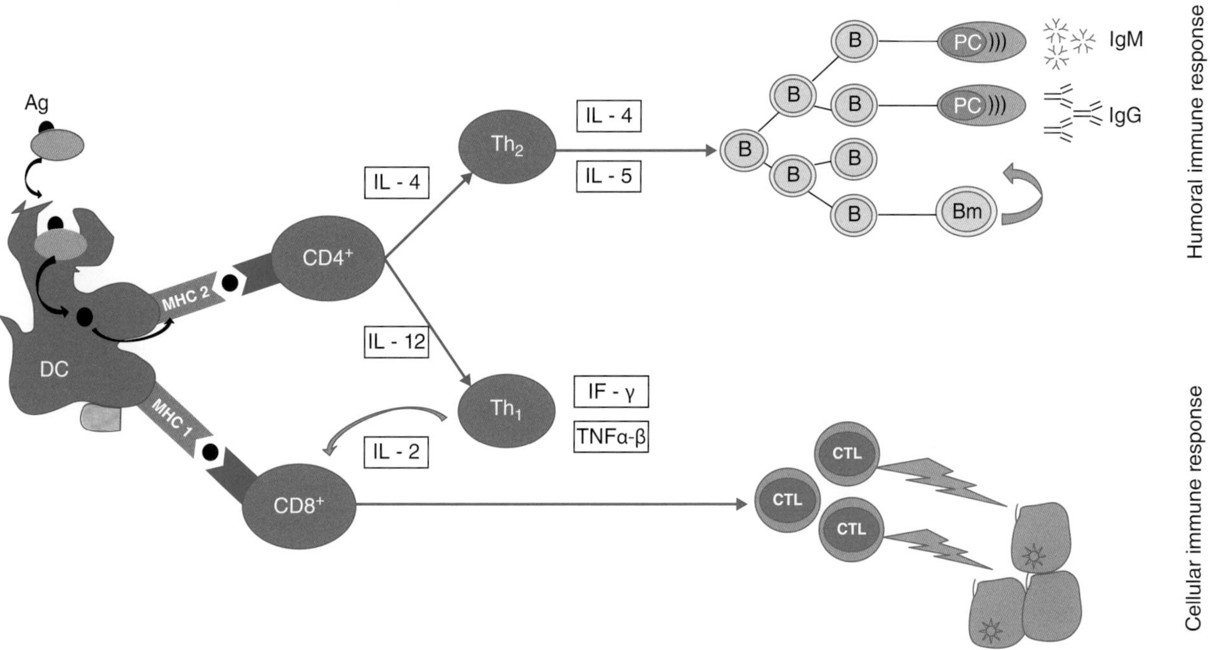

Figure 47.1 T-cell–dependent immune responses to immunization. Modified with permission from Heininger U: Impfratgeber, 10. Auflage, UNI-MED Verlag Bremen.

These T-cell–dependent immune responses are observed in response to protein antigens. In contrast, lipoprotein and particularly polysaccharide antigens illicit T-cell–independent immune responses.[3,4] Here, the antigen is directly recognized by B-cell surface molecules rather than presented by dendritic cells via MHC peptide complexes. This implies a rapid response, but only minimal memory and minimal switch from IgM to IgG such that a strong increase in IgG levels following re-exposure is absent (Fig. 47.3). This has important consequences for developing vaccines against organisms with virulence factors primarily comprised of polysaccharides (e.g., encapsulated *Haemophilus influenzae*, meningococci, pneumococci). Humoral immunity is the traditional hallmark of determining the immune response to vaccines.[5]

While cellular immunity—conferred by T cells recognizing antigens of viruses or intracellular bacteria presented on the surface of infected cells—may be the primary mechanism of neutralization and protection, measurement in the routine clinical setting remains challenging. In contrast, concomitant humoral immune responses against such organisms can be measured, and the level of some of these responses is taken as a surrogate marker of immunity once their correlation with vaccine effectiveness has been demonstrated.[6] Still, measure of individual protection is not part of routine immunization programs.

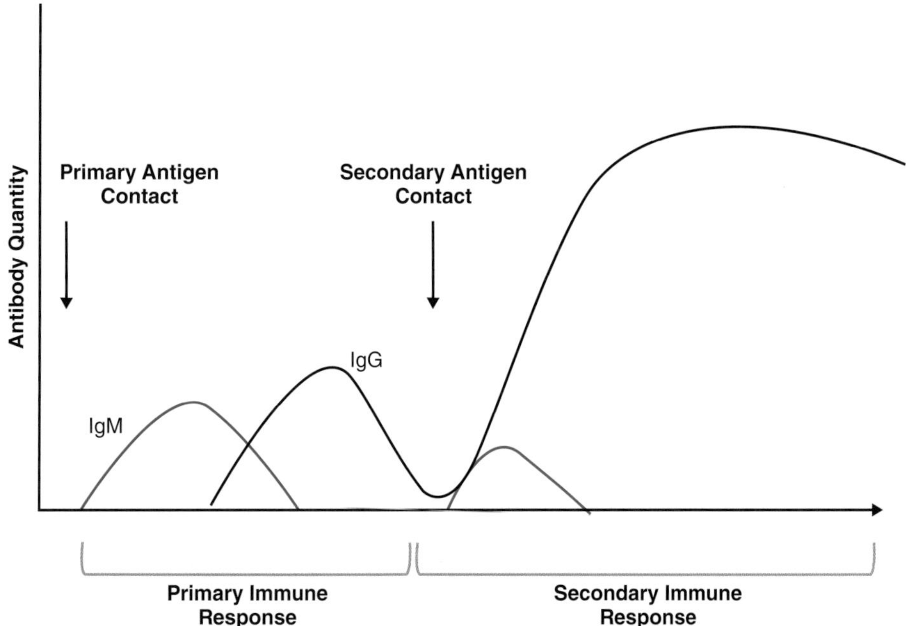

Figure 47.2 T-cell–dependent primary and secondary immune response. Modified with permission from Heininger U: Impfratgeber, 10. Auflage, UNI-MED Verlag Bremen.

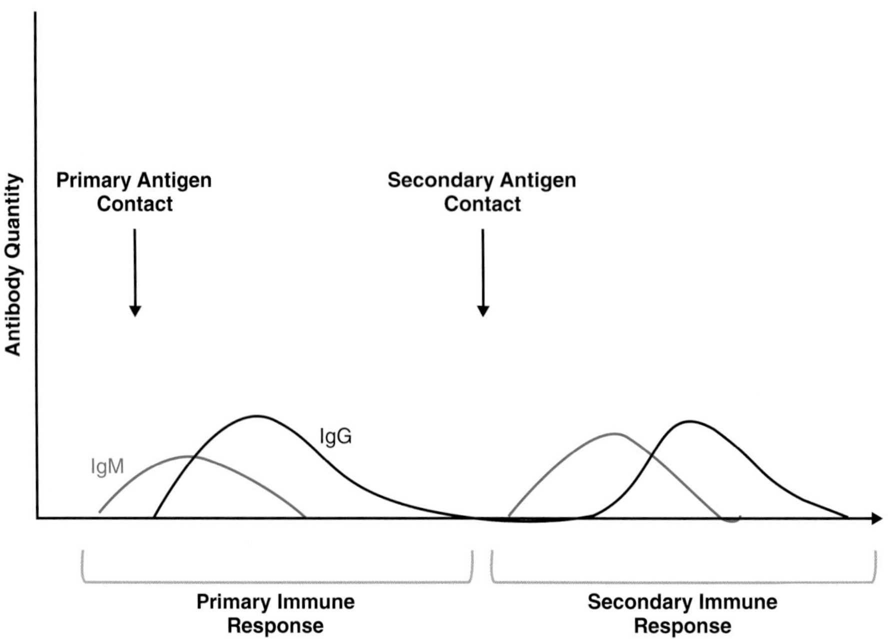

Figure 47.3 T-cell–independent primary and secondary immune response. Modified with permission from Heininger U: Impfratgeber, 10. Auflage, UNI-MED Verlag Bremen.

BASIC APPROACHES TO ACHIEVING VACCINE-INDUCED IMMUNITY

Immunization is the act of targeted, intentional, artificial induction of immunity, thereby providing protection against disease. There are two main approaches to achieve this aim: passive and active immunization. Passive immunization is defined by the transfer of antibodies into the organism to be temporarily protected. A natural example of passive immunization is the transplacental transfer of antibodies to the fetus, providing nest protection for the first 3 to 9 months of infant life. Typical indications for injected passive immunization are pre- and postexposure prophylaxis (PrEP and PEP) in individuals with limited immunity and increased risk of acquiring a specific illness. Standard human Igs are widely available. However, disease-specific antibody concentrations vary and may be insufficient. Preparations of disease-specific IgG derived from pooled plasma of either humans (homologous) or animals (heterologous) are available. An overview of available Igs and frequent indications is provided in Table 47.2.

Heterologous antibodies are only used for indications where no homologous donor is available (e.g., *Clostridium botulinum* and *Clostridium perfringens*). Prior to any application of heterologous Ig, a skin-prick test with the solution should be performed by applying a single drop of a 1:100 dilution (0.1 mL in 10 mL 0.9% NaCl) to the volar surface of the forearm puncturing the skin with a fine subcutaneous (SC) cannula through the drop. Should a local allergic reaction be noted, desensitization should be performed according to the recommendation of the American Academy of Pediatrics[7] (Table 47.3)

The duration of passive immunity is dose dependent, with an IgG half-life of about 6 weeks. The recommended dosing generally intends to provide immunity for 4 to 6 weeks. Thus, after 4 weeks, a follow-up dose may be necessary.

Active immunization is defined as a controlled infection, whereby antigens are induced into the organism to achieve long-lasting immunity. This is accomplished by appropriately activating the host's immune system to yield immune responses, resembling those against the respective wild-type infection. The determinants of effect and duration of immunity include

- the vaccine type (e.g., live vs. inactivated)
- the construct (e.g., polysaccharide vs. conjugated, or combination vaccine)
- the schedule (e.g., age at immunization, interval between doses, environmental factors)
- the route of administration

The recommended ages of immunization and intervals between doses in the various national immunization programs vary to align with other preventive health measures and programs for neonates and children in the respective country. For administration of doses outside the routine schedules, the minimal time of 4 weeks between primary doses and 4 months between prime and boost doses should generally be observed. Accelerated schedules are available for some vaccines (e.g., hepatitis B [HB], tick-borne encephalitis [TBE]).

Simultaneous immunization is defined by providing active and passive immunity simultaneously. This may be necessary in situations where immediate protection is required until adaptive immunity has emerged in response to active immunization. This approach is only possible with inactivated vaccines, for example, PEP of tetanus, HB, or rabies. Simultaneous immunization with live virus vaccines is not successful as the passively administered Igs would interfere with replication of the attenuated live vaccine organisms. For the same reason, following the administration of disease-specific antibodies or standard Ig, administration of live-attenuated vaccines [e.g., measles, mumps, and rubella (MMR)] needs to be postponed for at least 3 months, because the administered antibodies will inhibit replication and immune response to these vaccines.

TABLE 47.2 Immunoglobulins Used for Passive Immunization and Their Indications

Product	*Major Indications*
Immunoglobulin for i.m. injection	• Replacement therapy in primary immunodeficiency disorders • Hepatitis A prophylaxis • Measles prophylaxis
Intravenous immunoglobulin (IVIG)	• Replacement therapy in primary immunodeficiency disorders • Kawasaki disease • Pediatric HIV infection • Hypogammaglobulinemia in chronic B-lymphocyte lymphocytic leukemia • Immune-mediated thrombocytopenia • Hematopoietic stem cell transplantation in adults to prevent graft-versus-host disease and infection • May be useful in a variety of other conditions
Subcutaneous immunoglobulin	• Treatments of patients with primary immunodeficiencies
Hepatitis B immunoglobulin (i.m.)	• Postexposure prophylaxis • Prevention of perinatal infection in infants born to hepatitis B surface antigen–positive mothers
Rabies immunoglobulin (i.m.)	• Postexposure prophylaxis
Tetanus immunoglobulin (i.m.)	• Postexposure prophylaxis • Treatment of tetanus
Varicella-zoster immunoglobulin (i.m.) or IVIG	• Postexposure prophylaxis of susceptible people at high risk for complications from varicella
Cytomegalovirus IVIG	• Prophylaxis in seronegative transplant recipients
Vaccinia immunoglobulin (i.v.)	• Prevent or modify serious adverse events following smallpox vaccination caused by vaccinia replication
Botulism IVIG human	• Treatment of infant botulism
Diphtheria antitoxin, equine	• Treatment of diphtheria
Heptavalent botulinum antitoxin against all 7 (A-G) botulinum toxin types	• Treatments of food and wound botulism
Palivizumab (monoclonal antibody) (i.m.)	• Prophylaxis for infants against respiratory syncytial virus

i.m., intramuscularly; i.v., intravenous.

TABLE 47.3 Desensitization Prior to the Use of Heterologous Immunoglobulin by Route of Administration

Sequence[a]	*Dilution in 0.9% NaCl*	*Quantity in mL*	*Application*
1	1:1,000	0.1	i.d., i.v
2	1:1,000	0.3	i.d., i.v.
3	1:1,000	0.6	s.c., i.v.
4	1:100	0.1	s.c., i.v.
5	1:100	0.3	s.c., i.v.
6	1:100	0.6	s.c., i.v.
7	1:10	0.1	s.c., i.v.
8	1:10	0.3	s.c., i.v.
9	1:10	0.6	s.c., i.v.
10	Undiluted	0.1	s.c., i.v.
11	Undiluted	0.3	s.c., i.v.
12	Undiluted	0.6	i.m., i.v.
13	Undiluted	1.0	i.m., i.v.

[a]Every 15 minutes.
Desensitization before using heterologous immunoglobulins.
i.d., intradermally; s.c., subcutaneously; i.m., intramuscularly; i.v., intravenous.

VACCINE TYPES AND CONSTRUCTS

Vaccines are suspensions of immunizing agents. They contain either attenuated live microorganisms, killed organisms, fractions thereof, or nontoxic modifications of specific virulence factors, such as bacterial toxins (toxoids). The suspension is comprised of suspending fluid, adjuvants (variable), and other excipients. The suspending fluid is typically sterile water. This may also include substances of the biologic system in which the immunizing agent was manufactured [e.g., formaldehyde (<0.1 mg), neomycin (<0.15 mg), egg and yeasts proteins]. Adjuvants are constituents enhancing the immune response to the disease-specific antigens. Other excipients include preservatives used to prevent bacterial or fungal contamination, including phenol (<1.25 mg), 2-phenoxyethanol (< 5mg), thiomersal (<0.5 mg), and stabilizers used to promote temperature stability and prevent precipitation [e.g., $MgSO_4$, glycerin, gelatin (<14.5 mg)].[8]

Live vaccines are typically comprised of live organisms (mainly viruses, e.g., MMR, varicella-zoster, oral poliomyelitis, rotavirus) attenuated to replicate at such a low rate that a healthy immune system will mount immunity prior to manifestation of serious disease and its complications. These vaccines tend to induce lifelong protection similar to wild-type disease in those who respond. This typically takes one or two doses. Live vaccines do not need adjuvants, as the immunizing antigens are delivered in the natural context soliciting the necessary immune response.

Inactivated vaccines are typically comprised of inactivated whole organisms [e.g., hepatitis A or Japanese encephalitis (JE) viruses], extracted and purified components of the whole organism (e.g., acellular pertussis, HB, subunit influenza), toxoids (e.g., tetanus, diphtheria), or soluble components of encapsulated bacteria [e.g., *Haemophilus influenzae type b (Hib)*, meningococci, pneumococci]. Polysaccharide antigens (e.g., capsular bacterial components) are linked to carrier proteins (e.g., outer membrane proteins, tetanus toxoid) to convert T-cell–independent immune responses with limited duration of immunity to T-cell–dependent responses with durable immunity. Conjugation of polysaccharides to proteins frequently also reduces colonization by increasing effective transudation of IgG through mucosal membranes.[9] While IgA may be induced by some vaccines (e.g., oral polio, rotavirus) and they may reduce mucosal replication, immunity primarily correlates with IgG responses. Inactivated vaccines typically require a series of priming doses and a series of booster doses to provide long-time protection. This is even in spite of the inclusion of adjuvants.

Adjuvants are particularly used to enhance and modulate immune responses to vaccines. Adjuvants may be used for multiple purposes: increasing the primary response, the duration of immunity, widening cross-protection, and optimizing dose sparing for vaccines with limited supply (e.g., outbreak control of known and emerging diseases). This is particularly true for inactivated vaccines, because the complexity of the antigen is limited as compared to whole organisms.[10]

Adjuvants directly stimulate the host immune response and can be classified according to the receptor of action or their chemical properties: aluminum salts [e.g., hydroxide (Al-OH), hydroxide phosphate, hydroxyphosphate sulfate, potassium phosphate], toll-like receptor (e.g., TLR4, TLR9) agonists, saponins, and oil-in-water emulsions (e.g., MF59). Today's licensed adjuvanted diphtheria, tetanus, pertussis (DTP); *Hib*; pneumococcal; human papillomavirus (HPV); HB; and hepatitis A vaccines are generally adjuvanted with aluminum salts. Some influenza vaccines are adjuvanted with oil-in-water emulsions (e.g., squalene, tocopherol).

Aluminum salts have been used as adjuvants for almost a century, and billions of doses were administered. The mechanisms of action include slow release of antigen, leading to higher immune responses, improved antigen uptake by antigen-presenting cells, and direct activation of the Nalp3 inflammasome pathway and interaction with membrane lipids, resulting in direct CD4 T-cell activation.[11–13]

There have been reports of injection-site granulomas, as well as focal aluminum deposits associated with a diffuse syndrome named macrophagic myofasciitis (MMF). The presence of aluminum residues at the injection site is well documented, and temporary local foreign-body reactions may occur. However, the association of MMF with aluminum-containing vaccines was identified as a methodologic error in the hypothesizing study.[14] The aluminum content per dose is 0.2 to 0.85 mg per dose. While the route of administration may be different, comparison with the aluminum content in infant formula (0.2 mg per L), soy-based formula (0.4 to 0.9 mg per mL), and antacids (104 to 208 mg per tablet) is instructive.[15]

The more recent development of oil-in-water emulsions has virtually replaced the water-in-oil emulsions known for inducing injection-site granulomas and which are challenging to produce in a standardized and lot consistent manner. Oil-in-water emulsions are shown to locally recruit and activate antigen-presenting cells in direct conjunction with the antigen. Oil-and-water emulsions particularly demonstrated their benefits for H5N1 influenza campaign, when employed for antigen sparing. AS03 and MF59 are currently the two main emulsions used. Both have demonstrated excellent immunogenicity, including the observation of cross-neutralizing antibodies and increased antibody affinity.

When reused for the 2009/H1N1 global influenza pandemic, safety concerns were raised in relation to AS03-adjuvanted vaccines (see section on influenza vaccine). Further research is needed to elucidate whether causal relation can be established and whether ASO3 adjuvant may play a role.[16]

TLR agonists comprise a group of adjuvants binding to different TLR types, such as TLR4 agonists (e.g., MPL). Binding to the TLR4 activates two physiologic intracellular signaling pathways. AS04 (including MPL) has been used in a GSK manufactured HPV vaccine and has a well-established safety profile. Other TLR4 agonists are in development. TLR9 agonists make up most of the other TLR agonists used in late-stage clinical trials. These include the heterogeneous family of CpG-containing oligonucleotides. Some have been successfully tested in malaria, HIV, and next-generation HB, and pneumococcal vaccines. Other TLR ligands (e.g., TLR5, TLR7) and a rather large group of other adjuvants are being developed and evaluated in early-phase clinical trials. They are unlikely to emerge in licensed vaccines in the near future.

Combination vaccines contain antigens against multiple target diseases. This approach has become necessary to improve administration of the increasing number of vaccines and to facilitate their global dissemination and delivery without unduly increasing the number of injections and required health care contacts. Diphtheria, tetanus, and pertussis (previously with whole-cell pertussis components, DTP, since the mid-1990s with acellular pertussis components, DTaP/TdaP) were among the first combination vaccines. Polio (inactivated polio vaccine or IPV) and *H. influenzae* (*Hib*) were successively added to DTaP to form four-valent and five-valent vaccines, respectively. Finally, HB was added to achieve six-valent vaccines, of which three products are on the market in the Western world today. Of the live virus vaccines, MMR combination vaccine was one of the first and is still on the market. It has been expanded by the addition of varicella virus to make up MMRV combination vaccines, of which two are currently on the market.

In the past decades, the combination of vaccine antigens has been optimized, given the currently available technologies. In the near future, it will be challenging to add further antigens in the available constructs. Vaccines combining multiple serotypes of the same organism (e.g., pneumococci, meningococci) are generally not classified as combination vaccines, and yet, similar vaccine construct limitations occur. Thus, pharmacologists should be prepared to see novel technologies emerge with novel safety and effectiveness challenges.

The evaluation of the effectiveness of combination vaccines is complex. Yet, the currently marketed combination vaccines demonstrate satisfactory effectiveness for all antigens and demonstrate similar or favorable safety profile compared to the sum of individual vaccines. However, the local immune response may be increased, leading to increased reactogenicity of the combination vaccines as compared to the individual vaccines. In the light of fewer injections and thus an overall shorter time of exposure for possible local reactions, the use of combination vaccines in general is the preferred choice. The concern of immune system overload of combination vaccines has been raised ever since the availability of combination vaccines. As of today, the bulk of evidence including studies immunizing premature infants refutes this hypothesis.[17,18] To the contrary, there is increasing evidence that a high dose and combined antigen load is protective of autoimmune diseases and the development of allergies.[19–21]

CONTRAINDICATIONS AND PRECAUTIONS TO VACCINES

The vaccine manufacturer labels the products in line with the responsible regulatory authority. The national technical advisory committee [e.g., Advisory Committee on Immunization Practices (ACIP), in the United States] may provide modifications to both precautions and contraindications to meet population and health care professional needs. Table 47.4 outlines contraindications and precautions to common vaccine types. In general, other systemic or local adverse events neither require precautions nor represent contraindications.

Substantially immunocompromised patients are not recommended to receive live-attenuated vaccines. This includes individuals receiving greater than or equal to 2 mg per kg per day or greater than or equal to 20 mg per day of prednisone or equivalent doses of systemic corticosteroids for 2 weeks or longer or other immunosuppressive medication. This also includes severe combined immunodeficiency and severely immunocompromised patients with inborn errors of the immune system. Pregnancy is a contraindication for most live vaccines, yellow fever (YF) under certain circumstances being an exception.

EVALUATION OF ADVERSE EVENTS FOLLOWING IMMUNIZATION

Adverse events following immunization (AEFIs) are any untoward medical occurrences which follow but may not have a causal relationship with immunization. They are typically classified as local or systemic AEFI. Thus, they are either events at or near the injection site or single- or multiorgan systemic events.

Safety concerns increase with the increasing success of immunization programs. With a decreasing incidence of vaccine-preventable diseases, public attention shifts toward adverse events. When safety concerns are raised at a time when the target disease has disappeared, immunization rates will decrease with decreasing public confidence. A resurgence of disease is likely to follow. Therefore, maintaining the success of immunization programs critically relies on public confidence, which is based on public perception. Public perception depends on the quality of information provided. Therefore, information about

TABLE 47.4 Examples for Typical Contraindications and Precautions to Common Vaccine Types

Vaccine Type	*Precautions*		*Contraindication*	
DTaP/Tdap	Moderate or severe acute illness	Progressive neurologic disorders Seizure, hypotonic hyperresponsive episode, or persistent crying (≥3 h) within 3 d of DTaP History of Arthus reaction to tetanus toxoid	Severe allergic reaction to a vaccine component	Encephalopathy within 7d of DTaP
IPV		Pregnancy		
Hib		Age <6 wk		
HPV		Pregnancy		
HBV		Infant <2,000 g of HBsAg-negative women		
HAV				Pregnancy
PCV13/PPSV				
MCV4				
TIV/QIV				GBS <6 wk of TIV
LAIV		GBS <6 wk of TIV		Pregnancy Known severe immunodeficiency Selected chronic conditions defined by CDC.[22]
MMR/MMRV		History of thrombocytopenia		Pregnancy Known severe immunodeficiency
Varicella				Pregnancy Known severe immunodeficiency
Rotavirus		Immunocompromise Chronic gastrointestinal disease Spina bifida or bladder exstrophy History of intussusception		Known severe immunodeficiency

DTaP/Tdap, Diphtheria–tetanus–pertussis prime and boost doses; IPV, inactivated polio vaccine; *Hib, Haemophilus influenzae*, type b; HPV, human papillomavirus; HBV, hepatitis B virus; HAV, hepatitis A virus; PCV13/PPSV; 13-valent pneumococcal conjugate vaccine/pneumococcal polysaccharide vaccine; MCV4, tetravalent meningococcal vaccine; TIV/QIV, trivalent and quadrivalent inactivated influenza vaccine; LAIV, live-attenuated influenza vaccine; MMR/MMRV, measles–mumps–rubella/measles–mumps–rubella with varicella.

the safety of immunization needs to be placed on the most rigorous scientific basis possible. This requires high-quality data being collected and reported to the competent authorities. Withdrawal of the product from the market, modification of pertinent recommendations, or continued supply depends on rapid and thorough evaluation of patients with AEFI.

Introduction of new vaccines into national immunization programs should be accompanied by appropriate safety surveillance.[23]

VACCINE SAFETY CONCERNS OF INDIVIDUALS

As vaccines are highly standardized products delivered to a highly nonstandardized population across the globe, unanticipated responses to immunization may occur. While it is comforting to know that most children will not experience AEFI, some do, and we might learn from analyzing such cases more closely rather than disregarding them as part of statistical background noise. It is the study of these subgroups that will provide further insight into specific and nonspecific reactions to immunologic stimuli in terms of safety and immunogenicity.

AEFI presenting with a clinical syndrome above and beyond the normal response to vaccines should be evaluated, classified, and reported. Figure 47.4 outlines a proposed workflow for clinical pharmacologists in collaboration with the attending pediatrician.[24] Reporting of AEFI should follow the national regulations and international guidance. Publication of AEFI or safety data should follow international harmonization efforts

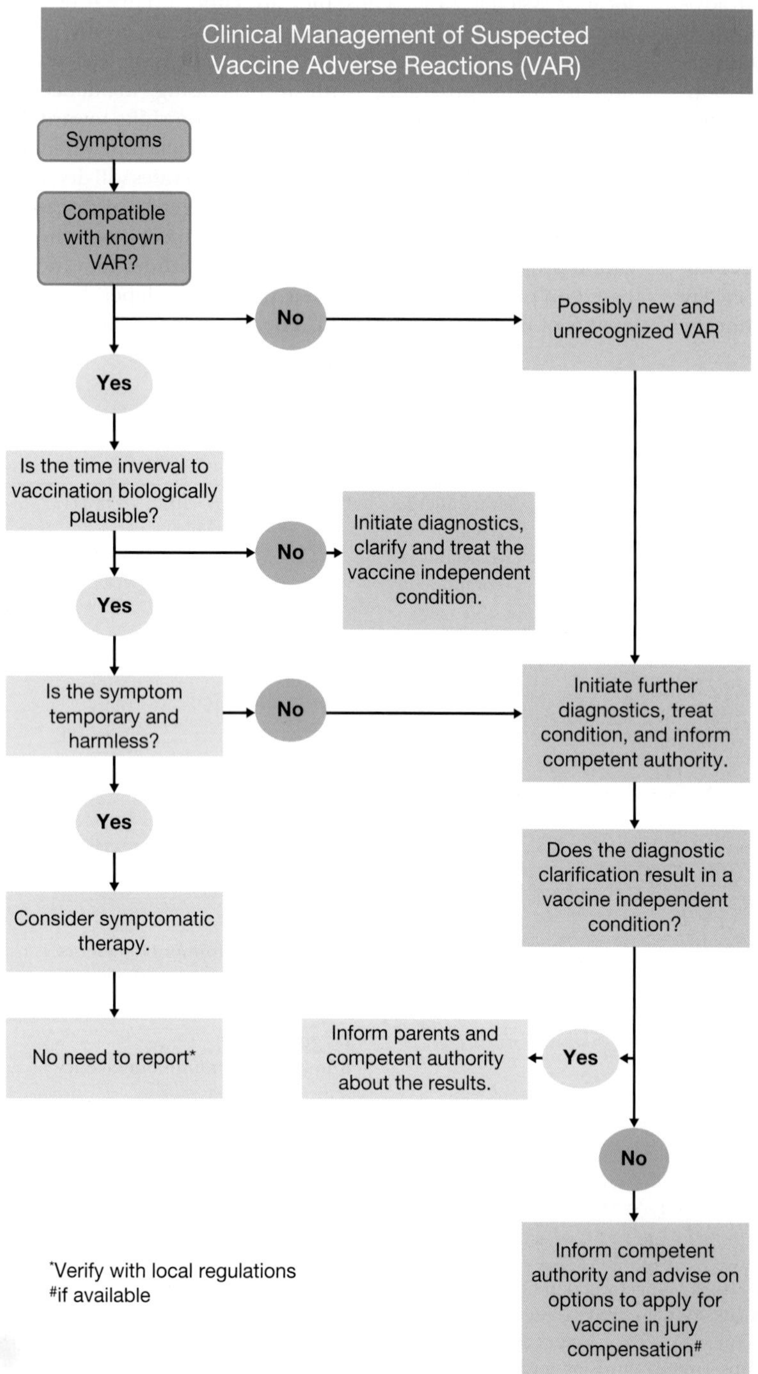

Figure 47.4 Flow diagram for the clinical evaluation of patients with adverse event following immunization. Modified with permission from Heininger U: Impfratgeber, 10. Auflage, UNI-MED Verlag Bremen.

and guidance, to give additional value to individual data by allowing data comparability, meta-analysis, or pooling in support of the overall scientific learning curve.

Although temporal association is a necessary condition, it is insufficient to establish a causal relation. Even a biologically plausible temporal association is not sufficient to assume a causal relation. In fact, assumed biologic plausibility has often been misleading and thus provided a more sophisticated variant of the *post hoc ergo propter hoc* fallacy. The term "vaccine adverse reaction" (VAR) or "side effect" should only be used if a causal relation between an AEFI and immunization has been established based on the appropriate Hill criteria (e.g., consistency, strength of association, specificity, temporality, biologic plausibility).[25,26] Table 47.5 outlines AEFI for which current scientific evidence does not support the hypothesis of a causal relation.

AEFIs causally related to immunization are called side effects or vaccine adverse reactions (VARs). Immunization is an induced, controlled stimulus to the immune system; thus, some adverse reactions can be expected. Immunization safety concerns have existed since the day of the first available vaccine, and the history of raving successes of immunization has been repeatedly clouded by outright vaccine safety disasters. Today, most VAR of currently licensed vaccines are transient and mild, and the health benefits of saving children from tragic outcomes of common infectious diseases by far outweigh the risks of immunizations.

Local reactions including injection-site swelling, redness, induration, and pain can be an expression of the intended immune response or maybe unduly severe. This is also true for systemic events, such as, fever. Beyond a mild, expected systemic response with, for example, low-grade fever and general discomfort and tiredness, the immune response may be so pronounced to cause high fever (>40°C) or to uncover underlying disease promoted by any febrile illness (e.g., febrile seizures, severe myoclonic epilepsy of infancy). VARs may occur within 3 days following inactivated vaccines or according to the incubation period of live-attenuated vaccines (e.g., 5 to 12 days following MMRV vaccination). The hypothetical risk window for autoimmune disease is generally deemed to be 6 weeks (e.g., Guillain–Barré syndrome or GBS). Table 47.6 outlines serious AEFI for which there is some scientific evidence in support

TABLE 47.5 AEFI for Which Current Scientific Evidence Does Not Support the Hypothesis of a Causal Relation with Immunization

Adverse Events Following Immunization	*Alleged Vaccine*
Atopic disease	Several
Autism	Measles–mumps–rubella
Crohn disease	Measles–mumps–rubella
Chronic arthritis	Rubella
Encephalopathy	Pertussis, measles
Ethyl-mercury toxicity	Several
Guillain–Barré syndrome	Meningococcal
Autoimmune diseases, various	Human papillomavirus
Insulin-dependent diabetes mellitus	*Haemophilus influenzae* type b Hepatitis B
Macrophagic myofasciitis	Aluminum-adjuvant–containing vaccines
Multiple sclerosis	Hepatitis B
Squalene toxicity	Influenza, anthrax
Sudden infant death syndrome	Several

AEFI, adverse event following immunization.

TABLE 47.6 AEFI for Which There is Some Scientific Evidence in Support of the Hypothesis of a Causal Relation with Immunization

Adverse Events Following Immunization	*Vaccine*	*Pathogenesis*
Anaphylaxis	• Measles–mumps–rubella • Varicella • Influenza • Polio, trivalent inactivated	Coombs type 1 (gelatin, neomycin, latex?)
Extensive limb swelling	• Diphtheria–tetanus–acellular pertussis (booster doses) • Pneumococcal conjugate • Influenza	Unknown (activation of memory CD4+ T-helper and Langerhans cells?)
Flaccid paralysis	Oral polio vaccine	Reversion of live-attenuated virus to pathogenicity
Guillain–Barré syndrome	Influenza	Unknown
Intussusception	Rotavirus	Unknown
Meningitis	Mumps (Urabe, Leningrad–Zagreb)	Unknown (insufficient attenuation of live virus?)
Oculo-respiratory syndrome	Influenza	Unknown (virion aggregates?)
Thrombocytopenia	• Measles–mumps–rubella • Varicella	Unknown (cross-reacting antibodies?)

AEFI, adverse event following immunization.

of the hypothesis of a causal relation with currently available immunizations.

Causality assessment is a critical part of pre- and postlicensure AEFI monitoring and comprises the systematic review of data about an AEFI case to determine the likelihood of a causal association between the event and the vaccine(s) received. The second edition of the user manual for the revised World Health Organization (WHO) causality classification includes a checklist and classification process in four categories: (a) inconsistent causal association with immunization, (b) consistent causal association to immunization, (c) indetermined, and (d) unclassifiable (Fig. 47.5).

PUBLISHED VACCINE SAFETY CONCERNS

Immunization safety concerns are different from concerns about other medical interventions, because they are administered to generally healthy individuals and the tolerance of adverse events is substantially lower compared to adverse events following medication for an existing illness. As successful vaccination programs span whole populations with everyone exposed and several generations over time, hardly any doctor, nurse, or parent may have ever seen the prevented diseases. Thus, it is an increasing challenge to evaluate and communicate the benefits of immunization in the apparent absence of disease and the presence of AEFIs, even if mild. Of concern, rare and serious AEFI suspected to be VAR and published as a vaccine safety concern rapidly spread by modern media and access to data.

Immunization safety concerns often follow a recognizable pattern: the alleged AEFI is a prevalent medical entity of increasing prevalence or unknown cause; the AEFI is suggested to be caused by immunization by some investigators; the methodology of the "index study" (and subsequent studies by the same study group) is inadequate (typically poorly or not controlled case series); public communication is made prematurely and resonating with individuals suffering from the medical entity, but underestimating the potential of harming those who could be protected by the vaccine; the results of the "index study" are not reproducible by other study groups; regaining public confidence thereafter is a slow process over several years as the evidence of an absent causal association and the rejection of the initial hypothesis takes years and is generally difficult to communicate. Particularly in the early phase of communicated AEFI, hypothesized to be VAR, methodologic scrutiny of the evidence base, prudent communication, and considering the advice of national vaccine advisory committees have proven to be beneficial. Useful online resources are provided in Table 47.7.

IMMUNIZATION IN SPECIAL CIRCUMSTANCES

IMMUNIZATION IN PREGNANCY

Until recently, immunization in pregnancy was considered a significant risk. However, this was primarily based on a lack of data and unfounded assumptions. The assessment of benefits and risks of vaccination in pregnancy has dramatically changed, due to increasing insights into the immunology of vaccines and the immune system in both the mother and the infant during and immediately after pregnancy.[27,28] There is now increasing evidence that vaccination in pregnancy with inactivated vaccines is

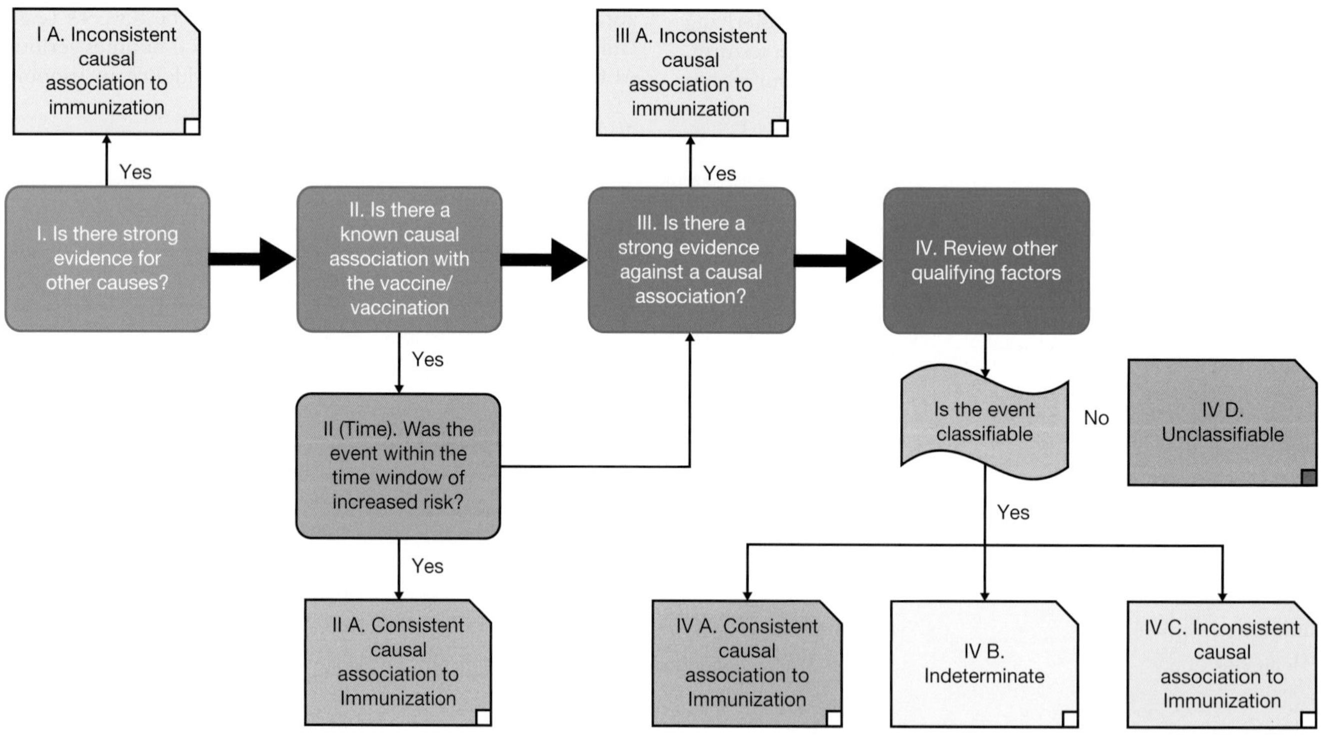

Figure 47.5 World Health Organization classification algorithm for causality assessment of adverse event following immunization.

TABLE 47.7 Organizations Providing Information Based on Highest Scientific Standards

Source	*Website*
World Health Organization	https://www.who.int/vaccine_safety/en/ https://www.vaccinesafetynet.org/
Centers for Disease Control and Prevention	www.cdc.gov/vaccines
American Academy of Pediatrics	www.aap.org/immunization
Institute for Vaccine Safety	www.vaccinesafety.edu
Immunization Action Coalition	www.immunize.org www.vaccineinformation.org
National Network for Immunization Information	www.immunizationinfo.org
Vaccine Education Center at The Children's Hospital of Philadelphia	https://www.chop.edu/centers-programs/vaccine-education-center
The Brighton Collaboration	www.brightoncollaboration.org
The Vaccine Page	www.vaccines.org

effective in addressing the U.N. Sustainable Development Goals of improving maternal health, reducing the rate of stillbirths, and decreasing neonatal mortality and morbidity.[29]

This is achieved by transfer of maternal antibody across the placenta to the fetus to result in protection from target diseases in the first few months of life when the respective diseases may be severe and preventable.

There is no evidence that any inactivated vaccine may cause harm in pregnancy, and there is an increasing global effort to optimize the quality of safety data as immunization programs are implemented globally.[30–32] Live virus vaccines inadvertently administered to pregnant women have not shown to harm either the mother or the fetus, with the exception of smallpox vaccine. In contrast, no cases of congenital rubella or varicella have been reported in infants born to women with inadvertent immunization during pregnancy.[33,34]

Today, immunization in pregnancy against DTP, influenza, and HB (risk based) is recommended in many countries worldwide. Assessment of rubella and varicella immunity and catch-up immunization in women of childbearing age are widely recommended. Evaluation in pregnancy and immunization immediately after birth are recommended for those susceptible during pregnancy. Further evidence on the possibly favorable safety profile of (postexposure) MMR immunization in pregnancy is needed to evaluate whether the potential risks of immunization outweigh the high risk of wild-type disease and its complications following confirmed exposure. Routine pregnancy testing of women of childbearing age before administering a live virus vaccine is not recommended.[35,36]

Further vaccines, including respiratory syncytial virus (RSV), group B streptococcus, and cytomegalovirus (CMV), are in clinical testing and may become available for use in pregnancy in the near future.

VACCINATION OF PRETERM INFANTS

Neonates constitute 45% of deaths among children under the age of 5 years worldwide.[37] Preterm and low birth weight infants are at increased risk of infections and suffer from an increased frequency and severity of vaccine-preventable infections. Twenty percent of hospitalized very low birth weight infants suffer from one or more systemic infections.[38] Over 50% of reported cases of pertussis occur in infants and low birth weight infants, and they are at almost double the risk when compared to normal birth weight infants [relative risk (RR) 1.86; 95% confidence interval (CI) 1.33–2.38].[39]

Transplacental maternal antibodies play an important role in protecting neonates in the first approximately 6 months of life. However, transfer of antibodies begins with 14 to 16 weeks of gestation and reaches effective levels by 32 weeks of gestation. Therefore, premature infants would benefit from either maternal or neonatal vaccination as their maternally derived antibody levels are lower and persist for a shorter time as compared to term infants.

A key challenge of immunizing infants, and particularly preterm infants, is that both B- and T-cell responses are subject to immune maturation.[40,41] The development of adaptive immunity may be divided into two phases: phase 1 is characterized by preventing alloimmune reactions between the mother and the fetus; $CD4^+$ differentiation is polarized toward Th2 and Th17 pathways, weak Th1 activation, and consecutively low interferon (IFN)-γ. This corresponds to susceptibility to typical neonatal bacterial, viral, and parasitic infections.[42]

Immunization and birth with Bacillus Calmette–Guérin (BCG), oral polio, and HB vaccine have proven the principle of successful early-life immunization programs.[43] Immune adaptation to extrauterine life starts at the time of birth rather than the expected date of delivery. Thus, following the routine schedule based on postnatal age rather than developmental age leads to protective immunity and is recommended in spite of the described immunologic differences between these age groups.[44] An exception to this rule are preterm infants with a birth weight of less than 2,000 g receiving hepatitis B virus (HBV) vaccine. Infants born to hepatitis B surface antigen (HBsAg)–positive mothers should receive simultaneous HBV vaccine and hepatitis B immunoglobulin (HBIG) within 12 hours of birth. This first dose of HBV vaccine should be supplemented by three additional doses in infants weighing less than 2,000 g at birth (0-1-2-12 month schedule).[45]

The safety of this schedule in preterm infants was demonstrated. Particularly the concern of an increased risk of apneas and bradycardias premature infants could not be verified.[46] However, as cardiorespiratory events are observed among preterm infants, a precautionary 48- to 72-hour hospitalization for the first dose is recommended for infants born less than 28 weeks of gestation. For those demonstrating bradycardias or apnea following the first dose, the same is recommended for the second dose.

VACCINATION OF IMMUNOCOMPROMISED INDIVIDUALS

Immunocompromised hosts are of increased risk of vaccine-preventable diseases, which may be life-threatening to them. This heterogeneous group of patients includes infants and children with primary and acquired immunodeficiency as well as those with immunosuppressive disease or treatment. In this group, inactivated vaccines are safe and recommended. Influenza vaccine is recommended also for its indirectly protective effect on invasive bacterial disease. Live vaccines are contraindicated as the attenuated organism may replicate uncontrolled. Therefore, immunization of household and health care contacts with injected live vaccines is recommended to provide herd protection. Oral polio vaccine should be replaced by IPV, and immunocompromised patients should avoid contact with stool from infants vaccinated with rotavirus vaccine for at least 14 days. Following confirmed exposure, passive immunization may be the only option to directly protect immunocompromised patients from diseases otherwise protected with live vaccines.

For HIV-positive infants and children, measles and varicella are likely to cause life-threatening illness. As an exemption, these children may be granted live measles vaccine if $CD4^+$ counts are above 25% in infants, above 20% in 12 to 35 months old, and above 15% in children older than 36 months. A second exemption form children with chronic granulomatous disease (CGD) and complement disorders. Both groups may receive MMR and varicella vaccines.[47]

Isolated IgA deficiency or IgG subclass defects do not represent a contraindication to immunization with any vaccine. Neither is the administration of oral corticosteroids of less than 2 mg prednisone per kg per day (max. 20 mg) for less than 2 weeks.

Patients with structural or functional asplenia may and should receive all routine immunizations, particularly including protection against encapsulated bacteria (i.e., pneumococci, meningococci, *Hib*).

Timing of immunization is critical for all immunocompromised individuals. Whenever possible, immunizations should be given prior to the onset of immunocompromise (e.g., elective splenectomy, solid organ or bone marrow transplant, start of immunosuppressive medication against chronic inflammatory disorders). If the course of disease does not allow such planning, immunization should start or resume as soon as possible after immunosuppression. The time interval and schedule vary depending on the underlying condition. Current recommendations are summarized in Table 47.8.

The German national vaccine advisory group "STIKO" has recently performed comprehensive literature reviews, summarizing all current evidence on safety and efficiency of immunizations in immunocompromised hosts.[48,49]

ALLERGIES

Patients with significant (type 1) allergies against vaccine components may not be immunized. Sensitization to egg protein (e.g., ovalbumin) is the most common form. It may be comprised in YF, influenza, MMR (most are propagated in chicken embryo cell cultures), TBE, and rabies vaccines. With the exception of YF vaccine, generally, no allergic reactions are observed in spite of preexisting sensitization. Allergic reactions following immunization may occur in one in a million doses. They are antigen specific, and neither will induce nor promote sensitization to environmental allergens. To the contrary, patients with atopic disease benefit from protection against infectious diseases.

MIGRANTS

Migrant health is an increasingly relevant immunization challenge. Often, immunizations are documented only at the health care provider in the home country, or the immunization record is lost by the time of arrival. As a rule, only documented immunizations count. Children should receive primary immunization according to the pediatric catch-up schedule or completion of the schedule—if further doses have been documented. Further, two doses of MMR and varicella vaccine are recommended, unless a reliable history of previous varicella (disease) can be obtained. Finally, influenza immunization should be offered.

TABLE 47.8 Vaccines Recommended for Patients with Acquired Immunocompromise

		Recommendation	
Condition	*Vaccine*	*Pre*	*Post*
Solid organ transplant	Inactivated	All routine immunizations prior to transplantation	Lack of evidence (continue with interval of at least 2 mo after transplant)
	Live		Contraindicated
Chronic inflammatory disorders	Inactivated	All routine immunizations prior to transplantation	Continue according to schedule, aim for treatment gap, if feasible
	Live		Contraindicated unless corticosteroid treatment <2 mg/kg/d (20 mg) prednisone
Stem cell transplant, allogenic	Inactivated	Immunity transferred by donor but waning	(6-) 12 mo after transplant (3-) 6 mo for flu and PCV Boost PCV at 12 mo if GVHD
	Live		>24 mo after transplant (schedule 0-6) Contraindicated if GVHD
Stem cell transplant, autologous	Inactivated	Immunity will be lost	>(4-) 6 mo after transplant.[50,51]
	Live		>24 mo after transplant (schedule 0-6)

GVHD, graft-versus-host disease; PCV, pneumococcal conjugate vaccine.

ROUTINE CHILDHOOD IMMUNIZATIONS

DIPHTHERIA–TETANUS–PERTUSSIS COMPONENT COMBINATION VACCINES

Illnesses

Diphtheria is a highly contagious disease caused by *Corynebacterium diphtheriae.* It typically presents with severe pharyngitis with the formation of white pseudomembranes. The toxin causes fatal damage of the respiratory epithelium, heart, and nerves and other organ systems. Without treatment, mortality is up to 20%.[52] The predominant route of transmission is by respiratory droplets.

Tetanus is a life-threatening illness caused by the bacterium *Clostridium tetani* and is characterized by severe muscle contractions and involuntary spasms, typically starting at the jaw and progressing to the rest of the body. The toxin affects the central nervous system and leads to dyspnea, cardiac arrhythmias, hyperthermia, and hypertension. Mortality is about 10%, the duration of disease may be months, and immunity in survivors is unreliable. The route of infection is typically via wounds or punctures in contact with contaminated soil or objects. There is no human-to-human transmission.

Pertussis is a cough illness caused by *Bordetella pertussis* bacteria. It typically presents with prolonged coughing paroxysms, ending with a deep forceful gasp (whoop) or vomiting. Encephalopathy occurs in 1 in 1,000 cases. In infants, it causes fatal pneumonia and apnea and contributes to the burden of sudden infant death. It is highly contagious and primarily transmitted by respiratory droplets.

Preparations

DTP vaccines comprise purified preparations of formalin-inactivated bacterial toxins (toxoids), antigenically uniform among all isolates. The tetanus toxoid content for children younger than 7 years is typically 5 to 12.5 Lf units per 0.5 mL dose, and the one for older children and adults 5 Lf units per 0.5 mL dose. The diphtheria toxoid content for children less than 7 years is typically 6.7 to 15 Lf units per 0.5 mL dose, and the one for older children and adults is typically 2 Lf units per 0.5 mL dose. To make this distinction, the abbreviation D is used for priming doses, and the abbreviation d is used for boosting doses with reduced antigen formulations (DTaP/Tdap). These are combined with pertussis toxoid (PT), and up to three further bacterial surface proteins, including pertactin (PRN), filamentous hemagglutinin (FHA), and fimbriae (FIM). Aluminum salts serve as adjuvants. Thiomersal-free products are widely available. It should be stored at 2° to 8°C, avoiding freezing.

No pertussis-only vaccine is available in the Western world. No diphtheria-only vaccine is available. Tetanus-only vaccines still exist and are only available with thiomersal.

Vaccine Usage

The recommended immunization schedule for infants and young children involves three to five doses. In a so-called "3+1" schedule, the priming doses are given at, for example, 2, 4, 6, or 2, 3, 4 months of age followed by one further dose at 12 (-15) months of age. In a so-called "2+1" schedule, priming doses are given at 2, 4, 12, or 3, 5, 11 (-12) months of age. Further booster doses are recommended variably at preschool and adolescent age. Tdap is recommended for pregnant women in an increasing number of countries worldwide.

Periodic booster doses are recommended variably. Some countries recommend them at 10 to 20 year intervals throughout life to maintain protection, others only as part of wound management. In the event of a contaminated wound, a tetanus booster is recommended if 5 years (some countries: 10) or more have passed since the previous dose, provided that adequate primary immunization was given. Including the diphtheria and pertussis components in these postexposure doses and regular boosters reduces the risk of diphtheria and the circulation of *B. pertussis* in the adult population and thus limits transmission to infants.

Tdap may be given at an interval shorter than 10 years since the last tetanus toxoid–containing vaccine to protect against pertussis, especially for the following:

- Pregnant women
- Adults who have or anticipate having close contact with an infant younger than 12 months should receive a single dose of Tdap and trivalent inactivated influenza vaccine. Ideally, the vaccines should be given at least 2 weeks before contact.
- Health care personnel who have direct patient contact should receive Tdap every 10 years.

Vaccine Effectiveness

Ever since the introduction of diphtheria and tetanus vaccines, these diseases have virtually disappeared in most countries with high coverage rates. Pertussis vaccines reduce the risk of disease by about 85%.

Tetanus immunization of women during pregnancy has virtually eliminated neonatal tetanus as a complication of unhygienic umbilical cord care.

Vaccine Adverse Reaction and Contraindications

These vaccines are well tolerated apart from causing mild-to-moderate injection-site inflammation and occasional low-grade fever. Booster doses may cause greater injection-site reaction with redness, swelling, and soreness. Extensive limb swelling is rare, but mainly associated with the fourth and fifth consecutive dose of acellular pertussis vaccine.

Immunization with tetanus toxoid as a combined form with DTP should not be used in subjects:

- with a history of a serious allergic reaction (such as anaphylaxis) to any of the vaccine components
- with a history of encephalopathy (e.g., coma or prolonged seizures) not attributable to an identifiable cause within 7 days of administration of a vaccine with pertussis components should not receive a pertussis-containing vaccine
- Tdap is not recommended to be administered within 4 weeks after the most recent tetanus toxoid–containing vaccine.

HAEMOPHILUS INFLUENZAE TYPE B VACCINES

Illness

Hib is a leading cause of life-threatening purulent invasive infections, including meningitis, epiglottitis, sepsis, pneumonia, and cellulitis in unvaccinated populations.

Preparations

Immunity depends on opsonic antibodies directed at the *Hib* capsular polysaccharide, polyribosyl ribitol phosphate (PRP). To overcome the T-cell–independent immune response patterns to purified PRP characteristic of children younger than 24 months, PRP is conjugated to either tetanus toxoid (PRP-T), genetically inactivated diphtheria toxin (PRP-CRM), or an outer membrane protein complex from *Neisseria meningitidis* (PRP-OMP).

The *Hib* vaccine is available as *Hib* only, in combination with DTaP-IPV, and in combination with DTaP-IPV and recombinant HBV vaccine.

Vaccine Usage

The recommended *Hib* immunization schedule for infants and young children involves two or three doses in the first year of life.

Vaccine Effectiveness

Prior to the introduction of *Hib* vaccines, 1 in 200 to 500 children had invasive *Hib* disease associated with high mortality. *Hib* meningitis was a leading cause of deafness. On completion of the priming series, 98% of infants have protective antibody levels. In countries with high infant vaccine coverage, *Hib*-associated disease and its complications have virtually disappeared.

Vaccine Adverse Reaction and Contraindications

Hib conjugates cause only minor adverse effects, such as fever and injection-site reactions, of short duration. Local reactions do not increase with successive doses. Allergy to the carrier protein and an anaphylactic reaction to a previous dose are contraindications.

HEPATITIS B VACCINES

Illness

HBV is a DNA virus causing acute and chronic hepatitis, cirrhosis, and liver cancer.

This virus can be transmitted through contact with infectious blood, semen, and other bodily fluids from having sex with an infected person, sharing contaminated needles to inject drugs, or from an infected mother to her newborn.

Preparations

HB vaccine contains purified HBsAg. This glycoprotein is expressed in recombinant yeast and mammalian cells and purified. The antigen is then adsorbed on aluminum hydroxide or aluminum phosphate. The preparations contain no more than 5% yeast protein.

Vaccine Usage

The HBV immunization schedule comprises three doses (0, 1, and 6 months) or is adapted to the DTaP schedule when used in combination vaccines. Rapid schedules requiring four doses are proposed by manufacturers and approved by some national regulatory authorities (i.e., 0, 1, 2, and 12 months or 0, 7, and 21 days with a booster at 12 months). HBV vaccine is also available as a combination with hepatitis A vaccine in various formulations. When HBV is not included in the infant immunization program but started in adolescence, two doses of the adult dose with a minimum 6 months interval are sufficient between the ages of 11 and 14 years. Thereafter, three doses of the adult formulation are required in a 0-1-6 month schedule. Accelerated schedules are available if rapid protection is required.

Management of infants born to women who are HBsAg positive or unknown status includes the following:

- Infants born to HBsAg-positive women should receive a single-antigen HB vaccine in the first 12 hours of life simultaneously with HBIG (0.5 mL) administered at different injection sites. The vaccine series should be completed according to a recommended schedule for infants born to HBsAg-positive mothers. The final dose in the vaccine series should not be administered before the age of 6 months.
- For preterm infants weighing less than 2,000 g, the initial vaccine dose (birth dose) should not be counted as part of the vaccine series because of the potentially reduced immunogenicity of HB vaccine in these infants; three additional doses of vaccine (for a total of four doses) should be administered beginning when the infant reaches the age of 1 month.
- Postvaccination testing for anti-HBs and HBsAg should be performed after completion of the vaccine series, at the age of 9 to 18 months—approximately 4 weeks after the final vaccine dose. However, testing should not be performed before the age of 9 months to avoid detection of anti-HBs from HBIG administered during infancy and to maximize the likelihood of detecting late HBV infection. Anti-HB core testing of infants is not recommended because passively acquired maternal anti-HB core might be detected in infants born to HBV-infected mothers until the age of 24 months.
  - HBsAg-negative infants with anti-HBs levels of 10 IU per L or more are protected and need no further medical management. Some countries recommend to achieve anti-HBs levels of 100 IU per L or more.
  - HBsAg-negative infants with anti-HBs levels of less than 10 IU per L should be revaccinated with a second three-dose series and retested 1 to 2 months after the final dose of vaccine.
  - Infants who are HBsAg-positive should receive appropriate follow-up.
- Infants of HBsAg-positive mothers may be breast-fed beginning immediately after birth.
- HBsAg-containing combination vaccines may be used for infants aged 6 weeks or older born to HBsAg-positive mothers to complete the vaccine series after receipt of the birth dose.
- Women admitted for delivery without documentation of HBsAg test results should have blood drawn and tested as soon as possible after admission.
- While test results are pending, all infants born to women without documentation of HBsAg test results should receive the first dose of single-antigen HB vaccine (without HBIG) within 12 hours after birth.
  - If the mother is then determined to be HBsAg positive, her infant should receive HBIG as soon as possible, but no later than the age of 7 days.
  - If the mother is determined to be HBsAg negative, the vaccine series should be completed according to a recommended schedule for infants born to HBsAg-negative mothers.
  - If the mother has never been tested to determine her HBsAg status, the vaccine series should be completed

according to a recommended schedule for infants born to HBsAg-positive mothers. Administration of HBIG is not necessary for these infants.

- If the mother's HBsAg status cannot be determined at 12 hours of birth or earlier, neonates weighing less than 2,000 g should receive both single-antigen HB vaccine and HBIG (0.5 mL). The birth dose of vaccine should not be counted as part of the three doses required to complete the vaccine series; three additional doses of vaccine (for a total of four doses) should be administered according to a recommended schedule on the basis of the mother's HBsAg test result.

Vaccine Effectiveness

A completed age-appropriate series of HB vaccine leads to protective antibody levels in over 95% of infants, children, and adolescents.

Vaccine Adverse Reaction and Contraindications

This vaccine is contraindicated in patients with previous hypersensitivity to any HB-containing vaccine, or hypersensitivity to any component of the vaccine, including yeast. Vaccination is not contraindicated in persons with a history of multiple sclerosis, GBS, autoimmune disease (e.g., systemic lupus erythematosus or rheumatoid arthritis), or other chronic diseases.

Pregnancy is not a contraindication to vaccination. Limited data indicate no apparent risk for adverse events to developing fetuses when HB vaccine is administered to pregnant women. Current vaccines contain noninfectious HBsAg and should cause no risk to the fetus.

HUMAN PAPILLOMAVIRUS VACCINES

Illness

HPV may cause genital and extragenital infections. Approximately 40 types are primarily sexually transmitted from person to person. Types 16 and 18 are the main genotypes for cervical intraepithelial neoplasia (CIN) and cause about 70% of cervical cancer.

Types 6 and 11 infections are the major cause of genital warts. These two types of HPV are responsible for more than 90% of genital warts. These types may also spread from mother to infants during pregnancy or delivery and can rarely cause warts in the upper respiratory tract (throat, larynx) of the child.

Preparations

Safe and effective virus-like particle-derived recombinant vaccines have been developed against several HPV types associated with cervical cancer and genital warts (genotypes 6, 11, 16, 18, 31, 33, 45, 52, and 58). Two vaccine preparations are currently on the market, a bivalent (Cervarix®) and a nonavalent (Gardasil® 9) formulation. They are aluminum salt adjuvanted (plus ASO_4 in the bivalent vaccine) and do not contain thimerosal.

Vaccine Usage

Each dose of the nonavalent HPV vaccine (0.5 mL) is administered intramuscularly (IM). It should be administered in a two-dose schedule (0 to 6 months) to males and females 9 to 14 years of age and as a three-dose schedule (0-2-6 months) from age 15 years onward. Coadministration with other age-appropriate vaccines, such as Tdap, Td, and MCV4, is possible (see package insert for up-to-date information). The bivalent vaccine is licensed for a two-dose schedule (0-5-13 months) in males and females 9 to 14 years of age and as a three-dose schedule (0-1-6 months) from age 15 years onward.

If a person already has chronic infection with one of the HPV types, the vaccine will not prevent disease from that type.

Vaccine Effectiveness

The efficacy of the HPV vaccine has been studied in adolescent women and men in multiple countries. In women who previously had not been exposed to the HPV types in the vaccine, the vaccine effectiveness was 90% for HPV 6/11/16/18 infection and genital warts, 45% for low-grade, and 85% for high-grade cytologic cervical abnormalities. Efficiency data in males are also available, primarily from Australia.[53,54]

Vaccine Adverse Reaction and Contraindications

The HPV vaccines are well tolerated, and there is consistent evidence of no increased risk of serious AEFI. A number of allegations of presumed autoimmune diseases and other entities induced by HPV vaccines have been raised. However, evaluation by the Global Advisory Committee for Vaccine Safety (GACVS) of WHO came to the conclusion that these allegations have no scientific basis.[55] Currently available HPV vaccines are not recommended for pregnant women since data on vaccination during pregnancy are limited. However, there is no evidence of risk to the fetus when a pregnant woman is inadvertently vaccinated.

MEASLES–MUMPS–RUBELLA VACCINES

Illnesses

Measles is a serious disease caused by a highly contagious virus spread by droplets. Measles typically begins with fever, followed by cough, runny nose, conjunctivitis, and malaise after a short fever interval. Measles encephalitis occurs in 1 per 1,000 cases of natural measles, frequently resulting in significant brain damage in the survivors. Approximately 5% of children with measles develop pneumonia. Mortality is 1 to 3 per 1,000 infected children. Death is more common in infants, malnourished children, and among immunocompromised persons such as those with leukemia and HIV infection.

Subacute sclerosing panencephalitis (SSPE) is a rare fatal illness caused by ongoing measles virus infection of the brain. Symptoms of brain damage usually begin 7 to 10 years after infection. Death occurs 1 to 3 years after the onset of symptoms. Risk factors for developing SSPE include developing measles infection at a young age. The incidence of SSPE is estimated to be between 7 and 11 per 100,000 cases of measles.

Measles has also been shown to lead to prolonged suppression of the immune system called "immune amnesia."[56]

Mumps is a viral infection of the salivary glands. Complications can include orchitis (in 20% to 50% of infected postpubertal males), brain involvement including aseptic meningitis (15% of cases), pancreatitis (2% to 5% of cases), and infection of ovaries (5% of postpubertal females). Permanent deafness may occur in about 1 per 2,000 cases.

Rubella virus may cause congenital rubella syndrome (CRS), a devastating disease that affects the infants of susceptible women exposed to rubella during their pregnancy. CRS can result in neonatal deafness, mental retardation, cataracts and other eye defects, heart defects, and hepatitis. Because of the risk of CRS, it is particularly important that postpubertal women be immune to rubella. Routine screening of pregnant women for rubella immunity is only recommended in the absence of immunization.

Preparations

MMR vaccine is a live-attenuated virus vaccine comprising the Moraten measles strain, the Jeryl-Lynn mumps strain, and the RA27/3 rubella strain. Several other vaccines with different vaccine strains are also available worldwide.

Vaccine Usage

MMR immunization for children and adolescence is recommended in a two-dose series, with the first dose between the ages of 9 and 12 months and the second dose at least 1 month after the first (but not before 12 months of age) with an interval of several months for optimal duration of immunity if epidemiologic pressure is low. Susceptible women should receive the rubella vaccine or MMR at least 28 days before getting pregnant to prevent CRS.

Because of the risk of CRS, it is particularly important that postpubertal women be immune to rubella.

Immunization of household members of pregnant or immunocompromised individuals is recommended and safe, as MMR cannot be transmitted by immunized individuals.

Vaccine Effectiveness

Today's MMR vaccines are highly effective against measles and rubella with greater than or equal to 95% response to the first dose. The second dose leads to greater than or equal to 98% seroconversion and is administered to address primary vaccine failure. Unfortunately, MMR is less effective against mumps, and a third dose can be considered for outbreak control.[57]

Vaccine Adverse Reaction and Contraindications

No serious side effects have been reported with mumps vaccine itself. Measles vaccine is not associated with SSPE. The rubella component is generally well tolerated.

The vaccine should not be used in subjects with serious allergies to gelatin or any of the other components of the vaccine. Inadvertent vaccination with MMR vaccines in pregnancy has been observed to be uneventful, and termination of pregnancy is not warranted. The vaccine should not be used in immunocompromised persons (with the exception of asymptomatic HIV-infected persons).

MENINGOCOCCAL VACCINES

Illness

N. meningitidis (or meningococcus) causes life-threatening invasive infections, primarily sepsis or meningitis. The serogroups A, B, C, Y, and W are the leading causes of invasive disease, with a case fatality rate of approximately 10% and long-term sequelae including deafness and other neurologic impairment. Human-to-human transmission is via respiratory droplets.

Preparations

Three quadrivalent (ACWY) meningococcal conjugate vaccines are available. They contain antigens of capsular polysaccharides of serogroups A, C, Y, and W-135 and are conjugated to diphtheria toxin derivatives (CRM197). A 0.5-mL dose of Menveo® consists of 10 µg of lyophilized meningococcal serogroup A (MenA) capsular polysaccharide conjugated to CRM197, and 5 µg each of capsular polysaccharide of serogroup C, W, and Y (MenCWY) conjugated to CRM197 in 0.5 mL of phosphate-buffered saline. A 0.5 mL dose of Menactra® contains 4 µg each of meningococcal A, C, W, and Y polysaccharides conjugated to approximately 48 µg of diphtheria toxoid protein carrier in sodium phosphate–buffered isotonic sodium chloride solution.

Nimenrix® contains 5 µg each of meningococcal A, C, W, and Y polysaccharides conjugated to approximately 44 µg of tetanus toxoid protein carrier in isotonic sodium chloride solution.

Two serogroup B meningococcal vaccines are available. One (Bexsero®) contains 50 µg each of recombinant proteins neisserial adhesin A (NadA), neisserial heparin-binding antigen (NHBA), and factor H–binding protein (fHbp) conjugated with 25 µg of outer membrane vesicles (OMV), 5 mg aluminum hydroxide (0.519 mg of Al^{3+}), and 776-mg histidine in buffered isotonic sodium chloride solution. This vaccine is licensed from 2 months of age onward. The other one (Trumenba®) comprises 60 µg each of two lipidated fHBP variants (total of 120 µg of protein), 0.018 mg of polysorbate 80, 25 mg of Al^{3+}, and 10 mM histidine-buffered saline at pH 6.0 and is currently licensed from 10 years of age onward. For the various schedules of these two innovative vaccines, see respective package inserts.

Furthermore, monovalent MenA (Africa) and MenC (Europe) conjugate vaccine formulations are in use.

Vaccine Usage

Recommendations are commonly adapted to local epidemiology and serogroup distributions. Therefore, usage of MenA, MenC, MenACWY, and MenB vaccines in general varies considerably from country to country as do recommendations for universal use (few) or high-risk indications (many) for each of the three available formulations.

Vaccine Effectiveness

The overall burden of meningococcal disease has declined significantly following introduction of the various immunization programs worldwide.[58–60]

Vaccine Adverse Reaction and Contraindications

Meningococcal conjugate vaccines are generally well tolerated. Minor adverse effects include fever and injection-site redness, swelling, and tenderness.

MenB vaccines induce fever in significant proportions of immunizations. Therefore, the United Kingdom recommends prophylactic use of antipyretics along immunization.[61,62] Anaphylactic reaction to a previous dose is a contraindication to further immunization.

PNEUMOCOCCAL VACCINES

Illness

Streptococcus pneumoniae (or pneumococcus) is a leading cause of life-threatening invasive bacterial infections in unvaccinated populations, especially in infants. Manifestations include otitis media, pneumonia, sepsis, and purulent meningitis. An average 30% of the population are colonized with *S. pneumoniae* in the upper respiratory tract. Invasive disease is facilitated by breakdown, for example, infection, of the mucosal membranes. Thus, upper respiratory tract infections are a major risk factor for invasive pneumococcal disease. Human-to-human transmission is via respiratory droplets.

Preparations

Immunity depends on antibodies against serotype-specific capsular polysaccharides. To overcome the unresponsiveness to purified polysaccharides of children younger than 24 months, they are conjugated to carrier proteins such as a nontoxic form of diphtheria toxin (CRM197) or tetanus toxoids. A 13-valent conjugate vaccine is available to protect against 13 leading serotypes of invasive pneumococcal disease: 1, 3, 4, 5, 6A, 6B, 7F, 9V, 14, 18C, 19A, 19F, and 23F. Each 0.5-mL dose of liquid suspension contains 30.8 μg of total polysaccharide and 32 μg of CRM_{197} protein, adsorbed on aluminum phosphate adjuvant, without preservative.

An alternative 10-valent conjugate vaccine is comprising capsular polysaccharide for serotypes 1, 5, 6B, 7F, 9V, 14, and 23F conjugated to nontypeable *H. influenzae* protein D (HiD), and capsular polysaccharide of serotypes 18C and 19F conjugated to tetanus and diphtheria toxoids, respectively. Each 0.5-mL dose of liquid suspension contains 1 to 3 μg of polysaccharide, adsorbed on aluminum phosphate adjuvant, without preservative.

Vaccine Usage

The infant pneumococcal conjugate vaccine (PCV) schedule comprises 2 to 3 priming and a booster dose, for example, 2, 4, 6, 12, or 2, 4, 12 months of age. PCV should be considered for all children up to 59 months of age. Immunized children have up to 20% less invasive disease as compared to control subjects and are less likely to be colonized.

Vaccine Effectiveness

Upon completion of the priming series, protective antibody levels are mounted against 97% of vaccine types and 89% of all serotypes.

Vaccine Adverse Reaction and Contraindications

The conjugate vaccines are generally well tolerated. Minor adverse effects include fever and injection-site redness, swelling, and tenderness. Anaphylactic reaction to a previous dose is a contraindication to further immunization.

POLIO VACCINE, INACTIVATED

Illness

Poliomyelitis is a highly contagious disease, leading to destruction of nerves and consecutive paralysis in 1 per 1,000 cases. It is caused by three serotypes. The route of transmission is by person-to-person contact, primarily via the fecal–oral route.

Preparations

Two types of polio vaccine have been available since the 1950s: oral (OPV) and inactivated (IPV). Both are highly effective in preventing polio. Initially, OPV was preferred for its stronger herd immunity. However, 1 in approximately 300,000 doses of all OPV was associated with vaccine-associated paralytic polio (VAPP). This has led to a replacement of OPV with IPV in most countries close to polio eradication. IPV contains purified formalin-inactivated polio viruses. Viral cultures are based on monkey kidney or human diploid cell strains. Streptomycin, polymyxin B, and/or neomycin may be present in small amounts from the cell culture medium. The preservative used is 2-phenoxyethanol (not thimerosal). In the Western world, IPV vaccines are available either alone or in combination with diphtheria and tetanus toxoids and acellular pertussis vaccines (DTaP-IPV). IPV products are injected SC in a dose of 0.5 mL. They should be stored at 2° to 8°C.

Vaccine Usage

The recommended IPV immunization schedule for infants and young children involves four to five doses, usually administered in combination and at the same time points as DTaP. Booster doses every 10 years are recommended for high-risk groups or during outbreaks. IPV can be used in pregnancy, if rapid immunity is required or as part of pertussis immunization in pregnancy. OPV is only used in a few remaining countries and for outbreak control.

Vaccine Effectiveness

Among children given three doses of IPV, 99% to 100% develop serum antibodies to all three types of poliovirus. More than 90% develop antibodies after two doses already. The Western Hemisphere has been declared polio free since 1994. Humans are the only host for polio virus. Thus, elimination of poliovirus is perceivable based on the successful global implementation of immunization programs.

Vaccine Adverse Reaction and Contraindications

IPV is generally well tolerated, causing minimal adverse effects. IPV should not be given to children who experienced an anaphylactic reaction to a previous dose of IPV or to streptomycin, polymyxin B, or neomycin. IPV can be given during pregnancy if immediate protection is required.

ROTAVIRUS VACCINE

Illness

Rotaviruses are intestinal viruses that infect virtually all children by 3 years of age. It is the most common cause of diarrhea in children, including hospital-acquired diarrhea; childcare center outbreaks are common. The illness often also includes fever and vomiting, lasting for a week or longer, and can cause persistent infection in immunocompromised people. Most rotavirus infections are mild, but about one in 50 cases develop severe dehydration.

Preparations

Two vaccines are currently available: *RV5* (*RotaTeq®*), a pentavalent live vaccine (G1, G2, G3, G4, P8), contains five reassortant types developed from human and bovine parent rotavirus strains and share neutralizing epitope identity with G1, G2, G3, G4, and P8. *RV1* (*Rotarix®*) is also a live-attenuated vaccine that contains one strain of live-attenuated human rotavirus, a G1 P(8) strain. RV1 shares neutralizing epitope identity with G1, G3, G4, and G9 through the P(8) VP4 protein. RV1 does not share neutralizing identity with G2 P(4) strains.

Vaccine Usage

RotaTeq requires a three-dose primary series, administered at 6 weeks of age with minimal intervals of 4 weeks for the two consecutive doses. Rotarix requires a two-dose primary series and is administered at greater than or equal to 6 weeks of age with a minimal interval of 4 weeks for the second dose. The final dose of rotavirus vaccine should be given before 6 months of age. Rotavirus vaccine may be given at the same time as other childhood vaccines.

Vaccine Effectiveness

Upon completion of the full series of RV5 or RV1 against rotavirus associated hospitalizations and emergency department visits were 84% (95% CI: 80–87%) and 83% (95% CI: 72–89%), respectively.[63] Vaccine introduction resulted in a median decline in rotavirus-associated hospitalizations and emergency department visits of 80% and 57%, respectively.

Vaccine Adverse Reaction and Contraindications

Historically, a previously available rotavirus vaccine (RotaShield®) was associated with an increased risk of intussusception. The intussusception hospitalization rates for infants in Canada have found no evidence of a change in rate after implementation of routine rotavirus immunization programs.[64]

VARICELLA VACCINE

Illness

Varicella (chickenpox) is a highly contagious moderately distressing illness, affecting 97% of the population until the 15th birthday in the Western world. Complications include cellulitis, necrotizing fasciitis, and encephalitis/cerebellitis. The virus may persist in nervous tissue and can cause zoster (shingles) decades after the primary infection.

In one European study, all countries presented the highest hospitalization incidences in children less than 5 years, with a range from 9 per 100,000 in Sweden to 75 per 100,000 in France, decreasing to less than 20 per 100,000 for all countries in the 5 to 9 years age group.[65]

Preparations

The vaccine consists of lyophilized, live-attenuated varicella-zoster virus (VZV). All currently licensed products are based on the Oka strain developed in Japan, but they differ slightly in potency and excipients. MMRV quadrivalent vaccines are also available.

Vaccine Usage

Varicella immunization recommendations for children and adolescence vary substantially in the Western world, where some countries have introduced universal childhood immunization programs (usually a two-dose series with the first dose between the ages of 9 and 12 months and the second dose at least 1 month after the first), while others rely on risk group immunization strategies.

When universally introduced, the use of live-attenuated varicella vaccine is recommended for the following:

- All children aged (9-) 12 months and older
- All older children and adults who have not had chickenpox and have not been vaccinated
- If someone who has never had chickenpox disease or received the vaccine is exposed to chickenpox, giving him or her the vaccine within 72 hours will probably prevent or significantly reduce the severity of the disease. It is recommended under such circumstances.

Transmission of vaccine strain varicella is possible, albeit rare and mild. Transmission of vaccine virus rarely occurs and has not been documented in the absence of rash. Immunization of household members of pregnant or immunocompromised individuals is recommended.

Vaccine Effectiveness

Varicella vaccine is 85% to 90% effective for prevention of varicella and 100% effective for prevention of moderate or severe disease. Breakthrough infections may occur but are generally mild. However, breakthrough varicella can be contagious.

Vaccine Adverse Reaction and Contraindications

Vaccine administration induces an infection that is generally subclinical, but 15% of children experience fever and 3% to 5% develop mild skin rash when infection peaks 2 to 3 weeks later. Infrequent adverse effects include anaphylaxis, thrombocytopenia, and encephalopathy. Delayed effects include vaccine-type herpes zoster, which is usually mild and rare.

The vaccine should not be given to subjects who have had a life-threatening allergic reaction to gelatin, to the antibiotic neomycin, or (for those needing a second dose) to a previous dose of the chickenpox vaccine; those who are receiving the MMR vaccine simultaneously should receive the injections contralaterally. Women should not become pregnant for at least 1 month after receiving the vaccine. However, to date, there are no reported cases of congenital varicella syndrome caused by the vaccine. In addition, the vaccine should not be given to persons with T-lymphocyte immunodeficiency, including those with leukemia, lymphoma, other malignancies affecting the bone marrow, and congenital T-cell abnormalities. The vaccine may be given to children with acute lymphocytic leukemia under study conditions, and HIV-infected persons who are immunocompetent may be vaccinated. Susceptible family members and other contacts of HIV-infected or immunodeficient persons should receive the chickenpox vaccine, because of the risk that natural chickenpox and its complications present for these patients.

INDICATION VACCINES

CHOLERA VACCINE

Illness

Vibrio cholerae infection may lead to severe diarrheal disease, accompanied by reduced fluid intake due to nausea and vomiting and rapidly leading to life-threatening dehydration. The global burden of disease is not well described. An annual incidence of one to four million infections and up to 140,000 deaths is estimated.[66] In cholera endemic regions, children less than 5 years of age are most affected. Incidence rates fluctuate in endemic areas and are accentuated by explosive local outbreaks. The severity is highlighted in cholera outbreaks in migrant camps, causing thousands of deaths within weeks.[67]

Preparations

Three oral cholera vaccines are available: Dukoral® (WC-rBS), a killed whole-cell monovalent (O1) vaccine with a recombinant B subunit of cholera toxin; Shanchol®; and Euvichol-Plus® (WC), killed modified whole-cell bivalent (O1 and O139) vaccines without the B subunit.

Vaccine Usage

WHO recommends cholera vaccine to be used in areas with endemic cholera, in humanitarian crises with high risk of cholera, and during cholera outbreaks, always in conjunction with other cholera prevention and control strategies.[68] Over 30 million doses were administered to date. Dukoral® is mainly used for travelers and can be given to individuals above 5 years of age in a two-dose schedule 1 to 6 weeks apart, whereas children under 5 years of age require three doses. Shanchol® and Euvichol-Plus® are available for children at least 1 year of age and stock piled for mass vaccination campaigns and can be given in two doses 2 weeks apart. Should the risk persist, revaccination of children aged 2 to 5 years with Dukoral® is recommended 6 months after the last dose. If more than 6 months have passed, the primary schedule should be repeated. Revaccination for Shanchol™ and Euvichol-Plus® is recommended 2 years after the last priming dose.

Vaccine Effectiveness

Vaccine effectiveness is 85% after two doses.[69,70] Duration of immunity is 6 months in children aged 2 to 5 years—otherwise 2 years.[71]

Vaccine Adverse Reaction and Contraindications

These vaccines are well tolerated and safe, including in pregnant women and HIV-positive individuals. An increased risk of serious AEFI was not observed. Known allergies to vaccine components constitute contraindications.

INFLUENZA VACCINE

Illness

Influenza is a highly contagious acute viral illness, primarily affecting the respiratory tract. Influenza A and B are the most common subtypes, leading to seasonal epidemic outbreak of mild-to-severe febrile upper respiratory tract infections, exacerbation of underlying disease, and secondary bacterial infection. Influenza is estimated to cause 300,000 to 650,000 deaths globally every year. This does not include the deaths due to influenza-related exacerbation of underlying disease (e.g., chronic respiratory, cardiovascular).

Preparations

There are many preparations of influenza vaccines available, usually licensed for use from 6 months of age onward. There are trivalent (two A and one B strains) and quadrivalent vaccines (two A and two B strains) available. Influenza viruses continuously change through genetic shift or drift of each strain. This necessitates seasonal adjustment of the candidate vaccine formulations. Three different manufacturing processes are employed: egg-based (i.e., live-attenuated candidate vaccine virus or purified antigens from candidate vaccine virus grown on fertilized hen eggs), cell-based (purified antigens from candidate vaccine virus grown in—egg-free—cell cultures), and recombinant (selected antigens are expressed synthetically in cell cultures) vaccines. Inactivated seasonal influenza vaccines for children are nonadjuvanted. Excipients may include antibiotics (e.g., neomycin, gentamicin) and stabilizers (e.g., gelatine). The preservative thiomersal is only used in multidose vials. Live-attenuated influenza vaccine (LAIV) is licensed and recommended preferentially in some countries (e.g., Germany) for children aged 24 months onward. It is administered nasally and cold adapted for safety reasons, that is, replication of the vaccine viruses takes place in the upper airways (usually nose), but not in the lower airways.

Vaccine Usage

The vaccine is indicated for immunization of risk groups. These include pregnant women; children aged 6 months to 5 years; elderly; individuals with underlying chronic diseases, including, but not limited to, cardiac, pulmonary, renal, metabolic, neurodevelopmental, liver, or hematologic diseases; and individuals with immunocompromised conditions. In addition, health care workers should be immunized because of increased exposure to the patients and risk of spread to vulnerable individuals. Seasonal vaccine is generally administered as a single dose. In children under 9 years of age, two doses at a 1-month interval are recommended when receiving the vaccine for the first time.

Vaccine Effectiveness

Vaccine effectiveness varies by season depending on how well the vaccine antigens are matched to the circulating strain. When the vaccine composition is similar to most of the circulating influenza viruses, effectiveness against physician visits and hospitalizations is in the range of 50% to 70%, with the higher estimate applying for children and the lower estimate for the elderly. While this may appear comparatively low, the number of deaths and disease complications averted are large, given the high burden of disease.

Vaccine Adverse Reaction and Contraindications

Influenza vaccine is generally safe. The annual reformulation, however, carries a risk of unexpected seasonal VAR (e.g., ocular respiratory syndrome in Canada in 2000, convulsive seizures in Australia in 2010). GBS is a recognized VAR in about 1 in 1,000,000 vaccinated. The risk of GBS following circulating wild-type virus is 7 to 20 times higher. An increased risk of narcolepsy following Pandemrix, one of the H1N1 vaccines used during the flu season 2009 to 2010, was described in observational studies. However, detection bias and exposure misclassification may have increased risk estimates, and other studies could not confirm the hypothesis.[72,73] Neither the pathogenesis of narcolepsy nor a causal relation with H1N1 immunization could be fully established to date.[74]

JAPANESE ENCEPHALITIS VACCINE

Illness

JE is the leading cause of viral encephalitis in Asia. It is acquired in rural areas, is mosquito borne, and leads to encephalitis in 1 in 20 to 1,000 infected individuals, with a case fatality rate of 25% and neuropsychiatric sequelae in 50% of survivors. The incidence rate of about 2 in 100,000 population translates to 70,000 cases of JE and approximately 14,000 to 20,000 death annually in the 24 countries with endemic JE.

Preparations

Over a dozen JE vaccines are in use today. They are based on the genotype 3 strain. The main vaccine types include inactivated Vero cell–derived vaccines, a live-attenuated vaccine, and a live-recombinant (chimeric) vaccine. Inactivated mouse brain–derived vaccines are being scaled back for the availability of the other safer constructs.[75]

The licensed Vero cell–derived vaccines (IXIARO®, JESPECT®), based on the SA14-14-2 strain, are aluminum hydroxide adjuvanted and contain excipients, including phosphate salts, formaldehyde, bovine albumin, host cell proteins, and host cell DNA. For the live-recombinant vaccine, the premembrane and envelope coding sequences from the 17D genome are exchanged with the respective sequences of the SA14-14-2 strain. The chimeric virus is then grown on Vero cells. The only live-attenuated vaccine, meeting WHO production standards, is developed by the Chengdu Institute of Biological Products in China and is based on the SA14-14-2 strain. It contains gelatin, sucrose, human albumin, gentamicin, and kanamycin.

Vaccine Usage

JE vaccine is recommended for children living in endemic areas. National schedules are variable. Live-attenuated vaccines are most commonly used in this setting at variable schedules. The Chengdu vaccine is generally given at 8 months and 2 years of age.

The inactivated Vero cell culture vaccine is widely available in nonendemic countries and administered in a two-dose schedule, with 0.25 mL 4 weeks apart in children aged 2 months to 2 years and with 0.5 mL for older children and adults. This JE vaccine is recommended for travelers planning to spend a month or longer in endemic areas during the JE virus transmission season and frequent travelers to endemic areas. It is also recommended for shorter term travelers with increased risk of JE exposure in rural areas during the transmission season. JE vaccine is not recommended for short-term travelers whose visit will be restricted to urban areas or outside the well-defined JE virus transmission season.

Vaccine Effectiveness

Live-attenuated JE vaccines may provide 99% seroconversion after one dose.[76] About 90% of subjects demonstrate seroprotection 6 months after primary vaccination with the Vero cell–derived vaccine.[77,78] About 95% of children mount protective antibody levels 1 month after live-chimeric vaccine.[79]

Vaccine Adverse Reaction and Contraindications

In large trials and postlicensure surveillance, the main JE vaccines were not associated with safety concerns.[80–83]

RABIES VACCINE

Illness

Rabies is an acute and almost uniformly fatal viral encephalitis. The number of deaths that rabies causes globally is estimated to be at least 50,000 to 70,000 cases, with over 95% of human deaths occurring in the Asia and Africa regions. The rabies virus is most often transmitted by a bite and/or saliva from an infected animal (e.g., bats, raccoons, skunks, foxes, ferrets, cats, or dogs, wolves, coyotes, jackals). Globally, 99% of infections are transmitted to humans by dog bites. In the United States, bats are the most common vector. Forty percent of human rabies cases occur in children younger than 15 years.[84]

Preparations

Cell culture vaccines constitute most available rabies vaccines today and follow five basic approaches:

- Human diploid cell vaccine (HDCV) contains the Pitman-Moore L503 or Flury strain of rabies virus grown on MRC-5 human diploid cell culture and is inactivated with β-propiolactone. It contains no preservative or stabilizer.
- Purified chick embryo cell vaccine (PCECV) is a sterile lyophilized vaccine obtained by growing the fixed rabies virus strain Flury LEP-25 in primary cultures of chick fibroblasts. The virus is inactivated with β-propiolactone.
- Purified Vero cell rabies vaccine (PVRV) contains the inactivated and lyophilized Wistar strain of rabies virus grown on Vero cell cultures in fermenters, allowing mass cultivation. These are inactivated by β-propiolactone.
- Primary Hamster Kidney Cell vaccine (PHKCV) uses the Beijing strain and is inactivated with formalin and adsorbed to aluminum hydroxide. It also contains 0.01% thiomersal and 10-mg human albumin.
- Purified duck embryo vaccine (PDEV) uses duck embryo cells as substrate. The virus is inactivated by β-propiolactone. PDEV contains thiomersal.

Nerve tissue vaccines (Semple, Fuenzalida) containing rabies virus–infected goat or sheep brain tissue were the first available vaccine types. Today, the less favorable safety profiles limit their use to only a small number of countries worldwide.

Vaccine Usage

PrEP is indicated for individuals with frequent contact with rabies virus or possibly rabid animals as well as travelers to endemic areas. For PrEP, licensed from birth, two (instead of three) doses are necessary [0 and (7-) 28 days].[85,86]

PEP is indicated for individuals following nibbling of uncovered skin, minor scratches, or transdermal bites of possibly infected animals. PEP consists of extensive washing and local treatment of the wound as soon as possible after exposure, plus a course of potent and effective rabies vaccine that meets WHO standards, plus administration of rabies immunoglobulin (RIG), if indicated. Active immunization as part of PEP in previously unvaccinated individuals follows the schedule 0, 3, 7, and 14 days. PEP in those who had received complete PrEP, no RIG but two further doses of vaccine (0 and 3 days) are recommended.

Vaccine Effectiveness

PrEP and PEP are associated with high immunogenicity and effectiveness.[87] Over 50 million individuals have received PrEP in the United States, and breakthrough rabies has not been described. Almost all individuals mount the recommended levels of rabies virus, neutralizing antibody following PEP with chick embryo cell vaccine.[88] About 30 million people worldwide receive PEP annually, preventing hundreds of thousands of rabies deaths annually.

Vaccine Adverse Reaction and Contraindications

The nerve tissue vaccines were associated with increased reactogenicity and serious neurologic AEFI, including meningoencephalomyelitis, ascending flaccid Landry paralysis, and transverse myelitis. In contrast, cell culture–based vaccines in use today are generally well tolerated and safe. An increased risk of serious AEFI has not been observed. Known allergies to vaccine components constitute contraindications.

TICK-BORNE ENCEPHALITIS VACCINE

Illness

TBE is a leading cause of viral central nervous system infections in endemic areas (see annually updated geomapping). In addition to local residents, such as outdoor active individuals, at least hundred-thousands of travelers visit these areas every year.

Ixodes ricinus in Europe and *Ixodes persulcatus* in the Far-East and Siberia are the main vector ticks. The proportion of infected ticks varies by region and may be up to 30% in some high-risk areas in Eastern Europe. Most infected tick bites lead to asymptomatic or mild flu-like disease. About 40% of patients experience serious illness with high fever, encephalitis, and paralyses. Lethality with infections by the European subtype is 0.5% to 2% and almost always affects adults. For the Far Eastern subtype, a 35% lethality rate is reported. In contrast, less severe aseptic meningitis is the main manifestation of TBE in children.[89] Neurologic sequelae are observed in 35% to 60% of pediatric patients (usually mild), and up to 80% of patients with TBE do not fully recover.[90,91]

Preparations

Two well-characterized TBE vaccines are in use today (FSME-Immun® and Encepur®). Both are produced on chicken embryonic fibroblast cells, inactivated by formaldehyde, and use aluminum hydroxide as adjuvant. Neither contains thiomersal. Both are available in pediatric (FSME-Immun Junior® 1 to 15 years of age; Encepur-Children®: 1 to 11 years of age) and adult formulations. Three additional vaccines are available today, two developed in Russia—neither has pediatric formulations—and one in China with limited available information.

Vaccine Usage

Immunization is recommended for individuals residing in endemic areas. Over 100 million doses were administered in the past 40 years. Both vaccines require a three-dose schedule for priming, with at least 1 month between doses 1 and 2 and 5 to 12 months between doses 2 and 3 (9 to 12 months for Encepur®). Both are suitable for accelerated schedules accelerating the second dose to day 14. Encepur® has also been licensed for an accelerated four-dose schedule (days 0, 7, and 21, followed by fourth dose 12 months later). Booster doses are recommended 3 years after the priming series followed by 5-year intervals.

Vaccine Effectiveness

The vaccine effectiveness is estimated to be 95% to 99% and has demonstrated dramatic reduction of TBE In highly endemic areas.[92,93]

Vaccine Adverse Reaction and Contraindications

The current formulations (adapted in 2001) are well tolerated and safe. Fever within 24 to 48 hours following immunization occurs frequently in young children (15% to 20%), especially after the first dose. No serious VAR are known today. Known allergies to vaccine components and anaphylaxis to hen eggs constitute contraindications. Persons with other forms of egg allergies should be vaccinated under appropriate medical supervision.

TUBERCULOSIS

Illness

Tuberculosis (TB) is a highly infectious disease caused by *Mycobacterium tuberculosis* transmitted by droplets and aerosols. The bacteria elicit a granulomatous immune response (tubercles) and primarily affect the lungs. However, most other organ systems may be affected. There are two forms of TB: latent TB infection and TB disease. About one-quarter of the world's population is infected. TB is the leading cause of death from a single infectious agent globally, leading to 1.5 million people dying annually of TB. Two forms of TB are life-threatening: TB meningitis and miliary TB. The latter being a systemic disease with bacterial spread throughout the lungs and into the bloodstream. While TB can be diagnosed and treated, multidrug-resistant TB is an increasing public health problem worldwide.

Preparations

BCG strains are the basis of *Mycobacterium bovis* live-attenuated bacterial vaccine. Multiple strains of BCG have evolved in various laboratories around the world. Each strain possesses different characteristics. Five main strains are used in more than 90% of the vaccines worldwide: Pasteur 1173 P2, the Danish 1331, the Glaxo 1077 (derived from the Danish strain), the Tokyo 172-1, the Russian BCG-I, and the Moreau RDJ strains (NIBSC and WHO, 2004). There is a lack of standardization in the manufacturing processes, and concentration of live particles in the vaccines ranges from 50,000 to 3 million per dose, according to the strains. Recombinant TB vaccines have not reached licensure so far.

Vaccine Usage

The WHO recommends BCG be given as a single dose to all children born in countries with a high incidence of TB and/or high leprosy burden. The use of available BCG vaccine is not recommended for neonates and children in the United States and many other high-income countries as it is not highly effective and increases the diagnostic challenge.[94] In countries without universal neonatal BCG programs, the following risk groups may be considered for selective immunization: neonates born to parents (or other close contacts/relatives) with current or previous TB or with leprosy, neonates born in households with contacts to countries with high incidence of TB and/or high leprosy burden, or neonates in any other locally identified risk group with TB and/or with leprosy disease.[95]

Vaccine Effectiveness

Strain and manufacturing variability led to widely differing data on immunogenicity, efficacy, and effectiveness. Effectiveness of vaccination in neonates and infants against pulmonary TB is estimated to be 60% and 75%, respectively. Effectiveness of neonatal immunization against miliary and meningeal TB is estimated to be 70% to 90%, respectively.[96,97] Duration of protection is estimated to be at least 15 years.[98] Revaccination does not demonstrate an added protective effect against TB. BCG vaccine was also shown to be effective against leprosy and non-TB mycobacteria.

Vaccine Adverse Reaction and Contraindications

Safety profiles are strain specific. Overall, the Glaxo 1077, Tokyo 172-1, or Moreau RDJ strains appear to have a more favorable safety profile compared to the Pasteur 1173 P2 and Danish 1331 strains. Local BCG-itis, regional (suppurative) lymphadenitis are frequent with 1 in 1,000 to 1 in 10,000 doses. Systemic BCG disease is a recognized VAR in immunocompromised individuals (e.g., up to 1% in HIV-positive infants), with a mortality rate of over 50%.[99] BCG related immune reconstitution syndrome in patients receiving treatment for immune-compromising condition (e.g., antiretroviral illness). As a result, the following WHO recommendations apply: neonates born to women of unknown HIV status should be vaccinated as the benefits of BCG vaccination outweigh the risks. Neonates of unknown HIV status born to HIV-infected women should be vaccinated if they have no clinical evidence suggestive of HIV infection, regardless of whether the mother is receiving antiretroviral therapy (ART). Although evidence is limited, for neonates with HIV infection confirmed by early virologic testing, BCG vaccination should be delayed until ART has been started and the infant confirmed to be immunologically stable (CD4 >25%). There is insufficient evidence of the safety in pregnancy.

TYPHOID FEVER VACCINE

Illness

Typhoid fever is an acute febrile illness caused by *Salmonella typhi*, with estimated 11 to 18 million infections globally every year. The case fatality rate of untreated typhoid fever was 10% to 20%. Antibiotic treatment has reduced mortality below 1% until multidrug-resistant typhoid fever emerged in Africa and South East Asia. High continued fever may lead to serious complications, including the central nervous system, heart, liver, and gallbladder.

Preparations

Several typhoid vaccines are available. These include two live oral vaccine (strain Ty21a), two Vi polysaccharide vaccines conjugated to tetanus toxoid, and seven nonconjugated Vi polysaccharide vaccines.[100,101]

Vaccine Usage

The nonconjugated Vi polysaccharide vaccines are administered as a single IM or SC dose in children aged 2 years and older. The conjugated Vi polysaccharide vaccines are recommended for children above 3 months of age as a two-dose IM schedule with the second dose 1 to 2 months following the first. The live oral vaccine (enteric-coated capsules) is recommended as a three-dose schedule with 2 days interval between doses. In the United States and Canada, a four-dose schedule given every other day is recommended.[102]

Typhoid fever vaccines are indicated for school-aged children in and travelers to endemic areas, military personnel, and medical and laboratory professionals exposed to or handling *S. typhi*.

Vaccine Effectiveness

Conjugated Vi vaccines have shown seroconversion rates of 92% to 99% and a protection rate of 87% in human challenge trials. Unconjugated Vi polysaccharide vaccine is not effective in children less than 2 years of age.

Vaccine Adverse Reaction and Contraindications

Highly purified Vi polysaccharide and oral vaccines are well tolerated and safe. Serious AEFIs are extremely rare with 1 in 200,000 to 300,000, and causal association could not be established. Postlicensure safety data of conjugated Vi vaccines are pending. Known allergies to vaccine components constitute contraindications.

YELLOW-FEVER VACCINE

Illness

YF is a mosquito-borne (*Aedes aegypti*) acute viral illness associated with hepatitis and hemorrhagic fever. YF is endemic and intermittently epidemic in 33 countries in Africa and 11 countries in South America. The global burden of disease is estimated to be 200,000 cases each year, with 30,000 deaths and 90% occurring in Africa. Case fatality rate of severe disease is 30% to 50%.

Preparations

Today, the seven available YF vaccines are all lyophilized live-attenuated viral vaccines based on the 17D strain. They are cultivated in embryonated hen eggs and vary in 17D substrains (17D-204 and 17DD), adjuvant and excipient (e.g., ovalbumin, gelatin, sorbitol) composition. No preservatives are added. A global YF vaccine stockpile coordinated by WHO is held for emergency response.

Vaccine Usage

The vaccine is administered as a single dose IM or SC. A booster dose is not necessary. In endemic countries, YF vaccine should be given at 9 to 12 months of age (e.g., at the same time as measles-containing vaccine). Vaccine should be offered to all unvaccinated travelers aged greater than 9 months, traveling to and from endemic areas.

Vaccine Effectiveness

Ninety nine percent of vaccine recipients develop protective levels of neutralizing antibodies within 10 days of vaccination. Duration of immunity is estimated to be at least 20 to 35 years and probably for life.[103,104] Vaccine failure is exquisitely rare but has been described.

Vaccine Adverse Reaction and Contraindications

Allergic responses to YF vaccine (e.g., ovalbumin, gelatine) occur in less than 1 in 1,000,000 doses and primarily in persons with known egg allergy. However, only 16% of subjects with egg allergy mount an allergic reaction. Skin testing has negative predictive value of 80% and a positive predictive value of 57% for allergic reactions.[105]

YF-associated neurologic disease (YF-AND) has two main manifestations: acute virolytic encephalitis, meningoencephalitis, and immune-mediated disease, including acute disseminated encephalomyelitis (ADEM) and GBS. The risk of encephalitis in less than 6 month of age (0.5 to 4 in 1,000 doses) led to the current age limitation in infants. The incidence in older individuals since then has been estimated to be around 0.4 per 100,000 doses.[106] YF-associated viscerotropic disease (YF-AVD) is an inflammatory syndrome involving the liver and viscera, resembling wild-type YF disease. It is estimated to occur at a rate of 0.4 in 100,000 doses. This risk is age dependent, and children have a much lower risk.[107] Overall, the risk of disease following wild-type infection is five to six logs higher than vaccination to serious VAR.

The vaccine is contraindicated in children aged 6 months and younger and is not recommended for those aged 6 to 8 months, except during epidemics when the risk of infection with the YF virus may be very high, and for breastfed infants. Known allergies to vaccine components and anaphylaxis to hen eggs constitute contraindications. Persons with other forms of egg allergies should be vaccinated under appropriate medical supervision. YF vaccine is contraindicated in individuals with immunomodulatory or suppressive treatment and immunodeficiencies (primary immunodeficiency, symptomatic HIV, $CD4^+$ T lymphocytes <200 per mm or <15%, <6 years of age).

REFERENCES

1. Maruyama M, Lam KP, Rajewsky K. Memory B-cell persistence is independent of persisting immunizing antigen. *Nature* 2000;407:636–642.
2. Marsden VS, Kappler JW, Marrack PC. Homeostasis of the memory T cell pool. *Int Arch Allergy Immunol* 2006;139:63–74.
3. Weintraub A. Immunology of bacterial polysaccharide antigens. *Carbohydr Res* 2003;338:2539–2547.
4. MacLennan IC, Toellner KM, Cunningham AF, et al. Extrafollicular antibody responses. *Immunol Rev* 2003;194:8–18.
5. Cooper NR, Nemerow GR. The role of antibody and complement in the control of viral infections. *J Invest Dermatol* 1984;83(Suppl 1):121s–127s.
6. Casadevall A. The methodology for determining the efficacy of antibody-mediated immunity. *J Immunol Methods* 2004;291:1–10.
7. Pickering LK, Baker CJ, Kimberlin DW, et al. *Red Book: 2009 Report of the Committee on Infectious Diseases*, 28th ed. Elk Grove Village, IL: American Academy of Pediatrics, 2009.
8. Offit PA, Jew RK. Addressing parents' concerns: do vaccines contain harmful preservatives, adjuvants, additives, or residuals? *Pediatrics* 2003;112(6 Pt 1):1394–1397. doi:10.1542/peds.112.6.1394.
9. Trotter CL, McVernon J, Ramsay ME, et al. Optimising the use of conjugate vaccines to prevent disease caused by *Haemophilus influenzae* type b, *Neisseria meningitidis* and *Streptococcus pneumoniae*. *Vaccine* 2008;26:4434–4445.
10. Coffman RL, Sher A, Seder RA. Vaccine adjuvants: putting innate immunity to work. *Immunity* 2010;33:492–503.
11. Flach TL, Ng G, Hari A, et al. Alum interaction with dendritic cell membrane lipids is essential for its adjuvanticity. *Nat Med* 2011;17:479–487.
12. Eisenbarth SC, Colegio OR, O'Connor W, et al. Crucial role for the Nalp3 inflammasome in the immunostimulatory properties of aluminium adjuvants. *Nature* 2008;453:1122–1126.
13. Kool M, Petrilli V, De Smedt T, et al. Cutting edge: alum adjuvant stimulates inflammatory dendritic cells through activation of the NALP3 inflammasome. *J Immunol* 2008;181:3755–3759.
14. WHO Vaccine Safety Advisory Committee. Macrophagic myofasciitis and aluminum-containing vaccines. *Wkly Epidemiol Rec* No 74, 1999:338–340.
15. Children's Hospital of Philadelphia. https://www.chop.edu/centers-programs/vaccine-education-center/vaccine-ingredients/aluminum. Accessed January 1, 2020.
16. Edwards K, Lambert PH, Black S. Narcolepsy and pandemic influenza vaccination: what we need to know to be ready for the next pandemic. *Pediatr Infect Dis J* 2019;38(8):873–876.
17. Offit PA, Quarles J, Gerber MA, et al. Addressing parents' concerns: do multiple vaccines overwhelm or weaken the infant's immune system? *Pediatrics* 2002;109:124–129.
18. Halsey NA. Combination vaccines: defining and addressing current safety concerns. *Clin Infect Dis* 2001;33(Suppl):S312–S318.
19. Stratton K, Wilson CV, McCormick MC. Immunization safety review: multiple immunizations and immune dysfunction. In *Immunization Safety Review Committee, Board on Health Promotion and Disease Prevention, Institute of Medicine.* Washington, DC: National Academy Press, 2002.
20. Bach J-F. The effect of infections on susceptibility to autoimmune and allergic diseases. *N Engl J Med* 2002;347:911–920.
21. Weiss ST. Eat dirt: the hygiene hypothesis and allergic diseases. *N Engl J Med* 2002;347:930–931.
22. CDC. Prevention and control of seasonal influenza with vaccines: recommendations of the Advisory Committee on Immunization Practices (ACIP), 2010. *Morbid Mortal Wkly Rep* 2010;59(RR-8):1–62.
23. CIOMS Working Group on Vaccine Safety. *CIOMS guide to active vaccine surveillance. Council for International Organizations of Medical Sciences.* Geneva, Switzerland: WHO Press, 2017.
24. Heininger U. *Impfratgeber. Impfempfehlungen für Kinder, Jugendliche und Erwachsene,* 10 ed. Bremen, Germany: Unimed Science, 2019.
25. Rothman KJ, Greenland S. Causation and causal inference in epidemiology. *Am J Public Health* 2005;95(Suppl 1):S144–S150.
26. Folb PI, Bernatowska E, Chen R, et al. A global perspective on vaccine safety and public health: the Global Advisory Committee on Vaccine Safety. *Am J Public Health* 2004;94:1926–1931.
27. Munoz FM, Jamieson DJ. Maternal immunization. *Obstet Gynecol* 2019;133(4):739–753. doi:10.1097/AOG.0000000000003161.
28. Keller-Stanislawski B, Englund JA, Kang G, et al. Safety of immunization during pregnancy: a review of the evidence of selected inactivated and live attenuated vaccines. *Vaccine* 2014;32(52):7057–7064. doi:10.1016/j.vaccine.2014.09.052.
29. Abu Raya B, Edwards KM, Scheifele DW, et al. Pertussis and influenza immunisation during pregnancy: a landscape review. *Lancet Infect Dis* 2017;17(7):e209–e222. doi:10.1016/S1473-3099(17)30190-1.
30. Bonhoeffer J, Kochhar S, Hirschfeld S, et al. Global alignment of immunization safety assessment in pregnancy—The GAIA project. *Vaccine* 2016;34(49):5993–5997. doi:10.1016/j.vaccine.2016.07.006.
31. Munoz FM, Eckert LO, Katz MA, et al. Key terms for the assessment of the safety of vaccines in pregnancy: results of a global consultative process to initiate harmonization of adverse event definitions. *Vaccine* 2015;33(47):6441–6452. doi:10.1016/j.vaccine.2015.07.112.
32. Jones CE, Munoz FM, Kochhar S, et al. Guidance for the collection of case report form variables to assess safety in clinical trials of vaccines in pregnancy. *Vaccine* 2016;34(49):6007–6014. doi:10.1016/j.vaccine.2016.07.007.
33. Mangtani P, Evans SJW, Lange B, et al. Safety profile of rubella vaccine administered to pregnant women: a systematic review of pregnancy related adverse events following immunisation, including congenital rubella syndrome and congenital rubella infection in the foetus or infant. *Vaccine* 2020;38(5):963–978. doi:10.1016/j.vaccine.2019.11.070.
34. Shields KE, Galil K, Seward J, et al. Varicella vaccine exposure during pregnancy: data from the first 5 years of the pregnancy registry. *Obstet Gynecol* 2001;98:14–19.
35. Centers for Disease Control and Prevention. Measles, mumps, and rubella: vaccine use and strategies for elimination of measles, rubella, and congenital rubella syndrome and control of mumps: recommendations of the Advisory Committee on Immunization Practices (ACIP). *MMWR Recomm Rep* 1998;47(RR-8):1–57.
36. Centers for Disease Control and Prevention. Prevention of varicella: recommendations of the Advisory Committee on Immunization Practices (ACIP). *MMWR Recomm Rep* 2007;56(RR-4):1–40.
37. WHO. Child mortality and causes of death. In *Global Health Observatory Data.* 2015. www.who.int/gho/child_health/mortality/en/. Accessed August 21, 2020..
38. Stoll BJ, Hansen N, Fanaroff AA, et al. Late-onset sepsis in very low birth weight neonates: the experience of the NICHD Neonatal Research Network. *Pediatrics* 2002;110:285–291.

39. Langkamp DL, Davis JP. Increased risk of reported pertussis and hospitalization associated with pertussis in low birth weight children. *J Pediatr* 1996;128:654–659.
40. Basha S, Surendran N, Pichichero M. Immune responses in neonates. *Expert Rev Clin Immunol* 2014;10:1171–1184. doi:10.1586/1744666X.2014.942288.
41. PrabhuDas M, Adkins B, Gans H, et al. Challenges in infant immunity: implications for responses to infection and vaccines. *Nat Immunol* 2011;12:189–194. doi:10.1038/ni0311-189.
42. Dowling DJ, Levy O. Ontogeny of early life immunity. *Trends Immunol* 2014;35:299–310. doi:10.1016/j.it.2014.04.007.
43. Saso A, Kampmann B. Vaccine responses in newborns. *Semin Immunopathol* 2017;39(6):627–642. doi:10.1007/s00281-017-0654-9.
44. Saari TN; American Academy of Pediatrics Committee on Infectious Diseases. Immunization of preterm and low birth weight infants. American Academy of Pediatrics Committee on Infectious Diseases. *Pediatrics* 2003;112(1 Pt 1):193–198. doi:10.1542/peds.112.1.193.
45. Waitz M, Hopfner R, Hummler HD, et al. Hepatitis B post-exposure prophylaxis in preterm and low birth weight infants. *AJP Rep* 2015;5:e67–e72.
46. Carbone T, McEntire B, Kissin D, et al. Absence of an increase in cardiorespiratory events after diphtheria-tetanus-acellular pertussis immunization in preterm infants: a randomized, multicenter study. *Pediatrics* 2008;121(5):e1085–e1090.
47. Pickering LK. Immunization in special clinical circumstances. In: *Red Book report of the Committee on Infectious Diseases*. 28th ed. Elk Grove Village, IL: American Academy of Pediatrics, 2009.
48. Niehues T, Bogdan C, Hecht J, et al. Impfen bei Immundefizienz: Anwendungshinweise zu den von der Ständigen Impfkommission empfohlenen Impfungen(I) Grundlagenpapier. *Bundesgesundheitsblatt Gesundheitsforschung Gesundheitsschutz* 2017;60(6):674–68.
49. Wagner N, Assmus F, Arendt G, et al. Impfen bei Immundefizienz: Anwendungshinweise zu den von der Ständigen Impfkommission empfohlenen Impfungen. (IV) Impfen bei Autoimmunkrankheiten, bei anderen chronisch-entzündlichen Erkrankungen und unter immunmodulatorischer Therapie. *Bundesgesundheitsblatt Gesundheitsforschung Gesundheitsschutz* 2019;62(4):494–515.
50. Ljungman P, Cordonnier C, Einsele H, et al. Vaccination of hematopoietic cell transplant recipients. *Bone Marrow Transplant* 2009;44:521–526.
51. Tomblyn M, Chiller T, Einsele H, et al. Guidelines for preventing infectious complications among hematopoietic cell transplantation recipients: a global perspective. *Biol Blood Marrow Transplant* 2009;15:1143–1238.
52. Baten J, Wagner A. Autarky, market disintegration, and health: the mortality and nutritional crisis in Nazi Germany 1933–1937. *Econ Hum Biol* 2003;1(1):1–28.
53. Harder T, Wichmann O, Klug SJ, et al. Efficacy, effectiveness and safety of vaccination against human papillomavirus in males: a systematic review. *BMC Med* 2018;16(1):110.
54. Brotherton JML, Giuliano AR, Markowitz LE, et al. Monitoring the impact of HPV vaccine in males-considerations and challenges. *Papillomavirus Res* 2016;2:106–111. doi:10.1016/j.pvr.2016.05.001.
55. Global Advisory Committee on Vaccine Safety, 7–8 June 2017. Safety update of HPV vaccines. *Wkly Epidemiol Rec* No 28, 2017;92:393–404
56. Behrens L, Cherry JD, Heininger U, et al. The susceptibility to other infectious diseases following measles during a three year observation period in Switzerland. *Pediatr Infect Dis J* 2020;39(6):478–482. doi:10.1097/INF.0000000000002599.
57. Albertson JP, Clegg WJ, Reid HD, et al. Mumps outbreak at a university and recommendation for a third dose of measles-mumps-rubella vaccine—Illinois, 2015–2016. *Morb Mortal Wkly Rep* 2016;65(29):731–734. doi:10.15585/mmwr.mm6529a2.
58. Borrow R, Miller E. Long-term protection in children with meningococcal C conjugate vaccination: lessons learned. *Expert Rev Vaccines* 2006;5(6):851–857.
59. Diomandé FVK, Djingarey MH, Daugla DM, et al. Public health impact after the introduction of PsA-TT: the first 4 years. *Clin Infect Dis* 2015;61(Suppl 5):S467–S472.
60. Ladhani SN, Andrews N, Parikh SR, et al. Vaccination of infants with meningococcal group B vaccine (4CMenB) in England. *N Engl J Med* 2020;382(4):309–317.
61. Kapur S, Bourke T, Maney JA, et al. Emergency department attendance following 4-component meningococcal B vaccination in infants. *Arch Dis Child* 2017;102(10):899–902. doi:10.1136/archdischild-2016-311020.
62. Dubus M, Ladhani S, Vasu V. Prophylactic paracetamol after meningococcal B vaccination reduces postvaccination fever and septic screens in hospitalized preterm infants. *Pediatr Infect Dis J* 2020;39(1):78–80.
63. Pindyck T, Tate JE, Parashar UD. A decade of experience with rotavirus vaccination in the United States—vaccine uptake, effectiveness, and impact. *Expert Rev Vaccines* 2018;17(7):593–606. doi:10.1080/14760584.2018.1489724.
64. Hawken S, Ducharme R, Rosella LC, et al. Assessing the risk of intussusception and rotavirus vaccine safety in Canada. *Hum Vaccin Immunother* 2017;13(3):703–710. doi:10.1080/21645515.2016.1240846.
65. Riera-Montes M, Bollaerts K, Heininger U, et al. Estimation of the burden of varicella in Europe before the introduction of universal childhood immunization. *BMC Infect Dis* 2017;17(1):353. doi:10.1186/s12879-017-2445-2.
66. Ali M, Nelson AR, Lopez AL, et al. Updated global burden of cholera in endemic countries. *PLoS Negl Trop Dis* 2015;9(6):e0003832. doi:10.1371/journal.pntd.0003832.
67. Siddique AK, Salam A, Islam MS, et al. Why treatment centres failed to prevent cholera deaths among Rwandan refugees in Goma, Zaire. *Lancet* 1995;345:359–361.
68. World Health Organization. Cholera vaccines: WHO position paper—August 2017. *Wkly Epidemiol Rec* No 34, 2017;92:477–500.
69. Lucas ME, Deen JL, von Seidlein L, et al. Effectiveness of mass oral cholera vaccination in Beira, Mozambique. *N Engl J Med* 2005;352(8):757–767.
70. Khatib AM, Ali M, von Seidlein L, et al. Effectiveness of an oral cholera vaccine in Zanzibar: findings from a mass vaccination campaign and observational cohort study. *Lancet Infect Dis* 2012;12(11):837–844.
71. Thiem VD, Deen JL, von Seidlein L, et al. Long-term effectiveness against cholera of oral killed whole-cell vaccine produced in Vietnam. *Vaccine* 2006;24:4297–4303.
72. Wijnans L, Dodd C, de Ridder M, et al. Pandemic influenza vaccine & narcolepsy: simulations on the potential impact of bias. *Expert Rev Vaccines* 2016;15(5):573–584.
73. Weibel D, Sturkenboom M, Black S, et al. Narcolepsy and adjuvanted pandemic influenza A (H1N1) 2009 vaccines—multi-country assessment. *Vaccine* 2018;36(41):6202–6211.
74. Edwards K, Hanquet G, Black S, et al. Meeting report narcolepsy and pandemic influenza vaccination: what we know and what we need to know before the next pandemic? A report from the 2nd IABS meeting. *Biologicals* 2019;60:1–7.
75. Halstead SB, Thomas SJ. New Japanese encephalitis vaccines: alternatives to production in mouse brain. *Expert Rev Vaccines* 2011;10(3):355–364.
76. Bista MB, Banerjee MK, Shin SH, et al. Efficacy of single-dose SA 14-14-2 vaccine against Japanese encephalitis: a case control study. *Lancet* 2001;358(9284):791–795.
77. Dubischar KL, Kadlecek V, Sablan JB, et al. Immunogenicity of the inactivated Japanese encephalitis virus vaccine IXIARO in children from a Japanese encephalitis virus-endemic region. *Pediatr Infect Dis J* 2017;36(9):898–904.
78. Jelinek T, Cromer MA, Cramer JP, et al. Safety and immunogenicity of an inactivated Vero cell_derived Japanese encephalitis vaccine (IXIARO® JESPECT®) in a pediatric population in JE non-endemic countries: an uncontrolled, open-label phase 3 study. *Travel Med Infect Dis* 2018;22:18–24.
79. Chokephaibulkit K, Sirivichayakul C, Thisyakorn U, et al. Safety and immunogenicity of a single administration of live-attenuated Japanese encephalitis vaccine in previously primed 2-to 5-year-olds and naive 12-to 24-month-olds: multicenter randomized controlled trial. *Pediatr Infect Dis J* 2010;29(12):1111–1117.
80. Tauber E, Kollaritsch H, von Sonnenburg F, et al. Randomized, double-blind, placebo-controlled phase 3 trial of the safety and tolerability of IC51, an inactivated Japanese encephalitis vaccine. *J Infect Dis* 2008;198(4):493–499.
81. Wu W, Liu D, Li K, et al. Post-marketing safety surveillance for inactivated and live-attenuated Japanese encephalitis vaccines in China, 2008–2013. *Vaccine* 2017;35(29):3666–3671.
82. Rabe IB, Miller ER, Fischer M, et al. Adverse events following vaccination with an inactivated, Vero cell culture-derived Japanese encephalitis vaccine in the United States, 2009–2012. *Vaccine* 2015;33(5):708–712.
83. Dubischar-Kastner K, Kaltenboeck A, Klingler A, et al. Safety analysis of a Vero-cell culture derived Japanese encephalitis vaccine, IXIARO (IC51), in 6 months of follow-up. *Vaccine* 2010;28(39):6463–6469.
84. Centers for Disease Control and Prevention. Compendium of animal rabies prevention and control. *MMWR Recomm Rep* 2006;55(RR-05):1–8.
85. WHO Expert Consultation on Rabies: third report: WHO technical report series N°1012. 2018. http://apps.who.int/iris/bitstream/handle/10665/272364/9789241210218-eng.pdf?ua=1. Accessed March 2, 2020.
86. Langedijk AC, de Pijper CA, Spijker R, et al. Rabies antibody response after booster immunization: a systematic review and meta-analysis. *Clin Infect Dis* 2018;67(12):1932–1947.
87. Denis M, Knezevic I, Wilde H, et al. An overview of the immunogenicity and effectiveness of current human rabies vaccines administered by intradermal route. *Vaccine* 2019;37(Suppl 1):A99–A106.
88. Preiss S, Chanthavanich P, Chen LH, et al. Post-exposure prophylaxis (PEP) for rabies with purified chick embryo cell vaccine: a systematic literature review and meta-analysis. *Expert Rev Vaccines* 2018;17(6):525–545.
89. Schuler M, Zimmermann H, Altpeter E, et al. Epidemiology of tick-borne encephalitis in Switzerland, 2005 to 2011. *Euro Surveill* 2014;19(13):pii:20756.
90. Kaiser R. Tick-borne encephalitis. *Infect Dis Clin North Am* 2008;22:561–575.
91. Kaiser R. Long-term prognosis of patients with primary myelitic manifestation of tick-borne encephalitis: a trend analysis covering 10 years [in German]. *Nervenarzt* 2011;82:1020–1025.
92. Kunz C. TBE vaccination and the Austrian experience. *Vaccine* 2003;21(Suppl 1):S50–S55.
93. Heinz FX, Holzmann H, Essl A, et al. Field effectiveness of vaccination against tick-borne encephalitis. *Vaccine* 2007;25:7559–7567.
94. Dierig A, Tebruegge M, Krivec U, et al. Current status of Bacille Calmette Guérin (BCG) immunisation in Europe—a ptbnet survey and review of current guidelines. *Vaccine* 2015;33:4994–4999.
95. World Health Organization. BCG vaccines: WHO position paper—February 2018. *Wkly Epidemiol Rec* 2018;93(8):73–96.
96. Roy A, Eisenhut M, Harris RJ, et al. Effect of BCG vaccination against *Mycobacterium tuberculosis* infection in children: systematic review and meta-analysis. *BMJ* 2014;349:g4643.
97. Mangtani P, Abubakar I, Ariti C, et al. Protection by BCG vaccine against tuberculosis: a systematic review of randomized controlled trials. *Clin Infect Dis* 2014;58(4):470–480.
98. Abubakar I, Pimpin L, Ariti C, et al. Systematic review and metaanalysis of the current evidence on the duration of protection by bacillus Calmette–Guérin vaccination against tuberculosis. *Health Technol Assess* 2013;17(37):1–372.
99. Hesseling AC, Johnson LF, Jaspan H, et al. Disseminated bacilli Calmette-Guérin disease in HIV-infected South African infants. *Bull World Health Organ* 2009;87(7):505–511.
100. Szu SC. Development of Vi conjugate—a new generation of typhoid vaccine. *Expert Rev Vaccines* 2013;12(11):1273–1286.
101. Milligan R, Paul M, Richardson M, et al. Vaccines for preventing typhoid fever. *Cochrane Database Syst Rev* 2018;5:CD001261.
102. Ferreccio C, Levine MM, Rodriguez H. Comparative efficacy of two, three, or four doses of Ty21a live oral typhoid vaccine in enteric-coated capsules: a field trial in an endemic area. *J Infect Dis* 1989;159:766–769.
103. Nnaji CA, Shey MS, Adetokunboh OO, et al. Immunogenicity and safety of fractional dose yellow fever vaccination: a systematic review and meta-analysis. *Vaccine* 2020;38(6):1291–1301.
104. Jean K, Donnelly CA, Ferguson NM, et al. A meta-analysis of serological response associated with yellow fever vaccination. *Am J Trop Med Hyg* 2016;95(6):1435–1439.
105. Miller JR, Orgel HA, Meltzer EO. The safety of egg-containing vaccines for egg-allergic patients. *J Allergy Clin Immunol* 1983;71(6):568–573.
106. Khromava AY, Eidex RB, Weld LH, et al. Yellow fever vaccine: an updated assessment of advanced age as a risk factor for serious adverse events. *Vaccine* 2005;23(25):3256–3263.
107. Lindsey NP, Schroeder BA, Miller ER, et al. Adverse event reports following yellow fever vaccination. *Vaccine* 2008;26:6077–6082.

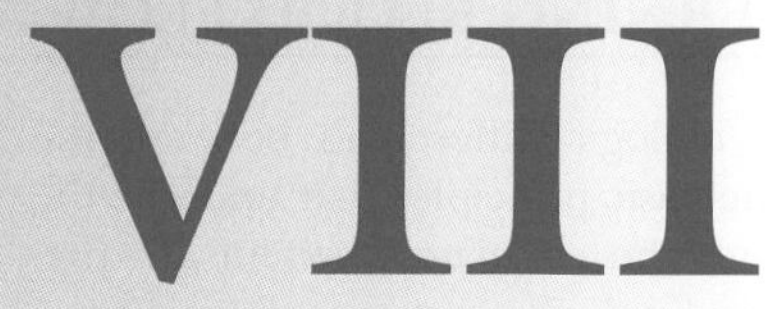

SECTION VIII

Cardiorenal Drugs

Regan E. Giesinger
A. R. Bischoff
Stephanie M. Boyd
Amy H. Stanford
Patrick J. McNamara

CHAPTER 48

Neonatal Cardiovascular Pharmacology

THE PRETERM MYOCARDIUM

Embryologically, the heart is the first organ to function, and it begins in the fourth week after conception when the needs of the growing embryo can no longer be met by diffusion from the placenta. It is initially a tubular structure formed from splanchnic mesoderm; however, it undergoes two stages of looping that result in the adult shape.[1] The fetus is exposed to a dramatically different environment than the adult and, as such, is physiologically adapted to a unique set of ambient conditions. Myocardial architecture, energy utilization, calcium handling, and catecholamine receptor development, therefore, develop progressively over time such that the immature heart at the limits of viability has different properties that become gradually more mature as the neonate develops into an infant and throughout its early childhood.

ARCHITECTURAL AND METABOLIC DEVELOPMENT

Myofibrils, which are the contractile element of the myocyte, are arranged in parallel in the adult myocardium and constitute 50% to 60% of the cellular volume.[2] The noncontractile tissue consists of cellular organelles and collagen, which exist in two primary forms: type I confers rigidity, and type III confers elasticity. Type III collagen is present in approximately 2× the concentration of type I.[3] Energy is supplied primarily by mitochondria that are oriented in rows between myofibrils, and glycogen makes up a relatively small proportion of cellular energy utilization.[2] In contrast, in the developing fetus, myofibrils are typically randomly oriented, peripherally located, and disorganized, with only a few sarcomeres in each segment. Because of the relatively low volume of myofibrils, collagen makes up a greater proportion of the myocyte and is made up of a preponderance of rigid type I collagen, and the premature heart continues to change until adult ratios are reached in late infancy.[3] Mitochondria are present but typically randomly distributed throughout the sarcoplasm and are in relatively low numbers until the late fetal or early postnatal period. Instead, glycogen is available in large pools within the sarcoplasm and fills the spaces between the myofibrils.[2] The relative lack of myofibrils, abundance of noncontractile tissue, and inefficient energy sources contribute to the reduced myocardial compliance that is clinically evident in the preterm myocardium.

MATURATIONAL CHANGES IN CALCIUM HANDLING

The movement of calcium is essential to the performance of cardiac muscle regardless of maturation. An initial influx of calcium into the cytosol via L-type calcium channels triggers the release of more calcium from the sarcoplasmic reticulum (SR). This free cytosolic calcium binds to troponin C that induces a conformational change in the regulatory complex. An actin molecule that is able to bind to the myosin ATPase is exposed, which facilitates the hydrolysis of ATP. The subsequent energy release triggers "sliding" of actin and myosin and shortening of the sarcomere. At the end of the contractile phase, calcium entry into the cell slows and an ATP-dependent calcium pump sequesters the cytosolic calcium into the SR. Thus, calcium moves off troponin C, and adenosine diphosphate (ADP) is displaced from the myosin head to be replaced by ATP and the sarcomere is returned to its original length. The SR, therefore, is an important player in excitation and relaxation, and its function across gestations is important. The SR in an adult makes up 1% to 5% of the cell volume, and although coupling between the SR and sarcolemma is evident in the early myocyte, both the activity and ultrastructure of SR are developmentally regulated.[2,4] The neonatal myocardium is relatively deficient in L-type calcium channels, and fetal sheep demonstrate a decreased ability to store transported calcium owing to an imbalance between calcium influx and efflux from the SR. Several studies suggest that this may be mediated by a greater density of calcium release channels in early development.[4,5] This difference supports the hypothesis that the immature myocardium is more dependent on trans-sarcolemmal calcium influx for contractility than the adult myocardium. Because calcium reuptake is important for muscle relaxation, immaturity of the SR may be a factor that contributes to the reduced ventricular compliance exhibited by preterm myocardium. The T-tubular system, which is important for rapid transit of calcium in the extracellular space, arises with increasing cell size and may also be immature at birth, particularly of preterm infants.[2]

DEVELOPMENTAL VARIATION IN ADRENERGIC RECEPTORS

Just as other aspects of biology mature with increasing gestation, the adrenergic system, which is the pathway most commonly leveraged to control postnatal cardiovascular well-being, changes with development.[6] At early gestations, there are few β_1 receptors but many active α_1 receptors[7] that may skew the response to nonspecific exogenously administered catecholamines to a vasoconstrictive rather than an inotropic profile. Studies in fetal mice have demonstrated a similar number of α receptors at 15 to 20 days' gestation as in the adult heart and a larger number in the early neonate.[8] Similarly, preterm piglet hearts exhibit an abundance of α_{1a} receptor mRNA and a higher proportion of α_{2a} receptor mRNA compared to term.[9] β receptors, in contrast, begin to increase in density at postgestation day 18 in the developing rat and reach adult levels during the second postnatal week.[6] Preterm piglets exhibit ~50% of the β receptor density as compared to term piglets. Despite lower density, functioning β receptors are essential in controlling the heart rate and, therefore, the survival of the fetus.[10] The behavior of β receptors when stimulated may compensate for their relative paucity. In contrast to the adult, in whom activation of the β receptor results in production of inhibitory G-proteins, neonatal β receptors exhibit sensitization. Stimulation of the β receptor G-protein by either β agonists or other molecules using a similar G-protein pathway (e.g., glucagon) results in an increase in adenylyl cyclase catalytic activity.[11,12] The biologic rationale for this is uncertain; however, it may be a fetal adaptive response to the surge of maternal catecholamines that occur during the labor and delivery process. It is important to note that small mammals (mice, rats, and rabbits) are born at an earlier stage of cardiac maturity, and development continues over the first postnatal days to weeks, as compared to larger animal models. Consequently, further characterization of these changes in large animal or human models may be useful.

FUNCTIONAL AND PHYSICAL PRINCIPLES GOVERNING BLOOD FLOW

Although there are many biologic differences between the preterm and adult heart, the basic principles that underlie the movement of blood through the circulatory system are preserved. Blood, like any other fluid, always moves down a pressure gradient. A variety of factors, which are governed by the Hagen–Poiseuille equation, more commonly referred to as Poiseuille's law, modify the efficiency, speed, and pattern of flow. The assumptions of this law, which are occasionally but only infrequently violated in the circulatory system, are that the fluid is incompressible and that flow is laminar through a vessel that is much longer than its diameter.

$$\Delta p = (8\mu LQ)/(\pi R^4)$$

In Poiseuille's law, flow (Q) varies proportionally with change in pressure (p), viscosity (μ), and length (L) and is inversely proportional to the fourth power of radius (R). Thus, the flow through the vasculature may be manipulated most efficiently by changing the vessel radius, but pressure gradient and viscosity are also important and potentially modifiable. Throughout the following chapter, we will discuss opportunities to modify flow in various disease conditions using manipulation of the components of Poiseuille's law such as transfusion of hemoglobin and manipulation of pulmonary vascular resistance (PVR) to limit transductal flow in the setting of a hemodynamically significant ductus arteriosus (DA). The circulatory system is adaptive and dynamic; however, there are a variety of other mechanisms beyond fluid mechanics by which aspects of cardiac function are modified by changing ambient conditions. There are important differences in these rules owing to the fundamental differences in ultrastructure previously discussed, which make the neonatal population unique as compared to the more mature cardiovascular system.

FRANK–STARLING LAW

In the healthy adult, as left ventricular (LV) filling increases so too does cardiac contractility. This is because organized myofibrils that are stretched to an increasing degree rebound with greater force. The neonatal myocardium, particularly following preterm delivery, has a different pattern of response. At very low atrial filling pressures, there is an incremental increase in contractility; with increasing filling pressures as the myocardium is stretched, myofibrils achieve their optimal conformation. Thereafter, however, there is little change in ventricular contractility as filling pressures continue to increase[13] (Fig. 48.1). This has important implications for the management, particularly of diseases associated with low left atrial preload, such as acute pulmonary hypertension. LV systolic function may be compromised by low pulmonary blood flow unless right-to-left atrial shunt compensates for low filling pressure. In contrast, when treating patients with impaired systemic blood flow, volume cannot be counted on to increase cardiac contractility unless the left atrium is critically underfilled. It is prudent to begin treatment with volume therapy; however, in the neonatal population, relatively early introduction of inotrope and/or vasopressor, as appropriate to the dominant physiology, is recommended.

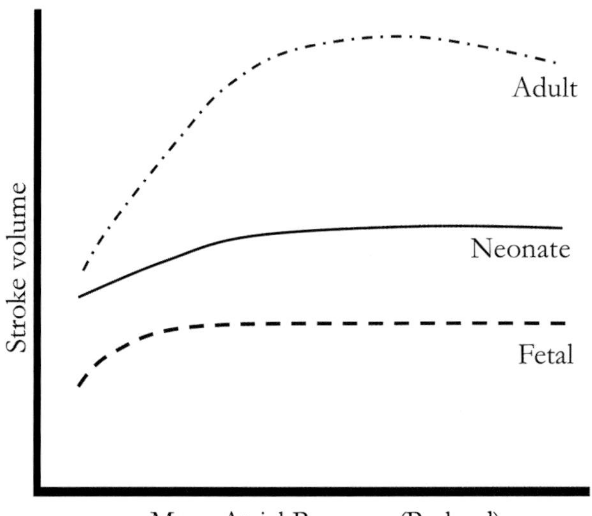

Figure 48.1 Schematic of the Frank–Starling curve according to maturity. (Adapted from Reller MD, Morton MJ, Reid DL, et al. Fetal lamb ventricles respond differently to filling and arterial pressures and to in utero ventilation. *Pediatr Res* 1987;22:621–626.)

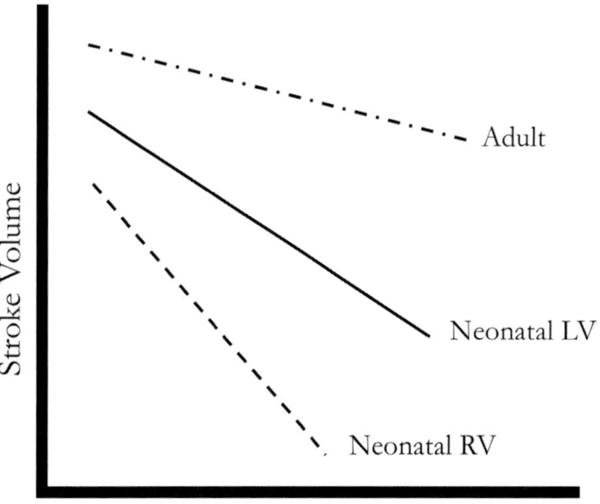

Figure 48.2 Schematic representing the relationship between afterload and cardiac contractility or stroke volume. Adults have the lowest decrement with increasing afterload when both the neonatal left ventricle (LV) and even more so the right ventricle (RV) experience a steep decline in cardiac performance as mean arterial pressure increases. (Data from Reller MD, Morton MJ, Reid DL, et al. Fetal lamb ventricles respond differently to filling and arterial pressures and to in utero ventilation. *Pediatr Res* 1987;22:621–626; and Pinson CW, Morton MJ, Thornburg KL. An anatomic basis for fetal right ventricular dominance and arterial pressure sensitivity. *J Dev Physiol* 1987;9:253–269.)

STRESS–VELOCITY RELATIONSHIP

The relationship between the velocity of isotonic shortening and the force developed was published in a classical study of cat papillary muscle in 1962 by Edmund Sonnenblick.[14] In the healthy heart, the velocity of circumferential fiber shortening, which reflects the speed at which the muscle cell shortens and therefore is a surrogate marker of contractility, is inversely proportional to the amount of afterload against which it is pumping. In the neonatal heart, the slope of the relationship between afterload and contractility is steeper than in the adult such that for every increase in afterload seen, there is a proportionally greater decline in contractility in comparison with the mature heart (Fig. 48.2). Because of geometric, adaptive, and metabolic differences, the neonatal left and right ventricles (RVs) also respond differently to afterload. When both ventricles are exposed to the same increase in afterload, the RV experiences greater wall stress and therefore has a greater decrement in myocardial performance.[13,15] Understanding the force–velocity relationship is fundamental to managing neonatal cardiovascular disease because many of the conditions that result in neonatal cardiovascular instability (e.g., transitional owing to the loss of low-resistance placenta, acute/chronic pulmonary hypertension, and surgical DA closure) are afterload-mediated diseases. The drugs appropriate for use in this population are largely those with positive inotropic properties and either neutral or with more minor vasoconstrictive effects. The use of vasoconstrictors to increase blood pressure should be restricted to select circumstances, such as when coronary perfusion pressure is critically low.

FORCE–FREQUENCY RELATIONSHIP

One of the fundamental laws that govern the coupling of cardiac performance to metabolic demand is the relationship between heart rate and contractility. Heart rate is driven to increase by neurohormonal control mechanisms intrinsic to the sympathetic nervous system in response to increased needs. The maximal change in heart rate is variable, but is approximately 2.5 to 3× magnitude (e.g., 60 to 180 beats per minute). In contrast, metabolic demand for oxygen with exercise may increase sevenfold to tenfold.[16] It is clear that heart rate alone is not sufficient to meet those needs and a corresponding increase in contractility to produce a greater stroke volume per beat is also required. At extremely high heart rate, however, further tachycardia becomes problematic. The interval between contractions shortens to a point that there is insufficient time for calcium to be cleared from the sarcolemma and sequestered into the SR; therefore, the force of the subsequent beats declines. This results in a U-shaped curve with the lowest contractility at both the lowest and highest extremes of heart rate (Fig. 48.3). The human neonate has a relatively flat force–frequency relationship (FFR) as compared to older infants and adults; however, it demonstrates a large increase in frequency-dependent acceleration of relaxation.[17] This difference may be a partial explanation for why neonatal animal models demonstrate a resilience to elevated heart rate. As compared to adult piglets, neonates experience a rightward shift of the FFR such that sustained moderate tachycardia may be better tolerated than a comparable rate among adult patients. This is likely related to differences in calcium handling and may partially explain why neonates with supraventricular tachycardia may present with cardiac dysfunction after a relatively prolonged tachycardia event that would be rapidly fatal in an adult. The consequence of this rightward deviation, however, is that resumption of normal heart rate may be associated with impaired myocardial performance until the "normal" relationship between heart rate and contractility is restored.[18]

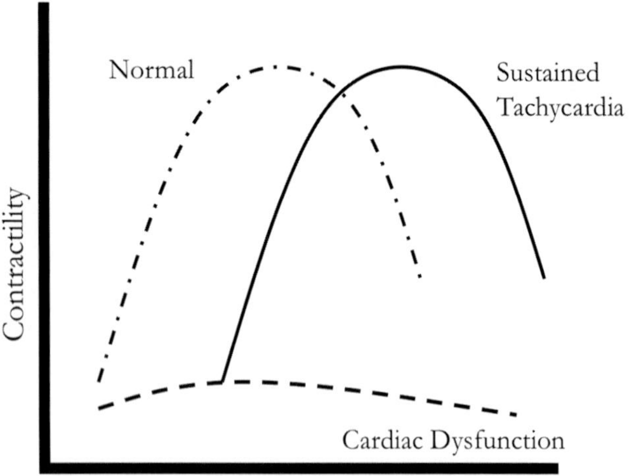

Figure 48.3 Force–frequency relationship differences between the normal myocardium, the neonate with sustained tachycardia, and the dysfunctional heart. (Data from Wiegerinck RF, Cojoc A, Zeidenweber CM, et al. Force frequency relationship of the human ventricle increases during early postnatal development. *Pediatr Res* 2009;65:414–419; and Schmidt MR, White PA, Khambadkone S, et al. The neonatal but not the mature heart adapts to acute tachycardia by beneficial modification of the force-frequency relationship. *Pediatr Cardiol* 2011;32:562–567.)

In patients with cardiac dysfunction regardless of age, the ability of the myocardium to respond to increasing heart rate with an associated increase in contractility and therefore stroke volume is blunted.[18] The normal U-shaped curve, therefore, becomes flat. This is an important principle in that many of the cardiovascular medications that are used as primary vasoconstrictors (e.g., dopamine and norepinephrine) are also chronotropes. If an increase in the heart rate is not associated with a concurrent increase in cardiac contractility, there may be negative consequences on filling time and myocardial metabolic requirements without any associated increase in stroke volume. This may be detrimental to the physiology, particularly of neonates with preexisting tachycardia (e.g., owing to shock, fever, poor LV preload, and other medications) who are receiving multiple β adrenergic agents.

RELATIONSHIP BETWEEN BLOOD PRESSURE AND BLOOD FLOW

Blood pressure is one of the core elements that make up a comprehensive cardiovascular clinical examination. It is easily measured, reproducible, and objective. A large body of literature has been dedicated to attempting to link various arbitrary definitions of "hypotension," which are primarily aimed at attaining a certain predefined mean pressure with neurologic outcomes (e.g., intraventricular hemorrhage [IVH]) and have produced conflicting results. Heterogeneity in methodology and population, lack of untreated controls, and an inconsistent definition of low blood pressure make the body of evidence difficult to interpret. In addition, it is important to note that low blood pressure is a symptom and not a disease in and of itself. It is not only possible but also frequent for neonates to have significant cardiovascular impairment in the presence of normal or high blood pressure, particularly when the underlying pathology is cardiac dysfunction secondary to afterload or a primary myocardial process. The underlying circulatory milieu is likely to have a substantial impact on how consequential low blood pressure becomes with respect to determining the impact on neurocognitive outcomes. For example, a preterm neonate with low mean blood pressure (MBP) because of diastolic runoff via the DA in the first 6 hours after birth with normal systemic perfusion and a low oxygen requirement is likely to have a very different prognosis than a preterm of comparable age with a comparable MBP because of failed transition, acute pulmonary hypertension, and with elevated serum lactate and hypoxemia. What is clear, however, is that low systemic blood flow is an important problem, particularly among neonates born preterm. In this population, low systemic blood flow has been documented in 35% of neonates born <30 weeks and 65% of neonates born <27 weeks.[19]

As a consequence of prematurity being an intrinsically abnormal state, frequent cardiovascular and respiratory comorbidities, and limited tools for evaluating actual physiology, there has been long-standing uncertainty as to what "normal" blood pressure truly is. A British Association of Perinatal Medicine position statement on best practices for the care of the neonate with respiratory distress syndrome published in 1992 the now widely cited expert opinion that MBP is usually around the gestational age (GA) of the well neonate.[20] Since that time, several groups have attempted to define normal blood pressure by developing percentiles for systolic, diastolic, and MBP in small populations of neonates.[21] Evidence supports the assertion that current definitions of low systemic pressure are not synonymous with low systemic blood flow, however. In a group of 126 preterm infants studied at 5 hours of age, superior vena cava flow (SVCF), as a surrogate for LV output, and blood pressure measurements were discordant 42% of the time.[22] Using MBP < GA, the most commonly used definition of hypotension,[23] in a different group of preterms, correctly categorized only 71% of neonates with low systemic blood flow and falsely identified 12% of neonates with high or normal systemic blood flow as hypotensive.[24] Using an MBP cutoff of 30 mmHg, regardless of GA, 64% of neonates with high or normal SVCF were erroneously classified as hypotensive. It is probable that there is no single threshold that applies to every neonate, and a composite of change from baseline, normative data, and evidence of poor perfusion should be used.

The use of the individual components of blood pressure may provide more direction as to the etiology of the underlying cardiovascular compromise. Systolic blood pressure is generated by the force exerted against the vessel when the aortic valve is open and varies directly with the magnitude of cardiac output.[25] Diastolic, in contrast, is the resting force of the blood against the vessel walls when the aortic valve is closed and, therefore, is reflective of the size (vascular tone) and number of vessels. Using systolic and diastolic separately to evaluate the most likely contributors to disease as opposed to the mean, which is a time-weighted average of the two, may be valuable in clinical practice (Fig. 48.4). Adjunct tools such as targeted neonatal echocardiography, near-infrared spectroscopy, and noninvasive cardiac output monitoring

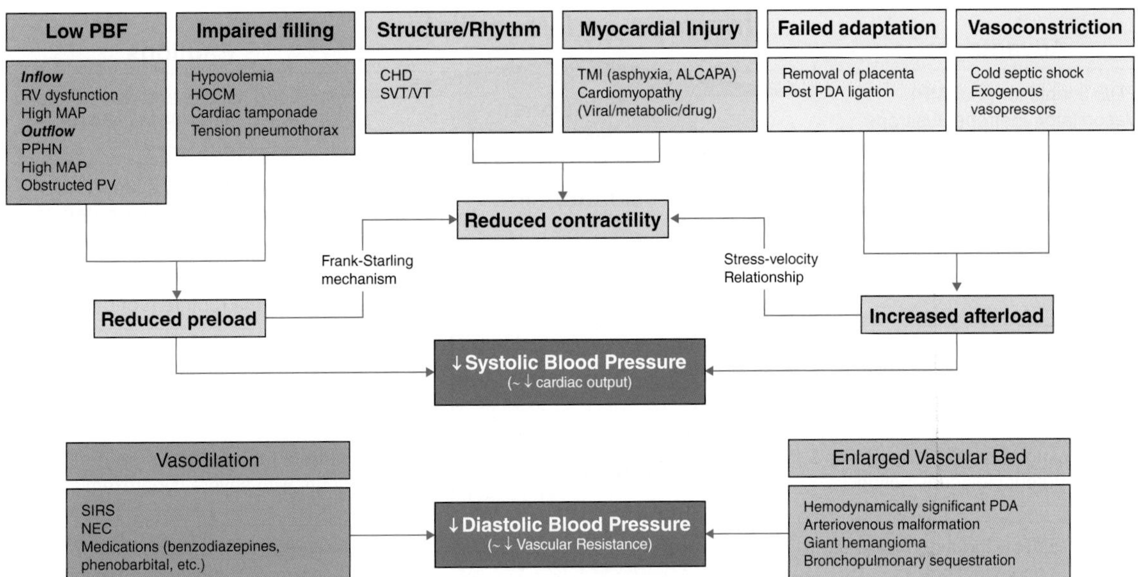

Figure 48.4 Physiologic approach to the appraisal of low systolic and low diastolic blood pressure based on relevant disease states. ALCAPA, anomalous left coronary artery to the pulmonary artery; CHD, congenital heart disease; HOCM, hypertrophic obstructive cardiomyopathy; MAP, mean airway pressure; NEC, necrotizing enterocolitis; PBF, pulmonary blood flow; PDA, patent ductus arteriosus; PPHN, persistent pulmonary hypertension; PV, pulmonary veins; SIRS, systemic inflammatory response syndrome; SVT, supraventricular tachycardia; TMI, transient myocardial ischemia; VT, ventricular tachycardia.

may be used to supplement clinical data and, in the case of targeted neonatal echocardiography, define the physiology more precisely.

SUPPORT FOR HEART FUNCTION

The support of heart function can be achieved by a combination of inotropes, medications that act on the myocyte to increase contractility, and vasodilators. Arterial vasodilation decreases ventricular wall tension and improves stroke volume and cardiac output. We hereby present the mechanisms of medications used for the support of newborn heart function: (a) predominant inotropes, including dobutamine and epinephrine; (b) inotropes with vasodilator effect, including milrinone and levosimendan; and (c) vasodilators such as sodium nitroprusside (SNP) and inhaled nitric oxide (iNO; Table 48.1).

PROPERTIES OF DRUGS WITH PREDOMINANT INOTROPIC ACTION

Dobutamine

Dobutamine is a synthetic catecholamine that promotes direct stimulation of myocardial adrenergic receptors.[26] It is a racemic mixture comprising two parts: the negative isomer is an α_1 receptor agonist that increases myocardial contractility and systemic vascular resistance (SVR), whereas the positive isomer is a β_1 or β_2 receptor agonist that increases myocardial contractility and heart rate and decreases SVR (Fig. 48.5). The activation of β_1 receptors on the myocytes initiates a cascade that generates cyclic adenosine monophosphate (cAMP) and ultimately increases intracellular calcium concentration that stimulates contractility.[27] In contrast, a process that includes phosphorylation increases the rate of calcium that is transported from the cytosol back into the SR during diastole, which helps promote relaxation of the cardiac muscle and ensures sufficient calcium

Table 48.1 Summary of Medications Impacting Heart Function in Neonates

Medication	*Mechanism of Action*	*Hemodynamic Effect*
Dobutamine	Negative isomer: α_1 receptor agonist Positive isomer: β_1 and β_2 receptor agonist	↑ inotropy and chronotropy ↓/ no effect on SVR
Epinephrine	β_1 and β_2 receptor agonist at low doses (0.01–0.1 μg/kg/min) Added α_1 receptor agonist effect at doses >0.1 μg/kg/min	↑ inotropy and chronotropy ↓/ no effect on SVR ↑ SVR at higher doses
Milrinone	Selective phosphodiesterase 3A inhibitor	↑ inotropy, lusitropy ↓↓ SVR and ↓↓ PVR
Levosimendan	Calcium-sensitizing agent	↑ inotropy, lusitropy ↓ SVR and ↓ PVR
Sodium nitroprusside	Release of NO, stimulates cGMP production	↓↓ SVR and ↓↓ PVR
Inhaled nitric oxide	Stimulates cGMP production	↓↓ PVR

cGMP, cyclic guanosine monophosphate; NO, nitric oxide; PVR, pulmonary vascular resistance; SVR, systemic vascular resistance.

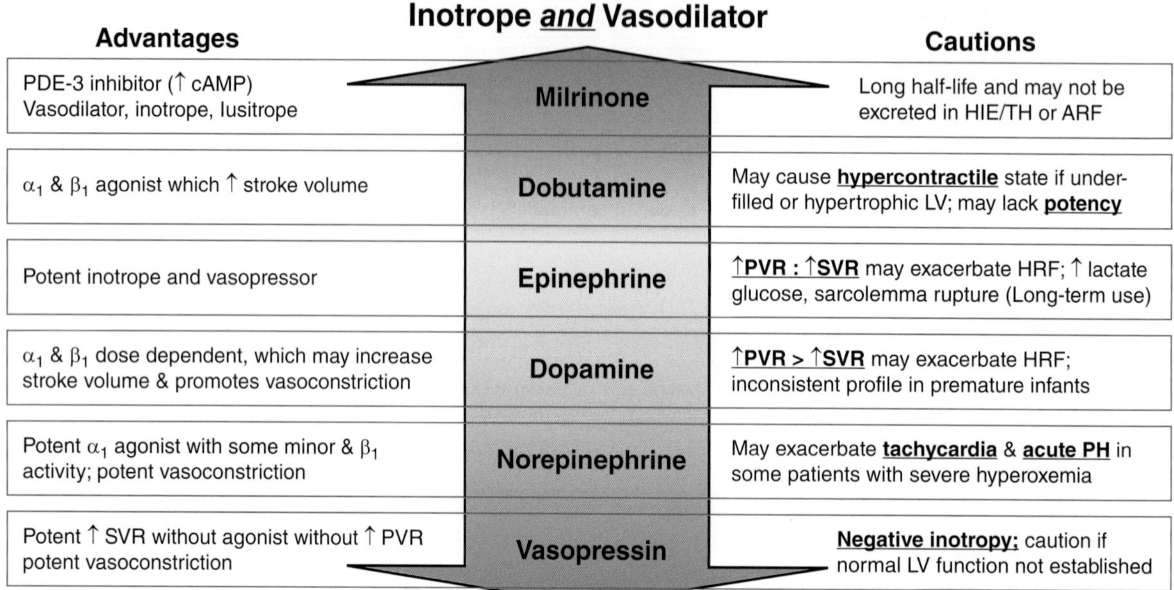

Figure 48.5 Spectrum of drug activity from inotropes with vasodilator properties at one extreme to pure vasopressors at the other end. Selected advantages and cautions are described. ARF, acute renal failure; cAMP, cyclic adenosine monophosphate; HIE, hypoxic ischemic encephalopathy; HRF, hypoxic respiratory failure; LV, left ventricle; PDE, phosphodiesterase; PH, pulmonary hypertension; PVR, pulmonary vascular resistance; SVR, systemic vascular resistance; TH, therapeutic hypothermia.

availability for the next cycle, improving cardiac excitation–contraction coupling.[27]

The resultant net hemodynamic effect is increased inotropy and chronotropy with either no effect or a decrease in SVR.[28,29] The expression of α and β adrenergic receptors is developmentally regulated and may affect both cardiac and vascular responses to dobutamine in newborns. In early development, α adrenergic receptor expression is upregulated, as compared to β adrenergic expression, such that premature infants may have attenuated decreases in SVR when compared to term infants.[28] Such characteristics make dobutamine a drug of choice in conditions where there is myocardial dysfunction such as the transitional period of preterm infants, acute pulmonary hypertension, and asphyxia, but not in those with concomitant low SVR where the vasodilatory properties may be disadvantageous.[28,30,31] Additionally, neonates with both cardiac dysfunction and severe hypotension may benefit from either a more potent combined inotrope/vasopressor (e.g., epinephrine) or a combination therapy of dobutamine and one of the predominant vasopressors (e.g., norepinephrine and vasopressin).

The hemodynamic effects of dobutamine have been extensively studied. Animal studies show a dose-dependent increases in heart rate and stroke volume, with increased cardiac output as a consequence.[32–34] Studies in neonatal ovine and porcine models suggest that the vasodilating effects of dobutamine are more obvious in the systemic as compared to pulmonary circulation.[34,35] In human neonates, the increase in cardiac output is determined mainly by increases in stroke volume,[36] and the effects on arterial pressure are somewhat controversial.[37–45] Importantly, dobutamine's effects in the peripheral circulation are neither potent nor reliable in situations that call for modification of vascular tone. A Cochrane review comparing the use of dopamine versus dobutamine in preterm infants concluded that dopamine was superior in increasing arterial pressure, with no differences in medium- to long-term outcomes of mortality, periventricular leukomalacia (PVL), or severe IVH.[38] There are, however, a number of studies that demonstrate a superior physiologic profile of dobutamine among patients without vasodilation as a main component of their disease pathology, such as improvements in SVCF[46] and LV output,[43] which are not present with dopamine.[46,47]

Dobutamine is administered as a continuous infusion, with doses usually ranging from 2 to 20 μg per kg per minute. A positive effect on LV performance has been shown at doses of 5 to 10 μg per kg per minute in preterm neonates,[37,40,41] with changes noted in cardiac output within the first 20 minutes of infusion and improvement in other markers of systemic blood flow after 8 to 10 hours.[39] Higher doses of dobutamine may decrease myocardial compliance and impact ventricular filling.[28,48] In addition, at doses above 12.5 to 15 μg per kg per minute, it is common to see tachycardia, without further benefit to contractility, which may negatively impact the FFR. Dobutamine is metabolized by the liver into 3-O-methyldobutamine and its conjugates and then excreted in the urine.[49] Wide variations in plasma concentrations are likely related to differences in plasma clearance rates that are independent of birth weight and GA.[37] Side effects may include tachycardia, arrhythmias, hypertension, and hypotension.[37,49]

Epinephrine

Epinephrine is an endogenous catecholamine released by the adrenal gland in response to stressful stimuli. It stimulates both α and β adrenergic receptors and exerts its cardiovascular effects in a dose-dependent manner. The β_1 and β_2 receptors in the cardiac muscle and vascular bed are stimulated at low doses (0.01 to 0.1 μg per kg per minute), leading to increased inotropy, chronotropy, and peripheral vasodilation.

The α_1 receptors become activated at doses higher than 0.1 μg per kg per minute, causing vasoconstriction and increased inotropy, whereas the vascular α_2 effects are less prominent.[50,51] The effects seen on the different vasculatures also appear to be dose dependent,[52,53] and the onset of action occurs in a few minutes.

In some patients, a significant increase in blood pressure and systemic blood flow may be seen secondary to its effects on vascular tone and cardiac output. Low-dose epinephrine is an alternative therapy for patients with cardiac dysfunction either when dobutamine has been ineffective or when both increased contractility and increased vascular tone (owing to either low diastolic or combined systolic and diastolic blood pressure) are required. In patients with low cardiac output secondary to impaired LV systolic performance but elevated blood pressure because of compensatory renovascular effects, low-dose epinephrine may have a positive inotropic effect that leads to improved systemic blood flow and a paradoxical normalization of blood pressure. Diseases in which epinephrine is commonly used include septic shock with cardiac dysfunction (e.g., cold shock) and diseases associated with severe cardiac dysfunction (e.g., myocarditis or ischemic cardiac injury in perinatal asphyxia). In myocardial impairment secondary to acute pulmonary hypertension, the combination of inotropy and vasoconstriction may improve RV perfusion pressure and cardiac output.[48] Caution is advised among patients with severe hypoxemia in the setting of acute pulmonary hypertension, however, because animal data suggest that epinephrine may also increase PVR and pulmonary artery pressure (PAP).[52]

Several studies have compared epinephrine to dopamine in a variety of patient populations. In animal models of hypoxia and pulmonary hypertension, epinephrine more effectively increases cardiac output and stroke volume, and dopamine is associated with a greater increase in PAP (higher PAP to systemic artery pressure [SAP]) as compared to epinephrine, making epinephrine the agent with the preferred side-effect profile as compared to dopamine in this patient population (see Fig. 48.5).[52–54] Studies in hypotensive newborns showed equivalence between the two drugs in terms of reversal of hypotension.[55,56] In a randomized trial of preterm infants weighing <1,750 g, dopamine was associated with reduced and epinephrine with increased LV output.[57] In general, however, epinephrine induced more tachycardia and higher plasma lactate and serum glucose.[55,56] These adverse effects are thought to be due to drug-induced stimulation of β_2 adrenoreceptors in the liver and skeletal muscle, with lower insulin release leading to hyperglycemia and increased glycogenolysis leading to higher lactate production. The rise in serum lactate seems to be independent of the improvement in hemodynamic status and requires careful interpretation.

Changes in cerebral hemodynamics with these drugs are variable according to GA in hypotensive preterm neonates[56] as are the effects of epinephrine in the coronaries. Isolated coronary artery preparations showed constriction of the vascular bed,[58] whereas systemic infusion reduced coronary vascular resistance and increased blood flow.[51] It is possible that the increase in coronary blood flow may surpass the increase in myocardial oxygen demand secondary to the inotropic and chronotropic effects; however, prolonged use of epinephrine should be avoided if possible. Epinephrine has been associated with impaired compliance via rupture of sarcolemma and deposition of calcium in the mitochondria, resulting in myocardial ischemia.[31,59] Epinephrine is the final end point of the catecholamine synthesis pathway. Norepinephrine, which is produced from dopamine, is metabolized into epinephrine via the enzyme phenylethanolamine-N-methyltransferase (PNMT) and broken down into dihydroxymandelic acid and metanephrine by monoamine oxidase (MAO) and catecholamine-O-methyltransferase (COMT), respectively. Ultimately, both norepinephrine and epinephrine are metabolized into the inactive metabolites vanillylmandelic acid (VMA) and 3-methyl-4-hydroxyphenyl-glycol (MHPG), which are excreted in the urine (Fig. 48.6).

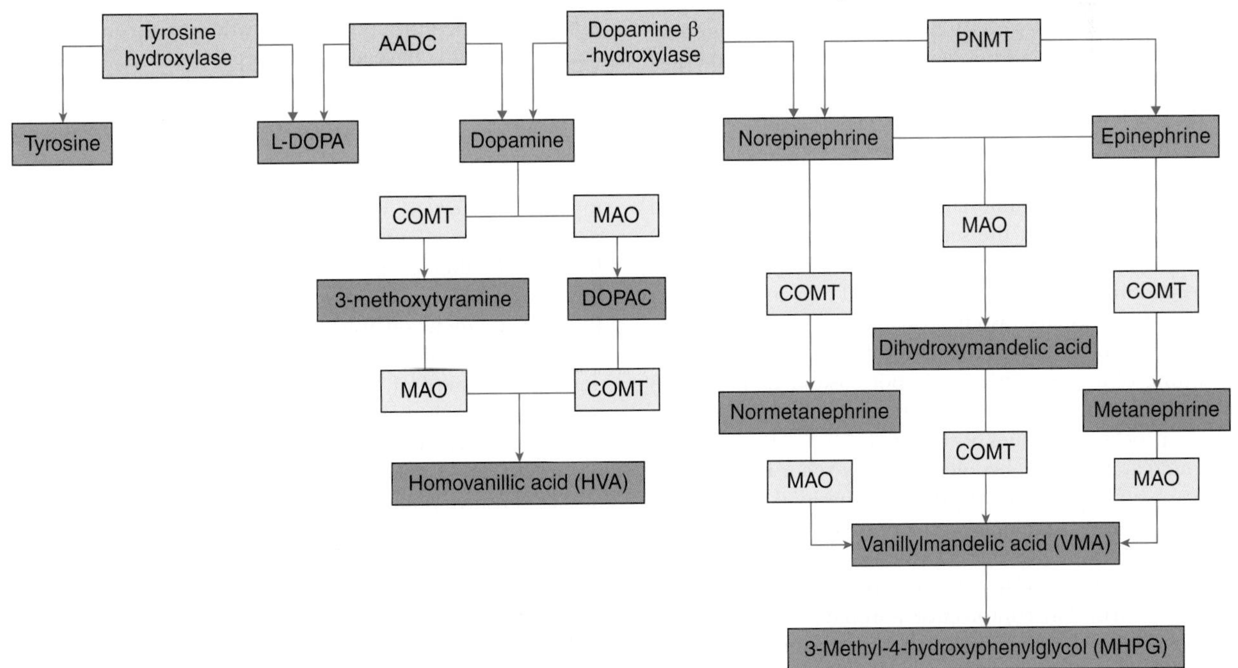

Figure 48.6 Catecholamine synthesis and metabolism. AADC, L-aromatic amino acid decarboxylase; COMT, catecholamine-O-methyltransferase; DOPA, dihydroxyphenylalanine; MAO, monoamine oxidase; PNMT, phenylethanolamine-N-methyltransferase.

PROPERTIES OF INOTROPES WITH VASODILATOR EFFECTS

Milrinone

Milrinone is a selective phosphodiesterase-3A (PDE-3A) inhibitor with vasodilator, inotropic,[60,61] and lusitropic[62] properties. The inhibition of intracellular PDE-3A decreases the hydrolysis rate of 3′,5′-cAMP, activating protein kinases that modulate L-type calcium channels to promote higher influx of calcium into the sarcoplasm.[31,63] The increased cytosolic calcium in turn triggers calcium release from the SR, resulting in the activation of contractile proteins.[63,64] Protein kinases activated by cAMP also have a role in the phosphorylation of phospholamban and troponin I, which are proteins found in the SR and a subunit of the troponin–tropomyosin complex, respectively. Both of these are implicated in accelerated removal of calcium from the cell via activation of Ca-ATPase and decreased affinity of troponin C to calcium. The net effect is a shortening of contraction time and thereby a longer relaxation period in the cardiac cycle (lusitropic effect).[63] In the smooth muscle cells of both systemic and pulmonary vasculature, increased cAMP modulates increased nitric oxide (NO) signaling and results in calcium-mediated vasodilation.[65] The inotropic effect of milrinone, in particular, seems to be developmentally regulated owing to differential expression of PDE isoforms between fetal and postnatal life[62] and variable mechanisms of calcium-mediated myocardial contraction as previously described (see section "Maturational Changes in Calcium Handling"). It is, therefore, probable that the primary mechanism by which milrinone is related to improved cardiac function, particularly in the preterm population, is mediated by afterload reduction with secondary improvement in cardiac output.[48]

The combination of afterload reduction in both the systemic and pulmonary vasculature, in addition to inotropic and lusitropic properties, improves the hemodynamics in a variety of cardiovascular conditions in the neonatal population. These include prophylaxis of low cardiac output syndrome in post-cardiac surgery and ligation of the patent DA,[64,66,67] acute pulmonary hypertension[68,69] with RV dysfunction,[70] and congenital diaphragmatic hernia.[71] Additionally, a direct myocardial effect may be beneficial in cases of LV dysfunction.[72] Milrinone use has been reported in heart dysfunction related to myocarditis[73] as well as in heart dysfunction after cardiac surgery, where afterload reduction and inotropy have additive effects in improving cardiac output.[64] In pulmonary hypertension, experimental evidence suggests that, in the setting of 100% oxygen administration, iNO upregulates PDE-3 expression.[74] Hence, theoretically, the coadministration of milrinone and iNO may augment cAMP-related pulmonary vasodilation.[48,75,76] Systemic hypotension has been associated with the use of milrinone, particularly in the setting of acute pulmonary hypertension. Its incidence is variable, which may be related to the nature of the underlying disease process and issues of clearance.[68,69,77,78] Patients with low PBF-mediated systolic hypotension may see a net increase in blood pressure because of improved LV preload and cardiac output.[69] In contrast, patients with preexisting borderline or low diastolic blood pressure or a primary vasodilating process may develop problematic hypotension owing to reduction in SVR. This, in turn, may compromise coronary perfusion pressure and exacerbate cardiac dysfunction. Caution is advised in these clinical situations.[69]

Milrinone is excreted by the kidneys with little to no metabolism, such that its plasma concentration is largely influenced by renal function and urinary output.[77,79] Studies suggest that newborns demonstrate lower clearance and higher volume of distribution when compared to older children and adults.[80–82] Among term infants, milrinone has a half-life of approximately 4 hours.[69] The half-life increases and the total clearance decreases with lower GA,[69,75,80] whereas clearance is directly proportional to chronologic age in older infants.[82,83] Among preterm infants, a half-life of 10 hours has been suggested,[80] although there is likely to be developmental differences across gestations. There are scarce reports on the pharmacokinetics of milrinone in the pediatric population with acute kidney injury, showing lower clearance when compared to adult and pediatric patients without renal impairment.[79,84–86] Although a pharmacokinetic study of near-term neonates reported that hypotension following milrinone administration was not related to plasma concentration,[77] this has not been studied in larger samples. Excretion is likely to be even longer in patients with prematurity, end-organ dysfunction, and hypoxic ischemic encephalopathy with or without therapeutic hypothermia.[31]

Milrinone administration is by continuous infusion usually started between 0.2 and 0.33 μg per kg per minute and titrated to a maximum of 1 μg per kg per minute to achieve desirable effect.[69,80] It can or cannot be preceded by a loading dose of 0.5 to 0.75 μg per kg per minute for the first 1 to 3 hours, and the onset of action is usually in 5 to 15 minutes. Among 10 preterm neonates born in 24 to 30 weeks' gestation studied in the first postnatal month, a 3-hour loading dose of 0.5 μg per kg per minute followed by a lower dose continuous infusion, which varied by GA (0.15 μg per kg per minute <27 weeks and 0.2 μg per kg per minute ≥27 weeks), was recommended.[67] Although this work supports the principle that an alternative dosing regime is required depending on maturity, this approach requires evaluation in a larger cohort. Coinfusion of a normal saline bolus of 10 to 15 mL per kg during the first hour of the infusion may aid in the prevention of low diastolic arterial pressure caused by vasodilation.[66,80] The most common side effect is hypotension, although tachyarrhythmias, thrombocytopenia, and hypokalemia have also been reported.[65]

Levosimendan

Levosimendan is a myofilament calcium-sensitizing agent with inotropic action as well as ATP-dependent potassium channel vasodilator effect.[27] It stabilizes the binding of calcium to troponin C, thereby prolonging the systolic interaction of actin–myosin filaments. Unlike other agents, levosimendan's action is dependent on intracellular calcium, making this agent capable of parallel enhancement of myocardial contractility and improvement of LV diastolic function without promoting arrhythmogenesis or alteration of myocardial oxygen demand.[27] At higher doses, it has also been associated with the inhibition of cardiac PDE-3. Vasodilation is most likely induced by opening of ATP-sensitive potassium channels in vascular smooth muscle cells of several vasculatures including coronary, pulmonary, renal, splanchnic, cerebral, and systemic arteries, as well as saphenous, portal, and systemic veins.[27]

The hemodynamic profile is similar to milrinone and may be beneficial in patients with myocardial dysfunction where afterload reduction improves cardiac output.[27] Its use has been described in adults with congenital heart failure,[87] as well as in neonates, infants, and children, particularly in the setting of postoperative cardiac surgery.[88–92] Further studies are required to assess efficacy, dosing, and safety of this medication in newborns and preterm infants. The application may be relevant in disease states where there is concomitant myocardial dysfunction and increased afterload such as prevention and/or treatment of postligation cardiac syndrome following patent DA closure and acute pulmonary hypertension of the newborn.

PROPERTIES OF PRIMARY VASODILATORS

Sodium Nitroprusside

SNP is a sodium salt that consists of ferrous ion, NO, and five cyanide anions.[93] It is a direct-acting vasodilator in the arterial and venous bed,[93] with no direct effect on myocardial contractility or heart rate.[93,94] In vivo, it functions as a prodrug and reacts with sulfhydryl groups on erythrocytes, albumin, and other proteins to release NO.[95] NO activates guanylate cyclase, which stimulates the production of cyclic guanosine monophosphate (cGMP). Vasodilation is independent of vascular endothelium[96] and results from cGMP-mediated decrease in intracellular calcium and protein kinase–mediated dephosphorylation of myosin light chains within vascular smooth muscle cells.[97–99] The main hemodynamic effect is reduced SVR, and therefore reduced afterload, as well as increased venous capacitance with decreased preload. Secondary to its vasodilator effects, SNP decreases ventricular filling pressures, reduces wall stress, and lowers myocardial oxygen demand. The net result is increased cardiac output and systemic tissue oxygenation provided that coronary perfusion pressure is maintained.[93,99,100]

The primary role of SNP is in diseases of either high afterload or primary left heart dysfunction. As a result, it has been extensively used in adults with hypertension, congestive heart failure, and cardiogenic shock.[93,101] In the pediatric population and among neonates, its use is less frequent; however, it has been used in hypertensive emergencies[102,103] as well as in pulmonary hypertension and shock.[101] There is also a potential role as an afterload reducer following cardiovascular surgery to increase systemic oxygen delivery and to decrease myocardial oxygen consumption.[99] As with many pharmacotherapies, animal studies using a hypoxia-induced pulmonary hypertension model suggest that response to SNP may be dependent on maturation. This may, in part, account for variable clinical responses to vasodilators in hypoxemic newborns.[104]

SNP has a very rapid onset of action (i.e., within 30 seconds), a peak effect in 2 minutes, and a cessation of effect after 3 minutes of discontinuation.[99] It is a highly effective agent in situations where rapid blood pressure lowering is indicated, such as heart failure induced by hypertensive crisis.[93,103] SNP is administered as a continuous intravenous (IV) infusion, typically initiated at 0.5 μg per kg per minute, and can be titrated rapidly to achieve the desired effect. There are limited data on pediatric and neonatal dosage that suggest a maximum dose of 2 μg per kg per minute, with higher doses reserved for short periods when urgent blood pressure control is required.[105,106] Because of its rapid effect, vigilant monitoring is recommended to avoid rapid and potentially life-threatening hypotension with systemic hypoperfusion. In addition, there are few reports on the potential application of SNP in nebulized form.[107–109] In piglets, nebulized SNP appears to have a selective effect in the pulmonary vasculature, with no effect on arterial blood pressure or heart rate.[109] The reduction in PAP has been shown to be of similar magnitude and timing to that of iNO in both animal and human studies.[107,108]

SNP metabolism results in the release of both NO and five molecules of cyanide. Four molecules of cyanide react with thiosulfates to produce thiocyanate in the liver, which is then excreted exclusively by the kidney with a mean elimination half-life of 3 to 7 days,[95,99] whereas the other molecule binds with a methemoglobin molecule to form cyanomethemoglobin. Exposure to light leads to photodegradation and subsequent rapid cyanide anion release.[93] Depletion of body storage of thiosulfate or cyanide production surpassing current thiosulfate stores leads to accumulation of cyanide, with subsequent toxicity related to increases in cyanomethemoglobin.[106] Toxicity usually occurs at higher dosages (described as more than 1.8 μg per kg per minute in pediatric patients[105]) or prolonged exposure (usually longer than 24 to 48 hours).[93,99] Cyanomethemoglobin is unavailable for oxygen binding that, at high levels, causes end-organ dysfunction and lactic acidosis.[93,110] Toxicity is detected by plasma thiocyanate levels above 2 μg per mL and can be treated by infusing thiosulfate or with hemodialysis.[106] Other signs of cyanide toxicity may include altered mental status, seizures, anorexia, fatigue, hypothyroidism, and muscle spasms,[93,101] and SNP is also associated with increased intracranial pressure.[102] Newborns are theoretically at higher risk for toxicity owing to relatively low stores of thiosulfate in the liver,[111] and the metabolites are more likely to accumulate in renal failure.

Inhaled Nitric Oxide

NO in its endogenous form derives from the enzymatic conversion of the amino acid L-arginine by endothelial nitric oxide synthase (eNOS). In vascular smooth muscle cells, NO activates guanylate cyclase and produces cGMP. Protein kinase activation results in decreased sensitivity of the myosin to calcium-induced contraction and lowers intracellular calcium concentration,[112] with consequent relaxation of the vascular smooth muscle.[113] NO is a volatile gas that can be therapeutically administered by inhalation with selective pulmonary vasodilator effects.[114] In contrast to nonselective vasodilators, which lower systemic blood pressure, iNO is an ideal agent for use in diseases of high PVR. In patients with low cardiac output, further reduction in SVR may compromise coronary blood flow and increase PVR/SVR ratio, which may result in further diversion of deoxygenated blood to the systemic circulation. Hence, targeted pulmonary vasodilation with iNO is the mainstay of treatment for patients with high PVR as a primary problem.

Neonates with acute pulmonary hypertension of the newborn, for instance, have a persistent elevation of PVR that compromises pulmonary blood flow and causes afterload-mediated RV dysfunction. In addition, LV filling is impacted by both pulmonary hypoperfusion and RV dilation that displaces the interventricular septum leftward. Contractile dysfunction of the LV results from interventricular interaction and poor preload. Particularly among newborns, the presence of intra- and extracardiac shunts further compromises oxygenation by diverting deoxygenated blood flow from the pulmonary to the systemic vasculature. Pulmonary vasodilation with iNO, therefore, is the primary target of therapy and is associated with improved cardiac function and reduced need for extracorporeal membrane oxygenation.[113] iNO improves oxygenation by reducing PVR, improving ventilation/perfusion matching within the lung, and decreasing right-to-left extrapulmonary shunt.[114] In many patients, improved pulmonary blood flow results in increased LV output even following iNO as monotherapy.[30]

iNO is typically administered through the circuit of an invasive mechanical ventilator, although recent reports show that it can be administered by noninvasive methods.[115] Starting doses usually range from 10 to 20 ppm, but can be as high as 80 ppm. For the 50% to 60% of neonates with hypoxemic respiratory failure that are responsive to iNO, the effects are typically seen within a couple of minutes of administration.[113] Weaning guidelines are not clearly delineated; however, dose reduction should occur gradually to avoid rebound hypoxemia or hypotension secondary to decreased cardiac output.[112] Echocardiography to ensure normal RV function prior to weaning may be advisable. In the bloodstream, iNO binds to heme and generates methemoglobin, which should be measured daily and should not exceed 2.5% of total hemoglobin. Toxicity related to methemoglobinemia is rare at doses less than 80 ppm,[116] unless iNO is used in conjunction with other medications that may cause similar toxicity, such as SNP.

SUPPORT FOR SYSTEMIC HYPOTENSION

Hypotension is a common symptom of cardiovascular instability in both term and preterm infants admitted to the neonatal intensive care unit (NICU). Neonatal hypotension has been linked to the subsequent development of deleterious consequences, such as IVH, renal and hepatic injury, necrotizing enterocolitis (NEC), periventricular white matter injury, and poor neurodevelopmental outcomes.[117] Although the association between correction of hypotension and improved long-term outcomes is not clear, timely correction of low organ perfusion pressure has the potential to improve short-term organ-level morbidities. An infant with hypotension requires frequent evaluation of vital signs, perfusion, urine output, plasma lactate, and neurologic status to monitor and tailor therapy. There are many potential contributors to systemic hypotension, however, and specific delineation of biventricular cardiac function, cardiac output, relative pulmonary and systemic pressures, and the role of shunts using echocardiography may be beneficial. In the absence of cardiac dysfunction, treatment of hypotension may include volume replacement, vasopressor support, and, in some situations, steroid therapy. In the following section, we will describe the properties of drugs that are primarily systemic vasoconstrictors (e.g., dopamine, vasopressin, norepinephrine, and phenylephrine) and glucocorticoids (see Fig. 48.5).

PROPERTIES OF PREDOMINANTLY VASOCONSTRICTING DRUGS

Dopamine

Dopamine is a naturally occurring catecholamine precursor to norepinephrine. Although it is the most commonly used vasoactive medication used to control low blood pressure regardless of indication,[23] this practice is questionable based on its pharmacologic properties. In animal models, older children, and adults, there is a known dose-dependent stimulation of the catecholamine system via α and β adrenergic receptors and action at dopaminergic receptors, resulting in its serotoninergic actions.[118] At low doses, dopamine (2 to 4 μg per kg per minute) improves renal and mesenteric blood flow by stimulating dopaminergic receptors, leading to vasodilation. At moderate doses (5 to 10 μg per kg per minute), dopamine increases myocardial contractility and heart rate by stimulating β_1 and β_2 as well as α_1 receptors. At high doses (10 to 20 μg per kg per minute), dopamine's α adrenergic stimulation causes an increase in SVR and PVR.[28]

Among neonatal patients, there are several differences that may result in a variable clinical response to dopamine, which is patient dependent and not necessarily dose dependent. As described earlier, the relatively earlier development of the α adrenergic system may contribute to a primarily vasoconstrictive response at lower doses as compared to adult or pediatric patients. Additionally, maturational differences in the adrenal enzyme systems utilized to convert dopamine into norepinephrine and epinephrine may create inconsistency. Approximately 50% of dopamine's biologic activity is attributable to metabolism into downstream vasoactive catecholamines. Dopamine is converted to norepinephrine and then to epinephrine by the enzymes dopamine beta-hydroxylase (DBH) and PNMT, respectively. Among fetal sheep, the activity of DBH, and therefore the metabolism of dopamine to norepinephrine, can be detected at a gestation equivalent to a 21-week human pregnancy.[119] In several models, the development of DBH has been shown to precede PNMT, resulting in an earlier appearance of adrenal norepinephrine as compared to epinephrine.[120,121] Primate and human data also suggest that the maturation of this enzyme system may still be occurring in many neonates born at the earliest viable GAs (22 to 26 weeks). In a study that included 31 human fetal adrenal glands aged ≤26 weeks' gestation, the earliest DBH activity was noted at 15 weeks and the earliest PNMT was found at 18 to 19 weeks' gestation. Only one 24-week fetus (3%), however, demonstrated the activity of both enzymes.[121] Additionally, several conditions common to pregnancies that end in preterm birth, including placental insufficiency[122] and chronic hypoxia,[123] are associated with abnormalities in the development of the adrenal medulla and delayed maturation of these pathways. An additional mechanism by which dopamine exerts its influence is via the release of stored norepinephrine from terminal synapses. Importantly, among premature neonates, these stores may be low and may become depleted in 8 to 12 hours.[28,118] Direct administration of norepinephrine may be an alternative approach to systemic vasoconstriction, which bypasses many of these issues.

Clinical evidence also suggests heterogeneity in dopamine response profile, particularly among immature infants. In a cohort of preterm infants with a mean gestation of 26 weeks, Zhang et al. showed two distinct patterns. Some neonates demonstrate increased LV output with a modest increase in MBP. Concerningly, despite a relatively low dose of 6 to 8 μg per kg per minute for both response patterns, other preterms exhibited a large increase in MBP and a concurrent reduction in LV output, suggesting a primary vasoconstrictive response.[47] Similarly, Roze et al. demonstrated increased SVR without a significantly improved cardiac output among hypotensive premature infants treated with dopamine.[43] In a randomized crossover trial of preterm patients, dopamine has been shown to produce a greater increase in blood pressure, whereas dobutamine produces a greater increase in systemic blood flow.[46] Dopamine has also been associated with increased pulmonary vascular tone and an increase in the PVR/SVR ratio.[52,124] This is particularly important among patients with acute pulmonary hypertension and concurrent low systemic blood pressure. Dopamine's pharmacologic profile may be detrimental to the physiology of these patients, and the use of alternate agents that do not preferentially constrict the pulmonary vascular bed (e.g., vasopressin) may be preferable. The physiologic responses to dopamine underscore its primary role as a systemic vasoconstrictor, which is most appropriately used to treat patients with low systemic vascular tone in the absence of clinically significant pulmonary hypertension.[29]

Dopamine is administered by continuous infusion with acceptable dosing range of 2 to 20 μg per kg per minute, although as described earlier, the effects may be variable both between doses and among patients. The imprecision of therapeutic efficacy and unpredictability of these effects, particularly at extremely low GAs, needs to be considered when making treatment decisions. The half-life of dopamine varies from 2 minutes at term up to 5 minutes in preterm infants. Because of immaturity of the autonomic nervous system, dopamine may produce some adverse responses at a high dose in neonates. An inadvertent dopamine overdose may precipitate short-lived reflex bradycardia, and the most common direct side effects are tachycardia and cardiac arrhythmias.[125] Dopamine is metabolized rapidly by both MAO in the liver and catechol-O-methyltransferase present in the circulating blood to 3,4-dihydroxyphenyl-acetic acid, 3-methoxytyramine, and homovanillic acid (HVA). Both HVA and small amounts of dopamine are directly conjugated and excreted in the sulfate or glucuronide form in the urine[125] (see Fig. 48.6).

Norepinephrine

Norepinephrine is a naturally occurring sympathomimetic amine. Its primary action is via nonselective activation of α receptors. In the myocardium, norepinephrine has a 20× greater affinity for β_1 as compared to β_2 receptors.[126] This is relevant because, although low in density, β_2 receptors have a much greater ability to activate intracellular signaling than do β_1 receptors. This translates into a relatively lower inotropic activity of norepinephrine, especially at low doses, compared to epinephrine, which potently activates both subtypes. This receptor profile underlies norepinephrine's clinical utility as a primary vasoconstrictor with relatively minor inotropic and chronotropic properties (see Fig. 48.5).

Norepinephrine remains the first-line agent in vasodilator shock in adult and pediatric patients.[127] Endogenous norepinephrine has a sentinel role in maintaining vascular tone, and dopamine, the most well-studied cardiovascular drug in the neonatal population, relies on norepinephrine as an essential intermediary. Theoretically, norepinephrine may improve tissue perfusion pressure and cardiac function both directly by minor positive inotropy and, more importantly, indirectly via enhanced coronary flow in the presence of increased diastolic pressure. Despite being a biologically plausible agent for neonates, where vasodilation is the predominant physiologic pattern, there remains little published evidence of norepinephrine efficacy in neonates. One study by Tourneux et al. demonstrated increased systemic blood pressure, increased urinary output, and decreased serum lactate concentration in term infants with shock refractory to volume, dopamine, and dobutamine.[128] Similarly, norepinephrine has been associated with increased systemic blood pressure among neonates <32 weeks' gestation.[129] Although treated neonates in this study had high mortality and survivors had a high rate of neurodevelopmental impairment, the role of selection bias is unclear, and further study in the preterm population is warranted.

In a similarly small study of term neonates with pulmonary hypertension and low systemic blood pressure, norepinephrine has been associated with decreased PAP to SAP ratio, better oxygenation, and improved LV output. Given that both PAP and SAP increased with its use, improved oxygenation was most likely mediated by a greater component of left-to-right shunt among patients with an open DA, rather than a direct impact on PAP.[130] Thus, in the subset of patients with vasodilator shock or those with pulmonary hypertension with sublevel or systemic level PAP, norepinephrine may be a reasonable agent. Caution is advised among patients with critical hypoxemia or suprasystemic pulmonary hypertension in which even marginally increased PAP may be dangerous.

In general, caution is recommended among patients with documented LV dysfunction as increased SVR with relatively minor cardiac support may negatively impact the stress–velocity relationship and be poorly tolerated. Similarly, norepinephrine should be avoided for patients with hypertrophic obstructive cardiomyopathy given its β adrenergic activity. Such patients benefit from low heart rate and are at risk of dynamic LV outflow tract obstruction with exposure to positive inotropy. Vasopressin remains the alternative vasoconstrictor of choice in patients with restrictive myocardial physiology.

Norepinephrine is administered by continuous infusion with an acceptable dosing range of 0.02 to 0.5 μg per kg per minute; however, the maximum published dose is 2 μg per kg per minute. It is commonly initiated at 0.02 to 0.04 μg per kg per minute and titrated every 30 minutes in 0.05 to 0.1 μg per kg per minute increments until the desired effect is reached. When clinical goals have been met, norepinephrine can be decreased by 0.05 to 0.1 μg per kg per minute.[131] Onset of action of norepinephrine is rapid, with peak effect occurring within 3 to 5 minutes of initiation of the continuous infusion. The half-life is approximately 1 to 2 minutes.[132] The most common side effects include reflex bradycardia in the setting of a sudden increase in SVR, cardiac arrhythmias, and peripheral ischemia.[31] Norepinephrine is metabolized by COMT and MAO. The principal end products are either VMA or a conjugated form of MHPG, both of which are thought to be biologically inactive and are excreted in the urine[133] (see Fig. 48.6).

Vasopressin

Vasopressin, also known as arginine vasopressin (AVP), is an endogenous neuropeptide antidiuretic hormone that is formed in the hypothalamus and secreted from the posterior pituitary gland. The primary function of vasopressin includes regulation of plasma osmolarity, circulating blood volume, and alteration of vascular tone. There are three subtypes of vasopressin receptor.[134] When acting via the V_1 receptor in vascular smooth muscle of the systemic and splanchnic circulations, vasopressin leads to an increase in intracellular calcium causing vasoconstriction.[135] In animal models, there is substantial variation in the degree of vasoconstriction in response to vasopressin. In the splanchnic circulation, vasopressin is a potent vasoconstrictor, whereas in the coronary, renal, and cerebral circulations,

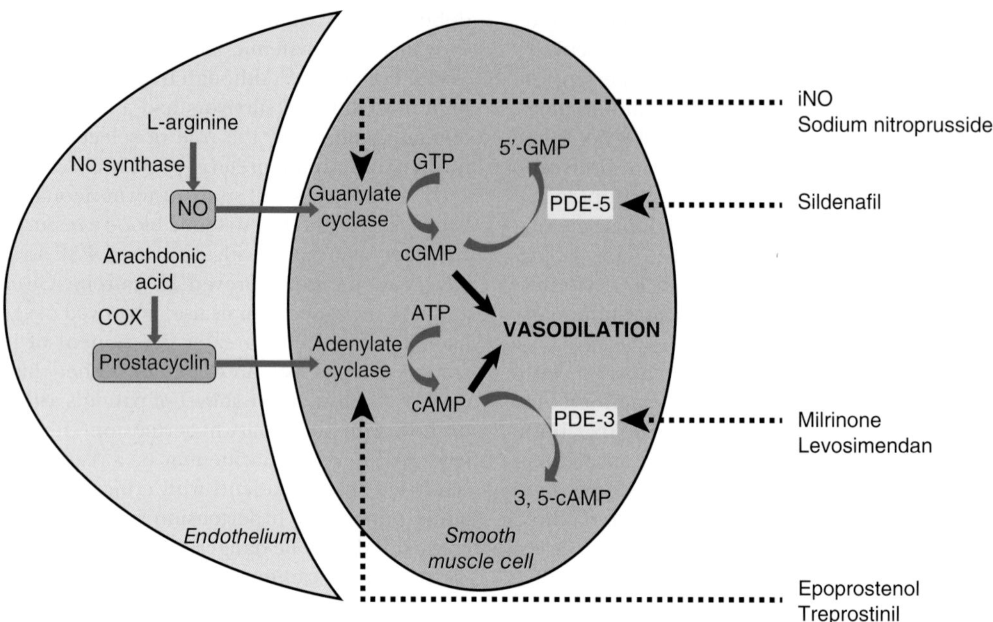

AQ1 **Figure 48.7** Target cellular pathways for medications with vasodilator properties. (a) L-arginine is converted into nitric oxide. In the smooth muscle cell, it activates guanylate cyclase. Inhaled nitric oxide and sodium nitroprusside target guanylate cyclase to promote the conversion of guanosine triphosphate (GTP) into cyclic guanosine monophosphate (cGMP), which in turn leads to vasodilation. cGMP is subsequently degraded by phosphodiesterase 5 (PDE-5) into its inactive form (5′-GMP). Sildenafil is a PDE-5 inhibitor. (b) Arachidonic acid gets converted by cyclooxygenase (COX) into prostacyclin, which in turn activates adenylate cyclase in the smooth muscle cell to convert ATM into cyclic adenosine monophosphate (cAMP). Epoprostenol and treprostinil stimulate this process. Phosphodiesterase 3 (PDE-3) promotes the degradation of cAMP into its inactive form (3′,5′-cAMP) and is the target for medications such as milrinone and levosimendan.

its effect is attenuated.[136] Variation in activity is primarily related to differences in endothelial V_1 receptor distribution (Fig. 48.8).[137] Stimulation of endothelial V_1 receptors triggers the release of NO and negates the vasoconstrictive effect of vasopressin.[138] This is particularly relevant in the pulmonary vascular bed, in which a high density of endothelial V_1 receptor activity may counteract calcium-mediated signaling and results in net neutral vascular tone (Fig. 48.8).[137] In the collecting duct of the kidney, vasopressin regulates water reabsorption by V_2 receptor–mediated regulation of aquaporins. These osmotic effects are helpful to defend against hypovolemia and hemorrhage, by increasing SVR and then an increase in blood pressure.[31] Vasopressin acting on V_3 receptors stimulates the release of adrenocorticotropic hormone (ACTH) and signals the production of cortisol from the adrenal glands.[134,139] Stimulation of the V_3 receptor in adults has been associated with reduced heart rate; however, this effect remains to be proven in neonates.

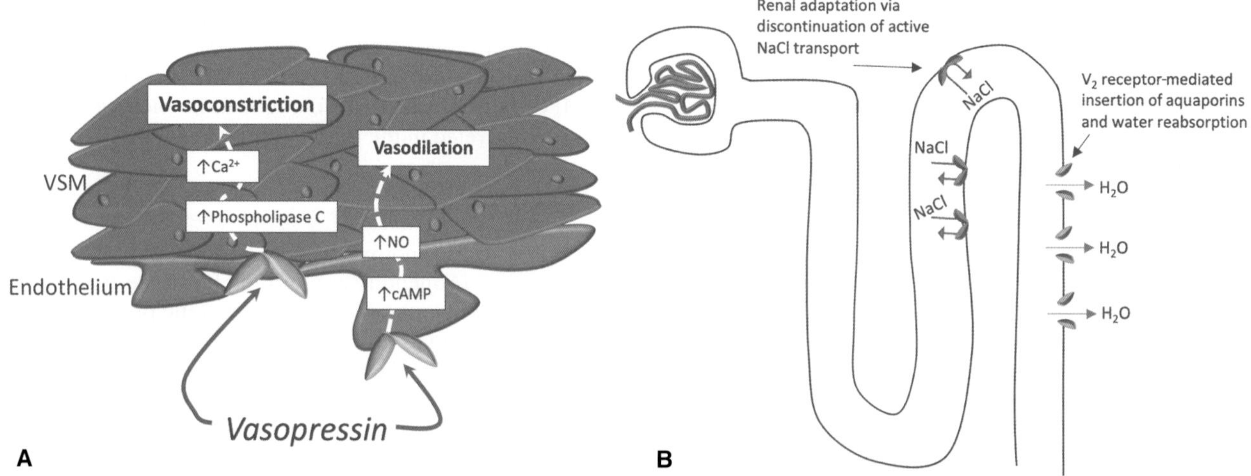

Figure 48.8 Schematic of biologic mechanisms of vasopressin. **A:** Via the V_1 receptor, vasopressin activates different intracellular second messenger systems depending on the binding site. **B:** Via the V_2 receptor, vasopressin inserts aquaporins in the collecting duct of the kidney, thereby reabsorbing water and concentrating urine. The healthy kidney adapts by reducing active reabsorption of NaCl ions, resulting in greater water retention within the nephron more proximally. The net result is natriuresis with accompanying water excretion. cAMP, cyclic adenosine monophosphate; VSM, vascular smooth muscle.

Vasopressin has been used effectively in neonates to increase blood pressure and reduce requirement for catecholamines in vasodilatory shock caused by inflammation such as septic shock.[140–142] It is associated with an increased urinary output owing to improved renal perfusion pressure in the early phase and then later owing to natriuresis.[143] The use of vasopressin in pulmonary hypertension to improve blood pressure and oxygenation has also been published.[144–146] Selective vasoconstriction in the systemic and splanchnic circulation with no vasoconstriction or minor vasodilation in the pulmonary vascular bed makes vasopressin a theoretically ideal agent for these patients. Alternative mechanisms may also be at play. In a rat model, vasopressin was associated with reduced PAP owing to the release of atrial natriuretic peptide.[147] Although not yet demonstrated in the neonate, vasopressin may also act synergistically with catecholamine therapy via its V_3 effects because vasopressin in the presence of ACTH is associated with an increase in adrenal cortisol secretion.[148] Because vasopressin has no inotropic properties, cardiac output may be compromised if the left heart is dysfunctional and not sufficiently supported by alternative therapies.[31]

The most clinically relevant side effect of vasopressin is via its V_2 effects on the kidney (see Fig. 48.8). The management of sodium and fluid balance when using vasopressin requires close attention. In the early phase, renal reperfusion owing to restored blood pressure may lead to increased urinary output, which may then become excessive if the patient is experiencing post–acute tubular necrosis polyuria. Insertion of aquaporins owing to the activation of V_2 receptors leads to reabsorption of water in the collecting duct of the kidney, which may lead to transient oliguria. The healthy kidney rapidly adapts to this, however, by stopping active reabsorption of sodium in the ascending loop, therefore increasing the osmotic drive for water to remain in the urine in the more proximal nephron. Patients who are being treated with vasopressin who are not oliguric (≤1 mL per kg per hour) should have regular monitoring of urinary sodium excretion to avoid natriuresis-mediated hyponatremia.[31] Sodium replacement at or above the levels being excreted in the urine is typically sufficient to avoid hyponatremia. Once vasopressin is discontinued, the hyponatremia resolves and rapid adjustment of delivered sodium and water is typically required to avoid iatrogenic hypernatremia.

Vasopressin is administered by continuous infusion with a therapeutic dose range of 0.1 to 1.2 mU per kg per minute. The recommended starting dose is 0.3 mU per kg per minute with titration up every 15 to 60 minutes, depending on the severity of illness, in intervals of 0.2 to 0.3 mU per kg per minute to achieve target arterial pressure. The half-life of vasopressin is 10 to 20 minutes, and therefore, dose changes every 30 to 90 minutes are reflected in the patients' condition.[149] Weaning of vasopressin should be done in increments of 0.1 to 0.2 mU per kg per minute every 2 to 3 hours until discontinued once clinical goals have been achieved. Vasopressin is a hormone that is endogenously secreted; therefore, prolonged administration of greater than 48 to 72 hours may result in renal suppression of endogenous production. Because of this suppression, vasopressin discontinuation may be associated with immediate polyuria, fluid dysregulation, and electrolyte derangement, so care must be taken to monitor urine output and electrolytes closely. If polyuria results in intravascular volume depletion despite replacement, vasopressin may be restarted at a dose of 0.05 mU per kg per minute for an additional 12 hours to reestablish fluid homeostasis.[31] Vasopressin is metabolized in the liver and kidneys, and a small proportion of vasopressin is eliminated in the urine.[139]

Phenylephrine

Phenylephrine is a pure α adrenergic agonist and therefore results in vasoconstriction with minor cardiac inotropy and no chronotropy.[150] In adults, phenylephrine is used for hypotension in the setting of hyperdynamic sepsis, neurologic disorders, and anesthesia-induced hypotension.[151] In neonates, phenylephrine may be used in infants with tetralogy of Fallot during a "tet spell" because it induces an increase in systemic blood pressure, which produces an increase in pulmonary blood flow.[152] Similar to vasopressin, however, one potential side effect is that phenylephrine may decrease stroke volume and therefore cardiac output if there is preexisting LV dysfunction.[153] Phenylephrine is rarely utilized in the neonate and premature infant,[154] and there is no published literature on its efficacy and safety in premature infants.

Phenylephrine is administered via continuous IV infusion with a usual initial range of 0.1 to 0.5 μg per kg per minute, which can then be titrated to desired response, and in cases of shock or intraoperative hypotension, doses up to 2 μg per kg per minute have been reported.[155] The observed effective half-life of IV phenylephrine is approximately 5 minutes. IV use of phenylephrine may cause severe bradycardia, most likely baroreflex mediated, and reduced cardiac output because of an increase in cardiac afterload, especially in patients with preexisting cardiac dysfunction.[156] Phenylephrine is metabolized primarily by MAO and sulfotransferase in the liver and excreted mainly in the urine.[155]

GLUCOCORTICOIDS

Hydrocortisone is a commonly used corticosteroid for cardiovascular dysfunction in the neonatal population. The mechanism of action of corticosteroids for the treatment of hypotension is multifactorial and complex (Fig. 48.9). First, hydrocortisone induces the final enzyme in the transformation of norepinephrine to epinephrine in the adrenal gland and may therefore upregulate the release of epinephrine into circulation if those enzyme systems have matured sufficiently to be active (see section "Dopamine" for details). Second, the repetitive stimulation of receptors by either endogenous production or exogenous administration of high-dose catecholamines may lead to uncoupling of receptors from intracellular signaling mechanisms and downregulation of response. This may be countered by hydrocortisone, which increases adrenergic receptor expression.[157] Third, hydrocortisone works to upregulate angiotensin II receptors and their second messenger systems, which play important roles in blood pressure regulation.[154] Fourth, inhibiting the expression of inducible NO synthase and vasodilatory prostaglandin action by hydrocortisone may improve vascular tone.[158,159] Finally, preterm infants or those infants with adrenal injury in the setting of hypoxic ischemic encephalopathy[160] and/or infection may be unable to mount an adequate cortisol response in the face of stressful stimulus. Adrenal insufficiency should be considered

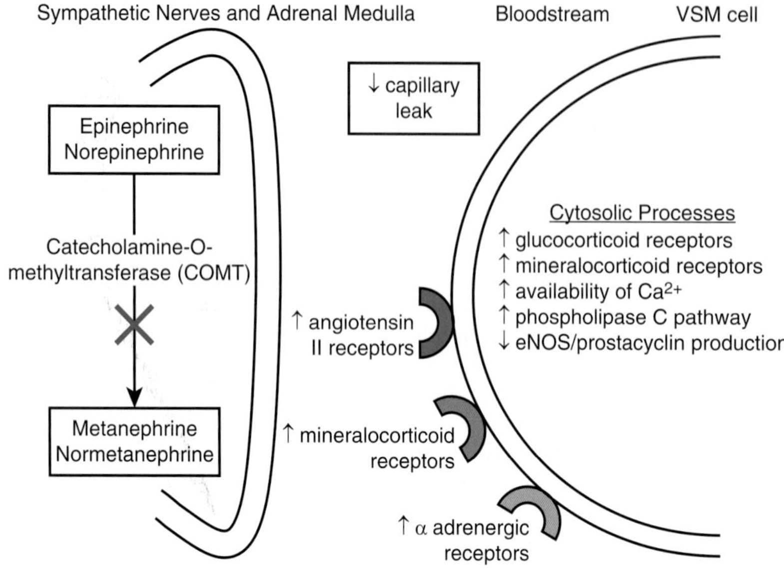

Figure 48.9 Schematic of biologic mechanisms of action of hydrocortisone. At the cellular level, hydrocortisone upregulates cell surface receptors for vasoactive substrate and modifies intracellular second messaging systems associated with vasoconstriction. In sympathetic nervous tissue, the rate-limiting enzyme in the breakdown of catecholamines (COMT) is inhibited, resulting in an increase in vasoconstrictive mediators. Capillary leak is reduced. Ca^{2+}, calcium ion; eNOS, endothelial nitric oxide synthase; VSM, vascular smooth muscle.

in a compatible clinical situation and/or after failure to respond to one or more catecholamine medications. In these situations, hydrocortisone can be considered as hormone replacement.[158]

The onset of action of hydrocortisone is 2 to 6 hours, and it has been associated with improved blood pressure over that time course among premature infants with hypotension refractory to catecholamine therapy.[161] It is also associated with increased urine output and cardiac output and the decreased need for vasopressor support among patients receiving other catecholamine therapy.[158,159] There are little data to support the use of hydrocortisone as a single first-line agent for hypotension. A small (n = 50) study randomizing preterm infants to hydrocortisone prophylaxis or placebo for the prevention of respiratory morbidity in the first week identified a survival advantage among hydrocortisone-treated infants (16% vs. 40% mortality), with a lower rate of new onset of hypotension following randomization. However, the study was underpowered owing to premature termination, and hypotension when it occurred was cotreated with dopamine.[162]

A typical hydrocortisone dose is to load with 1 to 2 mg per kg followed by 0.5 to 1 mg per kg IV every 6 to 12 hours. For infants greater than 35 weeks' gestation, the dosing interval is 6 to 8 hours, and for infants less than 35 weeks' gestation, the dosing interval is 8 to 12 hours owing to a half-life of 8 to 12 hours. Typical side effects of hydrocortisone include hyperglycemia, hypertension, thrombus formation, and a potential increased risk of infection.[163] Hypertrophic cardiomyopathy has been reported following hydrocortisone exposure in preterm infants,[163,164] and the effects on neurodevelopmental outcomes are unclear.[165] Hydrocortisone should not be used with indomethacin owing to the increased incidence of spontaneous intestinal perforation. Hydrocortisone is metabolized in the liver to inactive glucuronide and sulfate metabolites. Inactive metabolites and small amounts of unmetabolized hydrocortisone are excreted by the kidneys.[166]

TREATMENT OF A HEMODYNAMICALLY SIGNIFICANT PATENT DUCTUS ARTERIOSUS

DA is of vital physiologic importance during fetal life. Together with the foramen ovale, the DA is responsible for diversion of the majority of oxygenated placental blood to the systemic fetal circulation[167] (Fig. 48.10). In healthy term infants, functional closure of the DA occurs within 72 hours after birth,[168,169] facilitated by an increase in blood oxygen tension and the removal of placental circulation as the major source of prostaglandin E_2 (PGE_2).[170] Among preterm neonates, there is an increased risk of the DA remaining patent beyond the first few postnatal days. Up to 65% of extremely low birth weight neonates are affected,[171] and hemodynamically significant persistent DA (hsPDA) occurrence is inversely related to GA at birth.[172] Both anatomic immaturity of the DA[168] and altered prostaglandin metabolism[173] and responsiveness[174] have been implicated in hsPDA pathophysiology in preterm infants. There are widely varied philosophies on whether the hsPDA should be allowed to spontaneously resolve, although this may involve prolonged exposure to the consequences of shunt,[175,176] or to intervene to effect closure during the hospitalization. The timing of intervention among those who choose to treat also remains a highly controversial issue. For those who choose not to intervene early, conservative management includes strategies to modulate shunt by manipulating Poiseuille's law. Such strategies include permissive hypercapnia, maintenance of adequate oxygen carrying capacity via packed red cell transfusion as needed, and avoidance of agents that lower PVR such as high concentrations of oxygen.[177,178] Transfusion of red cells may also increase blood viscosity and reduce left-to-right shunt; this approach has been shown to reduce left-to-right shunting in the context of congenital heart disease[179] but has not been well studied in infants with hsPDA. It is not clear which patients may benefit

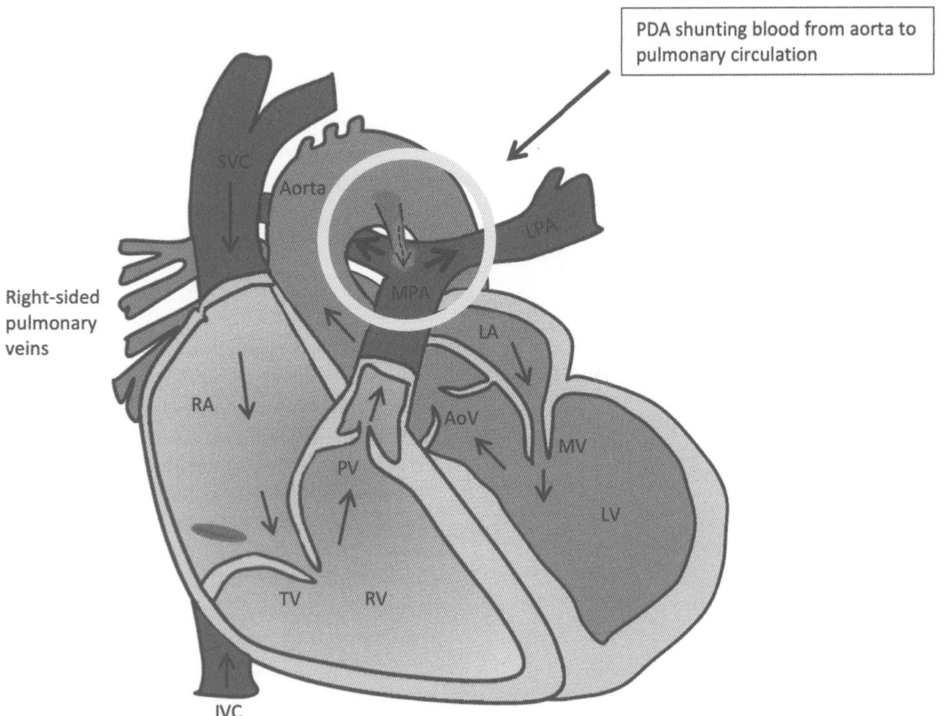

Figure 48.10 Anatomic location and blood flow via a patent ductus arteriosus. AoV, aortic valve; IVC, inferior vena cava; LA, left atrium; LPA, left pulmonary artery; LV, left ventricle; MPA, main pulmonary artery; MV, mitral valve; PV, pulmonary valve; RA, right atrium; RV, right ventricle; SVC, superior vena cava; TV, tricuspid valve.

from conservative treatment. Among patients in whom medical therapy is the chosen course of action, there are several possible pharmacologic interventions including indomethacin, ibuprofen, and acetaminophen, which have demonstrated variable efficacy.

FLUID MODULATION AND DIURETICS

Evidence for fluid restriction, though popular historically, is limited. Theoretically, reduction in overall circulating volume without modulating the proportion of cardiac output that is diverted to the lungs has the potential to exacerbate postductal hypoperfusion. A recent small observational study did not find beneficial effects on hemodynamics[180] and reaffirmed the risks associated with dehydration, reduced systemic perfusion, and inadequate nutritional intake. Avoidance of furosemide during pharmacologic therapy for hsPDA may also be prudent; furosemide is known to stimulate renal prostaglandin production,[181,182] and an animal model has shown that furosemide both delays PDA closure and dilates constricted DA vessels.[183] A randomized controlled trial in human neonates has shown an increased incidence of PDA in infants with respiratory distress syndrome with the use of furosemide, when compared with an alternative diuretic, chlorothiazide.[184]

The mainstay of pharmacologic treatment of PDA has been nonsteroidal anti-inflammatory drugs (NSAIDs), nonselective cyclooxygenase (COX)-1 and -2 inhibitors, ibuprofen, and indomethacin, with use first described for this purpose in 1976.[185,186] The two medications inhibit the COX-1 and COX-2 enzyme isoforms to differing degrees,[187] with relevant implications for their differing side-effect profiles. There is also increasing interest in the use of acetaminophen owing to the range of adverse effects observed with NSAIDs (Table 48.2) and growing evidence of the efficacy of acetaminophen for ductal closure.[188] Incomplete pharmacodynamic and pharmacokinetic data on NSAID use in preterm infants have contributed to the use of these medications in varying doses and by multiple different routes of administration.[189] Numerous regimens have been described in the literature and are summarized in recent meta-analyses[188,190] (Table 48.3). Serial bedside echocardiography enables the achievement of equivalent ductal closure rates with a reduction in total NSAID doses and a lower rate of adverse effects.[191,192] A recent review by the Cochrane Collaboration did not find sufficient evidence that echocardiography-guided PDA treatment reduces medication-related morbidity; however, research in this area is ongoing.[193]

PROPERTIES OF NONSTEROIDAL ANTI-INFLAMMATORY DRUGS

IV indomethacin and IV ibuprofen are the most frequently used pharmacologic treatment options for PDA,[189,205] although a recent meta-analysis of 60 studies involving over 4,000 infants suggests that oral ibuprofen in high doses may be associated with the greatest likelihood of PDA closure.[188] Increasing GA and birth weight are associated with a positive response to COX inhibitor treatment,[206] which may be related to increased sensitivity of the immature ductus to PGE_2.[207,208] Both ibuprofen and indomethacin interfere with the synthesis of prostaglandins from arachidonic acid by blocking the first step in the prostaglandin

TABLE 48.2 Reported Adverse Effects Associated with Pharmacologic Treatments for PDA

Adverse Effect	*Indomethacin*	*Ibuprofen*	*Acetaminophen*
Renal impairment (oliguria/anuria, elevated serum creatinine)	Yes; 10%–15%	Yes; risk lower than with indomethacin; occurs more frequently with high oral dose	No
Thrombocytopenia and/or impaired function	Yes	Yes	No
Hyponatremia	Yes	Yes, if renal impairment occurs	
Gastrointestinal bleeding	Yes	Yes	No
Spontaneous intestinal perforation	Yes, particularly with corticosteroid cotreatment	Possible, particularly with corticosteroid cotreatment	No
Necrotizing enterocolitis (NEC)	Weak	IV: Yes; risk lower than with indomethacin; treatment may confer lower risk than placebo/no treatment Oral: No[188]	No
Impaired coronary perfusion	Yes; clinical significance uncertain	No	No
Transient cerebral vasoconstriction	Yes[194]	No	No
Hyperbilirubinemia	No	Yes	No[a]
Abnormal liver function tests	No	No	Yes; uncommon
Acute pulmonary hypertension	No	Yes; uncommon	No

[a]Acetaminophen metabolism may be impaired in the setting of significant hyperbilirubinemia.
IV, intravenous; PDA, patent ductus arteriosus.

TABLE 48.3 Pharmacologic Treatment Modalities for PDA: Dosing Schedules and Pharmacokinetics

	Indomethacin	*Ibuprofen*	*Acetaminophen*
Dosing	• Intravenous: 0.1–0.2 mg/kg/dose over 30 min (q12–24h) • Usually 0.2 mg/kg followed by 0.1 mg/kg (up to 0.2 mg/kg; consider in infants >48 h of age) • *Short course*: 1–3 doses • *Long course*: 4–6 doses (generally given as one dose every 24 h)	• Intravenous or oral • *Low dose*: 10 mg/kg; then two doses of 5 mg/kg • *High dose*: 15–20 mg/kg; then two doses of 7.5–10 mg/kg • Doses q24h • Intravenous infusion over 15–30 min	• Intravenous or oral • 15 mg/kg q6h × 3–7 d or 20 mg/kg loading dose followed by 7.5 mg/kg every 6 h for 4 d • *Not currently recommended for PDA prophylaxis*
Pharmacokinetics			
Volume of distribution (Vd)	Vd = 0.22–0.86 L/kg	Vd = 0.35–0.36 L/kg	Vd = 1.07 L/kg
Clearance (Cl)	Cl = 0.13–0.28 mL/kg/min	Cl = 0.15–0.16 mL/kg/min	Cl = 2.3 mL/kg/min (28 wk) to 2.8 mL/kg/min (44 wk)
Half-life ($t_{1/2}$)	$t_{1/2}$ = 12–20 h (shorter end of range with increasing postnatal age and weight)	$t_{1/2}$ = 26.8–43.1 h (postnatal days 3–5, decreases with increasing postnatal age)	$t_{1/2}$ = 143 min (preterm) to 59 min (term) following single dose

PDA, patent ductus arteriosus.

Yaffe S, Friedman WF, Rogers D, et al. The disposition of indomethacin in preterm babies. *J Pediatr* 1980;97(6):1001–1006; Al Za'abi M, Donovan T, Tudehope D, et al. Orogastric and intravenous indomethacin administration to very premature neonates with patent ductus arteriosus: population pharmacokinetics, absolute bioavailability, and treatment outcome. *Ther Drug Monit* 2007;29(6):807–814; Smyth J, Collier PS, Darwish M, et al. Intravenous indomethacin in preterm infants with symptomatic patent ductus arteriosus: a population pharmacokinetic study. *Br J Clin Pharmacol* 2004;58(3):249–258; Pacifici G. Clinical pharmacology of indomethacin in preterm infants: implications in patent ductus arteriosus closure. *Paediatr Drugs* 2013;15(5):363–376; Pacifici G. Clinical pharmacology of ibuprofen in preterm infants: a meta-analysis of published data. *Med Express* 2014;1(2):55–61; Van Overmeire B, Touw D, Schepens PJ, et al. Ibuprofen pharmacokinetics in preterm infants with patent ductus arteriosus. *Clin Pharmacol Ther* 2001;70(4):336–343; Hirt D, Van Overmeire B, Treluyer JM, et al. An optimized dosing scheme for preterm neonates with patent ductus arteriosus, based on a population pharmacokinetic and pharmacodynamic study. *Br J Clin Pharmacol* 2008;65(5):629–636; Allegaert K, Palmer GM, Anderson BJ. The pharmacokinetics of intravenous paracetamol in neonates: size matters most. *Arch Dis Child* 2011;96(6):575–580; Cook S, Roberts JK, Samiee-Zafarghandy S, et al. Population pharmacokinetics of intravenous paracetamol (acetaminophen) in preterm and term neonates: model development and external evaluation. *Clin Pharmacokinet* 2016;55(1):107–119; Allegaert K, Van der Marei CD, Debeer A, et al. Pharmacokinetics of single dose intravenous propacetamol in neonates: effect of gestational age. *Arch Dis Child Fetal Neonatal Ed* 2004;89(1):F25–F28.

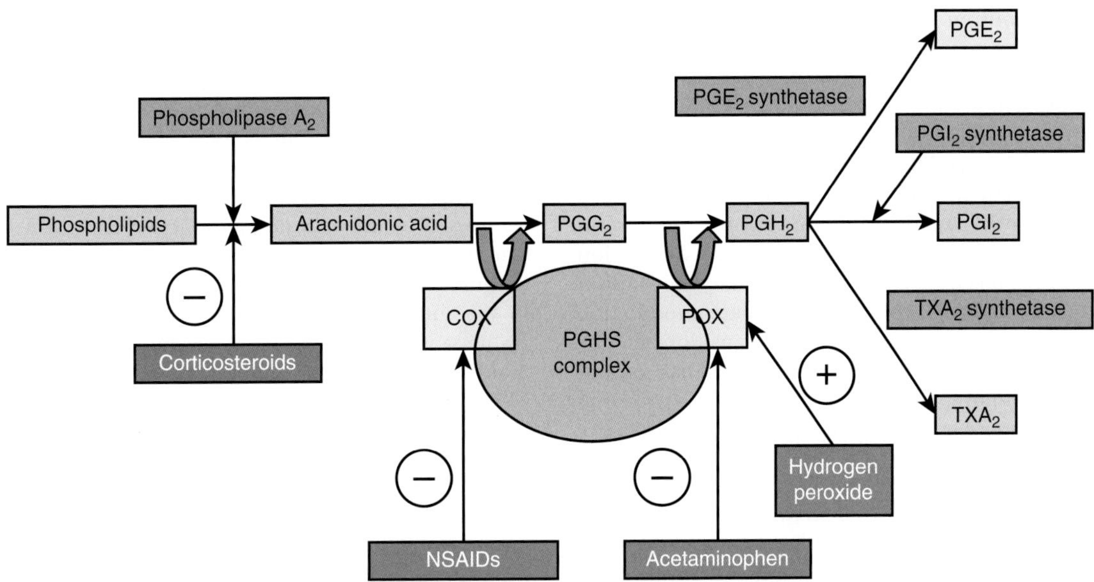

Figure 48.11 Schematic of prostaglandin synthesis pathway. COX, cyclooxygenase; NSAIDs, nonsteroidal anti-inflammatory drugs; PGE_2, prostaglandin E_2; PGG_2, prostaglandin G_2; PGH_2, prostaglandin H_2; PGHS, prostaglandin H_2 synthase complex; PGI_2, prostaglandin I_2; POX, peroxidase; TX, thromboxane.

H_2 synthase (PGHS) enzyme reaction[209] (Fig. 48.11). A clear relationship between measured prostaglandin levels and responsiveness to COX inhibitors for PDA closure has not been elucidated.[206] Inhibition of COX activity by ibuprofen and indomethacin is also associated with changes in alveolar epithelial sodium channel expression and increased clearance of lung water in an animal model of PDA, which may be an additional contributor to improved pulmonary mechanics.[210]

Side effects of NSAIDs in preterm infants appear to relate to peak concentrations, with lower rates of toxicity observed with continuous infusions compared with intermittent dosing.[188,211] Unfortunately, continuous administration has not been shown to be as efficacious for PDA closure, although the absence of loading doses and the low maintenance doses studied may have contributed to this finding.[212] There are also a number of practical limitations to continuous infusion in preterm neonates, including a requirement for a dedicated vascular access line, compatibility with other medications, and potential infection risks. For these reasons, intermittent bolus dosing is the preferred treatment method.

Indomethacin

Indomethacin, the most widely used medication for PDA closure,[213] exerts its effect via nonselective inhibition of COX-1 and COX-2[214] (also known as PGHS-1 and PGHS-2)[197] enzymes. Disruption of these enzymes results in decreased prostaglandins and constriction of the muscular DA wall.[214] Administration is generally via the IV route owing to unreliable intestinal absorption because oral bioavailability is only 13% in preterm infants.[198] Efficacy for a first course of indomethacin ranges from 60% to 80%[207,215–217] and is influenced by ductal flow velocity,[218] antenatal corticosteroid exposure,[219] and comorbidities such as infection[220] and respiratory distress syndrome.[221] In 15% to 35% of infants who initially respond to indomethacin, the DA will subsequently remanifest.[207,216] This is significantly more likely for infants born ≤26 weeks' gestation.[222] Success rates with subsequent treatment courses are lower; rates of 40% to 50% have been reported.[223,224] Although advanced GA has been cited as an adverse prognostic factor for response to a second treatment course,[213,225] there are likely genetic, disease-specific, and patient-specific characteristics beyond age, which have not been accounted for in the current literature and which have a significant impact on indomethacin responsiveness of chronologically older neonates. Both prolonged (four or more) and short (three) doses of indomethacin have been used. A meta-analysis comparing prolonged and short course treatment found no significant difference in rates of PDA closure, remanifestation, retreatment, or subsequent surgical treatment.[226] A longer course was associated with less renal impairment, but a greater risk of NEC. Accepted dosing schedules for indomethacin are outlined in Table 48.3.

Clearance and volume of distribution of indomethacin are significantly influenced by weight in preterm infants.[196] Clearance is lower than among adults, likely secondary to developmental immaturity of liver and renal function,[196] although this increases with postnatal age.[197] Volume of distribution and half-life are increased[196] (see Table 48.3). The plasma half-life of indomethacin is approximately 12 to 20 hours.[195–197] In preterm infants, indomethacin is 95% to 98% plasma protein bound, and there is no displacement of bilirubin.[227] There is no clear association between indomethacin plasma concentration and ductal closure, and significant interindividual variability in pharmacokinetics has been observed. Polymorphisms in genes encoding cytochrome P450 enzymes involved in indomethacin metabolism (specifically CYP2C9) have been associated with response to indomethacin for PDA closure[228] and may contribute to this variability.

A number of adverse effects of indomethacin use in preterm infants have been described. The most common of these is transient renal impairment, which occurs in 10% to 15% of treated infants[198] and is manifested by an increase in serum creatinine and oliguria.[229,230] Hyponatremia may ensue,[230] owing to the combination of increased renal vascular resistance, reduced renal blood flow, and enhanced vasopressin action.[231] Fluid restriction may be necessary in this instance until the recovery of urine output. Serum creatinine levels generally return to normal approximately 1 week after cessation of therapy.[198] Renal failure is therefore considered a contraindication to indomethacin use in preterm infants.[232] The drug also induces reversible cerebral vasoconstriction[233,234] and reduces renal and mesenteric blood flow in the first 2 hours after bolus dosing.[235] Prophylactic indomethacin use has been associated with a reduction in the risk of severe intraventricular hemorrhage and PVL.[194] Although direct cerebral vasoconstriction may play some role, it is unlikely to be the primary mechanism given the transient nature of this effect, and early modulation of ductal shunt is a plausible alternative. Transition may be characterized by a variable duration of low cardiac output state, particularly among extremely preterm infants, owing to impaired preload (e.g., failure of increase in pulmonary blood flow), elevated afterload (e.g., loss of the low-resistance placenta), or both. It has been shown that a low-flow state commonly precedes IVH, suggesting an ischemia–reperfusion mechanism.[236] Rapid escalation of left-to-right ductal shunt, which exposes the preductal circulation (e.g., the brain) to a rapid increase in perfusion pressure and flow, may occur in the setting of a large drop in PVR. Administration of prophylactic indomethacin may reduce the magnitude and/or velocity by which this escalation occurs and thereby lower the risk of reperfusion hemorrhage.

Although one retrospective cohort study suggested an association between antenatal tocolytic indomethacin and NEC in the first 15 postnatal days,[237] the evidence supporting such an association is weak. In contrast, in a large Israeli population of over 6,000 preterm neonates (24 to 34 weeks' gestation), the presence of hsPDA was significantly associated with NEC among both indomethacin-treated and nontreated patients.[238] In the same study, administration of indomethacin in the absence of hsPDA was not associated with NEC.[238] Spontaneous gastrointestinal perforation, in contrast, has been observed with indomethacin use, particularly during concomitant corticosteroid administration.[239,240] Cotreatment with indomethacin and corticosteroids is therefore not recommended. Impairment in coronary artery perfusion in the setting of hsPDA has also been reported,[240] the clinical significance of which is uncertain. Administration via syringe pump over 30 minutes has been recommended in order to minimize the adverse effects on cerebral, renal, and gastrointestinal blood flow.[198] Thrombocytopenia and platelet dysfunction can complicate indomethacin use in preterm infants, and the platelet count should be ascertained before the initiation of therapy.[230] Intercurrent ongoing acute hemorrhage (e.g., periventricular/intraventricular hemorrhage [P/IVH] and pulmonary hemorrhage) is generally considered a contraindication to indomethacin treatment.

Ibuprofen

Ibuprofen arose as an alternative to indomethacin for the treatment of hsPDA owing to adverse effects experienced with the latter medication. Ibuprofen works by binding reversibly and competitively with predominantly the COX-2 enzyme isoform,[241] with less COX-1 inhibition than indomethacin.[187] This inhibition results in a reduction in the generation of PGE_2 from arachidonic acid,[212] which promotes ductal closure (see Fig. 48.11). Reduced renal and cerebral side effects are observed with ibuprofen than with indomethacin.[242–244] A Cochrane review has recently reported equal efficacy with indomethacin[245]; however, other studies have reported lower efficacy, particularly of the IV formulation.[188,246] Reduced effectiveness at lower GAs has been reported.[247]

IV and oral ibuprofen are both composed of a racemic mixture of two enantiomers: (R−)-ibuprofen and (S+)-ibuprofen[212]; the (S+)-enantiomer is the more active component.[248] Following administration, 50% to 65% of the (R−)-ibuprofen is inverted by the enzyme methylacyl-coenzyme A racemase.[249] The majority of this action occurs in the liver; however, there is some suggestion that some transformation may also occur in the gut in orally administered ibuprofen. Metabolism is via hepatic cytochrome P450 enzymes, with CYP2C9 predominantly responsible for the breakdown of (R−)-ibuprofen and CYP2C8 for (S+)-ibuprofen.[212] The half-life in preterm infants is approximately 34 hours for (S+)-ibuprofen and 8 hours for (R−)-ibuprofen.[250] As with indomethacin, clearance increases and half-life decreases with increasing postnatal age.[201] The half-life on postnatal day 3 is 43.1 hours, and by the fifth day of life, it is 26.8 hours.[199] Pharmacokinetic data for ibuprofen in preterm neonates are detailed in Table 48.3.

Traditional ibuprofen dosing was via IV infusion once daily for 3 consecutive days, at doses of 10 mg per kg for the initial dose, followed by 5 mg per kg on each of the two subsequent days.[247] Increased effectiveness via the oral route may relate to a greater area under the curve (AUC)[251] and/or the longer half-life and duration of contact with the PDA[252] observed with oral ibuprofen treatment. It is also possible that conversion from the (R−)- to (S+)-stereoisomer may be more effective when administered enterally. Increased efficacy has been observed with a higher dose schedule of 20 mg per kg, followed by two doses of 10 mg per kg.[188,252] Oral ibuprofen at this higher dose range has recently been described as the more effective ibuprofen regimen with a more favorable side-effect profile than indomethacin; however, indomethacin has a substantially larger evidence base and remains commonly and safely used in many practices.[188] Accepted dosing schedules for ibuprofen in preterm infants are outlined in Table 48.3.

The impact of ibuprofen on renal,[243,253] mesenteric,[188,254] and cerebral blood flow[243] may be less than what is observed with indomethacin. This may relate to a more selective effect of ibuprofen on COX-2,[255] although other, yet to be identified mechanisms may be involved.[214] Ibuprofen is 99% protein bound and may displace bilirubin[256] in addition to affecting hepatic glucuronidation.[214] Because of this combination of factors, ibuprofen use has been associated with higher peak total serum bilirubin levels in some[257] but not all studies.[187] There are reports of pulmonary hypertension in association with ibuprofen treatment for PDA in preterm neonates,[258] and several deaths in the prophylaxis group resulted in early termination of a randomized trial of ibuprofen prophylaxis.[259,260] Caution is advised utilizing prophylactic agents that may result in ductal restriction in the setting of hypoxemia and/or situations of unknown heart function. As with other NSAIDs, ibuprofen inhibits platelet aggregation,[261] with an effect that is more short-lived than with indomethacin,[261] lasting between 6 and 24 hours after administration.[261] Platelet count should be established prior to initiating therapy, and active bleeding is regarded as a contraindication to treatment.

ACETAMINOPHEN

Acetaminophen, also known as paracetamol or N-acetyl-p-aminophenol (APAP), is widely used as an antipyretic and analgesic treatment for infants and children, including newborns.[209,262] The use of acetaminophen for hsPDA closure in preterm infants was first reported in 2011.[263] The nonselective COX inhibitors (COX-I) inhibit the COX site on the PGHS enzyme, catalyzing conversion of arachidonic acid to PGG_2 by oxidation.[209] There is an additional site on the PGHS enzyme known as the peroxidase (POX) site, which converts PGG_2 to PGH_2, which is the precursor to PGE_2 (see Fig. 48.11).[209] Whereas COX activity is dependent on POX activity,[209] POX activity is independent of COX.[264] Acetaminophen is believed to competitively inhibit the POX enzyme.[209] The specific mechanism whereby acetaminophen facilitates ductal closure is unclear; however, POX inhibition may play a role.[265] Evidence from an in vitro model suggests that doses of acetaminophen much higher than routine clinical use are needed to induce PDA closure.[266] Interestingly, acetaminophen may act as a potent pulmonary vasoconstrictor, which may limit the magnitude of the transductal flow according to Poiseuille's law.[267] Advantages of acetaminophen over NSAIDs include a favorable side-effect profile and similar efficacy to ibuprofen and indomethacin in achieving ductal closure.[263] The drug does not have significant antiplatelet activity[268] and is associated with minor or no adverse gastrointestinal effects.

Acetaminophen undergoes metabolism by the liver. In adults, this consists of both conjugation with glucuronide (glucuronidation) by glucuronyl transferase (acetaminophen glucuronide, comprising 52% to 57% of urinary metabolites) and sulfation by sulfotransferases (acetaminophen sulfate, comprising 30% to 44% of urinary metabolites).[269] A very small proportion (5% to 10%) is oxidized to the reactive metabolite N-acetyl-p-benzoquinone imine (NAPQI),[269] via CYP2E1,[265] which is chiefly responsible for acetaminophen-induced hepatotoxicity.[269] The majority of these metabolites are transported via the bloodstream to the kidneys.[269] Glucuronidation is not well developed in neonates,[270] although this increases with advancing GA.[271] As a result, a greater proportion of acetaminophen metabolism occurs via sulfation,[272] which may contribute to the lower rates of hepatotoxicity observed in neonates than in other age groups.[265] It is important to note, however, that potentially hepatotoxic downstream NAPQI metabolites have been identified in preterm neonates exposed to acetaminophen at therapeutic doses.[273] Acetaminophen clearance increases with postnatal age[273] (see Table 48.3) and is about one-third that observed in children and adults.[202] Both acetaminophen and bilirubin are metabolized by hepatic glucuronyl transferases, and dose reduction in the setting of unconjugated hyperbilirubinemia has been suggested; however, very limited data exist in the setting of hsPDA treatment.[274]

A number of studies have shown similar efficacy of acetaminophen to COX-I in achieving PDA closure, particularly in the first week of life,[188,275,276] although to date the number of neonates included in studies of acetaminophen for this indication is relatively small and the quality of these studies is variable. Long-term follow-up outcomes for infants treated with acetaminophen for PDA and controlled trial data for use in the most extremely preterm infants (<26 weeks) are awaited. Evidence to support the use of acetaminophen as a "rescue" therapy after unsuccessful COX inhibitor treatment is currently limited.[265] Because of the favorable side-effect profile of acetaminophen, this approach is gaining acceptance, particularly in infants being considered for surgical ligation.[265] The use of acetaminophen for PDA prophylaxis is not well established, which may be partly due to its inability to reduce the rates of P/IVH in published studies to date.[265] Also, although acetaminophen may produce more rapid PDA closure, it may be less effective in extremely preterm neonates.[265,276] In general, however, the number of neonates ≤24 weeks' gestation studied is small. A recent systematic review by the Cochrane Collaboration did not find sufficient evidence to enable recommendation of acetaminophen as a first-line therapy for hsPDA,[275] although research into this therapy is continuing to evolve.

Acetaminophen has high oral bioavailability (88%) and reaches peak blood concentrations within 90 minutes of enteral administration. Both oral and IV acetaminophen have been used for the treatment of hsPDA in preterm neonates.[276] As has been shown for ibuprofen, there is emerging evidence that the oral route may be more effective, although this requires further investigation.[276] Acetaminophen concentrations correlate with ductal closure and with postnatal age.[277] Data for steady state or trough levels have largely been extrapolated from target concentrations for analgesia, rather than for PDA treatment.[277] Levels of 10 to 20 mg per L have, however, been correlated with PDA closure rates of 71% to 83% and >20 mg per L with 100% closure rate in small samples of preterm infants, without adverse effects.[277–279] Doses of 10 mg per kg every 6 hours could be expected to achieve a mean plasma concentration of 11 mg per L in infants 34 to 44 weeks' gestation.[202] Dosing schedules described for acetaminophen in PDA treatment and pharmacokinetic data for acetaminophen in neonates are outlined in Table 48.3.

Acetaminophen use for PDA treatment is associated with lower rates of renal impairment, gastrointestinal bleeding, increased serum bilirubin, and thrombocytopenia than with COX-I.[280,281] As described earlier, developmental differences in metabolism of acetaminophen may contribute to a lower risk of liver toxicity with use in neonates. Transient elevations in liver transaminases have been reported in a small number of neonates receiving high-dose acetaminophen[276]; therefore, monitoring for hepatotoxicity during treatment is important.

CARDIOVASCULAR THERAPY AT ≤24 WEEKS' GESTATION

With increasing survival at 22 to 24^{+6} weeks' gestation, it is relevant to consider the impact of extrapolating evidence generated in an older preterm population to the limits of viability. As described earlier, there are significant differences between the myocardium, receptor profile, and responses to stimuli between preterm and term infants. Clearance and metabolism are impacted by organ function, volume of distribution, and protein characteristics. It is reasonable to conclude that the more immature, the more differences are likely to be identified. There are very little data to support specific pharmacokinetics and pharmacodynamics of neonates at these extremes of viability. What little is known, however (e.g., reduced clearance of milrinone, see section "Milrinone"[67,282]), suggests that maturity plays a role in drug activity. Further research in this patient population is required.

REFERENCES

1. Van Mierop LH. Embryology of the univentricular heart. *Herz* 1979;4:78–85.
2. Smolich JJ. Ultrastructural and functional features of the developing mammalian heart: a brief overview. *Reprod Fertil Dev* 1995;7:451–461.

3. Marijianowski MM, van der Loos CM, Mohrschladt MF, et al. The neonatal heart has a relatively high content of total collagen and type I collagen, a condition that may explain the less compliant state. *J Am Coll Cardiol* 1994;23:1204–1208.
4. Mahony L. Maturation of calcium transport in cardiac sarcoplasmic reticulum. *Pediatr Res* 1988;24:639–643.
5. Mahony L, Jones LR. Developmental changes in cardiac sarcoplasmic reticulum in sheep. *J Biol Chem* 1986;261:15257–15265.
6. Kojima M, Ishima T, Taniguchi N, et al. Developmental changes in beta-adrenoceptors, muscarinic cholinoceptors and Ca2+ channels in rat ventricular muscles. *Br J Pharmacol* 1990;99:334–339.
7. Chemtob S, Guest I, Potvin W, et al. Ontogeny of responses of rabbit aorta to atrial natriuretic factor and isoproterenol. *Dev Pharmacol Ther* 1991;16:108–115.
8. Yamada S, Yamamura HI, Roeske WR. Ontogeny of mammalian cardiac alpha 1-adrenergic receptors. *Eur J Pharmacol* 1980;68:217–221.
9. Kim MY, Finch AM, Lumbers ER, et al. Expression of adrenoceptor subtypes in preterm piglet heart is different to term heart. *PLoS One* 2014;9:e92167.
10. Portbury AL, Chandra R, Groelle M, et al. Catecholamines act via a beta-adrenergic receptor to maintain fetal heart rate and survival. *Am J Physiol Heart Circ Physiol* 2003;284:H2069–H2077.
11. Zeiders JL, Seidler FJ, Slotkin TA. Ontogeny of regulatory mechanisms for beta-adrenoceptor control of rat cardiac adenylyl cyclase: targeting of G-proteins and the cyclase catalytic subunit. *J Mol Cell Cardiol* 1997;29:603–615.
12. Sun LS. Regulation of myocardial beta-adrenergic receptor function in adult and neonatal rabbits. *Biol Neonate* 1999;76:181–192.
13. Reller MD, Morton MJ, Reid DL, et al. Fetal lamb ventricles respond differently to filling and arterial pressures and to in utero ventilation. *Pediatr Res* 1987;22:621–626.
14. Sonnenblick EH. Force-velocity relations in mammalian heart muscle. *Am J Physiol* 1962;202:931–939.
15. Pinson CW, Morton MJ, Thornburg KL. An anatomic basis for fetal right ventricular dominance and arterial pressure sensitivity. *J Dev Physiol* 1987;9:253–269.
16. Puglisi JL, Negroni JA, Chen-Izu Y, et al. The force-frequency relationship: insights from mathematical modeling. *Adv Physiol Educ* 2013;37:28–34.
17. Wiegerinck RF, Cojoc A, Zeidenweber CM, et al. Force frequency relationship of the human ventricle increases during early postnatal development. *Pediatr Res* 2009;65: 414–419.
18. Schmidt MR, White PA, Khambadkone S, et al. The neonatal but not the mature heart adapts to acute tachycardia by beneficial modification of the force-frequency relationship. *Pediatr Cardiol* 2011;32:562–567.
19. Paradisis M, Evans N, Kluckow M, et al. Randomized trial of milrinone versus placebo for prevention of low systemic blood flow in very preterm infants. *J Pediatr* 2009;154: 189–195.
20. Development of audit measures and guidelines for good practice in the management of neonatal respiratory distress syndrome. Report of a Joint Working Group of the British Association of Perinatal Medicine and the Research Unit of the Royal College of Physicians. *Arch Dis Child* 1992;67:1221–1227.
21. Northern Neonatal Nursing Initiative. Systolic blood pressure in babies of less than 32 weeks gestation in the first year of life. Northern Neonatal Nursing Initiative. *Arch Dis Child Fetal Neonatal Ed* 1999;80:F38–F42.
22. Kluckow M, Evans N. Low superior vena cava flow and intraventricular haemorrhage in preterm infants. *Arch Dis Child Fetal Neonatal Ed* 2000;82:F188–F194.
23. Stranak Z, Semberova J, Barrington K, et al. International survey on diagnosis and management of hypotension in extremely preterm babies. *Eur J Pediatr* 2014;173:793–798.
24. Osborn DA, Evans N, Kluckow M. Clinical detection of low upper body blood flow in very premature infants using blood pressure, capillary refill time, and central-peripheral temperature difference. *Arch Dis Child Fetal Neonatal Ed* 2004;89:168F–173F.
25. Kharrat A, Rios DI, Weisz DE, et al. The relationship between blood pressure parameters and left ventricular output in neonates. *J Perinatol* 2019;39(5):619–625.
26. Ruffolo RR Jr. The pharmacology of dobutamine. *Am J Med Sci* 1987;294:244–248.
27. Toller WG, Stranz C. Levosimendan, a new inotropic and vasodilator agent. *Anesthesiology* 2006;104;556–569.
28. Noori S, Seri I. Neonatal blood pressure support: the use of inotropes, lusitropes, and other vasopressor agents. *Clin Perinatol* 2012;39:221–238.
29. Seri I. Management of hypotension and low systemic blood flow in the very low birth weight neonates during the first postnatal week. *J Perinatol* 2006;26(Suppl 1):S8–S13;discussion S22–S23.
30. Evans N. Which inotrope for which baby? *Arch Dis Child Fetal Neonatal Ed* 2006;91:F213–F220.
31. Giesinger RE, McNamara PJ. Hemodynamic instability in the critically ill neonate: an approach to cardiovascular support based on disease pathophysiology. *Semin Perinatol* 2016;40:174–188.
32. Al-Salam Z, Johnson S, Abozaid S, et al. The hemodynamic effects of dobutamine during reoxygenation after hypoxia: a dose-response study in newborn pigs. *Shock* 2007;28:317–325.
33. Hinds JE, Hawthorne EW. Comparative cardiac dynamic effects of dobutamine and isoproterenol in conscious instrumented dogs. *Am J Cardiol* 1975;36:894–901.
34. Cheung PY, Barrington KJ, Bigam D. The hemodynamic effects of dobutamine infusion in the chronically instrumented newborn piglet. *Crit Care Med* 1999;27:558–564.
35. Smolich JJ, Sano T, Penny DJ. Blunting of pulmonary but not systemic vasodilator responses to dobutamine in newborn lambs. *Pediatr Res* 2000;47:107–113.
36. Schranz D, Stopfkuchen H, Jungst BK, et al. Hemodynamic effects of dobutamine in children with cardiovascular failure. *Eur J Pediatr* 1982;139:4–7.
37. Martinez AM, Padbury JF, Thio S. Dobutamine pharmacokinetics and cardiovascular responses in critically ill neonates. *Pediatrics* 1992;89:47–51.
38. Subhedar NV, Shaw NJ. Dopamine versus dobutamine for hypotensive preterm infants. *Cochrane Database Syst Rev* 2003;CD001242.
39. Robel-Tillig E, Knupfer M, Pulzer F, et al. Cardiovascular impact of dobutamine in neonates with myocardial dysfunction. *Early Hum Dev* 2007;83:307–312.
40. Stopfkuchen H, Queisser-Luft A, Vogel K. Cardiovascular responses to dobutamine determined by systolic time intervals in preterm infants. *Crit Care Med* 1990;18:722–724.
41. Stopfkuchen H, Schranz D, Huth R, et al. Effects of dobutamine on left ventricular performance in newborns as determined by systolic time intervals. *Eur J Pediatr* 1987;146:135–139.
42. Greenough A, Emery EF. Randomized trial comparing dopamine and dobutamine in preterm infants. *Eur J Pediatr* 1993;152:925–927.
43. Roze JC, Tohier C, Maingueneau C, et al. Response to dobutamine and dopamine in the hypotensive very preterm infant. *Arch Dis Child* 1993;69:59–63.
44. Klarr JM, Faix RG, Pryce CJ, et al. Randomized, blind trial of dopamine versus dobutamine for treatment of hypotension in preterm infants with respiratory distress syndrome. *J Pediatr* 1994;125:117–122.
45. Ruelas-Orozco G, Vargas-Origel A. Assessment of therapy for arterial hypotension in critically ill preterm infants. *Am J Perinatol* 2000;17:95–99.
46. Osborn D, Evans N, Kluckow M. Randomized trial of dobutamine versus dopamine in preterm infants with low systemic blood flow. *J Pediatr* 2002;140:183–191.
47. Zhang J, Penny DJ, Kim NS, et al. Mechanisms of blood pressure increase induced by dopamine in hypotensive preterm neonates. *Arch Dis Child Fetal Neonatal Ed* 1999;81: F99–F104.
48. Jain A, McNamara PJ. Persistent pulmonary hypertension of the newborn: advances in diagnosis and treatment. *Semin Fetal Neonatal Med* 2015;20:262–271.
49. Mahoney L, Shah G, Crook D, et al. A literature review of the pharmacokinetics and pharmacodynamics of dobutamine in neonates. *Pediatr Cardiol* 2016;37:14–23.
50. Noori S, Seri I. Evidence-based versus pathophysiology-based approach to diagnosis and treatment of neonatal cardiovascular compromise. *Semin Fetal Neonatal Med* 2015;20:238–245.
51. Barrington K, Chan W. The circulatory effects of epinephrine infusion in the anesthesized piglet. *Pediatr Res* 1993;33:190–194.
52. Cheung PY, Barrington KJ. The effects of dopamine and epinephrine on hemodynamics and oxygen metabolism in hypoxic anesthetized piglets. *Crit Care (London, England)* 2001;5:158–166.
53. Barrington KJ, Finer NN, Chan WK. A blind, randomized comparison of the circulatory effects of dopamine and epinephrine infusions in the newborn piglet during normoxia and hypoxia. *Crit Care Med* 1995;23:740–748.
54. Obaid L, Johnson ST, Emara M, et al. Epinephrine versus dopamine to treat shock in hypoxic newborn pigs resuscitated with 100% oxygen. *Shock* 2008;29:262–268.
55. Valverde E, Pellicer A, Madero R, et al. Dopamine versus epinephrine for cardiovascular support in low birth weight infants: analysis of systemic effects and neonatal clinical outcomes. *Pediatrics* 2006;117:e1213–e1222.
56. Pellicer A, Valverde E, Elorza MD, et al. Cardiovascular support for low birth weight infants and cerebral hemodynamics: a randomized, blinded, clinical trial. *Pediatrics* 2005;115:1501–1512.
57. Philipos EZ, Robertson MA. A randomized double blinded controlled trial of dopamine vs epinephrine for inotropic support in premature infants, 1750 grams [abstract]. *Pediatr Res* 2000;47:425A.
58. Hardin RA, Scott JB, Haddy FJ. Effect of epinephrine and norepinephrine on coronary vascular resistance in dogs. *Am J Physiol* 1961;201:276–280.
59. Caspi J, Coles JG, Benson LN, et al. Age-related response to epinephrine-induced myocardial stress. A functional and ultrastructural study. *Circulation* 1991;84:III394–III399.
60. LeJemtel TH, Scortichini D, Levitt B, et al. Effects of phosphodiesterase inhibition on skeletal muscle vasculature. *Am J Cardiol* 1989;63:27A–30A.
61. Silver PJ, Harris AL, Canniff PC, et al. Phosphodiesterase isozyme inhibition, activation of the cAMP system, and positive inotropy mediated by milrinone in isolated guinea pig cardiac muscle. *J Cardiovasc Pharmacol* 1989;13:530–540.
62. Akita T, Joyner RW, Lu C, et al. Developmental changes in modulation of calcium currents of rabbit ventricular cells by phosphodiesterase inhibitors. *Circulation* 1994;90:469–478.
63. Honerjager P. Pharmacology of positive inotropic phosphodiesterase III inhibitors. *Eur Heart J* 1989;10(Suppl C):25–31.
64. Ferrer-Barba A, Gonzalez-Rivera I, Bautista-Hernandez V. Inodilators in the management of low cardiac output syndrome after pediatric cardiac surgery. *Curr Vasc Pharmacol* 2016;14:48–57.
65. Samiee-Zafarghandy S, Raman SR, van den Anker JN, et al.; Best Pharmaceuticals for Children Act-Pediatric Trials Network Administrative Core Committee. Safety of milrinone use in neonatal intensive care units. *Early Hum Dev* 2015;91:31–35.
66. El-Khuffash AF, Jain A, Weisz D, et al. Assessment and treatment of post patent ductus arteriosus ligation syndrome. *J Pediatr* 2014;165:46.e41–52.e41.
67. Hallik M, Ilmoja ML, Tasa T, et al. Population pharmacokinetics and dosing of milrinone after patent ductus arteriosus ligation in preterm infants. *Pediatr Crit Care Med* 2019;20(7):621–629.
68. McNamara PJ, Laique F, Muang-In S, et al. Milrinone improves oxygenation in neonates with severe persistent pulmonary hypertension of the newborn. *J Crit Care* 2006;21:217–222.
69. McNamara PJ, Shivananda SP, Sahni M, et al. Pharmacology of milrinone in neonates with persistent pulmonary hypertension of the newborn and suboptimal response to inhaled nitric oxide. *Pediatr Crit Care Med* 2013;14:74–84.
70. James AT, Bee C, Corcoran JD, et al. Treatment of premature infants with pulmonary hypertension and right ventricular dysfunction with milrinone: a case series. *J Perinatol* 2015;35:268–273.

71. Patel N. Use of milrinone to treat cardiac dysfunction in infants with pulmonary hypertension secondary to congenital diaphragmatic hernia: a review of six patients. *Neonatology* 2012;102:130–136.
72. Duggal B, Pratap U, Slavik Z, et al. Milrinone and low cardiac output following cardiac surgery in infants: is there a direct myocardial effect? *Pediatr Cardiol* 2005;26:642–645.
73. Klugman D, Berger JT, Sable CA, et al. Pediatric patients hospitalized with myocarditis: a multi-institutional analysis. *Pediatr Cardiol* 2010;31:222–228.
74. Chen B, Lakshminrusimha S, Czech L, et al. Regulation of phosphodiesterase 3 in the pulmonary arteries during the perinatal period in sheep. *Pediatr Res* 2009;66:682–687.
75. Lakshminrusimha S, Steinhorn RH. Inodilators in nitric oxide resistant persistent pulmonary hypertension of the newborn. *Pediatr Crit Care Med* 2013;14:107–109.
76. Deb B, Bradford K, Pearl RG. Additive effects of inhaled nitric oxide and intravenous milrinone in experimental pulmonary hypertension. *Crit Care Med* 2000;28:795–799.
77. Giaccone A, Zuppa AF, Sood B, et al. Milrinone pharmacokinetics and pharmacodynamics in neonates with persistent pulmonary hypertension of the newborn. *Am J Perinatol* 2017;34:749–758.
78. James AT, Corcoran JD, McNamara PJ, et al. The effect of milrinone on right and left ventricular function when used as a rescue therapy for term infants with pulmonary hypertension. *Cardiol Young* 2016;26:90–99.
79. Gist KM, Goldstein SL, Joy MS, et al. Milrinone dosing issues in critically ill children with kidney injury: a review. *J Cardiovasc Pharmacol* 2016;67:175–181.
80. Paradisis M, Jiang X, McLachlan AJ, et al. Population pharmacokinetics and dosing regimen design of milrinone in preterm infants. *Arch Dis Child Fetal Neonatal Ed* 2007;92:F204–F209.
81. Zuppa AF, Nicolson SC, Adamson PC, et al. Population pharmacokinetics of milrinone in neonates with hypoplastic left heart syndrome undergoing stage I reconstruction. *Anesth Analg* 2006;102:1062–1069.
82. Bailey JM, Hoffman TM, Wessel DL, et al. A population pharmacokinetic analysis of milrinone in pediatric patients after cardiac surgery. *J Pharmacokinet Pharmacodyn* 2004;31:43–59.
83. Lindsay CA, Barton P, Lawless S, et al. Pharmacokinetics and pharmacodynamics of milrinone lactate in pediatric patients with septic shock. *J Pediatr* 1998;132:329–334.
84. Gist KM, Mizuno T, Goldstein SL, et al. Retrospective evaluation of milrinone pharmacokinetics in children with kidney injury. *Ther Drug Monit* 2015;37:792–796.
85. Ramamoorthy C, Anderson GD, Williams GD, et al. Pharmacokinetics and side effects of milrinone in infants and children after open heart surgery. *Anesth Analg* 1998;86:283–289.
86. Gist KM, Cooper DS, Wrona J, et al. Acute kidney injury biomarkers predict an increase in serum milrinone concentration earlier than serum creatinine-defined acute kidney injury in infants after cardiac surgery. *Ther Drug Monit* 2018;40:186–194.
87. Dickstein K, Cohen-Solal A, Filippatos G, et al. ESC guidelines for the diagnosis and treatment of acute and chronic heart failure 2008: the Task Force for the diagnosis and treatment of acute and chronic heart failure 2008 of the European Society of Cardiology. Developed in collaboration with the Heart Failure Association of the ESC (HFA) and endorsed by the European Society of Intensive Care Medicine (ESICM). *Eur J Heart Fail* 2008;10:933–989.
88. Moga MA, Nguyen N, Mazwi ML, et al. Pharmacological manipulation of peripheral vascular resistance in special clinical situations after pediatric cardiac surgery. *Curr Vasc Pharmacol* 2016;14:63–72.
89. Lechner E, Hofer A, Leitner-Peneder G, et al. Levosimendan versus milrinone in neonates and infants after corrective open-heart surgery: a pilot study. *Pediatr Crit Care Med* 2012;13:542–548.
90. Turanlahti M, Boldt T, Palkama T, et al. Pharmacokinetics of levosimendan in pediatric patients evaluated for cardiac surgery. *Pediatr Crit Care Med* 2004;5:457–462.
91. Bravo MC, Lopez P, Cabanas F, et al. Acute effects of levosimendan on cerebral and systemic perfusion and oxygenation in newborns: an observational study. *Neonatology* 2011;99:217–223.
92. Lechner E, Moosbauer W, Pinter M, et al. Use of levosimendan, a new inodilator, for postoperative myocardial stunning in a premature neonate. *Pediatr Crit Care Med* 2007;8:61–63.
93. Hottinger DG, Beebe DS, Kozhimannil T, et al. Sodium nitroprusside in 2014: a clinical concepts review. *J Anaesthesiol Clin Pharmacol* 2014;30:462–471.
94. Gmeiner R, Riedl J, Baumgartner H. Effect of sodium nitroprusside on myocardial performance and venous tone. *Eur J Pharmacol* 1975;31:287–291.
95. Ivankovich AD, Miletich DJ, Tinker JH. Sodium nitroprusside: metabolism and general considerations. *Int Anesthesiol Clin* 1978;16:1–29.
96. Rapoport RM, Murad F. Endothelium-dependent and nitrovasodilator-induced relaxation of vascular smooth muscle: role of cyclic GMP. *J Cyclic Nucleotide Protein Phosphor Res* 1983;9:281–296.
97. Levy JH. Management of systemic and pulmonary hypertension. *Tex Heart Inst J* 2005;32:467–471.
98. Fok H, Jiang B, Clapp B, et al. Regulation of vascular tone and pulse wave velocity in human muscular conduit arteries: selective effects of nitric oxide donors to dilate muscular arteries relative to resistance vessels. *Hypertension* 2012;60:1220–1225.
99. Mills KI, Costello JM, Almodovar MC. A review of systemic vasodilators in low cardiac output syndrome following pediatric cardiac surgery. *Curr Vasc Pharmacol* 2016;14:29–36.
100. Schlant RC, Tsagaris TS, Robertson RJ Jr. Studies on the acute cardiovascular effects of intravenous sodium nitroprusside. *Am J Cardiol* 1962;9:51–59.
101. Benitz WE, Malachowski N, Cohen RS, et al. Use of sodium nitroprusside in neonates: efficacy and safety. *J Pediatr* 1985;106:102–110.
102. Chandar J, Zilleruelo G. Hypertensive crisis in children. *Pediatr Nephrol* 2012;27:741–751.
103. Gordillo-Paniagua G, Velasquez-Jones L, Martini R, et al. Sodium nitroprusside treatment of severe arterial hypertension in children. *J Pediatr* 1975;87:799–802.
104. Getman CE, Goetzman BW, Bennett S. Age-dependent effects of sodium nitroprusside and dopamine in lambs. *Pediatr Res* 1991;29:329–333.
105. Moffett BS, Price JF. Evaluation of sodium nitroprusside toxicity in pediatric cardiac surgical patients. *Ann Pharmacother* 2008;42:1600–1604.
106. Thomas C, Svehla L, Moffett BS. Sodium-nitroprusside-induced cyanide toxicity in pediatric patients. *Expert Opin Drug Saf* 2009;8:599–602.
107. Schreiber MD, Dixit R, Rudinsky B, et al. Direct comparison of the effects of nebulized nitroprusside versus inhaled nitric oxide on pulmonary and systemic hemodynamics during hypoxia-induced pulmonary hypertension in piglets. *Crit Care Med* 2002;30:2560–2565.
108. Mestan KK, Carlson AD, White M, et al. Cardiopulmonary effects of nebulized sodium nitroprusside in term infants with hypoxic respiratory failure. *J Pediatr* 2003;143: 640–643.
109. Meadow W, Rudinsky B, Bell A, et al. Effects of nebulized nitroprusside on pulmonary and systemic hemodynamics during pulmonary hypertension in piglets. *Pediatr Res* 1998;44:181–186.
110. Meyer S, Baghai A, Sailer NL, et al. Lactic acidosis caused by sodium nitroprusside in a newborn with congenital heart disease. *Eur J Pediatr* 2005;164:253–254.
111. Friederich JA, Butterworth JF. Sodium nitroprusside: twenty years and counting. *Anesth Analg* 1995;81:152–162.
112. Griffiths MJ, Evans TW. Inhaled nitric oxide therapy in adults. *N Engl J Med* 2005;353:2683–2695.
113. Barrington KJ, Finer N, Pennaforte T, et al. Nitric oxide for respiratory failure in infants born at or near term. *Cochrane Database Syst Rev* 2017;1:CD000399.
114. Kinsella JP. Inhaled nitric oxide in the term newborn. *Early Hum Dev* 2008;84:709–716.
115. Sahni R, Ameer X, Ohira-Kist K, et al. Non-invasive inhaled nitric oxide in the treatment of hypoxemic respiratory failure in term and preterm infants. *J Perinatol* 2017;37:54–60.
116. Avila-Alvarez A, Del Cerro Marin MJ, Bautista-Hernandez V. Pulmonary vasodilators in the management of low cardiac output syndrome after pediatric cardiac surgery. *Curr Vasc Pharmacol* 2016;14:37–47.
117. Fanaroff JM, Wilson-Costello DE, Newman NS, et al. Treated hypotension is associated with neonatal morbidity and hearing loss in extremely low birth weight infants. *Pediatrics* 2006;117:1131–1135.
118. Seri I. Cardiovascular, renal, and endocrine actions of dopamine in neonates and children. *J Pediatr* 1995;126:333–344.
119. McMillen IC, Mulvogue HM, Coulter CL, et al. Ontogeny of catecholamine-synthesizing enzymes and enkephalins in the sheep adrenal medulla: an immunocytochemical study. *J Endocrinol* 1988;118:221–226.
120. Verhofstad AA, Hokfelt T, Goldstein M, et al. Appearance of tyrosine hydroxylase, aromatic amino-acid decarboxylase, dopamine beta-hydroxylase and phenylethanolamine N-methyltransferase during the ontogenesis of the adrenal medulla: an immunohistochemical study in the rat. *Cell Tissue Res* 1979;200:1–13.
121. Wilburn LA, Goldsmith PC, Chang KJ, et al. Ontogeny of enkephalin and catecholamine-synthesizing enzymes in the primate fetal adrenal medulla. *J Clin Endocrinol Metab* 1986;63:974–980.
122. Coulter CL, McMillen IC, Robinson JS, et al. Placental restriction alters adrenal medullary development in the midgestation sheep fetus. *Pediatr Res* 1998;44:656–662.
123. Ducsay CA, Hyatt K, Mlynarczyk M, et al. Long-term hypoxia modulates expression of key genes regulating adrenomedullary function in the late gestation ovine fetus. *Am J Physiol Regul Integr Comp Physiol* 2007;293:R1997–R2005.
124. Cheung PY, Barrington KJ, Pearson RJ, et al. Systemic, pulmonary and mesenteric perfusion and oxygenation effects of dopamine and epinephrine. *Am J Respir Crit Care Med* 1997;155:32–37.
125. Bhatt-Mehta V, Nahata MC. Dopamine and dobutamine in pediatric therapy. *Pharmacotherapy* 1989;9:303–314.
126. Kaumann AJ, Hall JA, Murray KJ, et al. A comparison of the effects of adrenaline and noradrenaline on human heart: the role of beta 1-and beta 2-adrenoceptors in the stimulation of adenylate cyclase and contractile force. *Eur Heart J* 1989;10(Suppl B):29–37.
127. Dellinger RP, Levy MM, Rhodes A, et al. Surviving sepsis campaign: international guidelines for management of severe sepsis and septic shock: 2012. *Crit Care Med* 2013;41:580–637.
128. Tourneux P, Rakza T, Abazine A, et al. Noradrenaline for management of septic shock refractory to fluid loading and dopamine or dobutamine in full-term newborn infants. *Acta Paediatr* 2008;97:177–180.
129. Rowcliff K, de Waal K, Mohamed AL, et al. Noradrenaline in preterm infants with cardiovascular compromise. *Eur J Pediatr* 2016;175:1967–1973.
130. Tourneux P, Rakza T, Bouissou A, et al. Pulmonary circulatory effects of norepinephrine in newborn infants with persistent pulmonary hypertension. *J Pediatr* 2008;153:345–349.
131. Kleinman ME, Chameides L, Schexnayder SM, et al. Part 14: pediatric advanced life support: 2010 American Heart Association Guidelines for Cardiopulmonary Resuscitation and Emergency Cardiovascular Care. *Circulation* 2010;122:S876–S908.
132. Lexicomp Online. *Pediatric and neonatal Lexi-drugs online: norepinephrine.* Riverwoods, IL: Wolters Kluwer Health, Inc.
133. Rang HP, Ritter J, Flower R, et al. Noradrenergic transmission. In: *Rang & Dale's pharamcology.* Amsterdam, The Netherlands: Elsevier Health Sciences, 2014:177–196.
134. Beaulieu MJ. Vasopressin for the treatment of neonatal hypotension. *Neonatal Netw* 2013;32:120–124.
135. Barrett LK, Singer M, Clapp LH. Vasopressin: mechanisms of action on the vasculature in health and in septic shock. *Crit Care Med* 2007;35:33–40.
136. Tamaki T, Kiyomoto K, He H, et al. Vasodilation induced by vasopressin V2 receptor stimulation in afferent arterioles. *Kidney Int* 1996;49:722–729.
137. Garcia-Villalon AL, Garcia JL, Fernandez N, et al. Regional differences in the arterial response to vasopressin: role of endothelial nitric oxide. *Br J Pharmacol* 1996;118:1848–1854.
138. Sai Y, Okamura T, Amakata Y, et al. Comparison of responses of canine pulmonary artery and vein to angiotensin II, bradykinin and vasopressin. *Eur J Pharmacol* 1995;282:235–241.

139. Treschan TA, Peters J. The vasopressin system: physiology and clinical strategies. *Anesthesiology* 2006;105:599–612;quiz 639–640.
140. Meyer S, Gottschling S, Baghai A, et al. Arginine-vasopressin in catecholamine-refractory septic versus non-septic shock in extremely low birth weight infants with acute renal injury. *Crit Care (London, England)* 2006;10:R71.
141. Meyer S, Loffler G, Polcher T, et al. Vasopressin in catecholamine-resistant septic and cardiogenic shock in very-low-birthweight infants. *Acta Paediatr* 2006;95:1309–1312.
142. Bidegain M, Greenberg R, Simmons C, et al. Vasopressin for refractory hypotension in extremely low birth weight infants. *J Pediatr* 2010;157:502–504.
143. Kaga M, Matsuda T, Watanabe T, et al. Renal vasodilatory action of arginine vasopressin in extremely low birth weight infants. *Tohoku J Exp Med* 2013;231:159–164.
144. Mohamed A, Louis D, Surak A, et al. *Outcomes of preterm neonates treated with vasopressin for refractory pulmonary hypertension: case series.* Baltimore, MD: Pediatric Academic Society, 2016.
145. Mohamed A, Nasef N, Shah V, et al. Vasopressin as a rescue therapy for refractory pulmonary hypertension in neonates: case series. *Pediatr Crit Care* 2014;15:148–154.
146. Shivananda S, Ahliwahlia L, Kluckow M, et al. Variation in the management of persistent pulmonary hypertension of the newborn: a survey of physicians in Canada, Australia, and New Zealand. *Am J Perinatol* 2012;29:519–526.
147. Jin HK, Chen YF, Yang RH, et al. Vasopressin lowers pulmonary artery pressure in hypoxic rats by releasing atrial natriuretic peptide. *Am J Med Sci* 1989;298:227–236.
148. Schneider EG. Effect of vasopressin on adrenal steroidogenesis. *Am J Physiol* 1988;255:R806–R811.
149. Lexicomp Online. *Pediatric and neonatal Lexi-Drugs online: vasopressin.* Riverwoods, IL: Wolters Kluwer Health, Inc.
150. Cooper BE. Review and update on inotropes and vasopressors. *AACN Adv Crit Care* 2008;19:5–13;quiz 14–15.
151. Mercier FJ, Auge M, Hoffmann C, et al. Maternal hypotension during spinal anesthesia for caesarean delivery. *Minerva Anestesiologica* 2013;79:62–73.
152. Tanaka K, Kitahata H, Kawahito S, et al. Phenylephrine increases pulmonary blood flow in children with tetralogy of Fallot. *Can J Anaesth* 2003;50:926–929.
153. Thiele RH, Nemergut EC, Lynch C, 3rd. The physiologic implications of isolated alpha(1) adrenergic stimulation. *Anesth Analg* 2011;113:284–296.
154. Rios DR, Moffett BS, Kaiser JR. Trends in pharmacotherapy for neonatal hypotension. *J Pediatr* 2014;165:697.e1–701.e1.
155. Wessel DL. Managing low cardiac output syndrome after congenital heart surgery. *Crit Care Med* 2001;29:S220–S230.
156. Goertz AW, Schmidt M, Lindner KH, et al. Effect of phenylephrine bolus administration on left ventricular function during postural hypotension in anesthetized patients. *J Clin Anesth* 1993;5:408–413.
157. Hausdorff WP, Caron MG, Lefkowitz RJ. Turning off the signal: desensitization of beta-adrenergic receptor function. *Faseb J* 1990;4:2881–2889.
158. Noori S, Friedlich P, Wong P, et al. Hemodynamic changes after low-dosage hydrocortisone administration in vasopressor-treated preterm and term neonates. *Pediatrics* 2006;118:1456–1466.
159. Seri I, Tan R, Evans J. Cardiovascular effects of hydrocortisone in preterm infants with pressor-resistant hypotension. *Pediatrics* 2001;107:1070–1074.
160. Kovacs K, Szakmar E, Meder U, et al. Serum cortisol levels in asphyxiated infants with hypotension. *Early Hum Dev* 2018;120:40–45.
161. Mizobuchi M, Yoshimoto S, Nakao H. Time-course effect of a single dose of hydrocortisone for refractory hypotension in preterm infants. *Pediatr Int* 2011;53:881–886.
162. Bonsante F, Latorre G, Iacobelli S, et al. Early low-dose hydrocortisone in very preterm infants: a randomized, placebo-controlled trial. *Neonatology* 2007;91:217–221.
163. Rohr SB, Sauer H, Gortner L, et al. Cardiovascular and metabolic side effects associated with hydrocortisone and dexamethasone use in VLBW infants: a single-centre experience. *Acta Paediatrica* 2013;102:e436.
164. Jiang J, Zhang J, Kang M, et al. Transient hypertrophic cardiomyopathy and hypertension associated with hydrocortisone in preterm infant: A case report. *Medicine* 2019;98:e16838.
165. Ibrahim H, Sinha IP, Subhedar NV. Corticosteroids for treating hypotension in preterm infants. *Cochrane Database Syst Rev* 2011;(12):CD003662.
166. Global Library of Women's Medicine. Hydrocortisone. In: von Dadelszen P, ed. London, England: Paula and David Bloomer.
167. Mielke G, Benda N. Cardiac output and central distribution of blood flow in the human fetus. *Circulation* 2001;103:1662–1668.
168. van Laere D, van Overmeire B, Gupta S, et al. Application of NPE in the assessment of a patent ductus arteriosus. *Pediatr Res* 2018;84:46–56.
169. Gentile R, Stevenson G, Dooley T, et al. Pulsed Doppler echocardiographic determination of time of ductal closure in normal newborn infants. *J Pediatr* 1981;98:443–448.
170. Coceani F, Baragatti, B. Mechanisms for ductus arteriosus closure. *Semin Perinatol* 2012;36:92–97.
171. Costeloe K, Hennessy E, Gibson AT, et al. The EPICure study: outcomes to discharge from hospital for infants born at the threshold of viability. *Pediatrics* 2000;106:659–671.
172. Kluckow M, Lemmers P. Hemodynamic assessment of the patent ductus arteriosus: beyond ultrasound. *Semin Fetal Neonatal Med* 2018;23:239–244.
173. Gournay V. The ductus arteriosus: physiology, regulation, and functional and congenital anomalies. *Arch Cardiovasc Dis* 2011;104:578–585.
174. Clyman R, Campbell D, Heymann MA, et al. Persistent responsiveness of the neonatal ductus arteriosus in immature lambs: a possible cause for reopening of patent ductus arteriosus after indomethacin-induced closure. *Circulation* 1985;71:141–145.
175. Semberova J, Sirc J, Miletin J, et al. Spontaneous closure of patent ductus arteriosus in infants ≤ 1500 g. *Pediatrics* 2017;140:e2014258.
176. Nemerofsky S, Parravicini E, Bateman D, et al. The ductus arteriosus rarely requires treatment in infants> 1000 grams. *Am J Perinatol* 2008;25:661–666.
177. Fajardo M, Claure N, Swminathan S, et al. Effect of positive end-expiratory pressure on ductal shunting and systemic blood flow in preterm infants with patent ductus arteriosus. *Neonatology* 2014;105:9–13.
178. Smith A, McNamara PJ, El-Khuffash AF. Non-pharmacological management of a hemodynamically significant patent ductus arteriosus. *Semin Fetal Neonatal Med* 2018;23: 245–249.
179. Lister G, Hellenbrand WE, Kleinman CS, et al. Physiologic effects of increasing hemoglobin concentration in left-to-right shunting in infants with ventricular septal defects. *N Engl J Med* 1982;306:502–506.
180. De Buyst J, Rakza T, Pennaforte T, et al. Hemodynamic effects of fluid restriction in preterm infants with significant patent ductus arteriosus. *J Pediatr* 2012;161:404–408.
181. Patak R, Fadem SZ, Rosenblatt SG, et al. Diuretic-induced changes in renal blood flow and prostaglandin E excretion in the dog. *Am J Physiol* 1979;263:F494–F500.
182. Friedman Z, Demers LM, Marks KH, et al. Urinary excretion of prostaglandin E following the administration of furosemide and indomethacin to sick low-birth-weight infants. *J Pediatr* 1978;93:512–515.
183. Toyoshima K, Momma K, Nakanishi T. In vivo dilatation of the ductus arteriosus induced by furosemide in the rat. *Pediatr Res* 2010;67:173–176.
184. Green T, Thompson TR, Johnson DE, et al. Furosemide promotes patent ductus arteriosus in premature infants with the respiratory distress syndrome. *N Engl J Med* 1983;308:743–748.
185. Heymann M, Rudolph AM, Silverman NH. Closure of the ductus arteriosus in premature infants by inhibition of prostaglandin synthesis. *N Engl J Med* 1976;295:530–533.
186. Friedman W, Hirschklau MJ, Printz MP, et al. Pharmacologic closure of patent ductus arteriosus in the preterm infant. *N Engl J Med* 1976;295:526–529.
187. Corff K, Sekar KC. Clinical considerations for the pharmacologic management of patent ductus arteriosus with cyclooxygenase inhibitors in preterm infants. *J Pediar Pharmacol Ther* 2007;12:147–157.
188. Mitra S, Florez ID, Tamayo ME, et al. Association of placebo, indomethacin, ibuprofen, and acetaminophen with closure of hemodynamically significant patent ductus arteriosus in preterm infants. *JAMA* 2018;319:1221–1238.
189. Mercanti I, Ligi I, Boubred F, et al. Ibuprofen in the treatment of patent ductus arteriosus in preterm infants: what we know, what we still do not know. *Curr Pharm Des* 2012;18:3007–3018.
190. Marconi E, Bettiol A, Ambrosio G, et al. Efficacy and safety of pharmacological treatments for patent ductus arteriosus closure: a systematic review and network meta-analysis of clinical trials and observational studies. *Pharmacol Res* 2019;148:104418.
191. Su B, Peng CT, Tsai CH. Echocardiographic flow pattern of patent ductus arteriosus: a guide to indomethacin treatment in premature infants. *Arch Dis Child Fetal Neonatal Ed* 1999;81:F197–F200.
192. Carmo K, Evans N, Paradisis M. Duration of indomethacin treatment of the preterm patent ductus arteriosus as directed by echocardiography. *J Pediatr* 2009;155:819–822.
193. Wyllie J, Gupta S. Prophylactic and early targeted treatment of patent ductus arteriosus. *Semin Fetal Neonatal Med* 2018;23:250–254.
194. Fowlie P, Davis PG. Prophylactic intravenous indomethacin for preventing mortality and morbidity in preterm infants. *Cochrane Database Syst Rev* 2002;3:CD000174.
195. Yaffe S, Friedman WF, Rogers D, et al. The disposition of indomethacin in preterm babies. *J Pediatr* 1980;97(6):1001–1006.
196. Al Za'abi M, Donovan T, Tudehope D, et al. Orogastric and intravenous indomethacin administration to very premature neonates with patent ductus arteriosus: population pharmacokinetics, absolute bioavailability, and treatment outcome. *Ther Drug Monit* 2007;29(6):807–814.
197. Smyth J, Collier PS, Darwish M, et al. Intravenous indomethacin in preterm infants with symptomatic patent ductus arteriosus: a population pharmacokinetic study. *Br J Clin Pharmacol* 2004;58(3):249–258.
198. Pacifici G. Clinical pharmacology of indomethacin in preterm infants: implications in patent ductus arteriosus closure. *Paediatr Drugs* 2013;15(5):363–376.
199. Pacifici G. Clinical pharmacology of ibuprofen in preterm infants: a meta-analysis of published data. *Med Express* 2014;1(2):55–61.
200. Van Overmeire B, Touw D, Schepens PJ, et al. Ibuprofen pharmacokinetics in preterm infants with patent ductus arteriosus. *Clin Pharmacol Ther* 2001;70(4):336–343.
201. Hirt D, Van Overmeire B, Treluyer JM, et al. An optimized dosing scheme for preterm neonates with patent ductus arteriosus, based on a population pharmacokinetic and pharmacodynamic study. *Br J Clin Pharmacol* 2008;65(5):629–636.
202. Allegaert K, Palmer GM, Anderson BJ. The pharmacokinetics of intravenous paracetamol in neonates: size matters most. *Arch Dis Child* 2011;96(6):575–580.
203. Cook S, Roberts JK, Samiee-Zafarghandy S, et al. Population pharmacokinetics of intravenous paracetamol (acetaminophen) in preterm and term neonates: model development and external evaluation. *Clin Pharmacokinet* 2016;55(1):107–119.
204. Allegaert K, Van der Marei CD, Debeer A, et al. Pharmacokinetics of single dose intravenous propacetamol in neonates: effect of gestational age. *Arch Dis Child Fetal Neonatal Ed* 2004;89(1):F25–F28.
205. Mercanti I, Boubred F, Simeoni U. Therapeutic closure of the ductus arteriosus: benefits and limitations. *J Matern Fetal Neonatal Med* 2009;22(Suppl 3):14–20.
206. Hu Y, Jin H, Jiang Y, et al. Prediction of therapeutic response to cyclooxygenase inhibitors in preterm infants with patent ductus arteriosus. *Pediatr Cardiol* 2018;39:647–652.
207. Gersony W, Peckham GJ, Ellison RC, et al. Effects of indomethacin in premature infant with patent ductus arteriosus: results of a national collaborative trial. *J Pediatr* 1983;102:895–906.
208. Clyman R, Mauray F, Roman C, et al. Effect of gestational age on ductus response to circulating prostaglandin E2. *J Pediatr* 1983;102:907–911.
209. Anderson B. Paracetamol (acetaminophen): mechanisms of action. *Paediatr Anaesth* 2008;18:915–921.

210. McCumin D, Seidner S, Chang LY, et al. Ibuprofen-induced patent ductus arteriosus closure;physiologic, histologic, and biochemical effects in the premature lung. *Pediatrics* 2008;121:954–956.
211. Hammerman C, Shchors I, Jacobson S, et al. Ibuprofen versus continuous indomethacin in premature neonates with patent ductus arteriosus: is the difference in the mode of administration? *Pediatr Res* 2008;64:291–297.
212. Flint R, Ter Heine R, et al. Simulation-based suggestions to improve ibuprofen dosing. *Eur J Clin Pharmacol* 2018;74:1585–1591.
213. Louis D, Wong C, Ye XY, et al. Factors associated with non-response to second course indomethacin for PDA treatment in preterm neonates. *J Matern Fetal Neonatal Med* 2018;31:1407–1411.
214. Cuzzolin L, Bardanzellu F, Fanos V. The dark side of ibuprofen in the treatment of patent ductus arteriosus: could paracetamol be the solution? *Expert Opin Drug Metab Toxicol* 2018;14:855–868.
215. Van Overmeire B, Van de Broek H, Van Laer P, et al. Early versus late indomethacin treatment for patent ductus arteriosus in premature infants with respiratory distress syndrome. *J Pediatr* 2001;138:205–211.
216. Narayanan M, Cooper B, Weiss H, et al. Prophylactic indomethacin: factors determining permanent ductus arteriosus closure. *J Pediatr* 2000;136:330–337.
217. Lee J, Rajadurai VS, Tan KW, et al. Randomized trial of prolonged low-dose versus conventional dose indomethacin for treating patent ductus arteriosus in very low birth weight infants. *Pediatrics* 2003;112:345–350.
218. Olsson K, Jonzon A, Sindelar R. A high ductal flow velocity is associated with successful pharmacological closure of patent ductus arteriosus in infants 22-27 weeks gestational age. *Crit Care Res Pract 2012*;2012;715265.
219. Chorne N, Jegatheesan P, Lin E, et al. Risk factors for persistent ductus arteriosus patency during indomethacin treatment. *J Pediatr* 2007;151:629–634.
220. Gonzalez A, Sosenko IR, Chandar J, et al. Influence of infection on patent ductus arteriosus and chronic lung disease in premature infants weighing 1000 grams or less. *J Pediatr* 1996;128:470–478.
221. Kim E, Kim EK, Choi CW, et al. Intrauterine inflammation as a risk factor for persistent ductus arteriosus patency after cyclooxygenase inhibition in extremely low birth weight infants. *J Pediatr* 2010;157:745–750.
222. Weiss H, Cooper B, Brook M, et al. Factors determining reopening of the ductus arteriosus after successful clinical closure with indomethacin. *J Pediatr* 1995;127:466–471.
223. Keller R, Clyman RI. Persistent Doppler flow predicts lack of response to multiple courses of indomethacin in premature infants with recurrent patent ductus arteriosus. *Pediatr* 2003;112:583–587.
224. Richards J, Johnson A, Fox G, et al. A second course of ibuprofen is effective in the closure of a clinically significant PDA in ELBW infants. *Pediatr* 2009;124:e287–e293.
225. McCarthy JS, Zies LG, Gelband H. Age-dependent closure of the patent ductus arteriosus by indomethacin. *Pediatrics* 1978;62:706–712.
226. Herrera C, Holberton J, Davis P. Prolonged versus short course of indomethacin for treatment of PDA in preterm infants. *Cochrane Database Syst Rev* 2007;2:CD003480.
227. Vert P, Bianchetti G, Marchal F, et al. Effectiveness and pharmacokinetics of indomethacin in premature newborns with patent ductus arteriosus. *Eur J Clin Pharmacol* 1980;18:83–88.
228. Smith C, Ryckman KK, Bahr TM, et al. Polymorphisms in CYP2C9 are associated with response to indomethacin among neonates with patent ductus arteriosus. *Pediatr Res* 2017;82:776–780.
229. Shaffer C, Gal P, Ransom JL, et al. Effect of age and birth weight on indomethacin pharmacodynamics in neonates treated for patent ductus arteriosus. *Crit Care Med* 2002;30:343–348.
230. Kumar R, Yu VY. Prolonged low-dose indomethacin therapy for patent ductus arteriosus in very low birthweight infants. *J Paediatr Child Health* 1997;33:38–41.
231. Romagnoli C, Zecca E, Papacci P, et al. Furosemide does not prevent indomethacin-induced renal side effects in preterm infants. *Clin Pharmacol Ther* 1997;62:181–186.
232. Allegaert K. The impact of ibuprofen or indomethacin on renal drug clearance in neonates. *J Matern Fetal Neonatal Med* 2009;22:88–91.
233. Lambru G, Manzoni GC, Torelli P, et al. Reversible cerebral vasoconstriction phenomena following indomethacin administration. *Headache* 2011;51:813–818.
234. Edwards A, Wyatt JS, Richardson C, et al. Effects of indomethacin on cerebral haemodynamics in very preterm infants. *Lancet (London, England)* 1990;335:1491–1495.
235. Christmann V, Liem KD, Semmekrot BA, et al. Changes in cerebral, renal and mesenteric blood flow velocity during continuous and bolus infusions of indomethacin. *Acta Paediatr* 2002;91:440–446.
236. Noori S, Seri I. Hemodynamic antecedents of peri/intraventricular hemorrhage in very preterm neonates. *Semin Fetal Neonatal Med* 2015;20:232–237.
237. Sood B, Lulic-Botica M, Holzhausen KA, et al. The risk of necrotizing enterocolitis after indomethacin tocolysis. *Pediatr* 2011;128:e54–e62.
238. Dollberg S, Lusky A, Reichman B. Patent ductus arteriosus, indomethacin and necrotizing enterocolitis in very low birth weight infants: a population-based study. *J Pediatr Gastroenterol Nutr* 2005;40:184–188.
239. Stark A, Carlo WA, Tyson JE, et al; National Institute of Child Health and Human Development Neonatal Research Network. Adverse effects of early dexamethasone in extremely-low-birth-weight infants. National institute of child health and human development. *N Eng J Med* 2001;344:95–101.
240. Watterberg K, Gerdes JS, Cole CH, et al. Prophylaxis of early adrenal insufficiency to prevent bronchopulmonary dysplasia. *Pediatrics* 2004;114:1649–1657.
241. Prusakiewicz J, Duggan KC, Rouzer CA, et al. Differential sensitivity and mechanism of inhibition of COX-2 oxygenation of arachidonic acid and 2-arachidonoylglycerol by ibuprofen and mefanamic acid. *Biochemistry* 2009;48:7353–7355.
242. Cuzzolin L, Dal Cere M, Fanos V. NSAID-induced nephrotoxicity from the fetus to the child. *Drug Safety* 2001;24:9–18.
243. Pezzati M, Vangi V, Biagiotti R, et al. Effects of indomethacin and ibuprofen on mesenteric and renal blood flow in preterm infants with patent ductus arteriosus. *J Pediatr* 1999;135:733–738.
244. Mosca F, Bray M, Lattanzio M, et al. Comparative evaluation of the effects of indomethacin and ibuprofen on cerebral perfusion and oxygenation in preterm infants. *J Pediatr* 1997;131:549–554.
245. Ohlsson A, Walia R, Shah SS. Ibuprofen for the treatment of patent ductus arteriosus in preterm or low birth weight (or both) infants. *Cochrane Database Syst Rev* 2018;9:CD003481.
246. Lin YJ, Chen CM, Rehan VK, et al. Randomized trial to compare renal function and ductal response between indomethacin and ibuprofen treatment in extremely low birth weight infants. *Neonatology* 2017;111:195–202.
247. Desfrere L, Zohar S, Morville P, et al. Dose-finding study of ibuprofen in patent ductus arteriosus using the continual reassessment method. *J Clin Pharm Ther* 2005;30:121–132.
248. Rainsford K. Ibuprofen: pharmacology, efficacy and safety. *Inflammopharmacology* 2009;17:275–342.
249. Mazaleuskaya LL, Theken KN, Gong L, et al. PharmGKB summary: ibuprofen pathways. *Pharmacogenet Genomics* 2015;25:96–106.
250. Gregoire N, Desfrere L, Roze JC, et al. Population pharmacokinetic analysis of ibuprofen enantiomers in preterm newborn infants. *J Clin Pharmacol* 2008;48:1460–1468.
251. Barzilay B, Youngster I, Batash D, et al. Pharmacokinetics of oral ibuprofen for patent ductus arteriosus closure in preterm infants. *Arch Dis Child Fetal Neonatal Ed* 2012;97:F116–F119.
252. Dani C, Vangi V, Bertini G, et al. High-dose ibuprofen for patent ductus arteriosus in extremely preterm infants: a randomized controlled study. *Clin Pharmacol Ther* 2012;91:590–596.
253. Van Overmeire B, Smets K, Lecoutere D, et al. A comparison of ibuprofen and indomethacin for closure of patent ductus arteriosus. *N Eng J Med* 2000;343:674–681.
254. Speziale M, Allen RG, Henderson CR, et al. Effects of indomethacin and ibuprofen on the regional circulation in newborn piglets. *Biol Neonate* 1999;76:242–252.
255. Vane J, Botting RM. Mechanism of action of anti-inflammatory drugs. *Scand J Rheumatol Suppl* 1996;102:9–21.
256. Thibaut C, Hazard A, Huon C, et al. Effect of ibuprofen on bilirubin-albumin binding during the treatment of patent ductus arteriosus in preterm infant. *J Matern Fetal Neonatal Med* 2011;24:7–9.
257. Zecca E, Ronagnoli C, De Carolis MP, et al. Does ibuprofen increase neonatal hyperbilirubinemia? *Pediatr* 2009;124:480–484.
258. Kim S, Shin SH, Kim HS, et al. Pulmonary arterial hypertension after ibuprofen treatment for patent ductus arteriosus in very low birth weight infants. *J Pediatr* 2016;179:49–53.
259. Gournay V, Roze JC, Kuster A, et al. Prophylactic ibuprofen versus placebo in very premature infants: a randomised, double-blind, placebo-controlled trial. *Lancet (London, England)* 2004;364:1939–1944.
260. Gournay V, Savagner C, Thiriez G, et al. Pulmonary hypertension after ibuprofen prophylaxis in very preterm infants. *Lancet (London, England)* 2002;359:1486–1488.
261. Garcia-Martin E, Martinez C, Tabares B, et al. Interindividual variability in ibuprofen pharmacokinetics is related to interaction of cytochrome P450 2C8 and 2C9 amino acid polymorphisms. *Clin Pharmacol Ther* 2004;76:119–127.
262. Cuzzolin L, Antonucci R, Fanos V. Paracetamol (acetaminophen) efficacy and safety in the newborn. *Curr Drug Metab* 2013;14:178–185.
263. Hammerman C, Bin-Nun A, Markovitch E, et al. Ductal closure with paracetamol: a surprising new approach to patent ductus arteriosus treatment. *Pediatrics* 2011;128:e1618–e1621.
264. Smith W, DeWitt DL, Garavito RM. Cyclooxygenases: structural, cellular, and molecular biology. *Annu Rev Biochem* 2000;69:145–182.
265. Jasani B, Weisz DE, McNamara PJ. Evidence-based use of acetaminophen for hemodynamically significant ductus arteriosus in preterm infants. *Semin Perinatol* 2018;42:243–252.
266. El-Khuffash A, Jain A, Corcoran D, et al. Efficacy of paracetamol on patent ductus arteriosus closure may be dose dependent: evidence from human and murine studies. *Pediatr Res* 2014;76:238–244.
267. Tamir Hostovsky L, Pan J, McNamara PJ, et al. Acetaminophen increases pulmonary and systemic vasomotor tone in the newborn rat. *Pediatr Res* 2020;87(7):1171–1176.
268. Graham G, Davies MJ, Day RO, et al. The modern pharmacology of paracetamol: therapeutic actions, mechanism of action, toxicity and recent pharmacological findings. *Inflammopharmacology* 2013;21:201–232.
269. Mazaleuskaya L, Sangkuhl K, Thorn CF, et al. PharmGKB summary: pathways of acetaminophen metabolism at therapeutic versus toxic doses. *Pharmacogenet Genomics* 2015;25:416–426.
270. Strassburg C, Strassburg A, Kneip S, et al. Developmental aspects of human hepatic drug glucuronidation in young children and adults. *Gut* 2002;50:259–265.
271. Krekels E, van Ham S, Allegaert K, et al. Developmental changes rather than repeated administration drive paracetamol glucuronidation in neonates and infants. *Eur J Clin Pharmacol* 2015;71:1075–1082.
272. Cook S, Stockmann C, Samiee-Zafarghandy S, et al. Neonatal maturation of paracetamol (acetaminophen) glucuronidation, sulfation, and oxidation based on a parent-metabolite population pharmacokinetic model. *Clin Pharmacokinet* 2016;55:1395–1411.
273. Flint R, Roofhooft DW, van Rongen A, et al. Exposure to acetaminophen and all its metabolites upon 10, 15, and 20 mg/kg intravenous acetaminophen in very-preterm infants. *Pediatr Res* 2017;82:678–684.
274. Palmer G, Atkins M, Anderson BJ, et al. I.V. acetaminophen pharmacokinetics in neonates after multiple doses. *Br J Anaesth* 2008;101:523–530.
275. Ohlsson A, Shah PS. Paracetamol (acetaminophen) for patent ductus arteriosus in preterm or low birth weight infants. *Cochrane Database Syst Rev* 2018;4:CD010061.
276. Terrin G, Conte F, Oncel MY, et al. Paracetamol for the treatment of patent ductus arteriosus in preterm neonates: a systematic review and meta-analysis. *Arch Dis Child Fetal Neonatal Ed* 2016;101:F127–F136.

277. Bin-Nun A, Fink D, Mimouni FB, et al. Paracetamol serum concentrations in neonates treated enterally for ductal closure: a pilot study. *J Pediatr* 2018;198:304–307.
278. Yurrtutan S, Oncel MY, Arayici S, et al. A different first-choice drug in the medical management of patent ductus arteriosus: oral paracetamol. *J Matern Fetal Neonatal Med* 2013;26:825–827.
279. Kessel I, Waisman D, Lavie-Nevo K, et al. Paracetamol effectiveness, safety, and blood level monitoring during patent ductus arteriosus closure: a case series. *J Matern Fetal Neonatal Med* 2014;27:1719–1721.
280. El-Mashad A, El-Mahdy H, El Amrousy D, et al. Comparative study of the efficacy and safety of paracetamol, ibuprofen, and indomethacin in closure of patent ductus arteriosus in preterm neonates. *Eur J Pediatr* 2017;176:233–240.
281. Bagheri M, Niknafs P, Sabsevari F, et al. Comparison of oral acetaminophen versus ibuprofen in premature infants with patent ductus arteriosus. *Iran J Pediatr* 2016;26:e3975.
282. Hallik M, Tasa T, Starkopf J, et al. Dosing of milrinone in preterm neonates to prevent postligation cardiac syndrome: simulation study suggests need for bolus infusion. *Neonatology* 2017;111:8–11.

Nikola Dragisic
Patrick J. McNamara
Ian H. Law
Luis A. Ochoa

CHAPTER 49

Antiarrhythmic Drugs: Disorders of Cardiac Rhythm and Pharmacologic Management

Arrhythmias in healthy children are relatively common, such as premature atrial contractions and sinus arrhythmias, but typically do not require treatment and are incidentally discovered during routine examinations or while being monitored during an illness. In the pediatric population, the overall incidence of arrhythmias has been reported to be low either by utilizing ambulatory heart rate monitors or hospital admissions.[1–3] Symptomatic arrhythmias necessitating hospital admissions account for 5% to 7% of total hospital admissions.[1] Similarly, cardiac arrhythmias are very common and occur frequently in the fetus and newborn. Arrhythmias occur in roughly 2% of pregnancies and up to 14% of newborns, with the highest incidence being in patients who have congenital heart disease.[4,5] During fetal life, the diagnosis of an arrhythmia is primarily dependent on echocardiography. After birth, the history, physical exam, and electrocardiogram (ECG) are crucial in making the diagnosis. The prognosis and management of an arrhythmia are dependent upon an accurate diagnosis and a thorough understanding of the underlying mechanism. Arrhythmias may be primary in nature such as inherent channelopathies (e.g., long QT syndrome), or secondary to structural heart disease, cardiomyopathies, infections (myocarditis), electrolyte abnormalities, acid–base disturbances, elevated catecholaminergic state, or iatrogenic (e.g., catheters in the heart). The majority of arrhythmias in these patient populations are benign and resolve spontaneously or require short-term antiarrhythmic medications. Approximately one-third of arrhythmias recur later in life, typically around adolescence.[4]

FETAL ARRHYTHMIAS

Fetal arrhythmias are found in 1% to 2% of all pregnancies.[6] The most common abnormal fetal rhythm results from premature atrial contractions.[7,8] The normal fetal heart rate, for a mid- to late gestational aged fetus, is between 120 and 160 beats per minute (bpm). A sustained fetal tachycardia has an incidence of roughly 1 in 1,000 pregnancies and is defined as a fetal heart rate greater than 180 bpm for greater than 50% of the fetal scan.[6] At baseline, the normal fetal heart is operating at near-maximum functional capacity and continues to do so as it grows and matures. A sustained fetal tachycardia is associated with significant morbidity and mortality due to the heart's relative immaturity and limited functional reserve to accommodate the sustained arrhythmia. The tachyarrhythmia will lead to an elevation in ventricular end-diastolic pressure, causing increased central venous pressure, which results in decreased venous return and, ultimately, decreased cardiac output.[9] Fetal hydrops develops in roughly half of these cases, and fetal demise occurs at a rate of about 9% if left untreated.[6,7,10] It is generally said that the more abnormal the heart rate and the younger the gestational age, the less likely that a fetus will tolerate a significant arrhythmia. Supraventricular tachycardia (SVT) and atrial flutter are the most common types of sustained fetal tachyarrhythmia.

ROLE OF FETAL ECHOCARDIOGRAPHY

Fetal arrhythmias present as either a fast or slow heart rate, an irregular rhythm, or a combination of both. A fetal echocardiogram allows us to evaluate the fetus' heart rate and rhythm. This can be done through either M-mode imaging or pulsed-wave Doppler imaging. M-mode imaging allows for the simultaneous assessment of atrial and ventricular wall motion (Fig. 49.1). Pulsed-wave Doppler can be used to assess either the relationship between mitral inflow and aortic outflow or between superior vena cava inflow and aortic outflow (Fig. 49.2). Both M-mode and pulsed-wave Doppler provide a chronologic sequence that allows for assessment of atrial and ventricular systole.[11,12] For there to be atrioventricular (AV) synchrony, each atrial event needs to be followed by a ventricular event with a normal amount of time between the two.[13] This form of analysis is limited to demonstrating mechanical systolic events and cannot provide any further information on the morphology, duration, or amplitude of electrical events.

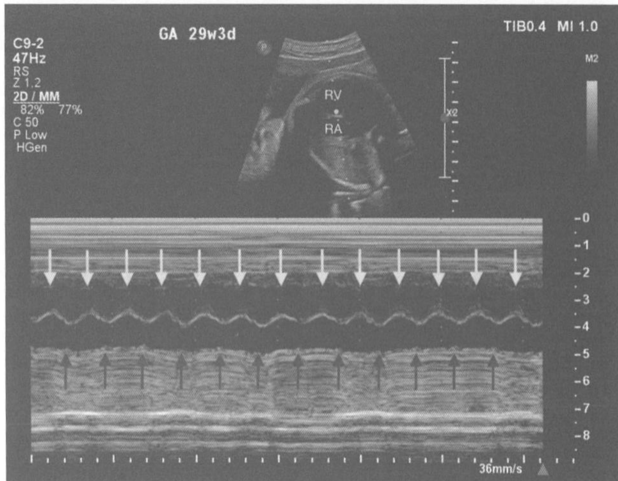

Figure 49.1 Fetal echocardiogram M-mode demonstrating 1:1 atrioventricular synchrony. The blue arrows are indicative of atrial contractions, while the white arrows depict ventricular contractions. GA, gestational age; RA, right atrium; RV, right ventricle.

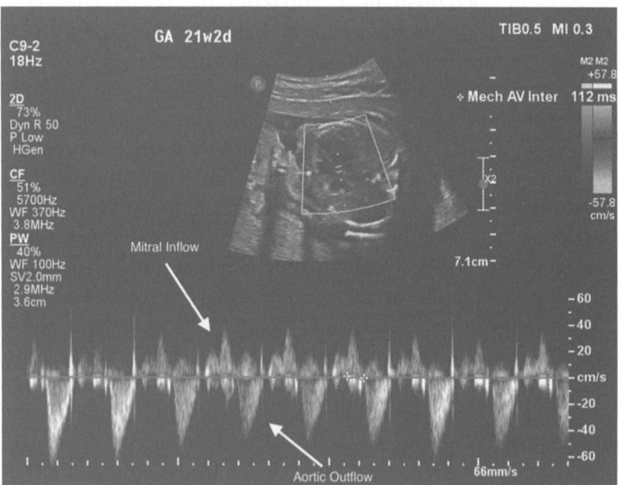

Figure 49.2 Fetal echocardiogram demonstrating pulsed-wave Doppler with 1:1 atrioventricular (AV) synchrony. The mitral inflow represents atrial systole, while the aortic outflow represents ventricular systole. GA, gestational age.

CARDIAC CONDUCTION SYSTEM

DEVELOPMENT OF THE CONDUCTION SYSTEM

Roughly 3 weeks following conception, the heart takes its first beat. The heart initially starts off as a primitive tubular structure and over the next 4 weeks of gestation it remodels. During this time, the cardiac conduction system is also developing, and by the end of the seventh week of gestation, if appropriately formed, the heart should be a four-chambered structure with sequentially synchronous contraction of the atrial and ventricular chambers. At this point, the heart rate is approximately 110 bpm.[4] By 9 to 10 weeks' gestational age, the sinoatrial (SA) node will assume primary pacemaker function, and the heart rate will reach up to 170 bpm. By 20 to 40 weeks' gestation, the heart rate will be regular in rhythm, ranging between 110 and 180 bpm, and typically have a maximum beat-to-beat variation of 15 bpm.[4,14] Postnatally, the heart rate slows further as the newborn continues to grow and develop.

CARDIAC CONDUCTION

All cardiac muscle cells have the ability and capacity to propagate action potentials between cells through specialized intracellular gap junction protein complexes.[15] A small subset of cardiomyocytes make up the subspecialized conduction system of the heart. This group of specialized cells includes the SA node, preferential atrial conduction pathways (e.g., Bachman bundle), the AV node, the bundle of His and its branches, and, finally, the ventricular network of Purkinje fibers. Normal cardiac conduction starts with the SA node which contains cells that are capable of spontaneous depolarization, making it the primary pacemaker of the heart. The electrical signal that is generated from the SA node is subsequently propagated across the atrial tissue to the AV node, then continuing down the His-Purkinje system and ventricular fascicles to depolarize the ventricles. This electrical propagation allows for sequential depolarization of the atria followed by the ventricles, thus producing the different stages of the cardiac cycle.

Cardiac myocytes are comprised of a vast variety of ion channels, connexins, and calcium-handling storage systems that are integral for action potential propagation.[15,16] Cardiomyocytes are divided into "pacemaker cells" or slow response cells (SA node, AV node, and Purkinje fibers) and "work" cells or fast response cells. The work cells have a large stable resting membrane potential and display a prolonged action potential with a plateau phase. Pacemaker cells are the opposite and have smaller unstable resting potentials and are capable of spontaneous depolarization, allowing them to generate the intrinsic electrical activity of the heart.

The cardiac action potential seen in work cells has five phases (Fig. 49.3A). During phase 0, membrane permeability to potassium decreases, while sodium permeability increases via voltage-gated fast sodium channels that open during this phase. The inward influx of positively charged sodium channels results in the production of a rapid depolarization from −90 to +10 mV. During phase 1, sodium permeability decreases, resulting in partial repolarization of the cell membrane. Phase 2, the plateau phase, occurs when there is a balance between inbound calcium and outbound potassium, producing a net neutral cell membrane. Membrane permeability to calcium decreases toward the end of this phase, but the plateau is still maintained partially by an influx in sodium ions via the sodium–calcium exchanger. Phase 3 ensues and is characterized by rapid repolarization secondary to an outward flux of potassium ions. The resting membrane potential phase 4 is restored and maintained by the selective permeability of the cell membrane to potassium and inward leak current likely carried by sodium.[16,17]

Pacemaker cells display automaticity and are capable of spontaneous depolarization (Fig. 49.3B). The pacemaker potential is characterized by three phases. Phase 4 is produced by a decrease in membrane permeability to potassium and a slow inward calcium current, leading to depolarization. Simultaneously, there is also an increase sodium current due to the presence of a sodium–calcium exchanger. Once the pacemaker threshold potential is reached (−35 mV), voltage-gated calcium channels open, allowing calcium to enter the cell and depolarization occurs constituting phase 0. Phase 3 represents repolarization and is secondary to an increase in potassium

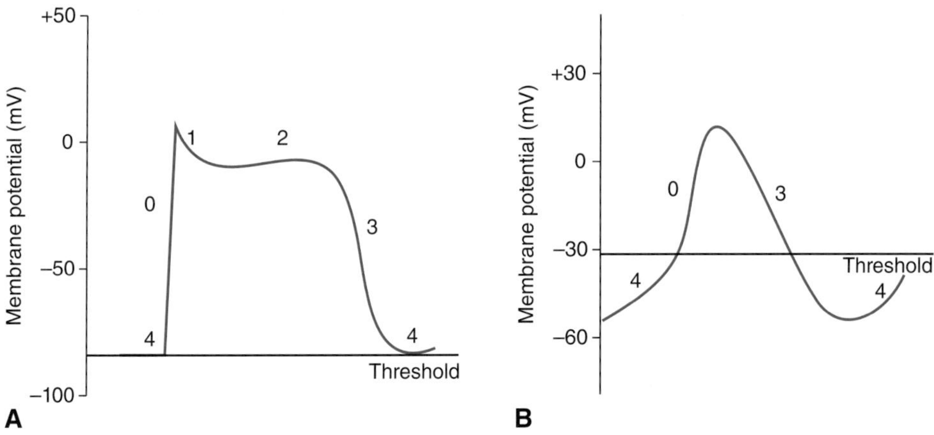

Figure 49.3 Cardiac action potentials. The cardiac action potential is shown in work cells (**A**) and pacemaker cells (**B**). Action potential in work cells includes phases 0 to 4: Phase 0, corresponds to depolarization of the membrane with opening of fast sodium channels; Phase 1, partial repolarization due to rapid decrease in sodium passage as the fast sodium channels close; Phase 2, known as the plateau phase, balances between calcium moving into the cell and potassium leaving the cell; Phase 3, final repolarization phase with inactivation of L-type calcium channels and increasing outward potassium current; Phase 4, resting membrane potential. Action potential in pacemaker cells consists of phases 4, 0, and 3: Phase 4, pacemaker potential with membrane becoming more positive due to slow inward calcium current until it reaches the threshold potential; Phase 0, depolarization with opening of voltage-gated calcium channels, allowing calcium influx; Phase 3, repolarization with inactivation of calcium channels and increase in potassium permeability.

permeability and inactivation of calcium channels. At the SA node, potassium permeability can be increased further by enhanced vagal stimulation, resulting in hyperpolarization of the cell and reducing the firing rate. As expected, sympathetic stimulation does the opposite.[17]

ARRHYTHMIA MECHANISMS

Arrhythmias occur when there are abnormalities in impulse formation, impulse propagation, or autonomic instability, resulting in abnormally slow or abnormally fast heart rates. Bradycardia may result from failure to initiate an impulse, such as in sick sinus syndrome, or failure to propagate an impulse, as in AV node block. Tachycardias, on the other hand, arise from reentry, triggered activity, or abnormal automaticity. Reentry is the most common mechanism of tachyarrhythmia.[18]

REENTRY

For reentry to occur, there must be a circuit around which an electrical impulse can travel. For the most common reentrant arrhythmias, this involves two pathways with discrepant conduction velocities and refractory periods. In the case of atrioventricular reentrant tachycardia (AVRT), the AV node is usually the antegrade limb and an accessory pathway is the retrograde limb such that the electrical impulse travels down the AV node into the ventricle, then returns back through the accessory pathway to the atrium, then back down the AV node, and so on. For AV node reentrant tachycardia (AVNRT), typically, one of the limbs of the circuit displays a relatively slow conduction with a short refractory period (deemed the "slow pathway"), while the other limb must have fast conduction pathway with a long refractory period ("fast pathway"). In AVNRT, the antegrade limb is typically the slow pathway, and the retrograde limb is the fast pathway. Both AVRT and AVNRT usually have a rapid onset and offset. These types of arrhythmias are terminated when one or both limbs of the tachycardia are in their refractory period. For atrial flutter, the circuit involves a loop of current traveling around nonconducting tissue, most commonly the tricuspid valve.

TRIGGERED ACTIVITY

Triggered activity is dependent on depolarizations that occur during or after the preceding action potential that, if large enough, may reach the threshold potential, leading to additional action potentials. Triggered activity may result from depolarizations that occur during phase 2 or 3 (early after depolarizations) or after full repolarization (delayed after depolarizations). These triggered events give rise to extrasystoles.

ABNORMAL AUTOMATICITY

Abnormal automaticity occurs when a group of cells gains the ability to spontaneously depolarize during electrical diastole (phase 4 of the action potential) reaching membrane threshold, resulting in a generated impulse. The pacemaker cells of the heart demonstrate this phenomenon inherently.[18] Atrial ectopic tachycardia (AET), junctional ectopic tachycardia, and accelerated idioventricular rhythm (AIVR) are examples of arrhythmias resulting from abnormal automaticity.

ANTIARRHYTHMIC MEDICATIONS

Antiarrhythmic pharmacotherapy is based on three major principles: (a) reducing conduction velocity, (b) reducing automaticity of pacemaker cells (including latent pacemaker cells), and (c) prolonging refractory periods. Antiarrhythmic medications typically have a narrow therapeutic index. This results in a significant overlap with their proarrhythmic effects. Drug–drug interactions must also be taken into consideration, such as when a medication effects drug metabolism. Due to these

TABLE 49.1 Antiarrhythmic Medication Induced Cellular Effect and ECG Changes

Medication	*Cellular Effect*	*Expected ECG Changes*
Class IA Antiarrhythmics (Sodium Channel Blockers)		
Quinidine	↑ERP/APD, ↓conduction	Prolongation of the QRS and QT intervals
Procainamide		
Class IB Antiarrhythmics (Sodium Channel Blockers)		
Lidocaine	↑ERP/APD	Possible shortening of the QT interval
Class IC Antiarrhythmics (Sodium Channel Blockers)		
Flecainide	↓Conduction, ↑APD	Prolongation of the QRS and PR intervals Possible shortening of the QT interval
Propafenone		
Class II Antiarrhythmics (β-Blockers)		
Propranolol	β-Adrenergic blockade	Decrease in heart rate Possible shortening of the QT interval Possible prolongation of the PR interval
Metoprolol		
Atenolol		
Esmolol		
Class III Antiarrhythmics (Potassium Channel Blockers)		
Sotalol	↑APD	Decrease in heart rate Prolongation of the QRS, QT, and PR intervals
Amiodarone		
Class IV Antiarrhythmics (Calcium Channel Blockers)		
Verapamil	Calcium channel blockade	Decrease in heart rate Increase in PR interval
Miscellaneous		
Digoxin	Vagolytic	Decrease in heart rate Increase in PR interval

APD, action potential duration; ECG, electrocardiogram; ERP, effective refractory period.
Data from Moffett BS, Salvin JW, Kim JJ. Pediatric cardiac intensive care society 2014 consensus statement: pharmacotherapies in cardiac critical care antiarrhythmics. *Pediatr Crit Care Med* 2016;17:S49–S58.

interactions, previously therapeutic doses may become toxic. Organ function and electrolytes must also be monitored and taken into consideration when administering antiarrhythmic medications.

The modified Vaughan-Williams classification system of antiarrhythmic medications is the most commonly used classification system. This system separates antiarrhythmic medications into (a) cardiac sodium channel blockers, (b) β-adrenergic receptor blockers, (c) repolarization-prolonging medications, and (d) calcium channel blockers. Antiarrhythmic medications are selected based on the patient's medical condition and arrhythmia. Table 49.1 summarizes antiarrhythmic-induced cellular effects and ECG changes. The most appropriate medication will ideally carry the lowest adverse event profile. Table 49.2 summarizes antiarrhythmic drug dosing in children. If the arrhythmia is not well controlled with the selected agent, then a different or additional agent may be warranted. *At present time, there are no definitive studies addressing medical management in premature infants.* However, the underlying arrhythmia mechanisms are the same, and, hence, the same medical therapies are utilized for this vulnerable patient population, although caution in treating premature infants should be taken due to potential hemodynamic compromise, drug–drug interactions, and impaired drug metabolism and excretion due to the immature hepatic and renal systems.

MODIFIED VAUGHAN-WILLIAMS CLASSIFICATION SYSTEM OF ANTIARRHYTHMIC MEDICATIONS

Class I: Sodium Channel Blockers

These drugs affect phase 0 of the cardiac myocyte action potential, resulting in prolongation of depolarization, also described as slowing conduction, resulting in a widening of the QRS complex on ECG. This class slows conduction in atrial, ventricular, and accessory pathway tissue. These drugs may be more effective in terminating or suppressing primary atrial tachycardias and may be effective for reciprocating tachycardias. There are three subclasses of class I antiarrhythmic medications: IA, IB, and IC.

IA: Quinidine, Procainamide, and Disopyramide

These medications have sodium channel–blocking properties, as well as a moderate amount of potassium channel–blocking activity. The potassium channel–blocking activity will result in prolonged repolarization (increase refractoriness), which may prolong the QTc on surface ECG. These drugs are contraindicated in congenital or acquired long QT syndromes. Class IA medications have use-dependent pharmacokinetics, meaning that at fast heart rates, there are more sodium channels open or activated, to which these medications have a higher affinity. This class is frequently used for conversion of atrial flutter/fibrillation

TABLE 49.2 Antiarrhythmic Drug Dosing in Children

Drug	Loading Dose/Initial Dose	Maintenance Dose	Frequency	Therapeutic Serum Concentration
Intravenous Administration				
Adenosine *(rapid flush is required immediately after administration)*	0.1 mg/kg (max. 6 mg) Dose can be progressively increased up to 0.3 mg/kg (max. 12 mg)			
Digoxin	20–50 μg/kg TDD (over 16–24 h)	5–10 μg/kg/d	q12h	0.7–2 μg/L
Esmolol	100–500 μg/kg per dose over 1–2 min	300–1,000 μg/kg/min	Continuous infusion	
Procainamide	3–6 mg/kg/dose (max. 100 mg per dose) OR 15 mg/kg Do not exceed 500 mg in 30 min	20–80 μg/kg/min OR 50–100 mg/kg/d	Continuous infusion OR q4h	Procainamide 4–8 mg/L Procainamide + NAPA 15-30 mg/L
Lidocaine	1 mg/kg	20–50 μg/kg/min	Continuous infusion	1.5–5 mg/L
Propranolol	0.1 mg/kg (over 5 min)	Repeat q2h PRN	q4h	50–100 μg/L
Verapamil	0.1–0.15 mg/kg	Repeat q15 min PRN		50–200 μg/L
Amiodarone	5 mg/kg per dose over 30–60 min, may repeat 1–2×	10–20 mg/kg/d Or 5–15 μg/kg/min	Continuous infusion	
Oral Administration				
Digoxin	30–50 μg/kg/TDD (over 16–24 h)	6–10 μg/kg/d	b.i.d., q.d.	Same as i.v. formulation
Quinidine	3–5 mg/kg/ q3h × 3 doses	15–60 mg/kg/d	q.i.d., t.i.d. (XR)	2–5 mg/L
Procainamide		50–125 mg/kg/d	q.i.d.	Same as i.v. formulation
Disopyramide		10–20 mg/kg/d	q.i.d., b.i.d. (XR)	2–5 mg/L
Mexiletine		2.5–5.0 mg/kg/q8h	t.i.d., b.i.d.	0.75–2.0 mg/L
Flecainide		2.0–4.0 mg/kg/d	b.i.d.	200–1,000 μg/L
Propafenone		150–600 mg/m²/d	t.i.d.	
Propranolol		2.0–6.0 mg/kg/d	q.i.d., q.d. (XR)	Same as i.v. formulation
Atenolol		0.7–1.4 mg/kg/d	b.i.d., q.i.d.	
Metoprolol		10–60 mg/kg/d	b.i.d., q.d.	
Verapamil		2–8 mg/kg/d	t.i.d.	
Amiodarone	10–15 mg/kg/d	5.0–10 mg/kg/d	q.d.	1.5–2.5 μg/L
Sotalol Children <2 years of age		30 mg/m²/dose OR 2 mg/kg/d OR 80–200 mg/m²/d	t.i.d.	0.5–2.0 g/L
Verapamil		4.0–8.0 mg/kg/d	t.i.d., q.d. (XR)	50–200 μg/L

AV, atrioventricular block; b.i.d., every 12 hours; i.v., intravenous; NAPA, *N*-acetyl procainamide; q.d., daily; q.i.d., every 6 hours; qxh or min = every × hours or minutes; t.i.d., every 8 hours; TDD, total digitalizing dose; XR, extended-release formulation.

and maintenance of sinus rhythm. Care should be taken when utilizing this class as they can suppress myocardial contractility, which can result in exacerbation of congestive heart failure.

Procainamide is indicated for the treatment of SVTs, such as atrial, reentrant, junctional, or ventricular tachycardias (VT), in the intensive care setting. Intravenous loading dose of procainamide can be achieved within 15 minutes, allowing for effective plasma concentrations of 4 to 8 μg/mL. Procainamide's half-life is approximately 1.7 hours in children.[19] The active metabolite, *N*-acetyl procainamide (NAPA), is produced by the liver and contributes to the antiarrhythmic action. Atrial conduction during atrial flutter may be slowed with the use of procainamide, which can lead to inadvertent fast AV node conduction converting a hemodynamically stable 2:1 conducting atrial flutter into a hemodynamically unstable 1:1 conducting atrial flutter. Caution should be taken in patients with hepatic or renal dysfunction.[20] Procainamide may cause lupus-like syndrome when given long term, with incidence of 15% to 20%.[21]

IB: Lidocaine and Mexiletine

Class IB antiarrhythmics have a higher affinity for fast sodium channels and are, therefore, more effective with tachyarrhythmias as they also shorten phase 3 of the action potential. Due to fast sodium channel blockade, lidocaine and mexiletine are used for ventricular arrhythmias with little effect on atrial tissue, SA and AV nodes.

Lidocaine has rapid onset of action within 1 to 2 minutes after bolus administration. The plasma half-life is 1 to 2 hours, and it is eliminated primarily by the liver.[20] Lidocaine clearance is reduced in congestive heart failure and hepatic dysfunction. In addition, β-adrenergic blockers and cimetidine may increase serum lidocaine levels. Lidocaine has no significant cardiosuppressive effects. Mexiletine is an oral medication that is structurally similar to lidocaine and is used for ventricular arrhythmias.[22] Unlike lidocaine with almost immediate onset of action, the onset of action for mexiletine ranges from 30 minutes to 2 hours, with plasma half-life of 10 to 12 hours. Central nervous system suppression is an adverse effect seen with the use of lidocaine and mexiletine.

IC: Flecainide and Propafenone

Class IC antiarrhythmics work on decreasing the slope of phase 0 of the action potential by inhibiting the slow sodium channels. They also inhibit the potassium repolarization current, resulting in QRS widening, slowing conduction through the His-Purkinje system and ventricular myocardium. Flecainide and propafenone have been indicated for atrial arrhythmias, primarily those with reentrant mechanisms, and junctional and ventricular arrhythmias.

Flecainide has been shown to be highly effective in isolation or in combination with amiodarone in the treatment of refractory pediatric SVT.[23] Careful screening and monitoring of patients treated with flecainide should be performed. The CAST study, which was performed in adults with ischemic heart disease, demonstrated that caution should be taken when administering flecainide to patients with acquired heart disease as it worsened survival.[24] Proarrhythmic events with flecainide use in pediatrics has been reported at 7.9%, with 1.9% experiencing cardiac arrest and death.[25] Recent studies have demonstrated an improved safety profile in pediatric patients and those with congenital heart disease.[23]

Flecainide is well absorbed and has a bioavailability of 90% to 95%. Milk and milk-based formulas may inhibit oral absorption. Typical onset of action is 1 to 2 hours, with serum half-life in newborns of 29 hours, infants 11 to 12 hours, and children 8 hours.[26] Flecainide is metabolized in the liver and eliminated in the urine; however, it is not dialyzable.

Propafenone is also sodium channel blocker in addition to having mild β-adrenergic, potassium, and L-type calcium channel–blocking properties.[27] Its properties allow it to be used for the treatment of supraventricular arrhythmias in addition to some ventricular arrhythmias. Like flecainide, propafenone can have proarrhythmic effects. Propafenone is well absorbed with peak concentration achieved in 2 to 3 hours and has a serum half-life of 2 to 8 hours. Metabolism occurs in the liver and can be affected by both “fast” and “slow” metabolizers.[20,27]

Class II: β-Blockers

β-Blockers are generally effective in tachyarrhythmias (SVT or VT) associated with an increased sympathetic β-adrenergic tone.[18] β-Blockers depress the activity of the SA node, AV node, and ectopic foci, while increasing the AV nodes effective refractory period. Their impact on anterograde and retrograde AV nodal conduction provides clinical utility in slowing the ventricular response during rapid atrial arrhythmias and terminating reentry supraventricular arrhythmias. Limited agents are available for intravenous treatment of tachyarrhythmias. In hemodynamically unstable patients, β-blockers should be used cautiously because of hypotension and potential sinus bradycardia. In pediatrics, the most commonly used β-blockers are propranolol, esmolol, and atenolol.

Propranolol is a noncardioselective β-blocker that does not possess intrinsic sympathomimetic activity.[28] Propranolol may be administered as either an intravenous or oral medication. When administered orally, it undergoes substantial first-pass metabolism by the liver and reaches peak serum concentrations about 6 hours following administration.[28] Through competitive inhibition of the β-adrenergic receptor, propranolol decreases conduction velocity through the SA and AV nodes and myocardial automaticity. This results in rate control, which can be used in the treatment of cardiac arrhythmias, allowing for an increase in systemic ejection time and an increase in cardiac volume. Propranolol also competitively inhibits β-adrenergic receptors within vascular smooth muscle, leading to its use in the treatment of hypertension. Propranolol is almost completely metabolized by the liver. Reported half-life elimination varies considerably among studies; however when dosed therapeutically, the half-life tends to range from 3.4 to 6 hours.[28] Adverse effects that may be seen with propranolol, as with other β-blockers, are bradycardia, hypotension, and hypoglycemia.

Esmolol is a cardioselective β-blocker that is administered intravenously for the treatment of arrhythmias and severe hypertension.[29] Esmolol has a rapid time of onset and a short duration of action. Esmolol's half-life is less than 10 minutes.[30] Like propranolol, esmolol is metabolized by the liver, and the metabolites are rapidly excreted by the kidneys. Adverse effects of esmolol include bradycardia, hypotension, fatigue, dizziness, depression, agitation, and confusion.

Atenolol is a cardioselective β-blocker that is administered either orally or intravenously for the treatment of arrhythmias and hypertension.[31] Its peak absorption after administration is seen at between 2 and 4 hours when administered orally. Unlike propranolol and esmolol, atenolol undergoes little or no metabolism by the liver and is renally excreted. The elimination half-life of atenolol is 6 to 7 hours.[32] Atenolol does not cross the blood–brain barrier. Adverse effects of atenolol include bradycardia, hypotension, fatigue, dizziness, depression, memory loss, and impotence. Atenolol has been associated with mild-to-moderate elevations of serum aminotransferase levels in 1% to 2% of patients.[31]

Class III: Potassium Channel Blockers

This class of medications blocks potassium channels and lengthens action potential durations and refractory periods. This results in QT interval prolongation on surface ECG. Class III medications can be used for a wide range of atrial and ventricular arrhythmias, typically used as second-line agents for those that are not responsive to conventional therapy. Typically, they require ECG monitoring due to potential proarrhythmic effects.

In addition to blocking potassium channels, amiodarone and sotalol are considered "mixed" because of their additional effects. Amiodarone has class I sodium channel–blocking effects at higher heart rates, class II inhibition of β-adrenergic receptors, and mild class IV calcium channel blocker effects. Amiodarone is an effective agent for the treatment of supraventricular and ventricular tachyarrhythmias in children.[33] Amiodarone may be administered either intravenously or orally; however, the oral preparation is slow to achieve a therapeutic response and is of limited usefulness for acute, life-threatening arrhythmias.[33] Studies have demonstrated that under these conditions, intravenous amiodarone may be administered safely in children and has been shown to be an effective antiarrhythmic agent.[33,34] Unfortunately, amiodarone does have numerous extracardiac side effects and toxicities. Amiodarone affects multiple organ systems, including the lungs, thyroid, liver and gastrointestinal tract, eyes, skin, and the neurologic system. Sinus bradycardia is a well-recognized adverse effect of amiodarone. Patients receiving intravenous amiodarone should have arterial pressure monitored and have back-up pacing available.[33,34] For this reason, it is also important to obtain baseline studies examining liver, kidney, and thyroid function prior to initiating therapy. Much of these side effects are related to the cumulative dose and can be reversible with drug discontinuation.[18] The elimination half-life of amiodarone is approximately 58 days, and this is felt to be secondary to being lipophilic with slow release from lipid-rich tissue.[35]

Sotalol may be administered intravenously or orally. Intravenous sotalol has demonstrated to be an effective agent for the treatment of active arrhythmias, including SVT and VT, in the pediatric population, with a median time to conversion being 33 minutes as demonstrated by Valdés et al.[36] Sotalol has both class II and class III antiarrhythmic effects. Sotalol has reverse-use dependence, where its effects are more pronounced at lower heart rates, resulting in increased risk of Torsades de pointes (TdP) with sinus bradycardia. Close rhythm, heart rate, and blood pressure monitoring should be performed with initiation of sotalol therapy. Furthermore, a baseline ECG should be obtained prior initiating therapy and with serial ECG monitoring thereafter closely monitoring for QTc prolongation. Renal function must also be monitored closely, since this is a renally excreted medication and can lead to fatal proarrhythmias if use is continued in patients with acute renal failure.[18] Other adverse effects may also include bradycardia and hypotension, given the β-blocker properties. Sotalol is eliminated primarily through the kidneys and has a half-life of 10 to 20 hours.[37]

Class IV: Calcium Channel Blockers

The calcium channel blockers are nondihydropyridine calcium channel blockers, and their antiarrhythmic properties are achieved through increasing the refractory period of the AV node. They are used to control the ventricular rate during atrial flutter and atrial fibrillation and for termination and prevention of SVTs dependent on the AV node. Due to negative inotropic effects, they are typically not administered in congestive heart failure patients, or in children younger than 1 year of age. They are also contraindicated in patients with ventricular preexcitation as they can accelerate anterograde conduction over the accessory pathway.

Verapamil slows AV node conduction and prolongs the effective refractory period within the AV node in a rate-related manner, via inhibition of the calcium influx through slow calcium channels. This results in a reduced ventricular rate, which can help with treatment of atrial flutter or atrial fibrillation. Verapamil undergoes extensive metabolism in the liver. Following intravenous infusion, verapamil has a half-life of about 2 to 5 hours.[38] Adverse effects of verapamil include bradycardia and hypotension. Concomitant use with other agents with similar adverse effect profile requires careful monitoring. Diltiazem has a similar drug profile, with a half-life of 3 to 4.5 hours.[39]

Miscellaneous

Digoxin does not fall within the modified Vaughan–Williams classification system. Digoxin works by blocking the sodium-potassium ATPase, which results in increased intracellular calcium and, ultimately, an increase in inotropy. It also enhances vagal tone, which results in inhibition of the SA and AV nodes. Digoxin has a narrow therapeutic index, which results in common manifestations of nausea, vomiting, diarrhea, and changes in color vision at supratherapeutic levels. At toxic levels, it can result in paroxysmal atrial tachycardia, AV block, or bidirectional VT. Digoxin is considered safe in pregnancy. Digoxin and other AV nodal–blocking antiarrhythmic medications such as calcium channel blockers may cause increase impulse propagation from the atria to the ventricle via the accessory pathway in patients with Wolff–Parkinson–White (WPW) syndrome, resulting in an accelerated ventricular response for patients in atrial fibrillation.[40] Instead, other medications, such as β-blockers and procainamide, can be used in WPW syndrome without the associated risk of enhanced antegrade conduction down the accessory pathway.[40]

Adenosine also does not fall within the modified Vaughan–Williams classification system. Adenosine opens adenosine-sensitive inward rectifier potassium channels, resulting in hyperpolarization and inhibition of the sinus and AV node. Its transient effect on the AV node makes it an ideal choice for treatment of reentry, nodal-dependent SVT, including that associated with WPW syndrome. However, it is absolutely contraindicated in patients with WPW syndrome who are in atrial fibrillation (preexcited atrial fibrillation) because it can potentially lead to more rapid conduction of atrial fibrillation to the ventricles via the accessory pathway by selectively inhibiting the AV node, resulting in ventricular fibrillation. Adenosine can be given safely to pregnant patients. Half-life of adenosine is less than 10 seconds since it is metabolized by red blood cells. For this reason, it is best to administer adenosine through an intravenous line that infuses rapidly, followed by a rapid saline flush. Adverse events are infrequent but can include severe bradycardia, asystole, atrial fibrillation, AV blocks, ventricular arrhythmias, and bronchospasm. A resuscitation cart should be readily available during administration in the event that an adverse event does occur.

TRANSPLACENTAL TREATMENT OF TACHYARRHYTHMIAS

Pharmacologic transplacental treatment of tachyarrhythmias was initially documented in the 1970s.[6] Recently, the American Heart Association (AHA) published a systemic review and meta-analysis that compared the efficacy, safety, and

TABLE 49.3 Medication Dose and Administration for Transplacental Management of Tachyarrhythmias

	Digoxin	*Flecainide*	*Procainamide*	*Sotalol*	*Amiodarone*
Dose	Oral load: 0.25–2 mg over 24–48 h	Oral: 100 mg b.i.d.	Oral load: 1 g	Oral: 80–160 mg b.i.d.	Load (oral or i.v.): 1,600–2,400 mg/d divided 2–4 times daily × 2–7 d.
	Oral maintenance: 0.375–1 mg/d	Maintenance: Increase up to 450 mg/d if there is no response	Oral maintenance: 200–500 mg every 3–6 h	Maintenance: can be increased up to 640 mg/d	Maintenance: 200–400 mg/d b.i.d.
	i.v. load: 1–2 mg i.v. maintenance: 0.5 mg daily		i.v. load: 100 mg over 2 min, then 1–6 mg/min		
	Targeted maternal drug levels of 1–2.5 ng/mL (upper therapeutic range)	Targeted maternal drug levels of 0.2–1 mu/mL	Targeted maternal drug levels of 4–10 mg/L		
Adverse events	Bradycardia, heart block, maternal nausea/vomiting, visual disturbances	Dizziness, headache, paresthesia, nausea, vomiting	Hypotension, nausea, blood dyscrasias, prolonged QT, lupus-like syndrome	Bradycardia, hypotension, hypoglycemia, prolonged QT, Torsade de Pointes	Bradycardia, hypotension, prolonged QT, Torsade de Pointes, hepatotoxicity, thyroid dysfunction, skin color alteration, corneal deposits, pulmonary fibrosis

b.i.d., every 12 hours; i.v., intravenous; t.i.d., every 8 hours.

fetal–maternal tolerance of first-line monotherapies for fetal SVT and atrial flutter, the two most common fetal tachyarrhythmias, with outcomes of interest being termination of the tachyarrhythmia, fetal demise, and maternal complications.[6] The four most commonly used medications that were compared were digoxin, flecainide, sotalol, and amiodarone.

Flecainide was found to be superior to digoxin and sotalol in cases of fetal SVT, specifically with cases of hydropic fetal SVT.[6] When hydrops is present, the bioavailability of digoxin decreases, leading to lower blood concentrations when compared to a nonhydropic fetus. Flecainide has an excellent bioavailability in hydropic fetuses and is thus a better agent to use than digoxin in this patient population.

For atrial flutter, there was no significant difference observed in termination between digoxin or sotalol, demonstrating both as good first-line therapies for atrial flutter. Duration of treatment required for conversion to sinus rhythm was longer with atrial flutter when compared to SVT. Unfortunately, there are cases of resistant fetal tachyarrhythmias that result in fetal demise despite multidrug therapy. Table 49.3 demonstrates antiarrhythmic drug dosing for transplacental management of tachyarrhythmias.

ANALYZING AND MANAGING RHYTHM ABNORMALITIES

An abnormal rhythm can be categorized into three broad categories: irregular, bradycardic, or tachycardic. Appropriate analysis and diagnosis of an abnormal rhythm is crucial in determining management and prognosis. Table 49.4 summarizes the characteristic ECG changes seen with abnormal perinatal rhythms.

IRREGULAR RHYTHMS

A premature beat is the most common type of arrhythmia witnessed during the perinatal period.[4] They can originate from the atria, the AV junction, or the ventricle, completely bypassing the SA node (Fig. 49.4).

Extrasystoles

Premature atrial complexes (PACs) account for about 90% of irregular rhythms found in fetuses and infants.[4,41] A PAC originates from an ectopic atrial focus that is capable of spontaneous depolarization (inherent or acquired automaticity), resulting in an ectopic or premature atrial contraction. A PAC that reaches the SA node may depolarize it, causing the SA node to "reset." If this happens, this results in a longer than normal interval prior to the next sinus beat known as the "postextrasystolic pause." If a PAC arrives early enough in the conduction cycle, it can result in AV conduction with aberrancy, usually with a right bundle branch morphology, since the right bundle branch has a longer refractory period than the left.[16] A PAC may be blocked secondary to AV nodal or infra-Hisian block, with the sinus node still resetting, resulting in a compensatory pause.

If the premature beat originates from the ventricle, it is known as a premature ventricular contraction (PVC). PVCs represent less than 2% of fetal premature beats. After birth, the incidence is highest in the neonatal period and then decreases rapidly thereafter, with an incidence of 18% and 6%, respectively.[41] PVCs can be unifocal or multifocal depending on the number of foci. Typically, the QRS complexes are broadened with an abnormal morphology and are followed by a full compensatory pause—the next atrial beat will arrive at an interval

TABLE 49.4 Electrocardiographic Presentation of Abnormal Rhythms

Atrioventricular Block	
First-degree AV block	Prolonged PR interval for age. Each atrial beat is conducted.
Second-degree AV block, Mobitz type I (Wenckebach)	Progressive increase in PR interval ending in a nonconducted atrial beat. Shortened PR interval of the first conducted atrial beat after the block.
Second-degree AV block, Mobitz type II	Sudden interruption of AV conduction. Fixed PR interval before and after the blocked atrial beat.
Third-degree AV block, complete heart block	Complete dissociation between atrial and ventricular contractions. Atrial rate must be faster than ventricular rate.
Supraventricular Tachycardias	
AV reentrant supraventricular tachycardia	Regular, narrow QRS complex tachycardia. Obligatory 1:1 AV conduction. P waves are obscured or buried in the ST segment.
AV nodal reentrant supraventricular tachycardia	Regular, narrow QRS complex tachycardia. Primarily 1:1 AV conduction but can have 2:1 AV conduction. P waves are obscured by the terminal QRS complex.
Atrial flutter	Rapid, saw-tooth flutter waves, with fixed or variable R-R intervals.
Permanent junctional reciprocating tachycardia	Narrow QRS complex tachycardia with VA association. Long RP interval. Typically inverted P waves in inferior leads.
Junctional tachycardia	Narrow QRS complex tachycardia with either AV association or AV dissociation.
Atrial ectopic tachycardia	Abnormal P-wave morphology with an inappropriately fast rate. Isoelectric baseline between atrial waves.
Ventricular Tachycardias	
Ventricular tachycardia	Three or more consecutive wide QRS complex beats of ventricular origin occurring at a faster rate than the underlying rhythm. VA dissociation is hallmark.

AV, atrioventricular; VA, ventriculoatrial.

that is equal or double the preceding R-R interval. Retrograde conduction to the atria may or may not occur following a PVC.

Both PACs and PVCs are mostly benign and remain self-limited, with spontaneous resolution seen in 95% of children by 1 year of age.[4] Before birth, PACs have been associated with less than 1% risk of fetal tachycardia and carry a slightly higher risk if atrial bigeminy or couplets are observed.[42,43] If there is a reassuring history and physical examination with no underlying congenital cardiac disease or serious myocardial disease, then no further investigation or monitoring is necessary. If an infant is clinically unwell and has extrasystoles, then other etiologies should be ruled out. It is important to evaluate for and treat any electrolyte and metabolic abnormalities, focusing on hypokalemia, hyperkalemia, hypercalcemia, hypoglycemia, hypomagnesemia, and

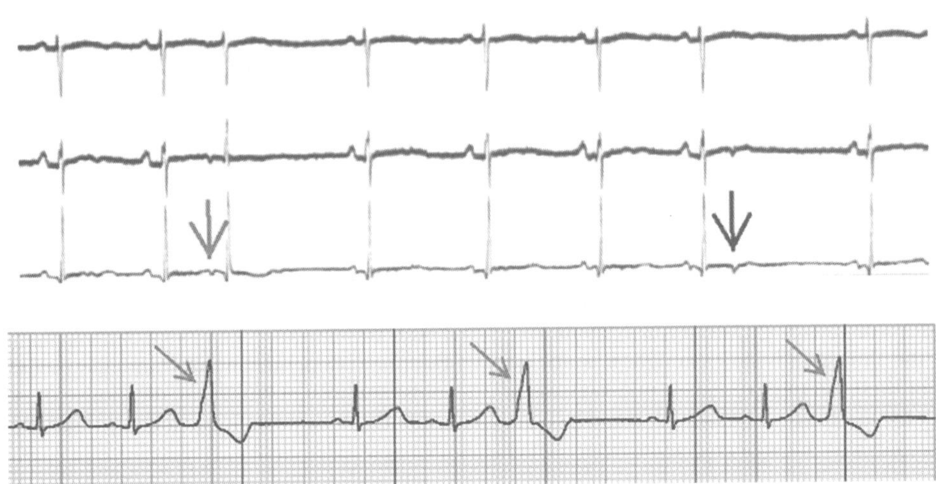

Figure 49.4 Extrasystoles. PACs (**A**) and PVCs (**B**). In **A**, there is a PAC (*left arrow*) within the T wave that is conducted, resulting in a QRS. There is an additional PAC that occurs in the T wave within the refractory period of the AV node, resulting in a nonconducted PAC (*right arrow*). Following both PACs, there is a compensatory pause noted. In **B**, PVCs are indicated by wide and premature QRS complexes without a preceding P wave (*arrows*). These PVCs are occurring in a trigeminal pattern with a noncompensatory pause as there was retrograde reset of the SA node. PACs, premature atrial complexes; PVCs, premature ventricular contractions; SA, sinoatrial.

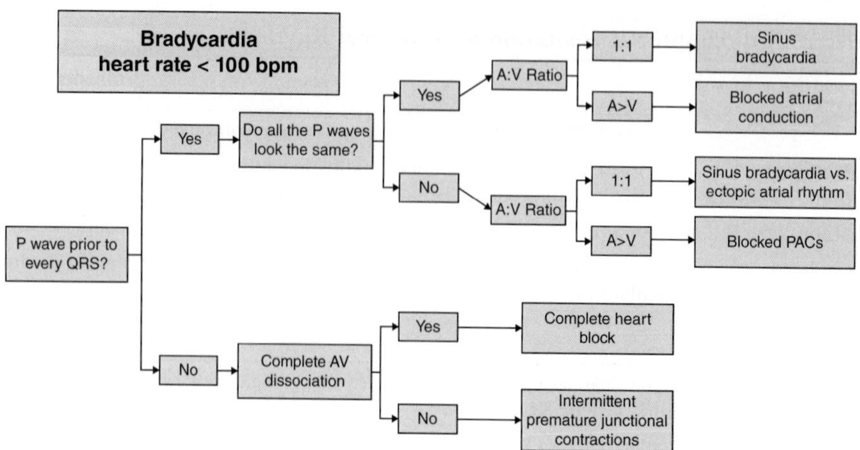

Figure 49.5 Bradycardia diagnosis flowsheet. A, atrial activity; AV, atrioventricular; PACs, premature atrial complexes; V, ventricular activity.

hypoxia. In the absence of these abnormalities, evaluation for atrial or ventricular distention, cardiac dysfunction, presence of a central venous line within the heart, underlying infection or inflammation, and iatrogenic causes should be carried out.

BRADYCARDIA

Normative values for heart rate in children are age dependent. In newborns, bradycardia is defined as a resting heart rate less than 95 bpm. Bradycardia can be a benign physiologic response secondary to increase parasympathetic or vagal tone. Bradycardia can also be abnormal, specifically if it is prolonged or persistent and compromising the cardiovascular state. Fetal bradycardia is considered as a heart rate less than 110 bpm. Bradycardia represents less than 5% of arrhythmias in fetuses and infants.[8] The main mechanisms of perinatal bradycardia include sinus bradycardia, complete heart block (CHB), and functional heart block/blocked premature atrial complexes (described previously in the PAC section). Figure 49.5 can be used as an algorithm to aid in analysis of bradycardic rhythms.

Sinus Bradycardia

Sinus bradycardia is the most common cause of low heart rate. It's typically transient and secondary to vagal stimulation (i.e., deep sleep, vomiting, or defecation in infants). Persistent sinus bradycardia is usually secondary to cardiac failure and hydrops in the fetus but may also be secondary to either maternal hypothermia or long QT syndrome.

Mechanism

The rhythm appropriately originates from the SA node, but it is slower than expected for the patient's age. Typically, at normal heart rates, the SA node will physiologically suppress latent pacemakers. However, if the sinus rate is slow enough, it is not uncommon to see one of these latent pacemakers take over as the dominant pacemaker for the heart. An example would be a low atrial rhythm originating from another group of cardiac cells in the atria that are capable of spontaneous depolarization. Other latent pacemaker cells include other cardiac cells with automaticity in and around the AV node and the His-Purkinje system.

Electrocardiogram Criteria

The heart rate is slower than expected for age with a P wave prior to every QRS complex. The P waves and the QRS complexes are of single morphology (Fig. 49.6).

Treatment

For all bradycardias, management depends on etiology and severity. Correction of electrolyte disturbance, hypoglycemia, hypothermia, and hypothyroidism can result in improved heart rates. If there is hemodynamic instability, acute pharmacologic management includes atropine or epinephrine boluses with isoproterenol or epinephrine infusion or temporary pacing as secondary therapies, while the underlying cause is corrected. Permanent pacing can be utilized as long-term therapy in refractory cases, such as sinus node dysfunction.

Fetal Considerations

Sinus bradycardia in the fetus is typically well tolerated. However, further investigation is often warranted since it may be secondary to fetal distress, sinus node dysfunction, congenital anomalies, long QT syndrome, or antibody mediated (anti-Ro antibodies).[8]

Fetal Echo Criteria

Normal mechanical atrial and ventricular systolic events are observed by echocardiogram at a slower rate than expected for the patient's age.

Fetal Treatment

Treatment depends on cause and may include no treatment, steroids/anti-inflammatory medications for myocarditis (anti-Ro antibodies), or premature delivery (fetal distress).

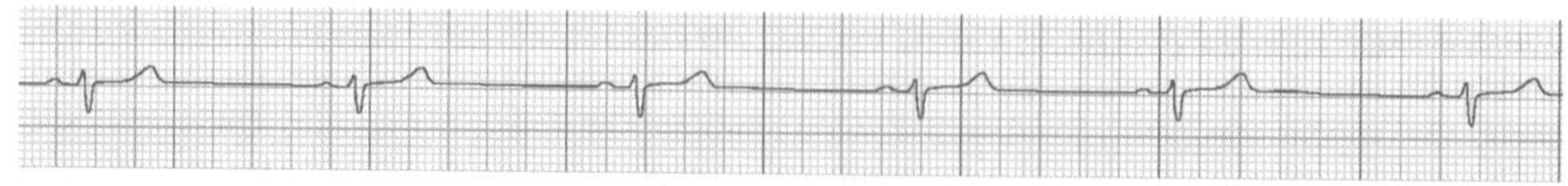

Figure 49.6 Sinus bradycardia at 43 bpm with a normal PR interval.

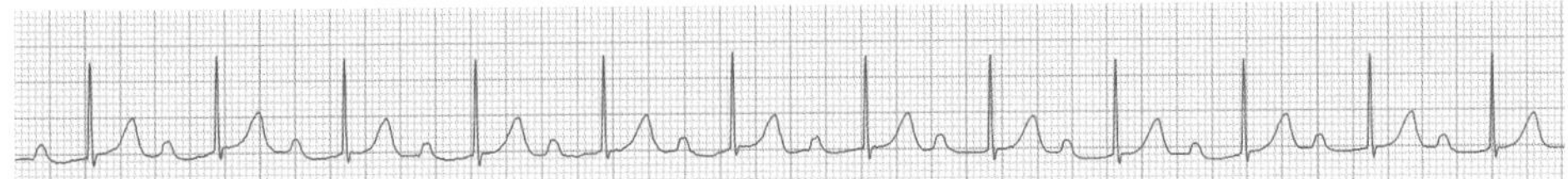

Figure 49.7 First-degree atrioventricular block. Sinus rhythm with a prolonged PR interval of 300 milliseconds is depicted.

First-Degree Atrioventricular Block

With first-degree AV block, there is successful conduction of each atrial beat but with delay to the ventricular myocardium. Diagnosis is made based on the measurement of a prolonged AV interval or PR interval for age on Doppler recording or ECG, respectively (Fig. 49.7). First-degree AV block is a benign condition and is well tolerated. It does not require any treatment.

Second-Degree Atrioventricular Block

The diagnosis is similar for all forms of AV block. This is accomplished by identifying the atrial and ventricular beats, measuring the PR interval, and noting the nonconducted atrial beats. There are two types of second-degree AV block, Mobitz type I and Mobitz type II (Fig. 49.8).

In Mobitz type I (Wenckebach), there is a sequential increase in AV conduction delay ending in a nonconducted atrial beat (Fig. 49.8A). It is usually a physiologic condition, frequently observed when vagal tone is more prominent, especially during sleep. Progression to higher degrees of AV block is possible, especially if it is related to maternal autoantibody exposition. An underlying cardiac condition is also possible and needs to be excluded during the prenatal ultrasound and after birth by the history and physical examination. A 24-hour ambulatory Holter is reasonable after birth to observe if the condition is only transient and related to periods of high vagal tone. If so, no further follow-up is necessary.

In Mobitz type II, there is no progressive lengthening of the AV conduction, but rather a sudden interruption of AV conduction (Fig. 49.8B). This is rare but more serious than type I, often related to either inflammation (maternal antibodies, myocarditis) or traumatic injury. There is a high risk of progression to complete AV block.

Complete Heart Block

CHB is the complete dissociation between atrial and ventricular contractions. Both the atria and the ventricles generate their own spontaneous contractions that are independent of each other, with the atrial rate being greater than the ventricular rate. If the ventricular rate is greater than the atrial rate, then this might be an accelerated junctional rhythm and does not necessarily imply CHB.

Mechanism

Prenatal CHB will be secondary to either congenital heart disease (seen with left isomerism, AV septal defects, corrected transposition of the great arteries) or maternal autoantibodies associated with autoimmune diseases, such as systemic lupus erythematosus.[7,8,12]

Postnatally, the majority of acquired CHB is following surgical repair for congenital heart disease or carditis (i.e., viral myocarditis). Idiopathic causes might be encountered as well.

Electrocardiogram Criteria

The atrial and ventricular impulses are occurring independent of each other. There is no propagation of impulse from either the atrial to the ventricle or ventricle to the atria (Fig. 49.9).

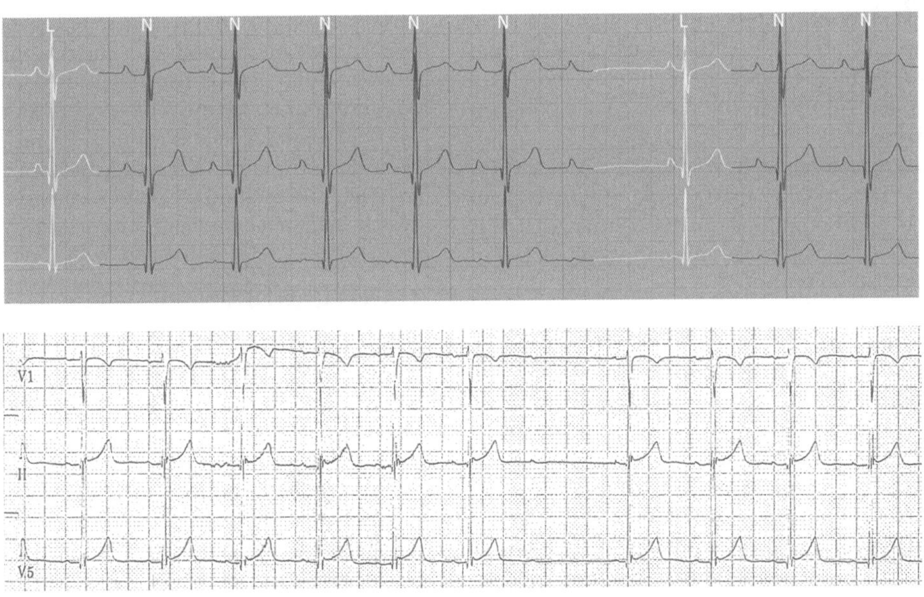

Figure 49.8 Second-degree atrioventricular block, Mobitz type I (**A**) and type II (**B**). **A:** There is progressive PR prolongation with eventual dropped QRS complex followed by a conducted sinus beat with a normal PR interval. **B:** There is a fixed PR interval until there is a P wave without a QRS complex. The subsequent beats once again have a fixed PR interval.

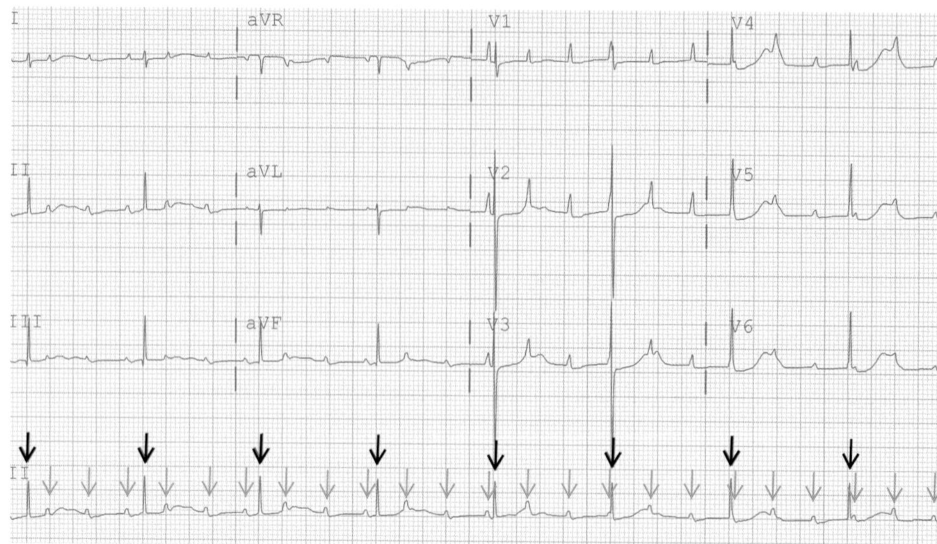

Figure 49.9 Complete heart block. There is complete atrioventricular dissociation as the sinus (atrial) rate is 165 bpm (*blue arrows*) with a ventricular rate of 60 bpm (*black arrows*). The narrow QRS complexes indicate a junctional escape origin. aVF, augmented vector foot; aVL, augmented vector left; aVR, augmented vector right.

Treatment

In comparison to fetal management, postnatal management is more clearly established due to the possibility of ultimately placing a pacemaker. Nonsurgical advanced second- or third-degree heart block might be followed conservatively if there is an appropriate ventricular rate that is capable of maintaining adequate cardiac output.[4]

If the patient is hemodynamically unstable, transcutaneous pacing or pharmacologic intervention to increase the ventricular rate should be performed. Postnatal isoproterenol infusion can be used to maintain an adequate ventricular output until implantation of a permanent epicardial pacemaker system can be placed. Under current American College of Cardiology/AHA guidelines, a permanent pacemaker implantation has class I indications if the patient has (a) symptomatic bradycardia, ventricular dysfunction, or low cardiac output; (b) wide complex QRS escape rhythm; or (c) a ventricular rate less than 55 bpm in the absence of congenital heart disease and a ventricular rate of less than 70 bpm in the presence of significant congenital heart disease.[44]

CHB with coexisting congenital heart disease carries a worse prognosis, with only 20% to 40% survival beyond the neonatal period.[45] The 1-year survival rate for isolated perinatal CHB is between 80% and 90%. Dilated cardiomyopathy is observed in approximately 25% of the survivors.[4,46]

Fetal Considerations

CHB is the most common congenital conduction abnormality and accounts for approximately 40% of all major arrhythmias prior to birth.[8] Approximately half of all fetal cases of CHB are associated with major structural heart disease. Heterotaxy syndrome, with left atrial isomerism, carries a high risk of intrauterine demise and is a common cause of CHB in the fetus. In the absence of major structural heart disease, CHB can be seen with fetal transplacental passage of anti-Ro antibodies.[47] In approximately 1% to 5% of exposes fetuses, the maternal antibodies can lead to CHB, sinus bradycardia, myocarditis, endocardial fibroelastosis, and/or dilated cardiomyopathy.[8] If severe, it can lead to low cardiac output, fetal hydrops, and death. Perinatal death is associated with bradycardia-associated heart block at rates less than 50 to 55 bpm.

Fetal Echo Criteria

Echocardiogram will demonstrate a normal mechanical atrial systole rate. Ventricular systole will be much slower and independent of atrial systole. Typical ventricular rate is between 40 and 80 bpm.

Fetal Treatment

When delivery is not an option, therapeutic choices are limited. There is no intrauterine treatment available to treat CHB, and there is currently no consensus on prenatal therapy for treatment of isolated CHB. However, if the heart block is secondary to severe immune-mediated myocardial inflammation, β-adrenergic medications, dexamethasone, and intravenous immunoglobulin (IVIG) have been used to improve cardiac output and improve chances of survival. Since having a heart rate below 55 bpm correlates with a poor prognosis, therapies have been aimed toward increasing the ventricular rate. Therapies are currently used on a case-by-case basis and initiated typically by maternal–fetal medicine subspecialists.

TACHYCARDIA

Tachycardia is defined as a heart rate greater than the normal age-appropriate heart rate for at least three consecutive beats, above 180 bpm in the fetus between 20 and 40 weeks of gestation and above 200 bpm in infants. A sustained tachycardia has a significant risk of hemodynamic compromise, heart failure, morbidity, and mortality. Possible mechanisms in pediatrics include sinus tachycardia, SVT (reentrant and automatic), permanent junctional reciprocating tachycardia (PJRT), atrial fibrillation, and, rarely, VT. To aid in appropriate analysis of tachycardic rhythms, refer to Figure 49.10.

In fetuses, 70% of the tachyarrhythmias are paroxysmal AVRT, 24% are primary atrial tachycardias (mostly atrial

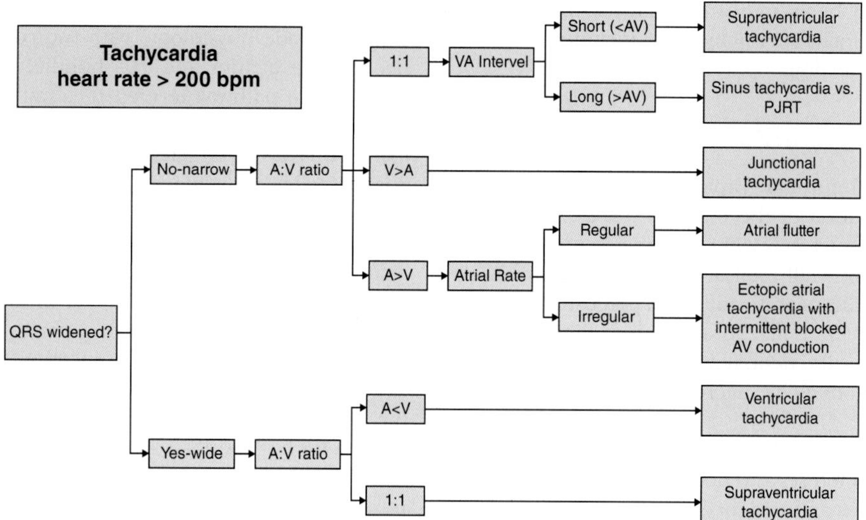

Figure 49.10 Tachycardia diagnosis flowsheet. A, atrial activity; AV, atrioventricular interval; PJRT, permanent junctional reciprocating tachycardia; V, ventricular activity; VA, ventriculoatrial interval.

flutter), and 6% are sinus tachycardia.[4] During infancy, 80% of nonsinus tachycardia are AVRT, 15% are primary atrial tachycardia (mostly atrial flutter), and 5% are AVNRT.[4,8]

Sinus Tachycardia

Sinus tachycardia is the most common cause of long RP tachycardia, and the heart rate usually gradually accelerates and slows down. Maternal fever, drug use, or hyperthyroidism and hypoxemia are the most frequent causes of sinus tachycardia in the fetus. During infancy, the same etiologies are encountered, but hypovolemia due to dehydration or shock is the leading cause.[48]

Mechanism

The rhythm appropriately originates from the SA node, but it is faster than expected for the patient's age (i.e., >200 bpm for the newborn and >180 bpm for the fetus).

Electrocardiogram Criteria

There is a P wave prior to every QRS complex with an appropriate AV conduction delay. The P waves and the QRS complexes are of single morphology (Fig. 49.11).

Treatment

Sinus tachycardia can be a normal physiologic response to exogenous catecholamines, anemia, thyrotoxicosis, fever, and infection. Treatment of underlying cause results in improved heart rate response. Inappropriate sinus tachycardia can occur, which can lead to ventricular dysfunction.

Fetal Considerations

Before birth, sinus tachycardia can be difficult to separate or distinguish from ectopic atrial tachycardia and PJRT. It is characterized by atrial rates of less than 200 bpm, normal AV conduction, and some variability of the fetal heart rate. If the rate is greater

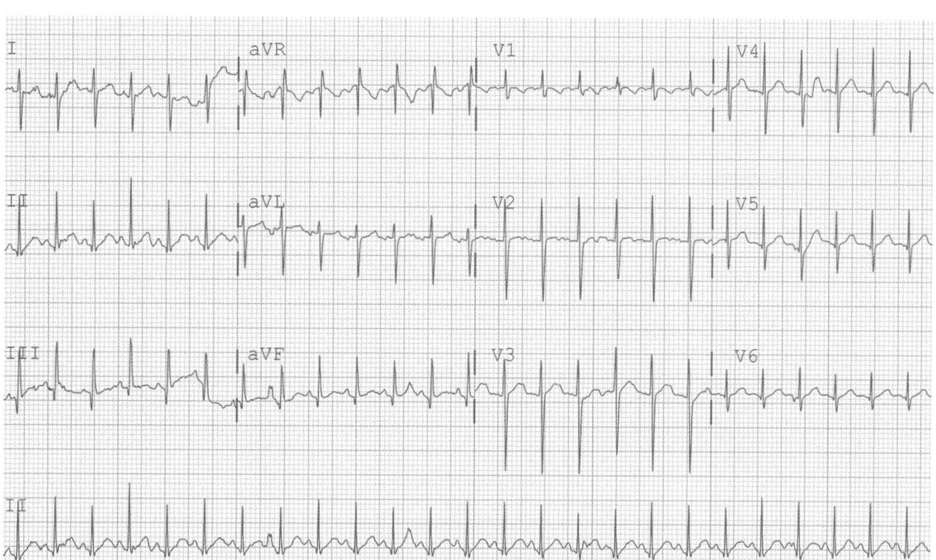

Figure 49.11 Sinus tachycardia at 190 bpm in a 3-month-old infant. aVF, augmented vector foot; aVL, augmented vector left; aVR, augmented vector right.

than 200 bpm, this may be an indication that the fetus is critically ill. Other cause of fetal sinus tachycardia includes maternal distress, anemia, and infection.

Supraventricular Tachycardia

SVT is defined as an abnormally rapid rhythm that originates proximal to the bifurcation of the bundle of His.[16] Fetal SVT has an incidence of about 1 in 3,700 pregnancies and accounts for roughly 5% to 10% of all fetal arrhythmias, but for more than 50% of the clinically significant ones.[4,49] Postnatally, the incidence ranges between 1 in 250 and 1 in 1,000 children, with a peak incidence in the neonatal period.[4] SVTs can utilize either a reentry or automaticity mechanism for initiation and propagation.

Accessory pathway-mediated tachycardia (AVRT) is the most common type of SVT in fetuses and neonates.[8] AVRT associated with WPW syndrome has an incidence of 0.1% to 0.5% among the general population and has a known association with congenital heart disease, ranging from 9% to 32%.[16] Structural cardiac diseases known to be associated with WPW syndrome include Ebstein anomaly of the tricuspid valve, congenitally corrected transposition of the great arteries, and hypertrophic cardiomyopathy. Infiltrative disease, such as Pompe disease, can also be associated with APMTs. Cardiac rhabdomyomas can bridge the AV gap, resulting in eccentric conduction.

Mechanism

In both AVRT and AVNRT, the mechanism of arrhythmia propagation is reentrant utilizing conduction tissue with different conduction velocities and refractory periods. In AVRT, the atrial tissue is "electrically" connected to the ventricular tissue via an epicardial AV accessory pathway that can have either antegrade or retrograde or both conducting properties, allowing for propagation of electrical stimulus propagating the tachycardia. In AVRT, the atrial and ventricular masses are coupled in the circuit resulting in 1:1 AV conduction. In AVNRT, there is "dual-AV node physiology" with two conducting pathways connecting the atrium and His bundle, thus forming a reentry circuit. One pathway termed the "fast" pathway, located in an anterosuperior position to the AV node, has fast conduction velocity with a long refractory period compared to the "slow" pathway located posteroinferior, which has slower conduction and a shorter refractory period. The difference is conduction velocities and refractory periods allows for a timely placed premature beat to enter the circuit, leading to AVNRT. In AVNRT, there is typically 1:1 AV conduction; however, there can also be 2:1 AV conduction as the ventricular tissue is not part of the circuit, unlike in AVRT. Both AVRT and AVNRT require a premature extrastimulus to occur during the vulnerable period of one of the limbs of the circuit to propagate. Onset and termination is sudden for both AVRT and AVNRT.

Electrocardiogram Criteria

A fast and regular narrow QRS complex tachycardia with no clear P waves is a typical ECG finding (Fig. 49.12). A retrograde (inverted) P wave may be seen immediately following a QRS complex in AVRT or in atypical "fast-slow" AVNRT. The QRS complex morphology is typically narrow, unless there is rate-related bundle branch block or there is antidromic reciprocating tachycardia (antegrade conduction through the accessory pathway and retrograde conduction through the AV node).

ECG findings in WPW syndrome consists of a short PR interval, a slurred upstroke of the QRS complex (the delta wave), and a QRS complex of longer duration than normal for age during sinus rhythm. These findings may not be evident in all the surface ECG leads; however, the most sensitive leads for detection are the mid-precordial V2 to V4 leads. Other clues include left-axis deviation, absent Q waves in lead V6, abnormally wide Q waves in the limb leads, a junctional escape beat with a different QRS morphology, and accentuation or loss of preexcitation with a PAC.

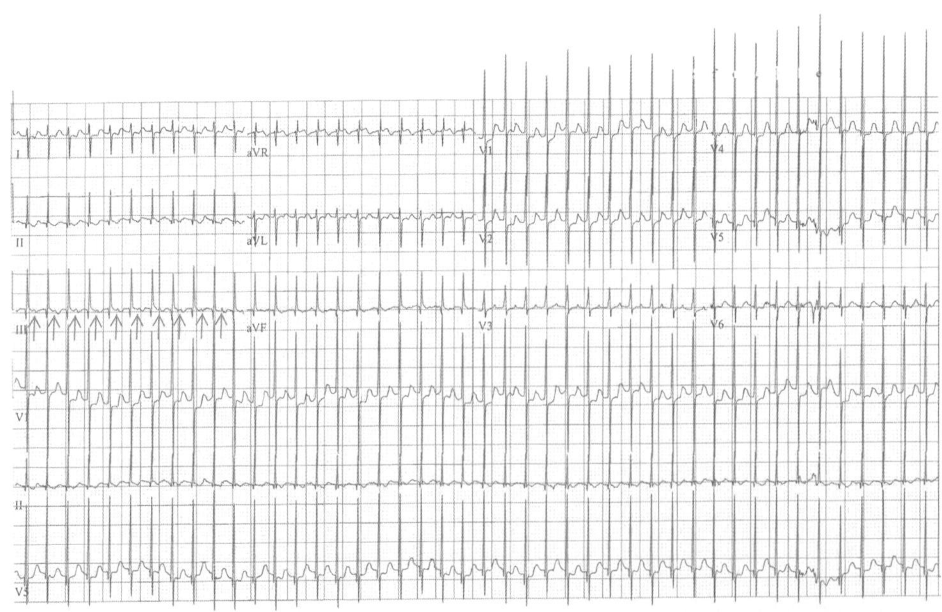

Figure 49.12 Supraventricular tachycardia. Regular narrow QRS complex tachycardia at 265 bpm. Retrograde P waves are seen best in lead III (*arrows*). This child had a concealed left-sided accessory pathway. aVF, augmented vector foot; aVL, augmented vector left; aVR, augmented vector right.

Treatment

Neonatal reentrant SVTs warrant treatment with either vagal maneuvers or medical cardioversion. Vagal maneuvers such as applying ice to the face can be successful. A mix of crushed ice with water in a plastic bag or glove should be applied to the infant face for 10 to 15 seconds, without compromising breathing. In stable patients, it can be repeated once. Carotid sinus massage and ocular pressure are not recommended due to prolonged asystole and potential retinal detachment, respectively. If vagal maneuvers fail to cardiovert, then a rapid intravenous bolus injection of adenosine (through proximal large vein) over 1 to 2 seconds immediately followed by a rapid saline flush can result in cardioversion. Alternatively, transesophageal pacing or antiarrhythmic medications may also be tried. Table 49.5 indicates first- and second-line pharmacotherapy. Electrical cardioversion is rarely required, but if the infant or child is hemodynamically unstable, then a synchronized electrical cardioversion utilizing 0.5 to 1 Joule per kg is indicated.

Fetal Considerations

Reentrant SVTs present as intermittent or persistent tachycardia with heart rates between 190 and 300 bpm. SVT can occur at any point in time during pregnancy following the first trimester.[8]

Fetal Echo Criteria

Analysis via fetal echocardiogram demonstrates a short V-A pattern, meaning that an atrial contraction occurs shortly after the ventricular contract. During this time, the AV valves are closed. This results in a pronounced *a* wave flow reversal in the precordial veins and the ductus venosus.

Fetal Treatment

If the SVT episodes are brief and infrequent, then close observation without medical treatment is appropriate and safe. Unfortunately, if there is incessant tachyarrhythmia, then the fetus is at risk of developing heart failure with hydrops if left untreated and risk for perinatal death is high.[8] Therefore, rapid pharmacologic cardioversion to a normal sinus rhythm is crucial and, if successful, may lead to resolution of fetal hydrops if sinus rhythm and appropriate cardiac function are maintained. Possible medications to treat fetal SVT are maternal digoxin, flecainide, or sotalol. They may be given either alone or in combination. If the SVT is resistant to these therapies, amiodarone may be used. As discussed previously, flecainide has an excellent bioavailability in hydropic fetuses and is thus a better agent to use than digoxin in this patient population. Very little data exist on the postnatal management for fetuses diagnosed with SVT, with the current two strategies being either discontinuation of all therapies at birth or to continue antiarrhythmics prophylactically for 6 to 12 months.

Atrial Flutter

Atrial flutter is a macro-reentrant arrhythmia that accounts for less than 1% of arrhythmias in the pediatric population. In infants with structurally normal hearts, atrial flutter is typically an isolated event. In older children, atrial flutter is typically associated with underlying heart disease.

Mechanism

Atrial flutter requires an isthmus of myocardial tissue with difference in conduction velocity and refractoriness bounded by

TABLE 49.5 Summary of Recommended Medical Therapies in Pediatrics Based on Observed Tachyarrhythmia

Arrhythmia	*Recommended Medical Therapy*		
Sinus tachycardia	Observation Address underlying etiology of sinus tachycardia (i.e., fever, anemia, hyperthyroidism).		
Reentry supraventricular tachycardia	First-line therapy	i.v.: adenosine, esmolol, procainamide	Oral: propranolol, digoxin (contraindicated if WPW syndrome)
	Second-line therapy	i.v.: amiodarone	Oral: sotalol, amiodarone, flecainide
Atrial flutter	First-line therapy	i.v.: esmolol (rate control), procainamide (rhythm control)	Oral: propranolol, digoxin
	Second-line therapy	i.v.: amiodarone (rhythm control)	Oral: metoprolol, atenolol (rate control); sotalol, amiodarone (rhythm control)
Permanent junctional reciprocating tachycardia	First-line therapy	i.v.: esmolol (rate control)	Oral: propranolol, atenolol, metoprolol, digoxin
	Second-line therapy	i.v.: amiodarone (rhythm control)	Oral: flecainide, sotalol, amiodarone, verapamil
Ectopic atrial tachycardia	First-line therapy	i.v.: esmolol, procainamide	Oral: propranolol, atenolol
	Second-line therapy	i.v.: amiodarone	Oral: propafenone, sotalol, flecainide, amiodarone
Ventricular tachycardia	First-line therapy	i.v.: amiodarone, procainamide	Oral: none
	Second-line therapy	i.v.: lidocaine	Oral: none
Torsades de Pointes	First-line therapy	i.v.: magnesium sulfate	Oral: none
Accelerated idioventricular rhythm	Observation If hemodynamically unstable, may consider rate control with i.v. propranolol or esmolol.		

i.v., intravenous; WPW, Wolff–Parkinson–White.
Data from Moffett BS, Salvin JW, Kim JJ. Pediatric cardiac intensive care society 2014 consensus statement: pharmacotherapies in cardiac critical care antiarrhythmics. *Pediatr Crit Care Med* 2016;17:S49–S58.

either structural or functional barriers, such as the tricuspid valve annulus, pulmonary veins, vena cava junctions, or crista terminalis.[50] A premature stimulus is required to enter the circuit, allowing for propagation. As opposed to other SVTs, the AV node is not part of the reentry circuit, thus allowing for variable AV conduction from 1:1 to 4:1.

Electrocardiogram Criteria

Typically, a regular and rapid atrial tachycardia with saw-tooth flutter waves is best seen in the inferior leads II, III, and augmented vector foot (aVF) (Fig. 49.13). There is a continuous atrial activation on ECG due to reentry mechanism, as opposed to an isoelectric segment between P waves seen in AETs. There is usually AV block, resulting in regular R-R intervals with AV conduction of 1:1 to 4:1. Atrial flutter rate typically 360 bpm or higher and ventricular rates are 200 to 300 bpm in infants.

Treatment

Neonatal recurrence of atrial flutter is unusual, and long-term therapy is rarely required. Postnatally, cardioversion is the first choice therapy either by transesophageal atrial overdrive pacing or via synchronize direct current cardioversion. If electrical cardioversion is not preferred and the patient is hemodynamically stable, medical cardioversion may be attempted, usually with a potassium-blocking antiarrhythmic agent.

Fetal Consideration

The typical atrial rate ranges between 300 and 500 bpm, which is commonly associated with 2:1 AV conduction but can also observe 3:1 and 4:1 AV conduction. In the absence of structural heart disease, atrial flutter is almost exclusively observed in fetuses during the third trimester or at birth. It is usually tolerated well, with fetal hydrops and death being uncommon.

Fetal Treatment

Sotalol and digoxin are the first-line medications for the treatment of fetal atrial flutter. Treatment is aimed to either suppress or slow the ventricular rate to a more normal heart rate. If it persists after birth, sinus rhythm can be restored by transesophageal atrial overdrive pacing, synchronized electrical cardioversion, or pharmacotherapy.

Junctional Tachycardia Including Permanent Junctional Reciprocating Tachycardia

The AV junction is comprised of essentially three parts, the atrial tissue approaching the AV node, the AV node itself, and penetrating portions of the His bundle. The AV junction possesses intrinsic automaticity, allowing it to serve as an ectopic pacemaker or as a site of reentry.[51] When the AV junction serves as an ectopic pacemaker, it can result in a junctional tachycardia. When the rate is greater than the 95th percentile for a normal heart rate in the newborn period, this is termed "congenital junctional ectopic tachycardia."[52] When the AV junction serves as a site of reentry, it can result in PJRT.

PJRT is an uncommon form of reentrant SVT in children. It is commonly incessant in children, and its persistence may lead to tachycardia-induced cardiomyopathy. Symptoms of congestive heart failure may be present in younger aged patients. Patients who are older at diagnosis typically have a slower tachycardia secondary to paroxysmal forms or age-dependent slowing of the tachycardia.[53] PJRT is typically not associated with structural heart disease.

Mechanism

Junctional tachycardia results from an ectopic automatic focus within the AV junction. If there is intact antegrade and retrograde conduction, then a beat arising from the AV junction will cause both atrial and ventricular depolarization.[51] This is evident on an ECG as retrograde P waves and narrow QRS complexes. If only antegrade conduction occurs, then the junctional rhythm will be characterized by narrow QRS complexes without atrial penetration since the impulse arises above the branching point of the His bundle. Junctional tachycardia is a common cause of AV dissociation resulting from a combination of physiologic interference in the AV node from the antegrade sinus impulse and the retrograde junctional impulse. In this case, the atrial

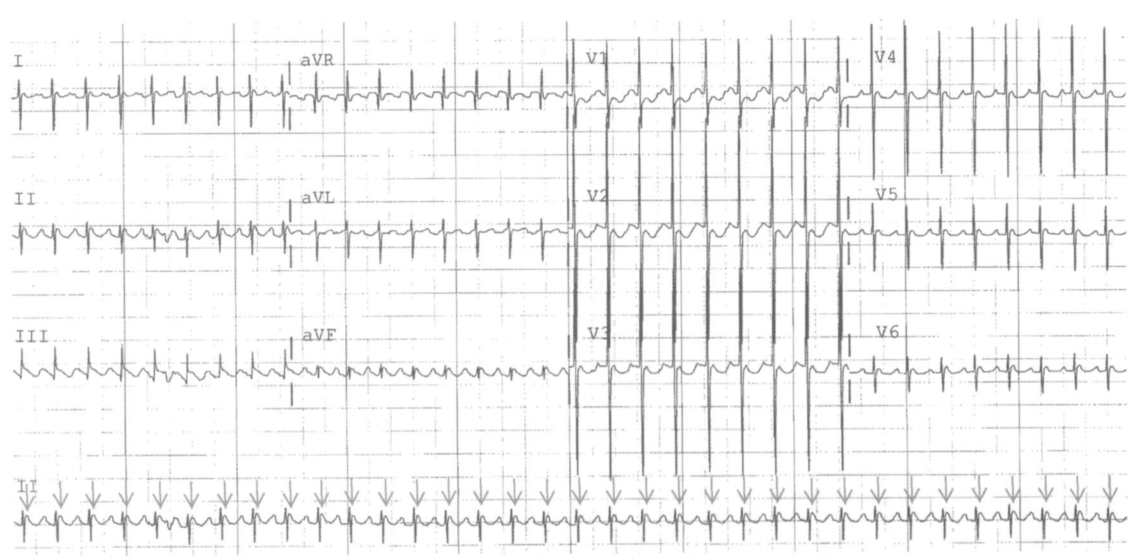

Figure 49.13 Atrial flutter with 2:1 atrioventricular conduction with an atrial rate of 400 bpm. There are atrial flutter waves within the terminal QRS complexes (*arrows*). aVF, augmented vector foot; aVL, augmented vector left; aVR, augmented vector right.

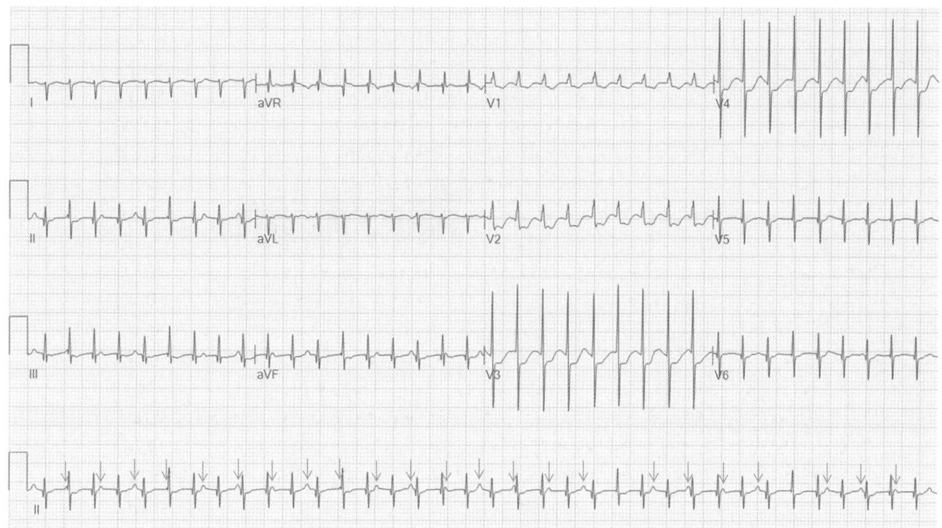

Figure 49.14 Junctional tachycardia. There is narrow QRS complex tachycardia with atrioventricular dissociation at 220 bpm. Arrows marking the P waves. aVF, augmented vector foot; aVL, augmented vector left; aVR, augmented vector right.

and ventricular rates are independent, with the ventricular rate being faster than the atrial rate.

PJRT is an orthodromic reentry tachycardia with antegrade conduction utilizing the AV node and retrograde conduction via a fairly slow and decremental concealed retrograde conducting accessory pathway, resulting in a long PR pattern. The slow and decremental conducting properties of the retrograde accessory pathway lead to the incessant tachycardia.

Electrocardiogram Criteria

For junctional tachycardia, the typical ECG patter is a narrow complex rhythm, unless there is a preexisting bundle branch block or rate-related aberrancy. Retrograde P waves may be present and can appear before, during, or after the QRS complex (Fig. 49.14). If there is AV dissociation, the ventricular rate is greater than the atrial rate.

For PJRT, the typical ECG pattern is that of an incessant tachycardia with long RP intervals and inverted P waves in the inferior leads II, III, and aVF (Fig. 49.15).

Treatment

Most infants with junctional tachycardia will require a combination of antiarrhythmic medications. The most commonly used antiarrhythmic for junction escape tachycardia is amiodarone.[52] Other antiarrhythmics include digoxin, β-blockers, flecainide, procainamide, and sotalol, among others. There are currently no specific guidelines for the treatment of perinatal junctional tachycardia.[52]

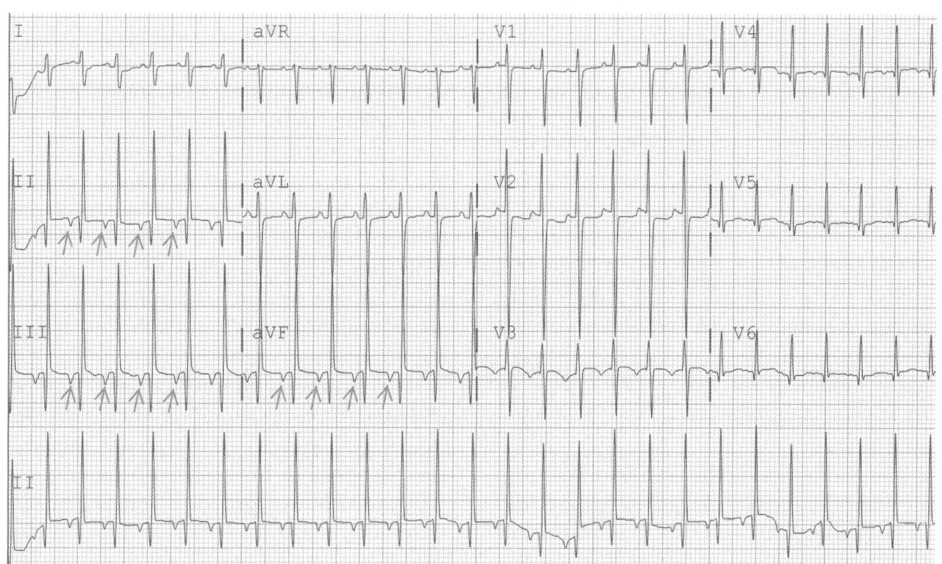

Figure 49.15 Permanent junctional reciprocating tachycardia. There are inverted P waves in the inferior leads (*arrows*). This is a long RP tachycardia with a regular and narrow QRS complex tachycardia at 197 bpm. aVF, augmented vector foot; aVL, augmented vector left; aVR, augmented vector right.

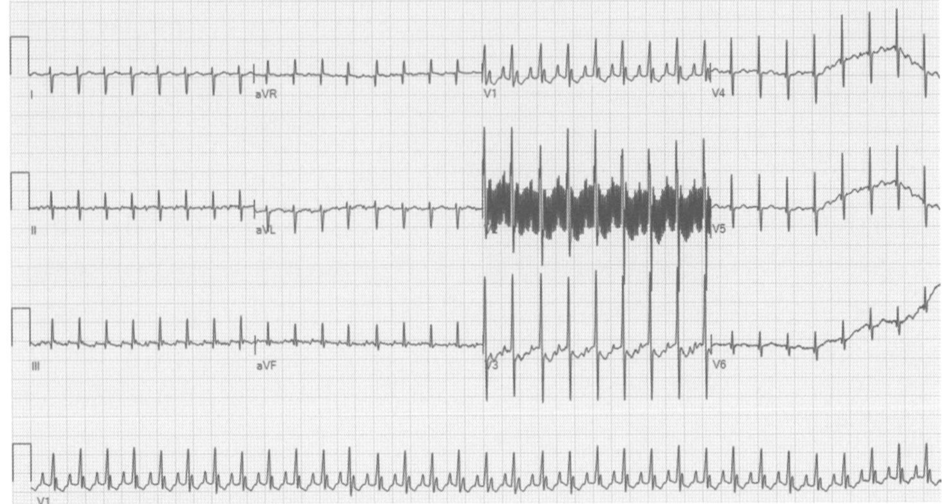

Figure 49.16 Atrial ectopic tachycardia. Regular narrow QRS complex tachycardia with prominent P waves best seen in lead V1. This is a long RP tachycardia. There is lead noise noted in lead V2. aVF, augmented vector foot; aVL, augmented vector left; aVR, augmented vector right.

Spontaneous resolution of PJRT is low. However, it has been reported to occur in 20% of cases.[53] Treatment of PJRT can be difficult due to high failure rate of medications, at times necessitating combination of antiarrhythmics. Flecainide has been demonstrated to be effective in 60% of cases and is often used as first-line agent.[54] However, a combination of flecainide and amiodarone may be necessary for rhythm control. Rate control can be tried, but definitive treatment of PJRT is possible with radiofrequency ablation of the accessory pathway in later life.

Fetal Considerations

Junctional tachycardias are extremely difficult to diagnosis in utero and, for this reason, are considered to be extremely rare.

Atrial Ectopic Tachycardia

AET is an uncommon cause of SVT in children. It is usually chronic and can be sustained. However, AET can have spontaneous resolution if diagnosed before 3 years of age, with 74% resolution if presenting in the first year of life.[55] Due to high-resolution rate at an early age, these children are typically treated with medical therapy. Unfortunately, progression to tachycardia-induced cardiomyopathy can occur, but it is often reversible with arrhythmia control.[55] AET usually occurs in children without structural heart disease.

Mechanism

AET arises from an atrial focus with enhanced automaticity. During AET, intermittent changes in tachycardia rate with warming up and cooling down may be observed. The tachycardia may be paroxysmal or sustained.

Electrocardiogram Criteria

Although the P-wave morphology and axis usually differ from sinus rhythm, AET foci near the sinus node make it hard to differentiate from sinus tachycardia. In AET, there is an isoelectric baseline, distinguishing it from atrial flutter (Fig. 49.16). There is typically 1:1 AV conduction, although the PR interval may be prolonged. The QRS complex is usually of normal morphology.

Treatment

Short-term antiarrhythmic treatment is often required for frequent, faster AETs until potential spontaneous resolution. Multiple antiarrhythmic medications or combination of medications have been used, with β-blockers being the most common first-line agent. Catheter ablation procedures have been effective in up to 81% of cases.[55]

Ventricular Tachycardia

VT is very rare in fetuses and infants. VT accounts for 1% of all tachyarrhythmias and with an incidence of 0.3 episodes per 100,000 infants.[4] Half of the pediatric cases of VT occur in patients with an underlying channelopathy such as long QT syndrome; structural heart disease such as hypertrophic cardiomyopathy, right ventricular dysplasia, and left ventricular noncompaction; or congenital heart disease.[4] Other causes can include electrolyte abnormalities, viral and anti-Ro antibody-mediated myocarditis, or cardiac tumors, or it can be idiopathic. The postnatal definition of VT is a ventricular rate that is greater than or equal to 120 bpm in adults or 25% greater than the normal sinus rate. A ventricular rate within approximately 125% of the sinus rate in asymptomatic patients is known as an accelerated idioventricular rhythm (AIVR). AIVR is a rare benign cause of broad QRS complex tachycardia in a neonate, characterized by a broad QRS on ECG with a ventricular rate higher than the prevailing sinus rate (Fig. 49.17). Spontaneous conversion to sinus rhythm might be observed in AIVR when the sinus rate rises due to the infant's agitation. AIVR is self-limited, benign, and typically does not require intervention.

TdP is an uncommon form of polymorphic VT and is characterized by a "twisting" of the QRS complexes around the isoelectric baseline. It is typically seen with channelopathies (i.e., Brugada or long QT syndrome) but may also result from myocarditis, myocardial ischemia, electrolyte abnormalities (particularly hypokalemia and/or hypomagnesemia), acid–base disturbances, and endocrine disorders. The episodes are typically paradoxical in nature and self-limiting. Longer episodes may result in ventricular fibrillation and rapid hemodynamic compromise and sudden cardiac death.[16]

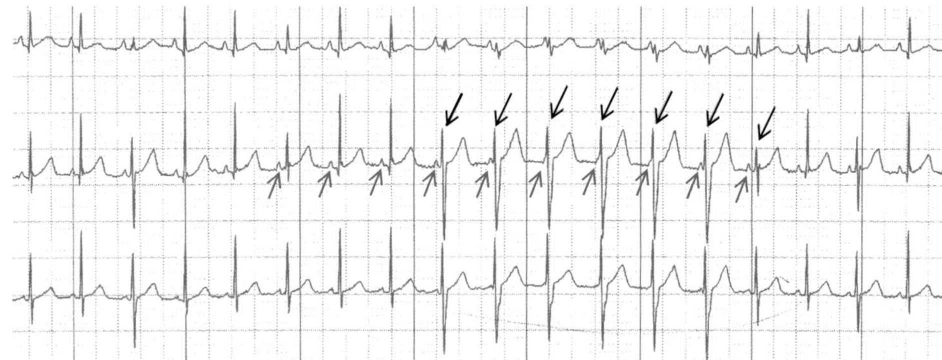

Figure 49.17 Accelerated idioventricular rhythm (AIVR). The sinus rate (*blue arrows*) is seen fusing into the accelerated ventricular rhythm (*black arrows*). AIVR is suppressed once the sinus rhythm increases beyond the ventricular rate.

Mechanism

VTs can arise from reentry, triggered activity, or automaticity mechanisms. VT utilizing a reentrant mechanism may occur around a scar. Triggered activity may result in TdP. Cardiac tumors may lead to automaticity.

Electrocardiogram Criteria

A postnatal ECG will demonstrate wide QRS complex beats with dissociation of the P wave from the QRS complex occurring at a faster rate than the underlying sinus rhythm (Fig. 49.18). In infants or children, there may be retrograde conduction, resulting in 1:1 ventriculoatrial (VA) conduction. It is also possible to have variations in the R-R interval due to sinus capture beats.

Treatment

Treatment and prognosis depend on the VT mechanism and pattern, the hemodynamic impact, and the associated conditions. Treatments to acutely control VT may include intravenous medications such as lidocaine, amiodarone, or procainamide, or oral medications such as β-blockers and/or mexiletine. In the absence of long QT syndrome, amiodarone, flecainide, or sotalol may be useful. If the patient is hemodynamically unstable, then management should follow the AHA PALS guidelines. Potassium channel blockers are contraindicated in long QT syndrome, with β-blockers as the gold standard. In long QT syndrome type 3 (mediated by a gain in function of the sodium channel), sodium channel blockers have been proven to be effective. Long-term management still has to be established, although VT resolution occurs with and without outpatient antiarrhythmic medication.[56]

The outcome for perinatal VT depends on the etiology. A poor prognosis is associated with patients who have congenital heart disease, cardiomyopathies, long QT syndrome, and cardiac tumors. The mortality rate is 36% in this patient population.[57] In otherwise healthy babies, VT is generally associated with a good prognosis.[4,56,57]

Fetal Consideration

Prenatally, the diagnosis can be challenging, but should be suspected if AV dissociation is observed and there are more ventricular contractions than atrial ones on the fetal echo.

Fetal Echo

The fetal echocardiogram shows a tachycardia less than 200 bpm that is often incessant on presentation. The ventricular rate is higher than the atrial rate, and there is no clear relationship between ventricular and atrial events (AV dissociation).

Fetal Treatment

Prior to birth, short-term maternal intravenous magnesium has been recommended as the first-line medication for VT greater than 200 bpm.[42] Prenatal treatments have also included β-blockers, flecainide, sotalol, lidocaine, and amiodarone. Unfortunately, there are limited studies with small patient populations;

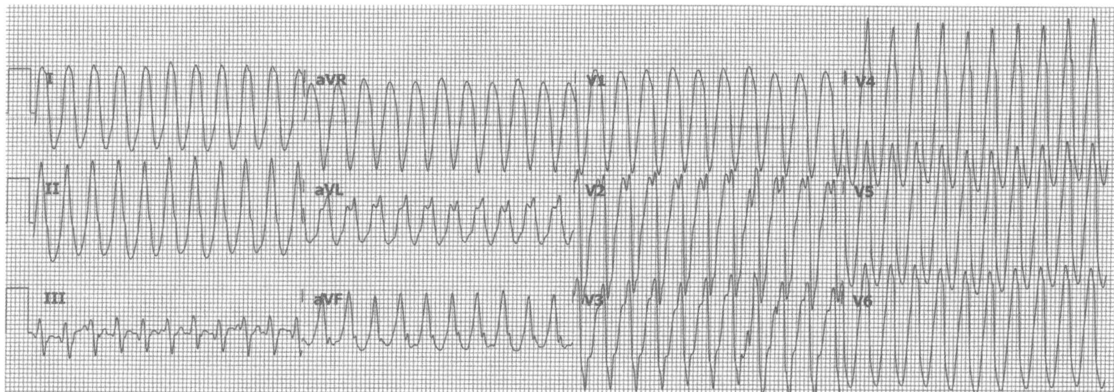

Figure 49.18 Ventricular tachycardia. Wide QRS complex tachycardia with left bundle branch morphology and no discernable P waves. aVF, augmented vector foot; aVL, augmented vector left; aVR, augmented vector right.

hence, a first-line therapy has yet to be established. Flecainide or propranolol has been recommended secondary to its ability to decrease QT interval and thus decrease the risk of inducing TdP.

REFERENCES

1. Strasburger JF. Cardiac arrhythmias in childhood diagnostic consideration and treatment. *Drugs* 1991;42:974–983.
2. Alfred Sacchetti VM, Baricella R, Cameron J, et al. Primary cardiac arrhythmias in children. *Pediatr Emerg Care* 1999;15:95–98.
3. Dickinson DF, Scott O. Ambulatory electrocardiographic monitoring in 100 healthy teenage boys. *Br Heart J* 1984;51:179–183.
4. Sekarski N, Meijboom EJ, Di Bernardo S, et al. Perinatal arrhythmias. *Eur J Pediatr* 2014;173:983–996.
5. Badrawi N, Hegazy RA, Tokovic E, et al. Arrhythmia in the neonatal intensive care unit. *Pediatr Cardiol* 2009;30:325–330.
6. Alsaied T, Baskar S, Fares M, et al. First-line antiarrhythmic transplacental treatment for fetal tachyarrhythmia: a systematic review and meta-analysis. *J Am Heart Assoc* 2017;6:e007164.
7. Kleinman CS, Nehgme RA. Cardiac arrhythmias in the human fetus. *Pediatr Cardiol* 2004;25:234–251.
8. Jaeggi E, Ohman A. Fetal and neonatal arrhythmias. *Clin Perinatol* 2016;43:99–112.
9. Sridharan S, Sullivan I, Tomek V, et al. Flecainide versus digoxin for fetal supraventricular tachycardia: comparison of two drug treatment protocols. *Heart Rhythm* 2016;13:1913–1919.
10. van Engelen AD, Weijtens O, Brenner JI, et al. Management outcome and follow-up of fetal tachycardia. *J Am Coll Cardiol* 1994;24:1371–1375.
11. Jaeggi E, Fouron JC, Fournier A, et al. Ventriculo-atrial time interval measured on M mode echocardiography: a determining element in diagnosis, treatment, and prognosis of fetal supraventricular tachycardia. *Heart* 1998;6:582–587.
12. Fouron JC. Fetal arrhythmias: the Saint-Justine hospital experience. *Prenat Diagn* 2004;24:1068–1080.
13. Nii M, Hamilton RM, Fenwick L, et al. Assessment of fetal atrioventricular time intervals by tissue Doppler and pulse Doppler echocardiography: normal values and correlation with fetal electrocardiography. *Heart* 2006;92:1831–1837.
14. Hornberger LK, Sahn DJ. Rhythm abnormalities of the fetus. *Heart* 2007;93:1294–1300.
15. Davis LM, Rodefeld ME, Green K, et al. Gap junction protein phenotypes of the human heart and conduction system. *J Cardiovasc Electrophysiol* 1995;6:813–822.
16. Allen HD, Penny DJ, Fraser CD. *Moss and Adams heart disease in infants, children, and adolescents: including the fetus and young adult.* Philadelphia, PA: Wolters Kluwer, 2016.
17. Pinnell J, Turner S, Howell S. Cardiac muscle physiology. *Contin Educ Anaesth Crit Care Pain* 2007;7:85–88.
18. Mankad P, Kalahasty G. Antiarrhythmic drugs: risks and benefits. *Med Clin North Am* 2019;103:821–834.
19. Moffett BS, Cannon BC, Friedman RA, et al. Therapeutic levels of intravenous procainamide in neonates: a retrospective assessment. *Pharmacotherapy* 2006;26:1687–1693.
20. Klotz U. Antiarrhythmics: elimination and dosage considerations in hepatic impairment. *Clin Pharmacokinet* 2007;46:985–996.
21. Borchers AT, Keen CL, Gershwin ME. Drug-induced lupus. *Ann NY Acad Sci* 2007;1108:166–182.
22. Schlepper M. Cardiodepressive effects of antiarrhythmic drugs. *Eur Heart J* 1989;10:73–80.
23. Hill AC, Silka MJ, Bar-Cohen Y. A comparison of oral flecainide and amiodarone for the treatment of recurrent supraventricular tachycardia in children. *Pacing Clin Electrophysiol* 2019;42:670–677.
24. Echt DS, Liebson PR, Mitchell LB, et al. Mortality and morbidity in patients receiving encainide, flecainide, or placebo. The cardiac arrhythmia suppression trial. *N Engl J Med* 1991;324:781–788.
25. Fish FA, Gillette PC, Benson DW. Proarrhythmia, cardiac arrest and death in young patients receiving encainide and flecainide. *J Am Coll Cardiol* 1991;18:356–365.
26. Perry JC, McQuinn RL, Smith RT Jr, et al. Flecainide acetate for resistant arrhythmias in the young: Efficacy and pharmacokinetics. *J Am Coll Cardiol* 1989;14:185–191.
27. Gillis AM, Kates RE. Clinical pharmacokinetics of the newer antiarrhythmic agents. *Clin Pharmacokinet* 1984;9:375–403.
28. Al-Majed AA, Bakheit AHH, Abdel Aziz HA, et al. Propranolol. In: Brittain HG, ed. *Profiles of drug substances, excipients and related methodology.* San Diego, CA: Academic Press, 2017: Vol 42, 287–338.
29. Esmolol. In: *LiverTox: clinical and research information on drug-induced liver injury.* Bethesda, MD: National Institute of Diabetes and Digestive and Kidney Diseases, 2012.
30. Esmolol. In: *Drugs and lactation database (LactMed).* Bethesda, MD: National Library of Medicine (US), 2006.
31. Atenolol. In: *LiverTox: clinical and research information on drug-induced liver injury.* Bethesda, MD: National Institute of Diabetes and Digestive and Kidney Diseases, 2012.
32. Gurpreet Singh Wander STC, Kaur K. Atenolol drug profile. *J Assoc Phys India* 2009;57:13–16.
33. Figa FH, Gow RM, Hamilton RM, et al. Clinical efficacy and safety of intravenous amiodarone in infants and children. *Am J Cardiol* 1994;74:573–577.
34. Perry JC, Fenrich AL, Hulse JE, et al. Pediatric use of intravenous amiodarone: efficacy and safety in critically III patients from a multicenter protocol. *J Am Coll Cardiol* 1996;27:1246–1250.
35. Siddoway LA. Amiodarone: guidelines for use and monitoring. *Am Fam Physician* 2003;68:2189–2196.
36. Valdés SO, Miyake CY, Niu MC, et al. Early experience with intravenous sotalol in children with and without congenital heart disease. *Heart Rhythm* 2018;15:1862–1869.
37. Hanyok JJ. Clinical pharmacokinetics of sotalol. *Am J Cardiol* 1993;72:A19–A26.
38. Exela Pharma Sciences. *Verapamil.* Silver Spring, MD: U.S. Food and Drug Administration, 2016.
39. Grace AA, Camm AJ. Voltage-gated calcium-channels and antiarrhythmic drug action. *Cardiovasc Res* 2000;45:43–51.
40. Moffett BS, Salvin JW, Kim JJ. Pediatric cardiac intensive care society 2014 consensus statement: pharmacotherapies in cardiac critical care antiarrhythmics. *Pediatr Crit Care Med* 2016;17:S49–S58.
41. Nagashima M, Matsushima M, Ogawa A, et al. Cardiac arrhythmias in healthy children revealed by 24-hour ambulatory ECG monitoring. *Pediatr Cardiol* 1987;8:103–108.
42. Donofrio MT, Moon-Grady AJ, Hornberger LK, et al. Diagnosis and treatment of fetal cardiac disease: a scientific statement from the American Heart Association. *Circulation* 2014;129:2183–2242.
43. Sonesson SE, Eliasson H, Conner P, et al. Doppler echocardiographic isovolumetric time intervals in diagnosis of fetal blocked atrial bigeminy and 2:1 atrioventricular block. *Ultrasound Obstet Gynecol* 2014;44:171–175.
44. Epstein AE, DiMarco JP, Ellenbogan KA, et al. ACC/AHA/HRS 2008 guidelines for device-based therapy of cardiac rhythm abnormalities: executive summary. *Heart Rhythm* 2008;5:934–955.
45. Lopes LM, Penha Tavares GM, Damiano AP, et al. Perinatal outcome of fetal atrioventricular block: one-hundred-sixteen cases from a single institution. *Circulation* 2008;118:1268–1275.
46. Villain E, Coastedoat-Chalumeau N, Marijon E, et al. Presentation and prognosis of complete atrioventricular block in childhood, according to maternal antibody status. *J Am Coll Cardiol* 2006;48:1682–1687.
47. Jaeggi E, Laskin C, Hamilton R, et al. The importance of the level of maternal anti-Ro/SSA antibodies as a prognostic marker of the development of cardiac neonatal lupus erythematosus a prospective study of 186 antibody-exposed fetuses and infants. *J Am Coll Cardiol* 2010;55:2778–2784.
48. Gimovsky ML, Nazir M, Hashemi E, et al. Fetal/neonatal supraventricular tachycardia. *J Perinatol* 2004;24:191–193.
49. Vergani P, Mariani E, Ciriello E, et al. Fetal arrhythmias: natural history and management. *Ultrasound Med Biol* 2005;31:1–6.
50. Waldo AL. Mechanisms of atrial flutter and atrial fibrillation: distinct entities or two sides of a coin? *Cardiovasc Res* 2002;54:217–229.
51. Rosen KM. Junctional tachycardia. Mechanisms, diagnosis, differential diagnosis, and management. *Circulation* 1973;47:654–664.
52. Collins KK, Van Hare GF, Kertesz NJ, et al. Pediatric nonpost-operative junctional ectopic tachycardia. *J Am Coll Cardiol* 2009;53:690–697.
53. Vaksmann G, D'Hoinne C, Lucet V, et al. Permanent junctional reciprocating tachycardia in children: a multicentre study on clinical profile and outcome. *Heart* 2006;92:101–104.
54. Lindinger A, Heisel A, von Bernuth G, et al. Permanent junctional re-entry tachycardia. A multicenter long-term follow up study in infants, children, and young adults. *Eur Heart J* 1998;19:936–942.
55. Kang KT, Etheridge SP, Kantoch MJ et al. Current management of focal atrial tachycardia in children: a multicenter experience. *Circ Arrhythm Electrophysiol* 2014;7:664–670.
56. Levin MD, Stephens P, Tanel RE, et al. Ventricular tachycardia in infants with structurally normal heart: a benign disorder. *Cardiol Young* 2010;20:641–647.
57. Roggen A, Pavlovic M, Pfammatter JP. Frequency of spontaneous ventricular tachycardia in a pediatric population. *Am J Cardiol* 2008;101:852–854.

CHAPTER

50

Thomas G. Wells

Antihypertensive Drugs

HYPERTENSION IN CHILDREN AND ADOLESCENTS

The detection, diagnosis, management, and prevention of hypertension in the pediatric population is a complex and challenging problem. Measurement of blood pressure, diagnostic testing, and nonpharmacologic therapy, while exceedingly important in the management of children and adolescents with elevated blood pressure and hypertension, are discussed in detail elsewhere.[1,2] Pharmacotherapy and its rational application to blood pressure control remains an important concern for those patients who have severe or resistant hypertension, target organ damage, or comorbid medical conditions.

Hypertension, defined as systolic or diastolic blood pressure ≥95th percentile for age, sex, and height is further classified by severity into stage 1 and stage 2. The new standards also define stage 1 hypertension in children aged 13 years and older when blood pressure falls between 130/80 and 139/89. Stage 2 hypertension is diagnosed in children aged 13 years and older when blood pressure is ≥140/90. More detailed definitions, including the new pediatric normative blood pressure data, are presented elsewhere.[2] The term "prehypertension" has been replaced by "elevated blood pressure." For those children aged 1 to less than 13 years, elevated blood pressure is diagnosed when blood pressure is ≥90th but less than the 95th percentile. The maximum "normal" blood pressure for children aged 1 to less than 13 years is less than 120/80 for those whose blood pressure is less than the 90th percentile. For adolescents (ages ≥13 years of age), the range for elevated blood pressure is 120 to 129/less than 80. As with the previous standards, the newer classifications have implications for treatment.

Elevated blood pressure or hypertension is observed in as many as 10% to 13% of children on a single measurement.[3,4] The prevalence of hypertension as well as elevated blood pressure in some pediatric subpopulations appears to be increasing.[5] However, recent evidence based on the National Health and Nutrition Examination Survey (NHANES) studies[6] and the newest blood pressure guidelines suggests that the prevalence of persistent hypertension is unchanged, occurring in approximately 2% to 4% of the pediatric population.[7] The prevalence of persistently elevated blood pressure is similar. However, a large, recent study provided evidence that hypertension and elevated blood pressure in children are underdiagnosed and the true prevalence may be higher.[8] Furthermore, in overweight and obese children, the prevalence of hypertension is significantly increased.[9]

PHYSIOLOGY OF BLOOD PRESSURE REGULATION

To select rational therapeutic options, a basic understanding of the physiology of blood pressure regulation and perturbations in these regulatory mechanisms is critical. Blood pressure is largely dependent on cardiac output and systemic vascular resistance (Fig. 50.1). Cardiac output is dependent on both stroke volume and heart rate. Homeostatic mechanisms and feedback loops control aspects of these parameters through complex interactions involving baroreceptors and chemoreceptors (detection), the central nervous system (coordination), and the parasympathetic and sympathetic nervous systems, renin–angiotensin–aldosterone axis, and neuroendocrine systems (effectors). Vascular resistance and heart rate can be altered in seconds, while expansion or contraction of intravascular volume requires minutes to hours or longer. Clinical disorders resulting in altered blood pressure regulation may arise via perturbation to one or more of these mechanisms. An understanding of the underlying pathophysiology of the disease or medical condition aids in choosing an effective agent from among the various classes of antihypertensive drugs. It is also important to note that the initial effect of a drug may be attenuated over time as compensatory mechanisms come into play.

Selection of appropriate therapy often depends on the suspected cause of hypertension. Secondary causes of hypertension, particularly obesity and renal and renovascular diseases, are commonly observed in preadolescent children (Table 50.1). During adolescence, secondary causes of hypertension continue to occur, but the prevalence of primary, or more precisely, uncharacterized hypertension also increases.[13,15] It is likely that insulin resistance and genetically determined factors contribute to the development of hypertension in some children and adolescents.[16–20] Both primary and secondary hypertension in

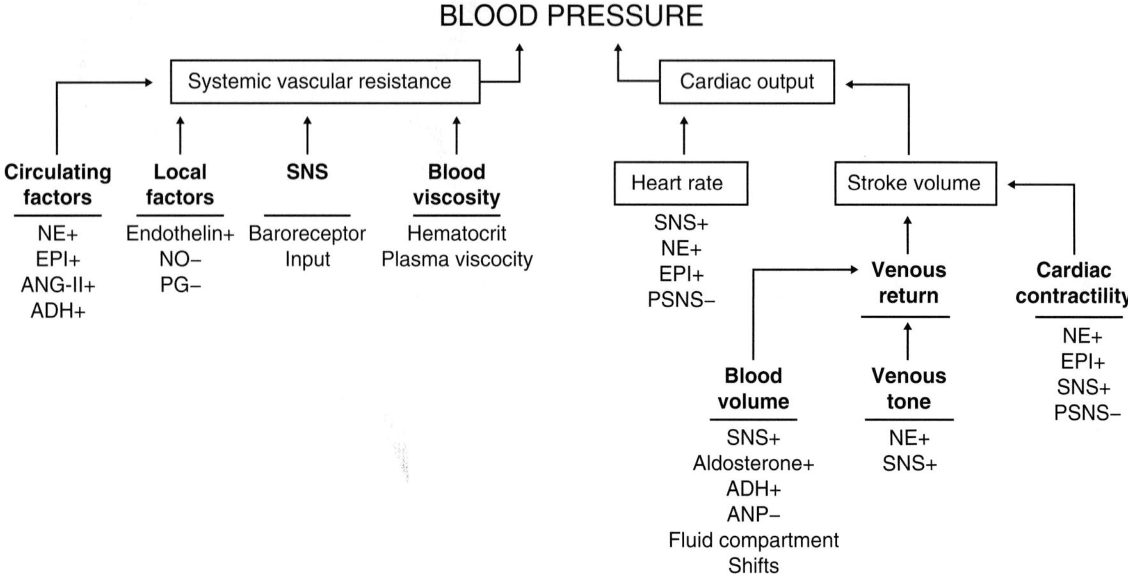

Figure 50.1 Blood pressure regulation: antihypertensive drugs act at various locations to alter numerous factors that determine blood pressure. ADH, vasopressin; Ang-II, angiotensin II; EPI, epinephrine; NE, norepinephrine; NO, nitrous oxide; PG, prostaglandin; PSNS, parasympathetic nervous system; SNS, sympathetic nervous system; +, stimulate; −, inhibit. (Illustration by Nick Wells.)

children and adolescents may result in significant target organ damage.[21–27]

Nonpharmacologic therapies, including weight reduction, dietary modifications, and regular aerobic exercise, are useful in the majority of hypertensive children and adolescents. These therapies may augment the effectiveness of drug therapy in both primary and secondary hypertension. In children, as in adults, most physicians have abandoned the older, stepped-care approach to therapy.[28] Individualized selection of therapeutic agents in children depends on many factors (Table 50.2).

TABLE 50.1 Causes of Hypertension in Children

Neonates (0–1 mo)	*Infants/Toddlers (1–24 mo)*	*Preschool (2–5 y)*	*School-Aged (6–11 y)*	*Adolescent (12–18 y)*
Renovascular[a]	Renal parenchymal diseases	Renal parenchymal diseases	Renal parenchymal diseases	Primary[b]
Coarctation of the aorta	Coarctation of the aorta	Coarctation of the aorta	Obesity	Obesity
Recessive polycystic kidney disease	Renovascular[c]	Renal artery stenosis	Renal artery stenosis	Renal parenchymal diseases
Miscellaneous renal/urologic conditions	Recessive polycystic kidney disease	Genetic disorders[d]	Genetic disorders[d]	Genetic disorders[d]
Abdominal wall defect closure	Bronchopulmonary dysplasia		Primary[b]	Renal artery stenosis
Drugs[e]	Drugs[f]	Drugs	Drugs[g]	Drugs[h]
All ages: fluid overload, pain, certain tumors, endocrine disorders (excessive endogenous aldosterone, 11β-hydroxylase deficiency, exogenous or endogenous thyroxine, corticosteroids, catecholamines), increased intracranial pressure, drugs (calcineurin inhibitors, corticosteroids, erythropoietin, etc.)				

[a]Renal artery thrombosis, renal artery hypoplasia, and renal vein thrombosis.
[b]Possibly due to a combination of genetic and environmental factors.
[c]Renal artery stenosis and renal vein thrombosis.
[d]Williams syndrome, Turner syndrome, neurofibromatosis, etc.
[e]Sympathomimetics, narcotic withdrawal (transplacental exposure).
[f]Adrenocorticotropic hormone.
[g]Decongestants and stimulants.
[h]Decongestants, stimulants, cocaine, amphetamines, caffeine, anabolic steroids, estrogens, and nicotine.
Data from references 10–14.

TABLE 50.2 Individualization of Antihypertensive Therapy in Children: Factors to Consider

1. Underlying etiology of hypertension
2. Severity of hypertension
3. Patient demographics
   a. Age
   b. Race
   c. Ethnicity
   d. Sex
4. Concurrent diseases or medical conditions
5. Concomitant drug therapy
6. Herbal or nontraditional therapies
7. Concurrent nonpharmacologic therapies
8. Available drug formulations
9. Patient compliance issues
   a. Dosing interval
   b. Adverse effects of treatments
   c. Supportive parent(s)/guardian
   d. School and activity schedules
   e. Self-motivation/reliability
   f. Stigma
   g. Cost of treatment
10. Athletic participation

CLASSIFICATION OF ANTIHYPERTENSIVE DRUGS

Antihypertensive agents are classified primarily by their site of action, which defines not only the mechanism through which they interfere with the blood pressure dysregulation but also certain predictable adverse effects. A scheme for classifying antihypertensive agents is presented in Table 50.3. Diuretics, although useful in the treatment of hypertension in children, are considered in detail elsewhere (see Chapter 51).

Although data concerning the pharmacokinetics, dosing, effectiveness, and safety of many antihypertensive agents used in children and adolescents are now available, large-scale, comparative trials similar to those conducted in adults are uncommon in children. Outcomes such as myocardial infarction and stroke, commonly employed in many large-scale, long-term trials conducted in adults, are unrealistic measures in children. Surrogate outcomes, such as blood pressure reduction, are useful but have limitations. Hence, in treating children with hypertension, choices among available therapeutic classes rely less on specific comparative trials in children and more on the suspected cause of the elevated blood pressure and the physiologic mechanisms known to underlie the condition. Other considerations include previous clinical experience, extrapolation from

TABLE 50.3 Classification of Antihypertensive Agents[a]

Class	*Subclass*	*Most Frequently Used Agents*
Diuretics	Thiazides	Hydrochlorothiazide, chlorothiazide, chlorthalidone
	Thiazide like	Indapamide
	Loop diuretics	Furosemide, bumetanide
	Potassium-sparing diuretics	Spironolactone, eplerenone, amiloride, triamterene
Adrenergic antagonists	Selective α-1	Prazosin, doxazosin, terazosin
	Selective α-2 (central antagonist)	Clonidine, guanfacine
	Nonselective α-1 and α-2	Phentolamine, phenoxybenzamine
	Selective β-1	Atenolol, bisoprolol, metoprolol, acebutolol, esmolol
	Nonselective β-1 and β-2	Propranolol, nadolol, pindolol, timolol
	α-1 and nonselective β	Labetalol, carvedilol
Dopaminergic partial agonist	D-1 partial agonist (moderate α-2 activity)	Fenoldopam
Calcium channel antagonists	Dihydropyridines	Nifedipine, amlodipine, nicardipine, felodipine, isradipine, nisoldipine
	Non-dihydropyridines	Diltiazem, verapamil
Angiotensin-converting enzyme inhibitors	Sulfhydryl group	Captopril
	Carboxyl group	Enalapril, lisinopril, ramipril, quinapril, benazepril, moexipril, perindopril, trandolapril
	Phosphate group	Fosinopril
Angiotensin II AT1-receptor antagonists		Losartan, irbesartan, candesartan, valsartan, azilsartan, olmesartan, telmisartan
Renin inhibitor		Aliskiren
Direct vasodilators	Predominately arterial dilation	Hydralazine, diazoxide, minoxidil
	Arterial and venous dilation	Nitroprusside

[a]Many older drugs (primarily centrally acting drugs with significant adverse effects) are no longer widely used in children and are not listed. Selective α-1 agents are not commonly used in children. Phentolamine and phenoxybenzamine are primarily used in children with hypertension caused by pheochromocytoma but have been used in other clinical settings (e.g., phentolamine for dermal extravasation of norepinephrine).

studies conducted in adults, and availability of pediatric-friendly drug formulations. Recommended dosing for children and adolescents (Table 50.4) and neonates (Table 50.5) is based on currently available information and may be subject to change depending on the outcome of ongoing and future clinical trials. Antihypertensive agents used in the treatment of hypertensive urgencies and emergencies are presented in Table 50.6.

DIURETICS AS ANTIHYPERTENSIVE THERAPY

The pharmacology of diuretic drugs is addressed elsewhere (see Chapter 51). Discussion here is limited to recent studies conducted in children where diuretics were specifically studied as treatment for hypertension.

Thiazide diuretics are frequently and successfully used to lower blood pressure in adults[29] and children. Because most thiazides are older drugs, there are few if any large, controlled trials in children. Dosing is based on adult data and accumulated experience with these agents. Similarly, loop diuretics are useful in hypertension secondary to fluid retention, but large, controlled trials using loop diuretics as a sole antihypertensive agent in children have not been conducted.

Potassium-sparing diuretics have been useful in selected disorders associated with hypertension, such as overproduction of

TABLE 50.4 Orally Administered Drug Therapy for Children and Adolescents with Chronic Hypertension[a]

	Initial Dose	*Dosing Interval (h)*	*Maximum Recommended Dose*
Thiazide diuretics			
Chlorothiazide	5–10 mg/kg/dose	12–24	20 mg/kg/d up to 1 g/d
Hydrochlorothiazide	12.5 mg 0.5–1 mg/kg/d	12–24	2 mg/kg/d up to 50 mg/d[b]
Chlorthalidone	0.3 mg/kg/d	24–48	2 mg/kg/d up to 50 mg
Potassium-sparing diuretics			
Amiloride	0.4–0.6 mg/kg/d	24	20 mg/d
Eplerenone	25 mg/d	12–24	100 mg/d
Spironolactone	1 mg/kg/d	6–24	3.3 mg/kg/d up to 200 mg/d[c]
Central α_2 agonists			
Clonidine	5–10 µg/kg/d	8–12	25 µg/kg/d up to 0.9 mg/d
Guanfacine[d]	0.5–1 mg	Start daily and increase as needed (immediate release); once daily (extended release)	Up to 3–4 mg (immediate release); up to 7 mg/d (extended release in adolescents)
α- and β-Adrenergic antagonists			
Labetalol	1–3 mg/kg/d	8–12	12 mg/kg/d up to 1,200 mg
β-Adrenergic antagonists			
Atenolol	0.5–1 mg/kg/d	24	2 mg/kg/d up to 100 mg/d
Metoprolol[e]	0.5–1 mg/kg/d	8–12	2 mg/kg/d up to 200 mg/d
Propranolol[e]	0.5–1 mg/kg/d	6–12	8 mg/kg/d up to 640 mg/d
Calcium channel antagonists			
Amlodipine[f]	0.1 mg/kg/d	24	0.6 mg/kg/d up to 10 mg/d
Felodipine	2.5 mg/d	24	10 mg/d
Isradipine[g]	0.1–0.2 mg/kg/d	6–12	0.8 mg/kg/d up to 20 mg/d
Nifedipine (extended release)	0.25–0.5 mg/kg/d	12–24	3 mg/kg/d up to 120 mg/d
Angiotensin-converting enzyme inhibitors			
Benazepril	0.1 mg/kg (5 mg)	24	0.6 mg/kg/d up to 40 mg/d

TABLE 50.4 Orally Administered Drug Therapy for Children and Adolescents with Chronic Hypertension[a] (*continued*)

	Initial Dose	*Dosing Interval (h)*	*Maximum Recommended Dose*
Captopril	0.3–0.5 mg/kg/dose	8–12	6 mg/kg/d up to 450 mg/d
Enalapril	0.08 mg/kg (5 mg)	24	0.6 mg/kg/d up to 40 mg/d
Fosinopril	0.1 mg/kg (10 mg)	24	0.6 mg/kg/d up to 40 mg/d
Lisinopril	0.07 mg/kg (5 mg)	24	0.6 mg/kg/d up to 40 mg/d
Ramipril	1.25–2.5 mg	24	20 mg
Quinapril	5–10 mg/d	12–24	80 mg
Angiotensin II–receptor antagonists			
Candesartan	<50 kg: 4–8 mg/d	12–24	<50 kg: 16 mg/d
	>50 kg: 8–16 mg/d		>50 kg: 32 mg/d
Irbesartan	6–12 years: 75 mg/d	24	6–12 years: 150 mg/d
	>12 years: 150 mg/d		>12 years: 300 mg/d
Losartan	0.7 mg/kg/d up to 50 mg	24	1.4 mg/kg/d up to 100 mg
Olmesartan	20–<35 kg: 10 mg/d	24	20 to <35 kg: 20 mg/d
	≥35 kg: 20 mg/d		≥35 kg: 40 mg/d
Telmisartan	1–2 mg/kg/d up to 40 mg/d	24	80 mg/d[h]
Valsartan[i]	1.3 mg/kg/d up to 40 mg/d	24	2.7 mg/kg/d up to 160 mg
Renin inhibitors			
Aliskiren	20–50 kg: 75 mg/d	24	20–50 kg: 150 mg/d
	>50 kg: 150 mg/d		>50 kg: 300 mg/d

[a]Many of these drugs have not been approved by the Food and Drug Administration for use in children. Some children benefit from dividing the total daily dose into two or three daily doses. Listed doses assume normal renal and hepatic function.
[b]The maximum daily dose when not used for hypertension is 200 mg. Doses above 50 mg are uncommon when used for primary hypertension.
[c]Some sources recommend up to 400 mg per day for children with primary aldosteronism.
[d]Use is very limited in hypertensive children; guanfacine is occasionally used in children with attention-deficit/hyperactivity disorder (ADHD) who also have hypertension when more traditional ADHD medications (including clonidine) are ineffective or not tolerated. Dosing in hypertension is not well established. Dosing is dependent on age and weight and may be limited by adverse effects.
[e]Metoprolol and propranolol are available as both tablets and extended-release tablets or capsules. Extended-release tablets or capsules are dosed once daily. Extemporaneous liquid formulations may be compounded.
[f]A commercial suspension (1 mg/mL) is now available.
[g]Isradipine is available as both a standard tablet and an extended-release preparation. Dosing for the extended release formulation is once daily.
[h]Doses up to 160 mg daily have been used in a pediatric clinical trial.
[i]In children aged 17 years and above, the starting dose may be increased to 80 mg per day, and the maximum dose should not exceed 320 mg per day.

aldosterone independent of stimulation by renin and angiotensin. Triamterene and amiloride reduce sodium reabsorption primarily in the collecting duct by inhibiting the egress of sodium from the luminal fluid through the epithelial Na^+ channel (ENaC), resulting in a reduction in sodium available to be exchanged for potassium through the Na^+/K^+–ATPase pump. The net result is a reduction in the reabsorption of sodium in exchange for potassium, causing a mild natriuresis and diuresis accompanied by a reduction in urinary loss of potassium. Although they are occasionally used (e.g., Liddle syndrome), these older agents have not been well studied in children with hypertension.

Spironolactone and eplerenone both bind to mineralocorticoid receptors effectively, blocking aldosterone from binding at these sites. Aldosterone is known to increase the number of ENaC sites and the activity of the Na^+/K^+–ATPase pump. The net effect is a mild natriuresis and diuresis with reduced urinary potassium loss similar to that seen with triamterene and amiloride.

The safety and effectiveness of eplerenone as an antihypertensive agent in children has been studied in a randomized,

TABLE 50.5 Drug Therapy for Hypertension in Neonates[a]

	Initial Dose	*Dosing Interval (hr)*	*Maximum Recommended Dose*	*Common Adverse Effects*
Diuretics				
Chlorothiazide	10–20 mg/kg/d	12	40 mg/kg/d	Electrolyte disorders; contraindicated in renal failure
Furosemide	0.5 mg/kg/dose	8–24	2 mg/kg/d	Electrolyte disorders, ototoxicity, nephrocalcinosis with chronic use
Adrenergic antagonists				
Esmolol	50–100 μg/kg/min	Continuous IV	200 μg/kg/min[b]	Hypotension, bradycardia, bronchoconstriction, lethargy, vomiting
Propranolol	0.25–1 mg/kg/dose	6–12	5 mg/kg/d	Bradycardia, bronchoconstriction, lethargy, vomiting
Calcium channel antagonists				
Amlodipine[c]	0.1 mg/kg/dose	24	Unknown	Peripheral edema, irritability, rash
Nicardipine	0.5 μg/kg/min	Continuous IV	3 μg/kg/min	Hypotension, flushing, tachycardia
ACEIs[d]				
Captopril	0.01 mg/kg/dose	6–12	0.5 mg/kg/dose (2 mg/kg/d)	Hypotension, oliguria, acute renal failure, hyperkalemia, seizures
Enalaprilat	5–10 μg/kg/dose	8–24	20 μg/kg/dose	Hypotension, oliguria, acute renal failure, hyperkalemia
Vasodilators				
Hydralazine	0.1–0.2 mg/kg/dose (IV)	4–6	1 mg/kg/dose	Tachycardia, hypotension, emesis, diarrhea, irritability, rash

[a]Few studies have been conducted in neonates, and dosing recommendations are based on published manuscripts mainly describing small case series, anecdotal experience, and retrospective reviews. Controlled trials are almost nonexistent for children <1 month of age.
[b]Doses above 200 μg per kg per min have been used in neonates, but an increase in adverse effects may be observed.
[c]Because of its long elimination half-life and prolonged duration of action, amlodipine should be used with caution. Amlodipine is a CYP3A4 substrate; coadministration with CYP3A4 inhibitors may result in an exaggerated effect. A commercial suspension is available.
[d]Although there is some published experience with ACEIs in neonates, the risk of hypotension, oliguria, and renal failure is significant. Use with extreme caution.
ACEIs, angiotensin-converting enzyme inhibitors; IV, intravenous.

TABLE 50.6 Drug Therapy for Hypertensive Urgencies and Emergencies in Children and Adolescents (Excluding Neonates)

	Initial Dose	*Dosing Interval*	*Time to Onset/ Duration of Action*	*Maximum Dose*
Diuretics[a]				
Furosemide	Single dose (IV): 0.5–2 mg/kg	4–24 h	15–30 min/2–4 h	6 mg/kg/d
	Continuous (IV): 0.1–0.2 mg/kg/h	Continuous infusion (often after a bolus dose)		
Central α_2 agonists				
Clonidine	2 μg/kg/dose	6–8 h	5–15 min/5–7 h	10 μg/kg/dose
β-Receptor antagonists				
Esmolol[b]	Loading dose: 500 μg/kg (optional); start infusion at 50–150 μg/kg/min	Continuous infusion	1–5 min/10–20 min	Titrate to effect Maximum dose: 500 μg/kg/min
Labetalol[b,c]	Bolus dose: 0.25–1 mg/kg/dose	Every 10 minutes until BP controlled OR	2–5 min/2–4 h	Bolus dose: 1 mg/kg/dose up to 40–80 mg/dose repeated every 10 minutes until BP is controlled or reaching 300 mg (cumulative dose)
	Infusion: 0.25–1 mg/kg/h	Continuous infusion		1 mg/kg/h

TABLE 50.6 Drug Therapy for Hypertensive Urgencies and Emergencies in Children and Adolescents (Excluding Neonates) (*continued*)

	Initial Dose	*Dosing Interval*	*Time to Onset/ Duration of Action*	*Maximum Dose*
Dopaminergic partial agonist				
Fenoldopam	0.2–0.5 μg/kg/min	Continuous infusion	5–20 min/≤30 min	0.8 μg/kg/min
Calcium channel antagonists				
Nifedipine	0.1–0.25 mg/kg/dose	4–6 h	10–30 min/3–6 h	0.25 mg/kg/dose (higher doses risk significant hypotension)
Isradipine	0.05 mg/kg/dose	6–8 h	15–30 min/4–6 h	0.1–0.15 mg/kg/dose
Nicardipine[b]	0.5–1 μg/kg/min	Continuous infusion	1 min/30–120 min[d]	4–5 μg/kg/min
Angiotensin-converting enzyme inhibitors				
Enalaprilat	0.05–0.1 mg/kg (Maximum initial dose: 1.25 mg)	6 h	15 min/4–24 h	5 mg every 6 h
Direct vasodilator				
Hydralazine[b]	0.1–0.2 mg/kg/dose	4–6 h	5–10 min	3.5 mg/kg/d
Minoxidil	Age <12 years: 0.2 mg/kg/d (Maximum initial dose: 5 mg)	12–24 h	20–30 min/12–24 h	Age <12 years: 1 mg/kg/d (Maximum dose: 50 mg/d)
	Age ≥12 years: 5 mg/d			Age ≥12 years: 1 mg/kg/d (Maximum dose: 100 mg/d)
Nitroprusside[b]	0.3–0.5 μg/kg/min	Continuous infusion	1–2 min/1–10 min	Titrate the dose every 5–10 min to a maximum dose of 10 μg/kg/min

[a]Used as adjunct therapy in hypertension secondary to severe volume overload; rarely used as a sole agent.
[b]Preferred agents for hypertensive emergencies in most situations.
[c]Combined α-1 and nonselective β-adrenergic inhibition.
[d]A 50% reduction in effect is observed within 30 minutes after the infusion ends. In adults, the α half-life is 2.7 minutes, and the β half-life is 44.8 minutes.
BP, blood pressure; IV, intravenous.

double-blind, dose–response study.[30] More than 300 children, ages 4 to 16 years, were enrolled into one of three groups [25 mg daily, 25 mg twice daily (BID), and 25 mg increasing to 50 mg BID]. After 6 weeks, the children were re-randomized to continue the dose that they had been receiving or to placebo. Blood pressure reduction was observed in all three groups, but there was no apparent dose–response observed (systolic blood pressure reduction was −7.66, −7.84, and −7.99 mmHg in the low-, middle-, and high-dose groups, respectively). Only the 50-mg BID dose was statistically superior to placebo ($p = 0.048$). Reduction in diastolic blood pressure was neither dose dependent nor different from placebo. The adverse events observed during the study were mainly mild and not related to the study drug.

Diuretics play an important role as adjunct therapy in hypertension and may augment the effectiveness of other antihypertensive agents [e.g., angiotensin-converting enzyme inhibitors (ACEIs)]. There are limited data on the use of diuretics as sole therapy in children and adolescents. However, for selected etiologies of hypertension, diuretics are useful first-line therapy.

ADRENERGIC AGENTS

The sympathetic division of the autonomic nervous system plays a key role in the regulation of blood pressure. At the postganglionic synapse, norepinephrine released from vesicles in the presynaptic membrane in response to sympathetic stimulation binds to receptors on postganglionic effector organs. Stimulation of sympathetic nerves terminating in the adrenal medulla results in release of epinephrine into circulating blood and, to a lesser extent, other catecholamines.

The effects of the adrenergic nervous system are mediated through α and β receptors, each of which has several recognized subtypes. The α_1 adrenoceptors are located primarily in the brain, skin, and smooth muscle. In vascular smooth muscle, stimulation of α_1 receptors by epinephrine, norepinephrine, or drugs like phenylephrine results in vasoconstriction, increased systemic vascular resistance, and increased blood pressure. Postjunctional α_1 receptors, stimulated by prejunctional norepinephrine release, mediate the sympathetic effects on smooth muscle. Stimulation of α_2 receptors, located mainly in the presynaptic junction of postganglionic neurons, inhibits further release of norepinephrine, resulting in a reduction in postjunctional α_1 stimulation, vascular relaxation, and reduced systemic vascular resistance. Both α_1 and α_2 receptors have subtypes distinguished by response to various stimulating and inhibiting drugs.

Like α receptors, β receptors have distinct subtypes based on their distribution and response to endogenous and exogenous compounds. β_1 receptors are located predominantly in the heart and respond to norepinephrine released by sympathetic nerves and to circulating epinephrine and norepinephrine, resulting in increased sinoatrial and atrioventricular activity, myocardial contractility, and heart rate. In the kidney, β_1 receptors stimulate the release of renin from juxtaglomerular cells. β_2 receptors are located in smooth muscle in the vasculature, bronchi, and other locations. Stimulation of these receptors causes smooth muscle to relax and, in the blood vessels, vascular tone decreases. β_2 receptors have a greater affinity for epinephrine than norepinephrine. In skeletal muscle, stimulation of β_2 receptors causes glycogenolysis and uptake of potassium. β_3 receptors are located primarily in adipose tissue, and stimulation results in lipolysis.

Adrenergic antagonists reversibly or irreversibly bind to α and β receptors. Receptor blockade antagonizes the effects of norepinephrine at the postganglionic synaptic membrane as well as the effects of circulating catecholamines at receptor sites. The resultant effects are complex and depend on the targeted receptors and the unique properties possessed by individual adrenergic antagonists.[31]

α-ADRENERGIC ANTAGONISTS

Chronic use of peripheral α-adrenergic receptor antagonists is uncommon in children. In adults, the prazosin arm of the large, comparative trial of several classes of antihypertensive drugs (ALLHAT) was stopped early because it was found to be inferior to other drugs.[29] Clonidine and guanfacine, which stimulate central α_2 receptors resulting in inhibition of sympathetic outflow from the vasomotor center in the brain, are occasionally used when selected comorbid conditions are present or when their adverse effects (primarily sedation and xerostomia) are absent or tolerable. Central sympatholytics are rarely considered first-line therapy in ambulatory children.

Phentolamine and phenoxybenzamine are used to treat acute, severely elevated blood pressure which occurs in conditions associated with excessive circulating catecholamines. Phentolamine is an intravenously administered competitive inhibitor of α_1 and α_2 receptors and is useful for short-term treatment of hypertension secondary to an excess of catecholamines as is seen in patients with a pheochromocytoma. Phenoxybenzamine irreversibly blocks α_1 and α_2 receptors but, unlike phentolamine, can be administered orally. Blockade of α receptors decreases systemic vascular resistance and lowers blood pressure, which can result in hypotension at higher doses. In patients with pheochromocytoma, tachycardia may also occur and can be treated with a β_2 antagonist, but only after blood pressure has been controlled with an α antagonist.

CENTRAL α AGONISTS

Clonidine is a centrally acting α-adrenergic agonist whose action is mediated primarily through attenuation of output from central α_2 receptors. Clonidine acts as a sympatholytic agent, resulting in reduced sympathetic output from the brainstem, causing an initial reduction in systemic vascular resistance, heart rate, cardiac output, and blood pressure. Clonidine has many therapeutic uses, among which is its use as an antihypertensive agent since the 1960s.

Clonidine is rapidly and completely absorbed from the gastrointestinal tract. It is largely metabolized in the liver to inactive metabolites. Metabolism is slower in neonates and gradually increases during the first year of life, with term infants reaching near adult metabolic capacity by the end of the first year of life.[32]

Clonidine is available in several formulations, including tablets, an intravenous preparation, and a transdermal patch. Initial and maintenance oral dosing are presented in Table 50.4. Transdermal dosing starts at 0.1 mg per day. The transdermal patch may be increased to 0.3 mg per day. It is applied once weekly to a flat, hairless, cleaned area of skin and usually takes several days to reach maximal effect.

Adverse effects are common and may include sedation, dry mouth, dizziness, constipation, dry eyes, irritability, and sleep disorders. When stopping clonidine, tapering the dose slowly is advisable since severe rebound hypertension may occur with abrupt cessation of therapy.

Guanfacine is a centrally acting α-adrenergic agonist like clonidine. It is rarely used to treat hypertension in children. It has many of the same adverse effects and cautions seen with clonidine. In addition, hallucinations have been reported in children taking guanfacine. Dosing is dependent on age, weight, and treatment-emergent adverse effects. Like clonidine, it must be tapered when stopping therapy or rebound hypertension may occur.

β-ADRENERGIC ANTAGONISTS

β-Adrenergic receptor antagonists are distinguished by selectivity for the β_1 adrenergic receptor (Table 50.7), the presence of intrinsic sympathomimetic activity, unique pharmacologic properties (Table 50.8), and the presence of α-adrenergic blocking activity. Cardioselective drugs have greater affinity for β_1-adrenergic receptors, while nonselective agents have significant affinity for both β_1 and β_2 receptors. However, at higher doses, cardioselective agents may demonstrate not only β_1 antagonist activity but some degree of β_2 antagonism. Some β-adrenergic antagonists, including acebutolol and pindolol, have small but significant β-agonist effects, known as intrinsic sympathomimetic activity. Because the agonist effect is significantly less than the antagonist effect, the antihypertensive properties of these agents are not compromised. Intrinsic sympathomimetic activity of β-adrenergic blockers helps reduce selected adverse effects resulting from β_1 antagonism (e.g., bradycardia).

Nonselective β-adrenergic antagonists were approved for the management of hypertension in the 1960s. These agents, and subsequent introduction of the more selective β_1-receptor antagonists, attenuate sympathetic stimulation through competitive antagonism of epinephrine and norepinephrine at β-adrenergic receptors. Reversible blockade of β-adrenergic receptors lowers blood pressure by several means. Proposed mechanisms for the antihypertensive effects of β-adrenergic antagonists include binding to cardiac nodal sites, conduction pathways, and individual myocytes, with the net effect of slowing conduction and reducing the force and rate of contraction; inhibition of β_1-adrenergic receptors located on the juxtaglomerular cells, thus inhibiting renin release[33,34]; and, for some agents, inhibition of β_2 receptors in the vascular wall has a slight vasoconstrictor effect, which is overshadowed by the more potent α-agonist–induced vasoconstriction.[35,36]

The predominant immediate systemic effects of β-adrenergic antagonists in hypertensive subjects are reduction in myocardial contractility, cardiac output, and heart rate. These effects

TABLE 50.7 Classification of β-Adrenergic Receptor Antagonists

Drug	*Intrinsic Sympathomimetic Activity*	*α-Adrenergic Activity*
β-1 Selective		
Acebutolol	Yes	No
Atenolol	No	No
Bisoprolol	No	No
Esmolol	No	No
Metoprolol	No	No
Nonselective		
Pindolol	Yes	No
Carvedilol	No	Yes
Labetalol	No	Yes
Nadolol	No	No
Propranolol	No	No
Timolol	No	No

are partially offset by an increase in systemic vascular resistance. With long-term use of β-adrenergic antagonists, heart rate and cardiac output are reduced. Long-term administration of β-adrenergic antagonists has been associated with a gradual reduction in total peripheral resistance.

Depending on the underlying pathophysiology present in individual patients and the unique properties on each drug, the initial and long-term effects may differ.[31] For example, β-adrenergic antagonists are useful in clinical situations where stress-induced increase in sympathetic activity predominates but less useful as single agents in hypertension secondary to salt and water overload. Patients treated with β-adrenergic antagonists that possess intrinsic sympathomimetic activity are less likely to experience drop in heart rate and cardiac output and generally manifest a lesser degree of reflex vasoconstriction.[37]

The β-adrenergic antagonists vary significantly in key characteristics that determine their absorption, metabolism, distribution, and clearance. Most lipophilic β-adrenergic antagonists are better absorbed after oral administration than hydrophilic agents.[31] However, lipophilic drugs are more likely to be subjected to first-pass metabolism; hence, oral bioavailability may be variable. More hydrophilic β-adrenergic antagonists, such as atenolol, are largely excreted in the urine as unchanged drug, while more lipophilic agents, such as metoprolol, are metabolized by hepatic P450 CYP2D6 enzymes. Genetic polymorphisms for cytochrome 2D6 may explain the exaggerated effect observed in poor metabolizers following administration of agents that are inactivated by this pathway. Selected pharmacologic characteristics of β-adrenergic antagonists commonly used in children are listed in Table 50.8. In adults, plasma concentrations of these drugs often correlate poorly with measurable physiologic effects,[38,39] but few concentration–effect data are available in children.

Clinical Use in Children

The β-adrenergic antagonists have been used to treat a wide variety of conditions in children. However, relatively few studies have focused on the use of these drugs to treat pediatric hypertension.[40–53] With the advent of newer drugs, β-adrenergic antagonists are used less often but still play an important role in the management of pediatric hypertension associated with several conditions and in children who have severe hypertension requiring multiple drugs.

Propranolol was the first β-adrenergic antagonist available for the treatment of hypertension in children. In one case series, nine children with severe hypertension were treated with daily doses of 0.6 to 6.4 mg per kg of propranolol.[40] Blood pressure decreased in all nine patients. The mean reduction in systolic and diastolic blood pressures was 26 and 20 mmHg, respectively. As expected, there was no correlation between pretreatment plasma renin activity and the magnitude of blood pressure reduction. In another study conducted in children with poorly controlled hypertension following renal transplantation, similar doses resulted in mean reduction in systolic and diastolic blood pressures of 12 and 15 mmHg, respectively.[43] Propranolol was also shown to effectively reduce paradoxical hypertension after repair of coarctation of the aorta.[44]

Despite the lack of double-blind, controlled trials in children, atenolol has been used to treat pediatric hypertension for many years. The pharmacokinetics of atenolol has been studied in children and young adults with Marfan syndrome and arrhythmias.[45,46] In the past, an extemporaneous formulation permitted use in young children where β_1 selectivity was desired, but presently, a commercial preparation is available.

TABLE 50.8 Pharmacology of β-Adrenergic Antagonists Commonly Used to Treat Hypertension in Children

	First-Pass Effect[a]	*Oral Bioavailability (%)*	T_{max} *(h)*	*Metabolism/ Elimination*[b]	*Elimination Half-life (h)*
Propranolol	Low	25–40	1–2	Hepatic	3–6
Atenolol	Low	50–60	2–4	Renal	3.5–7[c]
Bisoprolol	Moderate	~80	2–4	Hepatic and renal	9–12
Acebutolol	Moderate	30–50	2–4	Hepatic and renal	3–4
Metoprolol	High	~50	1–2	Hepatic	3–7[d]
Labetalol	High	~25	2–4	Hepatic	5–8

[a]Low <10%; moderate ~10% to 30%; high >30%.
[b]Primary route of elimination.
[c]Significantly prolonged in neonates.
[d]Elimination half-life in neonates is 5 to 10 hours.

Metoprolol was evaluated in 16 patients, ages 12 to 22 years, with primary or secondary hypertension.[47] Nine patients were concurrently treated with diuretic therapy. The initial dose of metoprolol was 50 mg BID and increased to 100 mg BID in nonresponders. Blood pressure decreased to less than the 90th percentile in all subjects within 3 to 12 months. No adverse effects were reported. The mean resting heart rate fell from 87 to 79 per minute in female patients and from 87 to 70 per minute in male patients.

Extended-release metoprolol succinate was studied in children aged 6 to 16 years.[53] The trial included a placebo group and three doses: 0.2, 1, and 2 mg per kg. There was a dose-dependent decrease in diastolic blood pressure (−7.5 mmHg for the highest dose group). No similar dose-dependent reduction was observed for systolic blood pressure (−7.7 mmHg for the middle-dose group compared with −6.3 mmHg in the highest dose group). Blood pressure fell to less than the 95th percentile in more than half of the subjects randomized to drug treatment compared with 26% of those randomized to placebo. The maximum reduction in heart rate was 6.5 per minute.

Bisoprolol combined with hydrochlorothiazide was compared with placebo in a randomized, double-blind study conducted in children aged 6 to 17 years.[48] A dose-escalation design was used to compare placebo to 2.5, 5, and 10 mg of bisoprolol combined with 6.25 mg of hydrochlorothiazide. Normalization of blood pressure to less than the 90th percentile occurred in 45% of the bisoprolol/hydrochlorothiazide-treated subjects compared with 34% of the subjects who received placebo. Significant reductions in systolic and diastolic blood pressures were observed in children aged 6 to 12 years, but not in those aged 13 to 17 years.

Esmolol, a β_1-selective adrenergic antagonist, has been used to treat arrhythmias and severe hypertension in children. It is administered by continuous infusion and has a very rapid onset of action and a terminal elimination half-life of 6.9 minutes.[54] In one study, esmolol was administered as a bolus infusion of 1,000 μg per kg followed by a continuous infusion of 300 μg per kg per min,[54] while others have used a lower bolus infusion (500 μg per kg) followed by a lower rate of infusion (25 to 200 μg per kg per min).[55] After discontinuation of the infusion, heart rate and blood pressure returned to baseline within 2 to 16 minutes. Neither study observed significant age-related differences in pharmacokinetics or pharmacodynamics of the drug.

Esmolol was used to treat hypertension in the postoperative period in 20 pediatric patients, ages 1 month to 12 years, who underwent cardiac surgery.[49] The mean (± standard deviation) rate of infusion was 700 ± 232 μg per kg per min. Blood pressure was successfully lowered to less than the 90th percentile in all subjects. During treatment, a significant reduction in heart rate was observed. In a randomized, double-blind trial, Tabbutt et al. compared three doses of esmolol in postoperative patients following repair of coarctation of the aorta (bolus doses of 125, 250, and 500 μg per kg per min, followed by infusions at the same rates) and noted a significant drop in blood pressure in this population, with no significant difference in blood pressure reduction between dosing levels or age groups.[56]

Adverse Effects

As a group, β-adrenergic antagonists appear to have a relatively high therapeutic index; however, several adverse effects may occur during therapy. Nonselective β-adrenergic antagonists have been associated with blockade of β_2 receptors in airway smooth muscle and may precipitate or exacerbate bronchospasm.[51,57] Blockade of β_1 receptors in the atria may result in bradycardia.[52] Antagonism of ventricular β_1 receptors reduces cardiac output and may result in dizziness or exercise intolerance, and, in more extreme cases, hypotension and congestive heart failure.[51] Blockade of β_1 and β_2 receptors in the gastrointestinal tract may cause constipation or dyspepsia.[51] The risk of adverse effects resulting from blockade of β_2 receptor may be reduced if cardioselective β antagonists are used at lower doses. However, at higher doses, β_2-antagonist activity may become evident even with β_1-selective antagonists.

Monotherapy with β-adrenergic antagonists has a variable effect on serum cholesterol and triglycerides. Propranolol, atenolol, and metoprolol tend to increase triglycerides and lower high-density lipoprotein (HDL) cholesterol while having less effect on total and low-density lipoprotein (LDL) cholesterol.[57] Treatment with labetalol or pindolol did not result in any significant change in serum lipids. Most selective β-adrenergic antagonists, especially those with partial agonist activity or combined α and β blockade, generally have less effect on serum HDL-cholesterol and triglycerides.[58,59]

Most β-adrenergic antagonists have minimal effect on serum glucose and carbohydrate metabolism.[60,61] However, patients with diabetes mellitus may have an exaggerated hypoglycemic response, and, in some patients, the warning signs of hypoglycemia are blunted. For those patients with labile glycemic control, β-adrenergic antagonists should be used with caution.

Occasionally, patients treated with β-adrenergic antagonists may experience depression, fatigue, sedation, and sleep disturbances, including insomnia and nightmares. The lipid solubility of β-adrenergic antagonists varies,[31] and penetration of lipophilic agents into the CNS may be higher than that observed for lipophobic agents. However, the observed central effects do not always correlate with higher lipid solubility. Patients report that β-adrenergic antagonists are also associated with male sexual dysfunction; this is difficult to substantiate as many other substances are associated with similar symptoms.

COMBINED α AND β ANTAGONISTS

Labetalol, an α_1-adrenergic and nonselective β-adrenergic antagonist, has been administered intravenously to treat acute hypertensive urgencies and emergencies in children.[62–64] Both intermittent and continuous intravenous administration have been used with monitoring in an intensive care setting. Continuous administration is often preferred. In one study of 15 subjects, infusion rates of 0.25 to 1.4 mg per kg per h were used for several days with few adverse effects.[62] There is some indication that young children with traumatic brain injury may develop significant hypotension, and, in this group, labetalol should be used with caution.[64]

CALCIUM CHANNEL ANTAGONISTS

Calcium channel antagonists are a heterogeneous group of compounds that block L-type calcium channels. These compounds exert their antihypertensive effect primarily through their action on voltage-sensitive calcium channels in vascular smooth muscle cell membranes, resulting in dose-dependent inhibition of the inward flux of calcium in the heart and vasculature.[65,66] Calcium channel antagonists also have a variable effect on the sinoatrial node pacemaker and on conduction through the atrioventricular node by altering the nodal-refractory period. The overall hemodynamic effect of these agents depends, in part, on their relative affinity for peripheral vascular myocytes or the myocardium. Agents with greater affinity for the heart may exhibit negative inotropic, chronotropic, and dromotropic effects.[65,66]

On the basis of molecular structure, pharmacodynamics, and clinical indications, calcium channel antagonists can be divided into four classes: dihydropyridines, phenylalkylamines, benzothiazepines, and benzimidazolyl-substituted tetralines.[67–70] All calcium channel antagonists cause dilation of peripheral resistance vessels, and the net physiologic effect is a decrease in total peripheral vascular resistance. In vitro, all calcium channel antagonists have a negative inotropic effect, but in humans, the dihydropyridine group triggers a strong baroreflex-mediated rise in sympathetic nerve activity that blunts the negative inotropic effect.[71] Due to their greater selectivity for vascular smooth muscle and minimal effect on cardiac smooth muscle, dihydropyridine calcium channel antagonists (e.g., amlodipine, nifedipine, nicardipine) are widely used to treat hypertension in children. Phenylalkylamines (e.g., verapamil) and benzothiazepines (e.g., diltiazem) have a depressive effect on cardiac conduction and have been used not only to lower blood pressure but also to control selected tachyarrhythmias. Benzimidazolyl-substituted tetralines (e.g., mibefradil) reduce the heart rate without much effect on cardiac contractility. However, mibefradil, a T-channel antagonist, was withdrawn from the market due to serious and sometimes fatal drug interactions.[72]

Administration of calcium channel antagonists initially improves glomerular filtration rate (GFR) and effective renal plasma flow (ERPF), but filtration fraction is unchanged.[70,73] These changes are thought to be related to afferent arteriolar dilation; but with improvement in hypertension, GFR and ERPF usually return to pretreatment levels within a few weeks,[73] although peripheral vascular resistance remains lower. Calcium channel antagonists, particularly the dihydropyridines, acutely increase renin release, but aldosterone usually does not rise. In some studies, the dihydropyridine calcium channel antagonists inhibited aldosterone production.[74] Calcium channel antagonists may induce an acute natriuresis and diuresis.[75,76] but clinically significant changes in serum electrolytes and body fluid composition are not acutely observed.[77] With prolonged use, some dihydropyridines may cause fluid retention, resulting in dependent edema.

Pharmacology

Many of the dihydropyridine derivatives are subject to a vigorous first-pass metabolic effect, reducing oral bioavailability (Table 50.9). With chronic use, oral bioavailability may increase. Peak serum concentrations are attained rapidly after administration of short-acting nifedipine, but not after administration of amlodipine or sustained-release preparations of nifedipine and isradipine. The primary route of metabolic degradation occurs via cytochrome P450 CYP3A4, and the metabolites are excreted in the urine or gastrointestinal tract. As there are many inducers and inhibitors of CYP3A4, coadministration with compounds that profoundly interfere with CYP3A4 activity should be considered carefully. The mean elimination half-life of nifedipine in children aged 5 to 68 months is 1.8 hours.[78] Amlodipine is unique in that it has a large volume of distribution and prolonged elimination half-life, approximating the 30- to 50-hour half-life in adults.[79] Verapamil and diltiazem have active metabolites (norverapamil and desacetyldiltiazem, respectively), but the potency of the metabolites appears to be less than that of the parent compounds.

NIFEDIPINE

Short-acting nifedipine has been widely used to treat hypertension in children,[80–83] although its use has diminished as safer options have become available. After administration of nifedipine in capsular form, the onset of action is apparent within 5 to 30 minutes, and the peak effect is observed in 30 to 60 minutes.[80–83] Sublingual administration leads to a slightly quicker onset of action, but onset after swallowing intact capsules is almost as rapid. The mean reduction in systolic and diastolic blood pressures was 27 to 45 and 32 to 37 mmHg, respectively, in several case series. The duration

TABLE 50.9 Pharmacology of Dihydropyridine Calcium Channel Antagonists

	Oral Bioavailability (%)	T_{max} *(h)*	*Protein Binding (%)*	*Metabolism*	*Primary (Secondary) Elimination Routes*	*Elimination Half-life (h)*
Amlodipine	64–90	6–12	93	Hepatic (CYP3A4)	Renal (hepatic)	30–50
Felodipine[a]	20	2.5–5	99	Hepatic (CYP3A4)	Renal (hepatic)	11–16
Isradipine[a]	15–24	1.5	95	Hepatic (CYP3A4)	Renal (hepatic)	8
Isradipine ER	15–24	7–18	95	Hepatic (CYP3A4)	Renal (hepatic)	8
Nifedipine	60–75	0.5–1	92–98	Hepatic (CYP3A4)	Renal (hepatic)	2
Nifedipine ER[b]	50–60	2.5–5	92–98	Hepatic (CYP3A4)	Renal (hepatic)	2
Nicardipine IV[c]	N/A	N/A	>95	Hepatic (CYP3A4)	Hepatic	2.7 min

[a]Felodipine and isradipine are absorbed well (>90%), but extensive first-pass metabolism significantly reduces oral bioavailability. Food reduces the rate, but not the extent of absorption for both felodipine and isradipine. Both drugs are metabolized to inactive metabolites, which are excreted in the urine and feces. An extended-release formulation is available for both drugs.
[b]Extended-release nifedipine slowly releases nifedipine over 12 to 24 hours. Once absorbed, metabolism occurs through the same hepatic biotransformation pathways as the rapid-release nifedipine capsules. The half-life may be as short as 60 minutes in some individuals.
[c]The α half-life is 2.7 minutes, and the β half-life is 44.8 minutes. The slow terminal elimination half-life is 14.4 hours.

of effect was generally 4 to 5 hours after administration of the capsules, although effective blood pressure control reportedly lasted up to 12 hours in a few patients. In several studies, mean heart rate increased significantly after acute administration.[80,83]

Because serious adverse effects have been reported, the use of short-acting nifedipine in children has become controversial.[74,84,85] To administer short-acting nifedipine capsules to small children, the liquid contents must be removed from a 10-mg capsule, often with a 1-mL syringe, leading to imprecise dosing. In a retrospective review, adverse effects in children included severe hypotension, oxygen desaturation, and neurologic events, such as deterioration in neurologic status and stroke.[85] Neurologic events were particularly seen after administration to patients with acute CNS injury. In contrast, in a retrospective review of 117 hypertensive patients, mean arterial pressure decreased by greater than or equal to 25% in 35% of the treated patients without any reported serious adverse effects.[86] If short-acting nifedipine is used in a monitored hospital setting to treat severe hypertension, the initial dose should not exceed 0.25 mg per kg (maximum initial dose: 10 mg). Many pediatricians have abandoned the use of short-acting nifedipine.

In contrast to short-acting nifedipine, sustained-release formulations of nifedipine are used in older pediatric patients who are able to swallow tablets. The sustained-release formulations slowly release nifedipine as the tablet traverses the intestinal tract, resulting in much lower peak plasma concentrations, thus avoiding the higher plasma concentrations and more rapid and brief effect seen with the short-acting form. No large, controlled trials of sustained-release nifedipine have been conducted in children. Dosing information, based largely on off-label use, suggests that initial doses up to 0.5 mg per kg per dose can be safely used. Because nifedipine, like the other dihydropyridine calcium channel antagonists, is metabolized by CYP3A4, dose adjustments for patients with renal failure are not needed.

FELODIPINE

Extended-release felodipine was evaluated in 133 children, ages 6 to 16 years, with essential hypertension.[87] The subjects were randomized to receive placebo or one of three doses (2.5, 5, or 10 mg) administered once daily. Subjects randomized to all three active treatment groups started at 2.5 mg daily. Children assigned to the 5- and 10-mg dose groups were titrated at weekly intervals, until the maximum dose was reached. The duration of the study was 3 weeks. A reduction in diastolic blood pressure was observed after 2 weeks on the 5-mg dose when compared with placebo, but the 2.5- and 10-mg groups were not significantly different from placebo. The systolic blood pressure was not statistically different from placebo at any of the three doses. In a 16-week open-label extension, children receiving the 10-mg dose failed to achieve any incremental antihypertensive effect. Responders, considered to be those whose systolic and diastolic blood pressures dropped to less than the 90th percentile, were 19.4% in the 10-mg dosing group and less in the other groups. There did not appear to be a dose response over the limited range of doses. Except for a lower incidence of edema, adverse effects were similar to those observed in adult trials.

ISRADIPINE

The use of isradipine for secondary or urgent hypertension in hospitalized children has been reviewed retrospectively.[88–90] Doses varied widely, but the mean (± standard deviation) in two reports was 0.36 ± 0.17 and 0.38 ± 0.22 mg per kg per day, respectively. The total daily dose of short-acting isradipine was divided and administered two to four times daily in the majority of patients. Mean reduction in blood pressure also was variable. In one report, systolic and/or diastolic blood pressures fell 10% or more in 81% of the treated patients.[89] An extemporaneous liquid formulation was prepared and used in younger children.[90] Adverse effects included dizziness, headache, flushing, reflex tachycardia, and palpitations. In one review, five patients experienced hypotension, and four of those required intervention with saline fluid boluses and/or dopamine.[88] Because of the short duration of action requiring frequent dosing, a sustained-release preparation of isradipine is currently available for the treatment of chronic hypertension.

AMLODIPINE

Amlodipine has been widely used in pediatric patients for longer term control of blood pressure.[75] The main advantage of amlodipine compared with other dihydropyridine calcium channel antagonists is a prolonged elimination half-life, maintaining blood pressure control for an extended period of time. The long half-life allows once-daily dosing in most children, but some require BID dosing.[91] Amlodipine is usually not associated with the large swings in blood pressure seen with dihydropyridines that have a shorter duration of action. Doses ranged from 0.02 to 0.63 mg per kg per day (mean dose = 0.17 mg per kg per day). Children aged 12 years and younger appeared to require higher doses than older children.[92] Recently, a commercial suspension (1 mg per mL) has been approved and is replacing the extemporaneous suspensions previously used.

A randomized, placebo-controlled study examining the effectiveness and safety of amlodipine was conducted in 268 children aged 6 to 16 years.[93] Reductions in systolic blood pressure were observed in children receiving either 2.5 mg or 5 mg of amlodipine when compared with placebo (−6.9 and −8.7 mmHg, respectively). Systolic blood pressure was reduced to less than the 95th percentile in 34.6% of the children. Diastolic blood pressure, a secondary outcome, was also lowered.

Adverse effects reported with amlodipine use include headaches, dizziness, fatigue, and flushing. Long-term use in children has been occasionally associated with gingival hypertrophy and lower extremity edema.[94]

NICARDIPINE

Nicardipine is available in oral and intravenous formulations. Intravenous use has been reported in hypertensive urgencies and emergencies[95–101] as well as intraoperatively (spinal fusions)[102] and postoperatively (repair of aortic coarctation).[103,104]

Children as young as 1.5 months have been treated with intravenous nicardipine in nonrandomized, uncontrolled case series. The initial dose of nicardipine ranged from 0.2 to 5.0 μg per kg per min, but the most common starting dose was 0.5 to 1.0 μg per kg per min. Blood pressure was controlled in 15 minutes in one series, but the infusion rate was higher than in patients reported in other studies.[100] Titration of the rate of infusion occurred every 15 to 30 minutes in one report.[98] Blood pressure control was achieved within hours using infusion rates from 0.3 to 5.5 μg per kg per min, but short-term use of up to 10 μg per kg per min has been reported.[96,98,100,101] Tachycardia was observed frequently, but because many other factors may have affected heart rate in these critically ill children, it is difficult to attribute the increase solely to nicardipine. Other reported adverse effects included clinically significant hypotension (treated with intravenous saline and calcium), flushing, palpitations, and thrombophlebitis at peripheral infusion sites.[99]

ANGIOTENSIN-CONVERTING ENZYME INHIBITORS

The renin–angiotensin–aldosterone system (RAAS) plays a key role in the regulation of blood pressure. As depicted in Figure 50.2, renin catalyzes the conversion of angiotensinogen, which is synthesized primarily in the liver, to angiotensin I (Ang-I). In the kidney, renin is secreted by the juxtaglomerular cells located along the glomerular afferent arterioles adjacent to the macula densa. Renin release is stimulated by at least three mechanisms: decreased movement of NaCl across the macula densa, reduction in hydrostatic pressure at the glomerular afferent arteriole, and stimulation of postganglionic sympathetic nerves.

Ang-I is a decapeptide that is rapidly cleaved by ACE to form the octapeptide Ang-II. ACE is structurally identical to kininase II, the enzyme that converts bradykinin, a potent vasodilator, to inactive metabolites (Fig. 50.2). Circulating Ang-I is converted to Ang-II primarily by ACE located in the pulmonary epithelial cells. Ang-II is further degraded at the N-terminal end to Ang-III by aminopeptidase A and Ang-IV. Ang-II and Ang-III are equally potent stimulators of aldosterone release, but Ang-III has less vasopressor activity. Ang-III may play a role in the central regulation of body fluid homeostasis as it has been purported to stimulate vasopressin release during hypovolemia.

Ang-II raises blood pressure by both rapid- and slow-onset mechanisms. The more rapid increase in blood pressure is mediated by direct vasoconstriction, stimulation of the sympathetic nervous system, and, to a lesser extent, adrenal release of catecholamines. These actions effectively raise blood pressure within seconds to minutes. Ang-II also acts directly on the proximal tubule to increase sodium reabsorption and stimulates aldosterone release from the zona glomerulosa in the adrenal cortex, resulting in increased sodium reabsorption in the distal nephron. These latter effects increase blood pressure by expanding the blood volume but require hours or days before a significant response is observed.

The RAAS is also active at the tissue level in the heart, brain, kidney, blood vessels, and adrenal gland. At the local level, the RAAS plays an important role in endothelial dysfunction, vascular remodeling, and ventricular hypertrophy.

PHARMACOLOGY OF ANGIOTENSIN-CONVERTING ENZYME INHIBITORS

ACEIs have been classified into three distinct groups that have different structural and pharmacologic profiles[105] (Table 50.10). Despite structural differences, all of these agents act to competitively inhibit binding of ACE to Ang-I, resulting in a rapid reduction in circulating Ang-II. All of the ACEIs, except captopril and lisinopril, are prodrugs that are rapidly absorbed in the gastrointestinal tract and then metabolized to form active metabolites, which are potent inhibitors of ACE. Once activated, the initial reduction in blood pressure primarily results from a direct decrease in systemic vascular resistance and reduced

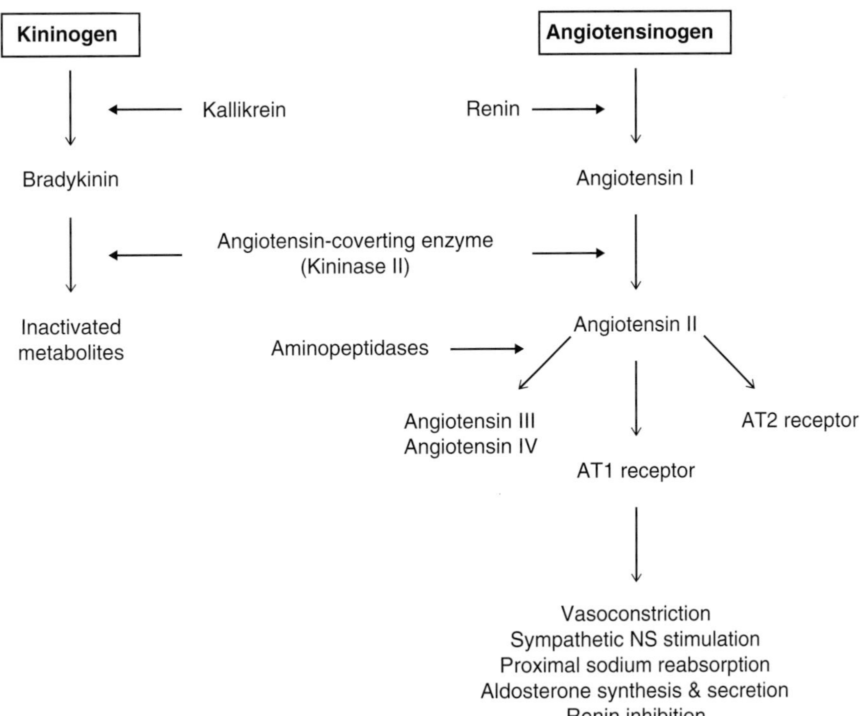

Figure 50.2 The renin–angiotensin–aldosterone system (RAAS): antihypertensive agents affect the RAAS at several points, primarily through inhibition of enzyme activity or interference with binding between substrates and receptors. AT1, angiotensin type 1; AT2, angiotensin type 2; NS, nervous system. (Illustration by Nick Wells.)

TABLE 50.10 Pharmacology of Orally Administered Angiotensin-Converting Enzyme Inhibitors

	Oral Bioavailability (%)	T_{max} *(h)*	*Protein Binding (%)*	*Major Metabolites*[a]	*Primary Elimination Routes*	*Elimination Half-life (h)*
Benazepril	35–40	0.5–1	97	Benazeprilat	Renal	0.4–0.8
Benazeprilat	<10	1–4	95	Glucuronides[b]	Renal	10–11
Captopril[c]	60–75	0.5–2	25–30	Cysteine-captopril disulfide; captopril dimer disulfide	Renal	2
Enalapril	60–70	0.5–1.5	NA	Enalaprilat	Renal	<2
Enalaprilat	<10	2–4	50	None	Renal	11–16
Fosinopril	35–40	1	NA	Fosinoprilat	Renal/hepatic	<2
Fosinoprilat	<10	3–4	99	Glucuronide, *p*-hydroxy metabolite	Renal	11–13
Lisinopril	28	5–6	0	No major metabolites	Renal	9–12
Quinapril	60	0.5–1.5	97	Quinaprilat	Renal	<2
Quinaprilat	<10	1.5–2.5	97	No major metabolites	Renal	25
Ramipril	50–60	1	73	Ramiprilat	Hepatic	<2
Ramiprilat	<10	2–4	56	Glucuronide, diketopiperazine ester, diketopiperazine acid	Renal/hepatic	13–17

[a]Metabolites of benazepril, enalapril, fosinopril, quinapril, and ramipril have greater antihypertensive activity and a longer duration of action than their prodrugs. Most of the active metabolites are further transformed in the liver by UDP-glucuronosyltransferase.[105]
[b]Glucuronidation is a minor elimination pathway for both benazepril and benazeprilat.
[c]Food reduces the extent of absorption.

sympathetic stimulation, which further reduces vascular resistance. In the longer term, ACE inhibition reduces aldosterone release and renal NaCl reabsorption. Some individuals display ACE escape phenomenon or aldosterone synthesis escape, resulting in blunting of the antihypertensive response and possibly contributing to ongoing tissue injury.[106] Circulating Ang-II is produced by ACE, but Ang-II generated in local tissue sites can be produced by ACE or tissue chymases.[107]

Under normal circumstances, ACEIs are not associated with reflex tachycardia or reduced cardiac output.[108] In children with congestive cardiomyopathy treated with captopril, cardiac index increased and the blood pressure was maintained, despite a significant drop in systemic vascular resistance.[109] However, in those children with restrictive cardiomyopathy, cardiac index did not increase, and significant hypotension was observed.

CAPTOPRIL

Captopril was the first ACEI approved for widespread clinical use. It has been studied extensively in children with proteinuria, renal and renovascular hypertension, and congestive heart failure.[109–116] Captopril effectively reduced blood pressure in the majority of children with severe hypertension, both in the short term[111,112] and over a longer period of time.[114,117]

The antihypertensive effect associated with captopril is evident quickly, often within 15 to 30 minutes, and the blood pressure nadir is usually achieved in 1 to 2 hours.[111,112] Maximum plasma concentrations (T_{max}) occurred between 0.5 and 2.0 hours in children with renal or renovascular hypertension as well as those with congestive heart failure.[111–113] Blood pressure returned to baseline after 6 to 10 hours,[111] suggesting that the dosing interval may need to be more frequent than twice daily in some patients. The elimination half-life in children with normal renal function was reported as 1 to 2 hours but was increased in those with reduced renal function or congestive heart failure.[111,112] These findings are similar to adults,[108] where, under normal circumstances, elimination is rapid and the duration of effective blood pressure control compared with other ACEIs is brief.

Captopril has been used extensively in neonates.[116,118–120] Renal blood flow in the newborn, especially premature newborns, is highly dependent on an intact RAAS.[121] As a result, newborns often exhibit a dramatic response to weight-based doses similar to those used in older children and adults. Attempts to use an initial dose of 0.3 to 0.5 mg per kg per dose resulted in profound hypotension in neonates accompanied by oliguria and, in some instances, renal failure.[120,121] Neurologic manifestations, including seizures, were temporally related to a 40% to 72% drop in systolic blood pressure after administration of captopril at a dose of 0.3 mg per kg.[122] Subsequently, the recommended initial dose in neonates was reduced to 0.01 mg per kg and titrated upward according to response.[119] No further episodes of profound hypotension were observed. The total dose of captopril required to control blood pressure was significantly lower in neonates than that in older children.[123] This has proven to be true for other ACEIs as well.

ENALAPRIL AND ENALAPRILAT

Enalaprilat, the active metabolite of enalapril maleate, is poorly absorbed from the gastrointestinal tract. In adults, addition of the ester group to enalaprilat to form enalapril maleate increased oral bioavailability from less than 10% to 55% to 75%.[108,124,125] Following absorption, enalapril maleate is rapidly hydrolyzed by hepatic esterases to form enalaprilat. The ACE inhibiting potency of enalapril is less than 1% of enalaprilat.[71] Enalapril has been available in tablet form and as an extemporaneously compounded solution for many years,[126] but a commercial oral solution was recently approved at a 1 mg per mL concentration.

Peak serum concentrations of enalapril occur within 30 to 90 minutes, but enalaprilat does not peak until approximately 4 hours after administration in adults.[124,127] The time to peak serum concentrations (T_{max}) is more variable in younger children. The median T_{max} is 6 hours in children aged 2 to 23 months compared with 4 hours in children aged 12 to 16 years.[128] In patients with severe liver disease, conversion of enalapril to enalaprilat may be delayed.[129]

Enalapril and enalaprilat are both eliminated in the urine. In children aged 2 to 16 years who received orally administered enalapril, combined urinary recovery of enalapril and enalaprilat over 24 hours was 47% to 86%, similar to that observed in adults.[128] Conversion of enalapril to enalaprilat in children was approximately 65% to 70%. The mean half-life for accumulation ranged from 14.6 hours in children aged 12 to 16 years to 16.3 hours in children aged 6 to 11 years.[128]

Enalapril and enalaprilat have been studied extensively in children with renal disease,[130–132] congestive heart failure,[133–136] and hypertension.[128,137–141] In children with hypertension, enalapril, administered once daily, effectively lowered blood pressure in children aged 6 to 16 years in a dose-dependent manner within 2 weeks.[138] The mean dose in the highest dosing group was 0.58 mg per kg per dose administered once daily. Recommended dosing for enalapril is presented in Table 50.4.

Neonates have been treated with both enalapril and enalaprilat.[133,139,140] Enalapril and enalaprilat appear to effectively lower blood pressure, but, as with captopril, dosage reductions are necessary to avoid hypotension, oliguria, and acute renal failure.[140,142] Enalaprilat has been especially useful in the short-term treatment of renal and renovascular hypertension and in those who do not tolerate orally administered medications. As with other ACEIs, enalapril and enalaprilat should not be used in children with bilateral renal artery stenosis or unilateral renal artery stenosis in a single kidney. Long-term administration of enalapril and other ACEIs in children with unilateral renal artery stenosis may result in reduced function in the affected kidney.

LISINOPRIL

Lisinopril is the lysine analog of enalaprilat. Unlike enalapril, lisinopril is readily absorbed from the intestinal tract and does not require activation by hepatic esterases. The oral bioavailability of lisinopril in adults[143] and children[144,145] is 20% to 50%. Lisinopril has been available in tablet form and as an extemporaneously compounded solution for many years, but a commercial oral solution was recently approved in a 1 mg per mL concentration.

In an open-label study, median time to peak plasma concentrations (T_{max}) in children aged 1 month to 15 years ranged from 5 to 6 hours.[144] This range is similar to values historically observed in adults.[143] Lisinopril, unlike other ACEIs, does not undergo metabolism and is eliminated unchanged in the urine. In 22 renal transplant patients with stable renal function, the mean T_{max} in three different dosing groups (0.1, 0.2, and 0.4 mg per kg daily) was 4.5 to 5.0 hours, and the mean terminal elimination half-life for lisinopril was 9.4 to 12.4 hours.[145] These values are similar to other studies conducted in adults, children, and adolescents.

The effectiveness and safety of lisinopril was demonstrated in a study involving 115 children aged 6 to 16 years.[146] Lisinopril was shown to reduce both systolic and diastolic blood pressures in a dose-dependent manner. Low doses (mean = 0.02 mg per kg daily) were not effective. A mean dose of 0.07 mg per kg administered once daily resulted in a reduction in systolic and diastolic blood pressures of 12.1 and 9.3 mmHg, respectively, after 2 weeks. Higher doses (mean = 0.61 mg per kg per dose administered once daily) resulted in corresponding reductions in systolic and diastolic blood pressures of 15.2 and 16.4 mmHg, respectively. The maximum daily dose was limited to 40 mg administered once daily. Lisinopril also appeared to effectively lower blood pressure in renal transplant recipients, but due to small numbers of subjects, a dose-dependent effect was not observed.[145]

OTHER ANGIOTENSIN-CONVERTING ENZYME INHIBITORS

Benazepril, fosinopril, moexipril, perindopril, quinapril, ramipril, and trandolapril are similar to enalapril, in that they all are prodrugs. Each prodrug is absorbed well from the gastrointestinal tract, then undergoes hydroxylation by hepatic esterases to active metabolites. Further biotransformation of these drugs varies, with some being converted to glucuronides by UDP-glucuronosyltransferase prior to renal elimination.[105] As with enalapril, biotransformation results in a delay in the appearance of active metabolites, a longer time to peak plasma concentrations, and a delay of 30 minutes or longer in the onset of action, making them less suitable for hypertensive urgencies than drugs that are more rapidly bioavailable.[108]

The single-dose pharmacokinetics of fosinopril was studied in 20 pediatric patients aged 6 to 16 years.[147] After a dose of 0.3 mg per kg, the mean area under the concentration–time curve (*AUC*) was similar to that seen in adults receiving an equivalent dose. Maximum peak plasma concentrations were also similar to those observed in adults. The mean terminal elimination half-life was 11 to 13 hours. A safety and efficacy trial was conducted in children aged 6 to 16 years with hypertension or high normal blood pressure.[148] Subjects were randomized to receive one of three doses of fosinopril (0.1, 0.3, or 0.6 mg per kg once daily). All three doses lowered blood pressure, but a dose–response relationship was not observed for either systolic or diastolic blood pressure. On average, both systolic and diastolic blood pressures decreased by 11 to 12 and 4 to 5 mmHg from baseline, respectively, after 4 weeks of therapy. Although fosinopril appeared to be effective, design flaws in the trial likely led to the failure to demonstrate a dose–response effect.[149] During the open-label phase of the trial, 83% of the subjects attained their target blood pressure.[148] As with other ACEIs, an antiproteinuric effect of fosinopril in children with steroid-resistant nephrotic syndrome has also been reported.[150]

The pharmacokinetics of quinapril were studied in 24 children aged 2.5 to 82 months.[151] Each subject received a 0.2 mg per kg dose of quinapril syrup. Quinapril was rapidly converted to quinaprilat, and peak plasma concentrations (C_{max}) for quinaprilat were observed at 1 to 2 hours. The mean half-life for quinaprilat was 2.3 hours and did not appear to be age dependent. The elimination half-life of quinaprilat was similar to adults with normal renal function.[152] The safety and effectiveness of quinapril has not been established in children.

Two randomized safety and effectiveness trials using ramipril were done in hypertensive children under a Written Request from the U.S. Food and Drug Administration. The first failed to show adequate efficacy, and the second was terminated early. Ramipril was shown to be effective and safe in the ESCAPE trial, conducted in 397 children aged 3 to 18 years with chronic renal failure.[153] A fixed dose of 6 mg per m^2 was given to all subjects for 6 months. Mean arterial pressure was reduced by 11.5 mmHg in subjects who initially had hypertension and by 4.4 mmHg in subjects whose blood pressure was initially normal. Mean urinary protein excretion was reduced by 50%.

The single-dose pharmacokinetics of benazepril in hypertensive children aged 0.7 to 16 years differs from published data in adults.[154] Benazepril is absorbed rapidly and hydrolyzed quickly to its active metabolite, benazeprilat. The mean time to maximum plasma concentrations (T_{max}) for benazeprilat is 1 to 2 hours.[155] The clearance of benazeprilat in children aged 2 to 5 years is twice that of adults. Clearance decreases throughout the remainder of the pediatric age range. Clearance in adolescents (13 to 17 years) was 27% more rapid than adults. The mean elimination half-life is approximately 5 to 5.5 hours in all pediatric age groups, which is less than half of that observed in adults. In a clinical study involving 107 children, benazepril was administered in doses from 0.1 to 0.6 mg per kg once daily.[156] Over this narrow dose range, no dose-dependent antihypertensive effect was observed, although blood pressure was reduced compared with children withdrawn to placebo.

ADVERSE EFFECTS OF ANGIOTENSIN-CONVERTING ENZYME INHIBITORS

Adverse effects related to ACEIs have been well documented.[114,138,146,157] In addition to hypotension, oliguria, and renal failure, hyperkalemia has been reported, especially in children with glomerular disease and renal failure. Headache and dizziness have been observed frequently in pediatric clinical trials. Rarely, cholestatic jaundice that may progress to hepatic failure has occurred.[158] Captopril has been associated with skin rash and leukopenia in a small number of patients.[114] A nonproductive cough, observed in approximately 1% to 4% of adults,[159] has been reported in children as well.[148,160,161] The cough subsides with discontinuation of ACEI therapy. Angioedema is an important but fortunately rare adverse effect and may be fatal.[161,162] More recently and of great concern to children who potentially may receive ACEIs for decades, an association between long-term use of ACEIs and the development of lung cancer has been reported in adults.[163,164] The association was evident after taking ACEIs for 5 years and appeared to increase as the duration of treatment increased. The overall risk was reported as 1.3 per 1,000 patient-years.[163]

ACEIs have been associated with fetal anomalies after prolonged in utero exposure during the second and third trimesters of pregnancy.[165,166] ACE fetopathy is characterized by renal tubular dysplasia, oligohydramnios, pulmonary hypoplasia, positional deformities of the limbs and face, decreased ossification of the skull, and postnatal renal failure. ACEIs should be avoided during pregnancy and should be stopped as soon as pregnancy is confirmed.

ANGIOTENSIN II–RECEPTOR ANTAGONISTS

Ang-II–binding sites include the angiotensin type 1 receptor (AT1R) and angiotensin type 2 receptor (AT2R), both of which bind Ang-II. Two additional binding sites are purported to bind Ang-II. These receptors have been studied less thoroughly and include MAS, an oncogene that is a putative receptor for the seven amino acid peptide degradation product of Ang-II and an Ang-IV–binding site.[167] The hypertensive effects of Ang-II appeared to be mediated primarily through the type 1 receptors. Evidence suggests that activation of the AT1R results in vasoconstriction, aldosterone synthesis and release, sodium reabsorption, and increased vasopressin release. Activation of AT1R may also cause vascular smooth muscle cell proliferation, vascular medial hypertrophy, and cardiac hypertrophy.[168] Stimulation of AT2Rs appears to oppose many of the effects associated with AT1R activation, resulting in vasodilation, inhibition of cellular growth, and promotion of cellular differentiation and tissue regeneration.[107,169]

PHARMACOLOGY OF ANGIOTENSIN II–RECEPTOR ANTAGONISTS

The Ang-II–receptor antagonists (ARBs) exert their effect through inhibition of binding of Ang-II to the AT1R and have a minimal direct effect on the AT2R. The affinity of ARBs for AT1Rs is approximately 1,000 times greater than their affinity for AT2Rs.[107] Unlike treatment with ACEIs, plasma levels of Ang-II increase during therapy with ARBs. However, ARBs inhibit binding of Ang-II to the AT1R, thus blunting the effect of higher Ang-II levels.

The absorption, metabolism, and elimination of ARBs vary among drugs. Candesartan cilexetil, olmesartan medoxomil, and azilsartan medoxomil are bioactivated by hydrolysis in the gastrointestinal tract during absorption. Losartan, irbesartan, valsartan, and telmisartan do not require gastrointestinal bioactivation. Losartan, irbesartan, and azilsartan are metabolized by CYP2C9, but the other ARBs are either cleared with minimal metabolism, undergo glucuronidation, or, in the case of azilsartan, are metabolized to inactive metabolites (Table 50.11). For drugs metabolized by CYP2C9, patients who also receive strong inhibitors of CYP2C9 (e.g., fluconazole) may have an exaggerated effect.

LOSARTAN

Losartan is a competitive inhibitor of the Ang-II AT1R. Losartan is rapidly absorbed from the gastrointestinal tract and metabolized by CYP2C9 to form an active metabolite, E-3174, a more potent, noncompetitive inhibitor of Ang-II binding to AT1. After an oral dose, peak serum concentrations of losartan and E-3174 are observed at 1 to 2 and 4 to 7 hours, respectively, in children aged 1 month to 15 years.[170] The multiple-dose pharmacokinetics of losartan in children aged 6 to 16 years was similar to that seen in adults. Losartan and E-3174 are excreted in the urine. In adults, renal clearance is reduced in patients with renal insufficiency.

To assess the antihypertensive effect of losartan, 177 children aged 6 to 16 years were treated using doses ranging from 2.5 to 100 mg.[171] A dose–response relationship was observed for diastolic blood pressure, but not for systolic blood pressure. Mean diastolic blood pressure after three weeks of treatment decreased by 6.0, 11.7, and 12.2 mmHg in the low (2.5/5 mg for children (<50 kg/ ≥50 kg), middle (25/50 mg), and high (50/100 mg) dose groups. Systolic blood pressure decreased by 4.4, 10.0, and 8.6 mmHg over the same time period, respectively.

TABLE 50.11 Pharmacology of Angiotensin II–Receptor Antagonists

	Oral Bioavailability (%)	*T_{max} (h)*	*Protein Binding (%)*	*Metabolism*	*Primary (Secondary) Elimination Routes*	*Elimination Half-life (h)*
Azilsartan	60	2–4	99	CYP2C9[a]	Hepatic (renal)	4–7
Candesartan[b]	15	4.3	99	O-demethylation (minor metabolic pathway)	Renal (biliary excretion)	5–7
Irbesartan	60–80	1.5–2	90	Glucuronidation	Biliary excretion (renal)	11–15
Losartan[c]	33	Losartan: 2.0 E-3174 (active metabolite): 4.1	99	CYP2C9 and CYP3A4	Renal and biliary excretion	Losartan: 2.3 ± 0.8 E-3174: 5.6 ± 1.2
Olmesartan[d]	26	2–4	99	Insignificant	Renal (biliary excretion)	8–9
Telmisartan	≈40–50	1.0–1.5	99	Glucuronidation	Biliary excretion	27–28
Valsartan	10–35	2	95	CYP2C9[e]	Biliary excretion (renal)	4–6

[a]Metabolites M-I and M-II are inactive.
[b]Candesartan cilexetil is rapidly converted to candesartan by ester hydrolysis during absorption from the gastrointestinal tract. Unchanged candesartan is excreted in the urine and bile. An inactive metabolite constitutes a minor pathway for clearance of the drug.
[c]Losartan undergoes first-pass metabolism and has an active carboxylic acid metabolite (E-3174) that is a noncompetitive antagonist of Ang-II. Several inactive metabolites are also formed. Losartan and the active metabolite are highly bound to plasma proteins. Both are excreted in the urine and feces.
[d]Like candesartan, olmesartan medoxomil is rapidly converted to olmesartan by ester hydrolysis during absorption from the gastrointestinal tract. The elimination half-life in adults is reported to be 13 hours.
[e]Valsartan appears to be a CYP2C9 substrate.

The effectiveness of losartan was confirmed when subjects were re-randomized to either continuation of active treatment or withdrawal to placebo.

Children (n = 101) aged 6 months to 6 years received losartan 0.1, 0.3, or 0.7 mg per kg once daily.[172] The dose in the high-dose group was titrated to 1.4 mg per kg (maximum dose 100 mg). Blood pressure reduction was confirmed, but dose dependence was not observed for systolic or diastolic blood pressure after 3 weeks of treatment. A 2-year open-label extension followed the randomized open-label phase. The incidence of treatment-emergent adverse effects related to losartan was low.

Losartan has been used in several other pediatric trials. Long-term antiproteinuric and renoprotective effects have been observed after treatment with losartan.[173,174] Losartan was shown to effectively reduced proteinuria over 3 years in children aged 1 to 17 years.[175] Losartan has also been used to slow aortic root dilation in children and young adults with Marfan syndrome[176] and in a pilot study to treat nonalcoholic fatty liver disease.[177]

IRBESARTAN

Irbesartan is rapidly absorbed after oral administration in both adults and children.[178] Median maximum serum concentrations (C_{max}) were observed at 2 hours in children aged 6 years and older after a single dose of 2 mg per kg and at steady state. Unlike losartan, irbesartan does not have an active metabolite. Only a small fraction of an administered dose is excreted unchanged in the urine. Biliary excretion represents the major elimination pathway.[179] The pharmacokinetics of irbesartan is similar in adults and children aged 6 years and older.[178] Based on the pharmacokinetic data, initial doses of 75 and 150 mg once daily were recommended in children aged 6 to 12 years and 13 to 17 years, respectively.[178]

Forty-four children aged 3.7 to 18 years were treated for 18 weeks with irbesartan.[180] The initial daily dose ranged from 2.2 to 2.9 mg per kg and was increased in nonresponders to a maximum daily dose of 5.0 mg per kg. Mean systolic and diastolic blood pressures decreased by 17 and 10 mmHg, respectively, after 18 weeks of treatment. Of the 36 patients who had arterial hypertension at the beginning of the trial, 20 were normotensive after 18 weeks. There was no apparent relationship between dose and reduction of blood pressure. Of the 20 patients who had proteinuria, 13 experienced a 25% or greater reduction in urine protein excretion during the study.

CANDESARTAN

Candesartan was studied in 93 hypertensive children aged 1 to 5 years.[181] A liquid suspension was administered to three dosing groups (0.05, 0.2, and 0.4 mg per kg daily). At 4 weeks, systolic blood pressure was reduced by 6, 9, and 12 mmHg, respectively, in the three groups. Diastolic blood pressure fell by 5, 8, and 11 mmHg, respectively, in the same three groups. Subjects continued in an extension trial and, at the end of 1 year, approximately 50% of the drug-treated subjects were normotensive. In those children with proteinuria, a 57% decline in albumin-to-creatinine ratio was observed.

The pharmacokinetics of candesartan in children aged 6 to 17 years was examined as part of a larger safety and effectiveness trial.[182] Children weighing less than 50 kg received placebo or one of three doses (2, 8, or 16 mg daily). Comparable doses in those weighing 50 kg or above were 4, 16, or 32 mg. Single-dose pharmacokinetics were obtained in 22 subjects. Mean T_{max} was

4.3 hours, and mean elimination half-life was 6.7 hours in children aged 6 to 11 years and 5.7 hours in adolescents aged 12 to 17 years. AUC_{0-24h} and C_{max} were similar in the two age groups. After 4 weeks of therapy, systolic and diastolic blood pressures were significantly lower than the placebo group, but a dose–response relationship was not observed. The largest drop in blood pressure was seen in the middle-dose group. In a 1-year extension study, 52% of the children were considered to have responded to candesartan (range: 50% to 63% at various time points during the year).

In an uncontrolled, short-term study of 11 hypertensive children who received an initial dose of 2 to 8 mg of candesartan, which was doubled if blood pressure response was inadequate, response was measured by casual blood pressures, ambulatory blood pressure monitoring, and home blood pressures.[183] Clinically significant reductions in blood pressure were observed by casual and ambulatory blood pressures, but no significant difference was seen in home blood pressure measurements.

VALSARTAN

The pharmacokinetics of valsartan was assessed in 26 children aged 1 to 16 years.[184] The mean T_{max} in all age groups was observed at approximately 2 hours after administration of the valsartan liquid suspension. The mean elimination half-life was 3.79 (ages 1 to <4 years), 3.95 (ages 4 to <6 years), 5.33 (ages 8 to <12 years), and 4.97 hours (ages 12 to 16 years). Normalized clearance and *AUC* were similar across all ages.

The safety and effectiveness of valsartan was assessed in 90 children aged 1 to 5 years with systolic hypertension.[185] Children were assigned to one of three dosing groups. The low-dose group received 5 mg of valsartan (weight <18 kg) or 10 mg (weight ≥18 kg), while children in the middle- and high-dose groups received 20/40 mg or 40/80 mg based on weight, respectively. Systolic and diastolic blood pressure decreased in each of the three groups, but a dose-dependent reduction was not observed. Following the dose–response phase of the study, half of the subjects were withdrawn to placebo, while the remainder continued on active treatment. Statistically significant differences in both systolic and diastolic blood pressures were observed, confirming the effectiveness of valsartan in young children.

Children (n = 261) aged 6 to 16 years were studied using a study design similar to that used in younger children.[186] Systolic and diastolic blood pressures in the low- (10/20 mg for children less than 35 kg/ ≥ 35 kg), middle- (40/80 mg) and high- (80/160 mg) dose groups decreased with therapy. The reduction in blood pressure was dose dependent, with reductions in systolic and diastolic blood pressures of 7.9/4.6 mmHg (low-dose groups), 9.6/5.8 mmHg (middle-dose groups), and 11.5/7.4 mmHg (high-dose groups). The effectiveness of valsartan was confirmed during a 2-week, double-blind study period where children were re-randomized to either continue on low-, medium-, or high-dose valsartan or switch to placebo.

OLMESARTAN

Olmesartan, like candesartan, is activated by ester hydrolysis during absorption in the gastrointestinal tract. The single-dose pharmacokinetics of olmesartan was studied in 24 hypertensive children aged 2 to 16 years.[187] Mean (± standard deviation) maximum serum concentrations were observed at 2.8 ± 1.3 and 2.5 ± 1.1 hours in children aged 6 to 12 years and 13 to 16 years, respectively. Clearance (Cl/F) and volume of distribution (V_d/F) were not significantly different between the two groups. Only four children less than 6 years of age were studied, and their data were not compared with data from older children due to the small sample size.

The safety and effectiveness of olmesartan in 302 children aged 6 to 16 years was studied in a randomized, double-blind, two-phase study.[188] During period 1, which lasted 3 weeks, children weighing less than 35 kg or 35 kg or above received either low dose (2.5 or 5 mg daily) or high dose (20 or 40 mg daily) of olmesartan medoxomil. After 3 weeks, both systolic and diastolic blood pressures were reduced in a dose-dependent manner. Black subjects had a slightly lesser reduction in blood pressure than non-blacks. In period 2, subjects were randomly withdrawn to either continue the same dose that they had been receiving during period 1 or switch to placebo. Blood pressure was lower in the group that continued olmesartan, but in the black subjects, the difference was not statistically significant.

OTHER ANGIOTENSIN-RECEPTOR ANTAGONISTS

Telmisartan and azilsartan have also been studied in children. Low (1 mg per kg) and high (2 mg per kg) doses of telmisartan were compared with placebo in 76 children aged 6 to 17 years.[189] The higher dose of telmisartan lowered blood pressure significantly better than placebo, but the low dose was not significantly different from placebo. The pharmacokinetics of azilsartan in children have been studied.[190,191] Results of a safety and effectiveness trial in pediatric subjects have not yet been published.

ADVERSE EFFECTS

As with most antihypertensive agents, dizziness and headaches have been reported in children treated with ARBs.[182,186,188] As expected, hypotension was occasionally reported.[173] In several studies, transient reduction in renal function accompanied by increased serum creatinine and blood urea nitrogen (BUN) has been observed.[175,186] Hyperkalemia has been reported with a frequency of 1% to 2%.
[185,186] Elevated uric acid was noted in the valsartan trial, especially at higher doses.[186] Neurocognitive effects were studied in a small group of children in the candesartan trial.[182] No consistent effect was observed on full-scale IQ testing.

As with ACEIs, angioedema may occur but appears to be less frequent in children and adults treated with ARBs. Children who demonstrate angioedema with ACEIs do not always have angioedema when switched to ARBs, but cross-reactivity has been observed. In adults, cross-reactivity has been estimated to be less than 10%.[192,193] Careful consideration of the risks and benefits of switching to ARBs in children who have experienced angioedema while taking ACEIs is advisable.

Adolescents and adults who are treated with ARBs and become pregnant may develop fetopathy similar to ACEI fetopathy.[195] Complications include oligohydramnios, hypotension, renal failure, pulmonary hypoplasia, and defects of the skull and limbs. Adolescents who are of childbearing potential should be cautioned about the risk of fetopathy should pregnancy occur. ARBs should be stopped as soon as pregnancy is confirmed, preferably during the first trimester. While fetopathy may occur with exposure to ACEIs and ARBs at any stage of pregnancy, the risk increases with exposure during the second and third trimesters.[194]

RENIN INHIBITORS

Aliskiren currently is the only nonpeptide, orally administered direct renin inhibitor approved in the United States and Europe for the treatment of hypertension. Aliskiren competitively binds to renin, thus reducing the conversion of angiotensinogen to Ang-I (see Fig. 50.2), causing a reduction in Ang-II production and, therefore, interfering with all of the downstream effects of Ang-II on the vascular system. Unlike ACEIs and ARBs, treatment with aliskiren does not cause a compensatory increase in plasma renin.

In adults, the oral bioavailability of aliskiren is very low (2.6%).[195,196] Single- and multiple-dose pharmacokinetics was assessed in children aged 6 to 17 years[197] who received weight-adjusted doses (2 and 6 mg per kg). Maximum plasma concentrations (T_{max}) of aliskiren were observed at 1 to 2 hours. As expected, both the maximum plasma concentration (C_{max}) and AUC_{0-24} were dose dependent. Aliskiren is eliminated primarily as unchanged drug via biliary excretion. In adults, a small amount is metabolized by CYP3A4. Approximately 1% is excreted in the urine.[198]

In 20 children aged 6 to 11 years, mean seated systolic and diastolic blood pressures decreased by 4.5 and 1.7 mmHg, respectively, after a 2 mg per kg dose, and 7.7 and 0 mmHg, respectively, after a 6 mg per kg dose.[199] In 19 children aged 12 to 17 years, mean seated systolic and diastolic blood pressures decreased 7.6 and 5.3 mmHg, respectively, after a 2 mg per kg dose, and 7.7 and 5.8 mmHg, respectively, after a 6 mg per kg dose.

Adverse effects have been infrequent. The most commonly observed treatment-emergent adverse events were headache, abdominal pain, and nausea.[197] In adults, diarrhea has been reported at higher doses. In children as in adults, there has been concern about coadministration of aliskiren and angiotensin-receptor antagonists.[200] In several patients, the combination resulted in a reduction in GFR.

While reports of fetopathy resulting from treatment with aliskiren during pregnancy are scarce, there is potential for fetopathy similar to that seen with ACEIs and ARBs to occur. As with ACEIs and ARBs, aliskiren should be avoided during pregnancy.[194]

DIRECT VASODILATORS

The direct vasodilators, such as hydralazine, minoxidil, diazoxide, and nitroprusside, relax vascular smooth muscle, resulting in vasodilation and reduced peripheral vascular resistance. Hydralazine, minoxidil, and diazoxide primarily affect arteriolar vessels. In addition to arteriolar dilation, nitroprusside also relaxes venous capacitance vessels, resulting in venous pooling.

Direct vasodilators are seldom used as sole agents to treat hypertension over prolonged periods of time. Reflex tachycardia, increased cardiac output, and sodium and water retention blunt their long-term effectiveness. Use of the intravenously administered direct vasodilators has diminished as safer and equally effective options have become available for use in hypertensive emergencies. Minoxidil is occasionally used in patients with difficult-to-control hypertension receiving multiple orally administered drugs, but widespread use is limited by its adverse effect profile.

HYDRALAZINE

Prior to the development of newer antihypertensive agents, hydralazine was often administered intravenously for hypertensive urgencies or emergencies and orally to patients unresponsive to diuretics and β-adrenergic antagonists.[28] After intravenous administration, the onset of antihypertensive effect usually begins in 5 to 10 minutes and lasts up to 6 hours. Onset of action is delayed after oral or intramuscular administration, but the duration of action is similarly brief.

The metabolism of hydralazine is complex.[201] Hydralazine is inactivated by acetylation in the gastrointestinal mucosa and the liver and is subject to a significant first-pass effect.[201] The slow acetylator phenotype is associated with a significant increase in oral bioavailability compared with fast acetylators.[202] However, after intravenous administration, the pharmacokinetics of hydralazine are similar in both slow and fast acetylators, but the predominant metabolites are different.[202]

The utility of hydralazine is limited by frequent adverse effects. In addition to those common to other direct vasodilators, hydralazine has been associated with a dose-dependent, lupus-like syndrome that may be due to accumulation of metabolites more often found in slow acetylators.[203] Acute and chronic administration of hydralazine often results in headaches, tachycardia, nausea, and vomiting, which can become intolerable.[204] Use of hydralazine has diminished as safer alternatives have become available.

NITROPRUSSIDE

Nitroprusside is used in the treatment of severe, symptomatic hypertension in children, especially in conditions where afterload reduction is desired.[205,206] Nitroprusside is administered intravenously by continuous infusion. Nitroprusside degrades over several hours in alkaline solutions or in the presence of fluorescent light. During administration, the drug must be placed in an opaque bag or syringe, and the tubing through which it is delivered must be covered with aluminum foil or other opaque material to reduce decomposition.

The onset of antihypertensive effect is evident within 1 to 2 minutes after the infusion begins. The recommended initial rate of infusion is 0.3 to 0.5 μg per kg per min.[207] The infusion can be titrated to desired effect at intervals of 5 to 10 minutes. Discontinuation of the infusion results in loss of effect within 3 to 10 minutes. The maximum recommended infusion rate is 8 to 10 μg per kg per min, but prolonged administration above 4 μg per kg per min is not generally needed and should be used with caution, especially in patients with renal failure. For treatment of hypertension, nitroprusside is usually not administered for more than 2 to 3 days, but it has been used safely in an 11-year-old child for 28 days.[208]

Twenty children, ages 7 to 17 years, with severe arterial hypertension and encephalopathy or cardiac failure were treated with nitroprusside for 8 to 240 hours.[205] All were judged to have an adequate response to therapy, and only three required nitroprusside for more than 48 hours. During treatment, infusion rates ranged from 0.5 to 3.5 μg per kg per min. The mean (range) reductions in systolic and diastolic blood pressures were 47 (30 to 80) and 49 (30 to 70) mmHg, respectively. Rapid improvement in cardiac function was noted in children who presented with congestive heart failure.

Nitroprusside combines with oxyhemoglobin to form methemoglobin and ultimately undergoes reduction to cyanide and nitric oxide, the latter likely initiating a cascade of intracellular events that results in vascular smooth muscle relaxation and vasodilation. Cyanide is converted to thiocyanate, and both compounds are excreted in the urine. Accumulation can occur in patients with renal insufficiency or those receiving very high rates of infusion for prolonged periods of time. Cyanide inhibits cytochrome oxidase and halts oxidative phosphorylation, resulting in shunting of pyruvate to lactate and the development of metabolic acidemia. Symptoms associated with cyanide and thiocyanate accumulation include tachypnea, headache, nausea, vomiting, and deteriorating mental status.[209] Progression to convulsions, coma, and death may occur without timely intervention. Sulfanegen, a new "antidote" for cyanide toxicity, has been tested in several animal models and may ultimately prove superior to currently available agents (thiosulfate- and hydroxyocobalamin-based treatments).[210–213]

Newer antihypertensive agents have largely supplanted nitroprusside for the management of most hypertensive emergencies in children. However, because nitroprusside reduces both capillary-wedge pressure and systemic vascular resistance, it is particularly useful in managing severe hypertension associated with congestive heart failure.[204]

MINOXIDIL

Minoxidil is a potent, orally administered vasodilator that is typically reserved for patients with severe hypertension not controlled by multiple other medications. It has been used effectively to treat acutely elevated blood pressure in children with chronic hypertension secondary to renal disease.[214]

Minoxidil is absorbed quickly and completely from the gastrointestinal tract. Peak serum concentrations are observed within 20 to 60 minutes after dosing.[215] Onset of action begins within 30 minutes in most patients, but maximal effect is not observed until 2 to 4 hours after administration.[215] Minoxidil undergoes both type I and type II biotransformation. It is activated in vivo by hepatic sulfotransferase. The inactive glucuronide metabolite is excreted in the urine. Because minoxidil has a relatively short half-life, it is usually administered at least twice daily.

Several prospective studies were conducted to determine the effectiveness of minoxidil in children with uncontrolled hypertension.[214,216–218] Initial dosing varied from 0.05 to 0.27 mg per kg daily, but most commonly initial doses were 0.1 to 0.2 mg per kg per 24 hours. Maximal dosing also varied widely, but few children received more than 1.0 mg per kg daily. Blood pressure was reduced effectively within 1 to 2 weeks in more than 80% of the reported patients.[214,218,219] All of the patients in each of these studies received at least one and typically two or more antihypertensives concurrently with minoxidil.

In children with chronic hypertension treated with multiple drugs, severe, acutely elevated blood pressure can be treated successfully with minoxidil.[214,220] Minoxidil lowered the blood pressure to less than the 95th percentile in 9 of 11 children who received at least 0.2 mg per kg daily, but only 5 of 12 when the dose was less than 0.2 mg per kg per 24 hours.[214] An antihypertensive effect was observed 1 hour after dosing and was maximal by 2 to 4 hours. Minoxidil may be used acutely, but because of significant adverse effects, chronic use is generally reserved for children with uncontrolled hypertension on three or more antihypertensive drugs, especially those with confirmed target organ lesions. Unless contraindicated, patients should be concurrently treated with a diuretic and a β-adrenergic antagonist. Minoxidil should be used with extreme caution if at all in children with stage 4 or 5 chronic kidney disease and is contraindicated in those with a pheochromocytoma.

Adverse effects related to minoxidil were frequent and included tachycardia, fluid retention, congestive heart failure, and pericardial effusion. With chronic therapy, hypertrichosis is often observed, typically on the forehead, trunk, and extremities. Abnormal hair growth disappeared within 3 months after discontinuation of the drug. Administration of minoxidil during pregnancy occasionally has been associated with fetal hirsutism and other congenital anomalies.[221]

RESISTANT HYPERTENSION

Hypertension that is "resistant" to drug therapy occurs frequently in children. "Resistant" hypertension is a failure to achieve expected therapeutic goals during active treatment. In adults, resistant hypertension is defined as "blood pressure of a hypertensive patient that remains elevated above goal despite the concurrent use of three antihypertensive agents of different classes".[222] The definition further states that "all agents should be administered at maximum or maximally tolerated doses and at the appropriate dosing frequency" and that "nonadherence in taking prescribed antihypertensive medications must also be excluded before resistant hypertension is diagnosed." Finally, patients with white-coat effect, which may occur in up to half of all children referred for evaluation of hypertension,[2] should not be included in the diagnosis of resistant hypertension.

Before a diagnosis of resistant hypertension is entertained, ambulatory blood pressure monitoring should be done when possible to exclude white-coat effect. This may not be possible in very young or uncooperative children. Verification of appropriate doses and doing intervals, assuring that maximally tolerated doses of at least three antihypertensive agents from distinct classes are in regular use, should be done. A thorough drug history, including pill counts and scrutiny of pharmacy dispensing records, should be conducted to assure optimal compliance with the prescribed drug regimen. A discussion of herbal or natural treatments should be undertaken.

There are many causes for apparent resistance, including patient-related, disease-specific, and drug-related factors (Table 50.12). Patient factors may include weight gain, rendering doses suboptimal, dietary factors, sleep apnea, malabsorption syndromes, and genetic variants associated with drug resistance.

Drug-related causes of apparent resistance to therapy include drugs that interfere with the absorption of orally administered antihypertensive agents, decrease intestinal transit time, or induce drug-activating or drug-metabolizing enzymes. Certain drugs are known to interfere with the effectiveness of antihypertensive drugs. For example, nonsteroidal anti-inflammatory drugs are known to interfere with the effectiveness of ACEIs, probably by reducing the production of vasodilatory prostaglandins.[224] Corticosteroids are commonly used to treat a variety of immune-mediated diseases that affect the kidneys in children and have been associated with the development or worsening of hypertension. Regular use of sympathomimetic agents,

TABLE 50.12 Causes of Resistance or Apparent Resistance to Antihypertensive Drug Therapy

Factors Involved	*Causes of Resistance or Apparent Resistance*
Patient-related factors	Gain in body mass Sleep apnea Volume overload Excessive sodium intake Excessive caffeine intake Genetic variants
Disease-specific factors	Worsening of underlying disease Missed diagnosis of secondary hypertension Relapsing and remitting diseases
Drug-related factors	Inadequate dose or inappropriate dosing interval Poor oral bioavailability Rapid inactivation or elimination (e.g., nifedipine) Inappropriate drug combinations Fluid retention secondary to vasodilatory therapy Concurrent interfering drug therapy (e.g., NSAIDs, sympathomimetics, stimulants, corticosteroids, calcineurin inhibitors)

NSAIDs, nonsteroidal anti-inflammatory drugs.

commonly included in over-the-counter or prescription decongestants, may cause vasoconstriction and increased blood pressure.[225,226] Calcineurin inhibitors (cyclosporine, tacrolimus), which are commonly used to prevent solid-organ rejection and graft-versus-host disease, may cause hypertension.[207,226] Abrupt discontinuation of clonidine or guanfacine has been associated with rebound hypertension, probably by increasing vasoconstriction.[207] There are many other examples of drug-related hypertension, including α- and β-receptor agonists, narcotic withdrawal, some oral contraceptives, erythropoietin, methylphenidate, cocaine, and amphetamines.[227]

Medical history, physical findings, and the addition or repetition of selected diagnostic tests may uncover previously undetected secondary disease, worsening of a known relapsing and remitting disease (e.g., vasculitis), or gastrointestinal disease that interferes with the absorption of orally administered drugs. Compliance with dietary restrictions may be assessed by taking a thorough dietary history coupled with measuring urinary electrolyte excretion in euvolemic patients who are not receiving diuretic therapy. Genetic screening for inherited diseases known to cause hypertension has become more widely available and should be considered in selected patients.

REFERENCES

1. Lurbe E, Agabiti-Rosei E, Cruickshank JK, et al. European Society of Hypertension guidelines for the management of high blood pressure in children and adolescents. *J Hypertens* 2016;34:1887–1920.
2. Flynn JT, Kaelber DC, Baker-Smith CM, et al. Clinical practice guideline for screening and management of high blood pressure in children and adolescents. *Pediatrics* 2017;140(3):e20171904.
3. Rames LK, Clarke WR, Connor WE, et al. Normal blood pressure and the evaluation of sustained blood pressure elevation in childhood: the Muscatine study. *Pediatrics* 1978;61(2):245–251.
4. Fixler DE, Laird WP. Validity of mass blood pressure screening in children. *Pediatrics* 1983;72(4):459–463.
5. Din-Dzietham R, Liu Y, Bielo MV, et al. High blood pressure trends in children and adolescents in national surveys, 1963 to 2002. *Circulation* 2007;116(13):1488–1496.
6. Kit BK, Kuklina E, Carroll MD, et al. Prevalence of and trends in dyslipidemia and blood pressure among US children and adolescents. *JAMA Pediatr* 2015;169(3):272–279.
7. Bell CS, Samuel JA, Samuels JP. Prevalence of hypertension in children: applying the new American Academy of Pediatrics guideline. *Hypertension* 2019;73:148–152.
8. Kaelber DC, Liu W, Ross M, et al. Diagnosis and medication treatment of pediatric hypertension: a retrospective cohort study. *Pediatrics* 2016;138(6):e20162195.
9. Sorof JM, Lai D, Turner J, et al. Overweight, ethnicity, and the prevalence of hypertension in school-aged children. *Pediatrics* 2004;113(3 Pt 1):475–482.
10. Task Force on Blood Pressure Control in Children; National Heart, Lung, and Blood Institute; National Institutes of Health. Report of the Second Task Force on Blood Pressure Control in Children—1987. *Pediatrics* 1987;79:1–25.
11. Nickavar A, Assadi F. Managing hypertension in the newborn infants. *Int J Prev Med* 2014;5(Suppl 1):S39–S43.
12. Dillon MJ. Secondary forms of hypertension in children. In: Portman RJ, Sorof JM, Ingelfinger JR, eds. *Pediatric hypertension.* Totowa, NJ: Humana Press, 2004:159–179.
13. Mattoo TK, Gruskin AB. Essential hypertension in children. In: Portman RJ, Sorof JM, Ingelfinger JR, eds. *Pediatric hypertension.* Totowa, NJ: Humana Press, 2004:181–211.
14. Stein DR, Ferguson MA. Evaluation and treatment of hypertensive crises in children. *Integr Blood Press Control* 2016;9:49–58.
15. National High Blood Pressure Education Program Working Group on High Blood Pressure in Children and Adolescents. The fourth report on the diagnosis, evaluation, and treatment of high blood pressure in children and adolescents. *Pediatrics* 2004;114(Suppl 2):555–576.
16. de Simone G, Mureddu GF, Greco R, et al. Relations of left ventricular geometry and function to body composition in children with high casual blood pressure. *Hypertension* 1997;30(3 Pt 1):377–382.
17. Lever AF, Harrap SB. Essential hypertension: a disorder of growth with origins in childhood? *J Hypertens* 1992;10(2):101–120.
18. Okasha M, McCarron P, McEwen J, et al. Determinants of adolescent blood pressure: findings from the Glasgow University student cohort. *J Hum Hypertens* 2000;14(2):117–124.
19. Sinaiko AR, Steinberger J, Moran A, et al. Relation of insulin resistance to blood pressure in childhood. *J Hypertens* 2002;20(3):509–517.
20. Ahn S-Y, Gupta C. Genetic programming of hypertension. *Front Pediatr* 2017;5:285. doi:10.3389/fped.2017.00285.
21. Urbina EM, Lande MB, Hooper SR, et al. Target organ abnormalities in pediatric hypertension. *J Pediatr* 2018;202:14–22.
22. Daniels SR, Loggie JM, Khoury P, et al. Left ventricular geometry and severe left ventricular hypertrophy in children and adolescents with essential hypertension. *Circulation* 1998;97(19):1907–1911.
23. Hanevold C, Waller J, Daniels S, et al. The effects of obesity, gender, and ethnic group on left ventricular hypertrophy and geometry in hypertensive children: a collaborative study of the International Pediatric Hypertension Association. *Pediatrics* 2004;113(2):328–333.
24. Lande MB, Carson NL, Roy J, et al. Effects of childhood primary hypertension on carotid intima media thickness: a matched controlled study. *Hypertension* 2006;48(1):40–44.
25. Lande MB, Kaczorowski JM, Auinger P, et al. Elevated blood pressure and decreased cognitive function among school-age children and adolescents in the United States. *J Pediatr* 2003;143(6):720–724.
26. Sorof JM. Prevalence and consequence of systolic hypertension in children. *Am J Hypertens* 2002;15(2 Pt 2):57S–60S.
27. Khoury M, Urbina EM. Cardiac and vascular target organ damage in pediatric hypertension. *Front Pediatr* 2018;6:148. doi:10:3389/fped.2018.00148.
28. Task Force on Blood Pressure Control in Children; National Heart, Lung, and Blood Institute; National Institutes of Health. Report of the Task Force on Blood Pressure Control in Children. *Pediatrics* 1977;59:797–820.
29. ALLHAT Officers and Coordinators for the ALLHAT Collaborative Research Group. Major outcomes in high-risk hypertensive patients randomized to angiotensin-converting enzyme inhibitor or calcium channel blocker vs diuretic: The Antihypertensive and Lipid-Lowering Treatment to Prevent Heart Attack Trial (ALLHAT). *JAMA* 2002;288(23):2981–2997.
30. Li JS, Flynn JT, Portman R, et al. The efficacy and safety of the novel aldosterone antagonist eplerenone in children with hypertension: a randomized, double-blind, dose-response study. *J Pediatr* 2010;157:282–287.
31. Frishman WH, Alwarshetty M. β-Adrenergic blockers in systemic hypertension. Pharmacological considerations related to the current guidelines. *Clin Pharmacokinet* 2002;41:505–516.
32. Potts AL, Larsson P, Eksborg S, et al. Clonidine disposition in children; a population analysis. *Paediatr Anaesth* 2007;17:924–933.
33. Buhler FR, Laragh JH, Baer L, et al. Propranolol inhibition of renin secretion. *N Engl J Med* 1972;287:1209–1214.
34. Keeton TK, Campbell WB. The pharmacologic alteration of renin release. *Pharmacol Rev* 1981;31:81–227.
35. Tarazi RC, Dustan HP. Beta-adrenergic blockade in hypertension. *Am J Cardiol* 1972;29:633–640.
36. Hansson L, Zweifler AJ, Julius S, et al. Hemodynamic effects of acute and prolonged beta-adrenergic blockade in essential hypertension. *Acta Med Scand* 1974;196:27–34.
37. Man in't Veld AJ. Vasodilation, not cardiodepression, underlies the antihypertensive effects of beta-adrenoceptor antagonists. *Am J Cardiol* 1971;67:13B–17B.
38. McDevitt DG, Shand DG. Plasma concentration and time course of beta blockade due to propranolol. *Clin Pharmacol Ther* 1975;18:708–713.
39. McAreavey D, Vermeulen R, Robertson JI. Newer beta-blockers and the treatment of hypertension. *Cardiovasc Drugs Ther* 1991;5:577–588.
40. Griswold WR, McNeal R, Mendoza SA, et al. Propranolol as antihypertensive agent in children. *Arch Dis Child* 1978;53:594–596.
41. Bachmann H. Propranolol versus chlorthalidone—a perspective therapeutic trial in children with chronic hypertension. *Helv Paediatr Acta* 1984;39:55–61.

42. Mongeau JG, Biron P, Pichardo LM. Propranolol efficacy in adolescent essential hypertension. In: New MI, Levine LS, eds. *Juvenile hypertension*. New York, NY: Raven Press, 1977:219–222.
43. Potter DE, Schambelan M, Salvatierra O Jr, et al. Treatment of high-renin hypertension with propranolol in children after renal transplantation. *J Pediatr* 1977;90:307–311.
44. Gidding SS, Rocchini AP, Beekman R, et al. Therapeutic effect of propranolol on paradoxical hypertension after repair of coarctation of the aorta. *N Engl J Med* 1985;312:1224–1228.
45. Phelps SJ, Alpert BS, Ward JL, et al. Absorption pharmacokinetics of atenolol in patients with Marfan syndrome. *J Clin Pharmacol* 1995;35:268–274.
46. Buck ML, Wiest D, Gillette PC, et al. Pharmacokinetics and pharmacodynamics of atenolol in children. *Clin Pharmacol Ther* 1989;46:629–633.
47. Falkner B, Lowenthal DT, Affrime MB. The pharmacodynamic effectiveness of metoprolol in adolescent hypertension. *Pediatr Pharmacol (New York)* 1982;2:49–55.
48. Sorof JM, Cargo P, Graepel J, et al. β-Blocker/thiazide combination for treatment of hypertensive children: a randomized double-blind, placebo-controlled trial. *Pediatr Nephrol* 2002;17:345–350.
49. Wiest DB, Garner SS, Uber WE, et al. Esmolol for the management of pediatric hypertension after cardiac operations. *J Thorac Cardiovasc Surg* 1998;115:890–897.
50. Decalmer PB, Chatterjee SS, Cruickshank JM, et al. Beta-blockers and asthma. *Br Heart J* 1978;40:184–189.
51. Frishman W, Silverman R, Strom J, et al. Clinical pharmacology of the new beta-adrenergic blocking drugs. Part 4. Adverse effects. Choosing a beta-adrenoceptor blocker. *Am Heart J* 1979;98:256–262.
52. Gillette P, Garson A Jr, Eterovic E, et al. Oral propranolol treatment in infants and children. *J Pediatr* 1978;92:141–144.
53. Batisky DL, Sorof JM, Sugg J, et al. Efficacy and safety of extended release metoprolol succinate in hypertensive children 6 to 16 years of age: a clinical trial experience. *J Pediatr* 2007;150(2):134–139, 139.e1.
54. Adamson PC, Rhodes LA, Saul JP, et al. The pharmacokinetics of esmolol in pediatric subjects with supraventricular arrhythmias. *Pediatr Cardiol* 2006;27(4):420–427.
55. Cuneo BF, Zales VR, Blahunka PC, et al. Pharmacodynamics and pharmacokinetics of esmolol, a short-acting beta-blocking agent, in children. *Pediatr Cardiol* 1994;15(6):296–301.
56. Tabbutt S, Nicolson SC, Adamson PC, et al. The safety, efficacy, and pharmacokinetics of esmolol for blood pressure control immediately after repair of coarctation of the aorta in infants and children: a multicenter, double-blind randomized trial. *J Thorac Cardiovasc Surg* 2008;136(2):321–328.
57. Wolinsky H. The effects of beta-adrenergic blocking agents on blood lipid levels. *Clin Cardiol* 1987;10:561–566.
58. Ames RP. The effects of antihypertensive drugs on serum lipids and lipoproteins. II. Non-diuretic drugs. *Drugs* 1986;32:335–357.
59. Weidmann P, Gerber A, Mordasini R. Effects of antihypertensive therapy on serum lipoproteins. *Hypertension* 1983;5(Suppl III):120–131.
60. Artman M, Grayson R, Boerth RC. Propranolol in children: safety–toxicity. *Pediatrics* 1982;70:30–31.
61. Wells TG, Ulstrom RA, Nevins TE. Hypoglycemia in pediatric renal allograft recipients. *J Pediatr* 1988;113:1002–1007.
62. Bunchman TE, Lynch RE, Wood EG. Intravenously administered labetalol for treatment of hypertension in children. *J Pediatr* 1992;120:140–144.
63. Mueller JB, Solhaug MJ. Labetalol in pediatric hypertensive emergencies. *Pediatr Res* 1988;23:543A.
64. Thomas CA, Moffett BS, Wagner JL, et al. Safety and efficacy of intravenous labetalol for hypertensive crisis in infants and small children. *Pediatr Crit Care Med* 2011;12(1):28–32.
65. Janis RA, Scriabine A. Sites of action of Ca^{2+} channel inhibitor. *Biochem Pharmacol* 1983;32:3499–3507.
66. Elliot WJ, Ram CVS. Calcium channel blockers. *J Clin Hypertens* 2011;13(9):687–689.
67. Struyker-Boudier HA, Smits JF, DeMey JG. The pharmacology of calcium antagonists: a review. *J Cardiovasc Pharmacol* 1990;15(Suppl 4):S1–S10.
68. Braunwald E. Mechanism of action of calcium-channel-blocking agents. *N Engl J Med* 1982;307:1618–1627.
69. Snyder SH, Reynolds IJ. Calcium-antagonist drugs. Receptor interactions that clarify therapeutic effects. *N Engl J Med* 1985;313:995–1002.
70. Bauer JH, Reams GP. The effects of antihypertensive therapy on renal function. In: Kaplan NM, Brenner BM, Laragh JH, eds. *Perspectives on hypertension. Vol. 3: New therapeutic strategies for hypertension.* New York, NY: Raven Press, 1989:253–287.
71. Brunton LL, Hilal-DanDan R, Knollmann BC, eds. *Goodman and Gilman's: The pharmacological basis of therapeutics,* 13th ed. New York, NY: McGraw-Hill, 2017.
72. SoRelle R. Withdrawal of Posicor from market. *Circulation* 1998;98:831–832.
73. Flynn JT. Nifedipine in the treatment of hypertension in children. *J Pediatr* 2002;140:787–788.
74. Ikeda K, Isaka T, Fujioka K, et al. Suppression of aldosterone synthesis and secretion by Ca(2+) channel antagonists. *Int J Endocrin* 2012;2012. doi:10.1155/2012/519467.
75. Moncica I, Oh PI, ul Qamar I, et al. A crossover comparison of extended release felodipine with prolonged action nifedipine in hypertension. *Arch Dis Child* 1995;73:154–156.
76. Rogan JW, Lyszkiewicz DA, Blowey D, et al. A randomized prospective crossover trial of amlodipine in pediatric hypertension. *Pediatr Nephrol* 2000;14:1083–1087.
77. Bauer JH, Sunderrajan S, Reams G. Effects of calcium entry blockers on renin-angiotensin-aldosterone system, renal function and hemodynamics, salt and water excretion and body fluid composition. *Am J Cardiol* 1985;56:62H–67H.
78. Johnson CE, Beekman RH, Kostyshak DA, et al. Pharmacokinetics and pharmacodynamics of nifedipine in children with bronchopulmonary dysplasia and pulmonary hypertension. *Pediatr Res* 1991;29:500–503.
79. Flynn JT Ludden T, Mahan JD, et al. Population pharmacokinetics of amlodipine in children with hypertension (abstract). *Pediatr Res* 2002;51:465A.
80. Dilmen U, Caglar MK, Senses A, et al. Nifedipine in hypertensive emergencies of children. *Am J Dis Child* 1983;137:1162–1165.
81. Lopez-Herce J, Dorao P, de la Oliva P, et al. Dosage of nifedipine in hypertensive crises of infants and children. *Eur J Pediatr* 1989;149:136–137.
82. Lopez-Herce J, Albajara L, Cagigas P, et al. Treatment of hypertensive crisis in children with nifedipine. *Intensive Care Med* 1988;14:519–521.
83. Siegler RL, Brewer ED. Effect of sublingual or oral nifedipine in the treatment of hypertension. *J Pediatr* 1988;112:811–813.
84. Grossman E, Messerli FH, Grodzicki T, et al. Should a moratorium be placed on sublingual nifedipine capsules given for hypertensive emergencies and psuedo-emergencies? *J Am Med Assoc* 1996;276:1328–1331.
85. Truttman AC, Zehnder-Schlapback S, Bianchetti MG. A moratorium should be placed on the use of short-acting nifedipine for hypertensive crisis. *Pediatr Nephrol* 1998;12:259–261.
86. Blaszak RT, Savage JA, Ellis EN. The use of short-acting nifedipine in pediatric patients with hypertension. *J Pediatr* 2001;139:34–37.
87. Trachtman H, Frank R, Mahan JD, et al. Clinical trial of extended-release felodipine in pediatric essential hypertension. *Pediatr Nephrol* 2003;18:548–553.
88. Miyashita Y, Peterson D, Rees JM, et al. Isradipine for treatment of acute hypertension in hospitalized children and adolescents. *J Clin Hypertens (Greenwich)* 2010;12(11):850–855.
89. Johnson CE, Jacobson PA, Song MH. Isradipine therapy in hypertensive pediatric patients. *Ann Pharmacother* 1997;31(6):704–707.
90. Flynn JT, Warnick SJ. Isradipine treatment of hypertension in children: a single-center experience. *Pediatr Nephrol* 2002;17(9):748–753.
91. Flynn JT, Smoyer WE, Bunchman TE. Treatment of hypertensive children with amlodipine. *Am J Hypertens* 2000;13:1061–1066.
92. Tallian KB, Nahata MC, Turman MA, et al. Efficacy of amlodipine in pediatric patients with hypertension. *Pediatr Nephrol* 1999;13:304–310.
93. Flynn JT, Newburger JW, Daniels SR, et al. A randomized, placebo-controlled trial of amlodipine in children with hypertension. *J Pediatr* 2004;145:353–359.
94. Pfammatter JP, Clericetti-Affolter C, Truttmann AC, et al. Amlodipine once daily in systemic hypertension. *Eur J Pediatr* 1998;157:618–621.
95. Tobias JD. Nicardipine to control mean arterial pressure in a pediatric intensive care unit population. *Am J Anesthesiol* 1996;23:109–112.
96. Gouyon JB, Geneste B, Semama DS, et al. Intravenous nicardipine in hypertensive preterm infants. *Arch Dis Child Fetal Neonatal Ed* 1997;76:F126–F127.
97. Michael J, Groshong T, Tobias JD. Nicardipine for hypertensive emergencies in children with renal disease. *Pediatr Nephrol* 1998;12:40–42.
98. Flynn JT, Mottes TA, Brophy PD, et al. Intravenous nicardipine for treatment of severe hypertension in children. *J Pediatr* 2001;139:38–43.
99. Tenney F, Sakarcan A. Nicardipine is a safe and effective agent in pediatric hypertensive emergencies. *Am J Kidney Dis* 2000;35:E20.
100. Tobias JD. Nicardipine to control mean arterial pressure after cardiothoracic surgery in infants and children. *Am J Ther* 2001;8:3–6.
101. Milou C, Debuche-Benouachkou V, Semama DS, et al. Intravenous nicardipine as first-line antihypertensive drug in neonates. *Intensive Care Med* 2000;26:956–958.
102. Tobias JD, Lowe S, Deshpande JK. Nicardipine: perioperative applications in children. *Paediatr Anaesth* 1995;5:171–176.
103. Mastropietro CW, Arango Uribe D. Nicardipine and hypertension following aortic coarctectomy or superior cavopulmonary anastomosis. *World J Pediatr Congenit Heart Surg* 2016;7(1):32–35.
104. Nakagawa TA, Sartori SC, Morris A, et al. Intravenous nicardipine for treatment of post-coarctectomy hypertension in children. *Pediatr Cardiol* 2004;25(1):26–30.
105. Zisaki A, Miskovic L, Hatzimanikatis V. Antihypertensive drugs metabolism: an update to pharmacokinetic profiles and computational approaches. *Curr Pharm Des* 2015;21(6):806–822.
106. Lakkis J, Lu WX, Weir MR. RAAS escape: a real clinical entity that may be important in the progression of cardiovascular and renal disease. *Curr Hypertens Rep* 2003;5(5):408–417.
107. Siragy HM. Angiotensin receptor blockers: How important is selectivity? *Am J Hypertens* 2002;15(11):1006–1014.
108. Raia JJ Jr, Barone JA, Byerly WG, et al. Angiotensin-converting enzyme inhibitors: a comparative review. *DICP* 1990;24(5):506–525.
109. Bengur AR, Beekman RH, Rocchini AP, et al. Acute hemodynamic effects of captopril in children with a congestive or restrictive cardiomyopathy. *Circulation* 1991;83(2):523–527.
110. Trachtman H, Gauthier B. Effect of angiotensin-converting enzyme inhibitor therapy on proteinuria in children with renal disease. *J Pediatr* 1988;112(2):295–298.
111. Sinaiko AR, Mirkin BL, Hendrick DA, et al. Antihypertensive effect and elimination kinetics of captopril in hypertensive children with renal disease. *J Pediatr* 1983;103(5):799–805.
112. Levy M, Koren G, Klein J, et al. Captopril pharmacokinetics, blood pressure response and plasma renin activity in normotensive children with renal scarring. *Dev Pharmacol Ther* 1991;16(4):185–193.
113. Pereira CM, Tam YK, Collins-Nakai RL. The pharmacokinetics of captopril in infants with congestive heart failure. *Ther Drug Monit* 1991;13(3):209–214.
114. Mirkin BL, Newman TJ. Efficacy and safety of captopril in the treatment of severe childhood hypertension: report of the International Collaborative Study Group. *Pediatrics* 1985;75(6):1091–1100.
115. Friedman AL, Chesney RW. Effect of captopril on the renin-angiotensin system in hypertensive children. *J Pediatr* 1983;103(5):806–810.
116. Hymes LC, Warshaw BL. Captopril. Long-term treatment of hypertension in a preterm infant and in older children. *Am J Dis Child* 1983;137(3):263–266.
117. Callis L, Vila A, Catala J, et al. Long-term treatment with captopril in pediatric patients with severe hypertension and chronic renal failure. *Clin Exp Hypertens A* 1986;8(4–5):847–851.
118. Bifano E, Post EM, Springer J, et al. Treatment of neonatal hypertension with captopril. *J Pediatr* 1982; 100(1):143–146.
119. O'Dea RF, Mirkin BL, Alward CT, et al. Treatment of neonatal hypertension with captopril. *J Pediatr* 1988;113(2):403–406.
120. Tack ED, Perlman JM. Renal failure in sick hypertensive premature infants receiving captopril therapy. *J Pediatr* 1988;112(5):805–810.

121. Guignard JP, Gouyon JB, John EG. Vasoactive factors in the immature kidney. *Pediatr Nephrol* 1991;5(4):443–446.
122. Perlman JM, Volpe JJ. Neurologic complications of captopril treatment of neonatal hypertension. *Pediatrics* 1989;83(1):47–52.
123. Sinaiko AR, Kashtan CE, Mirkin BL. Antihypertensive drug therapy with captopril in children and adolescents. *Clin Exp Hypertens A* 1986;8(4–5):829–839.
124. Kubo SH, Cody RJ. Clinical pharmacokinetics of the angiotensin converting enzyme inhibitors. A review. *Clin Pharmacokinet* 1985;10(5):377–391.
125. Riley LJ Jr, Vlasses PH, Ferguson RK. Clinical pharmacology and therapeutic applications of the new oral converting enzyme inhibitor, enalapril. *Am Heart J* 1985;109(5 Pt 1): 1085–1089.
126. Rippley RK, Connor J, Boyle J, et al. Pharmacokinetic assessment of an oral enalapril suspension for use in children. *Biopharm Drug Dispos* 2000;21(9):339–344.
127. Ulm EH, Hichens M, Gomez HJ, et al. Enalapril maleate and a lysine analogue (MK-521): disposition in man. *Br J Clin Pharmacol* 1982;14(3):357–362.
128. Wells T, Rippley R, Hogg R, et al. The pharmacokinetics of enalapril in children and infants with hypertension. *J Clin Pharmacol* 2001;41(10):1064–1074.
129. Larmour I, Jackson B, Cubela R, et al. Enalapril (MK421) activation in man: importance of liver status. *Br J Clin Pharmacol* 1985;19(5):701–704.
130. Proesmans W, Wambeke IV, Dyck MV. Long-term therapy with enalapril in patients with nephrotic-range proteinuria. *Pediatr Nephrol* 1996;10(5):587–589.
131. Webb N, Shahinfar S, Wells T, et al. Losartan and enalapril are comparable in reducing proteinuria in children with Alport syndrome. *Pediatr Nephrol* 2013;28(5):737–743.
132. Hari P, Sahu J, Sinha A, et al. Effect of enalapril on glomerular filtration rate and proteinuria in children with chronic kidney disease: a randomized controlled trial. *Indian Pediatr* 2013;50(10):923–928.
133. Nakamura H, Ishii M, Sugimura T, et al. The kinetic profiles of enalapril and enalaprilat and their possible developmental changes in pediatric patients with congestive heart failure. *Clin Pharmacol Ther* 1994;56(2):160–168.
134. Eronen M, Pesonen E, Wallgren EI, et al. Enalapril in children with congestive heart failure. Acta Paediatr Scand 1991; 80(5):555–558.
135. Frenneaux M, Stewart RA, Newman CM, et al. Enalapril for severe heart failure in infancy. *Arch Dis Child* 1989;64(2):219–223.
136. Lloyd TR, Mahoney LT, Knoedel D, et al. Orally administered enalapril for infants with congestive heart failure: a dose-finding study. *J Pediatr* 1989;114(4 Pt 1):650–654.
137. Miller K, Atkin B, Rodel PV Jr, et al. Enalapril: a well-tolerated and efficacious agent for the paediatric hypertensive patient. *J Hypertens Suppl* 1986;4(5):S413–S416.
138. Wells T, Frame V, Soffer B, et al. A double-blind, place-bocontrolled, dose–response study of the effectiveness and safety of enalapril for children with hypertension. *J Clin Pharmacol* 2002;42(8):870–880.
139. Schilder JL, Van den Anker JN. Use of enalapril in neonatal hypertension. *Acta Paediatr* 1995;84(12):1426–1428.
140. Wells TG, Bunchman TE, Kearns GL. Treatment of neonatal hypertension with enalaprilat. *J Pediatr* 1990;117(4):664–667.
141. Mason T, Polak MJ, Pyles L, et al. Treatment of neonatal renovascular hypertension with intravenous enalapril. *Am J Perinatol* 1992;9(4):254–257.
142. Dutta S, Narang A. Enalapril-induced acute renal failure in a newborn infant. *Pediatr Nephrol* 2003;18(6):570–572.
143. Lancaster SG, Todd PA. Lisinopril. A preliminary review of its pharmacodynamic and pharmacokinetic properties, and therapeutic use in hypertension and congestive heart failure. *Drugs* 1988;35(6):646–669.
144. Hogg RJ, Delucchi A, Sakihara G, et al. A multicenter study of the pharmacokinetics of lisinopril in pediatric patients with hypertension. *Pediatr Nephrol* 2007;22(5):695–701.
145. Trachtman H, Frymoyer A, Lewandowski A, et al. Pharmacokinetics, pharmacodynamics, and safety of lisinopril in pediatric kidney transplant patients: implications for starting dose selection. *Clin Pharmacol Ther* 2015;98(1):25–33.
146. Soffer B, Zhang Z, Miller K, et al. A double-blind, placebocontrolled, dose–response study of the effectiveness and safety of lisinopril for children with hypertension. *Am J Hypertens* 2003;16(10):795–800.
147. Wells T, Zhou SY, Hammet J, et al. Single-dose pharmacokinetics of an oral solution of fosinopril in children. *J Clin Pharmacol* 2003;43:1029.
148. Li JS, Berezny K, Kilaru R, et al. Is the extrapolated adult dose of fosinopril safe and effective in treating hypertensive children? *Hypertension* 2004;44(3):289–293.
149. Benjamin DK, Smith PB, Jadhav P, et al. Pediatric antihypertensive trial failures: Analysis of end points and dose range. *Hypertension* 2008;51:834–840.
150. Yi Z, Li Z, Wu XC, et al. Effect of fosinopril in children with steroid-resistant idiopathic nephrotic syndrome. *Pediatr Nephrol* 2006;21(7):967–972.
151. Blumer JL, Daniels SR, Dreyer WJ, et al. Pharmacokinetics of quinapril in children: assessment during substitution for chronic angiotensin-converting enzyme inhibitor treatment. *J Clin Pharmacol* 2003;43(2):128–132.
152. Olson SC, Horvath AM, Michniewicz BM, et al. The clinical pharmacokinetics of quinapril. *Angiology* 1989;40:351–359.
153. Wuhl E, Mehls O, Schaefer F, et al. Antihypertensive and antiproteinuric efficacy of ramipril in children with chronic renal failure. *Kidney Int* 2004;66:768–776.
154. Mishina EV. Clinical Pharmacology Review NDA19851 Lotensin, 10/16/2003. https://www.fda.gov/media/87097/download. Accessed November 6, 2019.
155. Benazepril package insert. Revised 7/2014. https://www.accessdata.fda.gov/drugsatfda_docs/label/2015/019851s045s049lbl.pdf. Accessed November 5, 2019.
156. Lotensin (benazepril hydrochloride) NDA19851/S-038, T2009-60 REV: June 2009. https://www.accessdata.fda.gov/drugsatfda_docs/label/2009/019851s038lbl.pdf. Accessed November 14, 2019.
157. Blowey DL. Safety of the newer antihypertensive agents in children. *Expert Opin Drug Saf* 2002;1(1):39–43.
158. Hagley MT, Hulisz DT, Burns CM. Hepatotoxicity associated with angiotensin-converting enzyme inhibitors. *Ann Pharmacother* 1993;27:228–231.
159. Simon SR, Black HR, Moser M, et al. Cough and ACE inhibitors. *Arch Intern Med* 1992;152(8):1698–1700.
160. Bianchetti MG, Caflisch M, Oetliker OH. Cough and converting enzyme inhibitors. *Eur J Pediatr* 1992;151(3):225–226.
161. Donati-Genet P, Bianchetti MG. Modulators of the renin–angiotensin–aldosterone system and cough in childhood. *Pediatr Nephrol* 1996;10(4):545–546.
162. Williams GH. Converting-enzyme inhibitors in the treatment of hypertension. *N Engl J Med* 1988;319(23):1517–1525.
163. Hicks BM, Filion KB, Yin H, et al. Angiotensin converting enzyme inhibitors and risk of lung cancer: population based cohort study. *BMJ* 2018;363:k4209. doi:10.1136/bmj.k4209.
164. Fenton DC. Angiotensin converting enzyme inhibitors and lung cancer. *BMJ* 2018;363:k4337. doi:10.1136/bmj.k4337.
165. Pryde PG, Sedman AB, Nugent CE, et al. Angiotensin-converting enzyme inhibitor fetopathy. *J Am Soc Nephrol* 1993;3(9):1575–1582.
166. Sedman AB, Kershaw DB, Bunchman TE. Recognition and management of angiotensin converting enzyme inhibitor fetopathy. *Pediatr Nephrol* 1995;9(3):382–385.
167. Singh KD, Karnik SS. Angiotensin receptors: structure, function, signaling and clinical applications. *J Cell Signal* 2016;1(2):111. doi:10.4172/jcs.1000111.
168. Kaschina E, Unger T. Angiotensin AT1/AT2 receptors: regulation, signaling and function. *Blood Press* 2003;12:70–88.
169. Unger T. Blood pressure lowering and renin-angiotensin system blockade. *J Hypertens Suppl* 2003;21(6):S3–S7.
170. Shaw W, Hogg R, Koch V, et al. Losartan and E-3174 pharmacokinetics in hypertensive children and infants. *J Am Soc Nephrol* 2002;13:149A.
171. Shahinfar S, Cano F, Soffer BA, et al. A double-blind, dose–response study of losartan in hypertensive children. *Am J Hypertens* 2005;18(2 Pt 1):183–190.
172. Webb NJA, Wells TG, Shahinfar S, et al. A randomized, open-label, dose-response study of losartan in hypertensive children. *Clin J Am Soc Nephrol* 2014;9:1441–1448.
173. Ellis D, Vats A, Moritz ML, et al. Long-term antiproteinuric and renoprotective efficacy and safety of losartan in children with proteinuria. *J Pediatr* 2003;143(1):89–97.
174. White CT, Macpherson CF, Hurley RM, et al. Antiproteinuric effects of enalapril and losartan: a pilot study. *Pediatr Nephrol* 2003;18(10):1038–1043.
175. Webb NJA, Shahinfar S, Wells TG, et al. Losartan and enalapril are comparable in reducing proteinuria in children. *Kidney Int* 2012;82:819–826.
176. Lacro RV, Dietz HC, Sleeper LA, et al. Atenolol versus losartan in children and young adults with Marfan's syndrome. *N Engl J Med* 2014;371:2061–2071.
177. Vos MB, Jin R, Konomi JV, et al. A randomized, controlled, crossover pilot study of losartan for pediatric nonalcoholic fatty liver disease. *Pilot Feasibility Stud* 2018;4:109. doi.org/10.1186/s40814-018-0304-4.
178. Sakarcan A, Tenney F, Wilson JT, et al. The pharmacokinetics of irbesartan in hypertensive children and adolescents. *J Clin Pharmacol* 2001;41:742–749.
179. Vachharajani NN, Shyu WC, Mantha S, et al. Oral bioavailability and disposition characteristics of irbesartan, an angiotensin antagonist, in healthy volunteers. *J Clin Pharmacol* 1998;38:702–707.
180. Franscini LMD, Von Vigier RO, Pfister R, et al. Effectiveness and safety of the angiotensin II antagonist irbesartan in children with chronic kidney disease. *Am J Hypertens* 2002;15:1057–1063.
181. Schaefer F, van de Walle J, Zurowska A, et al. Efficacy, safety and pharmacokinetics of candesartan cilexetil in hypertensive children from 1 to less than 6 years of age. *J Hypertens* 2010;28:1083–1090.
182. Trachtman H, Hainer JW, Sugg J, et al. Efficacy, safety, and pharmacokinetics of candesartan cilexetil in hypertensive children aged 6 to 17 years. *J Clin Hypertens* 2008;10:743–775.
183. Franks AM, O'Brien CE, Stowe CD, et al. Candesartan cilexetil effectively reduces blood pressure in hypertensive children. *Ann Pharmacother* 2008;42:1388–1395.
184. Blumer JL, Batisky DL, Wells T, et al. Pharmacokinetics of valsartan in pediatric and adolescent subjects with hypertension. *J Clin Pharmacol* 2009;49:235–241.
185. Flynn JT, Meyers KEC, Neto JP, et al. Efficacy and safety of the angiotensin receptor blocker valsartan in children with hypertension aged 1 to 5 years. *Hypertension* 2008;52(2)222–228.
186. Wells T, Blumer J, Meyers KEC, et al. Effectiveness and safety of valsartan in children aged 6 to 16 years with hypertension. *J Clin Hypertens* 2011;13:357–365.
187. Wells TG, Blowey DL, Sullivan JE, et al. Pharmacokinetics of olmesartan medoxomil in pediatric patients with hypertension. *Paediatr Drugs* 2012;14:401–409.
188. Hazan L, Hernandez Rodriguez OA, Bhorat AE, et al. A double-blind, dose-response study of the efficacy and safety of olmesartan medoxomil in children and adolescents with hypertension. *Hypertension* 2010;55:1323–1330.
189. Wells TG, Portman R, Norman P, et al. Safety, efficacy, and pharmacokinetics of telmisartan in pediatric patients with hypertension. *Clin Pediatr* 2010;49:938–946.
190. Enya K, Saji BT, Kato T, et al. Pharmacokinetics of a single dose of azilsartan in pediatric patients: a phase 3, open-label multicenter study. *Adv Ther* 2018;35:1181–1190.
191. Webb NJ, Wells T, Tsai M, et al. Single-dose pharmacokinetics and safety of azilsartan medoxomil in children and adolescents with hypertension as compared to healthy adults. *Eur J Clin Pharmacol* 2016;72:447–457. doi:10.1007/s00228-015-1987-8.
192. Macauley TE, Dunn SP. Cross-reactivity of ACE inhibitor-induced angioedema with ARBs. U.S. Pharmacist 2007; 32(2):HS17–HS23.
193. Haymore BR, Yoon J, Mikita CP et al. Risk of angioedema with angiotensin receptor blockers in patients with prior angioedema associated with angiotensin-converting enzyme inhibitors: a meta-analysis. *Ann Allergy Asthma Immunol* 2008;101:495–499.
194. Bullo M, Tschumi S, Bucher BS, et al. Pregnancy outcome following exposure to angiotensin-converting enzyme inhibitors or angiotensin receptor antagonists: a systematic review. *Hypertension* 2012;60:444–450.
195. Nussberger J, Wuerzner G, Jensen C, et al. Angiotensin II suppression in humans by the orally active renin inhibitor aliskiren (SPP100): comparison with enalapril. *Hypertension* 2002;39(1):E1–E8.

196. Bonanni L, Vestra, MD. Oral renin inhibitors in clinical practice: a perspective review. *Ther Adv Chronic Dis* 2012;3(4):173–181.
197. Sullivan JE, Keefe D, Zhou Y, et al. Pharmacokinetics, safety profile, and efficacy of aliskiren in pediatric patients with hypertension. *Clin Pediatr (Phila)* 2013;52(7):599–607.
198. de Gasparo M, Cumin F, Nussberger J, et al. Pharmacological investigations of a new renin inhibitor in normal sodium-unrestricted volunteers. *Br J Clin Pharmacol* 1989;27:587–596.
199. ClinicalTrials.gov, NCT00834041. https://www.clinicaltrials.gov/ct2/show/results/NCT00834041?view=results. Accessed August 8, 2020.
200. Kelland EE, McAuley LM, Filler G. Are we ready to use aliskiren in children? *Pediatr Nephrol* 2011;26:473–477.
201. Ludden TJ, McNay JL Jr, Shepherd AM, et al. Clinical pharmacokinetics of hydralazine. *Clin Pharmacokinet* 1982;7:185–205.
202. Reece PA, Cozamanis I, Zacest R. Kinetics of hydralazine and its main metabolites in slow and fast acetylators. *Clin Pharmacol Ther* 1980;28:769–778.
203. Timbrell JA, Facchini V, Harland SJ, et al. Hydralazine-induced lupus: is there a toxic metabolic pathway? *Eur J Clin Pharmacol* 1984;27:555–559.
204. Chun G, Frishman WH. Rapid-acting parenteral antihypertensive agents. *J Clin Pharmacol* 1990;30:195–209.
205. Gordillo-Paniagua G, Velasquez-Jones L, Martini R, et al. Sodium nitroprusside treatment of severe arterial hypertension in children. *J Pediatr* 1975;87:799–802.
206. Benitz WE, Malachowski N, Cohen RS, et al. Use of sodium nitroprusside in neonates: efficacy and safety. *J Pediatr* 1985;106:102–110.
207. Taketomo CK, Hodding JH, Kraus DM, eds. *Pediatric dosage handbook*, 11th ed. Hudson, OH: Lexi-Comp, 2004.
208. Luderer JR, Hayes AH, Dubynsky O, et al. Long-term administration of sodium nitroprusside in childhood. *J Pediatr* 1977;91:490–491.
209. Linakis JG, Lacouture PG, Woolf A. Monitoring cyanide and thiocyanate concentrations during infusion of sodium nitroprusside in children. *Pediatr Cardiol* 1991;12:214–218.
210. Hottinger DG, Beebe DS, Kozhimannil T, et al. Sodium nitroprusside in 2014: a clinical concepts review. *J Anesthesiol Clin Pharmacol* 2014;30(4):462–471.
211. Stutelberg MW, Monteil AR, Belani KG, et al. Pharmacokinetics of next generation cyanide antidote sulfanegen in rabbits. *Int J Pharmacokinet* 2017;2(2). doi.org/10.4155/ipk-2016-0021.
212. Brenner M, Kim JG, Sari JL, et al. Sulfanegen sodium treatment in a rabbit model of sub-lethal cyanide toxicity. *Toxicol Appl Pharmacol* 2010;248:269–276.
213. Belani K, Singh H, Beebe D, et al. Cyanide toxicity in juvenile pigs and its reversal by a new prodrug, sulfanegen sodium. *Anesth Analg* 2012;114(5):956–961.
214. Strife CF, Quinlan M, Waldo FB, et al. Minoxidil for control of acute blood pressure elevations in chronically hypertensive children. *Pediatrics* 1986;78:861–865.
215. Fleishaker JC, Andreadis NA, Welshman IR, et al. The pharmacokinetics of 2.5-to 10-mg oral doses of minoxidil in healthy volunteers. *J Clin Pharmacol* 1989;29:162–167.
216. Sinaiko AR, Mirkin BL. Management of severe childhood hypertension with minoxidil: a controlled clinical study. *J Pediatr* 1977;91:138–142.
217. Sinaiko AR, O'Dea RF, Mirkin BL. Clinical response of hypertensive children to long-term minoxidil therapy. *J Cardiovasc Pharmacol* 1980;2(Suppl 2):S181–S188.
218. Puri HC, Maltz HE, Kaiser BA, et al. Severe hypertension in children with renal disease: treatment with minoxidil. *Am J Kidney Dis* 1983;3:71–75.
219. Pennisi AJ, Takahashi M, Bernstein BH, et al. Minoxidil therapy in children with severe hypertension. *J Pediatr* 1977;90:813–819.
220. Halling SE, Asling-Monemi K, Herthelius M, et al. Minoxidil therapy in children and young adult patients with renal disease and refractory hypertension: value when multidrug regimens have failed to achieve blood pressure control. *J Human Hypertens* 2010;24(8)552–554.
221. Kaler SG, Patrinos ME, Lambert GH, et al. Hypertrichosis and congenital anomalies associated with maternal use of minoxidil. *Pediatrics* 1987;79:434–436.
222. Carey RM, Calhoun DA, Bakris GL, et al. Resistant hypertension: Detection, evaluation, and management: a scientific statement from the American Heart Association. *Hypertension* 2018;72:e53–e90. doi:10.1161/HYP.0000000000000084.
223. Hanevold CD. White coat hypertension in children and adolescents. *Hypertension* 2019;73:24–30.
224. Alper AB, Calhoun DA. Contemporary management of refractory hypertension. *Curr Hypertens Rep* 1999;1:402–407.
225. Hanna JD, Chan JC, Gill JR. Hypertension and the kidney. *J Pediatr* 1991;118:327–340.
226. Saken R, Kates GL, Miller K. Drug-induced hypertension in infancy. *J Pediatr* 1979;95:1077–1079.
227. Rossi GP, Seccia TM, Maniero C, et al. Drug-related hypertension and resistance to antihypertensive treatment: a call for action. *J Hypertens* 2011;29:2295–2309.

CHAPTER

51

Jean-Pierre Guignard
Silvia Iacobelli

Diuretics

INTRODUCTION

Diuretics promote the excretion of water and electrolytes. They are primarily used in states of inappropriate salt and water retention. Such states can be secondary to renal diseases (nephrotic syndrome, glomerulonephritis, chronic renal failure), congestive heart failure (CHF), and liver disease (cirrhosis). Diuretics are also used in a variety of clinical situations in which an increase in sodium excretion is not the primary goal of treatment. Such conditions include acute renal failure (ARF), electrolyte disturbances (hypokalemia or hyperkalemia, hypercalcemia, hypercalciuria) and nephrogenic diabetes insipidus. Effective therapeutic goals when using diuretics require thorough knowledge of the renal regulation of water and electrolytes.

RENAL FUNCTION

Urine formation starts by the ultrafiltration of plasma through the glomerular capillary wall. The glomerular filtration rate (GFR) is determined by the net filtration pressure across the glomerular capillaries and the glomerular ultrafiltration coefficient (K_f), which is the product of the surface area and the permeability of the glomerular capillaries:

$$GFR = K_f \times \text{net filtration pressure}$$

Changes in systemic arterial pressure, intrarenal arteriolar resistance, and the plasma oncotic pressure modulate GFR.[1] Both renal perfusion and GFR are controlled by hormones and autacoids such as angiotensin II, the prostaglandins, endothelin, bradykinin, and nitric oxide, and by the sympathetic nervous system. The filtration process does not produce significant changes in the concentration of small solutes. Modifications of the filtrate occur by the reabsorption and secretion of solutes across the renal tubular cells and by the reabsorption of water.

TRANSPORT OF SOLUTES

Reabsorption of solutes is achieved by active or passive transport across the tubular cell membranes, using a transcellular or a paracellular route. Primary active transport requires a source of metabolic energy, provided by adenosine triphosphate (ATP) hydrolysis. The most important active process in the nephron is the Na^+, K^+-ATPase located on the basolateral side of the tubular cells. Other primary active transport mechanisms include various ATPases: Ca^{2+}-ATPase, H^+-ATPase, and H^+, K^+-ATPase. Secondary active transport of solutes along (**symport**) or against (**antiport**) the Na^+ gradient created by its primary active transport occurs via specific protein carrier molecules (**transporters**). Some proteins in the cell membranes, termed **uniporters**, transport only a single substance down the concentration gradient. Such is the case for glucose moving across the basolateral membrane of proximal tubular cells. Finally, cell membranes contain channels allowing the rapid passage of specific ions (Na^+, K^+, Cl^-) across cellular membranes.[2] Transport via channels or uniporters is sometimes referred to as *facilitated diffusion*.

Water flows passively down the osmotic gradient created by the active transport of solutes. The water reabsorbed along the nephron carries solutes, a process termed *solvent drag*. Macromolecules are transported by *endocytosis*, a process also using the energy provided by the ATPases.

REABSORPTION OF SODIUM

The renal tubule can reabsorb up to 99% of the filtered load of sodium. Two-thirds are reabsorbed in the proximal tubule, 25% in the ascending limb of loop of Henle, and 10% in the distal tubule and collecting duct. The driving force for Na^+ reabsorption is the Na^+, K^+-ATPase in the basolateral membrane of the tubular cell. The gradient created by the active pumping of Na^+ out of the cell allows the passive entry of Na^+ at the luminal membrane, along its electrochemical gradient. The basolateral pump also provides energy for the secondary antiport or symport transport of solutes, such as Cl^-, HCO_3^-, Ca^{2+}, phosphate, glucose, urea, and amino acids.[1]

In the early proximal tubule, the reabsorption of Na^+ is coupled to that of HCO_3^- and a number of organic molecules. Many of these solutes are almost completely removed from the tubular fluid in the first part of the proximal tubule. In the second half of the proximal tubule, Na^+ is reabsorbed along with Cl^-.

The thick ascending limb of Henle's loop reabsorbs approximately 25% of the filtered load of Na^+. It is impermeable to water. The movement of Na^+ across the luminal membrane is mediated by the Na^+, $2Cl^-$, K^+ symporter. The Na^+ that is reabsorbed is deposited in the medullary interstitium, where it is trapped by the countercurrent multiplier mechanism, together with urea. The integrity of the Na^+, K^+-ATPase and of the Na^+, $2Cl^-$, K^+ cotransport is necessary for the generation of a hypertonic medulla required to concentrate the urine.

The early distal tubule forms part of the juxtaglomerular apparatus that provides the feedback control of single-nephron GFR. In this part of the nephron, which is also impermeable to water, the continuous avid reabsorption of Na^+ results in the dilution of urine. This segment is thus referred to as the *diluting segment*.

The late distal tubule and collecting duct are composed of two distinct cell types, the principal cells and the intercalated cells. The principal cells reabsorb Na^+ and water and secrete K^+, a process controlled by aldosterone. The intercalated cells reabsorb K^+ and secrete H^+ in the tubular lumen. These cells play an important role in regulating acid–base balance. In the distal tubule and collecting duct, part of sodium enters the luminal membrane via an epithelial Na^+ channel ($E_{NA}C$).

The medullary collecting duct reabsorbs approximately 3% of the filtered load of Na^+. Active H^+ secretion against steep concentration gradients occurs in this segment, which is essential for the excretion of fixed acids. The permeability of the collecting duct cells to water is under the influence of arginine vasopressin (AVP), also known as the antidiuretic hormone (ADH).[1]

TRANSPORT OF WATER

The proximal tubule is highly permeable to water, much of which passes through the cells via aquaporin 1 (AQP-1) water channels present in both the apical and the basolateral cell membranes.[3] While the descending limb of Henle's loop is highly permeable to water, the thin and thick ascending segments of the loop are almost totally impermeable. The permeability of the collecting duct to water is under the control of AVP. This hormone increases the permeability of the cortical tubular cells by incorporating AQP-2 water channels in the apical membrane.[3] In the presence of AVP, the permeability of this segment to water is thus increased, allowing the diffusion of free water out of the tubular lumen into the highly hypertonic interstitium.[1] AQP-3 is expressed along the connecting tubule and entire length of the collecting duct (in principal cells). Although this protein does not regulate short-term water movement by vesicular trafficking, it is under long-term influence of AVP and, therefore, integrally involved in urinary concentration.[3]

TRANSPORT OF OTHER CATIONS AND ANIONS (K^+, Ca^{2+}, Pi, Mg^{2+})

Potassium

The kidneys play a major role in maintaining K^+ balance. Two-thirds of the filtered K^+ are reabsorbed in the proximal tubule and 20% in the ascending limb of loop of Henle. The regulation of K^+ excretion occurs via the secretion of K^+ in the distal tubule and collecting duct. When the dietary intake of K^+ is too large, K^+ excretion can exceed the K^+ filtered load. Three major factors control the rate of distal K^+ secretion: (a) the activity of the Na^+, K^+-ATPase, (b) the electrochemical gradient for K^+ across the apical membrane, and (c) the permeability of the apical membrane to K^+. The excretion of K^+ is regulated by the plasma K^+ concentration, the acid–base balance, aldosterone, and AVP.

Calcium

Seventy percent of the filtered Ca^{2+} is reabsorbed in the proximal tubule, 20% in the thick ascending limb of loop of Henle, 9% in the distal tubule, and 1% in the collecting duct. In the proximal tubule, Ca^{2+} enters the apical membrane by diffusing through a paracellular route or Ca^{2+} channels, down the electrochemical gradient created by the primary and secondary active transport of Ca^{2+} out of the basolateral membrane (Ca^{2+}-ATPase; Na^+-Ca^{2+} antiport). Reabsorption of Ca^{2+} in the ascending limb is largely passive down the electrochemical gradient created by the active reabsorption of Na^+. The reabsorption of Na^+ and Ca^{2+} changes in parallel in both the proximal and the thick ascending limb of loop of Henle. This accounts for the occurrence of parallel changes in Ca^{2+} and Na^+ excretion. In the distal tubule, the reabsorption of Ca^{2+} is entirely active and independent from that of Na^+. The renal excretion of Ca^{2+} is regulated by parathyroid hormone, calcitriol, and calcitonin.[1]

Phosphate

The proximal tubule reabsorbs 80% of the filtered load of Pi and the distal tubule 10%. The remaining 10% is excreted in the urine. Pi enters the apical membrane by a $2Na^+$–Pi symporter and exits the cell across the basolateral membrane by a Pi–anion antiporter. The excretion of Pi is mainly regulated by parathyroid hormone. Extracellular fluid (ECF) volume expansion decreases the reabsorption of Pi. Other factors depressing the reabsorption of Pi include metabolic acidosis and the glucocorticoids.[1]

Magnesium

The kidney plays a major role in the defense of serum magnesium concentration, as the renal tubule matches the urinary magnesium excretion and the net entry of magnesium into the ECF. Of the magnesium filtered load, 10% to 15% are reabsorbed in the proximal convoluted tubule and 70% to 80% in the thick ascending limb of the loop of Henle. The distal convoluted tubule actively reabsorbs only a small fraction of the filtered load, depending on magnesium dietary supply. Many hormones and nonhormonal factors affect renal magnesium transport: parathyroid hormone, calcitonin, and insulin increase magnesium absorption in the loop of Henle, whereas metabolic acidosis and hypercalciuria lead to renal magnesium wasting.[4]

SECRETION OF ORGANIC CATIONS AND ANIONS

The proximal tubule reabsorbs solutes and water and also secretes various organic cations and anions, many of which are end products of metabolism. The transport mechanisms for both organic cations and anions are nonspecific, so that several cations and anions can compete for the cationic or the anionic secretory pathways. In addition to endogenous organic cations and anions, various exogenous drugs are also eliminated by secretion. Such is the case for the anionic diuretics (acetazolamide, thiazides, furosemide, bumetanide) or cationic diuretics (amiloride).[1]

REGULATION OF Na^+ AND WATER TRANSPORT

In addition to the glomerular tubular balance that via Starling forces adapts the reabsorption of Na^+ to its filtered load, Na^+ transport is regulated by various hormones and paracrine factors. Angiotensin II, aldosterone, the atrial natriuretic peptide (ANP), the prostaglandins, the catecholamines, and dopamine play major roles.[1]

Angiotensin II

Angiotensin II stimulates proximal Na^+ and water reabsorption by increasing the apical Na^+/H^+ exchange. It stimulates the secretion of aldosterone. By acting on the zona glomerulosa of the adrenal cortex to release aldosterone, it indirectly favors distal Na^+ reabsorption. Angiotensin II release is activated by a decrease in ECF volume and renal perfusion.

Aldosterone

Aldosterone stimulates the distal reabsorption of Na^+ by increasing the permeability of the collecting tubule luminal membrane to Na^+. Aldosterone also favors the secretion of K^+ and H^+ and increases the reabsorption of Cl^-. Aldosterone stimulates the Na^+, K^+-ATPase and the production of ATP. The secretion of aldosterone by the adrenal cortex is stimulated by angiotensin II, hyperkalemia, and severe hyponatremia.

Atrial Natriuretic Peptide

The heart produces two natriuretic peptides (NPs): the ANP stored in the atrial myocytes, and the brain natriuretic peptide (B-type natriuretic peptide or BNP) stored in the ventricular myocytes. Both peptides are released when the heart dilates. The kidneys produce a related NP termed *urodilatin.* In general, the NPs antagonize the actions of the renin–angiotensin–aldosterone system. The 28-amino-acid peptide is released when atrial stretch receptors sense an increase in the effective circulating volume. ANP stimulates the excretion of Na^+ by (a) increasing GFR via vasodilatation of the afferent arterioles, (b) inhibiting renin release and the secretion of aldosterone, (c) inhibiting the Na^+, K^+-ATPase in the inner medullary collecting duct, and (d) closing the $E_{NA}Cs$.

Prostaglandins

The prostaglandins, synthesized by the cyclooxygenases in the renal cortex, the medullary interstitium, and the collecting duct epithelial cells, increase Na^+ excretion. They do it by increasing GFR and by inhibiting Na^+ reabsorption in the collecting duct.

Norepinephrine and Epinephrine

Norepinephrine and epinephrine released from sympathetic nerves and the adrenal medulla, respectively, stimulate Na^+ reabsorption in the proximal tubule, the thick ascending limb of the loop of Henle, the distal tubule, and the collecting duct.

Dopamine

Dopamine, synthesized by proximal tubular cells and dopaminergic nerves, increases the excretion of Na^+ by inhibiting Na^+ proximal reabsorption.

Antidiuretic Hormone (Arginine Vasopressin)

Water following Na^+ passively, its reabsorption is increased by all the factors that stimulate Na^+ reabsorption. The hormone that really regulates water balance is AVP, a nonapeptide with a molecular weight of 1,099 Da.

Two main types of receptors mediate the actions of AVP: V1 (V1A and V1B) and V2. V_{1A} receptors are located on vascular smooth muscle and mediate vasoconstriction. V_{1B} receptors are present in the anterior pituitary gland and mediate the release of adrenocorticotropic hormone. The V_2 receptors are located in the renal distal tubule and collecting duct. AVP binding to the V_2 receptors leads to activation of an adenylyl cyclase with subsequent rise in intracellular cyclic adenosine monophosphate (cAMP). This second messenger mediates the translocation of intracellular vesicles containing the water channel AQP-2 into the apical plasma membrane[3] and increases the transcription of AQP-2. AVP-regulated AQP-2 shuttling is the primary determinant for water permeability of the collecting duct and, consequently, for the antidiuresis. In addition, AVP stimulates Na^+–K^+–$2Cl^-$ cotransport in the ascending limb of loop of Henle via V_2 receptors.

The release of AVP is rapid, its plasma half-life is short (10 to 15 minutes), thus allowing a fine regulation of the plasma osmolality. Small changes in P_{osm} (± 3 mOsm per kg H_2O) activate or inhibit AVP release. Osmoreceptors, located in the supraoptic nucleus of the hypothalamus, regulate the release of AVP. Voloreceptors and baroreceptors also affect AVP release. Because of the greater sensitivity of the osmoreceptors, their influence predominates when changes in osmolality and plasma volume are moderate. When large changes in plasma volume occur, however, the influence of the voloreceptors and baroreceptors predominates over that of the osmoreceptors, leading to "inappropriate" secretion of AVP, with consequent water retention and hemodilution. Nonosmotic stimulation or inhibition of AVP release occurs as a consequence of drugs (nicotine, morphine, barbiturates), pain, and respiratory or cerebral distress.[1]

BODY FLUID HOMEOSTASIS

The kidney is responsible for maintaining the ECF volume and osmolality constant in spite of large changes in salt and water intake.

Body Fluid Volume

NaCl, the major osmotically active solute in ECF, determines its volume. The balance between the intake and the renal excretion of Na^+ thus regulates ECF volume and, as a consequence, cardiac output and blood pressure. Long-term changes in Na^+ excretion are regulated by aldosterone. More rapid changes in Na^+ excretion are achieved by changes in GFR and/or by various intrarenal hormones that regulate Na^+ reabsorption.

ECF volume is closely related to plasma volume. Alterations in plasma volume are sensed on both the venous and the arterial sides of the circulation. Arterial sensors perceive the adequacy of blood flow in the arterial circuit, a parameter coined as *effective circulating volume.* This volume is also sensed by baroreceptors located in the juxtaglomerular apparatus of the kidney. A decrease in renal perfusion pressure activates the renin–angiotensin–aldosterone system. Changes in the effective circulating volume activate other intrarenal hormones that modulate Na^+ reabsorption either directly by an action on tubular transport or indirectly by changes in GFR.[1]

Body Fluid Osmolality

The plasma osmolality is maintained within narrow limits. A 2% to 3% increase in P_{osm} stimulates the osmoreceptors with the consequent release of AVP, leading to the reabsorption of free water in the collecting duct. Urine flow rate decreases, and the osmolality of the urine increases. The opposite happens when P_{osm} decreases by 2% to 3%. The concentration of urine can vary from 40 to 1,400 mOsm per kg H_2O, depending on whether AVP is completely absent or maximally stimulated. Concentration of the urine requires the presence of a hypertonic medullary interstitium. Impaired NaCl transport in the thick ascending limb of loop of Henle or defective countercurrent multiplier mechanisms results in a decrease in maximal urine osmolality.[1]

Developmental Aspects of Renal Function and Body Fluid Homeostasis

In the human fetus, urine formation starts around the 10th to 12th week of gestation. The urine is normally hypotonic, indicating that the kidney actively reabsorbs electrolytes and solutes from the glomerular ultrafiltrate. The fetal kidney responds to diuretics administered to the mother by increasing her urine flow rate. The full complement of nephrons is achieved around the 35th week of gestation. GFR and renal plasma flow increase progressively throughout gestation but remain relatively low. GFR at birth is equal to 20 mL per minute per 1.73 m^2 in term infants and doubles in the first 2 weeks of life. It reaches mature levels of 100 mL per minute per 1.73 m^2 by the 6th to 12th month of postnatal age. GFR is lower at birth in premature neonates and develops at a somewhat lower velocity.[5,6]

The reabsorption of filtered solute also undergoes maturational changes. Proximal Na^+ reabsorption increases in parallel with an increase in the activity of the Na^+, K^+-ATPase and in the number of the glucose- and bicarbonate-Na^+ cotransporters. Reabsorption in the loop of Henle also increases along with the activity of the Na^+, K^+-ATPase in this segment. Resistance of the distal tubule to aldosterone has been claimed to be partly responsible for Na^+ wasting in the first weeks of premature infants.[7]

In early postnatal life, several transporters and enzymes involved in the reabsorption of bicarbonate are weakly expressed, resulting in a relatively low HCO_3^- excretion threshold. The overall reabsorption of various electrolytes and solutes also undergoes maturational changes linked to the maturation of the transporters, symporters, and antiporters.

The distribution of water in the various compartments of the body varies with age. The ECF volume decreases from 60% body weight at 28 weeks of gestation to 42% at term and 20% at 3 months of age. These changes reflect the excretion of excessive ECF and a gradual increase in the amount of fat tissues. Although the volume of body fluid varies during growth, the tonicity of ECF is kept constant by the kidney, which excretes or retains appropriate amounts of water.[8]

The newborn, premature or at term, is able to decrease urine osmolality to values as low as 40 mOsm per kg H_2O. Free-water excretion depends on the distal reabsorption of Na^+ and hence on the amount of Na^+ delivered to the distal tubule. Because of the low GFR present in the newborn infant, the ability to excrete large amounts of free water is limited.[8]

The concentrating ability is limited in newborn infants, the more so in the preterm neonates. The relative ineffectiveness of the concentrating mechanism in the neonate has been ascribed to (a) a low corticomedullary concentration gradient, (b) shortness of the loops of Henle, (c) decreased formation of cAMP in response to ADH, and (d) interference of the elevated levels of prostaglandins with the vasopressin-stimulated cAMP synthesis.

In spite of elevated aldosterone levels, premature neonates frequently have difficulties in maintaining a positive Na^+ balance on a Na^+ intake of 1 to 2 mmol per kg per day on the 2nd to 4th week of life. Deficient proximal NaCl reabsorption and relative resistance to aldosterone have been claimed to be responsible for Na^+ wasting. Both the renin–angiotensin system and the osmoreceptors–voloreceptors control system of ADH are efficient in the early newborn period. Hyponatremia is frequently seen, however, as the consequence of inappropriate secretion of ADH secondary to respiratory or cerebral distress.[8,9]

CLINICAL USE OF DIURETICS

Diuretics are used in sodium-retaining states with or without the formation of edema, in situations of arterial hypertension or electrolyte imbalances, oliguric renal failure, and nephrogenic diabetes insipidus.[10–13] Diuretics can be used to test the integrity of distal tubular function.

EDEMATOUS STATES

Salt and water retention with edema formation can occur as a primary event or as a consequence of reduced effective circulating volume with secondary hyperaldosteronism. The use of diuretics can be life-saving when Na retention is associated with an expansion of the ECF volume. It may, on the contrary, further compromise the situation when sodium retention occurs in response to homeostatic mechanisms mobilized to defend the circulating volume. The use of diuretics, therefore, requires careful monitoring of the patient's hemodynamic states and an understanding of his or her underlying condition.[7,14]

Congestive Heart Failure

CHF is associated with an increase in pressure in the venous circulation. The increased capillary pressure favors the movement of fluid into the interstitium, resulting in the formation of edema. Failure of the heart to provide normal tissue perfusion is sensed as a decrease in effective circulating volume by the kidney, which is stimulated to retain NaCl and water. The presence of edema thus represents a side effect of the compensatory renal response to defend the effective circulating volume. The treatment of this condition consists in restoring normal cardiac output. By mobilizing the edematous fluid, diuretics improve the symptoms of CHF. The pulmonary edema secondary to left-sided heart failure requires the urgent use of diuretics to reduce the life-threatening pulmonary congestion.[12]

Nephrotic Syndrome

The nephrotic syndrome is characterized by an increase in the permeability of the glomerular barrier to proteins, heavy proteinuria, hypoproteinemia, and the formation of edema. Two pathogenic mechanisms have been proposed to explain the formation of edema. In the *underfill hypothesis*, decreased plasma oncotic pressure results in decreased effective circulating volume with consequent secondary hyperaldosteronism and hypervasopressinism, leading to progressive salt and water retention. In this situation, usually seen at the onset of the minimal changes in nephrotic syndrome, the hypovolemia is manifested by clinical signs such as tachycardia, abdominal pain, and poorly perfused limbs. Elevated hematocrit and very low urinary sodium (<10 mmol per L) confirm the state of hypovolemia. Diuretics should only be used with great caution in this condition and only after correction of the hypovolemia by albumin infusion.

In the *overfill theory*,[15] the edema is caused by the primary retention of Na^+ and water, with increased plasma volume, increased hydrostatic capillary pressure, and leak of fluid into the interstitium. The pathogenesis of saline retention in the overfill hypothesis is not yet clear. Decrease in the activity of the ANP has been claimed to be responsible for the increased Na^+ retention. These patients benefit from diuretic administration.

The *underfill* and the *overfill* theories are not necessarily exclusive. The predominance of a mechanism may depend on the stage and nature of the nephrotic syndrome, the rate of development of proteinuria, and the plasma oncotic pressure.[15,16]

Liver Diseases

The occurrence of edema in patients with liver disease is secondary to decreased albumin synthesis, decreased oncotic pressure, and decreased effective circulating volume. The kidney responds by increasing salt and water retention. As ascites develops, there is a rise in intra-abdominal pressure, a phenomenon that impairs venous drainage from the lower limbs. Although diuretic therapy for ascites fails to improve survival in children, it benefits quality of life and limits complications such as bacterial peritonitis.[17] Defective liver function also results in impaired inactivation of salt- and water-retaining hormones, such as aldosterone or vasopressin.

ARTERIAL HYPERTENSION

Arterial hypertension may be secondary to salt retention and expansion of the ECF volume. Na^+ retention may be directly related to excessive synthesis of aldosterone in primary hyperaldosteronism. In the renal vascular form of hypertension, increased formation of angiotensin II elevates the blood pressure by inducing vasoconstriction and by stimulating sodium reabsorption. In essential hypertension, the retention of Na^+ is not obvious. It has been recently hypothesized that impaired extrusion of Na^+ out of the cells, secondary to defective Na^+/Ca^{2+} countertransport could lead to an increase in intracellular Ca^{2+} with consequent increased vascular contractility.[18] By leading to ECF volume contraction, diuretics decrease the blood pressure, so they are often used as first-line drugs in the treatment of arterial hypertension.[19,20] Interestingly, the antihypertensive effects of thiazides persist after normalization of the ECF volume and are mediated by vasodilation.

In adults, low-dose diuretics (hydrochlorothiazide 12.5 mg; torasemide 2.5 mg) constitute effective once-daily monopharmacotherapies for mild-to-moderate uncomplicated essential hypertension,[18] and recent studies suggest chlorthalidone as the preferred thiazide diuretic for the treatment of hypertension, but studies on infants are not available.[21] The pediatric hypertension guidelines do not endorse a specific agent for initial treatment of children with primary hypertension.[22] Nonetheless, thiazide diuretics can be considered an appropriate choice as first-line therapy in children requiring pharmacologic intervention.[21] If diuretic therapy is initiated, it is recommended that therapy begin with low doses slowly titrating the dosage. Electrolyte abnormalities are the most common adverse effects associated with the use of thiazide diuretics for hypertension, and serial assessment of serum electrolytes and magnesium is warranted with chronic therapy. Thiazide and thiazide-like diuretic are contraindicated for competitive athletes and diabetic patients.[21]

ELECTROLYTE IMBALANCE

Diuretics can be used in various situations associated with dyselectrolytemia. They can increase K^+ excretion in hyperkalemic states (loop diuretics, thiazides), increase calcium excretion in hypercalcemia (loop diuretics), or decrease the rate of calcium excretion in hypercalciuric states (thiazides). Increased HCO_3^- excretion can be achieved by the acetazolamide, whereas increased H^+ excretion can be stimulated by loop diuretics.

NEPHROGENIC DIABETES INSIPIDUS

This condition is characterized by the resistance of the collecting duct to the action of ADH. It can be due either to an X-linked congenital defect in the V_2 receptors or to an autosomal recessive mutation in the AQP-2 molecule. The patient with diabetes insipidus excretes large amounts of dilute urine. The thiazides can reduce the extracellular space volume by impairing sodium distal reabsorption and increasing NaCl excretion. This decrease in ECF volume stimulates proximal salt and water retention, thus eventually leading to reduced urine flow rate. Prolonged treatment with hydrochlorothiazide–amiloride appears to be more effective and better tolerated than with just hydrochlorothiazide. Such treatment is as efficacious as the association hydrochlorothiazide–indomethacin, with fewer severe side effects.[23]

ACUTE RENAL FAILURE

Because they have been shown to variably increase total renal blood flow, loop diuretics are often administered to patients with oliguric renal insufficiency, in the hope of promoting diuresis and improving GFR and renal perfusion.[24] Although diuretic administration may convert oliguric ARF to nonoliguric ARF, there is no evidence that this treatment can ameliorate renal function or improve the outcome of patients with ARF.[24]

DIFFERENTIAL DIAGNOSIS OF CONGENITAL TUBULOPATHIES

Diuretics such as acetazolamide, furosemide, or hydrochlorothiazide can be used to test distal tubular acidification or distal sodium reabsorption defects.

CLASSIFICATION OF DIURETICS

Diuretics can be classified according to their site and mode of action (Fig. 51.1 and Table 51.1). They all increase sodium and water excretion and variably modify electrolyte excretion (Table 51.2). *Filtration diuretics* increase salt and water excretion by primarily increasing GFR. *Osmotic diuretics* depress salt and electrolyte reabsorption in the proximal tubule and loop of Henle. *Inhibitors of carbonic anhydrase* act primarily on the proximal tubule. The most commonly used diuretics inhibit Na^+ reabsorption either in the ascending limb of loop of Henle (*loop diuretics*), in the distal convoluted tubule (*thiazide and*

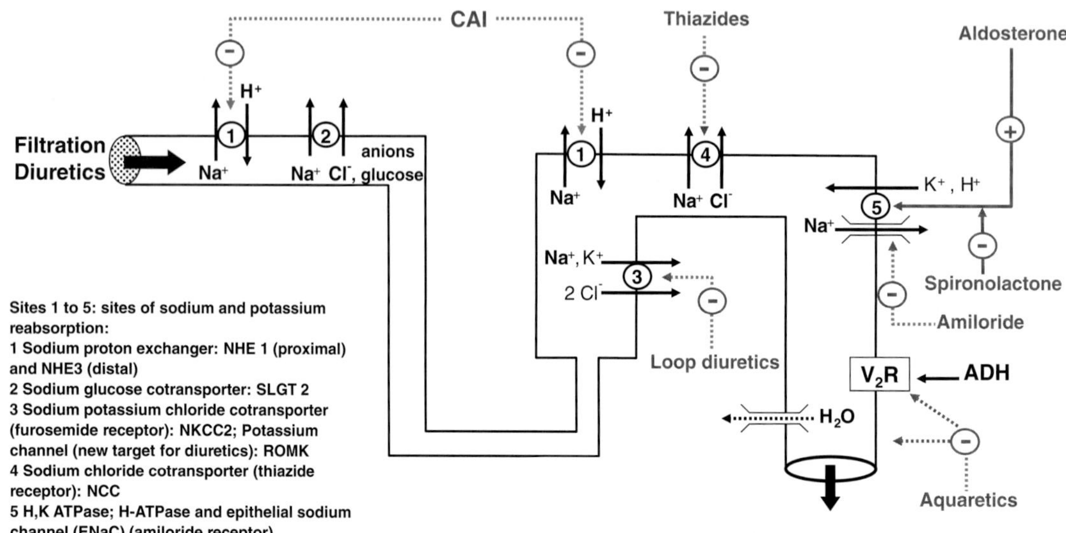

Figure 51.1 Sodium reabsorption along the nephron and sites of action of diuretic agents. ADH, antidiuretic hormone; CAI, carbonic anhydrase inhibitors.

thiazide-like diuretics), or in the late distal tubule and collecting duct (K^+-sparing diuretics).[13,11] New diuretics are being developed with different modes of action (*NPs, adenosine antagonists, vasopressin antagonists*). All diuretics share adverse effects, which are actually extension of their primary effects on electrolyte excretion (Table 51.3), as well as nonelectrolyte adverse effects (Table 51.4).

TABLE 51.1 Clinical Use of Diuretics

Type of Diuretic	*Clinical Uses*
Osmotic diuretics	Oliguric acute renal failure Cerebral edema Elevated intrarenal pressure
Carbonic anhydrase inhibitors	Acute mountain sickness Glaucoma Epilepsy Production of alkaline diuresis Assessment of distal urinary acidification
Loop diuretics	Edematous states Hypercalcemia Hyperkalemia Respiratory disorders in neonates Oliguric states and prerenal failure Nephrotic syndrome Severe hyponatremia Assessment of distal urinary acidification
Thiazides	Edematous states Arterial hypertension Hypercalciuria Bronchopulmonary dysplasia Nephrogenic diabetes insipidus Diagnosis of renal tubular hypokalemic disorders
Potassium-sparing diuretics	Adjunctive therapy with loop or thiazide diuretics Prevention of hypokalemia
Aquaretics	Promotion of free-water excretion Hyponatremic states, congestive heart failure

FILTRATION DIURETICS

Agents that increase diuresis by increasing GFR are sometimes called *filtration diuretics.* These agents include the glucocorticoids and theophylline, as well as inotropic agents such as isoproterenol, dopamine, and dobutamine. By increasing GFR, these drugs only moderately increase Na^+ excretion. Part of the natriuresis achieved by filtration diuretics reflects inhibition of tubular Na^+ reabsorption rather than an increase in the Na^+ filtered load only.

Dopaminergic Agents

Dopamine, a naturally occurring catecholamine, acts on the specific dopaminergic receptors DA_1 and DA_2, and also activates the α and the β adrenoreceptors. Dopamine may improve renal function by (a) increasing cardiac output through stimulation of the β-adrenergic receptors, (b) increasing blood pressure by inotropic and vasoactive mechanisms, (c) increasing renal perfusion via stimulation of the dopamine receptors in the renal vessels, and (d) directly inhibiting sodium reabsorption.[25] The beneficial effects of low-dose dopamine in oliguric states are variable and, when present, modest. Because of a great overlap in the response to dopamine and significant individual variation, no dose is clearly only a beneficial renal dose.[26] Even at low doses, dopamine may increase cardiac contractility and systemic vascular resistance and produce tachycardia, arrhythmia, tissue necrosis, and digital gangrene.[27] Dopamine also blunts hypoxic ventilatory drive and may increase pulmonary shunt fraction in critically ill patients. The effects of low-dose dopamine on urine output in very low birth weight (VLBW) infants or critically ill infants have been proved only in retrospective cohorts.[28] Until efficacy and safety are demonstrated in control prospective studies, the use of dopamine as a renal protective agent remains questionable.[29] The cost of the modest improvement in urine output and sodium excretion with dopamine may be too high.

The same conclusion applies to dopexamine, a dopaminergic agent devoid of action on the α receptors,[30] and probably also

TABLE 51.2 Acute Effects of Diuretics on Electrolyte Excretion[a]

	Na^+	K^+	Ca^{2+}	Mg^{2+}	H^+	Cl^-	HCO_3^-	$H_2PO_4^-$	*Uric Acid: Acute*	*Uric Acid: Chronic*
Osmotic diuretics	↑↑	↑	↑	↑↑	?	↑	↑	↑	↑	?
Carbonic anhydrase inhibitors	↑	↑↑	=	~	↓	(↑)	↑↑	↑↑	?	↓
Loop diuretics	↑↑	↑↑	↑↑	↑↑	↑	↑↑	↑	↑	↑	↓
Thiazide diuretics	↑	↑↑	~	ς↑	↑	↑	↑	↑	↑	↓
K^+-sparing diuretics	↑	↓	↓	↓	↓	↑	(↑)	=	?	↓

↑↑, marked increase; ↑, moderate increase; (↑), slight increase; ↓, decrease; =, no change; ~, variable effects; V↑, variable increase; ?, insufficient data.

[a]In the absence of significant volume depletion, which would trigger complex adjustments.

From Jackson EK. Diuretics. In: Goodman and Gilman's. In: Harman JG, Limbird LE, eds. *The pharmacological basis of therapeutics.* McGraw-Hill Med. Publ. Div., 10th ed. 2001:764, with permission.

TABLE 51.3 Electrolytes Disturbances Induced by Diuretics

	Osmotic	*Carbon Anhydrase Inhibitors*	*Loop*	*Thiazides*	*K^+-Sparing*
Hypovolemia	+++	–	+++	+	+
Hyponatremia	– –	–	– –	+++	–
Hypokalemia	– –	+	+++	– –	–
Hyperkalemia	–	–	–	–	– –
Hypercalciuria	+	–	– –	–	–
Hypercalcemia	–	–	–	+	–
Hypomagnesemia	+	–	+	+	–
Hypophosphatemia	+	–	+	+	–
Hyperuricemia	–	–	– –	– –	–
Metabolic acidosis	+	– –	–	–	+
Metabolic alkalosis	+	–	– –	– –	–

From Sherbotie JR, Kaplan B. Diuretics. In: Aranda J, Yaffé S, eds. Chapter 46. *Pediatr pharmacol*, Philadelphia, PA: WB Saunders Co, 1992:524–534, with permission.

TABLE 51.4 Nonelectrolyte Side Effects of Diuretics

Osmotic diuretics		Congestive heart failure and pulmonary edema, nausea, vomiting
Carbonic anhydrase inhibitors		Drowsiness, fatigue, central nervous system depression, paresthesia, calculus formation
Loop diuretics		Ototoxicity (usually reversible), nephrocalcinosis in neonates, patent ductus arteriosus in neonates, hyperuricemia, hyperglycemia, hyperlipidemia, hypersensitivity
Thiazides		Hyperglycemia, insulin resistance, hyperlipidemia, hypersensitivity (fever, rash, purpura, anaphylaxis, interstitial nephritis), hyperuricemia
K^+-sparing	Amiloride	Diarrhea, headache
	Triamterene	Glucose intolerance, interstitial nephritis, blood dyscrasias
	Spironolactone	Gynecomastia, hirsutism, peptic ulcers, ataxia, headache

to dobutamine, a dopaminergic agent that stimulates the β_1 adrenoreceptors, with little effect on the β_2 and the α receptors.[31]

Adenosine A_1 Receptor Antagonists

While not belonging stricto sensu to the group of filtration diuretics, adenosine antagonists are discussed in this section. Adenosine is produced in the kidney. In physiologic conditions, it participates in the regulation of GFR, renin secretion, and sodium reabsorption.[32] Adenosine acts on four types of receptors, the A_1, A_{2A}, A_{2B}, and A_3.[33] The A_1 receptors are widely distributed in the kidney and found in the renal vasculature, glomeruli, juxtaglomerular apparatus, cortical tubules, ascending limbs of loops of Henle, and collecting duct cells.[34] Stimulation of the A_1 receptors inhibits adenylate cyclase and activates K^+ channels. A_1 receptors participate in the tubuloglomerular feedback mechanism by vasoconstricting the afferent arteriole. Intact adenosine A_1 receptors are required for the diuretic and natriuretic action of theophylline and caffeine.[35,36] The A_2 receptors activate adenylate cyclase and vasodilate the efferent arteriole.[33] Stimulation of A3 receptors results in constriction of smooth muscle and relaxation of cardiac muscle.

Theophylline and caffeine are nonselective antagonists of adenosine receptors.[37] When used in low doses (0.5 mg per kg) in newborn rabbits, theophylline increased Na^+ and water excretion.[38] This natriuretic response, which occurs without significant change in GFR, could be mediated by blockade of the A_1 receptors. When used in oliguric acute hypoxemic vasomotor nephropathy in newborn animals, theophylline protects renal function and increases urine output.[38]

Since enhanced intrarenal adenosine levels lead to reduced GFR in several pathologic conditions, aminophylline and theophylline have been tested in randomized controlled trials (RCTs) for their prophylactic and curative use in the renal impairment in critically ill children, following severe respiratory distress syndrome (RDS), ischemia–reperfusion injury, and perinatal asphyxia in newborn infants.[39-43] A systematic review and meta-analysis showed that prophylactic theophylline compared to placebo significantly reduces the incidence of severe renal dysfunction in term infants following perinatal asphyxia.[44]

Recently, one retrospective cohort study on 200 infants undergoing pediatric cardiac surgery found that children who received aminophylline to treat intraoperative oliguria produced more postoperatively urine and needed less renal replacement therapy for acute kidney injury, compared to infants receiving intraoperative furosemide.[45]

OSMOTIC DIURETICS

Chemistry

Osmotic diuretics are agents that inhibit the reabsorption of solute and water by altering osmotic driving forces along the nephron. Osmotic diuretics include mannitol, glycerin, isosorbide, and urea. Mannitol, a hexahydric alcohol related to mannose, with a molecular weight of 182 Da, is most commonly used.[46]

Mechanisms and Sites of Action

Freely filtered and (mostly) not reabsorbed, osmotic diuretics increase the tubular fluid osmolality, thus impairing the diffusion of water out of the tubular lumen, as well as that of NaCl by a solvent drag effect. The osmotic diuretics act in the proximal tubule and the loop of Henle. By attracting water from the intracellular compartment, osmotic diuretics increase ECF volume and renal blood flow. Increased medullary blood flow washes out the hypertonic medulla, thus impairing the concentrating mechanism. By inhibiting NaCl reabsorption out of the water-impermeable thick ascending limb, osmotic diuretics also impair the dilution of urine. Osmotic diuretics increase nonspecifically the excretion of all electrolytes. The natriuresis induced by osmotic diuretics is only about 10% of the filtered load.

Pharmacokinetic Properties

While isosorbide and glycerin can be given orally, mannitol and urea must be administered intravenously (IV). Glycerin is mostly metabolized. Mannitol, urea, and isosorbide are excreted in the urine. The half-life of mannitol is 0.25 to 1.5 hours; it is prolonged in patients with renal failure.

Efficacy and Therapeutic Uses

Osmotic diuretics increase the excretion of Na^+, K^+, Cl^-, Mg^{2+}, Ca^{2+}, Cl^-, and HCO_3^-. They improve renal perfusion without significantly affecting GFR. Mannitol is used to increase urine flow rate in patients with prerenal failure, promote the excretion of toxic substances by forced diuresis, and reduce elevated intracranial and intraocular pressures. For drug dosages, see Table 51.5.

Specific Indications

Oliguric Prerenal Failure

Mannitol is infused in oliguric euvolemic patients at a dose of 2 to 5 mL per kg of body weight of 20% mannitol, IV over 5 minutes. The diuretic response appears within 1 to 3 hours. While mannitol may promote diuresis, it does not significantly protect GFR.[24] In patients receiving radiocontrast agents, mannitol does not appear better than simple hydration with 0.45% NaCl.[47] Mannitol is also sometimes used to prevent the occurrence of ARF in patients undergoing cardiac surgery.[48] In LBW infants, mannitol increases the risk of intraventricular (cerebral) hemorrhage; its use should, therefore, be avoided.[49]

Dialysis Disequilibrium

Mannitol can be used to prevent the occurrence of the dialysis disequilibrium syndrome. By compensating the decrease in plasma osmolality induced by dialytic removal of solutes during the dialysis session, mannitol prevents the occurrence of cerebral edema. Mannitol is infused in the second half of the dialysis session at a dose of 2 to 5 mL per kg of 20% mannitol.

Intracranial and Ocular Pressure

Osmotic diuretics are used to reduce cerebral edema and decrease intraocular pressure in glaucoma, as well as preoperatively in patients requiring ocular surgery.

Adverse Effects—Interactions

Circulatory overload and CHF can occur as a consequence of inadequate expansion of ECF volume. Fluid and electrolyte imbalance can occur after overuse of mannitol. Extravasation can lead to tissue necrosis.

INHIBITORS OF CARBONIC ANHYDRASE

Chemistry

Acetazolamide, a sulfonamide derivative, is the main inhibitor of carbonic anhydrase used in humans.

Mechanisms and Sites of Action

Inhibition of carbonic anhydrase, present in all tubular cells and the brush border of proximal tubular cells, results in depressed cellular formation and subsequent secretion of H^+. As a consequence, the HCO_3^- ions that are normally reabsorbed by combining with H^+ in the tubular lumen are excreted in the urine. Decreased H^+ secretion is associated with decreased Na^+ reabsorption. In the distal tubule, K^+ secretion is enhanced because of

TABLE 51.5 Dosages of Common Diuretics

Drug	*Route/Interval (q h)*	*Dosage (mg/kg/day)*	*Half-Life $t_{1/2}$ (h)*	*Comments*
Mannitol	i.v., 2–4	200–500	0.3–2	Risk of expansion of ECV
Acetazolamide	p.o., 6–8	5	6–9	Not effective at GFR <20[a]; self-limited action as plasma HCO_3^- falls
Furosemide	p.o., 12–24	1–2	~1.5	Effective at GFR <10[a]
	i.v., 12–24	0.5–1.5	~1.5	Doses may be increased up to 5 mg/kg in CRF
	c.i.v.i.	100–200 μg/kg/h		Hypokalemia; Mg, Ca depletion; ototoxicity; metabolic alkalosis
Torasemide	p.o.	0.5–1	~3.5	Longer $t_{1/2}$ and larger duration than furosemide; effective at GFR <10[a]; idem furosemide
Ethacrynic acid	p.o., 12–24	1–2	~1	Effective at GFR <10[a]; idem furosemide
Bumetanide	p.o., 12–24	0.01–0.10	~1	Effective at GFR <10[a]; idem furosemide
	i.v., 12–24	0.01–0.05		
	c.i.v.i.	5–10 μg/kg/h	~1	
Hydrochlorothiazide	p.o. 12–24	1–3	~2.5	Not effective at GFR <20[a]; hypokalemia, metabolic alkalosis
Chlorthalidone	p.o., 24–48	0.5–2.0	45	Not effective at GFR <20[a]; hypokalemia, metabolic alkalosis
Metolazone	p.o. 12–24	0.2–0.4	8–10	Effective at GFR <20[a]; hypokalemia
Spironolactone	p.o. 6–12	1–3	~1.6	Delayed effect. Avoid in CRF or K supplementation hyperkalemia, acidosis
Canrenoate-K	i.v. 24	4–10	~16	Single i.v. dose; hyperkalemia, acidosis
Triamterene	p.o. 12–24	2–4	~4.2	Avoid in CRF or K supplementation hyperkalemia, acidosis
Amiloride	p.o. 24	0.5	~21	Avoid in CRF or K supplementation hyperkalemia, acidosis

c.i.v.i., constant intravenous infusion; CRF, chronic renal failure; ECV, extracellular volume; i.v., intravenous; p.o., oral; q, every.
[a]GFR, glomerular filtration rate (mL per min per 1.73 m^2).

the increased delivery of Na^+ to the late distal tubule and because of reduced H^+ available for secretion in exchange with Na^+.[1] Carbonic anhydrase inhibitors are weak diuretics, at best producing the excretion of 5% of the Na^+ and water filtered load. The action of carbonic anhydrase inhibitors is self-limiting. The excretion of HCO_3^- decreases in parallel with the development of metabolic acidosis in response to carbonic anhydrase inhibition.

Pharmacokinetic Properties

Acetazolamide is readily absorbed; it has a 100% oral availability and a half-life of 6 to 9 hours. It is eliminated in the urine. Acetazolamide crosses the placental barrier and is secreted in breast milk.

Efficacy and Therapeutic Uses

Acetazolamide increases the urinary excretion of bicarbonate, sodium, and potassium, thus promoting alkaline diuresis. The mild metabolic acidosis induced by the continuous administration of acetazolamide limits the diuretic effects of the agent. Acetazolamide is consequently not used presently for its natriuretic effect. It may be useful to alkalinize the urine when necessary, as for instance, when chemotherapy is given. Acetazolamide has useful specific indications related to its ability to inhibit the carbonic anhydrase in different systems. Such indications are mountain sickness and glaucoma. Acetazolamide has been used for the management of chronic metabolic acidosis in neonates and infants with chronic respiratory insufficiency[50] or in pediatric intensive care unit (PICU) cardiac patients with metabolic alkalosis secondary to loop diuretic therapy.[51] Acetazolamide can be a beneficial adjunctive agent in the pharmacotherapy of refractory epilepsy.[52]

Specific Indications: Assessment of Distal Tubular Acidification

Acetazolamide can also be used to assess reliably the distal acidification ability by measuring the urine minus blood PCO_2 in alkaline urine.[53] For drug dosages, see Table 51.5.

Adverse Effects—Interactions

The occurrence of metabolic acidosis is common if the urinary losses of HCO_3^- are not substituted. Paresthesias, drowsiness, rash, and fever are not uncommon. Formation of renal calculi, rare blood dyscrasias, and hepatic failure are occasionally seen.

LOOP DIURETICS: INHIBITION OF NA^+, K^+, $2Cl^-$ SYMPORT

Chemistry

Loop diuretics form a group of diuretics with diverse chemical structures.[10,54] Furosemide and bumetanide are sulfonamide derivatives, torasemide is a sulfonylurea, and ethacrynic acid is a phenoxyacetic acid derivative.

Mechanisms and Sites of Action

Loop diuretics reach the proximal tubular lumen by glomerular filtration and/or following proximal tubular secretion via the organic acid pump. Afterward, they are transported to the thick ascending limb of loop of Henle where they block the Na^+, K^+, $2Cl^-$ symporter. So, loop diuretics are highly efficacious, as 25% of NaCl filtered load is reabsorbed in the thick ascending limb of Henle's loop, and only a small proportion of the filtered load of sodium that escapes reabsorption in the loop can be reabsorbed downstream.

By inhibiting NaCl reabsorption in Henle's loop, loop diuretics abolish the lumen-positive voltage and thus the driving force for Ca^{2+} and Mg^{2+} reabsorption. They consequently increase Ca^{2+} and Mg^{2+} excretion. Loop diuretics significantly increase K^+ excretion. Inhibition of NaCl transport upstream of the distal tubule results in increased Na^+ delivery to the late portion of the distal tubule and cortical collecting duct. This part of the nephron responds by increasing K^+ and H^+ secretion. This secretion is also stimulated by the state of secondary hyperaldosteronism usually present as a consequence of diuretic-induced decrease in ECF volume. By inhibiting NaCl reabsorption in the water-impermeable thick ascending limb of loop of Henle, loop diuretics interfere both with the diluting and the concentrating mechanism. Loop diuretics do not inhibit $HCO3^-$ reabsorption.

Pharmacokinetic Properties

The effect of loop diuretics is more closely related to their urinary excretion rate than to their plasma concentration. Therefore, pharmacokinetic factors that affect loop diuretic delivery to the thick ascending limb of the loop of Henle are major determinants of drugs response.[54] These factors include volume of distribution, protein binding, renal clearance, and nonrenal clearance.

Furosemide is rapidly absorbed from the gastrointestinal tract, with a bioavailability close to 60% to 70%. It is 99% bound to plasma albumin. Furosemide and ethacrynic acid displace bilirubin from albumin-binding sites.[11] Furosemide is mainly excreted unchanged in the urine. The diuretic response to loop diuretics appears within a few minutes after IV administration and within 30 to 60 minutes after oral administration. The effect does not last more than 2 hours after IV injection and 6 hours after oral administration. Nonrenal clearance is increased in patients with chronic renal failure. The half-life is prolonged in patients with renal and liver insufficiency. In premature neonates less than 32 weeks gestational age, GFR is the main determinant to deliver furosemide into the urine, whereas at term, active secretion by the proximal tubule cell is the main component of renal clearance.[55] Plasma half-life as long as 45 hours have been observed in premature and term neonates, and plasma half-life decreases with increasing postnatal age.[56,57]

Although the pharmacology of furosemide has been well studied in children[58] and neonates,[56] that of other loop diuretics is not as well defined. The pharmacokinetics and pharmacodynamics of bumetanide have been studied in critically ill children[59] and critically ill infants.[60] Diuretic efficiency of bumetanide was maximal at doses of 0.005 to 0.010 mg per kg.[61] The efficacy of torasemide has been assessed in immature animals,[62] and its efficacy and safety in children with heart failure. A significant improvement in heart failure was observed, along with a potassium-sparing effect that was subscribed to the anti-aldosterone properties of this agent.[63] Loop diuretics cross the placental barrier and are secreted in breast milk.

Efficacy and Therapeutic Uses

Loop diuretics are the most potent natriuretic agents, also markedly increasing Cl^-, K^+, Ca^{2+}, and Mg^{2+} excretion.[10] They have steep dose–response curves. They remain active in patients with advanced renal failure. Loop diuretics are the most frequently used diuretics in children, infants, and neonates. Specific indications include oliguric states associated with prerenal failure, various respiratory disorders such as RDS, bronchopulmonary dysplasia and asthma, indomethacin-associated oliguria, and hypercalcemic states. Loop diuretics can decrease blood pressure in hypertensive children, but their short duration of action makes them less suitable than the thiazides in this indication.

Continuous Intravenous Infusion of Loop Diuretics

Clinical trials in infants indicate that continuous infusion therapy of furosemide can produce more efficient and better-controlled diuresis with less fluid shifts and greater hemodynamic stability.[64,65] Several studies provide a strong evidence that in case of volume overload after cardiac surgery and in critically ill patients, continuous IV furosemide is preferable compared to intermittent doses,[66,67] although this may not necessarily be true for hemodynamically stable patients.[68] Despite this evidence, the dosing schedule for continuous furosemide infusion is largely empirical. In hemodynamically unstable infants after cardiac surgery, the administration of a loading dose (1–2 mg per kg) of the diuretic before starting the continuous infusion accelerates the diuretic response.[65] This loading dose, followed by a continuous infusion at 0.2 mg per kg per hour (adjusted according to a target urine output of 4 mL per kg per hour), appears a safe and effective treatment for volume overload.[69]

Only few retrospective studies have evaluated the continuous infusion of bumetanide in critically ill infants, showing that an infusion dose ranging from 1 to 10 μg per kg per h (mean 5.7 ± 2.2 μg per kg per h) was effective in achieving negative fluid balance.[70,71]

Indications

Edematous States

CHF is the most common indication to the use of loop diuretics in neonates and infants. In infants with severe CHF, the diuretic effect of furosemide is inversely related to serum aldosterone levels. The concomitant administration of a K^+-sparing diuretic improves the response to loop diuretics.[72] Furosemide increases the peripheral venous capacitance and can thus be useful independently from its diuretic effect. In adults, torasemide has been shown to be at least as effective as furosemide in reducing salt and water retention,[73] to have a longer duration of action, and to reduce overall treatment costs of CHF in comparison with furosemide.[74]

Nephrotic Syndrome

In hypovolemic patients with massive nephrotic edema, IV furosemide can be used to promote sodium and water excretion. In hypovolemic patients, furosemide (1–2 mg per kg) should be given only after the expansion of the extracellular space with IV albumin (5 mL per kg of 20% albumin in 60 min). This regimen usually results in a loss of 1% to 2% of body weight. The dose can be repeated. The effect is transient but may be useful in patients with severe ascites and/or pulmonary edema. The therapy may be associated with potentially serious complications, such as CHF or respiratory distress.[75] Coadministration of IV furosemide and mannitol (5 mL per kg of a 20% solution) could be a safe, inexpensive, and effective alternative to the classic furosemide–albumin regimen.[76] In hypervolemic patients, the use of furosemide alone appears safe and effective.[77]

Oliguric States

Furosemide is frequently used in oliguric states secondary to prerenal or renal failure, in the hope of promoting diuresis and improving renal function. Although furosemide may increase urine output and facilitate the clinical management of the patient, it is unlikely to improve GFR. By inducing diuresis and possibly hypovolemia, loop diuretics carry the risk of further stressing the oliguric kidney. There is as yet no clinical[24] or experimental[78] evidence that loop diuretics can prevent ARF or improve the outcome of patients with ARF. However, in patients undergoing cardiopulmonary bypass surgery, urine output response to furosemide administered intraoperatively predicts cardiac surgery–induced acute kidney injury development and other important morbidities.[79]

Respiratory Distress Syndrome

Furosemide administration has produced conflicting results in preterm neonates with RDS.[11] While furosemide usually acutely induces diuresis, and a transient improvement in pulmonary function, the more recent critical review of the literature[80] failed to support the routine administration of furosemide (or any diuretic) in preterm infants with RDS and concluded that elective administration of diuretics should be weighed against the risk of inducing cardiovascular complications. Diuretics cannot even be recommended as the treatment for transient tachypnea of the newborn at term.[81]

Preterm Infants with or Developing Chronic Lung Disease

Loop diuretics have been given to preterm infants with chronic lung disease (CLD), in the hope of decreasing the need for oxygen or ventilatory support. A critical review of the available data of the literature concluded that in preterm infants younger than 3 weeks developing CLD, furosemide had either inconstant effects or no detectable effects.[82] In infants older than 3 weeks with CLD, the acute IV administration of furosemide (1 mg per kg) improved lung compliance and airway resistance for 1 hour. Chronic administration of furosemide improved both oxygenation and lung compliance. A similar conclusion was drawn from studies on the effect of aerosolized furosemide in preterm infants with CLD. Although not enough information was available in preterm infants younger than 3 weeks, data in preterm infants older than 3 weeks with CLD showed that a single dose of aerosolized furosemide improved pulmonary mechanisms. But in view of the lack of data from randomized trials concerning the effects on important clinical outcomes, routine or sustained use of aerosolized loop diuretics in infants with or developing CLD cannot be recommended.[83] Recently, a multicenter observational cohort study of 835 extremely premature infants born 23 to 28 weeks of gestation—the Prematurity and Respiratory Outcomes Program (PROP) study—was conducted in order to determine whether daily respiratory status improved more in extremely low gestational age premature infants after diuretic exposure, compared with those not exposed. The results did not support the ability of diuretics to substantially improve the extremely premature infant's respiratory status.[84]

All the above results allow the conclusion that diuretics are no longer recommended for routine management of the early or late phases of RDS nor CLD. However, diuretics administration remains recommended in severe chronically ill patients for the management of accumulation of interstitial lung fluid, such as in cases of pulmonary edema which may occur in respiratory acute and chronic morbidities.[85]

Posthemorrhagic Ventricular Dilatation

A critical review of randomized trials in newborn infants with posthemorrhagic ventricular dilatation (PVD)[86] concluded that acetazolamide and furosemide therapy is neither effective nor safe in treating preterm infants with PVD. The largest trial in 177 infants showed that acetazolamide and furosemide treatment resulted in a borderline increase in the risk for motor impairment at 1 year and in an increased risk for nephrocalcinosis, without decreasing the risk for disability, chronic motor impairment, or death.[86]

Indomethacin-induced Oliguria

Oliguria occurs frequently after administration of indomethacin to close a patent ductus arteriosus (PDA). Inhibition of prostaglandin synthesis by indomethacin is responsible for the oliguria. Because furosemide increases prostaglandin production, it could potentially help prevent indomethacin-related toxicity and also decrease ductal response to indomethacin. Available studies indicate that furosemide increased urine output in all patients, leading to a 5% weight loss during a three-dose course. It increases creatinine clearance only in patients with initial blood urea nitrogen-to-creatinine ratio of less than 20 mg per mg. A critical review concluded that there was as yet not enough evidence to support the administration of furosemide to preterm infants treated with indomethacin for PDA.[87] Also noteworthy is the conclusion that there is as yet not enough evidence from randomized trials to show that there is any value in giving dopamine to prevent renal dysfunction in indomethacin-treated preterm infants.[88]

Hypercalcemic States

Loop diuretics can promote calcium excretion and decrease hypercalcemia. Isotonic saline must be infused concomitantly to prevent volume depletion.

Severe Hyponatremia

Severe hyponatremia can be treated by loop diuretics and the concomitant isovolumetric infusion of hypertonic saline.

Intratracheal Furosemide

Direct intratracheal administration of furosemide has been claimed to produce beneficial effects in children with asthma, infants with bronchopulmonary dysplasia, and toddlers with compromised lung mechanics after cardiac surgery. In the latter study, a systemic effect was observed within 15 minutes after intratracheal instillation of the agent.[89]

Assessment of Distal Renal Acidification

The simultaneous administration of furosemide and fludrocortisone has been shown to be an easy, effective, and well-tolerated alternative to standard ammonium chloride loading to assess urinary acidification and confirm the diagnosis of distal renal tubular acidosis.[90] For drug dosages, see Table 51.5.

Adverse Effects—Interactions

Because of their efficacy, common adverse effects including volume depletion, postural hypotension, dizziness and syncope, hyponatremia, and hypokalemia are commonly observed. These effects are dose dependent and often occur after overzealous use of large doses of diuretics or chronic administration.

Hypochloremic Metabolic Alkalosis

This condition occurs frequently as a consequence of direct stimulation by loop diuretics of H^+ secretion in the collecting tubule.

Hypercalciuria

Elevated Ca^{2+} urinary losses in response to loop diuretics are associated with a significant risk of *nephrocalcinosis* in premature infants,[91] secondary hyperparathyroidism, bone resorption, and rickets. When prolonged, hypercalciuria may lead to renal impairment.[92] Although thiazide diuretics decrease calcium and oxalate excretion, adding thiazides to loop diuretics did not appear beneficial.[93]

Patent Ductus Arteriosus

The suggestion that by stimulating prostaglandin synthesis furosemide could promote PDA has not been confirmed. On the contrary, in a large cohort of VLBW infants, furosemide exposure was recently associated with decreased odds of PDA treatment.[94]

Ototoxicity

The use of furosemide has been identified as an independent risk factor for sensorineural hearing loss in preterm infants.[95] Hearing loss may be transient or permanent. It is usually associated with elevated blood concentrations of loop diuretics. The coadministration of loop diuretics and aminoglycosides increases the risk of ototoxicity. By avoiding elevated peak concentrations of furosemide, the continuous infusion decreases the risk of ototoxicity.[54]

Chronic Use

Increased distal delivery of Na^+ as a consequence of loop diuretic administration leads to hypertrophy of distal nephrons with consequent hyper-reabsorption of Na^+.

Miscellaneous

Pancreatitis, jaundice, deterioration of glucose tolerance, thrombocytopenia, gastroesophageal reflux, increased fracture risk, and serious skin disorders occur occasionally.[96,97] The majority of adverse effects occur with the use of high doses.

In newborns infants receiving oral liquid furosemide formulations (which contain ethanol as excipient), blood acetaldehyde concentrations were dosed and appeared consistent with moderate alcohol exposure, so the risk of harms from acetaldehyde needs to be balanced against the likelihood of benefits from the active ingredient.[98]

Interactions

Drug interactions may occur with the coadministration of nephrotoxic antibiotics, nonsteroidal anti-inflammatory drugs, anticoagulants, and cisplatin.

DISTAL CONVOLUTED TUBULE: INHIBITORS OF Na^+, Cl^- SYMPORT

Chemistry

The benzothiadiazide derivatives are sulfonamides. They are weak diuretics that inhibit the reabsorption of NaCl at the diluting site in the early distal tubule. The main thiazides include chlorothiazide and hydrochlorothiazide. Thiazide-like agents such as chlorthalidone and metolazone belong to this group.

Mechanisms and Sites of Action

The thiazides are organic anions that gain access to the tubular lumen by filtration and secretion in the proximal tubule. They decrease NaCl reabsorption in the distal convoluted tubule by inhibiting the Na^+–Cl^- apical symporter. This symporter, sometimes called ENCC1 or TSC, is predominantly expressed in the epithelial cells of the distal convoluted tubule. Its expression is upregulated by aldosterone.[1] To reach their site of action on the luminal side of the tubular cells, the thiazides must be secreted by the anionic organic acid pathway in the proximal tubule. Approximately 4% to 5% of the Na^+ filtered load is being reabsorbed in the distal collecting duct, and inhibition of Na^+ reabsorption at this site can only modestly increase NaCl excretion. Some of the thiazides also slightly increase the excretion of HCO_3^- by weakly inhibiting the carbonic anhydrase. By increasing Na^+ delivery to the late distal tubule, the thiazides lead to increased reabsorption of Na^+ in the late distal tubule, in exchange for K^+ and H^+, which are lost in the urine. By inhibiting NaCl reabsorption in the early distal tubule, the thiazides blunt the ability to dilute the urine. They do not interfere with the concentrating mechanism. The thiazides stimulate Ca^{2+} reabsorption in the distal tubule, probably by opening the apical membrane Ca^{2+} channels. The thiazides (but not metolazone) are ineffective at GFRs below 30 mL per minute per 1.73 m^2.

Pharmacokinetic Properties

The thiazides are fairly rapidly absorbed after oral administration. They variably bind to plasma proteins. They are eliminated unchanged, exclusively (chlorothiazide, hydrochlorothiazide, chlorthalidone) or in great part (~80%) (metolazone) in the urine. Administration of thiazides initiates diuresis in 2 hours, an effect that lasts for 12 hours. The response to metolazone is somewhat more rapid (1 hour) and lasts longer (12 to 24 hours). The thiazides cross the placental barrier and are secreted in breast milk.

Efficacy and Therapeutic Uses

Thiazide diuretics moderately increase the excretion of Na^+, Cl^-, and water. All thiazides (chlorothiazide, hydrochlorothiazide) and thiazide-like diuretics have overall similar effects when used in maximal doses. When administered chronically, they decrease the excretion of Ca^{2+}, as well as that of uric acid, probably as a consequence of increased proximal reabsorption due to volume depletion. The excretion of Mg^{2+} is somewhat increased, as is the excretion of K^+ and fixed acids. Increased Na^+ delivery to the late distal tubule and collecting duct is responsible for the increased excretion of K^+ and fixed acids. Because of the risk of inducing hypokalemia, prophylactic coadministration of K^+-sparing diuretics may be indicated to prevent the occurrence of severe hypokalemia. Alternatively, potassium supplementation may be useful in patients at risk. Magnesium supplementation may also be necessary. The thiazides, but not metolazone, increase the excretion of HCO_3^-. In the absence of significant volume depletion, the thiazides do not normally influence renal hemodynamics and GFR. In contrast with the thiazides and chlorthalidone, metolazone remains effective at GFRs below 30 mL per minute per 1.73 m^2.

Indications

The main indications for the administration of thiazide diuretics include edematous states, hypertension, and a few specific indications.

Hypercalciuria

The thiazides decrease calcium excretion, and this effect may be useful in states of idiopathic hypercalciuria, as well as to prevent calcium losses in patients receiving glucocorticoids.[99] They have been associated with loop diuretics to decrease the risk of hypercalciuria and nephrocalcinosis in VLBW infants undergoing loop diuretic therapy, with disappointing results.[10] The thiazides have been used to prevent renal stone formation in susceptible patients. The use of thiazides has been associated with a rise in total serum cholesterol and in the low-density lipoprotein/high-density lipoprotein ratio, indicating that the risks and benefits of the thiazide therapy should be considered before starting treatment.[100] In children with X-linked hypophosphatemia on renal phosphate and vitamin D therapy, hydrochlorothiazide decreased the urinary excretion of calcium but did not reverse the nephrocalcinosis.[101]

Proximal Tubular Renal Acidosis

The thiazides have been used to raise the plasma bicarbonate concentration in proximal renal tubular acidosis. This effect is the consequence of volume contraction induced by the thiazides, a chronic condition that is deleterious for growth.

Nephrogenic Diabetes Insipidus

The thiazides have been successfully used in children with nephrogenic diabetes insipidus. They are safe and effective.[102] By inducing volume contraction, they enhance the proximal tubular reabsorption of water and electrolytes, thus significantly decreasing urine output. While usefully decreasing urine output, volume contraction may inhibit growth in young children with nephrogenic diabetes insipidus. The concomitant use of hydrochlorothiazide and amiloride obviates the need for the K^+ supplementation and has been shown useful as the standard treatment with hydrochlorothiazide and indomethacin[23,103] in reducing urine output.

Chronic Lung Disease

Thiazide and thiazide-like diuretics have been used in the hope of improving pulmonary mechanisms and clinical outcome in preterm infants with CLD. A critical analysis of available well-planned studies led to the conclusion that in preterm infants older than 8 weeks with CLD, a 4-week treatment with thiazide and spironolactone improved lung compliance and reduced the need for furosemide. However, the reviewers concluded that positive effects should be interpreted with caution as the numbers of patients studied were small.[104]

Diagnosis of Renal Tubular Hypokalemic Disorders

Assessment of the maximal diuretic response induced by the administration of hydrochlorothiazide (1 mg per kg, orally) allows to differentiate Gitelman from Bartter syndrome, the former presenting with a blunted response to the diuretic agent.[105] For drug dosage, see Table 51.5.

Adverse Effects—Interactions

Thiazides may adversely affect water balance and induce electrolyte imbalances (Table 51.3). Other side effects include gastrointestinal disturbances, hypersensitivity reactions, cholestatic jaundice, pancreatitis, thrombocytopenia, hyperglycemia in diabetic and susceptible patients, and hyperlipidemia. Precipitation of hepatic encephalopathy has been observed in patients with hepatic cirrhosis. The thiazides displace bilirubin from albumin and should be cautiously administered to patients with jaundice.

LATE DISTAL AND CORTICAL COLLECTING DUCT: K^+-SPARING DRUGS

Chemistry

Two types of diuretics form the group of K^+-sparing diuretics: (a) the inhibitors of a renal $E_{NA}Cs$ and (b) the antagonists of mineralocorticoid receptors. The overall effects of these two groups of diuretics differ only in their mode of action.

Mechanisms and Sites of Action

The antagonists of the action of aldosterone on the principal cells of the collecting duct increase Na^+ excretion and decrease K^+ and H^+ secretion. Spironolactone, the main agent in this group, competitively inhibits the binding of aldosterone to the mineralocorticoid receptor, thus decreasing the synthesis of aldosterone-induced proteins. The aldosterone antagonists have greater effects in situations of hyperaldosteronism. They do not modify the renal hemodynamics. Highly selective antagonists of the mineralocorticoid receptor are currently under investigation.[106]

The $E_{NA}C$ blockers amiloride and triamterene block the entry of Na^+ into the cell through the Na^+-selective channels ($E_{NA}C$) in the apical membrane. Because of changes in electrical profile across the apical membrane, the diffusion of both H^+ and K^+ from cells into tubular fluid decreases. Activation of the renin–angiotensin–aldosterone system by the diuretics also impairs the excretion of K^+, H^+, Ca^{2+}, and Mg^{2+}. $E_{NA}C$ blockers do not affect renal hemodynamics.

Pharmacokinetic Properties

Spironolactone is rapidly absorbed from the gastrointestinal tract, with a bioavailability close to 90%. It is 90% bound to plasma proteins and is excreted mainly in the urine and, to a lesser extent, in the feces. Spironolactone has a slow onset of action, requiring 2 to 3 days for maximum effect.

Canrenoate-potassium has similar actions to those of spironolactone. It is available for IV administration.

Amiloride is incompletely absorbed from the gastrointestinal tract, with a bioavailability of only 50%. It is not bound to plasma proteins and is excreted unchanged in the urine. Its half-life is 6 to 9 hours. It is prolonged in patients with hepatic or renal failure.

Triamterene is unreliably absorbed. It is metabolized by hepatic conjugation. One-fifth of the dose is excreted unchanged in the urine. Its half-life is 1 to 3 hours.

All K^+-sparing diuretics cross the placental barrier and are secreted in breast milk.

Efficacy and Therapeutic Uses

K^+-sparing diuretics are also often used in association with thiazide diuretics in the management of preterm infants with CLD. Although they certainly decrease the risk of hypokalemia and facilitate the clinical management of the infants, there is as yet no definite proof that their association to thiazide improves the long-term outcome of preterm infants with CLD.

The overall effects on electrolyte excretion are similar for spironolactone, amiloride, and triamterene. They are weak natriuretic agents that reduce the excretion of potassium and hydrogen ions. K^+-sparing diuretics are mainly used in Na^+-retaining states in association with loop or thiazide diuretics. They enhance the natriuretic effect while at the same time limiting K^+ losses. Refractory edema secondary to CHF, cirrhosis of the liver, and the nephrotic syndrome represent the most common indications for the use of K-sparing diuretics. In these conditions associated with secondary hyperaldosteronism, spironolactone is the first-choice agent, provided renal function is not impaired.[107] Because they induce K^+ retention, K^+-sparing diuretics should not be used in patients with impaired renal function or in those receiving K^+ supplementation. They should also be avoided in patients prone to develop metabolic acidosis. The respiratory function and sputum excretion of patients with cystic fibrosis have been improved by the inhalation of 10^{-3} M amiloride, possibly by the blocking effect of $E_{NA}C$ in pulmonary tissue.[108] A multicenter, randomized, double-blind, placebo-controlled trial has not confirmed the beneficial effect of aerosolized amiloride.[109] Amiloride has been successfully used in association with hydrochlorothiazide in patients with nephrogenic diabetes insipidus, obviating the need for using indomethacin.[23] For drug dosage, see Table 51.5.

Adverse Effects—Interactions

The main adverse effect of K^+-sparing diuretics is to increase the K^+ plasma concentration to harmful levels. Close monitoring of K^+ concentration is thus mandatory. Gastrointestinal disturbances, dizziness, photosensitivity, and blood dyscrasias have been reported after the use of triamterene.

Significant adverse effects have been observed with spironolactone: gynecomastia, hirsutism, impotence, and menstrual irregularities can occur. Gynecomastia in males is related to both the dose and duration of treatment. Breast enlargement and tenderness occur in women. The pathogenesis of the adverse effects of spironolactone on the endocrine system is probably related to an antiadrenergic action and reduced 17-hydroxylase activity.

K^+-sparing diuretics should not be used in patients receiving angiotensin-converting enzyme (ACE) inhibitors, as the association can worsen the risk of hyperkalemia.

The half-life of amiloride is prolonged in patients with hepatic or renal failure.

NEW DEVELOPMENT IN DIURETIC THERAPY

Two categories of diuretics are under development:

1. The Natriuretic Peptides
2. The Arginine Vasopressin Antagonists

Natriuretic Peptides

The ANP and BNP are two peptides with natriuretic and diuretic properties.[110] Both are released by cardiac cells in the atria in response to increased blood volume. ANP (28-amino-acid) and BNP (32-amino-acid) act via the natriuretic peptide receptor A (NPR-A). In addition to increasing the excretion of Na^+, both peptides inhibit the sympathetic system and the renin–angiotensin–aldosterone system. They also relax vascular smooth muscle. Both ANP and BNP are degraded by the metalloproteinase endopeptidase 24.11 also called neutral endopeptidase (NEP). Urodilatin is a noncirculating NP (32-amino-acid) secreted by distal tubular cells and is not degraded by the NEP located in the proximal tubular cells.[111]

ANP favors filtration by relaxing the afferent artery and the mesangial cells.[112] The NPs inhibit Na^+ proximal reabsorption and decrease distal Na^+ reabsorption indirectly by blunting angiotensin II and aldosterone synthesis and directly by inhibiting the thiazide-sensitive Na^+ channel. ANP increases diuresis by inhibiting the action of AVP on water permeability.

Enhancing the activity of the NPs could help patients presenting with inappropriate salt and water retention.[113] This can be achieved by (a) administration of exogenous ANP and BNP, (b) using nonpeptide antagonists of the NP-A receptor, and (c) using NEP inhibitors.

Studies with nesiritide, a BNP[114] has produced promising results in situations of heart failure in adults. Very few studies have reported the efficacy and safety of nesiritide infusion, either alone or in combination for treating decompensated hearth failure.[114,115] These studies have several limitations: retrospective design or small size cohorts.

The use of NEP also appears promising, resulting in significant natriuresis and diuresis. Because NEP also inhibits the degradation of angiotensin II, ACE inhibitors should be associated with NEP inhibitors in order to prevent vasoconstriction that may be secondary to stimulation of the renin–angiotensin–aldosterone system in response to loss of Na^+ and water. Drugs like omapatrilat, which inhibit both the ACE and the NEP, are being successfully investigated in adults presenting with chronic heart failure.[114] Sacubitril/valsartan (LCZ696) is an angiotensin-receptor neprilysin inhibitor approved for the treatment of adult heart failure. A large prospective RCT is ongoing in order to evaluate whether sacubitril/valsartan is superior to enalapril for treatment of pediatric patients with heart failure and reduced systemic left ventricular systolic function.[117]

Arginine Vasopressin Antagonists

AVP, the ADH, acts on three types of receptors: (a) the V_{1A} receptors mediating vasoconstriction, (b) the V_{1B} mediating the release of adrenocorticotropic hormone, and (c) the V_2 receptors mediating free-water reabsorption in the collecting duct.

AVP also stimulates $Na^+–K^+–2Cl^-$ cotransport in the ascending limb of loop of Henle via V_2 receptors.

Orally active nonpeptide-selective V_2 antagonists have been developed.[118,119] They include the following agents: lixivaptan, tolvaptan, and satavaptan. Experimental and adult human studies demonstrate that these agents increase the excretion of free water and decrease the urine osmolality in a dose-dependent manner. They may thus prove useful in treating hyponatremic states.[110,119]

Blockade of V_2 receptors results in increased levels of AVP. This can lead to stimulation of the V_1 receptors and result in vasoconstriction. Combined V_{1A} and V_2 receptors blockade may prevent this adverse hemodynamic response.[120]

Recent basic and clinical studies have shown that AVP-receptor antagonists, especially V_2-receptor antagonists, may have therapeutic potential for heart failure in adult patients. However, these agents have not been shown to improve short- or long-term morbidity or mortality in clinical studies.[121]

Based on currently available adult studies, oral or IV conivaptan, a dual $V_{1A} + V_2$–receptor antagonist, appears to be effective in inducing aquaresis to correct hyponatremia with short-term use in both hypovolemic and hypervolemic patients.[122] One of the most concerning issues with the use of any V_2-receptor antagonist in the treatment of hyponatremia is the rate of correction of serum sodium concentration. The occurrence of hypokalemia in up to 22% of patients is also of considerable concern. This hypokalemia could be due to renal potassium wasting secondary to increased diuresis with consequent facilitated potassium secretion.

Worth mentioning is the observation that AVP is a powerful modulator of cystogenesis. AVP V_2-receptor antagonists indeed inhibit the formation and growth of renal cysts in animal models of cystic kidney disease, presumably by downregulating cAMP signaling, cell proliferation, and chloride-driven fluid secretion. Clinical studies in patients with autosomal polycystic kidney disease (PKD) are presently being performed. Preliminary results of phase 2 and phases 2 to 3 clinical trials suggest that the antagonist tolvaptan is safe and well tolerated in autosomal dominant PKD.[123] These results provide further support for clinical trials of V_2-receptor antagonists in PKD.

The use of V_2- or $V_{1A} + V_2$–receptor antagonists has not been validated in neonates, infants, or children.

REFERENCES

1. Giebisch G, Windhager E. The urinary system. Part VI. In: Boron WF, Boulpaep EL, eds. *Medical physiology*. Philadelphia, PA: Saunders, 2003:735–876.
2. Garty H, Palmer LG. Epithelial sodium channels: function, structure, and regulation. *Physiol Rev* 1997;77:359–396.
3. Ikeda M, Matsuzaki T. Regulation of aquaporins by vasopressin in the kidney. *Vitam Horm* 2015;98:307–337.
4. Houillier P. Mechanisms and regulation of renal magnesium transport. *Annu Rev Physiol* 2014;76:411–430.
5. Guignard JP. Renal function in the newborn infant. *Pediatr Clin North Am* 1982;29:777–790.
6. Guignard JP, John EG. Renal function in the tiny, premature infant. *Clin Perinatol* 1986;13:377–401.
7. Guignard JP, Gouyon JB. Body fluid homeostasis in the newborn infant with congestive heart failure: effects of diuretics. *Clin Perinatol* 1988;15:447–466.
8. Guignard JP. Renal morphogenesis and development of renal function. In: Taeusch HW, Ballard RA, Gleason CA, eds. *Avery's diseases of the newborn*, 8th ed. Philadelphia, PA: WB Saunders Co, 2005:1257–1266.
9. Guignard JP. Postnatal development of glomerular filtration rate in neonates. In: Polin RA, Abman SH, Rowitch DH, Benitz WE, Fox WW, eds. Fetal and Neonatal Medicine, 5th ed, vol 2. Elsevier, Philadelphia, 2017:993-1002.
10. Brater DC. Diuretic therapy. *N Engl J Med* 1998;339:387–395.
11. Chemtob S, Kaplan BS, Sherbotie JR, et al. Pharmacology of diuretics in the newborn. *Pediatr Clin North Am* 1989;36:1231–1250.
12. Lowrie L. Diuretic therapy of heart failure in infants and children. *Prog Pediatr Cardiol* 2000;12:45–55.
13. Wells TG. The pharmacology and therapeutics of diuretics in the pediatric patient. *Pediatr Clin North Am* 1990;37:463–504.
14. Morrison RT. Edema and principles of diuretic use. *Med Clin North Am* 1997;81:689–704.
15. Schrier RW, Fassett RG. A critique of the overfill hypothesis of sodium and water retention in the nephrotic syndrome. *Kidney Int* 1998;53:1111–1117.
16. Vande Walle JG, Donckerwolcke RA. Pathogenesis of edema formation in the nephrotic syndrome. *Pediatr Nephrol* 2001;16:283–293.
17. Sabri M, Saps M, Peters JM. Pathophysiology and management of pediatric ascites. *Curr Gastroenterol Rep* 2003;5:240–246.
18. Reyes AJ. Diuretics in the therapy of hypertension. *J Hum Hypertens* 2002;16(Suppl 1):S78–S83.
19. Dupont AG. The place of diuretics in the treatment of hypertension: a historical review of classical experience over 30 years. *Cardiovasc Drugs Ther* 1993;7(Suppl 1):55–62.
20. Freis ED. The efficacy and safety of diuretics in treating hypertension. *Ann Intern Med* 1995;122:223–226.
21. Blowey DL. Diuretics in the treatment of hypertension. *Pediatr Nephrol* 2016; 31:2223–2233.
22. Lurbe E, Agabiti-Rosei E, Cruickshank JK, et al. European Society of Hypertension guidelines for the management of high blood pressure in children and adolescents. *J Hypertens* 2016;34(10):1887–1920.
23. Kirchlechner V, Koller DY, Seidl R, et al. Treatment of nephrogenic diabetes insipidus with hydrochlorothiazide and amiloride. *Arch Dis Child* 1999;80:548–552.
24. Kellum JA. Use of diuretics in the acute care setting *Kidney Int Suppl* 1998;66:S67–S70.
25. Seri I. Cardiovascular, renal, and endocrine actions of dopamine in neonates and children. *J Pediatr* 1995;126:333–344.
26. Dasta JF, Kirby MG. Pharmacology and therapeutic use of low-dose dopamine. *Pharmacotherapy* 1986;6:304–310.
27. Baldwin L, Henderson A, Hickman P. Effect of postoperative low-dose dopamine on renal function after elective major vascular surgery. *Ann Intern Med* 1994;120:744–747.
28. Crouchley JL, Smith PB, Cotten CM, et al. Effects of low-dose dopamine on urine output in normotensive very low birth weight neonates. *J Perinatol* 2013; 33(8):619-621.
29. Gambaro G, Bertaglia G, Puma G, et al. Diuretics and dopamine for the prevention and treatment of acute renal failure: a critical reappraisal. *J Nephrol* 2002;15:213–219.
30. Jaton T, Thonney M, Guignard JP. Failure of dopexamine to protect the hypoxemic newborn rabbit kidney. *Dev Pharmacol Ther* 1991;17:161–166.
31. Driscoll DJ, Gillette PC, Lewis RM, et al. Comparative hemodynamic effects of isoproterenol, dopamine, and dobutamine in the newborn dog. *Pediatr Res* 1979;13:1006–1009.
32. Di Sole F. Adenosine and renal tubular function. *Curr Opin Nephrol Hypertens* 2008;17:399–407.
33. Fredholm BB, Arslan G, Halldner, et al. Structure and function of adenosine receptors and their genes. *Naunyn Schmiedebergs Arch Pharmacol* 2000;362:364–374.
34. Welch WJ. Adenosine type 1 receptor antagonists in fluid retaining disorders. *Expert Opin Investig Drugs* 2002;11:1553–1562.
35. Wilcox CS, Welch WJ, Schreiner GF, et al. Natriuretic and diuretics actions of a highly selective adenosine A_1 receptor antagonist. *J Am Soc Nephrol* 1999;10:714–720.
36. Rieg T, Steigele H, Schnermann J, et al. Requirement of intact adenosine A_1 receptors for the diuretic and natriuretic action of the methylxanthines theophylline and caffeine. *J Pharmacol Exp Ther* 2005;313:403–409.
37. Biaggioni I, Paul S, Puckett A, et al. Caffeine and theophylline as adenosine receptor antagonists in humans. *J Pharmacol Exp Ther* 1991;258:588–593.
38. Gouyon JB, Guignard JP. Theophylline prevents the hypoxemia-induced renal hemodynamic changes in rabbits. *Kidney Int* 1988;33:1078–1083.
39. Huet F, Semama D, Grimaldi M, et al. Effects of theophylline on renal insufficiency in neonates with respiratory distress syndrome. *Intensive Care Med* 1995;21:511–514.
40. Jenik AG, Ceriani Cernadas JM, Gorenstein A, et al. A randomized, double-blind, placebo-controlled trial of the effects of prophylactic theophylline on renal function in term neonates with perinatal asphyxia. *Pediatrics* 2000;105(4):E45.
41. Bakr AF. Prophylactic theophylline to prevent renal dysfunction in newborns exposed to perinatal asphyxia—a study in a developing country. *Pediatr Nephrol* 2005;20:1249–1252.
42. Bhat MA, Shah ZA, Makhdoomi MA, et al. Theophylline for renal function in term neonates with perinatal asphyxia: a randomized, placebo-controlled trial. *J Pediatr* 2006;149:180–184.
43. Cattarelli D, Spandrio M, Gasparoni A, et al. A randomised, double blind, placebo controlled trial of the effect of theophylline in prevention of vasomotor nephropathy in very preterm neonates with respiratory distress syndrome. *Arch Dis Child Fetal Neonatal Ed* 2006;91:F80–F84.
44. Al-Wassia H, Alshaikh B, Sauve R. Prophylactic theophylline for the prevention of severe renal dysfunction in term and post-term neonates with perinatal asphyxia: a systematic review and meta-analysis of randomized controlled trials. *J Perinatol* 2013; 33(4):271–277.
45. Mirza Onder A, Rosen D, Mullett C, et al. Comparison of intraoperative aminophylline versus furosemide in treatment of oliguria during pediatric cardiac surgery. *Pediatr Crit Care Med* 2016;17(8):753–763.
46. Better OS, Rubinstein I, Winaver JM, et al. Mannitol therapy revisited (1940–1997). *Kidney Int* 1997;52:886–894.
47. Solomon R, Werner C, Mann D, et al. Effects of saline, mannitol, and furosemide to prevent acute decreases in renal function induced by radiocontrast agents. *N Engl J Med* 1994;331:1416–1420.
48. Rigden SP, Dillon MJ, Kind PR, et al. The beneficial effect of mannitol on post-operative renal function in children undergoing cardiopulmonary bypass surgery. *Clin Nephrol* 1984;21:148–151.
49. Gouyon JB, Guignard JP. Drugs and acute renal insufficiency in the neonate. *Biol Neonate* 1986;50:177–181.
50. Tam B, Chhay A, Yen L, et al. Acetazolamide for the management of chronic metabolic alkalosis in neonates and infants. *Am J Ther* 2014;21(6):477–481.

51. López C, Alcaraz AJ, Toledo B, et al. Acetazolamide therapy for metabolic alkalosis in pediatric intensive care patients. *Pediatr Crit Care Med* 2016;17(12):e551–e558.
52. Reiss WG, Oles KS. Acetazolamide in the treatment of seizures. *Ann Pharmacother* 1996;30:514–519.
53. Alon U, Hellerstein S, Warady BA. Oral acetazolamide in the assessment of (urine-blood) PCO_2. *Pediatr Nephrol* 1991;5:307–311.
54. Eades SK, Christensen ML. The clinical pharmacology of loop diuretics in the pediatric patient. *Pediatr Nephrol* 1998;12:603–616.
55. van den Anker, JN. Pharmacokinetics and renal function in preterm infants. *Acta Paediatr* 1996;85(12):1393–1399.
56. Mirochnick MH, Miceli JJ, Kramer PA, et al. Furosemide pharmacokinetics in very low birth weight infants. *J Pediatr* 1988;112(4):653–657.
57. Vert P, Broquaire M, Legagneur M, et al. Pharmacokinetics of furosemide in neonates. *Eur J Clin Pharmacol* 1982;22:39–45.
58. Prandota J. Clinical pharmacology of furosemide in children: a supplement. *Am J Ther* 2001;8:275–289.
59. Marshall JD, Wells TG, Letzig L, et al. Pharmacokinetics and pharmacodynamics of bumetanide in critically ill pediatric patients. *J Clin Pharmacol* 1998;38:994–1002.
60. Sullivan JE, Witte MK, Yamashita TS, et al. Pharmacokinetics of bumetanide in critically ill infants. *Clin Pharmacol Ther* 1996;60:405–413.
61. Sullivan JE, Witte MK, Yamashita TS, et al. Dose-ranging evaluation of bumetanide pharmacodynamics in critically ill infants. *Clin Pharmacol Ther* 1996;60:424–434.
62. Dubourg L, Mosig D, Drukker A, et al. Torasemide is an effective diuretic in the newborn rabbit. *Pediatr Nephrol* 2000;14:476–479.
63. Senzaki H, Kamiyama M, Masutani S, et al. Efficacy and safety of torasemide in children with heart failure. *Arch Dis Child* 2008;93:768–771.
64. Luciani GB, Nichani S, Chang AC, et al. Continuous versus intermittent furosemide infusion in critically ill infants after open heart operations. *Ann Thorac Surg* 1997;64:1133–1139.
65. van der Vorst MM, Ruys-Dudok van Heel I, Kist-van Holthe JE, et al. Continuous intravenous furosemide in haemodynamically unstable children after cardiac surgery. *Intensive Care Med* 2001;27:711–715.
66. Singh, NC, Kissoon,N, al Mofada, S, et al. Comparison of continuous versus intermittent furosemide administration in postoperative pediatric cardiac patients. *Crit Care Med* 1992;20(1):17–21.
67. Martin, SJ, Danziger, LH. Continuous infusion of loop diuretics in the critically ill: a review of the literature. *Crit Care Med* 1994;22(8):1323–1329.
68. Klinge JM, Scharf J, Hofbeck M, et al. Intermittent administration of furosemide versus continuous infusion in the postoperative management of children following open heart surgery. *Intensive Care Med* 1997;23:693–697.
69. van der Vorst MMG, Kist-van Holthe JE, den Hartigh J, et al. Absence of tolerance and toxicity to high-dose continuous intravenous furosemide in haemodynamically unstable infants after cardiac surgery. *Br J Clin Pharmacol* 2007;64:796–803.
70. McCallister KM, Chhim R, Briceno-Medina M et al. Bumetanide continuous infusions in critically ill pediatric patients. *Pediatr Crit Care Med* 2015;16(2):e19–e22.
71. Bulkley CF, Johnson PN, Henry E, et al. Bumetanide continuous-infusion dosing in critically ill pediatric patients. *Am J Health Syst Pharm* 2012;69(17):1458, 1460–1461.
72. Baylen BG, Johnson G, Tsang R, et al. The occurrence of hyperaldosteronism in infants with congestive heart failure. *Am J Cardiol* 1980;45:305–310.
73. Knauf H, Mutschler E. Clinical pharmacokinetics and pharmacodynamics of torasemide. *Clin Pharmacokinet* 1998;34:1–24.
74. Young M, Plosker GL. Torasemide: a pharmacoeconomic review of its use in chronic heart failure. *Pharmacoeconomics* 2001;19:679–703.
75. Haws RM, Baum M. Efficacy of albumin and diuretic therapy in children with nephrotic syndrome. *Pediatrics* 1993;91:1142–1146.
76. Lewis MA, Awan A. Mannitol and frusemide in the treatment of diuretic oedema in nephrotic syndrome. *Arch Dis Child* 1999;80:184–185.
77. Kapur G, Valentini RP, Imam AA, et al. Treatment of severe edema in children with nephrotic syndrome with diuretics alone—a prospective study. *Clin J Am Soc Nephrol* 2009;4:907–913.
78. Dubourg L, Drukker A, Guignard J-P. Failure of the loop diuretic torasemide to improve renal function of hypoxemic vasomotor nephropathy in the newborn rabbit. *Pediatr Res* 2000;47:504–508.
79. Borasino S, Wall KM, Crawford JH, et al. Furosemide response predicts acute kidney injury after cardiac surgery in infants and neonates. *Pediatr Crit Care Med* 2018;19(4):310–317
80. Stewart A, Brion LP, Soll RF. Diuretics for respiratory distress syndrome in preterm infants. *Cochrane Database Syt Rev* 2011;(1):CD001454.
81. Kassab M, Khriesat WM, Anabrees J. Diuretics for transient tachypnoea of the newborn. *Cochrane Database Syst Rev* 2015;(11):CD003064.
82. Brion LP, Primhak RA. Intravenous or enteral loop diuretics for preterm infants with (or developing) chronic lung disease: *Cochrane Database Syst Rev* 2002;(1):CD001453.
83. Brion LP, Primhak RA, Yong W. Aerosolized diuretics for preterm infants with (or developing) chronic lung disease. *Cochrane Database Syst Rev* 2006;(3):CD001694.
84. Blaisdell CJ, Troendle J, Zajicek A. Prematurity and respiratory outcomes program. acute responses to diuretic therapy in extremely low gestational age newborns: results from the prematurity and respiratory outcomes program cohort study. *J Pediatr* 2018;197:42-47.
85. Deakins KM. Bronchopulmonary dysplasia. *Respir Care* 2009; 54(9):1252–1262.
86. Whitelaw A, Kennedy CR, Brion LP. Diuretic therapy for newborn infants with posthemorrhagic ventricular dilatation. *Cochrane Database Syst Rev* 2001;(2):CD002270.
87. Brion LP, Campbell DE. Furosemide for symptomatic patent ductus arteriosus in indomethacin-treated infants. *Cochrane Database Syst Rev* 2001;(3):CD 001148.
88. Barrington K, Brion LP. Dopamine versus no treatment to prevent renal dysfunction in indomethacin-treated preterm newborn infants. *Cochrane Database Syst Rev* 2002;(3):CD 003213.
89. Aufricht C, Votava F, Marx M, et al. Intratracheal furosemide in infants after cardiac surgery: its effects on lung mechanics and urinary output, and its levels in plasma and tracheal aspirate. *Intensive Care Med* 1997;23:992–997.
90. Walsh SB, Shirley DG, Wrong OM, et al. Urinary acidification assessed by simultaneous furosemide and fludrocortisone treatment: an alternative to ammonium chloride. *Kidney Int* 2007;71:1310–1316.
91. Gimpel C, Krause A, Franck P, et al. Exposure to furosemide as the strongest risk factor for nephrocalcinosis in preterm infants. *Pediatr Int* 2010;52:51–56.
92. Downing GJ, Egelhoff JC, Daily DK, et al. Kidney function in VLBWI infants with furosemide-related renal calcifications at ages 1 to 2 years. *J Pediatr* 1992;120:599–604.
93. Campfield T, Braden G, Flynn-Valone P, et al. Effect of diuretics on urinary oxalate, calcium, and sodium excretion in VLBWI infants. *Pediatrics* 1997;99:814–818.
94. Thompson EJ, Greenberg RG, Kumar K. Association between furosemide exposure and patent ductus arteriosus in hospitalized infants of very low birth weight. *J Pediatr* 2018;199:231–236.
95. Borradori C, Fawer CL, Buclin T, et al. Risk factors of sensorineural hearing loss in preterm infants. *Biol Neonate* 1997;71:1–10.
96. Cotton R, Suarez S, Reese J. Unexpected extra-renal effects of loop diuretics in the preterm neonate. *Acta Pediatr* 2012;101(8):835–845.
97. Heo JH, Rascati KL, Lopez KN, et al. Increased fracture risk with furosemide use in children with congenital heart disease. *Pediatr* 2018;199:92–98.
98. Pandya HC, Mulla H, Hubbard M. Essential medicines containing ethanol elevate blood acetaldehyde concentrations in neonates. *Eur J Pediatr* 2016;175:841–847.
99. Lukert BP, Raisz LG. Glucocorticoid-induced osteoporosis: pathogenesis and management. *Ann Intern Med* 1990;112:352–364.
100. Reusz GS, Dobos M, Tulassay T. Hydrochlorothiazide treatment of children with hypercalciuria: effects and side effects. *Pediatr Nephrol* 1993;7:699–702.
101. Seikaly MG, Baum M. Thiazide diuretics arrest the progression of nephrocalcinosis in children with X-linked hypophosphatemia. *Pediatrics* 2001;108:E6.
102. Al Nofal A, Lteif A. Thiazide diuretics in the management of young children with central diabetes insipidus. *J Pediatr* 2015;167(3):658–661.
103. Knoers N, Monnens LA. Amiloride-hydrochlorothiazide versus indomethacin-hydrochlorothiazide in the treatment of nephrogenic diabetes insipidus. *J Pediatr* 1990;117:499–502.
104. Stewart A, Brion LP, Ambrosio-Perez I. Diuretics acting on the distal renal tubule for preterm infants with (or developing) chronic lung disease. *Cochrane Database Syst Rev* 2011;(7):CD001817.
105. Colussi G, Bettinelli A, Tedeschi S, et al. A thiazide test for the diagnosis of renal tubular hypokalemic disorders. *Clin J Am Soc Nephrol* 2007;2:454–460.
106. Delyani JA. Mineralocorticoid receptor antagonists: the evolution of utility and pharmacology. *Kidney Int* 2000;57:1408–1411.
107. Buck ML. Clinical experience with spironolactone in pediatrics. *Ann Pharmacother* 2005;39:823–828.
108. Hofmann T, Senier I, Bittner P, et al. Aerosolized amiloride: dose effect on nasal bioelectric properties, pharmacokinetics, and effect on sputum expectoration in patients with cystic fibrosis. *J Aerosol Med* 1997;10:147–158.
109. Pons G, Marchand MC, d'Athis P, et al. French multicenter randomized double-blind placebo-controlled trial on nebulized amiloride in cystic fibrosis patients. The amiloride-AFLM Collaborative Study Group. *Pediatr Pulmonol* 2000;30:25–31.
110. Costello-Boerrigter LC, Boerrigter G, Burnett JC Jr. Revisiting salt and water retention: new diuretics, aquaretics, and natriuretics. *Med Clin North Am* 2003;87:475–491.
111. Forssmann W, Meyer M, Forssmann K. The renal urodilatin system: clinical implications. *Cardiovasc Res* 2001;51:450–462.
112. Semmekrot B, Guignard J-P. Atrial natriuretic peptide during early human development. *Biol Neonate* 1991;60:341–349.
113. Colucci WS, Elkayam U, Horton DP, et al. Intravenous nesiritide, a natriuretic peptide, in the treatment of decompensated congestive heart failure. Nesiritide Study Group. *N Engl J Med* 2000;343:246–253.
114. Jefferies JL, Denfield SW, Price JF, et al. A prospective evaluation of nesiritide in the treatment of pediatric heart failure. *Pediatr Cardiol* 2006;27(4):402–407.
115. Bronicki RA, Domico M, Checchia PA et al. The use of nesiritide in children with congenital heart disease. *Cardiol Young* 2017;27(8):1577–1584.
116. Chen HH, Lainchbury JG, Burnett JC Jr. Natriuretic peptide receptors and neutral endopeptidase in mediating the renal actions of a new therapeutic synthetic natriuretic peptide *Dendroaspis* natriuretic peptide. *J Am Coll Cardiol* 2002;40:1186–1191.
117. Shaddy R, Canter C, Halnon N, Design for the sacubitril/valsartan (LCZ696) compared with enalapril study of pediatric patients with heart failure due to systemic left ventricle systolic dysfunction (PANORAMA-HF study). *Am Heart J* 2017;193:23–34.
118. Costello-Boerrigter LC, Boerrigter G, Burnett JC. Pharmacology of vasopressin antagonists. *Heart Fail Rev* 2009;14:75–82.
119. Kumar S, Berl T. Vasopressin antagonists in the treatment of water-retaining disorders. *Semin Nephrol* 2008;28:279–288.
120. Udelson JE, Smith WB, Hendrix GH, et al. Acute hemodynamic effects of conivaptan, a dual V(1A) and V(2) vasopressin receptor antagonist, in patients with advanced heart failure. *Circulation* 2001;104:2417–2423.
121. Hline SS, Pham PT, Pham PT, et al. Conivaptan: a step forward in the treatment of hyponatremia? *Ther Clin Risk Manag* 2008;4:315–326.
122. Izumi Y, Miura K, Iwao H. Therapeutic potential of vasopressin-receptor antagonists in heart failure. *J Pharmacol Sci* 2014;124(1):1–6.
123. Torres VE. Vasopressin antagonists in polycystic kidney disease. *Semin Nephrol* 2008;28:306–317.

SECTION

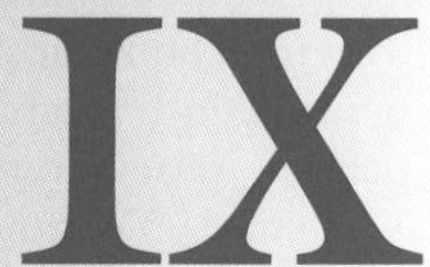

Gastrointestinal Pharmacology

CHAPTER

52

Suruchi Batra
Laurie S. Conklin

Gastrointestinal Drugs

INTRODUCTION

Gastrointestinal (GI) disorders such as gastroesophageal reflux disease (GERD), peptic ulcer disease (PUD), and intestinal dysmotility can occur in children, and a wide variety of drugs are used to treat these conditions. Left untreated, gastritis can progress to PUD, which can lead to complications such as bleeding, perforation, and obstruction. PUD in children is less common than in adults; in a 1-month study in 19 Europeans centers, a frequency of 8.1% of ulcers and/or erosions was found in children undergoing upper endoscopy.[1] The common causes of peptic ulcers include *Helicobacter pylori* (*H. pylori*), medication use (i.e., corticosteroids and nonsteroidal anti-inflammatory drugs), and stress-related gastric injury.[2] Stress ulcers and gastritis are common causes of GI bleeding in critically ill children. In a cohort of 1,006 consecutive admissions enrolled in a pediatric intensive care unit (ICU), 10.2% of pediatric participants had upper GI (UGI) bleeding and 1.6% had clinically significant UGI bleeding, resulting in hemodynamic instability and the need for red blood cell transfusion.[3] *H. pylori* is an infection acquired in childhood which increases the risk of PUD and gastric cancer.[4] *H. pylori*–associated gastritis without PUD rarely gives rise to symptoms or progresses to more serious disease complications during childhood. However, if *H. pylori* infection is identified, then treatment should be administered, and eradication confirmed due to delayed risk of gastric cancer.[5]

Children are commonly referred to as "therapeutic orphans" to reflect the paucity of drug studies performed in pediatric as opposed to adult populations. Although this term was coined more than 50 years ago, it remains relevant today; off-label use of GI drugs in children is particularly prominent.[6,7] One study demonstrated that 49% of medications were prescribed off-label by pediatric gastroenterologists to patients in an outpatient clinic.[8] Significant knowledge gaps remain in the pharmacology of these drugs in children, particularly for children younger than 1 year. However, Food and Drug Administration (FDA) regulations mandating study plans in children, as well as novel trial designs and methods of extrapolation, have resulted in more available pediatric prescribing information.[9] This chapter reviews the current pediatric knowledge of drugs utilized to treat nausea/vomiting, GERD, PUD, and dysmotility. When available, the specific pharmacokinetics and pharmacodynamics of these drugs in children are discussed.

NAUSEA AND VOMITING IN CHILDREN

Nausea and vomiting (emesis) occur in a wide variety of diseases and clinical settings. Nausea may be a prodrome to vomiting or may occur on its own. Emesis may be mediated through neurotransmitters (serotonin, dopamine, substance P, acetylcholine) in the GI tract and the central nervous system (CNS). Various clinical factors, such as the emetogenic potential of chemotherapeutic drugs, the etiology of vomiting, and the age of the child, may impact the efficacy of antiemetics. Because multiple neurotransmitters are involved in vomiting, several agents from various drug classes have been used to treat, as well as prevent, chemotherapy-induced nausea and vomiting (CINV), including muscarinic agents, cannabinoids, steroids, and antagonists of histamine, dopamine, and serotonin receptors.[10]

DOPAMINE (D2) RECEPTOR ANTAGONISTS

Dopamine receptors are found in the chemoreceptor trigger zone (CTZ), and dopamine receptor antagonists, that is, phenothiazines (i.e., prochlorperazine) and the butyrophenones (i.e., haloperidol) have been used as central-acting antiemetics. However, the use of these drugs is limited by the side effects of extrapyramidal reactions, sedation, and disorientation.[11] Thus, prochlorperazine is no longer recommended for use in the pediatric population for prevention of CINV.[12] Promethazine hydrochloride (Phenergan®) is a phenothiazine derivative with histamine H_1-receptor antagonist and anticholinergic properties. In 2004, a "boxed warning" was added to the labeling for Phenergan®, including a contraindication for use in children less than 2 years of age and a strengthened warning with regard to use in children aged 2 years or older, because of the potential for fatal respiratory depression.[13] Metoclopramide and domperidone are D2 antagonists that act centrally, but also have a prokinetic effect in the UGI tract (increasing gastric emptying). Because the action of metoclopramide is not specific for receptors in the CTZ but acts also on the dopaminergic system of different CNS areas, use may be associated with sedation, anticholinergic effects, and extrapyramidal symptoms. The incidence of extrapyramidal reactions with metoclopramide administration can be as high as 25% in pediatric and elderly patients.[14] In 2013, the European Medicines Agency (EMA) released a statement that the risk of neurologic adverse for metoclopramide outweighed the benefit when taken for a prolonged amount of time at a high dose. A similar warning was made by the FDA in 2009, and Health Canada issued a statement in 2015, declaring that metoclopramide is contraindicated in infants younger than 1 year due to its side effects. The risk of developing tardive dyskinesia increases when patients are maintained on metoclopramide for chronic administration (>12 weeks) and at high dosages.[14] Conversely, domperidone has a low incidence of extrapyramidal adverse events because the drug penetrates poorly into the CNS.[15] However, domperidone is associated with prolonged QT intervals in infants.[16] Domperidone was shown to be effective in reducing the need for intravenous (IV) fluid in children with acute gastroenteritis who fail oral rehydration therapy.[17] In the United States, domperidone is available only through an expanded access investigational new drug application from the FDA.

5-HYDROXYTRYPTAMINE-3 RECEPTOR ANTAGONISTS

The serotonin 5-hydroxytryptamine-3 (5-HT_3) antagonists are used for the management of anesthesia-, chemotherapy-, and radiation-related nausea and vomiting. 5-HT_3 antagonists block receptors in the enterochromaffin-like (ECL) cells of the intestinal mucosa, thereby decreasing vagal input to the vomiting center, although these agents may also block receptors in the CNS.[18]

The recommended agents for use in the pediatric population are granisetron, ondansetron, tropisetron (first-generation antagonists), and palonosetron (a second-generation compound).[12] Of the available drugs in this class, ondansetron has been most studied in children. In adults, the elimination half-lives for these compounds range from 3.9 to 10.6 hours.[19] The pharmacokinetic profile of ondansetron in children does not differ substantially from that of adults.[20] The terminal elimination half-life in younger children (3 to 12 years), adolescents, and adults varies between 2.5 and 4 hours, being slightly less in younger children.[20] Similarly, there are minor variations in the volume of distribution, area under the concentration versus time curve, and clearance. The 5-HT_3 antagonists are generally well absorbed (60%), although ondansetron undergoes a significant first-pass effect. Significant hepatic insufficiency may prolong the elimination of ondansetron, but toxicity has not been reported in this setting.[21] Palonosetron has shown to be more effective in delayed CINV compared to first-generation 5-HT_3 receptor antagonists, because it has a 30-fold higher binding affinity and a longer plasma half-life (40 hours vs. 4 to 6 hours of ondansetron).[22]

It is recommended that all pediatric patients receiving chemotherapy of high or moderate emetogenic potential should receive a combination of a 5-HT_3 receptor antagonist, plus dexamethasone and aprepitant (a neurokinin-1 receptor antagonist) as prophylaxis.[12] A 2016 Cochrane review concluded that granisetron or palonosetron may be more efficacious than ondansetron for CINV in childhood.[23]

Ondansetron may be effective in young children with vomiting related to acute gastroenteritis, though recent guidelines highlighted a need for safety studies.[24] In seven randomized controlled trials of ondansetron compared with placebo, ondansetron significantly increased the proportion of children with cessation of vomiting, reduced the need for IV fluid therapy, and the immediate hospital admission rate.[25,26] In a "black box" alert issued in 2011, the FDA recommended electrocardiogram monitoring in patients with electrolyte abnormalities who are receiving ondansetron because they may be at risk for developing prolongation of the QT interval. However, review of the literature and postmarketing studies failed to reveal any reports of arrhythmias developing in otherwise healthy patients after the administration of a single-oral ondansetron dose. Clinicians should be aware of ondansetron's potential to prolong the QT interval when administered IV, particularly in high doses and in high-risk patients.[27]

All drugs in this class are metabolized by cytochrome P450 (CYP450). Granisetron is primarily metabolized by CYP3A4. Ondansetron is metabolized by CYP2D6, CYP2E1, CYP3A, and CYP1A2.[19] The role of genetic variability in CYP2D6 activity has been examined as a determinant of drug efficacy. The potential benefit of using CYP2D6 genotype to guide ondansetron use is that patients with genotypes that are associated with a decreased response [e.g., CYP2D6 ultrarapid metabolizers (UMs)] may be identified, and alternative antiemetics administered. However, at this time, the evidence does not justify increasing the dose in CYP2D6 UMs because effect of dose adjustments based on CYP2D6 ultrarapid metabolism needs further study.[28]

GASTROINTESTINAL DYSMOTILITY IN CHILDREN

UGI dysmotility may manifest clinically as dysphagia, vomiting, or gastroesophageal reflux. Gastroesophageal reflux of gastric contents into the esophagus is a physiologic process. However, gastroesophageal reflux is referred to as gastroesophageal reflux disease, or GERD, when there are associated bothersome symptoms or complications. For most infants, gastroesophageal reflux resolves by 8 to 12 months of age and can be managed with nonpharmacologic therapies.[29] In some infants, GERD can lead to irritability, feeding aversion, and respiratory distress. Children who have other underlying medical conditions such as prematurity, neurologic impairment, and pulmonary problems, including cystic fibrosis, are at higher risk for GERD.[29] Neurogenic dysmotility is common in patients presenting with orthostatic intolerance and GI symptoms such as nausea, bloating, and abdominal pain.[30] Opiates, paralytics, and mechanical ventilation can affect gastric emptying, and prokinetic agents are used in up to 19.9% of critically ill children.[31] GI dysmotility is common in children with short-bowel syndrome secondary to necrotizing enterocolitis, intestinal atresia, volvulus, and gastroschisis.

PROKINETIC AGENTS

Prokinetic agents are utilized to improve gastric and intestinal dysmotility, though they are used off-label with limited evidence of effectiveness in pediatrics. Unfortunately, several prokinetic agents also have safety concerns in children. Cisapride is a serotonin 5-HT_4 receptor agonist that acts indirectly as a parasympathomimetic. Because of persistent concerns over its safety, cisapride was removed from the market in the United States and Canada. Domperidone and metoclopramide are not recommended for use in the treatment of GERD in infants and children. Bethanechol, an acetylcholine receptor agonist that has its greatest effect on the smooth muscle of the distal esophagus, has been studied in a few trials in pediatric GERD. However, the drug has uncertain efficacy and carries a high potential of side effects. Thus, bethanechol is not recommended for use in children.[29]

Baclofen, a derivative of γ-aminobutyric acid, has also been used extensively for the treatment of disorders involving muscular contraction. Baclofen reduces the frequency of transient lower esophageal sphincter relaxations, reduces acid reflux symptoms, and accelerates gastric emptying, but it has not been evaluated in controlled trials for the treatment of GERD in children.[29] Although baclofen may be efficacious in some children, its potential to cause muscle weakness, dizziness, fatigue, and lowered threshold for seizures may limit its use as a first-line therapy. However, based on expert opinion, baclofen can be considered prior to surgery in children in whom other pharmacologic treatments have failed.[29]

Metoclopramide, 2-methoxy-5-chloro-procainamide, is a D2 antagonist commonly used to treat motility disorders. Metoclopramide's mechanism of action is thought to result from a combination of central and peripheral dopamine antagonism. The drug's antiemetic effects are most likely mediated centrally at the dopamine D2 receptor. Peripherally, the augmentation of acetylcholine release from postganglionic nerve terminals is likely responsible for the drug's effect on GI smooth muscle.[30,31] In addition, metoclopramide appears to sensitize the muscarinic receptors of GI smooth muscle to acetylcholine.[32] This overall prokinetic effect is due to the drug's coordination of accelerated gastric emptying by increasing gastric tone, increasing the amplitude of antral contractions and relaxation of the pylorus and duodenum, while increasing the peristalsis of the jejunum, thus accelerating intestinal transit from the duodenum to the ileocecal valve.[30]

Metoclopramide is rapidly absorbed following oral administration, and substantial interindividual variation has been observed in maximal serum concentrations as well as in the drug's oral bioavailability (range, 32% to 97%).[31,33] This variation is most likely due to first-pass drug metabolism.[34,35] Approximately 40% of metoclopramide is bound to plasma protein, primarily α_1-acid glycoprotein.[36] The majority of metoclopramide is metabolized in the liver by sulfation, and approximately 20% of the dose is excreted unchanged in the urine. Its elimination half-life in adults ranges from 2.5 to 5 hours.[34,35]

Limited pharmacokinetic data are available to characterize the disposition of metoclopramide in children.[34,37,38] One study found that children, ages 7 to 14 years, had pharmacokinetic parameters that were similar to those of adults.[37] Kearns et al.[37,38] reported that the mean values for plasma clearance and volume of distribution were increased 1.4- and 2.1-fold in neonates, respectively, in comparison to values reported in adults. The mean value for elimination half-life in neonates was not significantly different from that in older infants, children, and adults.[34,38] However, interindividual variability for elimination half-lives was large in neonates and older infants.[37,38] Developmental or pharmacogenetic influences on drug metabolism, particularly in the sulfotransferase isoforms responsible for the N-4-sulfation of metoclopramide,[34,38] may contribute to this variability. The data support a starting oral dose of metoclopramide of 0.15 mg per kg administered every 6 hours in term newborns, infants, and children.[38]

Because of the effects of metoclopramide on gastric emptying and intestinal motility, it has the potential to alter the oral bioavailability and resulting serum concentration relationships (e.g., peak plasma concentration and time to peak plasma concentration) of many drugs. Studies of this potential drug interaction have yielded variable results, indicating an inconsistent effect of metoclopramide on the GI absorption of concurrently administered drugs.[33]

Erythromycin has been demonstrated to have prokinetic activity and is effective at doses less than those typically used for antimicrobial therapy.[39] The drug appears to have pharmacodynamics similar to the polypeptide hormone motilin, stimulating migrating motor complexes in the GI tract.[40,41] Erythromycin was found to increase the lower esophageal sphincter tone and the duration, but not the amplitude of contractions of the distal esophagus in adults with GER.[40] In a retrospective review evaluating data from 348 neonatal ICUs, of infants exposed to ≥ 1 dose of erythromycin or metoclopramide or both, metoclopramide was associated with increased risk of adverse events compared with erythromycin.[42]

The optimal dose of erythromycin for improved GI motility is 1 to 3 mg per kg. Higher doses (10 to 15 mg per kg), similar to those used in antimicrobial therapy, tend to cause continuous high-amplitude contractions or motor quiescence.[43] A dose-ranging study in healthy adults noted enhanced gastric motility, with increasing doses of 0.75, 1.5, and 3 mg per kg.[44] In a study of premature newborns, IV erythromycin at a dose of 0.75 mg per kg significantly increased gastric and duodenal contractions.[45]

The inhibitory effect of erythromycin on the CYPP450 system, especially CYP3A4, has been well described and is a significant factor for the development of adverse drug reactions. In addition, the rapid IV infusion of erythromycin lactobionate has been associated with bradycardia, hypotension, prolongation of the QTc interval, and ventricular arrhythmias.[46,47] Studies have demonstrated an association between postnatal erythromycin exposure and the development of infantile hypertrophic pyloric stenosis.[48] However, there is no evidence for an association between macrolide use during pregnancy or breastfeeding and the occurrence of infantile hypertrophic pyloric stenosis.[49]

GASTROESOPHAGEAL REFLUX DISEASE, PEPTIC ULCER DISEASE, AND *HELICOBACTER PYLORI* INFECTION IN CHILDREN AND INFANTS

Initial treatment of acid peptic disease includes discontinuation of offending agents and treatment of underlying etiologies. Acid suppression is an effective strategy to alleviate symptoms and promote ulcer healing. Available agents on the market include histamine 2 receptor antagonists (H2Ras) and proton pump inhibitors (PPIs).

ANTACIDS

In the past, antacids were used as prophylaxis for stress ulceration in ICUs and prior to surgical procedures. Antacids reduce and neutralize secreted gastric acid and have cytoprotective effects. Sodium bicarbonate and calcium carbonate are the most potent antacids, followed by magnesium- and then aluminum-containing products. Sodium bicarbonate and calcium carbonate are also rapid-acting antacids. However, chronic high exposure or high-dose ingestion of calcium carbonate can cause milk-alkali syndrome; a triad of hypercalcemia, alkalosis, and renal failure.[27] Chronic use of sodium bicarbonate is associated with fluid retention, systemic alkalosis, and the milk-alkali syndrome.[50,51] Diarrhea and hypermagnesemia are associated with the use of magnesium-containing antacids, particularly in patients with compromised renal function. Adverse events associated with the use of aluminum-containing antacids include constipation, hypophosphatemia, and hypocalcemia. Aluminum accumulation and the formation of bezoars have also been reported for aluminum-containing antacids, particularly in young infants with compromised renal function.[52,53] Thus, antacids have been largely replaced by other acid-modifying drugs (e.g., H_2-receptor antagonists, PPIs) due to safety and dosing concerns. Long-term therapy (>2 to 4 weeks) with antacids in infants and children should be closely monitored for adverse effects.

H_2-RECEPTOR ANTAGONISTS

H_2-receptor antagonists are some of the most commonly used drugs in children for reflux-related symptoms, treatment of gastric or duodenal ulcers, and treatment of prophylaxis against GI hemorrhage. Four H_2-receptor antagonists are available for clinical use in the United States (Table 52.1). However, only ranitidine and famotidine are approved for use in both children and adolescents. Nizatidine is approved for adolescents, but not for children younger than 12 years. H_2-receptor antagonists are frequently utilized in neonatal and pediatric ICUs as prophylaxis for gastric stress ulceration. However, their routine use in critically ill patients has been questioned due to the concern that alteration of gastric pH leads to gastric bacterial overgrowth of genera, including *Staphylococcus* and *Streptococcus*. Acid suppression also leads to changes in lung microflora. Additional studies are needed to determine whether acid suppression predicts clinical infection risk.[54]

The four H_2-receptor antagonists are similar to one another in efficacy but have different drug interaction and side-effect profiles, based on their respective chemical structures. The original H_2-receptor antagonist, cimetidine, contains an imidazole ring. Ranitidine contains an amino methyl furan moiety, which provides greater potency and a longer duration of action. Famotidine is a thiazole ring and is 10 to 15 times more potent than ranitidine and 40 to 60 times more potent than cimetidine in inhibiting gastric acid secretion. The longer elimination half-life of famotidine may be particularly desirable for use in children by allowing for less frequent dosing (twice daily as opposed to three to four times daily for ranitidine).

The H_2-receptor antagonists reduce gastric acid secretion by acting as competitive, reversible inhibitors of histamine at the histamine H_2 receptor. The effects of histamine are mediated by binding to H_1 and H_2 receptors, and binding of histamine to H_2 receptors stimulates gastric acid secretion. H_2-receptor antagonists do not have effects on other receptors, including the H_1 receptor, or the muscarinic, nicotinic, or sympathomimetic α- or β receptors.[55] H_2-receptor antagonists also decrease the acid-secretory response of the parietal cell to stimulated acid secretion from cholinergic agents, gastrin, food, and vagal stimulation.[55] However, the most prominent effects of H_2-receptor antagonists are on acid secretion; thus, they are particularly effective in suppressing nocturnal acid production. Because nocturnal acid secretion is an important factor in the development of duodenal ulcers, H_2-receptor antagonists may be particularly effective for the management of these patients. In addition, H_2-receptor antagonists are utilized in combination with PPIs in patients who have nocturnal gastric acid breakthrough.[56] Although most H_2-receptor antagonists are not thought to have direct effects on gastric motility, nizatidine has been reported to enhance GI activity, independent of its effects on altering gastric acid secretion.[57]

The oral bioavailability of H_2-receptor antagonists varies depending on the specific agent, and nizatidine has the highest bioavailability (~70%) of the four drugs. Antacids decrease the relative bioavailability of H_2-receptor antagonists by 12% to 25%.[58] For the most part, these drugs are not highly protein bound. Between 25% and 40% of cimetidine is metabolized. Between 60% and 80% of nizatidine, ranitidine, and famotidine are eliminated by the kidneys as unchanged drugs. Dose adjustment is indicated for the H_2-receptor antagonists in children and adolescents with renal failure[59] and in infants with developmentally determined alterations in renal clearance. The H_2-receptor antagonists are not removed to any significant extent by peritoneal or hemodialysis.

The pharmacokinetics of cimetidine, ranitidine, and famotidine has been well characterized in children.[60–63] Both glomerular filtration and tubular secretion contribute to the renal elimination of famotidine, ranitidine, and cimetidine, and these processes do not reach adult maturity until 5 to 12 months of age.[64,65] Consistent with the developmental profile for renal function in children during the first year of life, prolonged renal and plasma clearance for famotidine have been reported for children younger than 3 months.[62,66] A report (Table 52.1) describing the disposition of nizatidine in children (mean age, 8.0 ± 2.4 years) indicates that the pharmacokinetics is very similar to that previously reported in adults.[67]

The pharmacokinetics of ranitidine and famotidine has been characterized in infants (Table 52.2). Less information is available to guide the dosing of H_2-receptor antagonists in premature infants, but several pharmacodynamic studies have been performed in this population. Kuusela[68] studied 16 critically ill infants (mean gestational age, 33 weeks) and found

TABLE 52.1 Pharmacokinetics of H_2-Receptor Antagonists in Children (Mean ± SD)

	Age (y)	$t_{1/2}$ *(h)*	V_d *(L/kg)*	*Cl*	*References*
Cimetidine	9.0 (2.3)	1.4 (0.3)	1.2 (0.5)	10.4 mL/min/kg (4)	124
Ranitidine	12.6 (3.7)	1.8 (0.3)	2.3 (0.9)	795 mL/min/kg (334)	60
Famotidine	6.1 (4.9)	3.2 (3.0)	2.4 (1.7)	0.70 L/h/kg (0.34)	61,62
Nizatidine	8.0 (2.4)	1.2 (0.2)	3.2 (0.6)	1.23 L/h/kg (0.2)	67

Cl, clearance; $t_{1/2}$, elimination half-life; SD, standard deviation; V_d, volume of distribution.

TABLE 52.2 Pharmacokinetics of H_2-Receptor Antagonists in Infants (Mean ± SD)

	Age	$t_{1/2}$ *(h)*	V_d *(L/kg)*	*Cl*	*References*
Ranitidine	12 mo (6.9)	2.1 (1.3)	1.6 (1.0)	13.9 mL/min/kg (10.0)	68
Famotidine	6.6 d (4.4)	10.5 (5.4)	1.35 (0.42)	0.132 L/h/kg (0.061)	62
	0–3 mo	7.6 (4.6, 12.6)[a]	1.76 (1.43, 2.18)[a]	0.2 mL/min/kg (0.14, 1.27)[a]	66

Cl, clearance; $t_{1/2}$, elimination half-life; SD, standard deviation; V_d, volume of distribution.
[a]Ninety percent confidence interval.

that preterm infants required only twice-daily dosing (0.5 mg per kg per dose), whereas term infants required thrice-daily dosing (1.5 mg per kg per dose) to maintain a gastric pH of more than 4. Kelly et al.[69] found that continuous infusions of ranitidine of 0.0625 mg per kg per hour in premature infants (gestational age, 24 to 31 weeks) achieved a mean gastric pH of 4.9. Dose adjustments may be indicated in infants receiving ranitidine during extracorporeal membrane oxygenation (ECMO).[70] Wells et al.[71] reported that the elimination half-life of ranitidine was prolonged (6.6 ± 2.8 hours) in term infants receiving ECMO in comparison with data previously reported in other critically ill infants (3.5 ± 0.3 hours).[63]

In general, the H_2-receptor antagonists are well tolerated in children.[72] Adverse reactions are more common with cimetidine than with the other drugs of this class and have been reported to be as high as 4.5%.[73] GI symptoms, rash, and dizziness are the most common adverse effects associated with H_2-receptor antagonists.[74] CNS effects, including mania and seizures, have also been described with cimetidine. Elevated CNS-to-plasma ratios of cimetidine have been documented in adults with renal or hepatic insufficiency who experience CNS symptoms while receiving the drug.[75] Adverse effects related to the endocrine system include gynecomastia, galactorrhea, impotence, and, possibly, a decrease in spermatogenesis.[76] Elevations of serum prolactin have been associated with IV use of cimetidine. Thrombocytopenia and agranulocytosis are considered rare adverse effects of H_2-receptor antagonists.[76]

Drug interactions are more common with cimetidine than with the other H_2-receptor antagonist. This is secondary to the inhibitory effects of cimetidine on the cytochromes P450. Concurrent therapy of cimetidine and theophylline has resulted in the accumulation of theophylline and the development of seizures.[77] Reduced drug clearance has also been reported for the coadministration of cimetidine with warfarin, phenytoin, quinidine, caffeine, metronidazole, diazepam, imipramine, lidocaine, meperidine, procainamide, propranolol, and triamterene. Although ranitidine has been reported to bind to CYPP450, its binding affinity is approximately 10-fold lower than that of cimetidine. Clinically significant drug interactions for ranitidine, famotidine, and nizatidine are unusual.[78]

The H_2-receptor antagonists may be administered by oral, intramuscular, or IV routes. Oral formulations are available for all four drugs, and IV and intramuscular formulations are available for cimetidine, ranitidine, and famotidine. Liquid pediatric formulations are available for all four H_2-receptor antagonists.

PROTON PUMP INHIBITORS

The final common pathway for acid production within the parietal cells is the H^+/K^+ adenosine triphosphatase (ATPase) enzyme transport system, commonly referred to as the proton pump. Drugs that target this pathway are a class of substituted benzimidazole compounds referred to as proton pump inhibitors (PPIs). Omeprazole, the first PPI, was approved for human use in the United States in 1988. Subsequently, four PPIs have been approved by the FDA, including lansoprazole, pantoprazole, rabeprazole, and esomeprazole, the pure S isomer of omeprazole.[79] Although only pantoprazole lacks FDA-approved product labeling in pediatric patients, none of the PPIs have approved labeling for children younger than 1 year. It was not possible to evaluate the adult primary end point, mucosal healing assessed by endoscopy, in children. Thus, esomeprazole was approved by the FDA for use in children down to age 1, demonstrating similarity to adult pharmacokinetics and intragastric pH measurements.[80]

PPIs are substituted 2-pyridyl methyl sulfinyl benzimidazoles.[81] They are weakly basic compounds that differ from each other by molecular substituents attached to the benzimidazole and pyridine components of the molecule. All PPIs are prodrugs, given that protonation of the nitrogen on the pyridine group produces the active form of the drug, a cyclic sulfonamide. This intermediate is trapped within the acidic environment of the parietal cell canaliculi and binds covalently to exposed cysteine thiol groups on the luminal surface of the proton pump, thus disabling it. Differences in the pK_a of the various PPIs have been shown to affect their onset of action (rapid to slower: rabeprazole > omeprazole > lansoprazole > pantoprazole).[81,82] Table 52.3 provides an overview of pharmacokinetic parameters of the currently marketed PPIs. Esomeprazole and lansoprazole are the most bioavailable of the PPIs (Table 52.3).

Considerable variability exists for the plasma concentration profiles for the PPIs due, in part, to differences in their presystemic clearance (e.g., lowest bioavailability for those drugs that are metabolized by CYP3A4) and coadministration with food (lansoprazole > omeprazole > pantoprazole).[79] Lansoprazole, pantoprazole, and rabeprazole demonstrate dose proportionality [i.e., linearity between dose and resulting area under the curve (AUC)], in contrast with omeprazole and esomeprazole, where the extent of bioavailability increases with repeated dosing.[83] The PPIs are effective only if converted to their respective active moieties in the parietal cell canaliculi where active H^+ ion secretion is taking place.[79] Consequently, any condition or circumstance (e.g., administration of food, concomitant medications) that reduces H^+ ion secretion (and raises pH) by the parietal cell will prolong the time of onset of effect consequent to delayed prodrug activation (Table 52.3). Finally, examination of the average apparent oral clearance (*Cl/F*) data for the PPIs suggests possible differences among the respective drugs, with values for omeprazole and rabeprazole being generally higher than those for other compounds in the class (Table 52.3). It is important to note, however, that any apparent difference in *Cl/F* may simply reflect inter- or intrapatient differences in the extent of presystemic clearance of the drug.

TABLE 52.3 Comparative Average Pharmacokinetic Parameters of the Proton Pump Inhibitors in Adults

Parameter	*Omeprazole 20 mg*	*Esomeprazole 40 mg*	*Pantoprazole 40 mg*	*Lansoprazole 30 mg*	*Rabeprazole 20 mg*
AUC (mg/L/h)	0.2–1.2	12.6 (μmol/L/h)	2–5	1.7–5	0.8
C_{max} (mg/L)	0.08–8.0	NA	1.1–3.3	0.6–1.2	0.41
T_{max} (h)	1–3	1.6	2–4	6.3–2.2	3.1
Activation time (min)[a]	2.8/84	NA	4.6/282	2.0/90	6.3/7.2
$t_{1/2}$ (h)	0.6–1.0	1.2–1.5	0.9–1.9	0.9–1.6	1
Cl/*F* (L/h/kg)	0.45	NA	0.08–0.13	0.2–0.28	0.5
Bioavailability (%)	35–65	89–90	57–100	80–91	52
Protein binding (%)	95	97	98	97–99	95–98
Dose linearity	Nonlinear	Nonlinear	Linear	Linear	Linear

AUC, area under the plasma concentration–time curve; *Cl/F*, apparent total plasma clearance; C_{max}, peak plasma concentration; NA, not available; $t_{1/2}$, elimination half-life; T_{max}, time to peak plasma concentration.
[a]Value independent of dose at gastric pH values of 1.2/5.1, respectively.
References 61–63 and product information for respective agents.

In addition to tablets and capsules, several dosage forms are available that allow administration to children who cannot swallow a tablet or capsule. These include IV formulations, granules or powder for oral suspension, and oral disintegrating tablets (ODTs). Extemporaneous liquid formulations of these drugs have been prepared for pediatric use, although there are limited available data regarding their stability and/or bioavailability in infants and children. Given that formulation-specific differences have the potential to alter drug bioavailability in pediatric patients and, therefore, clinical efficacy, the impact of disrupting the integrity of a solid PPI dose form in making an extemporaneous preparation must be considered. The lansoprazole ODT is approved for use in pediatric patients[84] and affords the option of dissolution and administration via oral syringe or nasogastric tube.[84,85] Although not labeled for pediatric use, omeprazole is available as single-dose powder packets for suspension. Two studies have demonstrated good stability of the prepared suspension over time when stored at 3°C to 5°C. A 2 mg per mL suspension retained at least 98% of the initial concentration when stored for 45 days to 1 month.[86,87] Stability at room temperature was concentration dependent, with greater stability at higher concentrations.[87] Finally, esomeprazole and lansoprazole are both available as granules or powder for suspension.

As illustrated by the information contained in Table 52.3, all of the PPIs are extensively (>90%) bound to circulating plasma proteins (primarily albumin).[83] Thus, their apparent volume of distribution is limited to a physiologic space that is far less than total body water (i.e., 0.6 to 0.7 L per kg). Although drug–drug interactions between omeprazole and both phenytoin and warfarin have been reported,[88] there is no evidence that these are produced because of alterations in drug–protein binding.

The optimal activity of PPIs is achieved when they are administered on an empty stomach, preferably 30 to 60 minutes before meals. Taking PPIs on an empty stomach improves their absorption, but also ensures that their peak plasma levels align with the activation of proton pumps that are activated by the presence of food.[89] Some patients do not respond adequately to PPIs, or develop treatment-related adverse events. This variable response among patients is in part due to genotype variability of *CYP2C19*, the gene encoding the CYP450 (*CYP2C19*) isoenzyme responsible for the metabolism of PPIs.[90] It should be noted that rabeprazole is nonenzymatically metabolized, and thus, CYP2C19 variation does not impact patients receiving this drug.[91] CYP2C19 is polymorphically expressed in humans, and the phenotypic status of the CYP2C19-metabolizing activity is classified into ultrarapid, rapid, normal, intermediate, or poor metabolizer, depending on the genotype of an individual.[90] The poor metabolizer (PM) phenotype for CYP2C19 is produced by the inheritance of two recessive mutated alleles and is present in approximately 3% to 5% of Caucasians and African Americans and in approximately 15% to 20% of the Asian population. Although at least seven nonfunctional alleles for CYP2C19 have been identified to date (CYP2C19*2 to CYP2C19*8), the two most common variants, *CYP2C19*2* and *CYP2C19*3* result from single-nucleotide substitutions that convey a dramatic reduction in enzyme activity. PMs have a substantially higher exposure (i.e., increased plasma concentrations and AUC) from a therapeutic dose of a PPI, as reflected by recent data for omeprazole.[90] On the other hand, the CYP2C19*17 variant contributes to enhanced clearance of PPIs. This is a common polymorphism, with approximately 30% of individuals with European and African ancestry, and 2% to 4% of Asians carrying at least one copy of CYP2C19*17. Individuals with two copies of *17 are classified as UMs.[90]

In a randomized crossover study, Furuta et al.[92] assessed whether the effect of a PPI on intragastric pH correlated with CYP2C19 genotype status (i.e., a surrogate measure of phenotype). The investigators demonstrated a significant (r = 0.87, $p < 0.0001$) correlation between mean intragastric pH and the AUC for omeprazole (ng per mL per hour). This finding indicated an association between CYP2C19 phenotype and both pharmacokinetics and pharmacodynamics as well as a possible gene–dose effect, with individuals who have one functional CYP2C19 allele (i.e., the intermediate metabolizers) producing values between those from subjects who were homozygous UMs and PMs. The effect of the "intermediate metabolizer" phenotype for CYP2C19 on pantoprazole (single-dose administration) pharmacokinetics was examined by Kearns et al.[93] in a pediatric study. A statistically significant difference in dose-normalized AUC (i.e., ng per mL per hour per 1 mg per kg of drug) between EMs with one versus two functional alleles was found.

Standard therapy for *H. pylori* eradication requires triple therapy with two antibiotics and a PPI. If initial treatment fails, quadruple therapy may be used, which requires the addition of bismuth to the standard triple therapy regimen.[3] The utilization of a PPI is imperative to both treatment regimens. Increased gastric pH allows for enhanced stability of acid-labile antibiotics and may decrease transport of antibiotics from the stomach into the blood stream.[94] Consequently, PPI use ensures optimal antibiotic gastric concentration for *H. pylori* treatment.

Standard PPI dosing may not be sufficient for *H. pylori* infection eradication in individuals with the rapid metabolizer or UM genotype.[94–106] Thus, higher PPI dosing may be required to ensure effective *H. pylori* treatment. Furuta et al.[97] reported significant differences ($p < 0.001$) in cure rates for *H. pylori* infection in adults with different CYP2C19 genotypes treated with lansoprazole, clarithromycin, and amoxicillin (57.8%, 88.2%, and 92.3% for rapid metabolizers, intermediate metabolizers, and PMs, respectively).

Reviews examining the impact of ontogeny on drug disposition provide pharmacokinetic evidence to support reduced activity of CYP2C19 and CYP3A4 in neonates and young infants and the potential for increased activity (relative to adults) of these enzymes in the first 4 to 5 years of life.[98,99] Early data reporting the pharmacokinetics of oral omeprazole in infants and children supported a potential increase in the apparent plasma clearance in young children. These data prompted Hassall et al.[100] to suggest that developmental differences in omeprazole pharmacokinetics (i.e., increased clearance) were responsible for a greater dose requirement (mg per kg) of the drug in young children to ensure efficacy.

The pharmacokinetics of the PPIs has been studied in infants, children, and adolescents. A summary of the studies and pharmacokinetic parameters is provided in Table 52.4. Except for two studies that revealed a trend toward a more rapid clearance in infants and young children,[99,101] the pharmacokinetics of omeprazole, lansoprazole, and pantoprazole does not appear to be dependent on development in infants from approximately 1 month to 16 years of age. Infants and young children also appear to clear esomeprazole more rapidly than do adults and older children.[102,103]

PPIs are approved by the FDA for treatment/management of the following conditions in adults: duodenal ulcers and erosive esophagitis (treatment and maintenance), gastric ulcers, *H. pylori* infection, pathologic hypersecretory conditions, and GERD. Lansoprazole and esomeprazole have been approved for the prevention of gastric ulcers associated with nonsteroidal anti-inflammatory drugs; lansoprazole is also approved for the treatment of these ulcers. In recent years, all PPIs, except for pantoprazole, have received FDA approval for use in pediatric patients for the treatment of GERD. Esomeprazole and lansoprazole are also approved for the treatment of erosive esophagitis. However, PPIs still lack formal FDA approval for other pediatric conditions for which they are administered "off-label," including *H. pylori* infection, adjuvant therapy in patients with cystic fibrosis, as premedication for general anesthesia, extraesophageal symptoms associated with GERD (e.g., asthma, chronic cough, sinusitis, recurrent otitis media), and apnea and/or bradycardia associated with GER and/or increased gastric residual volumes in neonates.

Of all drugs in this class, omeprazole and lansoprazole have been studied most in children. Gibbons and Gold[79] summarized data from pediatric studies of omeprazole (8 trials involving 408 children) and lansoprazole (4 trials involving 184 children). Most subjects were older than 2 years. Collectively, these investigations demonstrated the following: a predictable time-dependent increase in gastric and esophageal pH associated with treatment, a greater than 80% symptomatic improvement while on therapy, histologic improvement/healing of gastric and esophageal lesions with maintenance therapy, an efficiency of treatment (both incidence of response and rate of onset) associated with dose escalation (e.g., omeprazole daily doses > 1.5 mg per kg and lansoprazole daily doses > 1.0 mg per kg), and a significant (>60%) relapse rate when treatment with a PPI was discontinued. More recent pediatric clinical trials of omeprazole and lansoprazole support these findings,[104,105] including children aged 2 years or younger. Omeprazole has

TABLE 52.4 Pharmacokinetic Parameters for Infants, Children, and Adolescents

References	*Drug*	*Patient Age*	*Dosing*	*AUC (μg/L/h)*	*Clearance (L/h/kg)*	$t_{1/2}$ *(h)*	*Findings/Interpretations*
125	Omeprazole i.v.	4.5–27 mo	0.56 mg/kg[a]	780[a]	0.68[a]		The AUC had positive correlation with the percentage of time pH > 4 in 24 h
			1.16 mg/kg[a]	3,950[a]	0.42[a]		
126	Lansoprazole p.o.	0.25–13 y	0.73 mg/kg[a]	2,034[b]	0.76[b]	0.77[b]	AUC significantly higher in responders vs. nonresponders
			1.44 mg/kg[b]	479[b]	2.94[b]	0.75[b]	
			1.36 mg/kg[b]	737[b]	2.26[b]	0.93[b]	
85	Lansoprazole p.o.	1–11 y	15 mg/d	1,707[b]		0.68[b]	Lower dose with weight <30 kg; profile similar to that of adults
			30 mg/d	1,883[b]		0.71[b]	
135	Lansoprazole p.o.	12–17 y	15 mg/d	1,017[b]		0.84[b]	Similar profile to adults
			30 mg/d	2,490[b]		0.95[b]	
127	Omeprazole i.v.	<10 d	0.4–1.2 mg/kg b.i.d.	ND	0.12–0.2	1.6–2.1	Infants <10 d of age metabolize omeprazole at a slower rate than infants (4.5–17 mo), whose metabolism is similar to that of adults
		4.5–17 mo	0.4–1.2 mg/kg b.i.d.				

(*continued*)

TABLE 52.4 Pharmacokinetic Parameters for Infants, Children, and Adolescents (*continued*)

References	*Drug*	*Patient Age*	*Dosing*	*AUC (μg/L/h)*	*Clearance (L/h/kg)*	$t_{1/2}$ *(h)*	*Findings/Interpretations*
128	Omeprazole p.o.	0–24 mo	1.0 mg/kg	658[b]		1.0[b]	Increased exposure to omeprazole in infants <5 mo of age
			1.5 mg/kg	346[b]		1.0[b]	
99	Omeprazole p.o.	1–6 y	1.3 mg/kg	2,003[a]		0.85[a]	Increasing metabolism with decreasing age to second year of life
		7–12 y	0.7 mg/kg	2,866[a]		1.74[a]	
		13–16 y	1.1 mg/kg	3,420[a]		1.58[a]	
101	Lansoprazole p.o.	18 d–14 y	17-mg single dose	3,503[b]		1.5[b]	Trend toward higher elimination rate in infants
129	Omeprazole p.o.	2–16 y	0.2–0.9 mg/kg	809.5[b]	1.76[b]	0.98[b]	No apparent association between age and elimination rate constant; no difference in AUC between CYP2C19 heterozygous and homozygous extensive metabolizers
93	Pantoprazole p.o.	6–16 y	20- or 40-mg single dose	4.3/45.5[c]	0.3/0.03[d]	0.6/5.8[e]	No apparent age association with oral clearance or elimination rate constant; significantly higher dose-normalized AUC in CYP2C19 homozygous versus heterozygous extensive metabolizers
130	Pantoprazole i.v.	2–16 y	0.8 or 1.6 mg/kg		7.6 L/h[b]	1.1[b]	No apparent age association with clearance
131	Rabeprazole p.o.	12–16 y	10-mg single dose	305[b]	0.75[b]	0.55[b]	Pharmacokinetics was similar to that observed in adults; possible accumulation with multiple doses of 20 mg
			10 mg/d	249.8[b]	0.61[b]	0.58[b]	
			20-mg single dose	557.8[b]		1.04[b]	
			20 mg/d	828.4[b]		0.97[b]	
102	Esomeprazole p.o.	1–24 mo	0.25 mg/kg	0.65[b,f]		0.77[b]	Exposure and percentage of time pH >4 related to dosage; 0.25 mg/kg did not reduce reflux episodes
			1 mg/kg	3.51[b,f]		0.95[b]	
103	Esomeprazole p.o.	1–5 y	5 mg/d	0.74[b,g]	1.01[b]	0.42[b]	Pharmacokinetics at steady state was dose and age dependent; younger children metabolized more quickly
		1–5 y	10 mg/d	4.83[b,g]	0.39[b]	0.74[b]	
		6–11 y	10 mg/d	3.70[b,g]	0.25[b]	0.88[b]	
		6–11 y	20 mg/d	6.28[b,g]	0.31[b]	0.76[b]	
132	Esomeprazole p.o.	12–17 y	20 mg single dose	1.58[b,g]	36.61 L/h[b]	0.55[b]	Pharmacokinetics was dose and time dependent; similar to adults
			20 mg/d	3.65[b,g]	15.88 L/h[b]	0.82[b]	
			40 mg single dose	5.57[b,g]	20.78 L/h[b]	0.86[b]	
			40 mg/d	13.86[b,g]	8.36 L/h[b]	1.22[b]	
133	Lansoprazole p.o.	13–24 mo	15 mg once or twice daily	1906[b,h]		0.66[b]	Results similar to older children and adults
134	Pantoprazole p.o.	5–16 y	20- or 40-mg single dose	9.44 mg/L/h[b]	0.26[b]	1.27[b]	Pharmacokinetics of p.o. and i.v. formulations was similar
	Pantoprazole i.v.	2–16 y	0.8- or 1.6-mg/kg single dose	8.95 mg/L/h[b]	0.20[b]	1.22[b]	

AUC, area under plasma concentration–time curve; b.i.d., twice daily; i.v., intravenously; ND, no data; p.o., orally; $t_{1/2}$, elimination half-life; CYP, cytochrome P450.
[a]Median values.
[b]Mean values.
[c]Mean values normalized as mg/L/h per 1 mg/kg for CYP2C19 extensive/poor metabolizers.
[d]Mean values as L/h/kg for CYP2C19 extensive/poor metabolizers.
[e]Mean values for CYP2C19 extensive/poor metabolizers.
[f]AUC for the dosing interval expressed as μmol/h/L.
[g]$AUC_{0-\infty}$ expressed as μmol/h/L.
[h]AUC_{0-24} h.

also been shown to be effective in the reduction of esophageal acid exposure in premature infants (34 to 40 weeks postmenstrual age) with symptoms of GERD.[106]

Clinical trials of esomeprazole in children with GERD ranging in age from 1 month to 17 years demonstrate dose-related acid suppression, decreased esophageal acid exposure, decreased symptoms, and healing of erosive esophagitis.[107] Pantoprazole has similarly been shown to be an effective treatment for GERD in children aged 5 to 16 years.[108–110]

PPIs are generally well tolerated in children. Headaches, nausea, and diarrhea are the most commonly reported adverse effects. A persistent, two- to fivefold rise in serum gastrin level, stimulation of ECL cells,[111] and histologic changes in parietal cells[112] are associated with the use of PPIs. However, a review of studies reporting long-term treatment with PPIs failed to identify an association between ECL hyperplasia and progression to dysplasia and carcinoid tumors, the development of fundic cysts and polyps associated with hypertrophic parietal cells, or increased infections consequent to prolonged periods of gastric hypochlorhydria.[113] Studies suggest an increased risk of GI and respiratory tract infections, vitamin B_{12} deficiency, hypomagnesemia, bone fractures, and rebound hyperacidity after discontinuation of PPIs in children. Further data are needed to characterize these risks in infants and children.[114]

PPIs can both inhibit and induce CYP enzymes and, consequently, have the potential to produce drug–drug interactions for selected pharmacologic agents.[115] Omeprazole and lansoprazole have been shown to competitively inhibit CYP2C9 (K_i of 40.1 and 52.1, respectively). Both drugs noncompetitively inhibit CYP3A4, but the inhibition is weak (K_i of 84.4 and 170.4, respectively).[116] There is strong competitive inhibition of CYP2C19 by omeprazole, lansoprazole, and rabeprazole. Rabeprazole, with a K_i of 9.2, is roughly three times less potent than omeprazole or lansoprazole (K_i of 3.1 and 3.2, respectively) in inhibiting CYP2C19. Omeprazole and lansoprazole can also weakly inhibit the activity of CYP2D6 (K_i of 240.7 and 44.7, respectively). Masubuchi et al.[117] compared the induction of CYP1A2 and CYP3A4 activity in humans for three PPIs. For CYP1A2, induction potential was highest with omeprazole, followed by lansoprazole and then pantoprazole. For CYP3A4, there were no apparent differences in induction potency among the three compounds.

The potential for metabolism-based drug–drug interactions can be assessed by determining whether and how extensively a compound inhibits or induces a CYP enzyme. It is important to evaluate whether drug concentrations in the body or at the site of action are close to levels known to affect the enzyme (i.e., comparison of the K_i values for inhibition with the plasma PPI concentrations associated with therapeutic drug administration). In humans, metabolic drug–drug interactions have been reported when omeprazole is coadministered with phenytoin, diazepam, carbamazepine,[116] St. John's wort,[118] tacrolimus,[119] saquinavir,[120] nelfinavir,[121] or indinavir.[122] Given that the S isomer of omeprazole has less affinity for CYP2C19, the drug interaction potential of esomeprazole would be expected to be less than that of the racemic mixture.[123] The absence of drug interactions reported with the other PPIs may simply reflect the larger extent to which omeprazole has been studied. Finally, evaluation of the interaction potential for the PPIs should center not only on therapeutic drugs but also on potential environmental toxicants that rely on the enzymes affected by the PPIs (e.g., heterocyclic hydrocarbons by CYP1A2) for their bioactivation.

DISCLOSURES

LSC is an employee of ReveraGen Biopharma and has stock options in ReveraGen.

ACKNOWLEDGMENTS

Dr. Conklin receives support from *NICHD* U54HD090254 Research in Pediatric Developmental Pharmacology Center.

Dr. Batra is supported by the NICHD T32HD087969 Postdoctoral Training in Pediatric Clinical Pharmacology.

REFERENCES

1. Kalach N, Bontems P, Koletzko S, et al. Frequency and risk factors of gastric and duodenal ulcers or erosions in children: a prospective 1-month European multicenter study. *Eur J Gastroenterol Hepatol* 2010;22(10):1174–1181.
2. Sierra D, Wood M, Kolli S, et al. Pediatric gastritis, gastropathy, and peptic ulcer disease. *Pediatr Rev* 2018;39:542–549.
3. Chaibou M, Tucci M, Dugas MA, et al. Clinically significant upper gastrointestinal bleeding acquired in a pediatric intensive care unit: a prospective study. *Pediatrics* 1998;102:933–938.
4. Amieva M, Peek RM Jr. Pathobiology of *Helicobacter pylori*-associated gastric cancer. *Gastroenterology* 2016;150:64–78.
5. Jones NL, Koletzko S, Goodman K, et al. Joint ESPGHAN/NASPGHAN guidelines for the management of *Helicobacter pylori* in children and adolescents (update 2016). *J Pediatr Gastroenterol Nutr* 2017;64(6):991–1003.
6. Shah SS, Hall M, Goodman DM, et al. Off-label use in hospitalized children. *Arch Pediatr Adolesc Med* 2007;1616(3):282–290.
7. Karesh A, Tomaino J, Mulberg AE. Off-label use of medicine in pediatrics: focus on gastrointestinal diseases. *Curr Opin Pediatr* 2013;25(5):612–617.
8. Dick A, Keady S, Mohamed F, et al. Use of unlicensed and off-label medications in paediatric gastroenterology with a review of the commonly used formularies in the UK. *Aliment Pharmacol Ther* 2003;17(4):571–575.
9. Dunne J, Rodriguez WJ, Murphy MD, et al. Extrapolation of adult data and other data in pediatric drug-development programs. *Pediatrics* 2011;128(5):e1241–e1249.
10. Navari RM. Management of chemotherapy-induced nausea and vomiting in pediatric patients. *Pediatr Drugs* 2017;19(3):213–222.
11. Lau Moon Lin M, Robinson PD, Flank J, et al. The safety of prochloroperazine in children: a systematic review and meta-analysis. *Drug Saf* 2016;39:509–516.
12. Dapuis LL, Sung L, Moassiotis A, et al. 2016 updated MASCC/ESMO consensus recommendations: prevention of chemotherapy-induced nausea and vomiting in children. *Support Care Cancer* 2017;25:323–331.
13. Starke PR, Weaver J, Chowdhury BA. Boxed warning added to promethazine labeling for pediatric use. *N Engl J Med* 2005;352:2653.
14. Lau Moon Lin M, Robinson PD, Flank J, et al. The safety of metoclopramide in children: a systematic review and meta-analysis. *Drug Saf* 2016;39(7):675–687.
15. Romano C, Dipasquale V, Scarpignato C. Antiemetic drug use in children: what the clinician needs to know. *J Pediatr Gastroenterol Nutr* 2019;68(4):466–471.
16. Djeddi D, Kongolo G, Lefaix C, et al. Effect of domperidone on QT interval in neonates. *J Pediatr* 2008;153(5):663–666.
17. Marchetti F, Bonati M, Maestro A, et al. Oral ondansetron versus domperidone for acute gastroenteritis in pediatric emergency departments: multicenter double blind randomized controlled trial. *PLoS One* 2016;11(11):e0165441.
18. Lindley C, Blower P. Oral serotonin type 3-receptor antagonists for prevention of chemotherapy-induced emesis. *Am J Health Syst Pharm* 2000;57(18):1685–1697.
19. Kovac AL. Prophylaxis of postoperative nausea and vomiting: controversies in the use of serotonin 5-hydroxytryptamine subtype 3 receptor antagonists. *J Clin Anesth* 2006;18(4):304–318.
20. Culy CR, Bhana N, Plosker GL. Ondansetron: a review of its use as an antiemetic in children. *Paediatr Drugs* 2001;3(6):441–479.
21. Roila F, Del Favero A. Ondansetron clinical pharmacokinetics. *Clin Pharmacokinet* 1995;29(2):95–109.
22. Tan J, Wang S, Liang X, et al. Palonosetron is nonsuperior to ondansetron in acute phase but provides superior antiemetic control in delayed phase for pediatric patients administered highly emetogenic chemotherapy. *Pediatr Blood Cancer* 2018;65(2). doi:10.1002/pbc.26815
23. Phillips RS, Friend AJ, Gibson F, et al. Antiemetic medication for prevention and treatment of chemotherapy-induced nausea and vomiting in childhood. *Cochrane Database Syst Rev* 2016;2:CD007786.
24. Guarino A, Ashkenazi S, Gendrel D, et al. European Society for Pediatric Gastroenterology, Hepatology, and Nutrition/European Society for Pediatric Infectious Diseases evidence-based guidelines for the management of acute gastroenteritis in children in Europe: update 2014. *J Pediatr Gastroenterol Nutr* 2014;59(1):132–152.
25. Tomasik E, Ziółkowska E, Kołodziej MI. Systematic review with meta-analysis: ondansetron for vomiting in children with acute gastroenteritis. *Aliment Pharmacol Ther* 2016;44:438–446.
26. Freedman SB, Ali S, Oleszczuk M, et al. Treatment of acute gastroenteritis in children: an overview of systematic reviews of interventions commonly used in developed countries. *Evid Based Child Health* 2013;8(4):1123–1137.

27. Freedman SB, Uleryk E, Rumantir M, et al. Ondansetron and the risk of cardiac arrhythmias: a systematic review and postmarketing analysis. *Ann Emerg Med* 2014;64:19–25.
28. Bell GC, Caudle KE, Whirl-Carrillo M, et al. Clinical pharmacogenetics implementation consortium (CPIC) guideline for CYP2D6 genotype and use of ondansetron and tropisetron. *Clin Pharmacol Ther* 2017;102(2):213–218.
29. Rosen R, Vandenplas Y, Singendonk M, et al. Pediatric gastroesophageal reflux clinical practice guidelines: joint recommendations of the North American Society for Pediatric Gastroenterology, Hepatology, and Nutrition and the European Society for Pediatric Gastroenterology, Hepatology, and Nutrition. *J Pediatr Gastroenterol Nutr* 2018;66(3):516–554.
30. McCallum RW. Review of the current status of prokinetic agents in gastroenterology. *Am J Gastroenterol* 1985;80(12):1008–1016.
31. Cohen S, Morris DW, Schoen HJ, et al. The effect of oral and intravenous metoclopramide on human lower esophageal sphincter pressure. *Gastroenterology* 1976;70(4):484–487.
32. Albibi R, McCallum RW. Metoclopramide: pharmacology and clinical application. *Ann Intern Med* 1983;98(1):86–95.
33. Lauritsen K, Laursen LS, Rask-Madsen J. Clinical pharmacokinetics of drugs used in the treatment of gastrointestinal diseases (Part I). *Clin Pharmacokinet* 1990;19(1):11–31.
34. Bateman DN. Clinical pharmacokinetics of metoclopramide. *Clin Pharmacokinet* 1983;8(6):523–529.
35. Ross-Lee LM, Eadie MJ, Hooper WD, et al. Single-dose pharmacokinetics of metoclopramide. *Eur J Clin Pharmacol* 1981;20(6):465–471.
36. Webb D, Buss DC, Fifield R, et al. The plasma protein binding of metoclopramide in health and renal disease. *Br J Clin Pharmacol* 1986;21(3):334–336.
37. Kearns GL, van den Anker JN, Reed MD, et al. Pharmacokinetics of metoclopramide in neonates. *J Clin Pharmacol* 1998;38(2):122–128.
38. Kearns GL, Butler HL, Lane JK, et al. Metoclopramide pharmacokinetics and pharmacodynamics in infants with gastroesophageal reflux. *J Pediatr Gastroenterol Nutr* 1988;7(6):823–829.
39. Curry JI, Lander TD, Stringer MD. Review article: erythromycin as a prokinetic agent in infants and children. *Aliment Pharmacol Ther* 2001;15(5):595–603.
40. Pennathur A, Tran A, Cioppi M, et al. Erythromycin strengthens the defective lower esophageal sphincter in patients with gastroesophageal reflux disease. *Am J Surg* 1994;167(1):169–172; discussion 172–173.
41. Jadcherla SR, Klee G, Berseth CL. Regulation of migrating motor complexes by motilin and pancreatic polypeptide in human infants. *Pediatr Res* 1997;42(3):365–369.
42. Ericson JE, Arnold C, Cheeseman J, et al. Use and safety of erythromycin and metoclopramide in hospitalized infants. *J Pediatr Gastroenterol Nutr* 2015;61(3):334–339.
43. Peeters TL. Erythromycin and other macrolides as prokinetic agents. *Gastroenterology* 1993;105(6):1886–1899.
44. Boivin MA, Carey MC, Levy H. Erythromycin accelerates gastric emptying in a dose–response manner in healthy subjects. *Pharmacotherapy* 2003;23(1):5–8.
45. Tomomasa T, Miyazaki M, Koizumi T, et al. Erythromycin increases gastric antral motility in human premature infants. *Biol Neonate* 1993;63(6):349–352.
46. Farrar HC, Walsh-Sukys MC, Kyllonen K, et al. Cardiac toxicity associated with intravenous erythromycin lactobionate: two case reports and a review of the literature. *Pediatr Infect Dis J* 1993;12(8):688–691.
47. Fichtenbaum CJ, Babb JD, Baker DA. Erythromycin induced cardiovascular toxicity. *Conn Med* 1988;52(3):135–136.
48. Murchison L, De Coppi P, Eaton S. Post-natal erythromycin exposure and risk of infantile hypertrophic pyloric stenosis: a systematic review and meta-analysis. *Pediatr Surg Int* 2016;32(12):1147–1152.
49. Abdellatif M, Ghozy S, Kamel MG, et al. Association between exposure to macrolides and the development of infantile hypertrophic pyloric stenosis: a systematic review and meta-analysis. *Eur J Pediatr* 2019;178(3):301–314.
50. Stiel JN, Mitchell CA, Radcliff FJ, et al. Hypercalcemia in patients with peptic ulceration receiving large doses of calcium carbonate. *Gastroenterology* 1967;53(6):900–904.
51. Texter EC Jr. A critical look at the clinical use of antacids in acid-peptic disease and gastric acid rebound. *Am J Gastroenterol* 1989;84(2):97–108.
52. Tsou VM, Young RM, Hart MH, et al. Elevated plasma aluminum levels in normal infants receiving antacids containing aluminum. *Pediatrics* 1991;87(2):148–151.
53. Portuguez-Malavasi A, Aranda JV. Antacid bezoar in a newborn. *Pediatrics* 1979;63(4):679–680.
54. Rosen R, Amirault J, Liu H, et al. Changes in gastric and lung microflora with acid suppression: acid suppression and bacterial growth. *JAMA Pediatr* 2014;168(10):932–937.
55. Wolfe MM, Soll AH. The physiology of gastric acid secretion. *N Engl J Med* 1988;319(26):1707–1715.
56. Xue S, Katz PO, Banerjee P, et al. Bedtime H_2 blockers improve nocturnal gastric acid control in GERD patients on proton pump inhibitors. *Aliment Pharmacol Ther* 2001;15(9):1351–1356.
57. Sun WM, Hasler WL, Lien HC, et al. Nizatidine enhances the gastrocolonic response and the colonic peristaltic reflex in humans. *J Pharmacol Exp Ther* 2001;299(1):159–163.
58. Bachmann KA, Sullivan TJ, Jauregui L, et al. Drug interactions of H_2-receptor antagonists. *Scand J Gastroenterol Suppl* 1994;206:14–19.
59. Maples HD, James LP, Stowe CD, et al. Famotidine disposition in children and adolescents with chronic renal insufficiency. *J Clin Pharmacol* 2003;43(1):7–14.
60. Blumer JL, Rothstein FC, Kaplan BS, et al. Pharmacokinetic determination of ranitidine pharmacodynamics in pediatric ulcer disease. *J Pediatr* 1985;107(2):301–306.
61. James LP, Marshall JD, Heulitt MJ, et al. Pharmacokinetics and pharmacodynamics of famotidine in children. *J Clin Pharmacol* 1996;36(1):48–54.
62. James LP, Marotti T, Stowe CD, et al. Pharmacokinetics and pharmacodynamics of famotidine in infants. *J Clin Pharmacol* 1998;38(12):1089–1095.
63. Fontana M, Massironi E, Rossi A, et al. Ranitidine pharmacokinetics in newborn infants. *Arch Dis Child* 1993;68(5 Spec No):602–603.
64. Hook JB, Bailie MD. Perinatal renal pharmacology. *Annu Rev Pharmacol Toxicol* 1979;19:491–509.
65. Arant BS Jr. Developmental patterns of renal functional maturation compared in the human neonate. *J Pediatr* 1978;92(5):705–712.
66. Wenning LA, Murphy MG, James LP, et al. Pharmacokinetics of famotidine in infants. *Clin Pharmacokinet* 2005;44(4):395–406.
67. Abdel-Rahman SM, Johnson FK, Manowitz N, et al. Single-dose pharmacokinetics of nizatidine (Axid) in children. *J Clin Pharmacol* 2002;42(10):1089–1096.
68. Kuusela AL. Long-term gastric pH monitoring for determining optimal dose of ranitidine for critically ill preterm and term neonates. *Arch Dis Child Fetal Neonatal Ed* 1998;78(2): F151–F153.
69. Kelly EJ, Brownlee KG, Ng PC, et al. The prophylactic use of ranitidine in babies treated with dexamethasone. *Arch Dis Child* 1992;67(4 Spec No):471.
70. Kanto WP Jr. A decade of experience with neonatal extracorporeal membrane oxygenation. *J Pediatr* 1994;124(3):335–347.
71. Wells TG, Heulitt MJ, Taylor BJ, et al. Pharmacokinetics and pharmacodynamics of ranitidine in neonates treated with extracorporeal membrane oxygenation. *J Clin Pharmacol* 1998;38(5):402–407.
72. Wiest DB, O'Neal W, Reigart JR, et al. Pharmacokinetics of ranitidine in critically ill infants. *Dev Pharmacol Ther* 1989;12(1):7–12.
73. Freston JW. Cimetidine: II. Adverse reactions and patterns of use. *Ann Intern Med* 1982;97(5):728–734.
74. Brogden RN, Carmine AA, Heel RC, et al. Ranitidine: a review of its pharmacology and therapeutic use in peptic ulcer disease and other allied diseases. *Drugs* 1982;24(4):267–303.
75. Schentag JJ, Cerra FB, Calleri G, et al. Pharmacokinetic and clinical studies in patients with cimetidine-associated mental confusion. *Lancet* 1979;1(8109):177–181.
76. Jensen RT, Collen MJ, Pandol SJ, et al. Cimetidine-induced impotence and breast changes in patients with gastric hypersecretory states. *N Engl J Med* 1983;308(15):883–887.
77. Powell JR, Donn KH. Histamine H_2-antagonist drug interactions in perspective: mechanistic concepts and clinical implications. *Am J Med* 1984;77(5B):57–84.
78. Smith SR, Kendall MJ. Ranitidine versus cimetidine. A comparison of their potential to cause clinically important drug interactions. *Clin Pharmacokinet* 1988;15(1):44–56.
79. Gibbons TE, Gold BD. The use of proton pump inhibitors in children: a comprehensive review. *Paediatr Drugs* 2003;5(1):25–40.
80. Earp JC, Mehotra N, Peters KE, et al. Esomeprazole FDA approval in children with GERD: exposure-matching and exposure-response. *J Pediatr Gastroenterol Nutr* 2017;65(3):272–277.
81. Kromer W, Kruger U, Huber R, et al. Differences in pH-dependent activation rates of substituted benzimidazoles and biological in vitro correlates. *Pharmacology* 1998;56(2):57.
82. Richardson P, Hawkey CJ, Stack WA. Proton pump inhibitors. Pharmacology and rationale for use in gastrointestinal disorders. *Drugs* 1998;56(3):307–335.
83. Stedman CA, Barclay ML. Review article: comparison of the pharmacokinetics, acid suppression and efficacy of proton pump inhibitors. *Aliment Pharmacol Ther* 2000;14(8):963–978.
84. Freston JW, Chiu YL, Mulford DJ, et al. Comparative pharmacokinetics and safety of lansoprazole oral capsules and orally disintegrating tablets in healthy subjects. *Aliment Pharmacol Ther* 2003;17(3):361–367.
85. Gremse DA, Donnelly JR, Kukulka MJ, et al. A novel option for dosing of proton pump inhibitors: dispersion of lansoprazole orally disintegrating tablet in water via oral syringe. *Aliment Pharmacol Ther* 2004;19(11):1211–1215.
86. Johnson CE, Cober MP, Ludwig JL. Stability of partial doses of omeprazole-sodium bicarbonate oral suspension. *Ann Pharmacother* 2007;41(12):1954–1961.
87. Burnett JE, Balkin ER. Stability and viscosity of a flavored omeprazole oral suspension for pediatric use. *Am J Health Syst Pharm* 2006;63(22):2240–2247.
88. Prichard PJ, Walt RP, Kitchingham GK, et al. Oral phenytoin pharmacokinetics during omeprazole therapy. *Br J Clin Pharmacol* 1987;24:543–545.
89. Hatlebakk JG, Katz PO, Camacho-Lobato L, et al. Proton pump inhibitors: better acid suppression when taken before a meal than without a meal. *Aliment Pharmacol Ther* 2000;14:1267–1272.
90. El Rouby N, Lima JJ, Johnson JA. Proton pump inhibitors: from CYP2C19 pharmacogenetics to precision medicine. *Expert Opin Drug Metab Toxicol* 2019;14(4):447–460.
91. Horn J. Review article: relationship between the metabolism and efficacy of the proton pump inhibitors—focus on rabeprazole. *Aliment Pharmacol Ther* 2004;20:11–19.
92. Furuta T, Ohashi K, Kosuge K, et al. CYP2C19 genotype status and effect of omeprazole on intragastric pH in humans. *Clin Pharmacol Ther* 1999;65(5):552–561.
93. Kearns G. Pantoprazole disposition in pediatrics. *Clin Pharmacol Ther* 2003;73:38.
94. Kuo CH, Lu CY, Shih HY, et al. CYP2C19 polymorphism influences *Helicobacter pylori* eradication. *World J Gastroenterol* 2004;20(43):16029–16036.
95. Deshpande N, Sharanya V, Ravi Kanth VV, et al. Rapid and ultra-rapid metabolizers with CYP2C19*17 polymorphism do not respond to standard therapy with proton pump inhibitors. *Meta Gene* 2016;9:159–164.
96. Jainan W, Vilaichone R. Effects of the CYP2C19 genetic polymorphism on gastritis, peptic ulcer disease, peptic ulcer bleeding and gastric cancer. *Asian Pac J Cancer Prev* 2014;15:10957–10960.
97. Furuta T, Sugimoto M, Shirai N, Ishizaki T. CYP2C19 pharmacogenomics associated with therapy of *Helicobacter pylori* infection and gastro-esophageal reflux diseases with a proton pump inhibitor. *Pharmacogenomics* 2007;8(9):1199–1210.
98. Alcorn J, McNamara PJ. Ontogeny of hepatic and renal systemic clearance pathways in infants: part II. *Clin Pharmacokinet* 2002;41(13):1077–1094.
99. Andersson T, Hassall E, Lundborg P, et al. Pharmacokinetics of orally administered omeprazole in children. International Pediatric Omeprazole Pharmacokinetic Group. *Am J Gastroenterol* 2000;95(11):3101–3106.

100. Hassall E, Israel D, Shepherd R, et al. Omeprazole for treatment of chronic erosive esophagitis in children: a multicenter study of efficacy, safety, tolerability and dose requirements. International Pediatric Omeprazole Study Group. *J Pediatr* 2000;137(6):800–807.
101. Tran A, Rey E, Pons G, et al. Pharmacokinetic–pharmacodynamic study of oral lansoprazole in children. *Clin Pharmacol Ther* 2002;71(5):359–367.
102. Omari T, Davidson G, Bondarov P, et al. Pharmacokinetics and acid-suppressive effects of esomeprazole in infants 1-24 months old with symptoms of gastroesophageal reflux disease. *J Pediatr Gastroenterol Nutr* 2007;45(5):530–537.
103. Zhao J, Li J, Hamer-Maansson JE, et al. Pharmacokinetic properties of esomeprazole in children aged 1 to 11 years with symptoms of gastroesophageal reflux disease: a randomized, open-label study. *Clin Ther* 2006;28(11):1868–1876.
104. Khoshoo V, Dhume P. Clinical response to 2 dosing regimens of lansoprazole in infants with gastroesophageal reflux. *J Pediatr Gastroenterol Nutr* 2008;46(3):352–354.
105. Fiedorek S, Tolia V, Gold BD, et al. Efficacy and safety of lansoprazole in adolescents with symptomatic erosive and non-erosive gastroesophageal reflux disease. *J Pediatr Gastroenterol Nutr* 2005;40(3):319–327.
106. Omari TI, Haslam RR, Lundborg P, et al. Effect of omeprazole on acid gastroesophageal reflux and gastric acidity in preterm infants with pathological acid reflux. *J Pediatr Gastroenterol Nutr* 2007;44(1):41–44.
107. Croxtall JD, Perry CM, Keating GM. Esomeprazole: in gastroesophageal reflux disease in children and adolescents. *Paediatr Drugs* 2008;10(3):199–205.
108. Tsou VM, Baker R, Book L, et al. Multicenter, randomized, double-blind study comparing 20 and 40 mg of pantoprazole for symptom relief in adolescents (12 to 16 years of age) with gastroesophageal reflux disease (GERD). *Clin Pediatr (Phila)* 2006;45(8):741–749.
109. Tolia V, Bishop PR, Tsou VM, et al. Multicenter, randomized, double-blind study comparing 10, 20 and 40 mg pantoprazole in children (5-11 years) with symptomatic gastroesophageal reflux disease. *J Pediatr Gastroenterol Nutr* 2006;42(4):384–391.
110. Madrazo-de la Garza A, Dibildox M, Vargas A, et al. Efficacy and safety of oral pantoprazole 20 mg given once daily for reflux esophagitis in children. *J Pediatr Gastroenterol Nutr* 2003;36(2):261–265.
111. Gunasekaran TS, Hassall EG. Efficacy and safety of omeprazole for severe gastroesophageal reflux in children. *J Pediatr* 1993;123(1):148–154.
112. Drut R, Altamirano E, Cueto Rua E. Omeprazole-associated changes in the gastric mucosa of children. *J Clin Pathol* 2008;61(6):754–756.
113. Song H, Zhu J, Lu D. Long-term proton pump inhibitor (PPI) use and the development of gastric pre-malignant lesions. *Cochrane Database Syst Rev* 2014;(12):CD010623.
114. De Bruyne P, Ito S. Toxicity of long-term use of proton pump inhibitors in children. *Arch Dis Child* 2018;103:78–82.
115. Kearns GL, Winter HS. Proton pump inhibitors in pediatrics: relevant pharmacokinetics and pharmacodynamics. *J Pediatr Gastroenterol Nutr* 2003;37(Suppl 1):S52–S59.
116. Ishizaki T, Horai Y. Review article: cytochrome P450 and the metabolism of proton pump inhibitors–emphasis on rabeprazole. *Aliment Pharmacol Ther* 1999;13(Suppl 3):27–36.
117. Masubuchi N, Li AP, Okazaki O. An evaluation of the cytochrome P450 induction potential of pantoprazole in primary human hepatocytes. *Chem Biol Interact* 1998;114(1–2):1–13.
118. Wang LS, Zhou G, Zhu B, et al. St John's wort induces both cytochrome P450 3A4-catalyzed sulfoxidation and 2C19-dependent hydroxylation of omeprazole. *Clin Pharmacol Ther* 2004;75(3):191–197.
119. Moreau C, Taburet AM, Furlan V, et al. Interaction between tacrolimus and omeprazole in a pediatric liver transplant recipient. *Transplantation* 2006;81(3):487–488.
120. Winston A, Back D, Fletcher C, et al. Effect of omeprazole on the pharmacokinetics of saquinavir-500 mg formulation with ritonavir in healthy male and female volunteers. *AIDS* 2006;20(10):1401–1406.
121. Fang AF, Damle BD, LaBadie RR, et al. Significant decrease in nelfinavir systemic exposure after omeprazole coadministration in healthy subjects. *Pharmacotherapy* 2008;28(1):42–50.
122. Tappouni HL, Rublein JC, Donovan BJ, et al. Effect of omeprazole on the plasma concentrations of indinavir when administered alone and in combination with ritonavir. *Am J Health Syst Pharm* 2008;65(5):422–428.
123. Andersson T, Hassan-Alin M, Hasselgren G, et al. Drug interaction studies with esomeprazole, the (S)-isomer of omeprazole. *Clin Pharmacokinet* 2001;40(7):523–537.
124. Lloyd CW, Martin WJ, Taylor BD. The pharmacokinetics of cimetidine and metabolites in a neonate. *Drug Intell Clin Pharm* 1985;19(3):203–205.
125. Faure C, Michaud L, Shaghaghi EK, et al. Intravenous omeprazole in children: pharmacokinetics and effect on 24-hour intragastric pH. *J Pediatr Gastroenterol Nutr* 2001;33(2):144–148.
126. Faure C, Michaud L, Shaghaghi EK, et al. Lansoprazole in children: pharmacokinetics and efficacy in reflux oesophagitis. *Aliment Pharmacol Ther* 2001;15(9):1397–1402.
127. Andersson T. Pharmacokinetics of intravenous omeprazole in neonates and infants [Abstract]. *J Pediatr Gastroenterol Nutr* 2001;33:424.
128. Andersson T. Pharmacokinetics and pharmacodynamics of oral omeprazole in infants [Abstract]. *J Pediatr Gastroenterol Nutr* 2001;33:416.
129. Kearns G. Omeprazole disposition in children following single-dose administration: relationship to CYP2C19 genotype. *J Clin Pharmacol* 2003;43(8):840–848.
130. Ferron GM. Pharmacokinetics of IV pantoprazole in pediatric patients [Abstract]. *Clin Pharmacol Ther* 2003;73:36.
131. James L, Walson P, Lomax K, et al. Pharmacokinetics and tolerability of rabeprazole sodium in subjects aged 12 to 16 years with gastroesophageal reflux disease: an open-label, single-and multiple-dose study. *Clin Ther* 2007;29(9):2082–2092.
132. Li J, Zhao J, Hamer-Maansson JE, et al. Pharmacokinetic properties of esomeprazole in adolescent patients aged 12 to 17 years with symptoms of gastroesophageal reflux disease: a randomized, open-label study. *Clin Ther* 2006;28(3):419–427.
133. Heyman MB, Zhang W, Huang B, et al. Pharmacokinetics and pharmacodynamics of lansoprazole in children 13 to 24 months old with gastroesophageal reflux disease. *J Pediatr Gastroenterol Nutr* 2007;44(1):35–40.
134. Kearns GL, Blumer J, Schexnayder S, et al. Single-dose pharmacokinetics of oral and intravenous pantoprazole in children and adolescents. *J Clin Pharmacol* 2008;48(11):1356–1365.
135. Gunasekaran T. Pharmacokinetics of lansoprazole in adolescents with GERD [Abstract]. *J Pediatr Gastroenterol Nutr* 2000;31:S97.

CHAPTER

53

Suruchi Batra
Laurie S. Conklin

Drugs in Inflammatory Bowel Diseases

INTRODUCTION

Inflammatory bowel diseases (IBDs) are chronic inflammatory diseases of the gastrointestinal tract, which include Crohn disease (CD) and ulcerative colitis (UC). About 10% to 15% of patients with IBD cannot be firmly diagnosed with CD or UC; hence, they are initially diagnosed as having inflammatory bowel disease unclassified (IBD-U).[1] The exact causal mechanisms of IBD are unclear, but pathogenesis of IBD involves a dysregulated mucosal immune response toward host commensal intestinal microbiota, in people who are genetically predisposed.[2] The nucleotide-binding oligomerization domain containing 2 (*NOD2*) gene has been implicated in severe phenotypes of CD. Furthermore, many IBD susceptibility gene variants, such as *NOD2*, regulate host–microbial interactions.[3,4] Microbial dysbiosis in IBD is well documented, but mechanisms by which specific bacterial groups play a causal role in conferring risk of developing IBD are not yet well understood.[5] The incidence of pediatric IBD is approximately 10 per 100,000 children in the United States and Canada.[6–8] About 10% to 20% of IBD patients present with the first signs of disease before 18 years of age.[9] Childhood IBD is the fastest growing age group affected.[10]

IBD follows a relapsing and remitting course; clinical manifestations, evolution of the disease, and prognosis are variable. Both CD and UC are systemic diseases, with extraintestinal manifestations affecting approximately one-third of patients.[11] Extraintestinal manifestations can be particularly burdensome to patients and include ankylosing spondylitis, iritis, primary sclerosing cholangitis, as well as other immune-mediated inflammatory diseases (i.e., erythema nodosum, arthritis). Some inflammatory extraintestinal conditions are associated with IBD but also may emerge as complications of therapy, including multiple sclerosis and psoriasis.[12] IBD is challenging for children and adolescents due to long-term complications, including malnutrition, impaired bone health, depression, and growth failure.[13–19] Insufficient control of inflammatory disease impacts quality of life for children and adolescents with IBD.[20]

In CD, disease may be localized anywhere along the gastrointestinal tract. Clinical manifestations can vary in severity; currently, physicians use the Pediatric Crohn's Disease Activity Index (PCDAI) to assess clinical severity[21] (Table 53.1). Endoscopic severity score may be categorized via utilization of the Simple Endoscopic Score for CD (SES-CD)[21] (Table 53.2). CD may manifest as one of three different subtypes: inflammatory, penetrating, or stricturing disease. The latter two types may result in life-altering complications, including fistulae, abscesses, bowel perforation, bowel obstruction, and intra-abdominal sepsis.[22] Most children with CD have inflammatory disease at the time of diagnosis, but up to one-third of children progress to intestinal complications during a period of less than 10 years of follow-up.[23] Moreover, surgery is required for CD in children within 5 years in 15% to 20% of patients.[24] Increasingly, studies of pediatric CD progression have highlighted the variable course of disease; patients at risk for severe disease or poor response to treatment may need more aggressive or targeted treatment.

The Pediatric RISK Stratification Study was a prospective inception cohort study of newly diagnosed children with CD. More than 1,800 patients, ages 6 to 17 years, were recruited at disease onset and prospectively followed for complications and response to therapies. Certain factors were positively correlated with development of severe CD, including African American race, older age, and seropositivity for the anti–*Saccharomyces cerevisiae* antibody (ASCA) and anti-flagellin (Cbir1) antibodies. Notably, patients with a stricturing phenotype were not responsive to early (defined as started in the first 90 days following diagnosis) anti–tumor necrosis factor α (anti-TNFα) therapy. In addition, gene expression signature from the terminal ileal biopsies of patients with stricturing disease showed increased extracellular matrix genes, implying a different biologic process in newly diagnosed stricturing CD.[22] Extracellular matrix protein 1 and other biomarkers of fibrosis may aid in identifying children at high risk of a stricturing phenotype.[25,26]

In contrast to CD, intestinal inflammation in UC is confined to the large intestine. Clinical manifestations of UC include hematochezia, anemia, and fatigue. Clinical, endoscopic, and histologic features are generally similar across the age spectrum. However, in treatment-naïve pediatric patients, UC can be distinguished from Crohn colitis by increased expression of genes associated with type 2 and type 17 immune responses.[27] More than 200 genetic loci are implicated in IBD, with 29 being UC specific.[28] Most loci have a very small effect size, except for the human leukocyte antigen loci on chromosome 6, with an association that is approximately twice as strong in pediatric

TABLE 53.1 Pediatric Crohn's Disease Activity Index

History			
Score	**0**	**5**	**10**
Abdominal pain	None	Mild; brief, does not interfere with activities	Moderate/severe; daily, longer lasting, affects activities, nocturnal
Patient functioning	No limitation	Occasional difficulty in maintaining activities	Frequent limitation of activity
Stools per day	0–1, liquid, no blood	0–2 semiformed or 2–5 liquid stools; small amount of blood	≥6 liquid stools, gross bleeding, nocturnal stooling
Physical Examination			
Score	**0**	**5**	**10**
Weight	Voluntary weight gain or stable weight	Involuntary weight stable, weight loss 1%–9%	Weight loss ≥10%
Height at diagnosis	<1 channel decrease	≥1, <2 channel decrease	>2 channel decrease
Height at follow-up	Height velocity ≥−1 SD	Height velocity <−1 SD, >−2 SD	Height velocity ≤−2 SD
Abdomen	No tenderness, no mass	Tenderness or mass without tenderness	Tenderness, involuntary guarding, or definite mass
Perirectal disease	None, asymptomatic tags	1–2 indolent fistula, scant drainage, no tenderness	Active fistula, drainage, tenderness or abscess
Laboratory			
Score	**0**	**5**	**10**
Hematocrit			
<10 y male or female	>33%	28%–32%	<28%
11–14 y male	≥35%	30%–34%	<30%
15–19 y male	≥37%	32%–36%	<32%
11–19 y female	≥34%	29%–33%	<29%
ESR (mm/h)	<20	20–55	>50
Albumin (g/dL)	>3.5	3.1–3.4	≤3.0
Extraintestinal Manifestations			
Fever ≥38.5°C for 3 d over past week, arthritis, uveitis, erythema nodosum, pyoderma gangrenosum			
Score	**0**	**5**	**10**
	None	1	≥2
Score <10 = inactive disease; 11–30 = mild disease; >30 = moderate-to-severe disease			
Change in 12.5 points shows significant improvement			

TABLE 53.2 Simple Endoscopic Score for Crohn Disease

Score	*0*	*1*	*2*	*0*
Size of ulcers	None	Aphthous ulcers (0.1–0.5 cm)	Large ulcers (0.5–2 cm)	Very large ulcers (>2 cm)
Ulcerated surface	None	<10%	10%–30%	>30%
Affected surface	Unaffected	<50%	50%–75%	>75%
Presence of narrowing	None	Single, can be passed	Multiple, can be passed	Cannot be passed
Score: <10 indicates remission				
Score per segment (rectum, sigmoid and descending colon, transverse colon, ascending colon, terminal ileum)				

UC as compared with adults.[29] The highest prevalence of UC is recorded in Western countries; newly industrialized countries document the greatest increases in incidence.[30] UC disease severity and response to therapy are heterogeneous in children.[31,32] Currently, UC is graded by a physician as mild, moderate, or severe, based on the Pediatric Ulcerative Colitis Activity Index (PUCAI), a clinical score which has been correlated with endoscopic assessments[33,34] (Table 53.3). These disease definitions are used clinically and to define clinical trial populations. However, these definitions may be changing as molecular data further defines subsets of disease. Endoscopic severity may be assessed using the Mayo endoscopic score.

The Predicting Response to Standardized Pediatric Colitis Therapy (PROTECT) study included 428 UC patients from 29 pediatric gastroenterology centers in North America.[31,32] In this trial, rectal biopsies from 206 patients underwent high-throughput RNA sequencing (RNAseq). A gene signature for severe disease (nonresponse to corticosteroids) was identified, which was enriched with cytokines and chemokines that promote activation of the innate immune system and recruitment of neutrophils. This signature showed substantial overlap with genes previously associated with nonresponse to other medications used to treat UC, thus likely identifying disease severity (not therapy-specific nonresponse). In the future, mucosal inflammatory state may define the likelihood of response to current treatment approaches with more accuracy than the clinical assessment of severity.[35]

TABLE 53.3 Pediatric Ulcerative Colitis Activity Index

Variable	*Severity*	*Score*
Abdominal pain	No pain	0
	Pain can be ignored	5
	Pain cannot be ignored	10
Rectal bleeding	None	0
	Small amount, <50% of stools	10
	Small amount with most stools	20
	Large amount, >50% of stools	30
Stool consistency of most stools	Formed	0
	Partially formed	5
	Completely unformed	10
Number of stools per 24 h	0–2	0
	3–5	5
	6–8	10
	>8	15
Nocturnal stool	No	0
	Yes	10
	No limitation	0
	Occasional limitation	5
Activity level	Severe restriction	10

Score <10 remission; 10–34 mild disease; 35–64 moderate disease; 65–85 severe disease

Change of ≥20 points indicates significant response

TREATMENT GOALS IN PEDIATRIC INFLAMMATORY BOWEL DISEASE—CURRENT LANDSCAPE

The primary goals of treatment of children and adolescents with IBD are induction and maintenance of symptomatic remission to improve quality of life, maintaining durable maintenance of remission, and prevention of complications caused by the disease and medications. The approach to treatment of pediatric IBD has changed over the past 10 years, and a growing number of therapeutics are available to physicians and patients (Table 53.4). Historically, the target of treating CD and UC was control of symptoms via a "step-up approach," with the use of corticosteroids and 5-aminosalicylates (5-ASA) in most patients at diagnosis. Symptoms were managed with additional courses of corticosteroids and maintenance treatment consistent of escalation to immunomodulators, biologics, or a combination of both. Surgical management was reserved for refractory patients.

However, the treatment target in pediatric CD and UC has evolved from predominantly symptom control to an emphasis on endoscopic remission in addition to symptom remission. Mucosal or endoscopic healing has been defined as lack of visible findings on colonoscopy as indicated by a Mayo score of 0 or 1[36] (Table 53.5). It is increasingly appreciated that improvement in endoscopic disease activity correlates with long-term outcomes for patients, including lower corticosteroid use, decreased hospitalizations, and reduced risk of structural bowel damage.[37–40] Histologic healing may be a more sensitive marker of disease activity, but further studies are needed to determine standardized definition of disease activity, healing, and evaluation before histology may be used as a clinical trial outcome.[41]

Disease response is thus based on clinical response or daily symptoms of disease, serum/fecal biomarkers, and endoscopic evaluation to assess endoscopic and histologic healing. Pediatric and adolescent patients with IBD disease are monitored regularly at outpatient clinical visits, at least three to four times per year. These visits allow for assessment of clinical symptoms and biomarkers. There is currently no established guideline regarding need for surveillance endoscopy and colonoscopy in pediatrics. However, more pediatric gastroenterologists are advocating for surveillance endoscopy and colonoscopy 6 to 12 months after treatment initiation, following the adult treat-to-target paradigm.[36,42]

It has been demonstrated that mucosal healing does not eliminate the possibility of progression to structural bowel damage; in children with CD, residual transmural inflammation observed on magnetic resonance imaging often persists despite mucosal healing on endoscopy.[43] Thus, there remains a need for novel medications that change the course of these diseases. In addition, growth and nutrition optimization, as well as preserving and treating bone and mental health, are important clinical outcomes for children and adolescents with IBD. Variation in disease course and response to therapy underscores the growing appreciation for an individualized treatment paradigm for pediatric IBD and need for careful objective assessment of disease following treatment. In addition, it highlights the need for additional therapies for children with refractory inflammatory, fibrotic, and stricturing disease.

TABLE 53.4 Medications Routinely Used in Pediatric Inflammatory Bowel Disease

Category	*Medications*	*Route of Administration*	*Dose*	*Side Effects*
Glucocorticoids	Prednisone	Oral or intravenous	1 mg/kg divided into 1 or 2 doses daily; maximum 40 mg daily for acute symptoms/flare, then taper until off	Glucose intolerance, adrenal insufficiency, Cushingoid features, striae, acne, gastritis, behavioral changes, sleep disturbances, cataracts, glaucoma, osteopenia, osteonecrosis, hypertension, and increased risk of opportunistic infections
	Budesonide	Oral	9 mg daily × 8 wk, then taper by 3 mg every 2 wk until off	
Mesalamine	NA	Oral	50–100 mg/kg/d divided into 2–4 doses daily	Nephrotoxicity
		Enema	4,000 mg once daily at bedtime	
		Suppository	500 mg once daily at bedtime	
Methotrexate	NA	Oral or subcutaneous	20–29 kg: 10 mg once weekly	Flu-like symptoms, pneumonitis, nausea, vomiting, abdominal pain, leukopenia, mucositis, stomatitis, immunosuppression, hypersensitivity reactions, myelosuppression, and teratogenicity
			30–39 kg: 15 mg once weekly	
			40–49 kg: 20 mg once weekly	
			≥50 kg; 25 mg once weekly	
Thiopurine[a]	Azathioprine	Oral	2–2.5 mg/kg daily; maximum 200 mg	Flu-like illness, increased risk of infection, pancreatitis, hepatotoxicity, and myelosuppression
	Mercaptopurine	Oral	1–1.5 mg/kg daily	
Infliximab[b]	Induction	Intravenous	5 mg/kg once, given at 0, 2, and 6 wk	Hypersensitivity reaction, antidrug antibody formation, immunosuppression, increased risk of malignancy, increased risk of postoperative complications
	Maintenance	Intravenous	5 mg/kg every 6–8 wk	
Adalimumab	Induction	Subcutaneous	17–40 kg: 80 mg, day 1; 40 mg, day 15	Hypersensitivity reaction, antidrug antibody formation, immunosuppression, increased risk of postoperative complications
			≥40 kg: 150 mg, day 1; 80 mg, day 15	
	Maintenance	Subcutaneous	17–40 kg: 20 mg every other week	
			≥40 kg: 40 mg every other week	
Vedolizumab	Induction	Intravenous	300 mg once, given at 0, 2, and 6 wk	Hypersensitivity reaction, antidrug antibody formation
	Maintenance	Intravenous	300 mg every 8 wk	
Ustekinumab	Induction	Intravenous	≤5 kg: 260 mg once	Hypersensitivity reaction, antidrug antibody formation, immunosuppression
			>55 kg–85 kg: 390 mg once	
			>85 kg: 520 mg once	
	Maintenance	Subcutaneous	90 mg every 8 wk	

[a]Thiopurine methyltransferase enzyme testing is recommended to guide dosing; individuals with intermediate enzyme activity may require dose reduction by 50%; thiopurines should be used with extreme caution in individuals with low enzyme activity.
[b]Dose escalation with higher dose of 10 mg/kg/ dose or more frequent infusions may be needed for patients with severe disease.

TABLE 53.5 Mayo Score—Endoscopic Score for Ulcerative Colitis

Score	*Disease Activity*	*Endoscopic Features*
Mayo Score		
0	Inactive	None
1	Mild	Erythema, decreased vascular pattern, mild friability
2	Moderate	Marked erythema, absent vascular pattern, friability, erosions
3	Severe	Spontaneous bleeding, ulceration
Score for rectosigmoid region		

THERAPEUTIC APPROACH TO PEDIATRIC CROHN DISEASE

Corticosteroids remain a first-line therapeutic option for the treatment of acute flares or inducing remission in pediatric CD. However, chronic corticosteroid use leads to complications that are already problematic in pediatric CD, including low bone mineral density, growth failure, and mood changes. Thus, corticosteroids are contraindicated as a maintenance medication in pediatric CD. Moreover, over half of pediatric patients with CD treated with corticosteroids become dependent upon corticosteroids, and less than one-third of patients achieve healing of the intestinal mucosa with this treatment approach.[44,45] Oral budesonide is a corticosteroid targeted to the intestinal mucosa with lower systemic bioavailability because of extensive (90%)

first-pass hepatic metabolism. In a randomized, double-blind, controlled multicenter trial of budesonide versus prednisolone in mild-to-moderate pediatric CD, budesonide induced less adrenal suppression, moon facies, and acne, while inducing remission at a similar rate.[46] However, its use is generally limited to 3 to 4 months in duration as the risk of adverse effects is not completely eliminated.[47]

There is a lack of data supporting use of 5-ASA in pediatric CD, and use for pediatric CD has dramatically decreased as other, more effective treatment options have become available.[48] Immunomodulators, including thiopurines and methotrexate, offer an alternative treatment option. Use of early thiopurines for maintenance of remission in CD (6-mercaptopurine, azathioprine) became more common practice in the 1990s, supported by some data in children.[49–51] Common adverse reactions to thiopurines include flu-like illness, increased risk of infection, pancreatitis, hepatotoxicity, and myelosuppression.[47] Myelosuppression is a dose-dependent side effect. Thiopurines are metabolized by thiopurine methyltransferase (TPMT); individuals with low TPMT activity are at risk for increased dose-dependent adverse effects.[52] Accordingly, utilization of TPMT enzyme testing and monitoring thiopurine metabolite levels are recommended.[53] Research in the past decade has established the increased risk of malignancy for IBD patients treated with thiopurines, including the risk for nonmelanoma skin cancers[54] and increased risk of lymphoproliferative disease (LPDs), frequently associated with Epstein–Barr virus (EBV)[55] A prospective, long-term registry of 5,000 pediatric patients with IBD suggests that malignancy and EBV-related LPDs have been associated with thiopurine use in the pediatric population[56] Thiopurine use in men younger than 35 years of age has been associated with risk for development of hepatosplenic T-cell lymphoma, an extremely rare, but aggressive and typically fatal malignancy.[57] Use of thiopurines as monotherapy has not been shown to decrease rates of surgery, nor improve growth in children with CD[58,59] Thus, use of thiopurines as monotherapy for pediatric CD has decreased.

Another immunomodulator, methotrexate, is a folate antagonist that is believed to have immunomodulator and anti-inflammatory properties when used for the treatment of CD. There is a paucity of studies of methotrexate as monotherapy for adult CD, and no randomized controlled or other interventional studies for the use of methotrexate among pediatric patients.[60] Possible adverse reactions include flu-like symptoms, pneumonitis, nausea, vomiting, abdominal pain, leukopenia, mucositis, stomatitis, immune suppression, hypersensitivity reactions, and myelosuppression.[47,61] Methotrexate administered subcutaneously versus orally may have improved bioavailability and be associated with less gastrointestinal side effects.[62] Moreover, side effects may be minimized with concomitant folic acid administration. Extreme caution is taken when initiating methotrexate therapy in females of childbearing age due to significant teratogenic risk.[63]

Development of infliximab, an intravenous, monoclonal anti-TNFα, dramatically changed the treatment approach to CD. Infliximab has been shown to induce and maintain both clinical remission and mucosal healing in pediatric and adult patients with IBD who are unresponsive or refractory to conventional therapies.[64] Perianal fistulas, an extraintestinal manifestation associated with CD, may be closed by infliximab treatment.[65] A randomized, multicenter, open-label study (the REACH trial) evaluated safety and efficacy of infliximab in the induction and maintenance of moderate-to-severe CD in children aged 6 to 17 years. Notably, in the REACH trial, subjects were required to be on a stable dose of azathioprine, 6-mercaptopurine, or methotrexate; 35% were also receiving corticosteroids at baseline.[66] A second anti-TNFα therapy was developed, adalimumab, which is administered subcutaneously. In the IMAgINE 1 trial of adalimumab in pediatric CD, over 80% of patients responded to therapy within 4 weeks of treatment. Infliximab-naive patients achieved greater remission and response rates than infliximab-experienced patients.[67] Adalimumab has been shown to maintain long-term remission in pediatric patients with CD.[68]

Anti-TNFα therapy has been associated with improvement in bone mineral density in younger and growing children with CD, suggesting that this therapy could offer particular benefit to patients with growth failure or low bone mineral density.[69] Complication-free survival and slower progression of bowel damage in children with inflammatory CD are increased by early anti-TNFα therapy.[22,70] In children with newly diagnosed CD, early monotherapy with biologic treatment, specifically anti-TNFα therapy, was demonstrated to be superior to early treatment with an immunomodulator and corticosteroids and facilitates catch-up growth.[71,72] Adverse reactions associated with anti-TNFα therapies include hypersensitivity and immune suppression, which increases the risk of opportunistic infections.[45] However, risk of serious infections in children on anti-TNFα is lower than that among pediatric patients treated with steroids, or among adults with IBD treated with anti-TNFα therapies.[73] Rare reports have associated the development of demyelinating disorders to anti-TNFα therapy.[74,75]

Ustekinumab is a monoclonal antibody that binds to the common subunit of interleukin 12 and interleukin 23, blocking these proinflammatory cytokines that modulate lymphocyte function.[76] Trials in adults with CD demonstrated safety and efficacy in moderate-to-severe CD.[77–79] Ustekinumab is not yet approved for use in children. However, off-label use is increasing in medically refractory children and adolescents; observational studies have been published reporting safety and efficacy in cohorts of children and adolescents with CD.[80–84]

Exclusive enteral nutrition (EEN) is an established form of dietary therapy in children with CD. In an inception cohort of 147 children, EEN was associated with higher remission rates than corticosteroids, but with similar relapse and complication rates in new-onset mild-to-moderate pediatric CD.[85] EEN induces clinical remission in about 80% of patients and has been shown to modulate the microbiome.[86] However, long-term acceptability of EEN is limited, and studies of EEN as a maintenance therapy are lacking. EEN has few side effects and provides an important option for CD management in lieu of, or in conjunction with, other medical therapies.

THERAPEUTIC APPROACH TO PEDIATRIC ULCERATIVE COLITIS

5-ASA medications (mesalamine most commonly), administered orally and/or rectally, are considered first-line treatment for mild-to-moderate UC in children. Symptomatic response is typically seen within weeks. When disease is more severe, corticosteroids or anti-TNFα agents are used to induce remission. How many children with UC require escalation to other therapies? In 213 children with UC treated with 5-ASA within 1 month of diagnosis, about 40% remained in remission without escalation of therapy at 1 year.[87] In the Predicting Response to Standardized Pediatric Colitis Therapy (PROTECT) study, a multicenter inception cohort study of children with UC, the goal was to determine rates and predictors of week 52 corticosteroid-free remission achieved with mesalamine maintenance therapy only. Mesalamine was recommended as induction and maintenance therapy for mild patients and as maintenance after corticosteroid-induced response in moderate patients. Ninety percent of participants had received mesalamine at some point in the first 12 weeks, and 75% for at least 8 weeks. At week 12, mesalamine was being used by 77% of patients either alone or in conjunction with oral corticosteroids.[31] However, similarly to findings in the Turner et al.'s study,[87] the majority needed more than mesalamine to maintain corticosteroid-free remission. Within 1 year of diagnosis, 19% of participants were treated with thiopurines, 31% were receiving anti-TNFα therapy, and 6% required a colectomy.[32] IBD patients receiving 5-ASA are at risk for rare nephrotoxicity, which most commonly manifests as interstitial nephritis.[88] Renal injury can be severe, but a majority of patients will recover after 5-ASA discontinuation and immunosuppressive therapy.[89]

Corticosteroids are commonly used for induction of remission and management of acute disease flares in UC. However, the duration of time for which they are utilized should be minimized due to numerous well-established side effects. Side effects associated with chronic corticosteroid use include glucose intolerance, adrenal insufficiency, Cushingoid features, striae, acne, gastritis, behavioral changes, sleep disturbances, cataracts, glaucoma, osteopenia, osteonecrosis, hypertension, and increased risk of opportunistic infections.[90] These side effects can occur with intravenous or oral administration. Glucocorticoids may be administered rectally via enema or suppository form, which allows for topical administration with minimal systemic side effects. There is evidence that an 8-week course of budesonide in a multimatrix form targeting the colon can induce remission in adults with a flare of UC.[91]

For chronic moderate-to-severe UC in children and adolescents, anti-TNFα therapies are used to safely induce and maintain remission.[92] In an open-label trial of infliximab in 60 children with moderate-to-severe UC, approximately one-third of children achieved remission at week 52; these results are similar to adult remission rates.[93] Notably, clinical trials of anti-TNFα therapies in pediatric IBD have been uncontrolled, as it is considered unethical to expose children to a placebo once efficacy was demonstrated in adult trials.[94,95] Treatment strategies have also evolved with an early step-up approach, shift of treatment target to mucosal healing, and therapeutic drug monitoring (TDM). Thus, remission rates in clinical practice may not align with those in clinical trials. A reduction in colectomy rates has been observed in pediatric UC since biologics have become available.[96]

Acute severe colitis (ASC), defined as a PUCAI ≥ 65, is an emergency condition due to risk of perforation, sepsis, and mortality. Intravenous corticosteroids are considered first-line therapy for ASC. Infliximab and calcineurin inhibitors (tacrolimus and cyclosporine) are used as second-line therapy for anti–TNFα-naïve children failing intravenous corticosteroids. Typically, cyclosporine and tacrolimus are used as rescue therapy, as a bridge to another long-term maintenance medication (i.e., vedolizumab). Failure rates of these secondary therapies are high, reaching 40% to 50% in the short term (within 3 months) and 70% in the long term (within 3 years), leading to colectomy in approximately 45% of adult patients within 5 years.[97] When infliximab is used as a second-line therapy in ASC, intensified dosing (higher and more frequent infusions) is often prescribed, due to rapid clearance of the drug.[98] There remains considerable uncertainty regarding the optimal dosing approach for infliximab to corticosteroid-refractory ASC. Though uncontrolled studies in adults suggest a benefit for infliximab dose optimization and intensification, the success of this strategy in avoiding colectomy compared with standard induction paradigms remains unclear and randomized trials are needed.[99,100] Generally, colectomy is recommended following failure of second-line medical therapy; however, sequential treatment with calcineurin inhibitors and infliximab is often considered in specialized centers. In such cases, extra precautions must be considered, such as *Pneumocystis jirovecii* pneumonia prophylaxis and physiologic steroids to avoid adrenal insufficiency.[101]

Vedolizumab is a humanized monoclonal antibody that specifically recognizes and binds to the integrin α4β7 heterodimer. The integrin α4β7 interacts with a gut-associated addressin, MadCAM, to direct trafficking of activated leukocytes to the intestinal mucosa. Vedolizumab blocks this process, leading to gut-specific anti-inflammatory activity. Vedolizumab has been shown to be safe and effective for induction and maintenance of remission in adults with active UC and CD.[102] Studies of vedolizumab in adults demonstrate a favorable safety profile, with low rates of serious infections, infusion reactions, and malignancies.[103] Few studies of vedolizumab have been performed in children with UC, though children are being treated with vedolizumab off-label.[104–106] Outcomes in trials of vedolizumab in adults with CD were more mixed.[107,108]

CURRENT CHALLENGES IN TREATING CHILDREN WITH INFLAMMATORY BOWEL DISEASE

A unique risk of biologic therapy is the development of antidrug antibodies (ADAs), which can decrease effectiveness and increase the risk of reactions. Maintaining adequate trough levels[109] and concomitant use of immunomodulators may decrease the risk of ADA.[52,110] Treatment with concomitant anti-TNFα and immunomodulator therapy has been shown to improve durability, increase drug concentrations, and reduce formation of antibodies to infliximab in young adults and children with IBD.[111,112] The Study of Biologic and Immunomodulator Naive Patients in Crohn Disease (SONIC) trial demonstrated improved efficacy of thiopurine and infliximab concomitant therapy in adults with CD, over monotherapy with either treatment.[113] Notably, post hoc evaluation showed that among patients with CD and similar serum concentrations of infliximab, combination therapy with azathioprine was not significantly more effective than infliximab monotherapy. Combination therapy with azathioprine appears to improve efficacy by increasing pharmacokinetic (PK) features of infliximab, not by synergistic effect.[114]

The Combination of Maintenance Methotrexate-Infliximab Trial (COMMIT) study did not demonstrate a treatment benefit of concomitant infliximab and methotrexate in adult patients with CD, but did demonstrate less immunogenicity and higher drug concentrations in those receiving both therapies.[115] There is no prospective study directly comparing thiopurine to methotrexate combination therapy for any anti-TNF α drug for either

CD or UC. In children with CD, concomitant treatment with an immunomodulator (methotrexate or thiopurine) for more than 6 months after starting infliximab increases the durability of response.[116] In North America, physicians seem to prefer use of concomitant methotrexate, secondary to risks of hepatosplenic T-cell lymphoma and risk of other malignancies in children with IBD treated with thiopurines. Despite evidence for improved efficacy of concomitant azathioprine, concerns regarding safety have lessened enthusiasm for the widespread acceptance of concomitant thiopurines in children. Indeed, the number of concomitantly administered IBD drugs is the main risk factor for drug-related adverse events necessitating treatment cessation.[117]

Proactive infliximab monitoring has also been shown to be a strategy to prevent antibody formation.[109] The PK of monoclonal antibodies is variable, and doses needed to achieve target serum levels are difficult to predict. TDM may be used to assess serum concentrations to guide dose adjustments. Several studies have established that consistent anti-TNFα serum concentrations are correlated with higher rates of clinical and endoscopic remission in children and adults.[118–120] The American Gastroenterology Association has established guidelines for target serum concentrations in adult IBD patients during maintenance of anti-TNFα treatment: infliximab serum concentration of ≥ 5 mg per dL and adalimumab serum concentration of ≥ 7.5 mg per dL.[53] One important challenge in the use of TDM is that target serum drug concentrations may vary with individual patient risk factors and severity of disease. For example, serum levels needed to close perianal fistulas in children are higher than the target for maintenance.[121] Patients with a higher inflammatory burden may require higher serum trough levels to achieve remission due to increased drug clearance.[122,123]

Recent research highlights how TDM may be used to optimize serum levels of biologic medication for individual patients. TDM may be used as a "reactive" measure for IBD patients undergoing biologic treatment who may present with concerns for disease flare. In this setting, TDM is used to assess whether the patient has a low drug trough concentration associated with the onset of symptoms. Minar et al. demonstrated the utility of reactive TDM trough assessment of 72 children with CD who presented with concern for loss of response to therapy. Of the 72 children, 25 (35%) had subtherapeutic levels and required dose escalation.[124] Subsequent to dose escalation, there was significant improvement in remission rates at 6 months. However, relying on reactive TDM may prevent the ability to proactively optimize PK of infliximab. In a pediatric cohort of 50 patients with IBD on infliximab therapy, only a minority had a target trough of 3 μg per mL at week 14. Most patients required more frequent infusions or higher dosing than standard therapy to achieve goal trough concentrations.[109]

Proactive TDM requires obtaining serum concentrations at set intervals during treatment, even in the absence of active symptoms. If levels are found to be suboptimal, then they are proactively optimized to ensure patients maintain a therapeutic drug level. The Trough Concentration Adapted Infliximab Treatment (TAXIT) trial was a prospective randomized controlled trial in adults with IBD in which enrolled patients were dose optimized during infliximab induction dosing. Then, patients were randomized to dosing based on the level or clinical status. After dose optimization, continued concentration-based dosing was not superior to clinically based dosing for achieving remission at 1 year, but was associated with fewer flares during the course of treatment. There is a concern that this 1-year study may not have been long enough in duration to detect a difference in outcomes.[125] In contrast, other studies of both infliximab and adalimumab have retrospectively found proactive TDM allowed for early identification of patients with low trough concentrations and better probability of patients remaining on drug in remission.[126,127] A recent meta-analysis found limited existing evidence to support an association between any TDM strategy and superior clinical remission rates, but does support a cost-saving benefit for reactive TDM, and suggests a potential benefit for anti-TNFα durability with proactive TDM. The authors concluded that further longer term studies are needed, particularly to evaluate proactive TDM and to generate data on other anti-TNFα therapies, drug levels during induction, and pediatric populations.[128] An important question is whether proactive TDM will be equal or better than use of combination therapy (biologics with immunomodulator) as a strategy to increase drug levels and prevent ADA formation due. Despite these strategies, early anti-TNFα therapy has not been shown to prevent surgery or complications in children who have the phenotype of stricturing CD.[22]

A growing area of interest is whether the utilization of biologic therapy increases the risk of postoperative complications in IBD patients undergoing surgical intervention. Current studies have relayed mixed results. Preoperative use of infliximab has been linked to an increased occurrence of postoperative complications.[129] However, subsequent studies did not find an increased risk with the preoperative use of anti-TNFα agents,[130] vedolizumab,[131,132] or ustekinumab.[133] Further pediatric studies are needed to guide clinical management.

A FORWARD VIEW TO THE TREATMENT OF PEDIATRIC INFLAMMATORY BOWEL DISEASE

Many novel drugs are being developed for IBD. Unfortunately, drug studies in pediatric IBD have been conducted long after approval has been granted for adults. This lag time leads to extensive off-label use, often without clear guidance on dosing.[95] A novel biologic being developed in adults with IBD is etrolizumab, an anti-β7 integrin antibody in phase 3 trials. A phase 1 PK-pharmacodynamic (PD) and long-term safety study in children with IBD has been initiated prior to adult approval, in hopes that earlier dosing information will be available (NCT03478956). PK-PD modeling studies have been done in adult trials and demonstrated a relationship between PK and PD (free β7 receptors on circulating intestinal-homing CD4+ T lymphocytes).[134] Such studies may allow for bridging exposure response from adult to pediatric trials.

Small molecule drugs are also being developed for IBD, offering advantages over biologics, including lower cost, lack of immunogenicity, and oral delivery. Tofacitinib is an inhibitor of the Janus kinases (JAK 1/3 and, to a lesser extent, JAK 2). JAKs are tyrosine kinases expressed in lymphocytes, granulocytes, macrophages, and many nonimmune cells that lead to intracellular phosphorylation of signal transducers and activation of transcription molecules impacting immune responses.[135] Tofacitinib has been approved for treatment of moderate-to-severe UC in adults. The drug has not yet been studied in pediatrics.[136]

Another novel small molecule drug in development for IBD is ozanimod, an oral agonist of the sphingosine-1-phosphate receptor subtypes 1 and 5. Ozanimod induces lymphocyte sequestration, potentially decreasing the number of activated lymphocytes circulating to the gastrointestinal tract. In a randomized, placebo-controlled, double-blind phase 2 study, 197 adult patients with moderately to severely active UC were tested for efficacy and safety of ozanimod. Different doses were tested (0.5 and 1.0 mg per day) for 8 weeks; the primary end point was clinical remission. Phase 3 studies are underway in adults with UC and CD.[137]

Due to dysbiosis associated with IBD, there is great interest in fecal microbiota transplantation (FMT) as a possible treatment. Comprehensive reviews of the FMT literature in IBD indicate 23% to 33% remission rates in UC and 56% to 78% remission rates in CD.[138] However, interpretation of studies is challenging due to lack of controls, variation in donor selection, modes of delivery, treatment protocols, and outcomes. Making clear conclusions from these studies, however, is challenged by their uncontrolled nature, variation in recipient and donor selection, mode of delivery, preparation dose, treatment protocols, and outcomes.[139] A direct causal relationship between dysbiosis and IBD has not been definitively established in humans, and it is not known whether dysbiosis is primary or secondary in IBD.[140] Thus, it is postulated that FMT in secondary dysbiosis will only be effective long term if persistently administered, or if the primary cause of the dysbiosis can be eliminated.[139]

The treatment of pediatric IBD is a rapidly advancing field, with novel immunologic and microbial approaches on the horizon. There is currently a focus on molecular phenotyping, risk stratification, achieving early remission, and dose optimization. It will be critical for well-planned studies to be conducted in pediatrics in order to clarify dosing before off-label use ensues. It will also be essential to monitor long-term safety of children treated with novel drugs, particularly as they are likely to be prescribed in series or concomitantly. PK monitoring has dramatically changed the clinical use of biologics in children and young adults. Use of PK-PD modeling from adult trial data will likely augment clinical trial data to demonstrate efficacy in pediatrics.

DISCLOSURES AND ACKNOWLEDGMENTS

Dr. Conklin is an employee of ReveraGen Biopharma and has stock options in ReveraGen. She receives support from NICHD U54HD090254 Research in Pediatric Developmental Pharmacology Center.

Dr. Batra is supported by the NICHD T32HD087969 Postdoctoral Training in Pediatric Clinical Pharmacology.

REFERENCES

1. Chandradevan R, Hofmekier T, Mondai K, et al. Evolution of pediatric inflammatory bowel disease unclassified (IBD-U): incorporated with serological and gene expression profiles. *Inflamm Bowel Dis* 2018;24:2285–2290.
2. Jostins L, Ripke S, Weersma RK, et al. Host-microbe interactions have shaped the genetic architecture of inflammatory bowel disease. *Nature* 2012;491:119–124.
3. Cho JH. The genetics and immunopathogenesis of inflammatory bowel disease. *Nat Rev Immunol* 2008;8:458–466.
4. Ogura Y, Bonen DK, Inohara N, et al. A frameshift mutation in NOD2 associated with susceptibility to Crohn's disease. *Nature* 2001;411:603–606.
5. Somineni HK, Kugathasan S. The microbiome in patients with inflammatory diseases. *Clin Gastroenterol Hepatol* 2019;17(2):243–255.
6. Benchimol EI, Fortinsky KJ, Gozdyra P, et al. Epidemiology of pediatric inflammatory bowel disease: a systematic review of international trends. *Inflamm Bowel Dis* 2011;17(1):423–439.
7. Abramson O, Durant M, Mow W, et al. Incidence, prevalence, and time trends of pediatric inflammatory bowel disease in Northern California, 1996 to 2006. *J Pediatr* 2010;157(2):233–239.
8. Adamiak T, Walkiewicz-Jedrzejczak D, Fish D, et al. Incidence, clinical characteristics, and natural history of pediatric IBD in Wisconsin: a population-based epidemiological study. *Inflamm Bowel Dis* 2013;19(6):1218–1223.
9. Cosnes J, Gower-Rousseau C, Seksik P, et al. Epidemiology and natural history of inflammatory bowel diseases. *Gastroenterology* 2011;140:1785–1794.
10. Benchimol E, Mack DR, Nguyen GC. Incidence, outcomes, and health services burden of very early onset inflammatory bowel disease. *Gastroenterology* 2014;147:803–813.
11. Jose FA, Garnett EA, Vittinghoff E, et al. Development of extraintestinal manifestations in pediatric patients with inflammatory bowel disease. *Inflamm Bowel Dis* 2009;15(1):63–68.
12. Bernstein CN, Benchimol EI, Bitton A, et al. The impact of inflammatory bowel disease in Canada 2018: extra-intestinal diseases in IBD. *J Can Assoc Gastroenterol* 2019;2(Suppl 1):S73–S80.
13. Shamir R, Phillip M, Levine A. Growth retardation in pediatric Crohn's disease: pathogenesis and interventions. *Inflamm Bowel Dis* 2007;13:620–628.
14. Pappa HM, Gordon CM, Saslowsky TM, et al. Vitamin D status in children and young adults with inflammatory bowel disease. *Pediatrics* 2006;118(5):1950–1961.
15. Pappa H, Thayu M, Sylvester F, et al. Skeletal health of children and adolescents with inflammatory bowel disease. *J Pediatr Gastroenterol Nutr* 2011;53(1):11–25.
16. Heuschkel R, Salvestrini C, Beattie RM, et al. Guidelines for the management of growth failure in childhood inflammatory bowel disease. *Inflamm Bowel Dis* 2008;14(6):839–849.
17. Paganelli M, Albanese C, Borelli O, et al. Inflammation is the main determinant of low bone mineral density in pediatric inflammatory bowel disease. *Inflamm Bowel Dis* 2007;13:416–423.
18. Sawczenko A, Ballinger AB, Savage MO, et al. Clinical features affecting final adult height in patients with pediatric-onset Crohn's disease. *Pediatrics* 2006;118:124–129.
19. Szigethy EM, Youk AO, Benhayon D, et al. Depression subtypes in pediatric inflammatory bowel disease. *J Pediatr Gastroenterol Nutr* 2014;58(5):574–581.
20. Karwowski CA, Keljo D, Szigethy E. Strategies to improve quality of life in adolescents with inflammatory bowel disease. *Inflamm Bowel Dis* 2009;15:1755–1764.
21. Hyams JS, Ferry GD, Mandel FS, et al. Development and validation of a pediatric Crohn's disease activity index. *J Pediatr Gastroenterol Nutr* 1991;12:439–447.
22. Kugathasan S, Denson LA, Walters TD, et al. Prediction of complicated disease course for children newly diagnosed with Crohn's disease: a multicenter inception cohort study. *Lancet* 2017;389(10080):1710–1718.
23. Duricova D, Fumery M, Annese V, et al. The natural history of Crohn's disease in children: a review of population-based studies. *Eur J Gastroenterol Hepatol* 2017;29:125–134.
24. Schaefer ME, Machan JT, Kawatu D, et al. Factors that determine risk for surgery in pediatric patients with Crohn's disease. *Clin Gastroenterol Hepatol* 2019;8:789–794.
25. Wu J, Lubman DM, Kugathasan S, et al. Serum protein biomarkers of fibrosis aid in risk stratification of future stricturing complications in pediatric Crohn's disease. *Am J Gastroenterol* 2019;114(5):777–785.
26. Ballengee CR, Stidham RW, Liu C, et al. Association between plasma level of collagen type III alpha 1 chain and development of strictures in pediatric patients with Crohn's disease. *Clin Gastroenterol Hepatol* 2018;17(9):1799–1806.
27. Rosen MJ, Karns R, Vallance JE, et al. Mucosal expression of type 2 and type 17 immune response genes distinguishes ulcerative colitis from colon-only Crohn's disease in treatment-naïve pediatric patients. *Gastroenterology* 2017;152(6):1345–1357.
28. Liu JZ, van Sommeren S, Huang H, et al. Association analyses identify 38 susceptibility loci for inflammatory bowel disease and highlight shared genetic risk across populations. *Nat Genet* 2015;47:979–986.
29. Venkateswaran S, Prince J, Cutler D, et al. Enhanced contribution of HLA in pediatric onset ulcerative colitis. *Inflamm Bowel Dis* 2018;24(4):829–838.
30. Ng SC, Shi HY, Hamidi N, et al. Worldwide incidence and prevalence of inflammatory bowel disease in the 21st century: a systematic review of population-based studies. *Lancet* 2018;390(10114):2769–2778.
31. Hyams JS, Davis S, Mack DR, et al. Factors associated with early outcomes following standardized therapy in children with ulcerative colitis (PROTECT): a multicentre inception cohort study. *Lancet Gastroenterol Hepatol* 2017;2(12):855–868.
32. Hyams JS, Thomas SD, Gotman N, et al. Clinical and biological predictors of response to standardized paediatric colitis therapy (PROTECT): a multicenter inception cohort study. *Lancet* 2019;393:1708–1720.
33. Turner D, Seow CH, Greenberg GR, et al. A systematic prospective comparison of noninvasive disease activity indices in ulcerative colitis. *Clin Gastroenterol Hepatol* 2009;7:1081–1088.
34. Turner D, Hyams J, Markowitz J, et al. Appraisal of the pediatric ulcerative colitis activity index (PUCAI). *Inflamm Bowel Dis* 2009;15:1218–1223.
35. Haberman Y, Karns R, Dexheimer PJ, et al. Ulcerative colitis mucosal transcriptomes reveal mitochondriopathy and personalized mechanisms underlying disease severity and treatment response. *Nat Commun* 2019;10(1):38.
36. Lega S, Dubinsky MC. What are the targets of inflammatory bowel disease management? *Inflamm Bowel Dis* 2018;24(8):1670–1675.
37. Kerur B, Litman HJ, Stern JB, et al. Correlation of endoscopic disease severity with pediatric ulcerative colitis activity index score in children and young adults with ulcerative colitis. *World J Gastroenterol* 2017;23(18):3322–3329.
38. Bossyut P, Baert F, D'Heygere F, et al. Early mucosal healing predicts favorable outcomes in patients with moderate to severe ulcerative colitis treated with golimumab: data from the real-life BE-SMART cohort. *Inflamm Bowel Dis* 2019;25(1):156–162.
39. Colombel JF, Rutgeerts P, Reinisch W, et al. Early mucosal healing with infliximab is associated with improved long-term clinical outcomes in ulcerative colitis. *Gastroenterology* 2011;141(4):1194–1201.

40. Schnitzler F, Fidder H, Ferrante M, et al., Mucosal healing predicts long-term outcome of maintenance therapy with infliximab in Crohn's disease. *Inflamm Bowel Dis* 2009;15:1295–1301.
41. Salem MS, Melmed GY. The role of histology in determining disease activity, treatment and prognosis: are we there yet? *Gastroint Endosc Clin N Am* 2019;29(3):437–446.
42. Peyrin-Biroulet L, Sandborn W, Sands BE, et al. Selecting therapeutic targets in inflammatory bowel disease (STRIDE): determining therapeutic goals for treat-to-target. *Am J Gastroenterol* 2015;110(9):1324–1338.
43. Weinstein-Nakar I, Focht G, Church P, et al. Associations among mucosal and transmural healing and fecal level of calprotectin in children with Crohn's disease. *Clin Gastroenterol Hepatol* 2018;16(7):1089–1097.
44. Tung J, Loftus EV Jr, Freese DK, et al. A population-based study of the frequency of corticosteroid resistance and dependence in pediatric patients with Crohn's disease and ulcerative colitis. *Inflamm Bowel Dis* 2006;12(12):1093–1100.
45. Modigliani R, Mary JY, Simon JF, et al. Clinical, biological, and endoscopic picture of attacks of Crohn's disease: evolution on prednisone. *Gastroenterology* 1990;98(4):811–818.
46. Escher JC, European Collaborative Research Group on Budesonide in Paediatric IBD. Budesonide versus prednisolone for the treatment of active Crohn's disease in children: a randomized, double-blind, controlled multicentre trial. *Eur J Gastroenterol Hepatol* 2004;16(1):47–54.
47. Baldwin K, Kaplan J. Medical management of pediatric inflammatory bowel disease. *Semin Pediatr Surg* 2017;26(6):360–366.
48. Guilcher K, Fournier N, Schoepfer A, et al. Change of treatment modalities over the last 10 years in pediatric patients with inflammatory bowel disease in Switzerland. *Eur J Gastroenterol Hepatol* 2018;30(10):1159–1167.
49. Markowitz J, Rosa J, Grancher K, et al. Long-term 6-mercaptopurine in treatment of adolescents with Crohn's disease. *Gastroenterology* 1990;99:1347–1351.
50. Perrault J, Greseth JL, Tremaine WJ. 6-Mercaptopurine therapy in selected cases of corticosteroid-dependent Crohn's disease. *Mayo Clin Proc* 1991;66:480–484.
51. Verhave M, Winter HS, Grand RJ. Azathioprine in the treatment of children with inflammatory bowel disease. *J Pediatr* 1990;117:809–814.
52. Voskuil MD, Bangma A, Weersma RK, et al. Predicting (side) effects for patients with inflammatory bowel disease: the promise of pharmacogenetics. *World J Gastroenterol* 2019;25(21):2539–2548.
53. Feuerstein JD, Nguyen GC, Kupfer SS, et al. American Gastroenterological Association guideline on therapeutic drug monitoring in inflammatory bowel disease. *Gastroenterology* 2017;153(3):827–834.
54. Peyrin–Biroulet L, Khosrotehrani K, Carrat F, et al. Increased risk for nonmelanoma skin cancers in patients who receive thiopurines for inflammatory bowel disease. *Gastroenterology* 2011;141(5):1621–1628.
55. Beaugerie L, Brosse N, Bouvier A, et al. Lymphoproliferative disorders in patients receiving thiopurines for inflammatory bowel disease: a prospective observational cohort study. *Lancet* 2009;374:1617–1625.
56. Hyams JS, Dubinsky MC, Baldassano RN, et al. Infliximab is not associated with increased risk of malignancy or hemophagocytic lymphohistiocytosis in pediatric patients with inflammatory bowel disease. *Gastroenterology* 2017;152(8):1901–1914.
57. Kotlyar D, Osterman M, Diamond R, et al. A systematic review of factors that contribute to hepatosplenic T-cell lymphoma in patients with inflammatory bowel disease. *Clin Gastroenterol Hepatol* 2011;9(1):36–41.
58. Panes J, Lopez-Sanroman A, Bermejo F, et al. Early azathioprine therapy is no more effective than placebo for newly diagnosed Crohn's disease. *Gastroenterology* 2013;145(4):766–774.
59. Pfefferkorn M, Burke G, Griffiths A, et al. Growth abnormalities persist in newly diagnosed children with Crohn disease despite current treatment paradigms. *J Pediatr Gastroenterol Nutr* 2009;48(2):168–174.
60. Colman RJ, Lawton RC, Dubinsky MC, et al. Methotrexate for the treatment of pediatric Crohn's disease: a systematic review and meta-analysis. *Inflamm Bowel Dis* 2018;24:2135–2141.
61. Guariso G, Gasparetto M. Treating children with inflammatory bowel disease: Current and new perspectives. *World J Gastroenterol* 2017;23(30):5469.
62. Vena G, Cassano N, Iannone F. Update on subcutaneous methotrexate for inflammatory arthritis and psoriasis. *Ther Clin Risk Manag* 2018;14:105–116.
63. Saibeni S, Bollani S, Losco A, et al. The use of methotrexate for treatment of inflammatory bowel disease in clinical practice. *Dig Liver Dis* 2012;44(2):123–127.
64. Hanauer S, Feagan BG, Lichtenstein GR, et al. Maintenance infliximab for Crohn's disease: the ACCENT I randomized trial. *Lancet* 2002;359:1541–1549.
65. Sands BE, Anderson FH, Bernstein CN, et al. Infliximab maintenance therapy for fistulizing Crohn's disease. *N Engl J Med* 2004;350(9):876–885.
66. Hyams J, Crandall W, Kugathasan S, et al. Induction and maintenance infliximab therapy for the treatment of moderate-to-severe Crohn's disease in children. *Gastroenterology* 2007;132(3):863–873.
67. Hyams JS, Griffiths A, Markowitz J, et al. Safety and efficacy of adalimumab for moderate to severe Crohn's disease in children. *Gastroenterology* 2012;143(2):365–374.
68. Faubion WA, Dubinsky M, Ruemmele FM, et al. Long-term efficacy and safety of adalimumab in pediatric patients with Crohn's disease. *Inflamm Bowel Dis* 2017;23(3):453–460.
69. Griffin LM, Thayu M, Baldassano RN, et al. Improvements in bone density and structure during anti-TNFα therapy in pediatric Crohn's disease. *J Clin Endocrinol Metab* 2015;100(7):2630–2639.
70. Panchal H, Wagner M, Chatterji M, et al. Earlier anti-tumor necrosis factor therapy of Crohn's disease correlates with slower progression of bowel damage. *Dig Dis Sci* 2019;64(11):3274–3283. doi:10.1007/s10620-018-5434-4.
71. Walters TD, Kim MO, Denson LA, et al. Increased effectiveness of early therapy with anti-tumor necrosis factor-α vs. an immunomodulator in children with Crohn's disease. *Gastroenterology* 2014;146(2):383–391.
72. Church PC, Guan J, Walters TD, et al. Infliximab maintains durable response and facilitates catch-up growth in luminal pediatric Crohn's disease. *Inflamm Bowel Dis* 2014;20(7):1177–1186.
73. Dulai PS, Thompson KD, Blunt HB, et al. Risks of serious infection or lymphoma with anti-tumor necrosis factor therapy for pediatric inflammatory bowel disease: a systematic review. *Clin Gastroenterol Hepatol* 2014;12(9):1443–1451.
74. Mohan N, Edwards E, Cupps T, et al. Demyelination occurring during anti-tumor necrosis factor therapy for inflammatory arthritides. *Arthritis Rheum* 2001;44(12):2862–2869.
75. Enayati P, Papadakis K. Association of anti-tumor necrosis factor therapy with the development of multiple sclerosis. *J Clin Gastroenterol* 2005;39(4):303–306.
76. Benson J, Peritt D, Scallon BJ, et al. Discovery and mechanisms of ustekinumab. *MAbs* 2011;36:535–545.
77. Feagan BG, Sandborn WJ, Gasink C, et al. Ustekinumab as induction and maintenance therapy for Crohn's disease. *N Engl J Med* 2016;375:1946–1960.
78. Sandborn WJ, Gasink C, Gao LL, et al.; CERTIFI Study Group. Ustekinumab induction and maintenance therapy in refractory Crohn's disease. *N Engl J Med* 2012;367(16);1519–1528.
79. Sandborn WJ, Rutgeerts P, Gasink C, et al. Long-term efficacy and safety of ustekinumab for Crohn's disease through the second year of therapy. *Aliment Pharmacol Ther* 2018;48:65–77.
80. Dayan JR, Dolinger M, Benkov K, et al. Real world experience with ustekinumab in children and young adults at a tertiary care pediatric inflammatory bowel disease center. *J Pediatr Gastroenterol Nutr* 2019;69:61–67.
81. Bishop C, Simon H, Suskind D, et al. Ustekinumab in pediatric Crohn's disease patients. *J Pediatr Gastroenterol Nutr* 2016;63:348–351.
82. Rinawi F, Rosenbach Y, Assa A, et al. Ustekinumab for resistant pediatric Crohn's disease. *J Pediatr Gastroenterol Nutr* 2014;11:1111.
83. Cameron FL, Garrick V, Russell RK. Ustekinumab in treatment of refractory Crohn disease. *J Pediatr Gastroenterol Nutr* 2016;62:e30.
84. Chavannes M, Martinez-Vinson C, Hart L, et al. Management of paediatric patients with medically-refractory Crohn's disease using ustekinumab: a multicentered cohort study. *J Crohn Colitis* 2019;13(5):578–584.
85. Cohen-Dolev N, Sladek M, Hussey S. et al. Differences in outcomes over time with exclusive enteral nutrition compared with steroids in children with mild to moderate Crohn's disease: results from the GROWTH CD study. *J Crohn's Colitis* 2018;12(3):306–312.
86. Swaminath A, Feathers A, Ananthakrishnan AN, et al. Systematic review with meta-analysis: enteral nutrition therapy for the induction of remission in paediatric Crohn's disease. *Aliment Pharmcacol Ther* 2017;46(7):645–656.
87. Turner D, Yerushalmi B, Kori M, et al. Once versus twice-daily mesalazine to induce remission in paediatric ulcerative colitis: a randomized controlled trial. *J Crohn's Colitis* 2017;11:527–533.
88. Gisbert J, González-Lama Y, Maté J. 5-Aminosalicylates and renal function in inflammatory bowel disease. *Inflamm Bowel Dis* 2007;13(5):629–638.
89. Corica D, Romano C. Renal involvement in inflammatory bowel diseases. *J Crohn's Colitis* 2016;10(2):226–235.
90. Oray M, Abu Samra K, Ebrahimiadib N, et al. Long-term side effects of glucocorticoids. *Expert Opin Drug Saf* 2016;15(4):457–465.
91. Rubin DT, Cohen RD, Sandborn WJ, et al. Budesonide multimatrix is efficacious for mesalamine-refractory, mild to moderate ulcerative colitis: a randomized, placebo-controlled trial. *J Crohn's Colitis* 2017;11(7):785–791.
92. Aloi M, Bramuzzo M, Arrigo S, et al. Efficacy and safety of adalimumab in pediatric ulcerative colitis: a real-life experience from the SIGENP-IBD registry. *J Pediatr Gastroenterol Nutr* 2018;66(6):920–925.
93. Hyams J, Damaraju L, Blank M, et al. Induction and maintenance therapy with infliximab for children with moderate to severe ulcerative colitis. *Clin Gastroenterol Hepatol* 2012;10(4):391–399.
94. Turner D, Koletzko S, Griffiths AM, et al. Use of placebo in pediatric inflammatory bowel diseases: a position paper from ESPGHAN, ECCO, PIBDnet, and the Canadian Children IBD Network. *J Pediatr Gastorentrol Nutr* 2016;62(1):183–187.
95. Turner D, Griffiths AM, Wilson D, et al. Designing clinical trials in paediatric inflammatory bowel diseases: a PIBDnet commentary. *Gut* 2020;69(1):32–41. doi:10.1136/gutjnl-2018-317987.
96. Bolia R, Rajanayagam J, Hardikar W, et al. Impact of changing treatment strategies on outcomes in pediatric ulcerative colitis. *Inflamm Bowel Dis* 2019;25(11):1838–1844. doi:10.1093/ibd/izz072.
97. Seah D, DeCruz P. Review article: the practical management of acute severe ulcerative colitis. *Aliment Pharmacol Ther* 2016;43:482–513.
98. Kevans D, Murthy S, Mould DR, et al. Accelerated clearance of infliximab is associated with treatment failure in patients with corticosteroid-refractory acute ulcerative colitis. *J Crohn's Colitis* 2018;12(6):662–669.
99. Hindryckx P, Novak G, Vandecasteele N, et al. Review article: dose optimization of infliximab for acute severe colitis. *Aliment Pharmacol Ther* 2017;45(5):617–630.
100. Nalagatla N, Falloon K, Tran G, et al. Effect of accelerated infliximab induction on short- and long-term outcomes of severe acute colitis. *Clin Gastroenterol Hepatol* 2019;17(3): 502.e1–509.e1. doi:10.1016/j.cgh.2018.06.031.
101. Turner D, Ruemmele F, Orlanski-Meyer E, et al. Management of paediatric ulcerative colitis, Part 2: acute severe colitis – an evidence-based consensus guideline from the European Crohn's and Colitis Organization and the European Society of Paediatric Gastroenterology, Hepatology, and Nutrition. *J Pediatr Gastroenterol Nutr* 2018;67(2):292–310.
102. Feagan BG, Rutgeerts P, Sands BE, et al. Vedolizumab as induction and maintenance therapy for ulcerative colitis. *N Engl J Med* 2013;369(8):699–710.
103. Colombel JF, Sands BE, Rutgeerts P, et al. The safety of vedolizumab for ulcerative colitis and Crohn's disease. *Gut* 2017;66(5):839–851.
104. Singh N, Rabizadeh S, Jossen J, et al. Multi-center experience of vedolizumab effectiveness in pediatric inflammatory bowel disease. *Inflamm Bowel Dis* 2016;22:2121–2126.
105. Schneider AM, Weghuber D, Hetzer B, et al. Vedolizumab use after failure of TNF-α antagonists in children and adolescents with inflammatory bowel disease. *BMC Gastroenterol* 2018;18(1):140.
106. Conrad MA, Stein RE, Maxwell EC, et al. Vedolizumab therapy in severe pediatric inflammatory bowel disease. *Inflamm Bowel Dis* 2016;22(10):2425–2431.

107. Sands BE, Feagan BG, Rutgeerts P, et al. Effects of vedolizumab induction therapy for patients with Crohn's disease in whom tumor necrosis factor antagonist treatment failed. *Gastroenterology* 2014;147(3):618–627.
108. Sandborn WJ, Feagan BG, Rutgeerts P, et al. Vedolizumab as induction and maintenance therapy for Crohn's disease. *N Engl J Med* 2013;369(8):711–721.
109. Lega S, Phan BL, Rosenthal CJ, et al. Proactively optimized infliximab monotherapy is as effective as combination therapy in IBD. *Inflamm Bowel Dis* 2019;25(1):134–141.
110. Cozijnsen M, Escher J, Griffiths A, et al. Benefits and risks of combining anti-tumor necrosis factor with immunomodulator therapy in pediatric inflammatory bowel disease. *Inflamm Bowel Dis* 2015;21(4):951–961.
111. Cheng J, Hamilton Z, Smyth M, et al. Concomitant therapy with immunomodulator enhances infliximab durability in pediatric inflammatory bowel disease. *Inflamm Bowel Dis* 2017;23(10):1762–1773.
112. Chi LY, Zitomersky NL, Liu E, et al. The impact of combination therapy on infliximab levels and antibodies in children and young adults with inflammatory bowel disease. *Inflamm Bowel Dis* 2018;24(6):1344–1351.
113. Colombel JF, Sandborn WJ, Reinisch W, et al. Infliximab, azathioprine, or combination therapy for Crohn's disease. *N Engl J Med* 2010;362(15):1383–1395.
114. Colombel JF, Adedokun OJ, Gasink C, et al. Combination therapy with infliximab and azathioprine improves infliximab pharmacokinetic features and efficacy: a post hoc analysis. *Clin Gastroenterol Hepatol* 2019;17(8):1525–1532.
115. Feagan BG, McDonald JWD, Panaccione R, et al. Methotrexate in combination with infliximab is no more effective than infliximab alone in patients with Crohn's disease. *Gastroenterology* 2014;146(3):681.
116. Grossi V, Lerer T, Griffiths A, et al. Concomitant use of immunomodulators affects the durability of infliximab therapy in children with Crohn's disease. *Clin Gastroenterol Hepatol* 2015;13(10):1748–1756.
117. Godat S, Fournier N, Safroneeva E, et al. Frequency and type of drug-related side effects necessitating treatment discontinuation in the Swiss Inflammatory Bowel Disease Cohort. *Eur J Gastroenterol* 2018;30(6):612–620.
118. Ungar B, Glidai Y, Yavzori M, et al. Association between infliximab drug and antibody levels and therapy outcome in pediatric inflammatory bowel diseases. *J Pediatr Gastroenterol Nutr* 2018;67(4):507–512.
119. Van Hoeve K, Dreesen E, Hoffman I, et al. Higher infliximab trough levels are associated with better outcome in paediatric patients with inflammatory bowel disease. *J Crohn's Colitis* 2018;12(11):1316–1325.
120. Vande Casteele N, Jeyerajah J, Jairath V, et al. Infliximab exposure-response relationship and thresholds associated with endoscopic healing in patients with ulcerative colitis. *Clin Gastroenterol Hepatol* 2019;17(9):1814–1821.
121. El-Matary W, Walters TD, Huynh HQ, et al. Higher postinduction infliximab serum trough levels are associated with healing of fistulizing perianal Crohn's disease in children. *Inflamm Bowel Dis* 2019;25(1):150–155.
122. Dotan I, Ron Y, Becker S, et al. Patient factors that increase infliximab clearance and shorten half-life in inflammatory bowel disease: a population pharmacokinetic study. *Inflamm Bowel Dis* 2014;20(12):2247–2259.
123. Fasanmade AA, Adedokun OJ, Blank M, et al. Pharmacokinetic properties of infliximab in children and adults with Crohn's disease: a retrospective analysis of data from 2 phase III clinical trials. *Clin Ther* 2011;33(7):946–964.
124. Minar P, Saeed SA, Afreen M, et al. Practical use of infliximab concentration monitoring in pediatric Crohn disease. *J Pediatr Gastroenterol Nutr* 2016;62(5):715–766.
125. Vande Casteele N, Ferrante M, Van Assche G, et al. Trough concentrations of infliximab guide dosing for patients with inflammatory bowel disease. *Gastroenterology* 2015;148(7):1320–1329.
126. Vaughn BP, Martinez-Vazquez M, Patwardhan VR, et al. Proactive therapeutic concentration monitoring of infliximab may improve outcomes for patients with inflammatory bowel disease: results from a pilot observational study. *Inflamm Bowel Dis* 2014;20(11):1996–2003.
127. Papamichael K, Juncadella A, Wong D, et al. Proactive therapeutic drug monitoring of adalimumab is associated with better long-term outcomes compared to standard of care in patients with inflammatory bowel disease. *J Crohn's Colitis* 2019;13(8):976–981. doi:10.1093/ecco-jcc/jjz018.
128. Ricciuto A, Dhaliwal J, Walters TD, et al. Clinical outcomes with therapeutic drug monitoring in inflammatory bowel disease: a systematic review with meta-analysis. *J Crohn's Colitis* 2018;12(11):1302–1315.
129. Billioud V, Ford A, Tedesco E, et al. Preoperative use of anti-TNF therapy and postoperative complications in inflammatory bowel diseases: a meta-analysis. *J Crohn's Colitis* 2013;7(11):853–867.
130. Mitsuya J, Gonzalez R, Thomas R, et al. The effect of biologics on postoperative complications in children with inflammatory bowel disease and bowel resection. *J Pediatr Gastroenterol Nutr* 2019;68(3):334–338.
131. Law C, Narula A, Lightner A, et al. Systematic review and meta-analysis: preoperative vedolizumab treatment and postoperative complications in patients with inflammatory bowel disease. *J Crohn's Colitis* 2018;12(5):538–545.
132. Lightner A, Tse C, Potter D, et al. Postoperative outcomes in vedolizumab-treated pediatric patients undergoing abdominal operations for inflammatory bowel disease. *J Pediatr Surg* 2018;53(9):1706–1709.
133. Shim H, Ma C, Kotze P, et al. Preoperative ustekinumab treatment is not associated with increased postoperative complications in Crohn's disease: a Canadian Multi-Centre Observational Cohort Study. *J Can Assoc Gastroenterol* 2018;1(3):115–123.
134. Wei X, Giblansky L, Wang Y, et al. Pharmacokinetic and pharmacodynamic modeling of serum etrolizumab and circulating β receptor occupancy in patients with ulcerative colitis. *J Clin Pharmacol* 2018;58(3):386–398.
135. Roskoski R Jr. Janus kinase (JAK) inhibitors in the treatment of inflammatory and neoplastic diseases. *Pharmacol Res* 2016;111:784–803.
136. Sandborn WJ, Su C, Sands BE, et al. Tofacitinib as induction and maintenance therapy for ulcerative colitis. *N Engl J Med* 2017;376(18):1723–1736.
137. Sandborn WJ, Feagan BG, Wolf DC, et al. Ozanimod induction and maintenance treatment for ulcerative colitis. *N Engl J Med* 2016;374(18):1754–1762.
138. Basso PJ, Camara NOS, Sales-Campos H. Microbial-based therapies in the treatment of inflammatory bowel disease-an overview of human studies. *Front Pharmacol* 2019;9:1571.
139. Kellermayer R. Fecal microbiota transplantation: great potential with many challenges. *Transl Gastroenterol Hepatol* 2019;4:40.
140. Ni J, Wu GD, Albenberg L, et al. Gut microbiota and IBD: causation or correlation? *Nat Rev Gastroenterol Hepatol* 2017;14(10):573–584.

SECTION

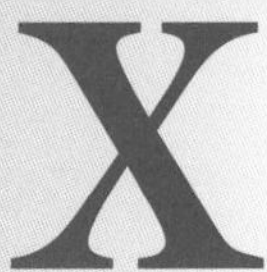

Endocrine and Hematologic Pharmacology

CHAPTER 54

Nicolas C. Nicolaides
Tomoshige Kino
George P. Chrousos

Glucocorticoids

INTRODUCTION

Glucocorticoids regulate a broad spectrum of physiologic functions essential for life and play an important role in the maintenance of basal and stress-related homeostasis.[1–3] Approximately 20% of the genes expressed in human leukocytes are regulated positively or negatively by glucocorticoids.[4] Glucocorticoids are involved in almost every cellular, molecular, and physiologic network of the organism and play a pivotal role in critical biologic processes, such as growth, reproduction, intermediary metabolism, immune and inflammatory reactions, as well as central nervous system (CNS) and cardiovascular functions.[1–4] Physiologic amounts of glucocorticoids are also essential for normal renal tubular function and thus for water and electrolyte homeostasis. Furthermore, glucocorticoids represent one of the most widely used therapeutic agents often employed in the treatment of inflammatory, autoimmune, and lymphoproliferative disorders.[1–3]

The adrenal glands consist of the adrenal cortex and the adrenal medulla. In the fetus, the adrenal cortex is divided into two zones, the outer definitive zone and the inner fetal zone. The latter represents approximately 80% of the adrenal volume and secretes weak androgens with the delta-5 configuration (dehydroepiandrosterone, DHEA). After birth, the fetal adrenal zone regresses rapidly during the first 2 weeks of life and disappears almost completely by the third month of life. A few islands of cells remain, which may later develop into androgen-secreting cells. During infancy and childhood, the definitive zone and perhaps remnants of the fetal zone evolve into the adult adrenal cortex, which consists of three anatomic zones: the outer *zona glomerulosa*, the intermediate *zona fasciculata*, and the inner *zona reticularis*. The *zona glomerulosa* is responsible for the production of aldosterone, the *zona fasciculata* for the production of cortisol, and the *zona reticularis* for the production of adrenal androgens. The adrenal medulla is functionally related to the sympathetic nervous system and secretes epinephrine and norepinephrine, both at basal conditions and in response to stress. The adrenal cortex and medulla are embryologically and functionally interdependent, influencing each other's organogenesis, growth, and function.[1,2]

PATHWAYS OF STEROID BIOSYNTHESIS

The synthesis of the glucocorticoid cortisol and the mineralocorticoid aldosterone is under the control of regulatory systems that largely function independently. The major regulation of the former is by the adrenocorticotropic hormone (ACTH), while the latter is regulated primarily by the renin–angiotensin system and circulating potassium ions. All steroid hormones produced by the adrenal cortex are derived from cholesterol. Low-density lipoprotein (LDL) cholesterol is the major source of cholesterol utilized in adrenal steroidogenesis; however, the adrenal cortices can synthesize cholesterol de novo. Proteolytic and lipolytic enzymes act on LDL to release cholesterol esters for storage in lipid droplets in the adrenal steroidogenic cells.[1–3]

In order for the adrenal cortex to synthesize active steroid hormones, a number of changes are required in the structure of cholesterol. Several of these reactions are catalyzed by the steroid hydroxylases, which are members of a superfamily of genes known collectively as cytochromes P450 (CYP). Adrenal steroidogenesis follows three distinct routes, which reflect the zonal differences in terms of function and regulation (Fig. 54.1).

The rate-limiting step in steroid biosynthesis is importation of cholesterol from cellular stores to the matrix side of the mitochondrial inner membrane, where the cholesterol side-chain cleavage (scc) system is located. This importation is controlled

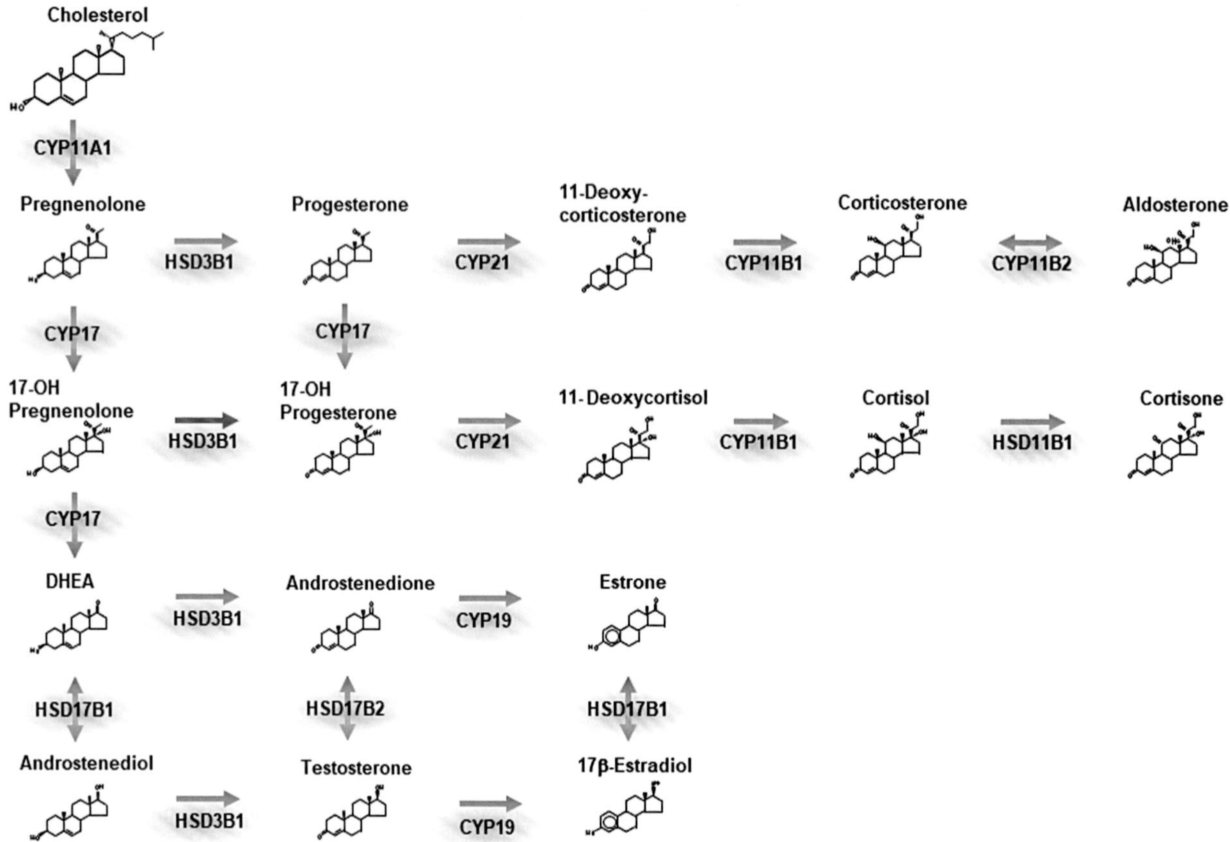

Figure 54.1 Schematic representation of adrenal steroidogenesis. DHEA, dehydroepiandrosterone.

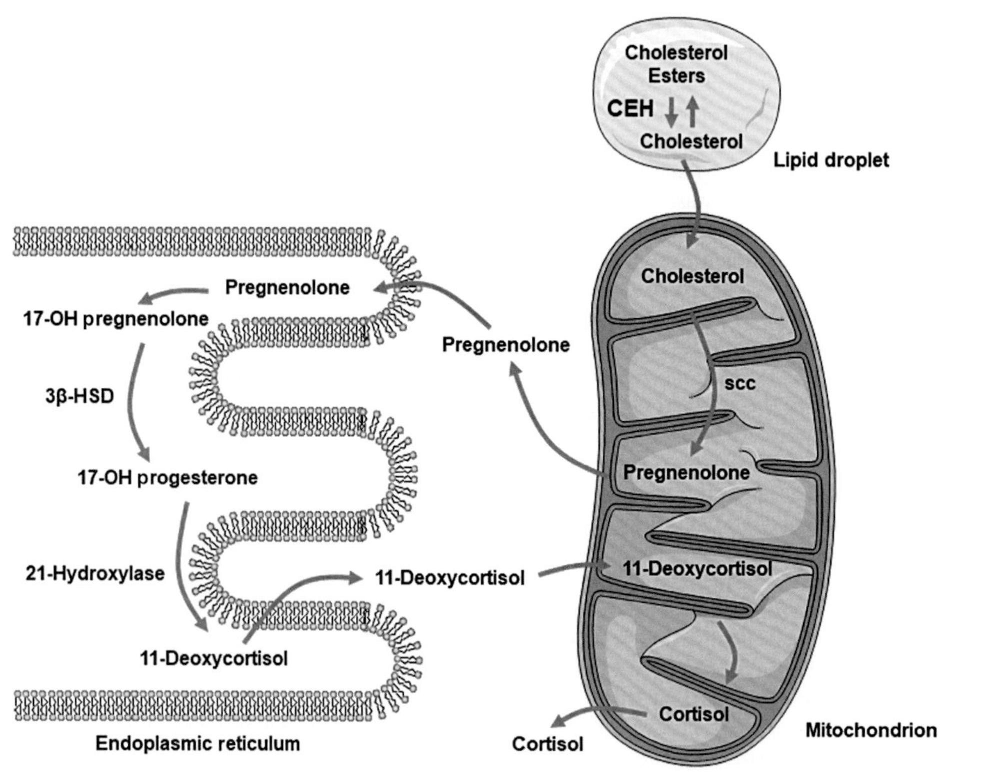

Figure 54.2 Pathway of biosynthesis of cortisol in the adrenal cortex. 3β-HSD, 3β-hydroxysteroid dehydrogenase; CEH, cholesteryl ester hydrolase; scc, side-chain cleavage. Modified from Nicolaides NC, Charmandari E, Chrousos GP. Adrenal Steroid Hormone Secretion: Physiologic and Endocrine Aspects. In *Reference Module in Biomedical Sciences*. Elsevier; 2014.

by the steroidogenic acute regulatory (StAR) protein, the synthesis of which is increased by trophic adrenocortical stimuli, such as ACTH.[3,5,6] In addition to StAR protein, cholesterol transfer is mediated by another protein, the peripheral benzodiazepine receptor.[7] The first enzymatic step in steroid biosynthesis common to all steroidogenic pathways takes place in the mitochondrion and leads to the cleavage of six carbon atoms from the side chain of cholesterol, converting this C_{27} compound to the C_{21} precursor steroid pregnenolone. This reaction is known as cholesterol scc and is catalyzed by the cytochrome P450 enzyme CYP11A (P450 scc, cholesterol desmolase, scc enzyme), which is an integral protein of the inner mitochondrial membrane.[1–3,8] Pregnenolone, the common precursor for all steroids, then passes by diffusion from the mitochondrion to the cytoplasm where it undergoes further metabolism by several other enzymes (Fig. 54.2).

To synthesize mineralocorticoids in the *zona glomerulosa*, the microsomal 3β-hydroxysteroid dehydrogenase (3β-HSD) converts pregnenolone to progesterone.[3,9] The latter is 21-hydroxylated in the cytoplasm by CYP21 (P450c21, 21-hydroxylase) to produce deoxycorticosterone (DOC). Aldosterone, the most potent 17-deoxysteroid mineralocorticoid compound, is produced by 11β-hydroxylation of DOC to corticosterone, followed by 18-hydroxylation and 18-oxidation of corticosterone (see Fig. 54.1). The final three steps in aldosterone synthesis are accomplished by a single mitochondrial P450 enzyme, CYP11B2 (P450aldo, aldosterone synthase).[10]

To produce cortisol, CYP17 (P450c17, 17α-hydroxylase/17,20-lyase) in the endoplasmic reticulum of the *zona fasciculata* and *zona reticularis* converts pregnenolone to 17α-hydroxypregnenolone.[3,11] 3β-HSD in the *zona fasciculata* utilizes 17α-hydroxypregnenolone as a substrate, producing 17α-hydroxyprogesterone. The latter is 21-hydroxylated by CYP21 to form 11-deoxycortisol, which is further converted to cortisol by CYP11B1 (P450c11, 11β-hydroxylase) in the mitochondria (see Fig. 54.2).

In the *zona reticularis* of the adrenal cortex and in the gonads, the 17,20-lyase activity of CYP17 converts 17α-hydroxypregnenolone to DHEA, a C_{19} steroid and sex steroid precursor. DHEA is further converted by 3β-HSD to androstenedione. In the gonads, androstenedione is reduced by 17β-HSD.[12] In pubertal ovaries, aromatase (CYP19, P450c19) can convert androstenedione and testosterone to estrone and estradiol, respectively.[13] Testosterone may be further metabolized to dihydrotestosterone by steroid 5α-reductase in androgen target tissues.[14]

The enzymatic differences between the *zona glomerulosa* and the *zona fasciculata* are summarized as the *zona glomerulosa* lacking P450c17α but have the ability to catalyze the 18-oxidation of corticosterone, the precursor of aldosterone. Interestingly, this activity has been shown to be a property of the 11β-hydroxylase, which appears to be capable of 18-hydroxylation and subsequent reduction to the aldehyde aldosterone.

REGULATION OF CORTISOL SECRETION

Plasma glucocorticoid concentrations are regulated in ways that reflect the varying physiologic needs for the hormones under basal conditions and in response to stress. Cortisol secretion is primarily regulated by ACTH, a 39-amino-acid peptide released from the anterior pituitary lobe in response to the hypothalamic neuropeptides corticotropin-releasing hormone (CRH) and arginine vasopressin (AVP). CRH is the strongest and probably the most important stimulator of ACTH secretion. AVP also activates secretion of ACTH and potentiates the effect of CRH on ACTH secretion. Catecholamines, angiotensin II, oxytocin, atrial natriuretic peptide, cholecystokinin, vasoactive intestinal polypeptide, and pituitary adenylate cyclase-activating polypeptide may also contribute to the secretion of ACTH.[1–3]

ACTH is synthesized as part of a large precursor molecule of 214-amino-acid, proopiomelanocortin. Depending on the cleavage enzymes, which are expressed in a tissue-specific manner, ACTH and several other peptides, for example, NH2-terminal peptide, joining peptide, β-lipotropin or γ-lipotropin, β-endorphin, α-melanocyte–stimulating hormone (αMSH), and corticotropin-like intermediate peptide, are produced. The first 18 amino acids of the N-terminus of ACTH are conserved through species and carry its biologic activity. Thus, synthetic ACTH (1 to 24) and ACTH (1 to 18) are often used for clinical purposes instead of the full-length ACTH. The sequence of αMSH, which is contained within the ACTH molecule, among other functions, stimulates the production of melanin by the melanocytes, causing skin and mucosal hyperpigmentation when secreted in excess.[1–3]

ACTH is secreted in regular pulses of variable amplitude over 24 hours, with peak concentrations attained in the early morning hours (04:00 AM to 08:00 AM), thus forming the basis of the circadian pattern of ACTH and cortisol secretion.[1–3,15] The acute action of ACTH is to increase the flux of cholesterol through the steroidogenic pathway, resulting in rapid production of steroids. ACTH also influences the remaining steps of steroidogenesis, as well as the uptake of cholesterol from plasma lipoproteins, thus ensuring a continuous supply of cholesterol to the mitochondria to meet the demands of activated pregnenolone biosynthesis. It also maintains the size of the adrenal glands.

CRH is the principal hypothalamic factor that stimulates the pituitary production of ACTH, while AVP plays a synergistic role.[16] Both neuropeptides are produced by parvocellular neurons of the paraventricular nuclei of the hypothalamus, but are also found in other parts of the CNS, as well as in peripheral non-CNS locations.[17] CRH and AVP are secreted in a pulsatile manner that results in the episodic secretion of ACTH and the circadian variation of cortisol secretion. The frequency of the hypothalamic pulsations of CRH and AVP is relatively constant, while the amplitude of these secretory episodes increases in the early morning hours and during stress, resulting in major changes in the plasma concentrations of cortisol. Therefore, it is the magnitude of each pulse of CRH/AVP and, consequently, ACTH that determines the total daily cortisol secretion. In addition to ACTH, other factors may also play an important role in the regulation of the adrenal cortex, including neural factors, medullary peptides, and immune system products.[18,19]

Cortisol is the primary negative regulator of basal hypothalamic–pituitary–adrenal (HPA) axis activity through negative feedback upon the pituitary, the hypothalamus, and suprahypothalamic centers, such as the hippocampus.[20] Thus, both ACTH and CRH secretion are inhibited by glucocorticoids. This effect is mediated by the classic glucocorticoid receptor α (GRα) in the pituitary and hypothalamus and by both GRα and the mineralocorticoid receptor (MR) in the hippocampus. The MR is in fact functioning as a GR, granted that the enzyme 11β-dehydrogenase type 2, which converts cortisol to the inactive cortisone, is not present in this tissue to protect it from the mineralocorticoid effects of cortisol. The concentrations of aldosterone are too low to compete with cortisol for the hippocampal MRs. Whether and to what extent direct glucocorticoid feedback on the adrenal cortex itself regulates cortisol synthesis is not clear.[21]

SECRETION AND METABOLISM

In normal subjects, the secretion of glucocorticoids follows a diurnal pattern, with peak concentrations observed between 06:00 AM and 08:00 AM and lowest concentrations around midnight.[22] The cortisol production rate is approximately 10 to 15 mg per m^2 per day.[23] More than 90% of circulating cortisol, and, to a lesser extent, aldosterone, is bound tightly to corticosteroid-binding globulin (CBG) or transcortin.[24] The remaining (10%) of the circulating cortisol is free or loosely bound to albumin. The free and albumin-bound fractions of cortisol represent the biologically active form of the hormone. When plasma cortisol concentrations exceed 20 μg per dL, CBG becomes fully saturated, and most of the excess cortisol is biologically active. CBG is synthesized in the liver. Estrogens, thyroid hormones, pregnancy, and oral contraceptives are associated with increased CBG concentrations,[24–26] whereas hypercortisolism, hepatic, or renal disease results in decreased CBG concentrations. In the presence of an intact HPA axis, alterations in CBG concentrations are likely not to affect circulating free cortisol concentrations.

The primary site of cortisol metabolism in humans is the liver, kidney, and a number of target tissues. Cytosolic and microsomal enzymes, including cytochrome P450, 5α/5β-reductase, 3α/3β-oxidoreductase, and 11β-HSD, play an important role in the hepatic metabolism of cortisol.[27–29] The major routes of hepatic metabolism involve A-ring and side-chain reduction followed by conjugation with glucuronic acid or sulfate.[30] The inactive glucuronide and sulfate metabolites are excreted by the kidneys, whereas only less than 1% of cortisol is excreted unchanged in the urine. Therefore, the metabolic clearance of cortisol is influenced primarily by factors altering hepatic clearance and, to a significant degree, by renal enzymes and factors affecting renal excretion.

11β-HSD modulates glucocorticoid action in tissues by altering the rate of conversion between cortisol and cortisone. There are two types of 11β-HSD: 11β-HSD type 1 (11β-HSD1) and 11β-HSD type 2 (11β-HSD2). 11β-HSD1 acts as a reductase, catalyzing the conversion of inactive cortisone to active cortisol, and may contribute to the tissue hypersensitivity to glucocorticoids. 11β-HSD1 is widely expressed in the liver, lung, adipose tissue, vascular components, ovary, and the CNS. Increased expression of 11β-HSD1 activity in splanchnic adipose tissue is associated with visceral obesity, indicating that 11β-HSD1 can enhance glucocorticoid action in local tissues.[29]

In contradistinction to 11β-HSD1, the physiologic importance of the other 11β-HSD2 is well documented. Patients harboring mutations in this enzyme develop symptoms of mineralocorticoid excess, while mice bearing a deletion in this gene demonstrate glucocorticoid-dependent mineralocorticoid excess. 11β-HSD2 acts as a dehydrogenase that converts cortisol to inactive cortisone and is expressed in classic aldosterone-sensitive tissues, such as the kidney, colon, sweat glands, and the placenta, where it protects the MR from the mineralocorticoid effects of cortisol, allowing the much lower aldosterone concentrations to exert such actions.[29]

MOLECULAR MECHANISMS OF GLUCOCORTICOID ACTION

At the cellular level, the actions of glucocorticoids are mediated by an intracellular receptor protein, the GR, which functions as a hormone-activated transcription factor that regulates the expression of glucocorticoid target genes.[1,31–33] The human GR (hGR) belongs to the superfamily of steroid/thyroid/retinoic acid receptor proteins.[31] The *hGR* gene consists of nine exons and is composed of a poorly conserved amino-terminal domain (NTD); a central, highly conserved DNA-binding domain (DBD); a hinge region (HR); and a carboxyl-terminal, ligand-binding domain (LBD).[1,31–33] The NTD contains a major transactivation domain, termed activation function (AF)-1, which is located at amino acids 77 to 262 of the hGR. The DBD spans over amino acids 420 to 480 and contains two zinc finger motifs through which the receptor binds to specific DNA sequences in the promoter region of target genes, the glucocorticoid response elements (GREs). The HR lies between the DBD and the LBD and provides the appropriate structural flexibility for the activated receptor to bind onto GREs. In addition, this region contains critical lysines that undergo acetylation by the transcription factor "circadian locomotor output cycle kaput" (CLOCK), which is involved in the circadian oscillations of gene expression.[34] The LBD contains a second transactivation domain, AF-2, as well as sequences important for interaction with heat shock proteins (HSPs), nuclear translocation, and receptor dimerization[35–37] (Fig. 54.3A and B).

Alternative slicing of the *hGR* gene in exon 9 generates two highly homologous receptor isoforms, termed α and β. These are identical through amino acid 727, but then diverge, with hGRα having an additional 50 amino acids and hGRβ having an additional, nonhomologous 15 amino acids[38] (Fig. 54.3A). hGRα is ubiquitously expressed in almost all human tissues and cells, resides primarily in the cytoplasm, and represents the classic GR that functions as ligand-dependent transcription factor. hGRβ is also ubiquitously expressed in tissues usually at lower concentrations than hGRα, with the exception of epithelial cells and neutrophils.[38] In contradistinction to hGRα, hGRβ resides primarily in the nucleus of cells independently of the presence of ligand, does not bind glucocorticoids, and exerts a dominant negative effect upon the wild-type hGRα.[32,39] Moreover, hGRβ might regulate the transcription of several target genes, independently of the hGRα-mediated transcriptional activity.[40]

In addition to alternative splicing, Lu and Cidlowski demonstrated that eight distinct receptor isoforms, termed GRα-A, GRα-B, GRα-C1, GRα-C2, GRα-C3, GRα-D1, GRα-D2, and GRα-D3, are generated through alternative initiation of GRα messenger RNA (mRNA) translation.[41] Although these isoforms have similar affinity for ligand binding and similar ability to bind onto the regulatory regions of glucocorticoid-responsive genes, they display different transcriptional activity.[42,43] Less than one in 10 target genes is commonly regulated by these receptor isoforms.[43] Furthermore, these isoforms are different in terms of subcellular localization and tissue expression.[41]

In the absence of ligand, hGRα resides primarily in the cytoplasm of cells as part of a large multiprotein complex, which consists of the receptor polypeptide, two molecules of hsp90, and several other proteins.[44] The hsp90 molecules are thought to sequester hGRα in the cytoplasm of cells by maintaining the receptor in a conformation that masks or inactivates its nuclear localization signals (NLSs). Upon hormone binding,

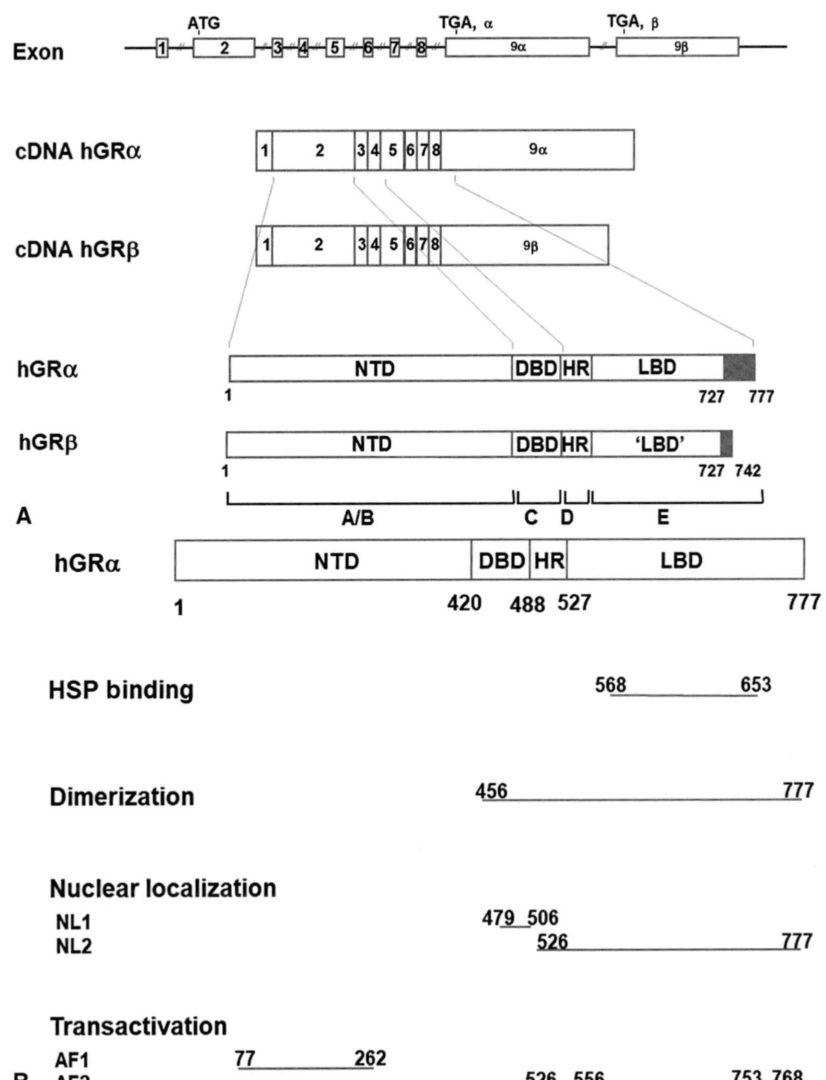

Figure 54.3 (A) Genomic and complementary DNA and protein structures of the human glucocorticoid receptor (hGR). The *hGR* gene consists of 10 exons. Exon 1 is an untranslated region, exon 2 codes for the amino-terminal domain **[A/B]**, exons 3 and 4 for the DNA-binding domain (DBD) **[C]**, and exons 5–9 for the hinge region **[D]** and the ligand-binding domain (LBD) **[E]**. The *GR* gene contains two terminal exons 9 (exon 9α and 9β) alternatively spliced to produce the classic hGRα isoform and an additional non–ligand-binding hGRβ isoform. **(B)** Functional domains of the GR. The functional domains and subdomains are indicated beneath the linearized protein structures. NL, nuclear localization; AF, activation function; cDNA, complementary DNA.

the receptor undergoes conformational changes, which result in dissociation from hsp90 and other proteins, unmasking of the NLSs and exposure of the ligand-binding pocket. In its new conformation, the activated, ligand-bound hGRα translocates into the nucleus, where it binds as homodimer to GREs located in the promoter region of target genes. hGRα then communicates with the basal transcription machinery and regulates the expression of glucocorticoid-responsive genes positively or negatively, depending on the GRE sequence and promoter context[44] (Fig. 54.4). The receptor can also modulate gene expression, as a monomer, independently of GRE binding, by physically interacting with other transcription factors, such as activating protein-1, nuclear factor (NF)-κB, and signal transducers and activators of transcription.[44]

Following binding to GREs, the activated hGRα enhances the expression of glucocorticoid-responsive genes by regulating the assembly of a transcriptional preinitiation complex at the promoter region of target genes. This is achieved by interaction of the liganded receptor with the basal transcription factors, a group of proteins composed of RNA polymerase II, TATA-binding protein (TBP), and a host of TBP-associated proteins (TAF_{II}s). The interaction between the activated receptor and the basal transcription factors is mediated by the coactivators, which are nucleoproteins with chromatin remodeling and other enzymatic activities[45,46] (Fig. 54.5).

In addition to transcriptional activation, the activated hGRα can suppress gene expression through binding to negative GREs (nGREs), which contains the consensus sequence CTCCn0-2GGAGA with the number of nucleotides between the half sites ranging from zero to two.[47] Upon binding to nGREs, the hGRα recruits both corepressors, such as NCoR1 and SMRT, as well as histone deacetylases, thereby repressing a number of glucocorticoid target genes.[48]

The response of a single cell exposed to glucocorticoids depends on the interplay between (a) the concentration of free hormone, (b) the relative potency of the hormone, and (c) the

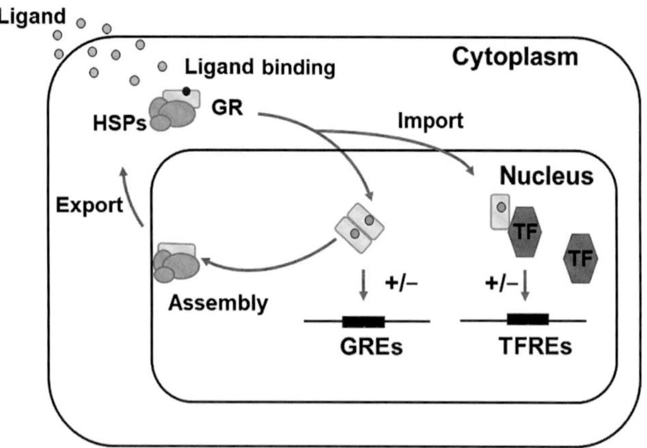

Figure 54.4 Nucleocytoplasmic shuttling of the glucocorticoid receptor. GR, glucocorticoid receptor; GRE, glucocorticoid response element; HSP, heat shock protein; TF, transcription factor; TFRE, transcription factor responsive element.

ability of the cell to receive and transduce the hormonal signal. The concentration of the free hormone is primarily under the control of the HPA axis but is also influenced by the plasma and tissue concentrations of CBG, whereas the relative potency of any endogenous or exogenous glucocorticoid is influenced by its bioavailability, affinity for hGR, and ability to retain the hGR in the nucleus.[44]

Glucocorticoids may exert an ever-increasing number of their effects within seconds or minutes, independently of transcription/translation processes. These "nongenomic" glucocorticoid effects are mediated by plasma membrane-anchored GRs that induce the activity of the mitogen-activated protein kinase (MAPK) or the phosphatidylinositol 3-kinase (PI3K).[49] The nature of membrane GRs still is under investigation.[50–52] Nevertheless, representative examples of nongenomic glucocorticoid actions are (a) some immunomodulatory glucocorticoid effects via disruption of the T-cell receptor (TCR) complex[53]; (b) the rapid inhibition of ACTH release from the pituitary gland by glucocorticoids[54]; (c) the vasorelaxation in cases of myocardial or brain ischemia via glucocorticoid-induced activation of endothelial nitric oxide synthase (eNOS) and other vasodilatory molecules[55]; and (d) the rapidly increasing frequency of excitatory postsynaptic potentials in the hippocampus during exposure to glucocorticoids.[56]

Glucocorticoids also influence directly the expression of mitochondrial genome via mitochondrial GR–GREs interactions.[57] Surprisingly, GRs have been detected within mitochondria, while GREs have been identified at several positions in the mitochondrial DNA. Furthermore, glucocorticoids regulate mitochondrial DNA expression indirectly through the expression of mitochondrial RNA-processing enzymes and transcription factors mostly via nuclear GR–GRE interactions (reviewed in Nicolaides and Charmandari[58]).

Tissue glucocorticoid sensitivity is also influenced by clock transcription factors. Nader and collaborators have demonstrated that the transcription factor CLOCK acetylates multiple lysine residues located in the HR of hGRα.[34] This CLOCK-mediated acetylation results in less DNA binding of the receptor, leading to reduced hGRα-mediated transcriptional activity (Fig. 54.6).

EFFECTS OF GLUCOCORTICOIDS

GROWTH AND DEVELOPMENT

Although small increases in cortisol concentrations exert a stimulatory effect on growth hormone (GH) secretion by increasing GH mRNA levels and enhancing GH gene expression,[59] significant chronic hypercortisolism results in reduced GH secretion and growth suppression,[60–62] attenuation of GH response to exogenous stimuli,[63,64] and inhibition of the effects of insulin-like growth factor 1 and other growth factors on target tissues.[60,61,65] Children with Cushing syndrome have delayed or arrested growth and achieve a final adult height that is, on average, 7.5 to 8.0 cm below their predicted height.[60,66]

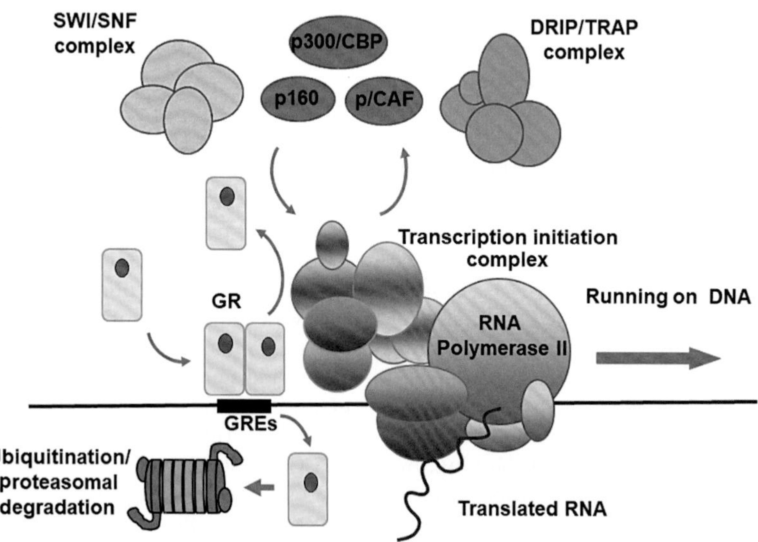

Figure 54.5 Schematic representation of the interaction of the glucocorticoid receptor with coactivators and other chromatin modulators. AF, activation function; CBP, cAMP-responsive element-binding protein (CREB)-binding protein; DRIP, vitamin D receptor-interacting protein; p/CAF, p300/CBP-associated factor; TRAP, thyroid hormone receptor-associated protein; SWI, mating-type switching; SNF, sucrose nonfermenting.

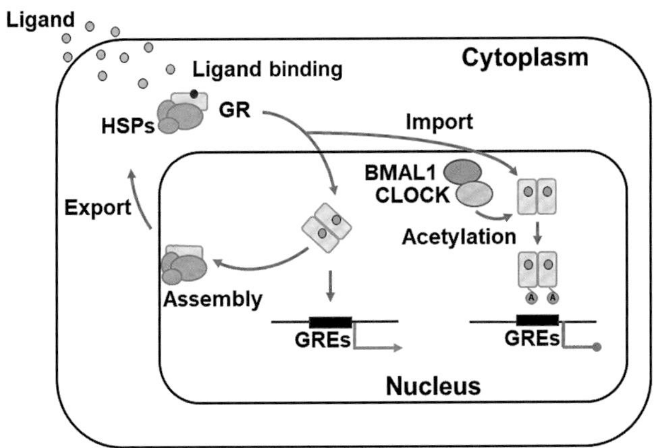

Figure 54.6 Acetylation of hGRα by the transcription factor CLOCK. In the deacetylated form, the activated hGRα binds onto the GREs, thereby influencing the expression of glucocorticoid target genes. Upon CLOCK-mediated acetylation of hGRα, the receptor displays less DNA binding, leading to decreased hGRα-mediated transcriptional activity. CLOCK, circadian locomotor output cycle kaput; hGR, human glucocorticoid receptor; GRE, glucocorticoid response element; HSP, heat shock protein.

Glucocorticoids play an important role in fetal development and lung maturation by stimulating the synthesis and release of surfactant proteins (SP-A, SP-B, SP-C).[67,68] The absence of functional GR in $GR^{-/-}$ knockout mice leads to severe neonatal respiratory distress syndrome and death within a few hours after birth.[69] Glucocorticoids also stimulate the enzyme phenylethanolamine *N*-methyltransferase, which converts norepinephrine to epinephrine in adrenal medulla and chromaffin tissue. $GR^{-/-}$ knockout mice do not develop an adrenal medulla.

CARBOHYDRATE AND LIPID METABOLISM

Glucocorticoids increase blood glucose concentrations through their action on glycogen, protein, and lipid metabolism. In the liver, glucocorticoids stimulate glycogen deposition, while in peripheral tissues (muscle, fat), they inhibit glucose uptake and utilization. In adipose tissue, lipolysis is activated, and free fatty acids are released into the circulation.[1–3] Glucocorticoids have a permissive effect on other hormones, such as catecholamines and glucagon, leading to insulin resistance and an increase in blood glucose concentrations at the expense of protein and lipid catabolism.

Glucocorticoids stimulate adipocyte differentiation and promote adipogenesis by enhancing the transcriptional activity of relevant important genes, including lipoprotein lipase, glycerol-3-phosphate dehydrogenase, and leptin.[1–3] Chronic hypercortisolism leads to increased deposition of visceral or central adipose tissue. The predilection for visceral obesity may be related to the increased expression of both the GR and type 1 isozyme of 11β-HSD in omental as opposed to subcutaneous adipose tissue.[70,71]

THYROID AND REPRODUCTIVE FUNCTION

Glucocorticoids suppress the thyroid axis most likely through a direct action on thyroid-stimulating hormone secretion, and they inhibit 5′-deiodinase activity, which converts thyroxin to triiodothyronine. They also act centrally to inhibit gonadotropin-releasing hormone pulsatility and release of luteinizing hormone and follicle-stimulating hormone (FSH).[1–3,66]

SKIN, MUSCLE, AND CONNECTIVE TISSUE; BONE AND CALCIUM METABOLISM

Glucocorticoids induce insulin resistance in the muscle and result in catabolic changes in muscle, skin, and connective tissue. They inhibit osteoblast function, thus explaining the osteopenia and osteoporosis associated with chronic glucocorticoid excess. Glucocorticoids also induce a negative calcium balance by inhibiting intestinal calcium absorption and increasing renal calcium excretion.[1–3]

WATER AND ELECTROLYTE HOMEOSTASIS

Glucocorticoids increase blood pressure via mechanisms that involve actions on the kidney and vasculature. In vascular smooth muscle, glucocorticoids increase sensitivity to pressor agents, such as catecholamines and angiotensin II, and reduce NO-mediated endothelial dilatation. They also increase angiotensinogen synthesis. In the kidney, cortisol acts on the distal nephron to cause sodium retention and potassium loss (mediated by the MR) depending on the activity of 11β-HSD2.[29] Elsewhere across the nephron, glucocorticoids increase glomerular filtration rate, proximal tubular epithelial sodium transport, and free water clearance.[1–3]

IMMUNE FUNCTION

Glucocorticoids have profound inhibitory effects on the immune/inflammatory response.[72,73] Therefore, glucocorticoids have become one of the most efficient therapeutic compounds for the management of allergic, inflammatory, and autoimmune diseases, as well as for suppressing the host immune reaction in organ transplantation. At the cellular level, the main anti-inflammatory and immunosuppressive effects of glucocorticoids include alterations in leukocyte traffic and function, decreases in production of cytokines and mediators of inflammation, and inhibition of their action on target tissues by the latter. These effects are exerted both at the resting, basal state and during inflammatory stress, when the circulating concentrations of glucocorticoids are elevated. Thus, a circadian activity of several immune factors has been demonstrated in reverse-phase synchrony with that of plasma glucocorticoid concentrations.[1–3,74] Glucocorticoids increase the risk for infection, including those of bacteria, viruses, fungi, and parasites.[1–3]

CENTRAL NERVOUS SYSTEM

The brain is an important target tissue for glucocorticoids. Both glucocorticoid and MRs are expressed in discrete regions of the brain, including hippocampus, hypothalamus, cerebellum, and cortex.[75] Glucocorticoids cause neuronal death mostly in the hippocampus, and this effect may underlie their role in cognitive function, memory, and neurodegenerative diseases. Chronic hypercortisolism has multiple effects on CNS functions, such as cognition, mood, behavior, memory, and sleep pattern. Glucocorticoids may cause frank and Korsakoff psychosis, major depression, schizophrenia, Alzheimer disease, anorexia nervosa, and cerebrovascular brain injury, as well as cognitive disturbances, including difficulties in attention and concentration, memory disturbance, and impaired thinking. Chronic hypercortisolism may also affect the anatomy of CNS, leading to reduction of hippocampal volume, ventricular enlargement, and cortical atrophy. On the other hand, physiologic doses of glucocorticoids appear to be necessary for memory and cognitive function, as well as other important functions of the CNS.[1–3]

The CNS contains two types of "glucocorticoid" receptors, which bind glucocorticoids and mediate their actions. One is the MR (type I) and the other is the classic GR (type II). The former is distributed predominantly in the limbic system, including the hippocampus, septum, septohippocampal nucleus, and amygdala, while the latter is wildly distributed in the entire CNS. Given that the CNS, and in particular the hippocampus, does not express 11β-HSD2, the MR may act as a high-affinity receptor for glucocorticoids in this region of the brain. It appears that the MR mediates the tonic effect of glucocorticoids on circadian fluctuations, the sensitivity of the stress response, and organization of the behavioral responses to stress, while the GR mediates the feedback inhibition of glucocorticoids on the HPA axis activity and facilitates memory storage.[1–3]

In the eye, glucocorticoids raise intraocular pressure through an increase in aqueous humor production and deposition of matrix within the trabecular meshwork, which inhibits aqueous drainage.[76]

GASTROINTESTINAL FUNCTION

Chronic administration of glucocorticoids increases the risk of developing peptic ulcer disease. Pancreatitis with fat necrosis is reported in patients with glucocorticoid excess. The GR is expressed throughout the gastrointestinal tract and the MR in the distal colon, and these mediate the corticosteroid control of epithelial ion transport.[1–3]

TREATMENT WITH GLUCOCORTICOIDS

Natural and synthetic glucocorticoids can be used for both endocrine and nonendocrine disorders. In endocrine practice, glucocorticoids are used in establishing the diagnosis and cause of Cushing syndrome, in the hormonal replacement therapy of adrenal insufficiency, and in the treatment of congenital adrenal hyperplasia, which consists of both glucocorticoid and/or mineralocorticoid substitution and suppression of excess androgen secretion. Glucocorticoids are also given in pharmacologic doses to treat patients with inflammatory, allergic, or immunologic disorders[1–3] (Table 54.1). Chronic therapy has many side effects, ranging from suppression of the HPA axis and Cushing syndrome to infections and changes in mental status. Factors that influence both the therapeutic and adverse effects of glucocorticoids include the pharmacokinetic properties of the glucocorticoid, daily dosage, timing of doses during the day, individual differences in steroid metabolism, as well as the duration of treatment.

GLUCOCORTICOID REPLACEMENT THERAPY

In cortisol and aldosterone deficiency states (primary adrenal insufficiency), physiologic replacement is best achieved with a combination of hydrocortisone and the mineralocorticoid fludrocortisone; hydrocortisone alone at replacement doses does not usually provide sufficient mineralocorticoid activity for complete replacement.[77]

In primary *Addison disease* or following bilateral adrenalectomy, hydrocortisone by mouth is usually required. This is given in two to three doses, the larger in the morning and the smaller in the evening, to mimic the normal diurnal rhythm of cortisol secretion. Recently, the U.S. Endocrine Society recommended a total daily dose of hydrocortisone ranging between 15 and 25 mg divided into two or three doses decreasing during the day.[78] Thus, the highest dose should be given in the morning, the second dose either 2 hours after lunch (in the case of two-dose regimen) or at noon, followed by a third dose, approximately 4 to 6 hours before bedtime.[78] The optimum daily dose is determined by the clinical response. Chronic glucocorticoid therapy is supplemented by fludrocortisone. The latter is titrated clinically and on the basis of normal plasma renin activity measurements.[77]

In *acute adrenocortical insufficiency* or *adrenal crisis*, the first-line management depends on fluid resuscitation and glucocorticoid replacement at stress doses.[79,80] Therefore, hydrocortisone is given intravenously (preferably as sodium succinate or phosphate) every 6 to 8 hours in sodium chloride intravenous infusion 0.9%.[77] If hydrocortisone is not available, methylprednisolone should be the second-line treatment, whereas dexamethasone should be administered as the least

TABLE 54.1 Therapeutic Indications of Corticosteroids

Disorders	*Examples*
Allergic reactions	Angioneurotic edema, asthma, urticaria
Endocrine	Replacement therapy in Addison disease, hypopituitarism, congenital adrenal hyperplasia
Gastrointestinal	Inflammatory bowel disease (ulcerative colitis, Crohn disease), chronic active hepatitis, liver transplantation/rejection
Hematologic	Leukemia, lymphoma, hemolytic anemia, idiopathic thrombocytopenic purpura
Infections	Meningococcal meningitis, septic shock
Muscular	Polymyalgia rheumatica, myasthenia gravis
Neurologic	Cerebral edema, raised intracranial pressure
Ophthalmologic	Acute uveitis, conjunctivitis, optic neuritis, choroiditis
Renal	Nephrotic syndrome, vasculitides, kidney transplantation/rejection
Respiratory	Angioedema, anaphylaxis, asthma, sarcoidosis, tuberculosis, respiratory distress syndrome
Rheumatologic	Systemic lupus erythematosus, polyarteritis nodosa, temporal arteritis, juvenile rheumatoid arthritis
Skin	Dermatitis, pemphigus, atopic dermatitis

preferred regiment.[81] According to the U.S. Endocrine Society guidelines, adults in adrenal crisis should be treated with an intravenous bolus of 100-mg hydrocortisone, which should be followed by 200 mg per 24 hour as a continuous infusion or 6-hourly injections and subsequently reduced to 100 mg per day the next day.[78,80] Hydrocortisone should be tapered to maintenance dosage in 1 to 3 days according to clinical manifestations.[82] In children, the stress dose depends on the age and size expressed as body surface area. For infants, the recommended stress dose is 25 mg per m^2, for preschool children 50 mg per m^2 and for children above the age of 12 years 100 mg per m^2.[78] Subsequently, the same dose is divided 6 hourly for 24 to 48 hours. Fluid resuscitation is achieved by a rapid bolus of 20 mL per kg of normal saline, while hypoglycemia should be corrected by 0.5 to 1 g per kg of intravenous dextrose.[78]

In *hypopituitarism*, glucocorticoids should be given as in adrenocortical insufficiency, but since the production of aldosterone is regulated by the renin–angiotensin system, a mineralocorticoid compound is not usually required. Additional replacement therapy with levothyroxine and sex hormones should be given as indicated by the pattern of hormone deficiency.[83] In case of thyroid and cortisol deficiency, cortisol should be given first, as hypothyroidism may mask severe cortisol deficiency, which might be unleashed upon thyroid replacement.[83]

In *congenital adrenal hyperplasia*, the anterior pituitary increases the secretion of corticotropin to compensate for the reduced secretion of cortisol; this results in increased adrenal androgen production. Therefore, in addition to cortisol replacement, hydrocortisone should be given to suppress androgen overproduction, thereby preventing virilization and ensuring optimal growth and fertility.[84] For these therapeutic purposes, hydrocortisone doses should be adjusted up to 15 mg per m^2 per day in early infancy and between 10 and 15 mg per m^2 per day after the first year of life.[80,85] Careful and continual dose titration is required to avoid growth retardation and toxicity. Salt-losing forms of congenital adrenal hyperplasia require parallel mineralocorticoid replacement. Mineralocorticoid replacement may be beneficial even when salt-losing symptoms are not evident, as it allows use of lower doses of hydrocortisone.[86]

GLUCOCORTICOID THERAPY

In comparing the relative potencies of corticosteroids in terms of their anti-inflammatory (glucocorticoid) effects, it should be borne in mind that high glucocorticoid activity is more advantageous when it is accompanied by relatively low mineralocorticoid activity, granted that high doses could be given without producing salt retention as a side effect. The mineralocorticoid activity of fludrocortisone at replacement doses, on the other hand, is appropriate, while its anti-inflammatory activity is of no clinical relevance. The equivalent anti-inflammatory doses of corticosteroids are given in Table 54.2.

The relatively high mineralocorticoid activity of *hydrocortisone* and its immediate precursor *cortisone* and the resulting fluid retention make them unsuitable for disease suppression on a long-term basis. Thus, although they are preferable for adrenal replacement therapy, we recommend synthetic glucocorticoids with intermediate- or long-term actions for treating diseases that require high (stress) doses of glucocorticoids. Hydrocortisone may be used on a short-term basis by intravenous injection for the emergency management of some conditions. The relatively moderate anti-inflammatory potency of hydrocortisone also makes it a useful topical corticosteroid for the management of mild inflammatory skin conditions, because side effects (both topical and systemic) are less marked than those of fluorinated synthetic glucocorticoids; cortisone is not active topically.

TABLE 54.2 Equivalent Anti-inflammatory Doses of Corticosteroids

	Equivalent Dose	*Plasma Half-Life (min)*	*Biologic Half-Life (h)*
Prednisolone	5 mg	90	18–36
≡ Betamethasone	750 µg	300	36–54
≡ Cortisone acetate	25 mg	80–118	8–12
≡ Dexamethasone	750 µg	200	36–54
≡ Hydrocortisone	20 mg	60	8–12
≡ Methylprednisolone	4 mg	180	18–36
≡ Triamcinolone	4 mg	30	18–36

This table takes no account of mineralocorticoid effects, nor does it take account of variations in duration of action.[59,86]

Prednisolone has predominantly glucocorticoid activity and is the corticosteroid most commonly used by mouth for long-term disease suppression. Prednisolone or, mainly, methylprednisolone can also be given parenterally. *Betamethasone* and *dexamethasone* have very high glucocorticoid activity but insignificant mineralocorticoid activity. This makes them particularly suitable for high-dose glucocorticoid therapy in conditions in which fluid retention would be a disadvantage (e.g., cerebral edema). Betamethasone and dexamethasone are fluorinated at the 9α position and have a long duration of action. The latter, coupled with their lack of mineralocorticoid action, makes them suitable for conditions that require suppression of ACTH secretion (e.g., hard-to-control congenital adrenal hyperplasia).

Some esters of betamethasone, beclomethasone, and dexamethasone exert a considerably marked topical effect (e.g., on the skin or the nasal or lung epithelium); use is made of this to obtain topical effects while minimizing systemic side effects (e.g., for skin applications and inhalations). The same steroids, however, may cause skin atrophy. *Deflazacort* is derived from prednisolone and has high glucocorticoid activity.[86]

ADMINISTRATION OF CORTICOSTEROIDS

Whenever possible, *local, compartmentalized treatment* with creams, intra-articular injections, inhalations, eye drops, or enemas should be used in preference to *systemic treatment*. The suppressive action of a corticosteroid on cortisol secretion is least when it is given as a single dose in the morning. In an attempt to reduce pituitary–adrenal suppression, the total dose for 2 days can sometimes be given as a single dose on alternate days; alternate-day administration has not been very successful in the management of asthma though. HPA axis suppression can also be reduced by means of intermittent therapy with short courses. In some conditions, it may be possible to reduce the dose of corticosteroid by adding a small dose of an immunosuppressant drug. Interestingly, when glucocorticoids are given in the context of severe stress, such as chemotherapy for leukemia, they produce very little HPA axis suppression.[87]

Dosage of corticosteroids varies widely in different diseases and in different patients and should always be individualized.

If the use of a corticosteroid can save or prolong life, as in acute leukemia or acute transplant rejection, high doses may need to be given, because the complications of therapy are likely to be less serious than the effects of the disease itself.

When long-term corticosteroid therapy is used in some chronic diseases, the adverse effects of treatment may become greater than the disabilities caused by the disease. To minimize side effects, the maintenance dose should be kept as low as possible.

When potentially less harmful measures are ineffective, corticosteroids are used topically for the treatment of inflammatory conditions of the skin. Corticosteroids are used both topically (by rectum) and systemically (by mouth or intravenously) in the management of ulcerative colitis and Crohn disease. Moderate-to-high doses of corticosteroids are given by intravenous injection in the acute respiratory distress syndrome and in the systemic inflammatory syndrome/septic shock. Corticosteroids are recommended in meningococcal meningitis and in the recently described severe acute respiratory distress syndrome (SARS).[88,89]

Dexamethasone and betamethasone have little, if any, mineralocorticoid action, and their long duration of action makes them particularly suitable for suppressing corticotropin secretion in hard-to-control congenital adrenal hyperplasia, where the dose should be tailored to clinical response and by measurement of primarily adrenal androgens (delta4-androstenedione and, rarely, 17-hydroxyprogesterone in serum or plasma).

In acute hypersensitivity reactions, such as angioedema of the upper respiratory tract and anaphylactic shock, corticosteroids are indicated as an adjunct to emergency treatment with adrenaline (epinephrine). In such cases, hydrocortisone (as sodium succinate) by intravenous injection may be required.

Corticosteroids are preferably used by inhalation in the management of asthma, but systemic therapy in association with bronchodilators is required for the emergency treatment of severe acute asthma. Corticosteroids may also be useful in conditions such as rheumatic fever, chronic active hepatitis, and sarcoidosis; they may also lead to remissions of acquired hemolytic anemia, idiopathic nephrotic syndrome in children, and thrombocytopenic purpura. Corticosteroids can improve the prognosis of serious conditions, such as systemic lupus erythematous, temporal arteritis, and polyarteritis nodosa; the effects of the disease process may be suppressed and symptoms relieved, but the underlying condition is not cured, although it may ultimately remit. It is usual to begin therapy in these conditions at fairly high doses and then to reduce the dose to the lowest dose that allows disease control.[86]

SIDE EFFECTS OF CORTICOSTEROIDS

Overdosage or prolonged use may exaggerate some of the normal physiologic actions of corticosteroids, leading to glucocorticoid and/or mineralocorticoid side effects.

Administration of corticosteroids may result in suppression of growth and may affect the development of puberty. It is important to use the lowest effective dose; alternate-day regimens may be appropriate and limit growth reduction.

Mineralocorticoid side effects include hypertension, sodium and water retention, and potassium loss. They are most marked with fludrocortisone but are significant with cortisone, hydrocortisone, corticotropin, and tetracosactide (tetracosactrin). Mineralocorticoid actions are negligible with the high-potency long-acting glucocorticoids, betamethasone, and dexamethasone and occur only slightly with the intermediate-acting methylprednisolone, prednisolone, and triamcinolone.

Glucocorticoid side effects include obesity, especially of the centripetal type; carbohydrate intolerance and/or diabetes type 2 and osteoporosis; avascular necrosis of the femoral head; mental disturbances (insomnia, hypomania, and depression may be induced, particularly in patients with a history of mental disorder); as well as muscle wasting (proximal myopathy) (Table 54.3). Corticosteroid therapy is also weakly linked with peptic ulceration. High doses of chronically administered corticosteroids must always be gradually tapered to avoid symptoms of acute glucocorticoid deficiency. In children, administration of corticosteroids may result in suppression of growth and delay of bone age. In general, chronic use of systemic glucocorticoids in children compromises their final stature to a varying degree. Other complications include increased susceptibility to infection, poor wound healing, and activation of latent tuberculosis.[86]

ADRENAL SUPPRESSION

During prolonged therapy with corticosteroids, adrenal atrophy develops and may persist for years after discontinuation of therapy. When a question about the presence of adrenal suppression is raised, the rapid Synacthen (or high-dose ACTH stimulation test) is mostly used.[90] A bolus of 250 μg of corticotropin 1 to 24 or a bolus of 10 μg per kg body weight is administered intravenously, and cortisol is measured after 30 or 60 minutes or both. Plasma cortisol concentrations over 18 or 20 μg per dL, respectively, at these times indicate adequate recovery of the HPA axis.[90] Abrupt withdrawal after a prolonged period may lead to acute adrenal insufficiency, hypotension, or death. Withdrawal may also be associated with anorexia, nausea, fever, myalgias, arthralgias, rhinitis, conjunctivitis, painful itchy skin nodules, abdominal pain, diarrhea, weight loss, and/or psychiatric manifestations.

To compensate for a diminished adrenocortical response caused by prolonged corticosteroid treatment, any significant intercurrent illness, trauma, or surgical procedure requires a temporary increase in corticosteroid dose, or, if already stopped, a temporary reintroduction of corticosteroid treatment. Therefore, anesthetists must know whether a patient is taking or has been taking a corticosteroid, to avoid a precipitous fall in blood pressure during anesthesia or in the immediate postoperative period.

Children on long-term corticosteroid treatment should wear an "Alert Bracelet" and carry a "Steroid Treatment Card" which gives guidance on minimizing risk and provides details of prescriber, drug, dosage, and duration of treatment, as well as an "Emergency Kit."[86]

INFECTIONS

Prolonged courses of corticosteroids increase susceptibility to and severity of infections; clinical presentation of infections may also be atypical. Serious infections, for example, *septicemia* or *tuberculosis*, may reach an advanced stage before being recognized, and *amebiasis* or *strongyloidiasis* may be activated or exacerbated (exclude before initiating a corticosteroid in those at risk or with

TABLE 54.3 Effects of Chronic Pharmacologic Use of Glucocorticoids

Category	*Side Effects*
Endocrine and metabolic	Suppression of HPA axis (adrenal suppression)
	Growth failure in children
	Carbohydrate intolerance
	Hyperinsulinism
	Insulin resistance
	Abnormal glucose tolerance test
	Diabetes mellitus
	Cushingoid features
	Moon facies, facial plethora
	Generalized and truncal obesity
	Supraclavicular fat collection
	Posterior cervical fat deposition (buffalo hump)
	Glucocorticoid-induced acne
	Thin and fragile skin, violaceous striae
	Impotence, menstrual disorders
	Decreased TSH and T_3
	Hypokalemia, metabolic alkalosis
Gastrointestinal	Gastric irritation, peptic ulcer
	Acute pancreatitis (rare)
	Fatty infiltration of liver (hepatomegaly; rare)
Hematopoietic	Leukocytosis
	Neutrophilia
	Increased influx from bone marrow and decreased migration from blood vessels
	Monocytopenia
	Lymphopenia
	Migration from blood vessels to lymphoid tissue
	Eosinopenia
Immunologic	Suppression of delayed hypersensitivity
	Inhibition of leukocyte and tissue macrophage migration
	Inhibition of cytokine secretion/action
	Suppression of the primary antigen response
Musculoskeletal	Osteoporosis, spontaneous fractures
	Aseptic necrosis of femoral and humoral heads and other bones
	Myopathy/muscle weakness
Ophthalmologic	Posterior subcapsular cataracts (more common in children)
	Elevated intraocular pressure/glaucoma
Neuropsychiatric	Sleep disturbances, insomnia
	Euphoria, depression, mania, psychosis
	Pseudotumor cerebri (benign increase in intracranial pressure)
Cardiovascular	Hypertension
	Congestive heart failure in predisposed patients

HPA, hypothalamic–pituitary–adrenal; TSH, thyroid-stimulating hormone secretion; T_3, triiodothyronine.

suggestive symptoms). Fungal or viral *ocular infections* may also be exacerbated.

Chickenpox

Unless they have had chickenpox, patients receiving oral or parenteral corticosteroids for purposes other than replacement should be regarded as being *at risk of severe chickenpox.* Manifestations of fulminant illness include pneumonia, hepatitis, and disseminated intravascular coagulation; rash is not necessarily a prominent feature. Passive immunization with varicella-zoster immunoglobulin is needed for exposed nonimmune patients receiving systemic corticosteroids or for those who have used them within the previous 3 months; varicella-zoster immunoglobulin should preferably be given within 3 days of exposure and no later than 10 days. Confirmed chickenpox warrants specialist care and urgent treatment. Corticosteroids should not be stopped, and dosage may need to be increased. Topical, inhaled, or rectal corticosteroids are less likely to be associated with an increased risk of severe chickenpox.

Measles

Patients taking corticosteroids should be advised to take particular care to avoid exposure to measles and seek immediate medical advice if exposure occurs. Prophylaxis with intramuscular normal immunoglobulin may be needed.[86]

INTERACTION OF GLUCOCORTICOIDS WITH OTHER DRUGS

The interactions of corticosteroids with other drugs are listed in Table 54.4.

PREGNANCY AND BREASTFEEDING

A review of the data on the safety of systemic corticosteroids used in pregnancy and breastfeeding has concluded the following:

- Corticosteroids vary in their ability to cross the placenta; betamethasone and dexamethasone cross the placenta readily, while most of hydrocortisone and 88% of prednisolone are inactivated by 11β-HSD2 as they cross the placenta.
- There is no convincing evidence that systemic corticosteroids increase the incidence of congenital abnormalities, such as cleft lip or palate.
- When administration is prolonged or repeated during pregnancy, systemic corticosteroids increase the risk of intrauterine growth retardation; there is no evidence of intrauterine growth retardation following short-term treatment (e.g., prophylactic treatment for neonatal respiratory distress syndrome).
- Usually, any adrenal suppression in the neonate following prenatal exposure resolves spontaneously after birth and is rarely clinically significant; however, it would be safe to perform a standard cortrosyn test in the neonate to exclude adrenal suppression (Table 54.3).
- Prednisolone appears in small amounts in breast milk, but maternal doses of up to 40 mg daily are unlikely to cause systemic effects in the infant; infants should be monitored for adrenal suppression if the mothers are taking higher doses.[86]

TABLE 54.4 Interactions of Corticosteroids with Other Drugs

Drug	*Interaction with Corticosteroids*
ACE inhibitors	Antagonism of hypotensive effect
Acetazolamide	Increased risk of hypokalemia
Adrenergic blockers	Antagonism of hypotensive effect
α-Blockers	Antagonism of hypotensive effect
Aminoglutethimide	Metabolism of corticosteroids accelerated (reduced effect)
Amphotericin	Increased risk of hypokalemia (avoid concomitant use unless corticosteroids needed to control reactions)
Angiotensin II–receptor antagonists	Antagonism of hypotensive effect
Antidiabetics	Antagonism of hypoglycemic effect
Aspirin (also benorilate)	Increased risk of gastrointestinal bleeding and ulceration
	Corticosteroids reduce plasma-salicylate concentration
Barbiturates and primidone	Metabolism of corticosteroids accelerated (reduced effect)
β-Blockers	Antagonism of hypotensive effect
Calcium-channel blockers	Antagonism of hypotensive effect
Carbamazepine	Accelerated metabolism of corticosteroids (reduced effect)
Carbenoxolone	Increased risk of hypokalemia
Cardiac glycosides	Increased risk of hypokalemia
Clonidine	Antagonism of hypotensive effect
Coumarins	Anticoagulant effect possibly altered
Diazoxide	Antagonism of hypotensive effect
Diuretics	Antagonism of diuretic effect
Diuretics, loop	Increased risk of hypokalemia
Diuretics, thiazide and related	Increased risk of hypokalemia
Erythromycin	Erythromycin possibly inhibits metabolism of corticosteroids
Estrogens	Oral contraceptives increase plasma concentration of corticosteroids
Hydralazine	Antagonism of hypotensive effect
Ketoconazole	Ketoconazole possibly inhibits metabolism of corticosteroids
Methotrexate	Increased risk of hematologic toxicity
Methyldopa	Antagonism of hypotensive effect
Mifepristone	Effect of corticosteroids (including inhaled corticosteroids) may be reduced for 3–4 d after mifepristone
Minoxidil	Antagonism of hypotensive effect
Moxonidine	Antagonism of hypotensive effect
Nonsteroidal anti-inflammatory drugs	Increased risk of gastrointestinal bleeding and ulceration
Nitrates	Antagonism of hypotensive effect
Nitroprusside	Antagonism of hypotensive effect
Phenytoin	Metabolism of corticosteroids accelerated (reduced effect)
Progestogens	Oral contraceptives increase plasma concentration of corticosteroids
Rifamycins	Accelerated metabolism of corticosteroids (reduced effect)
Ritonavir	Plasma concentration possibly increased by ritonavir
Somatropin	Growth-promoting effect may be inhibited
Sympathomimetics, β_2	Increased risk of hypokalemia with concomitant use of high doses
Theophylline	Increased risk of hypokalemia
Vaccines	High doses of corticosteroids impair immune response; avoid use of live vaccines
Deflazacort is a Corticosteroid and has the Following Interaction Information	
Antacids	Reduced absorption of deflazacort
Dexamethasone is a Corticosteroid and has the Following Interaction Information	
Ephedrine	Metabolism of dexamethasone accelerated
Indinavir	Possibly reduced plasma-indinavir concentration
Lopinavir	Possibly reduced plasma-lopinavir concentration
Ritonavir	Plasma concentration possibly increased by ritonavir
Saquinavir	Possibly reduced plasma-saquinavir concentration
Methylprednisolone is a Corticosteroid and has the Following Interaction Information	
Cyclosporin	Plasma-cyclosporin concentration increased by high-dose methylprednisolone (risk of convulsions)
Erythromycin	Erythromycin inhibits metabolism of methylprednisolone
Itraconazole	Itraconazole possibly inhibits metabolism of methylprednisolone
Ketoconazole	Ketoconazole inhibits metabolism of methylprednisolone
Prednisolone is a Corticosteroid and has the Following Interaction Information	
Cyclosporin	Increased plasma concentration of prednisolone
Ritonavir	Plasma concentration possibly increased by ritonavir
Beclomethasone, betamethasone, budesonide, cortisone, fludrocortisone, flunisolide, fluticasone, hydrocortisone, tetracosactide, and triamcinolone are corticosteroids but have no additional interaction information.	

The above-listed interactions do not generally apply to corticosteroids used for topical action (including inhalation).[63,91]
ACE, angiotensin-converting enzyme.

WITHDRAWAL OF CORTICOSTEROIDS

A *gradual* withdrawal of systemic corticosteroids should be considered in those subjects whose disease is unlikely to relapse and have

- recently received repeated courses (particularly if taken for longer than 3 weeks),
- taken a short course within 1 year of stopping long-term therapy,
- other possible causes of adrenal suppression,
- received more than 40 mg daily prednisolone (or equivalent) (in adults),
- been given repeat doses in the evening, and
- received more than 3 weeks' treatment.

Systemic corticosteroids may be stopped abruptly in those whose disease is unlikely to relapse *and* who have received treatment for 2 weeks or less *and* who are not included in the patient groups described above.[92]

During corticosteroid withdrawal, the dose may be reduced rapidly down to physiologic doses (equivalent to adult prednisolone dose of 5 mg daily) and then reduced more slowly. Assessment of the disease may be needed during withdrawal to ensure that relapse does not occur.[92]

RECENT ADVANCES IN SYNTHETIC GLUCOCORTICOIDS

The replication of natural circadian rhythms of cortisol and the minimization of side effects remain two challenging goals in the evolving field of novel synthetic glucocorticoids.[93,94] In an attempt to mimic the daily oscillations of cortisol concentrations, two novel and, one existing, glucocorticoid analogs have come to the fore.[95] Plenadren®, a combination of immediate- and delayed-release hydrocortisone, was compared with immediate-release hydrocortisone; the former was associated with body weight reduction and improvements in blood pressure, glucose metabolism, and quality of life.[96] The recent Dual Release Hydrocortisone *vs.* Conventional Glucocorticoid Replacement in Hypocortisolism (DREAM) study demonstrated that patients who were switched to modified-release hydrocortisone had a statistically significant body weight loss and an increase in $CD16^+$ natural killer cells compared to those who received regular hydrocortisone.[97] The latter effect might ameliorate the "low-grade systemic inflammatory state," thereby contributing to better quality of life scores.[95] Interestingly, the same investigators showed altered circadian expression of 19 of 68 genes in peripheral blood mononuclear cells compared to those receiving standard therapy in the same group of patients.[98]

Chronocort®, another modified-release hydrocortisone preparation, is administered on retiring to bed and on awakening, effectively reproducing the normal circadian oscillations of cortisol concentrations.[95] In a phase II clinical trial, patients with congenital adrenal hyperplasia, who received Chronocort, had increased suppression of 17-OH progesterone.[99] Neither Plenadren® nor Chronocort® have been licensed for use in pediatric patients. The TAIN (Treatment of Adrenal Insufficiency in Neonates) has developed Infacort, an immediate-release synthetic glucocorticoid analog, which consists of a microcrystalline core captured by a hydrocortisone layer that is further coated by several layers and an external "taste-making" one.[91] Recent clinical studies using Infacort® demonstrated promising beneficial results and no serious adverse effects.[100,101]

In addition to modified-release glucocorticoids, efforts have been made toward the design of novel glucocorticoid analogs with minimal adverse side effects.[94] As most glucocorticoid-induced side effects are mediated by GR transactivation, a logical approach has been to design the so-called "dissociated GR ligands," which could preferentially induce GR transrepression and/or GR interaction with the NF-κB. The latter is the predominant transcription factor activated during inflammatory conditions. An ever-increasing number of selective glucocorticoid receptor modulators (SGRMs), including CORT108297 and CORT118335, have been tested in many disease animal models.[102–106] Although there is promise for the future use of SGRMs in clinical practice, it still remains a big challenge to predict which molecular pathways and what types of tissues will be affected by these novel compounds. The evolving strong combination of molecular, cellular, and structural biology will provide us a deeper mechanistic understanding of selective GR actions.

REFERENCES

1. Stewart PM. The adrenal cortex. In: Larsen PR, Kronenberg HM, Melmed S, et al., eds. *Williams textbook of endocrinology*, 10th ed. Philadelphia, PA: Elsevier Science, 2003:491–551.
2. Miller WL. The adrenal cortex and its disorders. In: Brook CGD, Clayton P, Brown R, eds. *Brook's clinical pediatric endocrinology*, 5th ed. Oxford, UK: Blackwell Publishing Ltd., 2005:293–351.
3. Simpson ER, Waterman MR. Steroid biosynthesis in the adrenal cortex and its regulation by adrenocorticotropin. In: DeGroote LJ, Besser M, Burger HG, et al., eds. *Endocrinology*. Philadelphia, PA: W.B. Saunders, 1995:1630–1641.
4. Galon J, Franchimont D, Hiroi N, et al. Gene profiling reveals unknown enhancing and suppressive actions of glucocorticoids on immune cells. *FASEB J* 2002;16:61–71.
5. Stocco DM, Clark BJ. Regulation of the acute production of steroids in steroidogenic cells. *Endocr Rev* 1996;17:221–244.
6. Arakane F, Kallen CB, Watari H, et al. The mechanism of action of steroidogenic acute regulatory protein (StAR). StAR acts on the outside of mitochondria to stimulate steroidogenesis. *J Biol Chem* 1998;273:16339–16345.
7. Papadopoulos V. Structure and function of the peripheral-type benzodiazepine receptor in steroidogenic cells. *Proc Soc Exp Biol Med* 1998;217:130–142.
8. Nebert DW, Nelson DR, Coon MJ, et al. The P450 superfamily: update on new sequences, gene mapping, and recommended nomenclature. *DNA Cell Biol* 1991;10:1–14.
9. Cherradi N, Rossier MF, Vallotton MB, et al. Submitochondrial distribution of three key steroidogenic proteins (steroidogenic acute regulatory protein and cytochrome P450 scc and 3β-hydroxysteroid dehydrogenase isomerase enzymes) upon stimulation by intracellular calcium in adrenal glomerulosa cells. *J Biol Chem* 1997;272:7899–7909.
10. White PC, Curnow KM, Pascoe L. Disorders of steroid 11β-hydroxylase isozymes. *Endocr Rev* 1994;15:421–438.
11. Yanase T, Simpson ER, Waterman MR. 17α-hydroxylase/17,20-lyase deficiency: from clinical investigation to molecular definition. *Endocr Rev* 1991;12:91–108.
12. Penning TM. Molecular endocrinology of hydroxysteroid dehydrogenases. *Endocr Rev* 1997;18:281–305.
13. Simpson ER, Mahendroo MS, Means GD, et al. Aromatase cytochrome P450, the enzyme responsible for estrogen biosynthesis. *Endocr Rev* 1994;15:342–355.
14. Wilson JD, Griffin JE, Russell DW. Steroid 5α-reductase 2 deficiency. *Endocr Rev* 1993;14:577–593.
15. Wallace WH, Crowne EC, Shalet SM, et al. Episodic ACTH and cortisol secretion in normal children. *Clin Endocrinol (Oxf)* 1991;34(3):215–221.
16. Itoi K, Seasholtz AF, Watson SJ. Cellular and extracellular regulatory mechanisms of hypothalamic corticotropin-releasing hormone neurons. *J Endocr* 1998;45:13–33.
17. Habib KE, Gold PW, Chrousos GP. Neuroendocrinology of stress. *Endocrinol Metab Clin North Am* 2001;30(3):695–728.
18. Ehrhart-Bornstein M, Hinson JP, Bornstein SR, et al. Intraadrenal interactions in the regulation of adrenocortical steroidogenesis. *Endocr Rev* 1998;19(2):101–143.
19. Bornstein SR, Chrousos GP. Clinical review 104: adrenocorticotropin (ACTH)-and non-ACTH-mediated regulation of the adrenal cortex: neural and immune inputs. *J Clin Endocrinol Metab* 1999;84(5):1729–1736.
20. Keller-Wood ME, Dallman M. Corticosteroid inhibition of ACTH secretion. *Endocr Rev* 1984;5:1–24.
21. Reincke M, Beuschlein F, Menig G, et al. Localization and expression of adrenocorticotropic hormone receptor mRNA in normal and neoplastic human adrenal cortex. *J Endocrinol* 1998;156:415–423.
22. Krieger DT, Allen W, Rizzo F, et al. Characterization of the normal temporal pattern of plasma corticosteroid levels. *J Clin Endocrinol Metab* 1971;32(2):266–284.
23. Esteban NV, Yergey AL. Cortisol production rates measured by liquid chromatography/mass spectrometry. *Steroids* 1990;55(4):152–158.

24. Brien TG. Human corticosteroid binding globulin. *Clin Endocrinol (Oxf)* 1981;14(2):193–212.
25. Mataradze GD, Kurabekova RM, Rozen VB. The role of sex steroids in the formation of sex-differentiated concentrations of corticosteroid-binding globulin in rats. *J Endocrinol* 1992;132(2):235–240.
26. Stolk RP, Lamberts SW, de Jong FH, et al. Gender differences in the associations between cortisol and insulin in healthy subjects. *J Endocrinol* 1996;149(2):313–318.
27. Gower DB. Steroid catabolism and urinary excretion. In: Makin HLJ, ed. *Biochemistry of steroid hormones*. Oxford, UK: Blackwell Science Ltd., 1984:349–382.
28. Iyer RB, Binstock JM, Scwartz IS, et al. Human hepatic cortisol reductase activities: enzymatic properties and substrate specificities of cytosolic cortisol Δ4–5β-reductase and dihydrocortisol-3α-oxidoreductase(s). *Steroids* 1990;55:495–500.
29. Draper N, Stewart PM. 11beta-hydroxysteroid dehydrogenase and the pre-receptor regulation of corticosteroid hormone action. *J Endocrinol* 2005;186(2):251–271.
30. Abel SM, Maggs JL, Back DJ, et al. Cortisol metabolism by human liver *in vitro*—I. Metabolite identification and inter-individual variability. *J Steroid Biochem Mol Biol* 1992;43:713–719.
31. Carson-Jurica MA, Schrader WT, O'Malley BW. Steroid receptor family: structure and functions. *Endocr Rev* 1990;11(2):201–220.
32. Hollenberg SM, Weinberger C, Ong ES, et al. Primary structure and expression of a functional human glucocorticoid receptor cDNA. *Nature* 1985;318(6047):635–641.
33. Nicolaides NC, Galata Z, Kino T, et al. The human glucocorticoid receptor: molecular basis of biologic function. *Steroids* 2010;75(1):1–12.
34. Nader Chrousos GP, Kino T. Circadian rhythm transcription factor CLOCK regulates the transcriptional activity of the glucocorticoid receptor by acetylating its hinge region lysine cluster: potential physiological implications. *FASEB J* 2009;23(5):1572–1583.
35. Picard D, Yamamoto KR. Two signals mediate hormone-dependent nuclear localization of the glucocorticoid receptor. *EMBO J* 1987;6(11):3333–3340.
36. Hollenberg SM, Evans RM. Multiple and cooperative trans-activation domains of the human glucocorticoid receptor. *Cell* 1988;55(5):899–906.
37. Dalman FC, Scherrer LC, Taylor LP, et al. Localization of the 90-kDa heat shock protein-binding site within the hormone-binding domain of the glucocorticoid receptor by peptide competition. *J Biol Chem* 1991;266(6):3482–3490.
38. Oakley RH, Sar M, Cidlowski JA. The human glucocorticoid receptor beta isoform. Expression, biochemical properties, and putative function. *J Biol Chem* 1996;271(16):9550–9559.
39. Charmandari E, Chrousos GP, Ichijo T, et al. The human glucocorticoid receptor (hGR) beta isoform suppresses the transcriptional activity of hGRalpha by interfering with formation of active coactivator complexes. *Mol Endocrinol* 2005;19(1):52–64.
40. Kino T, Manoli I, Kelkar S, et al. Glucocorticoid receptor (GR) beta has intrinsic, GRalpha-independent transcriptional activity. *Biochem Biophys Res Commun* 2009;381(4):671–675.
41. Lu NZ, Cidlowski JA. Translational regulatory mechanisms generate N-terminal glucocorticoid receptor isoforms with unique transcriptional target genes. *Mol Cell* 2005;18(3):331–342.
42. Ramamoorthy S, Cidlowski JA. Corticosteroids: mechanisms of action in health and disease. *Rheum Dis Clin North Am* 2016;42(1):15–31.
43. Wu I, Shin SC, Cao Y, et al. Selective glucocorticoid receptor translational isoforms reveal glucocorticoid-induced apoptotic transcriptomes. *Cell Death Dis* 2013;4:e453.
44. Bamberger CM, Schulte HM, Chrousos GP. Molecular determinants of glucocorticoid receptor function and tissue sensitivity to glucocorticoids. *Endocr Rev* 1996;17(3):245–261.
45. McKenna NJ, O'Malley BW. Combinatorial control of gene expression by nuclear receptors and coregulators. *Cell* 2002;108(4):465–474.
46. Auboeuf D, Honig A, Berget SM, et al. Coordinate regulation of transcription and splicing by steroid receptor coregulators. *Science* 2002;298(5592):416–419.
47. Hudson WH, Youn C, Ortlund EA. The structural basis of direct glucocorticoid-mediated transrepression. *Nat Struct Mol Biol* 2013;20(1):53–58.
48. Surjit M, Ganti KP, Mukherji A, et al. Widespread negative response elements mediate direct repression by agonist-liganded glucocorticoid receptor. *Cell* 2011;145(2):224–241.
49. Groeneweg FL, Karst H, de Kloet ER, et al. Mineralocorticoid and glucocorticoid receptors at the neuronal membrane, regulators of nongenomic corticosteroid signalling. *Mol Cell Endocrinol* 2012;350(2):299–309.
50. Deng Q, Waxse B, Riquelme D, et al. Helix 8 of the ligand binding domain of the glucocorticoid receptor (GR) is essential for ligand binding. *Mol Cell Endocrinol* 2015;408:23–32.
51. Nicolaides NC, Kino T, Roberts ML, et al. The role of S-palmitoylation of the human glucocorticoid receptor (hGR) in mediating the nongenomic glucocorticoid actions. *J Mol Biochem* 2017;6(1):3–12.
52. Ayrout M, Simon V, Bernard V, et al. A novel non genomic glucocorticoid signaling mediated by a membrane palmitoylated glucocorticoid receptor cross talks with GnRH in gonadotrope cells. *Sci Rep* 2017;7(1):1537.
53. Löwenberg M, Verhaar AP, Bilderbeek J, et al. Glucocorticoids cause rapid dissociation of a T-cell-receptor-associated protein complex containing LCK and FYN. *EMBO Rep* 2006;7(10):1023–1029.
54. Hinz B, Hirschelmann R. Rapid non-genomic feedback effects of glucocorticoids on CRF-induced ACTH secretion in rats. *Pharm Res* 2000;17(10):1273–1277.
55. Hafezi-Moghadam A, Simoncini T, Yang Z, et al. Acute cardiovascular protective effects of corticosteroids are mediated by non-transcriptional activation of endothelial nitric oxide synthase. *Nat Med* 2002;8(5):473–479.
56. Karst H, Berger S, Turiault M, et al. Mineralocorticoid receptors are indispensable for nongenomic modulation of hippocampal glutamate transmission by corticosterone. *Proc Natl Acad Sci USA* 2005;102(52):19204–19207.
57. Psarra AM, Sekeris CE. Glucocorticoids induce mitochondrial gene transcription in HepG2 cells: role of the mitochondrial glucocorticoid receptor. *Biochim Biophys Acta* 2011;1813(10):1814–1821.
58. Nicolaides NC, Charmandari E. Novel insights into the molecular mechanisms underlying generalized glucocorticoid resistance and hypersensitivity syndromes. *Hormones (Athens)* 2017;16(2):124–138.
59. Miller TL, Mayo KE. Glucocorticoids regulate pituitary growth hormone-releasing hormone receptor messenger ribonucleic acid expression. *Endocrinology* 1999;138(6):2458–2465.
60. Magiakou MA, Mastorakos G, Chrousos GP. Final stature in patients with endogenous Cushing's syndrome. *J Clin Endocrinol Metab* 1994;79(4):1082–1085.
61. Magiakou MA, Mastorakos G, Gomez MT, et al. Suppressed spontaneous and stimulated growth hormone secretion in patients with Cushing's disease before and after surgical cure. *J Clin Endocrinol Metab* 1994;78(1):131–137.
62. Allen DB. Growth suppression by glucocorticoid therapy. *Endocrinol Metab Clin North Am* 1996;25(3):699–717.
63. Kaufmann S, Jones KL, Wehrenberg WB, et al. Inhibition by prednisone of growth hormone (GH) response to GH-releasing hormone in normal men. *J Clin Endocrinol Metab* 1988;67(6):1258–1261.
64. Miell JP, Corder R, Pralong FP, et al. Effects of dexamethasone on growth hormone (GH)-releasing hormone, arginine-and dopaminergic stimulated GH secretion, and total plasma insulin-like growth factor-I concentrations in normal male volunteers. *J Clin Endocrinol Metab* 1991;72(3):675–681.
65. Burguera B, Muruais C, Penalva A, et al. Dual and selective actions of glucocorticoids upon basal and stimulated growth hormone release in man. *Neuroendocrinology* 1990;51(1):51–58.
66. Charmandari E, Kino T, Souvatzoglou E, et al. Pediatric stress: hormonal mediators and human development. *Horm Res* 2003;59(4):161–179.
67. Iannuzzi DM, Ertsey R, Ballard PL. Biphasic glucocorticoid regulation of pulmonary SP-A: characterization of inhibitory process. *Am J Physiol* 1993;264(3 Pt 1):L236–L244.
68. Ballard PL, Ertsey R, Gonzales LW, et al. Transcriptional regulation of human pulmonary surfactant proteins SP-B and SP-C by glucocorticoids. *Am J Respir Cell Mol Biol* 1996;14(6):599–607.
69. Cole TJ, Blendy JA, Monaghan AP, et al. Targeted disruption of the glucocorticoid receptor gene blocks adrenergic chromaffin cell development and severely retards lung maturation. *Genes Dev* 1995;9(13):1608–1621.
70. Bronnegard M, Arner P, Hellstrom L, et al. Glucocorticoid receptor messenger ribonucleic acid in different regions of human adipose tissue. *Endocrinology* 1990;127(4):1689–1696.
71. Bujalska IJ, Kumar S, Stewart PM. Does central obesity reflect "Cushing's disease of the omentum"? *Lancet* 1997;349(9060):1210–1213.
72. Chrousos GP. The hypothalamic-pituitary-adrenal axis and immune-mediated inflammation. *N Engl J Med* 1995;332(20):1351–1362.
73. Boumpas DT, Chrousos GP, Wilder RL, et al. Glucocorticoid therapy for immune-mediated diseases: basic and clinical correlates. *Ann Intern Med* 1993;119(12):1198–1208.
74. DeRijk R, Michelson D, Karp B, et al. Exercise and circadian rhythm-induced variations in plasma cortisol differentially regulate interleukin-1 beta (IL-1 beta), IL-6, and tumor necrosis factor-alpha (TNF alpha) production in humans: high sensitivity of TNF alpha and resistance of IL-6. *J Clin Endocrinol Metab* 1997;82(7):2182–2191.
75. McEwen BS, De Kloet ER, Rostene W. Adrenal steroid receptors and actions in the nervous system. *Physiol Rev* 1986;66(4):1121–1188.
76. Wordinger RJ, Clark AF. Effects of glucocorticoids on the trabecular meshwork: towards a better understanding of glaucoma. *Prog Retin Eye Res* 1999;18(5):629–667.
77. Charmandari E, Nicolaides NC, Chrousos GP. Adrenal insufficiency. *Lancet* 2014;383(9935):2152–2167.
78. Bornstein SR, Allolio B, Arlt W, et al. Diagnosis and treatment of primary adrenal insufficiency: an endocrine society clinical practice guideline. *J Clin Endocrinol Metab* 2016;101(2):364–389.
79. Puar TH, Stikkelbroeck NM, Smans LC, et al. Adrenal crisis: still a deadly event in the 21st century. *Am J Med* 2016;129(3):339.e1–339.e9.
80. Oprea A, Bonnet NCG, Pollé O, et al. Novel insights into glucocorticoid replacement therapy for pediatric and adult adrenal insufficiency. *Ther Adv Endocrinol Metab* 2019;10:2042018818821294.
81. Øksnes M, Ross R, Løvås K. Optimal glucocorticoid replacement in adrenal insufficiency. *Best Pract Res Clin Endocrinol Metab* 2015;29(1):3–15.
82. Hahner S. Acute adrenal crisis and mortality in adrenal insufficiency: still a concern in 2018! *Ann Endocrinol* 2018;79:164–166.
83. Heidelbaugh JJ. Endocrinology update: hypopituitarism. *FP Essent* 2016;451:25–30.
84. Porter J, Blair J, Ross RJ. Is physiological glucocorticoid replacement important in children? *Arch Dis Child* 2017;102(2):199–205.
85. Clayton PE, Miller WL, Oberfield SE, et al. Consensus statement on 21-hydroxylase deficiency from the European Society for Paediatric Endocrinology and the Lawson Wilkins Pediatric Endocrine Society. *Horm Res* 2002;58(4):188–195.
86. British Medical Association & The Royal Pharmaceutical Society of Great Britain. *British National Formulary for Children* (Corticosteroids). 2006:421–430.
87. Kuperman H, Damiani D, Chrousos GP, et al. Evaluation of the hypothalamic-pituitary-adrenal axis in children with leukemia before and after 6 weeks of high-dose glucocorticoid therapy. *J Clin Endocrinol Metab* 2001;86(7):2993–2996.
88. Meduri GU, Tolley EA, Chrousos GP, et al. Prolonged methylprednisolone treatment suppresses systemic inflammation in patients with unresolving acute respiratory distress syndrome: evidence for inadequate endogenous glucocorticoid secretion and inflammation-induced immune cell resistance to glucocorticoids. *Am J Respir Crit Care Med* 2002;165(7):983–991.
89. So LK, Lau AC, Yam LY, et al. Development of a standard treatment protocol for severe acute respiratory syndrome. *Lancet* 2003;361(9369):1615–1617.
90. Nicolaides NC, Pavlaki AN, Magiakou MA, Chrousos GP. Glucocorticoid therapy and adrenal suppression. In: Feingold KR, Anawalt B, Boyce A, et al., eds. *Endotext [Internet]*. South Dartmouth, MA: MDText.com, Inc., 2000–2018.
91. British Medical Association & The Royal Pharmaceutical Society of Great Britain. *British National Formulary for Children* (Corticosteroids). 2006:767.
92. Nicolaides NC, Chrousos GP. Hypothalamic pituitary adrenal suppression. In: *Encyclopedia of endocrine diseases*, 2nd ed. Vol 3, 2018:83–89.
93. Scherholz ML, Schlesinger N, Androulakis IP. Chronopharmacology of glucocorticoids. *Adv Drug Deliv Rev* 2019;151–152:245–261.
94. Meijer OC, Koorneef LL, Kroon J. Glucocorticoid receptor modulators. *Ann Endocrinol (Paris)* 2018;79(3):107–111.

95. Stewart PM. Modified-release hydrocortisone: is it time to change clinical practice? *J Endocr Soc* 2019;3(6):1150–1153.
96. Johannsson G, Nilsson AG, Bergthorsdottir R, et al. Improved cortisol exposure-time profile and outcome in patients with adrenal insufficiency: a prospective randomized trial of a novel hydrocortisone dual-release formulation. *J Clin Endocrinol Metab* 2012;97(2):473–481.
97. Isidori AM, Venneri MA, Graziadio C, et al. Effect of once-daily, modified-release hydrocortisone versus standard glucocorticoid therapy on metabolism and innate immunity in patients with adrenal insufficiency (DREAM): a single-blind, randomised controlled trial. *Lancet Diabetes Endocrinol* 2018;6(3):173–185.
98. Venneri MA, Hasenmajer V, Fiore D, et al. Circadian rhythm of glucocorticoid administration entrains clock genes in immune cells: a DREAM trial ancillary study. *J Clin Endocrinol Metab* 2018;103(8):2998–3009.
99. Mallappa A, Sinaii N, Kumar P, et al. A phase 2 study of Chronocort, a modified-release formulation of hydrocortisone, in the treatment of adults with classic congenital adrenal hyperplasia. *J Clin Endocrinol Metab* 2015;100(3):1137–1145.
100. Whitaker MJ, Spielmann S, Digweed D, et al. Development and testing in healthy adults of oral hydrocortisone granules with taste masking for the treatment of neonates and infants with adrenal insufficiency. *J Clin Endocrinol Metab* 2015;100(4):1681–1688.
101. Neumann U, Whitaker MJ, Wiegand S, et al. Absorption and tolerability of taste-masked hydrocortisone granules in neonates, infants and children under 6 years of age with adrenal insufficiency. *Clin Endocrinol (Oxf)* 2018;88(1):21–29.
102. Kach J, Long TM, Selman P, et al. Selective glucocorticoid receptor modulators (SGRMs) delay castrate-resistant prostate cancer growth. *Mol Cancer Ther* 2017;16:1680–1692.
103. Pineau F, Canet G, Desrumaux C, et al. New selective glucocorticoid receptor modulators reverse amyloid-β peptide-induced hippocampus toxicity. *Neurobiol Aging* 2016;45:109–122.
104. Beaudry JL, Dunford EC, Teich T, et al. Effects of selective and non-selective glucocorticoid receptor II antagonists on rapid-onset diabetes in young rats. *PLoS One* 2014;9:e91248.
105. Hunt HJ, Ray NC, Hynd G, et al. Discovery of a novel non-steroidal GR antagonist with in vivo efficacy in the olanzapine-induced weight gain model in the rat. *Bioorg Med Chem Lett* 2012:1–5.
106. Meyer M, Gonzalez Deniselle MC, Hunt H, et al. The selective glucocorticoid receptor modulator CORT108297 restores faulty hippocampal parameters in Wobbler and corticosterone-treated mice. *J Steroid Biochem Mol Biol* 2014;143:40–48.

CHAPTER

55

Eda Cengiz
William V. Tamborlane

Insulin and Diabetes

Insulin has been named the "Miracle Drug" after its discovery in 1921 and transformed diabetes mellitus from a death sentence to a chronic disease with a demanding treatment regimen. Prior to the advent of insulin therapy, the life expectancy of children with type 1 diabetes mellitus (T1DM) was approximately 1 year from diagnosis. Referred to as the "Pissing Evile" in 17th-century England, this disease was known for its agonizing, unremitting progression to emaciation, coma, and death.[1]

In 1921, Banting, Best, Collip, and Macleod isolated insulin from beef pancreas and, in 1922, attempted to treat Leonard Thompson, a teenager with T1DM.[2] Once the effect of indulin on treating diabetes mellitus was demonstrated, the insulin preparation extracted from animal pancreas, containing numerous impurities and varying potency, was put in use immediately for the treatment of people with diabetes. Since then, insulin has been on the forefront of science, becoming one of the best-characterized vertebrate hormones, with a wealth of data on its crystalline structure and mechanism of action at the molecular, cellular, and organ levels. Its chemical structure was determined in 1951, which paved the way for insulin's chemical synthesis in 1960. The three-dimensional structure was determined by Dorothy Hodgkin in 1969, the insulin gene was cloned in 1980,[3] and recombinant insulin has been available commercially since this time. Insulin therapy has recently taken a turn toward the use of insulin analogs instead of native human insulin formulations, and there are continued studies on alternative routes of delivery.

TYPE 1 DIABETES MELLITUS

T1DM is characterized by varying degrees of absolute (not relative) insulinopenia due to T-cell–mediated autoimmune destruction of the pancreatic β cells. T1DM autoimmune markers include islet cell autoantibodies and autoantibodies to GAD (GAD65), insulin, the tyrosine phosphatases IA-2 and IA-2β, and ZnT8. A decline in insulin-secreting capacity for months or years precedes the clinical manifestation of diabetes, which usually occurs once 80% of the β cells have been destroyed. It can present at any age, ranging from infancy to mid-adulthood. The incidence of T1DM has increased worldwide in all age groups (even in the very young) postulated to be due to environmental factors.[4] In most countries, the highest incidence is found among children aged 10 to 14 years[5] and 3 to 6 years. Both sexes are affected in equal parts. In the past, T1DM was thought to occur more frequently in Caucasians. However, newer reports suggest that, in certain regions in the United States, African American children may be affected as frequently as Caucasian children.[6] Newly recognized cases are predominantly seen in the autumn and winter months, with many speculations as to the cause of this seasonal and long-term cyclical variation.[7–9] Furthermore, the natural regional proclivity for T1DM to the northern hemisphere (such as Finland and Sweden) as opposed to the southern hemisphere (Peru and Venezuela) remains unexplained.

Common symptoms at the time of presentation include a 2- to 3-week history of polyuria and polydipsia, weight loss, abdominal pain, anorexia, vomiting, and fatigue, reflecting the metabolic effects of insulin deficiency. Especially in young children, a history of abdominal pain and vomiting is often misinterpreted as part of a viral syndrome. Therefore, routine urine testing of glucose and ketones is warranted in any child who presents with these complaints. Although the presence of glucosuria is a good screening tool, the following criteria have been established to confirm the diagnosis: a random serum glucose level of 200 mg per dL or more (11.1 mmol per L) must accompany symptoms suggestive of diabetes. Alternatively, a fasting serum glucose level of 126 mg per dL or more (7 mmol per L) can also establish the diagnosis. HbA_{1c} is an indirect measure of average blood glucose levels and multiple factors, including age, race/ethnicity, and anemia/hemoglobinopathies, may impact hemoglobin glycation independently of glycemia. HbA_{1c} 6.5% (48 mmol per mol) or higher has been introduced as another metric to diagnose T1DM.[10] It remains unclear whether HbA_{1c} and the same HbA_{1c} cut-point should be used to diagnose diabetes in children and adolescents, given that the epidemiologic studies that formed the basis for recommending HbA_{1c} to diagnose diabetes included only adult populations. Only blood glucose criteria should be used to diagnose diabetes in conditions associated with increased red blood cell turnover, such as sickle cell disease, pregnancy (second and third trimesters), hemodialysis, recent blood loss or transfusion, or erythropoietin therapy. If a test result is suggestive of T1DM, it is recommended that the same test be repeated, or a different test be performed without delay using a new blood sample to confirm the diagnosis. If two different tests (such as HbA_{1c} and fasting plasma glucose) are both above the diagnostic threshold, this also confirms the diagnosis. On the other hand, if a patient has discordant results from two different tests, then the test result that is above the diagnostic cut-point should be repeated, with consideration of the possibility of HbA_{1c} assay interference.[10]

Glucosuria alone is not diagnostic of diabetes in children as it often accompanies a variety of renal tubular disorders.

Glucosuria (with mild hyperglycemia) may also be stress induced during severe infection or steroid therapy. In these cases, hyperglycemia is transient and remits after convalescence.

People with T1DM often present with acute symptoms of diabetes and markedly elevated blood glucose levels, and approximately one-third are diagnosed with life-threatening diabetic ketoacidosis (DKA). As soon as the diagnosis of diabetes is established, insulin therapy should be initiated promptly to prevent further metabolic decompensation and the development or worsening of DKA. After initiation of insulin therapy, there is a partial recovery of β-cell function. During this so-called honeymoon period, diabetes control is quite good and easy to achieve.[11] The duration of the honeymoon period is variable, lasting from weeks up to 2 years, after which the insulin secretory capacity of the β cell declines permanently.

T1DM is a manageable disease if treated appropriately. HbA_{1c} has been a well-established measure of glycemic control. A rising percentage of the glycosylated hemoglobin fraction, HbA_{1c}, indicates a higher-than-normal glucose exposure of the erythrocyte during its life span of 120 days; therefore, it is an objective measure of glycemic control over the past 2 to 3 months. HbA_{1c} level lower than 7.5% should be maintained to prevent acute and chronic complications of T1DM under the age of 19 years based on the International Society for Pediatric and Adolescent Diabetes (ISPAD) and the American Diabetes Association (ADA) guidelines.

Patients with T1DM are prone to other autoimmune disorders, such as Hashimoto thyroiditis, Graves disease, Addison disease, celiac disease, vitiligo, autoimmune hepatitis, myasthenia gravis, and pernicious anemia, and should be monitored for these autoimmune diseases.

INSULIN

Insulin is a globular protein containing two chains (Fig. 55.1): the A chain consists of 21 residues, and the B chain has 30 residues, and the molecule is linked by three disulfide bridges (two interchain: A7–B7 and A20–B19, and one intra–A chain: A6–A11).[12]

Insulin plays a central role in the regulation of vertebrate metabolism with a profound effect on carbohydrates. It also exerts significant control over lipid, protein, and mineral metabolism. The most pronounced insulin effect is found at its three target tissues: liver, fat, and muscle.

The liver is a key organ in maintaining a steady state of serum glucose levels, tightly controlled by the insulin-to-glucagon ratio in the portal circulation. There is minimal direct insulin effect on the hepatocyte glucose transporter 2 (GLUT2); instead, insulin indirectly promotes glucose uptake into the liver by stimulating enzymes involved in glucose metabolism and storage. In a fasting state, low insulin levels enhance gluconeogenesis from glucose precursors, while the relative glucagon predominance stimulates glycogenolysis. Both of these processes are synergistic in achieving a steady fasting hepatic glucose production rate of 2 mg per kg per minute in adults and averaged 5 to 7 mg per kg per minute in children.[13]

As soon as insulin levels rise postprandially, hepatic glucose production is suppressed, and glycogenesis and fatty acid synthesis are enhanced. Once the liver is saturated with glycogen, any additional glucose, under the presence of insulin, is shunted to the synthesis of fatty acids. The fatty acids are esterified with α-glycerol phosphate to produce triglycerides, which are then transported as the very low-density lipoprotein (VLDL) fraction to the adipocyte.

In the adipose tissue, insulin enhances the activity of lipoprotein lipase, which is found in the capillary endothelium. Lipoprotein lipase hydrolyzes the triglycerides of the VLDL fraction to fatty acids and monoglycerides. Fatty acids are membrane permeable and can easily enter the adipocyte, where they are re-esterified to triglycerides. Insulin plays a key role in creating these fat stores by directly enhancing glucose uptake into the adipocyte through stimulating glucose transporter 4 (GLUT4), which facilitates glucose entry into the cell (see "Insulin Receptor" section). Intracellular glucose in the adipocyte increases glycolysis, which increases the production of α-glycerol phosphate needed for fat esterification. Furthermore, insulin inhibits the breakdown of fat through inhibiting hormone-sensitive lipase, which induces lipolysis in the insulin-depleted state.

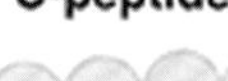

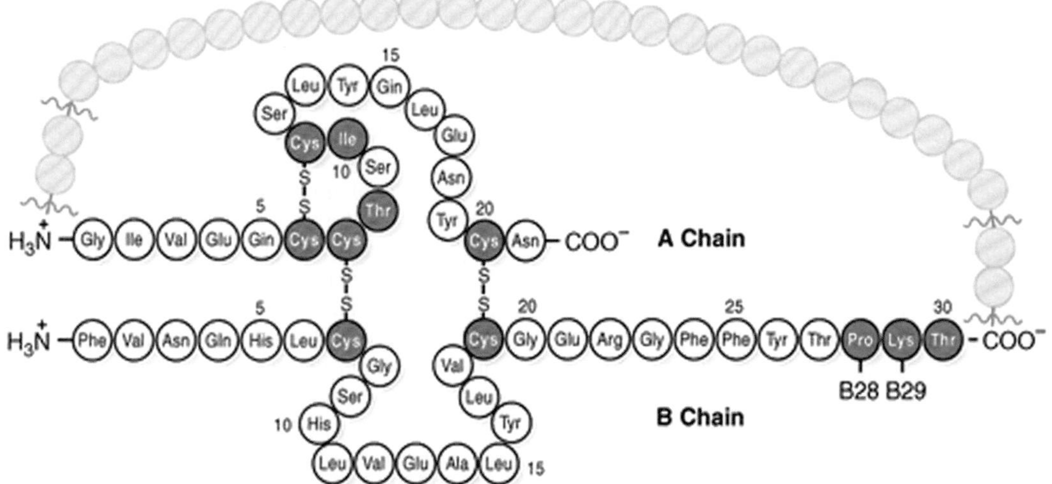

Figure 55.1 Insulin structure. (From Lieberman MA, Marks A, Peet A. *Marks' Basic Medical Biochemistry*. Philadelphia, PA: Lippincott Williams & Wilkins, 2013.)

In muscle, the main function of insulin is to facilitate glucose entry into the cell by binding to the insulin receptor, which then upregulates GLUT4. Once inside the muscle, glucose is used for immediate energy expenditure and for building up muscle glycogen stores. Insulin furthermore has an anabolic effect on the muscle, promoting positive nitrogen balance by enhancing amino-acid (especially branched chain amino acids) uptake, inhibiting protein breakdown, and, to a lesser extent, promoting protein synthesis. During fasting (low insulin state), glucose is mainly taken up by organs that do not depend on insulin for glucose transport, such as the brain.

Insulin also activates the sodium–potassium adenosine triphosphatase (ATPase) in many cells and, therefore, enhances potassium flux into the cell, even in the absence of glucose movement or pH changes.

The physiologic journey of insulin from its synthesis to its final destination in cells is summarized in the following sections.

SYNTHESIS OF INSULIN

Insulin synthesis is confined to the pancreatic islet β cells. The β cells make up the bulk of the Langerhans islet and reside in the center of the islet closest to the blood supply. Islets are surrounded by capillaries with small pores, the fenestrae, allowing permeability and unrestricted nutrient exchange. Consequently, β cells can sense the nutritional state of the circulation quickly and respond by releasing insulin that diffuses from the fenestrae in to the circulation.[14] Glucagon-secreting α cells surround the β cells in a circular pattern. The outmost layer of the islet cell is formed by somatostatin- and gastrin-secreting δ cells. Islets containing α, β, and δ cells are mostly found in the anterior lobe, body, and tail of the pancreas. They are connected through gap junctions, a feature that has been proposed in facilitating the paracrine effect of insulin on glucagon and somatostatin. Polypeptide-producing F cells are also found in a portion of islet cells. They are restricted to those islets located in the posterior lobe of the pancreas head and are supplied by a separate vascular system. Even though the Langerhans islets are the most powerful regulators of glucose metabolism, they comprise less than 1% of the pancreatic organ mass. The average person has about 1 million islets varying in size from 50 to 300 μm in diameter.

Insulin originates in the form of a large precursor, preproinsulin, that is synthesized in the ribosome of the β cell's rough endoplasmic reticulum. This 110-amino-acid peptide is encoded by a single gene located on chromosome 11.[15] Microsomal signal peptidases rapidly excise a terminal portion of the peptide chain, leaving 86-amino-acid proinsulin to be transported to the Golgi apparatus. There it is packaged into secretory vesicles, located close to the cell membrane. The 21 amino acids adjacent to the COOH terminus of the insulin protein are referred to as the α chain. The α chain is joined via a dipeptide bond to the 31-amino-acid c (connecting) peptide. Another dipeptide link connects the c-peptide chain further to the 30 amino acids of the β chain, leading up to the protein's NH_2 terminus. The tertiary structure of insulin is created by the folding and oxidation of the proinsulin in which two disulfide bridges are created between the α and β chain and another disulfide bridge within the α chain. In the secretory granules, c-peptide is split off from proinsulin, resulting in equimolar release of insulin and c-peptide. The insulin secretion process involves fusion of the cell membrane and secretory granules with subsequent exocytosis of not only insulin and c-peptide but also small amounts of proinsulin. Although c-peptide has no insulin-like effect, proinsulin has about 7% to 8% of the biologic activity of insulin.[16] Unlike most protein hormones, the insulin structure is highly conserved among the species. Porcine insulin differs from human insulin only by one amino acid in the β chain and bovine insulin by three amino-acid residues.

INSULIN SECRETION

Insulin secretion after carbohydrate intake is a highly dynamic process regulated by various factors and involves the fusion of insulin granules with the β-cell plasma membrane and exocytosis of granule content. Glucose is the main stimulator of insulin release from the β cell. The insulin release occurs in a characteristic biphasic pattern; an acute "first phase" that lasts only a few minutes with insulin secretion peaking at 1.4 nmol per minute, followed by a sustained "second phase" with the secreting rate at approximately 0.4 nmol per minute. The stimulation of insulin secretion is detectable at glucose concentrations as low as 54 mg/dl (3 mmol/L) and reaches a half-maximal stimulation at 108mg/dL (6 mmol/L).[17] Insulin is secreted directly into the portal vein and is immediately degraded by liver insulinases to approximately half of its original concentration. In serum, insulin levels rise to maximum levels 30 to 45 minutes after food ingestion and decline to basal levels by 2 to 3 hours postprandial. During prolonged fasting, both glucose and insulin levels will drop even further, but insulin levels will remain measurable between 2 and 5 μU per mL.[18]

Although glucose is the strongest stimulator of insulin secretion, other sugars (e.g., mannose), certain amino acids (e.g., arginine, leucine), other hormones and neurotransmitters, and vagal nerve stimulation also modulate insulin secretion, keeping glucose concentrations in a narrow range.

In the rodent, glucose is transported into the β cell by a high-capacity (GLUT2) glucose transporter.[19] GLUT2 is also the predominant glucose transporter in human pancreas and liver and is capable of bidirectional transport, allowing transport in either direction depending on the glucose concentration on each side of the membrane. Other GLUT isoforms (GLUT1 or GLUT3) that are ubiquitously present in most cells may also contribute to basal transport activity into the pancreas.

After uptake into the islet cell, glucose is phosphorylated to glucose-6-phosphate by glucokinase, the rate-limiting step of glucose metabolism in the islet cell.[20] Glucokinase serves as the islets' "glucose sensor," and its activity is tightly linked to glucose levels. Mutations in the glucokinase gene have been associated with defects in glucose sensing, necessitating higher glucose levels to stimulate insulin secretion. This defect is clinically referred to as MODY 2 (maturity-onset diabetes of youth, form 2), leading to mild hyperglycemia.[21,22]

Intracellular glucose metabolism raises ATP levels, which, in turn, close the potassium-dependent (K^-) ATP channels in the β-cell membrane. The subsequent suppression of potassium (K) efflux leads to a progressive depolarization of the plasma membrane and the firing of action potentials. A drop in voltage follows, opening the voltage-sensitive L-type calcium channels for an influx of calcium ions.[23] The rise of cytoplasmic calcium concentrations leads to a series of poorly defined reactions that culminate in the extrusion of insulin granules. Insulin assembles as a Zn^{2+}-coordinated hexamer in the human β cell[24] and functions in the bloodstream as a Zn^{2+}-free monomer.[25]

Each β cell contains thousands of K-ATP channels, which in fasting conditions are open, clamping the cell membrane potential at −70 mV. Sulfonylureas are hypoglycemic agents that are now known to modulate the K-ATP channel by attaching to a specific 145-kDa channel subunit named SUR.[26] Sulfonylureas attach to the receptor and inhibit the K-ATP channel. The subsequent cascade of membrane depolarization and calcium influx then leads to an insulin secretory effect that is independent of serum glucose levels. Loss-of-function mutations in the gene encoding the β-cell potassium channel result in persistent hyperinsulinemic hypoglycemia of infancy.[27,28] Gain-of-function mutations of the same gene results in certain types of neonatal diabetes mellitus that can respond to Sulfonylureas, and some patients can be taken off insulin.[29–31]

INSULIN RECEPTOR

Insulin action is mediated by the insulin receptor, a transmembrane glycoprotein present in virtually all vertebrates. Under healthy conditions, only a small proportion of the total available cell receptors are occupied to achieve maximal biologic effect. High ambient insulin levels downregulate the insulin receptor by reducing the number of available insulin receptors. Furthermore, saturation of the receptor with insulin leads to "negative cooperativity," a term used for reduced affinity for insulin in the adjacent receptor. The human insulin receptor was cloned in 1985,[32] and the gene maps to the short arm of chromosome 19.[33]

There are two insulin receptor isoforms, the insulin receptor isoform A (IRA) and the insulin receptor isoform B (IRB). These two isoforms are differentiated by an extracellular 12-amino-acid carboxy-terminal sequence and are associated with differential biologic functions driven by their differential expression in various tissues.[34] IRA is predominantly expressed in the brain, spleen, and cancerous cells and mediates the mitogenic activity of insulin,[35] and IRB is located in organs involved in glucose metabolism, such as the liver, and mediates the metabolic activity of insulin.[34] Insulin can exert some of its action through hybrid insulin receptors that are formed between IRA, IRB, and insulin-like growth factor 1 receptor (IGF1R) by heterodimeric associations.[35,36]

The structural components of the receptor are two extracellular α subunits that are linked to each other as well as to the two β subunits by disulfide bonds, forming a heterodimer. The α subunits are external to the cell membrane and contain the hormone-binding sites. The transmembrane-spanning β subunit has three domains: extracellular, transmembrane, and cytosolic. The cytosolic domain contains tyrosine protein kinase activity. The binding of insulin at the extracellular α subunit is transduced to the intracellular β subunits, leading to rapid onset of receptor autophosphorylation.[37] Among the proteins phosphorylated are the insulin receptor substrates 1 to 3 (IRS-1 to IRS-3). IRS-1 acts as a docking protein for other proteins, such as phosphatidylinositol 3 kinase (PI3 K). The cellular products created by PI3 K, in turn, appear to activate the translocation of glucose transport proteins (GLUT4) to the cell surface, facilitating glucose uptake. GLUT4 is available in the cytoplasm of all cells that have insulin-sensitive glucose transport across the cell membrane. Once insulin binds to the receptor, GLUT4 migrates to the cell surface, allowing the cell to efficiently take up glucose.

After binding to the receptor, the receptor–insulin complex is internalized and processed to release of free insulin and recycling of the receptor back to the cell membrane. Whether the internalization of insulin permits any special action of insulin at the level of the nucleus remains a speculation, and insulin action beyond receptor activation is incompletely defined.

INSULIN SIGNALING

Insulin's binding to its receptor stimulates signal transduction pathway that culminate in GLUT4 translocation to the plasma membrane. GLUT4 is responsible for glucose uptake in all cells whose glucose transport across the cell membrane is insulin dependent. Once insulin binds to the receptor, two distinct intracellular signal transduction pathways lead to a migration of GLUT4 to the cell surface, allowing the cell to efficiently take up glucose.

The first pathway is often referred to as the IRS/PI3 K/Akt pathway.[38,39] In this pathway, IRS-1 is tyrosine phosphorylated by the insulin-stimulated tyrosine kinase activity of the insulin receptor. This allows the regulatory unit (p85) of PI3 K to dock onto the IRS-1, which, in turn, activates PI3 K. This leads to a generation of phosphatidylinositol 3,4,5-triphosphate (PIP3), which, in turn, activates the Ser/Thr kinases Akt and atypical protein kinase C (aPKC). These kinases are essential in the process of GLUT4 translocation to the cell surface, facilitating glucose uptake. The second pathway is also referred to as the Cbl–CAP pathway.[40,41] Under the presence of the adapter protein CAP, the Cbl proto-oncoprotein is tyrosine phosphorylated.[40] The CAP–Cbl complex then dissociates from the insulin receptor and move to a lipid raft subdomain of the plasma membrane for a second route of GLUT4 translocation.[42]

EXOGENOUS INSULIN TREATMENT

Although normoglycemia is a fairly concise treatment goal in diabetes management, the clinical use of insulin is remarkably complex. With so many nutritional, hormonal, and lifestyle variables affecting glucose homeostasis, there is rarely a predictable treatment algorithm that applies to all patients, especially in children and adolescents with T1DM. Even in a single patient, treatment regiments remain under constant scrutiny warranting regular reassessments and fine-tuning. Therefore, insulin regimens are never absolute, but loose guidelines that mold with the patient throughout life.

In general, insulin requirements in a patient with newly diagnosed T1D are calculated based on the age, pubertal status, and the presence of ketonuria. Young children (toddlers) who do not present with ketoacidosis may only require 0.3 units per kg per day. The average prepubertal child will require 0.5 to 0.75 units per kg per day, possibly more in the presence of ketosis. Pubertal children will be more insulin resistant due to their higher physiologic levels of growth hormone and usually require 1 to 1.5 units per kg per day. Within 1 to 3 weeks of commencing therapy, insulin requirements usually decrease drastically as partial remission (honeymoon period) occurs. To maximize the duration of remission, it is recommended that a twice-daily insulin regimen is maintained (even at a low dose of 0.2 units per kg per day), as long as episodes of hypoglycemia do not ensue.

EVOLUTION OF INSULIN: ANIMAL AND HUMAN INSULIN PREPARATIONS

Following the discovery of insulin, animal-sourced insulin became the main source of supply for insulin treatment. Animal insulins had low purity, however maintained biologic function when applied to humans. Today animal insulins are obsolete in the management of diabetes mellitus. However, the different animal preparations with their various pharmacodynamics have become the prototype after which synthetic human insulins are modeled. They are, therefore, of exemplifying interest.

Shortly after the discovery of insulin, pork and beef insulin products became the treatment of choice for several decades. Early on in the commercial production, trace quantities of zinc were added to produce "regular" insulin, a more stable (crystalline zinc) insulin.[43] The duration of this regular insulin was on average 5 to 8 hours, often too short for overnight glucose control. Protamine, a basic fish (trout) protein, was added to slow down the absorption from the subcutis by decreasing the solubility at physiologic pH.[44] Combining both zinc and protamine further extended absorption time, leading to insulin action in excess of 24 hours.[45] In 1946, the Hagedorn Laboratories produced a protamine zinc insulin in which protamine was added in stoichiometric proportions to insulin, thereby reducing excess free protamine in solution. Hagedorn coined the name "isophane" (Greek: equal appearance) for the long-acting insulin, but the name did not stick and it became known as NPH (neutral protamine Hagedorn) insulin. Another method to prolongate insulin action without adding a protein was the creation of a zinc–insulin complex in the presence of large amounts of zinc and acetate buffer. Under careful pH adjustments, this insulin could be produced in a completely crystalline form (ultralente) or as an amorphous precipitate (semilente). The combination of these two zinc-acetate insulins (70% ultralente and 30% semilente) created lente insulin, with a similar duration to NPH. One of the major limitations of these animal insulins was their immunogenic potential, stemming from contamination with pancreatic extract impurities, such as animal c-peptide, proinsulin, glucagon, somatostatin, and pancreatic polypeptide.[46] Chromatographic purification techniques were used to produce purified animal insulin after 1974. The foreign amino-acid sequence itself was also proposed to contribute to immunogenicity, leading to insulin resistance.[47] To avoid the effect of a foreign protein sequence, a semisynthetic insulin was developed in which the human amino-acid sequence was created by switching out the differentiating amino acid in porcine insulin.[48]

The first synthesis of human insulin by recombinant DNA (rDNA) technology in 1978 represents a seminal milestone in the history of this hormone. Recombinant biosynthesis of insulin enabled production of virtually unlimited quantities of the human protein. Advances in peptide chemistry and rDNA-based macromolecule synthesis have enabled the synthesis of structurally optimized insulin analogs capable of delivering superior pharmacology by the production of completely synthetic human insulin in the 1980s. The initial process entailed separate production of the α and β chains from *Escherichia coli* with biochemical combination of the two chains to yield an intact molecule.[49] In 1986, human insulin could be produced in its entirety from synthetic proinsulin. This method includes the insertion of a synthetic proinsulin into the genome of baker's yeast with subsequent enzymatic yield of human insulin and c-peptide. This technique allows for natural post-translational folding of the peptide and ensures the appropriate three-dimensional structure of the molecule.[50,51]

Human insulins have been marketed as regular (short acting), NPH and lente (intermediate acting), and ultralente (long acting) with identical formulations as their animal counterparts in respect to content of auxiliary substances. They have very similar biologic potency to animal insulin when given intravenously.[52,53] However, subcutaneous (SC) administration of intermediate- or long-acting human insulin has a shorter time–action profile than animal insulin, and lente and ultralente insulins are no longer used in clinical practice.

CONTEMPORARY INSULIN TREATMENT REGIMENS

Exogenous insulin replacement consists of bolus and basal insulin. The bolus insulin is essential for prandial coverage and for supplemental correction doses to lower high blood glucose levels to a target range. Prandial insulin boluses attempt to mimic endogenous insulin secretion from the βcell in response to food intake that occurs in a rapid first phase followed by a sustained second phase with prolonged release of insulin in to the portal circulation. Correction insulin boluses can be given premeal or in between meals to normalize glycemia. Basal insulin controls hepatic glucose output and lipolysis (Fig. 55.2).

A common initial insulin regimen after diagnosis is a twice-daily injections of human intermediate-acting (NPH) or long-acting (detemir, glargine) insulin and injections of short-acting insulin (regular insulin) or rapid-acting insulin (RAI) (insulin lispro, insulin aspart, insulin glulisine). In

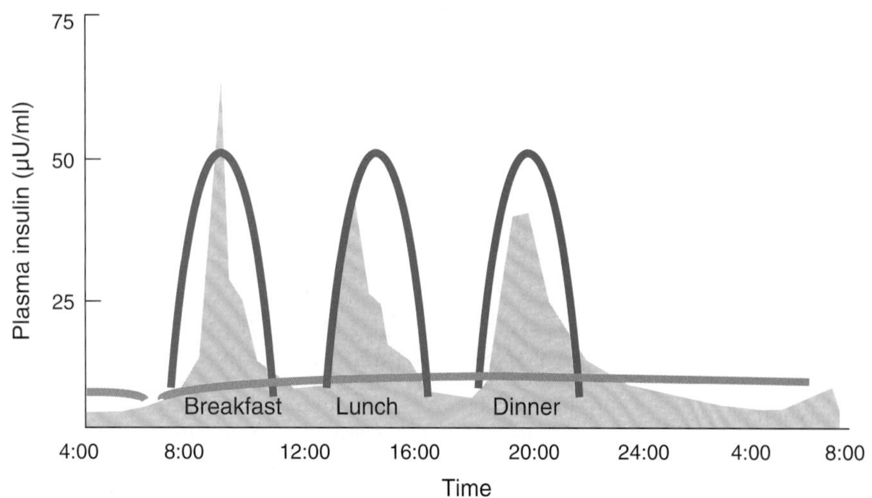

Figure 55.2 Basal-bolus insulin graph.

general, when patients are on an NPH or detemir insulin with an RAI regimen, two-thirds of the total dose is given before breakfast and one-third before dinner. The prebreakfast and predinner doses are composed of two-thirds intermediate-acting insulin and one-third short-acting insulin and given as a single (mixed) injection. Glargine is considered a 24-hour insulin, with some exceptions; therefore, patients receive a once-daily injection of glargine with RAI injection for each meal.

The twice-daily insulin injection regimen could be sufficient during the honeymoon period due to the fact that the endogenous insulin secretion provides much of the overnight basal insulin requirements, leading to normal fasting blood glucose values. Thus, increased and more labile prebreakfast glucose levels herald the loss of residual β-cell function, often necessitating a third injection. To contain rising morning blood glucose values, the predinner dose can be separated into an injection of short-acting insulin before dinner and long-acting insulin before bedtime, thereby delaying peak action to the early morning hours. Although theoretically sound, the challenge remains to achieve normoglycemia in the morning, while avoiding nocturnal hypoglycemia during the nighttime fast. The physiologic basis for this battle with morning hyperglycemia is the dawn phenomenon, an early morning surge of counterregulatory hormones, mainly growth hormone and cortisol. Dawn phenomenon must be differentiated from rebound hyperglycemia (Somogyi effect) that results from a counterregulatory hormone rise in response to an untoward nocturnal hypoglycemia. Most diabetes care providers have no hesitations switching to a variety of three-injection regimens, trying to match varying peak actions with the lifestyle of the patient and his or her family. Prefilled, disposable pen devices of one type of insulin have made it easier for patients to accept split-dose regimens or extra injections before lunch or before an afternoon snack. Various jet (transcutaneous pressure) injectors have also become available commercially over the past decade. Theoretically, they are indicated for children with needle phobia and are deemed to have the therapeutic advantage of increased accuracy and better SC dispersion with subsequent faster absorption. Because they are cumbersome to use and often traumatize the skin (causing greater discomfort), they have not penetrated the pediatric market very well. Disposable insulin pens with ultrafine short needles are by far the more popular alternative for a single insulin injection.

To gain better control, a third type of insulin, such as ultralente, was sometimes added to the morning or evening injection mixture to cover for waning NPH levels in the late afternoon and early morning. However, with the recent advent of the 24-hour peakless insulin glargine analog, such regimens became a managing style of the past. Insulin glargine has a flatter and longer time–activity profile than NPH or ultralente and, therefore, more closely mimics the basal insulin activity of the pancreas. The only disadvantage of insulin glargine in multiple injection regimens is that it cannot be mixed with other insulins, requiring a separate injection. Unlike other long-acting insulins that are cloudy in appearance, insulin glargine is clear like the short-acting insulins. There is concern that it would be easy to confuse the two types of insulin, leading to significant dosing and administration errors. However, the fact that insulin glargine is fully suspended in solution may decrease technical errors, as it does not require resuspension prior to administration. Disposable pens with premixed-intermediate (NPH) and short-acting (insulin lispro or regular) insulin are also available, but they are rigid in their composition and allow little flexibility in fine-tuning glycemic control. They are usually used in patients whose compliance with insulin administration is at stake and the simplest dosing regimen is maintained to avoid DKA. Sometimes, these premixed preparations are indicated if it is an impossible feat for the patient or caregiver to mix insulin, resulting in major dosing errors.

When interpreting blood glucose readings, a number of factors that affect injection therapy must be considered prior to making an actual insulin dose adjustment. First and foremost, compliance and administration technique must be considered. From a psychosocial aspect, children and adolescents will often painstakingly cover up missed injections. A review of skills is equally important in uncovering technical slips, which can lead to poor glycemic control. For example, the long-acting insulins such as NPH need to be resuspended prior to injection for concentration constancy between injections. Omitting this crucial step leads to great variability in glycemic control. Furthermore, the presence of hypertrophied injection sites, which results from local growth factor effect of repeated insulin injections into the same site, can slow down or decrease absorption. The site location is another factor that comes into the equation when fine-tuning insulin regimens. Insulin is absorbed most rapidly from the SC abdomen and less rapidly from the arms. Absorption is most delayed from the SC tissue in the legs. The depth of injection, the ambient temperature, or the state of perfusion at the injection site can also affect absorption.

An alternative to multiple-daily injection (MDI) that has revolutionized diabetes management is continuous subcutaneous insulin infusion (CSII) therapy, also referred to as insulin pump therapy. For many families, this is the preferred choice for achieving the goals of intensive therapy with increased lifestyle flexibility.

INSULIN ANALOGS

Insulin analogs are modified human insulin molecules with altered pharmacodynamic and physicochemical properties. Human insulin could be modified by changing the amino-acid sequence or by the addition of free fatty acid chains to the original molecule that primarily leads to altered absorption from the SC tissue (PMID: 26560137). The alteration could serve one of two main purposes: to accelerate insulin absorption for a rapid onset of action and shorter duration or to slow down the absorption to prolong the insulin action with a more stable glucodynamic action. The ultimate goal has been to create a formulation using molecular technology that could mimic endogenous insulin action as close as possible. Throughout the years, the clinical use of both rapid-and long-acting new insulin analogs has made achieving target glycemic control with less hypoglycemia a possibility despite the challenges with SC absorption particularly for RAI analogs.

Rapid-Acting Insulin Analogs

RAI analogs were developed with an intent to accelerate insulin absorption, thereby minimizing postprandial glucose (PPG) excursions more effectively. The change in amino-acid sequences, for instance, replacement of proline by lysine at B28 and lysine by proline at B29, led to the development of insulin lispro. Insulin glulisine was developed by replacing asparagine with lysine at B3 and replacing of lysine with glutamic acid at B29. Insulin aspart was produced by replacing proline by aspartic acid at B28.

These changes in B chain of insulin impaired the tendency of insulin chains to aggregate as dimers and hexamers, hence faster dissociation in the SC space after injection. Subsequently, monomeric form of insulin is absorbed more rapidly into circulation after SC injection with a more rapid onset on glucose-lowering action and less protracted insulin action.[54,55] Figure 55.3 shows the amino-acid substitutions in current RAIs.

New RAI analogs (lispro, aspart, glulisine) reduce PPG excursions as compared to regular insulin with their earlier absorption and action profiles. These RAI analogs permitted insulin injection closer to meal onset, allowing greater flexibility in daily life. Moreover, the risk of hypoglycemia for several hours after the meal has been reduced, given that regular insulin had prolonged duration of action after its injection. RAI analogs have also become the insulins of choice for use in CSII, where algorithms for bolus calculation and basal rate adaptations rely on the more rapid onset of action of these insulins. The convenience of taking the injection 15 minutes before or even with the meal as opposed to 30 to 40 minutes prior to the meal also led to better compliance with therapy. Faster onset of action, earlier peak activity, and higher peak concentrations of rapid-acting analogs have been particularly beneficial in overcoming problems associated with insulin resistance of puberty.

The first insulin analog in this group did not quite make it to clinical use because of one important side effect. Asp (B10) insulin was engineered by replacing the naturally occurring histidine with aspartic acid on residue 10 of the insulin β chain and was found to be absorbed twice as fast as regular insulin.[56] However, this simple amino-acid exchange altered the three-dimensional structure of insulin, leading to increased affinity of this molecule to the structurally related IGF1R. Furthermore, Asp (B10) insulin demonstrated extended activation of the insulin receptor with decreased dissociation and prolonged stimulation of cellular processing.[57,58] This mitogenic risk was confirmed in Sprague-Dawley rats that developed mammary tumors after supraphysiologic doses of this analog. Further human application of this analog has since then been halted.

In 1996, the first RAI analog, insulin lispro, was Food and Drug Administration (FDA) approved for clinical use. Insulin lispro received its name from its chemical structure in which the amino acid lysine at position 29 of the β chain was exchanged with the position 28 proline of the same chain. This amino-acid reversal decreases the tendency of insulin to self-associate, leading to faster absorption, higher peak levels, and shorter duration of action.[59] Studies comparing regular insulin and insulin lispro demonstrated no difference in affinity to the insulin receptor. There is a higher affinity to the IGF1R, but this did not cause a difference in growth-stimulating activity when compared to regular insulin.[60] Clinical trials have demonstrated that insulin lispro acts within 15 minutes, peaks at approximately 1 hour, and lasts 2 to 4 hours after SC injection.[59,61] Insulin lispro is stable in CSII systems and has been shown to improve PPG levels when CSII therapy was compared using regular human insulin.[62–64] There is no difference in the frequency of catheter occlusion or other site-related problems with insulin lispro as compared to buffered regular insulin.[63,64] However, there were recent reports of a few patients who developed marked lipoatrophy while using insulin lispro during CSII.[65,66] The basis of this lipoatrophy is unclear but was resolved with use of regular human insulin. In the past, lipoatrophy was seen with the use of less purified insulins and was assumed to have an immunologic basis. Contrasting are the reports of similar immunogenicity between insulin lispro and recombinant human regular insulin.[67] Also, insulin lispro has been a successful substitute for human regular insulin in several cases of presumed immunogenic insulin resistance.[68,69] A concern for the use of

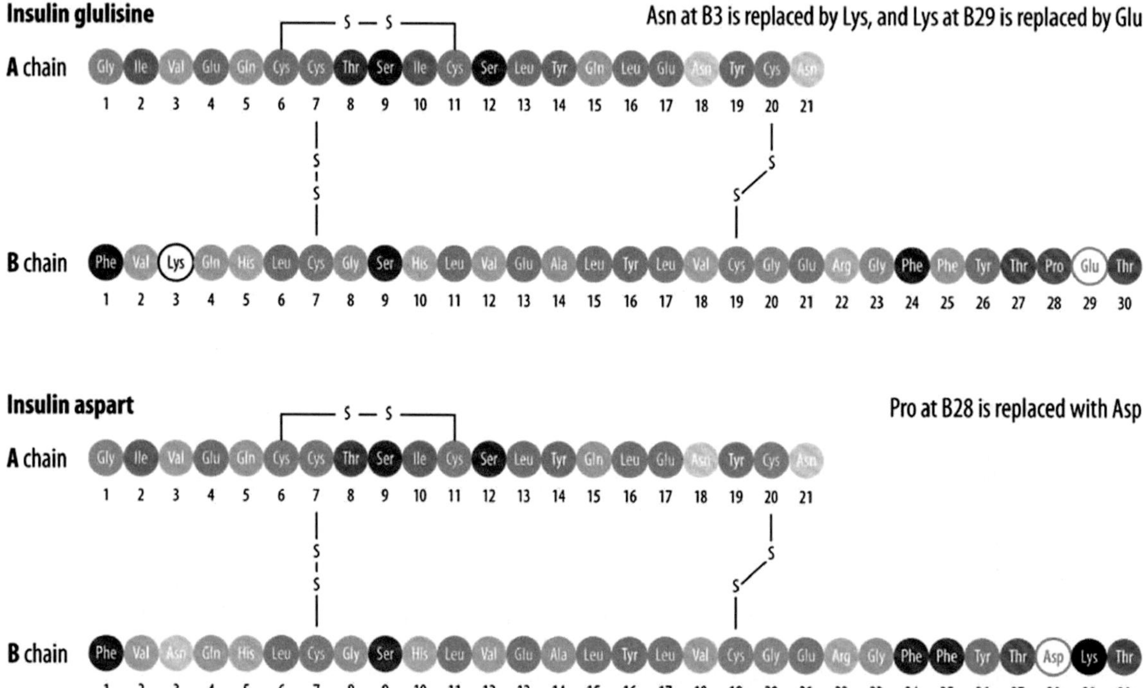

Figure 55.3 Diagram of amino acid substitutions in current rapid-acting insulin analogs. Presentation slide by Dr. Eda Cengiz.

insulin lispro (or any other RAI) in CSII is its short duration of action, possibly increasing the risk of DKA in cases of mechanical malfunction or catheter occlusion.[70]

Another synthetic insulin analog, insulin aspart, was approved for clinical use in the United States in June 2000. Preclinical studies have shown that the insulin aspart has the same insulin receptor and IGF1R interaction kinetics as human insulin, diminishing concerns about the mitogenic potential of insulin aspart. Similar to insulin lispro insulin, insulin aspart was conceptualized as a mealtime insulin. It is absorbed more rapidly than human regular insulin, reaches higher maximal concentrations postprandially, and has a shorter duration of action.[71–73] In a multicenter study, the risk of postprandial hypoglycemia requiring third-party intervention was reduced significantly without leading to deterioration of late postprandial blood glucose levels when insulin aspart was compared to regular insulin.[74]

Insulin glulisine has a similar pharmacokinetic, pharmacodynamic, and safety profile as compared to other RAI analogs and is formulated without the addition of zinc. It also has a different effect on activation of IRS-1 and IRS-2 with decreased activation of IRS1 shown by animal studies suggesting favorable effects on decreasing apoptosis.[75,76] It does not appear to accumulate in patients with renal impairment.[77] Insulin glulisine is comparable to other rapid-acting analogs with respect to glycemic control, and its somewhat faster absorption rate has questionable clinical significance.[78] Postmeal administration of glulisine was associated with a slight reduction of weight (−0.3 kg), while premeal administration was associated with minor weight gain (+0.3 kg).[62]

After the introduction of insulin, patients experienced cutaneous reactions directly related to insulin. These immunologic reactions and skin alterations were stemming from foreign proteins from animal insulins acting as allergens. Later on, preservatives such as metacresol or agents to prolong action such as zinc protamine were reported to be the culprit of these reactions. Prevalence of hypersensitivity reactions substantially declined from 60% to 50%.[79,80] Insulin therapy-related lipodystrophies are still not obsolete. This group encompasses lipohypertrophy and lipoatrophy. Lipohypertrophy is a result of the insulin anabolic effect, promoting adipose tissue differentiation and growth.[81] Lipoatrophy is a relatively uncommon allergic reaction mainly due to the impure insulin molecule. Fat atrophy is the result of lysosomal enzyme activity triggered by an immune-mediated inflammation.[82] Lipoatrophy is not merely a cosmetic issue since the absorption of insulin from these sites is erratic.[83] Local steroid injections, alternative methods of insulin delivery have been proposed for the management of lipoatrophic sites and achieved some success.[84,85]

In most diabetes centers, insulin lispro, insulin aspart, and insulin glulisine are used interchangeably when it comes to selecting a short-acting insulin/RAI for either CSII or as part of MDI regimens. Open-label, randomized, multicenter studies in pregnant women with T1DM found insulin lispro[86] and insulin aspart[87] to be safe for both mother and offspring. Congenital abnormalities do not appear to be more frequent with either lispro or aspart use during pregnancy.

Ultrarapid-Acting Insulin Analogs

The earliest secreted insulin is a necessary element of the normal mealtime insulin response, to offset the rapid rise in postprandial blood glucose and consequently optimal exogenous prandial insulin needs a rapid "on response" with a relatively powerful glucose-lowering effect. The development of RAI analogs allowed faster absorption of insulin into circulation from the SC injection site, and while near-normal glycemic control can be achieved by RAI, substantial limitations have become apparent as tight glycemic control has been accepted as standard-of-care diabetes treatment. Faster onset and offset of insulin action, replicating physiologic insulin action, is greatly desirable to provide greater glycemic control, minimize hypoglycemic episodes, and reduce weight gain; therefore, research and development for new-generation ultra-RAIs have been mothered by this necessity. There are a number of methods and new insulins already approved or in development that aim to achieve faster glucose-lowering insulin action.

Faster-Acting Insulin Aspart

Faster-acting insulin aspart (Flasp; Novo Nordisk) is insulin aspart in a new formulation which contains excipients, nicotinamide and L-asparaginase, that are naturally occurring entities and are considered as safe (GRAS) by the FDA and result in faster initial absorption after SC injection.[88,89] Compared with insulin aspart, faster-acting insulin aspart is associated with a faster onset of action and increased early exposure that, in turn, leads to a significantly greater early glucose-lowering effect. Furthermore, increased early exposure with faster-acting insulin aspart, compared with insulin aspart, led to improved glycemic control following a postmeal challenge in both the SC injection and CSII settings without an increase in hypoglycemia.[88]

Afrezza-Inhaled Insulin

Afrezza-inhaled insulin has become the fastest-acting exogenous insulin, given that the insulin is absorbed quickly from lungs eliminating the delays after SC injection (Fig. 55.4).[90] Technosphere® insulin (Afrezza®, MannKind Corporation) consists of human insulin adsorbed on to microparticles formed by fumaryl diketopiperazine (FDKP). In vitro studies have found no evidence that FDKP is cytotoxic to the human lung, and there was no indication of any effect on airway epithelial tight junction integrity, cell viability, or cell permeability.[91] Afrezza insulin is delivered by a thumb-sized inhaler device specifically designed for its delivery by inhalation. Once inhaled, Afrezza dissolves rapidly in the alveolar fluid of the deep lung and is rapidly absorbed into systemic circulation from the large surface area of the alveolar space with the added benefit of a thin alveolar barrier between air and blood.[91,92] It is packaged in single-use, color-coded cartridge dosages: 4 units (blue), 8 units (green), and 12 units (yellow). Afrezza insulin was approved for treating adult patients with T1DM and T2DM by the FDA in 2014, and clinical studies are underway for the pediatric indication (clinical trials.gov). The RAI to Afrezza insulin dose conversion formula has been revised, and a 1.5 conversion ratio has been approved by the FDA (multiply the RAI units by 1.5 to calculate the corresponding Afrezza units) and is currently used to calculate premeal and correction Afrezza insulin dosing. Afrezza is contraindicated in patients with asthma or chronic obstructive pulmonary disease, and it should not be recommended to patients who smoke. Basic spirometry testing should be done to assess forced expiratory volume in 1 second (FEV_1) at baseline, after 6 months of therapy and annually, even in the absence of pulmonary symptoms.

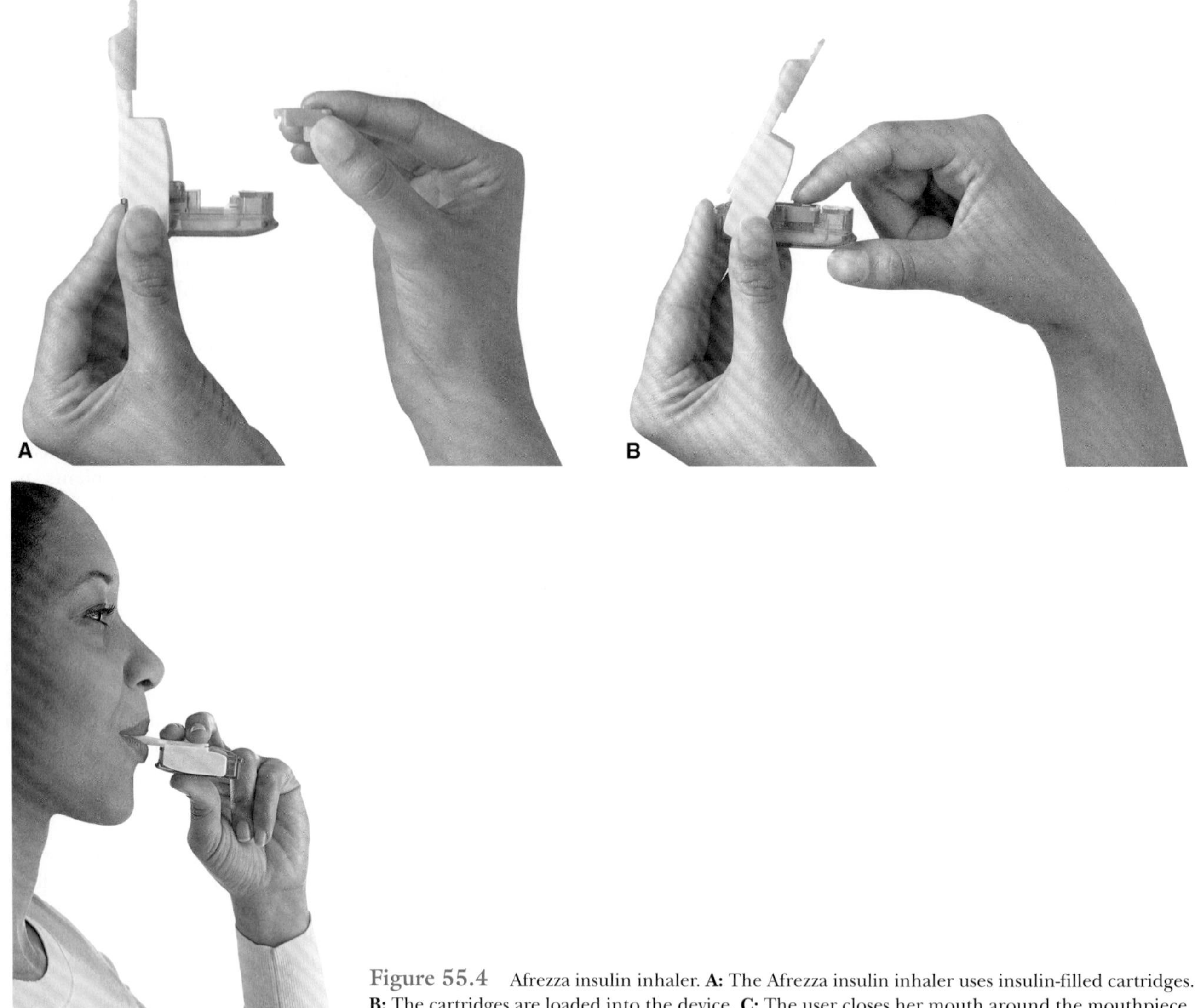

Figure 55.4 Afrezza insulin inhaler. **A:** The Afrezza insulin inhaler uses insulin-filled cartridges. **B:** The cartridges are loaded into the device. **C:** The user closes her mouth around the mouthpiece and inhales insulin deeply through the inhaler. With permission from https://afrezza.com/.

FUTURE DEVELOPMENTS

BioChaperone Lispro Insulin

BioChaperone® Lispro (Adocia) is a modified dextran molecule designed for fast absorption. In healthy subjects, this product was shown to have a similar pharmacokinetic and pharmacodynamic profile to faster insulin aspart. In subjects with T1D, BioChaperone Lispro demonstrated an earlier onset of action, earlier maximum action, and stronger metabolic effect in the first 2 hours after dosing, compared with insulin lispro, as shown by a 61% reduced PPG excursions.[93]

Ultrarapid Lispro

The ultrarapid lispro is designed by adding citrate and treprostinil to the original insulin lispro molecule. The insulin resorption from the SC tissue is more rapid by citrate's effect on increasing vascular permeability and treprostinil's effect on enhancing local vasodilatation at the injection site. While there are data suggestive of faster pharmacodynamic and pharmacokinetic profiles, clinical data have been limited.[94]

LONG-ACTING INSULIN ANALOGS

At the other end of the pharmacodynamic spectrum, insulin analogs are being developed to retard and stabilize the absorption kinetics profile to create prolonged and peakless activity by decreasing solubility at the site of injection and slow release of insulin into the circulation. A basal insulin analog is intended to mimic the steady, unprovoked secretion profile of a healthy pancreas. The primary strategy used in the discovery of superior basal insulin therapy relies upon decreased solubility at the site of injection, slow release of insulin into the circulation, or slow clearance rate from the circulation. The first slow-acting insulin was produced in 1936 using protamine and zinc. One of the first analogs developed synthetically to prolong absorption was NovoSol Basal insulin. Although intraindividual variability was improved, interindividual variability of insulin action remained high.[95] This insulin also demonstrated poor bioavailability, necessitating very high doses. NovoSol Basal was subsequently withdrawn from further studies. This was followed by other formulations, the NPH insulin in 1950 and the "lente" insulins in 1951. Ultralente and NPH fell short of the ideal basal insulin desired properties of low and constant plasma insulin levels in between meals and overnight without pronounced peak effects. This led to the investigation of new basal insulin preparations that replicate the endogenous insulin physiology.

In the spring of 2000, the FDA approved the use of insulin glargine (HOE 901), a long-acting insulin analog for use in patients with T1DM and T2DM. The analog resulted from the elongation of the β chain at position 30 by two arginine residues as well as by substitution of asparagine at the 21 position of the α chain with glycine to maintain chemical stability in the aqueous, acidic formulation. Elongation of the β chain raises the isoelectric point of the molecule from a pH of 5.4 to 6.7, increasing its solubility at acid pH and decreasing its solubility at neutral pH. Insulin glargine is, therefore, a stable solute in acid formulation, making it the first soluble long-acting insulin. When insulin glargine is injected into the SC tissue (neutral pH), it precipitates, slowing and stabilizing the absorption for a peakless insulin effect.[96] To enhance stabilization, the current commercial preparation of insulin glargine contains 30 mg per L of zinc, since higher concentrations of zinc did not have any added benefit.[97] Insulin glargine was initially reported to have a flat profile[98]; however, more recent studies demonstrate a gentle rise in effect with an unpronounced peak at 6 hours.[99,100] Despite the twice-daily use of glargine for some patients, not much benefit has been shown with this regimen as compared with the single-day injection as basal insulin.[101] Preclinical studies on insulin receptor binding and promotion of mitogenesis through "overstimulated" phosphorylation [as seen with Asp (B10) insulin] found that insulin glargine behaved like regular human insulin with respect to receptor binding, autophosphorylation, and phosphorylation of signaling elements.[102] In cardiac myocytes, there was no difference in IGF1R-mediated growth-promoting activity of insulin glargine as compared with native human insulin; however, there was a higher affinity of insulin glargine to the IGF1R.[103] A recent comparison of all insulin analogs confirmed a significantly greater affinity of insulin glargine for the IGF1R than human insulin.[104] To date, it is unclear whether these findings carry some unrecognized safety implications. Most studies so far have not evidenced increased tumor development with insulin glargine, and its metabolic characteristics resemble human insulin more closely than the oncogenic Asp (B10) insulin.[105] The major clinical benefit of a peakless basal insulin, especially for pediatric use, is the potential reduction of nocturnal hypoglycemia. In an adult study comparing nighttime hypoglycemia between NPH and insulin glargine, the frequency of hypoglycemia was reduced by 22% in the group using insulin glargine.[106] A similar study comparing glycemic control between the use of insulin glargine and NPH in children and adolescents found that overall fasting blood glucose levels were significantly lower, while there was a trend toward fewer episodes of severe nocturnal hypoglycemia.[107]

Insulin Glargine 300 (300 units of glargine insulin per mL) is another long-acting basal insulin that has been approved for use in T1D and T2D. It delivers the same dose of glargine in one-third of the volume with a slightly different pharmacokinetic and pharmacodynamic profile than Glargine 100 (100 units of glargine insulin per mL). Glargine 300 is released more gradually from the SC tissue precipitate than Glargine 100, giving a more constant pharmacokinetic profile with a less pronounced peak of action, low within-day variability, and low between-day variability.[108,109]

Insulin detemir was created by attaching a myristic acid to B29 and removing threonine from B30 of regular insulin molecule[110] to slow adsorption and facilitate extended plasma circulation through noncovalent albumin binding. This molecular change enhances albumin binding once it is injected SC, leading to a slow absorption from the site and prolongation of insulin action in the circulation. Its biologic duration of action is dose dependent lasting between 12 and 24 hours.[99,111] It has less of a peak glucose-lowering effect, which occurs later than seen in NPH insulin.[112,113] It has less intrasubject insulin absorption variability, better reproducibility, and less frequent episodes of hypoglycemia as compared with NPH.[114] So far, in vitro safety profiles of insulin detemir have been favorable, mostly because of its lower affinity to the IGF1R as compared with human insulin and glargine insulin.[104] Furthermore, no clinically significant drug-binding interference of insulin detemir albumin with other albumin-binding drugs has been noted on in vitro analysis.[115] Insulin detemir acts in the brain as well as in the peripheral tissue, which might lead to appetite suppression that can explain some of the reduced weight gain observed during treatment with detemir.[116] A clinical study comparing weight gain for patients on detemir versus glargine reported somewhat greater weight gain with the glargine group without any statistical significance.[111]

ULTRALONG-ACTING INSULIN ANALOGS

Ultralong-acting insulin is defined as insulin showing the clinically significant biologic action of a glucose-lowering effect beyond 24 hours after SC injection.[117] The concept of ultralong-acting insulins has been explored to mitigate the injection burden and to improve treatment compliance. Ultralong glucodynamic action profile coupled with lower day-to-day within-subject glucose-lowering variability and peakless insulin action have been key targets for ultralong-acting insulin formulations.

Insulin degludec is an ultralong-acting basal insulin with a modified structure that leads to the formation of soluble multihexamers upon SC injection, resulting in a depot from which IDeg is released slowly and continuously into the circulation.[118] It reversibly binds to serum protein albumin, resulting in a relatively high concentration of insulin degludec in the bloodstream that contributes to its prolonged kinetics.[119] The daily injected dose is equivalent to the daily eliminated amount of insulin (the steady state) after 2 to 3 days of once-daily administration.[119] Insulin degludec has a 42-hour duration of action with an even distribution of glucose-lowering activity and a terminal half-life of 25 to 26 hours once steady state is achieved.[120] It has been shown to have a lower day-to-day within-subject variability in glucose-lowering effect and similar effect in HbA_{1c} and weight reduction compared with Glargine 100.[121–123]

CONTINUOUS SUBCUTANEOUS INSULIN INFUSION

CSII, commonly referred as insulin pump treatment, was introduced more than 40 years ago, as a means to more closely simulate normal plasma insulin profiles than could be achieved by conventional injection regimens.[124]

The insulin pump is composed of an insulin reservoir that is attached to a programmable insulin delivery device. Plastic tubing connects the insulin reservoir to a catheter that is inserted SC into either the abdomen or the hip. The tubeless insulin pump, "Pod Pump," has a slightly different structure that has direct connection to the SC tissue through a catheter without any tubing. Typically, patch pumps require that a handheld device be connected to the pod via a wireless link to enable adjustments in insulin dosing and settings.

The pump is programmed to deliver a continuous "basal rate" of RAI throughout the day. Basal rates can be programmed to change each hour of the day, but it is unusual to need more than six basal rates throughout the day. Variations in basal rate can be particularly beneficial overnight, since basal rates can be programmed to decrease in the early part of the night to prevent hypoglycemia and increased in the hours before dawn to keep glucose from rising. During the day, the patient "dials up" an RAI bolus in accordance with the carbohydrate content of the meal. This allows more flexibility with the quantity and content of food intake. The continuous basal rate eliminates the need for the use of intermediate- or long-acting insulins, and therefore, meal planning does not have to center around peaking insulin action, as recommended with conventional insulin therapy.

Some of the limitations of CSII are possible encumbrance during intense exercise or contact sports. Since only RAI is used, any interruption in flow (catheter occlusion or disconnection) can lead to rapid deterioration of metabolic control, especially during sleeping hours. In addition, local infections at the site of catheter insertion can occur, especially if improper hygienic technique is employed or site changes are delayed. Local infection can interfere significantly with glycemic control during CSII.

The CSII introduced a new insulin basal-bolus treatment concept that was different from the insulin injection method and has emerged as an ideal tool to intensify insulin treatment while minimizing hypoglycemia. The initial devices (insulin pumps) were cumbersome to use, and there was uncertainty about the long-term benefits of intensive treatment. The results of the Diabetes Control and Complications Trial (DCCT) indicating that the long-term benefits of strict diabetes control outweigh the risks of severe hypoglycemia[125,126] resulted in a paradigm shift in diabetes treatment. As a result, intensive diabetes management has become the gold standard, and insulin pump therapy is promoted by expert diabetes care providers. Subsequently, new improvements in pump therapy led to advanced pump features, including multiple programmable basal/bolus rates and correction factors (sensitivity factor), ability to adjust basal and bolus doses in small increments, and bolus history function to assess missing bolus doses of insulin.

The usage of CSII has increased, and effects of CSII on glycemic control have been well investigated. A meta-analysis of randomized pediatric trials comparing CSII to MDI reported a modest reduction in HbA_{1c} and severe hypoglycemia rate in children and adults with CSII use.[127] Data analysis from a multinational database registry demonstrated that on average, the HbA_{1c} levels were significantly lower by 0.5 points among patients receiving insulin pump therapy as compared to patients on MDI. supporting research studies with real-life clinical data.[128] There is clinical evidence suggesting that patients with poor initial HbA_{1c} demonstrate better glycemic control when they switch from MDI to CSII therapy,[129,130] and CSII may reduce DKA risk and retinopathy and peripheral neuropathy in youth with T1D.[131–133] Furthermore, adolescents on CSII therapy has been shown to cope better with the psychosocial aspects of having diabetes.[134]

Insulin pump therapy has been suggested as the preferred mode of insulin delivery for children under 7 years of age, given the treatment flexibility and remote insulin bolusing.[135] Treatment guidelines by the Pediatric Endocrine Society (PES) define clinical indications for when to consider pump therapy for children as follows: patients with recurrent severe hypoglycemia, wide fluctuations in blood glucose levels regardless of HbA_{1c}, suboptimal glycemic control with above target HbA_{1c} levels, microvascular complications and/or risk factors for macrovascular complications, or insulin regimen that compromises lifestyle despite good glycemic control.[136,137] Fulfillment of one or more criteria is considered a possible indication for initiating pump therapy, provided that candidates have adequate understanding of this therapeutic tool. Same guidelines identify young children (especially infants and neonates), adolescents with eating disorders, children and adolescents with pronounced dawn phenomenon or with needle phobia, pregnant adolescents, ketosis-prone individuals, and competitive athletes as patient populations that might benefit from insulin pump use.[136,137]

The technology era has been revolutionizing insulin pump treatment during the past decade. Modern pump designs with enhanced technology features have become available. New and advanced insulin pump models have incorporated sophisticated pumping mechanisms, touchscreen feature, Bluetooth connectivity, and digitally enhanced systems into the CSII. Insulin pumps have become more advanced with multiple features and an interface with glucose meters, continuous glucose monitors (CGMs), and potentially other relevant devices.

MONITORING OF GLYCEMIC CONTROL

Self-monitoring of blood glucose is central to the management of diabetes. It provides instant feedback, enabling the patient to assume immediate intervention if necessary. Furthermore, the trend analysis of daily blood glucose values over the course of a few days supplies the diabetes care provider with crucial information when readjusting insulin regiments or contemplating therapeutic strategies. The newer glucose meters are very portable and require only a tiny drop of blood. Most have computerized memories to facilitate record-keeping.

Concurrent developments in materials science and microfabrication enabled the development of real-time blood glucose sensing and their integration into the insulin pump delivery systems. The glucose oxidase (GOx)–based electrochemical sensors for continuous, real-time monitoring of interstitial glucose levels have introduced the possibility of monitoring glucose continuously and real time. Commercially available CGM technology emerged over the past 15 years. The first-generation glucose monitor in the market was the Medtronic Continuous Glucose Monitoring System (CGMS), which stored glucose readings every 5 minutes up to 3 days. The blood glucose values were available only after downloading the sensor without the convenience of real-time values. Guardian Medtronic CGM, as the next CGM manufactured by Medtronics, had real-time alarm for hypoglycemia without actual real-time glucose values as an added feature. GlucoWatch G2 Biographer was the first

CGM with real-time glucose values. Inaccurate readings, false alarms, and local irritation on the insertion site with lack of improvement in glycemic control and hypoglycemic episodes destined GlucoWatch to become a part of CGM history rather than a popular device in use.[138]

Both the new-generation and old-generation CGM measure interstitial fluid glucose, however, with different methods. Many of the new-generation glucose sensors use needle-type catheter inserted in the SC area and has GOx at the tip. The electrochemical reaction produces an electric current directly proportional to the ambient glucose concentration that is read by the sensor and transmitted by wireless radio frequency telemetry to the receiver. Interference with glucose readings by the sensor can occur with certain substances. Glutathione, ascorbic acid, uric acid, acetaminophen/paracetamol, isoniazid, and salicylate may become co-oxidized at the sensor and lead to overestimation of glucose levels.[139,140] Recent advances in the sensor technology were reported to overcome this problem.[141,142]

Current CGM devices in use consist of four off-the-shelf FDA-approved brands. Guardian Connect displays glucose values between 40 and 400 mg per dL every 5 minutes with directional trends and rate of change illustrated by arrows. Start-up initialization is 2 hours. The sensor requires first calibration 2 hours after insertion with consequent calibrations every 12 hours. The Guardian CGM communicates with the compatible Medtronic insulin pump without the need of a separate monitor. The predictive alerts could be set to alarm 5, 10, 15, 20, 25, or 30 minutes before glucose limits have been reached or rate of change alerts when glucose levels are changing between 1.1 and 5 mg per dL per minute, in 0.1 increments. Customizable high and low alarm features are available in both. Sensors can be worn for 6 days. The sensor and pump data can be uploaded and retrospectively reviewed from a web-based data management system.

The Dexcom G6 CGM does not require calibration and could be used for 10 days after a 2-hour start-up initialization period. It has built-in hypo-hyperglycemia, trend, and predictive alerts. No finger-stick confirmation is required when making insulin treatment decisions. It could be integrated with Tslim and Omnipod insulin pumps. Dexcom G6 automatically and continuously sends data to the user's Dexcom Clarity smartphone application and web-based data management software for real-time data upload to the cloud and data-sharing options with up to five caregivers.

Eversense CGM is an implantable pill-sized sensor with a removable and rechargeable transmitter that sits on top of the skin. It provides CGM for up to 90 days after a 24-hour postinsertion warm-up period. It requires calibration every 12 hours and has interface with a smartphone application and web-based data management application.

The Freestyle Libre reads glucose levels through a sensor that is worn on the back of the upper arm for up to 14 days after a 1 hour postinsertion warm-up period. Libre does not communicate continuously with the reader; hence, there are no hyper-hypoglycemia alerts, and the user has to scan the sensor to get a reading that are displayed as number values as well as trends. Libre does not require calibration, and its data could be saved in a cloud-based diabetes management system to view reports and change reader settings.

Overall percentage of error has been reduced throughout the years and runs around 8% to 9% for the new-generation CGMs. As mentioned before, accuracy depends on multiple factors, such as current glucose concentration and rate of change of glucose values with poor correlation during hypoglycemia and during times of rapid change.

There is growing evidence that CGM use results in a significant HbA_{1c} reduction in patients with T1D without an increase in hypoglycemia whether they are on CSII or MDI treatment, provided that CGM is used ≥6 days per week.[143] Real-time CGM use is suggested for adults with T1D regardless of the glycemic control status, given that patients in good glycemic control also had a significant reduction in severe hypoglycemia and time spent in biochemical hypoglycemic range by CGM use.[31]

New metrics of glycemic control have been implemented into diabetes management after CGM use has become standard of care for diabetes management. Some of the proposed glycemic control metrics include (1) average glucose; (2) percentage of time in hypoglycemic ranges, that is, less than 54 mg per dL (level 2), 54 to 70 mg per dL (level 1)[75]; (3) percentage of time in target range, that is, 70 to 180 mg per dL (3.9 to 9.9 mmol per L); (4) percentage of time in hyperglycemic range, that is, ≥180 mg per dL, and are commonly used during clinical trials.[144] CGM data are used to generate standardized reports with visual cues to determine glycemic patterns and to guide treatment decisions.

The ultimate goal is to integrate the insulin pump and the CGM via a control algorithm that will enable insulin delivery automatically without involving the patient. This system, the artificial pancreas (AP), will revolutionize the diabetes management by providing a functioning bioelectronic β cell that mimics the physiologic function of pancreas. AP projects have gained significant momentum for the past decade with the advent in technology and continue to be one of the most promising areas of research in the field of diabetes management.

SENSOR-AUGMENTED INSULIN PUMP TREATMENT AND ARTIFICIAL PANCREAS SYSTEMS

The application of CGM with pumps has enabled real-time information on glucose levels to guide insulin dosing from the insulin pumps, facilitating the development of sensor-augmented insulin pump (SAP) treatment (Fig. 55.5). Multiple clinical trials clearly demonstrated the efficacy of using SAP, in improving glycemic controls as compared to MDI. The evolution of current pump and CGM technologies continued as sophisticated insulin delivery decision-making algorithms have been incorporated into the insulin pumps to adjust insulin delivery (suspend, increase, or decrease insulin infusion) based on CGM values. The early integrated SAP systems with low glucose suspend (LGS) feature that suspends insulin delivery when the CGM value reaches a set value was the first step in automated insulin delivery (AID). The LGS significantly lowered the risk of hypoglycemic events both in the adult and pediatric population, particularly at night. The next and advanced version, the predicted low glucose system (PLGS), suspends the insulin delivery in advance of a hypoglycemic episode, and results from clinical trials have shown reduction in hypoglycemia without any increase in hyperglycemia.[145]

Complete AID has been the ultimate goal for diabetes management to provide physiologic insulin delivery since the

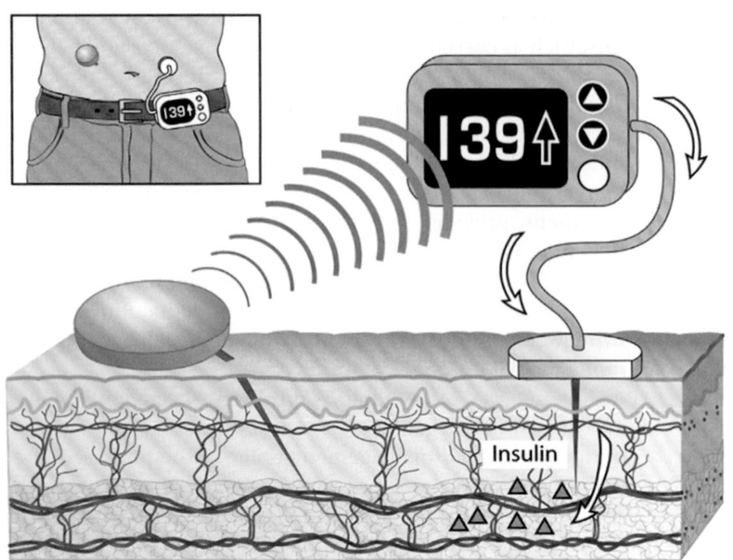

Figure 55.5 Continuous glucose monitor and sensor-augmented insulin pump. A schematic depiction of automated insulin delivery by continuous glucose sensor augmented insulin pump treatment. Reprinted from Cengiz E, Sherr JL, Weinzimer SA, Tamborlane WV. New-generation diabetes management: glucose sensor-augmented insulin pump therapy. *Expert Rev Med Devices.* 2011;8(4):449–458.

invention of insulin pump. Fully automated AID systems entail integrated insulin pump, CGM, and algorithm-based insulin delivery without any manual input from the user. Hybrid AID, also known as the hybrid AP system, has been adopted in first-generation AID. It requires users to count carbohydrates and bolus for meals and snacks while the system adjusts insulin delivery in the background, based on sensor glucose levels, after its safety and efficacy have been shown by a clinical trial (reduction of HbA_{1c} in adults from 7.3% ± 0.9% to 6.8% ± 0.6% and adolescents 7.7% ± 0.8% to 7.1% ± 0.6%).[146] A multitude of other AID systems are currently being investigated, including those with dual hormones and more advanced glucose sensor techniques.

NEW-GENERATION INSULIN TREATMENT

SMART INSULINS

Smart insulin is a chemically activated insulin in response to changes in blood glucose levels. It remains inactive until blood glucose is above a certain threshold, and its activity ceases when target blood glucose levels are attained. The development of smart insulins has been gaining significant momentum with initial prototypes now reaching the proof-of-concept stage.[147] The glucose sensing ability and insulin response to changing levels of blood glucose are essential factors for a safe and efficient smart insulin treatment. Glucose sensing is accomplished by one of three methods: a system based on the enzymatic conversion of glucose to gluconic acid by GOx, a system based on glucose detection derived from its affinity to concanavalin A (ConA), or a system based on the interaction between glucose and phenylboronic acid.[147] Once blood glucose levels are assessed accurately, glucose-dependent insulin release occurs from a storage that is capable of chemical or conformational change upon interaction with elevated glucose levels. There are multiple smart insulin projects that are being tested in animal models with a potential to investigate their efficacy and safety in human trials in the future.[148]

ADJUNCT TREATMENT METHODS

Several adjunctive therapies to insulin have been evaluated in patients with T1DM to improve glycemic control and reduce treatment burden. Adjunctive treatments could be classified into two major groups as physiologic and pharmacologic interventions.

Pramlintide, an amylin analog, is an FDA-approved physiologic injectable adjunctive treatment option for T1DM. It can improve glycemic control, primarily through lowering postprandial blood glucose levels. Weight loss and increased risk of hypoglycemia have been reported when pramlintide is used with insulin.[149] Incretins are hormones that augment insulin secretion after oral intake of glucose. Glucagon-like peptide (GLP)-1 and the glucose-dependent insulinotropic polypeptide (GIP) are responsible for the incretin effect in human body. GLP1 agonist use with insulin treatment has been associated with a 0.4 to 0.8 reduction in HbA_{1c} and average weight loss of 2.5 to 5 kg increase satiety. It has been postulated that GLP1-agonists adjunctively function to lessen the need for insulin through further reductions in body weight targeting obese patients with T1DM.[150]

Majority of the pharmacologic adjunctive treatment methods are investigational rather than FDA-approved treatments. Metformin used in obese patients with T1DM may demonstrate benefits on insulin dose and weight without increasing hypoglycemia risk. Its beneficial effects on lowering peripheral insulin sensitivity as a marker of reduction in cardiovascular disease risk are recently shown in overweight/obese youth with T1DM.[151] Sodium–glucose cotransporter-1 (SGLT-1) is the primary transporter for absorption of glucose and galactose in the gastrointestinal tract, and its inhibition blunts and delays PPG excursion. Sodium–glucose cotransporter-2 (SGLT2) inhibitors impair renal glucose reabsorption in an insulin-independent manner. SGLT2 inhibitor and dual SGLT1 and SGLT2 inhibitor adjunct use have been studied in T1DM[149] and showed improved glycemic control, a significant reduction both in body weight and systolic blood pressure, and treatment efficacy maintained in lower estimated glomerular filtration rate levels with no increased hypoglycemia.[152] Increased risk of euglycemic DKA has been associated with the use of all the approved SGLT2 inhibitors, and β-hydroxybutyrate monitoring should be performed when there is suspicion of ketosis despite normal blood glucose levels. The dual SGLT1 and SGLT2 inhibitors use for overweight (body mass index ≥ 27 kg per m^2) adult patients with T1D is recently approved for adjunct use in Europe.[153]

There is a significant need for innovative methods to attain target glycemic control for people with T1DM, and adjunctive therapies may offer alternative treatment solutions to reach glycemic goals while reducing insulin doses, promoting weight loss, and limiting hypoglycemia. Patients not reaching A_{1c} goals with insulin therapy and those who could benefit from weight loss are most likely to benefit from adjunctive therapy. Patient-specific characteristics should be assessed carefully when considering adjunctive treatments.

DIABETIC KETOACIDOSIS

DKA is a life-threatening catabolic state that occurs in the context of relative or absolute insulin deficiency. It is defined as hyperglycemia (a serum glucose of ≥300 mg per dL) and metabolic acidosis (a pH of <7.3 and a serum bicarbonate of <15 mEq per L).

Around 20% to 30% of DKA episodes occur in patients who had not been diagnosed with diabetes in the past.[154] In previously diagnosed children, DKA occurs with omission of insulin or under conditions that interfere with insulin action, such as the rise of counterregulatory hormones (epinephrine, norepinephrine, cortisol, growth hormone, and glucagon) and during infection, trauma, and emotional stress. Successful management of DKA requires clear comprehension of the pathophysiologic mechanisms that lead to the acid–base, fluid, and electrolyte imbalance that ensues.

On a cellular level, insulinopenia creates a state of starvation, as fuel substrates cannot be taken up by the cell. Peripheral tissues are resistant to the action of insulin, aggravating the insulinopenia in DKA. In muscle cells, this accelerates protein breakdown, resulting in free amino acids. In the liver, these amino acids are converted to glucose, perpetuating hyperglycemia. In light of perceived starvation, the liver further contributes to hyperglycemia by exaggerated glycogenolysis and gluconeogenesis with a rising glucagon-to-insulin ratio in the portal circulation. Hyperglycemia (above the renal threshold of 180 mg per dL) induces osmotic diuresis. Loss of water and electrolytes quickly results in hyperosmolar dehydration in these patients.

A lack of insulin in the adipose tissue activates hormone-sensitive lipoprotein lipase, releasing large amounts of fatty acids into the plasma, which are transformed to ketone bodies, such as acetoacetic acid, β-hydroxybutyrate, and acetone. The rising ketonemia leads to metabolic acidosis. Ketonuria further exacerbates dehydration and loss of electrolytes.

In defense against cell shrinkage, hyperosmolarity causes the intracellular accumulation of osmoprotective molecules (myoinositol, taurine, and glutamate), which occurs most importantly in the brain cells. Although this cell preservation mechanism is beneficial during hyperosmolar dehydration, it poses a risk for the development of cerebral edema during rehydration therapy. As water freely passes through the blood–brain barrier, it is then drawn into the intracellular space by the abundance of osmols, rapidly increasing cell volume, leading to brain swelling. Other mechanisms, including increased capillary permeability, may also contribute to cerebral edema in DKA.

MANAGEMENT OF DIABETIC KETOACIDOSIS

Once the diagnosis has been established, fluid resuscitation, electrolyte management, and insulin administration are the mainstay of therapy. Key to successful recovery from DKA is frequent electrolyte monitoring, clinical evaluations, and meticulous record-keeping. In the initial assessment, a complete history and physical examination should elicit any kind of precipitating infections, necessitating concomitant antibiotic therapy.

The first step in treatment of DKA is the administration of an isotonic (0.9% or normal) saline fluid bolus of 10 to 20 mL per kg of body weight (not to exceed 1 L) over 1 hour. If the patient is in shock, a 20-mL saline fluid bolus per kg body weight is rapidly administered and may be repeated to achieve hemodynamic stability. The infusion rate is then lowered to replace maintenance requirements and dehydration deficit over 36 to 48 hours. Since dehydration in DKA is intracellular, clinical measures of dehydration (such as pulse and perfusion) often underestimate the degree of deficit. A rule of thumb is to assume a 10% dehydration deficit in any child who presents in DKA. However, rehydration fluids are not to exceed 4 L per m^2 in 24 hours, as this has been associated with an increased risk of cerebral edema.[155] Once the fluid bolus has been given, results of initial laboratory studies are usually available to help tailor fluid and electrolyte replacement. It is important to be aware of the frequently seen initial drop in pH after volume replacement as a result of lactic acid mobilization. Fluid administration and urine output should be carefully monitored throughout the therapy.

SODIUM

At the time of presentation, patients may be hypernatremic or hyponatremic. When interpreting low-appearing sodium values from the electrolyte panel, one should be aware that they could be spuriously low due to an increase in serum glucose, lipids, and proteins. To correct for this pseudohyponatremia, 1.6 mEq per L is added to the sodium value for every 100 mg per dL of serum glucose above 100 mg per dL. This corrected sodium is then used to guide the interpretation. If corrected sodium is between 130 and 145 mEq per L, rehydration fluids can be continued with 0.45% saline (half of normal saline). Hypernatremia (>145 mEq per L) should be corrected with 0.675% saline (three-fourths of normal saline). A corrected sodium of less than 130 mEq per L requires 0.9% saline rehydration. When monitoring rehydration, the uncorrected serum sodium should always rise as the serum glucose is falling. A static uncorrected serum sodium in light of normalizing glucose levels is an ominous sign of overhydration and indicates a risk for the development of cerebral edema. When interpreting the calculated (corrected) serum sodium during fluid resuscitation, stable values are desirable, but falling values should prompt an immediate decrease in the fluid rate.

POTASSIUM

Despite total body depletion of potassium, initial potassium levels are usually normal or elevated. Insulin deficiency, acidosis, and dehydration all contribute to the relative high extracellular potassium level. Once insulin therapy is initiated, potassium is transported from the extracellular to the intracellular space, placing the patient at risk for a rapid drop in serum potassium, especially in light of total body depletion. As acidosis is corrected, each increase in serum pH by 0.1 further decreases serum potassium by 0.6 mEq per L. Therefore, close monitoring of serum potassium and administration of potassium at the time of initiation of insulin therapy will offset a precipitous drop in serum potassium. Hyperchloremic metabolic acidosis could be seen after administering potassium chloride (KCl) due to excessive chloride infusion. If the initial potassium level is more than 6.0 mEq per L, it is generally advised to hold off on adding potassium to intravenous hydration. However, once insulin infusion is started, serum potassium levels need to be monitored, and potassium is added to the hydration fluid once values fall below 6.0 mEq per L. Because a precipitous drop in potassium is expected with insulin therapy, normal or low potassium levels before initiation of insulin therapy warrant higher potassium supplementation.[156]

GLUCOSE

Bedside glucose measurements are not able to accurately measure the patient's glucose level above 500 mg per dL. Blood should be sent to the laboratory for accurate assessment. The preferable collection tube is a plasma separator tube, which inhibits glucose degradation. The concentration of the intravenous insulin dose (insulin drip) is based on the age of the patient. In children aged 3 years and younger, an insulin dose of 0.05 units of short-acting insulin per kilogram per hour is cautiously administered. In all other age groups, insulin therapy is initiated at 0.1 units of short-acting insulin per kilogram per hour. In general, glucose should not be lowered faster than 100 mg per dL over an hour. When serum glucose falls below 300 mg per dL, dextrose is added to the saline solution, but the insulin drip is continued until acidosis is substantially corrected. In patients with severe hyperglycemia (>1,000 mg per dL), dextrose should be added earlier to avoid a precipitous drop in blood sugar that may occur with improved glomerular filtration during hydration. Once the patient is able to resume oral intake with a pH of more than 7.3 and a serum bicarbonate level of more than 15 mEq per L, the intravenous insulin can be discontinued and replaced with SC injections.

BICARBONATE AND pH

In severe DKA, acidosis with a pH of less than 7.00 or a serum bicarbonate level of less than 5 mEq per L can occur. Although acidosis can be eventually corrected with insulin therapy and fluid resuscitation, bicarbonate treatment may be indicated in the ill-appearing patient, where acidosis may be impairing myocardial function. However, several caveats exist when administering bicarbonate in DKA. One of them is that the resulting rapid left shifts in the oxygen dissociation curve accelerate the entry of potassium into the cells. This could precipitate hypokalemia if potassium is not replete. It has been further stipulated that bicarbonate may worsen cerebral acidosis because it crosses the blood–brain barrier more slowly than carbon dioxide. A recent study suggests that of all the therapeutic interventions, only the administration of bicarbonate in DKA was associated with increased risk of cerebral edema.[157] It is, therefore, not surprising that the administration of bicarbonate remains one of the most debated treatments in DKA management, and if at all used, it is used sparingly (sodium bicarbonate at 1 mEq per kg given slowly over 1 to 2 hours and discontinued once pH approaches 7.1).

CALCIUM/MAGNESIUM/PHOSPHORUS

Phosphate levels are usually low, and phosphate can be replaced in the form of potassium phosphate, especially if PO_4 is less than 1.0 mg per dL. Since administering phosphate can lower serum calcium and magnesium, these levels should also be monitored. There are theoretical benefits to routinely using potassium phosphate instead of potassium chloride for rehydration. For example, it does not contribute to hyperchloremic metabolic acidosis, and it may also help to replenish stores of 2,3-diphosphoglycerate, which are important for tissue reoxygenation. However, these effects may not outweigh the risk of hypocalcemia during phosphate administration.

Acute cerebral edema remains to be an important complication of DKA. Young children, especially younger than 3 years, with new-onset diabetes are at higher risk to develop cerebral edema. Immediate intervention is utmost important if a patient develops neurologic deterioration and suggested treatment is mannitol at 1 g per kg of body weight.

OUTPATIENT MANAGEMENT OF TYPE 1 DIABETES MILETUS

Diabetes is a demanding disease requiring a multidisciplinary team approach, particularly for its outpatient management. The team ideally consists of a pediatric diabetologist, diabetes nurse specialist(s), social worker, dietician, and a psychologist who is experienced in the management of young patients and will focus on the needs of the patient and his or her family. The overall goal is to build a nonauthoritarian, collaborative relationship that will motivate the patients to be fully involved in their diabetes care, continue to assess the disease course, and prevent complications as much as possible.

In newly diagnosed patients, the first few weeks are critically important in the process of teaching self-management skills to the parent and child. In younger age groups, the parent is usually in daily contact with the diabetes clinical nurse specialist. Glucose levels, adjustment to diabetes, diet, and exercise are reviewed. The timing of the phone calls should be prearranged and ideally made to the same clinician. After making the insulin adjustment for the day, the rationale should be explained to the parent. Usually within 3 weeks, the parents are feeling more confident, and many are ready to attempt to make their own adjustments.

Once stabilized, regular follow-up visits on a two- to three-monthly basis are recommended for most patients. The main purpose of these visits is to ensure that the patient is achieving primary treatment goals. In addition to serial measurements of height and weight, particular attention should be paid to monitoring of blood pressure and examinations of the optic fundus, thyroid, and SC injection sites. Routine outpatient visits provide an opportunity to review glucose monitoring, to adjust the treatment regimen, and to assess child and family adjustment. Follow-up advice and support should be given by the nutritionist, diabetes nurse specialist, and psychologist or social worker. Use of the telephone, fax, or e-mail should be encouraged for adjustments in the treatment regimen between office visits.

Diet guidance for children with diabetes is best provided by a nutritionist who is an integral part of the treatment team and comfortable working with children. In addition to helping achieve optimal glucose levels and normal growth and development, nutritional management of diabetes is aimed at reducing the risk for other diseases, such as obesity, high blood cholesterol level, or high blood pressure. Underlying all of these is the establishment of sound eating patterns that include balanced, nutritious foods and consistent timing of food intake.[158]

The ADA dietary guidelines are used for dietary counseling. In addition to incorporating sound nutritional principles concerning the fat, fiber, and carbohydrate content, the importance of consistency in meal size and regularity in the timing of meals is emphasized. The prohibition of simple sugar in the diet has been de-emphasized, but it should still comprise no more than 10% of total carbohydrate intake. The success of the nutritional program may ultimately depend on the degree to which the meal planning is individualized and tailored to well-established eating patterns in the family. Moreover, flexibility can be enhanced if blood glucose monitoring results are used to evaluate the impact of change in dietary intake.

Carbohydrate counting is an increasingly popular way to increase flexibility in food intake that is commonly used by patients using insulin pumps or MDIs. It is based on matching the amount of RAI that is needed for each gram or serving of carbohydrate in the meal. With instructions on how to use nutritional labels on food packages, even children can become expert at counting carbohydrates. Some foods, like pizza, that cause a prolonged increase in blood glucose levels, may require higher insulin dosing with square or dual-wave bolus for insulin pump patients.

Regular exercise and active participation in organized sports have positive implications concerning the psychosocial and physical well-being of our patients. Parents and patients should be advised that different types of exercise may have different effects on blood glucose levels. For example, sports that involve short bursts of intensive exercise may increase rather than decrease blood glucose levels.[159] On the other hand, long-distance running and other prolonged activities are more likely to lower blood glucose levels. Parents also need to be warned that a long bout of exercise during the day may lead to hypoglycemia while the child is sleeping during the night, which may require a reduction in the dose of intermediate- and long-acting insulin or basal rates by 20% to 50%.

Severe hypoglycemia is a common problem in patients striving for strict glycemic control with intensive treatment regimens. In the DCCT, the risk of severe hypoglycemia was threefold higher in intensively treated patients than in conventionally treated patients, and being an adolescent was an independent risk factor for a severe hypoglycemic event. The majority of severe hypoglycemic events occur overnight due, in part, to sleep-induced defects in counterregulatory hormone responses to hypoglycemia.

Monitoring glucose level is critical to detect asymptomatic hypoglycemia, especially in the young child with diabetes. The older child is usually aware of symptoms, such as weakness, shakiness, hunger, or headache, and is encouraged to treat these symptoms as soon as they occur. The older child who can accurately recognize symptoms is taught to immediately treat with 15 g of carbohydrate (e.g., three to four glucose tablets, 4 oz of juice, or 15 g of a glucose gel) without waiting to check a glucose level. Each episode should be assessed to make proper adjustments if a cause can be identified. Every family should have a glucagon emergency kit at home to treat severe hypoglycemia.

Children with intercurrent illnesses, such as infections or vomiting, should be closely monitored for elevations in blood glucose levels and ketonuria. On sick days, blood glucose levels should be checked every 2 hours, and the urine should be checked for ketones with every void. Supplemental doses of RAI (0.1 to 0.3 units per kg) should be given every 2 to 4 hours for elevations in glucose and ketones. Because of its more rapid absorption, a RAI analog will lower plasma glucose faster than regular insulin. If the morning dose has not been given, and the child has a modestly elevated glucose level (150 to 250 mg per dL), small doses of NPH can be given to avoid a too rapid fall in plasma glucose levels. This works especially well in young children whose glucose levels fall quickly with RAI. Adequate fluid intake is essential to prevent dehydration. Fluids such as flat soda, clear soups, popsicles, and gelatin water are recommended to provide some electrolyte and carbohydrate replacement. If vomiting is persistent and ketones remain moderate or large after several supplemental insulin doses, arrangements should be made for parenteral hydration and evaluation in the emergency department.

Parents are told from the time of diagnosis that vomiting is a diabetes emergency and that they need to call for help after first checking blood glucose and urine ketone levels. This is especially true for children on pump therapy, since a catheter occlusion can throw the child into ketosis rapidly. If a pump-treated patient has elevated glucose and ketone levels, they are instructed to take a bolus injection of an RAI analog by syringe. The dose of insulin varies between 0.2 and 0.4 units per kg. They are then instructed to change their infusion set and to program a temporary basal rate at twice the usual basal rate for 4 to 5 hours. Blood glucose and urine ketone levels are rechecked every hour, and additional bolus doses can be given as needed. Once vomiting ceases and ketones become negative, the basal rate is returned to its usual setting. If the patient is not improving with these measures, the child should be seen by a clinician.

HOW CLOSE ARE WE TO A CURE? PANCREAS AND ISLET CELL TRANSPLANT AND IMMUNOMODULATION THERAPY

Until now, transplantation of whole vascular pancreas has been reserved for patients with end-stage renal failure who are also in need of a kidney transplant. Transplant prior to renal failure has been controversial because of the considerable risks involved in the surgery itself and the lifelong immunosuppression required to prevent graft rejection. However, a recent surgical review found that, with improved operating room techniques and new immunosuppressive protocols, patient and graft survival has improved. Whole pancreas transplant may, therefore, be a viable option for adults with poorly controlled diabetes, before the need for kidney transplantation arises.[160]

Nevertheless, the concept of whole pancreas transplant could become obsolete as protocols of islet cell transplantation are being developed. In the year 2000, the University of Alberta in Edmonton, Canada, published a minimally invasive procedure in which the portal vein is cannulated and then injected slowly with isolated islet cells. The so-called Edmonton Protocol was the first protocol to demonstrate that insulin independence could be achieved without entire pancreas transplant.[161] However, subsequent multicenter trials were not this successful, with only half of the 36 subjects achieving insulin independence after 1 year.[162]

The major stumbling blocks have been optimal immunosuppressive regimens. Undersuppression without corticosteroids was promoted by the Edmonton Protocol to enhance glycemic control. However, a recent study found that this might have contributed to the development of donor-specific antibodies.[163] Furthermore, tacrolimus and sirolimus, the preferred immunosuppressants of the Edmonton Protocol, may have worked against success by interfering with islet cell proliferation.[164] Other prohibitive factors are the need of up to four donor pancreases to harvest enough islets for transplant. As far as children are concerned, all such protocols pose an unacceptable risk of long-term immunosuppressive therapy—particularly in the area of growth and development.

The shortage of human donor pancreases has led researchers to seek out alternative ways to "grow" islet cells. Therefore, recent research has been directed toward the pluripotent stem cell of the early blastocyst, also referred to as embryonic stem cell. The first human embryonic stem cell lines were established in 1998. Although there is general consensus about the potential therapeutic benefits gained from studies with human stem cell lines, controversy still exists as to whether and how new human cell lines should be established. Efficient direct differentiation of human embryonic stem cells to glucose sensing and insulin-producing pancreatic β cells has been achieved in mice; however, outcomes have not been as successful in humans, and ongoing research projects are implemented to address some of the challenges.[165,166]

Autoimmune origin of T1DM has been known for years, and recent advances in immunomodulation therapy brought the possibility of prevention and cure of diabetes one step ahead. Target population for the prevention studies are subjects with positive autoantibodies (IAA, GAD65, IA-2, IA-2b, ZnT8) and/or early β-cell dysfunction, suggesting high risk of developing diabetes. Previous trials including nicotinamide (a component of vitamin B3), parenteral insulin use, or nasal insulin did not reveal promising results for the prevention of diabetes.[167,168] Secondary intervention studies to halt β-cell destruction with chronic use of immunosuppressant and immunomodulation therapies were tried without much success due to serious side effects and loss of effect after some time.[169,170] Current ongoing investigational therapies include combination of multiple immunomodulation treatments and plasmid-based treatments to prolong β-cell preservation.[171,172]

REFERENCES

1. Havcock P SD, Santiago JV, Skyler JS, et al. *History of insulin therapy. Intensive insulin therapy.* Princeton, NJ: Excerpta Medica; 1983:1–19.
2. Bliss M. Banting's, Best's, and Collip's accounts of the discovery of insulin. *Bull Hist Med* 1982;56:554–568.
3. Bell GI, Pictet RL, Rutter WJ, et al. Sequence of the human insulin gene. *Nature* 1980;284:26–32.
4. Variation and trends in incidence of childhood diabetes in Europe. EURODIAB ACE study group. *Lancet* 2000;355:873–876.
5. Karvonen M, Viik-Kajander M, Moltchanova E, et al. Incidence of childhood type 1 diabetes worldwide. Diabetes Mondiale (DiaMond) Project Group. *Diabetes Care* 2000;23:1516–1526.
6. Libman IM, LaPorte RE, Becker D, et al. Was there an epidemic of diabetes in nonwhite adolescents in Allegheny County, Pennsylvania? *Diabetes Care* 1998;21:1278–1281.
7. Atkinson MA. Molecular mimicry and the pathogenesis of insulin-dependent diabetes mellitus: still just an attractive hypothesis. *Ann Med* 1997;29:393–399.
8. Hiemstra HS, Schloot NC, van Veelen PA, et al. Cytomegalovirus in autoimmunity: T cell crossreactivity to viral antigen and autoantigen glutamic acid decarboxylase. *Proc Natl Acad Sci U S A* 2001;98:3988–3991.
9. Vaarala O, Hyoty H, Akerblom HK. Environmental factors in the aetiology of childhood diabetes. *Diabetes Nutr Metab* 1999;12:75–85.
10. American Diabetes Association. 2. Classification and diagnosis of diabetes: *Standards of Medical Care in Diabetes—2018. Diabetes Care* 2018;41:S13–S27.
11. Cengiz E, Connor CG, Ruedy KJ, et al. Pediatric diabetes consortium T1D new onset (NeOn) study: clinical outcomes during the first year following diagnosis. *Pediatr Diabetes* 2014;15:287–293.
12. Hua Q. Insulin: a small protein with a long journey. *Protein Cell* 2010;1:537–551.
13. Bier DM, Leake RD, Haymond MW, et al. Measurement of "true" glucose production rates in infancy and childhood with 6,6-dideuteroglucose. *Diabetes* 1977;26:1016–1023.
14. Fu Z, Gilbert ER, Liu D. Regulation of insulin synthesis and secretion and pancreatic Beta-cell dysfunction in diabetes. *Curr Diabetes Rev* 2013;9:25–53.
15. Owerbach D, Bell GI, Rutter WJ, et al. The insulin gene is located on the short arm of chromosome 11 in humans. *Diabetes* 1981;30:267–270.
16. Porterfield SP. *Endocrine physiology.* Saint Louis, MO: Mosby-Year Book, 1996.
17. Henquin JC, Dufrane D, Nenquin M. Nutrient control of insulin secretion in isolated normal human islets. *Diabetes* 2006;55:3470 -3477.
18. Kashyap S, Belfort R, Gastaldelli A, et al. A sustained increase in plasma free fatty acids impairs insulin secretion in nondiabetic subjects genetically predisposed to develop type 2 diabetes. *Diabetes* 2003;52:2461–2474.
19. Thorens B, Sarkar HK, Kaback HR, et al. Cloning and functional expression in bacteria of a novel glucose transporter present in liver, intestine, kidney, and beta-pancreatic islet cells. *Cell* 1988;55:281–290.
20. Matschinsky F, Liang Y, Kesavan P, et al. Glucokinase as pancreatic beta cell glucose sensor and diabetes gene. *J Clin Invest* 1993;92:2092–2098.
21. Froguel P, Vaxillaire M, Sun F, et al. Close linkage of glucokinase locus on chromosome 7p to early-onset non-insulin-dependent diabetes mellitus. *Nature* 1992;356:162–164.
22. Vionnet N, Stoffel M, Takeda J, et al. Nonsense mutation in the glucokinase gene causes early-onset non-insulin-dependent diabetes mellitus. *Nature* 1992;356:721–722.
23. Safayhi H, Haase H, Kramer U, et al. L-type calcium channels in insulin-secreting cells: biochemical characterization and phosphorylation in RINm5F cells. *Mol Endocrinol* 1997;11:619–629.
24. Blundell TL, Cutfield JF, Dodson GG, et al. The structure and biology of insulin. *Biochem J* 1971;125:50P–51P.
25. Dodson G, Steiner D. The role of assembly in insulin's biosynthesis. *Curr Opin Struct Biol* 1998;8:189–194.
26. Aguilar-Bryan L, Nichols CG, Wechsler SW, et al. Cloning of the beta cell high-affinity sulfonylurea receptor: a regulator of insulin secretion. *Science* 1995;268:423–426.
27. Kane C, Shepherd RM, Squires PE, et al. Loss of functional KATP channels in pancreatic beta-cells causes persistent hyperinsulinemic hypoglycemia of infancy. *Nat Med* 1996;2:1344–1347.
28. Thomas PM, Cote GJ, Wohllk N, et al. Mutations in the sulfonylurea receptor gene in familial persistent hyperinsulinemic hypoglycemia of infancy. *Science* 1995;268:426–429.
29. Babenko AP, Polak M, Cave H, et al. Activating mutations in the ABCC8 gene in neonatal diabetes mellitus. *N Engl J Med* 2006;355:456–466.
30. Gloyn AL, Pearson ER, Antcliff JF, et al. Activating mutations in the gene encoding the ATP-sensitive potassium-channel subunit Kir6.2 and permanent neonatal diabetes. *N Engl J Med* 2004;350:1838–1849.
31. Pearson ER, Flechtner I, Njolstad PR, et al. Switching from insulin to oral sulfonylureas in patients with diabetes due to Kir6.2 mutations. *N Engl J Med* 2006;355:467–477.
32. Ebina Y, Ellis L, Jarnagin K, et al. The human insulin receptor cDNA: the structural basis for hormone-activated transmembrane signalling. *Cell* 1985;40:747–758.
33. Seino S, Seino M, Nishi S, et al. Structure of the human insulin receptor gene and characterization of its promoter. *Proc Natl Acad Sci U S A* 1989;86:114–118.
34. Belfiore A, Malaguarnera R, Vella V, et al. Insulin receptor isoforms in physiology and disease: an updated view. *Endocr Rev* 2017;38:379–431.
35. Belfiore A, Frasca F, Pandini G, et al. Insulin receptor isoforms and insulin receptor/insulin-like growth factor receptor hybrids in physiology and disease. *Endocr Rev* 2009;30:586–623.
36. Pandini G, Frasca F, Mineo R, et al. Insulin/insulin-like growth factor I hybrid receptors have different biological characteristics depending on the insulin receptor isoform involved. *J Biol Chem* 2002;277:39684–39695.
37. Luo RZ, Beniac DR, Fernandes A, et al. Quaternary structure of the insulin-insulin receptor complex. *Science* 1999;285:1077–1080.
38. Bae SS, Cho H, Mu J, et al. Isoform-specific regulation of insulin-dependent glucose uptake by Akt/protein kinase B. *J Biol Chem* 2003;278:49530–49536.
39. Wang Q, Somwar R, Bilan PJ, et al. Protein kinase B/Akt participates in GLUT4 translocation by insulin in L6 myoblasts. *Mol Cell Biol* 1999;19:4008–4018.
40. Baumann CA, Ribon V, Kanzaki M, et al. CAP defines a second signalling pathway required for insulin-stimulated glucose transport. *Nature* 2000;407:202–207.
41. Pessin JE, Saltiel AR. Signaling pathways in insulin action: molecular targets of insulin resistance. *J Clin Invest* 2000;106:165–169.
42. Chiang SH, Baumann CA, Kanzaki M, et al. Insulin-stimulated GLUT4 translocation requires the CAP-dependent activation of TC10. *Nature* 2001;410:944–948.
43. Scott DA. Crystalline insulin. *Biochem J* 1934;28:1592–1602.
44. Hagedorn HC, Jensen BN, Krarup NB, et al. Landmark article Jan 18, 1936: protamine insulinate. By H.C. Hagedorn, B.N. Jensen, N.B. Krarup, and I. Wodstrup. *JAMA* 1984;251:389–392.
45. Scott DA, Fisher AM. Studies on insulin with protamine. *J Pharmacol Exp Ther* 1936;58:78–92.
46. Chance RE, Root MA, Galloway JA. The immunogenicity of insulin preparations. *Acta Endocrinol Suppl (Copenh)* 1976;205:185–198.
47. Davidson JK, DeBra DW. Immunologic insulin resistance. *Diabetes* 1978;27:307–318.
48. Morihara K, Oka T, Tsuzuki H. Semi-synthesis of human insulin by trypsin-catalysed replacement of Ala-B30 by Thr in porcine insulin. *Nature* 1979;280:412–413.

49. Goeddel DV, Kleid DG, Bolivar F, et al. Expression in *Escherichia coli* of chemically synthesized genes for human insulin. *Proc Natl Acad Sci U S A* 1979;76:106–110.
50. Raskin P, Clements RS Jr. The use of human insulin derived from baker's yeast by recombinant DNA technology. *Clin Ther* 1991;13:569–578.
51. Thim L, Hansen MT, Norris K, et al. Secretion and processing of insulin precursors in yeast. *Proc Natl Acad Sci U S A* 1986;83:6766–6770.
52. Brogden RN, Heel RC. Human insulin. A review of its biological activity, pharmacokinetics and therapeutic use. *Drugs* 1987;34:350–371.
53. Home PD, Alberti KG. Human insulin. *Clin Endocrinol Metab* 1982;11:453–483.
54. Brange J, Owens DR, Kang S, et al. Monomeric insulins and their experimental and clinical implications. *Diabetes Care* 1990;13:923–954.
55. Home PD. The pharmacokinetics and pharmacodynamics of rapid-acting insulin analogues and their clinical consequences. *Diabetes Obes Metab* 2012;14:780–788.
56. Nielsen FS, Jorgensen LN, Ipsen M, et al. Long-term comparison of human insulin analogue B10Asp and soluble human insulin in IDDM patients on a basal/bolus insulin regimen. *Diabetologia* 1995;38:592–598.
57. Bornfeldt KE, Gidlof RA, Wasteson A, et al. Binding and biological effects of insulin, insulin analogues and insulin-like growth factors in rat aortic smooth muscle cells. Comparison of maximal growth promoting activities. *Diabetologia* 1991;34:307–313.
58. Hamel FG, Siford GL, Fawcett J, et al. Differences in the cellular processing of AspB10 human insulin compared with human insulin and LysB28ProB29 human insulin. *Metabolism* 1999;48:611–617.
59. Howey DC, Bowsher RR, Brunelle RL, et al. [Lys(B28), Pro(B29)]-human insulin. A rapidly absorbed analogue of human insulin. *Diabetes* 1994;43:396–402.
60. Slieker LJ, Brooke GS, DiMarchi RD, et al. Modifications in the B10 and B26-30 regions of the B chain of human insulin alter affinity for the human IGF-I receptor more than for the insulin receptor. *Diabetologia* 1997;40(Suppl 2):S54–S61.
61. Torlone E, Fanelli C, Rambotti AM, et al. Pharmacokinetics, pharmacodynamics and glucose counterregulation following subcutaneous injection of the monomeric insulin analogue [Lys(B28),Pro(B29)] in IDDM. *Diabetologia* 1994;37:713–720.
62. Lougheed WD, Zinman B, Strack TR, et al. Stability of insulin lispro in insulin infusion systems. *Diabetes Care* 1997;20:1061–1065.
63. Renner R, Pfutzner A, Trautmann M, et al. Use of insulin lispro in continuous subcutaneous insulin infusion treatment. Results of a multicenter trial. German Humalog-CSII Study Group. *Diabetes Care* 1999;22:784–788.
64. Zinman B, Tildesley H, Chiasson JL, et al. Insulin lispro in CSII: results of a double-blind crossover study. *Diabetes* 1997;46:440–443.
65. Ampudia-Blasco FJ, Hasbum B, Carmena R. A new case of lipoatrophy with lispro insulin in insulin pump therapy: is there any insulin preparation free of complications? *Diabetes Care* 2003;26:953–954.
66. Griffin ME, Feder A, Tamborlane WV. Lipoatrophy associated with lispro insulin in insulin pump therapy: an old complication, a new cause? *Diabetes Care* 2001;24:174.
67. Fineberg NS, Fineberg SE, Anderson JH, et al. Immunologic effects of insulin lispro [Lys (B28), Pro (B29) human insulin] in IDDM and NIDDM patients previously treated with insulin. *Diabetes* 1996;45:1750–1754.
68. Hirsch IB, D'Alessio D, Eng L, et al. Severe insulin resistance in a patient with type 1 diabetes and stiff-man syndrome treated with insulin lispro. *Diabetes Res Clin Pract* 1998;41:197–202.
69. Kumar D. Lispro analog for treatment of generalized allergy to human insulin. *Diabetes Care* 1997;20:1357–1359.
70. Attia N, Jones TW, Holcombe J, et al. Comparison of human regular and lispro insulins after interruption of continuous subcutaneous insulin infusion and in the treatment of acutely decompensated IDDM. *Diabetes Care* 1998;21:817–821.
71. Lindholm A, McEwen J, Riis AP. Improved postprandial glycemic control with insulin aspart. A randomized double-blind cross-over trial in type 1 diabetes. *Diabetes Care* 1999;22:801–805.
72. Mudaliar SR, Lindberg FA, Joyce M, et al. Insulin aspart (B28 asp-insulin): a fast-acting analog of human insulin: absorption kinetics and action profile compared with regular human insulin in healthy nondiabetic subjects. *Diabetes Care* 1999;22:1501–1506.
73. Raskin P, Guthrie RA, Leiter L, et al. Use of insulin aspart, a fast-acting insulin analog, as the mealtime insulin in the management of patients with type 1 diabetes. *Diabetes Care* 2000;23:583–588.
74. Home PD, Lindholm A, Hylleberg B, et al. Improved glycemic control with insulin aspart: a multicenter randomized double-blind crossover trial in type 1 diabetic patients. UK Insulin Aspart Study Group. *Diabetes Care* 1998;21:1904–1909.
75. Garg SK. New insulin analogues. *Diabetes Technol Ther* 2005;7:813–817.
76. Garg SK, Ellis SL, Ulrich H. Insulin glulisine: a new rapid-acting insulin analogue for the treatment of diabetes. *Expert Opin Pharmacother* 2005;6:643–651.
77. Danne T, Becker RHA, Heise T, et al. Pharmacokinetics, prandial glucose control, and safety of insulin glulisine in children and adolescents with type 1 diabetes. *Diabetes Care* 2005;28:2100–2105.
78. Roach P. New insulin analogues and routes of delivery: pharmacodynamic and clinical considerations. *Clin Pharmacokinet* 2008;47:595–610.
79. Arkins JA, Engbring NH, Lennon EJ. The incidence of skin reactivity to insulin in diabetic patients. *J Allergy* 1962;33:69–72.
80. Paley RG, Tunbridge RE. Dermal reactions to insulin therapy. *Diabetes* 1952;1:22–27.
81. Fujikura J, Fujimoto M, Yasue S, et al. Insulin-induced lipohypertrophy: report of a case with histopathology. *Endocr J* 2005;52:623–628.
82. Richardson T, Kerr D. Skin-related complications of insulin therapy: epidemiology and emerging management strategies. *Am J Clin Dermatol* 2003;4:661–667.
83. Young RJ, Hannan WJ, Frier BM, et al. Diabetic lipohypertrophy delays insulin absorption. *Diabetes Care* 1984;7:479–480.
84. Kumar O, Miller L, Mehtalia S. Use of dexamethasone in treatment of insulin lipoatrophy. *Diabetes* 1977;26:296–299.
85. Whitley TH, Lawrence PA, Smith CL. Amelioration of insulin lipoatrophy by dexamethasone injection. *JAMA* 1976;235:839–840.
86. Wyatt JW, Frias JL, Hoyme HE, et al. Congenital anomaly rate in offspring of mothers with diabetes treated with insulin lispro during pregnancy. *Diabet Med* 2005;22:803–807.
87. Hod M, Damm P, Kaaja R, et al. Fetal and perinatal outcomes in type 1 diabetes pregnancy: a randomized study comparing insulin aspart with human insulin in 322 subjects. *Am J Obstet Gynecol* 2008;198:186.e1–186.e7.
88. Heise T, Pieber TR, Danne T, et al. A pooled analysis of clinical pharmacology trials investigating the pharmacokinetic and pharmacodynamic characteristics of fast-acting insulin aspart in adults with type 1 diabetes. *Clin Pharmacokinet* 2017;56:551–559.
89. Heise T, Zijlstra E, Nosek L, et al. Pharmacological properties of faster-acting insulin aspart vs insulin aspart in patients with type 1 diabetes receiving continuous subcutaneous insulin infusion: a randomized, double-blind, crossover trial. *Diabetes Obes Metab* 2017;19:208–215.
90. Heinemann L, Heise T. Review: current status of the development of inhaled insulin. *Br J Diabetes Vasc Dis* 2004;4:295–301.
91. Angelo RR, Rousseau K, Grant M, et al. Technosphere® insulin: defining the role of Technosphere particles at the cellular level. *J Diabetes Sci Technol* 2009;3:545–554.
92. Raskin P, Heller S, Honka M, et al. Pulmonary function over 2 years in diabetic patients treated with prandial inhaled Technosphere Insulin or usual antidiabetes treatment: a randomized trial. *Diabetes Obes Metab* 2012;14:163–173.
93. Andersen G, Meiffren G, Lamers D, et al. Ultra-rapid BioChaperone Lispro ameliorates postprandial blood glucose control compared to insulin lispro commercial formulation in subjects with type 1 diabetes mellitus. *Diabetes Obes Metab* 2018;20:2627–2632.
94. Kapitza C, Leohr, J, Liu, R, et al. EASD Abstract: A novel formulation of insulin lispro shows significantly faster absorption and improvement in postprandial glucose excursions versus insulin lispro in patients with type 2 diabetes. *Diabetologia* 2017;60:1–608.
95. Jorgensen S, Vaag A, Langkjaer L, et al. NovoSol Basal: pharmacokinetics of a novel soluble long acting insulin analogue. *BMJ* 1989;299:415–419.
96. Heinemann L, Linkeschova R, Rave K, et al. Time-action profile of the long-acting insulin analog insulin glargine (HOE901) in comparison with those of NPH insulin and placebo. *Diabetes Care* 2000;23:644–649.
97. Owens DR, Coates PA, Luzio SD, et al. Pharmacokinetics of 125I-labeled insulin glargine (HOE 901) in healthy men: comparison with NPH insulin and the influence of different subcutaneous injection sites. *Diabetes Care* 2000;23:813–819.
98. Lepore M, Pampanelli S, Fanelli C, et al. Pharmacokinetics and pharmacodynamics of subcutaneous injection of long-acting human insulin analog glargine, NPH insulin, and ultralente human insulin and continuous subcutaneous infusion of insulin lispro. *Diabetes* 2000;49:2142–2148.
99. Heise T, Nosek L, Ronn BB, et al. Lower within-subject variability of insulin detemir in comparison to NPH insulin and insulin glargine in people with type 1 diabetes. *Diabetes* 2004;53:1614–1620.
100. Porcellati F, Rossetti P, Busciantella NR, et al. Comparison of pharmacokinetics and dynamics of the long-acting insulin analogs glargine and detemir at steady state in type 1 diabetes: a double-blind, randomized, crossover study. *Diabetes Care* 2007;30:2447–2452.
101. Porcellati F, Rossetti P, Ricci NB, et al. Pharmacokinetics and pharmacodynamics of the long-acting insulin analog glargine after 1 week of use compared with its first administration in subjects with type 1 diabetes. *Diabetes Care* 2007;30:1261–1263.
102. Berti L, Kellerer M, Bossenmaier B, et al. The long acting human insulin analog HOE 901: characteristics of insulin signalling in comparison to Asp(B10) and regular insulin. *Horm Metab Res* 1998;30:123–129.
103. Bahr M, Kolter T, Seipke G, et al. Growth promoting and metabolic activity of the human insulin analogue [GlyA21,ArgB31,ArgB32] insulin (HOE 901) in muscle cells. *Eur J Pharmacol* 1997;320:259–265.
104. Kurtzhals P, Schaffer L, Sorensen A, et al. Correlations of receptor binding and metabolic and mitogenic potencies of insulin analogs designed for clinical use. *Diabetes* 2000;49:999–1005.
105. Home PD, Ashwell SG. An overview of insulin glargine. *Diabetes Metab Res Rev* 2002;18(Suppl 3):S57–S63.
106. Ratner RE, Hirsch IB, Neifing JL, et al. Less hypoglycemia with insulin glargine in intensive insulin therapy for type 1 diabetes. U.S. Study Group of Insulin Glargine in Type 1 Diabetes. *Diabetes Care* 2000;23:639–643.
107. Schober E, Schoenle E, Van Dyk J, et al. Comparative trial between insulin glargine and NPH insulin in children and adolescents with type 1 diabetes. *Diabetes Care* 2001;24:2005–2006.
108. Becker RH, Dahmen R, Bergmann K, et al. New insulin glargine 300 units mL^{-1} provides a more even activity profile and prolonged glycemic control at steady state compared with insulin glargine 100 units mL^{-1}. *Diabetes Care* 2015;38:637–643.
109. Becker RH, Nowotny I, Teichert L, et al. Low within and between-day variability in exposure to new insulin glargine 300 U/ml. *Diabetes Obes Metab* 2015;17:261–267.
110. Morales J. Defining the role of insulin detemir in basal insulin therapy. *Drugs* 2007;67:2557–2584.
111. Pieber TR, Treichel HC, Hompesch B, et al. Comparison of insulin detemir and insulin glargine in subjects with type 1 diabetes using intensive insulin therapy. *Diabet Med* 2007;24:635–642.
112. Brunner GA, Sendhofer G, Wutte A, et al. Pharmacokinetic and pharmacodynamic properties of long-acting insulin analogue NN304 in comparison to NPH insulin in humans. *Exp Clin Endocrinol Diabetes* 2000;108:100–105.
113. Heinemann L, Sinha K, Weyer C, et al. Time-action profile of the soluble, fatty acid acylated, long-acting insulin analogue NN304. *Diabet Med* 1999;16:332–338.
114. Kurtoglu S, Atabek ME, Dizdarer C, et al. Insulin detemir improves glycemic control and reduces hypoglycemia in children with type 1 diabetes: findings from the Turkish cohort of the PREDICTIVE observational study. *Pediatr Diabetes* 2009;10:401–407.
115. Kurtzhals P, Havelund S, Jonassen I, et al. Effect of fatty acids and selected drugs on the albumin binding of a long-acting, acylated insulin analogue. *J Pharm Sci* 1997;86:1365–1368.
116. Hordern SV, Wright JE, Umpleby AM, et al. Comparison of the effects on glucose and lipid metabolism of equipotent doses of insulin detemir and NPH insulin with a 16-h euglycaemic clamp. *Diabetologia* 2005;48:420–426.

117. Ooi CP, Ting TH, Loke SC. Ultra-long acting insulin versus long-acting insulin for type 1 diabetes mellitus. *Cochrane Database Syst Rev* 2018;2018:CD011102.
118. Heise T, Nosek L, Bottcher SG, et al. Ultra-long-acting insulin degludec has a flat and stable glucose-lowering effect in type 2 diabetes. *Diabetes Obes Metab* 2012;14:944–950.
119. Tambascia MA, Eliaschewitz FG. Degludec: the new ultra-long insulin analogue. *Diabetol Metab Syndr* 2015;7:57.
120. Heise T, Korsatko S, Nosek L, et al. Steady state is reached within 2-3 days of once-daily administration of degludec, a basal insulin with an ultralong duration of action. *J Diabetes* 2016;8:132–138.
121. Heller S, Buse J, Fisher M, et al. Insulin degludec, an ultra-long acting basal insulin, versus insulin glargine in basal-bolus treatment with mealtime insulin aspart in type 1 diabetes (BEGIN Basal-Bolus Type 1): a phase 3, randomised, open-label, treat-to-target non-inferiority trial. *Lancet* 2012;379:1489–1497.
122. Mathieu C, Hollander P, Miranda-Palma B, et al. Efficacy and safety of insulin degludec in a flexible dosing regimen vs insulin glargine in patients with type 1 diabetes (BEGIN: Flex T1): a 26-week randomized, treat-to-target trial with a 26-week extension. *J Clin Endocrinol Metab* 2013;98:1154–1162.
123. Meneghini L, Atkin SL, Gough SC, et al. The efficacy and safety of insulin degludec given in variable once-daily dosing intervals compared with insulin glargine and insulin degludec dosed at the same time daily: a 26-week, randomized, open-label, parallel-group, treat-to-target trial in individuals with type 2 diabetes. *Diabetes Care* 2013;36:858–864.
124. Tamborlane WV, Sherwin RS, Genel M, et al. Reduction to normal of plasma glucose in juvenile diabetes by subcutaneous administration of insulin with a portable infusion pump. *N Engl J Med* 1979:573–578.
125. Effect of intensive diabetes treatment on the development and progression of long-term complications in adolescents with insulin-dependent diabetes mellitus: Diabetes Control and Complications Trial. Diabetes Control and Complications Trial Research Group. *J Pediatr* 1994;125:177–188.
126. Nathan DM, Genuth S, Lachin J, et al. The effect of intensive treatment of diabetes on the development and progression of long-term complications in insulin-dependent diabetes mellitus. *N Engl J Med* 1993;329:977–986.
127. Yeh HC, Brown TT, Maruthur N, et al. Comparative effectiveness and safety of methods of insulin delivery and glucose monitoring for diabetes mellitus: a systematic review and meta-analysis. *Ann Intern Med* 2012;157:336–347.
128. Wong JC, Foster NC, Maahs DM, et al. Real-time continuous glucose monitoring among participants in the T1D Exchange clinic registry. *Diabetes Care* 2014;37:2702–2709.
129. Pickup JC, Kidd J, Burmiston S, et al. Determinants of glycaemic control in type 1 diabetes during intensified therapy with multiple daily insulin injections or continuous subcutaneous insulin infusion: importance of blood glucose variability. *Diabetes Metab Res Rev* 2006;22:232–237.
130. Retnakaran R, Hochman J, DeVries JH, et al. Continuous subcutaneous insulin infusion versus multiple daily injections: the impact of baseline A1c. *Diabetes Care* 2004;27:2590–2596.
131. Karges B, Schwandt A, Heidtmann B, et al. Association of insulin pump therapy vs insulin injection therapy with severe hypoglycemia, ketoacidosis, and glycemic control among children, adolescents, and young adults with type 1 diabetes. *JAMA* 2017;318:1358–1366.
132. Maahs DM, Hermann JM, Holman N, et al. Rates of diabetic ketoacidosis: international comparison with 49,859 pediatric patients with type 1 diabetes from England, Wales, the U.S., Austria, and Germany. *Diabetes Care* 2015;38:1876–1882.
133. Zabeen B, Craig ME, Virk SA, et al. Insulin pump therapy is associated with lower rates of retinopathy and peripheral nerve abnormality. *PLoS One* 2016;11:e0153033.
134. Boland EA, Grey M, Oesterle A, et al. Continuous subcutaneous insulin infusion. A new way to lower risk of severe hypoglycemia, improve metabolic control, and enhance coping in adolescents with type 1 diabetes. *Diabetes Care* 1999;22:1779–1784.
135. American Diabetes Association. 7. Diabetes Technology: *Standards of Medical Care in Diabetes—2019. Diabetes Care* 2019;42:S71–S80.
136. Eugster EA, Francis G. Position statement: Continuous subcutaneous insulin infusion in very young children with type 1 diabetes. *Pediatrics* 2006;118:e1244–e1249.
137. Ostrow D, Phillips N, Avalos A, et al. Mutational bias for body size in rhabditid nematodes. *Genetics* 2007;176:1653–1661.
138. Diabetes Research in Children Network (DirecNet) Study Group. Youth and parent satisfaction with clinical use of the GlucoWatch G2 Biographer in the management of pediatric type 1 diabetes. *Diabetes Care* 2005;28:1929–1935.
139. Heinemann L. Future directions for insulin therapy and diabetes treatment. *Endocrinol Metab Clin North Am* 2007;36(Suppl 2):69–79.
140. Koschinsky T, Heinemann L. Sensors for glucose monitoring: technical and clinical aspects. *Diabetes Metab Res Rev* 2001;17:113–123.
141. Weinstein RL, Schwartz SL, Brazg RL, et al. Accuracy of the 5-day FreeStyle Navigator Continuous Glucose Monitoring System: comparison with frequent laboratory reference measurements. *Diabetes Care* 2007;30:1125–1130.
142. Wilson DM, Beck RW, Tamborlane WV, et al. The accuracy of the FreeStyle Navigator continuous glucose monitoring system in children with type 1 diabetes. *Diabetes Care* 2007;30:59–64.
143. Battelino T, Conget I, Olsen B, et al. The use and efficacy of continuous glucose monitoring in type 1 diabetes treated with insulin pump therapy: a randomised controlled trial. *Diabetologia* 2012;55:3155–3162.
144. Danne T, Nimri R, Battelino T, et al. International consensus on use of continuous glucose monitoring. *Diabetes Care* 2017;40:1631–1640.
145. Forlenza GP, Li Z, Buckingham BA, et al. Predictive low-glucose suspend reduces hypoglycemia in adults, adolescents, and children with type 1 diabetes in an at-home randomized crossover study: results of the PROLOG Trial. *Diabetes Care* 2018;41:2155–2161.
146. Garg SK, Weinzimer SA, Tamborlane WV, et al. Glucose outcomes with the in-home use of a hybrid closed-loop insulin delivery system in adolescents and adults with type 1 diabetes. *Diabetes Technol Ther* 2017;19:155–163.
147. Zaykov AN, Mayer JP, DiMarchi RD. Pursuit of a perfect insulin. *Nat Rev Drug Discov* 2016;15:425–439.
148. Juvenile Diabetes Cure Alliance. Smart insulin: an overview of all projects. 2018. http://thejdca.org/2018-smart-insulin-an-overview-of-all-projects.
149. Harris K, Boland C, Meade L, et al. Adjunctive therapy for glucose control in patients with type 1 diabetes. *Diabetes Metab Syndr Obes* 2018;11:159–173.
150. Frandsen CS, Dejgaard TF, Madsbad S. Non-insulin drugs to treat hyperglycaemia in type 1 diabetes mellitus. *Lancet Diabetes Endocrinol* 2016;4:766–780.
151. Cree-Green M, Bergman BC, Cengiz E, et al. Metformin improves peripheral insulin sensitivity in youth with type 1 diabetes. *J Clin Endocrinol Metab* 2019;104:3265–3278.
152. Danne T, Biester T, Kordonouri O. Combined SGLT1 and SGLT2 inhibitors and their role in diabetes care. *Diabetes Technol Ther* 2018;20:S269–S277.
153. AJMC Staff. Sotagliflozin approved in EU for adults with type 1 diabetes. 2019. https://www.ajmc.com/newsroom/sotagliflozin-approved-in-eu-for-adults-with-type-1-diabetes.
154. Faich GA, Fishbein HA, Ellis SE. The epidemiology of diabetic acidosis: a population-based study. *Am J Epidemiol* 1983;117:551–558.
155. Duck SC, Wyatt DT. Factors associated with brain herniation in the treatment of diabetic ketoacidosis. *J Pediatr* 1988;113:10–14.
156. Hafeez W VP. CME: Managing diabetic ketoacidosis—a delicate balance. *Contemp Pediatr* 2000;6:72.
157. Glaser N, Barnett P, McCaslin I, et al. Risk factors for cerebral edema in children with diabetic ketoacidosis. The Pediatric Emergency Medicine Collaborative Research Committee of the American Academy of Pediatrics. *N Engl J Med* 2001;344:264–269.
158. Tamborlane W, Warshaw J. Diabetes. In: *Yale guide to children's nutrition.* New Haven, CT: Yale University Press, 1997:161–169.
159. Mitchell TH, Abraham G, Schiffrin A, et al. Hyperglycemia after intense exercise in IDDM subjects during continuous subcutaneous insulin infusion. *Diabetes Care* 1988;11:311–317.
160. Sutherland DE, Gruessner RW, Dunn DL, et al. Lessons learned from more than 1,000 pancreas transplants at a single institution. *Ann Surg* 2001;233:463–501.
161. Shapiro AM, Lakey JR, Ryan EA, et al. Islet transplantation in seven patients with type 1 diabetes mellitus using a glucocorticoid-free immunosuppressive regimen. *N Engl J Med* 2000;343:230–238.
162. Shapiro AM, Ricordi C, Hering BJ, et al. International trial of the Edmonton protocol for islet transplantation. *N Engl J Med* 2006;355:1318–1330.
163. Campbell PM, Senior PA, Salam A, et al. High risk of sensitization after failed islet transplantation. *Am J Transplant* 2007;7:2311–2317.
164. Nir T, Melton DA, Dor Y. Recovery from diabetes in mice by beta cell regeneration. *J Clin Invest* 2007;117:2553–2561.
165. Pagliuca FW, Millman JR, Gurtler M, et al. Generation of functional human pancreatic beta cells in vitro. *Cell* 2014;159:428–439.
166. Rezania A, Bruin JE, Arora P, et al. Reversal of diabetes with insulin-producing cells derived in vitro from human pluripotent stem cells. *Nat Biotechnol* 2014;32:1121–1133.
167. Krischer JP, Cuthbertson DD, Yu L, et al. Screening strategies for the identification of multiple antibody-positive relatives of individuals with type 1 diabetes. *J Clin Endocrinol Metab* 2003;88:103–108.
168. Näntö-Salonen K, Kupila A, Simell S, et al. Nasal insulin to prevent type 1 diabetes in children with HLA genotypes and autoantibodies conferring increased risk of disease: a double-blind, randomised controlled trial *Lancet* 2008;372:1746–1755.
169. Bougneres PF, Carel JC, Castano L, et al. Factors associated with early remission of type I diabetes in children treated with cyclosporine. *N Engl J Med* 1988;318:663–670.
170. Type 1 Diabetes TrialNet. Completed studies. 2019. https://www.trialnet.org/our-research.
171. ClinicalTrials.gov. Diabetes autoimmunity withdrawn in new onset and in established patients. 2019. https://www.trialnet.org/our-research
172. Type 1 Diabetes TrialNet. Prevention studies. 2019. https://www.trialnet.org/our-research.

CHAPTER

56

Jorge Mejia-Corletto
Paul H. Saenger

Growth Hormone

INTRODUCTION

The therapeutic use of growth hormone (GH), derived from human cadaveric pituitaries, was introduced in the late 1950s and early 1960s.[1] The production of pituitary GH slowly increased over the next two decades, but supplies did not meet the treatment needs of all patients believed to have GH deficiency (GHD) due to difficulties in obtaining sufficient cadaveric pituitaries. The recognition of Creutzfeldt–Jakob disease (CJD) in recipients of pituitary-derived GH in 1985 led to its immediate discontinuation in most countries. The past two decades have seen a dramatic increase in worldwide availability of natural sequence recombinant human GH (rhGH), with improvement in treatment protocols for children with GHD. GH has been used increasingly for short children with non-GHD conditions in childhood and adolescence, including idiopathic short stature (ISS), intrauterine growth retardation (IUGR) or small for gestational age (SGA) infants, chronic renal failure (CRF), and genetic syndromes such as Turner syndrome (TS), Prader–Willi syndrome (PWS), and SHOX deficiency. In addition, studies began in the 1990s on the adult population of childhood onset of GHD, as well as on adult-onset GHD.

GROWTH HORMONE SECRETION

GROWTH HORMONE–RELEASING HORMONE AND SOMATOSTATIN

GH secretion is pulsatile, with diurnal variation, and varies significantly with sleep, nutrition, hormonal milieu (e.g., glucocorticoids, sex steroids), and pubertal status, with tightly controlled feedback mechanisms. GH self-entrains the ultradian rhythm of episodic GH release.[2,3] The frequency of GH pulses is preserved across all species, occurring at approximately 3- to 4-hour intervals, with the largest spontaneous peaks occurring during onset of deep sleep. Somatostatin (SST) plays a critical role in the pulse frequency of GH release.[4] Historically, it has been considered that only two hypothalamic hormones, growth hormone–releasing hormone (GHRH) and SST, control GH secretion: the former stimulates and the latter inhibits pituitary somatotroph release of GH.[4,5] It is recognized that endogenous GHRH is required for the normal GH response to each of the following pharmacologic stimuli: L-dopa, arginine, insulin-induced hypoglycemia, clonidine, and glucagon. Macimorelin is a new oral GH secretagogue (GHS) that has been developed and may find its usefulness during provocative testing for GHD in adults.[6] Insulin-induced hypoglycemia is still considered the gold standard.

GROWTH HORMONE–RELEASING HORMONE RECEPTOR

GH-releasing hormone receptors (GHRHRs) are located on the pituitary somatotrophs; these receptors belong to the G-protein–coupled receptor family. Homozygous or compound heterozygous inactivating mutations in the GHRHR cause complete lack of functional GHRHR protein and lack of detectable increase in serum GH to all provocative stimuli.[7] These mutations cause severe familial isolated GH deficiency (IGHD type 1b), and patients have a profoundly short stature with decreased serum levels of insulin-like growth factors 1 and 2 (IGF-1 and IGF-2) and IGF-binding protein 3 (IGFBP-3). Magnetic resonance imaging (MRI) shows hypoplasia of the anterior pituitary.[8] As expected, these individuals respond appropriately to exogenous GH administration.

GROWTH HORMONE SECRETAGOGUES

GH-releasing peptides (GHRPs) and nonpeptide mimetics, collectively referred to as GH secretagogues (GHSs), are a family of synthetic peptide and nonpeptide compounds that are capable of inducing GH release in all species, including humans. A novel feature is that they can stimulate GH release when given by oral, intranasal, or parenteral route.[9] The coadministration of GHRP with GHRH produces a synergistic GH release. Children with classic GHD, and especially those with pituitary stalk interruption syndrome (PSIS) on MRI, have a markedly diminished GH response to GHRPs.[8] This has been interpreted as a chronic absence or diminution of endogenous GHRH secretion.

GROWTH HORMONE SECRETAGOGUE RECEPTOR

GHS receptor (GHSR) is a G-protein–coupled receptor expressed mainly in the somatotrophs of the anterior lobe of the pituitary, the hypothalamus, and the hippocampus and on GHRH neurons. It is selective for the specific GHS peptides, such as ghrelin, which is a 28-amino-acid peptide that is an endogenous ligand of GHSR. Activation of GHSR by synthetic ligands initiates and amplifies pulsatile GH release in animals, including humans, via the stimulated release of GHRH, which can be blocked by SST and GH.[10]

GHRELIN

Endocrine cells in the gastric mucosa produce ghrelin, but expression in the intestine, pancreas, hypothalamus, and testis has also been reported.[11] Ghrelin stimulates GH secretion in vivo and from anterior pituitary cells in vitro. At least two different types of ghrelin receptors have been identified; their activation is involved in the secretion of a variety of pituitary hormones, appetite, and long-term regulation of energy homeostasis.[12,13]

GROWTH HORMONE GENE

The human *GH* gene locus is on the long arm of chromosome 17 and encodes for both pituitary GH (hGH-N), a single polypeptide chain of 191-amino-acid residues that is secreted from the pituitary, as well as placental hGH (hGH-V).[14] The *GH* gene locus is close to the gene locus for chorionic somatotropin or human placental lactogen derived from the placenta. The primary full-length 22-kDa peptide is alternately spliced to yield a 20-kDa peptide that is cosecreted with and circulates at 5% to 10% of 22-kDa GH levels. IGHD attributed to *GH* gene mutations may be inherited as autosomal recessive, dominant, or X-linked, with the last entity being associated with hypogammaglobulinemia. Deletions of hGH-N produce very severe autosomal recessive growth failure after birth.[15]

GROWTH HORMONE RECEPTOR

GH exerts many of its physiologic functions by regulating the transcription of genes of a variety of proteins, including IGF-1, transcription factors, and metabolic enzymes.[16] The GH receptor (GHR) was cloned in 1987 and led to the study of GH signaling at a molecular level. The complementary DNA (cDNA) for the hGHR encodes a 638-amino-acid protein that has single extracellular, transmembrane, and cytoplasmic domains. It is a member of the cytokine/hematopoietin receptor superfamily that binds more than 25 ligands, including prolactin and leptin. In the working model of GH action, a single molecule of GH binds to two molecules of the GHR in a sequential manner to form a dimer, an event that is crucial to subsequent GH signaling events. During activation, the extracellular domain undergoes proteolytic cleavage to yield a soluble GH-binding protein in plasma or GHBP. GH binding to two receptor molecules increases the affinity of each receptor for a nonreceptor tyrosine kinase termed JAK2. Activation of JAK2 induces phosphorylation of itself and of tyrosine residues on the cytoplasmic domain of the GHR, initiating a cascade of signaling molecules that are beyond the purview of this chapter.[16]

Inactivating mutations of the *GHR* gene or downstream signaling pathways cause the GH-insensitivity syndrome (GHIS). Laron syndrome or classic GHIS is rare; its phenotype resembles that of GHD, except for the presence of high serum GH concentrations and low levels of IGF-1, IFG-2, and IGFBP-3. Subcutaneous injections of recombinant IGF-1 or recombinant IGF-1–recombinant IGFBP-3 complex offer some promise of significantly improving height growth.[17] A patient with a post-GHR defect in conjunction with a primary immunodeficiency was described, and a mutation in the *STAT5b* gene has been implicated.[18]

GROWTH HORMONE ACTIONS

GH is a powerful anabolic hormone and has a broader spectrum of action than implied by its original name. The growth-promoting effects and metabolic effects of GH are mediated via interaction with the specific GHR and through the important intermediary IGF-1 and its receptor.[16,19,20]

The GH–IGF-I target tissue axis is very complex and plays a very important role in many physiologic processes[21] (Fig. 56.1). The pulsatile secretion of GH sets a cascade in motion involving multiple organs and systems. Also, the factors determining normal growth depend on a child's age. For example, intrauterine growth is not dependent on GH since infants with congenital absence of the pituitary are born normal in size. Early postnatal growth up until 6 months of age is predominantly insulin dependent. After these first 6 months, GH becomes increasingly important in controlling longitudinal growth. Several studies have demonstrated that up to 60% of SGA children with insufficient catch-up growth show a reduction in physiologic 24-hour GH secretion and/or low GH peaks during provocation tests. The reason for this is unknown.

The effects of GH can be accomplished only in the presence of a normal functioning GHR. The *GHR* gene is located on chromosome 5, and there are two isoforms in humans: a full-length isoform and an isoform that lacks exon 3 (d3-GHR).[21]

Although some of the effects of GH are direct actions, most effects are mediated through the peptide hormone IGF-I. The IGF family includes IGF-I, IGF-II, three-membrane–bound receptors, several IGFBPs, and the acid-labile subunit (ALS). IGF-I and IGF-II are closely related, single-chain polypeptides, which share approximately 50% of their amino acid sequence. IGF-I, but especially IGF-II, plays a dominant role in early fetal development through binding to the IGF-IR. However, after organogenesis, GH-dependent IGF-I bioactivity becomes more important. The role of IGF-II during postnatal life remains unclear. In mice, the disruption of the paternally inherited *IGF-II* allele causes severe IUGR, whereas the disruption of the maternally inherited *IGF-II* allele has no effect on growth. There has been a report an *IGF-II* variant with evidence of pathogenicity in a multigenerational family with severe IUGR and postnatal growth restriction and a Silver–Russell syndrome phenotype.[21]

The majority of IGF-I is firmly bound to IGFBPs. IGFBPs play an important role in regulating the availability of IGF-I. These binding proteins act as carrier proteins, transporting IGF-I from the circulation to the target tissues and prolonging the half-life of IGF-I. Six IGFBPs have been identified, and they show similar organization, mostly at the NH2- and COOH-terminal domains. All of the IGFBPs have a similar or higher binding affinity for IGF-I than for the IGF-IR. This suggests that the formation of IGF-I–IGFBP complexes competes with binding of IGF-I to the IGF-IR. In healthy subjects, most of the serum IGF-I circulates in a 150-kD ternary complex with IGFBP-3 (and, to a much lesser extent, IGFBP-5) and ALS. Only 1% to 5% of IGF-I is unbound, with a short half-life of 10 to 12 minutes.

To date, no mutations have been reported in *IGFBP* genes. Animal *IGFBP* knockout studies demonstrated only minor effects on fetal and postnatal growth.[22] Studies in *IGFBP* transgenic mice revealed that the predominant effect of overexpression of the IGFBPs has been growth inhibition, as would be anticipated from inhibition of the actions of IGF-I and IGF-II.[23,24] This has also been described in children with chronic renal insufficiency. IGFBPs also bind non-IGF ligands

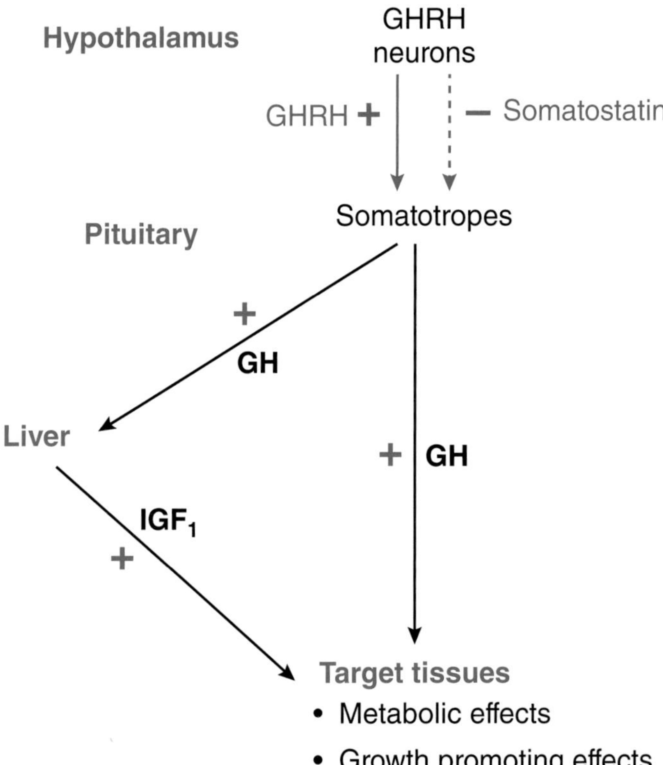

Figure 56.1 Schematic representation of the main components of the hypothalamic–pituitary–IGF-I axis. Hypothalamic neurons secrete GH releasing hormone (GHRH) in a pulsatile fashion which then stimulate anterior pituitary somatotrope cells to secrete GH into circulation. GH activates the GHR on the liver and various other target tissues. This may either result in direct, metabolic effects from GH or indirect actions being mediated through IGF-I. IGF-I can act in mainly an autocrine, paracrine, or endocrine fashion through binding to the IGF-IR which is expressed by nearly all cell types. IGF1 then exert negative feedback on GHRH and GH secretion and positive feedback on somatostatin release.

in the extracellular space, cell membrane, cytoplasm, and nucleus, thereby modulating cell proliferation, survival, and migration in an IGF-independent manner. In general, IGFBP activity is regulated by transcriptional mechanisms as well as by post-translational modifications and proteolysis. To our knowledge, only IGFBP-1, IGFBP-2, and IGFBP-3; ALS; and ternary complex formation have been studied specifically in short SGA children.[21]

When assessing responses to GH therapy, three general outcome measurements have been frequently assessed:

1. In childhood, auxologic measures provide parameters of linear growth response to GH: height standard deviation score (HT SDS), height velocity (HV), weight, pubertal progression, skeletal maturation, and attainment of adult final height (FH). One must distinguish between short-term changes in growth velocity and the attainment of adult FH, which may not be concordant. Thus, increased HV over intervals of less than 1 year and predictions of FH are not reliable predictors of increased adult height attainment.[25–27] Age, initial HT SDS, delayed bone age, GH-secretory capacity, and GH dosage are important general predictors of a good growth response in children.[26,27]
2. In both children and adults, biochemical indices have been utilized to predict and/or monitor GH effects on cellular and tissue metabolism. GH increases protein synthesis, leading to retention of nitrogen; enhanced skeletal growth; increased sodium, phosphate, and calcium excretion; increased glucose and amino acid transport; and decreased lipogenesis. Indices of bone and mineral metabolism include calcium, phosphate, bone alkaline phosphatases, osteocalcin, propeptides of procollagen type I and type III, and bone mineral content.[19] GH is the most important regulator of IGFs in all body tissues. In children and adults, there is a dose-related increase in both serum IGF-1 and IGF-II with acute GH administration.[28] IGF-I increases more rapidly and to a relatively greater extent than IGF-II. For this reason, serum IGF-I levels have become the most commonly utilized measurement for assessing adequacy of GH secretion and monitoring the status of patients with GHD or excess.
3. Body mass index (BMI), percentage total body fat, total body or extracellular water, and bone mineral density are used most frequently to assess body composition.[19] GH action on the adipocyte leads to reduction of body fat due to both decreased lipogenesis and increased lipolysis. Modest acute changes with wide variability have been observed with most of these body composition measurements.

GH dose exerts a very significant positive influence on all parameters used to assess effects on growth and metabolism. Few of the tests just described can reliably predict and/or monitor response to GH therapy. Of these, serum IGF-1 appears to offer the best indicator of the action of GH throughout all age groups. Lack of GH action is seen in children with classic GHD. In these patients, there is a decrease in serum GH, IGF-1, and IGFBP-3; decreased HT SDS and growth velocity; delayed skeletal maturation; delayed pubertal onset; and increased abdominal adiposity. These are reversed with GH therapy. Excessive GH action is classically seen in patients with acromegaly, who demonstrate increased serum GH not suppressed with glucose, increased serum IGF-1 and IGFBP-3, increased BMI, and acral enlargement. With treatment of acromegaly, clinical improvement is usually best correlated with reductions in serum levels of GH and IGF-1.

THE ROLE OF THE GROWTH HORMONE–INSULIN-LIKE GROWTH FACTOR AXIS ON FETAL GROWTH REGULATION

The fetal endocrine milieu of hormones and growth factors is likely of secondary importance in the regulation of human fetal growth due to redundancy and the ability of several different systems to interact to protect fetal viability.[29] In this context, GHD is relatively less important than GHI, and the paracrine/autocrine system of growth control involving local regulatory factors such as the IGFs and the IGFBPs becomes significant. IGF-1 and IGF-2 are endocrine, paracrine, and autocrine modulators of fetal growth and metabolism. In the human, circulating levels of the IGFs increase in both maternal and fetal serum during gestation, with IGF-2 present in two- to fivefold higher amount than IGF-1.[29,30] Animal gene knockout models support a predominant role for IGF-2 in fetal growth regulation.[29] Therefore, IGF-2 may well be particularly important in early gestation, where it may dictate the size of the placenta and its ability to transport nutrients, both of which could profoundly affect fetal size.[31]

In the human genetic model of GHIS or Laron syndrome due to mutations of the GHR, there is a marked decrease in fetal serum IGF-1 and IGF-2, despite markedly elevated serum GH and very low serum GHBP. The neonates are small at birth.[32]

THE DIAGNOSIS OF GROWTH HORMONE DEFICIENCY AND OTHER GROWTH DISORDERS

Initial Assessment: Clinical Evaluation

Despite the complexity and multiplicity of potential causes, several diagnoses can be established by a carefully elicited medical history and a comprehensive physical examination[33,34] (Table 56.1).

TABLE 56.1 Specific Diagnostic Findings and Key Points in Medical History and Physical Examination of Children with Short Stature

Findings and Key Points	*Interpretations and Applications*
Medical history	
Birth length, weight, head circumference, gestational age	Classification as SGA or AGA
Previous growth data	Height velocity and growth pattern analysis
Age at start of pubertal signs	Early, normal, or delayed puberty
Previous diseases, surgeries, and medication use (special attention to the use of glucocorticoids)	To identify organic or iatrogenic causes
Medical history of the various systems	To identify chronic and systemic diseases
Feeding and nutrition history	To identify states of malnutrition or child neglect
Neuropsychomotor development delay and/or intellectual disability	Syndromes, chromosomal disorders, metabolic disorders
Family history of similar cases, consanguinity or family from isolated community families; draw the family pedigree	To identify monogenic disorders with autosomal dominant or recessive inheritance
Parental height (measured)	To estimate the target height
Parents' age at the start of puberty	To assess likelihood of a familiar pattern of delayed puberty
Physical examination	
Length or height SDS	To assess the severity of growth deficit
Body proportions (sitting height:total height ratio SDS; arm span)	To identify altered sitting height:height ratio as a suggestive sign of skeletal dysplasia
Weight-for-height or BMI showing underweight	Weight more affected than height, low weight-for-height and low BMI are suggestive of malnutrition
Weight-for-height or BMI showing overweight or obesity	Hypothyroidism, Cushing syndrome, GH deficiency, pseudohypoparathyroidism
Head circumference SDS	Microcephaly and macrocephaly are important findings, indicating potential diagnosis
Dysmorphic features	Syndromes
Pubertal stage	Early, normal, or delayed puberty
General physical examination	Search for chronic and systemic diseases

AGA, adequate for gestational age; BMI, body mass index; GH, growth hormone; SDS, standard deviation score; SGA, small for gestational age.
From Collett-Solberg PF, Jorge AA, Boguszewski MC, et al. Growth hormone therapy in children; research and practice—a review. *Growth Horm IGF Res* 2019;44:20–32.

This process aims to recognize the presence of signs and symptoms that indicate a specific condition causing growth failure and thus guide further investigation. During the clinical evaluation, it is usually possible to distinguish children with short stature associated with chronic disease states or with syndromic conditions from those who are apparently healthy[34] (Fig. 56.2).

A key point is a detailed description of the child's growth pattern, including the time when the growth deficit was first observed. Birth characteristics must be evaluated (gestation and delivery conditions or complications; gestational age, birth weight, length, and head circumference), assessing if the growth impairment had a prenatal or postnatal onset. Medical history must be assessed, with a focus on neuropsychomotor development, nutritional status, medication use, and cardiac, renal, pulmonary, neurologic, and gastrointestinal symptoms/complaints.[33,35]

Physical examination should include the description of anthropometric measurements, dysmorphic features, and any other clues for one of the many causes of short stature[34] (Table 56.1). In children younger than 2 to 3 years, supine length, weight, weight-for-length, and head circumference should be measured, and fontanelles as well as dentition should be evaluated. In older children, erect height, arm span, sitting height (SH), head circumference, and weight should be measured.[33] BMI and HT:H ratio should be calculated. The pubertal status should be assessed. Evaluation of a child's height must be done in the context of standards for sex and age. Such standards can be either cross sectional (by calculation of HT SDS) or longitudinal (by plotting in growth charts). Serial measurements with a minimum interval of 6 months are necessary to determine the HV. Because genetic factors are important determinants of growth and height, sibling and parental height and pubertal pattern should be noted.

Many abnormal growth states are characterized by disproportionate growth, which is suggestive of skeletal dysplasia. Therefore, body proportion measurements should be part of the evaluation of short stature. The use of SH:H ratio for age and sex, which can also be expressed in SDS, according to published standards,[36] allows for the observation of body proportion changes throughout development. Children with short stature and an increased SH:H ratio for age and sex have a disproportional short stature caused by limb abnormalities, while children with short stature and a decreased SH:H ratio for age and sex have a disproportional short stature caused by axial segment abnormalities.[37]

Human Growth Hormone Measurement

One of the most relevant aspects for standardization when diagnosing GH-secretory disorders[38] (i.e., GHD, among others) relates to changes in *international reference preparations* (IRPs).[39] The first IRP for hGH (IRP 66/217) in 1969 was of pituitary origin, with a designated specific activity of 2 IU per mg.[40] A subsequent IRP (IRP 80/505) was based on purified pituitary GH, with a specific activity of 2.6 IU per mg, but the first and second biosynthetic GH IRPs (IRP 88/624 and 98/574) were purified 22-kDa rhGH with an assigned potency of 3 IU per mg (World Health Organization International Biological Reference Preparations).[40] Thus, before 1982, 20 μIU hGH was equivalent to 10 ng, but it is only equivalent to 6.7 ng today.[40] In addition, different antibodies have been used in immunoassays. Initially, these antibodies were polyclonal and directed against all epitopes of pit-GH, but after the 1990s, either polyclonal or monoclonal antibodies directed against different epitopes of monomeric 22-kDa rhGH were applied.[40] The latter approach may lead to lower hGH levels in human plasma.

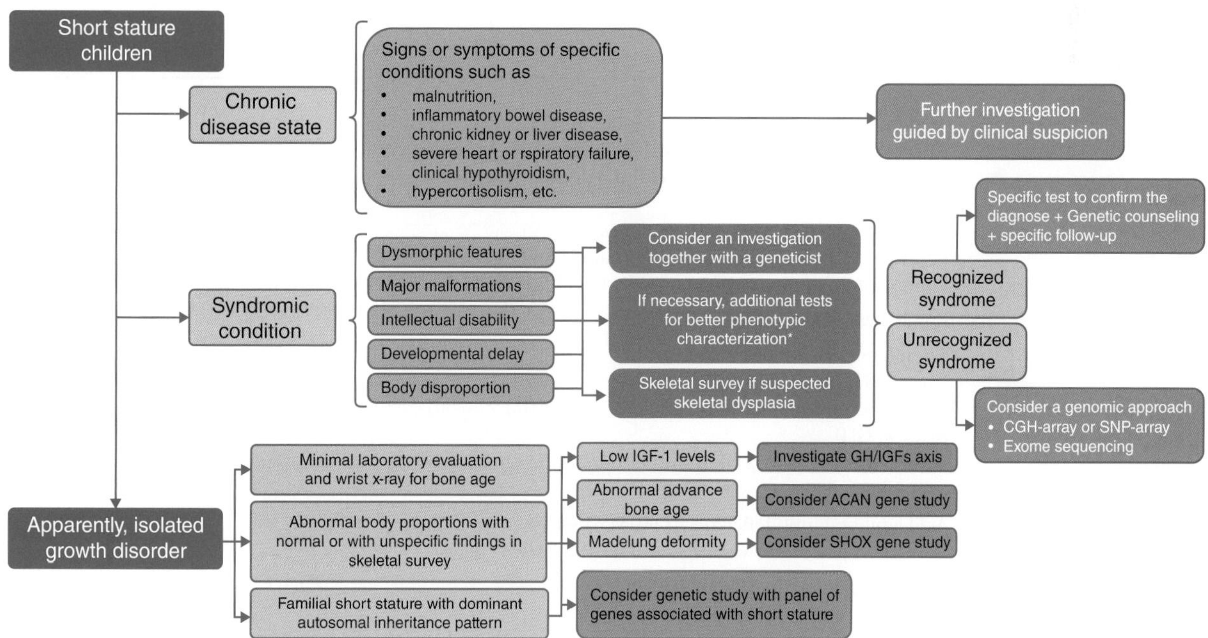

Figure 56.2 Overview of the investigation of children with short stature. CGH, comparative genomic hybridization; GH, growth hormone; IGF, insulin-like growth factor; SNP, single-nucleotide polymorphism. (Adapted from Collett-Solberg PF, Jorge AA, Boguszewski MC, et al. Growth hormone therapy in children; research and practice—a review. *Growth Horm IGF Res* 2019;44:20–32.)

Subsequent Assessment: Diagnostic Testing

Depending on specific clinical findings from the medical history and physical examination, special investigations are required to confirm the initial clinical impression. When a skeletal dysplasia is suspected, mainly for children with body disproportion abnormalities or skeletal deformities, skeletal survey analysis, including the skull, spine, pelvis, and upper and lower limbs, should be obtained for a more precise diagnosis.[41] Likewise, when dysmorphic features are suggestive of syndromic causes, diagnostic investigations should prioritize those possibilities. When a specific syndrome is recognized by clinical evaluation, the patient should be specifically tested. On the other hand, if no syndrome is clinically recognizable, patients with short stature associated with dysmorphic features should undergo genetic testing, including molecular karyotyping [single-nucleotide polymorphism array (SNPa) or array comparative genomic hybridization (aCGH)][42] and/or whole-genome sequencing (WGS).[43,44] In this scenario, it is important to consider referring to a geneticist, dysmorphologist, and/or pediatric endocrinologist group specializing in growth disorders for a more detailed evaluation. The majority of short children evaluated for short stature are apparently healthy, and their medical history and physical examination do not bring any specific clue to guide further laboratory or imaging examinations. Fewer than 1% of short apparently healthy children will have a pathologic condition.[45] In patients with a low pretest probability of disease, one must be careful regarding the interpretation of any abnormal test. The diagnostic workup should include tests for a group of diseases that can be associated with short stature with minimal other signs and symptoms.[46,47] Most clinicians consider a radiograph of the left hand and wrist (to assess the bone age) a useful test. There are two main standards to evaluate the bone age: Greulich and Pyle[48] and Tanner et al.[49] The most commonly used method for height prediction based on bone age is the Bayley and Pinneau's method.[50] More recently, an automated method to determine skeletal maturity became available.[51] This new methodology decreases the variability so common in manual methods of bone age assessment. Advanced bone age in relation to chronologic age, especially in prepubertal children, suggests defects in the *ACAN* gene.[52] Mild and nonspecific findings on hand and wrist x-ray, such as short metacarpals or short middle phalanges, can suggest defects in genes involved in growth plate maturation (*GNAS*, *NPR2*, *NPPC*, and *IHH*).[22,37,53] Even though most conditions that affect growth cause bone age delay, the most common cause of delayed bone age is constitutional. There are few evidence-based studies that support a list of minimal laboratory evaluations that should be systematically performed in all children with short stature.[23,45] In an apparently healthy short child, the laboratory tests could include serum concentrations of IGF-1 and thyroid-stimulating hormone (TSH)/free T4 and initial screening tests for celiac disease.[23,33,35,45] IGFBP-3 measurement in children younger than 3 years may improve the assessment of the GH–IGF-1 axis.[24] In childhood survivors of neoplasias, particularly those who received cranial radiotherapy, the accuracy of serum levels of IGF-I/IGFBP-3 is decreased.[54] Blood count, C-reactive protein, and erythrocyte sedimentation rate can help detect inflammatory states. It is a common practice to also include renal function tests and liver function tests in the evaluation. Additionally, it is generally advised to request a conventional or molecular (SNPa or aCGH) karyotype for short girls, even in the absence of typical signs of TS.[55] The inclusion of additional laboratory tests increases the cost of the investigation, and one should be aware that there is a relatively low probability of establishing a pathologic diagnosis in asymptomatic short children.[45] Defects of GH–IGF-1 axis should be investigated in patients with suggestive clinical findings. This is a heterogeneous group of conditions with a distinct phenotype[56,57] (Table 56.2). GHD is by far the most common defect in the GH–IGF-1 axis, although its frequency is only 1% to 2% in a nonselected group of short stature children.[34] More recently, it was suggested that

TABLE 56.2 Disorders of the GH–IGF Axis Associated with Short Stature

Type of Disorder	*Disorder*
GH deficiency	Idiopathic Acquired (craniopharyngioma, pituitary tumors, autoimmune diseases, granulomatous diseases, central nervous system infections, postradiotherapy, head trauma) Congenital: associated with structural defects Genetic GH secretion (*GH1* and *GHRHR* genes) Pituitary cell differentiation (*POU1F1* and *PROP1* genes) Pituitary development (*HESX1*, *GLI2*, *OTX2*, *LHX3*, *LHX4*, and *SOX3* genes)
Bioinactive GH	Kowarski syndrome (OMIM 262650)
GH insensitivity (GHI)	Complete GHI (OMIM 262500) Partial GHI (OMIM 604271) GHI associated with immune dysfunction (OMIM 245590) Atypical GHI Secondary or acquired GHI (anti-GH antibodies, malnutrition, liver disorders, poorly controlled diabetes mellitus, uremia)
Ternary complex defects	Acid-labile subunit deficiency (OMIM 615961) Defects on proteolytic cleavage of IGFBPs (*PAPPA2* gene)
IGF deficiency	IGF-1 deficiency (OMIM 608747) IGF-2 deficiency (OMIM 616489)

GH, growth hormone; IGF, insulin-like growth factor; IGFBP, insulin-like growth factor–binding protein; OMIM, Online Mendelian Inheritance in Man. From Collett-Solberg PF, Jorge AA, Boguszewski MC, et al. Growth hormone therapy in children; research and practice—a review. *Growth Horm IGF Res* 2019;44:20–32.

IGF-1R defects leading to variable degree of IGF-1 insensitivity can be present in 2% of children born SGA and without catch-up growth.[58] Long-standing short stature caused by GHD (except in the presence of precocious puberty) is accompanied by at least 1 to 2 years delay in bone age; therefore, children older than 3 years with a bone age equal to or above chronologic age may not be investigated for GHD[58,59]; however, this is controversial. The determination of IGF-1 levels is usually the first step to assess GH–IGF-1 axis[60] (Fig. 56.3). Children with IGF-1 serum levels above the mean for age and gender are unlikely to have defects in the GH–IGF axis,[58] except for IGF-1 insensitivity and PAPPA2 deficiency.[61] Children with low/low-normal serum levels of IGF-I should be further investigated for GHD.

The next step is to assess the production of GH. Since there is a physiologic circadian variation in serum levels of GH, random levels are not useful, except in the neonatal period, where levels tend to be high all day.[62,63] During the first week of life, a single random GH level less than 7 ng per mL confirms the diagnosis of GHD.[63] GHD due to congenital hypopituitarism is diagnosed without provocative testing in a newborn with hypoglycemia who does not attain a serum GH concentration above 7 ng per mL and the brain imaging is abnormal (ectopic posterior pituitary, pituitary hypoplasia, or abnormal stalk). GH stimulation tests have been used for decades to measure the response of the hypothalamus/pituitary gland to various stimuli. Even though they are considered the gold-standard test to diagnose GHD, there are several problems with them: (a) there is variable reproducibility, meaning that the same test in the same person on different days can give completely different results and different tests in the same individual can also produce different results; (b) there are different laboratory methods to measure GH; and the results between different methods may not be similar; (c) different laboratories using the same methods find different results for the same samples; and (d) there are no agreed-upon normal cutoffs points, and since different stimuli lead to different GH peaks, there may be a need for stimulus-specific cutoff points.[24,64–67]

In the 1980s, the cutoff point used to define GHD was 5 ng per mL, using polyclonal antibody assays. This means that if the highest GH level after a stimulus was below 5 ng per dL, the child was considered to have GHD, and if the value was above that, the child was considered not to have GHD. Later, the cutoff point was raised to 7 ng per mL and then to 10 ng per mL, and now, most assays use monoclonal antibodies that lead to varying apparent GH concentrations.[39,65,68] Raising the cutoff limit increases the number of children diagnosed with partial GHD, but it also increases the likelihood of diagnosis of GHD in children without the condition. The ideal cutoff point to identify most children with GHD without classifying non-GHD children as GHD and how to improve the accuracy of the diagnosis of GHD and non-GHD are topics still under debate.[60,65]

Another issue is that adolescents, due to their exposure to sex steroids, have a higher GH response to stimuli. Some clinicians suggest that all children should receive sex steroid priming prior to stimulation tests to decrease the number of false-positive diagnoses,[69] while others suggest that priming should be done only for peripubertal individuals[70] or only for prepubertal children already at pubertal age (delayed puberty).[71] However, conflicting published data show that priming induces higher values of GH levels but does not necessarily improve the accuracy of diagnosing GHD. Furthermore, sex steroid priming may not discriminate between those who are likely to have a clinically significant improvement in adult height after rhGH treatment from those who are not going to have a significant change; priming may also have side effects, such as priapism and testicular pain.[72] A recent systematic review on the diagnosis of GHD as a late effect of radiotherapy reported that there are no studies evaluating the use of sex steroid priming in childhood cancer survivors.[54] The use of priming is one more tool that can be used by the pediatric endocrinologist in selected cases. In summary, the diagnosis of GHD should be based on a combination of factors, including auxologic data (HT SDS and growth velocity), radiologic data (delayed bone age, with some exceptions, and pituitary imaging), laboratory data (IGF-1/IGFBP-3 and GH stimulation tests), and clinical expertise.

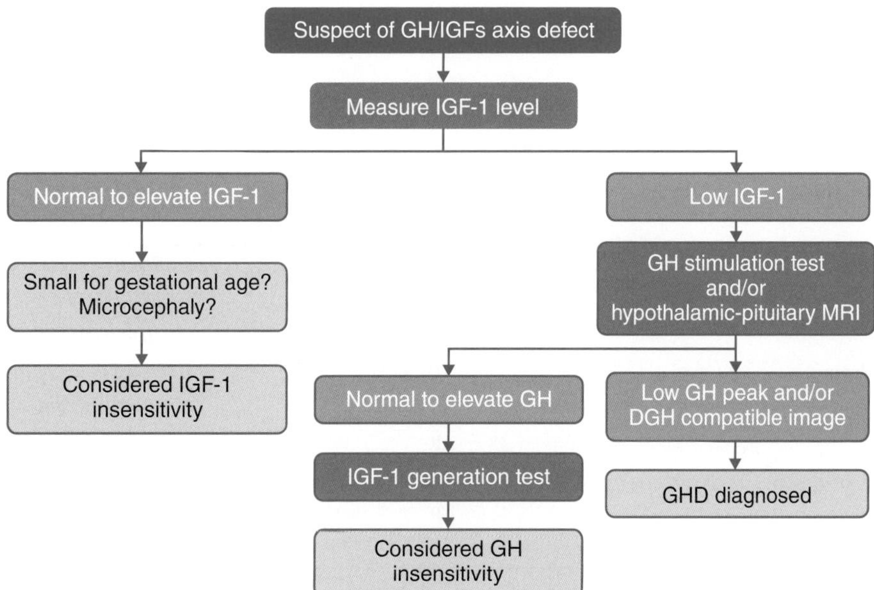

Figure 56.3 Overview of the investigation of GH–IGF-1 axis defects. GH, growth hormone; GHD, growth hormone deficiency; IGF-1, insulin-like growth factor 1; MRI, magnetic resonance imaging. (Adapted from Collett-Solberg PF, Jorge AA, Boguszewski MC, et al. Growth hormone therapy in children; research and practice—a review. *Growth Horm IGF Res* 2019;44:20–32.)

Recommendations for Genetic Testing

Genetic tests are being progressively introduced into clinical practice in all fields of medicine, including the evaluation of children with short stature. There are more than 1,000 conditions in the OMIM® database (https://www.omim.org/) associated with short stature with a known molecular basis.[56] They can be organized as conditions involving GH–IGF defects (Table 56.2), conditions causing skeletal dysplasia (reviewed in Bonafe et al.[73]), or conditions associated with syndromic presentations (Table 56.3). The diagnosis of several of these conditions can be made based on clinical and complementary

TABLE 56.3 Examples of Genetic Conditions Associated with Short Stature Organized According to Their Primary Mechanism

Disorder	*Inheritance*	*Gene*	*OMIM*
Associated with Skeletal Dysplasia			
DISORDERS AFFECTING PARACRINE FACTORS IN THE GROWTH PLATE			
• **Achondroplasia**	AD	*FGFR3*	100800
• **Hypochondroplasia**	AD	*FGFR3*	146000
• **Acrocapitofemoral dysplasia**	AR	*IHH*	607778
• **Albright hereditary osteodystrophy**	AD	*GNAS*	103580
• **Acromesomelic dysplasia, Maroteaux type**	AR	*NPR2*	602875
• **Geleophysic dysplasia 1**	AR	*ADAMTSL2*	231050
Defects affecting cartilage extracellular matrix			
• **Acromicric dysplasia**	AD	*FBN1*	102370
• **Geleophysic dysplasia 2**	AD	*FBN1*	614185
• **Pseudoachondroplasia**	AD	*COMP*	177170
• **Spondyloepiphyseal dysplasia congenital l**	AD	*COL2A1*	183900
• **Spondyloepimetaphyseal dysplasia aggrecan type**	AD	*ACAN*	612813
• **Spondyloepiphyseal dysplasia type Kimberley**	AD	*ACAN*	608361
Defects affecting intracellular pathways			
• **Langer mesomelic dysplasia**	AR	*SHOX*	249700
• Léri–Weill dyschondrosteosis	AD	*SHOX*	127300
• Campomelic dysplasia	AD	*SOX9*	114290
Associated with syndromic short stature			
DEFECTS AFFECTING INTRACELLULAR PATHWAYS			
• **Noonan syndrome**	AD	Several	163950
• **Neurofibromatosis type 1**	AD	*NF1*	162200
• **Kabuki syndrome 1**	AD	*KMT2D*	147920
• **Kabuki syndrome 2**	XLD	*KDM6A*	300867
• **Kenny–Caffey syndrome type 1**	AR	*TBCE*	244460
• **Kenny–Caffey syndrome type 2**	AD	*FAM111A*	127000
Defects in fundamental cellular processes			
• **Floating–Harbor syndrome**	AD	*SRCAP*	136140
• **KBG syndrome**	AD	*ANKRD11*	148050
• **CHARGE syndrome**	AD	*CHD7, SEMA3E*	214800
• **Cornelia de Lange syndrome**	AD/XLD	Several	122470
• **Rubinstein–Taybi syndrome**	AD	*CREBBP, EP300*	180849
• **Bloom syndrome**	AR	*RECQL3*	210900
• **Fanconi anemia**	AR/XLR	Several	227650
• **Three-M syndrome**	AR	*CUL7, BSL1, CCDC8*	273750
• **MOPD**	AR	*RNU4ATAC, PCNT*	210710

AD, autosomal dominant; AR, autosomal recessive; CHARGE, coloboma of the eye, heart defects, atresia of the choanae, retardation of growth and development, and ear abnormalities and deafness; MOPD, microcephalic osteodysplastic primordial dwarfism; OMIM, Online Mendelian Inheritance in Man; XLD, X-linked dominant; XLR, X-linked recessive.

From Collett-Solberg PF, Jorge AA, Boguszewski MC, et al. Growth hormone therapy in children; research and practice—a review. *Growth Horm IGF Res* 2019;44:20–32.

examinations[43,56,74,75] (see Fig. 56.2), with genetic testing serving to confirm the diagnosis. A candidate gene approach is used in these situations. However, due to the diversity, clinical variability, and rarity of these conditions, the clinical diagnosis can be challenging.[76–79]

In the past decade, the development of genetic techniques, primarily array-based genomic copy number analyses (or molecular karyotype) and whole-exome sequencing (WES)/WGS, has led to an increase in the diagnosis of patients with unrecognized rare genetic conditions.[80–83] The use of these methodologies as the first line of investigation of genetic conditions has been shown to yield a high rate of success to establish the etiologic diagnosis and to be cost-effective in selected situations.[80,81,83,84]

In the field of growth disorders, the prevalence of pathogenic copy number variation (CNV), especially when associated with developmental delay, intellectual disability, or additional major malformations, is 13% [95% confidence interval (CI) 10.4%–15.5%].[42] Array-based CNV analyses, such as aCGH or SNPa, should be used to aid in the diagnosis in these children[43,74,75] (see Fig. 56.1).

When there is a high degree of suspicion that the short stature is due to a monogenic condition, based on the history of consanguinity, clear autosomal dominant inheritance pattern, syndromic cases, and severe short stature, WES should be used. The usefulness of WES in growth disorders was demonstrated in several case reports,[36,77,85] in cohorts of patients with severe short stature,[86,87] and in the investigation of specific subtype of short stature children (as GHI).[88]

There are specific situations where genetic investigation gains importance due to the prevalence of the condition or due to the influence of the correct diagnosis in the treatment decision process. As already mentioned, every girl with short stature of undetermined cause needs a conventional or molecular karyotyping due to the possibility of TS.[54] Additionally, genetic investigation is more relevant when there is clinical suspicion of a cancer predisposition condition, such as neurofibromatosis type 1, Noonan syndrome, Fanconi anemia, or Bloom disease.[79,89,90] In typical cases, the genetic test leads to little change in the diagnostic or therapeutic approach, but for atypical or mild cases, a molecular confirmation of the diagnosis has an obvious impact on genetic counseling, decision to use rhGH therapy, and patient follow-up.

The sheer number of genes involved in growth disorders and the number of possible tests to investigate them are beyond the scope of this chapter.[91] Public databases such as GeneReview (https://www.ncbi.nlm.nih.gov/books/NBK1116/), Genetics Home Reference (https://ghr.nlm.nih.gov/), and OMIM (https://www.omim.org/) are useful in assisting the decision-making process regarding the use of a given genetic test.

The majority of children with HT SDS less than −2.0 have isolated short stature and are labeled as ISS. In these children, the absence of other clinical signs or the presence of nonspecific findings currently makes the gene candidate approach impracticable. There are no clear recommendations for when and how to do genetic investigation in children with isolated short stature. Since height is one of the most heritable human characteristics[92] and many children with short stature have parents with short stature, it is expected that the cause of a large proportion of these children is genetic. It has been accepted that there is a polygenic influence determining short stature,[93,94] but recent studies have challenged this dogma. Several studies demonstrated that a significant portion of healthy short children have a monogenic cause that explains their growth deficit.[95] A proportion of these children are at the mild end of the phenotypic spectrum of a known syndromic disorder associated with short stature,[86,87] such as Noonan syndrome or DiGeorge syndrome. Additionally, several studies have associated specific genes with the isolated short stature phenotype, including heterozygous pathogenic variants in *GHR*[96] and *SHOX*[97] in children classified as ISS, and other studies have broadened the genes involved[34] (Table 56.4). The most consistent and frequent findings in children originally classified as ISS are heterozygous variants in genes involved in growth plate development: *SHOX*,[37] *ACAN*,[52] *NPR2*,[53,98] *NPPC*,[99] and *IHH*.[22] Each of these genes accounts for a low proportion of cases of short stature (1% to 2% or less), but the percentage may be significantly higher in familial short stature.[98] Defects in these genes cause a variable degree of short stature with nonspecific phenotypes and are usually inherited in an autosomal dominant manner. This lack of specific characteristics makes it difficult to recognize without a molecular genetic study. For this reason, it is not effective to apply a candidate gene analysis, so a multiple-gene testing approach using next-generation sequencing (NGS) or the use of WES is preferable. The choice between the two will depend on the availability and cost–benefit evaluation. However, the approach with WES has been presented as more advantageous.[100] Even when using the WES approach, the analysis of these patients should prioritize the genes already associated with the isolated short stature phenotype and genes associated with syndromic conditions with great phenotypic variability that are already documented (Table 56.4).

At present, most patients will not have a conclusive result after genetic analysis. It will be important to learn if there is a relationship between a given genetic diagnosis and the response to rhGH treatment[37,52,101] or long-term health consequences.[52] It is likely that with the increased availability of genetic studies, the primary way to investigate short stature patients will change. In the near future, genetic testing may become the standard method of investigation of children with isolated short stature.[95] As genetic screening of short children in the future by NGS will be facilitated by its increasing availability and decreasing costs, it will be feasible to perform genetic testing of children who have been treated with GH under the indications of SGA or ISS. This will enable attainment of a better insight of GH efficacy and safety in children with specific genetic disorders.[39]

GROWTH HORMONE TREATMENT

The foremost aims of GH treatment in children are the normalization of height during childhood, attainment of a timely and normal pubertal growth, and the achievement of an adult height that is normal for the population and genetic target, in conjunction with normalization of other aspects (body composition, metabolism, and quality of life).[39]

The approved indications for the use of rhGH and the year of first approval are summarized in Table 56.5.[39]

PRODUCTS AND DOSAGE

Following the unfortunate occurrence of CJD in 1985, pituitary-derived GH was removed from production. Since then, the exclusive product has been the natural sequence recombinant

TABLE 56.4 Genes Associated with Isolated Short Stature Phenotype

Gene	*First Report*	*Inheritance Pattern*	*Frequency*[a]	*Evidence of Association*[b]	*Observation*	*Reference*
GHR	1995	AD	NA	Limited	Mild GH insensitivity phenotype (low IGF-1 and GHBP levels)	Goddard et al.[96]
SHOX	1997	AD	1%–16%	Definitive	Mild body disproportion	Rao et al.[97]
GH1	2003	AD	NA	Limited		Millar et al.[102]
IGF1R	2003	AD	NA	Moderate	Majority born SGA and elevated IGF-1 levels	Abuzzahab et al.[103]
IGFALS	2004	AR	NA	Moderate	Severe IGF-1 and IGFBP-3 deficiency disproportionate with mild height deficit	Domené et al.[104]
GHSR	2006	AD/AR	NA	Limited	It may be associated with GHD in the same family	Pantel et al.[105]
IGF1	2013	AD	NA	Limited		Batey et al.[106]
ACAN	2014	AD	1.4%–2.1%	Strong	Advanced bone age	Cohen et al.[107]
NPR2	2014	AD	1.2%–3.4%	Strong		Vasques et al.[108]
FGF3R	2015	AD	NA	Limited		Kant et al.[109]
PAPPA2	2016	AR	NA	Limited	Elevated IGF-1 and IGFBP-3 levels	Dauber et al.[61]
IHH	2018	AD	1.6%	Moderate	Shortening of the middle phalanx of second and fifth finger	Vasques et al.[22]
NPPC	2018	AD	NA	Limited	Mild brachydactyly	Hisado-Oliva et al.[99]
STAT5B	2018	AD	NA	Limited	Mild GH insensitivity phenotype with eczema	Klammt et al.[110]

[a]Frequency observed in studies that evaluated unselected children with isolated short stature (ISS or nonsyndromic SGA).
[b]Strength of evidence that changes in this gene are associated with the isolated short stature phenotype.
AD, autosomal dominant; AR, autosomal recessive; GH, growth hormone; GHBP, growth hormone–binding protein; GHD, growth hormone deficiency; IGF, insulin-like growth factor; IGFBP, insulin-like growth factor–binding protein; NA, not available; SGA, small for gestational age.
From Collett-Solberg PF, Jorge AA, Boguszewski MC, et al. Growth hormone therapy in children; research and practice—a review. *Growth Horm IGF Res* 2019;44:20–32.

GH peptide, which is distributed worldwide by several manufacturers. These products currently have a potency of 3 IU per mg and are usually administered by daily (six to seven injections per week) subcutaneous injections. These are usually given at bedtime to mimic endogenous GH secretion. The recommended doses are detailed in Table 56.6, varying from 0.18 to 0.40 mg per kg per week (0.5 to 1.2 IU per kg per week), depending on the diagnostic category. Larger GH doses are usually recommended in non-GHD children, as nonphysiologic pharmacologic doses are needed to overcome postulated "GH insensitivity" (GHI).

TABLE 56.5 Approved Indications for Recombinant Human Growth Hormone

Year of First Approval	*Indication*	*Region*
1985	Childhood GHD	The United States,[a] Europe, and Japan
1993	Chronic renal insufficiency	The United States,[a] Europe, and Japan
1996	Turner syndrome	The United States,[a] Europe, and Japan
1996	Adult GHD	The United States,[a] Europe, and Japan
1996	HIV-wasting syndrome	The United States[a] and Europe
1997	Achondroplasia	Japan[a]
2000	Prader–Willi syndrome	The United States,[a] Europe, and Japan
2001	SGA	The United States,[a] Europe, and Japan
2003	ISS	The United States[a]
2004	Short-bowel syndrome	The United States[a] and Europe
2005	GHD in transition	The United States[a] and Europe
2006	*SHOX* haploinsufficiency	The United States[a] and Europe
2007	Noonan syndrome	The United States[a]

[a]Country of first approval.
GHD, growth hormone deficiency; ISS, idiopathic short stature; SGA, small for gestational age.
From Ranke MB, Wit JM. Growth hormone—past, present and future. *Nat Rev Endocrinol* 2018;14(5):285–300.

TABLE 56.6 Cost-Effectiveness of Adult Height Gain in Various Treatment Categories

Study Category	*Gender*	*Untreated Adult Height (cm)*	*GH Dose (mg/kg/wk)*	*GH Treated Final Height (cm)*	*Cost/cm (1,000 USD)*[a]
Normal	M	178	—	—	—
	F		—	—	—
GHD	M	134–146[b]	0.18–0.35	168	10
	F	128–134[b]	0.18–0.35	155	10
PWS	M	154	0.23–0.35	+10[c]	11
	F	145–149	0.23–0.35	+10[c]	11
CRF	M	156	0.30–0.35	162–165	11–38
	F	152	0.30–0.35	151–155	11–38
ISS	M	150–170	0.20–0.40	164	22–43
	F	137–156	0.20–0.40	155	25–43
TS	F	143	0.375	146	25–28

Approximate mean values are expressed. For normal adult men, −2 SDS or approximate 5th percentile is 164 cm and for women, −2 SDS is 152 cm.

[a]The author converted U.K. estimates into U.S. dollars (USD).

[b]Estimated from small patient numbers. Den Ouden et al. reported six adult patents with untreated multiple pituitary hormone deficiencies, who achieved heights of 148 to 193 cm[111]

[c]Data reported from only one small study with methodologic concerns.

CRF, chronic renal failure; F, female; GH, growth hormone; GHD, growth hormone deficiency; ISS, idiopathic short stature; M, male; PWS, Prader–Willi syndrome; SDS, standard deviation score; TS, Turner syndrome.

Data from Bryant J, Care C, Mihaylova B, et al. Clinical effectiveness and cost effectiveness of growth hormone in children: as systematic review and economic evaluation. *Health Technol Assess* 2002;6(18):1–168.

GROWTH HORMONE TREATMENT OF CHILDREN WITH GROWTH HORMONE DEFICIENCY

The 60-year world experience concerning FH attainment with the use of GH to treat thousands of children with GHD has been reported.[27] It is to be stressed that the criteria used for the diagnosis of GHD varied considerably, and highly variable assay methodology was used for the determination of GH values in the reported studies. In addition, the GH doses and frequency of administration were quite disparate. This makes comparisons among published studies very problematic. In addition, the vast majority of reported studies are uncontrolled, and no randomized controlled trials have been published for subjects with GHD for obvious ethical reasons.

The long-term growth response of children with GHD to pituitary GH showed an impressive mean gain of 1.9 SDS, but GHD patients still ended up near the 3rd percentile (−2.3 SDS), likely due to the late onset of less than optimal GH therapy associated with extreme short stature (−4.2 SDS) at diagnosis. GHD patients treated almost exclusively with rhGH had less height deficit at onset and achieved greater adult height than those treated with pituitary GH, with a mean additional gain of 0.9 SDS (−1.4 vs. −2.3 SDS). Although they did not achieve mean target height, the majority of GHD patients treated with rhGH achieved a normal adult height.[27] This may be attributed to the fact that these patients received rhGH at larger doses, more frequently, and usually for a longer mean duration.

FH in children with GHD arising from central nervous system (CNS), craniospinal, or total body irradiation may be further compromised by radiation-induced skeletal damage, resulting in the inability to fully respond to GH.[112] These individuals may sustain additional deficiencies, such as hypothyroidism or inability to undergo puberty, which may, in turn, limit height growth.[112]

Patients who were younger and who had the greatest deficit in height achieved the greatest total height gain on rhGH. Delayed pubertal induction and midparental height are major factors influencing FH during rhGH treatment of children with GHD.

GROWTH HORMONE TREATMENT OF THE NON-GROWTH HORMONE–DEFICIENT SHORT CHILD

Despite the paucity of published controlled data that clearly indicate benefit, GH has become the most widely employed and most controversial therapeutic agent in the non-GH–deficient short child.[26,27] The use of GH for the child with ISS and TS represents a significant proportion of total use, averaging from 23% to 58% in the larger series.[27]

GROWTH HORMONE TREATMENT IN IDIOPATHIC SHORT STATURE

Many uncontrolled short-term studies indicate that GH administration accelerates HV in some normal short children. However, in a review of 413 short normal children treated with GH with variable doses for over 5 years, the overall mean FH gain over predicted adult height was only 2.7 cm, or +0.4 SDS.[27] This resulted in a mean FH SDS of −1.7 SDS, which is nearly identical to the observed FH with spontaneous growth in 229 children with ISS (−1.5 SDS for boys and −1.6 SDS for girls).[113,114] Thus, a very significant regression toward the mean takes place, and not all short children end up being short adults.

A recent meta-analysis evaluated all randomized controlled trials assessing the impact of GH on linear growth in children with ISS; three studies included a placebo-treated control group.[115] Only one trial evaluated final adult height, and another compared near-final adult height in girls. Both trials had small numbers of children, many dropping out over the study interval for unspecified reasons. The first study demonstrated an apparent gain in height of 3.7 cm or 0.57 SDS (95% CI, 0.03–1.10) in the GH-treated group compared with controls.[116] The second trial assessing FH or near FH demonstrated a 6 to 7 cm gain for those treated with GH compared with controls.[117] Of note, all children still ended up relatively short in both trials.

A recent publication, not included in this meta-analysis, reported on the FH outcomes of a randomized controlled study of physiologic and twice physiologic dose of GH for short non-GHD peripubertal children.[118] This study was again significantly hampered because approximately 30% of those enrolled were nonadherent to the protocol, as well as the fact that the etiology was heterogeneous for the short stature and included children with SGA. If the data of all of the children were analyzed by intent to treat, then those treated with physiologic doses of GH (0.033 mg per kg per day) had similar FHs compared to the controls (-2.0 ± 0.8 FH SDS vs. -2.1 ± 0.8 FH SDS, $p = 0.053$), whereas there was a modest increase in the higher dose group versus controls (-1.5 ± 0.9 FH SDS vs. -2.1 ± 0.8 FH SDS, $p < 0.01$). The data when analyzed "per protocol" or including only those children who adhered the results would suggest modest benefit from both doses of GH; of note, many GH-treated children still ended up at less than −2 SDS.[118]

In the one trial that evaluated this question, children with ISS did not have lower health-related quality of life scores than the normal population, except for social functioning.[55] Treated children did not report improvements in these scores and at times had worse health-related quality of life scores than the controls.[119] A reevaluation of the psychological status of both referred and population-based short children has also concluded that short stature does not appear to be associated with clinically significant psychological morbidity.[119,120]

A recent statement by the Lawson Wilkins Pediatric Endocrine Society and the European Society for Paediatric Endocrinology reviewed how best to evaluate the causes of short stature, alternatives to GH therapy, many of which are not fully vetted, FH post-GH use, as well as cost–benefit analysis for this relatively expensive therapy.[107]

In summary, it would thus appear from the data that the conclusion about the effect of GH and FH in children with ISS is tenuous. Prescription of GH remains a contentious issue in this otherwise healthy, well-adjusted group.[121]

GROWTH HORMONE TREATMENT IN TURNER SYNDROME

TS is not related to GHD, and the GH dose recommended, 0.375 mg per kg per week, is supraphysiologic. A recent world survey of FH in girls with TS treated with GH indicated considerable variation in the treatment protocols as to dose and age of onset of GH therapy, and in the concomitant use of estrogens or anabolic steroids.[27] The mean age of onset for GH therapy varied from 10 to 15 years, with doses from 0.18 to 0.70 mg per kg per week. The mean FH of 2,211 girls with TS treated with GH was 150.0 cm, which is 5.8 cm above the predicted adult height, with considerable individual variability in all studies.[27] An additional report of GH treatment, at a median GH dose of 0.29 mg per kg per week, of 188 TS patients from 96 German centers from 1987 to 2000 noted a similar gain of 6.0 (−1.3 to +13) cm above the projected adult height.[121] In the only randomized controlled trial of GH treatment to FH in TS reported from Canada, GH treatment significantly increased the mean FH of 69 girls: 141.4 ± 4.7 cm (mean $\pm$ 1 SD) in controls and 146.2 ± 6.5 cm in the GH group.[122] It can be concluded that girls with TS *as a diagnostic group* do benefit in adult FH with GH treatment.[27,122,123] However, all studies showed a poor outcome in some girls. A more efficacious intervention appears to be associated with a younger age of onset of GH treatment, larger doses of GH for longer periods, and a delay in estrogen administration until growth was nearly completed. It is critical that appropriate randomized controlled trials and meta-analyses assess which of these variables are most critical and, more importantly, best for the patient.[124,125]

GROWTH HORMONE TREATMENT OF CHILDREN BORN WITH INTRAUTERINE GROWTH RETARDATION OR SMALL FOR GESTATIONAL AGE

In approximately 15% to 20% of strikingly short children, postnatal growth failure is related to decreased prenatal growth velocity or IUGR, resulting in infants who are SGA. Most studies indicate that it is the low birth length that is most critical in the 10% to 15% of SGA infants who end up with persistent short stature during childhood and adulthood.[116,117] There have been many studies assessing short-term effects of GH on children with SGA. Simon et al. reviewed the seven published trials assessing final or near-final adult height in approximately 350 children; only one was a controlled study.[126] In this trial, the adolescents started with a mean HT SDS of -3.2 ± 0.7; there were twice as many treated children as controls. After approximately 2.7 years, FH was obtained in all those still followed in the trial; this represented 89% of the treated and 70% of the placebo group. Both had increased their HT SDS to -2.1 ± 1 versus -2.7 ± 0.9; the increases in those given GH at 0.067 mg per kg per day were significant compared with placebo ($p < 0.005$). Uncontrolled studies, particularly in prepubertal children often using doses of 0.067 mg per kg per day for 4 to 8 years, document more significant gains in FH SDS and without altering the age of onset of puberty; unfortunately, these were not controlled. It would appear that rhGH might normalize height if started early and using supraphysiologic doses, but additional randomized controlled studies are required for confirmation.

GROWTH HORMONE TREATMENT IN CHILDREN WITH CHRONIC RENAL FAILURE

Approximately 60% of patients with CRF have congenital disorders, and growth failure is significant from an early age.[107] This is felt to be due to malnutrition, renal bone disease, acidosis, and GHI.[127] The estimated mean height is −2.4 SDS from birth to 10 years, and FH is below the 3rd percentile in 33% of patients with CRF. Unlike rhGH indications for other non-GH–deficient disorders, GH is often given over shorter time intervals to increase body size pretransplant to facilitate transplantation, as well as post-transplant with the objective to improve FH. The usual rhGH dose is 0.30 to 0.35 mg per kg per week given in six to seven daily subcutaneous injections.

Results from randomized controlled studies as well as NAPRTCS (North American Pediatric Renal Transplantation Cooperative Study) have demonstrated an improvement of approximately 0.5 to 1.7 SDS compared with controls, which have mean SDS of −2.9.[128,129] Post-treatment, adult height has been reported as −1.7 SDS, or 164 cm in boys and 151 to 156 cm in girls.[130] Since normalization of growth and catch-up growth have also been reported with improved dialysis, the optimal approach to this multifactorial growth impairment remains to be clarified.[127]

GROWTH HORMONE TREATMENT IN PRADER–WILLI SYNDROME

Most patients with PWS have deletions or an inactive portion of chromosome 15. Children with PWS have body compositions that resemble those with GHD, with mean adult height of 154 cm in men and 147 cm in women.[130] The cause of the short stature is unknown, although abnormalities of the GH–IGF axis have been proposed, because reduced GH secretion has been observed. However, this interpretation is confounded by the known reduction in GH secretion seen in non-PWS obesity. Because of similarities between PWS and GHD, GH has been administered at doses of 0.20 to 0.35 mg per kg per week in the hope of increasing adult FH and improving body composition.[130,131] Although increased short-term HV has been observed, reliable adult FH has not been reported. This patient population is prone to develop a number of typical adverse events with rhGH. In particular, serious concern has recently arisen because of multiple unexplained sudden deaths in PWS children early in the course of their GH treatment program.

RECOMBINANT HUMAN GROWTH HORMONE DOSE ADJUSTMENTS

Dose adjustments can be made using the GH response at 6 and 12 months of therapy (through delta HT SDS or HV). In combination with IGF-1 measurement, the growth response may provide information about treatment efficacy, adherence, and, theoretically, safety. Prediction models can also be used to guide rhGH dosing and should be further validated in prospective studies.[55,132,133] The strongest predictive variable for adult height is the year 1 growth response in relation to the dose.

Measurements of IGF-1 levels should be considered after dose changes and annually. Trials using IGF-1–based dosing provide data to optimize rhGH therapy in GHD and ISS.[132,134] The use of IGF-1–based rhGH dosing may result in dose sparing.[135,136] With respect to making dose adjustments, the target level of IGF-1 should in general be close to 0 SDS in GHD, but individual adjustments can be considered. A 20% rhGH dose adjustment leads to a 1 SDS change in IGF-1 concentration in GHD patients.[137] Once catch-up growth in patients with GHD is achieved, consideration can be given to reducing the rhGH dose with close monitoring for continued normal HV.[135]

In non-GHD conditions, such as ISS, rhGH dose can be adjusted with a goal of an IGF-1 level of approximately +1 SDS, but the target should be adjusted on an individual basis. When consecutive IGF-1 levels are above +2 SDS, consideration should be given to reducing the rhGH dose to achieve long-term IGF-1 levels in the normal range, unless IGF-1 insensitivity is likely. In certain conditions characterized by partial IGF-1 insensitivity (Silver–Russell syndrome/SGA,[96] PWS,[137] IGF-1R defects[138]), IGF-1 levels above +2 SDS may be needed for effective growth. This is also true in some children with TS.[134] There is no upper limit of IGF-1 in children that has been demonstrated to be associated with GH treatment-related safety issues,[139] although long-term data are lacking. It may be important to counsel patients and caregivers about this dosing strategy, particularly when high IGF-1 levels are targeted.

There is no compelling evidence to support the use of IGFBP-3, free IGF-1, ALS levels, of IGF-1/IGFBP-3 ratio in monitoring of rhGH therapy. In patients with GHD and syndromes that increase cancer risk, including cancer survivors, IGF-1 target below the mean may be preferred.[140] However, this remains theoretical, as there is no evidence that such a goal reduces the risk of cancer recurrence or second malignancy.

DEFINITION AND MANAGEMENT OF SUBOPTIMAL RESPONSE TO RECOMBINANT HUMAN GROWTH HORMONE

An inadequate response after initiation of rhGH therapy in patients with GHD is often defined by one or more of the following criteria: delta HV less than 2 cm per year, HV SDS less than 0, or delta HT SDS less than 0.3 per year during the first 6 to 12 months of therapy,[141] but there is considerable variation according to age. Clinicians should use age, gender, and etiology-specific (including for GHD) response charts to assess individual growth responses after starting rhGH therapy.[142–144] In addition, prediction models can aid in assessing low initial responses, and the rhGH dose being used should also be taken into consideration.[55]

TRANSITION TO ADULT CARE

Only those children treated for GHD may be eligible to continue GH once their epiphyses have fused. One to 3 months after discontinuation of GH, they need to undergo repeat GH testing, and the cutoff to determine deficiency is more stringent.[145] The GH doses typically used are about one-tenth those used in GHD children; regular IGF-1 monitoring has been advocated to maintain these concentrations in the normal range adjusted for age and sex.

SAFETY OF RECOMBINANT HUMAN GROWTH HORMONE IN CHILDREN

Side effects caused by rhGH therapy are quite rare. There is a paucity of data linking the rhGH dose to treatment-related adverse events in children. In addition, there is no upper limit of IGF-1 that has been associated with treatment-related safety issues. There are some genetic conditions, such as TS, associated with an increased risk for adverse events, as detailed in the GRS Growth Hormone Safety Workshop Position Paper.[146]

GH therapy is considered to be safe with the exception of CJD, which developed from GH and extracted from human pituitary tissue. Approximately 26 cases of this disease have been identified among the 7,700 people in the United States who received hGH from the National Hormone Pituitary Program (NHPP). An additional six overseas (National Institute of Diabetes and Digestive and Kidney Diseases, Office of Communication, March 2008) patients who received GH from U.S. labs that produced the hormone for NHPP have also developed CJD. Unfortunately, the web page of the European and Allied Countries Collaborative Study Group of CJD (EUROCJD;

http://www.eurocjd.ed.ac.uk/) reported that as of March 2008, there have been many more cases of CJD related to GH therapy in France ($n = 100$) and the United Kingdom ($n = 44$).

Adverse events associated with rhGH therapy include pseudotumor cerebri, slipped capital femoral epiphysis (SCFE), fluid retention, insulin resistance resulting in hyperglycemia, diabetes mellitus, and/or hyperlipidemia. Some of these issues arise more frequently in children with specific indications for rhGH therapy (see later Wilson et al.[121]).

Because GH raises serum IGF-1 concentrations, which is mitogenic, ongoing surveillance of children with GHD arising secondary to a CNS neoplasm is closely monitored for regrowth of original tumor or the diagnosis of a second neoplasm. The literature is still controversial on these points. In a recent investigation as to whether the development of a second neoplasm was more likely in childhood cancer survivors treated with rhGH versus untreated survivors, the rate ratio was 2.15 (95% CI, 1.3–3.5; $p < 0.002$) for those treated versus those untreated. Meningiomas were the most common second neoplasm diagnosed in treated group.[147] Recurrence of the original tumor postinitiation of rhGH therapy is of considerable interest, and the literature does not provide yet a definitive answer as to whether there is an increased risk.[148]

For those children treated with supraphysiologic doses, additional scrutiny would appear to be warranted. Those treated with rhGH for ISS have few reported additional adverse events; however, this may be because relatively few children have been treated and/or the follow-up period is relatively short.[112] Girls with TS treated in the National Cooperative Growth Study appear to suffer more intracranial hypertension, SCFE, scoliosis, and pancreatitis compared with children treated for other conditions.[149]

Being born SGA already predisposes to insulin resistance, diabetes mellitus, the metabolic syndrome, and an apparent increased mortality attributed to coronary heart disease and stroke.[150] The addition of supraphysiologic rhGH would intuitively worsen insulin sensitivity. To date, this has not been observed using our current diagnostic tools. However, the long-term risk of prolonged GH therapy has not yet been determined.[151]

Pretransplant, children with CRF have increased insulin values with rhGH therapy but do not appear to have an increased risk of developing diabetes mellitus, except if the underlying diagnosis is cystinosis.[152] Post-transplant, the additive use of glucocorticoids and other antirejection medications such as tacrolimus with rhGH could further predispose to glucose intolerance, and monitoring for hyperglycemia is warranted. Perhaps, more worrisome is the issue as to whether GH increases the risk of acute rejection; the literature is still unclear on this matter.[129]

Since 2002, 25 GH-treated children with PWS have died, on average 4 months after GH initiation. More than two-thirds were due to respiratory causes, such as infections. The deaths occurred predominantly in obese males and those known to have sleep apnea (32% of deaths). Caution has been raised about prescribing GH to obese individuals with PWS, and recommendations about performing baseline and surveillance somnopolygrams have been promulgated in an attempt to reduce additional deaths.[153] Of course, issues of hyperglycemia-impaired insulin action and pseudotumor cerebri with rhGH also arise in this population.

The absolute risk of each of these potential complications is likely to be very small. However, the use of increased doses of GH in children with nonendocrine short stature (>0.35 mg per kg per week or >1.0 IU per kg per week), which are twice those required to promote growth acceleration in most patients with "classic" GHD, has the potential to increase the usual risk factors. Nevertheless, when recombinant GH is administered for an approved indication at an approved dosage, it is remarkably safe.[154–156]

THE USE OF GROWTH HORMONE TO INCREASE ADULT HEIGHT: HAS THE OUTCOME ACHIEVED EXPECTATIONS?

Children with short stature who begin GH treatment have the expectation of achieving not just target height but also normal adult height and all the benefits that they and their families expect from this attainment. Unfortunately, this expectation has not been fulfilled for many children.[27,130] Despite being treated daily with GH for many years, at considerable individual total cost, the majority of patients with classic GHD; children with ISS, SGA, CRF, or PWS; and girls with TS have not achieved "normal" adult height if the mean is used as reference[130] (Table 56.5). However, individual patients have shown dramatic responses and have surpassed target height expectations. The majority of patients with IGHD, who begin GH therapy at an earlier age, with daily administration of recombinant rather than pituitary GH at doses of 0.2 to 0.35 mg per kg per week, can be expected to achieve an FH in the normal range, with relatively normal psychosocial function.

In the past two decades, there has been expanded administration of GH to short children with normal GH secretion, to the extent that they have become the largest GH treatment category in many countries. The outcome of this increased use has been the promotion of certain legitimacy to the use of GH for the "normal short child." However, there has been inadequate debate about the reported lack of demonstrated long-term benefit in terms of either growth or psychological status and the potential for negative impact that an unfulfilled expectation may have on a short child and his or her family. The published literature on the use of GH is largely uncontrolled and does not support the view that a significant benefit will arise in the majority of idiopathic short children who have normal GH secretion by appropriate current criteria. The challenge is to develop methodology that will identify all short children, including those with genetic syndromes, who will most likely benefit from the administration of GH over a prolonged period of time. It is to be hoped that the next decade of GH research will provide additional insight to make this a truly cost-effective and globally available treatment for the majority of patients who really do require treatment with GH.

In a controversial ruling in June 2003, the U.S. Food and Drug Administration (FDA) approved an application to begin marketing synthetic hGH for a new pediatric "indication": ISS.[157] This new indication restricts therapy to children who are more than 2.25 SD below the mean for age and sex, or the shortest 1.2% of all children. In addition, treatment is offered to boys predicted to be less than 5 ft 3.5 in. (161 cm) tall by 18 years of age and to girls likely to be shorter than 4 ft 11 in. (150 cm). The FDA approval was based on two randomized, multicenter trials that enrolled approximately 300 children with ISS, only one of which was controlled. There are a number of criticisms of these and other trials for ISS, which has created significant discussion among pediatric endocrinologists. In response to the FDA decision, the Lawson Wilkins Pediatric Endocrinology Society (LWPES) Drug and Therapeutics Committee has advised a cautionary approach.[122]

EMERGING DIAGNOSTIC TOOLS AND THERAPEUTIC APPROACHES FOR SHORT STATURE

New therapeutic approaches for disorders of the GH–IGF-1 axis and various forms of short stature are likely to originate from a novel understanding of their pathophysiology.[39] However, new therapeutic approaches within the frame of our current knowledge have already emerged. These emerging approaches include new tools for diagnosis, optimizing treatment with conventional rhGH, long-acting hGH, treatment of achondroplasia with future perspective in ISS, the prospect of gene therapy, and GH–GHR antagonists, which are discussed briefly as follows.

Diagnostic Testing Approaches

Although there has been significant progress in the treatment of children with growth failure, the diagnostic categorization of these children remains a challenge. Application of genomic, proteomic, and metabolomic testing may improve our ability to categorize poorly growing children and predict which one will respond well to treatment.[34]

New agents for GH stimulation tests, such as Macimorelin, an oral ghrelin receptor agonist, may improve the diagnostic accuracy of provocative tests in children, adolescents during the transition period, and in adults. Macimorelin was approved in 2017 by the FDA for the diagnosis of GHD during adult life with accuracy comparable with that of the insulin tolerance test, and it was shown to be safe and convenient.[6] No studies in children are yet available.

Optimal Use of Daily Recombinant Human Growth Hormone

With regard to optimizing and individualizing GH therapy in terms of linear growth in children, prediction algorithms and IGF-1–guided therapies have been proposed by several groups.[136] Predictions models and mathematical algorithms derived from data on variables associated with the GH response obtained from large cohorts and attempt to describe predicted growth response of an individual with a certain disorder (GHD, TS, SGA, or ISS) during a specific growth phase (prepubertal, pubertal, or total growth from start of the treatment to adult height), with the smallest possible error.

Long-Acting Growth Hormone

Extensive reviews of the emerging field of long-acting growth hormone (LAGH) have recently been published, including the authors of this chapter.[158–160]

The approaches taken for the development of LAGH preparations vary and can influence the pharmacokinetics and/or the pharmacodynamics of rhGH. To date, LAGH preparations have been developed using various approaches to prolong GH action, including forming emulsions (using gelatine and triglycerides), GH encapsulation (using degradable microspheres), GH pegylation, GH conjugation (to albumin or amino acid "tails"), and GH fusion proteins (by means of linking an inert peptide with rhGH at a region that does not interact with the GHR).[158,160]

As the era of LAGH approaches, we need to consider whether there will be additional safety risks of LAGH compared to daily rhGH. In this regard, we need to consider issues related to the persistent elevation of GH and GH-related biomarkers, such as IGFeI, as well as issues related to the mechanisms of making GH long acting. Depending upon the structure of LAGH, there may be off-target effects due to components of the LAGH not present in rhGH. Treatment with daily rhGH given at bedtime attempts to mimic the normal daily profile of increased GH production overnight. However, daily rhGH is a single peak of GH action which differs from physiologic GH production of multiple GH pulses of different duration and intensity. Thus, our current daily rhGH treatment regimen does not provide a physiologic GH profile. LAGH products will likely have differing pharmacokinetic profiles of GH release from the injection site into the bloodstream, to the target tissue and to the GHR. The peak and trough levels of IGF-I during daily rhGH and LAGH therapy have been an area of intense debate. The goal of GH therapy has been increasing the IGF-I to promote growth. It remains to be determined whether LAGH will achieve similar or better growth than daily rhGH and whether individualizing LAGH therapy to target an IGF-I in the upper part of the normal range would improve efficacy without decreasing safety. Due to the differing pharmacodynamics profile of different forms of LAGH, it will be important to determine the best time to measure IGF-I for safety and efficacy.[34]

The Prospect of Gene Therapy

Gene therapy, a technique to replace, edit, silence, or inhibit a pathologic gene mutation, offers new approaches to treatment. There have been developments at the level of basic research regarding a cure for some forms of GHD. Using in vitro systems, mouse stem cells can be transformed into hormone-producing pituitary cells.[161] In IGHD type II, the misspliced 17.5-kDa GH isoform exerts a dominant-negative effect on the secretion of normal GH43. Its accumulation in the cytosol of somatotrophs can lead to other pituitary hormone deficiencies, a process that cannot be prevented by treatment with rhGH. Experiments with rat pituitary cells have shown that by modulation of the *GH1* splicing pattern, an increase in the normal 22-kDa GH isoform can be achieved.[162]

GH–GHR Antagonists

The artificial substitution of a single amino acid residue (Gly-120Lys; glycine substituted for lysine at position 120) in hGH was shown to transform the structure of the second GHR-binding site such that effective receptor binding was prevented.[163] The subsequently developed GH analog pegvisomant (Somavert) was shown to be a GHR antagonist in animal models and humans and has become part of the standard treatment (by means of daily injections) for acromegaly.[164] The effect observed in rodents of an LAGHR antagonist, with amino acid changes in the GH-binding domain and fused to GHBP, will probably be evaluated for its efficacy and safety in humans with poorly controlled acromegaly.[21] Using similar or novel approaches, antagonists, superagonists, or even analogs with cell-specific actions of GH, GHRH, SST, ghrelin, and other components of the GH system might be designed in the future.[39]

REFERENCES

1. Grumbach M, Bin-Abbas B, Kaplan S. The growth hormone cascade: progress and long-term results of growth hormone treatment in growth hormone deficiency. *Horm Res* 1998;49(Suppl 2):41–57.
2. Albertsson-Wikland K, Rosberg S, Kalberg J, et al. Analysis of 24-hour growth hormone profiles in healthy boys and girls of normal stature: relation to puberty. *J Clin Endocrinol Metab* 1994;78:1195–1201.
3. Miller J, Tannenbaum G, Colle E, et al. Day-time pulsatile growth hormone secretion during childhood and adolescence. *J Clin Endocrinol Metab* 1982;55:9889–9994.
4. Tannenbaum G, Ling N. The interrelationship of growth hormone (GH)-releasing factor and somatostatin in generation of the ultradian rhythm of GH secretion. *Endocrinology* 1984;115:1952–1957.
5. Tzanella M, Guyda H, Van Vliet G, et al. Somatostatin pre-treatment enhances GH responsiveness to GHRH: a potential new diagnostic approach to GH deficiency. *J Clin Endocrinol Metab* 1996;(7):2494.
6. Garcia JM, Biller BMK, Korbonits M, et al. Macimorelin as a diagnostic test for adult GH deficiency. *J Clin Endocrinol Metab* 2018;103(8):3083–3093.
7. Salvatori R, Serpa MG, Parmigiani G, et al. GH response to hypoglycemia and clonidine in the GH-releasing hormone resistance syndrome. *J Endocrinol Invest* 2006;29(9):805–808.
8. Aguiar-Oliveira M, Gill M, de A Barretto E, et al. Effect of severe growth hormone (GH) deficiency due to a mutation in the GH-releasing hormone receptor on insulin-like growth factors (IGFs), IGF-binding proteins, and ternary complex formation throughout life. *J Clin Endocrinol Metab* 1999;84(11):4118–4126.
9. Bach M, Gormley G. Clinical use of growth hormone secretagogues. In: Smith R, Thorner M, eds. *Human growth hormone: research and clinical practice (contemporary endocrinology).* Totawa, NJ: Humana Press, 2000.
10. Howard A, Feighner S, Smith R, et al. Molecular characterization of growth hormone secretagogue receptors. In: Smith R, Thorner M, eds. *Human growth hormone: research and clinical practice (contemporary endocrinology).* Totawa, NJ: Humana Press, 2000.
11. Broglio F, Arvat E, Benso A, et al. Ghrelin: endocrine and non-endocrine actions. *J Pediatr Endocrinol Metab* 2002;15:1219–1227.
12. Muccioli G, Baragli A, Granata R, et al. Heterogeneity of ghrelin/growth hormone secretagogue receptors. *Neuroendocrinology* 2007;86:147–164.
13. Tritos N, Kokkotou M. The physiology and potential clinical applications of ghrelin, a novel peptide hormone. *Mayo Clin Proc* 2006;81(5):653–660.
14. Waxman P, Frank S. Growth hormone action. In: Conn P, Means A, eds. *Principles of molecular regulation.* Totawa, NJ: Humana Press, 2000.
15. Bona G, Paracchini R, Giordano M, et al. Genetic defects in GH synthesis and secretion. *Eur J Endocrinol* 2004;151:S3–S9.
16. Herrington J, Carter-Su C. Signaling pathway activated by GH receptor. *Trends Endocrinol Metab* 2001;12(6):252–255.
17. Savage MO, Attie KM, David A, et al. Endocrine assessment, molecular characterization and treatment of growth hormone insensitivity disorders. *Nat Clin Pract Endocrinol Metab* 2006;2(7):395–407.
18. Rosenfeld RG, Kofoed E, Little B, et al. Growth hormone insensitivity resulting from post-GH receptor defects. *Growth Horm IGF Res* 2004;14:S35–S38.
19. Guyda H. How do we best measure growth hormone action? *Horm Res* 1997;48(Suppl 5):1–10.
20. Wollmann H, Ranke M. Metabolic effects of growth hormone in children. *Metabolism* 1995;44(10):97–102.
21. Wilkinson IR, Pradhananga SL, Speak R, et al. A long-acting GH receptor antagonist through fusion to GH binding protein. *Sci Rep* 2016;6:35072.
22. Vasques GA, Funari MFA, Ferreira FM, et al. IHH gene mutations causing short stature with nonspecific skeletal abnormalities and response to growth hormone therapy. *J Clin Endocrinol Metab* 2008;103(2):604–614.
23. Grote FK, Oostdijk W, de Muinck Keizer-Schrama SMPF, et al. Growth monitoring and diagnostic work-up of short stature: an international inventorization. *J Pediatr Endocrinol Metab* 2011;18(11):1031–1038.
24. Sizonenko PC, Clayton PE, Cohen P, et al. Diagnosis and management of growth hormone deficiency in childhood and adolescence. Part1: diagnosis of growth hormone deficiency, *Growth Horm IGF Res* 2001;11(3)137–165.
25. Allen DB, Brook C, Bridges N, et al. Therapeutic controversies: growth hormone (GH) treatment of non-GH deficient subjects. *J Clin Endocrinol Metab* 1994;79:1–10.
26. Guyda H. Use of growth hormone in children with short stature and normal growth hormone release: a growing problems. *Trends Endocrinol Metab* 1994;5(8):334–340.
27. Guyda H. Four decades of GH therapy for short children: what have we achieved? *J Clin Endocrinol Metab* 1999;84(12):4307–4316.
28. Grant M, Schmetz I, Russell B, et al. Changes in IGF-I and IGF-II and their binding proteins after a single injection of growth hormone. *J Clin Endocrinol Metab* 1986;63(4):981–984.
29. Deal C, Guyda H. Regulation of fetal growth and the GH-IGF-I axis: lessons for mouse to man. *Int Growth Monit* 1994;4:2–12.
30. Gluckman P. The endocrine regulation of fetal growth in late gestation: the role of insulin-like growth factors. *J Clin Endocrinol Metab* 1995;80(4):1047–1050.
31. Roberts C, Owens J, Sferruzzi-Perri A. Distinct actions of insulin-like growth factors (IGFs) on placental development and fetal growth: lessons from mice and guinea pigs. *Placenta* 2008;29(Suppl A):S42–S47.
32. Savage MO, Blum W, Ranke M, et al. Clinical features and endocrine status in patients with growth hormone insensitivity (Laron syndrome). *J Clin Endocrinol Metab* 1993;77:1465–1471.
33. Rogol AD, Hayden GF. Etiologies and early diagnosis of short stature and growth failure in children and adolescents. *J Pediatr* 2014;164(5):S1.e6–14.e6.
34. Collett-Solberg PF, Jorge AA, Boguszewski MC, et al. Growth hormone therapy in children; research and practice—A review. *Growth Horm IGF Res* 2019;44:20–32.
35. Oostdijk W, Grote FK, de Muinck Keizer-Schrama SM, et al. Diagnostic approach in children with short stature. *Horm Res* 2009;72:206–217.
36. Fredriks AM, van Buuren S, van Heel WJ, et al. Nationwide age references for sitting height, leg length, and sitting height/height ratio, and their diagnostic value for disproportionate growth disorder. *Arch Dis Child* 2005;90:807–812.
37. Malaquias AC, Scalco RC, Fontenele EG, et al. The sitting height/height ratio for age in healthy and short individuals and its potential role in selecting short children for SHOX analysis. *Horm Res Paediatr* 2013;80:449–456.
38. Junnila RK, Strasburger CJ, Bidlingmaier M. Pitfalls of insulin-like growth factor-i and growth hormone assays. *Endocrinol Metab Clin North Am* 2015;44:27–34.
39. Ranke MB, Wit JM. Growth hormone—past, present and future. *Nat Rev Endocrinol* 2018;14(5):285–300.
40. Bristow AF. International standards for growth hormone. *Horm Res* 1999;51(1):7–12.
41. Kant SG, Grote F, de Ru MH, et al. Radiographic evaluation of children with growth disorders. *Horm Res* 2007;68:310–315.
42. Homma TK, Krepischi ACV, Furuya TK, et al. Recurrent copy number variants associated with syndromic short stature of unknown cause. *Horm Res Paediatr* 2018;89(1):13–21.
43. Dauber A, Rosenfeld RG, Hirschhorn JN. Genetic evaluation of short stature. *J Clin Endocrinol Metab* 2014;99(9):3080–3092.
44. Tan TY, Dillon OJ, Stark Z, et al. Diagnostic impact and cost-effectiveness of whole-exome sequencing for ambulant children with suspected monogenic conditions. *JAMA Pediatr* 2017;171(9):855–862.
45. Sisley S, Trujillo MV, Khoury J, et al. Low incidence of pathology detection and high cost of screening in the evaluation of asymptomatic short children. *J Pediatr* 2013;163(4):1045–1051.
46. Tofts L, Das S, Collins F, et al. Growth charts for Australian children with achondroplasia. *Am J Med Genet Part A* 2017;173:2189–2200.
47. Grote FK, van Dommelen P, Oostdijk W, et al. Developing evidence-based guidelines for referral for short stature. *Arch Dis Child* 2008;93:212–217.
48. Greulich WW, Pyle SY, eds. *Radiographic atlas of skeletal development of the hand and wrist,* 2nd ed. Stanford, CA: Stanford University Press, 1959: xvi.(256p).
49. Tanner JM, Healy MJR, Cameron N, et al. *Assessment of skeletal maturity and prediction of adult height (TW3 Method),* 3rd ed. London, UK: W.B. Saunders, 2001.
50. Bayley N, Pinneau SR. Tables for predicting adult height from skeletal age: revised for use with the Greulich-Pyle hand standards. *J Pediatr* 1952;40(4):423–441.
51. Thodberg HH. Clinical review: an automated method for determination of bone age. *J Clin Endocrinol Metab* 2009;94(7):2239–2244.
52. Gkourogianni A, Andrew M, Tyzinski L, et al. Clinical characterization of patients with autosomal dominant short Stature due to aggrecan mutations. *J Clin Endocrinol Metab* 2017;102(2):460–469.
53. Vasques GA, Arnhold IJ, Jorge AA. Role of the natriuretic peptide system in normal growth and growth disorders. *Horm Res Paediatr* 2014;82:222–229.
54. Sfeir JG, Kittah NE, Tamhane SU, et al. Diagnosis of growth hormone deficiency as a late effect of radiotherapy in survivors of childhood cancers. *J Clin Endocrinol Metab* 2018:103(8):2785–2793.
55. Gravholt CH, Andersen NH, Conway GS, et al. Clinical practice guidelines for the care of girls and women with Turner syndrome: proceedings from the 2016 Cincinnati International Turner Syndrome Meeting. *Eur J Endocrinol* 2017;177(3):G1–G70.
56. Wit JM, Oostdijk W, Losekoot M, et al. Mechanisms in endocrinology: novel genetic causes of short stature. *Eur J Endocrinol* 2016;174(4):R145–R173.
57. Walenkamp MJ, Wit JM. Genetic disorders in the GHIGF-I axis in mouse and man. *Eur J Endocrinol* 2007;157(1):S15–S2.
58. Savage MO, Burren CP, Rosenfeld RG. The continuum of growth hormone-IGFI axis defects causing short stature: diagnostic and therapeutic challenges, *Clin Endocrinol (Oxf)* 2010;72(6):721–728.
59. Blum WF, Alherbish A, Alsagheir A, et al. The growth hormone-insulin-like growth factor-I axis in the diagnosis and treatment of growth disorders. *Endocr Connect* 2018;7(6):R212–R222.
60. Shen Y, Zhang J, Zhao Y, et al. Diagnostic value of serum IGF-1 and IGFBP-3 in growth hormone deficiency: a systematic review with meta-analysis. *Eur J Pediatr* 2015;174(4):419–427.
61. Dauber A, Muñoz-Calvo MT, Barrios V, et al. Mutations in pregnancy-associated plasma protein A2 cause short stature due to low IGF-I availability. *EMBO Mol Med* 2016;8(4):363–374.
62. Growth Hormone Research Society. Consensus guidelines for the diagnosis and treatment of growth hormone (GH) deficiency in childhood and adolescence: summary statement of the GH Research Society. *J Clin Endocrinol Metab* 2000;85(11):3990–3993.
63. Binder G, Weidenkeller M, Blumenstock G, et al. Rational approach to the diagnosis of severe growth hormone deficiency in the newborn. *J Clin Endocrinol Metab* 2010;95(5):2219–2226.
64. Wit JM, Clayton PE, Rogol AD, et al. Idiopathic short stature: definition, epidemiology and diagnostic evaluation. *Growth Horm IGF Res* 2008;18(2):89–110.
65. Rosenfeld RG, Albertsson-Wikland K, Cassorla F, et al. Diagnostic controversy: the diagnosis of childhood growth hormone deficiency revisited. *J Clin Endocrinol Metab* 1995;80(5):1532–1540.
66. Chalerv EA, Ballerini GA, Lazzati JM, et al. Cut-off values of serum growth hormone (GH) in pharmacological stimulation tests (PhT) evaluated in short-statured children using a chemiluminescent immunometric assay (ICMA) calibrated with the International Recombinant Human GH Standard 98/574. *Clin Chem Lab Med* 2013;51(5):e95–e97.
67. Secco A, di Iorgi N, Napoli F, et al. The glucagon test in the diagnosis of growth hormone deficiency in children with short stature younger than 6 years. *J Clin Endocrinol Metab* 2009;94(11):4251–4257.
68. Tanaka T, Cohen P, Clayton PE, et al. Diagnosis and management of growth hormone deficiency in childhood and adolescence—part 2: growth hormone treatment in growth hormone deficient children. *Growth Horm IGF Res* 2002;12(5)323–341.

69. Lodefalk M, Nilsson O. To prime or not to prime–is that still a question? A comment on the US guidelines on growth hormone and insulin-like growth factor-1 treatment in children and adolescents. *Horm Res Paediatr* 2017;88(2):179–180.
70. Grimberg A, DiVall SA, Polychronakos C, et al. Guidelines for growth hormone and insulin like growth factor-I treatment in children and adolescents: growth hormone deficiency, idiopathic short stature, and primary insulin-like growth factor-I deficiency. *Horm Res Paediatr* 2016;86(6)361–397.
71. Lazar L, Phillip M. Is sex hormone priming in peripubertal children prior to growth hormone stimulation tests still appropriate? *Horm Res Paediatr* 2010;73(4): 299–302.
72. Albrecht A, Penger T, Marx M, et al. Short-term adverse effects of testosterone used for priming in prepubertal boys before growth hormone stimulation test. *J Pediatr Endocrinol Metab* 2018;31(1):21–24.
73. Bonafe L, Cormier-Daire V, Hall C, et al. Nosology and classification of genetic skeletal disorders:2015 revision. *Am J Med Genet* 2015;167 (12):2869–2892.
74. Seaver LH, Irons M; American College of Medical Genetics (ACMG) Professional Practice and Guidelines Committee. ACMG practice guideline: genetic evaluation of short stature. *Genet Med* 2009;11(6):465–470.
75. Wit JM, Kiess W, Mullis P. Genetic evaluation of short stature. *Best Pract Res Clin Endocrinol Metab* 2011;25(1):1–17.
76. Dauber A, Stoler J, Hechter E, et al. Whole exome sequencing reveals a novel mutation in CUL7 in a patient with an undiagnosed growth disorder. *J Pediatr* 2013;162(1):202. e1–204.e1.
77. de Bruin C, Finlayson C, Funari MF, et al. Two patients with severe short stature due to a FBN1 mutation (p.Ala1728Val) with a mild form of acromicric dysplasia. *Horm Res Paediatr* 2016;86(5):342–348.
78. Wang SR, Carmichael H, Andrew SF, et al. Large-scale pooled next-generation sequencing of 1077 genes to identify genetic causes of short stature. *J Clin Endocrinol Metab* 2013;98(8):E1428–E1437.
79. Renes JS, Willemsen RH, Wagner A, et al. Bloom syndrome in short children born small for gestational age: a challenging diagnosis. *J Clin Endocrinol Metab* 2013;98(10):3932–3938.
80. Stark Z, Tan TY, Chong B, et al. A prospective evaluation of whole-exome sequencing as a first-tier molecular test in infants with suspected monogenic disorders. *Genet Med* 2016;18(11):1090–1096.
81. Yang Y, Muzny DM, Xia F, et al. Molecular findings among patients referred for clinical whole-exome sequencing. *JAMA* 2014;312(18):1870–1879.
82. Miller TD, Adam MP, Aradhya S, et al. Consensus statement: chromosomal microarray is a first-tier clinical diagnostic test for individuals with developmental disabilities or congenital anomalies. *Am J Hum Genet* 2010;86(5):749–764.
83. Stark Z, Schofield D, Alam K, et al. Prospective comparison of the cost-effectiveness of clinical whole-exome sequencing with that of usual care overwhelmingly supports early use and reimbursement. *Genet Med* 2017;19(8):867–874.
84. Vissers LELM, van Nimwegen KJM, Schieving JH, et al. A clinical utility study of exome sequencing versus conventional genetic testing in pediatric neurology. *Genet Med* 2017;19(9):1055–1063.
85. Freire BL, Homma TK, Funari MFA, et al. Homozygous loss of function BRCA1 variant causing a Fanconi-anemia-like phenotype, a clinical report and review of previous patients. *Eur J Med Genet* 2018;61(3):130–133.
86. Guo MH, Shen Y, Walvoord EC, et al. Whole exome sequencing to identify genetic causes of short stature. *Horm Res Paediatr* 2014;82(1):44–52.
87. Hauer NN, Popp B, Schoeller E, et al. Clinical relevance of systematic phenotyping and exome sequencing in patients with short stature. *Genet Med* 2018;20 (6):630–638.
88. Shapiro L, Chatterjee S, Ramadan DG, et al. Whole-exome sequencing gives additional benefits compared to candidate gene sequencing in the molecular diagnosis of children with growth hormone or IGF-1 insensitivity. *Eur J Endocrinol* 2017;177(6):485–501.
89. Bizzarri C, Bottaro G. Endocrine implications of neurofibromatosis 1 in childhood. *Horm Res Paediatr* 2015;83(4):232–241.
90. Romano AA, Allanson JE, Dahlgren J, et al. Noonan syndrome: clinical features, diagnosis, and management guidelines. *Pediatrics* 2010;126(4):746–759.
91. Forlenza GP, Calhoun A, Beckman KB, et al. Next generation sequencing in endocrine practice. *Mol Genet Metab* 2015;115(2–3):61–71.
92. Silventoinen K, Sammalisto S, Perola M, et al. Heritability of adult body height: a comparative study of twin cohorts in eight countries. *Twin Res* 2003;6(5):399–408.
93. Durand C, Rappold GA. Height matters—from monogenic disorders to normal variation. *Nat Rev Endocrinol* 2013;9(3):171–177.
94. Marouli E, Graff M, Medina-Gomez C, et al. Rare and low-frequency coding variants alter human adult height. *Nature* 2017;542(7640):186–190.
95. Murray PG, Clayton PE, Chernausek SD. A genetic approach to evaluation of short stature of undetermined cause. *Lancet Diabetes Endocrinol* 2018;6(7):564–574.
96. Goddard AD, Covello R, Luoh SM, et al. Mutations of the growth hormone receptor in children with idiopathic short stature. The Growth Hormone Insensitivity Study Group. *N Engl J Med* 1995;333(17):1093–1098.
97. Rao E, Weiss B, Fukami M, et al. Pseudoautosomal deletions encompassing a novel homeobox gene cause growth failure in idiopathic short stature and Turner syndrome. *Nat Genet* 1997;16(1):54–63.
98. Wang SR, Jacobsen CM, Carmichael H, et al. Heterozygous mutations in natriuretic peptide receptor-B (NPR2) gene as a cause of short stature. *Hum Mutat* 2015;36(4): 474–481.
99. Hisado-Oliva A, Ruzafa-Martin A, Sentchordi L, et al. Mutations in C-natriuretic peptide (NPPC): a novel cause of autosomal dominant short stature. *Genet Med* 2018;20(1):91–97.
100. Dillon OJ, Lunke S, Stark Z, et al. Exome sequencing has higher diagnostic yield compared to simulated disease-specific panels in children with suspected monogenic disorders. *Eur J Hum Genet* 2018;26(5):644–651.
101. Vasques GA, Hisado-Oliva A, Funari MF, et al. Long-term response to growth hormone therapy in a patient with short stature caused by a novel heterozygous mutation in NPR2. *J Pediatr Endocrinol Metab* 2017;30(1):111–116.
102. Millar DS, Lewis MD, Horan M, et al. Novel mutations of the growth hormone 1 (GH1) gene disclosed by modulation of the clinical selection criteria for individuals with short stature. *Hum Mutat* 2003;21(4);424–440.
103. Abuzzahab MJ, Schneider A, Goddard A, et al; Intrauterine Growth Retardation (IUGR) Study Group. IGF-I receptor mutations resulting in intrauterine and postnatal growth retardation. *N Engl J Med* 2003;349(23):2211–2222.
104. Domené HM, Bengolea SV, Martínez AS, et al. Deficiency of the circulating insulin-like growth factor system associated with inactivation of the acid-labile subunit gene. *N Engl J Med* 2004;350(6):570–577.
105. Pantel J, Legendre M, Cabrol S, et al. Loss of constitutive activity of the growth hormone secretagogue receptor in familial short stature. *J Clin Invest* 2006;116(3):760–768.
106. Batey L, Moon JE, Yu Y, et al. A novel deletion of IGF1 in a patient with idiopathic short stature provides insight into IGF1 haploinsufficiency. *J Clin Endocrinol Metab* 2014;99(1):E153–E159.
107. Cohen P, Rogol AD, Deal CL, et al; ISS Consensus Workshop participants. Consensus statement on the diagnosis and treatment of children with idiopathic short stature: a summary of the Growth Hormone Research Society, the Lawson Wilkins Pediatric Endocrine Society, and the European Society for Paediatric Endocrinology Workshop. *J Clin Endocrinol Metab* 2007; 93(11):4210–4217.
108. Vasques GA, Amano N, Docko AJ, et al. Heterozygous mutations in natriuretic peptide receptor-B (NPR2) gene as a cause of short stature in patients initially classified as idiopathic short stature. *J Clin Endocrinol Metab* 2013;98(10):E1636–E1644.
109. Kant SG, Cervenkova I, Balek L, et al. A novel variant of FGFR3 causes proportionate short stature. *Eur Endocrinol* 2015;172(6):763–770.
110. Klammt J, Neumann D, Gevers EF, et al. Dominant-negative STAT5B mutations cause growth hormone insensitivity with short stature and mild immune dysregulation. *Nat Commun* 2018;9(1):2105.
111. Den Ouden D, Kroon M, Hoogland P, et al. A 43-year old male with untreated panhypopituitarism due to absent of pituitary stalk: from dwarf to giant. *J Clin Endocrinol Metab* 2002;87:5430–5434.
112. Hindmarsh P, Dattani M. Use of growth hormone in children. *Nat Clin Pract* 2006;2(5):260–268.
113. Strasburger C, Bidlingmaier M. How robust are laboratory measures of growth hormone status? *Horm Res* 2005;64(Suppl 2):1–5.
114. Tillman V, Buckler J, Kibirige M, et al. Biochemical tests in the diagnosis of childhood growth hormone deficiency. *J Clin Endocrinol Metab* 1997;82:531–535.
115. Bryant J, Baxter L, Cave C, et al. Recombinant growth hormone for idiopathic short stature in children and adolescents. *Cochrane Library* 2008(3):1–31.
116. Leschek E, Rose S, Yanovski J, et al. Effect of growth hormone treatment on adult height in peripubertal children with idiopathic short stature: a randomized, double-blind, placebo-controlled trial. *J Clin Endocrinol Metab* 2004;89:3140–3148.
117. Cowel C. Effects of growth hormone in short, slowly growing children without growth hormone deficiency. Australian Paediatric Endocrine Group. *Acta Paediatr Scand* 1990;326(Suppl):29–30.
118. Albertsson-Wikland K, Aronson A, Gustafsson J, et al. Dose-dependent effect of growth hormone on final height in children with short stature without growth hormone deficiency. *J Clin Endocrinol Metab* 2008;93(11):4342–4350.
119. Theunissen N, Kamp G, Koopman H, et al. Quality of life and self-esteem in children treated for idiopathic short stature. *J Pediatr* 2002;140:507–515.
120. Sandberg D. Quality of life and self-esteem in children treated for idiopathic short stature. *J Pediatr* 2003;143(5):691.
121. Wilson TA, Rose SR, Cohen P, et al. Update of guidelines for the use of growth hormone in children: the Lawson Wilkins Pediatric Endocrinology Society Drug and Therapeutics Committee. *J Pediatr* 2003;143:415–421.
122. Ranke M, Partsch C, Lindberg A, et al. Adult height after GH therapy in 188 Ullrich–Turner syndrome patients: results of the German IGLU Follow-up Study 2001. *Eur J Endocrinol* 2002;147(5):625–633.
123. Canadian GH Advisory Committee. GH treatment to final height in Turner syndrome: a randomized controlled trial. *Horm Res* 1998;50(Suppl 3):25.
124. Taback S, Guyda H, Van Vliet G. Pharmacological manipulation of height: qualitative review of study populations and design. *Clin Invest Med* 1999;22(2):53–59.
125. Baxter L, Bryant J, Cave C, et al. Recombinant growth hormone for children and adolescents with Turner syndrome. *Cochrane Library* 2008(3):1–28.
126. Simon D, Leger J, Carel J. Optimal use of growth hormone therapy for maximizing adult height in children born small for gestational age. *Best Pract Res Clin Endocrinol Metab* 2008;22(3):525–537.
127. Tom A, McCauley L, Rodd C, et al. Maintenance of growth with aggressive hemodialysis therapy in children with chronic renal insufficiency. *J Pediatr* 1999;134:464–467.
128. Mehls O, Wuhl E, Tonshoff B, et al. Growth hormone treatment in short children with chronic kidney disease. *Acta Paediatr* 2008;97:1159–1164.
129. Fine R, Stablein D. Long-term use of recombinant human growth hormone in pediatric allograft recipients: a report of the NAPRTCS Transplant Registry. *Pediatr Nephrol* 2005;20:404–408.
130. Bryant J, Care C, Mihaylova B, et al. Clinical effectiveness and cost effectiveness of growth hormone in children: as systematic review and economic evaluation. *Health Technol Assess* 2002;6(18):1–168.
131. Carrel A, Myers S, Whitman B, et al. Benefits of long-term GH therapy in Prader–Willi syndrome: a 4 year study. *J Clin Endocrinol Metab* 2002;87(4):1581–1585.
132. Richards S, Aziz N, Bale S, et al. Standards and guidelines for the interpretation of sequence variants: a joint consensus recommendation of the American College of Medical Genetics and Genomics and the Association for Molecular Pathology. *Genet Med* 2015;17(5):405–424.
133. Pollard S, Sun S, Regier DA. Balancing uncertainty with patient autonomy in precision medicine. *Nat Rev Genet* 2019;20(5):251–252.

134. Schrier L, de Kam ML, McKinnon R, et al. Comparison of body surface area versus weight-based growth hormone dosing for girls with Turner syndrome. *Horm Res Paediatr* 2014;81(5):319–330.
135. Hughes IP, Harris M, Cotterill A, et al. Comparison of weight-vs body surface area-based growth hormone dosing for children: implications for response. *Clin Endocrinol (Oxf)* 2014;80(3):384–394.
136. Wit JM, Ranke MB, Albertsson-Wikland K, et al. Personalized approach to growth hormone treatment: clinical use of growth prediction models. *Horm Res Paediatr* 2013;79(5):257–270.
137. Deal CL, Tony M, Höybye C, et al. Growth Hormone Research Society workshop summary: consensus guidelines for recombinant human growth hormone therapy in Prader-Willi syndrome. *J Clin Endocrinol Metab* 2013;98(6):E1072–E1087.
138. Netchine I, Azzi S, Houang M, et al. Partial primary deficiency of insulin-like growth factor (IGF)-I activity associated with IGF1 mutation demonstrates its critical role in growth and brain development. *J Clin Endocrinol Metab* 2009;94(10):3913–3921.
139. Schönau E, Westermann F, Rauch F, et al. A new and accurate prediction model for growth response to growth hormone treatment in children with growth hormone deficiency. *Eur J Endocrinol* 2001;144(1):13–20.
140. Cohen P, Rogol AD, Howard CP, et al. Insulin growth factor-based dosing of growth hormone therapy in children: a randomized, controlled study. *J Clin Endocrinol Metab* 2007;92(7):2480–2486.
141. Cohen P, Germak J, Rogol AD, et al. Variable degree of growth hormone (GH) and insulin-like growth factor (IGF) sensitivity in children with idiopathic short stature compared with GH-deficient patients: evidence from an IGF-based dosing study of short children. *J Clin Endocrinol Metab* 2010;95(5):2089–2098.
142. Cohen P, Weng W, Rogol AD, et al. Dose-sparing and safety-enhancing effects of an IGF-I-based dosing regimen in short children treated with growth hormone in a 2-year randomized controlled trial: therapeutic and pharmacoeconomic considerations. *Clin Endocrinol (Oxf)* 2014;81(1):71–76.
143. Cohen P, Rogol AD, Weng W, et al. Efficacy of IGF-based growth hormone (GH) dosing in nonGH-deficient (nonGHD) short stature children with low IGF-I is not related to basal IGF-I levels. *Clin Endocrinol (Oxf)* 2013;78(3):405–414.
144. Decker R, Albertsson-Wikland K, Kriström B, et al. GH dose reduction maintains normal prepubertal height velocity after initial catch-up growth in short children. *J Clin Endocrinol Metab* 2019;104(3):835–844.
145. Molitch ME, Clemmons DR, Malozowski S, et al; Growth Hormone Guideline Task Force. Evaluation and treatment of adult growth hormone deficiency: an Endocrine Society Clinical Practice Guideline. *J Clin Endocrinol Metab* 2006;91:1621–1634.
146. Allen DB. Safety of growth hormone treatment of children with idiopathic short stature: the US experience. *Horm Res Paediatr* 2011;76(Suppl 3):45–47.
147. Ergun-Longmire B, Mertens A, Mitby P, et al. Growth hormone treatment and risk of second neoplasms in the childhood cancer survivor. *J Clin Endocrinol Metab* 2006;91:3494–3498.
148. Darendeliler F, Karagiannis G, Wilton P, et al. Recurrence of brain tumours in patients treated with growth hormone: analysis of the KIGS (Pfizer International Growth Database). *Acta Paediatr* 2006;95:1284–1290.
149. Bolar K, Hoffman A, Maneatis T, et al. Long-term safety of recombinant human growth hormone in Turner syndrome. *J Clin Endocrinol Metab* 2008;93(2):344–351.
150. van Parren Y, Mulder P, Houdijk M, et al. Adult height after long-term, continuous growth hormone (GH) treatment in short children born small for gestational age: results of a randomized, double-blind, dose-response GH trial. *J Clin Endocrinol Metab* 2003;88:3584–3590.
151. Poduval A, Saenger P. Safety and efficacy of growth hormone treatment in small for gestational age children. *Curr Opin Endocrinol Diabetes Obes* 2008;15(4):376–382.
152. Mahan J, Warady B. Assessment and treatment of short stature in pediatric patients with chronic renal disease: a consensus statement. *Pediatr Nephrol* 2006;21:917–930.
153. Tauber M, Diene G, Molinas C, et al. Review of 64 cases of death in children with Prader–Willi Syndrome (PWS). *Am J Med Genet A* 2008;146A:881–887.
154. Wilton P. Adverse events during GH treatment: 10 years' experience in KIGS, a pharmacoepidemiological survey. In: Ranke M, Wilton P, eds. *Growth hormone therapy in KIGS—10 year's experience.* Heidelberg, Germany: Barth, 1999.
155. Nishi Y, Takana T, Takano K, et al. Recent status of the occurrence of leukemia in GH-treated patients in Japan. *J Clin Endocrinol Metab* 1999;80(4):1961–1965.
156. Blethen L, Allen D, Graves D, et al. Safety of recombinant deoxyribonucleic acid-derived growth hormone. The national cooperative growth study experience. *J Clin Endocrinol Metab* 1996;81:1704–1710.
157. FDA. FDA approves Humatrope for short stature. Available at: www.accessdata.fda.gov/drugsatfda_docs/label/2008/021908s005lbl.pdf-2009-03-3 Accessed September 1, 2020.1.
158. Saenger PH, Mejia-Corletto J. Long-acting growth hormone: an update. *Endocr Dev* 2016;30:79–97.
159. Yuen KCJ, Miller BS, Biller BMK. The current state of long-acting growth hormone preparations for growth hormone therapy. *Curr Opin Endocrinol Diabetes Obes* 2018;25(4):267–273.
160. Christiansen JS, Backeljauw PF, Bidlingmaier M, et al. Growth Hormone Research Society perspective on the development of long-acting growth hormone preparations. *Eur J Endocrinol* 2016;174(6):C1–C8.
161. Suga H. Making pituitary hormone-producing cells in a dish. *Endocr J* 2016;63(8):669–680.
162. Miletta MC, Petkovic V, Eblé A, et al. Rescue of isolated GH deficiency type II (IGHD II) via pharmacologic modulation of GH-1 splicing. *Endocrinology* 2016;157(10):3972–3982.
163. Kopchick JJ. Discovery and development of a new class of drugs: GH antagonists. *J Endocrinol Invest* 2003;26(10 Suppl):16–26.
164. Trainer PJ, Drake WM, Katznelson L, et al. Treatment of acromegaly with the growth hormone-receptor antagonist pegvisomant. *N Engl J Med* 2000;342(16):1171–1177.

Aditi Khokhar
Sheila Perez-Colon
Vatcharapan Umpaichitra
Vivian L. Chin
Delbert A. Fisher

CHAPTER 57

Thyroid Hormones

Thyroid hormones are critically important to normal growth and development during infancy, childhood, and adolescence. Thyroid hormone deficiency during fetal life and infancy leads to mental retardation, and hypothyroidism during childhood and adolescence leads to growth and developmental retardation. In addition, there are significant effects of thyroid hormones on energy metabolism and on the metabolism of nutrients and inorganic ions, and these actions are important in the maintenance of normal metabolic homeostasis. In the present chapter, we review thyroid hormone physiology and the pharmacology of the drugs and chemicals used in the diagnosis and management of disorders of thyroid function.

THYROID HORMONE SYNTHESIS AND RELEASE

Thyroid hormones and analogs are tyrosine derivatives. Their structures are summarized in Figure 57.1. The only source of thyroxine (tetraiodothyronine, T_4) is the thyroid gland. The major substrates for T_4 synthesis are iodide and tyrosine.[1,2] Tyrosine is not rate limiting, but iodine is a trace element, the limitation of which can severely impair thyroid hormone synthesis. The steps in thyroid hormone synthesis by the thyroid gland include iodide trapping, synthesis of thyroglobulin (Tg), organification of trapped iodide, storage of iodinated Tg in follicular colloid, endocytosis and hydrolysis of Tg to release thyroid hormones, and deiodination of monoiodotyrosine (MIT) and diiodotyrosine (DIT) with intrathyroidal recycling of the iodide[1,2] (Fig. 57.2).

The transport of iodide across the thyroid cell membrane is the first and rate-limiting step in thyroid hormone biosynthesis. The salivary glands, gastric mucosa, uterus, mammary glands, small intestine, and placenta are also able to concentrate iodide; however, they are not capable of iodothyronine synthesis. Normally, the thyroid follicular cell generates a thyroid/serum concentration gradient of 30- to 40-fold. This gradient increases markedly when stimulated by iodine deficiency, thyroid-stimulating hormone (thyrotropin; TSH), or thyroid-stimulating immunoglobulins (TSIs), or by drugs that impair the efficiency of hormone synthesis. Several inorganic

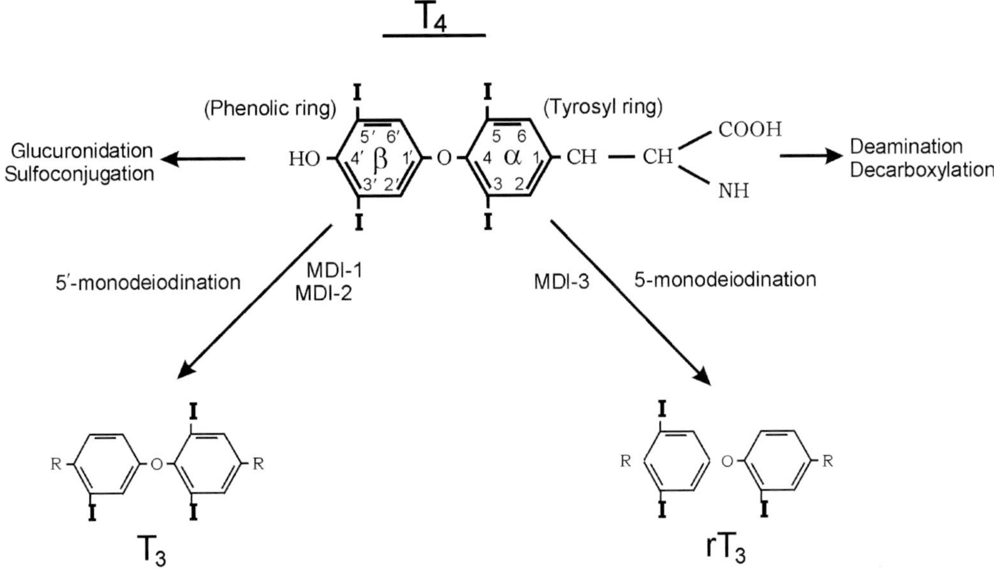

Figure 57.1 The metabolism of thyroxine (tetraiodothyronine). The major metabolic pathway is progressive monodeiodination by the three iodothyronine deiodinase enzymes, MDI-1, MDI-2, and MDI-3. Outer (phenolic) ring 5′-monodeiodination produces active 3,5,3′-triiodothyronine. Inner (tyrosyl) ring 5-monodeiodination produces inactive reverse (3,3′,5′) triiodothyronine. MDI-1 is also capable of inner-ring monodeiodination. The alanine side chain of the tyrosyl ring is subject to deamination and decarboxylation. Sulfoconjugation and glucuronide conjugation reactions at the 4′-phenolic–ring site occur in liver tissue.

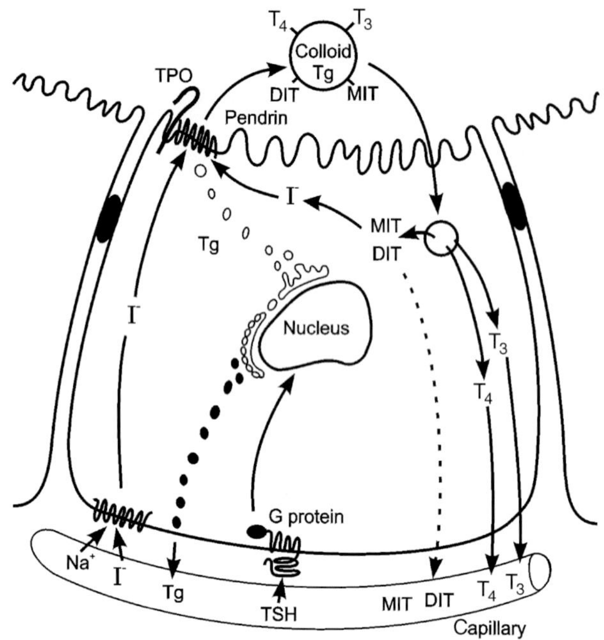

Figure 57.2 Drawing of the thyroid follicular cell illustrating thyroid hormone synthesis and secretion. Thyroid-stimulating hormone (TSH) regulates the process through the G-protein–linked plasma membrane TSH receptor. TSH binding stimulates thyroglobulin (Tg) synthesis and sodium iodide symporter uptake of circulating iodide. Small amounts of Tg are secreted, presumably from the endoplasmic reticulum into the thyroid lymphatics. The tyrosine residues of Tg are iodinated at the apical cell membrane catalyzed by thyroid peroxidase, the organification enzyme. The pendrin protein, a chloride/iodide transporter located at the apical cell membrane, facilitates organification. The resulting monoiodotyrosine (MIT) and diiodotyrosine (DIT) moieties with appropriate spatial orientation couple to form thyroxine (T_4) and triiodothyronine (T_3) within the stored Tg molecule. TSH also stimulates endocytosis of colloid droplets and progressive Tg proteolysis within the resulting phagolysosomes. The released T_4 and T_3 are secreted into the circulation. The uncoupled MIT and DIT are deiodinated by iodotyrosine deiodinase to release iodide, which is largely recycled within the follicular cell.

anions are capable of competitively inhibiting iodide transport; these include bromide (Br), nitrate (NO_2), thiocyanate (SCN), and perchlorate (ClO_4).

The predominant protein in thyroid colloid is Tg, a large 660-kD homodimer. The oxidation of iodide to an active intermediate is followed by iodination of Tg-bound tyrosyl residues. The thyroid gland normally contains 50 to 100 mg Tg for every 1 g of gland. The tyrosyl residues, which are the iodine acceptors of Tg, comprise about 3% of the weight of the protein, and about two-thirds of these are spatially oriented to be susceptible to iodination. Iodination of Tg tyrosyl residues forms MIT and DIT. These iodotyrosines then couple to form the iodothyronines T_3 and T_4; DIT + DIT couple to form T_4, while MIT + DIT coupling forms T_3. The relative proportions of T_3 and T_4 formed depend on the amount of iodide available. About 30% of the Tg iodoprotein is iodothyronine, with a T_4/T_3 ratio of 10:1 to 20:1.

The first step in thyroid hormone release is the endocytosis of stored colloid. The ingested colloid droplets fuse with proteolytic enzyme containing lysosomes to form phagolysosomes in which Tg is digested to release free iodothyronines into the cytoplasm for diffusion into the blood (Fig. 57.2). The MIT and DIT released during hydrolysis of Tg are largely deiodinated by a thyroidal iodotyrosine deiodinase.[1,2] The free iodide enters the intracellular iodide pool and is reutilized for new hormone synthesis (Fig. 57.2). A defect in thyroidal iodotyrosine deiodinase leads to a release of iodotyrosines into the circulation and their excretion in the urine. The loss from the thyroid gland of this normally recycled iodine, amounting to 70% to 80% of the daily thyroidal iodine supply, can significantly compromise thyroid hormone synthesis.

Some Tg is released into the circulation or the perivascular compartment during the process of synthesis, and there is good evidence that Tg reaches the general circulation via thyroidal lymphatics. Circulating Tg levels are high in premature infants during the first weeks of life, and values decrease with age throughout infancy and childhood.[2–4] Circulating Tg concentrations in normal children range from 2 to 70 ng per mL. Values increase after TSH administration and decrease during thyroid hormone administration.

REGULATION OF THYROID FUNCTION

Thyroid follicular cell function is regulated largely by circulating TSH and iodide levels.[1–3] TSH stimulates the production of intracellular cyclic adenosine monophosphate (cAMP), which appears to mediate most of the effects of TSH on thyroid metabolism. Pituitary TSH secretion is modulated by hypothalamic thyrotropin-releasing hormone (TRH)[5] and negative feedback action of thyroid hormones. TRH stimulates TSH release and increases TSH synthesis as well as TSH glycosylation. Feedback control is mediated via pituitary cell T_3 nuclear receptors that modulate TSH synthesis and pituitary cell membrane TRH-receptor binding. Increased thyroid hormone levels inhibit and decrease concentrations of pituitary TSH synthesis. The rate of pituitary TSH release is the net effect of the stimulation by TRH and the inhibitory effect of T_3 (see Fig. 57.3). Hypothalamic TRH production is modulated by environmental temperature via both peripheral and central (hypothalamic) thermal receptors. Decreasing environmental and body temperatures increases TRH production and increases the tonic level of TSH release. Thyroid hormones also modulate TRH synthesis within the hypothalamus.

The TRH neurons in the paraventricular hypothalamic nucleus receive input from other regions of the brain and from the circulation.[3] The major afferent links to these neurons include the catecholamine neurons in the brainstem and neurons from the arcuate nucleus. The former likely mediates upregulation of the *TRH* gene during cold exposure, while the latter mediates downregulation during starvation and illness.[3] Administration of the adipocyte hormone leptin, the production of which falls during fasting, prevents the fasting-induced fall in TSH. In addition, central administration of α-melanocyte–stimulating hormone (α-MSH) prevents the fasting-induced suppression of TSH. Agouti-related peptide and neuropeptide are orexigenic peptides that are downregulated by leptin and upregulated during fasting. When administered centrally, both can suppress TRH and TSH secretion. Thus, the arcuate nucleus integrates leptin signaling and assists in the regulation of *TRH* gene expression as well as food intake and energy expenditure.[3]

The average level of plasma iodide is also an important factor in the control of thyroid gland function.[1,2] Variation in iodine intake in the physiologic range regulates thyroid membrane

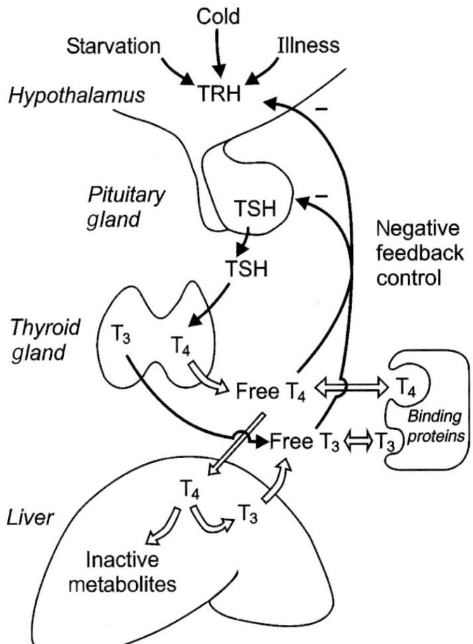

Figure 57.3 Drawing of the hypothalamic–pituitary–thyroid axis. Hypothalamic thyrotropin-releasing hormone (TRH) stimulates pituitary thyroid-stimulating hormone (TSH) production, which increases thyroid follicular cell activity and thyroid hormone secretion. Most T_3 is produced in peripheral tissues (here shown as liver) from T_4 catalyzed by iodothyronine deiodinase enzymes. The deiodination process produces approximately similar amounts of T_3 and reverse (inactive) T_3 or rT_3 (see Fig. 58.1). Most circulating T_4 and T_3 are protein bound. The free fractions act via a negative feedback loop to inhibit TRH and TSH maintaining serum-free hormone levels within a narrow physiologic range. TSH secretion is regulated by negative feedback of thyroid hormones on hypothalamic TRH secretion and pituitary TSH synthesis and secretion. This feedback is mediated via TRβ thyroid receptors. Cold exposure, starvation, or fasting, and nonthyroidal illness also modulate TRH and TSH secretion. See text for details.

iodide trapping, and in pharmacologic doses, iodide will block thyroid hormone synthesis. At least one important mechanism for these effects is the inhibitory action of iodide on the stimulation of cAMP by TSH.

METABOLISM OF THYROID HORMONES

The thyroid gland is the sole source of T_4, but most of the T_3 in the blood is derived from nonglandular sources via monodeiodination of T_4 in peripheral tissues[1,2] (see Fig. 57.3). Both T_3 and T_4 in the blood are associated with plasma proteins; the binding affinities of these proteins are greater for T_4 than T_3, and the concentration of T_4 in human blood is 50 to 100 times greater than that of T_3.[5] The concentrations of both are relatively constant in the steady state. The plasma half-life of T_4 in adult humans approximates 5 days, while the half-life of T_3 approximates 1 day. The circulating thyroid hormone–binding proteins include T_4-binding inter-α globulin (TBG), transthyretin (T_4-binding prealbumin), and albumin. TBG is the most important carrier protein for T_4; TBG and albumin seem equally important for T_3. The euthyroid steady-state concentrations of free T_4 and free T_3 approximate 0.02% and 0.20%, respectively, of the total thyroid hormone concentrations. Absolute mean free T_4 and T_3 concentrations approximate 1.5 and 0.3 ng per dL, respectively. In adolescents and adults, the plasma concentrations of the several binding proteins are 1 to 4 mg per dL for TBG, 10 to 20 mg per dL for transthyretin, and 2 to 5 g per dL for albumin. TBG levels are higher in children than in adults and decrease progressively to adult levels during adolescence.

Two major extravascular kinetic pools of T_3 and T_4 probably exist, one in which plasma–tissue interchange is rapid (chiefly the liver, kidney, and lung) and one in which exchange is slow (chiefly the skeletal, muscle, and skin).[6] An additional pool, chiefly in the gut and bone, with an intermediate exchange rate has been suggested. Peak T_4 concentrations after single-pulse doses of labeled hormone occur in these "pools" in minutes, hours, and days, respectively. Total body T_4 distribution in adults has been estimated as follows: about 20% in plasma, 30% in fast tissues, 45% in slow tissues, and 5% in intermediate tissues.

Deiodination is the major pathway of thyroid hormone metabolism in humans. The first step in T_4 metabolism is conversion either to T_3 or to reverse T_3[1,2,7] (Fig. 57.1). Monodeiodination of the β or outer (hydroxyl) ring produces T_3, which has three to four times the metabolic potency of T_4. Monodeiodination of the α or inner ring produces rT_3, which is metabolically inactive. Two types of outer-ring iodothyronine monodeiodinase (MDI) have been described (Fig. 57.1). MDI-1, predominantly expressed in the liver, kidney, and thyroid, is a high K_m enzyme, inhibited by propylthiouracil (PTU), and stimulated by thyroid hormone. MDI-1 is also capable of inner-ring monodeiodination, particularly of T_4 sulfate (to rT_3 sulfate) and T_3 sulfate (to T_2 sulfate).[7,8] MDI-2, predominantly located in the brain, pituitary, placenta, skeletal muscle, heart, thyroid, and brown adipose tissues (BATs), is a low K_m enzyme insensitive to PTU and inhibited by thyroid hormone. Both MDI-1 and MDI-2 contribute to circulating T_3 production, while MDI-2 acts as well to increase local tissue levels of T_3.[7,8] A third inner (tyrosyl)-ring iodothyronine monodeiodinase (MDI-3) has been characterized in most tissues, including the brain, placenta, uterus, and fetal skin. This enzyme system catalyzes the conversion of T_4 to rT_3 and T_3 to diiodothyronine.

Approximately 70% to 90% of circulating T_3 is derived from peripheral conversion and 10% to 25% from the thyroid gland. The relative values for rT_3 are 96% to 98% and 2% to 4%. Progressive tissue monodeiodination reactions degrade T_3 and rT_3 to diiodothyronine, monoiodothyronine, and noniodinated thyronine. Conjugation of the phenolic-ring hydroxyl group to sulfate or glucuronide produces glucuronide or sulfate analogs of the iodothyronines.[7,8] These are inactivating reactions because the analogs formed do not bind to thyroid hormone receptors and are rapidly metabolized by MDI-1 or excreted in the bile.[7,8] The exception is T_3 sulfate which demonstrates some 20% of native T_3 bioactivity when injected into hypothyroid rats. This presumably is due to the action of tissue sulfatases or bacterial sulfatases in the intestine.[8]

The alanine side chain of the inner ring of the hormones is also subject to degradative reactions, including deamination and decarboxylation.[7,8] Pyruvic acid analogs and small amounts of lactic acid analogs have been observed in urine and bile; these have minimal biologic activity. Two enzymes, L-amino acid oxidase and thyroid hormone aminotransferase, catalyze the deamination of T_4 and T_3 to their acetic acid analogs tetraiodothyroacetic acid (tetrac) and triiodothyroacetic acid (TRIAC).[7,8] TRIAC binds to the T_3 nuclear receptor with greater avidity than T_3 and demonstrates significant biologic activity when injected into animals or humans. However, relatively large doses are required because of rapid clearance and degradation via deiodination and glucuronidation.[7,8] TRIAC has been utilized in the treatment of thyroid hormone resistance. T_4 and T_3 are potent proangiogenic agents in the chick chorioallantoic membrane model of angiogenesis and in human dermal microvascular endothelial cell assays.[9] These actions are mediated via a plasma membrane hormone receptor site on integrin $\alpha_v\beta_3$. Tetrac has been shown to block this binding and to inhibit thyroid hormone action on tumor cell proliferation. Tetrac has no agonist activity at the hormone receptor site.[9] Two thyroid hormone derivatives, 3-iodothyronamine (T1AM) and thyronamine (T0AM), products of combined thyroid hormone decarboxylation and deiodination, have been shown in mice to induce transient hypothermia, decrease aortic pressure, block carbohydrate utilization, and increase fat utilization.[10,11] These molecules are present in mammalian brain, peripheral organs, thyroid gland, and blood serum. T1AM is strongly protein bound, and circulating concentrations are in the microgram per deciliter range similar to T_4.[12] It has been proposed that these thionamines act via thyronamine G-protein–coupled receptors, such as trace amine–associated receptors (TAAR1), adrenergic receptors (particularly α2), and 5-hydroxytryptophan receptors.[10,13]

THYROID HORMONE ACTIONS

Thyroid hormone effects are mediated predominantly by means of nuclear thyroid hormone protein receptors (TRs), which act as DNA-binding transcription factors regulating gene transcription. Two mammalian genes code for TR, Trα and TRβ, and alternative splicing of expressed messenger RNA (mRNA) species leads to production of the major isoforms Trα1, Trα2, TRβ1, and TRβ2.[14–17] In rodent species, hepatic TR-binding activity matures during the first 3 to 5 weeks of extrauterine life. Trα binding in brain and pituitary cells appears during fetal life, whereas TRβ isoforms increase during the early neonatal period.[14] In the fetal/neonatal rat, thyroid hormone effects on thermogenesis, hepatic enzyme activities, skin and brain maturation, and growth hormone (GH) metabolism mature largely during the first 4 postnatal weeks.[15,18]

In the human fetus, low levels of T_4 binding have been detected in brain tissue at 10 weeks of gestational age, and hepatic, cardiac, and lung TR binding are observed at 16 to 18 weeks.[15] Information is limited regarding the timing of appearance of thyroid hormone postreceptor effects in the human fetus. The length, weight, appearance, behavior, biochemical parameters, extrauterine adaptation, and early neonatal course of the athyroid human neonate are usually normal.[15] Growth of the human fetus is programmed independent of thyroid hormones by a complex interplay of genetic, nutritional, hormonal, and growth factors.

Postnatal thermogenesis is mediated through BAT, prominent in subscapular and perirenal areas in the mammalian fetus and neonate. Heat production in BAT is stimulated by catecholamines by means of β-adrenergic receptors and is thyroid hormone dependent. The uncoupling protein thermogenin, or UCP-1, unique to BAT, is located on the inner mitochondrial membrane and uncouples phosphorylation by dissipating the proton gradient created by the mitochondrial respiratory chain. An iodothyronine deiodinase (MDI) in BAT mediates local T_4 to T_3 conversion. Full thermogenin expression in BAT requires both catecholamine and T_3 stimulation.[19,20] UCP-2 is found in many tissues, but does not appear to be regulated by β-adrenergic agonists or thyroid hormone. UCP-3 has been cloned and is expressed in muscle and white adipose tissue as well as BAT.[20] Muscle UCP-3 is regulated by β_3-adrenergic stimulation and thyroid hormone and probably contributes to nonshivering thermogenesis in adult rats and presumably humans. UCP-3 mRNA levels are also regulated by dexamethasone, leptin, and starvation, but the regulation differs in BAT and muscle.[20] TR-mediated thyroid hormone actions also include the synthesis of selected enzymes and proteins in liver; stimulation of myogenin, α-actin, and myosin synthesis in cardiac tissue; promotion of mammary gland development and gene expression; and stimulation of growth and development and central nervous system (CNS) maturation.

Studies in the rat model have characterized a profound effect of thyroid hormones on GH secretion and action.[14,21] Hypothyroidism decreases pituitary GH content, impairs the pituitary GH response to GH-releasing hormone (GHRH), reduces basal and pulsatile GH secretion, and decreases circulating GH levels. Similar effects have been observed in hypothyroid human subjects. Hypothyroid patients show limited GH responses to insulin hypoglycemia, arginine, and GHRH; reduced nocturnal GH secretion; and reduced circulating levels of insulin-like growth factor 1 (IGF-1), IGF-2, IGF-binding protein-3, GH-binding protein, and bioactive IGF.[22–24] There is also evidence that thyroid hormones stimulate production of other growth factors, including epidermal growth factor, nerve growth factor, and erythropoietin. Thyroid hormones have direct actions on bone, potentiating the cartilage response to IGF-1 and stimulating osteoblastic bone resorption and remodeling.[25–27]

These hormonal and growth factor deficiencies contribute to the disordered growth of hypothyroid infants and children, including the decreased long bone growth, delayed bone maturation, delayed tooth eruption, and anemia. The actions of thyroid hormones and GH are synergistic. GH administered to neonatal hypophysectomized rats increases body weight, but it has a limited effect on skeletal growth; in contrast, thyroxine accelerates skeletal growth and potentiates the GH effects. Combined treatment optimizes growth and development. The vast majority of infants with congenital hypothyroidism (CH) are born with normal or increased length and weight, and early adequate thyroid hormone treatment prevents development of growth retardation. There may be a transient period of growth deceleration during the early weeks of treatment,[27] but even in infants with severe CH, manifested by very low serum T_4 concentrations and delayed bone maturation at birth, early, adequate treatment results in mean height and body mass index equal to or greater than values in normal children.[28,29] Bone age values are also normalized by 2 to 3 years.[30,31] Bone mineral density and metabolism are also normal in treated children given adequate nutrition.[32]

The effects of thyroid hormones on growth and physical development extend through most of the second decade, and delayed or inadequate replacement therapy during childhood or adolescence can reduce adult height.[33] Thyroxine treatment in children with growth retardation due to a prolonged period of untreated hypothyroidism usually induces marked catch-up growth, but in some instances, this is inadequate to normalize adult height.[33,34] Adult height is generally inversely correlated with the duration of untreated hypothyroidism prior to the advent of puberty.[33] This is thought to be due to the onset of puberty, limiting the chance to achieve full growth catch-up before epiphyseal fusion. Suppression of pubertal development by administration of gonadotropin-releasing hormone plus GH was shown to improve height gain in a juvenile hypothyroid patient.[33]

The critical role of thyroid hormones in CNS maturation has long been recognized. The first phase of fetal CNS maturation (neuronal multiplication, migration, and organization) occurs during the second trimester of gestation. A second phase (glial cell multiplication, migration, and myelinization) occurs during the perinatal period and extends through 3 to 4 postnatal years.[15] Available evidence suggests that deficiency or excess of thyroid hormones alters the timing or synchronization of the CNS developmental program, presumably by altering critical homeobox gene cascades and other genetic CNS maturation events.[15] Prior to activation of fetal thyroid function by the fetal hypothalamic–pituitary complex at midgestation, the fetus is dependent on maternal thyroid hormone that crosses the placenta in limited amounts. Several studies have shown that maternal hypothyroidism, often due to Hashimoto's thyroiditis, impairs the subsequent neuropsychological development of the offspring; even mild maternal hypothyroidism has been shown to reduce offspring IQ by 4 to 7 points.[34,35]

Severe iodine deficiency with combined maternal and fetal hypothyroidism results in severe neurologic impairment,[36] and mild endemic iodine deficiency, producing mild maternal and childhood hypothyroxinemia, has been shown to reduce the mean IQ of children.[35] Sixty percent to 70% of postnatal brain growth and differentiation occurs during the first 2 years of life, and it is during this period that the CNS effects of hypothyroidism are most devastating.[37] Untreated, severe CH is associated with an IQ deficit of 4 to 6 points per month during the first 5 to 7 months of postnatal life.[18,35] Such infants treated promptly at birth have minimal IQ impairment, being protected in utero by the limited amounts of maternal thyroxine crossing the placenta.[38,39] However, overall, a mean 6-point IQ deficit has been shown in a meta-analysis of published treatment outcome papers. This deficit is largely due to infants with severe disease with intrauterine hypothyroidism manifest as delayed bone maturation at birth. These data, summarized in Table 57.1, emphasize the critical role of thyroid hormones in CNS development both in utero and during infancy and early childhood.

TABLE 57.1 Effects of Thyroid Hormone Deficiency Relative to Phase of Central Nervous System Development

Cause of Thyroid Hormone Deficiency	*Phase of CNS Development*[a]	*Severity of CNS Damage to Child*[b]
Maternal hypothyroidism	I	+
Congenital hypothyroidism		
Untreated	I + II	++++
Newborn treated	I	± to +
Combined maternal–fetal hypothyroidism (newborn treated)	I	--
Endemic iodine deficiency (no treatment)		
Mild to moderate	I + II	+ to --
Severe	I + II	++++

[a] Phase I: neuronal multiplication, migration, and organization during the second trimester of gestation; phase II: glial cell multiplication, migration, and myelinization during perinatal period and extending through 3–4 years of age.
[b] +, 4–7 IQ points; ++++, 30–40 IQ points; -- not significantly affected.

RELATIVE EFFECTS OF THYROID HORMONES VERSUS AGE

Thyroid hormone actions vary with age. Thyroid hormone deficiency during human fetal life has minimal untoward effects. Somatic growth and development and linear bone growth proceed normally in the athyroid fetus, and bone maturation is normal or minimally retarded (3 to 6 weeks) at birth.[40,41] The reason(s) for the relative lack of thyroid hormone effect on fetal somatic growth is not clear. Likely explanations include low levels of active thyroid hormone in fetal serum and tissues and/or immaturity of thyroid hormone receptor responsiveness at the transcription, translation, or action levels.[18,42]

The developmental effects of thyroid hormones, such as the CNS effects, are most obvious during infancy and early childhood. Somatic growth, bone growth and maturation, and tooth development and eruption are thyroid dependent. After 3 to 4 years of age, thyroid hormone deficiency is not associated with mental retardation, but delayed somatic and linear bone growth and delayed eruption of permanent dentition are prominent. Bone maturation, measured as bone age, is also delayed, diaphyseal bone growth is reduced, and epiphyseal growth and mineralization largely cease.[2,27] Hypothalamic and anterior pituitary function may also be abnormal in hypothyroid children. Although, in most children, thyroid hormone deficiency leads to a delayed sexual development, occasional children manifest precocious sexual maturation with increased levels of circulating gonadotropins.[43–45] Precocious puberty is observed only rarely, so it is possible that these patients have genetic variants of the gonadotropin receptors, which can be stimulated by the increased TSH levels.[46] Similar findings have been reported for TSH and follicle-stimulating hormone (FSH) receptor variants stimulated by β human chorionic gonadotropin (βhCG).[46,47] Van Wyk and Grumbach reported the association of multicystic ovaries with hypothyroidism and precocious puberty. This pathology is more frequently seen in girls. Precocious puberty is always isosexual and is characterized by breast enlargement, multicystic ovaries, and menstrual bleeding. It is believed that high levels of TSH interact with the FSH receptors, inducing FSH-like effects on the gonads.[48] When the hypothyroid state is alleviated, the manifestations of sexual precocity regress, and normal puberty ensues when the general level of maturity has progressed appropriately.

In female patients, serum prolactin levels also tend to be increased, and galactorrhea may occur if serum estrogen levels are high enough to permit breast development and milk production. These changes seem to occur in children with high serum TSH levels, and enlargement of the sella turcica has been observed. The increased serum prolactin levels are probably explained by the fact that TRH stimulates both TSH and prolactin release from the pituitary.

During childhood and adolescence and until epiphyseal closure, thyroid hormone deficiency leads to reduced somatic growth, reduced linear bone growth, and delayed bone maturation. In addition, epiphyseal dysgenesis is commonly observed.[27,49] The effects of thyroid hormone deficiency on dental development are less profound, but delay in eruption of second dentition may occur. Abnormalities of hypothalamic–pituitary function secondary to hypothyroidism are also common in adolescence.[2,27] Puberty is often delayed or incomplete. In normal women, menstrual cycles are commonly nonovulatory, and bleeding may be irregular. This pattern is usually more prolonged in hypothyroid female adolescents. In addition, menorrhagia or hypomenorrhea may occur.

THYROID FUNCTION DURING INFANCY AND CHILDHOOD

IODINE METABOLISM

During prepubertal and pubertal periods of growth and development, there is a progressive growth of the thyroid gland, a progressive increase in thyroid Tg and iodothyronine stores, and a progressive increase in T_4 production rate, measured in micrograms per day.[2] Measured as microgram per gram thyroid or as production relative to body mass, T_4 production decreases progressively, roughly in parallel with metabolic rate (calorie intake) (Fig. 57.4). The iodide space (on a body weight basis)

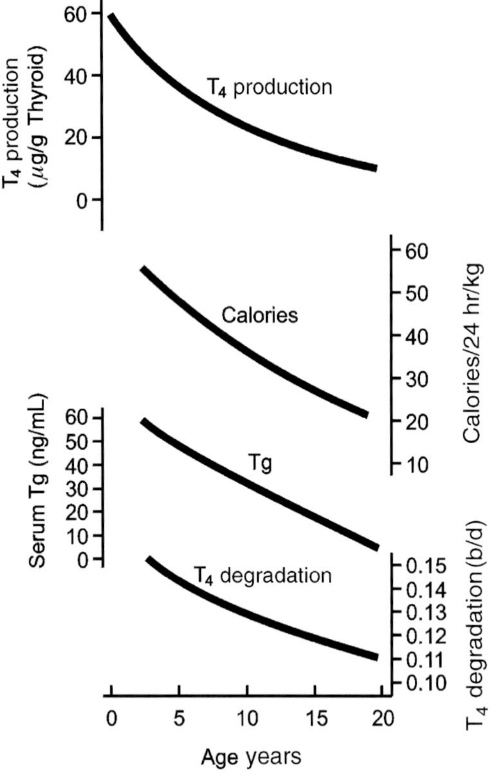

Figure 57.4 Thyroid function during childhood is characterized by a progressive increase in thyroid gland size and thyroid hormone production in microgram per day. However, interpreted as µg/g thyroid gland or T_4 degradation rate (fraction of the thyroxine pool degraded daily), T_4 production decreases roughly in parallel with the decrease in metabolic rate (as calories/kg/d). The serum thyroglobulin (Tg) concentration decreases reflecting the relative decreases in T_4 secretion.

in infants is relatively larger than that in older children, adolescents, or adults, and the thyroid iodide clearance rate is nearly three times that of adults.[2] Renal iodide clearance is also high in infants and decreases progressively with age. The progressive decrease in thyroid iodide clearance may be, at least in part, secondary to the change in renal iodide clearance.

During childhood, the growth of the thyroid gland in residents of iodine-sufficient areas roughly parallels body growth. The gland volume, measured by ultrasound, increases in size from about 1 g at birth to a mean of about 5 g at 10 years of age. Average thyroid iodine content increases from 0.3 mg at birth to 16 mg in adolescents and adults.[2,50,51] In areas of severe iodine deficiency, the thyroid weight in newborns may be 2 to 3 g, and iodine content may be as low as 40 µg. The iodide space also increases progressively in volume with age; however, the relative size (in liters per kilogram, expressed as percentage of body weight) decreases from about 50% of body weight at birth to 40% in 30-kg children (at about age 10 years).[2,52,53] These values can be compared with the 33% body weight values in 65-kg adults.

Radioiodine uptake and clearance during childhood and adolescence vary with diet and iodine intake. Values during the first two decades have been reported to decrease progressively or remain relatively stable.[2,54] This discrepancy is presumably caused by variations in iodine intake. The data showing a decrease with age were from areas of low-iodine intake in Europe and Australia. A relatively high-iodine intake could tend to mask differences in uptake with age. Thyroid iodine clearance (per gram of thyroid tissue) decreases progressively with age, associated with a progressive decrease in T_4 production rate (or turnover) on a microgram per kilogram per day basis.

SERUM THYROID HORMONE CONCENTRATIONS AND T_4 PRODUCTION

Serum total T_4 and T_3 concentrations decrease gradually with age.[2] The decrease in serum total T_4 and T_3 result largely from a decrease in serum TBG concentrations that is progressive from early childhood through 15 to 16 years of age, when the mean serum TBG concentration is about the same as in adults. Reciprocal changes occur in serum transthyretin concentrations. These changes presumably reflect the effects of gonadal steroids, but other factors such as nutrition may be involved.[55]

Serum-free T_4 concentrations decrease slightly during childhood and adolescence.[2,56,57] The percentage of iodine-131–labeled protein-bound iodine appearing in blood (percentage of dose per liter per kilogram of body weight) after labeling of the thyroid gland also decreases with age during the first two decades, as does T_4 turnover and production rate on a body weight basis (microgram per kilogram per day).[2,52] Estimated T_4 turnover or production rate values are 5 to 6 µg per kg per day in infants, 4 µg per kg per day in children aged 1 to 3 years, 2 to 3 µg per kg per day in children aged 3 to 9 years, and 1 µg per kg per day in adults.

The serum concentration of rT_3 remains unchanged or increases slightly during childhood and adolescence. The serum-free rT_3 index (total rT_3 × fractional T_3 resin uptake) remains stable or increases slightly. Because circulating rT_3 is derived predominantly from peripheral deiodination of T_4, these observations and the fact that the mean calculated ratios of serum rT_3/serum T_4 and the free rT_3 index/free T_4 index increase progressively with age suggest that the relative rate of T_4 deiodination to rT_3 increases with age during childhood and adolescence.[58] The decreases with age in the ratios of serum T_3/serum rT_3 and the free T_3 index/free rT_3 index suggest a progressive decrease in the relative conversion of T_4 to T_3 with age during the first two decades.[58] Reverse T_3 may be elevated in nonthyroidal illnesses.

The progressive decrease in thyroid gland T_4 production (microgram per gram), T_4 turnover, serum Tg, and thyroidal radioiodine uptake indicates a progressive relative decrease in thyroid function with age.[2] The decreasing serum TSH concentration with age suggests that these decreases are mediated primarily by reduced TSH secretion. Whether this reflects decreased TRH secretion or a non-TRH mechanism is not clear. A progressive reduction in thyroid gland TSH responsiveness might also be involved.

THYROID HORMONE PREPARATIONS

The thyroid hormones, as shown in Figure 57.1, are iodine-containing amino acid derivatives of thyronine.[1,2] The structural requirements for bioactivity have been well defined. The two aromatic rings are essential, as is the ether linkage. The alanine side chain in position 1; halogen or methyl groups in positions 3, 5, and 3′; and the hydroxyl group in position 4 are all necessary for optimal activity. The natural hormones are levorotatory; the dextrorotatory isomers have 10% or less of the bioactivity of the L-isomers. The D-T_4 isomer had been utilized clinically in the past as a cholesterol-lowering agent but has no role in replacement therapy. TRIAC binds to the thyroid hormone receptor as effectively as T_3 in vitro but has a much shorter half-life in vivo. The potential clinical usage of thyroacetic acids has been investigated.

Several preparations of thyroid hormones are available, as summarized in Table 57.2. Na-l-thyroxine (T_4) and Na-l-triiodothyronine (T_3) are synthetic preparations of the natural hormones. These hormones are also available in combination in a 4:1 ratio of T_4 to T_3. Thyroid U.S. Pharmacopeia (USP) is a dried and powdered preparation of porcine or bovine thyroid gland.

Na-l-thyroxine is the drug of choice for replacement therapy. It is uniform in potency, is easily measured in serum, and provides physiologic serum T_3 levels, since most of the circulating T_3 is normally derived from T_4 by monodeiodination in tissues. Most synthetic T_4 preparations have been reformulated since 1982 to guarantee specified hormone concentrations.[59]

TABLE 57.2 Preparation and Relative Potencies of Thyroid Hormone Preparations

Preparation	*Source*	*Equivalent Dosage*
Na-l-thyroxine	Synthetic	100 µg
Na-l-triiodothyronine	Synthetic	25 µg
Na-l-thyroxine (80%) + Na-l-triiodothyronine (20%)	Synthetic	50–62.5 µg
Thyroid (USP)	Natural	60 mg

USP, U.S. Pharmacopeia.

Absorption of the hormone is variable, ranging from 50% to 100%; average absorption approximates 80%.[59]

There is only limited application for Na-l-triiodothyronine (T_3) in thyroid therapy. Absorption of T_3 is nearly complete after oral administration, but the serum half-life is short (1 day vs. 5 days for T_4). Blood levels are more variable and more difficult to stabilize. In adult patients with hypothyroidism, it has been suggested that partial substitution of triiodothyronine for thyroxine replacement therapy may improve mood and neuropsychological function, and it has been shown in hypothyroid adult rats that such dual treatment more reliably reproduces normal tissue levels of thyroxine and triiodothyronine.[60,61] However, there is no consensus favoring combined therapy at the present time, and serum and tissue levels of T_3 are normalized with T_4 therapy alone.[62,63] T_3 may be useful in the early treatment of severe hypothyroidism in older children or for short-term suppression studies. It may also be useful in the management of TSH-dependent hyperthyroidism.

THERAPY WITH THYROID HORMONES

CONGENITAL HYPOTHYROIDISM

Infants with CH usually have thyroid dysgenesis due to abnormal thyroid gland embryogenesis. They may have agenesis or have a residual hypoplastic gland in the normal or an ectopic location. Ten percent to 15% have an inborn abnormality in TSH secretion or response (hypothalamic–pituitary hypothyroidism) or in thyroid hormone synthesis.[15,18,56] Less commonly, transient neonatal hypothyroidism can be caused by exposure to an antithyroid drug or an antithyroid antibody derived transplacentally from the mother.

In infants with CH, initial treatment with 10 to 15 µg per kg T_4 daily is desirable to consistently normalize the serum T_4 concentration (to >10 µg per dL) within 2 to 4 weeks, particularly in infants with severe CH.[15,18,38,64] This amounts to an initial treatment dose of 50 µg daily in most term infants. Crushed tablets are preferred over liquid formulation for young infants and children since there is no reliable liquid formulation. It can be given with a small amount of water, breast milk, or formula. Soy formula, iron, calcium, and vitamins should not be given at the same time. It is now clear that the major source of brain cell T_3, the receptor-active hormone, is serum T_4. Some 70% of T_3 in the cerebral cortex of neonatal rats is derived from local monodeiodination of T_4.[65,66] Thus, institution of replacement T_4 in a dose adequate to rapidly normalize the serum T_4 concentration is essential to minimize the period of CNS T_4 deficiency and help ensure optimal brain development. Replacement therapy with T_3 or mixtures of T_4 and T_3 is not recommended.

Careful monitoring of individual infants and dosage adjustment are necessary during the early weeks and months of life to guarantee adequate treatment and prevent prolonged hyperthyroxinemia. Premature synostosis with and without brain dysfunction has been reported in association with neonatal thyrotoxicosis or with excessive thyroid hormone doses in the treatment of CH.[67,68] In the latter cases, the T_4 doses were in the 200 to 300 µg per day range throughout most of infancy.[68] The threshold and duration of T_4 secretion or dosage required to produce premature synostosis is not clear, but the modest doses recommended with careful monitoring produce little risk. It is useful to obtain serum levels 12 to 24 hours after the last T_4 dose to avoid the effect of transient and variable absorption.

TABLE 57.3 Dose of Oral Thyroxine for Replacement Therapy of Infants and Children

Age	*Daily Dose (μg/kg/d)*	*Range of Dose (μg)*
1–6 mo	7–15	30–50
6–12 mo	4–8	50–100
1–5 y	5–6	75–150
5–10 y	3–4	100–200
10–20 y	1.5–3	100–250

The serum TSH concentration may be inappropriately elevated in infants with CH and may not be suppressed to normal levels with treatment.[36,63,69] Adequate treatment probably should suppress serum TSH values to less than 15 mU per L by 1 to 2 months.[38,64] Although the early weeks and months of treatment are critical for infants with CH, the CNS is thyroid hormone dependent for 2 to 4 years, and growth is thyroid hormone dependent during the first two decades of life.[2,27] Thus, careful monitoring of treatment is required throughout childhood and adolescence. The total dosage of T_4 increases progressively to 200 to 250 μg daily in adolescence (Table 57.3). The dosage on a kilogram body weight basis decreases progressively to the adult value of 1.5 μg per kg per day.

Clinical evidence of normal growth and development and lack of signs and symptoms of toxicity judges adequacy of therapy. Growth in length and weight should be plotted monthly during the first 3 months and at 2- to 3-month intervals thereafter during the first year. Measurements of circulating hormone concentrations are essential to assess adequacy of treatment. Measurements of free T_4 and TSH are helpful. It is recommended to maintain TSH in the age-specific reference range (but to avoid undetectable TSH < 0.05 mU per L) and serum concentrations of T_4 or free T_4 in the upper half of the age-specific reference range.[70] If hypothyroidism is secondary, due to hypothalamic–pituitary dysfunction, treatment with adrenal corticosteroids and GH may be necessary as deficiencies of adrenocorticotropic hormone (ACTH) and GH could also be present.[71] Adrenal insufficiency may be manifested as failure to thrive and/or hypoglycemia in the neonatal period. GH deficiency may also contribute to hypoglycemia and may impair growth.[71]

ACQUIRED HYPOTHYROIDISM

Acquired hypothyroidism before age 5 to 6 years most commonly results from delayed failure of the thyroid remnant in infants with thyroid dysgenesis, but inborn defects in thyroid hormone synthesis, ingested goitrogens, chronic thyroiditis, or hypothalamic–pituitary disease may be involved. After 5 to 6 years of age, hypothyroidism is usually due to chronic lymphocytic thyroiditis. Surgery or radioiodine treatment also can result in hypothyroidism.[2]

Irreversible brain damage is not a likely result of hypothyroidism acquired after 2 to 3 years of age. By this time, CNS growth is largely complete. Delayed growth, however, may be marked and most commonly is manifest as delayed tooth development and eruption, delayed skeletal growth and maturation, and linear growth retardation. Aberrations in pubertal development and menstrual irregularities are common.[2] These manifestations are reversible with adequate replacement therapy. As in infants, the treatment of choice is oral Na-l-thyroxine. The replacement dose on a body weight basis decreases progressively with age (Table 57.3). The dosage should be adjusted at 2- to 4-month intervals to a level that maintains the serum-free T_4 concentration in the midrange of normal together with normal TSH concentrations. Initial administration of the total daily estimated replacement dose will result in a gradual increase in serum-free T_4 concentrations over a 3- to 4-week period. If cardiac disease is suspected, more gradual replacement may be indicated.

Treatment of secondary hypothyroidism in childhood or adolescence may require simultaneous replacement with adrenal corticosteroids, GH, and gonadal steroid(s). Hashimoto's thyroiditis is the most common cause of acquired hypothyroidism.[2] It is an autoimmune disease associated with progressive autoimmune damage to thyroid follicular cells. The disease most frequently involves only the thyroid gland. Occasionally, however, Hashimoto's thyroiditis is associated with other endocrine gland autoimmune deficiencies.[72,73] These include diabetes mellitus, adrenal insufficiency, hypoparathyroidism, or hypogonadism. Autoimmune gastritis with pernicious anemia and cutaneous moniliasis are sometimes associated. Treatment of these other endocrine gland deficiencies may be necessary.

Hashimoto's thyroiditis presents early as a mild-to-moderate euthyroid goiter. The disease remits spontaneously in about one-third of children,[2] while the remainder gradually develop hypothyroidism. One key to diagnose Hashimoto's thyroiditis is determining the presence of elevated antithyroid antibody titers, which include anti-Tg antibodies (anti-TgAbs) and/or antimicrosomal/antithyroid peroxidase antibodies (TPOAb). The presence of elevated TPOAb titers in patients with subclinical hypothyroidism helps predict progression to overt hypothyroidism, 4.3% per year with TPOAb versus 2.6% per year without elevated TPOAb titers.[74,75] In cases of euthyroidism with the presence of antibodies, treatment is not needed, but such patients should be followed up periodically.

NONTOXIC DIFFUSE GOITER

Nontoxic diffuse goiter in childhood is often referred to as simple colloid goiter.[2] It is most common during adolescence in female patients, where it has been referred to as adolescent goiter. These patients are euthyroid with mild-to-moderate goiters, characterized histologically by large thyroid follicles rimmed by flattened epithelial cells. The glands are usually diffusely enlarged and of nearly normal consistency, but nodularity can occur. The etiology is unclear, but some of these patients manifest multinodular goiter as adults.[76] The natural history is for spontaneous reduction with time, and treatment with thyroxine is not indicated. In a long-term study on 20-year follow-up, 60% of patients were normal, 20% were unchanged, and a few (10%) developed thyroiditis.[77]

THYROID NODULES

Suppressive therapy with T_4 is sometimes used to differentiate benign from malignant thyroid nodules. Diagnostic procedures usually include thyroid scanning and/or fine-needle biopsy (FNA).[2] In the occasional patient with an inconclusive biopsy result, a trial of suppressive T_4 therapy may be useful. In this instance, the end point is a decrease in size of the nodule or a failure of further growth over a period of 6 to 12 months. The dose of T_4 is adjusted to suppress serum TSH concentrations to the very low or undetectable level (<0.02 U per mL) using a highly sensitive TSH assay method. This may require T_4 doses 30% to 50% higher than replacement doses. T_3 is not usually used for suppression because the half-life of serum levels is relatively short, and T_4 provides more reliable TSH suppression.

ANTITHYROID DRUGS

Many compounds and chemicals have been shown to inhibit the synthesis and/or metabolism of thyroid hormones. The most important of these are the thioureylenes, the iodinated organic radiographic-contrast agents, iodide, and radioactive iodine (RAI).

THIOUREYLENES

Astwood and colleagues in the 1940s characterized a series of thioureylene drugs that inhibit thyroid hormone synthesis via a thiocarbamide group (S = C–N).[78] Several compounds have been utilized for the treatment of hyperthyroidism.[78] These include thiourea, thiouracil, methylthiouracil, PTU, methimazole (MMI), and carbimazole (CBI). The drugs currently used to treat hyperthyroidism include PTU, MMI, and CBI.[79] CBI acts by conversion to MMI. The thioureylene drugs act by inhibiting the organification of iodine via inhibition of thyroid peroxidase activity. Inhibition of hormone synthesis results in depletion of the thyroid stores of iodinated Tg and a progressive decrease in thyroid stores of iodinated Tg and a progressive decrease in thyroid hormone secretion from the thyroid gland. In addition to blocking hormone synthesis, PTU inhibits the peripheral conversion of T_4 to T_3; MMI does not share this action.[79] Effective amounts of the drugs are absorbed within 30 to 60 minutes after an oral dose. The half-life of PTU in plasma approximates 2 hours and that of MMI 6 to 13 hours. The drugs are concentrated within the thyroid, and metabolites are excreted largely in urine. They cross the placenta and appear in breast milk.

There is a significant incidence of toxic reaction to all thioureylene drugs.[79,80] The incidence of major and minor toxicities is summarized in Table 57.4. The most common minor reaction is a purpuric, papular rash, which is usually mild and subsides spontaneously. Other minor reactions include nausea, headache, paresthesias, hair loss, and joint pain and stiffness. Agranulocytosis, the most serious reaction, is observed in 1 in 500 to 1 in 1,000 cases. It usually develops during the first few months of treatment and may develop rapidly. Mild granulocytopenia may be due to thyrotoxicosis or may be an early sign of serious drug toxicity. Drug fever, hepatitis, nephritis, and a lupus-like reaction are rare complications. Antineutrophil cytoplasmic antibodies are relatively common in PTU-treated patients (4% to 46%), while the incidence of ANCA-associated vasculitis is much lower (0% to 1.4%).[80]

Should granulocytopenia be observed, frequent leukocyte counts are indicated to rule out serious drug toxicity. Routine blood counts are not helpful, since agranulocytosis can develop after several months and may appear rapidly. The U.S. Food and Drug Administration reports severe liver injury and acute renal failure in children and adults treated with PTU. They recommend reserving PTU for those who cannot tolerate other treatments, including MMI, RAI, or surgery.

IODIDE

Iodide is the oldest antithyroid drug. In large doses (>0.1 mg per kg per day), it inhibits thyroid iodide transport, iodothyronine synthesis, and thyroid hormone release.[79] As a result, there is a rapid fall in serum thyroid hormone levels that may persist several weeks. Eventually, there is an "escape" from the thyroid iodide blockade mediated in part by the inhibition of thyroid cell membrane iodide transport and a reduction in intrathyroidal iodide concentrations. Thus, iodide is usually restricted to short-term therapy (several weeks). Iodide treatment has been used in the immediate preoperative period to prepare patients for thyroidectomy and for the treatment of severe thyrotoxicosis or thyroid crisis in conjunction with thioureylene drugs.

Toxic reactions to iodide are observed occasionally.[79] Acute life-threatening angioedema and laryngeal edema may occur with or without a cutaneous hemorrhagic rash. Serum sickness–like manifestations have also been observed with fever, arthralgia, eosinophilia, and lymphadenopathy. Chronic intoxication (iodism) is also described, including soreness of the teeth and gums, increased salivation, nasal irritation, swelling of the eyes, headache, and chronic cough. Acneiform skin lesions, gastric irritation, and diarrhea may occur. These signs and symptoms disappear within a few days after discontinuing iodide ingestion.

Iodide preparations include strong iodine solution (Lugol solution) for oral use and sodium iodide for intravenous use. Lugol solution is formulated as 5% iodine and 10% potassium iodide. The iodine is reduced to iodide in the intestine before absorption. Intravenous NaI is available as a 10% solution.

RADIOACTIVE IODINE

There are several clinically useful isotopes of radioiodine.[81] These include I^{131}, I^{125}, and I^{123}. The half-lives are 8 days, 60 days, and 13 hours, respectively. Gamma ray–emitting isotopes are used for scanning, whereas β radiation is desirable for tissue radiation treatment. All three isotopes are γ emitters and are

TABLE 57.4 Characteristics of Commonly Used Thioureylene Drugs

				Toxic Reactions	
Drug	*Blood Half-Life (h)*	*Initial Dose (mg/kg/dose)*	*Maintenance Dose (mg/kg/d)*	*Major (%)*	*Minor (%)*
Propylthiouracil	2	5–8	1–3	0.9	2.2
Methimazole	6–13	0.5–0.7	0.1–0.3	1.4	4.5
Carbimazole	5	0.5–0.7	0.1–0.3	0.9	2.2

used for thyroid scanning. ^{125}I and ^{123}I are preferred because they provide lower thyroid radiation doses. I^{131} is used for treatment because of its β radiation; the average absorbed β dose per gram tissue is approximately 10 rad per day per Ci. Other isotopes of iodine are not in general clinical use.

TREATMENT OF HYPERTHYROIDISM

CHILDHOOD THYROTOXICOSIS

Hyperthyroidism in childhood is usually due to Graves' disease but can be secondary to Hashimoto's thyroiditis, hyperfunctioning thyroid nodule(s), or an activating mutation of the TSH receptor. Treatment of Graves' disease may be accomplished with antithyroid drugs, surgery, or radioiodine. Antithyroid drug treatment is considered the first-line treatment, with MMI being the drug of choice.[82]

The dose of MMI is 0.2 to 0.5 mg per kg per day, with a range of 0.1 to 1.0 mg per kg per day (maximal dose typically does not exceed 30 mg per day), but higher doses can be used for thyroid storm. The dose is increased if improvement is not observed within 2 to 3 weeks. MMI has longer half-life than PTU, and some patients will maintain effective blockade of thyroid hormone synthesis with once-daily drug administration, particularly after remission has been induced. PTU is reserved for children who are allergic to or who develop an adverse effect from MMI that necessitates drug discontinuation or when RAI or surgery is not a suitable option. PTU is still used for life-threatening thyroid storm, because of its ability to act rapidly and inhibit the peripheral conversion of T_4 to T_3, and in women in the first trimester of pregnancy due to the risk of embryopathy, including aplasia cutis, with use of methimazole.[83] The recommended PTU dosage is 5.7 mg per kg per day. After initiation of MMI therapy, thyroid function tests are generally repeated in 2 weeks and then monthly until values normalize. Once the patient becomes euthyroid, the dose of antithyroid medication is reduced by 50% or more. Depending on disease severity, thyroid function tests may not normalize for several months. After normalization of thyroid hormone concentrations, thyroid function tests should be monitored every 3 to 4 months. Measurements of serum T_3 concentration may be useful when the clinical assessment and serum T_4 measurements are in disagreement; on occasion, the antithyroid medication will be adequate to inhibit T_4, but not T_3 secretion, and the patient will appear euthyroid or even hyperthyroid, with low levels of serum T_4 and elevated serum T_3 concentrations. Measurements of thyroid-stimulating antibody levels are useful in predicting remission and are helpful in assessing drug-induced hypothyroidism.

β-Blockers, such as propranolol, are recommended for children who have palpitations and tremors and in those with tachycardia and/or hypertension, until thyroid hormone levels decline in response to the antithyroid drug therapy. Propranolol, at a dose of 0.5 to 2.0 mg per kg daily, is divided into three or four doses daily.[84] In patients with severe disease or distressing cardiovascular symptoms, propranolol can be increased to 4 to 6 mg per kg per day. β-Receptor blockade is potentially dangerous in patients with asthma, cardiac failure, or arrhythmias. Cardioselective β-blockers such as atenolol should be used in children with reactive airway disease at a dose of 1 to 2 mg per kg daily instead of propranolol.[83]

Potassium iodide in large doses potentiates the action of thioureylene drugs. Therapeutic doses for hyperthyroidism range from 2 to 4 mg per kg per day, usually given as strong iodine solution or a saturated solution of potassium iodide. The inhibitory effect on hormone synthesis and/or release usually persists 10 to 40 days. As indicated earlier, potassium iodide is most useful for short-term treatment of severe disease and for preoperative preparation of patients for surgery.

Two approaches to long-term treatment have been used: (a) continue adjusting the antithyroid drug dose to maintain a euthyroid state or (b) provide a blocking dose of drugs and treat the patient with exogenous T_4. The latter approach is not generally recommended because it has been shown to result in a higher rate of antithyroid medication side effects.[85] A patient is considered to be in remission if he or she has had a normal serum TSH, free T_4, and total T_3 for 1 year after discontinuation of antithyroid drug therapy. The reported remission rates vary considerably between geographical areas ranging from 20% to 68% from across the world.[86]

If drug toxicity ensues, the drug becomes ineffective either for patient or for pharmacologic reasons, or if the goiter is large and unresponsive to a reasonable drug treatment regimen, alternative treatment may be considered. Near-total thyroidectomy for Graves' disease in children is safe and effective when performed by experienced thyroid surgeons.[87,88] In addition to relief of systemic symptoms, the majority of patients presenting with Graves' ophthalmopathy experienced improvement of their ocular disease after operation. In 5% of patients, surgical management has allowed for detection and treatment of clinically occult thyroid malignancies. Total or near-total thyroidectomy is recommended for patients with large thyroid glands (100 g or larger).[87,88]

RAI therapy (I^{131}) is an effective alternative treatment for older children and adolescents with Graves' disease. It is not recommended in children younger than 5 years of age. It has been observed that the young thyroid gland may be particularly sensitive to radiation, raising the concern that young children might have an increased risk of thyroid cancer after radiation exposure.[86] Relatively higher doses of RAI (i.e., 200 to 300 μCi per g of thyroid tissue) are recommended now in pediatric population than previously used. For children between the ages of 5 and 10 years, the total dose should be limited to <10 mCi.[86,89] This dose leads to permanent resolution of the hyperthyroidism in a high percentage of patients. In addition, ablation of the gland will likely reduce the risk of future thyroid tumor development. This dose will lead to hypothyroidism in most patients, necessitating lifelong thyroid hormone replacement.

NEONATAL THYROTOXICOSIS

Neonatal Graves' disease is due to transplacental passage of a thyroid-stimulating hormone receptor antibody (TRAb) from a mother with active or inactive Graves' disease.[90,91] It is a rare condition, probably due to the low incidence of thyrotoxicosis in pregnancy (1 to 2 cases per 1,000 pregnancies) and the fact that the neonatal disease occurs in only about 1 in 70 cases of thyrotoxic pregnancy.[18,90,91] The usual clinical manifestations include irritability, flushing, tachycardia, hypertension, poor weight gain, thyroid enlargement, and exophthalmos. Thrombocytopenia, hepatosplenomegaly, jaundice, and hypoprothrombinemia have also been observed. Arrhythmias, cardiac failure, and death may occur if the thyrotoxicity is severe and the treatment is inadequate. Mortality approaches 25% in disease severe enough to be diagnosed.[18,87]

Current guidelines recommend TRAb determination early in pregnancy and during the second half of gestation, with close monitoring with fetal ultrasounds if TRAb levels exceed two to three times the upper limit of the normal range.[92,93] Fetal hyperthyroidism can be prevented by administering antithyroid medications to the mother. PTU (preferred during the first trimester) and methimazole cross the placenta and are equally effective for treating hyperthyroidism in pregnancy. Methimazole is the preferred medication period for infants with neonatal Graves' (0.5 to 1 mg per kg per day, depending on the initial severity of the disease, in three divided doses). Propranolol (2 mg per kg per day, in two divided doses) can also be used to control tachycardia during the first 1 to 2 weeks of treatment. The methimazole dose can be progressively titrated down based on the thyroid hormone levels. The disease is transient and may last from 1 to 3 months, until maternal TRAbs are infant's cleared from the infant.[94]

Rare cases of neonatal thyrotoxicosis have been reported due to an activating mutation of the TSH receptor.[18,95,96] Management with iodide and/or antithyroid drugs has been successful, but the thyrotoxicosis is not transient as is the case in neonatal Graves' disease. Long-term management experience is limited in such children, and surgery or radioiodine therapies must be eventually considered.

THYROTROPIN-DEPENDENT HYPERTHYROIDISM

Hyperthyroidism with diffuse goiter and elevated serum levels of TSH has been reported in some patients without pituitary enlargement.[2,97–99] These patients manifest a defect in the feedback control of T_3 on TSH release, such that a new set point is established with hypersecretion of TSH, hypersecretion of thyroid hormone, and mild-to-moderate tissue hyperthyroidism. The rare patients with activating mutations of the TSH receptor appear clinically similar but have suppressed serum TSH concentrations. In contrast to patients with TSH-secreting tumors, the TSH-α subunit is not elevated and the TSH response to TRH is augmented.

Treatment is difficult and not generally satisfactory. Thyroid ablation by surgery or radioiodine controls the hyperthyroidism but aggravates the TSH hypersecretion and increases the risk of development of a pituitary adenoma. Suppression of TSH by exogenous supraphysiologic doses of thyroid hormone may aggravate the hyperthyroidism. However, this approach has been at least partially successful,[97–99] and treatment with TETRAC has been proposed.[99] TRIAC is an experimental drug. Treatment with TRIAC has been employed in children and adults in a daily dose of 1.4 to 2.8 mg, but is not always efficacious. Dextrothyroxine, also an experimental drug, has been shown to be successful in some cases.[97] When these compounds fail, the dopaminergic agent bromocriptine or somatostatin (octreotide acetate) has been employed with variable effectiveness.[97,100]

SPORADIC TOXIC THYROID HYPERPLASIA

Toxic thyroid hyperplasia is a rare syndrome of childhood-onset hyperthyroidism caused by activating mutations of the thyrotropin receptor.[96] The mutations in the childhood-onset cases produce a milder phenotype than the more severe neonatal cases and tend to be sporadic rather than familial.[95,96] Diagnosis is based on elevated serum-free thyroxine with suppressed TSH levels in children with diffuse goiter. Management is similar to that in children with Graves' disease.

AUTONOMOUS TOXIC ADENOMAS

Autonomous functioning thyroid nodules are uncommon in childhood and adolescence. Rarely, single or multiple autonomously functioning nodules may be associated with clinical hyperthyroidism.[101–105] The major causes of toxic thyroid nodules are activating mutations of the thyrotropin receptor or the intracellular-linked Gsα protein. Such nodules are true follicular adenomas and nearly always benign; the incidence of thyroid carcinoma in functioning nodules is less than 1%. It is generally felt that function in a thyroid nodule essentially excludes a diagnosis of thyroid carcinoma. Small functional nodules usually do not produce clinical thyrotoxicosis; large nodules (>3 cm diameter) are more likely to do so. Nodular autonomy is usually discerned by thyroid radioiodine scan and confirmed if the serum TSH concentration measured by a highly sensitive TSH method is suppressed and/or is unresponsive to TRH stimulation.[102,103]

The natural history of functioning thyroid nodules in the individual patient is variable. Such patients, if euthyroid, will usually remain euthyroid, but there may be a gradual increase in thyroid hormone production with development of clinical evidence of hyperthyroidism. Nodule enlargement or thyrotoxic symptoms may create the need for ablative therapy. Functioning nodules producing clinical and chemical thyrotoxicosis require surgical removal. Radioiodine treatment now tends to be reserved for older patients (>40 years of age). Antithyroid drug therapy is considered only for short-term management.

THYROID NODULES AND CANCER

THYROID NODULES

Thyroid nodules in children are significant for three reasons: they may herald underlying thyroid disease, they may be hyperfunctioning nodules and produce hyperthyroidism, or they may represent carcinoma.[2,104] In the first instance, the approach is to address the basic disease, often Hashimoto's thyroiditis. Functioning nodules producing clinical and chemical thyrotoxicosis require treatment, as indicated in the previous section. Thyroid nodules are more likely to be malignant in children than adults referred for evaluation of nodular thyroid disease (22% to 26% vs. ~5%).[106–108] Childhood cancer survivors who were treated for their primary malignancy with radiation therapy, especially survivors of Hodgkin lymphoma, leukemia, and CNS tumors, are at high risk of developing thyroid nodule.[109,110]

Thyroid carcinoma is the most common endocrine-related cancer in children, which typically presents with a nodule. Papillary thyroid cancer (PTC) accounts for 90% or more of all childhood thyroid malignancy.[111] It tends to be bilateral and multifocal with metastasis to the neck lymph nodes. Follicular thyroid cancer (FTC) is uncommon. This type of cancer tends to be unifocal and tends to metastasize via blood to the lungs and bones. Medullary thyroid cancer (MTC), poorly differentiated tumors, and undifferentiated (anaplastic) thyroid carcinomas are rare in young patients.

For evaluation, ultrasound characteristics and clinical context should be used to identify nodules that warrant FNA. Ultrasound features such as hypoechogenicity, irregular margins, and increased intranodular blood flow are more common in malignant lesions. In addition, the presence of microcalcifications and abnormal cervical lymph nodes increase the likelihood of malignancy.[112,113] All FNA in children should be performed under ultrasound guidance.[114]

The Bethesda classification system is used to report thyroid cytopathology risk based on FNA sample result. The result is usually reported as malignant, indeterminate/suspicious, inadequate/nondiagnostic, or benign. The treatment for thyroid cancer varies depending on the type of cancer and localization/extension. Surgery is indicated if the FNA report indicates a malignant or suspicious lesion. Many consider that surgery is also indicated for a prior history of therapeutic radiation to the head or neck, a hard nodule, evidence of tracheal invasion (dysphagia, hoarseness, or cough), vocal cord paralysis, adjacent lymph node involvement, or distant metastases.

LEVOTHYROXINE SUPPRESSION FOR BENIGN NODULES

Levothyroxine (LT_4) suppression therapy has been evaluated for its efficacy to reduce nodule size or to reduce the risk of subsequent nodule formation. However, there are only minimal data regarding long-term safety and potential side effects of LT_4 therapy.[115,116] LT_4 therapy has been prescribed to reduce the size of benign thyroid nodules, but the clinical benefit of a small to modest reduction in size is not clear.[117]

MANAGEMENT OF PAPILLARY THYROID CANCER

For the majority of children with PTC, total thyroidectomy is recommended. A surgeon who performs at least 30 or more cervical endocrine procedures annually should ideally perform the surgery. A comprehensive neck ultrasound to evaluate all regions of the neck is required prior to surgery in order to optimize the preoperative surgical plan. Prophylactic central neck dissection should be done. Lateral neck dissection is recommended in cases of cytology-proven metastasis. Routine prophylactic lateral neck dissection is not recommended. Imaging by magnetic resonance imaging (MRI) or computed tomography (CT) with contrast should be considered in patients with large or fixed thyroid masses, vocal cord paralysis, or bulky metastatic lymphadenopathy in order to optimize surgical planning. Iodine 131 (I^{131}) therapy is indicated for the treatment of iodine-avid persistent locoregional or nodal disease that cannot be resected as well as for iodine-avid distant metastases.[114]

Iodine I^{131} ablation is used in some cases depending on the risk level, as defined by the American Thyroid Association (ATA). On those cases, which are postsurgery and on thyroid hormone replacement, the thyroid hormone replacement should be stop for 2 to 3 weeks prior to the iodine administration for better absorption.

Following surgery or surgery plus radioiodine, the patient is maintained on full suppression doses of exogenous LT_4 to suppress endogenous TSH. Metastatic tumor growth is assessed by serial measurements of circulating TSH-stimulated Tg. Recurrences are usually managed with repeat surgery or I^{131} treatment depending on individual patient risks and the presence or absence of distant metastases.[114]

FOLLICULAR CARCINOMA

Follicular thyroid cancer is rare in children, representing about 5% to 10% of all pediatric thyroid cancer diagnoses. The major histopathologic variants of FTC are the oncocytic (Hürthle cell) and clear cell variants. Depending on the extent of invasion, FTC is currently subdivided into two major groups: minimally invasive FTC and widely invasive FTC. Therapeutic approach is similar to papillary thyroid cancer. Prognosis for most patients is good.[118]

MEDULLARY CARCINOMA

MTC represents neoplasia of the parafollicular “C” cells and is associated with excessive secretion of calcitonin.[2,104,119] Other secretory products can include ACTH, MSH, histaminase, serotonin, prostaglandins, SRIF, and endorphin. MTC represents 4% to 10% of all malignant thyroid neoplasia: 75% of cases are sporadic and 25% familial. The prognosis is generally guarded because lymph node involvement occurs early, even when the tumor is small. Sporadic cases appear as a noniodide-concentrating (cold) thyroid nodule; the diagnosis is confirmed or suspected on the basis of needle biopsy or open biopsy. Thyroidectomy is the only current approach to treatment of medullary carcinoma, since “C” cells do not concentrate radioiodine.

Prior to 1987, the only available test for early detection of MTC in genetically at-risk patients was measurement of serum calcitonin with or without stimulation. Since then, DNA diagnosis has become the procedure of choice.[2,100,119] Identification of an activating germline mutation in the RET proto-oncogene indicates that the affected individual has a greater than 90% probability of developing MTC. The optimal treatment in children at genetic risk with *RET* gene mutation is early thyroidectomy before malignant transformation occurs.[2,100,119] There is now a large experience correlating RET mutations with MTC aggressiveness, and high-risk mutations are ranked 1 to 3, with 3 being highest risk. It is now recommended that children with the highest risk mutations undergo prophylactic thyroidectomy before 6 months of age. Thyroidectomy before 5 years of age for level 2 risk patients and at 5 to 10 years of age for level 1 risk patients is recommended.[2,100]

It is not possible to determine a priori whether an individual with apparent sporadic MTC has hereditary or sporadic disease. Available information indicates that 6% to 7% of apparent sporadic MTC patients have germline mutations of the RET proto-oncogene. It is important to identify these individuals so that screening can be provided to other family members. For this reason, it is now recommended by the American Society of Clinical Oncology and the National Comprehensive Cancer Network as well as ATA that all patients with apparently sporadic MTC be tested for germline *RET* gene mutations.[120]

THYROTROPIN-RELEASING HORMONE

TRH is the first hypothalamic peptide characterized and synthesized nearly simultaneously by Guillemin and Schally.[121,122] It is a tripeptide (pyroglutamyl-histidyl-proline amide) secreted by the hypothalamus into the hypothalamic–pituitary portal vascular system to stimulate TSH release from anterior pituitary thyrotroph cells. TRH acts on these cells via a specific plasma membrane receptor. TRH stimulates prolactin release and, in selected circumstances, can evoke GH release.[123] TRH is also present in extrahypothalamic brain tissue and in extraneural tissues, such as the pancreas. TRH is synthesized as a 225-amino-acid precursor (prepro-TRH) containing five TRH progenitor sequences.[124] Processing of prepro-TRH results in cleavage of several larger peptides as well as TRH.[125] The significance of these is not clear. TRH is metabolized via a pyroglutamyl amino peptidase to a cyclized metabolite, histidyl-proline diketopiperazine or cyclo.[126] Cyclo[126] is also widely distributed in brain tissue and appears to have unique bioactivities different from TRH. TRH is also deaminated, and the free acid may have bioactivity.[123]

The major bioactivity of TRH is the modulation, with T_3, of TSH release. TRH as the synthetic tripeptide is commercially available as a sterile, lyophilized powder (500-µg vials). The plasma half-life is very short (several minutes). The minimal intravenous dose required to evoke an increase in serum TSH is about 0.2 µg (200 ng) per kg. The TSH response increases progressively with increasing dose to plateau at 5 to 6 µg per kg. The peak rise in serum TSH is seen within 15 to 30 minutes; a secondary increase in serum T_3 levels occurs within 90 to 150 minutes.[123] TRH is also active orally, but doses 20 to 40 times greater are required.

THYROTROPIN-RELEASING HORMONE TESTING

TRH, though not currently available, was used for testing pituitary TSH reserve. An intravenous dose of TRH (7 µg per kg) is injected, and measurements of serum TSH are usually conducted at 30 to 60 minutes. The TSH response, in general, is proportional to the basal TSH level. Thus, patients with primary hypothyroidism have augmented responses. Patients with hyperthyroidism have inhibited responses. The test has been utilized (a) to confirm a diagnosis of thyrotoxicosis in patients with borderline serum T_4 and T_3 concentrations (an absent TSH response to TRH supports a diagnosis of hyperthyroidism) and (b) to differentiate hypothalamic and pituitary etiologies for TSH deficiency in patients with hypothyroidism and low TSH levels.[71] A normal TSH response to TRH indicates normal pituitary TSH secretory capacity and implies a hypothalamic TRH deficiency. An absent TSH response supports a diagnosis of pituitary TSH deficiency. Measurements of serum T_3 before and after 4 hours of TRH administration provide information regarding thyroid gland responsiveness. TRH has been injected intravenously in pregnant women to stimulate fetal thyroid function near term.[127] A dose of 400 µg induced a marked increase in cord blood TSH within 20 minutes and evoked significant increases in cord blood T_4 and T_3 levels as well.

THYROTROPIN

Thyrotropin (TSH) is a 28- to 30-kD glycoprotein synthesized in the pituitary gland in response to TRH stimulation.[128] It is a member of the glycoprotein hormone family, which includes FSH, luteinizing hormone, and hCG. All consist of a common α subunit and a unique β subunit. The α subunits are composed of 92 amino acids. Recombinant human TSH is now available for clinical use to stimulate thyroid cell function for diagnostic and therapeutic purposes[128,129] (Table 57.5). Recombinant human TSH (Thyrogen®, Genzyme Inc., Cambridge, MA) has replaced sterile, lyophilized TSH from animal sources for human use. It is available as a sterile, lyophilized product in kit form (two 1.1-mg vials, and two 10-mL vials of sterile water for injection). The usual dosage is 0.9 mg intramuscularly every 24 hours for two doses or every 72 hours for three doses (1.1 mg is reconstituted in 1.2-mL sterile water: 1-mL solution contains 0.9 mg TSH).

TABLE 57.5 Clinical Applications of Recombinant Human TSH

Clinical Use	*Diagnostic or Therapeutic Purpose*
TSH stimulation test	Testing thyroid reserve Confirming diagnosis of thyroid hemiagenesis Identifying "warm" thyroid nodules
Differentiated thyroid cancer management	Stimulation of thyroglobulin secretion to identify residual thyroid tissue Stimulation of radioiodine uptake in residual thyroid tissue prior to whole-body scanning Stimulation of remnant thyroid tissue iodide uptake prior to therapeutic dosing with radioiodine

TSH, thyroid-stimulating hormone.

REFERENCES

1. Larsen PR, Davies TF, Schlumberger MJ, et al. Thyroid physiology and diagnostic evaluation of patients with thyroid disorders. In: Larsen PR, Kronenberg HM, Melmed M, Polonsky KS, eds. *Williams textbook of endocrinology*, 11th ed. Philadelphia, PA: Saunders Elsevier, 2008:299–332.
2. Fisher DA, Grueters A, eds. *Pediatric endocrinology*, 3rd ed. Philadelphia, PA: Saunders Elsevier, 2008:227–253.
3. Hollenberg AN. Regulation of thyrotropin secretion. In: Braverman LE, Utiger RD, eds. *The thyroid, a fundamental and clinical text*, 9th ed. Philadelphia, PA: Lippincott Williams & Wilkins, 2005:197–213.
4. De Nayer PH, Cornette C, Vanderschueren M, et al. Serum thyroglobulin levels in preterm neonates. *Clin Endocrinol (Oxf)* 1984;321:148–153.
5. Benvenga S. Thyroid hormone transport proteins and the physiology of protein binding. In: Braverman LE, Utiger RD, eds. *The thyroid, a fundamental and clinical text*, 9th ed. Philadelphia, PA: Lippincott Williams & Wilkins, 2005:97–108.
6. De Stefano JJ, Bray GA, eds. *The thyroid, physiology and treatment of disease*. Oxford, UK: Pergamon Press, 1979:47–82.
7. Wu SY, Green WL, Huang WS, et al. Alternate pathways of thyroid hormone metabolism. *Thyroid* 2005;15:943–958.
8. St. Germain DL. Thyroid hormone metabolism. In: DeGroot LJ, Jameson JL, eds. *Endocrinology*, 5th ed. Philadelphia, PA: Elsevier Saunders, 2005:1861–1871.
9. Mousa SA, Bergh J, Dier E, et al. Tetraiodothyroacetic acid, a small molecule integrin ligand, blocks angiogenesis induced by vascular endothelial growth factor and basic fibroblast growth factor. *Angiogenesis* 2008;11:183–190.
10. Doyle KO, Suchland KL, Ciesielski TMP, et al. Novel thyroxine derivatives, thionamine and 3-iodothyronamine, induce transient hypothermia and marked neuroprotection against stroke injury. *Stroke* 2007;38:2569–2576.
11. Braulke LJ, Klingenspor M, DeBarber A, et al. 3-Iodothyronamine: a novel hormone controlling the balance between glucose and lipid utilization. *J Comp Physiol B* 2008;178:167–177.
12. Geraci T, Field C, Colasurdo V, et al. 3-iodothyronamine (T1AM) levels in human serum and tissues. Program at the American Thyroid Association Meeting; October 1–5, 2008; Chicago, IL: 126.
13. Chiellini G, Bellusci L, Sabatini M, et al. Thyronamines and analogues—the route from rediscovery to translational research on thyronergic amines. *Mol Cell Endocrinol.* 2017;458:149–155.
14. Forrest D, Golarai G, Connor J, et al. Genetic analysis of thyroid hormone receptors in development and disease. *Recent Prog Horm Res* 1996;51:1–22.
15. Brown RS, Huang S, Fisher DA. The maturation of thyroid function in the perinatal period and during childhood. In: Braverman LE, Utiger RD, eds. *The thyroid, a fundamental and clinical text*, 9th ed. Philadelphia, PA: Lippincott Williams & Wilkins, 2005:1013–1028.
16. Yen PM. Genomic and nongenomic actions of thyroid hormones. In: Braverman LE, Utiger RD, eds. *The thyroid, a fundamental and clinical text*, 9th ed. Philadelphia, PA: Lippincott Williams & Wilkins, 2005:135–150.
17. Munoz A, Bernal J. Biological activities of thyroid hormone receptors. *Eur J Endocrinol* 1997;137:433–445.
18. Fisher DA, Grueters A, eds. *Pediatric endocrinology*, 3rd ed. Philadelphia, PA: Elsevier Saunders, 2008:198–226.
19. Silva JE, Rabelo R. Regulation of the uncoupling gene expression. *Eur J Endocrinol* 1997;136:251–264.

20. Gong DW, He Y, Karas M, et al. Uncoupling protein-3 is a mediator of thermogenesis regulated by thyroid hormone, β3 adrenergic agonists, and leptin. *J Biol Chem* 1997;272:24129–24132.
21. Glasscock GF, Nicoll CS. Hormonal control of growth in the neonatal rat. *Endocrinology* 1981;109:176–184.
22. Snyder PJ. The pituitary in hypothyroidism. In: Braverman LE, Utiger RD, eds. *The thyroid*, Philadelphia, PA: Lippincott-Raven, 1995:836–840.
23. Meill J, Taylor A, Zini M, et al. Effects of hypothyroidism and hyperthyroidism on insulin-like growth factors (IGFs) and growth hormone and IGF binding proteins. *J Clin Endocrinol Metab* 1993;76:950–955.
24. Chernausek SD, Turner R. Attenuation of spontaneous nocturnal growth hormone secretion in children with hypothyroidism and its correlation with plasma insulin-like growth factor-I concentrations. *J Pediatr* 1989;114:968–972.
25. Britto J, Fenton A, Holloway W, et al. Osteoblasts mediate thyroid hormone stimulation of osteoclastic bone resorption. *Endocrinology* 1994;134:169–176.
26. Huang SM, Chan SH, Wu TJ, et al. Effect of thyroid hormone on urinary excretion of epidermal growth factor. *Eur Surg Res* 1997;29:222–228.
27. Fisher DA. Growth and development of hypothyroid infants. In: Stabler B, Bercu BB, eds. *Therapeutic outcome of endocrine disorders*, New York, NY: Springer Verlag, 2000:221–234.
28. Bucher H, Prader A, Illig R. Head circumference, height, bone age and weight in 103 children with congenital hypothyroidism before and during thyroid hormone replacement. *Helv Paediatr Acta* 1985;30:305–316.
29. Aronson R, Ehrlich R, Bailey JD, et al. Growth in children with congenital hypothyroidism detected by neonatal screening. *J Pediatr* 1990;116:33–37.
30. Heyerdahl S, Kase B, Stake G. Skeletal maturation during thyroxine treatment in children with congenital hypothyroidism. *Acta Paediatr* 1994;83:618–622.
31. Chiesa A, de Papendieck LG, Keselman A, et al. Growth follow-up in 100 children with congenital hypothyroidism before and during treatment. *J Pediatr Endocrinol* 1994;7:211–217.
32. Leger J, Ruiz JC, Guibourdenche J, et al. Bone mineral density and metabolism in children with congenital hypothyroidism after prolonged L-thyroxine therapy. *Acta Paediatr* 1997;86:704–710.
33. Boersma B, Otten BJ, Stoelings GBA, et al. Catch-up growth after prolonged hypothyroidism. *Eur J Pediatr* 1996;155:362–367.
34. Haddow JE, Palomaki G, Allan WC, et al. Maternal thyroid deficiency during pregnancy and subsequent neuropsychological development of the child. *N Engl J Med* 1999;341:549–555.
35. Glinoer D, Delange F. The potential repercussions of maternal, fetal, and neonatal hypothyroxinemia on the progeny. *Thyroid* 2000;10:871–887.
36. Sato T, Suzuki Y, Taetani T, et al. Age related change in the pituitary threshold for TSH release during thyroxine replacement therapy for cretinism. *J Clin Endocrinol Metab* 1977;44:553–559.
37. Dobbing J. The later growth of the brain and its vulnerability. *Pediatrics* 1974;53:2–6.
38. Bongers-Schokking JJ, Koot HM, Wiersma D, et al. Influence of timing and dose of thyroid hormone replacement on development of infants with congenital hypothyroidism. *J Pediatr* 2000;136:292–297.
39. Derksen-Lubsen G, Verkerk PH. Neuropsychological development in early treated congenital hypothyroidism: analysis of literature data. *Pediatr Res* 1996;39:561–566.
40. Price DA, Ehrlich RM, Walfish PG. Congenital hypothyroidism, clinical and laboratory characteristics of infants detected by neonatal screening. *Arch Dis Child* 1981;56:845–851.
41. Letarte J, LaFranchi S, Dussault JH, eds. *Congenital hypothyroidism*, New York: Marcel Dekker, 1983:351–383.
42. Fisher DA, Polk DH, Wu SY. Fetal thyroid metabolism: a pluralistic system. *Thyroid* 1984;4:367–371.
43. Chattopadhyay A, Kumar V, Marulaiah M. Polycystic ovaries, precocious puberty and acquired hypothyroidism: the Van Wyk and Grumbach syndrome. *J Pediatr Surg* 2003;38:1390–1392.
44. Anasti JN, Flack MR, Frochlich J, et al. A potential novel mechanism for precocious puberty in juvenile hypothyroidism. *J Clin Endocrinol Metab* 1995;80:276–279.
45. Hemady ZS, Siler-Khodr TM, Najjar S. Precocious puberty in juvenile hypothyroidism. *Pediatrics* 1978;92:55–59.
46. Rodien P, Bremonte C, Sanson MLR, et al. Familial gestational hyperthyroidism caused by a mutant thyrotropin receptor hypersensitive to human chorionic gonadotropin. *N Engl J Med* 2008;339:1823–1826.
47. Montanelli M, Delbaere A, Di Carlo C, et al. A mutation in the follicle-stimulating hormone receptor as a cause of familial spontaneous ovarian hyperstimulation syndrome. *J Clin Endocrinol Metab* 2004;89:1255–1258.
48. Van Wyk JJ, Grumbach MM. Syndrome of precocious menstruation and galactorrhoea in juvenile hypothyroidism: an example of hormonal overlap in pituitary feedback. *J Pediatr* 1960;57:416–435.
49. Reilly WA, Smyth FS. Cretinoid epiphyseal dysgenesis. *J Pediatr* 1937;11:786–796.
50. Delange F, Becker G, Caron P, et al. Thyroid volume and urinary iodine in European school children: standardization of values for assessment of iodine deficiency. *Eur J Endocrinol* 1997;136:180–187.
51. Chanoine JP, Toppet V, Lagasse R, et al. Determination of thyroid volume by ultrasound from the neonatal period to late adolescence. *Eur J Pediatr* 1991;150:395–399.
52. Fisher DA, Oddie TH, Wait JC. Thyroid function tests: findings in Arkansas children and young adults. *Am J Dis Child* 1964;107:282–287.
53. Ponchon G, Beckers C, DeVisscher M. Iodine kinetic studies in newborns and infants. *J Clin Endocrinol Metab* 1966;21:1392–1394.
54. Beckers C, Malvaux P, De Visscher M. Quantitative aspects of the secretion and degradation of thyroid hormones during adolescence. *J Clin Endocrinol Metab* 1966;26:202–206.
55. Ingenbleek Y, Bernstein LH. Plasma transthyretin as a biomarker of lean body mass and catabolic states. *Adv Nutr* 2015;6(5):572–580.
56. Delange F, Fisher DA, eds. *Clinical paediatric endocrinology*, 3rd ed. Oxford, UK: Blackwell Science, 1995:397–433.
57. Nelson JC, Clark SJ, Borot DL, et al. Age related changes in serum free thyroxine, during childhood and adolescence. *J Pediatr* 1993;125:899–905.
58. Fisher DA, Sack J, Oddie TH, et al. Serum T4, TBG, T3 uptake, T3, reverse T3 and TSH concentrations in children 1 to 15 years of age. *J Clin Endocrinol Metab* 1977;45:191–198.
59. Fish LH, Schwartz HL, Cavanaugh J, et al. Replacement dose, metabolism and availability of levothyroxine in the treatment of hypothyroidism. *N Engl J Med* 1987;316:764–770.
60. Bunevicius R, Kazanavicius G, Zalinkevicius R, et al. Effects of thyroxine as compared with thyroxine plus triiodothyronine in patients with hypothyroidism. *N Engl J Med* 1999;340:424–429.
61. Escobar-Morreale HF, del Ray F, Obregon MJ, et al. Only the combined treatment with thyroxine and triiodothyronine ensures euthyroidism in all tissues of the thyroidectomized rat. *Endocrinology* 1996;137:2490–2502.
62. Eisenberg M, Samuels M, Distefano JJ. Extension, validation, and clinical applications of a feedback control system simulation of the hypothalamic–pituitary thyroid axis. *Thyroid* 2008;18:1071–1085.
63. Fisher DA, Schoen EJ, LaFranchi S, et al. The hypothalamic–pituitary–thyroid negative feedback control axis in children with treated congenital hypothyroidism. *J Clin Endocrinol Metab* 2000;85:2722–2727.
64. Selva KA, Mandel SH, Rien L, et al. Initial treatment dose of L-thyroxine in congenital hypothyroidism. *J Pediatr* 2002;141:786–792.
65. Crantz FR, Silva JE, Larsen PR. An analysis of the sources and quantity of 3,5,3′ triiodothyronine specifically bound to nuclear receptors in rat cerebral cortex and cerebellum. *Endocrinology* 1982;110:367–375.
66. Morreale De Escobar G, Obregon MJ, Ruiz De Ono C, et al. Transfer of thyroxine from the mother to the rat fetus near term: effects on brain 3,5,3′-triiodothyronine deficiency. *Endocrinology* 1988;122:1521–1531.
67. Daneman D, Howard NJ. Neonatal thyrotoxicosis, intellectual impairment and craniosynostosis in later years. *J Pediatr* 1980;97:257–259.
68. Penfold JL, Simpson DA. Premature craniosynostosis, a complication of thyroid replacement therapy. *J Pediatr* 1975;86:360–363.
69. McCrossin RB, Sheffield LJ, Robertson EF. Persisting abnormality in the pituitary–thyroid axis in congenital hypothyroidism. In: Nagataki S, Stockigt JHR, eds. *Thyroid research VIII*. Canberra, Australia: Australian Academy of Sciences, 1980:37–40.
70. Leger J, Olivieri A, Donaldson M, et al. European Society for Paediatric Endocrinology consensus guidelines on screening, diagnosis, and management of congenital hypothyroidism. *Horm Res Paediatr* 2014;81(2):80–103.
71. Van Tijn DA, de Vijlder JJM, Vulsma T. Role of thyrotropin releasing hormone stimulation test in diagnosis of congenital central hypothyroidism in infants. *J Clin Endocrinol Metab* 2008;93:410–419.
72. Weetman AP. Autoimmune thyroid disease. In: DeGroot LJ, Jameson JL, eds. *Endocrinology*, 5th ed. Philadelphia, PA: Elsevier Saunders, 2005:1979–1993.
73. Brent GA, Larsen P, Davies TE. Hypothyroidism and thyroiditis, In: Kronenberg HM, Melmed S, Polonsky KS, et al, eds. *Williams textbook of endocrinology*, 11th ed. Philadelphia, PA: Elsevier Saunders, 2008:377–409.
74. Vanderpump MP, Tunbridge WM, French JM, et al. The incidence of thyroid disorders in the community: a twenty-year follow-up of the Whickham Survey. *Clin Endocrinol (Oxf)*. 1995;43(1):55–68.
75. Huber G, Staub JJ, Meier C, et al. Prospective study of the spontaneous course of subclinical hypothyroidism: prognostic value of thyrotropin, thyroid reserve, and thyroid antibodies. *J Clin Endocrinol Metab* 2002;87(7):3221–3226.
76. Tajtakova M, Langer P, Gonsornikova V, et al. Recognition of a subgroup of adolescents with rapidly growing thyroids under iodine replete conditions: seven year follow-up. *Eur J Endocrinol* 1998;138:674–680.
77. Rallison ML, Dobyns BM, Keating FR, et al. Occurrence and natural history of chronic lymphocytic thyroiditis in childhood. *J Pediatr* 1975;86(5):675–682.
78. Astwood EB, Bissell A, Hughes AM. Further studies on the chemical nature of compounds which inhibit the function of the thyroid gland. *Endocrinology* 1945;37:456–481.
79. Farwell AP, Braverman LE, Limberg LE, eds. *Goodman and Gilman's the pharmacological basis of therapeutics*, 10th ed. New York, NY: McGraw Hill, 2001:1563–1596.
80. Panamonta O, Sumethkul V, Radinahmed P, et al. Propylthiouracil associated antineutrophil cytoplasmic antibodies in patients with childhood onset Graves' disease. *J Pediatr Endocrinol Metab* 2008;21:539–543.
81. Links JM. Radiation physics. In: Braverman LE, Utiger RD, eds. *The thyroid*, 8th ed. New York, NY: JB Lippincott, 2000:333–344.
82. Bansal S, Umpaichitra V, Desai N, PerezColon S. Pediatric Graves' disease. *Int J Endocr Metab Disord* 2015;1(1).
83. Srinivasan S, Misra M. Hyperthyroidism in children. *Pediatr Rev* 2015;36(6):239–248.
84. Birrell G, Cheetham T. Juvenile thyrotoxicosis; can we do better? *Arch Dis Child* 2004;89(8):745–750.
85. Cooper DS. Antithyroid drugs. *N Engl J Med* 2005;352(9):905–917.
86. Ross DS, Burch HB, Cooper DS, et al. American Thyroid Association guidelines for diagnosis and management of hyperthyroidism and other causes of thyrotoxicosis. *Thyroid* 2016;26(10):1343–1421.
87. Rivkees SA. Hypothyroidism and hyperthyroidism in children. In: Pescovitz OH, Eugster E, eds. *Pediatric endocrinology*, Philadelphia, PA: Lippincott Williams & Wilkins, 2004:508–521.
88. Sherman J, Thompson GB, Lteif A, et al. Surgical management of Graves' disease in childhood and adolescence: an institutional experience. *Surgery* 2006;140:1056–1062.
89. Rivkees SA, Dinauer C. An optimal treatment for pediatric Graves' disease is radioiodine. *J Clin Endocrinol Metab* 2007;92(3):797–800.
90. Zakarija M, McKenzie JM, Hoffman WH. Prediction and therapy of intrauterine and late onset neonatal hyperthyroidism. *J Clin Endocr Metab* 1986;62:368–371.
91. Smallridge RC, Wartofsky L, Chopra IJ, et al. Neonatal thyrotoxicosis: alterations in serum concentrations of LATS protector, T4, T3, reverse T3 and 3,3′ T2. *J Pediatr* 1978;93:118–120.

92. De Groot L, Abalovich M, Alexander EK, et al. Management of thyroid dysfunction during pregnancy and postpartum: an Endocrine Society clinical practice guideline. *J Clin Endocrinol Metab* 2012;97(8):2543–2565.
93. Luton D, Le Gac I, Vuillard E, et al. Management of Graves' disease during pregnancy: the key role of fetal thyroid gland monitoring. *J Clin Endocrinol Metab* 2005;90(11):6093–6098.
94. Leger J. Management of fetal and neonatal Graves' disease. *Horm Res Paediatr* 2017;87(1):1–6.
95. Gruters A, Schoneberg T, Biebermann H, et al. Severe congenital hyperthyroidism caused by a germ-line neo mutation in the extracellular portion of the thyrotropin receptor. *J Clin Endocrinol Metab* 1998;83:1431–1436.
96. Vassart G. Thyroid stimulating hormone receptor mutations. In: DeGroot LJ, Jameson JL, eds. *Endocrinology*, 5th ed. Philadelphia, PA: Elsevier Saunders, 2005:2191–2199.
97. Gurnell M, Beck-Peccoz P, Chatterjee VK. Resistance to thyroid hormone. In: DeGroot LJ, Jameson LJ, eds. *Endocrinology*, 5th ed. Philadelphia, PA: Elsevier Saunders, 2005:2227–2238.
98. Rosler A, Litvin Y, Hoge C, et al. Familial hyperthyroidism due to inappropriate thyrotropin secretion successfully treated with triiodothyronine. *J Clin Endocr Metab* 1982;54:76–82.
99. Beck-Peccoz P, Piscitelli G, Cattaneo MG, et al. Successful treatment of hyperthyroidism due to non-neoplastic pituitary TSH secretion with 3,5,3′-triiodothyroacetic acid (TRIAC). *J Endocrinol Invest* 1983;6:217–223.
100. Isales CM, Tamborlane W, Gertner JM, et al. Effect of short-term somatostatin and long-term triiodothyronine administration to a child with nontumorous inappropriate thyrotropin secretion. *Pediatrics* 1988;112:51–57.
101. Bauer AJ, Tuttle RM, Francis GL. Thyroid nodules and thyroid cancer in children and adolescents. In: Pescovitz OH, Eugster EA, eds. *Pediatric endocrinology*, Philadelphia, PA: Lippincott Williams & Wilkins, 2004:522–547.
102. Abe K, Konno M, Sato T, et al. Hyperfunctioning thyroid nodules in children. *Am J Dis Child* 1980;134:961–963.
103. Osbourne RC, Goren E, Bybee DE, et al. Autonomous thyroid nodules in adolescents: clinical characteristics and results of TRH testing. *J Pediatr* 1982;100:383–386.
104. Pacini F, DeGroot LJ, Jameson JL, eds. *Endocrinology*, 5th ed. Philadelphia, PA: WB Saunders, 2005:2147–2180.
105. Schlumberger MJ, Filetti S, Hay ID. Nontoxic diffuse and nodular goiter and thyroid neoplasia. In: Kronenberg HM, Melmed S, Polonsky KS, et al, eds. *Williams textbook of endocrinology*, 11th ed. Philadelphia, PA: Elsevier Saunders, 2008:441–442.
106. Gupta A, Ly S, Castroneves LA, et al. A standardized assessment of thyroid nodules in children confirms higher cancer prevalence than in adults. *J Clin Endocrinol Metab* 2013;98(8):3238–3245.
107. Niedźiela M. Pathogenesis, diagnosis and management of thyroid nodules in children. *Endocr Relat Cancer* 2006;13(2):427–453.
108. Gharib H, Papini E, Garber JR, et al. American Association of Clinical Endocrinologists, American College of Endocrinology, and Associazione Medici Endocrinologi Medical guidelines for clinical practice for the diagnosis and management of thyroid nodules—2016 update. *Endocr Pract* 2016;22(5):622–639.
109. Sklar C, Whitton J, Mertens A, et al. Abnormalities of the thyroid in survivors of Hodgkin's disease: data from the Childhood Cancer Survivor Study. *J Clin Endocrinol Metab* 2000;85(9):3227–3232.
110. Meadows AT, Friedman DL, Neglia JP, et al. Second neoplasms in survivors of childhood cancer: findings from the Childhood Cancer Survivor Study cohort. *J Clin Oncol* 2009;27(14):2356–2362.
111. Halac I, Zimmerman D. Thyroid nodules and cancers in children. *Endocrinol Metab Clin North Am* 2005;34(3):725–744, x.
112. Lyshchik A, Drozd V, Demidchik Y, et al. Diagnosis of thyroid cancer in children: value of gray-scale and power Doppler US. *Radiology* 2005;235(2):604–613.
113. Leboulleux S, Girard E, Rose M, et al. Ultrasound criteria of malignancy for cervical lymph nodes in patients followed up for differentiated thyroid cancer. *J Clin Endocrinol Metab* 2007;92(9):3590–3594.
114. Francis GL, Waguespack SG, Bauer AJ, et al. Management guidelines for children with thyroid nodules and differentiated thyroid cancer. *Thyroid* 2015;25(7):716–759.
115. Corrias A, Mussa A, Wasniewska M, et al. Levothyroxine treatment in pediatric benign thyroid nodules. *Horm Res Paediatr* 2011;75(4):246–251.
116. Faber J, Galloe AM. Changes in bone mass during prolonged subclinical hyperthyroidism due to L-thyroxine treatment: a meta-analysis. *Eur J Endocrinol* 1994;130(4):350–356.
117. Sdano MT, Falciglia M, Welge JA, et al. Efficacy of thyroid hormone suppression for benign thyroid nodules: meta-analysis of randomized trials. *Otolaryngol Head Neck Surg* 2005;133(3):391–396.
118. Vaisman F, Corbo R, Vaisman M. Thyroid carcinoma in children and adolescents-systematic review of the literature. *J Thyroid Res.* 2011;2011:845362.
119. Koovaraki MA, Shapiro SE, Perrier ND, et al. RET protooncogene: a review of and update of genotype–phenotype correlations in hereditary medullary thyroid cancer and associated endocrine tumors. *Thyroid* 2005;15:531–544.
120. Wells SA Jr, Asa SL, Dralle H, et al. Revised American Thyroid Association guidelines for the management of medullary thyroid carcinoma. *Thyroid* 2015;25(6):567–610.
121. Guillemin R. Peptides in the brain. The new endocrinology of the neuron. *Science* 1978;202:390–402.
122. Schally AV. Aspects of the hypothalamic regulation of the pituitary gland: its implication for the control of reproductive processes. *Science* 1978;202:18–28.
123. Jackson IMD. Thyrotropin releasing hormone. *N Engl J Med* 1982;306:145–155.
124. Lechan RM, Wu P, Jackson IMD, et al. Thyrotropin releasing hormone precursor: characterization in rat brain. *Science* 1986;231:159–161.
125. Wu P, Lechan RM, Jackson IMD. Identification and characterization of thyrotropin releasing hormone precursor peptides in rat brain. *Endocrinology* 1986;121:108–111.
126. Iruichijima T, Prasad C, Wilber JF, et al. Thyrotropin releasing hormone and cyclo (His–Pro)-like immunoreactivities in the cerebrospinal fluids of normal infants and adults and patients with various neuropsychiatric and neurologic disorders. *Life Sci* 1987;41:2419–2428.
127. Roti E, Gnudi A, Braverman LE. The placental transport, synthesis and metabolism of hormones and drugs with affect thyroid function. *Endocr Rev* 1983;4:131–149.
128. Weintraub BD, Kazlauskaite R, Grossman M, et al. Thyroid stimulating hormone and regulation of the thyroid axis. In: DeGroot LJ, Jameson JL, eds. *Endocrinology*, 4th ed. Philadelphia, PA: WB Saunders, 2001:1345–1360.
129. Torres MST, Ramirez L, Simkin PH, et al. Effect of various doses of recombinant human thyrotropin on the thyroid radioactive iodine uptake and serum levels of thyroid hormones and thyroglobulin in normal subjects. *J Clin Endocrinol Metab* 2001;86:1660–1664.

CHAPTER

58

Sarah E. Kolnik
Kendell R. German
Sandra E. Juul

Hematologic Agents

INTRODUCTION

The bone marrow of a healthy growing fetus produces billions of cells each day. The challenge is greater in neonates than in adults because the marrow must produce enough cells to maintain a stable cell number per body mass as the baby grows. Preterm birth or illness in the newborn period is associated with additional hematologic stressors, which can result in anemia or neutropenia. This chapter addresses multiple mechanisms of anemia and neutropenia in the newborn and reviews the use of available recombinant growth factors to treat these conditions.

In addition to its hematopoietic effects, much of the recent research on erythropoietic-stimulating agents is focused on their potential neuroprotective effects. These nonhematologic effects are also reviewed in this chapter.

ERYTHROPOIETIN

PHYSIOLOGIC AND PHARMACOLOGIC EFFECTS

Erythropoietin (Epo) is an endogenous glycoprotein that regulates erythrocyte production.[1,2] Since the US Food and Drug Administration (FDA) approval in 1989, many randomized controlled trials have been done to test the safety and efficacy of recombinant human (r)Epo as an erythropoietic agent. Given that rhEpo has been proven to decrease the need for transfusions in children and adults,[3] rhEpo is now widely used to treat or prevent anemia due to a variety of causes.

Humans have four main sites of embryonic and fetal erythropoiesis: yolk sac, ventral aspect of the aorta, liver, and bone marrow. Epo production mirrors this, beginning in the yolk sac, moving to the liver as the primary source during most of fetal life, and then switching to renal production around term birth. Factors regulating this switch are still not fully understood.[4,5] Growth factors important for definitive erythropoiesis include Epo, stem cell factor (c-kit ligand), interleukin (IL)-3 and IL-6, granulocyte–macrophage colony-stimulating factor (GM-CSF), and, possibly, insulin and insulin-like growth factor 1 (IGF-1), both of which act as nonessential survival factors for CD34+ cells[6,7] and have been shown to increase Epo production in animal models.[8] Epo maintains red cell production during fetal, neonatal, and adult life by inhibiting apoptosis of erythroid progenitors and by stimulating their proliferation and differentiation into normoblasts.[9] Epo receptor (EpoR) density is highest in the burst-forming units erythroid and colony-forming units erythroid (Fig. 58.1). In addition to increasing and maintaining erythrocyte progenitors, Epo increases the synthesis of hemoglobin, membrane proteins, and transferrin receptors. Epo can be considered the primary growth factor in the process of erythropoiesis, as in its absence, definitive erythropoiesis does not occur: both Epo and EpoR null mutation mice die on the 13th day of intrauterine development due to the absence of secondary erythropoiesis.[10] Since Epo does not cross the placenta, Epo concentrations measured in the fetus reflect fetal synthesis.[11]

During development, the EpoR is present on many nonhematopoietic cell types, including liver stromal cells,[12] smooth muscle cells,[13] myocardiocytes,[14] endothelial cells,[15] enterocytes,[16] renal tubular cells, epithelial cells in the lung, retinal cells,[16] placental tissues,[17] Leydig cells,[18] and cells specific to the central nervous system.[19–21] The role of Epo in these tissues is under investigation.

To maintain the increase in red cell volume associated with fetal growth, it is estimated that approximately 50×10^9 erythrocytes per day must be produced. When compared with adult Epo concentrations present at the time of acute anemia, measured fetal Epo concentrations seem low in the face of such production requirements. It has, therefore, been proposed that Epo is more efficient in the stimulation of erythropoiesis during fetal development, that it acts as a paracrine factor during hepatic hematopoiesis, and/or that other growth factors synergize with Epo. Candidate factors include hepatic growth factor, thrombopoietin, and IGF-1.[22,23] Production of Epo is stimulated by hypoxia-inducible factors 1 and 2 and is regulated by requirements for tissue oxygenation. Elevated Epo concentrations (up to 8,000 mU per mL) have been reported in pathologic states, such as fetal hypoxia, anemia, and placental insufficiency, and in infants of diabetic mothers.[24,25] Amniotic fluid levels of Epo have been correlated with intrauterine hypoxia, markers of oxidative stress, and adverse fetal outcomes.[26–28] Elevated cord blood and early postnatal elevations of endogenous Epo have also been associated with increased risk of intraventricular hemorrhage (IVH) and low mental and motor scores on the Bayley examination, likely reflecting prolonged intrauterine hypoxia.[29,30] In the NEAT-O trial, baseline Epo concentrations (drawn in the first 24 hours after birth) for infants diagnosed with moderate or severe hypoxic–ischemic encephalopathy (HIE) ranged from less than 0.31 (limit of the assay) to 5,047 mU per mL.[31]

In healthy term infants, serum Epo concentrations decrease following birth to reach a nadir between 4 and 6 weeks

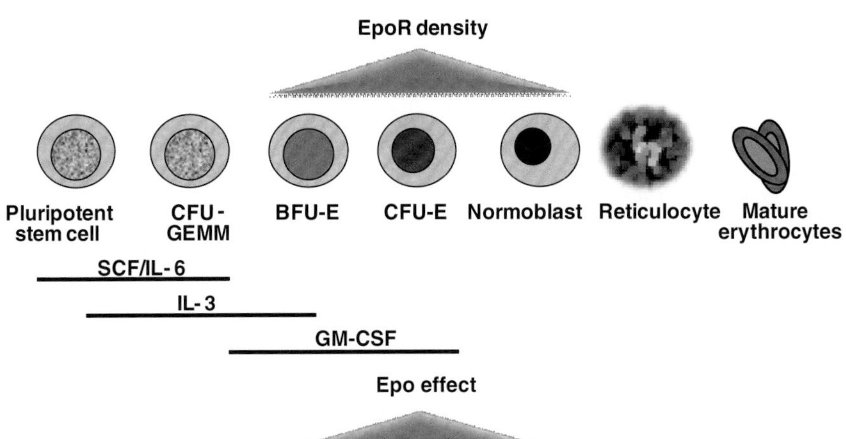

Figure 58.1 Lineage development of erythrocytes, with emphasis on growth factors and timing of erythropoietin effect. BFU-E, burst-forming unit erythroid; CFU-E, colony-forming unit erythroid; CFU-GEMM, colony-forming unit granulocyte, erythrocyte, monocyte, megakaryocyte; Epo, erythropoietin; EpoR, erythropoietin receptor; GM-CSF, granulocyte–macrophage colony-stimulating factor; IL-6, interleukin-6; SCF, stem cell factor.

of life, which correlates with the physiologic nadir of anemia. By 10 to 12 weeks of life, they reach adult concentrations (~15 mU per mL).

CLINICAL TRIALS IN NEWBORN INFANTS

Preterm infants remain among the most highly transfused patient populations despite attempts to limit phlebotomy losses, the implementation of transfusion guidelines, and the use of rhEpo. Common contributors to anemia in the hospitalized preterm infant include phlebotomy loss (which may exceed the infant's circulating blood volume), short red blood cell life span (70 days vs. 120 days in adults), high growth requirements, iron deficiency, inflammatory states, and anemia of prematurity. When measured, circulating Epo concentrations in this population are low relative to the degree of anemia.[32] Other forms of anemia in neonates include Rh-hemolytic disease of the newborn and a variety of anemias that are associated with chronic lung disease.

Anemia of Prematurity

The majority of erythrocyte transfusions administered to very low-birth-weight (VLBW, birth weight <1,500 g) neonates are given during the first 3 weeks of life, largely due to phlebotomy losses in the face of a small blood volume.[33,34] Transfusion rate, number, cumulative volume, and donor exposures increase with decreasing gestational age. While not approved for use in children younger than 1 month, many randomized controlled trials have been done to test the safety and efficacy of erythropoietic agents (rhEpo and Darbepoetin) in preterm infants.[35–37] rhEpo has been shown to reduce both volume and number of packed red blood cell transfusions in this population, but has not been widely adapted, since most studies do not show a reduction in donor exposure. This is most likely due to the common practice of aliquoting a single adult unit of blood and reserving the aliquots for one patient[3] combined with variability in clinical practice: transfusion guidelines differ in stringency, phlebotomy practices vary by institution, and the timing and dosing of both rhEpo and iron vary widely.[38,39]

One reasonable approach to managing anemia in the extremely preterm infant is to decrease phlebotomy and combine the use of iron supplementation, blood transfusion, and rhEpo therapy with the goal of one donor exposure per infant maximum. Contemporary blood preservatives have extended the use of stored blood up to 42 days. One adult unit of blood can be divided into multiple aliquots and assigned to one infant. The infant can be transfused with these aliquots as needed during the first 6 weeks of life (one donor exposure). Iron status should be optimized. rhEpo with iron can be used to prevent further transfusions if the infant remains significantly anemic with low reticulocyte counts.

Hyporegenerative Anemia of Neonates with Rh-Hemolytic Disease

Infants with Rh-hemolytic disease can develop a late anemia at 1 to 3 months of life secondary to diminished erythrocyte production. The incidence of late anemia seems to be much higher in infants who receive intrauterine transfusions.[40–42] In these infants, the anemia is characterized by low plasma concentrations of Epo, while erythroid progenitors remain highly responsive to rhEpo in vitro.[42] Studies evaluating the use of rhEpo as a potential treatment for hematologic diseases that lead to hemolytic or hypoproliferative anemia are in their early stages, and no consensus guidelines are available.[43–46]

Anemia of Bronchopulmonary Dysplasia

The anemia associated with bronchopulmonary dysplasia (BPD) is normocytic, normochromic, and hyporegenerative with marrow normoblast iron stains that are distinct from those observed in the anemia of chronic disorders and the anemia of prematurity.[47] In a study of 15 neonates with the anemia of BPD randomized to receive 200 U per kg of rhEpo per day subcutaneously for 10 consecutive days or placebo, treated infants had increased reticulocytes and hematocrits and required fewer transfusions than placebo recipients.[48]

A retrospective study was conducted by Rayjada et al. to evaluate the association between rhEpo and the reduced incidence of

BPD in preterm infants. They showed a significant correlation between rhEpo and reduced incidences of BPD in preterm infants where rhEpo was initiated within the first month of life. They speculate that the ability of Epo to mobilize circulating endothelial progenitor cells and improve lung repair in animal models may be the mechanism underpinning this association.[43] In contrast, in a study of 433 preterm infants 26 0/7 to 31 6/7 weeks' gestation who received three doses of 3,000 U per kg per dose ($n = 229$) versus placebo ($n = 219$), no difference in BPD was noted.[49]

Neonates with Congenital Heart Disease and Those Requiring Surgery

Infants with certain varieties of congenital heart disease often experience prolonged hospitalization, multiple invasive procedures, and significant phlebotomy losses. These neonates frequently receive multiple blood transfusions. Neonates with congenital heart disease awaiting heart transplantation who received 200 U per kg per day of rhEpo had a significant increase in hematocrit and a decrease in transfusions.[50]

A limited number of studies have evaluated the role of rhEpo as an alternative to transfusions in neonates awaiting cardiac surgery. In Japan, a study evaluated the effect of three doses of rhEpo (300 U per kg) on transfusion requirements of infants undergoing cardiac surgery.[51] A beneficial effect of rhEpo has been reported among neonates who underwent open heart surgery and in those whose parents are Jehovah's Witnesses.[52] Further studies evaluating the use of rhEpo to reduce transfusion requirements in neonates with congenital heart disease are needed. Neonates who undergo surgery are at risk for needing multiple transfusions, especially since their ability to regenerate blood is limited by their blunted endogenous production of Epo. A small study where neonates requiring surgery were randomized to receive rhEpo (200 units per kg per day) or placebo for 14 days demonstrated an improvement in those neonates who receive rhEpo by increasing reticulocyte counts and maintaining hematocrit.[53] Thus, the erythropoietic-stimulating effect of rhEpo has promising implications in improving hematologic indices in this neonatal population.

STRUCTURE, DOSE, ROUTES, AND REGIMENS

Epoetin Hospira is produced by recombinant technology in Chinese Hamster Ovary (CHO) cells transfected with the human EPO gene as a 165-amino-acid glycoprotein with a molecular weight of 30.4 kDa. The human recombinant form of Epo is commercially available as epoetin alfa (rhEpo) (Epogen, Amgen, Thousand Oaks, CA; Procrit, Ortho Biotech, Raritan, NJ).

Darbepoetin alfa (Darbe), a synthetic protein closely related to rhEpo, is also commonly used as an erythropoietic-stimulating agent in the neonatal population. It is also a 165-amino-acid glycoprotein but contains five *N*-linked oligosaccharide chains, rather than the three contained in rhEpo.[54] These two additional glycosylation sites increase the molecular weight to 37.0 kDa and increase the terminal half-life threefold as determined in adult patients.[55] Darbe is available from Amgen and is formulated for intravenous and subcutaneous administration.

A wide range of rhEpo dosing schedules have been used for hyporegenerative anemia in the preterm infant (50 to 700 U per kg per dose).[56] Garcia et al. showed that for every 500 U per kg per week increase in rhEpo dosing, the average number of transfusions per patient decreased by three-fourths of a transfusion.[57] We recommend subcutaneous administration of rhEpo 400 U per kg three times per week, or daily intravenous rhEpo 200 U per kg per day, for a minimum of 2 weeks.[58] Alternatively, rhEpo can be administered in a continuous intravenous infusion such as parenteral nutrition, using a dose of 200 U per kg per day.[59] To promote effective erythropoiesis, iron must be given concomitant with rhEpo. Patients on enteral feedings of at least 100 mL per kg per day who are receiving rhEpo should receive 6 to 8 mg per kg per day of elemental iron. Alternatively, parenteral iron may be given at 1 mg per kg per day.[58] The adequacy of iron supplementation should be assessed at least every 2 weeks while giving erythropoietic-stimulating agents, due to the elevated iron needs associated with increased heme production. This is particularly critical in order to prevent iron deficiency in the brain, which may lead to adverse neurodevelopmental outcomes as iron is shunted preferentially for erythropoiesis. Zinc protoporphyrin-to-heme (ZnPP/H) ratios and ferritin measurements are markers of iron sufficiency commonly used in the neonatal intensive care unit (NICU). While low ferritin levels reliably indicate iron deficiency, ferritin is known to be elevated in the setting of inflammation and thus is not a reliable indicator of iron sufficiency when elevated. Given that ferritin is more significantly affected by common inflammatory events encountered in the neonatal population, such as sepsis and transfusion, ZnPP/H ratio may be a more reliable marker of iron status in this population.[60] Reticulocyte hemoglobin concentration may also be a useful marker of iron sufficiency.[61–63]

Darbe has the advantage of a single once-weekly injection rather than the thrice-weekly dosing of rhEpo.[54] This is particularly important for infants without intravenous access who must receive subcutaneous injections. The pharmacokinetics, safety, and efficacy of Darbe doses ranging from 1 to 10 μg per kg have been well studied.[37,64–66]

PHARMACOKINETIC PROPERTIES IN NEWBORN INFANTS

rhEpo can be administered by intravenous infusion or subcutaneous injection. The pharmacokinetics of intravenous doses ranging from 500 to 2,500 U per kg was studied in preterm infants weighing less than 1,000 g.[67] Nonlinear kinetics were noted, with the half-life ranging from 5.4 to 8.7 hours as dosing increased, and clearance decreased. A similar study was done in term infants with HIE, with doses ranging from 250 to 2,500 U per kg per dose.[68,69] Compared with adults, neonates require higher doses of rhEpo per kilogram and more frequent dosing to achieve an equivalent hematopoietic response, due to their greater plasma clearance, high volume of distribution, and short fractional elimination time.[70–72] The precise mechanism for Epo elimination has not been established in neonates, but it has been speculated that rhEpo is eliminated by irreversible binding to its receptors on erythroid progenitor cells with subsequent internalization.[73]

ADVERSE EFFECTS, TOXICITY, AND PRECAUTIONS

Known adverse effects of chronic rhEpo treatment in adults include hypertension,[74] thrombus formation,[75] polycythemia, and red cell aplasia secondary to anti-Epo antibodies.[76] Hypertensive leukoencephalopathy has also been reported in a few adult patients requiring long-term rhEpo for anemia due to dialysis-dependent renal failure.[77] An FDA warning was released in 2008 for patients with chronic kidney failure who receive rhEpo at higher than recommended doses, as an increased risk of blood clots, strokes, heart attacks, and death have been identified. In preterm neonates, rhEpo use for the treatment of anemia has been very safe, with none of the adverse effects noted in adult populations.[3,49,56]

Previously, researchers were concerned that use of rhEpo in the preterm population might increase the risk for retinopathy of prematurity (ROP). ROP is characterized by the pathophysiologic growth of immature blood vessels as the retina is vascularized, which can trigger retinal detachment and loss of vision if unchecked.[78] The disease primarily affects LBW (<1,250 g) and preterm infants born less than 31 weeks' gestation.[79] Retinal vascularization occurs from 16 weeks' gestation to birth,[80] and in infants born prematurely, this process can be disrupted. Early investigators hypothesized that the angiogenic properties of Epo might increase the proliferative phase of ROP. While one early meta-analysis showed an increased risk of ROP with early use of rhEpo and iron for erythropoiesis,[81] subsequent animal and prospective studies have failed to show this association.[49,82,83]

NONHEMATOPOIETIC EFFECTS OF ERYTHROPOIETIN

Following the observations of EpoR expression in brain and other organs[16,84] and the capacity for Epo production by astrocytes,[85] a broader concept of Epo as a neuroprotective molecule has emerged.[86] Neuroprotection by high-dose rhEpo has been demonstrated in neonatal and adult animal models of injury, including hypoxia–ischemia, stroke, and hemorrhage.[87–89] rhEpo improves both short- and long-term outcomes following unilateral neonatal brain injury in neonatal rats, decreasing structural and behavioral deficits.[90–92] Brief courses (5 days) of high-dose rhEpo have also been shown to be safe in neonatal rats, with no long-term negative consequences.[93] Neuroprotective effects of rhEpo have also been demonstrated in preterm sheep[94] and near-term nonhuman primates.[95] Thus, rhEpo may provide an important adjunct to neuroprotective therapy in neonates. The mechanisms by which rhEpo provides neuroprotection are complex and include direct neuronal effects and indirect systemic effects, as well as both early and late effects. Early effects of rhEpo include antiapoptotic,[96–98] anti-inflammatory,[89,99] and antioxidant effects[89,97,100–103] and increased resistance to excitotoxicity.[104,105] Late rhEpo effects that improve brain recovery include increased neurogenesis, angiogenesis, and migration of regenerating neurons.[106,107] rhEpo is directly involved in prevention of oxidative stress with generation of antioxidant enzymes, inhibition of nitric oxide production, and decrease of lipid peroxidation.[108] These properties of rhEpo may be relevant in therapeutic prevention of injury in developing brain of premature infants, where antioxidant systems are immature, or for the treatment of hypoxic–ischemic brain injury in term infants.[109,110]

Clinical Studies of Neonatal Neuroprotection with Erythropoietin

The bulk of ongoing research in the field of erythrocyte-stimulating agents involves the investigation of its potential neuroprotective effects. Several phase I/II clinical trials and meta-analyses have suggested an improvement in neurodevelopmental outcome in preterm infants treated with prophylactic high-dose rhEpo.[68,111–113] Multicenter phase III studies are ongoing for the use of rhEpo or Darbe for prophylaxis of preterm infants, or treatment of IVH, and for term infants with HIE or stroke.[110,114–116] The use of high-dose rhEpo for neuroprotection should be discouraged until results from these trials are available.

More information is needed regarding the ideal population to target for neuroprotection, the optimal rhEpo dose, and duration of therapy. It is also unclear whether rhEpo has a role as a prophylactic measure for at-risk extremely preterm infants, or whether it should only be used as a rescue treatment following stroke, intracranial hemorrhage, or perinatal asphyxia in term infants. Similarly, for term infants with perinatal brain injury, more data are needed. Since therapeutic hypothermia is now the standard of care in high-resource settings, rhEpo must be tested in conjunction with this therapy to determine additive efficacy.[68] It may also be considered as monotherapy in lower resource settings.[117]

Potential Side Effects of High-Dose Recombinant Erythropoietin for Neuroprotection

rhEpo is a potent erythropoietic growth factor. Thus, we can expect that using high doses of rhEpo as neuroprotective treatment will have hematopoietic effects. These will likely include increasing erythropoiesis and, possibly, clinically insignificant higher white counts and lower platelet counts, as seen in the study by Fauchere et al.[49] In the neonatal population where anemia is ubiquitous, the increase in erythropoiesis is unlikely to be a negative consequence but rather a beneficial side effect. It is unknown, however, how this potential increase in hematopoiesis might affect iron balance. This is important because preterm infants are at high risk for iron deficiency, since the bulk of iron transfer occurs in the third trimester. Iron is essential for normal growth and development because it is an important component of proteins and enzymes required for oxygen transport, cell division, neurotransmitter synthesis, myelination, and cellular oxidative metabolism.[118] Iron deficiency can lead to adverse neurodevelopmental consequences, with deficits in executive function and memory.[119] Because of this, Epo or Darbe treatment should be accompanied by iron supplementation.

The role of Epo in the developing gastrointestinal tract is being defined. The EpoR is present in the developing gut, but its role is not well described.[16] Increases in villous height and crypt depth, as well as improved barrier function have been reported in animal models following the enteral administration of rhEpo.[16,120–122] Systemic absorption following enteral administration in rodents has been reported[123]; however, in preterm infants given up to 1,000 U per kg per dose rhEpo, no increase in circulating Epo nor any erythropoietic effects were noted.[124,125] A retrospective study showed the incidence of necrotizing enterocolitis was lower in neonates who received rhEpo[126]; however, no such difference was noted in a larger prospective study.[49,127]

GRANULOCYTE COLONY-STIMULATING FACTOR

PHYSIOLOGIC AND PHARMACOLOGIC EFFECTS

Granulocyte colony-stimulating factor (G-CSF) is a physiologic regulator of neutrophil production and function.[128] It is produced in vivo by multiple cell types, including monocytes, macrophages, fibroblasts, and endothelial cells. G-CSF has multiple effects on white cell maturation and function, as well as other, more recently described, nonhematopoietic functions.[129] These effects include clonal maturation of committed myeloid progenitors, release of neutrophils from the bone marrow to the blood, and enhancement of neutrophil functions, including chemotaxis, phagocytosis, superoxide production, and bactericidal activity. Administration of recombinant G-CSF (rG-CSF) has long been used to prevent infections in patients with nonmyeloid malignancies receiving anticancer drugs and suffering febrile neutropenia. In addition, rG-CSF is used to facilitate hematopoietic recovery following bone marrow transplantation and to mobilize peripheral blood progenitor cells in healthy donors.[130] In neonates, it has been used in the setting of active infection or as prophylaxis against infection in infants with severe neutropenia from a variety of etiologies. Although the circulating neutrophil counts of term neonates resemble those of adults, their bone marrow reserves tend to be lower and easily exhausted, leading many neonates to become neutropenic in the setting of infection rather than neutrophilic. Further, the chemotactic, phagocytic, and respiratory burst activity of preterm neonates is low within the first few weeks of life.[131] However, recent studies evaluating the use of rG-CSF in this population have, in general, failed to show an outcome benefit to supplemental rG-CSF with the possible exception of severe chronic neutropenia, often caused by an underlying genetic syndrome.[131]

CLINICAL TRIALS IN NEWBORN INFANTS

Neonates with Bacterial Sepsis

Neonatal sepsis is often associated with neutropenia,[132] and the neutrophil function of neonates is low in comparison with adults.[131] Given that rG-CSF increases neutrophil counts, it was hypothesized that rG-CSF administration to neonates with bacterial sepsis might improve mortality. Unfortunately, both retrospective and prospective clinical studies have failed to show any mortality benefit.[133–136] Enrollment in a prospective randomized, double-masked, placebo-controlled trial by Miura et al. aimed at examining the use of rG-CSF for treatment of early-onset sepsis in preterm neonates was halted early as preliminary analysis of 44 patients failed to show any mortality benefit with rG-CSF treatment, and the oversight committee felt it would be extremely unlikely that further enrollment would show any benefit.[134] Similarly, prospective randomized trials examining the use of prophylactic rG-CSF in preterm neonates by Carr et al. and Kuhn et al. failed to show any disease-free survival benefit.[137,138] Based on these randomized trials as well as a meta-analysis by the Cochrane review, there is inadequate evidence to support the use of rG-CSF for treatment of bacterial sepsis or neutropenia in the neonatal population.[136]

Small for Gestational Age Neonates

Early neutropenia (as well as thrombocytopenia) is more common in infants born small for gestational age (SGA) (<10th percentile). The underlying etiology for this is hypothesized to be decreased neutrophil production in the setting of intrauterine hypoxia.[139] In a large, retrospective analysis, Christensen et al., showed that while necrotizing enterocolitis was more common among SGA infants with neutropenia [odds ratio (OR) 4.01, 95% confidence interval (CI), 2.08–7.35, $p < 0.001$], treatment with rG-CSF or intravenous immunoglobulin did not show a significant benefit.[139]

Neonates Born to Mothers with Pregnancy-Induced Hypertension

Neutropenia can be severe in neonates born to women who have pregnancy-induced hypertension (PIH).[140–142] Neutropenia associated with PIH (mediated by a circulating inhibitor to granulocytopoiesis)[140,143,144] can occur in up to 50% of exposed infants and generally resolves by 1 to 2 weeks of life. In preterm infants, neutropenia is approximately three times as common in PIH-exposed infants as compared with those unexposed and may last longer than 2 weeks.[142] SGA infants also appear to be more significantly affected (33.3% of infants with SGA plus maternal PIH have neutropenia vs. 22.5% for appropriate for gestational age infants with maternal PIH).[145]

Although some studies have shown an improvement in neutrophil count with rG-CSF, given that neutropenia is typically self-resolved, treatment is not usually indicated. However, if the neutropenia is severe (<500 per μL) and prolonged, other diagnoses should be entertained, and rG-CSF could be considered.

Neonates with Alloimmune Neutropenia

In alloimmune neutropenia, the mother becomes immunized to paternal granulocyte antigens present on fetal neutrophils.[146] Maternal immunoglobulin crosses the placenta and binds to fetal neutrophils. The severity of the neutropenia is influenced by the antibody titer and the immunoglobulin G subclass involved.[147] Although most neonates with alloimmune neutropenia do not require treatment, those with severe and prolonged neutropenia generally respond very well to rG-CSF therapy in doses from 5 to 10 μg per kg per day for 3 to 5 days.[58] Additional doses can be given to adjust the absolute neutrophil count (ANC) so that it remains greater than 1,000 per μL. The response is clinically evident within 24 to 48 hours.

Neonates with Autoimmune Neutropenia

Autoimmune neutropenia is analogous to autoimmune hemolytic anemia and thrombocytopenia. The etiologic mechanisms remain unclear, but associations have been reported with parvovirus B 19 infection and β-lactam antibiotics.[147] Neutrophil antibodies may adversely affect the function of neutrophils even in the absence of neutropenia.[148] Neonates with autoimmune neutropenia respond well to rG-CSF at 10 μg per kg per day given by intravenous or subcutaneous routes. The duration of treatment is based on the resolution of the neutropenia with an ANC greater than 1,000 per μL.[58]

Neonates with Chronic Idiopathic Neutropenia

Long-term observational studies in children indicate that chronic idiopathic neutropenia (CIN) often lasts for 3 to 5 years in children, then spontaneously remits, but it rarely remits in adult cases. Most recent data suggest that CIN and acute idiopathic neutropenia (AIN) are immune-mediated diseases, but there are no new clinical or genetic tests to aid in diagnosis. Treatment with rG-CSF is effective to increase blood neutrophils in almost all cases. However, this treatment should be reserved for patients with both neutropenia and evidence of recurrent fevers, inflammatory symptoms and infections. There is little or no evidence to indicate that rG-CSF treatment predisposes to myeloid malignancies neonates. It is important to recognize CIN and AIN, the most common causes of chronic neutropenia in both children and adults. If the neutropenia is not severe, that is more than 0.5 × 10 per L, most patients can be observed and not treated with antibiotics or a growth factor. When neutropenia is severe, treatment with rG-CSF may be beneficial.[149]

CIN occurs in extremely preterm infants who have no evidence of antibody-mediated neutropenia, no history of PIH, and no features that result in a specific diagnosis.[142,150,151] Although these infants are generally well appearing, the ANC can fall below 500 per μL for many weeks or months. This type of neutropenia can respond to rG-CSF but remits spontaneously remits, so treatment is generally not necessary.[150,151]

The use of rG-CSF in neonates requires further studies to define the precise indications, doses, and intervals to be used.

STRUCTURE, DOSE, ROUTES, AND REGIMENS

G-CSF was first recognized and purified in the mouse and then in humans in 1986.[152] Four different commercially available forms of G-CSF exist: filgrastim (Neupogen) and filgrastim with sustained duration (Neulasta) available in the United States and Ro 25-8315 (Nartograstim) and lenograstim (Granocyte) available only in Europe.[153,154]

The recommended dose of rG-CSF is 5 to 10 μg per kg per day.[58] Both the intravenous and subcutaneous routes of administration are used. In general, for the treatment of neutropenia in neonates with sepsis, rG-CSF has been given once a day for 3 to 5 consecutive days.[155] Longer dosing duration may be needed for the treatment of alloimmune and autoimmune neutropenia. In neonates with either of the latter conditions, the length of therapy should be tailored to the individual patient, as variability in antibody titers among individuals can make specific recommendations difficult.

PHARMACOKINETIC PROPERTIES IN NEWBORN INFANTS

In neonates with presumed sepsis, the half-life of filgrastim is 4.4 ± 0.4 hours, and the peak serum concentrations are dose dependent (1 μg per kg, 2,040 ± 1,340 pg per mL; 5 μg per kg, 20,000 ± 6,260 pg per mL; 10 μg per kg, 126,750 ± 22,570 pg per mL) and occur 2 hours following intravenous administration.[156] Two of the subjects in this study were neutropenic, which may affect the pharmacokinetics.

In a study of 10 neutropenic neonates (five secondary to reduced neutrophil production with PIH and intrauterine growth retardation and five as a result of accelerated neutrophil usage with sepsis and shock), extremely high baseline G-CSF serum and urine concentrations were measured in neutropenic patients with sepsis and shock (20,028 to 98,280 pg per mL) compared with those without (65 to 210 pg per mL).[157] This might be due to an upregulation of G-CSF production during infection or to saturation of G-CSF receptors (G-CSF-Rs) by endogenous G-CSF. Alternatively, expression of G-CSF-R by tumor necrosis factor α (TNF-α) or other mediators during sepsis might contribute to high circulating G-CSF concentrations.[158] In vitro studies of incubations of granulocytes with TNF-α have shown a 70% reduction in the number of G-CSF-R within 10 minutes. TNF-α serum concentrations are elevated in infants with sepsis.[158]

Traditional pharmacokinetic measurements can be flawed when applied to rG-CSF because of the unique manner in which G-CSF is cleared.[157] Ericson et al. reported a linear relationship ($R^2 = 0.85$) between the blood neutrophil count and the rG-CSF clearance with repeated dosing.[159] Kuwabara and colleagues concluded that the clearance of rG-CSF is inversely related to the dose administered and that with repeated dosing, the clearance increases.[160] Both postulated that rG-CSF clearance was dependent principally on saturable receptor binding, but that at very high doses, glomerular filtration and elimination in the urine become a process for nonsaturable clearance. An additional factor that complicates the analysis of rG-CSF elimination in neonates is the presence of the G-CSF-R on nonhematopoietic tissues.[161]

The PEGylation of filgrastim into the form known as Neulasta extends the half-life.[162] When a single PEG group is attached to the N-terminal residue of rG-CSF, the circulation time increases with no effect on activity.[163] Studies in animals suggest that the average elimination half-life of PEGylated rG-CSF is two to four times longer than rG-CSF.[164] PEGylation of filgrastim decreases its renal clearance so that clearance is almost entirely dependent on receptor-mediated elimination.[165] No studies have been reported on the pharmacokinetics of Neulasta in either preterm or term neonates.

ADVERSE EFFECTS, TOXICITY, AND PRECAUTIONS

Adverse effects have rarely been described when rG-CSF is used to treat neonates with sepsis. In a 2-year follow-up of neonates who received rG-CSF for 3 days, Rosenthal et al. reported normal hematologic, immunologic, and neurologic development.[166] Reductions in platelet counts have been reported after septic neonates or children were treated with rG-CSF[167,168]; however, this may have been due to the underlying septic condition. Donadieu and colleagues reported thrombocytopenia after rG-CSF administration to children with chronic neutropenia in the absence of sepsis.[169] Gilmore et al. noted irritability in one infant after two doses, possibly secondary to bone pain.[170] No studies have evaluated the safety or efficacy of either of the PEGylated forms of rG-CSF in neonates.

This meta-analysis evaluated the impact of G-CSF added to chemotherapy on treatment outcomes, including survival and disease recurrence in patients with acute myeloid leukemia (AML). Treatment with chemotherapy plus G-CSF appears to provide better survival and treatment responses compared with chemotherapy alone, particularly for patients with previously untreated AML.[171]

Long-term rG-CSF treatment may result in an increased risk of myelodysplastic syndrome (MDS) or AML, possibly due to increased marrow stress resulting in telomere shortening. Glycogen storage disease patients with prolonged rG-CSF exposure may be at an increased risk of MDS/AML states associated with rG-CSF–induced shortened telomeres.[172] Development of Kawasaki syndrome after treatment with rG-CSF has also been reported.[173]

Concerns exist that prolonged exposure to rG-CSF might predispose neonates to MDS or to osteoporosis. Some children with Kostmann syndrome have developed leukemia while receiving rG-CSF.[174] Other factors in addition to the use of rG-CSF certainly contribute to their increased risk of leukemia, including structural abnormalities of the G-CSF-R.[175] Neonates with Kostmann syndrome or any form of severe prolonged neutropenia who are receiving chronic rG-CSF should be monitored for the development of abnormal cytogenetics. Some children have developed osteoporosis on long-term rG-CSF therapy. However, it is unclear whether the risks of this adverse event are related to the primary disease or to the rG-CSF therapy.[176,177] The administration of rG-CSF is contraindicated in any patients with known hypersensitivity to *Escherichia coli*–derived proteins or any component of the product.

NONHEMATOPOIETIC EFFECTS OF RECOMBINANT GRANULOCYTE COLONY-STIMULATING FACTOR

As with EpoR, G-CSF-R expression is not limited to the hematopoietic system. G-CSF-R expression occurs in a variety of cell types, including endothelial cells, glia, and neurons.[178] Both G-CSF and its receptor are expressed on neuronal cells.[179,180] Recent work, primarily in adult models of ischemia, has demonstrated that rG-CSF has important neuroprotective properties.[181,182] However, the precise mechanisms of action of C-CSF in the brain remain unclear.

Long-term neuroprotection afforded by rG-CSF in both morphologic and functional parameters after a hypoxic–ischemic event in the neonate provides a rationale for exploring clinical translation.[183]

rG-CSF displays anti-inflammatory properties by reducing blood–brain barrier disruption and decreasing the number of infiltrating neutrophils in the infarct penumbra.[178] rG-CSF increases neurogenesis[181] and enhances angiogenesis following an ischemic insult.[184] Whether rG-CSF can decrease neuronal injury by mobilization of hematopoietic stem cells into damaged brain areas is currently a matter of discussion.[185]

Expanding evidence on the antiapoptotic effect of rG-CSF comes from several in vitro and in vivo studies. rG-CSF exerts its antiapoptotic effect by interference with various apoptotic signaling pathways, such as activation of the antiapoptotic target Bcl-X_L and PI3K/phosphoinositide-dependent kinase/Akt pathway controlling neuronal survival.[181]

However, data from adult studies may not be transferable to neonates. In contrast to the neuroprotective effects of G-CSF in adult models, the systemic administration of rG-CSF and stem cell factor surprisingly worsened excitotoxic brain injury in newborn mice.[186]

GRANULOCYTE–MACROPHAGE COLONY-STIMULATING FACTOR

PHYSIOLOGIC AND PHARMACOLOGIC EFFECTS

GM-CSF acts on multiple cell lineages, including macrophages, eosinophils, and, to a lesser extent, neutrophils. Given its ability to stimulate circulating granulocyte production, it has been used in animal studies, neonates, and adult trials to treat neutropenia and sepsis (particularly in the setting of neutropenia). However, limited studies exist, particularly in the neonatal population, to assess its effects on morbidity and mortality. Although rGM-CSF appears safe for use in the neonatal population, given the lack of evidence to support patient benefit, most authors argue that its use is not indicated in the neonatal population.[187,188]

CLINICAL TRIALS IN NEWBORN INFANTS

Neonatal Sepsis and Sepsis Prophylaxis

Although not as widely studied as rG-CSF, some small studies examine the use of rGM-CSF as prophylaxis for neonatal sepsis. Carr et al. conducted a single-blind, multicenter, randomized trial evaluating the use of rGM-CSF as prophylaxis for sepsis in 280 preterm neonates. They administered 10 μg per kg of rGM-CSF subcutaneously to neonates for 5 days starting within 72 hours of birth. Although they showed a significant increase in neutrophil counts following trial entry, there was no difference in 14-day sepsis-free survival.[137] In regard to potential nonhematologic effects of rGM-CSF, 5-year outcomes of Carr's trial[189] showed no difference in neurodevelopmental outcome between the rGM-CSF- and placebo-treated groups, suggesting that there is no benefit to rGM-CSF in regard to neuroprotection. (Though this study was not powered to evaluate neuroprotective effects; therefore, these results are inconclusive.)

STRUCTURE, DOSE, ROUTES, AND REGIMENS

GM-CSF is a protein with 127 amino acids and a molecular weight of 18 to 22 kDa. rGM-CSF is marketed as Leucomax (Novartis, UK) and Leukine (Immunex, Seattle, WA). rGM-CSF is produced by many cell types and promotes the growth of precursors of several myeloid and megakaryocyte lines.[190] The physiologic characteristics of rGM-CSF are somewhat similar to those of rG-CSF, but GM-CSF has a wider spectrum of action.[191] As a result, monocyte, macrophage, and eosinophil counts generally increase more after rGM-CSF therapy than following rG-CSF treatment (Fig. 58.2). In addition, rGM-CSF enhances monocyte function and has a greater effect on chemotaxis and the bactericidal function of neutrophils than does rG-CSF.[192,193] Interactions between rG-CSF and rGM-CSF remain to be fully elucidated.

Neutropenia is a relatively frequent condition in SGA and/or LBW neonates. CSFs, namely, rG-CSF and rGM-CSF, have been proposed for prophylaxis and therapy of severe infections in this condition. Available data do not support the use of these substances for prophylaxis of infections in the presence of neutropenia. On the contrary, there might be space for their use, mainly for rG-CSF, in case of severe infectious complications in severely neutropenic neonates (absolute polymorphonuclear neutrophil count <500 per μL) and/or in the presence of specific hematologic diseases causing neutropenia.[187]

rGM-CSF has been dosed intravenously at 5 to 10 μg per kg per day in human newborn infants for prophylaxis against nosocomial infection.[164] Published dosing schedules have included once a day for 7 days, twice a day for 7 days, daily for 5 days, and daily for 7 days, followed by every other day for a total of 21 days.[136,187,194,195]

PHARMACOKINETIC PROPERTIES IN NEWBORN INFANTS

The distribution half-life of rGM-CSF administered intravenously is 5 to 15 minutes, and the elimination half-life is 1.4 ± 0.8 to 3.9 ± 2.8 hours.[164] Peak concentrations, which occurred at the end of a 2-hour intravenous infusion, were dose dependent and were undetectable by 24 hours. After subcutaneous injection, the elimination half-life was 2.9 hours, with a peak concentration at 4 hours.

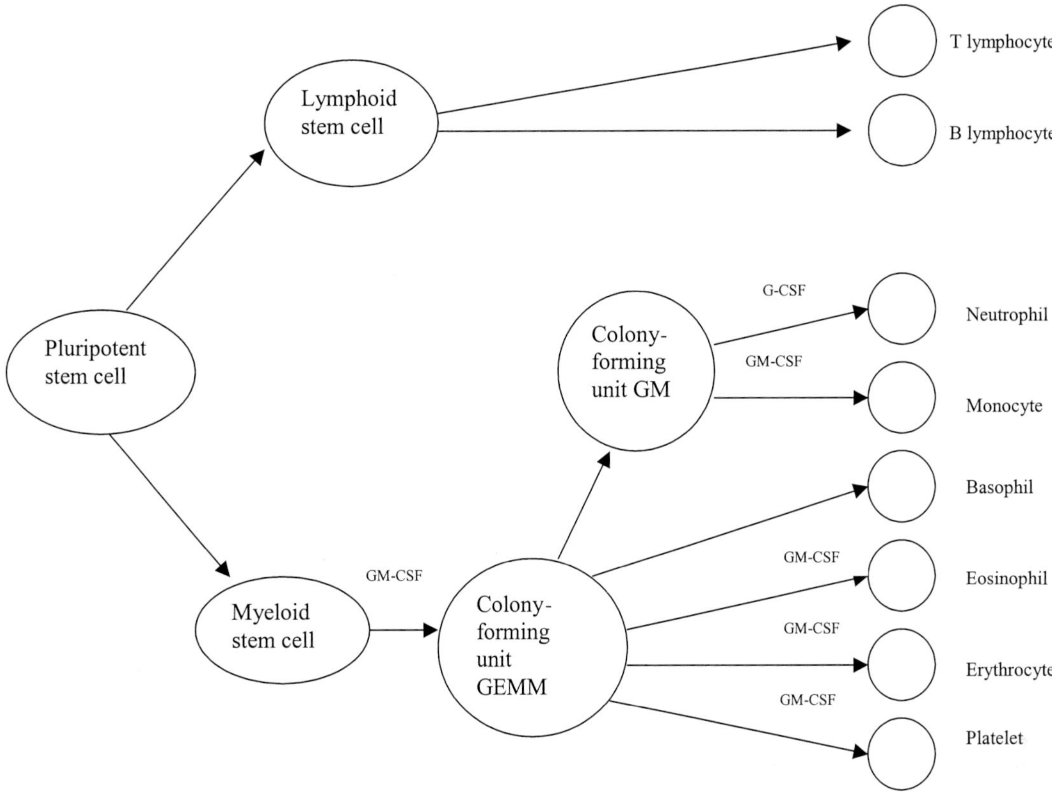

Figure 58.2 Lineage development of peripheral blood cells from pluripotent stem cell. CSF, colony-stimulating factor; G-CSF, granulocyte colony-stimulating factor; GEMM, granulocyte, erythrocyte, monocyte, megakaryocyte; GM-CSF, granulocyte–macrophage colony-stimulating factor. (Redrawn from Steward WP. Granulocyte and granulocyte–macrophage colony-stimulating factors. *Lancet* 1993;342:153–155, with permission.)

ADVERSE EFFECTS, TOXICITY, AND PRECAUTIONS

Serious adverse effects of rGM-CSF treatment of newborns have not been reported. Five-year outcomes of infants treated with rGM-CSF versus placebo were evaluated from the PROGRAMS trial. Although no neuroprotective effects were seen, no adverse effects of treatment with rGM-CSF were reported.[189]

REFERENCES

1. Goldwasser E, Krantz SB, Wang FF. Erythropoietin and erythroid differentiation. *Symp Fundam Cancer Res* 1984;37:103–107.
2. Lai PH, Everett R, Wang FF, et al. Structural characterization of human erythropoietin. *J Biol Chem* 1986;261(7):3116–3121.
3. Ohlsson A, Aher SM. Early erythropoietin for preventing red blood cell transfusion in preterm and/or low birth weight infants. *Cochrane Database Syst Rev* 2014;(4):CD004863.
4. Zanjani ED. Liver to kidney switch of erythropoietin formation. *Exp Hematol* 1980;8(Suppl 8):29–40.
5. Dame C, Juul SE. The switch from fetal to adult erythropoiesis. *Clin Perinatol* 2000;27(3):507–526.
6. Muta K, Krantz SB, Bondurant MC, et al. Distinct roles of erythropoietin, insulin-like growth factor I, and stem cell factor in the development of erythroid progenitor cells. *J Clin Invest* 1994;94(1):34–43.
7. Ratajczak J, Zhang Q, Pertusini E, et al. The role of insulin (INS) and insulin-like growth factor-I (IGF-I) in regulating human erythropoiesis. Studies in vitro under serum-free conditions—comparison to other cytokines and growth factors. *Leukemia* 1998;12(3):371–381.
8. Masuda S, Chikuma M, Sasaki R. Insulin-like growth factors and insulin stimulate erythropoietin production in primary cultured astrocytes. *Brain Res* 1997;746(1–2):63–70.
9. Goldwasser E. The action of erythropoietin as the inducer of erythroid differentiation. *Prog Clin Biol Res* 1985;184:77–84.
10. Wu H, Liu X, Jaenisch R, et al. Generation of committed erythroid BFU-E and CFU-E progenitors does not require erythropoietin or the erythropoietin receptor. *Cell* 1995;83(1):59–67.
11. Widness JA, Schmidt RL, Sawyer ST. Erythropoietin transplacental passage—review of animal studies. *J Perinat Med* 1995;23(1–2):61–70.
12. Ohneda O, Yanai N, Obinata M. Erythropoietin as a mitogen for fetal liver stromal cells which support erythropoiesis. *Exp Cell Res* 1993;208(1):327–331.
13. Morakkabati N, Gollnick F, Meyer R, et al. Erythropoietin induces Ca2+ mobilization and contraction in rat mesangial and aortic smooth muscle cultures. *Exp Hematol* 1996;24(2):392–397.
14. Wu H, Lee SH, Gao J, et al. Inactivation of erythropoietin leads to defects in cardiac morphogenesis. *Development* 1999;126(16):3597–3605.
15. Ribatti D, Presta M, Vacca A, et al. Human erythropoietin induces a pro-angiogenic phenotype in cultured endothelial cells and stimulates neovascularization in vivo. *Blood* 1999;93(8):2627–2636.
16. Juul SE, Yachnis AT, Christensen RD. Tissue distribution of erythropoietin and erythropoietin receptor in the developing human fetus. *Early Hum Dev* 1998;52(3):235–249.
17. Sawyer ST, Krantz SB, Sawada K. Receptors for erythropoietin in mouse and human erythroid cells and placenta. *Blood* 1989;74(1):103–109.
18. Mioni R, Gottardello F, Bordon P, et al. Evidence for specific binding and stimulatory effects of recombinant human erythropoietin on isolated adult rat Leydig cells. *Acta Endocrinol (Copenh)* 1992;127(5):459–465.
19. Konishi Y, Chui D-H, Hirose H, et al. Trophic effect of erythropoietin and other hematopoietic factors on central cholinergic neurons in vitro and in vivo. *Brain Res* 1993;609(1–2):29–35.
20. Tabira T, Konishi Y, Gallyas F Jr. Neurotrophic effect of hematopoietic cytokines on cholinergic and other neurons in vitro. *Int J Dev Neurosci* 1995;13(3–4):241–252.
21. Juul SE, Yachnis AT, Rojiani AM, et al. Immunohistochemical localization of erythropoietin and its receptor in the developing human brain. *Pediatr Dev Pathol* 1999;2(2):148–158.
22. Iguchi T, Sogo S, Hisha H, et al. HGF activates signal transduction from EPO receptor on human cord blood CD34+/CD45+ cells. *Stem Cells* 1999;17(2):82–91.
23. Akahane K, Tojo A, Urabe A, et al. Pure erythropoietic colony and burst formations in serum-free culture and their enhancement by insulin-like growth factor I. *Exp Hematol* 1987;15(7):797–802.
24. Buescher U, Hertwig K, Wolf C, et al. Erythropoietin in amniotic fluid as a marker of chronic fetal hypoxia. *Int J Gynaecol Obstet* 1998;60(3):257–263.
25. Stangenberg M, Legarth J, Cao HL, et al. Erythropoietin concentrations in amniotic fluid and umbilical venous blood from Rh-immunized pregnancies. *J Perinat Med* 1993;21(3):225–234.
26. Mikovic Z, Mandic V, Parovic V, et al. Erythropoietin in amniotic fluid as a potential marker in distinction between growth restricted and constitutionally small fetuses. *J Matern Fetal Neonatal Med* 2014;27(11):1134–1137.

27. Teramo KA, Widness JA. Increased fetal plasma and amniotic fluid erythropoietin concentrations: markers of intrauterine hypoxia. *Neonatology* 2009;95(2):105–116.
28. Escobar J, Teramo K, Stefanovic V, et al. Amniotic fluid oxidative and nitrosative stress biomarkers correlate with fetal chronic hypoxia in diabetic pregnancies. *Neonatology* 2013;103(3):193–198.
29. Bhandari V, Buhimschi CS, Han CS, et al. Cord blood erythropoietin and interleukin-6 for prediction of intraventricular hemorrhage in the preterm neonate. *J Matern Fetal Neonatal Med* 2011;24(5):673–679.
30. Korzeniewski SJ, Allred E, Logan JW, et al. Elevated endogenous erythropoietin concentrations are associated with increased risk of brain damage in extremely preterm neonates. *PLoS One* 2015;10(3):e0115083.
31. Massaro AN, Wu YW, Bammler TK, et al. Plasma biomarkers of brain injury in neonatal hypoxic-ischemic encephalopathy. *J Pediatr* 2018;194:67.e1–75.e1.
32. Ohls RK, Harcum J, Li Y, et al. Serum erythropoietin concentrations fail to increase after significant phlebotomy losses in ill preterm infants. *J Perinatol* 1997;17(6):465–467.
33. Valieva OA, Strandjord TP, Mayock DE, et al. Effects of transfusions in extremely low birth weight infants: a retrospective study. *J Pediatr* 2009;155(3):331.e1–337.e1.
34. Widness JA. Pathophysiology of anemia during the neonatal period, including anemia of prematurity. *Neoreviews* 2008;9(11):e520.
35. Juul S. Neuroprotective role of erythropoietin in neonates. *J Matern Fetal Neonatal Med* 2012;25(Suppl 4):105–107.
36. Warwood TL, Ohls RK, Lambert DK, et al. Intravenous administration of darbepoetin to NICU patients. *J Perinatol* 2006;26(5):296–300.
37. Patel S, Ohls RK. Darbepoetin administration in term and preterm neonates. *Clin Perinatol* 2015;42(3):557–566.
38. Aher SM, Ohlsson A. Late erythropoiesis-stimulating agents to prevent red blood cell transfusion in preterm or low birth weight infants. *Cochrane Database Syst Rev* 2019;2:CD004868.
39. Ohlsson A, Aher SM. Early erythropoiesis-stimulating agents in preterm or low birth weight infants. *Cochrane Database Syst Rev* 2017;11:CD004863.
40. Dallacasa P, Ancora G, Miniero R, et al. Erythropoietin course in newborns with Rh hemolytic disease transfused and not transfused in utero. *Pediatr Res* 1996;40(2):357–360.
41. al-Alaiyan S, al Omran A. Late hyporegenerative anemia in neonates with rhesus hemolytic disease. *J Perinat Med* 1999;27(2):112–115.
42. Koenig JM, Ashton RD, De Vore GR, et al. Late hyporegenerative anemia in Rh hemolytic disease. *J Pediatr* 1989;115(2):315–318.
43. Rayjada N, Barton L, Chan LS, et al. Decrease in incidence of bronchopulmonary dysplasia with erythropoietin administration in preterm infants: a retrospective study. *Neonatology* 2012;102(4):287–292.
44. Warwood TL, Lambert DK, Henry E, et al. Very low birth weight infants qualifying for a 'late' erythrocyte transfusion: does giving darbepoetin along with the transfusion counteract the transfusion's erythropoietic suppression? *J Perinatol* 2011;31(Suppl 1):S17–S21.
45. Zuppa AA, Alighieri G, Calabrese V, et al. Recombinant human erythropoietin in the prevention of late anemia in intrauterine transfused neonates with Rh-isoimmunization. *J Pediatr Hematol Oncol* 2010;32(3):e95–e101.
46. Zuppa AA, Cardiello V, Alighieri G, et al. Anti-Rh(c), "little c," isoimmunization: the role of rHuEpo in preventing late anemia. *J Pediatr Hematol Oncol* 2013;35(6):e269–e271.
47. Christensen RD, Hunter DD, Goodell H, et al. Evaluation of the mechanism causing anemia in infants with bronchopulmonary dysplasia. *J Pediatr* 1992;120(4 Pt 1):593–598.
48. Ohls RK, Hunter DD, Christensen RD. A randomized, double-blind, placebo-controlled trial of recombinant erythropoietin in treatment of the anemia of bronchopulmonary dysplasia. *J Pediatr* 1993;123(6):996–1000.
49. Fauchere JC, Koller BM, Tschopp A, et al. Safety of early high-dose recombinant erythropoietin for neuroprotection in very preterm infants. *J Pediatr* 2015;167(1):52.e1–e3–57.e1–e3.
50. Shaddy RE, Bullock EA, Tani LY, et al. Epoetin alfa therapy in infants awaiting heart transplantation. *Arch Pediatr Adolesc Med* 1995;149(3):322–325.
51. Ootaki Y, Yamaguchi M, Yoshimura N, et al. The efficacy of preoperative administration of a single dose of recombinant human erythropoietin in pediatric cardiac surgery. *Heart Surg Forum* 2007;10(2):E115–E119.
52. Holt RL, Martin TD, Hess PJ, et al. Jehovah's Witnesses requiring complex urgent cardiothoracic surgery. *Ann Thorac Surg* 2004;78(2):695–697.
53. Bierer R, Roohi M, Peceny C, et al. Erythropoietin increases reticulocyte counts and maintains hematocrit in neonates requiring surgery. *J Pediatr Surg* 2009;44(8):1540–1545.
54. Egrie JC, Browne JK. Development and characterization of novel erythropoiesis stimulating protein (NESP). *Br J Cancer* 2001;84(Suppl 1):3–10.
55. Overbay DK, Manley HJ. Darbepoetin-alpha: a review of the literature. *Pharmacotherapy* 2002;22(7):889–897.
56. Juul S. Erythropoietin in anemia of prematurity. *J Matern Fetal Neonatal Med* 2012;25(Suppl 5):80–84.
57. Garcia MG, Hutson AD, Christensen RD. Effect of recombinant erythropoietin on "late" transfusions in the neonatal intensive care unit: a meta-analysis. *J Perinatol* 2002;22(2):108–111.
58. Calhoun DA, Christensen RD, Edstrom CS, et al. Consistent approaches to procedures and practices in neonatal hematology. *Clin Perinatol* 2000;27(3):733–753.
59. Ohls RK, Christensen RD. Stability of human recombinant epoetin alfa in commonly used neonatal intravenous solutions. *Ann Pharmacother* 1996;30(5):466–468.
60. German K, Vu PT, Grelli KN, et al. Zinc protoporphyrin-to-heme ratio and ferritin as measures of iron sufficiency in the neonatal intensive care unit. *J Pediatr* 2018;194:47–53.
61. Kakimoto-Shino M, Toya Y, Kuji T, et al. Changes in hepcidin and reticulocyte hemoglobin equivalent levels in response to continuous erythropoietin receptor activator administration in hemodialysis patients: a randomized study. *Ther Apher Dial* 2014;18(5):421–426.
62. Lorenz L, Arand J, Büchner K, et al. Reticulocyte haemoglobin content as a marker of iron deficiency. *Arch Dis Child Fetal Neonatal Ed* 2015;100(3):F198–F202.
63. Al-Ghananim RT, Nalbant D, Schmidt RL, et al. Reticulocyte hemoglobin content during the first month of life in critically ill very low birth weight neonates differs from term infants, children, and adults. *J Clin Lab Anal* 2016;30(4):326–334.
64. Ohls RK, Christensen RD, Kamath-Rayne BD, et al. A randomized, masked, placebo-controlled study of darbepoetin alfa in preterm infants. *Pediatrics* 2013;132(1): e119–e127.
65. Keller F, Ludwig U, Czock D. Pharmacokinetic and pharmacodynamic considerations on the erythropoietin effect and adverse events of darbepoetin. *Expert Opin Drug Metab Toxicol* 2015;11(1):139–147.
66. An G, Ohls RK, Christensen RD, et al. Population pharmacokinetics of darbepoetin in infants following single intravenous and subcutaneous dosing. *J Pharm Sci* 2017;106(6):1644–1649.
67. Juul SE, McPherson RJ, Bauer LA, et al. A phase I/II trial of high-dose erythropoietin in extremely low birth weight infants: pharmacokinetics and safety. *Pediatrics* 2008;122(2):383–391.
68. Wu YW, Mathur AM, Chang T, et al. High-dose erythropoietin and hypothermia for hypoxic-ischemic encephalopathy: a phase II trial. *Pediatrics* 2016;137(6):e20160191.
69. Frymoyer A, Juul SE, Massaro AN, et al. High-dose erythropoietin population pharmacokinetics in neonates with hypoxic-ischemic encephalopathy receiving hypothermia. *Pediatr Res* 2017;81(6):865–872.
70. Widness JA, Veng-Pedersen P, Peters C, et al. Erythropoietin pharmacokinetics in premature infants: developmental, nonlinearity, and treatment effects. *J Appl Physiol* 1996;80(1):140–148.
71. Krishnan R, Shankaran S, Krishnan M, et al. Pharmacokinetics of erythropoietin following single-dose subcutaneous administration in preterm infants. *Biol Neonate* 1996;70(3):135–140.
72. Kumar P, Shankaran S, Krishnan RG. Recombinant human erythropoietin therapy for treatment of anemia of prematurity in very low birth weight infants: a randomized, double-blind, placebo-controlled trial. *J Perinatol* 1998;18(3):173–177.
73. Widness JA, Veng-Pedersen P, Schmidt RL, et al. In vivo 125I-erythropoietin pharmacokinetics are unchanged after anesthesia, nephrectomy and hepatectomy in sheep. *J Pharmacol Exp Ther* 1996;279(3):1205–1210.
74. Ismail N, Ikizler TA. Erythropoietin-induced hypertension. *J Med Liban* 1997;45(1):25–30.
75. Wolf RF, Gilmore LS, Friese P, et al. Erythropoietin potentiates thrombus development in a canine arterio-venous shunt model. *Thromb Haemost* 1997;77(5):1020–1024.
76. Casadevall N. Pure red cell aplasia and anti-erythropoietin antibodies in patients treated with epoetin. *Nephrol Dial Transplant* 2003;18(Suppl 8):37–41.
77. Delanty N, Vaughan C, Frucht S, et al. Erythropoietin-associated hypertensive posterior leukoencephalopathy. *Neurology* 1997;49(3):686–689.
78. Tasman W, Patz A, McNamara JA, et al. Retinopathy of prematurity: the life of a lifetime disease. *Am J Ophthalmol* 2006;141(1):167–174.
79. Palmer EA, Flynn JT, Hardy RJ, et al. Incidence and early course of retinopathy of prematurity. The Cryotherapy for Retinopathy of Prematurity Cooperative Group. *Ophthalmology* 1991;98(11):1628–1640.
80. Ashton N. Oxygen and the retinal blood vessels. *Trans Ophthalmol Soc UK* 1980;100(3): 359–362.
81. Ohlsson A, Aher SM. Early erythropoietin for preventing red blood cell transfusion in preterm and/or low birth weight infants. *Cochrane Database Syst Rev* 2006;3:CD004863.
82. Xu XJ, Huang HY, Chen HL. Erythropoietin and retinopathy of prematurity: a meta-analysis. *Eur J Pediatr* 2014;173(10):1355–1364.
83. Slusarski JD, McPherson RJ, Wallace GN, et al. High-dose erythropoietin does not exacerbate retinopathy of prematurity in rats. *Pediatr Res* 2009;66(6):625–630.
84. Li Y, Juul SE, Morris-Wiman JA, et al. Erythropoietin receptors are expressed in the central nervous system of mid-trimester human fetuses. *Pediatr Res* 1996;40(3):376–380.
85. Masuda S, Okano M, Yamagishi K, et al. A novel site of erythropoietin production. Oxygen-dependent production in cultured rat astrocytes. *J Biol Chem* 1994;269(30): 19488–19493.
86. Brines M, Cerami A. Emerging biological roles for erythropoietin in the nervous system. *Nat Rev Neurosci* 2005;6(6):484–494.
87. Brines ML, Ghezzi P, Keenan S, et al. Erythropoietin crosses the blood-brain barrier to protect against experimental brain injury. *Proc Natl Acad Sci U S A* 2000;97(19):10526–10531.
88. Demers EJ, McPherson RJ, Juul SE. Erythropoietin protects dopaminergic neurons and improves neurobehavioral outcomes in juvenile rats after neonatal hypoxia-ischemia. *Pediatr Res* 2005;58(2):297–301.
89. Sun Y, Calvert JW, Zhang JH. Neonatal hypoxia/ischemia is associated with decreased inflammatory mediators after erythropoietin administration. *Stroke* 2005;36(8):1672–1678.
90. van der Kooij MA, Groenendaal F, Kavelaars A, et al. Neuroprotective properties and mechanisms of erythropoietin in in vitro and in vivo experimental models for hypoxia/ischemia. *Brain Res Rev* 2008;59(1):22–33.
91. Pett GC, Juul SE. The potential of erythropoietin to treat asphyxia in newborns. *Res Rep Neonatol* 2014;4:195–207.
92. Rangarajan V, Juul SE. Erythropoietin: emerging role of erythropoietin in neonatal neuroprotection. *Pediatr Neurol* 2014;51(4):481–488.
93. McPherson RJ, Demers EJ, Juul SE. Safety of high-dose recombinant erythropoietin in a neonatal rat model. *Neonatology* 2007;91(1):36–43.
94. Wassink G, Davidson JO, Dhillon SK, et al. Partial white and grey matter protection with prolonged infusion of recombinant human erythropoietin after asphyxia in preterm fetal sheep. *J Cereb Blood Flow Metab* 2017;37(3):1080–1094.
95. Traudt CM, McPherson RJ, Bauer LA, et al. Concurrent erythropoietin and hypothermia treatment improve outcomes in a term nonhuman primate model of perinatal asphyxia. *Dev Neurosci* 2013;35(6):491–503.
96. Kumral A, Genc S, Ozer E, et al. Erythropoietin downregulates bax and DP5 proapoptotic gene expression in neonatal hypoxic-ischemic brain injury. *Biol Neonate* 2006;89(3):205–210.
97. Sun Y, Zhou C, Polk P, et al. Mechanisms of erythropoietin-induced brain protection in neonatal hypoxia-ischemia rat model. *J Cereb Blood Flow Metab* 2004;24(2):259–270.
98. Spandou E, Soubasi V, Papoutsopoulou S, et al. Erythropoietin prevents hypoxia/ischemia-induced DNA fragmentation in an experimental model of perinatal asphyxia. *Neurosci Lett* 2004;366(1):24–28.

99. Villa P, Bigini P, Mennini T, et al. Erythropoietin selectively attenuates cytokine production and inflammation in cerebral ischemia by targeting neuronal apoptosis. *J Exp Med* 2003;198(6):971–975.
100. Sakanaka M, Wen TC, Matsuda S, et al. In vivo evidence that erythropoietin protects neurons from ischemic damage. *Proc Natl Acad Sci U S A* 1998;95(8):4635–4640.
101. Bryl E, Myśliwska J, Debska-Slizień A, et al. The influence of recombinant human erythropoietin on tumor necrosis factor alpha and interleukin-10 production by whole blood cell cultures in hemodialysis patients. *Artif Organs* 1998;22(3):177–181.
102. Chattopadhyay A, Choudhury TD, Bandyopadhyay D, et al. Protective effect of erythropoietin on the oxidative damage of erythrocyte membrane by hydroxyl radical. *Biochem Pharmacol* 2000;59(4):419–425.
103. Bany-Mohammed FM, Slivka S, Hallman M. Recombinant human erythropoietin: possible role as an antioxidant in premature rabbits. *Pediatr Res* 1996;40(3):381–387.
104. Keller M, Yang J, Griesmaier E, et al. Erythropoietin is neuroprotective against NMDA-receptor-mediated excitotoxic brain injury in newborn mice. *Neurobiol Dis* 2006;24(2):357–366.
105. Kawakami M, Iwasakia S, Sato K, et al. Erythropoietin inhibits calcium-induced neurotransmitter release from clonal neuronal cells. *Biochem Biophys Res Commun* 2000;279(1):293–297.
106. Tsai PT, Ohab JJ, Kertesz N, et al. A critical role of erythropoietin receptor in neurogenesis and post-stroke recovery. *J Neurosci* 2006;26(4):1269–1274.
107. Wang L, Zhang Z, Wang Y, et al. Treatment of stroke with erythropoietin enhances neurogenesis and angiogenesis and improves neurological function in rats. *Stroke* 2004;35(7):1732–1737.
108. Solaroglu I, Solaroglu A, Kaptanoglu E, et al. Erythropoietin prevents ischemia-reperfusion from inducing oxidative damage in fetal rat brain. *Childs Nerv Syst* 2003;19(1):19–22.
109. Juul SE, Pet GC. Erythropoietin and neonatal neuroprotection. *Clin Perinatol* 2015;42(3):469–481.
110. Juul SE, Comstock BA, Heagerty PJ, et al. High-dose erythropoietin for asphyxia and encephalopathy (HEAL): a randomized controlled trial—background, aims, and study protocol. *Neonatology* 2018;113(4):331–338.
111. Fischer H, Reibel NJ, Bührer C, et al. Prophylactic early erythropoietin for neuroprotection in preterm infants: a meta-analysis. *Pediatrics* 2017;139(5):e20164317.
112. Wang H, Zhang L, Jin Y. A meta-analysis of the protective effect of recombinant human erythropoietin (rhEPO) for neurodevelopment in preterm infants. *Cell Biochem Biophys* 2015;71(2):795–802.
113. Garg B, Sharma D, Bansal A. Systematic review seeking erythropoietin role for neuroprotection in neonates with hypoxic ischemic encephalopathy: presently where do we stand. *J Matern Fetal Neonatal Med* 2018;31(23):3214–3224.
114. Juul SE, Mayock DE, Comstock BA, et al. Neuroprotective potential of erythropoietin in neonates; design of a randomized trial. *Matern Health Neonatol Perinatol* 2015;1:27.
115. Ruegger CM, Hagmann CF, Bührer C, et al. Erythropoietin for the repair of cerebral injury in very preterm infants (EpoRepair). *Neonatology* 2015;108(3):198–204.
116. Benders MJ, van der Aa NE, Roks M, et al. Feasibility and safety of erythropoietin for neuroprotection after perinatal arterial ischemic stroke. *J Pediatr* 2014;164(3):481.e1–e2–486.e1–e2.
117. Malla RR, Asimi R, Teli MA, et al. Erythropoietin monotherapy in perinatal asphyxia with moderate to severe encephalopathy: a randomized placebo-controlled trial. *J Perinatol* 2017;37(5):596–601.
118. Dallman PR. Biochemical basis for the manifestations of iron deficiency. *Annu Rev Nutr* 1986;6:13–40.
119. Lozoff B, Jimenez E, Hagen J, et al. Poorer behavioral and developmental outcome more than 10 years after treatment for iron deficiency in infancy. *Pediatrics* 2000;105(4):E51.
120. Juul SE, Joyce AE, Zhao Y, et al. Why is erythropoietin present in human milk? studies of erythropoietin receptors on enterocytes of human and rat neonates. *Pediatr Res* 1999;46(3):263–268.
121. Juul SE, Ledbetter D, Joyce A, et al. Erythropoietin acts as a trophic factor in neonatal rat intestine. *Gut* 2001;49(2):182–189.
122. Shiou SR, Yu Y, Chen S, et al. Erythropoietin protects intestinal epithelial barrier function and lowers the incidence of experimental neonatal necrotizing enterocolitis. *J Biol Chem* 2011;286(14):12123–12132.
123. Kling PJ, Willeitner A, Dvorak B, et al. Enteral erythropoietin and iron stimulate erythropoiesis in suckling rats. *J Pediatr Gastroenterol Nutr* 2008;46(2):202–207.
124. Juul SE, Christensen RD. Absorption of enteral recombinant human erythropoietin by neonates. *Ann Pharmacother* 2003;37(6):782–786.
125. Juul SE. Enterally dosed recombinant human erythropoietin does not stimulate erythropoiesis in neonates. *J Pediatr* 2003;143(3):321–326.
126. Ledbetter DJ, Juul SE. Erythropoietin and the incidence of necrotizing enterocolitis in infants with very low birth weight. *J Pediatr Surg* 2000;35(2):178–181.
127. El-Ganzoury MM, Awad HA, El-Farrash RA, et al. Enteral granulocyte-colony stimulating factor and erythropoietin early in life improves feeding tolerance in preterm infants: a randomized controlled trial. *J Pediatr* 2014;165(6):1140.e1–1145.e1.
128. Cairo MS. Review of G-CSF and GM-CSF. Effects on neonatal neutrophil kinetics. *Am J Pediatr Hematol Oncol* 1989;11(2):238–244.
129. Xiao BG, Lu CZ, Link H. Cell biology and clinical promise of G-CSF: immunomodulation and neuroprotection. *J Cell Mol Med* 2007;11(6):1272–1290.
130. Bensinger W, Appelbaum F, Rowley S, et al. Factors that influence collection and engraftment of autologous peripheral-blood stem cells. *J Clin Oncol* 1995;13(10):2547–2555.
131. Del Vecchio A, Christensen RD. Neonatal neutropenia: what diagnostic evaluation is needed and when is treatment recommended? *Early Hum Dev* 2012;88(Suppl 2):S19–S24.
132. Cairo MS. Neutrophil storage pool depletion in neonates with sepsis. *J Pediatr* 1989;114(6):1064–1065.
133. Lee JA, Sauer B, Tuminski W, et al. Effectiveness of granulocyte colony-stimulating factor in hospitalized infants with neutropenia. *Am J Perinatol* 2017;34(5):458–464.
134. Miura E, Procianoy RS, Bittar C, et al. A randomized, double-masked, placebo-controlled trial of recombinant granulocyte colony-stimulating factor administration to preterm infants with the clinical diagnosis of early-onset sepsis. *Pediatrics* 2001;107(1):30–35.
135. Carr R, Modi N, Doré C, et al. A randomized, controlled trial of prophylactic granulocyte-macrophage colony-stimulating factor in human newborns less than 32 weeks gestation. *Pediatrics* 1999;103(4 Pt 1):796–802.
136. Carr R, Modi N, Doré C. G-CSF and GM-CSF for treating or preventing neonatal infections. *Cochrane Database Syst Rev* 2003(3):CD003066.
137. Carr R, Brocklehurst P, Doré CJ, et al. Granulocyte-macrophage colony stimulating factor administered as prophylaxis for reduction of sepsis in extremely preterm, small for gestational age neonates (the PROGRAMS trial): a single-blind, multicentre, randomised controlled trial. *Lancet* 2009;373(9659):226–233.
138. Kuhn P, Messer J, Paupe A, et al. A multicenter, randomized, placebo-controlled trial of prophylactic recombinant granulocyte-colony stimulating factor in preterm neonates with neutropenia. *J Pediatr* 2009;155(3):324.e1–330.e1.
139. Christensen RD, Yoder BA, Baer VL, et al. Early-onset neutropenia in small-for-gestational-age infants. *Pediatrics* 2015;136(5):e1259–e1267.
140. Koenig JM, Christensen RD. Incidence, neutrophil kinetics, and natural history of neonatal neutropenia associated with maternal hypertension. *N Engl J Med* 1989;321(9):557–562.
141. Koenig JM, Christensen RD. The mechanism responsible for diminished neutrophil production in neonates delivered of women with pregnancy-induced hypertension. *Am J Obstet Gynecol* 1991;165(2):467–473.
142. Juul SE, Haynes JW, McPherson RJ. Evaluation of neutropenia and neutrophilia in hospitalized preterm infants. *J Perinatol* 2004;24(3):150–157.
143. Fraser SH, Tudehope DI. Neonatal neutropenia and thrombocytopenia following maternal hypertension. *J Paediatr Child Health* 1996;32(1):31–34.
144. Brazy JE, Grimm JK, Little VA. Neonatal manifestations of severe maternal hypertension occurring before the thirty-sixth week of pregnancy. *J Pediatr* 1982;100(2):265–271.
145. Bizerea TO, Stroescu R, Rogobete AF, et al. Pregnancy induced hypertension versus small weight for gestational age: cause of neonatal hematological disorders. *Clin Lab* 2018;64(7):1241–1248.
146. Maheshwari A, Christensen RD, Calhoun DA. Immune-mediated neutropenia in the neonate. *Acta Paediatr Suppl* 2002;91(438):98–103.
147. Maheshwari A, Christensen RD, Calhoun DA. Immune neutropenia in the neonate. *Adv Pediatr* 2002;49:317–339.
148. Lejkowski M, Maheshwari A, Calhoun DA, et al. Persistent perianal abscess in early infancy as a presentation of autoimmune neutropenia. *J Perinatol* 2003;23(5):428–430.
149. Dale DC, Bolyard AA. An update on the diagnosis and treatment of chronic idiopathic neutropenia. *Curr Opin Hematol* 2017;24(1):46–53.
150. Juul SE, Calhoun DA, Christensen RD. "Idiopathic neutropenia" in very low birthweight infants. *Acta Paediatr* 1998;87(9):963–968.
151. Juul SE, Christensen RD. Effect of recombinant granulocyte colony-stimulating factor on blood neutrophil concentrations among patients with "idiopathic neonatal neutropenia": a randomized, placebo-controlled trial. *J Perinatol* 2003;23(6):493–497.
152. Nagata S, Tsuchiya M, Asano S, et al. Molecular cloning and expression of cDNA for human granulocyte colony-stimulating factor. *Nature* 1986;319(6052):415–418.
153. Martin-Christin F. Granulocyte colony stimulating factors: how different are they? how to make a decision? *Anti-Cancer Drugs* 2001;12(3):185–191.
154. van der Auwera P, Platzer E, Xu ZX, et al. Pharmacodynamics and pharmacokinetics of single doses of subcutaneous pegylated human G-CSF mutant (Ro 25-8315) in healthy volunteers: comparison with single and multiple daily doses of filgrastim. *Am J Hematol* 2001;66(4):245–251.
155. Christensen RD, Calhoun DA, Rimsza LM. A practical approach to evaluating and treating neutropenia in the neonatal intensive care unit. *Clin Perinatol* 2000;27(3):577–601.
156. Gillan ER, Christensen RD, Suen Y, et al. A randomized, placebo-controlled trial of recombinant human granulocyte colony-stimulating factor administration in newborn infants with presumed sepsis: significant induction of peripheral and bone marrow neutrophilia. *Blood* 1994;84(5):1427–1433.
157. Calhoun DA, Lunøe M, Du Y, et al. Granulocyte colony-stimulating factor serum and urine concentrations in neutropenic neonates before and after intravenous administration of recombinant granulocyte colony-stimulating factor. *Pediatrics* 2000;105(2):392–397.
158. Gessler P, Neu S, Brockmann Y, et al. Decreased mRNA expression of G-CSF receptor in cord blood neutrophils of term newborns: regulation of expression by G-CSF and TNF-alpha. *Biol Neonate* 2000;77(3):168–173.
159. Ericson SG, Gao H, Gericke GH, et al. The role of polymorphonuclear neutrophils (PMNs) in clearance of granulocyte colony-stimulating factor (G-CSF) in vivo and in vitro. *Exp Hematol* 1997;25(13):1313–1325.
160. Kuwabara T, Kobayashi S, Sugiyama Y. Pharmacokinetics and pharmacodynamics of a recombinant human granulocyte colony-stimulating factor. *Drug Metab Rev* 1996;28(4):625–658.
161. Calhoun DA, Donnelly WH Jr, Du Y, et al. Distribution of granulocyte colony-stimulating factor (G-CSF) and G-CSF-receptor mRNA and protein in the human fetus. *Pediatr Res* 1999;46(3):333–338.
162. Gaertner HF, Offord RE. Site-specific attachment of functionalized poly(ethylene glycol) to the amino terminus of proteins. *Bioconjug Chem* 1996;7(1):38–44.
163. Kinstler OB, Brems DN, Lauren SL, et al. Characterization and stability of N-terminally PEGylated rhG-CSF. *Pharm Res* 1996;13(7):996–1002.
164. Tanaka H, Satake-Ishikawa R, Ishikawa M, et al. Pharmacokinetics of recombinant human granulocyte colony-stimulating factor conjugated to polyethylene glycol in rats. *Cancer Res* 1991;51(14):3710–3714.
165. Johnston E, Crawford J, Blackwell S, et al. Randomized, dose-escalation study of SD/01 compared with daily filgrastim in patients receiving chemotherapy. *J Clin Oncol* 2000;18(13):2522–2528.
166. Rosenthal J, Healey T, Ellis R, et al. A two-year follow-up of neonates with presumed sepsis treated with recombinant human granulocyte colony-stimulating factor during the first week of life. *J Pediatr* 1996;128(1):135–137.
167. Bedford Russell AR, Emmerson AJ, Wilkinson N, et al. A trial of recombinant human granulocyte colony stimulating factor for the treatment of very low birthweight infants with presumed sepsis and neutropenia. *Arch Dis Child Fetal Neonatal Ed* 2001;84(3): F172–F176.

168. Barak Y, Leibovitz E, Mogilner B, et al. The in vivo effect of recombinant human granulocyte-colony stimulating factor in neutropenic neonates with sepsis. *Eur J Pediatr* 1997;156(8):643–646.
169. Donadieu J, Boutard P, Bernatowska E, et al. A European phase II study of recombinant human granulocyte colony-stimulating factor (lenograstim) in the treatment of severe chronic neutropenia in children. Lenograstim Study Group. *Eur J Pediatr* 1997;156(9):693–700.
170. Gilmore MM, Stroncek DF, Korones DN. Treatment of alloimmune neonatal neutropenia with granulocyte colony-stimulating factor. *J Pediatr* 1994;125(6 Pt 1):948–951.
171. Feng X, Lan H, Ruan Y, et al. Impact on acute myeloid leukemia relapse in granulocyte colony-stimulating factor application: a meta-analysis. *Hematology* 2018;23(9):581–589.
172. Li AM, Thyagu S, Maze D, et al. Prolonged granulocyte colony stimulating factor use in glycogen storage disease type 1b associated with acute myeloid leukemia and with shortened telomere length. *Pediatr Hematol Oncol* 2018;35(1):45–51.
173. Ueno K, Nomura Y, Arata M, et al. Development of Kawasaki syndrome in autoimmune neutropenia after treatment with granulocyte colony-stimulating factor. *Pediatr Int* 2011;53(3):388–390.
174. Bonilla MA, Dale D, Zeidler C, et al. Long-term safety of treatment with recombinant human granulocyte colony-stimulating factor (r-metHuG-CSF) in patients with severe congenital neutropenias. *Br J Haematol* 1994;88(4):723–730.
175. Germeshausen M, Skokowa J, Ballmaier M, et al. G-CSF receptor mutations in patients with congenital neutropenia. *Curr Opin Hematol* 2008;15(4):332–337.
176. Cottle TE, Fier CJ, Donadieu J, et al. Risk and benefit of treatment of severe chronic neutropenia with granulocyte colony-stimulating factor. *Semin Hematol* 2002;39(2):134–140.
177. Dale DC, Bolyard AA, Schwinzer BG, et al. The Severe Chronic Neutropenia International Registry: 10-year follow-up report. *Support Cancer Ther* 2006;3(4):220–231.
178. Schabitz WR, Kollmar R, Schwaninger M, et al. Neuroprotective effect of granulocyte colony-stimulating factor after focal cerebral ischemia. *Stroke* 2003;34(3):745–751.
179. Schneider A, Kuhn HG, Schabitz WR. A role for G-CSF (granulocyte-colony stimulating factor) in the central nervous system. *Cell Cycle* 2005;4(12):1753–1757.
180. Solaroglu I, Cahill J, Jadhav V, et al. A novel neuroprotectant granulocyte-colony stimulating factor. *Stroke* 2006;37(4):1123–1128.
181. Schneider A, Krüger C, Steigleder T, et al. The hematopoietic factor G-CSF is a neuronal ligand that counteracts programmed cell death and drives neurogenesis. *J Clin Invest* 2005;115(8):2083–2098.
182. Gibson CL, Bath PM, Murphy SP. G-CSF reduces infarct volume and improves functional outcome after transient focal cerebral ischemia in mice. *J Cereb Blood Flow Metab* 2005;25(4):431–439.
183. Fathali N, Lekic T, Zhang JH, et al. Long-term evaluation of granulocyte-colony stimulating factor on hypoxic-ischemic brain damage in infant rats. *Int Care Med* 2010;36(9):1602–1608.
184. Lee ST, Chu K, Jung K-H, et al. Granulocyte colony-stimulating factor enhances angiogenesis after focal cerebral ischemia. *Brain Res* 2005;1058(1–2):120–128.
185. Komine-Kobayashi M, Zhang N, Liu M, et al. Neuroprotective effect of recombinant human granulocyte colony-stimulating factor in transient focal ischemia of mice. *J Cereb Blood Flow Metab* 2006;26(3):402–413.
186. Keller M, Simbruner G, Górna A, et al. Systemic application of granulocyte-colony stimulating factor and stem cell factor exacerbates excitotoxic brain injury in newborn mice. *Pediatr Res* 2006;59(4 Pt 1):549–553.
187. Castagnola E, Dufour C. Role of G-CSF GM-CSF in the management of infections in preterm newborns: an update. *Early Hum Dev* 2014;90(Suppl 2):S15–S17.
188. Shane AL, Sanchez PJ, Stoll BJ. Neonatal sepsis. *Lancet* 2017;390(10104):1770–1780.
189. Marlow N, Morris T, Brocklehurst P, et al. A randomised trial of granulocyte-macrophage colony-stimulating factor for neonatal sepsis: childhood outcomes at 5 years. *Arch Dis Child Fetal Neonatal Ed* 2015;100(4):F320–F326.
190. Lau AS, Lehman D, Geertsma FR, et al. Biology and therapeutic uses of myeloid hematopoietic growth factors and interferons. *Pediatr Infect Dis J* 1996;15(7):563–575.
191. Carr R, Modi N. Haemopoietic colony stimulating factors for preterm neonates. *Arch Dis Child Fetal Neonatal Ed* 1997;76(2):F128–F133.
192. Sullivan GW, Carper HT, Mandell GL. The effect of three human recombinant hematopoietic growth factors (granulocyte-macrophage colony-stimulating factor, granulocyte colony-stimulating factor, and interleukin-3) on phagocyte oxidative activity. *Blood* 1993;81(7):1863–1870.
193. Sreenan C, Osiovich H. Myeloid colony-stimulating factors: use in the newborn. *Arch Pediatr Adolesc Med* 1999;153(9):984–988.
194. Ray M, Mukhopadhyay K, Narang A. Granulocyte macrophage-colony stimulating factor (GM-CSF) in neonatal neutropenia. *Indian J Pediatr* 2000;67(1):67–68.
195. Wolach B, Gavrieli R, Pomeranz A. Effect of granulocyte and granulocyte macrophage colony stimulating factors (G-CSF and GM-CSF) on neonatal neutrophil functions. *Pediatr Res* 2000;48(3):369–373.

Stacey L. Berg
Jennifer H. Foster
Lisa R. Bomgaars

CHAPTER 59

Clinical Pharmacology of Antineoplastic Drugs

Safe administration of antineoplastic therapy to children remains a challenge. Among the most critical issues are the toxicity of antineoplastic drugs and the developmental heterogeneity of the pediatric population. Antineoplastic agents have the lowest therapeutic index of any drugs in clinical use. Because cancer is life-threatening, clinicians and patients are willing to tolerate toxicity from anticancer agents that would be unacceptable for any other class of drugs. Furthermore, these agents are virtually always used in combination, even when the interactions among the agents selected are poorly understood. Children of any age, from newborn to adolescent, may require therapy, yet the impact of developmental factors on the pharmacology of antineoplastic drugs is seldom known. In particular, neonates and young infants, who are most likely to differ physiologically from older children and adults, represent such a small number of pediatric cancer cases that there is relatively little opportunity to study the clinical pharmacology of drugs in this population, despite the critical importance of the data to be obtained.

In this chapter, we apply general principles of pharmacology, including absorption, distribution, metabolism, and elimination, to an overview of the antineoplastic drugs commonly used to treat childhood cancer. Because these agents do not comprise one homogeneous class, we consider mechanism of action as a general characteristic that must be understood about each drug before the pharmacology of the agent can be fully appreciated. We illustrate the way that each basic pharmacologic principle may be applied to antineoplastic agents using specific drugs as examples, then discuss the way that understanding individual drugs can be used to design the combination chemotherapy regimens that are the cornerstone of anticancer treatment for children. Finally, we review special considerations in the pharmacology of antineoplastic drugs in infants and younger children.

MECHANISMS OF ACTION

Understanding drug mechanism of action is useful in making rational decisions about the dose and administration schedule for individual drugs as well as about logical ways to combine drugs into multiagent regimens. For example, antimetabolites are considered cell-cycle phase specific because they produce cytotoxicity during S phase, when they can be incorporated as fraudulent substrates into replicating DNA. Thus, these agents are often administered by prolonged infusion or in multiple daily doses to increase the likelihood that drug will be present when cells are passing through S phase. Similarly, logical combinations of agents may be based on nonoverlapping mechanisms of resistance or nonoverlapping toxicities, but they may also take advantage of mechanism of action by inhibiting the same intracellular process at different points in its pathway, or by taking advantage of lesions induced by one drug to potentiate the activity of another (as discussed later).[1] Some commonly used anticancer drugs and their mechanisms of action are listed in Table 59.1.

Many anticancer drugs work by interfering at some stage with the synthesis or function of DNA and RNA in tumor cells. These disruptions usually induce apoptosis as the final common pathway of cell death and are not tumor specific.[2–5] In the past, potential anticancer drugs were usually identified in general screens for cytotoxicity, such as the National Cancer Institute panel of tumor cell lines.[6,7] More recently, however, drug development has focused on agents that target specific molecular aberrations in tumor cells that drive the cancer phenotype.

The antimetabolites, structural analogs of normal intracellular molecules, act as fraudulent substrate enzymes in critical biochemical pathways. Antimetabolites are among the oldest anticancer agents in clinical use, and they can be viewed as rationally synthesized agents because they are specifically designed to take advantage of well-characterized biochemical pathways, although the pathways are not specific to tumor cells. Many antimetabolites act as prodrugs that require metabolic activation; this feature is discussed in detail in the section on biotransformation. Antimetabolites exert their cytotoxicity by inhibiting enzymatically catalyzed steps in the synthesis of nucleic acids or by being incorporated into DNA or RNA, resulting in defective products. The antimetabolites most commonly used in children include cytarabine (Ara-C), 6-mercaptopurine (MP), thioguanine (TG), and methotrexate. Other antimetabolites with activity in pediatric cancers include nelarabine (Ara-G) in T-cell malignancies,[8–11] clofarabine in relapsed acute lymphoblastic leukemia,[12,13] and gemcitabine in sarcomas.[14–16]

Many conventional anticancer agents exert their cytotoxicity by producing interstrand and intrastrand cross-links or strand

TABLE 59.1 Mechanism of Action of Commonly Used Anticancer Drugs

Drug Class	*Examples*	*Mechanism of Action*
Alkylating agents	Cyclophosphamide	Forms DNA cross-links
	Ifosfamide	
	Cisplatin	
	Carboplatin	
	Temozolomide	
Anthracyclines	Daunomycin Doxorubicin Idarubicin	Intercalates into DNA; inhibits topoisomerase-II
Epipodophyllotoxins	Etoposide (VP-16)	Inhibits topoisomerase-II
	Teniposide (VM-26)	
Antimetabolites	Methotrexate	Inhibits dehydrofolate reductase
	Cytarabine	Forms fraudulent substrates
	6-Mercaptopurine	
Vinca alkaloids	Vincristine	Inhibits microtubule assembly
Taxanes	Paclitaxel	Stabilizes microtubules
	Docetaxel	
Camptothecin analogs	Topotecan	Inhibits topoisomerase-I
	Irinotecan	
Molecularly targeted agents	Imatinib mesylate (Gleevec)	Inhibits bcr–abl tyrosine kinase, c-Kit, and PDGF-R pathways
Receptor tyrosine kinase inhibitors	Larotrectinib, entrectinib	Inhibit *trk*, *alk*, *ros* pathways
Immunotherapy	Tisagenlecleucel, blinatumomab	Anti-CD19 CAR-T cell, antibody

CAR, chimeric antigen receptor; PDGF-R, platelet-derived growth factor receptor.

breaks in DNA. Alkylating agents, such as cyclophosphamide and ifosfamide, form covalent bonds with intracellular molecules, including DNA as the primary target.[17] Although cisplatin and carboplatin are not classical alkylating agents, they also undergo similar chemical reactions to form covalent bonds and cross-links like those formed by alkylating agents.[18]

The anthracycline antitumor antibiotics doxorubicin, daunomycin, and idarubicin and the related compound actinomycin D have planar multiring structures that can intercalate into the double helix of DNA, interfering with its replication and transcription. The cytotoxicity of the anthracyclines results from DNA strand breaks that are mediated by the enzyme topoisomerase-II.[19,20] The anthracyclines also undergo enzymatic reduction to form free radicals. It is not known whether these highly reactive compounds contribute to the antitumor effect of the anthracyclines, but they may contribute in part to their well-known cardiac toxicity via direct damage or through effects on mitochondria and calcium signaling.[19,21–23] Anthracycline toxicity can be ameliorated by coadministration of the iron-chelating agent dexrazoxane.[24]

The epipodophyllotoxins etoposide (VP-16) and teniposide (VM-26) also interact with topoisomerase-II to produce DNA strand breaks, but they do not intercalate into DNA. Topoisomerase-II is normally responsible for opening and rejoining DNA during replication, but in the presence of an epipodophyllotoxin, the strand-closing reaction is blocked.[25,26] The camptothecin analog irinotecan inhibits topoisomerase-I, a nuclear enzyme involved in DNA uncoiling during replication.[27] Treatment with camptothecins leads to the formation of DNA–topoisomerase-I adducts and single-strand DNA breaks.[27]

Tubulin, a structural protein that polymerizes to form microtubules, which are critical for successful completion of mitosis, is the intracellular target for several classes of anticancer agents. The *Vinca* alkaloids vincristine and vinblastine bind to tubulin, thus blocking microtubule assembly, preventing the formation of the mitotic spindle and inhibiting mitosis.[25] In contrast, the taxanes paclitaxel and its semisynthetic analog docetaxel also interact with microtubules, but these agents block mitosis by stabilizing microtubules, preventing their normal disassembly.[28–30] Although taxanes have well-defined roles in the treatment of adult cancers, they appear to have limited utility in pediatric tumors and are not widely used.

The bacterial enzyme L-asparaginase, first identified in the 1950s in guinea pig serum,[31] depletes the circulating pool of the amino acid L-asparagine, which is nonessential in mammals. Lymphoblasts, however, lack the enzyme that converts aspartic acid to asparagine and, therefore, are dependent on the presence of L-asparagine to maintain protein synthesis.[32] L-Asparaginase therapy is an important component of lymphoblastic leukemia treatment. Because it is a foreign protein, administration often results in production of antibodies. While overt allergic reactions are clinically significant, development of the so-called "silent antibodies" may also be important as it results in altered pharmacokinetics, with rapid inactivation of drug potentially leading to decreased efficacy.[33,34]

Although the cytotoxic agents discussed above remain the backbone of anticancer therapy, the development of molecularly targeted agents is revolutionizing oncology. Proof of principle is the tyrosine kinase inhibitor imatinib mesylate (Gleevec). This agent inhibits the bcr–abl tyrosine kinase that results from the Philadelphia (9,22) chromosome translocation in chronic myelogenous leukemia (CML).[35,36] It also inhibits platelet-derived growth factor receptor (PDGF-R), stem cell factor (SCF) receptor, and c-*kit*–mediated signaling.[37–39] Imatinib mesylate is active in most patients with CML as well as in some patients with Philadelphia chromosome–positive acute lymphocytic leukemia (Ph + ALL).[36,40–47] Imatinib also provides the prototypical example of resistance conferred by a point mutation in the molecular target[48] and the ability to restore therapeutic effect with a similar inhibitor that is not affected by the mutation.[49,50] Imatinib, dasatinib, and nilotinib are approved for the treatment of pediatric Ph + ALL. Other molecularly targeted agents are rapidly entering therapeutic use in pediatric cancer. Larotrectinib, a receptor tyrosine kinase inhibitor, is highly active in neurotrophin tropomyosin receptor kinase (trk) fusion–driven sarcomas.[51,52] Entrectinib is also under investigation for *trk-*, *alk-*, and *ros*-mutated tumors.[53] Similarly, the anaplastic lymphoma kinase (ALK) inhibitor crizotinib has shown activity in pediatric lymphoma, inflammatory myofibroblastic tumor, as well as neuroblastoma.[54] The activity of these agents heralds an era in which treatment may be selected in a histology-agnostic manner based on the presence of molecular targets in tumors.

In addition to small molecules, immunotherapy may target specific tumor alterations. For example, both the anti-CD19 chimeric antigen receptor (CAR)-T-cell product tisagenlecleucel (Kymriah) and the bispecific T-cell engager antibody construct blinatumomab target CD19 on leukemic blasts and produce a high-response rate in pediatric ALL.[55,56] As with tyrosine kinase inhibitors, a single mutation, in this case loss of the CD19 antigen from leukemic blasts, may be sufficient to confer resistance.[57] CD22-targeted CAR-T cells may be effective when lymphoblasts lose CD19 expression.[58] Another form of immunotherapy with documented activity in pediatric cancer is the monoclonal antibody dinutuximab, which targets the disialoganglioside GD2 on the surface of neuroblastoma cells.[59] Conversely, checkpoint inhibitors, such as nivolumab and ipilimumab, which have been paradigm shifting in adult cancer treatment, have not shown marked activity in early pediatric testing, perhaps because the relatively low mutation burden of pediatric cancer results in a low level of nonspecific, neoantigen expression.[60–62]

PHARMACOKINETICS

Pharmacokinetics is the study of drug absorption, distribution, metabolism, and excretion. Understanding these processes may help to determine the proper dose, schedule, and route of administration for anticancer agents. In addition, modeling the pharmacokinetic behavior of a drug may yield important insights into relationships among things like dose and toxicity and response. In children, this understanding is particularly important because developmental physiologic differences between children and adults, such as the degree of drug absorption, plasma protein or tissue binding, distribution of drug in the various tissues of the body, and excretory organ function, may mean that the appropriate dose and schedule of administration of a given drug might be quite different in children from adults. In addition, understanding drug elimination pathways can be helpful when recommending dose adjustments for patients with hepatic or renal dysfunction.[63]

Among the most important pharmacokinetic concepts is systemic drug exposure, quantified by determining the area under the plasma concentration–time curve, or AUC. Measuring systemic drug exposure can be labor-intensive and often involves collaborative research efforts. For drugs administered by prolonged continuous infusion, determination of the steady-state plasma drug concentration is adequate. For drugs administered intermittently, determination of the AUC generally requires sampling at multiple points over a prolonged period. However, detailed pharmacokinetic modeling may permit development of a limited sampling strategy in which the AUC can be predicted from a small number of pharmacokinetic samples after drug distribution is thoroughly described in a relatively small initial group of patients.[64–66] This has been an effective strategy for targeting of busulfan AUCs in pediatric bone marrow transplant.[67] In addition, parameters other than AUC should also be evaluated for clinical correlations. For example, methotrexate toxicity depends more on the time that drug concentrations stay above certain levels than on the AUC (as discussed later).

ABSORPTION

Absorption refers to the movement of an agent from a peripheral site into the systemic circulation. Because oral administration is the most important nonintravenous route of anticancer drug administration, it is important to consider limitations produced by the gastrointestinal tract. After oral administration, drugs may be degraded by acids in the stomach, adsorbed by food or other medications, metabolized by enzymes in gut luminal cells, extracted by the liver in first-pass metabolism before a systemic effect can be produced, or simply not absorbed due to physicochemical characteristics of the drug molecule. The rate and extent of drug absorption after oral compared with intravenous administration is referred to as bioavailability. Before a drug can be incorporated into anticancer treatment regimen, its bioavailability must be understood. The most reliable way to study bioavailability is to compare plasma AUCs after oral and intravenous administration in the same patient; bioavailability is usually expressed as the fraction of the AUC after intravenous administration produced by oral administration.

The two agents most commonly administered by mouth in childhood anticancer therapy are methotrexate and mercaptopurine (MP), which are used in nearly all maintenance regimens for ALL. Both these agents exhibit considerable variation in bioavailability.[68–73] Concomitant food administration diminishes the absorption of both agents.[74,75] There may also be diurnal variation in the absorption or elimination of these drugs, as suggested by the observation that children who take oral methotrexate and MP in the evening appear to have lower risk of relapse than those who take them in the morning.[76–79]

Bioavailability of methotrexate at low doses (7.5 to 40 mg per m^2) is quite variable. In one study, absorption ranged from 23% to 95%.[68] Furthermore, methotrexate absorption appears to be saturable, with a plateau in AUC observed at doses of 30 mg per m^2.[68,80,81] Therefore, the relationship between dose and AUC is not linear for oral methotrexate. To overcome these limitations, intramuscular administration is sometimes used instead of oral administration of methotrexate. In one study of children with ALL, intramuscular injection of methotrexate resulted in approximately twice the bioavailability of oral administration, and at doses exceeding 40 mg per m^2, intramuscular absorption did not show the same nonlinearity as oral administration.[81]

Oral administration of MP also results in variable systemic exposure. MP undergoes extensive first-pass metabolism in the liver and gut mucosa by the enzyme xanthine oxidase.[73,82] In addition, there is considerable interpatient variability of plasma MP concentrations even when the dose is administered under fasting conditions.[71–73] Intrapatient variability has also been observed with repeated monitoring of individual patients.[73]

Other agents may have more predictable bioavailability after oral administration. The absorption of prednisone and dexamethasone is greater than 80%,[83,84] although variability in the absorption of prednisone has been reported in children.[85] Oral busulfan is rapidly absorbed, with a bioavailability of 70% in children.[86,87] Interestingly, there appears to be circadian variation in busulfan plasma concentrations, with the highest troughs occurring in the early morning.[88]

DISTRIBUTION

Distribution of a drug refers to its transfer among various tissues, blood, tumor, and any other compartments. Although it is possible to measure drug concentrations in different tissues under laboratory conditions, it is not feasible to do so in most clinical settings. Drug concentrations in various compartments can be estimated using pharmacokinetic modeling techniques, but the compartments referred to in models do not usually correlate directly with physiologic compartments. However, the use of pharmacokinetic models, in addition to preclinical studies, permits some conclusions to be drawn about the distribution of most anticancer agents. For example, the pharmacokinetic behavior of both the anthracyclines and the *Vinca* alkaloids is consistent with extensive tissue binding. Disappearance of these drugs from plasma drug during the distributive phase is extremely rapid, with a distribution half-life of less than 10 minutes. These agents also exhibit volumes of distribution that are much larger than the circulatory volume (several hundred L per m^2) as well as a prolonged terminal half-lives.[89,90] In addition, tissue levels of anthracyclines, which bind extensively to DNA, are 10- to 500-fold higher than plasma concentrations of the drugs.[19]

Methotrexate distributes widely in total body water.[91] This is important in relationship to drug toxicity because methotrexate distributes freely into extravascular fluid collections such as pleural effusions or ascites. These fluid collections can contain substantial amounts of methotrexate after high-dose administration and can act as depots that release drug slowly back to other tissues, resulting in prolonged systemic drug exposure and increased toxicity.[92] Thus, methotrexate should be administered with caution to patients with ascites or pleural effusions, and consideration should be given to draining such fluid collections prior to methotrexate therapy.

Distribution of drugs into the central nervous system (CNS) represents a special challenge in anticancer therapy. Both primary and metastatic CNS tumors are very common in children, and drugs must cross the blood–brain barrier (BBB) to gain access to these tumors. In many tumors, the BBB is at least partially disrupted by the tumor itself.[93] In other cases, the BBB is relatively intact. Drugs that are poorly soluble in lipids, undergo significant ionization in plasma, or are highly protein bound are unlikely to penetrate extensively across the BBB.[94–96] Most anticancer drugs in clinical use do not cross the intact BBB to any significant extent. Because it is very difficult to measure drug penetration into tumor or brain tissue, the concentration of drug in the cerebrospinal fluid (CSF) is often used as a surrogate marker for CNS penetration, which is most accurately expressed as the ratio of drug AUC in CSF to drug AUC in plasma. CSF-to-plasma ratios for the *Vinca* alkaloids, anthracyclines, and epipodophyllotoxins are less than 10%. A few agents, such as thiotepa and the nitrosoureas, penetrate well. Several useful agents, such as cytarabine and methotrexate, do not penetrate well but can be administered in such high systemic doses that even though the CSF-to-plasma ratio is low, the CSF concentration is still cytotoxic.[97–103] However, such high-dose systemic approaches produce significant systemic toxicity. The most common approach to overcome this problem is the direct intrathecal administration of anticancer agents. Methotrexate and cytarabine remain the mainstay of intrathecal therapy, although other agents, such as thiotepa,[104] DepoCyt (liposomally encapsulated cytarabine),[105–108] topotecan,[109] gemcitabine,[110,111] and busulfan,[112] are used occasionally.

BIOTRANSFORMATION

Biotransformation, or metabolism, of anticancer drugs can result in the production of active agents or inactivation of the agents. Some commonly administered anticancer agents are really prodrugs that require metabolic transformation before they have antitumor activity (Table 59.2). Other drugs are active in the form administered, but undergo metabolism to additional active species that may contribute importantly to activity or toxicity. For these agents, all active moieties must be considered in evaluating the relationship between pharmacokinetic parameters such as AUC or half-life and pharmacodynamic parameters such as response or toxicity. Drug activation most commonly occurs in the liver, where the bulk of drug metabolism takes place. Some drugs, especially antimetabolites, may be activated in their target tissues as they are incorporated into DNA, RNA, or other macromolecules. A few drugs, such as alkylating agents, undergo spontaneous chemical decomposition in solution to cytotoxic reactive intermediates. Interpatient variability in metabolic activation may be an important part of interpatient variability in drug activity or especially toxicity at a given dose. Saturation of drug-metabolizing enzymes at high-dose levels may lead to nonlinear dose–response curves. Interaction or competition with other drugs for a metabolic pathway, or even a drug's induction of its own metabolic pathways, could also result in unexpected alterations in exposure to active species. In designing plans for regional therapy, such as intrathecal or intra-arterial drug administration, it is important to remember that agents requiring activation at a distant site will not be useful.

TABLE 59.2 Agents That Function as Prodrugs or Have Active Metabolite Species

Class of Drug	*Prodrug*	*Active Species*
Antimetabolites	Cytarabine	Arabinosylcytidine triphosphate
	Methotrexate	Methotrexate; methotrexate polyglutamates
	Mercaptopurine	Thioguanine nucleotides
	Thioguanine	
Alkylating agents	Cyclophosphamide	4-Hydroxymetabolites
	Ifosfamide	
Anthracyclines	Idarubicin	Idarubicin; idarubicinol
Topoisomerase inhibitors	Irinotecan	SN-38

As mentioned, most antimetabolites are activated at their target sties. For example, after entering cells, cytarabine is converted to the active nucleotide arabinosylcytidine triphosphate (Ara-CTP) in three phosphorylation steps catalyzed by deoxycytidine kinase, deoxycytidylate kinase, and nucleoside diphosphate kinase.[113,114] Ara-CTP then acts as a fraudulent substrate for DNA replicative and repair enzymes. The pharmacokinetic parameters of the active intracellular metabolites are more predictive of response than plasma levels of the parent drug. For example, studies have shown little correlation between the pharmacokinetic parameters of cytarabine in plasma and leukemic cell concentrations of Ara-CTP. Ara-CTP retention in blasts correlates with response better than plasma drug concentrations.[115–117] Furthermore, decreased deoxycytidine kinase activity, resulting in decreased accumulation of Ara-CTP, is a primary mechanism of Ara-C resistance.[118–121] Similarly, thioguanine nucleotides accumulate in red blood cells, and accumulation of these nucleotides can be used as a marker of medication compliance.[122]

The antimetabolite methotrexate is not strictly a prodrug, since its parent form strongly inhibits dihydrofolate reductase

(DHFR) and blocks the conversion of naturally occurring folates to their active, chemically reduced form. This, in turn, results in depletion of purines and thymidylate, and eventually to inhibition of DNA synthesis.[123,124] However, intracellular polyglutamation of methotrexate enhances the drug's inhibitory effect on several critical synthetic enzymes in both the purine and the pyrimidine synthetic pathways, as well as increasing its intracellular retention. The enzyme responsible for polyglutamation of folates and methotrexate, folylpolyglutamate synthetase (FPGS), is expressed in higher amounts in the leukemic blasts from children with ALL than in those from children with acute nonlymphoblastic leukemia. In addition, higher FPGS activity in B-cell leukemic blasts compared with T-cell blasts may also partially explain the better response to methotrexate-based maintenance therapy in B-lineage leukemias, as these cells accumulate methotrexate polyglutamates to a significantly greater extent.[125,126]

The oxazaphosphorines, cyclophosphamide and ifosfamide, are prodrugs that require hepatic activation. Hydroxylation of the 4-carbon position on the ring yields the primary 4-hydroxyl metabolites, which are in spontaneous equilibrium with the open-ring aldehydes. The 4-hydroxyl metabolites are cytotoxic in vitro and are believed to be the transport forms of the active alkylating species, phosphoramide mustard and ifosfamide mustard, which are formed by spontaneous elimination of acrolein from the open-ring aldehydes.[17,127,128] After administration of the same dose, activated cyclophosphamide metabolites are present at about three times the concentration of activated ifosfamide metabolites.[129] In addition, the activation of ifosfamide is saturable near the MTD,[127] whereas saturable elimination of cyclophosphamide becomes apparent only at very high doses (4 to 6 g per m^2) used in bone marrow transplant regimens.[130]

The primary metabolites of the anthracyclines are the corresponding alcohols doxorubicinol, daunomycinol, and idarubicinol, formed by the action of carbonyl reductases or aldoketoreductases.[131] The AUCs of daunomycinol and idarubicinol exceed those of the parent drug after intravenous administration, whereas the AUC of doxorubicin exceeds that of doxorubicinol.[19,132–135] Doxorubicinol and daunomycinol are less cytotoxic than the parent drugs, but idarubicinol is equitoxic to idarubicin in vitro and may contribute importantly to overall drug activity.[136,137] Some data suggest that anthracycline-induced cardiac toxicity may be mediated by the alcohol metabolites and not by parent drug.[138–141]

ELIMINATION

The role of biotransformation in the elimination of drugs from the body is even more important than its role in drug activation. Metabolism, along with renal or biliary excretion, is the primary pathway for drug clearance. Clearance determines the systemic exposure to a drug. Because drug exposure is often related to toxicity, delayed elimination can lead to increased toxicity. Therefore, understanding the route of elimination is important in understanding potential toxicities in patients with organ dysfunction, especially renal or hepatic dysfunction.

Because hepatic or renal clearance plays an important role in the elimination of most drugs, it would appear to make sense to reduce the dose administered in patients with evidence of hepatic and renal dysfunction.[63] Unfortunately, there are no tests of hepatic and renal function that are clearly predictive of delayed drug elimination, and for most recommended dose modifications, there is little pharmacokinetic or clinical data available to validate the recommendations. For most agents, therapeutic monitoring, or measurement of plasma drug concentrations to predict toxicity or guide further dosing, is not available. Complicating the problem is the concern that empiric dose modifications, while avoiding toxicity, might compromise anticancer effect in patients with mild-to-moderate organ dysfunction.[142] For young children, in whom developmental changes in organ function are overlaid on drug- or disease-related organ dysfunction, the dilemma of dose modification is even more acute. Rational guidelines for dose modification or therapeutic monitoring will only be developed through systematic study of anticancer drug pharmacokinetics in children with varying degrees of organ dysfunction.

The anticancer drug for which therapeutic monitoring is most commonly used is methotrexate. One reason for this is that, in contrast to most other anticancer drugs, methotrexate toxicity is related to the length of time that drug concentration exceeds a specific threshold concentration, rather than to the drug AUC. This greatly simplifies monitoring because it is easier to measure a drug's concentration at a particular moment than to predict a drug's AUC in real time. Furthermore, even though it is obviously not possible to reduce the methotrexate dose retrospectively in the face of toxic levels, this is the one agent for which reliable antidotes exist that can lessen toxicity. As discussed previously, methotrexate works by inhibiting DHFR, resulting in depletion of reduced folate pools. Leucovorin (folinic acid) provides an exogenous source of reduced folates and effectively rescues cells from methotrexate toxicity.[91,143–145]

Seventy percent to 90% of a methotrexate dose is renally excreted through glomerular filtration and tubular secretion and reabsorption.[92,146,147] Methotrexate clearance is delayed in patients with significant renal dysfunction, which can result in significant toxicity even after a relatively low dose of the drug. Adequate renal function should be confirmed prior to administration of high-dose methotrexate therapy. Serum methotrexate concentration and renal function should be monitored during and after the dose. Patients with delayed methotrexate clearance should receive leucovorin until the plasma methotrexate concentration falls below 0.1 μmol per L (10^{-7} M). In addition, the leucovorin dose may have to be adjusted according to the serum concentration of methotrexate.[148] In patients with significant renal dysfunction after methotrexate or with the life-threatening emergency of intrathecal methotrexate overdose, the administration of glucarpidase (formerly carboxypeptidase G2), an enzyme that cleaves methotrexate to inactive metabolites, can reduce methotrexate concentrations rapidly and appears to ameliorate toxicity significantly.[149–151]

Aside from methotrexate, most antimetabolites are metabolized by the same degradative pathways as their endogenous counterparts. Cytarabine is rapidly deaminated to uridine arabinoside (Ara-U), which is not cytotoxic, by the ubiquitous enzyme cytidine deaminase. Similarly, MP and fluorouracil are catabolized through purine and pyrimidine degradative pathways to inactive metabolites. MP is also inactivated through S-methylation, which is catalyzed by thiopurine methyltransferase (TPMT). TPMT activity is inversely related to the amount of active thioguanine nucleotides formed from MP and TG.[152] A common polymorphism in the *TPMT* gene results in a trimodal distribution of enzyme activity.[152] One in 300 patients has very low TPMT activity and is extremely sensitive to thiopurines, and erythrocyte thioguanine nucleotide levels in these

TPMT-deficient patients are markedly elevated.[153,154] Even a short course of therapy can result in profound myelosuppression in TPMT deficiency.[155–157] *TPMT* genotype is often used to guide dosing for MP as well as thioguanine and the related compound azathioprine.[158]

The primary mechanism of clearance for chemically reactive agents like nitrogen mustard is spontaneous chemical decomposition to inactive intermediates. This mechanism does not depend on normal hepatic or renal function; therefore, dose modification for these agents is not usually predicated on organ dysfunction. Similarly, cisplatin, in its active, unbound form, is "eliminated" by equation followed by formation of covalent bonds to plasma or tissue proteins. Once bound to proteins, the drug is inactive. Approximately 25% of the dose is eliminated through renal excretion.[159–161] However, even in patients with no renal function, full-dose cisplatin is tolerated,[162] and the terminal half-life is not prolonged,[163] presumably because the active platinum species bind rapidly with plasma and tissue proteins. Nonetheless, cisplatin dosing is routinely modified in patients with renal dysfunction because cisplatin is nephrotoxic and renal function could be further impaired.

Carboplatin is less chemically reactive than cisplatin, and renal excretion rather than tissue binding is the primary route of carboplatin elimination.[164] Plasma carboplatin exposure is linearly related to glomerular filtration rate (GFR). Formulas have been developed to adjust the carboplatin dose based on the GFR to achieve either a target AUC[165–168] or a desired level of thrombocytopenia.[169]

The anthracyclines are eliminated primarily by hepatic biotransformation and biliary excretion. In addition, enzymatic reduction of the anthraquinone ring produces free radical forms that then spontaneously eliminate the sugar moiety, giving rise to inactive deoxyaglycone metabolites.[19] Delayed clearance of doxorubicin with increased toxicity was reported in early studies in both adults and children with hepatic dysfunction.[170,171] However, other studies have shown no significant difference in plasma pharmacokinetics or toxicity in patients with mild hepatic dysfunction compared with those with normal hepatic function.[142] In a study in patients with acute nonlymphocytic leukemia incorporating decreased doses of doxorubicin in patients with abnormal liver function tests, dose modification was associated with lower plasma drug levels, less toxicity, and a diminished duration of response and survival.[172] The usual recommendation is to reduce the doxorubicin dose in patients with direct bilirubin elevations, although some patients with hyperbilirubinemia may not require dose modification.[173–177] The anthracyclines can also be conjugated with a sulfate or glucuronide group as a further detoxification step. Decreased clearance of doxorubicinol, an active metabolite of doxorubicin, has been reported in children with more than 30% body fat.[178]

The oxazaphosphorines, which, as noted, require oxidation by hepatic microsomal enzymes at the 4-position for activation, are also inactivated by further oxidation at the same site. This reaction is catalyzed by aldehyde dehydrogenase. Enzymatic cleavage of the chloroethyl side chain of these compounds yields the potentially toxic by-product chloroacetaldehyde. This pathway is more important for ifosfamide than cyclophosphamide metabolism, and chloroacetaldehyde has been implicated in toxicities that are more common with ifosfamide, including its neurotoxic and nephrotoxic effects.[127,179]

The epipodophyllotoxin analogs, etoposide and teniposide, are both extensively metabolized, but the renal elimination of these two drugs differs. Renal excretion accounts for 30% to 40% of the total systemic clearance of etoposide,[180,181] but only 10% of teniposide clearance.[182,183] The greater protein binding of teniposide probably explains this difference, as only unbound drug is renally excreted. In one study, a statistically significant correlation between etoposide clearance and creatinine clearance was reported, whereas abnormal liver function did not appear to affect clearance.[184] These studies have led to the recommendation that etoposide dose should be reduced in patients with renal dysfunction, but dose modification may not be necessary in those with abnormal liver function tests.

The metabolism of the *Vinca* alkaloids is poorly understood despite the common use of these agents, especially in childhood cancer. Part of the reason is that assays for measuring parent drug or metabolites have been difficult to develop. Recent data suggest that the CYP3A4 and CYP3A5 pathways have a role in the metabolism of these agents.[185,186]

Variability among individuals produced by genetic polymorphisms of drug-metabolizing enzymes is increasingly being recognized as a major factor in anticancer drug therapy. This field is developing very quickly, and many single-nucleotide polymorphisms (SNPs) in enzymes affecting drug metabolism and chemosensitivity have been identified, such as the cytochrome P-450 system, pathways responsible for conjugation reactions, including acetylation, sulfation, glucuronidation, and methylation, and DNA repair pathways.[187–194] In a large review of the PharmGKB database for gene–drug associations in pediatric oncology,[195] strong evidence for gene–drug interactions were identified for thiopurines and cisplatin. As discussed previously, *TPMT* is one of the best-studied genetic polymorphism affecting anticancer drug metabolism. Appreciation of the effect of *TPMT* polymorphisms and their relationship to toxicity led to inclusion of this information in in the drug label in 2004. In addition, polymorphisms in the *NUTD15* gene are also associated with increased thiopurine toxicity.[196] Ototoxicity from cisplatin is also linked to variants in several genes, including *XPC*.[197] Unlike *TPMT*, however, no dosing adjustments are suggested based on this variant.

Fluorouracil is metabolized by a gene with well-described polymorphism, dihydropyrimidine dehydrogenase (DPD), and patients with DPD deficiency are at risk for severe fluorouracil toxicity.[198] Patients with polymorphisms in the UGT1A1 promoter have reduced glucuronidation of the active irinotecan metabolite SN-38 and are at increased risk for neutropenia.[199] The pharmacogenomics of anthracycline metabolism are complex, and polymorphisms in various genes have been associated with altered anthracycline disposition, with potential implications for cardiotoxicity.[200–202] Other chemotherapeutic agents with moderate gene–drug associations but insufficient evidence for dosing recommendations in most circumstances include carboplatin, methotrexate, cyclophosphamide, and irinotecan.[195] Evaluation of the pharmacogenetics and pharmacogenomics of anticancer agents is an active area of research and is likely to continue having a major impact on individualization of anticancer drug dosing in the future.[203–206]

COMBINATION CHEMOTHERAPY

Anticancer agents are almost always used in combinations, not administered singly. Both clinical experience and experimental models support this approach. For example, in the early days of chemotherapy for children with ALL, single-agent therapy produced disease remission in many cases, but these remissions were brief. When drugs were combined, however, both the number of patients entering remission and the duration of the remissions improved.[207,208] These observations are consistent with the Goldie-Coldman, or somatic mutation, model of drug resistance in which resistance to a particular drug arises from a spontaneous genetic mutation in a single tumor cell. The chance of a tumor's acquiring resistance to multiple drugs in a combination, however, is orders of magnitude lower because the probability of multiple mutations all taking place in a single cell is the product of the probabilities of all the single mutations. Thus, even if a cell or subpopulation is resistant to one agent in the combination, other agents should still be effective.[209,210] The Goldie-Coldman hypothesis, however, does not take into account multidrug resistance, in which a single genetic mutation, such as amplification of the *mdr1* gene, confers resistance to a broad range of antineoplastic agents, including drugs to which the tumor has never been exposed.[211–219]

In general, drugs selected for combinations are all demonstrate single-agent activity against the tumor type for which the combination is designed. Where possible, drugs are also selected for "non–cross-resistance," meaning that the known mechanisms by which tumors acquire resistance to the drugs are different for the different agents being combined. In addition, the mechanisms of antitumor action of the drugs should differ. Ideally, agents would be synergistically active and, in the case of molecularly targeted drugs, would "hit" the same pathway in different places. In a few instances, known drug interactions can be advantageous in combination therapy. For example, although the folate analog leucovorin has no independent antitumor activity, it increases the cytotoxic effect of fluorouracil by enhancing the binding of fluorouracil to its target, thymidylate synthase.[38,220] Finally, the agents selected for a combination should have nonoverlapping toxicities whenever possible to permit the administration of all the agents at their maximum tolerated doses. Some of the commonly used drug combinations are listed in Table 59.3.[221–228] Clearly, a thorough knowledge of the clinical pharmacology of individual anticancer drugs is required in the design of optimal combination regimens.

TABLE 59.3 Some Common Combination Chemotherapy Regimens

Nickname	*Components*
VAC	Vincristine
	Dactinomycin
	Cyclophosphamide
VAdriaC	Vincristine
	Doxorubicin
	Cyclophosphamide
VP/Ifos	Ifosfamide
	Etoposide
CHOP	Cyclophosphamide
	Doxorubicin
	Vincristine
	Prednisone
ICE	Ifosfamide
	Carboplatin
	Etoposide

SPECIAL CONSIDERATIONS IN INFANTS AND YOUNGER CHILDREN

Critical developmental changes in body composition, renal and hepatic function, and other determinants of drug disposition are discussed in other chapters of this book. Antineoplastic agents are affected by these changes, just as other classes of drugs are. Because the therapeutic index of chemotherapy drugs is so low, understanding developmental issues is particularly critical for pediatric oncologists. Unfortunately, data directly related to the effects of these issues on anticancer drug pharmacokinetics and pharmacodynamics are scanty. Most drugs have been insufficiently studied, especially in infants, to provide conclusive recommendations about age-specific dosing regimens or other modifications.

Anticancer drug doses for children and adults are usually based on body surface area (BSA). First, "[i]t is natural to proportion dosage according to size of patient,"[229] and second, BSA is a better predictor than weight of excretory organ function.[230] However, it is common for anticancer drug AUC to vary as much as 10-fold among children even if the same dose is administered.[174] Calculation of BSA using formulas that incorporate height and weight is intrinsically inaccurate.[231] In adult oncology, there is surprisingly little evidence that BSA-based dosing offers any advantage over simply choosing a fixed dose for use in all adults.[232,233] In addition, for many anticancer drugs, there is a poor correlation between dose (normalized to BSA) and pharmacokinetic parameters or toxicity.[234–237]

Further confounding this issue is the fact that the ratio of weight to BSA is not constant in young children but varies from approximately 18 kg per m^2 at 1 month of age to nearly 40 kg per m^2 by adulthood (Fig. 59.1).[238] Thus, if a uniform BSA-based dose is given to all children, infants receive a much higher weight-based dose (Fig. 59.2).[238] Based on observations of increased toxicity in infants less than 1 year of age receiving actinomycin D or vincristine doses based on BSA, many protocols utilize weight-based dosing for infants and young children.[239–241] When an arbitrary predefined milestone is reached, such as age

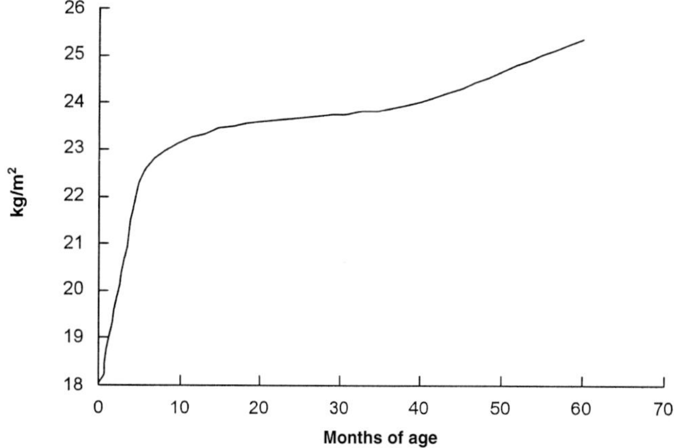

Figure 59.1 Ratio of body weight to body surface area from birth to 70 months of age.

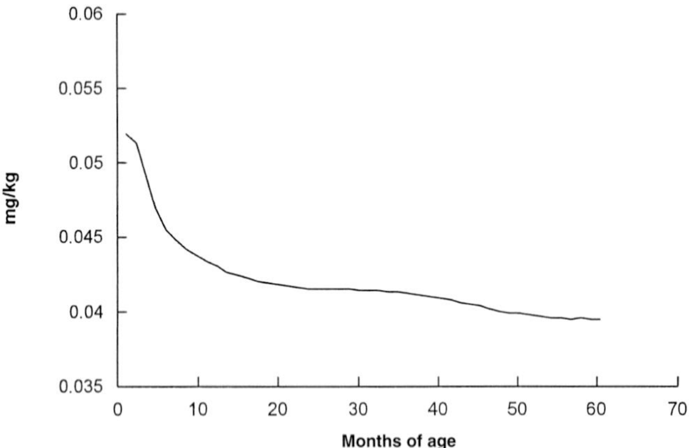

Figure 59.2 Change in dose of drug per kilogram of body weight after administration of a fixed dose per square meter of body surface area from birth to 70 months of age.

greater than 12 months or weight over 12 kg, the patient is then switched to BSA-based dosing. The drawback of this method is that the new dosing method often results in an abrupt increase in the patients' dose. BSA-based "dose banding" has, therefore, been incorporated in the Children's Oncology Group treatment protocols. This method uses predefined BSA ranges to determine a patient's dose, resulting in smoothly increasing doses rather than sharp increases at an arbitrary point in time.[242]

In contrast to the difficulty of dosing systemically administered anticancer agents, there is relative clarity over dosing intrathecal chemotherapy, where only age is considered. The CSF volume approaches adult size by about 3 years of age, whereas BSA obviously does not do so until the late teenage years. Bleyer[243] demonstrated that there was a direct correlation between patient age and CSF methotrexate concentration when intrathecal methotrexate was dosed based on BSA. Older patients were more likely to have neurotoxicity, whereas younger patients were more likely to have ineffective therapy when a BSA-based dose of 12 mg per m^2 was given.[243] In contrast, when methotrexate was given at a constant 12 mg dose to all patients older than 3 years regardless of size, methotrexate levels were significantly less variable and meningeal relapse became less frequent in younger children.[243,244] In contrast to BSA or weight-based calculations for doses of systemically administered drugs, the dose for intrathecal chemotherapy is based on patient age, regardless of body size.

CONCLUSIONS

Anticancer drug therapy in children is remarkably effective: the cure rate for all children with cancer now approaches 85%.[245] Nonetheless, therapy for some tumors, such as brain tumors, lags behind, and for all cancer treatment in children, both acute and long-term morbidity of therapy remains a difficult problem. Further improvements will only come about through pharmacologically guided preclinical research and clinical trials.

ACKNOWLEDGMENTS

The authors acknowledge David G. Poplack for his contribution to the previous editions of this chapter.

REFERENCES

1. Wittes RE, Goldin A. Unresolved issues in combination chemotherapy. *Cancer Treat Rep* 1986;70:105–125.
2. Fisher DE. Apoptosis in cancer therapy: crossing the threshold. *Cell* 1994;78:539–542.
3. Kerr JF, Winterford CM, Harmon BV. Apoptosis. Its significance in cancer and cancer therapy. *Cancer* 1994;73:2013–2026.
4. Kohn KW, Jackman J, O'Connor PM. Cell cycle control and cancer chemotherapy. *J Cell Biochem* 1994;54:440–452.
5. Sachs L, Lotem J. Control of programmed cell death in normal and leukemic cells: new implications for therapy. *Blood* 1993;82:15–21.
6. Cragg GM. Natural product drug discovery and development: the United States National Cancer Institute role. *P R Health Sci J* 2002;21:97–111.
7. Cragg GM, Newman DJ. Discovery and development of antineoplastic agents from natural sources. *Cancer Invest* 1999;17:153–163.
8. Berg SL, Blaney SM, Devidas M, et al. Phase II study of nelarabine (compound 506U78) in children and young adults with refractory T-cell malignancies: a report from the Children's Oncology Group. *J Clin Oncol* 2005;23:3376–3382.
9. Kisor DF, Plunkett W, Kurtzberg J, et al. Pharmacokinetics of nelarabine and 9-beta-D-arabinofuranosyl guanine in pediatric and adult patients during a phase I study of nelarabine for the treatment of refractory hematologic malignancies. *J Clin Oncol* 2000;18:995–1003.
10. Kurtzberg J, Ernst TJ, Keating MJ, et al. Phase I study of 506U78 administered on a consecutive 5-day schedule in children and adults with refractory hematologic malignancies. *J Clin Oncol* 2005;23:3396–3403.
11. Lambe CU, Averett DR, Paff MT, et al. 2-Amino-6-methoxypurine arabinoside: an agent for T-cell malignancies. *Cancer Res* 1995;55:3352–3356.
12. Bonate PL, Arthaud L, Cantrell WR Jr, et al. Discovery and development of clofarabine: a nucleoside analogue for treating cancer. *Nat Rev Drug Discov* 2006;5:855–863.
13. Jeha S, Gaynon PS, Razzouk BI, et al. Phase II study of clofarabine in pediatric patients with refractory or relapsed acute lymphoblastic leukemia. *J Clin Oncol* 2006;24:1917–1923.
14. Abbruzzese JL. Phase I studies with the novel nucleoside analog gemcitabine. *Semin Oncol* 1996;23:25–31.
15. Plunkett W, Huang P, Searcy CE, et al. Gemcitabine: preclinical pharmacology and mechanisms of action. *Semin Oncol* 1996;23:3–15.
16. Plunkett W, Huang P, Xu YZ, et al. Gemcitabine: metabolism, mechanisms of action, and self-potentiation. *Semin Oncol* 1995;22:3–10.
17. Colvin M, Chabner BA. Alkylating agents. In: Chabner BA, ed. *Cancer chemotherapy principles and practice*. Philadelphia, PA: Lippincott; 1990:276–313.
18. Reed E, Kohn KW. Platinum analogues. In: Chabner BA, ed. *Cancer chemotherapy principles and practice*. Philadelphia, PA: Lippincott; 1990:465–490.
19. Myers CE, Chabner BA. Anthracyclines. In: Chabner BA, ed. *Cancer chemotherapy principles and practice*. Philadelphia, PA: Lippincott; 1990:356–381.
20. Pommier Y, Leo E, Zhang H, et al. DNA topoisomerases and their poisoning by anticancer and antibacterial drugs. *Chem Biol* 2010;17:421–433.
21. Bachur NR, Gordon SL, Gee MV. A general mechanism for microsomal activation of quinone anticancer agents to free radicals. *Cancer Res* 1978;38:1745–1750.
22. Gianni L, Herman EH, Lipshultz SE, et al. Anthracycline cardiotoxicity: from bench to bedside. *J Clin Oncol* 2008;26:3777–3784.
23. Wallace KB. Adriamycin-induced interference with cardiac mitochondrial calcium homeostasis. *Cardiovasc Toxicol* 2007;7:101–107.
24. Lipshultz SE, Rifai N, Dalton VM, et al. The effect of dexrazoxane on myocardial injury in doxorubicin-treated children with acute lymphoblastic leukemia. *N Engl J Med* 2004;351:145–153.
25. Bender RA, Hamel E, Hande KR. Plant alkaloids. In: Chabner BA, ed. *Cancer chemotherapy principles and practice*. Philadelphia, PA: Lippincott; 1990:253–275.
26. van Maanen JM, Retel J, de Vries J, et al. Mechanism of action of antitumor drug etoposide: a review. *J Natl Cancer Inst* 1988;80:1526–1533.
27. Slichenmyer WJ, Rowinsky EK, Donehower RC, et al. The current status of camptothecin analogues as antitumor agents. *J Natl Cancer Inst* 1993;85:271–291.
28. Ringel I, Horwitz SB. Studies with RP 56976 (taxotere): a semisynthetic analogue of taxol. *J Natl Cancer Inst* 1991;83:288–291.
29. Schiff PB, Fant J, Horwitz SB. Promotion of microtubule assembly in vitro by taxol. *Nature* 1979;277:665–667.
30. Schiff PB, Horwitz SB. Taxol stabilizes microtubules in mouse fibroblast cells. *Proc Natl Acad Sci U S A* 1980;77:1561–1565.
31. Broome J. Evidence that the L-asparaginase activity of guinea pig serum is responsible for its antilymphoma effects. *Nature* 1961;191:1114–1115.
32. Holcenberg JS. Enzymes as drugs. *Annu Rev Pharmacol Toxicol* 1977;17:97–116.
33. Avramis VI, Panosyan EH. Pharmacokinetic/pharmacodynamic relationships of asparaginase formulations: the past, the present and recommendations for the future. *Clin Pharmacokinet* 2005;44:367–393.
34. Tong WH, Pieters R, Kaspers GJ, et al. A prospective study on drug monitoring of PEGasparaginase and Erwinia asparaginase and asparaginase antibodies in pediatric acute lymphoblastic leukemia. *Blood* 2014;123:2026–2033.
35. Deininger MW, Goldman JM, Lydon N, et al. The tyrosine kinase inhibitor CGP57148B selectively inhibits the growth of BCR-ABL-positive cells. *Blood* 1997;90:3691–3698.
36. Druker BJ, Tamura S, Buchdunger E, et al. Effects of a selective inhibitor of the Abl tyrosine kinase on the growth of Bcr-Abl positive cells. *Nat Med* 1996;2:561–566.
37. Buchdunger E, Cioffi CL, Law N, et al. Abl protein-tyrosine kinase inhibitor STI571 inhibits in vitro signal transduction mediated by c-kit and platelet-derived growth factor receptors. *J Pharmacol Exp Ther* 2000;295:139–145.
38. Carroll M, Ohno-Jones S, Tamura S, et al. CGP 57148, a tyrosine kinase inhibitor, inhibits the growth of cells expressing BCR-ABL, TEL-ABL, and TEL-PDGFR fusion proteins. *Blood* 1997;90:4947–4952.

39. Heinrich MC, Griffith DJ, Druker BJ, et al. Inhibition of c-kit receptor tyrosine kinase activity by STI 571, a selective tyrosine kinase inhibitor. *Blood* 2000;96:925–932.
40. Champagne MA, Capdeville R, Krailo M, et al. Imatinib mesylate (STI571) for treatment of children with Philadelphia chromosome-positive leukemia: results from a Children's Oncology Group phase 1 study. *Blood* 2004;104:2655–2660.
41. Druker BJ, Talpaz M, Resta DJ, et al. Efficacy and safety of a specific inhibitor of the BCR-ABL tyrosine kinase in chronic myeloid leukemia. *N Engl J Med* 2001;344:1031–1037.
42. Johnson JR, Bross P, Cohen M, et al. Approval summary: imatinib mesylate capsules for treatment of adult patients with newly diagnosed Philadelphia chromosome-positive chronic myelogenous leukemia in chronic phase. *Clin Cancer Res* 2003;9:1972–1979.
43. Kantarjian HM, Cortes JE, O'Brien S, et al. Imatinib mesylate therapy in newly diagnosed patients with Philadelphia chromosome-positive chronic myelogenous leukemia: high incidence of early complete and major cytogenetic responses. *Blood* 2003;101:97–100.
44. Kantarjian HM, O'Brien S, Cortes JE, et al. Treatment of Philadelphia chromosome-positive, accelerated-phase chronic myelogenous leukemia with imatinib mesylate. *Clin Cancer Res* 2002;8:2167–2176.
45. Kantarjian HM, Talpaz M. Imatinib mesylate: clinical results in Philadelphia chromosome-positive leukemias. *Semin Oncol* 2001;28:9–18.
46. Kantarjian HM, Talpaz M, O'Brien S, et al. Imatinib mesylate for Philadelphia chromosome-positive, chronic-phase myeloid leukemia after failure of interferon-alpha: follow-up results. *Clin Cancer Res* 2002;8:2177–2187.
47. Kolb EA, Pan Q, Ladanyi M, et al. Imatinib mesylate in Philadelphia chromosome-positive leukemia of childhood. *Cancer* 2003;98:2643–2650.
48. Roumiantsev S, Shah NP, Gorre ME, et al. Clinical resistance to the kinase inhibitor STI-571 in chronic myeloid leukemia by mutation of Tyr-253 in the Abl kinase domain P-loop. *Proc Natl Acad Sci U S A* 2002;99:10700–10705.
49. Breccia M, Cannella L, Nanni M, et al. Nilotinib can override dasatinib resistance in chronic myeloid leukemia patients with secondary resistance to imatinib first-line therapy. *Acta Haematol* 2007;118:162–164.
50. Hochhaus A, Kantarjian HM, Baccarani M, et al. Dasatinib induces notable hematologic and cytogenetic responses in chronic-phase chronic myeloid leukemia after failure of imatinib therapy. *Blood* 2007;109:2303–2309.
51. DuBois SG, Laetsch TW, Federman N, et al. The use of neoadjuvant larotrectinib in the management of children with locally advanced TRK fusion sarcomas. *Cancer* 2018;124:4241–4247.
52. Laetsch TW, Hawkins DS. Larotrectinib for the treatment of TRK fusion solid tumors. *Expert Rev Anticancer Ther* 2018;19:1–10.
53. Pacenta HL, Macy ME. Entrectinib and other ALK/TRK inhibitors for the treatment of neuroblastoma. *Drug Des Devel Ther* 2018;12:3549–3561.
54. Mosse YP, Voss SD, Lim MS, et al. Targeting ALK with crizotinib in pediatric anaplastic large cell lymphoma and inflammatory myofibroblastic tumor: a Children's Oncology Group Study. *J Clin Oncol* 2017;35:3215–3221.
55. Grupp SA, Kalos M, Barrett D, et al. Chimeric antigen receptor-modified T cells for acute lymphoid leukemia. *N Engl J Med* 2013;368:1509–1518.
56. Maude SL, Laetsch TW, Buechner J, et al. Tisagenlecleucel in children and young adults with B-cell lymphoblastic leukemia. *N Engl J Med* 2018;378:439–448.
57. Ruella M, Maus MV. Catch me if you can: leukemia escape after CD19-directed T cell immunotherapies. *Comput Struct Biotechnol J* 2016;14:357–362.
58. Fry TJ, Shah NN, Orentas RJ, et al. CD22-targeted CAR T cells induce remission in B-ALL that is naive or resistant to CD19-targeted CAR immunotherapy. *Nat Med* 2018;24:20–28.
59. Ozkaynak MF, Gilman AL, London WB, et al. A comprehensive safety trial of chimeric antibody 14.18 with GM-CSF, IL-2, and isotretinoin in high-risk neuroblastoma patients following myeloablative therapy: children's Oncology Group Study ANBL0931. *Front Immunol* 2018;9:1355.
60. Yarchoan M, Hopkins A, Jaffee EM. Tumor mutational burden and response rate to PD-1 inhibition. *N Engl J Med* 2017;377:2500–2501.
61. Chan TA, Yarchoan M, Jaffee E, et al. Development of tumor mutation burden as an immunotherapy biomarker: utility for the oncology clinic. *Ann Oncol* 2019;30:44–56.
62. Lawrence MS, Stojanov P, Polak P, et al. Mutational heterogeneity in cancer and the search for new cancer-associated genes. *Nature* 2013;499:214–218.
63. Powis G. Effects of disease states on pharmacokinetics of anticancer drugs. In: Ames MM, Powis G, Kovach JS, eds. *Pharmacokinetics of anticancer agents in humans*. Amsterdam, Netherlands: Elsevier; 1983:365–397.
64. Bomgaars LR, Bernstein M, Krailo M, et al. Phase II trial of irinotecan in children with refractory solid tumors: a Children's Oncology Group Study. *J Clin Oncol* 2007;25:4622–4627.
65. Egorin MJ, Forrest A, Belani CP, et al. A limited sampling strategy for cyclophosphamide pharmacokinetics. *Cancer Res* 1989;49:3129–3133.
66. Ratain MJ, Vogelzang NJ. Limited sampling model for vinblastine pharmacokinetics. *Cancer Treat Rep* 1987;71:935–939.
67. Zao JH, Schechter T, Liu WJ, et al. Performance of Busulfan dosing guidelines for pediatric hematopoietic stem cell transplant conditioning. *Biol Blood Marrow Transplant* 2015;21:1471–1478.
68. Balis FM, Savitch JL, Bleyer WA. Pharmacokinetics of oral methotrexate in children. *Cancer Res* 1983;43:2342–2345.
69. Kearney PJ, Light PA, Preece A, et al. Unpredictable serum levels after oral methotrexate in children with acute lymphoblastic leukaemia. *Cancer Chemother Pharmacol* 1979;3:117–120.
70. Koren G, Solh H, Klein J, et al. Disposition of oral methotrexate in children with acute lymphoblastic leukemia and its relation to 6-mercaptopurine pharmacokinetics. *Med Pediatr Oncol* 1989;17:450–454.
71. Lennard L, Keen D, Lilleyman JS. Oral 6-mercaptopurine in childhood leukemia: parent drug pharmacokinetics and active metabolite concentrations. *Clin Pharmacol Ther* 1986;40:287–292.
72. Sulh H, Koren G, Whalen C, et al. Pharmacokinetic determinants of 6-mercaptopurine myelotoxicity and therapeutic failure in children with acute lymphoblastic leukemia. *Clin Pharmacol Ther* 1986;40:604–609.
73. Zimm S, Collins JM, Riccardi R, et al. Variable bioavailability of oral mercaptopurine. Is maintenance chemotherapy in acute lymphoblastic leukemia being optimally delivered? *N Engl J Med* 1983;308:1005–1009.
74. Pinkerton CR, Welshman SG, Glasgow JF, et al. Can food influence the absorption of methotrexate in children with acute lymphoblastic leukaemia? *Lancet* 1980;2:944–946.
75. Riccardi R, Balis FM, Ferrara P, et al. Influence of food intake on bioavailability of oral 6-mercaptopurine in children with acute lymphoblastic leukemia. *Pediatr Hematol Oncol* 1986;3:319–324.
76. Balis FM, Jeffries SL, Lange B, et al. Chronopharmacokinetics of oral methotrexate and 6-mercaptopurine: is there diurnal variation in the disposition of antileukemic therapy? *Am J Pediatr Hematol Oncol* 1989;11:324–326.
77. Koren G, Ferrazzini G, Sohl H, et al. Chronopharmacology of methotrexate pharmacokinetics in childhood leukemia. *Chronobiol Int* 1992;9:434–438.
78. Koren G, Langevin AM, Olivieri N, et al. Diurnal variation in the pharmacokinetics and myelotoxicity of mercaptopurine in children with acute lymphocytic leukemia. *Am J Dis Child* 1990;144:1135–1137.
79. Rivard GE, Infante-Rivard C, Hoyoux C, et al. Maintenance chemotherapy for childhood acute lymphoblastic leukaemia: better in the evening. *Lancet* 1985;2:1264–1266.
80. Balis FM, Mirro J Jr, Reaman GH, et al. Pharmacokinetics of subcutaneous methotrexate. *J Clin Oncol* 1988;6:1882–1886.
81. Teresi ME, Crom WR, Choi KE, et al. Methotrexate bioavailability after oral and intramuscular administration in children. *J Pediatr* 1987;110:788–792.
82. Zimm S, Collins JM, O'Neill D, et al. Inhibition of first-pass metabolism in cancer chemotherapy: interaction of 6-mercaptopurine and allopurinol. *Clin Pharmacol Ther* 1983;34:810–817.
83. Duggan DE, Yeh KC, Matalia N, et al. Bioavailability of oral dexamethasone. *Clin Pharmacol Ther* 1975;18:205–209.
84. Pickup ME. Clinical pharmacokinetics of prednisone and prednisolone. *Clin Pharmacokinet* 1979;4:111–128.
85. Green OC, Winter RJ, Kawahara FS, et al. Plasma levels, half-life values, and correlation with physiologic assays for growth and immunity. *J Pediatr* 1978;93:299–303.
86. Hassan M, Ljungman P, Bolme P, et al. Busulfan bioavailability. *Blood* 1994;84:2144–2150.
87. Regazzi MB, Locatelli F, Buggia I, et al. Disposition of high-dose busulfan in pediatric patients undergoing bone marrow transplantation. *Clin Pharmacol Ther* 1993;54:45–52.
88. Vassal G, Challine D, Koscielny S, et al. Chronopharmacology of high-dose busulfan in children. *Cancer Res* 1993;53:1534–1537.
89. Groninger E, Meeuwsen-de Boar T, Koopmans P, et al. Pharmacokinetics of vincristine monotherapy in childhood acute lymphoblastic leukemia. *Pediatr Res* 2002;52:113–118.
90. Robert J. Anthracyclines. In: Grochow L, Ames M, eds. *A clinician's guide to chemotherapy pharmacokinetics and pharmacodynamics*. Baltimore, MD: Williams & Wilkins; 1998:93–173.
91. Pratt CB, Roberts D, Shanks EC, et al. Clinical trials and pharmacokinetics of intermittent high-dose methotrexate-"leucovorin rescue" for children with malignant tumors. *Cancer Res* 1974;34:3326–3331.
92. Allegra CJ. Antifolates. In: Chabner BA, ed. *Cancer chemotherapy principles and practice*. Philadelphia, PA: Lippincott; 1990:110–153.
93. Strother D, Pollack I, Fisher P, et al. Tumors of the central nervous system. In: Pizzo PA, Poplack DG, eds. *Principles and practice of pediatric oncology*. 4th ed. Philadelphia, PA: Lippincott Williams & Wilkins; 2002:751–824.
94. Koch-Weser J, Sellers EM. Binding of drugs to serum albumin (first of two parts). *N Engl J Med* 1976;294:311–316.
95. Mellett LB. Physicochemical considerations and pharmacokinetic behavior in delivery of drugs to the central nervous system. *Cancer Treat Rep* 1977;61:527–531.
96. Poplack D, Bleyer W, Horowitz M. Pharmacology of antineoplastic agents in cerebrospinal fluid. In: Wood J, ed. *Neurobiology of cerebrospinal fluid*. New York, NY: Plenum Press; 1980:561–578.
97. Balis FM, Savitch JL, Bleyer WA, et al. Remission induction of meningeal leukemia with high-dose intravenous methotrexate. *J Clin Oncol* 1985;3:485–489.
98. Donehower RC, Karp JE, Burke PJ. Pharmacology and toxicity of high-dose cytarabine by 72-hour continuous infusion. *Cancer Treat Rep* 1986;70:1059–1065.
99. Evans WE, Hutson PR, Stewart CF, et al. Methotrexate cerebrospinal fluid and serum concentrations after intermediate-dose methotrexate infusion. *Clin Pharmacol Ther* 1983;33:301–307.
100. Frick J, Ritch PS, Hansen RM, et al. Successful treatment of meningeal leukemia using systemic high-dose cytosine arabinoside. *J Clin Oncol* 1984;2:365–368.
101. Frick JC, Hansen RM, Anderson T, et al. Successful high-dose intravenous cytarabine treatment of parenchymal brain involvement from malignant lymphoma. *Arch Intern Med* 1986;146:791–792.
102. Morra E, Lazzarino M, Brusamolino E, et al. The role of systemic high-dose cytarabine in the treatment of central nervous system leukemia. Clinical results in 46 patients. *Cancer* 1993;72:439–445.
103. Shapiro WR, Young DF, Mehta BM. Methotrexate: distribution in cerebrospinal fluid after intravenous, ventricular and lumbar injections. *N Engl J Med* 1975;293:161–166.
104. Grossman SA, Finkelstein DM, Ruckdeschel JC, et al. Randomized prospective comparison of intraventricular methotrexate and thiotepa in patients with previously untreated neoplastic meningitis. Eastern Cooperative Oncology Group. *J Clin Oncol* 1993;11:561–569.
105. Bomgaars L, Geyer JR, Franklin J, et al. Phase I trial of intrathecal liposomal cytarabine in children with neoplastic meningitis. *J Clin Oncol* 2004;22:3916–3921.
106. Glantz MJ, Jaeckle KA, Chamberlain MC, et al. A randomized controlled trial comparing intrathecal sustained-release cytarabine (DepoCyt) to intrathecal methotrexate in patients with neoplastic meningitis from solid tumors. *Clin Cancer Res* 1999;5:3394–3402.
107. Glantz MJ, LaFollette S, Jaeckle KA, et al. Randomized trial of a slow-release versus a standard formulation of cytarabine for the intrathecal treatment of lymphomatous meningitis. *J Clin Oncol* 1999;17:3110–3116.
108. Jaeckle KA, Phuphanich S, Bent MJ, et al. Intrathecal treatment of neoplastic meningitis due to breast cancer with a slow-release formulation of cytarabine. *Br J Cancer* 2001;84:157–163.

109. Blaney SM, Heideman R, Berg S, et al. Phase I clinical trial of intrathecal topotecan in patients with neoplastic meningitis. *J Clin Oncol* 2003;21:143–147.
110. Bernardi RJ, Bomgaars L, Fox E, et al. Phase I clinical trial of intrathecal gemcitabine in patients with neoplastic meningitis. *Cancer Chemother Pharmacol* 2008;62:355–361.
111. Chen YM, Chen MC, Tsai CM, et al. Intrathecal gemcitabine chemotherapy for non-small cell lung cancer patients with meningeal carcinomatosis—a case report. *Lung Cancer* 2003;40:99–101.
112. Gururangan S, Petros WP, Poussaint TY, et al. Phase I trial of intrathecal spartaject busulfan in children with neoplastic meningitis: a Pediatric Brain Tumor Consortium Study (PBTC-004). *Clin Cancer Res* 2006;12:1540–1546.
113. Chabner BA. Cytidine analogues. In: Chabner BA, Collins JM, eds. *Cancer chemotherapy principles and practice*. Philadelphia, PA: Lippincott; 1990:154–179.
114. Kufe DW, Spriggs DR. Biochemical and cellular pharmacology of cytosine arabinoside. *Semin Oncol* 1985;12:34–48.
115. Estey E, Plunkett W, Dixon D, et al. Variables predicting response to high dose cytosine arabinoside therapy in patients with refractory acute leukemia. *Leukemia* 1987;1:580–583.
116. Liliemark JO, Plunkett W, Dixon DO. Relationship of 1-beta-D-arabinofuranosylcytosine in plasma to 1-beta-D-arabinofuranosylcytosine 5′-triphosphate levels in leukemic cells during treatment with high-dose 1-beta-D-arabinofuranosylcytosine. *Cancer Res* 1985;45:5952–5957.
117. Plunkett W, Iacoboni S, Estey E, et al. Pharmacologically directed ara-C therapy for refractory leukemia. *Semin Oncol* 1985;12:20–30.
118. Bergman AM, Pinedo HM, Peters GJ. Determinants of resistance to 2′,2′-difluorodeoxycytidine (gemcitabine). *Drug Resist Updat* 2002;5:19–33.
119. Hagenbeek A, Martens AC, Colly LP. In vivo development of cytosine arabinoside resistance in the BN acute myelocytic leukemia. *Semin Oncol* 1987;14:202–206.
120. Kees UR, Ford J, Dawson VM, et al. Development of resistance to 1-beta-D-arabinofuranosylcytosine after high-dose treatment in childhood lymphoblastic leukemia: analysis of resistance mechanism in established cell lines. *Cancer Res* 1989;49:3015–3019.
121. Stam RW, den Boer ML, Meijerink JP, et al. Differential mRNA expression of Ara-C-metabolizing enzymes explains Ara-C sensitivity in MLL gene-rearranged infant acute lymphoblastic leukemia. *Blood* 2003;101:1270–1276.
122. Lennard L, Welch J, Lilleyman JS. Intracellular metabolites of mercaptopurine in children with lymphoblastic leukaemia: a possible indicator of non-compliance? *Br J Cancer* 1995;72:1004–1006.
123. Chu E, Allegra C. Antifolates. In: Chabner B, Longo D, eds. *Cancer chemotherapy and biotherapy principles and practice*. Philadelphia, PA: Lippincott-Raven; 1996:109–148.
124. Goldman ID, Matherly LH. The cellular pharmacology of methotrexate. *Pharmacol Ther* 1985;28:77–102.
125. Barredo JC, Synold TW, Laver J, et al. Differences in constitutive and post-methotrexate folylpolyglutamate synthetase activity in B-lineage and T-lineage leukemia. *Blood* 1994;84:564–569.
126. Galpin AJ, Schuetz JD, Masson E, et al. Differences in folylpolyglutamate synthetase and dihydrofolate reductase expression in human B-lineage versus T-lineage leukemic lymphoblasts: mechanisms for lineage differences in methotrexate polyglutamylation and cytotoxicity. *Mol Pharmacol* 1997;52:155–163.
127. Brade WP, Herdrich K, Varini M. Ifosfamide—pharmacology, safety and therapeutic potential. *Cancer Treat Rev* 1985;12:1–47.
128. Grochow LB, Colvin M. Clinical pharmacokinetics of cyclophosphamide. *Clin Pharmacokinet* 1979;4:380–394.
129. Wagner T, Heydrich D, Jork T, et al. Comparative study on human pharmacokinetics of activated ifosfamide and cyclophosphamide by a modified fluorometric test. *J Cancer Res Clin Oncol* 1981;100:95–104.
130. Chen TL, Passos-Coelho JL, Noe DA, et al. Nonlinear pharmacokinetics of cyclophosphamide in patients with metastatic breast cancer receiving high-dose chemotherapy followed by autologous bone marrow transplantation. *Cancer Res* 1995;55:810–816.
131. Piska K, Koczurkiewicz P, Bucki A, et al. Metabolic carbonyl reduction of anthracyclines—role in cardiotoxicity and cancer resistance. Reducing enzymes as putative targets for novel cardioprotective and chemosensitizing agents. *Invest New Drugs* 2017;35:375–385.
132. Gil P, Favre R, Durand A, et al. Time dependency of adriamycin and adriamycinol kinetics. *Cancer Chemother Pharmacol* 1983;10:120–124.
133. Greene RF, Collins JM, Jenkins JF, et al. Plasma pharmacokinetics of adriamycin and adriamycinol: implications for the design of in vitro experiments and treatment protocols. *Cancer Res* 1983;43:3417–3421.
134. Huffman DH, Bachur NR. Daunorubicin metabolism in acute myelocytic leukemia. *Blood* 1972;39:637–643.
135. Reid JM, Pendergrass TW, Krailo MD, et al. Plasma pharmacokinetics and cerebrospinal fluid concentrations of idarubicin and idarubicinol in pediatric leukemia patients: a Childrens Cancer Study Group report. *Cancer Res* 1990;50:6525–6528.
136. Kuffel MJ, Ames MM. Comparative resistance of idarubicin, doxorubicin and their C-13 alcohol metabolites in human MDR1 transfected NIH-3T3 cells. *Cancer Chemother Pharmacol* 1995;36:223–226.
137. Reid J, Kuffel M. Cytotoxic concentrations of idarubicinol, the alcohol metabolite of idarubicin, are present in CSF following administration of idarubicin to children with relapsed leukemia. *Proc Am Assoc Cancer Res* 1989;30:250.
138. Cusack BJ, Young SP, Driskell J, et al. Doxorubicin and doxorubicinol pharmacokinetics and tissue concentrations following bolus injection and continuous infusion of doxorubicin in the rabbit. *Cancer Chemother Pharmacol* 1993;32:53–58.
139. de Jong J, Schoofs PR, Snabilie AM, et al. The role of biotransformation in anthracycline-induced cardiotoxicity in mice. *J Pharmacol Exp Ther* 1993;266:1312–1320.
140. Olson RD, Mushlin PS, Brenner DE, et al. Doxorubicin cardiotoxicity may be caused by its metabolite, doxorubicinol. *Proc Natl Acad Sci U S A* 1988;85:3585–3589.
141. Stewart DJ, Grewaal D, Green RM, et al. Concentrations of doxorubicin and its metabolites in human autopsy heart and other tissues. *Anticancer Res* 1993;13:1945–1952.
142. Sulkes A, Collins JM. Reappraisal of some dosage adjustment guidelines. *Cancer Treat Rep* 1987;71:229–233.
143. Frei E 3rd, Jaffe N, Tattersall MH, et al. New approaches to cancer chemotherapy with methotrexate. *N Engl J Med* 1975;292:846–851.
144. Hitchings GH, Burchall JJ. Inhibition of folate biosynthesis and function as a basis for chemotherapy. *Adv Enzymol Relat Areas Mol Biol* 1965;27:417–468.
145. Stoller RG, Hande KR, Jacobs SA, et al. Use of plasma pharmacokinetics to predict and prevent methotrexate toxicity. *N Engl J Med* 1977;297:630–634.
146. Huffman DH, Wan SH, Azarnoff DL, et al. Pharmacokinetics of methotrexate. *Clin Pharmacol Ther* 1973;14:572–579.
147. Liegler DG, Henderson ES, Hahn MA, et al. The effect of organic acids on renal clearance of methotrexate in man. *Clin Pharmacol Ther* 1969;10:849–857.
148. Bleyer WA. Antineoplastic agents. In: Yaffe SJ, ed. *Pediatric pharmacology: therapeutic principles in practice*. New York, NY: Grune & Stratton; 1980:349–377.
149. Widemann BC, Balis FM, Murphy RF, et al. Carboxypeptidase-G2, thymidine, and leucovorin rescue in cancer patients with methotrexate-induced renal dysfunction. *J Clin Oncol* 1997;15:2125–2134.
150. Widemann BC, Balis FM, Shalabi A, et al. Treatment of accidental intrathecal methotrexate overdose with intrathecal carboxypeptidase G2. *J Natl Cancer Inst* 2004;96:1557–1559.
151. Ramsey LB, Balis FM, O'Brien MM, et al. Consensus guideline for use of glucarpidase in patients with high-dose methotrexate induced acute kidney injury and delayed methotrexate clearance. *Oncologist* 2018;23:52–61.
152. Lennard L, Lilleyman JS, Van Loon J, et al. Genetic variation in response to 6-mercaptopurine for childhood acute lymphoblastic leukaemia. *Lancet* 1990;336:225–229.
153. Evans WE, Horner M, Chu YQ, et al. Altered mercaptopurine metabolism, toxic effects, and dosage requirement in a thiopurine methyltransferase-deficient child with acute lymphocytic leukemia. *J Pediatr* 1991;119:985–989.
154. Lennard L, Van Loon JA, Weinshilboum RM. Pharmacogenetics of acute azathioprine toxicity: relationship to thiopurine methyltransferase genetic polymorphism. *Clin Pharmacol Ther* 1989;46:149–154.
155. Marra CA, Esdaile JM, Anis AH. Practical pharmacogenetics: the cost effectiveness of screening for thiopurine S-methyltransferase polymorphisms in patients with rheumatological conditions treated with azathioprine. *J Rheumatol* 2002;29:2507–2512.
156. McLeod HL, Coulthard S, Thomas AE, et al. Analysis of thiopurine methyltransferase variant alleles in childhood acute lymphoblastic leukaemia. *Br J Haematol* 1999;105:696–700.
157. McLeod HL, Krynetski EY, Relling MV, et al. Genetic polymorphism of thiopurine methyltransferase and its clinical relevance for childhood acute lymphoblastic leukemia. *Leukemia* 2000;14:567–572.
158. Relling MV, Gardner EE, Sandborn WJ, et al. Clinical Pharmacogenetics Implementation Consortium guidelines for thiopurine methyltransferase genotype and thiopurine dosing. *Clin Pharmacol Ther* 2011;89:387–391.
159. Jacobs C, Kalman SM, Tretton M, et al. Renal handling of cis-diamminedichloroplatinum(II). *Cancer Treat Rep* 1980;64:1223–1226.
160. Reece PA, Stafford I, Davy M, et al. Disposition of unchanged cisplatin in patients with ovarian cancer. *Clin Pharmacol Ther* 1987;42:320–325.
161. Vermorken JB, van der Vijgh WJ, Klein I, et al. Pharmacokinetics of free and total platinum species after rapid and prolonged infusions of cisplatin. *Clin Pharmacol Ther* 1986;39:136–144.
162. Gouyette A, Lemoine R, Adhemar JP, et al. Kinetics of cisplatin in an anuric patient undergoing hemofiltration dialysis. *Cancer Treat Rep* 1981;65:665–668.
163. Belt RJ, Himmelstein KJ, Patton TF, et al. Pharmacokinetics of non-protein-bound platinum species following administration of cis-dichlorodiammineplatinum(II). *Cancer Treat Rep* 1979;63:1515–1521.
164. van der Vijgh WJ. Clinical pharmacokinetics of carboplatin. *Clin Pharmacokinet* 1991;21:242–261.
165. Bin P, Boddy AV, English MW, et al. The comparative pharmacokinetics and pharmacodynamics of cisplatin and carboplatin in paediatric patients: a review. *Anticancer Res* 1994;14:2279–2283.
166. Calvert AH. Dose optimisation of carboplatin in adults. *Anticancer Res* 1994;14:2273–2278.
167. Marina NM, Rodman J, Shema SJ, et al. Phase I study of escalating targeted doses of carboplatin combined with ifosfamide and etoposide in children with relapsed solid tumors. *J Clin Oncol* 1993;11:554–560.
168. Newell DR, Pearson AD, Balmanno K, et al. Carboplatin pharmacokinetics in children: the development of a pediatric dosing formula. The United Kingdom Children's Cancer Study Group. *J Clin Oncol* 1993;11:2314–2323.
169. Egorin MJ, Van Echo DA, Tipping SJ, et al. Pharmacokinetics and dosage reduction of cis-diammine(1,1-cyclobutanedicarboxylato)platinum in patients with impaired renal function. *Cancer Res* 1984;44:5432–5438.
170. Benjamin RS, Wiernik PH, Bachur NR. Adriamycin chemotherapy—efficacy, safety, and pharmacologic basis of an intermittent single high-dosage schedule. *Cancer* 1974;33:19–27.
171. Evans WE, Crom WR, Sinkule JA, et al. Pharmacokinetics of anticancer drugs in children. *Drug Metab Rev* 1983;14:847–886.
172. Brenner DE, Wiernik PH, Wesley M, et al. Acute doxorubicin toxicity. Relationship to pretreatment liver function, response, and pharmacokinetics in patients with acute nonlymphocytic leukemia. *Cancer* 1984;53:1042–1048.
173. Chang PC, Brenner DE, Riggs CE, et al. Adriamycin toxicity: preliminary guidelines for dosage reduction. *Clin Res* 1979;27:382A.
174. Crom WR, Glynn-Barnhart AM, Rodman JH, et al. Pharmacokinetics of anticancer drugs in children. *Clin Pharmacokinet* 1987;12:168–213.
175. Cupp MJ, Higa GM. Doxorubicin dosage guidelines in a patient with hyperbilirubinemia of Gilbert's syndrome. *Ann Pharmacother* 1998;32:1026–1029.
176. Gurevich I, Akerley W. Treatment of the jaundiced patient with breast carcinoma: case report and alternate therapeutic strategies. *Cancer* 2001;91:660–663.
177. Kaye SB, Cummings J, Kerr DJ. How much does liver disease affect the pharmacokinetics of adriamycin? *Eur J Cancer Clin Oncol* 1985;21:893–895.

178. Thompson PA, Rosner GL, Matthay KK, et al. Impact of body composition on pharmacokinetics of doxorubicin in children: a Glaser Pediatric Research Network study. *Cancer Chemother Pharmacol* 2008;64:243–251.
179. Pratt CB, Green AA, Horowitz ME, et al. Central nervous system toxicity following the treatment of pediatric patients with ifosfamide/mesna. *J Clin Oncol* 1986;4:1253–1261.
180. Allen LM, Creaven PJ. Comparison of the human pharmacokinetics of VM-26 and VP-16, two antineoplastic epipodophyllotoxin glucopyranoside derivatives. *Eur J Cancer* 1975;11:697–707.
181. Hande KR, Wedlund PJ, Noone RM, et al. Pharmacokinetics of high-dose etoposide (VP-16-213) administered to cancer patients. *Cancer Res* 1984;44:379–382.
182. D'Incalci M, Rossi C, Sessa C, et al. Pharmacokinetics of teniposide in patients with ovarian cancer. *Cancer Treat Rep* 1985;69:73–77.
183. Holthuis JJ, de Vries LG, Postmus PE, et al. Pharmacokinetics of high-dose teniposide. *Cancer Treat Rep* 1987;71:599–603.
184. D'Incalci M, Rossi C, Zucchetti M, et al. Pharmacokinetics of etoposide in patients with abnormal renal and hepatic function. *Cancer Res* 1986;46:2566–2571.
185. Dennison JB, Jones DR, Renbarger JL, et al. Effect of CYP3A5 expression on vincristine metabolism with human liver microsomes. *J Pharmacol Exp Ther* 2007;321:553–563.
186. Dennison JB, Kulanthaivel P, Barbuch RJ, et al. Selective metabolism of vincristine in vitro by CYP3A5. Drug Metab Dispos 2006;34:1317–1327.
187. Carlini EJ, Raftogianis RB, Wood TC, et al. Sulfation pharmacogenetics: SULT1A1 and SULT1A2 allele frequencies in Caucasian, Chinese and African-American subjects. *Pharmacogenetics* 2001;11:57–68.
188. Iyer L, King CD, Whitington PF, et al. Genetic predisposition to the metabolism of irinotecan (CPT-11). Role of uridine diphosphate glucuronosyltransferase isoform 1A1 in the glucuronidation of its active metabolite (SN-38) in human liver microsomes. *J Clin Invest* 1998;101:847–854.
189. Iyer L, Whitington P, Roy S, et al. Genetic basis for the glucuronidation of SN-38: role of UGT*1 isoform. *Clin Pharmacol Ther* 1997;61:164.
190. Kuehl P, Zhang J, Lin Y, et al. Sequence diversity in CYP3A promoters and characterization of the genetic basis of polymorphic CYP3A5 expression. *Nat Genet* 2001;27:383–391.
191. Raftogianis RB, Wood TC, Otterness DM, et al. Phenol sulfotransferase pharmacogenetics in humans: association of common SULT1A1 alleles with TS PST phenotype. *Biochem Biophys Res Commun* 1997;239:298–304.
192. Ratain MJ, Mick R, Berezin F, et al. Paradoxical relationship between acetylator phenotype and amonafide toxicity. *Clin Pharmacol Ther* 1991;50:573–579.
193. Reid J, Buckner J, Schaaf L, et al. Anticonvulsants alter the pharmacokinetics of irinotecan (CPT-11) in patients with recurrent glioma. *Proc Am Soc Clin Onocl* 2000;19:A160.
194. Weinshilboum RM, Otterness DM, Szumlanski CL. Methylation pharmacogenetics: catechol O-methyltransferase, thiopurine methyltransferase, and histamine N-methyltransferase. *Annu Rev Pharmacol Toxicol* 1999;39:19–52.
195. Mlakar V, Huezo-Diaz Curtis P, Satyanarayana Uppugunduri CR, et al. Pharmacogenomics in pediatric oncology: review of gene-drug associations for clinical use. *Int J Mol Sci* 2016;17.
196. Moriyama T, Nishii R, Perez-Andreu V, et al. NUDT15 polymorphisms alter thiopurine metabolism and hematopoietic toxicity. *Nat Genet* 2016;48:367–373.
197. Caronia D, Patino-Garcia A, Milne RL, et al. Common variations in ERCC2 are associated with response to cisplatin chemotherapy and clinical outcome in osteosarcoma patients. *Pharmacogenomics J* 2009;9:347–353.
198. Diasio RB, Beavers TL, Carpenter JT. Familial deficiency of dihydropyrimidine dehydrogenase. Biochemical basis for familial pyrimidinemia and severe 5-fluorouracil-induced toxicity. *J Clin Invest* 1988;81:47–51.
199. Innocenti F, Undevia SD, Iyer L, et al. Genetic variants in the UDP-glucuronosyltransferase 1A1 gene predict the risk of severe neutropenia of irinotecan. *J Clin Oncol* 2004;22:1382–1388.
200. Lal S, Mahajan A, Chen WN, et al. Pharmacogenetics of target genes across doxorubicin disposition pathway: a review. *Curr Drug Metab* 2010;11:115–128.
201. Blanco JG, Sun CL, Landier W, et al. Anthracycline-related cardiomyopathy after childhood cancer: role of polymorphisms in carbonyl reductase genes—a report from the Children's Oncology Group. *J Clin Oncol* 2012;30:1415–1421.
202. Visscher H, Ross CJ, Rassekh SR, et al. Pharmacogenomic prediction of anthracycline-induced cardiotoxicity in children. *J Clin Oncol* 2012;30:1422–1428.
203. Huang RS, Ratain MJ. Pharmacogenetics and pharmacogenomics of anticancer agents. *CA Cancer J Clin* 2009;59:42–55.
204. Nagasubramanian R, Innocenti F, Ratain MJ. Pharmacogenetics in cancer treatment. *Annu Rev Med* 2003;54:437–452.
205. Relling MV, Dervieux T. Pharmacogenetics and cancer therapy. *Nat Rev Cancer* 2001;1:99–108.
206. Watters JW, McLeod HL. Cancer pharmacogenomics: current and future applications. *Biochim Biophys Acta* 2003;1603:99–111.
207. Henderson EH, Samaha RJ. Evidence that drugs in multiple combinations have materially advanced the treatment of human malignancies. *Cancer Res* 1969;29:2272–2280.
208. Poplack DG. Acute lymphoblastic leukemia and less frequently occurring leukemias in the young. In: Levine A, ed. *Cancer in the young.* New York, NY: Masson; 1982:405–460.
209. Goldie JH, Coldman AJ. The genetic origin of drug resistance in neoplasms: implications for systemic therapy. *Cancer Res* 1984;44:3643–3653.
210. Goldie JH, Coldman AJ. Application of theoretical models to chemotherapy protocol design. *Cancer Treat Rep* 1986;70:127–131.
211. Fojo AT, Ueda K, Slamon DJ, et al. Expression of a multidrug-resistance gene in human tumors and tissues. *Proc Natl Acad Sci U S A* 1987;84:265–269.
212. List AF. Non-P-glycoprotein drug export mechanisms of multidrug resistance. *Semin Hematol* 1997;34:20–24.
213. Michieli M, Damiani D, Ermacora A, et al. P-glycoprotein (PGP), lung resistance-related protein (LRP) and multidrug resistance-associated protein (MRP) expression in acute promyelocytic leukaemia. *Br J Haematol* 2000;108:703–709.
214. Moscow JA, Schneider E, Ivy SP, et al. Multidrug resistance. *Cancer Chemother Biol Response Modif* 1997;17:139–177.
215. Pastan I, Gottesman M. Multiple-drug resistance in human cancer. *N Engl J Med* 1987;316:1388–1393.
216. Roninson IB, Abelson HT, Housman DE, et al. Amplification of specific DNA sequences correlates with multi-drug resistance in Chinese hamster cells. *Nature* 1984;309:626–628.
217. Roninson IB, Chin JE, Choi KG, et al. Isolation of human mdr DNA sequences amplified in multidrug-resistant KB carcinoma cells. *Proc Natl Acad Sci U S A* 1986;83:4538–4542.
218. Scotto KW, Biedler JL, Melera PW. Amplification and expression of genes associated with multidrug resistance in mammalian cells. *Science (New York, NY)* 1986;232:751–755.
219. Shen DW, Fojo A, Chin JE, et al. Human multidrug-resistant cell lines: increased mdr1 expression can precede gene amplification. *Science (New York, NY)* 1986;232:643–645.
220. Grem JL. Fluorinated pyrimidines. In: Chabner BA, Collins JM, eds. *Cancer chemotherapy principles and practice.* Philadelphia, PA: Lippincott; 1990:180–224.
221. Burgert EO. Ewing's sarcoma. *Curr Concepts Oncol* 1986;8:11–17.
222. Dahl GV, Rivera GK, Look AT, et al. Teniposide plus cytarabine improves outcome in childhood acute lymphoblastic leukemia presenting with a leukocyte count greater than or equal to 100 x 10(9)/L. *J Clin Oncol* 1987;5:1015–1021.
223. Geyer JR, Pendergrass TW, Milstein JM, et al. Eight drugs in one day chemotherapy in children with brain tumors: a critical toxicity appraisal. *J Clin Oncol* 1988;6:996–1000.
224. Hays DM. Rhabdomyosarcoma: management in children and young adult. *Curr Concepts Oncol* 1986;8:3–10.
225. Magrath IT, Janus C, Edwards BK, et al. An effective therapy for both undifferentiated (including Burkitt's) lymphomas and lymphoblastic lymphomas in children and young adults. *Blood* 1984;63:1102–1111.
226. Maurer HM, Beltangady M, Gehan EA, et al. The intergroup rhabdomyosarcoma study-I. A final report. *Cancer* 1988;61:209–220.
227. Miser JS, Kinsella TJ, Triche TJ, et al. Ifosfamide with mesna uroprotection and etoposide: an effective regimen in the treatment of recurrent sarcomas and other tumors of children and young adults. *J Clin Oncol* 1987;5:1191–1198.
228. Reaman GH, Ladisch S, Echelberger C, et al. Improved treatment results in the management of single and multiple relapses of acute lymphoblastic leukemia. *Cancer* 1980;45:3090–3094.
229. Dawson W. Relations between age and weight and doses of drugs. *Ann Intern Med* 1940;13:1594–1613.
230. Pinkel D. The use of body surface area as a criterion of drug dosage in cancer chemotherapy. *Cancer Res* 1958;18:853–856.
231. Gurney H. Dose calculation of anticancer drugs: a review of the current practice and introduction of an alternative. *J Clin Oncol* 1996;14:2590–2611.
232. Hempel G, Boos J. Flat-fixed dosing versus body surface area based dosing of anticancer drugs: there is a difference. *Oncologist* 2007;12:924–926.
233. Mathijssen RH, de Jong FA, Loos WJ, et al. Flat-fixed dosing versus body surface area based dosing of anticancer drugs in adults: does it make a difference? *Oncologist* 2007;12:913–923.
234. Baker SD, Verweij J, Rowinsky EK, et al. Role of body surface area in dosing of investigational anticancer agents in adults, 1991-2001. *J Natl Cancer Inst* 2002;94:1883–1888.
235. Grochow LB, Baraldi C, Noe D. Is dose normalization to weight or body surface area useful in adults? *J Natl Cancer Inst* 1990;82:323–325.
236. Gurney HP, Ackland S, Gebski V, et al. Factors affecting epirubicin pharmacokinetics and toxicity: evidence against using body-surface area for dose calculation. *J Clin Oncol* 1998;16:2299–2304.
237. Ratain MJ. Body-surface area as a basis for dosing of anticancer agents: science, myth, or habit? *J Clin Oncol* 1998;16:2297–2298.
238. McLeod HL, Relling MV, Crom WR, et al. Disposition of antineoplastic agents in the very young child. *Br J Cancer Suppl* 1992;18:S23–S29.
239. Green DM, Finklestein JZ, Norkool P, et al. Severe hepatic toxicity after treatment with single-dose dactinomycin and vincristine. A report of the National Wilms' Tumor Study. *Cancer* 1988;62:270–273.
240. Green DM, Norkool P, Breslow NE, et al. Severe hepatic toxicity after treatment with vincristine and dactinomycin using single-dose or divided-dose schedules: a report from the National Wilms' Tumor Study. *J Clin Oncol* 1990;8:1525–1530.
241. Woods WG, O'Leary M, Nesbit ME. Life-threatening neuropathy and hepatotoxicity in infants during induction therapy for acute lymphoblastic leukemia. *J Pediatr* 1981;98:642–645.
242. Balis FM, Womer RB, Berg S, et al. Dosing anticancer drugs in infants: current approach and recommendations from the Children's Oncology Group's Chemotherapy Standardization Task Force. *Pediatr Blood Cancer* 2017;64.
243. Bleyer AW. Clinical pharmacology of intrathecal methotrexate. II. An improved dosage regimen derived from age-related pharmacokinetics. *Cancer Treat Rep* 1977;61:1419–1425.
244. Bleyer WA, Coccia PF, Sather HN, et al. Reduction in central nervous system leukemia with a pharmacokinetically derived intrathecal methotrexate dosage regimen. *J Clin Oncol* 1983;1:317–325.
245. Noone A, Howlader N, Krapcho M, et al. *SEER cancer statistics review, 1975-2015.* Bethesda, MD: National Cancer Institute. https://seer.cancer.gov/csr/1975_2015/, based on November 2017 SEER data submission, posted to the SEER web site, April 2018.

SECTION

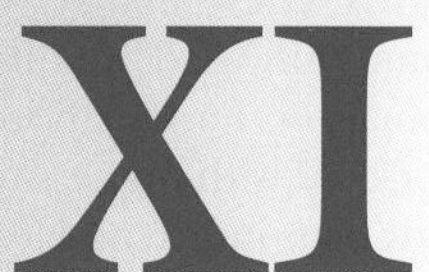

Nutritional Pharmacology, Pharmacotoxidromes, Adverse Drug Reactions, and Interactions

CHAPTER 60

Mary Frances Picciano
Michelle K. McGuire
Paul M. Coates

Nutrient Supplements

Reprinted with updates in memory of Dr. Mary Frances Picciano

INTRODUCTION

During infancy and childhood, patterns of healthy growth and development are generally predictable and orderly. Although these growth trajectories are primarily determined by genetics, environmental influences such as nutritional status can also be important. This is especially true during the most rapid periods of growth, such as those which occur in infancy and adolescence. A good example of this is proteins. During early infancy, protein requirements are estimated to be 1.52 g per kg per day; this decreases gradually through childhood until it reaches 0.8 g per kg per day.[1] Although obtaining adequate amounts of the essential nutrients *from foods* during periods of growth is considered most desirable, sometimes, this becomes difficult, and supplementation is warranted. This is especially true for several of the micronutrients (vitamins and minerals), which are the main focus of this chapter.

Vitamins and minerals are essential for myriad functions related to growth, differentiation, and development. Vitamins can also regulate the expression of genes involved in cell proliferation and tissue specification. Minerals primarily act as enzymatic cofactors and stabilizers for enzymes and transcription factors, although some are also critical for structural purposes. Because of the far-reaching functions of vitamins and minerals, micronutrient deficiencies can have negative impacts during periods of growth and development as well as long-term effects on structural integrity. Early malnutrition may also predispose an individual to increased risk for chronic degenerative diseases (e.g., cardiovascular disease) later in life.

Because of the importance of nutritional adequacy during early life, dietary recommendations for the pediatric population are relatively well delineated, and supplementation with vitamins and minerals is sometimes used to prevent or treat nutrient inadequacies.[2] The main objective of this chapter is to review a selected group of micronutrients that are most frequently provided to infants and children as dietary supplements. These include vitamin A (and the carotenoids), vitamin D, vitamin E, vitamin K, calcium, iron, zinc, iodine, and fluoride. We also comment briefly on a group of lipids referred to as the "ω-3 fatty acids." For each of these, we discuss their biologic forms and functions, dietary sources, dietary reference intake (DRI) values, signs and symptoms of deficiencies and toxicities, and the most current recommendations for supplementation. We also review the definition of a dietary supplement, how these products are regulated by the Food and Drug Administration, and statistics related to supplement use—especially in children.

WHAT IS A DIETARY SUPPLEMENT?

Although dietary supplements have long been available to the U.S. consumer, they were not officially defined until 1994 when the U.S. Congress passed the Dietary Supplement Health and Education Act (DSHEA).[3] Since that time, a "dietary supplement" has been defined as a product that meets the following requirements:

- Intended to supplement the diet or contain one or more of the following: vitamin, mineral, herb or other plant-derived substance (e.g., ginseng, garlic), amino acid, concentrate, metabolite, constituent, or extract.
- Intended for ingestion in pill, capsule, tablet, or liquid form.
- Not represented for use as a conventional food or as the sole item of a meal or diet.

The DSHEA was the first legislation to clearly define dietary supplements *as foods* (as opposed to drugs) having implications for both manufacturers and consumers in terms of what was needed (or not needed) for evidence of efficacy, safety, and quality of dietary supplement products. For example, similar to how food products are handled, manufacturers are required to have evidence to support claims of efficacy and safety. However, unlike what pharmaceutical companies are required to do for drugs, food manufacturers are generally not required to seek premarket approval of their claims by the Food and Drug Administration.

DIETARY SUPPLEMENT USE IN AMERICAN CHILDREN

The use of dietary supplements in the United States is strong and growing, and it is estimated that revenue from sales of dietary supplements was more than $21 billion in 2005.[4]

Of the dietary supplements available, vitamins and minerals—as well as combinations thereof—are the most widely used types. Most (65%) of these supplements are purchased from retail establishments, such as natural, health food, grocery, or drug stores; only 7% are obtained from a health practitioner.

Of special interest to this chapter is dietary supplement use among children. Ervin and colleagues compiled data from the National Health and Nutrition Examination Survey conducted between 1988 and 1994 (before the passage of the DSHEA) and reported that children aged 1 to 5 years were major users of dietary supplements.[5] The supplements most commonly taken by children aged 2 months to 11 years were multivitamins or combinations of multiple vitamins and minerals. Slightly less than 10% of children were taking two or more supplements.

Dietary supplement use by infants and children between 1999 and 2002 (after passage of the DSHEA) has also been reported.[6] In this study, the investigators used nationally representative data from the National Health and Nutrition Examination Survey, studying children (n = 10,136) from birth through 18 years. Their data indicate that 31.8% of children used dietary supplements, with the lowest use reported among infants younger than 1 year (11.9%), followed by teenagers 14 to 18 years (25.7%). Highest use was among 4- to 8-year-old children (48.5%). In an ethnic comparison, supplement consumption was found to be greatest in non-Hispanic white and Mexican American participants; lowest use was among non-Hispanic black participants. There appeared to be no difference in intake between boys and girls. These analyses suggest that the type of supplement most commonly used by children is a multivitamin/multimineral combination. Furthermore, supplement use was reported to be associated with higher income, a smoke-free environment, lower body mass index, and less daily recreational "screen time." The highest use was in children who were underweight or at risk for becoming underweight.

In summary, the use of dietary supplements and more specifically those containing vitamins and minerals is common in the pediatric American population. In the next sections, we discuss several micronutrients that are sometimes recommended as dietary supplements during infancy and childhood. We address their physiologic importance, recommended intakes, signs and symptoms of deficiency and toxicity, and, when possible, recommendations for supplementation.

VITAMIN A AND THE CAROTENOIDS

The term "vitamin A" (or retinoid) refers to a group of fat-soluble compounds that all contain a complex 20-carbon structure with a methyl-substituted cyclohexenyl ring and a tetrene side chain. These compounds differ among themselves in that they can contain a hydroxyl group (retinol), aldehyde group (retinal), carboxylic acid group (retinoic acid), or ester group (retinyl ester).

The term "vitamin A" is also used to describe a series of dietary compounds (called carotenoids) that can be converted in the body to retinol, some of which are shown in Figure 60.1. These dietary substances are also called "provitamin A carotenoids" to distinguish them from other carotenoids that cannot be converted to vitamin A. Carotenoids, which usually contain 40-carbon atoms with conjugated double bonds and one or two cyclic structures, function mainly as antioxidants. Of the 600 or more carotenoids that exist in nature, β-carotene, α-carotene, and cryptoxanthin are the primary provitamin A forms. There is growing interest in both non-provitamin A and provitamin A carotenoids, because higher dietary intakes of some forms have been associated with decreased risk for macular degeneration and cataracts, some cancers, and some cardiovascular events.[7]

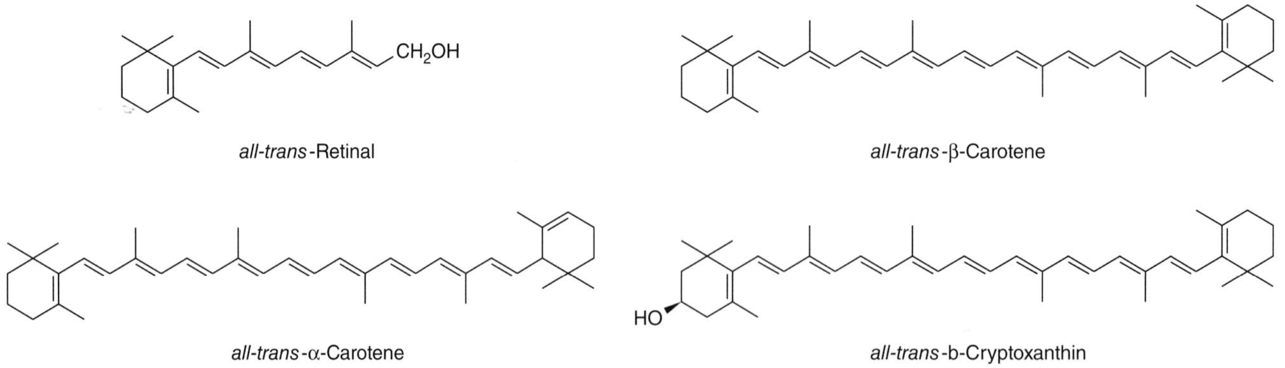

CH_2OH

all-trans-Retinal

all-trans-β-Carotene

all-trans-α-Carotene

HO

all-trans-b-Cryptoxanthin

Figure 60.1 Structures of retinol and provitamin A carotenoids. (Modified from Institute of Medicine, Food and Nutrition Board. *Dietary reference intakes for vitamin C, vitamin E, selenium, and carotenoids*. Washington, DC: National Academy Press, 2000, with permission.)

METABOLISM OF VITAMIN A

Regardless of whether it is consumed as preformed vitamin A or a provitamin A carotenoid, retinoids are metabolized in many organs (liver, intestine, kidney, and skin), being converted to different forms with specific functions. For example, retinal can be reversibly reduced to retinol and irreversibly oxidized to retinoic acid.[8] Retinoids, bound to retinoid-binding proteins and receptors, are transported to specific sites for metabolic transformations both within the plasma and the cell.

PHYSIOLOGIC ROLES OF VITAMIN A

Perhaps, the most thoroughly understood function of vitamin A (specifically retinal and retinoic acid) in the body is the role it plays in vision. Specifically, retinal is required for the transduction of light into neural signals necessary for vision, whereas retinoic acid is needed to maintain normal differentiation of the cornea and conjunctional membranes. However, vitamin A is also needed for a variety of other functions. For instance, during embryonic development, retinoic acid as well as specific retinoid receptors (retinoic acid receptor and retinoid X receptor) and retinol-binding proteins are postulated to be involved in the development of the vertebrae and spinal cord. Retinoic acid also functions in limb development and formation of the heart, eyes, and ears.[8]

Retinoic acid also appears to be involved in the genesis of tissue specificity, directing undifferentiated stem cells to stop proliferating and assume a differentiated phenotype.[8] In addition, retinoic acid regulates the expression of various genes that encode structural proteins involved in maintaining epithelial cell integrity (e.g., skin keratins), extracellular matrix proteins (e.g., laminin), and retinol-binding proteins and receptors. Retinoic acid is also needed to maintain adequate circulating levels of natural killer cells, increase macrophage phagocytic activity, and increase cytokines that mediate T- and B-lymphocyte production.[9]

DIETARY SOURCES OF VITAMIN A

Preformed vitamin A is found in some animal-derived foods, such as liver, dairy products, and fish. Provitamin A carotenoids tend to be plentiful in colorful fruits and vegetables, such as cantaloupe, carrots, broccoli, spinach, and some oily plants (e.g., avocado and red palm oil). The primary dietary form of provitamin A is β-carotene, which is cleaved to form free retinol in the small intestine. Note that the vitamin A content of foods or biologic tissues is measured using a unit referred to as a retinol activity equivalent (RAE); 1 RAE is equivalent to 1 µg of all-*trans*-retinol, 2 µg of supplemental all-*trans*-β-carotene, 12 µg of dietary all-*trans*-*β*-carotene, or 24 µg of other dietary provitamin A carotenoids.*

*Historically, vitamin A activity was described in international units (IU), with 1 µg of retinol equivalent to 3.33 IU.

DIETARY REFERENCE INTAKE VALUES FOR VITAMIN A

DRIs have been set for vitamin A during infancy. Like all of the adequate intake (AI) levels for young infants (0 to 6 months), that for vitamin A is based on the vitamin A intake of infants primarily fed human milk. The AI for this essential nutrient from 0 to 6 months is 400 µg of RAE per day; from 7 to 12 months, it is 500 µg of RAE per day. Recommended dietary allowances (RDAs) for children aged 1 to 3 and 4 to 8 years are 300 and 400 µg of RAE per day, respectively, after which time they increase. Because vitamin A toxicity can occur, tolerable upper intake levels (ULs) have also been set. These values are 600 µg of RAE per day for the first 3 years of life, 900 µg of RAE per day from 4 to 8 years, 1,700 µg per day from 9 to 13 years, and 2,800 µg per day from 14 to 18 years. The AI and UL values for vitamin A (as well as the other micronutrients discussed in this chapter) during infancy are listed in Table 60.1; the AI/RDA and UL values during childhood and adolescence can be found in Table 60.2.

CONSEQUENCES OF INADEQUATE VITAMIN A INTAKE AND EFFECT OF SUPPLEMENTATION

Because human milk, bovine milk, and infant formulas are good sources of vitamin A, vitamin A deficiency in the United States is rare in infancy and childhood. However, vitamin A deficiency can occur in infants and children with fat malabsorption.[2] Furthermore, vitamin A concentration in milk from mothers delivering prematurely is very low and may not provide recommended amounts.[10] Thus, vitamin A nutriture may be inadequate in this subpopulation, even in developed countries.

The most common signs and symptoms of vitamin A deficiency progress from night blindness to xerosis (dryness and wrinkling of the conjunctiva) and the development of Bitot spots, to corneal xerophthalmia, keratopathy, and, finally, loss of vision. In developing countries (especially Asia and Africa), vitamin A deficiency is not only the leading cause of preventable blindness, but it also elevates the risk of disease and death from severe infections, such as diarrhea and measles.[11,12] For example, children with mild xerophthalmia are at increased risk of respiratory tract infections and diarrhea, and mortality rates are up to four times greater among children with than without mild xerophthalmia. Experts estimate that between 100 and 140 million children are vitamin A deficient worldwide, 250,000 to 500,000 of whom become blind annually; half of these affected children are thought to die within 12 months of losing their sight.[13] Other factors in developing countries that can influence a child's requirement for vitamin A are the presence and severity of infection with parasites, inadequate iron status, low intakes of dietary fat, and protein energy malnutrition.

Fortunately, high-dose vitamin A supplementation can reduce the incidence of morbidity, including night blindness in children.[13] However, vitamin A supplementation may be able to reverse the process at its early stages.[14] There is also growing evidence that the risk of severe morbidity and mortality diminishes with vitamin A repletion. For example, a meta-analysis of controlled trials in several developing countries suggests a 23%

to 30% reduction in mortality of young children older than 6 months after vitamin A supplementation.[15] Similarly, a recent randomized trial conducted in Bangladesh showed a 15% reduction in all-causal mortality when newborns received a single oral supplement of vitamin A (50,000 IU) at birth.[16]

Vitamin A supplementation may also help prevent mortality and morbidity in very low-birth-weight (VLBW) infants. In support of this, a recent Cochrane review utilized data from eight randomized controlled trials that compared the effects of supplemental vitamin A with standard vitamin A regimes in VLBW infants.[17] These authors concluded that supplementing VLBW infants with vitamin A was associated with a reduction in death or oxygen requirement at 1 month of age and oxygen requirement among survivors at 36 weeks, with the latter outcome being confined to infants with birth weight less than 1,000 g.

Improvement in vitamin A status of preterm infants is also associated with decreased incidence of and morbidity from bronchopulmonary dysplasia, indicating that vitamin A supplementation may prevent lung injury and promote healing.[18] Vitamin A supplementation may be especially beneficial for extremely LBW infants. Ambalavanan and colleagues determined whether vitamin A supplementation in extremely LBW infants ($n = 807$) during the first month after birth affects survival without neurodevelopmental impairment.[19] Although they found no evidence that neonatal vitamin A supplementation reduced hospitalizations or pulmonary problems after discharge, those provided with supplementation had reduced bronchopulmonary dysplasia.

Many recent studies have reported positive effects of vitamin A supplementation on overall infant and child health, especially in areas of endemic vitamin A deficiency, although others show no effect and sometimes even detrimental outcomes.[20–22] An example is a randomized clinical trial of 147 severely anemic children living in Zanzibar who were being treated with the antimalarial drug sulfadoxine pyrimethamine.[23] The authors hypothesized that both vitamin A (100,000 or 200,000 IU depending on age) and sulfadoxine pyrimethamine treatments

TABLE 60.1 Representative Values for Nutrient Content of Mature Human Milk and Reference Intake Values for Selected Nutrients During Infancy and Childhood

			DRI[a]		
Nutrient	*Milk Content Per Liter*[b]	*Estimated Infant Intake Per Day*[c]	*Age (mo)*	*AI*	*UL*
Retinol (μg)	300–600	200–500	0–6	400	600
			7–12	500	600
Carotenoids (mg)	0.2–0.6	0.2–0.5	–	–	–
Vitamin D (μg)[d]	0.33	0.26	0–6	5	25
			7–12	5	25
Vitamin E (mg)	3.0–8.0	2.3–6.2	0–6	4	ND
			7–12	5	ND
Vitamin K (μg)	2–3	1.6–2.3	0–6	2	ND
			7–12	2.5	ND
Calcium (mg)	200–250	156–195	0–6	210	ND
			7–12	270	ND
Iron (mg)	0.3–0.9	0.2–0.7	0–6	0.27	40
			7–12	11	40
Zinc (mg)	1.0–3.0	0.8–2.3	0–6	2	4
			7–12	3	5
Iodine (μg)	113–150	88–117	0–6	110	ND
			7–12	130	ND
Fluoride (μg)	4–15	3–12	0–6	10	700
			7–12	500	900

[a]From Institute of Medicine, Food and Nutrition Board. *Dietary reference intakes for vitamin C, vitamin E, selenium, and carotenoids.* Washington, DC: National Academy Press, 2000; Institute of Medicine, Food and Nutrition Board. *Dietary reference intakes for calcium, phosphorus, magnesium, vitamin D, and fluoride.* Washington, DC: National Academy Press, 1997; Institute of Medicine, Food and Nutrition Board. *Dietary reference intakes for vitamin A, vitamin K, arsenic, boron, chromium, copper, iodine, iron, manganese, molybdenum, nickel, silicon, vanadium, and zinc.* Washington, DC: National Academy Press, 2001.

[b]Data from Jensen RG, ed., *Handbook of milk composition.* San Diego, CA: Academic Press, 1995; Picciano MF. Nutrient composition of human milk. *Pediatr Clin North Am* 2001;48:53–67.

[c]Estimated intake based on milk intake of 0.78 L/d for the first 6 months of life.

[d]The American Academy of Pediatrics recommends all breastfed infants be supplemented with 400 IU/d vitamin D beginning within the first few days of life. Formula-fed infants receiving less than 1 L/d vitamin D–fortified formula also need an alternative way to get 400 IU/d vitamin D, such as through vitamin supplements.[2]

AI, adequate intake; DRI, dietary reference intakes; ND, no data available; UL, tolerable upper intake level.

TABLE 60.2 Dietary Reference Intakes (Per Day) of Nutrients Likely to be Limiting in Diets of Children

Nutrient	*Age (y)*	*RDA/AI*[a]	*UL*	*Dietary Sources*
Retinol (μg)	1–3	**300**	600	Liver, dairy products, fish
	4–8	**400**	900	
	9–13	**600**	1,700	
	14–18	**900,700**	2,800	
Vitamin D (μg)[b]	1–3	5	50	Fish liver oils, animal products from animals-fed vitamin D, fortified milk, and cereals
	4–8	5	50	
	9–13	5	50	
	14–18	5	50	
Vitamin E (mg)	1–3	**6**	200	Vegetable oils, unprocessed cereal grains, nuts, fruits, vegetables, meats
	4–8	**7**	300	
	9–13	**11**	600	
	14–18	**15**	800	
Vitamin K (μg)	1–3	30	ND	Green vegetables, Brussel sprouts, cabbage, plant oils, margarine
	4–8	55	ND	
	9–13	60	ND	
	14–18	75	ND	
Calcium (mg)	1–3	500	2,500	Dairy products, calcium-set tofu, legumes, Chinese cabbage, kale, broccoli
	4–8	800	2,500	
	9–13	1,300	2,500	
	14–18	1,300	2,500	
Iron (mg)	1–3	**7**	40	Fruits, vegetables, and fortified cereals (nonheme), meat and poultry (heme)
	4–8	**10**	40	
	9–13	**8**	40	
	14–18	**11, 15**	45	
Zinc (mg)	1–3	**3**	7	Red meats, poultry, seafoods, beans, nuts, legumes, fortified cereals
	4–8	**5**	12	
	9–13	**8**	23	
	14–18	**11, 9**	34	
Iodine (μg)	1–3	**90**	200	Sea products, processed foods, dairy products, iodized salt
	4–8	**90**	300	
	9–13	**120**	600	
	14–18	**150**	900	
Fluoride (mg)	1–3	0.7	1.3	Fluoridated water, teas, marine fish, fluoridated dental products
	4–8	1	2.2	
	9–13	2	10	
	14–18	3	10	

[a]For boys and girls.
[b]The American Academy of Pediatrics recommends that all children and teens consume 400 IU per d vitamin D from fortified foods or supplements.[2]
AI, adequate intake; ND, no data available; RDA, recommended dietary allowance (in bold type); UL, tolerable upper intake level.
From Institute of Medicine, Food and Nutrition Board. *Dietary reference intakes for vitamin C, vitamin E, selenium, and carotenoids.* Washington, DC: National Academy Press, 2000; Institute of Medicine, Food and Nutrition Board. *Dietary reference intakes for calcium, phosphorus, magnesium, vitamin D, and fluoride.* Washington, DC: National Academy Press, 1997; Institute of Medicine, Food and Nutrition Board. *Dietary reference intakes for vitamin A, vitamin K, arsenic, boron, chromium, copper, iodine, iron, manganese, molybdenum, nickel, silicon, vanadium, and zinc.* Washington, DC: National Academy Press, 2001.

rapidly stimulate erythropoietin production. However, while it did reduce inflammation (as measured by C-reactive protein) and mobilized iron from stores, vitamin A supplementation decreased erythropoietin concentrations. There is also evidence of a differential response to vitamin A supplementation between boys and girls.[24,25] and this interaction between vitamin A supplementation and sex on vitamin A–related outcomes warrants further study.

Because low vitamin A status has been shown to be a risk factor for maternal-to-child human immunodeficiency virus (HIV) transmission, there has also been considerable interest in whether vitamin A supplementation may be beneficial. Several intervention trials have been conducted, some of them (but not all) suggesting a positive outcome of supplementation.[26] However, unease about potential negative outcomes associated with large-dose maternal or neonatal vitamin A supplementation on infant mortality in HIV-endemic areas is considerable.[27] Emerging data suggest that there may exists a gene–environment interaction between having the mannose-binding lectin (*MBL-2*) gene and vitamin A intake in terms of HIV transmission during infancy.[28]

CONSEQUENCES OF EXCESSIVE INTAKE OF VITAMIN A

Commonly recognized signs and symptoms of vitamin A toxicity (hypervitaminosis A) in infants and young children include skeletal abnormalities, bone tenderness and pain, increased intracranial pressure, desquamation, brittle nails, mouth fissures, alopecia, fever, headache, lethargy, irritability, weight loss, vomiting, and hepatomegaly.[29] As little as 1,800 μg RAE per day can produce serious toxic effects in children. Although vitamin A toxicity is typically associated with excessive consumption of supplemental vitamin A, toxic effects have also been reported in young children fed large amounts of chicken liver daily (90 μg per g RAE) for 1 month or longer.[30]

Experimental data indicate that β-carotene, even when ingested in extremely large doses, is not carcinogenic, mutagenic, embryotoxic, or teratogenic. Instead, it results in a benign disorder referred to as *hypercarotenemia*, characterized by elevated concentrations of carotenoids in serum and liver and carotenoid deposits in skin and underlying subcutaneous adipose, causing the skin to become yellowish orange in color.[31]

RECOMMENDATIONS FOR VITAMIN A SUPPLEMENTATION DURING INFANCY AND CHILDHOOD

The International Vitamin A Consultative Group, the World Health Organization (WHO), and the United Nations Children's Fund recommend oral doses of vitamin A for infants and young children in vitamin A–deficient populations. Specifically, the International Vitamin A Consultative Group recommends that three 50,000 IU doses of vitamin A should be given at the same time as infant vaccines during the first 6 months of life in all populations where vitamin A deficiency is an important public health problem.[32] High-dose vitamin A treatment is also recommended for infants and young children with xerophthalmia, severe malnutrition, or measles. The WHO recommends broad-based prophylaxis with vitamin A in vitamin A–deficient children who suffer from xerophthalmia, measles, prolonged diarrhea, wasting malnutrition, and other acute infections.

Specifically, if a child shows any ocular signs of deficiency, it is recommended that he/she receive vitamin A on days 1, 2, and 14 and then repeatedly throughout the first year of life.[33] The American Academy of Pediatrics (AAP) does not make any special recommendations concerning dietary supplementation with vitamin A during infancy and childhood other than those associated with using appropriate human milk fortifiers and proprietary formulas when needed. However, there is some evidence that supplemental vitamin A may be indicated for LBW preterm infants.[10,17]

VITAMIN D

Vitamin D (technically referred to as calciferol) and its metabolites constitute a group of fat-soluble sterols that are essential for proper growth and development of the skeletal system. Vitamin D exists in two major physiologically relevant forms: vitamin D_2 (ergocalciferol) and vitamin D_3 (cholecalciferol) (Fig. 60.2). Ergosterol, the precursor to vitamin D_2, is synthesized by plants; 7-dehydrocholesterol, the precursor of vitamin D_3, is synthesized by humans and other mammals in their skin. Conversion

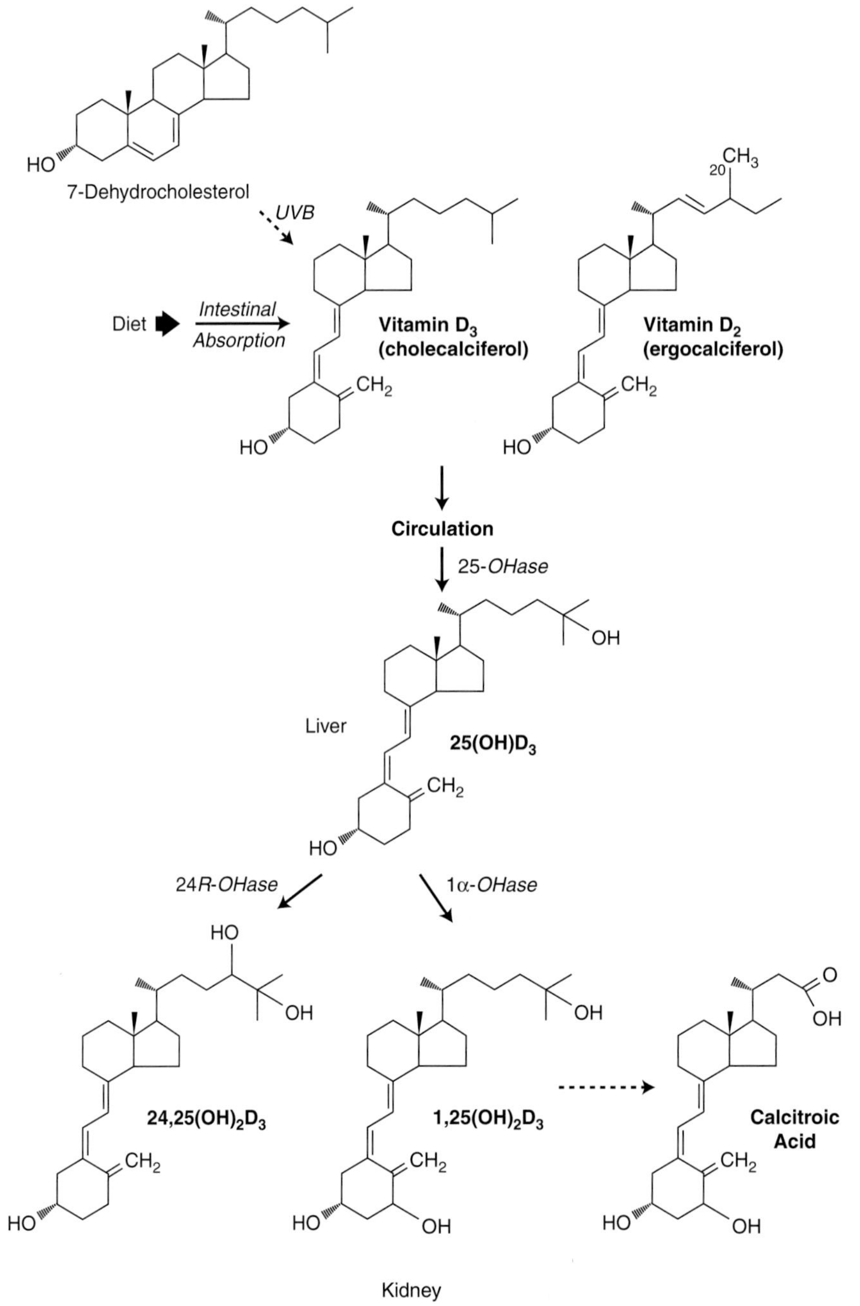

Figure 60.2 Metabolic pathways for vitamin D_3. Vitamin D_2 originates from ergosterol. Major metabolic steps in vitamin D_2 metabolism are similar to those in vitamin D_3 metabolism. 25-OHase, vitamin D 25-hydroxylase; 24R-OHase, 25(OH)D-24R-hydroxylase; 1α-OHase, 25-OH-D-1α-hydroxylase; UVB, ultraviolet B light. (Modified from Holick MF. Vitamin D. In: Olso NJA, Shike M, Ross AC, et al., eds. *Modern nutrition in health and disease.* Baltimore, MA: Williams & Wilkins, 1999:347–362, with permission.)

of both precursors to active vitamin D initially requires cleavage via ultraviolet B light (UVB; 290 to 320 nm). It is because of this that vitamin D is sometimes referred to as the "sunshine vitamin" and why vitamin D deficiency is more common in areas of the world where exposure to sunlight is limited (e.g., Scandinavian countries). The availability and metabolism of vitamin D is complex, involving endogenous synthesis, sunlight exposure, dietary intake, and biotransformation to active and inactive metabolites (Fig. 60.2). Briefly, circulating vitamin D_3 is converted in the liver to 25-hydroxyvitamin D_3 and then again hydroxylated principally in the kidney to the biologically active form, 1,25-dihydroxyvitamin D_3 (calcitriol).

PHYSIOLOGIC ROLES OF VITAMIN D

Vitamin D has many roles in the body, although the most well studied relates to its importance in skeletal growth and maturation. For instance, the active metabolite (calcitriol) functions as a hormone along with parathyroid hormone (PTH) in small intestine, bone, and kidney tissues to maintain serum calcium and phosphate concentrations within physiologically optimal ranges. In addition to enhancing dietary absorption of calcium and phosphorus in the small intestine, 1,25-dihydroxy-vitamin D_3 functions with PTH to mobilize calcium from bone and increase renal resorption of calcium when blood calcium is low. Other recently recognized functions of vitamin D include immunomodulation, control of other hormone systems, inhibition of cell growth, and induction of cell differentiation.[34–36]

SOURCES OF VITAMIN D AND FACTORS AFFECTING VITAMIN D STATUS

As described, the body can synthesize vitamin D, given adequate precursor material and sunlight. In this way, vitamin D is often considered a conditionally essential nutrient or prohormone, instead of an essential nutrient. Nonetheless, vitamin D can be obtained from dietary sources and is, therefore, a nutrient. Like vitamin A, the amount of vitamin D in a food or biologic material is measured by the amount of biologic activity it provides. In the case of vitamin D, the IU, the biologic activity of 1 μg of vitamin D is said to be 40 IU.[37] One International Unit of vitamin D activity is equivalent to 5 ng of 25-hydroxyvitamin D_3 and 1 ng of 1,25-dihydroxyvitamin D_3.

Egg yolks, butter, whole milk, fatty fish, fish oils, and mushrooms are some of the few foods that naturally contain vitamin D, and even these foods are not especially rich sources. Therefore, obtaining an AI of vitamin D solely from nonfortified foods is seldom possible.[38] However, most liquid and dried milk products as well as breakfast cereals are fortified with this vitamin, and, in fact, most dietary vitamin D comes from these foods in the United States. Human milk is relatively low in vitamin D (0.33 μg per L IU), unless the mother is given supraphysiologic doses of the vitamin.[39]

Dietary vitamin D intake can influence an individual's vitamin D status. However, perhaps more than any other nutrient, other environmental and lifestyle factors are also important. One of these factors is latitude.[37] Changes in season and dark skin pigmentation also affect vitamin D status. Compared with their lighter skin counterparts, individuals with darker skin require longer periods of sun exposure to produce similar amounts of vitamin D.

REFERENCE INTAKE VALUES FOR VITAMIN D AND RECOMMENDATIONS FOR SOLAR EXPOSURE

The AI for vitamin D during infancy, childhood, and adolescence is 5 μg per day (Tables 60.1 and 60.2). Experts now agree that the dietary intake of vitamin D recommended to prevent vitamin D deficiency in normal infants cannot be met with human milk as the sole source of vitamin D. The same is likely true for dietary sources for children and adolescents. Thus, additional vitamin D must be obtained from endogenous production (via sunlight exposure) and/or supplements. Recommendations for solar exposure are discussed here, whereas recommendations for supplementation are provided in a subsequent section.

The amount of solar exposure needed to furnish adequate vitamin D is difficult to define because the amount of UVB light that penetrates skin depends on many factors, such as latitude, time of day, level of air pollution, extent of skin pigmentation, sunscreen usage, and habitual dress. Nonetheless, Specker et al. suggested sun exposure of 30 minutes per week was adequate for white infants wearing only a diaper and living in Cincinnati, Ohio (USA), or 2 hours per week if they were fully clothed without a hat.[40] However, dietary or supplemental sources of vitamin D become essential during the winter months at northern latitudes because intensity of and exposure to UVB radiation is insufficient to meet the needs for endogenous synthesis.

Because vitamin D toxicity can occur, ULs for this nutrient have also been set. Based on measurement of linear growth[41] and hypercalcemia,[42] the UL for infants is 25 μg (1,000 IU) of vitamin D per day for the first 12 months of life; this doubles to 50 μg of vitamin D per day for children aged 1 to 18 years[37] (Tables 60.1 and 60.2).

CONSEQUENCES OF INADEQUATE VITAMIN D STATUS

Vitamin D deficiency during early life can result in a serious disease called rickets, which results from inadequate synthesis of 1,25-dihydroxyvitamin D_3. Rickets is characterized by impaired skeletal mineralization at the epiphyseal growth plates, causing deformities and poor linear growth of the long bones. Clinical signs of advanced rickets include craniotabes, frontal skull bossing, rachitic rosary (enlarged costochondral junctions), widened ribs, bowed legs, and muscle weakness. Subclinical vitamin D deficiency occurs months before signs of rickets become obvious and is assessed by measuring plasma 25-hydroxyvitamin D_3 concentration. Vitamin D deficiency later in life can result in osteomalacia, and emerging evidence suggests that low vitamin D status may be a risk factor to the development of various chronic diseases, including cardiovascular disease, hypertension, diabetes mellitus, some inflammatory and autoimmune diseases, and cancer.[43–45]

Until recently, rickets resulting from vitamin D deficiency was believed to be almost nonexistent in the United States. However, many cases of rickets due to low vitamin D intake and inadequate endogenous synthesis in the skin have recently been reported in the United States as well as in other Western countries such as Canada, Greece, and the United Kingdom.[46–50] Vitamin D–deficiency rickets is also common in breastfed infants of Arab and south Asian countries.[51] One recent estimate suggests that the annual incidence of vitamin D–deficiency rickets in developed countries ranges between 2.9

and 7.5 cases per 100,000 children.[52] Other data suggest that lesser degrees of vitamin D insufficiency are also widespread.[53] Vitamin D–deficiency rickets has also been reported recently in adolescence, thus making the issue of vitamin D deficiency crucial during the entire period of growth.[54–56]

Infants and children with dark skin pigmentation, living at northern latitudes, or who are exclusively breastfed are at highest risk for developing vitamin D deficiency. Vitamin D–deficiency rickets is also more common in children whose mothers observe the Islamic custom of covering their entire bodies with clothing; practice prolonged breastfeeding without vitamin supplementation or addition of vitamin D–fortified dairy products in their infants' diet; or do not themselves consume vitamin D–fortified dairy products.

CONSEQUENCES OF EXCESSIVE VITAMIN D INTAKE

Large oral doses of vitamin D lead to excessive calcium absorption by the intestine, increased bone resorption, and hypercalcemia. This condition, referred to as *hypervitaminosis* D, is characterized by elevated levels of 25-hydroxyvitamin D_3 ranging from 160 to 500 ng per mL.[37] Hypercalcemia associated with hypervitaminosis D disrupts normal kidney function, resulting in polydipsia and polyuria. Anorexia, nausea, and vomiting have also been reported in individuals taking 50,000 to 200,000 IU of vitamin D per day. It is noteworthy that doses of 1,800 to 6,300 IU of vitamin D per day were reported decades ago to inhibit linear growth.[37] However, that finding was not confirmed in a later study conducted over a longer period of time and with a larger number of infants.[41]

RECOMMENDATIONS FOR VITAMIN D SUPPLEMENTATION

Because of growing concerns of widespread vitamin D deficiency in infants and children—especially those with dark skin—several organizations now recommend routine vitamin D supplementation in these groups. Data from studies conducted in China, the United States, and Norway show that consumption of at least 200 IU of vitamin D per day prevents clinical signs of vitamin D deficiency and maintains serum 25-hydroxyvitamin D_3 at or above 27.5 nmol per L (11 ng per mL). Indeed, this value is consistent with the current AI for vitamin D during infancy.[37] However, it is clear that 25-hydroxyvitamin D_3 concentrations of more than 50 nmol per L can be maintained in exclusively breastfed infants with supplements of 400 IU of vitamin D per day, which is the amount contained in one teaspoon of cod liver oil and for which there is historic precedence of safety and prevention and treatment of rickets.[57–59]

In light of the AAP recommendation that infants be kept out of direct sunlight and wear protective clothing and sunscreen when exposed to sunlight,[60] it is important that special efforts be directed toward supplementing populations at increased risk of developing rickets and vitamin D deficiency. Therefore, the AAP recommends that all breastfed infants be supplemented with 400 IU of vitamin D per day beginning within the first few days of life.[60] Formula-fed infants receiving less than 1 L of vitamin D–fortified formula per day also need an alternative way to get 400 IU of vitamin D per day, such as through vitamin supplements. This level of supplementation should be continued through childhood. Adolescents who do not obtain 400 IU of vitamin D per day through vitamin D–fortified milk (100 IU per 8 oz serving) and vitamin D–fortified foods should receive a vitamin D supplement of 400 IU per day.

VITAMIN E

The term "vitamin E" refers to all tocol and tocotrienol chemical derivatives that exhibit biologic activity similar to that of α-tocopherol, the most abundant and active form of vitamin E. Vitamin E occurs in eight naturally occurring forms: four tocopherols and four tocotrienols (Fig. 60.3). As shown in Figure 60.3, tocopherols have similar chromanol structures, which vary only in the number and position of methyl groups on the chromanol ring: trimethyl (α), dimethyl (β or γ), and mono (δ). Tocotrienols differ from tocopherols in that they have an unsaturated side chain.

The most biologically active form of vitamin E occurs naturally in foods and thus is often referred to as "natural" α-tocopherol or, more technically, *RRR*-α-tocopherol.† Synthetic vitamin E is a mixture of eight stereoisomers of α-tocopherol and is designated all-*rac*-α-tocopherol (often termed d,l-α-tocopherol). Compared with *RRR*-α-tocopherol, other stereoisomers of all-*rac*-α-tocopherol have lower (21% to 90%) biologic activity. Absorption of α-tocopherol from natural and synthetic sources is similar. Synthetic vitamin E is preferentially degraded over the natural forms; thus, it is postulated that *RRR*-α-tocopherol has a specific regulatory role in a system that sorts, distributes, and degrades the different forms of vitamin E.[62]

PHYSIOLOGIC ROLES OF VITAMIN E

Vitamin E has many functions in the body, the first recognized being that of reproduction. In fact, the name *tocopherol* was derived from the Greek *tokos* (childbirth) and *phero* (to bear). In general, this vitamin functions as a chain-breaking antioxidant to prevent free radical damage.[63] Specifically, vitamin E typically carries out its antioxidant function within membranes. This antioxidant protection is especially important in cells that are exposed to oxygen, such as those in the lungs and red blood cells. Recent evidence also suggests a protective effect of vitamin E in the eye, such that cataract formation may be decreased with vitamin E supplementation.[64]

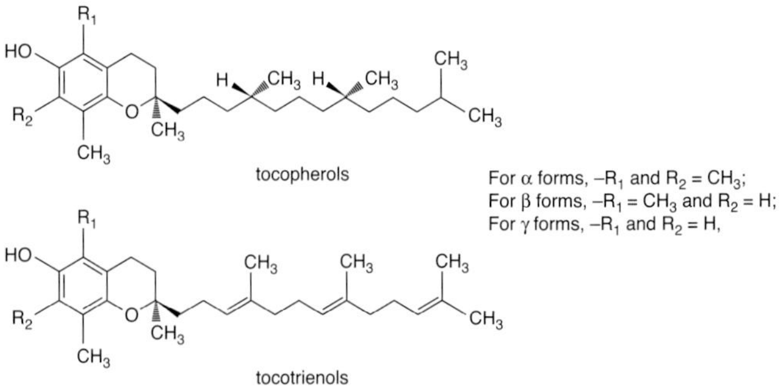

tocopherols

tocotrienols

For α forms, $-R_1$ and $R_2 = CH_3$;
For β forms, $-R_1 = CH_3$ and $R_2 = H$;
For γ forms, $-R_1$ and $R_2 = H$,

Figure 60.3 Parent forms of tocopherols and tocotrienols. (Modified from Traber MG, Sies H. Vitamin E in humans: demand and delivery. *Ann Rev Nutr* 1996;16:321–347, with permission.)

†*RRR*-α-tocopherol was formerly called "d-α-tocopherol."

DIETARY SOURCES OF VITAMIN E

Natural α-tocopherol is obtained largely from dietary sources, such as whole grains, nuts, vegetable oils, and meats. The *RRR*-α-tocopherol content is especially high in wheat germ, safflower oil, and sunflower oil. Vitamin E in the diet is typically associated with polyunsaturated fatty acids (PUFAs), in particular linoleic acid. Vitamin E supplements, such as those widely consumed in the United States, are sold in the retinyl ester form and can contain natural *RRR*-α-tocopherol or the synthetic all-*rac*-α-tocopherol.

A common unit is used to express the total vitamin E activity of a food, diet, or biologic sample. Traditionally, the IU for vitamin E was based on the biologic activity as determined by a rat fetal resorption assay. However, current convention is to report the vitamin E activity of a substance using units of milligrams of *RRR*-α-tocopherol, or *RRR*-α-tocopherol equivalents (αTE). For purposes of calculating vitamin E intakes in αTE, γ-tocopherol is assumed to substitute for α-tocopherol with an efficiency of 10%, β-tocopherol with an efficiency of 50%, and α-tocotrienol with an efficiency of 30%. Note that 1 mg of α-tocopherol (αTE) is equal to 1.49 IU of vitamin E.

Experts generally agree that human milk supplies an amount of vitamin E adequate to meet the requirements of term infants. Values in human milk for α-tocopherol equivalents, composed mainly of α-tocopherol, range from 3.0 to 8.0 mg per L, and the vitamin E content of milk from mothers of preterm infants is similar to that from mothers of term infants (Table 60.1).[39] Maternal tocopherol intake via supplements does not appear to have a major influence on the vitamin E content of human milk.[65]

REFERENCE INTAKE VALUES FOR VITAMIN E

The AI for vitamin E is 4 mg per day from 0 to 6 months and 5 mg per day from 7 to 12 months (Table 60.1). The RDA increases progressively to 15 mg per day during childhood and adolescence (Table 60.2). ULs for vitamin E increase from 200 to 800 during infancy, childhood, and adolescence. These values apply to any form of supplemental vitamin E, fortified foods, or a combination of the two, but not to vitamin E from natural forms.

CONSEQUENCES OF INADEQUATE VITAMIN E INTAKE

Vitamin E deficiency is rare in the United States but can occur in situations related to fat malabsorption. An example of rather widespread vitamin E deficiency occurred in the 1960s and the 1970s when some infant formulas contained high levels of PUFAs and low levels of vitamin E. Because PUFAs are easily damaged (oxidized) by free radicals, consumption of these formulas caused infants to have an increased need for antioxidant nutrients such as vitamin E. This event led to vitamin E fortification of infant formulas. Symptoms of vitamin E deficiency include peripheral neuropathy, hemolytic anemia, and abnormalities in platelet function.

CONSEQUENCES OF EXCESSIVE VITAMIN E INTAKE

Excessively high doses of vitamin E consumed as supplements or given as intravenous solutions have resulted in toxicity in adults and preterm infants. For instance, intravenous administration of all-*rac*-α-tocopherol acetate (E-Ferol; 15 to 30 mg) to VLBW preterm infants caused pulmonary deterioration, thrombocytopenia, and liver and renal failure.[66] Other reports of toxicity associated with pharmacologic oral or parenteral doses of vitamin E include increased risk of necrotizing enterocolitis, sepsis, and retinal hemorrhages.[63] When serum vitamin E concentrations are less than 3.5 mg per dL, adverse reactions of vitamin E supplementation are not reported in preterm infants; however, at greater concentrations, adverse reactions are not uncommon.[67]

RECOMMENDATIONS FOR VITAMIN E SUPPLEMENTATION

Because the vitamin E concentration in human milk is viewed to be sufficient to meet the needs of term infants, there is no evidence to support vitamin E supplementation for breastfeeding mothers and their healthy infants. However, in conditions of fat malabsorption, supplemental doses of 25 IU per kg per day of vitamin E are required to prevent deficiency. In these situations, the water-soluble form of vitamin E is preferable.[2]

The usefulness of vitamin E supplementation in preterm infants is somewhat controversial.[10] Some experts have suggested that LBW preterm infants receive 6 to 12 IU per kg per day of vitamin E enterally because vitamin E levels in human milk decline as lactation proceeds and because preterm infants have low stores at birth, poor absorption of fat, and increased risk of oxidative stress.[65] However, the AAP does not recommend pharmacologic doses of vitamin E for the prevention or treatment of retinopathy of prematurity, bronchopulmonary dysplasia, and intraventricular hemorrhage.[2]

VITAMIN K

Vitamin K is a fat-soluble vitamin that functions as a coenzyme for the synthesis of biologically active proteins involved in blood coagulation and bone metabolism. For example, vitamin K–dependent carboxylase, a liver microsomal enzyme, uses vitamin K as a substrate to catalyze the posttranslational conversion of specific glutamyl residues to γ-carboxylglutamyl (Gla) residues in a number of proteins.[68] Biologically activated proteins dependent on vitamin K include the clotting factors plasma prothrombin (factor II), VII, IX, and Xm as well as proteins C and S, which have anticoagulant activity. In the absence of vitamin K, hemorrhage results from the formation of biologically inactive clotting factors. Other vitamin K–dependent proteins—such as bone Gla protein (also called "osteocalcin") and matrix Gla protein—are postulated to function in the mineralization of bone, but their mechanisms of action remain unclear.

SOURCES AND FORMS OF VITAMIN K

Vitamin K found in the body is obtained from two sources—diet and synthesis by intestinal microbiota. Naturally occurring vitamin K exists in two forms: vitamin K_1 (phylloquinone), synthesized by and found in plants, and vitamin K_2 (menaquinone), synthesized by higher organisms, including intestinal bacteria. A third synthetic form is called menadione (Fig. 60.4).

Most foods contain little vitamin K, and the vitamin K content of human milk is also low (2 to 3 µg per L; Table 60.1).[39] Food sources of this vitamin include green leafy vegetables

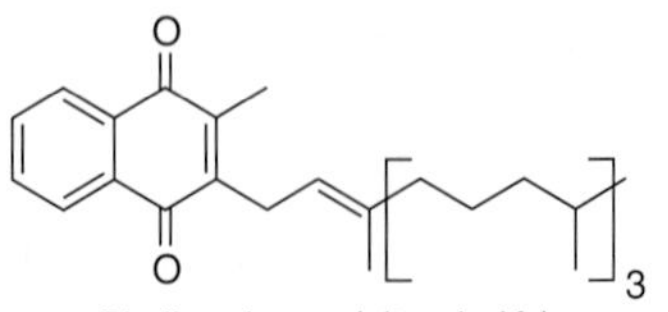

Figure 60.4 Biologically active forms of vitamin K. (Modified from Suttie JW. Vitamin K and human nutrition. *J Am Diet Assoc* 1992;92:585–590, with permission.)

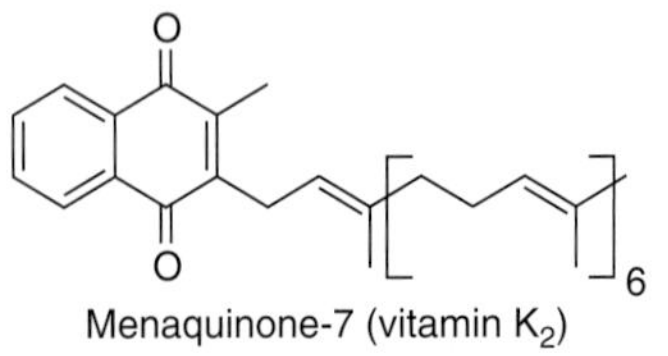

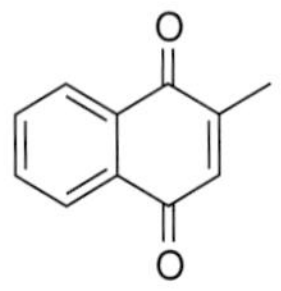

(e.g., collards, spinach, salad greens), vegetable oils, and margarine.[69] Although the combination of dietary vitamin K intake and intestinal synthesis in adults is typically thought to be sufficient, adequate dietary intake of vitamin K for infants aged 0 to 12 months is less likely. Aside from low levels in human milk,[39] inadequate stores of vitamin K resulting from poor placental transport also contribute to the low vitamin K status in some newborn infants. In fact, serum vitamin K concentration is low or undetectable in cord blood.

REFERENCE INTAKE VALUES FOR VITAMIN K

Establishment of DRI values for vitamin K was challenging because the dietary requirements and metabolism of vitamin K are poorly understood. This is, in part, because of the lack of sensitive methods to assess vitamin K status.[69] For example, although serum phylloquinone concentration reflects dietary intake over the previous 24 hours, it is not a good indicator of chronic vitamin K status.[69]

Nonetheless, recommended intake values of this vitamin in early life have been established. The AI for infants 0 through 6 months of age was determined to be 2.0 µg of vitamin K per day and assumes that infants also receive prophylactic vitamin K at birth in amounts suggested by the American and Canadian pediatric societies (as discussed next). The AI increases to 2.5 µg per day from 7 to 12 months of life and then again to 30 and 55 µg per day at 1 and 4 years, respectively. The AI for 9- to 18-year-olds is 60 to 75 µg per day. Data on adverse effects from high vitamin K intakes are not sufficient for a quantitative risk assessment, and no adverse effects have been reported with high intakes of this vitamin. Thus, UL values have not been set.

CONSEQUENCES OF INADEQUATE VITAMIN K INTAKE

Poor vitamin K status at birth associated with bleeding during the first weeks of life is now termed *vitamin K–deficiency bleeding* (VKDB) and is categorized as early, classic, and late.[70‡] The early form occurs in the first 24 hours of life and is characterized by cephalic hematoma and intracranial and intra-abdominal hemorrhage. Early VKDB is sometimes noted in infants born to mothers treated with anticoagulants or anticonvulsants during pregnancy. In the classic form, hemorrhage occurs between 2 and 7 days of life, with bleeding occurring from the umbilical cord stump, gastrointestinal tract, or circumcision site. Late VKDB presents between 7 days and 3 months of life, often resulting in intracranial hemorrhage and sometimes death.

VKDB occurs almost exclusively in breastfed infants who have not received vitamin K prophylaxis or have gastrointestinal disorders associated with fat malabsorption.[71] Furthermore, researchers have found that most cases of late VKDB are found in infants not receiving prophylactic vitamin K treatment at birth.

CONSEQUENCES OF EXCESSIVE VITAMIN K INTAKE

Vitamin K toxicity is rare, and no adverse effects have been associated with excessive vitamin K consumption from food or supplements in recent years. An earlier report, however, of increased risk of cancer and leukemia developing during childhood raised concern about vitamin K prophylaxis.[72] As a result of methodologic limitations of that study, multiple large case-cohort studies were conducted; no relationship was found between vitamin K given intramuscularly at birth and development of cancer and leukemia in children.[73,74]

RECOMMENDATIONS FOR VITAMIN K SUPPLEMENTATION

The efficacy of parenteral vitamin K prophylaxis in prevention of classic VKDB is well established, and several recommendations for vitamin K supplementation and/or injection during infancy have been put forth. Both American and Canadian pediatric societies recommend that newborns receive vitamin K as phylloquinone in a single intramuscular dose of 0.5 to 1.0 mg.[2,75] If this is not possible, an oral dose of 1 to 2 mg should be administered at birth, 1 to 2 weeks of age, and 4 weeks of age. Oral supplements of vitamin K are not presently licensed for newborn infants in the United States, although several researchers recommend that they be developed.[76,77]

The situation for preterm infants is less well defined. Kumar et al.[70] found that premature infants given 1 mg of vitamin K intramuscularly at birth plus 60 to 130 µg per day parenterally exhibited plasma vitamin K levels directly reflective of vitamin K intakes and adequate vitamin K status. Consequently, these authors suggest that 10 µg per kg per day of vitamin K via the parenteral route of administration is more than adequate to maintain adequate vitamin K status in preterm infants. The AAP recommends that preterm infants receive 0.5 mg vitamin K as a single intramuscular dose. In conditions associated with fat malabsorption, supplemental doses of 2.5 to 5 mg two to seven times per week may be required to prevent vitamin K deficiency.[2]

Maternal supplementation with vitamin K may be an alternative for parents not wishing their newborns to receive intramuscular vitamin K prophylaxis. In exclusively breastfed infants

‡VKDB was previously termed "hemorrhagic disease of the newborn."

not receiving intramuscular phylloquinone at birth, vitamin K status was improved by maternal oral supplements of 5 mg per day of phylloquinone through the first 12 weeks postpartum.[78]

CALCIUM

Calcium is the most abundant mineral in the body, being the main structural component of the skeletal system. Whereas approximately 99% of the body's calcium is in bones and teeth, the other 1% is also critical for health, being found in plasma and soft tissues where it functions in vasoconstriction, vasodilation, muscle contraction, nerve impulse transmission, and hormone secretion. Recent evidence also suggests that calcium may play a role in regulating body composition, although not all studies are in agreement.[79–81] Regulation of serum calcium concentration is orchestrated by the actions of several hormones, including PTH and calcitonin.

The most commonly used index of calcium homeostasis is serum total calcium concentration, but this does not reflect dietary intake because it is tightly regulated. In fact, low serum calcium concentrations usually imply abnormal parathyroid function or kidney failure—not primary calcium deficiency. Indirect indicators of calcium adequacy, such as measurement of bone mineral content and/or density, are often used clinically to assess calcium status.

DIETARY SOURCES OF CALCIUM AND FACTORS INFLUENCING ITS BIOAVAILABILITY

Dietary calcium is found mainly in dairy products, dark green vegetables, legumes, and fortified foods. The concentration of calcium in human milk remains relatively constant at 200 to 250 mg per L through the first 6 months postpartum and is thought to be sufficient for exclusively breastfed infants.[39] Indeed, human milk satisfies infant calcium requirements, as there are no reports of calcium deficiency in vitamin D–replete, full-term infants who are exclusively breastfed.[37]

Many factors influence calcium bioavailability. For example, intestinal calcium absorption depends on the availability of 1,25-dihydroxyvitamin D_3 and its intestinal receptors. The bioavailability of dietary calcium also varies approximately inversely with intake, although the absolute quantity of calcium absorbed continues to increase with intake.[82] Myriad dietary constituents—in addition to vitamin D availability—also affect calcium absorption and excretion. For instance, oxalates and phytates, found mainly in vegetables and grains, inhibit absorption. Intestinal transit time and mucosal mass also affect fractional calcium absorption,[83] and decreased stomach acid can reduce the solubility of insoluble calcium salts, thus decreasing absorption unless they are given with a meal. Consequently, the absorption of calcium from supplements improves when they are taken with food. Life stage also influences calcium absorption, with the highest fractional absorption seen in infancy (60%) and in early puberty (34%). Racial differences in calcium metabolism have been noted in both children and adults. For example, African American girls have greater absorption efficiencies than do white girls after menarche.[84] Metabolic differences may contribute to the widely observed higher bone mass in African American children, but implications for "race"-specific requirements remain unclear.[37]

DIETARY REFERENCE INTAKES FOR CALCIUM

Note that because sufficient data do not exist, only AIs (not RDAs) for calcium exist. The AI for calcium is 210 mg per day from 0 to 6 months; this increases to 270 mg per day from 7 to 12 months (Table 60.1). Intake of calcium from infant formulas may need to be greater than that from human milk in order to achieve the same retention, since absolute fractional absorption of calcium from bovine milk or other formula may be lower than from human milk.[85] The AI for children aged 1 to 3 years increases to 500 mg per day, for children aged 4 to 8 years it is 800 mg per day, and for children aged 9 to 18 years it is 1,300 mg per day (Table 60.2). These values are based on intake levels which appear to support optimal bone health, recognizing that other factors such as genetics, hormones, and physical activity all interact to affect this important outcome variable.

There is little information concerning primary calcium toxicity, and the available data on the adverse effects of excess calcium intake primarily concern calcium intake from nutrient supplements. For infants 0 through 12 months of age, further studies are needed before a UL can be established. Although the Food and Nutrition Board (FNB) recognizes that the safety of excess calcium intake in children aged 1 through 18 years has yet to be studied adequately, a UL for this age group has been established as 2,500 mg per day. This amount reflects that obtained from both diet and supplements (Table 60.2).

CONSEQUENCES OF INADEQUATE CALCIUM INTAKE

Inadequate calcium intake during infancy and childhood can have many negative effects. In LBW infants, inadequate enteral intakes of calcium result in biochemical abnormalities (e.g., hypophosphatemia), low net mineral retention, low rates of bone mineralization, and reduced linear growth.[86] Low calcium intake can also contribute to the development of rickets in infants and children, especially those consuming very restrictive diets. Data also support the possibility that low bone mass may be a contributing factor to some fractures in children.[87,88]

Average dietary intakes for calcium by children in the United States decline dramatically after the second year of life and are well below recommended intakes.[89] In fact, only about 10% of girls and 25% of boys aged 9 to 17 years consume the AI values.[90] This is important, because chronic calcium deficiency resulting from inadequate intake or poor intestinal absorption is one cause of reduced bone mass and subsequent osteoporosis. Some evidence suggests that suboptimal intakes of calcium in children and adolescents may be related to the replacement of milk intake by soft drinks and fruit juices and/or fruit drinks.[91] Lactose intolerance may also impact calcium intake in some ethnic groups.[2] Although there are some data to suggest that calcium supplementation may increase bone mineral content in adolescents, other data suggest that these effects are short-lived.[92,93]

CONSEQUENCES OF EXCESSIVE CALCIUM INTAKE

Data on adverse effects of excess calcium intake are lacking for infants and children. In adults, however, adverse effects of excess calcium are kidney stone formation, the syndrome of hypercalcemia and renal insufficiency with and without alkalosis, and the interaction of calcium with other minerals. Hypercalcemia results in poor muscle tone, constipation, excessive urine loss, nausea, and, when most severe confusion, coma and death. Although calcium can interfere with iron and zinc absorption, human studies fail to show cases in which iron and zinc depletion occurs as a result of high calcium intake. Small children may be at risk of iron and zinc deficiency when calcium intake is excessive, but no dose–response data exist.

RECOMMENDATIONS FOR CALCIUM SUPPLEMENTATION

Although human milk or infant formula provides sufficient calcium to the healthy full-term infant, premature infants have higher calcium requirements than do full-term infants. The AAP recommends that these infants' calcium requirements be met by using either human milk fortified with additional minerals or specially designed formulas for premature infants.[2] Similarly, LBW infants should receive human milk fortified with additional minerals or formulas specially designed for premature infants.[2]

Most experts recommend that children and teens should get as much calcium as possible *from food* because calcium-rich foods also tend to furnish other nutrients involved in calcium utilization. However, the AAP recognizes that, for children and adolescents who cannot or will not consume adequate amounts of this mineral from preferred dietary sources, the use of calcium supplements should be considered.[94]

It is especially noteworthy that the AAP strongly recommends that pediatricians actively support the goal of achieving calcium intakes in children and adolescents by asking questions about dietary calcium intake and providing information about specific sources of dietary calcium that are also low in fat, such as low-fat dairy products. Establishing these healthy eating practices in childhood (as opposed to simply providing a calcium supplement) is important so that they will be followed throughout the life span.

IRON

Iron, an essential mineral, is a constituent of several classes of proteins: heme proteins (e.g., hemoglobin), iron–sulfur or other nonheme enzymes (e.g., flavoproteins), and those involved in iron storage and transport (e.g., transferrin).[95] The iron–heme complex in hemoglobin is required for the transport of oxygen from lungs to tissues, and in myoglobin, it is required for the storage of oxygen for use during muscle contraction. Iron is also a cofactor in a variety of heme-containing enzymes, such as cytochrome oxidase, catalase, and peroxidase. Nonheme, iron-containing enzymes such as aconitase (an iron–sulfur protein) and metalloflavoproteins such as ferredoxins are involved in oxidative metabolism. Iron also plays a role in DNA synthesis as a component of the enzyme ribonucleotide reductase.

IRON HOMEOSTASIS

Iron homeostasis is primarily maintained through the coordinated regulation of absorption and transport, and recent studies have shed considerable light on its absorption and metabolism in infancy and childhood.[96] Briefly, dietary iron is solubilized in the stomach and absorbed in the duodenum in the ferrous (Fe^{2+}) form. Absorption of iron is influenced by age, iron status, state of health, form of iron ingested, gastric and luminal acidity, and several dietary components (described below). Iron uptake into the luminal surface of the mucosal epithelium is believed to be facilitated by various cell membrane proteins; however, it is unclear how such interactions determine iron bioavailability.[95,97]

Iron is taken up in the small intestine by divalent metal transporter-1 and is either stored by ferritin inside the mucosal cell or transported to the systemic circulation by ferroportin, while being oxidized by hephaestin to be incorporated into transferrin.[95] Hepcidin, a small peptide synthesized by the liver, can sense iron stores and regulated iron transport by inhibition of ferroportin. Note that regulation of iron transporters is immature in infants, and this may possibly explain some of the adverse effects of iron supplementation described later in this section.

Excess iron is stored intracellularly as ferritin and also hemosiderin in the reticuloendothelial system of the liver, spleen, bone marrow, and other organs. The molecular regulation of intestinal iron absorption and transport, with transcriptional, posttranscriptional, and posttranslational control mechanisms, is an ongoing area of active research. Nonetheless, it is clear that iron-regulatory proteins modulate the use of messenger RNA (mRNA)–encoding proteins that are involved in the transport, storage, and use of iron.[98]

DIETARY SOURCES AND BIOAVAILABILITY OF IRON

Most dietary iron is in the plant-based nonheme form found in grains, fruits, and vegetables. This type of iron is less bioavailable than heme iron found in foods of animal origin. Dietary components known to inhibit iron absorption are calcium, phytates (such as those in legumes, rice, and grains), and polyphenols found in tea and coffee. Promoters of iron absorption include ascorbic acid (vitamin C), organic acids, and certain animal proteins.

Noteworthy is the fact that human milk is a source of highly bioavailable iron, providing 0.3 to 0.9 mg per L.[39] Iron contained in cow milk and bovine-based formula is less well absorbed and, for this and other reasons, is not recommended until 1 year of age.[2] In addition, full-term infants are born with considerable iron stores, and these stores are mobilized during infancy. However, even these infants must eventually rely on exogenous sources because stores endowed at birth are generally depleted by 6 months.

REFERENCE INTAKES FOR IRON

Like other AIs in infancy, that for iron reflects the observed mean iron intake of infants principally fed human milk (Table 60.1); for the first 6 months of life, the AI is 0.27 mg per day. However, for reasons outlined by the FNB, there should be no expectation that an average intake of 0.27 mg per day is adequate to meet the needs of almost all individual infants (such as those fed formula), and the use of the AI as an intake goal should be applied with extreme care. From 7 to 12 months, the RDA for iron increases to 11 mg per day. Recommended intakes for children then decrease to 7 mg per day at 1 year, increasing to 11 and 15 mg per day during adolescence for boys and girls, respectively (Table 60.2).

There is considerable concern about iron overload, and the UL for infants and children is 40 mg per day and is based on gastrointestinal complications of iron supplementation (Table 60.2). This value increases to 45 mg per day for adolescents. The FNB recognizes that under some circumstances, individuals receiving intermittent doses of iron supplements may exceed the UL. However, the effects of intermittent dosing on gastrointestinal side effects have not been studied adequately.

CONSEQUENCES OF INADEQUATE IRON INTAKE AND EFFECT OF SUPPLEMENTATION

Iron deficiency is the most common nutritional deficiency worldwide, with the best-known consequence being anemia. It is estimated that 50% of the world's anemia burden is attributable to iron deficiency and that iron deficiency accounts for 841,000 deaths and more than 35 million disability-adjusted life years lost.[99] Even otherwise healthy, full-term infants are prone to iron deficiency in the first year of life; between 3% and 30% of full-term infants develop iron deficiency during infancy, usually from 6 to 12 months of age.[100] The incidence (26% and 86%) is even higher in preterm infants.[101] This is partly because iron stores are especially low in preterm infants, and total-body iron content has to increase at an accelerated rate postnatally. Thus, compared with term infants, preterm infants require more iron both in absolute amount and on a body weight basis.

There are many biochemical markers of mild, moderate, and severe iron deficiency. For example, chronic iron deficiency is often identified by depleted iron stores (low serum ferritin and transferrin receptor). Early functional iron deficiency can be evaluated by measuring elevated free erythrocyte protoporphyrin, decreased transferrin saturation, and/or decreased mean corpuscular volume. Iron deficiency anemia is often assessed via decreased hemoglobin and hematocrit values. Ideally, these laboratory tests should be used in combination to identify the evolution of iron deficiency through these three stages.

Diagnosis of iron deficiency during infancy is complex and lacks uniform diagnostic criteria. As in other age groups, anemia occurs after the storage, and nonstorage tissue iron pools are depleted. Indicators of iron status currently most frequently used in this population are serum ferritin, transferrin receptor, percent transferrin saturation, erythrocyte protoporphyrin, mean corpuscular volume, hemoglobin concentration, and hematocrit.[102] Regardless of iron supplementation during early life in otherwise healthy, breastfed infants can positively influence many of these indicators of iron status.[103]

Aside from the effects of frank iron deficiency on anemia, there are also important effects of more moderate deficiency levels. For example, moderate anemia is associated with mental and motor developmental delays in children, and longitudinal studies indicate that children who were anemic in early childhood continue to have poor cognitive and motor development and depressed school achievement into middle childhood.[104,105] There is also compelling evidence that iron supplementation in early life—especially in iron-deficient areas—provides benefits in terms of motor development and social-emotional behavior.[106] For children older than 2 years, iron supplementation has also been associated with improvements in cognition.[107] There is also some evidence that early iron supplementation may enhance physical performance in childhood and adolescence.[108] However, some (but not all) studies suggest that early iron supplementation may increase the risk for infectious disease in some populations—including those at highest risk for malaria.[109,110] Furthermore, iron supplementation may have small but significant negative effects on growth in some iron-replete infants and children.[111,112] Thus, there is general consensus that a single strategy for ensuring adequate iron nutrition in young children in different parts of the world is not likely satisfactory.

Another consequence of iron deficiency is enhanced heavy metal absorption and inadequate oxygen delivery. For example, clinical and epidemiologic studies have shown that absorption of lead increases with the severity of iron deficiency. Inadequate oxygen delivery during exercise and abnormal enzyme function in tissues also result from anemia. An association between iron deficiency and immune function has also been proposed.[113]

CONSEQUENCES OF EXCESSIVE IRON INTAKE

Possible adverse effects of excessive dietary iron intake include promotion of cellular oxidation, impaired resistance to infection, interference with absorption or metabolism of other nutrients, and adverse reactions manifested by gastrointestinal abnormalities or behavioral disturbances. Reports of acute toxicity resulting from clinical overdoses of medicinal iron have been reported for young children,[114–116] and accidental iron overdose is the most common cause of poisoning deaths in children younger than 6 years in the United States.[117] And, as previously mentioned, some (but not all) studies suggest that iron supplementation may increase the disease risk in some endemic populations.

RECOMMENDATIONS FOR IRON SUPPLEMENTATION

The AAP recommends that healthy, full-term, breastfed infants receive a supplemental source of iron (~1 mg per kg per day) starting at 4 to 6 months of age preferably from complementary foods.[2] Iron-fortified infant cereal and/or meats are a good source of iron for initial introduction of an iron-containing food. For breastfed preterm or LBW infants, an oral iron supplement in the form of drops once a day at 2 mg per kg per day starting at 1 month should be given until 12 months of age. Note that the dose of iron (1 mg per kg) in a vitamin preparation with iron is not likely to provide sufficient iron for the preterm breastfed infant. For all infants younger than 12 months, only iron-fortified formula should be used for weaning or supplementing breast milk. Because current preterm infant and preterm discharge formulas supply only 1.8 mg per kg per day iron to the average preterm infant, formula-fed preterm infants may benefit from an additional 1 mg per kg per day iron administered as drops or in a vitamin preparation with iron. The AAP also suggests supplementation of some young children with iron during the second year, especially if the child does not have a source of meat-based iron in the diet. Common over-the-counter preparations used for iron supplementation are described in Table 60.3.

It is important to note that these recommendations may not apply to infants living in areas of endemic malaria, and the reader is urged to follow the development of recommendations for these populations as they are put forth.[118] Currently, the WHO recommends that caution should be exercised in settings where the prevalence of malaria and other infectious diseases is high and that iron supplementation be targeted to those who are anemic and at risk of iron deficiency.[119]

TABLE 60.3 Selected Over-the-Counter Products Used for Iron Supplementation in Infants and Children

Product	*Iron Concentration (mg/mL)*	*Usual Daily Dose*
Baby vitamin drops with iron (Goldline Laboratories, Miami, FL)	10	1 mL
Ferrous sulfate drops (Fer-In-Sol, Mead Johnson, Evansville, IN, and various generic brands)	25 (125 mg/mL ferrous sulfate)	2–6 mg/kg/d
Poly-Vi-Sol with iron drops (Mead Johnson, Evansville, IN)	10	1 mL
Polyvitamin drops with iron (various brands)	10	1 mL
Tri-Vi-Sol with iron drops (Mead Johnson, Evansville, IN)	10	1 mL
Vi-Daylin ADC vitamins + iron drops (Ross Laboratories, Columbus, OH)	10	1 mL

Modified from Kleinman RE, ed. *American Academy of Pediatrics' Pediatric nutrition handbook*, 6th ed. Elk Grove Village, IL: American Academy of Pediatrics, 2008.

ZINC

Zinc is an essential trace mineral that has a multitude of physiologic and biochemical functions, notably in embryogenesis and growth. Zinc functions as a catalytic, structural, and/or regulatory component of nearly 300 enzymes in which it maintains structural integrity and plays a role in regulation of gene expression.[120] Although the biochemical and molecular genetics of zinc function is relatively well developed, the relationships of these genetic events to zinc deficiency or toxicity and the specific functions for which zinc is particularly critical remain to be established.[121] As such, explanations for depressed growth, immune dysfunction, increased diarrhea, altered cognition, host–defense properties, defects in carbohydrate utilization, teratogenesis, and numerous other clinical outcomes of mild and severe zinc deficiency are not well established. This is, in part, due to lack of a sensitive and functional indicator of zinc nutritional status, although investigations into this are ongoing.[122]

Zinc is primarily (95%) an intracellular ion, being found in all organs, tissues, fluids, and secretions of the body. Zinc concentrations are particularly high in the bone, skeletal muscle, skin, liver, brain, kidney, heart, hair, and plasma. However, plasma zinc is tightly regulated and does not reflect changes in dietary intake until severe and prolonged deficiency prevails.

Homeostatic regulation of zinc metabolism is achieved principally through coordination of absorption and secretion of endogenous reserves.[121] This involves adaptive mechanisms influenced by dietary zinc intake. Zinc absorption is mainly in the small intestine and is influenced by the solubility of the zinc compounds and zinc status. Zinc secretion into and excretion out of the intestine provide the major route of zinc excretion. Zinc depletion in humans is accompanied by reduced endogenous zinc losses from both pancreatic and intestinal cell secretions. Regulation of zinc absorption may provide a gross control of body zinc content, whereas endogenous zinc release provides fine control to maintain homeostasis.

DIETARY SOURCES AND BIOAVAILABILITY OF ZINC

Zinc is found not only primarily in foods of animal sources (e.g., oysters, red meats, poultry, liver) but also in plant foods (e.g., beans, nuts, whole grains, fortified cereals, legumes) and supplements. Like iron, zinc absorption from a diet containing animal-based foods is greater than that from a purely vegetarian diet, and many dietary factors can enhance or inhibit its bioavailability. For example, large-molecular-weight compounds (e.g., phytates) and competing divalent cations (e.g., iron) inhibit zinc absorption. Conversely, low-molecular-weight ligands (e.g., cysteine) and other organic acids promote zinc absorption. Zinc depletion also increases the efficiency of intestinal absorption.

The mechanism by which zinc enters the mucosal cell is unknown. However, once inside, zinc is bound to metallothionein and is held within the cell or passes through the cell for use in zinc-dependent processes. In plasma, newly absorbed zinc circulates bound to albumin. Zinc in human milk is highly bioavailable, and its concentration declines as lactation progresses.[18] Like iron, the bioavailability of zinc in human milk is higher than that in bovine milk. Consequently, most formulas are supplemented with zinc to contain 5 to 7 mg per L; preterm formulas generally contain 5 to 10 mg per L.

DIETARY REFERENCE INTAKES FOR ZINC

An AI for zinc is 2.0 mg per day for infants from 0 to 6 months (Table 60.1). However, the FNB notes that the zinc bioavailability from soy formulas is significantly lower than that from milk-based formulas and that the absorption from human milk is greater than all types of proprietary formula products. The RDA for zinc is 3 mg per day for infants and children aged 7 months to 3 years, 5 mg per day from 4 to 8 years, 8 mg per day from 9 to 13 years, and 9 to 11 mg per day, depending on sex, from 14 to 18 years (Table 60.2). Based on a single study by Walravens and Hambidge who fed 68 healthy, full-term infants a formula containing 5.8 mg per L zinc with no documented adverse effects, the UL for infants has been set at 4 mg per day from 0 to 6 months and 5 mg per day from 7 to 12 months.[123] This value increases to 7, 12, 23, and 34 mg per day zinc at 1, 4, 9, and 14 years of age, respectively.

CONSEQUENCES OF INADEQUATE ZINC INTAKE AND EFFECT OF SUPPLEMENTATION

Zinc deficiency is difficult to detect because clinical features and laboratory indicators are not always consistent, and a reliable sensitive functional indicator of zinc is lacking. Nonetheless, in the 1970s, mild zinc deficiency was described in formula-fed infants consuming a zinc-poor formula.[123] Fortification of the formula led to normal growth. Severe zinc deficiency is seen in patients with acrodermatitis enteropathica and those provided total parenteral nutrition lacking sufficient amounts of this mineral. Characteristics of severe zinc deficiency are growth retardation, alopecia, diarrhea, delayed sexual maturation and impotence, eye and skin lesions, and loss of appetite.

More recently, there has been considerable scientific attention given to the potential impact of zinc supplementation on behavior (including attention-deficit/hyperactivity disorder or ADHD) and a variety of childhood illnesses, such as diarrhea and respiratory illness. However, the experimental data are conflicting and suggest a complex set of interactions that likely impact the effect of zinc nutrition on these outcomes. For instance, two separate meta-analyses have found that zinc supplementation reduced frequency and severity of diarrhea and respiratory illnesses as well as the duration of diarrheal morbidity.[124,125] Another study found that zinc supplementation (70 mg per week) resulted in fewer incidents of pneumonia and decreased incidence of diarrhea; importantly, there were fewer pneumonia-related deaths in the group given zinc supplements than in the placebo group.[126] However, results are not consistent across studies.[127–129] This is highlighted in a study conducted in Peru in which morbidity was greater after supplementation with zinc plus multivitamins and minerals than it was after supplementation with zinc alone.[130] Results of studies designed to test the effect of zinc supplementation on behavioral outcomes in children are also mixed.[131,132] It is likely that other factors, such as psychosocial stimulation, interact with zinc nutrition to influence psychological outcomes.[133]

CONSEQUENCES OF EXCESSIVE ZINC INTAKE

Adverse effects associated with chronic intake of excessive supplemental zinc include suppression of immune response, decreased high-density lipoprotein cholesterol, and reduced copper status. Typical signs of acute zinc toxicity include epigastric pain, diarrhea, nausea, and vomiting. In adults, acute toxicity has been associated with a dose of 225 to 450 mg of zinc as zinc sulfate.[134] Chronic ingestion of zinc supplements (100 to 300 mg per day for several months) induces secondary copper deficiency caused by the competitive interaction between these elements during intestinal absorption. Zinc supplements as low as 25 mg per day have also been shown to induce copper deficiency in adults.[135]

RECOMMENDATIONS FOR ZINC SUPPLEMENTATION

Because human milk may not always meet the infant's need for zinc, those fed human milk may benefit from zinc supplementation after 6 months of age, when complementary foods are introduced, particularly if such foods are low in zinc and the diet includes inhibitors of zinc absorption.[136] Many premature infants fed human milk may become zinc depleted, although frank zinc deficiency may not be apparent.[137]

Consequently, zinc supplements may help meet growth needs during infancy and childhood,[136] particularly for infants and children at high risk of zinc deficiency.[137] Addressing the apparent relationship between zinc nutrition and diarrhea, the WHO recommends zinc supplementation (10 mg per day) once a day for 10 to 14 days when an infant (less than 6 months old) has diarrhea; the recommended dosage increases to 20 mg per day for older infants.[138] For preterm infants, the AAP recommends a zinc intake of 1 to 3 mg per kg per day.[2] This level of intake can be achieved through the use of term or preterm formulas and human milk fortifiers. Additional supplementation is not recommended.

During the second half year of life, zinc requirements are high. Thus, zinc requirements of early childhood during the transition from milk to solid foods are also difficult to meet. Complementary foods (e.g., 50 to 70 g of lean beef per day or 40 g of dry fish per day) must provide 84% to 89% of zinc required by infants between the ages of 6 and 24 months.[136] Zinc intakes by infants[137] and children in the United States and less developed countries[139] suggest that zinc supplementation may be useful for infants and children with diets low in animal products and phytate-rich cereals and legumes. Some experts recommend that, instead of turning to supplemental forms of the mineral, parents should consider meat and/or liver instead of cereal as a "first food" for infants.[140] Older infants and children who are fed a strict vegan diet may need zinc supplements because bioavailability from plants foods is low.[134,141]

IODINE

Iodine is a nonmetallic trace mineral essential to humans for synthesis of the thyroid hormones thyroxine (T_4) and triiodothyronine (T_3). Thyroid hormones are necessary for regulation of human growth, development, metabolism, and reproductive function. Most iodine is concentrated in the thyroid gland; other target organs are the developing brain, muscle, heart, pituitary, and kidney. In target tissues, the physiologically active form (T_3) binds to nuclear receptors where it regulates gene expression.

Iodine is rapidly absorbed and removed from the circulation by the thyroid gland and kidneys. Iodine can also be absorbed through the skin from topical iodine applications or from iodine vapors from cleaning agents and fossil fuel combustion. The hypothalamus and pituitary are involved in the regulation of iodine metabolism. Thyrotropin-releasing hormone, a hypothalamic hormone, stimulates the release of thyroid-stimulating hormone (TSH), which, in turn, stimulates uptake of iodine by the thyroid gland, synthesis of thyroxine hormones, and secretion of T_3 and T_4 into the circulation. Persistently elevated levels of TSH in response to low circulating levels of T_3 and T_4 can lead to hypertrophy of the thyroid gland and, ultimately, goiter formation. Excess iodine is excreted in urine, and urinary iodine is often used as an indicator of iodine status.

DIETARY SOURCES OF IODINE

The iodine content of foods depends on the iodine content of the soil and water used to grow them. Ocean fish and mollusks tend to contain high amounts of iodine because they concentrate iodine found in seawater into their tissues. However, most of the iodine in our diet comes from iodized salt, which contains about 77 µg per g of this mineral in the form of potassium iodide. Iodine concentration of human milk depends on maternal intake; typical values range from 113 to 150 µg per L.[39] Nonetheless, infants fed human milk generally consume adequate quantities of this mineral. Because bovine milk is a rich source of iodine, milk-based infant formulas are also good sources.

DIETARY REFERENCE INTAKES FOR IODINE

Based on intake of iodine by exclusively breastfed infants, the AI for this mineral during the first half year of life is 110 µg per day, increasing to 130 µg per day from 7 to 12 months. The DRI committee noted, however, that there have been no studies in which the bioavailability of iodine in infant formulas and human milk has been compared. Thus, it is unknown whether this amount is actually sufficient for formula-fed infants. The RDAs for iodine are of 90 µg per day for children aged 1 to 8 years, 120 µg per day for children aged 9 to 13 years, and 120 µg per day for older children and adolescents (Table 60.2). The committee was not able to establish a UL for iodine during the first year of life, but the ULs were set at 200 µg per day for children aged 1 to 3 years, 300 µg per day from 4 to 8 years, 600 µg per day from 9 to 13 years, and 900 µg per day from 14 to 18 years.

CONSEQUENCES OF INADEQUATE IODINE INTAKE AND IODINE SUPPLEMENTATION

Although iodine intake remains a public health concern worldwide, endemic iodine deficiency was a significant problem in the United States at the beginning of the 20th century, being eliminated largely by aggressive programs encouraging the consumption of iodine-fortified salt.[142] Currently, there is some controversy as to whether iodine intake is adequate in the United States, but most data indicate that it is.[143,144] Nonetheless, continued nutritional monitoring of iodine intake in the United States is warranted.[145]

There is no controversy, however, that iodine deficiency remains one of the most common nutrient deficiencies worldwide.[146] Manifestations of iodine deficiency take on many forms, which are collectively called *iodine deficiency disorders*. Iodine deficiency disorders include mental retardation, hypothyroidism, goiter, cretinism, and growth and developmental abnormalities. The most severe form, called cretinism, occurs when a baby is born to an iodine-deficient mother. Cretinism causes severe mental retardation, poor growth, infertility, and increased risk for mortality. When iodine deficiency occurs in childhood or later, TSH secretion greatly increases, causing the thyroid gland to grow and develop into a goiter.

Although it has long been established that iodine supplementation during pregnancy and the postnatal period could prevent cretinism and childhood goiter, more recent research suggests that it may have more far-reaching effects. Unfortunately, there are no long-term data on the effect of iodine supplementation on infant development. However, a meta-analysis of studies (n = 37; 12,291 children) conducted in China suggested that iodine supplementation (via food fortification) resulted in greater intellectual development of children who were mildly iodine deficient.[147] Furthermore, data from well-controlled studies indicate that iodine repletion in moderately iodine-deficient school-aged children can improve cognitive and motor function, increase concentrations of insulin-like growth factor 1 (IGF-1) and insulin-like growth factor-binding protein 3, and improve growth.[148,149]

CONSEQUENCES OF EXCESSIVE IODINE INTAKE

As mentioned, consequences of excess iodine intake for infants for the first year have not been studied sufficiently. However, to prevent high intakes of iodine, it is recommended that the only source of intake for infants in their first year of life should be food and formula.[39] For older individuals, chronic excessive intakes of iodine may compromise thyroid function and also contribute to development of goiter, hypothyroidism (due to feedback inhibition of thyroid hormone synthesis), and hyperthyroidism (also called iodine-induced hyperthyroidism).[2]

RECOMMENDATIONS FOR IODINE SUPPLEMENTATION

Because human milk contains sufficient iodine as do proprietary infant formulas, the AAP does not recommend iodine supplementation during infancy.[2] Furthermore, because children in the United States get an ample supply of iodine, supplementation is not recommended during childhood and adolescence. However, in areas of the world where iodine is less available either naturally or because iodized salt is not routinely used, iodine supplementation may be important.

FLUORIDE

Fluoride, although not technically an essential nutrient, is a dietary mineral associated with the prevention of dental caries and, more recently, stimulation of new bone formation.[37] Fluoride exists as the fluoride ion or as hydrofluoric acid in body fluids. Fluoride is incorporated into tooth enamel as fluorapatite during the preeruptive stage of enamel formation, and approximately 99% of total-body fluoride is found as fluorohydroxyapatite in mineralized tissues. Present in saliva and dental plaque, fluoride helps prevent dental caries by three mechanisms: it inhibits plaque formation and decreases bacterial acid production, prevents demineralization by incorporation into tooth surface crystals, and enhances remineralization of enamel.[150] At one time, fluoride was thought to provide protection of preeruptive teeth via systemic mechanisms, but it is now generally accepted that its main effect is instead via topical use.

Fluoride is absorbed in the stomach and small intestine and excreted mainly via the kidney. For young children, as much as 80% of fluoride intake can be retained by the developing skeleton and teeth.[151] Body fluid and tissue concentrations of fluoride are proportional to the level of chronic intake; in other words, they are not homeostatically regulated.[37]

SOURCES AND BIOAVAILABILITY OF FLUORIDE

Few foods contain fluoride naturally, with some teas and marine fish being the main exceptions. Instead, fluoride is available mainly from artificially fluoridated water supplies. Highlighting the importance of municipal water fluoridation is the fact that the Centers for Disease Control and Prevention (CDC) has named this practice one of the top 10 public health achievements in the 20th century. In the United States, communities with fluoridated water have fluoride concentrations of 0.7 to 1.11 mg per L; nonfluoridated water typically contains less than 0.4 mg per L.[37] Sources of fluoride in the diet include beverages, formulas, and foods made with fluoridated water; casual ingestion of fluoride toothpaste and mouth rinses; and fluoride supplements. Fluoride has high bioavailability when sodium fluoride is ingested with water. If ingested with milk, formula, or foods that contain high concentrations of calcium or other divalent ions that form insoluble compounds, absorption may be reduced by 10% to 25%.

Fluoride intake by infants can vary widely depending on whether the infant is fed human milk or formula and whether the formula is ready to feed or requires reconstitution with water. Fluoride concentration of human milk typically is 4 to 15 μg per L, which results in intakes of 3 to 12 μg per day. Note that, depending on what type of water is used to reconstitute infant formula, fluoride intake by formula-fed infants can be as high as 1.0 mg per day. This is, however, highly variable. The CDC recommends that parents concerned about the effect that mixing their infant's formula with fluoridated water may have in developing enamel fluorosis can lessen this exposure by mixing formula with low-fluoride water most or all of the time.[152] Bottled water known to be low in fluoride is labeled as being purified, deionized, demineralized, distilled, or prepared by reverse osmosis.

DIETARY REFERENCE INTAKES FOR FLUORIDE

The AI for fluoride is 10 μg per day for infants from 0 to 6 months and 0.5 mg per day from 7 to 12 months (Table 60.1). This value increases to 0.7 mg per day from 1 to 3 years and 1 mg per day from 4 to 8 years. The UL for infants from 0 to 6 months is 0.7 mg per day and from 7 to 12 months is 0.9 mg per day. For children 1 to 3 years of age, the UL is 1.3 mg per day, and from 4 to 8 years, it is 2.2 mg per day (Table 60.2).

CONSEQUENCES OF INADEQUATE FLUORIDE INTAKE AND EFFECTS OF SUPPLEMENTATION

Inadequate intake of fluoride at any age places the individual at risk for dental caries.[153] As such, fluoride supplements are typically beneficial to children living in fluoride-deficient areas where water fluoridation is not practiced. Furthermore, the earlier children are exposed to fluoridated water or dietary fluoride supplements, the greater the reduction in dental caries in both the primary and permanent teeth. As part of the Iowa Fluoride Study, Hamasha and colleagues documented patterns of dietary fluoride supplement use and found that 11.2% of 12-month-old infants were taking them.[154] This percentage decreased to 6.3% and further to 4.7% at 12 and 96 months, respectively, and mean dosage gradually increased from 0.25 to 0.75 mg per day during this period.

CONSEQUENCES OF EXCESSIVE FLUORIDE INTAKE

Administration of supplemental fluoride must be done judiciously, because ingestion of excess fluoride can result in various degrees of fluorosis.[155] Enamel fluorosis is caused by excessive fluoride intake during the preeruptive development of teeth. After the enamel has completed maturation, it is no longer susceptible to fluorosis. Thus, it is recommended by some that tooth brushing with fluoride-containing toothpastes should not begin until the age of 2 years and that no more than a pea-sized portion be used.[156] Consequences of moderate-to-severe forms of fluorosis are cosmetic, being characterized by an increasing porosity, which causes the enamel to appear opaque and mottled. Mild fluorosis has no effect on tooth function and may render the enamel more resistant to caries. Clinical features include changes ranging from barely discernible to fine white lines running across the teeth and finally to entirely chalky white teeth.

TABLE 60.4 Fluoride Supplementation Schedule

	Fluoride Concentration in Local Water Supply (ppm)		
Age	*<0.3*	*0.3–0.6*	*>0.6*
Birth to 6 mo	0.00	0.00	0.00
6 mo–3 y	0.25	0.00	0.00
3–6 y	0.50	0.25	0.00
6 to at least 16 y	1.00	0.50	0.00

Must know the fluoride concentration in the patient's drinking water before prescribing fluoride supplements; all values are mg/d of fluoride supplement.

Modified from Kleinman RE, ed. *American Academy of Pediatrics' Pediatric nutrition handbook*, 6th ed. Elk Grove Village, IL: American Academy of Pediatrics, 2008.

RECOMMENDATIONS FOR FLUORIDE SUPPLEMENTATION

Dietary fluoride supplements in the form of tablets, lozenges, or liquids (including fluoride–vitamin preparations) have been used throughout the world since the 1940s. Most supplements contain sodium fluoride as the active ingredient. The CDC, American Dental Association, AAP, and Canadian Pediatric Society all recommend dietary fluoride supplementation aimed primarily at populations drinking suboptimally fluoridated water.[2,150,157] The AAP's fluoride schedule is provided in Table 60.4. To maximize the topical effect of fluoride, tablets and lozenges are intended to be chewed or sucked for 1 to 2 minutes before being swallowed. For infants, supplements are available as a liquid and used with a dropper. Note that, to use this schedule effectively, one must know the fluoride level of the municipal water supply. This can be easily determined by contacting the local water department or visiting the CDC's website at https://nccd.cdc.gov/doh_mwf/Default/Default.aspx.

Because dietary fluoride supplements are intended to compensate for fluoride-deficient drinking water, the dosage schedule requires knowledge of the fluoride content of the child's primary drinking water. Consideration should also be given to other sources of water (e.g., home, child care settings, school, or bottled water) and to other sources of fluoride (e.g., toothpaste or mouth rinse), which can complicate the prescribing decision.

ω-3 FATTY ACIDS

Perhaps, the most recently considered dietary components in terms of supplementation during infancy and childhood are the ω-3 (or n-3) fatty acids, which include the dietary essential α-linolenic acid (ALA; 18:3ω-3) as well as its longer chain polyunsaturated fatty acid (LCPUFA) metabolites eicosapentaenoic acid (EPA; 20:5ω-3) and docosahexaenoic acid (DHA; 22:6ω-3). It has long been known that the ω-3 fatty acids are important in terms of visual and neurologic development. More recent work, however, now suggests a host of additional physiologic roles for these compounds including being critical for optimal immune function, protecting from inflammation, and decreasing the risk for a variety of chronic degenerative diseases, such as cardiovascular events. Of particular importance to pediatric nutrition is the fact that plasma and erythrocyte DHA concentrations are higher in breastfed than in formula-fed infants.[158] Although this finding was initially interpreted as suggesting that infants cannot synthesize enough DHA to meet their needs, it is now clear that both term and preterm infants have this capability.[159] Nonetheless, because of the importance of LCPUFA to neural development, there has been considerable interest in determining the potential importance of supplementing the infant's diet with these compounds, especially if formula feeding is practiced.

DIETARY SOURCES OF THE ω-3 FATTY ACIDS

ALA is found naturally in some vegetable oils such as canola and flax seed, whereas the LCPUFAs synthesized from this essential fatty acid are found primarily in oily fish. Smaller amounts are also present in meats and eggs. Human milk contains a variety of ω-3 fatty acids, and their concentration depends greatly on the maternal diet. Because infant formulas are generally made with corn, coconut, safflower, and soy oils, unless they are fortified with LCPUFAs, they contain very low levels of them. Relatively recent suggestions by some that formula-fed infants consume LCPUFA-fortified formulas, however, have resulted in these types of formulas being widely available in the United States.

DIETARY REFERENCE INTAKES FOR THE ω-3 FATTY ACIDS

The AI for the ω-3 LCPUFAs during the first year of life is 0.5 g per day. After this time, the AIs refer instead to recommended intakes for ALA. Recommended intakes are 0.7 and 0.9 g per day ALA from 1 to 3 and 4 to 8 years, respectively. During the preteen years, reference intakes are slightly higher for boys than for girls (1.2 and 1.0 g per day, respectively), increasing even more during adolescence (1.6 and 1.1 g per day, respectively). There are no ULs established for this class of fatty acids.

CONSEQUENCES OF INADEQUATE ω-3 FATTY ACID INTAKE AND EFFECT OF SUPPLEMENTATION

Documentation of ω-3 fatty acid deficiency in infants and children is scant. However, there is a report of a 6-year-old child who had been maintained for several weeks on a parenteral nutrition product lacking ALA.[160] This resulted in numbness, weakness, blurred vision, and inability to walk, which were reversed when ALA was added to the diet. Nonetheless, because of the intense recent interest in the possibility that the ω-3 fatty acids might be conditionally essential during infancy, many studies have been conducted to investigate the effect of supplementation during early life. Specifically, most of these investigations have focused mostly on cognitive–behavioral development and visual acuity, and their results have been mixed. A meta-analysis published in 2000 that included randomized studies of term infants fed DHA-supplemented versus unsupplemented formula found an advantage of DHA consumption on behaviorally based tests of visual acuity at 2 months of age, but not any other age.[161] This same meta-analysis found no effect when electrophysiologic methods of assessment were considered. Recent Cochrane reviews have concluded that there is likely no consistent effect of consumption of DHA-supplemented formula on visual acuity of term or preterm infants.[162,163] However, other recent analyses suggest that there is "reasonably compelling" evidence of a beneficial effect in preterm, but not in term infants.[164] Similarly, studies designed to test the effect of long-chain ω-3 fatty acid intake during infancy on cognitive–behavioral development also provide some evidence of a potential benefit, but again the results are mixed.[165,166] This area of research represents one of active scrutiny and investigation.

CONSEQUENCES OF EXCESSIVE Ω-3 FATTY ACID INTAKE

Although there was some concern that excessive ω-3 fatty acid intake during infancy may have detrimental effects on growth, a recent meta-analysis of 21 studies found no evidence of such an effect on term infants.[167] Thus, the AAP has concluded that there is no need for concern that supplementation of the infant diet with these compounds will stunt growth.[2] There is also concern that overconsumption of long-chain ω-3 fatty acids might increase the risk of conditions related to oxidative damage such as necrotizing enterocolitis and bronchopulmonary dysplasia. Presently, there are not sufficient data to support or refute these possibilities.

RECOMMENDATIONS FOR ω-3 FATTY ACID SUPPLEMENTATION

The AAP has no official position on supplementation of term or preterm infant formulas with LCPUFAs in general or ω-3 LCPUFAs in particular.[2] Similarly, the Life Science Research Organization Expert Panel on Nutrient Composition of Term Infant Formulas recommends neither a minimum nor maximum amount of these lipids for term infant formulas.[168] The Life Science Research Organization has, however, specified a maximum (but not minimum) amount of DHA for preterm formulas.[169]

SUMMARY

In summary, it is clear that supplementation of the diet with selected micronutrients and fatty acids may improve health in some infants and children. This is particularly true in the most at-risk children such as those born prematurely or of LBW, or those living in areas of endemic nutrient deficiencies. However, evolving data suggest complex webs of interactions more multifarious than previously recognized, and health professionals must often consider confounding factors when determining whether dietary supplementation is warranted. One of the best examples of this that has recently surfaced is that of iron supplementation, which may increase morbidity and mortality in areas with endemic malaria. Thus, caution should always be used when determining whether dietary supplementation should be recommended, and altering nutrient adequacy of the diet should generally be considered carefully first. As research in this area is ongoing, remaining attentive of new recommendations from expert groups such as the AAP and WHO is critical.

REFERENCES

1. Institute of Medicine, Food and Nutrition Board. *Dietary reference intake for energy, carbohydrate, fiber, fat, fatty acids, cholesterol, protein, and amino acids.* Washington, DC: National Academy Press, 2005.
2. Kleinman RE, ed. *American Academy of Pediatrics pediatric nutrition handbook,* 6th ed. Elk Grove Village, IL: American Academy of Pediatrics, 2008.
3. U.S. Congress. Pub L No. 103-417. *Dietary supplement health and education act (DSHEA).* Washington, DC: U.S. Government Printing Office, 1994.
4. Nutrition Business Journal. *NBJ's supplement business report 2006.* San Diego, CA: New Hope Natural Media, 2006.

5. Ervin RB, Wright JD, Kennedy-Stephenson J. Use of dietary supplements in the United States, 1988–94. *J Vital Health Stat* 1999;244:1–14.
6. Picciano MF, Dwyer JT, Radimer KL, et al. Dietary supplement use among infants, children, and adolescents in the United States, 1999–2002. *Arch Pediatr Adolesc Med* 2007;161:978–985.
7. Institute of Medicine, Food and Nutrition Board. *Dietary reference intakes for vitamin C, vitamin E, selenium, and carotenoids.* Washington, DC: National Academy Press, 2000.
8. Ross AC. Vitamin A and carotenoids. In: Shils ME, Shike M, Ross AC, et al., eds. *Modern nutrition in health and disease,* 10th ed. Baltimore, MA: Williams & Wilkins, 2005.
9. Zhao Z, Ross AC. Retinoic acid repletion restores the number of leukocytes and their subsets and stimulates natural cytotoxicity in vitamin A-deficient rats. *J Nutr* 1995;125:2064–2073.
10. Greer FR. Fat-soluble vitamin supplements for enterally fed preterm infants. *Neonatal Netw* 2001;20(5):7–11.
11. West KP Jr. Vitamin A deficiency disorders in children and women. *Food Nutr Bull* 2003;24:S78–S90.
12. World Health Organization. *Global prevalence of vitamin A deficiency (Micronutrient Deficiency Information System Working Paper).* Geneva, Switzerland: World Health Organization, 1995.
13. Katz J, West KP Jr, Khatry SK, et al. Impact of vitamin A supplementation on prevalence and incidence of xerophthalmia in Nepal. *Invest Ophthalmol Vis Sci* 1995;36:2577–2583.
14. World Health Organization. *Vitamin A supplements: a guide to their use in the treatment of vitamin A deficiency and xerophthalmia.* Geneva, Switzerland: World Health Organization, 1997.
15. Fawzi WW, Chalmers TC, Herrera MG, et al. Vitamin A supplementation and child mortality. A meta-analysis. *JAMA* 1993;269:898–903.
16. Klemm RD, Labriqu AB, Christian P, et al. Newborn vitamin A supplementation reduced infant mortality in rural Bangladesh. *Pediatrics* 2008;122:242–250.
17. Darlow BA, Graham PJ. Vitamin A supplementation to prevent mortality and short and long-term morbidity in very low birth-weight infants. *Cochrane Database Syst Rev* 2007;(4):CD000501.
18. Jensen RG, ed. *Handbook of milk composition.* San Diego, CA: Academic Press, 1995.
19. Ambalavanan N, Tyson JE, Kennedy KA, et al. Vitamin A supplementation for extremely low birth weight infants: outcome at 18 and 22 months. *Pediatrics* 2005;114:e249–e254.
20. Brown N, Roberts C. Vitamin A for acute respiratory infection in developing countries: a meta-analysis. *Acta Paediatr* 2004;93:1437–1442.
21. Chen H, Zhuo Q, Yuan W, et al. Vitamin A for preventing acute lower respiratory tract infections in children up to seven years of age. *Cochrane Database Syst Rev* 2008;(5):CD006090.
22. Grotto I, Mimouni M, Gdalevich M, et al. Vitamin A supplementation and childhood morbidity from diarrhea and respiratory infections: a meta-analysis. *J Pediatr* 2003;142:297–304.
23. Cusick SE, Tielsch JM, Ramsan M, et al. Short-term effects of vitamin A and antimalarial treatment on erythropoiesis in severely anemic Zanzibari preschool children. *Am J Clin Nutr* 2005;82:406–412.
24. Diness BR, Fisker AB, Roth A, et al. Effect of high-dose vitamin A supplementation on the immune response to Bacille Calmette-Guerin vaccine. *Am J Clin Nutr* 2007;86:1152–1159.
25. Benn CS, Martins C, Rodrigues A, et al. Randomized study of effect of different doses of vitamin A on childhood morbidity and mortality. *BMJ* 2005;331:1428–1432.
26. Wisonge CS, Shey MS, Sterne JA, et al. Vitamin A supplementation for reducing the risk of mother-to-child transmission of HIV infection. *Cochrane Database Syst Rev* 2005;(4):CD003648.
27. Humphrey JH, Iliff PF, Marinda ET, et al. Effects of a single large dose of vitamin A, given during the postpartum period to HIV-positive women and their infants, on child HIV infection, HIV-free survival, and mortality. *J Infect Dis* 2006;193:860–871.
28. Kuhn L, Coutsoudis A, Trabattoni D, et al. Synergy between man-nose-binding lectin gene polymorphisms and supplementation with vitamin A influences susceptibility to HIV infection in infants born to HIV-positive mothers. *Am J Clin Nutr* 2006;84:610–615.
29. American Academy of Pediatrics Committee on Infectious Diseases. Vitamin A treatment of measles. *Pediatrics* 1993;91:1014–1015.
30. Mahoney CP, Margolis MT, Knauss TA, et al. Chronic vitamin A intoxication in infants fed chicken liver. *Pediatrics* 1980;65:893–897.
31. Underwood BA. The role of vitamin A in child growth, development and survival. *Adv Exp Med Biol* 1994;352:201–208.
32. Ross DA. Recommendations for vitamin A supplementation. *J Nutr* 2001;131:2902S–2906S.
33. World Health Organization. Treatment of associated conditions. https://www.who.int/maternal_child_adolescent/documents/management_childhood_conditions/en/. . Accessed August 18, 2020.
34. Holick MF. Vitamin D. In: Shils ME, Shike M, Ross AC, et al., eds. *Modern nutrition in health and disease,* 10th ed. Baltimore, MA: Williams & Wilkins, 2005.
35. Arnson Y, Amital H, Shoenfeld Y. Vitamin D and autoimmunity: new aetiological and therapeutic considerations. *Ann Rheum Dis* 2007;66:1137–1142.
36. Prentice A, Goldberg GR, Schoenmakers I. Vitamin D across the lifecycle: physiology and biomarkers. *Am J Clin Nutr* 2008;88:500S–506S.
37. Institute of Medicine, Food and Nutrition Board. *Dietary reference intakes for calcium, phosphorus, magnesium, vitamin D, and fluoride.* Washington, DC: National Academy Press, 1999.
38. Ovesen L, Brot C, Jakobsen J. Food contents and biological activity of 25-hydroxyvitamin D: a vitamin D metabolite to be reckoned with? *Ann Nutr Metab* 2003;47:107–113.
39. Picciano MF. Nutrient composition of human milk. *Pediatr Clin North Am* 2001;48:53–67.
40. Specker BL, Valanis B, Hertzberg V, et al. Sunshine exposure and serum 25-hydroxyvitamin D concentrations in exclusively breast-fed infants. *J Pediatr* 1985;107:372–376.
41. Fomon SJ, Younoszai MK, Thomas LN. Influence of vitamin D on linear growth of normal full-term infants. *J Nutr* 1966;88:345–350.
42. Graham S. Idiopathic hypercalcemia. *Postgrad Med* 1959;25:67–72.
43. Cushman KD. Vitamin D in childhood and adolescence. *Postgrad Med J* 2007;83:230–235.
44. Harris SS. Vitamin D in type I diabetes prevention. *J Nutr* 2005;135:323–325.
45. Holick MF. Sunlight and vitamin D for bone health and prevention of autoimmune diseases, cancers, and cardiovascular disease. *Am J Clin Nutr* 2004;80:1678S–1688S.
46. Ward LM. Vitamin D deficiency in the 21st century: a persistent problem among Canadian infants and mothers. *CMAJ* 2005;172:769–770.
47. Kreiter SR, Schwartz RP, Kirkman HN Jr, et al. Nutritional rickets in African American breast-fed infants. *J Pediatr* 2000;137:153–157.
48. Hatun S, Ozkan B, Orbak Z, et al. Vitamin D deficiency in early infancy. *J Nutr* 2005;135:279–282.
49. Lapatsanis S, Moulas A, Cholevas V, et al. Vitamin D: a necessity for children and adolescents in Greece. *Calcif Tissue Int* 2005;77:348–355.
50. Pal BR, Shaw NJ. Rickets resurgence in the United Kingdom: improving antenatal management in Asians. *J Pediatr* 2001;139:337–338.
51. Dawodu A, Agarwal M, Hossain M, et al. Hypovitaminosis D and vitamin D deficiency in exclusively breast-feeding infants and their mothers in summer: a justification for vitamin D. *J Pediatr* 2003;142:169–173.
52. Kimball S, Fuleihan Gel H, et al. Vitamin D: a growing perspective. *Crit Rev Clin Lab Sci* 2008;45:339–414.
53. Rovner AJ, O'Brien KO. Hypovitaminosis D among healthy children in the United States: a review of the current evidence. *Arch Pediatr Adolesc Med* 2008;162:513–519.
54. Schnadower D, Agarwal C, Oberfield SE, et al. Hypocalcemic seizures and secondary bilateral femoral fractures in an adolescent with primary vitamin D deficiency. *Pediatrics* 2006;118:2226–2230.
55. Harkness LS, Cromer BA. Vitamin D deficiency in adolescent females. *J Adolesc Health* 2005;37:75.
56. Pettifor JM. Rickets and vitamin D deficiency in children and adolescents. *Endocrinol Metab Clin North Am* 2005;34:537–553.
57. Park EA. The therapy of rickets. *JAMA* 1940;115:370–379.
58. Mozolowski W. Jedrzej Sniadecki (1768–1883) on the cure of rickets. *Nature* 1939;143:131.
59. Rajakumar K, Thomas SB. Reemerging nutritional rickets: a historical perspective. *Arch Pediatr Adolesc Med* 2005;159:335–341.
60. American Academy of Pediatrics Committee on Environmental Health. Ultraviolet light: a hazard to children. *Pediatrics* 1999;104:328–333.
61. Wagner CL, Greer FR; American Academy of Pediatrics Section on Breastfeeding; American Academy of Pediatrics Committee on Nutrition. Prevention of rickets and vitamin D deficiency in infants, children, and adolescents. *Pediatrics* 2008;122:1142–1152.
62. Brigelius-Flohe R, Traber MG. Vitamin E: function and metabolism. *FASEB J* 1999;13:1145–1155.
63. Traber MG, Packer L. Vitamin E: beyond antioxidant function. *Am J Clin Nutr* 1995;62:1501S–1509S.
64. Christen WG, Liu S, Glynn RJ, et al. Dietary carotenoids, vitamins C and E, and risk of cataract in women: a prospective study. *Arch Ophthalmol* 2008;126:102–109.
65. Gross SJ. Vitamin E. In: Tsang RC, Lucus A, Uauy R, et al., eds. *Nutritional needs of the preterm infant: scientific basis and practical guidelines.* Baltimore, MA: Williams & Wilkins, 1993.
66. Arrowsmith JB, Faich GA, Tomita DK, et al. Morbidity and mortality among low birth weight infants exposed to an intravenous vitamin E product, E-Ferol. *Pediatrics* 1989;83:244–249.
67. Bell EF. Upper limit of vitamin E in infant formulas. *J Nutr* 1989;119(Suppl 12):1829–1831.
68. Suttie JW. Vitamin K and human nutrition. *J Am Diet Assoc* 1992;92:585–590.
69. Booth SL, Suttie JW. Dietary intake and adequacy of vitamin K1. *J Nutr* 1998;128:785–788.
70. Kumar D, Greer FR, Super DM, et al. Vitamin K status of premature infants: implications for current recommendations. *Pediatrics* 2001;108:1117–1122.
71. Greer FR. Are breast-fed infants vitamin K deficient? *Adv Exp Med Biol* 2001;501:391–395.
72. Golding J, Greenwood R, Birmingham K, et al. Childhood cancer, intramuscular vitamin K, and pethidine given during labour. *Br Med J* 1992;305:341–346.
73. McKinney PA, Juszczak E, Findlay E, et al. Case-control study of childhood leukaemia and cancer in Scotland: findings for neonatal intramuscular vitamin K. *Br Med J* 1998;316:173–177.
74. Parker L, Cole M, Craft AW, et al. Neonatal vitamin K administration and childhood cancer in the north of England: retrospective case-control study. *Br Med J* 1998;316:189–193.
75. American Academy of Pediatrics Fetus and Newborn Committee. Routine administration of vitamin K to newborns. *Pediatrics* 2003;112:191–192.
76. American Academy of Pediatrics Vitamin K Ad Hoc Task Force. Controversies concerning vitamin K and the newborn. *Pediatrics* 1993;91:1001–1003.
77. Sutor AH. New aspects of vitamin K prophylaxis. *Semin Throm Hemost* 2003;29:373–376.
78. Greer FR, Marshall SP, Foley AL, et al. Improving the vitamin K status of breastfeeding infants with maternal vitamin K supplements. *Pediatrics* 1997;99:88–92.
79. Winzenberg T, Shaw K, Fryer J, et al. Calcium supplements in healthy children do not affect weight gain, height, or body composition. *Obesity (Silver Spring)* 2007;15:1789–1798.
80. Teegarden D. The influence of dairy product consumption on body composition. *J Nutr* 2005;135:2749–2752.
81. Lanou AJ, Barnard ND. Dairy and weight loss hypothesis: an evaluation of the clinical trials. *Nutr Rev* 2008;66:272–279.
82. Heaney RP, Weaver CM, Fitzsimmons ML. Influence of calcium load on absorption fraction. *J Bone Min Res* 1990;5:1135–1138.
83. Weaver CM, Heaney RP. Calcium. In: Shils ME, Shike M, Ross AC, et al., eds. *Modern nutrition in health and disease,* 10th ed. Baltimore, MA: Williams & Wilkins, 2005.
84. Abrams SA, O'Brien KO, Stuff JE. Changes in calcium kinetics associated with menarche. *J Clin Endocrinol Metab* 1996;81:2017–2020.
85. Fomon SJ, Nelson SE. Calcium, phosphorus, magnesium, and sulfur. In: Fomon SJ, ed. *Nutrition of normal infants.* St. Louis, MO: Mosby-Year Book, Inc., 1993.
86. Schanler RJ, Rifka M. Calcium, phosphorus and magnesium needs for the low-birth-weight infant. *Acta Paediatr Suppl* 1994;405:111–116.
87. Bailey DA, Wedge JH, McCulloch RG, et al. Epidemiology of fractions of the distal end of the radius in children as associated with growth. *J Bone Joint Surg Am* 1989;71:1225–1231.
88. Parfitt AM. The two faces of growth: benefits and risks to bone integrity. *Osteoporos Int* 1994;4:382–398.
89. American Academy of Pediatrics Committee on Nutrition. Calcium requirements of infants, children, and adolescents. *Pediatrics* 1999;104:1152–1157.
90. Cromer B, Harel Z. Adolescents: at increased risk for osteoporosis? *Clin Pediatr (Phila)* 2000;39:565–574.
91. American Academy of Pediatrics, Committee on Nutrition. The use and misuse of fruit juice in pediatrics. *Pediatrics* 2001;107:1210–1213.
92. Wosje KS, Specker BL. Role of calcium in bone health during childhood. *Nutr Rev* 2000;58:253–268.
93. Lambert HL, Eastell R, Karnik K, et al. Calcium supplementation and bone mineral accretion in adolescent girls: an 18-mo randomized controlled trial with 2-y follow-up. *Am J Clin Nutr* 2008;87:455–462.

94. Greer FR, Krebs NF. Optimizing bone health and calcium intakes of infants, children, and adolescents. *Pediatrics* 2006;117:578–585.
95. Lonnerdal B, Kelleher SL. Iron metabolism in infants and children. *Food Nutr Bull* 2007;28:S491–S499.
96. Domellof M. Iron requirements, absorption and metabolism in infancy and childhood. *Curr Opin Clin Nutr Metab Care* 2007;10:329–335.
97. Wood RJ, Ronnenberg AG. Iron. In: Shils ME, Shike M, Ross AC, et al., eds. *Modern nutrition in health and disease*, 10th ed. Baltimore, MA: Williams & Wilkins, 2005.
98. Eisenstein RS, Ross KL. Novel roles for iron regulatory proteins in the adaptive response to iron deficiency. *J Nutr* 2003;133:1510S–1516S.
99. Stolzfus RJ. Iron deficiency: global prevalence and consequences. *Food Nutr Bull* 2003;24:S99–S103.
100. Looker AC, Dallman PR, Carroll MD, et al. Prevalence of iron deficiency in the United States. *JAMA* 1997;277:973–976.
101. Borigato EV, Martinez FE. Iron nutritional status is improved in Brazilian preterm infants fed food cooked in iron pots. *J Nutr* 1998;128:855–859.
102. Yip R. The changing characteristics of childhood iron nutritional status in the United States. In: Filer LJ, ed. *Dietary iron: birth to two years*. New York, NY: Raven Health Care Communications, 1989.
103. Friel JK, Aziz K, Andrews WL, et al. A double-masked, randomized control trial of iron supplementation in early infancy in healthy term breastfed infants. *J Pediatr* 2003;143:582–586.
104. Eden AN. Iron deficiency and impaired cognition in toddlers: an underestimated and undertreated problem. *Paediatr Drugs* 2005;7:347–352.
105. Zlotkin S. Clinical nutrition: 8. The role of nutrition in the prevention of iron deficiency anemia in infants, children and adolescents. *Can Med Assoc J* 2003;168:59–63.
106. Lozoff B. Iron deficiency and child development. *Food Nutr Bull* 2007;28:S560–S571.
107. Grantham-McGregor S, Ani C. A review of studies on the effect of iron deficiency on cognitive development in children. *J Nutr* 2001;131:649S–668S.
108. Gera T, Sachdev HP, Nestel P. Effect of iron supplementation on physical performance in children and adolescents: systematic review of randomized controlled trials. *Indian Pediatr* 2007;44:15–24.
109. Lynch S, Stoltzfus R, Rawat R. Critical review of strategies to prevent and control iron deficiency in children. *Food Nutr Bull* 2007;28:S610–S620.
110. Stolzfus RJ, Heidkamp R, Kenkel D, et al. Iron supplementation of young children: learning from the new evidence. *Food Nutr Bull* 2007;28:S572–S584.
111. Majumdar I, Paul P, Talib VH, et al. The effect of iron therapy on the growth of iron-replete and iron-deplete children. *J Trop Pediatr* 2003;49:84–88.
112. Lind T, Seswandhana R, Persson LA, et al. Iron supplementation of iron-replete Indonesian infants is associated with reduced weight-for-age. *Acta Paediatr* 2008;97:770–775.
113. Maggini S, Wintergerst ES, Beveridge S, et al. Selected vitamins and trace elements support immune function by strengthening epithelial barriers and cellular and humoral immune responses. *Br J Nutr* 2007;8:S29–S35.
114. Anderson AC. Iron poisoning in children. *Curr Opin Pediatr* 1994;6:289–294.
115. Banner W Jr, Tong TG. Iron poisoning. *Pediatr Clin North Am* 1986;33:393–409.
116. Vermylen C. What is new in iron overload? *Eur J Pediatr* 2008;167:377–381.
117. Food and Drug Administration. Federal Register 62 FR 2217. https://www.fda.gov/food/guidance-documents-regulatory-information-topic-food-and-dietary-supplements/dietary-supplements-guidance-documents-regulatory-information. Accessed August 18, 2020.
118. Allen L, Black RE, Brandes N, et al. Conclusions and recommendations of a WHO expert consultation meeting on iron supplementation for infants and young children in malaria endemic areas. *Med Trop (Mars)* 2008;68:182–188.
119. World Health Organization. WHO statement: iron supplementation of young children in regions where malaria transmission is intense and infectious disease highly prevalent. http://www.who.int/child_adolescent_health/documents/pdfs/who_statement_iron.pdf. Accessed November 13, 2008.
120. Cousins RJ. Metal elements and gene expression. *Annu Rev Nutr* 1994;14:449–469.
121. King JC, Cousins R. Zinc. In: Shils ME, Shike M, Ross AC, et al., eds. *Modern nutrition in health and disease*, 10th ed. Baltimore, MD: Williams & Wilkins, 2005.
122. Fischer Walker CL, Black RE. Functional indicators for assessing zinc deficiency. *Food Nutr Bull* 2007;28:S454–S479.
123. Walravens PA, Hambidge KM. Growth of infants fed a zinc supplemented formula. *Am J Clin Nutr* 1976;29:1114–1121.
124. Aggarwal R, Sentz J, Miller MA. Role of zinc administration in prevention of childhood diarrhea and respiratory illnesses: a meta-analysis. *Pediatrics* 2007;119:1120–1130.
125. Lukacik M, Thomas RL, Aranda JV. A meta-analysis of the effects of oral zinc in the treatment of acute and persistent diarrhea. *Pediatrics* 2008;121:325–363.
126. Brooks WA, Santosham M, Naheed A, et al. Effect of weekly zinc supplements on incidence of pneumonia and diarrhoea in children younger than 2 years in an urban, low-income population in Bangladesh: randomised controlled trial. *Lancet* 2005;366:999–1004.
127. Boron P, Tokuc G, Vagas E, et al. Impact of zinc supplementation in children with acute diarrhoea in Turkey. *Arch Dis Child* 2006;91:296–299.
128. Sazawal S, Black RE, Ramsan M, et al. Effect of zinc supplementation on mortality in children aged 1–48 months: a community-based randomized placebo-controlled trial. *Lancet* 2007;369:927–934.
129. Brown KH, Lopez de Romana D, Arsenault JE, et al. Comparison of the effects of zinc delivered in a fortified food or a liquid supplement on the growth, morbidity, and plasma zinc concentrations of young Peruvian children. *Am J Clin Nutr* 2007;85:538–547.
130. Penny ME, Marin RM, Duran A, et al. Randomized controlled trial of the effect of daily supplementation with zinc or multiple micronutrients on the morbidity, growth, and micronutrient status of young Peruvian children. *Am J Clin Nutr* 2004;79:457–465.
131. Black MM. The evidence linking zinc deficiency with children's cognitive and motor functioning. *J Nutr* 2003;133:1473S–1476S.
132. Arnold LE, DiSilvestro RA. Zinc in attention-deficit/hyperactivity disorder. *J Child Adolesc Psychopharmacol* 2005;15:619–627.
133. Gardner JM, Powell CA, Baker-Henningham H, et al. Zinc supplementation and psychosocial stimulation: effects on the development of undernourished Jamaican children. *Am J Clin Nutr* 2005;82:399–405.
134. Mangels AR, Messina V. Considerations in planning vegan diets: children. *J Am Diet Assoc* 2001;101:670–677.
135. Fosmire GJ. Zinc toxicity. *Am J Clin Nutr* 1990;51:225–227.
136. Allen L. Zinc and micronutrient supplements for children. *Am J Clin Nutr* 1998;68:495S–498S.
137. Krebs NF, Westcott J. Zinc and breastfed infants: if and when is there a risk of deficiency? *Adv Exp Med Biol* 2002;503:69–75.
138. World Health Organization. Treatment of Diarrhea. https://www.who.int/maternal_child_adolescent/documents/9241593180/en/. Accessed August 18, 2020.
139. Murphy SP, Calloway DH, Beaton GH. School children have similar predicted prevalences of inadequate intakes as toddlers in village populations in Egypt, Kenya, and Mexico. *Eur J Clin Nutr* 1995;49:647–657.
140. Hambidge KM, Krebs NF. Zinc deficiency: a special challenge. *J Nutr* 2007;137:1101–1105.
141. Messina V, Mangels AR. Considerations in planning vegan diets: infants. *J Am Diet Assoc* 2001;101:661–669.
142. Bleichrodt N, Shrestha RM, West CE, et al. The benefits of adequate iodine intake. *Nutr Rev* 1996;54:S72–S78.
143. Pennington JA. Intakes of minerals from diets and foods: is there a need for concern? *J Nutr* 1996;126:2304S–2308S.
144. Pearce EN. National trends in iodine nutrition: is everyone getting enough? *Thyroid* 2007;17:823–827.
145. Hollowell JG, Staehling NW, Hannon WH, et al. Iodine nutrition in the United States. Trends and public health implications: iodine excretion data from National Health and Nutrition Examination Surveys I and III (1971–1974 and 1988–1994). *J Clin Endocrinol Metab* 1998;83:3401–3408.
146. Maberly GJ, Haxton DP, van der Haar F. Iodine deficiency: consequences and progress toward elimination. *Food Nutr Bull* 2003;24:S92–S98.
147. Qian M, Wang D, Watkins WE, et al. The effects of iodine on intelligence in children: a meta-analysis of studies conducted in China. *Asia Pac J Clin Nutr* 2005;14:32–42.
148. Zimmerman MB. The adverse effects of mild-to-moderate iodine deficiency during pregnancy and childhood: a review. *Thyroid* 2007;17:829–835.
149. Zimmermann MB, Connoly K, Bozo M, et al. Iodine supplementation improves cognition in iodine-deficient schoolchildren in Albania: a randomized, controlled, double-blind study. *Am J Clin Nutr* 2006;83:108–114.
150. Canadian Paediatric Society Nutrition Committee. The use of fluoride in infants and children. *Paediatr Child Health* 2002;7:569–572.
151. Ekstrand J, Fomon SJ, Ziegler EE, et al. Fluoride pharmacokinetics in infancy. *Pediatr Res* 1994;35:157–163.
152. Centers for Disease Control and Prevention. CDC Community water flourine: infant formula. https://www.cdc.gov/fluoridation/faqs/infant-formula.html. Accessed August 18, 2020.
153. Centers for Disease Control and Prevention. Recommendations for using fluoride to prevent and control dental caries in the United States. *MMWR Morb Mortal Wkly Rep* 2001;50(RR14):1–42.
154. Hamasha AA, Levy SM, Broffitt B, et al. Patterns of dietary fluoride supplement use in children from birth to 96 months of age. *J Public Health Dent* 2005;65:1–13.
155. American Dental Association, American Academy of Pediatric Dentistry, American Academy of Pediatrics. Dosage schedule for dietary fluoride supplements. Proceedings of a workshop. Chicago, Illinois, USA. January 31–February 1, 1994. *J Public Health Dent* 1999;59:203–281.
156. Brown D, Whelton H, O'Mullane D. Fluoride metabolism and fluorosis. *J Dent* 2005;33:177–186.
157. Adair SM. Overview of the history and current status of fluoride supplementation schedules. *J Public Health Dent* 1999;59:252–258.
158. Innis SM, Akrabawi SS, Diersen-Schade DA, et al. Visual acuity and blood lipids in term infants fed human milk or formulae. *Lipids* 1997;32:63–72.
159. Uauy R, Mena P, Wegher B, et al. Long chain polyunsaturated fatty acid formation in neonates: effect of gestational age and intrauterine growth. *Pediatr Res* 2000;47:127–135.
160. Holman RT, Johnson SB, Hatch TF. A case of human linolenic acid deficiency involving neurological abnormalities. *Am J Clin Nutr* 1982;35:617–623.
161. SanGiovanni JP, Berkey CS, Dwyer JT, et al. Dietary essential fatty acids, long-chain polyunsaturated fatty acids, and visual resolution acuity in healthy full-term infants: a systematic review. *Early Hum Dev* 2000;57:165–188.
162. Simmer K, Schulzke SM, Patole S. Longchain polyunsaturated fatty acid supplementation in preterm infants. *Cochrane Database Syst Rev* 2008;(1):CD000375.
163. Simmer K, Patole SK, Rao SC. Longchain polyunsaturated fatty acid supplementation in infants born at term. *Indian Pediatr* 2009;46:783–784.
164. Gibson RA, Chen W, Makrides M. Randomized trials with polyunsaturated fatty acid interventions in preterm and term infants: functional and clinical outcomes. *Lipids* 2001;36:873–883.
165. Jensen CL, Voigt RG, Prager TC, et al. Effects of maternal docosahexaenoic acid intake on visual function and neurodevelopment in breastfed term infants. *Am J Clin Nutr* 2005;82:123–132.
166. Malcolm CA, McCulloch DL, Montgomery C, et al. Maternal docosahexaenoic acid supplementation during pregnancy and visual evoked potential development in term infants: a double blind, prospective, randomized trial. *Arch Dis Child Fetal Neonatal Ed* 2003;88:F383–F390.
167. Makrides M, Gibson RA, Udell T, et al. Supplementation of infant formula with long-chain polyunsaturated fatty acids does not influence the growth of term infants. International LCPUFA Investigators. *Am J Clin Nutr* 2005;81:1094–1101.
168. Raiten DJ, Talbot JM, Waters JH. LSRO Report: assessment of nutrient requirements for infant formulas. *J Nutr* 1998;128:2059S–2293S.
169. Klein CJ. Nutrient requirements for preterm infant formulas. *J Nutr* 2001;132:1395S–1577S.

CHAPTER

61

Wayne R. Snodgrass
Susan C. Smolinske

Herbal Drugs in Children

This chapter addresses issues surrounding the use of herbal products in children. These included descriptions of herbal products, reasons why persons use such products, the most commonly used herbals in the United States and their use during pregnancy and breastfeeding, adverse effects, drug interactions, and regulatory issues. It is clear that children are being given herbal products in the United States. It is also clear for both children and adults that too many herbal products currently do not meet good manufacturing practices, that many herbal products are unpredictable in their concentrations of active ingredients, that many herbal products lack high-quality studies of efficacy, that labeling of most herbal products is not adequate, and that many herbal products pose a risk of toxicity. The benefit-to-risk ratio of most herbal products remains unknown. Because of the great demand by the public for herbal products, greater efforts and resources should be devoted to high-quality research to determine the effectiveness and safety of herbal products.

INTRODUCTION

The use of herbal products by children is a growing area of interest and concern. Only very limited information regarding therapeutic efficacy and risk of adverse reactions to herbal products in adults is published in peer-reviewed medical and scientific journals. Even less is known regarding herbal products usage, efficacy, and risks in children.

OBJECTIVES

The objectives in this chapter are to describe what herbal products are, why patients and parents use them, and their adverse effects and drug interactions and to discuss some approaches to evaluating data and clinical trials, the lack of quality control of manufacture of some herbal products, the issue of standardization of dose and active ingredients, the lack of full dose–response curve data, and the lack of high-quality clinical trials.

DEFINITION OF HERBAL PRODUCTS

Herbal products are drugs. They are complex mixtures of chemicals prepared from plants,[1,2] or are parts of raw, uncooked plants. The identified or suspected active ingredients are often multichemical in nature.[3] Herbal products are not required to be proven either safe or effective prior to marketing.[4] The Food and Drug Administration (FDA) has minimal to no regulatory authority regarding the safety and efficacy of herbal products. The burden of proof for safety is on the FDA, not the manufacturer.[5] This is the opposite situation to that of food additives and drugs. This situation likely results in an increased risk to the general public, and, unfortunately, it has been established by law. The 1994 Dietary Supplement Health and Education Act (DSHEA) categorizes herbal products as "dietary supplements." Thus, consumers have little protection against misleading or fraudulent claims made by herbal manufacturers.[6,7]

Herbal products are rarely sold in child-resistant packaging[8] and are exempt from regulations that mandate imprint code identification markings. Lack of product uniformity even among batches of product from a single manufacturer has been documented. Some herbal products may contain pesticides, heavy metals, or other chemicals leached from the ambient soil media.[9] There is no guarantee even on the correct identity of herbal products being sold, and ingredients may be changed frequently without notification to FDA. Herbal products may be contaminated or misidentified at any stage from harvesting through packaging.[4] Some herbal products (e.g. , aconite roots), may vary greatly in their alkaloid content depending on the origin, the time of harvest, and the method of processing.[10] There is a lack of quality control of manufacture of many herbal products, with standards in some cases far below what is generally recognized as necessary for therapeutic drugs.[11,12] Standardization of dose and active ingredients is unknown for many, and perhaps most, herbal products. For example, St. John's wort is "standardized" by its hypericin content, but hyperforin is the active ingredient. "Standardized" typically is not defined or the method stated on either the product label or a product monograph, assuming a monograph or package insert exists. Labels for dietary supplements (herbal products) may contain statements of nutrition support without preauthorization by the FDA.[13,14] On June 22, 2007, the FDA passed a final rule that established a set of good manufacturing practices (GMPs) for certain dietary supplements. Bulk suppliers and some individual practitioners are exempt; thus, this may not have prevented some of the large-scale contamination issues. Because most herbal products have no high-quality clinical trial studies, there is a lack of full dose–response data. Even if a dose range is recommended, typically, there is no dose–response information.

Children may have a different dose response than adults, as has been well established for some therapeutic drugs. Therapeutic indices vary for herbal products and may be unpredictable, particularly in children.[15] Children's doses cited by many herbal guides are strictly anecdotal.[15]

About 7,000 species of plants are used in China as herbal remedies,[10] and there are more than 5,000 kinds of Chinese medicinal herbs. There are more than 700 patent Chinese medicine factories, and there are more than 1,500 factories producing Chinese herbal pills and other dose forms.[16] It is estimated that there are more than 20,000 herbal products on the market.[17]

EPIDEMIOLOGY

An estimated 30% to 35% of adult Americans use herbal products.[18] Estimates for children are based on very limited data. Approximately 11% of parents used some form of alternative medicine for their children, based on a questionnaire sent to 2,000 parents with a 96% response rate.[19] It has been stated that up to 50% of children with autism in the United States probably are being given some form of complementary/alternative medicine.[20] One survey of emergency department visits identified that 14.5% of women used herbal products during pregnancy and 23.5% of children younger than 16 years were given herbal preparations.[21] Among teenagers who use complementary and alternative therapies, nearly 75% use herbs.[6] In 142 families that brought their children to an emergency department in 2001, 45% of caregivers reported giving their children an herbal product.[22]

An estimated 15% of Americans visited a provider of herbal medicine in 1998. Approximately 25% of Western drugs are isolated from plants, and another approximately 25% are modifications of substances derived from plants. Internationally, approximately 120 prescription drugs are produced directly from plant extracts. The U.S. commercial market for herbal products was projected to be $5 billion in the year 2000.[23]

Historically, the use of plants for medicinal purposes is documented in Chinese texts of the Yellow Emperor Huang Di in 2697 B.C.E. and in the Ebers Papyrus in 1550 B.C.E. (>800 remedies, mostly botanical). Hippocrates (466 to 377 B.C.E.) used plants in his practice of medicine.

REASONS WHY ADULTS USE HERBAL PRODUCTS

Typical adult users of herbal products are educated, middle class, white, and between the ages of 25 and 49.[24] They have a holistic belief in the integration of body, mind, and spirit. They report poorer perceived health status compared with matched nonusers of herbal products. They are not more dissatisfied with and are not more distrustful of conventional medical care. Some of these persons may be somatizers.[24]

REASONS WHY CHILDREN AND ADOLESCENTS USE HERBAL PRODUCTS

One potential use of herbal products by children and adolescents is to attempt to enhance sports performance, similar to the abuse of steroids, growth hormone analogs, and supplements such as creatine.[25] One published source recommends, for treatment of attention deficit hyperactivity disorder in children, use of St. John's wort, kava kava, catnip, and kola nut, singly or in combination.[15] A voluntary recall of ginseng products occurred after teachers reported that students were drinking ginseng extract that contained up to 24% alcohol.[15] Other reports document the use of alternative medicine and/or herbal products in children for diagnoses such as juvenile arthritis, infant colic, enuresis, postoperative pain, agitation, and plantar warts.[26–32]

Adolescent abuse of herbal blends, purchased over the Internet, or in local alternative stores, has become epidemic. These products are possibly manufactured in China, with common brand names of "Spice" or "Serenity." While labeled to contain a variety of herbal plants with psychoactive activity, chemical analysis has uniformly shown them to have none of the labeled content, but instead to contain "designer" drugs that act on the THC receptor, sometimes 100 times as potent. These appear to cause a higher degree of toxicity and tolerance than THC, thus posing an emerging threat.[33]

High-quality clinical trials can provide valid scientific evidence of the efficacy of herbal products, both for pediatric and adult therapeutic uses. One prospective, double-blind, clinical trial supported the potential efficacy of one herbal tea preparation in the treatment of infant colic[34]; this study is worthy of confirmation and is an example of an herbal product clinical trial that may provide useful and scientifically valid information. However, much more additional safety information is required before this product could be recommended for widespread use and incorporated into routine treatment recommendations.

U.S. PHARMACOPEIA DESIGNATION

In order to obtain a U.S. Pharmacopeia (USP) designation and to place the letters "USP" on a label, a manufacturer must submit its product for testing by the USP and must fulfill the standards set by the USP. Most herbal products do not have a USP designation, and it is likely that many herbal products would not meet USP standards because of factors such as batch-to-batch variability, lack of stability, and/or contaminants. A designation of NF (National Formulary) on a product without a USP designation means that the product fulfills the manufacturing quality standards set by the USP but does not have USP or FDA endorsement for the intended use.[5] Most herbal products currently do not have an NF designation. The USP has instituted a program to certify herbal products that meet its standards, including a label designation to inform the consumer that an herbal product has met USP standards. Only a small number of herbal products have received certification by the USP.

NATIONAL CENTER FOR COMPLEMENTARY AND ALTERNATIVE MEDICINE AND OFFICE OF CANCER COMPLEMENTARY AND ALTERNATIVE MEDICINE

The National Center for Complementary and Alternative Medicine (NCCAM) is a part of the National Institutes of Health (NIH), and the Office of Cancer Complementary and Alternative Medicine (OCCAM) is at the National Cancer Institute, also part of the NIH. These units provide information and support research involving herbal products and other types of complementary/alternative medicine.[35] The website for NCCAM is http://www.nccam.nih.gov.

MOST COMMONLY USED HERBAL PRODUCTS IN THE UNITED STATES

The most commonly used herbal products in the United States are chamomile, *Echinacea*, feverfew, garlic, ginger, ginkgo, ginseng, kava, saw palmetto, St. John's wort, and valerian. The commercial claims for therapeutic benefit for these herbal products typically are not substantiated by prospective, randomized, placebo-controlled, double-blind clinical trials. The claims for therapeutic use include chamomile for gastric ulcers and as a sedative, *Echinacea* for the common cold, feverfew for migraine headache prevention, garlic for hyperlipidemia and hypertension, ginger as an antiemetic, ginkgo for dementia and claudication, ginseng as a "tonic," kava for anxiety, saw palmetto for prostate hypertrophy, St. John's wort for mild endogenous depression, and valerian as a sedative. There has been a surge in recent years of the use of foods, candies, or beverages promoted as energy enhancement products to adolescents. These products typically contain caffeine derived from guarana or cola nut, in doses of up to 300 mg per serving, along with other ingredients, such as ginseng, vitamins, amino acids, and *Ginkgo biloba*.[36]

HERBAL PRODUCTS' ADVERSE EFFECTS

A number of adverse effects of herbal products have been reported.[37,38] Some of these adverse effects are severe and potentially life-threatening.[39,40] Some herbal products' adverse effects have resulted in death. The World Health Organization Collaborating Center for International Drug Monitoring in Uppsala, Sweden, has had more than 5,000 reports of suspected adverse reactions that involve herbal medicines.[10] Exposures reported to poison centers in the United States involving dietary supplements have increased 46% from 2000 to 2012, with the majority (70%) in children under the age of 6 years.[41]

A study looking at adverse effects in children reported to the FDA from dietary supplements evaluated 977 single-supplement events. Products marketed for muscle building, energy, and weight loss had almost three times the risk for severe outcomes compared with vitamins.[42]

Examples of herbal products' adverse effects (some of which are based on animal or in vitro studies) include *Aconitum*-related cardiac arrhythmias and death, *Aristolochia*-related renal failure, chaparral-related hepatotoxicity, comfrey-related hepatotoxicity and carcinogenicity, ma huang–related hypertension and/or cerebral vascular accident (i.e., stroke) and/or cardiac arrhythmias, pokeroot-related aplastic anemia sometimes resulting in death, *Sassafras*-related carcinogenicity, Chuen-Lin–related neonatal hyperbilirubinemia,[16,43,44] and berberine-related neonatal hyperbilirubinemia.[45] Other adverse effects of herbal products in children include fatal hepatic veno-occlusive disease in an infant due to pyrrolizidine alkaloids in an herbal tea,[46] central nervous system depression in infants due to an herbal tea,[47] multiple excessive ovarian follicular development,[48] aplastic anemia in a 12-year-old boy treated with an herbal product for an upper respiratory illness,[49] and gynecomastia in three prepubertal boys who chronically applied topical products containing lavender or tea tree oil.[50] Compared to other chemical exposures, some herbal products may be taken at doses that are relatively close to their toxic range, and they may be taken chronically.[51]

Reporting of adverse effects of herbal products was formerly not mandatory for manufacturers or distributors.[52] By contrast, reporting of adverse effects of therapeutic drugs is mandatory for manufacturers.[3] Data from one study suggest that users of herbal products may be less likely to consult a physician for a suspected adverse reaction to an herbal product compared with a similar adverse reaction to a conventional nonprescription medicine.[53] On December 22, 2006, an amendment to the Food, Drug, and Cosmetic (FD&C) Act was enacted that requires a manufacturer to report a serious adverse reaction to a dietary supplement to the FDA in the same manner as that to an over-the-counter (OTC) drug and to include labeling with reporting instructions.[54]

Rating of herbs by the FDA as unsafe, undefined safety, and safe is based primarily on anecdotal data and has some value as a starting point for evaluating specific herbs.[55]

An indirect form of adverse effects of herbal products is the serious harm that has occurred in children with cancer when traditional chemotherapy was replaced with unproven herbal therapies.[56]

HERBAL PRODUCTS–DRUG INTERACTIONS

Examples of drug interactions include aloe plus digoxin or aloe plus a diuretic resulting in hypokalemia, feverfew plus warfarin resulting in increased bleeding, garlic plus warfarin resulting in increased bleeding, ginger plus warfarin resulting in increased bleeding, gingko plus warfarin resulting in increased bleeding, ginseng plus digoxin resulting in increased plasma levels of digoxin, ginseng plus furosemide resulting in a decreased diuresis, ginseng plus warfarin resulting in a decreased international normalized ratio, kava plus sedatives resulting in central nervous system depression, ma huang plus β-blockers resulting in decreased β-blockade effect, ma huang plus monoamine oxidase inhibitors resulting in increased toxicity, ma huang plus theophylline resulting in increased toxicity, ma huang plus decongestants resulting in increased toxicity, St. John's wort plus adrenergic drugs resulting in hypertension, St. John's wort plus antidepressants resulting in serotonin syndrome, St. John's wort plus lithium resulting in increased lithium toxicity, St. John's wort plus angiotensin-converting enzyme inhibitors resulting in hypertension, and valerian plus central nervous system depressants resulting in increased sedation.

An extremely serious drug interaction between cyclosporine and St. John's wort is important to note. Cyclosporine is metabolized by cytochrome P-450 isoenzyme 3A4 (CYP3A4). Because of enzyme induction of CYP3A4 by St. John's wort (twofold induction of CYP3A4 by St. John's wort; threefold induction of CYP3A4 by rifampin), acute heart rejection occurred in two heart transplant patients who started St. John's wort while receiving cyclosporine.[57]

HERBAL PRODUCTS, PREGNANCY, AND BREASTFEEDING

Approximately 26 herbs are cited for restricted use in pregnancy.[58] Approximately 11 herbs are contraindicated during lactation. Most information on herbal products and breastfeeding is anecdotal and not based on scientific research.[59] The herbs to avoid in pregnant women and/or women of childbearing age include abortifacient herbs (>16 are known), emmenagogues (herbs that promote menstruation), nervous system stimulants, stimulant laxatives, berberine-containing herbs, pyrrolizidine alkaloid–containing herbs, and herbs with a high-volatile oil content.

The herb blue cohosh is contraindicated during pregnancy. This herb has been used near the end of pregnancy to induce uterine contractions. Two newborn infants with severe toxicity due to maternal use of blue cohosh have been described. One infant was born with severe congestive heart failure, cardiogenic shock, and anterolateral myocardial infarction.[60] Another infant was born with severe seizures, encephalopathy, and renal failure.[61] One newborn developed extensive petechiae and purpura after exposure in utero to evening primrose for 1 week in an attempt to ripen the mother's cervix to ease labor.[62]

Some midwives encourage the use of certain herbs as "tonics" or teas for use during pregnancy and/or lactation and also the use of some herbal products during labor and delivery.[63–65] This practice has not been well studied; the risks for mother, fetus, and infant mostly are unknown. Some herbs are known animal teratogens (e.g., hellebore, hemlock, tragacanth).[66,67] Some herbs are known human fetal toxins (e.g., blue cohosh).[66] The reported prevalence of use of Chinese herbal medicines by pregnant women in Hong Kong is 54%.[44] The reasons cited for this high prevalence of use of herbal products by pregnant women included ideas such as "to ensure firm implantation of the fetus in the uterus"![44]

The Teratology Society emphasizes the following recommendations: dietary supplements cannot be assumed to be safe for the embryo or fetus; dietary supplements should not be labeled for use in pregnancy unless they have been shown to be safe by standard scientific methods; all dietary supplements should carry a warning that their safety in pregnancy is unknown, unless safety has been established by standard scientific means; the FDA should consider all pregnancy-related conditions to be potential "diseases" in terms of the 1994 DSHEA; and the FDA should work with the U.S. Congress to amend the DSHEA of 1994 to ensure appropriate protection for the human embryo and fetus.[66]

AN EXAMPLE: *ECHINACEA*

More detailed consideration of one herbal product, *Echinacea*, will illustrate various issues regarding herbal products, such as their safety versus efficacy and the lack of high-quality, prospective, controlled clinical trials.

Echinacea is also known as the purple coneflower, a member of the daisy family of plants, and is native to North America. It is the most popular herb in the United States. Estimated sales are $300 million annually. It is sold in various forms, such as liquid extracts, tinctures, and solid dose forms. It is marketed in the United States for prevention or treatment of common cold (coryza).

Echinacea contains a variety of chemical compounds that have been identified as active constituents. These components include alkylamides, alkaloids, arabinogalactan, cichoric acid, flavonoids, isobutylamides, polyenes, and polysaccharides.

Echinacea has been approved only as "supportive therapy" by the Federal Health Agency in Germany for upper respiratory illnesses (URIs), urogenital infections, and wounds. There are approximately 26 published controlled clinical trials regarding the efficacy of *Echinacea*.[68] None of these clinical trials are of sufficient methodologic quality to be conclusive. Deficiencies in most of these studies include treatment assignment not being randomized and treatment assignment not being blinded. One randomized, double-blind, placebo-controlled clinical trial for URI showed a statistically significant decrease in symptoms and duration of "flulike" illness in 180 subjects.[69] The effects were dose dependent and occurred at a dose of 3.6 mL per day or 180 drops per day. Another randomized, double-blind, placebo-controlled clinical trial of *Echinacea* in recurrent URIs showed less frequent recurrences of URIs, less severe recurrences of URIs, and a 14% relative risk reduction in URIs. However, both of these two clinical trials had deficits of inadequate use or description of diagnostic criteria, randomization procedures, treatment interventions, methods for assessment of outcomes, assurance of blinding, details of results, and quality of the statistical analysis. Another randomized, double-blind, placebo-controlled clinical trial in 302 volunteers did not show a prophylactic effect for *Echinacea*.[70]

It is of note that information sources for *Echinacea*, as well as for other herbal products, vary in the depth of analysis and evaluation. For example, *Echinacea* is said to appear safe for use in children for colds, although there was no information on dose or duration of therapy. On the other hand, the duration of use for *Echinacea* is typically restricted to 2 weeks or less. Use exceeding 8 weeks has led to immunosuppression. A warning on the bottle label that use exceeding 8 weeks may lead to immunosuppression may not be stated for many or even most products containing *Echinacea*. This latter situation is related directly to the lack of authority for the FDA to regulate herbal products as determined by the 1994 DSHEA law passed by the U.S. Congress.

Adverse effects of *Echinacea* include the following: in persons with asthma, atopy, or allergic rhinitis, there is increased risk of severe allergic reactions, dyspnea, and/or anaphylaxis; in persons with diabetes, there may be a worsening of metabolic control. In addition, *Echinacea* is not recommended in persons with tuberculosis, human immunodeficiency virus infection, multiple sclerosis, and autoimmune diseases.

Flavonoids in *Echinacea* inhibit CYP3A4, an enzyme which has most of its activity in the liver and which metabolizes approximately 40% of all drugs marketed in the United States that are cleared by the liver. Thus, it is predictable that several drug interactions with *Echinacea* are likely to occur.

APPROACHES TO EVALUATING DATA AND CLINICAL TRIALS

Principles of rational therapy apply to herbal products just as they do to therapeutic drugs. These principles include establishing a working diagnosis, understanding the disease to be treated, choosing the best drug (considerations of benefit-to-risk ratio), individualizing treatment, choosing end points to follow to evaluate therapeutic response, and having a therapeutic contract with the patient or parent.

For a physician, evaluating therapeutic data and clinical trial data includes considerations such as the following: Was the assignment of patients to treatments really randomized?

Were all clinically relevant outcomes reported? Were the study patients recognizably similar to those patients you treat? Were both statistical and clinical significance considered in the reported data? Is the therapeutic maneuver feasible in your practice? Were all patients who entered the study accounted for at its conclusion? Published checklists for evaluating clinical trial data and published studies of clinical trials may be helpful in evaluating drug therapies and herbal product therapies.

An *N* of one randomized clinical trial may be done in an outpatient office or clinic medical practice when the patient (parent) insists on taking (giving) a treatment that the physician thinks is useless or potentially harmful, when neither the physician nor the patient (parent) is confident of the optimal dose, and when treatment is for a chronic illness or disease.

HERBAL PRODUCTS INFORMATION SOURCES

The quality of information sources available from manufacturers for herbal products varies widely and is typically far below that available from manufacturers of marketed therapeutic drugs. In addition, lay public sources of information may be incomplete, erroneous, or even contain potentially harmful information or recommendations. For example, for herbal products containing ginger, a lay magazine article states that though ginger has not been studied in children, it is considered safe. In other words, this is simply an opinion not based on data because there are no published data on the safety of ginger in children. The same article goes on to recommend chiropractic adjustment for chronic ear infections in children, a recommendation that has no basis in biologic function or disease process.[71]

The German E Commission monographs are cited widely as a reliable source of herbal information. These monographs are a compilation of the evaluations of an expert committee using the data available to them. There are few randomized, prospective, controlled clinical trial data cited or available. The German E Commission's findings are based for the most part on standardized pharmaceutical preparations found in Germany and may not necessarily be extrapolated to less-regulated products on the U.S. market.

The Internet is a source of information on herbal products, with a wide variation in the quality of the information available. As of April 1999, there were more than 10,000 commercial Internet sites for ginkgo, 11,000 for St. John's wort, and more than 20,000 for ginseng.[72]

The Dietary Supplement Label Database (DSLD) is a joint project of the NIH Office of Dietary Supplements and the National Library of Medicine and contains continuously updated label information for more than 75,000 products.[73]

FUTURE RESEARCH NEEDS

Future research needs related to herbal products include quantitative epidemiologic studies of the prevalence and the incidence of the use of herbal products in infants and children, the development of laboratory methods for the assay of herbal components and the synthesis of herbal ingredients, and high-quality clinical trials in children of the efficacy and safety of very carefully selected single-chemical entities found in herbal products.

CONCLUSION

Herbal products possibly may offer some potential benefits to some children. However, insufficient quality control in manufacture despite stronger GMPs regulations and lack of consistency of many, if not most, herbal products prevent results of any high-quality clinical trial being extrapolatable to other products or possibly even to other batches of the same product from the same company. Thus, before clinical trials of herbal products are carried out, consistent quality and reproducibility of herbal products must be achieved. Then, careful selected clinical trials in adults, followed later by clinical trials in children, may be done. With this approach, the benefits of herbal products in children, if any, may be established, while the risks and adverse effects, if any, may be identified.

More immediately, epidemiologic studies of the current use of herbal products in children should be carried out; these epidemiologic studies should include collection of data regarding adverse effects of herbal products being used in children. As a first step, this would assist in identifying those herbal products posing a risk to children.

REFERENCES

1. Kemper KJ. Seven herbs every pediatrician should know. *Contemp Pediatr* 1996;13:79–93.
2. Kemper KJ. Separation or synthesis: a holistic approach to therapeutics. *Pediatr Rev* 1996;17(8):279–283.
3. Boullleta JL, Nace AM. Safety issues with herbal medicine. *Pharmacotherapy* 2000;20(3):257–269.
4. O'Hara M, Kiefer D, Farrell K, et al. A review of 12 commonly used medicinal herbs. *Arch Fam Med* 1998;7:523–536.
5. Bauer BA. Herbal therapy: what a clinician needs to know to counsel patients effectively. *Mayo Clin Proc* 2000;75:835–841.
6. Gardiner P, Kemper KJ. Herbs in pediatric and adolescent medicine. *Pediatr Rev* 2000;21:44–57.
7. Zeisel SH. Regulation of "nutraceuticals." *Science* 1999;285:1853–1854.
8. Houlder AM. Herbal medicines should be in child resistant containers. *Br Med J* 1995;310:1473.
9. Ernst E. Harmless herbs? A review of the recent literature. *Am J Med* 1998;104:170–178.
10. Chan TY. Monitoring the safety of herbal medicines. *Drug Saf* 1997;17:209–215.
11. Liberti LE, Der Marderosian A. Evaluation of commercial ginseng products. *J Pharm Sci* 1978;67:1487–1489.
12. Heptinstall S, Awang DV, Dawson BA, et al. Parthenolide content and bioactivity of feverfew. Estimation of commercial and authenticated feverfew products. *J Pharm Pharmacol* 1992;44:391–395.
13. Anonymous. Commission on dietary supplement labels issues final report. *J Am Diet Assoc* 1998;98:270.
14. Food and Drug Administration, HHS. Current good manufacturing practice in manufacturing, packaging, labeling, or holding operations for dietary supplements; final rule. *Fed Regist* 2007;72(121):34751–34958.
15. Turow V. Herbal therapy for children. *Pediatrics* 1998;102:1492.
16. Borins M. The dangers of using herbs. What your patients need to know. *Postgrad Med* 1998;104:91–99.
17. Buck ML, Michel RS. Talking with families about herbal therapies. *Pediatrics* 2000;136:673–678.
18. Eisenberg DM, Kessler RC, Foster C, et al. Unconventional medicine in the United States: prevalence, costs, and patterns of use. *N Engl J Med* 1993;328:246–252.
19. Spigelblatt L, Laîné-Ammara G, Pless IB, et al. The use of alternative medicine by children. *Pediatrics* 1994;94:811–814.
20. Sandler AD, Brazdziunas D, Cooley WC, et al. Counseling families who choose complementary and alternative medicine for their child with chronic illness or disability. *Pediatrics* 2001;107:598–601.
21. Kristoffersen SS, Atkin PA, Shenfield GM. Uptake of alternative medicine. *Lancet* 1996;347:972.
22. Lanski SL, Greenwald M, Perkins A, et al. Herbal therapy use in a pediatric emergency department population. *Pediatrics* 2003;111:981–985.
23. Bouldin AS, Smith MC, Garner SL. Pharmacy and herbal medicine in the U.S. *Soc Sci Med* 1999;20(3):257–269.
24. Astin JA. Why patients use alternative medicine. Results of a national study. *JAMA* 1998;279:1548–1553.
25. Bucci LR. Selected herbals and human exercise performance. *Am J Clin Nutr* 2000;72(Suppl):624S–636S.
26. Cavalcanti FS, de Freitas GG. Alternative medicine in a patient with juvenile chronic arthritis. *J Rheumatol* 1992;19:1827–1828.

27. Southwood TR, Malleson PN, Roberts-Thomson PJ, et al. Unconventional remedies used for patients with juvenile arthritis. *Pediatrics* 1990;85:150–154.
28. Klougart N, Nilsson N, Jacobsen J. Infantile colic treated by chiropractors: a prospective study of 316 cases. *J Manipulative Physiol Ther* 1989;12:281–288.
29. Leboeuf C, Brown P, Herman A, et al. Chiropractic care of children with nocturnal enuresis: a prospective outcome study. *J Manipulative Physiol Ther* 1991;14:110–115.
30. Alibeu JP, Jobert J. Aconite in homeopathic relief of post-operative pain and agitation in children. *Pediatrie* 1990;45:465–466.
31. Anonymous. Canadian Pediatric Society Statement. Megavitamin and megamineral therapy in childhood. *Can Med Assoc J* 1990;143:1009–1013.
32. Labrecque M, Audet D, Latulippe LG, et al. Homeopathic treatment of plantar warts. *Can Med Assoc J* 1992;146:1749–1753.
33. European Monitoring Centre for Drugs and Drug Addiction. Understanding the spice phenomenon. Thematic Paper. Lisbon, Portugal: European Monitoring Centre for Drugs and Drug Addiction, 2009:1–37. www.emcdda.europa.eu.
34. Weizman Z, Alkrinawi S, Goldfarb D, et al. Efficacy of herbal tea preparation in infantile colic. *J Pediatr* 1993;122:650–652.
35. Muscat M. National Cancer Institute's OCCAM partners with NCCAM to expand research on unconventional cancer treatments. *Altern Ther Health Med* 1999;5(4):26–30.
36. Clauson KA, Shields KM, McQueen CE, et al. Safety issues associated with commercially available energy drinks. *J Am Pharm Assoc* 2008;48(3):e55–e63.
37. Shannon M. Alternative medicines toxicology: a review of selected agents. *Clin Toxicol* 1999;37:709–713.
38. Klepser TB, Klepser ME. Unsafe and potentially safe herbal therapies. *Am J Health Syst Pharm* 1999;56:125–138.
39. Anonymous. Herbs hazardous to your health. *Am Pharm* 1984;NS24(3):20–21.
40. Furbee B, Wermuth M. Life-threatening plant poisoning. *Crit Care Clin* 1997;13:849–888.
41. Rao N, Spiller HA, Hodges NL, et al. An increase in dietary supplement exposures reported to US poison control centers. *J Med Toxicol* 2017;13(3):227–237.
42. Or F, Kim Y, Simms J, et al. Taking stock of dietary supplements' harmful effects on children, adolescents, and young adults. *J Adolesc Health* 2019;65(4):455–461. doi:10.1016/j.jadohealth.2019.03.005.
43. Yeung CY, Lee FT, Wong HN. Effect of a popular Chinese herb on neonatal bilirubin protein building. *Biol Neonate* 1990;58:98–103.
44. Chan TY. The prevalence, use, and harmful potential of some Chinese herbal medicines in babies and children. *Vet Hum Toxicol* 1994;36:238–240.
45. Chan E. Displacement of bilirubin from albumin by berberine. *Biol Neonate* 1993;63:201–208.
46. Roulet M, Laurini R, Rivier L, et al. Hepatic veno-occlusive disease in a newborn infant of a woman drinking herbal tea. *J Pediatr* 1998;112:433–436.
47. Rosti L, Nardini A, Bettinelli ME, et al. Toxic effects of an herbal tea mixture in two newborns. *Acta Pediatr* 1994;83:683.
48. Cahill DJ, Fox R, Wardle PG, et al. Multiple follicular development associated with herbal medicine. *Hum Reprod* 1994;9:1469–1470.
49. Nelson L, Shih R, Hoffman R. Aplastic anemia induced by an adulterated herbal medication. *Clin Toxicol* 1995;33:467–470.
50. Henley DV, Lipson N, Korach KS, et al. Prepubertal gynecomastia linked to lavender and tea tree oils. *N Engl J Med* 2007;356:479–485.
51. Anonymous. Herbal health. *Environ Health Perspect* 1998;106(12):A590–A592.
52. Angell M, Kassirer JP. Alternative medicine: the risks of untested and unregulated remedies. *N Engl J Med* 1998;339:839–841.
53. Barnes J, Mills SY, Abbot NC, et al. Different standards for reporting adverse drug reactions to herbal remedies and conventional over-the-counter medicines: face-to-face interviews with 515 users of herbal remedies. *Br J Clin Pharmacol* 1998;45:496–500.
54. Food and Drug Administration. The Dietary Supplement and Nonprescription Drug Consumer Protection Act, Public Law 109–462, 2006.
55. Marderosian AD. *Natural product medicine*. Philadelphia, PA: George F. Stickley, 1988:96–104.
56. Coppes MJ, Anderson RA, Egeler RM, et al. Alternative therapies for the treatment of childhood cancer. *N Engl J Med* 1998;339:846–847.
57. Ruschitzka F, Meier PJ, Turina M, et al. Acute heart transplant rejection due to St. John's wort. *Lancet* 2000;355:548–549.
58. Blumenthal M, Werner B. *German Commission E Monographs. Therapeutic monographs on medicinal plants for human use*. Austin, TX: American Botanical Council, 1998.
59. Kopec K. Herbal medications and breastfeeding. *J Hum Lact* 1999;15:157–161.
60. Jones TK, Lawson BM. Profound neonatal congestive heart failure caused by maternal consumption of blue cohosh herbal medication. *J Pediatr* 1998;13:79–93.
61. Wright IM. Neonatal effects of maternal consumption of blue cohosh. *J Pediatr* 1999;134:384–385.
62. Belew C. Herbs and the childbearing woman. Guidelines for midwives. *J Nurse Midwifery* 1999;44(3):231–252.
63. Wedig KE, Whitsett JA. Down the primrose path: petechiae in a neonate exposed to herbal remedy for parturition. *J Pediatr* 2008;152:140–143.
64. Lee L. Introducing herbal medicine into conventional health care settings. *J Nurse Midwifery* 1999;44(3):253–266.
65. McFarlin BL, Gibson MH, O'Rear J, et al. A national survey of herbal preparation use by nurse-midwives for labor stimulation. Review of the literature and recommendations for practice. *J Nurse Midwifery* 1999;44:205–216.
66. Friedman JM. Teratology society. Presentation to the FDA public meeting on safety issues associated with the use of dietary supplements during pregnancy. *Teratology* 2000;62:134–137.
67. Panter KE, Keeler RF, Buck WB. Congenital skeletal malformations induced by maternal ingestion of *Conium maculatum* in newborn pigs. *Am J Vet Res* 1985;46:2064.
68. Melchart D, Linde K, Worku F, et al. Immunomodulation with echinacea: a systematic review of controlled trials. *Phytomedicine* 1994;1:245–254.
69. Braunig B, Dorn M, Knick E. *Echinacea purpurea* radix: zur starkung der korpereigenen abwehr bei grappalen infekten. *Z Phytother* 1993;13:7–13.
70. Melchart D, Walther E, Linde K, et al. Echinacea root extracts for the prevention of upper respiratory tract infections. A double-blind placebo-controlled randomized trial. *Arch Fam Med* 1998;7:541–545.
71. Zintl A. Natural cures for kids. *Ladies Home* 1998;56–62.
72. Nowak D, Zlatic T. Herbal products and the Internet: a marriage of convenience. *J Am Pharm Assoc* 1999;39:241–242.
73. Gahche JJ, Bailey RL, Potischman N, et al. Federal monitoring of dietary supplement use in the resident, civilian, noninstitutionalized US Population, National Health and Nutrition Examination Survey.. *J Nutr* 2018;148(Suppl 2):1436S–1444S.

SUGGESTED READINGS

American Academy of Pediatrics, Committee on Children with Disabilities. Counseling families who choose complementary and alternative medicine for their child with chronic illness or disability. *Pediatrics* 2001;107:598–601.

Ang-Lee MK, Moss J, Yuan CS. Herbal medicines and perioperative care. *JAMA* 2001;286:208–216.

Anonymous. International Conference on Harmonization of Technical Requirements for Registration of Pharmaceuticals for Human Use. ICH harmonized tripartite guideline: clinical investigation of medicinal products in the pediatric population. 2002. http://www.ich.org/LOB/media/MEDIA487.pdf.

Anonymous. Problems with dietary supplements. *Med Lett Drugs Ther* 2002;44:84–86.

Brue AW, Oakland TD. Alternative treatments for attention-deficit/hyperactivity disorder: does evidence support their use? *Altern Ther Health Med* 2002;8:68–74.

Cala S, Crismon ML, Baumgartner J. A survey of herbal use in children with attention-deficit-hyperactivity disorder or depression. *Pharmacotherapy* 2003;23:222–230.

Crawley FP, Kurz R, Nakamura H. Testing medications in children. *N Engl J Med* 2003;348:763–764.

Dockrell TR, Leever JS. An overview of herbal medications with implications for the school nurse. *J Sch Nurs* 2000;16:53–58.

Eisenberg DM, Davis RB, Ettner SL, et al. Trends in alternative medicine use in the United States, 1990–1997: results of a follow-up national survey. *JAMA* 1998;280:1569–1575.

Ernst E. Serious adverse effects of unconventional therapies for children and adolescents: a systematic review of recent evidence. *Eur J Pediatr* 2003;162:72–80.

Evans WE, McLeod HL. Drug therapy: pharmacogenomics—drug disposition, drug targets, and side effects. *N Engl J Med* 2003;348:538–549.

Friedman T, Slayton WB, Allen LS, et al. Use of alternative therapies for children with cancer. *Pediatrics* 1997;100:6. www.pediatrics.org/cgi/content/full/100/6/e1.

Geissler PW, Harris SA, Prince RJ, et al. Medicinal plants used by Luo mothers and children in Bondo district, Kenya. *J Ethnopharmacol* 2002;83:39–54.

Grimm W, Müller HH. A randomized controlled trial of the effect of fluid extract of *Echinacea purpurea* on the incidence and severity of colds and respiratory infections. *Am J Med* 1999;106:138–143.

Haller CA, Benowitz NL. Adverse cardiovascular and central nervous system events associated with dietary supplements containing ephedra alkaloids. *N Engl J Med* 2000;343:1833–1838.

Heuschkel R, Afzal N, Wuerth A, et al. Complementary medicine use in children and young adults with inflammatory bowel disease. *Am J Gastroenterol* 2002;97:382–388.

Hofmann D, Hecker M, Völp A. Efficacy of dry extract of ivy leaves in children with bronchial asthma: a review of randomized controlled trials. *Phytomedicine* 2003;10:213–220.

Madsen H, Andersen S, Nielsen RG, et al. Use of complementary/alternative medicine among pediatric patients. *Eur J Pediatr* 2003;162:334–341.

Marcus DM, Grollman AP. Botanical medicines—the need for new regulations. *N Engl J Med* 2002;347:2073–2076.

Moore C, Adler R. Herbal vitamins: lead (Pb) toxicity and developmental delay. *Pediatrics* 2000;106:600–602.

Neuhouser ML, Patterson RE, Schwartz SM, et al. Use of alternative medicine by children with cancer in Washington State. *Prev Med* 2001;33:347–354.

Ottolini MC, Hamburger EK, Loprieato JO, et al. Complementary and alternative medicine use among children in the Washington, DC area. *Ambul Pediatr* 2001;1:122–125.

Pitetti R, Singh S, Hornyak D, et al. Complementary and alternative medicine use in children. *Pediatr Emerg Care* 2001;17:165–169.

Samenuk D, Link MS, Homoud MK, et al. Adverse cardiovascular events temporally associated with ma huang, an herbal source of ephedrine. *Mayo Clin Proc* 2002;77:12–16.

Sarrell EM, Cohen HA, Kahan E. Naturopathic treatment for ear pain in children. *Pediatrics* 2003;111:e574–e579.

Shenfield G, Lim E, Allen H. Survey of the use of complementary medicines and therapies in children with asthma. *J Paediatr Child Health* 2002;38:252–257.

Sikand A, Laken M. Pediatrician's experience with and attitudes toward complementary/alternative medicine. *Arch Pediatr Adolesc Med* 1998;152:1059–1064.

Simpson N, Roman K. Complementary medicine use in children: extent and reasons. A population-based study. *Br J Gen Pract* 2001;51:914–916.

Steinbrook R. Testing medications in children. *N Engl J Med* 2002;347:1462–1470.

Talalay P. The importance of using scientific principles in the development of medicinal agents from plants. *Acad Med* 2001;76:238–247.

Tani M, Nagase M, Nishiyama T, et al. The effects of long-term herbal treatment for pediatric AIDS. *Am J Chin Med* 2002;30:51–64.

Tomassoni AJ, Simone K. Herbal medicines for children: an illusion of safety? *Curr Opin Pediatr* 2001;13:162–169.

Vessey JA, Rechkemmer A. Natural approaches to children's health: herbals and complementary and alternative medicine. *Pediatr Nurs* 2001;27:61–67.

Webb NJ, Pitt WR. Eucalyptus oil poisoning in childhood: 41 cases in southeast Queensland. *J Paediatr Child Health* 1993;29:368–371.

Woolf AD. Herbal remedies and children: do they work? Are they harmful? *Pediatrics* 2003;112:240–246.

CHAPTER

62

Bram A. Dolcourt

Pediatric Poisonings and Antidotes

OVERVIEW

Poisoning is one of the most common pediatric medical emergencies. In 2018, the American Association of Poison Control Centers' (AAPCC) National Poison Data System (NPDS) reported 925,347 toxic exposures in children younger than 6 years and 1,231,486 in children younger than 20 years. This represented 58.65% of all calls to poison control centers. This report included 51 fatalities in children younger than 6 years and 188 fatalities in those younger than 20 years, representing 6.4% of all fatal exposures reported. Nine hundred and three of the exposures in those younger than 6 years resulted in a "major" outcome (life-threatening or resulted in significant residual disability or disfigurement).[1] Data in the NPDS rely on information collected by poison control centers and consequently under-capture the true incidence of poisoning and overdose in the United States. The degree of under-reporting is not known. For comparison, in 2017, the Web-based Injury Statistics Query and Reporting System (WISQARS) database of the Centers for Disease Control and Prevention (CDC) reports 93 fatalities in those younger than 6 years and 1,101 in those younger than 20 years, while the NPDS reported 25 and 141 in the same age groups.[2,3]

Overall, poisoning episodes are largely exposures, and only 12.5% of exposures in children aged 5 years or younger lead to hospitalization. The majority were managed and monitored at home. Poison centers are staffed by skilled professionals who, contacted early, can treat most children at home.[1] Beyond their ability to provide immediate first aid advice and reassurance to caregivers of poisoned children, poison centers have added value. They positively affect the utilization of health care resources,[4,5] and they uniformly compile data that provide real-time disease surveillance and drive safety initiatives.[1] They actively carry out poison prevention activities for the public and for health care professionals. Poison centers provide caregivers and health care providers in all 50 United States, Puerto Rico, and the District of Columbia universal access to specially trained pharmacists, nurses, and physicians via a toll-free number. This uniform nationwide number, 1-800-222-1222, is the result of collaboration among the AAPCC, the CDC, and the Health Resources and Services Administration.[1]

The peak age for poisoning is age 1 to 3 years. Children younger than 3 years were involved in approximately 39% of exposures, and approximately 44% occurred in children younger than 6 years. A male predominance is found among recorded cases involving children younger than 13 years, but this gender distribution is reversed in teenagers.[1]

The most common agents involved in toxic exposures in children younger than 6 years are substances that are found in and around the home. Carbon monoxide has been the most common cause of fatal poisoning in children aged 12 years and younger. Analgesics, including acetaminophen and opioids, are the most common fatal medications. An unintentional error is the most reason for overdose in this group. The most common exposures minimally in this age group are cosmetics, cleaning products, and analgesics.[1,3]

Current trends suggest that during adolescence, suicide is a leading reason for fatal poisoning. Over the past 10 years, there has been a steady increase in the number of adolescent completed/attempted suicides reported to poison control centers. From 2011 to 2018, clonidine, bupropion, antihypertensive medication, and amitriptyline were most associated with morbidity (death and major outcomes) in the adolescent age group. The most rapidly increasing medications associated with morbidity in this age group are selective serotonin reuptake inhibitors (SSRIs), nonsteroidal anti-inflammatory drugs (NSAIDs), acetaminophen, antihistamines, and sedative hypnotics. These patterns are likely due to availability and may change as prescribing patterns change.[1]

Differences between pediatric and adult poisoning exist. Most toxic exposures in children younger than 6 years are accidental or unintentional. Young children often ingest or are exposed to a single substance.[1] Furthermore, the time to discovery is brief. Most (73%) exposures in young children are reported within 10 minutes, and children arrive to the emergency department sooner than adults. Because the child is often found with the substance, exact ingredient identification is more feasible and reliable. Generally, a smaller amount of substance is ingested by children compared with adults. Even so, one may be seriously misguided by the universal assumption that children "only ingest small amounts of pills" or "will not ingest things that are malodorous or bad tasting."

Why does pediatric poisoning continue to occur? As just noted, most exposures in young children are accidental and unintentional. These occur as toddlers explore their environment and exhibit normal hand-to-mouth activity. Other factors include caregivers' underestimation of the developmental skills of their child, imitative behavior (watching parents take medication), "look-alike" substances or containers (similarities between the intoxicant and familiar candy or beverages), and poor packaging. Concerning packaging, the use of child-resistant containers has dramatically decreased the number and severity of pediatric exposures.[6,7] Nonetheless, carelessness or distraction on the part of the caregiver while the product is in use limits the effectiveness of this safety feature.[8] Lack of grandparent awareness about the safe storage of their own medication is another cause for pediatric poisoning.[9] Often, these exposures are serious because they involve highly toxic pharmaceuticals, such as cardiovascular agents or antidiabetics.[10] Grandparent's handbags, bedside stands, kitchen tables, and day-of-the-week pill dispensers are all potentially hazardous. Another important cause of poisoning, therapeutic error, constituted 13% of toxic exposures across all ages in 2018 and accounts for 7% of poisoning deaths in children younger than 6 years. Across age groups, the most common therapeutic errors result from double dosing. Other therapeutic errors in children commonly result from dispensing-cup errors, ten-fold dosing errors, and drug interactions. Intentional poisoning may result from suicidal intent, home stressors, or substance abuse and, unfortunately, should be considered as early as age 6 years. The most common reasons for poisoning fatality in 13- to 19-year-olds, a group with a steadily increasing fatality rate, are suicide, followed by abuse.[1]

Risk factors for pediatric poisoning have been examined; however, several studies are decades old, and their current applicability is uncertain.[11–13] Studies on stress and pediatric poisoning have reached inconsistent conclusions.[14] Recurrent poisoning may occur in up to 30% of children with a history of previous ingestion.[15] Pica is associated with lead poisoning and may be a risk factor for other ingestions.[16] A parental factor that is common among unintentional poisoning in younger children is that the event occurs during a period of reduced supervision.[15,17]

APPROACH TO THE POISONED CHILD

THE ABCDs OF STABILIZATION

As with all emergencies, the initial priority in management of poisoning is stabilization. This may be accomplished by following the "ABCD" principles, or a management approach that prioritizes *a*irway, *b*reathing, *c*irculation, and neurologic *d*isability assessment. Confirmation that protective airway reflexes are intact (and if not, securement of the airway) takes precedent over all other aspects of care. The narrow-caliber pediatric airway is easily obstructed, making ingestions of corrosives, houseplants, and foreign bodies of particular concern.[18] The airway may be further compromised or aspiration may occur during subsequent gastric decontamination procedures, such as gastric lavage or the administration of charcoal.[19,20] Elective intubation in the obtunded child is always preferable to the "crash" situation. This is especially relevant when central nervous system (CNS) depressants or proconvulsants have been ingested. Next, adequate breathing must be ensured. Children more rapidly develop respiratory depression and apnea from CNS depressants than do adults.[18] Furthermore, the classic phases seen with certain drug intoxications (respiratory alkalosis during early salicylism) may not be present, or progression to respiratory acidosis may occur more rapidly than expected. While pulse oximetry assesses oxygenation, blood gas analysis is necessary to assess adequacy of ventilation and tidal volume. Pulse oximetry will not detect carboxyhemoglobinemia and may underestimate the degree of methemoglobinemia present.

Adequacy of circulation should be clinically assessed through cardiac monitoring and blood pressure and capillary refill measurement. Intravenous (IV) access is ideally obtained quickly, while the child is well perfused, rather than after the onset of hypotension, when this becomes technically more difficult. Children are more likely to have significant volume depletion from poisoning because they are less tolerant of volume losses from sweating, diarrhea, vomiting, and cathartic use. Other "Cs" to remember include aggressive cooling in the setting of hyperthermia (as occurs with the use of anticholinergics) and complete disrobing, to reveal signs of trauma, burns, or other clues regarding the substance involved.

The "Ds" of patient stabilization include assessment of neurologic disability and decontamination. Seizures that occur as a result of poisoning should be treated with benzodiazepines or barbiturates. Phenytoin does not effectively control drug-related seizures.[21] In patients with depressed mental status, reversible causes for coma should be sought. If CNS or respiratory depression is present, especially in the presence of miosis, naloxone, a narcotic antagonist, should be administered. The pediatric dose is 0.1 mg per kg or 2 mg IV. Unfortunately, opioids are widely available in many homes and account for a large and growing course of pediatric poisoning exposure.[1] A rapid glucose determination should be carried out. If this is not feasible, dextrose should be administered empirically as a 10% solution in neonates and 25% solution in infants at doses of 0.25 to 1.0 g per kg IV. Children experience glycogen depletion after only a few hours of fasting and are more prone to hypoglycemia than adults following the ingestion of agents such as ethanol. Ethanol-induced hypoglycemia may occur at blood ethanol levels as low as 20 mg per dL. Flumazenil may be used to reverse the CNS-depressant effects of benzodiazepines in the setting of known single-drug benzodiazepine ingestion or conscious sedation. The pediatric dose is 0.01 mg per kg by slow IV administration. This antidote is to be avoided if the child has a history of seizures, is taking benzodiazepines therapeutically, has possibly coingested proconvulsants, or is suspected to have increased intracranial pressure.[22] Thiamine, while typically reserved for adults with altered mental status, may be considered for lethargic children with a history of malnutrition, anorexia, on chemotherapy, or on total parenteral nutrition.

DECONTAMINATION

Dermal decontamination is carried out to decrease the level of patient exposure to the intoxicant and, in some cases, to prevent secondary spread to health care providers. Children's skin is much thinner than that of adults; therefore, both the dermal absorption of toxins and chemical burns occur more readily.[18] Ocular chemical exposures should be of the highest priority and should be treated with immediate tepid water irrigation that begins at the scene and continues until medical evaluation is underway. The skin should be thoroughly washed with mild soap and tepid water, with attention to wounds, skin folds, hair, and nails. Close temperature monitoring is necessary in infants and young children, who may become hypothermic during the skin decontamination process.

The role of gastrointestinal (GI) decontamination is an area of great controversy. Demonstrating improved outcome in poisoned patients through gastric emptying procedures is difficult, given the low associated poisoning mortality. This major drawback limits the translation of the available evidence to strict practice guidelines.

Syrup of ipecac reliably produces vomiting in 85% of patients. It was previously recommended as an early treatment for poisoning, especially in the prehospital environment. A 2004 joint position paper by the AAPCC, American Academy of Clinical Toxicology (AACT), and the American College of Medical Toxicology (ACMT) recommended against the routine use of syrup of ipecac for accidental or intentional poisoning.[23] This followed a 2003 position from the American Academy of Pediatrics (AAP), recommending that ipecac should not be kept in the home or routinely administered.[24] Previously, studies had demonstrated no benefit from ipecac use and risks of aspiration.[25] At this time, ipecac is not recommended, except in consultation with a medical toxicologist or poison control center.

Gastric lavage may be considered in patients presenting within 60 minutes of the ingestion of a potentially toxic amount of a toxic substance, or for those critically ill patients for whom the time of ingestion is unknown. The procedure involves the orogastric placement of a 24- to 32-Fr Ewald tube with the patient lying in the left lateral decubitus position. Repeated instillation and removal of 50- to 100-mL aliquots of half-normal or normal saline is carried out until the lavage fluid is clear. The use of cold tap water in small children may result in hyponatremia or hypothermia. Lavage solutions employed in the past such as sodium bicarbonate or sodium phosphate are not recommended. Scant evidence exists to suggest more than minimal benefit. Gastric lavage should not be performed in patients with inadequate airway protective reflexes or in those with corrosive substance ingestion. Serious potential complications from the procedure include upper airway obstruction, pulmonary aspiration, and GI tract perforation. There is no role for routine use of gastric lavage in poisoning, and it should only be used in carefully selected patients.[19]

Activated charcoal is frequently administered orally to patients who have recently overdosed; however, the recommendation from AAPCC, ACMT, and European Association of Poison Control Centers since 1999 is that it should not be routinely administered to poisoned patients unless (a) the substance is amenable to charcoal therapy, (b) 1 hour or less has elapsed from the time of ingestion, and (c) there are no contraindications to charcoal administration (Table 62.1).

When administered within 1 hour of ingestion, activated charcoal may reduce toxin absorption by up to 75%.[20,26] The usual dose is ten times that of the estimated dose of toxic substance. When the amount of the substance is unknown, charcoal is dosed empirically at 0.5 to 1 g per kg of body weight. It is administered as well-mixed slurry of charcoal and water. Sorbitol is frequently added to promote GI motility. It can be administered via a nasogastric tube; however, the risk and benefits need to be assessed on a case-by-case basis. Palatability may be improved through the use of a commercial cherry-flavored product, additives such as chocolate or fruit syrup, or disguising in an opaque container/opaque straw.[20]

TABLE 62.1 Charcoal Use in Acute Poisoning

Potential Benefit from Single-Dose–Activated Charcoal[26,27]	*No Benefit from Single-Dose–Activated Charcoal*
Acetaminophen	Metals (lithium, lead)
ACE inhibitors	Strong acids (hydrochloric acid, HF)
Amphetamines	Strong alkaline (lye)
Antidepressants	Inorganic salts
Antihistamines	Alcohols
Carbamazepine,[a] phenytoin	Inorganic salts
Aspirin	
Atropine	
Barbiturates (phenobarbital[a])	
Benzodiazepines	
β-Blockers	
Calcium channel blockers	
Chloroquine	
Dapsone[a]	
Digoxin, digitoxin	
Furosemide	
Neuroleptics	
NSAIDs, aspirin[a]	
Sulfonylureas, esp. glipizide	
Opioids	
Theophylline,[a] caffeine[a]	
Quinine,[a] quinidine[a]	

[a]Potential benefit from multidose-activated charcoal (MDAC).[28]
ACE, angiotensin-converting enzyme; HF, hydrogen fluoride; NSAIDs, nonsteroidal anti-inflammatory drugs.

Administration of activated charcoal has not been shown to improve patient outcome, although trials have generally been inadequate to show meaningful patient-centered outcomes. The rationale for its administration is based on a number of theoretical benefits. These include the direct adsorption of the toxic material, prevention of systemic absorption, and interruption of enterohepatic recirculation of specific drugs or their metabolites.[20] In addition, based on the immense surface area of the intestinal villi, which lie in close proximity to intestinal capillaries, continuous forward movement of charcoal through the intestines may create a concentration gradient that allows systemically circulating drug to diffuse back into the gut lumen and adsorb to charcoal. This concept has been termed "gut dialysis." For some ingestions, charcoal is administered in a pulse-dosed manner.[27] During such practice, cathartics should be given only with the first dose of charcoal each day to prevent fluid and electrolyte imbalance. In addition, the status of intestinal activity must be monitored closely to prevent ileus-induced charcoal impaction, especially in patients with anticholinergic poisoning. Not all agents adsorb to activated charcoal. For example, metals such as iron and lithium, some pesticides, some corrosives, and some alcohols are poorly bound.[27]

Cathartics have not been shown to improve outcome following drug overdose, but they are commonly administered with the first dose of activated charcoal. They are classified as saline (magnesium citrate, magnesium sulfate) and saccharide (sorbitol). Based on their high osmolarity, they cause fluid to enter the GI tract and bowel peristalsis to increase. Magnesium sulfate may stimulate the release of cholecystokinin, increasing motor and secretory action in the GI tract. Sorbitol has been demonstrated to be the most rapidly acting cathartic in terms of "time to first stool" as compared with saline cathartics. Overly aggressive use of cathartics can cause pediatric dehydration and hypermagnesemia, and they are, therefore, typically not used in infants. The dose in older children is 20% magnesium sulfate, 250 mg per kg; 6% magnesium citrate, 4 mL per kg; or sorbitol, 0.5 to 1 g per kg. Sorbitol is not recommended for children younger than 12 months.[29]

Contraindications to charcoal administration include lack of a protected airway and evidence of GI tract obstruction or perforation. Between 6% and 27% of patient who are given charcoal will experience an episode of vomiting; however, the substance ingested may influence the risk of vomiting. Charcoal pneumonitis is an infrequent, but potentially serious adverse event associated with charcoal administration and is reported in 1.6% of cases.[20,26] Charcoal should not be given to patients who ingest corrosive agents, as it will obscure endoscopy, unless there is another systemic toxin that is amenable to charcoal therapy.[20]

Whole-bowel irrigation (WBI) is a technique employed to rid the GI tract of ingested substances that do not adsorb to charcoal, such as iron or lithium. The procedure involves continuous GI administration of balanced solution of electrolytes and polyethylene glycol at a relatively high volume. These solutions are isosmotic and allow for mechanical cleansing of the gut without the risk of fluid or electrolyte imbalance, even in young children. WBI may also be considered in patients who are suspected to have concretions or who have ingested lead-based paint chips, massive amounts of a toxic substance, sustained-release preparations (e.g., calcium channel blockers), or drug packets. Polyethylene glycol solution is given as 20 to 40 mL per kg per hour in children. This typically requires nasogastric tube insertion. While WBI may speed the transit time for some substances, there is no evidence of clinical benefit. Risks include vomiting, which can be exacerbated by GI obstruction or ileus. WBI is not recommended in patients with abnormal GI anatomy.[30]

HISTORY AND PHYSICAL

Once stabilization of the patient has been accomplished, a complete history should be obtained along with a complete physical examination. Historical elements should include the substance or substances involved, when the child was last known to be normal, the suspected time of ingestion, and other substances available. When inquiring about other substances, it is important to cast a broad net, including over-the-counter medications, previous "leftover" prescriptions, supplements, herbal/nonallopathic medications, substances of abuse, abusable research chemicals (such as "spice," U-44700, "smart drugs," and other products available online), and other household/industrial products that may be in the home. The amounts of available substances and an estimation potential dose should be obtained. It is important to assume the worst-case scenario when calculating dose estimation. Detailed interviews with multiple caregivers may be necessary to accomplish this. The original containers or pictures of the containers and substances may be helpful. A retrospective search of the home may be useful because children may find items that may be hidden from adult view, such as pills on the floor or discarded containers in wastebaskets. Despite thorough questioning, history of poisoning or drug ingestion may be lacking. The clinician should always place poisoning in the differential diagnosis for children with the risk factors for poisoning, multiple organ system involvement, or a confusing clinical picture.[18,31]

Many exposures in children involve nontoxic or minimally toxic products. It is important to note that a nontoxic exposure may still be of concern as it could represent a suicidal gesture, a sign of caretaker distress, and indicate inadequate supervision or an unsafe environment. In addition, symptoms that occur in the setting of "nontoxic" exposure may suggest unrelated diagnoses, incorrectly identified substances, or product tampering. While less common, clinicians should be aware substances that may be potentially fatal in small or single-unit doses.[32,33] Substances generally considered to be minimally toxic are listed in Table 62.2, and substances that are of significant toxicity are highlighted in Table 62.3.

A meticulous physical examination should search to uncover the presence of a toxidrome. The examination should focus on abnormalities of vital signs, mental status, pupils/fundi, mucous membrane hydration, corrosive effect on the mucous membranes and skin, bowel sounds, bladder distension, and reflexes. The presence of odors, bullae, cyanosis, or other skin discolorations should be noted. Miosis, bradycardia, and hypertension are unusual in pediatric patients and should point to possible drug effect.[18] The clinical features of several toxidromes are outlined in Table 62.4.

Poisoning may be a warning sign of child abuse or neglect.[35,36] Suspicions should be raised when poisoning occurs in children younger than 6 months or in those without the developmental capability to access the substance in question. Other

TABLE 62.2 Minimally Toxic or Nontoxic Substances
Silica gel
Vitamins A and D ointment
Blackboard or sidewalk chalk
Lipsticks and noncamphor lip balms
Watercolor paints
Handwashing or dishwashing detergents (not dishwasher or laundry detergent or ethanol-based hand scrubs)
Calamine lotion (excluding products with antihistamines)
Clay (play)
Crayons
Diaper rash creams/ointments
Fabric softener sheets
Glow products
Glue (white arts and crafts)
Household plant food
Oral contraceptives
Pen ink
Pencils
Starch/sizing
Throat lozenges without local anesthetics
Topical antibiotics/topical steroids
Water-based paints

TABLE 62.3 Drugs and Toxins That Can Cause Severe Toxicity to a 10-kg Child after a Small Dose

Antiarrhythmics
Benzocaine
β-Blockers
Bupropion
Calcium channel blockers
Camphor
Chloroquine
Chlorpromazine
Clonidine
Diphenhydramine
Diphenoxylate
Ethylene glycol
Hydroxychloroquine
Imidazolines (tetrahydrozoline, oxymetazoline, xylometazoline, naphazoline)
Lindane
Methanol
Methyl salicylate
Orphenadrine
Opioids
Quinine
Theophylline
Thioridazine
Tricyclic antidepressants
Selenious acid (gun bluing)
Sulfonylureas

Data from Matteucci MJ. One pill can kill: assessing the potential for fatal poisonings in children. *Pediatr Ann* 2005;34:964–968; and Chomchai C, Sirisamut T, Silpasupagornwong U. Pediatric fatality from gun bluing solution: the need for a chemical equivalent of the one-pill-can-kill list. *J Med Assoc Thai* 2012;95:821–824.

situations suggestive of possible abuse include those in which the history provided changes or is inconsistent between caregivers. Ingestions by older children (>5 years) and ingestions of psychotropic agents, drugs of abuse, sedative hypnotics, and ethanol are all potentially of concern. A long interval between the time of ingestion and the time to presentation for medical evaluation is also suspicious. It is prudent to review previous medical records of children with poisoning. The incidence is unclear; however, evidence suggests that abused children often have previous emergency department visits.[37] Children with accidental ingestions may have repeat exposures and are potentially at risk for other injuries.[38] Munchausen syndrome by proxy is an extremely rare condition that should be suspected in children with recurrent unexplained illness whose parent is a medical professional, is very willing to provide detailed data on unusual illnesses, and is overly friendly or helpful.[37]

LABORATORY

Toxicology screens are of limited value in children with the witnessed ingestion of a single substance. Such screens may be negative even in the face of serious toxicity.[39,40] Routine chemistries, blood gas analysis, osmolality, ketones, and lactate levels are all useful in the evaluation of metabolic acidosis, which is the most common laboratory finding. Agents that are typically available for relatively rapid results usually include medications that require therapeutic monitoring or are used for other evaluation and treatment. These include frequently available tests, anticonvulsants (phenytoin, carbamazepine, valproic acid, phenobarbital), iron, methanol, salicylates, caffeine, ethanol, digoxin, lead, lithium, methemoglobin, methotrexate, and theophylline. Methanol, ethylene glycol, carboxyhemoglobin, and acetaminophen are also frequently available.[40] Critical

TABLE 62.4 Toxidromes

	Opioids	*Anticholinergic*	*Cholinergic*	*Sympathomimetic*
Pulse	Decreased	Increased	Decreased	Increased
Blood pressure	Decreased	Increased	Variable	Increased
Respirations	Decreased	Variable	Variable	Increased
Temperature	Decreased	Increased	Decreased	Increased
Bowel sounds	Decreased	Decreased	Hyperactive	Normal
Skin	Sweaty	Dry, red, hot	Sweaty	Sweaty
Mental status	Depressed	Agitated delirium/seizures	Depressed/agitated	Delirium/seizures
Pupils	Miosis	Mydriasis	Miosis	Mydriasis
Other	Track marks	Urinary retention, no axillary sweat	Fasciculations Weakness, bronchospasm, bronchorrhea, (?) garlic odor/pesticides	Bruxism
Examples	Codeine	Antihistamines	Organophosphates	Cocaine
	Other nonopioids (clonidine, γ-hydroxybutyrate)			
	Heroin	Antipsychotics	Carbamates	Amphetamines
	Methadone	Scopolamine		Theophylline
	Oxycodone	Atropine		

Data from Calello DP, Henretig FM. Pediatric toxicology: specialized approach to the poisoned child. *Emerg Med Clin North Am* 2014;32:29–52.

early interventions may be indicated for the appropriate management of intoxication resulting from these substances, depending on specific serum or blood levels. In addition, tests in the older child or adolescent with a suspected intentional drug overdose should include routine acetaminophen and salicylate levels and consideration of a pregnancy test. Other laboratory testing should be individualized and may include a complete blood count, calcium test, liver function test, and urinalysis. Urine drug of abuse testing should not be routine and instead should be individualized to the clinical situation.[39] More comprehensive drug testing with modalities such as gas chromatography/mass spectroscopy may seem attractive, but still needs to be obtained within the appropriate clinical scenario. Testing often takes significant time, may lead to false conclusions, and cannot be relied upon to detect all medications and substances.[41]

RADIOGRAPHS

Radiographs are of limited diagnostic value, but may be helpful in some instances. Few medications are radiopaque; however, calcium salts, chloral hydrate, iron, iodine-containing products, phenothiazines (i.e., haloperidol), enteric-coated tablets, and halogenated solvents (i.e., chloroform, methylene chloride) all may be visible on plain radiographs. The absence of substance does not rule out ingestions, however. Radiographs may be useful to follow GI burden during decontamination efforts, such as in the setting of ingested lead chips or other foreign body.[42] Other radiograph studies such as chest radiographs and computed tomography should be individualized.

ENHANCED ELIMINATION

The elimination of absorbed, circulating toxic substances may be enhanced through a number of methods. The renal excretion of a few drugs that are weak acids can be increased by alkalinization of the urine and ion trapping the ionized form of the drug in the renal tubule. This method prevents renal tubular reabsorption of drugs, such as salicylates, phenobarbital, chlorpropamide, and 2,4-dichlorophenoxyacetic acid. This is different than inducing high urine volumes with excess IV fluids ("forced diuresis"). The most important factor in the enhancement of renal elimination of drugs is the urinary pH and not the volume of urine output. The target urinary pH is 7.5 to 8.0 and should be monitored hourly, along with close monitoring of electrolytes and calcium. A Foley catheter is generally required.[43,44]

Hemodialysis is a method that increases the elimination of a few specific substances. Its use was reported in children younger than 6 years only four times in 2017 and 131 times in all patients aged 19 years or younger.[3] The physical characteristics of the intoxicant determine whether it will be amenable to removal by hemodialysis. Specifically, the drug must be able to freely cross the dialysis membrane. With high-flux, high-efficiency dialysis, substance up to 10,000 Da is potentially amenable to extracorporeal clearance. While low protein binding and low volume of distribution make a substance more amenable to hemodialysis, patient intoxicated by some highly protein-bound and high volume of distribution substances show benefit with hemodialysis.[45] Although hemodialysis has been anecdotally reported to enhance the elimination of a wide variety of intoxicants, there are published guidelines for acetaminophen,[46] salicylates,[47] phenobarbital,[48] methanol,[49] lithium,[50] carbamazepine,[51] theophylline,[52] valproic acid,[53] and thallium.[54] Dialysis is helpful to control refractory acidosis associated with metformin intoxication.[55] Hemodialysis can also be used for ethylene glycol intoxication,[56] some metals, and a few other renally excreted drugs, but the indications are less clear. Hemodialysis is at times technically difficult in hemodynamically unstable patients and in neonates. Alternatively, exchange transfusion has been employed for the management of severe neonatal theophylline or salicylate intoxication.

Multidose-activated charcoal is another method used to enhance drug elimination. Its use is warranted for the treatment of serious intoxications with phenobarbital, theophylline, carbamazepine, dapsone, and quinine.[28,57] It may be considered for salicylate, colchicine, and amatoxin (mushroom) toxicity. Multidose charcoal is commonly recommended for the treatment of phenytoin toxicity based on volunteer data showing decreased elimination half-lives. A beneficial outcome for phenytoin-poisoned patients, however, has not been demonstrated.[57]

ANTIDOTES

Antidote use in children, as in adults, is rarely required. Good supportive care is the most important treatment modality. Most poisonings are managed with the stabilization, decontamination, and supportive care processes outlined earlier. When their use is necessary, however, the therapeutic indications for antidotes are generally the same as for adults. In 2017, the most commonly used antidote was naloxone.[3] When antidotes are used, treatment is aimed at neutralizing the intoxicant, and dosing may not be weight based in children. For example, if a child ingests 0.25 mg of digoxin and develops a cardiac dysrhythmia, digoxin-Fab fragments will be administered at the dose needed to neutralize the estimated amount of digoxin that is bioavailable.[58] In the setting of crotaline (rattlesnake) envenomation, antivenin is based on the clinical severity of the envenomation and not the child's weight.[59] Other trends in antidote use include the use of lipid emulsion to treat local anesthetic and other cardiovascular poisons,[60] large doses of insulin to treat β-blocker and calcium channel blocker overdose,[61] and the use of octreotide following pediatric sulfonylurea poisoning.[62] Commonly used antidotes are listed in Table 62.5.

REFRACTORY SHOCK

Venoarterial extracorporeal membrane oxygenation (ECMO) is an emerging therapy for the treatment of refractory shock in poisoned adults as a bridge to recovery. There are limited data on its use; however, published case series and reports show promise. In 2018, ECMO use in the treatment for poisoning was reported to NPDS on 10 patients younger than 6 years.[1] It should be considered a salvage therapy for the poisoned child who is not responding to treatment and is at risk of death.[64,65]

PREVENTION

Educating caregivers on poisoning prevention has been demonstrated to improve medication storage practices. Examples of primary messages that clinicians should provide to caregivers are listed in Table 62.6. The most important of these is to avoid bringing toxic substances into the home. Cleaning products, personal care products, and medications should be kept out of

TABLE 62.5 Antidotes for Poisoning

Antidote	*Toxicant*
Antivenin	Crotalids (rattlesnakes)
	North American coral snake
	Exotic snake species
	Black widow spider
	Scorpion
	Sea wasp or box jellyfish
Atropine	Organophosphates
	Carbamates
	Physostigmine
	Clitocybe, Inocybe mushrooms
Benztropine/diphenhydramine	Dystonic reaction from neuroleptic medication
Calcium	Hydrofluoric acid
	Calcium channel blocker
Chelators	
Calcium disodium ethylenediaminetetraacetic acid	Lead, cadmium, copper, zinc
Deferoxamine	Iron, aluminum
Dimercaprol	Arsenic, lead, gold, inorganic mercury
D-Penicillamine	Investigational for copper, lead, mercury, arsenic, and bismuth
Dimercaptosuccinic acid (succimer)	Lead, mercury
Cyanide antidote kit	Cyanide
	Hydrogen sulfide
Digoxin-specific antibodies	Digoxin/digitoxin
	Cardiac glycoside–containing plants such as oleander, foxglove, lily of the valley
Ethanol	Methanol
	Ethylene glycol
	Glycol ethers
4-Methylpyrazole (Antizol)	Ethylene glycol
Flumazenil (Romazicon)	Benzodiazepines
Folic acid (Leucovorin)	Methanol
	Methotrexate
	Trimethoprim
Glucagon	β-Blockers
	Calcium channel blockers
	Insulin/oral hypoglycemic agents
Glucose	Insulin/oral hypoglycemic agents
Methylene blue	Drugs causing methemoglobinemia
Hydroxocobalamin	Cyanide
Insulin	β-Blockers
	Calcium channel blockers
Lipid emulsion	Local anesthetics (bupivacaine)
N-Acetylcysteine	Acetaminophen
	Pennyroyal oil
	Cyclopeptide mushrooms
	Carbon tetrachloride
Naloxone	Opiates/narcotics
	Clonidine
	Dextromethorphan

(continued)

TABLE 62.5 Antidotes for Poisoning (*continued*)

Antidote	*Toxicant*
Octreotide	Sulfonylureas
Oxygen	Carbon monoxide
Prothrombin complex	Warfarin
	Direct-acting oral anticoagulants
Pralidoxime chloride	Organophosphates
	Carbamates
Protamine	Heparin
Pyridoxine (vitamin B6)	Isoniazid
	Gyromitra esculenta
	Ethylene glycol
	Disulfiram
	Carbon disulfide
Thiamine	Ethanol
	Ethylene glycol
Vitamin K1	Warfarin
	Long-acting warfarins (rat poisons)

Data from Dart RC, Borron SW, Caravati EM, et al. Expert consensus guidelines for stocking of antidotes in hospitals that provide emergency care. *Ann Emerg Med* 2009;54:386–394.e1. doi:10.1016/j.annemergmed.2009.01.023.

TABLE 62.6 Pediatric Poisoning Prevention

Avoid bringing chemicals or medications into the home
If toxic substances must be kept in the home, keep all medications/cleaning products out of sight, on a top shelf, in a locked cabinet, or closet
Remember: out of reach ≠ out of sight
Keep regional poison control center phone sticker on each phone
Up to 30% of children who have toxic ingestions will be repeaters and are at risk for other injuries
Visitors' purses/backpacks should be kept out of reach/out of sight
Bedside stands are hazardous—do not keep medications in this location
Do not keep medications, vitamins, or iron supplements on kitchen tables or countertops
Use only child-resistant containers
Do not take medication in front of children
Never refer to medication as candy
Flush old medications down the toilet
Do not store cleaning products or pesticides near food or in food or beverage containers
Keep all products in their original container
Rinse out all containers thoroughly prior to disposal into the wastebasket
Double-bag (unbroken) mercury thermometers in lockable plastic baggies and take to community hazardous disposal waste site; for broken thermometers, call regional poison control center
Do not bring chemicals or products home from the workplace
Contact regional poison control center at 1-800-222-1222 for brochures on poison proofing the home and toxic plants

Data from Wynn PM, Zou K, Young B, et al. Prevention of childhood poisoning in the home: overview of systematic reviews and a systematic review of primary studies. *Int J Inj Contr Saf Promot* 2016;23:3–28.

sight, on a high shelf, ideally in a locked cabinet or closet.[66] Labeling products as hazardous with brightly colored stickers may improve safety; however, the evidence is weak.[67]

Medication packaging and other regulatory changes can have a significant impact in the rate of poisoning from different substances. In response to publications showing a significant number of adverse events and deaths in children aged 4 years and younger, the Food and Drug Administration (FDA) pressured manufacturers to remove cough and cold products for this age group from stores.[68] Historically, iron was one of the major causes of poisoning death in children.[69] In 2003, the FDA required that higher dose iron tablets be sold in unit dose, "blister," packs to reduce the risk of overdose. Even after the iron packaging requirements were successfully challenged in court, the rate of poisoning from these substances has diminished substantially.[1]

Pediatric THC and opioid exposures have been generally rising, likely due to availability.[10,70] Analgesics, including opioids, resulted in the greatest number of pediatric deaths in 2017. This continues a long-term trend.[1,3] The CDC, FDA, National Institute on Drug Abuse (NIDA), and AAP all have resources available to help combat accidental opioid and drug overdose in young children and abuse in older children.[71–74]

REFERENCES

1. Gummin DD, Mowry JB, Spyker DA, et al. 2018 Annual Report of the American Association of Poison Control Centers' National Poison Data System (NPDS): 36th Annual Report. *Clin Toxicol* 2019;57:1220–1413. doi:10.1080/15563650.2019.1677022.
2. Centers for Disease Control and Prevention. National Center for Injury Prevention and Control (2020) Web-based Injury Statistics Query and Reporting System (WISQARS). www.cdc.gov/injury/wisqars.
3. Gummin DD, Mowry JB, Spyker DA, et al. 2017 Annual Report of the American Association of Poison Control Centers' National Poison Data System (NPDS): 35th Annual Report. *Clin Toxicol* 2018;56(12):1213–1415.
4. LoVecchio F, Curry SC, Waszolek K, et al. Poison control centers decrease emergency healthcare utilization costs. *J Med Toxicol* 2008;4:221–224. doi:10.1007/BF03161204.
5. Blizzard JC, Michels JE, Richardson WH, et al. Cost-benefit analysis of a regional poison center. *Clin Toxicol* 2008;46:450–456. doi:10.1080/15563650701616145.
6. Walton WW. An evaluation of the Poison Prevention Packaging Act. *Pediatrics* 1982;69:363–370.
7. Paul IM, Reynolds KM, Delva-Clark H, et al. Flow restrictors and reduction of accidental ingestions of over-the-counter medications. *Am J Prev Med* 2019;56:e205–e213. doi:10.1016/j.amepre.2018.12.015.
8. Lembersky RB, Nichols MH, King WD. Effectiveness of child-resistant packaging on toxin procurement in young poisoning victims. *Vet Hum Toxicol* 1996;38:380–383.
9. McFee RB, Caraccio TR. "Hang Up Your Pocketbook"—an easy intervention for the granny syndrome: grandparents as a risk factor in unintentional pediatric exposures to pharmaceuticals. *J Am Osteopath Assoc* 2006;106:405–411.
10. Burghardt LC, Ayers JW, Brownstein JS, et al. Adult prescription drug use and pediatric medication exposures and poisonings. *Pediatrics* 2013;132:18–27. doi:10.1542/peds.2012-2978.
11. Jensen GD, Wilson WW. Preventive implications of a study of 100 poisonings in children. *Pediatrics* 1960;25:490–495.
12. Sibert R. Stress in families of children who have ingested poisons. *Br Med J* 1975;3:87–89. doi:10.1136/bmj.3.5975.87.
13. Sobel R. The psychiatric implications of accidental poisoning in childhood. *Pediatr Clin North Am* 1970;17:653–685. doi:10.1016/s0031-3955(16)32458-0.
14. Schmertmann M, Williamson A, Black D, et al. Risk factors for unintentional poisoning in children aged 1–3 years in NSW Australia: a case–control study. *BMC Pediatr* 2013;13:88. doi:10.1186/1471-2431-13-88.
15. Schwebel DC, Evans WD, Hoeffler SE, et al. Unintentional child poisoning risk: a review of causal factors and prevention studies. *Child Health Care* 2017;46:109–130. doi:10.1080/02739615.2015.1124775.
16. Leung AKC, Hon KL. Pica: a common condition that is commonly missed—an update review. *Curr Pediatr Rev* 2019;15:164–169. doi:10.2174/1573396315666190313163530.
17. Schillie SF, Shehab N, Thomas KE, et al. Medication overdoses leading to emergency department visits among children. *Am J Prev Med* 2009;37:181–187. doi:10.1016/j.amepre.2009.05.018.
18. Calello DP, Henretig FM. Pediatric toxicology: specialized approach to the poisoned child. *Emerg Med Clin North Am* 2014;32:29–52. doi:10.1016/j.emc.2013.09.008.
19. Benson BE, Hoppu K, Troutman WG, et al. Position paper update: gastric lavage for gastrointestinal decontamination. *Clin Toxicol (Phila)* 2013;51:140–146. doi:10.3109/15563650.2013.770154.
20. Chyka PA, Seger D, Krenzelok EP, et al. Position paper: single-dose activated charcoal. *Clin Toxicol (Phila)* 2005;43:61–87. doi:10.1081/clt-200051867.
21. Chen H-Y, Albertson TE, Olson KR. Treatment of drug-induced seizures. *Br J Clin Pharmacol* 2016;81:412–419. doi:10.1111/bcp.12720.
22. Shannon M, Albers G, Burkhart K, et al. Safety and efficacy of flumazenil in the reversal of benzodiazepine-induced conscious sedation. *J Pediatr* 1997;131:582–586. doi:10.1016/S0022-3476(97)70066-0.
23. American Academy of Clinical Toxicology. Position paper: ipecac syrup. *J Toxicol Clin Toxicol* 2004;133–143. doi:10.1081/clt-120037421.
24. American Academy of Pediatrics Committee on Injury, Violence and Poison Prevention. Poison treatment in the home. American Academy of Pediatrics Committee on Injury, Violence, and Poison Prevention. *Pediatrics* 2003;112:1182–1185. doi:10.1542/peds.112.5.1182.
25. Bond GR. Home syrup of ipecac use does not reduce emergency department use or improve outcome. *Pediatrics* 2003;112(5):1061–1064. doi:10.1542/peds.112.5.1061.
26. Juurlink DN. Activated charcoal for acute overdose: a reappraisal. *Br J Clin Pharmacol.* 2016;81(3):482–487. doi:10.1111/bcp.12793.
27. Zellner T, Prasa D, Färber E, et al. The use of activated charcoal to treat intoxications. *Dtsch Arztebl Int* 2019;116:311–317. doi:10.3238/arztebl.2019.0311.
28. Ahari S, Schult R, Wiegand TJ. Use of multidose activated charcoal in the toxic registry. *J Med Toxicol* 2014. doi:10.1007/s13181-013-0376-x.
29. Position paper: cathartics. *J Toxicol Clin Toxicol* 2004;42:243–253. doi:10.1081/clt-120039801.
30. Thanacoody R, Caravati EM, Troutman B, et al. Position paper update: whole bowel irrigation for gastrointestinal decontamination of overdose patients. *Clin Toxicol (Phila)* 2015;53:5–12. doi:10.3109/15563650.2014.989326.
31. Madden MA. Pediatric toxicology: emerging trends. *J Pediatr Intensive Care* 2015;4:103–110. doi:10.1055/s-0035-1556753.
32. Matteucci MJ. One pill can kill: assessing the potential for fatal poisonings in children. *Pediatr Ann* 2005;34:964–968. doi:10.3928/0090-4481-20051201-12.
33. Koren G. Medications which can kill a toddler with one tablet or teaspoonful. *J Toxicol Clin Toxicol* 1993;31:407–413. doi:10.3109/15563659309000409.
34. Chomchai C, Sirisamut T, Silpasupagornwong U. Pediatric fatality from gun bluing solution: the need for a chemical equivalent of the one-pill-can-kill list. *J Med Assoc Thai* 2012;95:821–824.
35. Stauffer SL, Wood SM, Krasowski MD. Diagnostic yield of hair and urine toxicology testing in potential child abuse cases. *J Forensic Leg Med* 2015;33:61–67. doi:10.1016/j.jflm.2015.04.010.
36. Gauthey M, Capua M, Brent J, et al. Poisoning with malicious or criminal intent: characteristics and outcome of patients presenting for emergency care. *Clin Toxicol* 2019;57:628–631. doi:10.1080/15563650.2018.1546009.
37. Dine MS, McGovern ME. Intentional poisoning of children—an overlooked category of child abuse: report of seven cases and review of the literature. *Pediatrics* 1982;70:32–35.
38. Baraff LJ, Guterman JJ, Bayer MJ. The relationship of poison center contact and injury in children 2 to 6 years old. *Ann Emerg Med* 1992;21:153–157. doi:10.1016/S0196-0644(05)80150-7.
39. Hoffman RJ, Nelson L. Rational use of toxicology testing in children. *Curr Opin Pediatr* 2001;13(2):183–188.
40. Archer JRH, Wood DM, Dargan PI. How to use toxicology screening tests. *Arch Dis Child Educ Pract Ed* 2012;97:194–199. doi:10.1136/archdischild-2012-301792.
41. Wiley JF. Difficult diagnoses in toxicology: poisons not detected by the comprehensive drug screen. *Pediatr Clin North Am* 1991;38:725–737. doi:10.1016/S0031-3955(16)38127-5.
42. Dolcourt B, Paxton J, Bora K, et al. Pennies for your thoughts: a case series of pancytopenia due to zinc-induced copper deficiency in the same patient. *Clin Pract Cases Emerg Med* 2019;3(4):341–344. doi:10.5811/cpcem.2019.7.43697.
43. Proudfoot AT, Krenzelok EP, Vale JA. Position paper on urine alkalinization. *J Toxicol Clin Toxicol* 2004;42(1):1–26.
44. Proudfoot AT, Krenzelok EP, Vale JA, et al. AACT/EAPCCT position paper on urine alkalinization. *J Toxicol Clin Toxicol* 2002.
45. Ghannoum M, Nolin TD, Lavergne V, et al. Blood purification in toxicology: nephrology's ugly duckling. *Adv Chronic Kidney Dis* 2011;18(3):160–166.
46. Gosselin S, Juurlink DN, Kielstein JT, et al. Extracorporeal treatment for acetaminophen poisoning: recommendations from the EXTRIP workgroup. *Clin Toxicol* 2014;52(8):856–867. doi:10.3109/15563650.2014.946994.
47. Juurlink DN, Gosselin S, Kielstein JT, et al. Extracorporeal treatment for salicylate poisoning: systematic review and recommendations from the EXTRIP workgroup. *Ann Emerg Med* 2015;66(2):165–181.
48. Mactier R, Laliberté M, Mardini J, et al. Extracorporeal treatment for barbiturate poisoning: recommendations from the EXTRIP workgroup. *Am J Kidney Dis* 2014;64(3):347–358. doi:10.1053/j.ajkd.2014.04.031.
49. Lavergne V, Nolin TD, Hoffman RS, et al. The EXTRIP (EXtracorporeal TReatments In Poisoning) workgroup: guideline methodology. *Clin Toxicol* 2012;50(5):403–413.
50. Decker BS, Goldfarb DS, Dargan PI, et al. Extracorporeal treatment for lithium poisoning: systematic review and recommendations from the EXTRIP workgroup. *Clin J Am Soc Nephrol* 2015;10(5):875–887. doi:10.2215/CJN.10021014.
51. Ghannoum M, Yates C, Galvao TF, et al. Extracorporeal treatment for carbamazepine poisoning: systematic review and recommendations from the EXTRIP workgroup. *Clin Toxicol* 2014;52(10):993–1004.
52. Ghannoum M, Wiegand TJ, Liu KD, et al. Extracorporeal treatment for theophylline poisoning: systematic review and recommendations from the EXTRIP workgroup. *Clin Toxicol* 2015;53(4):215–229.
53. Ghannoum M, Laliberté M, Nolin TD, et al. Extracorporeal treatment for valproic acid poisoning: systematic review and recommendations from the EXTRIP workgroup. *Clin Toxicol* 2015;53(5):454–465. doi:10.3109/15563650.2015.1035441.
54. Ghannoum M, Nolin TD, Goldfarb DS, et al. Extracorporeal treatment for thallium poisoning: recommendations from the EXTRIP workgroup. *Clin J Am Soc Nephrol* 2012;7(10):1682–1690. doi:10.2215/CJN.01940212.
55. Calello DP, Liu KD, Wiegand TJ, et al. Extracorporeal treatment for metformin poisoning: systematic review and recommendations from the extracorporeal treatments in poisoning workgroup. *Crit Care Med* 2015;43:1716–1730. doi:10.1097/CCM.0000000000001002.
56. Iliuta I-A, Lachance P, Ghannoum M, et al. Prediction and validation of the duration of hemodialysis sessions for the treatment of acute ethylene glycol poisoning. *Kidney Int* 2017;92:453–460. doi:10.1016/j.kint.2017.02.018.
57. Position statement and practice guidelines on the use of multi-dose activated charcoal in the treatment of acute poisoning. *J Toxicol Clin Toxicol* 1999;37:731–751. doi:10.1081/CLT-100102451.
58. Woolf AD, Wenger T, Smith TW, et al. The use of digoxin-specific fab fragments for severe digitalis intoxication in children. *N Engl J Med* 1992;326:1739–1744. doi:10.1056/NEJM199206253262604.
59. Lavonas EJ, Ruha A-M, Banner W, et al. Unified treatment algorithm for the management of crotaline snakebite in the United States: results of an evidence-informed consensus workshop. *BMC Emerg Med* 2011;11:2. doi:10.1186/1471-227X-11-2.
60. Presley JD, Chyka PA. Intravenous lipid emulsion to reverse acute drug toxicity in pediatric patients. *Ann Pharmacother* 2013;47:735–743. doi:10.1345/aph.1R666.
61. Arroyo AM, Kao LW. Calcium channel blocker toxicity. *Pediatr Emerg Care* 2009;25:532–538. doi:10.1097/PEC.0b013e3181b0a504.
62. Glatstein M, Scolnik D, Bentur Y. Octreotide for the treatment of sulfonylurea poisoning. *Clin Toxicol* 2012;50:795–804. doi:10.3109/15563650.2012.734626.
63. Dart RC, Borron SW, Caravati EM, et al. Expert consensus guidelines for stocking of antidotes in hospitals that provide emergency care. *Ann Emerg Med* 2009;54:386.e1–394.e1. doi:10.1016/j.annemergmed.2009.01.023.
64. de Lange DW, Sikma MA, Meulenbelt J. Extracorporeal membrane oxygenation in the treatment of poisoned patients. *Clin Toxicol* 2013;51:385–393. doi:10.3109/15563650.2013.800876.
65. Gupta V, Wander GS. ECMO in poisoning. *J Card Crit Care TSS* 2017;1:82–88. doi:10.1055/s-0038-1626679.
66. Wynn PM, Zou K, Young B, et al. Prevention of childhood poisoning in the home: overview of systematic reviews and a systematic review of primary studies. *Int J Inj Contr Saf Promot* 2016;23:3–28. doi:10.1080/17457300.2015.1032978.
67. Cox EP, Wogalter MS, Stokes SL, et al. Do product warnings increase safe behavior? A meta-analysis. *J Public Policy Mark* 1997;16:195–204. doi:10.1177/074391569701600201.

68. American Academy of Pediatrics. Cough and cold medicine—not for children. https://www.aap.org/en-us/about-the-aap/aap-press-room/aap-press-room-media-center/Pages/Cough-and-Cold-Medicine-Not-for-Children.aspx. Accessed January 30, 2020.
69. Litovitz T, Manoguerra A. Comparison of pediatric poisoning hazards: an analysis of 3.8 million exposure incidents. A report from the American Association of Poison Control Centers. *Pediatrics* 1992;89(6 Pt 1):999–1006.
70. Whitehill JM, Harrington C, Lang CJ, et al. Incidence of pediatric cannabis exposure among children and teenagers aged 0 to 19 years before and after medical marijuana legalization in Massachusetts. *JAMA Netw Open* 2019;2:e199456. doi:10.1001/jamanetworkopen.2019.9456.
71. CDC Tips to Prevent Poisonings. https://www.cdc.gov/homeandrecreationalsafety/poisoning/preventiontips.htm. Accessed January 30, 2020.
72. Research F and DAC for DE and Drug Safety Priorities 2018. https://www.fda.gov/media/124681/download.
73. NIDA opioids. https://www.drugabuse.gov/drugs-abuse/opioids. Accessed January 30, 2020.
74. Pediatrics AA of American Academy of Pediatrics resources to address the opioid epidemic. https://www.aap.org/en-us/advocacy-and-policy/aap-health-initiatives/Substance-Use-and-Prevention/Pages/opioid-epidemic-resources.aspx. Accessed January 30, 2020.

Michael Rieder
Abdelbaset Elzagallaai
Bruce Carleton

CHAPTER 63

Adverse Drug Reactions in Newborns and Children

DRUG THERAPY AND CHILDREN

Historically, childhood has been a dangerous time, with the average mortality rate for children under 5 years being 25%, that is, one in four children would die before their fifth birthday, usually from infectious diseases.[1] This changed dramatically in the early 20th century due to three seminal events, including public sanitation, vaccination, and the development of specific drug therapy.[2–4] While penicillin is commonly believed to be the first antibiotic, in fact the first widely used antimicrobial drug was sulfanilamide, whose efficacy against bacterial infection in patients was demonstrated by Dr. Gerhard Domagk in 1935.[3,5] The introduction of effective antimicrobial therapy had an immediate and profound impact on child health, with children who had previously required lengthy hospital stays being treated with antimicrobials at home. It was also the beginning of the Therapeutic Revolution that has resulted in an explosive availability of effective therapies beginning with small molecules and now moving into biologics, factor, and cell-based therapies associated with radical changes in the nature, location, and delivery of care.

The widespread introduction of specific drug therapy had both positive and negative effects, a true "double-edged sword."[6] While clinicians now had effective and potent therapy, it soon became clear that potent therapy could have potent adverse effects. This was perhaps most clearly illustrated by the Elixir of Sulfanilamide tragedy in 1937, when a liquid preparation of sulfanilamide was formulated by Massengill using diethylene glycol—a potent nephrotoxin—as a solvent.[7] No premarketing testing was done, and as a consequence, more than 100 children died of renal failure while thousands of other suffered renal injuries. The public outrage over this event resulted in the passage of the 1938 Food, Drug, and Cosmetic Act, which among other things required premarketing safety testing and submission of these findings to the Food and Drug Administration (FDA) prior to approving drugs for marketing.[7]

The drug approval process has evolved in response to other tragedies, many among children such as the chloramphenicol gray baby syndrome and the thalidomide disaster. These changes have not always favored children; an unintended consequence of the Kefauver-Harris amendments to the Food and Drug Act passed in 1962 in response to the thalidomide disaster—which in setting standards for efficacy and safety that were supposed to ensure that drug therapy in children would be guided by evidence in fact resulted in children being excluded from investigation into new therapeutic agents, an exclusion that was reflected in product monographs and product labeling.[8,9] This led over time to the vast majority of drugs used in children being used off-label, a situation summarized by Dr. Harry Shirkey as children being "The Therapeutic Orphan."[10,11]

While changes in legislation and advocacy have changed this situation somewhat over time, this points to the importance of adverse drug reactions (ADRs) not only to the individual patient but also to the health care system.[6] An important additional consideration is the increasing complexity of child health care. A common myth is that medications are infrequently prescribed, and when they are, these are primarily antibiotics. Our group explored this issue in a cohort of one million Canadian children for a year and found that, in fact on average, there were four prescriptions written per year per child and, while antibiotics were the commonest drugs prescribed, in fact there was a very wide range of drugs used, with more than 2,500 different drugs being prescribed.[12] The fact that drugs are commonly used in children and that they come from a wide variety of classes has been subsequently confirmed in other studies from other jurisdictions.[13–18]

Germane to the issue of ADRs, two facts emerge from the data. First, the drugs used commonly for adults and children are quite different. Second, in addition to different drugs, patterns of drug use are quite different. While drug use in adults is largely driven by age as a primary determinant—that is, the older you are, the more drugs you are likely to receive—such that as age increases, drug use becomes more nearly universal. In contrast, drug use in children is often bimodal, in the sense that most children receive prescription medication infrequently if at all, while children with complex or chronic disease—who can make up to 20% of the population—receive medication frequently and often receive numbers of different prescription medications.[12,15] These include children in acute care units such as the neonatal or pediatric intensive care unit (NICUs), children with cancer, and children with chronic problems, such as epilepsy or arthritis. This is highly germane to the issue of adverse drug events as many of these children have multiple risk factors for ADRs.

ADVERSE DRUG REACTIONS AND CHILDREN

While the fact that drugs can cause untoward effects was appreciated since well before the dawn of specific therapy in 1935, this issue was brought into sharp focus in 1998 by the work of Lazarou *et al.*, who demonstrated that ADRs were the fourth commonest cause of death in the United States.[19–22] This work and the work of others stimulated an increased appreciation for the potential impact of ADRs on health care and outcomes, notably as estimates are that up to 100,000 patients per year die in the United States due to adverse drug effects.[21,22] As well, the cost of treating and monitoring for ADRs runs into the billions of dollars, being a major burden to the health care system. Work on ADRs initially focused on adults, notably given the common myth that ADRs were less common in children than adults.[20] Over the past two decades, this has been challenged as it has become apparent that the risk for ADRs in children is similar to that of adults and, in some cases, may be higher.[23–32]

The reasons for this become apparent when we consider the known risk factors for ADRs (Table 63.1).[33] Many of these risk factors apply to children who are receiving the largest amount of drugs. One example is premature infants in the NICU unit, where the combination of being at the extremes of age, polypharmacy, and developmental immaturity of the liver and kidney places these very vulnerable infants at a high risk of developing an ADR; indeed, it has been suggested that if a premature infant stays in the NICU long enough, the chance of an ADR approaches 100%.[34,35] Children with complex chronic problems are at increased risk of an ADR for many of the same reasons. In this context, having had a general anesthetic is probably a marker for more serious or more complicated disease.[32,33]

In the case of infants and children—notably infants—there are additional factors that impact on the changing risk for ADRs across childhood. A very important consideration is developmental ontogeny, in that there are significant changes in drug disposition over childhood.[36–38] Developmentally determined changes in the classic tenets of drug disposition—absorption, distribution, metabolism, and excretion (ADME)—can profoundly alter drug and drug metabolite concentrations in children, notably for preterm infants. This, in turn, can substantially increase the risk for ADRs. As well, the enhanced metabolic capacity of toddlers compared with adults puts them at increased risk for activation-associated ADRs.[20]

As noted above, the burden of ADRs includes significant risk for mortality and substantial morbidity. An additional burden associated with ADRs in children is the potential for long-term effects, which can be manifested in adult life as decreased health-related quality of life and a shortened life span. This has been appreciated for some time in the case of premature neonates and is increasingly recognized as a major problem for other groups of children, such as children with cancer, for whom adverse effects of chemotherapy are the second commonest cause of death.[39–43]

A final consideration with respect to risk of ADRs in children relates to the changing face of therapy. While drug therapy for children has historically primarily involved classic small drug molecules, over the past decade, there has been an incremental and substantial increase in the use of biologic and other novel therapies, which have introduced new therapeutic approaches, but have also brought in new sets of adverse effects.[44] Some of these adverse events are both common and severe; chimeric antigen receptor therapy, a remarkably effective therapy for certain treatment-unresponsive cancers, is associated with a very high risk for cytokine storm, a very serious adverse effect.[45]

ADRs are a major health care problem for infants, children, and youth for a number of reasons. First, they are a source of mortality—in some cases, a major source. Second, they are a major contributor to morbidity. The cost and consequences of ADRs are also a major burden for patients and the health care system. Patients are frequently mislabeled as to ADR risk, which is known to be associated with the use of less effective therapeutic agents, prolonged hospital stay, and increased risk of therapeutic failure. Monitoring for potential ADRs costs the health

TABLE 63.1 Risk Factors for Adverse Drug Reactions

Risk Factor	*Comments*
History of adverse drug reactions	ADRs are more frequent in patients who previously suffered an ADR or drug allergy—regardless of the class of drug to which they had experienced an adverse event to.
Polypharmacy	Administering multiple medications correlates with a synergistic rather than additive risk for ADRs; when patients take eight or more medications, the chance of an ADR increases logarithmically.
Organ impairment	Liver, kidney, and heart diseases may increase risk for ADRs, presumably by reducing the rate of drug clearance; in infants, developmental immaturity of hepatic and renal function markedly reduces clearance of certain drugs.
Extremes of age	Neonates and the elderly are at higher risk of experiencing ADRs due to hepatic enzyme immaturity and abnormality, respectively, reduced renal drug elimination capacity as well as increased chance of polypharmacy.
Female sex	Women experience a higher percentage of ADRs than do men.
Certain genetic polymorphisms	Certain genetic polymorphisms may increase the risk of experiencing ADRs.
Large doses	The chance of developing certain types of ADRs, notably drug hypersensitivity, appears to be greater among drugs used in higher doses.
Requirement for general anesthetic	Administration of a general anesthetic may be a marker for organ impairment or polypharmacy.

Data from Gallagher RM, Bird KA, Mason JR, et al. Adverse drug reactions causing admission to a paediatric hospital: a pilot study. *J Clin Pharm Ther* 2011;36(2):194–199 and Rieder MJ. Adverse drug reactions across the age continuum: epidemiology, diagnostic challenges, prevention, and treatments. *J Clin Pharmacol* 2018;58(Suppl 10):S36–S47.

care system billions of dollars. Finally, premarketing clinical trials often do not include infants, children, or youth, and the ADRs described in the product monograph may not be reflective of the risk for infants and children. Thus, unexpected and often severe ADRs occur in infants and children postmarketing.

DEFINITION AND CLASSIFICATION OF ADVERSE DRUG REACTIONS

Important steps in addressing a clinical problem include definition, identification, and classification. While there are a number of different definitions for ADRs, commonly used definitions include the World Health Organization (WHO) definition and that of Edwards and Aronson (Table 63.2).[19,33] Essentially, an ADR is a harm produced by a drug. An important differentiation is between adverse drug event and ADRs.[33,46] The concept of adverse drug events is broad and includes issues such as drug error (a relatively frequent problem in child health care) and other system issues, while ADRs are more commonly reflective of adverse outcomes associated with administration of the desired drug, typically in the desired dose.

It is important to acknowledge a major nosological issue with respect to popular designation of adverse events associated with therapy, an issue shared by both patients and health care providers. There is a common and regrettable use of the word "allergy" to apply as a blanket descriptor for all adverse events that occur in temporal relationship to drug therapy. This is both inaccurate and misleading. Although allergy in popular usage is considered to be sensitivity to a drug or chemical, in fact, allergy is a very specific term, which a purist might define as an immunoglobulin E–mediated adverse event, but which is more commonly considered as an adverse reaction to a drug known to be mediated by the immune system. The latter definition is much more useful, as it both speaks to mechanism and helps to guide clinical decision-making as to diagnosis and therapy.

While there are also several systems for classification of ADRs, the most clinically useful system for classifying ADRs is that described by Rawlins and Thompson, who, in 1977, proposed that ADRs should be considered to be predictable or unpredictable (Table 63.3).[47] While other classification systems have been proposed, many of them retain the core precepts of Rawlins and Thompson's system.[48]

Rawlins and Thompson grouped ADRs into a number of classifications; of most relevance to children's care are predictable and unpredictable ADRs (Table 63.3). In the broadest sense, predictable ADRs are those that can be predicated based on a comprehensive knowledge of the pharmacology of the drug in question and are typically dose related. In the original classification system of Rawlins and Thompson, predictable ADRs were known as type A or augmented, as they represent an augmentation of the pharmacologic activity of the drug. Unpredictable ADRs are in contrast not predictable based on the known pharmacology of the drug and are typically not dose related and were originally known as type B or bizarre. Predictable or type A ADRs are much more common than type B and are often less severe.

Within the groupings of predictable and unpredictable ADRs, there are a number of subtypes (Table 63.3). The approach and management of ADRs in these subtypes is variable depending on the mechanism(s) of the ADR in question, severity of symptoms, severity of the disease under treatment, and availability of therapeutic options, highlighting the importance of accurate diagnosis and classification in ensuring optimal management.[20]

MECHANISMS OF ADVERSE DRUG REACTIONS AND DEVELOPMENTAL PHARMACOLOGY

The mechanisms producing ADRs are dependent on the type of ADR, as outlined above. In the case of side effects, the mechanism is often via off-target effects of the desired pharmacologic response, for example, in a different organ than the one at which therapy is directed. Drug–drug, drug–food, and drug–disease interactions are typically based on an exaggerated or diminished pharmacologic response based on changes in drug clearance.

In the case of unpredictable ADRs, mechanisms are often complex, unknown, or poorly understood. An example is intolerance that clearly occurs in susceptible populations, but the mechanism(s) of how these evolve and identification of those at highest risk remains unclear. Idiosyncratic ADRs mechanism(s) often remain poorly defined, although recent work has suggested that in some cases, risk can be quantified by genetic evaluation of patients, notably as to haplotype.[49–52] In the case

TABLE 63.2 Definitions of Adverse Drug Reactions

"A response to a drug that is noxious and unintended and occurs at doses normally used in man for the prophylaxis, diagnosis or therapy of disease, or for modification of physiological function"
World Health Organization, International drug monitoring: the role of national centres. *Rep Ser WHO* 1972, no 498.

"An appreciably harmful or unpleasant reaction, resulting from an intervention related to the use of a medicinal product, which predicts hazard from future administration and warrants prevention or specific treatment, or alteration of the dosage regimen, or withdrawal of the product."
Edwards IR, Aronson JK. Adverse drug reactions: definitions, diagnosis, and management. *Lancet* 2000;356:1255–1259.

"Any noxious, unintended, and undesired effect of a drug after doses used in humans for prophylaxis, diagnosis, or therapy including noxious and unintended effects resulting not only from the authorized use of a medicinal product at normal doses, but also from medication errors and uses outside the terms of the marketing authorization, including the misuse and abuse of the medicinal product."
A. Vi, Guideline on Good Pharmacovigilance Practices (GVP) Module VI–Management and Reporting of Adverse Reactions to Medicinal Products (Rev.1), 2014, Date for coming into effect of first version Date for coming into effect of Revision 1, 3.

Modified from Rieder MJ. Adverse drug reactions across the age continuum: epidemiology, diagnostic challenges, prevention, and treatments. *J Clin Pharmacol* 2018;58(Suppl 10):S36–S47.

TABLE 63.3 Classification of Adverse Drug Reactions

Type of Reaction	*Definition*
Predictable	These adverse effects are predicated by the drug's known pharmacology. They are dose related and often diminish over time.
Side effects	Undesired effects of a drug's pharmacologic action, often on off-target sites, for example, fine hand tremor associated with the initiation of inhaled β-agonist therapy, which often fades over time. Side effects can be troublesome but are rarely severe and often diminish over time.
Secondary effects	Indirect consequences of a drug's pharmacologic action, often predictable, but not inevitable, for example, pseudomembranous colitis following lincosamide therapy, which occurs in a minority of patients treated with lincosamides as the development of colitis requires overgrowth of *Clostridium difficile,* production of toxin by the bacteria, damage to the mucosa of the gastrointestinal tract by the toxin and the host response to the toxin and mucosal damage.
Interactions	Undesired effects of a drug caused by an interaction with another drug, disease, or food, for example, renal toxicity of cyclosporine during concomitant therapy with clarithromycin due to inhibition of cyclosporine metabolism or lightheadedness and flushing when nifedipine is taken with grapefruit juice, as grapefruit juice inhibits the intestinal metabolism of nifedipine, resulting in higher serum nifedipine concentrations and more potent pharmacologic effects.
Toxicity	Undesired effects of a drug produced when the drug is present in excessive concentrations, often by mechanisms different from those producing the desired pharmacologic effect, for example, renal toxicity produced by aminoglycoside overdose as manifested by acute tubular necrosis produced by altered phospholipid metabolism as well as effects on renal blood flow, while the antimicrobial effects of aminoglycoside are due to binding to bacterial ribosomes.
Unpredictable	These adverse effects are not predicated or predictable by the drug's known pharmacology. Their mechanism is often complex or poorly understand, they are not dose related, and their effect also often do not diminish over time.
Intolerance	Undesired consequences of therapy that occur in susceptible patients, often at low or therapeutic drug concentrations, often characterized as severe side effects despite usual doses and usual therapeutic concentrations, for example, tinnitus in a small number of patients on conventional doses of aspirin.
Allergic/ Pseudoallergic	Undesired consequences of a drug mediated by the immune system or having characteristics suggestive of an immune-mediated pathogenesis, for example, anaphylaxis associated with penicillin allergy, which is mediated by IgE, or reactions to iodinated-contrast media, which appear to be immune mediated but have not had a clear mechanism defined as yet.
Idiosyncratic	Undesired consequences of therapy that are uncommon and not associated with the known pharmacology of the drug in question, whose mechanisms appear to often complex and involve multiple stages, such as initial bioactivation followed by a misdirected immune response, for example, Stevens-Johnson syndrome associated with sulfonamide therapy.
Psychogenic	Poorly defined adverse events in which patients develop disabling symptoms to a number of drug, often associated with symptoms, but possibly not signs, for example, multidrug sensitivity in adults.

Modified from Rieder MJ. Novel approaches to adverse drug reactions in children. *Pediatr Clin North Am* 2012;59:1001–1004 and Rawlins MD, Thompson JW. Pathogenesis of adverse drug reactions. In: Davies DM, ed. *Textbook of adverse drug reactions.* Oxford, UK: Oxford University Press, 1977:10.
IgE, immunoglobulin E.

of allergic/pseudoallergic ADRs, while mechanism(s) are often poorly understood, there are some examples (such as immediate hypersensitivity to penicillin) when the mechanisms are understood in a good degree of detail.[53–55]

There is one unique aspect to ADRs in infants and children—notably infants—that merits further consideration, that being developmental pharmacology. Simply put, the disposition of medications in children is subject to ontogeny, in that developmental changes in key pharmacologic parameters impact substantially on the fate of drugs in infants and children.[36–38,56] The admonition that "children are not small adults" is true across childhood, but nowhere is this more important than in the first year of life, especially among infants born prematurely. In terms of the classic pharmacologic rubric for orally administered drugs of ADME, variations exist across all four domains, each having potential impacts on risk for ADRs.

ABSORPTION

In common with adults, the vast majority of drugs used in the therapy of children are administered orally. There are well-described developmental differences in oral and gastrointestinal physiology between infants and older children and adults.[57–59] These changes include the near-neutral pH of the newborn's stomach compared with the acidic stomach pH seen in adults and older children, delayed gastric emptying seen for the first 6 months of life, variable intestinal transit time, immature intestinal function, and altered capacity for both intestinal wall metabolism and transport. Many of these changes, notably with respect to metabolism and transporter function, remain poorly understood. The overall impact of these changes on the fate of and risk for ADRs is, for most drugs, minor. However, for some drugs, such as phenytoin, the marked differences between absorption in infants and older children place infants at an increased risk for both therapeutic failure and ADRs.[60] In addition to changes in oral administration, drug absorption via the intramuscular and pulmonary routes can vary greatly in infants versus older children, related to diminished muscular mass and muscular blood flow and to differences in pulmonary function between infants and adults.[61,62] As well, the skin of newborns demonstrates transient, but significant, increase in percutaneous drug absorption compared with the skin of older infants, who, in turn, have enhanced percutaneous drug absorption compared with adults.[56,63] This can be associated with toxicity for drugs that are not normally toxic by the cutaneous route in adults, especially if administered in large amounts.[64]

DISTRIBUTION

Drug distribution is heavily dependent on body composition, and there are substantial differences in body composition between infants and adults, with infants having 80% body water compared with 55% in adults and extracellular water of 45% in infants compared with 20% in adults.[65] Thus, drugs that are distributed through body water have a larger volume of distribution in infants than in older children and adults. Another major determinant of drug disposition is plasma protein binding. Plasma protein binding in infants is less extensive than in adults, which appears to be due to a mixture of relatively reduced binding capacity as well as relatively reduced binding affinity.[59,65] Finally, the blood–brain barrier of the infant is less well developed than that of adults and is more porous.[59] Thus, drugs that are highly protein bound may have a somewhat larger volume of distribution in infants than in adults, while drugs that normally do not cross the blood–brain barrier may be able to do so in infants. That being said, the impact of these changes on risk for ADRs is, overall, quite small.

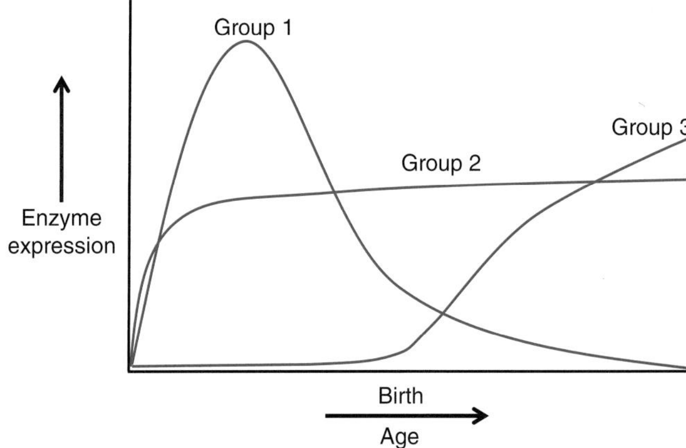

Figure 63.1 A schematic representation of the three major patterns of enzyme ontogeny, with group 1 being enzymes that are primarily expressed during the first and second trimesters, group 2 being those enzymes that are expressed relatively constantly during gestation, and group 3 being those enzymes whose expression increases dramatically after birth. Examples of group 1 enzymes include CYP3A7, FMO1, SULT1A3/4, and SULT1E1. Examples of group 2 enzymes include CYP2C19, CYP3A5, and SULT1A1. Examples of group 3 enzymes include CYP1A2, CYP2C9, CYP2D6, CYP2E1, CYP3A4, FMO3, ADH1B, ADH1C, and SULT2A1. (Hines RN. The ontogeny of drug metabolism enzymes and implications for adverse drug events. *Pharmacol Ther* 2008;118:250–267.)

METABOLISM

It is well recognized that infants, notably preterm infants, have substantial differences in metabolic capacity and metabolic pathways when compared with older children and adults.[36,56,65] This difference in metabolism has translated into therapeutic disaster on numerous occasions. One of the first, and among the most notable, was the chloramphenicol gray baby syndrome.[66–69] In the late 1950s, a syndrome characterized by cardiovascular instability with rapid progression to death was noted among infants being treated with chloramphenicol for potential sepsis.[67] It has subsequently been appreciated that this was due to developmental limitations of chloramphenicol glucuronidation, with the consequence of immature glucuronidation being accumulation of chloramphenicol producing dose-dependent mitochondrial toxicity manifested by impaired mitochondrial metabolism evidenced clinically as cardiac failure.[68] This tragedy illustrated how developmental immaturity in drug metabolism capacity places neonates—especially premature neonates—at special risk.[69]

It is also now appreciated that developmental expression of metabolic capacity is not uniform. Hines has described an overview that, although by his own admission somewhat simplistic, is also very useful in considering the potential impact of enzyme ontogeny on risk for ADRs (Fig. 63.1).[69] In this context, the three groups proposed are likely representative of enzymes that have substantially different biologic roles. As an illustration, it is most likely that the enzymes represented in group 1, whose peak expression occurs during the first and second trimesters of intrauterine life, have important roles in tissue differentiation and fetal development. The enzymes represented by group 2 are those that appear to have relatively consistent expression, whereas the enzymes in group 3—the largest group of enzymes—are those that have little or no function during intrauterine and early infant life and whose expression increases over the first several years of life (Fig. 63.1). Of key relevance to the risk for ADRs, the third group includes CYP2C9, CYP2D6, and CYP3A34, the major isozymes of cytochrome P450 most commonly associated with phase 1 metabolism and human drug oxidation. One key example is the CYP3A7 to CYP3A4 switch, in which the primary isoform of CYP3A in the human fetus is CYP3A7 while the primary isoform of CYP3A in children and adults is CYP3A4.[70–72] Thus, infants may be at special risk when treated with drugs whose elimination is primarily dependent on these metabolic pathways. It should also be emphasized that there is considerable variation between and within enzymatic pathways as to the rate of maturation.[36,69–72] Although the field of enzyme ontogeny still has many unknowns, there is now good-quality data for modeling to be done to predict possible dose ranges and concentrations in infants when well-characterized drugs are used, and this modeling is becoming of increasing significance in safety pharmacology as part of the drug development process.[73] These considerations apply to drugs given directly to the infant but also can apply to drugs delivered to the infant by breastfeeding.[74]

The issue of developmental alterations in drug metabolism is more complex than the issue concentration-dependent or predictable ADRs due to impaired drug clearance. There are a number of enzymes whose activity, on a per kilogram or per metered square dose, is much more in toddlers than in adults.[36,65,69,75] This has the potential to alter the risk for unpredictable ADRs, notably idiosyncratic ADRs, such as drug hypersensitivity for which there is a reasonable body of evidence that drug bioactivation is a critical first step in initiating an immune response that ultimately determines the clinical characteristics of drug hypersensitivity.[76] Thus, the enhanced metabolic capacity of toddlers—more specifically with respect to drug oxidation—may lead to metabolic bioactivation of drugs to a greater extent than among adults, placing the toddler at unique risk for activation-induced ADRs. There is a small but compelling body of evidence supporting this; as an illustration, the risk of having a severe cutaneous reaction to lamotrigine is three times higher in children than in adults.[77,78] Similarly, there is a 10-fold increase in risk for valproic acid–induced hepatotoxicity among toddlers compared with adults, while there also appears to be a 10-fold increase in the risk for cefaclor-induced serum sickness–like reactions in children compared with adults.[79] Although the overall rate is still fairly low (1:500 for valproic acid–induced hepatotoxicity and 1:100 for cefaclor-induced serum sickness–like reactions), these represent serious and potentially life-threatening ADRs; as well, they are significantly more common than among adults (in the case of cefaclor, 1:100 in toddlers vs. 1:5,000 for adults). Among children with cancer, serious ADRs are also often more common than among adults, again for reasons which currently are often not well understood.[80,81] It will be important to better understand the pathophysiology of these adverse events to pursue the goal of safer drug therapy for children.

EXCRETION

As for drug metabolism, renal drug elimination is also subject to developmental expression in a manner that parallels the development of renal function.[82,83] During intrauterine life, nephrons begin to form at week 5 and by week 8 become functional.[82,83] Glomerular filtration can be appreciated early in intrauterine life and slowly increases during gestation, peaking at between 32 and 35 weeks of gestational age, while nephrogenesis ends at about 36 weeks of intrauterine life.[83] At birth, glomerular filtration rate (GFR) is approximately 4 mL per minute per 1.73 m^2 body surface area; this doubles over the first several weeks of life and then rises to achieve adult values at about the end of the first year of life.[83] Significantly, over the toddler years, the GFR on a relative basis is higher than in adults, resulting in enhanced clearance for drugs eliminated via the renal route compared with adults.[83] Thus, the developmental pharmacology of renal drug elimination is characterized by a duality, with infants—especially preterm infants—having markedly less ability to eliminate drugs via the kidney, while toddlers have an enhanced ability to do so.[82] This enhanced ability to eliminate drugs in toddlers may also be associated with an enhanced metabolic ability of the kidney to activate drugs.[84,85]

The impact of this on drug elimination in the preterm infant has been appreciated for some time, with the reduced ability to eliminate drugs and drug metabolites by the kidney, placing newborn infants at increased risk for concentration-dependent toxicity. As an illustration, there is a substantial and robust literature on the need for altered aminoglycoside dosing—notably with respect to dosing interval—when treating newborns of different gestational ages with aminoglycoside antibiotics.[86,87] Clinicians caring for newborns are typically aware of these issues and use drugs that are eliminated principally by the kidney with caution, including using, when possible, therapeutic drug monitoring to individualize therapy and reduce the risk of concentration-dependent toxicity.[86,87]

It has been less well appreciated that the enhanced activity of the kidney in the toddler years may, as noted above, also be associated with an increased risk for other types of ADRs. One aspect of kidney function that has been somewhat underappreciated with respect to drug is renal drug metabolism.[85] Although the metabolic capacity of the liver clearly overshadows that of the kidney, the kidney has substantial inherent capacity for the metabolism of many crucial molecules, one example being vitamin D metabolism, such as calcitriol (1,25-dihydroxycholecalciferol), is formed in the kidney by the metabolism of 25-dihydroxycholecalciferol. It has been appreciated for some time that toddlers are at increased risk for nephrotoxicity from drugs such as ifosfamide, an alkylating agent widely used in the therapy of solid tumors.[85] Work in our laboratory and elsewhere has suggested that this may be due to chloroacetaldehyde, which is formed in equimolar amounts to the active metabolite, ifosfamide mustard, when the parent drug ifosfamide undergoes ring hydroxylation and chloroethyl side oxidation.[88] In toddlers, unbalanced production of chloroacetaldehyde by side-chain oxidation as opposed to ring hydroxylation producing ifosfamide mustard may then lead to renal cellular injury and functional renal damage.[85,88] The relevance of this hypothesis is that this offers the possibility of intervention, and pilot work has suggested that concurrent therapy with ifosfamide and the thiol donor *N*-acetylcysteine prevents the development of ifosfamide-induced nephrotoxicity in a rat model.[89]

Thus, alterations in renal function in children can occur in both directions, interestingly both being associated with enhanced risk for ADRs. Strategies to reduce risk for ADRs in these cases diverge sharply, in the former case being dose monitoring and dose reduction, while in the latter case, it is possible that concurrent therapy and other risk reduction models may provide an effective and alternative approach to reducing the risk of ADRs.

DRUG TRANSPORTERS

It has now been clearly demonstrated that the influx and efflux of many drugs into and out of tissues and cells are dependent on the presence of active transport systems, conventionally referred to as drug transporters.[90,91] These systems are often key determinants of the drug concentration at level of the target tissue and, as such, are of considerable importance in determining variability in drug response. Although a number of drug transporters have been found and characterized, there has been very little work on the ontogeny of drug transporters.[92–94] What little work has been done suggests that there may be substantial differences in transporter expression and activity in children compared with adults; a recent animal model has demonstrated that there was very little expression of organic anion transporter 1 (OAT1), a key renal drug transporters, in fetal kidney.[95] There was a sharp increase in expression of OAT1 after birth.[95] The regulation of these changes, potential impact on drug response, and potential effect(s) on drug safety have yet to be elucidated. Given the large number and complexity of drug transporters, there is considerable research that needs to be done before we can have the same degree of confidence in appreciating impacts on drug safety as we have with the conventional pharmacokinetic concepts of ADME.[92,93]

PHARMACODYNAMICS AND DRUG RECEPTORS

Although pharmacokinetics is an important determinant of how much drug is available to the therapeutic target, the biologic response is often dictated by ligand–receptor interactions.[96] The interaction between a drug and a drug receptor is the fundamental determinant of many of the effects of commonly used and therapeutically vital drugs, such as bronchodilation produced by β agonists interacting with the β receptor or analgesia produced by morphine interacting with the μ receptor, both classic cell-surface G-protein–coupled receptors, to anti-inflammatory effects produced by prednisone interacting with the glucocorticoid receptor in the cytosol. As in the case of drug transporters, there has been very little work done to explore the ontogeny of drug receptors, and consequently, the impact of altered receptor density or affinity on drug response in children is not well understood.[97] This is an obvious area where clarity could provide considerable insights into variability in drug response in children. Again, much research needs to be done before we can approach our understanding of potential developmental changes in drug receptor expression or activity on the desired and adverse effects of drug therapy in children. Given advances in molecular and cellular biology, genetics, and advanced imaging, it is likely that over the next decade, there will be a number of new insights into drug receptor ontogeny, efficacy, and affinity in infants and children that can better direct therapy, help us understand undesired drug effects, and guide therapeutic innovation.

IDENTIFICATION OF POTENTIAL ADVERSE DRUG REACTIONS AND PHARMACOVIGILANCE

An important challenge in developing an approach to ADRs in infants and children on the part of both the individual clinician and the health care system is recognition of drug-related adverse events. This is a special challenge for infants and children, in that historically premarketing clinical trials have not included infants and children and ADR data were extrapolated from adult data.[8,10,98] In the case of severe unpredictable ADRs such as drug hypersensitivity, their relatively uncommon occurrence means that the vast majority of unpredictable ADRs are not described until the drug in question has gone through the development process and has been approved for general use. As an example, the majority of drugs are evaluated in 5,000 to 20,000 patients under tightly controlled circumstances prior to marketing.[99-102] Many serious drug hypersensitivities occur at an incidence of 1:5,000 patients, an incidence that has potential impacts on public policy and drug regulation.[76] There is essentially no chance that a hypersensitivity reaction that occurs at this rate will be detected prior to drug approval and entry into the market, given the usual number of participants in phase 1 to 3 clinical trials. This has significant implications, in that serious hypersensitivity information would, therefore, become part of the product monograph either late or never.[76]

This is highly germane for drug safety issues in infants and children as ADRs that are identified and characterized during the drug development process are included in the product monograph and enter diagnostic consideration when evaluating untoward events occur during therapy. Historically, phase I to III trials conducted premarketing have usually only included adults. In the case of infants and children, many important and severe ADRs have only been described after the drug in question has been approved for routine clinical use and marketed, given that this was not studied premarketing.[103,104] While this is changing in certain jurisdictions due to the enactment of pediatric regulations, the increasing development of "niche" pharmaceuticals and targeted phase III studies would suggest that in some form, this problem will persist. Thus, the identification and characterization of unexpected or previously undescribed ADRs is a key component of drug safety strategies for children. Pharmacovigilance can be defined as the detection and assessment of adverse event associated with drug therapy, derive from the Greek *pharmakon* (drug) and the Latin *vigilare* (to keep watch).[105,106]

The granting of market approval for a drug is often followed by the requirement for the manufacturer to report unexpected adverse events to the appropriate drug regulatory agency, for example, the FDA Adverse Event Reporting System (FAERS) which is a computerized database operated by and evaluated by the FDA'S Center for Drug Evaluation and Research (CDER).[107] When received by the drug regulatory agency, the reports are analyzed and, if a concern is found, can result in a number of actions, ranging from issuing a warning (such as the FDA "black box" warnings) to withdrawing the drug from the market.[108,109]

There are a number of problems that make evaluation of potential ADRs problematic. The first is that most postmarketing surveillance systems are passive and rely on voluntary reporting.[110] This is known to result in very significant under-reporting of putative ADRs, such that, in some cases, signal for a suspected ADR—such as pemoline-associated hepatotoxicity—may have been noted for as long as two decades before regulatory action was taken.[111] This has been recognized as a problem, and new directions in drug safety for infants and children have included the creation of child-specific networks for focused active surveillance and evaluation of adverse events associated with drug therapy.[110,112] An advantage of this approach is the ability not only to identify previously underappreciated ADRs in infants and children but also to investigate these ADRs on a mechanistic basis.[83,113] As well, the focused approach provides the opportunity to address those possible ADRs that are most common or which can produce most harm.[114] This approach also facilitates characterizing ADRs by phenotypic constancy, as a frequent problem in assessment of untoward events associated with drug therapy has been variability in identification and characterization of the phenotype of the adverse event in question.[114] Phenotypic inconstancy has made mechanistic study of ADRs difficult and, in some cases, impossible.[110]

The next set of problems is the evaluation of the event itself. Given that therapy does not occur in a vacuum, key considerations include the patient and disorder being treated. Are there unique characteristics of the patient that must be taken into account? What is the natural history of the disease in question? Are there other comorbid conditions that may impact on signs and symptoms or produce their own set of signs and symptoms? The nature, timing, and evolution of the event in question are critical facts that must be determined in as much detail as possible. This is a particular problem for infants and children, in that many putative ADRs are manifested clinically, while many of the disorders being treated have their own set of cutaneous manifestations. As an example, when a child develops a rash while being treated with amoxicillin for otitis media—an event that happens thousands of times a year—is the rash due to amoxicillin or is it due to the viral infection commonly preceding acute otitis media?

The nature of the ADR is also an area of some debate. This is notably the case when the ADR is identified in the laboratory. To illustrate, is a transient elevation in transaminases after the initiation of therapy an ADR or is this perhaps a predictable pharmacologic effect of the drug on hepatic metabolism with no clinical consequences? This remains an area of active discourse.

Then, there is the issue of causation. Causality analysis for adverse drug effects is difficult, complex, and, rarely, conclusive. A number of systems have been devised to assist in the determination of causation, but they are both rarely definitive and often not suitable for infants and children.[20] A commonly used system is the Naranjo Scale, developed by Dr. Claudio Naranjo and his team to evaluate adverse events associated with the use of psychotropic medication in adults.[115] While a useful guide to direct thinking as to the possible role of medications in untoward events, in many circumstances, the sensitivity and positive predictive value are low, and the applicability to children and to current clinical practice unclear.[20,116] Specific instruments have subsequently been developed for certain populations, such as neonates, while investigators at the University of Liverpool have developed an assessment tool for ADRs in infants and children based on work conducted at the Alder Hey Children's Hospital.[117,118] There has been promising work on the use of *in vitro* assays to assess risk for ADRs, but these assays require validation and clinical conformation and remain largely a research domain.[67] Despite the development of new instruments and assays designed for infants and children, definitive proof of causality remains elusive, and the mainstay of ADR evaluation remains the clinical assessment by astute health care providers.

ADVERSE DRUG EVENTS

While the focus of this discussion has been on ADRs infants and children, it should be remembered that infants and children are at increased risk for adverse drug effects, such as 10-fold overdose and drug error. Historically, problems such as 10-fold error have been attributed to child-unfriendly medications, lack of familiarity with pediatric dosing, and mathematical skills issues in certain personnel.[119] It was hoped that systems solutions such as the electronic medical record (EMR) would be useful in reducing these types of adverse drug events.

While there was considerable optimism as to the potential for EMRs to enhance drug safety, objective analysis would suggest that it remains uncertain if this is true, notably for infants and children.[120–123] While EMRs can and do certainly reduce certain types of errors, such as simple mathematical miscalculation, they introduce the possibility of other error types, notably when the EMR is primarily designed for adult patients. Issues such as alert fatigue and problems with drop-down menus remain problematic for many EMRs. As EMRs evolve and linkages between child-specific clinical decision tools and prescribing platforms evolve, it is hoped that the EMR will reach its potential in reducing adverse drug events on a system-wide basis.

THE CLINICAL APPROACH TO A SUSPECTED ADVERSE DRUG EVENT IN AN INFANT OR CHILD

An organized approach is helpful for any clinical problem, few more pressing than the assessment of an undesired event occurring during the course of drug therapy. In addition to the signs and symptoms that may be attributed to the drug in question, the natural history and response to therapy of the disease of interest are also highly germane to determining whether the event in question is drug related or is part of the evolution of the disease process driving therapy. In the case of children, a further complication is the fact that children at highest risk for ADRs are also those most likely to be treated with more than one drug, raising issues such as drug–drug interactions.

In the case of suspected ADRs, the approach is almost entirely clinical, with the laboratory typically providing supporting evidence, if anything at all. An organized clinical approach is thus all the more important (Table 63.4).

APPRECIATION

The first step in the evaluation of an untoward event occurring in the context of therapy is to appreciate that the event may be drug related. To paraphrase, one cannot diagnose what one cannot imagine. This is of special relevance when infants or children are being treated with new or novel therapies, especially when these therapies were created and evaluated primarily in adults. As noted above, many serious drug hypersensitivities occur in an incidence that will never be detected in conventional phase I to III trials, yet will be seen when the drug is marketed and used by tens of thousands if not millions of patients worldwide.

ASSESSMENT

As noted above, a careful and comprehensive clinical assessment is the key to the evaluation of suspected ADRs. Key elements of history include the details of the disorder being treated, including the stage and history of the disease, the drug in question, dose and route, and the timing of dosing. The history of the

TABLE 63.4 Clinical Approach to a Possible Adverse Drug Reaction

Appreciation	*Is it possible that the untoward event in question is drug related?*
Assessment	What is the presentation and evolution of the event in question? What are the characteristics of drug use, the disorder being treated, other therapies, and the patient being treated?
Analysis	Is the event in question related to drug therapy, the disorder being treated, or to considerations unique to this patient?
Assistance	Can therapy be continued, or does therapy need to be stopped? Does alternate therapy need to be put into place? Is there active therapy for the event in question? Will symptomatic therapy be helpful?
Aftermath	What is the impact of the event in question on future therapy with the drug of interest or similar agents? Do the patient and family fully appreciate this, and will this impact on adherence with future therapy? Have all the health care providers in the circle of care been so informed? In the case of a new therapeutic agent or a previously undescribed ADR, has the appropriate drug regulatory agency been notified?

Modified from Rieder MJ. Adverse drug reactions across the age continuum: epidemiology, diagnostic challenges, prevention, and treatments. *J Clin Pharmacol* 2018;58(Suppl 10):S36–S47.

event under study must include the timing, presentation, and evolution of the event. The details of concurrent therapy and other exposures are very important as is the history of the patient, including previous ADRs, comorbidities, and other conditions of relevance.

ANALYSIS

The next step—and a crucial one—is the decision as to whether the event in question is due to a drug or not. This decision is more problematic than one might expect as a key part of decision-making is up to date and reliable drug information. Most physicians prescribe from fairly limited lists of drugs, in the range of 120 to 160 drugs. As one can imagine, the list of drugs is practice specific, but even among generalists, the list is not all that long. Among these drugs, the physician is often quite familiar with both common and severe ADRs to these agents. However, worldwide, there are more than 2,500 licensed pharmaceutical products world wise and more than 11,000 novel drug molecules, a number that increases annually. Thus, it is very important to have an updated and reliable drug information source—such as an academic health sciences center Drug Information Center—to provide data on drugs that the health care team is unfamiliar with. The role of an expert drug information pharmacist in this process cannot be understated.

Confirmation of the ADR is rarely possible, and as noted above, determination of causation is at best problematic. There are some specific diagnostic assays available for certain drugs—such as skin testing for penicillin allergy or rechallenge for less severe reactions—and while diagnostic tests for other drugs are under development, the cornerstone of ADR diagnosis remains clinical.

ASSISTANCE

If the event in question is indeed drug related, then there are a series of decisions to be made. The first—and often one that clinicians end at—is whether therapy should be stopped. While this seems obvious, it, in many cases, is not. If, as an example, the disorder being treated has not been adequately controlled, then consideration needs to be made as to whether the ADR is sufficiently severe and will of sufficient duration to justify stopping therapy. If the disorder being treated has been controlled—for example, otitis media that has resolved—cessation of therapy is entirely appropriate. In the case of side effects, an option is treating through, especially when therapy is vitally important—for example, antiretroviral therapy for HIV infection—and when side effects are self-limited and diminish over time. If this is the plan moving forward, it is critical that the patient and family are fully aware of and agree with this decision. Finally, if the disorder in question is not adequately controlled and the ADR is sufficiently severe or likely to be prolonged, then cessation of therapy and selection of an alternate treatment are necessary. Again, this needs to be clearly communicated to the patient and family.

In terms of therapy for the ADR itself, in most cases, therapy is supportive and symptomatic. An example is the use of antihistamines for urticaria due to penicillin therapy. It is important for the patient and family to appreciate how long symptoms may persist and when to seek follow-up. In the case of severe ADRs, active and aggressive management may be needed, for example, drug-induced anaphylaxis.[54,124] For very serious idiosyncratic ADRs such as Stevens-Johnson syndrome and toxic epidermal necrolysis, excellent supportive care is key to reduce mortality.[125] As well, emerging evidence suggests that immunomodulation with corticosteroids, intravenous immunoglobulin, or immunosuppressant drugs such as cyclosporine may reduce the duration and severity of the ADR.[76,125,126]

AFTERMATH

The fact of having sustained an ADR has a number of consequences, some that are often not fully appreciated. In terms of the impact on the patient, fortunately, many ADRs do not have long-term consequences on the physical health of the patient. However, some serious ADRs have long-term and very impactful effects on health, for example, anthracycline-associated cardiotoxicity manifesting as heart failure in later life.[42] In addition to these impacts, ADRs can produce psychological effects that impact on health-related quality of life.[127]

Some of these impacts include the effect on the patient–physician relationship. It would be naïve not to anticipate that having prescribed a medication that produced an adverse effect might not alter the patient–physician relationship, notably with respect to compliance with future therapy. In order to minimize this impact, very clear dialogue and communication about the nature of the ADR is important, including treating it as a distinct clinical entity and fully exploring how this would impact on future therapy.

The impact of an ADR on future therapy is a very important consideration. In addition to the patient and family, other health care providers in the circle of care need to be informed of the fact of an ADR and which drugs should be avoided in the future. This is especially germane in child health care, as those children at highest risk for ADRs are those with the most complex disease who are likely to be cared for by multiple health care providers.

It is now increasingly clear that labeling a patient with an ADR—notably an allergy—has long-term consequences on their health care that are more substantial than had been appreciated. This has been best described in the context of penicillin allergy, in which being identified as penicillin allergic is associated with the use of less effective and sometimes more expensive alternate therapies which is associated with increased hospital stay, greater health care cost, and increased risk of bad outcomes, including increased mortality.[128–132] Thus, care should be taken to be accurate in the diagnosis of ADRs and to be specific as to which drugs can and cannot be used in the future. When possible confirmation with tests such as penicillin, skin testing or rechallenge should be undertaken by health care providers expert in this area.

Finally, it is very important—especially for ADRs to new therapeutic agents or for unique or novel ADR patterns—that this be reported, both to the appropriate regulatory authority and in the peer-reviewed literature. Given the drug approval process and how this is applied for drugs used in infants and children, this is especially germane. Essentially, all serious drug hypersensitivities in infants and children have been described in the peer-reviewed literature by astute clinicians following drug approval.

LOOKING TO THE FUTURE

Shakespeare famously described the future as "the Undiscovered Country," and while this is certainly applicable for ADRs, the evolving Therapeutic Revolution in innovative therapies and advances in technology provide some insights into at least the direction the future is likely to take. Drug approval patterns have changed dramatically over the past decade, and as many as half of new molecular entities are biologic, with an increasing number of cellular therapies. Thus, it is likely that there will be new and potentially severe ADRs emerging as these agents enter into the therapeutic arena.

In addition to new therapeutic agents, it is likely that there will be new diagnostic approaches to ADRs. Many of these assays are likely to be based on genetics, and currently, a number of drug regulatory agencies recommend haplotype assessment before starting therapy with specific drugs, for example, determination whether a patient of Han Chinese ancestry has the HLA allele HLA-B*1502 prior to staring therapy with carbamazepine.[50–53,133] This has been shown to reduce the risk of serious skin reactions, such as Stevens-Johnson syndrome, among patients who have this allele. Although the decrease in risk is dramatic and the sensitivity and specificity are in the range of 90% and 80%, respectively, equally dramatic is the fact that the vast majority of patients with this allele can tolerate therapy with carbamazepine, as the positive predictive value is in the range of 1% to 3%.[50–52] Given this, it is likely that the future of biomarkers for ADRs will rely on panels of multiple biomarkers, including the use of different omics technologies, to provide robust and reliable risk assessment for ADRs and to assist in diagnosis.[133] It will be very important that well-designed studies be conducted to evaluate this approach in the evaluation of untoward events occurring during therapy in infants and children.

REFERENCES

1. Bideau A, Desjardins B, Pérez Brignoli H, eds. *Infant and child mortality in the past*. Oxford, UK: Claredon Press, 1997.
2. Bonnani P. Demographic impact of vaccinations: a review. *Vaccine* 1999;17(Suppl 3):S120–S125.
3. Weinshilboum RM. The therapeutic revolution. *Clin Pharmaocl Ther* 1987;42:481–484.
4. Thomas L. *The youngest science: notes of a medicine watcher*. New York, NY: Viking Press, 1983.
5. Domagk GJ. Ein Beitrag zur Chemotherapie der bakteriellen infektionen. *Dtsch med Wochenschr* 1935;61:250–253.
6. Elzagallaai AA, Greff M, Rieder MJ. Adverse drug reactions in children: the double-edged sword of therapeutics. *Clin Pharmcol Ther* 2017;101:725–735.
7. Wax PM. Elixirs, diluents, and the passage of the 1938 Federal Food, Drug and Cosmetic Act. *Ann Intern Med* 1995;122:456–461.
8. Rieder M. If children ruled the pharmaceutical industry: the need for pediatric formulations. *Drug News Perspect* 2010;23:1–8.
9. Kauffman RE. Status of drug approval processes and regulation of medicines for children. *Curr Opin Pediatr* 1995;7:195–198.
10. Shirkey HC. Editorial comment: therapeutic orphans. *J Pediatr* 1968;72:119–120.
11. Gore R, Chugh PK, Tripathi CD, et al. Pediatric off-label and unlicensed drug use and its implications. *Curr Clin Pharmacol* 2017;12:18–25.
12. Rieder MJ, Matsui D, MacLeod S: Myths and challenges—drug utilization by Canadian children. *Paed Child Health* 2003;8:7A–8A.
13. Lasky T. Estimates of pediatric medication use in the United States: current abilities and limitations. *Clin Ther* 2009;31:436–445.
14. Turner MA, Lewis S, Hawcutt DB, et al. Prioritising neonatal medicines research: UK Medicines for Children Research Network scoping survey. *BMC Pediatr* 2009;9:50.
15. Vernacchio L, Kelly JP, Kaufman DW, et al. Medication use among children <12 years of age in the United States: results from the Slone Survey. *Pediatrics* 2009;124:446–454.
16. Clavenna A, Bonati M. Drug prescriptions to outpatient children: a review of the literature. *Eur J Clin Pharmacol* 2009;65:749–755.
17. Chai G, Governale L, McMahon AW, et al. Trends of outpatient prescription drug use in US children, 2002-2010. *Pediatrics* 2012;130:23–31.
18. Rosli R, Dali AF, Abd Aziz N, et al. Drug utilization on neonatal Wards: a systematic review of observational Studies. *Front Pharmacol* 2017;8:27.
19. Edwards IR, Aronson JK. Adverse drug reactions: definitions, diagnosis and management. *Lancet* 2000;356:1255–1259.
20. Rieder MJ. Novel approaches to adverse drug reactions in children. *Pediatr Clin North Am* 2012;59:1001–1004.
21. Lazarou, J, Pomeranz BH, Corey PN. Incidence of adverse drug reactions in hospitalized patients: a meta-analysis of prospective studies. *JAMA* 1998;279:1200–1205.
22. Shepherd G, Yacoub K, May DW. Adverse drug reaction deaths reported in United States vital statistics, 1999–2006. *Ann Pharmacother* 2012;46:169–175.
23. Impicciatore P, Choonara I, Clarkson A, et al. Incidence of adverse drug reactions in paediatric in/out-patients: a systematic review and meta-analysis of prospective studies. *Br J Clin Pharmacol* 2001;52:77–83.
24. Mitchell AA, Lacouture PG, Sheehan JE, et al. Adverse drug reactions in children leading to hospital admission. *Pediatrics* 1988;82:24–29.
25. Thiesen S, Conroy EJ, Bellis JR, et al. Incidence, characteristics and risk factors of adverse drug reactions in hospitalized children—a prospective observational cohort study of 6,601 admissions. *BMC Med* 2013;11:237.
26. Posthumus AA, Alingh CC, Zwaan CC, et al. Adverse drug reaction-related admissions in paediatrics, a prospective single-centre study. *BMJ Open* 2012;2:1–6.
27. Martinez-Mir I, García-López M, Palop V, *et al.* A prospective study of adverse drug reactions in hospitalized children. *Br J Clin Pharmacol* 1999;47:681–688.
28. Jonville-Bera AP, Giraudeau B, Blanc P, et al. Frequency of adverse drug reactions in children: a prospective study. *Br J Clin Pharmacol* 2002;53:207–210.
29. Gholami K, Babaie F, Shalviri G, et al. Pediatric hospital admission due to adverse drug reactions: Report from a tertiary center. *J Res Pharm Pract* 2015;4:212–215.
30. Gallagher RM, Bird KA, Mason JR, et al. Adverse drug reactions causing admission to a paediatric hospital: a pilot study. *J Clin Pharm Ther* 2011;36(2):194–199.
31. Langerova P, Vrtal J, Urbanek K. Adverse drug reactions causing hospital admissions in childhood: a prospective, observational, single-centre study. *Basic Clin Pharmacol Toxicol* 2014;115:560–564.
32. Gallagher RM, Bird KA, Mason JR, et al. Adverse drug reactions causing admission to a paediatric hospital. *PLoS One* 2012;7:e50127.
33. Rieder MJ. Adverse drug reactions across the age continuum: epidemiology, diagnostic challenges, prevention, and treatments. *J Clin Pharmacol* 2018;58(Suppl 10):S36–S47.
34. Aranda JV, Portuguez-Malavasi A, Collinge J, et al. Epidemiology of adverse drug reactions in the newborn. *Dev Pharmacol Ther* 1982;5:173–184.
35. Allegaert K, van den Anker J. Adverse drug reactions in neonates and infants: a population-tailored approach is needed. *Br J Clin Pharmacol* 2015;80:788–795.
36. Kearns GL, Abdel-Rahman SM, Alander SW, et al. Developmental pharmacology—drug disposition, action, and therapy in infants and children. *N Engl J Med* 2003;349:1157–1167.
37. Blake MJ, Castro L, Leeder JS, et al. Ontogeny of drug metabolizing enzyme in the neonate. *Semin Fetal Neonatal Med* 2005;10:123–138.
38. Van den Anker J. Developmental pharmacology. *Dev Disabil Res Rev* 2010;16:233–238.
39. Rosoff PM. The two-edged sword of curing childhood cancer. *N Engl J Med* 2006;355:1522–1523.
40. Jones B, Spunt SL, Green D, et al. Renal late effects in patients treated for cancer in childhood: A report from the Children's Oncology Group. *Pediatr Blood Cancer* 2008;51:724–731.
41. Jiménez-Triana CA, Castelán-Martinez OD, Rivas-Ruiz R, et al. Cisplatin nephrotoxicity and longitudinal growth in children with solid tumors. *Medicine (Baltimore)* 2015;94:e1413.
42. Aminkeng F, Ross CJ, Rassek SR, et al. Recommendations for genetic testing to reduce the incidence of anthracycline-induced cardiotoxicity. *Br J Clin Pharmacol* 2016;82:683–695.
43. Sulciner ML, Serhan CN, Gilligan MM, et al. Resolvins suppress tumor growth and enhance cancer therapy. *J Exp Med* 2018;215:115–140.
44. Stacknik J, Gabay M. Biologics in pediatrics. In: Field MJ, Boat TF, eds. *Committee on Pediatric Studies Conducted Under the Best Pharmaceuticals for Children Act (BPCA) and the Pediatric Research Equity Act (PREA); Board on Health Sciences Policy; Institute of Medicine.* Washington, DC: National Academies Press (US), 2012.
45. June CH, Sadelain M. Chimeric antigen receptor therapy. *N Engl J Med* 2018;379:64–73.
46. Bates DW, Cullen DJ, Laird N, et al. Incidence of adverse drug events and potential adverse drug events. Implications for prevention. ADE Prevention Study Group. *JAMA* 1995;274:29–34.
47. Rawlins MD, Thompson JW. Pathogenesis of adverse drug reactions. In: Davies DM, ed. *Textbook of adverse drug reactions*. Oxford, UK: Oxford University Press, 1977:10.
48. Aronson JK, Ferner RE. Joining the DoTS: new approach to classifying adverse drug reactions. *BMJ* 2003;327:1222–1225.
49. Rieder MJ, Carleton B. Pharmacogenomics and adverse drug reactions in children. *Front Genet* 2014;5(78):1–11.
50. Karnes JH, Miller MA, White KD, et al. Applications of immunopharmacogenomics: predicting, preventing and understanding immune-mediated adverse drug reactions. *Ann Rev Pharmacol Toxicol* 2019;59:463–486.
51. Jung JW, Kim JY, Park IW, et al. Genetic markers of severe cutaneous adverse reactions. *Korean J Intern Med* 2018;33:867–875.
52. Usui T, Naisbitt DJ. Human leukocyte antigen and idiosyncratic adverse drug reactions. *Drug Metabol Pharmacokinet* 2017;32:21–30.
53. Pichichero ME, Zagursky R. Penicillin and cephalosporin allergy. *Ann Allergy Asthma Immunol* 2014;112:404–412.
54. Trubiano JA, Stone CA, Grayson LM, et al. The three Cs of antibiotic allergy—classification, cross-reactivity and collaboration. *J Allergy Clin Immunol Pract* 2017;5:1532–1542.
55. Pongdee T, Li JT. Evaluation and management of penicillin allergy. *Mayo Clin Proc* 2018;93:101–107.

56. Lu H, Rosenbaum S. Developmental pharmacokinetics in pediatric populations. *J Pediatr Pharmacol Ther* 2014;19:262–276.
57. Strolin Benedetti M, Baltes EL. Drug metabolism and disposition in children. *Fundam Clin Pharmacol* 2003;17:281–299.
58. Bartelink IH, Rademaker MA, Schobben AF, et al. Guidelines on paediatric dosing on the basis of developmental physiology and pharmacokinetic considerations. *Clin Pharmacokinet* 2006;45:1077–1097.
59. Lenfestey MW, Neu J. Gastrointestinal development: implications for management of preterm and term infants. *Gastroenterol Clin North Am* 2018;47:773–791.
60. Cheng A, Banwell B, Levin S, et al. Oral dosing requirements for phenytoin in the first three months of life. *J Popul Ther Clin Pharmacol* 2010;17:e256–e261.
61. American Academy of Pediatrics. Committee on Drugs. Alternate routes of drug administration: advantages and disadvantages. *Pediatrics* 1997;100:143–152.
62. Tetelbaum M, Finkelstein Y, Nava-Ocampo AA, et al. Back to basics: understanding drugs in children: pharmacokinetic maturation. *Pediatr Res* 2005;26:321–328.
63. Furue M, Terao H, Rikihisa W, et al. Clinical dose and adverse effects of topical steroids in daily management of atopic dermatitis. *Br J Dermatol* 2003;148:128–133.
64. Rincon E, Baker RL, Iglesias AJ, et al. CNS toxicity after topical application of EMLA cream on a toddler with molluscum contagiosum. *Pediatr Emerg Care* 2000;16:252–254.
65. Batchelor HF, Marriott JF. Paediatric pharmacokinetics: key considerations. *Br J Clin Pharmacol* 2013;79:395–404.
66. Choonara I, Rieder MJ. Drug toxicity and adverse drug reactions in children—a brief historical review. *Paediatr Perinat Drug Ther* 2002;5:12–18.
67. Sutherland JM. Fatal cardiovascular collapse in infants receiving large amounts of chloramphenicol. *AMA J Dis Child* 1959;97:761–767.
68. de Wildt SN, Kearns GL, Leeder JS, et al. Glucuronidation in children. *Clin Pharmacokinet* 1999;36:439–452.
69. Hines RN. The ontogeny of drug metabolism enzymes and implications for adverse drug events. *Pharmacol Ther* 2008;118:250–267.
70. Leeder JS. Developmental pharmacogenetics: a general paradigm for application to neonatal pharmacology and toxicology. *Clin Pharmacol Ther* 2009;195:1–5.
71. Blake MJ, Gaedigk A, Pearce RE, et al. Ontogeny of dextromethorphan *O*- and *N*-demethylation in the first year of life. *Clin Pharmacol Ther* 2007;81:510–516.
72. Kearns GL, Robinson PK, Wilson JT, et al.; Pediatric Pharmacology Research Unit Network. Cisapride disposition in neonates and infants: in vivo reflection of cytochrome P450 3A4 ontogeny. *Clin Pharmacol Ther* 2003;74:312–325.
73. Alcorn J, McNamara PJ. Using ontogeny information to build predictive models for drug elimination. *Drug Discov Today* 2008;13:507–512.
74. Madadi P, Koren G. Pharmacogenetic insights into codeine analgesia: implications to pediatric codeine use. *Pharmacogenomics* 2008;9:1267–1284.
75. Strolin Benedetti M, Whomsley R, Baltes EL. Differences in absorption, distribution, metabolism and excretion of xenobiotics between the paediatric and adult populations. *Expert Opin Drug Metab Toxicol* 2005;1:447–471.
76. Elzagallaai AA, Rieder MJ. In vitro testing for diagnosis of idiosyncratic adverse drug reactions: implications for pathophysiology. *Br J Clin Pharmacol* 2015;80:889–900.
77. Hirsch LJ, Weintraub DB, Buchsbaum R, et al. Predictors of lamotrigine-associated rash. *Epilepsia* 2006;47(2):318–322.
78. Levi N, Bastuji-Garin S, Mockenhaupt M, et al. Medications as risk factors of Stevens–Johnson syndrome and toxic epidermal necrolysis in children: a pooled analysis. *Pediatr* 2009;123:e297–e304.
79. Kearns GL, Wheeler JG, Rieder MJ, et al. Serum sickness-like reaction to cefaclor: lack of in vitro cross-reactivity with loracarbef. *Clin Pharmacol Ther* 1998;63:686–693.
80. Ross CJ, Katzov-Eckert H, Dubé MP, et al.; the CPNDS Consortium. Genetic variants in TPMT and COMT are associated with hearing loss in children receiving cisplatin chemotherapy. *Nat Genet* 2009;41:1345–1349.
81. Hausner E, Fiszman ML, Hanig J, et al. Long-term consequences of drugs on the paediatric cardiovascular system. *Drug Saf* 2008;31:1083–1096.
82. Chen N, Aleksa K, Woodland C, et al. Ontogeny of drug elimination by the human kidney. *Pediatr Nephrol* 2006;21:160–168.
83. Upadhyay KK, Silverstein DM. Renal development: a complex process dependent on inductive interaction. *Curr Pediatr Rev* 2014;10:107–114.
84. Solhaug MJ, Bolger JM, Jose PA. The developing kidney and environmental toxins. *Pediatr* 2004;113:1084–1091.
85. Hanly L, Chen N, Rieder M, et al. Ifosfamide nephrotoxicity in children: a mechanistic base for pharmacological prevention. *Exp Opin Drug Saf* 2009;8:155–168.
86. Nielsen EI, Sandström M, Honoré PH, et al. Developmental pharmacokinetics of gentamicin in preterm and term neonates: population modelling of a prospective study. *Clin Pharmacokinet* 2009;48:253–263.
87. Sherwin CM, Svahn S, Van der Linden A, et al. Individualised dosing of amikacin in neonates: a pharmacokinetic/pharmacodynamic analysis. *Eur J Clin Pharmacol* 2009;65:705–713.
88. Chen N, Aleksa K, Woodland C, et al. The effect of *N*-acetylcysteine on ifosfamide-induced nephrotoxicity: in vitro studies in renal tubular cells. *Transl Res* 2007;150:51–57.
89. Chen N, Aleksa K, Woodland C, et al. *N*-Acetylcysteine prevents ifosfamide-induced nephrotoxicity in rats. *Br J Pharmacol* 2008;153:1364–1372.
90. Degorter MK, Kim RB. Hepatic drug transporters, old and new: pharmacogenomics, drug response, and clinical relevance. *Hepatology* 2009;50:1014–1016.
91. Kim RB. Transporters and drug discovery: why, when, and how. *Mol Pharmacol* 2006;3:26–32.
92. Brouwer KL, Aleksunes LM, Brandys B, et al. Human ontogeny of drug transporters: review and recommendations of the Pediatric Transporter Working Group. *Clin Pharmacol Ther* 2015;98:166–187.
93. Elmorsi U, Barber J, Rostami-Hodjegan A. Ontogeny of hepatic drug transporters and relevance to drugs used in pediatrics. *Drug Metabol Dispos* 2016;44:992–998.
94. Johnson TN, Thomson M. Intestinal metabolism and transport of drugs in children: the effects of age and disease. *J Pediatr Gastroenterol Nutr* 2008;47:3–10.
95. Sekine T, Endou H. Children's toxicology from bench to bed—drug-induced renal injury (3): drug transporters and toxic nephropathy in childhood. *J Toxicol Sci* 2009;34(Suppl 2):SP259–SP265.
96. Maehle AH, Prull CR, Halliwell RF. The emergence of the drug receptor theory. *Nat Rev Drug Dis* 2002;1:637–641.
97. Sloboda DM, Moss TJ, Li S, et al. Expression of glucocorticoid receptor, mineralocorticoid receptor, and 11beta-hydroxysteroid dehydrogenase 1 and 2 in the fetal and postnatal ovine hippocampus: ontogeny and effects of prenatal glucocorticoid exposure. *J Endocrinol* 2008;197:213–220.
98. Zisowsky J, Krause A, Dingemanse J. Drug development for pediatric populations: regulatory aspects. *Pharmaceutics* 2010;2:364–388.
99. Mittmann N, Knowles SR, Gomez M, et al. Evaluation of the extent of under-reporting of serious adverse drug reactions: the case of toxic epidermal Necrolysis. *Drug Saf* 2004;27:477–487.
100. Rzany B, Mockenhaupt M, Baur S, et al. Epidemiology of erythema exsudativum multiforme major, Stevens-Johnson syndrome and toxic epidermal Necrolysis in Germany (1990-1992): structure and results of a population-based registry. *J Clin Epidemiol* 1996;49:769–773.
101. Stephenson T. How children's responses to drugs differ from adults. *Br J Clin Pharmacol* 2005;59:670–673.
102. Castro-Pastrana LI, Ghannadan R, Rieder MJ, et al. Cutaneous adverse drug reactions in children: an analysis of reports from the Canadian Pharmacogenomics Network for Drug Safety (CPNDS). *J Popul Ther Clin Pharmacol* 2011;18:e106–e120.
103. Onakpoya IJ, Heneghan CJ, Aronson JK. Delays in the post-marketing withdrawal of drug to which deaths have been attributed: a systemic investigation and analysis. *J Chem Int Model* 2013;53:1689–1699.
104. Rocca E, Copeland S, Ralph Edwards I. Pharmacovigilance as scientific discovery: an argument for trans-disciplinarity. *Drug Saf* 2019;42:1115–1124.
105. Osimani B, Mignini F. Causal assessment of pharmaceutical treatments: why standards of evidence should not be the same for benefits and harms. *Drug Saf* 2015;15:1–11.
106. Landes J, Osimani B, Poellinger R. Epistemology of causal inference in pharmacology: towards a framework for the assessment of harms. *Eur J Phiolos Sci* 2018;8:3–49.
107. U.S. Food & Drug Administration. MedWatch: the FDA safety information and adverse event reporting program. [cited 2017 Dec 08]. https://www.fda.gov/safety/medwatch-fda-safety-information-and-adverse-event-reporting-program
108. Solotke MT, Dhruva SS, Downing NS, et al. New and incremental FDA black box warnings from 2008 to 2015. *Expert Opin Drug Saf* 2018;17:117–123.
109. Pinnow E, Amr S, Bentzen SM, et al. Postmarket safety outcomes for new molecular entities (NME) drugs approved by the Food and Drug Administration between 2002 and 2014. *Clin Pharmacol Ther* 2018;104:390–400.
110. Ross CJ, Visscher H, Sistonen J, et al.; CPNDS Consortium. The Canadian Pharmacogenomics Network for Drug Safety: a model for safety pharmacology. *Thyroid* 2010;20:681–687.
111. Etwel FA, Rieder MJ, Bend JR, et al. A surveillance method for the early identification of idiosyncratic adverse drug reactions. *Drug Saf* 2008;31:169–180.
112. Tanoshima R, Khan A, Biala AK, et al. Analysis of adverse drug reactions-nationwide active surveillance network: Canadian Pharmacogenomics Network for Drug Safety Database. *J Clin Pharmacol* 2019;59:356–363.
113. Aminkeng F, Bhavsar AP, Visscher H, et al. A coding variant in RARG confers susceptibility to anthracycline-induced cardiotoxicity in childhood cancer. *Nat Genet* 2015;47:1079–1084.
114. Shaw K, Amstutz U, Castro-Pastrana L, et al. Pharmacogenomic investigation of adverse drug reactions (ADRs): the ADR prioritization tool, APT. *J Pop Ther Clin Pharm* 2013;20(2):e110–e127.
115. Naranjo CA, Sellers EM, Sandor P, et al. A method for estimating the probability of adverse drug reactions. *Clin Pharmacol Ther* 1981;30:239–245.
116. Garcia-Cortes M, Lucena MI, Pachkoria K, et al. Evaluation of Naranjo adverse drug reactions probability scale in causality assessment of drug-induced liver injury. *Aliment Pharmacol Ther* 2008;27:780–789.
117. Du W, Tutag Lehr V, Lieh-Lai M, et al. An algorithm to detect adverse drug reactions in the neonatal intensive care unit: a new approach. *J Clin Pharmacol* 2013;53:87–95.
118. Bracken LE, Nunn AJ, Kirkham JJ, et al. Development of the Liverpool adverse drug reaction avoidability assessment tool. *PLos One* 2017;12:e0169393.
119. Wong IC, Wong LY, Cranswick NE. Minimizing medication errors in children. *Arch Dis Child* 2009;94:161–164
120. Scott IA, Pillans PI, Barras M, et al. Using EMR-enabled computerized decision support systems to reduce prescribing of potentially inappropriate medications: a narrative review. *Ther Adv Drug Saf* 2018;9:559–573.
121. Keasberry J, Scott IA, Sullivan C, et al. Going digital: a narrative overview of the clinical and organizational impacts of eHealth technologies in hospital practice. *Aust Health Rev* 2017;41:646–664.
122. Yang JH, Kim M, Park YT, et al. The effect of the introduction of a nationwide DUR system where local DUR systems are operating—the Korean experience. *Int J Med Inform* 2015;84:912–919.
123. Harrington L, Kennerly D, Johnson C. Safety issues related to the electronic medical record (EMR): synthesis of the literature from the last decade, 2000–2009. *J Healthc Manag* 2011;56:31–43.
124. Lieberman P, Nicklas RA, Oppenheimer J, et al. The diagnosis and management of anaphylaxis practice parameter: 2010 update. *J Allergy Clin Immunol* 2010;126:477–480.

125. Schwartz RA, McDonough PH, Lee BW. Toxic epidermal necrolysis: Part II. Prognosis, sequelae, diagnosis, differential diagnosis, prevention and treatment. *J Am Acad Dermatol* 2013;69:187.e1–187.e16.
126. Meng X, Yerly D, Naisbitt D. Mechanisms leading to T-cell activation in drug hypersensitivity. *Curr Opin Allergy Clin Immunol* 2018;18:317–324.
127. Del Pozzo-Magana BR, Rieder MJ, Lazo-Langner A. Quality of life in children with adverse drug reactions: a narrative and systematic review. *Br J Clin Pharmacol* 2015;80:827–833.
128. Conway EL, Lin K, Selick JA, et al. Impact of penicillin allergy on time to first dose of antimicrobial therapy and clinical outcomes. *Clin Ther* 2017;39:2276–2283.
129. Krishna MT, Huissoon AP, Li M, et al. Enhancing antibiotic stewardship by tackling "spurious" penicillin allergy. *Clin Exp Allergy* 2017;47:1362–1373.
130. Sousa-Pinto B, Cardoso-Fernandes A, Arajuo L, et al. Clinical and economic burden of hospitalizations with registration of penicillin allergy. *Ann Allergy Asthma Immunol* 2018;120:190–194.
131. Trublano JA, Grayson ML, Thursky KA, et al. How antibiotic allergy labels may be harming our most vulnerable patients. *Med J Austral* 2018;208:469–470.
132. Sakoulas G, Geriak M, Nizet V. Is a reported penicillin allergy sufficient grounds to forgo the multidimensional antimicrobial benefits of b-lactam antibiotics? *Clin Infect Dis* 2019;68:157–164.
133. Carr DF, Pirmohamed M. Biomarkers of adverse drug reactions. *Exp Biol Med* 2018;243:291–299.

CHAPTER

64

L. M. Hanff

Medication Errors in Children

DEFINITIONS

A *medication error* is defined as any preventable event that may cause or lead to inappropriate medication use or patient harm while the medication is in the control of the healthcare professional, patient, or consumer [definition by National Coordinating Council for Medication Error Reporting and Prevention (NCC MERP)]. Essentially, the right drug must be given to the right patient, in the right route, at the right dose, and at the right time (five rights).[1] Figure 64.1 illustrates the relationship among medication errors and potential, preventable, or unpreventable adverse drug events (ADEs).[2,3] ADEs are any injuries due to medications.[4] Preventable ADEs are medication errors that harm patients, whereas unpreventable ones are considered adverse drug reactions (ADRs) and not errors. Errors can be acts of commission or omission.

INTRODUCTION

In recent years, the realization that medication errors exert a high toll on patient safety and healthcare costs has resulted in increased attention for preventive measures. Studies on the efficacy of interventions, both in adult and in pediatric care, have been performed, and guidelines to improve medication safety have been developed.

The 2007 Institute of Medicine (IOM) report on prevention of medication errors estimates that a hospital patient may be subjected to at least one medication error per day.[5] Importantly, the pediatric population has been shown to be three times more likely to be harmed when medication errors occur.[29]

The opportunities for error are staggering when one considers that hundreds of medication orders are prescribed each day in larger neonatal units. Each medication use process has five steps beginning with conception to prescription, transcription, preparation/dispensing, administration, and ends with monitoring of effects (Fig. 64.2); each step has subprocesses that must get all five earlier mentioned rights correct. In total, a single antibiotic order will have at least a dozen error opportunities, assuming that no process variations exist. However, medication use processes operate frequently in the midst of certain barriers that will, no doubt, produce process variation and greatly increase error opportunities. For example, distractions may cause a physician to prescribe the wrong dose; a ward clerk, nurse, or pharmacist to transcribe a written prescription incorrectly onto the pharmacy's queue; the pharmacist to make a calculation error or prepare or dispense the wrong medication; or the patient's nurse to administer the drug to the wrong patient or to the right patient at the wrong time. In the outpatient setting, the patient's parent or caregiver may measure the dose incorrectly. Finally, in a patient with a deteriorating clinical condition (e.g., organ failure), the patient may start therapy with the correct drug and dose, but inadequate monitoring of serum creatinine concentrations could subsequently prevent the necessary dosage adjustment should renal function decline.

Most errors fall into the commission category in which the correct medication plan is executed incorrectly. Omission errors are those in which the wrong medication plan (including

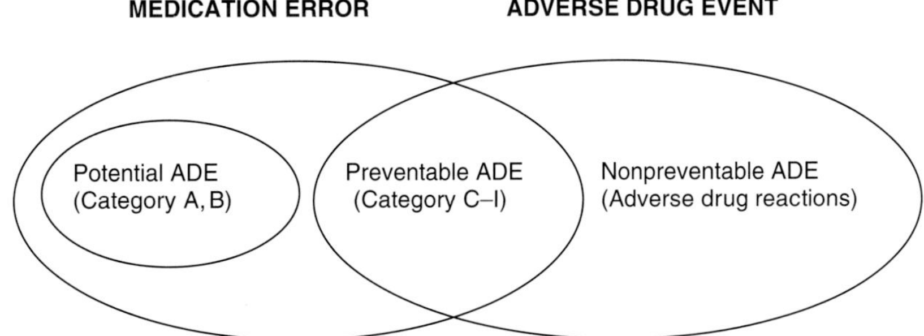

Figure 64.1 Relationship among medication errors, adverse drug events (ADE), and adverse drug reactions. (Adapted from Gandhi TK, Seger DL, Bates DW. Identifying drug safety issues: from research to practice. *Int J Qual Health Care* 2000;12(1):69–76; National Coordinating Council for Medication Error Reporting and Prevention. Factsheet 2015. https://www.nccmerp.org/sites/default/files/nccmerp_fact_sheet_2015-02-v91.pdf.

Prescription
Handwritten or computer prescriber order typically entered by physician, nurse practitioner, or trainee.

Transcription
Critical prescription information is transferred onto the patient's medication administration record either manually or electronically.

Preparation and dispensing
Pharmacist prepares, labels, and dispenses the final drug product. Many pediatric doses require extemporaneous compounding from stock containers.

Administration
The nurse or medication technician administers the medication. In the outpatient setting, the patient or caregiver is responsible for drug administration. In either case, the five rights of medication administration should be achieved (right patient, drug, dose, time, and route)

Monitor for effects
Patients are monitored for drug reactions. Laboratory values such as plasma drug concentrations, serum creatinine concentrations, and hepatic function should be checked and drug dose or administration schedule adjusted as indicated.

Figure 64.2 Typical steps involved in the medication use process.

no treatment) is executed. Propagation errors are "passive" in the sense that the usual safeguards (i.e., five rights checklist) are not used to stop an error committed earlier in the use process from reaching the patient. Workflows producing these errors involve complex human and environmental factors. The IOM report "To Err Is Human" attributes most patient injuries not to culpable individuals but to systemic factors such as poor communication systems and unrealistic dependency on human memory and vigilance.[6]

DETECTING MEDICATION ERRORS

Reports on medication error rates vary widely depending on the reporting mechanism.[7–9] Somewhat structured written "incident reports" are most commonly used through a voluntary reporting system. Significant underreporting exists, especially for near misses. This is partly due to a hesitancy to report errors given the traditional approach to medication error management of blaming the responsible individual(s) rather than focusing on correcting a flaw in the medication delivery system that allowed the error to occur. The IOM committee, in its "Preventing Medication Errors" publication, comments that the reports of about 400,000 preventable ADEs annually are likely to be underestimates. Detection methods include review of written orders, prompt reporting, chart review, electronic record extraction, and direct participation in clinical care.[5] Jha et al. emphasized the complementary effect of using three methods, computerized surveillance of medical records, chart review, and voluntary reporting, together to find errors.[10] Trigger-based detection methods, such as the Institute for Healthcare Improvement global trigger tool, have been shown to be effective in identifying error clues in retrospective chart reviews.[11] Its success has prompted adapting its use for other medical errors in clinical care.

Accurate error identification and accounting is critical to improve processes in medication management systems in order to reduce medication errors and improve patient safety. Traditional strategies for identifying and analyzing medication errors are based primarily on incident reporting or root cause analysis.[12,13] Institution-wide incident reporting systems are a requirement for all hospitals in the United States accredited by The Joint Commission on Accreditation of Healthcare Organizations (JCAHO) and include adverse events (e.g., ADEs), no-harm events, and near misses.[12] Event reporting remains voluntary within hospitals.[14]

In the ambulatory setting, it is estimated that four invalid doses per 100 immunizations are given to children, or 36% of children are being immunized at least one invalid dose during childhood.[15] Too much immunization happens in approximately 21% of patients.[16] In two emergency room reports, 10 and 3.9 errors per 100 patients happen in the prescribing and administering phases, respectively.[17] In the hospital setting, where most of the reports have been generated, approximately 47% of medication errors are medication related.

In summary, medication error rates are underreported. Reporting standards need further specifications. Nevertheless, reported error rates are unacceptably high and can be used to track the effectiveness of medication error prevention programs and help to focus efforts.

COMMON TYPES OF MEDICATION ERRORS

It is estimated that at least 380,000 to 450,000 preventable ADEs occur in U.S. hospitals annually.[18,19] Many reported ADEs were preventable (27% to 50%) and occurred in the prescription and administration stages (39% and 38%, respectively).[20] Prescription error types were predominately wrong dose, known allergy, wrong frequency, and drug–drug interaction. In the Bates et al. study, 53% of the prescription errors were missing doses; of the remaining 250 medication errors, 31% were dose errors, 31% wrong frequency, 10% wrong route of drug administration, 6% illegible prescription handwriting, and 4% drug administration to a patient with a documented allergy to the agent, numbers that more closely resemble the percentages reported by the other studies listed in Table 64.1.[4,8,17,21,22] Leape et al.[20] analyzed 264 preventable and potential ADE events and identified the three top proximal causes of error as lack of knowledge of the drug, lack of information about the patient, and rules violations (22%, 14%, and 10%, respectively). Most errors occurred in the prescription and administration phase (39% and 38%, respectively). They found that poor access to information accounted for 78% of the errors, with the top three system failures being drug knowledge dissemination, dose and identity checking, and patient information availability (29%, 12%, and 11%, respectively). Studies also suggest that overdoses are the most common type of dosing error, with the majority of errors occurring at the drug ordering state.[22–24] Not surprisingly, the drug classes most often involved in medication errors are the ones most often prescribed to hospitalized patients (Table 64.2).[4,21,22] Antibiotics are most often associated with medication errors in the hospitalized patients, accounting for approximately 20% to 40% of all medication errors. Other drug classes commonly involved in medication errors include cardiovascular agents, gastrointestinal agents, vitamin or mineral products, electrolyte concentrates, and nonnarcotic and narcotic analgesics.

TABLE 64.1 Common Types of Medication Errors, as a Percentage of Total Medication Errors Identified in Each Respective Study

Study	Total Number of Errors (% All Orders)	Wrong Dose (%)	Wrong Schedule (%)	Wrong Route (%)	Wrong Drug or Patient (%)	Missing Dose	Known Allergy	Incomplete Order (%)
Bates et al.[4]	530 (5.3)	14.5	8.1	4.9	2.1	53	2.1	—
Lesar et al.[21]	905 (0.31)	46.5	—	3.4	6.6	—	6.7	22.3
Lesar et al.[22]	696 (0.39)	58.3	—	3.3	5.4	—	12.9	—
Simborg and Derewicz[17]	105 (7.4)[a]	72.4[a]	—	1.9[a]	17.1[a]	—	—	—
	20 (1.6)[b]	35[b]		5[b]	25[b]			
Blum et al.[8]	1,012 (1.3)[c]	45[c]	27[c]	—	—	—	—	17[c]
	1,277 (2.7)[d]	58[d]	28[d]					4[d]

[a]Traditional multidose system with handwritten physician orders.
[b]Unit dose system with computerized physician order entry.
[c]Adult teaching hospital.
[d]Pediatric hospital.

TABLE 64.2 Drug Classes Most Often Involved in Medication Errors, as a Percentage of Total Medication Errors Identified in Each Respective Study

Study	Total Number of Errors (% All Orders)	Antimicrobials (%)	Cardiovascular Agents (%)	Gastrointestinal Agents (%)	Analgesics (%)	Vitamins/ Electrolytes (%)
Bates et al.[4]	530 (5.3)	19	8	—	7	10
Lesar et al.[21]	905 (0.31)	23.1	10.2	10.4	8.5	5.7
Lesar et al.[22]	696 (0.39)	39.7	17.5	7.3	10.2	3

Underutilization of medications (errors of omission) deserves mention and is reported mostly by the adult literature. Most studies report a wide variation in compliance with "in time treatment" of acute myocardial infarction (MI), antibiotic prophylaxis, and thromboembolic prophylaxis. Depending on the exact treatment (error of omission), MI was at 51% to 93%, surgical antibiotic prophylaxis was at 70% to 98%, and thromboembolic prophylaxis was at 5% to 90%.[25–28]

MEDICATION ERRORS IN PEDIATRIC PATIENTS

Kaushal and associates investigated the frequency of medication errors, ADEs, and potential ADEs in 1,120 inpatients ranging in age from neonates through adulthood at two teaching medical centers.[29] Of 10,778 prescriptions written during the study, 616 medication errors were identified for a rate of 5.7 errors per 100 orders written. In this study, medication errors occurred at a higher rate in adult patients (8.6 errors per 100 hospital admissions) than in any other age group studied with 6.2, 4.1, 4.8, 5.8, and 6.3 medication errors per 100 admissions, respectively, in the neonatal, infant, preschool, school-aged, and adolescent cohorts ($p = 0.006$). In contrast, potential ADEs were identified at a significantly higher rate in neonates (2.0 potential ADEs per 100 hospital admissions) than in any other age group with 0.5, 0.8, 1.2, 1.1, and 1.4 potential ADEs per 100 admissions, respectively, in the infant, preschool, school-aged, adolescent, and adult cohorts ($p < 0.001$). The results of the study were also compared with those of a similar study conducted by Bates and colleagues in adult inpatients.[2] Recently, the high frequency of ADE-related admissions to the pediatric emergency unit was again confirmed.[30]

Although most studies[23,31–34] but not all[29] suggest that medication error rates are similar between pediatric and adult medicine, medication errors are more likely to harm children than adults, with 30% of pediatric errors leading to disability lasting for more than 6 months and 15% leading to death.[35] Several factors contribute to a higher risk of ADEs in pediatric patients when medication errors do occur (Table 64.3).[32,36–38] The Joint Commission summarized reasons for increased harm in pediatrics as (a) most medications need to be altered for pediatric use and requires pediatric-specific dosage calculations and processes that increase error opportunities; (b) many healthcare facilities, especially emergency rooms, lack the necessary staff orientation to pediatric care, protocols and safeguards, and reference materials; (c) children are usually less tolerant to the physiologic impact of medication errors; and (d) children, especially infants, cannot communicate adverse effects effectively.[39] Neonates and young infants may be less capable physiologically of coping with a medication error such as a drug overdose due to immaturity of critical body processes.[29,36,37] For example, in comparison with healthy adults, the heart of newborn infants is characterized by decreased ventricular compliance, a lower ratio of contractile to noncontractile myocardial proteins, and a higher resting heart rate.[40,41] Neonates therefore have a lower

TABLE 64.3 Factors That Increase the Risk of Adverse Drug Reactions in Pediatric Patients

1. Greater pharmacokinetic variability: Pharmacokinetic variables are age related and can change rapidly in young neonates, necessitating frequent drug dose and schedule adjustments; pharmacokinetic differences are magnified in preterm neonates such as in:
   a. Gastrointestinal drug absorption in neonates with increased gastric pH, delayed gastric emptying, and reduced biliary function
   b. Drug distribution in neonates with increased total body water and extracellular fluid, decreased total body fat, and decreased plasma protein binding
   c. Drug metabolism in neonates with decreased phase I and phase II drug-metabolizing and transporter enzyme activity; both the level of activity and the rate of maturation are isozyme specific
   d. Drug excretion in neonates with decreased glomerular filtration and renal tubular secretion
2. Dependence on individualized dosage calculations where calculations need to account for patient age, body weight or surface area, organ function, and disease state
3. Lack of appropriate pediatric dosage forms since younger patients often cannot or will not take oral tablets or capsules, necessitating the extemporaneous compounding of oral solutions or suspensions for many medications
4. Lack of FDA/EMA-approved pediatric labeling
5. Dependence on precise measurement and delivery devices: Doses of oral solutions and suspensions must be measured accurately; parenteral drug products are often delivered in smaller volumes in young neonates and infants, necessitating the use of precise infusion or syringe pumps
6. Children and infants cannot communicate adverse drug effects effectively

EMA, European Medicines Agency; FDA, Food and Drug Administration.
From Folli HL, Poole RL, Benitz WE, et al. Medication error prevention by clinical pharmacists in two children's hospitals. *Pediatrics* 1987;79:718–722; Evans RS, Pestolnik SL, Classen DC, et al. Preventing adverse drug events in hospitalized patients. *Ann Pharmacother* 1994;28:523–527.

preload preserve and cannot tolerate volume loading as well as adults do. The higher baseline heart rate means that neonates are less capable of augmenting cardiac output by increasing heart rate without compromising diastolic filling.

It is not surprising that most harmful errors involve the wrong drug dose or happen during administration. Pharmacokinetic processes are widely variable and age specific, with highly variable age-related differences in drug absorption, distribution, metabolism, and excretion in children.[42,43] The variability in pharmacokinetic processes is several fold greater in children than in adults.[42,43] Age-related differences in drug pharmacodynamics and pharmacokinetics are discussed in depth in previous chapters. From birth to adulthood, the greatest amount of pharmacokinetic variability occurs during the neonatal period.[42,43] These processes can change rapidly and dramatically during the first 4 weeks of postnatal life, as excess total body water is lost, renal and hepatic function begin to mature, and plasma protein binding begins to normalize, necessitating frequent drug dose and schedule adjustments. For example, the mean (standard deviation) total body clearance of theophylline has been shown to increase threefold between the postconceptual age of 35.5 ± 2.9 weeks and 63.2 + 14.4 weeks (21.5 + 6.9 vs. 60.7 + 14.4 mL per kg per hour, respectively).[44] This change is attributed primarily to maturation of the principal metabolic pathway in the liver, cytochrome P-450 IA2 (CYP1A2). CYP1A2 activity approaches normal by approximately 55 weeks of postconceptual age, followed by above average levels of activity during childhood and a decrease to adult levels during puberty in a gender-specific fashion.[45] The effect of this change in CYP1A2 activity on the elimination half-life of theophylline is dramatic, as the half-life decreases approximately 10-fold during infancy. The mean (range) half-life in premature infants (25 to 32 weeks of gestational age and 3 to 15 days of postnatal age), children (1 to 4 years of age), and adults (23 to 79 years of age) has been reported to be 30.2 (14.4 to 57.7), 3.4 (1.9 to 5.5), and 6.7 (3.6 to 12) hours, respectively.[46]

Pediatric drug therapy is also frequently complicated by the larger variability in patient's body weight or body surface area (BSA) and renal or hepatic function when attempting to appropriately individualize the patient's drug dose.[36] This process requires accurate and current patient-specific information and accurate dosage calculation. As Table 64.4 illustrates, dosing errors are the most common type of medication errors identified in pediatric patients.[29–33] When calculating dosages based upon bodyweight, attention needs to be paid for older children to the absolute limit of the dosage, which usually equals the adult dosage. Also, depending on the source of information, pediatric dosages can be displayed in many different ways, such as mg per kg per day or mg per kg per dosage or µg per kg per hour, which makes prescribing for children even more complex.

TABLE 64.4 Common Types of Medication Errors in Pediatric Inpatients, as a Percentage of Total Medication Errors Identified in Each Respective Study

Study	*Total Number of Errors (% All Orders)*	*Wrong Dose (%)*	*Wrong Schedule (%)*	*Wrong Route (%)*	*Wrong Drug or Patient (%)*	*Known Allergy*	*Incomplete Order (%)*
Kaushal et al.[29]	616 (5.7)	28	9.4	18	1.5	1.3	2.3
Folli et al.[32]	479 (0.47)	85	—	1.9	5.6	0.4	—
Kozer et al.[23]	271 (—)	49.1	43.2	2.6	1.8	—	—
Raju et al.[33]	315 (—)	13.7	21.6	4.1	13.3	—	—

Instead of kg, pounds are sometimes used as weight parameter or BSA, which introduces more possibilities for errors.

The risk of medication errors in pediatric patients can also be increased by the lack of an appropriate pediatric dose form. Solid oral dose forms are often inappropriate for younger children, yet suitable oral solutions or suspensions are not available for many drugs used to treat pediatric illnesses. As a result, pharmacists are often required to extemporaneously compound and dispense appropriate formulations for pediatric patients. Not only does this increase the risk of error by requiring additional calculations, in many instances critical information related to the stability and bioavailability of these products is not available.[36]

Many drugs commonly used in pediatric medicine also continue to lack Food and Drug Administration (FDA)-approved labeling or European Medicines Agency (EMA) labeling.[36] As a result, the optimal dose and schedule for these agents, based on the results of clinical trials, are lacking. This not only increases the risk of ADEs but also increases the likelihood of suboptimal therapy.

Pediatric patients may have a higher rate of medication errors due to unique challenges with respect to drug delivery.[36] Intravenous drug formulations intended for use in neonates and young infants must often be delivered in very small volumes, requiring precise, and in many instances unique, compounding procedures and specialized delivery devices such as infusion or syringe pumps. Because the drug concentration is generally higher than in the corresponding adult formulation, the risk for an ADE may be higher if a medication error is made with respect to the infusion rate. The frequent need for oral solutions or suspensions necessitates careful and precise measurement of each dose. The latter problem is complicated even further if the product is administered on an outpatient basis because the patient's parent or caregiver is generally dependent on the available device to measure and prepare for each dose.[14,36]

PREVENTING MEDICATION ERRORS

Preventing medication errors requires a multilevel, multidisciplinary patient-centered effort. Simultaneous engagement from all levels is critical: (a) government and state funding to help institutions implement national safe practice guidelines, (b) institutional culture transformation from one of distrust and secrecy to one of trust and teamwork, (c) self-policing individuals who hold genuine ownership and responsibility for not only the patients' clinical care but also their safe passage through the medical system, (d) focus on systemic causes of errors rather than individual blame, and (e) patients who actively participate in their medication management. At each of these levels, the focus would be at each medication management phase: prescribing, transcribing, preparation/dispensing, administering, and monitoring. Lastly, the prevention strategy requires a detailed preimplementation evaluation of the intervention's potential impact on local processes and anticipation of existing adoption barriers. According to an FMEA (failure mode and effects analysis) by Kunac and Keith looking at neonatal intensive care unit (NICU) medication safety, the top failure step was "lack of awareness of medicine safety issues."[47] The next 27 failure steps occurred in the administration stage, including environment stressors, lack of accountability, no protocols, unsafe storage of medications, dose calculation mistakes, and not checking patient identity. Similar findings were reported in another FMEA done by Williams and Tally in a U.S. hospital, suggesting that these causes are not unique to the NICU.[48] Studies also suggest that overdoses are the most common type of dosing error, with the majority of errors occurring at the drug ordering state.[22–24]

This section discusses interventions for preventing medication errors at each stage of drug ordering and delivery process.[49–51] However, our understanding of optimal interventions and the effectiveness of individual strategies is still limited.[52,53]

PREVENTING PRESCRIBING ERRORS

Studies in both adult and pediatric inpatients suggest that prescription errors, most commonly the wrong dose, frequency of administration, or route of administration, account for approximately 50% of all medication errors.[18,29,54] Opportunities identified to improve prescribing safety include computerized physician order entry (CPOE) by using clinical decision support, developing a standard formulary for pediatric patients while limiting variability of medication concentrations, using of clinical pharmacist support,[55] and enhancing training of medical professionals.[56]

The CPOE systems are widely proposed as a means of reducing these errors.[29,57,58] Basic CPOE eliminates many of the problems associated with handwritten prescriptions, such as incomplete prescriptions or illegible handwriting, and obviate the need for dose calculation. Most systems also include some form of clinical decision support software (CDSS).[57] CDSS can provide critical drug, patient, and laboratory information to the physician at the time of order entry, thereby reducing the risk of error. Critical components of an effective CPOE/CDSS system have been suggested.[36] The system should generate computerized medication administration records (MARs) from a database shared by the prescriber and pharmacy, which can reduce transcription errors. The system should provide the prescriber, at the time of order entry, with patient-specific information (e.g., age, weight or BSA, drug allergies, and pertinent laboratory variables) and a complete list of current medications. The software should be capable of not only calculating appropriate age- and weight-based doses but also incorporating important clinical data such as vital signs and laboratory values. Thus, the various patient weights entered into an electronic health information system should be standardized across vendors and clear to healthcare providers as to which weight is used for drug calculations. In some countries, the issue of performing medication calculations based on pounds instead of the recognized standard of kilograms may introduce errors. The system should have high usability scores,[59] minimizing user-clicks and decision branch points to reduce potential process variations and "work-arounds." The system should provide unsolicited alerts regarding critical potential drug–drug or drug–food interactions. Although many current vendor systems can do this, most still require extensive modifications to the architectural technical framework to optimize the efficiency of their alert capabilities. For example, if a physician interfaced with a CPOE/CDSS system to order gentamicin for a 3-month-old infant, the system could provide the patient's current weight and serum creatinine, along with the recommended weight-based dose and administration interval based on the infant's age and level of renal function. The system could also provide a complete list of the patient's positive culture and sensitivity results, along with all concomitant medications and any patient allergies. Equally important is that the system generates a standardized, complete prescription in a format that minimizes confusion once the prescription is reviewed by the pharmacist or nurse. For example, with respect to drug doses, the use of leading zeroes should be standard for all doses less than "1" (e.g., 0.1 mg rather than .1 mg), whereas the use of trailing zeroes should be strictly prohibited for whole numbers (e.g., 1 mg rather than 1.0 mg).[60] However, CPOE is not a panacea, particularly in pediatric practice, where a system must have the flexibility to account for rapid and ongoing large changes in patient weight or organ function.[29]

In pediatrics, the use of non-licensed, off-label, or extemporaneously manufactured products is still common, because of the lack of licensed products or adequate drug formulations for all age groups. This limits the use of an effective CPOE/CDSS system, because the backbone of these systems, a validated and up-to-date drug library, cannot always be applied in pediatrics, due to the underuse of commercial, licensed products.

The use of a standard formulary for pediatric patients has been advocated. An example of such a formulary has been successfully implemented in the Netherlands and has been embraced by the Dutch Associations of Pediatricians, pharmacists, and general practitioners. The formulary allows for consistent pharmacotherapy and dosage guidelines among all healthcare providers in the Netherlands and provides pharmacotherapeutic education for starting professionals.[61]

Drug reconciliation is another intervention, known to reduce medication errors at admission and discharge.[62] Drug reconciliation has been defined as: the process of creating the most accurate list possible of all medications a patient is taking, including the name of the medication, dose, directions, frequency, and route, and comparing this against the physician's admission, transfer, and discharge orders with the aim of providing the right medications to the patient at all transition points within the hospital. This intervention is implemented in several countries both for adult and pediatric settings, and has been shown to effectively reduce medication discrepancies.

Effective physician training is also critical in eliminating prescription errors. Simulations have shown promise in effectively training residents in a safe environment to increase competence and skill.[63] Dedicated pediatric training for medical, pharmaceutical, and nursing staff should include content such as common medication errors in children, systems-improvement tools to avoid or abate errors, and the effects of developmental differences in pediatric patients. Comprehensive and repetitive testing of dosage calculations and calculation of BSA and conversion to metric height and weight measurements should be practiced and competency should be demonstrated.[51]

PREVENTING PREPARATION AND DISPENSING ERRORS

Because so many medications used in pediatric patients require calculations and individual preparation including dilution steps, all nonemergency medications should preferably be prepared, labeled, and dispensed by the pharmacy. With traditional ward stock systems, the nurse is responsible for preparing and labeling each dose using a stock drug container stored on the patient ward. Because the nurse is also responsible for drug administration, bypassing the pharmacy removes an important safety check from the drug delivery system, not to mention increasing the workload of the nursing staff. In a national survey of hospital medication–dispensing systems conducted in 1998, 50% of responding hospitals continued to use drug distribution systems that bypassed the pharmacy.[64]

The pharmacy must directly verify all questionable or nonstandard drug doses or administration schedules with the prescriber prior to dispensing. In institutions utilizing handwritten prescriptions, the prescriber should be careful to include all required components of the prescription (Table 64.5) and write legibly.[36] Again, the pharmacist must verify any questionable information with the prescriber before dispensing the drug.

CPOE systems should be designed to share a common patient database between the prescriber and the pharmacy. The system should be capable of providing the pharmacist with current patient-specific information such as weight, serum creatinine, or liver enzyme values. The pharmacist should recalculate and verify all drug doses and verify the appropriateness of the dosing regimen based on current renal or hepatic function before dispensing.

Pharmacists are increasingly active members of the healthcare team, present in the patient care area and interacting with the prescriber when the prescription is written, or write out orders themselves within their agreed scope of care. Kaushal and colleagues concluded that the presence of a clinical pharmacist on work rounds could have prevented 94% of the potential ADEs observed in their study.[29] A separate study conducted in an adult intensive care unit showed a 66% decrease in preventable ADEs with the active participation of a clinical pharmacist during rounds.[65]

Prevention of Preparation Errors

In pediatrics, the use of standardized or rounded off dosages is not always feasible to the large continuum of dosages ranging for premature neonates to obese adolescents. Preferably, the pharmacy prepares the medication for individual patients,

TABLE 64.5 Recommended Components of a Prescription

1. Patient-specific information: Information should include full name, age or date of birth, current body weight, and known drug allergies
2. Drug name, strength, dose form, and number or amount to be dispensed: Generic drug names should be used exclusively and should be listed in metric units; leading zeroes should always be used for doses or less than "1" unit (e.g., 0.1 mg rather than .1 mg), whereas trailing zeroes should never be used for drug doses off whole number units (e.g., 1 mg rather than 1.0 mg)
3. Daily mg per kg drug dose: This will facilitate verification of the dose by the pharmacist and/or nurse
4. Name and contact number (pager or telephone) of prescriber
5. Complete patient instructions: Instructions should include indication for drug use, dosing instructions (dose, frequency and route of administration, and duration of therapy), and the number of authorized refills should be included; for drug products intended for outpatient use the instructions should include easily recognizable units of measure (e.g., "15 mL") and should be accompanied in parenthesis with an adequate device

From Fernandez CV, Gillis-Ring J. Strategies for the prevention of medical error in pediatrics. *J Pediatr* 2003;143(2):155–162.

including all parenteral drugs. The use of supporting, validated software to aid the technicians during the preparation procedures is helpful in monitoring the preparation process and preventing mistakes, especially in a high throughput setting. Current preparation software includes identification of vials by barcode scanning of the label, gravimetric checks during preparation, and automatic printing of individual labels.

However, individual preparation by the pharmacy in emergency settings or stocking of all medications in all possible dosage ranges at the ward is not feasible in many pediatric settings. Therefore, preparation and use of stock containers at the ward cannot be avoided completely. Procedures need to be in place to assist the healthcare professional with correct calculations and dilution steps during preparation and adequate checks need to be performed.

Preventing Administration Errors

The nurse is generally responsible for actual medication administration in hospitalized patients, and provides the critical last check of the dose and prescription prior to drug administration.[36] They have the arduous task of avoiding errors as well as preventing the propagation of errors committed earlier in the medication management from reaching the patient. Leape et al.[20] identified several systemic factors associated with medication errors, including deficient staffing and high workload. Both in the adult setting and in the pediatric setting, the use of a barcode medication administration system (BCMA) has been advocated to reduce administration errors, including wrong time administration. Evidence regarding the reducing effect of BCMA on preventable ADEs in pediatrics has been increasing, although robust implementation resulting in prevention of all potential errors in pediatric administration is still difficult.[66]

The inability to communicate with (very) young patients poses an additional risk for errors. Young children are generally not capable of acting as their own advocate. Parents or caregivers should participate as active members of the healthcare team, providing critical patient-specific information and monitoring throughout the therapy for the appearance of adverse effects.

PREVENTING MEDICATION ERRORS AT HOME

Few studies have been published regarding the frequency of medication errors in the outpatient setting, although it has been estimated that 5% to 35% of outpatients experience at least one ADE annually.[67,68] The frequency of medication errors by caregivers in infants discharged from the NICU was 66.3% as shown by Solanki et al.[69] Dose administration error (measurement of a dose different from what was prescribed) was the most common error (54%).

In pediatric outpatients, the aforementioned need with many medications to measure liquid doses from stock containers increases the potential for human error, as well as the lack of age-suitable formulations. Suboptimal drug labeling and medication packaging have been identified as key contributors to outpatient medication errors.[70] Matching dosing tools more closely with prescribed dose volumes has been identified as an important strategy for reducing pediatric medication errors. The American Academy of pediatrics (AAP) therefore supports a policy on the use of milliliter-only dosing for liquid medications used in the home and suggests that standardized delivery devices be distributed.[71]

The United States Pharmacopeia Center for the Advancement of Patient Safety has issued a list of recommendations for parents designed to reduce the risk of medication errors in hospitalized pediatric patients.[72] On admission, parents should provide the pharmacy during drug reconciliation and/or the physician with a complete list of all prescription medications, over-the-counter medications, and dietary supplements the child is currently receiving. Parents should also know their child's current height and weight and inform the physician of any drug or food allergies. If the child has potentially fatal allergy, a MedicAlert bracelet should be worn at all times while in the hospital. Because dosage calculation errors are a common cause of pediatric medication errors, parents should know their child's metric weight and verbally confirm this with physician when each prescription is written. Parents should be given both verbal and written information about each of the child's medications including possible adverse effects. To safely monitor the child's medication use, the parents should know each drug, dose and dose form, and which drug is being given, and closely monitor and report any potential adverse effect. Finally parents should be discouraged from using household measuring devices (tablespoons, etc.) when measuring doses of liquid or suspension medications. An appropriate measuring device should be supplied with the medication, and the parent instructed on the proper use of the device, including a demonstration by the parent of measuring competency. Before discharge home for this first time after diagnosis with outpatient medications, the home caretakers must demonstrate to the hospital staff the caretakers' ability to obtain, dose, and administer the home medications to the patient.

SUMMARY

Medication error prevention in pediatric patients presents a formidable challenge to the healthcare community. Infants and children are considered to be at higher risk for error-related ADEs because of the complexity of prescribing and dose calculations, based upon individual factors such as age, weight, maturation of metabolic organ systems, and renal function. Furthermore, the limited physiologic reserve, the narrow therapeutic range of some drugs, and the inability to communicate with young patients add to the increased risk. Effective strategies to prevent these errors must continue to focus on effective, accurate reporting and dissemination of medication errors and near misses to identify correctable deficiencies in the medication ordering and delivery system. Proposed interventions, such as clinical decision support, calculation aids, alerts in cases of underdosage or overdosage, educational interventions and close monitoring are only useful if specifically targeted on pediatric pharmacotherapy. Aside from technical innovations like CPOE and BCMA, nontechnical calculation aids and alerts must be subjects of investigation to support professionals in countries where high-tech applications are not feasible. As drug treatment is increasingly important in many pediatric diseases, minimizing or eliminating medication errors can make a real difference in the quality of healthcare and the safety of infants and children undergoing drug treatment.

ACKNOWLEDGMENT

Many thanks to Manon de Boer for her valuable efforts in the technical preparation of this manuscript.

REFERENCES

1. Nicholas PK, Agius CR. Towards safer IV medication administration. *Am J Nurs* 2005;105(3):25–30.
2. Gandhi TK, Seger DL, Bates DW. Identifying drug safety issues: from research to practice. *Int J Qual Health Care* 2000;12(1):69–76.
3. National Coordinating Council for Medication Error Reporting and Prevention. Factsheet 2015. https://www.nccmerp.org/sites/default/files/nccmerp_fact_sheet_2015-02-v91.pdf.
4. Bates DW, Boyle DL, WanderVilet MB, et al. Relationship between medication errors and adverse drug events. *J Gen Intern Med* 1995;10:199–205.
5. Aspden P, Julie A, Wolcott J, et al.; Institute of Medicine; Committee on Identifying and Preventing Medication Errors, eds. *Preventing medication errors: quality chasm series.* Washington, DC: National Academies Press, 2006.
6. Kohn LT, Corrigan JM, Donaldson MS. *To err is human: building a safer health system.* Washington, DC: National Academies Press, 1999.
7. O'Shea E. Factors contributing to medication errors: a literature review, *J Clin Nurs* 1999;8:496–504.
8. Blum KV, Abel SR, Urbanski CJ, et al. Medication error prevention by pharmacists. *Am J Hosp Pharm* 1988;45(9):1902–1903.
9. Griffin JP, Weber JC. Voluntary systems of adverse reaction reporting—part II. *Adverse Drug React Acute Poisoning Rev* 1986;5:23–25.
10. Jha AK, Kuperman GJ, Ritternberg E, et al. Identifying hospital admissions due to adverse drug events using a computer-based monitor. *Pharmacoepidemiol Drug Saf* 2001;10(2):113–119.
11. Griffin FA, Resar RK. *IHI global trigger tool for measuring adverse events. IHI innovation series white paper.* Cambridge, MA: Institute for Healthcare Improvement, 2007.
12. Wald H, Shojania KG. Incident reporting. In: Shojania KG, Duncan BW, McDonals KM, et al., eds. *Making healthcare safer: a critical analysis of patient safety practices.* Rockville, MD: Agency for Healthcare Research and Quality, 2001:41–50.
13. Wald H, Shojania KG. Root cause analysis. In: Shojania KG, Duncan BW, McDonals KM, et al., eds. *Making healthcare safer: a critical analysis of patient safety practices.* Rockville, MD: Agency for Healthcare Research and Quality, 2001:51–56.
14. Huynh C, Wong IC, Correa-West J, et al. Paediatric patient safety and the need for aviation black box thinking to learn from and prevent medication errors. *Pediatr Drugs* 2017;19:99–105.
15. Butte AJ, Shaw JS, Bernstein H. Strict interpretation of vaccination guidelines with computerized algorithms and improper timing of administered doses. *Pediatr Infect Dis J* 2001;20(6):561–565.
16. Feikema SM, Klevens RM, Washington ML, et al. Extraimmunization among U.S. children. *JAMA* 2000;283(10):1311–1317.
17. Simborg DW, Derewicz HJ. A highly automated hospital medication system. Five years' experience and evaluation. *Ann Intern Med* 1975;83(3):342–346.
18. Bates DW, Cullen DJ, Laird N, et al. Incidence of adverse drug events and potential adverse drug events. Implications for prevention. *JAMA* 1995;274:35–43.
19. Classen DC, Pestotnik SL, Evans RS, et al. Adverse drug events in hospitalized patients. Excess length of stay, extra costs, and attributable mortality. *JAMA* 1997;277(4):301–306.
20. Leape LL, Bates DW, Cullen DJ, et al. Systems analysis of adverse drug events. ADE Prevention Study Group. *JAMA* 1995;274(1):35–43.
21. Lesar TS, Briceland LL, Delcoure K, et al. Medication prescribing errors in a teaching hospital. *JAMA* 1990;263:2329–2334.
22. Lesar TS, Briceland L, Stein DS. Factors related to errors in medication prescribing. *JAMA* 1997;277:312–317.
23. Kozer E, Scolnic D, Macpherson A, et al. Variables associated with medication errors in pediatric emergency medicine. *Pediatrics* 2002;110:737–742.
24. Lesar TS. Errors in the use of medication dosage equations. *Arch Pediatr Adolesc Med* 1998;152:340–344.
25. Bedouch P, Labarere J, Chirpaz E, et al. Compliance with guidelines on antibiotic prophylaxis in total hip replacement surgery: Results of a retrospective study of 416 patients in a teaching hospital. *Infect Control Hosp Epidemiol* 2004;25(4):302–307.
26. Aujesky D, Guignard E, Pannatier A, et al. Pharmacological thromboembolic prophylaxis in a medical ward: room for improvement. *J Gen Intern Med* 2002;17(10):788–791.
27. Sanborn TA, Jacobs AK, Frederick PD, et al. Comparability of quality-of-care indicators for emergency coronary angioplasty in patients with acute myocardial infarction regardless of on-site cardiac surgery (report from the National Registry of Myocardial Infarction). *Am J Cardiol* 2004;93(11):1335–1339.
28. Chopard P, Dorffler-Melly J, Hess U, et al. Venous thromboembolism prophylaxis in acutely ill medical patients: definite need for improvement. *J Intern Med* 2005;257(4):353–357.
29. Kaushal R, Bates DW, Landrigan C, et al. Medication errors and adverse drug events in pediatric inpatients. *JAMA* 2001;285:2114–2120.
30. Carvalho IV, de Sousa VM, Visacri MB, et al. Adverse drug event-related admissions to a pediatric emergency unit. *Pediatr Emerg Care* 2018. doi:10.1097/PEC.0000000000001582.
31. Fortescue EB, Kaushal R, Landigran CP, et al. Prioritizing strategies for preventing medication errors and adverse drug events in pediatric inpatients. *Pediatrics* 2003;111:722–729.
32. Folli HL, Poole RL, Benitz WE, et al. Medication error prevention by clinical pharmacists in two children's hospitals. *Pediatrics* 1987;79:718–722.
33. Raju TN, Kecskes S, Thorton JP, et al. Medication errors in neonatal and paediatric intensive-care units. *Lancet* 1989;2:374–376.
34. Slonim AD, LaFleur BJ, Ahmed W, et al. Hospital-reported medical errors in children. *Pediatrics* 2003;111:617–621.
35. Fernandez CV, Gillis-Ring J. Strategies for the prevention of medical error in pediatrics. *J Pediatr* 2003;143(2):155–162.
36. Levine SR, Cohen MR, Blanchard NR, et al. Guidelines for preventing medication errors in pediatrics. *J Pediatr Pharmacol Ther* 2001;6:426–442.
37. Gupta A, Waldhauser LK. Adverse drug reactions from birth to early childhood. *Pediatr Clin North Am* 1997;44:79–92.
38. Evans RS, Pestolnik SL, Classen DC, et al. Preventing adverse drug events in hospitalized patients. *Ann Pharmacother* 1994;28:523–527.
39. The Joint Commission. Preventing pediatric medication errors. 2008. http://www.jointcommission.org/sentinelevents/sentineleventalert/sea_39.htm.
40. Steinberg C, Notterman DA. Pharmacokinetics of cardiovascular drugs in children. *Clin Pharmacokinet* 1994;27:345–367.
41. Perloff WH. Physiology of the heart and circulation. In: Swedlow DB, Raphaely RC, eds. *Cardiovascular problems in pediatric critical care.* New York, NY: Churchill Livingstone, 1986:1–86.
42. Stewart CF, Hampton EM. Effect of maturation on drug disposition in pediatric patients. *Clin Pharm* 1987;6:548–564.
43. Crom WR. Pharmacokinetics in the child. *Environ Health Perspect* 1994;102(Suppl 11):111–118.
44. Kraus DM, Fischer JH, Reitz SJ, et al. Alterations in theophylline metabolism during the first year of life. *Clin Pharmacol Ther* 1993;54:351–359.
45. Evans C, Lambert GH, Tucker M, et al. The effects of gender on P4501A2 activity in the human adult. *Cancer Epidemiol Biomarkers Prev* 1995;4:529–533.
46. Aranda JV, Sitar DS, Parsons WD, et al. Pharmacokinetic aspects of theophylline in premature newborns. *N Engl J Med* 1976;295:413–416.
47. Kunac DL, Reith DM. Identification of priorities for medication safety in neonatal intensive care. *Drug Saf* 2005;28(3):251–261.
48. Williams E, Tally R. The use of failure mode effect and criticality analysis in a medication error subcommittee. *Hosp Pharm* 1994;29:331–332, 334–336, 339.
49. Bannan DF, Tully MP. Bundle interventions used to reduce prescribing and administration errors in hospitalized children: a systematic review. *J Clin Pharm Ther* 2016;41:246–255.
50. Manias E, Kinney S, Cranswick N, et al. Interventions to reduce pediatric medication errors in pediatric intensive care. *Ann Pharmacother* 2014;48(10):1313–1331.
51. Benjamin L, Frush K, Shaw K, et al. Pediatric medication safety in the emergency department. *Pediatrics* 2018;141(3):e20174066.
52. Rinke ML, Bundy DG, Velasquez CA, et al. Interventions to reduce pediatric medication errors: a systematic review. *Pediatrics* 2014;134:338.
53. Maaskant JM, Vermeulen H, Apampa B, et al. Interventions for reducing medication errors n children in hospital. *Cochrane Database Syst Rev* 2015;(30):CD006208.
54. Ghaleb MA, Barber N, Franklin BD, et al. The incidence and nature of prescribing and medication administration errors in paediatric patients. *Arch Dis Child* 2010;95:113–118.
55. Wang JK, Herzog NS, Kaushal R, et al. Prevention of pediatric medication errors by hospital pharmacists potential benefit of computerized physician order entry. *Pediatrics* 2007;119;e77.
56. Johnson KB, Lehmann CU. Electronic prescribing in pediatrics: toward safer and more effective medication management. *Pediatrics* 2013;131(4):1350–1356.
57. Kaushal R, Bates DW. Computerized physician order entry (CPOE) with clinical decision support systems (CDSSs). In: Shojania KG, Duncan BW, McDonals KM, et al., eds. *Making healthcare safer a critical analysis of patient safety practices.* Rockville, MD: Agency for Healthcare Research and Quality, 2001:59–69.
58. Bates DW, Teich J, Lee J, et al. The impact of computerized physician order entry on medication error prevention. *J Am Med Inform Assoc* 1999;6:313–321.
59. Hortman PA, Thompson CB. Evaluation of user interface satisfaction of a clinical outcomes database. *Comput Inform Nurs* 2005;23(6):301–307.
60. Lilley LL, Guanci R. Careful with the zeroes! How to minimize one of the most persistent causes of gross medication errors. *Am J Nurs* 1997;97:14.
61. Van der Zanden TM, de Wildt SN, Liem Y, et al. Developing a paediatric drug formulary for the Netherlands. *Arch Dis Child* 2017;102(4):357–361.
62. Huynh C, Wong IC, Tomlin S, et al. Medication discrepancies at transitions in pediatrics: a review of the literature. *Pediatr Drugs* 2013;15:203–215.
63. Jeffrey H, Bermann M, Chen B, et al. Incorporation of a computerized human simulator in critical care training: a preliminary report. *J Trauma* 2002;53(6):1064–1067.
64. Ringold DJ, Santell JP, Schneider PJ, et al. ASHP national survey of pharmacy practice in acute care settings: prescribing and transcribing—1998. *Am J Health Syst Pharm* 1999;56:142–157.
65. Leape LL, Cullen DJ, Clap MD, et al. Pharmacist participation on physician rounds and adverse drug events in the intensive care unit. *JAMA* 1999;282:267–270.
66. Morriss FH, Abramowitz PW, Nelson SP, et al. Effectiveness of a barcode medication administration system in reducing preventable adverse drug events in a neonatal intensive care unit: a prospective cohort study. *J Pediatr* 2009;154:363–368.
67. Hutchinson TA, Flegel KM, Kramer MS, et al. Frequency, severity and risk factors for adverse drug reactions in adult out-patients: a prospective study. *J Chronic Dis* 1986;39:533–542.
68. Hanlon JT, Schmader KE, Koronkowski MJ, et al. Adverse drug events in high risk older outpatients. *J Am Geriatr Soc* 1997;45:945–948.
69. Solanki R, Mondal N, Mahalakshmy T, et al. Medication errors by caregivers at home in neonates discharged from the neonatal intensive care unit. *Arch Dis Child* 2017;102:651–654.
70. Yin HS, Parker RM, Sanders LM, et al. Pictograms, units and dosing tools, and parent medication errors: a randomized study. *Pediatrics* 2017;140(1):e20163237.
71. American Academy of Pediatrics, Committee on Drugs. Metric units and the preferred dosing of orally administered liquid medications. *Pediatrics* 2015;135(4):784–787.
72. United States Pharmacopoeia, Center for the Advancement of Patient Safety. *Tips for parents: preventing medication errors.* Rockville, MD: United States Pharmacopoeia, Center for the Advancement of Patient Safety, 2003.

CHAPTER

65

Kelly P. Shaw
Shannon Manzi

Drug Interactions in Newborns and Children

INTRODUCTION

The administration of multiple drugs to one patient is a common occurrence, in particular when the patient is a critically or chronically ill newborn or child. Drug–drug interactions can be classified into two principal groups: pharmacokinetic, involving absorption, distribution, metabolism, or elimination; and pharmacodynamics, affecting either receptor function, biologic or physiologic control processes, or an additive or opposed pharmacologic effect.[1] The risk of drug interactions increases relative to the number of medications administered. In addition to drug–drug interactions, more is understood about drug–herb, drug-dietary supplement, and drug–food interactions. These interactions can range in severity from theoretical to clinically significant, including prolonged morbidity and even mortality. This chapter reviews key information concerning the properties and mechanisms of drug–drug interactions.

ABSORPTION/ADMINISTRATION

Simultaneous administration of enterally administered drugs sets the stage for potentially clinically significant drug–drug interactions. Absorption of drugs from the gastrointestinal (GI) tract is complex and may be impacted in a variety of ways. Numerous factors are accountable in determining the amount of drug that is absorbed by the body, including age, hydrochloric acid secretion, gastric emptying time, intestinal motility, and bile acid secretion. The primary mechanism of absorption is passive diffusion of nonionized drug molecules via the lipophilic GI mucosa.[2] Subsequently, drugs that change the pH, gastric emptying time, or GI motility will interact with the absorption of other medications. Drug interactions related to GI absorption generally fall into one of eight categories: adsorption, complexation or chelation, resin binding, increased GI motility, decreased GI motility, increased gastric pH, decreased intestinal flora, and the modification of metabolism within the GI tract.[3,4]

Interactions of adsorption are best described with activated charcoal. The large surface area of activated charcoal allows for adsorption of other drugs, and this feature is utilized advantageously in the treatment of toxic exposures and overdose.

It is well documented that some antibiotics such as fluoroquinolones and tetracyclines will bind to iron, calcium, calcium-fortified foods, and antacids if given concomitantly.[5,6] This insoluble complex puts the patient at risk for potential treatment failure based on little or no systemic absorption and may lead to the development of resistant organisms. Phenytoin is another example wherein enterally administered drug may also bind to heavy metals, as well as enteral tube feedings.[7,8] When these interactions go unrecognized, subtherapeutic phenytoin levels and a subsequent loss of seizure control may result. To best avoid such interactions, the iron, calcium, and antacids must be given either 2 hours before or 2 hours after the dose of the interacting drug. The temporary halting of continuous enteral feeding for 2 hours before and 2 hours after phenytoin administration is typically suggested.

Cholestyramine and sucralfate will physically bind other medications, such as fluoroquinolones, ketoconazole, phenytoin, warfarin, valproic acid, and digoxin. In some circumstances, administering the drug 2 hours before cholestyramine or sucralfate and monitoring for effects will be adequate. In other cases, the combination may be best avoided entirely, such as with cholestyramine and warfarin.

Increased motility can decrease drug absorption. Erythromycin, a macrolide antibiotic, is known to increase gut motility and, in recent years, has been exploited for this property as an alternative to cisapride. Cisapride was removed from the market secondary to life-threatening arrhythmias and torsades de pointes (TdP) that occurred when combined with other drugs that inhibited the cytochrome P3A4 (CYP3A4) isoenzyme, depleted electrolytes, or prolonged QT interval.[9] Historically, there was a concern regarding the impact of increasing gut motility and a potential decrease in the extent of drug absorption—for example, it was reported that the bioavailability of a digoxin tablet formulation (not *Lanoxin*) was reduced when taken concomitantly with metoclopramide therapy.[10] More recently, however, reports of the opposite effect have surfaced where tacrolimus toxicity was associated with concomitant metoclopramide therapy.[11] This drug–drug interaction is likely the result of enhanced absorption of tacrolimus secondary to metoclopramide, whereby coadministration of the metoclopramide substantially improves gastric motility and promotes the delivery of tacrolimus to the absorption sites in the small intestine. Drugs that delay gastric emptying will usually slow the transition of a drug into the small intestine, thus delaying and, possibly, decreasing absorption.

Other interactions can be exploited to enhance the absorption of a drug. Didanosine liquid is prepared with an antacid suspension to ensure adequate pH for optimal stability.[12] The role of pH in the absorption of ketoconazole is well described, as an acidic medium is required for dissolution and subsequent absorption.[13] Administration of ketoconazole in the presence of proton-pump inhibitors, H_2-blockers, or antacids severely hinders ketoconazole bioavailability. Ferrous sulfate is converted to the more absorbable ferric state in the presence of vitamin C. Many medications should be taken with food to enhance absorption, whereas some drugs should be given on an empty stomach. Often, the presence of food will delay the absorption, but not impact the overall bioavailability of the drug. Consistency, either with or without food, should be the aim for patients taking medications having the potential for fluctuations in serum levels and resultant toxicities, such as phenytoin, propranolol, and warfarin.

Intestinal flora plays an important role in body homeostasis. These bacteria, present widely in the large intestine, may have a role in drug interactions for medications that are recirculated back into the intestine after initial absorption, as in the case of enteral contraceptives. Oral contraceptives are absorbed undergoing a significant first-pass effect, are conjugated in the liver, and are subsequently eliminated via the bile.[14] Intestinal flora hydrolyzes the eliminated drug, yielding free estrogen that can then be reabsorbed. The presence of the intestinal flora is essential to maintain adequate serum concentrations of estrogen to prevent pregnancy. Although there is some controversy regarding this interaction, when a woman taking enteral contraceptives is also subject to antibiotic treatment, if intestinal flora is compromised, the estrogen level may drop, putting her at risk for unintended pregnancy.[15]

Also, P-glycoprotein, a genetically encoded and widely distributed drug transporter, has been described in significant drug interactions. P-glycoprotein is highly expressed in normal tissues throughout the body that function as barriers to drug absorption (apical border of intestinal epithelial cells), enhance drug elimination from the body (biliary canalicular or renal tubular epithelial cells), or on capillary endothelial cells at "sanctuary sites" (blood–brain barrier, testes, and placenta).[16,17] Induction and inhibition of intestinal P-glycoprotein are reported to play a role in several drug interactions.[16] For example, paclitaxel bioavailability rises in the presence of cyclosporine and clarithromycin, both potent inhibitors of P-glycoprotein, suggesting that P-glycoprotein serves as an intestinal barrier preventing paclitaxel absorption.[18] Likewise, P-glycoprotein inhibition by verapamil has been associated with improved digoxin absorption and elevated digoxin levels.[16] Drugs that modify the activity of P-glycoprotein are of particular interest in predicting the effect on direct oral anticoagulants (DOAC) as both rivaroxaban and dabigatran are known P-glycoprotein substrates.[19,20]

Drug interactions occurring during the administration phase are not only limited to the enteral route. Intravenous aminoglycoside antibiotics can be inactivated if given within 30 minutes of a penicillin derivative. Postexposure prophylaxis that requires both passive immunoglobulin and active vaccine immunization should be given at distinct injection sites on different extremities to avoid diminishing the immune response to the vaccine.

Similar to taking advantage of enteral drug interactions to enhance a drug effect, injectable drug interactions can, at times, be useful. Epinephrine, a potent vasoconstrictor, will decrease blood flow to an area. When added to a local anesthetic during laceration treatment, the epinephrine creates a more visible working environment. The lack of blood flow reduces plasma concentrations and thus minimizes the possibility of systemic toxicity. Additionally, the reduction in blood flow enhances the efficacy by slowing the clearance of anesthetic from the nerve.[21]

DISTRIBUTION

Distribution of medications is dependent on total body water, extracellular fluid, percentage of adipose tissue, and the capacity to bind to plasma proteins. Alterations in total body water and extracellular fluid become relevant for medications that are not significantly protein bound, such as in a patient with ascites. Albumin and α-1 glycoprotein are the primary circulating plasma proteins to which drugs bind. Albumin is the predominant plasma protein and binds in particular to acidic and neutral drugs, whereas α-1 glycoprotein preferentially binds basic drugs.[22] Variations in plasma protein concentration are seen secondary to certain disease states and can influence free drug concentration. Drug interactions occur because of competition for binding sites on these proteins. In effect, one drug displaces the other off the binding site, or occupies the site, not allowing the other drug to bind.

An interaction will not be clinically significant unless the involved drugs are highly protein bound (>90%) or have very narrow therapeutic indices. A classic example is phenytoin, which is not only involved in physical binding interactions discussed previously, as well as cytochrome P450 (CYP450) interactions to be discussed later, but is also generally between 89% and 93% protein bound with a very narrow therapeutic window. Concurrent administration with salicylates or valproic acid will increase the free fraction of phenytoin because of competition for the same plasma protein–binding sites.[23] Should the free fraction of phenytoin rise above 2 μg per dL, toxicity is generally seen consisting of ataxia, nystagmus, increased seizure activity, and, if high enough, coma.

METABOLISM

The liver is the most important organ involved in drug metabolism, although metabolism also occurs to a more limited extent in the blood, GI tract, kidney, lung, skin, and placenta. Drug metabolism is divided into three categories, phase I (oxidation, reduction, hydrolysis), phase II (conjugation), and phase III (drug transporters).[24] Phase I reactions generally result in a compound that is less toxic and more hydrophilic, allowing for efficient excretion. At times, phase I reactions lead to the metabolism of a parent compound or prodrug into the active metabolite (e.g., acetaminophen, methanol, enalapril). Mixed function oxidases, or the CYP450 system of enzymes, are responsible for the bulk of phase I reactions. Phase II reactions generally terminate the biologic activity of the drug and prepare it for elimination through conjugation with glucuronide, sulfate, or glycine; although the compounds have a larger molecular weight, they are more water soluble. Phase III pathways include the use of drug transporters such as P-glycoprotein, organic anion transporting polypeptides (OATPs), organic anion transporters (OATs), and organic cation transporters (OCTs).[24]

The CYP450 enzymes are unique isoenzymes found primarily in the liver and are responsible for the metabolism of many drugs and toxins (Table 65.1). The enzymes are so named

TABLE 65.1 Cytochrome P450 Substrates, Inhibitors, and Inducers

1A2	*2B6*	*2C8*	*2C9*	*2C19*	*2D6*	*2E1*	*3A3/4*
				Substrates			
Acetaminophen	Alfentanil	Amiodarone	Amitriptyline	Amitriptyline	Amitriptyline	Acetaminophen	Alfentanil
Amitriptyline	Bupropion	Amodiaquine	Candesartan	Bupropion	Amphetamine	Benzene	Alprazolam
Caffeine	Cyclophosphamide	Buprenorphine	Celecoxib	Carisoprodol	Atomoxetine	Caffeine	Amiodarone
Clomipramine	Diazepam	Carbamazepine	Diclofenac	Citalopram	Carvedilol	Chlorzoxazone	Amitriptyline
Clozapine	Efavirenz	Cerivastatin	Diltiazem	Clomipramine	Chlorpheniramine	Dapsone	Amlodipine
Cyclobenzaprine	Ifosfamide	Chloroquine	Fluoxetine	Clopidogrel	Chlorpromazine	Dextromethorphan	Atorvastatin
Duloxetine	Ketamine	Cyclophosphamide	Flurbiprofen	Cyclophosphamide	Clomipramine	Eszopiclone	Bromocriptine
Estradiol	Propofol	Dapsone	Fluvastatin	Diazepam	Clozapine	Ethanol	Budesonide
Fluvoxamine	Selegiline	Diclofenac	Glipizide	Escitalopram	Codeine	Enflurane	Bupropion
Haloperidol	Sertraline	Fluvastatin	Glyburide	Esomeprazole	Desipramine	Halothane	Buspirone
Imipramine	Tamoxifen	Ibuprofen	Ibuprofen	Fluoxetine	Dextromethorphan	Isoflurane	Caffeine
Melatonin	Valproic acid	Ifosfamide	Irbesartan	Imipramine	Diltiazem	Isoniazid	Calcium channel blockers
Mexiletine	Verapamil	Methadone	Ketoprofen	Indomethacin	Duloxetine	Sevoflurane	Carbamazepine
Naproxen		Montelukast	Losartan	Lansoprazole	Encainide	Theophylline	Cisapride
Olanzapine		Morphine	Montelukast	Nelfinavir	Flecainide	Venlafaxine	Citalopram
Ondansetron		Paclitaxel	Naproxen	Omeprazole	Fluoxetine	Verapamil	Clarithromycin
Pentazocine		Repaglinide	Phenytoin	Pantoprazole	Fluvoxamine	Zopiclone	Clomipramine
Propranolol		Rosiglitazone	Piroxicam	Phenobarbital	Haloperidol		Clonazepam
Ropivacaine		Sorafenib	Rosiglitazone	Phenytoin	Hydrocodone		Cocaine
Tacrine		Troglitazone	Sildenafil	Primidone	Imipramine		Codeine
Tamoxifen		Torsemide	Sulfamethoxazole	Progesterone	Lidocaine		Cyclophosphamide
Theophylline		Verapamil	Tamoxifen	Proguanil	Methadone		Cyclosporine
TCAs		Zopiclone	Terbinafine	Propranolol	Metoclopramide		Dapsone
Tizanidine			Torsemide	Teniposide	Metoprolol		Dexamethasone
Verapamil			Tolbutamide	TCAs	Mexiletine		Dextromethorphan
R-Warfarin			*S*-Warfarin	*R*-Warfarin	Mirtazapine		Diazepam
Zileuton			Verapamil		Nifedipine		Diltiazem
Zolmitriptan					Nortriptyline		Disopyramide
					Olanzapine		Docetaxel
					Ondansetron		Doxorubicin
					Oxycodone		Doxycycline
					Paroxetine		Ergotamine
					Perphenazine		Erythromycin
					Propafenone		Ethinyl estradiol
					Propranolol		Ethosuximide
					Risperidone		Etoposide
					Sertraline		Fentanyl
					Tamoxifen		Finasteride
					Thioridazine		Fluconazole
					Timolol		Fluoxetine
					Tramadol		Haloperidol
					Trazodone		Ifosfamide
					TCAs		Imatinib
					Venlafaxine		Imipramine
							Indinavir
							Isradipine
							Itraconazole
							Ketoconazole
							Lansoprazole
							Lidocaine
							Loratadine
							Losartan
							Lovastatin (not pravastatin)
							Methadone
							Midazolam
							Mirtazapine
							Montelukast
							Nefazodone

(continued)

TABLE 65.1 Cytochrome P450 Substrates, Inhibitors, and Inducers (*continued*)

1A2	*2B6*	*2C8*	*2C9*	*2C19*	*2D6*	*2E1*	*3A3/4*
				Substrates			
							Nicardipine
							Nifedipine
							Nimodipine
							Omeprazole
							Ondansetron
							Paclitaxel
							Paroxetine
							Pimozide
							Progesterone
							Protease inhibitors
							Quetiapine
							Quinidine
							Quinine
							Rifabutin
							Rifampin
							Risperidone
							Ritonavir
							Salmeterol
							Saquinavir
							Sertraline
							Sildenafil
							Simvastatin
							Tacrolimus
							Tamoxifen
							Theophylline
							Trazodone
							Triazolam
							TCAs
							Venlafaxine
							Verapamil
							Vinca alkaloids
							Warfarin
							Zolpidem
				Inhibitors			
Amiodarone	Clopidogrel	Abiraterone	Amiodarone	Cimetidine	Amiodarone	Disulfiram	Amiodarone
Cimetidine	Mifepristone	Amitriptyline	Cimetidine	Delavirdine	Bupropion	Methylpyrazole	Boceprevir
Ciprofloxacin	Thiotepa	Gemfibrozil	Clopidogrel	Efavirenz	Celecoxib		Cimetidine
Clarithromycin	Ticlopidine	Ketoconazole	Efavirenz	Esomeprazole	Chloroquine		Ciprofloxacin
Erythromycin		Lapatinib	Fenofibrate	Felbamate	Chlorpheniramine		Clarithromycin
Estrogens		Montelukast	Fluconazole	Fluconazole	Chlorpromazine		Clotrimazole
Fluoxetine		Terfenadine	Fluorouracil	Fluoxetine	Cimetidine		Cobicistat
Fluvoxamine		Teriflunomide	Fluoxetine	Fluvoxamine	Citalopram		Cyclosporine
Gatifloxacin		Triazolam	Fluvastatin	Indomethacin	Clemastine		Diltiazem
Grapefruit juice		Trimethoprim	Fluvoxamine	Isoniazid	Clomipramine		Erythromycin
Interferon			Isoniazid	Ketoconazole	Cocaine		Fluconazole
			Lovastatin	Lansoprazole	Diphenhydramine		Fluoxetine
			Metronidazole	Omeprazole	Doxorubicin		Fluvoxamine
			Miconazole	Paroxetine	Duloxetine		Grapefruit juice
			Paroxetine	Ritonavir	Eliglustat		Imatinib
			Phenylbutazone	Ticlopidine	Escitalopram		Indinavir
			Probenecid	Topiramate	Fluoxetine		Itraconazole
			Ritonavir	Voriconazole	Haloperidol		Itraconazole
			Sertraline		Hydroxyzine		Ketoconazole
			Sulfadiazine		Imatinib		Lopinavir/Ritonavir
			Sulfamethoxazole-trimethoprim		Indinavir		Miconazole
			Teniposide		Methadone		Nefazodone
			Valproate		Metoclopramide		Nifedipine
			Voriconazole		Paroxetine		Omeprazole
			Zafirlukast		Perphenazine		Propoxyphene
					Propoxyphene		Protease inhibitors

TABLE 65.1 Cytochrome P450 Substrates, Inhibitors, and Inducers (*continued*)

1A2	*2B6*	*2C8*	*2C9*	*2C19*	*2D6*	*2E1*	*3A3/4*
					Quinidine		Saquinavir
					Quinine		Telaprevir
					Ranitidine		Tipranavir/Ritonavir
					Ritonavir		Verapamil
					Sertraline		Voriconazole
					Terbinafine		Zafirlukast
					Thioridazine		
					Ticlopidine		
					Tipranavir/Ritonavir		
Inducers							
Broccoli	Carbamazepine	Cortisol	Aprepitant	Carbamazepine	Pregnancy	Chronic ethanol	Armodafinil
Brussels sprouts	Efavirenz	Dabrafenib	Carbamazepine	Norethindrone		Isoniazid	Bosentan
Carbamazepine	Nevirapine	Dexamethasone	Ethanol	Phenobarbital		Ritonavir	Carbamazepine
Charbroiled food	Phenobarbital	Phenobarbital	Phenobarbital	Phenytoin		Tobacco	Dexamethasone
Cigarette smoke	Phenytoin	Rifampin	Phenytoin	Prednisone			Efavirenz
Modafinil	Rifampin		Primidone	Rifampin			Griseofulvin
Nafcillin	Ritonavir		Rifabutin	St. John's wort			Modafinil
Omeprazole			Rifampin	Tipranavir/Ritonavir			Nafcillin
Phenobarbital			Secobarbital				Nevirapine
Phenytoin							Phenobarbital
Rifampin							Phenytoin
Ritonavir							Prednisone
Tobacco							Primidone
							Rifabutin
							Rifampin
							Ritonavir
							St. John's wort
							Sulfinpyrazone
							Troglitazone

Data from http://medicine.uipui.edu/flockhart/table.htm; Shannon M. Drug-drug interactions and the cytochrome P450 system: an update. *Pediatr Emerg Care* 1997;13(5):350–353; Totah RA, Terrie AE. Cytochrome P450 2C8: substrates, inhibitors, pharmacogenetics, and clinical relevance. *Clin Pharm Ther* 2005;77:341–352; Taketomo CK, Hodding JH, Kraus DM. *Pediatric dosage handbook*, 10th ed. Cleveland, OH: Lexicomp Inc, 2003–2004; and Flockhart DA. Drug interactions: cytochrome P450 drug interaction table. Indiana University School of Medicine, 2007. https://drug-interactions.medicine.iu.edu/MainTable.aspx. Accessed May 26, 2020.
TCAs, tricyclic antidepressants.

because of the absorption of light at a wavelength of 450 nm and are grouped into families 1, 2, and 3 and then divided into subfamilies A to E.[25] The individual member enzymes are then further designated by a number (e.g., 3A4, 2D6). These enzymes are genetically encoded and, therefore, are associated with interpatient variability and the subject of the study of pharmacogenomics (PGx). While we will touch on PG influences below, an in-depth discussion is outside the scope of this chapter. Age-related development of CYP450 enzymes after the age of 6 months matures and even surpasses adult capacity during the first year of life.[26]

Inducers are drugs that are capable of enhancing CYP450 enzyme activity by increasing enzyme synthesis. These drugs will augment the enzyme's metabolizing capacity, speeding up substrate drug metabolism, and decreasing the object drug effect.[27] The time onset of enzyme induction is dependent on the half-life of the inducing drug. An inducer such as phenobarbital, with a long half-life, can take up to a week to have an impact. In contrast, a decrease in the concentration of a drug metabolized by CYP2C9 can occur within 24 hours after the initiation of rifampin, a rapid and potent inducer.[28]

The inhibition of CYP450 enzymes may occur secondary to competitive binding between two drugs or permanent inactivation.[29] Generally, inhibition begins after the first dose of the inhibitor, and the duration of inhibition correlates with the half-life of the drug. Most commonly, these interactions result in the slowdown of substrate drug metabolism, yielding increased plasma concentrations, increased drug effect, and thereby increased risk of adverse events. Drugs have been intentionally combined to exploit CYP450 inhibition; the protease inhibitor ritonavir, a potent CYP3A4 inhibitor, is added to lopinavir and elvitegravir to boost serum levels in patients with human immunodeficiency virus.[30,31]

CYP1A2

Nearly 10% of medications used today are metabolized by cytochrome 1A2 (CYP1A2), most notably caffeine, theophylline, lidocaine, tricyclic antidepressants, and warfarin as well as endogenous compounds such as melatonin and estradiol.[32] The activity of CYP1A2 can be induced by cigarette smoke, charbroiled foods, and cruciferous vegetables (e.g., cabbage, broccoli). Several medications can also affect CYP1A2 activity. Phenobarbital, carbamazepine, and rifampin induce CYP1A2 as well as several other enzymes, leading to clinically relevant drug interactions. Inhibitors of CYP1A2 include cimetidine, ciprofloxacin, erythromycin, fluvoxamine, and grapefruit juice. Omeprazole and ritonavir simultaneously induce CYP1A2 and inhibit one or more other enzymes.

CYP2A6

The role of CYP2A6 has more recently begun to be understood and has gained increasing interest. The enzyme is involved in the metabolism of several clinically relevant substrates, most notably nicotine, caffeine, letrozole, and efavirenz.[33] The gene encoding CYP2A6 is highly polymorphic, with greater than 40 variants identified. Most of the polymorphisms occur more commonly in Caucasians and Africans, while a few variants are more frequent among Asians and Alaskan Natives. In addition to CYP2A6 genetics creating variable expression, the enzyme is known to be induced by drugs, such as phenobarbital, dexamethasone, estrogen, and rifampin.[33] Both methoxsalen and selegiline inhibit CYP2A6 through irreversible binding. Current interest in CYP2A6 is driven in part by the impact on nicotine metabolism. As the primary enzyme responsible for nicotine conversion to the inactive cotinine, it appears to play a role in modulating smoking behaviors.

CYP2B6

While 2B6 is the principal isoform for drug metabolism in the CYP2B family, even at full maturity, 2B6 is expressed at low levels relative to other CYP enzymes. The significance of cytochrome 2B6 (CYP2B6) in drug metabolism is still not completely known. CYP2B6 is genetically polymorphic and is implicated in the metabolism of a growing number of clinically important drugs. It is estimated that nearly 8% of drugs on the market are metabolized via CYP2B6, and this has been on the rise with the continued introduction of new drugs.[34,35] Clinically used drugs that are known to be metabolized by CYP2B6 include chemotherapeutics such as cyclophosphamide, ifosfamide, the antiestrogen tamoxifen, as well as efavirenz, ketamine, propofol, and diazepam.[36,37] Ritonavir, a protease inhibitor, is known to be a CYP2B6 inducer, which may explain the increased elimination of several drugs as demonstrated with bupropion.[38] Genetic polymorphisms resulting in poor metabolizer status occur in approximately 3% of Caucasians and up to 20% of African Americans. This phenotype seems to predict a more complicated clinical course and higher risk of toxicity-driven drug discontinuation.[34]

CYP2C8

Cytochrome 2C8 (CYP2C8) has been recognized as an enzyme of greater importance over the past decade due in part to the recognition of serious adverse events associated with gemfibrozil, a potent inhibitor of 2C8.[39] Comprising approximately 7% of total microsomal CYP content in the liver, it carries out oxidative metabolism in nearly 5% of drugs cleared via phase I processes.[40] Therapeutic agents metabolized by CYP2C8 include paclitaxel, amiodarone, rosiglitazone, cerivastatin, and fluvastatin. Known inhibitors of CYP2C8 consist of trimethoprim, gemfibrozil, montelukast, and ketoconazole, as well as several known CYP3A4 substrates—amitriptyline, terfenadine, and triazolam—causing up to 50% inhibition of CYP2C8 activity.[40] Of note, drugs that were approved for use prior to the role of 2C8 recognition may have deficient or incorrect product information about their potential for drug interactions.[41] Several genetic polymorphisms have been identified with CYP2C8, the most common of which is seen in roughly 18% of African Americans and rarely in Caucasians.

CYP2C9

Cytochrome 2C9 (CYP2C9) is the most abundant enzyme among the CYP2C subfamily and is a major factor in drug metabolism. Responsible for the metabolism of several common medications, including ibuprofen, carvedilol, celecoxib, losartan, phenytoin, glyburide, and warfarin, CYP2C9 contributes to the metabolism of roughly 15% of all drugs utilizing the P450 pathways.[28,42] Rifampin and rifabutin are powerful inducers of CYP2C9 activity and will, therefore, decrease serum concentrations of the above substrates. Other inducers include carbamazepine, ethanol, and phenobarbital. Warfarin is produced as a racemic mixture of *R*-warfarin and *S*-warfarin, with the *S*-enantiomer being responsible for the predominance of pharmacologic activity. *S*-Warfarin is principally metabolized via CYP2C9; inhibition of this enzyme pathway results in a clinically significant drug–drug interaction, such that the Food and Drug Administration approved updated labeling for warfarin in 2007 remarking on this pharmacogenetic issue.[43] More recently, in 2014, the Clinical Pharmacogenetics Implementation Consortium (CPIC) released a guideline on dosing phenytoin/fosphenytoin based on CYP2C9 variants.[44] Known inhibitors of CYP2C9 include fluconazole, ketoconazole, metronidazole, amiodarone, lovastatin, and even several flavonoids, secondary metabolites of many plants consumed by humans in a typical diet.[45] Genetic polymorphisms occur in up to one-third of Caucasians, contributing to abnormally decreased enzyme activity in these individuals.[46]

CYP2C19

Like several other monoamine oxidases, cytochrome 2C19 (CYP2C19) has been shown to exhibit a genetic polymorphism; 3% to 6% of Caucasians, 15% to 20% of Japanese, and 10% to 20% of African Americans are poor metabolizers.[47,48] Medications metabolized by CYP2C19 include several benzodiazepines, citalopram, tricyclic antidepressants, omeprazole, and certain selective serotonin reuptake inhibitors (SSRIs), as well as the antiepileptics clobazam, phenobarbital, and valproic acid.[49,50] The isoenzyme is of major relevance to antineoplastic and antiepileptic drug interactions. Induction or inhibition of CYP2C19 can cause a decrease in antineoplastic drug concentrations. Similarly, enzyme inhibition or induction by antineoplastic drugs may lead to toxicity or loss of seizure control. This complex relationship is important, particularly in the treatment of patients with brain cancer, however, the role of 2C19 in the metabolism of newer drugs to market has become of less relevance.[35,46] Known inducers of CYP2C19 include carbamazepine, phenytoin, rifampin, and phenobarbital, whereas inhibitors include fluoxetine, sertraline, fluvoxamine, omeprazole, ritonavir, and isoniazid.[51]

CYP2D6

Cytochrome 2D6 (CYP2D6) is an extensively studied polymorphic drug-metabolizing enzyme. Although it comprises a relatively small percentage (2% to 6%) of the total CYP450 in the liver, it is involved in the metabolism of many drugs, up to 25% of all drugs.[52] Greater than 160 medications rely on CYP2D6 for metabolism, including β-blockers, analgesics, antidepressants, and antiemetics, though fewer drugs approved in the recent years rely heavily on this pathway.[35,53] Approximately 7% to 10% of Caucasians are poor metabolizers of medications utilizing CYP2D6; these patients are then at risk for drug accumulation and toxicity from substrates of this enzyme, such as amitriptyline, flecainide, metoprolol, paroxetine, and risperidone.[28] The conversion of codeine to the active form, morphine, is catalyzed by CYP2D6; therefore, patients with low enzyme activity demonstrate a poor analgesic response, and those with an ultrarapid metabolizer phenotype can experience severe life-threatening episodes of apnea. The predictability of this response has prompted discussion in favor of genotype-influenced rational prescribing.[54]

Unlike other CYP450 enzymes, there are no known inducers of this activity, except pregnancy. Several medications inhibit CYP2D6; the most potent include cimetidine, diphenhydramine, fluoxetine, haloperidol, paroxetine, and codeine.

CYP2E1

Although cytochrome 2E1 (CYP2E1) metabolizes a relatively small fraction of medications, approximately 1.5% metabolic activity in the liver, this enzyme plays a significant role in the activation and inactivation of toxins.[48] CYP2E1 metabolizes primarily small organic molecules (e.g., ethanol, carbon tetrachloride) as well as acetaminophen and dapsone. The product of acetaminophen's CYP2E1 metabolism is a highly reactive intermediate, *N*-acetyl-*p*-benzoquinoneimine (NAPQI), a hepatotoxin that must be detoxified by conjugation with glutathione. Chronic ethanol use, as seen in patients with alcohol dependence, results in increased risk for hepatotoxicity secondary to acetaminophen due to the ethanol induction of CYP2E1 as well as a secondary depletion of glutathione stores.[55] Induction of CYP2E1 leads to a greater percentage of acetaminophen being metabolized to NAPQI. Research continues to explore the benefits of using inhibitors such as disulfiram to prevent the toxicity associated with some CYP2E1 metabolites.[55]

CYP3A3/4

Cytochrome 3A (CYP3A) is both the most abundant and clinically significant family of CYP450 enzymes. CYP3A4's role as the major metabolic pathway for medications has increased from 40% in the established drug list to 64% in the newly approved drug list.[56] The CYP3A family comprises four major enzymes: CYP3A4, CYP3A5, CYP3A7, and CYP3A43. CYP3A4 is the most common and is frequently referenced in drug interaction references. Because these enzymes are so closely related (most are 97% similar), they are often referred to as the subfamily name, CYP3A. Close to 60% of the liver's total CYP450 is CYP3A, and the presence of CYP3A in the small intestine results in decreased bioavailability of many drugs.[57] Among the many significant CYP3A inhibitors are grapefruit juice, the macrolides erythromycin and clarithromycin, the antifungals ketoconazole and itraconazole, the antidepressants fluoxetine and fluvoxamine, the anti-HIV agent ritonavir, and calcium channel blockers such as verapamil.

Clopidogrel, an enteral antiplatelet medication, is metabolized to an active thiol metabolite by the CYP3A4 enzyme. Variability in patient response has led to the investigation of the mechanism, which has been at least partly attributed to drug–drug interactions in some patients.[58] Intake of calcium channel blockers, known to inhibit CYP3A, has been associated with reduced efficacy of clopidogrel to inhibit platelet aggregation. It is, however, this same interaction, inhibition of CYP3A that permits the use of ritonavir as a boosting agent for other protease inhibitors.[59,60]

CYP3A inducers include dexamethasone, rifampin, carbamazepine, phenobarbital, and phenytoin. Following the resurgence of tuberculosis (TB) in the United States in the late 1980s through early 1990s, the annual rate of TB has declined steadily. Unfortunately, however, that decrease has now slowed, and the proportion of multidrug-resistant TB cases contributed by foreign-born persons continues to rise.[61] Given these data, it is not surprising that rifampin, an inducer of the CYP3A subfamily, continues to play a role in clinically relevant drug interactions. Of particular clinical significance is the potential reduction of enteral contraceptive efficacy by rifampin, since estradiol levels can be reduced by rifampin-mediated CYP3A induction.[47]

N-ACETYLTRANSFERASE

Acetylation is a unique, non-CYP pathway of drug metabolism. Dapsone, hydralazine, isoniazid, procainamide, and sulfonamides are examples of drugs metabolized via acetylation. Acetylation polymorphisms, being discovered nearly 70 years ago, are well described.[62] Variants in the alleles coding for the conjugating *N*-acetyltransferase enzymes occur in nearly half of Americans, resulting in slow acetylators. Slow acetylator phenotypes occur in 60% to 70% of Northern Europeans and 5% to 10% of Asians.[63] These slow acetylators demonstrate enhanced toxicity but longer drug effectiveness. The fast acetylator phenotypes may not demonstrate the desired therapeutic response to treatment. Genotype-based dosing for isoniazid has been shown to decrease the risk of drug-induced liver injury (DILI) while not resulting in increased treatment failure.[64]

HUMAN ETHER-A-GO-GO–RELATED GENE

The human ether-a-go-go-related (*hERG*) gene is responsible for the potassium channels mediating ventricular repolarization.[65] Drug-induced cardiac arrhythmias, specifically TdP, are of considerable concern, in particular in patients genetically predisposed to long QT syndrome. Genetic abnormalities predispose patients to either long QT syndrome or short QT syndrome, both of which could result in fatal cardiac arrhythmia.[66] The potassium channel is also sensitive to drug binding, as well as changes in extracellular potassium levels, both of which may give rise to decreased channel function and subsequent acquired long QT syndrome. Drugs that can cause QT prolongation include antiarrhythmics (especially Class 1A and Class III), antipsychotics, quinolones, and macrolide antibiotics. The administration of drugs metabolized by CYP3A4 oxidases, such as terfenadine, cisapride, pimozide, and astemizole, are particularly vulnerable when coadministered with agents that inhibit CYP3A4, such as ketoconazole, erythromycin, and clarithromycin.[67]

ELIMINATION/EXCRETION

Elimination and excretion of drugs occur primarily via the kidneys. Biliary secretion, plasma esterases, and other minor pathways are important routes, albeit less common than renal elimination. Renal elimination is dependent on multiple factors, such as glomerular filtration rate, tubular secretion, and tubular reabsorption.

Glomerular filtration hinges upon the protein-binding characteristics of the drug and the glomerular filtration rate. Changes in glomerular filtration rate are often the result of changes in blood pressure or glomerular hydrostatic pressure—both of which can be the result of drug therapy.[68] Drug interactions occurring under these circumstances are considered indirect interactions, as it is the nephrotoxicity induced by one drug that causes the adverse effects of the object drug. For example, excessive antihypertensive therapy may result in diminished renal blood flow. In such a case, drugs primarily eliminated via glomerular filtration will accumulate and have the potential to cause toxicity.[69]

Urinary alkalinization or acidification by some medications can cause others to be more (or less) readily excreted. Other agents can inhibit renal tubular secretion and assist in maintaining higher serum concentrations than the body would otherwise allow. A classic example is the use of probenecid and penicillin, secondary to probenecid blocking the tubular secretion of β-lactams.[70] More recently, probenecid has been studied for use with the antiviral oseltamivir for treatment and prophylaxis in the event of an influenza pandemic.[71] Oseltamivir is administered as a prodrug, which is rapidly hydrolyzed to its active metabolite, which is then subject to excretion via glomerular filtration and renal tubular secretion. Administration of probenecid results in marked reductions in renal clearance and subsequent elevations in plasma area under the curve. Researchers are hopeful that this interaction can be exploited to allow for considerable dose saving.[28] In contrast, probenecid has also become an integral part of the regimen for decreasing the nephrotoxic effects of cidofovir by limiting the exposure of renal proximal tubular cells to the drug.[72] Finally, probenecid should not be used with sulfonamides, ketorolac, or methotrexate because of increased serum concentrations and half-life, resulting in increased toxicity.[73]

An additional interaction involving renal tubular secretion that can be potentially detrimental is that of methotrexate and the proton-pump inhibitor omeprazole. By inhibiting hydrogen ions (protons) in the renal tubules, omeprazole may also inhibit methotrexate elimination as it is actively secreted in the distal tubules with hydrogen ions via the H^+/K^+-ATPase pump.[74] A more recent trial supports this interaction via another mechanism: here, four proton-pump inhibitors were analyzed and demonstrated a significant inhibition of breast cancer resistance protein-mediated transport of methotrexate for elimination.[75] These interactions can result in prolonged elevated serum concentrations, particularly concerning after treatment with a high-dose regimen for cancer therapy.

Interactions involving the use of potassium-sparing diuretics such as spironolactone with drugs or herbal supplements that can increase serum potassium levels are also concerning. Here serum potassium escalates secondary to a drug-induced impairment of the renin–angiotensin–aldosterone system that regulates potassium excretion.[76] Following the publication of the findings that mortality was significantly lowered in patients on spironolactone in the Randomized Aldosterone Evaluation Study (RALES), reports of hyperkalemia climbed.[76,77] Impaired renal function and the addition of several other medications are thought to compound the retention of potassium. For this reason, when combined with spironolactone, the following agents can increase potassium, possibly leading to hyperkalemia and cardiac arrest if not intercepted: nonsteroidal anti-inflammatory drugs, COX-2 inhibitors, angiotensin-converting enzyme inhibitors, angiotensin II receptor antagonists, β-blockers, cyclosporine, tacrolimus, heparin, ketoconazole, trimethoprim, and pentamidine.[78–80] Patients receiving these medications with spironolactone warrant intensive monitoring of renal function and potassium levels.

OATPs, OATs, AND OCTs: THE ORGANIC ANION AND CATION TRANSPORTERS OF THE *SLCO* AND *SLC22A* GENE SUPERFAMILIES

Many drugs stem from organic anions or cations whose disposition and elimination rely on the function of specific drug transporters that belong to two major superfamilies. Individual members of these superfamilies are expressed in nearly every epithelium within the body. OATPs, of which several have been identified, mediate a wide range of compounds, including bile acids and steroid conjugates. OATP1A2 is thought to play a role in the absorption, distribution, and elimination of xenobiotics. OAT2A1 has been identified throughout the body with action as a prostaglandin transporter. OATP substrates include a number of medications, such as statins, sartans, antibiotics, and some anticancer drugs.[81] OATPs are recognized as potential pathways for drug–drug interactions; for example, cyclosporine is a strong inhibitor of OATP-mediated transport and has been associated with elevated levels of statin drugs.[82]

OATs mediate the transport of a wide range of low-molecular weight substrates that include various drugs and toxins as well as steroid hormone conjugates. Early evidence suggests that OATs may be stimulated by agents that activate protein kinase A (PKA). Studies elucidating the relationships between drugs that stimulate PKA and the further effect on OATs and drugs mediated by OATs will be important. Probenecid is a known inhibitor of OAT3 and OAT1 action, the precise transporters utilized by methotrexate for elimination.[83] OAT transport is understood to increase in an acidic pH, and it is believed that the higher urinary pH in the presence of probenecid is responsible for a decrease in OAT1- and OAT3-mediated clearance and renal elimination of β-lactam antibiotics.[84]

OCTs are also multispecific uptake transporters that are expressed in epithelia throughout the body. As with the OATPs and OATs, it appears that a potential risk associated with the system is that of drug–drug interactions. OCT1 variations have been associated with altered pharmacokinetics of both metformin and imatinib.[81,85] Serotonin uptake into the liver is essential for its elimination; this uptake, mediated by OCT1, has been shown to be inhibited with the coadministration of other commonly prescribed medications, including diphenhydramine, fluoxetine, and verapamil.[86] Further study will likely uncover OATP, OAT, and OCT involvement in the mechanism of additional drug–drug interactions.

SUMMARY

The mechanisms of drug interactions are varied, typically including object and subject drugs though may include herbal supplements and foods. As the knowledge of drug interactions increases, it is important to have on-hand drug interaction

TABLE 65.2 Questions to Help the Clinician Detect Drug Interactions

1. Identification of the nature of the interaction
- Is there a potential interaction between a drug and another drug, disease, food, nutrition, or a combination of any of these factors?

2. Understanding the mode of action of the interaction
- Can the pharmacokinetic interaction be explained in terms of absorption, distribution, metabolism, or elimination of the drug?
- Is the interaction pharmacodynamic?
- What is the time course of the interaction? Several factors will affect the time course of the interaction, such as the mechanism of the interaction, the pharmacokinetics of the object drug, the nature of the interacting drug (inhibitor, inductor, substrate), the sequence of prescription, and the baseline concentration of the target drug.[a]
- Is this interaction well documented in published work, or are there strong suspicions (theoretical or clinical) to expect that an adverse drug interaction might take place?
- Would the potential interaction appear when a drug is added or discontinued?

3. Identification of potential or real clinical outcomes for the patient
- What are the short- and long-term clinical outcomes for the patient?
- Is the patient having new problems (e.g., falls and gait difficulties, bleeding, blood pressure changes, confusion) that can be explained by a drug interaction?
- Does the patient have risk factors that might increase the likelihood of an adverse outcome (e.g., with regard to comorbidities, other drugs that are taken, dose and duration of treatment, pharmacogenetics)?[b]

4. Monitoring and follow-up for potential drug interactions
- Is an appropriate monitoring plan in place—e.g., INR, serum drug concentration, electrolytes, blood pressure, glucose concentration, and who is responsible for the follow-up to promote continuity of care? Does this plan account for the estimated time course of the interaction?[c]
- Are caregivers vigilant to monitor for the appearance of new symptoms after any changes to drug treatment?
- Has the drug interaction been documented in the patient's medical record?

[a] For example, a patient on chronic treatment with a drug that induces CYP3A4, (e.g., rifampicin) who is then given a CYP3A4 substrate will experience little or no effect from the CYP3A4 substrate, starting with the very first dose of the substrate. If, however, the same two drugs are given, but the inducer is added to the substrate, the interaction will take much longer to develop. Another example would be a patient who is just on the verge of toxic effects from drug A when an inhibitor of drug A's metabolism is added (drug B). Drug A might normally take days to achieve a new steady-state serum concentration when drug B (inhibitor of drug A) is added. In most people, the interaction would be delayed. However, if the patient was only a few drug molecules away from toxicity, he may develop toxic effects in less than 24 hours.
[b] For example, a patient on warfarin who is started on thyroid supplement for hypothyroid is at higher risk of over-anticoagulation and bleeding than a patient on chronic thyroid supplement treatment who is started on warfarin.
[c] For example, it can take 7 to 10 days for the international normalized ratio (INR) to stabilize after a patient on warfarin starts taking a CYP2C9 inhibitor.
Reproduced from Mallet L. The challenge of managing drug interactions in elderly people. *Lancet* 2007;370:185–191, with permission.

resources available to ensure patient safety. Being informed about the potential for drug interactions is the best way to prevent them from occurring. Moreover, understanding the mechanisms of drug interactions will assist all clinicians in avoiding these serious, often, preventable events (Table 65.2). It is important to bear in mind that although interactions follow a predictable pattern, there is often interpatient variability. Any potential interaction must be evaluated using patient-specific data to best determine the most beneficial course of action.

REFERENCES

1. Palleria C, Di Paolo A, Giofre C, et al. Pharmacokinetic drug-drug interaction and their implication in clinical management. *J Res Med Sci* 2013;18(7):601–610.
2. Peck T, Hill S, Williams M. Drug passage across the cell membrane. In: Peck T, Williams M, *eds. Pharmacology for anesthesia and intensive care*, 3rd ed. New York, NY: Cambridge University Press, 2008.
3. Tripathi J, Thapa P, Maharjan R, et al. Current state and future perspectives on gastroretentive drug delivery systems. *Pharmaceutics* 2019;11(4). doi:10.3390/pharmaceutics11040193.
4. Lopes CM, Bettencourt C, Rossi A, et al. Overview on gastroretentive drug delivery systems for improving drug bioavailability. *Int J Pharm* 2016;510:144–158.
5. Wallace AW, Victory JM, Amsden GW. Lack of bioequivalence when levofloxacin and calcium-fortified orange juice are coadministered to healthy volunteers. *J Clin Pharmacol* 2003;43(5):539–544.
6. Neuhofel AL, Wilton JH, Victory JM, et al. Lack of bioequivalence of ciprofloxacin when administered with calcium-fortified orange juice: a new twist on an old interaction. *J Clin Pharmacol* 2002;42(4):461–466.
7. Au Yeung SC, Ensom MH. Phenytoin and enteral feedings: does evidence support an interaction? *Ann Pharmacother* 2000;34(7–8):896–905.
8. Faraji B, Yu PP. Serum phenytoin levels of patients on gastrostomy tube feeding. *J Neurosci Nurs* 1998;30:55–59.
9. Cisapride withdrawn because of cardiac side effects. *Pharm J* 2000;265:152. https://www.pharmaceutical-journal.com/cisapride-withdrawn-because-of-cardiac-side-effects/20002355.article?firstPass=false.
10. Manninen V, Melin J, Apajalahti A, et al. Altered absorption of digoxin in patients given propantheline and metoclopramide. *Lancet* 1973;301:398–400.
11. Prescott WA Jr, Callahan BL, Park JM. Tacrolimus toxicity associated with concomitant metoclopramide therapy. *Pharmacotherapy* 2004;24(4):532–537.
12. Videx (Didanosine) package insert. Princeton, NJ: Bristol Meyers Squibb, 2018.
13. Nizoral (Ketoconazole) package insert. Titusville, NJ: Janssen Pharmaceuticals Inc. 2013.
14. Bolt HM. Interactions between clinically used drugs and oral contraceptives. *Environ Health Perspect* 1994;102(Suppl 9):35–38.
15. Summers A. Interaction of antibiotics and enteral contraceptives. *Emerg Nurs* 2008;16(6):20–21.
16. Lin JH, Yamazaki M. Role of P-glycoprotein in pharmacokinetics. *Clin Pharmacokinet* 2003;42(1):59–98.
17. Mealey KL, Fidel J. P glycoprotein mediated drug interactions in animals and humans with cancer. *J Vet Intern Med* 2015;29:1–6.
18. Patel K, Patil A, Mehta M, et al. Oral delivery of paclitaxel nanocrystal (PNC) with dual Pgp-CYP3A4 inhibitor: preparation, characterization and antitumor activity. *Int J Pharm* 2014;472(1–2):214–223.
19. Vazquez SR. Drug-drug interactions in an era of multiple anticoagulants: a focus on clinically relevant drug interactions. *Hematology Am Soc Hematol Educ Program* 2018;2018(1):339–347. doi:10.1182/asheducation-2018.1.339.
20. Kawabata M, Yokoyama Y, Sasano T, et al. Bleeding events and activated partial thromboplastin time with dabigatran in clinical practice. *J Cardiol* 2013;62:121–126.
21. Sinnott CJ, Cogswell LP, Johnson A, et al. On the mechanism by which epinephrine potentiates lidocaine's peripheral nerve block. *Anesthesiology* 2003;98:181–188.
22. Kremer JM, Wilting J, Janssen LH. Drug binding to human alpha-1-acid glycoprotein in health and disease. *Pharmacol Rev* 1988;40(1):1–47.
23. Perucca E, Hebdige S, Frigo GM, et al. Interaction between phenytoin and valproic acid: plasma protein binding and metabolic effects. *Clin Pharmacol Ther* 1980;28(6):779–789.
24. Almazroo OA, Miah MK, Venkataramanan R. Drug metabolism in the liver. *Clin Liv Dis* 2017;21(1):1–20.

25. Guengerich FP, Waterman MR, Egli M. Recent structural insights into cytochrome P450 function. *Trends Pharmacol Sci* 2016;37(8):625–640.
26. Kearns GL, Abdel-Rahman SM, Alander SW, et al. Developmental pharmacology—drug disposition, action, and therapy in infants and children. *N Engl J Med* 2003;349:1157–1167.
27. Li GC, Yang L, Zhou SF. Interactions between Chinese herbal medicines and drugs. *Aust J Acupunct Chin Med* 2007;2(1):17–24.
28. Lynch T, Price A. The effect of cytochrome P450 metabolism on drug response, interactions, and adverse effects. *Am Fam Physician* 2007;76:391–396.
29. Shannon M. Drug-drug interactions and the cytochrome P450 system: an update. *Pediatr Emerg Care* 1997;13(5):350–353.
30. Molto J, Barbanoh MJ, Miranda C, et al. Simultaneous population pharmacokinetic model for lopinavir and ritonavir in HIV-infected adults. *Clin Pharmacokinet* 2008;47(10):681–692.
31. Mathias AA, West S, Hui J, et al. Dose-response of ritonavir on hepatic CYP3A activity and elvitegravir enteral exposure. *Clin Pharm Ther* 2009;85(1):64–70.
32. Zhou SF, Wang B, Yang LP, et al. Structure, function, regulation and polymorphism and the clinical significance of human cytochrome P450 1A2. *Drug Metab Rev* 2010;42(2):268–354.
33. Tanner J-A, Tyndale RF. Variation in CYP2A6 activity and personalized medicine. *J Pers Med* 2017;7(4):18. doi:10.3390/jpm7040018.
34. Nolan D, Phillips E, Mallal S. Efavirenz and CYP2B6 polymorphism: implications for drug toxicity and resistance. *Clin Infect Dis* 2006;42:408–410.
35. Yu J, Zhou Z, Owens KH, et al. What can be learned from recent new drug applications? A systematic review of drug interaction data for drugs approved by the US FDA in 2015. *Drug Metab Dispos* 2017;45:86–108.
36. Turpeinen M, Raunio H, Pelkonen O. The functional role of CYP2B6 in human drug metabolism: substrates and inhibitors in vitro, in vivo and in silico. *Curr Drug Metab* 2006;7(7):705–714.
37. Hodgson E, Rose RL. The importance of cytochrome P450 2B6 in the human metabolism of environmental chemicals. *Pharmacol Ther* 2007;113:420–428.
38. Kharasch ED, Mitchell D, Coles R, et al. Rapid clinical induction of hepatic cytochrome P450B6 activity by ritonavir. *Antimicrob Agents Chemother* 2008;52(5):1663–1669.
39. Backman JT, Filppula AM, Niemi M, et al. Role of cytochrome P450 2C8 in drug metabolism and interactions. *Pharmacol Rev* 2016;68:168–241.
40. Totah RA, Terrie AE. Cytochrome P450 2C8: substrates, inhibitors, pharmacogenetics, and clinical relevance. *Clin Pharm Ther* 2005;77:341–352.
41. Filppula AM, Laitila J, Neuvonen PJ, et al. Reevaluation of the microsomal metabolism of montelukast: major contribution by CYP2C8 at clinically relevant concentrations. *Drug Metab Dispos* 2011;39(5):904–911.
42. Daly AK, Rettie AE, Fowler DM, et al. Pharmacogenomics of CYP2C9: functional and clinical considerations. *J Pers Med* 2018;8(1).doi:10.3390/jpm8010001.
43. Huang S-M, Temple R. Is this drug or dose for you?: impact and consideration of ethnic factors in global drug development, regulatory review, and clinical practice. *Clin Pharm Ther* 2008;84(3):287–294.
44. Caudle KE, Rettie AE, Whirl-Carrillo M, et al. Clinical pharmacogenetics implementation consortium guidelines for CYP2C9 and HLA-B genotypes and phenytoin dosing. *Nature* 2014;96:542–548.
45. Si D, Wang Y, Guo Y, et al. Mechanism of CYP2C9 inhibition by flavones and flavonols. *Drug Metab Dispos* 2009;37:629–634.
46. Lee C, Goldstein JA, Pieper JA. Cytochrome P450 2C9 polymorphisms: a comprehensive review of the in-vitro human data. *Pharmacogenetics* 2002;12:251–263.
47. Cupp MJ, Tracy TS. Cytochrome P450: new nomenclature and clinical implications. *Am Fam Physician* 1998;57(1):107–116.
48. Wijnen PA, Op den Buijshc RA, Drent M, et al. Review article: the prevalence and clinical relevance of cytochrome P450 polymorphisms. *Aliment Pharmacol Ther* 2007;26(Suppl 2):211–219.
49. Yap KY, Chui WK, Chan A. Drug interactions between chemotherapeutic regimens and antiepileptics. *Clin Ther* 2008;30(8):1385–1407.
50. Uno T, Sugimoto K, Sugawara K, et al. The effect of CYP2C19 genotypes on the pharmacokinetics of warfarin enantiomers. *J Clin Pharm Ther* 2008;33:67–73.
51. Guidance for Industry: Drug development and drug interactions: Table of substrates, inhibitors and inducers. U.S. Food and Drug Administration (FDA), Maryland USA. https://www.fda.gov/drugs/drug-interactions-labeling/drug-development-and-drug-interactions-table-substrates-inhibitors-and-inducers#table5-2. Accessed May 11, 2019.
52. Goetz MP, Kamal A, Ames MM. Tamoxifen pharmacogenomics: the role of CYP2D6 as a predictor of drug response. *Clin Pharmacol Ther* 2008;83(1):160–166.
53. He Z-X, Chen X-W, Zhou Z-W, et al. Impact of physiological, pathological and environmental factors on the expression and activity of human cytochrome P450 2D6 and implications in precision medicine. *Drug Metab Rev* 2015;47(4):470–519.
54. Lanfear DE, McLeod HL. Pharmacogenetics: using DNA to optimize drug therapy. *Am Fam Physician* 2007;76:1179–1182.
55. Lin JH. CYP induction-mediated drug interactions: in vitro assessment and clinical implications. *Pharm Res* 2006;23(6):1089–1116.
56. Saravanakumar A, Sadighi A, Ryu R, et al. Physiochemical properties, biotransformation, and transport pathways of established and newly approved medications: a systematic review of the top 200 most prescribed drugs vs. the FDA-approved drugs between 2005 and 2016. *Clin Pharmacokinet* 2019;58(10):1281–1294. doi:10.1007/s40262-019-00750-8.
57. Manzi SF, Shannon M. Drug interactions—a review. *Clin Pediatr Emerg Med* 2005;6:93–102.
58. Siller-Matula JM, Lang I, Christ G, et al. Calcium-channel blockers reduce the antiplatelet effect of clopidogrel. *J Am Coll Cardiol* 2008;52:1557–1563.
59. Zhou SF, Xue CC, Yu XQ, et al. Clinically important drug interactions potentially involving mechanism-based inhibition of cytochrome P450 3A4 and the role of therapeutic drug monitoring. *Ther Drug Monit* 2007;29(6):687–710.
60. Mathias AA, West S, Hui J, et al. Dose-response of ritonavir on hepatic CYP3A activity and elvitegravir enteral exposure. *Clin Pharmacol Ther* 2009;85(1):64–70.
61. Pratt R, Robinson V, Navin T, et al. Trends in tuberculosis—United States, 2007. *Morb Mortal Wkly Rep* 2008;57(11):281–285.
62. Spielberg SP. N-acetyltransferases: pharmacogenetics and clinical consequences of polymorphic drug metabolism. *J Pharmacokinet Biopharm* 1996;24(5):509–519.
63. Wilkinson G. Pharmacokinetics. In: Hardman JG, Limbird LE, Gillman AG, eds. *Goodman & Gilman's the pharmacologic basis of therapeutics*, 10th ed. New York, NY: McGraw-Hill, 2001.
64. Azuma J, Ohno M, Kubota R, et al. NAT2 genotype guided regimen reduces isoniazid-induced liver injury and early treatment failure in the 6-month four-drug standard treatment of tuberculosis: a randomized controlled trial for pharmacogenetics-based therapy. *Eur J Clin Pharmacol* 2013;69(5):1091–1101.
65. Shepard PD, Canavier CC, Levitan ES. Ether-a-go-go-Related gene potassium channels: what's all the buzz about? *Schizophr Bull* 2007;33(6):1263–1269.
66. Hancox JC, McPate MJ, Harchi AE, et al. The hERG potassium channel and hERG screening for drug-induced torsades de pointes. *Pharmacol Ther* 2008;119:118–132.
67. Zhou SF. Drugs behave as substrates, inhibitors and inducers of human cytochrome P450 3A4. *Curr Drug Metab* 2008;9(4):310–322.
68. Weir MR. Renal effects of nonselective NSAIDs and coxibs. *Cleve Clin J Med* 2002;69(Suppl 1):S153–S158.
69. Hansten PD, Horn JR. *Drug interactions analysis and management 2008*. St. Louis, MO: Wolters Kluwer Health, 2008.
70. Brown GR. Cephalosporin-probenecid drug interactions. *Clin Pharmacokinet* 1993;24(4):289–300.
71. Wattanagoon Y, Stepniewska K, Lindegardh N, et al. Pharmacokinetics of high dose oseltamivir in healthy volunteers. *Antimicrob Agents Chemother* 2009;53:945–952.
72. Cundy KC. Clinical pharmacokinetics of the antiviral nucleotide analogs cidofovir and adefovir. *Clin Pharmacokinet* 1999;36(2):127–143.
73. Watson Laboratories Inc. Probenecid package insert. 2003.
74. Beorlegui B, Aldaz A, Ortega A, et al. Potential interaction between methotrexate and omeprazole. *Ann Pharmacother* 2000;34:1024–1027.
75. Suzuki K, Doki K, Homma M, et al. Co-administration of proton pump inhibitors delays elimination of plasma methotrexate in high-dose methotrexate therapy. *Br J Clin Pharmacol* 2009;67(1):44–49.
76. Hauben M, Reich L, Gerrits CM, et al. Detection of spironolactone-associated hyperkalemia following the Randomized Aldactone Evaluation Study (RALES). *Drug Saf* 2007;30(12):1143–1149.
77. Juurlink DN, Mamdani MM, Lee DS, et al. Rates of hyperkalemia after publication of the Randomized Aldactone Evaluation Study. *N Engl J Med* 2004;351:543–551.
78. Saklayen MG, Gyebi LK, Tasosa J, et al. Effects of additive therapy with spironolactone on proteinuria in diabetic patients already on ACE inhibitor or ARB therapy: results of a randomized, placebo-controlled, double-blind, crossover trial. *J Investig Med* 2008;56(4):714–719.
79. Svensson M, Gustafsson F, Glatius S, et al. Hyperkalemia and impaired renal function in patients taking spironolactone for congestive heart failure: a retrospective study. *BMJ* 2003;327:1141–1142.
80. Palmer BF. Managing hyperkalemia caused by inhibitors of the renin-angiotensin-aldosterone system. *N Engl J Med* 2004;351:585–592.
81. Roth M, Obaidat A, Hagenbuch B. OATPs, OATs and OCTs: the organic anion and cation transporters of the SLCO and SLC22A gene superfamilies. *Br J Pharmacol* 2012;165:1260–1287.
82. Neuvonen PJ, Niemi M, Backman JT. Drug interactions with lipid-lowering drugs: mechanisms and clinical relevance. *Clin Pharm Ther* 2006;80:565–581.
83. Nozaki Y, Kusuhar H, Kondo T, et al. Species difference in the inhibitory effect nonsteroidal anti-inflammatory drugs on the uptake of methotrexate by human kidney slices. *J Pharmacol Exp Ther* 2007;322(3):1162–1170.
84. Ahn S-Y, Eraly SA, Tsigelney I, et al. Interaction of organic cations with organic anion transporters. *J Biol Chem* 2009;284(45):31422–31430.
85. McCreight LJ, Bailey C, Pearson ER. Metformin and the gastrointestinal tract. *Diabetologia* 2016;59:426–435.
86. Boxberger KH, Hagenbuch B, Lampe JN. Common drugs inhibit human organic cation transporter 1 (OCT1)-mediated neurotransmitter uptake. *Drug Metab Dispos* 2014;42:990–995.

APPENDIX

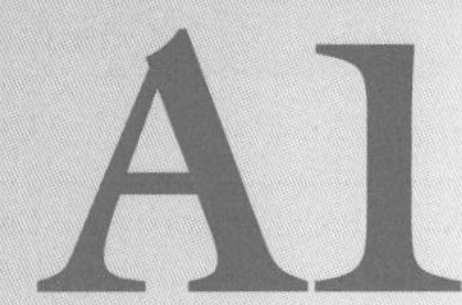

Densley Francois
Mirjana Lulic-Botica
Thomas J. Duggan
Jacob V. Aranda

Neonatal Drug Formulary

TABLE A1.1 Commonly Used Medications in a Newborn Intensive Care Unit

Medication	*Dosage*	*Comments*
Acetaminophen (Tylenol)	10–15 mg/kg/dose q6–8 h p.o./p.r., max 75 mg/kg/d (term neonate) 60 mg/kg/d (preterm neonate)	• Contraindicated in G6PD deficiencies • Caution in liver failure
Acyclovir (Zovirax)	20 mg/kg/dose i.v. q8 h (neonatal HSV)	• Infuse over 1 h: monitor BUN, SCr, liver enzymes, CBC • For 14–21 d in HSV infection • Dose adjust with elevated serum creatinine levels *Serum Creatinine Level (mg/dL)* / *Dose (mg/kg/dose)* / *Interval (h)* 0.8–1.1 / 20 / q12 1.2–1.5 / 20 / q24 >1.5 / 10 / q24
Adenosine (Adenocard)	50 μg/kg rapid i.v.p. over 1–2 s Increase dose by 50 μg/kg increments q2 min until return of sinus rhythm; max 250 μg/kg	• Flush with saline immediately postdose • Adenosine 6 mg/2 mL vial size: Dilute 1 mL adenosine vial with 18 mL of normal saline for final concentration of 300 μg/mL • After converting SVT to normal sinus rhythm, give digoxin or propranolol • Decreased effect when theophylline/caffeine onboard due to competitive antagonism
Albumin 5%/25%	5%: 0.5 g/kg (10 mL/kg) i.v. over 20–30 min 25%: 1 g /kg i.v. over 2–3 h	• Administer through 5-μm filter • Isotonic crystalloid solutions should be used first line (*Neonatal Resuscitation guidelines 2015* states that an isotonic crystalloid rather than albumin is the solution of choice for volume expansion in the delivery room [Class IIb; LOE 7]) • May be placed in TPN when treating fluid overload due to third spacing • Too rapid of an infusion may result in vascular overload • 25% concentration should be avoided secondary to possible risk of hemolysis and IVH in preterm neonates • If 25% concentration required secondary to renal failure and fluid restriction, it must be Y-in to main i.v. or TPN so that final concentration is ≤5% • Albumin infusions should be administered within 6 h of preparation

(*continued*)

TABLE A1.1 Commonly Used Medications in a Newborn Intensive Care Unit (*continued*)

Medication	*Dosage*	*Comments*
Alteplase (TPA) (Activase)	**For catheter occlusion:** 0.5–1 mg via catheter; dwell time 2 h Aspirate out of catheter. DO NOT INFUSE. May repeat in 1 h for one more dose **Thrombolytic therapy:** **Dose:** 0.1–0.6 mg/kg/h for 6 h	• Note: Syringes are frozen, so allow for thaw time • Contraindicated: bleeding • **Chest 2012 guidelines regarding thrombolytic therapy in neonates**: "We recommend against thrombolytic therapy for neonatal VTE unless major vessel occlusion is causing critical compromise of organs or limbs (Grade 2C)"
Amikacin	Postnatal age: <14 d <800 g: 16 mg/kg/dose i.v. q48 h 801–1,200 g: 16 mg/kg/dose i.v. q42 h 1,201–2,800 g: 15 mg/kg/dose i.v. q36 h >2,800 g: 15 mg/kg/dose i.v. q30 h Postnatal age: >14 d <800 g: 20 mg/kg/dose i.v. q42 h 801–1,200 g: 20 mg/kg/dose i.v. q36 h 1,201–200 g: 18 mg/kg/dose i.v. q30 h >2,000 g: 18 mg/kg/dose i.v. q24 h	• Reserved for tobramycin-resistant gram-negative pathogens • **Therapeutic levels**: peak 20–30 µg/mL, trough <4 µg/mL • Monitor BUN, SCr, UO
Aminophylline	Loading dose: 5 mg/kg/dose i.v. over 30 min Maintenance dose: 1.5–3 mg/kg/dose i.v. q8–12 h Aminophylline drip—start at 0.2 mg/kg/h i.v. 6 wk–6 mo: 0.5 mg/kg/h 6 mo–1 y: 0.6–0.7 mg/kg/h	• Apnea level 7–12 µg/mL • BPD level: 10–15 µg/mL • Half-life is variable per age: Premature 20–30 h Term 10–25 h <6 mo 14 h >6 mo 5 h • Serum levels reduced in neonates because of decreased binding of theophylline to fetal albumin, resulting in greater free drug. • Draw theophylline level 3 d after therapy initiated or changed • Adjust frequency of theophylline dosing in anticipation of change of half-life • Toxic levels can result in tachycardia, PVC, seizures • Increases theophylline level: erythromycin, furosemide, hypothyroid • Decreases theophylline level: phenobarbital, phenytoin, rifampin, high-protein diet • In preterm infants, ~30% of aminophylline or theophylline is converted to caffeine
Amiodarone (Cordarone)	Loading dose: 5 mg/kg slow i.v.p. over 20–60 min Maintenance dose: 5–15 µg/kg/min Max: 15 µg/kg/min	• Standard continuous concentrations: 1 mg/mL, 2 mg/mL, 4 mg/mL • Vials contain polysorbate, which may cause hypotension on rapid infusion • Limited data available in neonates; safety and efficacy not established • Class II antiarrhythmic which inhibits adrenergic stimulation and decreases AV conduction • Contains benzyl alcohol • NOT compatible with heparin, sodium bicarbonate • Monitor for signs of hypothyroidism/hyperthyroidism (contains 37% iodine by weight) • Inhibits cytochrome P450 isoenzyme: increases plasma levels of digoxin, theophylline, and phenytoin
Amoxicillin (Amoxil)	30 mg/kg/d p.o. div q12 h 10–20 mg/kg p.o. q.d. for prophylaxis due to hydronephrosis	• Prophylaxis to continue until VCUG (voiding cystourethrography) completed • Powder for oral suspension is stable for 14 d under refrigeration after reconstitution
Amoxicillin/clavulanic acid (Augmentin)	30 mg/kg/d p.o. div q12 h	• Clavulanic acid binds and inhibits β-lactamases which inactivate amoxicillin • Administer with feeds to decrease GI side effects

TABLE A1.1 Commonly Used Medications in a Newborn Intensive Care Unit (*continued*)

Medication	*Dosage*	*Comments*
Amphotericin B (conventional)	Dose: 1 mg/kg i.v. over 2–3 h Bladder irrigation: 5–15 mg/100 mL. Instill 10 mL/kg via catheter; clamp for 60–120 min; perform irrigation t.i.d.–q.i.d. for 2–4 d	• Total cumulative dose 15 mg/kg • Total cumulative dose 20–25 mg/kg for persistent fungemia or CNS involvement • Binds to ergosterol altering cell membrane permeability, causing leaking of cell components • Monitor BUN, SCr, liver enzymes, electrolytes (hypokalemia, hypomagnesemia), and CBC • DO NOT FLUSH WITH ANY SOLUTIONS CONTAINING SALINE • Final concentration 0.1 mg/mL • Fluid-restricted patients may concentrate up to 0.5 mg/mL in D5W/D10W through a CVC • Poor CSF penetration
Amphotericin B lipid complex (Abelcet)	5 mg/kg/dose i.v. q24 h infuse over 2 h (may be dosed up to 7.5–10 mg/kg in refractory cases per infectious disease recommendation)	• Restricted criteria at most institutions and may require approval by infectious disease specialist • Exhibits nonlinear kinetics with high tissue concentration in the liver, spleen, and lung • Empirical antifungal therapy for suspected candidiasis has been shown to improve mortality and morbidity • DO NOT use lipid complex Amphotericin B (ABLC) for *Candida lusitaniae* and *Candida guilliermondii* • Compatible in D5W/D10W • DO NOT ADD HEPARIN • Monitor renal, hepatic, electrolyte, and hematologic status • Final concentration: 1 mg/mL • Max concentration of 2 mg/mL may be used in fluid-restricted patients • No guidelines regarding dose adjustment requirement in renal failure
Amphotericin B liposomal (Ambisome)	3–5 mg/kg/dose i.v. q24 h, infuse over 2 h (may be dosed up to 7 mg/kg in refractory cases per infectious disease recommendation)	• Restricted criteria at most institutions and may require approval by infectious disease specialist • Exhibits nonlinear kinetics with high tissue concentration in the liver, spleen, and lung • Empirical antifungal therapy for suspected candidiasis has been shown to improve mortality and morbidity • Compatible in D5W/D10W • Monitor renal, hepatic, electrolyte, and hematologic status • Final concentration: 1 mg/mL • Max concentration of 2 mg/mL may be used in fluid-restricted patients • No guidelines regarding dose adjustment required in renal failure
Ampicillin	Postnatal age <7 d <2 kg: 50 mg/kg/dose i.v./i.m. q12 h >2 kg: 50 mg/kg/dose i.v./i.m. q8 h Postnatal age >7 d <2 kg: 75 mg/kg/dose i.v./i.m. q12 h >2 kg: 50 mg/kg/dose i.v./i.m. q8 h GBS meningitis Postnatal age <7 d: 300 mg/kg/d i.v. div q8 h Postnatal age >7 d: 300 mg/kg/d i.v. q6 h	• Incompatible with TPN
Ampicillin/sulbactam (Unasyn)	Premature neonate: 100 mg ampicillin/kg/d div q12 h Full-term neonate: 100 mg/kg/d i.v. div q8 h Pediatric dosing/meningitis: 200–400 mg ampicillin/kg/d div q6 h	• Limited data in neonates • Sulbactam is a β-lactamase inhibitor • Dosed based on ampicillin component

(*continued*)

TABLE A1.1 Commonly Used Medications in a Newborn Intensive Care Unit (*continued*)

Medication	*Dosage*	*Comments*
Atenolol (Tenormin)	0.8–1 mg/kg/dose p.o. q.d. MAX: 2 mg/kg/d	• Selective β1-blocker • 2 mg/mL oral solution compounded from tablets • Monitor BP, heart rate, and respiratory rate
Atropine	Bradycardia: 0.02 mg/kg/dose i.v./i.m./s.c./e.t. May repeat q5 min up to 1 mg total dose	• Treatment of sinus bradycardia • 0.25 mg/5 mL (0.05 mg/mL)
Azithromycin (Zithromax)	<6 mo: 10 mg/kg/dose i.v. q.d. for 5 d (pertussis)	• No dosing guidelines for treatment of ureaplasma infections
Aztreonam (Azactam)	≤2 kg 60 mg/kg/d i.v. div q12 h >2 kg 90 mg/kg/d i.v. div q8 h	• Treatment for multidrug-resistant aerobic gram-negative infections
Beractant (Survanta)	4 mL/kg intratracheal q6 h for up to 4 doses if required	• Criteria: FiO_2 > 0.3 and MAP >7 • 25 mg/mL (4 mL, 8 mL)
Sodium citrate/citric acid (Bicitra)	2–3 mEq/kg/d div q6–8 h p.o.	• Each mL contains 1 mEq of bicarbonate and 1 mEq sodium • Monitor serum Na, K, $HCO3^-$, urine pH • Conversion to bicarbonate may be impaired with hepatic failure • Polycitra contains 2 mEq/mL bicarbonate, 1 mEq/mL potassium, and 1 mEq/mL sodium • Polycitra K contains 2 mEq/mL bicarbonate and 2 mEq/mL potassium
Bumetanide (Bumex)	0.01–0.05 mg/kg/dose p.o./i.v. q24–48 h	• Monitor serum electrolytes, renal function, UO
Calcitriol (Rocaltrol)	Hypoparathyroidism: 0.02–0.06 µg/kg/d Hypocalcemia (premature infants): 1 µg p.o. q.d. for 5 d	• Oral solution 1 µg/mL
Calcium salts	Hypocalcemia: 50–150 mg/kg/d div q4–6 h (expressed as elemental calcium)	
Calcium gluconate	Symptomatic hypocalcemia: 100–200 mg/kg/dose i.v. q6 h	• 10% gluconate contains 9 mg/mL elemental calcium • Order 2–4 doses for symptomatic hypocalcemia • Avoid giving via UAC • Not recommended for infusion with TPN due to Ca-PO_4 ratio limitations • Ionized calcium is preferred measurement due to poor correlation between serum ionized calcium (free) and total serum calcium, especially with low albumin states and acid/base imbalances • Initiate as bolus for true hypocalcemia only • Normal calcium levels: • Preterm <1 wk 6–10 mg/dL • Term <1 wk 7–12 mg/dL • Total corrected calcium in low albumin states: Total corrected Ca: = Total serum Ca + 0.8 (4 − measured serum albumin) • Calcium corrections based on the above calculations may be inaccurate in the neonatal population • Ionized calcium level should be obtained if hypocalcemia is considered to be clinically significant.
Caffeine citrate (Cafcit) (specify caffeine citrate on order)	Loading dose: 20 mg/kg i.v./p.o. Maintenance dose: 5 mg/kg/d i.v./p.o.	• Measuring serum concentrations is not necessary. If performed, trough level: 5–25 µg/mL • Consider switching to p.o. as soon as possible due to cost • Caffeine citrate is ½ caffeine base • Order dose as caffeine citrate • May require larger maintenance dose for preterm infants
Captopril (Capoten)	Premature neonates: 0.01 mg/kg/dose p.o. q8–12 h Term neonates: 0.05–0.1 mg/kg/dose p.o. q8–24 h; titrate up to 2 mg/kg/d	• Administer 1 h before feeding • Management of CHF, HTN • ACE inhibitor which decreases angiotensin II, which increases plasma renin activity and decreases aldosterone secretion • Monitor BP, serum creatinine, CBC, serum potassium

TABLE A1.1 Commonly Used Medications in a Newborn Intensive Care Unit (*continued*)

Medication	*Dosage*	*Comments*
Carbamazepine (Tegretol)	10–20 mg/kg/d p.o. div b.i.d.–t.i.d. Max 35 mg/kg/d	• Therapeutic range: 4–12 μg/mL • Adjust dose to clinical response and levels • Adjuvant agent in neonates not responding to conventional therapy • Cytochrome P450 isoenzyme: may induce metabolism of midazolam, phenytoin, theophylline, VPA, and topiramate
Carnitine	20 mg/L standard in TPN for all neonates ≤5 kg Dose of 10–20 mg/kg/d have been used in preterm infants whose triglyceride levels remain high	• Prevention and treatment of carnitine deficiency • Facilitates transport of long-chain fatty acids into mitochondria
Caspofungin (Cancidas)	2 mg/kg i.v. over 2 h	• Safety and efficacy not established in children • Reserved for last-line therapy secondary to refractory fungemia • Infectious disease approval only • FDA approved for aspergillosis, invasive refractory candidiasis, esophageal candidiasis • Noncompetitive inhibitor of β-1,3-glucan synthase in the echinocandin class • Dilute to final concentration of 0.2 mg/mL • Monitor for increase in liver enzymes, infusion-related reactions (thrombophlebitis) • DO NOT USE DILUENTS/FLUSHES CONTAINING DEXTROSE • Restricted criteria at most institutions and may require approval by infectious disease specialist
Cefazolin (Ancef)	<7 d <2 kg: 25 mg/kg/dose i.v. q12 h >2 kg: 50 mg/kg/dose i.v. q12 h >7 d <2 kg: 25 mg/kg/dose i.v. q8 h >2 kg: 50 mg/kg/dose i.v. q8 h	• Infuse over 30 min
Cefdinir (Omnicef)	>6 mo–1 y: 7 mg/kg/dose p.o. q12 h for 10 d	• Third-generation oral cephalosporin
Cefepime (Maxipime)	50 mg/kg/dose i.v. q12 h Febrile neutropenia: 50 mg/kg/dose i.v. q8 h	• Reserve for ceftazidime-resistant gram-negative pathogens • Monitor closely for increases in bilirubin, especially in preterm infants • Fourth-generation cephalosporin • Dose adjust in renal impairment
Cefpodoxime (Vantin)	>6 mo: 5 mg/kg/dose p.o. q12 h	• Third-generation oral cephalosporin • Monitor CBC, liver enzymes
Cefotaxime (Claforan)	0–4 wk <1,200 g: 50 mg/kg/dose i.v./i.m. q12 h >1 kg and >7 d: 50 mg/kg/dose q8 h	• Manufacturer discontinued in the United States • Compatible with TPN • Third-generation cephalosporin • Used for empiric coverage of late-onset sepsis with vancomycin • When not available, other third- or fourth-generation cephalosporins such as ceftazidime and cefepime have been considered as alternatives after review of local susceptibility and resistance patterns.
Ceftaroline	6 mg/kg/dose i.v. q8 h	• Limited data in neonates, this dosing only studied in neonates >34 wk' gestation • Usage may require infectious disease approval • Duration of therapy is variable, typically 5–14 d, dependent on severity of infection and clinical response
Ceftazidime (Fortaz)	50 mg/kg/dose i.v. q12 h >1 kg and >7 d: 50 mg/kg/dose i.v. q8 h Meningitis: 50 mg/kg/dose i.v. q8 h	• Compatible with TPN • Third-generation cephalosporin

(*continued*)

TABLE A1.1 Commonly Used Medications in a Newborn Intensive Care Unit (*continued*)

Medication	*Dosage*	*Comments*
Ceftriaxone (Rocephin)	Gonococcal prophylaxis: 25–50 mg/kg i.m./i.v. × one dose (NOT to exceed 125 mg)	• Third-generation cephalosporin • Good penetration into CSF (meningitis) • Generally not used in the neonatal population for indications other than gonococcal prophylaxis secondary to potential bilirubin displacement • NOT compatible with calcium or calcium-containing solutions (TPN). Immediate precipitation will result
Cephalexin (Keflex)	25–50 mg/kg/d p.o. div q6–8 h Severe infections: 50–100 mg/kg/d p.o. div q6–8 h Otitis media: 75–100 mg/kg/d p.o. div q6 h	• 250 mg/5 mL oral suspension
Cholestyramine 5%	5% cream: apply t.i.d.–q.i.d. to diaper rash area	• Reserved for severe diaper rash • Compounded by pharmacy
Chlorothiazide (Diuril)	10–40 mg/kg/d p.o. div q8–12 h 5–20 mg/kg/d i.v. div q12 h	• Monitor electrolytes at initiation of therapy • May require sodium supplementation for diuretic-induced hyponatremia • Generally initiated for babies >1 mo
Ciprofloxacin (Cipro)	Preterm: 10 mg/kg/dose p.o./i.v. q12 h Term: 15 mg/kg/dose p.o./i.v. q12 h	• Ciprofloxacin is not considered a first-line agent in the neonatal population secondary to reported adverse events related to joints and/or surrounding tissues (cartilage in animals) • Reserved for documented multidrug-resistant aerobic gram-negative bacilli
Clindamycin (Cleocin)	<7 d and <2,000 g: 5 mg/kg/dose i.v. q12 h >2,000g: 5 mg/kg/dose i.v. q8 h >7 d: <1,200 g: 5 mg/kg/dose i.v. q12 h 1,200–2,000 g: 5 mg/kg/dose i.v. q8 h >2,000 g: 20–30 mg/kg/d i.v. div q6–8 h	• Compatible with TPN • Infuse slowly over 30 min • Contains benzyl alcohol • Preferred agent for *Mycoplasma hominis* cultured from endotracheal tube
Cloxacillin (Tegopen)	>1 mo: 50–100 mg/kg/d p.o. div q6	• Use with MSSA • Oral antistaphylococcal penicillin
Colistimethate (Colistin)	2.5–5 mg/kg/d i.v. div q6–12 h	• Restricted criteria at most institutions and may require approval by infectious disease specialist • Safety and efficacy in neonates has not been established. • Should be reserved for use for life-threatening infections caused by organisms resistant to traditional antimicrobials • Adjust dose in renal impairment • Does NOT penetrate CSF • Monitor for nephrotoxicity and neurotoxicity
Cosyntropin (Cortrosyn)	0.015 mg/kg/dose i.v./i.m.	• Diagnostic agent for adrenocortical insufficiency • i.m. concentration 0.25 mg/mL • i.v.p.: administer in 2–5 mL of normal saline over 2 min
Cyclopentolate 1% (Cyclogyl Tropicamide)	ROP examination: one drop into each eye 10–30 min prior to examination May repeat × 1 dose in 5 min	• Used in diagnostic procedures requiring mydriasis and cycloplegia • Monitor BP and heart rate
Cysteine	40 mg cysteine per gram of amino acids (Trophamine) 3 g/kg/d of amino acids provide 120 mg/kg/d of cysteine	• Supplement to Trophamine amino acid solution • Monitor BUN, SCr, acid–base balance • MAX 120 mg/kg/d • Addition of cysteine to TPN solutions enhances the solubility of calcium and phosphate but can increase the need for acetate in the TPN
Desmopressin (DDAVP)	0.1 mg p.o. q.d. (range 0.1–0.5 mg p.o. q.d. per endocrinology) 5 µg/d intranasally div once daily to b.i.d. (range 5–30 µg/d)	• Treatment for diabetes insipidus • Crush tablet in Ora-sweet to make 0.1 mg/mL

TABLE A1.1 Commonly Used Medications in a Newborn Intensive Care Unit (*continued*)

<table>
<tr><th>Medication</th><th>Dosage</th><th>Comments</th></tr>
<tr><td>Dexamethasone (Decadron)</td><td>Airway edema/extubation: 0.5–2 mg/kg/d i.v. div q6 for 4 doses (begin 24 h prior to extubation) CLD: DART (Dexamethasone A Randomized Trial) protocol
0.15 mg/kg/d i.v. div q12 h × 3 d
0.1 mg/kg/d div q12 h × 3 d
0.05 mg/kg/d div q12 h × 2 d
0.02 mg/kg/d div q12 h × 2 d
<table>
<tr><th>Glucocorticoid</th><th>Approximate Equivalent Dose (mg)</th></tr>
<tr><td>Short acting</td><td></td></tr>
<tr><td>Hydrocortisone</td><td>20</td></tr>
<tr><td>Intermediate acting</td><td></td></tr>
<tr><td>Methylprednisolone</td><td>4</td></tr>
<tr><td>Prednisolone</td><td>5</td></tr>
<tr><td>Prednisone</td><td>5</td></tr>
<tr><td>Long acting</td><td></td></tr>
<tr><td>Dexamethasone</td><td>0.75</td></tr>
</table></td><td>• Monitor BP, glucose metabolism, GI bleed, weight loss
• Consider concomitant ranitidine therapy (total daily dose of ranitidine may be placed in TPN)
• Use of dexamethasone is controversial in CLD, and the AAP statement in Pediatrics states "the routine use of systemic dexamethasone for the prevention or treatment of CLD in infants with VLBW is not recommended" and "current use of dexamethasone should be limited to infants on maximal ventilator and oxygen support"
Before treatment, the parents should be informed of the potential life-saving benefit and the uncertain additional risk of neurologic injury, and informed consent should be obtained</td></tr>
<tr><td>Dexmedetomidine (Precedex)</td><td>Loading dose optional: 0.1–0.5 μg/kg/dose over 10–20 min (bolus with caution)
Initial infusion: 0.1–0.3 μg/kg/h (rates up to 1.5 μg/kg/h reported in literature)</td><td>• Bolus dosing associated with hypotension/bradycardia in neonates
• Metabolized by glucuronidation, an immature pathway in neonates, therefore prolonged half-life in neonates
• Manufacturer label use for up to 24 h; most studied reports use dexmedetomidine for longer than 24 h</td></tr>
<tr><td>Diazoxide (Proglycem)</td><td>10–15 mg/kg/d p.o. div q8–12 h</td><td>• Inhibits pancreatic insulin release
• For hypoglycemia due to hyperinsulinemia
• Peak hyperglycemic effect within 1 h</td></tr>
<tr><td>Dicloxacillin</td><td>25–50 mg/kg/d p.o. div q6 h</td><td>• Monitor for elevated liver enzymes, thrombocytopenia, and eosinophilia</td></tr>
<tr><td>Osteomyelitis</td><td>50–100 mg/kg/d div q6 h</td><td>• Food decreases rate and extent of absorption</td></tr>
<tr><td>Digoxin (Lanoxin)</td><td>
<table>
<tr><th></th><th colspan="2">TDD (μg/kg)</th><th colspan="2">Main Dose (μg/kg)</th></tr>
<tr><th></th><th>p.o.</th><th>i.v.</th><th>p.o.</th><th>i.v.</th></tr>
<tr><td>Preterm</td><td>20–30</td><td>15–25</td><td>5–7.5</td><td>4–6</td></tr>
<tr><td>Full-term</td><td>25–5</td><td>20–30</td><td>8–10</td><td>5–8</td></tr>
</table></td><td>• Give ½ TDD as initial dose, then ¼ TDD for 2 doses q6–12 h
• Adjust dose for renal impairment
• Therapeutic range 0.8–2 ng/mL
• Draw trough level just prior to next dose
• Half-life:
Preterm: 61–70 h
Term: 35–45 h</td></tr>
<tr><td>Diltiazem (Cardizem)</td><td>1.5–2 mg/kg/d p.o. div t.i.d.–q.i.d.</td><td>• Management of paroxysmal supraventricular tachycardia (PSVT), atrial fibrillation, atrial flutter
• i.v. form reserved as antiarrhythmic
• Cytochrome P450 isoenzyme
• Diltiazem may increase serum concentrations of carbamazepine, digoxin, and midazolam and increase effect of fentanyl and rifampin.</td></tr>
<tr><td>Diphenhydramine (Benadryl)</td><td>5 mg/kg/d p.o./i.v. div q6–8 h</td><td>• Additive sedative when given concomitantly with other CNS depressants</td></tr>
</table>

(*continued*)

TABLE A1.1 Commonly Used Medications in a Newborn Intensive Care Unit (*continued*)

Medication	*Dosage*	*Comments*
Dobutamine	2–20 µg/kg/min i.v. continuous titrate to response	• Standard continuous concentrations: 0.8 mg/mL, 1.6 mg/mL, 3.2 mg/mL • Compatible with TPN • Half-life = 2 min • DO NOT infuse through UAC • Stimulates β1-adrenergic receptors and increases heart rate, increases contractility • Little effect on β2 or α receptors • Treat extravasations with phentolamine • Consider double-concentrating infusion drip, especially in the ELBW neonate to minimize volume occupied by continuous drip infusions

Rate (mL/h) = Factor × Weight (kg)

Desired dose (µg/kg/min)	*Concentration*		
	0.8 mg/Ml	*1.6 mg/mL*	*3.2 mg/mL*
2	0.15	0.075	0.037
3	0.225	0.112	0.056
4	0.3	0.15	0.075
5	0.375	0.187	0.093
6	0.45	0.225	0.112
7	0.525	0.262	0.131
8	0.6	0.3	0.15
9	0.675	0.337	0.169
10	0.75	0.375	0.188
11	0.825	0.412	0.206
12	0.9	0.45	0.225
13	0.975	0.487	0.243
14	1.05	0.525	0.262
15	1.125	0.562	0.281
16	1.2	0.6	0.3
17	1.275	0.637	0.319
18	1.35	0.675	0.338
19	1.425	0.712	0.356
20	1.5	0.75	0.375

Medication	*Dosage*	*Comments*
Dopamine	5–20 µg/kg/min i.v. continuous Titrate to response	• Standard continuous concentrations: 0.8 mg/mL, 1.6 mg/mL, 3.2 mg/mL • SEE above table for quick rate calculation • Half-life = 2 min • DO NOT infuse through UAC • Treat extravasation with phentolamine • LOW DOSE: stimulates dopaminergic receptors—renal and mesenteric vasodilatation • INTERMEDIATE DOSE: stimulates both dopaminergic and β1-adrenergic ↑HR/clearance • HIGH DOSE: stimulates α-adrenergic receptors; ↑BP and vasoconstriction
Enalapril (Vasotec)	0.1 mg/kg/d p.o. q24 h 5–10 µg/kg/dose i.v. q8–24 h	• Injection contains benzyl alcohol as preservative • Use with caution in preterm neonates • Adjust dose in renal impairment • Indicated for mild to severe hypertension, CHF, and asymptomatic left ventricular dysfunction

TABLE A1.1 Commonly Used Medications in a Newborn Intensive Care Unit (*continued*)

<table>
<tr><th>Medication</th><th>Dosage</th><th>Comments</th></tr>
<tr><td>Enoxaparin (Lovenox)</td><td>Prophylaxis: 0.75 mg/kg/dose s.c. q12 h
Treatment: 1.5 mg/kg/dose s.c. q12 h</td><td>Treatment or prophylaxis of thromboembolic disorders
• Potentiates the action of antithrombin III and inactivates coagulation factor Xa.
• Monitor: CBC, platelets, stool occult tests, and other signs of excessive bleeding or bruising
• Closely monitor platelet decreases of <100,000 or >50% from baseline
• Required therapeutic doses as high as 2.5 mg/kg/dose s.c. q12 reported in literature for preterm neonates
• Can be reversed with protamine, but not completely; only 60%–75% of aXa activity can be reversed
• Monitor anti–factor Xa levels:
<table>
<tr><th>aXa Level</th><th>Level Interpretation</th><th>When to Repeat Levels</th></tr>
<tr><td><0.35 units/mL</td><td>↑ Dose by 25%</td><td>4 h after next dose</td></tr>
<tr><td>0.35–0.49 units/mL</td><td>↑ Dose by 10%</td><td>4 h after next dose</td></tr>
<tr><td>0.5–1 units/mL</td><td>Continue same dose</td><td>Next day, repeat in 1 wk, and then every month</td></tr>
<tr><td>1.1–1.5 units/mL</td><td>↓ Dose by 20%</td><td>Before next dose</td></tr>
<tr><td>1.6–2 units/mL</td><td>Hold dose for 3 h and then ↓ dose by 30%</td><td>Before next dose, then 4 h after next dose</td></tr>
<tr><td>>2 units/mL</td><td>Hold doses until aXa level is ≤0.5 units/mL and then decrease dose by 40%</td><td>Before next dose and every 12 h until level <0.5 units/mL</td></tr>
</table>
Adapted from Monagle P, Chan AKC, Goldenberg NA, et al. Antithrombotic therapy in neonates and children: antithrombotic Therapy and Prevention of Thrombosis: American College of Chest Physicians Evidence-Based Clinical Practice Guidelines (9th Edition). Chest 2012;141(2 Suppl):e737S–e801S.</td></tr>
<tr><td>Epinephrine</td><td>Bradycardia:
0.01 mg/kg/dose i.v. 0.03 mg/kg/dose intratracheal (0.1–0.3 mL/kg/dose using 0.1 mg/mL concentration)
May repeat every 3–5 min as needed.
Hypotension (inotrope): 0.05–1 μg/kg/min. Titrate dose to desired effect</td><td>• Standard continuous concentrations: 1 mg/100 mL, 5 mg/100 mL
• Half-life = 2 min
• DO NOT infuse through UAC
• Treat extravasation with phentolamine</td></tr>
</table>

(*continued*)

TABLE A1.1 Commonly Used Medications in a Newborn Intensive Care Unit (*continued*)

Medication	*Dosage*	*Comments*

Desired dose (μg/kg/min)	*Rate (mL/h) = Factor × Weight (kg) Concentration*	
	0.01 mg/mL	*0.05 mg/mL*
0.05	0.3	0.06
0.1	0.6	0.12
0.15	0.9	0.18
0.2	1.2	0.24
0.25	1.5	0.3
0.3	1.8	0.36
0.35	2.1	0.42
0.4	2.4	0.48
0.45	2.7	0.54
0.5	3	0.6
0.55	3.3	0.66
0.6	3.6	0.72
0.65	3.9	0.78
0.7	4.2	0.84
0.75	4.5	0.9
0.8	4.8	0.96
0.85	5.1	1.02
0.9	5.4	1.08
0.95	5.7	1.14
1	6	1.2

Medication	*Dosage*	*Comments*
Erythromycin	10 mg/kg/dose i.v./p.o. q6 h Ethylsuccinate: for chlamydial conjunctivitis and pneumonia: 12.5 mg/kg/dose p.o. q6 h × 14 d	• Compatible with TPN • Reduces theophylline clearance; monitor levels
Erythropoietin (Epogen)	50–200 units/kg/dose s.c. q. MWF Or 100 units/kg/dose s.c. 5 times/wk Or 200 units/kg/dose s.c. every other day for 10 doses i.v. route requires an increase of 30%–50% of dose	• Supplement with iron concurrently to provide for increased requirements during expansion of red cell mass
Esmolol (Brevibloc)	SVT Loading dose: 100–500 μg/kg over 1 min Maintenance dose: 200 μg/kg/min Titrate 50–100 μg/kg/min q5–10 min (range: 300–1,000 μg/kg/min)	• Standard continuous concentrations: 5 mg/mL, 10 mg/mL, 20 mg/mL • Class II antiarrhythmic for SVT • Blocks response to β1-adrenergic stimulation • Use in extreme caution in patients with hyperreactive airway disease • DO NOT administer through UAC line
Fentanyl (Sublimaze)	Sedation/analgesia: 1–4 μg/kg/dose q2–4 h Continuous: 0.5–2 μg/kg bolus, then 0.5–1 μg/kg/h	• Standard continuous concentrations 5 μg/mL, 10 μg/mL, 40 μg/mL • Compatible with TPN • Adjust dose in renal failure • Reverse with naloxone • Slow i.v.p. over 3–5 min to prevent chest wall rigidity • Less histamine effect (more suitable in CLD with less airway narrowing) • Less GI motility impairment, less urinary retention • Decreases peripheral vascular resistance which is potentially useful in PPHN

Dose desired (μg/kg/h)	*Rate (mL/h) = Factor × Weight (kg) Concentration*	
	5 μg/mL	*10 μg/mL*
0.5	0.1	0.05
1	0.2	0.1
2	0.4	0.2
3	0.6	0.3
4	0.8	0.4
5	1	0.5

TABLE A1.1 Commonly Used Medications in a Newborn Intensive Care Unit (*continued*)

Medication	*Dosage*	*Comments*
Ferrous sulfate (Fer-in-sol)	2–4 mg elemental iron/kg/d div q12–24 h Max 15 mg/d = 0.6 mL/d	• Fer-in-sol contains 25 mg elemental iron/mL • Delaying initiating iron supplementation for infant until 1 mo of age since oral iron may reduce vitamin E absorption • Iron-fortified formulas contain 12-mg iron/L, providing ~2 mg/kg/d
Filgrastim (Neupogen)	5–10 μg/kg/d i.v./s.c. once daily for 3–5 d	• For neutropenic neonates with sepsis • Discontinue filgrastim when ANC >1,000/mm^3 for 3 d
Fluconazole (Diflucan)	Systemic fungal infection: 12–25 mg/kg loading dose, then 6–12 mg/kg/dose i.v. q24 h Prophylaxis regimen: 3–6 mg/kg/dose i.v./p.o. (see dosing interval table below)	• ANC = (neutrophils + bands) (WBC × 10) • Second-line agent at our institution for infections with *Candida* species after persistent positive blood culture taken at 48–72 h while on lipid complex amphotericin B (ABLC) • DO NOT use fluconazole for *Candida krusei* • Monitor liver enzymes • Adjust for renal failure • Oral bioavailability >90% • Prophylaxis regimen provides targeted short-term fluconazole prophylaxis for VLBW infants at highest risk for invasive fungal infections (IFIs) during periods of broad-spectrum antibiotic administration • Criteria for prophylaxis: <1,000 g, <6 wk postnatal AND with one of the following: Central venous access Parenteral nutrition Endotracheal intubation History of NEC

Postmenstrual Age (wk)	*Postnatal Age (d)*	*Dosing Interval (h)*
≤29	0–14	72
	>14	48
30–36	0–14	4
	14	24
37–44	0–7	48
	>7	24
≥45	>0	24

Medication	*Dosage*	*Comments*
Flucytosine (Ancobon)	25–100 mg/kg/d div q12–24 h	• Therapeutic level: 25–100 μg/mL • Draw level 2 h postdose on or after day 4 • Good CNS penetration • Not to be used as monotherapy • Monitor liver enzymes, bone marrow suppression, BUN, SCr, and crystalluria
Flumazenil (Romazicon)	0.01 mg/kg i.v. over 15 s; repeat every minute for cumulative dose of 0.05 mg/kg or total of 1 mg whichever is lower	• Treatment of benzodiazepine overdose • Onset of action within 1–3 min
Fosphenytoin (Cerebyx)	Loading dose for status epilepticus: 15–20 mg PE/kg i.v. over 10 min Maintenance dose: 4–6 mg PE/kg/d i.v.	• DOSE expressed as phenytoin sodium equivalents (PE) • Phenytoin 1 mg = fosphenytoin 1 mg PE • MAX 3 mg/PE/kg/min • Monitor phenytoin serum concentrations
Furosemide (Lasix)	1–2 mg/kg/dose q12–24 h i.v./p.o./i.m.	• Monitor electrolytes • Poor oral bioavailability • Compatible with TPN
Ganciclovir (Cytovene)	Congenital CMV infections: 6 mg/kg/d i.v. q12 h for 6 wk	• Congenital CMV infections as recommended by infectious disease specialist and manifests with hearing loss and learning disabilities • CMV IgM (+) indicates current/recent exposure • Adjust dose in renal failure • Monitor CBC, platelets, UO, SCr, and liver enzymes • Handle and dispose of as chemotherapeutic agent
Gentamicin	For early-onset sepsis PMA age <29 wk <7 d: 5 mg/kg/dose i.v. q48 h >7 d: 4 mg/kg/dose i.v. q36 h PMA age 30–34 wk <7 d: 4.5 mg/kg/dose i.v. q36 h >7 d: 4 mg/kg/dose i.v. q24 h PMA age >35 wk: 4 mg/kg/dose i.v. q24 h	• Therapeutic level • Peak 6–12 μg/mL • Trough 0.5–1.2 μg/mL • Concentration-dependent killing • Desired peak level = Eight times *MIC* • Target synergy peak level is 3–4 μg/mL
Glucagon	Hypoglycemia: 0.02–0.03 mg/kg i.v./i.m. × 1 dose. May repeat × 1 dose in 20 min if needed	• Dilute with manufacturer-provided diluent to final concentration of 1 mg/mL

(*continued*)

TABLE A1.1 Commonly Used Medications in a Newborn Intensive Care Unit (*continued*)

<table>
<tr><th>Medication</th><th>Dosage</th><th>Comments</th></tr>
<tr><td>Glycopyrrolate (Robinul)</td><td>p.o. 40–100 µg/kg/dose t.i.d.–q.i.d.
i.m./i.v. 4–10 µg/kg/dose q3–4 h</td><td>• Decreases oral secretions
• Oral absorption is poor
• Contains benzyl alcohol as preservative and should, therefore, be used with caution in neonates when given parenterally</td></tr>
<tr><td>Heparin flush</td><td>10 units q24 h as heparin flush for CVC (Broviac) catheter</td><td>• See attached guideline on use of heparin to maintain line patency in the neonatal intensive care unit</td></tr>
<tr><td>Heparin</td><td>Loading dose 75 units/kg over 10 min
Maintenance dose 28 units/kg/h
Adjust to APTT of 60–85 s
<table>
<tr><th>APTT (s)</th><th>Dose Adjustment</th><th>Time to Repeat APTT</th></tr>
<tr><td><50</td><td>50 units/kg bolus, increase infusion rate by 10%</td><td>4 h after infusion change</td></tr>
<tr><td>50–59</td><td>Increase infusion rate 10%</td><td>4 h after infusion change</td></tr>
<tr><td>60–85</td><td>Continue same rate</td><td>4 h after infusion change</td></tr>
<tr><td>86–95</td><td>Decrease infusion rate 10%</td><td>4 h after infusion change</td></tr>
<tr><td>96–120</td><td>Hold infusion 30 min; then ↓infusion rate by 10%</td><td>4 h after infusion change</td></tr>
<tr><td>>120</td><td>Hold infusion 60 min; then ↓infusion rate by 15%</td><td>4 h after infusion change</td></tr>
</table></td><td>• Standard continuous concentrations: 10 units/mL, 50 units/mL, 100 unit/mL
• Treatment of thrombosis
• Obtain APTT 4 h after initiation of infusion and every 4 h after infusion rate change
• Monitor for signs of bleeding
• Contraindicated in IVH, GI bleed, platelets <50,000
Adapted from Monagle P, Chan AKC, Goldenberg NA, et al. Antithrombotic therapy in neonates and children: Antithrombotic Therapy and Prevention of Thrombosis: American College of Chest Physicians Evidence-Based Clinical Practice Guidelines (9th Edition). Chest 2012;141(2 Suppl):e737S–e801S.</td></tr>
<tr><td>Homatropine (Isopto-Homatropine) 2%</td><td>Uveitis:
One drop b.i.d.–t.i.d. into affected eye(s)</td><td>• Anticholinergic agent producing cycloplegia and mydriasis</td></tr>
<tr><td>Hyaluronidase (Amphadase)</td><td>Inject 150 units (1 mL) div as five separate 0.2 mL s.c./intradermal injections around the periphery of the extravasation site at the leading edge</td><td>• See attached guideline on the management of neonatal extravasations
• Initiate immediately and ideally within 1 h of extravasation
• Initiate for stage III/IV infiltrate
• Do not inject i.v.</td></tr>
<tr><td>Hydralazine (Apresoline)</td><td>0.1–0.2 mg/kg/dose i.v. q6–8 h
Max 3.5 mg/kg/d i.v.
0.25–1 mg/kg/dose p.o. q6–8 h
Max 5 mg/kg/d p.o.</td><td>• Low bioavailability when given p.o.</td></tr>
<tr><td>Hydrocortisone (Solu-Cortef)</td><td>Hypotension: 2 mg/kg i.v. × 1 dose then 1 mg/kg/dose i.v. q6 h
Anti-inflammatory or immunosuppressive: 1–5 mg/kg/d i.v.
CLD:
0.5 mg/kg/dose i.v. q6 h × 3 d, then
0.5 mg/kg/dose i.v. q8 h × 3 d, then
0.5 mg/kg/dose i.v. q12 h × 3 d, then
0.5 mg/kg/dose i.v. q24 h × 1 d
(total cumulative dose: 14 mg/kg over 10 d)
OR
0.5 mg/kg/dose i.v. q12 h for 12 d, then
0.25 mg/kg/dose i.v. q12 h for 3 d
(total cumulative dose: 13.5 mg/kg over 15 d)</td><td>• Third-line agent for treatment of hypotension in neonates not responding to inotropes for a short-course therapy (up to 5 d)
• Studies have shown that preterm neonates with critical cardiovascular compromise will respond to hydrocortisone treatment; evidence that VLBW neonates have impaired cortisol production in response to stress or endogenous or exogenous corticotropin
• Extended therapy will require slow tapering
• Monitor for edema, hypokalemia, hyperglycemia, growth suppression, suppression of HPA function
• Physiologic replacement doses of hydrocortisone are ~14 mg/m^2/d in the neonate
• Corticosteroids may facilitate extubation in ventilator-dependent neonates with established or evolving BPD
• Early, low-dose hydrocortisone treatment does not appear to be associated with increased cerebral palsy.
• Before treatment, the parents should be informed of the potential life-saving benefit and the uncertain additional risk of neurologic injury, and informed consent should be obtained</td></tr>
</table>

<table>
<thead>
<tr><th colspan="3">TABLE A1.1 Commonly Used Medications in a Newborn Intensive Care Unit (continued)</th></tr>
<tr><th>Medication</th><th>Dosage</th><th>Comments</th></tr>
</thead>
<tbody>
<tr><td>Ibuprofen (Motrin, Advil)</td><td>Analgesic:
4–10 mg/kg/dose p.o. q6–8 h
MAX 40 mg/kg/d
Intravenous (for PDA treatment):
Neonates 500–1,500 g and ≤32 wk gestational age
Initial dose of 10 mg/kg/dose i.v. × 1 dose followed by 5 mg/kg/dose i.v. q24 h × 2 doses (three-dose course)
High dose: 20 mg/kg/dose i.v. × 1 dose followed by 10 mg/kg/dose i.v. q24 h × 2 doses (three-dose course)</td><td>• Analgesic/antipyretic
• Use with caution with impaired renal or hepatic function
• Criteria for initiation of treatment in PDA: Echo confirmation of PDA with left-to-right shunting, check IVH status, check UO and serum creatinine, check platelet count
• Hold subsequent i.v. dose if UO decreases to <0.6 mL/kg/h
• A second course of treatment may be given if the ductus arteriosus fails to close or reopens
• Infuse through dedicated line over 15 min
• Monitor BUN, SCr, platelets, UO
• Contraindications: active bleeding, significant thrombocytopenia (platelets <60k), BUN > 30, SCr >1.4, UO <1 mL/kg/h coagulation defects, NEC
• 2018 meta-analysis comparing ibuprofen, indomethacin, and acetaminophen for closure of PDA found high-dose oral ibuprofen to offer the highest likelihood of success</td></tr>
<tr><td>Imipenem/cilastatin (Primaxin)</td><td>0–4 wk, <1,200 g: 20 mg/kg/dose i.v. q18–24 h
≤7 d: 1,200–1,500 g: 20 mg/kg/dose i.v. q12 h
≤7 d: >1,500 g: 25 mg/kg/dose i.v. q12 h
>7 d 1,200–1,500 g: 20 mg/kg/dose i.v. q12 h >1,500 g: 25 mg/kg/dose i.v. q8 h
1–3 mo: 25 mg/kg/dose i.v. q6 h</td><td>• Restricted criteria at most institutions and may require approval by an infectious disease specialist
• Reserved for more serious or refractory gram-negative infections with documented resistance to all other β-lactams
• Monitor for seizures
• Dose adjust in renal impairment</td></tr>
<tr><td>i.v. immunoglobulin (IVIG)</td><td>500–1,000 mg/kg/dose i.v. for 1 dose over 2–6 h</td><td>• Infuse via dedicated line
• Restricted criteria at most institutions:
Neonatal platelet alloimmunization
May require approval by hematology disease specialist</td></tr>
<tr><td>Indomethacin (Indocin)</td><td>Treatment of PDA: (i.v.):
<table>
<tr><th>Age at First Dose</th><th>Dose #1</th><th>Dose #2</th><th>Dose #3</th></tr>
<tr><td><48 h</td><td>0.2 mg/kg</td><td>0.1 mg/kg</td><td>0.1 mg/kg</td></tr>
<tr><td>2–7 d</td><td>0.2 mg/kg</td><td>0.2 mg/kg</td><td>0.2 mg/kg</td></tr>
<tr><td>>7 d</td><td>0.2 mg/kg</td><td>0.25 mg/kg</td><td>0.25 mg/kg</td></tr>
</table>
Dosing regimen q12 h. Consider q24 regimen in the ELBW neonate or with UO <1 mL/kg/h.</td><td>• Change to q24 in the ELBW neonate or if UO <1 mL/kg/h
• Decreases renal and GI blood flow
• Hold dose with oliguria UO <0.6 mL/kg/h
• Monitor BUN, SCr, platelets, UO
• Incompatible with TPN and lipids
• Use immediately after reconstitution
• Indomethacin is tightly bound to albumin and may displace bilirubin
• Contraindicated: active bleeding, significant thrombocytopenia (platelets <60k), BUN > 30 SCr >1.6 (as high as 1.8 reported), coagulation defects, NEC
• Do not administer via UAC.</td></tr>
<tr><td>Insulin (Insulin R)</td><td>0.05–0.2 units/kg/h continuous i.v. infusions
0.05–0.2 units/kg s.c. q6–12 h</td><td>• Standard continuous concentrations: 0.5 units/mL, or 1 unit/mL
• Use for persistent glucose intolerance in ELBW
• Compatible with or in TPN
• Preterm infants are insulin resistant
• Treatment for hyperkalemia requires glucose load of 5 mg/kg/min
• Flush ~10 mL through tubing to saturate binding sites of tubing
• Will require multiple dilutions for dose preparation in the ELBW neonate</td></tr>
<tr><td>Insulin, aspart (Novolog)</td><td>0.05–0.2 units/kg s.c. q6–12 h</td><td>• High-alert medication
• Rapid-acting insulin
• Will require multiple dilutions for dose preparation in the ELBW neonate</td></tr>
</tbody>
</table>

(continued)

TABLE A1.1 Commonly Used Medications in a Newborn Intensive Care Unit (*continued*)

Medication	*Dosage*	*Comments*
Iron dextran	Anemia of prematurity: 0.4–1 mg/kg/d i.v. continuous infusion (in TPN) With (concomitant) erythropoietin therapy: 20 mg/kg/wk i.v.	• Can be added to TPN • Will discolor TPN (rust color) • Monitor for rust color precipitates
Isoniazid	Treatment: 10–15 mg/kg/d p.o. q.d. or div q12 h Prophylaxis: 10 mg/kg/d p.o. once a day	• Monitor liver enzymes • Cytochrome P450 inhibitor—may increase concentrations of phenytoin, carbamazepine, and diazepam
Isoproterenol	0.05–2 μg/kg/min	• Standard continuous concentrations: 20 μg/mL, 40 μg/mL • Do not administer through UAC • Indicated for ventricular arrhythmia secondary to AV nodal block
Lansoprazole (Prevacid)	0.7–1.66 mg/kg/dose p.o. once daily	• Incompatible with TPN
Levothyroxine (Synthroid)	10–15 μg/kg/d p.o. 5–8 μg/kg/d i.v.	• Administer i.v. dose immediately after reconstitution • Give oral dose on empty stomach • i.v. dose = 50%–75% of oral dose
Lidocaine 1%	2–5 mg/kg s.c. 0.5–1 mg/kg endotracheally	• Use s.c. for ring or nerve blocks • Consider adding sodium bicarbonate to buffer lidocaine to decrease pain • Lidocaine also available as topical spray
Lidocaine/prilocaine (EMLA)	Topical agent: 0.5–2 g under occlusive dressing 1 h prior to procedure (1 g = 1 mL)	• Apply 2 g = 2 mL for term infants and 0.5 g = 0.5 mL for preterm infants • Appears safe in preterm infants when applied in small amounts once daily
Linezolid (Zyvox)	10 mg/kg/dose i.v./p.o. q8 h (Use q12 h in neonates <1,200 g and <7 d)	• Restricted criteria at most institutions and may require approval by an infectious disease specialist • Reserved for documented vancomycin-resistant *Enterococcus* (VRE) or documented infection with vancomycin-resistant *Staphylococcus aureus* or vancomycin-resistant *coagulase-negative staphylococci* • Monitor CBC/platelets for pancytopenia; ALT, optic neuropathy (long-term treatment), renal function • Enhanced vasopressor effects (dopamine, epinephrine) when given concomitantly with linezolid • Oral bioavailability 100%
Loperamide (Imodium)	0.08–0.24 mg/kg/d p.o. div b.i.d.–t.i.d. MAX 2 mg/dose	• Acts directly on intestinal muscles to inhibit peristalsis and prolong transit time • Used in neonates with high output stoma post small-bowel resections • May increase risk of bacterial overgrowth • Use caution in hepatic dysfunction
Lorazepam (Ativan)	Status epilepticus: 0.05 mg/kg i.v. over 2–5 min May repeat in 10–15 min Anxiety/sedation 0.05–0.1 mg/kg/dose i.v.p. q4–8 h	• Preparation contains benzyl alcohol and, therefore, use with caution, especially in preterm infants due to neurotoxicity and myoclonus • Dilute with sterile water 1:1 prior to infusion • Should be infused in a dedicated line (drug-compatibility issues) • Incompatible with TPN • Slow i.v.p. over 2 min
Magnesium sulfate	Hypomagnesemia: 25–50 mg/kg/dose **magnesium sulfate i.v.** q8–12 h for 2–3 doses Infuse slowly over 2–4 h	• 25–50 mg/kg/dose magnesium sulfate = 0.2–0.4 mEq magnesium/kg/dose • 1 g of magnesium sulfate = 98.6 mg **elemental** magnesium = 8.12 mEq magnesium • Do not exceed 1 mEq/kg/h
Medium-chain triglyceride (MCT oil)	Supplement with feeding to add an additional 10 kcal/kg/d Preterm neonates: 0.2–0.3 mL per feed (every 3 h)	• MCTs are composed of fatty acids with chain length varying from 6 to 12 carbon atoms • 1 mL = 7.7 calories • DOES NOT provide any essential fatty acids since it contains ONLY saturated fats

TABLE A1.1 Commonly Used Medications in a Newborn Intensive Care Unit (*continued*)

Medication	*Dosage*	*Comments*
Meropenem (Merrem)	Postnatal 0–7 d: 20 mg/kg/dose i.v. q12 h Postnatal >7 d: 1,200–2,000 g: 20 mg/kg/dose i.v. q12 h >2,000 g: 20 mg/kg/dose i.v. q8 h Meningitis: 40 mg/kg/dose i.v. q8 h	• Restricted criteria at most institutions and may require approval by an infectious disease specialist • Treatment of multidrug-resistant gram-negative and gram-positive aerobic and anaerobic pathogens • Safety and efficacy in children <3 mo of age have not been established • Adjust dose in renal impairment
Methadone	Neonatal abstinence syndrome: 0.05–0.2 mg/kg/dose i.v./p.o. q12–24 h taper dose by 10%–20%/wk	• Extended elimination half-life and, therefore, difficult to taper doses. Consider alternative agents • Cytochrome P450 isoenzyme substrate • Carbamazepine, phenytoin, nevirapine, nelfinavir, and rifampin may increase the metabolism of methadone and precipitate withdrawal • Methadone may increase zidovudine serum concentrations
Methylprednisolone (Solu-Medrol)	Status asthmaticus: 2 mg/kg i.v. × 1 loading dose, then 1 mg/kg/dose i.v. q6 h	• ONLY sodium succinate salt can be given i.v. • Short-course burst in preterm neonates for 5 d to assist in weaning off the ventilator when settings are no longer weanable and oxygenation not maintained
Metoclopramide (Reglan)	0.1 mg/kg/dose i.v./p.o. q6 h	• Monitor for extrapyramidal reactions: tardive dyskinesia, dystonia • Potent dopamine receptor antagonist • Increases gastric emptying time
Metronidazole (Flagyl)	0–4 wk, <1,200 g: 15 mg/kg/dose i.v. q48 h <2 kg: 7.5 mg/kg i.v. q12 h >2 kg, <7 d: 7.5 mg/kg/dose i.v./p.o. q8 h >2 kg, >7 d: 10 mg/kg/dose i.v./p.o. q8 h	• Do not refrigerate since precipitation may occur • Use with caution in patients with liver impairment
Micafungin (Mycamine)	10 mg/kg/dose i.v. q.d. (based on preliminary pharmacokinetic data)	• Restricted criteria at most institutions and may require approval by an infectious disease specialist • Add a third agent (echinocandin) for infections with all *Candida* species if persistent fungemia and repeat blood culture taken at 48–72 h remains positive despite combination therapy with ABLC and fluconazole • Appears that neonates have increased clearance requiring a higher dose • Monitor CBC, platelets, liver enzymes, and bilirubin levels • No adjustment required in renal impairment
Midazolam (Versed)	0.05–0.15 mg/kg slow i.v.p. q2–4 h 0.1–0.3 mg/kg/dose intranasal 0.15–0.45 mg/kg/dose p.o. Continuous infusion: Initial 0.03–0.06 mg/kg/h = 0.5–1 μg/kg/min).	• Standard continuous concentrations: 0.5 mg/mL, 1 mg/mL, and 5 mg/mL • Sedative/hypnotic • NO analgesic properties • Use preservative-free vials
Milrinone (Primacor)	Loading dose: 50 μg/kg i.v. over 15 min Maintenance dose: 0.5 μg/kg/min (reported range: 0.25–1 μg/kg/min)	• Standard continuous concentrations: 0.1 mg/mL, 0.2 mg/mL • Inhibits PDE3 which increase cAMP • Short-term treatment of acute decompensated heart failure • Incompatible with furosemide • Use caution in renal dysfunction
Morphine sulfate	0.05–0.2 mg/kg/dose i.v.p./s.c./i.m. q4 h p.r.n. 0.15–0.6 mg/kg p.o. q4 h p.r.n. 0.03–0.1 mg/kg/dose p.o. q3–4 h Continuous infusion: 0.01–0.03 mg/kg/h = 10–30 μg/kg/h Neonatal abstinence syndrome: 0.04 mg/kg = 0.1 mL/kg p.o. q3–4 h (reported range 0.03–0.1 mg/kg/dose) Increase dose by 0.02 mg/kg = 0.05 mL/kg/dose as needed until desired response is achieved Taper 10%–20% per day as tolerated	• Standard continuous concentrations: 0.2 mg/mL, 0.5 mg/mL • Monitor for respiratory depression, O_2 saturation, urinary retention, decreased bowel sounds • Continuous infusion for >5 d will likely develop withdrawal with an abrupt discontinuation • Use preservative-free product • Rate of morphine elimination is much slower in the neonate due to decrease in clearance rates resulting in higher serum concentrations

(*continued*)

TABLE A1.1 Commonly Used Medications in a Newborn Intensive Care Unit (*continued*)

Medication	*Dosage*	*Comments*
Multivitamin (Poly-Vi-Sol) (AquADEK)	Term infant: 1 mL/d Preterm infant: 1 mL/d div q6–12 h	• AquADEKs multivitamin drops differ from Poly-Vi-Sol in terms of a higher concentration of vitamins A, C, E, B_6, B_{12}, and C. ADEK also contains 400 μg vitamin K, 15 μg biotin, 5 mg zinc, 3 mg β-carotene, niacin, pantothenic acid, selenium, β-carotene, and coenzyme Q10.
Nafcillin	0–4 wk, <1,200 g: 25–50 mg/kg/dose q8–12 h ≤7 d, 1,200–2,000 g: 25 mg/kg/dose i.v. q12 h ≤7 d, >2,000 g: 25 mg/kg/dose i.v. q8 h >7 d, 1,200–2,000 g: 25 mg/kg/dose i.v. q8 h >7 d, >2,000 g: 25 mg/kg/dose i.v. q6 h	• Use for MSSA. Use caution in severe hepatic impairment
Naloxone (Narcan)	0.1 mg/kg i.v./i.m./s.c. Repeat every 2–3 min as needed for recurrent apnea and hypoventilation	• Management of neonatal opioid-induced depression • Should be avoided in babies whose mothers are suspected of having had long-term exposure to opioids (Class indeterminate)
Nevirapine (Viramune)	Prevention of maternal–fetal HIV transmission if higher risk of transmission: ≥32 k gestation at birth: 3 doses, given within 48 h of birth, 48 h after the first dose and 96 h after the second dose Birth weight 1.5–2 kg: 8 mg/dose p.o.; no calculation is required for this dose; **this is the actual dose, not a mg/kg dose** Birth weight >2 kg: 12 mg/dose p.o.; no calculation is required for this dose; **this is the actual dose, not a mg/kg dose**	• 2020 Perinatal HIV Guidelines • Non-nucleoside reverse transcriptase inhibitor • Use with 6-wk zidovudine prophylaxis to infant • Bioavailability >90% • 50 mg/5 mL oral suspension • Cytochrome P450 isoenzyme substrate inducer and inhibitor • Look-alike, sound-alike medication: may be confused with nelfinavir (Viracept)
Nystatin	Oral candidiasis: 100,000 units p.o. q.i.d. (50,000 units to each side of cheek)	• Shake suspension well before use • Concentration: 100,000 units/mL
Octreotide (Sandostatin)	Persistent hyperinsulinemic hypoglycemia: 2–10 μg/kg/d i.v. div q12 h Increase dose per patient response MAX 40 μg/kg/d Chylothorax: 0.5–4 μg/kg/h continuous infusion for 1–2 wk. Titrate to response Reported range: 0.3–4 μg/kg/h	• Only Sandostatin injection may be i.v., i.m., and s.c. • Dilute continuous infusion in 50–200 mL of dextrose 5% or normal saline
Omeprazole (Prilosec)	1 mg/kg/d once daily or b.i.d. p.o.	• Proton-pump inhibitor which decreases the acid produced in the stomach • Used in neonates for severe reflux
Opium tincture, diluted (Laudanum)	0.08–0.2 mg/dose p.o. q3–4 h p.r.n. DO NOT CONFUSE WITH CAMPHORATED TINCTURE OF OPIUM (PAREGORIC)	• Treatment of neonatal narcotic abstinence • Initiate dose at 0.08 mg for term infants every 3 h ATC; may be titrated to response slowly wean as tolerated • Monitor respiratory and cardiac status, abdominal distension and loss of bowel sounds, and decreased UO
Oxacillin	0–4 wk, <1,200 g: 25 mg/kg/dose i.v. q12 h <7 d: 1,200–2,000 g: 25–50 mg/kg/dose i.v. q12 h >2 kg: 25–50 mg/kg/dose i.v. q8 h >7 d: 1,200–2,000 g: 25–50 mg/kg/dose i.v. q8 h >2,000 g: 25–50 mg/kg/dose i.v. q6 h	• Monitor liver enzymes, bilirubin, CBC, BUN, SCr
Pancuronium (Pavulon)	0.1 mg/kg i.v.p. q1 h p.r.n. 0.02–0.04 mg/kg/h (0.4–0.6 μg/kg/min) continuous i.v. infusion	• Standard continuous concentrations: 0.1 mg/mL, 0.5 mg/mL • Monitor BP; infant must be intubated and sedated • Adjust in renal impairment • Continuous infusions are used rarely in the neonatal population when adequate and appropriate sedation is provided • Consider use of muscle relaxant to facilitate acute respiratory failure or hyperventilation ventilator management (PPHN) • Prolonged skeletal muscle paralysis in the preterm neonate is not advised

TABLE A1.1 Commonly Used Medications in a Newborn Intensive Care Unit (*continued*)

Medication	*Dosage*	*Comments*
Penicillin G, aqueous	Proven or highly probably congenital syphilis: 50,000 units/kg/dose i.v. q12 h × 7 d, then 50,000 units/kg/dose i.v. q8 h thereafter for a total of 10 d	• Compatible with TPN and lipid • 10-D treatment for congenital syphilis
Penicillin G benzathine	50,000 units/kg × 1 dose i.m.	• One dose i.m. only for asymptomatic congenital syphilis in neonates >1,200 g
Penicillin G procaine	50,000 units/kg/d i.m. q24 h × 10 d	• i.m. only • Use with caution in neonates due to procaine toxicity and sterile abscesses
Phenobarbital	Loading dose: 15–20 mg/kg/dose i.v./p.o. Maintenance dose: 5 mg/kg/d i.v./p.o. div q12 h	• Therapeutic level: 15–40 μg/mL • Half-life in neonates 45–200 h • Obtain trough level just before next dose • May give additional 5 mg/kg boluses q15 min until seizure controlled. MAX 40 mg/kg
Phentolamine (Regitine)	Dilute 5 mg vial with 10 mL preservative-free normal saline Administer 0.1 mL injections s.c. around the periphery of the extravasation site at the leading edge Do not exceed a max dose of 0.1 mg/kg or 2.5 mg total	• Use for extravasations with α-adrenergic drugs
Phenylephrine 2.5%	One drop 15–30 min prior to ROP examination	• Use only the 2.5% ophthalmic solution in neonates • Apply pressure to the lacrimal sac postadministration to minimize systemic absorption

Phenytoin (Dilantin)	Loading dose: 15–20 mg/kg i.v./p.o. × 1 dose
	Maintenance dose: 5 mg/kg/d maintenance dose div q12 h (reported range: 5–8 mg/kg/d)
		• Max infusion rate 0.5–1 mg/kg/min
		• Initiate maintenance dose 12 h after loading dose
		• Therapeutic range: 8–15 μg/mL
		• Therapeutic free (unbound) range: 1.5–2.5 μg/mL (up to 20% free)
		• Oral loading doses should be div in 2–3 doses q2 h to ensure complete oral absorption
		• Monitor free and total serum concentrations in patients with hyperbilirubinemia, hypoalbuminemia, renal dysfunction, and uremia
		• Neonates have increased free fraction due to decreased protein binding
		• Follows dose-dependent Michaelis–Menten pharmacokinetics
		• Draw trough level just before next dose
		• Postload/peak: 1 h after end of infusion
		• Give oral dose 2 h before feeds if possible
		• Drug interactions:
		  • Phenytoin can decrease serum concentrations of theophylline, dopamine
		  • Phenytoin serum concentrations can be decreased by zidovudine, continuous nasogastric feeds

Phosphate, Na/K	Low dose: 0.08 mmol/kg Intermediate dose: 0.16–0.24 mmol/kg for serum level 0.5–1 mg/dL High dose: 0.36 mmol/kg for serum level <0.5 mg/dL	• Infuse slowly over 1–2 h (max: 0.06 mmol/kg/h) • Peripheral line max concentration: 0.05 mmol/mL • Central line max concentration: 0.12 mmol/mL • Neonates are in positive phosphate balance, and only 60% of phosphate absorbed from diet is excreted in the urine • High serum phosphate level in neonates is NOT a manifestation of a lower GFR but of a higher proximal tubular reabsorption capacity • Normal serum phosphate levels in a neonate are 4.8–8.2 mg/dL
Phytonadione (Vitamin K)	Hemorrhagic disease of newborn: 0.5 mg s.c./i.m., birth weight <1,500 g 1 mg s.c./i.m., birth weight >1,500 g	• s.c. is the preferred route • Vitamin K deficiency due to malabsorption, decreased synthesis of vitamin K, and drug interactions
Piperacillin	≤7 d: 50 mg/kg/dose i.v. q8 h >7 d: 50 mg/kg/dose i.v. q6 h	• Synergy with aminoglycosides • Adjust with renal dysfunction

(*continued*)

TABLE A1.1 Commonly Used Medications in a Newborn Intensive Care Unit (*continued*)

Medication	*Dosage*	*Comments*
Piperacillin/tazobactam (Zosyn)	150–300 mg/kg/d of piperacillin component i.v. div q6–8 h	• Restricted criteria at most institutions and may require approval by an infectious disease specialist • Adjust dose for renal dysfunction • Tazobactam prevents degradation of piperacillin by binding to β-lactamases • Tazobactam component does not provide any additional coverage for *Pseudomonas aeruginosa*
Plasma protein fraction (Plasmanate)	10 mL/kg i.v. over 30–60 min. May repeat dose if needed	• Isotonic crystalloid solutions should be used first line [Neonatal Resuscitation guidelines 2005 states that an isotonic crystalloid rather than albumin is the solution of choice for volume expansion in the delivery room. (Class IIb; LOE 7)]. • Avoid 25% concentration in preterm neonates because of increased risk for IVH
Poractant alfa (Curosurf)	Intratracheal: Initial dose: 2.5 mL/kg/dose (200 mg/kg/dose), then 1.25 mL/kg/dose (100 mg/kg/dose) q12 h for up to 2 additional doses MAX 5 mL/kg	• Treatment of respiratory distress syndrome (RDS) in premature infants • Criteria: FiO_2 >0.3 and MAP >7 • Unused AND unopened vials warmed to room temperature may be returned to refrigerator within 24 h (warming: ONCE ONLY). • 80 mg/mL (1.5 mL, 3 mL)
Potassium supplements	0.5–1 mEq/kg/dose slow i.v. (max 1 mEq/kg/h) Hypokalemia secondary to diuretics: 1–2 mEq/kg/d p.o. q.d. or div q12 h	• Infuse 0.3–0.5mEq/kg/h (max rate: 1 mEq/kg/h) • MUST be diluted prior to i.v. administration • Peripheral line concentration: 0.08 mEq/mL • Central line concentration 0.15 mEq/mL • p.o. formulation should also be diluted prior to administration • Normal daily requirement 2–6 mEq/kg/d
Prednisolone	Asthma exacerbations: 1–2 mg/kg/d div b.i.d.	• Look-alike sound-alike medication; may be confused with PredniSONE
Prednisone	Asthma exacerbations 1–2 mg/kg/d div b.i.d.	• Look-alike sound-alike medication; may be confused with PrednisoLONE
Propranolol (Inderal)	0.25 mg/kg/dose p.o. q6–8 h up to max of 5 mg/kg/d 0.01 mg/kg slow i.v.p. over 10 min. Repeat every 6–8 h up to max of 0.15 mg/kg/dose i.v. q6–8 h	• Do not abruptly discontinue therapy. Taper over 2 wk • Cytochrome P450 isoenzyme and substrate
Prostaglandin E1 (Alprostadil) (Prostin VR)	0.05–0.1 µg/kg/min (up to 0.4 µg/kg/min has been reported) *Final Concentration* — *Rate Calculation (Multiply Factor × Weight [kg])* 5 µg/mL — 0.6–1.2 mL/kg/h 10 µg/mL — 0.3–0.6 mL/kg/h	• Max 0.4 µg/kg/min • Standard continuous concentrations: 5 µg/mL, 10 µg/mL • Monitor for apnea, hypocalcemia, hypoglycemia, and hypokalemia • Infuse through UVC at ductal opening • Therapeutic response indicated with increase in pH and increase with systemic BP. Once stable, the rate may be decreased by 50% • Long-term use of prostaglandin E1 can lead to gastric outlet obstructions, cortical hyperostosis • Observe closely for extravasations secondary to high osmolarity
Pyridoxine (vitamin B_6)	Pyridoxine-depended seizures: 10–100 mg p.o./i.m./i.v.	• Prevention and treatment of pyridoxine-dependent seizures in infants
Ranitidine (Zantac)	<2 wk: 1 mg/kg/dose i.v./p.o. q12 h >1 mo: 2–4 mg/kg/d i.v. div q6–8 h 2–4 mg/kg/d p.o. div q12 h Continuous: 0.0625 mg/kg/h (range 0.04–0.1 mg/kg/h)	• Compatible with TPN and lipids • Safety and effectiveness of use in neonates <1 mo has not been established • Use with caution when thrombocytopenia present • H2-blocker use as been associated with late-onset sepsis and NEC. It should be discontinued as soon as possible • There is wide variability among institutions in patterns of use of ranitidine and other similar medications. Randomized controlled trials are needed to develop a consistent evidence-based approach • Dose adjust in renal impairment

TABLE A1.1 Commonly Used Medications in a Newborn Intensive Care Unit (*continued*)

Medication	*Dosage*	*Comments*
Rifampin (Rifadin)	10–20 mg/kg/d p.o./i.v. div q12 h	• Causes red/orange discoloration of body secretions • Used with vancomycin for synergy for *staphylococcal* infections • Slow i.v. over 30 min • May need to increase dose of theophylline, digoxin if given concomitantly • Monitor liver enzymes, CBC, bilirubin, platelets
Rocuronium	Rapid sequence intubation: 0.5 mg/kg over 30 s Maintenance of relaxation Intermittent dose: 0.075–0.15 mg/kg over 30 s Continuous infusion: 7–10 μg/kg/min	• Moderate increase in half-life in liver disease, minimal increase in renal disease • Histamine release at high doses • Longer acting in neonates compared to older children
Sildenafil (Revatio)	Pulmonary hypertension: 0.25–1 mg/kg/dose p.o. q8–12 h (Wide range of doses has been reported. Further studies are needed to determine optimal dose in the neonatal population)	• PDE5 inhibitor • Monitor BP closely due to vasodilator effects • Monitor platelets, ROP, loss of hearing • Cytochrome P450 isoenzyme and substrate
Silver sulfadiazine (Silvadene)	Apply once daily or b.i.d.	• Acts on bacterial cell wall and cell membrane
Sodium bicarbonate	HCO_3 needed (mEq) = Base deficit (mEq/L) × 0.3 × Weight (kg)	• Max concentration 0.5 mEq/mL • Infuse through dedicated line and monitor closely for extravasation • Tissue necrosis can occur due to the hyperosmolarity of sodium bicarbonate. (4.2% = 0.5 mEq/mL = 900 mOsm/L) • Not compatible with calcium or any calcium-containing solution. Immediate precipitation will result • Not compatible with TPN • Administer slowly at max rate of 10 mEq/min or 1 mEq/kg/h
Sodium chloride	Correction of hyponatremia: mEq sodium needed = (desired sodium [mEq/L] − actual sodium [mEq/L]) × 0.6 × Weight (kg)	• Maintenance requirements: Preterm: 2–8 mEq/kg/d Term: 1–4 mEq/kg/d • Serum/plasma levels: Preterm: 132–140 mEq/L Term: 133–142 mEq/L >2 mo: 135–145 mEq/L
Sodium polystyrene sulfonate (Kayexalate)	1 g/kg/d p.o./p.r. q6 h	• 1 g of resin binds ~1 mEq potassium • Use with caution in neonates, especially in preterm neonates with rectal route secondary to reported perforations • Does NOT rapidly reverse hyperkalemia • Sodium content ~100 mg/g
Spironolactone (Aldactone)	1–3 mg/kg/dose p.o. div q12–24 h	• Monitor electrolytes, BUN, SCr
Sulfacetamide (Bleph-10)	1–2 drops q1–3 h × 7–10 d (during daytime) Ointment: once daily to q.i.d. and at bedtime	• Treatment and prophylaxis of conjunctivitis
Sulfamethoxazole/trimethoprim (Bactrim)	>2 mo: Mild–moderate infections: 6–12 mg TMP/kg/d i.v. div q12 h	• Cytochrome P450 inhibitor • Bioavailability 90%–100% • Dose recommendations are based on the trimethoprim (TMP) component • Dose adjust in renal impairment
Theophylline	See aminophylline	
Ticarcillin/clavulanate (Timentin)	200–300 mg ticarcillin component/kg/d div i.v. q6–8 h	• Restricted criteria at most institutions and may require approval by an infectious disease specialist • Antibacterial activity is synergistic when given concomitantly with aminoglycosides • Adjust dose in renal dysfunction • Monitor BUN, SCr, liver enzymes, CBC

(*continued*)

TABLE A1.1 Commonly Used Medications in a Newborn Intensive Care Unit (*continued*)

Medication	*Dosage*	*Comments*

Tobramycin (Tobrex)	PMA age <29 wk
	<7 d: 5 mg/kg/dose i.v. q48 h
	>7 d: 4 mg/kg/dose i.v. q36 h
	PMA age 30–34 wk
	<7 d: 4.5 mg/kg/dose i.v. q36 h
	>7 d: 4 mg/kg/dose i.v. q24 h
	PMA age >35 wk: 4 mg/kg/dose i.v. q24 h
		• Therapeutic levels:
		  • Peak 4–12 μg/mL
		  • Trough 0.5–1.2 μg/mL
		• Reserved for gentamicin-resistant gram-negative pathogens
		• Concentration-dependent killing
		• Peak level desired is 8 times the *MIC*

Topiramate (Topamax)	1–3 mg/kg/dose p.o. q.d. (max 25 mg) Increase weekly by 1–3 mg/kg/d div p.o. b.i.d. (Maintenance dose: 5–9 mg/kg/d p.o. div b.i.d.)	• Cytochrome P450 inhibitor • Topiramate may increase phenytoin levels and phenytoin, and carbamazepine may decrease topiramate levels
Trace metals (PTE-5)	Product that is used in TPN: 0.2 mL/kg/d of PTE-5 Contents per mL of PTE-5 *Cr* | *Cu* | *I* | *Mn* | *Se* | *Zn* 1 μg | 0.1 mg | … | 25 μg | 15 μg | 1 mg	• Metals may accumulate in conditions of renal failure or biliary obstruction • Must be diluted prior to use • Remove copper and manganese for biliary obstruction with marked increase in liver enzymes
Tropicamide 1% (Mydriacyl)	Cycloplegia: 1–2 drops (1%) May repeat in 5 min	• Eye examination must be performed within 30 min • Apply pressure to lacrimal sac postadministration to minimize systemic absorption
Ursodiol (Actigall) (UDCA)	Biliary atresia: 10–15 mg/kg/d once daily TPN-induced cholestasis 10 mg/kg/dose p.o. t.i.d.	• Treatment of cholestasis associated with TPN, biliary atresia, and cystic fibrosis • Monitor direct biliary levels • Hydrophobic bile acid that decreases both secretion of cholesterol from liver and its intestinal absorption
Valproic acid (Depakene, Depakote)	i.v.: 10–15 mg/kg/d div q6 h Increase by 5–10 mg/kg/d weekly until therapeutic level obtained p.o.: 10–15 mg/kg/d div q.d.–t.i.d. Increase by 5–10 mg/kg/d weekly until therapeutic level obtained Rectal: Loading dose: 17–20 mg/kg Maintenance dose: 10–15 mg/kg/dose q8 h	• Monitor trough concentrations closely • Therapeutic range: (increased free fraction in neonates) Total: 40–80 μg/mL Free: <15–20 μg/mL • Neonates will have an increased free fraction due to decreased protein binding • Monitor liver enzymes, bilirubin, CBC, platelets, serum ammonia • Monitor above closely secondary to reports of hepatic failure, pancreatitis, and hyperammonemic encephalopathy. Contraindicated in severe hepatic dysfunction • VPA is a CYP2D6 isoenzyme inhibitor: will increase levels of phenobarbital and can displace phenytoin from protein-binding sites • Reserved agent as recommended by neurology for refractory uncontrolled seizures in neonates not responding to more standard treatment modalities

Vancomycin	15 mg/kg/dose i.v.
	PMA age <29 wk
	<14 d: q18 h
	>14 d: q12 h
	PMA age 30–36 wk
	<14 d: q12 h
	>14 d: q8 h
	PMA age >37 wk:
	<7 d: q12 h
	>7 d: q8 h
		• Therapeutic levels:
		  • Peak: 25–40 μg/mL
		  • Trough 5–15 μg/mL
		• More aggressive target peak and trough serum concentrations for vancomycin may be required in certain disease states such as endocarditis, meningitis, and osteomyelitis
		• Neonates: Postnatal age >14 d and <1,200 g may eliminate vancomycin at a quicker rate at this later postnatal age requiring a shorter frequency dosing regimen. Consider q12–18 h dosing interval
		• Desired trough level should be 4× *MIC*
		• Obtain levels if course >3 d and every 7 d as therapy continues
		• Monitor BUN, SCr 2–3 times a week
		• Incompatible with heparin >1:1
		• Time-dependent killing > *MIC*

TABLE A1.1 Commonly Used Medications in a Newborn Intensive Care Unit (*continued*)

Medication	*Dosage*	*Comments*
Vecuronium	Initial dose: 0.03–0.15 mg/kg over 30 s Continuous infusion: 1.5–2.5 μg/kg/min	• Prolonged half-life in renal or hepatic disease secondary to active metabolite • Longer acting in neonates compared to older children
Vitamin A (Aquasol A)	5,000 international units i.m. every MWF	• 12 doses total or up to postnatal age of 28 d • Protect from light • Studies have shown a decrease in CLD among ELBW infants, decrease in sepsis, and increase overall survival (NNT = 13)
Vitamin D (Ergocalciferol)	400–1,200 IU p.o. once a day	• Monitor alkaline phosphatase levels • 8,000 IU/mL
Vitamin E	25–50 IU p.o. once a day	• Routine administration for ROP or BPD secondary to O_2 therapy is not recommended by AAP
Zidovudine (Retrovir)	**<30 wk gestation at birth** Birth to age 4–6 wk: 2 mg/kg/dose p.o. q12 h **≥30–<35 wk gestation at birth** Birth to age 2 wk: 2 mg/kg/dose p.o. q12 h Age 2 wk to 4–6 wk: 3 mg/kg/dose p.o. q12 h **≥35 wk gestation at birth:** 4 mg/kg/dose p.o. q12 h	• Length of therapy: 6 wk • Monitor CBC • Formerly known as AZT

AAP, American Academy of Pediatrics; ABLC, amphotericin B lipid complex; ACE, angiotensin-converting enzyme; ANC, absolute neutrophil count; APTT, activated partial thromboplastin time; ATC, around the clock; AV, atrioventricular; b.i.d., twice daily; BP, blood pressure; BPD, bronchopulmonary dysplasia; BUN, blood urea nitrogen; CBC, complete blood count; CHF, chronic heart failure; CI, cardiac index; CLD, chronic lung disease; CMV, cytomegalovirus; CNS, central nervous system; CSF, cerebral spinal fluid; CVC, central venous catheter; div, divided; D5W, dextrose 5% in water; D10W, dextrose 10% in water; ELBW, extremely low birth weight; FDA, Food and Drug Administration; G6PD, glucose 6 phosphate dehydrogenase deficiency; GA, gestational age; GBS, group B streptococcus; GI, gastrointestinal; HPA, hypopituitary axis; HSV, herpes simplex virus; HTN, hypertension; i.m., intramuscular; IVH, intraventricular hemorrhage; i.v.p., intravenous push; MAP, mean arterial pressure; *MIC*, minimum inhibitory concentration; MSSA, methicillin-sensitive *Staphylococcus aureus*; MWF, Monday, Wednesday, and Friday; NEC, necrotizing enterocolitis; NNT, number needed to treat; PDA, patent ductus arteriosus; PDE, phosphodiesterase; plat, platelets; PMA, premenstrual age; p.o., orally; PPHN, persistent pulmonary hypertension in newborns; p.r., rectal; p.r.n., as needed; PVC, premature ventricular contraction; q.d., daily; q.i.d., four times a day; ROP, retinopathy of prematurity; s.c., subcutaneous; SCr, serum creatinine;
SVT, supraventricular tachycardia; TDD, total digitalizing dose; t.i.d. thrice daily; TPA, tissue plasminogen activator; TPN, total parenteral nutrition; UAC, umbilical artery catheter; UO, urinary output; UVC, umbilical venous catheter; VLBW, very low birth weight; VPA, valproic acid; VTE, venous thromboembolism.

TABLE A1.2 Recommended Childhood Immunization (0–6 Year) Schedule for the United States 2009[a]

	Birth	*2 mo*	*4 mo*	*6 mo*	*6–12 mo*	*12–15 mo*	*15–18 mo*	*19–23 mo*	*2–3 y*	*4–6 y*
Diphtheria, tetanus, acellular pertussis		X	X	X			X			X
Haemophilus influenzae type B		X	X	X		X				
Hepatitis A							(Two doses)			
Hepatitis B	X	X			X					
Influenza						GIVE YEARLY INFLUENZA VACCINE				
Meningococcal									MCV	
MMR						X				X
Pneumococcal—conjugated 13		X	X	X		X				
Polio virus—inactivated		X	X		X				X	
Rotavirus		X	X	X						
Varicella						X				X

[a]Use of combination vaccine products is encouraged at initiation of 2-month vaccine administration to decrease number of required injections. See Table A1.4 for combination products available.
MCV, meningococcal conjugated vaccine; MMR, measles, mumps, rubella.

TABLE A1.3 Hepatitis B Surface Antigen Status

Mother's HepBsAg Status	*Hepatitis B Vaccine Schedule*	*Hepatitis B Immunoglobulin (HBIG) Schedule*
Positive	Dose #1 @ birth (≤12 h) Dose #2 @ 1–2 mo Dose #3 @ 6 mo	HBIG Dose @ birth (≤12 h)
Negative	Dose #1 @ birth (before discharge)[a] Dose #2 @ 1–2 mo Dose #3 @ 6–18 mo	Not required
Unknown	Dose #1 @ birth (≤12 h) Dose #2 @ 1–2 mo Dose #3 @ 6 mo	Determine the mother's HepBsAg status as soon as possible postdelivery. Preterm neonates (<2 kg): Dose @ birth (≤12 h) Mother's HepBsAg status must be determined within 12 h postdelivery for the preterm infant. If not determined within 12 h, the HBIG must be given due to less reliable immune response Term neonates Administer HBIG within 7 d if mother tests HepBsAg positive

[a]The first dose of hepatitis B vaccine should be administered at the time of birth for term infants. Preterm infants should receive the first dose of hepatitis B vaccine at the time of discharge or by 1 month chronologic age, regardless of weight. This initial vaccine, however, should not be counted in the required three doses to complete the immunization series.

TABLE A1.4 Vaccines

Vaccines	*Dosage*	*Notes*
Diphtheria, tetanus, and acellular pertussis (DTaP) (Infanrix, Tripedia)	0.5 mL i.m.	• The fourth dose may be administered as early as 12 mo as long as 6 mo has elapsed since the third dose • Administer final dose in the series at 4–6 y
DTaP/IPV/HIB (Pentacel)	0.5 mL i.m.	• The vaccine is approved for use in infants and children aged 6 wk through 4 y • Four doses given at 2, 4, 6, and 15–18 mo of age
Haemophilus B conjugate vaccine PedvaxHIB (Act-HIB)	0.5 mL i.m.	• Minimum age of 6 wk • The conjugate HIB vaccines licensed for use in infants are interchangeable • Act-HIB: Previously unvaccinated infants aged 2 through 6 mo should receive 3 doses of vaccine administered 2 mo apart, followed by a booster dose at age 12–15 mo • PedvaxHIB: Unvaccinated children aged 2 through 11 mo should receive 2 doses of vaccine 2 mo apart, followed by a booster dose at 12–15 mo of age
Hepatitis A (Havrix) (Vaqta)	0.5 mL i.m. administered as two injections 6–12 mo apart	• Minimum age of 12 mo for first dose
Hepatitis B vaccine (Recombivax HB, Engerix-B)	0.5 mL i.m. Strength for each brand is different: 10 µg = 0.5 mL = Engerix-B 5 µg = 0.5 mL = Recombivax HB	• Administer the first dose within 24 h of birth for all medically stable infants ≥2,000 g • For infants <2,000 g: administer 1 dose at chronologic age 1 mo or hospital discharge • Mothers HepBsAg unknown should receive the vaccine within 12 h of birth. Preterm infants should receive HBIG as well if status is not determined within 12 h • Thimerosal-free vaccine • Four doses of Hep B to infants are permissible when combination vaccines are administered after the birth dose

TABLE A1.4 Vaccines (*continued*)

Vaccines	*Dosage*	*Notes*
Hepatitis B vaccine/DTaP/IPOL Combination vaccine (Pediarix)	0.5 mL i.m.	• This combination vaccine should not be used in infants younger than 6 wk. Therefore, it should be initiated at 2 mo immunization schedule • Use of this combination vaccine at each routine immunization schedule will result in administration of a fourth dose of hepatitis B vaccine (accepted on routine schedule)
Hepatitis B vaccine/haemophilus B conjugate Combination vaccine (Comvax)	0.5 mL i.m.	• This combination vaccine should not be used in infants younger than 6 wk. Therefore, it should be initiated at 2 mo immunization schedule
Influenza vaccine (inactivated) (Fluzone)	TIV: • 6–35 mo: 0.25 mL i.m. • >3 y old: 0.5 mL i.m.	• Minimum age of 6 mo [trivalent inactivated influenza vaccine (TIV)] • Minimum age of 2 y for live, attenuated influenza vaccine (LAIV) • Administer annually to children aged 6 mo to 18 y • Administer 2 doses at least 4 wk apart in children <9 y old who have received the influenza vaccine for the first time
Measles/mumps/rubella (MMR)	0.5 mL i.m.	• Minimum age of 12 mo
Pneumococcal, conjugated 13-valent (Prevnar)	0.5 mL i.m.	• Minimum age of 6 wk for pneumococcal conjugate vaccine (PCV) and minimum of 2 y for pneumococcal polysaccharide vaccine (PPSV)
Polio vaccine, enhanced inactivated (IPOL)	0.5 mL i.m./s.c.	• This vaccine contains all three serotypes of polio vaccine virus
Rotavirus live (pentavalent) (Rotateq) (Rotarix)	2 mL p.o.	• ORAL vaccine • Administer the first dose before 15 wk and final dose by 8 mo • Fecal shedding of vaccine virus was evaluated in a subset of persons enrolled in the phase III trials. Vaccine virus was shed by 9% of 360 infants after dose 1, but none of 249 and 385 infants after doses 2 and 3, respectively • Fecal shedding of rotavirus antigen was evaluated in all or a subset of infants from seven studies in various countries. After dose 1, rotavirus antigen shedding was detected by ELISA in 50%–80% (depending on the study) of infants at ~day 7 and 0%–24% at ~day 30. After dose 2, rotavirus antigen shedding was detected in 4%–18% of infants at ~day 7 and 0%–1.2% at ~day 30. The potential for transmission of vaccine virus to others was not assessed • Administer to hospitalized infants AT THE TIME OF DISCHARGE due to fecal shedding of vaccine virus (up to 15 d)
Varicella live (Varivax)	0.5 mL i.m.	• Minimum age of 12 mo • Avoid use of salicylates for 6 wk following vaccination due to potential increase risk of Reye syndrome

Report all serious adverse reactions to the U.S. Department of Health and Human Services (DHHS) Vaccine Adverse Event Reporting System (VAERS): 1-800-822-7967.

HepBsAg, hepatitis B surface antigen; HBIG, hepatitis B immunoglobulin; i.m., intramuscular; p.o., orally; s.c., subcutaneous.

TABLE A1.5 Immunoglobulins

Immunoglobulins	*Dosage*	*Notes*
Hepatitis B immunoglobulin (HBIG)	0.5 mL i.m.	• HepBsAg-positive mothers: Administer within 12 h of birth • Efficacy decreases significantly if treatment is delayed > 48 h • HepBsAg unknown mothers: Administer HBIG and hepatitis B vaccine to preterm infants within 12 h of life. Administer hepatitis B vaccine to term infants within 12 h of life and HBIG within 7 d of life.
Palivizumab (Synagis)	15 mg/kg i.m.	• Give monthly throughout RSV season for a total course of 5 doses or until the end of the RSV season, whichever occurs first (November to March for Midwest) • Eligibility criteria: • Infant with chronic lung disease of prematurity • Infants born before 29 wk of gestation • Infants with hemodynamically significant congenital heart disease • The updated recommendations of palivizumab administration and major policy changes include: • Modification of recommendations for initiation and cessation of RSV prophylaxis based on current CDC descriptions of seasonality (geographical regions in the United States) • Max of 5 doses in all geographic areas
Varicella immunoglobulin (VariZIG)	<2 kg: 62.5 units i.m. 2.1–10 kg: 125 units i.m.	• Administer to infants whose mothers have an onset of varicella 5 d or less prior to delivery or in the first 48 h after delivery • Or if <32 wk of gestation and exposed to varicella • Most effective if given within 48–96 h of exposure

CDC, Centers for Disease Control and Prevention; HepBsAg, hepatitis B surface antigen; i.m., intramuscular; IND, investigational new drug; RSV, respiratory syncytial virus.

TABLE A1.6 Respiratory Medications

Respiratory Medication	*Dosage*	*Notes*
Acetylcysteine (Mucomyst)	0.5 mL of 20% t.i.d./q.i.d. nebulized	• Use for patients with abnormal or viscous mucous secretions • Exerts mucolytic action through its free sulfhydryl group which opens up the disulfide bonds in mucoproteins and ↓viscosity
Albuterol (Ventolin)	0.5–1 mg inh in 2 mL 0.9% sodium chloride q4–6 h 0.1–0.45 mg/kg/h continuous nebulization	• Monitor for tachycardia, CNS, hypokalemia, tremor • May administer more often in severe cases • Continuous infusion: nebulized at constant rate of 2 mL/h in the newborn • Dose calculated/100 mL = dose (mg/kg/h) × weight (kg) × 50 • Tachyphylaxis with prolonged use
Budesonide (Pulmicort)	0.25 mg inh daily b.i.d.	• Used on a limited basis in neonatal population for infants who have developed chronic lung disease and remain on respiratory support • Does not work immediately. Allow for minimum of 2–3 wk of therapy to determine any potential benefits in terms of decreasing respiratory support • Up to 39% of oral inhalation is systemically absorbed • Monitor for growth suppression, adrenal suppression, hypokalemia, growth of *Candida* in mouth/nares
Cromolyn (Intal)	>2 y old: 20 mg inh q.i.d.	• Generally not recommended for neonates and preterm infants • Prevents mast cell release of histamine, leukotrienes • Monitor for wheezing, congestion, and lacrimation • Does not work immediately—need to be on consistent regimen for 2–4 wk
Ipratropium (Atrovent)	Neonates: 25 μg/kg/dose inh t.i.d. Infants: 125–250 μg inh t.i.d.	• Blocks the action of acetylcholine at parasympathetic sites in bronchial smooth muscle causing bronchodilation • Additive effects with anticholinergics
Vaponephrine (Racepinephrine)	0.25–0.5 mL of 2.25% racemic epinephrine in 2 mL 0.9% sodium chloride nebulized q6 h	• For stridor (short-term treatment)

b.i.d., twice daily; CNS, central nervous system; inh, inhaled; q, every; q.d., daily; q.i.d., four times daily; t.i.d., thrice daily.

TABLE A1.7 Infusion of Medications Through the Umbilical Artery Catheter (UAC)

Drugs that should not be routinely administered through the UAC include any agents that are
- Hyperosmolar agents (osmolality > serum 281–289 mOsm/L)
- Vasoconstrictor agents
- Irritants
- Alkalinic agents

Complications (rates reported: 1.5%–23%)
- Vascular: thrombus, emboli, vasospasms, and hypertension
- Infections: colonizations of 39% reported after 6 d of UAC placement, systemic infections
- Perforation
- Miscellaneous

Placement:
- HIGH: catheter tip high in the aorta at T4–T11 levels
- LOW: catheter tip at L4

Medications that CAN be infused through the UAC:

Medications and flushes should be infused slowly over 20–30 min, be dilute and isotonic as possible
- Albumin
- Aminophylline
- Ampicillin
- Blood products
- Cefotaxime (Cephalosporins)
- Dexamethasone
- Dextrose (max 15%)
- Digoxin
- Furosemide
- Gentamicin
- Heparin
- Hydrocortisone
- Maintenance i.v.p. with dextrose
- Electrolytes
- Pancuronium
- Penicillin G
- Phentolamine
- Sodium bicarbonate—consider diluting
- Total parenteral nutrition (TPN)

Medications that CANNOT be infused through the UAC
- Acyclovir
- Alprostadil
- Amphotericin B
- Caffeine
- Calcium gluconate (or any salt)
- Diazepam
- Dobutamine
- Dopamine
- Epinephrine
- Fat emulsion
- Immunoglobulin
- Indomethacin
- Isoproterenol
- Lorazepam
- Metoclopramide
- Norepinephrine
- Phenobarbital[a]
- Phenytoin
- Potassium boluses
- Propranolol
- Tromethamine (THAM)
- Vancomycin[a]

[a] Relative contraindication with reported vasospasm and skin blanching.

TABLE A1.8 Neonatal Intravenous Push Medications

Medication	*Dose*	*Comments*
Adenosine (Adenocard)	50–100 µg/kg rapid i.v.p. over 1–2 s Increase dose by 50–100 µg/kg increments q1–2 min until return of normal sinus rhythm MAX 300 µg/kg or until termination of PSVT	• Flush with saline immediately post each dose administration • Adenosine 6 mg/2 mL vial: Take 1 mL of adenosine and dilute with 0.9% NS 9 mL for a final concentration of 300 µg/mL • Half-life: <10 s
Albumin 5% (Buminate)	0.5–1 g/kg/dose i.v. (5–10 mL/kg/dose) i.v.p. over 10 min MAX 2–4 mL/min	• Administer through 5-µm filter • Consider NS as colloid. (Neonatal Resuscitation guidelines 2015: An isotonic crystalloid rather than albumin is the solution of choice for volume expansion in the delivery room [Class IIb; LOE 7])
Atropine	0.01–0.03 mg/kg/dose over 1 min	
Calcium gluconate	100–200 mg/kg/dose i.v.p. over 10–30 min	• Do NOT administer through UAC line
Dextrose	1–2 mL/kg of D10W i.v.p. over 1 min	
Digoxin (Lanoxin)	Preterm neonate: Loading dose: 15–25 µg/kg/dose slow i.v.p. over 5–10 min Maintenance dose: 4–6 µg/kg/dose slow i.v.p. over 5 min Term neonate: Loading dose: 20–30 µg/kg/dose slow i.v.p. over 5–10 min Maintenance dose: 5–8 µg/kg/dose slow i.v.p. over 5 min	• Therapeutic range 0.8–2 ng/mL • Half-life varies: • Preterm neonate 61–70 h • Term neonate 35–45 h
Epinephrine (1:10,000)	0.01–0.03 mg/kg/dose rapid i.v.p. (0.1–0.3 mL/kg of 1:10,000 solution) 0.3–1 mL/kg/dose endotracheally (ET)	• Repeat every 3–5 min p.r.n. • Do NOT administer through UAC line

TABLE A1.8 Neonatal Intravenous Push Medications (*continued*)

Medication	*Dose*	*Comments*
Fentanyl (Sublimaze)	1–4 μg/kg/dose i.v.p. slowly over 3–5 min	• Slow i.v.p. over 3–5 min to prevent chest wall rigidity • Reverse with naloxone • Less histamine release (more suitable in CLD due to less airway narrowing) • Less GI motility impairment, less urinary retention • Decreases peripheral vascular resistance which is potentially useful in PPHN
Furosemide (Lasix)	1–2 mg/kg/dose i.v.p. over 2–4 min Max rate 0.5 mg/kg/min (4 mg/min)	• Monitor electrolytes • Rapid administration associated with ototoxicity
Hydralazine (Apresoline)	0.1–0.2 mg/kg/dose q4–6 h p.r.n.	• Max 3.5 mg/kg/d divided q4–6 h • Administer i.v.p. over 1 min • (Max 0.2 mg/kg/min)
Lorazepam	0.05–0.1 mg/kg/dose i.v.p. over 2–5 min May repeat subsequent doses in 10–15 min	• Preparation contains benzyl alcohol and, therefore, should be used with caution in the preterm infant due to potential neurotoxicity, myoclonus, and "gasping syndrome" • Dilute with sterile water or NS 1:1 prior to administration • Infuse through dedicated line.
Midazolam (Versed)	0.05–0.15 mg/kg/dose i.v.p. over 5 min	• No analgesic properties • CNS side effects include paradoxical excitement, rhythmic myoclonic jerking (in preterm infants ~8% incidence), tonic–clonic movements
Morphine sulfate	0.05–0.2 mg/kg/dose i.v.p. over 5 min	• Monitor for respiratory depression, O_2 saturation, urinary retention, decreased bowel sounds
Naloxone	0.1 mg/kg/dose rapid i.v.p. Repeat every 2–3 min p.r.n.	• Use with caution in infants of opioid-dependent mothers
Pancuronium (Pavulon)	0.1 mg/kg/dose i.v.p. over 1 min	• Monitor BP; neonate must be intubated and sedated • Adjust dose in renal impairment
Phenobarbital	Loading dose: 20 mg/kg/dose i.v.p. over 20 min Additional 5–10 mg/kg bolus doses may be required until seizure controlled max of 40 mg/kg total Max infusion rate of 1 mg/kg/min	• Therapeutic level: 15–40 μg/mL • Half-life in neonates: 45–200 h • Do NOT administer through UAC line
Phenytoin (Dilantin)	Loading dose 20 mg/kg/dose i.v.p. over 20 min Max infusion rate 0.5–1 mg/kg/min	• Do NOT administer through UAC line
Plasma protein fraction (Plasmanate)	10–15 mL/kg/dose i.v.p. over 10 min	• Use 0.9% NS when possible: • 0.9% NS 500 mL: <$1 • Plasmanate/albumin 50 mL: $62 • Isotonic crystalloid solutions should be used first line for acute volume expansion (Neonatal Resuscitation guidelines 2015 states that albumin-containing solutions are not the fluid of choice for initial volume expansion secondary to increased risk of infections and associated increased mortality [Class IIb; LOE 7].)
Sodium bicarbonate	1–2 mEq/kg/dose i.v. over at least 30 min. Max 1 mEq/kg/h	• Infuse through dedicated line and monitor closely for extravasation. Tissue necrosis can occur because of the hyperosmolarity of sodium bicarbonate. (4.2% = 0.5 mEq/mL = 900 mOsm/L) • Not compatible with calcium or any calcium-containing solution. Immediate precipitation will result • Sodium bicarbonate is not a recommended therapy in the neonatal resuscitation guidelines and, therefore, rapid i.v. infusions are **not** administered

BP, blood pressure; CLD, Chronic lung disease; CNS, central nervous system; D10W, dextrose 10% in water; GI, gastrointestinal; i.v.p., intravenous push; NS, normal saline; PPHN, persistent pulmonary hypertension in newborns; p.r.n., as needed; PSVT, paroxysmal supraventricular tachycardia; UAC, umbilical artery catheter.

TABLE A1.9 Therapeutic Drug Monitoring (TDM) and Drug Sampling Times

Drug	*Infusion Time*	*Therapeutic Range*	*When to Draw Levels*	*Comments*
Amikacin	0.5 h	Peak: 20–30 μg/mL Trough: <4 μg/mL	Trough: ½ h prior to dose Peak: ½ h after end of infusion	Reserved for tobramycin-resistant gram-negative bacteria Dose 7.5 mg/kg/dose i.v. × 1 in renal failure patients—draw random level in 24 h and redose when level is <4 μg/mL
Caffeine (Cafcit)	0.5 h	5–25 μg/mL	Draw trough level just prior to next dose	Long half-life: 45–100 h. Draw trough level at steady state after day 5 of therapy
Carbamazepine (Tegretol)	NA	4–12 μg/mL	Just prior to next dose	ORAL form only Carbamazepine may be administered rectally if required: Give same total daily dose but give in small diluted multiple doses (dilute with water)
Digoxin (Lanoxin)	Slowly over 5–10 min	0.8–2 ng/mL	Draw trough level just prior to next dose or at least 6 h after dose given	Give ½ TDD as initial dose, then 1/4 TDD times 2 doses q6–12 h apart Half-life: Preterm 61–70 h Term 35–45 h
Enoxaparin (Lovenox)	NA	Anti–factor Xa level: 0.5–1 unit/mL is therapeutic	4 h postdose	Initiate dose at 1.5 μg/kg/dose s.c. q12 and titrate per aXa levels Monitor for signs of bleeding Repeat level if extremely low or high prior to dose change
Flucytosine (Ancobon)	NA	25–100 μg/mL Trough: 25–50 μg/mL Peak: 50–100 μg/mL	Trough: just prior to dose Peak: 2 h postdose after at least 4 d of therapy	ORAL form only Good CNS penetration Not to be used as monotherapy
Gentamicin	0.5 h	Peak: 3–10 μg/mL Trough: <1.2 μg/mL	Trough: ½ h prior to dose Peak: ½ h after end of infusion	Gent levels for synergy: Peak 3–4 μg/mL Trough <1 μg/mL Levels not routinely done Dosing in renal failure patients 2 mg/kg/dose i.v. × 1—draw random in 24 h and redose when level is ≤1.2 μg/mL
Heparin	Continuous infusion	APTT 60–85 s	Obtain APTT 4 h after initiation of continuous infusion and every 4 h after infusion rate change	Loading dose: 75 units/kg, then maintenance dose: 28 units/kg/h
Levetiracetam (Keppra)	0.5 h	Trough: 5–30 μg/mL	Trough: just before dose	Exact dosing in neonates not established. Second- or third-line agent used in refractory seizures. Loading dose: 10–20 mg/kg/dose, then 5–10 mg/kg/d divided in 2–3 doses. May increase by 10 mg/kg/d if tolerated to max of 60 mg/kg/d
Phenobarbital	Slow i.v.p. over 20 min Max infusion rate 1 mg/kg/min	15–40 μg/mL	Draw trough level just prior to next dose Postload/peak: 1 h after end of infusion	Initiate maintenance dose 12 h after loading dose
Phenytoin (Dilantin)	Slow i.v.p. over 20 min Max infusion rate of 0.5–1 mg/kg/min	Total: 8–15 μg/mL Free: 1.5–2.5 μg/mL	Draw trough level just prior to next dose Postload/peak: 1 h after end of infusion	Initiate maintenance dose 12 h after loading dose Oral loading dose should be administered in 2–3 doses q2 h to ensure complete oral absorption

(*continued*)

TABLE A1.9 Neonatal Intravenous Push Medications (*continued*)

Drug	*Infusion Time*	*Therapeutic Range*	*When to Draw Levels*	*Comments*
Theophylline (Aminophylline is an i.v. product)	Aminophylline 0.5 h	AOP: 7–12 µg/mL BPD: 10–15 µg/mL	Draw trough level just prior to next dose Peak: 1 h postdose Continuous infusion: 16–24 h after initiation of infusion	Apnea 7–12 µg/mL BPD 10–15 µg/mL $t_{1/2}$ variable by age: Premature 20–30 h Term 10–25 h <6 mo 14 h >6 mo 5 h Draw level 3 d after therapy initiated or changed Adjust frequency and dosing in anticipation of change of half-life
Tobramycin	0.5 h	Peak: 3–10 µg/mL Trough: <1.2 µg/mL	Trough: ½ h prior to dose Peak: ½ h after end of infusion	Reserve for documented *Pseudomonas aeruginosa* or other gram-negative pathogen resistant to gentamicin Dosing in renal failure patients 2 mg/kg/dose i.v. × 1—draw random in 24 h and redose when level is ≤1 µg/mL
Valproic acid (Depacon)	1 h	Total: 40–80 µg/mL Free: <15 µg/mL	Draw trough level just before next dose	Increase in free fraction in neonates Consult neurology prior to initiation Side effects: hyperammonemic encephalopathy, pancreatitis, thrombocytopenia, ↑liver enzymes, and liver failure
Vancomycin	1 h	Peak: 25–40 µg/mL Trough: 5–20 µg/mL	Trough: ½ h prior to dose Peak: 1 h after infusion	No need for levels for empiric 3 d rule outs Desired trough level should be 4× *MIC* Target higher trough levels with *MIC* >1 as tolerated Peaks do not signify efficacy and are of little value, except to understand more about the patient-specific pharmacokinetic profile More aggressive target trough concentrations are required in disease states, such as meningitis, endocarditis, pneumonia, and osteomyelitis Obtain levels if course of therapy >3 d and every 7 d as therapy continues

AOP, apnea of prematurity; BPD, bronchopulmonary dysplasia; CNS, central nervous system; i.v., intravenous; i.v.p., intravenous push; *MIC*, minimum inhibitory concentration; NA, not applicable; $t_{1/2}$, half-life; TDD, total digitalizing dose.

TABLE A1.10 Drug Compatibility with Neonatal TPN and Fat Emulsion at Y-Site (Terminal Injection Site)

Medication	*Compatibility with TPN*	*Compatibility with Lipids*	*Comments*
Acyclovir	N	N	
Albumin	Y	Y	
Alprostadil	Y	NI	
Amikacin	Y	N	Incompatible with heparin at concentrations >1 unit/mL
Aminophylline	Y	Y	1 mg/mL concentration ONLY compatible. 5 mg/mL is incompatible with Trophamine
Amphotericin B	N	N	
Amphotericin B lipid complex	N	N	
Ampicillin	N	N	More stable in NS/SW than dextrose

TABLE A1.10 Drug Compatibility with Neonatal TPN and Fat Emulsion at Y-Site (Terminal Injection Site) (*continued*)

Medication	*Compatibility with TPN*	*Compatibility with Lipids*	*Comments*
Ampicillin/sulbactam (Unasyn)	Y	Y	
Amiodarone (Cordarone)	N	NI	
Atropine	Y	NI	
Azithromycin	Y	NI	
Bumetanide	Y	Y	
Caffeine	Y	Y	
Calcitriol	NI	NI	
Calcium gluconate	Y	Y	Potential for precipitation based on specific TPN and the Ca-PO_4 ratio. Infuse bolus doses over 30 min NOT with TPN when possible so as to avoid precipitation and decrease osmolality.
Caspofungin	N	N	
Cefazolin	Y	Y	
Cefepime	Y	Y	
Cefotaxime	Y	Y	
Cefoxitin	Y	Y	
Ceftazidime	Y	Y	
Ceftriaxone	N	Y	Concomitant use with i.v. calcium-containing solutions in neonates (≤28 d) is CONTRAINDICATED due to fatal lung and kidney damage associated with calcium-ceftriaxone precipitates in preterm and term neonates
Chlorothiazide	N	NI	
Clindamycin	Y	Y	
Colistimethate (Colistin)	NI	NI	
Dexamethasone	Y	Y	
Digoxin	Y	Y	
Dobutamine	Y	Y	
Dopamine	Y	Y	
Enalaprilat	Y	NI	
Epinephrine	Y	N	
Erythromycin	Y	Y	
Esmolol	N	NI	
Fentanyl	Y	Y	
Fluconazole	Y	N	
Furosemide	Y	Y	Furosemide must be administered i.v. push; Dex/AA will degrade furosemide when mixed together for several hours
Ganciclovir	N	N	Concentration-dependent compatibility
Gentamicin	Y	N	Incompatible with heparin at concentrations >1 unit/mL
Glucagon	NI	NI	
Glycopyrrolate	N	NI	
Heparin	Y	Y	Not compatible at concentrations >100 units/mL
Hydralazine	Y	N	
Hydrocortisone	Y	Y	
Ibuprofen	NI	NI	
Imipenem–cilastatin	Y	Y	
Indomethacin	N	NI	
Insulin, regular	Y	Y	
Iron dextran	Y	N	Usually placed in TPN. Mix only in Dex/AA solutions containing at least 2% amino acids
Isoproterenol	Y	Y	

(*continued*)

TABLE A1.10 Drug Compatibility with Neonatal TPN and Fat Emulsion at Y-Site (Terminal Injection Site) (*continued*)

Medication	*Compatibility with TPN*	*Compatibility with Lipids*	*Comments*
Levetiracetam	NI	NI	
Levothyroxine	N	N	
Lidocaine	Y	Y	
Linezolid	Y	NI	
Lorazepam	Y	N	
Magnesium sulfate	Y	N	
Meropenem	Y	Y	
Methylprednisolone	Y	Y	
Metoclopramide	Y	Y	
Metronidazole	Y	N	
Micafungin	Y	Y	
Midazolam	N	N	Damage to emulsion integrity
Milrinone	Y	NI	
Morphine	Y	Y	
Nafcillin	Y	Y	
Oxacillin	Y	Y	
Pancuronium	Y	NI	
Penicillin G	Y	N	
Phenobarbital	N	N	
Phenytoin	N	N	Incompatible with heparin at concentrations >1 unit/mL
Phosphates	N	N	
Phytonadione	Y	NI	
Piperacillin	Y	Y	
Piperacillin/tazobactam	Y	Y	
Potassium salts	Y	Y	
Propranolol	NI	NI	
Pyridoxine	NI	Y	
Ranitidine	Y	Y	
Rifampin	N	NI	
Sodium bicarbonate	N	Y	
Ticarcillin	Y	Y	
Ticarcillin–clavulanate	Y	Y	(Timentin)
Tobramycin	Y	Y	Incompatible with heparin at concentrations >1 unit/mL
Trimethoprim/sulfamethoxazole	Y	Y	(Bactrim, Septra)
Valproic acid	N	N	
Vancomycin	Y	N	Incompatible with heparin at concentrations >1 unit/mL
Zidovudine	Y	Y	

i.v., intravenous; N, no; NI, no information; NS, normal saline; SW, sterile water; Y, yes.
NI should be treated as incompatible.

GUIDELINES FOR HEPARIN USE TO MAINTAIN LINE PATENCY IN THE NEONATAL INTENSIVE CARE UNIT

ISSUE

The overuse of heparin is a risk factor to the neonate. Heparin is a risk factor for neonatal candidiasis. Other risk factors for neonatal candidiasis include extremely low gestational age, thrombocytopenia, use of skin emollients, intralipids, enclosed humid environment, lack of breast milk feeds, lack of enteral feeds, hyperglycemia-insulin therapy, use of cephalosporins, hydrocortisone, and heparin.

Other risk factors related to heparin include increased risk of heparin-induced thrombocytopenia (HIT), bleeding, and long-term effects on bones.

Type of Line	*Can the i.v. Site be Locked?*	*Recommendations for Flush When Locking the i.v. Site*	*Should Heparin be Added to i.v. Fluids?*	*Recommendation for the Addition of Heparin to i.v. Fluids*	*Recommended Minimum Volume to be Infused in Line*
Peripheral	Yes	0.5 mL preservative-free normal saline (0.9% sodium chloride) every 8 h	No	None	1 mL/h
PICC (any gauge)	No	None	Yes	Heparin 0.5 units/mL for rates: <2 mL/h May exclude the ELBW critically ill neonate	1 mL/h
Hickman–Broviac, CVC	Yes	Heparin 10 units daily	No	None	2 mL/h
UAC	No	None	Yes	Heparin 0.5 units/mL	0.5 mL/h
UVC	No	None	No	None	1 mL/h
Secondary UVC (Double lumen)	Yes	Heparin 10 units daily	No	None	No minimum
Femoral	Yes	Heparin 10 units daily	No	None	No minimum

CVC, central venous catheter; ELBW, extremely low birth weight; i.v., intravenous; PICC, peripherally inserted central catheter; UAC, umbilical artery catheter; UVC, umbilical venous catheter.

RECOMMENDATIONS FOR USE OF HEPARIN

1. The use of heparin will be reserved on the basis of the above guidelines. Normal saline (NS) locks will be flushed with 0.9% sodium chloride.
2. If the total intravenous (IV) infusion rate is less than 2 mL per hour for peripherally inserted central catheter (PICC) line, add heparin 0.5 units per mL to total parenteral nutrition (TPN) or maintenance IV fluid.
   a. The extremely low birth weight (ELBW) neonate may be excluded in the first few days of life since the initial total fluid goals are low and concomitant continuous infusions may be infusing. The addition of heparin based on rate is under the assumption that the neonate has adequate oral intake with heparin added to maintain patency of line for a short duration until that oral fluid goal is achieved.
3. It is not necessary to add heparin to every IV fluid that is being coinfused with TPN or the main IV fluid.
4. Umbilical artery catheter (UAC) minimum infusion rates of 0.5 mL per hour should be reserved for the ELBW infant.

INFILTRATE MANAGEMENT FOR THE NEONATE

BACKGROUND

Neonates are more prone to extravasations secondary to smaller veins, more reactive veins which vasoconstrict more readily, and immature skin structure.

PURPOSE

To provide prompt, appropriate management of extravasation from agents that may cause severe tissue damage when infiltrated (outside the blood vessel).

DEFINITIONS

Extravasation: Discharge or escape of drug from a blood vessel into the tissue which can cause pain, burning, inflammation, necrosis, sloughing, or ulceration of the tissue.

CLASSES OF AGENTS THAT MAY CAUSE EXTRAVASATION

A. Vesicant—an agent that produces blistering or tissue damage (necrosis) on exposure
   a. Chemotherapeutic agents

B. Hyperosmolar—an agent that alters cellular fluid balance and may lead to cell damage or death
   a. Acyclovir, alprostadil (prostaglandin E1), aminophylline, calcium chloride, calcium gluconate, contrast media, dextrose greater than 10% concentration, diazepam, indomethacin, ibuprofen, lorazepam, phenytoin, potassium chloride, sodium bicarbonate, sodium chloride 0.9%, thiopental, TPN/lipid emulsion

C. Vasoconstrictor—an agent that restricts local blood flow and may lead to ischemic necrosis
   a. Dobutamine, dopamine, epinephrine, norepinephrine, phenylephrine, vasopressin

SIGNS AND SYMPTOMS OF EXTRAVASATION

Swelling
Pain
Erythema

POTENTIAL EXTRAVASATION OUTCOMES

Vessel damage
Necrosis

Skin sloughing
Discoloration
Gangrene
Surgical repair/amputation
Scarring

ASSESSMENT: STAGING OF EXTRAVASATION

STAGING OF IV INFILTRATES

Stage	*Characteristics of Infiltrate*
Stage I	Painful i.v. site, NO erythema, NO swelling, NO drainage. Flushes with ease
Stage II	Painful i.v. site, slight swelling (0%–20%), redness, NO blanching, good pulse below site, 1–2 s capillary refill below site
Stage III	Painful i.v. site, marked swelling (30%–50%), blanching, skin cool to touch, good pulse below infiltration site, 1–2 s capillary refill below infiltration site
Stage IV	Painful i.v. site, severe swelling (>50%), blanching, skin cool to touch, decreased or absent pulse,[a] capillary refill >4 s,[a] skin breakdown or necrosis.[a]

[a]The presence of any one of these characteristics constitutes a stage IV infiltrate.

Adapted from Flemmer L, Chan JS. A pediatric protocol for management of extravasation. *Pediatr Nurs.* 1993;19(4):355–358; Millam DA. IV therapy: when to change tubings and sites. *Nursing.* 1988;18(7):65–67; Montgomery LA, Hanrahan K, Kottman K, Otto A, Barrett T, Hermiston B. *Guideline for I.V. infiltrations in pediatric patients.* 1999;25(2):167–169,173–180.

EXTRAVASATION TREATMENT

TREATMENT FOR EXTRAVASATION OF HYPEROSMOLAR AGENTS

1. Minimize tissue exposure.
   a. Discontinue administration of medication immediately.
   b. Remove catheter.
   c. Notify physician or neonatal nurse practitioner (NNP).
   d. Determine stage of infiltrate.
   e. Stage III and IV infiltrates require antidote treatment.
2. Minimize inflammation, swelling, and discomfort.
   a. Avoid applying pressure to site.
   b. DO NOT apply warm or cold compresses.
   c. Elevate extremity if possible and if tolerated.
   d. Observe site for pain, erythema, swelling, induration, progression of lesion size, signs of skin breakdown every 30 minute for 1 hour and then every hour for 4 hours.
3. Administer antidote—hyaluronidase (Amphadase).
   a. Hyaluronidase is a mucolytic enzyme which modifies the normal intercellular tissue barrier/permeability through hydrolysis of hyaluronic acid. This allows for the rapid dispersion of extravasated fluid through tissues.
   b. Initiate immediately and ideally within 1 hour of extravasation.
   c. Initiate for stage III/IV infiltrate.
   d. Inject 150 units (1 mL) as five separate 0.2 mL subcutaneous/intradermal injections around the periphery of the extravasation site at the leading edge.
   e. Use 26-gauge needle and change needle after each injection.

TREATMENT OF EXTRAVASATION OF VASOCONSTRICTOR AGENTS

1. Minimize tissue exposure.
   a. Discontinue administration of medication immediately.
   b. Assess and document pulse and circulation distal to the extravasated area.
   c. Notify physician.
   d. Determine stage of infiltrate.
      i. Stage III and IV infiltrates require antidote treatment.
2. Minimize inflammation, swelling, and discomfort.
   a. Elevate extremity as patient tolerates if possible.
   b. DO NOT apply warm or cold compresses.
   c. Observe site for pain, erythema, swelling, induration, progression of lesion size, signs of skin breakdown every 30 minutes for 1 hour and then every hour for 4 hours.
3. Administer antidote—phentolamine (Regitine).
   a. Phentolamine is an α-adrenergic blocking agent that produces peripheral vasodilation. Phentolamine reverses dermal necrosis produced by vasopressor (α-adrenergic) infiltration.
   b. Prepare diluted phentolamine with final concentration of 0.5 mg per mL. (Dilute 5 mg in 10 mL preservative-free 0.9% NaCl).
   c. Administer 0.1 mL injections subcutaneously around the periphery of the extravasation site at the leading edge.
   d. Use 26-gauge needle and change needle after each injection site.
   e. Do not exceed a maximum dose of 0.1 mg per kg or 2.5 mg.
   f. Generally only 2 to 3 injections required.
   g. Monitor vital signs every 15 minutes for 2 hours and watch for complications of hypotension and tachycardia.

TABLE A1.11 Intravenous Extravasation Medications

Extravasated Drug	*Antidote*	*Dilution*	*Intervention*
Hyperosmolar agents: Acyclovir Alprostadil—(Prostaglandin E1) Aminophylline Calcium chloride Calcium gluconate Contrast media Dextrose >10% Diazepam Indomethacin Ibuprofen Lorazepam Phenytoin Potassium chloride Sodium bicarbonate Sodium chloride >0.9% Thiopental TPN and lipids	Hyaluronidase (Amphadase)	Draw up 150 units (1 mL) into syringe	1. Notify physician or NP 2. Determine stage of infiltrate. Stage III or IV extravasations meet criteria for hyaluronidase administration 3. Physician/NP to inject 150 units (1 mL) as five separate 0.2 mL subcutaneous injections around the periphery of the extravasation site at the leading edge 4. Use 26-gauge needle and change needle after each injection site 5. Physician or NP to document description of wound and procedure in the progress note section of infant's medical record 6. Document medication administration
Vasoconstrictor agents: Dobutamine Dopamine Epinephrine Norepinephrine Phenylephrine Vasopressin	Phentolamine (Regitine)	Dilute phentolamine to final concentration of 0.5 mg/mL. (Dilute 5 mg in 10 mL preservative-free 0.9% NaCl.)	1. Notify physician or NP 2. Determine stage of infiltrate. Stage III or IV extravasation meets criteria for phentolamine administration 3. Physician/NP to administer 0.1 mL injections subcutaneously around the periphery of the extravasation site at the leading edge 4. Use 26-gauge needle and change needle after each injection site 5. Do not exceed a max dose of 0.1 mg/kg or 2.5 mg 6. Generally, only two to three injections required 7. Monitor for signs of hypotension and tachycardia

NP, nurse practitioner; TPN, total parenteral nutrition.
Data from Beall V, Hall B, Mulholland JT, et al. Neonatal extravasation: an overview and algorithm for evidence-based treatment. *Newborn Infant Nurs Rev* 2013;13(4):189–195.

POSTEXTRAVASATION WOUND HEALING—USE OF HYDROGELS

1. Initiate therapy upon collaboration with the physician.
2. Draw up 10 mL of preservative-free NS into a 10 mL syringe. In another 10-mL syringe, squeeze the contents of the hydrogel tube. Place both syringes in the isolette to warm their contents. Warming may take 15 to 20 minutes.
3. Measure the size of the wound, that is, length and width, and record findings.
4. Put on sterile gloves. Irrigate the affected area with the warmed preservative-free NS. Do not touch the wound with the syringe tip.
5. Place the affected limb into a sterile polyethylene bag forming a "glove" or "boot." A sterile urine collection bag may be used. The mouth of the bag may need to be cut to allow for placement over the extremity. Leave a small opening where the syringe filled with the hydrogel will be injected. Make sure that glove/boot is large enough to allow for full extension of the affected extremity.
6. Squirt hydrogel into the bag to completely cover the wound forming a thin layer between bag and wound. Use 5 to 10 mL from the syringe containing the hydrogel, depending on the size of the extravasation.
7. Ensure that wound is covered at all times and that the bag does not come in contact with the wound surface.
8. The neck of the bag is closed using surgical tape.
9. An additional bag may be placed over the polyethylene bag to minimize disruption of applied thick layer of gel. Secure the bag with surgical tape, taking care to avoid making the tape too tight around the extremity.
10. A splint may be applied to the extremity to support the weight of the gel.
11. Dressing may be left on for 3 days.
12. Monitor for signs of infection with each dressing change.
13. Do dressing changes every 3 days. Slide bag off limb and irrigate with NS. No contact as rubbing or patting of the wound site is required.
14. Monitor for signs of infection.
15. During healing, a pale yellow, semisolid fibrinous layer may develop, but this does not affect the healing process. Do not disturb this layer.
16. Healing process is dramatic but slow and may require five to seven dressing changes.
17. Document interventions and neonate's responses each shift with the nursing assessment.

NEONATAL INTENSIVE CARE UNIT INTRAVENOUS ELECTROLYTE SUPPLEMENTATION GUIDELINES

BACKGROUND

Blood/serum osmolarity 300 to 310 mOsm per L
Isotonic solution 280 to 310 mOsm per L

The tonicity of a solution dictates whether it should be infused peripherally or centrally. When solutions with extremes of tonicity are infused, fluids shift into or out of cells. This resulting change in cell size of the vein wall will cause the inflammatory and clotting process to occur, which can lead to phlebitis and thrombophlebitis.

PERIPHERAL INTRAVENOUS MAXIMUM OSMOLARITY: 900 MOSM PER L FOR NON–TOTAL PARENTERAL NUTRITION SOLUTIONS

Ability of peripheral veins to dilute parenteral infusions is compromised when osmolarity is greater than 900 mOsm per L.

Hypotonic solutions such as 0.2% NS (1/4 NS) can cause the red blood cell to swell and burst and can result in hemolytic anemia.

DEFINITIONS

1. **Osmolarity**
   The concentration of the solute in a solution per unit of solvent, usually mmol solute per liter.
2. **Tonicity**
   Frequently used in place of osmotic pressure or tension is related to the number of particles found in solution. Osmolarity is most often used when referring to blood, and tonicity is most often used when referring to IV fluid, but the terms may be used interchangeably.
3. **Isotonic**
   Of equal tension. Denoting a solution having the same tonicity as another solution with which it is compared.
4. **Hypertonic**
   Having a higher concentration of solute particles per unit volume than a comparison solution, regardless of kinds of particles. A solution in which cells shrink due to efflux of water.
5. **Hypotonic**
   Having a lower concentration of solute particles per unit volume than a comparison solution, regardless of kinds of particles. A solution in which cells expand because of influx of water.

TABLE A1.12 Osmolarity of Common Intravenous Admixture Fluids in NICU

Solution Type	*Osmolarity (mOsm/L)*
0.2% NS	77
0.45% NS	154
0.9% NS	308
Dextrose 5% in water	252
Dextrose 10% in water	505
D5W/0.2% NS	321
D5W/0.45% NS	406
D5W/0.9% NS	560
D10W/0.2% NS	573
D10W/0.45% NS	661
D10W/0.9% NS	817
D5W/0.2% NS/20KCl/L	360
D10W/0.2% NS/20KCl/L	613
D5W/0.2% NS/20KCl/L/calcium 560 mg/L elemental	401
D10W/0.2% NS/20KCl/L/calcium 560 mg/L elemental	654
D5W/0.9% NS/20KCl/L	604
D10W/0.9% NS/20KCl/L	857
D5W/0.9% NS/20KCl/L/calcium 560 mg/L elemental	645
D10W/0.9% NS/20KCl/L/calcium 560 mg/L elemental	898

NICU, neonatal intensive care unit; NS, normal saline.

TABLE A1.13 Osmolarity of Common Electrolyte Additives

Electrolyte	*Strength*	*Osmolarity per mL (mOsm/mL)*
NaCl	2.5 mEq/mL	5
Na acetate	2 mEq/mL	5
Potassium chloride/acetate	2 mEq/mL	4
Magnesium sulfate	125 mg/mL	4.06
Calcium gluconate	100 mg/mL	0.308
Phosphate—as potassium	3 mmol/mL	7.4
Phosphate—as sodium	4 mEq/mL	12

POTASSIUM REPLACEMENT GUIDELINES

INDICATION

Serum potassium less than 3 mEq per L

Incorporate into maintenance IV solution for serum levels greater than or equal to 3 mg per dL; intermittent IV potassium administration should be reserved for severe depletion.

DOSE

0.5 to 1 mEq per kg per dose potassium chloride **IV slowly** over 1 to 2 hours × one dose

PREPARATION

Peripheral	0.08 mEq per mL final concentration
Central	0.15 mEq per mL final concentration

Potassium must always be diluted.

DAILY REQUIREMENTS

Term infant:	1 to 2 mEq per kg per day
Preterm infant:	2 to 6 mEq per kg per day

REFERENCE RANGE

3.4 to 5 mEq per L

(Note that electrolytes obtained by heel stick in this population will often be hemolyzed and result in an artificially high potassium level. A suspected true elevation of the potassium level may result in electrocardiographic changes and will require confirmation with a repeat level obtained arterially.)

CONCOMITANT DRUG THERAPIES THAT MAY REQUIRE LARGER MAINTENANCE POTASSIUM

Continuous albuterol respiratory treatment; amphotericin B, diuretics, and caspofungin.

NOTES

Infuse slowly over 1 to 2 hours. Continuous cardiac monitoring (may cause cardiac arrhythmias) is required during infusion.

Monitor site closely during infusion since infiltrations can cause severe tissue damage.

MAGNESIUM REPLACEMENT GUIDELINES

INDICATION

Serum magnesium less than 1.5 mEq per L

DOSE

Magnesium sulfate 25 to 50 mg per kg per dose **IV** q8 to 12 hours for two to three doses
Infuse slowly over 2 to 4 hours

PREPARATION

125 mg per mL

DAILY REQUIREMENTS

Term infant: 0.125 to 0.25 mEq per kg per day (1.6 to 3.1 mg per kg per day)[1]
Preterm infant: 0.25 to 0.5 mEq per kg per day (3.1 to 6.3 mg per kg per day)[2]

REFERENCE RANGE

1.5 to 2.3 mEq per L

CONCOMITANT DRUG THERAPIES THAT MAY REQUIRE LARGER MAINTENANCE MAGNESIUM

Amphotericin B

NOTES

Infuse slowly over 2 to 4 hours. Hypotension may result with rapid IV administration. Monitor blood pressure and monitor for cardiac arrhythmia and respiratory and central nervous system depression.

Overdoses may be treated with calcium gluconate.

1 mg elemental magnesium.
2 mg elemental magnesium.

PHOSPHATE REPLACEMENT GUIDELINES

INDICATION

Exact treatment in terms of dosing of severe hypophosphatemia may be difficult since the extent of total body deficits and response to therapy may be difficult to predict. Aggressive doses of phosphate may result in a transient serum elevation, followed by redistribution into intracellular compartments or bone tissue.

Intestinal absorption by the oral route is unreliable, and large doses of phosphate may cause diarrhea.

Low dose	When losses are recent and uncomplicated
Intermediate dose	Serum phosphate 0.5–1 mg/dL
High dose	Serum phosphate <0.5 mg/dL

(Note: These guidelines for dose replacement are based on adult serum phosphate levels. The renal handling of phosphate by the neonatal kidney is different than the adult. Adults maintain a neutral phosphate balance by excreting the same amount of phosphate as they absorb by the gastrointestinal tract. Neonates are in positive phosphate balance, and only 60% of phosphate absorbed from diet is excreted in the urine. This high serum phosphate level in neonates is NOT a manifestation of a lower glomerular filtration rate but of a higher proximal tubular reabsorption capacity. Normal serum phosphate levels in a neonate are 4.8 to 7.2 mg per dL and in an adult are 2.3 to 5 mg per dL.)

DOSE

Replacement

i.v., intravenous.

Low dose	0.08 mmol/kg sodium phosphate **i.v.** × 1 dose Infuse slowly over 4–8 h
Intermediate dose	0.16–0.24 mmol/kg sodium phosphate **i.v.** × 1 dose Infuse slowly over 4–8 h
High dose	0.36 mmol/kg sodium phosphate **i.v.** × 1 dose Infuse slowly over 4–6 h

PREPARATION

Peripheral: 0.05 mmol per mL
Central: 0.12 mmol per mL

DAILY REQUIREMENTS

Term: 25 to 40 mg per kg per day[3]
Preterm: 60 to 140 mg per kg per day[4]

3 mg elemental phosphorus.
4 mg elemental phosphorus.

REFERENCE RANGE

Newborn: 4.2 to 9 mg per dL (Note that range is higher for infants than for adults)
6 weeks to 18 months: 3.8 to 6.7 mg per dL

NOTES

Non-TPN maintenance IV solutions containing phosphate CANNOT contain calcium. These solutions in the absence of buffering agents such as amino acids and cysteine placed in TPN are NOT COMPATIBLE.

Infuse slowly over 2 to 4 hours. Monitor for hypocalcemia and hypotension.

CALCIUM REPLACEMENT GUIDELINES

INDICATION

Serum calcium (<7 mg per dL)

Note that the direct correlation between serum ionized calcium and total serum calcium is poor, especially in states of low albumin or acid/base imbalances. Direct measurement of ionized calcium is recommended.

Total corrected calcium (with low albumin) = Total serum calcium + 0.8 (4 − measured serum albumin)

DOSE

Replacement

200 to 800 mg per kg per day IV divided q6 h as calcium gluconate

MAINTENANCE

IV solutions containing calcium that wish to match the current TPN concentration are expressed as "elemental calcium of 560 mg per L as calcium gluconate," which is then 3,000 mg per L.

Note that calcium and phosphorus content will be halved if amino acid concentration is less than 15 g per L or if neonate is greater than 2 kg with a total fluid goal of greater than 120 mL per kg per day.

PREPARATION

50 mg per mL for doses less than 150 mg
100 mg per mL (straight drug)

DAILY REQUIREMENTS

Term: 0.5 to 2.5 mEq per kg per day
Preterm: 4 to 5 mEq per kg per day

REFERENCE RANGE

Newborns 7 to 12 mg per dL

NOTES

Non-TPN maintenance IV solutions containing calcium CANNOT contain phosphate. These solutions in the absence of buffering agents such as amino acids and cysteine placed in TPN are NOT COMPATIBLE.

Monitor IV sites closely for infiltration. Rapid IV administration can cause bradycardia and arrhythmias.

SODIUM REPLACEMENT GUIDELINES

INDICATION

Serum sodium less than 130 mEq per L

DOSE

Correction of hyponatremia:

mEq sodium needed = Desired sodium (mEq per L) − actual sodium (mEq per L) × 0.6 × Weight (kg)

Replace sodium gradually. Replace half the calculated amount over 12 to 24 hours.

MAINTENANCE

Standard TPN solution contains 26 mEq per L Na.

IV maintenance solutions wishing to match the TPN concentration should contain 0.3% NS = 26 mEq per L.

PREPARATION

1/2 NS (0.45%) = 77 mEq per L
NS (0.9%) = 154 mEq per L
Hypertonic saline (3%) = 513 mEq per L (reserved for only acute life-threatening symptomatic hyponatremia)

DAILY REQUIREMENTS

Premature neonates: 2 to 8 mEq per kg per day
Term neonates: 1 to 4 mEq per kg per day

REFERENCE RANGE

Premature neonates: 132 to 140 mEq per L
Term neonates: 133 to 142 mEq per L
Infants older than 2 months: 135 to 145 mEq per L

NOTES

Hypertonic 3% saline should be reserved in life-threatening emergencies (1,025 mOsm per L) and can cause phlebitis (administer via central line only).

Excessive dosage or too rapid administration rate can cause pulmonary edema and lead to sudden increases in serum osmolality that may result in central nervous system hemorrhage.

DISCLAIMER/NOTICE

Drug information is constantly evolving because of ongoing research, clinical experience, and government regulations. It is often subject to interpretation and evaluation by the clinician. Although great care has been taken to ensure the accuracy of the information presented, the reader is advised that the authors, editors, reviewers, and contributors cannot be held responsible for the continued currency of the information or for any errors, omissions, or applications of this information, or for any consequences arising subsequently. The decisions regarding drug therapy must be based on the independent judgment of the clinician, changing information about a drug (e.g., as reflected in the literature, the manufacturer's most current product information), and changing medical practices. This appendix is intended for use in conjunction with other necessary information and is not intended to be solely relied upon by any user.

SUGGESTED READINGS

Ankola PA, Atakent YS. Effect of adding heparin in very low concentration to the infusate to prolong the patency of umbilical artery catheters. *Am J Perinatol* 1993;10(3):229–232.

Beall V, Hall B, Mulholland JT, et al. Neonatal extravasation: an overview and algorithm for evidence-based treatment. *Newborn Infant Nurs Rev* 2013;13(4):189–195.

Bryant BG. Drug, fluid, and blood products administered through the umbilical artery catheter: complications experiences from one NICU. *Neonatal Netw* 1990;9(1):27–46.

Butler-O'Hara M, Buzzard CJ, Reubens L, et al. A randomized trial comparing long-term and short-term use of umbilical venous catheters in premature infants with birth weights of less than 1251 grams [published online ahead of print June 19, 2006]. *Pediatrics* 2006;118(1):e25–e35.

Centers for Disease Control and Prevention. Recommended Child and Adolescent Immunization Schedule for ages 18 years or younger. https://www.cdc.gov/vaccines/schedules/downloads/child/0-18yrs-child-combined-schedule.pdf. Accessed March 27, 2020.

Chloral Hydrate: Is It Still Being Used? Are there safer alternatives? Institute for safe medication practices website. https://www.ismp.org/resources/chloral-hydrate-it-still-being-used-are-there-safer-alternatives. Updated November 3, 2016. Accessed March 27, 2020.

Emery EF, Fok TF, Ng PC, et al. Randomized controlled trial of colloid infusions in hypotensive preterm infants. *Arch Dis Child* 1992;67:1185–1188.

Escobedo MB, Aziz K, Kapadia VS, et al. 2019 American Heart Association focused update on neonatal resuscitation: an update to the American Heart Association Guidelines for Cardiopulmonary Resuscitation and Emergency Cardiovascular Care. *Circulation* 2019;140(24):e922–e930.

FDA Drug Safety Communication: FDA restricts use of prescription codeine pain and cough medicines and tramadol pain medicines in children; recommends against use in breastfeeding women. FDA website. https://www.fda.gov/drugs/drug-safety-and-availability/fda-drug-safety-communication-fda-restricts-use-prescription-codeine-pain-and-cough-medicines-and. Updated April 20, 2017. Accessed March 27, 2020.

Fletcher MA, Brown DR, Landers S, et al. Umbilical arterial catheter use: report of an audit conducted by the study group for complication of perinatal care. *Am J Perinatal* 1994;11(2):94–99.

Furdon SA, Horgan MJ, Bradshaw WT, et al. Nurses' guide to early detection of umbilical arterial catheter complications in infants. *Adv Neonatal Care* 2006;6(5):242–256; quiz 257–260.

Green C, Yohanna MD. Umbilical arterial and venous catheters: placement, use and complications. *Neonatal Netw* 1998;17(6):23–27.

Havranek T, Johanboeke P, Madramootoo C, et al. Umbilical artery catheters do not affect intestinal blood flow responses to minimal enteral feedings [published online ahead of print March 29, 2007]. *J Perinatol* 2007;27(6):375–379.

Hodding JH. Medication administration via the umbilical arterial catheter: a survey of standard practices and review of the literature. *Am J Perinatol* 1990;7(4):329–332.

Jacob M, Chappell D, Conzen P, et al. Small-volume resuscitation with hyperoncotic albumin: a systematic review of randomized clinical trials. *Crit Care* 2008;12(2):R34.

Lexi-Drugs. Lexicomp. Riverwoods, IL: Wolters Kluwer Health, Inc. http://online.lexi.com. Accessed March 27, 2020.

Manzoni P, Esposito S, Gallo E, et al. Switch therapy in full-term neonates with presumed or proven bacterial infection. *J Chemother* 2009;21(1):68–73.

Micromedex. Neofax database. Greenwood Village, CO: Truven Health Analytics. http://micromedex.com/. Accessed March 27, 2020.

Mitra S, Florez ID, Tamayo ME, et al. Association of placebo, indomethacin, ibuprofen, and acetaminophen with closure of hemodynamically significant patent ductus arteriosus in preterm infants: a systematic review and meta-analysis. *JAMA* 2018;319(12):1221–1238.

Monagle P, Chan AKC, Goldenberg NA, et al. Antithrombotic therapy in neonates and children: Antithrombotic Therapy and Prevention of Thrombosis, 9th ed: American College of Chest Physicians Evidence-Based Clinical Practice Guidelines. Chest 2012;141(2 Suppl):e737S–e801S.

Oca MJ, Nelson M, Donn SM. Randomized trial of normal saline versus 5% albumin for the treatment of neonatal hypotension. *J Perinatol* 2003;23:473–476.

Panel on Treatment of Pregnant Women with HIV Infection and Prevention of Perinatal Transmission. Recommendations for use of antiretroviral drugs in transmission in the United States. http://aidsinfo.nih.gov/contentfiles/lvguidelines/PerinatalGL.pdf. Accessed March 27, 2020.

Phelps SJ, Hagemann TM, Lee KR, et al. *Pediatric injectable drugs: the teddy bear book*, 11th ed. Bethesda, MD: American Society of Health System Pharmacists; 2018.

Robertson CMT, Bork KT, Tawfik G, et al. Avoiding furosemide ototoxicity associated with single-ventricle repair in young infants. *Pediatr Crit Care Med* 2019;20(4):350–356.

Smith L, Dills R. Survey of medication administration through umbilical arterial and venous catheters. *Am J Health Syst Pharm* 2003;60:1569–1572.

So KW, Fok TF, Ng PC, et al. Randomized controlled trial of colloid or crystalloid in hypotensive preterm infants. *Arch Dis Child Fetal Neonatal Ed* 1997;76:F43–F46.

Stocker M, Berger TM. Arterial and central venous catheters in neonates and infants. *Anaesthesist* 2006;55(8):873–882.

Sutton AM, Turner TL, Cockburn F, et al. Pharmacokinetic study of sulbactam and ampicillin administered concomitantly by intraarterial or intravenous infusion in the newborn. *Rev Infect Dis* 1986;8(Suppl 5):518–522.

Trissel's 2™. Lexicomp database. Riverwoods, IL: Wolters Kluwer Health, Inc. http://online.lexi.com. Accessed March 27, 2020.

Updated guidance for palivizumab prophylaxis among infants and young children at increased risk of hospitalization for respiratory syncytial virus infection. *Pediatrics.* 2014;134(2):415–420.

Wyckoff MH, Aziz K, Escobedo MB, et al. Part 13: neonatal resuscitation: 2015 American Heart Association Guidelines update for cardiopulmonary resuscitation and emergency cardiovascular care. *Circulation.* 2015;132(18 Suppl 2):S543–S560.

APPENDIX

A2

Shannon F. Manzi

Pediatric Drug Formulary

DISCLAIMER

This version of the Boston Children's Hospital formulary supported by Lexicomp platform has been edited for content and length. The nature of drug information is constantly evolving because of ongoing research and clinical experience and is often subject to interpretation. Although great care has been taken to ensure the accuracy of the information presented, the reader is advised that the authors, editors, reviewers, contributors, and Boston Children's Hospital cannot be held responsible for the continued currency of the information or for any errors, omissions, or applications of this information, or for any consequences arising subsequently.

Because of the dynamic nature of drug information, readers are advised that decisions regarding drug therapy must be based on the independent judgment of the clinician, changing information about a drug (e.g., as reflected in the literature and the manufacturer's most current product information), and changing medical practices. Therefore, these data are intended to be used in conjunction with other necessary information and are not intended to be solely relied upon by any user.

TABLE A2.1 Pediatric Drug Formulary

Medication	*Dosage*	*Comments*
Abacavir (Ziagen)	8 mg/kg/dose p.o. b.i.d.; max dose: 300 mg b.i.d.	• HLA-B*57:01 testing required prior to use. Hypersensitivity in 5%—DO NOT rechallenge
Acetaminophen (Tylenol)	Pre-op loading dose: 30 mg/kg/dose p.r. for 1 dose ED: high dose (may only be prescribed by attending or fellow) 40 mg/kg/dose p.r. for 1 dose 10–15 mg/kg/dose p.o./p.r. q4 h p.r.n. Not to exceed max of 3.75 g/d or 75 mg/kg/d, whichever is less	• Infants and children with continued fever, viral illness, dehydration, nausea, and vomiting may be at a higher risk for hepatic injury
Acetazolamide (Diamox)	20 mg/kg/d i.v./p.o. div q6 h; increase by 25 mg/kg/d; a max dose of 100 mg/kg/d has been used	• Adjust dosing interval in renal impairment
Acetylcysteine (Acetadote, Mucomyst)	Acetaminophen poisoning: • Oral: 140 mg/kg, followed by 17 doses of 70 mg/kg q4 h; repeat dose if emesis occurs within 1 h of administration • Intravenous: If approved by toxicology, 150 mg/kg i.v. over 60 min followed by 50 mg/kg i.v. over 4 h then 100 mg/kg over 16 h. Secretion management, inhalation: • Infants: 1–2 mL of 20% solution or 2–4 mL of 10% solution via nebulizer t.i.d.–q.i.d. • Children: 3–5 mL of 20% solution or 6–10 mL of 10% solution via nebulizer t.i.d.–q.i.d. • Adolescents: 5–10 mL of 10%–20% solution via nebulizer t.i.d.–q.i.d. Renal protection for radiographic contrast agent-induced reductions in renal function: oral, 10 mg/kg/dose up to 600 mg p.o. b.i.d. on day prior to and day of procedure Meconium ileus equivalent: oral, rectal irrigation, 5–30 mL of 10%–20% solution 3–6 times/d for at least 24 h and symptom improvement	• Injection: restricted to toxicology • Treatment should still be considered in patients presenting late; minimize free water in pediatric patients, dilute to no less than 30 mg/mL in D5W • Patients should receive an aerosolized bronchodilator 10–15 min prior to INH acetylcysteine
Acyclovir (Zovirax)	Herpes simplex virus encephalitis: 60 mg/kg/d i.v. div q8 h Varicella zoster virus and herpes simplex virus: 30 mg/kg/d i.v. div q8 h 80 mg/kg/d p.o. div 3–5 times/d Oral max: 3,200 mg/d	• Adequate hydration required to prevent nephrotoxicity: 1.5 times maintenance IVF per day recommended, or 2 times maintenance 1 h before and during, and 1 h after, acyclovir infusion; carefully monitor urine output (must be ≥1.5 mL/kg/h) • Dose for obese patients should be based on ideal body weight
Adenosine (Adenocard)	Children <50 kg: • Neonates: 0.05 mg/kg i.v. × 1 dose; if not effective within 2 min, increase dose by 0.05-mg/kg increments q2 min to a max dose of 0.25 mg/kg or until termination of PSVT • Infants and children: PALS dose for treatment of SVT 0.1 mg/kg (max: 6 mg); if not effective, give 0.2 mg/kg (max: 12 mg) Children and adolescents weighing ≥50 kg and adults: 6 mg; if not effective within 1–2 min, 12 mg may be given; may repeat 12 mg × 1	• May need to use higher dose for refractory SVT • Administer simultaneously with NS flush, may use three-way stopcock
Albuterol (Proventil, Ventolin)	0.5% inhalation solution INH q1–6 h p.r.n.: • <10 kg: 0.25 mL/dose • 10–30 kg: 0.5 mL/dose • >30 kg: 1 mL/dose Inhalation: MDI: 90 µg/actuation • Children <12 y: 1–2 inhalations q.i.d. • Children ≥12 y to adults: 2–4 inhalations q4–6 h Maximum 12 inhalations/day during maintenance therapy Status asthmaticus: • < 10 kg: 4 puffs • 10–30 kg: 6 puffs • ≥30 kg: 8 puffs • Intensive care patients: continuous nebulized albuterol at 0.5 mg/kg/h	• Aerosolized: dilute 0.5% solution with 1–2 mL of NS and administer with appropriate small-volume nebulizer • Suggested β_2-agonist total max: 20 mg/h

(*continued*)

TABLE A2.1 Pediatric Drug Formulary

Medication	*Dosage*	*Comments*
Allopurinol (Aloprim)	Prevention of acute uric acid nephropathy in myeloproliferative neoplastic disorders: Children ≤10 y: • Intravenous: 100 mg/m^2/dose i.v. q8 h; max dose: 600 mg/d • Oral: <6 y: 50 mg p.o. t.i.d.; 6–10 y: 100 mg p.o. t.i.d. Children >10 y and adults: • Intravenous: 200–400 mg/m^2/d i.v. in 1–3 div doses; max: 600 mg/d • Oral: 600–800 mg/d p.o. in 2–3 div doses	• Begin 1–2 d before chemotherapy • Adjust dose in renal impairment • Daily doses >300 mg should be administered in div doses
Alprazolam (Xanax)	Children <18 y: initial doses of 0.005 mg/kg or 0.125 mg p.o., increase by increments of 0.125–0.25 mg/dose; max of 0.02 mg/kg/dose or 0.06 mg/kg/d Adults: 0.25–0.5 mg p.o. b.i.d.–t.i.d., titrate dose upward; max dose: 10 mg/d	• Adequate studies in children have not been completed
Alprostadil (Prostin)	Neonates and infants: 0.05–0.1 µg/kg/min; maintenance 0.01–0.4 µg/kg/min	• With therapeutic response, rate is reduced to lowest effective dosage
Alteplase (tPA) (Activase)	Catheter clearance: • <10 kg: 0.5 mg • ≥10 kg: Non-port CVL 1 mg • ≥10 kg: Port CVL 2 mg in clogged port for 20 min–2 h, then withdraw Systemic thrombolytic therapy: 0.05–0.5 mg/kg/h i.v. × 6 h Max: 0.2 mg/kg/h for non–life- or limb- threatening clots	• Central venous catheter occlusion: Dose listed is per lumen; for multilumen catheters, treat one lumen at a time • Consult hematology service for all continuous infusions
Amikacin (Amikin)	15–22.5 mg/kg/d i.v. div q8 h	• Restricted to ID service • Check trough level prior to third dose; check peak level after third dose • Goal: pre, <10 µg/mL; post, 15–30 µg/mL
Aminocaproic acid (Amicar)	Load: 50–100 mg/kg i.v. × 1 Maintenance: continuous infusion of 30 mg/kg/h i.v. OR 100 mg/kg/dose i.v./p.o. q6 h Max dose: 30 g/d	

Aminophylline	All doses based on aminophylline
	Apnea of prematurity:
	• Loading dose: 5 mg/kg p.o./i.v. × 1
	• Maintenance: initial: 5 mg/kg/d p.o. div q12 h; increased doses may be indicated as liver metabolism matures (usually >30 d of life)
	Treatment of acute bronchospasm:
	• Loading dose (in patients not currently receiving aminophylline or theophylline): 6 mg/kg (based on aminophylline) given i.v. over 20–30 min
	• Approximate i.v. maintenance dosages are based on continuous infusions; intermittent dosing (often used in children <6 mo of age) may be determined by multiplying the hourly infusion rate by 24 h and dividing by the desired number of doses/d (usually in 3–4 doses/d):
	  • 6 wk–6 mo: 0.5 mg/kg/h
	  • 6 mo–1 y: 0.6–0.7 mg/kg/h
	  • 1–9 y: 1–1.2 mg/kg/h
	  • 9–12 y and young adult smokers: 0.9 mg/kg/h
	  • 12–16 y: 0.7 mg/kg/h
		• Monitor serum levels to determine appropriate doses
		• Theophylline levels should be initially drawn after 3 d of therapy; repeat levels are indicated 3 d after each increase in dose or weekly if on a stabilized dose

Amiodarone (Cordarone)	VF/VT arrest: 5 mg/kg i.v./i.o. rapid push, may repeat up to max 15 mg/kg Dysrhythmia (unstable): 5 mg/kg i.v./i.o. over 20–60 min Max: 300 mg/dose	• Dilute in D5W only • Use 0.22-µm filter inline • Glass container only for large-volume parenteral

TABLE A2.1 Pediatric Drug Formulary (*continued*)

Medication	*Dosage*	*Comments*
Amitriptyline (Elavil)	1–3 mg/kg/d p.o. div t.i.d., max 200 mg/d Migraine prophylaxis: start 0.25 mg/kg/dose before bedtime, increase by 0.25 mg/kg/d every 14 d, max 1 mg/kg/d.	• Use caution in hepatic impairment
Amlodipine (Norvasc)	0.1 mg/kg p.o. once daily max 10 mg/d	• Can be compounded into liquid
Amoxicillin (Amoxil)	40–120 mg/kg/d p.o. div q8 h; max: 3 g/d	• Usual 80 mg/kg/d
Amoxicillin/clavulanic acid (Augmentin)	Augmentin tablets: 40 mg/kg/d p.o. div q8 h Augmentin ES-600 liquid: 40–90 mg/kg/d p.o. div q8 h Max: 3 g as amoxicillin/d	• Dosed as amoxicillin • Usual 90 mg/kg/d for otitis media • Diarrhea associated w/higher doses of clavulanic acid
Amphetamine and dextro-amphetamine (Adderall)	3–5 y: 2.5 mg/d p.o., increase by 2.5 mg/d each week until response; max 40 mg/d in div doses ≥6 y: 5 mg/d p.o. div once daily to b.i.d., increase by 5 mg each week until response, max 40 mg/d in div doses	• Controlled substance
Amphotericin B (Fungizone)	0.5–1 mg/kg/dose i.v. q.d., max: 1.5 mg/kg/d CF: 15 mg INH b.i.d. Bladder irrigation: 50 µg/mL in sterile water irrigation solution, 15–60 mL per installation, clamp 60–120 min and drain. Repeat b.i.d.–q.i.d. for 2–5 d.	• Max concentration for fluid-restricted patients 0.2 mg/mL via central line
Amphotericin B liposomal (Ambisome)	3 mg/kg/d i.v. q.d., max: 5 mg/kg/d (neonates may require up to 7 mg/kg/d)	• ID approval required
Ampicillin	200–400 mg/kg/d i.v. div q6 h; max: 12 g/d	
Ampicillin/sulbactam (Unasyn)	200 mg/kg/d i.v. div q6 h Max: 8 g/d as ampicillin May add extra ampicillin for total 12 g/d	• Dose based on ampicillin component
Aprepitant (Emend)	<40 kg: 3 mg/kg (max 125 mg) p.o. day 1, then 2 mg/kg (max 80 mg) p.o. on days 2–4 ≥40 mg: 125 mg p.o. on day 1, 80 mg p.o. on days 2–4	• Administer first dose 1 h prior to chemotherapy • Use with 5HT3 antagonist and steroid
Aripiprazole (Abilify)	2.5–5 mg/d, may increase up to a max of 30 mg/d	• Titrate to sedation, GI side effects • Significant drug–drug interactions
Aspirin	10–15 mg/kg/dose p.o. q4–6 h p.r.n. Acute myocardial infarction (AMI): 324 mg p.o. (chewed) × 1 dose Kawasaki disease: 80–100 mg/kg/d p.o. div q6 h until fever resolves, then 3–5 mg/kg/d p.o. q.d.	• Use 4–81 mg chewable aspirin for AMI if available
Atenolol (Tenormin)	Initial: 0.8–1 mg/kg/dose p.o. q.d. Range: 0.8–1.5 mg/kg/dose p.o. q.d. Max: 2 mg/kg/dose p.o. q.d.	
Atomoxetine (Strattera)	≤70 kg: 0.25–0.5 mg/kg/d p.o. increase every 3 d (or greater), max 1.4 mg/kg/d or 100 mg/d (whichever is less)	• Significant drug–drug interactions
Atovaquone (Mepron)	Treatment: 40 mg/kg/d p.o. div q12 h; max: 1,500 mg/d Prophylaxis: 30–45 mg/kg/d p.o. q.d.	
Atropine	Bradycardia: 0.02 mg/kg/dose i.v./i.o.; may repeat × 1 p.r.n. max: 1 mg/dose Organophosphate poisoning: <10 kg: 0.5 mg i.m. (use autoinjector if available) ≥10 kg: 2 mg i.m. (use autoinjector if available) Repeat p.r.n., doses are frequently in g/d.	• If giving via ETT, dose is 2–10 × i.v. dose • Dilute ETT dose in 3–5 mL of NS and follow with several positive-pressure breaths
Azathioprine (Imuran)	Initial: 2–5 mg/kg/dose p.o./i.v. q.d. Maintenance: 1–3 mg/kg/dose p.o./i.v. q.d.	• TPMT/NUDT15 testing strongly recommended before use

(*continued*)

TABLE A2.1 Pediatric Drug Formulary (*continued*)

Medication	*Dosage*	*Comments*
Azithromycin (Zithromax)	Otitis media: 30 mg/kg (max: 1,500 mg/dose) p.o. × 1 dose GABHS pharyngitis: 12 mg/kg/d q.d. × 5 d OR 10 mg/kg/dose p.o. q.d. × 1 d, then 5 mg/kg/dose p.o. q.d. × 4 d CAP: 10 mg/kg/dose i.v./p.o. q.d. × 1 d (max: 500 mg/dose), followed by 5 mg/kg/dose p.o./i.v. q.d. (max: 250 mg/dose) × 4 d *Chlamydia* prophylaxis postsexual assault: 1,000 mg p.o. × 1 dose	
Aztreonam (Azactam)	90–120 mg/kg/d i.v. div q6–8 h CF: 50 mg/kg/dose i.v. div q6–8 h (max 200 mg/kg/d); max: 8 g/d Perioperative prophylaxis: 30 mg/kg × 1 dose within 60 min of incision. Redose q4 h while inter-op.	• Adjust dose in renal impairment
Baclofen (Lioresal)	Oral: • 2–7 y: initial 10–15 mg/d div q8 h; max: 40 mg/d • >8 y: titrate dosage as above, max: 60 mg/d • Adults: 5 mg t.i.d., max: 80 mg/d Continuous intrathecal infusion dose µg/h = daily dose div by 24 h Average daily intrathecal dose: • Children ≤12 y: 100–300 µg/d (4.2–12.5 µg/h); doses as high as 1,000 µg/d have been used • Children >12 y and adults: 300–800 µg/d (12.5–33 µg/h); doses as high as 2,000 µg/d have been used	• Titrate dose q3 d in increments of 5–15 mg/d • Further adjustments in infusion rate may be done q24 h p.r.n.; for spinal cord–related spasticity, increase in 10%–30% increments/24 h; for spasticity of cerebral origin, increase in 5%–10% increments/24 h
Basiliximab (Simulect)	Children <35 kg: renal transplantation: 10 mg i.v. within 2 h prior to transplant surgery, followed by a second 10-mg dose i.v. 4 d after transplantation Children ≥35 kg and adults: renal transplantation: 20 mg i.v. within 2 h prior to transplant surgery, followed by a second 20-mg i.v. dose 4 d after transplantation	• The second dose should be withheld if complications occur (including severe hypersensitivity reactions or graft loss)
Benztropine (Cogentin)	Drug-induced extrapyramidal reaction: • >3 y: 0.02–0.05 mg/kg/dose p.o./i.m./i.v. q.d.–b.i.d. • Adults: 1–4 mg/dose p.o./i.m./i.v. q.d.–b.i.d. • Parkinsonism: 0.5–6 mg/d p.o. in 1–2 div doses; begin with 0.5 mg/d; increase in 0.5-mg increments at 5- to 6-d intervals to achieve the desired effect	• Use in children <3 y should be reserved for life-threatening emergencies
Beractant (Survanta)	Prophylactic treatment: give 4 mL/kg as soon as possible; as many as 4 doses may be administered during the first 48 h of life, no more frequently than 6 h apart Rescue treatment: give 4 mL/kg as soon as the diagnosis of RDS is made; may repeat if needed, no more frequently than q6 h to a max of 4 doses	• The need for additional doses is determined by evidence of continuing respiratory distress or if the infant is still intubated and requiring at least 30% inspired oxygen to maintain a PaO_2 ≤80 torr
Bisacodyl (Dulcolax)	Oral: • 3–12 y: 5–10 mg or 0.3 mg/kg/d p.o. q.d. • ≥12 y and adults: 5–15 mg/d p.o. q.d. Rectal: • 2–11 y: 5–10 mg/d p.r. q.d. • ≥12 y and adults: 10 mg/d p.r. q.d.	• <2 y: 5 mg/d p.r. q.d.

TABLE A2.1 Pediatric Drug Formulary (*continued*)

Medication	*Dosage*	*Comments*
Botulinum toxin type A (Botox)	Strabismus: Children 2 mo–12 y: • Horizontal or vertical deviations <20 prism diopters: 1.25 units into any one muscle • Horizontal or vertical deviations 20–25 prism diopters: 1–2.5 units into any one muscle • Persistent VI nerve palsy of ≥1 mo duration: 1–1.25 units into the medial rectus muscle Children ≥12 y and adults: • Horizontal or vertical deviations <20 prism diopters: 1.25–2.5 units into any one muscle • Horizontal or vertical deviations 20–50 prism diopters: 2.5–5 units into any one muscle • Persistent VI nerve palsy of ≥1 mo duration: 1.25–2.5 units into the medial rectus muscle Spasticity associated with cerebral palsy, children >18 mo to adolescents: small muscle, 1–2 units/kg; large muscle, 3–6 units/kg; max dose per injection site 50 units; max dose for any one visit 12 units/kg, up to 400 units; no more than 400 units should be administered during a 3-mo period	• For strabismus, reexamine patient 7–14 d after each injection to assess effects; dose may be increased up to twofold of the previously administered dose; do not exceed 25 units as a single injection for any one muscle
Budesonide (Pulmicort Turbuhaler, Pulmicort Respules)	Intranasal: children ≥6 y and adults, Rhinocort: initial, 8 sprays (4 sprays/nostril) per day (256 μg/d); after symptoms decrease (usually by 3–7 d), reduce dose slowly q2–4 wk to the smallest effective dose Nebulization: children 12 mo–8 y, Pulmicort Respules: • Previously treated with bronchodilators alone: initial, 0.25 mg b.i.d. or 0.5 mg once daily; max dose: 0.5 mg/d • Previously treated with INH corticosteroids: initial, 0.25 mg b.i.d. or 0.5 mg once daily; max dose: 1 mg/d • Previously treated with oral corticosteroids: initial, 0.5 mg b.i.d. or 1 mg once daily; max dose: 1 mg/d Oral inhalation, children ≥6 y: • Previously treated with bronchodilators alone or with INH corticosteroids: initial, 200 μg (1 puff) b.i.d.; max dose: 400 μg (2 puffs) b.i.d. • Treated with oral corticosteroids: initial, 400 μg (2 puffs) b.i.d. (max dose)	• Administer via a nebulizer medication system with filter; requires no further dilution
Bumetanide (Bumex)	Neonates: 0.01–0.05 mg/kg/dose i.v./i.m./p.o. q24–48 h Infants and children: 0.015–0.1 mg/kg/dose i.v./i.m./p.o. q6–24 h (max dose: 10 mg/d)	
Bupropion (Wellbutrin)	Children and adolescents: 1.4–6 mg/kg/d p.o. q.d.	• Pay attention to dose formulation • Adjust doses in renal and hepatic dysfunction
C1 inhibitor (Cinryze, Berinert)	Treatment: 20 units/kg i.v. Prophylaxis (adolescents/adults): 1,000 units every 3–4 d	• Use Cinryze within 3 h of reconstitution (8 h for Berinert) • May repeat Berinert dose for treatment, note significant thrombotic events reported at doses > 100 units/kg
Caffeine citrate	Apnea of prematurity: p.o./i.v.: • Loading dose: 10–20 mg/kg as caffeine citrate (5–10 mg/kg as caffeine base) • Maintenance dose: 5–10 mg/kg/d as caffeine citrate (2.5–5 mg/kg/d as caffeine base) once daily starting 24 h after the loading dose Spinal puncture headache: • Adults 300 mg p.o./i.v. as a single dose	• If theophylline has been administered to the patient within the previous 5 d, a full or modified loading dose (50%–75% of a loading dose) may be given at the discretion of the physician • Maintenance dose is adjusted based on patient's response (efficacy and adverse effects) and serum caffeine concentrations

(*continued*)

TABLE A2.1	Pediatric Drug Formulary (*continued*)	
Medication	*Dosage*	*Comments*
Calcitriol (Rocaltrol)	Management of hypocalcemia in patients with chronic renal failure: Hemodialysis patients: Intravenous: • Children: 0.01–0.05 μg/kg i.v. 3 times/wk • Adults: 0.5 μg (0.01 μg/kg) i.v. 3 times/wk; may increase dose by 0.25- to 0.5-μg increments at 2- to 4-wk intervals until an optimal response is achieved; range 0.5–3 μg (0.01–0.05 μg/kg) Oral: • Children: 0.25–2 μg/d p.o. q.d. • Adults: 0.25 μg p.o. q.d.; may increase in 0.25-μg increments at 4- to 8-wk intervals; range 0.5–1 μg/d Nonhemodialysis patients: moderate-to-severe renal failure (CrCl 15–55 mL/min; corrected for surface area in children): oral: • Children <3 y: 0.01–0.015 μg/kg p.o. once daily • Children ≥3 y and adults: 0.25 μg/d p.o. q.d. (max dose: 0.5 μg/d) Hypoparathyroidism/pseudohypoparathyroidism: oral (evaluate dose at 2- to 4-wk intervals): • Children <1 y: 0.04–0.08 μg/kg p.o. q.d. • Children 1–5 y: 0.25–0.75 μg p.o. q.d. • Children >6 y and adults: 0.5–2 μg p.o. q.d. Vitamin D–dependent rickets: children and adults, oral: 1 μg p.o. once daily Vitamin D–resistant rickets (familial hypophosphatemia): children and adults, oral: • Initial: 0.015–0.02 μg/kg p.o. once daily • Maintenance: 0.03–0.06 μg/kg p.o. once daily • Max dose: 2 μg p.o. once daily Hypocalcemia in premature infants: oral, 1 μg p.o. once daily for 5 d Hypocalcemic tetany in premature infants: i.v., 0.05 μg/kg i.v. once daily for 5–12 d	• Maintain calcium levels of 9–10 mg/dL
Calcium carbonate	Recommended daily allowance (dose is in terms of elemental calcium): • <6 mo: 400 mg/d • 6–12 mo: 600 mg/d • 1–10 y: 800 mg/d • 11–24 y: 1,200 mg/d • Adults >24 y: 800 mg/d Hypocalcemia (dose depends on clinical condition and serum calcium level): oral (dose expressed in mg of elemental calcium): • Neonates: 50–150 mg/kg/d p.o. in 4–6 div doses; not to exceed 1 g/d • Children: 45–65 mg/kg/d p.o. in 4 div doses • Adults: 1–2 g/d or more p.o. in 3–4 div doses	
Calcium chloride	10–20 mg/kg/dose central i.v./i.o., slowly, max 2 g/dose	• 10% solution = 100 mg/mL • Must further dilute prior to administration
Calcium gluconate	100–200 mg/kg/dose i.v./i.o., slowly Max: 3 g/dose Continuous infusion: 200–500 mg/kg/d	• 10% solution = 100 mg/mL • Central line preferred, but not required
Cannabidiol (Epidiolex)	Dravet or Lennox–Gastaut syndrome: ≥2 y: 2.5 mg/kg/dose p.o. b.i.d., increase weekly by 2.5 mg/kg dose p.r.n.; max 20 mg/kg/d titrate to side effects	• Baseline LFTs required • Significant drug–drug interactions, particularly CYP2C19 substrates • Do not administer via PVC enteral tubes
Captopril (Capoten)	Neonates: 0.05–0.1 mg/kg/dose p.o. t.i.d. Children: 0.3–0.5 mg/kg/dose p.o. t.i.d. Adults: 6.25–25 mg/dose p.o. t.i.d.	

TABLE A2.1 Pediatric Drug Formulary (*continued*)

Medication	*Dosage*	*Comments*
Carbamazepine (Tegretol, Carbatrol)	10–35 mg/kg/d p.o. div b.i.d.–t.i.d.	• Consider HLA-B*15:02 and HLA-A*31:01 testing prior to initiation • Dose individualized based on levels • Suppositories made by pharmacy
Carnitine (Carnitor)	Primary carnitine deficiency: oral: • Children: 50–100 mg/kg/d p.o. div b.i.d.–t.i.d., max: 3 g/d • Adults: 330–990 mg/dose p.o. b.i.d.–t.i.d. Valproic acid toxicity: prophylaxis: 50–100 mg/kg/d p.o. div b.i.d.–t.i.d. Active hepatotoxicity/overdose: • Oral: 150–500 mg/kg/d p.o. div b.i.d.–t.i.d., max: 3 g/d • Intravenous: 50 mg/kg i.v. load, followed (in severe cases) by 50 mg/kg/d infusion; maintenance: 50 mg/kg/d i.v. div q4–6 h, increase p.r.n. to a max of 300 mg/kg/d ESRD patients on hemodialysis: • Intravenous: adults, predialysis carnitine levels below normal (30–60 µmol): 10–20 mg/kg i.v. after each dialysis session; maintenance doses as low as 5 mg/kg may be used after 3–4 wk of therapy depending on response (carnitine level) Supplement to parenteral nutrition: neonates, 10–20 mg/kg/d in parenteral nutrition solution	• Dosage must be individualized based on patient response; higher doses have been used
Caspofungin (Cancidas)	For patients weighing <15 kg: • Loading dose: 1.5 mg/kg i.v. × 1 (max: 70 mg) • Daily dose: 1 mg/kg/d i.v. q.d. (max: 50 mg) For patients weighing >15 kg: • Loading dose: 70 mg/m^2 i.v. × 1 (max: 70 mg) • Daily dose: 50 mg/m^2/d i.v. q.d. (max: 50 mg)	• Adjust dose in hepatic dysfunction
Cefazolin (Kefzol, Ancef)	50–150 mg/kg/d i.v. div q8 h Max: 12 g/d	• Usual adult 2 g/dose
Cefdinir (Omnicef)	Infants and children (≥6 mo–12 y): • Otitis media or pharyngitis/tonsillitis: 14 mg/kg/d p.o. div q12 h for 5–10 d or 14 mg/kg/d p.o. q.d. for 10 d • Skin and soft-tissue infection: 14 mg/kg/d p.o. div b.i.d. for 10 d • Acute maxillary sinusitis: 14 mg/kg/d p.o. div q12 h for 10 d or 14 mg/kg/d p.o. q.d. for 10 d Children >12 y and adults: • Acute exacerbations of chronic bronchitis or pharyngitis/tonsillitis: 600 mg p.o. q.d. for 10 d or 300 mg p.o. q12 h for 5–10 d • Skin and soft-tissue infection or CAP: 300 mg p.o. q12 h for 10 d • Acute maxillary sinusitis: 600 mg p.o. q.d. for 10 d or 300 mg p.o. q12 h for 10 d	• Max: 600 mg/d • Adjust dose in renal impairment
Cefepime (Maxipime)	150–200 mg/kg/d i.v. div q8 h; max: 6 g/d	• Adjust dose in renal impairment
Cefoxitin (Mefoxin)	80–160 mg/kg/d i.v. div q6–8 h; max: 12 g/d	• Adjust dose in renal impairment
Ceftaroline (Teflaro)	Serious MRSA infection: <40 kg: 15 mg/kg i.v. q8 h ≥40 kg: 600 mg i.v. q8 h CAP or skin/soft-tissue infection: >2 mo and < 2 yr: 8 mg/kg/dose i.v. q8 h ≥2 yr and < 18 yr: 12 mg/kg/dose (max 400 mg/dose) i.v. q8 h	• ID approval required • Adjust dose in renal impairment

(*continued*)

TABLE A2.1 Pediatric Drug Formulary (*continued*)

Medication	*Dosage*	*Comments*
Ceftazidime (Fortaz)	150 mg/kg/d i.v. div q8 h, max: 6 g/d CF: 150–200 mg/kg/d i.v. div q8 h (max: 6 g/d)	• Adjust dose in renal impairment
Ceftriaxone (Rocephin)	50–100 mg/kg/d i.v./i.m. q12–24 h, max: 4 g/d Postsexual assault (gonorrhea prophylaxis): 125 mg i.m. × 1	• Do not use in infants with hyperbilirubinemia
Celecoxib (Celebrex)	Adolescents: oral, initial dose 400 mg, followed by an additional 200 mg if needed on day 1; maintenance dose 200 mg b.i.d. p.r.n.	
Cephalexin (Keflex)	25–100 mg/kg/d p.o. div q.i.d.; max: 4 g/d	
Cetirizine (Zyrtec)	2–5 y: 2.5–5 mg/d p.o. div q.d.–b.i.d. ≥6 y: 5–10 mg/d p.o. div q.d.–b.i.d.	
Charcoal, activated	1 g/kg/dose p.o./n.g. × 1 dose; max: 60 g/dose	• Do not use sorbitol-containing product for repetitive dosing • May repeat dose as necessary (q4–6 h) for agents with enterohepatic recirculation or bezoar formation • Single dose: 1 g absorbs 100–1,000 mg of poison
Chloramphenicol	25–50 mg/kg i.v. q12–24 h Meningitis: 75–100 mg/kg/d i.v. div q6 h; max 4 g/d	• Restricted to ID • Monitor serum levels closely
Chlorothiazide (Diuril)	20–40 mg/kg/d i.v./p.o. div q12 h	
Ciprofloxacin (Cipro)	20–30 mg/kg/d i.v. div q12 h; max: 800 mg/d Severe *Pseudomonas aeruginosa*: 30 mg/kg/d i.v. div q12 h; max: 1.2 g/d 20–30 mg/kg/d p.o. div q12 h; max: 1.5 g/d CF: 40 mg/kg/d p.o. div q12 h; max: 2 g/d	
Cisatracurium (Nimbex)	Children 2–12 y: initial 0.2 mg/kg i.v., followed by maintenance dose of 0.03 mg/kg i.v. p.r.n. Children >12 y to adults: initial 0.15–0.2 mg/kg i.v., followed by maintenance dose of 0.03 mg/kg i.v. q40–60 min p.r.n. Continuous infusion 0.1–0.2 mg/kg/h i.v.	• Reserved for patients with renal dysfunction
Citalopram (Celexa)	Children and adolescents: OCD (unlabeled use): 10–40 mg/d p.o.	
Clarithromycin (Biaxin)	15 mg/kg/d p.o. div b.i.d.; max: 1 g/d	• Significant drug–drug interactions
Clindamycin (Cleocin)	25–40 mg/kg/d i.v. div q8 h, max: 4.8 g/d; 10–30 mg/kg/d p.o. div q8 h, max: 1.8 g/d	
Clobazam (Onfi)	< 2 y: 0.25–1 mg/kg/d 2–16 y: initial 5 mg/d, increase no more frequently than q5 d, to a max of 40 mg/d	• Dose adjustment required for CYP2C19 poor metabolizers • Significant drug–drug interactions • Do not use in severe hepatic impairment
Clonazepam (Klonopin)	Infants and children <10 y or 30 kg: • Initial: 0.01–0.03 mg/kg/d (max: 0.05 mg/kg/d) p.o. div b.i.d.–t.i.d.; increase by no more than 0.5 mg every third day until seizures are controlled or adverse effects seen • Maintenance: 0.1–0.2 mg/kg/d p.o. div t.i.d.; not to exceed 0.2 mg/kg/d Children ≥10 y (>30 kg) and adults: • Initial daily dose not to exceed 1.5 mg p.o. div t.i.d.; may increase by 0.5–1 mg every third day until seizures are controlled or adverse effects seen • Maintenance: 0.05–0.2 mg/kg/d p.o. div t.i.d.; do not exceed 20 mg/d	• Note: This is frequently confused with clonidine. Please use caution.

TABLE A2.1 Pediatric Drug Formulary (*continued*)

Medication	*Dosage*	*Comments*
Clonidine (Catapres, Duraclon)	Hypertension: oral, initial 5–10 µg/kg/d p.o. div q8–12 h; increase gradually, if needed, to 5–25 µg/kg/d in div doses q6 h; max dose: 0.9 mg/d ADHD: oral, initial: 0.05 mg/d p.o. q.d., increase q3–7 d by 0.05 mg/d to 3–5 µg/kg/d p.o. div t.i.d.–q.i.d.; usual max dose: 0.3–0.4 mg/d Clonidine tolerance test (test of growth hormone release from the pituitary): oral, 0.15 mg/m^2 or 4 µg/kg p.o. as a single dose Analgesia: epidural (continuous infusion), reserved for cancer patients with severe intractable pain, unresponsive to other analgesics or epidural or spinal opiates; initial, 0.5 µg/kg/h; adjust with caution, based on clinical effect; do not exceed adult doses Transdermal: children may be switched to the transdermal delivery system after oral therapy is titrated to an optimal and stable dose; a transdermal dose approximately equivalent to the total oral daily dose may be used	• Clonidine patches may be cut if necessary to provide appropriate dose • 8 µg/kg/d has been used for ADHD • Note this has been confused with clonazepam (Klonopin). Please use caution.
Colistimethate (Coly-Mycin)	Children and adults: 2.5–5 mg/kg/d i.v./i.m. div b.i.d.–q.i.d. Inhalation: 75 mg + 3 mL NS (4 mL total) via nebulizer b.i.d.	• Adjust i.v. dose in renal dysfunction
Corticotropin (Acthar-HP)	Infantile spasms: • 150 units/m^2 i.m. q.d. × 2 wk • 30 units/m^2 i.m. q.d. × 3 d • 15 units/m^2 i.m. q.d. × 3 d • 10 units/m^2 i.m. q.d. × 3 d • 10 units/m^2 i.m. q.o.d. × 6 d	• Monitor blood pressure, electrolytes
Cromolyn (Gastrocrom)	Oral solution: < 2 y: 20 mg/kg/d p.o. div q.i.d., max 30 mg/kg/d 2–12 y: 100 mg p.o. q.i.d., do not exceed 40 mg/kg/d 12 y: 200 mg p.o. q.i.d.	
Cyclosporine (Neoral, Gengraf, Sandimmune)	Intravenous: • Initial: 5–6 mg/kg/dose i.v. administered 4–12 h prior to organ transplantation • Maintenance: 2–10 mg/kg/d i.v. in div doses q8–24 h; patients should be switched to oral cyclosporine as soon as possible Oral: solution or soft gelatin capsule (Sandimmune): • Initial: 14–18 mg/kg/dose p.o. administered 4–12 h prior to organ transplantation • Maintenance, postoperative: 5–15 mg/kg/d p.o. div q12–24 h; maintenance dose is usually tapered to 3–10 mg/kg/d Oral: solution or soft gelatin capsule in a microemulsion (Gengraf, Neoral): based on the organ transplant population • Initial: same as the initial dose for solution or soft gelatin capsule OR • Renal: 9 mg/kg/d (range 6–12 mg/kg/d) • Liver: 8 mg/kg/d (range 4–12 mg/kg/d) • Heart: 7 mg/kg/d (range 4–10 mg/kg/d)	• Brands NOT interchangeable, order must specify brand name • Cyclosporine doses should be adjusted to maintain whole-blood HPLC trough concentrations in the reference range • A 1:1 ratio conversion from Sandimmune to Neoral or Gengraf has been recommended initially; however, lower doses of Neoral or Gengraf may be required after conversion to prevent overdose

(*continued*)

TABLE A2.1 Pediatric Drug Formulary (*continued*)

Medication	*Dosage*	*Comments*
Cyproheptadine (Periactin)	Allergic conditions: • Children: 0.25 mg/kg/d or 8 $mg/m^2/d$ p.o. in 2–3 div doses OR • 2–6 y: 2 mg q8–12 h (not to exceed 12 mg/d) • 7–14 y: 4 mg q8–12 h (not to exceed 16 mg/d) • Adults: 4–20 mg/d div q8 h (not to exceed 0.5 mg/kg/d) Appetite stimulation (anorexia nervosa): >13 y, 2 mg p.o. q.i.d.; may be increased gradually over a 3-wk period to 8 mg p.o. q.i.d. Migraine headaches: • Children: 4 mg p.o. b.i.d.–t.i.d. • Adults: 4–8 mg p.o. t.i.d. • Spasticity associated with spinal cord damage: ≥12 y, 4 mg p.o. q.h.s.; increase by 4 mg/dose q3–4 d; average daily dose 16 mg in div doses; not to exceed 36 mg/d	• Reduce dose in patients with significant hepatic dysfunction
Dantrolene (Dantrium, Ryanodex)	Oral: 0.5 mg/kg/dose p.o. b.i.d., increase frequency up to q.i.d. at weekly intervals, then increase dose, max 3 mg/kg/dose or 400 mg/d Intravenous: Crisis: 2.5 mg/kg i.v. over 1 min, repeat p.r.n. up to 10 mg/kg; reassess and repeat regimen if needed Postcrisis: 1 mg/kg i.v. or 2 mg/kg p.o. q.i.d. for 1–3 d	• Prepare and store injection kits in areas where malignant hyperthermia may occur
Dapsone	Prophylaxis for first episode of opportunistic infection: *Toxoplasma gondii*: children ≥1 mo of age, 2 mg/kg or 15 mg/m^2 (max dose: 25 mg) p.o. once daily in combination with pyrimethamine 1 mg/kg p.o. once daily and leucovorin 5 mg p.o. q3 d Primary and secondary PCP prophylaxis: 2 mg/kg/d p.o. once daily, max dose: 100 mg/d, or 4 mg/kg/dose p.o. once weekly, max dose: 200 mg/dose Leprosy: 1–2 mg/kg/d p.o. given once daily in combination therapy; max dose: 100 mg/d	• Do not use in patients with G6PD deficiency
Desmopressin (DDAVP)	Diabetes insipidus: • Oral: 0.05 mg p.o. b.i.d.; titrate to desired response; range 0.1–1.2 mg p.o. div b.i.d.–t.i.d. • Intranasal: children 3 mo–≥12 y, initial (using 100 µg/mL nasal solution) 5 µg/d (0.05 mL/d) div once daily to b.i.d., range 5–30 µg/d (0.05–0.3 mL/d); children >12 y and adults, initial (using 100-µg/mL nasal solution) 5–40 µg (0.05–0.4 mL) div once daily to t.i.d. • Intravenous, subcutaneous: children >12 y and adults, 2–4 µg/d in 2 div doses or 1/10 of the maintenance intranasal dose Hemophilia: • Intravenous, subcutaneous: children ≥3 mo and adults, 0.3 µg/kg beginning 30 min before procedure; may repeat dose if needed • Intranasal: children >12 y and adults, using high-concentration Stimate nasal spray: ≥50 kg: 150 µg (1 spray) >50 kg: 300 µg (1 spray each nostril) Nocturnal enuresis: • Intranasal: children ≥6 y (using 100-µg/mL nasal solution), initial 20 µg (0.2 mL) q.h.s., range 10–40 µg; it is recommended that 1/2 of the dose be given in each nostril • Oral: children >12 y, 0.2–0.4 mg p.o. once before bedtime	• Adjust morning and evening doses separately for an adequate diurnal rhythm of water turnover • The nasal spray pump delivers doses of 10 µg (0.1 mL) or multiples thereof; other doses must be given via the rhinal tube • Repeat use of the nasal spray in hemophilia is determined by the patient's clinical condition and laboratory work; if using preoperatively, administer 2 h before surgery

TABLE A2.1 Pediatric Drug Formulary (*continued*)

Medication	*Dosage*	*Comments*
Dexamethasone (Decadron)	Croup: 0.6 mg/kg/dose i.m./p.o. × 1, max: 16 mg/dose Inflammation: 0.5–2 mg/kg/d i.v./p.o. div q6–8 h	• Dexamethasone 1 mg = methylprednisolone 5 mg
Dexmedetomidine (Precedex)	Initial: 0.2–0.5 µg/kg/h, max 2 µg/kg/h Bolus doses: 0.5 µg/kg over 10 min Pre-op: 1–2 µg/kg i.m.	• ED, ICU, OR only
Dextroamphetamine (Dexedrine)	ADHD: • <3 y: not recommended • 3–5 y: initial, 2.5 mg/d p.o. given every morning; increase by 2.5 mg/d at weekly intervals until optimal response is obtained, usual range is 0.1–0.5 mg/kg/dose every morning with max of 40 mg/d given in 1–3 div doses per day • 6 y: 5 mg p.o. once or b.i.d.; increase in increments of 5 mg/d at weekly intervals until optimal response is reached, usual range is 0.1–0.5 mg/kg/dose every morning (5–20 mg/d) with max of 40 mg/d given in 1–3 div doses per day Narcolepsy: • Children 6–12 y: initial 5 mg/d, may increase at 5-mg increments at weekly intervals until optimal response is obtained; max dose: 60 mg/d • Children >12 y and adults: initial 10 mg/d, may increase at 10-mg increments at weekly intervals until optimal response is obtained; max dose: 60 mg/d Exogenous obesity: >12 y and adults, 5–30 mg/d p.o. in div doses of 5–10 mg given 30–60 min before meals	
Dextrose	0.5–1 g/kg i.v./i.o.	• D50W 1–2 mL/kg • D25W 2–4 mL/kg • D10W 5–10 mL/kg • Max concentration for peripheral continuous infusions: D12.5W
Diazepam (Valium, Diastat)	Rectal: • Gel, <5 y: 0.5 mg/kg/dose p.r. q2 h p.r.n. • Gel, 6–11 y: 0.3 mg/kg/dose p.r. q2 h p.r.n. • Gel, ≥12 y: 0.2 mg/kg/dose p.r. q2 h p.r.n. • Injection given p.r. 0.5 mg/kg p.r. × 1 Intravenous: 0.05–0.2 mg/kg/dose i.v. q2–4 h p.r.n., max: 10 mg/dose Oral: 0.1–0.8 mg/kg/d p.o. div q6–8 h, max: 10 mg/dose	• May use undiluted injectable preparation rectally • Max i.v. 0.6 mg/kg per 8-h period
Didanosine (Videx)	90–120 mg/m^2/dose p.o. b.i.d.; max: 200 mg/dose	

(*continued*)

TABLE A2.1 Pediatric Drug Formulary (*continued*)

Medication	*Dosage*	*Comments*
Digoxin (Lanoxin)	Loading (see note for frequency): Oral: • Neonates: 20–35 μg/kg p.o. • 1 mo–2 y: 35–60 μg/kg p.o. • 2–5 y: 30–40 μg/kg p.o. • 5–10 y: 20–30 μg/kg p.o. • >10 y: 10–15 μg/kg p.o. • Adult: 0.75–1 mg p.o. Intravenous: • Neonates: 15–30 μg/kg i.v. • 1 mo–2 y: 30–50 μg/kg i.v. • 2–5 y: 25–35 μg/kg i.v. • 5–10 y: 15–30 μg/kg i.v. • >10 y: 8–12 μg/kg i.v. • Adult: 0.5–1 mg i.v. Maintenance: Oral: • Neonates: 2.5–5 μg/kg/dose p.o. b.i.d. • 1 mo–2 y: 5 μg/kg/dose p.o. b.i.d. • 2–10 y: 2.5–5 μg/kg/dose p.o. b.i.d. • >10 y: 2.5–5 μg/kg/dose p.o. q.d. • Adult: 0.125–0.25 mg p.o. q.d., max: 0.5 mg/d Intravenous: • Neonates: 2–4 μg/kg/dose i.v. q12 h • 1 mo–2 y: 3.5–6 μg/kg/dose i.v. q12 h • 2–10 y: 3–4 μg/kg/dose i.v. q12 h • >10 y: 2–3 μg/kg/dose i.v. q24 h • Adult: 0.1–0.4 mg i.v. q24 h	• Loading dose should be divided to provide ½ the total dose at initial dose, then give ¼ of the dose at 6- to 12-h intervals × 2 doses • Adjust dose in renal dysfunction • Dose on lean body weight
Diphenhydramine (Benadryl)	1 mg/kg/dose i.v./p.o. q6 h p.r.n.; max 300 mg/d	• Usual adult 25–50 mg/dose
Dobutamine	2.5–20 μg/kg/min i.v.	• Central line preferred
Docusate (Colace)	5 mg/kg/d p.o. in 1–4 div doses OR • <3 y: 10–40 mg/d p.o. in 1–4 div doses • 3–6 y: 20–60 mg/d p.o. in 1–4 div doses • 6–12 y: 40–150 mg/d p.o. in 1–4 div doses • Adolescents and adults: 50–400 mg/d p.o. in 1–4 div doses	• May use several drops of the liquid in ear canal to remove cerumen buildup
Dopamine	2.5–20 μg/kg/min i.v.	• If starting in shock state, begin at 10 μg/kg/min • Central line preferred
Dornase alfa (Pulmozyme)	>5 y: 2.5 mg/d INH q.d.–b.i.d.	• Select nebulizers in conjunction with a Pulmo-Aide or a Pari-Proneb compressor • b.i.d. dosing may be beneficial in some patients, especially older than 21 y or with forced vital capacity >85%
Dronabinol (Marinol)	Antiemetic: 5 mg/m^2/dose p.o. 1–3 h before chemotherapy, then give 5 mg/m^2/dose p.o. q2–4 h after chemotherapy for a total of 4–6 doses/d; dose may be increased up to a max of 15 mg/m^2 per dose if needed	• Dose may be increased in 2.5 mg/m^2 increments
Doxycycline	2–4 mg/kg/d p.o./i.v. div q12–24 h; max: 200 mg/d	
Efavirenz (Sustiva)	• 10–15 kg: 200 mg p.o. q.d. • 15–20 kg: 250 mg p.o. q.d. • 20–25 kg: 300 mg p.o. q.d. • 25–32.5 kg: 350 mg p.o. q.d. • 32.5–40 kg: 400 mg p.o. q.d. • 40 kg: 600 mg p.o. q.d. Max: 600 mg/d	• Take at bedtime to improve tolerability of CNS side effects
Emtricitabine and tenofovir (Truvada)	Postexposure prophylaxis: • 17–22 kg: 100/150 tablet p.o. q.d. • 22–28 kg: 133/200 tablet p.o. q.d. • 28–35 kg: 167/250 tablet p.o. q.d. • >35 kg: 200/300 tablet p.o. q.d.	• Adjust dose in renal impairment

TABLE A2.1 Pediatric Drug Formulary (*continued*)

Medication	*Dosage*	*Comments*
Enalapril (Vasotec)	Initial: 0.1 mg/kg/d p.o. div q.d.–b.i.d., titrate up to max 0.5 mg/kg/d Usual adult: 10–40 mg/d p.o. div q.d.–b.i.d. Max: 40 mg/d	• Adjust dose in renal dysfunction
Enoxaparin (Lovenox)	DVT treatment: • PMA < 37 wk and <2 mo = 2 mg/kg/dose s.c. q12 h • PMA ≥ 37 wk and <2 mo = 1.7 mg/kg/dose s.c. q12 h • ≥2 mo = 1 mg/kg/dose s.c. q12 h DVT prophylaxis: • PMA < 37 wk and <2 mo = 1 mg/kg/dose s.c. q12 h • PMA ≥ 37 wk and <2 mo = 0.85 mg/kg/dose s.c. q12 h • ≥2 mo and < 60 kg = 0.5 mg/kg/dose s.c. q12 h • ≤13 y and > 60 kg = 30 mg s.c. q12 h • ≥14 y and 60–90 kg = 40 mg s.c. once a day • ≥14 y and obese >90 kg = 40 mg s.c. q12 h	• For treatment, check LMWH level 4 h after dose • Goal, anti–factor Xa depends on risk level, general goal is 0.5–1 unit/mL standard risk, 0.4–0.6 unit/mL high risk
Epinephrine	Intramuscular (1 mg/mL): 0.01 mL/kg/dose (0.01 mg/kg) i.m.; 10–25 kg: 0.15 mg, >30 kg: 0.3 mg; max: 0.5 mL/dose Intravenous (0.1 mg/mL): 0.1 mL/kg/dose (0.01 mg/kg) i.v./i.o. q3–5 min Continuous infusion: 0.05–2 µg/kg/min i.v. ETT (1 mg/mL): 0.1 mL/kg/dose (0.1 mg/kg) ETT q3 min	• Dilute ETT dose in 3–5 mL of NS and follow with several positive-pressure breaths • Central line preferred for continuous infusion
Erythromycin	15–50 mg/kg/d i.v. div q6 h; max: 4 g/d 30–50 mg/kg/d p.o. div q6 h; max: 3.2 g/d Prokinetic: • Children: initial 3 mg/kg/dose i.v. infused over 60 min followed by 20 mg/kg/d p.o. in 3–4 div doses before meals, or before meals and at bedtime • Adults: initial 200 mg i.v. followed by 250 mg p.o. t.i.d. 30 min before meals	
Erythropoietin alfa (Epogen)	Anemia of prematurity: 25–100 units/kg/dose i.v./s.c. 3 times/wk or 100 units/kg/dose i.v./s.c. 5 times/wk or 200 units/kg/dose q.o.d. for 10 doses Anemia in cancer patients: 150 units/kg/dose i.v./s.c. 3 times/wk; max: 1,200 units/kg/wk Anemia in chronic renal failure: 50–150 units/kg/dose i.v./s.c. 3 times/wk	
Esmolol (Brevibloc)	500 µg/kg i.v. × 1 over 1 min; then continuous infusion 50 µg/kg/min i.v. If no response in 4 min, repeat 500 µg/kg i.v. × 1 over 1 min, then continuous infusion 100 µg/kg/min i.v. Max: 200 µg/kg/min	• Some cardiology centers use lower initial dosing (50 µg/kg/dose × 1)
Ethambutol (Myambutol)	Tuberculosis: 15–25 mg/kg/d p.o. once daily OR 50 mg/kg/dose p.o. twice weekly, not to exceed 2.5 g/dose Nontuberculous mycobacterial infection: 15 mg/kg/d p.o. q.d., not to exceed 1 g/d	
Ethosuximide (Zarontin)	<6 y: initial 15 mg/kg/dose p.o. div b.i.d., max: 250 mg/dose; titrate q4–7 d; usual maintenance 15–40 mg/kg/d, max: 1.5 g/d >6 y: initial 250 mg/dose p.o. b.i.d., increase by 250 mg per dose q4–7 d, up to 1.5 g/d	• Give with food • Goal: trough 40–100 µg/mL
Etomidate (Amidate)	RSI: 0.3 mg/kg/dose i.v. × 1 dose	• One dose only; not for continuous infusion
Fentanyl (Sublimaze)	1–2 µg/kg/dose i.v. q1 h p.r.n. Acute pain: 1–2 µg/kg intranasal (max 100 µg); give ½ to each nare, no more than 1 mL per nare Procedural sedation: 1–2 µg/kg/dose i.v. × 1 (max: 100 µg/dose); repeat dose 1 µg/kg/dose (max: 50 µg/dose) q3 min p.r.n. sedation; total max 5 µg/kg	• Usual adult 100 µg/dose • Adjust dose in renal dysfunction

(*continued*)

TABLE A2.1 Pediatric Drug Formulary (*continued*)

Medication	*Dosage*	*Comments*
Ferrous sulfate	Severe iron-deficiency anemia: 4–6 mg elemental iron/kg/day p.o. in 3 div doses Mild-to-moderate iron-deficiency anemia: 3 mg elemental iron/kg/d p.o. in 1–2 div doses Prophylaxis: 1–2 mg elemental iron/kg/d p.o.	• Dose expressed in terms of elemental iron
Filgrastim (Neupogen)	Neonates: 5–10 µg/kg/d s.c./i.v. once daily for 3–5 d has been administered to neutropenic neonates with sepsis Children and adults: 5–10 µg/kg/d s.c./i.v. (~150–300 µg/m^2/d) once daily for up to 14 d until ANC = 10,000/mm^3 Cancer patients receiving bone marrow transplant: 5–10 µg/kg/d s.c./i.v. administered ≥24 h after cytotoxic chemotherapy and ≥24 h after bone marrow infusion	• Dose escalations of 5 µg/kg/d may be required in some individuals when response at 5 µg/kg/d is not adequate • If administering i.v., add albumin 2 mg/mL to D5W prior to adding filgrastim
Fluconazole (Diflucan)	Load: 6–12 mg/kg i.v./p.o. × 1 dose Maintenance: 3–12 mg/kg/dose i.v./p.o. q.d. Max: 800 mg/d	
Flucytosine (Ancobon)	100–150 mg/kg/d p.o. div q6 h	• Monitor levels: pre >25 µg/mL; post 40–60 µg/mL
Flumazenil (Romazicon)	Benzodiazepine reversal: 0.01 mg/kg/dose i.v., max: 0.2 mg/dose; may repeat p.r.n. to 0.05 mg/kg or 1 mg total, whichever is less	• Do not use in patients on chronic benzodiazepines for seizure disorders
Fluoxetine (Prozac)	Children 5–18 y: initial doses of 5–10 mg/d (or 10 mg given 3 times a week) may result in fewer adverse effects; dose is titrated upward p.r.n.; usual dose 20 mg/d	• Some studies have reported 20–40 mg/d in older children with OCD and Tourette syndrome • Use caution in children, increased risk of suicidal ideation
Fluticasone (Flovent, Flonase)	Asthma: Inhalation: • Children ≥4–11 y: dosing based on previous therapy: Flovent, Diskus, and Rotadisk; bronchodilator alone: recommended starting dose 50 µg b.i.d.; highest recommended dose 100 µg b.i.d. INH corticosteroids: recommended starting dose 50 µg b.i.d.; highest recommended dose: 100 µg b.i.d.; a higher starting dose may be considered in patients previously requiring higher doses of INH corticosteroids • Children 11 y: dosing based on previous therapy: Flovent, Diskus, and Rotadisk; bronchodilator alone: recommended starting dose 100 µg b.i.d.; highest recommended dose 500 µg b.i.d. INH corticosteroids: recommended starting dose 100–250 µg b.i.d.; highest recommended dose 500 µg b.i.d.; a higher starting dose may be considered in patients previously requiring higher doses of INH corticosteroids Flovent MDI: dosing based on previous therapy Bronchodilator alone: recommended starting dose 88 µg b.i.d.; highest recommended dose: 440 µg b.i.d. INH corticosteroids: recommended starting dose 88–220 µg b.i.d.; highest recommended dose 440 µg b.i.d.; a higher starting dose may be considered in patients previously requiring higher doses of INH corticosteroids Oral corticosteroids: recommended starting dose 880 µg b.i.d.; highest recommended dose 880 µg b.i.d.; starting dose is patient dependent; in patients on chronic oral corticosteroid therapy, reduce prednisone dose no faster than 2.5 mg/d on a weekly basis; begin taper after ≥1 wk of fluticasone therapy Rhinitis: intranasal, children ≥4 y and adolescents: initial 1 spray (50 µg/spray) per nostril once daily; patients not adequately responding or patients with more severe symptoms may use 2 sprays (100 µg) per nostril; depending on response, dosage may be reduced to 100 µg q.d.; total daily dose should not exceed 2 sprays in each nostril (200 µg/d); dosing should be at regular intervals	• Titrate to the lowest effective dose once asthma stability is achieved; children previously maintained on Flovent Rotadisk may require dosage adjustments when transferred to Flovent Diskus

TABLE A2.1 Pediatric Drug Formulary (*continued*)

Medication	*Dosage*	*Comments*
Fluticasone/salmeterol (Advair)	Children ≥12 and adults: oral inhalation, one inhalation b.i.d., morning and evening, 12 h apart Max dose: fluticasone 500 µg/salmeterol 50 µg, one inhalation b.i.d. See package insert for detailed information on transitioning patients from fluticasone or budesonide	• Dosing for <12 y not approved, although single inhaler products of fluticasone and salmeterol have been used • Advair Diskus is available in three strengths, initial dose prescribed should be based on previous asthma therapy • Dose should be increased after 2 wk if adequate response is not achieved
Folic acid	Deficiency: • Infants: 15 µg/kg/dose i.v./i.m./s.c./p.o. q.d., max: 50 µg/d • 1–10 y: 1 mg/d i.v./i.m./s.c./p.o. initial, then 0.1–0.4 mg/d • >11 y: 1 mg/d i.v./i.m./s.c./p.o. initial, then 0.5 mg/d	• Normal total folate 5–15 ng/mL
Fomepizole (Antizol)	Methanol, ethylene glycol, propylene glycol toxicity: 15 mg/kg i.v. loading dose × 1, then 10 mg/kg/dose i.v. q12 h; at 48 h, increase dose to 15 mg/kg/dose i.v. q12 h; if on hemodialysis, interval should be changed to q6 h	• Also referred to as 4-MP
Fosphenytoin (Cerebyx)	20 mg PE/kg i.v. load; in status epilepticus run at 3 mg PE/kg/min, max: 150 mg PE/min; then 5–8 mg PE/kg/d i.v./i.m. div q12 h	• PE = phenytoin equivalents • Hypotension may occur during bolus infusion, slow rate • Trough level: total = 10–20 µg/mL, free = 0.4–1.4 µg/mL
Furosemide (Lasix)	1 mg/kg/dose i.v./p.o. q6 h Continuous infusion 0.05–0.1 mg/kg/h	• Suggested max: 6 mg/kg/d
Gabapentin (Neurontin)	Initial dose 5 mg/kg/d p.o. q.d., usual dose 8–35 mg/kg/d p.o. div t.i.d., max dose up to 90 mg/kg/d (or 3,600 mg/d) has been reported Adult: initial dose 300 mg p.o. q.d., increase by 300 mg each day; usual dose 900–1,800 mg/d p.o. div t.i.d., max dose of 3,600 mg/d has been well tolerated	• Liquid must be refrigerated
Ganciclovir (Cytovene)	10 mg/kg/d i.v. div q12 h, then may switch to oral: • Children: maintenance dose, prophylaxis of CMV disease in solid-organ transplant patients: oral, 500 mg/m^2/dose p.o. q8 h OR 30 mg/kg/dose q8 h with food, max: 1,000 mg/dose • Adults: maintenance 1,000 mg p.o. t.i.d. or 500 mg p.o. 6 times/d q3 h during waking hours	• Follow chemotherapy precautions • Dose adjustment required in renal dysfunction
Gentamicin	• <35 wk GA: <30 d old: 3 mg/kg i.v. q24 h • ≥35 wk GA: <30 d old: 4 mg/kg i.v. q24 h • >1 mo–10 y: 7.5 mg/kg i.v. q24 h or div q8 h • >10 y: 6 mg/kg i.v. q24 h or div q8 h	• Check peak/trough with third dose • Exclusions from extended interval program include CrCl <60 mL/min/1.73 m^2; febrile neutropenia; CF; endocarditis; patients with rapid fluid shifts • Dose in obese patients based on adjusted body weight: AdjBW = 0.4 × (ABW − IBW) + IBW, where ABW is actual body weight, IBW is ideal body weight
Glucagon	Hypoglycemia <20 kg: 0.015–0.03 mg/kg i.m./s.c./i.v., max 0.5 mg ≥20 kg: 1 mg i.m./s.c./i.v.	• Use immediately after reconstitution
Glycopyrrolate (Robinul)	Secretory control: • Oral: 40–100 µg/kg/dose p.o. t.i.d.–q.i.d. • Intravenous: 4–10 µg/kg/dose i.v. t.i.d.–q.i.d.	• May use injectable product p.o.
Guanfacine	Older children: initial 0.5 mg p.o. q.h.s., increase as tolerated every 3–14 d, usual 1.5–3 mg/d p.o. div t.i.d.; max 4 mg/d	
Haloperidol (Haldol)	Behavioral emergency: 0.025–0.075 mg/kg/dose i.m. q6 h; followed by ½ initial dose q2 h p.r.n.; max: 10 mg/dose; i.v. use reserved for ICU Oral: 0.05–0.15 mg/kg/d p.o. div b.i.d. or t.i.d. Post-op refractory nausea and vomiting: >12 y and >40 kg: 0.02 mg/kg/dose (max 1 mg) i.v. × 1 dose	• Use caution with other antipsychotic agents • Can prolong QTc, obtain EKG when possible

(*continued*)

TABLE A2.1 Pediatric Drug Formulary (*continued*)

Medication	*Dosage*	*Comments*
Heparin	Therapeutic: 75 units/kg i.v. × 1, then continuous infusion as follows: • $<$1 y: 28 units/kg/h i.v. • ≥1 y: 20 units/kg/h i.v.	• Adjust based on heparin levels
Hydralazine (Apresoline)	0.1–0.5 mg/kg/dose i.v. q4–6 h p.r.n.	• Usual adult 20 mg/dose
Hydrocortisone (Solu-Cortef)	Emergent: 1–2 mg/kg i.v. × 1; max 100 mg/dose Stress dose: 50 mg/m^2 i.v. × 1, then 50 mg/m^2/d i.v. div q6–8 h Maintenance dose: 10–20 mg/m^2/d i.v./p.o. div q6–8 h	
Hydromorphone (Dilaudid)	Acute pain (moderate to severe): • Children ≥6 mo and $<$50 kg: • Oral: 0.03–0.08 mg/kg/dose p.o. q3–4 h p.r.n. • Intravenous: 0.015 mg/kg/dose i.v. q3–6 h p.r.n. • Children $>$50 kg and adults: opiate-naive, 1–2 mg p.o./s.c./i.v. q3–4 h p.r.n.; usual adult 2 mg, some adults may require 4 mg; patients with prior opiate exposure may require higher initial doses	• Use caution in opiate-naïve patients. Use lowest dose possible.
Hydroxocobalamin (Cyanokit)	70 mg/kg i.v. (max 5,000 mg) over 15 min; may repeat 35 mg/kg i.v. (max 2,500 mg) infused over 15–120 min if needed	• Requires dedicated i.v. line, incompatible with many medications
Hydroxyzine (Atarax, Vistaril)	Oral: 2 mg/kg/d p.o. div q6–8 h p.r.n. Intramuscular: 0.5–1 mg/kg/dose i.m. q4–6 h p.r.n.	• Has been used i.v. with caution
Hypertonic saline 3%	4 mL/kg i.v. over 20 min if seizing secondary to hyponatremia; continuous infusion 1–2 mL/kg/h i.v.	• Ensure gradual correction if nonacute hyponatremia
Ibuprofen (Motrin)	10 mg/kg/dose p.o. q6 h p.r.n.	• Usual adult 600–800 mg/dose
Imipenem/cilastatin (Primaxin)	• $<$3 mo: 100 mg/kg/d i.v. div q6 h • $>$3 mo: 60–100 mg/kg/d i.v. div q6 h Max: 4 g/d	
Infliximab (Remicade)	Crohn disease: moderately to severely active: 5 mg/kg i.v. as a single infusion over a minimum of 2 h Fistulizing: 5 mg/kg i.v. as an infusion over a minimum of 2 h; dose repeated at 2 and 6 wk after the initial infusion Rheumatoid arthritis (in combination with methotrexate therapy): 3 mg/kg i.v. followed by an additional 3 mg/kg at 2 and 6 wk after the first dose; then repeat q8 wk thereafter	• Dosing has ranged from 3 to 10 mg/kg i.v. infusion repeated at 4- or 8-wk intervals • Infusion reactions common, may need to premedicate
Indinavir (Crixivan)	350–500 mg/m^2/dose p.o. t.i.d.; alternatively, adults 800 mg p.o. b.i.d. plus ritonavir booster; max: 800 mg p.o. t.i.d.	• Administer on empty stomach • Adjust dose in hepatic dysfunction
Insulin (regular) (Humulin R)	Acute symptomatic hyperkalemia: 0.1 units/kg i.v./s.c. × 1; DKA: continuous infusion 0.1 units/kg/h i.v.	• Prime tubing 15 min prior to infusion to ensure adequate dosing • Do not use bolus dosing for DKA
Ipratropium (Atrovent)	Nebulization: • $<$10 kg: 0.25 mg INH q20 min × 3 doses with albuterol • $>$10 kg: 0.5 mg INH q20 min × 3 doses with albuterol MDI: • 3–12 y: 1–2 puffs t.i.d., max: 6 puffs/24 h • $>$12 y: 2 puffs q.i.d., max: 12 puffs/24 h	• No benefit seen in acute asthma with continuing treatment after initial ED doses
Isoniazid	10–20 mg/kg/d p.o. q.d.; max: 300 mg/d	• Consider prophylactic pyridoxine therapy
Ivacaftor (Kalydeco)	CF: ≥6 y: 150 mg p.o. q12 h	• Must have documentation of CFTR variant • Adjust doses for CYP3A4 inhibitors

TABLE A2.1 Pediatric Drug Formulary (*continued*)

Medication	*Dosage*	*Comments*
Ketamine (Ketalar)	Acute pain: 0.5 mg/kg intranasal, may repeat × 1 in 15 min Procedural sedation: 1–2 mg/kg/dose i.v. × 1 (max: 100 mg/dose), repeat dose 0.5 mg/kg/dose i.v. (max: 50 mg/dose) q2–5 min p.r.n. sedation, max: 5 mg/kg or 500 mg; OR 4–5 mg/kg/dose i.m. with atropine 0.02 mg/kg/dose (max: 0.5 mg) × 1, may repeat ketamine 2 mg/kg i.m. × 1 if inadequate sedation in 10 min RSI: 0.5–2 mg/kg/dose i.v.; OR 3–7 mg/kg/dose i.m. × 1	• Drug of choice for RSI in status asthmaticus • Laryngospasm and emergence reactions can occur
Ketorolac (Toradol)	• 8–12.5 kg: 4 mg i.v. q6 h × 24–72 h • 12.5–25 kg: 7.5 mg i.v. q6 h × 24–72 h • >25–50 kg: 15 mg i.v. q6 h × 24–72 h • >50 kg: 30 mg i.v. q6 h × 24–72 h	• Absolute max: 5 d of therapy
Labetalol (Normodyne, Trandate)	0.25–1 mg/kg/dose i.v. q4–6 h, max: 20 mg/dose Continuous infusion 0.25–1 mg/kg/h, max: 3 mg/kg/h	
Lacosamide (Vimpat)	≥3 y: 1 mg/kg/d p.o./i.v. div b.i.d. (max 50 mg/dose); increase weekly by 1 mg/kg/d to a max of 10 mg/kg/d (max 400 mg/d)	• Adjust dose for hepatic impairment
Lactulose	Constipation: • Children: 7.5–15 mL/d p.o. div q.d.–b.i.d. • Adults: 15–30 mL/d p.o. div q.d.–b.i.d. Max: 60 mL/d	
Lamivudine (Epivir)	4 mg/kg/dose p.o. b.i.d.; max: 150 mg b.i.d.	• Also referred to as 3TC • May be administered with food • Do not use with zidovudine • Adjust dose in renal dysfunction
Lamotrigine (Lamictal)	Not recommended for children <17 kg Regimens containing valproic acid: • Weeks 1 and 2: 0.15 mg/kg/d p.o. in 1–2 doses, round down to nearest 5 mg • Weeks 3 and 4: 0.3 mg/kg/d p.o. in 1–2 doses, round down to nearest 5 mg • After week 4, titrate to effect, increase q1–2 wk by 0.3 mg/kg/d, rounded down to nearest 5-mg dose; usual maintenance 1–5 mg/kg/d in 1–2 doses (max: 200 mg/d) Regimens containing enzyme-inducing AEDs without valproic acid: • Weeks 1 and 2: 0.6 mg/kg/d p.o. div b.i.d., rounded down to nearest 5 mg • Weeks 3 and 4: 1.2 mg/kg/d p.o. div b.i.d., rounded down to nearest 5 mg • After week 4, titrate to effect, increase q1–2 wk by 1.2 mg/kg/d, rounded down to nearest 5 mg; usual maintenance 5–15 mg/kg/d p.o. div b.i.d. (max: 400 mg/d) Dosage, adult and children >12 y: Regimens containing valproic acid • Weeks 1 and 2: 25 mg p.o. q.o.d. • Weeks 3 and 4: 25 mg p.o. q.d. • After week 4, titrate to effect, increase q1–2 wk by 25–50 mg/d; usual maintenance 100–400 mg/d p.o. div b.i.d.; usual dose 100–200 mg/d if on valproic acid ONLY Regimens containing enzyme-inducing AEDs without valproic acid: • Weeks 1 and 2: 50 mg p.o. q.d. • Weeks 3 and 4: 100 mg/d p.o. div b.i.d. • After week 4, titrate to effect, increase q1–2 wk by 100 mg/d; usual maintenance 300–500 mg/d p.o. div b.i.d.	• Titrate slowly • Educate patients to report appearance of rash immediately

(*continued*)

TABLE A2.1 Pediatric Drug Formulary (*continued*)

Medication	*Dosage*	*Comments*
Lansoprazole (Prevacid)	0.5–1.6 mg/kg p.o. q.d. GERD, erosive esophagitis: children 1–11 y: • ≤30 kg: 15 mg p.o. q.d. • >30 kg: 30 mg p.o. q.d. Duodenal ulcer: children ≥12 y and adults, 15 mg p.o. q.d. for 4 wk; maintenance therapy 15 mg p.o. q.d. Primary gastric ulcer (and also associated with NSAID use): children ≥12 y and adults, 30 mg p.o. q.d. for up to 8 wk Pathologic hypersecretory conditions: children ≥12 y and adults, initial 60 mg p.o. q.d.; adjust dose based on patient response; doses of 90 mg p.o. b.i.d. have been used; administer doses >120 mg/d in div doses Reflux esophagitis: children ≥12 y and adults, 30–60 mg p.o. q.d. for 8 wk *Helicobacter pylori*–associated antral gastritis: 30 mg p.o. b.i.d. for 2 wk (in combination with 1 g amoxicillin and 500 mg clarithromycin given b.i.d. for 14 d)	• Limited data in children
Levetiracetam (Keppra)	13–30 mg/kg/d p.o. div q.d.–b.i.d.; max: 4 g/d Loading dose: 30 mg/kg/dose i.v. × 1 over 15 min, 10–100 mg/kg/d	• Doses over 300 mg/kg/d have been used
Levonorgestrel (Plan B)	1.5 mg p.o. × 1	• Package includes both tablets and patient instructions
Levothyroxine (Levoxyl, Synthroid)	Oral: • 0–6 mo: 8–10 µg/kg or 25–50 µg p.o. q.d. • 6–12 mo: 6–8 µg/kg or 50–75 µg p.o. q.d. • 1–5 y: 5–6 µg/kg or 75–100 µg p.o. q.d. • 6–12 y: 4–5 µg/kg or 100–150 µg p.o. q.d. • >12 y: 2–3 µg/kg or ≥150 µg p.o. q.d. • Growth and puberty complete: 1.6 µg/kg p.o. q.d.	• Conversion to i.v. or i.m.: use 50%–75% of the oral dose
Lidocaine	1–2 mg/kg i.v./i.o. × 1; continuous infusion 20–50 µg/kg/min i.v./i.o. Prevention of ICP spikes during suctioning: 1 mg/kg via ETT × 1 prior to suctioning	• If giving via ETT, dose is 2–4 × i.v. dose • Dilute ETT dose in 3–5 mL of NS and follow with several positive-pressure breaths
Linezolid (Zyvox)	• <12 y: 30 mg/kg/d i.v./p.o. div q8 h (max: 1.8 g) • >12 y: 20 mg/kg/d i.v./p.o. div q12 h (max: 1.2 g)	• Acts as weak MAOi—watch for potential drug–drug and drug–food interactions
Lisinopril	≥6 y: 0.07 mg/kg p.o. once daily (max initial dose 5 mg); increase every 1–2 weeks; max 40 mg/d.	• Decrease dose by 50% if patient has hyponatremia, hypovolemia, severe CHF, decreased renal function or receiving diuretics
Lithium (Eskalith, Lithobid)	15–60 mg/kg/d p.o. div t.i.d.–q.i.d., max: 2.4 g/d If using sustained-release preparation, give total daily dose in 2 div doses	• Adjust dose in renal dysfunction • Avoid NSAIDs and thiazide diuretics
Loperamide (Imodium)	Acute diarrhea: Initial doses (in first 24 h): • 2–5 y: 1 mg t.i.d. • 6–8 y: 2 mg b.i.d. • 8–12 y: 2 mg t.i.d. After initial dosing, 0.1 mg/kg doses after each loose stool, but not exceeding initial dose Chronic diarrhea: 0.08–0.24 mg/kg/d div b.i.d.–t.i.d., max: 2 mg/dose Traveler's diarrhea: treat for no more than 2 d: • 6–8 y: 1 mg after first loose stool followed by 1 mg after each subsequent stool; max: 4 mg/d • 9–11 y: 2 mg after first loose stool followed by 1 mg after each subsequent stool; max: 6 mg/d • 12 y to adults: 4 mg after first loose stool followed by 2 mg after each subsequent stool; max: 8 mg/d	

TABLE A2.1 Pediatric Drug Formulary (*continued*)

Medication	*Dosage*	*Comments*
Lopinavir/ritonavir (Kaletra)	• 7–15 kg: 12 mg lopinavir/3 mg ritonavir/kg/dose p.o. b.i.d. • 15–40 kg: 10 mg lopinavir/2.5 mg ritonavir/kg/dose p.o. b.i.d. • >40 kg: 400 mg lopinavir/100 mg ritonavir p.o. b.i.d.	• Administer with food • Refrigerate capsules and oral solution
Loratadine (Claritin)	• 2–5 y: 5 mg p.o. q.d. • ≥6 y: 10 mg p.o. q.d.	
Lorazepam (Ativan)	0.05–0.1 mg/kg/dose i.v./p.o. q4–8 h p.r.n., max: 4 mg/dose Status epilepticus: 0.1 mg/kg/dose i.v./i.m. q5–15 min (max 4 mg/dose) × 2–3 doses	• Use caution in patients susceptible to propylene glycol toxicity
Lumacaftor and ivacaftor (Orkambi)	CF: ≥6–11 y: lumacaftor 100 mg/ivacaftor 125 mg, 2 tablets p.o. q12 h ≥12 y: lumacaftor 200 mg/ivacaftor 125 mg, 2 tablets p.o. q12 h	• Must have documentation of CFTR variant • Bronchospasm can occur after dose
Magnesium sulfate	Asthma: 40 mg/kg i.v. slow over 20 min Torsades de pointes: 25–50 mg/kg/dose i.v. slow Max: 2 g/dose	
Mannitol 20%	0.5–1 g/kg/dose i.v. over 20 min for increased ICP/cerebral edema, then 0.25–1 g/kg/dose i.v. q4–6 h p.r.n.	• Use filter during administration • Never give as continuous infusion
Megestrol (Megace)	Cachexia: 4–8 mg/kg/d p.o. in 2–4 div doses	
Meropenem (Merrem)	60–120 mg/kg/d i.v. div q8 h; max 6 g/d	• Usual course of therapy is 3–6 wk
Mercaptopurine	Dose based on indication, consult local protocols. Usual induction: 2.5–5 mg/kg/d p.o. once daily; usual maintenance: 1.5–2.5 mg/kg/d p.o. once daily	• Also referred to as 6-MP • TPMT/NUDT15 testing strongly recommended prior to initiation
Mesalamine (Asacol)	Capsules 50 mg/kg/d p.o. div q6–12 h; tablets 50 mg/kg/d p.o. div q8–12 h	• Oral products are formulated to slowly release therapeutic quantities of drug throughout the GI tract
Methadone	0.025–0.1 mg/kg/dose p.o./i.v. q4–12 h p.r.n.	• Increase dosing interval after 2–3 doses to prevent accumulation
Methylphenidate (Ritalin, Ritalin XR, Metadate, Concerta)	≥6 y: 0.3 mg/kg/dose p.o. before breakfast and lunch, max: 5 mg/dose, increase by 0.1 mg/kg/dose every week p.r.n.; usual dose: 0.3–1 mg/kg/d, max: 2 mg/kg/d or 60 mg/d, whichever is less	• Some patients may require t.i.d. dosing • If using sustained-release products, titrate with regular product and convert based on 8-h increments
Methylprednisolone (Solu-Medrol)	Asthma, anti-inflammatory: 2 mg/kg × 1 dose load (max 125 mg), then 1 mg/kg/dose i.v. q6–12 h Pulse therapy: 30 mg/kg/d i.v. for 1–5 d, max 1.5 g/d	• Administer doses >1 g over at least 1 h
Metoclopramide (Reglan)	0.1–0.2 mg/kg/dose i.v./p.o. q6 h p.r.n., max: 10 mg/dose High-dose regimen: 1 mg/kg/dose (max: 50 mg/dose) i.v./p.o. q6 h p.r.n. nausea with acetaminophen overdose or chemotherapy	• If using high-dose regimen, consider adding diphenhydramine
Metolazone (Zaroxolyn)	0.2–0.4 mg/kg/d p.o. div q12–24 h	
Metronidazole (Flagyl)	30 mg/kg/d i.v./p.o. div q6 h, max: 4 g/d Postsexual assault: 2 g p.o. × 1 dose	• Counsel patients to avoid alcohol
Midazolam (Versed)	0.05–0.1 mg/kg/dose i.v./i.m. q1–2 h p.r.n., max: 10 mg/dose Continuous infusion 0.05–0.1 mg/kg/h i.v. Procedural sedation: • Intravenous: 0.05–0.1 mg/kg/dose i.v. × 1 (max: 2 mg/dose), may repeat q3 min at 0.05 mg/kg (total max: 0.3 mg/kg or 10 mg, whichever is less) • Oral: 0.25–0.75 mg/kg/dose p.o., max: 12 mg/dose • Intranasal: 0.2 mg/kg/dose (max 10 mg) for seizure; 0.5 mg/kg/dose (max 10 mg) for sedation	• Use preservative free for continuous infusions in neonates
Milrinone (Primacor)	50 µg/kg i.v. × 1, then 0.25–1 µg/kg/min i.v.	
Minocycline (Minocin)	4 mg/kg p.o./i.v. followed by 2 mg/kg/dose p.o./i.v. q12 h	

(*continued*)

TABLE A2.1 Pediatric Drug Formulary (*continued*)

Medication	*Dosage*	*Comments*
Montelukast (Singulair)	• 2–5 y: 4 mg/d • 6–14 y: 5 mg/d • >14 y: 10 mg/d	
Morphine	• <6 mo: 0.05 mg/kg/dose i.v./s.c. q2–4 h p.r.n. • >6 mo: 0.05–0.1 mg/kg/dose i.v./s.c. q2 h p.r.n. Continuous infusion: 0.05–0.1 mg/kg/h i.v. Oral dosing: 0.1–0.2 mg/kg/dose p.o. (usual max 15 mg IR/dose) q4 h p.r.n.	• Usual adult 10 mg/dose i.v.
Nalbuphine (Nubain)	Opiate-induced pruritus: 10–20 μg/kg/dose i.v. q3–6 h p.r.n. Pain: 0.1–0.15 mg/kg/dose i.v. q3–6 h p.r.n.	
Nalmefene (Revex)	Opioid reversal: 0.25 μg/kg/dose i.v. q2 min (max: 40 μg/dose) to a max of 1 μg/kg	• Total max dose: 0.5 mg
Naloxone (Narcan)	Opioid reversal: • Full reversal: 0.1 mg/kg/dose intranasal/i.v./i.m./ETT • Graded reversal: 1–10 μg/kg/dose intranasal/i.v./i.m. Max: 2 mg/dose • Continuous infusion for pruritus: 0.25 μg/kg/h (max 1 μg/kg/h) • Continuous infusion for opioid overdose: 2.5–160 μg/kg/h, titrate to avoid rebound, taper when discontinuing	If giving via ETT, dose is 2–10 × i.v. dose • Dilute ETT dose in 3–5 mL of NS and follow with several positive-pressure breaths • Note that higher doses must be used in buprenorphine overdoses
Neostigmine (Prostigmin)	Nondepolarizing paralytic reversal: 0.07 mg/kg i.v. × 1; max: 5 mg total	• Premed first with glycopyrrolate 5–15 μg/kg/dose i.v.
Nifedipine (Procardia)	0.25–0.5 mg/kg/dose p.o. q6 h; max: 10 mg/dose	• Must withdraw liquid from capsule for doses <10 mg, use "Easter egg" method by poking holes in both ends prior to withdrawing
Nitazoxanide	Diarrhea: • 12–47 mo: 100 mg p.o. q12 h for 3 d • 4–11 y: 200 mg p.o. q12 h for 3 d	
Nitrofurantoin (Macrodantin)	5–7 mg/kg/d p.o. div q6 h; max: 400 mg/d UTI prophylaxis: 1–2 mg/kg/d p.o. q.d., max: 100 mg/d	• Note the b.i.d. formulation should be ordered as the combination of macrocrystals and monohydrate
Nitroglycerin	0.5–5 μg/kg/min i.v.	
Nitroprusside	0.5–10 μg/kg/min i.v.	• Check cyanide and thiocyanate levels, especially if dose >4 μg/kg/min or if used for >3 d
Norepinephrine (Levophed)	0.05–1 μg/kg/min i.v.	• Central line preferred
Nortriptyline (Pamelor)	Depression: 1–3 mg/kg/d p.o. div t.i.d.–q.i.d., max: 150 mg/d Nocturnal enuresis: • 20–25 kg: 10 mg p.o. q.h.s. • 25–35 kg: 10–20 mg p.o. q.h.s. • 35–54 kg: 25–35 mg p.o. q.h.s.	• Give 30 min prior to bedtime for nocturnal enuresis • Adjust dose in hepatic insufficiency
Octreotide (Sandostatin)	Bolus: 1–2 μg/kg i.v./s.c., max: 50 μg/dose Continuous infusion: 1–2 μg/kg/h i.v., max: 50 μg/h	
Omeprazole (Prilosec)	1 mg/kg p.o. q.d., may increase to b.i.d.; usual adult 20 mg/d; max: 3.3 mg/kg/d	
Ondansetron (Zofran)	Nononcology nausea and vomiting: • <5 kg: 0.5 mg i.v./p.o. q8 h p.r.n. • 5–30 kg: 1 mg i.v./p.o. q8 h p.r.n. • ≥30 kg: 2 mg i.v./p.o. q8 h p.r.n. Chemotherapy-associated nausea and vomiting: 0.45 mg/kg/d i.v./p.o. q24 h or div q8 h	

TABLE A2.1 Pediatric Drug Formulary (*continued*)

Medication	*Dosage*	*Comments*
Oseltamivir (Tamiflu)	Treatment: • <15 kg: 30 mg p.o. b.i.d. • 15–23 kg: 45 mg p.o. b.i.d. • >23–40 kg: 60 mg p.o. b.i.d. • >40 kg: 75 mg p.o. b.i.d. Prophylaxis • <15 kg: 30 mg p.o. q.d. • 15–23 kg: 45 mg p.o. q.d. • >23–40 kg: 60 mg p.o. q.d. • >40 kg: 75 mg p.o. q.d.	
Oxacillin	150–200 mg/kg/d i.v. div q4–6 h; max: 12 g/d	• Adjust dose in renal dysfunction
Oxcarbazepine (Trileptal)	20–75 mg/kg/d p.o. div b.i.d.–q.i.d.; max: 5.4 g/d	
Oxybutynin (Ditropan)	0.1–0.2 mg/kg/dose p.o. q6–12 h; max: 5 mg/dose	
Oxycodone	Immediate release 0.05–0.15 mg/kg/dose p.o. q4–6 h p.r.n.; usual max: 10 mg/dose	• If using sustained-release OxyContin, divide total daily dose b.i.d.–t.i.d.
Palivizumab (Synagis)	15 mg/kg/dose i.m. every month during RSV season in high-risk patients	
Pamidronate (Aredia)	0.5–1 mg/kg i.v. q.d. for 3 d, may repeat in 4–6 mo intervals	
Pancuronium (Pavulon)	0.1 mg/kg/dose i.v. q1–2 h p.r.n.; continuous infusion: 0.1 mg/kg/h i.v.	
Pantoprazole (Protonix)	0.5–1 mg/kg/d i.v./p.o. div q.d.–b.i.d.; adult 40 mg i.v. q.d.	• Use within 2 h of reconstitution
Penicillin G (aqueous)	100,000–400,000 unit/kg/d i.v. div q4–6 h; max: 24 mU/d	
Penicillin G Benzathine	50,000 unit/kg i.m. × 1; max: 1.2 mU/dose	• i.m. ONLY
Penicillin VK	25–50 mg/kg/d p.o. div q6–8 h; max: 2 g/d	
Pentamidine (Pentam 300)	Treatment of PCP: 4 mg/kg/d i.v./i.m. (i.v. preferred) once daily for 14–21 d Prophylaxis for PCP: load 4 mg/kg/dose i.v. q.d. for 3 d then 4 mg/kg/dose i.v./i.m. q2–4 wk OR Inhalation every month via nebulizer: • Infants <1 y: 2.27 mg/kg × nebulizer output (L/min) × weight (kg) divided by alveolar ventilation (L/min) • Children <5 y: some institutions have used a dose of 8 mg/kg INH every month • Children ≥5 y: 300 mg/dose INH every month Treatment of trypanosomiasis: 4 mg/kg/d i.m. once daily for 10 d Treatment of visceral leishmaniasis: 2–4 mg/kg/d i.m. once daily or q2 d for up to 15 doses	• Aerosolized pentamidine is administered at doses adjusted for minimum ventilation and weight
Pentobarbital (Nembutal)	Procedural sedation: • Intravenous: 1–2 mg/kg/dose (max: 100 mg/dose) i.v. q5 min until asleep (total max: 6 mg/kg or 300 mg, whichever is less) • Oral: 2–6 mg/kg/dose p.o. × 1 Refractory status epilepticus 1 mg/kg/h i.v., max 8 mg/kg/h; most patients will require vasopressor support	
Phenazopyridine (Pyridium)	12 mg/kg/d p.o. div t.i.d. for 2 d; max: 200 mg/dose	
Phenobarbital	20 mg/kg i.v. load, then 5 mg/kg/d i.v./p.o. div q12–24 h	• Trough level 15–40 µg/mL
Phentolamine (Regitine)	Treatment of pressor extravasation: dilute 2.5–5 mg phentolamine in 5–10 mL NS, infiltrate area with ~1 mL within 12 h of extravasation, max: 0.1 mg/kg or 2.5 mg, whichever is less Diagnosis of pheochromocytoma: 0.05–0.1 mg/kg/dose i.v. × 1 dose, max: 5 mg/dose	

(*continued*)

TABLE A2.1 Pediatric Drug Formulary (*continued*)

Medication	*Dosage*	*Comments*
Phenylephrine (Neo-Synephrine)	0.1–0.5 μg/kg/min i.v.	• Central line preferred
Phenytoin (Dilantin)	5–8 mg/kg/d p.o. div q.d.–t.i.d.	• Dose individualized based on levels
Phytonadione (vitamin K_1)	1–5 mg/dose s.c. q24 h × 3 d 2.5–5 mg/dose p.o. q24 h; may also be given 3 times/wk	• Must be given SLOWLY if using i.v. route
Piperacillin/tazobactam (Zosyn)	200–300 mg/kg/d i.v. div q6 h CF: 300–500 mg/kg/d i.v. div q6 h Max: 18 g as piperacillin/d	• Dosed as piperacillin
Potassium chloride	Intravenous: 0.25–1 mEq/kg/dose i.v. over at least 1 h Oral: 2–5 mEq/kg/d p.o. div b.i.d.–q.i.d.	• Potassium level within previous hour • PIV max: 80 mEq/L • CVL max: 200 mEq/L • Patient must be placed on CV monitor if >0.25 mEq/kg/h • Patient must be in ICU if >0.5 mEq/kg/h • Dilute oral solution prior to administration
Prednisone/prednisolone (Deltasone, Prelone, Orapred)	Asthma: 2 mg/kg p.o. × 1, then 2 mg/kg/d p.o. div q12 h Anti-inflammatory: 0.5–2 mg/kg/d div q.d.–q.i.d. Max: 80 mg/dose	
Primidone (Mysoline)	10–25 mg/kg/d p.o. div b.i.d.–q.i.d.; max: 2 g/d	• Therapeutic range 5–12 μg/mL
Procainamide (Procan)	• <1 y: load 3–7 mg/kg i.v. over 30 min; then 20–80 μg/kg/min • >1 y: load 5–15 mg/kg i.v. over 30 min; then 20–80 μg/kg/min	• Final concentration for maintenance infusion 2–8 mg/mL
Prochlorperazine (Compazine)	0.4 mg/kg/d p.o./p.r. div q6 h p.r.n., 0.13 mg/kg/dose i.m. q6 h p.r.n.; max: 10 mg/dose	• Use i.v. with caution
Propranolol (Inderal)	Hypertension/arrhythmias: Oral: • Neonates: 0.25 mg/kg/dose p.o. q6–8 h • Children: initial: 0.5–1 mg/kg/d p.o. div q6–8 h; maintenance 1–5 mg/kg/d p.o. div q6–8 h Intravenous: • Neonates: 0.01 mg/kg/dose i.v. q6–8 h p.r.n. (max: 1 mg/dose) • Children: 0.01–0.1 mg/kg/dose i.v. q6–8 h p.r.n. (max: 3 mg/dose) Migraine headache prophylaxis: 0.6–1.5 mg/kg/d p.o. div q8 h, max: 4 mg/kg/d	
Protein Complex Concentrate (KCentra)	Vitamin K antagonist reversal: • INR 2 to <4: 25 units/kg (max 2,500 units) • INR 4–6: 35 units/kg (max 3,500 units) • INR >6: 50 units/kg (max 5,000 units) Factor Xa inhibitor induced bleeding: • 25–50 units/kg (max 5,000 units)	• Do not infuse with other medications
Pseudoephedrine (Sudafed)	• <2 y: 1 mg/kg/dose p.o. q6 h p.r.n. • 2–5 y: 15 mg p.o. q6 h p.r.n. • 6–12 y: 30 mg p.o. q6 h p.r.n. • >12 y: 60 mg p.o. q6 h p.r.n.	
Pyrazinamide	20–30 mg/kg/d p.o. q.d.; max: 2 g/d	
Racemic epinephrine (Vaponefrin)	2.25% inhalation solution: 0.25 mL (<5 kg), 0.5 mL (>5 kg) INH q1 h p.r.n.	• May use epinephrine injection equivalent dose: racemic epinephrine 10 mg = L-epinephrine 5 mg
Ranitidine (Zantac)	3 mg/kg/d i.v. div q8 h, max 180 mg/d; 4–6 mg/kg/d p.o. div q12 h, max 300 mg/d; continuous infusion 0.15 mg/kg/h i.v.	
Rasburicase (Elitek)	0.15–0.2 mg/kg/dose i.v. once daily for up to 5 d	• Contraindicated in G6PD

TABLE A2.1 Pediatric Drug Formulary (*continued*)

Medication	*Dosage*	*Comments*
Rifabutin (Mycobutin)	*Mycobacterium avium* complex (MAC): 5–6 mg/kg/d p.o. q.d. (max: 75 mg/d) Prophylaxis for first episode of MAC in human immunodeficiency virus (HIV)–infected patients: • Children <6 y: 5 mg/kg once daily • Children ≥6 y: 300 mg once daily Prophylaxis for recurrence of MAC in HIV-infected patients: 5 mg/kg p.o. once daily (max: 300 mg/d) in combination with clarithromycin	• Limited studies in children • In patients who experience GI upset, rifabutin can be administered 150 mg b.i.d. with food
Rifampin (Rifadin)	10–20 mg/kg/d p.o. div q.d.–b.i.d.; max: 1.2 g/d	
Risperidone (Risperdal)	Pervasive developmental disorder (unlabeled use): initial 0.25 mg b.i.d.; titrate up to 0.25 mg/d q5–7 d; optimal dose range 0.75–3 mg/d Autism (unlabeled use): initial 0.25 mg q.h.s.; titrate to 1 mg/d (0.1 mg/kg/d) Schizophrenia: initial 0.5 mg b.i.d.; titrate as necessary up to 2–6 mg/d Bipolar disorder (unlabeled use): initial 0.5 mg; titrate to 0.5–3 mg/d Tourette disorder (unlabeled use): initial 0.5 mg; titrate to 2–4 mg/d	
Ritonavir (Norvir)	350–450 mg/m^2/dose p.o. b.i.d.; booster dose 100–200 mg/m^2/dose p.o. b.i.d.; max: 600 mg/dose b.i.d.	• Administer with food • Oral solution may be mixed with milk, pudding, or formula
Rocuronium (Zemuron)	RSI: 0.6–1.2 mg/kg/dose i.v./i.m. × 1 dose	• Use higher end of dosing range if giving i.m.
Rufinamide (Banzel)	10 mg/kg/d p.o. div b.i.d; increase by 10 mg/kg increments q.o.d. to a tare of 45 mg/kg/d p.o. div b.i.d. Max 3,200 mg/d.	• Decrease dose with valproic acid
Sertraline (Zoloft)	• 6–12 y: initial 25 mg/d p.o. q.d., titrate at weekly intervals until effect, max: 200 mg/d • >12 y: initial 50 mg/d p.o. q.d., titrate at weekly intervals until effect, max: 200 mg/d	• Use caution in children, increased risk of suicidal ideation
Sirolimus	• ≥13 y, <40 kg: loading dose 3 mg/m^2 (day 1), followed by a maintenance of 1 mg/m^2/d • Adults ≥40 kg: loading dose: for de novo transplant recipients, a loading dose of 3 times the daily maintenance dose should be administered on day 1 of dosing; maintenance dose 2 mg/d; doses should be taken 4 h after cyclosporine and should be taken consistently either with or without food	• Adjust dose in hepatic impairment
Sodium bicarbonate	• 1 mEq/kg = 1 mL/kg i.v./i.o. slow • Tumor lysis syndrome: D5W with 75 mEq/L sodium bicarbonate at 125 mL/m^2/h to maintain urine pH 7–8 and SG ≤ 1.010 Overdose: 100 mEq in 1,000 mL D5W, 1 mEq/kg/h i.v.; titrate	• Use 0.5 mEq/mL concentration for neonates
Sodium chloride	Maintenance: • Premature neonates: 2–8 mEq/kg/d p.o./i.v. div q.d.–t.i.d. • Term neonates: 1–4 mEq/kg/d p.o./i.v. div q.d.–t.i.d. • Children: 3–4 mEq/kg/d p.o./i.v. div q.d.–t.i.d. Severe hyponatremia: see hypertonic saline	
Sodium polystyrene (Kayexalate)	1 g/kg/dose (max: 15 g/dose) p.o. q6 h OR 1 g/kg/dose (max: 50 g/dose) p.r. q2–6 h	Avoid sorbitol-containing preparations for the p.r. route
Spironolactone (Aldactone)	1–3 mg/kg/d p.o. div q12–24 h	
Succinylcholine (Quelicin)	RSI: 1–2 mg/kg/dose i.v. × 1 dose; 3–4 mg/kg/dose i.m. × 1 dose; max: 150 mg/dose	• Premed with atropine <7 y • Use 2 mg/kg/dose i.v. if <1 y • Contraindicated in hyperkalemia, myopathies, trauma > 24 h

(*continued*)

TABLE A2.1 Pediatric Drug Formulary (*continued*)

Medication	*Dosage*	*Comments*
Sucralfate (Carafate)	40–80 mg/kg/d p.o. div q6 h; max: 1 g/dose	• Multiple drug–drug interactions
Sugammadex (Bridion)	Immediate reversal of rocuronium or vecuronium: 16 mg/kg i.v. as soon as possible	• Not for reversal of other paralytic agents
Sulfamethoxazole/trimethoprim (Bactrim)	8–20 mg TMP/kg/d i.v./p.o. div q6–12 h Treatment of PCP: 20 mg TMP/kg/day i.v. div q6 h	• Dose based on TMP component
Tacrolimus (Prograf, Protopic)	Oral: 0.15–0.3 mg/kg/d p.o. div q12 h Intravenous: 0.05–0.15 mg/kg/d i.v. continuous infusion Topical: 0.03% ointment applied b.i.d.	• Oral dose conversion is 4–5 times the i.v. dose • Titrate to levels of 5–10 ng/mL in stem cell transplant • Children require higher doses than adults
Terbutaline (Brethine)	10 μg/kg i.v./s.c. × 1, then 0.4–6 μg/kg/min i.v.	• Suggested max total β_2-agonist dose = 20 mg/h
Tetracycline	>8 y: 25–50 mg/kg/d p.o. div q6 h; max: 3 g/d	• For patients >8-y-old
Thiamine (vitamin B_1)	Neonatal seizures: 100 mg i.v. × 1 dose Mitochondrial defect: 100–200 mg p.o. q.d.	
Tiagabine (Gabitril)	Initial dose 0.1 mg/kg/d p.o. (max: 4 mg/dose) q.d. for 1 wk; then increase by 0.1 mg/kg/d (max: 4 mg) for wk 2, then by 0.1–0.2 mg/kg/d (max 8 mg) weekly thereafter; titrate to effect Usual dose is 0.3–1.25 mg/kg/d p.o. div t.i.d.; max dose: 32 mg/d Adult: initial dose 4 mg/d p.o. q.d. for 1 wk; then increase by 4–8 mg/d each week div b.i.d.–q.i.d., titrate to response; max dose: 56 mg/d	• t.i.d. dosing may be better tolerated
Tobramycin (Nebcin)	See gentamicin TOBI nebs: 300 mg INH b.i.d. CF: 10–12 mg/kg/d i.v. div q8–12 h	• CF patients require higher dosing • Individualize dose based on levels and *MIC* of organism
Topiramate (Topamax)	Initial dose 0.5–1 mg/kg/d p.o. div b.i.d. for 1 wk; then increase by 0.5–1 mg/kg/d each week; titrate to effect Adult: initial dose 50 mg/d p.o. q.d. for 1 wk; then 100 mg/d p.o. div b.i.d. for 1 wk, increase by 50 mg/d each week, titrate to response Usual dose 200 mg p.o. b.i.d.; max dose: 1,600 mg/d	• Usual minimally effective dose is 6 mg/kg/d div b.i.d.; doses as high as 50 mg/kg/d have been used in children receiving other enzyme-inducing AEDs
Ursodiol (Actigall)	Biliary atresia: 10–15 mg/kg/d p.o. q.d. TPN-induced cholestasis: 30 mg/kg/d p.o. div t.i.d. CF: 30 mg/kg/d p.o. div q.d.–t.i.d. Max: 300 mg/dose	• Use oral suspension formulation without sorbitol to avoid diarrhea
Valacyclovir (Valtrex)	Treatment (not prophylaxis): 45–50 mg/kg/d p.o. div t.i.d.; max: 3 g/d	
Valganciclovir (Valcyte)	• <15 kg: induction 15 mg/kg/dose p.o. b.i.d. for ~14 d; maintenance 15 mg/kg/dose p.o. q.d. • >15 kg: induction: 500 mg/m^2/dose p.o. b.i.d. for ~14 d; maintenance 500 mg/m^2/dose p.o. q.d.	
Valproic acid (Depacon, Depakote, Depakene)	20 mg/kg i.v./p.o. load × 1 dose Initial: 15 mg/kg/d i.v. div q6 h; 15 mg/kg/d p.o. div q8 h Usual range: 20–100 mg/kg/d in div doses	• In status epilepticus, administer at 5 mg/kg/min • Routine i.v. doses, administer over 1 h • May require up to 100 mg/kg/d if on enzyme-inducing AEDs • Desired trough 50–100 μg/mL • May add carnitine for liver protection with high doses
Vancomycin	40–60 mg/kg/d i.v. div q6–8 h Use 60 mg/kg/d i.v. div q6 h for CNS infection Antibiotic-associated pseudomembranous colitis: • Children: 40 mg/kg/d p.o. in div doses q6 h for 7–10 d; not to exceed 2 g/d • Adults: 0.5–2 g/d p.o. in div doses q6–8 h	• Usual adult dose 2 g/d i.v. div q12 h • Check trough with third dose, trough 5–15 μg/mL • Adjust dose in renal dysfunction
Vasopressin (Pitressin)	Diabetes insipidus: 0.5 mU/kg/h i.v., double dose q30 min p.r.n. to effect (UO < 2 mL/kg/h) to max 10 mU/kg/h GI bleed: 2–5 mU/kg/min i.v., titrate p.r.n.; once no bleeding × 12 h taper off over 24–48 h	

TABLE A2.1 Pediatric Drug Formulary (*continued*)

Medication	*Dosage*	*Comments*
Vecuronium (Norcuron)	0.1 mg/kg/dose i.v. q1 h p.r.n. Continuous infusion 0.05–0.07 mg/kg/h i.v. RSI 0.3 mg/kg i.v. × 1 dose	• Not routinely used for RSI due to long duration of effect
Voriconazole (Vfend)	Loading dose 12 mg/kg/d p.o./i.v. div q12 h for 1 d, then 6–8 mg/kg/d p.o./i.v. div q12 h; max: 600 mg/d	• Do not use i.v. formulation in patients with CrCl <50 mL/min/1.73 m^2
Warfarin (Coumadin)	Load on day 1: 0.2 mg/kg p.o. × 1 (max: 10 mg); further loading and maintenance dosing based on INR; usual maintenance 0.1 mg/kg/d with great variation	• Counsel patients on drug–food interactions
Zidovudine (Retrovir)	Neonates: 2 mg/kg/dose p.o. q.i.d. OR 1.5 mg/kg/dose i.v. q6 h Children: 160 mg/m^2/dose p.o. t.i.d. OR 120 mg/m^2/dose i.v. q6 h Max: oral 200 mg/dose t.i.d. Continuous infusion 20 mg/m^2/h i.v.	• Also referred to as AZT • May be administered with food • Adjust dose in severe renal and hepatic dysfunction
Zonisamide (Zonegran)	Initial 2–4 mg/kg/d p.o. div q.d.–t.i.d.; usual 4–8 mg/kg/d p.o. div q.d.–t.i.d.. Recommended max is 12 mg/kg/d Adult: initial 100–200 mg/d p.o. div q.d.–t.i.d. (titrate to 200–400 mg/d over 2 wk) Max dose: 600 mg/d	• Studies have used up to 20 mg/kg/d for infantile spasms

i.o., intraosseous; i.m., intramuscular; i.v., intravenous; n.g., nasogastric; p.o., oral; p.r., rectal: s.c., subcutaneous.
b.i.d., twice daily; div, divided; p.r.n., as needed; q, every; q.d., daily; q.h.s., at bedtime; q.i.d., four times a day; q.o.d., every other day; t.i.d., thrice daily.
ADHD, attention deficit and hyperactivity disorder; AED, antiepileptic drug; ANC, absolute neutrophil count; CAP, community-acquired pneumonia, CF, cystic fibrosis; CHF, congestive heart failure; CMV, cytomegalovirus; CNS, central nervous system; CrCl, creatinine clearance; CV, cardiovascular; CVL, central venous line; D5W, dextrose 5% in water; D10W, dextrose 10% in water; D25W, dextrose 25% in water; DVT, deep vein thrombosis; ED, emergency department; ESRD, end-stage renal disease; ETT, endotracheal tube; GA, gestational age; GABHS, group A β-hemolytic streptococcus; GERD, gastroesophageal reflux disease; GI, gastrointestinal; HPLC, high-performance liquid chromatography; ICP, intracranial pressure; ICU, intensive care unit; ID, infectious disease; INH, inhaled; INR, international normalized ratio; IVF, intravenous fluid; LMWH, low-molecular-weight heparin; MAOi, monoamine oxidase inhibitor; MDI, metered dose inhaler; *MIC*, minimum inhibitory concentration; NS, normal saline; NSAIDs, nonsteroidal anti-inflammatory drugs; OCD, obsessive–compulsive disorder; OR, operating room; PaO_2, partial pressure of oxygen in arterial blood; PALS, pediatric advanced life support; PCP, *Pneumocystis carinii* pneumonia; PIV, peripheral intravenous (line, catheter); PMA, postmenstrual age, PSVT, paroxysmal supraventricular tachycardia; RDS, respiratory distress syndrome; RSI, rapid-sequence intubation; RSV, respiratory syncytial virus; SCI, spinal cord injury; SG, specific gravity; SVT, supraventricular tachycardia; TMP, trimethoprim; TPN, total parenteral nutrition; UO, urine output; UTI, urinary tract infection; VF/VT, ventricular fibrillation/ventricular tachycardia.

Index

Note: Page numbers followed by *f* and *t* indicate figures and tables respectively.

D